Barker, Burton and Zieve's

PRINCIPLES OF Ambulatory Medicine

SEVENTH EDITION

Edited by

NICHOLAS H. FIEBACH, M.D.
Professor of Clinical Medicine
College of Physicians and Surgeons, Columbia University
Director, Medical House Staff Training Program
Columbia University Medical Center
New York Presbyterian Hospital
New York, New York

DAVID E. KERN, M.D., M.P.H.
Associate Professor of Medicine
Johns Hopkins University School of Medicine
Director, Division of General Internal Medicine
Johns Hopkins Bayview Medical Center
Baltimore, Maryland

PATRICIA A. THOMAS, M.D.
Associate Professor of Medicine
Associate Dean for Curriculum
Johns Hopkins University School of Medicine
Baltimore, Maryland

ROY C. ZIEGELSTEIN, M.D.
Professor of Medicine
The Johns Hopkins University School of Medicine
Executive Vice Chairman, Department of Medicine
Director, Residency Program in Internal Medicine
Johns Hopkins Bayview Medical Center
Baltimore, Maryland

Consulting Editors

L. RANDOL BARKER, M.D., SC.M., M.A.C.P.
Professor of Medicine
Johns Hopkins University School of Medicine
Division of General Internal Medicine
Johns Hopkins Bayview Medical Center
Baltimore, Maryland

PHILIP D. ZIEVE, M.D.
Professor of Medicine
Johns Hopkins University School of Medicine
Senior Advisor to the Medical Center
Johns Hopkins Bayview Medical Center
Baltimore, Maryland

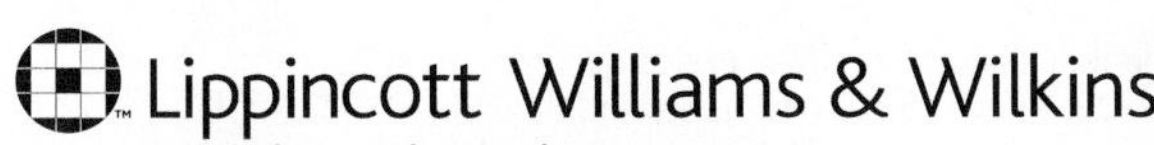
Lippincott Williams & Wilkins
a Wolters Kluwer business
Philadelphia • Baltimore • New York • London
Buenos Aires • Hong Kong • Sydney • Tokyo

Acquisitions Editor: Sonya Seigafuse
Managing Editor: Nancy Winter
Developmental Editor: Leah Hayes
Project Manager: Alicia Jackson
Senior Manufacturing Manager: Benjamin Rivera
Marketing Manager: Angela Panetta
Design Coordinator: Steve Druding
Cover Designer: Larry Didona
Production Service: TechBooks
Printer: Quebecor World-Taunton

Printed in the USA

Library of Congress Cataloging-in-Publication Data

Principles of ambulatory medicine / editors, L. Randol Barker . . . [et al.]—7th ed.
p. ; cm.
Includes bibliographical references and index.
ISBN 0-7817-6227-8
1. Family medicine. 2. Ambulatory medical care. I. Barker, L. Randol (Lee Randol).
[DNLM: 1. Ambulatory Care. WX 205 P957 2007]
RC46.P894 2007
616—dc22 2006011532

To purchase additional copies of this book, call our customer service department at (800) 638-3030 or fax orders to (301) 223-2320. International customers should call (301) 223-2300.

Visit Lippincott Williams & Wilkins on the Internet: at LWW.com. Lippincott Williams & Wilkins. Customer service representatives are available from 8:30 am to 6 pm, EST.

10 9 8 7 6 5 4 3 2 1

PRINCIPLES OF Ambulatory Medicine

SEVENTH EDITION

CONTRIBUTORS

Unless otherwise indicated, hospital appointments are at Johns Hopkins Bayview Medical Center, Baltimore, Maryland, and faculty appointments are at the Johns Hopkins University School of Medicine.

Ross E. Andersen, Ph.D.
Associate Professor of Medicine

John E. Anderson, M.D.
Assistant Professor of Medicine

Andrew F. Angelino, M.D.
Assistant Professor of Psychiatry and Behavioral Sciences
Medical Director—Acute Psychiatry Service

Frank C. Arnett, Jr., M.D.
Professor of Internal Medicine
Division of Rheumatology and Clinical Immunogenetics
University of Texas—Houston Medical School
Houston, Texas

Bimal H. Ashar, M.D., M.B.A.
Assistant Professor of Medicine

Paul G. Auwaerter, M.D., M.B.A.
Associate Professor of Medicine

Jennifer E. Axilbund, M.S., C.G.C.
Senior Genetic Counselor
Research Associate in Oncology

Carlos A. Bagley, M.D.
Senior Resident of Neurosurgery

L. Randol Barker, M.D., Sc.M., M.A.C.P.
Professor of Medicine
Division of General Internal Medicine

William H. Barker, M.D., F.R.C.T, EDIN
Professor Emeritus
Department of Preventive Medicine and Gerontology
University of Rochester Medical Center
Rochester, New York

Linda F. Barr, M.D.
Assistant Professor of Medicine
Pulmonary and Critical Care Associates of Baltimore
Towson, Maryland

R. Graham Barr, M.D., Dr. P.H.
Florence Irving Assistant Professor
Departments of Medicine and Epidemiology
Columbia University Medical Center
New York, New York

Shehzad Basaria, M.D.
Assistant Professor of Internal Medicine and Endocrinology

Joan M. Bathon, M.D.
Professor of Medicine

Michele F. Bellantoni, M.D.
Associate Professor of Medicine
Medical Director

O. Joseph Bienvenu, III, M.D., Ph.D.
Assistant Professor of Psychiatry
Associate Director, Anxiety Disorders Clinic

James H. Black, III, M.D.
Assistant Professor of Surgery
Attending Surgeon,
Vascular/Endovascular Surgery

David W. Blodgett, M.D., M.P.H.
Adjunct Faculty
Department of Health Policy and Management
Johns Hopkins Bloomberg School of Public Health

David G. Borenstein, M.D.
Clinical Professor of Medicine
George Washington University Medical Center
Washington, D.C.

Gary R. Briefel, M.D.
Associate Professor of Medicine
Chief, Division of Renal Medicine

Robert E. Bristow, M.D.
Associate Professor and Director of Obstetrics and Gynecology

Anne E. Burke, M.D.
Assistant Professor of Obstetrics and Gynecology

Arthur L. Burnett, M.D.
Professor of Urology

Ronald P. Byank, M.D.
Associate Professor of Orthopedic Surgery

Hugh Calkins, M.D., B.A.
Professor of Medicine
Professor of Pediatrics
Director, Arrhythmia Service and Clinical Electrophysiology Laboratory
Director, ARVD Program

Nisha Chandra-Strobos, M.D.
Professor of Medicine
Director, CUU
Director, Clinical Cardiovascular Services

Colleen Christmas, M.D.
Assistant Professor of Medicine

Jeanne M. Clark, M.D., M.P.H.
Assistant Professor of Medicine and Epidemiology
The Johns Hopkins University School of Medicine and Bloomberg School of Public Health

Karan A. Cole, Sc.D.
Assistant Professor of Medicine
Division of General Internal Medicine
Director, Med-Psych Rotation
Director, JHU Faculty Development Program and Teaching Skills

Eugene C. Corbett, Jr., M.D.
Bernard B. and Anne L. Brodie Professor of Medicine
Professor of Nursing
General Medicines, Geriatrics, and Palliative Care
University of Virginia Health Science Center
Charlottesville, Virginia

Grace A. Cordts, M.D., M.H.P., M.S.
Assistant Professor of Medicine

Rima J. Couzi, M.D., M.B., B.C.H., M.H.S.
Assistant Professor of Oncology

Leonard R. DeRogatis, Ph.D.
Associate Professor of Psychiatry
Director, Center for Sexual Health and Medicine

Christopher J. Earley, M.D., Ph.D.
Associate Professor of Neurology

Peter J. Fagan, Ph.D.
Associate Professor of Medical Psychology

Clare H. Ferrigno, M.S.N., F.N.P., C.R.N.P.
NP/Program Coordinator
Division of Medical Oncology

Nicholas H. Fiebach, M.D.
Professor of Clinical Medicine
Columbia University College of Physicians and Surgeons
Director, Medical House Staff Training Program
New York Presbyterian Hospital
Columbia University Medical Center
New York, New York

Michael I. Fingerhood, M.D.
Associate Professor of Medicine

Thomas E. Finucane, M.D.
Professor of Medicine
Chair, Ethics Committee

Paul S. Fishman, M.D., Ph.D.
Professor of Neurology
University of Maryland Medical School
Baltimore, Maryland

John A. Flynn, M.D., M.B.A.
Associate Professor of Medicine
Clinical Director, Division of General Internal Medicine

Howard W. Francis, M.D.
Associate Professor of Otolaryngology—Head and Neck Surgery

David S. Friedman, M.D., M.P.H.
Associate Professor of Opthalmology
Wilmer Eye Institute

Ira M. Garonzik, M.D.
Assistant Professor of Neurosurgery
Director, Baltimore Neurosurgery and Spine Center

Steve N. Georas, M.D.
Associate Professor of Medicine
Medical Director, Respiratory Care Department

Robert L. Giuntoli, II, M.D.
Assistant Professor of Gynecology/Obstetrics
Attending Physician, Department of Gynecology/Obstetrics

Sheldon H. Gottlieb, M.D.
Associate Professor of Medicine
Senior Cardiologist

Constance A. Griffin, M.D.
Associate Professor of Pathology, Oncology, and Medicine

Richard J. Gross, M.D., Sc.M.
Associate Professor of Medicine
Acting Physician, Department of Medicine

Uzma J. Haque, M.D.
Assistant Professor of Rheumatology

John W. Harmon, M.D.
Professor of Surgery
Staff Surgeon, Department of Surgery

David B. Hellmann, M.D., M.A.C.P.
Vice Dean
Mary Betty Stevens Professor of Medicine
Chairman, Department of Medicine

H. Franklin Herlong, M.D.
Associate Professor of Medicine

Glenn A. Hirsch, M.D.
Instructor of Medicine, Division of Cardiology

George R. Huggins, M.D.
Professor of Obstetrics and Gynecology

Nada S. Jabbur, M.D.
Associate Professor
Department of Ophthalmology
Johns Hopkins at Green Spring Station
Lutherville, Maryland

Nathaniel W. James, IV, M.D.
Assistant Professor of Medicine
University of Vermont College of Medicine
Burlington, Vermont
Attending Physician
Maine Medical Center
Portland, Maine

Roxanne M. Jamshidi, M.D., M.P.H.
Assistant Professor of Gynecology/Obstetrics

Suzanne M. Jan de Beur, M.D.
Assistant Professor of Medicine
Chief, Division of Endocrinology

Constance J. Johnson, M.D.
Associate Professor of Neurology
Vanderbilt University
Nashville, Tennessee

Peter W. Kaplan, M.B.,B.S.
Professor of Neurology
Director of Epilepsy and Nerve Physiology

Matthew L. Kashima, M.D., M.P.H.
Assistant Professor of Otolaryngology Head and Neck Surgery
Chief of Service, Department of Otolaryngology Head and Neck Surgery

David E. Kern, M.D., M.P.H.
Associate Professor of Medicine
Director, Division of General Internal Medicine

Edward S. Kraus, M.D.
Associate Professor of Medicine
Associate Medical Director, Adult Kidney Transplant Program

Bruce S. Lebowitz, D.P.M
Instructor of Orthopedic Surgery

Frederick A. Lenz, M.D., Ph.D.
Professor of Neurosurgery
Attending Neurosurgeon

Shari M. Ling, M.D.
Assistant Professor of Rheumatology and Geriatric Medicine and Gerontology
Staff Clinician, Clinical Research Branch, NIA
Harbor Hospital
Baltimore, Maryland

Mark C. Liu, M.D.
Associate Professor of Medicine
Johns Hopkins Asthma and Allergy Center
Staff Physician

Rafael H. Llinas, M.D.
Assistant Professor of Neurology
Medical Director, Neurology Service

Sara Love-Schlessman, C.R.N.P.
Certified Nurse Practioner
Otolaryngology—Head and Neck Surgery

Meredith B. Loveless, M.D.
Instructor of Obstetrics/Gynecology

Douglas K. MacLeod, D.M.D.
Former Chairman, Department of Dentistry
Baltimore City Hospitals
Private Practice
Raleigh, North Carolina

Jeffrey L. Magaziner, M.D.
Assistant Professor of Medicine

Joseph E. Marine, M.D.
Assistant Professor of Medicine
Division of Cardiology
Director of Electrophysiology

Susan A. Mayer, M.D.
Assistant Professor of Medicine
Director, Echocardiography Laboratory

Una D. McCann, M.D.
Associate Professor of Psychiatry and Behavioral Sciences
Director, Anxiety Disorders Clinic

Simon C. Mears, M.D., Ph.D.
Assistant Professor of Orthopaedic Surgery
Chief, Division of Total Joint Arthroplasty and Trauma

Esteban Mezey, M.D.
Professor of Medicine

Myron Miller, M.D.
Professor of Medicine

Redonda G. Miller, M.D., M.B.A.
Associate Professor of Medicine

Mack C. Mitchell, Jr., M.D.
Associate Professor of Medicine
Director, Division of Gastroenterology

Francis M. Mondimore, M.D.
Assistant Professor of Psychiatry and Behavioral Sciences

Patrick A. Murphy, M.D., Ph.D.
Professor of Medicine
Attending Physician

David N. Neubauer, M.D.
Assistant Professor of Psychiatry and Behavioral Sciences
Associate Director, Johns Hopkins Sleep Disorder Center

John K. Niparko, M.D.
George T. Nager Professor of Otolaryngology

Eric L. Nuermberger, M.D.
Assistant Professor of Medicine
Attending Physician

Irina Petrache, M.D.
Assistant Professor of Medicine and Pathology
Attending Physician

Michael J. Polydefkis, M.D.
Assistant Professor of Neurology
Director, EMG Laboratory
Co-Director, Cutaneous Nerve Laboratory

Gregory P. Prokopowicz, M.D., M.P.H.
Assistant Professor of Medicine

Michael J. Purtell, M.D., Ph.D.
Assistant Professor of Oncology

Peter V. Rabins, M.D., M.P.H.
Professor of Psychiatry

Darius A. Rastegar, M.D.
Assistant Professor of Medicine

Robert P. Roca, M.D., M.P.H.
Associate Professor of Psychiatry
Vice President and Medical Director
Sheppard Pratt Health System
Towson, Maryland

Annabelle Rodriguez-Oquendo, M.D.
Assistant Professor of Medicine
Director, Diabetes Management Service

Linda C. Rogers, C.R.N.P.
Assistant, Department of OB/GYN

Glen S. Roseborough, M.D.
Assistant Professor of Surgery

Alvin M. Sanico, M.D.
Assistant Professor of Medicine
Medical Director, Asthma Sinus Allergy Program at Greater Baltimore Medical Center
Baltimore, Maryland

Larry N. Scherzer, M.D., M.P.H., Sc.D
Department of Pediatrics
University of Connecticut
East Hartford, Connecticut

Chester W. Schmidt, Jr., M.D.
Professor of Psychiatry
Chairman, Department of Psychiatry and Behavioral Sciences

Stephen D. Sears, M.D., M.P.H.
Adjunct Associate Professor of Community and Family Medicine
Dartmouth Medical School
Chief Medical Officer
Maine General Medical Center
Augusta, Maine

Edward P. Shapiro, M.D.
Professor of Medicine
Director, Noninvasive Cardiology

Philip L. Smith, II, M.D.
Professor of Medicine
Professor, Asthma and Allergy Center

Sharon D. Solomon, M.D.
Assistant Professor of Ophthalmology

David A. Spector, M.D.
Associate Professor of Internal Medicine
Director, Nephrology Program

Robert J. Spence, M.D.
Associate Professor of Surgery
Director, Burn Reconstruction

Kerry J. Stewart, Ed.D.
Professor of Medicine
Director, Clinical and Research Exercise Physiology

Michael B. Streiff, M.D.
Assistant Professor of Medicine
Medical Director, Anticoagulation Management Services

Patricia A. Thomas, M.D.
Associate Professor of Medicine
Associate Dean for Curriculum

Varsha K. Vaidya, M.D.
Assistant Professor of Psychiatry and General Internal Medicine
Director, Consultation Liaison Psychiatry

Mark F. Walker, M.D.
Assistant Professor of Neurology

Larry Waterbury, M.D.
Associate Professor of Oncology and Medicine

Robert S. Weinberg, M.D.
Chairman, Department of Ophthalmology

Laura S. Welch, M.D.
Adjunct Professor of Environmental and Occupational Health
George Washington University
Medical Director, Center to Protect Workers Rights
Silver Spring, Maryland

Karen A. Wendel, M.D.
Assistant Professor
Division of Infectious Diseases
University of Colorado Health Science Center
Denver, Colorado

S. Elizabeth Whitmore, M.D., Sc.M.
Associate Professor of Dermatology

John H. Wilckens, M.D.
Assistant Professor of Orthopaedics
Chairman, Department of Orthopaedics

Robert A. Wise, M.D.
Professor of Pulmonary and Critical Care Medicine

Christopher L. Wolfgang, M.D., Ph.D.
Assistant Professor of Surgery
Attending Surgeon

E. James Wright, M.D.
Assistant Professor of Urology
Chief, Department of Urology

Jean Wu, M.D., M.H.S.
Instructor of Medicine

Paul M. Yen, M.D.
Associate Professor of Medicine
Division of Endocrinology

Jonathan M. Zenilman, M.D.
Professor of Medicine
Chief, Infectious Diseases Division

Roy C. Ziegelstein, M.D.
Professor of Medicine
Executive Vice Chairman
Director, Residency Program in Internal Medicine

Philip D. Zieve, M.D.
Professor of Medicine
Senior Advisor

Acknowledgment

The Editors wish to acknowledge Ms. Susan McFeaters, who has provided skillful and dedicated assistance on all editions of this book and, for the seventh edition, has become the Johns Hopkins administrative coordinator for the entire book.

CONTENTS

SECTION 7: HEMATOLOGIC PROBLEMS *817*

SECTION 8: PULMONARY PROBLEMS *867*

SECTION 9: CARDIOVASCULAR PROBLEMS *947*

SECTION 10: MUSCULOSKELETAL PROBLEMS *1123*

SECTION 11: METABOLIC AND ENDOCRINOLOGIC PROBLEMS *1291*

PREFACE

This book is directed to practitioners who care for ambulatory adult patients. The purposes of the book are (a) to provide an in-depth account of the evaluation, management, and long-term course of common clinical problems that are addressed in the ambulatory setting, and (b) to provide guidance for recognizing problems that require either referral for specialized care or hospitalization and for appreciating the expected course of those problems.

Three principles have guided the preparation of each edition of *Principles of Ambulatory Medicine*.

1. Practitioners working in a busy practice need to know about *probabilities* related to the occurrence, course, evaluation, and treatment of their patients' problems.
2. The patient makes most decisions in ambulatory care, and the quality of those decisions depends on the *patient–practitioner relationship* and *patient education*.
3. The practitioner and the patient should incorporate a *preventive point of view* into all actions taken to address the patient's health.

With the seventh edition, Doctors Nicholas H. Fiebach, David E. Kern, Patricia A. Thomas, and Roy C. Ziegelstein have become the Editors, and Doctors L. Randol Barker and Philip D. Zieve have become Consulting Editors. All four of the Editors served as Associate Editors for the sixth edition. They played major roles in the expansion and reorganization of that edition, including the addition of seventeen new chapters and many new authors.

For the seventh edition, updating and revising of all chapters have been based on evidence from recent clinical trials, on current consensus-based recommendations for many conditions, and on the comments of those who have used the book. There are new sections on Bioterrorism, the Family and Medical Leave Act, and eye surgery for refractive errors.

Principles of Ambulatory Medicine is extensively cross-referenced both to avoid redundancy and to facilitate access to useful information contained elsewhere in the book. In addition, for easy reference, the key topics in each chapter are presented in outline form at the beginning of the chapter. For the seventh edition, Specific References cited in the text are listed at the end of each chapter, and General References, many of them websites, are found at the following internet address: www.hopkinsbayview.org/PAMreferences.

SECTION 1

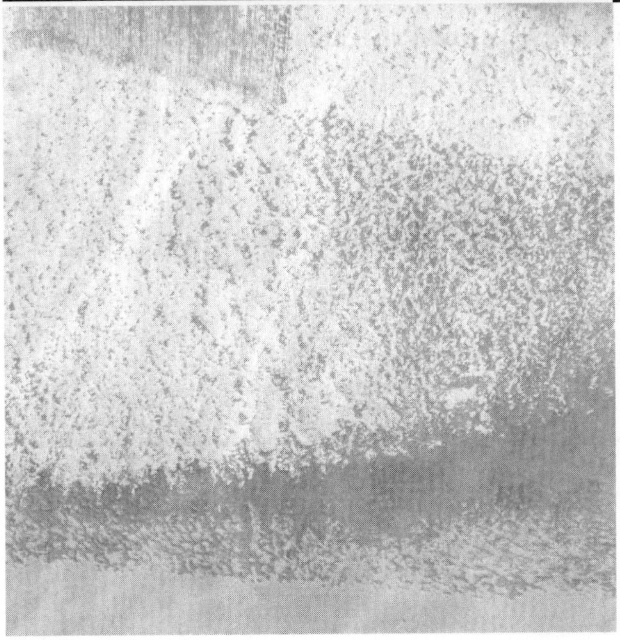

Issues of General Concern in Ambulatory Medicine

Chapter 1

Ambulatory Care: Territory and Core Proficiencies

L. Randol Barker

A fundamental tenet of this book is that ambulatory care has distinctive characteristics that should shape practitioners' approaches to patients. This chapter describes the territory of ambulatory care in the United States, as well as some of the proficiencies that are central to ambulatory practice.

THE TERRITORY OF AMBULATORY PRACTICE

Who provides ambulatory care? What patients make ambulatory care visits? What problems do patients present at their visits? What ambulatory care is provided for these problems? To answer these questions, the United States National Ambulatory Medical Care Survey (NAMCS), started in 1973, has collected information periodically from a representative sample of physicians' offices.

Office-Based Practitioners

Table 1.1 shows the distribution by specialty of the approximately 890 million visits to physicians' offices in the United States during 2002. Of these visits, 18% were to the offices of internists and 24% were to the offices of general or family practitioners; 3% of all visits were to physician's assistants or nurse practitioners (1). This book is directed primarily to those physicians and other practitioners who provide primary care for adult patients.

Ambulatory Patients

The NAMCS *definition of an ambulatory patient* is "an individual presenting for personal health services who is neither bedridden nor currently admitted to any health care institution." A critical expansion of this definition is that ambulatory or homebound patients (or members of their households) have most of the responsibility for carrying out their own care: They must administer treatments, monitor symptoms and functional status, adapt to the constraints imposed by illness, and decide how to deal with new problems when they arise. These characteristics have important implications for the care of ambulatory patients, as discussed later in this chapter and throughout this book.

Table 1.2 shows the age and sex distribution of the patients who made ambulatory visits to physicians' offices in 2002. In that year, the annual number of office visits by adults ranged from 1.8 for people 15 to 24 years old to 7.2 for people age 75 years and older (1).

Problems of Ambulatory Patients

What types of problems are seen in ambulatory practice? Using the *International Classification of Diseases, 9th Revision, Clinical Modification* (ICD-9-CM), participants in NAMCS were asked to name the principal reasons for the visits by patients. Table 1.3 lists the 20 most common diagnoses named in 2002. Because comorbidity, especially the coexistence of physical and mental morbidity, is very common in ambulatory patients, this list of principal reasons

TABLE 1.1 Number, Percent Distribution, and Annual Rate of Office Visits by Selected Physician Practice Characteristics: United States, 2002

Physician Practice Characteristics	*Number of Visits in Thousands*	*Percent Distribution (%)*	*Number of Visits per 100 Persons per Year*
All visits	889,980	100.0	314.4
General and family practice	215,466	24.2	76.1
Internal medicine	156,692	17.6	55.4
Pediatrics	120,018	13.5	198.1
Obstetrics and gynecology	70,324	7.9	60.9
Ophthalmology	49,937	5.6	17.6
Orthopedic surgery	38,028	4.3	13.4
Dermatology	32,227	3.6	11.4
Psychiatry	21,659	2.4	7.7
Cardiovascular diseases	20,822	2.3	7.4
Urology	17,133	1.9	6.1
Otolaryngology	17,080	1.9	6.0
General surgery	17,000	1.9	6.0
Neurology	9,622	1.1	3.4
All other specialties	103,974	11.7	36.7

From Woodwell DA, Cherry DK. National Ambulatory Medical Care Survey: 2002 Summary. Advance Data for Vital and Health Statistics No. 346. Hyattsville, MD: National Center for Health Statistics, August 26, 2004.

for visits tells only part of the story. Furthermore, at least half of ambulatory care visits are for symptoms, and a diagnosis that explains these symptoms is infrequently found (2). Ongoing research on common symptoms will contribute critical information for addressing the needs of ambulatory patients (see Kroenke and Laine, *Investigating Symptoms,* at www.hopkinsbayview.org/PAMreferences).

Ambulatory Care

In 2002, ambulatory care for adult patients provided by physicians who identified themselves as the patient's primary care provider had the following general characteristics (1):

Average number of visits per week	92
Average time with physician	16 to 20 minutes
≥6 visits in past year (% of patients)	24%
Status of patient (% of visits)	
Established patient	91%
New problem	33%
Drug mentions (% of visits)	74% to 77%
Average number of drug mentions per visit	2 drugs

Table 1.4 shows the proportion of ambulatory care visits reimbursed by each of the primary sources of payment in the United States for the year 2002.

In addition to office visits, *telephone and e-mail encounters and house calls* are important in the care of ambulatory patients. Telephone and e-mail encounters enable physicians and patients to handle many problems efficiently. (See Reisman and Stevens, www.hopkinsbayview.org/PAMreferences.) Home visits are helpful for providing care to patients who are too frail to make office visits and for learning facts about patients' home conditions that may facilitate management of their problems at future office visits. In 2002, primary care physicians practicing in the United States reported the following regarding nonoffice encounters with patients (1).

	Office Visits	*Telephone Consultation*	*E-mail Consultation*	*Home Visits*
Percent of physicians		73%	7%	19%
Average number per week	92	26	6	11

Self-Care and Alternative Care

Before making visits to physicians, patients usually attempt to diagnose and treat their own symptoms. Additionally, in the past decade an increasing number of patients in the United States report using one or more of the many types of complementary and alternative care medicines that are described in Chapter 5 (3).

Classic studies of self-care in a number of countries show that at any one time approximately 30% of persons are taking nonprescribed medications or are engaged in self-care for a problem for which they have not consulted a physician (4). Over-the-counter (OTC) medications now account for the majority of medicines taken in the United States (5). The frequency distribution of conditions managed by self-care was estimated by Fry (6), on the basis of many years of general practice in a community well

TABLE 1.2 Number, Percent Distribution, and Annual Rate of Office Visits by Patient's Age, Sex, and Race: United States, 2002

Patient's Age (Years), Sex, and Race	*Number of Visits in Thousands*	*Percent Distribution (%)*
All visits	889,980	100.0
Age		
Younger than 15 years	159,235	17.9
15–24 years	71,865	8.1
25–44 years	192,359	21.6
45–64 years	242,142	27.2
65–74 years	109,331	12.3
75 years and over	115,049	12.9
Sex and Age		
Female	529,075	59.4
Under 15 years	76,382	8.6
15–24 years	44,909	5.0
25–44 years	128,743	14.5
45–64 years	144,205	16.2
65–74 years	61,819	6.9
75 years and over	73,017	8.2
Male	360,905	40.6
Younger than 15 years	82,853	9.3
15–24 years	26,956	3.0
25–44 years	63,616	7.1
45–64 years	97,937	11.0
65–74 years	47,512	5.3
75 years and over	42,032	4.7
Race		
White	766,096	86.1
Black or African American	89,455	10.1
Asian	26,341	3.0
Native Hawaiian or other Pacific Islander	3,430	0.4
American Indian or Alaska Native	2,237	0.3
Multiple races	2,421	0.3

From Woodwell DA, Cherry DK. National Ambulatory Medical Care Survey: 2002 Summary. Advance Data for Vital and Health Statistics No. 346. Hyattsville, MD: National Center for Health Statistics, August 26, 2004.

TABLE 1.3 The 20 Most Common Primary Diagnoses in Ambulatory Care Visits: United States, 2002

Primary Diagnosis Group	*Number of Visits in Thousands*	*Percent Distribution (%)*
All visits	889,980	100.0
Essential hypertension	48,180	5.4
Routine infant or child health check	35,935	4.0
Acute upper respiratory infections, excluding pharyngitis	30,141	3.4
Diabetes mellitus	24,877	2.8
Arthropathies and related disorders	23,725	2.7
General medical examination	22,362	2.5
Spinal disorders	20,444	2.3
Rheumatism, excluding back	17,766	2.0
Normal pregnancy	17,585	2.0
Otitis media and eustachian tube disorders	16,702	1.9
Malignant neoplasms	15,651	1.8
Chronic sinusitis	14,197	1.6
Allergic rhinitis	14,101	1.6
Asthma	12,692	1.4
Gynecologic examination	11,883	1.3
Disorder of lipoid metabolism	11,767	1.3
Heart disease, excluding ischemic	11,670	1.3
Ischemic heart disease	10,970	1.2
Acute pharyngitis	10,090	1.1
Follow-up examination	9,995	1.1
All other diagnoses	509,248	57.2

From Woodwell DA, Cherry DK. National Ambulatory Medical Care Survey: 2002 Summary. Advance Data for Vital and Health Statistics No. 346. Hyattsville, MD: National Center for Health Statistics, August 26, 2004.

known to him, as 25% upper respiratory tract infections, 20% musculoskeletal symptoms, 20% emotional problems, 10% acute gastrointestinal symptoms, 5% skin rashes, and 20% miscellaneous other symptoms. Both the changing status of drugs from prescription to OTC formulations and the availability of herbal remedies without a prescription (see Chapter 5) have expanded the "formulary" that patients can access for self-care.

Table 1.5, adapted from NAMCS data, shows the time interval between the onset of a new problem and the decision to go to a physician (i.e., the duration of self-care) for a number of common conditions. Not surprisingly, patients with lacerations presented within 1 day, patients with symptoms of acute infection and chest pain tended to present within 1 week, and patients with most other problems tended to present after at least 1 week of self-care.

Self-care before professional care is an important way in which the patient, not the practitioner, makes the decisions in the domain of ambulatory medicine. The patient's primary role in carrying out the plan of care after an office visit has already been emphasized. These two features confirm the primacy of the patient's actions in determining the course of events in ambulatory medicine.

Temporal Dimension of Ambulatory Medicine

The information from the NAMCS does not illuminate the longitudinal nature of ambulatory care. Table 1.6 shows

TABLE 1.4 Number and Percent Distribution of Office Visits by Primary Expected Source of Payment: United States, 2002

Primary Expected Source of Payment	*Number of Visits in Thousands*	*Percent Distribution (%)*
All visits	889,980	100.0
Private insurance	525,520	59.0
Medicare	188,207	21.1
Medicaid/SCHIP (State Children's Health Insurance Program)	67,110	7.5
Self-pay	39,526	4.4
Workers' compensation	14,658	1.6
No charge/charity	2,485	0.3
Other	21,456	2.4
Unknown/blank	31,018	3.5

From Woodwell DA, Cherry DK. National Ambulatory Medical Care Survey: 2002 Summary. Advance Data for Vital and Health Statistics No. 346. Hyattsville, MD: National Center for Health Statistics, August 26, 2004.

the 5-year profile of care for an elderly woman. This patient's story illustrates each of the following important questions, for which only the passage of time provides the answers:

- *What is the significance of a recent symptom* (e.g., the temporal headache for 1 year reported in 1975, subsequently not a serious problem)?
- *What is the advisability of initiating a referral for a problem* (e.g., cataract identified but asymptomatic in 1975; evaluated when more symptomatic in 1978 and classified as not mature)?
- *How well will the patient adhere to recommended treatment* (e.g., the digoxin prescribed in 1975 for heart failure, taken reliably for 5 years)?
- *What is the impact of a new treatment on the patient's health* (e.g., addition of a diuretic in 1978, with heart failure gradually improving during the next month)?
- *What is the impact of intercurrent medical problems on the patient's functional status?* (The answer to this question varied over time and was dependent on intercurrent problems: Although the patient's ambulation deteriorated greatly during the 5 years, other valued activities, such as crocheting and canning, did not.)
- *What is the impact of the patient's illness on family members in the same household?* (The answer to this question also varied over time; "exhaustion" at one point did not predict transfer to a long-term care facility.)

Goals of Ambulatory Care

Patient Expectations

The goals of ambulatory care are strongly influenced by the expectations of patients for their day to day activities in the community. When they make office visits, ambulatory patients are seeking help to relieve symptoms or to cure, ameliorate, or prevent illness, so that they can maintain or resume valued activities. Depending on the severity of their problems, outpatients may be greatly, moderately, or not at all constrained from attaining their expectations. By virtue of living in the community, they (or other caregivers) play an active role in how these expectations are addressed, in contrast to the more passive role played by hospitalized patients.

Implications for Practice

To determine how any patient is doing, it is helpful to be aware of the patient's particular expectations and how well the patient is meeting them. This usually involves learning about the makeup of the patient's current household and

TABLE 1.5 Percentage Distribution of New Problem Office Visits by Time Since Onset of Complaint or Symptom, According to Selected Principal Reasons for Visit: United States, 1977

		Time Since Onset of Complaint or Symptom (days)					
Principal Reason for Visit	*Total*	*1*	*1–6*	*7–21*	*30–90*	*>90*	*Not Applicable*
All new problem visits	100.0	8.2	37.3	15.6	10.3	13.9	14.8
Symptoms of throat	100.0	6.9	77.9	10.6	2.3	1.9	0.4
Cough	100.0	3.3	73.0	18.6	2.9	2.1	0.2
Head cold, upper respiratory tract infection	100.0	6.2	72.5	16.5	3.0	1.1	0.7
Fever	100.0	17.6	76.4	4.7	0.2	1.0	
Headache	100.0	5.1	35.6	19.0	16.5	19.7	3.2
Back symptoms	100.0	6.5	37.6	26.4	11.8	16.2	1.5
Chest pain	100.0	7.6	45.8	22.6	9.3	13.6	1.2
Laceration, upper extremity	100.0	70.4	15.4	7.8	3.0	2.1	1.3

From National Ambulatory Medical Care Survey: 1977 Summary. Hyattsville, MD: National Center for Health Statistics.

TABLE 1.6 Profile of 5 Years in the Care of an Elderly Patient (each problem *italicized*)

	Year				
Feature	***1975***	***1976***	***1977***	***1978***	***1979***
Encounters	Initial visit, four office visits, many phone calls	Three office visits, many phone calls	Five office visits, two hospital admissions, one home visit, many phone calls	Four office visits, many phone calls	Four office visits, many phone calls
Principal medical problems	*Acute myocardial infarction* (mild congestive heart failure; digitalized; home management by patient's choice)	Stable (digoxin)	Stable (digoxin)	*Congestive heart failure* (diuretic added)	Stable (digoxin, diuretic)
	Degenerative joint disease (knees for years; cervical spine for years)	Waxes and wanes (aspirin, Motrin)	Same (coated aspirin)	Same (coated aspirin)	Same (coated aspirin)
	Temporal headaches for 1 year (erythrocyte sedimentation rate, 30)	Rarely	Rarely	Rarely	Rarely
	Hearing loss (ear, nose, and throat examination: senile high frequency deficit, no prescription)	Stable	Stable	Stable	Stable
	Bilateral cataracts	Stable	Stable	Referred (not mature)	Stable
	Leukoplakia, mouth (biopsy: not malignant)	Stable	Stable	Stable	Referred for change in appearance (biopsy: not malignant)
	Hematocrit, 35 (guaiac-negative)	Stable	Stable	Stable	Stable
	Constipation (for years)	Waxes and wanes (OTC laxative as needed)	Same (OTC laxative as needed)	Same (OTC laxative as needed and stool softener)	Same (OTC laxative as needed and stool softener)
		Leg cramps (quinine at bedtime)	Minimal (quinine at bedtime)	Same (quinine at bedtime)	Same (quinine at bedtime)
		Left cerebral transient ischemic attack	*Left CVA* (hospital, physical therapy)	Stable (right hemiparesis)	*Recurrent left CVA* (home management)
			Dog bite (cellulitis)	No recurrence	No recurrence
			Rectal bleeding (hospital, negative workup)	No recurrence	No recurrence
			Dysuria (culture negative)	*Family temporarily "exhausted"*; (Visiting Nurses Association)	Family doing well
				Painful toe	Persists (codeine)
				Appetite lost temporarily	No recurrence
Overall profile	87-year-old widow living with daughter's family, ambulatory and independent in the home, mentally intact, crochets and cans food; weight, 166; multiple medical problems identified at initial visit	88 years old, status the same; weight, 160; two new problems	89 years old, ambulation with walker assistance after CVA; weight, 151; four new problems, hospitalized twice	90 years old, status the same; weight, 140; three new problems	91 years old; ambulation more impaired after second CVA; mentally intact, crochets and cans food; weight, 139; no new problems

CVA, cerebrovascular accident; OTC, over-the-counter.

TABLE 1.7 Factors to Consider in the Family Life Cycle State of One's Patient

Family Life Cycle State	Developmental Tasks
Leaving home	Differentiate self in relation to family Develop intimate peer relationships Establish oneself in work
Couples and pairing	Form a committed relationship Realign relationships with extended family to include partner
Pregnancy and childbirth	Make room for children in the family Become parents while remaining spouses
Family with young children	Form a parent team Negotiate relationships with extended family to include parenting and grandparenting roles
Family with adolescents	Shift parent-child relationship to permit adolescent to move in and out of system
Adulthood and middle years	Refocus on marital and career issues Deal with disabilities and death in grandparents Deal with own aging and mortality
Graying of the family	Maintain functioning in face of physiologic decline
Death and grieving	Deal with loss of spouse, siblings, and peers Prepare for own death

Adapted from Carter CA, McGoldrick M, eds. The family life cycle: a framework for family therapy. New York: Gardner Press, 1980.

the patient's usual role in the family, the patient's occupation and level of formal education, and the patient's valued activities. It is also helpful to be aware of the developmental tasks that may be relevant to a patient's family. Table 1.7 lists tasks that are typical of the various stages in the *life cycle of a family*. The significance of this information can be illustrated by the common example of a middle-aged man who has had an uncomplicated myocardial infarction. After 3 months, the patient might be assessed as "status postmyocardial infarction—doing well." If he has resumed work and other valued activities, then he is probably "doing well." If he is not back at work, is financially stressed, and his wife reports that he has become irritable, then he is not doing well and the situation requires evaluation.

Awareness of a patient's life circumstances is particularly important in *preventive care* (see Chapter 14), in which the patient's degree of wellness, rather than degree of illness, is assessed. Assessing wellness means determining a patient's goals, learning whether a patient engages in health-promoting behaviors and identifying what health risks the patient has. For example, a 45-year-old mother who seeks balance between her professional and family life, is happily married, is free of chronic disease, has stopped smoking, has had periodic negative Papanicolaou (Pap) smears, exercises regularly, and drinks alcohol only socially would be assessed as very well. If everything was the same except that the patient smoked two packs of cigarettes daily, she would be assessed as only moderately well because of the major risk posed by heavy tobacco exposure. If she was feeling quite aimless, was recently divorced, had stopped seeing friends, and was smoking and drinking heavily, she would be assessed as not very well, even though she might not complain of any particular symptoms or have objective evidence of any disease.

The approach to addressing the goals of ambulatory patients described here was recently summarized as shifting one's focus from a disease orientation to a focus on the meanings that patients attach to their illness, which typically consists of multiple diseases and symptoms in chronically ill patients (7).

CORE PROFICIENCIES FOR AMBULATORY PRACTICE

Information such as that provided by the NAMCS (discussed earlier) has implications for several core proficiencies needed in the practice of ambulatory medicine. These core proficiencies include medication prescribing, documentation of care, coordination of care, discharge planning, cost containment, evidence-based decision making, patient-centered communication, patient education and promotion of healthy behavior, and integration of prevention into practice. Chapters 2, 3, 4, and 14, respectively, address in depth the latter four areas.

Medication Prescribing

Clinical pharmacology is the source for the many details needed for appropriate prescribing of medications. Apart from the impact of a medication on a patient's condition, it is important to be aware of the following aspects of each drug that one prescribes:

- *Practical information about initiating the drug:* appropriate starting dosage and schedule; modifications in dosage and schedule dictated by patient age, concurrently administered drugs, and the presence of diseases affecting drug metabolism; time interval for the effects of the drug to become apparent; duration of a course of the drug (when not a maintenance drug); how to assess the impact of the drug; potential interaction with other drugs the patient is taking; approximate cost to the patient of the drug; and whether the patient can afford it.
- *The major side effects of the drug:* when to anticipate them and how to detect, monitor for, and manage them.
- *The major reasons for inadequate response to a drug:* nonadherence, insufficient dosage of drug, antagonism of the drug by patient behavior or use of concurrent drugs,

and primary refractoriness to the drug; how to recognize and manage each of these problems.

- *Practical information about adjusting the dosage:* minimum and maximum dosages that can be tried and the time intervals that are appropriate for adjusting dosages and assessing impact.

Because prescription of medications is the single most common action taken by nonsurgical clinicians in ambulatory practice (see above), rapid access to this practical information through published or electronic resources is particularly important.

Documentation of Care

Documentation of care in the ambulatory record serves several purposes. It provides for rapid access by practitioners to the information they need for clinical decision making at serial visits; justification of the level of care for which payers are billed; and data accessibility for a quality-of-care audit. Documentation of care also stands as legal evidence of a practitioner's actions. Both paper and electronic records can be designed to meet these purposes. In 2002, approximately 18% of primary care physicians used electronic clinical records (1). For a number of compelling reasons, the implementation of electronic health records, with connectivity between users, is regarded as a national priority in the United States (8).

A well-structured primary care record, either paper or electronic, includes the following components and information:

- *A primary care front sheet* (Fig. 1.1) that includes a social profile (information about the patient's living situation, marital status, family makeup, occupation, education, social and recreational environment), a problem list that is prominently displayed and facilitates awareness of the patient's problems, and other information that should be readily findable, such as the patient's allergic history, past hospitalizations and operations, and the status of advance directives.
- *A treatment and clinical/laboratory flow sheet* that is prominently displayed and makes important past and current information accessible for decision making (Fig. 1.2).
- *A preventive care profile and flow sheet* that documents the patient's risk factors (including family history of illness) and promotes the appropriate provision of periodic preventive care (for an example, see Fig. 14.3).
- *Encounter forms,* including forms for telephone encounters, that allow clear documentation of information, thinking, and plans.
- Dividers, color-coded forms, and *standardized locations for various types of information* such as consultants' letters and laboratory reports, to increase the accessibility of clinical data.

To document patient education, prescriptions, and work slips, it is helpful to use forms that make duplicates for mounting in the patient's record.

Coordination of Care

Another proficiency important in ambulatory practice is skill in coordinating the patient's care. Coordination of care refers to referral for, awareness of, and interpretation of the services that a patient may need or receive. The availability of many diagnostic and consultative services requires generalists (1) to be prudent in recommending them and in using the information they provide, and (2) to be aware of the cost of a service, the nature of the experience the patient will undergo, and the likelihood that the service will be of value to the patient.

The services recommended for patients may involve permanent, temporary, or partial transfer of responsibility for the patient's care (e.g., to a surgeon), or they may be strictly consultative, meaning that they provide information to be used by the referring physician or practitioner (ranging from diagnostic test results to a consultant's suggestions).

Approximately 7.3% of office visits include *referral of the patient to another physician* (1). The following general guidelines are important in coordinating the care of a patient who is referred for consultation:

- Assure that the necessary information is transmitted to the person who will provide the service. For example, there should be clear communication of the facts generally needed by consultants (Table 1.8).
- Ensure that the patient understands the reason for the recommended services, arrange to obtain information promptly after a service has been performed, and ensure that the patient learns, as soon as it is appropriate, the meaning of this information.

The finding in a 2003 survey that in one of seven primary care office visits information critical for decision making is missing, speaks to the challenge presented by the coordinating role of the generalist practitioner (9). As noted above, the wider use of interconnected electronic clinical records has the potential to greatly streamline this role.

Patients sometimes obtain services for medical problems without referral by their personal physician. These most often include visits to emergency departments, to specialists such as ophthalmologists, or to alternative practitioners (3). Being aware of these visits is another way in which generalists coordinate their patients' care. When they obtain services elsewhere, patients can play an essential role by requesting that information be sent to their personal physicians.

Discharge Planning

Admission of the patient to the hospital follows approximately 0.5% of office visits (1). For each admission,

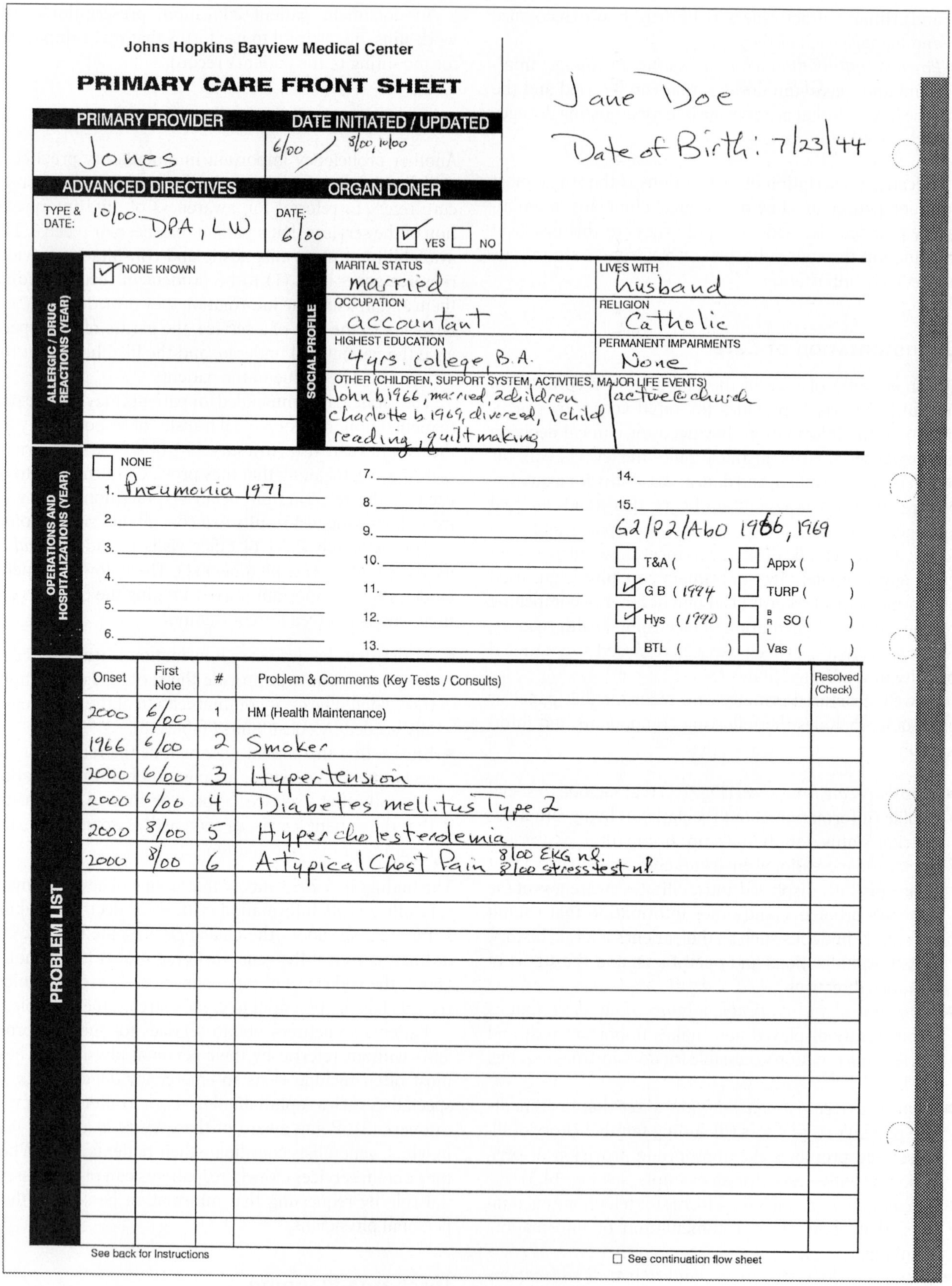

Johns Hopkins Bayview Medical Center

PRIMARY CARE FRONT SHEET

Jane Doe

Date of Birth: 7/23/44

PRIMARY PROVIDER	DATE INITIATED / UPDATED
Jones	6/00 / 8/00, 10/00

ADVANCED DIRECTIVES	ORGAN DONER
TYPE & DATE: 10/00 DPA, LW	DATE: 6/00 ☑ YES ☐ NO

ALLERGIC / DRUG REACTIONS (YEAR)

☑ NONE KNOWN

SOCIAL PROFILE

MARITAL STATUS	LIVES WITH
married	husband
OCCUPATION	**RELIGION**
accountant	Catholic
HIGHEST EDUCATION	**PERMANENT IMPAIRMENTS**
4yrs. college, B.A.	None

OTHER (CHILDREN, SUPPORT SYSTEM, ACTIVITIES, MAJOR LIFE EVENTS)
John b.1966, married, 2 children
Charlotte b.1969, divorced, 1 child
reading, quilt making
active @ church

OPERATIONS AND HOSPITALIZATIONS (YEAR)

☐ NONE

1. Pneumonia 1971
2.
3.
4.
5.
6.
7.
8.
9.
10.
11.
12.
13.
14.
15.

G2/P2/Ab0 1966, 1969

☐ T&A ( ) ☐ Appx ( )
☑ GB (1994) ☐ TURP ( )
☑ Hys (1990) ☐ BRL SO ( )
☐ BTL ( ) ☐ Vas ( )

PROBLEM LIST

Onset	First Note	#	Problem & Comments (Key Tests / Consults)	Resolved (Check)
2000	6/00	1	HM (Health Maintenance)	
1966	6/00	2	Smoker	
2000	6/00	3	Hypertension	
2000	6/00	4	Diabetes mellitus Type 2	
2000	8/00	5	Hypercholesterolemia	
2000	8/00	6	Atypical Chest Pain 8/00 EKG nl. 8/00 stress test nl.	

See back for Instructions

☐ See continuation flow sheet

FIGURE 1.1. Example of a primary care front sheet.

Johns Hopkins Bayview Medical Center
CLINICAL FLOW SHEET
(over for guidelines)

Jane Doe

Date of Birth: 7/23/44

Height (Date) 5'5", 170cm (6/00)

CHRONIC MEDICATIONS & NON-DRUG THERAPY

Date	6/00	8/00	10/00	1/01	5/01	11/01						
Pill Size, Dose, & Schedule (Insert R for refill, specific # disp. for DEA Rx; Insert Y, N, +/- for compliance)												
cong. estrogens	0.625 mg/d	→	→	→	→	Y→						
metformin 6/00		500 mg qd	500 mg bid	Y→	→	Y→						
lisinopril 8/00			10 mg qd	10 mg bid	→	Y→						
atorvastatin 8/00			10 mg qd	Y→	→	Y→						
smoking	1PPD	1PPD	1PPD	½PPD	⊖	2-5 cigs/d						
exercise	⊖	walks T.I.W	+/- →	Y→	→	Y→						
low salt, low chol, low sat fat, diabetic diet		→	+/- →	→	→	+/- →						

RESULTS →

CLINICAL & LABORATORY DATA

Weight lb/kg	185/84	186/85	184/84	182/83	181/82	179/81						
BP	154/95	158/100	142/88	134/79	130/65	127/75						
BMI / HgbA1C	29/8.2	/7.5	/7.2	/6.9		28/6.8						
fasting / random glucose	210/	160/	135/	127/		129/						
Cholesterol / fasting triglyceride	265/230	258/208	179/182	164/175	194/190	176/182						
HDL / LDLc	45/174	48/168	46/97	46/83	43/113	47/93						
Microalbumen U/A	18/NL											
BUN / Cr	18/0.8				19/0.7							
Foot Exam	NL				NL							
Eye Exam			9/00 NL			9/02 NL						
AST / ALT / CK		28/19	24/26	26/21 / 76	/18	/24						

130-656-186N (10/00) ☐ **Check if Clinical and Laboratory Data Flow Sheet continued on reverse**

FIGURE 1.2. Example of a clinical flow sheet, which aligns treatments and clinical/laboratory parameters.

TABLE 1.8 Information that Subspecialty Consultants Generally Need from the Referring Physician

The specific reason for the consultation
Relevant current medical problems
Relevant current medications
Relevant diagnostic tests already completed
What the patient has been told about the referral
Patient's attitude about the problem (if relevant)
Patient's address or telephone number

hospital discharge usually means the return of the patient to ambulatory care by the patient's primary physician. Each of the generic proficiencies described earlier is especially important when patients make the transition from dependence on hospital personnel to dependence on themselves or their families for management of their medical problems.

Beginning with the implementation of the federal prospective payment systems in the 1980s, and continuing with the growth of managed care in the 1990s, very short hospital stays have become the norm in the United States. By the beginning of the 21st century, inpatient care by hospitalists had become common and had been shown to add to the efficiency of hospital care (10). These changes have drawn attention to the elements of effective discharge planning, such as ensuring that patients and their families have a good understanding of the plan of care, ensuring that a concise discharge summary goes promptly to the practitioner or to the setting responsible for postdischarge care, and using home health services or other community-based services to help patients complete care that was previously carried out during prolonged hospital stays. Chapter 9 provides detailed information about home health services.

Cost Containment and Managed Care

Because of the extraordinary increase in available medical services in the past three decades and because of the parallel increase in the cost and the use of these services, cost containment in medical care is generally recognized as a national imperative. Managed care—that is, health care in which delivery and financing of care are linked in a variety of models—has emerged as a major strategy for containing costs. Managed care plans make arrangements with physicians ranging from directly employing them (staff-model HMOs) to contracting with them (group-model, network-model, and independent practice association–model) (11). Based on the 2002 NAMCS data from primary care physicians, 40% have 3 to 10 and 35% have more than 10 managed care contracts (1).

The goals of containing costs while providing high-quality care have critical implications for generalist physicians and practitioners, because it is they who coordinate much of the medical care provided in our society (12). These goals can be addressed in a number of ways, including the following:

- Taking a history carefully and allowing some time to pass before embarking on an extensive diagnostic workup of a new symptom;
- Keeping well informed about the impact on health outcomes of costly diagnostic procedures and therapies;
- Avoiding additional tests that will not alter one's decisions;
- Devoting sufficient time to educating patients about their conditions (especially about conditions that often lead to inappropriate and costly doctor shopping by the patient);
- Prescribing only necessary medications and selecting the least-expensive preparations;
- Using home health services and other community services, including innovative programs focused on high-cost conditions such as congestive heart failure, to forestall the need for hospital admission or to shorten the length of hospitalization.

Before the era of managed care, fee-for-service reimbursement tended to foster excessive use of laboratory tests and costly procedures. There were few external incentives for practitioners to engage in the inquiry, observation, counseling, and decision making that would have obviated much inappropriate use of health services. Besides fostering more appropriate spending of health care dollars, managed care may foster inappropriately low use of laboratory tests and costly procedures. Fortunately, direct incentives to practitioners to reduce the use of such services have been banned in most settings. To the extent that managed care rewards physicians for cognitive services—and does not overburden them with administrative hurdles or force upon them unreasonable productivity expectations—it has the potential both to promote the health of patients and to reduce the unnecessary use of costly services.

SPECIFIC REFERENCES

1. Woodwell DA, Cherry DK. National Ambulatory Medical Care Survey: 2002 Summary. Advance Data for Vital and Health Statistics No. 346. Hyattsville, MD: National Center for Health Statistics, August 26, 2004.
2. Kroenke K. Studying symptoms: sampling and measurement issues. Ann Intern Med 2001; 134:844.
3. Eisenberg DM, Davis RB, Ettner SL, et al. Trends in alternative medicine use in the United States, 1990–1997. JAMA 1998;280:1569.
4. Kohn R, White KL, eds. Health care. New York: Oxford University Press, 1976.
5. Google Fact Sheet, 2005. The Use of Over-the-Counter Medicines.

6. Fry J. Common diseases: their nature, incidence and care. 2nd ed. Philadelphia: Lippincott, 1979.
7. Tinetti ME, Fried T. The end of the disease era. Am J Med 2004;116:179.
8. Institute of Medicine, Committee on the Data Standards for Patient Safety. Key Capabilities of an Electronic Health Record System. Washington, DC: Institute of Medicine, 2003.
9. Smith PC, Araya-Guerra R, Bublitz C, et al. Missing clinical information during primary care visits. JAMA 2005;293:565.
10. Wachter RM, Goldman L. The hospitalist movement 5 years later. JAMA 2002;287:487.
11. Gold MR, Hurley R, Lake T, et al. A national survey of the arrangements managed-care plans make with physicians. N Engl J Med 1995;333:1678.
12. Bodenheimer T, Fernandez A. High and rising health care costs. Part 4: can costs be controlled while preserving quality? Ann Intern Med 2005;143:26.

*For annotated **General References** and resources related to this chapter, visit www.hopkinsbayview.org/PAMreferences.*

Chapter 2

Practicing Evidence-Based Medicine

*Darius A. Rastegar**

GENERAL APPROACH

Clinicians are increasingly (and appropriately) asked to provide both scientifically sound and cost-effective medical care. These expectations have given rise to an emphasis on *evidence-based medicine* (EBM), which is defined as the conscientious, explicit, and judicious use of current best evidence in making decisions about the care of individual patients (1). EBM focuses on issues integral to day-to-day patient care: assessment of risks, prevention, screening, diagnosis, prognosis, treatment, and management of the increasing amount of medical information that confronts health care practitioners.

Evidence-based decision making is especially important in ambulatory practice because this is the setting where patients are most likely to present with undifferentiated problems. It is also the setting where most clinical decisions are made.

The following steps are considered to be indispensable to practicing EBM:

Step 1: Formulate specific questions that are relevant to a patient's care and identify the type of information that is needed (e.g., efficacy or harm of a treatment, accuracy of a diagnostic test).
Step 2: Identify and retrieve the relevant data.
Step 3: Critically appraise the relevant information.
Step 4: Apply the valid information to the patient whose presentation initiated the inquiry, taking into account the patient's values and wishes.

The importance of *step 1,* formulation of specific questions, can be understood by considering two similar questions that might be generated when a practitioner sees a patient with hepatitis C who asks whether antiviral therapy, which the patient has read about in the newspaper, should be initiated:

- Question A: How effective is interferon and ribavirin for the treatment of hepatitis C?
- Question B: For Mr. B, the 48-year-old man with type 2 hepatitis C whose transaminases and liver function tests have been normal during the last 9 months, what is the evidence regarding the efficacy and safety of interferon and ribavirin in preventing cirrhosis and other complications?

The second question is more specific and will better help to tailor the search effort (step 2) to the clinical outcomes that are most relevant to the practitioner and the patient.

The successful completion of *step 2* requires efficient and effective searching skills. Most medical libraries offer brief hands-on tutorials to teach clinicians how to search databases such as MEDLINE and the Internet to find the current best evidence. The National Library of Medicine (see www.hopkinsbayview.org/PAMreferences) provides access to PubMed (MEDLINE) and multiple health and science databases. It also offers full-text versions of many articles, eliminating the need for additional steps to retrieve the desired manuscripts.

*Scott M. Wright contributed to an earlier version of this chapter.

Step 3, critical appraisal, is likely to be most difficult and time-consuming for clinicians. The two components of this step are (a) *deciding whether the results are valid* and (b) *deciding whether the results are relevant* to the specific question being asked.

It is more efficient to resolve the second component first, which can usually be done fairly quickly. If the results are neither relevant nor clinically important, then one can avoid the time and effort spent judging the validity and quality of the information. There are numerous books and articles published in the medical literature (e.g., the Users' Guides to the Medical Literature series published by the *Journal of the American Medical Association*) that aim to teach clinicians the core skills of critical appraisal. Having confidence in one's ability to critically appraise manuscripts on a wide variety of topics (e.g., diagnosis, treatment, cost-effectiveness), and which use a myriad of study designs, may take time, practice, and even additional training. Such training can be found in workshops at regional and national meetings or through medical libraries.

Step 4 involves integrating the important and valid newly found information into the care of one's patient. This step can be the most satisfying component of practicing EBM. Educating patients that a particular diagnostic approach or treatment is supported by current medical research may instill a sense of confidence about the practitioner's knowledge and expertise in finding new data. However, even after completing all these steps, choosing the best course of action is not always straightforward, and the patient's values and wishes should determine the ultimate course of action. For example, a patient may wish to forgo a treatment that may prolong their life but will likely worsen their quality of life (e.g., chemotherapy for metastatic cancer) or a patient may be unwilling to trade a short-term risk for the possibility of a long-term benefit (e.g., carotid endarterectomy for asymptomatic carotid stenosis).

It would be impractical to assume or recommend that primary care practitioners embark on these fundamental steps of EBM every time a clinical question comes up. However, when critical queries arise that are likely to recur or are particularly important to an individual patient, this version of "self-directed continuing medical education" is likely to be helpful to both practitioners and patients. Some barriers to practicing EBM include skepticism by practitioners, information overload and feeling overwhelmed by the growth of medical knowledge, lack of time, and lack of appropriate resources, skills, or motivation to implement EBM (2). Furthermore, for some clinical questions, high-quality data is lacking.

All dedicated and committed clinicians, however, practice EBM to some degree. To counterbalance the barriers to practicing EBM, the following facilitating behaviors have been proposed: (a) reading and keeping up-to-date with the medical literature (see Keeping Up); (b) refining one's EBM skills (practice makes perfect); (c) collaborating with colleagues so that valuable clinical evidence is shared among practitioners; (d) writing down specific clinical questions (step 1) when they come up so that the process can continue when time permits; (e) setting up one's computer (e.g., bookmarking relevant websites) and one's office (e.g., acquiring access to high-quality information) so as to find information efficiently; and (f) making friends with the librarian at the nearest medical library.

The remainder of this chapter discusses the core principles of EBM that apply to issues most relevant to primary care practice: diagnosis, prognosis, treatment, risk or potential harm, and cost-effectiveness. Strategies for keeping up are also discussed. Chapter 14 discusses principles that apply to prevention and screening.

DIAGNOSIS

How Clinicians Formulate a Diagnosis

Diagnostic assessment begins the moment one meets a patient. Behavioral scientists have described at least four ways in which clinicians formulate diagnoses: pattern recognition, algorithm, exhaustion, and hypothesis-deduction.

Pattern Recognition

Many diagnoses are made instantly because clinicians have learned to recognize patterns specific to certain diseases, such as the face of a patient with Down syndrome or the elbows of a patient with psoriasis. The certainty of these types of diagnoses is so great that further testing often is unnecessary.

Algorithm

Algorithms are growing more common as a result of the growth of clinical practice guidelines, which, when grounded scientifically, can be extremely helpful. The drawbacks of algorithms are that they must be constructed before the patient is seen, and they must account for every possibility in a workup.

Exhaustion

As Sackett pointed out (see Sackett et al., *Clinical Epidemiology,* at www.hopkinsbayview.org/PAMreferences), medical students should be taught how to do a complete history and physical examination, and then be taught never to do one again. On occasion, however, clinicians do resort to comprehensive histories and examinations, as much to buy time to think as to uncover hidden disease.

Hypothesis–Deduction

Clinicians usually diagnose by forming hypotheses and testing them, as is done in scientific experimentation. On hearing that a patient has chest pain, the practitioner builds a short list of hypotheses, invites further description, and then asks focused questions that help confirm or rule out the hypotheses. The questions in the interview and each maneuver in the examination are as much diagnostic tests as the electrocardiogram or the chest radiograph. Studies of clinicians' behavior reveal that the short list of hypotheses usually does not exceed three or four diagnoses. Typically, new hypotheses are added as others are discarded, but the eventual goal is to narrow the list and reduce the uncertainty about which diagnosis is most likely. Studies of clinicians in ambulatory practice showed that hypotheses were generated, on average, 28 seconds into the interview, and that correct diagnoses of standard problems were made 6 minutes into 30-minute workups; the correct diagnoses were made in 75% of the encounters (3).

The hypothesis–deduction model reveals a truth common to all methods of diagnosis: Rarely can a clinician be absolutely certain of any diagnosis. Clinicians live with uncertainty, and the role of all diagnostic tests—the interview, the physical examination, the laboratory evaluation, trials of empiric treatments, allowing time to pass (expectant observation)—is to narrow the uncertainty enough to place a diagnostic label on a patient's problem. How narrow the uncertainty must be depends on the practitioner's and the patient's tolerance of uncertainty, the severity of the suspected disease, the "treatability" of the suspected disease, and the benefits and risks of possible treatments.

Steps in the Hypothesis–Deduction Process

Evidence shows that clinicians implicitly use common sense and their medical knowledge to reach a diagnosis with adequate certainty. Explicitly, the diagnostic process follows certain steps.

Step 1: Form a Hypothesis and Estimate Its Likelihood

The estimate of likelihood is called the *pretest probability* (or *prior probability*); it simply represents the estimate of prevalence of the disease in a group of people similar to the patient at hand. Each hypothesized diagnosis and the estimate of its likelihood comes initially from evidence collected during the interview and physical examination and from the practitioner's fund of knowledge from sources such as other patients, colleagues, textbooks, and journals. More recently, computer programs have been developed to aid clinicians in making this estimate; these programs have the potential to become a powerful tool in clinical decision making.

Step 2: Decide How Certain the Diagnosis Must Be

If the hypothesized disease is easily and safely treated, one might have to be less certain than if the disease has an ominous prognosis or demands complex, risk-laden treatment. For example, a 75% certainty that a patient has streptococcal pharyngitis might be sufficient to prescribe an antibiotic, whereas a much higher level of certainty is needed before diagnosing and treating a patient with suspected leukemia. If the pretest probability is above the threshold for a hypothesized disease (e.g., greater than 75% for streptococcal pharyngitis), further tests are unnecessary and treatment is prescribed. Conversely, if one is adequately certain that the patient does not have the hypothesized disease (e.g., 90% probability that the patient does not have streptococcal pharyngitis), no further tests are required and the patient can be reassured and educated. However, if the level of uncertainty remains between these two extremes, further testing (e.g., a throat culture) can help move the case toward one extreme or the other. Diagnostic testing usually is most helpful between the two extremes of certainty, whereas further testing generally has little impact on the posttest probability if the pretest probability is very high or very low.

Step 3: Choose a Diagnostic Test

Which test to choose depends on many factors, including its safety, its *accuracy* (e.g., how closely an observation or a test result reflects the true clinical state of a patient), how easily it can be done, its cost, and, not least, the patient's preferences and values regarding tests, especially those that carry risks. Accuracy includes both reliability and validity. *Reliability* of a test, also called reproducibility or precision, is the extent to which repeated measurements of a stable phenomenon give results close to one another. *Validity* is the degree to which a test measures what it is supposed to measure. A test can be reliable but not valid (i.e., it reliably measures the wrong phenomenon), or it can be valid but not reliable (i.e., it measures the phenomenon of interest, but with wide scatter).

When considering a test, one needs to reflect on each of these factors. Table 2.1 summarizes practical guidelines to assess and critically appraise reported studies of diagnostic tests. When selecting a test for a patient, the crucial questions to ask are, "Will the results of the test change my plan?" and "Will my patient be better off from having had the test?" (*the utility of the test*). If the answer to these questions is "No," the test should not be performed.

TABLE 2.1 Guidelines for Assessing a Study of a Diagnostic Test

Was there an independent blind comparison with a gold standard?
Was the test evaluated in a sample of patients that included an appropriate spectrum of disease (mild to severe, treated and untreated) plus patients with commonly confused disorders?
Was the setting for the evaluation adequately described?
Were the reproducibility of the test result (precision) and its interpretation (observer variation) determined?
Was the term *normal* defined sensibly?
Were the methodologies for conducting the test described well enough for their exact replication?
Was the utility of the test determined (i.e., were the patients better off for having had the test)?

Adapted from Sackett DL, Haynes RB, Guyatt GH, et al. Clinical epidemiology: a basic science for clinical medicine. 2nd ed. Boston: Little, Brown, 1991.

Step 4: Be Aware of the Test's Performance Characteristics

Every diagnostic test has a sensitivity and specificity for each disease it tests for. *Sensitivity* and *specificity* have become common terms in medical discussion, but they are often misunderstood. The sensitivity of a test (the *true positive rate*) is equal to the number of study subjects with a given disease who have a positive test divided by all study subjects with the disease. The specificity of a test (the *true negative rate*) is the number of study subjects without the disease who have a negative test divided by all those without the disease. The 2 × 2 table in Fig. 2.1 reveals much about these and related terms.

Tests with high sensitivity have a low false-negative rate and are useful for "ruling out" a diagnosis (when they are negative). Conversely, tests with high specificity have a low false-positive rate and are useful for "ruling in" a diagnosis (when they are positive). One way of remembering this is with the mnemonics SnNOut (high sensitivity, negative result rules out) and SpPIn (high specificity, positive result rules in). However, it should be pointed out that these rules of thumb do not always hold up in actual practice; the ability of a sensitive test to rule out a diagnosis is reduced when the specificity is low (4).

"Diseased" and "not diseased" are labels that reflect a best test or a definition of a certain disease: the so-called *gold standard.* For pulmonary embolus, for example, the gold standard is the pulmonary angiogram. For angina, there is no sure test, so a case definition becomes the gold standard. Skepticism must be used in evaluating gold

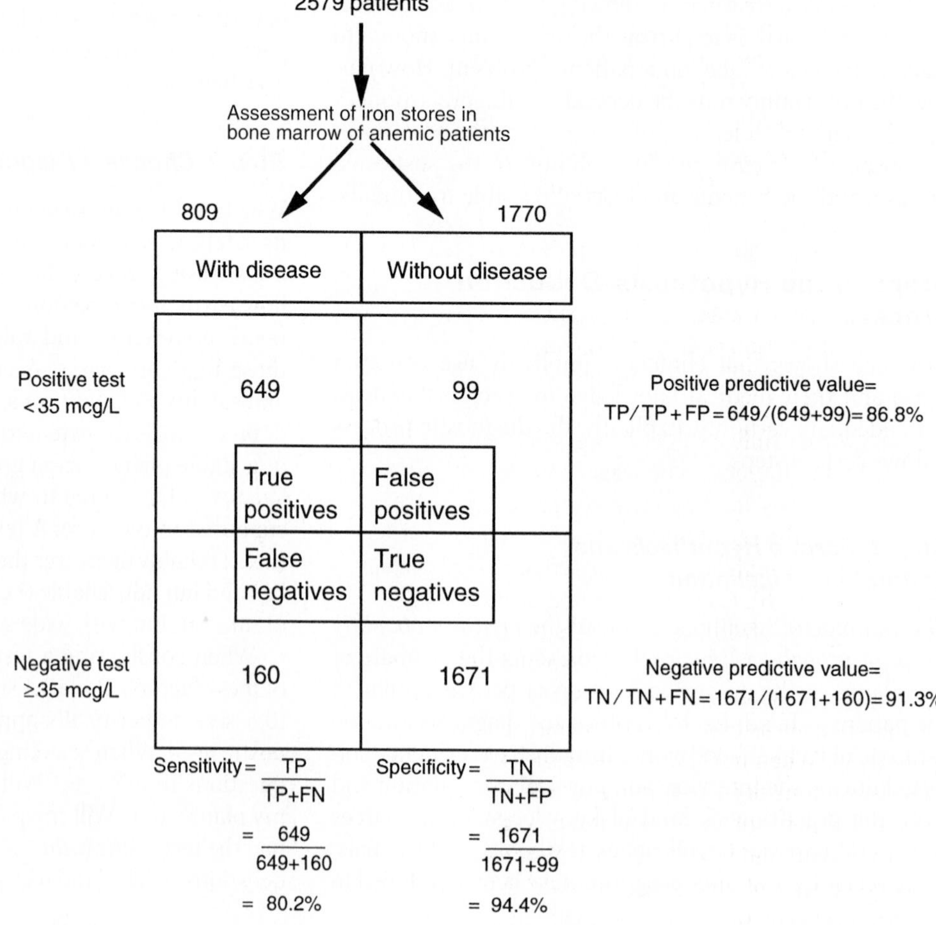

FIGURE 2.1. Test performance determined by research. Researcher identifies diseased and nondiseased patients using a gold standard and then determines the performance characteristics (sensitivity and specificity) of another test. *Example:* Iron-deficiency anemia determination using bone marrow aspirate/biopsy as the gold standard and serum ferritin measurement as the screening test. (Data from Guyatt GH, Patterson C, Ali M, et al. Diagnosis of iron deficiency in the elderly. Am J Med 1990;88:205.)

TABLE 2.2 Tradeoff between Sensitivity and Specificity when Diagnosing Iron-Deficiency Anemia: Likelihood Ratios

Serum Ferritin Level to be Used as the Cutoff Value (μg/L)	*Sensitivity (%)*	*False-Negative Rate (1− sensitivity, %)*	*Specificity (%)*	*False-Positive Rate (1− specificity, %)*	*Positive Likelihood Ratio (sensitivity/false-positive rate)*	*Negative Likelihood Ratio (false-negative rate/specificity)*
<15	58.6	41.4	98.9	1.1	53.3	0.42
<35	80.2	19.8	94.4	5.6	14.3	0.21
<65	90.4	9.6	84.7	15.3	5.9	0.11
<95	94.1	5.9	75.3	24.7	3.8	0.08

Adapted from Guyatt GH, Patterson C, Ali M, et al. Diagnosis of iron deficiency in the elderly. Am J Med 1990;88:205, and from Sackett DL, Haynes RB, Guyatt GH, et al. Clinical epidemiology: a basic science for clinical medicine. 2nd ed. Boston: Little, Brown, 1991.

standards, for they often have their own limitations. For example, when gallbladder ultrasonography was tested for use in the diagnosis of cholelithiasis, it initially seemed to be a poor test in comparison with the gold standard (oral cholecystogram), not because of problems with the new test, but because, as was later shown, the gold standard was itself a poor test (5). Studies of diagnostic testing may have other problems, including *verification bias* (when those with a positive test result are more likely to have further evaluation), *spectrum bias* (when the population tested does not reflect those in whom the test will be used), and *incorporation bias* (when the results of the test under study are included among criteria to establish the reference standard).

Sensitivity and specificity are not static properties of a test. As the cutoff value for an abnormal result is made more extreme, the test's sensitivity decreases and its specificity increases. Table 2.2, where progressively lower ferritin levels are used to characterize elderly patients as having iron-deficiency anemia (IDA), illustrates this principle (6). This illustration matches the common-sense conclusion that as a patient's test result becomes more abnormal, one can be more certain that the patient has disease—although never fully certain. If one selects a very low ferritin level for the cutoff between normal and abnormal (Table 2.2), many iron-deficient people will remain undiagnosed (i.e., the sensitivity will be low), but almost all of those diagnosed will be truly iron deficient (i.e., the specificity will be high). Conversely, if one decides to label patients as having IDA based on a ferritin level well within the normal range (e.g., 75 μg/L), one will not miss much disease (higher sensitivity), but will falsely label numerous anemic patients as being iron deficient who are not (lower specificity). When interpreting the results of a test, a clinician must consider the severity of disease, the potential risks and benefits of treatment, and changing information about the risks and benefits of treatment.

Another way of showing the relationship (and tradeoff) between sensitivity and specificity is to plot a *receiver operating curve* (ROC); the true-positive rate (sensitivity) is plotted on the vertical axis and the false-positive rate (1 − specificity) on the horizontal axis. Figure 2.2 shows a plot of the values provided in Table 2.2. Receiver operating curves can be a useful tool to compare different diagnostic tests; in general, the closer the curve is to the left-upper-hand corner (100% sensitivity and specificity), the better the test performs.

Step 5: Determine a Posttest Probability of Disease

The perfect test (100% sensitivity and specificity) would yield a "yes" or "no" answer to the question "Does my patient have disease or not?" However, because no test is perfect, the more appropriate question is: "Given the result of this test, what is the posttest probability that my patient has (or does not have) disease?" Posttest probability takes into account both the performance characteristics (sensitivity and specificity) of the test and the pretest (prior) probability of disease in a group of patients similar to the patient in question.

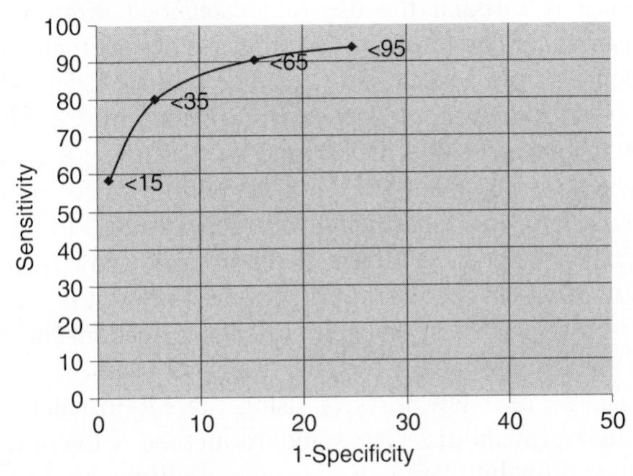

FIGURE 2.2. Receiver operating curve (ROC) of serum ferritin for iron-deficiency anemia.

One method for determining posttest probability is through the use of *predictive values.* Predictive values can be calculated from the known sensitivity and specificity of a test and the estimated pretest probability of disease. Sensitivity and specificity are generally transferable from study to practice settings, provided the diseased and nondiseased populations in the study and in the practice settings are similar. Sensitivity and specificity usually are not influenced by the prevalence, or pretest probability, of disease. However, predictive values must be recalculated for each patient or population from the estimated pretest probability or prevalence of disease in that particular group. *Positive predictive value* is the probability of disease in a patient who has an abnormal test result. *Negative predictive value* is the probability of no disease in a patient for whom a test result is normal. Figure 2.1 illustrates the calculation of posttest probability, based on pretest probability, sensitivity, and specificity.

The lower the pretest probability of disease, the lower the positive predictive value of a test, the lower the posttest probability of disease, and the more likely it is that a positive test result is falsely positive. This influence of pretest probability on posttest probability makes intuitive sense. For example, when a seasoned clinician encounters an unexpected positive test result in a patient with a very low likelihood of disease, the clinician is suspicious of the finding and either repeats the test, suspecting laboratory error, or orders another, more specific test to confirm or refute the finding.

Published information is available that can be helpful in estimating pretest probability, and therefore the predictive value of test results, in patients with selected characteristics. Examples of how such information can be used to interpret test results and determine diagnostic strategies are illustrated elsewhere in this book for deep vein thrombosis (see Chapter 57) and renovascular hypertension (see Chapter 67).

Another method of calculating posttest probability of disease is through the use of a *likelihood ratio* (LR). This number combines the relationships of sensitivity and specificity into a single number. The positive LR (+LR) is the *true-positive rate* (sensitivity) divided by the *false-positive rate* (1 − specificity), and the negative LR (–LR) is the *false-negative rate* (1 − sensitivity) divided by the *true-negative rate* (specificity). LR ranges from 0 to infinity; when the positive LR is between 0 and 1, a positive test result *decreases* the posttest probability; when it is >1, it *increases* the posttest probability; a LR of 1 does not change the posttest probability (i.e., the test is not useful).

There are a few ways of using the LR to calculate posttest probabilities. The standard method is to convert pretest probability into an *odds ratio*, multiply this by the likelihood ratio to determine posttest odds ratio, and then convert the posttest odds ratio to a probability:

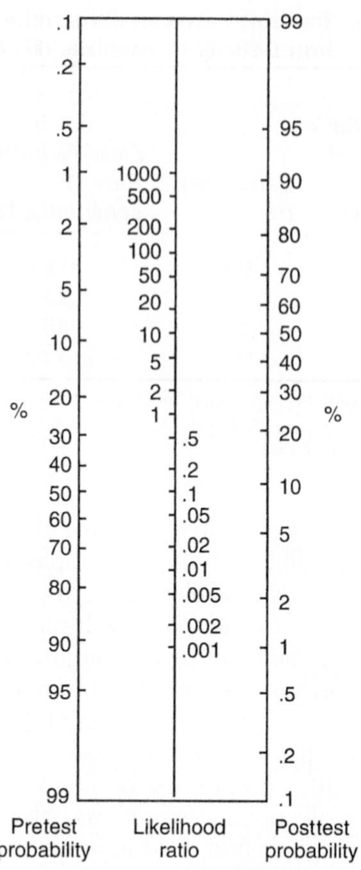

FIGURE 2.3. Nomogram for interpreting test results using likelihood ratios. *Example from text:* An elderly male patient with anemia has a pretest probability of having IDA equal to 33%. His serum ferritin level is 33 μg/L, which is associated with a positive LR of 14.3. Extending a straight line through the pretest probability of 33% and the LR of 14.3 results in a posttest probability of 88%. (Adapted from Fagan TJ. Nomogram for Bayes' theorem. N Engl J Med 1975;293:257.)

1. Pretest Probability ÷ (1 − Pretest Probability) = Pretest Odds
2. Pretest Odds × Likelihood Ratio = Posttest Odds
3. Posttest Odds ÷ (1 + Posttest Odds) = Posttest Probability

Another method is to use a nomogram (Fig. 2.3) that allows conversion of pretest to posttest probabilities, given a known LR, without having to convert back and forth between probabilities and odds. This alternative is quick, is easy to use, and decreases the chances of calculation error.

However, converting probabilities to odds ratios and back can be cumbersome, and most of us do not carry nomograms in our pockets. For this reason, it may be simpler to use a method of estimating posttest probabilities (7). This method is fairly accurate when the pretest probability is between 10% and 90% (i.e., neither very high nor very low). Table 2.3 summarizes the approximate change

TABLE 2.3 Simplified Posttest Probability Estimates Based on Likelihood Ratio*

Likelihood Ratio	*Approximate Change in Probability*
1/10 (0.1)	−45%
1/5 (0.2)	−30%
1/2 (0.5)	−15%
1	0%
2	+15%
5	+30%
10	+45%

*These estimates are only applicable if the pretest probability is between 10% and 90%.
From McGee S. Simplifying likelihood ratios. J Gen Intern Med 2002;17:646.

in probability associated with a range of LRs. One can simply remember that positive LRs of 2, 5, 10 are associated with approximate posttest probability *increases* of 15%, 30% and 45% respectively. Conversely, LRs of 1/2 (0.5), 1/5 (0.2), and 1/10 (0.1) *decrease* the posttest probability by 15%, 30% and 45% respectively.

For example, suppose the clinician is faced with a 67-year-old male patient who has increasing fatigue and is found to be anemic. Knowing that the baseline prevalence (pretest probability) of IDA among anemic elderly patients is 31% (6), one might consider this man's pretest probability of IDA to be approximately 33%, for an odds of 1:2, or 0.5. If the serum ferritin is 33 μg/L, we can see from Table 2.2 that when a cutoff of <35 μg/L is used, the positive LR is 14.3:

$$\text{Pretest odds of IDA} \times (+)\text{LR} = \text{Posttest odds,} \quad \text{or } 0.5 \times 14.3 = 7.16$$

So the odds of the patient having IDA based on this test result are 7:1. Converting back to probability, the patient has a posttest probability of IDA of about $7 \div (1 + 7) = 7 \div 8 = 88\%$. Given this posttest probability, further diagnostic workup (e.g., colonoscopy) to identify the cause of the IDA is appropriate.

Using the nomogram and a straightedge, the posttest probability is approximately 85%. Finally, if we use the simplified estimation method outlined earlier, we know that the likelihood ratio is >10; consequently, we should add at least 45% to the pretest probability of 31%, yielding a posttest probability of >76%, which is probably close enough to the actual value to help us in our decision making.

PROGNOSIS

Often, the information that is most important to a patient who has a new diagnosis is the prognosis ("What is going to happen to me?"). In choosing therapy, one decides what one can do for the patient's disease. Yet, predicting what will happen to a particular patient usually is not possible, and clinicians must rely on probabilities. Sometimes, specific characteristics ("prognostic factors") such as demographic factors, disease-specific factors, and comorbidities can help further delineate a patient's prognosis. Clinical prediction rules that take these factors into account can help practitioners arrive at more accurate estimates of prognosis.

Prognosis can be addressed in two ways: the *natural history* of a disease and the *clinical course* of a disease. Because few diseases today progress without medical intervention, less is being learned about natural history and more is being learned about clinical course. For example, the natural history of diabetes in the late 20th century is unknown because virtually no diagnosed patients go without some type of therapy, yet through many studies, more is known about the course of treated diabetes.

Most information about prognosis comes from prospective cohort studies in which patients with a disease are monitored over time. Cohort studies may include only untreated subjects (natural history of a disease), only treated subjects, or a combination of both treated and untreated subjects (clinical course of a disease). Cohort studies are simple in design, yet they are often costly in time and money. They are susceptible to biases, such as *sampling bias,* in which the group of patients being monitored is not representative of all patients with that condition. Table 2.4 summarizes suggested guidelines for assessing studies of prognosis.

TREATMENT

Once a diagnosis is made, treatment becomes the focus of care. Before embarking on a treatment plan, one must decide on the goals of treatment (to cure, delay complications, relieve acute distress, reassure, or comfort). Clearly, more than one goal may be chosen. For example, when

TABLE 2.4 Guidelines for Assessing a Study of Prognosis

Was a representative and well-defined sample of patients (at a similar point in disease course) assembled?
Are these patients similar to my own?
Was followup sufficiently long and complete?
Were objective and relevant outcome criteria developed and used?
Was the outcome assessment "blind"?
Was adjustment for important prognostic factors carried out?

Adapted from Laupacis A, Wells G, Richardson WS, et al. User's guides to the medical literature. V: how to use an article about prognosis. JAMA 1994:272:234.

diagnosing and treating type 2 diabetes, one may seek to cure (counsel weight loss and exercise), to delay or prevent complications (seek tight glucose control), and to relieve distress, reassure, and comfort (listen to the patient's fears, reassure the patient that diabetes is a treatable disease and that he or she will not be abandoned).

Once the goals have been set, treatments are chosen. Unfortunately, many treatments have never been tested scientifically in ways that answer the questions that are of interest to clinicians and their patients (e.g., probability of benefit, size of benefit, onset time and duration of response, frequency of complications of treatment), and many aspects of treatment are difficult to measure through scientific experiments. Fortunately, drugs and procedures are increasingly being subjected to clinical trials, and measures of quality of life are being included in the evaluation of therapies.

The *clinical trial* is the current standard for assessment of drugs and therapeutic procedures. The strongest clinical trials are randomized, double-blinded controlled trials. The strength of a *randomized controlled trial* (RCT) is that the study groups are likely to be similar with respect to known determinants of outcome, as well as those determinants that are unknown. However, randomization is often difficult to accomplish in the real world, where patients are free to join or refuse to join a clinical trial and where money to support research is limited. Theoretically, in a trial that is *double blinded* (meaning that neither the patient nor the researcher knows who is receiving the experimental treatment), the researchers' and patients' assessment of outcome is not biased by prior knowledge of their assignment (e.g., to placebo or to active treatment). However, studies may not be truly blinded; for example, in a trial of β-blockers against placebo, patients and clinicians can measure pulse rates. Nonetheless, the clinical trial is the least-biased method currently available for researchers to test how well drugs and other interventions work in ideal situations (*efficacy*) and in the real world (*effectiveness*). Table 2.5 lists guidelines that clinicians can use when assessing the results of a clinical trial. As illustrated in the table, there are important questions to ask of a clinical trial that reports benefits to treated subjects. Were clinically relevant outcomes, such as measures of patient health (e.g., morbid events, functional status) reported, and not just surrogate end points (e.g., reduction of blood pressure)? Was all-cause mortality, not just mortality caused by the disease in question (e.g., colon cancer), reported? In addition to reporting the *statistical significance* of findings (the probability that the findings are true), did the study discuss or clarify the *clinical significance* of the findings (whether the benefits were clinically meaningful)? As the size of a study increases, there is an increased likelihood that clinically small or nonmeaningful benefits, which are nonetheless statistically significant, will be demonstrated.

TABLE 2.5 Guidelines for Assessing a Study of Treatment (Clinical Trials)

Was the assignment of patients to treatments really randomized?
Were all clinically relevant outcomes reported?
Were the study patients recognizably similar to my own?
Were both statistical and clinical significance considered?
Is the treatment feasible for patients in my practice?
Was the analysis performed on an intention-to-treat basis?
Were all patients who entered the study accounted for at its conclusion?

Adapted from Sackett DL, Haynes RB, Guyatt GH, et al. Clinical epidemiology: a basic science for clinical medicine. 2nd ed. Boston: Little, Brown, 1991.

Moreover, one must pay close attention to the followup of the subjects enrolled in trials; *intention-to-treat* analysis is a strategy for analyzing data in which all study participants are analyzed in the group to which they were assigned, regardless of whether they dropped out, were noncompliant, or crossed over to another treatment or nontreatment group. Such an analysis may weaken the ability of a study to demonstrate the effect of a treatment, but it prevents selection biases caused by differences in participants who drop out from a treatment compared with those who remain.

Researchers often report treatment outcomes in terms of the *relative risk reduction* (RRR), which is the difference in the event rate between control and experimental groups of patients expressed as a proportion of the event rate in the control group: RRR = (control event rate − experimental event rate) ÷ control event rate. The difference between the control and experimental event rates is the *absolute risk reduction* (ARR): ARR = control event rate − experimental event rate. RRR can alternatively be expressed as the ARR divided by the control event rate: RRR = ARR ÷ control event rate. RRR is only meaningful in the context of absolute risk and can be misleading when applied to individual patients. If someone is at very low risk for an adverse outcome, a treatment with even a high RRR will have negligible effect on their absolute risk. On the other hand, for someone who is at high risk for an adverse event, even a small RRR can have a significant impact on their absolute risk. One method of incorporating absolute risk into an assessment of an intervention's impact, besides stating ARR, is to calculate the *number needed to treat* (NNT). This refers to the number of persons who need to be treated for one person to benefit and is a more useful measure for a clinician than the RRR. The calculation for NNT is simply 100%/ARR, with ARR expressed as a percentage, or 1/ARR, with ARR expressed as a fraction (e.g., 0.10 for an ARR of 10%).

These concepts can be illustrated using the results of two trials of beta-hydroxy-beta-methylglutaryl-coenzyme A (HMG-CoA) reductase inhibitors ("statins") for the

TABLE 2.6 Use of Data to Estimate Clinical Consequences of Treatment: Comparison of Two Trials

	Fatal or Non-fatal MI after 5 years		*RRR*	*ARR*	*NNT to Benefit One Patient*
Trial	*Control (placebo)*	*Treatment (statin)*	*(Control – Treatment) ÷ Control*	*Control – Treatment*	*100% ÷ ARR*
4S (1)	22%	14%	(22% – 14%) ÷ 22% = 36%	22% – 14% = 8%	100% ÷ 8% = 12 patients
CAPS (2)	2.9%	1.7%	(2.9% – 1.7%) ÷ 2.9% = 41%	2.9% – 1.7% = 1.2%	100% ÷ 1.2% = 83 patients

ARR, Absolute risk reduction; NNT, number needed to treat; RRR, relative risk reduction.
Data from (1) Scandinavian Simvastatin Survival Study. Randomised trial of cholesterol lowering in 4444 patients with coronary heart disease. Lancet 1994;344:1383, and (2) Downs JR, Clearfield M, Weis S, et al. Primary prevention of acute coronary events with lovastatin in men and women with average cholesterol levels: results of AFCAPS/TexCAPS. Air Force/Texas Coronary Atherosclerosis Prevention Study. JAMA 1998;279:1615.

prevention of myocardial infarction. The Scandinavian Simvastatin Survival Study (4S) included subjects with high cholesterol levels and a history of coronary heart disease (8). In contrast, the Air Force/Texas Coronary Atherosclerosis Prevention Study (AFCAPS/TexCAPS) trial included a lower-risk group of individuals with average cholesterol levels and no known heart disease (9). Table 2.6 provides the rates of myocardial infarction (fatal and non-fatal) in each trial and shows how to calculate the RRR, ARR, and NNT. Although treatment with a statin in both trials yielded similar *relative* risk reductions (≈40%), the *absolute* risk reductions and numbers needed to treat are quite different. This illustrates the importance of understanding an individual's risk when trying to gauge the impact of a therapeutic intervention; a practitioner (on average) would need to treat 83 patients with average cholesterol levels and no history of heart disease with a statin for 5 years to prevent a myocardial infarction, while only 12 patients with high cholesterol levels and heart disease would need to be treated to prevent one event.

There are a few caveats about clinical trials. Although the RCT is the best study design for assessing the value of a treatment, one should be cautious about relying on the results of any single study, even one that was done well. Systematic reviews and meta-analyses, which combine the results a number of studies, are discussed later in this chapter (see Keeping Up). Sometimes clinical trials have not been performed. In this situation, the clinician may need to rely on cohort, case-control, or cross-sectional studies. These types of studies are more commonly used to assess risk or harm and are discussed in the next section.

RISK OR POTENTIAL HARM

Practitioners are frequently called on to make assessments and judgments regarding risk or potential harm resulting from either medical interventions or environmental exposures. Table 2.7 summarizes some of the guidelines for assessing evidence of harm. Ideally, these questions would be answered in a RCT; however, for obvious ethical reasons, RCTs are not undertaken with the intent of studying a harmful exposure. Sometimes, a potentially beneficial intervention is unexpectedly found to be harmful in a clinical trial, or there may be both benefits and harms associated with the intervention.

More commonly, harm is addressed through observational studies. One kind of observational study is a *cohort study,* in which exposed and unexposed patients are identified and monitored for a period of time, and outcomes in the two groups are compared. For example, a cohort of cigarette smokers and nonsmokers could be monitored and the incidence of lung cancer in both groups measured. In these studies, the two groups may be different with respect to important determinants of outcome other than the exposure being studied (*confounding variables*). Researchers often can statistically adjust for these factors,

TABLE 2.7 Guidelines for Assessing a Study of Harm

What type of study was reported: a prospective cohort study (with or without comparison group); a retrospective case-control study; a cross-sectional study; a case series; or a case report?
Were comparison groups clearly identified and similar with respect to potential determinants of outcome, other than the one of concern? If not, were differences in potential determinants controlled for in the analysis of data?
Were outcomes measured the same way in the groups compared (and was the assessment objective and blinded)?
Was followup sufficiently long and complete?
Was there a temporal relationship between exposure and harm?
Was there a dose–response gradient?
What was the magnitude of the risk, and how precise is this estimate?

Adapted from Levine M, Walter S, Lee H, et al. User's guides to the medical literature. IV: how to use an article about harm. JAMA 1994;271:1615.

but there may be other contributing factors of which they are unaware.

Another method of assessing harm is through *case-control studies*. In these studies, patients with an outcome of interest (cases) are identified and compared with others who are similar in respects other than the outcome (controls). Exposure rates in the case and control groups are then compared to look at the association between the exposure and the outcome. For example, the smoking rate in a group of patients with lung cancer may be compared with a group of patients without lung cancer who are otherwise similar. These studies are subject to *recall bias*: patients with an illness may be more likely to recall or report an unusual exposure than those who are not ill. In addition, like cohort studies, they are limited by the possibility of differences in unidentified risk factors between the groups.

Cohort and case-control studies can also be used to assess potentially beneficial associations, as was done in studies that suggested a cardiovascular benefit of hormone replacement therapy. However, this benefit was not demonstrated when studied in an RCT (10), calling the purported benefit into question and highlighting the limitations of observational data.

Weaker designs for identifying risk or harm include cross-sectional studies, case series, and case reports. *Cross-sectional studies* can establish associations but not causal links. They are strengthened by statistical methods that control for confounding variables (potential determinants of harm other than the one of concern). Temporal relationships, however, are usually not established. In *case reports* or *case series,* adverse outcomes associated with a particular exposure are reported in a single patient or group of patients. These reports are useful for identifying potentially harmful exposures to be studied further, but they are weak evidence for a causal relationship by themselves. However, if the outcome is very harmful and otherwise rare, this kind of evidence may be sufficient to take action. This might occur, for example, when severe adverse reactions associated with a particular medication are reported, especially if safer alternatives exist. A recent example is troglitazone, which was taken off the market after case reports of severe hepatotoxicity associated with its use.

COST-EFFECTIVENESS

In ambulatory practice, cost considerations arise frequently. Cost-effectiveness analyses evaluate health care outcomes in relation to cost. The primary goals are to determine the most efficient use of resources and to minimize the costs associated with the achievement of health goals and objectives. A common strategy for cost-effectiveness studies is to compare a novel approach or therapy with the current practice or standard of care. The time frame of the study should be long enough to allow for costs and long-term benefits to be realized. The perspective of the analysis takes into account who benefits from the intervention as well as who pays for it (society, the payer, or the patient). Cost-effectiveness analyses often rely on a number of assumptions, and small variations in one or more of these parameters can have a significant effect on the conclusions; a *sensitivity analysis* can help determine how sensitive the outcomes are to changes in the parameters.

TABLE 2.8 Guidelines for Assessing a Study with an Economic Analysis of Clinical Practice

Did the analysis provide a full economic comparison of health care strategies?
Were the costs and outcomes appropriately measured and valued?
Were the estimates of costs and outcomes related to the baseline risk in the treatment population?
Was a sensitivity analysis performed that included a range of estimates for important assumptions? Are the findings consistent across reasonable ranges of assumptions, or do they change as the assumptions vary within reasonable ranges?
What were the incremental costs and outcomes of each strategy?
Are treatment benefits worth the harms and costs?

Adapted from Drummond MF, Richardson WS, O'Brien BJ, et al. User's guides to the medical literature. XIII: how to use an article on economic analysis of clinical practice. JAMA 1997;277:1552.

Whether decisions are being made for a population (e.g., frequency of screening colonoscopy, drugs to be added to a formulary) or for a particular patient (e.g., choice of antihypertensive medicine), the potential benefits should be weighed against the resources used and money spent. Table 2.8 summarizes some guidelines for assessing evidence in studies performing economic analyses.

In *cost-effectiveness analyses,* costs usually are measured in monetary units (e.g., dollars) and a single clinical outcome is considered (e.g., mortality). In *cost-utility analyses,* multiple clinical outcomes, including quality of life, are represented and result in the calculation of "quality-adjusted life years (QALY)." In both types of analyses, alternative diagnostic or therapeutic approaches are studied with a primary emphasis placed on economic considerations.

KEEPING UP

One of the major challenges to clinicians is keeping one's personal fund of medical knowledge current. Studies suggest that older practitioners are often "out of date" and tend to provide lower-quality care (11). For primary care practitioners who are expected to know about a wide array of clinical topics, keeping up-to-date can be particularly difficult. It has been suggested that each practitioner should develop a personal mission as to the extent of "up-to-datedness" he or she hopes to achieve and maintain. Two questions that may help to better define this territory are (a) "What information do I need to have in my head to be satisfied with my knowledge base for the performance of my job?" and (b) "What information would I be embarrassed not to know?" (12).

One author estimated that if clinicians tried to keep up with the medical literature by reading one article each day, they would be 55 centuries behind in their reading after 1 year (see Sackett et al., *Clinical Epidemiology,* at www.hopkinsbayview.org/PAMreferences). In a seminal study, experienced clinicians in ambulatory practice said they had about two clinical questions per week that went unanswered; however, when shadowed in day-to-day practice, they were found to actually have about two unanswered questions for every three patients seen (13). Moreover, although these clinicians said that their main sources of information were textbooks and journals, their behavior showed that they got most of their clinical information from colleagues and drug retailers. Fortunately, in ambulatory medicine, some *high-quality secondary* or *abstracting publications* exist that produce abstracts and often provide expert commentary on clinical articles believed to be of particular importance (approximately 2% to 3% of articles screened from hundreds of journals) (14). Examples are the *ACP Journal Club* and *Evidence-Based Medicine*.

Scheduling of time to obtain and find relevant reading material is a critical step in keeping up-to-date. The actual reading of the pulled material can occur either in the scheduled time or when a lull presents itself (e.g., a patient no-show). *Proactive* scanning or browsing through a small number of peer-reviewed journals that regularly yield articles relevant to one's clinical practice is an integral part of keeping up. *Reactive* learning (also called problem-focused learning) is stimulated by clinical encounters or questions from patients or medical learners and requires searching to find the appropriate materials (steps 1 and 2 of the core EBM skills described at the beginning of this chapter). Sackett described the *"educational prescription"* as a means of phrasing and keeping track of questions as they arise with the goal and intent of searching for the best available evidence to answer these queries at some time later. A combination of proactive and reactive approaches is thought to represent the ideal balance for dealing with the evolution of medical knowledge. Several additional ideas have been suggested by authors who have pondered the challenge of keeping clinically up-to-date (Table 2.9) (15).

Although original research articles continue to be an excellent source for new information, other types of publications can also be helpful in the quest to stay current. One common source of medical information is the *overview.* The chapters of this book (and other textbooks) are one example of an overview; review articles in medical journals are another. These types of overviews are easy to access (especially if the textbook is at hand) and easy to use; they require little work or effort to obtain needed information. However, they are limited by the biases and limitations of the authors and typically do not explain how the information was gathered or how conclusions were reached.

Systematic reviews and *meta-analyses* published in peer-reviewed journals with detailed methods describing specifically the literature search and the inclusion/exclusion criteria of the original articles can be invaluable. Critical appraisal methods for these two article types have been developed and can be applied to evaluate the quality of the work (16); Table 2.10 summarizes these methods. Some of the limitations that need to be considered

TABLE 2.9 Elements of an Information Plan

Browse at least one general journal regularly.
Maintain surveillance on new information.
Establish reliable ways of looking up common facts.
Identify a set of ways to look up obscure facts.
Develop critical appraisal skills.
Set aside high-quality time regularly to deal with information needs.
Invest time to discover new sources of useful information.

From Fletcher RH, Fletcher SW. Keeping clinically up-to-date. J Gen Intern Med 1997;12:S5.

TABLE 2.10 Guidelines for Assessing a Review Article

Are the results of the study valid?
Did the review address an explicitly described, focused clinical question?
Were appropriate criteria (inclusion and exclusion) used for selecting studies for review?
Were search strategies explicitly described, thorough, and appropriate? Is it unlikely that important, relevant studies were missed?
Was the validity of the included studies appraised and accounted for?
Were assessments of the studies reproducible?
Were results similar from study to study?
If data from different studies were combined quantitatively, were the methods explicit and reasonable?
What are the results?
What are the overall results of the review?
How precise are the results?
Are the results presented in a manner that permits comparison and synthesis of the key features and findings of the studies reviewed?
Will the results help me in caring for my patients?
Can the results be applied to my patient care?
Were all clinically important outcomes (benefits and harms) considered?
Are the benefits worth the harms and costs?

Adapted from Oxman AD, Cook DJ, Guyatt GH. Users' guides to the medical literature. VI: how to use an overview. Evidence-Based Medicine Working Group. JAMA 1994;272:1367.

include the heterogeneity of studies (with regard to populations studied and outcomes assessed) and the fact that small studies with negative results are less likely to be published than those with positive results (*publication bias*). Authors often try to correct for these limitations, but meta-analyses have sometimes yielded results and conclusions that were discordant with subsequent large RCTs (17). Nevertheless, meta-analysis can be a powerful tool to synthesize the available evidence in an unbiased fashion. In addition to those published in medical journals, the *Cochrane Collaboration* (and the Cochrane Library—see www.hopkinsbayview.org/PAMreferences) represents an international endeavor to develop, maintain, and disseminate systematic reviews on clinical and health-related topics.

Guidelines are systematically developed statements that offer recommendations to assist with decision making in specific situations. It has been found that clinicians often do not employ effective interventions (e.g., prescribing beta-blockers to patients after a myocardial infarction). Guidelines serve the dual purpose of offering easily accessible recommendations for practitioners and publicizing these recommendations to practitioners and the general public. Guidelines typically are developed by expert panels. They are best when they employ explicit criteria for gathering the evidence and making recommendations and acknowledge the level of evidence for each recommendation. Guidelines may be biased by the composition of the expert panel, and sometimes conflicting guidelines are disseminated by different organizations. For example, the American Urological Association recommends offering prostate-specific antigen (PSA) determinations to screen for prostate cancer, whereas the United States Preventive Services Task Force does not. Table 2.11 lists some suggestions for evaluating practice guidelines.

Each information source has strengths and weaknesses. Colleagues may be misinformed. Drug retailers have a product to sell, making them biased. Textbooks are often out of date by the time they are printed. Traditional continuing medical education courses provide variable degrees of evidence-based education and have been shown to have little effect on practice.

TABLE 2.11 Guidelines for Assessing a Practice Guideline

Was a recent, reproducible, and comprehensive review of the literature carried out?
Were the methods of the review explicit and strong? Specifically, were inclusion and exclusion criteria explicit and reasonable? Were methods of synthesizing the data explicit and reasonable? Was each recommendation assigned a level of evidence supporting it and a strength based on an explicit synthesis of all considerations?
How does this guideline compare to other guidelines? Does the group issuing this guideline have biases or conflicts of interest?
Have important studies been conducted subsequent to the guideline that would alter the recommendations?
Does the burden of the problem addressed warrant implementation of the guideline?
Would implementation of the guideline be cost-effective and feasible?

Adapted from Sackett DL, Straus SE, Richardson WS, et al. Evidence-based medicine: how to practice and teach EBM. 2nd ed. Edinburgh: Churchill Livingstone, 2000.

Because "keeping up" with the medical literature represents a colossal challenge, some authors have provided some direction for how to optimize the chance that one's time investment will result in a reasonable return (18,19). They suggest that the usefulness of medical information for a given provider is proportional to its relevance, validity, and accessibility. *Relevance* relates to the frequency with which the provider encounters the topic. *Validity* refers to the quality of the information and the likelihood that the information is true. *Accessibility* connotes the ease with which the information source can be retrieved. These authors recommend that practitioners seek out information sources that are relevant, valid, and easily accessible.

Finally, *medical librarians* can be extraordinary helpful in keeping clinicians in touch with changes in the medical literature, and they most are happy to meet with clinicians to make them aware of new resources. Befriending one's medical librarian is a critical component of a "keeping up" strategy and can pay huge dividends in the pursuit of evidence-based medical practice.

SPECIFIC REFERENCES*

1. Sackett DL, Rosenberg WM, Gray JAM, et al. Evidence-based medicine: what it is and what it isn't. BMJ 1996;312:71.
2. Wilkinson EK, Bosanquet A, Salisbury C, et al. Barriers and facilitators to the implementation of evidence-based medicine in general practice: a qualitative study. Eur J Gen Pract 1999;5:66.
3. Barrows HS, Norman GR, Neufeld VR, et al. The clinical reasoning of randomly selected physicians in general medical practice. Clin Invest Med 1982;5:49.
4. Pewsner D, Battaglia M, Minder C, et al. Ruling a diagnosis in or out with "SpPIn" and "SnNOut": a note of caution. BMJ 2004;329:209.
5. Shea JA, Berlin JA, Escarce JJ, et al. Revised estimates of diagnostic test sensitivity and specificity in suspected biliary tract disease. Arch Intern Med 1994;154:2573.
6. Guyatt GH, Patterson C, Ali M, et al. Diagnosis of iron deficiency in the elderly. Am J Med 1990; 88:205.
7. McGee S. Simplifying likelihood ratios. J Gen Intern Med 2002;17:646.
8. Scandinavian Simvastatin Survival Study Group. Randomised trial of cholesterol lowering in 4444 patients with coronary heart disease. Lancet 1994;344:1383.
9. Downs JR, Clearfield M, Weis S, et al. Primary prevention of acute coronary events with lovastatin in men and women with average cholesterol levels. JAMA 1998;279:1615.
10. Hulley S, Grady D, Bush T, et al. Randomized trial of estrogen plus progestin for secondary prevention of coronary heart disease in postmenopausal women. JAMA 1998;280:605.
11. Choudhry NK, Fletcher RH, Soumerai SB. Systematic review: the relationship between

*Bold numerals denote published controlled clinical trials, meta-analyses, or consensus-based recommendations.

clinical experience and quality of health care. Ann Intern Med 2005;142:260.
12. Laine C. How can physicians keep up to date? Annu Rev Med 1999;50:99.
13. Covell DG, Uman CG, Manning PR. Information needs in office practice: are they being met? Ann Intern Med 1985;103:596.
14. Wyatt JC. Reading journals and monitoring the published work. J R Soc Med 2000;93:423.
15. Fletcher RH, Fletcher SW. Evidence-based approach to the medical literature. J Gen Intern Med 1997;12:S5.
16. Oxman AD, Cook DJ, Guyatt GH. Users' guides to the medical literature: VI. How to use an overview. Evidence-Based Medicine Working Group. JAMA 1994;272:1367.
17. Borzak S, Ridker PM. Discordance between meta-analyses and large-scale randomized controlled trials: examples from the management of acute myocardial infarction. Ann Intern Med 1995;123:873.
18. Smith R. What clinical information do clinicians need? BMJ 1996;313:1062.
19. Shaughnessy AF, Slawson DC, Bennett JH. Becoming an information master: a guidebook to the medical information jungle. J Fam Pract 1994;39:489.

For annotated ***General References*** *and resources related to this chapter, visit www.hopkinsbayview.org/PAMreferences.*

Chapter 3

The Practitioner–Patient Relationship and Communication during Clinical Encounters

L. Randol Barker

Each practitioner–patient relationship is established through person-to-person interactions in which the practitioner's goals are to obtain accurate and critical information from the patient and reach a valid formulation of the patient's problem or status; to provide information to the patient and ensure that the patient comprehends it; to decide on a management plan with the patient; to facilitate patient adherence to agreed-on plans; to attain mutual satisfaction with the relationship; and to alleviate the patient's symptoms. Achievement of these goals depends on the practitioner's knowledge of medicine, respect for the patient's participation in the interaction, and skills in communication and patient education. This chapter and Chapter 4 address the latter two issues.

THE PRACTITIONER–PATIENT RELATIONSHIP

Types of Relationships

Our society's concept of the practitioner–patient relationship has evolved through the years. In 1951, Parsons described the patient's role as essentially passive (1). Later Szasz and Hollender (2) outlined the following three types of interactions between practitioner and patient: the *active–passive relationship,* in which the practitioner has all authority (similar to Parson's conceptualization); the *guidance–cooperation relationship,* in which the practitioner still is somewhat directive and the patient cooperates; and *mutual participation,* in which there is active collaboration between patient and practitioner, and patients assume more responsibility for their care. The consumer movement of the 1960s and 1970s promoted the mutual participation relationship between practitioners and patients.

In the 1990s, the term *patient-centered care* was introduced to emphasize the primacy of the patient in the mutual participation model. It has been pointed out that the following are indicators of patient-centeredness (3–5):

- Practitioner's goals that include learning and valuing the patient's personal illness story and reaching agreement with the patient on the meaning of the illness and on the management plan.
- Grounding of the law and medical ethics in the concept of patient autonomy.

- Quality assessment that includes the patient's perspective as a fundamental component.
- Consideration of these factors in planning health care education and research.

More recently, the term *relationship-centered care* was promulgated to delineate a relationship that integrates the perspectives and roles of both patients and practitioners and that broadens that relationship to include the dimension of self-awareness (6–8).

Ethical Aspects of the Relationship

The mutual participation model is central to *the principles of medical ethics that have been delineated in the past two decades* (9). These principles define a practitioner–patient relationship in which the practitioner respects the sanctity of the individual person and believes that that person's goals should be the basis for medical decisions. In practice, these principles require that practitioners learn what their patients' expectations and goals are and that patients (or their surrogates) participate as fully as possible in decisions about their health care. Such participation requires that the patient be competent to consider a specific decision; that the patient receive sufficient information regarding available options, demonstrate comprehension of that information, and be given sufficient time to consider the options; and that the patient's decision be voluntary, that is, free from constraints imposed by the interests of other persons. Additional ethical principles that are critical in a respectful practitioner–patient relationship are truthfulness and protection of confidentiality.

Adherence to each of the principles of patient-centered medical ethics is not always possible or appropriate in ambulatory practice. For example, although patients generally want to be well informed, many still prefer to have their practitioner recommend choices (10). In addition, a practitioner's personal beliefs and standards of practice must be considered. If a patient requests a course of action that is contrary to the practitioner's beliefs or standards or that endangers others, the practitioner must indicate this to the patient and, if the patient's wishes cannot be accommodated, care should be transferred to another practitioner or to the court system. Challenging situations such as these are not uncommon in ambulatory practice (11).

For situations that involve patient competence, truth telling, confidentiality, and patient behaviors that may harm others, a practitioner–patient relationship that has been developed over time may make both prevention and resolution of problems more feasible. For example, an elderly patient may agree to discontinue driving and propose satisfactory alternatives in the context of a trusting relationship.

Problems caused by *external factors,* particularly the ground rules governing services covered under managed care plans, may also be amenable to resolution through the practitioner–patient relationship. Encouraging patients to become informed about the processes and guidelines of their health care insurance and offering other options when patients make unreasonable requests are examples of ways to include the patient in addressing such externally imposed challenges (see Managed Care and the Practitioner–Patient Relationship).

Involvement with Family Members and Significant Others

Commonly, a spouse, family members, or friends—especially those who are close to the patient during a period of illness—both want to know about the patient's condition and are affected by the patient's illness. Significant others may play an important role in determining the course of the patient's illness by sharing in decision making, providing support, or, at times, creating barriers. Consequently, developing a relationship with those close to the patient is a predictable and important aspect of the care of many patients. A practitioner's involvement with others may range from the brief exchanges that occur at the beginning or end of office visits to interactions during a planned family meeting (12). The skills for use in the traditional practitioner–patient dyad, described later, are the skills appropriate when others are included.

Special considerations for relating to family members and friends include the following:

- Recognizing the impact on the patient's illness of patient–family dynamics and practitioner–family dynamics.
- Avoiding breach of confidentiality by ensuring that the patient consents to inclusion of others in a visit; then, when appropriate, including others during all or part of the encounter.
- Learning about and acknowledging the distress that the patient's illness has caused for those close to the patient.
- Providing information and engaging in problem solving that will facilitate the roles of others in promoting the patient's health.
- When appropriate, including family members in decision making.

Additional details about the positive and negative influences of family on a patient's health are found elsewhere in this text (see Social Support in Chapter 4).

Planned Family Meetings

There are a number of situations in which it is helpful to convene the members of a patient's family and, at times, others such as a nurse or social worker. Common examples include addressing end-of-life issues (see Chapter 13); addressing poor control of a chronic illness; decisions

TABLE 3.1 Tasks to Consider for Planning and Conducting a Family Meeting

Premeeting Tasks
Clarify the purposes for the meeting.
Establish which family members, friends, or professionals should attend.
Set up the appointment, specifying the planned duration and location.
Develop a strategy for conducting the meeting, including specific questions, observations, or tasks that will facilitate addressing the purpose of the meeting.

The Five Phases of a Family Meeting

Phase 1: Socialize (Approximately 5 Minutes)
Greet each person attending the meeting.
State the purpose for the meeting, provide any crucial information that all need to know up front, and check briefly with each family member about themselves, their work, their relation to the patient, etc.

Phase 2: Set the Goals (Approximately 5 Minutes)
Ask the group, "What would you like to make sure we accomplish today?"
Restate each goal so it is clear, concise, and realistic; propose any important goals that the family has not mentioned.
Set priorities among the goals.

Phase 3: Discuss the Illness or Issue (Approximately 15 Minutes)
Elicit each participant's view of the illness or issue. Ask about past experiences or recent changes that could impact the issue of concern, such as moves, occupational changes, other illnesses, and deaths. Observe repetitive family interactional patterns. Final plans should not go against these patterns, unless specifically negotiated.
Encourage the patient and family to ask questions.
Ask how the family has dealt with similar illness or issues in the past.

Phase 4: Identify Resources and Ideas (Approximately 10 Minutes)
Identify family strengths and resources of all kinds.
Identify medical resources and community resources.

Phase 5: Establish a Plan (Approximately 10 Minutes)
Include resources and ideas that family members have suggested.
Negotiate a formal or an informal contract with the family. Have each person state what he or she will do.
Discuss any referrals, if relevant, at this point.
Offer to write down key information for family members.
Ask for any final questions.
Summarize the plan.
Thank everyone for coming and participating in the meeting.

Postmeeting Tasks
Write up a report of the meeting, including the attendance, the problem list, a global assessment of individual and family functioning, the family's strengths and resources, and the plan (both the medical regimen and the roles to be played by the patient and family members).

Adapted from McDaniel S, Campbell T, Seaburn D. Family oriented primary care: a manual for medical providers. New York: Springer-Verlag, 1990.

regarding a long-term care plan; substance abuse (see Family Intervention in Chapter 28); and marital or sexual difficulties or other family dysfunction (see Family Counseling in Chapter 20). Table 3.1 describes specific tasks that one should consider when planning and conducting a family meeting.

Sociocultural Diversity, Health Literacy, and the Practitioner–Patient Relationship

Sociocultural Diversity

A classic paper published in 1978 points out that predictably there are differences in the ways in which a practitioner and a patient think about and respond to the patient's medical problems (13). The sources of these differences range from the unique ideas of individual patients, not infrequently based on transgenerational family stories of illness (14), to ideas and behaviors particular to the social or cultural groups to which patients belong. The composition of the United States population in the year 2000, summarized in Table 3.2, indicates that patients with diverse cultural traditions are likely to make up an important proportion of the patients cared for by most practitioners. Many of these patients will be recent immigrants; Chapter 41 provides information about the regulations related to health assessment of new immigrants to the United States and about important considerations related to the health care experiences, traditions, and expectations

TABLE 3.2 Profile of General Demographic Characteristics: United States, 2000

Subject	Number	Percent
Total population	281,421,906	100.0
Sex		
Male	138,053,563	49.1
Female	143,368,343	50.9
Race[a]		
One race	274,595,6768	97.6
White	211,460,626	75.1
Black or African American	34,658,190	12.3
American Indian and Alaska Native	2,475,956	0.9
Asian	10,242,998	3.6
Native Hawaiian and other Pacific Islander	398,835	0.1
Some other race	15,359,073	5.5
Two or more races	6,826,228	2.4
Hispanic or Latino (of any race)	35,305,818	12.5

[a]The concept of race as used by the Census Bureau reflects self-identification by people according to the race or races with which they most closely identify. These categories are sociopolitical constructs and should not be interpreted as being scientific or anthropologic in nature. Furthermore, the race categories include both racial and national-origin groups.
From U.S. Census Bureau, Census 2000.

of immigrants. In addition, the 2000 census found that approximately 18% of the United States population speaks a language other than English at home (15) and that 4.2% speak English poorly or not at all: 28% of Hispanics, 23% of Asian or Pacific Islanders, and 13% of Indo-Europeans (16).

Health Literacy

Health literacy was recently recognized as a major factor in the quality of health and health care in the United States. Health literacy is defined as "the degree to which individuals have the capacity to obtain, process, and understand basic health information and services needed to make appropriate health decisions" (17). A review of existing data suggests that limited health literacy is common—a prevalence of 22% to 29% for low health literacy and 16% to 23% for marginal health literacy (18). Limited health literacy is consistently associated with low education level, older age, and ethnicity (18). In 2004, in recognition of the importance of the issue, a national research program was initiated to determine the association of health literacy and quality of health and health care, and to delineate ways to identify and address limited health literacy (19).

Implications for the Practitioner–Patient Relationship

In a number of ways, the effectiveness of the practitioner–patient relationship may be enhanced, or diminished, depending on awareness of and response to *differences between patient and practitioner.* The following general approaches can enhance the relationship:

- Learning and inquiring explicitly about the beliefs, values, and behaviors of the sociocultural group to which one's patient belongs. Common sources of group-determined beliefs and behaviors are religious tenets related to illness, traditional roles of family members in medical decisions, and folk healers. It has been pointed out that culture-based values regarding the following five factors may be fundamental to a person's health-related behavior: status bestowed on practitioners or family members, personal privacy, fatalism, importance of the individual and the group, and access to information. Additionally, patients may bring cultural preferences regarding communication content (e.g., topics appropriate to discuss, nonverbal cues) and style (e.g., directness, distance, touch, degree of formality, forms of address, pace, voice pitch) (see Gardenswartz and Rowe, *Managing Diversity in Health Care,* at www.hopkinsbayview.org/PAMreferences).
- Recognizing and reflecting about one's own beliefs, biases, and emotional reactions toward cultural and individual differences, and suspending judgment when possible.
- Ensuring that an interpreter is present when there is a language barrier (see Chapter 41 for information about telephone access to interpreters).
- Including culture-friendly objects and patient materials in medical offices, such as artwork that reflects different races, ethnicities, or sexual orientations, and patient instructional or educational materials written in different languages.
- Inquiring of those at risk (e.g., low education level, elderly, ethnic subgroups) in a nonjudgmental way about health literacy, using phrases such as "Many people need the help of others to read or understand information about their medical care . . . instructions on medicine bottles, appointment letters, written materials about their illness and so forth. How often do you need help like that?" For those who report a need for help or who have limited health literacy, ensuring that they have access to someone, ideally a family member, who can read information that is important to their medical care.
- Learning about, explicitly inquiring about, and accommodating patients' explanatory models for their illnesses.

Patients' explanatory models for their illnesses address the same issues as practitioners' explanatory models: etiology, name of the illness, pathophysiology ("what is wrong"), expected course, treatment, and response to treatment (13). Often, there are differences in the two models based on the difference in perspective between patients and practitioners (Table 3.3). Both parties may inhibit the

TABLE 3.3 Summary of Common Differences in Explanatory Models between Western-Trained Practitioners and Traditional Ethnic Patients

Aspect of Model	Western Practitioner	Ethnic Patient
Etiologic Beliefs		
Social causes of illnesses	Usually limited to stress model or attributed to paranoia	Many social indiscretions can cause illness; blaming of self or others for symptoms is common
Environmental causes of illnesses	Exposure to known pathogens, toxins, and social stress may cause symptoms	"Hot–cold" imbalance in the body caused by dietary indiscretions or drafts may cause symptoms
Belief that conditions of the blood cause illness	Limited to specific hematologic disorders or hypertension	Many "conditions" of blood can cause illness (e.g., "too thick," "too slow," "too little")
Symptom Interpretation and Presentation		
Altered states of consciousness (trance, visions, etc.)	Usually considered abnormal	Often considered normal, desirable
Attitudes toward pain expression	Stoicism expected unless complaints are congruent with clear organic pathology	Either total stoicism or emotional expression of pain is healthy and expected
Focus on physical symptoms (somatization)	May be considered as a psychiatric syndrome	Expected, proper way of expressing distress
Treatment Expectations		
Who is the patient?	Individual is the focus of decision making and care	Family must be involved in decision making
Beliefs about self-medication and alternative practitioners	Considered potentially dangerous, undesirable	Common

From Johnson TM, Hardt EJ, Kleinman A. Cultural factors in the medical interview. In: Lipkin M Jr, Putnam SM, Lazare A, eds. The medical interview: clinical care, education, and research. New York: Springer-Verlag, 1995.

development of an effective relationship—practitioners by focusing only on abstract disease formulations to address each of these issues, and patients by dwelling on their own formulation of what is wrong and resenting their practitioner's apparent inattention to that formulation. By recognizing or exploring patients' own explanatory models (and, at times, learning of conflicting beliefs about the illness held by others close to the patient), then coming up with mutually acceptable ways of accounting for and addressing the illness, practitioners are more likely to help patients who bring strongly held personal or cultural beliefs to the encounter.

Racial and language concordance between patient and practitioner appears to correlate with more collaborative relationships (20) or better health care outcomes (21). This finding points to the importance of more diversity in the makeup of the practitioner workforce as well as the need for all practitioners to enhance their commitment to and skills for relating to patients in the context of sociocultural differences.

Managed Care and the Practitioner–Patient Relationship

The ways in which managed care may affect the practitioner–patient relationship have received much attention. Table 3.4 contains a summary of potential improvements and threats to the relationship that are associated with managed care. The authors considered the impact on factors key to the relationship (the six Cs): patient *choice*, practitioner *competence*, practitioner–patient *communication*, practitioner *compassion* for the patient, *continuity* of practitioners, and *avoidance of conflict* of interest (22).

In a thoughtful essay, Shorey captures much about the change that managed care has brought to the practitioner–patient relationship: From the need to build trust in the context of a dyad (practitioner and patient), practitioners need now to inspire trust in a context (managed care) in which they value dyadic relationships but also consider the health of all patients in their panels (23). A number of other authors have written helpful analyses of this topic (see www.hopkinsbayview.org/PAMreferences). In 2004, a working group of stakeholders (patients, physicians, managed care representatives, and medical ethicists) published a multicomponent statement of ethical principles for managed care (see Povar at www.hopkinsbayview.org/PAMreferences).

COMMUNICATION DURING CLINICAL ENCOUNTERS

The Functions of the Medical Interview

The following three functions, delineated by Lazare, Putnam, and Lipkin (24), are widely accepted as ways to describe what happens in medical interviews:

TABLE 3.4 The Effects of Managed Care on the Physician–Patient Relationship

Potential Improvements	Potential Threats
Choice	
■ Expanded choice of managed care plans, particularly in areas with low managed care penetration	■ "Cherry picking" increasing the number of uninsured Americans
■ Expanded choice of preventive and pediatric services	■ Employers restricting patients' choice of managed care plans and physicians ■ Price competition forcing patients to choose between continuing with their current physicians or switching to a cheaper plan ■ Financial failures of managed care plans forcing change in managed care plan without choice ■ Restrictions by managed care plans of choice of specialists and particular services
Competence	
■ Development and use of measures to assess quality of physicians and managed care plans	■ Underuse of specialists and specialized facilities
■ Greater use of preventive medical care	■ Unreliable and non–risk-adjusted quality measures providing a distorted view of competence
Communication	
■ Increased number of generalists and primary care providers	■ Productivity requirements creating shorter office visits, reduced telephone access, and other access barriers to physicians
■ Creation of physician–nonphysician provider teams to provide a broader range of providers knowledgeable about the patient's condition	■ Advertising creating inflated patient expectations
Compassion	
	■ Less time for interaction with patients during stressful decisions
Continuity	
■ Selection of a primary care provider encouraged (for patients who may never have had continuity of care by a single provider)[a]	■ Price competition forcing patient choice of continuity at a higher price vs. the cheapest plan ■ "Deselection" of physicians, disrupting existing physician–patient relations ■ Frequent changes by employer of managed care plans forcing changes of physician
(No) Conflict of Interest	
■ No incentive to overuse or overtreat as exists in fee-for-service environment[a]	■ Linking practitioner salary incentives and bonuses to reduced use of tests and procedures for patients

[a]Added by the author.
Adapted from Emanuel EJ, Dubler NN. Preserving the physician–patient relationship in the era of managed care. JAMA 1995;273:323.

- *Determining and monitoring the nature of the patient's problems*
- *Developing, maintaining, or concluding the therapeutic relationship*
- *Carrying out patient education and implementing a treatment plan*

More recently, an overarching fourth function, *partnership building*, has been delineated (25). Partnership building refers to the many ways in which the patient's input is enlisted and respected in information gathering and decision making during a practitioner–patient interaction. One or more of these broad functions is central to all of the skills for practitioner–patient communication described in this chapter and in Chapter 4.

Importance of Effective Communication

The importance of effective communication has been confirmed in a variety of studies of the practitioner–patient relationship. A large body of published research shows that effective communication skills correlate with obtaining valid information, getting patients to disclose fully the reasons for their visits, reported satisfaction with the practitioner, improved patient adherence to medical regimens, a reduced risk of being sued for malpractice (see Lipkin et al., *The Medical Interview,* at www.hopkinsbayview.org/PAMreferences), and higher physician satisfaction (26). A smaller body of literature also exists in which experimental studies, using control and intervention subjects, document the positive impact of effective communication skills on patient outcomes, including emotional health, symptom resolution, patient function, blood pressure and glucose control, and pain control (27).

Although gathering and providing of information may appear to be the primary reason for direct communication with patients, the *therapeutic nature of the interaction* is perhaps the factor that is most important to the health of the patient. As summarized by Reiser and Schroder (28):

> Repeatedly, practitioners will feel the power of something intangible, yet unmistakable, in the nature of the practitioner–patient relationship that helps a sick person to get better. It is hard to overestimate the potency and curative potential of this very unique and special relationship. For all our technical advances, this relationship remains one of medicine's most powerful therapeutic tools.

The skills that establish the therapeutic nature of *every* medical encounter are described here and in Chapter 4. Chapter 20 describes the important phenomenon of transference and additional skills that are useful when the primary purpose of the encounter is to deal with psychosocial problems.

The Patient's Experience during Ambulatory Encounters

The impact of communication during an ambulatory encounter is determined by the way both parties think about the encounter in advance and afterward and by the communication skills used during the encounter. The latter can be seen as skills that are useful for organizing the flow of the visit and skills that are useful throughout the visit (see next section).

Recognizing What the Patient Experiences

An interaction with a patient is likely to be more effective when, as much as possible, the practitioner recognizes the feelings and concerns that the patient brings to the visit *and* voices this to the patient. As discussed earlier (see Sociocultural Diversity and the Practitioner–Patient Relationship), this may include being aware of traditional beliefs and behaviors of patients from diverse cultural backgrounds (13).

It is important to realize what it is like for a patient to go to a practitioner. The way in which most patients think about a visit to the practitioner has been described as "expectant trust" (see Chapter 20). Patients may come with anxieties concerning what the practitioner will find wrong with them; they may come expecting the practitioner to help them solve one or more problems; or they may have any of a number of other types of expectations about the visit. Patients know that their practitioners have busy schedules, and some may be reluctant to ask what they think the practitioner will regard as trivial questions. Social distance often exists between practitioner and patient and, when combined with the practitioner's special knowledge, gives the practitioner considerable authority. As a result, patients may be reluctant to contradict or correct their practitioners' statements, may misrepresent their thoughts or feelings to provide answers they think the practitioner wants to hear, or may not ask for clarification despite being confused by medical terminology. During the physical examination, some patients feel embarrassment at being exposed, and this may further inhibit disclosure of important concerns. Most patients, even those who have had a long-standing relationship with their practitioner, experience some of these types of discomfort during an office visit. It can help to ask oneself, "If I were this patient, how would I be feeling during this visit?" It is equally telling to ask oneself, after a visit, "If I were that patient, how would I be feeling about the visit when I have reached home?"

As discussed later (see Challenging Situations and Practitioner Self-Care), practitioners also bring expectations and vulnerabilities to encounters with patients. Awareness of these factors can be seen as an important skill that may determine the quality of communication during a visit.

Rapport

An aspect of the practitioner–patient relationship that especially facilitates disclosure of concerns by patients and readies them to make decisions is the development and maintenance of rapport. Rapport is a mixture of harmony and affinity felt between two or more people. Rapport is fostered with a knowing look or by voicing awareness of the patient as someone unique (e.g., "How's everything going since you moved from your house to an apartment?"). Rapport also develops when a patient feels that his or her input is *respected* and that the practitioner has *empathy* for the patient (see Addressing Emotions).

Skills for Organizing the Flow of the Visit

Given the limited time available for ambulatory visits, it helps to have a scheme for organizing the flow of a visit. The scheme described here emphasizes relationship-centered skills that are useful for each of the stages of a visit. The next section describes skills that may be helpful in any part of the visit.

Planning the Visit

It is helpful to review critical information in the patient's record before starting the visit. For an established patient, record review could include checking on the patient's social history, on preventive care due at this visit, or on issues addressed at the previous visit. This can be done before seeing the patient or just after the greeting ("Before we start, let me take a minute to get right up-to-date with what is in your chart."). This planning ensures that the practitioner knows information that will help set the agenda for the visit, and it limits the need to look through the chart in the presence of the patient.

Opening the Interaction

Greeting a patient, shaking the patient's hand, using the patient's name, and, if it is a first visit, introducing oneself all make the patient feel welcome. The first few moments of first or second encounters are crucial because the practitioner and the patient are sizing up one another, and nonverbal behavior often takes precedence over what is being said. Both practitioner and patient are paying attention to physical features, type of handshake, voice tone and pitch, age, dress, and overall demeanor.

The *seating arrangement* of the office can affect the development of rapport. When the patient's and the practitioner's chairs are arranged so that the two are facing one another without the full breadth of a desk interposed, a patient may feel less intimidated than when facing a practitioner across a desk.

Exploratory Information Gathering

For gathering information about a patient's problems, it helps to begin with an *exploratory approach* and to ensure that the patient knows that this is one's intent. Exploratory interviewing combines *open-ended phrasing of questions* and *allowing a patient to respond without being interrupted.* An exploratory approach is the most efficient way to learn what the patient knows, and it indicates interest in the patient from the outset. Asking the patient, "How have you been doing since your last visit?" is an appropriate open-ended question for a planned followup visit. For a new-patient visit or a visit requested by the patient, the practitioner will want to explore the reason for the visit by saying, "Please tell me what brings you in today." This type of phrasing provides an opportunity for the patient to describe the reasons for the visit and does not imply that there is a problem.

Agenda Setting

In response to the opening inquiry, the patient's response might be, "Well, I haven't been doing so well lately. My shoulder has been giving me a problem." Before exploring the first problem mentioned, it is helpful to establish whether there are other issues that the patient wants to address during the visit (e.g., "Before we talk about your shoulder, is there anything else?"). If one assumes that the patient wishes to discuss only one problem and proceeds to explore that problem, the patient may mention other problems whenever there is an opportunity, often when one is preparing to close the visit. The practitioner should also name items to be added to the agenda (e.g., "I also want to get up-to-date on your smoking."), then restate the issues to be addressed during the visit. If too many issues are identified, it is appropriate to ask, "Which problems seem to be bothering you the most?" and mutually to prioritize those issues to be addressed at the visit.

Getting the Patient's Story

After agreement on the agenda for the visit, the practitioner continues to explore the problems one at a time. "Tell me about the shoulder pain" would be a clear invitation to the patient to describe the problem in his or her own words. When patients give the history in their own words, the length of the interview does not increase (29) and they are more likely to explain why a problem concerns them (e.g., "With spring coming, I'm thinking that I might have to give up tennis altogether because of the pain.").

If an exploratory approach is maintained, a patient's medical problem usually emerges as part of a meaningful personal story (4,30). For example, the patient's concern that a shoulder pain means that he or she will never play tennis again may be founded in the experience of the patient's father years before—a personal story that would clarify the importance of the symptom to the patient and would be crucial to consider in the closing part of the visit (see later discussion). In addition to bringing out important information, an interview that allows emergence of a patient's personal story invariably contributes to the development of rapport.

Exploratory questions can be used throughout the interaction. When the patient produces information that needs clarifying, additional exploratory questions are helpful to establish a common meaning. For example, if the patient has named "constipation" as a new concern, it helps to explore what this means to the patient (e.g., "Tell me what you mean by constipation?"). One may discover that the patient has a bowel movement every other day and yet believes that this means constipation.

Clarifying and Hypothesis Testing

Not visible to the patient, but constantly operating during an interview, is hypothesis testing by the practitioner. Because exploratory inquiry rarely provides all of the information needed to evaluate a problem, it is usually necessary to use focused questions to fill in gaps and narrow the differential diagnosis. Table 3.5 lists generic information that is important in assessing most problems.

Direct or focused questions are questions phrased to clarify specific facts, such as, "When did you first notice the pain?" or "What words would you use to describe the pain?" or "Can you show me with your hand where the pain is?" When seeking such specific information, it is important to *avoid asking leading questions*—questions that

TABLE 3.5 Generic Information Important in Assessing Most Problems

Chronology of symptoms
Onset of problem: since when?
Frequency
Duration of an episode
Temporal trend: unchanging, better, worse
Past history of similar problem: when, etc.?
Quality of symptoms
Severe to not severe
Quality consistent or variable
Location, radiation (if pertinent)
Patient's own words to describe quality
Description of one episode (for recurring symptom)
Associated additional symptoms
Factors, circumstances that aggravate symptoms
Factors, circumstances that alleviate symptoms
Remedies or measures tried
Impact of symptoms on valued activities
Patient's explanatory model for symptoms[a]
Fears or concerns caused by symptoms

[a]See page 29 and Table 3.3.

tend to elicit predetermined answers, usually in the form of a simple "yes" or "no." For example, the following question, presumably related to a hypothesis that has occurred to the practitioner, is a leading question: "You don't have the pain every day, do you?" This leading question gives the message to the patient that the practitioner does not expect the pain to occur every day. Patients who are somewhat passive may agree to whatever their practitioner suggests, even if the answer is inaccurate. Once a patient has responded inaccurately, the patient may become distracted and forget to report important information.

When a patient cannot provide needed information, it sometimes helps to offer a number of *choices from which to select*. For example, if the patient reports chest pain but is unable to provide accurate information about whether the pain radiates, the practitioner might ask, "Does the pain seem to go anywhere else, such as to your back, one of your arms, your neck, or your legs?" Although the practitioner may have an idea of the likely response, this will not be obvious to the patient because the patient is given several choices. In contrast, a question such as, "Does the pain move to your left arm?" is a leading question, giving the patient the impression that this is the correct answer.

A patient will at times give a vague, aggregate description of an episodic symptom. In this situation, it is helpful to have the patient *describe in detail a single episode*, for example: "Tell me about the last time you felt the nausea and crampy pain." This technique clarifies the nature of the symptoms, and, importantly, it often brings to light social or environmental factors important to the problem (e.g., "Well, the last bad headache was Saturday. Yeah, my teenage son had stayed out all night.").

When asking direct questions, it is important to *ask only one question at a time* and to phrase each question so that it refers to one piece of information. Thus, when the patient responds, the practitioner knows to what the patient is referring. For example, to questions such as, "Are you having any problems sleeping or eating?" or "Are you constipated or do you have diarrhea?" a positive response may not reveal which is the problem. Conversely, a negative response may refer to only one of these problems.

While responding to questions, the *patient may give verbal cues* related to the discussion or concerning other issues that need exploration. At times it is appropriate to pursue a verbal cue when it is uttered; at other times it is more appropriate to acknowledge it and let the patient know that you will return to it later. If a verbal cue is pertinent to the present discussion, it is helpful to repeat the patient's words or to explore what the patient means. For example, in response to a question about pain, a patient may respond, "Well, it seems to have gotten worse lately, but maybe it's just my nerves." Here, an appropriate response would be an open-ended question such as "Your nerves?" or "What do you mean?" The following response to a question about sleep quality in a patient with pain is an example of a verbal cue that one would explore separately: "Sometimes I wake up in the middle of the night, but it isn't because of the pain." Depending on the hypothesis that one is testing regarding the patient's pain, it might be more appropriate to pursue the sleep problem later in the interaction.

A patient's *nonverbal cues* can also provide important information. A patient's *vocal message*—including pitch, tone, and tempo—may confirm or contradict the content of the patient's verbal message. Nonverbal cues also include *body language*. Elements of body language that can be observed are the patient's sitting position (e.g., sitting on the edge of the chair suggests apprehension, facing away from the practitioner suggests mental discomfort), head position (e.g., held back in defiance, anxiety, or fear; held down or turned away in sadness, shame, or denial), facial expression (eyes, eyebrows, and forehead show the greatest range of emotions, including surprise, fear, anger, happiness, disgust, sadness), hands (e.g. wringing or rubbing of hands can show anxiety; clenched fists may signify anger), and arms and legs (e.g., crossing of the legs, and especially the arms, can signify resistance, defensiveness, or discomfort). At times, incongruity between what the patient says and the patient's voice quality or body language is the only indicator of an important problem that the patient is hesitant to disclose.

Carrying Out Patient Education, Choosing a Treatment Plan, and Closing

Telling the patient one's formulation of a medical problem and reaching consensus on next steps are the final phases of an ambulatory encounter. Because ambulatory patients are by definition quite autonomous, the skills needed in these phases are uniquely important in ambulatory care. Chapter 4, in the section entitled "Patient Education and Promotion of Healthy Behaviors," describes in detail the principles and skills for addressing this part of the visit.

At the close of a visit, it is important to accomplish a number of concrete tasks:

- Schedule a followup visit at a mutually agreed to interval.
- Instruct the patient to telephone back (or tell the patient that you or someone from the office will telephone) when this is indicated.

At this point, the physician should reemphasize his or her interest in the patient. Actions such as shaking the patient's hand or touching the patient on the shoulder, using the patient's name, ensuring that the patient has one's professional card, reminding the patient of night and weekend coverage, and encouraging telephone contact for interval problems convey the physician's interest to the patient.

Skills Useful throughout the Visit

A number of communication skills, described here, may be useful in any part of an ambulatory visit.

"Road Signs," Summarizing, Vocabulary

"Road signs," summarizing, and affirmative vocabulary help patients to participate effectively in the visit. These may include the following:

- *Using orienting and transitional statements* to ensure that the patient understands when the focus of the interview is changing (e.g., "At this point, I would like to learn more about your day-to-day activities.").
- Naming, then addressing, *one problem or issue at a time* (e.g., "Now, about your shoulder pain . . ." or "The medicine that I will prescribe . . .").
- *Summing up and checking periodically* (e.g., "So far, what I understand about your trouble sleeping is that . . ."), which lets patients know that one has heard what they said and gives them the chance to clarify or expand on important information.
- Using *vocabulary consistent with the patient's background* and avoiding formulations that may confuse the patient (e.g., telling a patient that test results are "negative" may convey to the patient that something is wrong).

Noting the Patient's Educational Needs

Patient education can be addressed most efficiently by *ascertaining the patient's educational needs throughout the interview*—by hearing or asking what the patient knows or wants to know about issues as they come up—but *deferring the process of providing information and working out a plan* to the latter part of the visit. It helps to give the patient a road sign (e.g., "When we finish up your visit, we will go over several things you can do to lose the weight you have gained."). (See details in the schemes described in Chapter 4.)

Using Eye Contact

The eyes are a primary medium of expression, and they often tell more about a person's message than words do. Maintaining eye contact and communicating with one's eyes at the same level as the patient's (e.g., both parties seated) are basic to patient comfort. Looking at one's watch or at the chart while discussing a patient's problem may indicate to the patient that the practitioner is not listening, is not interested, or is too busy to answer questions that the patient may already be reluctant to ask. Although eye contact is one of the best ways to convey interest, staring can be uncomfortable and should be avoided.

Addressing Emotions

Predictably, patients experience one or more emotions before, during, and after visits to the practitioner. During visits, patients may or may not disclose their feelings. Empiric studies show that patients usually do not express emotions directly but through verbal or nonverbal clues (e.g., "It's been kind of different for me lately"; looking down or away when emotions are present) (30,31). A number of communication skills can facilitate disclosure and addressing of emotions (Table 3.6). Three basic reasons for addressing emotions are that patients usually feel better when they know that the practitioner is aware of their feelings; patients may be more able to concentrate and make decisions after an emotional state such as anxiety, sadness, or anger has been addressed, even briefly; and expressing emotions may be therapeutic for a patient.

Skills Related to Physical Examination and Documentation

Physical Examination

Appropriate communication during the physical examination includes describing what one is doing, obtaining further history when examining the location of a symptom, and avoiding the tendency to give important information (diagnosis and plan) during the physical examination or when the patient is getting dressed; in both instances the patient is distracted and cannot be expected to focus on the practitioner's message or to formulate questions as well.

TABLE 3.6 Skills for Addressing a Patient's Emotions

Skills for Facilitating Disclosure of Feelings

Explicitly Ask or Encourage Patient to Express/Clarify Feelings/Concerns
Restate patient's words about how the patient feels (e.g., "You feel down . . .?" repeated immediately after the patient says these words).
Acknowledge or probe feelings that seem to be present or just under the surface (e.g., "I notice you're getting tearful." or "How do you feel about . . .?").
Clarify or check feelings that patient has disclosed (e.g., "Let me see if I can better understand what you are feeling.").

Allow Patient to Express Feelings/Concerns
Be attentive, do not interrupt.
Allow silence while patient prepares response or experiences emotional reaction.

Skills for Responding to and Supporting Patient

Convey Concern for and Interest in the Patient
Explicitly by saying so (e.g., "My concern is to help you get well.").
Implicitly by remaining attentive, facilitating disclosure, indicating that the patient has been heard (e.g., by mentioning aspects of patient's life affected by an illness or by changing facial expression and vocal tone).

Communicate Understanding of Patient's Feelings (Empathize)
Name patient's feelings/situation (e.g., "Sounds as if you are pretty angry.").
Check accuracy of naming (e.g., "Is this the way you experience it?").
Use facilitative utterances (e.g., lower voice, use appropriate utterances such as "uh huh" that indicate that the patient is being attended to).

Legitimize Patient's Feelings/Thoughts/Actions
Indicate that patient's emotions/thoughts/actions are understandable and "normal" under the circumstances (e.g., "It's understandable that you feel this way." "Many would have done as you did.").

Convey Respect for the Patient's Efforts, Ideas
Compliment patient for whatever patient is doing well or plans to do (e.g., "Your decision to join Weight Watchers sounds good to me." "I can see that you have given a lot of thought to. . . .").

Respond Nonjudgmentally
Do not impose your own bias, values, or assumptions on patient characteristics or actions that evoke negative stereotypes or disappointment.
Nonverbally: Do not give negative message (e.g., nodding head disapprovingly, sighing in frustration, when a patient reports noncompliance).
Verbally: Do not imply that patient is "flawed or bad" (e.g., "That's alcoholism for you. . . ." or "Didn't you realize that if you ate crabs you'd put yourself into heart failure again?"). Instead, acknowledge that you have heard the patient's story.

Respond Nondefensively
Do not respond to patient anger or criticism by defense of performance; instead, acknowledge anger/criticism and try to address the reasons for the patient's behavior and concerns.
Admit mistakes, apologize when appropriate, be open to considering second opinions, and avoid self-righteousness.

Use Self-Disclosure Effectively[a]
Reveal information about yourself, when appropriate, to convey support or empathy to the patient (e.g., "I felt the same way after I lost my mother.").

Assure Partnership/Support
Make statements using the first person that assure support to the patient and convey the sense of partnership (e.g., "I will be with you throughout this illness.").

[a] Preliminary findings from a large sample of primary care visits suggest that some patients may rate the visit less positively when physician self-disclosure occurs (32).

Documentation

Dictating or writing a visit note can be done in a way that does not diminish rapport with the patient. It is helpful to point out that one will be making a few notes during the visit. It is equally helpful to suspend the interaction briefly while focusing on one's note, because this is a time that requires thought as well as writing or dictating. Dictating the note with the patient present may contribute to the goal of including the patient in all aspects of the encounter. In addition, offering to provide to the patient a copy of the encounter note has been suggested as a means of strengthening the practitioner–patient partnership (33).

Challenging Situations

All practitioners have been faced with challenging patients in medical practice. Patients may be challenging to care for because of their style of communicating; because of the overwhelming nature of their problems; because of their failure to adhere to health-promoting treatment or

TABLE 3.7 Common Negative Responses of Physicians to Difficult Patients and Strategies to Cope with These Responses

Physician's Emotional or Behavioral Reaction	*Coping Strategies*[a]
Avoidance	Analyze why; attempt to understand and master feelings that lead to avoidance; stay with the patient; discuss with colleagues.
Identification with patient	Recognize, avoid tendency to deny seriousness of disease or to give way to despair; stay with the patient.
Hostility/rejection	Acknowledge and analyze; do not attempt to like the unlikable patient; use behavioral approaches; if situation is intolerable, transfer patient to another physician.
Feelings of impotence, inadequacy (e.g., in caring for dying patient)	Discover areas in which help and comfort can be rendered, both physical and emotional; be realistic about limitations to medicine; give the patient time to go through the stages of dying or bereavement.
Feelings of loss of control or threatened authority	Acknowledge and analyze; be realistic about personal limitations and actual range of influence and authority; be aware that patient's need for control over his or her own body may conflict with physician's urge to control the situation.
Frustration, confusion, uncertainty about dealing with the patient; coping strategies not effective	Request psychiatric consultation/referral.
Anxiety, guilt, frustration about meeting patient's recognized emotional needs	Allocate time realistically according to need; request consultation/referral.

[a] See also skills in Table 3.6 and Psychosocial Treatment Techniques in Chapter 20.
From Gorlin R, Zucker HD. Physicians' reaction to patients. N Engl J Med 1983;308:1059.

behavior; because they present psychosocial distress through somatic symptoms; because they do not respond positively to the practitioner's efforts; or because they have lifelong maladaptive personalities. Approaches to dealing with situations that may be difficult for practitioners are covered in Section 3 of this book, "Psychiatric and Behavioral Problems," and in chapters describing patients who do not adhere to health-promoting behaviors (Chapter 4); adolescent and geriatric patients (Chapters 11 and 12, respectively); patients who have illnesses that create major psychosocial stress, such as cancer (Chapter 10), terminal illness (Chapter 13), human immunodeficiency virus infection (Chapter 39), diabetes (Chapter 79), or epilepsy (Chapter 88); and patients with myocardial infarction (Chapter 63) or stroke (Chapter 91).

Practitioners predictably react emotionally to difficult patients and situations. Often, these reactions are evoked by patients' feelings that seem to be directed personally at the practitioner; at times they are caused by recapitulation of aspects of the practitioner's own relationships (see discussion of countertransference, Chapter 20). Awareness of these feelings sometimes provides clues to a patient's diagnosis (e.g., sadness or feeling drained—depression, frustration—somatoform disorder) and provide the opportunity for reflection and behavior adjustments that can improve practitioner–patient rapport and optimize management (7,34).

Table 3.7 summarizes common negative responses of practitioners to patients and strategies for dealing with these responses. Most of the strategies require one to take time for self-exploration, one of several strategies that practitioners identify as healthy adaptations to stress (see next section).

PRACTITIONER SELF-CARE

An unstated assumption about the practitioner–patient relationship is that a practitioner is always ready to respond with skill and concern to a patient's distress. Because of the extraordinary needs of sick patients and the demands of running a practice, most practitioners are at risk for experiencing excessive stress themselves, beginning during training and spanning their professional careers. Substance abuse, mental illness, family dysfunction, and loss of satisfaction are well-recognized accompaniments of practitioner stress. To counterbalance the risk of excessive stress and to increase the likelihood that they will be skillful, caring, and satisfied in their professional relationships, practitioners need to address the care of themselves.

When asked about their healthy approaches to stress, practitioners identify the following personal strategies, each of which should be available to most practitioners (34,35).

Values Clarification and Time Management. This strategy, although it is implicitly present in each person's life, can be especially helpful when it is undertaken explicitly by professionals such as practitioners, whose working days often bring more demands than they can reasonably meet. The process of thinking about and writing down one's core values can help to identify activities that do or do not reflect those core values and to rearrange one's priorities. A common example of the impact of value clarification is the decision of an overcommitted professional to refuse, delegate, or discontinue low-priority activities so that more time can be allocated to valued family activities and personal life.

Self-Awareness and Sharing Feelings with Others. These strategies may be important for addressing stressful situations, which may range from patient care encounters that evoke negative responses (Table 3.7) to family tension caused by the demands of one's professional life. One can incorporate these strategies by reserving time to reflect privately or to write a personal journal. And if one has a group of like-minded colleagues, one can schedule regular meetings at which to share, in confidence, one another's dilemmas and joys (35) and to better recognize feelings and responses, such as those listed in Table 3.7. The latter strategy is especially helpful for dealing with the negative effects of reflecting alone on stressful issues.

Personal Health Care. The strategies in this section can be seen as ways to promote and protect one's mental well-being. It is equally important for practitioners to identify goals for their physical health and to address these goals with concrete measures such as exercising regularly, getting adequate sleep, avoiding harmful health habits, selecting and visiting a personal practitioner, and taking sick time when not well enough to work.

A 1997 multiauthor paper provides extensive information related to practitioner self-awareness and self-care (34).

SPECIFIC REFERENCES

1. Parsons T. The social system. New York: Free Press, 1951.
2. Szasz T, Hollender MH. A contribution to the philosophy of medicine: the basic models of the practitioner–patient relationship. Arch Intern Med 1956;97:585.
3. Laine C, Davidoff F. Patient-centered medicine. JAMA 1996;275:152.
4. Smith RC, Hoppe RB. The patient's story: integrating the patient- and physician-centered approaches to interviewing. Ann Intern Med 1991;115:470.
5. Stewart M, Brown JB, Weston WW, et al. Patient-centered medicine: transforming the clinical method. Beverly Hills, CA: Sage, 1995.
6. Roter D. The enduring and evolving nature of the patient-physician relationship. Patient Educ Couns 2000;39:5.
7. Epstein RM. Mindful practice. JAMA 1999;282: 833.
8. Wylie JL, Wagenfeld-Heintz E. JHQ 138-Development of relationship-centered care. National Association of Healthcare Quality (NAHQ). Available at: www.nahq.org/journal/ce/article.html.
9. Arnold R, Forrow L, Barker LR. Medical ethics and practitioner–patient communication. In: Lipkin M, Putnam SM, Lazare A, eds. The medical interview: a textbook on medical interviewing. New York: Springer-Verlag, 1995;345.
10. Levinson W, Kao A, Kuby A, Thisted RA. Not all patients want to participate in decision making: a national study of public preferences. J Gen Intern Med 2005;20:531.
11. Connelly JE, DalleMura S. Ethical problems in the medical office. JAMA 1988;260:812.
12. Doherty WJ, Baird MA. Developmental levels in family-centered medical care. Fam Med 1986; 18:153.
13. Kleinman A, Eisenberg L, Good B. Culture, illness, and care: clinical lessons from anthropologic and cross-cultural research. Ann Intern Med 1978;88:251.
14. Seaburn DB, Lorenz A, Kaplan D. The transgenerational development of chronic illness meanings. Fam Syst Med 1992;10:385.
15. U.S. Bureau of the Census. Profile of Selected Social Characteristics: 2000 (Table DP-2). Available at: http://factfinder.census.gov.
16. U.S. Bureau of Census. Ability to Speak English: 2000 (Table QT-P17). Available at: http://factfinder.census.gov.
17. Ratzan SC, Parker RM. Introduction. In: Selden CR, Zorn M, Ratzan SC, et al., eds. National Library of Medicine Current Bibliographies in Medicine: Health Literacy. Vol NLM, Pub no. CBM 2000-1. Bethesda, MD: National Institutes of Health, U.S. Department of Health and Human Services, 2000. Available at: www.nlm.nih.gov/pubs/cbm/hliteracy.html. Last accessed January 15, 2004.
18. Paasche-Orlow MK, Parker RM, Gazmararian JA, et al. The prevalence of limited health literacy. J Gen Intern Med 2005; 20:175.
19. Berkman ND, Dewalt DA, Pignone MP, et al. (RTI International-University of North Carolina Evidence-Based Practice Center): Literacy and health outcomes: evidence report/technology assessment number. Available at: www.ahrq.gov/clinic/litinv.htm. Last accessed February 13, 2004.
20. Cooper-Patrick L, Gallo JJ, Gonzales JJ, et al. Race, gender, and partnership in the patient–physician relationship. JAMA 1999;282:583.
21. Napoles-Springer A, Perez-Stable EJ. The role of culture and language in determining best practices. J Gen Intern Med 2001;16: 493.
22. Emanuel EJ, Dubler NN. Preserving the physician–patient relationship in the era of managed care. JAMA 1995;273:323.
23. Shorey JM. Research in practitioner–patient communication within a managed care era: a physician's perspective. Med Encounter 1997;13(2).
24. Lazare A, Putnam SM, Lipkin M Jr. Three functions of the medical interview. In: Lipkin M Jr, Putnam SM, Lazare A, eds. The medical interview: clinical care, education, and research. New York: Springer-Verlag, 1995;3.
25. Roter D. The medical visit context of treatment decision making and the therapeutic relationship. Health Expect 2000;3:17.
26. Roter DL. The enduring and evolving nature of the patient-physician relationship. Patient Educ Couns 2000;39:5.
27. Stewart MA. Effective physician–patient communication and health outcomes: a review. CMAJ 1995;152:1423.
28. Reiser DE, Schroder AK. Patient interviewing: the human dimension. Baltimore: Williams & Wilkins, 1980.
29. Putnam SM, Stiles WB, Jacab MC, et al. Teaching the medical interview: an intervention study. J Gen Intern Med 1988;3:38.
30. Suchman A, Markakis K, Beckman HB, et al. A model of emphatic communication in the medical interview. JAMA 1997;277:678.
31. Levinson W, Goraware-Bhat R, Lamb J. A study of patient clues and physician responses in primary care and surgical settings. JAMA 2000; 284:1021.
32. Beach MC, Roter D, Rubin H, et al. Is physician self-disclosure related to patient evaluation of office visits? J Gen Intern Med 2004;19:905.
33. Delbanco T, Berwick DM, Boufford JI, et al. Healthcare in a land called PeoplePower: nothing about me without me. Health Expect 2001;4:144.
34. Novack DH, Suchman AL, Clark W, et al. Calibrating the physician: personal awareness and effective patient care. JAMA 1997;278:502.
35. Quill TE, Williamson PR. Healthy approaches to physician stress. Arch Intern Med 1990;150: 1857.
36. Williamson PR. Support groups: an important aspect of physician education [editorial]. J Gen Intern Med 1991;6:179.

*For annotated **General References** and resources related to this chapter, visit www.hopkinsbayview.org/PAMreferences.*

Chapter 4

Patient Education and the Promotion of Healthy Behaviors

Karan A. Cole and David E. Kern

One meaning of the word *doctor* is "teacher." Through teaching, practitioners can help patients understand their conditions, be reassured, and adopt new treatment regimens. Most of the elements of communication during a visit, described in Chapter 3, contribute to effective teaching. Developing trust, identifying the patient's information needs and psychosocial context, and involving the patient in developing a plan are as important for successful outcomes as providing information.

PATIENT EDUCATION

Definition

Patient education occurs when the health practitioner uses a combination of educational assessment and intervention strategies that influence the patient's knowledge, attitudes, or health behaviors. *Health behaviors* encompass a wide range of activities that relate to health, including seeking health advice; keeping health care appointments; taking medications; undertaking preventive measures; modifying existing patterns of eating, exercising, or substance use; and solving problems. Patient education is sometimes completed during one practitioner–patient interaction, but more often it is an ongoing process that occurs over the course of several visits.

The Practitioner–Patient Relationship

Patient education takes place in the context of a practitioner–patient relationship, which influences the nature of the educational process. As discussed in Chapter 3, the relationship between practitioner and patient can be conceptualized as a spectrum that ranges from active–passive to mutual participation. In an *active–passive relationship,* the practitioner, as expert, is responsible for explaining and prescribing and the patient is responsible for following orders. This type of relationship presumes an *authoritative approach* to patient education and behavior change. In a *mutual participation relationship,* the patient and practitioner actively collaborate and patients take more responsibility for their care. This type of relationship assumes that most patients are capable of participating with the practitioner in the development of their own management plans. It incorporates an *empowerment approach* to patient education and behavior change, during which the practitioner facilitates patient involvement in goal identification, problem solving, and planning (1). Practitioners assume the role of mentor, consultant, and expert in medical knowledge.

Effective patient education does not involve the exclusive use of either an authoritative or an empowerment approach. Approaches often are combined, and the balance of authoritative and empowerment approaches within a given practitioner–patient interaction is determined by practitioner and patient attitudes and skills and by patient needs.

recommendations may be more amenable to intervention than those who do not (46).

The manner of asking influences the accuracy of patient response and the degree of patient comfort. Some questioning techniques can provide reasonably valid estimates of patient health-related behaviors (47). It is generally agreed that patients should be questioned about their behavior in an *open-ended, facilitative, nonthreatening, nonjudgmental, yet detailed and specific* way. Questioning should continue until the patient has provided information about what medicines are being taken and how often, how often doses are missed, and what nonpharmacologic modes of treatment are being used. Patients should specifically be asked about health-related behaviors on the day of and the day preceding their visit. (For example, some diabetic patients routinely omit all drugs, including insulin, at the time of a morning visit; *24-hour recalls* are more accurate than general reports, which tend to be idealized.) Using such techniques, the practitioner will be able to identify 50% or more of those patients who are not following a negotiated regimen (and all of those who have not followed through because they did not understand the regimen). On occasion, more accurate information may be obtained by asking family or household members. In certain cross-cultural interactions, the practitioner may need to use an implicit or indirect approach to determining patient behavior.

Example: Ineffective Method

PRACTITIONER: Now, Mrs. Smith, are you taking your medications as prescribed? [judgmental and leading question, permits a Yes/No answer and promotes a Yes answer, confines response to medications]

PATIENT: Yes, every day.

RESULT: The practitioner raises the dosage or adds a new medication because the patient's blood pressure is still inadequately controlled. The patient becomes frustrated.

Example: Effective Method

PRACTITIONER: Now, Mrs. Smith, can you tell me what you are doing to control your blood pressure? [open-ended, nonjudgmental, focuses responsibility on the patient, does not confine response to medications]

PATIENT: Well, I've stopped adding salt to my food and have pretty much cut out all salted snacks. I do occasionally have a frozen dinner when I'm alone. And, of course, I'm taking the medication.

PRACTITIONER: Uh, huh. [facilitative]

PATIENT: Yes, that blue pill.

PRACTITIONER: And how are you taking it? [directive, not leading]

PATIENT: Twice a day.

PRACTITIONER: Any other medications? [directive, not leading]

PATIENT: No. I stopped the fluid pill when we started the blue one.

PRACTITIONER: And did you take the blue one this morning? [directive]

PATIENT: No, I never take my medicine the day I come to the office!

PRACTITIONER: What about yesterday? [directive, not leading]

PATIENT: Yes ... at least in the morning. Yesterday afternoon was so hectic! You know how busy my days are!

PRACTITIONER: I guess it's hard to take that afternoon dose? [facilitative, empathetic, nonjudgmental]

PATIENT: Yes, because my schedule varies so much.

PRACTITIONER: What did you decide about starting on an exercise program? [directive, nonjudgmental, focuses responsibility on the patient]

PATIENT: Thought about it, but haven't done anything yet. Do you really think it's important?

RESULT: The practitioner congratulates (positively reinforces) the patient on salt restriction, tailors a medication regimen to the patient's schedule, explains why the patient should take her medication on the day of an office visit, provides more information on the value of regular exercise, and provides written instructions and a contract to which both agree. The practitioner decides not to restart the diuretic because the patient has restricted her salt and because the current blood pressure reading does not reflect the effect of the patient's current medication regimen. If the dietary history had been less convincing or the patient had gained weight, the patient might have been asked for a 24-hour diet recall (which is more accurate than general questioning) on this and subsequent visits.

Medication Counts

Medication counts (pill counts) are a form of indirect behavioral monitoring that provides a more objective measure of how patients are following prescribed medication regimens than does simply asking. They have been used to demonstrate the lack of reliability of patient-reported medication-taking behavior. Results are usually expressed in terms of percentages. The ability to measure sequential behavior depends on the use of short intervals between counts, which is usually infeasible. Although more accurate than reported behavior, medication counts do have limitations. If patients are suspicious of being monitored, they can remove medicines from containers without ingesting them. Overestimates of medication usage can also occur if other people are using medicine from the same container. Medication usage may be underestimated if the patient is using two or more medication containers but makes only one available for counting. Many patients do not bring their medication containers with them to the practitioner's office despite reminders. Finally, some patients might take offense at having their medications counted, resulting in deterioration of the practitioner–patient relationship.

The medication count can be approximated by the more practical and less intrusive method of prescribing quantities of medication that should be consumed within a reasonable interval of time, and then observing the *frequency with which prescription renewals are requested.*

Ingenious medication dispensers have been devised that monitor not only the amount but also the regularity with which medicine is removed (48). They are emerging as a new gold standard for the assessment of medication-taking behavior, but currently they are used primarily in research trials, are expensive, and are not generally available for use in clinical practice.

Assays

An objective but indirect method of assessing medication-taking behavior involves testing drug levels in blood, urine, breath, or saliva. Drug levels correlate with compliance determined by other methods as well as by outcome. Marked variation in drug levels may reflect inconsistencies in medication taking. Monitoring drug levels and relaying results to the patient might improve medication-taking behavior.

However, there are limitations to this method. Assays can be expensive. For accurate assessment, multiple measurements are required over an extended period. There is the possibility that patients who know they are being monitored may take medicine immediately before the collection of specimens but not at other times. More important may be differences in drug absorption, distribution, metabolism, and excretion among individuals, which make it impossible to decide whether a low level represents ineffective medication-taking behavior or inadequate dosage in the individual patient. The absence of any drug in the specimen suggests failure to take any of the medication, assuming the specimen has been collected appropriately. The practitioner should have a working knowledge of the pharmacokinetics of the medicine being assayed so that the collection of specimens can be timed correctly. Short-acting drugs, which are rapidly cleared from the blood and excreted, are difficult to monitor by assay techniques because of the difficulty in collecting specimens at appropriate times. Finally, assays are not available for many medications.

Assays can also be used to assess *abstention* from alcohol, drugs, and smoking (see Chapters 27 through 29).

Outcomes

Another objective but more indirect method of assessing health-related behaviors is to monitor expected therapeutic or physiologic outcomes. For example, blood pressure can be monitored in a patient who is taking antihypertensive medication, weight in a patient on a weight-reduction diet, and pulse rate in a patient prescribed a β-blocker. *Review of the longitudinal relationship between a specific therapeutic regimen and outcome measures* can provide clues to health-related behaviors (e.g., the review may disclose widely varying blood pressures on a constant regimen). Such a review can be expedited by the presence and maintenance of a treatment versus outcome flow sheet (see Chapter 1). Feedback about outcomes to patients can also serve to motivate them to change their behavior or positively reinforce changes they have made.

Many of the limitations of drug assays also pertain to assessment of health-related behaviors by the monitoring of outcomes. Outcomes can be influenced by variations in drug bioavailability, absorption, distribution, and excretion; multiple measurements are required. Furthermore, additional factors can influence outcome. For example, a reduction in stress may lower blood pressure, or the presence of concomitant heart disease might be responsible for bradycardia.

Observation

An additional approach to assessing health-related behaviors is to observe patients directly, or indirectly through others, such as family members, household members, or visiting nurses. Patient self-monitoring reports can also serve as a form of indirect monitoring. They have the additional benefit of providing feedback to the patient, which can motivate the patient to change behaviors or positively reinforce changes that have been made.

An extension of this approach involves the *comparison of drug levels or outcomes of therapy during observed versus unobserved periods of a targeted behavior* such as medication consumption. Observations and measurements can be accomplished either in the office, at home, or during hospitalization, depending on the pharmacokinetics of a medication, insurance coverage, and the availability of home care resources. A specific example of this methodology is the 5-hour office blood pressure check in patients who have resistant hypertension, during which the patients take their medication under supervision, then have their blood pressure measured at regular intervals for several hours (49).

Inspection of all pill bottles is a commonly used and important form of observation. Having patients routinely bring all medication containers to the office (including those for both prescribed and over-the-counter medications) may provide invaluable information. What a patient is actually taking is often different from what is recorded in the chart. Other health care providers may have added or subtracted a medication, for which the patient does not remember the name or dose. Sometimes the practitioner discovers that a patient is still taking a discontinued medication or is taking two different preparations of the same drug. Having patients bring medication bottles to each visit is particularly important for patients with cognitive impairment and for those on complicated medication regimens.

INTERVENTION

General Principles

Once an educational assessment has been made, the practitioner is well positioned to help the patient acquire the information, attitudes, skills, and behaviors needed to deal with the medical problem. It is helpful to keep in mind some general principles (Table 4.3) when designing and implementing an educational intervention for a given patient.

- Whenever possible, *ground the educational intervention in a practitioner–patient relationship that promotes patient trust in the practitioner* (see Practitioner–Patient Relationship earlier in this chapter and Chapter 3 for the characteristics of and methods for developing such a relationship). The successful past management of problems also enhances trust in the practitioner.
- *Target the intervention* to:
  - Address the stage of the patient's readiness for change, which has been identified as part of the educational assessment process described earlier (Fig. 4.1).
  - Meet the patient's educational needs—including knowledge, attitudinal, behavioral, and environmental needs—that were identified by using the assessment approaches described earlier (see Background Information).

TABLE 4.3 Intervention: General Principles

Start with a practitioner–patient relationship that promotes patient trust in the practitioner.
Target the educational intervention to
  Address patient-identified readiness to change (Fig. 4.1)
  Meet the patient's specific educational needs
Use specific measurable objectives to focus each interaction; use instructional, behavioral, and motivational/empowerment strategies, mechanical aids, and resources within and beyond the practice as a menu of options to achieve objectives.
Prioritize and limit objectives and material to be covered at each interaction.
Remain patient-centered and interactive.
Avoid premature education before relevant information has been collected and synthesized.
Check for patient comprehension and agreement.

- *Develop specific, measurable objectives* that can be used to focus the educational strategies. The numerous instructional, behavioral, and motivational/empowerment strategies; mechanical aids; and resources within and beyond one's practice, which are discussed later, then can be viewed as a menu of options that can be used to help achieve the objectives.

Examples

OBJECTIVE: Between this visit and the next, the patient will adhere to a medication regimen, agreed upon by him and me.

or

OBJECTIVE: By the end of this visit, the patient will be reassured that her malaise and weight loss are unlikely to be caused by cancer (her fear) and will entertain the possibility of depression as a cause.

- *Prioritize and limit the objectives and material to be covered* at each interaction, so that they do not overwhelm the patient and can be accomplished within available time limits.
- *Remain patient-centered and interactive* (e.g., by accommodating or addressing the patients' routines, beliefs, values, and expectations and including them in the plan). This permits the practitioner to continually adapt educational strategies to meet the patient's needs. It enhances patient understanding, retention, and adoption of treatment regimens and agreed-upon lifestyle changes.
- *Avoid premature education.* Except for simple responses to answerable questions, it is generally preferable to provide patient education *after* relevant historical and physical examination data are collected, information synthesized, an educational assessment made, and a tentative plan formulated. Premature education can result in the giving of misinformation, which will require later correction. It can be ineffective or inefficient if it is not based on adequate assessment or if it is inappropriately focused and prioritized. It is also inefficient because it provides information early in an encounter that will usually be repeated at the close of the encounter.
- *Check for patient comprehension and agreement* with explanations and management plans. Checking helps the practitioner gauge the success of an intervention.

Examples

PRACTITIONER: I know we covered a lot today. It would help if you could tell me in your own words what you are going to do between now and the next visit.

or

PRACTITIONER: Last visit we discussed treatment options for your angina. I also gave you a handout on angina. I wonder what your thoughts are now about the options and my recommendations?

Applying these general principles to practitioner–patient educational interactions should enhance patients' understanding, satisfaction, and adoption of desired health-related behaviors. Specific educational and behavioral change methods are discussed later in this chapter. They should be viewed as a menu of options that can be used in implementing the general principles that were discussed in this section and summarized in Table 4.3.

Efficacy of Educational and Behavioral Change Interventions

Educational and behavioral change interventions can be classified as instructional, behavioral, motivational/empowerment, mechanical aids, or organizational strategies. Successful interventions have increased adherence rates by amounts that range from <10% to almost 70%, averaging between 25% and 30% (percentage change equals percentage of adherent patients in the experimental group minus percentage of adherent patients in the control group). Adherence-improving interventions can also be cost-effective (3). A combination of instructional and behavioral/motivational interventions is more effective than instruction alone (50).

Instructional Strategies

Some sort of explanation or communication of information is a part of almost every practitioner–patient interaction. Sometimes the explanation is an end in itself (e.g., explaining to a patient the expected course of a condition for which there is no treatment, clarifying a patient's unfounded fears about a laboratory test). In other situations, it promotes adherence by providing patients with a rationale for treatment and clarifying a treatment regimen (40). The patient education content related to specific problems and diagnostic procedures is described in later chapters of this book (see especially Patient Experience examples related to procedures). Instructional strategies that enhance understanding, retention, and adherence are displayed in Table 4.4 and discussed next.

Information is most effective when it is *targeted* to the needs of the patient, provides an *explanatory framework* understandable and acceptable to the patient, and *addresses misconceptions and potential barriers* to adherence. The use of medical jargon should be avoided, and the use of language should be tailored to the educational and cultural background of the patient.

To improve retention, verbal instructions should be *clear, concise, and explicit,* with *important features emphasized and repeated*. When there is a large or complex body of information to be conveyed, it is helpful to break it down into understandable categories, as in "I am going to tell you what I think is causing your symptoms, what tests I am going to suggest, and the treatment that should help you. Now, what I think is causing these symptoms. . . ." This technique has been shown to improve retention of information when compared with a less organized recitation of facts (40). An *interactive* approach to communicating information encourages patients to ask questions and have their questions answered. It permits ongoing targeting of the educational message and assessment of patient understanding. It should also increase retention.

TABLE 4.4 Intervention: Instructional Strategies

Target information to meet educational needs.
Provide explanatory framework that is understandable and acceptable to patient.
Address patient misconceptions, fears, and barriers.
Use language appropriate to educational and cultural background of patient; avoid medical jargon.
Use verbal communication methods that increase understanding and retention.
Be clear
Be concise
Be explicit
Repeat important content
Categorize
Use dialogue, as opposed to monologue
Test for comprehension.
Give written instructions.
Give printed educational material that is written at the appropriate reading level.

Because patient factors such as anxiety and reluctance to ask questions can interfere with understanding, it is useful to *check for patient understanding and retention* of the essentials of the information that has been communicated. Furthermore, because patients tend to recall the diagnosis better than the treatment plan (40), it is important to ascertain retention of the essentials of the treatment plan. For example, for a streptococcal throat infection, determine whether the patient understands that penicillin will be taken for a full 10 days (not the exact dosage or schedule, which will be transcribed onto the pill bottle). So as not to offend the patient when checking for comprehension, it is helpful to use an approach such as, "We covered a lot today, and I'm not sure whether I have explained things clearly. It would help me if you would tell me what you understand to be the plan," rather than directly ordering the patient, "Now tell me what the plan is."

Written instructions further enhance adherence (40), and are an important adjunct to verbal instruction. They can be documented on self-duplicating forms (Fig. 4.3). The duplicate portion can be attached to a visit note or a specially constructed educational flow sheet for documentation and future reference. Providing patients with understandable charts that list medications and display

INSTRUCTIONS for: Jane Smith

(1) Reduce lisinopril (10mg) from 2 to 1 pill per day.

(2) Other medications the same

(3) Call me in 2 days to let me know if dizziness is better.

(4) Record blood pressure twice weekly. Call me if BP averages over 150 systolic or over 95 diastolic

(5) Next appointment October, 2005.

6/13/05 DATE — L. B. Jones, MD PROVIDER SIGNATURE

PATIENT'S COPY | RECORD COPY

FIGURE 4.3. Patient instruction form. (The form makes a copy for the patient's record.)

the schedule for each medication enhances adherence to prescribed regimens (51). Legible written or printed instructions provide a remedy for forgetfulness and can be reviewed at leisure in the less stressful environment of the patient's home.

Because it usually requires time to make sense out of information about one's condition (e.g., newly diagnosed hepatitis), because patients retain only about one-half of the essential information communicated at a visit (34,40), and because practitioner–patient communication is usually focused and time-limited, *printed educational materials* can be used to reinforce and expand on what the patient has been told. When printed materials are given to a patient, the practitioner can personalize them by underlining important points, writing down additional important information, and writing the day's date on it.

Complicating patient education and the promotion of healthy behaviors is the growing recognition that a surprisingly high percentage of patients have low literacy skills and a majority have difficulty understanding and implementing medical recommendations (25). Thus it behooves practitioners to assess the literacy level of their patients and to appropriately tailor educational interventions and written informational materials. Resources for patient educational materials and screening them for literacy level are discussed below under "Organizing a Practice for Patient Education."

Behavioral Strategies

Communication of information is necessary but often insufficient to ensure the adoption and maintenance of health-related behaviors by a patient. This is particularly true in the setting of chronic disease, probably because most patients have already learned their prescribed regimen and have learned something about their disease. Behavioral strategies (Table 4.5) attempt to directly influence the adoption or maintenance of certain behaviors. Strategies that incorporate various combinations of patient involvement, alterations in the treatment regimen (simplification, tailoring, shaping), use of behavioral stimuli and reinforcements, and supervision have been shown to improve patient adherence to chronic and short-term therapeutic regimens.

Mechanisms of *enhancing patient involvement* include facilitating patient question asking, negotiating a treatment plan with the patient (rather than dictating a treatment plan to the patient), signing a contract with the patient, and encouraging patient self-monitoring, such as the measuring of glucose levels or taking of blood pressure readings at home. All of these measures increase patients' responsibility for their own care, increase patient confidence, and enhance patient motivation to adopt healthy behaviors. Several studies have demonstrated that these measures improve health outcomes (28–30,41). Self-monitoring may also move patients from precontemplation to contemplation to action in the readiness for change

TABLE 4.5 Intervention: Behavioral Strategies

Involve patients in
Developing management plans
Self-monitoring
Simplify treatment regimen.
Tailor treatment regimen to fit patients characteristics and environment.
Implement complex treatment regimen in a stepwise or graduated manner (shaping).
Manage behavioral stimuli (cues).
Use reinforcements.
Enlist support from family, friends, workplace.
Increase supervision.

cycle (Fig. 4.1), and may motivate problem solving in cases in which the patient is not following through with a treatment plan.

Simplification of the treatment regimen refers to minimizing the number of medications, minimizing the duration of treatment (for short-term regimens), minimizing the frequency of dosing (e.g., once instead of three times daily), and synchronizing the dosing (e.g., three medicines twice daily instead of one medicine twice daily, the second medicine three times daily, and the third medicine four times daily). The less complex the regimen, the greater the adherence rate. This is a particularly important strategy both because of its effectiveness and its ease of implementation.

Tailoring is a process whereby the therapeutic regimen is fitted to the patient's characteristics and environment. Effective tailoring requires knowledge of patients as persons—their beliefs, lifestyles, social and family support systems, and, specifically, any barriers to adopting healthy behaviors. Forgetful patients may benefit from linking medication taking or prescribed activities to daily routines such as eating meals, brushing teeth, getting up in the morning, or going to bed at night. In addition, medication should be kept available where it is taken (e.g., at the breakfast table). If possible, patients should avoid taking medication at times of the day when their activities are variable or when they are likely to be distracted (e.g., at work). Other examples of tailoring include involving patients who like to be in control in planning and monitoring their own therapy; substituting liquid medication for patients who have difficulties swallowing tablets or capsules; increasing supervision and peer support for patients who are having difficulty on their own following a desired regimen (e.g., a weight-reduction diet); and recommending exercise programs that can be incorporated into the schedules of extremely busy, time-pressured patients and that eliminate travel, waiting time, and the need for special scheduling. When cost is a factor, less expensive regimens can be prescribed or financial assistance sought. When a patient's health belief or explanatory model of disease interferes, it can sometimes be accommodated. For example, Hispanic patients who subscribe to the hot–cold theory of health and disease avoid the use of hot substances during pregnancy and therefore may refuse to take hot medications such as iron and vitamins. Adherence in this situation may be obtained by encouraging the patient to neutralize the hot properties of these medications with cool substances such as fruit juices or herb teas. *Language barriers* can be addressed by involving translators or by using written, computerized, or automated voice messaging systems that match patients' languages.

When a regimen is particularly complex or difficult, behavior change may be facilitated by *graduated regimen implementation, or shaping,* whereby parts of the regimen are implemented and the patient is initially rewarded for adhering to only part of the regimen. Once the first part has been achieved, additional components of the regimen are added in stepwise fashion, with rewards being given when there is adherence to both previously accomplished and newly added components. Patient involvement in identifying the steps and the rewards further facilitates the process.

In addition to adjusting the therapeutic regimen to meet the patient's needs, patient and practitioner can work together to identify and manage *behavioral stimuli (cues) and reinforcements* that promote or diminish desired behaviors. Watching television, for example, may be an environmental cue for patients who have learned the habit of eating when they watch television, even when they are not hungry. To eliminate this behavior, the practitioner and the patient might reach an agreement whereby a patient eats only at the dining room table with the television off. Another behavioral cue might be the presence of cigarettes or a friend smoking. In preparation for a smoking cessation effort, a patient might want to remove all cigarettes from the house or to negotiate an agreement with the friend to refrain from smoking in the patient's presence. Patient involvement is critical, because almost all environmental stimuli exist in the patient's environment outside the practitioner's office and because something that might work from the practitioner's perspective might not work at all for the patient. Involvement of family and friends can be helpful in supporting the management of behavioral cues in the patient's environment. Alternatively, family and friends may be a barrier if they refuse to cooperate.

Reinforcement consists of feedback that can either promote or discourage specified behaviors. Reporting back to the patient the results of drug-level assays and therapeutic outcomes (e.g., decrease in blood pressure, cholesterol, or weight) is an example of a practitioner-controlled reinforcement. Together with the patient, the practitioner can identify existing reinforcements, support or initiate those that promote, and attempt to eliminate or diminish those that discourage desired behaviors. Because positive feedback is more effective than punishment in helping patients adopt new behaviors, measures and outcomes that indicate adoption of desired behaviors should be praised, otherwise rewarded, or viewed by the patient as rewards in themselves. When measures or outcomes suggest that the patient is not following the regimen, the problem should be discussed. Rewards should be appropriate to the goals (e.g., eating an ice cream cone would be an inappropriate reward for having followed a diet) and can be increased as the patient gets closer to achieving the goals.

Education and the use of *family, friends, and employers* may be required to optimize rewards for desired behaviors or to reduce the rewards for undesired behaviors at home and in the community. Two common indications for such an intervention are reversal of reinforced psychosocial disability in the physically capable patient after myocardial infarction and maintenance of abstention in the detoxified alcoholic patient.

Increased supervision is a specific form of stimulus management and reinforcement that has been shown to improve adherence. It includes the scheduling of more frequent provider–patient contacts, the use of reminders, the use of drug assays, the use of automated voice messaging, and the eliciting of family or community support to assist in administering and monitoring treatment. For example, the practitioner may request more frequent blood pressure values in a hypertensive patient. The blood pressure readings can be taken by either a nurse at the practitioner's office, a nurse at work, a family member, or the patient. The direct supervision of medication administration is an option that is especially helpful for ensuring adherence in situations where it is known to be low, such as with patients who are forgetful or unreliable, have impaired intellectual or psychological functioning (e.g., patients with alcoholism, dementia, or schizophrenia), or have challenging psychosocial situations. Examples include the use of a single, intramuscular, long-acting penicillin dose rather than 10 days of an oral preparation, intermittent supervised oral antituberculosis therapy, and use of long-acting parenteral drugs in the ambulatory management of schizophrenia.

TABLE 4.6 Intervention: Motivation and Empowerment Strategies

- Help the patient adopt appropriate new beliefs, attitudes, and values.
  - Target education to fill gaps in knowledge base, correct misconceptions, provide explanations that are understandable and acceptable to the patient, and motivate the patient in the context of the patients value systems.
  - Use fear-and-benefit messages appropriately (relevant, accurate, connected to a treatment plan that is effective and feasible for patient).
  - Point out current/past patient beliefs, attitudes, and behaviors that are congruent with the desired new beliefs, attitudes, and values.
- Set agreed-upon goals.
- Enhance patient self-perceptions (self-efficacy, locus of control).
  - Project a positive attitude about patients abilities to change.
  - Emphasize past and present behaviors that demonstrate self-control.
  - Help the patient take credit for changes that have been accomplished.
  - Reframe "failures" as successes.
- Facilitate new skill development.
  - Involve the patient in the development of management strategies.
  - Facilitate problem solving by the patient.
  - Facilitate the development of specific, achievable behavioral objectives by the patient.
  - Facilitate the development of self-monitoring skills.

Motivation and Empowerment Strategies

Adoption of healthy behaviors tends to decay toward baseline after the cessation of many successful interventions. One explanation for the failure of most adherence-improving interventions to have enduring impact is their reliance on actions and supports that are *external* to the patient. Based on reviews of the relevant adherence, psychological, sociologic, and behavioral literature, DiMatteo et al. suggested *approaches that promote internalization of the patient's motivation and ability to adhere* (see DiMatteo and DiNicola, *Achieving Patient's Compliance*, www.hopkinsbayview.org/PAMreferences). These approaches include helping patients to adopt new beliefs, attitudes, or values; setting agreed-upon goals; enhancing patients' perceptions of their self-efficacy; and facilitating new skill development in patients (Table 4.6).

Patients may have to adopt new beliefs, attitudes, or values and abandon others. Because practitioners are a major source of health information for most Americans (34), they can assist in this process. They are more likely to succeed if they have earned the patient's trust and if they incorporate empowerment strategies that involve the patient in setting goals, solving problems, and planning for the intervention (see Practitioner–Patient Relationship). As previously mentioned, the first step in promoting change in health attitudes is to explore the patient's present knowledge, beliefs, attitudes, and values, as well as the patient's social and cultural norms. Education about the patient's diseases and regimens then can be tailored to correct misconceptions, fill in gaps in the patient's knowledge base, provide explanations that are understandable and acceptable to the patient, and motivate the patient in the context of the patient's value, social, and cultural systems. Simply taking time for discussion will raise the salience in the patient's mind of the issue being discussed. Threat or fear messages can motivate behavioral change, but they should not be too strong (i.e., so strong as to cause patient denial or paralysis) or too weak. Furthermore, they should be combined with a positive message about a feasible (for the patient) and effective therapeutic regimen. Because patients are often more present-oriented than future-oriented, short-term as well as long-term benefits of any regimen should be stressed. Because behavior can influence attitudes, and vice versa, the practitioner should point out the patient's own behaviors that support the attitude being promoted. One can help integrate the new attitude into the patient's total system of beliefs by noting how it correlates with other beliefs the patient has. One can also note how the new attitude adheres to cultural and social norms. Of course, new attitudes and beliefs need positive reinforcement, as previously discussed.

Mutually negotiating agreed-upon goals can be motivational and can provide direction for the patient. Patient involvement in, and preferably initiation of, goal setting is a crucial component of this step. For goals to be most effective, they must be "owned" by the patient. Goals should be set at two levels. The first level is long-term goals such as, "I want to quit smoking in 6 months." The second level is short-term, or proximal, goals. These goals refer to the specific actions that will be required to meet the long-term goal, such as, "I will begin using Nicorette gum at a 4-mg dosage next Monday, and I will reduce this to 2 mg in 6 weeks." These goals are actually more helpful to the patient because they are easier to achieve and can be measured more directly. To be effective, they should be specific, measurable, realistic, and achievable. Having the patient sign a contract can further increase the likelihood of success.

Patients with unhealthy *self-perceptions* or perceived low self-efficacy may need to be convinced that they can indeed effect a change in their lives (a process sometimes called *cognitive restructuring*). The practitioner can help by emphasizing the patient's past and present behaviors that demonstrated self-control, by enhancing the patient's feelings of responsibility for accomplished changes, by pointing out inaccuracies in the patient's negative self-perceptions, and by having and projecting a positive attitude to the patient about his or her ability to change.

Examples

PRACTITIONER: On one hand, you say you have no self-control. On the other, you tell me you stopped smoking for the entire period of your second pregnancy. That demonstrates to me that you can exhibit tremendous self-control.

PRACTITIONER: Two months ago you told me that you would never be able to manage insulin. Now you are monitoring your own blood sugars and calling me to propose changes in your insulin schedule. What does that tell you about yourself?

Patients and their practitioners often view partial successes as failures (e.g., the patient who has started drinking or smoking after a period of abstinence, the patient who has cut caffeine intake in half). In the office, practitioners can promote patients' self-esteem and sense of self-efficacy by *reframing these "failures" as successes,* as important steps along the way to accomplishing important health goals.

Example

PRACTITIONER: It's great you were able to stop smoking for a month! That really increases your chances of being able to quit for good. Did you know that most people who stop smoking require more than one attempt?

In addition, patients can learn how to shift their own self-perceptions during vulnerable moments at home, when negative thoughts may interfere with following through with a plan. In anticipation, patients can be asked about potential "sticking points." In response to having experienced these sticking points, they can be encouraged to reflect on and contrast their thoughts during the times they have been successful versus the times they have not. Using these "awarenesses," they can reframe a failure into a partial success in the moment, or they can use previously effective positive self-statements (e.g., "I can do this"). Patients can take this one step further by *posting positive statements or images as reminders* where they can often see them, or at places where they are likely to be tempted to not follow through with a treatment plan. Family members can be enlisted as verbal sources of positive statements or to help patients reframe their negative thoughts. It is essential, however, that patients consider this as helpful and not as overinvolvement or an attempt by the family to control their behaviors.

New skills can also be taught to patients, an empowerment approach that enhances their ability, as well as motivation, to initiate and maintain adherence to a difficult regimen. Patients can learn problem-solving skills by analyzing, with the practitioner, the health problem, treatment alternatives, and the advantages and disadvantages of potential actions. They can participate in the development of overall treatment goals. They can be tutored in developing specific, feasible, and measurable behavioral objectives for themselves and in breaking down large tasks into several small, manageable steps. When patients have adopted new attitudes, beliefs, or behaviors, they can be taught to anticipate and prepare themselves for likely challenges.

Examples

PRACTITIONER TO THE RECOVERING ALCOHOLIC: What challenges do you expect to your new sobriety? How are you going to handle it when people try to get you to drink at your niece's wedding this weekend?

PRACTITIONER TO THE HYPERTENSIVE PATIENT WHO IS SENSITIVE TO BEING VIEWED AS ILL BY OTHERS: How are you going to respond when one of your colleagues at work sees you taking your medication and says, "Oh, you have to take medicine now! What's wrong with you?"

Patients can also be taught to analyze and learn from past failures to enhance the likelihood of future success.

Examples

PRACTITIONER: Why has it been difficult for you to take the second dose?

PRACTITIONER: Exactly how did it occur, when you started smoking again? What does that tell you?

Practitioner: If you could overcome that problem, your chances for success would be really high! Any ideas?

Efforts to help patients adopt appropriate health-promoting beliefs, attitudes, values, skills, and behaviors can be integrated into ongoing care and usually should span several office visits. Once patients have experienced success in implementing changes in one health-related behavior, their sense of efficacy increases, and they are more likely to be successful in changing other behaviors.

Mechanical Aids

Medication-taking behavior can also be improved by the use of a number of mechanical aids. These include well-labeled medication containers (52), medication charts (51), pill calendars (devices on which patients keep track of their medication taking), special pharmaceutical packaging designed to aid memory (e.g., the packaging of birth control pills), and pill dispensers (devices that can be purchased for laying out medications in advance by day and, when necessary, by time of day). Well-designed forms can promote the use and effectiveness of written instructions (Fig. 4.3) (52) and patient adherence to self-monitoring (e.g., by providing patients with flow sheets for recording blood pressure or blood sugar values and asking the patients to bring the sheets with them to their next visit).

Appointment Keeping

A number of factors have been shown to improve appointment keeping by patients (53). Table 4.7 lists the strategies that can be used to improve appointment-keeping behavior.

Telephone and mail reminders, in which patients receive messages several days before their scheduled visits informing them of the dates and times of their appointments or messages inviting patients to reschedule after missed appointments, have consistently improved adherence, usually by 10% to 20%. The impact of the reminders may attenuate over time, however (54), and it may be possible to discontinue reminders without a subsequent increase in missed appointments (55). Wording of the message may be influential. In one study of high-risk patients (56), postcards with a persuasive educational message resulted in a significantly higher adherence rate for influenza vaccination than postcards with a neutral message that simply announced the availability of the vaccine.

The introduction of *individual instead of block appointment systems* and the *substitution of a single provider for multiple providers* have resulted in decreased waiting time and improved appointment keeping. Individual appointment systems give each patient a precise time for an appointment; block systems schedule several or all patients for the same time, usually at the beginning of office hours.

Techniques that the practitioner can use to improve appointment keeping for individual patients include logically *bridging to the next visit* by discussing its purpose with the patient (e.g., monitoring for recurrence, review of test results, decision about therapy); *negotiating a visit interval* that is mutually acceptable; *tailoring the appointment time* to the patient's needs; *obtaining a verbal agreement* from the patient to follow through; and *scheduling the appointment* instead of asking the patient to call for an appointment. Bridging and scheduling were tested successfully in a clinical trial (57).

Because *missed appointments* could presage dropouts from treatment, the charts or names of patients who miss their appointments should be reviewed daily by the patient's practitioner or by a nurse familiar with the patient. When indicated, the patient can be contacted by telephone, letter, or postcard. This review method helps prevent dropping out by patients given a followup appointment at the time of the previous visit, but it fails to identify dropouts who were instructed to call for their next appointment.

If referral is required, educating the patient about the purpose of referral, minimizing the elapsed time between the referral and the referral appointment, providing secretarial assistance to facilitate scheduling and transportation, and referring the patient to a specific practitioner and not simply to a specialty group or clinic have also been shown to improve appointment keeping for diagnostic studies and specialty consultations.

TABLE 4.7 Intervention: Improving Appointment Keeping Behavior

Logically "bridge" to the next appointment.
Negotiate appointment time and interval with patient.
Refer to specific doctors rather than to clinics.
Educate patient about the purpose of referral.
Reach agreement with or obtain verbal commitment from patient.
Schedule appointment for patient rather than having patient call for one.
Use individual, as opposed to block, appointment systems.
Minimize waiting time.
Use telephone or mailed reminders.
Establish review system for missed appointments.

Organizing a Practice for Patient Education

Patient education and adoption of healthy behaviors can be further enhanced through the implementation of effective practice operations. *Practice support staff* often have considerable interest in patient education, and involving them in this effort can save practitioner time and enhance the effectiveness of care. Many office practices involve nursing staff in educating patients about preventive measures such as immunizations, breast cancer screening, and family planning, and in working with patients who have newly diagnosed chronic illnesses such as diabetes mellitus, asthma, or hypertension. In these instances, it is important to agree in advance which aspects of patient education will be covered by the practice's support staff and which will be covered by the practitioner.

Mailing test results or providing this information to patients through the use of automated voice messaging are services that can be incorporated into routine office operations. Depending on the situation, additional information (e.g., norms and goals for test results, changes in regimen based on test results) can be included.

A collection of preselected *printed patient educational materials* can be maintained in an office file or on an office computer and distributed at the discretion of the practitioner or nursing staff. The materials should be available in languages and reading levels that are appropriate for the patient populations that the practice serves. Patient handouts for specific conditions are available via the Internet from government and health organizations and are cited in subsequent chapters of this book (also see below, *Web-based resources* under Using Resources Beyond the Practice). Patient handouts on a variety of subjects are also available via Internet services used primarily by institutions (e.g., Krames on Demand) and in the periodically updated book and CD-ROM *Griffith's Instructions for Patients* (see www.hopkinsbayview.org/PAMreferences). It is important to provide handouts at a reading level that matches the patient's literacy level. The reading level for printed material can be calculated by using a readability index such as the Fog Index, the Flesch Reading Ease Scale, or the Flesch-Kincaid Grade Level; formulas can be found using Internet search engines.

A certain amount of general patient education can be promoted in the *waiting room* by setting up a *pamphlet rack* containing 10 to 15 of the most commonly applicable printed materials. These might include pamphlets on age- and gender-appropriate preventive measures, smoking cessation, weight reduction, low-salt diets, exercise, and other topics of interest to patients and their families. Some practices have found it helpful to have a *bulletin board* with newspaper clippings about current health topics.

Other possibilities include the *delivery of health messages* to patients on telephone hold and the use of office newsletters, audiovisual materials, and computerized interactive programs (58). Automated voice messaging can be used to send messages to patients, as well as to receive patient questions and respond to them (59).

Finally, *medical records and related forms* can be structured in ways that promote the education and monitoring of patients. As mentioned earlier, self-duplicating forms for written instructions (Fig. 4.3) facilitate both the provision of written instructions to the patient and followup by the practitioner at the next visit. Preprinted forms can be used to facilitate or to assist the practitioner in the mailing of diagnostic test results to patients. A flow sheet that chronologically aligns chronic medications and nondrug therapies with clinical and laboratory data (Fig. 1.2) facilitates review of the relationship between a specific therapeutic regimen and associated clinical or laboratory parameters. A *method for keeping track of prescription renewals* can be incorporated into the patient record, such as the attachment of duplicate copies of all written prescriptions to a flow-carrier sheet. Such a method allows the practitioner to ascertain quickly when the patient is due for a refill. This is especially helpful when prescriptions are filled by more than one practitioner in the practice.

Using Resources beyond the Practice

Resources beyond the practitioner's practice can provide information, support, and skills training for patients. The use of such resources is particularly helpful when the practitioner's practice has limited resources or when the educational task is time-consuming or complex. In such situations, the practitioner's efforts should be supplemented by referral to

- *Health professionals who specialize in disease-specific management* (e.g., health educators for diabetic or asthma management);
- *Those who specialize in treatment-specific management* (e.g., nutritionists, physical therapists, trainers, exercise physiologists);
- *Specific treatment programs* (e.g., postmyocardial infarction rehabilitation, smoking cessation programs);
- *Organizations* that provide education and support for specific problems (e.g., American Diabetes Association, Alzheimer's Association);
- *Support groups* that expose patients to others with similar problems (e.g., community or Internet asthma, postmyocardial infarction, ostomy, and mastectomy groups; Alcoholics Anonymous);
- *Web-based resources* that provide patient education (e.g., www.Medlineplus.com and the Karolinska Institute [www.mic.ki.se/Diseases/index.html]) or interactive computer software for self-management.

Volunteer patients who are followed regularly in one's practice, or provided by outside organizations, and who have successfully managed their chronic illness can serve as important resources to patients newly diagnosed with the same condition. *Telephone hotlines* can provide immediate access to patients who are in distress or in need of immediate information (60) (e.g., patients who are victims of domestic violence). Patients can also be referred to specific *Internet sites* or provided with *audiovisual or CD-ROM interactive tutorials*. These have the advantages of

Chapter 5

Complementary and Alternative Medicine

Bimal H. Ashar

Over the past decade, the use of alternative medicine in the United States has skyrocketed. In 2002, an estimated 62% of patients reported using at least one type of alternative medicine therapy during the previous year (1). Yearly, out-of-pocket expenditures relating to alternative medicine by individuals in the United States are estimated at approximately $27.0 billion, roughly equivalent to the out-of-pocket expenditures for all U.S. allopathic physician services (2). *Alternative medicine* is broadly defined as approaches not routinely used by conventional practitioners. The term *complementary medicine* evolved in an effort to foster a positive relationship between allopathic and nonallopathic medicine. The idea that nonconventional therapies can serve as an adjunct to established Western medical practices has received increasing attention from patients, physicians, and governmental agencies. The National Center for Complementary and Alternative Medicine (NCCAM) was established by the National Institutes of Health (NIH) in 1999 to foster research, education, and the dissemination of evidence-based knowledge regarding alternative medicine. In an attempt to simplify these tasks, NCCAM has classified complementary and alternative medicine (CAM) practices into five major categories that encompass hundreds of individual modalities (Table 5.1). This chapter provides the clinician with an overview of some of the more popular CAM modalities currently used by patients. It will serve as a guide to enhance discussion between physicians and their patients.

UNDERSTANDING THE USE OF COMPLEMENTARY AND ALTERNATIVE MEDICINE

The Patient's Perspective

Before a discussion of specific CAM modalities is undertaken, a general understanding of some of the factors

TABLE 5.1 National Institutes of Health Classification of Complementary and Alternative Therapies

Category	*Examples*
Mind–body interventions	Meditation, biofeedback, prayer, aromatherapy
Alternative medical systems	Homeopathy, Ayurveda, traditional Chinese medicine
Manipulative and body-based methods	Chiropractic, massage, craniosacral therapy
Biologic-based therapies	Dietary therapy, herbal medicine, megavitamins, shark cartilage
Energy therapies	Therapeutic touch, qigong, bioelectric field manipulation, Reiki

From The National Center for Complementary and Alternative Medicine. Available at: http://nccam.nih.gov/health/whatiscam/.

TABLE 5.2 Reasons for Use of Complementary and Alternative Therapies

Belief that natural is better and safer
Failure of conventional medicine
Distrust in conventional medicine
Time constraints on the conventional physician
Media hype
Product advertising
Dissemination of information via the Internet

that may be responsible for the patient-driven alternative medicine movement is necessary (Table 5.2). A general theme underlying a majority of CAM therapies is their emphasis on "natural" modes of healing. Acupuncture, chiropractic, massage therapy, and homeopathy are purported to stimulate and invigorate the body's natural potential for preventing and treating disease. Similarly, herbs serve as natural supplements that many patients assume are milder and safer than human-derived medications. This desire of the public to return to nature has been bolstered by media hype, product advertising, and the widespread availability of information (and misinformation) over the Internet.

Additionally, the status of the conventional physician has changed over the past 25 years. Distrust in the medical profession has developed, in part because of conventional medicine's failure to provide effective and safe therapies for a number of common ailments. Diseases such as chronic fatigue syndrome, fibromyalgia, and other pain syndromes have been defined with little understanding of their pathophysiology and without any specific therapy for their treatment. Patients with these conditions represent a large subset of seekers of alternative modalities of care.

The Physician's Role

Despite the widespread prevalence of CAM use among the general population, most patients do not inform their physicians of such use (2). It is imperative that clinicians incorporate an "alternative medicine" history into their routine patient evaluations. Information regarding the types of therapies the patient is using, as well as the reasons for choosing such therapies, should be sought. Further discussions should center on the patient's experiences (positive or negative), and on efficacy data (if available), cost, and potential toxicity of the patient-chosen therapies. Physicians should encourage correspondence with CAM providers in an attempt to develop referral networks. These steps should serve to strengthen the patient–physician relationship and ensure monitoring of potential untoward effects. Specific approaches to obtaining a CAM history are described elsewhere (3).

ACUPUNCTURE

Technique

Acupuncture is a system of medicine derived primarily from ancient Asian practices. It involves the insertion of fine needles into the skin in order to restore the balance of energy, or *qi* (pronounced "chee"), in the body. Qi flows through channels called meridians that are distinct from neurologic dermatomal patterns.

Patient Experience. An initial acupuncture evaluation begins with the history and physical examination. Conventional allopathic techniques are combined with an in-depth musculoskeletal examination designed to identify potential sensitive areas (trigger points). Additional parts of the examination may include detailed inspections of the tongue, radial pulse, and ear. Once a treatment plan is developed, the patient is placed in the supine or prone position on a flat table. Thin needles ranging from 0.1 to 3.5 mm in diameter (Fig. 5.1) are then inserted into defined points to affect the flow of qi. The needles traverse to a depth of 0.5 to 8 cm, depending

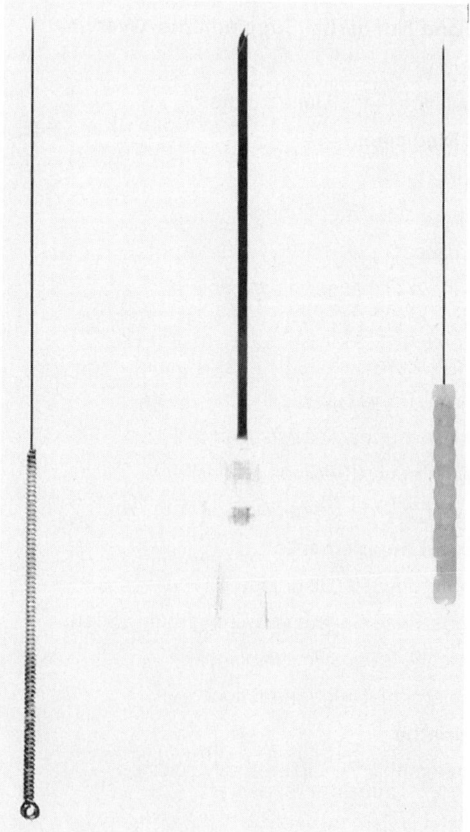

FIGURE 5.1. A 20-gauge needle (*center*) compared with two typical acupuncture needles (*left and right*).

on their location. Additional modalities, such as manual manipulation of the needles, heating of the needles with mugwort (moxibustion), or electrical stimulation, may be employed to assist in the movement of energy (4). The pain experienced by the patient depends on the skill of the practitioner, the thickness of the needle, the depth of insertion, the needle location, and patient sensitivity. Determination of a patient's response usually requires 8 to 12 weeks of therapy. The need for maintenance therapy usually is determined by the chronicity and severity of the underlying condition.

History of Acupuncture in the United States

Although the acupuncture movement seems to have only recently gained popularity, its origins in the United States date back to the 19th century. In the first edition of *Principles and Practice of Medicine,* Sir William Osler described acupuncture as the "most efficient treatment" for acute lumbago (5). In more modern editions of that text, however, references to acupuncture do not appear, reflecting a subsequent lack of confidence in acupuncture as a treatment modality. In 1971, reporter James Reston described how the use of acupuncture successfully relieved his postoperative pain after an appendectomy (6). His article served to stimulate interest among physicians, the public, and the government. More recently, the NIH released a consensus statement that validated the use of acupuncture for certain conditions and strongly encouraged further research (7).

Mechanism of Action

The reluctance of Western medicine to accept acupuncture as a therapeutic tool stems from a lack of knowledge regarding the pathophysiology of the acupuncture response. Studies show alterations in a number of biologic mediators, including endorphins, neurotransmitters, and neurohormones (7). Functional magnetic resonance imaging studies suggest a correlation between specific acupuncture points and regionally specific brain cortical activation (8). Blood flow is also affected by acupuncture needling (9,10). Despite these studies, no unifying mechanism has arisen to completely explain the purported benefits of acupuncture.

Efficacy and Safety

More than 9,000 articles are indexed in Medline under the search term "acupuncture." Yet, only a few of these papers describe clinical trials on the efficacy of acupuncture therapy. Most of the trials that have been done suffer from small sample sizes and methodologic flaws. Many challenges exist to the performance of meaningful acupuncture research. One major study barrier is the lack of standardization of the acupuncture field. There are many different types of acupuncture practiced today. Traditional Chinese acupuncture, auricular acupuncture, five-elements acupuncture, and hand acupuncture are just a few examples that would use unique points for similar conditions. Even among individuals who practice the same type of acupuncture, great variation may exist in actual point selection based on the practitioner's history, physical examination, and personal style. In the United States, many physician-acupuncturists have been instructed in a more disease-oriented approach that attempts to standardize treatments. Acupuncturists trained in the Chinese tradition typically spend 3 years learning to individualize treatments. In addition, they frequently use Chinese herbs in combination with acupuncture techniques to obtain a response. A major criticism of negative acupuncture studies by traditionalists is the abandonment of holism and individualization of care. Another major obstacle to acupuncture research is the difficulty in blinding practitioners and subjects. The use of "sham" acupuncture (needling inactive points) has been used in many trials, but has also been criticized because the flow of qi is still theoretically affected.

Despite their limitations, randomized controlled trials have been performed for a number of clinical conditions. The NIH consensus report stated that there is strong evidence to support the use of acupuncture for postoperative and chemotherapy-induced nausea and vomiting (7). Additional evidence exists for its efficacy for the treatment of chronic low back pain, although it has not been shown to be superior to other therapies (11,12) and its usefulness for acute low back pain has not yet been proven (11). Systematic reviews of the literature suggest the potential for positive effects on lateral epicondylitis and osteoarthritis of the knee (13,14). Equivocal evidence exists for the use of acupuncture for chronic pain depression and asthma (15–17). There is also strong evidence *against* the use of acupuncture for conditions such as smoking cessation and tinnitus (18,19).

The use of acupuncture is associated with very few serious adverse effects. There are case reports linking acupuncture therapy with pneumothorax, organ puncture, hepatitis, and skin infections; however, these events were usually attributable to improper sterilization of needles or practitioner negligence. Side effects, such as needle pain, tiredness, localized bleeding, and vasovagal syncope, are more commonly seen, but without serious sequelae (20).

CHIROPRACTIC

Chiropractic is a branch of Western medicine that has fought for professional respect since its inception in the late 1890s. Today, it is probably incorrect to classify chiropractic as a form of "alternative" medicine. Just under 10% of the population are estimated to have sought out chiropractic care for an underlying ailment, usually musculoskeletal in origin (1,21). Chiropractors are licensed in all 50 states. Most third-party payers, including Medicare, cover many of the services chiropractors provide.

Chiropractic Principles

Chiropractic philosophy places the nervous system at the center of health and well-being. Disease is considered to be fostered by imbalances in the neurophysiology of the body. This imbalance can be corrected by diagnosing and correcting mechanical abnormalities or subluxations in the spine. Although much variation exists in technique and adjunctive treatments, spinal manipulation remains at the core of the chiropractic approach to disease. It is a holistic form of health care in that it relies on the body's ability to ultimately restore physiologic balance after manipulation.

Patient Experience. A careful history and physical examination is performed by the chiropractor. Specific emphasis is placed on diagnosing spinal dysfunction. Areas along the spine are inspected and palpated for abnormalities in symmetry, tenderness, tone, and temperature. Passive and active range of motion are assessed carefully. Radiographs, ultrasonography, heat-sensing devices, and other tests may be employed to aid in diagnosis. After the diagnosis of a spinal abnormality, the patient may be placed with the side of the spinal restriction upward. The doctor's hands are then placed on certain points of the body so as to deliver a high-velocity, short-amplitude thrust to that spinal joint. This is typical of manipulation by direct contact (short-lever technique). In the long-lever technique, the spine is manipulated by thrusts to areas linked to the spine (e.g., a thrust to the thigh moves the vertebrae in the lower spine). Frequently, the patient experiences a cracking or popping noise. Possible adjuncts to therapy include massage, heat application, and trigger-point deactivation (22,23).

Efficacy and Safety

The most common condition treated by chiropractors is low back pain. Similar to the trials on acupuncture, chiropractic research generally suffers from methodologic flaws and difficulties in design. A recent meta-analysis of randomized controlled trials suggested that spinal manipulation appears to be more effective than sham therapy for acute or chronic low back pain, but not superior to other standard treatments such as analgesics, physical therapy, and back exercises (24). Although chiropractic for low back pain may not be the most cost-effective strategy (25), patient satisfaction seems to be higher than for nonmanual treatments (26).

Chiropractic has been used for a number of other conditions, including neck pain and headache syndromes. The data on efficacy are contradictory based on a few well-designed clinical trials (27,28). Some patients also turn to their chiropractor for the treatment of other disorders, such as menstrual pain, hypertension, asthma, and fibromyalgia. Again, no definitive conclusions regarding efficacy can be drawn because of the lack of research.

A number of serious adverse effects of chiropractic have been reported. Vertebrobasilar vascular accidents with subsequent infarction, vertebral fracture, diaphragmatic paralysis, internal carotid artery dissection, and tracheal rupture have been described and attributed primarily to cervical manipulation (23). The incidence of such severe complications is unknown but is thought to be rare. Serious complications of lumbar spine manipulation are also thought to be quite uncommon, and consist primarily of cauda equina syndrome (23). Minor complications, such as localized pain, are common but transient.

It is important for the primary physician to recognize *contraindications to spinal manipulation.* Patients with a coagulopathy, whether from illness or from medication, should be advised to refrain from chiropractic treatments. Additionally, patients with osteoporosis, rheumatoid arthritis, spinal infections, spinal neoplasms, spinal instability, or an absent odontoid process should avoid such therapy. Open communication between the patient, chiropractor, and the primary physician is vital to avoid serious complications.

HERBAL AND NONHERBAL SUPPLEMENTS: OVERVIEW

Extent of Use

Of all the fields encompassed by the category of CAM, none has grown more rapidly in recent years than the use of over-the-counter supplements. An estimated 19% of the population used over-the-counter natural products in 2002 (1). Billions of dollars are spent each year by consumers searching for natural substances to foster and maintain their health. The reasons for the popularity of supplements are easy to understand. These are easily accessible, relatively inexpensive, "natural" substances that are purported to improve a number of conditions. Many patients use them to fill the void created by the dearth of available preventive medications. Others see them as a quick, hassle-free cure to an underlying problem. There is potential for gain without the need for practitioner visits, lifestyle changes, or unpleasant procedures. To many physicians, however, supplements are unproven, unregulated, potentially dangerous "drugs" that offer limited benefits to their patients. The roles of various supplements in allopathic medicine will most likely change rapidly as issues of safety, efficacy, and regulation are settled.

Regulation in the United States

The U.S. Food and Drug Administration (FDA) historically regulated dietary supplements as foods, to ensure premarket safety and truthful labeling. In 1994, Congress passed the Dietary Supplements Health and Education Act (DSHEA), which served to expand the definition of "dietary supplements" and to deregulate the industry to meet the concerns of consumers and manufacturers. Vitamins, minerals, amino acids, herbs, and other botanicals are now all considered dietary supplements. Premarket testing for safety or efficacy is no longer required. Supplements are assumed to be safe unless proven otherwise by the FDA. The DSHEA attempted to place restrictions on labeling, however. Manufacturers can make claims only regarding the supplement's effects on a "structure or function" of the body (e.g., "for prostate health"). They cannot claim that their product is "intended to diagnose, treat, cure, or prevent any disease" (e.g., "for the treatment of benign prostatic hyperplasia"). Claims regarding structure and function are not required to be approved by the FDA before marketing. Despite the media attention given to the DSHEA, approximately one-third of Americans who use dietary supplements regularly believe that supplements are currently regulated by the government (29).

The lack of regulation of herbal and nonherbal supplements poses a number of problems. There are presently no standards in place to guarantee homogeneity among different products. For example, a patient may wish to take ginkgo biloba to potentially improve his memory. At the store he may choose from a number of different ginkgo products that vary tremendously in their composition. There is no assurance that the active ingredient or ingredients from the plant are even present in a given preparation. Variation also exists among batches from the same manufacturer owing to differences in plant composition, handling, and preparation. In many instances, the active ingredients are unknown, making standardization impossible.

The sale and distribution of herbs depends on proper identification of plants. A number of case reports have described breakdowns in this process. More than 40 cases of Chinese herb nephropathy were caused in Belgium by the inadvertent substitution of the nephrotoxic herb *Aristolochia fangchi* for *Stephania tetrandra,* an herb used in weight-reduction pills. Many of the affected patients went on to develop urothelial carcinoma (30). Cases of adulteration of Chinese herbal products with steroids, benzodiazepines, nonsteroidal anti-inflammatory drugs, and diuretics have also been described. Reports of contamination of herbal products with heavy metals also exist (31).

HERBAL MEDICINES

In general, adequate evidence is lacking to support many of the herbs marketed today. A number of herbal products rely on anecdotal evidence to support their use. Many of the clinical trials in the literature are small-scale, nonrandomized, and/or nonblinded. Large-scale randomized controlled trials are not cost-efficient for manufacturers because herbs are not patentable. Organizations like the Cochrane Collaboration have attempted to pool study data to draw conclusions from meta-analyses. Many of the analyses have been equivocal. The herbs listed in this section and in Table 5.3 represent a few of the more popular herbs

TABLE 5.3 Common Herbal Medications

Common Name	*Indications for Use*	*Suggested Dosage*	*Potential Toxicity*
Black cohosh	Menopausal symptoms	40–80 mg b.i.d. (4–8 mg triterpene glycosides)	Gastrointestinal discomfort
Cranberry	Urinary infections	300 mL of juice daily; 400-mg capsule twice daily	Nephrolithiasis
Echinacea	Upper respiratory tract infections	Varies widely depending on preparation	Hypersensitivity reactions
Feverfew	Migraine prophylaxis	50–100 mg of dried leaf preparation	Hypersensitivity reactions
Garlic	Cardiovascular protection	900 mg/d of 1.3% allicin content product	Gastrointestinal upset, bleeding
Ginkgo biloba	Dementia, claudication, tinnitus	40 mg t.i.d. of ginkgo leaf extract	Gastrointestinal upset, headache, bleeding, seizure
Ginseng	Fatigue, exercise performance, diabetes	Varies widely (100 mg/d to 3 g/d)	Mastalgia, insomnia, vaginal bleeding, hypertension
Kava-kava	Anxiety	60–210 mg of kava lactones per day	Rash, sedation, hepatitis, liver failure
Saw palmetto	Prostatic hyperplasia	160 mg b.i.d.	Mild gastrointestinal effects
St. John's wort	Depression, anxiety	300 mg t.i.d.	Headache, dry mouth, insomnia, fatigue, photosensitivity

*Supplement–Drug Cautions

used by Americans today. The suggested dosage usually is based on historical usage rather than specific safety or toxicity testing and may be quite variable.

Cranberry

Folklore has for years perpetuated the use of cranberry for the treatment of urinary tract infections (UTIs). Basic science research has suggested that the proanthocyanidins present in cranberries may inhibit the adherence of *Escherichia coli* to urinary tract epithelial cells. To date, no clinical trials have been done to suggest efficacy of cranberry juice or cranberry extract for the *treatment* of urinary tract infections. However, a recent systematic review of the use of cranberry for the prevention of UTI suggested efficacy, although the number of trials available for review were limited (32). Although cranberry supplementation is generally accepted to be quite safe, the possibility of inducing nephrolithiasis exists (33).

Ephedra and Bitter Orange

Traditional Chinese medicine has for centuries touted the use of ephedra for the treatment of asthma, congestion, and bronchitis. Also known as ma huang, it consists predominantly of two alkaloids, ephedrine and pseudoephedrine. In the United States, ephedra had become a popular ingredient in over-the-counter weight-loss preparations. When combined with caffeine, ephedrine caused significant weight loss over a 6-month period (34). However, as use of the dietary supplement increased, so did the number of adverse event reports. Hypertension, arrhythmias, myocardial infarction, stroke, and death have all been attributed to the use of ephedra products. This led to its eventual ban by the FDA in April 2004.

The prohibition of the sale of ephedra products, has led to the development and sale of a number of "ephedra-free" supplements for weight loss. Many of these supplements are marketed as safer alternatives, despite little evidence of safety or efficacy. One herb that has now become commonly used in such products is *Citrus aurantium*. Also known as bitter orange or zhi shi, this herb contains synephrine, a sympathomimetic amine that can theoretically raise pulse and blood pressure. To date, there is little efficacy data supporting its use for weight loss (35). Case reports have begun to emerge linking its use to myocardial infarction (36), QT prolongation and syncope (37), and ischemic stroke (38).

Echinacea

Echinacea is one of the most popular herbs in use. It is used primarily to prevent and treat upper respiratory tract infections. Although the plant genus *Echinacea* consists of a number of different species, medicinal use has centered predominantly on three of them (*Echinacea purpurea, Echinacea angustifolia,* and *Echinacea pallida*). These herbs have been thought to boost the immune system by stimulating cytokine activity. A number of clinical trials have demonstrated a positive effect on prevention and treatment of upper respiratory tract infections. Yet, definitive conclusions regarding efficacy have been difficult to make owing to study limitations (39). More rigorously designed trials seem to have negative results (40). There also exists great variation in species of plant studied, parts of the plant used (root, leaf, flower, seed), and extraction methods, further complicating interpretation of trials. Echinacea is thought to be quite safe for short-term use. No serious side effects have been reported, although hypersensitivity reactions can occur. Because of its ability to stimulate the immune system, echinacea is not recommended for patients with autoimmune disease or human immunodeficiency virus infection for fear of worsening disease. This concern remains a theoretical risk rather than an established fact. No long-term data on the safety of chronic use are presently available.

Feverfew (*Tanacetum parthenium*)

Feverfew has been used for centuries for a variety of conditions. It is commonly used for the prevention of migraine headaches. It is thought to inhibit prostaglandin synthesis, histamine release from mast cells, and degranulation of platelets. Additionally, it may have direct vasodilatory effects. There is currently very little evidence to support the use of feverfew migraine headache prophylaxis (41). If the leaves of the plant are chewed directly, mouth ulceration may occur. Otherwise, it is considered safe. Because of its effects on platelets, a theoretical concern about bleeding exists, although no cases have been reported to date.

Garlic (*Allium sativum*)

Garlic is one of the most highly studied herbal medications available. It has been thought to possess antimicrobial, anti-inflammatory, antifungal, antiprotozoal, antioxidant, and antineoplastic properties that make its use as a general tonic attractive. More recently, focus has shifted to garlic's effects on cardiovascular diseases and risk factors. A meta-analysis suggested that garlic supplementation may decrease levels of total cholesterol and low-density lipoproteins modestly, but only in the short-term. Platelet aggregation is significantly reduced, but the clinical importance of this finding remains elusive. No significant effects on blood pressure or glucose levels have been noted (42). Additionally, garlic has not been shown to improve symptomatic peripheral vascular disease (43). Garlic toxicity is usually mild and consists of gastrointestinal upset and body odor. Case reports of spontaneous bleeding and interactions with anticoagulants have been described (31).

Ginkgo biloba

Ginkgo biloba use has skyrocketed over the last few years based on reports and claims of its use for improving memory and treating dementia, peripheral vascular disease, and tinnitus. It is thought to have a number of biologic effects, including increasing blood flow, inhibiting platelet-activating factor, altering neuronal metabolism, and working as an antioxidant. Although overall data is limited, modest improvements in cognitive performance and social functioning in patients with Alzheimer disease or multi-infarct dementia have been seen with the use of ginkgo extract Egb 761 (44). However, there is currently no evidence that *Ginkgo biloba* is effective for the *prevention* of memory loss or dementia. Ginkgo has a modest effect on symptoms of intermittent claudication (45) but little effect on tinnitus (46). Side effects are rare and usually consist of gastrointestinal complaints or headaches. Cases of spontaneous bleeding (47) and seizures (48) have been reported. Because of the possible potentiation of anticoagulant effects, *Ginkgo biloba* use should probably be avoided in patients who are taking warfarin.

Ginseng (*Panax* species)

Ginseng is thought of by many as a virtual panacea. Asian ginseng (*Panax ginseng*) has been used for centuries as a general tonic, stimulant, and stress reliever. In Chinese medicine, American ginseng (*Panax quinquefolius*) has been used, but it is thought to possess less stimulant activity. Siberian ginseng (*Eleutherococcus senticosus*) has also gained popularity but belongs to a different plant species. The mechanism of action for ginseng is unknown but is thought to involve the concentration of ginsenosides, which are believed to act as an antioxidant and on a number of tissue receptors. Although small studies have suggested some improvement in mental performance and diabetic control, a systematic review of clinical trials failed to provide compelling evidence for advocating ginseng for improving physical performance, psychomotor performance, cognitive function, or for treating diabetes (49). In general, ginseng is considered safe. Reports of hypertension, insomnia, vomiting, headache, vaginal bleeding, Stevens–Johnson syndrome, and mastalgia have been cited (50). The possibility of an interaction with warfarin (reduced international normalized ratio [INR]) has also been raised (51). Care should be taken in patients who are taking anticoagulants.

Kava-kava (*Piper methysticum*)

Kava has been used for thousands of years by inhabitants of South Pacific islands. It is usually ingested as a mildly intoxicating beverage distinct from alcohol. Current interest in kava has centered on its use as an anxiolytic agent. Its mechanism of action on the central nervous system is unknown. Its effects seem to be independent of benzodiazepine-binding sites. A review of randomized, double-blind, clinical trials suggested that kava extract is superior to placebo for short-term treatment of anxiety (52). Undesired effects usually consist of mild gastrointestinal upset and allergic skin reactions. Eye irritation and a yellow, scaly, dry rash (kavaism) has been described with heavy, chronic use (50). Although rare and idiosyncratic, case reports of hepatitis, fulminant hepatic failure, and death have also been reported (53). These reports have prompted many European countries and Canada to ban its sale. Concomitant use with other anxiolytics or alcohol should be avoided to protect against excess sedation. Patients using kava should also have their liver function tests monitored periodically.

Saw Palmetto (*Serenoa repens*)

Benign prostatic hyperplasia is a common clinical condition among elderly men. Despite numerous conventional treatment options, many men choose against therapy because of the potential for adverse effects. This has led to the popularity of saw palmetto as an agent to treat symptoms associated with an enlarged prostate. A number of short-term studies show it to be effective in improving urologic symptoms and flow measures (54). Its exact mechanism of action is unknown, but may be related in part to inhibition of 5α-reductase. In a head-to-head trial, saw palmetto was shown to be equivalent to finasteride and tamsulosin in improving symptoms associated with benign prostatic hyperplasia. Fewer sexual side effects and no change in levels of prostate-specific antigen were seen in the group receiving the herbal treatment (55,56). However, saw palmetto has not yet been shown to prevent the complications of benign prostatic hyperplasia (e.g., acute urinary retention). Side effects reported with the use of saw palmetto have been mild and rare, although adequate data on long-term use are lacking. It should be noted that there is no known clinical evidence to support its use for the *prevention* of benign prostatic hyperplasia or prostate cancer.

St. John's Wort (*Hypericum perforatum*)

St. John's wort has been used extensively by Americans for self-diagnosed depression and dysphoria. It is the most widely *prescribed* antidepressant medication in Germany. Its mechanism of action and active ingredients have yet to be conclusively defined. However, data suggest that preparations of *Hypericum* extract may inhibit monoamine oxidase activity as well as synaptic neurotransmitter reuptake (57). The results of trials on St. John's wort for major depression are quite heterogeneous. A number of studies show minimal beneficial effects compared to placebo, whereas others suggest efficacy equivalent to a number of currently prescribed antidepressants (58). Clearly, lack of product standardization is an issue. In general, side effects of St. John's wort are mild and infrequent. The most commonly reported reactions include gastrointestinal irritations, allergic reactions, fatigue, dizziness, dry mouth, and headache. There are reports of photosensitization (57). Rare cases of serotonin syndrome have been reported with the combined use of St. John's wort and selective serotonin reuptake inhibitors (31). Therefore, caution must be exercised by patients taking prescription antidepressants. Most of the safety concerns regarding St. John's wort have revolved around potential drug–herb interactions, primarily as a consequence of its effect on the cytochrome P450 system (see below, Supplement-Drug Interactions and Table 5.4).

NONHERBAL SUPPLEMENTS

A number of nonherbal supplements have gained popularity over the past decade. These products consist predominantly of molecules normally found in the body. Vitamins, minerals, amino acids, and metabolic intermediates are just a few of the substances encompassed within this category. A manipulation of the concentrations of these molecules is thought to produce beneficial effects toward the prevention and treatment of disease. The efficacy, safety, and regulatory issues that surround herbal medications similarly apply to these supplements. The following paragraphs describe a few of the more popular products in this category.

Coenzyme Q10 (Ubiquinone)

Coenzyme Q10 is a substance produced by the body (and found in some foods) that is structurally similar to vitamins E and K. It is considered to be an antioxidant and also plays a major role in mitochondrial oxidative phosphorylation. It has gained popularity for the prevention and treatment for various cardiac disorders. To date, most of the trials on coenzyme Q10 have focused on its use in the treatment of congestive heart failure. A multicenter Italian study showed a reduction in hospitalizations and serious complications in patients with New York Heart Association class III and class IV heart failure treated with coenzyme Q10 (59). Other studies, however, have failed to show positive results (60,61). A recent review of the data concluded that there was no convincing evidence for or against the use of coenzyme Q10 for cardiac conditions (62). There is presently no evidence to either suggest that it reduces cardiac mortality or to support its use for the primary prevention of cardiac disease.

Supplementation with coenzyme Q10 has also been suggested to prevent beta-hydroxy-beta-methylglutaryl-coenzyme A (HMG-CoA) reductase inhibitor (statin)-induced myotoxicity. This assertion is based upon the demonstration of reduced levels of *circulating* coenzyme Q10 levels in patients taking statins. However, it is unclear whether this documented decrease is a true marker of tissue levels of coenzyme Q10. Additionally, if tissue levels are truly decreased, it is not known whether supplementation would restore these levels or result in clinical benefit (63). Coenzyme Q10 is also being used for a variety of other conditions, including hypertension, human immunodeficiency virus (HIV), and migraine headaches. There is very limited evidence to support its use for these conditions. There has been some promising data on the use of high-dose (>1000 mg/day) coenzyme Q10 in Parkinson disease (64), although it is premature to make definitive recommendations. The most commonly reported side effects with coenzyme Q10 administration are nausea, heartburn, and diarrhea. Its structural similarity to vitamin K has been suggested as the cause of a decrease in responsiveness to warfarin when administered concurrently (65,66). Typical doses for the treatment of cardiac disease are 50 to 200 mg/day.

Glucosamine Sulfate and Chondroitin Sulfate

Glucosamine and chondroitin are two of the most widely accepted supplements currently available. Even though they have not lived up to their initial claims as a "cure" for arthritis, they have provided many patients with some degree of relief from chronic joint pain. Glucosamine is an amino sugar that is a substrate for the production of glycosaminoglycans and proteoglycans, which are essential building blocks of connective tissue. Chondroitin is a glycosaminoglycan that may inhibit enzymatic destruction of synovial tissue and serve as an anti-inflammatory agent in addition to its role in structural cartilage formation. Meta-analyses of clinical trials have concluded that glucosamine–chondroitin preparations result in symptomatic and functional benefits for patients with osteoarthritis of the knees or hips and may slow the progression of joint space narrowing (67,68). Such effects may not be as pronounced with glucosamine alone (69,70). Both glucosamine and chondroitin are generally well tolerated. Mild gastrointestinal side effects are rarely seen. The recommended doses of glucosamine sulfate and chondroitin sulfate are, respectively, 500 mg three times daily and 400 mg three times daily. Treatment effect may not be seen for up to 8 weeks after beginning therapy. No significant drug interactions have been noted, although a theoretical risk of bleeding with concurrent administration of chondroitin sulfate and anticoagulants exists owing to chondroitin's structural homology with a small component of certain heparinoids (71). There is also theoretical concern about glucosamine inducing hyperglycemia. However, studies in type II diabetics have failed to demonstrate clinically significant rises in blood glucose or glycosylated hemoglobin (72).

SAMe (*S-Adenosylmethionine*)

S-adenosylmethionine (SAMe) is a common metabolic intermediary produced in the body through the interaction of methionine and adenosine triphosphate (ATP). It is considered to be vital to appropriate cellular functioning and survival. Because of its role in numerous metabolic pathways, it is suggested to be beneficial for a wide array of diseases, the best studied of which is osteoarthritis. A number of small clinical trials have suggested that its ability to improve the symptoms of osteoarthritis is equivalent to that of nonsteroidal anti-inflammatory drugs but with fewer side effects (73,74). A number of small studies on the use of SAMe for the treatment of depression show positive results (73,75). Many of these studies were conducted using a parenteral rather than oral form of medication because of the poor oral bioavailability of the medication. Studies on oral SAMe have typically used doses between 1200 and 1600 mg/day. Nausea and abdominal discomfort have been described rarely with the use of SAMe. In a number of depression trials, subsets of patients experienced hypomania (76). Additionally, there is concern for interactions with tricyclic antidepressants (77,78); consequently, concomitant use should be avoided. A major limitation to the use of SAMe is its cost. At its suggested dose of 400 to 1,600 mg/day, a 1-month supply can amount to well over $200 in out-of-pocket expense.

Supplement–Drug Interactions

It is estimated that one of every five adults taking prescription medications is also using over-the-counter supplements (2). Given that many of the supplements in use today have not been rigorously studied, little is known about their potential interactions with prescription medications. A number of case reports suggest that some herbal and nonherbal products may directly interact with certain drugs to inhibit or enhance their effects. Additionally, supplements may indirectly potentiate or oppose medication effects through independent mechanisms. Table 5.4 lists some potential problems when mixing prescription medications and supplements. Most of the cited cautions are based on case reports and theoretical concerns. It is

TABLE 5.4 Supplement–Drug Cautions

Supplement	*Drug*	*Reaction (Ref. No.)*
Astragalus membranaceus	Cyclosporine	Interference with immune suppression (79)
Capsaicin (chili pepper)	ACE inhibitors	Induce cough (80)
Chondroitin sulfate	Anticoagulants	Theoretic increased risk of bleeding
Coenzyme Q10	Warfarin	Decreased INR (65,66)
Dong quai	Warfarin	Increased INR (81)
Feverfew	Anticoagulants	Increased risk of bleeding
Garlic	Anticoagulants	Increased risk of bleeding
	Protease inhibitors	Decreased drug levels (82)
Ginkgo biloba	Anticoagulants	Increased risk of bleeding
Ginseng (*Panax*)	MAO inhibitors	Headache, tremor (83), mania (84)
	Warfarin	Decreased INR (51)
Kava-kava	Benzodiazepines	Increased sedation and lethargy (85)
Licorice	Oral contraceptives	Hypokalemia, hypertension, edema (86)
SAMe	Tricyclic antidepressants	Potentiation of effect and toxicity (77,78)
Siberian ginseng	Digoxin	Increased digoxin level (87)
St. John's wort	Cyclosporine	Decreased cyclosporine levels (88)
	Digoxin	Decreased digoxin levels (89)
	Protease inhibitors	Decreased indinavir levels (90)
	Oral contraceptives	Breakthrough bleeding (91)
	SSRIs	Serotonin syndrome (92)
	Statins	Decreased effectiveness of atorvastatin, lovastatin, simvastatin (93)
	Theophylline	Decreased theophylline levels (94)
	Warfarin	Decreased INR (91)
Yohimbe	MAO inhibitors	Potentiation of effects (95)
	Tricyclic antidepressants	Hypertension (96)

ACE, angiotensin-converting enzyme; INR, international normalized ratio; MAO, monoamine oxidase; SAMe, *S*-adenosylmethionine; SSRIs, selective serotonin reuptake inhibitors.

imperative that physicians discuss the possibility of interactions with their patients and report any suspected cases to the FDA. The MedWatch program has been set up to monitor the safety of drugs, devices, biologics, and dietary supplements. Physicians should report any significant adverse reactions or supplement–drug interactions to this program. Reporting can be done over the Internet (at the MedWatch website, www.fda.gov/medwatch) or by telephone (1-800-FDA-1088).

HOMEOPATHY

The principles of homeopathy were first publicized by Samuel Hahnemann in the late 1700s. Since then, it has generated much controversy and experienced waxing and waning popularity. Common diagnoses currently treated by homeopaths include otitis media, depression, allergy, hypertension, arthritis, and headache. In the United States, an estimated 3.6% of the population uses homeopathic remedies (1). This has occurred despite criticism from many scientists who believe that the homeopathic effect is nothing more than a placebo response. Much of the opposition stems from the inability to scientifically validate the basic tenets of this unique medical treatment system.

Homeopathic Principles and Medicines

The basis of homeopathy relies on two concepts: the law of similars and the use of dilutions. The law of similars suggests that patients with certain sets of symptoms can be cured of their ailments by administration of a drug that induces those symptoms in a healthy individual. An example of this principle in conventional medicine is the use of digoxin to treat arrhythmias, which it is capable of causing. The principle of dilutions suggests that substances retain their biologic activity even when they are diluted to levels at which no molecules of the original substance remain.

Homeopaths tend to focus on subjective symptoms and sensations rather than objective medical diagnoses. Thus a wide variety of medications can be used for the same diagnosis, depending on the clinical presentation. Various encyclopedias of homeopathic remedies exist (called *materia medica*) that describe symptoms produced by various diluted medications when administered to healthy individuals (provings). The patient's symptom complex is matched with the drug provings to determine the optimal therapeutic regimen. Treatment frequency can range from one or two doses to chronic daily dosing. Typically, patients are observed weeks later to determine progress and the need for alterations in the treatment plan.

Homeopathic medicines are usually derived from plant, mineral, or animal sources. They are regulated by the FDA under the Food, Drug, and Cosmetic Act of 1938. Most remedies are sold over the counter and require labeling information that includes ingredients, recommended dose, indications for use, and dilution. Homeopathic medications are typically exempt from requirements related to expiration dating and finished product testing because they contain little or no active ingredients. Additionally, these remedies are not restricted to the 10% alcohol limit of conventional drugs (97).

Efficacy and Safety

A number of clinical trials have been done on a variety of homeopathic remedies. Many of them, however, are of low methodologic quality. Three systematic reviews of placebo-controlled trials suggest that the effects of homeopathy are superior to those of placebo, whereas one review failed to support such a positive finding (98). Yet, analysis of individual conditions and treatments are less supportive. Reviews of homeopathic remedies for the treatment of osteoarthritis (99), asthma (100), dementia (101), and the prevention and treatment of influenza (102) are inconclusive. An examination of eight trials done on a specific homeopathic medication (*Arnica montana*) used for postoperative recovery failed to show efficacy beyond that of placebo (103). As with most other CAM therapies, systematic and rigorous research is needed to definitively prove effect.

Although serious toxicity from the use of homeopathic medicines is rare, unpleasant effects are quite common. "Aggravation reactions" occur when a patient's symptoms worsen acutely after starting a remedy. Homeopathic physicians view these reactions as desirable and as prognostic of a favorable outcome. Patients, however, may equate aggravations with side effects. As with herbal products, the potential for contamination and adulteration of homeopathic medications exists because these preparations are exempt from standard finished product testing.

A more serious problem exists when patients choose to defer effective conventional therapy for an unproven homeopathic remedy. Such cases have occurred with a number of CAM therapies. Additionally, some homeopaths discourage the use of conventional drugs because they are thought to hinder the effectiveness of homeopathic remedies. Many homeopathic physicians are also opposed to immunization and may influence patients against proven preventive health measures (104).

MISCELLANEOUS COMPLEMENTARY AND ALTERNATIVE THERAPIES

Massage Therapy

Therapeutic massage is defined as the manipulation of soft tissues so as to improve the overall health of the body.

TABLE 5.5 Techniques Used in Swedish Massage

Technique	Description
Effleurage	Deep or superficial stroking along the length of a muscle
Friction	Deep muscle stimulation applied by compression with fingertips or palm of hand
Pétrissage	Kneading of muscles in a circular pattern
Tapotement	Light slapping, beating, or chopping movements
Vibration	Rapid, to-and-fro, shaking movements of fingers by the hands

It is commonly used to relieve stress and anxiety, to promote relaxation, and to treat certain pain disorders. There are a number of different types of massage (e.g., Swedish, deep-tissue, neuromuscular, shiatsu). Massage therapists commonly combine various methods during a typical session. Swedish massage is the most common form currently practiced. It consists of a number of different techniques (Table 5.5) designed to relieve muscle tension and improve circulation. Aromatic oils are frequently employed as lubricants during treatments. Acupressure or shiatsu massage consists of the application of heavy pressure for extended periods at particular pressure points on the body. It is designed to affect the flow of energy and consequently to restore balance to the body. In deep-tissue massage, increasing amounts of pressure are applied to structurally align the body. Rolfing (structural integration) is a form of deep-tissue massage designed to improve muscular function through manipulation of fascial planes.

Efficacy and Safety

Massage therapy is used primarily as a relaxation technique. It has been shown subjectively and objectively to assist in stress reduction, although the intensity and duration of the response can be quite variable. Small studies support the use of massage for a number of conditions, including fibromyalgia, chronic fatigue, anxiety, and depression, but there is insufficient evidence to make definitive recommendations for its routine use for the treatment of these conditions. However, a review of three clinical trials of massage therapy for chronic low back pain suggested that it is useful for this condition and more cost-effective than other CAM therapies, such as acupuncture or spinal manipulation (105). Massage is generally considered to be safe. Care needs to be taken in patients with coagulation disorders, especially with the use of deep-tissue techniques.

Aromatherapy

Most people experience pleasant and unpleasant smells on a daily basis. Some odors may make us happy, while others may be irritating. The impact that these odors have on our bodies as a whole forms the basis for aromatherapy. In this CAM therapy, plant-derived essential oils are used to induce changes in emotion and health. Jasmine, chamomile, and lavender are just a few of the oils used to induce a positive relaxation response. Aromatherapy has been used alone or in combination with massage therapy for stress reduction. Evidence for its use for specific medical conditions, including anxiety, is presently inconclusive (106). No serious adverse effects are attributed to this therapy, although allergic responses may occur.

SPECIFIC REFERENCES*

1. Barnes PM, Powell-Griner E, McFann K, et al: Complementary and alternative medicine use among adults: United States, 2002. Advance Data for Vital and Health Statistics No. 343. Hyattsville, MD: National Center for Health Statistics, 2004. http://www.cdc.gov/nchs/data/ad/ad343.pdf.
2. Eisenberg DM, Davis RB, Ettner SL, et al. Trends in alternative medicine use in the United States, 1990–1997. JAMA 1998;280:1569.
3. Eisenberg DM. Advising patients who seek alternative medical therapies. Ann Intern Med 1997;127:61.
4. Helms JM. An overview of medical acupuncture. Altern Ther Health Med 1998;4:35.
5. Osler W. Principles and practice of medicine. New York: D. Appleton & Co, 1892.
6. Reston J. Now about my operation in Peking. New York Times 1971;July 26:1,6.
7. National Institutes of Health. Consensus statement.1997;15(5):1–34.
8. Cho ZH, Chung SC, Jones JP, et al. New findings of the correlation between acupoints and corresponding brain cortices using functional MRI. Proc Natl Acad Sci U S A 1998; 95: 2670.
9. Yuan X, Hao X, Lai Z, et al. Effects of acupuncture at fengchi point (GB 20) on cerebral blood flow. J Tradit Chin Med 1998;18:102.
10. Sandberg M, Lindberg LG, Gerdle B. Peripheral effects of needle stimulation (acupuncture) on skin and muscle blood flow in fibromyalgia. Eur J Pain 2004;8:163.
11. Manheimer E, White A, Berman B, et al. Meta-analysis: acupuncture for low back pain. Ann Intern Med 2005;142:651.
12. Furlan AD, van Tulder MW, Cherkin DC, et al. Acupuncture and dry-needling for low back pain. The Cochrane Database of Systematic Reviews 2005, Issue 1. Art. No: CD001351. DOI: 10.1002/14651858.CD001351.pub2.
13. Trinh KV, Phillips SD, Ho E, et al. Acupuncture for the alleviation of lateral epicondyle pain: a systematic review. Rheumatology 2004;43:1085.
14. Ezzo J, Hadhazy V, Birch S, et al. Acupuncture for osteoarthritis of the knee: a systematic review. Arthritis Rheum 2001;44:819.
15. Ezzo J, Berman B, Hadhazy VA, et al. Is acupuncture effective for the treatment of chronic pain? A systematic review. Pain 2000; 86:217.
16. Smith CA, Hay PPJ. Acupuncture for depression. The Cochrane Database of Systematic Reviews 2004, Issue 3. Art. No: CD004046.
17. McCarney RW, Brinkhaus B, Lasserson TJ, et al. Acupuncture for chronic asthma. The Cochrane Database of Systematic Reviews 2003, Issue 3. Art. No: CD000008. DOI: 10.1002/14651858.CD000008.pub2.
18. White AR, Rampes H, Ernst E. Acupuncture for smoking cessation. The Cochrane Database of Systematic Reviews 2002, Issue 2. Art. No.: CD000009. DOI: 10.1002/14651858.CD000009.
19. Park J, White AR, Ernst E. Efficacy of acupuncture as a treatment for tinnitus: a systematic review. Arch Otolaryngol Head Neck Surg 2000;126:489.
20. Ernst E, White AR. Prospective studies of the safety of acupuncture: a systematic review. Am J Med 2001;110:481.
21. Tindle HA, Davis RB, Phyllis RS, et al. Trends in use of complementary and alternative medicine by U.S. adults: 1997-2002. Altern Ther Health Med 2005;11:42.
22. Lawrence DJ. Chiropractic medicine. In: Jonas WB, Levin JS, eds. Essentials of alternative and complementary medicine. Philadelphia: Lippincott Williams & Wilkins, 1999:275.
23. Kaptchuk TJ, Eisenberg DM. Chiropractic: origins, controversies, and contributions. Arch Intern Med 1998;158:2215.
24. Assendelft WJ, Morton SC, Yu EI, et al. Spinal manipulative therapy for low back pain: a

*Bold numerals denote published controlled clinical trials, meta-analysis, or consensus-based recommendations.

meta-analysis of effectiveness relative to other therapies. Ann Intern Med 2003;138:871.
25. Kominski GF, Heslin KC, Morgenstern H, et al. Economic evaluation of four treatments for low-back pain: results from a randomized controlled trial. Med Care 2005;43: 428.
26. Cherkin DC, Deyo RA, Battie M, et al. A comparison of physical therapy, chiropractic manipulation, and provision of an educational booklet for the treatment of patients with low back pain. N Engl J Med 1998;339:1021.
27. Ernst E. Chiropractic spinal manipulation for neck pain: a systematic review. J Pain 2003;4: 417.
28. Astin JA, Ernst E. The effectiveness of spinal manipulation for the treatment of headache disorders: a systematic review of randomized clinical trials. Cephalgia 2002;22:617.
29. Blendon RJ, DesRoches CM, Benson JM, et al. Americans' views on the use and regulation of dietary supplements. Arch Intern Med 2001; 161:805.
30. Nortier JL, Martinez MC, Schmeiser HH, et al. Urothelial carcinoma associated with the use of a Chinese herb (*Aristolochia fangchi*). N Engl J Med 2000;342:1686.
31. Fugh-Berman A. Herb-drug interactions. Lancet 2000;355:134.
32. Jepson RG, Mihaljevic L, Craig J. Cranberries for preventing urinary tract infections. The Cochrane Database of Systematic Reviews 2004, Issue 2. Art. No: CD001321. DOI: 10.1002/14651858.CD001321.pub3.
33. Terris MK, Issa MM, Tacker JR. Dietary supplementation with cranberry concentrate tablets may increase the risk of nephrolithiasis. Urology 2001; 57:26.
34. Astrup A, Breum L, Toubro S, et al. The effect of an ephedrine/caffeine compound compared to ephedrine, caffeine and placebo in obese subjects on an energy restricted diet: a double blind trial. Int J Obes 1992;16:269.
35. Bent S, Padula A, Neuhaus J. Safety and efficacy of citrus aurantium for weight loss. Am J Cardiol 2004;94:1359.
36. Nykamp DL, Fackih MN, Compton AL. Possible association of acute lateral-wall myocardial infarction and bitter orange supplement. Ann Pharmacother 2004;38:812.
37. Nasir JM, Durning SJ, Ferguson M, et al. Exercise-induced syncope associated with QT prolongation and ephedra-free Xenadrine. Mayo Clin Proc 2004;79:1059.
38. Bouchard NC, Howland MA, Greller HA, et al. Ischemic stroke associated with use of an ephedra-free dietary supplement containing synephrine. Mayo Clin Proc 2005; 80:541.
39. Melchart D, Linde K, Fischer P, et al. Echinacea for preventing and treating the common cold. The Cochrane Database of Systematic Reviews 1999, Issue 1. Art. No: CD000530. DOI: 10.1002/14651858.CD000530.
40. Caruso TJ, Gwaltney JM. Treatment of the common cold with echinacea: a structured review. Clin Infect Dis 2005;40:807.
41. Pittler MH, Ernst E. Feverfew for preventing migraine. The Cochrane Database of Systematic Reviews 2004, Issue 1. Art. No: CD002286. DOI: 10.1002/14651858. CD002286.pub2.
42. Ackermann RT, Mulrow CD, Ramirez G, et al. Garlic shows promise for improving some cardiovascular risk factors. Arch Intern Med 2001;161:813.
43. Jepson RG, Kleijnen J, Leng GC. Garlic for peripheral arterial occlusive disease. The Cochrane Database of Systematic Reviews 1997, Issue 2. Art. No: CD000095. DOI: 10.1002/ 14651858.CD000095.
44. Birks J, Grimley Evans J. Ginkgo biloba for cognitive impairment and dementia. The Cochrane Database of Systematic Reviews 2002, Issue 4. Art. No: CD003120. DOI: 10.1002/14651858.CD003120.
45. Pittler MH, Ernst E. Ginkgo biloba extract for the treatment of intermittent claudication: a meta-analysis of randomized trials. Am J Med 2000;108:276.
46. Hilton M, Stuart E. Ginkgo biloba for tinnitus. The Cochrane Database of Systematic Reviews 2004, Issue 2. Art. No: CD003852. DOI: 10.1002/ 14651858.CD003852.pub2.
47. Bent S, Goldberg H, Padula A, et al. Spontaneous bleeding associated with ginkgo biloba: a case report and systematic review of the literature. J Gen Intern Med 2005;20:657.
48. Gregory PJ. Seizure associated with *Ginkgo biloba*? Ann Intern Med 2001; 134:344.
49. Vogler BK, Pittler MH, Ernst E. The efficacy of ginseng: a systematic review of randomized clinical trials. Eur J Clin Pharmacol 1999;55:567.
50. Miller LG. Herbal medicinals: selected clinical considerations focusing on known or potential drug-herb interactions. Arch Intern Med 1998; 158:2200.
51. Yuan CS Wei G, Dey L, et al. American ginseng reduces warfarin's effect in healthy patients: a randomized controlled trial. Ann Intern Med 2004;141:23.
52. Pittler MH, Ernst E. Kava extract versus placebo for treating anxiety. The Cochrane Database of Systematic Reviews 2003, Issue 1. Art. No: CD003383. DOI: 10.1002/14651858.CD003383.
53. Clouatre DL. Kava kava: examining new reports of toxicity. Toxicol Lett 2004;150:85.
54. Wilt T, Ishani A, Mac Donald R. Serenoa repens for benign prostatic hyperplasia. The Cochrane Database of Systematic Reviews 2002, Issue 3. Art. No: CD001423. DOI: 10.1002/14651858. CD001423.
55. Carraro JC, Raynaud JP, Koch G, et al. Comparison of phytotherapy (Permixon) with finasteride in the treatment of benign prostate hyperplasia: a randomized international study of 1,098 patients. Prostate 1996;29:231.
56. Zlotta AR, Teillac P, Raynaud JP, et al. Evaluation of male sexual function in patients with lower urinary tract symptoms (LUTS) associated with benign prostatic hyperplasia (BPH) treated with a phytotherapeutic agent (Permixon), tamsulosin or finasteride. Eur Urol 2005;48:269.
57. Greeson JM, Sanford B, Monti DA. St. John's wort (*Hypericum perforatum*): a review of the current pharmacological, toxicological, and clinical literature. Psychopharmacology (Berl) 2001;153:402.
58. Linde K, Mulrow CD, Berner M, et al. St John's wort for depression. The Cochrane Database of Systematic Reviews 2005, Issue 3. Art. No: CD000448. DOI: 10.1002/14651858. CD000448.pub2.
59. Morisco C, Trimarco B, Condorelli M. Effect of coenzyme Q10 therapy in patients with congestive heart failure: a long-term multicenter randomized study. Clin Invest 1993;71:S134.
60. Khatta M, Alexander BS, Krichten CM. The effect of coenzyme Q10 in patients with congestive heart failure. Ann Intern Med 2000;132:636.
61. Permanetter B, Rossy W, Klein G, et al. Ubiquinone (coenzyme Q10) in the long-term treatment of idiopathic dilated cardiomyopathy. Eur Heart J 1992;13:1528.
62. Shekelle P, Morton SC, Hardy M, et al: Effect of supplemental antioxidants vitamin C, vitamin E, and coenzyme Q10 for the prevention and treatment of cardiovascular disease. Evid Rep Technol Assess 2003;83:1.
63. Nawarskas JJ. HMG-CoA reductase inhibitors and coenzyme Q10. Cardiol Rev 2005;13:76.
64. Shults CW, Oakes D, Kieburtz K, et al. Effects of coenzyme Q10 in early Parkinson disease: evidence of slowing of the functional decline. Arch Neurol 2002;59:1541.
65. Landbo C, Almdal TP. Interaction between warfarin and coenzyme Q10. Ugeskr Laeger 1998;160:3226.
66. Spigset O. Reduced effect of warfarin caused by ubidecarenone. Lancet 1994;344:1372.
67. McAlindon TE, LaValley MP, Gulin JP, et al. Glucosamine and chondroitin for treatment of osteoarthritis: a systematic quality assessment and meta-analysis. JAMA 2000;283:1469.
68. Richy F, Bruyere O, Ethgen O, et al: Structural and symptomatic efficacy of glucosamine and chondroitin in knee osteoarthritis: a comprehensive meta-analysis. Arch Intern Med 2003;163:1514.
69. Reginster JY, Deroisy R, Rovati LC, et al. Long-term effects of glucosamine sulphate on osteoarthritis progression: a randomised, placebo-controlled clinical trial. Lancet 2001; 357:251.
70. Towheed TE, Maxwell L, Anastassiades TP, et al. Glucosamine therapy for treating osteoarthritis. The Cochrane Database of Systematic Reviews 2005, Issue 2. Art. No: CD002946. DOI: 10.1002/ 14651858.CD002946.pub2.
71. Acostamadiedo JM, Iyer UG, Owen J. Danaparoid sodium. Expert Opin Pharmacother 2000;1:803.
72. Scroggie DA, Albright A, Harris MD. The effect of glucosamine-chondroitin supplementation on glycosylated hemoglobin levels in patients with type 2 diabetes mellitus: a placebo-controlled, double-blinded, randomized clinical trial. Arch Intern Med 2003;163:1587.
73. Hardy M, Coulter I, Morton SC, et al: *S*-adenosyl-L-methionine for treatment of depression, osteoarthritis, and liver disease. Evidence Report/Technology Assessment no. 64. 2002;AHRQ publication no. 02-E034:1.
74. Di Padova C. *S*-adenosylmethionine in the treatment of osteoarthritis: review of the clinical studies. Am J Med 1987;83(5A):60.
75. Williams AL, Girard C, Jui D, et al. *S*-adenosylmethionine (SAMe) as treatment for depression: a systematic review. Clin Invest Med 2005;28:132.
76. Echols JC, Naidoo U, Salzman C. SAMe (*S*-adenosylmethionine). Harvard Rev Psychiatry 2000;8:84.
77. Iruela LM, Minguez L, Merino J, et al. Toxic interaction of *S*-adenosylmethionine and clomipramine. Am J Psychiatry 1993;150:522.
78. Berlanga C, Ortega-Soto HA, Ontiveros M, et al. Efficacy of *S*-adenosyl-L-methionine in speeding the onset of action of imipramine. Psychiatry Res 1992;44:257.
79. Chu DT, Wong WL, Mavligit GM. Immunotherapy with Chinese medicinal herbs. II: reversal of cyclophosphamide-induced immune suppression by administration of fractionated *Astragalus membranaceus* in vivo. J Clin Lab Immunol 1998;25:125.
80. Hakas JF. Topical capsaicin induces cough in patient receiving ACE inhibitor. Ann Allergy 1990;65:503.
81. Page RL, Lawrence JD. Warfarin potentiation by dong quai. Pharmacotherapy 1999;19:870.
82. Piscitelli SC, Burstein AH, Welden N, et al. The effect of garlic supplements on the pharmacokinetics of saquinavir. Clin Infect Dis 2002;34:234.
83. Shader RI, Greenblatt DJ. Phenelzine and the dream machine: ramblings and reflections. J Clin Psychopharmacol 1985;5:65.
84. Jones BD, Runikis AM. Interaction of ginseng with phenelzine. J Clin Psychopharmacol 1987; 7:201.
85. Almeida JC, Grimsley EW. Coma from the health food store: interaction between kava and alprazolam. Ann Intern Med 1996;125: 940.

86. de Klerk GJ, Nieuwenhuis MG, Beutler JJ. Hypokalemia and hypertension associated with use of liquorice flavoured chewing gum. BMJ 1997;314:731.
87. McRae S. Elevated serum digoxin levels in a patient taking digoxin and Siberian ginseng. CMAJ 1996;155:293.
88. Mai I, Kruger H, Budde K, et al. Hazardous pharmacokinetic interaction of Saint John's wort (*Hypericum perforatum*) with the immunosuppressant cyclosporin. Int J Clin Pharmacol Ther 2000;38:500.
89. Johne A, Brockmoller J, Bauer S, et al. Pharmacokinetic interaction of digoxin with an herbal extract from St. John's wort (*Hypericum perforatum*). Clin Pharmacol Ther 1999;66:338.
90. Piscitelli SC, Burstein AH, Chaitt D, et al. Indinavir concentrations and St. John's wort. Lancet 2000;355:547.
91. Yue QY, Bergquist C, Gerden B. Safety of St John's wort (*Hypericum perforatum*). Lancet 2000;355:576.
92. Lantz MS, Buchalter E, Giambanco V. St. John's wort and antidepressant drug interactions in the elderly. J Geriatr Psychiatry Neurol 1999;12:7.
93. Sugimoto K, Ohmori M, Tsuruoka S, et al. Different effects of St. John's wort on the pharmacokinetics of simvastatin and pravastatin. Clin Pharmacol Ther 2001;70:518.
94. Nebel A, Schneider BJ, Baker RK, et al. Potential metabolic interaction between St. John's wort and theophylline. Ann Pharmacother 1999;33:502.
95. McGuffin M, Hobbs C, Upton R, et al: Botanical safety handbook. Boca Raton, FL: CRC Press, 1997.
96. Lacomblez L, Bensimon G, Isnard F, et al. Effect of yohimbine on blood pressure in patients with depression and orthostatic hypotension induced by clomipramine. Clin Pharmacol Ther 1989; 45:241.
97. Stehlin I. Homeopathy: real medicine or empty promises? FDA Consumer 1996;30. Available at: www.fda.gov/fdac/features/096`home.html. Last accessed September 10, 2005.
98. Jonas WB, Kaptchuk TJ, Linde K. A critical overview of homeopathy. Ann Intern Med 2003; 138:393.
99. Long L, Ernst E. Homeopathic remedies for the treatment of osteoarthritis: a systematic review. Br Homeopath J 2001;90:37.
100. McCarney RW, Linde K, Lasserson TJ. Homeopathy for chronic asthma. The Cochrane Database of Systematic Reviews 2004, Issue 1. Art. No: CD000353. DOI: 10.1002/14651858.CD000353.pub2.
101. Mccarney R, Warner J, Fisher P, et al. Homeopathy for dementia. The Cochrane Database of Systematic Reviews 2003, Issue 1. Art. No: CD003803. DOI: 10.1002/14651858.CD003803.
102. Vickers AJ, Smith C. Homoeopathic oscillococcinum for preventing and treating influenza and influenza-like syndromes. The Cochrane Database of Systematic Reviews 2004, Issue 1. Art. No: CD001957. DOI: 10.1002/14651858.CD001957.pub2.
103. Ernst E, Pittler MH. Efficacy of homeopathic arnica: a systematic review of placebo-controlled clinical trials. Arch Surg 1998;133:1187.
104. Lee AC, Kemper KJ. Homeopathy and naturopathy: practice characteristics and pediatric care. Arch Pediatr Adolesc Med 2000; 154:75.
105. Cherkin DC, Sherman KJ, Deyo RA, et al. A review of the evidence for the effectiveness, safety, and cost of acupuncture, massage therapy, and spinal manipulation for back pain. Ann Intern Med 2003;138:898.
106. Cooke B, Ernst E. Aromatherapy: a systematic review. Br J Gen Pract 2000;50:493.

For annotated **General References** *and resources related to this chapter, visit www.hopkinsbayview.org/PAMreferences.*

Chapter 6

Sexual Disorders: Diagnosis and Treatment

Leonard R. Derogatis, Arthur L. Burnett, Linda C. Rogers, Chester W. Schmidt, Jr., and Peter J. Fagan

The past decade has seen dramatic changes in the management of male sexual disorders, particularly the sexual dysfunctions, as increasing numbers of safe, effective, pharmacologic agents have become available to practitioners to treat these conditions. Similar innovations in the treatment of female sexual dysfunctions also appear imminent, as a number of promising new drugs move closer to regulatory approval. In this environment, it is tempting to characterize sexual disorders in terms of a biogenic versus psychogenic dichotomy regarding both etiology and treatment. We believe, however, that such a polarized approach is both inaccurate and counterproductive in determining accurate diagnosis and effective treatment for sexual dysfunctions. Instead, we urge clinicians to adopt a posture that integrates biologic, psychological, and relational elements in their formulations of the majority of sexual disorders. Sexual problems accompany physical or mental illnesses, can be the result of endocrine deficiencies or imbalances, and are often secondary to side effects of medications or a result of the abuse of drugs. They may also be expressions of interpersonal conflict, intrapsychic distress, or cultural proscriptions that conflict with mainstream customs. Frustration, fatigue, and self-doubt can complicate the sexual life of a person who is aging, as well as those who are ill or recovering from surgery, and relational tensions and distrust can often interfere with the sexual response in a healthy adult. Conceptualizing these conditions in terms of multiple perspectives (1) greatly enhances our capacity to understand them in a comprehensive manner. While the primary care physician may not be in a position to explore all related perspectives, viewing sexual disorders as simultaneously biologic, psychological, and relational phenomena significantly improves our diagnostic acumen, and our potential for effective treatment.

Ultimately, the task of the primary care clinician is to ensure that the patient's sexual disorder is diagnosed accurately and treated effectively, weighing all of the factors that can be identified at the time. Given the pharmacologic developments in recent years, many patients' problems can be effectively addressed in the office of the primary care clinician. However, if either the psychological or somatic factors are too complex, the primary care clinician may wish to refer the patient to a specialist, a maneuver which at this point in time may be more demanding than referrals for other conditions. If available, a reliable Center for Sexual Medicine should be a first choice; however, good working relationships with urologists, gynecologists, or mental health professionals with an expressed interest and expertise in sexual medicine can often lead to an equally effective resolution of the problem. The encouraging news is that although effectiveness data for treatment outcomes in primary care are limited, the information available suggests that outcomes for reversible sexual problems are usually good, with clinically significant improvement seen in a majority of cases.

HUMAN SEXUAL RESPONSE CYCLE

To assess sexual disorders rapidly and accurately, it is helpful to be familiar with the human sexual response (HSR) cycle and the major physiologic factors that mediate each phase of the cycle. The HSR cycle is traditionally divided into four phases: desire, arousal, orgasm, and resolution. It is important to view the HSR as a construct to understand sexual behavior. In practice, many dysfunctions coexist and do not occur in the neat sequential order implied by the HSR cycle.

The Four Phases

The *first phase* of the HRS cycle is *one of desire* and consists of fantasies and wishes to engage in sexual activity. This response is psychic in origin, but the psychic stimulation is mediated, in all probability, by circulating androgens.

The *second phase is the arousal phase.* It consists of a number of physiologic changes plus the subjective sense of sexual pleasure and excitement. In both sexes there is an increase in heart and breathing rates, and development of muscular tension throughout the body, which is most pronounced in the pelvic area and thighs. For both sexes, the major physiologic change is the development of vascular congestion in the genital area. For females, the manifestations of vasocongestion are vaginal lubrication and swelling of the external genitalia. In males, vasocongestion leads to erection. These changes may be mediated by either of two neurologic pathways: (a) a local reflex pathway initiated by tactile stimulation of the penis or clitoris and mediated by sensory fibers entering the dorsal root ganglia, or (b) a cortical pathway initiated by psychic stimuli and mediated by sympathetic fibers. Each pathway promotes rapid inflow and retention of blood in the penis and the vulva. In addition to neurologic pathways, erection in the male and vasocongestion of the vulva and vagina in the female depend on intact arterial blood flow from the right and left internal pudendal arteries.

The third phase is orgasm. Subjectively, for both sexes, orgasm is a peaking of sexual pleasure accompanied by a sense of release from sexual tension. Physiologically in the male, the most obvious manifestation of orgasm is ejaculation. Ejaculation is mediated by the sympathetic nervous system and consists of two processes: emission, resulting from contraction of the vas deferens, prostate, and seminal vesicles; and actual ejaculation, resulting from rhythmic contraction of the muscles of the pelvic floor and from closure of the internal sphincters of the bladder (preventing retrograde ejaculation). In the female, the rhythmic contractions take place within the musculature of the outer third of the vagina and in the perineal muscles. The subjective component of orgasm is a cortical sensory phenomenon; it can be experienced without peripheral correlates such as ejaculation or bladder neck closure in men and vaginal contractions in women.

The fourth phase is termed *resolution,* which subjectively is accompanied by a sense of pleasure, warmth, well-being, and relaxation. Physiologically there is a gradual return of heart rate, breathing rate, and muscle tension to the baseline state. Most men are refractory to entering another cycle of sexual activity for some time (minutes in younger men, an hour or longer in middle-aged and older men). Women are not subject to this refractory period and may have multiple orgasms after continued or additional stimulation.

Alternative Model for Women

Recently, there has been much debate about whether the traditional HSR model is appropriate for all women in all circumstances (2). A less linear, more cyclic, model of sexual response may more accurately reflect the experience of many women, particularly those in long-term relationships. Many sexually satisfied women report that they seldom have spontaneous thoughts about sex but are able to express responsive desire to sexual cues from their partner. Desire for them is typically experienced subsequent to arousal, and the two states become mutually enhancing. Motivational factors include a desire for intimacy with the partner, and emotional and physical satisfaction, beyond specific sexual desire, which may or may not augment the experience. At times, men's sexual desire patterns may also fit this model. Under such a model, patients should not be considered candidates for a diagnosis of desire disorder even if they experience few spontaneous sexual thoughts and fantasies as long as their capacity for "responsive desire" is intact.

COMMON SEXUAL DISORDERS

The nomenclature and criteria used to classify sexual disorders in this chapter are based primarily on the American Psychiatric Association's *Diagnostic and Statistical Manual of Mental Disorders,* 4th edition (DSM-IV) (3). More recent work, which is highly consonant with the DSM-IV paradigm, but further refines and explicates certain criteria and definitions, has also been integrated into the model (4,5). The assessment and management of sexual desire disorders, sexual arousal disorders, orgasmic disorders, and sexual pain disorders across multiple etiologies are discussed here.

Tripartite Model of Etiology

As alluded to earlier, current thinking about the etiology of sexual dysfunctions tends to represent causality as deriving from multiple perspectives (1). Biologic/medical factors, psychological/intrapsychic issues, and relationship/interpersonal conflicts, among other influences, may play causal roles in these disorders. Obviously, the primary care provider is not equipped to evaluate an exhaustive list of potential causal agents, nor to weigh their relative contributions. For this reason we recommend a tripartite model for conceptualizing the etiology of sexual dysfunctions, one with three principal aspects: a *biogenic* aspect, a *psychogenic* aspect, and a *relational* aspect. Basically, this "three-legged stool" model describes a three-dimensional Cartesian coordinate system that locates each patient within the space of the primary axes, and identifies any discernible factors on a particular axis that may play an etiologic role. Once identified, putative causal factors (e.g., diabetes, performance anxiety, marital conflict) can be noted and a relative weight can be tentatively assigned by the physician. The primary care professional can then discuss findings with the patient, and decide which aspects (if any) of the case should be treated in the primary care office, and which are better referred to a specialist.

Example

Mrs. W, a 56-year-old married school teacher presented to the clinic with a primary complaint of complete loss of sexual desire. She indicated that she had noticed a slight reduction in her sexual desire upon entering menopause at the age of 49 years, but over the last 5 years her loss of desire has been extreme. She was very distressed by her situation, indicating that she had been a very sexual person throughout her life, and now is left simply going through the motions—sexually speaking, a shell of the woman she was. When she was age 52 years, the patient's father, to whom she was very strongly attached, died suddenly without warning. Her grief was profound, and within 6 months she was diagnosed with a Major Depressive Disorder. After several trials with a variety of antidepressant medications the psychiatrist to whom she was referred by her gynecologist selected an effective selective serotonin reuptake inhibitor (SSRI) regimen. She responded very well to treatment, and when seen in our clinic was essentially in complete remission from her depression. Her gynecologist had also prescribed a hormone replacement therapy (HRT) regimen to which she responded positively. Although the patient could achieve moderate levels of sexual arousal, and somewhat muted orgasms, her desire for sex was completely absent. The patient questioned why, after having done so well with other aspects of her treatment for depression, her sexual desire could not be restored.

An evaluation of the primary axes of the tripartite system revealed no problems in the patient's marital relationship (an excellent marriage of 25 years), and no other familial conflicts. All evidence indicated that Mrs. W was currently free of depressive disorder and clearly in remission, with psychological conflicts appearing minimal. These facts directed focus to the *biogenic* axis. The patient did remain on a maintenance dose of SSRIs; however, she indicated that she had not noticed a further decline in her sexual desire associated with treatment with antidepressants at initial therapeutic doses. Because her very first awareness of a decline in her sex drive was attendant upon the beginning of her menopause, an endocrine assay was ordered to establish her endocrine status. Total serum testosterone and free testosterone were observed to be in the "low" range. The patient was in remission from her depression, was on maintenance doses of SSRIs, and was free of potential marital conflicts, all possible

TABLE 6.1 Medical Conditions That Can Affect Sexual Response in Either Sex

Organic Factor	Sexual Disorders
Alcoholic neuropathy	Hypoactive arousal, hypoactive orgasm
Angina pectoris or recent myocardial infarction	Hypoactive desire
Any chronic systemic disease	Hypoactive desire, hypoactive arousal
Chronic pain	Hypoactive desire
Degenerative arthritis and disc disease of lumbosacral spine	Hypoactive desire, hypoactive arousal
Diabetes mellitus	Hypoactive arousal, retrograde ejaculation (men); hypoactive orgasm (women)
Endocrine disorders (thyroid deficiency states, Addison disease, androgen deficiency, Cushing disease, hypopituitarism, hyperprolactinemia)	Hypoactive desire, variable effect on arousal and orgasm
Multiple sclerosis	Hypoactive desire, hypoactive arousal, hypoactive orgasm
Cord lesions	
Low lesion	Hypoactive reflex arousal (psychogenic arousal and reflex ejaculation may be preserved)
High lesion	Hypoactive psychogenic arousal (reflex arousal and ejaculation may be preserved)
Radical pelvic surgery	Hypoactive arousal, hypoactive orgasm
Temporal lobe lesions	Hypoactive or increased desire
Vascular disease	
Large vessel (Leriche syndrome)	Hypoactive arousal
Small vessel (pelvic vascular insufficiency)	Hypoactive arousal

causal factors in her desire disorder. Discontinuation of her SSRI was a treatment option. However, because she was responding well to a recent serious episode of major depression, and neither she nor her psychiatrist wanted to risk a recurrence, we did not choose this option. We recommended a trial with a regimen of exogenous testosterone in the form of percutaneous topical gel (2%). After 4 weeks of treatment the patient reported a definite awakening of her libidinal drive, as well as increased feelings of energy and well-being. By the fifth week of treatment Mrs. W reported feeling "sexually restored."

In the case of Mrs. W, a biologic etiologic agent emerged as the fundamental cause of her desire disorder, a problem shared by many women during the perimenopausal and postmenopausal transition. Although not true in this instance, even when biologic problems are clearly central in the case, it is important to be aware that secondary relational (e.g., partner frustration) and/or intrapsychic (e.g., diminished self-concept) conflicts can serve as ancillary contributors to the problem. Tables 6.1 through 6.4 list medical conditions and medications that affect sexual response.

TABLE 6.2 Medical Conditions That Can Affect Sexual Response: Men Only

Organic Factor	Sexual Disorders
Dyspareunia (genital pain during intercourse)	Hypoactive desire, hypoactive arousal, and hypoactive orgasm
Disturbed penile anatomy (chordee, Peyronie disease, traumatic fracture, traumatic amputation)	
Penile skin infections	
Prostatic infections	
Testicular disease (orchitis, epididymitis, tumor, trauma)	
Urethral infections (gonorrhea, nonspecific urethral infections)	
Hypogonadal androgen-deficient states (Klinefelter syndrome, testicular agenesis, Kallmann syndrome, testicular tumors, orchitis, hyperprolactinemia, castration)	Hypoactive desire, hypoactive arousal, hypoactive orgasm
Mechanical problems (inguinal hernia, hydrocele)	Hypoactive arousal
Surgical procedures	
Abdominoperineal bowel resection	Hypoactive arousal
Lumbar sympathectomy	Hypoactive orgasm
Radical perineal prostatectomy	Hypoactive arousal

TABLE 6.3 Medical Conditions That Can Affect Sexual Response: Women Only

Organic Factor	*Sexual Disorders*
Complications of surgery Ovarian approximation to vagina Posthysterectomy scarring Shortened vagina Androgen Insufficiency Dyspareunia (painful intercourse) Agenesis of the vagina Clitoral phimosis Imperforate hymen, rigid hymen, tender hymenal tags Infections of external genitalia: herpes genitalis, labial cysts, furuncles, Bartholin cyst infections Infections of the vagina: herpes genitalis, *Candida albicans, Trichomonas* Injuries as a consequence of birth trauma: episiotomy scars, tears, uterine prolapse Irritations of the vagina: chemical dermatitis (douches), atrophic vaginitis, intercourse with insufficient lubrication Miscellaneous pelvis problems Cystitis, urethritis, urethral prolapse Endometriosis, ectopic pregnancy, pelvic inflammatory disease, ovarian cysts and tumors, pelvic tumors Intrauterine device complications	Hypoactive desire, hypoactive arousal, hypoactive orgasm, and vaginismus may occur with any of the organic factors listed at the left

TABLE 6.4 Common Drugs and Substances That Can Affect Sexual Response[a]

Drug(s)	*Sexual Disorders Reported*
Alcohol and sedatives (high dose)	Hypoactive desire, hypoactive arousal, delayed orgasm
Amiodarone	Hypoactive desire
Androgens	Increased desire (women)
Anticonvulsants	
Carbamazepine	Hypoactive arousal
Phenytoin	Hypoactive desire, hypoactive arousal
Antidepressants	Hypoactive desire, arousal, orgasm
Selective serotonin reuptake inhibitors	Hypoactive desire, hypoactive orgasm
Tricyclics	Hypoactive or increased desire and/or hypoactive arousal
Antihypertensives	
Centrally acting (beta blockers, clonidine, guanabenz, methyldopa, reserpine)	Hypoactive desire, hypoactive arousal, (?) hypoactive orgasm
Beta blockers, hydralazine	Hypoactive arousal
Peripherally acting (guanethidine, guanadrel)	Retrograde ejaculation, hypoactive desire
Antipsychotics	Hypoactive or increased desire, hypoactive arousal, retrograde ejaculation (Mellaril)
Digoxin	Hypoactive desire, hypoactive arousal
Disopyramide	Hypoactive arousal
Disulfiram	Hypoactive arousal, delayed ejaculation
Diuretics	Hypoactive arousal
Estrogens, progesterone	
Men	Hypoactive desire, hypoactive arousal, hypoactive orgasm
Women	Hypoactive desire
H_2 blockers (cimetidine, famotidine, ranitidine)	Hypoactive desire, hypoactive arousal
L-Dopa	Increased desire (elderly men)
Lithium	Hypoactive desire, hypoactive arousal
Marijuana (high dose)	Hypoactive arousal (low dose may produce increased desire in men)
Metoclopramide	Hypoactive desire, hypoactive arousal
Narcotics	Hypoactive desire, hypoactive arousal, hypoactive orgasm
Stimulants, high dose (cocaine, amphetamines)	Hypoactive desire, hypoactive arousal, hypoactive orgasm (low dose may produce increased desire)
Verapamil	Hypoactive arousal

[a] See also Crenshaw TL, Goldberg JP. Sexual pharmacology: drugs that affect sexual function. New York: WW Norton, 1996.

TABLE 6.5 Prevalence Ranges of Sexual Dysfunctions among Women and Men

Sexual Dysfunction	Prevalence	Source (Ref. No.)
Women		
Hypoactive sexual desire disorder	33% last 12 mo	U.S. random sample, 1994 (6)
Female sexual arousal disorder	19% last 12 mo	U.S. random sample, 1994 (6)
Female orgasmic disorder	24% last 12 mo	U.S. random sample, 1994 (6)
Dyspareunia	14% last 12 mo	U.S. random sample, 1994 (6)
Vaginismus	0.5%–1% last 12 mo	Two large population samples in Europe, 1998 (4), 1999 (5)
Men		
Hypoactive sexual desire disorder	16% last 12 mo	U.S. random sample, 1994 (6)
Male sexual arousal disorder (erectile disorder)	Current: 16%	Multinational (8 countries), 2004
		8% in age group 20–29 y to 37% in age group 70–75 y; community samples
	10% last 12 mo	U.S. random sample, 1994 (6);
	Current: minimal, 17%; moderate, 25%; complete, 10%	Older (range, age 40–70 y; median, 54 y) community samples, 1994 (7)
Premature ejaculation	29% last 12 mo	U.S. random sample, 1994 (6)
Male orgasmic disorder	8% last 12 mo	U.S. random sample, 1994 (6)
Dyspareunia	4% last 6 mo	Medical clinic sample, 1998 (8)

General Characteristics

Frequency

The data in Table 6.5 suggests that the prevalence of sexual disorders in the general population of the United States is substantial, and swells to even more dramatic proportions in clinical and aging populations. This being the case, screening for such conditions deserves the attention of the primary care physician. The table describes the prevalence of sexual dysfunction in surveys conducted in the United States as well other countries. Queries address the prevalence of *problems* analogous to the sexual dysfunctions discussed in this chapter, and use time frames of either *currently,* or *within the past 12 months or less*. The primary source for these data is the National Health and Social Life Survey (NHSLS) conducted with a randomly selected and stratified sample of 18- to 59-year-old participants in 1992 (6).

Age at Onset of Common Sexual Disorders

Psychological and behavioral antecedents of sexual disorders can sometimes be found in both adolescent and childhood sexual experiences and fantasies; however, a common age at onset is early adulthood. Menopause is also a peak time of onset for women's sexual dysfunctions, often as a result of dramatic changes in endocrine levels associated with this life epoch. There is also a well-defined relationship between aging and the prevalence of erectile disorder (ED) in men. Nowhere is this more clearly demonstrated than the Massachusetts Male Aging Study (7), which shows an increase in prevalence of ED from 8% among 40-year-old men to 40% among men age 69 years. Onset can basically occur at any time during adult life, particularly for dysfunctions associated with medical conditions or use of drugs or other substances, and for those dysfunctions that are situational or transient.

Predisposing Personality Factors

In general, effective and satisfying sexual function is usually considered to be associated with a healthy and adaptive personality development. Consequently, defects in personality structure accompanied by maladaptive personality traits (see Chapter 23) or psychopathology can certainly affect sexual function. However, such additional psychiatric problems are neither necessary nor sufficient conditions for the development of sexual problems. A study done in our clinic involving 288 patients, who were referred to us because of a diagnosis of a sexual dysfunction, revealed that only 30% of the sample fulfilled criteria for an additional psychiatric disorder (8) beyond the sexual dysfunction.

Course and Severity

The course of sexual dysfunctions varies. Dysfunctions may develop after a period of normal functioning or they may be lifelong. They may be generalized, occurring with all partners and in all contexts, or situational, limited to specific partners or contexts. There are differing degrees of impairment, from partial or intermittent to total and unremitting. Usually, early age at onset and total functional compromise indicate chronicity and predict a poorer treatment outcome. Conversely, a history of prior adequate sexual function, situational symptoms, and partial impairment are predictive of a more limited course for the disorder and a higher probability of a favorable treatment outcome.

Related Problems

Fundamentally, the major complications of sexual dysfunctions are disrupted marital or sexual relationships. In addition, presence of the dysfunction, particularly one of an unremitting nature, may give rise to a variety of negative emotions such as depression, anxiety, guilt, shame, frustration, and anger. These affect states not only affect the patient but also may intrude into many of the patient's broader life relationships. Most sexual dysfunctions of a substantial nature or duration also have a disparaging effect on the individual's self-concept, as they serve to undermine the individual's feelings of psychological integration and well-being.

General Approach to the Patient

Most patients do not feel comfortable initiating discussion with their primary care provider about their sexual activities and any sexual problems they may be having. For this reason it is very important to inquire about sexual function as a systematic part of the primary care workup of each patient. Table 6.6 outlines interviewing approaches that may be useful in this inquiry. One should not presume exclusive heterosexuality in a new patient but should ask questions that are gender neutral until orientation has been established. In patients who name a problem, the history of the present problem may be imprecise. Therefore, sufficient time should be set aside with the patient to obtain a clear account of the difficulty. For patients whose difficulties involve a partner or a spouse, it is important to have the partner's view of the problem. Sometimes the more-functional partner will seek help to gain support for bringing the less-functional partner into the evaluation.

The evaluation should be organized to obtain information about the onset and duration of the problem; about factors that make the problem better or worse; about concurrent events such as birth of children, changes in relationships or vocation, or onset of physical or emotional illness; and about use of new medications. Also, it is always important to elicit from patients their ideas about the cause of sexual problems and their expectations of treatment.

If it is determined that a referral to a specialist in sexual medicine is appropriate, the clinician should advise the patient to consult with his or her health insurance program to ascertain whether such treatment of sexual dysfunction or disorders is a covered benefit. Most plans do not cover marital therapy, and many exclude sexual therapy

TABLE 6.6 Suggested Questions Regarding Sexual Practices and Problems

Suggested Opening (Legitimizing Statement)
"Something that I ask each of my patients about is their sexual activity. Is that all right with you?"

Suggested Initial Question
(Open-ended question) "So, how are things going sexually?"
(Closed, somewhat leading question) "Have you noticed any problems in your ability to have and enjoy sexual relations?"
or
(Closed but facilitative question) "Do you have any problems or questions related to your current sexual activities?"

Screening Questions for Sexual Dysfunction (Ask for Clarification of Any Positive Response)
(Both sexes) "Have you noticed any loss of interest in having sex?"
(Men) "Any problems having an erection?"
(Women) "Any problems with becoming aroused, that is, getting sexually excited or 'turned on'?"
(Both sexes) "Any problems having an orgasm?"
(Both sexes) "Any pain during intercourse?"

Screening Questions Regarding Sexual Orientation
(Both sexes) "Have you ever had sex with men, women, or both?"
or
(Men) "Do you ever have sex with another man?"
(Women) "Do you ever have sex with another woman?"

Screening Questions for Risk of or History of Sexually Transmitted Disease[a]
(Both sexes) "In the past few years, about how many partners have you had for sexual relations?"
(Both sexes) "Have you ever had any kind of infection that you got from having sex?"

Open Question to Obtain Additional Information
"Is there any other information or any other questions about your sexual activities that you would like to discuss with me?"

[a]See information on safe and unsafe sexual practices and instructions for use of a condom in Chapter 39.

(especially nonmedical) as a covered benefit. Diagnostic medical procedures, including laboratory assays, are typically covered, however.

Female Sexual Disorders

Hypoactive Sexual Desire Disorder

Hypoactive sexual desire disorder (HSDD) is defined as, "the persistent or recurrent deficiency (or absence) of sexual fantasies, thoughts and desire for [or receptivity to] sexual activity." The judgment of deficiency or absence is made by the clinician, taking into account factors that affect sexual functioning, such as age, sex, and the context of the person's life. The disturbance causes the patient marked distress or interpersonal difficulty, and it does not occur exclusively during the course of another axis I disorder nor is it caused exclusively by the direct physiologic effects of a substance (e.g., drugs of abuse, medication) or a general medical condition.

Assessment

A multitude of factors can be involved in the loss or reduction of sexual desire in a woman. Age, menopausal status, psychiatric status, and quality of relationship should all be established as potentially important parameters in an attempt to understand the patient's condition. The presence of medical disorders, surgical interventions, specific pharmacologic therapies, or any substances of abuse should also be established and evaluated for etiologic potential.

In terms of prevalence, HSDD is the most prevalent of the female sexual dysfunctions (6). Among postmenopausal women, the condition is even more prevalent. Although many experts believe loss of desire peri- and postmenopause is related to the marked reduction in circulating androgens associated with this stage of life, a definitive causal relationship has not yet been established. HSDD will almost certainly be the most frequent sexual complaint that primary care providers will see, with perhaps 35% to 40% of postmenopausal women experiencing a clinically meaningful loss in levels of sexual desire.

As just discussed, although desire disorders are the most prevalent female sexual dysfunctions, with numerous possible origins, the clinician must take care to ensure that the complaint of low desire is a *primary* condition. At times, complaints of low desire are actually *secondary* results of cumulative frustration and loss of sexual interest because of repeated failures to become aroused, or to achieve orgasm. Facility with language can also play a role in these instances, in that many women are not familiar with, or do not fully understand, the term *sexual arousal* and as a result will use the phrase "loss of sexual interest" to communicate the global sexual experience as opposed to a specific symptomatic manifestation, that is, problems with sexual arousal.

Treatment of Hypoactive Sexual Desire

In deciding on a plan of treatment, the clinician must first establish what he or she believes is the primary etiologic agent, recognizing that there may be multiple causal factors in HSDD. Addressing the biogenic axis first, the presence of numerous diseases, surgical interventions, or medical conditions needs to be evaluated for a potential causal role (Tables 6.1 and 6.3). If a drug (Table 6.4) is suspected of interfering with sexual desire, several questions should be addressed. Is it possible to put the patient on a drug "holiday" for several weeks as a diagnostic challenge? If not, will an adjustment in dose be sufficient to effect a therapeutic change? Can a different pharmacologic agent be substituted for the drug of concern to see if any changes ensue? Finally, in some instances the addition of a known prosexual agent (e.g., adding bupropion hydrochloride [Wellbutrin] to an SSRI antidepressant regimen) can counteract the effects of the problem drug sufficiently to restore functioning. In a related vein, if loss of sexual drive is secondary to alcohol or substance abuse, treatment should be aimed at controlling the abuse (see Chapters 28 and 29).

Turning to the psychogenic and relational aspects of HSDD, transient hypoactive sexual desire disorders that are a consequence of *psychological factors,* such as stress or anger, or interpersonal problems can usually be managed effectively with short-term counseling. This assumes, however, that normal levels of sexual desire were present prior to the problem. If problems with sexual desire are long-term or lifetime in nature, then resolution of the problem is apt to be more complex and prolonged. When alcoholism, depression, or another psychosocial disorder is the primary problem, specific treatment for that disorder should accompany the counseling. Many cases of depression, even those that do not appear to be of a profound nature, can have a negative impact on sexuality. The design of a counseling program should include an agreement between the patient or couple and the clinician to meet for a specified number of sessions (usually two to five) for approximately 30 minutes per session.

Pharmacologic Treatments for HSDD

There are currently no drugs specifically approved by the U.S. Food and Drug Administration (FDA) for the treatment of the female sexual dysfunctions, including HSDD. In spite of this fact, off-label treatment of HSDD has been ongoing for about 40 years. Principal among the agents employed for this purpose are various androgens, principally testosterone, administered through a variety of modalities. Testosterone can be administered orally (in methyltestosterone and undecanoate preparations), intramuscularly, subcutaneously, via transdermal patch, and in a variety of gel applications. Of these, the only FDA-approved application is Estratest, a combination of methyltestosterone (MT) and esterified estrogen (EE), which is available in several doses. Estratest is officially approved for the treatment of moderate to severe vasomotor symptoms associated with menopause, and has been successfully used with both surgically and naturally menopausal women. Another regimen that has become popular is the use of testosterone 2% percutaneous gel, which is applied to the tissues of the vulva for 2 weeks and subsequently applied to the inner thigh. Response times to these courses of therapy are variable, but it is not uncommon to take 4 to 5 weeks of application before a restoration of desire is experienced. Adverse effects tend to be minimal in the large majority of patients, consisting primarily of minor androgenic skin effects, such as acne and hirsutism.

Although testosterone remains unapproved by the FDA for the treatment of sexual desire disorders, a recent review of a large number of clinical trials concluded it has clearly demonstrated efficacy in restoring libido and the capacity for sexual arousal and sexual satisfaction, with few safety concerns (9). Two recent, large, randomized clinical trials, one with surgically menopausal and the second with naturally menopausal women, both reported obvious efficacy and minimal adverse events (10,11).

Although there is a dearth of FDA-approved pharmacologic agents available to treat female desire disorders, there is no scarcity of investigational agents under development, most of them in Phase II or Phase III clinical trials. The transdermal testosterone patch Intrinsa and the testosterone gel application Tostrelle are both well along in development, as are a number of nonhormonal agents. The dopamine agonist apomorphine is under development as a treatment for HSDD in men and women, using both sublingual and inhaler delivery systems, and an inhaled form of the melanocortin-stimulating hormone PT-141 is in Phase II trials. Also, several sponsors are about to move into Phase III trials with drugs that can be best characterized as "atypical" antidepressants that have shown prosexual effects on libido. In addition, it is worth noting that several drugs not accurately labeled as "investigational" are also being studied for their therapeutic potential in this area. The atypical antidepressant bupropion (Wellbutrin) has shown consistent evidence of having a modest therapeutic influence on sexual desire (12,13), and the HRT drug tibolone (Livial), a synthetic steroid with androgenic as well as estrogenic and progestogenic properties, is also in U.S. trials, with a focus on postmenopausal women with HSDD (14). How soon any of these drugs will become approved by the FDA for this indication depends on numerous scientific, regulatory, and commercial factors; however, the fact that the level of activity in this area has grown almost geometrically in the past decade suggests that it will be sooner rather than later.

Female Sexual Arousal Disorders

Diagnostic Classification

Female sexual arousal disorder (FSAD) is defined as the absence or markedly diminished feelings of sexual arousal (i.e., sexual excitement or sexual pleasure) from any type of sexual stimulation. In addition, there may also be present a persistent or recurrent inability to attain, or to maintain until completion of sexual activity, an adequate vaginal lubrication–swelling response of sexual excitement. The disturbance causes marked distress or interpersonal difficulty, and is not better accounted for by another axis I disorder (except another sexual dysfunction) or caused by the direct physiologic effects of a substance (e.g., drugs of abuse, a medication) or a general medical condition.

Assessment

Problems with sexual arousal are common in women and may actually be at the root of many other sexual dysfunctions. As an example, orgasmic dysfunction is frequently secondary to difficulty with arousal, and if arousal disorder becomes chronic, it can lead to a loss of interest in sexual activities. Coitus with insufficient arousal can also play a role in the etiology of a variety of pain syndromes, in some instances because of a lack of vaginal lubrication and in others because of a failure of the "tenting" response of the distal vagina during intercourse.

The traditional focus in arousal disorder has been on genital changes in the arousal process in women as a corollary of the erection process in men. Recently, there has been a recognition that arousal in women is much more complex. Because women's genital changes are less obvious than men's, women can be completely unaware of them. They may attend far more to other somatic changes, such as heart rate, muscle tension, or breast sensations, or to their own subjective state of arousal (5).

Several research methodologies that reflect changes in blood flow in the vaginal walls or labia are used to study women's genital reactions to sexually arousing stimuli. Studies consistently find a lack of correlation between women's feelings of subjective arousal and the genital changes associated with arousal. For instance, women frequently react to a sexual stimulus with changes in genital blood flow, but they may be unaware of the changes, often do not feel aroused subjectively, and in fact may feel negatively about the stimulus (15).

Inability to attain and maintain levels of arousal that permit a smooth and trouble-free progression from the beginning of a sexual experience to its completion can be caused by both external and internal psychological events that may interfere with the patient's ability to focus on the physical and psychological stimuli that maintain sexual arousal. A vivid example of an external event is the ringing of a telephone during the sexual experience. An internal psychological event might be a recurring thought about how long one's partner may be able to sustain his erection. Often patients complaining of arousal disorders will report that they have great difficulty staying focused on the sexual experience and staying in the moment. For these women a combination of factors acts to render them easily distractible and unable to concentrate on the pleasure inherent in the sexual experience. The history and assessment should be structured to uncover the presence of external events and the specific content of psychological events when present. A common finding is a persistent preoccupation and anxiety about the patient or partner performing successfully. This problem may be primary, or it may occur as a secondary response to the frustration associated with organic dysfunction. When partner dysfunction is an issue, worry about a successful partner performance can become increasingly absorbing during the course of the sexual experience, so that the concern crowds out the patient's capacity to focus on the sexual stimuli that maintain the arousal response. When such patients realize arousal is diminishing, they try all the harder, shutting off completely their ability to respond to sexual stimuli. This process is called *spectatoring*, a term coined by William Masters and Virginia Johnson (16). The term describes a process whereby patients, through observation of their performance, psychologically take themselves out of the experience. The mental process is guaranteed to result in loss of sexual arousal. Typically it may begin after one or two failed experiences secondary to external events or stresses. Once the process begins, it becomes internally reinforcing, leading to further worry and further failure. When this process is suspected, the history should focus on the patient's mental experiences during sexual intercourse.

Other common causes of psychologically inhibited sexual arousal are *stressful life situations*. Patients who have recently lost a job, lost a relative, are concerned about retirement, or have developed an illness, may be unable to clear their minds of their worries during a sexual experience and therefore cannot respond. Similarly, negative emotions, feelings of anger or resentment directed toward the sexual partner can interfere with the ability to become sexually aroused. All women have difficulties becoming sexually aroused at some times in their lives; it is the persistent and chronic nature of poor arousal that is the hallmark of FSAD.

Treatments for Female Sexual Arousal Disorder

Psychological Treatments for FSAD

The strategy for management of sexual arousal disorders with psychological or relational etiologies is the same in both sexes and depends on whether the patient has had the dysfunction for a sustained period or whether the dysfunction has appeared recently and there is a history of competent sexual functioning. As discussed earlier, transient inhibition of sexual excitement is often secondary to stressful life situations or marital discord. These clinical situations often respond to brief counseling. The role of the therapist is to help the couple recognize the effect of the stress on their relationship as well as the effect of their feelings (often anger) on their ability to relate sexually. Encouragement of collaborative contingency planning for resolving problems reduces anxiety and anger, often helping the couple to return to their baseline level of sexual function. The same principles and steps are applicable to an individual patient.

When spectatoring is a major factor and does not remit after open discussion, referral to a professional skilled in sex therapy usually brings excellent results. Sensate focus therapy, first developed by Masters and Johnson, combines cognitive and behavioral techniques to replace spectatoring with appropriate sexual focus and behavior.

The following factors favor a *good prognosis* after treatment for psychogenic arousal disorder: history of adequate prior sexual functioning, acute instead of insidious onset, short duration of sexual impairment, stable social situation, high motivation for treatment, presence of sexual desire, partner willing to participate in treatment, absence of severe marital conflicts, and absence of significant concurrent psychopathology.

Even in patients for whom excellent function can be expected to return, sexual arousal may be impaired by worry and hesitation. This is especially true when impaired arousal has been present for more than a few weeks, which is often the case. Such patients may be invited to discuss this situation freely and given permission and encouragement to experiment with their partner in one or more ways (e.g., masturbation, erotic pictures or movies, new techniques) in order to test or promote their sexual functions. Of course, such advice should be consistent with the patient's personal beliefs.

Patients who have experienced a sexual arousal disorder over a long period, or who have never functioned competently (lifetime), may be given a trial of short-term counseling (see Chapter 20). If the counseling does not result in reasonable improvement, referral for more expert help should be considered.

Oral Pharmacologic Treatments for FSAD

Fresh with the flush of success accompanying the introduction of the phosphodiesterase type 5 (PDE 5) inhibitors (e.g., sildenafil) for the treatment of arousal disorders (erectile dysfunction) in men, pharmaceutical sponsors were encouraged to investigate the same drugs for the treatment of arousal disorder in women. Unfortunately, several large, controlled, clinical trials did not demonstrate an equivalent consistent efficacy in treating FSAD. As a result, the programs in this area (e.g., the female Viagra program) were discontinued. It is now clear that a significant reason for this failure was that the definitions of FSAD used in the inclusion criteria for clinical trials were too broad, and many patients were entered into the trials with arousal *symptoms* but not true arousal *disorder*. In these patients, many of whom were probably suffering from hormonal insufficiencies as a primary etiology, there would be no reason to expect that a PDE 5 inhibitor alone would be effective. In spite of these negative results, there is evidence that the PDE 5 inhibitors work in FSAD (17). It appears important, however, that the presentation be relatively uncomplicated, with explicit appreciation of genital symptoms and an absence of comorbid symptoms of desire disorder (18). In addition, there is also some evidence indicative of efficacy in arousal disorders for tibolone, the synthetic steroid (19).

Other Somatic Treatments for FSAD

The somatic treatment of biogenic arousal disorder in women follows the threefold goals of stabilizing disease process, reversing any medication side effects, and improving the genital environment. Any form of estrogen therapy will benefit atrophic vaginal tissue, but local applications (creams or a vaginal ring) are particularly effective. Women receiving estrogen-replacement therapy may also benefit from the addition of vaginal estrogen, especially in the early menopausal years. Estrogen improves lubrication, makes the vaginal epithelium thicker, and may improve vaginal sensitivity. Absorption from the vaginal mucosa is good, so if the uterus is intact a progestin must be used either continuously or cyclically to protect the endometrium.

There are some concerns that hysterectomy may affect sexual functioning. However, such concerns remain unsubstantiated. Clinical investigations have suggested that hysterectomy often produces no change in sexual function for the majority of women or in some cases may even enhance sexual functioning (20). Nonetheless, theoretical concerns that radical extirpative pelvic surgery in women may compromise the nerve supply involved in optimal sexual functioning have led to the development of techniques to preserve genital innervation.

In April 2000, the FDA approved an innovative device for the treatment of arousal problems in women known as Eros-CTD (Urometrics, St. Paul, MN). This is a battery-operated suction device that applies suction to the clitoris and improves sensation, lubrication, and orgasmic capacity. The erectile tissue of the clitoris was recently found to be more extensive than previously described in anatomy texts, through research by an Australian team who performed a series of cadaver dissections on women of various ages (21).

Female Orgasmic Disorder

In the NHSLS, 74% of women in the 18- to 29-year-old age group reported being *usually* orgasmic during sex, as opposed to 78% of women in the 40- to 49-year-old age group. The study also found that only 29% of women overall reported *always* having an orgasm during sex, and that 40% of women reported feeling extremely physically pleased, with 39% reporting feeling extremely emotionally satisfied (6).

Diagnostic Classification

Orgasm disorders caused by medical conditions or medications should be diagnosed as symptoms associated with the responsible conditions or medications (Tables 6.1, 6.3, and 6.4).

Female orgasmic disorder (FOD) is defined as a persistent or recurrent delay in or absence of orgasm following a normal sexual arousal phase, and an adequate course of sexual stimulation. Women exhibit wide variability in the type and intensity of stimulation that triggers orgasm. The diagnosis of female orgasmic disorder should be based on the clinician's judgment that the woman's orgasmic capacity is less than would be reasonable for her age, her sexual experience, and the adequacy of sexual stimulation she receives In addition, the disturbance must cause marked distress or interpersonal difficulty for the patient, and not be better accounted for by another axis I disorder (except another sexual dysfunction) and is not caused exclusively by the direct physiologic effects of a substance (e.g., a drug of abuse, a medication) or a general medical condition.

Organic conditions that affect orgasm comprise for the most part hormonal deficiencies, neurologic disorders, drugs that affect the autonomic system, and surgical or traumatic interruptions of the involved neural pathways (Tables 6.1, 6.3, and 6.4). History taking and physical examination should focus on these possibilities. In women, diabetic autonomic neuropathy is one of the most common organic causes of orgasm disorders, although certainly other neurologic diseases have sexual effects (22).

Psychologically caused orgasmic disorder is a common problem in women. Studies estimate that up to 25% of the female population has orgasm problems, and 30% to 50% of all women are sometimes anorgasmic with intercourse. Assessment should focus on the duration of the problem, a history of sexual functioning, the status of the relationship with the spouse or partner, and the presence of a stressful situation. A history of recent onset, competent past functioning, and identifiable precipitating stresses predicts a good response to treatment. Patients who have been anorgasmic for many years and are seeking help because of a change in their relationship or life situations are more difficult to treat.

Some women complain of anorgasmia, but evaluation reveals that the patient is actually experiencing a sexual arousal disorder. Because treatment may differ for these disorders, clarification of the phase in which the dysfunction is operating may be important.

Treatment for Female Orgasm Disorders

As with biogenic arousal disorder, the somatic treatment of biogenic orgasmic disorder in women follows a similar strategy. In patients with known neuronal damage, including diabetic neuropathy, the goal of therapy should be to help the patient adjust to the permanent loss or decrease of sexual responsiveness. This can be done by helping the patient value the role of sensual pleasuring, as distinct from sexual pleasuring that has as its single goal intercourse and orgasm.

Transient forms of anorgasmia caused by psychogenic factors are amenable to treatment with counseling. A history of previous orgasmic response is a good prognostic indicator. The block in orgasmic response is often caused by the process of spectatoring. The interfering process is usually secondary to stressful life situations or marital discord. Counseling for married women and others who have a regular sexual partner should include the partner, provided that this is agreeable to the patient. Counseling should be aimed primarily at resolving the dominant problems, which are usually life stresses or interpersonal strife. With the single patient, counseling should be directed at helping the patient suppress or remove the psychological events (i.e., spectatoring) that are occurring at a critical time, when the patient has reached a high plateau level of excitement and is prepared for orgasmic release. The interfering psychological events may be removed by having the patient focus to the best of her ability on the physical stimuli that she is experiencing during the excitement phase.

Women with anorgasmia of long duration can be given a trial of counseling. If counseling does not result in substantial improvement, referral for additional evaluation and treatment should be made.

Directed Masturbation

Orgasmic difficulty in women can be regarded as a skill deficit, and books are available that give women instructions on how to have an orgasm by using masturbation or a vibrator, and then to "bridge" this ability to coitus with a partner. This method is described well in two commonly used books, which can be recommended to patients (23,24). Success rates reported with this method are high; in one study, 95% of patients were able to achieve orgasm through masturbation, 85% with the direct stimulation of a sexual partner, and 40% with penile–vaginal intercourse (25).

Antidepressant-Related Side Effects

Sexual dysfunction caused by treatment with a SSRI antidepressant is a frequent complaint. Decreased libido and orgasmic dysfunction are the most common problems, but arousal difficulties are also reported. The incidence ranges from approximately 35% to 75% of patients treated. SSRIs probably impair sexual function because of a blockade of the 5-hydroxytryptamine 2 (5-HT_2) receptor, which is believed to inhibit dopaminergic function in the areas of the brain that are involved with sexual function. Peripheral mechanisms have also been postulated, such as effects on cholinergic receptors or on nitric oxide (26).

The common strategies for dealing with antidepressant-related sexual dysfunction were evaluated in a review article by Zajecka (27). Gradual reduction of the dose of the SSRI may be helpful, but the patient must be observed closely for the re-emergence of depressive symptoms. Some clinicians wait for tolerance to develop, but only 19% of patients reported any improvement over 4 to 6 months (26). Skipping doses of the antidepressant for 48 hours was helpful in improving sexual function for 50% of patients on the shorter-acting SSRIs, such as sertraline or paroxetine (28). Patients at risk for noncompliance should not be encouraged to try this strategy. Many agents have been used as antidotes for sexual dysfunction, but little well-controlled research has been done, and most recommendations are based on case reports or observational studies (Table 6.7). One placebo-controlled trial found that 59% of patients receiving buspirone augmentation had improved sexual function, as opposed to 30% of patients receiving placebo. Another strategy is to switch the patient to an antidepressant that does not block reuptake at the 5-HT_2 receptor, such as nefazodone, buproprion, or perhaps escitalopram (29).

Antidepressant-related sexual dysfunction is frequently a difficult problem and can lead to early discontinuation of antidepressant therapy. Because there are potential problems associated with all of the strategies mentioned, the best approach may be to choose an antidepressant that is less likely to cause sexual dysfunction in patients for whom this is an important concern (see Chapter 24). It is critical, when initiating antidepressant therapy, to assess baseline sexual functioning and to consider the potential impact of sexual dysfunction on that patient's recovery. If the patient is warned about the possibility of sexual dysfunction when started on an SSRI, it may be easier for the patient to bring it up if it does occur.

Female Sexual Pain Disorders

Diagnostic Classification

Dyspareunia. Dyspareunia is defined as recurrent or persistent genital pain associated with sexual intercourse in either a male or a female. The disturbance causes marked distress or interpersonal difficulty for the individual, and is not caused exclusively by vaginismus or lack of lubrication, is not better accounted for by another axis I disorder (except another sexual dysfunction), and is not caused exclusively by the direct physiologic effects of a substance (e.g., a drug of abuse, a medication) or a general medical condition.

Vaginismus. Is defined as a recurrent or persistent involuntary spasm of the musculature of the outer third of

TABLE 6.7 Antidotes for Selective Serotonin-Reuptake Inhibitor-Related Sexual Dysfunction

Drug	Trade Name	Usual Dose	Available Strengths	Comments
Cyproheptadine	Periactin	4–12 mg q.h.s.	4 mg	Sedating antihistamine
Amantadine	Symmetrel	100 mg b.i.d.	100 mg	Dopaminergic; caution with patients with psychosis
Methylphenidate	Ritalin	5–40 mg/d	5, 10, 20, 20 SR	May also be used p.r.n.; abuse potential
Bethanechol	Urecholine	10–50 mg p.r.n.	5, 10, 25, 50 mg	Cholinergic
Granisetron	Kytril	1 mg p.r.n.	1 mg	5-HT_3 antagonist
Yohimbine	Yocon	5.4 mg t.i.d.	5.4 mg	Can be anxiogenic; α_2-adrenergic antagonist
	Yohimex			
Sildenafil	Viagra	25–100 mg p.r.n. 0.5–4 h before intercourse	25, 50, 100 mg	Contraindicated with nitrates
Ginkgo biloba	No FDA-approved products	40–80 mg t.i.d.	Active ingredient varies with brand	Can increase clotting time, flatulence
Buspirone	BuSpar	7.5–30 mg b.i.d.	5, 10, 15, 30 mg	May potentiate antidepressant efficacy
Bupropion	Wellbutrin	75–150 mg q.d. or b.i.d.	75, 100 mg IR; 100, 150 mg SR	May potentiate antidepressant efficacy
Nefazodone	Serzone	50–100 mg/d	50, 100, 150, 200, 250 mg	Blocks 5-HT_2 postsynaptic receptor
Mirtazapine	Remeron	15–45 mg/d	15, 30, 45 mg	Blocks 5-HT_2 postsynaptic receptor

IR, immediate release; SR, sustained release.

the vagina that interferes with sexual intercourse. The disturbance causes marked distress or interpersonal difficulty for the individual, is not better accounted for by another axis I disorder (e.g., somatization disorder), and is not caused exclusively by the direct effects of a general medical condition.

Assessment and Treatment

In both sexes, the complaint of discomfort or pain during intercourse requires a careful history, physical examination, and laboratory testing. The most common causes are infections or atrophic vaginitis in women, and urethral or prostatic infection in men. As is true of the dysfunctions discussed previously, it is probably counterproductive to consider dyspareunia as either psychogenic or physical, because it is now recognized that nearly all cases have elements of both physical and psychological causes. Genital pain disorders are different from pain disorders elsewhere in the body only because the activity affected is frequently more emotionally charged than other activities. In fact, the term *sexual pain disorder* has been criticized by some because it focuses on the activity affected by the pain rather than on the anatomical location of the pain, or on the pain itself (30). This may have contributed to the long-held assumptions of many that painful sex was largely a psychological problem, an assumption that has undoubtedly contributed to the fact that only recently have these disorders begun to be rigorously studied. On the other hand, because sexual difficulties have an impact on one's self-esteem and relationships with partners, most patients with sexual pain disorders can benefit from counseling with an experienced mental health provider. This suggestion is sometimes met with resistance from the patient, but should be persistently encouraged by the provider.

Dyspareunia. Pain with vaginal intercourse is characterized as introital (or insertional), vaginal, or deep (pelvic pain with penile thrusting). Deep dyspareunia can be caused by almost any type of pelvic pathology and is addressed in Chapter 102. Dyspareunia can also be caused by insufficient arousal. With adequate arousal, there is engorgement of clitoral erectile tissue surrounding the anterior distal vagina, vaginal lubrication, ballooning of the vaginal apex, and uterine elevation. These changes all facilitate pain-free penetration. Women frequently recognize the lack of lubrication with insufficient arousal and may use a lubricant, but are unaware of the vaginal changes that accompany arousal. It is important, when discussing the use of a vaginal lubricant, to caution women and their partners not to abbreviate the arousal phase, because lubrication often is not enough to prevent pain with penetration. The experience of pain can then lead to the expectation of pain, which causes muscle tension and less arousal, creating a painful cycle.

Introital dyspareunia is quite common. A recent population-based survey found that 16% of female respondents reported histories of chronic burning, knifelike pain, or pain on contact that lasted for at least 3 months or longer, and nearly 7% were experiencing the problem at the time of the survey (31).

When a patient complains of introital dyspareunia, a careful examination, including wet preparation and pH (see Chapter 102), should be done to look for vaginal infections or dermatologic conditions. A vulvar biopsy is often required to assess skin changes, and fungal cultures should be sent on any patient without an obvious cause for vulvar burning or pruritus because the vaginal wet preparation is only approximately 50% sensitive for the diagnosis of a candidal infection (32). The vulva is typically also examined with the cotton swab test in which a moistened cotton swab is touched lightly to points around the vulvar vestibule and then to other areas on the vulva and perineum. The patient is asked to rate her pain on a scale of 0 (no pain) to 10 (severe pain). A diagram and a pain map can be used to document and track the pain.

The importance of evaluating the pelvic floor muscles in any patient with dyspareunia cannot be overstated. Muscular hypertonicity and trigger points are frequently contributing factors. A physical therapist with specialized training in pelvic floor treatments is a vital part of the treatment for many types of dyspareunia.

Women with dyspareunia are often unknowingly participating in behaviors that may cause or exacerbate their pain. A study of 503 women with "benign vulvar disease" found that 69% remained sexually active in spite of arousal failure and unlubricated and painful intercourse. The reasons given were timidity, unassertiveness, feeling guilty if they refused, and habitual passive compliance. Sixty-eight percent of patients participated in "potentially harmful hygiene or self-treatment" (33). Soaps and over-the-counter vaginal treatments are frequent causes of irritant or allergic reactions. A careful history is necessary to discover any possible contributing factors. Soaps with perfume or antibacterial components should be eliminated (sometimes even for the partner), fabric softener sheets should not be used in the dryer, douching should be stopped, and products applied to the vulva should be carefully reviewed for the potential to cause a reaction.

A frequent cause of dyspareunia in perimenopausal, menopausal, and in postpartum or lactating women is *atrophic vaginitis*. This can usually be treated quite easily with topical low-dose estrogen, and is covered more fully in Chapter 102.

Vulvodynia. Vulvar burning, irritation, soreness, rawness, or stinging in the absence of objective clinical and microbiologic abnormalities that has been present for 3 months or more can be diagnosed as vulvodynia. Other terms that have been used for this disorder are vestibular adenitis, vulvar vestibulitis, and vestibulodynia. Friedrich first described and defined this condition in 1987 (34), but it is, unfortunately, still unrecognized by many providers. In Harlow's 2003 population-based survey, 60% of patients saw three or more physicians for this condition, many of whom could not provide a diagnosis (31). These patients may also present to mental health providers after being told that there is "nothing wrong" physically. This condition is now understood as a form of neuropathic pain and is described more fully in Chapter 102.

Vaginismus. Vaginismus and vulvodynia are frequently comorbid, and can be difficult to distinguish from each other. The diagnosis of vaginismus is typically made with a pelvic exam, by palpating a spasm or by an involuntary muscle contraction in the distal vagina. The salient characteristic of vaginismus has been described as a muscle spasm or involuntary contraction, but some recent studies have found that electromyelogram (EMG) measurements in vaginistic women do not differ from vulvodynia patients or from normal controls. Other studies have found more hypertonicity and muscle spasms in women with vaginismus than in other women. Patients with vaginismus often have hyperesthesia at the introitus, or in the distal vagina, as well as in the hypertonic muscles. To complicate the diagnosis further, vaginismus may be situational and can be present only during sexual activity, or only with pelvic exams, or with both. A study by Reissing et al. (35) found that the characteristics that best differentiated vaginismus from vulvodynia were the degree of distress exhibited during the pelvic examination and the level of interference with coitus. More than 70% of women with vaginismus reported never having experienced vaginal penetration, whereas all of the women with vulvodynia had experienced coitus.

There are no good estimates of the prevalence of vaginismus, and much of the research that has been done has involved clinic populations and has not included control groups. Vaginismus is a difficult disorder to study because women are often phobic about pelvic examinations and are reluctant to come in for treatment or for research studies.

The cause of vaginismus is unknown. Many of the older theories about causation are largely discredited, including unconscious conflicts and extreme religiosity. Studies looking for histories of sexual abuse are conflicting, but a recent study by Reissing found an increased incidence of "sexual interference" prior to age 13 years in vaginismus patients (36). Vaginismus may begin as an appropriate response to a painful sensation, but then become self-perpetuating. Theories about the etiology of other chronic pain syndromes may provide the best explanations for this disorder, such as central or peripheral sensitization, catastrophization, and illness attribution (30). Many women with severe vaginismus have satisfactory relationships with their partners, and they frequently have satisfactory sexual relationships with noncoital sex. Many have no orgasmic difficulties.

A useful way to explain vaginismus to a patient is to compare a vaginistic patient's response to vaginal penetration to the typical, automatic, protective response of a person trying to put a contact lens in for the first time. The muscle contractions around the eye are quite involuntary at first, but can be eliminated with practice.

The most effective treatments for vaginismus are behavioral, and success rates of 80% or greater are frequently reported (37,38). However, dropout rates are frequently high, and very few studies actually consider coital pleasure after treatment. Success in treatment is highly dependent on the motivation of the woman, and the desire for pregnancy may be a more effective motivator than the desire to function sexually. Vaginal dilators are generally used, and the patient is taught to do the exercises at home. The vagina is not actually "dilated" during this process, but rather there is a deconditioning of the pelvic floor and pelvic muscles' response to vaginal penetration.

Treatment usually begins in the office, so that the patient can be taught to insert the dilators. Soft silicone vaginal dilators are usually purchased, but other cylindrically shaped objects can be used, such as culturette tubes, candles, or syringes with the needle tips cut off. Relaxation techniques and Kegel exercises are also taught. The patient is instructed to practice inserting the dilator regularly at home, and then to use progressively larger dilators. Vaginismus patients are often very uncomfortable with their own genitalia and may find it helpful to initially use a mirror, or to wear gloves for their practice sessions. Followup visits in the office are important to motivate the patient to practice consistently. She should be re-examined periodically for introital tenderness or muscle tenderness, because recovery will necessitate treatment of these problems as well.

Dilation exercises can be done by women themselves, or they can be incorporated into the couple's sexual activity. Most patients want to keep the dilation exercises under their own control at first, but some patients are comfortable having their partners insert the dilators, or may use the partner's fingers.

Medication is sometimes helpful. Antidepressant medications can be quite useful to diminish general anxiety, or benzodiazepines can be used for practice sessions. Some antidepressants such as tricyclics or venlafaxine may have the dual benefit of reducing anxiety and of helping to treat any comorbid vulvodynia. Topical lidocaine (2% to 5%) gel or cream can be used for vaginal or introital hyperesthesia. There are case reports of the successful use of botulinum toxin for vaginismus, but there are no published studies to date.

Sexual Aversion Disorder

Diagnostic Classification

Sexual aversion disorder is characterized as a persistent or recurrent extreme aversion to and avoidance of all or almost all genital sexual contact with a sexual partner. The disturbance causes marked distress or interpersonal difficulty, and it is not caused by another axis I disorder (except another sexual dysfunction).

Assessment

Certain patients may give a history of *aversion to or avoidance of all forms of genital contact* with a sexual partner, in contrast to a history of gradual or sudden loss of sexual desire. The complaint is often of long standing but may be of recent onset. The aversion may be so severe as to be associated with panic attacks should the patient find herself confronted with a sexual experience. It is important to recognize that fundamentally this disorder is an anxiety–phobic disorder in which the sexual expression serves as a focus for extreme anxiety. Sometimes the patient's presentation will minimize the anxiety component of the condition, making it appear to be a case of loss of sexual desire or chronic sexual disinterest. In these instances, the clinician must probe the respondent in some detail as to the nature and course of the problem to establish the anxiogenic nature of the condition.

Treatment of Sexual Aversion Disorder

Treatment usually requires a course of individual and couple treatment by a skilled sex therapist. The treatment goal is to replace the negative affect and avoidant behaviors associated with phobic-like stimuli with relaxation and pleasure in mutual sexual expression. The treatment of any associated panic attacks may be augmented with low-dosage antidepressant medication (see Chapter 22).

Male Sexual Disorders

Hypoactive Sexual Desire Disorder

Diagnostic Classification

As is the case with females, HSDD in the male is defined as the persistent or recurrent deficiency or absence of sexual fantasies thoughts or desire for sexual activity. The judgement of deficiency or absence is made by the clinician, taking into account factors that affect sexual functioning (e.g., age, presence of a partner, health status). As with women, the condition must cause the individual marked distress or interpersonal difficulty, and not occur exclusively during the course of another axis I disorder, nor be caused by a pharmacologic substance or another medical condition.

Assessment

As seen in Tables 6.1, 6.2, and 6.4, many medical conditions and drugs have the potential to decrease or eliminate sexual desire. In practice, many of these conditions are well known and easily diagnosed by the patient's physician. Numerous factors can be involved in the loss or reduction of sexual desire in males. Unlike women, however, it is extremely rare to see lifetime absence of sexual desire in a man, except in the case of specific endocrinopathies or other explicit medical conditions. The presence of medical disorders, trauma, surgical interventions, pharmacologic therapies for other medical conditions, and substance abuse are all potential etiologic agents and should be reviewed and ruled out. A laboratory assay of endocrine levels, including free, total, and biologically active testosterone, as well as sex hormone-binding globulin (SHBG), is often useful in gaining further insight into the nature of the basis for the condition. In some instances the physician may also want to request prolactin levels to rule out the presence of a pituitary microadenoma, which affects both men and women.

It is also important to bear in mind that beginning at about age 30 years, serum testosterone levels in males decrease approximately 1.6% per year. The sources of this decrease are both central and peripheral, and it occurs over a period when serum levels of SHBG are rising as a consequence of the aging process. This combination of effects can result in an androgen-deficiency syndrome, referred to as ADAM (androgen deficiency in aging men) (40).

In addition to low or absent sexual desire, men in this hypogonadal state manifest losses in strength, bone density, and muscle mass; experience fatigue and loss of well-being; and report a loss of initiative and confidence in themselves. Such a clinical presentation with a total testosterone level of <300 ng/dL is often associated with ADAM, and is estimated to have a prevalence of $>20\%$ in men older than age 60 years (41,42). Some in the field refer to this condition as *andropause;* however, many believe this term is inappropriate and a misnomer because the analogy with menopause in women fails at a number of levels.

Depression is also an extremely common cause of reduced sexual desire in both genders, and is itself a highly prevalent clinical condition. In addition, many of the drugs used to treat depression (e.g., the SSRIs) are themselves etiologic in desire disorders, with rates as high as 60% to 70% being reported (26) (Table 6.4).

Treatment

Effective treatment of HSDD in men greatly depends on correct identification of the underlying cause of the condition. If an androgen deficiency syndrome is found to be present, there are numerous options for testosterone replacement. Although other modalities exist testosterone gel and patches best approximate the normal circadian cycle. Both are available in a variety of doses, and once treatment has begun, total and free serum testosterone should be evaluated at 3, 6, and 12 months after initiation.

If it is determined that a loss of desire is secondary to the initiation of treatment of a clinical depression with SSRIs, a number of alternatives are available. As discussed earlier under Treatment for Female Orgasmic Disorder, the physician can try reducing the dose, switching to another less-problematic antidepressant, looking into the possibility of drug "holidays," or adding a prosexual agent (e.g., bupropion) to the therapeutic regimen. Usually, with patient cooperation, some experimentation will result in a favorable outcome.

Finally, it is worth noting that some patients present with a complaint of loss of sexual desire that is actually a secondary manifestation of another primary sexual dysfunction, usually ED. Repeated attempts resulting in erectile failure often humiliate and frustrate the patient to the point that he loses interest in sex, to some extent as an ego defense against his inability to perform. Care must be taken when interviewing the patient presenting with loss of sexual desire to ascertain that the condition is primary, and not the secondary result of another more central problem.

Male Erectile Disorder

Diagnostic Classification

A. Persistent or recurrent inability to attain or maintain an adequate erection until completion of sexual activity.
B. The disturbance causes marked distress or interpersonal difficulty.
C. The dysfunction is not better accounted for by another axis I disorder (other than a sexual dysfunction) and is not caused exclusively by the direct physiologic effects of a substance (e.g., a drug of abuse, a medication).

Assessment

Early detection and screening are useful actions in many patients, particularly those considered to be at high risk for erectile dysfunction. For instance, patients who have a sedentary lifestyle or are heavy cigarette users may be identified as at-risk individuals. Patients with medical histories consistent with cardiovascular disease, including diabetes, dyslipidemia, and hypertension, could also suffer from erectile dysfunction and benefit from intervention. Patient self-reported questionnaires that inquire about and rate levels of attainment and maintenance of erection, confidence in sexual performance, and even sexual satisfaction can be used. Although such tools were designed primarily for clinical trial use, they may serve as screening devices, if not as a means to monitor treatment responses in individual patients. As an example, the Sexual Health Inventory for Men, an abridged version of the International Index of Erectile Function, is commonly used for this purpose (43).

Diagnostic assessment begins with defining the presenting condition and then taking a thorough medical (including medications), surgical, and social history followed by appropriate laboratory testing. Confirmation of the problem adheres precisely to its definition as the inability to attain or maintain an erection sufficient for satisfactory sexual performance or intercourse (44). The

TABLE 6.8 Clinical Features Differentiating Predominantly Psychogenic from Predominantly Organic Erectile Dysfunction

Feature	*Psychogenic*	*Organic*
Onset	Usually abrupt, with temporal relationship to specific stress (e.g., marital difficulties, loss of job, bereavement, fatigue)	Usually insidious decline from previous competency (90%–95% of cases)
Course	Selective, intermittent, episodic, transient	Usually persistent, with progressive deterioration
Degree of impairment	Evidence of potential to respond to erotic stimuli and fantasies, with masturbation, other partner	Unable to obtain erection with masturbation, erotic stimuli, other partner
Nocturnal or morning erection	Generally present	Generally absent or reduced in frequency, intensity

Vliet LW, Meyer JK. Erectile dysfunction: progress in evaluation and treatment. Johns Hopkins Med J 1982;151:246.

initial history may lead to its attribution as either organic or predominantly psychogenic. Organic etiologies include neurogenic, hormonal, vascular, or medication-associated erectile dysfunction, whereas psychogenic etiologies include depression, stress, performance anxiety, relationship issues, and sexual arousal difficulties. Table 6.8 lists features of the clinical history that may be helpful in supporting this distinction. Physical examination may cover all aspects of the patient's health, although particular focus should be given to the neurologic and vascular systems, as well as to the genitourinary system. The patient's genitalia should be examined for any unusual characteristics, such as deformity, scarring, or angulation of the penis suggestive of Peyronie disease or prior trauma. Laboratory testing is purposefully done to confirm or exclude underlying disease and is generally tailored to the individual clinical presentation. Tests may include blood glucose, lipid profile, urinalysis, and complete blood count. An endocrine assessment, such as morning-time total testosterone measurement, may be performed when hypogonadism is suspected. Other endocrine tests, such as thyroid-stimulating hormone measurement, may be carried out if there is clinical suspicion of thyroid disease.

Subsequent management should be goal-oriented, in recognition that patients' preferences and expectations regarding management options for erectile dysfunction vary greatly. Accordingly, patient and partner involvement in such clinical decisions is a critical component of the full evaluation and treatment process.

Depending on the complexity of the clinical presentation, a referral to a urologist or erectile dysfunction specialist for additional tests may be appropriate. The contemporary role of such specialists has been reduced as a consequence of the recent introduction of effective first-line oral therapies for erectile dysfunction, which can be administered and evaluated for therapeutic success irrespective of the organic or psychogenic etiologic distinction. However, referral would be warranted prior to initiation of second- or third-line therapies, which are considered to be semi-invasive and possibly nonreversible. Recommended tests may include combined penile injection of vasodilators and sexual stimulation, duplex ultrasonography, cavernosography, pelvic-penile arteriography, nocturnal penile tumescence testing, and/or neurologic tests. A patient who presents with an atypical presentation, such as an adolescent or young adult with primary erectile dysfunction, is a reasonable candidate for referral. In addition, some patients may request referral for assurance that the problem has received an appropriate and comprehensive evaluation. Cases having medicolegal ramifications may also be subject to extensive diagnostic testing.

Treatment

Consistent with the principle of goal-directed assessment for the evaluation of erectile dysfunction, a similar principle may guide its treatment practices. It is imperative to consider what the patient (and partner) actually wants or expects to accomplish through treatment. Patients vary in their level of acceptance of their sexual disorders, and some may not wish to pursue treatment beyond easily administered, minimally invasive options. At the same time, a more significant, invasive intervention may be provided, depending on the extent of the problem and the manner of satisfaction derived with treatment. For instance, penile prosthesis surgery may be promptly pursued as a definitive option in patients desirous of this intervention despite the understanding that it is invasive and nonreversible.

First-Line Therapy. Management of erectile dysfunction is most commonly initiated by a combination of pharmacologic therapy (Table 6.9) and counseling, along with a modification of lifestyle habits. Patients should be counseled to modify any detrimental behaviors, such as cigarette smoking, excessive alcohol use, recreational drug use, lack of exercise, and uncontrolled diabetes, so as to improve their sexual ability or prevent progression of the problem. If a medication is viewed to be the offending element, the medication regimen may need to be adjusted. Psychosexual counseling is often appropriate, even when the etiology is largely organic, as psychosocial overlays

TABLE 6.9 Pharmacotherapies for Erectile Dysfunction

Drug	*Trade Name*	*Usual Dose Range*	*Available Strengths*	*Selected Side Effects and Comments*	*Efficacy*[a]
Oral Route					
Phosphodiesterase Type 5 Inhibitors					
Sildenafil	Viagra	25, 50, or 100 mg 1 h before sexual activity	25, 50, 100 mg	Headaches, flushing, dyspepsia, nasal congestion, visual disturbances	46%–69%
Vardenafil	Levitra	5–20 mg	5, 10, 20 mg		
Tadalafil	Cialis	5–20 mg	5, 10, 20 mg	Presence of sexual stimulation is required for efficacy Contraindicated for men receiving nitrate therapy in any form that in combination may produce severe hypotension Age, hepatic impairment, renal impairment, and use of drugs that are concurrently metabolized by the cytochrome P450 3A4 isoenzyme pathway in the liver necessitate lower dosing	
α-Adrenoceptor Antagonists					
Yohimbine	Yocon	5.4 mg t.i.d. for 1 mo	5.4 mg	Anxiety, nausea, palpitations, nervousness, hypertension, headache Modest results suggest its role is limited to men with psychogenic erectile dysfunction	~30%
Intraurethral Route					
Alprostadil	MUSE	125, 250, 500, or 1,000 μg, on demand	125, 250, 500, 1,000 μg	Local urogenital pain (29%), minor urethral bleeding (5%), dizziness (4%), hypotension (3%) In-office instruction and titration is highly recommended Contraindicated for patients with priapism histories	~40%
Intracavernosal Route				Priapism (1%), penile fibrosis (5%–10%), penile pain (10%) In-office instruction and titration is highly recommended Contraindicated for patients with histories of priapism and severe coagulopathy	
Alprostadil	Caverject, Edex	10 or 20 μg, on demand	5–60 μg		~70%
Alprostadil + phentolamine	Bi-mix	20 μg/mL + 0.5 mg/mL on demand	Variable		~90%
Papaverine + phentolamine	Bi-mix (Androskat)	30 mg/mL + 0.5 mg/mL on demand	Variable		~90%
Alprostadil + papaverine + phentolamine	Tri-mix	10 μg/mL + 30 mg/mL + 1.0 mg/mL on demand	Variable		~90%

[a]The outcome measure pertains to the subjective degree of success with sexual intercourse using patient and partner questionnaires.

coexist in many patients. Interventions regarding anxiety management, cognition, and/or behavioral interventions may be beneficial.

Androgen-replacement therapy constitutes first-line treatment when hormonal factors are judged to be involved in the presentation, although it is also recognized that this therapy is mainly useful for libidinal issues. The therapy is arguably worth implementing even in the presence of confounding etiologies. Androgen therapy may have other recognizable benefits other than sexual function restoration, with indications for decreased muscle mass, lethargy, depression, and osteoporosis, all of which are linked to reduced androgen levels. It is particularly noteworthy that risk associations, should be discussed, and a risk-to-benefit evaluation should be considered prior to implementing therapy.

PDE 5 inhibitors, a relatively new class of vasoactive drugs, currently represent the centerpiece of erectile dysfunction treatment. The PDE 5 enzyme is highly expressed in the smooth muscle of the corpora cavernosa and hydrolyzes cyclic guanosine monophosphate (cGMP), which is the intracellular mediator of the nitric oxide signaling pathway. Nitric oxide causes relaxation of the smooth muscle, enabling the vasodilation necessary for erection to occur. Selective inhibition of PDE 5, which prevents the breakdown of cGMP, represents a mechanistic approach to facilitate penile erection. Currently, three commercial, FDA-approved PDE 5 agents are available for treatment of erectile dysfunction in the United States: sildenafil citrate (Viagra), tadalafil (Cialis), and vardenafil (Levitra). Their biochemical potencies and selectivities are relatively similar, although slight differences exist with regard to maximal serum concentration, time to maximal concentration, bioavailability, clearance, and protein binding. The most salient difference among these agents is the longer half-life of elimination described for tadalafil (17.5 hours, compared with 3 to 5 hours for sildenafil and 4 to 5 hours for vardenafil) (45–47). Differences in molecular structure of tadalafil may account for this distinction. In healthy men, peak serum levels of the medications after oral ingestion occur at 1 hour for sildenafil and vardenafil and 2 hours for tadalafil, suggesting time intervals needed for optimal efficacy. Common to all drugs of this classification is the need for sexual stimulation to induce nitric oxide release, upon which the therapy acts pharmacologically.

Current published reports on the efficacy of the PDE 5 inhibitors describe comparative analyses with placebo and not to each other, such that a true comparative basis to judge the superiority of one agent relative to the other is not possible. Trial parameters and patient characteristics may vary between studies. The treatment end point of most relevance from the patient's perspective—success in completing sexual intercourse—is similar across studies of the PDE 5 inhibitors, ranging from 61% to 71% for the recommended starting dose for each (48–51). Success with the PDE 5 inhibitors is heightened through patient–partner involvement in treatment decisions, as well as modification of existing risk factors that influence the patient's ability to achieve an erection. In patients with comorbidities, if the condition is optimized, success rates of responsiveness to PDE 5 inhibitors are elevated; for example, 85% for treated hypogonadism (vs. 75% for untreated hypogonadism) and 62% for controlled diabetes (vs. 44% for uncontrolled diabetes) (52).

Special considerations with PDE 5 inhibitors exist based on drug metabolism, drug interactions, and cardiac risk. Because they are commonly metabolized by the cytochrome P450 3A4 isoenzyme pathway in the liver, a lower dose should be prescribed initially for patients who are taking medications that are also metabolized by this pathway, such as cimetidine, erythromycin, ketoconazole, nifedipine, saquinavir/ritonavir, and the statins. A lower starting dose should also be prescribed in instances of older age (>65) hepatic impairment, and renal impairment because of the increasing serum levels that may result from these factors. Adverse effects reported with the use of PDE 5 inhibitors include headache, flushing, and dyspepsia, which are discernibly vasodilatory and vasorelaxant responses occurring in other parts of the body that express PDE 5 (package insert references). Sildenafil-treated patients have also reported nasal congestion, visual disturbances, and diarrhea; vardenafil-treated patients have also reported rhinitis, sinusitis, and flulike symptoms; tadalafil-treated patients have also reported nasal congestion, back pain, and myalgia. All three PDE 5 inhibitors have been shown to potentiate the hypotensive effects of organic nitrates and are therefore contraindicated in patients using nitrate therapy, such as nitroglycerin and amyl nitrate "poppers." Although there were early concerns in relation to the cardiac safety of PDE 5 inhibitors, long-term studies have not shown increased myocardial infarction or death rates. However, the drugs are contraindicated in patients for whom sexual activity is inadvisable because of underlying cardiovascular disease, unless appropriate cardiovascular intervention has been performed (53).

A long-touted erectogenic and aphrodisiac agent, yohimbine (Yocon) has been rigorously evaluated to establish its role as an orally delivered agent for the treatment of erectile dysfunction (54,55). The medication is an alkaloid derived from the bark of the yohimbe tree and is reported to exert central effects on the mediation of penile erection as an α_2-adrenergic receptor antagonist. Conventionally, the medication is used at an oral dosage of 5.4 mg three times daily with clinical observation for at least 1 month to assess responsiveness. Although some evidence suggests that the medication may be more effective than placebo, its efficacy beyond placebo has not been affirmed in patients with confirmed organic erectile dysfunction. Adverse effects appear to be relatively infrequent but include hypertension, anxiety, tachycardia, and headache. Although yohimbine may be well tolerated, its modest results suggest that the medication is best limited to men with psychogenic erectile dysfunction.

Second-Line Therapy. When first-line therapies are ineffective or contraindicated, patients may be best directed to consider second-line therapies such as intraurethral therapy, intracavernosal therapy, and vacuum constriction devices. These options are understood to be more intrusive and invasive than first-line therapies.

Intraurethral pharmacotherapy, which implies the administration of vasoactive drugs via the urethral channel of the penis, offers a potentially less-invasive procedure for local pharmacotherapeutic intervention than intracavernosal pharmacotherapy, as the latter requires needle injections. A synthetic formulation of prostaglandin E_1

(alprostadil) can be delivered through a novel transurethral drug delivery system known as medicated urethral system for erection, or MUSE (56,57). Several technical points optimize success of the treatment, including the patient's properly depositing and manually distributing the medication into the penis and then standing for several minutes after its application to increase penile engorgement. A final responder rate to the medication is documented at approximately 40%, with typical responses including tumescence without full rigidity. The combined use of an adjustable penile constriction band (ACTIS), designed and FDA-approved to enhance the local retention and effect of the medication, improves response to this treatment (58). The most common side effects of MUSE include local urogenital pain associated with metabolism of the medication and minor urethral bleeding associated with traumatic delivery of the medication.

Intracavernosal pharmacotherapy requires needle injection of vasoactive medication into the corpus cavernosum (59). Three medications are regularly used, either individually or in combination: prostaglandin E_1, phentolamine, and papaverine. In-office titration is recommended because of the technical demands of this therapy, and because of the need to determine the dosage that yields an erection of sufficient rigidity for sexual intercourse yet lasts no more than 1 hour. Rates of successful sexual intercourse range between 70% and 90% (60). The treatment is contraindicated for men with psychological instability, a history of or risk for priapism, sickle cell disease, locally advanced pelvic or hematologic malignancy, histories of severe coagulopathy or unstable cardiovascular disease, or reduced manual dexterity (although the partner can be trained in the injection technique). Risks of complications include priapism (1% of men), penile fibrosis at the penile injection site (5% to 10% of men), local trauma such as hematoma (10% of injections), and penile pain (10% of men) (60).

Vacuum constriction devices offer a nonpharmacologic, mechanical means to produce an erection (61). A cylinder is temporarily placed externally around the penis with a seal that allows the creation of negative pressure for blood engorgement of the penis. The erection is maintained by placement of a constricting elastic ring around the base of the penis, after which the cylinder is removed and the erectionlike state allows sexual intercourse to occur. The treatment is generally pursued with instructional videotape or in-office teaching. The erectionlike state is achieved in at least 95% of applications. Significant complications are rare, with typical concerns related to cumbersomeness, coldness of the erect penis, and local penile trauma, such as petechiae and ecchymosis.

Third-Line Therapy. Penile prosthesis surgery is an alternative treatment for erectile dysfunction, often applied after nonsurgical options have been found ineffective or unacceptable (62,63). The devices are surgically implanted within the corporal bodies of the penis. The two main varieties of devices are semirigid malleable devices and hydraulic inflatable devices. Use of the devices requires basic instruction. They reliably produce penile rigidity permitting sexual intercourse. Because their immediate use circumvents issues of lack of spontaneity, high satisfaction rates are frequently reported. Potential complications (<5% at 5 years) include infection, erosion, and malfunction of the device, and usually require device removal or replacement (63). Penile revascularization surgery is beneficial to a minority of patients with a confirmed vascular lesion of probable traumatic origin amenable to vascular bypass techniques (62).

Premature Ejaculation

Diagnostic Classification

There are three DSM-IV diagnostic criteria for premature ejaculation (PE): (a) persistent or recurrent ejaculation with minimal sexual stimulation before, on, or shortly after penetration and before the person wishes it; (b) the disturbance causes marked distress or interpersonal difficulty; and (c) the disturbance is not exclusively caused by a substance (e.g., withdrawal from opioids).

Assessment

A fundamental aspect of the assessment of premature ejaculation is its accurate differentiation from other sexual dysfunctions. Of primary importance is the evaluation for erectile dysfunction, as many men may profess premature ejaculation when, instead, the actual problem is the patient's haste to achieve orgasm before the failure of erection. In such cases, successful treatment of erectile dysfunction may resolve the complaint of secondary premature ejaculation. Subsequent focus is given to sexual and psychosocial history. Key elements of the history taking is the determination of level of distress experienced by both the patient and his partner, discussion of the patient's perception of ejaculatory control, and inquiry into the onset and duration of premature ejaculation. The latter has importance to establish whether the condition is primary or secondary. Psychosocial aspects of the patient history, such as a history of childhood physical or sexual abuse, are relevant and may establish a need for psychotherapy as part of the treatment approach. A comprehensive medical history may lead to the identification of certain medical conditions that are associated with ejaculatory dysfunctions, such as diabetes and other neuropathies (64,65).

Treatment

Approaches to managing premature ejaculation are conventionally divided into two broad categories: psychotherapeutic–behavioral and pharmacotherapeutic. The former has long been advocated, mainly because of the paucity of other effective therapies. The strategy is to promote the patient's understanding of his progression through the human sexual response cycle and then, with his partner, practice one of two behavioral control techniques: the "squeeze" and "stop–start" techniques. The squeeze technique requires the partner to place her thumb and first two fingers around the coronal ridge of the penis and press firmly for 10 seconds. The pressure results in a 10% to 25% loss of erection and a decrease in the subjective sense of arousal. The technique teaches the couple a method of control that can be practiced well before the patient reaches high levels of sexual arousal. The stop–start method accomplishes the same result by discontinuing all forms of stimulation. The patient and his partner alternately stimulate and practice control with these techniques until they are confident of their ability to exercise control. At this point, they progress to coitus interrupting the experience with the behavioral techniques as necessary. Requirements of these techniques include a stable relationship and time to learn and use them. Reports are mixed with regard to their practicality and long-term efficacy.

An alternative approach is to use pharmacotherapies that strategically serve to reduce sensory input to the penis, prevent penile detumescence after ejaculation, and suppress apparent ejaculatory reflex mechanisms. Topical anesthetics, such as the lidocaine–prilocaine combination, as well as some herbal preparations, such as the Korean product SS-cream, are applied to the glans penis, diminishing sensitivity and delaying the threshold for ejaculation (66). Advantages are their simplicity and low cost. However, some of these preparations can cause local irritation as well as penile hypoanesthesia. Additional possible adverse effects include vaginal numbness and female anorgasmia, unless a condom is used. Pharmacostimulation of erection, such as oral PDE 5-inhibitor treatment and intracavernosal pharmacotherapy, has been used to promote the erectile response, perhaps even enabling erection after ejaculation has occurred, but such treatment has not been convincingly shown to delay ejaculation per se or operate through any direct mechanism of action to control the ejaculatory response. Oral retardants of ejaculation constitute the most common pharmacologic approach. Most of the currently used medications are centrally acting antidepressant drugs that involve central 5-hydroxytryptamine neurotransmission. These include clomipramine, a tricyclic antidepressant, and SSRIs such as fluoxetine, sertraline, and paroxetine. Clomipramine use is limited by drowsiness and significant anticholinergic side effects such as dry mouth and blurred vision. Although SSRIs are better tolerated, they often require long-term dosing regimens to be effective and they are also associated with nausea, drowsiness, cognitive impairments, and sexual side-effects, including decreased libido and erectile dysfunction. Pharmacotherapies currently in development may come closer to the ideal characteristics of well-tolerated, on-demand oral therapy for this very common male sexual dysfunction.

Male Orgasmic Disorder

Diagnostic Classification

There are three DSM-IV diagnostic criteria for male orgasmic disorder: (a) persistent or recurrent delay in, or absence of, orgasm following a normal sexual excitement phase, taking into account the patient's age; (b) the disturbance causes marked distress or interpersonal difficulty; and (c) the disturbance is not caused by another axis I disorder or exclusively by a substance (e.g., a drug of abuse or medication) or a medical condition.

Assessment

Although anorgasmia is a rather uncommon disorder in men, certain organic and psychogenic associations can be explored in evaluating this presentation. The organic conditions that affect orgasm comprise, for the most part, neurologic disorders, drugs that affect the autonomic nervous system or lower genitourinary tract, and surgical or traumatic interruptions of the invoked neural pathways for ejaculation (67). Clinical history taking and physical examination should focus on these possibilities. Accordingly, the workup may reveal such associations as the presence of diabetes, SSRI or alpha-blocker medication use, prior retroperitoneal lymph node dissection for malignancy, or radical pelvic surgery. It is important to evaluate ejaculatory ability and orgasm separately, because they do not necessarily coincide. The disorder referred to as *anejaculation,* or failure to ejaculate, is associated with disruption of the sympathetic nerve supply to the accessory male reproductive tract structures, primarily causing failure of emission, although orgasm may still be experienced because of the intact somatic innervation of the striated musculature of the pelvic floor. Distinct from this problem, *retrograde ejaculation* involves dysfunction of the internal urinary sphincter mechanism such that the ejaculate readily enters the bladder following sexual stimulation as a consequence of a drug or transurethral surgery. In this entity, subjective sensation of orgasm is typically preserved. Psychogenic anorgasmia in men is a rare disorder associated with personality disturbances. Obsessive–compulsive, avoidant and, infrequently, sadomasochistic traits are observed. Commonly, anorgasmia is restricted to penile–vaginal intercourse whereas other forms of sexual stimulation, for example, masturbation, permit orgasm.

Treatment

Treatment of orgasmic disorders in men centers mainly on correcting reversible causes when possible. This objective may most feasibly apply to the situation in which a drug is associated and can be changed. Treatment of anejaculation is generally indicated to restore fertility and targets mechanisms that achieve seminal emission. Adrenergic receptor agonists, such as ephedrine sulfate, pseudoephedrine hydrochloride, and imipramine hydrochloride, have been used for this purpose. However, their roles have been limited because of their variable success and their causing sympathomimetic side effects such as dizziness, weakness, nausea, and sweating (68). Electroejaculation and other assistive reproductive techniques are mostly employed for this management. Penile vibratory stimulation has also been described as a technique to treat idiopathic orgasmic dysfunction.

Sexual Disorders Resulting from Medical Conditions or Substance Abuse

There are two additions to the diagnostic nomenclature in the DSM-IV (3) for sexual dysfunction: *Sexual Dysfunction due to a General Medical Condition* and *Substance-Induced Sexual Dysfunction*. As one might expect from the labels, these two diagnostic categories address specific organic etiologies of sexual dysfunctions, the former reflecting effects of a general medical condition, the latter based on findings of a connection between sexual dysfunction and substance intoxication or medication use. The DSM-IV sets the following criteria:

Sexual Dysfunction due to ... (Indicate the General Medical Condition)

A. Clinically significant sexual dysfunction that results in marked distress or interpersonal difficulty predominates in the clinical picture.
B. There is evidence from the history, physical examination, or laboratory findings that the sexual dysfunction is fully explained by the direct physiologic effects of a general medical condition.
C. The disturbance is not better accounted for by another mental disorder (e.g., Major Depressive Disorder).

Substance-Induced Sexual Dysfunction

A. Clinically significant sexual dysfunction that results in marked distress or interpersonal difficulty predominates in the clinical picture.
B. There is evidence from the history, physical examination, or laboratory findings that the sexual dysfunction is fully explained by substance use as manifested by either (1) or (2):
   1. The symptoms in criterion A developed during, or within 1 month of, substance intoxication.
   2. Medication use is etiologically related to the disturbance.

GENDER IDENTITY DISORDERS

The essential feature of the gender-identity disorders is cross-gender identification. The hallmark is the desire to be, or the insistence that one is, the opposite gender and significant, persistent distress about one's biologic sex. There are childhood and adult forms of the disorder. Children manifest symptoms by rejecting stereotypical dress, play activities, and behaviors associated with being a "boy" or a "girl." The adoption of cross-gender roles is persistent, and attempts by parents to change the behaviors are met with strong resistance and emotional displays of anger and tearfulness.

Adolescents and adults are generally more circumspect about revealing or expressing their cross-gender identification, at least early in the process of coming to an understanding about their cross-gender desires. The consequences of expressing a cross-gender identification in childhood can be significantly adverse, especially for boys who are teased, physically abused, and ostracized by their peers. Coping with the disorder in adulthood has the potential of being extraordinarily disruptive to relationships, education, and professional/vocational development as the desire for cross-gender living, hormonal/surgical reassignment, and social acceptance in the cross-gender role becomes the central focus of the patient's existence. In the past decade, individuals with gender identity disorder have presented wanting to be a blend of both the male and female phenotype, presumably to match the gender-blending identity they strive to assume.

Etiology and Prevalence

No known genetic or biologic predisposing factors have as yet been elucidated. There is limited evidence from studies of families that cross-gender identification in children can be reinforced within the context of the parent–child relationship. Clinical studies of adults continue to reveal no specific pathologic personality features or psychiatric symptom clusters associated with the disorder. The disorders are rare. European epidemiologic studies reveal that 1 in every 30,000 adult males and 1 in every 100,000 adult females seek treatment for these disorders.

Course

Parents usually seek evaluation when the affected child enters school because the cross-gender identification and behaviors become public. One prospective study (69) found that almost 75% of the boys with this disorder reported a homosexual or bisexual orientation by adolescence or early adulthood, without any signs or symptoms of a gender identity disorder. One or two percent reported a gender identity disorder, and the remainder were heterosexual without evidence of a gender identity disorder. The course for girls is not known.

The course in adults is variable. For some it is chronic and unremitting, with the persistent, dedicated drive for living and functioning in the cross-gender role with or without hormonal/surgical reassignment. The ability to achieve the goal of surgical reassignment is usually more dependent on the intellectual and professional competencies and financial resources of the individual than on the influence of medical decision making. For the majority of adults, the combination of limited resources and a waxing-and-waning intensity of the desire to live and function in the cross-gender role leads to an on-again–off-again course.

Complications

The problems associated with the childhood form of the disorder have been noted. Adults who are thwarted in their attempts to achieve cross-gender living may become depressed; some have committed suicide, and males, on rare occasion, have attempted self-castration. The more common problems for adults are the disruption of marriage, social relationships, and vocational function associated with a change in gender role.

Assessment

For both children and adults, a complete medical and psychiatric evaluation is recommended. No specific laboratory tests are indicated. Adult patients may benefit from a personality assessment, such as the Neuroticism, Extroversion, and Openness–Personality Index Revised (NEO-PI-R) (70), more for treatment planning purposes than for diagnosis. The psychiatric or psychological component of the evaluation is best performed by professionals who have experience with patients with gender identity disorders.

Treatment

Children and adults who express dissatisfaction with their gender should be referred to professionals with expertise in these disorders. Therapy with children who are diagnosed with gender identity disorder is family oriented, with the goals of treatment being to explore the nature and characteristics of the child's or adolescent's gender identity, ameliorate comorbid problems in the patient's life, and help the patient and family make difficult decisions related to the management of the patient's gender identity. The treatment of adolescents and adults combines aspects of psychotherapy (for consideration of the decision to pursue reassignment), counseling (logistics of cross-gender living, referred to as "the real-life test"), endocrinology management (fully and partially reversible hormone therapy), and surgical management (surgical reassignment, age 18 years and older). The latter two medical interventions are available when the patient meets criteria, such as those of the Harry Benjamin International Gender Dysphoria Association (see www.hopkinsbayview.org/PAMreferences), which sets standards of care that are more or less accepted by most physicians in the United States.

PARAPHILIAS

The paraphilias are sexual disorders with the following essential features in DSM-IV (3): recurrent, intense sexually arousing fantasies, sexual urges, or behaviors involving nonhuman objects, the suffering or humiliation of oneself and/or one's sexual partner, or children, or other nonconsenting persons that occur over a period of at least 6 months.

Exhibitionism

Exhibitionism involves the displaying of one's genitals to a nonconsenting person. Sometimes the individual masturbates during the episode; more commonly the person later employs the memory of the episode as a masturbatory stimulus. There usually is no attempt to have contact, sexual or otherwise, with the victim.

Fetishism

Fetishism is the use of objects for sexual arousal. Common fetishistic objects are women's underpants, bras, slips, stockings, shoes, or certain textures such as silk or rubberized material. The person usually masturbates while fondling or smelling the object. Some fetishistic behaviors involve body parts such as feet.

Frotteurism

Frotteurism involves touching or rubbing up against a nonconsenting person, usually in a crowded space. The person attempts to rub his genitals or hand against the breast, genitals, or buttocks of the victim. Orgasmic release usually occurs after the episode, with the fantasy of the experience being the sexual stimulus.

Pedophilia

Pedophilia involves sexual activity with prepubescent children. Individuals diagnosed with pedophilia must be at least 16 years of age, and their victim must be at least 5 years younger. Most individuals diagnosed with pedophilia are male, although there are cases of females who sexually abuse children. In most states, the discovery by health providers of sexual abuse of children mandates reporting to local child protective services.

Sadism and Masochism

Sadism and masochism involve sexual activities during which arousal and gratification depend on either inflicting psychological and/or physical pain (sadism) or experiencing it (masochism). These paraphilias include a broad range of fantasies and behaviors, from awareness of potential cruelty or suffering to extreme physical injury and murder. Aspects of both sadism and masochism are often found in the same person, even though one or the other paraphilia is dominant.

Voyeurism

The essential feature of voyeurism involves the act of observing (peeping) unsuspecting victims disrobing or engaging in sexual activity. Orgasmic release is usually achieved through masturbation during or just after the episode of "peeping."

Transvestitic Fetishism

The focus of this paraphilia involves cross-dressing by males in female attire accompanied by sexual arousal and orgasmic release through masturbation. Middle-aged transvestites often experience a decrease or disappearance of sexual arousal and report a "calming" or "anxiety reduction" effect associated with cross-dressing. The paraphilia can be differentiated from the cross-dressing associated with gender identity disorders and from the dramatic displays of homosexual "drag queens," which usually do not result in sexual arousal. The transvestite experience often includes the fantasy that the patient is a woman, with singular focus on specific body parts (e.g., legs, breasts, lips).

Treatment of Paraphilia and Nonparaphilic Sexual Compulsion

Ideally, the goal of any therapeutic intervention is the elimination of the paraphilic behavior. Achievement of that goal is difficult because these behaviors are enjoyable or are positively reinforced by sexual gratification, or both. Often the best that can be done is continuous control of the behaviors using pharmacotherapy (antiandrogens) in combination with individual (cognitive–behavioral) psychotherapy and/or group therapy. Reports (71) indicate that the SSRI antidepressants may be helpful in some cases, in combination with individual or group therapy, especially among those with nonparaphilic, sexually compulsive behaviors. Based on the concept of paraphilia as similar to a sexual addiction, 12-step treatment programs are available for the control of paraphilias. Although these behaviors were once considered untreatable, combinations of the interventions described demonstrate that they can be controlled in compliant patients.

SEXUALITY AND SPECIAL POPULATIONS

Homosexuality

General Characteristics

The American Psychiatric Association removed homosexuality from its list of mental disorders in 1973. The diagnostic term *Sexual Disorder, Not Otherwise Specified* may be used for patients who experience persistent and marked distress about their sexual orientation.

The NHSLS population-based study of sexual practices in the United States (6) reported that 2.8% of men and 1.4% of women identified themselves as homosexual or bisexual. These numbers are at variance with Kinsey's historic percentages of 10% male and 5% female self-reported homosexuality. The authors of the more recent study are quick to point out there are no easy answers to questions about the prevalence of homosexuality.

Predisposing Factors

Various attempts to relate homosexuality to abnormal pituitary and sex hormone function have been unsuccessful. The evidence to support the contention that homosexuality is genetically determined is scant. Many theories about the cause of homosexuality involving psychosocial predisposition have been proposed. However, no studies clearly demonstrate psychosocial precipitants. At this time, it is prudent to consider a multifactorial model in the genesis of homosexual behaviors.

Development

Most people who accept a homosexual orientation continue that orientation throughout life. Some homosexuals are socially open about their lifestyle; many are covert, largely because of negative attitudes (homophobia) that are common in American communities. Aspects of life as a homosexual that are predictably stressful include the process of discovering one's sexual orientation, disclosure to others (coming out), and the threat of hate crimes.

Psychosocial Consequences

In the past, but possibly to a lesser degree at the present time, the principal risk to homosexual individuals (aside from human immunodeficiency virus infection in men) was the social stigma. More recently, many American communities have enacted or are considering legislation that explicitly protects homosexuals from job, housing, and other forms of discrimination. On the other hand, some jurisdictions and many fundamentalist religious groups support legal and moral discrimination against homosexuality. In most states, but not all, criminal penalties for homosexual acts have been eliminated for consenting adults. The principal legal difficulty currently is for people who are promiscuous and who use public facilities for their sexual activities. Homosexuality is entirely compatible with the development of sustained, affectionate, long-term relationships. A series of recent studies do suggest, however, that young homosexuals are at greater risk for mood disorders, anxiety disorders, substance abuse, and suicidal symptoms, including suicide attempts (72–74).

Assessment and Management

Most gay men prefer their personal physician to know of their homosexuality and indicate that they are more satisfied with the care they obtain when their physician is aware of their orientation (75). Studies of lesbians show that many are reluctant to disclose their sexual orientation to their physicians because of fear of judgmental attitudes (76). Obviously those who do not disclose at-risk sexual behaviors pose a difficult management problem for the physician.

Homosexual men require special considerations in their routine medical care. Those who have multiple partners should always be asked about their knowledge of safe sex practices (see Chapter 39) and of symptoms of sexually transmitted diseases, including human immunodeficiency virus infection (see Chapter 39), and they should be screened periodically for type B hepatitis (Chapter 47), syphilis (Chapter 37), and gonorrhea (Chapter 37). Men who practice receptive anal intercourse are subject to both infectious and traumatic anorectal conditions (see Chapter 98).

Most sexually transmitted diseases occur less frequently in lesbian patients, with the exception of three forms of vaginitis—candidiasis, trichomoniasis, and nonspecific vaginitis—each of which should be considered when a known lesbian patient has a vaginal discharge (76) (see Chapter 102). It is possible that the risk of breast cancer is increased in lesbians. In the absence of adequate information, cancer-screening recommendations for lesbians should be the same as those for other women according to age group (76) (see Chapters 14, 104 and 105).

Assessment of patients who express concerns about homosexual fantasies or experiences should focus on the frequency of the experience, on the patients' decisions to continue with homosexual experiences, and on whether they feel comfortable with those decisions. Patients who ultimately identify with a homosexual orientation and are comfortable with that identity do not present problems. However, patients who are anxious or depressed about their homosexual inclinations may need therapy. Adolescents or adults who anxiously report isolated episodes of homosexual experiences or fantasies may need brief supportive counseling (see Chapter 20).

Aging Patients

Aging people do not lose their capacity for sexual function on the basis of the aging process alone. It is important to invite questions regarding sexual function in the general care of older patients, because they are often embarrassed to bring up this aspect of their health. Patients who have any of the sexual disorders discussed previously should be evaluated in the same manner as a younger patient. The predictable changes associated with aging are slower arousal phase, increased ability to stay at plateau levels of arousal, and, in men, a longer refractory period. Women commonly experience dyspareunia as a result of atrophic vaginitis after menopause; Chapter 102 describes the management of this treatable problem.

Dementia is more often marked by decreased sexual desire than by occasional inappropriate sexual behavior. Partners of demented individuals report that the sexual interaction has lost most of its intimate quality and that the partner has become impersonal and mechanical in sexual activity.

With 1.6 million elderly persons residing in 20,000 nursing homes in the United States, there is need of institutional sensitivity to their sexual needs as well as appropriate strategies for those occasions when sexual behaviors become problematic. A growing body of literature addresses these two seemingly contradictory issues (77).

Children

It is unusual for children to complain of sexual difficulties. However, parents occasionally ask their own physicians questions about the developing sexuality of their children. Parents may express concern about the appearance of sexual behavior in children, such as mutual exploration of playmates' genitalia or masturbation. Parents can be reassured that such behaviors are normal and should be discouraged in a nonpunitive fashion. Failure to control the behavior may require further evaluation of both the child and the family. Sexual behavior that is coercive, inflicts pain, or involves a significant discrepancy in age should receive professional attention (78).

Occasionally, a physician recognizes the presence of sexual abuse within a family, either on the basis of physical findings or from information disclosed by a child during a medical visit. If someone outside the family has committed the abuse, both the child and the parents may require supportive counseling to help them vent their fear and anger about the experience. Discovery of sexual abuse within a family should be fully evaluated. This procedure should be initiated by reporting the problem to the division of protective services of the local department of social services. The health care professional should be cognizant of the requirements of the reporting laws within his or her jurisdiction, and of the limitations of those laws as they have been interpreted and implemented.

Adolescents

Adolescents with sexual difficulties (see Chapter 11) may be brought to the attention of the physician by either the adolescent or the adolescent's parents. Adolescents who are sexually active may have questions about their sexual function, birth control, venereal disease, or abortion. In most states, a physician may provide services for sex-related problems to an adolescent with or without parental consent.

Adolescents may request consultation about isolated homosexual experiences or homosexual fantasies. In most cases, the physician's role is to inform the adolescent that these experiences are not necessarily indicative of the development of lifelong homosexuality but may be expressions of adolescent sexual exploration. Adolescents who have developed a homosexual orientation or who are in the process of doing so may be brought to the physician by parents who are disturbed at the discovery of homosexual activities. In these instances, counseling should be given to the parents to help them accept the adolescent's orientation. Adolescents who are older than 17 years of age are unlikely to change their orientation. Younger adolescents have not yet consolidated their personality development and should be offered referral for psychiatric evaluation and possible treatment.

SPECIFIC REFERENCES*

1. Fagan, P. Sexual disorders: perspectives on diagnosis and treatment. Baltimore: Johns Hopkins Press, 2004.
2. Basson R. The female sexual response: a different model. J Sex Marital Ther 2000;26:51.
3. American Psychiatric Association. Diagnostic and statistical manual of mental disorders. 4th ed. Washington, DC: American Psychiatric Association, 1994.
4. Basson, R, Burnett, A, Derogatis, LR, et al. Report of the international consensus conference on female sexual dysfunction: definitions and classifications. Urology 2000;163:888.
5. Basson R, Leiblum S, Brotto L, et al. Revised definitions of women's sexual dysfunction. J Sex Med 2004;1:40.
6. Laumann EO, Gagnon JH, Michael RT, et al. The social organization of sexuality: sexual practices in the United States. Chicago: The University of Chicago Press, 1994.
7. Feldman HA, Goldstein I, Hatzichristou DG, et al. Impotence and its medical and psychosocial correlates: results of the Massachusetts Male Aging Study. J Urol 1994;151:54.
8. Fagan PJ, Schmidt CW, Wise TN, et al. Sexual dysfunction and dual psychiatric diagnoses. Compr Psychol 1988;29:278.
9. Bolour S, Braunstein G. Testosterone therapy in women: a review. Int J Impot Res 2005;10:1.
10. Buster JE, Kingsberg SA, Davis SR, et al. Testosterone patch for low sexual desire in postmenopausal women: a randomized trial. Obstet Gynecol 2005;105:944.
11. Braunstein GD, Sundwall DA, Katz M, et al. Safety and efficacy of a testosterone patch for the treatment of hypoactive sexual desire disorder in surgically menopausal women: a randomized, placebo-controlled trial. Arch Intern Med 2005;165:1582.
12. Segraves RT, Croft H, Kavoussi R, et al. Bupropion sustained release (SR) for the treatment of hypoactive sexual desire disorder (HSDD) in nondepressed women. J Sex Marital Ther 2001;27:303.
13. Segraves RT, Clayton A, Croft H, et al. Bupropion sustained release for the treatment of hypoactive sexual desire disorder in premenopausal women. J Clin Psychopharmacol 2004;24:339.
14. Modelska K, Cummings S. Tibolone for postmenopausal women: systematic review of randomized trials. J Clin Endocrinol Metab 2002;87:16.
15. Laan E, Everaerd W. Determinants of female sexual arousal: psychological theory and data. Annu Rev Sex Res 1995;6:32.
16. Masters WH, Johnson VE. Human sexual inadequacy. New York: Little, Brown, 1970.
17. Caruso S, Intelisano G, Lupo L, et al. Premenopausal women affected by sexual arousal disorder treated with sildenafil: a double blind, cross-over, placebo-controlled study. Br J Obstet Gynecol 2001;108:623.
18. Berman JR, Berman L, Toler SM. Safety and efficacy of sildenafil citrate for the treatment of female arousal disorder: a double-blind, placebo controlled study. J Urol 2003;170:2333.
19. Modelska K, Cummings S. Female sexual dysfunction in postmenopausal women: systematic review of placebo controlled trials. Am J Obstet Gynecol 2003;188:286.
20. Rhodes JC, Kjerulff KH, Langenberg PW, et al. Hysterectomy and sexual functioning. JAMA 1999;282:1934.
21. O'Connell HE, Huston JM, Anderson CR, et al. Anatomical relationship between urethra and clitoris. J Urol 2001;156:1892.
22. Yang CC. Female sexual function in neurologic disease. J Sex Res 2000;37:205.
23. Barbach LG. For yourself: the fulfillment of female sexuality. New York: New American Library, 1991.
24. Heiman J, Lopiccolo J. Becoming orgasmic: a sexual and personal growth program for women. New York: Simon and Schuster, 1988.
25. Lopicollo J, Stock WE. Treatment of sexual dysfunction. J Consult Clin Psychol 1986;54: 158.
26. Montejo-Gonzalez AL, Llorca G, Izquierdo JA, et al. SSRI-induced sexual dysfunction: fluoxetine, paroxetine, sertraline, and fluvoxamine in a prospective, multicenter, and descriptive clinical study of 344 patients. J Sex Marital Ther 1997; 23:176.
27. Zajecka J. Strategies for the treatment of antidepressant-related sexual dysfunction. J Clin Psychol 2001;62[Suppl 3]:35.
28. Rothschild AJ. Selective serotonin reuptake inhibitor-induced sexual dysfunction: efficacy of a drug holiday. Am J Psychiatry 1995;152:1514.
29. Ashton AK, Mahmood A, Iqbal F. Improvements in SSRI/SNRI-induced sexual dysfunction by switching to escitalopram. J Sex Marital Ther 2005;31:257.
30. Binik YM, Meana M, Berkely K, et al. The sexual pain disorders: is the pain sexual or is the sex painful? Annu Rev Sex Res 1999;86:135.
31. Harlow BL, Stewart EG. A population-based assessment of chronic unexplained vulvar pain: have we underestimated the prevalence of vulvodynia? J Am Med Womens Assoc 2003;58:82.
32. Bornstein J, Lakovsky Y, Lavi I, et al. The classic approach to diagnosis of vulvovaginitis: a critical analysis. Infect Dis Obstet Gynecol 2001;9:105.
33. Marin MG, King R, Sfameni S, et al. Adverse behavioral and sexual factors in chronic vulvar disease. Am J Obstet Gynecol 2000;183:34.
34. Friedrich EG Jr. Vulvar vestibulitis syndrome. J Reprod Med 1987;32:110.
35. Reissing ED, Binik YM, Khalife S, et al. Etiological correlates of vaginismus: sexual and physical abuse, sexual knowledge, sexual self schema and relationship adjustment. J Sex Marital Ther 2003;29:47.
36. Reissing ED, Binik YM, Khalife S, et al. Vaginal spasm, pain and behavior: an empirical investigation of the diagnosis of vaginismus. Arch Sex Behav 2004;33:5.
37. Idama TO, Pring DW. Vaginal dilator therapy—an outpatient gynaecological option in the management of dyspareunia. J Obstet Gynaecol 2000;20:303.
38. Zukerman Z, Roslik Y, Orvieto R. Treatment of vaginismus with the Paula Garburg sphincter muscle exercises. Harefuah 2005;144:246,303.
39. Shehzad, B, Dobbs, A. Hypogonadism and androgen replacement therapy in elderly men. Am J Med 2001;110:563.
40. Morales A, Heaton JP, Carson CC. Andropause: a misnomer for a true clinical entity. J Urol 2000; 163:705.
41. Morales A, Buvat J, Gooren LJ. Endocrine aspects of men sexual dysfunction. In: Lue TF, Basson R, Rosen R, eds. Sexual medicine: sexual

*Bold numerals denote published controlled clinical trials, meta-analyses, or consensus-based recommendations.

dysfunctions in men and women. Paris: World Health Organization, 2004:345.
42. Harman SM, Metter EJ, Tobin JD, et al. Longitudinal effects of aging on serum total and free testosterone levels in healthy men: Baltimore longitudinal study of aging. J Clin Endocrinol Metab 2001;86:724.
43. Rosen RC, Cappelleri JC, Smith MD, et al. Development and evaluation of an abridged, 5-item version of the International Index of Erectile Function (IIEF-5) as a diagnostic tool for erectile dysfunction. Int J Impot Res 1999; 11:319.
44. NIH Consensus Conference. Impotence. NIH Consensus Development Panel on Impotence. JAMA 1993;270:83.
45. Viagra [package insert]. New York: Pfizer, 2003.
46. Levitra [package insert]. Research Triangle Park, NC: GlaxoSmithKline, 2004.
47. Cialis [package insert]. Indianapolis, IN: Lilly, 2005.
48. Goldstein I, Lue TF, Padma-Nathan H, et al. Oral sildenafil in the treatment of erectile dysfunction. Sildenafil Study Group. N Engl J Med 1998;338:1397.
49. Padma-Nathan H, Steers WD, Wicker PA. Efficacy and safety of oral sildenafil in the treatment of erectile dysfunction: a double-blind, placebo-controlled study of 329 patients. Sildenafil Study Group. Int J Clin Pract 1998;52:375.
50. Brock GB, McMahon CG, Chen KK, et al. Efficacy and safety of tadalafil for the treatment of erectile dysfunction: results of integrated analyses. J Urol 2002;168:1332.
51. Porst H, Rosen R, Padma-Nathan H, et al. The efficacy and tolerability of vardenafil, a new, oral, selective phosphodiesterase type 5 inhibitor, in patients with erectile dysfunction: the first at-home clinical trial. Int J Impot Res 2001;13:192.
52. Guay AT, Perez JB, Jacobson J, et al. Efficacy and safety of sildenafil citrate for treatment of erectile dysfunction in a population with associated organic risk factors. J Androl 2001;22:793.
53. Kostis JB, Jackson G, Rosen R, et al. Sexual dysfunction and cardiac risk (the Second Princeton Consensus Conference). Am J Cardiol 2005;96:313.
54. Montague DK, Barada JH, Belker AM, et al. Clinical guidelines panel on erectile dysfunction: summary report on the treatment of organic erectile dysfunction. The American Urological Association. J Urol 1996;156:2007.
55. Ernst E, Pittler MH. Yohimbine for erectile dysfunction: a systematic review and meta-analysis of randomized clinical trials. J Urol 1998;159:433.
56. Padma-Nathan H, Hellstrom WJ, Kaiser FE, et al. Treatment of men with erectile dysfunction with transurethral alprostadil. Medicated Urethral System for Erection (MUSE) Study Group. N Engl J Med 1997;336:1.
57. Hellstrom WJ, Bennett AH, Gesundheit N, et al. A double-blind, placebo-controlled evaluation of the erectile response to transurethral alprostadil. Urology 1996;48:851.
58. Lewis RW. Transurethral alprostadil with MUSE (medicated urethral system for erection) vs intracavernous alprostadil—a comparative study in 103 patients with erectile dysfunction. Int J Impot Res 1998;10:61.
59. Virag R. Intracavernous injection of papaverine for erectile failure. Lancet 1982;2:938.
60. Barada JH, McKimmy RM. Vasoactive pharmacotherapy. In: AH Bennett, ed. Impotence. Philadelphia: WB Saunders, 1994: 229.
61. Witherington R. Vacuum constriction device for management of erectile impotence. J Urol 1989;141:320.
62. Jonas U, Evans C, Krishnamurti S, et al. Surgical treatment and mechanical devices. In: Jardin A, Wagner G, Khoury S, et al, eds. Erectile dysfunction. Plymouth, UK: Health Publication, 1999:357.
63. Lewis RW. Long-term results of penile prosthetic implants. Urol Clin North Am 1995;22:847.
64. Screponi E, Carosa E, Di Stasi SM, et al. Prevalence of chronic prostatitis in men with premature ejaculation. Urology 2001;58:198.
65. El-Sakka AI. Premature ejaculation in non-insulin-dependent diabetic patients. Int J Androl 2003;26:329.
66. Choi HK, Jung GW, Moon KH, et al. Clinical study of SS-cream in patients with lifelong premature ejaculation. Urology 2000;55:257.
67. Vale J. Ejaculatory dysfunction. BJU Int 2001; 83:557.
68. Master VA, Turek PJ. Ejaculatory physiology and dysfunction. Urol Clin North Am 2001;28:363.
69. Green R. The "sissy boy syndrome" and the development of homosexuality. New Haven, CT: Yale University Press, 1987.
70. Costa PT, McRae RR. The NEO-PI-R: professional manual. Odessa, FL: Psychological Assessment Resources, 1992.
71. Kafka M. Psychopharmacologic treatments for nonparaphilic compulsive sexual behaviors. CNS Spectrums. In J Neuropsychiatric Med 2000;49.
72. Fergusson DM, Horwood LJ, Beautrais AL. Is sexual orientation related to mental health problems and suicidality in young people? Arch Gen Psychiatry 1999;56:876.
73. Herrell R, Goldberg J, True WR, et al. Sexual orientation and suicidality: a co-twin control study in adult men. Arch Gen Psychiatry 1999; 56:867.
74. Sandfort TG, de Graaf R, Bijl RV, et al. Same-sex sexual behavior and psychiatric disorders: findings from the Netherlands Mental Health Survey and Incidence Study (NEMESIS). Arch Gen Psychiatry 2001;58:85.
75. Dardick L, Grady KE. Openness between gay persons and health professionals. Ann Intern Med 1980;93:115.
76. White J, Levinson W. Primary care of lesbian patients. J Gen Intern Med 1993;8:41.
77. Kamel HK. Sexuality in aging: focus on institutionalized elderly. Ann Long Term Care 2001;9:64.
78. Johnson TC. Assessment of sexual behavior problems in preschool-aged and latency-aged children. Child Adolesc Psychiatr Clin N Am 1993;2:431.

For annotated ***General References*** *and resources related to this chapter, visit www.hopkinsbayview.org/PAMreferences.*

Chapter 7

Sleep Disorders

David N. Neubauer, Philip L. Smith, III, and Christopher J. Earley

EPIDEMIOLOGY AND OVERVIEW

Increasingly, disorders of sleep and wakefulness are being recognized as pervasive throughout our society. The magnitude of the public health implications was emphasized in a report of the National Commission on Sleep Disorders Research (1). It noted that about 40 million Americans have chronic sleep–wake disorders, and that many of those people are undiagnosed and untreated. The report also emphasized the vital role of primary care physicians in recognizing, treating, and helping to educate the vast majority of those patients experiencing symptoms related to their sleep–wake cycles. Even though sleep-related complaints are common in general medical practice, a Gallup survey (2) showed that only a small minority of sleep-disturbed people bring their concerns to the attention of their physicians.

The sleep disorders represent a wide spectrum of symptoms. The inability to sleep at the desired time and the inability to remain awake during appropriate hours make up the majority of patient concerns. Abnormal behaviors and movements also may be associated with sleep. The *International Classification of Sleep Disorders,* 2nd edition (ICSD-2) (3), developed by the American Academy of Sleep Medicine in collaboration with other international sleep associations, reflects 7 major categories of sleep disorders and nearly 70 individual diagnoses. The major categories are insomnia, sleep-related breathing disorder, hypersomnia of central origin, circadian rhythm sleep disorder, parasomnias, sleep-related movement disorders, isolated symptoms, apparently normal variants, and unresolved issues, and other sleep disorder.

Appropriate diagnosis and effective treatment of sleep disorders can result in significant improvement in quality of life for patients. In addition, it may allow a reduction in the morbidity and mortality associated with excessive sleepiness, and help avert consequences of persistent insufficient sleep. An exploration of sleep–wake patterns and possible sleep disorders is an important component of any general review of systems. Sleep disturbances can exacerbate other medical conditions, and, conversely, many medical illnesses and medications can affect sleep patterns.

BASIC SLEEP PHYSIOLOGY

Daytime alertness and nighttime sleepiness are natural drives for most people leading normal lives. The fundamental sleep–wake cycle is maintained by at least two physiologically distinct control processes:

The *homeostatic mechanism* represents the balance between wake and sleep time over several days. This time balance varies greatly with species, but for adult humans is set at about one third sleep and two thirds waking. Sleep deprivation leads to increased sleepiness; however, the relationship is not exactly linear. Many people have had the experience of getting a second wind of alertness the morning after a night without sleep. This phenomenon is caused by the prominent circadian rhythm driving sleepiness and alertness.

The *circadian oscillator* establishes a sleep propensity variation over the normal 24-hour day. This oscillator also modulates core temperature and the activity levels of a large number of physiologic functions (e.g., certain neurotransmitters and hormone levels). Without time cues, especially the day–night, light–dark cycle, this circadian mechanism has a periodicity slightly greater than 24 hours and therefore must be reset daily. Light exposure during the daytime and darkness at night synchronize the rhythm. Neural pathways including the retina, suprachiasmatic nucleus, and pineal gland are well established, and these mechanisms promote the cycle of sleepiness and alertness and usually are in stable harmony. Although homeostatic sleepiness increases throughout the day, circadian alertness peaks in the evening. Under normal circumstances these rhythms allow one to remain alert for 16 hours and then fall asleep rapidly at one's habitual bedtime.

Normal sleep includes two major physiologically distinct states: *rapid eye movement* (REM) sleep and *nonrapid eye movement* (NREM) sleep. Initially, sleep may consist of the four successively deeper stages of NREM sleep. During each of these four stages, there is decreased fluctuation in heart rate, blood pressure, and respiration. This contrasts with REM sleep, where greater lability is noted. The presleep wake stage and the NREM sleep stages have additional distinctive clinical and electroencephalographic (EEG) characteristics.

- Presleep Wake Stage (Sleep Latency Period). As a person begins to fall asleep, eye blinks, limb movements, and moderate tone in skeletal muscles are accompanied by either low-voltage, mixed-frequency EEG signals or the characteristic alpha pattern (basic posterior rhythm).
- Stage 1. This represents light sleep with slow, rolling, eye movements. The alpha pattern disappears with lower frequency and usually higher voltage than the wake EEG. Sudden limb jerks normally may occur episodically, particularly during early stage 1 sleep.
- Stage 2. Eye movements become infrequent or absent and muscle tone usually is reduced. The EEG shows the stage-defining sleep spindle bursts, vertex sharp waves, K complexes, and some slow waveforms.
- Stages 3 and 4. EEG high-voltage, slow-wave activity predominates. These stages are defined according to the percentage of slow-wave activity present. Muscle tone is variable. Arousal is difficult from these deeper sleep stages.
- Rapid Eye Movement Sleep. At 1 to 2 hours after sleep onset, the first period of REM sleep occurs, with a characteristic marked decrease in muscle tone and bursts of rapid eye movements. During REM sleep there is a paralysis of major skeletal muscles punctuated by occasional episodes of muscle twitches. Hypercapnic and hypoxic respiratory drives are decreased, thermoregulation is decreased, heart rate and blood pressure are extremely variable, and penile erections occur. Dreaming is also most closely related to REM sleep, but it may occur, usually less vividly, at other times.

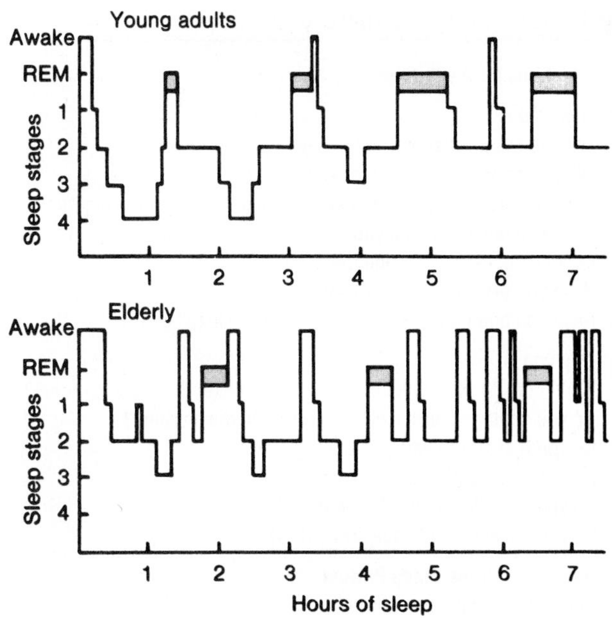

FIGURE 7.1. Normal sleep cycles in healthy young and elderly subjects.

On a typical night, a subject passes through three to five cycles of NREM and REM sleep. Figure 7.1 shows characteristic sleep patterns for healthy young adults and elderly people. With aging, there generally is a decrease in slow-wave sleep (stages 3 and 4), with an earlier sleep onset and waking time and more frequent awakenings during the night. The apparently decreased arousal threshold in older people is the most prominent difference between sleep at age 50 years and that at age 80 years. During the day, young adults require 10 to 15 minutes to fall asleep for a nap; older adults fall asleep more easily. As discussed later in the next section, Table 7.1, and subsequent sections on specific disorders, the recognition and deviations from the normal sleep cycles are helpful at times in establishing the correct diagnosis for a sleep disorder.

CLINICAL PRESENTATIONS OF SLEEP DISORDERS

The full evaluation of sleep complaints requires a general consideration of the patient's sleep–wake cycle, as well as specific questions that focus on the presenting symptoms. Table 7.1 lists questions that may yield information to support a diagnostic hypothesis.

INSOMNIA

Insomnia is the perception of not sleeping well, and it is the most common sleep complaint. It is estimated that 10% to 15% of the U.S. adult population have frequent

TABLE 7.1 Sleep History

Questions for the Patient
Nighttime
When do you get sleepy in the evening?
What time do you attempt to fall asleep?
How long do you believe it takes you to fall asleep most nights?
Once you fall asleep, do you sleep soundly through the night?
Do you feel restless during the evening?
Have you been told that you snore?
Have you been told that you move in your sleep?
Daytime
What time do you awaken (work days, weekends, and vacations)?
Do you need an alarm clock to awaken in the morning?
Do you feel rested when you get up?
Are you tired during the daytime?
Do you nap? (What time? How long?)
Do you fall asleep at undesired times?
Questions for the Sleep Partner
Does your bed partner snore?
Does your bed partner seem to stop breathing at times?
Does your bed partner kick or jerk his or her legs during sleep?

or chronic difficulty with insomnia. Almost everyone experiences some degree of insomnia during his or her lifetime. Moreover, people of all ages may experience disrupted sleep; there is a general increase in frequency with age. Men and women are affected equally until middle age. From their mid-forties on, women are much more likely to complain of difficulty sleeping (2).

Insomnia may involve difficulty falling asleep, awakening too early, or experiencing disrupted sleep throughout the night. The presentation also may include the report of unrefreshing sleep. Often, the patient complains of fatigue, poor concentration, and low productivity. In properly diagnosing complaints of poor sleep, it is important to realize that insomnia is a symptom that may result from a wide variety of processes. An essential initial consideration is the duration of the disturbance.

Episodes of insomnia may be acute or chronic. They may be described in terms of the timing of the sleep disturbance (e.g., initiating and maintaining sleep), duration, severity, and pattern over time. For some patients insomnia is a nightly problem. For others, disrupted sleep may be seemingly random or predictable, as with premenstrual insomnia, travel, or with anxiety on Sunday nights in anticipation of the work week. The ICSD-2 includes an Adjustment Insomnia diagnosis to represent the acute response to an identifiable stressor. Several different diagnoses may be associated with chronic insomnia, which generally is considered to be at least 1 month in duration. An initial precipitant often is recognizable in the history, but other perpetuating factors may promote the persistent symptoms (4). Complaints of marked sleep difficulty that have

TABLE 7.2 Causes of Chronic Insomnia

Poor sleep hygiene and behavioral patterns
Circadian rhythm disturbances
Psychiatric disorders
Medical and neurologic illnesses
Sleep disorders (e.g., sleep-disordered breathing)
Medications
Substance abuse
Environmental factors

continued for several years are not uncommon. Although the cause of chronic insomnia is often multifactorial, it is useful to consider the individual factors that may be associated with long-standing symptoms (Table 7.2).

Most *psychiatric disorders* can cause disturbed sleep. Symptoms of depression and anxiety often are associated with insomnia and may be precipitating and perpetuating causes. Early morning awakening is a characteristic of major depressive disorder; however, difficulties falling and staying asleep commonly are present as well. Difficulty sleeping is typical of patients with generalized anxiety disorder, posttraumatic stress disorder, panic disorder, schizophrenia, personality disorders, and dementia. Acute sleep changes often are seen with adjustment disorders. Each of these psychiatric disorders is described in detail in Section 3 of this book.

A broad range of *physical conditions* can cause difficulty sleeping. Pain and discomfort are common factors; however, other pathophysiologic processes may play important contributory roles. The more common medical problems associated with chronic insomnia are arthritic disorders; peptic ulcer disease and gastroesophageal reflux; asthma and chronic obstructive pulmonary disease; cardiovascular disease; hyperthyroidism; and renal failure. Orthopnea and nocturia cause fragmented sleep. Patients with fibromyalgia (see Chapter 74) often complain of unrefreshing sleep. Insomnia is common during normal physiologic stress such as pregnancy, especially during the first and third trimesters.

Among the *neurologic disorders* more commonly associated with insomnia are Parkinson disease and other movement disorders, stroke, epilepsy, and cerebral degenerative processes. Head trauma can cause long-standing sleep disturbance.

Several hundred *medications* can cause insomnia. Stimulants, ranging from caffeine to amphetamines, predictably decrease the ability to sleep. Correspondingly, withdrawal from sedating medications, including hypnotics, can be associated with a temporary sleep disruption. Bronchodilators, corticosteroids, and some antihypertensives, antiarrhythmics, calcium channel blockers, antiparkinson agents, anticonvulsants, antidepressants, and nonsteroidal anti-inflammatory drugs can cause insomnia. It is important to consider over-the-counter preparations as causes of disrupted sleep, particularly diet and cold and allergy products, because they may contain stimulating compounds such as caffeine.

Substance abuse can promote acute and chronic disturbances of sleep. Cocaine and other stimulants inhibit or fragment sleep. Paradoxically, narcotics such as heroin and morphine can have arousing effects that disturb sleep. The acute sedating effect of alcohol is well known; however, although sleep onset may be enhanced, the withdrawal-related catecholamine release often causes sleep disruption. This may occur after a single episode of moderate drinking. Heavier drinking can impair sleep markedly. Symptoms may persist during months to years of abstinence.

The influence of *circadian rhythms* on the sleep–wake cycle becomes apparent (usually transiently) with acute changes in the sleep schedule. Rapid transmeridian travel causes symptoms of jet lag, and changes in shift-work schedules may promote acutely disturbed sleep. Constantly changing work shifts or permanent night work schedules often inhibit effective entrainment and thereby cause chronic insomnia.

Delayed sleep phase syndrome is a disorder of circadian rhythms characterized by difficulty attaining sleep until about 3 to 6 a.m. Affected individuals tend to sleep until late morning or into the afternoon. Occupational or educational requirements may demand a more socially acceptable wake-up time that effectively truncates the sleep period and causes chronic sleep insufficiency. These people feel out of synchronization with the rest of society and usually come to the physician because of their inability to fall asleep at a more conventional hour. At the opposite end of the spectrum are people with *advanced sleep phase syndrome* who may experience sleepiness from 6 p.m. until 2 a.m., then complain of an inability to remain asleep throughout the night. Generally, the delayed pattern is more common among young people, whereas the advanced pattern occurs more often in the elderly. A rare circadian rhythm disturbance occurs in certain completely sightless people who are not entrained to a 24-hour cycle. They move in and out of phase with the day–night cycle and therefore have periodic symptoms of insomnia every few weeks.

Symptoms of insomnia may be associated with other sleep disorders in which the primary problems are breathing irregularity or excessive body muscle movements during sleep (see later discussions).

Consideration of the *sleeping environment* is an important component of the evaluation of patients with insomnia. Excessive light or disruptive noise can be arousing. Living near an airport or another source of loud noise may be detrimental to sleep in vulnerable patients. Temperature extremes can disrupt sleep continuity. Discomfort in bed may result from a poor mattress or a snoring bed partner. Household and neighborhood characteristics (e.g., loud televisions, city noises) also may be significant. A sense of insecurity or fear may promote sleeplessness.

TABLE 7.3 Sleep Hygiene Measures

Try to maintain a regular sleep–wake schedule. It is particularly important to get up at about the same time every day.
Avoid afternoon or evening napping if you have difficulty getting to sleep at night.
Allow yourself enough time in bed for adequate sleep duration (e.g., 11 p.m. to 7 a.m.).
Develop a relaxing evening routine for the hours as bedtime approaches.
Spend some idle time reflecting on the day's events before going to bed. Make a list of concerns and how some might be resolved.
Reserve the bed for sleep and sex. Do not do homework, pay bills, or engage in serious domestic discussions in bed.
Avoid evening alcohol.
Avoid caffeine in the afternoon and evening.
Minimize annoying noise, light, or temperature extremes.
Consider a light snack before bedtime.
Exercise regularly, but not late in the evening.
Do not try harder and harder to fall asleep. If you are unable to sleep, do something else out of bed and in another room, if possible.
Avoid smoking.

Issues related to sleep hygiene (Table 7.3) are important for all patients with insomnia complaints. Even when there is another reason that sleep is disturbed, behavioral patterns that affect sleep commonly play a role in perpetuating the disorder. Irregularity of bedtime and wake time may undermine the underlying circadian drive for sleepiness and alertness at the appropriate hours. Patients may have unrealistic expectations of their ability to change their sleep schedule markedly and then sleep effectively. Some patients nap in the daytime to make up for lost nighttime sleep and thereby further diminish their propensity to fall asleep at the desired hour.

Chronic insomniacs may spend excessive amounts of time in bed in the hope of maximizing their total sleep time, thereby further fragmenting their sleep. Remaining in bed during extended sleepless periods may reinforce the association between being in bed and being awake. Often, frustration and anxiety are integral to this repeated experience and further prolong wakefulness. Subsequently, sleep becomes less attainable.

In *psychophysiologic insomnia*, perpetuating factors predominate after the initial stimulating precipitants have subsided. A conditioned pattern of anxiety and tension has become established. The patient may report increasing tiredness during the evening but tortured wakefulness on getting in bed. Alternatively, what might have been a minor nighttime awakening becomes an exaggerated emotional response that further inhibits a rapid return to sleep.

TABLE 7.4 Complaints Associated with Excessive Daytime Sleepiness

Sleepiness
Tiredness, fatigue
Poor concentration
Forgetfulness
Decreased motivation
Irritability
Depressed mood
Workplace mistakes
Vehicular accidents or near-accidents

In summary, the history may identify one or more precipitating or perpetuating conditions that promote chronic insomnia. Practical approaches to the management of these conditions are described later in this chapter (see Management of Sleep Disorders).

EXCESSIVE DAYTIME SLEEPINESS

Clinical Features

Up to 5% of the population has problems with excessive daytime sleepiness (EDS) or related symptoms (Table 7.4). The younger and older age groups tend to experience more EDS than the middle-age group. Also, shift workers complain more of being tired and of various other problems associated with EDS than do nonshift workers. Some people do not perceive that their problems are sleep-related and therefore may not mention being sleepy during the day. The degree or severity of reported sleepiness can be judged by identifying which situations are most likely to produce sleep, by determining how often and how pervasively sleepiness occurs throughout the day, and by learning how disruptive this situation is to family, job, and personal well-being.

In determining the severity of sleepiness, one needs to ask patients under what conditions they are most likely to fall asleep. Table 7.5 classifies sleepiness severity according to the situations in which sleep may occur. If the situations listed are not associated with falling asleep, it is unlikely that EDS is the problem. If patients awaken from sleep feeling tired, they should be questioned further about their nighttime sleep habits. Patients' perceptions of sleepiness vary and depend on the environment, level of activity, and degree of motivation. Sitting in a dark room or listening to an uninteresting lecture may unmask sleepiness. Some individuals may be so busy and active all day that they have no sense of tiredness despite the fact they have not slept in more than 36 hours. As noted in Table 7.4, such people may not complain of being tired but may have problems with concentration or stamina. They may be fatigable or forgetful or have decreased motivation. They may have accidents either on the job or on the highway. Their job performance may suffer. Increased irritability or depression may be noted by family or friends.

TABLE 7.5 Sleepiness Severity

Severity	*Falls Asleep While*
Mild	Watching television
	Reading
	Attending lectures
	Riding in a car
	Sitting in church
Moderate	Socializing with family and friends
	Working
	Driving for an extended time
Severe	Driving locally or at a stop light
	Having a conversation
	Eating a meal

Animal and human studies show that with insufficient sleep, the EEG identifies brief but frequent disturbances in the ongoing wakeful state. If frequent, these brief intrusions may lead to inattention and poor concentration before sleepiness is perceived. The problems of EDS often are insidious. However, EDS can be identified by appropriately questioning the patient.

Differential Diagnosis

Once it is established that the patient has EDS, the cause must be identified. One first needs to determine whether drugs (e.g., alcohol, benzodiazepines, antidepressants, antipsychotics, antihistamines, some antihypertensive drugs) or medical conditions (e.g., chronic renal failure, cirrhosis, hypothyroidism) might be the cause of the EDS. After considering these causes, one should attempt to identify patients with disturbed nocturnal sleep. Disorders that are likely to cause sleep disruption and therefore EDS were discussed earlier (see Insomnia). Chronic insufficient sleep, chronic fatigue, narcolepsy, and idiopathic hypersomnia are discussed in this section; the sleep apneas are discussed in the next section.

A common cause of transient daytime fatigue is cessation of caffeine consumption (5). The *caffeine withdrawal syndrome* may occur after the discontinuation of even relatively low daily amounts of caffeine, such as 100 mg from one cup of coffee or two to three sodas. Withdrawal effects are more likely at higher doses but can occur after short-term use. The average daily caffeine consumption in adults in the United States is about 250 to 300 mg. Because caffeine use is so widespread, it often is not considered as influencing alertness, sleepiness, and fatigue. The caffeine withdrawal syndrome typically evolves over 12 to 24 hours, and it can persist for several days. It is alleviated by resumed caffeine consumption, even at considerably lower levels. The withdrawal effects can be minimized with a gradual reduction in the daily intake. Aside from fatigue, caffeine withdrawal most typically is associated with headache. Other effects may include irritability, nausea, and flulike symptoms.

Chronic Insufficient Sleep

The most common cause of EDS is chronic insufficient sleep. The primary problem is that patients do not achieve enough sleep to satisfy their body's requirement. The most common causes are personal lifestyles (e.g., shift workers, medical/surgical residents) and poor sleep habits (e.g., watching television until midnight and then getting up for work at 6 a.m.). Such individuals rarely have problems falling asleep or staying asleep. They may wake up feeling tired and may have symptoms of EDS. A detailed history of the amount of sleep per night over the past several months is important. If someone is getting 7 hours of sleep each night and is still tired, 8 or 9 hours may be needed. Questioning patients about weekend or holiday patterns of sleep, or about how they slept when they were younger or had a different lifestyle, may help to determine what the normal amount of sleep is for them. To establish the diagnosis and treat the problem, an 8-hour sleeping pattern must be established. Patients need to *keep a written record* of when they go to sleep (not when they go to bed but when they think they fall asleep) and when they awaken. The record should be completed for at least 1 month, after which the patient, with the diary in hand, should return for reassessment. If the patient is feeling better after the forced 8-hour sleep schedule, the diagnosis of chronic insufficient sleep is established. If the patient still complains of EDS and the diary indicates 8 or more hours of sleep per night, a referral to a sleep specialist should be offered.

Chronic Fatigue

Psychiatric disorders, especially depression and certain life events (e.g., death of family member, divorce, job loss, marital discord) often are associated with insomnia. Occasionally there is no clear-cut insomnia but only what appears to be symptoms of EDS. The patient may complain of increased fatigue, lack of motivation, poor concentration, or feeling tired all the time. These patients may sleep in the afternoon, but if they consistently sleep for long periods during the day, they invariably will have disturbed sleep at night and thus experience insomnia. The severity of sleepiness (Table 7.5) is important in differentiating fatigue from sleepiness. Although there may be complaints of tiredness, often there are no clear and consistent episodes of falling asleep. More often, the complaints are more severe than the actual degree of reported sleepiness. Finally, when lack of motivation overshadows all other complaints, one should consider chronic fatigue syndrome (see Chapter 58) or depression (see Chapter 24). There is no defined treatment for chronic fatigue other than treating the underlying problem. If a clear distinction between sleepiness and fatigue cannot be made, referral to a sleep specialist is appropriate.

Narcolepsy

The prevalence of narcolepsy in the United States is approximately 0.05% to 0.09%. The disorder may start in childhood, but the peak incidence is in the second decade. The diagnosis can be made on clinical grounds; however, a daytime sleep laboratory study (the multiple sleep latency test [MSLT], see Patient Experience) may be valuable when the clinical picture is not clear. Objective support for the diagnosis of narcolepsy is established by an average sleep latency on the MSLT of less than 5 minutes and the presence of two or more naps with REM activity (6). Normal results from this testing include an average sleep latency period of longer than 15 minutes and no REM sleep during these brief daytime naps.

Several clinical features constitute the syndrome of narcolepsy (Table 7.6). The most common of these are problems of attention and concentration and episodes of falling asleep. People with narcolepsy often have little difficulty related to sleepiness when they are physically active. It is when they are engaged in sedentary activities and repetitive or boring tasks that they experience great problems with attention and concentration and uncontrolled bouts of sleepiness. The degree of inattention may be so severe that the individual carries out complex tasks (e.g., driving) but has no recollection of the behaviors. This phenomenon, referred to as an *automatic behavior*, is rarely associated with other disorders. In contrast to individuals who have chronic sleep insufficiency, those with narcolepsy usually benefit greatly from brief naps.

Cataplexy and sleep paralysis are present in some patients with narcolepsy. Both of these conditions are

TABLE 7.6 Clinical Features of Narcolepsy

Altered Levels of Alertness and Attentiveness
Sleepiness
Poor concentration
Memory difficulty
Automatic behavior
Blurred or poorly focused vision
REM-Related Disturbances
Cataplexy
Sleep paralysis
Hypnagogic hallucinations
Sleep Disturbance
Frequent awakenings
Vivid dreams
Sleep terrors

REM, rapid eye movement sleep.

associated with paralysis in the context of full consciousness. Cataplexy occurs only with narcolepsy. Accordingly, a history of cataplexy and excessive daytime sleepiness leads to the diagnosis of narcolepsy. Cataplexy occurs when the patient is awake and is characterized by a sudden onset of paralysis precipitated by an acute emotional response. Although fear, anger, and excitement can cause a cataplexy, the most reliable historical indicator is its occurrence during laughter. Cataplexy can affect any muscle group in the face, trunk, or limbs but is symmetric in its effect. The simplest type of cataplexy is a drop of the jaw, which can affect speech, and cataplexy may make it difficult to hold one's head up for several minutes. However, the most dramatic are the episodes associated with loss of tone throughout the postural musculature. As the episode evolves, those experiencing cataplexy usually are able to lower themselves to a chair or to the floor, but injury may occur. There is full alertness during these episodes, but occasionally a patient falls asleep during the cataplexy. In general, cataplexy resolves spontaneously within a few minutes.

Sleep paralysis occurs just before falling asleep or just after awakening. The patient cannot move and usually cannot speak, but breathing is undisturbed. There may be a high degree of anxiety or terrifying hallucinations. The paralysis lasts seconds or minutes and resolves spontaneously. Because sleep paralysis can occur alone as an idiopathic condition, it does not confirm the presence of narcolepsy. In fact, sleep paralysis is more likely to be seen in patients who are chronically deprived of sleep.

Another cardinal feature of narcolepsy is *hallucinations*. These are vivid and sometimes very realistic sensory experiences that occur before one falls asleep (hypnagogic) or on awakening (hypnopompic). The experiences may be in any sensory modality (e.g., visual, auditory, tactile) and may range from simple to complex in presentation. For example, there may be a sense of something crawling on the legs, a well-formed visual hallucination, or an out-of-body experience. The phenomenon is comparable to dreaming with one's eyes open and being fully alert. Some patients have hypnagogic hallucinations and no other components of the narcolepsy syndrome.

Disturbed nocturnal sleep often is seen with narcolepsy. The most common complaint is that after sleeping for 3 to 4 hours, the patient awakens fully alert. After about 45 to 60 minutes, the patient again becomes tired and falls back to sleep. Sometimes there are multiple awakenings throughout the night. Patients may experience vivid dreams or hallucinations with these awakenings. The vivid dreams can be terrifying and nightmarish in content. The patient starts the day tired and unrested, which only worsens the underlying daytime problems. The management of narcolepsy is described later (see Management of Sleep Disorders).

Idiopathic Hypersomnia

This syndrome manifests as excessive daytime sleepiness; however, the REM-related clinical features seen with narcolepsy (Table 7.6) are absent. The symptoms are similar to those experienced by anyone who has chronic sleep insufficiency; however, these individuals sleep much more. They wake up tired and remain tired. Often they are very difficult to arouse and, when awake, may stumble around in a semistuporous state, which is referred to as sleep drunkenness. In contrast to narcolepsy, naps are long and unrefreshing. Daytime sleep studies (see discussion of the MSLT under Patient Experience) demonstrate very short sleep latencies, similar to narcolepsy, without REM episodes. The management of idiopathic hypersomnia is described later (see Management of Sleep Disorders).

SLEEP-DISORDERED BREATHING (SLEEP APNEA)

The sleep apneas are relatively common disorders that involve physiologic and psychological functioning with profound potential consequences. They are characterized by breathing abnormalities that vary from reduction (hypopnea) to complete cessation (apnea) of airflow associated with either an arousal or desaturation in blood oxyhemoglobin, or both. The sleep apneas include central apnea that is associated with cessation of respiratory effort, and obstructive apnea that is associated with occlusion of the upper airway and continued respiratory effort. The number of apneas and hypopneas are collated as the number of events per hour of sleep and are reported in various forms, such as the apnea–hypopnea index (AHI), the sleep-disordered breathing (SDB) index, or the respiratory disturbance index (RDI). The assessment of patients with nonapneic snoring is described in Chapter 111.

Epidemiology

A 1993 study of working men and women 30 to 60 years old reported a prevalence of clinically significant SDB of 9% among women and 24% among men (7). The authors estimated that approximately 2% of the women and 4% of the men met criteria for the sleep apnea syndrome. The prevalence may even be higher among obese people. Because of increased public awareness and the availability of diagnostic facilities, breathing problems during sleep are now being recognized in the very young and very old.

The typical patient who presents with *obstructive sleep apnea* is a middle-aged, mild to moderately obese man. However, it is important to recognize that severe obstructive sleep apnea may be diagnosed in individuals of all ages and body types. Obstructive apneas occasionally are associated with specific abnormalities of the upper airway

TABLE 7.7 Disorders Associated with Sleep-Disordered Breathing

Obstructive sleep apnea
Upper airway abnormalities
Oral (tonsillar hypertrophy, acromegaly)
Bony (micrognathia)
Medical conditions
Obesity
Cardiovascular (congestive heart failure)
Renal failure, dialysis
Acquired immunodeficiency syndrome
Hypothyroidism
Steroid treatment
Central sleep apnea
Cerebral disorder (stroke)
Brainstem–spinal disorder (polio, infarction, neoplasia, surgery)
Congestive heart failure (increased circulation time)

or with various medical conditions (Table 7.7). In general, patients with medical disorders that contribute to the development of obstructive SDB demonstrate overt symptoms and signs of their underlying medical problem. For example, patients with cardiomyopathy present with typical signs of severe congestive heart failure and a reduced ejection fraction on echocardiogram. Patients with renal failure and SDB are usually on dialysis. There are exceptions to this general rule. Patients with hypothyroidism often go undetected because their complaints of fatigue and sleepiness are ignored. Importantly, obesity (body mass index [BMI] $\geq$30), and even mild obesity (BMI of 26 to 30), continues to be recognized as the major contributor to the development of sleep apnea. This is especially true with adiposity of the visceral (truncal) distribution that is frequently seen in patients taking steroids or on highly active antiretroviral therapy.

In contrast with obstructive sleep apnea, *central sleep apnea* occurs most commonly in infants or patients older than 65 years of age (8). Central apnea may occur as a result of major cerebral disease, brainstem and spinal disorders, or cardiovascular disease (Table 7.7). The Cheyne-Stokes respiratory pattern is one example of central sleep apnea.

Presentation

Characteristically, patients with obstructive SDB present with significant snoring, or daytime hypersomnolence, or both (9). The snoring is loud, intermittent, and often punctuated by respiratory efforts unaccompanied by obvious airflow. A *bed partner* may observe that the apneas are associated with a struggling effort (obstructive apnea) or a lack of effort (central apnea). Because apnea, or any form of periodic breathing, usually is associated with both oxyhemoglobin desaturation and a brief arousal, sleep becomes fragmented and leads to daytime sleepiness. Initially, the patient may experience a subtle decrease in alertness toward the end of the day or when engaged in sedentary activities. As the apnea progresses in severity because of weight gain or age, more obvious signs of hypersomnolence, such as napping in the daytime, difficulties driving a car, and even severe sleepiness during normal waking activities, may occur (Table 7.5). Because most patients are unaware of their breathing pattern and often underestimate the severity of daytime hypersomnolence, it is essential that a bed partner or other observer be questioned regarding the patient in whom sleep apnea is suspected. Additional clinical features, such as choking or gasping episodes at night, evidence of systemic or pulmonary hypertension, and, in severe cases, cor pulmonale, may also suggest the underlying diagnosis. In general, the presenting symptoms of patients with both obstructive and central apnea are indistinguishable.

The *physical examination* usually is not diagnostic in patients with obstructive apnea, although patients with narrowing of the upper airway are at significantly higher risk. In particular, sleep-disordered breathing should be suspected in children and adults who demonstrate a compatible history and marked tonsillar hypertrophy or retrognathia. The BMI should be calculated and recorded (see Chapter 83), because visual estimation of whether someone is overweight or obese will lead to significant underestimation of the severity of obesity and the risk of the disorder. In elderly patients with *central sleep apnea*, the physical examination is normal, whereas patients with neurologic or cardiovascular pathology usually demonstrate obvious localizing neurologic signs (e.g., stroke) or cardiomegaly.

Course

The course of obstructive SDB is chronic and progressive because of the typical weight gain seen in a sedentary, aging population. Some patients develop progressive cardiopulmonary decompensation manifested by worsening hypercarbia and hypoxemia, which can be associated with cor pulmonale and life-threatening arrhythmias (10). Nevertheless, these complications are the exception and tend to occur in the severely obese patients (BMI >40) after many years of disease. By contrast, the course of central apnea is determined by the underlying pathologic process. Thus, if reversible central nervous system or cardiovascular disease exists, central apnea may resolve entirely. In normal elderly patients with central apnea, the course and prognosis are unknown.

Diagnosis

A working diagnosis of SDB can be made by direct observation of the patient during sleep, either at home or in a general hospital. However, even with ideal observation, clinically significant apnea may not be appreciated. The occurrence of five or more SDB events per hour constitutes an abnormal number of events. Although an SDB rate of more than five events per hour and daytime sleepiness are the minimal criteria that define the sleep apnea syndrome, there is good evidence that the sleepiness is correlated with the severity of the SDB rate and the degree of hypoxemia (11). Definitive diagnosis requires a sleep study (see Patient Experience) that quantitates the severity of SDB, including the degree of desaturations and the alteration in sleep architecture.

Other screening laboratory studies, such as determination of arterial blood gases and routine pulmonary function studies, provide information about mechanical abnormalities or problems with waking gas exchange that may be useful in therapy but not in diagnosis. Awake flow-volume curves (see Fig. 60.2) may demonstrate fluttering during expiration associated with evidence of variable extrathoracic obstruction in patients with obstructive apnea. However, this test is neither specific nor sensitive; consequently, it is not recommended for screening purposes. Home monitoring of arterial oxygen saturation (SaO_2) appears to be specific but not sensitive in the detection of sleep-disordered breathing. Although computed tomography or magnetic resonance imaging may demonstrate narrowing of the upper airway in patients with obstructive sleep apnea, it is presently unclear how this information can best be used in management. The management of SDB is described later (see Management of Sleep Disorders).

RESTLESS LEGS SYNDROME AND PERIODIC LEG MOVEMENTS IN SLEEP

Restless legs syndrome (RLS) is a disorder of sensation of unknown etiology. It occurs in 2% to 5% of the adult population, and in 10% to 15% of individuals 65 years of age or older. The prevalence is increased in conditions of iron deficiency, pregnancy, chronic renal failure, or peripheral neuropathy. It may be induced or aggravated by dopamine antagonists.

RLS is a clinical diagnosis based on the following criteria. First, there is a sensation that usually is characterized as a deep, uncomfortable feeling that occurs in one or both legs, either independently or concomitantly. Occasionally the sensation additionally involves the hands, arms, or trunk. The feeling may be reported as "aching," as "something moving," as "little insects," as "crazy legs," or in other ways. The description of the feeling is highly variable but is usually not that of pain. If pain is a prominent component, an alternative or coexisting disorder is suggested, such as a neuropathy. Along with the deep, uneasy feeling is a compulsion or urge to move. The urge to move may be so strong that the legs will seemingly jump on their own. Therefore, the patient is constantly moving or rubbing the legs or walking to relieve the sensation. The second feature is that the sensation is brought on with sitting or lying. Third, the uncomfortable sensation is relieved with movement and should be absent during walking. The sensation may return as soon as the individual sits or lies down again. Fourth, the sensation is the worst in the late evening or at bedtime. Typically, it is not present during the early morning. However, as the disorder progresses with time, symptoms appear earlier in the daytime, sometimes to the point that RLS symptoms exist throughout the day. Most commonly, the symptoms appear as soon as the person tries to relax in the late evening or gets into bed at night. Because of this sensory disturbance, the affected person cannot rest comfortably. Travel by any means is not possible if the person's ability to move is limited. Patients commonly cannot relax long enough to sit through a movie or to read without having to shuffle or pace compulsively. At night, the sensation can prevent sleep. Some patients spend several hours at night pacing until exhaustion induces sleep.

An associated component of RLS is the presence of semi-involuntary leg movements while awake or semirhythmic leg movements during sleep. When observing the patient during sleep, brief leg and foot movements occur periodically. The leg movements are called periodic leg movements of sleep (PLMS), and occur in association with many other conditions (Table 7.8). Occasionally, PLMS occur in the absence RLS symptoms and an obvious medical condition. Under these circumstances, the condition is referred to as periodic leg movement disorder (PLMD) and is considered a variant of RLS. The periodic leg movements may cause significant repeated arousals from sleep. The patient usually is unaware of the arousals and complains of awakening feeling tired and of being excessively sleepy during the day. Sometimes the leg kicks cause a complete awakening several times throughout the night, even though patients rarely recognize that the leg movements are the cause.

RLS is diagnosed on the basis of the clinical history, whereas PLMS is identified either by the history given by the bed partner or by polysomnographic recording (see Patient Experience). The polysomnographic recording is

TABLE 7.8 Causes of Periodic Limb Movements of Sleep

Restless legs syndrome
Sleep-disordered breathing
Antidepressant medications
Aging
Neurodegenerative disorders
Narcolepsy
Idiopathic periodic leg movement disorder (PLMD)

needed to make the diagnosis of PLMS or PLMD, but not RLS. The deep, uneasy feelings of RLS must be differentiated from arthralgia, myalgia, or sensory neuropathy. The absence of frank pain, the history of relief with movement, the compulsion to move, and normal results on neurologic, muscle, and joint examination help in the differential diagnosis. The presence of an initial sensory component and the voluntary nature of the movements should differentiate the secondary movements of RLS from those of myoclonus or dyskinesia. Nocturnal seizures, sleep-related dystonia, myoclonus, sleep apnea, primary insomnia, and PLMS are part of the differential diagnosis when a patient presents with a history of disturbed sleep associated with movements during sleep. If the clinical history is insufficient to establish the diagnosis, the patient should be referred to a sleep disorder clinic. The management of RLS is described later (see Management of Sleep Disorders).

ABNORMAL BEHAVIORS EMANATING FROM SLEEP (PARASOMNIAS)

Restful sleep may be punctuated by behaviors that may or may not awaken the patient. Sleep-related behaviors usually can be divided into the slow-wave sleep and REM-associated symptom complexes. *Nocturnal enuresis*, discussed below under Enuresis, is not associated with a particular sleep stage. In rare instances, sleep-related behaviors can be shown to be complex partial seizures (see Chapter 88). The parasomnias tend to occur in <10% of the population. These behaviors can range from the benign to the dramatic and may be violent. Several distinct syndromes have been recognized. Factors that can help distinguish the causes include the timing of the behavior, the likelihood of awakening from the episode, the degree of confusion present, and the patient's memory of the events. Sleep laboratory recordings may associate the various types of episodes with different sleep stages.

Arousal Disorders

Three types of sleep-related behaviors are classified as arousal disorders (3): sleepwalking, sleep terrors, and confusional arousals. They share an association with *slow-wave sleep* and thereby tend to occur during the first third of the night. The prevalence is greatest in childhood, but the disorders may persist in adulthood. A familial association has been noted in some cases. The frequency of episodes may range from several times per night to less than once a year. Commonly there is *amnesia for the event.* Typically the individual does not awaken spontaneously and is difficult to arouse. The patient may become aware of the events because of residual evidence such as relocated furniture or food left out on a table. Resistance to full awakening is characteristic, and marked confusion may be evident. Behaviors may be inappropriate, such as urinating in a closet or searching for nonexistent intruders.

Sleepwalking most commonly is simple and characterized by the patient walking around the room or house but rarely going outside. Generally sleepwalkers do not put themselves or others in a dangerous situation; however, dramatic exceptions have been reported. In some cases, there is an overlap with sleep terror symptoms, in which the person aggressively attempts to escape from, or protect against, an imagined threat.

By definition, *sleep terrors* are dramatic events. Evidence of autonomic discharge may be pronounced. Often, the person sits up and screams loudly and commonly is unarousable. The patient may return to sleep after several minutes and have no recollection of the incident the following morning. Patients who do awaken report an intense sense of fear associated with a distinct threat, but generally they do not offer a lengthy, dreamlike narrative. The sleep terror may lead to forceful escape behavior, which can injure the patient or someone else perceived to be an obstacle. Injury may result from leaping out of bed or colliding with furniture. Rarely, people have jumped through windows in an attempt to escape.

Confusional arousals involve persistent disorientation and incomplete awakening after an arousing stimulus that occurs while the person is in slow-wave sleep. Behaviors and speech content may be meaningless or inappropriate. A typical example would be a person responding to a ringing telephone 1 hour after sleep onset. The person may reach for other objects or may make little sense when talking. Amnesia for these episodes is common. Factors promoting deeper sleep increase the likelihood of such incomplete awakening. These may include sleep deprivation and use of sedating substances such as alcohol and central nervous system depressants.

Nightmares

Nightmares usually result in full awakenings and generally are not associated with prolonged confusion or sleep-related behaviors. Typically the patient can recount an extended dream narrative and can describe the frightening aspects of the story. In contrast to arousal disorders, nightmares are most common during REM sleep and tend to occur during the latter part of the night. Nightmares also are more likely to be remembered in the morning.

Dreams may be related to physical activity during sleep in *REM behavior disorder* (3). This disorder is more common in elderly persons. Normally there is skeletal muscle atonia during REM sleep; however, in this disorder, the active inhibition of motor impulses is incomplete. The dreamer may physically act out dream content, which may include kicking, punching, or leaping from the bed. Violent behaviors causing injury to the patient or to his or her bed partner have been reported. Most cases are idiopathic; however, neurologic diseases, toxic and metabolic processes, and medications have been implicated in promoting the symptoms. An association with the future development of Parkinson disease has been reported.

Management of the parasomnias is discussed in the next section.

MANAGEMENT OF SLEEP DISORDERS

Insomnia

A comprehensive sleep history from a patient with insomnia establishes the duration of the symptoms and explores possible predisposing, precipitating, and perpetuating factors. *Multifactorial causes are common* with insomnia. Treatment of the primary cause of the insomnia may be important, but reinforcing factors should also be addressed. Identified medical and psychiatric illnesses must be treated. Attention to sleep hygiene, behavioral programs, relaxation techniques, psychotherapy, environmental manipulations, and the use of hypnotic medications can play important roles in management. The objective of treatment is development by the patient of new behaviors and routines that allow a renewed sense of confidence in the ability to sleep effectively. This is achieved by a therapeutic alliance wherein the patient plays an active role in exploring potential sleep-inhibiting factors. Considerable experimentation may be necessary.

Although the quality of clinical studies has been highly variable, critical reviews of the published literature support the conclusion that both behavioral and pharmacologic approaches reduce the time it takes to fall asleep by 15 to 30 minutes and the number of awakenings by one to three per night (see Kupfer and Reynolds, *Management of Insomnia*, at www.hopkinsbayview.org/PAMreferences).

Sleep Hygiene Measures

Recommendations about sleep hygiene are beneficial to most patients with insomnia, regardless of the duration of their symptoms (Table 7.3). These basic guidelines address factors that directly cause disturbed sleep and inhibit recovery. They take into account fundamental physiologic and psychological understanding of the sleep process.

It is important to *take full advantage of the underlying circadian rhythm,* described previously, that promotes nighttime sleepiness and daytime alertness. Attempts to sleep at various times throughout the 24-hour cycle may perturb the rhythm. Daytime or evening napping can inhibit the onset of sleep at night. A consistent wake-up time is important because this is when the system is most sensitive to daily reinforcement.

Some people with insomnia spend excessive time in bed (e.g., 9 p.m. to 9 a.m.) in the hope of getting a little more sleep. Generally this is counterproductive. Physiologically there may be less-effective support of the circadian pattern. Because continuous sleep is unlikely, a situation is created in which failure is inevitable. Extended wakeful periods may be self-reinforcing. Sleep restriction (see Sleep Restriction Therapy) is a treatment modality that specifically addresses the problem of excessive time in bed without sleep.

It is useful to consider the extent to which a patient develops *negative associations with the bed and bedtime routines.* Good general advice includes reserving the bed for sleeping and sexual relations. Anxiety-provoking activities performed in bed may promote residual tension when sleep is attempted. Stressful behaviors may include studying for tests, paying bills, having domestic discussions, or watching violent television drama or news programs. These negatively stimulating activities should be replaced with relaxing behaviors.

Some patients find significantly improved sleep with the *elimination of stimulants* such as nicotine and caffeine, especially during the hours leading up to bedtime. Late-evening alcohol consumption should be avoided because of the potential for stimulation related to withdrawal later in the night.

A *comfortable bedroom environment* is important. Temperature extremes, particularly a warm room, can promote sleep disruption. Outside noises may be blocked out by white noise machines or wax ear plugs. Generally, people should not try to fall asleep with the television or radio playing. This tends to inhibit deep sleep and can cause awakenings.

Dietary habits may need to be addressed. Late, heavy meals may produce abdominal discomfort or reflux symptoms. On the other hand, hunger may interfere with sleep onset. A light snack may be an appropriate solution.

Regular exercise (see Chapter 16) is recommended to promote improved sleep at night (12). However, to prevent excessive stimulation, aerobic exercises should be avoided in the hours leading up to bedtime. For this reason, patients should be warned against wearing themselves out at night in the hope of falling asleep quickly.

Behavioral Management

Behavioral approaches are important in the treatment of chronic insomnia.

Relaxation Techniques

Relaxation techniques may have a permissive effect by reducing arousal, thereby allowing sleep onset (4). Relaxation may be achieved through the use of progressive relaxation, meditation, or biofeedback (see Chapter 22). Two other techniques—stimulus control therapy and sleep restriction therapy—involve specific instructions regarding nighttime routines and sleep–wake schedule hours.

TABLE 8.9 Summary of Bioterrorism Agents, Key Characteristics, and Treatment

Agent	*Signs and Symptoms*	*Incubation Period (Range)*	*Transmission*	*Infection Control*	*Diagnosis*	*Treatment for Adults*	*Post Exposure Prophylaxis for Adults*
Anthrax *Bacillus anthracis* A. Inhalation B. Cutaneous C. Gastrointestinal	A. Flulike symptoms (fever, fatigue, muscle aches, dyspnea, nonproductive cough, headache), chest pain; possible 1–2 day improvement, then rapid respiratory failure and shock B. Intense itching followed by painless papular lesions, then vesicular lesions, developing into eschar surrounded by edema C. Abdominal pain, nausea and vomiting, severe diarrhea	A. 1–6 days (up to 6 wks) B. 1–12 days C. 1–7 days	A. None B. Direct contact with skin lesions may result in cutaneous infection C. None	A. Standard precautions B. Contact precautions C. Standard precautions	A. Chest radiograph evidence of widening mediastinum; obtain sputum and blood culture B. Peripheral blood smear may demonstrate gram-positive bacilli C. Culture blood and stool	A. and C. Combined IV/PO therapy for 60 days Ciprofloxacin 500 mg q12h or doxycycline 100 mg q12h, and 1 or 2 additional drugs: vancomycin, rifampin, clindamycin, chloramphenicol, clarithromycin, penicillin, or ampicillin B. 7–10 day course of: ciprofloxacin 500 mg PO q12h or doxycycline 100 mg PO q2h	Prophylaxis for 60 days: ciprofloxacin 500 mg PO q12h or doxycycline 100 mg PO q12h Alternative: amoxicillin 500 mg PO q8h
Botulism; botulinum toxin	Afebrile, excess mucus in throat, dysphagia, dry mouth and throat, dizziness, then difficulty moving eyes, mild pupillary dilation and nystagmus, intermittent ptosis, indistinct speech, unsteady gait, extreme symmetric descending weakness, flaccid paralysis; generally normal mental status	Inhalation: 12–80 h Foodborne: 12–72 h (2–8 d)	None	Standard precautions	Obtain serum, stool, gastric aspirate, and suspect foods prior to administering antitoxin; differential diagnosis includes polio, Guillain-Barré, myasthenia, tick paralysis, CVA	Limited supply of antitoxins; supportive care and ventilatory support; avoid clindamycin and aminoglycosides	Limited supplies of antitoxins

(continued)

TABLE 8.9 (Continued) Summary of Bioterrorism Agents, Key Characteristics, and Treatment

Agent	*Signs and Symptoms*	*Incubation Period (Range)*	*Transmission*	*Infection Control*	*Diagnosis*	*Treatment for Adults*	*Post Exposure Prophylaxis for Adults*
Pneumonic plague *Yersinia pestis*	High fever, cough, hemoptysis, chest pain, nausea and vomiting, headache; advanced disease: purpuric skin lesions, copious watery or purulent sputum production; respiratory failure in 1–6 d	2–3 d (2–6 d)	Yes, droplet aerosols	Droplet precautions until 48 h of effective antibiotic therapy	A presumptive diagnosis may be made by Gram, Wayson, or Wright stain of lymph node aspirates, sputum, or cerebrospinal fluid with gram-negative bacilli with bipolar staining	10 d of therapy with: streptomycin 1 g IM q12h or gentamicin 2 mg/kg, then 1.0–1.7 mg/kg IV q8h Alternatives: doxycycline 200 mg PO load, then 100 PO mg q12h or ciprofloxacin 400 mg IV q12h	7-day course of doxycycline 100 mg PO q12h or ciprofloxacin 500 mg PO q12h
Pneumonic Tularemia; *Francisella tularensis*	Sudden onset of acute febrile illness, progressing to pharyngitis, bronchiolitis, pleuropneumonitis, hilar lymphadenitis. Initially flulike syndrome with fever (100.4–104°F, 38–40°C), chills, headache, coryza, sore throat. Dry or slightly productive cough, substernal tightness, pleuritic pain; hemoptysis rare. Radiograph with bronchopneumonia, often with pleural effusions and hilar lymphadenopathy. Other forms of disease: glandular, oculoglandular, pharyngeal, typhoidal ulceroglandular	3–5 d (1–14 d)	None; laboratory personnel potentially at risk: use BSL-2 for routine diagnostic procedures, BSL-3 if aerosol or droplet production possible	Standard precautions	Culture using selective media (BCY, cysteine or S-H enhanced). Blood (rarely positive), sputum, pharyngeal washings; Gram stain may show poorly stained, pleomorphic, gram-negative coccobacillus. Serology preferred confirmatory test. Rapid diagnostic tests available	Treatment for 10–14 d: streptomycin 1 g IM q12h or gentamicin 5 mg/kg/d IV Alternatives: doxycycline 100 mg IV q12h × 14 d or chloramphenicol 15 mg/kg IV q6h × 14 d or ciprofloxacin* 400 mg IV q12h × 10 d May change to PO when clinically improved	Prophylaxis for 14 d: doxycycline 100 mg PO q12h or ciprofloxacin 500 mg PO q12h

Viral hemorrhagic fevers *Filovirus* Ebola hemorrhagic fever Marburg hemorrhagic fever *Arenavirus* Lassa fever Junin (Argentinian) Machupo (Bolivian) Others	Distinguish a classification of viruses thought to have potential for use as a bioterrorism agent. All hemorrhagic fever viruses can cause capillary leak syndromes. Malaise, fever, myalgias, prostration, conjunctival injection, petechiae, ecchymoses, shock, diffuse hemorrhage, neurologic dysfunction, and pulmonary collapse	Ebola: 2–21 d Marburg: 3–14 d Lassa 6–15 d (5–21 d) Junin and Machupo 7–16 d	Transmissible via contact and droplet exposure from blood and body fluids; rare airborne transmission. Follow BSL-4 practices	Private room preferred; airborne precautions with N95 respirators or PAPRs. Contact precautions	Early postexposure nasal swabs and induced respiratory secretions for hemorrhagic fever RT-PCR, ELISA EM, and viral isolation (requires BSL-4 laboratory)	Aggressive supportive care and management of hypotension; blood replacement products for disseminated intravascular coagulation	None available at present; research is ongoing
Smallpox variola virus	Prodromal period with malaise, fever, rigors, vomiting, headache, and backache. After 2–4 d, skin lesions appear and progress uniformly from macules to papules to vesicles and pustules, mostly on face, palms, and soles, and subsequently the trunk	12–14 d (7–17 d)	Yes, airborne droplet nuclei or direct contact with skin lesions until all scabs fall off (3–4 wk)	Airborne (includes N95 mask) and contact precautions	Swab culture of vesicular fluid or scab, send to BSL laboratory	Supportive care	Early vaccine critical (in <4 d); call CDC for vaccinia. Vaccinia immune globulin in special cases

BSL, biosafety level. See CDC website, http://www.cdc.gov/od/ohs/biosfty/bmb14/bmb1453.htm for guidelines for biosafety in microbiological and biomedical laboratories (BMBL).

PAPRs, power air purifying respirators; RT-PCR, reverse transcriptase-polymerase chain reaction; ELISA, enzyme-linked immunosorbent assay; CDC, Center for Disease Control.

This table is based on information from the following references: Bartlett J, Henderson D, Inglesby T, et al. Smallpox as a biological weapon: medical and public health management. JAMA 1999;281(22):2127–2137; Borio L, Inglesby TV, Peters CJ, et al. Hemorrhagic fever as a biological weapon: medical and public health management. JAMA 2002;287:2391–2405; Dennis DT, Henderson DA, Inglesby TV, et al. Botulinum toxin as a biological weapon: medical and public health management. JAMA 2001;285:1059–1070; Dennis DT, Henderson DA, Inglesby TV, et al. Plague as a biological weapon: medical and public health management. JAMA 200;283:2281–2290; Dennis DT, Henderson DA, Inglesby TV, et al. Tularemia as a biological weapon: medical and public health management. JAMA 2001;285:2763–2773; Henderson DA, Inglesby TV, O'Toole T, et al. Anthrax as a biological weapon: medical and public health management. JAMA 2002;287:2236–2252.

TABLE 8.10 Recognizing and Treating Poisoning by Chemical Agents

Agent Type	*Agent Names*	*Mechanism of Action*	*Key Characteristics*	*Signs and Symptoms*	*Treatment*	*Further Considerations*
Nerve agents	Cyclohexyl sarin (GF) Sarin (GB) Soman (GD) Tabun (GA) VX Some insecticides (cholinesterase inhibitors) Novichok agents/Soviet V	Inactivate acetylcholinesterase enzymes, causing both muscarinic and nicotinic effects	SLUDGE -**S**alivation -**L**acrimation -**U**rination -**D**efecation -**G**astric -**E**mptying Pinpoint pupils Seizures	Miosis (pinpoint pupils) Blurred/dimmed vision Headache Nausea, vomiting, diarrhea Copious secretions/sweating Muscle twitching/ fasciculations Dyspnea Seizures Loss of consciousness	Decontamination Atropine Pralidoxime (2-PAM) chloride	Onset of symptoms from dermal contact may be delayed Repeat antidote administration may be necessary
Asphyxiant/blood agents	Arsine Cyanogen chloride Hydrogen cyanide	Arsine: causes intravascular hemolysis/ resulting renal failure Cyanogen chloride/hydrogen cyanide: cyanide binds with iron in cytochrome a_3 preventing intracellular oxygen utilization Increased anaerobic metabolism, creates excess lactic acid with resulting metabolic acidosis	Possible cherry-red skin (40%) Possible cyanosis Possible frostbite	Confusion Nausea Patients may gasp for air, similar to asphyxiation but more abrupt onset Seizures prior to death Metabolic acidosis	Decontamination Oxygen For cyanide, use antidotes: sodium nitrite, if available, then sodium thiosulfate Arsine has no specific antidote Supportive care	Arsine and cyanogen chloride may cause delayed pulmonary edema
Choking/pulmonary-damaging agents	Chlorine Hydrogen chloride Nitrogen oxides Phosgene	Acids or acid-forming agents that react with cytoplasmic proteins and destroy cell structure	Chlorine is a greenish-yellow gas with pungent odor Phosgene gas smells like newly mown hay or grass	Eye and skin irritation Airway irritation Dyspnea, cough Sore throat Chest tightness Wheezing Bronchospasm	Decontamination Remove from scene Semi-upright position If signs of respiratory distress are present, oxygen with or without positive airway pressure may be needed No specific antidote	May cause delayed pulmonary edema, even following a symptom-free period that varies in duration with the amount inhaled May lead to acute respiratory distress syndrome

Blistering/vesicant agents	Mustard/sulfur mustard (HD, H) Nitrogen mustard (HN-1, HN-2, HN-3) Lewisite (L) Phosgene oxime (CX)	Exact mechanisms are unknown Mustard: forms metabolites that bind to enzymes, proteins and other cellular components Lewisite: Binds to thiol groups in many enzymes	Mustard (HD) has an odor like horseradish, burning garlic, or mustard Lewisite (L) has an odor like geranium Phosgene oxime (CX) has a pepperish or pungent odor	Severe skin, eye, and mucosal irritation Skin erythema and blistering Tearing, conjunctivitis, corneal damage Mild respiratory distress to marked airway damage	Decontamination Oxygen p.r.n. British anti-Lewisite (BAL) may decrease systemic effects of Lewisite Mustard has no specific antidote	Possible pulmonary edema Mustard has an asymptomatic latent period Lewisite has immediate burning pain, blisters later Phosgene oxime causes immediate pain Monitor electrolyte balance Neutropenia and sepsis
Incapacitating/ behavior-altering agents	Agent 15/BZ	Competitively inhibits acetylcholine, which disrupts muscarinic transmission in central and peripheral nervous systems (atropinelike action)	May appear as mass drug intoxication with erratic behaviors, shared realistic and distinct hallucinations, disrobing and confusion Hyperthermia Mydriasis	Dry mouth and skin Initial tachycardia Altered consciousness, delusions, denial of illness, belligerence Hyperthermia Ataxia (lack of coordination) Hallucinations Mydriasis (dilated pupils)	Decontamination Evaluate mental status Restraints as needed Monitor core temperature carefully Specific antidote physostigmine may be available	Hyperthermia and self-injury are greatest risks Hard to detect because it is an odorless and non irritating substance Possible serious arrhythmias
Cytotoxic protein agents	Ricin Abrin	Inhibit protein synthesis	Exposure by inhalation or injection causes more dramatic course	Latent period of 4–8 h, followed by flulike signs and symptoms Progress within 18–24 h to nausea, cough, dyspnea, pulmonary edema (inhalation); gastrointestinal hemorrhage with emesis and bloody diarrhea; hepatic, splenic and renal failure (ingestion)	Decontamination Maintain fluid/electrolyte balance Maintain adequate oxygenation Provide pain management	Rapid progression of signs and symptoms Death possible within 36–48 h 5-d survival indicates recovery is likely

This table is based on information from Brennan RJ, Waeckerle JF, Sharp TW, et al. Chemical warfare agents: emergency medical and emergency public health issues. Ann Emerg Med 1999;34(2):191–204; Sidell FR. Chemical agent terrorism. Ann Emerg Med 1996;28:223–224; and Sidell F, Patrick WC, Dashiell TR. Jane's chem-bio handbook. Alexandria, VA: Jane's Information Group, 1998.

Those treating chemical or radiologic exposures must not become victims themselves. Under no circumstances should contaminated patients be brought into regular patient treatment areas such as emergency departments or hospitals prior to decontamination. Chemical agents that are most likely to be used in an attack can be classified according to mechanism of action. Table 8.10 summarizes these agents, including a sketch of their characteristics and treatment modalities.

When a radioactive weapon is used in an attack, ionizing radiation presents the highest threat to health beyond the initial blast. Ionizing radiation can be alpha or beta particles, or X or gamma rays. The lowest lethal dose of radiation exposure is approximately 200 rem. With appropriate medical care, the lethal dose increases to about 360 rem.

Proper decontamination and shielding procedures can minimize the effects of external exposure to radioactive agents. Internal exposure, primarily from alpha and beta particles taken into the body by breathing particles in the air, absorption through the skin, or by ingesting in water, soil, or food, must also be addressed. Internal contamination can be treated using chelating or blocking agents. Potassium iodide is a blocking agent; it prevents end-organ uptake of radioactive iodine. Chelating agents bind metals into complexes, preventing tissue uptake and promoting urinary excretion. Calcium disodium edetate and penicillamine are used to treat radioactive lead poisoning. Pentetate calcium trisodium (CaDTPA) and pentetate zinc trisodium (ZnDTPA) are used for americium, curium, and plutonium poisoning.

The Larger Emergency Response Picture

As part of the overall Federal National Response Plan (NRP), public health officials and the medical community have the primary responsibility to prepare for and respond to bioterrorism events. This responsibility is included under emergency support function (ESF) number 8 in the NRP. Each hospital is now required to maintain a current Emergency Operations Plan (EOP) that details how the institution will operate in emergency situations.

National syndromic surveillance projects collect emergency department visit data on cases with descriptor "syndromes" that might indicate a terrorist event. Additionally, over-the-counter sales data is collected to monitor medication use for syndromes associated with bioterrorism agents.

The Strategic National Stockpile (SNS) is a national repository of antibiotics, vaccines, and emergency medical equipment maintained by the CDC. The SNS is designed for delivery within 12 hours to any location in the United States. Current plans call for local responders to "go it alone" for the initial 72 hours after an event. Pre-event planning becomes critical to effectively respond to future emergency situations.

SPECIFIC REFERENCES

1. Steenland K, Burnett C, Lalich N, et al. Dying for work: the magnitude of U.S. mortality from selected causes of death associated with occupation. Am J Ind Med 2003;43:461.
2. Markowitz SB, Fischer E, Fahs MC, et al. Occupational disease in New York state: a comprehensive examination. Am J Ind Med 1989;16:417.
3. Pransky G, Snyder T, Dember A, et al. Under-reporting of work-related disorders in the workplace: a case study and review of the literature. Ergonomics 1999;42:171.

*For annotated **General References** and resources related to this chapter, visit www.hopkinsbayview.org/PAMreferences.*

Chapter 9

Selected Special Services and Programs: Disability Insurance, Vocational Rehabilitation, Family and Medical Leave Act, and Home Health Services

L. Randol Barker

Maintenance of a patient's overall health often requires efforts beyond those of the physician and the patient. Assistance often comes from community-based programs to which physicians may refer their patients. Many of these programs provide services for patients with specific types of illnesses; the roles of such categorical community services are described in the appropriate chapters in this book. Other services or programs are designed to assist patients or their families regardless of illness type. This chapter describes four of these: Social Security programs for disabled people; vocational rehabilitation; family and medical leave; and home health services. This chapter explains eligibility for these services and programs, the nature of the benefits, and the role of physicians in enabling their patients to participate in them. Chapter 8 provides similar information about another noncategorical program, workers' compensation, which is designed to provide coverage for health care costs and income support to people with work-related diseases.

SOCIAL SECURITY PROGRAMS FOR DISABLED PEOPLE

Loss or decrease of a person's ability to earn a living accompanies many illnesses. Beginning with the 1954 amendments to the Social Security Act, income support for medically disabled people has been available in the United States. Further modifications since 1954 have led to the program that exists today. Three fundamental benefits are currently available through the Society Security Administration: disability insurance (DI), Supplemental Security Income (SSI), and Medicare (health insurance for DI recipients). Medicaid is a federally and state-administered health insurance program that is available automatically in many states for people who receive SSI and for mothers of dependent children whose incomes are below the poverty level. Detailed information about each of these services is available from any local Social Security office.

Definition of Medical Disability

The Social Security Act defines disability as the "inability to engage in any substantial gainful activity by reason of a medically determinable physical or mental impairment that can be expected to result in death or has lasted or can be expected to last for a continuous period of not less than 12 months."

Disability Insurance (Title II of the Social Security Act)

Eligibility

To be eligible for DI payments, a disabled worker must have paid into the Social Security program for a minimum period of time before becoming disabled; in addition, there is a requirement for coverage during 5 of the 10 years before the onset of disability. Today, 9 of 10 workers and their employers pay the Social Security tax (Federal Insurance Contributions Act, or "FICA"). For younger workers (up to age 31 years), there are modified requirements to meet insured status.

Disabled dependents of a fully insured worker who is retired, disabled, or deceased may be eligible for DI payments in two situations: *a child* who became disabled before age 22 years (eligible for DI payments at the time that the child's parent retires, becomes disabled, or dies; payments may begin as early as age 18 years and continue as long as the child's disability lasts) and *a widow or widower* who is between 50 and 59 years of age and who did not work under Social Security but who became medically disabled before or within 7 years of the death of a fully insured spouse.

Benefits

DI payments go to disabled workers before the age of 65 years (after age 65 years, Social Security Retirement Income replaces disability payments) and to eligible children, widows, or widowers as long as they remain disabled. The first monthly DI check is not paid for the first 5 months after the onset of the worker's disability (e.g., a patient who is certified as disabled 6 calendar months after becoming disabled immediately becomes eligible for a check covering the 1 month in excess of the required 5-month wait). SSI (see Supplemental Security Income) is often awarded to people who are found to be "presumptively disabled," effective the first day of the month that follows the month in which they apply for benefits. Income from DI for a disabled worker is the same amount as the retirement income the worker would receive if he or she were age 65 years.

In 2003, the average monthly payments were $862 to disabled workers and $888 to nondisabled widows and widowers. In that year, 5.8 million disabled workers and 1.6 million spouses and children were receiving DI benefits. The leading causes of disability for disabled workers were mental disorders that do not involve retardation and musculoskeletal conditions. Approximately 10% had circulatory conditions or diseases of the nervous system (1).

In addition to income support, disabled people younger than age 65 years receive Medicare (Social Security Health Insurance) after they have been eligible for disability benefits for 24 months. Patients with end-stage renal disease receive Medicare coverage effective when they begin long-term dialysis.

Process of Disability Determination

There are a number of steps in the process of determining medical disability.

- The patient completes a detailed application at a local Social Security office. The patient must not be gainfully employed at the time of application. In 2005, *gainful employment* was defined as an activity that yields a monthly income of $830 or more for those with impairments other than blindness and $1,380 for people who are blind (2). Most patients initiate disability claims by themselves, but at times a physician or social worker suggests application to a patient who is not aware that his or her condition qualifies as a medical disability.
- The patient's physician receives a request for medical information and returns this report to the state Disability Determination office. The report sent by the patient's physician should be succinct and precise and should provide objective data regarding the condition for which disability is being claimed. It should be divided into the following subheadings: history, physical, laboratory reports, diagnosis, treatment, and response. The report should also describe the individual's ability to perform work-related activities (e.g., sitting, standing, walking, lifting, carrying, handling objects, hearing, speaking, and traveling; for mentally impaired persons, the ability to understand, to remember instructions, or to respond appropriately to supervision). The information provided should permit claim reviewers to determine both the severity and the duration of the patient's condition. If malingering is suspected, the report should describe the circumstances that raise doubts rather than recording this assessment without supporting information. The most helpful guide for completing these medical reports is the booklet *Disability Evaluation Under Social Security* (available free from any Social Security office or the state Disability Determination office). This manual, which was most recently revised in 2005, lists, with criteria that must be met, most conditions that are so severe they automatically qualify an individual for DI. These are referred to as Medical Listings. Tables 9.1 through 9.4 illustrate the criteria listed for four common conditions: chronic obstructive pulmonary disease, cerebrovascular accident, epilepsy caused by major motor seizures, and arthritis of a major weight-bearing joint. The conditions in the Medical Listings are the basis for most DI allowances made by disability claim reviewers. Since 1980 the Social Security Administration has paid a small fee to physicians for medical reports for the DI program; a small fee has also been paid for SSI reports since the inception of that program in 1974. Previously, patients were expected to pay for these

TABLE 9.1 Impairments Qualifying a Person with Chronic Obstructive Pulmonary Disease for Medical Disability Under Social Security

Height without Shoes (cm)	*Height without Shoes (inches)*	*FEV_1 Less than (L)*
154 or less	60 or less	1.05
155–160	61–63	1.15
161–165	64–65	1.25
166–170	66–67	1.35
171–175	68–69	1.45
176–180	70–71	1.55
181 or more	72 or more	1.65

FEV_1, forced expiratory volume in 1 second.
Chronic obstructive pulmonary disease due to cause, with the FEV_1 equal to or less than the values specified in this table corresponding to the person's height without shoes. (In cases of marked spinal deformity, see 3.00E.)
From Disability Evaluation Under Social Security, 2005. Available at www.hopkinsbayview.org/PAMreferences and also www.ssa.gov/disability/professionals/bluebook, and www.socialsecurity.gov/disability/professionals/bluebook/general-Information and-Introl-2005.pdf.

TABLE 9.2 Impairments Qualifying a Person with Central Nervous System Vascular Accident for Medical Disability Under Social Security

Central nervous system vascular accident, with one of the following more than 3 months postvascular accident: A. Sensory or motor aphasia resulting in ineffective speech or communication, or B. Significant and persistent disorganization of motor function in two extremities, resulting in sustained disturbance of gross and dexterous movements or gait and station.

From Disability Evaluation Under Social Security, 2005. Available at www.hopkinsbayview.org/PAMreferences and also www.ssa.gov/disability/professionals/bluebook, and www.socialsecurity.gov/disability/professionals/bluebook/general-Information and-Introl-2005.pdf.

reports. In some states, doctors also have access to a free teledictation service for dictating their reports.

- The information provided by the patient and the physician (the disability claim) is reviewed by the state Disability Determination Service (DDS) by a team comprised of a disability claims examiner and a physician. If deemed necessary, an independent medical examination is purchased by the DDS. In keeping with the 1974 Freedom of Information Act, patients can access their disability claim files.

If an insured worker has an impairment that does not meet the standard criteria for disability but nevertheless claims inability to do his or her usual job, the DDS obtains additional information to determine the claimant's residual functional capacity to perform past work despite the impairment(s). If the past work was such that the impairment would prevent performing the work, DDS proceeds to a last step to determine if the claimant can do other work. Limitations of age, education, training, and work experience are considered by the DDS team in establishing whether a worker is able to perform "other work."

TABLE 9.3 Impairments Qualifying a Person with Convulsive Epilepsy for Medical Disability Under Social Security

Epilepsy–convulsive epilepsy (grand mal or psychomotor), documented by detailed description of a typical seizure pattern, including all associated phenomena: occurring more frequently than once a month, despite at least 3 months of prescribed treatment[a] with A. Daytime episodes (loss of consciousness and convulsive seizures), *or* B. Nocturnal episodes manifesting residuals that interfere significantly with activity during the day.

[a]Adherence to therapy must be objectively confirmed by measurements of drug levels that are in the therapeutic range.

From Disability Evaluation Under Social Security, 2005. Found at www.hopkinsbayview.org/PAMreferences and also www.ssa.gov/disability/professionals/bluebook, and www.socialsecurity.gov/disability/professionals/bluebook/general-Information and-Introl-2005.pdf.

TABLE 9.4 Impairments Qualifying a Person with Major Dysfunction of a Joint(s) (due to any cause) for Medical Disability Under Social Security

Arthritis of a major weight-bearing joint (due to any cause) with history of persistent joint pain and stiffness with signs of marked limitation of motion or abnormal motion of the affected joint on current physical examination with A. Gross anatomic deformity of hip or knee (e.g., subluxation, contracture, bony or fibrous ankylosis, instability) supported by x-ray evidence of either significant joint space narrowing or significant bony destruction *and* markedly limiting ability to walk or stand, OR B. Reconstructive surgery or surgical arthrodesis of a major weight-bearing joint and return to full weight-bearing status did not occur, or is not expected to occur, within 12 months of onset.

From Disability Evaluation Under Social Security, 2005. Found at www.hopkinsbayview.org/PAMreferences and also www.ssa.gov/disability/professionals/bluebook, and www.socialsecurity.gov/disability/professionals/bluebook/general-Information and-Introl-2005.pdf.

Appeals Process

If the initial claim of disability has been denied, the claimant may file for reconsideration within 60 days of receiving a denial notice. The case is then reevaluated by a different DDS team. If the claim is denied at this reconsideration, the claimant has 60 days to file a request for a hearing. Hearings are conducted by administrative law judges. If the claim is again denied, the claimant may make an additional appeal for review by the Appeals Council. After that, the case may be taken to the United States District Court.

A patient's personal physician can be instrumental in ensuring that the patient gets the fullest consideration throughout the disability determination process. If the physician believes there are aspects of the patient's illness that make it more severe than the criteria indicate, the physician should communicate this information in writing, together with support for this opinion, to the Disability Determination office.

Periodic Review and Return to Work Incentives

All claims are reviewed for referral to vocational rehabilitation (see Vocational Rehabilitation) at the time the disability decision is made. In addition, every person with a permanent impairment is re-evaluated every 5 to 7 years. Those expected to improve are reviewed 6 to 8 months after the DI decision is made, and those in whom improvement is possible but less predictable are reviewed about every 3 years. Even if the original impairment is judged not to be severe on review, payments are continued for those who have started a vocational rehabilitation program because of improvement in their medical condition; benefits continue until the rehabilitation services are completed or until the person stops receiving these services. The purpose of these processes, and the following conditions, is to encourage disabled people to return to work.

- Disabled beneficiaries may test their ability to work for 9 months while continuing to receive benefits. After this trial work period, a determination is made about whether the work constitutes *substantial gainful activity* (defined in 2005 as an activity that yields a monthly income of $830 or more); if it does, benefits are suspended after an additional 3-month adjustment period (2).
- If a person who still has a disabling impairment stops work again within 36 months after Social Security payments have been suspended because of substantial gainful activity, the monthly DI benefits can be resumed, usually without a new application.
- A worker can usually continue to have Medicare coverage for at least 39 months after his or her DI benefits stop because of return to substantial gainful activity. If a worker starts receiving DI benefits again within 5 years after the DI was stopped and if the patient was previously entitled to Medicare, that protection resumes immediately.
- Work expenses related to the impairment that are paid for by a disabled person may be deducted from the patient's earnings in determining whether these constitute substantial gainful activity. This is true even if these expenses also apply to needs for daily living (e.g., a wheelchair).

In addition to disabled workers, workers' children who became disabled before the age of 22 years and disabled widows and widowers can also have a trial work period.

Supplemental Security Income

SSI is a federal program that was introduced in 1974 under Title XVI of the Social Security Act. It is paid for out of general funds rather than Social Security funds, but it is administered by the same state agencies that administer the Disability Determination program. The application process is similar to that described above for Social Security DI. Applications are filed at a local Social Security office, and the same criteria are used to evaluate SSI disability claims as are used for DI claims.

The basic differences between SSI and Social Security benefits are as follows:

- *Eligibility.* SSI is available for two groups of people when they are not insured by Social Security: those younger than age 65 years who are medically disabled and all uninsured people older than age 65 years. SSI for people older than age 65 years is similar in purpose to Social Security retirement income. In addition to these two groups, people who have presumptive disability (claim for total disability being processed) and disabled people who are in the 5-month waiting period for their DI payments to begin may be eligible for SSI. Eligibility in all these groups is based on need (total resources found to be below a certain defined level) and the absence of gainful employment (defined as earned monthly income of $830 or more).
- There is no waiting period. A person becomes eligible for the first SSI payment the first day of the month after he or she files a disability claim.

In most states, people approved for SSI are also eligible for Medicaid and other social services provided by their state. All people receiving SSI are reviewed once each year to determine whether their income and other resources still make them eligible to receive SSI. Like DI recipients, they are reviewed every 3 to 7 years to establish whether their disability is still present (see Periodic Review and Return to Work Incentives).

The maximal monthly income from SSI in 2005 was $579 for an individual and $869 for a couple. In 2003 there were 6.9 million recipients of SSI on the basis of disability, blindness, and age (older than age 65 years and without Social Security). Most had a mental disorder (1). As described for DI, the report of a patient's physician must be received before income support under SSI can be initiated.

VOCATIONAL REHABILITATION

State vocational rehabilitation agencies existed before the federal Disability Determination program was created in 1954. In many states, these agencies administer the Disability Determination program in addition to providing vocational rehabilitation services.

Eligibility

To be eligible for vocational rehabilitation, a person must have an impairment that interferes with his or her capacity to obtain suitable employment, or that is a threat to his or her present career; this does not mean that the person has to meet the criteria for medical disability discussed earlier. The person must have a reasonable chance of being able to engage in a suitable occupation after vocational rehabilitation services are provided. A suitable occupation would include being a homemaker provided that vocational rehabilitation would enable the person to remain in his or her own home instead of requiring institutional care.

Services

The services provided by vocational rehabilitation agencies vary among states. However, they usually include the following:

- *A medical examination.* A complete medical examination is provided to determine the extent of a person's disability.

- *Counseling and guidance.* A trained rehabilitation counselor is assigned to guide each client through the rehabilitation process.
- *Physical aids.* Items such as artificial limbs, braces, hearing aids, eyeglasses, and wheelchairs may be provided if needed.
- *Job training.* Training for the proper job is provided when necessary. This may be given at a vocational school, college or university, rehabilitation facility, or in the home.
- *Help with transportation expenses.*
- *Equipment and licenses.* Tools, equipment, and licenses necessary for getting started in the right job may be provided.
- *Job placement.* Placement in the right job is an important part of the rehabilitation process. The abilities of each client are carefully matched to job requirements.
- *Followup.* The counselor follows up on each placement to make sure that the client's job is suitable.

Physician's Role

As noted earlier, all people applying for Social Security disability benefits are screened for referral to vocational rehabilitation. For those people, the report of the patient's physician (see Process of Disability Determination) may be used by the vocational rehabilitation agency. For people who are not applying for medical disability, the physician is often asked to provide a general medical report for the vocational rehabilitation agency. An important role of physicians is to encourage patients to apply for vocational rehabilitation and to maintain continued interest in their progress. It has been estimated that every $1,000 spent for vocational rehabilitation increases by $35,000 the lifetime earnings of those who are rehabilitated.

FAMILY AND MEDICAL LEAVE ACT

Eligibility

The purpose of the Family and Medical Leave Act (FMLA), passed in 1993, is to grant temporary medical leave to employees under certain circumstances. Employers covered by the Act are (a) any employer who employs 50 or more employees for each working day during each of 20 or more calendar work weeks in the current or preceding calendar year and (b) all public agencies, which are covered without regard to the number of employees. Public as well as private elementary and secondary schools are included in this second category.

Under the FMLA, employers must grant an eligible employee up to a total of 12 work weeks of unpaid leave during any 12-month period for one or more of the following reasons:

1. For the birth and care of the newborn child of the employee.
2. For placement with the employee of a son or daughter for adoption or foster care.
3. To care for an immediate family member (spouse, child, or parent) with a serious health condition.
4. To take medical leave when the employee is unable to work because of a serious health condition.

Any employee who takes leave under FMLA is entitled, on return from such leave, to be restored to the position he or she held when the leave commenced or to an equivalent position with equivalent pay and benefits. During the leave the employer must maintain the employee's health coverage under any group health plan of the employer; and the leave will not result in the loss of any employment benefit accrued before the leave commenced.

Physician's Role

An employer may require that a request for leave for situations under items 3 and 4 above be supported by certification documented by the health care provider of the eligible employee or of the son, daughter, spouse, or parent of the employee, as appropriate. Sufficient certification, documented on the FMLA form, includes the following information:

- The date on which the serious health condition commenced.
- The probable duration of the condition.
- The appropriate medical facts within the knowledge of the health care provider regarding the condition.
- For purposes of leave under item 3 above, a statement that the eligible employee is needed to care for the family member and estimate of the amount of time that the employee is needed to provide care.
- For purposes of leave under item 4 above, a statement that the employee is unable to perform the functions of his or her position.
- In the case of certification for intermittent leave, or leave on a reduced work schedule, the expected duration of the intermittent leave or reduced leave schedule.

The four-page FMLA form and additional details regarding FMLA can be obtained from one's employer or at the website of the Department of Labor (www.dol.gov).

HOME HEALTH SERVICES

A consequence of illness as distressing to the patient as the loss of the ability to earn an income is the temporary or permanent loss of the ability to remain at home. Most people require acute hospital care one or more times in their adult lives, and a small proportion also require long-term institutional care. The principal objectives of home health services are to minimize the need for admission to acute or long-term care facilities and to decrease length of stay and associated costs in these facilities.

National Trends

Home health care is the sector of the health care industry that grew the most in the end of the 20th century (3). Growth in home health initially accelerated after passage of the Omnibus Reconciliation Acts of 1980 and 1981, which increased funding for home health services by Medicare and Medicaid. Between 1980 and 1995, the number of patients served per year grew from about 0.9 million to approximately 3.6 million for Medicare and from about 0.4 million to approximately 1.4 million for Medicaid. More recently, cost-effectiveness initiatives from the managed care industry have further promoted home care as an alternative to hospital care.

Range of Services and Providers

Home health services provided include basic care provided by informal caregivers (family members and friends); home food services available at a nominal cost to the patient (Meals-on-Wheels); care provided by physicians or their associates who make home visits; services provided by the personnel of home health agencies; specimen collection and performance of diagnostic procedures such as radiographs and electrocardiograms by clinical laboratories; and delivery/rental by medical suppliers of infusion equipment, medications, and durable medical equipment such as hospital beds. Even when professional help is involved, most of the responsibility for carrying out care is assumed by the patient or a member of the patient's family; as noted in Chapter 1, it is the assumption of responsibility by patients and their families that most distinguishes ambulatory care from institutional care.

Overall coordination of the home care provided by home health agencies is usually provided by a nurse case manager. A substantial proportion of the care is often carried out by home health aides, analogous to nursing aides on hospital wards, under the supervision of the nurse. In recent years, nurse practitioners, enterostomal therapists, and clinical pharmacy consultants have been added to the staffs of many home health agencies, so that more sophisticated care can be provided. In addition to nursing, home care services may include physical, occupational, and speech therapy; nutritional, behavioral, and social work counseling; and mental health services. Home health agencies provide the professional services of *hospice programs* (see Chapter 13) in many communities, or may have their own hospice programs. In addition, *maternal and child health programs* have been developed to respond to the needs created by rapid discharge of mothers and newborns.

TABLE 9.5 Problems Most Commonly Referred for Home Health Services

Postsurgical wound care (teach or provide dressing changes)
Orthopedic problems (rehabilitation after hospitalization)
Congestive heart failure (monitor for change in status, provide dietary counseling, assess medication compliance)
Diabetes (e.g., supervise insulin technique, provide dietary counseling, teach blood or urine monitoring of glucose, care of the lower extremities)
Incurable cancer and AIDS (provide dietary counseling, intravenous therapies, psychological support, and other aspects of hospice care)[a]
Stroke and other incapacitating neurologic problems (provide physical and occupational therapy)
Decubitus and stasis ulcers (teach or provide debridement and dressing changes)
Dementia in an older person living alone (assess environment for health hazards)
Chronic obstructive pulmonary disease (assess home for oxygen therapy, teach energy-conservation strategies)

AIDS, acquired immunodeficiency syndrome.
[a]See details in Chapter 13.

In recent years, home health agencies and suppliers have added services that require skilled use of equipment traditionally used only in hospitals. These services include the administration of *intravenous therapies,* ranging from short-term normal saline and electrolyte infusions to courses of antibiotics, cancer chemotherapy, cardiac medications, and total parenteral nutrition, and the care of *ventilator-dependent patients* at home. These initiatives have emerged in response to efforts to reduce the length of costly hospitalization for patients who prefer home care to hospital care for parenteral therapy that may have to be administered for 1 week or more. Day-to-day supervision of the overall care of patients receiving in-home parenteral therapy or ventilator support is usually not provided by the company that supplies and monitors the equipment; consequently, this responsibility is assumed by a nurse case manager who knows the physician's comprehensive plan for the patient and is in close contact with the supplier. Table 9.5 lists the types of clinical problems most commonly referred to home health agencies.

Criteria for Third-Party Reimbursement

Any patient or patient's family may purchase services from a home health agency. During the past 30 years, much of the cost of home care has been covered by Medicare, Medicaid, other third-party payers, and managed care organizations. The number and types of services authorized are being more tightly controlled today as part of cost-containment efforts. Beginning in 2001, Medicare changed from a cost-based to a prospective payment approach, similar to the diagnosis-related group approach to paying for

TABLE 9.6 Criteria for Third-Party Reimbursement for Home Health Services

Medicare[a,b]

Part A pays 100% for all covered services (skilled nursing, home health aide, social work, physical, occupational, and speech therapy). Care must be provided by a certified home health agency and must be medically necessary. The following conditions must be met to qualify for reimbursement:

1. Patient is *homebound* (i.e., the patient's condition interferes with the normal ability to leave the home or leaving the home would require a considerable effort).
2. Need for *intermittent* skilled nursing, physical therapy, or speech therapy. (One of these three services must be needed to qualify for reimbursement for the other services provided by home health agencies, i.e., social work, occupational therapy, home health aide, and nutrition services.)
3. Physician must sign renewal of orders every 60 days.

Medicaid (Coverage for home health services varies by state.)

Veterans Administration (Available for veterans who are homebound because of chronic illness.)

Home care from hospital-based programs[c]

Blue Cross and other private health insurance[c]

[a]Note that since 1981, Part A Medicare has covered patients even if they have not been recently hospitalized.
[b]See Chapter 13 for details regarding hospice criteria and benefits.
[c]Coverage for home health services varies by plan.

hospital care. These changes have promoted the development of detailed care guidelines and increased focus on instructing patients and family members to carry out care plans. Patients must meet the generic criteria listed in Table 9.6 for services to be reimbursed by Medicare and other third-party payers.

Medicare pays for "intermittent" home care services, defined as no more than 35 hours per week. There must be a documented goal of care that has a finite end point. Because of the Medicare criterion that the patient must have a medical problem requiring skilled care, payment for the services of a home health aide is often denied after the active problem becomes stable, even when the home health aide's services are important in maintaining the patient's health. In some instances, Medicaid funding is available for ongoing personal care services, provided in lieu of nursing home care.

Physician's Role

For home health services that are reimbursed, the patient's physician must approve and sign orders for all services and revisions of services. Medicare requires an extensive report and newly signed orders every 60 days.

The quality of the communication between physicians and home care providers often determines how much the patient will benefit from home health services. When physicians provide clear and complete initial information and both physicians and home care providers can reach each other easily when needed, patients who would otherwise require in-hospital care can receive excellent care in their homes.

The American Academy of Home Care Physicians (www.aahcp.org) is an organization of physicians and other home care professionals, founded in the late 1980s, that is dedicated to improving the quality of home care. The organization's newsletter, other publications, and annual meeting focus on the evaluation of and education about home health care ideas and programs.

SPECIFIC REFERENCES

1. Annual Statistical Report on the Social Security Disability Insurance Program, 2004. Available at www.ssa.gov/policy/docs/statcomps/di_asr/2004/index.htm/.
2. Society Security Online Electronic Fact Sheet, Update 2005. Available at: www.ssa.gov/pubs/10003.html.
3. Basic statistics about home care 1996. Washington, DC: National Association for Home Care, October 1996.

For annotated **General References** *and resources related to this chapter, visit www.hopkinsbayview.org/PAMreferences.*

Chapter 10

Care of the Patient with Cancer

Michael J. Purtell and Larry Waterbury

This chapter examines the role of the generalist in caring for patients who have cancer. Common cancers are discussed in other chapters (breast, Chapter 105; gastrointestinal, Chapter 45; gynecologic, Chapter 104; lung, Chapter 61; prostate, Chapter 53; skin, Chapter 114). Figure 10.1 depicts the estimated distribution of newly diagnosed cancers and cancer deaths for 2005. After initial diagnostic evaluation, the location of the primary cancer is unidentified in some patients with metastatic disease. The most common primary cancers that are eventually identified in such patients are cancers of the pancreas, lung, kidney, and colon (1). However, for 15% of such patients a primary is never identified after initial screening (syndrome of cancer with unknown primary). For these situations, an extensive search for the primary is not usually clinically useful. Therapy is based on the pattern of the metastases, and on the morphologic and immunochemical characteristics of the diagnostic tissue in conjunction with empiric guidelines derived from clinical trials testing various chemotherapy combinations. In the future, profiling the tissue with deoxyribonucleic acid (DNA) microarrays or selecting therapy with the use of proteomics, as well as further defining the extent of the cancer with such imaging modalities as positron emission tomography (PET) may become important (2,3).

GENERAL ASPECTS OF CARE

Communicating the Diagnosis

A patient's primary care provider is the one who is most likely to initiate diagnostic evaluation for cancer and to communicate the diagnosis to the patient. During these initial steps, the following elements are important: promptly scheduling tests and notifying the patient of results; communicating clearly; allowing the patient ample time to react to bad news. Almost always a referral to an oncologist should be considered. Treatment options and prognoses may change with new developments of which only the specialist may be aware. In the case of older (≥65; <75) patients, it is important that the primary care doctor does not unduly use age as a selection criteria when deciding if and to what subspecialty the patient should be referred. For example, it has been noted that whereas "fit" elderly (≥75) patients tolerate thoracic surgery as well as younger (<65) patients, many younger patients with early-stage lung cancer are referred to a thoracic surgeon, whereas the majority of elderly patients of similar potentially curable stage cancers are sent to the radiation oncologist, despite the underlining assumption that for early-stage lung cancer, surgery is the better option (4). Similarly, age should not be the major criteria when deciding between referral for hospice care or palliative chemotherapy (5). Irrespective of these considerations, it should be the role of the primary physician to promptly outline and explain, based on the type and extent of the cancer, what the patient's general options are and what the primary physician would recommend; to check the patient's understanding of information that has been given; and to include family members who the patient selects in all discussions regarding diagnosis, options, and prognosis. Chapters 3 and 4 discuss in detail approaches to communication with patients and their family members.

Initial Referral and Treatment

When possible, one should refer patients to oncologists whom one trusts and knows to be helpful, considerate clinicians. Multimodality treatment regimens involving the combined efforts of surgical, medical, and radiation oncologists may result in a bewildered patient without a

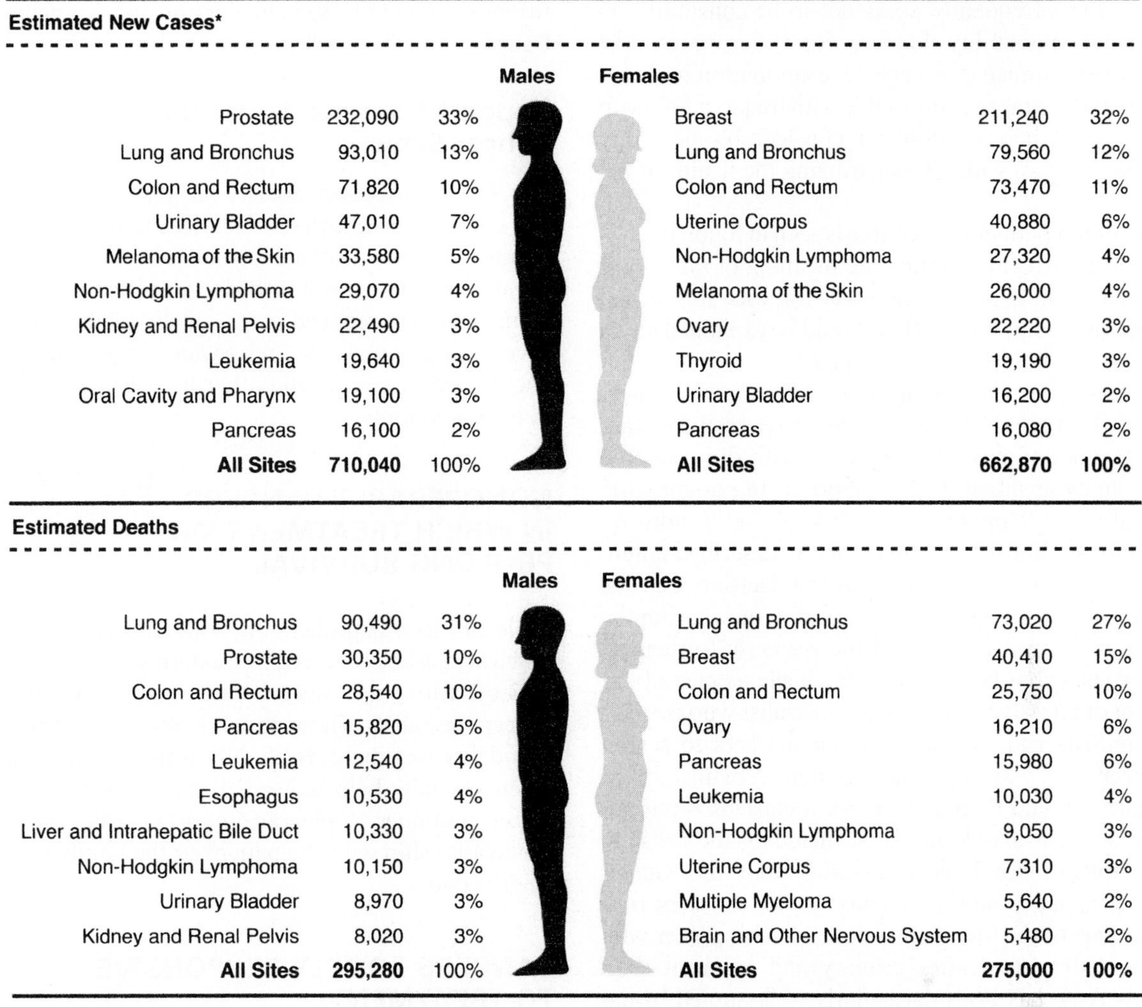

Estimated New Cases*

Males			Females		
Prostate	232,090	33%	Breast	211,240	32%
Lung and Bronchus	93,010	13%	Lung and Bronchus	79,560	12%
Colon and Rectum	71,820	10%	Colon and Rectum	73,470	11%
Urinary Bladder	47,010	7%	Uterine Corpus	40,880	6%
Melanoma of the Skin	33,580	5%	Non-Hodgkin Lymphoma	27,320	4%
Non-Hodgkin Lymphoma	29,070	4%	Melanoma of the Skin	26,000	4%
Kidney and Renal Pelvis	22,490	3%	Ovary	22,220	3%
Leukemia	19,640	3%	Thyroid	19,190	3%
Oral Cavity and Pharynx	19,100	3%	Urinary Bladder	16,200	2%
Pancreas	16,100	2%	Pancreas	16,080	2%
All Sites	**710,040**	100%	**All Sites**	**662,870**	**100%**

Estimated Deaths

Males			Females		
Lung and Bronchus	90,490	31%	Lung and Bronchus	73,020	27%
Prostate	30,350	10%	Breast	40,410	15%
Colon and Rectum	28,540	10%	Colon and Rectum	25,750	10%
Pancreas	15,820	5%	Ovary	16,210	6%
Leukemia	12,540	4%	Pancreas	15,980	6%
Esophagus	10,530	4%	Leukemia	10,030	4%
Liver and Intrahepatic Bile Duct	10,330	3%	Non-Hodgkin Lymphoma	9,050	3%
Non-Hodgkin Lymphoma	10,150	3%	Uterine Corpus	7,310	3%
Urinary Bladder	8,970	3%	Multiple Myeloma	5,640	2%
Kidney and Renal Pelvis	8,020	3%	Brain and Other Nervous System	5,480	2%
All Sites	**295,280**	100%	**All Sites**	**275,000**	**100%**

FIGURE 10.1. Estimated new cancer cases **(A)** and estimated cancer deaths **(B)** in 10 leading sites by sex, United States, 2005; excludes basal and squamous cell skin cancers and carcinoma in situ, except bladder. (From Jemal A, Murray T, Ward E, et al. Cancer statistics 2005. Ca Cancer J Clin 2005;55:10, with permission.)

clinician who accepts the primary responsibility for care. The patient's primary care practitioner should either coordinate care or identify who will be the coordinator for the patient's care and who will be accessible to the patient to answer questions, provide support, and ensure that necessary information is communicated. By receiving up-to-date and complete information about the diagnostic and therapeutic plans and the patient's evolving status, the primary care practitioner may be able to assess the overall picture and, as time goes on, identify when problems resulting from treatment (e.g., side effects, expense, family disruption, and deteriorating psychological status of patient) appear to outweigh the likely benefits of continued therapy. The treating oncologists will welcome such insights and consequently will consider a modification of the treatment regimen or will suggest a referral to a hospice program.

Followup Care

Most oncologists welcome participation of the patient's primary care practitioner in continuing care. This is particularly important when treatment is given in an oncology center in a distant city. Some less-toxic ambulatory treatment regimens and, particularly, symptom-management strategies may even be handled by the primary care practitioner under the direction of the specialist.

The followup of treated patients requires knowledge of the common sites and manifestations of tumor recurrence, the appropriate timing of followup examinations and tests, and a great deal of sensitivity in recognizing the feelings of the patient and the patient's family. Chapters elsewhere in this book on specific cancers discuss what is known and what is not known about the usefulness of followup assessments. Some patients function better if they are scheduled to be seen less frequently, so as not to be constantly reminded of the possibility of recurrence. Others require the constant reassurance of a negative examination and normal tests and are more comfortable with frequent followup visits. Usually there is room for considerable flexibility in a followup plan without jeopardizing the health of the patient.

Whenever a patient with cancer is seen in followup, it is important to explain carefully the meaning of symptoms or physical findings and the rationale for tests. If tests will take several days to return, that should be explained and a time for a telephone followup arranged.

It is possible in the future that *tumor markers* measured in the patient's serum—either to screen for cancer or to monitor therapy in patients with disseminated cancer—may be shown to be important in patient care. A critical analysis published in 1991 (6) and a more recent National Cancer Institute report (7) described potential roles for tumor markers in clinical decision making. Although tumor markers can be useful in monitoring the progress of known disease and the response to therapy, these are uses that benefit patients chiefly as part of the care plan of an oncologist or other specialist who is treating them. The routine use of tumor markers to screen for cancer in the asymptomatic patient remains potentially harmful, and there is no current consensus regarding any of the available markers, including the prostate specific antigen (see Table 14.2 and Chapter 53). Generally, it is inappropriate to monitor tumor markers routinely as part of the followup of patients with cancer who are potentially cured after primary and adjuvant therapy. This issue has been particularly well studied in patients with breast cancer (8). There are exceptions such as the use of the carcinoembryonic antigen (CEA) in colon cancer, the cancer antigen (CA)-125 in ovarian cancer, or β-human chorionic gonadotropin (β-hCG) in testicular cancers. The National Cancer Comprehensive Network publishes guidelines for the followup strategies of most cancers. These are available at its website: www.nccn.org/professionals/physician_gls/license_agreement.asp. Recommendations are ranked based on evidence-based criteria and degree of consensus among contributing experts.

Family Concerns

The crises attending evaluation for possible cancer and the diagnosis and care for cancer profoundly affect the spouses and families of patients. Common dilemmas for family members include emotional strain, physical demands in caring for the patient, altered roles and lifestyles, finances, and uncertainty about prognosis (9). In addition, there may be questions about the likelihood of cancer occurring in other members of the family. Each of these issues may require consideration by the patient's primary care practitioner (for details, see chapters on specific cancers and Chapters 13, 17, and 20).

Support from the American Cancer Society

The American Cancer Society has chapters in each state and can provide a variety of services to patients and their families. Services vary among states but may include loan of supplies (e.g., hospital beds), transportation to treatment facilities, reduced costs for chemotherapy, respite coverage for caregivers, and a wide range of information about support groups and other help available in the patient's community.

NONOPERABLE CANCERS IN WHICH TREATMENT MAY PROLONG SURVIVAL

Table 10.1 lists a number of nonoperable cancers in which survival may be prolonged by modern treatment regimens; patients with such cancers need ongoing followup with cancer specialists. These patients often benefit from multimodality treatment. Even within this group of cancers, when specialty help is needed, the primary care practitioner continues to play an important role, especially if the relationship with the patient or the family has been a lengthy one.

CANCERS POORLY RESPONSIVE TO TREATMENT

Table 10.2 lists a number of nonoperable cancers that are less responsive to therapy, where the impact of therapy on survival is unproven or minimal. Diagnosis and initial therapy for limited stage disease usually require surgery,

TABLE 10.1 Some Nonoperable Cancers for which Treatment May Be Curative or May Dramatically Prolong Survival[a]

Acute leukemia
Hodgkin disease
Lymphoma
Metastatic testicular cancer
Metastatic ovarian cancer
Small cell carcinoma of the lung
Metastatic breast cancer
Metastatic large bowel cancer
Chronic myelocytic leukemia
Chronic lymphocytic leukemia
Multiple myeloma

[a]Patients with these cancers require specialized multimodality therapy. Bone marrow and stem cell transplantation have a role in the treatment of some of these cancers.

TABLE 10.2 Some Cancers in which Treatment May Provide Palliation or a Modest Effect on Survival

Non–small cell lung cancer (unresectable)
Metastatic stomach cancer
Metastatic pancreatic cancer
Metastatic malignant melanoma
Metastatic soft-tissue sarcomas
Metastatic cervical cancer
Metastatic endometrial cancer
Metastatic renal cell carcinoma
Hormone refractory metastatic prostate cancer

TABLE 10.3 Factors Affecting Palliative Treatment Recommendations in Patients with Cancer

Natural history of the untreated cancer
Proven effect of treatment on the natural history
Likely effects on survival, morbidity, and quality of life
Toxicity of treatment
Functional status of the patient
Ability of the patient to comprehend the implications of treatment
Psychological state and philosophical position of the patient
Emotional strength and attitudes of immediate family
Financial situation, health coverage status

but when metastasis is proven, the effect of systemic therapy, radiotherapy, or both, is at most palliative. In such situations, patients often expect their primary care practitioners to help them select or recommend treatment plans. Several questions come up at this juncture.

Should palliative chemotherapy be recommended? Although it is difficult to generalize, several factors must be considered in attempting to help patients and their families decide whether the patient is likely to benefit from palliative chemotherapy. More than age, the functional status of the patient must be considered in such therapeutic decisions. The infirm, ill, poorly functional patient with widely disseminated and rapidly progressive disease may be more harmed than benefited by the side effects and discomforts of palliative treatment, especially if response rates are small and toxicity of treatment is high. Weight loss before therapy correlates closely with poor response rates in clinical chemotherapy trials in these less-responsive cancers (10). Other patients, even if elderly, who are in good functional status are much more suitable candidates for attempts at palliation (11). For example, elderly patients with metastatic lung cancer, but otherwise in good health, given systemic chemotherapy appear to maintain their quality of life longer than similar elderly patients given only supportive care. These findings mirror those observed with younger patients (4,5). The patient who believes that any chance of response is worth the price of toxicity and who cannot feel comfortable unless attempting some therapy, should generally be offered treatment.

If some attempt at palliative treatment seems worthwhile, should it be conventional therapy or experimental protocol therapy? Every oncology center has current protocols for the metastatic cancers listed in Table 10.2. Clinical protocols designed to seek improved methods of treatment are important for advances that may improve the outlook and the comfort of future patients. However, experimental therapy may have undesirable consequences for the individual patient. Sometimes, such protocols involve the investigation of treatments with more toxicity than current conventional therapies. They may require more frequent visits to the clinician and more frequent diagnostic tests, because of the necessity to document precisely the objective response. They may therefore also involve increased expense to the patient. The patient's insurance may or may not cover the specific experimental therapy being considered. Patients agreeing to experimental protocol therapy—and their practitioners—must be well informed about the side effects and likely benefits of therapy (12,13). The helpful consultant should describe the current conventional treatment for the patient's disease and tailor the recommendation to the specific patient. No treatment, conventional palliative chemotherapy or radiotherapy, or experimental therapy are appropriate choices for individual patients depending on their situations and preferences. Table 10.3 lists the major factors for patient and clinician in selecting among these options.

RADIOTHERAPY

Patient Experience. The patient with cancer often has misconceptions about and limited knowledge of radiotherapy. It is thus important to explain radiotherapy to the patient in terms of the rationale, patient experience, and likely benefits and side effects of this treatment modality. The initial visit usually includes a complete history and physical examination by the radiotherapist. Further diagnostic tests (e.g., radiographs and computed tomography) may be obtained. If the therapist agrees that treatment is appropriate and urgent, the radiotherapy ports may be determined at the first visit and the patient may receive his or her first treatment at that time. The patient is told that skin tattoos may be placed to facilitate the uniformity of subsequent treatments. It is important to explain that the therapy machines are bulky and somewhat overwhelming in appearance. Some patients are frightened by the experience. This may be particularly so with techniques such as stereotactic-based radiosurgery (i.e., gamma knife), which rely on extremely accurate targeting of the tumor. To achieve or maintain the necessary precision, the patient is immobilized in a brace to prevent undue motion. These procedures will become more commonplace as studies supporting their benefits—already shown for the treatment of brain metastases—become available (14). If the referring clinician appreciates this, it is useful to contact the radiotherapist and to explain the particular fears of the patient ahead of time. Therapists often give patients and their families a tour of the radiotherapy treatment rooms before starting therapy and spend extra time answering questions about the treatment and its benefits and complications. The patient should be aware that the treatments themselves are not painful. The initial consultation is usually time-consuming (several hours), but subsequent treatments are usually scheduled precisely and frequently require only a small amount of time (15 to 30 minutes). Treatments are usually given several days a week and the entire course may take several weeks to complete. The patient usually does not see the radiotherapist at the time of each treatment but is seen by a radiotherapy nurse or technician. Consequently, the patient needs to know precisely with whom to communicate to address side effects or questions during radiotherapy.

Time Until Symptomatic Response

In addition to the timing and types of side effects that may be experienced, it is important for the patient to know that the response to treatment is often delayed and that sometimes the maximal effect is noted a few weeks after the course of radiotherapy is completed. For example, radiotherapy is useful in the palliation of pain secondary to local bony metastases, but 2 to 3 weeks may elapse before improvement occurs and improvement may not be maximal until a few weeks after treatment is discontinued. Some responses are more rapid, occurring after only a few days of therapy (e.g., relief of superior vena cava obstruction and neurologic deficits from spinal cord obstruction or central nervous system metastasis).

An excellent booklet, *Radiation Therapy and You: A Guide to Self-Help During Treatment,* is available free from the National Institutes of Health to patients undergoing radiotherapy (see www.hopkinsbayview.org/PAMreferences). It is helpful to have copies of this booklet available for patients and families to read when radiotherapy is being considered.

Side Effects

Table 10.4 describes important side effects of radiotherapy. The patient will be most concerned by the common side effects that occur during treatment and by those that may remain for a few weeks after treatment is discontinued.

TABLE 10.4 Important Side Effects of Radiotherapy

Dermatitis: Less common with newer high-energy machines; avoid sunlight and extreme cold.
Acute radiation pneumonitis: Transient, usually occurring 6–12 wk after treatment; precipitated by corticosteroid withdrawal, concomitant chemotherapy; clinical manifestations include nonproductive cough, dyspnea, fever, leukocytosis with parenchymal infiltrates on radiograph in the area of the radiation ports; may respond to steroid treatment.
Pulmonary fibrosis: Occurs 6–12 mo after treatment; not responsive to steroids.
Esophagitis: Usually occurs during treatment; particularly severe when radiotherapy and chemotherapy are administered together.
Nausea, vomiting, and diarrhea: Occur during treatment with most abdominal radiotherapy, usually self-limited.
Enteritis: Rare, more likely with very high-dose treatment; small bowel more sensitive than large bowel and stomach; occurs weeks to years after radiotherapy; manifestations include obstruction, bleeding, perforation; pelvic irradiation (e.g., in the treatment of bladder or prostate cancer) may cause acute *proctitis*, which occasionally becomes chronic, sometimes leading to bleeding or stricture formation.
Pericarditis: Occurs months to years after radiation, usually resolves, occasionally progresses to constrictive pericarditis or tamponade requiring pericardiectomy. There is also an increased incidence of coronary artery disease seen years after mediastinal irradiation.
Neurologic side effects: Transverse myelitis, very rare; side effects from CNS irradiation in adults are rare. Lhermitte sign (the sensation of electric shocks passing down the body when the head is flexed) seen in 10% of patients undergoing mantle irradiation for Hodgkin disease; after radiotherapy, herpes zoster is common.
Hypothyroidism: Common in patients treated for Hodgkin disease with mantle field; may develop years after treatment.
Sterility: Usually temporary.
Growth retardation in children: Occurs both from direct skeletal effects and from hypopituitarism from CNS irradiation.
Oral and dental side effects: Dry mouth and partial or complete loss of taste or smell are common. Severe dental problems are common after head and neck irradiation because of decrease in saliva formation, increased sensitivity to caries. Osteonecrosis is a rare but serious side effect of head and neck irradiation.
Cystitis: Occurs during treatment with pelvic irradiation; clinical manifestations include urgency dysuria and hematuria occurring usually during the third and fourth weeks of treatment; usually self-limited and treated symptomatically with fluids and phenazopyridine (Pyridium), 200 mg four times a day; chronic bladder fibrosis is a rare late complication manifested usually by painless hematuria.
Second cancers: Breast, sarcoma, and lung in patients treated for Hodgkin disease with mantle field; may develop years after treatment.

CNS, central nervous system.
See references 17, and 23–27.

Dermatitis secondary to radiotherapy is less common than it used to be because of the use of the modern high-energy machines. Severe burning requiring specialized treatment is uncommon; however, skin discoloration may occur. The patient should be told that the radiation field should not be exposed to sunlight or extreme cold, that total but temporary hair loss will usually occur in the areas being radiated and that complete return of hair, after high-dose radiation, may take many months or may not occur.

The most troublesome side effects that occur during radiotherapy are *gastrointestinal.* Patients receiving radiation to the chest or upper back often experience symptoms of radiation esophagitis (odynophagia and sometimes reflux symptoms that may respond to elevation of the head of the bed and to antacids). Severe esophagitis is more likely to occur when radiotherapy has been used in patients who have had prior chemotherapy, especially with such agents as doxorubicin, bleomycin, or *cis*-platinum. *Candida* superinfection of the irritated esophagus is not unusual, especially in patients who are receiving steroids. This usually responds well to treatment with fluconazole (100 mg daily). Patients should improve with a 1-week course of therapy. Abdominal irradiation can cause diarrhea that may persist to some degree during the entire course of treatment. In addition to replacing fluids and electrolytes, some dietary maneuvers may minimize diarrhea; these are listed in Table 10.5. Nausea and anorexia are the most troublesome side effects of abdominal irradiation and are discussed separately later in this chapter.

Patients who receive radiotherapy to the head or neck are subject to *oral and dental complications.* Before treatment, all patients should have a complete dental examination by a dentist experienced in the treatment of patients who have undergone radiotherapy. Damage to the teeth, gums, and bone, plus the xerostomia that results from high-dosage radiotherapy to the oral mucous membranes and salivary glands, may result in severe problems. Many of these can be prevented by appropriate prophylaxis (aggressive treatment of periodontal disease and infected teeth before radiation) and an ongoing program during and after radiotherapy, which should be strictly followed. The use of artificial saliva (Saliva Substitute, Roxane Laboratories) may be helpful for patients with xerostomia.

TABLE 10.5 Dietary Maneuvers for Therapy-Induced Diarrhea

Clear liquids (warm or at room temperature)
Avoid fiber (roughage) in the diet
Take smaller amounts of food more often
Avoid fatty foods
Avoid highly spiced foods
Avoid carbonated drinks, beans, cabbage, broccoli, cauliflower, and corn

Corticosteroids and Radiotherapy

The patient's primary care practitioner may sometimes be involved with the early treatment of central nervous system metastases or spinal cord compression, using corticosteroids in conjunction with radiotherapy. Multiple regimens are used. A common regimen consists of dexamethasone (Decadron), 4 to 25 mg four times a day, continued until the patient has received several courses of radiotherapy and then slowly tapered over 2 to 3 weeks. Steroids decrease the local edema that occurs in these situations and help protect against radiation-induced edema during the first few days of therapy. Despite the use of steroid, a patient receiving spinal radiation for a cord compression syndrome may rarely experience sudden neurologic deterioration during the initial period of treatment because of radiation-induced edema. This demands an emergent evaluation by a neurosurgeon for possible decompression laminectomy.

Cumulative Dosage

A maximal cumulative dosage of radiotherapy can safely be given to any one site without the risk of significant permanent tissue damage. This dosage varies for each organ system. If ports do not overlap, definitive full-dose radiotherapy can be given to multiple sites either concomitantly or sequentially. Problems occur when ports are contiguous or overlapping. For example, it is often more beneficial to give palliative total spine irradiation to patients with several isolated spine metastases than to treat only focal symptomatic areas, which may preclude later palliative radiotherapy to symptomatic contiguous areas.

CHEMOTHERAPY

Patient Experience. The chemotherapy experience for the patient is so varied (depending on the disease being treated) that it is hard to give a general description. The medical oncologist giving therapy can best explain to the patient the specifics of treatment, including how it is administered, the frequency of treatment, the hoped-for response, and the side effects. The most common troublesome side effects for the patient are hair loss and nausea and vomiting. The frequency and degree of hair loss vary with the treatment regimen, but it is helpful for the patient to know that hair will regrow once the treatment is discontinued. The treatment of nausea and vomiting is discussed later in this chapter (see Nausea, Vomiting, and Anorexia). Table 10.6 lists other acute and chronic side effects of various chemotherapeutic agents. Knowledge of the long-term side effects of various agents is particularly important for the primary care practitioner, who may be responsible for followup care of patients with good prognoses after chemotherapy.

TABLE 10.6 Common Side Effects of Chemotherapy*

Hair loss: Alkylating agents, vincristine, vinblastine, adriamycin, mithramycin daunomycin, taxanes, gemcitabine. Hair regrowth occurs once chemotherapy is discontinued.
Hypercalcemia: Estrogens, antiestrogens (tamoxifen).
Fluid retention: Estrogens, androgens, steroids, taxanes, gemcitabine.
Skin darkening: Adriamycin (nails), 5-FU, bleomycin, busulfan, methotrexate. May improve slowly over time.
Dermatitis: Methotrexate, alkylating agents, vinblastine, 6-MP, 6-thioguanine bleomycin (may be delayed), tyrosine kinase inhibitors (TKIS).
Marrow depression: Almost all chemotherapy agents, except for vincristine and bleomycin. Nitrosoureas may be associated with delayed thrombocytopenia.
Neurologic: cis-Platinum (deafness), oxaliplatin (peripheral neuropathy), vincristine, vinblastine, methotrexate, hexamethylmelamine, 5-FU (ataxia), procarbazine, ifosphamide (encephalopathy seizures), taxanes, vinorelbine. Neurologic deficits occur during treatment and sometimes gradually improve, but sometimes are permanent.
Diarrhea: 5-FU, irinotecan, TKIS.
Gastrointestinal ulcerations: Methotrexate, 5-FU, bleomycin (mucocutaneous), adriamycin.
Cardiomyopathy: Adriamycin, daunorubicin, mitoxantrone, infusional 5-FU, Herceptin.
Pulmonary fibrosis: Bleomycin, alkylating agents, mitomycin-C, gemcitabine. Occurs gradually during treatment or may be delayed.
Renal damage: cis-Platinum, methotrexate, streptozotocin, ifosphamide, nitrosoureas.
Red urine: Adriamycin, daunomycin.
Hepatic toxicity: Mithramycin, methotrexate, nitrosoureas, cytosine arabinoside, 6-MP, taxanes.
Sexual and gonadal dysfunction: Many drugs and regimens.
Secondary neoplasm: Alkylating agents, especially when combined with radiotherapy. Occurrence is delayed years.
Flulike symptoms, malaise: Biologics (IL-2, interferon, monoclonal antibodies) gemcitabine, taxanes, cladribine.
Fever: Bleomycin, biologics.
Hypersensitivity reaction: Taxanes, etoposide, monoclonal antibodies.

5-FU, 5-fluorouracil; 6-MP, 6-mercaptopurine; IL-2; interleukin-2.
*Modified from reference 28.

An excellent free booklet, *Chemotherapy and You: A Guide to Self-Help During Treatment,* written for patients, is available through the National Institutes of Health (see www.hopkinsbayview.org/PAMreferences). It is helpful to have this booklet available for patients and families to read when chemotherapy is being considered.

Chemotherapy-Induced Granulocytopenic Fever

The most common side effect of cytotoxic chemotherapy is myelosuppression and the associated risk of systemic infection (15). Granulocytopenia is defined as an absolute neutrophil count of <1,000 cells/mm^3. However, a significant risk of infection is not incurred until the concentration falls below 500 cells/mm^3. In particular, the incidence of culture-proven septicemia correlates best with the number of days a patient remains with a neutrophil count below 100 cells/mm^3. The nadir of the white count, and hence the largest risk of serious infection, usually occurs 10 to 14 days after chemotherapy is administered. It is the responsibility of the treating oncologist to monitor the neutrophil counts and to instruct patients when to check their temperatures and when to seek help if a fever or other signs (e.g., malaise, chills, cough) of infection develop. However, there may be circumstances when the patient's primary care practitioner may be contacted by the patient.

It has been dogma that any granulocytopenic patient is at great risk for gram-negative bacteremia, especially *Pseudomonas,* and that all febrile neutropenic patients need immediate hospitalization with appropriate empiric antibiotic coverage. For the primary care practitioner, who may not have the patient's latest hemogram and who may not have followed the recent course of the patient, this still may be the best guideline. On admission the patient should have blood and urine cultures and a chest radiograph. A history of new symptoms and an examination guided by symptoms, but always including attention to the mouth, skin, and perirectal area, may reveal a source. Unlike unimpaired patients, immunocompromised patients can have a life-threatening septicemia with few or no focal signs or symptoms. Therefore, instead of watching and waiting at the time of admission, one should initiate treatment with broad-spectrum antibiotics such as a semisynthetic penicillin and an aminoglycoside or third- or fourth-generation cephalosporin to which *Pseudomonas* is sensitive. In recent years, the incidence of *Pseudomonas* bacteremia has markedly decreased in these patients; *Escherichia coli* and *Klebsiella pneumoniae* remain the most common infections, and the incidence of gram-positive infections, especially coagulase-negative staphylococci, has risen, probably because of the increased use of indwelling venous access devices. On occasion, when the patient is not sick and the expected length of neutropenia is short, the experienced oncologist may elect to treat the febrile neutropenic patient as an outpatient. The quinolones are most commonly used. When gram-positive infections are suspected, clindamycin and amoxicillin/potassium clavulanate are frequently used.

NAUSEA, VOMITING, AND ANOREXIA

Nausea and vomiting can be the most troublesome side effects of radiotherapy and chemotherapy. In the past, the symptomatic treatment of nausea was only moderately effective, and vomiting was particularly troublesome with therapies containing *cis*-platinum. However, antiemetic regimens combining corticosteroids (dexamethasone, 10 to 20 mg either intravenously or orally) with an HT_3 serotonin blocker (e.g., ondansetron, 15 to 30 mg intravenously or orally) have greatly reduced the incidence of nausea and vomiting in the first 24 hours after therapy with *cis*-platinum and other strongly emetic regimens (16; NCCN website at: www.nccn.org). Oral serotonin blockers can be helpful for ongoing nausea from radiotherapy and chemotherapy. Lorazepam may have a role in relaxing the anxious patient before chemotherapy, and because of its interference with short-term memory, it may also lessen the chance of a patient developing anticipatory nausea (17). The nausea of less emetogenic regimens usually can be controlled with a 10- to 20-mg dose of dexamethasone and a lower dose of an HT_3 serotonin inhibitor. Prochlorperazine, preferably 10 mg intravenously, can be effective for acute emesis; 10 mg orally or 25 mg rectally can be used for more chromic nausea. Nausea that begins 1 or 2 days after the administration of the chemotherapy and lasts for a week or more is still a difficult problem to treat, especially after administration of *cis*-platinum. Attempts to treat with a short course of oral dexamethasone (8 to 12 mg/day) or with prochlorperazine (one or two 10-mg capsules orally or a 25-mg suppository every 4 to 6 hours) are only moderately successful. Once developed, delayed nausea is usually not helped by oral serotonin blockers. However with the recent introduction of the antiemetic aprepitant (an inhibitor of neurokinin 1 receptors) and of palonosetron, a serotonin $5HT_3$ receptor inhibitor with a prolonged biologic half-life, delayed nausea and vomiting are less of a problem (18). In addition to pharmacologic palliation, the patient with marked nausea will find that it is often helpful to be extremely still, lying down in a quiet room without external stimuli. Even with the improvements in therapy for chemotherapy-induced nausea, patients still consider nausea and vomiting among the most troublesome side effects of chemotherapy (19).

A number of *dietary maneuvers* may be helpful to the patient experiencing nausea and vomiting after therapy. The patient who experiences severe nausea and vomiting after therapy should probably drink only clear liquids until the symptoms are decreased. In general, it is more helpful to take smaller portions of food frequently than to take larger meals less often, to take foods that are low in fat, and to avoid overly sweet foods. Mild nausea, especially that experienced before therapy or in anticipation of therapy, may be helped by taking dry toast or crackers in small quantities. It is recommended that patients not lie down just after eating. Some patients find also that it is helpful not to drink liquids with their food (because this may increase their feeling of bloating and subsequent nausea). Many patients become nauseated at the smell of food cooking, and it may be helpful for them to go to another part of the house or to stay out of the house when food is being prepared. Greasy and fried foods seem to be the worst offenders in this regard and are best avoided.

A major problem with intensive cancer therapy is *general anorexia,* which is often associated with alterations in taste and smell and which may result in considerable nutritional problems and weight loss (20). Consultation with a dietitian may be helpful in such a situation. Oral progesterone (Megace) in large doses (300 to 800 mg/day) may be helpful for the patient with persistent anorexia (21). Dexamethasone in dosages of 2 to 4 mg twice per day can also be used. The steroid side effects restricts its use to acute brief episodes or end-of-life situations. Some studies show that oxandrolone, a weak anabolic steroid, preserves muscle mass better than other agents. Because it does not have any immunosuppressive properties, it may be more suited for those patients still receiving chemotherapy (22). Its expense limits its use.

An excellent free booklet, *Eating Hints for Cancer Patient: Before, During, and After Treatment,* is available through the National Cancer Institute (see www.hopkins bayview.org/PAMreferences). It contains all sorts of dietary advice for patients with cancer, including many recipes.

TERMINAL CARE

The primary care practitioner who has participated in various phases of cancer care and who has an ongoing relationship with the patient and his or her family is often in the best position to help during a patient's terminal illness. The practitioner who develops some expertise in this regard can find enormous gratification from this role. Chapter 13 deals with many of the issues important in caring for terminally ill patients and their families, including the very important issues of pain control, hospice care, and bereavement. An excellent publication, *Coping with Cancer: A Resource for the Health Professional,* is available free of charge from the National Institutes of Health (see www.hopkinsbayview.org/PAMreferences). In addition to other useful information, it lists organizations and agencies that provide useful services that may aid the practitioner in providing support for the dying patient.

SPECIFIC REFERENCES*

1. Le Chevalier T, Cvitkovic E, Caille P, et al. Early metastatic cancer of unknown primary origin at presentation: a clinical study of 302 consecutive autopsied patients. Arch Intern Med 1988; 148:2035.
2. Varadhachary GR, Abbruzzese JL, Lenzi R. Diagnostic strategies for unknown primary cancer. Cancer 2004;100:1776.
3. Chorost MI, Lee C, Yeoh CB, et al. Unknown primary. J Surg Oncol 2004;87:191.
4. Hurria A, Kris MG. Management of lung cancer in older adults. Ca Cancer J Clin 2003;53:325.
5. Gridelli C, Aapro M, Ardizzoni A, et al. Treatment of advanced non–small-cell lung cancer in the elderly: results of an international expert panel. J Clin Oncol 2005;23:3125.
6. Bates SE. Clinical applications of serum tumor markers. Ann Intern Med 1991;115:623.
7. National Cancer Institute. Tumor markers. National Cancer Institute Cancer website. Available at: http://cancerweb.ncl.ac.uk/cancernet/600518.html. Last accessed September 30, 2005.
8. ASCO Breast Cancer Surveillance Expert Panel. Recommended breast cancer surveillance guidelines. J Clin Oncol 2000;17:1080.
9. Lewis FM. The impact of cancer on the family: a critical analysis of the research literature. In: Patient education and counseling. Limerick, Ireland: Elsevier Scientific Publishers, 1986:269.
10. Dewys WD. Prognostic effect of weight loss prior to chemotherapy in cancer patients. Am J Med 1980;69:491.
11. Yancik R, Ganz A, Varricchio GA, et al. Perspectives on comorbidity and cancer in older patients: approaches to expand the knowledge base. J Clin Oncol 2001;19:1147.
12. Penman DT. Informed consent for investigational chemotherapy: patients' and physicians' perceptions. J Clin Oncol 1984;2:849.
13. van Kleffens T, van Baarsen B, van Leeuwen E. The medical practice of patient automy and cancer treatment refusals: a patients' and physicians' perspective. Soc Sci Med 2004; 58:2325.
14. Andrews DW, Scott CB, Sperduto PW, et al. Whole brain radiation therapy with one to three metastases: phase III results of the RTOG 9508 randomized trial. Lancet 2004;363:1665.
15. Hughes WT, Armstrong D, Bodey GP, et al. Guidelines for the use of antimicrobial agents in neutropenic patients with unexplained fever. Clin Infect Dis 2002;34:730.
16. Gralla RJ, Osoba D, Krfis MG, et al. Recommendations for the use of antiemetics: evidence-based, clinical practice guidelines. J Clin Oncol 1999;17:2971.
17. Franzen P, Nyman J, Hagberg H, et al. A randomized placebo controlled study with ondansetron in patients undergoing fractionated radiotherapy. Ann Oncol 1996;7:587.
18. Warr DG, Grunberg SM, Gralla RJ, et al. The Oral NK (1) Antagonist aprepitant for the prevention of acute and delayed chemotherapy-induced nausea and vomiting: pooled data from 2 randomized, double-blind placebo controlled trials. Eur J Cancer 2005; 41:1278.
19. Griffin AM, Butow PN, Coates AS, et al. On the receiving end—patient perception of the side effects of cancer chemotherapy, 1993. Ann Oncol 1996;7:189.
20. Ottery FD. Supportive nutrition to prevent cachexia and improve quality of life. Semin Oncol 1995;22(Suppl 2):98.
21. Berenstein EG, Ortiz Z. Megestrol acetate for the treatment of anorexia-cachexia Syndrome. Cochrane Database Syst Rev 2005, Issue 2. Art. No: CD004310.pub2. DOI: 10.1002/14651858.CD004310.pub2.
22. Langer CJ, Hoffman JP. Clinical significance of weight loss in cancer for the use of anabolic agents in the treatment of cancer-related cachexia. Nutrition 2001;17(1 Suppl):S1.
23. Myer JL, Jerome MV. Radiation injury: advances in management and prevention. In: Myer JL, ed. Frontiers of radiation therapy and oncology. Vol. 32. Basel: Karger, 1999.
24. Zimmerman RP, Mark RJ, Tran LM, et al. Concomitant pilocarpine during head and neck RT is associated with decreased posttreatment xerostomia. Int J Radiat Oncol Biol Phys 1997; 37:571.
25. Berk L. An overview of radiotherapy trials for the treatment of brain metastases. Oncology 1995;9:1205.
26. Blayney DW, Longo D. Radiation-induced pericarditis. N Engl J Med 1982;306:550.
27. Gross NJ. Pulmonary effects of radiation therapy. Ann Intern Med 1997;86:81.
28. Perry MC, ed. Toxicity of chemotherapy. Semin Oncol 1992;19:453.

*Bold numerals denote published controlled clinical trials, meta-analyses, or consensus-based recommendations.

For annotated ***General References*** *and resources related to this chapter, visit www.hopkinsbayview.org/PAMreferences.*

loss. For all obese patients, one wishes to achieve a change in long-term eating patterns.

Some adolescents overeat because of unresolved psychological difficulties. If there are expressions of problems in peer, school, or parental relationships, these should be explored further. However, obesity alone is not an indication of psychopathology.

Anorexia Nervosa and Bulimia

Anorexia nervosa is serious disorder of growth in adolescents and adults. It is marked by voluntary suppression of appetite and loss of weight (at least 15% of the baseline weight) that is not attributable to a medical or psychiatric illness ordinarily associated with weight loss (i.e., inflammatory bowel disease or a major affective disorder). Patients characteristically exhibit an intense fear of becoming obese even when very thin and have a distorted body image, so they still consider themselves overweight (Table 11.3).

Anorexia nervosa is most commonly a disease of young adolescent girls (approximately 90% of cases), but it affects boys and older girls as well. Most often, the problem develops in children of upper-middle-class families. Before their illness, the patients typically are considered model children who do well in school and are obedient to their parents.

It would be wrong to consider anorexia and bulimia purely adolescent problems. These conditions extend into adulthood, and, indeed, anorexia is touted by some as a socially acceptable and fashionable lifestyle. Adults in professions where thinness is a professional requirement, such as athletes, actors, dancers, models, and TV personalities, are at special risk for eating disorders.

The cause of the disease is unknown. Although many theories have been proposed to explain it, none is entirely satisfactory. Often, there has been some stress in the family (divorce, death, change of location) before the onset of the illness.

No simple treatment can be recommended for patients with anorexia nervosa. Help should be sought from a psychiatrist who has experience with eating disorders. The best results seem to be achieved by involving the patient and the patient's family in an intensive program in which counseling and behavior modification are used to restructure the patient's eating habits and attitude toward food. Very ill patients should be hospitalized so that a proper program of nutrition can be instituted.

Complete remission of anorexia nervosa is unusual, but approximately 75% of patients achieve an acceptable

TABLE 11.3 DSM-IV Criteria for Diagnosing Eating Disorders

Anorexia Nervosa	*Bulimia Nervosa*
1. Refusal to maintain body weight at or above a minimally normal weight for age and height (e.g., weight loss leading to maintenance of body weight less than 85% of that expected, or failure to make expected weight gain during period of growth, leading to body weight less than 85% of that expected). 2. Intense fear of gaining weight or becoming fat, even though underweight. 3. Disturbance in the way in which one's body weight or shape is experienced, undue influence of body weight or shape on self-evaluation, or denial of the seriousness of the current low body weight. 4. In postmenarchal females, amenorrhea (i.e., the absence of at least three consecutive menstrual cycles). (A woman is considered to have amenorrhea if her periods occur only after hormone, e.g., estrogen, administration.) Specify type Restricting type: During the episode of anorexia nervosa, the person does not regularly engage in binge eating or purging behavior (i.e., self-induced vomiting or the misuse of laxatives or diuretics). Binge eating/purging type: During the episode of anorexia nervosa, the person regularly engages in binge eating or purging behavior (i.e., self-induced vomiting or the misuse of laxatives or diuretics).	1. Recurrent episodes of binge eating. An episode of binge eating is characterized by both of the following: a. Eating, in a discrete period of time (e.g., within any 2-hour period), an amount of food that is definitely larger than most people would eat during a similar period of time and under similar circumstances. b. A sense of lack of control over eating during the episode (e.g., a feeling that one cannot stop eating or control what or how much one is eating). 2. Recurrent inappropriate compensatory behavior to prevent weight gain, such as self-induced vomiting, misuse of laxatives, diuretics, or other medications; fasting; or excessive exercise. 3. The binge eating and inappropriate compensatory behaviors both occur, on average, at least twice a week for 3 months. 4. Self-evaluation is unduly influenced by body shape and weight. 5. The disturbance does not occur exclusively during episodes of anorexia nervosa. Specify type Purging type: The person regularly engages in self-induced vomiting or the misuse of laxatives or diuretics. Nonpurging type: The person uses other inappropriate compensatory behaviors, such as fasting or excessive exercise, but does not regularly engage in self-induced vomiting or the misuse of laxatives or diuretics.

From Diagnostic and statistical manual of mental disorders, 4th ed. (DSM-IV). Washington, DC: American Psychiatric Association, 1994, with permission.

improvement in both their physical and emotional states. The rest remain chronically undernourished and maladapted. With current treatment, mortality has been reduced to between 2% and 8% (3). Cause of death is equally attributable to overt suicide and medical complications of starvation. Poor prognosis is associated with long duration of illness, disturbed parent–child relationships, concomitant personality disorder, and the presence of vomiting (more common in bulimia). The degree of weight loss generally is unrelated to prognosis (4). The more persistent the behavior and the later in life these conditions are diagnosed and treated, the poorer the outcome in terms of maintaining a healthy weight. Adults who are grossly underweight have a mortality risk that is three times normal (3). Anorexic patients may have electrolyte deficiencies that can predispose to cardiac arrhythmia. With their obsession with excessive exercise, these patients dehydrate quickly.

Bulimia is a second eating disorder seen in adolescents and young adults. Most bulimic patients are female; bulimic symptoms have been reported by up to 10% of young women interviewed in community surveys (5). Characteristically, patients with bulimia periodically gorge themselves, only to follow this by self-induced vomiting and by further self-reprisals through abstinence from food (Table 11.3). As the disease progresses, patients may become withdrawn and depressed, leading to further appetite suppression. Amenorrhea is common in these patients, and it may be the presenting complaint. Some patients have a history of both anorexia and bulimia. Treatment of a patient with severe bulimia requires the help of a professional skilled in the management of eating disorders. Self-help groups such as Overeaters Anonymous may play an important role in the patient's long-term handling of bulimia.

SEXUAL DEVELOPMENT

Normal Patterns and Concerns

A major difference between the child and the adolescent is the development of the teen into a sexual being. The onset of puberty is associated with an intensification of sexual feelings and desires that lead to sexual exploration. With the liberalization of sexual mores in recent years, the problems of adolescent pregnancy and venereal diseases have grown to epidemic proportions.

The *staging of physical sexual development* of adolescents established by Tanner is a widely accepted method of following the physical changes of puberty (Tables 11.4 and 11.5 and Fig. 11.2). As the adolescent enters puberty, he or she also assumes a role as a sexual being who must

TABLE 11.4 Typical Progression of Female Adolescent Sexual Development (see also Fig. 11.2)

Stage 1 There is no pubic hair present, and there is no breast development. The ovaries have begun to enlarge. The external genitalia are preadolescent or those of a child.
Stage 2 Breast bud formation usually begins before pubic hair growth. A small mound is formed by the elevation of the breast and papilla. Areolar diameter increases. The adolescent height spurt begins, and there is an acceleration in the deposition of total body fat. The adult female habitus emerges as the breasts enlarge and the hips widen.
Stage 3 There is further spread of pubic hair and further enlargement of breasts and areola, with no separation of their contours. The vagina enlarges and the vaginal epithelium, responding to estrogen stimulation from the maturing ovaries, increases in thickness, with considerable deposition of glycogen. The height spurt usually reaches a peak early in stage 3, before menarche.
Stage 4 If menarche has not occurred late in stage 3, it should occur during stage 4. Axillary hair appears just before or after menarche, usually in early stage 4. There is a projection of the areola and papilla to form a secondary mound above the level of the breast. The areolar mound may be absent (25% of females). The breasts and pubic hair progress. The ovaries continue to enlarge. Ovulation may occur just after menarche, but it is usually delayed until stage 5.
Stage 5 Pubic hair and breast development resemble those of the adult female; the areola has recessed to the general contour of the breast. Height increase has decelerated since menarche; height may increase 2 to 4 inches after menarche. By 2 years after menarche, regular ovulation may be expected.
Stage 6 In 10% of females there is a further spread of pubic hair.

From Tanner JM. Growth at adolescence. New York: Appleton-Century-Crofts, 1966, with permission.

TABLE 11.5 Typical Progression of Male Adolescent Sexual Development

Stage 1 The male has no pubic hair or increase in size of the penis. This describes the male as a preadolescent or child. However, the testes are beginning to mature. Usually there is considerable acceleration in height and weight gain along with changes in body composition (especially more body fat).
Stage 2 There is early growth of the testes and scrotum before pubic hair appears. The height spurt accelerates; the male physique begins to change as fat and muscle are added, and the areola of the breast increases in size and darkens slightly.
Stage 3 There is further enlargement of the testes and scrotum, enlargement of the penis (mainly in length), and spreading and darkening of the pubic hair. Facial hair first appears at the corners of the upper lip. The height spurt accelerates further; there is broadening of the shoulders relative to the hips and generalized increased molding of the body, with considerable increase in muscle mass relative to fat. Hair appears in the perineum. Facial expression is significantly altered and appears more adult. The cartilage of the larynx enlarges, and the voice may begin to deepen. There is transient gynecomastia with slight projection of the areola.
Stage 4 Axillary hair first appears. There is continued enlargement of the scrotum, testes, and penis (the last, mainly in breadth). The pubic hair begins to appear adult. Facial hair is still limited to upper lip and chin. The first ejaculation, indicating considerable growth of the prostate gland, occurs early in stage 4. Sebaceous glands are approaching adult size and function. The voice deepens further.
Stage 5 Genital size and pubic hair distribution are adult in appearance. Hairs are present on the sides of the face. Gynecomastia has disappeared. The height spurt has decelerated and the physique is that of the mature male.
Stage 6 Some adolescents have a further spread of pubic hair up the linea alba, which may be described as stage 6. This later development, often not reached until the early twenties, occurs in 80% of males.

From Tanner JM. Growth at adolescence. New York: Appleton-Century-Crofts, 1966, with permission.

begin to meet expectations of society, family, and peer group and who is pushed into sexual propriety and conformity. These expectations are transmitted to the teen by multiple messages that are often conveyed poorly, and many teens remain ignorant and insecure about sexual issues.

Early adolescence is characterized by a bisexual period, in which close friendships are formed with members of the same sex but heterosexual attitudes develop. Young teens often develop best-buddy relationships. These relationships may even be physically intimate, but they are not considered characteristic of adult homosexuality. However, the teen (particularly male) may fear being a homosexual, and the frequent name-calling of this period (in which people are called "gay" or "queer" with little provocation) may be taken too seriously. Boys who have developed noticeable gynecomastia may be particularly confused about their sexual identity. Such boys need to be reassured of the normality of these concerns. Masturbation tends to be a frequent practice in this period, and there may be associated guilt that increases as the sex drive stimulates the teen to continue the practice. Again, where appropriate, problems associated with masturbation should be met with reassurance of its normality.

In mid to late adolescence, dating and heterosexual activities begin in earnest. By age 15 years, one in four girls and one in three boys has had sexual intercourse (6). Often, teens rush into sexual activity before they fully understand their own feelings about it. It is often part of the dating relationship—a prerequisite to communication, rather than vice versa. It may be part of thrill-seeking behavior for some teens, and others use it to escape from loneliness and depression.

Short Stature and Delayed Sexual Maturation

A common problem that comes to the attention of physicians is the teenager with short stature or delayed puberty. These two symptoms are often interrelated, and the medical investigation is similar, so they are discussed together. However, the presence of one does not necessarily indicate a problem with the other.

Most of these patients simply are at one end of the spectrum of normal development (7). Many teenage boys may not appreciate the fact that some people fall into the 10th percentile of a normal curve, and they may not accept a cursory dismissal of their concerns about size. Some may be helped by looking at normal growth curves that indicate the predicted ultimate height for people in their percentile (Fig. 11.1). Patients may need detailed discussion to comprehend fully and to cope with normal findings.

Assessment of short stature and delayed puberty by the generalist consists of the following steps:

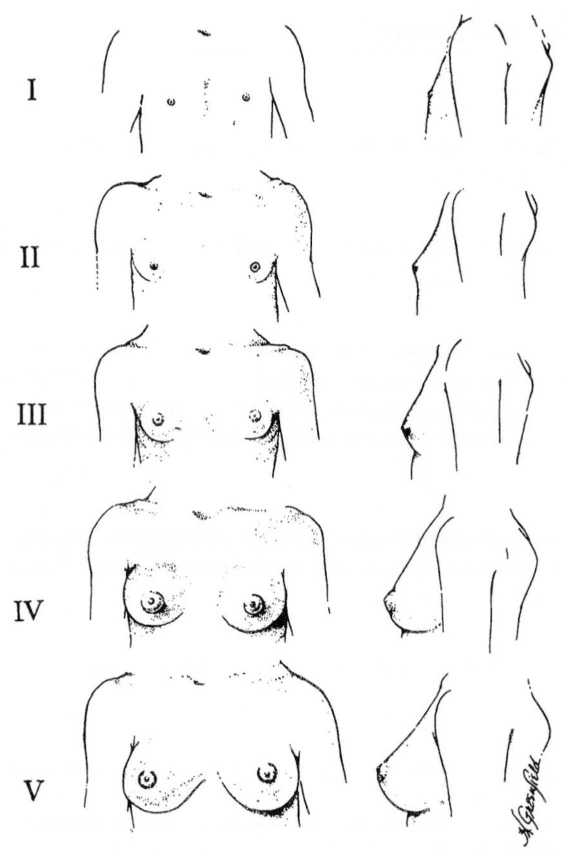

FIGURE 11.2. Diagrammatic representation of Tanner stages I to V of human breast maturation. (Adapted from Marshall WA, Tanner JM. Variations in pattern of pubertal changes in girls. Arch Dis Child 1969;44:291.)

1. A history of the onset of puberty and of the height of siblings, parents, and grandparents should be obtained. In particular, a history of several short family members (boys under 5′6″, girls under 5′0″) should be noted.

2. Growth records of the patient should be reviewed. Heights and weights should be plotted on an appropriate growth curve (Fig. 11.1). If a child has followed a single curve throughout life, a significant metabolic reason for this short stature is unlikely. However, if there is a falling away from a growth line, a metabolic problem is more likely.

3. The medical history should be reviewed, including a prenatal and neonatal history. A history of operations, head injuries, or chronic medical conditions that could predispose the patient to failure to thrive should be noted. If the child had a low birth weight, a review of underlying factors may disclose a possible chromosomal abnormality or toxic exposure (e.g., maternal cigarette smoking or alcohol use) that could produce long-term growth delay.

4. A developmental and psychosocial history may indicate possible familial problems or emotional neglect that could predispose to constitutional growth delay (so-called psychosocial dwarfism).

5. Inquiries into the teen's general health and daily habits may reveal problems needing investigation, such as poor appetite, frequent infections, drug abuse, chronic abdominal pain, or general fatigue and listlessness.

A *physical examination* is essential, including an accurate height and weight and Tanner stage assessment (Tables 11.4 and 11.5). If the testes are softening and show enlargement or if breast budding is present, there usually will be a normal sexual development. Unusual facies or ears, unusual hand creases, clinodactyly (deviation or deflection of the fingers), obesity, or delayed intellectual development may suggest a recognizable hereditary syndrome.

The initial *laboratory investigation* should include urinalysis; measurement of serum urea nitrogen, creatinine, and electrolytes; and radiographs of the hands and wrists to assess skeletal growth. More *specific laboratory investigations* may be suggested by the history and physical examination. Examples are thyroid enlargement (testing for hypothyroidism); normal physical examination and appearance but markedly short stature that is falling away from growth lines (testing for growth hormone deficiency); girls with delayed puberty, heights under the third percentile, associated with a short webbed neck, a systolic murmur, or widely spaced nipples (buccal smears performed to rule out Turner syndrome, i.e., X-O chromosomes); and striking pubertal delay without a history of similar delay in other family members (testing for gonadal failure including measurement of serum follicle-stimulating and luteinizing hormones, estradiol or testosterone, and urinary 17-ketosteroids and 17-hydroxysteroids; vaginal smear for maturation index and buccal smear for sex chromatin analysis or blood chromosome analysis).

Definitive diagnosis and planning for adolescents with suspected endocrine, metabolic, genetic, or psychological reasons for maturation delay require referral to an appropriate specialist. Families whose children have genetic disorders that affect growth and fertility will benefit from genetic counseling. The availability of biosynthetic growth hormone has raised possibilities for the management of teens with familial short stature. It is unclear whether growth hormone will increase the final adult height of normal children, although for some the rate of growth increases. Weighed against its questionable efficacy, growth hormone treatment is very expensive (often costing $5,000 to $10,000 per year).

Sexually Transmitted Disease

Sexually transmitted diseases (STDs) are epidemic in 15- to 19-year-olds. For example, more than 500,000 adolescents in the United States contract gonorrhea each year (6). The high frequency of STDs is partially caused by more casual attitudes toward sex and frequent changes of sex partners. Sex education programs have had little impact on the problem. Fear of infection apparently does not deter some teens, who seem irresponsible, impulsive, and emotionally insecure and who appear to have little respect for others. Often, parents fail to provide basic information about sex and the risks of infection and pregnancy that accompany it.

In most states, adolescents have a legal right to receive treatment for STDs without the parents' knowledge; it is important to be receptive to the teen seeking treatment. Visits for treatment should also be used to explain the mechanism of acquiring venereal infection and to explain and encourage the use of condoms to prevent reinfection. The diagnosis and treatment of various STDs are discussed elsewhere in this book (see Chapters 37 and 102).

The high rates of sexual intercourse and adolescent pregnancy in the 1980s and 1990s raised concerns about acquisition of infection with the human immunodeficiency virus (HIV) in this age group. Given the long incubation period of HIV infection, data showing that 21% of all acquired immunodeficiency syndrome cases occur in people 20 to 25 years of age suggest strongly that adolescence is an important period of acquisition of HIV infection (9). Other data suggest that a frequent route of spread of the virus in adolescence is by heterosexual transmission, rather than intravenous drug abuse, blood products, or homosexual contacts. Furthermore, many cases of HIV infection in infants may be linked to maternal acquisition of the virus during adolescence. It is imperative that teenagers, especially sexually active teens, be counseled about high-risk behaviors that may expose them to HIV infection and about safe sex practices. This information and details about the ambulatory care of HIV-infected patients are described in Chapter 39.

Pregnancy

Each year in the United States, almost 1 million teenage women—10% of all women age 15 to 19 years and 19% of those who have had sexual intercourse—become pregnant, accounting for 13% of all U.S. births. Seventy-eight percent of teen pregnancies are unplanned, accounting for about one-fourth of all accidental pregnancies annually (6). More than half (56%) of the 905,000 teenage pregnancies in 1996 ended in births, and nearly 4 in 10 teen pregnancies (excluding those ending in miscarriages) were terminated by abortion (8). Many of these pregnancies are associated with serious medical risks for the mother and the fetus. Mothers younger than age 14 years have particularly high risks of toxemia, anemia, prematurity, infants with low birth weight, prolonged labor, and postpartum complications. Many of these problems can be prevented by good obstetric care, so that the first goal in adolescent pregnancy should be early diagnosis and entry into a comprehensive treatment program.

There are multiple social and behavioral reasons for the high number of teenage pregnancies. For many adolescents, pregnancy may be part of a maladaptive attempt to solve psychological issues, such as independence from a clinging mother or manipulation of a boyfriend. Such patients may have previously engaged in other maladaptive activities, such as drug abuse or delinquency. They may also be ignorant about methods and availability of birth control (see Chapter 100), including emergency contraception (see below).

The teenager herself may be ambivalent about her pregnancy. Often, the manipulations that led to the pregnancy (e.g., the promise of a prolonged relationship) did not succeed and the patient feels abandoned. Furthermore, the pregnancy may result in hostility from the family when the teenager is in greatest need of help from her parents.

Clearly, the teenager about to make important decisions about herself and her pregnancy needs counseling. It can be provided by her primary physician or, commonly, by a staff member of a counseling agency such as Planned Parenthood. In either case, the patient's primary physician should be aware of programs in the community, including public schools that accommodate the needs of teenagers who choose to have their babies, and should be available for any problems that a pregnant teenager may wish to discuss. In many states, adolescents have the right to treatment for pregnancy-related events, including abortion, without parental consent or knowledge. If the teenager decides to continue with the pregnancy, she should be prepared to assume a parenting role. Furthermore, she should be educated about future pregnancies and given medical assistance for the pediatric care needed for her infant. If possible, daycare, vocational, and educational services should be available for the mother so that she may continue her education after the birth of her child. As an integral part of counseling, a stable caring person should be identified (a parent, if possible) who can assist the teen emotionally and financially and who can help her see the future for herself and her baby in a realistic manner.

Rape

Rape is a sexual act, usually intercourse, with a nonconsenting victim. The most common type of adolescent rape has been called acquaintance rape, and it is probable that most instances are never reported. Acquaintance rape occurs when the victim is sexually misused by a boyfriend during a date, or by a casual friend, or when a trusting teen accompanies her friends to a strange place where she is gang raped.

Teens, in exploring sexuality, may not have set limits to their petting, or if limits have been set unilaterally, they may afford little protection for the victim, especially when the assailant is an adolescent for whom limit setting has not been successful in other areas. Some teens may also, in their uncertainty, present themselves in provocative pseudomature ways (e.g., by wearing clothing that may be viewed as sexually inviting by male acquaintances).

There is a tendency in dealing with adolescent rape victims to imply that the victim may have invited the assault. This viewpoint inappropriately diverts attention from the fact that rape should always be treated as a very serious problem for the victim who reports it.

Initial care for the rape victim should be handled by a physician, with followup by a rape counseling service if one exists in the community. Often, a physician who is already acquainted with the patient can provide the best care.

The following are important considerations when caring for the rape victim:

- Rape is a crime of violence, as well as a sexual act.
- Above all else, the adolescent reporting rape has usually had a very frightening experience and needs short-term counseling either by her regular physician (see Chapter 20) or, ideally, through the auspices of a rape victims' support program. She will usually have a number of questions about the physical meaning of her experience, and it is important to ensure that she obtains answers to them.
- She should be examined carefully for evidence of trauma, both to the pelvic organs and to the rest of her body, and the information should be carefully recorded.
- She must decide whether she wishes to report the rape to the police. Many states have a "rape kit" to assist physicians in obtaining fluids and samples for forensic laboratory analysis. Primary care physicians may wish to refer victims to rape crisis teams, established in many communities, which are experienced in the forensic examination of rape victims.
- Most rape victims will need ongoing counseling by their physician or a counselor for a number of months to discuss persisting anxieties and questions.
- When it is not possible to exclude (by identifying and testing the rapist) exposure to HIV, the rape victim should be offered surveillance for HIV infection following a protocol similar to that described in Chapter 39 for accidental needlesticks in health care personnel.
- If sexual intercourse occurred within 72 hours of the examination, the rape victim should be offered emergency STD prophylaxis and contraception.
- *STD prophylaxis* in adolescents and adults after sexual assault is as follows:
  Ceftriaxone 125 mg intramuscularly in a single dose, *plus*
  Metronidazole 2 g orally in a single dose, *plus*
  Doxycycline 100 mg orally twice a day for 7 days.
  Consider Hepatitis B vaccination if nonimmune.
- *Pregnancy prophylaxis* (emergency contraception) in adolescents and adults after sexual assault is as follows:

Norgestrel or levonorgestrel plus ethinyl estradiol pills (oral contraception pills) within 72 hours of assault and again 12 hours later.

Brand	Color	First Dose	Second Dose
Ovral	White	2 pills	2 pills
Lo/Ovral	White	4 pills	4 pills
Levlen	Light orange	4 pills	4 pills
Nordette	Light orange	4 pills	4 pills
Tri-Levlen	Yellow	4 pills	4 pills
Triphasil	Yellow	4 pills	4 pills

- Serum pregnancy test should be obtained and proven negative. If a woman is pregnant, there is a risk of fetal urogenital malformations if emergency contraception fails.
- Nausea is a common side effect of treatment.
- Informed consent should be obtained.

PSYCHOSOCIAL DEVELOPMENT

Normal Patterns and Concerns

The major psychosocial developmental task for the adolescent as adulthood approaches is to increase independence from their parents and to establish a positive identity congruent with social norms. In early adolescence, the young teen is faced with the dilemma of seeking independence from parents while at the same time relying on them for emotional and physical support. The conflict over independence is evidenced by contradiction and ambivalence. For example, a teen may refuse to listen to parents' suggestions about study habits but blame mediocre grades on the fact that the parents did not help with homework assignments.

As teens enter middle and late adolescence, they demonstrate a remarkable resourcefulness in coping with anxiety over separation and in learning more mature behavior. Much assistance comes through peer relationships. Teens support each other by experimenting with adult roles that mirror societal expectations of behavior; a sense of moral responsibility begins to take shape. In this period, individual identity tends to be blunted by the seeking of independence from the family. Peers tend to look alike, dress alike, date alike, and experiment with drugs and sex alike. Later, as teens address their concerns about careers, a greater differentiation of personalities takes shape and individual identities emerge.

Normal development also requires the example of secure healthy parents in an environment in which the teen can feel secure. Thus, parents who are preoccupied with their own psychological problems at work, in their marriage, or with their own families may have difficulties helping and coping with the development of their adolescent offspring. Often such parents have not previously succeeded at their own adolescent tasks and so are unable to proceed with the task of adulthood—they have not developed the ability for intimacy, close personal feelings, the sharing of feelings and thoughts with others, and adhering to reasonable limits.

One clear fact about adolescent development is that its *emotional course is variable,* even among normal adolescents. The idea that adolescence is usually a time of crisis, in which persistent neurotic behavior is essential for development of a personal identity, has not been borne out by longitudinal research. On the other hand, it has been found that at least 20% of first-year college students have psychological problems, usually personality disorders of the compulsive, schizoid, or passive–aggressive type (see Chapter 23) expressed as difficulties in academic, social, and psychosexual functioning (10). Furthermore, adolescents are more likely than people in other age groups to be hospitalized for psychiatric conditions (11). A longitudinal study of teenage boys (12) points out that achievement of identity is a long-term process. Subjects were first studied in the first year of high school and were followed for 7 years. At the end of this interval, most subjects had yet to consolidate their identities to the point where they could develop an intimate relationship, one of the best indicators of progress to adulthood. Despite this, self-satisfaction and parental satisfaction were the norm. For many, adolescence is a crisis, but an internalized noiseless one.

Generally, the teen must succeed in the other spheres of development to meet tasks in the psychosocial sphere successfully. In children with retardation, physical disabilities, or chronic illness, the dependence–independence struggle may persist, impairing the development of self-esteem needed to develop a sense of identity.

Juvenile Delinquency

Juvenile delinquency is a legal term for youthful behavior that violates the law and would be adjudicated and punished if it had been committed by an adult. It is a major social problem and is sometimes brought to the attention of the practitioner, who is asked whether there is an underlying psychological cause for the delinquent behavior. To put delinquency in a statistical perspective, data from the Bureau of Justice Statistics National Crime Victimization Survey indicates that youths between ages 12 and 20 years were involved in more than 1 million arrests for serious crimes (assaults, threatened assaults, and robberies) in 2003 in the United States. If runaways, drug violations, curfew violations and other, less violent acts are included, there were more than 2.6 million juvenile arrests in the United States in 2003 (13).

Weiner (14) distinguishes between three broad categories of delinquency: sociologic delinquency, characterologic delinquency, and neurotic delinquency. *Sociologic delinquency* refers to illegal acts organized by a subcultural group (e.g., street gang). The delinquent acts are adaptive in that the teen receives the approval of his or her peers. The following four features of the clinical history suggest sociologic delinquency: first, the delinquent acts are performed with valued companions, rather than alone or with strangers; second, these teens see themselves as accepted and integral members of their peer group and rarely exhibit feelings of alienation or inadequacy; third, sociologic delinquents give little evidence of neurotic symptom formation or basic character flaws; and fourth, these delinquents often have had supportive family relationships during early childhood, although there may have been more recent problems that have led to their current activities. Often, involvement in other positive group activities changes the delinquent orientation of these teens.

Characterologic delinquents reflect a basically antisocial attitude toward life. Their acts do not evoke in them any guilt or remorse. Such teens are often loners who have not established a strong relationship of basic trust in their life. Their history suggests a series of problems, with a flurry of destructive acts such as fighting, fire setting, and cruelty to animals preceding their more destructive delinquent activity. Such children often require long-term psychiatric treatment. Chapter 23 provides additional details about the course and management of patients with an antisocial personality.

The *neurotic delinquent* commits destructive acts as an atypical (for him or her) behavior pattern to illustrate and emphasize certain needs. These acts may reflect feelings of being ignored by family or peers or indicate that the teen is suffering from some form of psychological distress, most often depression. The acts are committed in such a way that the teen is caught in the process or gives himself or herself away soon after; generally, if concealment of illegal acts is repetitive and successful, a neurotic basis of the delinquency is unlikely. There is rarely a history of early behavioral problems, and typically the delinquent has enjoyed a loving relationship with parents and family members. Occasionally, however, some recent family stress may trigger the delinquent act. In general, neurotic delinquency may be treated through short-term counseling (see Chapter 20).

Violence and Violence Prevention

Recent shootings in schools in the United States by children and adolescents have brought to the forefront the issue of youth aggression and violence. Professionals who work with youth must work to define their roles and develop skills to address the risk factors and warning signs of violent behavior.

Violence (homicide and suicide) is the major cause of death and morbidity, outside of accidents, for teens and young adults. Deaths caused by firearms among adolescents ages 15 years to 19 years in the United States in 2001 was 12.4 per 100,000, of which 7.5 per 100,000 were a consequence of firearm homicide. However, deaths caused by firearms among black teens ages 15 years to 19 years in the United States in 2001 was 60.5 per 100,000, of which 52.0 per 100,000 were a consequence of firearm homicide (15). Youths have continuing exposure to violence, sex, and drug use through television, movies, and music videos; one estimate suggests that young people may view 10,000 acts of violence a year (16). Research suggests that a cause-and-effect relationship exists between media violence and aggression (17). Of deeper concern is the exposure of young teens to actual violence and aggression. One large cross-sectional study stated that almost 30% of 6th to 10th graders reported that they had participated in bullying, been bullied, or both (18). This study went on to suggest that bullies and those who are bullied both have a range of concurrent conduct, and school, emotional, and physical problems. As adults, bullies are likely to exhibit criminal behavior, and those who have been bullied have higher rates of depression and poor self-esteem. It is disturbing that the perpetrators of the violence in Littleton, Colorado, Pearl, Mississippi, and Santee, California may have been bullying victims.

The American Academy of Pediatrics Task Force on Violence has suggested a number of age-appropriate interventions (19), including promoting appropriate parenting skills by querying and counseling about discipline at home, substance abuse, violence and abuse exposure—physical, sexual, and verbal—at school and home, dating and dating behavior, and how conflicts are resolved at home. Most importantly, practitioners should have knowledge of community- and school-based resources where at-risk youth may be referred. Practitioners who are very interested in violence prevention may work with communities to help design curricula, advocate for increased services, promote preventive activities, and foster community attitudes that affect the risk and incidence of violence. These may include promoting gun safety and reducing child access to guns, working with child abuse teams, and designing school curricula that include violence prevention. Practitioners can also work through advocacy groups to affect laws and regulations that are pertinent to violence prevention, such as gun safety requirements, prohibition of corporal punishment in schools, visitation programs for isolated families and new parents, and after-school programs for children and teens.

Substance Abuse

Although substance abuse, including tobacco use, is a major problem of adult life, it often begins during the adolescent years. By age 11 years, 1 in 5 adolescents has smoked cigarettes and approximately 1 in 11 adolescents has had his or her first drink of alcohol; by the age of 15 years, 1 in 7 adolescents smokes on a daily basis and more than 1 in 3 adolescents has drunk excessively at least once (6). Experimenting with substances of abuse may be viewed as a rite of passage bridging the gap between childhood and adulthood or as a condition for belonging to peer groups or organizations. Advertising or exposure to images that appear to link the use of cigarettes and alcohol to life successes, popularity, and sex can be important inducements for adolescents to try alcohol or tobacco. A major concern is to identify the adolescent abuser—one whose life is being disrupted by aberrant activities. This teenager is most likely to continue to abuse alcohol or drugs in adult life.

The routine evaluation of a teen should include questioning about the use of alcohol and of drugs. Substance use should be explored using nonthreatening questions such as those listed in Table 11.6. The presence of drug abuse and its impact on a teenager can also be uncovered by asking the parents questions such as those in Table 11.7. If the use of a substance is excessive and hazardous, factors that might have led to abuse should be explored. Drugs and alcohol are often abused as a response to some psychosocial problem, and it is only by identifying the problem that the abuse may be stopped. Lecturing on the dangers of alcohol, drugs, or tobacco seems to have little impact on adolescents. Unfortunately, teens who drive and use alcohol and drugs may endanger others, so it still behooves

TABLE 11.6 Sample Questions Concerning Drug Use for Adolescents

I know that many schools have drug problems. Does your school have such a problem?
Do most of your friends drink alcohol or smoke marijuana at parties?
Do any of your friends use drugs other than alcohol or marijuana?
Where do most young people obtain drugs?
Do you smoke cigarettes? How many per day?
Have you ever tried alcohol? Marijuana? Other drugs?
Have you ever been ill as a result of using drugs or drinking?
Have you ever been in trouble with the law as a result of drugs or alcohol?
Do your parents know that you've used alcohol or drugs?
What would (did) they say?
Have you ever worried about your alcohol or drug use?
Have you ever been drunk or stoned and driven a car (or motorcycle)?

From Schonberg SK, ed. Substance abuse: a guide for health professionals. Elk Grove Village, IL: American Academy of Pediatrics, 1988, with permission.

TABLE 11.7 Questions for Interviewing the Parents of the Adolescent Suspected of or Known to Be Abusing Drugs or Alcohol

1. Does your son/daughter spend many hours alone in his/her bedroom apparently doing nothing?
2. Does your son/daughter resist talking to you or persistently isolate himself/herself from the family?
3. Has your daughter's/son's taste in music had a dramatic change to hard rock music?
4. Has there been a definite change in your son's/daughter's attitude at school? With his/her friends? At home?
5. Has your daughter/son shown recent pronounced mood swings with increased irritability and angry outbursts?
6. Does your son/daughter always seem to be unhappy and less able to cope with frustration than he/she used to be?
7. Has your daughter's/son's personality changed from being a considerate and caring person to being selfish, unfriendly, and unsympathetic?
8. Does your son/daughter always seem to be confused or "spacey"?
9. Have money or valuable articles recently disappeared from your home?
10. Has your daughter/son begun to neglect household chores or homework?
11. Has there been a change in your son's/daughter's friends from age-appropriate friends to older "unacceptable" associates?
12. Has there been a change in your daughter's/son's appearance (i.e., sloppy dress and poor grooming and hygiene)?
13. Have there been excuses and alibis made and has there been lying to avoid confrontation or not to get caught?
14. Do you feel you have lost control of your son/daughter?
15. Has your daughter/son begun lying to cover up sources of money and possessions?
16. Have there been episodes of "ditching" or "skipping" school? Has your son/daughter lied to cover up bad report cards?
17. Have there been stealing, shoplifting, or encounters with the police?
18. Has your daughter/son become a "con artist"?
19. Have you noticed a marked increase in your son's/daughter's interest in drugs, drug literature, and the drug "culture" (i.e., clothing and accoutrements, paraphernalia, belt buckles, and tee shirts with a drug theme)?
20. Has your daughter/son recently quit a sport or dropped out of school clubs or social groups, stopped music lessons, quit the band or orchestra, or lost interest in a hobby?
21. Has there been a deterioration of school performance, frequent truancy, or conflict with coaches or teachers?
22. Do you feel your daughter/son has become untrustworthy, insincere, and distrustful ("paranoid")?
23. Has he/she become unpredictable or rebellious?
24. Has your son/daughter been verbally abusive to you or your spouse?
25. Has your daughter/son been physically abusive to you or your spouse?
26. Has your son/daughter tried to introduce any of your other children to drugs or alcohol?
27. Has your daughter/son talked about suicide or running away?
28. Is your son/daughter more argumentative lately? Does he/she tend to blame others for his/her problems?
29. Is there a paranoid flavor to all of your daughter's/son's relationships with adults, siblings, and authority figures?

From Schonberg SK, ed. Substance abuse: a guide for health professionals. Elk Grove Village, IL: American Academy of Pediatrics, 1988, with permission.

practitioners to discuss substance abuse with teens who deny personal drug use.

Occasionally, the serious abuser of hazardous substances develops physiologic symptoms that are dramatic enough to come to the physician's attention. Hospitalization for observation is almost always indicated for the teenager presenting with drug intoxication, even if emergency room evaluation indicates no immediate medical risks. The possibility of attempted suicide may be real and must be explored. Even if this is not a factor, there is still concern about the teen's ability to control his or her own drug abuse behavior.

How to intervene in teenage drug abuse behavior is a difficult question. Practical approaches to patients with substance abuse are contained in Chapters 27, 28, and 29.

Depression and Suicide

A behavioral hallmark of adolescents is mood shifts, from the peaks of elation to the depths of despair. Depressive symptoms are normal parts of psychosocial development. The quest for identity is balanced by a sense of loss once independence is achieved. Similarly, rejections by peers (e.g., first loves) may be felt very deeply. It is not unusual, as part of these depressions, for the adolescent to contemplate suicide. More than 1 in 4 adolescents in grades 9 through 12 has thought seriously about suicide, and 1 in 12 adolescents has actually attempted suicide (6).

Mattsson (20) describes five depressive states of adolescence:

1. Normal depressive mood swings represent transient reactions to personal disappointments or family difficulties. They rarely affect other life functions.

2. Acute depressive reactions are more severe states, often lasting weeks or months. They are normal reactions, similar to states of grief (see Chapter 24), often related to separation or loss of a close friend, relative, or teacher.

3. The adolescent who does not successfully work through grief and who becomes increasingly depressed and incapacitated by loss suffers from a depressive neurosis. Such teens withdraw from their normal functioning, are chronically sad, and begin to entertain suicidal ideation. This is a fairly severe level of depression and demands professional intervention.

4. The masked depressions of adolescence can be viewed as a subgroup of the depressive neuroses. Such teens cannot tolerate their painful feelings and express them through a variety of somatic or behavioral complaints. They may be frequent visitors to the primary care physician, suffering from ill-defined atypical symptoms without a clear organic basis. Their behavior may include overeating, delinquent acts, exhibitionist acts resulting in accidental self-destruction, and drug and alcohol abuse.

5. Psychotic depressive disorders are marked by impaired reality testing, thought disorders, paranoia, and suicidal intention, in addition to depressive symptomatology.

Primary care physicians are sometimes asked to evaluate depressed or suicidal adolescents. In taking the history, one should try to uncover recent events that may have precipitated the depressive disorder: any long-standing family, school, or peer problems; possibilities of organic brain disease or drug abuse that may mimic depressive symptoms; symptoms of cognitive or reality disturbances, suggesting a psychosis; and symptoms suggesting a masked depression. Openness in inquiry about depression usually puts the adolescent at ease and conveys that the physician truly understands what he or she may be feeling. A physical examination helps to rule out physical problems, and communication with the school may provide additional observations about the teen's current level of functioning. Considering the high prevalence of depressive symptoms and clinically significant depression during adolescence (estimated to be as high as 15% and 5%, respectively), there may be value to screening adolescents for depression. This is particularly important prior to transition periods, such as entry into high school or college, as social and academic stressors may lead depressed teens who may have been masking their symptoms to go into crisis. Such instruments as the Columbia Diagnostic Interview Schedule for Children (DISC) Depression Scale (21) or the Beck Depression Inventory (22) are relatively fast screening questionnaires that can be administered in an office setting and help clinicians identify depressed teens.

Adolescents with depressive symptoms need some counseling. If one believes medication is necessary and is unfamiliar with the use of psychoactive drugs in adolescents, conjoint treatment with a psychiatric consultant may prove helpful. Patients with long-standing depressive symptoms, which suggest thought disturbances, and possible suicide attempts should be referred for psychiatric intervention. Additional details about the office assessment and management of depression are found in Chapter 24.

INTELLECTUAL DEVELOPMENT

Normal Patterns and Concerns

In adolescence, a major change occurs with respect to education and intellect. Schools differentiate students, placing them into vocational or academic tracks. The emphasis shifts from the learning of tasks (e.g., basic reading, writing, and arithmetic) to the accumulation of facts and the ability to think abstractly. As teens prepare for college, learning becomes a competitive task. For some teens and families with high aspirations, the competitive nature of academic rankings and the pressure to be admitted into very selective colleges may isolate the child and interfere with social development. Career choices become limited as an individual's abilities and talents become manifest. Upon entering college, a greater amount of independence and responsibility is expected. Symbolically, the university begins to resemble the workplace in terms of both potential rewards and potential pressures.

Scholastic Failure

Academic achievement is strongly related to parental aspirations, socioeconomic status, and intellectual ability. Occasionally, a child cannot meet parental expectations, and the resultant crisis may lead to a visit to the physician. Failure in school may also be a symptom of a physical impairment, mental retardation, substance abuse, specific learning disabilities, or emotional stress. By making an accurate diagnosis of the underlying problem, a caring practitioner can help such children.

First, a history is necessary to determine the nature of the school difficulties. When did they begin? Has educational achievement been a problem throughout a school career, as with a global intellectual deficit, or is it specific to certain subjects or tasks, as with learning disorders? Is there a family history of poor school performance, as is seen with familial dyslexics? How does the teen act with family and peers? Is there evidence of disturbed behavior outside school, as with emotional disorders? Is the family structure stable or has there been separation, divorce, or death of a parent or grandparent? Is there evidence of substance abuse or physical abuse on the part of the teen or a member of the family? Is there daytime hypersomnolence that suggests a sleep disorder? What has the family done to try to work through problems?

Second, a physical examination, including neurologic examination, is indicated, with emphasis on signs of minimal cerebral dysfunction, such as difficulty with right–left discrimination or spatial orientation, or overt signs of cerebral palsy (23). In such patients, there may be suggestions of a neurologic problem in the medical history, the birth may have been abnormal, or the patient may have shown hyperactivity or attention deficits as a child. Vision testing and office assessment for slight or moderate hearing loss (see Chapter 110) are also particularly important.

Third, some specific intelligence testing is indicated. Children with mental retardation tend to show low intelligence quotient scores, and achievement tests show a delay of several grades in math and reading levels. Children with dyslexia have a normal intelligence quotient but show a wide scatter of scores on subtests, indicating a nonglobal deficit. Achievement tests may also show a difference between abilities in reading and mathematics.

Some learning problems may appear late in a school career (23). The recent criticism of the ability of some college students to write well has given credence to the notion of expressive language disorders, which may not become manifest until adolescence. Some people with fine perceptual problems may not reveal difficulties until geometry or drafting is studied in high school.

In 1974, Congress passed federal law 94-142, ensuring a free, appropriate, educational placement for all children up to age 21 years. Thus, adolescents with specific learning problems, retardation, or emotional difficulties are entitled to be placed in a classroom setting where they will learn. The physician who suspects an unrecognized problem in one of these spheres may help by referring the teen and the teen's parents for evaluation, which is usually available through the school or the local education system. Unfortunately, problems remain unrecognized for many children and they may, out of frustration, drop out of school.

Attention Deficit Hyperactivity Disorder

Attention deficit hyperactivity disorder (ADHD) may be one of the most common disorders of childhood, with prevalence rates ranging from 3% to 6% of prepubertal children. Although data on prevalence and persistence in adolescents and adults are limited, long-term followup studies show that critical symptoms of ADHD—impairment of attention and regulation of activity and poor impulse control—often persist into adulthood, and many adults with ADHD remain distractible, impulsive, inattentive, and disruptive throughout life. On average, symptoms of ADHD diminish by approximately 50% every 5 years between the ages of 10 and 25 years. Adolescents with ADHD may have impaired school performance, a disorganized approach to tasks, limited participation in extracurricular activities, increased risk of delinquency, and harmful social relationships and family interactions. In adults, ADHD is often linked with psychiatric illness, incarceration, job failures, marital discord, and divorce (24).

Diagnosis

ADHD is diagnosed, usually at serial visits using information from multiple sources. Table 11.8 lists the criteria for the diagnosis. The diagnostic challenge in adolescents and adults is to detect the more subtle presentations of symptoms in these stages of life. For example, in teens and adults, symptoms of hyperactivity may be confined to fidgetiness or an inner feeling of jitteriness or restlessness. Current nomenclature differentiates ADHD into three types: predominantly inattentive, predominantly impulsive, and combined.

There has been increasing attention to ADHD in adult patients and more adults are seeking treatment for this disorder. There are screening instruments that are geared toward the diagnosis in adult patients, including the Copeland Symptom Checklist for Adult ADHD, the Wender Utah Rating Scale, and the Brown Adult Attention Deficit Disorder Scale (25). Wender developed a set of adult ADHD criteria, in addition to a history suggestive of childhood ADHD, that includes hyperactivity (restlessness, feeling on edge, difficulty relaxing) and poor concentration (forgetting appointments and social commitments) plus two of five additional symptoms: affective lability, hot temper, inability to complete tasks and disorganization (difficulty prioritizing tasks), stress intolerance, and impulsivity (such as blurting out rude or insulting remarks).

The physical examination usually is noncontributory in diagnosing ADHD but may be useful to rule out other conditions that are characterized by hyperactivity or short attention spans (see below). In teens, it is helpful to examine results of intellectual testing and academic achievement testing. A symptom checklist (Connor Scale, Child Behavior Checklist) that can be completed by teachers and parents is also helpful to identify and quantify symptoms that teens may be demonstrating in their classrooms and homes (25).

Comorbidity

Up to 65% of adolescents with ADHD have one or more comorbid conditions, such as learning disabilities, mood disorders (10% to 20%), substance abuse, and alcoholism, and may also be confused with other conditions that have hyperactivity as a feature, such as hyperthyroidism, Gilles de la Tourette syndrome, adjustment or oppositional disorders, affective disorders with manic features, social or personality difficulties, and medication-induced attention problems (e.g., substance abuse) (24). These patients have difficulty in the workplace, in school, and in social relations. They have more cognitive difficulties, poor performance in school, and significant difficulties with social skills and appropriate behavior. As a result, they tend to be underachievers with personalities that may be intrusive, immature, or negative.

Treatment

ADHD is treated best with a multimodal combination of medication and counseling. On the basis of placebo-controlled trials, it has been found that stimulant drugs

TABLE 11.8 Diagnostic Criteria for Attention Deficit Hyperactivity Disorder

A. Either 1 or 2
1. Six (or more) of the following symptoms of inattention have persisted for at least 6 months to a degree that is maladaptive and inconsistent with developmental level.
   Inattention
   a. Often fails to give close attention to details or makes careless mistakes in schoolwork, work, or other activities.
   b. Often has difficulty sustaining attention in tasks or play activities.
   c. Often does not seem to listen when spoken to directly.
   d. Often does not follow through on instructions and fails to finish schoolwork, chores, or duties in the workplace (not because of oppositional behavior or failure to understand instructions).
   e. Often has difficulty organizing tasks and activities.
   f. Often avoids, dislikes, or is reluctant to engage in tasks that require sustained mental effort (such as schoolwork or homework).
   g. Often loses things necessary for tasks or activities (e.g., toys, school assignments, pencils, books, or tools).
   h. Is often easily distracted by extraneous stimuli.
   i. Is often forgetful in daily activities.
2. Six (or more) of the following symptoms of hyperactivity–impulsivity have persisted for at least 6 months to a degree that is maladaptive and inconsistent with developmental level.
   Hyperactivity
   a. Often fidgets with hands or feet or squirms in seat.
   b. Often leaves seat in classroom or in other situations in which remaining seated is expected.
   c. Often runs about or climbs excessively in situations in which it is inappropriate (in adolescents or adults, may be limited to subjective feelings of restlessness).
   d. Often has difficulty playing or engaging in leisure activities quietly.
   e. Is often "on the go" or often acts as if "driven by a motor."
   f. Often talks excessively.
   Impulsivity
   a. Often blurts out answers before questions have been completed.
   b. Often has difficulty awaiting turn.
   c. Often interrupts or intrudes on others (e.g., butts into conversations or games).

B. Some hyperactive–impulsive or inattentive symptoms that caused impairment were present before age 7 years.
C. Some impairment from the symptoms is present in two or more settings (e.g., at school [or work] and at home).
D. There must be clear evidence of clinically significant impairment in social, academic, or occupational functioning.
E. The symptoms do not occur exclusively during the course of a pervasive developmental disorder, schizophrenia, or other psychotic disorder and are not better accounted for by another mental disorder (e.g., mood disorder, anxiety disorder, dissociative disorder, or a personality disorder).

Diagnosis is:
Attention deficit hyperactivity disorder, combined type if both criteria A1 and A2 are met for the past 6 months.
Attention deficit hyperactivity disorder, predominantly inattentive type if criterion A1 is met but criterion A2 is not met for the past 6 months.
Attention deficit hyperactivity disorder, predominantly hyperactive–impulsive type if criterion A2 is met but criterion A1 is not met for the past 6 months.
For individuals (especially adolescents and adults) who currently have symptoms that no longer meet full criteria, "in partial remission" should be specified.

From Diagnostic and statistical manual of mental disorders, 4th ed. (DSM-IV). Washington, DC: American Psychiatric Association, 1994, with permission.

greatly reduce the core symptoms of ADHD, hyperactivity, impulsivity, and inattentiveness (24). It is estimated that 70% to 80% of children and 60% of adults have improvement in academic and social behaviors and in cognition and a reduction of disruptive and negative behaviors. Long-term improvement in academic outcome has not been found, however. Most patients with ADHD are treated pharmacologically with psychostimulant medications, such as methylphenidate or dextroamphetamine, although a small number respond well to antidepressant agents, such as desipramine. Table 11.9 summarizes practical information regarding these medications. Medication should be titrated carefully and should be used on days when focus and attention may be needed (e.g., for long-distance drives, school or work days). Medication should be prescribed to cover learning and work-related needs, such as homework and examination preparation times. With short-acting stimulant medications such as methylphenidate, holiday periods off medication may be permitted. Counseling interventions include psychoeducational counseling, behavioral management, school-based interventions, family therapy, and social competence training. In many communities patients and their families have access to the Children and Adults with Attention

TABLE 11.9 Medications for Attention Deficit Disorder with Hyperactivity (ADHD) in Adolescents and Adults

Drug	*Available Strengths (mg)*	*Dosage*	*Comments*
Methylphenidate (Ritalin, Concerta)	Tabs: 5, 10, 20 (3–6-h duration) Slow-release tabs: 20 (6–8-h duration) Concerta: 18, 36, 54 (8–12-h duration)	Initial: 0.25 mg/kg/dose given with breakfast and lunch Maintenance: 1–2 mg/kg/24h Maximum: 60 mg daily	Begin with initial dose. May double dosage weekly until desired clinical effect is achieved or maintenance dosage is reached. Stop if no improvement in 1 month. May give after-school dose for homework. Use cautiously in patients with hypertension, epilepsy. Contraindicated in patients with glaucoma, Gilles de la Tourette syndrome, monoamine oxidase inhibitor use. Commonly causes insomnia, anorexia. If full-day medication needed (e.g., after-school activities, homework) can use Concerta, which releases methylphenidate for up to 12 h ; usually start with 36 or 54 mg.
Dextroamphetamine (Dexedrine) or Adderall (combination of amphetamine with dextroamphetamine)	Tabs: 5, 10 (4–6-h duration) Elixir: 5 mg/5 mL (4–6-h duration) Sustained-release caps: 5, 10, 15 (6–8-h duration) Caps: 15 (4–6-h duration) Adderall: 5, 10, 20, 30 (4–8-h duration)	Initial: 10 mg/24 h in morning Maximum: 60 mg daily	Begin with initial dose. May increase by 10 mg/wk until maximum dose. Same guidelines as methylphenidate. Side effects more common than with methylphenidate because of longer duration of action. Adderall may start 5 mg b.i.d. and work up by 5 mg per dose.
Desipramine (Norpramin)	Tabs: 10, 25, 50, 100, 150 (up to 24-h duration)	Initial: 10 mg/24 h in morning Maximum: 100 mg daily	Begin at lowest dose for adolescent. Increase according to tolerance and response. Usual dosage 25–50 mg/d for adolescents. Must obtain electrocardiogram when using medication to look for signs of prolongation of QRS and QT intervals. For this reason, desipramine is a poor choice in patients with cardiovascular disease, congenital heart disease, hypertension, etc. Occasional behavioral side effects noted, especially if manic–depressive illness not recognized. May cause leukopenia, especially during febrile illness.

Deficit/Hyperactivity Disorder (www.chadd.org) and to the ADHD Association (www.add.org) support groups.

APPROACH TO THE ADOLESCENT PATIENT IN THE OFFICE SETTING

When interviewing teens, it is helpful to keep in mind that the transitional nature of adolescence makes it a time of great experimentation and risk taking (see Sexual Development and Substance Abuse sections, above).

Each adolescent approaches the developmental pressures of this period of life with his or her particular skills and emotions. From a health perspective, adolescents can be responsible partners in maintaining their well-being and complying with medical care, or they can be infantile, dependent, uncommunicative, aggressive, or irresponsible. It is important to interview adolescents in private. Adolescents need to believe they are the patient and that their problems are being listened to and taken seriously. It is often useful to also talk to the parents separately.

Interviewing the Patient

Some adolescent patients are difficult to interview. An uncommunicative patient may have been sent to a physician involuntarily or may lack verbal skills needed for coherence. One must be verbally active with such patients and watch for any nonverbal cues to use as wedges in trying to get the patient to speak. Examples of nonverbal cues are a look of interest or initiation of eye contact when a subject is mentioned that the patient would like to discuss, a clenched fist when an anger-provoking subject is raised, and frequent position change and fidgeting when the patient is anxious about a specific subject or about the visit to the physician in general. Because adolescents are often reticent about their major concerns, open-minded invitations to share information (e.g., "Is there anything else you wanted to talk about?") should be included in each office contact. The initial comprehensive interview may require several sessions. At the first visit, warmth and interest in the adolescent may open the way to better communication in future sessions.

Some adolescents respond more honestly to *written questionnaires* rather than to interviews. It may be a useful strategy to preface an interview with a form questionnaire for both the adolescent and the parent. As part of this questionnaire, ground rules can be outlined, such as assurances of confidentiality. In general, an adult-oriented questionnaire, with reviews of systems, is inappropriate for younger teens and should be reserved for teens age 18 years or older. The questionnaire should not take the place of the personal interview but can guide the interview to address issues of concern of the patient in greater detail.

Many adolescents continue to go to a pediatrician for medical care until they enter college, take a job, or marry. Because of this long-term association, their relationship may be almost like that of a parent and child: warm, intense, and comradely. These feelings cannot be transferred easily to a new physician, and it is unwise to attempt to transfer them.

Practitioners can most effectively surmount problems in communicating with adolescents by explaining their modus operandi in advance, emphasizing that they will be primarily the adolescent's physician rather than an agent of the patient's parents, as had been the case previously. The adolescent should also be encouraged to initiate patient–practitioner contacts. It is important to guard against paternalistic advice giving and to avoid showing disapproval or surprise when the adolescent attempts to impress one with tales of sexual exploits or the use of vulgar language. *Sexuality* is an important topic to address with teens, but one should not impose judgment on a teen's sexual activities, gender preferences, or other characteristics. Instead, one should address how a teen's sexuality may create health risk and focus screening and health education efforts on these risks.

It is wise to *establish certain ground rules* with adolescents. Patient–doctor confidentiality, for example, can be assured to adolescents only insofar as they do not reveal that they are contemplating harmful acts, such as running away or committing suicide. However, certain privileged communications should be kept confidential from parents. In particular, adolescent minors have the right to be seen for STDs or for sex offense-related examinations without the prior consent of a parent. The teen may also wish to keep some health-related or emotional problems, such as drug experimentation, from a parent's knowledge.

Interviewing the Parents

Whenever possible, parents should be involved with and concerned about the health of the teen. A separate interview with parents, immediately before or after the examination, may prove helpful and can emphasize particular concerns downplayed or denied by the patient. The parents of adolescent patients may be useful in providing emotional support and ensuring compliance with therapy; therefore, informing them about the adolescent's problems and needs is important.

Some parents ask physicians to take on the role of health educator or counselor for their adolescent child. Usually, these requests are for anticipatory guidance about birth control or drug usage. At times, the physician is asked to help the teen work through an upcoming family crisis, such as divorce, serious illness, or death. Often, adolescents welcome the opportunity to discuss these issues in private. Their knowledge in these areas is often found wanting, and a sensitive physician may help the adolescent grasp realities and make intelligent decisions. A number of books on these subjects are directed to an adolescent and young adult audience, and it may be useful to make these titles available (see www.hopkinsbayview.org/PAMreferences).

Parents often have questions about specific adolescent behavior. A particular episode or issue may come to the parents' attention, and they may ask the physician whether they should exert control over it. In such instances, one should not offer specific advice but should try to discern any moral or behavioral conflicts between the parents and the adolescent. When the parents' behavior is inconsistent with the parents' own stated values, adolescents often act in opposition to those values. Miller (26) suggests that parents are not helped in this instance by being told how to behave. Advice either increases the parents' uncertainty when faced with later difficulties or implies that the parents' own opinions are inappropriate. Adolescents probably turn out mentally healthier when presented with models of adult behavior with which their parents are comfortable, whether consistent with societal norms or not. However, parents must be prepared to make allowances so that their children have freedom to make their own mistakes. Family counseling is a technique that a general physician can use when several members of a household are involved (see Chapter 20).

Health Assessment and Preventive Care

The initial interview(s) should be comprehensive enough to ensure that the adolescent is meeting *appropriate developmental tasks*. Inquiries should be made into teenagers' relationships and functioning with their families, at school, and with peers. It is important to determine whether teenagers are establishing positive personal identities (Do they have hobbies? Do they voice their own opinions? Can they choose their own friends or must friends be approved by the parents? Do they have plans for the future?); whether they are accepting their sexuality and adjusting to adult sexual roles (Do they date? Are they sexually active? Do they have a knowledge of contraception? Is contraception used?); whether they are establishing independence from the family (Do they drive? Do they earn money on their own? What sort of hours do they keep?); whether they are working toward a career (What are their plans after high school? What subjects in school do they like? What are their grades? Do they plan to go to college? Are their goals realistic and are they supported by the family?); whether they have established good health habits (What are their views about nutrition? Do they have an adequate source of calcium and iron in their diet [see Chapter 15]? Do they eat breakfast? Is eating done on the run, in isolation, or with friends and family? Have they experimented with alcohol, tobacco, or other recreational drugs? What drugs? Have they ever been drugged or high when driving or when attending school?); and whether affective swings are interfering with functioning (Do they often feel down? What makes them happy? Have sad feelings ever made them consider harming themselves?).

Adolescents visit physicians infrequently. When they do, few receive counseling on critical adolescent health issues. In an analysis of the National Ambulatory Medical Care Survey between 1995 and 1997, Merenstein and colleagues found that counseling about any of seven areas studied (diet and nutrition, exercise, weight reduction, cholesterol reduction, HIV transmission, injury prevention, and tobacco use) was documented in 15.8% of family physician visits and 21.6% of pediatrician visits (27). However, the Youth Risk Behavior Surveillance statistics published by the Centers for Disease Control and Prevention suggest that more than half of all teens self report behaviors that may seriously jeopardize future health, including not using a bike helmet or a seat belt; alcohol, tobacco, marijuana, and drug use; unsafe sex practices and sexuality concerns; lack of physical exercise and sport participation; too much time watching television or playing computer games; attempts to lose or gain weight through purging or fad diets; poor nutritional habits, including lack of calcium intake, unusual diets, and failure to eat sufficient fruits and vegetables; use of nutritional additives and steroids for rapid muscle development; violent behavior and victimization; and mood and emotional concerns.

As part of the *review of systems before examination*, a self-administered medical questionnaire may be useful and time saving. Such a questionnaire should be brief, with language simple enough to be understood by teens with poor reading skills. Positive answers must be explored further.

A *physical examination* should be performed in the absence of parents. Teenage girls examined by male physicians may be more comfortable with a female adult in the room with them. Some parts of the physical examination occasionally omitted by physicians but essential for adolescent patients include blood pressure measurement and examination of the entire integument, the spine (for scoliosis), and the external genitalia (for signs of venereal disease and for assessment of sexual development using Tanner staging [Tables 11.4 and 11.5]). All sexually active adolescent girls should have a pelvic examination, including gonorrheal cultures and a Papanicolaou (Pap) smear (see Chapter 104). If one is uncomfortable doing this examination, the teen should be referred to a gynecologist (preferably female) who is used to dealing with adolescents.

There are *several important adjuncts to the physical examination of the healthy adolescent,* including testing for myopia and hyperopia (using a Snellen chart) and screening for deafness (by pure tone audiometry). Adolescence is a period marked by noise pollution in the form of loud music that can cause permanent damage to the eighth nerve (see Chapter 110). Adolescents who have difficulty in school should be screened for learning disorders. Having a teenager read a newspaper paragraph aloud or do some simple arithmetic may reveal a previously undetected learning disability.

Laboratory screening tests for healthy adolescents are remarkably few. Screening for anemia with a hematocrit or hemoglobin determination may be limited to menstruating young women. Tuberculosis screening with purified protein derivative should be performed only if there are family or community risk factors. Screening for hyperlipidemia is controversial during adolescence. The chance of diagnosing a problem severe enough to require pharmacologic therapy is small, whereas the benefits of a diet low in total fat and cholesterol may be universal. The decision to screen adolescents may be influenced by family history of myocardial infarction or stroke in a person younger than age 55 years or by personal opinion about whether an abnormal lipid profile may influence a patient's dietary practices. One may wish to screen teens for thyroid disorders if there is a positive family history for thyroid disease, with thyroid-stimulating hormone (TSH), thyroxine (T4), and, if thyroiditis is suspected, antithyroid antibodies. Urinalysis, blood chemistry screens, chest radiographs, and electrocardiograms are not indicated in healthy adolescents.

Healthy adolescents may require tests, immunizations, and/or physical examinations for special needs, such as travel, sports, camp, and college entry. In addition, there may be optional vaccines or tests that will need to be coordinated with the routine health schedule, such as varicella vaccine for students entering college or chest radiographs for students who have had bacillus Calmette-Guérin (BCG) vaccine and a positive purified protein derivative test.

Recommended Preventive Services

Figure 11.3 summarizes the consensus American Medical Association Guidelines for Adolescent Preventive Services. Some offices find it useful to keep this table, as

<table>
<tr><th></th><th colspan="11">Age of adolescent</th></tr>
<tr><th></th><th colspan="4">Early</th><th colspan="3">Middle</th><th colspan="4">Late</th></tr>
<tr><th>Procedure</th><th>11</th><th>12</th><th>13</th><th>14</th><th>15</th><th>16</th><th>17</th><th>18</th><th>19</th><th>20</th><th>21</th></tr>
<tr><td>Health guidance</td><td></td><td></td><td></td><td></td><td></td><td></td><td></td><td></td><td></td><td></td><td></td></tr>
<tr><td>Parenting*</td><td colspan="4">——■——</td><td colspan="3">——■——</td><td></td><td></td><td></td><td></td></tr>
<tr><td>Development</td><td>■</td><td>■</td><td>■</td><td>■</td><td>■</td><td>■</td><td>■</td><td>■</td><td>■</td><td>■</td><td>■</td></tr>
<tr><td>Diet & physical activity</td><td>■</td><td>■</td><td>■</td><td>■</td><td>■</td><td>■</td><td>■</td><td>■</td><td>■</td><td>■</td><td>■</td></tr>
<tr><td>Healthy lifestyles**</td><td>■</td><td>■</td><td>■</td><td>■</td><td>■</td><td>■</td><td>■</td><td>■</td><td>■</td><td>■</td><td>■</td></tr>
<tr><td>Injury prevention</td><td>■</td><td>■</td><td>■</td><td>■</td><td>■</td><td>■</td><td>■</td><td>■</td><td>■</td><td>■</td><td>■</td></tr>
<tr><td>Screening history</td><td></td><td></td><td></td><td></td><td></td><td></td><td></td><td></td><td></td><td></td><td></td></tr>
<tr><td>Eating disorders</td><td>■</td><td>■</td><td>■</td><td>■</td><td>■</td><td>■</td><td>■</td><td>■</td><td>■</td><td>■</td><td>■</td></tr>
<tr><td>Sexual activity***</td><td>■</td><td>■</td><td>■</td><td>■</td><td>■</td><td>■</td><td>■</td><td>■</td><td>■</td><td>■</td><td>■</td></tr>
<tr><td>Alcohol & other drug use</td><td>■</td><td>■</td><td>■</td><td>■</td><td>■</td><td>■</td><td>■</td><td>■</td><td>■</td><td>■</td><td>■</td></tr>
<tr><td>Tobacco use</td><td>■</td><td>■</td><td>■</td><td>■</td><td>■</td><td>■</td><td>■</td><td>■</td><td>■</td><td>■</td><td>■</td></tr>
<tr><td>Abuse</td><td>■</td><td>■</td><td>■</td><td>■</td><td>■</td><td>■</td><td>■</td><td>■</td><td>■</td><td>■</td><td>■</td></tr>
<tr><td>School performance</td><td>■</td><td>■</td><td>■</td><td>■</td><td>■</td><td>■</td><td>■</td><td>■</td><td>■</td><td>■</td><td>■</td></tr>
<tr><td>Depression</td><td>■</td><td>■</td><td>■</td><td>■</td><td>■</td><td>■</td><td>■</td><td>■</td><td>■</td><td>■</td><td>■</td></tr>
<tr><td>Risk for suicide</td><td>■</td><td>■</td><td>■</td><td>■</td><td>■</td><td>■</td><td>■</td><td>■</td><td>■</td><td>■</td><td>■</td></tr>
<tr><td>Physical assessment</td><td></td><td></td><td></td><td></td><td></td><td></td><td></td><td></td><td></td><td></td><td></td></tr>
<tr><td>Blood pressure</td><td>■</td><td>■</td><td>■</td><td>■</td><td>■</td><td>■</td><td>■</td><td>■</td><td>■</td><td>■</td><td>■</td></tr>
<tr><td>BMI</td><td>■</td><td>■</td><td>■</td><td>■</td><td>■</td><td>■</td><td>■</td><td>■</td><td>■</td><td>■</td><td>■</td></tr>
<tr><td>Comprehensive exam</td><td colspan="4">——■——</td><td colspan="3">——■——</td><td colspan="4">——■——</td></tr>
<tr><td>Tests</td><td></td><td></td><td></td><td></td><td></td><td></td><td></td><td></td><td></td><td></td><td></td></tr>
<tr><td>Cholesterol</td><td colspan="4">——1——</td><td colspan="3">——1——</td><td colspan="4">——1——</td></tr>
<tr><td>TB</td><td colspan="4">——2——</td><td colspan="3">——2——</td><td colspan="4">——2——</td></tr>
<tr><td>GC, Chlamydia, Syphilis & HPV</td><td colspan="4">——3——</td><td colspan="3">——3——</td><td colspan="4">——3——</td></tr>
<tr><td>HIV</td><td colspan="4">——4——</td><td colspan="3">——4——</td><td colspan="4">——4——</td></tr>
<tr><td>Pap smear</td><td colspan="4">——5——</td><td colspan="3">——5——</td><td colspan="4">——5——</td></tr>
<tr><td>Immunizations</td><td></td><td></td><td></td><td></td><td></td><td></td><td></td><td></td><td></td><td></td><td></td></tr>
<tr><td>MMR</td><td colspan="2">—■—</td><td></td><td></td><td></td><td></td><td></td><td></td><td></td><td></td><td></td></tr>
<tr><td>Td</td><td colspan="2">—■—</td><td></td><td></td><td></td><td></td><td></td><td></td><td></td><td></td><td></td></tr>
<tr><td>HepB</td><td colspan="2">—■—</td><td></td><td></td><td colspan="3">——6——</td><td colspan="4">——6——</td></tr>
<tr><td>HepA</td><td colspan="4">——7——</td><td colspan="3">——7——</td><td colspan="4">——7——</td></tr>
<tr><td>Varicella</td><td colspan="4">——8——</td><td colspan="3">——8——</td><td colspan="4">——8——</td></tr>
</table>

1. Screening test performed once if family history is positive for early cardiovascular disease or hyperlipidemia.

2. Screen if positive for exposure to active TB or lives/works in high-risk situation, e.g., homeless shelter, health care facility.

3. Screen at least annually if sexually active.

4. Screen if high-risk for infection.

5. Screen annually if sexually active or if 18 years or older.

6. Vaccinate if high risk for hepatitis B infection.

7. Vaccinate if at risk for hepatitis A infection.

8. Vaccinate if no reliable history of chicken pox.

** A parent health guidance visit is recommended during early and middle adolescence.*

*** Includes counseling regarding sexual behavior and avoidance of tobacco, alcohol, and other drug use.*

**** Includes history of unintended pregnancy and STD.*

FIGURE 11.3. Preventive health services for adolescents by age and procedure. (From American Medical Association. AMA guidelines for adolescent preventive services [GAPS]. Updated April 2001, with permission.)

TABLE 11.10 Sports Participation Health History

This evaluation is only to determine readiness for sports participation. It should not be used as a substitute for regular health maintenance exams.

Name__________ Grade__________ Sports__________

	YES	NO
1. Have you ever had an illness that		
a. Required you to stay in the hospital?	____	____
b. Lasted longer than a week?	____	____
c. Caused you to miss 3 days of practice or a competition?	____	____
d. d. Is related to allergies (e.g., hay fever, hives, asthma, insect stings)?	____	____
e. Required an operation?	____	____
f. Is chronic (e.g., asthma, diabetes)?	____	____
2. Have you ever had an injury that		
a. Required you to go to an emergency room or see a doctor?	____	____
b. Required you to stay in the hospital?	____	____
c. Required x-rays?	____	____
d. Caused you to miss 3 days of practice or a competition?	____	____
e. Required an operation?	____	____
3. Do you take any medication or pills?		
4. Have any members of your family under age 50 had a heart attack or heart problems, or died unexpectedly?		
5. Have you ever		
a. Been dizzy or passed out during or after exercise?	____	____
b. Been unconscious or had a concussion?	____	____
6. Are you unable to run 1/2 mile (2 times around the track) without stopping?		
7. Do you		
a. Wear glasses or contacts?	____	____
b. Wear dental bridges, plates, or braces?	____	____
8. Have you ever had a heart murmur, high blood pressure, or a heart abnormality?		
9. Do you have any allergies to any medicines?		
10. Are you missing a kidney?		
11. When was your last tetanus booster?		
12. For women		
a. At what age did you experience your first menstrual period?	____	____
b. In the last year, what was the longest time you have gone between periods?	____	____

EXPLAIN ANY "YES" ANSWERS

Signature of parent__________

Signature of athlete__________

Date__________

INTERIM HEALTH HISTORY

This form should be used during the interval between participation evaluations. Positive responses should prompt a physical exam.

1. Over the next 12 months, I wish to participate in the following sports:
   a. __________
   b. __________
   c. __________
   d. __________
2. Have you missed more than 3 consecutive days of participation in usual activities because of an injury this past year?
   YES______ NO______
3. Have you missed more than 5 consecutive days of participation in usual activities because of an illness, or have you had a medical illness diagnosed that has not resolved in the past year?
   YES______ NO______
   If yes, please indicate type of illness:______
4. Have you had a seizure or concussion, or been unconscious for any reason in the last year?
   YES______ NO______
5. Have you had surgery or been hospitalized in this past year?
   YES______ NO______
   If yes, please indicate
   a. Reason for hospitalization______
   b. Type of surgery______
6. List all medications you are currently taking and what condition the medication is for.
   a. __________
   b. __________
   c. __________
   d. __________
7. Are you worried about any problem or condition at this time?
   YES______ NO______
   If yes, please explain:______

Signature of athlete__________

Signature of athlete__________

Date__________

From Committee on Sports Medicine and Fitness, American Academy of Pediatrics. Sports medicine: health care for young athletes, 2nd ed. Elk Grove Village, IL: American Academy of Pediatrics, 1991, with permission.

a prompt and for documenting completed actions, in the records of adolescent patients. Since publication of this report, there has been a recommendation for universal vaccination of adolescents with meningococcus conjugate vaccine, a single dose between ages 11 and 18 years. This replaces the optional meningococcus polysaccharide vaccine that had been suggested prior to college entry. In addition, the Tetanus-diphtheria (Td) vaccine is being replaced with a diphtheria, tetanus toxoids, and acellular pertussis (DTaP) vaccine between ages 12 and 14 years. (See Centers for Disease Control at www.hopkinsbayview.org/PAMreferences.)

TABLE 11.11 Medical Conditions and Sports Participation

Condition	*May Participate?*	*Explanation*[a]
Atlantoaxial instability	Qualified yes	Condition common with Down syndrome. Athlete needs evaluation to assess risk of spinal cord injury during sports participation.
Bleeding disorder	Qualified yes	Athlete needs evaluation.
Cardiovascular diseases[b]		
Carditis	No	Carditis may result in sudden death with exertion.
Hypertension	Qualified yes	With essential hypertension, avoid weight and power lifting, body building, and strength training. Those with secondary hypertension or severe essential hypertension need evaluation.
Congenital heart disease	Qualified yes	Those with mild forms may participate fully. Those with moderate or severe forms, or who have undergone surgery, need evaluation.
Dysrhythmia	Qualified yes	Those with symptoms (chest pain, syncope, dizziness, shortness of breath or other) or evidence of mitral valve prolapse (regurgitation) need evaluation. All others may participate fully.
Mitral valve prolapse	Qualified yes	Those with symptoms (chest pain, symptoms of possible arrhythmia) or evidence of mitral regurgitation on physical examination need evaluation. All others may participate fully.
Heart murmur	Qualified yes	If the murmur is innocent, full participation is permitted. Otherwise, the athlete needs evaluation.
Cerebral palsy	Qualified yes	Athlete needs evaluation.
Diabetes mellitus	Yes	All sports can be played with proper attention to diet, blood glucose concentration, hydration, and insulin therapy. Particular attention is needed for activities that last 30 minutes or more. Blood glucose concentration should be monitored every 30 minutes during continuous exercise and 15 minutes after discontinuation of exercise.
Diarrhea	Qualified no	Unless disease is mild, no participation is permitted because diarrhea may increase the risk of dehydration and heat illness. See "Fever."
Eating disorders		
Anorexia nervosa Bulimia nervosa	Qualified yes	These patients need both medical and psychiatric assessment before participation.
Eyes: functionally one-eyed athlete, loss of any eye, detached retina, previous eye surgery or serious eye injury	Qualified yes	A functionally one-eyed athlete has a best-corrected visual acuity of less than 20/40 in the worse eye. These athletes would suffer significant disability if the better eye were seriously injured, as would those with loss of an eye. Some athletes who have undergone eye surgery or had a serious eye injury may have an increased risk of injury because of weakened eye tissue. Availability of eye guards approved by the American Society for Testing and Materials (ASTM) and other protective equipment may allow participation in most sports, but this must be judged on an individual basis.
Fever	No	Fever can increase cardiopulmonary effort, reduce maximum exercise capacity, make heat illness more likely, and increase orthostatic hypotension during exercise. Fever may rarely accompany myocarditis or other infections that make exercise dangerous.
Heat illness, history of	Qualified yes	Because of the increased likelihood of recurrence, the athlete needs individual assessment to determine the presence of predisposing conditions and arrange a prevention strategy.
Human immunodeficiency virus infection	Yes	Because of the apparent minimal risk to others, all sports may be played that the state of health allows. In all athletes, skin lesions should be properly covered, and athletic personnel should use universal precautions when handling blood or body fluids containing visible blood.
Kidney, absence of one	Qualified yes	Athlete needs individual assessment for contact/collision and limited contact sports.
Liver		
Enlarged liver	Qualified yes	If the liver is acutely enlarged, participation should be avoided because of the risk of rupture. If the liver is chronically enlarged, individual assessment is needed before collision/contact or limited contact sports are played.

TABLE 11.11 (Continued) Medical Conditions and Sports Participation

Condition	May Participate?	Explanation[a]
Hepatitis	Yes	Because of the apparent minimal risk to others, all sports may be played that the athlete's state of health allows. In all athletes, skin lesions should be covered properly, and athletic personnel should use universal precautions when handling blood or body fluid with visible blood.
Malignancy	Qualified yes	Athlete needs individual assessment.
Musculoskeletal disorders	Qualified yes	Athlete needs individual assessment.
Neurologic conditions		
History of serious head or spine trauma, severe or repeated concussions, or craniotomy	Qualified yes	Athlete needs individual assessment for collision or limited contact sports and for noncontact sports if there are deficits in judgment or cognition. Research supports a conservative approach to management of concussion.
Seizure disorder, well controlled	Yes	Risk of seizure during participation is minimal.
Seizure disorder, poorly controlled	Qualified yes	Athlete needs individual assessment for collision, contact, or limited contact sports. Avoid the following noncontact sports: archery, riflery, swimming, weight or power lifting, strength training, or sports involving heights. In these sports, occurrence of a seizure may be a risk to self or others.
Obesity	Qualified yes	Because of the risk of heat illness, obese athletes need careful acclimatization and hydration.
Organ transplant recipient	Qualified yes	Athlete needs individual assessment.
Ovary, absence of one	Yes	Risk of severe injury to the remaining ovary is minimal.
Respiratory		
Pulmonary compromise including cystic fibrosis	Qualified yes	Athlete needs individual assessment, but generally all sports may be played if oxygenation remains satisfactory during a graded exercise test. Patients with cystic fibrosis need acclimatization and good hydration to reduce the risk of illness.
Asthma	Yes	With proper medication and education, only athletes with the most severe asthma will need to modify their participation.
Acute upper respiratory	Qualified yes	Upper respiratory obstruction may affect pulmonary function. Athlete needs individual assessment for all but mild disease. See "Fever."
Sickle cell disease	Qualified yes	Athlete needs individual assessment. In general, if status of the illness permits, all but high-exertion collision/contact sports may be played. Overheating, dehydration, and chilling must be avoided.
Sickle cell trait (AS)	Yes	It is unlikely that athletes with sickle cell trait have an increased risk of sudden death or other medical problems during athletic participation except during the most extreme conditions of heat, humidity, and possibly increased altitude. These patients, like all athletes, should be carefully conditioned, acclimatized, and hydrated to reduce any possible risk.
Skin: boils, herpes simplex, impetigo, scabies, molluscum contagiosum	Qualified yes	While the patient is contagious, participation in gymnastics with mats, martial arts, wrestling, or other collision/contact or limited contact sports is not allowed.
Spleen, enlarged	Qualified yes	Patients with acutely enlarged spleens should avoid all sports because of risk of rupture. Those with chronically enlarged spleens need individual assessment before playing collision/contact or limited contact sports.
Testicle, absent or undescended	Yes	Certain sports may require a protective cup.

[a]"Needs evaluation" means that a physician with appropriate knowledge and experience should assess the safety of a given sport for an athlete with the listed medical condition. Unless otherwise noted, this is because of the variability of the severity of the disease or of the risk of injury among specific sports.

[b]Cardiac causes of sudden death in sports: hypertrophic cardiomyopathy, aortic rupture secondary to Marfan syndrome, congenital coronary artery anomalies, atherosclerotic coronary artery disease, and aortic stenosis. Most are rarely diagnosed during routine physical examination, although presence of marfanoid body habitus or characteristic heart murmur could aid early detection. Examiner needs to be alert to patients with positive family histories of early heart disease, hyperlipidemia, early sudden death, and Marfan syndrome.

From Andrews JS. Making the most of the sports physical. Contemp Pediatr 1997;14:183–205, and American Academy of Pediatrics, Committee on Sports Medical Fitness. Medical conditions affecting sports participation. Pediatrics 2001;107:1205, with permission.

Examining the Adolescent Athlete

The examination of adolescent athletes requires an evaluation of their health and consideration of their functional ability, growth, and maturation. The purpose of the preparticipation health evaluation is to identify medical conditions that might preclude safe and effective athletic participation, including those that might become worse by participation in sports activities. It can also serve the purpose of facilitating and encouraging safe sports participation. Often, the sports exam is the only health encounter that a teen may have with a physician. A brief screening questionnaire (Table 11.10) along with information already known to the physician will identify most conditions that may disqualify an adolescent from participation in various types of sports (Table 11.11). However, there are lengthier forms that serve as a general health review, both to identify injury potential and to further good health and training practices for young athletes (see Matheson at www.hopkinsbayview.org/PAMreferences).

As athletes become more experienced, the most commonly encountered problems are residuals of previous sports injuries, most of them musculoskeletal problems. Common exercise-related musculoskeletal injuries that can be managed in the office are described in Section 10: Musculoskeletal Problems of this book.

SPECIFIC REFERENCES*

1. America's Children 2005: key national indicators of well-being 2005. Available at: www.childstats.gov.
2. Centers for Disease Control and Prevention (CDC), National Center for Health Statistics (NCHS). National Health and Nutrition Examination Survey Data. Hyattsville, MD: U.S. Department of Health and Human Services, Center for Disease Control and Prevention, 2004. Available at www.cdc.gov/nchs/about/major/nhanes/datatblelink.htm, or in abridged form at www.childstats.gov/americaschildren/hea3.asp.
3. Neilson S. Epidemiology and mortality of eating disorders. Psychiatr Clin North Am 2001;24:201.
4. Kreipe RE. Eating disorder among children and adolescents. Pediatr Rev 1995;16:370.
5. Pope HG, Hudson JI, Yurgelun-Todd D. Anorexia nervosa and bulimia among 300 suburban women shoppers. Am J Psychiatry 1984;141:292.
6. American Medical Association. AMA guidelines for adolescent preventive services (GAPS): recommendations and rationale. Baltimore: Williams & Wilkins, 1994.
7. Kogut MD. Growth and development in adolescents. Pediatr Clin North Am 1973;20:789.
8. AGI: Teenage pregnancy; overall trends and state-by-state information. New York: Alan Guttmacher Institute, 1999.
9. Hein K. Commentary on adolescent acquired immune deficiency syndrome: the next wave of the human immunodeficiency virus epidemic? J Pediatr 1989;114:144.
10. Kysar JR, Zaks MS, Schuchman HP, et al. Range of psychological functioning in normal late adolescents. Arch Gen Psychiatry 1969;21:515.
11. Burns BJ, Taube CA. Mental health service for adolescents: assessment background paper for U.S. Congress, Office of Technology Assessment. In: Adolescent health I: summary and policy options. OTA-H-468. Washington, DC: U.S. Government Printing Office, 1991.
12. Offer D, Marcus D, Offer JL. A longitudinal study of normal adolescent boys. Am J Psychiatry 1970;126:917.
13. U.S. Department of Justice, Office of Justice Programs, Bureau of Justice Statistics. Available at: www.ojp.usdoj.gov/bjs/ibrs.htm.
14. Weiner IB. Delinquent behavior. In: Psychological disturbance in adolescence. New York: Wiley, 1992.
15. Federal Interagency Forum on Child and Family Statistics. America's children: key national indicators of well-being 2005. Available at: www.childstats.gov.
16. Donnerstein E, Slaby R, Eron L. The mass media and youth aggression. In: Eron L, Gentry J, Schlegel P, eds. Reason to hope: a psychological perspective on violence and youth. Washington, DC: American Psychological Association, 1995.
17. Strassburger V, Donnerstein E. Children, adolescents and the media: issues and solutions. Pediatrics 1999;103:129.
18. Nansel T, Overpeck M, Pilla R, et al. Bullying behaviors among U.S. youth. Prevalence and association with psychosocial adjustment. JAMA 2001;185:2094.
19. American Academy of Pediatrics Task Force on Violence. The role of the pediatrician in youth violence prevention in clinical practice and at the community level. Pediatrics 1999;103:173.
20. Mattsson A. Adolescent depression and suicide. In: Hockelman RA, Blatman S, Bounell PA, et al, eds. Principles of pediatrics. New York: McGraw-Hill, 1978 .
21. DISC Depression Group of Columbia University, 2002. Available from Columbia DISC Development Group, 1051 Riverside Drive, New York, NY, 10032.
22. Net version available at: www.lifelineeap.com/TheBeckDepressionInventory.htm.
23. Levine MD, Zallen BG. The learning disorders of adolescence: organic and non-organic failure to thrive. Pediatr Clin North Am 1984;31:345.
24. Goldman LS, Genel M, Bezman RJ, et al. Diagnosis and treatment of attention-deficit/hyperactivity disorder in children and adolescents. JAMA 1998;279:1100.
25. Murphy KR, Adler LA. Assessing attention-deficit/hyperactivity disorder in adults: Focus on rating scales. J Clin Psychiatry 2004; 65(Suppl 3):12.
26. Miller D. Adolescent crisis: challenge for patient, parent, and internist. Ann Intern Med 1973; 79:435.
27. Merenstein D, Green LA, Fryer GE, et al. Shortchanging adolescents: room for improvement in preventive care by physicians. Fam Med 2001;33:120.

*Bold numerals denote published controlled clinical trials, meta-analyses, or consensus-based recommendations.

For annotated ***General References*** *and resources related to this chapter, visit www.hopkinsbayview.org/PAMreferences.*

Chapter 12

Geriatric Medicine: Special Considerations

Colleen Christmas and Thomas E. Finucane

Geriatric patients differ from younger patients in ways that impact on their medical care. First, much of the ambulatory health care of geriatric patients is focused on management of chronic problems. Data from 1999 Medicare claims indicate that more than 75% of all Medicare beneficiaries suffer from at least one, and approximately 33% suffer from four or more, chronic conditions (1). Almost 50% of the population older than age 65 years has osteoarthritis, 40% has hypertension, nearly 33% has chronic heart disease, and more than 25% suffers from hearing impairment. Although seniors comprise approximately 13% of the population, they consume nearly 33% of all prescription medications.

Second, aging is accompanied by a decreasing ability to tolerate disturbances in homeostasis (so-called homeostenosis). Disease in the elderly may present as a change in functional or cognitive status rather than with the typical presentation seen in younger patients. This concept is also important to consider in contemplating the responses to therapies and in weighing the risks of treatments.

Third, because of disease burden and aging changes, many syndromes of old age, such as frailty, falls, and delirium, result from the cumulative effects of many factors. Because most geriatric syndromes are multifactorial in etiology, they often benefit from multifactorial interventions involving multidisciplinary teams of care providers addressing the biologic, psychological, spiritual, and social needs of the individual.

Finally, while quality of life is important at all ages, the contribution of this value to decision making in older individuals may be relatively greater than in younger individuals.

DEMOGRAPHIC CHANGES

In 2000 there were approximately 35 million people in the United States age 65 years or older; by 2030 this number is expected to double. Ambulatory adult medicine in the United States is already geriatric medicine to a great extent, and it is likely to become increasingly geriatric in the next several decades. On average, seniors visit a physician nine times a year, a rate that is nearly double that of younger adults. In 1999, a quarter of primary care physician's visits were from patients older than age 65 years, and the rate of growth of outpatient visits to specialists had started to outpace those to generalists (2).

These observations result from two distinct phenomena. First, at every age, life expectancy is increasing (Table 12.1). In 1980, a 65-year-old American could expect, on average, to live another 16.4 years. By 1997, this number has increased to 17.6 years. An 85-year-old woman today has a life expectancy of 6.6 years, 1 more year than a man at the same age. The "oldest old," older than age 85 years, are a special challenge to society as a whole and to physicians in particular. They are predominantly women, and as a group they are exceedingly frail, requiring a great deal of medical and social support. Of people 65 years old in 1980, 25% are expected to survive to age 90. By the year 2050, more than 40% will survive to age 90, based on moderately optimistic assumptions about mortality rates (3,4).

The second important phenomenon is the postwar baby boom of children born between 1945 and 1965. From 2010 to 2030, the U.S. population ages 65 to 84 years will

TABLE 12.1 Life Expectancy of Older Americans in 1900, 1950, and 1997

	1900	1950	1997
Life expectancy at birth (years)			
Total	49.2	68.1	76.5
Men	47.9	65.5	73.6
Women	50.7	71.0	79.4
Life expectancy at age 65 (additional years)			
Total	11.9	13.8	17.7
Men	11.5	12.7	15.9
Women	12.2	15.0	19.2
Life expectancy at age 85 (additional years)			
Total	4.0	4.7	6.3
Men	3.8	4.4	5.5
Women	4.1	4.9	6.6

Adapted from Federal Interagency Forum on Aging-Related Statistics. Older Americans 2004: Key indicators of well-being. Federal Interagency Forum on Age-Related Statistics. Washington, DC: U.S. Government Printing Office. November 2004.

increase 80%, whereas the population younger than age 65 years will increase only 7%. Thereafter, baby boomers will become "old," older than age 85 years. In 1990 there were 3 million old Americans. In 2010 there will be 6 million, and in 2050, 19 million people will be older than age 85 years (3).

The challenge for physicians will be sharpened by three additional effects: the increasing rates of disability, poverty, and ethnic diversity among the elderly. Disability arises from concomitant chronic medical illnesses, cognitive deficits, and depressive symptoms, in addition to underlying frailty. The percentage of people who need assistance with everyday activities rises steeply with age. Among the "young old," age 65 to 75 years, approximately 10% require assistance, whereas among the old, nearly 50% do. These figures are higher for African American and Hispanic elders. Thus, although large numbers of caregivers will be needed at the same time, data suggests that the number of available caregivers is declining. Defining poverty in the United States is arbitrary, but 2002 Census Bureau data showed that 7.8% of men and 14.1% of women age 75 and older were poor. On the average, in 2001, out-of-pocket health care spending totaled 22% of income in the lowest income quintile of households headed by an older person (4). Fifty-six percent of this spending was for the purchase of prescription drugs. All aspects of the U.S. population are becoming increasingly ethnically diverse. Whereas whites comprised 84%, blacks 8%, Asians and Pacific Islanders 2%, and Hispanics 6% of the elderly population in 2000, by 2050 the projections for these demographics are 64%, 12%, 7%, and 16%, respectively (5).

Care of the old, and especially the very old, requires special awareness of the progressive socioeconomic and physiologic vulnerability of old age. More than knowledge of specific disease states, awareness of the extreme frailty of the very old defines clinical geriatrics.

PUBLIC POLICY

Medicare

Medicare was intended as hospital insurance for the elderly, regardless of income, covering a period of acute illness and subsequent convalescence. Eligibility depends on age or other qualifying condition (e.g., end-stage renal disease) but not on income. In general, Part A pays institutions for hospital inpatient care, brief posthospital care (whether institutional or provided by a home health agency), and Medicare hospices. Part B pays physicians and providers of outpatient services, such as independent laboratories, mental health services, and rehabilitation services. Durable medical equipment is also covered by Part B. Some preventive services are covered under Medicare, including influenza and pneumococcal vaccines, screening mammograms every 12 months, screening Papanicolaou (Pap) smears every 3 years, colonoscopy every 10 years, and dual-energy x-ray absorptiometry (DEXA) bone mineral density measurements every 2 years. In January 2006, the largest change to occur in Medicare since its inception began when Medicare enrollees became eligible for various forms of prescription drug benefits. It is yet too soon to understand the impact of this change in Medicare. The most up-to-date information about the prescription drug plans available through Medicare is found at www.medicare.gov.

In 1996 Medicare indicated that it would cover inpatient hospital admissions for symptom palliation in terminally ill patients (6). For their services, hospice programs receive a prearranged payment to cover medical care, medications, and supplies related to the terminal diagnoses in the dying patient. Much of the debate about the most recent reform proposals has been driven by the escalating costs of health care; this is emphasized by the name Balanced Budget Act of 1997. This Act has had widespread fundamental effects on medical care in America. Its implementation has meant changes to Medicare support of graduate medical education, attempts at increasing choices for health care plans (Medicare health maintenance organizations), and the restructuring of reimbursement schedules for physician services and home health care (7). On the other hand, long-term care will likely remain beyond Medicare's purview. Chronically ill patients in nursing homes are generally not covered. Short-term stays for rehabilitation after hospitalization are reimbursed, but Medicare coverage ends, as a rule, once the patient stops improving.

Medicare has grown in size (to more than 34 million beneficiaries) and in complexity since its inception in 1965. More changes are anticipated in the coming years.

Effective care of the geriatric population entails continual efforts at keeping up-to-date with these and future amendments to Medicare. Detailed information on Medicare benefits for individuals is available from the federal government (see Preretirement Counseling and Planning later in this chapter).

Medicaid

Both Medicare and Medicaid are federally funded with oversight from the Center for Medicare and Medicaid Services (formally Health Care Financing Administration). However, unlike Medicare, Medicaid administration is left largely to the individual states. Each state sets its own policies within certain federal guidelines. To be eligible for Medicaid, it is necessary, but not sufficient, to be impoverished; age and other criteria such as disability must be met. In general, Medicaid offers more benefits than those covered by Medicare and traditional insurance plans. These benefits can include prescription drugs, prosthetics, hearing aids, and both inpatient and outpatient services. Although more than 41.3 million Americans participate in this program, with many now enrolled in Medicaid managed-care plans, less than half of poor Americans are actually covered by Medicaid. In 1997 alone, $159.9 billion dollars were spent for its services (8).

Most Medicaid dollars are spent on long-term care in nursing homes, and about half of nursing home revenue comes from Medicaid. Eligibility for nursing home placement is defined by the states and depends on functional disability and medical illness. Medicaid pays for nursing home care only if the person is indigent. Thus, a person with assets may qualify in one of two ways. He or she may spend the assets on nursing home care until impoverished or divest the assets by giving them to adult children. Rules about divestment are changing, but a "look back" period is common: Any assets given away in the previous 30 months, for example, may be counted as current assets. The issue of divestment is extremely divisive, as it is mainly the well off who can plan ahead to this extent. Increased authority and responsibilities have been parceled to the states since welfare reform. Because the program is in a period of change, practitioners should seek specific advice about nursing home placement and Medicaid eligibility from state and local sources.

Home Health Care

Home health care refers, broadly, to care, formal or informal, provided in the home. Nonetheless, this term is often used to refer to a specific Medicare benefit.

Part A Medicare certifies home health agencies and pays them for in-home care, primarily by nurses and aides. In keeping with Medicare philosophy, the program was intended to facilitate hospital discharge planning and to manage episodes of acute illness at home, thus shortening, or even preventing, some hospital admissions.

During chronic illness, spouses, adult children, other relatives, and sometimes friends have assumed most of the caregiving responsibilities for community-dwelling adults. In recent years, families have shared more of these tasks with help from paid formal home care. Increased caregiver stress, increased family and occupational responsibilities of caretakers, and perhaps some overall increase in the financial resources of older adults, may have played roles in this trend.

From 1988 to 1997, home health agency reimbursements grew from $2 billion to more than $17 billion. By 1997, 1 in 10 Medicare recipients had received home health care, accumulating an average of 80 home visits (7). Although the intent of the home health care program was to substitute or complement acute hospital care, 61% of all visits were to enrollees receiving services for 6 months or more. In fact, geographic areas with high rates of home care use do not have lower rates of hospitalization or shorter lengths of stay (9). The need for chronic care among community-dwelling elderly, along with several other factors, simply was not foreseen in the original design of Medicare. The criteria for Medicare coverage for homebound patients with unstable medical conditions and for hospice patients are summarized in Chapters 9 and 13, respectively.

Public policy about medical care of the elderly, especially the poor and frail elderly, is in flux. Out-of-pocket costs are rising, as are government expenditures. Federal scrutiny and demands on provider documentation will continue as definitions of eligible services become more refined. A broad-based plan for efficacious health care in the home may one day inspire more physician house calls (already reimbursable under Medicare) and perhaps usher in the concept of the home-based hospital (10).

Agencies on Aging

The Administration on Aging was born in 1965 out of President Johnson's Great Society program, with the purpose of establishing federal legislative agendas to serve the needs and improve the quality of life of Americans age 60 years and older. Through the Older American Act and its subsequent amendments, the Administration on Aging has since mandated the establishment of Units on Aging within all states. These Units allocate federal moneys to Area Agencies on Aging. Today there are 57 Units on Aging; they oversee more than 655 Area Agencies on Aging and 223 tribal organizations that help patients access resources within communities. The challenge has been to provide appropriate guidance to an increasingly diverse elderly population. For the more functional elders, services include assistance with finding employment and locating senior activity centers. Frail elderly are eligible for services such as home-delivered meals, advice on planning for long-term care, and support for caregivers. It is likely that comprehensive primary care of elderly patients will increasingly rely on referrals to the Area Agencies on Aging (11).

EVALUATING OLDER PATIENTS

Several aspects of the clinical evaluation of older patients deserve emphasis. When possible, *old records* should be obtained before the first visit. If it is not possible to obtain them before the first visit, they should be requested at the first visit. Patients should routinely bring all their *medications* to appointments, including over-the-counter medications and herbal supplements; these should be carefully reviewed for continued indication, tolerance, and adherence.

Attention should be paid to the *physical environment*. Bright, direct light is often uncomfortable for patients with cataracts. Prolonged sitting on a backless examining table or in a chilly room can be uncomfortable. Making a patient comfortable probably improves the quality of the medical history. For patients with presbycusis, it is more important to face the patient and speak slowly and clearly than it is to speak loudly. Also, the practitioner should have an assistive listening device (see Chapter 110) available for use by the patient when needed. Patients with marked kyphosis can often lie down more comfortably if a rolled-up sheet is placed on the pillow under the occiput.

Some form of *mental status examination* should be included in the initial evaluation of every older patient (see Chapter 26). Clinicians' impressions have been shown to be insensitive in detecting mild cognitive impairment (12). The incidence of Alzheimer disease increases greatly with age, from approximately 1% per year at ages 60 to 65 years to 6.5% per year in the 85-years-and-older age group (13). Because symptoms of disease in the elderly may be absent, atypical, muted, or ignored by the physician, subtle deterioration of cognitive or functional capacity, which may be the only indication of a serious pathologic condition, should be actively sought out.

In general, *more time* is needed for the evaluation of an elderly patient than for a younger patient. The former often has multiple problems, including sensory and mobility impairments that require a slower evaluation. Diagnostic testing should be highly selective. Stressful tests (which may include radiographic studies for a frail person with a mobility disorder) should have an expected therapeutic implication and should be explained thoroughly to the patient and, when applicable, to the caregiver. Extensive evaluation may require several visits. The highly streamlined evaluations so characteristic of modern medicine are simply too stressful and unrevealing for many ill elderly patients. Empathy and compassion are essential in high-quality care for a frail older patient. Several 30- or 60-minute visits may be more easily tolerated than a single, longer encounter, provided it is not too difficult for the patient and family to come to the office. However, too short an encounter (e.g., 10 to 20 minutes) may be disappointing, inadequate for proper care, and difficult for many elders, particularly those who have difficulty communicating their needs or understanding explanations and instructions. Patients with communication challenges may benefit from having a trusted family member or friend accompany them to the visit and the provision of written instructions for the plan of care.

Standardized Approaches to Functional Assessment

The traditional problem-oriented approach to medical care focuses primarily on medical diagnoses. Functional assessment is intended to measure the impact of disease and aging on a patient's ability to care for him- or herself, to live in the community, and to accomplish goals that are meaningful to the patient.

Frailty

The syndrome of frailty has many definitions, including decreased resilience in the face of external stress, difficulty in maintaining homeostasis, and vulnerability to adverse events. Declines in lean body mass, strength, endurance, balance, and walking performance and lower levels of activity are observed in frail older adults. A proposed definition is that individuals are frail if they meet three or more criteria related to weight loss, weakness, endurance, slowness, or low level of activity (Table 12.2) (14). Frail

TABLE 12.2 Characteristics of Frailty[a]

Trait	*Measure*
Shrinking Weight loss (unintentional) Sarcopenia (loss of muscle mass)	>10-lb weight loss (loss of ≥5% of body weight over the previous year)
Weakness	Grip strength: lowest 20% of population at baseline, adjusted for gender and body mass index
Poor endurance	Self-report of exhaustion
Slowness	Walking time/15 feet: slowest 20% of population (by gender, height)
Low activity	Lowest 20% of population in terms of energy expenditure: <383 kcals/wk (males) <270 kcals/wk (females)

[a]Presence of three or more of the listed criteria in an individual points to presence of the frailty phenotype. Adapted from Fried LP, Tangen CM, Walston JB, et al. Frailty in older adults: evidence for a phenotype. J Gerontol 2001;56A:M146.

TABLE 12.3 Areas and Levels of Assessment in the Katz Index of Independence in Activities of Daily Living

Bathing	Receives no assistance
	Receives assistance in bathing only one part
	Receives assistance in bathing more than one part
Dressing	Selects clothes and dresses without assistance
	Needs assistance in tying shoes only
	Needs assistance greater than above or stays undressed
Toileting	Needs no assistance
	Needs assistance only in getting to toilet room or in cleaning self
	Does not go to toilet room
Transferring	Needs no assistance from another person
	Needs assistance with transferring
	Does not get out of bed
Continence	Continent
	Occasional accident
	Needs supervision, uses catheter, or is incontinent
Feeding	Needs no assistance
	Needs assistance in cutting meat or buttering bread
	Needs more assistance or is tube or intravenously fed

Modified from Katz S, Ford AB, Moskowitz RW, et al. Studies of illness in the aged: the index at ADL: standardized measures of biological and psychosocial function. JAMA 1963;185:94, with permission.

individuals have higher rates of disability, hospitalization, and mortality, and are more likely to have coexisting cardiovascular diseases. This phenotype of frailty may represent a unique physiologic syndrome. Related biochemical markers and immunologic correlates of frailty are being sought. Targeted interventions that improve outcomes in frail patients may emerge (14).

Disability

Living independently requires the performance of certain basic activities. Essential goals of caring for an elderly person are to identify and minimize his or her dependence on others for these activities. The *Katz index of activities of daily living* (ADLs) outlines tasks that are fundamental to independent living (Table 12.3). A patient's ability to bathe, dress, toilet, transfer, feed, and maintain continence enables a clinician to deploy targeted interventions that meet the patient's current functional needs. Comparing ADL scores obtained before and after certain interventions (e.g., physical and occupational therapy for a patient after a stroke) allows the clinician to track the degree of functional improvement. Improvement in ADL scores, however, is not realistic in some patients. Poor performance of the Katz ADLs correlates with increased mortality, nursing home placement, and inadequate recovery from hip fracture (15,16). The *Barthel index* is another instrument with well-documented reliability and validity that has been used to quantify (via a 0 to 100 scoring scale) degrees of disability. Scores from the Barthel index correlate with recovery from stroke. Physicians caring for ambulatory patients often underestimate or overlook important disabilities in their patients (17).

Instrumental ADLs require a higher level of function and include abilities to travel outside the home, shop, prepare meals, do housework, or handle finances (18). Fried and Guralnik have elegantly summarized the evidence base for the assessment, natural history, demography, and impact of disability, and for interventions to prevent disability (19).

Overall understanding of a patient's level of functional ability, as well as the patient's capability to function in home, can enrich a physician's understanding of the goals of treatment for that patient. Several tools are available to assist with this task (20).

Geriatric Assessment

Comprehensive *geriatric assessment* is usually a multidisciplinary and always a multidimensional assessment of frail elderly patients and their support systems. It is occasionally confused with functional assessment, which was described in the prior section. Although it has received a great deal of favorable attention, geriatric assessment lacks a precise definition, and data supporting its usefulness are conflicting. The referral source and initial characteristics of patients, the nature of interventions (e.g., whether inpatient, in the office, or in the home, and whether consultation or ongoing therapy), and the measured outcomes have varied from study to study (21–24). In terms of outcomes, caregivers and clinicians often do not agree on perceived goals of care for frail elderly patients (25). Despite these limitations, outpatient and home assessments of elderly patients seem to have some benefits. Studies of outpatient geriatric evaluation and management (24), case finding and surveillance (26), postdischarge assessment (27), and pharmacy assessment (28) done in the home have demonstrated improved outcomes in terms of functional ability, duration of hospital stays, nursing home admissions, and medication errors, respectively.

Table 12.4 lists the central elements of geriatric assessment. Assessments performed in the above-cited studies generally contain these elements. Medicare currently does not provide specific compensation for multidisciplinary comprehensive geriatric assessment.

MEDICATION USE IN THE ELDERLY

One way of conceptualizing the aging process is as a gradual decline in the organism's ability to respond to perturbation and stress. At rest, for example, the body temperature, serum sodium, glucose, and heart rate of healthy younger

TABLE 12.4 Some Important Components of the Initial Geriatric Assessment

Cognitive assessment
- History from family often vital
- Mental status screening may involve Folstein Mini-Mental State Examination (see Table 26.1) (82)

Functional Assessment
- Inventory of functional status may include
  - Katz activities of daily living (Table 12.3)
  - Instrumental activities of daily living
- Fall risk assessment
  - Assessing history of falls, usual activity level
  - Observing patient rise unassisted from chair, walk several paces, turn, and return to the chair

Psychosocial assessment
- Depression screening may include Yesavage Geriatric Depression Scale (83)
- Consider assessment of
  - Driving skills
  - Risk for elder abuse
  - Available social support system
  - Adequacy of current living situation
  - Other barriers to ability to safe living
  - Caregiver stress

Outlook assessment
- Raise the issue of advanced directives (see Chapter 13)

Medications review
- Explicitly justify each prescription drug to ensure benefits exceed risks
- Evaluate the usefulness of alternative/complementary medicines based on available data

Preventive health care
- Recommend appropriate vaccinations
- Perform dental, vision, and hearing screen
- Recommend appropriate cancer screening

patients are about the same as those of older patients. When stressed by environmental temperature extremes, free-water load, glucose challenge, or exercise, however, the older patient will have a wider excursion from normal, will take longer to recover equilibrium, and is more likely to get sick, even in the absence of underlying disease. Medications can be seen as a perturbation. Most younger people can recover from this perturbation safely, but the elderly are more likely to have adverse effects as a result.

Elderly Americans take large numbers of drugs. Although some drugs are clearly beneficial, many others have little or no evidence of efficacy. Risks to the elderly patient from imprecise drug use can be substantial. A majority of physicians are inaccurate in reporting what medications their patients are taking, even when questioned in clinic or using the clinic chart to determine the medication regimen (29,30). In an epidemiologic study of over-the-counter medication use in the United States, 87% of independent elderly were taking at least one nonprescription medication and 6% were taking five or more (31). Complementary and alternative medications are popular (see Chapter 5). A useful clinical strategy is to insist that all medications, including over-the-counter and complementary medications, are brought to each visit and then to consider the justification for each drug.

Studies of drug disposition in the elderly demonstrate wide heterogeneity in several important physiologic functions. Although drug absorption is unimpaired in general, distribution within the body compartments may be different in older than in younger subjects. In older subjects, muscle mass, bone mass, body water, and some serum proteins are lower, whereas body fat content is higher. Hepatic drug clearance, in simplest terms, depends on hepatic blood flow, serum protein binding, and the intrinsic capacity of the hepatocyte mass. The first two of these factors may decrease with age, resulting in impaired drug metabolism in some patients. Renal glomerular rate can fall approximately 30% from the third decade to the eighth. The fall in glomerular filtration rate may not be accompanied by a rise in serum creatinine because muscle mass is falling concomitantly. Because of variability among subjects, prediction of drug levels from dosage is unreliable.

In many cases, *very low dosages* of medication may be effective, such as 12.5 mg of hydrochlorothiazide per day and beginning dosages of 0.25 mg haloperidol or 10 mg imipramine or nortriptyline per day. Unless the clinical situation requires otherwise, drugs should be started at low dosages in the elderly and titrated carefully upward during frequent, early followup. When available, drug levels are useful in monitoring the patient.

New drugs pose particularly serious risks for the elderly. In general, the U.S. Food and Drug Administration (FDA) approves new drugs after safety has been demonstrated in relatively small trials (32). Once the drugs are released, however, they are often used widely by the frail elderly, and serious but uncommon toxicities become apparent. Approximately 10% of all new drugs are withdrawn or have a "black box" warning added in the year they are placed on the market. Because older individuals are more often harmed by adverse drug reactions, new drugs should be tried carefully in older patients only after more standard drugs have been tried unsuccessfully or when the new drug presents a significant proven therapeutic advancement. Older drugs have more well-established safety profiles and are generally less expensive. Claims about the safety or the lack of side effects of newly released drugs should be viewed simply as advertising techniques.

Some specific drugs, selected because of their widespread use in the elderly, are considered here. Guiding principles of prescribing are avoid giving a medication to treat the side effects of another medication or where nonpharmacologic alternatives are available and strive to reach the least number and lowest doses of medications effective for each patient. Specific medications to avoid in the elderly have also been described (33).

Neuroleptics

Neuroleptics are often used to treat the behavioral complications of dementia, although the evidence base behind this approach is lacking. Of 100 demented patients treated with standard neuroleptics, 18 could be expected to benefit beyond placebo, according to a meta-analysis, and no one neuroleptic has been shown to be more effective than another (34), yet prices vary widely. The newer "atypical" antipsychotics are very expensive and large-scale randomized trials of their use for dementia are not available, although they are no more effective than standard neuroleptics in treatment of schizophrenia (35). Furthermore, a retrospective cohort study of the use of atypical antipsychotics for dementia failed to demonstrate a significant reduction in parkinsonism over standard neuroleptics (36). In 2005, the FDA placed a black box warning on atypical antipsychotics, citing a consistent finding of 60% to 70% increased risk of death in patients taking these drugs compared to placebo. However a recent retrospective study suggested that typical and atypical antipsychotics may pose equal risks of mortality in the elderly (37). If neuroleptic drugs are prescribed, evidence of good effect should be sought. If they provide nothing more than sedation (assuming sedation is desirable), other drugs should be used instead, such as short-acting benzodiazepines, although their use is also problematic in this age group. The properties of available antipsychotic drugs are described in Chapter 25, and the practical use of psychoactive drugs in the elderly is discussed fully in Chapter 26.

Nonsteroidal Anti-Inflammatory Drugs

For treatment of inflammatory conditions, nonsteroidal anti-inflammatory drugs (NSAIDs) are an excellent choice, although they can present serious toxicity in this age group and thus should only be used short-term, if at all. When they are used as analgesia for noninflammatory chronic pain, their considerable toxicities may outweigh their benefit. Current users of NSAIDs are almost five times more likely to have a fatal upper gastrointestinal hemorrhage when compared with former users or subjects who have never used them (38). Frail, elderly, white women are especially at risk. Renal and central nervous system toxicities are well known (see Chapter 77 for a full discussion on NSAIDs). In many cases of pain with or without underlying inflammation, acetaminophen may have a superior risk-to-benefit profile. Where the risk outweighs the benefit of NSAIDs and acetaminophen is ineffective, low-dose narcotic analgesics should be considered (potentially accompanied by a bowel regimen).

The cyclooxygenase-2 (COX-2)-specific NSAIDs have been heavily advertised, widely prescribed, and are extremely expensive. In recent years, some have been removed from the market because of demonstrated cardiovascular risks associated with their use. They should largely be avoided unless their safety profile is more firmly established. The FDA does not allow the claim that they are more effective than conventional NSAIDs.

Cold Remedies

There is no cure for the common cold, but there is a multimillion-dollar market in remedies. Common treatments bring the risk of antihistaminic or narcotic sedation, sympathomimetic stimulation, or a combination of the two. Decongestants and antihistamines are occasionally discovered to have fatal toxicities, as with phenylpropanolamine and terfenadine. Substantial amounts of alcohol are often included: Vicks NyQuil, for example, is 50 proof. Many common combinations are irrational, even contradictory. Clinicians should discourage their elderly patients, who are likely to be susceptible to anticholinergic and sympathomimetic effects, from buying these nostrums, many of which contain a variety of useless ingredients. Treatments for the common cold are discussed in Chapter 33.

Sleeping Pills

Disrupted sleep is common in old age (see Fig. 7.1), and the electroencephalogram of a normal elderly patient looks very different from that of a normal younger patient. In addition, some of the cognitive changes that occur in old age resemble the changes of sleep deprivation, such as slowed reaction time and slower learning of new material. It is unreasonable to expect, and it is not true, that any sedative hypnotic can convert the blunted and simpler sleep electroencephalogram of an older person to the complex and delicate electroencephalogram of a younger person. In fact, no sleeping pill improves alertness or daytime problem solving when given to patients with insomnia. This is true of even the newest sleeping pills available in 2005. The side effects can be very serious. Both benzodiazepine and nonbenzodiazepine sedatives are strongly associated with an increase risk of hip fracture (39). A randomized trial showed that teaching about sleep hygiene is as effective as giving sleeping pills and has more long-lasting effect (40). Cognitive behavioral therapy may be even more effective (41). Despite these findings, efforts to increase sales of hypnotics are vigorous. When insomnia is a symptom of depression, sleep quality does improve with treatment of the depression.

Drug–Drug Interactions

Elderly patients who take many medications are at high risk for drug–drug interactions. The strongest independent risk factor for an adverse drug event is the total number of drugs concurrently prescribed (42). Physicians should become familiar with and use a small number of medications. Warfarin (Coumadin) is increasingly used in elderly patients and its effect on coagulation can be affected by many drugs (see Chapter 57).

NEGLECT AND ABUSE IN THE ELDERLY

Most dependent elderly live in the community and are cared for by relatives. In most of these cases, excellent loving care is provided. In some cases, however, there is frank abuse or neglect, and in some the situation is ambiguous. The number of older Americans who are abused is likely to increase. This is thought to be partly a result of the national trend toward smaller families, as well as the rapidly increasing numbers of the very old, who are no longer wage earners and are more likely to be frail and dependent. Clear-cut examples of physical and emotional violence, sexual abuse, financial exploitation, and harmful neglect of frail elderly people have been reported.

Defining abuse can be difficult. Victims are often competent adults who choose to continue living in a suboptimal relationship with a caregiver. Neglect is also often difficult to define, especially in a relationship in which the caregiver has no legally defined responsibility. Furthermore, some situations offer only tragic options. If a single working mother cares for her demented mother who repeatedly wanders or urinates in closets, is it abuse if the daughter uses physical restraints? Suppose neither mother nor daughter will accept a nursing home and employment of professional caregivers is not financially feasible. Is it abuse if the daughter uses physical restraints?

Diagnosis is difficult because both abuser and victim may deny or minimize abuse. Consequently, diagnosis is often inferential. Treatment may be problematic in all but extreme cases. Remedies might include an alternative environment that is healthy, supportive, and acceptable to the victim or the provision of services that can relieve a stressed caregiver. Such treatment is often unavailable. Table 12.5 lists the risk factors for abuse (43,44).

TABLE 12.5 Risk Factors for Elder Abuse

Characteristics of the victim
Lives with related relative, not spouse
Cognitive impairment
Advanced age
Race
Poverty
Behavior problem
Medically ill
Functional disability
Characteristics of the abuser
Has provided long-term care
Stressed significantly by care of the victim
Under severe external stress
Abused as a child
Expresses frustration
Uses recreational drugs, including alcohol

Clinicians may be reluctant to become involved in a situation in which there is little reward, poor reimbursement, and potential liability. State statutes vary in defining the physician's responsibility and liability. The Council on Scientific Affairs of the American Medical Association has published a useful report on this subject. The report outlines several strategies for prevention and intervention (43). (The full report is available by writing to the Council on Scientific Affairs, AMA, 535 N. Dearborn St., Chicago, IL 60610.) In severe cases, however, legal advice should be sought and state and local agencies, such as Adult Protective Services, should be involved.

FALLS

Falls are common in the elderly and often have serious consequences, including death. It is estimated that 35% to 40% of community-dwelling adults age 65 years and older have at least one fall annually.

Falls are a typical geriatric syndrome: their etiology is often multifactorial and treatments are most effective when targeting several of these factors. Risk factors, such as the environment, medications, sensory impairment, dementia, depression, and deconditioning—as well as specific neurologic, cardiovascular, or musculoskeletal diseases—can be identified (45).

At least once yearly assessment of falls has been advocated. Evaluation should focus on the number of falls, events leading up to and after the falls, and environmental circumstances surrounding the falls. Moreover, the practitioner should screen for known intrinsic and extrinsic risk factors. This screening includes an assessment of prescription and alternative medicines; examination of vision, gait, balance, strength and flexibility of lower extremity; and evaluation of cardiovascular, neurologic, and other medical problems that may have caused the patient to fall. Mobility function may be determined by observing the patient as he or she stands up from a chair without assistance, walks several steps, turns, and returns to sit in the chair (46,47). Environmental factors such as dim lighting, steep stairs, loose carpeting, or small pets should be sought and, when possible, remedied.

Those who have fallen or have risk factors for falls are candidates for further interventions. For example, some exercise programs, particularly those including balance exercise (e.g., tai chi), reduce risk of falls by 10% to 17% (48). Home environmental assessments and subsequent modifications are also effective, as are treatment of cataracts, participation in a physical therapy program, and review and modification of medication regimens of those who have fallen (especially if they take more than four medications). A multifactorial intervention program targeting four specific risk factors in a vulnerable population reduced falls during 1 year of followup from 47% to 35% (49). The risk factors were postural hypotension, use of sedatives, use of four or more prescription medications, and impairment in arm or leg strength or range of motion, transfer skills, or gait skills (49). Finally, hip protectors and identification and treatment of osteoporosis may be helpful adjuncts in preventing potentially serious fractures, although there are other important consequences of falls (such as prolonged psychological impact and decrements in physical functioning) that are not benefitted. In a randomized controlled study that recruited ambulatory frail elderly persons, those who wore hip protectors had their risk for hip fractures after a fall reduced by 66% over an 18-month period. Once convinced to wear them, study participants kept them on 50% of the possible time (74% had them on during the falls) (50). These protectors are becoming commercially available, but compliance remains problematic. Whether vitamin D supplementation reduces fractures is debated, but many authorities advise supplementation with calcium and vitamin D for those who are at risk for falls and fractures. For a careful review of falls in elderly outpatients see King and Tinetti (51).

NUTRITION

For a variety of reasons, precise definition of dietary requirements for ambulatory elderly people is difficult. The elderly are physiologically and metabolically an extremely diverse group with a variety of illnesses, taking a variety of medicines. Absorptive function in the aging gut is poorly studied. However, recommended daily allowances for the elderly are extrapolated from data collected in studies of younger people. Recommended daily allowances based on age alone are imprecise. Basic principles of nutrition for persons of all ages are discussed in Chapter 15.

Two general principles have been demonstrated. First, most elderly Americans who seek medical attention are not undernourished. Second, desirable body weight for the elderly may be somewhat heavier than previously determined on the basis of insurance company tables of mortality and body mass index (BMI). These tables do not consider age. Based on independent analysis of insurance company data, Andres (52) calculated mortality ratios in various age groups according to BMI. This analysis suggests that the BMI associated with the lowest mortality rate varies with age. The older the age group, the higher the BMI associated with the longest survival. For example, the BMI associated with the lowest mortality among 25-year-old men is 21.4. For a 6-foot-tall man, this corresponds to a weight of 158 pounds. For a 65-year-old man, the best BMI is 26.6, 196 pounds for the same 6-foot-tall man. Roughly speaking, these tables allow a gain of approximately 1 pound per year throughout adult life. Several studies of long-term weight change tend to confirm that modest weight gain during adult life is associated with lower mortality (53). These tables do not apply to patients with diseases that are related to weight. For patients with type II diabetes mellitus, osteoarthritis, hypertension, and hyperlipidemia, weight loss is often a central part of treatment.

The pattern of body fat distribution is associated with several important diseases and with mortality. In women, high waist-to-hip circumference ratio is more strongly associated with death than is BMI (see Chapter 83) (54).

A variety of psychosocial factors (e.g., isolation, alcoholism, depression, low income) and physiologic changes (e.g., diminished taste and smell sensation, dental problems, dementia, dysphagia, side effects of medications) may contribute to a diminished intake of nutritious meals. The effects of multivitamin supplements are unknown. Trials of supplementation with certain specific vitamins (carotene and tocopherol) have shown no benefit (55,56). Although risks are low when vitamins are taken in moderation, costs can be high. Data are inconclusive about canned "complete" nutritional products provided to alert patients as a supplement to or substitute for regular food. Several studies suggest that intake of canned oral nutritional products offsets the intake of food at meals. These products are more costly than food, and unlikely to be superior to it.

Weight loss can result from a variety of causes, some trivial and some lethal. In general, the known causes of weight loss can be classified as decreased intake, reduced absorption, and increased use. Involuntary weight loss can be troubling in the elderly. In approximately 25% of cases, no cause is discovered despite intensive evaluation (57). Almost all the remaining causes can be found with a careful history and physical examination and judicious use of the laboratory. In the elderly, decreased intake should be carefully sought, with particular attention to medications, problems accessing food, depression, and oral hygiene. The search for malignancy during a careful history and physical examination and the exclusion of hyperthyroidism with appropriate laboratory investigation are also an important part of the evaluation. A chest radiograph may be useful if the patient has ever been a smoker, but nonspecific computerized tomography (CT) scans are not cost-effective and are low yield.

When inflammatory illness and cachexia are present, there are very few data to show that increasing nutrient intake benefits the patient. So-called markers of nutritional status, while frequently linked to poor outcome, may simply signal the presence of inflammatory illness rather than a situation that is improved with enhanced nutritional intake. As with oral nutritional supplements, appetite stimulants have not been shown to provide functional benefit or improved survival for patients with undiagnosed involuntary weight.

EXERCISE AND THE ELDERLY

Benefits from exercise are now incontrovertible and include improvements in bone density, sleep (58), risk of falls (48), disability and pain from knee arthritis (59), cardiovascular risk factors and disease (60), weight reduction (61), and rate of disability (14). Although not yet demonstrated in the elderly, studies in younger adults show that moderate exercise improves mood in depressed individuals. Moderate levels of resistive and aerobic exercises confer benefit. In fact, leisure-time physical activities ranging from walking to yard work and tai chi or calisthenics may suffice. Nonetheless, as with other age groups, older Americans as a whole maintain a relatively sedentary lifestyle. Barriers to attaining the above goals range from realistically grounded concerns (e.g., unsafe neighborhood, fear of exacerbating underlying illness) to attitudes and preferences (e.g., lack of time). Exploring these barriers in the sedentary older person and assessing the level of motivation seem to be reasonable initial steps in encouraging exercise in the sedentary older adult. Adherence to an exercise prescription may also correlate with activities that are enjoyable to the individual, take place in a preferred setting, and fit into his or her schedule.

For those who are inactive, it is reasonable to begin by finding ways to reduce inactivity (e.g., reducing time spent watching television) and suggesting some ways to augment baseline activities (e.g., taking stairs rather than escalator, establishing the habit of taking walks). Gradually, the intensity and duration of physical activities may be increased. The adage for medications applies here as well: start low, go slow. Two suggestions may be useful. First, the pace of walking should be slow enough that the elderly person can converse comfortably. Second, competition between walkers should be specifically discouraged. Shopping malls are good places to walk. The goal for the initially sedentary person is 30 *cumulative* minutes a day of moderately intense activities on most days of the week (61,62). This may be achieved, for example, by several 10-minute walks. For older adults who exercise already, emphasis might be placed on injury prevention and proper exercise techniques (e.g., avoidance of inadvertent Valsalva maneuvers that may induce hypotension) and benefits of both aerobic and resistive (strength training) programs. Fruitful followup visits usually incorporate continual encouragement, assessment and reassessment of attainable goals, careful questioning for symptoms of ischemic heart disease, and attention to any concerns of pain and injuries (61).

Patients with cardiac risk factors or established cardiovascular disease require careful evaluation, and perhaps in part for medicolegal reasons, a stress test should be considered before engaging in moderate or vigorous exercise. Lifestyle modification (i.e., reducing sedentariness) can safely be incorporated without any special cardiac testing. Those with an abnormal cardiac response to exercising (abnormally high blood pressure of >250/120 mm Hg, decrease in systolic blood pressure of >20 mm Hg, heart rate increase >90% of age-specific maximum) are not suited for moderate or vigorous exercise programs (63). The risk of an exercise-related cardiac event has been evaluated in those older than age 70 years (64). As expected, the rate of myocardial infarction occurrence is higher after vigorous exercise than after moderate exercise in those older than age 75 years. Although vigorous exercise does incur a higher relative risk of ensuing myocardial infarction than moderate exercise in those older than age 70 years, this relative risk was not significantly different from those who were younger than age 70 years. Nonetheless, most previously sedentary seniors age 75 years and older do not begin and seldom end up with a high-intensity aerobic program (65).

The value of *exercise testing* for apparently healthy elderly patients who want to begin an exercise program remains uncertain. Routine testing of all healthy older persons wanting to exercise may prove to be expensive, and the cost may be an unexpected barrier to starting an exercise program. Both the American Heart Association and the American College of Sports Medicine recommend exercise stress testing for sedentary older people before starting a *vigorous* exercise program, even in the absence of suspected or known underlying cardiovascular disease. In the case of moderate exercise for these individuals, the American College of Sports Medicine recommends testing if certain symptoms and signs suggestive of underlying cardiovascular disease (but otherwise relatively nonspecific) are present (66). However, neither organization addresses the usefulness of exercise stress testing before *resistive* exercise programs. Meaningful interpretation of treadmill testing is often undermined by the resting electrocardiogram abnormalities commonly seen in older persons. Moreover, the ability to successfully complete the exercise stress test diminishes with age; compared with 30% of those between ages 75 and 79, only 9% of those older than age 85 years who agreed to undergo exercise stress testing completed the test. If available guidelines were followed, one might expect a high rate of additional followup cardiac testing, potentially exposing patients to the inherent risks and costs of these procedures (61).

A reasonable *approach to preexercise assessment* starts with a complete history and physical. The physician should first screen for patients with overt cardiac disease or potential contraindications to exercising outside of a monitored setting (i.e., overt congestive heart failure, uncontrolled hypertension, angina, or myocardial infarction within the previous 6 months). This may be followed by an assessment of resting electrocardiogram (for new Q waves, ST-T segment abnormalities) and cardiac reserve before prescribing exercise regimens. Simple office-based maneuvers were previously proposed to evaluate cardiac reserve, including getting up and down from the clinic examination table, walking a distance of 15 m, climbing a flight of stairs, and cycling in the air for 60 seconds while sitting or lying on the examination table. In the absence of worrisome findings, a prescription for an exercise program may then be given, tailored to the interested individual (61).

ELDERLY DRIVERS

Physicians are increasingly asked to provide guidance on the issue of driving to older adults and their families. Driving helps keep elderly persons connected to friends and resources. It may impart a sense of independence. For some (especially rural dwellers), driving may be the sole means of transportation. Public transportation may be limited, unreliable, or unsafe for others.

Drivers older than age 65 years can be a potential safety concern. They are involved in 8% of all nonfatal traffic accidents and account for 12% of traffic fatalities. Rather than high speed and alcohol intoxication as in younger drivers, the causes of accidents at the hands of older drivers are frequently related to turning (especially to the left), lane changes, backing up, and nonobservance of traffic signs. The per mile fatality rate of those older than age 75 years is higher than that of any other adult age group; this rate is highest in drivers older than age 85 years, exceeding even that recorded for teens. Older drivers who sustain similar injuries as their counterparts also are more likely to die as a result. Unlike those involving younger drivers, accidents with older drivers occur at intersections, close to home, and usually take place during the day in good weather (67).

Potential barriers for the older driver include age-associated physiologic changes such as slower reaction time, lower visual acuity, and decreased joint mobility. Use of alcohol and some medications increases the risk of accidents. Several common chronic illnesses (such as Alzheimer dementia, depression, arthritis, diabetes mellitus, and cerebrovascular accidents) are associated with an increased likelihood of motor vehicle accidents (68). Many older adults avoid accidents by driving shorter distances, stopping more on longer trips, and picking less busy thoroughfares. Some may avoid driving on unfamiliar roads, or during rush hour, nighttime, and inclement weather. Others simply stop driving voluntarily. Women are more likely than men to do this. Those who no longer drive tend to be older, nonwhite, and have vision and/or functional impairments (69).

An office assessment of the older driver should elicit data to identify risks for underlying driving impairment. This may include screening for alcohol or substance abuse, causes of daytime somnolence (some medications, sleep apnea), and predisposition to hypoglycemic episodes, seizures, and syncopal events. Moreover, one should note that visual acuity below 20/50 falls below legal limits in many states. Predictors of adverse driving outcomes include impaired ability to copy a design on the Mini Mental State Examination, walking less than a block per day, foot and leg abnormalities (toe deformities, bunions, knee contractures, slowed toe tapping, or impaired toe walk), heart disease, and hearing deficit (70). The use of long-acting benzodiazepines has been associated with an increased risk of motor vehicle crash among the elderly (71). Concerns about driving ability are often first voiced by family members rather than patients. Asking them and the patient to recount specific incidences of problematic driving and traffic violations add to the understanding of the issues at hand. Seat belt use, whether as a driver or passenger, should be encouraged.

Some physicians have used office- or hospital-based computerized simulators to help tailor their assessment. Unfortunately, there is, as yet, no available standardization of these models, and they cannot realistically be expected to gauge all necessary skills required on the road. Other physicians screen for higher risk drivers and send them to occupational therapy-based assessment programs when available. These programs attempt to assess the impact of physical or cognitive deficits on driving. Therapies are then tailored with the goal of modifying underlying deficits via rehabilitation and fitting of adaptive equipment. Medicare reimbursement of these programs is uncertain.

Which 90-year-old drivers are more dangerous than 16-year-old drivers? When should the freedom to drive be coercively limited? These are complex questions. Medical, legal, and ethical considerations interact, and laws vary from state to state. The American Geriatrics Society and the American Association of Retired Persons cosponsor the 55 Alive Driver Safety Program. Information is available at AARP 55 Alive, 601 E. Street NW, Washington, DC 20049 (1-888-227-7669 to find a nearby class or www.aarp.org/drive for more information on safe driving tips and the driving programs).

HOSPITALIZATION

In planning a course of care for a sick elderly patient, hospitalization is often an option. However, the incidence of adverse events in hospitalized patients is well documented, and elderly patients are at particular risk. Patients older than age 65 years have more than twice the risk of adverse effects in the hospital compared with those ages 16 to 44 years. These patients also have the highest rates of adverse effects caused by negligence among all age groups (72). Moreover, rates for every category of procedure-related and drug-related adverse event are highest in patients older than age 65 years (72). In one study, iatrogenic causes comprised 11% of the admissions to an intensive care unit, with older age and higher number of drugs being the main risk factors (73).

The in-hospital *effects of prolonged immobilization* on ventilation, bone metabolism, plasma volume, and muscle strength and the risks of sensory deprivation, and physical restraints, have been well described (74). Bedsores, diminished functional status, nosocomial infection with resistant organisms, delirium, weight loss from hospital diets, and trauma are all further risks of hospitalization. Falls are common, and commonly harmful, immediately after hospital discharge (75). Efforts to take care of many moderately ill elderly patients at home are likely to develop further, independent of payer considerations.

PREVENTIVE GERIATRICS

Rowe and Kahn distinguish usual from successful aging (76). In a group of usual aging Americans, for example, bone and muscle mass fall and glucose tolerance worsens with age. However, regular exercise is associated with improved glucose metabolism, increased bone mass, and muscle strength and thus modifies "usual" aging.

Although available data do not permit clear-cut recommendations, most authorities believe that the well elderly should receive periodic testing similar to that of younger patients (see Chapter 14), particularly when the projected life expectancy is estimated to be more than 5 years. Elderly patients with marked cognitive impairment or severe chronic diseases make up a separate group of patients for whom the value of screening is less certain. Decisions about cancer screening for very frail elderly people are particularly complex. Life expectancy, quality of life, willingness and ability to accept treatments, and burdens of testing and subsequent treatments, as well as patient preferences, should be factored into the decision whether or not to initiate screening. Moreover, one should also consider the impact of the target disease if diagnosed late versus the overall effects of treatment regimens if the target disease is diagnosed early. Consent for screening and treatment of newly identified diseases from a cognitively impaired patient is a particularly vexing problem.

Data show that although elderly women visit physicians more often than younger women, they are less likely to have a pelvic examination and Pap smear and less likely to be diagnosed with uterine, ovarian, or cervical cancer in a localized (and potentially curable) stage (77). The prevalence of abnormal Pap smears among elderly women was 13.5 per 1,000 in one study, and the death rate from cervical cancer is highest in women older than age 65 years (78). Chapters 14 and 104 provide guidelines for gynecologic cancer screenings. A discussion of the controversy concerning screening for prostate disease in men is provided in Chapter 53; current guidelines are presented in Chapters 14 and 53. Life expectancy, rates of cancer death, and number needed to screen to prevent one death have been tabulated in a highly useful format for various types of cancer (79).

In patients at high risk for vertebral compression or hip fracture and for those with established kyphosis, a survey of the house for environmental hazards is recommended; such patients also should not lift heavy objects, including grandchildren. Adjunctive DEXA scanning may confirm osteoporosis, which can be treated with pharmacologic and nonpharmacologic interventions. Prevention of falls is discussed earlier in this chapter, and specific treatment of osteoporosis is discussed in Chapter 103.

Screening for and treating hyperlipidemia in elderly patients is a controversial topic; it is discussed in Chapter 82. Screening methods for visual loss and hearing loss are discussed in Chapters 107 and 110, respectively.

The benefits of discontinuing cigarette smoking among the elderly are probably substantial. Although several studies of smoking cessation among the elderly show little effect on primary prevention of coronary heart disease, smoking cessation reduces the risk of myocardial infarction and death in those with established disease (80). Cessation is a key step in the primary prevention of lung and other cancers and the primary or secondary prevention of obstructive lung disease, peripheral vascular disease, and peptic ulcer disease. Reducing the number of cigarettes smoked daily leads to a measurable reduction in the risk of lung cancer as well (81). A full discussion of strategies for smoking cessation is presented in Chapter 27.

The routine use of aspirin in older women continues to provoke considerable scrutiny. Its efficacy in reducing coronary events in older men is well established. Immunization information is provided in Chapter 18.

PRERETIREMENT COUNSELING AND PLANNING

Several problems related to retirement can be minimized if they are anticipated and planned for well in advance. Books are available to help the older person in planning (see General References). Large corporations, senior citizen centers, and several colleges offer courses in preretirement counseling and planning. Fee-for-service care management services are mushrooming across the country, touting their expertise in coordinating home services; serving as a conduit between patients, families, and care providers; and helping with the search for appropriate senior housing and institutions. The Administration on Aging has a wide range of materials to assist in such planning. Information is available at: www.aoa.gov/eldfam/Money_Matters/Money_Matters.asp.

Important topics for the older person to consider include anticipated economic changes, preparation of wills and estate planning, changes in tempo and nature of activities, the importance of developing hobbies and activities for leisure time, health care resources, and systems of health care and social support. As noted in Chapter 13, advance directives guiding medical therapy in the event of debilitating illness can be extremely valuable and are important for every adult to consider. Long-term care insurance is becoming more available, although there are disparities in cost, eligibility, and scope of coverage from one company policy to the next. An understanding of the Medicare program is important for every elderly citizen. Medicare's website (www.medicare.gov) is a comprehensive, user-friendly source of consumer information about the Medicare program. However, Medicare covers only 44% of total health expenditures for the elderly, so the aging patient and his or her family will need sound advice to plan properly for potential health care needs. The physician should encourage young elderly patients to investigate all these resources before they attain the age at which frailty is more common.

SPECIAL HOUSING AND OTHER COMMUNITY-BASED PROGRAMS

Housing programs that are primarily for the elderly are increasingly available. Many states or local governments have developed programs in the setting of a congregate facility in which support services such as eating programs or housekeeping are provided. These programs may be called *sheltered housing* or *elder housing* and are generally available only to people who are able to satisfy an economic means test. Information regarding such programs can be obtained through the state or regional office on aging.

Continuing care retirement communities are increasingly available. These require that an elder move (usually while still functionally independent) to a residential community. Several types of retirement communities exist. Some provide comprehensive services, including nursing home, personal care, and medical service, meals, and programs for an inclusive entrance and monthly fee. Others provide only housing and access to additional services that may be purchased on an a la carte basis. Cost varies tremendously. Patients who ask about entering such a community should be advised to analyze carefully the services included in the fee, review the record of the community with the state office on aging, and review the contract with a lawyer before agreeing to sign it. Some people are exuberant about such retirement communities, arguing that they provide excellent socialization and the reassurance that providing care in the event of dependency will never be a direct burden to one's family members. Others describe these retirement communities as simply ghettos for the frail elderly. Because of the expense, only a small portion of the elderly population could ever consider such an option.

In part because of the high cost of community care retirement communities, programs are being developed to provide similar support services while patients remain in their own homes. Such programs, typically called *social health maintenance organizations* or *life care at home programs*, are still experimental. One such model, On Lok, developed in the late 1970s in San Francisco, is now being replicated at a number of sites around the country. This *program for all-inclusive care for the elderly* provides comprehensive care on a capitated basis for individuals who are dually eligible for Medicare and Medicaid, features adult medical daycare, and, in many sites, special housing programs.

Medical and social daycare centers are available in many communities. The state, county, or city Area Office of Aging will have information about these programs. Generally, such programs provide an opportunity for daytime socialization or medical care and surveillance. Importantly, they also provide an opportunity for caregivers to have a respite from their care responsibilities. Unfortunately, medical daycare programs are not covered by most private insurance programs or Medicare (except for those who receive it under a Medicare/Medicaid waiver, e.g., via the Program for All-Inclusive Care for the Elderly). Medicaid does provide reimbursement for medical daycare services in some states, but with means testing. For others, medical daycare is an out-of-pocket expense that, although expensive, is usually about half the cost of nursing home care. Social daycare programs (sometimes known as senior centers) are less expensive but usually require that a person be functionally totally independent and often do not provide transportation services to the facility. Social daycare programs (as opposed to medical daycare) are often sponsored by churches, local government, or other organizations, which usually help offset the cost.

Assisted living facilities are a popular option for seniors. In addition to housing arrangements, they usually offer some additional services such as transportation, social activities, and prepared meals. Basic nursing support is sometimes available. Some facilities are built with the intention of serving cognitively impaired seniors. All 50 states have some form of regulations and licensure requirements for these facilities, and proposals for a national standard for quality are being devised. Quality of care and scale of operation vary greatly. Well-run operations may be found in a variety of settings, from modified homes operated by individual providers to gated communities with a multitude of amenities constructed by large corporations. As a whole, residents of assisted living facilities have multiple medical problems yet wish to maintain some levels of independence in a residential type of community. These facilities may increasingly become a viable arena for physicians interested in providing home-based medical care to the elderly.

TABLE 12.6 Some Helpful Internet Resources

Websites	Agency or Organization
www.aoa.gov	U.S. Administration on Aging
Helpful information on area agencies on aging, statistics on the elderly population, and descriptions of some national programs related to care of the elderly. Many links to other useful resources available.	
www.mfaaa.org/AreaAging.aspx	Mid-Floride Area Agency on Aging
Provides search for Area Agencies on Aging for every state, which are helpful in locating local resources for the elderly. Programs and public policies concerning older Americans.	
www.medicare.gov	Center for Medicare and Medicaid Services
Official U.S. government site on Medicare; relevant material on coverage, participating providers, updates on policies, and contact numbers (available in English, Spanish, and Chinese).	
www.americangeriatrics.org	American Geriatrics Society
Information of interest for practicing geriatricians.	
www.aarp.org	American Association of Retired Persons
Designed for the public; outlines issues related to senior living and health.	
www.alz.org	Alzheimer's Association
Sections for patients, caregivers, medical communities, and the media. Very useful resources for caregivers.	
www.arthritis.org	The Arthritis Foundation
Resources, educational materials, and available discussion groups for those with arthritis.	

OTHER IMPORTANT PROBLEMS OF THE ELDERLY PATIENT

The following problems are discussed in detail elsewhere in this book: constipation (Chapter 46), diverticular disease (Chapter 46), musculoskeletal problems (Section 10), menopause (Chapter 106), osteoporosis (Chapter 103), hearing loss (Chapter 110), skin problems (Section 17), dental problems (Chapter 112), disorders of the feet (Chapter 73), hypertension (Chapter 67), cataracts and macular degeneration (Chapter 107), psychiatric illnesses of old age such as dementia and delirium (Chapter 26), depression (Chapter 24), bereavement (Chapters 13 and 24), and urinary problems such as infection (Chapter 36), retention (Chapter 53), and incontinence (Chapter 54).

ADDITIONAL INFORMATION AND RESOURCES

Table 12.6 lists some governmental agencies and other organizations that offer information and resources to health care providers, caregivers, and the elderly.

SPECIFIC REFERENCES*

1. Berenson RA, Horvath J. Confronting the barriers to chronic care management in Medicare. Health Aff 2003;(Suppl);W3:37.
2. Warshaw GA, Bragg EJ, Shaull RW. Geriatric medicine training and practice in the United States at the beginning of the 21st century. New York: The Association of Directors of Geriatric Academic Programs Longitudinal Study of Training and Practice in Geriatric Medicine, 2002.
3. Hobbs FB, Damon BL. U.S. Bureau of the Census. Current Population Reports, Special Studies, P23-190, 65+ in the United States. Washington, DC: U.S. Government Printing Office, 1996.
4. Federal Interagency Forum on Aging-Related Statistics. Older Americans 2004: Key Indicators of Well Being. Federal Interagency Forum on Aging-Related Statistics. Washington, DC: U.S. Government Printing Office, November 2004.
5. Administration on Aging website. Available at www.aoa.gov.
6. Cassel CK, Vladeck BC. ICD-9 code for palliative or terminal care. N Engl J Med 1996;335:1232.
7. Iglehart JK. The American health care system: Medicare. N Engl J Med 1999;340:403.
8. Iglehart JK. The American health care system: Medicaid. N Engl J Med 1999;340:327.
9. Welch HG, Wennberg DE, Welch WP. The use of Medicare home health care services. N Engl J Med 1996;335:324.
10. Oldenquist GW, Scott L, Finucane TE. Home care: what a physician needs to know. Cleve Clin J Med 2001;68:433.
11. Stupp H. Area agencies on aging: a network of services to maintain elderly in their communities. Care Manage J 2000;2:54.
12. Boustani M, Peterson B, Hanson L, et al. Screening for dementia in primary care: a summary of the evidence for the U.S. Preventive Services Task Force. Ann Intern Med 2003; 138:927.
13. Kawas C, Gray S, Brookmeyer R, et al. Age-specific incidence rates of Alzheimer's disease: the Baltimore Longitudinal Study of Aging. Neurology 2000;54:2072.
14. Fried LP, Tangen CM, Walston JB, et al. Frailty in older adults: evidence for a phenotype. J Gerontol 2001;56:146.
15. Katz S, Stoud MW. Functional assessment in geriatrics: a review of progress and directions. J Am Geriatr Soc 1987;37:267.
16. Lichtenstein MJ, Federspiel CF, Schaffner W. Factors associated with early demise in nursing home residents: a case-control study. J Am Geriatr Soc 1985;33:315.
17. Calkins DR, Rubenstein LV, Cleary PD, et al. Failure of physicians to recognize functional disability in ambulatory patients. Ann Intern Med 1991;114:451.
18. Fillenbaum GG. Screening the elderly: a brief instrumental activities of daily living measure. J Am Geriatr Soc 1985;33:698.
19. Fried LP, Guralnik JM. Disability in older adults: evidence regarding significance, etiology, and risk. J Am Geriatr Soc 1997;45:92.
20. Fleming KC, Evans JM, Weber DC, Chutka DS. Practical functional assessment of elderly persons: a primary care approach. Mayo Clin Proc 1995;70:890.
21. Rubenstein LZ, Josephson KR, Wieland GD, et al. Effectiveness of a geriatric evaluation unit:

*Bold numerals denote published controlled clinical trials, meta-analyses, or consensus-based recommendations.

at home. If hospice is involved, the hospice team should be notified. In instances where hospice is not involved, the practitioner should be aware of the local jurisdictional laws on whether the police or only the funeral home need to be notified. Families should be instructed to make funeral arrangements ahead of time if they are able. If not, it is helpful if they at least contact their preferred funeral director. Information on hospice care in the United States is provided by both the National Hospice and Palliative Care Organization and the Hospice Association of America (see www.nhpco.org).

MANAGEMENT OF GRIEF

End-of-life care presents practitioners with three different aspects of grieving: grief of patients who have experienced a loss of a loved one; grief over losses that patients face when dying; and a practitioner's own grief reaction to the loss of a patient. This section addresses these three areas.

Bereavement research is beginning to help us understand the different reactions to loss and outline appropriate treatments. Even so, there are many questions still unanswered.

We do know there is a normal grief process that people go through adjusting to life without the person. Most people will adapt with only a minimal change in their daily lives lasting about 1 to 2 months (19). These people respond to support from friends and relatives. Health care providers can normalize the grief process for these patients. Some bereaved patients may need short-term medication for relief of anxiety and insomnia. A benzodiazepine or hypnotic (see Chapter 7) at bedtime if needed for sleep, or one of the anxiolytic benzodiazepines as needed for anxiety, should be considered for 1 to 2 weeks in the management of normal grief. Prolonged use of a benzodiazepine can interfere with the normal grief process. Many patients may be satisfied with an empathetic and supportive health care practitioner.

Abnormal grief reactions include bereavement-related depression and complicated grief reaction. It is important to distinguish complicated grief reaction, as it does not respond to interventions appropriate for major depression. Patients who meet *Diagnostic and Statistical Manual of Mental Disorders,* 4th edition (DSM-IV) criteria for major depression may need short-term counseling and antidepressant medication (Chapter 24). Health care providers can engage the patient in short-term counseling or refer as appropriate. Individuals at high risk for complicated grief reaction are younger (<46 years of age), have a sudden or unexpected loss, are without social supports, have pre-existing psychopathology, are suffering from multiple losses, or have lost a child (20).

A complicated grief reaction is suggested when patients present with 6 months of symptoms such as searching for the deceased, loneliness, preoccupation with thoughts of the deceased, and feelings of disbelief, distrust, anger, shock, detachment from others, and expressing similar somatic symptoms of the deceased (21). These bereaved individuals have an increased rate of physical symptoms, doctor visits, use of medication, disability, use of alcohol, hospitalization, and mortality (22).

It is estimated that approximately 10% to 20% of persons will develop a complicated grief reaction (23). Efficacious bereavement treatment for complicated grief requires intervention specifically directed at complicated grief (23). Health care providers will need to refer patients with complicated grief to appropriate bereavement treatment.

Research in bereavement has clinical implications for health care practitioners. Practitioners should not automatically refer all family members for bereavement counseling. Practitioners are in a unique position to normalize the grieving process for families and identify persons who might be at high risk for developing a complicated grief reaction.

The second aspect of managing grief deals with a patient's grief over current and anticipated losses of health, the future, physical abilities, and roles and relationships (1). The dying person has grief and other issues to work through and should be given the opportunity to function at his or her highest level in order to do so. Spiritual support can be critically important for many during this time. It is important to determine religious or spiritual practices or preferences, if any, and involve others who can minister to the person's needs in these areas to enhance quality of life and meaning (24,25).

Complicated grieving on the part of the dying person is a challenge for any care provider. Anger, fear, and other cognitive–emotional–spiritual crises can show themselves in somatic complaints. Terminally ill patients can have various emotional reactions to death. Kubler-Ross's five-stage model is one construct to describe and understand the grieving process (26). The stages are denial, anger, bargaining, depression, and acceptance. Patients do not go through these stages sequentially nor do they necessarily go through all five stages. Patients fluctuate in their ability to handle grief—confronting then avoiding. Some will never accept the situation and some seem to embrace their death. For the most part, people oscillate between acceptance and denial. The patient's grief should be acknowledged and expressed. It is best if patients are helped to express their grief of losses early in the disease. This helps patients cope more effectively as they face more losses as the disease progresses (27).

People who are dying often have existential questions such as "why me?" Often significant others, friends, and caregivers may not be able to discuss these issues because of fear of not being able to handle the emotional reactions the patient might have. A practitioner can and should

TABLE 13.4 Grief versus Depression in Terminal Illness

Issue	Grief	Depression
Definition	Feelings and behaviors resulting from a major loss	Depressed mood, decreased interest and pleasure, appetite/sleep disturbance, psychomotor agitation or retardation, loss of energy, feelings of worthlessness, guilt, decreased concentration, thoughts of death, with significant impairment in functioning over a 2-week period
Prevalence	Normal, expected	Not normal
	Associated with disease progression	Prevalence of major depression 1%–53%, increased prevalence (as high as 77%) with advanced disease
		Pain is a major risk factor and is also exacerbated by depression
Symptoms and signs	Somatic distress, sleep and appetite disturbances, decreased concentration, social withdrawal, sighing	Hopelessness, helplessness, feeling of worthlessness, guilt, and suicidal ideation are the most useful diagnostic clues
		Somatic distress, sleep and appetite disturbances, decreased concentration, social withdrawal are also common
Other differentiating symptoms and signs	Patient retains capacity for pleasure	Nothing is enjoyable
	Comes in waves	Constant, unremitting
	Passive wishes for death to come quickly	Intense and persistent suicidal ideation
	Able to look forward to the future	No sense of a positive future

Adapted from Block SD. Perspectives on care at the close of life. Psychological considerations, growth, and transcendence at the end of life: the art of the possible. JAMA 2001;285:2898.

encourage patients and caregivers to discuss their feelings, fears, and hopes. This helps the patient and loved ones come to terms with death and can help the survivors with their bereavement.

Practitioners can and should do the following interventions for grieving patients (28):

- Encourage open communication
- Encourage completion of unfinished business
- Encourage and foster hope
- Allow opportunity to discuss fears
- Validate and normalize feelings
- Provide physical presence
- Listen empathetically

It is challenging at times to distinguish normal grieving from depression in a patient who is dying. Table 13.4 compares the clinical presentations of each. If depression is diagnosed, treatment can improve quality of life. (For therapy, see Symptom Management in End-Stage Illnesses: Depression below.)

The care of dying patients and their families is rewarding but practitioners also grieve for their patients. Practitioners should be cognizant of their own emotional reactions to their dying patients and attend to their own emotional needs. Talking about their reactions to a death can be helpful. Practitioners who work exclusively in caring for dying persons are at risk for burnout if they do not attend to their own needs. Some activities that can be helpful, although not systematically studied, are writing condolence letters (29) and attending funerals of patients (30). In a 2005 *Annals of Internal Medicine* feature, "Words that Make a Difference," Back et al. discuss the benefits of saying goodbye to patients (31). This includes the patient's sense of contributing to others and the practitioner's opportunity to integrate their own reactions to their patient's pending death. The authors outline a seven-step approach to saying goodbye, which is shown in Table 13.5. They note that this will work best for practitioners already comfortable in communication skills and that not all patient relationships lend themselves to saying goodbye.

SYMPTOM MANAGEMENT IN END-STAGE ILLNESSES

Symptom management is an important aspect of end-of-life care. Untreated symptoms impact on quality of life and functional status. These symptoms can interfere with patient's ability to address spiritual and psychological issues at the end of life. Primary care practitioners should

TABLE 13.5 An Approach to Saying Goodbye

1. Choose an appropriate place and time.
2. Acknowledge the end of your routine contact and uncertainty about future contact.
3. Invite the patient to respond, and use that response as a piece of data about the patient's state of mind.
4. Frame the goodbye as an appreciation.
5. Give space for the patient to reciprocate, and respond empathetically to the patient's emotion.
6. Articulate an ongoing commitment to the patient's care.
7. Later, reflect on your work with this patient.

Adapted from Back AL, Arnold RM, Tulsky JA, et al. On saying goodbye: acknowledging the end of the patient–physician relationship with patients who are near death. Ann Intern Med 2005;142:682.

TABLE 13.6 Commonly Used Opioids

Name	Initial Dose (mg)[a] Oral	Initial Dose (mg)[a] IM/IV	Usual Dose Range[b] Oral	Usual Dose Range[b] IM/IV	Dose Interval (hr)	Dose Adjustments Needed	Preparations Available[c]
Morphine	15–30	10	30–90 mg	10–30 mg	3–4	Renal failure	IV/SQ, IR, PR, liq, liq conc
Morphine SR	15–30	n/a	30–200 mg	—	8–12	Renal/hepatic failure	SR, PR
Morphine SR	30	n/a	30–1600 mg	—	24	Renal/hepatic failure	SR
Hydromorphone	4–8	1.5	2–8 mg	1–2	4	Hepatic failure	IV/SQ, IR, PR
Hydromorphone SR	12	n/a	12 mg	—	24	Hepatic failure	SR
Oxycodone	10	n/a	5–15 mg	—	3–4	Renal failure	IR, liq, liq conc, PR
Oxycodone SR	10	n/a	10–80 mg	—	12	Renal/hepatic failure	SR
Fentanyl[d]	n/a	25 mcg/hr	—	—	72	Hepatic failure	Transdermal (dosage range 50–300 μg)
Fentanyl	200 μg	n/a	200–1600 μg	—	2		Transmucosal
Methadone	5	2.5	2.5–20 mg daily	2.5–10 mg	6–8	Renal/hepatic failure	IV/SQ, IR, liq, PR
Oxymorphone	n/a	1	—	—	3–4	Renal failure	IV/SQ, PR
Meperidine (Demerol)[e]	N/R	N/R	—	—	N/R	Renal failure	IV, IR

[a]For patients weighing over 110 pounds who have moderate to severe pain.
[b]Higher doses are needed in patients who develop tolerance; there is no ceiling dose for narcotics; maximum dose limited by side effects.
[c]Preparations abbreviations: IR, oral, immediate-release; IV, parenteral suitable for intravenous use; liq, liquid, liq conc, concentrated liquid solution; N/R, not recommended; PR, per rectum via commercial or custom-made suppository or microenema (Davis et al., 2002); SQ, subcutaneous; SR, oral sustained-release.
[d]Not an optimal choice for opioid-naive patient as 25 μg fentanyl transdermal equals approximately 50 mg morphine.
[e]Not recommended for use other than for a limited time.
Adapted from Miaskowski C, Clearly J, Burney R, et al. Guidelines for the management of cancer pain in adults and children. APS Clinical Practice Guidelines Series, No. 3. Glenview, IL, American Pain Society, 2005. See also www.ampainsoc.org.

evaluate and treat these symptoms to improve a patient's quality of life and functional status.

Pain Management

Successful pain management involves thoroughly assessing pain, then matching the treatment to the type of pain that is being experienced. Underlying causes of pain should be treated if possible and then appropriate pharmacologic and non-pharmacologic treatments should be initiated. This section focuses on pharmacologic interventions. Non-pharmacologic approaches include physical therapy, ice, heat, massage, acupuncture, hypnoses, relaxation training, guided imagery, and distraction techniques. Several of these approaches are outlined in Chapter 22. The pharmacologic approach includes narcotic medications (Table 13.6) and non-narcotic or adjuvant medications (Table 13.7).

In general, pain can be divided into two types: nociceptive and neuropathic. Nociceptive pain occurs when primary afferent nerve fibers, which are generally located in the skin, organs, muscles, and joints, are stimulated. This occurs with direct injury to an area such as through cuts, sprains, and inflammation. Pain can be acute or chronic. Nociceptive pain is further divided into somatic pain and visceral pain. Somatic pain is localized and described as aching, throbbing, or stabbing. Visceral pain, which occurs in areas of the body enclosed within a cavity, results in more generalized pain, described as cramping, gnawing, or boring and is involved with referred pain as well.

Neuropathic or nerve pain is frequently described as burning, throbbing, or "pins and needles" sensation that may or may not be associated with numbness and tingling. The etiology of nerve pain is multifactorial including nerve damage from radiation, surgery, or particular chemotherapeutic agents (e.g., oxaliplatin, paclitaxel, docetaxel, and vincristine), as well as nerve entrapment from solid tumors, or diabetic neuropathies. Nerve pain may worsen with movement, but frequently persists even at full rest and may be worse at night.

Somatic and Visceral Pain

Somatic and visceral pain organ and soft-tissue discomforts in end-stage conditions are generally managed with the use of narcotics. To optimize outcome and minimize side effects, there are a few basic rules to remember when using narcotics.

TABLE 13.7 Adjuvant Analgesic and Symptom Management Drugs for Adults and Children Weighing 50 kg or More

Class and Drug	Approximate Dosage Range	Administration	Use
Corticosteroids			
Dexamethasone	8–96 mg/d	Oral/intravenous	Pain associated with brain metastases and cord compression
Prednisone	40–80 mg/d	Oral	Dyspnea, bone pain
Anticonvulsant agents			
Carbamazepine	200–1,600 mg/d	Oral	Neuropathic pain (especially trigeminal neuralgia), seizures
Gabapentin	300–1000 mg/d	Oral	Neuropathic pain, seizures
Phenytoin	300–500 mg/d	Oral	Neuropathic pain, seizures
Antidepressant agents			
Amitriptyline	25–150 mg/d	Oral	Neuropathic pain, depression with sleeplessness
Doxepin	25–150 mg/d	Oral	Depression with sleeplessness
Imipramine	20–100 mg/d	Oral	
Neuroleptic agents			
Methotrimeprazine	40–80 mg/d	Intramuscular	Analgesia, sedation, and antiemetic (not available in United States)
Antihistamines			
Hydroxyzine	300–450 mg/d	Intramuscular	Adjuvant to opioids for pain; relief of itching, anxiety, insomnia, nausea
Cetirizine	5–10 mg d	Oral	Urticaria, itch
Fexofenadine	60–90 mg b.i.d.	Oral	Urticaria, itch
Loratadine	10 mg	Oral	Urticaria, itch
Local anesthetic and antiarrhythmic agents			
Lidocaine	5 mg/kg/d[a]	Intravenous, subcutaneous, topical	Neuropathic pain. Topical patches are excellent for postherpetic neuralgias
Psychostimulants			
Dextroamphetamine	5–10 mg/d	Oral	To improve opioid analgesia and decrease sedation
Methylphenidate	10–15 mg/d	Oral	

[a]The dosage given is per kilogram of body weight per day.
Adapted from Agency for Health Care Policy and Research (AHCPR). Management of Cancer Pain: Clinical Practice Guideline. Publication No. 940592, 1994.

1. Long-acting formulations of narcotics should be used for long-term pain control (Table 13.6).
2. Avoid using multiple long-acting formulations.
3. Short-acting narcotic formulations should be used when titrating narcotics for acute pain relief but should be converted to long-acting formulations when baseline dose is established (Table 13.6).
4. Short-acting formulations should be used for rescue dose or breakthrough pain, be one-fourth to one-third of the 12-hour long-acting dose, and be available every 2 to 3 hours (Tables 13.6 and 13.7).
5. Avoid narcotic combination products; the combination product limits dose escalation because acetaminophen and ibuprofen, often in these combination products, have a maximum dose whereas narcotics have no ceiling.
6. Always start a bowel regimen with narcotics unless contraindicated.
7. Assess the adequacy of pain relief after 24 hours of a change in a long-acting medication.
8. If patients are using "rescue doses" more than three times a day the long-acting medication should be increased. Calculate the new daily dose by adding the total long-acting pain medication with the amount of the rescue dose used in 24 hours. The new 24-hour requirement can then be converted to the appropriate long-acting dose and the breakthrough dosing increased if needed.

Examples

Long-acting: 90 mg morphine sulfate (MS Contin) q8h.
Rescue dosing: 20 mg liquid morphine q4h p.r.n; used six doses in the last 24 hours.
$90 \times 3 = 270$
$20 \times 6 = 120$

Numerical Scale

0	1	2	3	4	5	6	7	8	9	10
No Pain										Unbearable Pain

Visual Analog Scale

No Pain No pain________________worst possible pain Worst Pain

Directions: Ask the patient to indicate on the line where the pain is in relation to the two extremes. Qualification is only approximate; for example, a midpoint mark would indicate that the pain in approximately half of the worst possible pain.

Representative samples of pain intensity rating scales.

Adapted from Whaley L, Wong D. Nursing Care of Infants and Children, 3rd ed, CV Mosby Company, 1987:1070.

FIGURE 13.1. Representative samples of pain intensity rating scales. (Adapted from Whaley L, Wong D. Nursing care of infants and children. 3rd ed. St. Louis: CV Mosby, 1987:1070.)

Total: = 390 mg: Because MS Contin can be given every 8 or 12 hours, the new dose could be 200 mg q12h or 130 mg q8h.
Rescue dose is calculated on one-fourth of the 12-hour dose, or 50 mg. Increase rescue dose to 40–60 mg q4h p.r.n.

9. The oral route is the preferred route of administration. Intermittent intramuscular injections should be avoided. When an oral route is unavailable, transmucosal, transdermal, rectal, and subcutaneous, and intravenous routes are available (Table 13.6).
10. In evaluating pain control outcome, pain scales can provide an ongoing record of effectiveness of pain treatment. Several scales are available and illustrated in Fig. 13.1.
11. Use a table that lists equianalgesic doses when switching opiate medications (Table 13.8).

Managing Bone Pain

Bone pain can arise from primary bone cancers and metastatic cancer sites, as well as from arthritis and fractures. This pain is frequently described as a generalized or limb-specific achelike pain that worsens with movement or at night. In many instances, the degree of bone pain is increased by the presence of edema and inflammation. Additionally, there is an interaction between the tumor and the host, which causes the release of various growth factors and cytokines, some of which (e.g., endothelin-1) have been implicated in the etiology of cancer-related bone pain. Agents that specifically target these substances are currently in clinical trials.

TABLE 13.8 Commonly Used Opioids: Equianalgesic Doses

Drug	*Oral/Rectal Dose (mg)*	*Parenteral Dose (mg)*
Morphine	30	10
Hydromorphone	7.5	1.5
Oxycodone	20	n/a
Methadone	10	5
Oxymorphone	n/a	1
Meperidine[1]	300	75

Conversion Between Fentanyl Transdermal Patch and Parenteral or Oral Morphine

	Morphine (mg/24 hr)	
Fentanyl (μg/hr)	*Oral*	*IM/IV*
25	50	17
50	100	33
75	150	50
100	200	67
125	250	83
150	300	100

IM, intramuscular; IV, intravenous; n/a, not available in this form.
Adapted from American Pain Society. Principles of analgesic use in the treatment of acute pain and cancer pain. 5th ed. Glenview, IL, American Pain Society, 2003.

Inflammation responds well to the use of steroids and nonsteroidal anti-inflammatory medications (NSAIDs); consequently, NSAIDs are particularly useful in bone pain. Dexamethasone (Decadron) at doses of 4 to 12 mg two to three times a day and prednisone 10 to 40 mg per day are beneficial in combating bone pain. NSAIDs are an excellent tool for palliation and remain effective even when combined with narcotic pain relievers in minimizing distress from bone pain. Most NSAIDs come in oral form; ketorolac, however, is also available as an intravenous or intramuscular injection. Ketorolac dose should be limited (all forms) to a total of 5 days of treatment.

In the setting of bony metastasis, intravenous bisphosphonates, such as zoledronic acid (Zometa) 3 to 4 mg monthly or pamidronate (Aredia) 30 to 90 mg monthly, are useful to improve pain control and to decrease risk of pathologic fractures. For uncontrolled pain from osteoblastic bony lesions, strontium-89 or samarium-153 radionuclide therapy can be considered. These are given as a single intravenous injection. Side effects can include an initial flare in bone pain about a week after injection, which lasts a few days, as well as thrombocytopenia and anemia, which are greatest at 5 to 6 weeks after treatment. Relief is generally obtained in 7 to 21 days. Subsequent retreatments should be at least 12 weeks apart and only after blood counts have returned to baseline. Contraindications include a life expectancy less than 3 months, severe myelosuppression, urinary incontinence, or severe renal insufficiency (32).

Neuropathic Pain

Narcotics have some impact on nerve pain (33). However, research shows poor consistency in achieving adequate pain control with narcotics alone (34,35). This is theorized, in part, from a phenomenon known as windup. Windup occurs when the secondary afferent pain receptors become permanently turned on causing chronic pain and stimulating an intermediary receptor called N-methyl-D-aspartate (NMDA). Methadone is inhibitory to NMDA making it a good choice for neuropathic pain. Neural changes, which can occur with prolonged pain, may change the type of binding sites making narcotics less useful. These changes also contribute to escalating pain scenarios with minimal increase in stimuli. Fortunately, research does support the usefulness of other treatment modalities in managing neuropathic pain (36).

Topical lidocaine patches applied over areas of discomfort from postherpetic neuralgia is useful (37). Up to three may be applied and left on for 12 hours at a time, every 24 hours. Conflicting research exists for topical capsaicin, which was found to be helpful for diabetic neuropathy, but not for neuropathies of other etiologies (38).

Adjuncts such as tricyclic antidepressants (TCAs) and antiepileptics have shown benefit in relieving the symptoms of nerve pain (38–40). Although TCAs are effective, they frequently cause dry mouth, constipation, orthostasis, arrhythmias, and other side effects that can detract from quality of life. A growing body of research continues to support the use of antiepileptic drugs such as gabapentin and carbamazepine in managing neuropathies of various etiologies (34,35,38–40). Side-effect profiles of antiepileptics can include dry mouth and somnolence, but these are usually dose dependent. Other medications, such as baclofen, are also being investigated (36).

Transcutaneous electrical nerve stimulation (TENS) units are another adjunct to managing nerve pain, especially in association with soft-tissue discomfort. The units are small (about the size of a pager or wallet), battery operated, and have small wires with electrodes that are placed on the skin around the painful area or between the pain source and the spine (not over the spine, neck, or head). TENS should be avoided in people with pacemakers or automated internal defibrillators.

Although multiple modalities exist to improve nerve pain, in some cases, sufficient relief is still not obtained. When a combination of these interventions still fails to produce adequate control of neuropathic pain, nerve blocks should be considered.

Addiction and Tolerance

Inadequate pain relief can be caused by patients' and practitioners' misconceptions of narcotics. Because of fear on the part of the health care provider of inducing addiction, patients may receive dosages of narcotics that are too small or too infrequent to relieve pain adequately. Some patients are hesitant to use narcotics fearing addiction or that the medication will not be beneficial when they are "really in pain." Addiction is not a common problem when narcotics are used in this setting. Explaining to patients the difference between physical dependence, psychological dependence (addiction), and tolerance can be helpful to overcome patient fears. Physical dependence refers to the withdrawal syndrome that occurs with abrupt withdrawal of narcotic. Tolerance refers to the need to increase the dose of narcotic to get the same amount of relief. Psychological dependence or addiction involves the use of narcotics for nonmedical purposes with no improvement in quality of life.

Managing Side Effects of Narcotics

Narcotic analgesics and disease progression may both cause the following: respiratory depression; nausea and vomiting; constipation; sedation; urinary spasms, retention, and incontinence; myoclonus; and pruritus or rash. These side effects, whether from narcotics or the disease process are treated similarly.

Respiratory Depression

Respiratory depression is unlikely if narcotics are titrated appropriately. There may be a rare occasion to reverse narcotic-induced respiratory depression. When possible, one should simply withhold the next scheduled dose. If quick reversal is needed, this can be achieved with small doses of naloxone (Narcan) (0.1 to 0.2 mg) intravenously every few minutes. Unfortunately, the use of naloxone severely increases the risk of acute withdrawal and severe pain, which precipitates acute vomiting, as well as severe abdominal cramping, agitation, and perspiration, consistent with acute narcotic withdrawal seen in other populations.

Nausea

Nausea can occur with the use of narcotics, especially in the first 2 weeks, and should be treated aggressively. Nausea and vomiting can also result from tumor invasion, gastroparesis, bowel obstruction, and side effects of other treatment regimens. Multiple strategies exist to decrease nausea and vomiting while improving associated symptoms. Table 13.9 lists strategies to control nausea and vomiting.

Chemotherapy and radiation treatments can also produce nausea and vomiting. Chapter 10 provides more in-depth information on chemotherapy and radiation-induced nausea and vomiting.

Constipation

Narcotics cause constipation. Unless contraindicated, every person who is on a narcotic should be on a bowel

TABLE 13.9 Nausea and Vomiting Interventions

Intervention	Dose	Comments
Change to another opioid at comparable dose		This may eliminate nausea and vomiting completely.
Take narcotics with food		May diminish or prevent nausea.
Prochlorperazine (Compazine)	5–10 mg PO q4-6h 15 mg spansule q6-12h 25 mg suppository q4-6h	Compazine causes less sedation and hypotension than chlorpromazine. May cause acute extrapyramidal symptoms (e.g., dystonic reactions) that usually respond to diphenhydramine 1–2 mg/kg (adults) up to a maximum of 50 mg intramuscular or slow intravenous push followed by a maintenance dose for 48–72 hours.
Haloperidol (Haldol)	0.5–2 mg orally or subcutaneously q6-8h	Especially helpful if agitation is also a concern.
Lorazepam (Ativan)	0.5–2.0 mg orally q8h	Helpful in the presence of anxiety or agitation as well.
Megestrol acetate (Megace)	160–800 mg orally, maximum daily 60 mg	Has no effect on quality of life or survival.
Metoclopramide (Reglan)	10–20 mg orally or intramuscularly before meals	Useful for gastric fullness.
Dexamethasone (Decadron)	2–4 mg q8-24h	Improves overall sense of well-being; potentiates Reglan.
Hyoscyamine (Levsin)	1–2 tablets q4h	Decreases upper airway secretions.
Octreotide (Sandostatin)	50–250 μg subcutaneously or intravenously q8h	Useful in intestinal obstruction by decreasing gastrointestinal secretions. More costly than other measures.
Scopolamine patch	1.5-mg patch behind ear; change every 3 days	Decreases upper airway secretions.

regimen to prevent constipation. Bulk laxatives require an adequate intake of food and fluid to be effective and may have little use in the terminally ill patient with poor oral intake. A stool softener alone is rarely effective for narcotic-induced constipation. Combination strategies are the most useful. An example of a basic bowel regimen would include two senna with 200 mg of docusate sodium, twice a day, with the addition of 1 ounce of lactulose, sorbitol, or milk of magnesia daily as needed. The goal is to produce a bowel movement every 1 to 3 days. Table 13.10 lists strategies to manage and prevent constipation.

Sedation

Sedation is a concern for some people on narcotics. Oversedation can significantly impair quality of life. Sleepiness is not the same thing as pain control. By combining various pain management modalities and appropriate classes of pain medications to target particular pain sources, sedation can be reduced and quality of life improved. An example of this is the use of NSAIDs, narcotics, and a TENS unit to control a combination of nerve and soft-tissue discomfort. When successful pain management cannot be achieved without sedation, the use of methylphenidate (Ritalin) may be helpful to combat the lethargy associated with analgesics. When pain control is achieved, patients often sleep for an extended period. This should not be confused with sedation from the narcotics.

Urinary Spasms, Retention, and Incontinence

Urinary spasms can cause leakage of urine without pain or leakage with discomfort. Oxybutynin and tolterodine can be helpful for spasms alone. The associated discomfort from bladder spasms can be improved by using phenazopyridine (Pyridium), lorazepam, or low-dose diazepam. The use of an indwelling urinary catheter for continual bladder drainage may also be helpful in relieving bladder spasms without using additional pharmacotherapies. Urinary retention is caused directly by the effect of narcotics on the bladder, or indirectly by causing constipation. Decreasing the narcotic dose can help, as can aggressively treating constipation. An indwelling urinary catheter might be necessary in end-stage disease for comfort of the patient.

Myoclonus

Metabolites of narcotics (especially hydromorphone, morphine, and oxycodone) can build up and become neurotoxic causing myoclonus and hyperalgesia (41). This is most common with high-dose opiates. The resulting spasms increase pain causing the person to take more pain medication, seeking relief. This, in turn, causes a further build-up of metabolites and a worsening of spasms, resulting in more pain, for which additional pain medications are taken. This relentless cycle can greatly hamper quality of life and cause lethal seizures if it is not interrupted (42).

TABLE 13.10 Strategies to Manage and Prevent Constipation

Intervention	Starting Dose	Dose Range	Comments
1. Senokot (senna) Part of daily bowel regimen	1–2 pills by mouth twice a day	Up to 4 pills twice a day	Daily usage; take with a glass of liquid; works well combined with Colace
Colace (docusate sodium) Part of daily bowel regimen	100–200 mg twice a day	Up to 4 pills twice a day	Daily usage; take with a glass of liquid; works well combined with Senokot
2. Lactulose	30–60 mL daily as needed	Up to 30–60 mL four times a day	Causes excessive gas and cramping in those who are lactose intolerant
Sorbitol	30–60 mL daily as needed	30–60 mL four times a day	Can be used alone or in addition to senna and Colace for bowel regimen
Milk of magnesia (MOM)	30–60 mL daily as needed	30–60 mL twice a day	May use once daily (single agent) or with senna and Colace for constipation relief
3. Check for impaction			If Colace, senna, and either lactulose, sorbitol, or MOM are not beneficial after 24–48 hours
4. Dulcolax suppository (bisacodyl)	1 suppository daily		Can cause cramping; do not use with an impaction
5. Fleet enema (or other soap suds enema)	1 daily as needed	2 daily for *constipation*	Can be used with an impaction; not to be used as daily bowel regimen
6. Magnesium citrate	120 mL daily as needed	Up to 240 mL at one time	Use for constipation relief, not as daily bowel regimen
7. GoLYTELY (polyethylene glycol)	120 mL daily by mouth	Up to 500 mL per day	Can cause electrolyte imbalances
8. Milk and molasses enema (use ONLY when all other methods have failed)	120 mL molasses added to 480 mL of milk	MAX: equal parts of milk and molasses	NEVER USE FOR CHILDREN; warm to 103°F; ONLY USE WITH AN INTACT BOWEL

Myoclonus is an easily reversible symptom. Benzodiazepines such as lorazepam (Ativan) (1 to 2 mg orally or sublingually every 8 hours) and diazepam (Valium) (2–10 mg orally every 6 to 8 hours) work well to initially break the cycle (43). The dose of opiate should be decreased by 10% to 20% (or more) to allow for the clearance of metabolites. Sometimes it is necessary to change to a different opiate. Calculating equal analgesia should involve decreasing the dose of the new narcotic by approximately 30% until it is determined how the patient tolerates this new regimen (42). People who have been experiencing uncontrolled pain, especially with myoclonus and hyperalgesia, can become frightened and anxious when they hear their medication dosages are going to be decreased. Careful explanation of the mechanism of their myoclonus and hyperalgesia and of the additional measures being initiated to improve their comfort is required to allay their fears.

When pain cannot be controlled without myoclonus and hyperalgesia, the initiation of intravenous midazolam (Versed) can be used. This will require an inpatient setting.

Pruritus and Rash

Narcotics, renal and hepatic failure, as well as other disease- and treatment-related concerns can cause skin rashes and itching. Treatments that add minimal side effects are often best. Pruritus can be managed by emollient creams, aloe vera gels, anti-itch lotions (e.g., Sarna lotion), and topical diphenhydramine (Benadryl). Rashes should be treated according to their offending source if identified. Fungal rashes often respond to topical antifungal creams applied in a thin coating twice daily. In areas of high moisture, fungal rashes may be difficult to manage. Anecdotal evidence supports the use of 15 g of Nystatin powder (100,000 USP U/g concentration) mixed into a 16-ounce jar of zinc oxide. This can be applied to the affected skin daily or twice daily. Resistant rashes, hives, and itching can also be relieved by nonsedating antihistamines such as cetirizine, fexofenadine, and loratadine.

Insomnia

When insomnia is a problem, a benzodiazepine hypnotic can be used to induce sleep (see Chapter 7). Another consideration is the use of trazodone, which is beneficial for sleep and depression. Newer medications such as zolpidem (Ambien) are very useful to induce sleep and have less morning sedation, which can detract from quality of life.

Anxiety and Agitation

Concern on part of practitioners and other caregivers to the needs of the dying person may be all that is necessary to relieve early anxiety in the dying patient. Anxiolytic drugs also can be of some help in the management of these patients. Alprazolam (Xanax) 0.5 to 2 mg may be given every

8 hours either as needed or around the clock. Maximal dosing is up to 6 mg in 24 hours. Lorazepam (Ativan) 0.5 to 2 mg can be used every 6 to 12 hours. The sedating antihistamine hydroxyzine (Atarax, Vistaril), 25 to 50 mg by mouth three times daily, may also help patients who have anxiety associated with pain. A number of psychologic approaches (hypnosis, relaxation training, guided imagery, distraction techniques) are also useful for the cancer patient with pain and anxiety (see Nonpharmacologic Approaches in Chapter 22).

Terminal Anxiety

Terminal anxiety refers to the anxiety and frequent movement that may occur in the final days or hours prior to death. It can be distressing for caregivers who may be physically fatigued from the requirements of care or who may perceive their loved one to be suffering. Increased movement and agitation may also worsen pain. To minimize this anxiety, low-dose lorazepam (Ativan) at 0.5 to 2.0 mg every 4 to 12 hours is useful. If the anxiety and agitation do not respond well to lorazepam, haloperidol at 1 to 5 mg every 6 to 12 hours may be used instead of or in addition to lorazepam.

Depression

Many people experience transient depression when they learn they have a terminal prognosis. In some instances, the support of practitioners, as well as of family and friends, is all that is necessary for them to adjust to the mental, physical, emotional, and spiritual challenges they experience. For others, the diagnosis and prognosis will overload their present ability to cope, resulting in clinical depression. It is wrong to assume that depression will pass on its own without some level of intervention from present support systems, hospice support services, or the use of antidepressants. Managing pain is an essential part to minimizing terminal depression. Some patients, however, develop severe depression, particularly after a brief stage of anger. Loss of self-esteem, guilt feelings, psychomotor retardation, early morning awakening with a diurnal variation in mood, and even suicidal thoughts may appear in this setting. Discussion of suicide, even in a terminally ill and suffering patient, should raise the question of depression. When a number of these and other indicators of a major depression are present, antidepressants may bring relief. Standard depression medications are useful with consideration to their particular side effects. For instance, mirtazapine (Remeron) given at night is an excellent choice to improve sleep and stimulate appetite, while sertraline (Zoloft) is a good choice to be more awake during the day. There is a detailed discussion of the use of these drugs in Chapter 24.

Delirium

Periodic or persistent delirium (inattentiveness, inaccessibility, inability to recognize loved ones, gross confusion) is very common in the final days or weeks of terminal disease (44,45). In fact, most terminal cancer patients die in delirium (45). However, most of these patients do not have an agitated delirium, and their course is characterized by increasing withdrawal and somnolence. Some patients continue in a state of agitated delirium and require chronic medication. Haloperidol was more useful than benzodiazepines and phenothiazines in the treatment of agitated delirium (46). Risperidone has also been shown to be beneficial in case reports (47). There are conflicting data to support the use of hydration to improve terminal delirium (45,48). If an identifiable cause can be isolated, it should be treated to improve quality of life. Loss of clear communication as a result of delirium may be distressing to the patient's family. Management of easily reversible causes is therefore important except in the patient whose death is imminent. A list of the principal causes of delirium is found in Chapter 26.

Dyspnea

Dyspnea, best described as difficult or uncomfortable breathing, is a common and distressing symptom for the dying patient. It is important to focus on the patient's symptoms and not the observer's interpretation of physical findings when evaluating and treating dyspnea. Patients who are tachypneic may not feel dyspneic, yet patients breathing normally may indeed experience dyspnea.

Physical impediments to breathing and psychologic fears and discomfort are often commingled when a patient is near death. In this situation, a number of approaches can be combined for maximal effect. First, position the patient for maximal comfort and ease of breathing. For many this will be upright in bed or in a chair. Administering oxygen (if the patient is hypoxic) is useful (49), but not always necessary. Patients may feel better if air is circulated past them from a fan or an open window. The addition of low-dose opiates in the narcotic-naive patient is also beneficial. Morphine doses of 2–10 mg or oxycodone 2–5 mg (by mouth or sublingually), every 2 to 4 hours is generally effective to relieve dyspnea without respiratory suppression. For those already on narcotics for pain control, increasing the long-acting dose or frequency of rescue dosing may alleviate symptoms. The beneficial effects of narcotics on dyspnea are usually shorter than their effect on pain, requiring the administration of morphine in small doses, hourly in some instances.

The usefulness of nebulized morphine is controversial. It has been found equally effective as subcutaneous morphine in dyspnea from cancer (50), but was found to cause more hypercapnia and respiratory depression for those with chronic obstructive pulmonary disease (COPD) (51). Other trials have had mixed support, whereas some have failed to find it more useful than placebo (52,53). Bronchodilators are useful in relieving dyspnea, and there is evidence that these are underused in dying patients (52,53).

Steroids are helpful for dyspnea related to radiation pneumonitis, lymphangitic pulmonary metastases, exacerbation of COPD, or chemotherapy-induced hypersensitivity lung disease. Phenothiazines such as chlorpromazine and promethazine decrease dyspnea associated with chronic lung disease, probably because of their sedative effects, as does buspirone (52).

If patients have rapidly recurring pleural effusions, a small-diameter tube (pigtail catheter) can be placed in the radiology suite, left in for days to weeks, and managed at home without the discomfort associated with chest tube placement and sclerosis.

Hydration

Whether or not to supplement oral fluid intake in the dying patient is a complex issue and lacks randomized studies to help in the decision. Research demonstrates a weak relationship between the experience of thirst and the patient's actual state of hydration (54). Thirst occurs in some patients who are dying and can almost always be alleviated by good oral hygiene and a modest amount of oral fluids (55). It does not appear that thirst is a reason to consider parenteral fluids. Studies are lacking to know if intravenous or subcutaneous hydration is helpful in improving symptoms at the end of life. A small placebo-controlled trial demonstrated improvement in myoclonus and sedation in a group of patients with advanced cancer, dehydration, and decreased fluid intake given normal saline intravenously or subcutaneously (56). This study indicates the need for further studies with larger number of patients to resolve this issue.

SPECIFIC REFERENCES

1. Block SD. Perspectives on care at the close of life. Psychological considerations, growth, and transcendence at the end of life: the art of the possible. JAMA 2001;285:2898.
2. Fox E, Landrum-Mcniff K, Zhong Z, et al. Evaluation of prognostic criteria for determining hospice eligibility in patients with advanced lung, heart, or liver disease. Support investigators. Study to understand prognoses and preferences for outcomes and risks of treatments. JAMA 1999;282:1638.
3. Lynn J, Harrell F Jr, Cohn F, et al. Prognoses of seriously ill hospitalized patients on the days before death: implications for patient care and public policy. New Horiz 1997;5:56.
4. Lubitz JD, Riley GF. Trends in medicare payments in the last year of life. N Engl J Med 1993;328:1092.
5. O'connor CM, Gottlieb S, Bourque JM, et al. Impact of nonfatal myocardial infarction on outcomes in patients with advanced heart failure and the effect of bucindolol therapy. Am J Cardiol 2005;95:558.
6. Winton T, Livingston R, Johnson D, et al. Vinorelbine plus cisplatin vs. observation in resected non–small cell lung cancer. N Engl J Med 2005;352:2589.
7. Teno J, Lynn J, Wenger N, et al. Advance directives for seriously ill hospitalized patients: effectiveness with the patient self-determination act and the support intervention. Support investigators. Study to understand prognoses and preferences for outcomes and risks of treatment. J Am Geriatr Soc 1997;45:500.
8. Hofmann JC, Wenger NS, Davis RB, et al. Patient preferences for communication with physicians about end-of-life decisions. Support investigators. Study to understand prognoses and preference for outcomes and risks of treatment. Ann Intern Med 1997;127:1.
9. Teno JM, Stevens M, Spernak S, Lynn J. Role of written advance directives in decision making: insights from qualitative and quantitative data. J Gen Intern Med 1998;13:439.
10. Hopp FP, Duffy SA. Racial variations in end-of-life care. J Am Geriatr Soc 2000;48:658.
11. Mebane EW, Oman RF, Kroonen LT, et al. The influence of physician race, age, and gender on physician attitudes toward advance care directives and preferences for end-of-life decision-making. J Am Geriatr Soc 1999;47:579.
12. Carrese JA, Rhodes LA. Western bioethics on the Navajo reservation. Benefit or harm? JAMA 1995;274:826.
13. Wenrich MD, Curtis JR, Shannon SE, et al. Communicating with dying patients within the spectrum of medical care from terminal diagnosis to death. Arch Intern Med 2001; 161:868.
14. von Gunten CF, Ferris FD, Emanuel LL. The patient–physician relationship. Ensuring competency in end-of-life care: communication and relational skills. JAMA 2000;284:3051.
15. Fischer GS, Tulsky JA, Arnold RM. Communicating a poor prognosis. In: Portenoy RK, Bruera E, eds. Topics in palliative care. New York: Oxford University Press, 2000.
16. Buckman R. How to break bad news: a guide for heathcare professions. Baltimore, MD: Johns Hopkins University Press, 1992.
17. Koenig BA. Cultural diversity in decision making about care at the end of life. In: Field MJ, Cassel CK, eds. Approaching death: improving care at the end of life. Washington DC: National Academy Press, 1997:363.
18. Quill TE. Perspectives on care at the close of life. Initiating end-of-life discussions with seriously ill patients: addressing the "elephant in the room." JAMA 2000;284:2502.
19. Bonanno GA. Loss, trauma, and human resilience: have we underestimated the human capacity to thrive after extremely aversive events? Am Psychol 2004;59:20.
20. Schum JL, Lyness JM, King DA. Bereavement in late life: risk factors for complicated bereavement. Geriatrics 2005;60:18,24.
21. Pregerson HG, Jacos SC. Traumatic grief as a distinct disorder: a rationale, consensus criteria, and a preliminary empirical test. In: Stroebe M, Hansson R, Schut H, et al, eds. Handbook of bereavement research: consequences, coping and care. Washington DC: American Psychological Association, 2002:613.
22. Stroebe M, Hansson R, Stroebe W, et al. Handbook of bereavement: consequences, coping and care. 3rd ed. Washington DC: American Psychological Association, 2002.
23. Shear K, Frank E, Houck PR, et al. Treatment of complicated grief: a randomized controlled trial. JAMA 2005;293:2601.
24. Daaleman TP, Vandecreek L. Placing religion and spirituality in end-of-life care. JAMA 2000;284:2514.
25. Weaver AJ, Flannelly KJ. The role of religion/spirituality for cancer patients and their caregivers. South Med J 2004;97:1210.
26. Kubler-Ross E. On death and dying. New York: Macmillan, 1969:38.
27. Parkes CM. The dying adult. BMJ 1998;316:1313.
28. Zeitlin SV. Grief and bereavement. Prim Care 2001;28:415.
29. Bedell SE, Cadenhead K, Graboys TB. The doctor's letter of condolence. N Engl J Med 2001;344:1162.
30. Irvine P. The attending at the funeral. N Engl J Med 1985;312:1704.
31. Back AL, Arnold RM, Tulsky JA, et al. On saying goodbye: acknowledging the end of the patient-physician relationship with patients who are near death. Ann Intern Med 2005;142:682.
32. Finlay IG, Mason MD, Shelley M. Radioisotopes for the palliation of metastatic bone cancer: a systematic review. Lancet Oncol 2005;6:392.
33. Watson CP, Moulin D, Watt-Watson J, et al. Controlled-release oxycodone relieves neuropathic pain: a randomized controlled trial in painful diabetic neuropathy. Pain 2003;105:71.
34. Galer BS. Neuropathic pain of peripheral origin: advances in pharmacologic treatment. Neurology 1995;45(12 Suppl 9):S17.
35. Harden RN. Chronic neuropathic pain. Mechanisms, diagnosis, and treatment. Neurologist 2005;11:111.
36. Brookoff D. Chronic pain: 1. A new disease? Hosp Pract (Off Ed) 2000;35:45,59.
37. Argoff CE. Conclusions: chronic pain studies of lidocaine patch 5% using the neuropathic pain scale. Curr Med Res Opin 2004;20(Suppl 2):S29.
38. Wolfe GI, Trivedi JR. Painful peripheral neuropathy and its nonsurgical treatment. Muscle Nerve 2004;30:3.
39. Beniczky S, Tajti J, Timea VE, et al. Evidence-based pharmacological treatment of neuropathic pain syndromes. J Neural Transm 2005;112:735.
40. Vinik A. Use of antiepileptic drugs in the treatment of chronic painful diabetic neuropathy. J Clin Endocrinol Metab 2005; 90:4936.
41. Smith MT. Neuroexcitatory effects of morphine

and hydromorphone: evidence implicating the 3-glucuronide metabolites. Clin Exp Pharmacol Physiol 2000;27:524.
42. Hagen N, Swanson R. Strychnine-like multifocal myoclonus and seizures in extremely high-dose opioid administration: treatment strategies. J Pain Symptom Manage 1997;14:51.
43. Ferris DJ. Controlling myoclonus after high-dosage morphine infusions. Am J Health Syst Pharm 1999;56:1009.
44. Massie MJ, Holland J, Glass E. Delirium in terminally ill cancer patients. Am J Psychiatry 1983;140:1048.
45. Pereira J, Hanson J, Bruera E. The frequency and clinical course of cognitive impairment in patients with terminal cancer. Cancer 1997; 79:835.
46. Breitbart W, Marotta R, Platt MM, et al. A double-blind trial of haloperidol, chlorpromazine, and lorazepam in the treatment of delirium in hospitalized AIDS patients. Am J Psychiatry 1996;153:231.
47. Bourgeois JA, Hilty DM. Prolonged delirium managed with risperidone. Psychosomatics 2005;46:90.
48. Morita T, Tei Y, Inoue S. Agitated terminal delirium and association with partial opioid substitution and hydration. J Palliat Med 2003;6:557.
49. Bruera E, De Stoutz N, Velasco-Leiva A, et al. Effects of oxygen on dyspnoea in hypoxaemic terminal-cancer patients. Lancet 1993;342: 13.
50. Bruera E, Sala R, Spruyt O, et al. Nebulized versus subcutaneous morphine for patients with cancer dyspnea: a preliminary study. J Pain Symptom Manage 2005;29:613.
51. Foral PA, Malesker MA, Huerta G, et al. Nebulized opioids use in COPD. Chest 2004; 125:691.
52. Lagman RL, Davis MP, Legrand SB, et al. Common symptoms in advanced cancer. Surg Clin North Am 2005;85:237.
53. Ripamonti C, Fulfaro F, Bruera E. Dyspnea in patients with advanced cancer: incidence, causes and treatments. Cancer Treat Rev 1998;24:69.
54. Musgrave CF, Bartal N, Opstad J. The sensation of thirst in dying patients receiving I.V. hydration. J Palliat Care 1995;11:17.
55. Mccann RM, Hall WJ, Groth-Juncker A. Comfort care for terminally ill patients. The appropriate use of nutrition and hydration. JAMA 1994;272: 1263.
56. Bruera E, Sala R, Rico Ma, et al. Effects of parenteral hydration in terminally ill cancer patients: a preliminary study. J Clin Oncol 2005;23:2366.

For annotated **General References** *and resources related to this chapter, visit www.hopkinsbayview.org/PAMreferences.*

SECTION 2

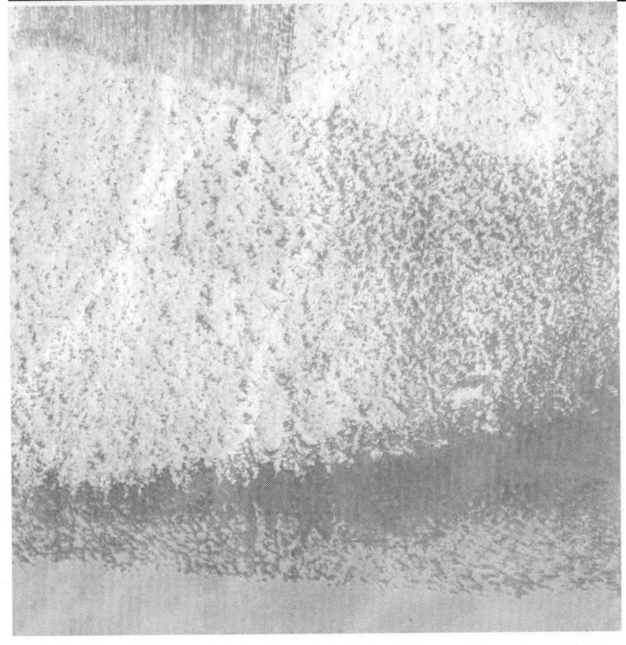

Preventive Care

Chapter 14

Integrating Prevention into Ambulatory Practice

Gregory P. Prokopowicz and David E. Kern

Prevention is a central part of patient care (1). Medical organizations, government agencies, insurance companies, and patients themselves expect practitioners to offer preventive services (2,3). Practitioners are in an important position to help reduce the burden of disease that affects society and its members. Evidence suggests that a health practitioner's advice can beneficially influence patient behavior (4,5). Increasingly, practitioners are being trained to interpret risks to health, to effectively communicate this information to patients, and to assist patients in desired behavior changes.

Three characteristics distinguish preventive from curative care:

1. *Preventive care aims to protect health prospectively*. In contrast to treatment, which tries to return a patient to a previous state of health, prevention attempts to maintain an existing state of health. This is true even for a chronically ill patient, for whom prevention might mean maintaining a limited functional status at home rather being admitted to a hospital or nursing home for a preventable worsening of illness.
2. *The practitioner, not the patient, usually initiates preventive care*. Although patients increasingly request preventive services, more often it is the practitioner who is aware of the need for such interventions.
3. In preventive care, *the practitioner must be more certain that an intervention is effective than in the care of established disease or symptomatic conditions*. Uncertainty is inherent in medicine. When ill patients seek treatment, the practitioner often must make a best guess regarding treatment. In prevention, however, patients are usually healthy and will remain so in the proximate future regardless of whether they undertake preventive measures. Consequently, there is an ethical obligation for the practitioner to have a high degree of certainty that suggested preventive interventions are likely to result in more good than harm (6).

Several considerations underlie the importance of prevention in routine office practice. First, approximately 50% of mortality from the 10 leading causes of death in the United States can be traced to alterable behavior (life-style) (7). Second, early detection and treatment of a number of common disorders, such as cervical carcinoma in situ and hypertension, effectively reduce mortality and morbidity from these conditions. Third, although infectious diseases have, to a large extent, been controlled in developed countries by public health measures such as immunization, outbreaks of pneumococcal disease continue to occur, and influenza remains a major preventable cause of death, especially among the elderly and immunocompromised (8,9). Fourth, the value of a comprehensive approach to prevention is suggested by the improvement in heath care outcomes attributable to prenatal care (10,11) and comprehensive geriatric assessment (12–15).

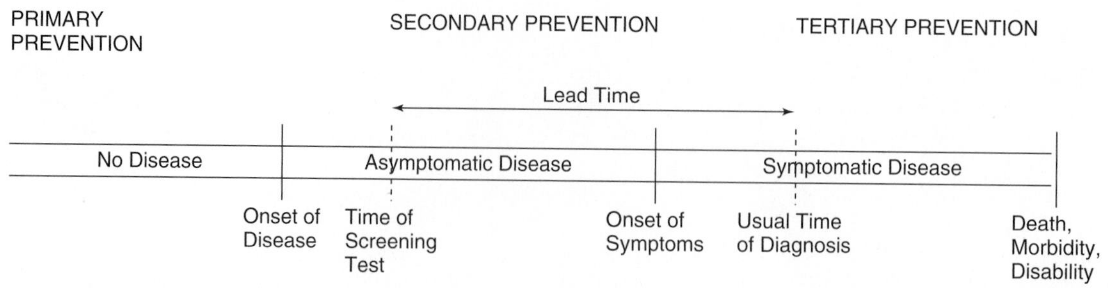

FIGURE 14.1. Primary, secondary, and tertiary prevention in the spectrum of a disease (see text for definitions).

TERMINOLOGY

Prevention can be divided into three stages according to the timing of the intervention (Fig. 14.1). *Primary prevention* occurs before the start of the disease process. For example, smoking cessation decreases the likelihood that a patient will develop coronary artery disease or lung cancer, barrier contraception or abstinence prevents the development of cervical dysplasia, and immunization prevents various infectious diseases. *Secondary prevention* detects early disease before it has become clinically apparent. Breast, cervical, and colon cancer screening to identify and remove occult malignancies, and thereby to improve outcome, represents secondary prevention. *Tertiary prevention* seeks to stop further complications after a disease has become clinically evident. Treatment after myocardial infarction with aspirin, beta blockers, angiotensin-converting enzyme (ACE) inhibitors, and statins represents tertiary prevention.

Although conceptually useful, the distinctions between primary, secondary, and tertiary prevention can become blurred in clinical practice. The early detection and treatment of asymptomatic hypertension, for example, would be considered tertiary prevention if one considers hypertension a disease and considers congestive heart failure, stroke, and renal failure complications of that disease. On the other hand, hypertension can be considered a risk factor for congestive heart failure, stroke, and renal failure, so that detection and treatment of hypertension to prevent these diseases from occurring can be considered primary prevention. Also, the terminology is not always used consistently. In the cardiology literature, for example, secondary prevention is commonly used to refer to the prevention of complications after the occurrence of a clinical event (such as myocardial infarction); this would be considered tertiary prevention using the conceptualization described here.

Several other terms are relevant to the practice of prevention. *Screening* is the process of identifying patients with unrecognized diseases or risk factors by the application of examinations, tests, or other procedures. A positive test is usually not diagnostic but requires further testing. *Mass screening* is screening applied to a large group, and *multiphasic screening* is simultaneous screening for various diseases, such as blood pressure and cholesterol measurement done at health fairs. *Case finding* occurs in a practitioner's practice when the clinician screens for disease unrelated to the symptom for which the patient has come.

EVALUATING PREVENTIVE MEASURES FOR USE IN AMBULATORY PRACTICE

The first step in integrating preventive care into office practice is deciding which measures to offer patients routinely. In deciding which measures to recommend, one should consider the burden of suffering attributable to each preventable condition, in terms of its prevalence and severity; the efficacy, cost, and safety of available screening tests; the efficacy and complications of treatment; and the effectiveness of each measure in routine office practice (Table 14.1). Recommendations that are periodically published by organizations such as the U.S. Preventive Services Task Force (USPSTF), Canadian Task Force on Preventive Health Care (CTF), the American Cancer Society, the American College of Physicians, the American Medical Association, the Centers for Disease Control and Prevention, and others can be consulted. For some measures, however, the recommendations are conflicting. The reports of the USPSTF and the CTF are firmly grounded in clinical epidemiology and provide the most scientific and least biased framework to date for evaluating which preventive health measures should be included in routine care (see www.hopkinsbayview.org/PAMreferences).

In evaluating a given measure, it is important to be aware of certain terms, concepts, pitfalls, and special considerations. The terms *sensitivity, specificity, prevalence,* and *predictive value,* which help define the value of a screening test, are defined in Chapter 2. *Efficacy* describes how well a test or maneuver performs under ideal circumstances. *Effectiveness* describes how well a test or maneuver performs under real-world circumstances. The effectiveness of a test or maneuver is usually somewhat less

TABLE 14.1 Questions to Ask in Evaluating a Recommended Preventive Measure

What is the burden of suffering attributable to the targeted condition?
What is the prevalence and/or incidence of the condition?
What is the size of the attributable morbidity?
What is the mortality rate?
Do efficacious screening tests exist?
Do they have acceptable sensitivity, specificity, and predictive value?[a]
Are they reliable?[a]
Are they practical and reasonably priced?
Are the side effects of screening acceptable?
Is preventive intervention efficacious in research settings?
Is the intervention efficacious in study groups?
Are compliance levels in study situations acceptable?
Are side effects acceptable?
Is intervention in the asymptomatic stage more beneficial than intervention after onset of symptoms?
Would use of the measure be effective in routine office practice?
Have suitable field trials been conducted?
Is the measure effective in reducing morbidity and mortality in nonstudy situations?
Are the compliance levels in nonstudy situations acceptable?
Are side effects in nonstudy situations acceptable?
What are the reliability, sensitivity, specificity, and predictive value of screening tests in one's own setting?[a]
Is the measure cost-effective?

[a] See Chapter 2 for a discussion of reliability, sensitivity, specificity, and predictive value.

than its efficacy. *Efficiency* describes how well the test or maneuver optimizes the use of limited resources. A *risk factor* is anything that, if present, increases the likelihood of disease. The proportion of a specific disease that can be accounted for by a risk factor is called the *attributable risk*.

Lead time (Fig. 14.1) is the period between the early detection of disease and its usual time of diagnosis. In the evaluation of the efficacy of early detection and treatment, lead time must be subtracted from overall survival time in screened patients to avoid *lead time bias*. Otherwise, early detection might appear to increase survival time, when in reality it is only increasing the duration of patients' awareness of their disease. Numerous cancer screening procedures have been thought to improve survival until lead time was addressed (16). *Length bias* (also called length-time bias, or length-biased sampling) occurs because tumors progress at different rates in different individuals. Screening tests preferentially find slow-growing tumors with long presymptomatic stages and better prognoses, but may miss fast-growing cancers with short presymptomatic stages, which can progress to become clinically apparent between screening intervals. Thus, survival may be better for patients detected by screening because of the characteristics of their tumors (less aggressive, lower grade), while overall mortality in screened and unscreened populations remains identical. A related concept is *pseudodisease*. This refers to indolent disease that would not have become clinically apparent during the lifetime of the subject had they not undergone screening, for example, a slow-growing prostate cancer in an elderly man. *Selection bias* occurs when patients undergoing a preventive measure differ from those with whom they are compared in a manner that affects the likelihood of their developing disease or affects the natural history of their disease. Volunteers, for example, may have more healthful lifestyles than those who do not volunteer. It is because of these biases that randomized controlled trials are important in evaluating preventive interventions.

The process of screening itself can cause morbidity. The test itself may carry a risk of complications (e.g., perforation from colonoscopy). The test may label some people as having a disease when they are in fact healthy (*false positives*), thereby causing anxiety or other suffering in the absence of disease. False positives refer to the identification of disease that is entirely absent, or to the identification of disease that is clinically inconsequential to the patient (*pseudodisease*) (17). If the disease is rare, or if the screening test does not have a high specificity, false-positive results may constitute a large fraction of all positive test results (see Chapter 2). For this reason, positive screening tests are usually followed by more specific diagnostic tests, and these may carry additional risks. On the other hand, a screening test with a low sensitivity (see Chapter 2) will inappropriately label some diseased patients as healthy (*false negatives*); this may induce them not to seek care even when they become symptomatic.

The advent of genetic testing and of highly sensitive imaging modalities (e.g., multislice spiral computerized tomography [CT]) has the potential to generate findings that are difficult to interpret for patient and practitioner alike (18–20). Direct-to-consumer marketing of such tests has raised additional concerns (21,22). The identification of disease or pathophysiologic abnormality in an otherwise healthy person can lead to adverse consequences from the *labeling effect* (23–25). For example, one study showed that absenteeism from work increased after workers were found to be hypertensive (24). Additionally, there may be implications for the patient with respect to insurance or employment. Practitioners can minimize such problems by choosing screening tests judiciously and by explaining risks and benefits to the patient, including the need for confirmatory testing and followup.

Caution should be used in adopting recommendations or guidelines that are based on demonstrations of efficacy in limited clinical trials. This is especially important with new technologies, where equipment and expertise may vary widely between institutions. For example, CT of the colon (virtual colonoscopy) has been variously reported to have a sensitivity of 59% and 90% (26). This discrepancy is probably a result of differences in equipment, protocols, and operator experience. As a result, the relevance of these data for the community practitioner considering CT colonography for his or her patient is questionable. The rise of freestanding radiology centers that advertise directly to the public may exacerbate the problem by increasing demand for unproven technologies (27).

Despite these precautions, there is sufficient evidence to support the integration of a number of primary and secondary preventive measures into office practice. Failure to do so reflects an inadequacy in the provision of primary care.

COMPONENTS OF PREVENTIVE CARE

General Examination and Baseline Data

Most practitioners perform a baseline general examination (history, physical, and selected laboratory tests) for some or all of their ambulatory patients. In addition, many practitioners repeat all or part of this examination on a periodic basis, in the form of an annual checkup. In contrast to the provision of selected preventive care measures discussed below, no firm scientific evidence links most of the general examination to reductions in morbidity and mortality (3). The question of whether, and how often, to perform a general physical examination remains a topic of debate. Most patients still expect annual examinations (28), however, and many clinicians find that periodic visits enhance the doctor–patient relationship and permit updating of the medical, social, and family history. Furthermore, periodic general examinations are sometimes required for people in high-risk occupations (e.g., airline pilots).

Provision of Selected Measures for Asymptomatic Patients (Primary and Secondary Preventive Care)

It is generally recommended that practitioners offer asymptomatic patients certain preventive care measures, selected on the basis of their likely benefits versus harm (see above and Table 14.1). Table 14.2 summarizes the preventive measures that are often considered for inclusion in the care of asymptomatic nonpregnant adults. For each preventive measure, the table provides the following information:

1. The *patient population* to which the measure should be applied (age, sex, risk status);
2. Recommended *time interval* between preventive interventions;
3. *Year of the recommendation*;
4. *Strength of the recommendation* for including or excluding the preventive measure in the care of asymptomatic patients, classified using the rating systems developed by the U.S. Preventive Services Task Force (USPSTF) and the Canadian Task Force on Periodic Health Examination (CTF).

The USPSTF rating system, which was revised in 2001 (29), assigns a grade (A through D, or I) to each preventive intervention as follows:

Grade Definition

A. The USPSTF strongly recommends that clinicians routinely provide the service to eligible patients. (The USPSTF found good evidence that the service improves important health outcomes and concludes that benefits substantially outweigh harms.)

B. The USPSTF recommends that clinicians routinely provide the service to eligible patients. (The USPSTF found at least fair evidence that the service improves important health outcomes and concludes that benefits outweigh harms.)

C. The USPSTF makes no recommendation for or against routine provision of the service. (The USPSTF found at least fair evidence that the service can improve health outcomes but concludes that the balance of the benefits and harms is too close to justify a general recommendation.)

D. The USPSTF recommends against routinely providing the service to asymptomatic patients. (The USPSTF found at least fair evidence that the service is ineffective or that harms outweigh benefits.)

I. The USPSTF concludes that the evidence is insufficient to recommend for or against routinely providing the service. (Evidence that the service is effective is lacking, of poor quality, or conflicting, and the balance of benefits and harms cannot be determined.)

The CTF uses the following rating system, revised in 2003 (30), for its recommendations:

Grade Definition

A. The CTF concludes that there is *good* evidence to recommend the clinical preventive action.

B. The CTF concludes that there is *fair* evidence to recommend the clinical preventive action.

C. The CTF concludes that the existing evidence is *conflicting* and does not allow making a recommendation for or against use of the clinical preventive action; however, other factors may influence decision making.

D. The CTF concludes that there is *fair* evidence to recommend against the clinical preventive action.

E. The CTF concludes that there is *good* evidence to recommend against the clinical preventive action.

I. The CTF concludes that there is *insufficient* evidence (in quantity and/or quality) to make a recommendation; however, other factors may influence decision making.

To determine the appropriate letter grade, both task forces assess the quality of evidence and the magnitude

TABLE 14.2 Preventive Measures to Consider in the Care of Asymptomatic Nonpregnant Adults

Preventive Measure	*Patient Population (Sex, Age [Years], Risk Status)*	*Time Interval*	*Year of Recommendation*	*Strength of Recommendation*[a,b]	*Chapter(s) to See for Details*
Good Evidence to Include					
Aspirin for primary prevention of cardiovascular events, discussion of benefits/risks[c]	M, F at high risk[c]	5 y	2002[a]	A	57, 62, 91
Blood pressure	All M, F ≥18[a] or 21[b]	1–2 y	2003[a], 1994[b]	A[a], B[b]	67
Breast cancer screening					
Mammography, with (preferable) or without clinical breast examination by health care practitioner	All F 50–69[d]	1–2 y	2002[a], 1998[b]	B[a,e], A[b,e]	105
Cervical cytology (Papanicolaou [Pap] test)	All F who have a uterus, onset of sexual activity, or age 18[b]–21[a] (whichever comes earlier) to age 65[a]–69[b] (if previous 2 Pap smears are normal)	1 y × 2, then 3 y[f]	2003[a], 1994[b]	A[a], B[b]	104
Chlamydia screening	F[g] at high risk	Discretionary, recommend at time of Pap smears[h]	2001[a], 1996[b]	A[a], B[b]	37, 102
Cholesterol, nonfasting total cholesterol (TC) and HDL cholesterol levels with further evaluation and treatment of those found to have high TC or low HDL[i]	All M ≥35; all F ≥45	5 y	2001[a]	A[a]	82
Colorectal cancer screening: fecal occult blood testing (FOBT), sigmoidoscopy, or colonoscopy	All M, F ≥50, normal risk	1 y (FOBT), 5 y (sigmoidoscopy), 10 y (colonoscopy)[j]	2002[a], 2001[b]	A[a,b]	45
Folate prophylaxis	F, previously affected pregnancy (neural tube deficit) or planning pregnancy	Beginning 1–3 mo before conception through 1st trimester	1996[a], 1994[b]	A[a,b]	100
Gonococcal culture	F at high risk[k] only[a] or M, F[b]	Discretionary[h]	2005[a], 1994[b]	B[a], A[b]	37, 102
Hepatitis B vaccination	All young adults not previously immunized and high-risk M, F of all ages[l]	Three doses, at 0, 1, and 6 mo	1996[a]	A[a]	18, 39, 47
HIV antibody testing	M, F[m] at high risk	Discretionary	2005[a], 1994[b]	A[a,b]	39
Influenza vaccination	All M, F ≥65; high-risk M, F of all ages[n]; health care providers for high-risk patients	1 y	1996[a], 1994[b]	A[a], B[b]	18

(continued)

TABLE 14.2 (Continued) Preventive Measures to Consider in the Care of Asymptomatic Nonpregnant Adults

Preventive Measure	Patient Population (Sex, Age [Years], Risk Status)	Time Interval	Year of Recommendation	Strength of Recommendation[a,b]	Chapter(s) to See for Details
Measles, mumps, rubella (MMR) vaccination (live)	All M and nonpregnant F born after 1956 who lack evidence of immunity to measles[o]	Once, or 2 doses ≥1 month apart[o]	1996[a]	A[a]	18
Pneumococcal vaccination	M, F[p] at high risk (see below for others)	Once, consider repeat dose at 5 y	1996[a], 1998[b]	B[a], A[b]	18
Smoking/tobacco use, counseling	All M, F	1–5 y	2003[a], 1994[b]	A[a,b]	27
Syphilis (serology), screening	M, F[q] at high risk	Discretionary	2004[a]	A[a]	37, 39, 102
Tetanus/diphtheria vaccination	All M, F	10 y or once after age 50 y (boosters); primary series at 0, 2, and 6–14 mo if not previously immunized	1996[a]	A[a]	18
Tuberculin skin test	M, F[r] at high risk	Discretionary	1996[a], 1994[b]	A[a,b]	34, 39
Travel to developing countries: immunization, prophylactic medications, counseling regarding preventive health practices	M, F at risk	Varies		A[h]	41
Fair Evidence to Include					
Abdominal aortic aneurysm, screening ultrasonography	M 65–75 who have ever smoked	Once	2005[a]	B[a]	94
Alcohol use, screening, with counseling of patients with problem drinking and counseling/referral of alcohol-dependent patients	All M, F	Discretionary	2004[a], 1994[b]	B[a,b]	28
Birth control counseling to reduce unwanted pregnancies	All sexually active M, F of childbearing age, especially adolescents	Discretionary	1996[a], 1994[b]	B[a,b]	100
Bone densitometry	All F >65; F >60[a] or postmenopausal F[b] at high risks[s]	Discretionary, >2 y	2002[a], 2004[b]	B[a], B[b]	103
Breast cancer screening					
Mammography with or without clinical breast examination by health care practitioner	All F 40–49	1–2 y	2002[a], 2001[b]	B[a,e], C[b]	105
Genetic counseling with or without BRCA gene testing	Adult F with strong family history of breast cancer	once	2005[a]	B[a]	17, 105

TABLE 14.2 (Continued) Preventive Measures to Consider in the Care of Asymptomatic Nonpregnant Adults

Preventive Measure	Patient Population (Sex, Age [Years], Risk Status)	Time Interval	Year of Recommendation	Strength of Recommendation[a,b]	Chapter(s) to See for Details
Cholesterol, nonfasting TC and HDL cholesterol	M 20–35, F 20–45 with risk factors[t]	5 y	2001[a]	B[a]	82
levels, with further evaluation and treatment of those found to be have high TC or low HDL[i]	M 20–35, F 20–45 without risk factors[t]	5 y	2001[a]	C[a]	82
Colorectal cancer screening: sigmoidoscopy[j]	All M, F ≥50, normal risk	3–10 y	2001[b]	B[b]	45
Depression, screening	All M, F	Discretionary	2002[a], 2005[b]	B[a,b]	24, 26
Diabetes mellitus, screening (e.g., with fasting plasma glucose)	M, F with hypertension or hyperlipidemia	Discretionary	2003[a], 2005[b]	B[a,b]	79
Diet: routine behavioral counseling	All M, F	Ongoing	2003[a], 1994[b]	I[a], B[b]	15, 82
Exercise, inquiry and counseling[u]	All M, F	Discretionary	2002[a], 1994[b]	I[a], B[a b]	12, 16, 63, 83, 103
Fall prevention	All M, F admitted to long-term care facilities	Discretionary	2005[b]	B[b]	12
Hearing impairment, screening	All M, F >65	Discretionary	1996[a], 1994[b]	B[a,b]	110
Obesity: screening (weight and height, BMI calculation)	All M, F[v]	Periodic	2003[a], 1999[b]	B[a], C[b]	
Pneumococcal vaccination	All M, F ≥65 (see above for others)	Once	1996[a], 1998[b]	B[a], C[b]	18
Rubella vaccination (or MMR) or rubella antibody screening and vaccination of those susceptible[w]	All nonpregnant F of childbearing age without documentation of previous rubella vaccination	Once, or 2 doses ≥1 mo apart[w]	1996[a], 1994[b]	B[a,b]	18
Seatbelt use, counseling	All M, F	Discretionary	1996[a], 1994[b]	B[a,b]	—
Skin inspection to detect skin cancer	M, F[x] at high risk	Discretionary	2001[a], 1994[b]	I[a], B and C[b]	114
Varicella vaccination	Susceptible adolescents and adults	2 doses given 4–8 wk apart	2001[b]	B[b]	18
Visual acuity testing	All M, F >65	Discretionary	1994, 1995[b]	B[b]	107
Insufficient Evidence to Include or Exclude					
Abdominal aortic aneurysm, screening ultrasonography	M 65–75 who have never smoked[a], asymptomatic individuals[b]	Once	2005[a], 1994[b]	C[a,b]	94
Aspirin therapy for the primary prevention of cardiovascular disease	All M 40–84 All F 50–84	Not applicable	1996[a], 1994[b] 1996[a], 1994[b]	C[a,b] C[a,b]	57, 62, 91
Breast self-examination, teaching/encouraging	All F ≥20	1 mo	2001[a,b]	I[a], D[b]	105

(continued)

TABLE 14.2 (Continued) Preventive Measures to Consider in the Care of Asymptomatic Nonpregnant Adults

Preventive Measure	Patient Population (Sex, Age [Years], Risk Status)	Time Interval	Year of Recommendation	Strength of Recommendation[a,b]	Chapter(s) to See for Details
Carotid artery stenosis, screening					
Auscultation or ultrasonography	All M, F >40–60 or at high risk for atherosclerotic cardiovascular disease	Discretionary Discretionary	1996[a], 1994,[b] 1996[a]	I[a], D[b] C[a]	91
Clinical breast examination by health care practitioner	All F ≥40	1–2 y	2002[a]	I[a]	105
Colorectal cancer, screening: CT colonography (virtual colonoscopy), colonoscopy[j]	All M, F ≥50	5–10 y	1996[a], 2001[b]	I[a], C[b]	45
Dementia (cognitive impairment) screening	All M, F ≥65–75	Discretionary	2003[a], 2001[b]	I[a], C[b]	26
Dental hygiene, primary care practitioner screening (for periodontal disease) or counseling (regarding brushing, flossing, fluoride, diet, and regular dental visits)[y]	All M, F	Discretionary	1996[a], 1994[b], 1995[b]	C[a,b]	112
Diabetes mellitus, screening (e.g., with fasting plasma glucose)	All M, F	Discretionary	2003[a], 1994[b]	I[a], D[b]	79
Domestic violence, screening	All F and elderly	Discretionary	2004[a], 2003[b]	I[a,b]	28
Driving while impaired by alcohol or drugs, counseling	All M, F	Discretionary	1996[a], 1994[b]	C[a,b]	28, 29
Drug abuse, screening	All M, F	Discretionary	1996[a]	C[a]	29
Coronary artery disease:					
Resting ECG, exercise treadmill, electron-beam CT scanning	M, F at high risk	Discretionary	2004[a]	I[a]	16, 62
Falls prevention, counseling[z]	All M, F ≥70–75	Discretionary	1996[a], 1994[b]	C[a,b]	12
Firearms at home, counseling[aa]	All M, F	Discretionary	1996[a], 1994[b]	C[a,b]	—
Glaucoma: tonometry or other methods	M, F ≥65	Discretionary	2005[a], 1995[b]	I[a], C[b]	108
Gonococcal culture	M at high-risk[k]	Discretionary	2005[a]	I[a]	37
Helmets, bicycle or motorcycle, counseling[bb]	All M, F	Discretionary	1996[a], 1994[b]	C[a,b]	—
Homocysteine, screening with fasting or postmethionine load plasma total homocysteine to detect and treat patients with high levels	M ≥35, F ≥45 at normal or high risk for coronary artery disease	Once	2000[b]	C[b]	62

TABLE 15.1 Sample USDA Food Guide and the DASH Eating Plan at the 2,000-Calorie Level[a]

Amounts of various food groups that are recommended each day or each week in the USDA Food Guide and in the DASH (Dietary Approaches to Stop Hypertension) Eating Plan (amounts are daily unless otherwise specified) at the 2,000-calorie level. Also identified are equivalent amounts for different food choices in each group. To follow either eating pattern, food choices over time should provide these amounts of food from each group on average.

Food Groups and Subgroups	*USDA Food Guide Amount[b]*	*DASH Eating Plan Amount*	*Equivalent Amounts*
Fruit Group	2 cups (4 servings)	2–2.5 cups (4–5 servings)	½ cup equivalent is: ½ cup fresh, frozen, or canned fruit; 1 med fruit; ¼ cup dried fruit USDA: ½ cup fruit juice DASH: ¾ cup fruit juice
Vegetable Group	2.5 cups (5 servings)	2–2.5 cups (4–5 servings)	½ cup equivalent is: ½ cup of cut-up raw or cooked vegetable; 1 cup raw leafy vegetable USDA: ½ cup vegetable juice DASH: ¾ cup vegetable juice
Dark green vegetables	3 cups/wk		
Orange vegetables	2 cups/wk		
Legumes (dry beans)	3 cups/wk		
Starchy vegetables	3 cups/wk		
Other vegetables	6.5 cups/wk		
Grain Group	6 ounce-equivalents	7–8 ounce-equivalents (7–8 servings)	1 ounce-equivalent is: 1 slice bread; 1 cup dry cereal; ½ cup cooked rice, pasta, cereal DASH: 1 oz dry cereal (½–1¼ cup depending on cereal type—check label)
Whole grains	3 ounce-equivalents		
Other grains	3 ounce-equivalents		
Meat and Beans Group	5.5 ounce-equivalents	6 ounces or less meat, poultry, fish 4–5 servings per wk nuts, seeds, and dry beans[c]	1 ounce-equivalent is: 1 ounce of cooked lean meats, poultry, fish; 1 egg USDA: ¼ cup cooked dry beans or tofu; 1 Tbsp peanut butter; ½ oz nuts or seeds DASH: 1½ oz nuts; ½ oz seeds; ½ cup cooked dry beans
Milk Group	3 cups	2–3 cups	1 cup equivalent is: 1 cup low-fat/fat-free milk, yogurt; 1.5 oz of low-fat or fat-free natural cheese; 2 oz of low-fat or fat-free processed cheese
Oils	27 g (6 tsp)	8–12 g (2–3 tsp)	1 tsp equivalent is: DASH: 1 tsp soft margarine; 1 Tbsp low-fat mayonnaise; 2 Tbsp light salad dressing; 1 tsp vegetable oil
Discretionary Calorie Allowance	267 calories	~2 tsp of added sugar (5 Tbsp per wk)	1 Tbsp added sugar equivalent is: DASH: 1 Tbsp jelly or jam; ½ oz jelly beans; 8 oz lemonade
Example of distribution:			
Solid fat[d]	18 g		
Added sugars	8 tsp		

[a]All servings are per day unless otherwise noted. USDA vegetable subgroup amounts and amounts of DASH nuts, seeds, and dry beans are per week.

[b]The 2,000-calorie USDA Food Guide is appropriate for many sedentary males 51 to 70 years of age, sedentary females 19 to 30 years of age, and for some other gender/age groups who are more physically active. See Table 15.3 for information about gender/age/activity levels and appropriate calorie intakes. See Appendices A-1, A-2 and A-3 at www.health.gov/dietaryguidelines/dga2005/document for more information on the food groups, amounts, and food intake patterns at other calorie levels.

[c]In the DASH Eating Plan, nuts, seeds, and dry beans are a separate food group from meat, poultry, and fish. The DASH diet generally recommends less sugar and fat, and more calcium, magnesium and potassium than the standard Food Guide (see text).

[d]The oils listed in this table are not considered to be part of discretionary calories because they are a major source of the vitamin E and polyunsaturated fatty acids, including the essential fatty acids, in the food pattern. In contrast, solid fats (i.e., saturated and *trans* fats) are listed separately as a source of discretionary calories.

From Dietary Guidelines for Americans 2005, available at www.health.gov/dietaryguidelines/dga2005/document. Last accessed December 18, 2005.

made with synthetic ingredients or sewage sludge, bioengineering, or ionizing radiation. Before a product can be labeled "organic," a government-approved certifier inspects the farm where the food is grown to make sure the farmer is following all the rules necessary to meet USDA organic standards. Companies that handle or process organic food before it gets to your local supermarket or restaurant must be certified, too (8).

TABLE 15.2 Comparison of Selected Nutrients in the Dietary Approaches to Stop Hypertension (DASH) Eating Plan[a], the USDA Food Guide[b], and Nutrient Intakes Recommended per Day by the Institute of Medicine (IOM)[c]

Estimated nutrient levels in the DASH Eating Plan and the USDA Food Guide at the 2,000-calorie level, as well as the nutrient intake levels recommended by the Institute of Medicine for females 19–30 years of age.

Nutrient	*DASH Eating Plan (2,000 kcals)*	*USDA Food Guide (2,000 kcals)*	*IOM Recommendations for Females 19–30 Years of Age*
Protein, g	108	91	RDA: 46
Protein, % kcal	21	18	AMDR: 10–35
Carbohydrate, g	288	271	RDA: 130
Carbohydrate, % kcal	57	55	AMDR: 45–65
Total fat, g	48	65	—
Total fat, % kcal	22	29	AMDR: 20–35
Saturated fat, g	10	17	—
Saturated fat, % kcal	5	7.8	ALAP[d]
Monounsaturated fat, g	21	24	—
Monounsaturated fat, % kcal	10	11	—
Polyunsaturated fat, g	12	20	—
Polyunsaturated fat, % kcal	5.5	9.0	—
Linoleic acid, g	11	18	AI: 12
Alpha-linolenic acid, g	1	1.7	AI: 1.1
Cholesterol, mg	136	230	ALAP[d]
Total dietary fiber, g	30	31	AI: 28[e]
Potassium, mg	4,706	4,044	AI: 4,700
Sodium, mg	2,329[f]	1,779	AI: 1,500; UL: $<$2,300
Calcium, mg	1,619	1,316	AI: 1,000
Magnesium, mg	500	380	RDA: 310
Copper, mg	2	1.5	RDA: 0.9
Iron, mg	21	18	RDA: 18
Phosphorus, mg	2,066	1,740	RDA: 700
Zinc, mg	14	14	RDA: 8
Thiamin, mg	2.0	2.0	RDA: 1.1
Riboflavin, mg	2.8	2.8	RDA: 1.1
Niacin equivalents, mg	31	22	RDA: 14
Vitamin B_6, mg	3.4	2.4	RDA: 1.3
Vitamin B_{12}, μg	7.1	8.3	RDA: 2.4
Vitamin C, mg	181	155	RDA: 75
Vitamin E (AT)[g]	16.5	9.5	RDA: 15.0
Vitamin A, μg (RAE)[h]	851	1,052	RDA: 700

[a] DASH nutrient values are based on a 1-week menu of the DASH Eating Plan. NIH publication No. 03–4082. Available at www.nhlbi.nih.gov.
[b] USDA nutrient values are based on population-weighted averages of typical food choices within each food group or subgroup.
[c] Recommended intakes for adult females 19–30 years of age; AI, adequate intake; AMDR, acceptable macronutrient distribution range; RDA, recommended dietary allowance; UL, upper limit.
[d] As low as possible (ALAP) while consuming a nutritionally adequate diet.
[e] Amount listed is based on 14 g dietary fiber/1,000 kcal.
[f] The DASH Eating Plan recommends $<$1,500 mg of sodium per day for individuals with hypertension, blacks, and middle-aged and older adults.
[g] AT, mg D-α-tocopherol.
[h] RAE, retinol activity equivalents.
From Dietary Guidelines for Americans 2005. Available at www.health.gov/dietaryguidelines/dga2005/document. Last accessed December 18, 2005.

In a more recent promulgation, the USDA allows for four categories of food labeling, depending on the organic purity of the foods produced: "100% Organic," "Organic" (at least 95% organic ingredients), "Made With Organic Ingredients" (at least 75% organic ingredients), and "Made With Some Organic Ingredients" (less than 70% but more than 30% organic ingredients). The USDA makes no claim that organically produced food is safer or more nutritious than conventionally produced food.

TABLE 15.3 Estimated Calorie Requirements (in Kilocalories) for Each Gender and Age Group at Three Levels of Physical Activity[a]

Estimated amounts of calories needed to maintain energy balance for various gender and age groups at three different levels of physical activity. The estimates are rounded to the nearest 200 calories and were determined using the Institute of Medicine (IOM) equation.

		Activity Level[b,c,d]		
Gender	***Age (Years)***	***Sedentary[b]***	***Moderately Active[c]***	***Active[d]***
Child	2–3	1,000	1,000–1,400[e]	1,000–1,400[e]
Female	4–8	1,200	1,400–1,600	1,400–1,800
	9–13	1,600	1,600–2,000	1,800–2,200
	14–18	1,800	2,000	2,400
	19–30	2,000	2,000–2,200	2,400
	31–50	1,800	2,000	2,200
	51+	1,600	1,800	2,000–2,200
Male	4–8	1,400	1,400–1,600	1,600–2,000
	9–13	1,800	1,800–2,200	2,000–2,600
	14–18	2,200	2,400–2,800	2,800–3,200
	19–30	2,400	2,600–2,800	3,000
	31–50	2,200	2,400–2,600	2,800–3,000
	51+	2,000	2,200–2,400	2,400–2,800

[a]These levels are based on estimated energy requirements (EER) from the *Institute of Medicine Dietary Reference Intakes Macronutrients Report* (2002), calculated by gender, age, and activity level for reference-sized individuals. "Reference size," as determined by IOM, is based on median height and weight for ages up to age 18 years of age and median height and weight for that height to give a body mass index (BMI) of 21.5 for adult females and 22.5 for adult males.
[b]Sedentary means a lifestyle that includes only the light physical activity associated with typical day-to-day life.
[c]Moderately active means a lifestyle that includes physical activity equivalent to walking about 1.5 to 3 miles per day at 3 to 4 miles per hour, in addition to the light physical activity associated with typical day-to-day life.
[d]Active means a lifestyle that includes physical activity equivalent to walking more than 3 miles per day at 3 to 4 miles per hour, in addition to the light physical activity associated with typical day-to-day life.
[e]The calorie ranges shown are to accommodate needs of different ages within the group. For children and adolescents, more calories are needed at older ages. For adults, fewer calories are needed at older ages.
From Dietary Guidelines for Americans 2005. Available at www.health.gov/dietaryguidelines/dga2005/document. Last accessed December 18, 2005.

TABLE 15.4 Physical Activity and Caloric Expenditure[a]

Physical Activity	***Calories Expended (Kcal/Hour[a])***
Rest	90
Sitting	120
Stand and move	252
Walk 2 mph	198
Walk 4 mph	396
Cycle 5 mph	180
Cycle 10 mph	396
Swim 20 yds/min	294
Swim 40 yds/min	594
Run 5 mph	564
Run 10 mph	1128
Hike with pack	420
Tennis, singles	468
Basketball	462
Racquetball	606

[a]Calculated from Appendix C tables in Williams MH. Nutrition for health, fitness and sport. 5th ed. Boston: McGraw-Hill, 1999:425–431.5

Survey Data on Nutritional Patterns

Because the study of nutrition and its relationship to health status has become increasingly important, national nutritional surveillance surveys were begun in the United States in 1970 (9). *National Health and Nutrition Examination Surveys* (NHANES) have been conducted three times—1971, 1976, and 1988—by the National Center for Health Statistics of the Centers for Disease Control and Prevention (NCHI/CDC). These population-based surveys use a probability sample of 25,000 to 35,000 individuals, using 24-hour dietary recall and food frequency questionnaires. Physical examination and a battery of clinical measurements and tests are also performed on all individuals in the sample. The NHANES data are used to establish food consumption patterns and nutritional status by both demographic and nutrient-specific criteria.

In 1995, the USDA initiated the *Healthy Eating Index* to measure how well American diets conform to recommended healthful eating patterns such as those included

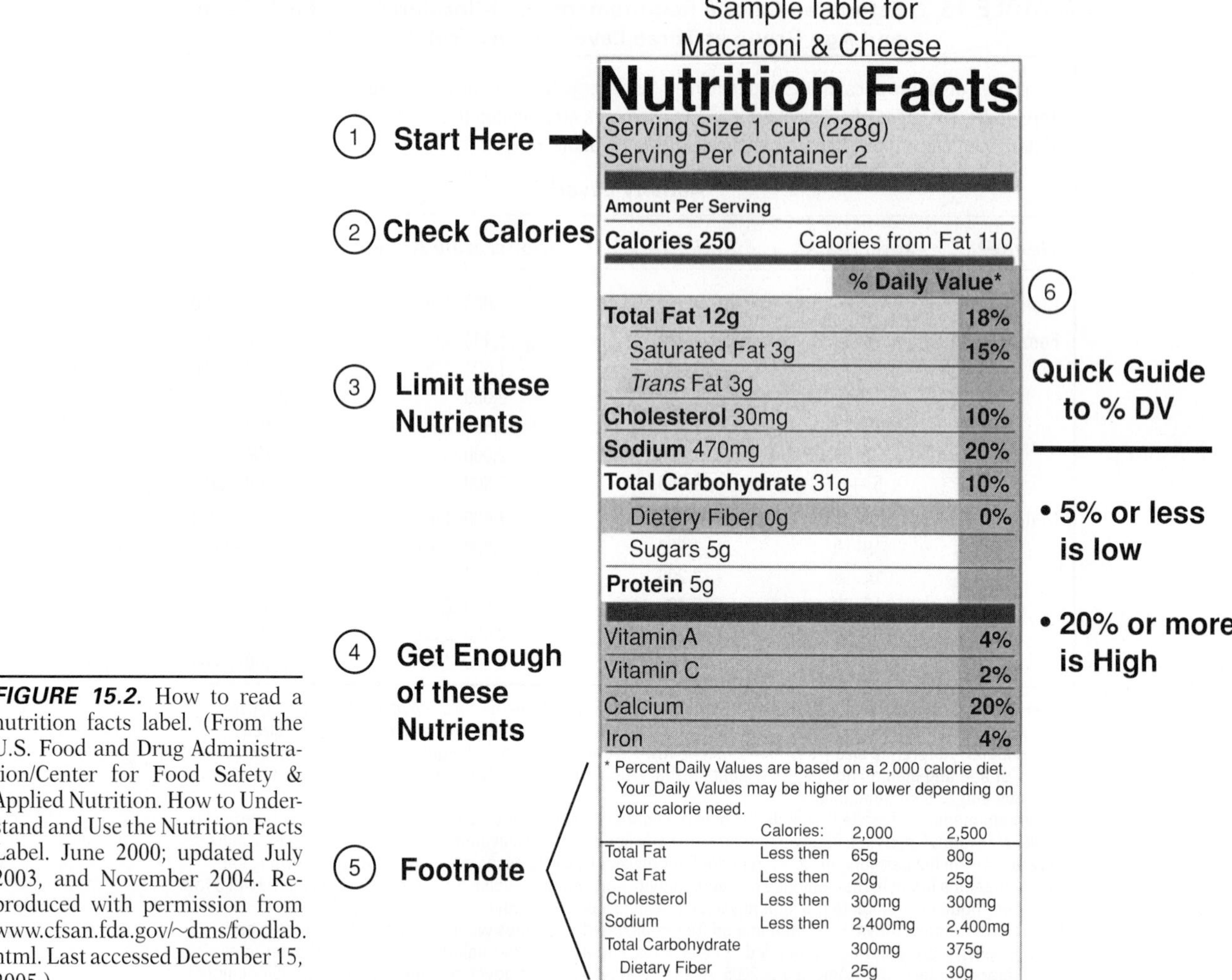

FIGURE 15.2. How to read a nutrition facts label. (From the U.S. Food and Drug Administration/Center for Food Safety & Applied Nutrition. How to Understand and Use the Nutrition Facts Label. June 2000; updated July 2003, and November 2004. Reproduced with permission from www.cfsan.fda.gov/~dms/foodlab.html. Last accessed December 15, 2005.)

in the Food Guide Pyramid. The 10 components of this index include grains, vegetables, fruits, milk, meat, total fat, saturated fat, cholesterol, sodium, and food variety. For two studies done in 1989 and 1990, a 3-day dietary intake was obtained using a sample size of approximately 4,000 individuals 2 years of age and older. The maximum score for the 10-component index is 100 points. Average overall scores for the 1989 and 1990 data were 63.8 and 63.9, respectively. Approximately 12% of persons had an index score above 80, and 15% were at 50 or below. The majority of individuals studied had diets that were rated as "Needs Improvement" (10).

NUTRITIONAL ASSESSMENT

Although primary care practitioners may refer patients to nutritionists for detailed assessments of dietary habits and for assistance in managing patients with nutritionally related disease such as obesity, atherosclerosis, diabetes, and renal failure, much general dietary counseling can be and is done by primary care practitioners. Useful dietary counseling requires a practical approach to nutritional assessment that helps to identify dietary deficiencies and excesses. The two steps of a practical approach to assessment include (a) taking a nutritional history and assessing nutrient intake and (b) recognizing manifestations of nutritional deficiency or excess.

Table 15.2 shows the important human macronutrients and micronutrients. Macronutrients are consumed in readily observed forms. Micronutrients, on the other hand, are less visible constituents of the major food groups. They include *vitamins* (organic compounds that are required in small amounts) and *minerals*.

The *portion sizes* used in this chapter, which may vary considerably from individual to individual, are based on a standard reference that is widely used by nutrition professionals (11).

TABLE 15.5 Disease–Nutrient Associations

Disease	Associated Nutrients
Atherosclerosis	Saturated fat, cholesterol
Diarrheal disease	Water, electrolytes, most nutrients
Liver disease	Alcohol
Cancer	Fat, antioxidants (A, C, E)
Diabetes mellitus	Fat, sugar, total energy, alcohol
Renal disease	Water, electrolytes, protein
Osteoporosis	Calcium, vitamin D
Hypertension	Sodium, potassium, calcium
Malnutrition	Many nutrients
Congestive heart failure	Sodium, water, potassium
Anemia	Iron, folate, vitamin B_{12}
Obesity	Fat, carbohydrate, total energy
Breast Disease	Vitamin E, caffeine

Obtaining Information about a Patient's Nutrition

Importance of Nutritional History Taking

The initial step in identifying dietary influence in the routine care of the patient is to collect information that provides a database for each individual with respect to important nutrients. From this, a judgment can then be made about whether these nutrients are deficient or excessive in the patient's diet. The nutrient history can be obtained by the health care practitioner directly or by another staff member. A practitioner-directed history has the advantage that the practitioner can simultaneously assess the patient's willingness to discuss his or her eating habits and make a judgment as to the veracity of the information. Additionally, the patient is more likely to conclude that personal nutrition has value comparable with other data that one seeks in the clinical interview. Given the major impact that diet has upon the etiology, pathogenesis, and course of many diseases, such a dialogue is important in current prevention and treatment strategies. Table 15.5 lists the nutrients associated with the most common contemporary diseases of people (12,13).

Practical Assessment of Nutrient Intake

Formal nutritional intake information is usually obtained with the use of either food frequency (FFQ) or daily food intake questionnaire. The latter may be done on the basis of a 24-hour dietary recall (past 24 hours) or by having the patient complete a daily food diary over a specified period of time.

Table 15.6 contains a list of questions that represent a suggested narrative for nutritional assessment. It combines elements of *specific 24-hour dietary recall* with that of *general questioning* about a patient's eating habits. It has the advantage of validating an individual's self-perception of personal nutrition with 24-hour eating recall information and includes specific inquiry about between-meal intake. When inconsistency in responses occur, discussion of them may lead to a better understanding of a patient's pattern of food consumption and of the type of exceptions that the patient makes in the day-to-day personal rules for eating. Although a single 24-hour hour dietary recall may be atypical, repeated 24-hour recalls can provide a fairly reliable assessment of average dietary intake.

An alternative, more time-efficient way to assess 24-hour intake is to give the patient a readable table of information about food groups such as Table 15.1, and have the patient fill in the number of servings of each food group consumed in the prior day. Because food intake reporting methods have been shown to collect information that often underestimates actual food consumption (2), it is wise to interpret any food intake report as representing *minimal food consumption at best*. Nevertheless, such information

TABLE 15.6 Sample Clinical Nutrition History That Combines Specific Dietary Recall and General Information

Meal-Oriented Questioning:

1. How many meals do you generally eat on a daily basis? How many *yesterday* or today?
2. What do you generally eat for breakfast? What did you eat *this morning*?
3. What do you generally eat for lunch? What did you actually eat for lunch *today or yesterday*?
4. Do you ever eat or drink anything between breakfast and lunch? What might you have had between breakfast and lunch *today or yesterday*?
5. What do you generally have for dinner/supper? What did you have *today or yesterday*?
6. Do you normally eat or drink between lunch and dinner/supper? If so, what do you have? Did you do so *today or yesterday*?
7. What do you generally eat or drink between dinner/supper and bedtime? What did you have then either *today or yesterday*?
8. Do you generally snack? If so, what are your preferred snacks? How often do you snack?

Selected Nutrient Questioning:

1. What liquids do you generally consume? What and how much did you drink in the past 24 hours? Do you drink water by itself? How often/how much?
2. Do you add salt to your food at the table? Do you cook with salt?
3. What fats do you generally cook with? What did you use *yesterday*?
4. Do you ever eat sweets? Daily? How often? What do you usually reach for in a snack? Do you add sugar to coffee or tea?
5. Do you consume foods with caffeine? Coffee? Tea? Soda? Chocolate? Quantities?
6. Do you know what fiber-containing foods you eat on a daily basis? Fresh vegetables? Fresh fruits? Salad? Fiber supplements?
7. Do you know how much cholesterol-related foods you eat on a daily basis? Red Meat? Saturated fats?
8. What and how much dairy products do you eat daily? Dark greens? Calcium supplements?

TABLE 15.7 Micronutrient Laboratory Tests

Nutrient	Test	Normal Range[a]
Calcium	Serum calcium Bone mineral density	8.2–10.0 mg/dL radiologic reference
Folate	Serum folate Red cell folate	2.6–17.0 ng/mL 150–450 ng/mL
Iron	Serum iron % Saturation Transferrin Ferritin	40–160 μg/dL 20–55% 213–360 mg/dL 18–311 ng/mL
Magnesium	Serum Mg	1.9–2.7 mg/dL
Potassium	Serum K^+ 24-hr urinary excretion	3.6–5.0 mEq/L 25–125 mEq/d (varies with diet)
Sodium	Serum sodium 24-hr urinary excretion	135–145 mEq/L 20–250 mEq/d (varies with diet)
Vitamin A	Serum retinol	35–70 μg/dL
Vitamin B_{12}	Serum B_{12}	251–911 pg/mL
Vitamin C	Serum ascorbic acid	0.6–2.0 mg/dL
Vitamin D	25-OH vitamin D 1,25$(OH)_2$ vitamin D	15–80 ng/mL 18–62 pg/mL
Vitamin E	Serum tocopherol	0.5–1.2 mg/dL

[a]Reference values vary with laboratories.

is essential in developing a starting point for discussion of an individual's food consumption behavior.

Once information about the average daily food intake is collected, an estimate of actual macronutrient and micronutrient element consumption can be made using the basic information in Tables 15.1 and 15.2.

Micronutrient intake is generally assessed by an analysis of food type consumption. It can also be inferred from serum biochemical testing (Table 15.7). Table 15.8 contains additional information about selected micronutrients that is pertinent to assessment regarding sufficient intake. It includes the recommended daily DRI, the type of food that generally provides each nutrient (vegetal, meat, dairy), and the food servings that would provide all of the RDA. The amount of each micronutrient which is contained in a standard over-the-counter multivitamin or pill supplement is also shown. Finally, when considering micronutrient dietary adequacy, it is helpful to know the amount that is stored in the body, the estimated duration of use of the body's storage amount, and amount lost daily (Table 15.9) (6).

Recognizing Clinical Manifestations of Nutritional Deficiency and Excess

In addition to the nutrition history, physical examination offers important clues to both macro- and micronutrient-related abnormalities. Tables 15.10 and 15.11 summarize some of the more important signs of nutrient deficiency and excess.

CONSIDERATIONS RELATED TO SELECTED NUTRIENTS

Certain nutrients are particularly important in their relationship to health and disease; some because they constitute the basic components of a selective diet (e.g., a vegetarian diet), some because of their influence upon caloric intake, some because of refinement in the processing of foods in the past century, and others because they contribute to commonly experienced symptoms.

TABLE 15.8 Micronutrient Dietary Sources (Recommended Amounts May Vary with Age and Gender)

Nutrient	Dietary Reference Intake	Food Source	Food Servings	Standard Over-the-Counter Preparation
Calcium	1,200 mg	Dairy, vegetal	1 qt milk	200–1000 mg
Folate	400 μg	Vegetal	5	400 μg
Iron	15 mg	Meat, vegetal	6	15 mg
Magnesium	400 mg	Vegetal > meat	6	100 mg
Potassium	4,700 mg	Most foods	8	80 mg
Sodium	< 2,300 mg	Most foods	8	None
Vitamin A	800 μg	Vegetal, dairy,	4	800 μg
		liver	<1	
Vitamin B_{12}	2.4 μg	Meat, fish	1	6 μg
Vitamin C	80 mg	Vegetal	2	80 mg
Vitamin D	400 IU	Dairy	1 qt milk	400 IU
Vitamin E	15 mg	Vegetal oil	3 tbsp	15 mg
		Most foods	6	

From Dietary Reference Intakes (DRIs): Recommended Intakes for Individuals. Food and Nutrition Board, Institute of Medicine, National Academies. Available at www.iom.edu/Object.File/Master/21/372/0.pdf.

TABLE 15.9 Micronutrient Storage Capacity and Daily Losses

Nutrient	*Storage Capacity*	*Supply Duration*	*Average Daily Loss*
Calcium	1,200 g (1% extraskeletal)	Years	200 mg
Folate	4,000 μg	60 days	60 μg
Iron	500 mg	>1 year	male: 1 mg; female: 1.5 mg
Magnesium*	2,500 mg	100 days	150 mg
Potassium*	180,000 mg (4,500 mEq)	~1 wk	800 mg (20 mEq)
Sodium[a]	>100,000 mg (>4,400 mEq)	Years	<230 mg (10 mEq)
Vitamin A	500,000 μg	>1 year	1,000 μg
Vitamin B_{12}	>2,000 μg	>3 years	2 μg
Vitamin C	1,500 mg	30+ days	>30 mg
Vitamin D[b]	?	Unknown	100 IU (2.5 μg)
Vitamin E[c]	?	?	?

[a]Electrolytes in storage serve active biologic functions.
[b]Vitamin D is one of the nonessential vitamins.
[c]Vitamin E deficiency is rare.
Modified from Food and Nutrition Board, National Research Council. Recommended Daily Allowances, 10th ed. Washington, DC: National Academy Press, 1989.

Vegetarian Diets

Vegetarian diets are increasingly popular. One of the more obvious reasons is the current epidemic of hypercholesterolemia and atherosclerosis related to the intake of saturated fats and the cholesterol content in animal protein foods. Secondly, evidence that vegetal sources of protein contain sufficient amounts of the ten essential amino acids is debunking the long-held myth that vegetarian eating does not provide as complete a protein source as animal meats (14). An important example is the demonstration that soybeans contain an amino acid content equivalent to that of egg albumin, the long-held standard referent for an ideal protein source (15).

Finally, it is increasingly appreciated that vegetarian eating not only can sustain health, but it can lead to improved health status. For example, studies show that vegetarian diets are consistently associated with lower rates of ischemic heart disease (16–21). In addition, studies of Seventh-Day Adventists reveal that their vegetarian-oriented lifestyle is also associated with decreased rates of cancer and all-cause mortality (22). Vegetarian diets contain higher amounts of fiber, antioxidants, folic acid, and phytochemicals, all of which are receiving increasing attention in modern dietary recommendations.

The vegetarian tradition is Asian in origin, particularly among Hindu populations. It currently includes a number of variations along a continuum of vegetarian purity. A *vegan* diet is considered the strictest diet. It excludes all forms of animal products including dairy and honey. A *lactovegetarian* diet includes dairy products, and *ovolactovegetarian* allows for the inclusion of both eggs and dairy. Many individuals use the term *partial-vegetarian* to indicate that they occasionally use animal products. A *macrobiotic* diet derives from East Asian traditions and in its most traditional form, involves the practice of a gradual change from a balanced vegetarian diet to one that primarily consists of grain, all in the interest of progressive nutritional and spiritual purity. Generally it emphasizes brown rice, fruits, and vegetables. Cooking is preferred over raw foods. Processed foods are avoided, as are tomatoes and potatoes. Fish is permitted.

The Food Guide Pyramid (Fig. 15.1) includes vegetarian eating in its general design and recommended food selections. The U.S. Department of Agriculture website

TABLE 15.10 Clinical Manifestations Related to Macronutrients

Macronutrient	*Signs of Deficiency*	*Signs of Excess*
Carbohydrate, total	Weight loss, asthenia, urinary ketosis	Obesity, weight gain
Carbohydrate, fiber	Constipation	Frequent stooling, abdominal bloating
Carbohydrate, starch	Weight loss, asthenia	Obesity, weight gain, insulin resistance, glucose intolerance
Carbohydrate, sugar	None	Obesity, weight gain, insulin resistance, glucose intolerance, halitosis, dental caries
Carbohydrate–alcohol	None	Facial plethora, alcoholic breath, large parotid glands, hepatitis, cirrhosis, cerebellar abnormalities
Total fat	Weight loss, asthenia, vitamin D deficiency (see Table 15.10)	Obesity, weight gain, xanthelasma, atherosclerosis
Saturated fat	Unknown	Hypercholesterolemia, atherosclerosis, corneal arcus
Cholesterol	Unknown	Hypercholesterolemia, atherosclerosis, corneal arcus
Protein	Weight loss, edema, infection, lethargy, hypoalbuminemia (kwashiorkor)	None
Water	Dehydration, high urine specific gravity, many organ system abnormalities	Hyponatremia (unusual)

TABLE 15.11 Clinical Manifestations Related to Micronutrients

Micronutrient	Signs of Deficiency	Signs of Excess
Calcium	Osteoporosis, kyphosis, hypocalcemia	Constipation, hypercalcemia, hypercalciuria, urolithiasis
Folate	Macrocytic anemia, neurologic birth defects	Unknown
Iron	Microcytic anemia	Hemochromatosis
Magnesium	Muscle weakness, low serum Mg, hypokalemia, long QT interval	Unknown
Potassium	Neuromuscular symptoms, ECG U-wave prominence	Cardiac arrhythmia, ECG peaked T waves
Salt	Neuromuscular symptoms, hyponatremia, hypotension	Hypertension, edema
Vitamin A	Impaired night vision, xerophthalmia, follicular hyperkeratosis, dry skin	Headache, desquamation, alopecia, osteosclerosis, splenomegaly
Vitamin B_{12}	Macrocytic anemia, glossitis, peripheral neuropathy	Unknown
Vitamin C	Scurvy, malaise	Diarrhea
Vitamin D	Hypocalcemia, rickets, osteomalacia	Hypercalcemia, hypercalciuria, calcinosis
Vitamin E	Reproductive failure, neuromuscular dysfunction (chronic malabsorption states)	Excesses may contribute to cardiovascular morbidity

ECG, electrocardiogram.

contains more detailed information on vegetal choice (see www.hopkinsbayview.org/PAM). Complete sources of amino acids are obtained in diets that include a combination of legumes (beans, peas, lentils, soybeans) and grain. Tofu is a particularly versatile soybean-based product used in the preparation of many vegetarian dishes.

In addition to alternative protein sources, vegetarian diets differ from meat-based diets in that they contain lower fat content and little saturated fat. They also have less iron, little if any vitamin B_{12}, and less calcium and zinc. However, they contain more fiber and antioxidant vitamins, more magnesium, and more folate (23,24). In addition, they potentially limit vitamin D availability in wintry months when sun exposure is limited. Although years can pass before people who become vegans develop B_{12} deficiency, breast-fed infants of strict vegetarian mothers have been reported to develop B_{12} deficiency (25). As well, milk-free diets can lead to rickets in young children (26). Significant nutrient deficiency is unusual in nonvegan vegetarian individuals. When eggs and dairy are avoided, however, supplementation with vitamin B_{12}, calcium, and vitamin D is recommended.

Calories

Caloric nutrient excess has reached epidemic proportions in the United States today. Obesity rates approach 40% of the adult population in this country and are increasing in many other countries (see Chapter 83). The increasing availability of energy-dense foods coupled with more sedentary lifestyles together contribute to this phenomenon. Furthermore, the epidemic of type II diabetes is associated with chronic caloric excess, sedentary lifestyle, and obesity.

The word *calorie* is derived from the Latin word *calor* meaning warm. The term is used as a measure of heat energy in food. Specifically, it refers to the amount of heat required to raise the temperature of 1 kg of water 1°C. In common food-related usage, the word *calorie* is used, although technically the term *kilocalorie* is the more correct designation. Table 15.12 shows the caloric value of the four major energy-containing nutrients.

Once ingested, more than 99% of caloric foods are absorbed. Very little of ingested caloric content is excreted in urine or stool under normal conditions. An exception is alcohol, which can be excreted unmetabolized in the urine. Ketones, which represent the incompletely metabolized combustion products of fat breakdown, are the other exception to this rule. Thus, most caloric intake is destined for either immediate metabolic use or storage as either glycogen (liver, muscle) or triglyceride (adipose cells).

The absorption and metabolic processing of caloric nutrients require energy. The incremental amount of caloric energy required in providing for metabolic processing varies from nutrient to nutrient (27,28). Table 15.13 shows average estimates for the metabolic cost of caloric macronutrient processing and storage. The *net* amount of calories stored for an equivalent (100 calories) amount of ingested carbohydrate, fat, or protein is shown. The last column of the table gives an estimate of the comparative annual weight that might be gained if an *extra 100 kcal per day* were eaten for each nutrient.

TABLE 15.12 Energy Contained in Caloric Nutrients

Nutrient	Energy (Kcal/g)
Protein	4
Carbohydrate	4
Alcohol	7
Fat	9

TABLE 15.13 Caloric Processing and Storage

Caloric Nutrient	% Calories Expended in Processing and Storage	Net Calories Stored[a] from 100 Ingested	Weight Gain Per Year[b] in Pounds
Fat	3%	97	9.7
Carbohydrate	25%	75	7.5
Protein	25–50%	50–75	5–7

[a]Assuming that calories (kcal) eaten exceed those needed for metabolic use.
[b]Weight gain if an extra 100 calories (kcal) per day is eaten of nutrient = net excess calories stored per day × 365 days/3,500 calories per pound as stored triglyceride.

Salt

Sodium chloride is the major osmotic constituent of the extracellular vascular and interstitial spaces. It is also the major component of intravenous fluids. From a dietary perspective, it is also a nutrient that can be deficient or excessive in the diet. Excessive salt can contribute to expansion of the extracellular space and influence the development of hypertension and congestive heart failure. In an otherwise healthy individual, diet-related salt deficiency is rare.

The normal human is capable of adapting to a very wide range of salt intake. Under conditions of limited salt intake, the kidney will excrete less than 230 mg (10 mEq) of sodium per day. This represents about one-tenth of a teaspoon of salt. On the other hand, among certain Oriental cultures, an intake of more than 25 g per day has been documented. The renin–angiotensin–aldosterone system adjusts salt excretion to match salt intake.

In U.S. surveys, daily sodium intake ranges from 3.8 to 7.5 g (29). In a workplace study of urinary 24-hour sodium excretion, a large range (4 to 24 g) was observed (30). Approximately 50% of salt intake is that added by the consumer for seasoning. For example, 1 teaspoon of salt contains 1,800 mg of sodium. Because of its importance in common health problems, quantitative information about the amount of sodium is required for standard nutritional labeling (see Fig. 15.2). The maximum amount of sodium per day that is recommended is 2,400 mg (6 g of salt) (5). Table 15.14 lists the sodium and salt content of selected intake sources.

TABLE 15.14 Sodium–Salt Equivalents

Intake	Sodium (mg)	Sodium (mEq)	Salt (g)
Milk, 1 pint	150	6.5	0.375
French fries 4 oz	220	10	0.550
Minimal intake	250	11	0.625
Low-sodium diet	500	22	1.5
Hamburger	530	23	1.3
Soup 8 oz	1,000	43	2.5
Big Mac	1,010	44	2.5
1 tsp salt	1,800	78	4.5
Recommended daily value	2,400	104	6.0
1 L lactated Ringer solution	3,100	134	7.75
1 L 0.9% normal saline	3,500	154	8.75
Average U.S. intake	5,000	217	12.0
125 mL/hr of normal saline ×24 hr	10,600	462	26.25

1 mEq Na = 23 mg; 2.5 mg NaCl contains 1 mg Na.

Sugar

The consumption of sugar in the American diet increased throughout the 20th century, continuing a trend that began in the 19th century when inexpensive methods of sugar production developed. The average annual per capita consumption was estimated to be 75 pounds in 1909, rising to approximately 130 pounds today. Sugar comprises approximately 25% of the total energy consumption in the U.S. diet. As an energy-dense nutrient that is easily consumed, it contributes to excess caloric intake and thus influences the development of obesity and diabetes. It also contributes to the development of dental caries.

Three-fourths of dietary sugar is sucrose, the type found in refined sugars; the remaining dietary sugars (fructose, maltose, lactose) come from natural foods such as fruit, honey, and milk. Sugar is added to many manufactured foods, including products not thought of as "sweet," such as salad dressings, mayonnaise, catsup, bread, crackers, and chips. Table 15.15 lists the sugar and caloric content of a variety of modern foodstuffs.

TABLE 15.15 Sugar Content of Selected Foods

Food Item	Sugar Content (g)	Total Sugar Calories	Total Serving Calories[a]
Teaspoon of sugar	4.5	18	18
Soda, 12 oz[b]	40	160	160
Ice cream, 1 cup	32	128	340
Yogurt, 4 oz	29	116	130
Juice, 8 oz	26	104	104
Chocolate bar, 1.6 oz	22	88	230
Cookie, 1 oz	21	84	120
Crackers, 5	16	64	70

[a]Includes sugar and nonsugar calories.
[b]Diet sodas contain less than 10 calories per 12 oz.

TABLE 15.16 Fiber Content of Selected Foods

Food Serving	Fiber Content (g)
Lettuce	0.5
White bread slice	0.6
Tomato	1.4
Wheat bread slice	2.0
Green beans	2.0
Oatmeal	2.6
Broccoli	2.7
Granola	3.0
Orange	3.1
Apple	3.7
Popcorn	4.0
Raisin Bran	6.0
Chili beans	6.0

Fiber

Since the 1960s, the importance of fiber in the diet has become more appreciated. It had been considered an inert ingredient until clinical studies revealed an association between colonic disease and the lack of fiber in the diet, and a favorable effect of fiber on blood sugar control in diabetes.

There are six vegetal fiber constituents: gum, mucilage, pectin, hemicellulose, lignin, and cellulose. All but the latter two are at least partially digested by human colonic bacteria. The term *bran* generally refers to the form of fiber that passes unaltered through the digestive tract, usually consisting of cellulose, hemicellulose, and lignin. Dietary fiber has hydrophilic activity and increases the water content of small intestinal and colonic stool. These factors explain why fiber increases stool bulk and diminishes bowel transit time (31). Dietary fiber also slows gastric emptying time and moderates carbohydrate absorption rates (32). Fiber can increase the fecal loss of nutrients, but this effect has not been associated with overt nutritional deficiency. Table 15.16 shows the fiber content of common foods.

SPECIFIC REFERENCES*

1. McGinnis JM, Foege WH. Actual causes of death in the United States. JAMA 1993;270:2207.
2. National Research Council. Nutrient adequacy: Assessment using food consumption surveys. Report of the subcommittee on Criteria for Dietary Evaluation, Food and Nutrition Board, Commission on Life Services. Washington, DC: National Academy Press, 1986.
3. USDA/USDHHS. Dietary Guidelines for Americans 2005. 6th ed. 2005. Available at www.healthierus.gov/dietaryguidelines. Last accessed December 17, 2005.
4. Food and Nutrition Board, Institute of Medicine. Food labeling, toward national unity. Washington, DC: National Academy Press, 1992.
5. Nutrition Labeling of Food. Food and Drugs. 21 C.F.R. 101.9, 1996.
6. Food and Nutrition Board, National Research Council: Recommended daily allowances. 10th ed. Washington, DC: National Academy Press, 1989.
7. Institute of Medicine. Dietary Reference Intakes website. Available at www.iom.edu/Object.File/Master/21/372/0.pdf. Last accessed December 18, 2005.
8. Organic Food Standards and Labels: The National Organic Program. Available at www.ams.usda.gov/nop/Consumers/brochure.html and www.ams.usda.gov/nop/NOP/Policy Statements/OrgProdIngre. html. Both last accessed December 18, 2005.
9. National Center for Health Statistics. National Health and Nutrition Examination Survey. Available at http://www.cdc.gov/nchs/nhanes.htm.
10. Center for Nutrition Policy and Promotion, U.S. Department of Agriculture. The Healthy Eating Index. Available at warp.nal.usda.gov/fnic/HEI/hlthyeat.pdf. Last accessed December 18, 2005.
11. Pennington JAT, Douglass JS. Bowes & Church's food values portions community used. 18th ed. Philadelphia: Lippincott Williams & Wilkins, 2005.
12. Murray CJL, Lopez AD. Mortality by cause for eight regions of the world: global burden of disease study. Lancet 1997;349:1269.
13. Murray CJL, Lopez AD. Global mortality, disability, and the contribution of risk factors: global burden of disease study. Lancet 1997; 349:1436.
14. Young VR, Pellett PL. Plant proteins in relation to human protein and amino acid nutrition. Am J Clin Nutr 1994;59:1203S.
15. Young VR. Soy protein in relation to human protein and amino acid nutrition. JADA 1991; 91:823.
16. Key TJ, Fraser GE, Thorogood M, et al. Mortality in vegetarians and non-vegetarians: detailed findings from a collaborative analysis of five prospective studies. Am J Clin Nutr 1999; 70:516S.
17. Appleby PN, Thorogood M, Mann JI, et al. The Oxford vegetarian study. Am J Clin Nutr 1999; 70:525S.
18. Joshipura KJ, Hu FB, Manson JE, et al. The effect of fruit and vegetable intake on risk for coronary heart disease. Ann Intern Med 2001; 134:1106.
19. Mozaffarian D, Kumanyika SK, Lemaitre RN, et al. Cereal, fruit, and vegetable fiber intake and the risk of cardiovascular disease in elderly individuals. JAMA 2003;289:1659.
20. Pereira MA, O'Reilly E, Augustsson K, et al. Dietary fiber and risk of coronary heart disease: a pooled analysis of cohort studies. Arch Intern Med 2004;164:370.
21. Singh RB, Dubnov G, Niaz MA, et al. Effect of an Indo-Mediterranean diet on progression of coronary artery disease in high risk patients (Indo-Mediterranean Diet Heart Study): a randomized single-blind study. Lancet 2002; 360:1455.
22. Fraser GE. Associations between diet and cancer, ischemic heart disease and all-cause mortality in non-Hispanic white California Seventh-Day Adventists. Am J Clin Nutr 1999;70:532S.
23. Dwyer JT. Vegetarian eating patterns: science, values and food choices—where do we go from here? Am J Clin Nutr 1994;59:1255S.
24. Haddad EH, Berk LS, Kettering JD, et al. Dietary intake and biochemical, hematologic and immune status of vegans compared to non-vegetarians. Am J Clin Nutr 1999;70:586S.
25. Higginbottom MC, Sweetman L, Nyhan WL. A syndrome of methylmalonic aciduria, homocystinuria, megaloblastic anemia and neurologic abnormalities in a vitamin B_{12}-deficient breast-fed infant of a strict vegetarian. N Engl J Med 1978;299:317.
26. Dwyer JT, Dietz WM, Huss G, et al. Risk of nutritional rickets among vegetarian children. Am J Dis Child 1979;133:134.
27. Anderson GH, Rolls BJ, Steffen DG. Nutritional implications of macronutrient substitutes. Ann N Y Acad Sci 1997;819:51.
28. Westerterp-Plantenga MS, Fredix EWHM, Steffens AB, et al. Food intake and energy expenditure. Boca Raton, FL: CRC Press, 1994: 247–250.
29. Fregley MJ. Attempts to estimate sodium intake in humans. In: Horan MJ, Blaustein M, Dunbar JB, eds. National Institute of Health workshop on nutrition and hypertension. New York: Biomedical Information, 1985: 93–112.
30. Dahl LK, Love RA. Etiological role of sodium chloride intake in essential hypertension in humans. JAMA 1957;164:397.
31. Burkitt DP, Walker ARP, Printer NS. Effect of dietary fiber on stools and transit times, and its role in the causation of disease. Lancet 1972; 2:1408.
32. Holt S, Heading, RC, Carter DC, et al. Effect of gel, fibre or gastric emptying on absorption of glucose and paracetamol. Lancet 1979;1:636.

*Bold numerals denote published controlled clinical trials, meta-analyses, or consensus-based recommendations.

For annotated **General References** *and resources related to this chapter, visit www.hopkinsbayview.org/PAMreferences.*

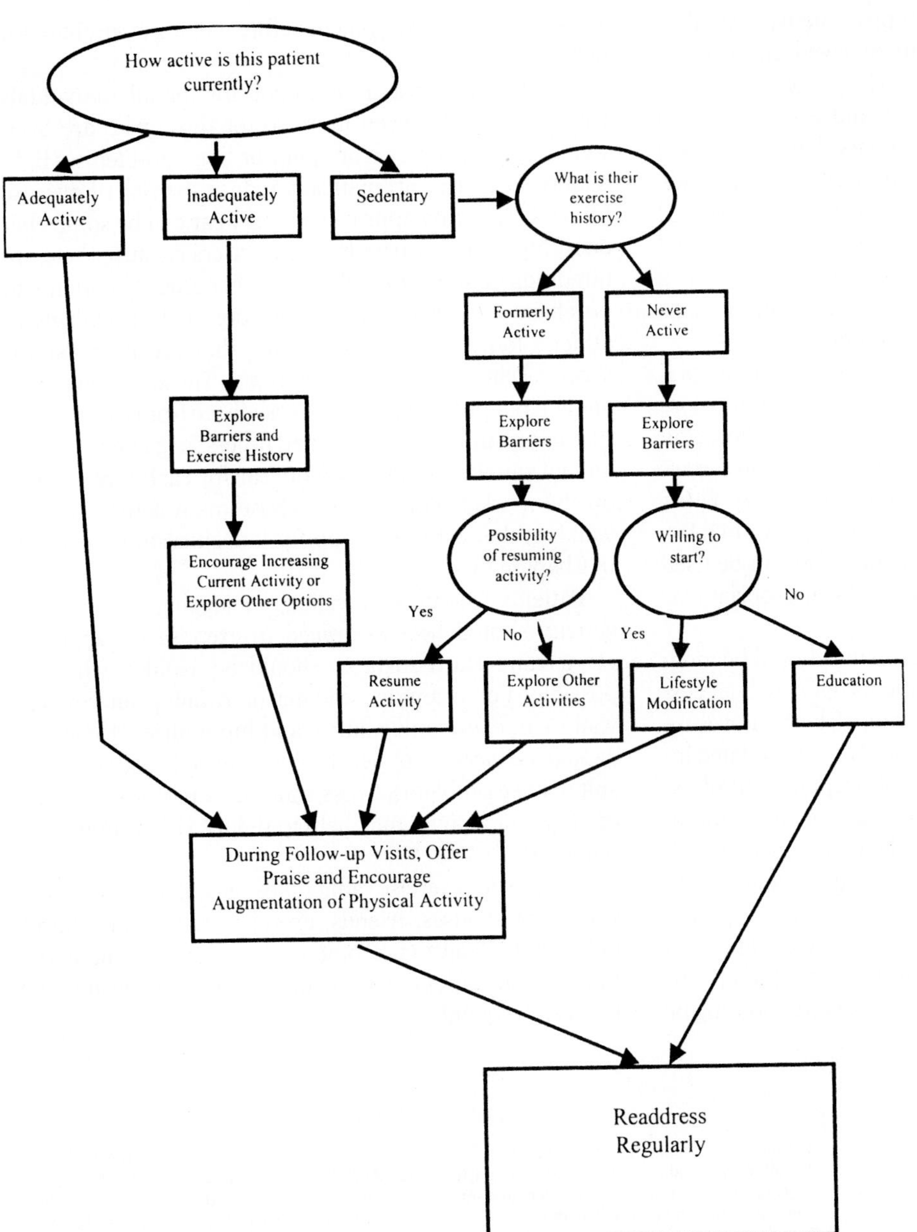

FIGURE 16.2. A framework for physicians to initiate discussion about exercise and physical activity. (From Christmas C, Andersen RE. Exercise and older patients: guidelines for the clinician. J Am Geriatr Soc 2000;48:318, with permission.)

TABLE 16.5 Barriers to and Predictors of Exercise Adherence

Predictor	*Barrier*
Physician's suggestion	Time interruption
Time-efficient routine	Lack of interest in exercise
Freedom from injury	Musculoskeletal injury
Instruction	Lack of knowledge
Feedback on fitness progress	Inadequate leadership
Spouse and peer approval	Lack of spousal support
Group participation	Poor progress awareness
Past participation	Boredom
Risk of disease	High-intensity exercise
Regular routine	Inclement weather

It is also important to capitalize on the fact that persons who are aware of the health benefits of exercise are more likely to become regular exercisers (45). Printed materials and lists of suggested reading can help the patient to self-educate and may also enhance adherence (Table 16.2).

A *lack of time* is one of the most common reasons cited by adults for not exercising. Let patients know that three programmed workouts per week for a minimum of 20 minutes is optimal but that doing something is much better than no activity at all because the greatest gains to health, as described earlier, are derived by moving from being totally sedentary to a moderate level of fitness. In many cases, patients are able to find more time for exercising once they become active and notice results from the program.

Periodic *feedback* on health improvements related to lifestyle improvement can lead to renewed enthusiasm. Recording prescribed physical activity in patient charts can help with followup office visits and exercise-related discussions. Office-based measurements that can be used as measures of success are reductions in resting heart rate, blood pressure, and body mass index and an improved lipid profile. At home, the individual should be encouraged to monitor their exercise performance (i.e., time to walk a mile, number of steps per day) body weight, and perhaps more important, their waist circumference.

Choosing the intensity level is important. Sedentary persons who begin exercising at moderate intensities are more likely to adhere to their programs than those who begin vigorously. Excessive frequencies (e.g., more than 5 days per week) or intensities that the patient perceives as being "hard" may also lead to higher dropout rates (43,45). The Borg Rating of Perceived Exertion scale can be used to help patients understand and select the appropriate exercise intensities (46).

To *reduce the risk of injury*, progression should be moderate as well, because sedentary patients who are unaccustomed to regular activity are at greater risk of an overuse injury from starting out too vigorously. Exercise-related injuries predictably increase the risk of dropping out of exercise programs. A 5% per week increase in the duration or intensity of training sessions will help to reduce the risk of injury. Individuals who use exercise equipment should also be encouraged to learn how to adjust the equipment to minimize injury risk. For example, a bicycle seat that is set too low may result in knee pain. Patients should consider a trial membership at a health club before joining or as a way of trying equipment before making a purchase for home use.

Appropriate footwear is important for all individuals who exercise, but even more so for those who are overweight or who suffer from joint or bone problems. High-quality shoes can dramatically reduce the risk of overuse injuries. Selecting appropriate footwear can be somewhat daunting for many beginning exercisers because there are hundreds of shoes to pick from. Encouraging patients to purchase their shoes from a vendor that specializes in athletic footwear will ensure that they receive a "sport-specific" shoe that is properly fitted. Those patients with known foot problems should seek advice from a podiatrist. Popular running magazines and fitness magazines publish annual ranking of the top footwear for each type of shoe on the market. For persons whose main activity will be walking, the features of appropriate shoes are illustrated in Chapter 73.

Patients who choose walking or jogging as a mode of activity should be encouraged to exercise on appropriate terrain. Hard surfaces should be avoided whenever possible. For example, walking or running on concrete walks can cause ankle, knee, and hip injuries. Uneven or canted surfaces (e.g., beaches or crowned roads) may result in knee problems. Cross-training or performing different types of activity may help to reduce risk of injury and boredom.

Long-term exercise adherence is enhanced by *support* from spouses, friends, exercise leaders, and family (42,43,47). Health care practitioners can become a vital link in their patient's social support network, even if contact is infrequent.

SPECIFIC REFERENCES*

1. U.S. Department of Health and Human Services. Physical Activity and Health: A Report of the Surgeon General. Atlanta, GA: U.S. Department of Health and Human Services, Centers for Disease Control and Prevention, National Center for Chronic Disease Prevention and Health Promotion, 1996.
2. Crespo CJ, Keteyian SJ, Snelling A, et al. Prevalence of no leisure-time physical activity in persons with chronic disease. Clin Exerc Physiol 2000;1:68.
3. Crespo CJ, Smit E, Andersen RE, et al. Race/ethnicity, social class and their relation to physical inactivity during leisure time: results from the Third National Health and Nutrition Examination Survey, 1988–1994. Am J Prev Med 2000;18:46.
4. Ma J, Urizar GG Jr, Alehegn T, et al. Diet and physical activity counseling during ambulatory care visits in the United States. Prev Med 2004;39:815.
5. Thompson PD, Buchner D, Pina IL, et al. Exercise and physical activity in the prevention and treatment of atherosclerotic cardiovascular disease: a statement from the Council on Clinical Cardiology (Subcommittee on Exercise, Rehabilitation, and Prevention) and the Council on Nutrition, Physical Activity, and Metabolism (Subcommittee on Physical Activity). Circulation 2003;107:3109.
6. U.S. Department of Health and Human Services. Healthy People 2010. 2nd ed. Washington, DC: U.S. Government Printing Office, November, 2000. Also available at www.healthypeople.gov/. Last accessed September 11, 2005.
7. Stewart KJ, Bacher AC, Turner K, et al. Exercise and risk factors associated with metabolic syndrome in older adults. Am J Prev Med 2005; 28:9.
8. Blair SN, Kohl HW, Paffenbarger RS. Physical fitness and all-cause mortality: a prospective study of healthy men and women. JAMA 1989; 262:2395.
9. Hu FB, Willett WC, Li T, et al. Adiposity as compared with physical activity in predicting mortality among women. N Engl J Med 2004;351:2694.
10. Crespo CJ, Palmieri MR, Perdomo RP, et al. The relationship of physical activity and body weight with all-cause mortality: results from the Puerto Rico Heart Health Program. Ann Epidemiol 2002;12:543.
11. Bauman AE. Updating the evidence that physical activity is good for health: an epidemiological review 2000–2003. J Sci Med Sport 2004;7:6.
12. Paffenbarger RS Jr, Kampert JB, Lee I-M, et al. Changes in physical activity and other lifestyle patterns influencing longevity. Med Sci Sports Exerc 1994;26:857.
13. Gregg EW, Cauley JA, Stone K, et al. Relationship of changes in physical activity and mortality among older women. JAMA 2003; 289:2379.
14. American College of Sports Medicine, Whaley MH, Brubaker PH, Otto RMV, et al., eds. ACSM's guidelines for exercise testing and prescription. 7th ed. Philadelphia: Lippincottt Williams & Wilkins, 2006.
15. Eden KB, Orleans CT, Mulrow CD, et al. Does counseling by clinicians improve physical activity? A summary of the evidence for the U.S. Preventive Services Task Force. Ann Intern Med 2002;137:208.
16. Jakicic JM, Winters C, Lang W, et al. Effects of intermittent exercise and use of home exercise equipment on adherence, weight loss, and fitness in overweight women: a randomized trial. JAMA 1999;282:1554.
17. Dunn AL, Andersen RE, Jakicic JM. Lifestyle physical activity interventions: history, short- and long-term effects, and recommendations. Am J Prev Med 1998;15:398.
18. Blair SN. 1993 C.H. McCloy research lecture:

*Bold numerals denote published controlled clinical trials, meta-analyses, or consensus-based recommendations.

physical activity, physical fitness, and health. Res Q Exerc Sport 1993;64:365.
19. Blair SN. Living with exercise. Dallas, TX: American Health, 1991.
20. Tudor-Locke C, Bassett DR Jr. How many steps/day are enough? Preliminary pedometer indices for public health. Sports Med 2004;34:1.
21. Saris WH, Blair SN, Van Baak MA, et al. How much physical activity is enough to prevent unhealthy weight gain? Outcome of the IASO 1st stock conference and consensus statement. Obes Rev 2003;4:101.
22. Katzmarzyk PT, Church TS, Janssen I, et al. Metabolic syndrome, obesity, and mortality: impact of cardiorespiratory fitness. Diabetes Care 2005;28:391.
23. Blair SN. Evidence for success of exercise in weight loss and control. Ann Intern Med 1993;119:702.
24. Lee CD, Blair SN, Jackson AS. Cardiovascular fitness, body composition, and all-cause and cardiovascular disease mortality in men. Am J Clin Nutr 1999;69:373.
25. Stewart KJ, Bacher AC, Turner KL, et al. Effect of exercise on blood pressure in older persons: a randomized controlled trial. Arch Intern Med 2005;165:756.
26. American College of Sports Medicine. Recommended quantity and quality of exercise for developing and maintaining cardiorespiratory and muscular fitness in healthy adults. Med Sci Sports Exerc 1990;22:265.
27. Pollock ML, Wilmore JH. Exercise in health and disease: evaluation and prescription for prevention and rehabilitation. 2nd ed. Philadelphia: WB Saunders, 1997.
28. Fiatorone MA, O'neill EF, Ryan ND, et al. Exercise training and nutritional supplementation for physical frailty in very elderly people. N Engl J Med 1994;330:1769.
29. Fletcher GF, Balady G, Blair SN, et al. Statement on exercise: benefits and recommendations for physical activity programs for all Americans. A statement for health professionals by the committee on exercise and cardiac rehabilitation of the council on clinical cardiology, American Heart Association. Circulation 1996;94:857.
30. Cress ME, Schechtman KB, Mulrow CD, et al. Relationship between physical performance and self-perceived physical function. J Am Geriatr Soc 1995;43:93.
31. Fiatorone MA, Marks EC, Ryan ND, et al. High-intensity strength training in nonagenarians. JAMA 1990;263:3029.
32. Nelson ME, Fiatorone MA, Morganti CM, et al. Effects of high-intensity strength training on multiple risk factors for osteoporotic fractures. A randomized controlled trial. JAMA 1994;272: 1909.
33. Liu-Ambrose T, Khan KM, Eng JJ, et al. Resistance and agility training reduce fall risk in women aged 75 to 85 with low bone mass: a 6-month randomized, controlled trial. J Am Geriatr Soc 2004;52:657.
34. Weaver FJ, Herrick KL, Ramirez AG et al. Establishing a community data-base for cardiovascular health education programs. Health Values 1978;2:249.
35. Woodwell DA, Cherry DK. National ambulatory medical care survey: 2002 summary. Adv Data 2004;346:1–44. Available at www.cdc.gov/nchs/about/major/ahcd/ahcd1.htm. Last accessed September 11, 2005.
36. Campbell MK, Devellis BM, Strecher VJ, et al. Improving dietary behavior: the effectiveness of tailored messages in primary care settings. Am J Public Health 1994;84:783.
37. Strecher VJ, O'Malley MS, Villagra VG, et al. Can residents be trained to counsel patients about smoking? Results from a randomized trial. J Gen Intern Med 1991;6:9.
38. Strecher VJ, Kreuter M, Boer DJ, et al. The effects of computer tailored smoking cessation messages in family practice settings. J Fam Pract 1994;39:262.
39. Strecher VJ, Seijts GH, Kok GJ, et al. Goal setting as a strategy for health behavior change. Health Educ Q 1995;22:190.
40. Patrick K, Sallis JF, Long B, et al. A new tool for encouraging activity: Project PACE. Physician Sports Med 1994;22:245.
41. Kohl HW, III, Powell KE, Gordon NF, et al. Physical activity, physical fitness, and sudden cardiac death. Epidemiol Rev 1992;14:37.
42. Dishman RK. Determinants of participation in activity. In: Bouchard C, Shephard RJ, Stephens T, et al., eds. Exercise, fitness, and health: a consensus of current knowledge. Champaign, IL: Human Kinetics, 1990: 75–101.
43. King AC, Blair SN, Bild DE, et al. Determinants of physical activity and interventions in adults. Med Sci Sports Exerc 1992;24:S221.
44. Marcus BH, Pinto BM, Clark MM, et al. Physician-delivered physical activity and nutrition interventions. Med Exerc Nutr Health 1995;4:325.
45. Rohm-Young D, King AC. Exercise adherence: determinants of physical activity and applications of health behavior change theories. Med Exerc Nutr Health 1995;4:335.
46. Borg GAV. Psychological bases of perceived exertion. Med Sci Sports Exerc 1982;14:377.
47. Dishman RK. Supervised and free-living physical activity: no differences in former athletes and nonathletes. Am J Prev Med 1988;4:153.

For annotated ***General References*** *and resources related to this chapter, visit www.hopkinsbayview.org/PAMreferences.*

Chapter 17

Genetic Testing and Counseling

Jennifer E. Axilbund and Constance A. Griffin

Numerous genes present in normal-appearing individuals can affect an individual's susceptibility to disease or contribute to the way an individual metabolizes particular drugs. Generalist clinicians need to be able to recognize genetic syndromes that may have a significant impact on their patients' future health. This chapter provides an overview of basic genetics, summarizes currently recognized genetic syndromes important in the practice of adult medicine, and describes the role of genetic testing and counseling in today's medical practice.

PRIMER OF BASIC GENETICS AND INHERITANCE

Genetic Code

The genetic code is spelled out in our deoxyribonucleic acid (DNA). DNA is built of a combination of nucleotides, including purines (adenine [A], guanine [G]), and pyrimidines (cytosine [C], thymine [T]). DNA is further arranged in a double helix, held together by hydrogen bonds between the complementary bases (A pairs with T, C pairs with G). The 20 amino acids found in the proteins of humans are spelled out using the four nucleotide bases. A sequence of three bases is called a *codon;* each codon codes for a specific amino acid. Because 64 combinations of bases are possible ($4 \times 4 \times 4$), the code is redundant, meaning that some amino acids are coded for by several different combinations of bases. The gene specified by the DNA is transcribed into messenger ribonucleic acid (RNA) and then translated into specific proteins. Not all DNA codes for proteins. Some DNA codes for "worker" RNA. Other DNA has structural functions at parts of the chromosomes called centromeres. The function of much of the DNA remains unknown. The process of translating the code from our DNA to the specified gene product (i.e., protein) is complex and requires editing functions that are specified in the code itself.

DNA is packaged into *chromosomes,* which are physical structures in the cell nucleus consisting of DNA and associated proteins. Humans have 46 chromosomes, arranged in 23 pairs. Twenty-two of these pairs are *autosomes,* meaning they are found in both males and females. The 23rd pair, consisting of XX or XY, specifies the individual's sex. During production of germline cells, namely eggs or sperm, the chromosomes undergo a reduction to haploidy, or a single set of chromosomes. When fertilization occurs, diploidy (two sets) is restored by the combination of one set of chromosomes from the mother and one set from the father.

In the process of duplicating our DNA, copy changes can occur. *Polymorphisms* are alterations that occur in the genetic code for a protein but that do not result in loss of function of the protein. The term *mutation* is generally reserved for changes in DNA sequence that alter the coded protein significantly. Types of mutations observed range from single base-pair substitutions, such as insertions or deletions of one or a few bases, to mutations that cause a shift in the DNA reading frame, resulting in a premature stop of protein translation.

Types of Inheritance

Gregor Mendel described the basic types of inheritance, and from his name comes the term "mendelian inheritance." This term describes single-gene inheritance. Individuals have two copies (alleles) of each gene and receive one copy of each gene from the germ cells of each parent. *Autosomal dominant disease* requires only a single abnormal copy of the gene to manifest disease. Examples of autosomal dominant diseases include Huntington disease and many of the recognized cancer predisposition syndromes. *Autosomal recessive diseases* require the inheritance of an abnormal copy of the gene from both the mother and the father. Cystic fibrosis is a well-known example in which phenotypically normal parents are only recognized to be carriers of a mutant allele when they have a child who has inherited the dysfunctional forms of the gene from both parents. *Sex-linked disease* means that the disease gene is located on a sex chromosome. Most sex-linked diseases are linked to the X chromosome. With X-linked inheritance, women typically do not manifest disease even when they inherit a mutant gene because the normal copy of the gene on their other X chromosome compensates. Men, with only a single copy of the X chromosome, are not protected by a normal gene copy and therefore manifest disease. Duchenne muscular dystrophy and hemophilia A are examples of sex-linked diseases.

Other disorders, including common diseases such as diabetes mellitus and hypertension, may involve the interactive effects of multiple genes. This is referred to as *polygenic or multifactorial inheritance,* and simple rules of mendelian inheritance seem not to apply. *Mitochondrial inheritance* describes yet another form of inheritance, because mitochondria, and, therefore, the genome of the mitochondria, are inherited only from the egg of the mother. Mitochondrial diseases include oxidative phosphorylation disorders, and widely varying manifestations can include specific types of cardiomyopathy, deafness, skeletal myopathy, and renal tubular acidoses, to name just a few.

The term *genotype* describes the genetic composition of an individual, whereas the term *phenotype* refers to the physical manifestations of a given genetic blueprint. Similar phenotypes can result from mutations in different genes presumably in related pathways; the specific molecular alteration in a gene may also relate to the phenotype observed. *Penetrance* of a gene refers to the likelihood that an abnormal form of a gene will be observed to cause an abnormal phenotype during an individual's lifetime. Some genes are high penetrance, such as those causing the hereditary forms of breast and ovarian cancer. Such individuals have a lifetime risk of developing breast cancer that is as high as 85%. Other genes are of relatively low penetrance, such as the I1307K mutation in the *APC* gene. This mutation is found in approximately 6% of the Ashkenazi Jewish population and is correlated with a lifetime colon cancer risk estimated to be between 10% and 30%. The interaction of environmental exposure, mutation repair, and the presence of other modifier genes presumably combine to affect the expression of disease.

CORE COMPETENCIES IN GENETICS

Health care professionals ordering genetic testing must be adequately trained to provide genetic counseling, obtain informed consent, and correctly interpret test results. Because availability of specialized genetics services is still limited, the generalist may be called upon to provide genetic counseling as part of routine care. The Core Competency Working Group of the National Coalition for Health Professional Education in Genetics has proposed a set of core competencies in genetics, of which the major components are listed here. The original publication describes the competencies in their entirety (1).

All health professionals should understand the following:

- The basic patterns of biologic inheritance and variation within families and populations;
- How identification of disease-associated genetic variations facilitates development of prevention, diagnosis, and treatment options;
- The difference between clinical diagnosis of disease and identification of genetic predisposition to disease;
- The influence of ethnicity, culture, related health beliefs, and economics in the client's ability to use genetic information and services;
- The potential physical and/or psychosocial benefits, limitations, and risks of genetic information for individuals, family members, and communities;
- The ethical, legal, and social issues related to genetic testing and recording of genetic information;
- The resources available to assist clients seeking genetic information or services;
- One's own professional role in the referral to genetic services or provision, followup, and quality review of genetic services.

All health professionals should be able to:

- Gather genetic family history information, including an appropriate (a minimum of three generations) family history;
- Identify clients who would benefit from genetic services;
- Explain basic concepts of probability and disease susceptibility and the influence of genetic factors in maintenance of health and development of disease;
- Seek assistance from and refer to appropriate genetics experts and peer support resources;
- Obtain credible current information about genetics for self, clients, and colleagues;
- Recognize the importance of delivering genetic education and counseling fairly, accurately, and without coercion or personal bias;
- Seek coordination and collaboration with an interdisciplinary team of health professionals;
- Recognize the limitations of their own genetics expertise.

The need for these competencies is illustrated in a study by Giardiello et al. (2), who examined physicians' ordering and interpretation of genetic testing for familial adenomatous polyposis (FAP). Eighty-three percent of tests were ordered for valid indications, but only 18.6% of patients received genetic counseling, only 16.9% of patients provided written consent, and 31.6% of test results were misinterpreted by the ordering physician.

MENDELIAN GENETIC DISORDERS

In contrast to genetic diseases recognized in childhood such as cystic fibrosis or Duchenne muscular dystrophy, a number of other genetic disorders, in addition to hereditary cancer, may not be recognized until the person is an adult. Some, such as Marfan syndrome, have major clinical phenotypic manifestations and very specific diagnostic criteria (see General References, Useful Websites, Online Mendelian Inheritance in Man). Genetic testing is available for many of these disorders, a subset of which is illustrated in Table 17.1. In contrast, a number of inherited diseases lack specific phenotypic features but may present with abnormal laboratory values or with common clinical events such as venous thrombosis (see examples in Table 17.2).

Profile of a Common Inherited Disease: Hemochromatosis

Hereditary hemochromatosis is a genetic disease with significant implications for the generalist. It is an autosomally recessively inherited disease, in which early diagnosis and treatment can lead to a normal to near-normal life span; the phenotypic manifestations are not usually apparent before significant iron overload has occurred. The causative gene is *HFE*, and mutations can result in inappropriately high absorption of iron by the gastrointestinal tract. Excess iron stores in the liver, pancreas, heart, skin, and other organs first produce only nonspecific symptoms, but left untreated, ultimately patients develop hepatic fibrosis or cirrhosis, diabetes mellitus, congestive heart failure, and other problems. Symptoms usually develop between ages 40 and 60 years in males, and somewhat later in females, after menopause.

Diagnosis in patients with symptoms is usually based on a serum transferrin iron saturation of greater than 60% for men and greater than 50% for women on at least two different determinations, in the absence of other causes of primary and secondary iron overload disorders. *Heterozygotes* (individuals carrying one copy of normal allele and one copy of mutant allele) do tend to have serum iron and

TABLE 17.1 Examples of Genetic Diseases with Specific Phenotypic Features for Which Genetic Testing Is Available

Disease	*Characteristics*	*Gene(s) Involved*	*Type of Inheritance*	*Clinical Management*	*Prevalence*
Marfan syndrome	Systemic disorder of connective tissue; high variability. Tall, thin, with long limbs, hands, feet	*FBN1*	AD	At risk for dislocated lens, aortic root dilation, mitral valve prolapse, scoliosis	1/5,000–10,000
Fragile X syndrome	Moderate mental retardation in males; mild mental retardation in affected females; abnormal faces	*FMR* (triple repeat expansion)	X-linked dominant (mothers of affected individuals carry presymptomatic gene expansion	Supportive care; genetic counseling for family members	Full mutation: males 1/3,600; females 1/4,000–6,000 Premutation: males 1/800; females 1/250
Huntington disease	Progressive motor, cognitive, psychiatric disorder	*HD* (triple repeat expansion)	AD	Only symptomatic treatment; genetic counseling of family members	1/20,000
Cystic fibrosis	Extensive airway damage, pancreatic insufficiency with malabsorption	*CFTR*	AR	Vigorous pulmonary intervention including antibiotics, mucolytics, chest physiotherapy; oral pancreatic enzyme replacement	Disease prevalence: whites, 1/3,200; African Americans, 1/15,000; Asian Americans, 1/31,000 Carrier frequency: whites, 1/28; African Americans, 1/61; Asian Americans, 1/88

AD, autosomal dominant; AR, autosomal recessive disease.

TABLE 17.2 Examples of Genetic Diseases without Specific Phenotypic Features for Which Genetic Testing Is Available

Disease	*Characteristics*	*Gene(s) Involved*	*Type of Inheritance*	*Clinical Management*	*Prevalence*
Hereditary hemochromatosis	Excessive iron storage in liver, heart, pancreas, other organs; penetrance >90% for homozygotes	*HFE*	AR	Diagnosis of clinical disease requires clinical, biochemical, histologic, and gene studies; removal of excess iron by phlebotomy	Disease prevalence: 1/400 Carrier frequency: 1/8–10
Factor V Leiden	Increased risk for venous thrombosis	*F5* ("Leiden" mutation is a specific single-base change)	AD	Prolonged anticoagulation following thrombotic event	Whites, 1/19; African Americans, 1/83; Asian Americans, 1/222 (mutation found in 15%–20% of patients with one DVT; 50% with repeated DVTs)
Long QT syndrome	ECG: QTc interval prolonged; hallmark arrhythmia *torsade de pointes*; primary presenting symptom is syncope	SCN5A, KCNE1, KCNH2, KCNE2, KCNQ1 (account for 70% of detectable mutations)	AD	Medication (beta blockers), pacemakers, implantable cardiac defibrillators	1/5,000–10,000

AD, autosomal dominant disease; AR, autosomal recessive disease; DVT, deep venous thrombosis; ECG, electrocardiogram.

ferritin and transferrin saturation levels that exceed normal but do not develop clinical iron overload. Confirmatory tests after the elevated transferrin iron saturation include liver biopsy or genetic testing for the two mutations that have been observed. Between 60% and 90% of patients with hereditary hemochromatosis (varies with the population) are *homozygotes* (individuals in whom both alleles of a gene are mutant) for the missense mutation C282Y. Approximately 3% are *compound heterozygotes:* they have one copy of the C282Y mutation and their second copy of the *HFE* gene contains a different missense mutation (H63D). The remainder of individuals with clinical manifestations of hereditary hemochromatosis have other mutations in the *HFE* gene or no identifiable mutation in the *HFE* gene. Molecular identification of the type(s) of mutations present in an affected individual is important, because C282Y homozygotes have greater degrees of iron overload than do compound heterozygotes. Identification of mutation in affected individuals allows predictive testing in their at-risk siblings and children. Treatment of hereditary hemochromatosis is by phlebotomy at regular intervals.

One in nine individuals in the population carries a mutant *HFE* allele, and the prevalence of individuals with two disease-causing mutations is estimated at approximately 1 in 400. Although the biochemical penetrance of disease (i.e., elevated serum transferrin) is particularly high in C282Y homozygotes, it is not 100%. Precise risk estimates are unknown, but clinical manifestation of iron overload, such as diabetes and cirrhosis, is low. Overall disease penetrance is higher in men than in women, attributed in large part to the regular blood loss associated with menstruation.

Identifying Patients at Risk for Hereditary Cancer

Most cancers are sporadic or nonhereditary in origin. However, approximately 5% to 10% of all cancers are believed to be caused by inherited mutations in cancer-related genes. The characteristics of hereditary cancer include one or more of the following:

- Two or more family members affected with the same type of cancer;
- More than one person in a single generation affected with the same type of cancer;
- Relatives in more than one generation affected with the same type of cancer;
- Ages at diagnosis younger than those seen in the general population;
- A single individual with more than one primary cancer;
- Clustering of two or more types of cancer known to be linked to a particular syndrome (e.g., breast and ovarian; colon and uterine);
- Male breast cancer.

Table 17.3 contains information about selected neoplasias for which genetic testing is available. Several excellent reviews describe the currently recognized cancer predisposition syndromes (3,4). Those identified thus far are those that are strongly influenced by a single gene. The role of additional genes, each of which might contribute a more moderate risk for cancer development, will undoubtedly be elucidated in the future.

COMPLEX GENETIC DISORDERS

Unlike mendelian genetic disorders where the pattern of inheritance is clear, risk assessment is usually more difficult with complex disorders. They are often multifactorial, and phenotypic manifestation is dependent upon numerous variables. The causative genes are more elusive, and genetic testing is seldom available. Thus, family history is the best way to recognize individuals at increased risk for complex genetic disorders. Documentation of family history is made easier through the development of tools, such as those by the American Medical Association and the Surgeon General of the United States (see General References, Useful Websites).

Diabetes Mellitus

Diabetes mellitus is widespread in the United States, and includes type 1, type 2, and gestational diabetes (5). With the exception of maturity-onset diabetes of the young (MODY), which is an autosomal dominant form of non–insulin-dependent diabetes diagnosed prior to age 25 years, diabetes is predominantly thought to be polygenic and multifactorial. Thus, it is caused by the interaction of many genetic and environmental factors, each contributing modestly to the eventual disease presentation. This makes it difficult to identify predisposing genetic factors in the majority of cases.

Almost half of type 1 diabetes is believed to be associated with the major histocompatibility complex human leukocyte antigens (HLAs), but even individuals who possess the highest risk genotype only develop disease 8% of the time (5). Prevention trials are underway, and are focusing on identifying environmental triggers of disease, as well as ways to suppress immunity and slow disease progression. Predictive genetic testing for type 1 diabetes is currently limited to research studies, including the potential for newborn screening.

Type 2 diabetes is strongly associated with obesity; 70% of type 2 diabetics are overweight. However, only 30% of obese Americans have the disease (5). Relatives of nonobese type 2 diabetics are at particularly increased risk. This provides evidence that obesity is an environmental trigger of the underlying genetic predisposition, although the responsible genes remain elusive. As a result, family

TABLE 17.3 Examples of Hereditary Neoplasias for Which Genetic Testing Is Available

Disease	*Characteristics*	*Gene(s) Involved*	*Type of Inheritance*	*Clinical Management*	*Prevalence*
Hereditary nonpolyposis colon cancer (HNPCC)	Early onset colon cancer, uterine cancer, other cancers; 80% penetrance	*MLH1, MSH2, PMS2, MSH6*	AD	Yearly colonoscopy minimizes chance of developing invasive colon cancer	1/500 (accounts for approximately 3% of colon cancer)
Familial adenomatous polyposis (FAP)	Colonic polyposis results in early-age colon cancer, 100% penetrance	*APC*	AD	Screening begins at puberty; eventual prophylactic colectomy	1/33,000 (accounts for approximately 0.5% of colon cancer)
Hereditary breast cancer	Early onset breast/ovarian cancer; male breast cancer	*BRCA1, BRCA2*	AD	Frequent breast and ovarian surveillance	1/500–1,000
Multiple endocrine neoplasia (MEN) type 1	Parathyroid, pancreatic islet, and pituitary tumors; parathyroid adenomas in 90% of patients	*MEN1*	AD	Screening in family with MEN1 begins at ages 5–10 yr	1/30,000
MEN type 2a, 2b	Medullary thyroid cancer, pheochromocytoma, parathyroid hyperplasia	*RET*	AD	Screening and prophylactic thyroidectomy as early as age 5 yr	1/30,000

AD, autosomal dominant disease; AR, autosomal recessive disease.

history remains the best way to identify at-risk individuals so that lifestyle changes and medication may be introduced to prevent disease, or at least slow its progression.

One current public health initiative is to develop an adequate tool to identify individuals at high risk to develop diabetes. Family history intake should include (a) relatives who have diabetes; (b) age of onset; (c) associated conditions, such as obesity or hypertension; and (d) specific disease complications. The latter area is of particular importance, as diabetic complications, such as nephropathy and retinopathy, tend to cluster in families. Ultimately, pharmacogenomics (for a definition, see Future Roles of Genetics in Patient Care) may play a vital role in management of this disease.

Heart Disease

As the leading cause of death in industrialized countries, understanding the genetic risks for coronary artery disease could have significant impact on preventive measures. However, this complex disorder is affected by many risk factors, both genetic and nongenetic, and is thought to result from a combination of several factors. More than 30 single-gene disorders include significant risk for coronary artery disease or myocardial infarction at a young age (6). The mode of inheritance varies with each specific disorder and includes autosomal dominant, autosomal recessive, and polygenic inheritance. Ultimately, most heart disease is multifactorial, and caused by the combination of multiple genetic and environmental factors. The personal and family histories are the most important clues to identifying individuals at risk. The greatest benefit of preventive measures may be for those with a strong genetic predisposition to coronary artery disease.

Hypertrophic cardiomyopathy is the most frequent cause of sudden death from cardiac causes in children and adolescents (7). The incidence is estimated to be 1/500 young adults based on population studies. Inheritance is autosomal dominant, with mutations identified in at least ten different sarcomeric proteins. The clinical course and degree of cardiac dysfunction is highly variable. Genes that predispose to arrhythmia have also been identified; these affect cardiac ion channels (7) and include long QT syndrome, idiopathic ventricular fibrillation, and cardiac conduction disease. Clinical genetic testing is not generally available for the diagnosis of monogenic cardiac disease and diagnosis currently relies on physical examination and clinical testing.

GENETIC COUNSELING AND TESTING FOR HEREDITARY CANCER

The impact of genetic testing on the health of patients has not yet been subjected to extensive clinical trials. In the coming decade, it is likely that much will be learned about

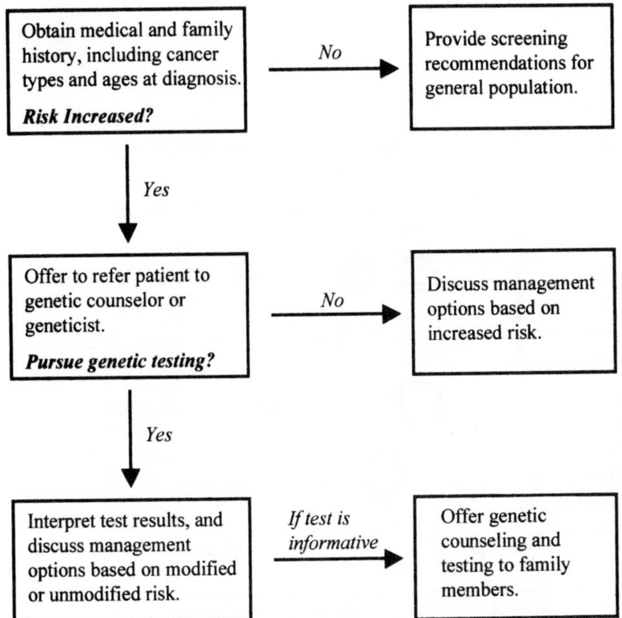

FIGURE 17.1. Recommended approach for a patient contemplating genetic testing for hereditary cancer.

this evolving area of preventive medicine. The approach to testing for genetic susceptibility to disease begins with genetic counseling. The flow diagram in Figure 17.1 illustrates the decisions in this process, beginning with the generalist clinician's recognition of a possible genetic disorder and the decision to offer referral for genetic counseling. Because much of the currently available genetic testing and counseling in adults is cancer related, Fig. 17.1 and the following sections describe the approach to an individual or family in which there may be a hereditary predisposition to cancer. The same approach would pertain to evaluation of other inherited diseases, infertility, and in prenatal diagnostics.

Overview of Counseling and Testing

To ensure that genetic tests are ordered appropriately and interpreted accurately, it is important, whenever possible, to enlist the help of a practitioner trained in cancer genetics. *Genetic counselors* are health care professionals who typically hold a masters-level graduate degree in the field of genetics, and most are certified by the American Board of Genetic Counseling. The National Society of Genetic Counselors maintains a directory of genetic counselors and their affiliated institutions. The cost of a genetic counseling visit usually ranges from $150 to $350. Depending on the problem, patients may need to return for one or more followup visits.

Genetic counseling is generally undertaken in a nondirective fashion (8). Because the decision to undergo genetic testing has family, societal, and insurance implications, it must be an informed decision made by the person who will be tested. Except for the few hereditary cancer syndromes that have onset in childhood and for which treatment is available, testing is not performed on children. The exceptions currently include familial adenomatous polyposis, which requires colon screening beginning at puberty, and multiple endocrine neoplasia type 2, which necessitates thyroidectomy in childhood (Table 17.3).

When a patient schedules a genetic counseling session, a detailed medical and family history is obtained. Relevant information includes type and location of the cancer, age at diagnosis, how the cancer was diagnosed, stage at diagnosis, whether or not the cancer was bilateral, history of other cancers, history of other chronic medical conditions, and history of exposures to carcinogens. Pathology reports are extremely useful when obtaining personal or family history, because patients often have difficulty distinguishing specific cancer types, or primary cancers versus recurrences or metastases.

The *proband* is the individual who comes for consultation. The *consultant* is the parent(s) who comes for consultation when the proband is a minor. The family history is the key to identifying a hereditary pattern of cancer within a family. Information about the proband and his or her parents, grandparents, aunts, uncles, first cousins, siblings, and children is obtained and diagrammed into a three-generation *pedigree* (9) (Fig. 17.2). This diagram makes traits inherited in a mendelian manner easier to recognize. Included is information about unaffected and affected relatives. For each family member, detailed medical history is necessary. It is important to recognize that in some diseases, such as FAP, the rate of new germline mutations is high (approximately 30%), and there may be no family history of disease. However, an individual with a new germline mutation can still pass on the disease to his or her children.

If the medical and family history is suspicious for inherited cancer susceptibility, the patient is educated on specific disease characteristics, basic genetic information, and the pattern of inheritance. If applicable, the risks, benefits, and limitations of genetic testing are reviewed, and the most informative approach to testing is determined. In addition, the patient is told about possible genetic discrimination and about the most current legal decisions regarding genetic testing.

Peripheral blood is usually the specimen of choice for genetic testing. Although some specific testing can be performed on paraffin-embedded formalin-fixed pathology specimens, the preservation of DNA in the specimen may be inadequate for the technical requirements of many of the analytical processes currently in use. The specific type of laboratory test that is performed is related to the type of alteration being sought. Some disease-causing mutations tend to occur in one area or a small number of areas of a gene, and testing can be confidently limited to those regions. An example is multiple endocrine neoplasia type 2b in which more than 90% of cases have the same

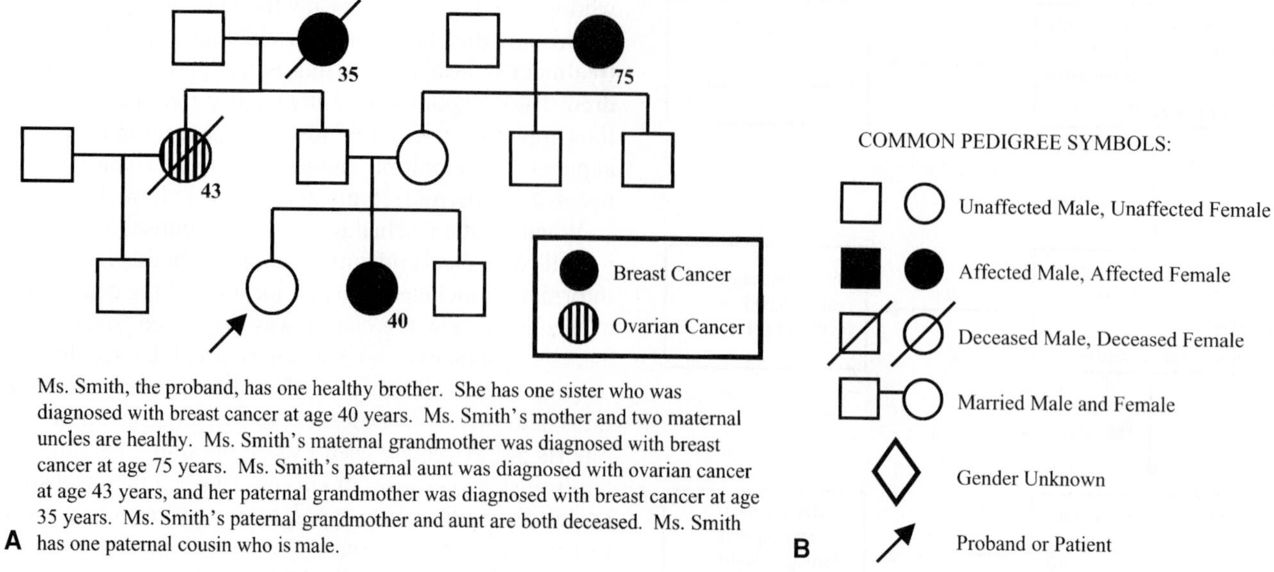

FIGURE 17.2. **A:** Example of a patient's family history diagrammed as a pedigree. **B:** Common pedigree symbols.

mutation. For other genetic disorders, such as hereditary nonpolyposis colon cancer (HNPCC) and BRCA-linked breast cancer, mutations in the relevant genes can occur over many thousands of base pairs. For these disorders, more comprehensive testing, such as DNA sequencing, is necessary. Recent advances also show that large rearrangements account for a significant proportion of genetic abnormalities. Such mutations are typically only detectable using techniques like Southern blot analysis. For these reasons, genetic testing ideally begins with an affected individual, so that one can define the mutation in the family.

If genetic testing detects a specific disease-causing mutation in an affected individual, this is termed *positive*. Other family members can then be tested for that specific mutation and receive definitive (*positive* or *true negative*) results. The test is deemed *inconclusive* if an affected individual is tested but no mutation is found. It is also inconclusive if the affected individual is not available for testing and testing of the at-risk unaffected individual does not identify a known disease-causing mutation. In the latter case, the at-risk person might not have a detectable mutation because he or she did not inherit it; alternatively, the cause of disease in the family may be an undiscovered gene or one for which testing has not been performed. Consequently, to prove that a person has not inherited a specific mutation, it is necessary that such a mutation be detectable using current technology and that it actually exists in the family. Finally, test results are also considered inconclusive if the laboratory detects an alteration in the DNA but is unable to classify it as clearly disease-causing or as a benign polymorphism. This is termed a "variant of uncertain significance." Typically, at-risk relatives are not tested for these variants as their impact on risk is unknown.

Genetic testing for cancer syndromes costs from $250 to more than $3,000, depending on how many laboratories perform a particular test and the technology employed. Many insurance companies cover some or all of the cost if the individual's personal or family history is suggestive of an inherited predisposition and medical necessity can be demonstrated. Very often, test availability is a function of patents or licenses on particular genetic tests. Some testing techniques are more sensitive than others, again based primarily on the type(s) of genetic abnormalities being sought. Depending on test complexity, days to months may elapse before a genetic test result is reported. A genetic test, in general, is classified as a high-complexity test under current Public Health Service Clinical Laboratory Improvement Act of 1988 guidelines. Quality control programs for genetic testing are under development, but at this time, these tests are not specifically regulated. Therefore, choice of a testing laboratory is best left to professionals with experience with specific laboratories.

Management of cancer risk is discussed by the genetic counselor, both with patients interested in genetic testing and those who prefer not to pursue such an analysis. Because genetic test results can drastically alter management, patients are often asked to return after the results are known for final recommendations. Management options include increased surveillance, chemoprevention, prophylactic surgery, and lifestyle alterations. For some disorders, consideration of prophylactic surgery may be indicated, whereas for others, a specific surveillance regimen is more appropriate. This usually depends on the lifetime cancer risk and the efficacy of available screening methods. There is virtually no evidence-based data regarding the impact of preventive behaviors, such as low-fat diet, exercise, and so forth, on the development of cancer in mutation-positive individuals. Because the disorders most often discussed are hereditary, some patients also seek information regarding various reproductive options or genetic testing recommendations for other family members.

Psychosocial Issues

Genetic testing not only impacts the individual patient but other family members as well. Consequently, patients may experience emotions different from those regularly encountered in the clinical setting (10). Positive results can evoke fear, anxiety, or uncertainty. Some patients experience guilt at having potentially passed a mutation to a child or anger for having inherited the mutation from a parent in the first place. Negative results can lead to relief and happiness, but also to survivor's guilt over having been "spared" from the disease that affected family members. Thus, genetic testing may lead to strained familial relationships. Still, some patients report a feeling of relief, regardless of whether the result is positive or negative, because cancer risk to themselves and their family members is better defined and better able to be managed.

It should be noted that each individual has a different perception of high risk versus low risk. To some patients, a 45% risk is still "less than half," whereas others view a 5% to 10% risk as frighteningly high. Therefore, before embarking on genetic testing, it is important to explore the patient's viewpoints. Particular attention should be paid to risk perception, ability to handle a positive or negative result, and patient communication with family members. It is also advantageous to discuss which management options the patient may prefer, knowing that decisions may ultimately be shaped by the results of the genetic testing.

Ethical and Legal Concerns

When involved in genetic testing, it is important to be familiar with ethical, social, and legal issues. As previously addressed, genetic testing provides information about other family members in addition to the individual seeking testing. This raises the ethical dilemma of "duty to warn." In short, is a health care professional required to notify relatives of a patient if a genetic disorder is detected in the family? Thus far, legal decisions on this matter are in conflict, because disclosure of information may violate confidentiality, whereas failure to disclose may be viewed as endangerment. Consequently, the impact of genetic information on family members must be clearly explained to patients.

Another issue is potential discrimination by insurance companies or employers. Currently, the concern is that genetic information will be viewed as evidence for a preexisting condition that insurers will refuse to cover or that will render an individual unemployable. Federal laws, such as the Health Insurance Portability and Accountability Act, provide some protection for individuals who are covered under a group health insurance plan. Many states have enacted protective laws as well. As of now, however, there is no federal legislation regarding patients who have individual health insurance coverage. There is also no protection from discrimination relating to life insurance or disability insurance.

Informed Consent

Because the implications of genetic testing are far-reaching, informed consent is vital. Proper informed consent includes a thorough discussion of the risks, benefits, and limitations of testing. Among other details, the patient should be made aware of what information can and cannot be obtained by the particular test in question. The sensitivity of the test must be clearly explained as well, and the patient should understand that the test may not be informative, meaning that it may not provide information that is useful for risk modification. The patient should also be aware that genetic testing is a personal decision and the patient should not be pressured into obtaining such testing.

In practice, genetic counseling should occur before testing for mutations in cancer-predisposition genes, as discussed above. In contrast, informed consent and extensive counseling before ordering tests for alterations in coagulation predisposition genes, such as factor V Leiden, are uncommon. This may reflect a decreased perception of risk for discrimination or the fact that the mutation in factor V is a simpler, less expensive, more widely available test.

FUTURE ROLES OF GENETICS IN PATIENT CARE

Testing for genetically determined responses to drugs and screening for a broad array of genetic susceptibility to disease may soon be available for use in clinical decision making. As is true of all tests used in clinical preventive medicine, expanded genetic testing and counseling will require critical assessment of their impact on patients' health before they become standards of care.

Pharmacogenomics describes the concept of individualized choice of drug therapy based on knowledge of the differences in drug absorption, metabolism, and excretion as determined by variation in the relevant genes (11). For example, a polymorphism in the gene *NAT2* (*N*-acetyltransferase 2) determines whether an individual is a rapid or slow acetylator of many drugs such as hydralazine and isoniazid. Adverse drug reactions, such as the increased risk for peripheral neuropathy caused by isoniazid, occur more frequently in individuals who are slow acetylators. Identification of increasing numbers of polymorphisms in genes that affect drug metabolism will allow health care practitioners to prescribe some drugs on the basis of the genetic profile of individual patients. This will only occur if testing for such genetic alterations can be performed quickly and inexpensively.

Technologic advances, such as the development of *microarray technology*, offer a way to screen for multiple genetic changes quickly and cheaply. Commonly known as "chips," these are high-density assemblies of oligonucleotides or complementary DNAs on a membrane or glass substrate. Specific DNA sequences can be sought by annealing with fluorescent dye-labeled RNA or DNA in solution and read with the assistance of computer programs. The Human Genome Project, which completed the sequencing of the human genome in 2001, is providing the information needed to develop such diagnostic technology. The day may not be far off when an individual with high blood pressure can be rapidly screened for specific genetic changes that affect blood pressure and the drugs that could be used to treat it, resulting in prescription of individualized rational drug therapy.

Prior to the widespread use of genetic information for clinical decision making, it will be necessary not only to develop efficient and affordable technologies, but also to assess the impact of the introduction of such technologies on clinical outcomes while simultaneously addressing the concerns discussed above regarding privacy and potential discrimination.

SPECIFIC REFERENCES*

1. Core Competency Working Group of the National Coalition for Health Professional Education in Genetics. Recommendations of core competencies in genetics essential for all health professionals. Genet Med 2001; 3:155.
2. Giardiello FM, Bresinger JD, Petersen GM, et al. The use and interpretation of commercial *APC* gene testing for familial adenomatous polyposis. N Engl J Med 1997;336:823.
3. Eng C, Hampel H, de la Chapelle A. Genetic testing for cancer predisposition. Annu Rev Med 2000;52:371.
4. Lindor NM, Greene MH. Mayo Familial Cancer Program. Special article: the concise handbook of family cancer syndromes. J Natl Cancer Inst 1998;90:1039.
5. Newell AM. Genetics for targeting disease prevention: diabetes. Prim Care 2004;31: 743.
6. Scheuner MT. Clinical application of genetic risk assessment strategies for coronary artery disease: genotypes, phenotypes, and family history. Prim Care 2004;31:711.
7. Nabel EG. Cardiovascular disease. N Engl J Med 2003;349:60.
8. Johnson KA, Brensinger JD. Genetic counseling and testing: implications for clinical practice. Nurs Clinic North Am 2000;35:615.
9. Bennett RL, Steinhaus KA, Uhrich SB, et al. Recommendations for standardized human pedigree nomenclature. Pedigree Standardization Task Force of the National Society of Genetic Counselors. Am J Hum Genet 1995; 56:745.
10. Grady C. Ethics and genetic testing. Adv Intern Med 1999;44:389.
11. Weinshilboum R. Inheritance and drug response. N Engl J Med 2003;348:529.

*Bold numerals denote published controlled clinical trials, meta-analyses, or consensus-based recommendations.

For annotated ***General References*** *and resources related to this chapter, visit www.hopkinsbayview.org/PAMreferences.*

Chapter 18

Immunization to Prevent Infectious Disease

William H. Barker

Protection against infectious diseases can be conferred by active immunization with vaccines and by passive immunization with immune globulin (Ig) preparations. Additional vaccines will become available in the next few years, and additional information will be generated to improve our understanding of the mechanisms of immune response to vaccines. Thus it can be expected that recommendations appropriate today will be revised in the future. This chapter describes vaccines and Ig preparations available in the United States, focusing on several questions commonly considered in practice: Who should receive what specific immunization? When should they receive it? What are the common side effects or adverse reactions? Chapter 41 provides similar information on immunization for travelers to developing countries.

PATIENT ASSESSMENT

History

A history of immunizations should be obtained from all patients. In young adults, this information may be readily available, but in older persons, it is often hard to obtain. Patients may or may not keep personal records that are of use. People who have served in the military will have received routinely recommended immunizations and several additional vaccines not generally administered to the general population. People who travel abroad frequently should have this information recorded on their International Vaccination Card. Immunization history is particularly important in determining whether to give tetanus toxoid or antitoxin after an injury, whether diphtheria should be seriously considered in the diagnosis of acute pharyngitis (see Chapter 33), and what immunizations are needed by patients who plan to travel outside the United States (see Chapter 41).

A history of *allergic reactions* or other untoward reactions to vaccines or their components should always be excluded before giving an immunization. Most modern vaccines are highly purified, and allergic reactions after their use are rare. However, a history of a severe adverse reaction to a vaccine is a contraindication to its further use. Anyone with a history of severe allergic reactions after eating eggs should not receive vaccines made in eggs (e.g., influenza and yellow fever vaccines). Viral vaccines prepared in tissue culture often contain small amounts of antibiotics (especially neomycin) to which some patients may be allergic. For patients with previous allergic reactions to any vaccine, the contents of each vaccine should be determined from the package insert before administration.

Immunization with live virus vaccines is generally contraindicated in patients with known *immunodeficiency syndromes* or recent treatment with *immunosuppressive drugs*. Patients known to be infected with the human immunodeficiency virus (HIV) may be at increased risk when receiving live vaccines, although adverse effects have been documented infrequently. Chapter 39 outlines current recommendations for vaccines in HIV-infected persons. *Pregnant women*, in whom a vaccine virus might pose a risk to the fetus, should generally not be given live vaccines. In addition to ascertaining by history that a woman of childbearing age is not pregnant, it is important to counsel the patient to use contraceptive practices to prevent pregnancy for 3 months after immunization with a live vaccine (see Chapter 100). Prophylactic use of Ig and the various hyperimmune globulin preparations is considered safe in pregnancy. Pregnancy is not a contradiction to administering live vaccine to children with whom a pregnant woman (e.g., mother or classroom teacher) will come in contact.

Recent administration of Ig preparations requires that the use of live virus vaccines be postponed because passively acquired immunity can interfere with the active response to the vaccine (1). Ig preparations should not be administered earlier than 2 weeks after live virus vaccine so that the vaccine virus can stimulate an active immune response. Yellow fever is an exception because interference does not occur.

Minor illness (e.g., upper respiratory infection with or without a low-grade fever) is not a contraindication to necessary immunization. A patient with moderate or *severe acute illness* should generally not be immunized until after the illness has resolved, both because vaccine side effects might add to the patient's morbidity and because the effectiveness of the vaccination may be diminished.

Physical and Laboratory Evaluation

When immunization is contemplated, physical examination and laboratory testing usually add little to the assessment of the patient. Pregnancy or an acute illness (see above) may be confirmed on examination if the history suggests one of these, and findings suggestive of an immunodeficiency syndrome should be pursued with appropriate clinical laboratory studies.

Serologic tests are useful in deciding whether to immunize adults in selected situations. When considering the use of rubella vaccine in a woman of childbearing age, the presence of antibodies to rubella virus obviates the need for vaccination. When considering the use of hyperimmune globulin preparations or hepatitis B vaccine for protection against hepatitis B, the demonstration of preexisting antibody to hepatitis B makes additional protection superfluous. The decision regarding screening for antibodies before vaccination should be based on the estimated prevalence of markers for hepatitis B infections in the population from which the patient comes and the cost of serologic testing (see below).

IMMUNIZATION PROCEDURES

The package insert for a vaccine always includes information about dosage, route, site of administration, interval between immunizations, common and uncommon side effects, contraindications, potential trace contaminants that may cause hypersensitivity reactions, and appropriate storage conditions for the vaccine.

Many widely used vaccines can be given simultaneously. The Advisory Committee on Immunization Practices (ACIP) of the Centers for Disease Control and Prevention lists the following guidelines for simultaneous vaccine administration: Inactivated vaccines can be administered simultaneously at separate sites or at the same site with combination preparations. Tetanus and diphtheria toxoids (Td) are most effectively given together as a combined vaccine. However, when vaccines commonly associated with side effects are given together, the side effects may be accentuated and consideration should be given to vaccinating on separate occasions. An inactivated vaccine and a live attenuated virus vaccine can be administered simultaneously at separate sites. Some live virus vaccines, such as measles, mumps, and rubella (MMR), are routinely given in combination.

Patients should be informed of the risks and benefits associated with any vaccine in understandable lay terms. The range of common side effects and appropriate symptomatic therapies should be explained. Because of the rare possibility of anaphylactic reactions, patients receiving any immunization should be observed for about 15 minutes after vaccine administration. Finally, patients should be clearly informed of the name of the immunizations they have received and encouraged to keep a written record of them. Official immunization cards are available in every state for this purpose.

Physicians and other health care providers are required to maintain permanent records of immunizations and to report certain adverse effects to the U.S. Department of Health and Human Services (2). These recording requirements are summarized in the U.S. Food and Drug Administration Drug Bulletin (3). A preventive care flowsheet, kept in the patient's office record, is an ideal location for vaccine history (see Fig. 14.3).

CURRENT RECOMMENDATIONS FOR VACCINES

Table 18.1 summarizes the major vaccines approved for use in adults in the United States; annual updates of this table may be accessed at website of the Immunization Action Coalition (www.immunize.org; go to Favorites from IAC, Summary of Adult Rules). The table is based on recommendations of the ACIP (see *www.hopkinsbayview.org/PAMreferences*). Chapter 11 provides similar information for adolescents (4). The following sections provide practical information on selected infectious diseases for which immune protection of adults is most likely to be undertaken in ambulatory practice.

DELIVERY SYSTEMS AND CONTINUING MEDICAL EDUCATION FOR PROVIDERS

Underuse and missed opportunities to provide indicated vaccination among adults enrolled in medical practices have been repeatedly documented, particularly among

TABLE 18.1 Summary of Recommendations for Adult Immunization

Vaccine Name and Route	*For Whom Vaccination Is Recommended*	*Schedule for Vaccine Administration (Any Vaccine Can Be Given with Another)*	*Contraindications and Precautions (Mild Illness Is Not a Contraindication)*
Influenza trivalent inactivated influenza vaccine (TIV) *Give IM*	■ Persons age 50 yrs and older. ■ Persons with medical problems (e.g., heart disease, lung disease, diabetes, renal dysfunction, hemoglobinopathy, immunosuppression) and/or people living in chronic-care facilities. ■ Persons with any condition that compromises respiratory function or the handling of respiratory secretions or that can increase the risk of aspiration (e.g., cognitive dysfunction, spinal cord injury, seizure disorder, or other neuromuscular disorder) ■ Persons working or living with at-risk people. ■ Women who will be pregnant during the influenza season. ■ All health care workers and other persons who provide direct care to at-risk people. ■ Household contacts and out-of-home caregivers of children ages 0–23 m. ■ Travelers at risk for complications of influenza who go to areas where influenza activity exists or who may be among people from areas of the world where there is current influenza activity (e.g., on organized tours). ■ Persons who provide essential community services. ■ Students or other persons in institutional settings (e.g., dormitory residents). ■ Anyone wishing to reduce the likelihood of becoming ill with influenza.	■ Given every year. ■ October through November is the *optimal* time to receive annual influenza vaccination to maximize protection; however vaccination may occur in December and throughout the influenza season (typically December through March) or at other times when the risk of influenza exists.	**Contraindication** ■ Previous anaphylactic reaction to this vaccine, to any of its components, or to eggs. **Precaution** ■ Moderate or severe acute illness.
Influenza live attenuated influenza vaccine (LAIV) *Give intranasally*	■ Healthy, nonpregnant women age 49 yrs and younger who meet any of the conditions listed below. - Working or living with at-risk people as listed in the section above. - Health care workers or other persons who provide direct care to at-risk people (excluding persons in close contact with severely immunosuppressed persons). - Household contacts and out-of-home caregivers of children ages 0–23 m. - Travelers who may be among people from areas of the world where there is current influenza activity (e.g., on organized tours). - Persons who provide essential community services. - Students or other persons in Institutional settings (e.g., dormitory residents). - Anyone wishing to reduce the likelihood of becoming ill with influenza.		**Contraindications** ■ Previous anaphylactic reaction to this vaccine, to any of its components, or to eggs. ■ Pregnancy, asthma, reactive airway disease or other chronic disorder of the pulmonary or cardiovascular system; an underlying medical condition, including metabolic disease such as diabetes, renal dysfunction, and hemoglobinopathy; a known or suspected immune deficiency disease or receiving immunosuppressive therapy; history of Guillain-Barré syndrome. **Precaution** ■ Moderate or severe acute illness.

(continued)

TABLE 18.1 (Continued) Summary of Recommendations for Adult Immunization

Vaccine Name and Route	*For Whom Vaccination Is Recommended*	*Schedule for Vaccine Administration (Any Vaccine Can Be Given with Another)*	*Contraindications and Precautions (Mild Illness Is Not a Contraindication)*
Pneumococcal polysaccharide (PPV23) *Give IM or SC*	■ Persons age 65 yrs and older. ■ Persons who have chronic illness or other risk factors, including chronic cardiac or pulmonary disease, chronic liver disease, alcoholism, diabetes, CSF leak, as well as people living in special environments or social settings (including Alaska Natives and certain American Indian populations). Those at highest risk of fatal pneumococcal infection are persons with anatomic asplenia, functional asplenia, or sickle cell disease; immunocompromised persons including those with HIV infection, leukemia, lymphoma, Hodgkin disease, multiple myeloma, generalized malignancy, chronic renal failure, or nephrotic syndrome; persons receiving immunosuppressive chemotherapy (including corticosteroids); and those who received an organ or bone marrow transplant and candidates for or recipients of cochlear implants.	■ Routinely given as a one-time dose; administer if previous vaccination history is unknown. ■ One-time revaccination is recommended 5 yrs later for persons at highest risk of fatal pneumococcal infection or rapid antibody loss (e.g., renal disease) and for persons age 65 yrs and older if the 1st dose was given prior to age 65 and 5 yrs or more have elapsed since the previous dose.	**Contraindication** ■ Previous anaphylactic reaction to this vaccine or to any of its components. **Precaution** ■ Moderate or severe acute illness. Note: Pregnancy and breastfeeding are not contraindications to the use of this vaccine.
Hepatitis B (Hep B) *Give IM* Brands may be used interchangeably	■ All adolescents. ■ High-risk persons, including household contacts and sex partners of HBsAg-positive persons; injecting drug users; heterosexuals with more than one sex partner in 6 months; men who have sex with men; persons with recently diagnosed STDs; patients receiving hemodialysis and patients with renal disease that may result in dialysis; recipients of certain blood products; health care workers and public safety workers who are exposed to blood; clients and staff of institutions for the developmentally disabled; inmates of long-term correctional facilities; and certain international travelers. ■ Persons with chronic liver disease. Note: Provide serologic screening for immigrants from endemic areas. When HBsAg-positive persons are identified, offer appropriate disease management. In addition, screen their sex partners and household members, and give the first dose of vaccine at the same visit. If found susceptible, complete the vaccine series.	■ Three doses are needed on a 0, 1, 6 m schedule. ■ Alternative timing options for vaccination include 0, 2, 4 m and 0, 1, 4 m. ■ There must be 4 wks between doses #1 and #2, and 8 wks between doses #2 and #3. Overall, there must be at least 16 wks between doses #1 and #3. ■ Schedule for those who have fallen behind: If the series is delayed between doses, DO NOT start the series over. Continue from where you left off.	**Contraindication** ■ Previous anaphylactic reaction to this vaccine or to any of its components. **Precaution** ■ Moderate or severe acute illness. Note: Pregnancy and breastfeeding are not contraindications to the use of this vaccine.

Hepatitis A (Hep A) *Give IM* Brands may be used interchangeably	■ Persons who travel or work anywhere except the U.S., Western Europe, New Zealand, Australia, Canada, and Japan. ■ Persons with chronic liver disease, including persons with hepatitis B and C; illegal drug users; men who have sex with men; people with clotting-factor disorders; persons who work with hepatitis A virus in experimental lab settings (not routine medical laboratories); and food handlers when health authorities or private employers determine vaccination to be cost effective. ■ Anyone wishing to obtain immunity to hepatitis A. Note: Prevaccination testing is likely to be cost effective for persons older than age 40 yrs, as well as for younger persons in certain groups with a high prevalence of hepatitis A virus infection.	For Twinrix™ (hepatitis A and B combination vaccine [GSK]), three doses are needed on a 0, 1, 6 m schedule. Recipients must be age 18 yrs or older. ■ Two doses are needed. ■ The minimum interval between dose #1 and #2 is 6 m. ■ If dose #2 is delayed, do not repeat dose #1. Just give dose #2.	**Contraindication** ■ Previous anaphylactic reaction to this vaccine or to any of its components. **Precautions** ■ Moderate or severe acute illness. ■ Safety during pregnancy has not been determined, so benefits must be weighed against potential risk. Note: Breastfeeding is not a contraindication to the use of this vaccine.
Td (Tetanus, diphtheria) *Give IM* Note: As of 8/24/05, ACIP has not issued recommendations for the use of acellular pertussis combination vaccines (Tdap). See note in next column.	■ All adolescents and adults. ■ After the primary series has been completed, a booster dose is recommended every 10 yrs. Make sure your patients nave received a primary series of 3 doses. ■ A booster dose for wound management may be needed as early as 5 yrs after receiving a previous dose, so consult ACIP recommendations.* ■ Use Td, not tetanus toxoid (TT), for all indications. Note: Two Tdap products, Boostrix (GSK) and Adacel (sanofi pasteur), were licensed by the FDA in 2005 for use in adults and/or adolescents. Consult package inserts for more information. It is anticipated that ACIP will issue recommendations for these products in late 2005.	■ Give booster dose every 10yrs after the primary series has been completed. ■ For those who are unvaccinated or behind, complete the primary series (spaced at 0, 1–2 m, 6–12 m intervals). Don't restart the series, no matter how long since the previous dose.	**Contraindication** ■ Previous anaphylactic or neurologic reaction to this vaccine or to any of its components. **Precautions** ■ Moderate or severe acute illness. ■ Guillain-Barré syndrome within 6wks of receiving a previous dose of tetanus toxoid-containing vaccine. Note: Pregnancy and breastfeeding are not contraindications to the use of this vaccine.
Polio (IPV) *Give IM or SC*	Not routinely recommended for persons age 18 yrs and older. Note: Adults living in the U.S. who never received or completed a primary series of polio vaccine need not be vaccinated unless they intend to travel to areas where exposure to wild-type virus is likely. Previously vaccinated adults can receive one booster dose if traveling to polio endemic areas.	■ Refer to ACIP recommendations* regarding unique situations, schedules, and dosing information.	**Contraindication** ■ Previous anaphylactic or neurologic reaction to this vaccine or to any of its components. **Precautions** ■ Moderate or severe acute illness. ■ Pregnancy. Note: Breastfeeding is not a contraindication to the use of this vaccine.

(continued)

TABLE 18.1 (Continued) Summary of Recommendations for Adult Immunization

Vaccine Name and Route	*For Whom Vaccination Is Recommended*	*Schedule for Vaccine Administration (Any Vaccine Can Be Given with Another)*	*Contraindications and Precautions (Mild Illness Is Not a Contraindication)*
Varicella (Var) (Chickenpox) *Give SC*	All susceptible adults and adolescents should be vaccinated. It is especially important to ensure varicella immunity among household cntacts of immunosuppressed persons and among health care workers. Note: At its June 2005 meeting, ACIP voted to regard birth in the U.S. in 1965 or earlier as presumptive evidence of varicella immunity, with or without a history of having had chickenpox. Persons's born in 1966–1997 with a reliable history of chickenpox (such as self or parental report of disease) can be assumed to be immune. For persons who have no reliable history, serologic testing may be cost effective, since most persons with a negative or uncertain history of varicella are immune.	■ Two doses are needed. ■ Dose #2 is given 4–8 wks after dose #1. ■ If varicella vaccine an MMR are both needed and are not administered on the same day, space them at least 4 wks apart. ■ If the second dose is delayed, do not repeat dose #1. Just give dose #2.	**Contraindications** ■ Previous anaphylactic reaction to this vaccine or to any of its components. ■ Pregnancy or possibility of pregnancy within 4 wks (use contraception). ■ Persons immunocompromised because of malignancies and primary or acquired cellular immunodeficiency including HIV/AIDS. (See *MMWR* 1999, Vol. 48, No. RR-6.) Note: For those on high-dose immunosuppressive therapy, consult ACIP recommendations regarding delay time.* **Precautions** ■ If blood, plasma, and/or immune globulin (IG or VZIG) were given in past 11m, see ACIP statement *General Recommendations on Immunization** regarding time to wait before vaccinating. ■ Moderate or severe acute illness. Note: Breastfeeding is not a contraindication to the use of this vaccine.
Meningococcal Conjugate vaccine (MCV4) Give IM— Polysaccharide vaccine (MPSV4) *Give SC*	■ College freshmen living in dormitories. ■ Adolescents and adults with anatomic or functional asplenia or with terminal complement component deficiencies. ■ Persons who travel to or reside in countries in which meningococcal disease is hyperendemic or epidemic (e.g., the "meningitis belt" of Sub-Saharan Africa during the dry season [Dec–June]). ■ Microbiologists who are routinely exposed to isolates of *N. meningitidis.* ■ Military recruits.	■ MCV4 is preferred over MPSV4 for persons age 55 yrs and younger, although MPSV4 is an acceptable alternative. ■ Give one dose to persons with risk factors; revaccinate after 5 yrs if risk of disease continues and previous vaccine was MPSV4.	**Contraindication** ■ Previous anaphylactic or neurologic reaction to this vaccine or to any of its components, including diphtheria toxoid (for MCV4). **Precaution** ■ Moderate or severe acute illness. Note: Pregnancy and breastfeeding are not contraindications to the use of either vaccine.

MMR (Measles, mumps, rubella) *Give SC*	■ Persons born in 1957 or later (including those born outside the U.S.) should receive at least one dose of MMR if there is no serologic proof of immunity or documentation of a dose given on or after the first birthday. ■ Persons in high-risk groups, such as health care workers, students entering college and other post high school educational institutions, and international travelers, should receive a total of two doses. ■ Persons born before 1957 are usually considered immune, but proof of immunity may be desirable for health care workers. ■ Women of childbearing age (i.e., adolescent girls and premenopausal adult women) who do not have acceptable evidence of rubella immunity or vaccination. ■ Special attention should be given to immunizing women born outside the U.S. in 1957 or later.	■ One or two doses are needed. ■ If dose #2 is recommended, give it no sooner than 4 wks after dose #1. ■ If varicella vaccine and MMR are both needed and are not administered on the same day, space them at least 4 wks apart. ■ If a pregnant woman is found to be rubella susceptible, administer MMR postpartum.	**Contraindications** ■ Previous anaphylactic reaction to this vaccine or to any of its components. ■ Pregnancy or possibility of pregnancy within 4 wks (use contraception). Persons immunocompromised because of cancer, leukemia, lymphoma, immunosuppressive drug therapy, including high-dose steroids or radiation therapy. Note: HIV positivity is NOT a contraindication to MMR except for those who are severely immunocompromised. **Precautions** ■ If blood, plasma, and/or immune globulin were given in past 11 m, see ACIP statement *General Recommendations on Immunization** regarding time to wait before vaccinating. ■ Moderate or severe acute illness. ■ History of thrombocytopenia or thrombocytopenic purpura. Note: Breastfeeding is not a contraindication to the use of this vaccine. Note: MMR is not contraindicated if a tuberculin skin test (i.e., PPD) was recently applied. IF PPD and MMR not given on same day, delay PPD for 4–6 wks after MMR.

*For specific ACIP recommendations, refer to the official ACIP statements published in *MMWR*. To obtain copies of these statements, call the CDC-INFO Contact Center at (800) 232-4636; visit CDC's website at www.cdc.gov/nip/publications/ACIP-list.htm; or visit the Immunization Action Coalition (IAC) website at www.immunize.org/acip.

This table is revised yearly. Visit IAC's website at www.immunize.org/adultrules to make sure you have the most current version. IAC thanks William Atkinson, MD, MPH, from CDC's National Immunization Program, and Linda Moyer, RN, from CDC's Division of Viral Hepatitis, for their assistance. For more information, contact IAC at 1573 Selby Avenue, St. Paul, MN 55104, (651) 647-9009, or email admin@immunize.org.

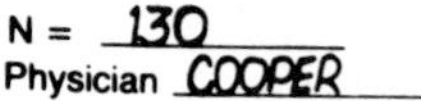

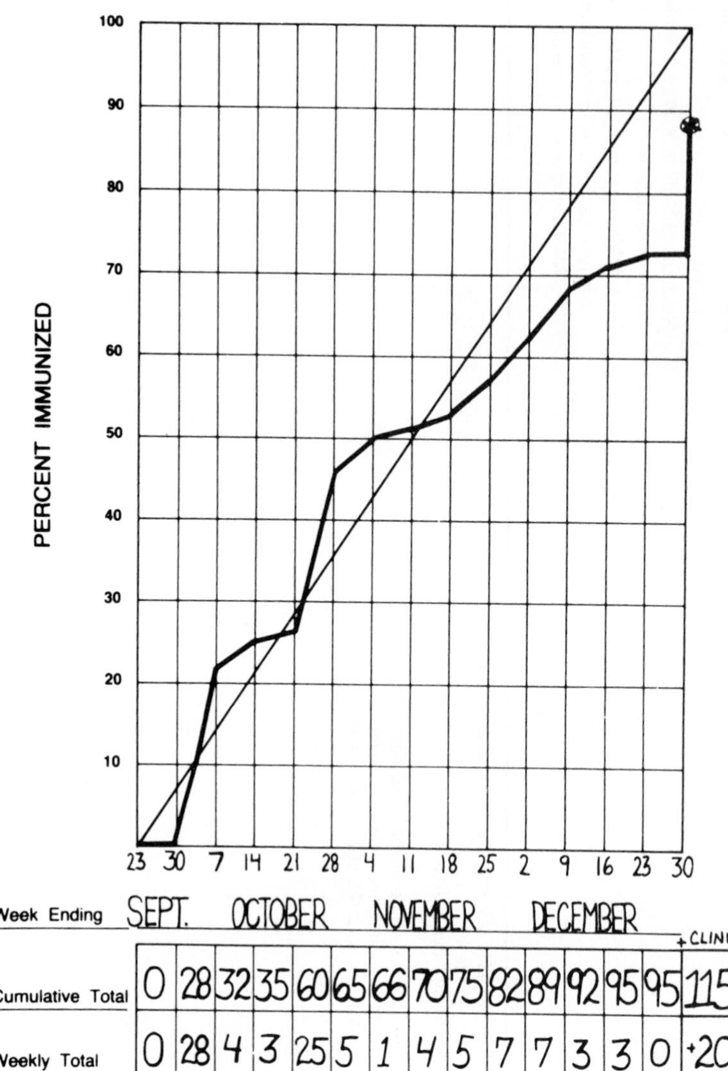

FIGURE 18.1. Completed poster displayed in an office practice. Year refers to the immunization season and *N* is the target population of patients 65 years old and older. The weekly and cumulative numbers of immunizations are tallied below the graph, and the percentage of the target population immunized is plotted weekly. (From Buffington J, Bell KM, LaForce FM, et al. A target-based model for increasing influenza immunizations in private practice. J Gen Intern Med 1991;6:204, with permission.)

minority groups (5). A variety of simple techniques for improving vaccination delivery, including reminder mailings, standing orders, staff nurse roles, and tracking systems, has been shown to be effective in both private office and clinic settings (6–9). Figure 18.1 illustrates a novel strategy for tracking and promoting provision of annual influenza immunization to target patients in a practice population. *Continuing medical education* on such techniques for use in adult vaccination may be accessed from the Association of Teachers of Preventive Medicine at www.atpm.org (9).

PROTECTION AGAINST SELECTED INFECTIONS

Diphtheria

Fewer than five cases of diphtheria are reported each year in the United States. People who have never received diphtheria toxoid should be immunized, and diphtheria toxoid should be given as booster doses with tetanus toxoid whenever tetanus toxoid is indicated (10).

For unimmunized adults, *adult type* tetanus and diphtheria toxoids are used. This preparation contains only approximately 25% of the diphtheria toxoid contained in the pediatric diphtheria and tetanus toxoids and no pertussis antigen to minimize the risk of local reactions in sensitized adults. Primary immunization in adults consists of an initial dose, a 1-month dose, and a third dose at 6 to 12 months. A Td booster is recommended every 10 years to ensure protection. There is a 25% to 50% incidence of local soreness, swelling, and itching after Td injections; fever occurs in less than 10%, and urticaria in approximately 2%, of individuals. Serious reactions (swelling of the whole arm or anaphylaxis) occur rarely.

For *asymptomatic unimmunized contacts of patients with diphtheria*, management includes prophylactic practitioner-diagnosed mumps (22). Most people born before 1957 can be considered immune. Because the mumps virus can cause severe illness in adults (orchitis, meningitis, or pancreatitis), there is good reason to provide protection to young adults who may be susceptible. Outbreaks of mumps have been reported among college and university students, and this group merits special attention. A single dose of mumps vaccine, alone or in MMR, yields durable protection in approximately 90% of recipients.

Rubella

Since 1970, live attenuated rubella virus vaccine has been administered routinely to children 1 year of age and older (22). The major rationale for use of this vaccine is prevention of the spread of rubella virus to pregnant women and thus reduction of the incidence of the congenital rubella syndrome (CRS). Reported cases of CRS remained constant at 50 to 60 from 1970 to 1980 and then fell dramatically to 1 in 1988; but in 1990 and 1991 a resurgence of rubella was observed, and there were more than 40 cases of CRS reported in the United States. Since 2001, rubella has ceased to be endemic in the United States and only four CRS cases were reported during 2001 to 2004.

Anyone working in a medical facility who does not have documentation of past rubella vaccination or serologic evidence of immunity should be vaccinated against rubella (MMR vaccine, see below) (22). Adults, and especially nonpregnant adolescent girls and women in the childbearing age group, should be offered rubella vaccine if they have not received vaccine or are not known to have serologic evidence of immunity. Serologic testing before vaccination is unnecessary because prior immunity does not increase the risks of vaccination. Vaccinated women should be cautioned against becoming pregnant (see Chapter 100) for the 3 months after receiving rubella vaccine because of the theoretical possibility of fetal damage. However, no cases of congenital abnormalities have been observed in more than 300 women who received rubella vaccine just before or during pregnancy, and the theoretical risk is less than 1%. Approximately 25% of postpubertal women receiving rubella vaccine experience arthralgias in the first 1 to 3 weeks after immunization. Frank arthritis is much less common and all symptoms are usually mild and transient.

Measles, Mumps, and Rubella Vaccine

In most cases, MMR is the vaccine of choice when any of its components is indicated, although the three vaccines are available separately. *A two-dose schedule is now highly recommended for all children* (22). The first dose of MMR should be administered at 12 to 15 months of age; the second dose is now recommended at 4 to 6 years, before school entry, but may be given at 11 to 12 years of age. The measles component is associated with the occurrence of fever or mild rash within 7 to 12 days after injection. MMR or its component vaccines should not be given to pregnant women. Anaphylaxis or other serious systematic adverse reactions are rare with MMR or any of the three individual component vaccines.

Most adults born before 1957 are assumed to be immune to mumps, measles, and rubella. *Adults born in 1957 or later* who do not have a medical contraindication should receive at least one dose of MMR vaccine unless they have documentation of vaccination or other acceptable evidence of immunity to these three diseases: laboratory evidence of immunity or health care practitioner documented diagnosis of the disease. Furthermore, it is now recommended that adolescents and college students who have no documentation of live MMR vaccinations or other acceptable evidence of immunity should receive a two-dose course of MMR vaccine, with the second dose administered no sooner than 1 month after the initial dose. Students with medical contraindications to vaccination with MMR and any of its component vaccines should be given a letter of explanation to present to the health officials of their educational institution.

Meningococcal Disease

Meningococcal disease is a serious potentially fatal infection that usually occurs sporadically, with the highest incidence in infants. Occurrence is relatively rare among the general population, but the incidence is increased among healthy young adults living in congregated circumstances, particularly military recruits in barracks and college students in dormitories (23). Two meningococcal vaccines for serotypes A, C, Y, and W-135 produced by Sanofi Pasteur are licensed for use in the United States. MPSV4, a polysaccharide vaccine (Menomune) is administered as a single subcutaneous injection that elicits protective antibody within 2 weeks. MCV4, a polysaccharide-protein conjugate vaccine (Menactra), licensed for use in the United States in 2005, is administered as a single intramuscular dose and elicits a more enduring immune response. Both vaccines cause sore arm at injection site in a small percent of recipients. Effective 2005, the ACIP recommended meningococcal vaccination for all adolescents, preferably at routine preadolescent health exam at 11 to 12 years of age, to all college freshmen living in dormitories, and to other high-risk groups (Table 18.1) (24). *Vaccination is also recommended to control community outbreaks*, defined as three or more cases within less than 3 months that result in an attack rate of 10 or more per 100,000 population at risk.

Chemoprophylaxis is recommended for close contacts of a patient with invasive meningococcal disease

TABLE 18.6 Schedule for Administering Chemoprophylaxis Against Meningococcal Disease

Drug	Age Group	Dosage	Duration and Route of Administration[a]
Rifampin[b]	Children aged <1 mo	5 mg/kg body weight every 12 hrs	2 days
	Children aged ≥1 mo	10 mg/kg body weight every 12 hrs	2 days
	Adults	600 mg every 12 hrs	2 days
Ciprofloxacin[c]	Adults	500 mg	Single dose
Ceftriaxone	Children aged <15 yrs	125 mg	Single IM[d] dose
Ceftriaxone	Adults	250 mg	Single IM dose

[a]Oral administration unless indicated otherwise.
[b]Not recommended for pregnant women because it is teratogenic in laboratory animals. Because the reliability of oral contraceptives might be affected by rifampin therapy, consideration should be given to using alternative contraceptive measures while rifampin is being administrated.
[c]Not usually recommended for persons aged <18 years or for pregnant and lactating women because it causes cartilage damage in immature laboratory animals. Can be used for chemoprophylaxis of children when no acceptable alternative therapy is available. Recent literature review identified no reports of irreversible cartilage toxicity or age-associated adverse events among children and adolescents (Source: Burstein GR, Berman SM, Blumer JL, Moran JS. Ciprofloxacin for the treatment of uncomplicated gonorrhea infection in adolescents: dose the benefit outweigh the risk? Clin infect Dis 2002;35:S191-9).
[d]Intramuscular.
From Recommendations of the Advisory Committee on Immunization Practices (ACIP). Prevention and control of meningococcal disease. MMWR Recomm Rep 2005;54(RR-7):1–21.

(Table 18.6) (24). Close contacts are defined as household members, child-care center contacts, anyone directly exposed to the patient's oral secretions (e.g., kissing, mouth-to-mouth resuscitation), and travelers who have had direct contact with respiratory secretions from an index-patient for a prolonged time (e.g., flight lasting longer than 8 hours).

Polio

Wild poliovirus and new-onset poliomyelitis have been eradicated from the Western hemisphere and Europe, and global eradication is anticipated within several years. With a view to eliminating vaccine-associated paralytic polio (VAPP) caused by oral polio vaccine (OPV), which was accounting for all new domestically acquired polio in the United States, national vaccination policy changed in 1997 from first line use of OPV to a sequential schedule of inactivated poliovirus vaccine (IPV) followed by OPV (25). In 2000, an exclusively IPV schedule was adopted (26). No further cases of VAPP have occurred in the United States.

Polio vaccination for adults in the United States is recommended for travelers to remaining polio endemic parts of the world (see Chapter 41). Adult travelers who have previously completed a primary OPV or IPV series require a single booster dose of IPV; unvaccinated adults require a primary vaccination series with IPV (25).

Rabies

Indigenously acquired human rabies is rare in the United States. Theoretically, all clinical cases of rabies are preventable if protective treatment is given promptly after exposure. The incubation period is usually 2 to 8 weeks, but it may be as short as 10 days or as long as 1 year or more.

Since 1982, inactivated rabies virus vaccine produced in human diploid cells has been in use in the United States. It causes fewer and milder reactions than the older duck embryo-derived vaccine. Formulations for intramuscular or intradermal injection are available, as is a hyperimmune globulin derived from human sera (human rabies immune globulin [HRIg]).

For *postexposure prophylaxis* after an animal bite (see Chapter 32), the recommended treatment schedule is as follows (27): on day 1, simultaneous administration of HRIg (20 IU/kg, up to half infiltrated into the wound and the remainder intramuscularly), and the first dose of vaccine, also given intramuscularly; additional vaccine doses are given on days 3, 7, 14, and 28. The effectiveness of this regimen in protecting humans from rabies has been well established. Adverse reactions (urticaria, anaphylaxis, transient headache, and fever) occur in less than 0.5% of persons receiving this vaccine.

For *preexposure prophylaxis*, people working in areas where rabies is enzootic or in occupations where potential for rabies exposure is high (e.g., veterinarians) should be vaccinated before exposure. In this situation, the appropriate formulation may be given intradermally in 0.1-mL doses or intramuscularly in 1.0-mL doses on days 0, 7, and 21 or 28 with booster doses every 2 years (see Chapter 41 for details regarding frequency of vaccine for those living in high-risk areas outside of the United States).

personal inadequacy in the face of life circumstances. By the time such patients acknowledge their distress to the doctor, their usual problem-solving methods have failed and their usual sources of support have been exhausted. Demoralization can be formulated as the product of *interactions between environmental stressors and personal vulnerabilities.* Environmental stressors may be remediable (e.g., temporary unemployment) or irremediable (e.g., conjugal bereavement). Personal vulnerabilities may be constitutional (e.g., mental retardation) or learned (e.g., excessive dependency or perfectionism). Particular personal vulnerabilities make individuals susceptible to particular stressors. For example, an exceedingly dependent person may be especially sensitive to the death of a spouse; rigid, controlling parents may be especially distressed by the rebelliousness of their adolescent children.

Psychotherapy may be viewed as an interactive process intended to restore morale. It involves both cognitive and relational tasks. The primary *cognitive task* is to develop a working formulation of patients' difficulties as products of environmental stressors and personal vulnerabilities, to appreciate the personal strengths and resources available to patients for problem-solving and amelioration of emotional distress, and to help patients apply these strengths and resources to regain a sense of mastery over life problems. Some strategies useful for these purposes are described in later sections of this chapter (see Psychosocial Treatment Techniques and Forms of Counseling).

The *relational task* is to promote in patients what Jerome Frank has called *"expectant trust"* (see Frank, at *www.hopkinsbayview.org/PAMreferences*). This describes an attitude on the part of patients that their practitioner cares about them, is competent to help, is confident of their recovery, and is committed to remain available until relief is obtained. Expectant trust is an important element in psychotherapeutic success, and it is enhanced by several of the techniques described in this chapter. Its effective mobilization also requires an understanding of the concepts of transference and countertransference.

Transference

Patients' expectations of their doctors have complex psychosocial roots. In part, they grow out of patients' experiences with their parents in circumstances of fear, pain, and other forms of distress. As a result of these experiences, patients consciously and unconsciously may come to expect that new people in their lives, particularly caretakers, will treat them as their parents did. These expectations are known as transference phenomena: *patients transfer expectations onto their health care practitioners.* When the transferred expectations are positive (*positive transference*), practitioners have at their disposal a powerful resource in their work to help their patients feel better. Positive transference may partly explain placebo responses and must be borne in mind when the effects of new therapeutic interventions are being evaluated.

Not all transference phenomena are positive. Everyone experiences anger, frustration, and other painful emotions in response to the disappointments and deprivations that invariably accompany growing up. These experiences sometimes leave emotional residua that may contaminate the relationship of the patient with caretakers or authority figures such as their health care practitioner. For example, patients who were abandoned by their parents may unconsciously expect that their practitioner will also abandon them and may therefore cling to the doctor with pathologic dependency. Other sorts of early life experiences may lead to passivity, hostility, and compulsiveness. Negative expectations (negative transference), as well as positive expectations, may be transferred onto health care practitioners and may give rise to maladaptive reactions that complicate the practitioner–patient relationship and interfere with therapeutic success if not properly managed.

In psychotherapy, transference phenomena are regarded as tools and opportunities as well as potential obstacles. Psychological distress is often the result of interpersonal problems with family, friends, and associates. Transference phenomena create, in the presence of the psychotherapist, modified but reasonably accurate representations of patients' current and past relationships. As patients, through transference, begin to treat the therapist as a significant person from the past, the therapist gains valuable insight into the roots of patients' interpersonal difficulties and may ultimately use these insights to help patients improve their relationships.

The type and intensity of the transference and the opportunities for its use in treatment vary with the intensity of the therapeutic relationship and the frequency of visits. In short-term counseling, intense therapeutic relationships generally do not develop, and the transference is predominantly positive.

Countertransference

Health care practitioners, like their patients, must endure the tribulations of childhood and adolescence and may thereby develop positive and negative *expectations that are transferred onto other people, including patients.* These expectations, called countertransference, may compromise the ability of the practitioner to care for particular patients. For example, the practitioner son of an abusive alcoholic father may have such a personal emotional stake in promoting the abstinence of his male alcoholic patients that he becomes enraged and ineffective with them when they relapse. It is the responsibility of the practitioner to be aware of countertransference phenomena and to resist their intrusion into the doctor–patient relationship, particularly in the context of counseling. The practitioner may find psychotherapy helpful for this purpose.

PSYCHOSOCIAL TREATMENT TECHNIQUES

Because the simple disclosure of emotional distress and its causes may bring considerable relief to patients, the process of psychosocial evaluation often has therapeutic value in itself. Chapter 19 describes general aspects of evaluation for psychosocial problems. This section describes the principal techniques used in counseling, and the following section describes the forms of planned counseling useful in office practice.

Establishing a Therapeutic Relationship

As noted earlier (see Transference), the therapeutic relationship recapitulates to some extent the parent–child relationship. Several elements are generic to an effective therapeutic relationship. The patient must trust the health care practitioner. Practitioners earn trust by showing interest consistently, accepting sensitive information without being judgmental, taking patients' concerns seriously, and controlling inappropriate reactions to difficult patients (see Table 3.7 in Chapter 3). In addition to establishing trust, practitioners should ensure that their patients understand how to gain access to them and recognize limits regarding access during ongoing treatment. It is useful to reflect on whether these trust-promoting and condition-setting actions have been accomplished before embarking on counseling, and whether the access policies already established by the practitioner's office are appropriate to the counseling situation.

Identifying and Addressing Information Needs

Misinformation or lack of information causes much distress. Patients often come to the office with an unfounded fear of dread illness or a significant misunderstanding of an established condition. At times, a patient's own "explanatory model" of what is wrong dominates the picture (see Chapter 4). When careful interviewing reveals the need for information and explanation, health care practitioners provide a vital service by tailoring their teaching to patients' needs and taking care to confirm that the information has been received and understood. Clear explanations of normal physiology, disease processes, and treatment regimens are often overlooked as powerful aids in counseling. Besides providing information, such explanations draw patients into collaborative relationships with their practitioners.

The following interventions are often therapeutic in themselves:

- Providing information regarding a *feared physical disorder*. For example,

  The son of a recently deceased diabetic patient thinks he also has diabetes and is greatly relieved by a negative workup for diabetes and a brief explanation of the implications of the result.

  A woman with mitral valve prolapse who has adopted unnecessary activity limitations is greatly reassured to learn that her condition is benign and that she may resume valued activities.

- Explaining the possible impact of *psychophysiologic processes on somatic symptomatology*. For example,

  A man with panic disorder is relieved to learn how hyperventilation may lead to neurologic symptoms.

- Explaining how *a psychosocial stressor may produce physical symptoms*. For example,

  A man with an anxiety disorder is helped to recognize that his symptoms are being intensified by an expected job layoff, alleviating his fear that he is "going crazy."

- Presenting the patient with a working diagnosis, a plan of care, and the likely prognosis. For example,

  A woman with major depression is greatly relieved when she is told the diagnosis, the plan to use gradually increasing doses of antidepressants, and the likelihood of significant improvement after a few weeks.

Eliciting and Responding to Feelings

It is critical for health care practitioners to be skillful in the management of emotions. Central to emotional management are a willingness to allow patients to discuss feelings in the office and an ability to listen empathically.

Empathic Listening

Patients are grateful when their practitioners take an obvious interest in what they are saying and the feelings that they are experiencing. Granting the patient time to reflect, remembering details of the history, responding with appropriate affect to situations described by the patient, and indicating what one has observed or heard about the patient's feelings are all actions that demonstrate concern, diminish the isolation that accompanies unexpressed feelings, and enhance the patient's self-esteem. For example,

A man with generalized anxiety disorder feels better after his practitioner listens to his account of his worries, summarized what he heard, and indicates that he understands how distressing the patient's symptoms are.

Legitimizing Feelings

Patients may feel embarrassed, isolated, or overwhelmed by their emotions. Legitimizing or normalizing emotions can be a powerful morale-enhancing intervention. For example,

"Most people in your situation have similar reactions. Yours is both normal and completely understandable."

Encouraging the Expression of Feelings

Patients who have "held in" strong feelings about past or current experiences usually feel better after giving voice to these feelings. The practitioner can encourage a therapeutic expression of feelings by noting that the patient looks tense, angry, or depressed or by commenting that the experience that the patient has just described must have made the patient feel upset.

Problem-Solving

Demonstrating Respect and Facilitating Choice

When counseling a patient, the practitioner should obviously avoid a condescending, patronizing, or overbearing tone. As noted earlier (see Demoralization), patients usually attempt to resolve their problems on their own before seeking professional help. Furthermore, they may describe themselves as usually able to handle problems. Inquiring about and acknowledging previous efforts, even when they have been unsuccessful, and supporting any voiced characterization of themselves as problem-solvers, can help prepare patients to take on current problems. The fundamental strategies for facilitated problem-solving involve helping the patient recognize assets (e.g., supportive people, enjoyed activities), identify options, and make reasonable choices. It is occasionally necessary to be more directive.

Encouraging Contingency Planning

Patients sometimes cannot see obvious solutions to distressing problems. Once becoming familiar with the pertinent facts, the practitioner may be able to help the patient make plans to deal with anticipated problems. In making contingency plans, it is useful to present hypothetical situations and to have the patient propose potential solutions. For example,

A woman who lives alone is distraught because her only child has hinted that she may not be able to get home for Christmas. The woman's practitioner encourages her to make alternative Christmas plans so that she will not be alone for the holiday if her daughter is in fact unable to come to visit. She telephones later in the week to say that she still does not know whether her daughter will be able to come for Christmas but has invited friends to her home for Christmas dinner, and feels much better.

Advising (Persuading)

The health care practitioner is considered by the patient to be an expert and should be willing to take advantage of that status under appropriate circumstances. Concrete recommendations may be especially helpful to patients whose decision-making ability may be impaired. For example,

A middle-aged man with major depression who is unrealistically dissatisfied with his job performance is tactfully persuaded to defer his decision about early retirement until his mood has improved.

MANAGING ABNORMAL ILLNESS BEHAVIOR

Abnormal illness behavior is present when the patient's symptoms or impairments, and associated health-care seeking behavior, are disproportionate to detectable disease. Mild forms of such behavior are commonplace in medical practice. In its more chronic, severe and disabling manifestations, abnormal illness behavior forms the core of the *somatoform disorders* (see Chapter 21), conditions in which patients express emotional distress and psychological conflict in terms of somatic complaints and convictions of serious illness. The following general strategies are useful when psychosocial problems present mainly as abnormal illness behavior.

Redirecting the Patient–Practitioner Interaction to Include Relevant Psychosocial Issues

For patients with abnormal illness behavior, it is helpful to address relevant psychosocial issues, such as functional status, in addition to physical complaints. The following strategies are recommended:

1. *Do not reinforce abnormal illness behavior.*
   - a. Avoid unnecessary testing.
   - b. Avoid unnecessary prescribing.
   - c. Avoid unnecessary referral to specialists.
   - d. Schedule regular visits (i.e., do not make visits contingent on a new or worsening symptom) and stay within a time frame agreed upon for visits.
   - e. Encourage decisions that improve functioning, despite symptoms. For example:

     The mood and physical well-being of a woman with long-standing depression (dysthymic disorder) and physical complaints improve after she is encouraged to take a job as a companion and housekeeper for an elderly woman who had a stroke.
2. *Do not expect to eradicate all symptoms* (i.e., do not view elimination of symptoms as an essential goal).

3. *Encourage the patient to talk about his or her life situation and not just about somatic symptoms*. For example,

A patient with somatization disorder (see Chapter 21) and an unremarkable recent urinalysis states that she plans to see the urologist who took care of her friend's bladder problem. She is instead persuaded to come for brief weekly visits to her primary practitioner. At the weekly visits, the practitioner addresses briefly the urinary symptoms, but focuses primarily on the patient's efforts to keep her teenage daughter in school. He commends her for her successful handling of these and other domestic problems. Her urinary complaints gradually resolve.

Involving Family and Friends

Family members and close friends are potentially valuable clinical resources. When including family members and others in the care of a patient, it is vital to respect the patient's right to confidentiality. It is important to obtain the patient's permission to speak with others and, when appropriate, to include the patient in meetings with family members (see Table 3.1 in Chapter 3). The following are common interventions that may enhance the usefulness of these meetings.

Meeting the Family's Information Needs

Family and close friends may suffer greatly as a result of their loved one's illness and often have the same informational needs as the patient (see Identifying and Addressing Information Needs section). These needs must be met if they are to understand the needs and feelings of the patient and to participate in providing aftercare. For example,

A 70-year-old man with major depression tells his primary care practitioner that his son will probably call to ask for information. The son calls the practitioner and expresses concern that his father has been angrily criticizing his young grandchildren for petty reasons and that this is not the way he used to treat the children. Furthermore, the son is worried that his father must have an ulcer because he leaves the table rubbing his stomach and shaking his head after eating a few bites. The practitioner empathizes with the patient's son and explains that the behavior change is typical for a depressed man, that the antidepressant medication that has just been started should lead to some improvement within 2 to 3 weeks, that the history and physical examination did not reveal evidence of an ulcer, and that it is likely that his father will recover entirely within 2 to 4 months. The son is relieved and expresses the hope that things will go the way the practitioner predicts.

Enlisting the Family's Help

For some conditions in which the patient demonstrates a failure to make choices favoring improvement, the family may be instrumental in persuading the patient to accept needed treatment. For example,

The family of an alcoholic patient agrees to participate in a family intervention (see Chapter 28) to get the patient to accept alcoholism treatment.

Knowing and Using Community Resources

Support groups, recreational or vocational programs, and home health services are among the community resources that may be helpful to patients. A practitioner's awareness of and enthusiasm for a community resource can greatly influence its impact. For example,

The depressed and anxious wife of an alcoholic man experiences marked improvement in her symptoms after she becomes active in Al-Anon, a resource suggested by her practitioner.

At the suggestion of her practitioner, an elderly woman attends a medical day care program. This resource enables the patient to remain at home with her family and alleviates the patient's resentment toward family members who felt compelled to check on her frequently during the day.

FORMS OF COUNSELING

The treatment techniques described earlier in this chapter help at times in the care of all patients. Several forms of planned counseling, each of which integrates a number of these treatment techniques, are helpful in the care of selected patients.

Supportive Therapy

The purpose of supportive therapy is to help a patient cope with both ongoing medical problems and stressful life circumstances. Unlike short-term counseling (see next section), the duration of supportive therapy is open ended, and it is often incorporated into the routine management of a chronic disease.

Example: Supportive Therapy

A practitioner decides that supportive psychotherapy will be helpful in the long-term treatment of a diabetic patient with a history of poor compliance and multiple family problems. The patient is seen once a month for 20 minutes to monitor the patient's diabetes, enhance compliance, and review family problems. The verbal exchange during the visits includes a review of the medical regimen and glucose monitoring, check for new symptoms, brief review of what has occurred in the patient's life since the last visit, elicitation and acknowledgment of feelings, and discussion of ways to cope with existing family problems. In this manner, a significant supportive service is provided in the context of management of the patient's chronic disease.

Short-Term Counseling

This form of intervention is especially useful in the treatment of the patient who accepts a psychological formulation for symptoms and who wants help in resolving a crisis related to those symptoms. The goals of treatment are to strengthen the patient's emotional defenses and to relieve symptoms without attempting to deal with long-standing intrapsychic conflicts.

It is usually important at the outset of counseling to establish a *therapeutic contract,* specifying the purpose, length, frequency, and cost (when relevant) of the sessions. These details form the boundaries within which the treatment will take place and may become significant during the course of treatment. Patients may react to the boundaries in terms of transference (see Transference section) by objecting to them or by attempting to change or violate them. Although there are exceptions, the boundaries generally should not be modified, because a change in the relationship between the patient and practitioner may arise as a result of transference. Most mental health professionals feel that the above contractual arrangements are important and should remain stable throughout the course of treatment, to enhance clarity and protect both the patient and provider.

The realities of practice usually require that sessions be brief (15 to 20 minutes) and limited in number (5 to 10). The short-term nature of treatment helps limit the emergence of negative transference and inappropriate dependency. Patients are usually seen individually, although at times, couples and families may be treated together (see Family Counseling). The aim of such short-term treatment is restoration of morale and relief of emotional distress, not personality change. Treatment should focus on problems that are conscious (i.e., readily accessible, not repressed) and current; one should gently divert patients from repeated recitations of past experiences and injuries. The interactive style should be natural and conversational rather than remote and analytical, and it should be tailored to enhance expectant trust (see Demoralization section). When appropriate, one should point out that the patient's emotional state is an understandable and valid reaction to difficult life circumstances, and that it will subside. In most cases, the practitioner's role is to facilitate problem-solving, not to prescribe solutions. To promote problem-solving, one should be prepared to help patients identify their strengths and resources, praise their demonstrations of adaptiveness, and help them explore how they might build on their strengths to solve problems. Patients should be encouraged to try options identified in the sessions by means of homework assignments carried out between sessions.

Throughout the course of short-term counseling, it is important to listen and screen for evidence of a complicating major psychiatric disorder, such as panic disorder, major depression, or alcoholism, because in these conditions, psychotherapy may need to be supplemented by pharmacotherapy or other interventions (see Chapters 22, 24, and 28).

Example: Short-Term Counseling

A 25-year-old woman came for evaluation because of severe leg pain. She had suffered a severe burn injury 1 year before and had experienced leg pain intermittently since then. The practitioner commented that she appeared tired and tense. At this, she became tearful and said that she and her husband had separated and that, although she felt this was for the best, she was extremely anxious and uncertain that she could manage on her own. She had frightened herself during the previous week by thinking that she might be better off dead.

The assessment revealed that she was not suicidal and did not meet criteria for major depression or panic disorder. The practitioner viewed the patient as demoralized and sought to identify the pertinent personal vulnerabilities and environmental stressors. On the basis of a long relationship, the practitioner knew the patient to be a quiet, self-conscious woman who depended on attractiveness as a source of self-esteem. She was also ambitious and hard-working and had enjoyed considerable occupational success. Her major stressor had been the burn injury. She had been spared facial disfigurement but had considerable scarring on her trunk and lower extremities, which she kept covered at all times. Another stressor was the dissolution of her marriage. She regarded this as a positive development, yet she became tearful when discussing it. When the practitioner pointed this out, she revealed that she was apprehensive about dating again. She felt certain that the scarring from her burns would make her unattractive to men and that she would therefore remain alone, unable to remarry and have children.

The practitioner responded that her distress was very understandable in view of the problems she had identified, especially her fears of future loneliness. The practitioner also told her that these fears might be premature and needed to be examined and proposed meeting weekly for five visits, 20 minutes each, to talk about her choices and assumptions. She agreed.

During the next session she complained about her dissolving marriage. After 5 to 10 minutes the practitioner praised her for having stuck with it as long as she had and for managing to hold a demanding job so successfully at the same time. She then spoke of compliments given her by coworkers, one of whom had always paid special attention to her. She was grateful for this now but insisted that no one would take an interest in her if he knew of her injuries. The practitioner asked her how she knew this, reiterated the position that her assumptions warranted exploration, and asked how she might comfortably undertake such an exploration. She considered some options and over the course of several weeks tried several of them, initially simply discussing her injury with others to assess people's responses to the news and finally allowing some friends to see her scarring. The practitioner praised her for her courage as she proceeded with these explorations and empathized with her as she dealt with feelings generated by recalling the accident and risking rejection by testing people's responses to her.

By the end of the allotted 5 weeks, she was no longer convinced that the future was hopeless. Although still anxious about the ongoing separation and her potential opportunity to date again, she was no longer feeling overwhelmed and believed herself capable of overcoming her self-consciousness about the injury. The practitioner acknowledged her progress and offered future support.

Family Counseling

The goals of this form of counseling are to facilitate effective communication among family members, bring to their awareness maladaptive patterns of behavior that may be destructive to one or more members of the family, and have family members develop more constructive patterns of behavior. The specific techniques are similar to those used in individual counseling.

Example: Family Counseling

A couple asked their family practitioner for help in dealing with their adolescent daughter, who was continually misbehaving at school and at home. Evaluation of the problem revealed that the parents considered the girl the "black sheep" of the family and had been inconsistent in setting behavioral limits. Counseling for the whole family was recommended. During the first session family members demonstrated their usual conflictual pattern of interaction in the presence of the practitioner: both parents and the other siblings attacked the daughter, blaming her for all of the family's troubles. The practitioner interrupted the attack and proposed that this exchange must resemble what goes on at home, indicated that the situation seemed uncomfortable for all who were present, and ventured that they would probably like to do something about it. After everyone concurred with these points, the practitioner shifted the focus to the development of a contract between the parents and their daughter designed to define the rules they expected her to follow and the consequences of violating the rules. The next session was a review of the parents' and daughter's adherence to the contract. The parents reported that the daughter broke the contract by misbehaving, but one of the older siblings pointed out that the parents were inconsistent in their enforcement of the rules. This observation helped the family recognize that the girl's behavior was a shared responsibility within the family. Over the remaining sessions, the practitioner continued to encourage the family to establish fair rules to which all could adhere consistently. By focusing on the behavior of the entire family, the pressure on the daughter was relieved, destructive patterns of interacting were interrupted, and more constructive patterns were introduced.

Behavior Modification

The impact of office psychotherapy and the impact of the strategies for managing many medical problems described in this book depend on the elements essential to any change in a patient's behavior: being concerned about one's problem, becoming motivated to make a change, taking action to make a change, and maintaining the change. Chapter 4 describes the conceptual bases for promoting behavior change and skills for facilitating behavior change. Skills and interventions useful for addressing specific conditions are described in most of the chapters of this book.

EFFICACY OF PSYCHOTHERAPY

There is good empirical support for the effectiveness of psychotherapy conducted by specially trained clinicians in the treatment of depression among outpatients. Studies of brief psychological treatments, primarily cognitive behavioral and interpersonal therapies, have shown rates of remission comparable to those associated with antidepressant medication in selected outpatients with depressive symptoms of mild to moderate severity (1,2). Moreover, there is evidence that psychotherapy enhances the effectiveness of antidepressant pharmacotherapy when both interventions are provided simultaneously (3). Although there has been little research on the effectiveness of psychotherapy conducted in primary care settings by primary care practitioners, at least one study has demonstrated that teaching primary care physicians communication skills and knowledge related to patients' psychosocial issues resulted in a change, not only in their communication with patients, but a reduction in their patients' emotional distress for as long as 6 months (4).

SPECIFIC REFERENCES*

1. Casacalenda N, Perry JC, Looper K. Remission in major depressive disorder: a comparison of pharmacotherapy, psychotherapy, and control conditions. Am J Psychiatry 2002;159:1354.
2. Churchill R, Hunot V, Corney R, et al. A systematic review of controlled trials of the effectiveness and cost-effectiveness of brief psychological treatments for depression. Health Technol Assess 2001;5:1.
3. Thase ME, Greenhouse JB, Frank E, et al. Treatment of major depression with psychotherapy, or psychotherapy-pharmacology combinations. Arch Gen Psychiatry 1997;54;1009.
4. Roter DL, Hall JA, Kern DE, et al. Improving physicians' interviewing skills and reducing patients' emotional distress: a clinical trial. Arch Intern Med 1995;155:1877.

*Bold numerals denote published controlled clinical trials, meta-analyses, or consensus-based recommendations.

For annotated ***General References*** *and resources related to this chapter, visit www.hopkinsbayview.org/PAMreferences.*

Chapter 21

Somatization

Robert P. Roca

ILLNESS BEHAVIOR AND SOMATIZATION

People who consult health care practitioners are expected to have discernible pathologic or pathophysiologic abnormalities (i.e., disease) accounting for their symptoms. The magnitude of their complaints and the associated disability are expected to be proportional to the disease diagnosed. They are supposed to pursue and cooperate with medical care and to resume normal social functioning as soon as possible. This sequence of responses is called *normal illness behavior* (1).

Sometimes there is a discrepancy between diagnosable disease and the magnitude and duration of symptoms and disability. Patients may complain of weakness or pain in the absence of objective findings. They may have pseudoseizures. They may visit their health care practitioners repeatedly with fears of having acquired immunodeficiency syndrome (AIDS) despite several negative human immunodeficiency virus (HIV) serology results and normal physical examinations. Such responses are examples of *abnormal illness behavior.*

Explaining discrepancies between objective evidence of disease and the subjective experience of symptoms is a major concern of psychosomatic medicine and an active area of research. It is speculated that "unexplained somatic symptoms" may in some cases result from functional disturbances of the central nervous system that may be possible to demonstrate in the future using functional central nervous system (CNS) imaging techniques (2). It is also believed that some patients with unexplained somatic symptoms may be manifesting *somatization,* a phenomenon in which physical symptoms are linked to psychological factors or conflicts. Its mechanisms are incompletely understood, but factors promoting somatization can often be discovered in individual cases.

WHY PATIENTS SOMATIZE

Explanations of somatization come from at least four distinct perspectives: Somatization may be viewed as a product of disease, a manifestation of personality, a modeled or reinforced behavior, or an understandable product of a patient's life story. Each perspective calls for different observations and illuminates different aspects of the phenomenon of somatization.

Somatization as a Symptom of Disease

Somatization may occur as a symptom of a psychiatric disorder, particularly major depression, panic disorder, schizophrenia, or dementia. Sometimes somatic symptoms are the only complaints that patients with these conditions present to their health care practitioners (3).

As noted above, unexplained physical symptoms may in some cases be caused by as yet uncharacterized "functional disturbances of the nervous system" (2); this is a speculative proposal without firm empirical support at this time. There is no doubt that unexplained symptoms may also be caused by clear-cut medical conditions that have simply not yet been diagnosed—even when the symptoms seem to be expressing a psychological conflict or need. Studies of one subset of somatizing patients—those originally diagnosed as hysterics—have shown that up to 30% may ultimately be found to have medical or neurologic disorders that, in retrospect, explain the presenting hysterical symptoms (4). On the other hand, a general tendency to complain of somatic symptoms may be *negatively* correlated with the presence of particular specific pathologic entities (e.g., coronary artery disease [CAD]) (5). Furthermore, the greater the number of unexplained somatic symptoms (e.g., pain complaints), the greater the likelihood of a diagnosable psychiatric disorder such as major depression (6).

Somatization as a Manifestation of Personality

The concept of personality implies enduring attitudes and habitual patterns of response. Personalities may be viewed as approximations of ideal prototypes (e.g., histrionic, obsessive-compulsive) or as clusters of individual traits (e.g., dependency, assertiveness), as discussed in Chapter 23. Somatization has been associated with personality viewed in both of these ways. Patients with a histrionic or an obsessive-compulsive personality type may be predisposed to develop, respectively, somatization disorder or hypochondriasis (see later sections on these disorders). Patients with prominent traits of introspectiveness (i.e., tendancy to devote diffuse attention to thoughts and feelings about the self) (7) or neuroticism (i.e., emotionally unstable, vulnerable to stress, and self-conscious) (8) are particularly likely to experience and report unexplained physical symptoms.

Somatization as Reinforced Behavior

Somatization may be viewed as behavior modeled or reinforced by the patient's environment (9). This perspective prompts exploration for a history of similar symptoms in the patient or a close contact and encourages a search for evidence of social benefit associated with the patient's current symptoms.

Case Example

A 20-year-old woman was evaluated in the office for back pain. The physical examination was unimpressive, and an extensive workup was unrevealing. Discussions with the family disclosed that the patient's father was about to lose his disability income and that financial hardship was expected. Environmental reinforcements related to possibly becoming eligible for disability, thereby ameliorating the family's anticipated financial crisis, probably contributed to the continuation of this patient's symptoms.

Somatization and the Life Story

Somatization may be viewed as a maladaptive but understandable expression of, or response to, difficulties originating in early life experiences. This perspective is at least as old as the concept of "hysterical conversion," introduced in 1795 by John Ferrier and elaborated upon by Freud and Breuer in the late 19th century (10), and its validity is supported by abundant evidence that persons with histories of childhood abuse have higher rates of unexplained physical symptoms and medical services utilization (11,12). Although particular formulations are difficult to prove in individual cases, they may help clinicians comprehend and manage illness behavior that is otherwise irritating and baffling. For example, patients who suffer parental abuse and neglect may carry into adulthood potent mixtures of hostility and dependency that are activated in relationships with health care practitioners. Such patients may develop physical symptoms without diagnosable disease and pursue unrevealing medical evaluations. Sometimes hostile and demanding, they may demean the competence and the commitment of their health care practitioners, even as they crave medical attention and insist on even more care. Such behaviors may be seen as expressions of angry disappointment with their earliest caretakers, who did not adequately meet their dependency needs, now displaced onto the practitioner. Other patients may have childhood memories of experiencing attention and caring only when they were ill, or they may have come from families or cultures in which it was customary to express emotional distress as physical symptoms. Such formulations may help clinicians respond to such patients without anger and permit the development of a constructive doctor–patient relationship. Other formulations of this type are discussed elsewhere (13).

Reaching a Working Formulation and Making a Diagnosis

Thus the development of a working formulation requires consideration of the relative merits of the four distinct explanatory points of view in a particular case. Once the clinician has determined that the unexplained symptoms are not because of a previously undiagnosed medical disorder, there are four fundamental questions:

1. Does the patient have a psychiatric disorder of which somatization is a symptom?
2. Does the patient have personality traits or a personality type predisposing to somatization?
3. Is the patient's abnormal illness behavior modeled or reinforced by some aspect of the patient's environment?
4. Is this behavior empathically understandable as a product of the patient's unique life history and current predicament?

As shown later, the working formulation often carries specific therapeutic implications.

Somatizing patients may fall into defined diagnostic groups (Table 21.1). The diagnostic classification of somatization is presently under review, and there are proposals

TABLE 21.1 Psychiatric Disorders Associated with Somatization

Mental disorders
- Mood disorders, especially major depression
- Anxiety disorders, especially panic disorder
- Schizophrenia

Personality disorders, especially histrionic, dependent, and obsessive-compulsive

Adjustment disorder with anxiety or depression

Psychological factors affecting medical conditions

Somatoform disorders
- Somatization disorder
- Undifferentiated somatoform disorder
- Hypochondriasis
- Conversion disorder
- Somatoform pain disorder
- Body dysmorphic disorder

Disorders with voluntary symptom production
- Factitious disorder with physical symptoms
- Malingering

for radical revision (14). Despite these controversies, there is agreement that unexplained somatic symptoms account for a substantial proportion of both primary care and specialist visits and that the formal somatoform disorders (e.g., conversion disorder, somatization disorder, hypochondriasis) and factitious disorders account for only a small proportion of these cases (14). Many more patients have incomplete forms of these conditions (e.g., somatoform disorder not otherwise specified; undifferentiated somatoform disorder), adjustment disorders with anxiety or depression partly manifested by somatic symptoms, or actual medical conditions whose manifestations are influenced by psychosocial factors (see Psychological Factors Affecting Medical Conditions section).

This chapter reviews adjustment disorders, psychological factors affecting medical conditions, the primary somatoform disorders, and disorders in which symptom production is deliberate. Mood disorders (Chapter 24), anxiety disorders (Chapter 22), schizophrenia (Chapter 25), and personality disorders (Chapter 23) are discussed in detail elsewhere in this book.

ADJUSTMENT DISORDERS

Description

Adjustment disorders are reactive emotional states resulting from difficulty meeting the demands of life. Patients feel overwhelmed by illness, marital discord, or other problems and become demoralized. While adjustment disorders are classified according to the patient's predominant psychological symptomatology (e.g., depression, anxiety), sometimes the patient's most prominent complaints are somatic symptoms. It is in these cases that patients with adjustment disorders are most likely to present to their general health providers. This is because (1) somatic complaints legitimize a visit to the doctor and (2) emotional distress precipitated by stressful experiences can amplify bodily symptoms and lead patients to become convinced that they are seriously ill. When emotional and somatic symptoms arise in response to psychosocial problems, a diagnosis of adjustment disorder should be considered (see Table 24.1 in Chapter 24).

Case Example

A shy 26-year-old parochial school teacher was evaluated for dizziness, abdominal cramps, nausea, excessive urination, and a sensation of fullness in the bladder. When physical examination and laboratory tests revealed no physiologic disturbance, a more detailed history was taken. It showed that the patient's symptoms began shortly after a confrontation with his school principal over his attempt to organize a teacher's union and his criticism of school policies. (Diagnosis: adjustment disorder with anxiety and physical symptoms.)

Patients such as this one are often unaware of the relationship between their psychological distress and somatic symptoms.

As illustrated in the following example, diagnosis may be difficult when the symptoms precipitated by psychosocial stress resemble those of a patient's established disease process.

Case Example

A 54-year-old widow recovering from a myocardial infarction complained to her primary care practitioner of fatigue, breathlessness, and pleuritic chest pain unrelated to exertion. Her physical examination and electrocardiographic findings were unchanged. Questioning revealed that the patient was forced to leave her job after her heart attack and was barely able to afford necessary medications. She tearfully revealed that, although her son had offered to help pay for her medications, her daughter-in-law hinted that they could not really afford to help. This proud and formerly self-sufficient woman, who was initially reluctant to accept any help, now felt even more vulnerable and inadequate, and she acknowledged that the periodic symptoms in her chest invariably occurred while she was thinking about these difficulties. (Diagnosis: adjustment disorder with mixed emotional features and physical symptoms.)

In this case, emotional distress produced symptoms suggesting cardiac disease. The correct diagnosis was made when the relevant history was elicited.

Management

Three strategies are important in evaluating patients who may have adjustment disorders:

1. *Elicit the relevant history.* Asking the patient open-ended questions such as, "How are things at home (or at work)?" invites patients to expand on their history and often reveals potential sources of psychosocial distress. Most patients are grateful for a clinician's interest, respect time limits, and go on to solve the precipitating problem themselves. Even before the practitioner has taken a psychosocial history, patients may provide verbal and nonverbal cues suggesting distress (e.g., saying "Things aren't the way they used to be," wringing hands and looking away when describing a new somatic symptom) (15). Many patients who are initially reluctant to acknowledge psychosocial distress eventually open up in response to gentle, persistent encouragement from a trusted clinician.
2. *Rule out major depression.* Patients who attribute their low mood to identifiable psychosocial stressors do not necessarily have an adjustment disorder. Such symptoms as persistently depressed mood, loss of interest in usual activities, poor concentration, reduced energy, diminished appetite, and disturbed sleep suggest a major depressive disorder for which antidepressant medication usually is indicated (see Chapter 24). The presence of an apparent psychosocial precipitant should never deter the physician from inquiring about such symptoms.
3. *Temper the workup.* Patients should be examined and appropriate laboratory tests ordered; however, extensive workups to exclude improbable diagnoses should be undertaken only after careful consideration and after allowing some time to elapse, because such workups may imbed patients in the sick role and prolong their disability.
4. *Work with the patient to understand and accept the link between somatic symptoms and psychosocial stress.* Patients do not like to hear the doctor say "It's all in your head." But most patients can accept the proposal that stressful life events can produce or exacerbate physical discomfort, particularly when the physician has listened closely to their complaints, examined them carefully, and ordered appropriate laboratory tests, if indicated. Sometimes it is helpful to offer a simple illustration of how emotional stimuli can lead to physical manifestations ("You have noticed how the hair on a cat's back will stand up when the cat sees a dog. In a similar way, we may undergo physiological changes in response to stress, and these changes can make us sick."). This is an example of what has been called "the coconstruction of the meaning of distress," a critical task of the clinical encounter in these cases (16).

The identification of a psychosocial basis for patients' somatic complaints is often sufficient to allow them to marshal their own resources for coping (17). When these measures fail, the patient may need goal-focused short-term counseling (see Chapter 20). In selected cases, short-term prescription of anxiolytic or hypnotic medications may be helpful.

There have been only a few reports of outcomes of minor mood disturbances managed by generalists (17–19). From these studies, the following tentative conclusions can be stated:

- A large proportion of patients get better after just one office visit. Most often, this visit includes empathic listening, a partial physical examination, and reassurance that the patient does not have a serious physical problem.
- Short-term prescribing of drugs for anxiety or insomnia may not increase the proportion of patients who show significant improvement (about two thirds of patients) on re-evaluation after 1 month (18). This conclusion derives from a single careful study in which patients with minor mood disturbances were allocated at random to receive brief counseling plus a benzodiazepine drug or brief counseling only.

Several practical considerations regarding longitudinal management are suggested by these findings:

- It is generally prudent to determine the impact of an initial visit on a patient's distress (by a brief telephone or office followup visit within 1 week) before considering a psychotropic drug for an adjustment disorder.
- About one third of patients who seem to have an adjustment disorder do not respond to the aforementioned strategies. At followup visits, such patients should be reinterviewed systematically to look for evidence of panic disorder (Chapter 22), major depression (Chapter 24), alcoholism (Chapter 28), chemical dependency (Chapter 29), and domestic violence (Chapter 28) affecting themselves or a member of their household, or one of the somatoform disorders described later in this chapter. For all of these problems, specific treatment in addition to office psychotherapy is indicated.

PSYCHOLOGICAL FACTORS AFFECTING MEDICAL CONDITIONS

Description

Psychological factors can exacerbate somatic symptoms caused by a concurrent physical disorder. The resulting symptoms are sometimes called *psychophysiologic.* Table 21.2 lists the most common conditions in which such symptoms may occur. When the features listed in Table 21.3 are present, the diagnosis from the *Diagnostic and*

TABLE 21.2 Common Conditions in Which Psychophysiologic Symptoms Are Important

Physiologic System	*Symptomatic Condition*	*Chapter with Further Information*
Cardiovascular	Migraine headache	87
	Vasovagal syndrome (fainting)	89
	Hypertension (usually asymptomatic)	67
	Supraventricular tachycardia	64
	Angina	62
Gastrointestinal	Irritable bowel syndrome	44
	The following symptoms may occur singly or together: anorexia, nausea, vomiting, abdominal cramps, diarrhea, constipation, aerophagia, acid-peptic symptoms	42–46
Genitourinary	Menstrual disturbance	101
	Difficulties in micturition: frequency (in both sexes), retention (females), hesitancy (in males)	36, 53
	Sexual disorders	6
	Dyspareunia	
	Anorgasmia	
	Inhibited sexual excitement	
	Delayed ejaculation, premature ejaculation	
Musculoskeletal	Pain secondary to increased muscle tension: occipital or bitemporal headaches, backaches, myalgia in various muscle groups	71, 74, 87
	Fatigue	
	Tremor	90
	Rheumatoid arthritis	77
Respiratory	Hyperventilation syndrome	22
	Bronchospasm	60
	Dyspnea	59
Skin	Hyperhidrosis	
	Pruritus	

Statistical Manual of Mental Disorders, 4th Edition (DSM-IV), is Psychological Factors Affecting Medical Condition.

Most of the conditions listed in Table 21.2 may occur with or without a significant psychological component; detailed descriptions of most of these conditions are found elsewhere in this book, as indicated in the table. For a patient's symptoms to be interpreted as psychophysiologic, they should bear a temporal relationship to a stressful life situation and should subside when the stressful situation abates.

TABLE 21.3 Diagnostic Criteria for Psychological Factors Affecting Physical Condition

A. A general medical condition (coded on axis III) is present.
B. Psychological factors adversely affect the general medical condition in one of the following ways:
   1. The factors have influenced the course of the general medical condition as shown by a close temporal association between the psychological factors and the development or exacerbation of, or delayed recovery from, the general medical condition.
   2. The factors interfere with the treatment of the general medical condition.
   3. The factors constitute additional health risks for the individual.
   4. The factors elicit stress-related physiologic responses that precipitate or exacerbate symptoms of a general medical condition (e.g., chest pain or arrhythmia in a patient with CAD).

Conversion symptoms (see Conversion Disorder section) are differentiated from psychophysiologic symptoms by the absence of a pathophysiologic condition in the former. Psychophysiologic problems are closely related to adjustment disorders, but they are distinguishable from them in that the somatic symptoms are caused by a recognized pathophysiologic condition and the same symptoms may occur in the absence of psychosocial stressors. This diagnosis is also used when psychological factors interfere with the treatment of a general medical condition (e.g., when strong denial of illness interferes with adherence to medication regimens).

Management

When initiation or exacerbation of a physical condition is related to environmental stressors, management is the same as that described for adjustment disorder.

SOMATOFORM DISORDERS

As a group, the somatoform disorders are characterized by the occurrence of physical symptoms that lack an organic basis and are linked, by positive evidence or strong presumption, to psychological factors or conflicts. They may be acute or chronic, mild or severely disabling. Because patients with these disorders believe themselves to be physically ill, they are treated primarily by nonpsychiatrists and generally do not accept psychiatric referral. In addition to the management strategies described here, the strategies for managing abnormal illness behavior, described in Chapter 20, usually are helpful.

Somatization Disorder

Description

The best-studied disorder in this group is somatization disorder, formerly known as hysteria or Briquet syndrome. This is a chronic disorder beginning before 30 years of age in which the patient seeks treatment for multiple, widely distributed symptoms lacking any known pathologic basis or pathophysiologic mechanism. To meet *DSM-IV* criteria for this disorder, the patient must have a history of at least eight such symptoms, drawn from the four symptom subgroups listed in Table 21.4: Pain symptoms (at least four), gastrointestinal (GI) symptoms (two or more), sexual symptoms (at least one), and pseudoneurologic symptoms (at least one). Accurate diagnosis often requires review of old records and careful history-taking to determine that a sufficient number of unexplained symptoms have been presented for evaluation and treatment or have caused the patient to take over-the-counter (OTC) remedies or alter his or her lifestyle. *Seven symptoms are especially useful in screening*: shortness of breath without exertion, dysmenorrhea, burning sensations in sexual organs, difficulty swallowing (lump in throat), amnesia, vomiting, and pain in extremities. The presence of three of these symptoms without adequate physical explanation identifies somatization disorder with a sensitivity of 87% and specificity of 95% (20). Symptoms are often described in dramatic and colorful terms, but details tend to be vague and contradictory.

Somatization disorder occurs in 0.2% to 2.0% of women in the general population, but it is much more common among women seen in clinical settings (21). It is rare in men. Histrionic personality traits may be present. Somatization disorder occurs in 10% to 20% of female first-degree relatives of women with somatization disorder; alcoholism and antisocial personality disorder occur frequently among their male relatives.

Common complications include substance abuse and iatrogenic illness. One classic study found that women with hysteria undergo more than three times as many operations as control women and lose, by weight, more than three times the mass of organs (22).

The disorder is chronic. In a retrospective study of 49 patients, almost 70% of women were still symptomatic 15 years after diagnosis (23). However, the mortality rate of women with somatization disorder is the same as that of normal women (24), and the likelihood of developing another medical or psychiatric disorder explaining the symptoms is only 10% in long-term followup (25).

TABLE 21.4 Diagnostic Criteria for Somatization Disorder

A. History of many physical complaints beginning before 30 years of age, occurring over a period of several years, and resulting in treatment being sought or significant impairment in social or occupational functioning.

B. Each of the following criteria must have been met at some time during the course of the disorder.
  1. Four pain symptoms: A history of pain related to at least four different sites or functions (such as head, abdomen, back, joints, extremities, chest, rectum, during sexual intercourse, during menstruation, or during urination)
  2. Two GI symptoms: A history of at least two GI symptoms other than pain (such as nausea, diarrhea, bloating, vomiting other than during pregnancy, or intolerance of several different foods)
  3. One sexual symptom: A history of at least one sexual or reproductive symptom other than pain (such as sexual indifference, erectile or ejaculatory dysfunction, irregular menses, excessive menstrual bleeding, vomiting throughout pregnancy)
  4. One pseudoneurologic symptom: A history of at least one symptom or deficit suggesting a neurologic disorder not limited to pain (conversion symptoms such as blindness, double vision, deafness, loss of touch or pain sensation, hallucinations, aphonia, impaired coordination or balance, paralysis or localized weakness, difficulty swallowing, difficulty breathing, urinary retention, seizures; dissociative symptoms such as amnesia, or loss of consciousness other than fainting)

C. Either of the following must have been met:
  1. After appropriate investigation, each of the symptoms in criterion B cannot be fully explained by a known general medical condition, or the direct effects of a substance (e.g. a drug of abuse, a medication).
  2. When there is a related general medical condition, the physical complaints or resulting social or occupational impairment are in excess of what would be expected from the history, physical examination, or laboratory findings.

D. The symptoms are not intentionally produced or feigned (as in Factitious Disorder or Malingering).

Reprinted with permission from Diagnostic and statistical manual of mental disorders. 4th Edition. Washington, DC: American Psychiatric Association, 1994.

Case Example

A 43-year-old married woman was referred for psychiatric evaluation by her internist who, noting her presentation with ill-defined symptoms, was requesting help with management. She complained of generalized muscle aching and periodic sensations throughout her body described as "how you feel when someone scratches his fingers on a blackboard." She also complained of skin lesions on her back and stated that she was hypothyroid and suffered from a chronic urinary tract infection. Her history included tonsillectomy, groin lymph node biopsy (twice), hysterectomy, bladder suspension (twice), rectocele repair, removal of abdominal adhesions, multiple cystoscopies, appendectomy, and removal of a tongue papilloma. The patient stated she had Ménière disease and episodes of sudden shortness of breath. She also carried a diagnosis of fibrositis, for which she had taken steroids in the past, and restless legs syndrome. She had stopped having sexual intercourse with her husband because of "pain that 10 gynecologists could not cure." Her current medicines included a benzodiazepine, a nonsteroidal anti-inflammatory agent, and a belladonna alkaloid. She mentioned that she had always been ill and that she hated men. Her psychosocial history included marriage to an alcoholic who abused her and a positive family history of suicide. In presenting her symptoms, the patient was extremely vague and interjected facts about her emotional life with an inappropriate laugh. She believed that her symptoms were caused by food allergy. She had stopped eating and at the time of her initial visit to her internist had ingested only distilled water for 4 days. Physical examination and laboratory test results were normal.

Management

Because these patients adhere firmly to the idea that they are physically ill, they usually do not accept psychiatric referral, and their treatment lies largely in the hands of nonpsychiatrists. Guidelines for management include the following:

1. *Review past medical records* to determine the range of symptomatic complaints brought to health care practitioners and the adequacy of documented evaluations.
2. *Respond to physical symptoms appropriately* by taking a careful history and doing the appropriate physical examination. Recognize that the history, as a diagnostic test, will have comparatively low specificity for physical disease (see Chapter 2) and that questioning techniques that diminish the likelihood of false positive findings, such as the use of open-ended and nonleading questions (see Chapter 3), are particularly important for such patients. Avoid hospitalizations, specialty consultations, and invasive laboratory tests unless objective indications exist (see Managing Abnormal Illness Behavior, in Chapter 20).
3. *Review the four explanatory perspectives* (see Why Patients Somatize) for factors that might be promoting the development of somatization: psychiatric disease (especially major depression), personality disorder (especially histrionic type), behavioral model (e.g., sick family members), and environmental reinforcers (e.g., increased attention from parents) supporting the sick role, as well as aspects of the patient's life story (e.g., poor attention to early childhood dependency needs) that make the patient's symptoms (e.g., endless recitation of complaints that keep the patient under very close medical scrutiny) understandable. When possible, address the apparently etiologic factors in the treatment plan (e.g., treat major depression with antidepressants; counsel family members to give attention for healthy behavior but to refrain from rewarding illness behavior).
4. *Work with the patient to understand and accept the link between somatic symptoms and psychosocial stress* (see above under Adjustment Disorder, Management).
5. Do not expect symptoms to remit entirely, and *do not promise cure or complete resolution of symptoms*.
6. *Promote the performance of normal function despite symptoms,* and praise the patient for carrying out specific activities and for being productive in the face of discomfort.
7. Assure the patient of your continuing availability, and *schedule regular, brief visits* so that access to medical attention does not require the development of new symptoms.
8. *Help the family* of the patient recognize that, despite the abundance and persistence of symptoms, no serious disease has been found, and encourage them to support a strategy that de-emphasizes expensive and elaborate diagnostic tests and stresses maintenance of function in the face of symptoms.
9. *Try "mining for gold"* (26). Because these patients focus on physical symptoms, which usually are not explained by physical disease and do not resolve with treatment, the clinician is likely to spend each visit investigating the physical symptoms of concern, performing unrevealing diagnostic tests, and becoming frustrated. By spending some time during each visit "mining for gold" (i.e., getting to know in depth the person who is the patient) the clinician may discover previously unrecognized admirable and likeable aspects of the patient, forge a mutually satisfactory practitioner–patient relationship, and be able to facilitate more effectively the patient's maintenance of health and functional status despite symptoms.

The usefulness of measures such as these in the management of somatization disorder has been demonstrated in a randomized, controlled study (27).

TABLE 21.5 Diagnostic Criteria for Undifferentiated Somatoform Disorder

A. One or more physical complaints (e.g., fatigue, loss of appetite, GI or urinary complaints)
B. Either of the following:
 1. After appropriate investigation, the symptoms cannot be explained by a known general medical condition or pathophysiologic mechanism (e.g., the effects of injury, medication, drugs, or alcohol).
 2. When there is a related general medical condition, the physical complaints or resulting social or occupational impairment are grossly in excess of what would be expected from the physical findings.
C. The symptoms cause clinically significant distress or impairment in social, occupational, or other important areas of functioning.
D. The duration of the disturbance is at least 6 months.
E. The disturbance is not better accounted for by another mental disorder (e.g., another somatoform disorder, sexual dysfunction, mood disorder, anxiety disorder, sleep disorder, or psychotic disorder).
F. The symptoms are not intentionally produced or feigned (as in Factitious Disorder or Malingering).

Reprinted with permission from Diagnostic and statistical manual of mental disorders. 4th Edition. Washington, DC: American Psychiatric Association, 1994.

Undifferentiated Somatoform Disorder and Multisomatoform Disorder

Undifferentiated somatoform disorder is a residual category designed to accommodate patients who do not fully meet criteria for somatization disorder (Table 21.5). Symptoms must be present for at least 6 months for the diagnosis to be made. There need be no identifiable precipitant. Although the disorder has not been well studied, it is believed to be much more common than somatization disorder. Its prognosis and clinical course are unknown.

Multisomatoform disorder is a term that does not appear in *DSM-IV*. It has been proposed as an alternative to "undifferentiated somatoform disorder" for patients with a 2-year history of apparent somatoform symptoms and at least three current somatoform symptoms, reported from a 15-symptom checklist (28). Of 1,000 participants in the Primary Care Evaluation of Mental Disorders (PRIME-MD) (29) study, 82 (8.2%) met criteria for this condition. These patients had significantly greater numbers of disability days and doctor visits as well as impairments in health-related quality of life and were far more likely than patients with other psychiatric conditions to be judged "difficult" by their physicians.

Although there are no studies of treatment for these specific disorders, there is evidence that techniques useful in full-fledged somatization disorder (see Somatization Disorder, Management) are helpful for long-term somatizing patients who do not meet all of the diagnostic criteria for somatization disorder (30).

TABLE 21.6 Diagnostic Criteria for Conversion Disorder

A. One or more symptoms or deficits affecting voluntary motor or sensory function suggesting a neurologic or general medical condition.
B. Psychological factors are judged to be associated with the symptom or deficit because the initiation or exacerbation of the symptom or deficit is preceded by conflicts or other stressors.
C. The symptom or deficit is not intentionally produced or feigned (as in Factitious Disorder or Malingering).
D. The symptom of deficit cannot, after appropriate investigation, be fully explained by a neurologic or general medical condition, and is not a culturally sanctioned behavior or experience.
E. The symptom or deficit causes clinically significant distress or impairment in social, occupational, or other important areas of functioning; or warrants medical evaluation.
F. The symptom or deficit is not limited to pain or sexual dysfunction, does not occur exclusively during the course of somatization disorder, and is not better accounted for by another mental disorder.

Reprinted with permission from Diagnostic and statistical manual of mental disorders. 4th Edition. Washington, DC: American Psychiatric Association, 1994.

Conversion Disorder

Description

Conversion disorder is a disorder in which an unexplained loss or alteration of body functioning develops in the presence of evidence that the symptoms solve or express a psychological conflict or need (Table 21.6). The symptoms often simulate neurologic disease but conform to the patient's notion of body function rather than to the rules of neuroanatomy, and medical evaluation yields no evidence of diagnosable disease. Amnesia, aphonia, blindness, paralysis, numbness, and seizures are among the most common conversion symptoms. The disorder probably occurs more often in women than in men, and it usually begins in adolescence or early adulthood. Patients may have histrionic or dependent personalities and may exhibit remarkable serenity (*"la belle indifference"*) in the face of their impairments.

Conversion disorder is unique among *DSM-IV* somatoform disorders in that the definition not only describes the diagnostic criteria but also proposes psychological mechanisms as explanations. A mechanism called *secondary gain* is invoked when unexplained symptoms allow the patient to avoid onerous tasks or undesirable duties (see Somatization as Reinforced Behavior).

Case Example

A 15-year-old girl with a history of migraine headache and transient visual field cuts was evaluated for a new visual field cut that had developed without headache over the previous 24 hours. On examination, the visual defect was found to "split the macula."

At the time of psychiatric interview she revealed that she expected her visual problems to prevent her from obtaining a driver's license when she turned 16. She went on to say that she was afraid to drive, that no other woman in her family drove, and that she would be called upon by everyone to provide transportation. She was referred to a pediatric neurology service, where she received physical therapy and daily psychotherapy. Her field defect resolved.

A second mechanism, *primary gain,* is invoked when conversion symptoms appear to resolve an internal conflict created by a feeling, impulse, or wish that the individual finds frightening or morally unacceptable.

Case Example

A 50-year-old man was admitted to the hospital because of amnesia. He spoke normally and was otherwise neurologically intact, although he could not remember his name or any other details of personal history. After about 24 hours he began speaking freely about anger related to the recent dissolution of his marriage. Particularly upsetting had been news that his boss was dating his wife. Immediately before the development of amnesia he had thought that he might be provoked to violence if he discovered them together. His amnesia completely resolved in 2 days, and he was discharged from the hospital. He briefly participated in outpatient psychotherapy. The working formulation was that the amnesia had served to remove unacceptable violent intentions from his awareness and to protect him from acting on them.

Acute conversion symptoms have a good prognosis for recovery, especially if the patient has no other psychiatric disorder.

Management

Guidelines for the treatment of patients with conversion disorder include the following:

1. Be certain that the patient has had an *adequate medical evaluation,* because some patients with conversion symptoms have an undiagnosed medical disorder (4).
2. *Review the various explanatory perspectives for factors that might be promoting the development of conversion symptoms* (see Why Patients Somatize): e.g., environmental reinforcers supporting the sick role (e.g., not having to drive) or aspects of the patient's life story (e.g., violent feelings toward an abusive alcoholic father) that make the symptoms understandable (e.g., visual impairment that prevents driving; paralysis of the hand that prevents violent revenge against the father). When possible, address specific interventions to the etiologic factors identified (e.g., refer the angry child of an alcoholic to Al-Anon).
3. Emphasize the evidence that no serious disease is present, and express optimism about the prospect of full recovery. Consider physical therapy or some other physical rehabilitative intervention to *help the patient save face* during recovery.
4. *Do not bluntly confront the patient with the psychological origins of the symptoms,* but stress that emotional factors can exacerbate such problems. Review the patient's current life circumstances and difficulties, and consider undertaking a course of short-term counseling (see Chapter 20).

Hypochondriasis

Description

Hypochondriacal concerns that are relieved by evaluation, explanation, and reassurance are common in medical practice. Hypochondriasis, however, is a chronic disorder in which unrealistic interpretation of physical symptoms leads the patient to fear the presence of a serious illness in the face of repeated reassurances based on adequate medical evaluation (Table 21.7). Onset is usually in the third decade but may occur later. Both sexes are equally affected. Obsessive-compulsive personality traits are often observed. Anxiety, depression, drug dependence, and iatrogenic disease are common complications. The disorder tends to be chronic, with waxing and waning intensity. Symptomatic exacerbations occur in response to psychosocial stresses and to stimuli that provoke bodily preoccupation and fear of disease.

TABLE 21.7 Diagnostic Criteria for Hypochondriasis

A. Preoccupation with fears of having, or the idea that one has, a serious disease based on the person's misinterpretation of bodily symptoms.
B. The preoccupation persists despite appropriate medical evaluation and reassurance.
C. The belief (in criterion A) is not of delusional intensity (as in Delusional Disorder, Somatic type) and is not restricted to a circumscribed concern about appearance (as in Body Dysmorphic Disorder).
D. The preoccupation causes clinically significant distress or impairment in social, occupational, or other important areas of functioning.
E. The duration of the disturbance is at least 6 months.
F. The preoccupation does not occur exclusively during the course of generalized anxiety disorder, obsessive-compulsive disorder, panic disorder, major depressive episode, separation anxiety, or another somatoform disorder.

Specify if with poor insight: if, for most of the time during the current episode, the person does not recognize that the concern about having a serious illness is excessive or unreasonable.

Reprinted with permission from Diagnostic and statistical manual of mental disorders. 4th Edition. Washington, DC: American Psychiatric Association, 1994.

Case Example

A 30-year-old accountant had always been self-conscious about his physical appearance, a concern that he attempted to allay by weight lifting. After his father died of a heart attack, he became concerned that he might have heart disease and was fearful about the implication of insignificant chest pains. He also worried about his blood pressure, which was transiently elevated at the time of his yearly physical examinations. His most recent examination revealed insignificant liver enzyme elevations, a finding over which he fretted for weeks. Despite these concerns, he rarely missed a day of work. He was not sure that he did not have a serious disease but thought he had best trust his health care provider.

Management

Because patients with hypochondriasis believe that they are physically ill, they often refuse psychiatric treatment. Guidelines for management by generalists are similar to those for other chronic somatoform disorders and include the following:

1. *Review past medical records* to determine the range of symptomatic complaints brought to health care practitioners and the adequacy of documented evaluations.
2. *Respond to physical symptoms appropriately* by taking a careful history and doing the appropriate physical examination. Reassurances cannot be given to the patient if the physical complaints are not investigated. At the same time, recognize that the history, as a diagnostic indicator, may have comparatively low specificity for physical disease (see Chapter 2), and that questioning techniques that diminish the likelihood of false positive findings, such as the use of open-ended and nonleading questions (see Chapter 3), are particularly important in such patients. Avoid hospitalization, inappropriate specialty consultations, and invasive laboratory tests unless objective indications exist (see Managing Abnormal Illness Behavior, in Chapter 20).
3. *Review the four explanatory perspectives* (see Why Patients Somatize) for factors that might be promoting hypochondriasis: psychiatric illness (especially major depression and anxiety disorders), personality disorder (especially obsessive-compulsive type), behavioral models or environmental reinforcers supporting the role (e.g., family members who were excessively concerned about patient's childhood health and lavished attention in response to minor ailments), and aspects of the patient's life story (e.g., religious upbringing with particular emphasis on sexual morality and punishment of sinners) that make the symptoms empathically understandable (e.g., hypochondriacal fear of AIDS in a man with repeatedly negative HIV antibody tests who had a single extramarital encounter 5 years before). When possible, address specific interventions to etiologic factors identified (e.g., counsel family members to give attention for healthy behavior but refrain from rewarding illness behavior). It is especially important to consider treating concurrent major depression and anxiety disorders with antidepressant medications, because the amelioration of major mood and anxiety symptoms often greatly improves the receptivity of hypochondriacal patients to reassurance about their physical health.
4. Do not expect symptoms to remit entirely, and *do not promise cure or complete resolution of symptoms* (see Managing Abnormal Illness Behavior, in Chapter 20).
5. *Promote the performance of normal functions despite symptoms,* and praise the patient for carrying out specific activities and being productive in the face of discomfort.
6. Reassure the patient of your continuing availability, and *schedule regular, brief visits* so that access to medical attention does not depend on the development of new symptoms.
7. *Work with the patient to understand and accept the link between somatic symptoms and psychosocial stress* (see above under Adjustment Disorder, Management).
8. *Help the family* of the patient recognize that despite the persistence of symptoms no serious disease has been found, and encourage them to support a strategy deemphasizing expensive and elaborate diagnostic tests and stressing maintenance of function in the face of symptoms.
9. *Try "mining for gold"* (26) (see above under Somatization Disorder, *Management*).
10. Some patients may accept *short-term counseling* (see Chapter 20). Formal cognitive-behavioral therapy has been shown to be effective, at least when provided to willing patients by experienced therapists (31,32). "Explanatory therapy," a similar but less technical approach originally described by Kellner (33), has also been shown to reduce hypochondriacal fears, emotional distress, and health care utilization, but it is not presently of proven benefit when administered by nonspecialists (34).

Pain Disorder

Description

Somatoform pain disorder is a chronic disorder characterized by unexplained or amplified complaints of pain (Table 21.8). It usually has its onset in the fourth or fifth decade and is associated with marked functional disability. The diagnosis is most useful when psychological factors can be linked to the onset and maintenance of pain. A typical scenario begins with lower back pain, which often develops on the job and is initially diagnosed as a sprain. The patient may see his or her primary care practitioner and attempt

TABLE 21.8 Diagnostic Criteria for Pain Disorder

A. Pain in one or more anatomic sites is the predominant focus of the clinical presentation and is of sufficient severity to warrant clinical attention.
B. The pain causes clinically significant distress or impairment in social, occupational, or other important areas of functioning.
C. Psychological factors are judged to have an important role in the onset, severity, exacerbation, or maintenance of the pain.
D. The symptoms are not intentionally produced or feigned (as in Factitional Disorder or Malingering).
E. The pain is not better accounted for by a mood, anxiety, or psychotic disorder and does not meet criteria for dyspareunia.

Reprinted with permission from Diagnostic and statistical manual of mental disorders. 4th Edition. Washington, DC: American Psychiatric Association, 1994.

to return to work. Soon thereafter the pain recurs, sometimes after apparent reinjury. Specialty consultations (e.g., orthopedic, neurosurgical) ensue. Conservative treatments (e.g., physical therapy) are ineffective. Surgery may be performed, perhaps with transient benefit, but soon there is a resurgence of symptoms described as worse than ever. After 6 to 12 months of illness the patient is out of work, socially isolated, physically inactive, dependent on narcotic analgesics, angry, and demoralized. He or she may believe that health professionals and family members do not regard the pain as real.

Management

Treatment of somatoform pain disorder is similar to the management of other somatoform disorders:

1. *Review past medical records* to determine the timing and extent of prior evaluations and treatments.
2. Respond to pain complaints with a *thorough history and physical examination* and determine that adequate medical, surgical, and neurologic evaluations have been done, but avoid procedures and hospitalization in the absence of clear indications.
3. *Review the four explanatory perspectives* (see Why Patients Somatize) for factors that might be promoting unexplained or amplified pain complaints, and design a treatment plan that addresses specific etiologic factors identified: major psychiatric disease (especially major depression and chemical dependency, both of which are common in patients with somatoform pain), personality traits (especially exaggerated dependency), environmental reinforcers (e.g., financial compensation, relief from work responsibility, sympathy from family and friends), and aspects of life history that make the pain complaints empathically understandable (e.g., abusive or negligent parenting leading to a yearning to be cared for in a passive-dependent way that is often hidden behind a defiant facade).
4. Convey optimism that improvement is likely, but *do not promise cure or complete resolution of symptoms*.
5. *Promote the performance of functions that are reasonable for the patient to perform despite symptoms,* and praise patients for carrying out specific activities and being productive in the face of discomfort.
6. Reassure the patient of your continuing availability, and *schedule regular, brief visits* so that access to medical attention does not require exacerbation of symptoms.
7. *Consider topical treatments and physical therapy* because of their intrinsic value, safety, and symbolic value as indicators that the physical reality of the patient's pain is recognized.
8. Generally, *avoid prescribing benzodiazepines and narcotic analgesics,* and persuade addicted patients to pursue detoxification. In selected patients who are functional on a stable opioid regimen, it is reasonable to maintain the regimen as part of a contractual plan for the management of chronic pain (see Chapter 29). Antidepressant medication may be of use in some patients, especially if the pain is neuropathic in nature (see Chapter 13) or if there is concomitant anxiety (see Chapter 22) or depression (see Chapter 24).
9. *Work with the patient to understand and accept the link between somatic symptoms and psychosocial stress* (see above under Adjustment Disorder, Management).
10. *Attempt to direct the patient to discuss life problems, especially interpersonal conflicts and disappointments.*
11. *Enlist the support of the patient's family* in an effort to reinforce maintenance of function in the face of symptoms rather than persistence of disability.
12. Consider referral to a center specializing in the *multidisciplinary care* of patients with chronic pain syndromes.
13. *Try "mining for gold"* (26) (see above under Somatization Disorder, *Management*).

Body Dysmorphic Disorder

Description

Body dysmorphic disorder is a disorder characterized by an excessive or completely unfounded preoccupation with a defect in personal appearance (Table 21.9). The prevalence of the disorder is unknown. Onset typically occurs between adolescence and age 30 years. Perceived facial imperfections, such as the shape of the nose or jaw, are the most common sources of concern.

Case Example

A 60-year-old man entered into psychiatric treatment for chronic depression. He reported long-standing attitudes and patterns of behavior suggesting obsessionality and extreme

TABLE 21.9 Diagnostic Criteria for Body Dysmorphic Disorder

A. Preoccupation with an imagined defect in appearance. If a slight physical anomaly is present, the person's concern is markedly excessive.
B. The preoccupation causes clinically significant distress or impairment in social, occupational, or other important areas of functioning.
C. The preoccupation is not better accounted for by another mental disorder (e.g., dissatisfaction with body shape and size in Anorexia Nervosa).

Reprinted with permission from Diagnostic and statistical manual of mental disorders. 4th Edition. Washington, DC: American Psychiatric Association, 1994.

self-consciousness. He also reported a preoccupation beginning in adolescence with the shape of his jaw. He had undergone elaborate surgical treatment for this but continued to feel that other people were put off by his appearance, a belief contributing to his social discomfort. The examining psychiatrist found nothing remarkable about the appearance of his face. The patient's preoccupation with this perceived defect was partially ameliorated by antidepressant treatment, but he continued to regard himself as misshapen.

Management

Little is known about the treatment and prognosis of the disorder. Some authors believe it should be regarded as a symptom, not as a distinct condition. Generally, patients should be discouraged from pursuing surgical solutions, especially when their concerns are entirely unfounded. Otherwise, many of the management guidelines described earlier for other chronic somatoform disorders are applicable. In particular, it is useful to review the four explanatory perspectives for factors promoting the development and maintenance of the symptoms and to treat any specific etiologic factor identified: an associated major psychiatric illness (usually major depression), personality types predisposing to the disorder (especially obsessive-compulsive and avoidant types—see Chapter 23), behavioral models for these concerns (e.g., parents who were dissatisfied with similar physical attributes in themselves), and aspects of the life story that make the symptoms empathically understandable (e.g., early experiences with critical parents leading the patient to feel unwanted or unacceptable).

DISORDERS WITH VOLUNTARY SYMPTOM PRODUCTION

The fundamental feature of disorders with voluntary symptom production is the deliberate simulation of physical symptoms. This characteristic distinguishes patients with these disorders from those with chronic somatoform

TABLE 21.10 Diagnostic Criteria for Factitious Disorder with Physical Symptoms

A. Intentional production or feigning of physical or psychological signs or symptoms.
B. The motivation for the behavior is to assume the sick role.
C. External incentives for the behavior (such as economic gain, avoiding legal responsibility, or improving physical well-being, as in Malingering) are absent.

Reprinted with permission from Diagnostic and statistical manual of mental disorders. 4th Edition. Washington, DC: American Psychiatric Association, 1994.

disorders, described earlier, in which symptom genesis is not deliberate.

Factitious Disorder with Physical Symptoms

Description

Factitious illness is characterized by the deliberate simulation of physical symptoms for the sole purpose of assuming the sick role (35). When this behavior is chronic and leads to multiple hospitalizations, it is known as chronic factitious disorder with physical symptoms (Table 21.10) or *Munchhausen syndrome.* When there is deliberate simulation of a psychiatric syndrome, it is designated as Factitious Disorder with Psychological Symptoms.

Patients may report invented symptoms (e.g., severe right lower quadrant abdominal pain), or they may deliberately produce physical signs by heating thermometers, tying tourniquets around their legs, or ingesting anticoagulant drugs. The history may be dramatic but vague in medically relevant detail. Onset is usually in early adulthood, often shortly after hospitalization for a *bona fide* physical illness. Job stability, family life, and other interpersonal relationships suffer profoundly as a result of multiple lengthy hospitalizations.

Management

The main goals of management are to prevent unnecessary hospitalizations and to avoid invasive procedures. The management of the hospitalized patient may be facilitated by early psychiatric consultation to assist in diagnosis, determine whether other treatable psychiatric disorders are present, help plan tactful confrontation of the patient with the diagnosis, and attempt to persuade the patient to accept psychiatric hospitalization.

Malingering

Description

Malingering is the deliberate simulation of physical (or psychological) symptoms to achieve a specific benefit. It is an important and common problem in settings where sickness is rewarded with certain benefits (e.g., avoidance of military service or court appearances, financial compensation for injuries). Malingering comprises three types (see Ford, at www.hopkinsbayview.org/PAMreferences):

1. Pure malingering, in which there is deliberate deception by the description or production of nonexistent symptoms or signs (rare)
2. Partial malingering, which involves the conscious and voluntary exaggeration of symptoms of a real disease
3. Deliberate attribution of an actual disability to an injury or accident that did not cause it

The diagnosis of malingering should be suspected whenever symptoms or disabilities greatly exceeding objective disease are accompanied by obvious social or financial benefit. Other observations suggesting the diagnosis include inconsistency of symptoms (e.g., a blind person detected reading), unusually vague or markedly exaggerated reports of symptoms, and the expression of indignant anger in response to gentle confrontation.

Malingering must be distinguished from factitious disorders, in which the patient has no goal aside from achieving patienthood, and from conversion disorders, in which symptom production is not conscious or intentional.

Management

The goal of management is to persuade malingering patients to give up their symptoms. Patients should gradually and tactfully be made aware that malingering is suspected, and the gratifications associated with the sick role should be removed. Reports of symptoms should be given minimal attention. If psychiatric disorders are thought to underlie or complicate apparent malingering, psychiatric consultation should be obtained.

SPECIFIC REFERENCES*

1. Mechanic D. The concept of illness behavior: culture, situation, and personal disposition. Psychol Med 1986;16:1.
2. Sharpe M, Carson A. "Unexplained" somatic symptoms, functional syndromes, and somatization: do we need a paradigm shift? Ann Intern Med 2001;134:926.
3. Simon GE, VonKorff M, Piccinelli M, et al. An international study of the relation between somatic symptoms and depression. N Engl J Med 1999;341:1329.
4. Lazare A. Conversion symptoms. N Engl J Med 1983;305:745.
5. O'Malley PG, Jones DL, Feuerstein IM, et al. Lack of correlation between psychological factors and subclinical coronary artery disease. N Engl J Med 2000;343:1298.
6. Dworkin SF, Von Korff M, LeResche L. Multiple pains and psychiatric disturbance. An epidemiologic investigation. Arch Gen Psychiatry 1990;47:239.
7. Hansell S, Mechanic D. Introspectiveness and adolescent symptom reporting. J Hum Stress 1985;11(Winter):165.
8. Costa PT, McCrae RR. Hypochondriasis, neuroticism, and aging. Am Psychol 1985; 40:19.
9. Lipowski ZJ. Somatization: the concept and its clinical application. Am J Psychiatry 1988;145:1358.
10. Taylor GJ: Somatization and conversion: distinct or overlapping constructs?. J Am Acad Psychoanal 2003;31:487.
11. Arnow BA. Relationships between childhood maltreatment, adult health and psychiatric outcomes, and medical utilization. J Clin Psychiatry 2004;65 (supp 12):10.
12. Katon W, Sullivan M, Walker E. Medical symptoms without identified pathology: relationship to psychiatric disorders, childhood and adult trauma, and personality traits. Ann Intern Med 2001;134:917.
13. Barsky AJ, Klerman GL. Overview: hypochondriasis, bodily complaints, and somatic styles. Am J Psychiatry 1983;140:273.
14. Mayou R, Kirmayer LJ, Simon G, et al. Somatoform disorders: time for a new approach in DSM-V. Am J Psychiatry 2005;162:847.
15. Drossman DA. The problem patient: evaluation and care of medical patients with psychosocial disturbances. Ann Intern Med 1978;88:366.
16. Kirmayer LJ, Groleau D, Looper KJ, et al. Explaining medically unexplained symptoms. Can J Psychiatry 2004;49:663.
17. Johnstone A, Goldberg D. Psychiatric screening in general practice. Lancet 1976;1:605.
18. Catalan J, Bath D, Edmonds G, et al. The effects of non-prescribing of anxiolytics in general practice: I. Controlled evaluation of psychiatric and social outcome. Br J Psychiatry 1984; 144:593.
19. Catalan J, Bath D, Bond A, et al. The effects of nonprescribing of anxiolytics in general practice: II. Factors associated with outcome. Br J Psychiatry 1984;144:603.
20. Othmer E, DeSouza C. A screening test in somatization disorder (hysteria). Am J Psychiatry 1985;142:1146.
21. Manu P, Lane TJ, Matthews DA. Screening for somatization disorder in patients with chronic fatigue. Gen Hosp Psychiatry 1989;11:294.
22. Cohen ME, Robins E, Purtell JJ, et al. Excessive surgery in hysteria. JAMA 1953;151:977.
23. Coryell W, Norten SG. Briquet's syndrome (somatization disorder) and primary depression: comparison of background and outcome. Compr Psychiatry 1981;22:249.
24. Coryell W. Diagnosis-specific mortality. Primary depression and Briquet's syndrome (somatization disorder). Arch Gen Psychiatry 1981;38:939.
25. Perley MJ, Guze SB. Hysteria: the stability and usefulness of clinical criteria. N Engl J Med 1962;266:421.
26. Levinson W. Mining for gold. J Gen Intern Med 1993;8:172.
27. Smith GR, Monson RA, Ray DC. Psychiatric consultation in somatization disorder: a randomized controlled study. N Engl J Med 1986;314:1407.
28. Kroenke K, Spitzer RL, deGruy FV, et al. Multisomatiform disorder: an alternative to undifferentiated somatoform disorder for the somatizing patient in primary care. Arch Gen Psychiatry 1997;54:352.
29. Spitzer RL, Williams JBW, Kroenke K, et al. Utility of a new procedure for diagnosing mental disorders in primary care: the PRIME-MD 1000 study. JAMA 1994;272:1749.
30. Smith GR, Rost K, Kashner TM. A trial of the effect of a standardized psychiatric consultation on health outcomes and costs in somatizing patients. Arch Gen Psychiatry 1995;52:238.
31. Warwick HMC, Clark DM, Cobb AM, et al. A controlled trial of cognitive-behavioral treatment of hypochondriasis. Br J Psychiatry 1996; 169:189.
32. Barsky AJ, Ahern DK. Cognitive behavior therapy for hypochondriasis; a randomized controlled trial. JAMA 2004;291:1464.
33. Kellner R. Psychotherapeutic strategies in hypochondriasis: a clinical study. Am J Psychother 1982;36:146.
34. Fava GA, Grandi S, Rafanelli C, et al. Explanatory therapy in hypochondriasis. J Clin Psychiatry 2000;61:317.
35. Krahn LE, Li Hongzhe, O'Connor MK. Patients who strive to be ill: factitious disorder with physical symptoms. Am J Psychiatry 2003; 160:1163.

*Bold numerals denote published controlled clinical trials, meta-analyses, or consensus-based recommendations.

*For annotated **General References** and resources related to this chapter, visit www.hopkinsbayview.org/PAMreferences.*

Chapter 22

Anxiety and Anxiety Disorders

Una D. McCann and O. Joseph Bienvenu, III

Anxiety is the term applied to a psychophysiologic state characterized by worry (apprehensive expectation), muscle tension, autonomic hyperactivity, and hypervigilance. Anxiety may improve performance in response to danger or challenge and, thus, may serve an adaptive function. However, when excessive or inappropriate in form or context, it leads to subjective distress and impairment in social and occupational functioning. Anxiety can be caused by a number of medical illnesses (e.g., hyperthyroidism, pheochromocytoma), and the presence of anxiety can prolong or exacerbate medical conditions (e.g., irritable bowel syndrome [IBS]). There is also some evidence that anxiety, like depression, may be an independent risk factor for the development of certain conditions, such as cardiovascular disease, hypertension, irritable bowel syndrome, and migraine headaches (1,2).

NORMAL ILLNESS-RELATED ANXIETY

Patients visiting their health care providers or awaiting the results of tests are often anxious. Although such anxiety may be understandable and realistically related to concerns about the meaning of symptoms and consequences of disease, it nonetheless requires recognition and management because it may interfere with medical care. For example, it has been found that survivors of myocardial infarction (MI) and their spouses recollect little of the information given to them during in-hospital convalescence, partly as a result of anxiety (3). Such findings highlight the importance of detecting normal illness-related anxiety and treating it skillfully. The following approaches are helpful:

- Assume that patients with new symptoms have concerns about serious illness. It is helpful to ask patients for their ideas about the causes of their symptoms. Often, a relative or friend has had a similar symptom related to a serious disease.
- Avoid comments or jargon that might sensitize or frighten patients (e.g., commenting, while examining a skin lesion, "It's been a long time since I've seen one like that.").
- Prepare the patient for painful or unfamiliar procedures with explanations. Assume that any procedure may be frightening to a patient.
- Assume that any patient recovering from serious illness is anxious about the future; determine whether any unnecessary disability in such patients is caused by fear or inadequate education. Hospitalized patients often get incomplete explanations of their illnesses at the time of discharge.

DRUG-RELATED ANXIETY

When evaluating patients with symptoms of anxiety, it is important to identify all medications or substances taken during or just before the onset of symptoms of anxiety. Prescribed drugs, over-the-counter (OTC) preparations, caffeine, ephedra-containing cold medications or dietary supplements, "herbal" preparations, alcohol, and other substances can all cause symptoms similar to those found in the primary anxiety disorders described later in this chapter. Licit and illicit stimulants, such as methylphenidate, amphetamine, cocaine, and 3,4-methylenedioxymetham phetamine (MDMA or "ecstasy") can produce symptoms indistinguishable from those of idiopathic anxiety disorders. Table 22.1 lists common examples of such compounds.

When considering the role of *caffeine* in producing anxiety, it is helpful to know the approximate amount of caffeine in commonly consumed beverages and substances:

- Coffee (1 cup): brewed, 60 to 180 mg; instant, 30 to 120 mg; decaffeinated, 2 to 5 mg
- Tea (1 cup): brewed U.S. brands, 20 to 90 mg; imported brands, 25 to 100 mg
- Soft drinks (6 oz): 15 to 23 mg
- Dark chocolate (1 oz): 5 to 35 mg

TABLE 22.1 Drugs and Other Substances That May Exacerbate (or Produce) Anxiety

Anticholinergic drugs
Corticosteroids
Drugs of abuse[a]
Amphetamines and amphetamine derivatives
Cocaine
Hallucinogens
Inhalants
Marijuana and other drugs that alter perception
Methylenedioxymethamphetamine (MDMA, "Ecstasy")
Phencyclidine (PCP)
Sympathomimetic agents
β_2 bronchodilators
Decongestants (found in most OTC cold remedies)
Ephedra-containing dietary supplements and "energy boosters"
Weight-reduction agents
Thyroid hormone
Xanthine-containing drugs, foods, and beverages
Bronchodilators with theophylline
Caffeine (use and discontinuation)[b]
Many OTC cold and arthritis remedies
Withdrawal symptoms
Alcohol
Sedative-hypnotics
Tobacco

[a]See Chapter 29.
[b]See text for approximate amount of caffeine in common beverages.

Patients who experience prominent anxiety, panic attacks, obsessions, or compulsions in relation to the ingestion of these substances are classified by the American Psychiatric Association as having a substance-induced anxiety disorder. However, because individuals with an anxiety disorder, particularly panic disorder, are more susceptible to the anxiogenic effects of stimulants (4), the clinician should be vigilant for an underlying idiopathic pre-existing anxiety disorder in patients with substance-induced anxiety.

ANXIETY DISORDERS

The anxiety disorders are a group of psychiatric conditions in which anxiety is the predominant symptom. Anxiety causes distress and dysfunction because it is *excessive, unrealistic,* or *inappropriate in form or context.* The five major anxiety disorders are panic disorder, obsessive-compulsive disorder (OCD), phobia (specific, social, or agoraphobia), posttraumatic stress disorder (PTSD), and generalized anxiety disorder (GAD). As a group, the anxiety disorders are the most common psychiatric illnesses in the United States, affecting an estimated 19 million American adults (5). In addition to existing in their "pure" forms, individual anxiety disorders are frequently comorbid with other psychiatric conditions, including other anxiety disorders, affective disorders (Chapter 24), somatoform disorders (Chapter 21), substance use disorders (Chapters 28 and 29), and eating disorders (Chapter 11). Although adjustment disorder with anxiety is not classified as an anxiety disorder, this condition is frequently encountered by primary physicians and should be considered in the differential diagnosis of anxiety. Therefore, a brief description of adjustment disorder with anxiety is provided here before the anxiety disorders are reviewed.

Adjustment Disorder with Anxiety

Description

The term *adjustment disorder with anxiety* is used when excessive and maladaptive anxiety occurs in response to a recent, identifiable stressor. This "reactive" anxiety resolves when the stressor remits or when the patient reaches a new level of adaptation or adjustment. Chapter 24, Table 24.1 lists American Psychiatric Association criteria.

Case Study

A 55-year-old married man presented to the office because of non-exertional chest pain, dizziness, and breathlessness. He had suffered a heart attack 3 months before but had recovered uneventfully. A recent stress test had shown no signs of coronary insufficiency or serious arrhythmia. His wife reported that the patient had not been himself since leaving the hospital and that "every little thing gets on his nerves." Although he had formerly been "on the go all of the time," he was now afraid to go out of the house. Physical examination now showed no evidence of heart failure, and the electrocardiogram (ECG) was unchanged. The physician reviewed the encouraging results of the ECG and treadmill test, reassured the patient about his symptoms, explained that anxiety is common after MI, and asked the patient to enroll in a cardiac rehabilitation program, to telephone in 1 week to report on his symptoms, and to return to the office in 2 weeks for followup examination and a review of his progress. The physician also demonstrated some simple relaxation techniques (see Nonpharmacologic Approaches, Self-Regulation Techniques) and gave the patient a small supply of lorazepam to be used on an as-needed basis.

Epidemiology, Origins, and Natural History

Estimates of the point prevalence of adjustment disorder are highly variable, ranging from 5% to 20%, dependent upon the population evaluated. Adjustment disorder is believed to be equally common in males and females. By definition, an adjustment disorder with anxious mood must begin within 3 months of a precipitating stressor and last no longer than 6 months after the stressor (or its consequences) ceases.

Treatment

Management includes the following steps:

- Advise the patient to moderate or eliminate use of caffeine and other stimulants.
- Consider short-term counseling (see Chapter 20) to meet the patient's informational needs, assist in problem-solving, provide encouragement, and restore morale.
- Offer training in relaxation and other techniques of self-regulation (see later discussion).
- Consider instituting a time-limited (1 to 2 weeks) course of anxiolytic medication, usually a benzodiazepine (see Pharmacologic Treatments).

Panic Disorder

Description

The hallmark feature of panic disorder is the occurrence of panic attacks—discrete episodes of extreme anxiety—accompanied by a variety of physical and emotional symptoms. To meet the criteria for a *panic attack,* the episode must comprise at least four symptoms in addition to intense fear or discomfort. Symptoms of panic include palpitations, sweating, trembling, shortness of breath, feeling of choking, chest pain or discomfort, nausea or abdominal distress, dizziness, derealization (feelings of unreality) or depersonalization (feeling detached from oneself), paresthesias, chills or hot flushes, fear of losing control or going crazy, and fear of dying. In addition to the involvement of panicky feeling and physical/emotional symptoms, panic attacks must reach peak intensity within 10 minutes after their onset.

The presence of repeated, unexpected panic attacks is necessary but not sufficient for the diagnosis of *panic disorder.* As described later, a number of other anxiety disorders as well as mood disorders are sometimes associated with panic attacks. In contrast to other disorders, panic disorder requires that, after the experience of a panic attack (or attacks), the affected individual is persistently (for at least 1 month) worried about having another panic attack or concerned about the significance or consequences of the panic attack.

Patients with panic disorder have significantly increased *utilization* of both outpatient and inpatient general medical services. *Utilization of primary care services* by patients with panic disorder is approximately three times higher than that of the average patient and is higher than that of patients with other psychiatric illnesses, such as major depression (2,6). The prevalence of panic disorder may be increased in several medical conditions, including labile hypertension (7), mitral valve prolapse (8), asthma (9,10), chronic obstructive pulmonary disease (COPD) (11), and migraine headache (12,13).

Approximately one third of individuals with panic disorder develop *agoraphobia*, or fear and avoidance of places and situations where a panic attack might occur or escape would be difficult (14). If the agoraphobia is left untreated, the number and extent of avoided situations can expand and generalize, rendering the patient housebound. Agoraphobia can occur in the absence of panic attacks (agoraphobia without history of panic disorder in *Diagnostic and Statistical Manual of Mental Disorders, 4th Edition [DSM-IV]*); but the latter condition is less commonly encountered in psychiatric clinics than panic disorder with agoraphobia (15). Among patients with panic disorder, those most likely to develop agoraphobia are women who have persistent panic attacks (i.e., no history of clinical remissions), a high degree of interpersonal sensitivity, and a history of anxiety or depression in childhood (15). Table 22.2 summarizes American Psychiatric Assocation diagnostic criteria for panic disorder without and with agoraphobia.

Case Study

A 24-year-old graduate student was referred by the emergency department for recurrent episodes of substernal chest pain, some of which had occurred during sleep. Chest pain was associated with abdominal pain, shortness of breath, and dizziness. Medical workup had revealed no cardiac or endocrine source for the patient's symptoms. The patient reported that during the last semester of graduate school she began experiencing these episodes "out of the blue." Her first episode took place when she was "pulling an all-nighter studying for her dissertation presentation." She acknowledged drinking quite a bit of coffee during that period, but since then she had experienced panic attacks while not using caffeine heavily. Although she admitted to some life stressors, such as starting a new job and moving to a new city, she viewed these stressors as positive. The patient reported that since she first began to have panic attacks she had become "obsessed" with the thought that she had some sort of heart condition that would kill her.

The patient stated that she would be agreeable to both medication treatment and "talking therapy." She was started on a low dose of a selective serotonin reuptake inhibitor (SSRI) and was referred to a cognitive behavioral therapist for short-term (12-week) symptom-focused therapy. Within 6 weeks the patient reported that her anticipatory anxiety had diminished significantly, as had the intensity and frequency of her panic attacks. Within 3 months, she was panic free. She continued taking the SSRI for 18 months, after which it was slowly tapered.

Epidemiology, Origins, and Natural History

The case study illustrates a number of characteristic features of panic disorder. It typically begins in late adolescence or early adulthood, with the median age at onset of 24 years (16). It has a prevalence of 1% to 2% and is twice as common in women as in men (14,16). Many patients with panic disorder experience panic-free remissions,

TABLE 22.2 Diagnostic Criteria for Panic Disorder without and with Agoraphobia

Without Agoraphobia

A. Both 1 and 2:
   1. Recurrent unexpected panic attacks.
   2. At least one of the attacks has been followed by a month or more of (a) persistent concern about having additional attacks, (b) worry about the implications of the attack or its consequences (e.g., losing control, having a heart attack, "going crazy"), or (c) a significant change in behavior related to the attacks.

B. Absence of agoraphobia (defined below).

C. The panic attacks are not because of the direct effects of a substance (e.g., drugs of abuse, medication) or a general medical condition (e.g., hyperthyroidism).

D. The anxiety is not better accounted for by another mental disorder, such as Obsessive-Compulsive Disorder (e.g., fear of contamination), Posttraumatic Stress Disorder (e.g., in response to stimuli associated with a severe stressor), Separation Anxiety Disorder, or Social Phobia (e.g., fear of embarrassment in social situations).

With Agoraphobia

A. Both 1 and 2:
   1. Recurrent unexpected panic attacks.
   2. At least one of the attacks has been followed by a month or more of (a) persistent concern about having additional attacks, (b) worry about the implications of the attack or its consequences (e.g., losing control, having a heart attack, "going crazy"), or (c) a significant change in behavior related to the attacks.

B. The presence of agoraphobia, that is, anxiety about being in places or situations from which escape might be difficult (or embarrassing) or in which help may not be available in the event of having an unexpected or situational predisposed panic attack. Agoraphobic fears typically involve characteristic clusters of situations that include being outside the home alone, being in a crowd or standing in a line, being on a bridge, and traveling in a bus, train, or car. Note: Consider the diagnosis of Specific Phobia if limited to one or only a few specific situations, or Social Phobia if the avoidance is limited to social situations.

C. Agoraphobic situations are avoided (e.g., travel is restricted), or else endured with marked distress or with anxiety about having a panic attack, or require the presence of a companion.

D. The panic attacks are not due to the direct effects of a substance (e.g., drugs of abuse, medication) or a general medical condition (e.g., hyperthyroidism).

E. The anxiety or phobic avoidance is not better accounted for by another mental disorder, such as Specific Phobia (e.g., avoidance limited to a single situation like elevators), Separation Anxiety Disorder (e.g., avoidance of school), Obsessive-Compulsive Disorder (e.g., fear of contamination), Posttraumatic Stress Disorder (e.g., avoidance of stimuli associated with a severe stressor), or Social Phobia (e.g., avoidance limited to social situations because of fear of embarrassment).

Reprinted with permission from Diagnostic and statistical manual of mental disorders. 4th Edition. Washington, DC: American Psychiatric Association, 1994.

particularly after treatment. However, panic disorder is typically a chronic, lifelong condition, and those patients who achieve remission often experience relapses (15). Frequently associated psychiatric conditions include major depression, social phobia, PTSD, GAD, agoraphobia, OCD, and substance abuse (14,17–19).

Patients with panic disorder present special differential diagnostic challenges to generalists and cardiologists. Although panic symptoms are often difficult to distinguish from angina and may lead to unnecessary cardiac catheterization (20), patients with panic disorder have an increased cardiovascular mortality rate (21–23). Other studies, which were limited by the fact that they included male subjects only, revealed that the risk of sudden cardiac death in patients with panic-like symptoms is as much as six times higher than in patients with low anxiety levels, even when known risk factors for cardiac death (e.g., cholesterol level, tobacco use, family history) are taken into account (2). Additionally, panic symptoms may be simulated by a number of noncardiac medical disorders, including alcohol and sedative-hypnotic drug withdrawal, marijuana use, pheochromocytoma, hyperthyroidism, hypoglycemia, and temporal lobe epilepsy.

Studies support the view that panic disorder is *primarily a biologic disorder.* Genetic factors have been implicated by family studies demonstrating a tenfold increase in panic disorder among first-degree relatives of panic probands (24) and a higher concordance rate for panic disorder among monozygotic than among dizygotic twins (25). Lactate infusion (26) and hyperventilation (27) may stimulate panic attacks in people with panic disorder, suggesting the existence of specific biologic triggers. Pharmacologic treatments may by themselves dramatically reduce the frequency of panic episodes (see Evaluation and Treatment). Although the neurobiology of panic disorder is not clearly established, preclinical models of conditioned fear, in concert with clinical pharmacologic and neuroimaging studies, have implicated a number of brain regions and neurotransmitters or neuromodulators in the symptoms of anxiety and panic. With regard to brain regions, there are considerable data suggesting that the central nucleus of the amygdala, the orbitofrontal cortex/anterior insula, and the anterior cingulate cortex are involved in the expression of fear and anxiety. Among the endogenous neural substances that are believed to be involved in anxiety are norepinephrine, serotonin, corticotrophin-releasing factor, gamma-aminobutyric acid (GABA), and substance P.

There are also *learning (or conditioning) theories* to explain panic disorder. These propose that panic attacks develop when physical sensations occurring at times of stress are interpreted as signs of grave illness, giving rise to panic. The physical sensations of arousal become conditioned phobic stimuli, provoking the panic symptomatology (conditioned response) (28). Conditioning models have been particularly persuasive in accounting for the development and maintenance of agoraphobia (29).

Evaluation and Treatment

A systematic approach to the evaluation and treatment of panic disorder includes the following steps:

- Take a history and perform a focused physical examination, looking for evidence of a medical disorder that could simulate panic disorder (e.g., insulin-induced hypoglycemia, temporal lobe seizures, cardiac ischemia, or dysrhythmias).
- Inquire about the use of caffeine-containing beverages, stimulant drugs, alcohol, marijuana, and other substances associated with anxiety or panic symptoms (Table 22.1).
- Inquire about sleeping habits. Studies have demonstrated that the symptoms of panic disorder worsen with sleep deprivation, so erratic sleep–wake schedules should be avoided.
- Inquire about life stressors, and facilitate the patient's solving of problems (see Chapter 20). Although this may not eliminate panic attacks, it will help reduce the levels of generalized anxiety that often develop in patients with panic disorder.
- *Use pharmacologic means* to reduce the frequency and intensity of panic attacks. The first-line treatment for new-onset idiopathic panic disorder is the use of an SSRI (30,31). Although most antidepressants are effective in the treatment of panic disorder, the SSRIs have a favorable side-effect profile compared with either the tricyclic antidepressants or the monoamine oxidase inhibitors. A number of new-generation antidepressants with excellent side effect profiles appear also to be effective in the treatment of panic disorder but do not yet have the track record established by the SSRIs. High-potency benzodiazepines used to be a popular method for treating panic disorder, and they have the advantage of rapid onset of action compared with the antidepressants. However, given the potential risks of tolerance and dependence, they should not be considered a first- or second-line treatment option.

Regardless of the type of antidepressant used for treatment, patients with panic disorder are notoriously sensitive to a variety of medications. It is quite common for a patient with panic disorder, if treated with a "typical" starting dose of an antidepressant (e.g., 50 mg of sertraline or 20 mg of fluoxetine) to develop what is commonly referred to as the "jitteriness syndrome." Patients report feeling keyed up, or on edge, or as if they had consumed excessive amounts of caffeine. Some patients actually note an increase in the number of panic attacks early in the course of treatment. To avoid severe jitteriness and consequent noncompliance, it is important to educate the patient about this phenomenon in advance and to initiate dosing at lower than typical dosages (i.e., 25 mg sertraline or 10 mg fluoxetine). Doses should not be increased until jitteriness totally resolves. Some patients experience an increase in jitteriness each time the dose is increased, but typically this is a short-lived phenomenon (1 to 2 weeks).

Panic disorder is a chronic, recurring illness. In new-onset panic disorder, it is generally accepted that pharmacotherapy should continue for at least 1 year, at which time medications can be tapered over a 4- to 6-month period for a drug-free trial period (32). It is clear, however, that many patients relapse after medications are discontinued. Patients who have experienced more than one previous relapse should be considered for long-term antidepressant treatment, which has been shown to be effective in preventing relapse (33,34).

Once widely accepted as a first-line therapy for the treatment of panic disorder, benzodiazepines now are generally viewed as a short-term adjunct to therapy by most anxiety disorder experts in this country. Patients who are significantly impaired by their symptoms of anxiety during the period before stabilization on antidepressant are sometimes treated with benzodiazepines as a "bridge" (35). However, this strategy is not always fully successful, because more than 50% of patients have difficulty discontinuing benzodiazepines (36).

Controlled clinical research studies have also demonstrated the efficacy of cognitive behavior therapy (CBT) in the treatment of panic disorder (37). Indeed, CBT has been found, in most studies, to be equally or more efficacious than medication treatment alone, and it can be quite cost-effective. The biggest drawback to CBT, assuming that the patient is willing to make the time commitment to participate, is the paucity of well-trained therapists skilled in administering CBT effectively. As suggested by its name, CBT comprises both cognitive and behavioral therapeutic techniques and is typically administered in 12 sessions over a 12-week period. During this time, patients systematically learn to recognize and correct cognitive distortions associated with their panic attacks (e.g., "When I feel my heart beat quickly, it means that I have a fatal heart problem") and master relaxation methods to use in the face of mounting anxiety. Because hyperventilation is a frequent feature of panic attacks that exacerbates some panic symptoms (and can lead to acroesthesia), most CBT programs for panic involve breathing retraining, wherein patients learn diaphragmatic breathing techniques and how to decrease their respiratory rate when anxious. Finally, CBT often involves interoceptive exposure (i.e., producing physical symptoms, such as dizziness, that are associated with panic and distorted cognitions). If a patient has concomitant agoraphobia, the therapist may also employ exposure therapy techniques, gradually exposing the patient to feared situations as he or she learns to employ cognitive and behavioral methods of panic control.

As with most psychiatric illnesses, an important aspect of the treatment of panic disorder is education of the patient and significant others regarding the nature of this condition. Usually, patients are relieved to learn that panic disorder is a common, treatable disease with a biologic basis. Education by the clinician, supplemented by readily available books written for the lay person, may help reduce the patient's sense of isolation and embarrassment and provide practical advice about managing panic symptoms. The National Institutes of Health (NIH) has an up-to-date website with comprehensive information about all of the anxiety disorders as well as a list of books, web links, and national organizations suitable for professionals and laypersons (see *www.hopkinsbayview.org/PAMreferences*).

Obsessive-Compulsive Disorder

Description

As suggested by its name, the essential features of OCD are obsessions—recurrent, persistent, intrusive thoughts (e.g., "Touching this doorknob will give me a disease")—and compulsions—purposeful but senseless behaviors or rituals (e.g., washing hands 17 times each morning). The obsessive thoughts are distressing to the patient, who usually is aware that the thoughts are illogical and unreasonable. In an individual patient, obsessions and compulsions are often related, and the compulsive behaviors are conducted in an effort to reduce the anxiety brought on by the obsessive thoughts. However, it is not uncommon for a patient to have a variety of obsessions that have no thematic relationship. It is the presence of obsessions and/or compulsions that distinguishes OCD from obsessive-compulsive *personality* disorder (see Chapter 23), a personality type characterized by meticulousness, perfectionism, and rigidity. Table 22.3 lists the American Psychiatric Association diagnostic criteria for OCD.

Case Study

An 83-year-old widow was referred for evaluation because of disabling fears of contamination. She was a retired mathematics teacher who liked her subject because 1 and 1 always equal 2: "I

TABLE 22.3 Diagnostic Criteria for Obsessive–Compulsive Disorder

A. Either obsessions or compulsions:
   Obsessions as defined by 1, 2, 3, and 4:
   1. Recurrent and persistent thoughts, impulses, or images that are experienced, at some time during the disturbance, as intrusive and inappropriate, and cause marked anxiety or distress.
   2. The thoughts, impulses, or images are not simply excessive worries about real-life problems.
   3. The person attempts to ignore or suppress such thoughts or impulses or to neutralize them with some other thought or action.
   4. The person recognizes that the obsessional thoughts, impulses, or images are a product of his or her own mind (not imposed from without as in thought insertion).

   Compulsions as defined by 1 and 2:
   1. Repetitive behaviors (e.g., hand washing, ordering, checking) or mental acts (e.g., praying, counting, repeating words silently) that the person feels driven to perform in response to an obsession, or according to rules that must be applied rigidly.
   2. The behaviors or mental acts are aimed at preventing or reducing distress or preventing some dreaded event or situation; however, these behaviors or mental acts either are not connected in a realistic way with what they are designed to neutralize or prevent, or are clearly excessive.
B. At some point during the course of the disorder, the person has recognized that the obsessions or compulsions are excessive or unreasonable. Note: This does not apply to children.
C. The obsessions or compulsions cause marked distress, are time-consuming (take more than an hour per day), or significantly interfere with the person's normal routine, occupational functioning, or usual social activities or relationships with others.
D. If another axis I disorder is present, the content of the obsessions or compulsions is not restricted to it (e.g., preoccupation with food in the presence of an eating disorder, hair pulling in the presence of trichotillomania, concern with appearance in the presence of body dysmorphic disorder, preoccupation with drugs in the presence of a substance use disorder, preoccupation with having a serious illness in the presence of hypochondriasis, or guilty ruminations in the presence of major depressive disorder).[a]
E. Not due to the direct effects of a substance (e.g., drugs of abuse, medication) or a general medical condition.

[a]See Chapter 19 for definition of axis I and axis II disorders.
Reprinted with permission from Diagnostic and statistical manual of mental disorders. 4th Edition. Washington, DC: American Psychiatric Association, 1994.

like the certainty." A practicing Catholic, she recalled that during adolescence she had once delayed disposing of a sanitary napkin because she had sneezed over it after returning home after Mass and worried that bits of the communion wafer might have lodged in it. She had received psychiatric treatment several times for obsessive-compulsive symptoms but had recently been doing well until she was forced to change apartments. After the move she became preoccupied with worries about contamination with germs. Especially vexing was deciding when she had adequately washed her hands after defecating; she was consumed by uncertainty about how long she should wash and how she could safely dispose of the towel after drying her hands. Her main fear was that others might be contaminated and become ill as a result of her carelessness. As a result of these ideas, she washed her hands excessively, did not leave her apartment, ate poorly (so that she would defecate less), and was unable to engage in normal conversation. Treatment consisted of a form of CBT called "response prevention" and the use of an SSRI (see Evaluation and Treatment). Within 2 weeks she showed improvement, and by the end of 8 weeks she was able to dispel obsessive ideas effortlessly and felt no compulsion to wash excessively.

Epidemiology, Origins, and Natural History

One to two percent of people in the community (38) and in the general medical clinic (39) meet criteria for OCD. Its prevalence is slightly higher among women and tends to decline with age. Symptoms usually have their onset in adolescence or early adulthood. In one study of patients with OCD (40), the most common obsessions were fear of contamination (55%), fear of acting aggressively (50%), and fear of performing unacceptable sexual activities (32%). Somatic obsessions were present in 34% of patients, including a woman who performed breast self-examinations 100 times per day to reassure herself that she had not developed breast cancer (40), and 36% had obsessive thoughts involving the need for symmetry. The most common compulsions involved checking, cleaning, and counting. In most cases the symptoms were chronic and continuous, with some tendency for symptomatic worsening during times of stress. Associated psychiatric diagnoses included major depression (30%), simple phobia (7%), and panic disorder (5%).

Explanations for OCD have been advanced from several perspectives. Psychoanalytic writers have viewed obsessive-compulsive symptoms as products of reaction formation against unacceptable wishes and impulses, often related to aggression and sexuality. Behavioral theorists and practitioners have stressed the anxiety-reducing effects of compulsive rituals and have proposed that compulsions are maintained precisely because of their positively reinforcing ameliorating effects on conditioned anxiety. The importance of personality traits in the development of OCD is suggested by data showing that preexisting obsessive traits (e.g., meticulousness, perfectionism, indecisiveness) are very common in clinical samples of patients with OCD (40) and that people who are obsessional, anxious, or self-conscious may be especially vulnerable to the emergence of OCD in response to life change (41).

Other research suggests that OCD has *biologic origins*. The importance of genetic factors is supported by studies showing high rates of OCD among first-degree relatives of patients with OCD (42) and evidence for a major gene in segregation analyses (43). Clinical studies linking OCD with head trauma (44) and other neurologic disorders (45) add support to the conception that OCD may be a manifestation of brain disease. Of all the anxiety disorders, OCD has been most extensively studied with neuroimaging techniques. Available neuroimaging data, considered together, implicate abnormalities within the cortico-striato-thalamo-cortical network (46). Particularly, patients with OCD tend to have hyperactive orbitofrontal, anterior cingulate, and caudate activity that is further activated during symptom provocation and that is attenuated with treatment (47). It has been proposed that the primary lesion of OCD is located in the corpus striatum (48), an hypothesis that is supported by the finding that autoimmune processes known to damage the striatum can be associated with new-onset OCD (49). Results of functional neuroimaging studies, considered together with genetic, epidemiologic, and pharmacologic data, have led to the hypothesis that prefrontal–basal ganglia–thalamic–prefrontal circuits are particularly important in the pathophysiology of OCD (50). Of great theoretical and practical importance is the demonstration that numerous antidepressants that prevent uptake of serotonin into presynaptic neurons are effective in the treatment of OCD (51). This observation strongly implicates a role for central serotonergic neuronal systems in the pathophysiology of this disorder.

Evaluation and Treatment

A systematic approach to the evaluation and treatment of OCD involves the following steps:

- In the history and physical examination, look for evidence of medical conditions, medications, or dietary practices that may simulate or exacerbate symptoms of anxiety. It has been found that some individuals develop OCD after a streptococcal infection and subsequent autoimmune damage to the corpus striatum (49), so the relationship between symptom onset and a possible streptococcal infection should be explored.
- Consider *use of cognitive behavioral therapy*. Most experts recommend CBT as a first-line treatment for every patient who is willing to participate (52). This suggestion follows from the view that compulsions are maintained by their temporary amelioration of conditioned

anxiety. Patients are taught to control their obsessive ruminations by commanding themselves to stop ruminating when obsessive ideas arise (thought stopping), and they are exhorted to resist carrying out their compulsive acts so that they can learn that there are no dire consequences associated with nonexecution of the rituals (response prevention). These techniques are often helpful if patients can be persuaded to practice them.

- Consider use of *antidepressant medications* that have been shown to have specific efficacy in OCD. First-line drugs, all of which are significantly more effective than placebo, include the tricyclic clomipramine and the SSRIs (53–55). Although clomipramine may be somewhat more effective than the SSRIs in OCD, it also has a higher, more problematic side-effect profile. As with all anxiety disorders, when initiating treatment with an SSRI, medication dosages should gradually be titrated upward. Patients should receive treatment for 10 to 12 weeks with an SSRI in adequate doses before alternative therapy is considered (56). For reasons that are not entirely clear, patients with OCD often require dosages of SSRI in excess of those used to treat depression or other anxiety disorders, and even on the highest tolerated dose, up to 25% of patients are unresponsive to treatment (57,58). As with depression and other anxiety disorders, initial responses may not be apparent until 4 to 6 weeks into treatment, and it can take months before optimal treatment effects are reached. Treatment should be continued for at least 6 to 12 months and then tapered slowly, if a drug-free trial is desired. If symptoms of OCD reappear during the course of the drug taper, medication doses should be restored to pre-taper levels (56). For patients with chronic severe symptoms, long-term maintenance treatment should be considered, because it has been shown that medications can protect against relapse (59). Chapter 24 has practical information about antidepressant drugs.
- Consider short-term *problem-solving counseling* (see Chapter 20). Although this may not bring total relief, it is clear that symptomatic exacerbations of this chronic disorder tend to come at times of stress and change, and short-term counseling may help reduce the impact of such influences. On the other hand, insight-oriented, introspective psychotherapies have generally been ineffective in the treatment of OCD.

Generalized Anxiety Disorder

Description

GAD is characterized by persistent and excessive worry that is present more days than not for at least a 6-month period. In addition to excessive, inappropriate, or unrealistic worry, the patient must experience at least three of six physical symptoms, including restlessness, easy fatigability, difficulty concentrating, irritability, muscle tension, and sleep disturbance. Table 22.4 lists American Psychiatric Association criteria.

TABLE 22.4 Diagnostic Criteria for Generalized Anxiety Disorder

A. Excessive anxiety and worry (apprehensive expectation), occurring more days than not for at least 6 months, about a number of events or activities (such as work or school performance).
B. The person finds it difficult to control the worry.
C. The anxiety and worry are associated with at least three of the following six symptoms (with at least some symptoms present for more days than not for the past 6 months):
   1. Restlessness or feeling keyed up or on edge
   2. Being easily fatigued
   3. Difficulty concentrating or mind going blank
   4. Irritability
   5. Muscle tension
   6. Sleep disturbance (difficulty falling or staying asleep, or restless unsatisfying sleep)
D. The focus of the anxiety and worry is not confined to features of an axis I disorder, e.g., the anxiety or worry is not about having a panic attack (as in Panic Disorder), being embarrassed in public (as in Social Phobia), being contaminated (as in Obsessive-Compulsive Disorder), being away from home or close relatives (as in Separation Anxiety Disorder), gaining weight (as in Anorexia Nervosa), or having a serious illness (as in Hypochondriasis), and is not part of Posttraumatic Stress Disorder.[a]
E. The anxiety, worry, or physical symptoms cause clinically significant distress or impairment in social, occupational, or other important areas of functioning.
F. Not due to the direct effects of a substance (e.g., drugs of abuse, medication) or a general medical condition (e.g., hyperthyroidism), and does not occur exclusively during a mood disorder, psychotic disorder, or pervasive developmental disorder.

[a] See Chapter 19 for definition of axis I and axis II disorders.
Reprinted with permission from Diagnostic and statistical manual of mental disorders. 4th Edition. Washington, DC: American Psychiatric Association, 1994.

Case Study

A 50-year-old woman came to her physician complaining of difficulty swallowing, insomnia, tremor, and loose stools. She reported that she'd been a "worrier" since her 20s, but that this characteristic had increased in the year since her husband died, and she became responsible for managing all aspects of the household. Three of her adult children, one of whom had mental retardation, lived at home, and she continued to prepare their meals and do their laundry. She admitted that she was "scared of everything," generally tense ("Little things make me jump"), and often experienced feelings of shakiness, diaphoresis, and fluttering in the chest, usually in response to contemplating driving by herself or engaging in another feared activity. She did not describe discrete intense panic episodes (see Panic Disorder). She did report feeling blue for the past several months, and that she had difficulty enjoying things. Physical examination, ECG, and exercise stress test results were normal. Although she was reluctant to take medications, she agreed to try treatment with venlafaxine XR, beginning at a dose of 75 mg per day. Additionally, she agreed to meet with her physician on a monthly basis for 12 months for counseling. During counseling sessions she learned simple relaxation techniques (see later discussion), helped construct a program of systematic desensitization regarding driving, and developed a plan to request that her children participate more consistently in the running of the household. At the end of 1 year she was greatly improved. She was driving regularly to visit friends across town with growing confidence.

Epidemiology, Origins, and Natural History

GAD is one of the more common anxiety disorders, with an estimated lifetime prevalence of 5.1% (60). Patients frequently initially present to their general practitioner with a variety of somatic complaints, for which no medical basis is discovered (61). Like all of the anxiety disorders except OCD, GAD is more common in women and usually begins in the early twenties. GAD is a chronic illness that often persists for several decades (61,62). It is relatively uncommon for GAD to exist in isolation; the majority of patients also meet criteria for major depression, another anxiety disorder, or alcohol abuse (63).

The causes of GAD are not fully understood. A number of studies have indicated that there is a mild genetic component to GAD (25,64). A large-scale study in female twins suggested that GAD and major depression share a common genetic basis, possibly explaining the frequent comorbidity of these two illnesses (65). Twin research also suggests that the personality trait neuroticism (a general tendency to experience negative emotions) also shares genetic underpinnings with GAD (66). Traumatic early life experiences, especially the death of a parent (67), may be a predisposing factor, although patients with this disorder do not characterize their childhoods as more difficult than nonanxious people do (68). Events in later life, especially unexpected events perceived as important and negative (69), may also play a role in the emergence of symptoms.

Evaluation and Treatment

A systematic approach to the evaluation and treatment of the patient with GAD includes the following steps:

- Take a medical history, and perform a focused physical examination to look for evidence of medical disorders (e.g., hyperthyroidism, pheochromocytoma, hypoglycemia) that may manifest with concomitant somatic symptoms and anxiety.
- Inquire about consumption of alcohol, caffeine-containing beverages, and other drugs (e.g., diet pills), and counsel the patient to eliminate the ingestion of caffeine and other stimulants and to moderate alcohol consumption.
- Inquire about life stresses, and encourage the patient to find solutions to problems; anxious patients are often demoralized and benefit from short-term counseling (see Chapter 20) aimed at solving problems and restoring self-esteem.
- Instruct the patient in *self-regulation techniques* such as progressive muscle relaxation (see Nonpharmacologic Approaches, Self-Regulation Techniques), and encourage regular practice.
- Consider the use of an *antidepressant medication*. There is growing evidence that a variety of antidepressants may be effective for the treatment of GAD (70–72) (see Table 24.4 in Chapter 24). The newer antidepressants, such as the SSRIs and venlafaxine, have favorable side effect profiles in comparison to tricyclic antidepressants and are a good first-line option, particularly in patients with comorbid depression or another anxiety disorder. In contrast to benzodiazepines, antidepressants must be taken for several weeks before they become effective, and they carry little risk of tolerance or dependence. Patients should be treated for at least 1 year before tapering and discontinuation of medication is considered.
- Consider a trial of *buspirone* (72,73). It is well tolerated and effective in the treatment of GAD, particularly for the core symptoms of worry and apprehensive expectation, although its onset of action is slower than that of benzodiazepines, and it may not be particularly effective in patients with a history of long-term benzodiazepine use. It carries essentially no risk of tolerance or dependency. Effective therapy is continued for at least 6 to 12 months.
- Be reluctant to prescribe *benzodiazepines*. Unfortunately, many patients receive benzodiazepines as their first treatment for GAD because of their ability to treat symptoms of arousal, autonomic hyperactivity, and muscle tension. Given that there are numerous other medication options, these drugs should not be considered as a first treatment option. Benzodiazepines commonly cause symptoms such as drowsiness and sedation, and they can also cause ataxia, dizziness, and uncoordination (74). Because patients with GAD are at increased risk for substance abuse, benzodiazepines should be prescribed only with caution and for the short term.
- No response to treatment or relapse should lead to reassessment of the diagnosis, examination for medical and psychiatric comorbidity (especially major depression), and possible psychiatric referral.
- GAD tends to be a chronic condition with only 38% complete and 47% partial remission at 5 years (75,76). Therefore, the need for ongoing treatment is likely.

Phobias

Description

As a group, phobias are enduring fears of harmless objects or situations (phobic stimuli) that lead patients to avoid contact with them (phobic avoidance). Patients with *specific phobia* fear discrete objects and situations, such as animals, heights, air travel, needles, and visits to the doctor, whereas patients with *social phobia* have fears of social humiliation and the scrutiny of others. People with *agoraphobia* fear being in situations from which escape is difficult or where help may not be available in the event of an anxiety-provoking episode, such as in open or public spaces (literally, fear of the *agora* or marketplace). Although phobic patients generally recognize their fears to be excessive and unreasonable, they nonetheless seek to avoid the phobic stimulus because exposure provokes intense anxiety. The diagnosis of phobia is made only if avoidance of the feared object or situation leads to social or occupational impairment or if the patient experiences great distress as a result of the symptom.

Tables 22.5 and 22.6, respectively, list American Psychiatric Association criteria for specific phobia and social phobia. Agoraphobia can be seen in a number of anxiety disorders (e.g., social phobia, PTSD) and is described in the section on panic disorder.

TABLE 22.5 Diagnostic Criteria for Specific Phobia

A. Marked and persistent fear that is excessive or unreasonable, cued by the presence or anticipation of a specific object or situation (e.g., flying, height, animals, receiving an injection, seeing blood).
B. Exposure to the phobic stimulus almost invariably provokes an immediate anxiety response, which may take the form of a situationally bound or situationally predisposed panic attack. Note: In children, the anxiety may be expressed by crying, tantrums, freezing, or clinging.
C. The person recognizes that the fear is excessive or unreasonable. Note: In children, this feature may be absent.
D. The phobic situation is avoided or else endured with intense anxiety or distress.
E. The avoidance, anxious anticipation, or distress in the feared situations interferes significantly with the person's normal routine, occupational (academic) functioning, or social activities or relationships with others, or there is marked distress about having the phobia.
F. The anxiety, panic attacks, or phobic avoidance associated with the specific object or situation are not better accounted for by another mental disorder, such as Obsessive-Compulsive Disorder (e.g., fear of contamination), Posttraumatic Stress Disorder (e.g., avoidance of stimuli associated with a severe stressor), Separation Anxiety Disorder (e.g., avoidance of school), Social Phobia (e.g., avoidance of social situations because of fear of embarrassment), Panic Disorder with Agoraphobia, or Agoraphobia without history of panic disorder.

Adapted with permission from Diagnostic and statistical manual of mental disorders. 4th Edition. Washington, DC: American Psychiatric Association, 1994.

TABLE 22.6 Diagnostic Criteria for Social Phobia

A. A marked and persistent fear of one or more social or performance situations in which the person is exposed to unfamiliar people or to possible scrutiny by others. The individual fears that he or she will act in a way (or show anxiety symptoms) that will be humiliating or embarrassing. Note: In children, there must be evidence of capacity for social relationships with familiar people and the anxiety must occur in peer settings, not just in interactions with adults.
B. Exposure to the feared social situation almost invariably provokes anxiety, which may take the form of a situationally bound or situationally predisposed panic attack. Note: In children, the anxiety may be expressed by crying, tantrums, freezing, or withdrawal from the social situation.
C. The person recognizes that the fear is excessive or unreasonable. Note: In children, this feature may be absent.
D. The feared social or performance situations are avoided or else endured with intense anxiety or distress.
E. The avoidance, anxious anticipation, or distress in the feared social or performance situation interferes significantly with the person's normal routine, occupational (academic) functioning, or social activities or relationships with others, or there is marked distress about having the phobia.
F. The fear or avoidance is not due to the direct effects of a substance (e.g., drugs of abuse, medication) or a general medical condition, and is not better accounted for by Panic Disorder with or without Agoraphobia, Separation Anxiety Disorder, Body Dysmorphic Disorder, a Pervasive Developmental Disorder, or Schizoid Personality Disorder.
G. If a general medical condition or other mental disorder is present, the fear in criterion A is unrelated to it; for example, the fear is not of stuttering, trembling (in Parkinson disease) or of exhibiting abnormal eating behavior (in Anorexia Nervosa or Bulimia Nervosa).

Adapted with permission from Diagnostic and statistical manual of mental disorders. 4th Edition. Washington, DC: American Psychiatric Association, 1994.

Case Study

A 50-year-old married business executive sought treatment because of an addiction to chlordiazepoxide. In his early 20s he had first become aware of his discomfort in large groups, particularly when he was the focus of attention. On occasion, he would experience panic attacks during these large social gatherings. He discovered that regular use of chlordiazepoxide improved his general level of comfort, and by age 50 he was using 80 mg per day routinely. In addition to feeling anxious in large groups, the patient was anxious in small groups when he was the center of attention. He avoided writing checks in public because he was afraid that his hand would tremble or that he would hold up a check-out line. His job required that he occasionally make professional presentations before clients and supervisors. In the days preceding a presentation, he would experience substantial anticipatory anxiety associated with the fear that he would be unable to recall what he wanted to say, or that his throat would close up, preventing him from speaking. In response to this fear, he would increase his daily chlordiazepoxide dosage by 50% to 100%. On the day of the presentation he would take 200 to 300 mg and would perform well. He was dissatisfied with this practice because he now felt depressed and believed that the medication might be playing a role. His diagnosis at the time of evaluation was social phobia and benzodiazepine dependence. A slow chlordiazepoxide taper was undertaken and completed within 6 months. At the same time, the patient participated actively in a structured CBT group and was prescribed an SSRI. His social anxiety declined, and his confidence grew as he succeeded in attending parties and giving talks.

Epidemiology, Origins, and Natural History

In recent years, the distinctions among the various types of phobias have received increased scrutiny (77). These include *specific phobia* (e.g., fear of heights, snakes, blood, insects), *circumscribed social phobia* (fear of one type of social situation, such as public speaking) and *generalized social phobia* (fear of a number of different social situations). Of the various types of phobia, generalized social phobia is associated with the greatest impairment and is more likely to be present with other psychiatric disorders. Family and twin studies support a genetic contribution in each type of phobia (25).

Specific phobias are characterized by excessive fear of specific objects or situations. When confronted with the feared object or situation, a patient with a specific phobia becomes extremely anxious and may experience a situation-bound panic attack. Most adults with specific phobias recognize that their fear is irrational, but despite this realization, they avoid the object or endure exposure with great difficulty. One survey found that among eight common phobias, the most common fear in women was that of animals, and the most common in men was that of heights (78). Other common phobias relate to enclosed places, blood, snakes, spiders, and various forms of transportation, such as flying in airplanes. Approximately 8% of the adult population suffer from one or more specific phobias during a 1-year period (79). Most adult phobias are chronic, and they generally do not remit without treatment.

Social phobia, also known as social anxiety disorder, is characterized by excessive and persistent anxiety in social situations, including performances and public speaking (80). The basis of the anxiety is that patients are afraid that they will humiliate or embarrass themselves. Often patients are concerned that people will notice certain embarrassing physical symptoms, such as perspiration, blushing, trembling, or tremulous voice. When placed in unavoidable social situations, patients with social phobia can have panic attacks. In contrast to panic disorder, the panic attacks in social phobia are not "out of the blue." Further, although patients with panic disorder are concerned about the symptoms of the panic attack (e.g., believe they are having a heart attack), patients with social phobia are concerned that others will notice that they are having a panic attack. Like both panic disorder and specific phobias, social phobia is often characterized by significant anticipatory anxiety. Social phobics can suffer for days or weeks before the feared social interaction.

The lifetime prevalence of social phobia is approximately 13.3% (60). This number includes both patients with circumscribed and those with generalized social phobia. Like most anxiety disorders, social phobia is more common in women than in men and typically begins in childhood or adolescence. It is frequently comorbid with other psychiatric illnesses, including the affective disorders (41.4%), other anxiety disorders (56.9%), and substance abuse disorders (39.6%) (79). As with panic disorder, patients with social phobia have an increased risk of certain medical conditions (e.g., peptic ulcers) and make more frequent use of medical resources than others in the general population (81). Generalized social phobia is a chronic, often lifelong condition (81).

Patients with social phobia may become addicted to alcohol or to sedative-hypnotics as a result of self-directed efforts to ameliorate their social anxiety. Furthermore, phobias and phobic anxiety may be risk factors for ischemic heart disease and other forms of cardiovascular morbidity. There is a significant association between measures of phobic anxiety (fears of enclosed spaces, illness, going out alone, heights, and crowds) and the probability of subsequent ischemic cardiac events (82). Such relationships may be mediated by anxiety-related hyperventilation, which has been shown to cause coronary vasospasm and cardiac ischemia (83), or by anxiety-induced arrhythmia (84).

Treatment

Approaches to treatment of specific phobia are based on the notion that phobic avoidance is maintained by the anxiety-preventing consequences of the avoidance. The treatment of phobias has advanced greatly with the development of behavioral therapies aimed at extinguishing phobic anxiety and phobic avoidance. Three commonly used techniques are desensitization, participant modeling, and social skills training.

Systematic *desensitization* begins with the gradual exposure of the patient to increasingly vivid and anxiety-provoking mental images of the phobic stimulus. As anxiety is generated, the patient induces relaxation by use of a relaxation technique (see Non-pharmacologic Approaches, Self-Regulation Techniques). By exercising a response incompatible with anxiety (i.e., relaxation) in reaction to the phobic stimulus, the patient gradually extinguishes the phobic anxiety. This treatment occurs over a series of sessions until the patient is comfortable enough to encounter the stimulus *in vivo*. Related to systematic desensitization is *flooding* or *implosion*, in which the imagery is presented suddenly rather than gradually.

In vivo desensitization involves gradual, stepwise exposure of the patient to the feared stimulus in real life. The patient is often initially accompanied by the therapist or a trained family member. Progress from less to more anxiety-producing tasks is accomplished by mastering anxiety at each level. The basis for the technique is that repeated exposure leads to extinction of phobic anxiety.

Participant modeling is a form of *in vivo* desensitization in which the therapist models the desired interaction with the feared object. This kind of procedure may be useful with patients who have a severe needle phobia and whose avoidance of needles may be potentially life-threatening (e.g., in patients requiring insulin). Therapy involves the following steps (85):

- Education aimed at providing realistic information about the feared object
- Response modeling, in which the therapist handles the feared object
- Joint performance, in which the patient and therapist are both exposed to the phobic stimulus
- Self-directed practice (e.g., inserting a needle into an orange)

Behavioral techniques such as these have been used successfully to treat phobias related to hemodialysis and needles. They may be carried out by nonphysicians and are usually effective within 15 sessions or less. Among patients treated by these techniques, phobias, hypochondriacal symptoms, and work adjustment often improve within 6 months, and visits to health care providers decrease markedly (86,87).

Social skills training is not always an appropriate treatment for phobias, including social phobia. Cognitive behavioral treatment of social phobia often involves exposure to social situations. The issue is not necessarily lack of social competence; rather, it is getting over unrealistic anxiety regarding humiliation and embarrassment.

Specific phobias are typically treated with the CBT methods described previously. Some patients with prominent sympathomimetic symptoms (e.g., tremor, diaphoresis, palpitations) in isolated performance situations benefit from treatment with β-adrenergic blockers, administered the day of the performance situation. These individuals should always initially take low doses (e.g., 25 to 50 mg of atenolol) and should have a test dose days or weeks before use in the performance situation. This "practice" dose serves to reassure the patient that he or she will not experience untoward effects and that the dose is not excessive (e.g., associated with disabling drops in blood pressure). Social phobia can be effectively treated by either use of CBT (individual or group) or medications. CBT for social phobia involves correcting distorted cognitions (e.g., "The audience will see me perspire and blush and will think I am incompetent") and teaching behavioral techniques (e.g., progressive muscle relaxation) to use in the face of social anxiety. As with most forms of CBT, treatment for social phobia is time limited (typically 12 weeks) and focuses on the symptoms of social phobia rather than interpersonal conflicts or long-standing psychological issues.

At present, the first-line medication treatment for generalized social phobia is an SSRI, although monoamine oxidase inhibitors (MAOIs), high-potency benzodiazepines, and the anticonvulsant gabapentin have also been demonstrated to be efficacious (88–90). Some of the newer-generation antidepressants also show significant promise for the treatment of generalized social phobia, although they have a less well-established track record than the SSRIs do (91).

Posttraumatic Stress Disorder

Description

People who have been exposed to a traumatic event that involved *potential death or serious injury to themselves or another* sometimes develop a syndrome characterized by intrusive recollections or dreams of the event, avoidance of stimuli provoking memories of the event, and a heightened level of arousal. Such symptoms are relatively common immediately after a severe trauma. However, if the symptoms persist at least 1 month at a fairly severe level, a diagnosis of PTSD is appropriate. Table 22.7 summarizes American Psychiatric Association criteria.

Case Study

A 45-year-old mechanic sustained burns on the arms and thorax when an engine exploded during repair. He had no history of psychiatric disorder. His surgical treatment was successful, leaving him with little residual physical disability. However, after discharge he experienced marked sleep disturbance, generalized anxiety, and loss of interest in usual activities. He avoided proximity to fire in any form and could not tolerate listening to reports about fires on the radio. Treatment with an SSRI aided sleep, improved his mood, and reduced the frequency of his intrusive memories and recurrent dreams, but it did not affect his avoidance behavior. On the anniversary of his injury he would not leave his room because he could not be persuaded that it was safe to do so.

Epidemiology, Origins, and Natural History

About 3.6% of U.S. adults ages 18 to 54 years (5.2 million people) have PTSD during the course of a given year (NIMH, *www.hopkinsbayview.org/PAMreferences*). In men, the full syndrome is usually found among war veterans who were injured in combat; in women, the most

TABLE 22.7 Diagnostic Criteria for Posttraumatic Stress Disorder

A. The person has been exposed to a traumatic event in which both of the following have been present:
  1. The person has experienced, witnessed, or been confronted with an event or events that involve actual or threatened death or serious injury, or a threat to the physical integrity of oneself or others.
  2. The person's response involved intense fear, helplessness, or horror. Note: In children, it may be expressed instead by disorganized or agitated behavior.

B. The traumatic event is persistently re-experienced in at least one of the following ways:
  1. Recurrent and intrusive distressing recollections of the event, including images, thoughts, or perceptions. Note: In young children, repetitive play may occur in which themes or aspects of the trauma are expressed.
  2. Recurrent distressing dreams of the event. Note: In children, there may be frightening dreams without recognized content.
  3. Acting or feeling as if the traumatic event were recurring (includes a sense of reliving the experience, illusions, hallucinations, and dissociative flashback episodes, including those that occur upon awakening or when intoxicated). Note: In young children, trauma-specific reenactment may occur.
  4. Intense psychologic distress at exposure to internal or external cues that symbolize or resemble an aspect of the traumatic event.
  5. Physiologic reactivity upon exposure to internal or external cues that symbolize or resemble an aspect of the traumatic event.

C. Persistent avoidance of stimuli associated with the trauma and numbing of general responsiveness (not present before the trauma), as indicated by at least three of the following:
  1. Efforts to avoid thoughts, feelings, or conversations associated with the trauma
  2. Efforts to avoid activities, places, or people that arouse recollections of the trauma
  3. Inability to recall an important aspect of the trauma
  4. Markedly diminished interest in participation in significant activities
  5. Feeling of detachment or estrangement from others
  6. Restricted range of affect (e.g., unable to have loving feelings)
  7. Sense of a foreshortened future (e.g., does not expect to have a career, marriage, children, or a normal life span)

D. Persistent symptoms of increased arousal (not present before the trauma), as indicated by at least two of the following:
  1. Difficulty falling or staying asleep
  2. Irritability or outbursts of anger
  3. Difficulty concentrating
  4. Hypervigilance
  5. Exaggerated startle response

E. Duration of the disturbance (symptoms in B, C, and D) is more than 1 month.

F. The disturbance causes clinically significant distress or impairment in social, occupational, or other important areas of functioning.

Acute: if duration of symptoms is less than 3 months
Chronic: if duration of symptoms is 3 months or longer
Delayed Onset: if onset of symptoms is at least 6 months after the stressor

Reprinted with permission from Diagnostic and statistical manual of mental disorders. 4th Edition. Washington, DC: American Psychiatric Association, 1994.

common precipitant is physical assault. Individual posttraumatic stress symptoms (particularly nightmares, feelings of jitteriness, and sleep disturbances) are much more common, occurring in approximately 15% of the population. Combat, physical assault, seeing someone being hurt or die, and experiencing a serious threat or close call are the most common traumatic experiences associated with such symptoms (92). The highest rates of poststress disorder are found among women who are victims of violent crime, especially rape (93). For reasons that are not entirely clear, PTSD is more common in women than men (94,95).

People with PTSD are twice as likely as people without PTSD to have another psychiatric disorder, particularly OCD, dysthymia, substance abuse, bipolar affective disorder, or antisocial personality. There is also an increased risk of PTSD among people with a history of childhood behavioral problems, especially lying, stealing, truancy, vandalism, and school expulsion. Among people with a history of four such behaviors, 6% met formal criteria for PTSD and 29% reported at least one symptom (92).

National Comorbidity Survey respondents who met criteria for PTSD had 40% elevated odds of high school and college failure, 30% elevated odds of teenage child-bearing, 60% elevated odds of marital instability, and 150% elevated odds of unemployment at the time of the survey, compared with people without PTSD (95,96). Some of these correlates could reasonably be expected to be a *result* of PTSD.

Explanations of PTSD have been advanced from several perspectives. From the behavioral viewpoint, the posttraumatic symptoms (e.g., hyperarousal, intrusive recollections) are viewed as products of classically conditioned linkages between innocuous stimuli (e.g., a news report about a fire) and the original traumatic event (e.g., painful injury in a fire). The avoidance symptoms are explained in terms of operant conditioning: Avoidance of stimuli reminiscent of the traumatic event is reinforced by resulting protection of the patient from the symptoms of phobic anxiety (i.e., hyperarousal). Biologic theorists have proposed explanations involving changes in central adrenergic autonomic arousal (97) and in cerebral mechanisms regulating sleep cycles (98). Neuroimaging studies implicate right cerebral limbic and paralimbic areas in the symptoms of PTSD, with hyperreactivity of the amygdala in response to reminders of the trauma (47). Potential roles for personality traits and early life experiences have been suggested by observations of burn patients and other trauma victims demonstrating relationships between maladaptive personality traits, early life loss, trauma, behavioral problems, and poor posttraumatic adjustment (92,99).

Treatment

Behavioral, psychotherapeutic, and pharmacologic treatment approaches have all been advocated for the treatment of PTSD. *Behavioral treatments* such as desensitization are generally required to help patients overcome the conditioned avoidance of stimuli reminiscent of the traumatic event. *Psychotherapy* is virtually always needed to assist patients in dealing with anger about the injury, guilt about survival, and similar themes common among people with PTSD. There is some evidence that early cognitive-behavior therapy diminishes subsequent PTSD symptoms, if not the disorder (100,101).

Antidepressant and anxiolytic medications have been used with variable efficacy. Tricyclic antidepressants and monoamine oxidase inhibitors may be effective in ameliorating hyperarousal, intrusion, and avoidance symptoms and in relieving concurrent major depression (102,103). Several studies have demonstrated the utility of SSRIs for the treatment of PTSD (104). Benzodiazepines are sometimes used, but there is no empiric evidence for their effectiveness in this setting, and they are relatively contraindicated in patients who are at high risk for chemical dependency. Neuroleptic drugs are almost never indicated.

TREATMENT OF ANXIETY DISORDERS: GENERAL MEASURES

Specific treatments have been described for each specific anxiety disorder. This section describes nonpharmacologic and pharmacologic measures that may be of use in several of the anxiety disorders.

Nonpharmacologic Approaches

A variety of cognitive and behavioral interventions are useful in the treatment of anxiety disorders, some of which are listed here.

Education and Explanation

Patients with panic attacks, obsessions and compulsions, posttraumatic distress symptoms, social anxiety, and generalized anxiety often feel different, isolated from others, and confused about the nature of their malady. They benefit greatly from learning that they have a diagnosable disorder, that they are not alone in their suffering, and that there are effective treatments. Patients should be encouraged to contact the NIMH (see *www.hopkinsbayview.org/PAMreferences*) for free and up-to-date science-based information on the anxiety disorders.

Self-Regulation Techniques

Many patients benefit from learning specific techniques that reduce motor tension, hyperarousal, and autonomic hyperactivity. These self-regulation techniques include muscle relaxation, diaphragmatic breathing, biofeedback, self-hypnosis, and meditation exercises (105). Interested generalists can develop skills in teaching these techniques to their patients. Alternatively, patients can be referred to behavioral therapists for instruction.

In progressive muscle relaxation and diaphragmatic breathing (Table 22.8), patients learn to ameliorate anxiety by sequential contraction and relaxation of muscle groups or by slow inhalation using the diaphragm. With regular practice, patients can apply these techniques in times of distress and achieve considerable relief. Commercially available audiotapes are available to help guide patients through the procedure (see *www.hopkinsbayview.org/PAMreferences*); the book, *The Relaxation Response* (106), is written for the layperson and may also be useful.

In *biofeedback* training (107), patients learn to control anxiety with the aid of electromyographic information provided to them in the form of visual or auditory messages. During treatment sessions, electrodes are placed in a muscle (e.g., frontalis) or muscle group. Patients then attempt to reduce muscle tension, receive immediate feedback about the effectiveness of their efforts (e.g., reduction in amplitude of a tone fed back to them through earphones), and learn to alter their technique to achieve more complete electromyographic (and clinical) relaxation.

Self-hypnosis training often begins with office-based sessions during which the therapist uses a standard hypnotic induction technique and then, for example, asks the patient to notice a warm, tingling feeling starting in the legs and feet and spreading slowly throughout the body. Pleasant, peaceful mental images might be suggested. Patients are taught to induce these states on their own and are advised to practice them regularly, reinforced by periodic office visits for reassessment and further practice. Clinicians may develop skills in performing hypnosis by attending seminars such as those sponsored by the Society for Clinical and Experimental Hypnosis.

TABLE 22.8 Essential Steps in Progressive Muscle Relaxation, Rapid Muscle Relaxation Techniques, and Diaphragmatic Breathing Exercises

A. Progressive muscle relaxation[a]	
Forehead/scalp	Raise the eyebrows high; hold; feel strain; relax.
Forehead	Scowl or frown; bunch eyebrows with nose upward; relax.
Eyes	Squeeze eyes shut; hold; feel strain in temples; relax.
Mouth	Smile broadly until mouth quivers slightly; relax; press lips tightly inward; hold; relax.
Jaw	Grit teeth gently but firmly; hold; relax; part lips slightly.
Neck/arm/shoulder	Press head back against right hand; relax; repeat exercise with left hand.
Neck/arm/shoulder	Press head forward against right hand placed on forehead; relax; repeat with left hand.
Back/legs/abdomen	Sitting, grip chair sides firmly; raise legs slightly; lift buttocks 1 inch from chair; point toes forward, then backward; relax.
Hands/arm	Make fist; clench tightly; relax.
B. Rapid Relaxation[b]	
1. Sit or lie down. The quieter the place, the better.	
2. Take a deep breath through your mouth, hold it for 10 seconds, and exhale slowly.	
3. Mentally repeat the word "relax" four times in a calm manner.	
4. Gradually space out repeating "relax" until each repetition takes about 7 seconds.	
5. Keep practicing until you achieve the level of relaxation you desire.	
C. Diaphragmatic breathing—While sitting or lying down with a pillow at the small of your back	
1. Breathe in slowly and deeply by pushing your stomach out.	
2. Say the word "relax" silently to yourself before exhaling.	
3. Exhale slowly, letting your stomach come in.	
4. Repeat entire procedure 10 times consecutively, with emphasis on slow, deep breaths.	
Practice should take place five times per day, 10 consecutive diaphragmatic breaths each sitting. Time for mastery is after 1–2 wk of daily practice.	

[a]Subject is instructed to practice this exercise while seated comfortably or reclining.
[b]For immediate relaxation in everyday stressful situations.

Meditation techniques, such as Zen, yoga, or transcendental meditation, have been practiced for centuries. They have recently become popular treatments for anxiety because they favorably alter anxiety-related physiologic variables such as respiratory rate, oxygen consumption, and galvanic skin response, a measure of autonomic activity. Meditation techniques that are effective in ameliorating anxiety include or encourage the following elements (108):

- *A mental device:* There should be a constant stimulus, such as a sound, word, or phrase repeated silently or audibly or fixed gazing at an object.
- *Passive attitude:* If distracting thoughts occur during the repetition or gazing, they should be disregarded and attention should be redirected to the chosen stimulus. The patient should not worry about the quality of performance.
- *Decreased muscle tone:* The patient should be in a comfortable position so that minimal muscular work is required.
- *Quiet environment:* An environment with minimal distractions should be chosen. If visual fixation on an object is not used, the patient's eyes should be closed.

Pharmacologic Treatments

Individual pharmacologic treatments for the various anxiety disorders have already been discussed. Generally, the SSRIs are a reasonable first-line treatment choice for all of the anxiety disorders, with the possible exception of GAD, for which buspirone may be an acceptable first choice. However, data demonstrating the efficacy of venlafaxine in the treatment of GAD suggest that it may be an excellent first-line choice as well (71,72). Also, given that GAD is commonly comorbid with depression and other anxiety disorders, the combination of buspirone with an SSRI or other antidepressant may be indicated.

Guidelines for use of SSRIs and antidepressants are described elsewhere in this text (see Chapter 24). As noted earlier, when treating new-onset panic disorder or GAD, clinicians often prescribe benzodiazepines as a bridge to help relieve anxiety in patients during the period of titration of antidepressant therapy. Typically, high-potency benzodiazepines such as lorazepam or clonazepam are used for this purpose. Generally, the initial dosages should be low (e.g., 0.25 mg lorazepam every 8 hours or 0.25 mg clonazepam twice daily). Patients should be warned not to drink alcohol or engage in activities such as driving when first using benzodiazepines. Some patients develop a central nervous system (CNS) toxicity even at low dosages of these drugs, and patients should be vigilant for this adverse effect. Although pharmaceutical manufacturers and the U.S. Food and Drug Administration (FDA) recommend that benzodiazepines be used only on a short-term basis (i.e., days to weeks) (109), approximately 90% of benzodiazepines sold in the United States in 1990 were used by people reporting daily use for 4 months or longer (110). This may be related to reports indicating that long-term benzodiazepine users have difficulty discontinuing medication and use benzodiazepines to avoid withdrawal (111). Because of the risk of tolerance and dependence, clinicians should limit the duration of benzodiazepine use to the minimal period required for adequate relief of acute anxiety symptoms. Table 22.9 displays usual dosages and pharmacokinetic properties of the various benzodiazepines.

In recent years, the popularity of herbal remedies and "natural" dietary supplements has grown significantly (see Chapter 5). A number of these dietary supplements are purported to relieve symptoms of anxiety, including kava-kava, valerian root, and St. John's wort. Although none of these alternative treatments has yet been proved effective by FDA standards, there is growing acceptance that they may be useful for the treatment of anxiety disorders, particularly in less severe cases. Patients often do not view these substances as "medications" and may not report their use to their primary caregiver. Therefore, the primary care physician should inquire about use of herbal dietary supplements, particularly before initiating treatment with pharmaceutical-grade medications. "Natural" herbal supplements can be psychoactive and are often metabolized by pathways similar to those of pharmaceutical medications. Drug interactions (occasionally severe) and additive effects have been reported in patients who simultaneously used prescription drugs and herbal or non-herbal supplements (see Chapter 5, Table 5.4). Therefore, caution should be exercised in prescribing drugs to patients who are taking supplements. Patients taking kava-kava who are prescribed anxiolytics and patients taking St. John's wort who are prescribed SSRIs should be advised to taper their herbal supplement before initiating treatment with the prescribed medication.

During the next few years, several new agents may become available for the treatment of anxiety disorders. Among these are corticotropin-releasing factor antagonists and substance P antagonists, both of which have shown promise in preclinical models of anxiety. Several pharmaceutical companies are developing these agents for potential use in anxiety disorders and depression.

TABLE 22.9 Usual Dosage and Pharmacokinetics of Anxiolytic Benzodiazepines

Drug (Trade Name), Year Introduced	*Onset of Effect After Oral Dose*[a]	*Available Strengths (mg)*	*Oral Daily Dosage Range Divided Two or Three Times a Day (mg)*	*Active Metabolites Present*	*Elimination Half-Life*[b] *(hr)*
Alprazolam[c] (Xanax), 1981	Intermediate	0.25, 0.5, 1 (scored tablets)	0.75–6	No	8–16
Chlordiazepoxide[c] (Librium; Libritabs), 1960	Intermediate	5, 10, 25 (capsules); 5, 10, 25 (tablets)	15–100	Yes	5–30
Clonazepam[d] (Klonopin), 1990	Intermediate	0.5, 1, 2 (tablets)	1.5–20	Yes	18–50
Clorazepate dipotassium[c] (Tranxene; Tranxene SD), 1972	Rapid	3.75, 7.5, 15 (capsules); 11.25, 22.5 (tablets)	15–60 4.25, 22.5 (single doses are intended for patients stabilized on 3.75 or 7.5 mg t.i.d.)	Yes Yes	36–200 36–200
Diazepam[c] (Valium), 1961	Rapid	2, 5, 10 (tablets)	4–40	Yes	20–50
Diazepam (Valrelease), 1982	Slow	15 (capsules)	15–30 (single dose of 15 is equivalent to 5 mg of Valium t.i.d.)	Yes	20–50
Halazepam (Paxipam), 1981	Slow to intermediate	20, 40 (tablets)	80–160	Yes	50–100
Lorazepam[c] (Ativan), 1977	Intermediate	0.5, 1, 2 (tablets)	1–6	No	10–20
Oxazepam[c] (Serax), 1963	Slow to intermediate	10, 15, 30 (capsules) 15 (tablets)	30–120 30–120	No	5–10
Prazepam (Centrax), 1977	Slow	5, 10 (capsules)	20–60	Yes	36–200

[a]Drugs with more rapid onset of action are those more rapidly absorbed.
[b]Elimination half-life of lipophilic activity.
[c]Generic available.
[d]Clonazepam is not approved by the U.S. FDA for treatment of anxiety. It is approved as an anticonvulsant, and for short-term use in panic disorder.

SPECIFIC REFERENCES*

1. Kubzansky LD, Kawachi I, Weiss ST, et al. Anxiety and coronary heart disease: a synthesis of epidemiological, psychological and experimental evidence. Ann Behav Med 1998;20:47.
2. Zaubler TS, Katon W. Panic disorder in the general medical setting. J Psychosom Res 1998;44:25.
3. Mayou R, Williamson B, Foster A. Attitudes and advice after myocardial infarction. BMJ 1976;1:1577.
4. Gorman JM, Kent JM, Sullivan GM, et al. Neuroanatomical hypothesis of panic disorder, revised. Am J Psychiatry 2000;157:493.
5. **5.** Anxiety Disorders. NIH Publication No. 00-3879. Bethesda, MD: National Institutes of Health, 1994. Reprinted 1995, 1997, and 2000.
6. Katon W. Panic disorder: relationship to high medical utilization, unexplained physical symptoms and medical costs. J Clin Psychiatry 1996;57[Suppl 10]:11.
7. Zaubler TS, Katon W. Panic disorder and medical comorbidity: a review of the medical and psychiatric literature. Bull Menninger Clin 1996;2[Suppl A]:A12.
8. Margraff J, Ehlers A, Roth WT. Mitral valve prolapse and panic disorder: a review of their relationship. Psychosom Med 1988;50:93.
9. Shavitt RG, Gentil V, Mandetta R. The association of panic/agoraphobia and asthma: contributing factors and clinical implications. Gen Hospital Psychiatry 1992;14:420.
10. Yellowlees PM, Haynes S, Potts N, et al. Psychiatric morbidity in patients with life-threatening asthma: initial report of a controlled study. Med J Austr 1988;149:246.
11. Spinhoven P, Ros M, Westgeest A, et al. The prevalence of respiratory disorders in panic disorder, major depressive disorder and V-code patients. Behav Res Ther 1994;32:647.
12. Merikangas KR, Angst J, Isler H. Migraine and psychopathology: results of the Zurich cohort study of young adults. Arch Gen Psychiatry 1990;47:849.
13. Breslau N, Davis GC. Migraine, physical health and psychiatric disorder: a prospective epidemiologic study in young adults. J Psychiatric Res 1993;27:211.
14. Regier DA, Rae DS, Narrow WE, et al. Prevalence of anxiety disorders and their comorbidity with mood and addictive disorders. Br J Psychiatry 1998;[Suppl 34]:24.
15. Aronson TA, Logue CM. On the longitudinal course of panic disorder: developmental history and prediction of phobic complications. Compr Psychiatry 1987;28:344.
16. Robins LN, Regier DA, eds. Psychiatric disorders in America: the Epidemiologic Catchment Area Study. New York: The Free Press, 1991.
17. Breier A, Charney DS, Heninger GR. Major depression in patients with agoraphobia and panic disorder. Arch Gen Psychiatry 1984;41:1129.
18. Breier A, Charney DS, Heninger GR. The diagnostic validity of anxiety disorders and their relationship to depressive illness. Am J Psychiatry 1985;142:787.
19. Breier A, Charney DS, Heninger GR. Agoraphobia with panic attacks. Arch Gen Psychiatry 1986;43:1029.
20. Bass C, Cawley R, Wade C, et al. Unexplained breathlessness and psychiatric morbidity in patients with normal and abnormal coronary arteries. Lancet 1983;1:605.
21. Coryell W, Noyes R, Clancy J. Excess mortality in panic disorder: a comparison with primary unipolar depression. Arch Gen Psychiatry 1982;39:701.
22. Kawachi I, Colditz GA, Ascherio A, et al. Prospective study of phobic anxiety and risk of coronary heart disease in men. Circulation 1994;89:1992.
23. Kawachi I, Sparrow D, Vokonas PS, et al. Symptoms of anxiety and risk of coronary heart disease: the Normative Aging Study. Circulation 1994;90:2225.
24. Pauls DL, Slymen P. A family study of panic disorders. Arch Gen Psychiatry 1983;40:1065.
25. **25.** Hettema JM, Neale MC, Kendler KS. A review and meta-analysis of the genetic epidemiology of anxiety disorders. Am J Psychiatry 2001;158:1568.
26. Gorman JM, Dillon D, Fyer AJ, et al. The lactate infusion model. Psychopharmacol Bull 1985;21:428.
27. Clark DM, Salkovskis PM, Chalkley AJ. Respiratory control as a treatment for panic attacks. J Behav Ther Exp Psychiatry 1985;16:23.
28. Barlow DH. Behavioral conception and treatment of panic. Psychopharmacol Bull 1986;22:802.
29. Goldstein AJ, Chambless DL. A reanalysis of agoraphobia. Behav Res Ther 1978;9:47.
30. **30.** Zohar J, Westenberg HG. Anxiety disorders: a review of tricyclic antidepressants and selective serotonin reuptake inhibitors. Acta Psychiatr Scand 2000;403[Suppl]:39.
31. **31.** Oehrberg S, Christiansen PE, Behnke K. Paroxetine in the treatment of panic disorder: a randomized, double-blind, placebo-controlled study. Br J Psychiatry 1995;167:374.
32. Sheehan DV. Current concepts in the treatment of panic disorder. J Clin Psychiatry 1999; 60[Suppl 18]:16.
33. Davidson JRT. Long-term treatment of panic disorder. J Clin Psychiatry 1998;49[Suppl 8]:17.
34. Le Crubier Y, Judge R. Long-term evaluation of paroxetine, clomipramine and placebo in panic disorder. Acta Psychiatr Scand 1997;95:153.
35. **35.** American Psychiatric Associating. Practice guideline for the treatment of patients with panic disorder. Am J Psychiatry 1998:155[Suppl 5]:1.
36. Gorman JM. The use of newer antidepressants for panic disorder. J Clin Psychiatry 1997; 58[Suppl 14]:54.
37. Otto MW, Pollack MH, Maki KM. Empirically supported treatments for panic disorder: costs, benefits, and stepped care. J Consult Clin Psychol 2000;68:556.
38. Myers JK, Weissman MM, Tischler GL, et al. Six-month prevalence of psychiatric disorders in three communities. Arch Gen Psychiatry 1984;41:959.
39. Van Korff M, Shapiro S, Burke JD, et al. Anxiety and depression in a primary care clinic. Arch Gen Psychiatry 1987;44:152.
40. Rasmussen SA, Tsuang MT. Clinical characteristics and family history in DSM-III obsessive-compulsive disorder. Am J Psychiatry 1986;143:317.
41. McKeon J, Roa B, Mann A. Life events and personality traits in obsessive-compulsive neurosis. Br J Psychiatry 1984;144:185.
42. Nestadt G, Samuels J, Riddle M, et al. A family study of obsessive-compulsive disorder. Arch Gen Psychiatry 2000;57:358.
43. Nestadt G, Lan T, Samuels J, et al. Complex segregation analysis provides compelling evidence for a major gene underlying obsessive-compulsive disorder and for heterogeneity by sex. Am J Hum Genet 2000; 67:1611.
44. McKeon J, McGuffin P, Robinson P. Obsessive-compulsive neurosis following head injury: a report of four cases. Br J Psychiatry 1984;144:190.
45. Grimshaw L. Obsessional disorder and neurological illness. J Neurol Neurosurg Psychiatry 1964;27:229.
46. Saxena S, Brody AL, Schwartz JM, et al. Neuroimaging and frontal-subcortical circuitry in obsessive-compulsive disorder. Br J Psychiatry 1998;173[Suppl 35]:26.
47. Rauch SL. Neuroimaging research and the neurobiology of obsessive-compulsive disorder: where do we go from here? Biol Psychiatry 2000;47:168.
48. Rauch SL, Whalen PJ, Dougherty DD, et al. Neurobiological models of obsessive compulsive disorders. In: Jenike MA, Baer L, Minichiello WE, eds. Obsessive-compulsive disorders: practical management. St. Louis: Mosby, 1998: 222.
49. Swedo SE, Leonard HL, Garvey M, et al. Pediatric autoimmune neuropsychiatric disorders associated with streptococcal infections: clinical description of the first 50 cases. Am J Psychiatry 1998;155:263.
50. Insel TR. Toward a neuroanatomy of obsessive-compulsive disorder. Arch Gen Psychiatry 1992;49:739.
51. Stein DD. Neurobiology of the obsessive-compulsive spectrum disorders. Biol Psychiatry 2000;47:296.
52. **52.** March JS, Frances A, Carpenter D, et al. The expert consensus guideline series: treatment of obsessive-compulsive disorder. J Clin Psychiatry 1997;58[Suppl 4]:1.
53. **53.** Greist JH, Jefferson JW, Kobak KA, et al. Efficacy and tolerability of serotonin transport inhibitors in obsessive-compulsive disorder: a meta-analysis. Arch Gen Psychiatry 1995; 52:53.
54. **54.** Thoren P, Asberg M, Cronholm B, et al. Clomipramine treatment of obsessive-compulsive disorder: I. A controlled clinical trial. Arch Gen Psychiatry 1980;37:1281.
55. **55.** Ackerman DL, Greenland S. Multivariate meta-analysis of controlled drug studies for obsessive-compulsive disorder. J Clin Psychopharmacol 2002;22:309.
56. Rasmussen SA, Eisen JL. Treatment strategies for chronic and refractory obsessive-compulsive disorder. J Clin Psychiatry 1997;58[Suppl 13]:9.
57. Goodman WK. Obsessive-compulsive disorder: diagnosis and treatment. J Clin Psychiatry 1999;60:S27.
58. Vythilingum B, Cartwright C, Hollander E. Pharmacotherapy of obsessive-compulsive disorder: experience with the selective serotonin reuptake inhibitors. Int Clin Psychopharmacol 2000;15[Suppl 2]:S7.
59. **59.** Romano S, Goodman W, Tamura R, et al. Long-term treatment of obsessive-compulsive disorder after an acute response: a comparison of fluoxetine versus placebo. J Clin Psychopharmacol 2001;21:46.
60. Kessler RC, McGonagle KA, Zhao S, et al. Lifetime and 12-month prevalence of DSM-III-R psychiatric disorders in the United States: results from the National Comorbidity Survey. Arch Gen Psychiatry 1994;51:8.
61. Barlow DH, Blanchard EB, Vermylyea JA, et al. Generalized anxiety and generalized anxiety disorder: description and reconceptualization. Am J Psychiatry 1986;143:40.
62. Yonkers KA, Warshaw MG, Massion AO, et al. Phenomenology and course of generalized anxiety disorder. Br J Psychiatry 1996;168:308.
63. Brawman-Mintzer O, Lydiard RB. Generalized anxiety disorder: issues in epidemiology. J Clin Psychiatry 1996;57 [Suppl 7]:3.

*Bold numerals denote published controlled clinical trials, meta-analyses, or consensus-based recommendations.

64. Noyes R Jr, Clarkson C, Crowe R, et al. A family study of generalized anxiety disorder. Am J Psychiatry 1987;144:1019.
65. Kendler KS. Major depression and generalized anxiety disorder: same genes, (partly) different environments—revisited. Br J Psychiatry 1996;[Suppl 30]:68.
66. Hettema JM, Prescott CA, Kendler KS. Genetic and environmental sources of covariation between generalized anxiety disorder and neuroticism. Am J Psychiatry 2004;161:1581.
67. Torgersen S. Childhood and family characteristics in panic and generalized anxiety disorders. Am J Psychiatry 1986;143:630.
68. Hoehn-Saric R. Characteristics of chronic anxiety patients. In: Klein DF, Rabkin J, eds. Anxiety: new research and changing concepts. New York: Raven Press, 1981.
69. Blazer D, Hughes D, George LK. Stressful life events and the onset of a generalized anxiety syndrome. Am J Psychiatry 1987;144:1178.
70. Kapczinski F, Lima MS, Souza JS, et al. Antidepressants for generalized anxiety disorder. The Cochrane Database of Systematic Reviews 2003, Issue 2. Art. No.: CD003592. DOI: 10.1002/14651858.CD003592.
71. Boyer P, Mahe V, Hackett D. Social adjustment in generalised anxiety disorder: a long-term placebo-controlled study of venlafaxine extended release. Eur Psychiatry 2004;19:272–279.
72. Davidson JR, DuPont RL, Hedges D, et al. Efficacy, safety and tolerability of venlafaxine extended release and buspirone in outpatients with generalised anxiety disorder. J Clin Psychiatry 1999;60:528.
73. Sramek JJ, Tansman M, Suri A, et al. Efficacy of buspirone in generalized anxiety disorder with coexisting mild depressive symptoms. J Clin Psychiatry 1996;57:287.
74. American Psychiatric Association. Benzodiazepines: dependence, toxicity and abuse. A task force report of the American Psychiatry Association. Washington, DC: American Psychiatric Association, 1991.
75. Kessler RD, Wittchen HU. Patterns and correlates of generalized anxiety disorder in community samples. J Clin Psychiatry 2002; 63(Suppl 8):4.
76. Yonkers KA, Dyck IR, Warshaw M, et al. Factors predicting the clinical course of generalised anxiety disorder. Br J Psychiatry 2000;176:544.
77. Kessler RC, Stein MB, Berglund P. Social phobia subtypes in the National Comorbidity Survey. Am J Psychiatry 1998;155:613.
78. Curtis GC, Magee WJ, Eaton WW, et al. Specific fears and phobias: epidemiology and classification. Br J Psychiatry 1998;173: 212.
79. Magee WJ, Eaton WW, Wittchen HU, et al. Agoraphobia, simple phobia and social phobia in the National Comorbidity Survey. Arch Gen Psychiatry 1996;53:159.
80. Ballenger JC, Davidson JR, Lecrubier Y, et al. Consensus statement on social anxiety disorder from the International Consensus Group on Depression and Anxiety. J Clin Psychiatry 1998; 59[Suppl 17]:54.
81. Davidson JRT, Hughes DL, George LK, et al. The epidemiology of social phobia: findings from the Duke Epidemiological Catchment Area Study. Psychol Med 1993;23:709.
82. Haines AP, Imeson JD, Meade TW. Phobic anxiety and ischaemic heart disease. BMJ 1987;295:297.
83. Rasmussen K, Henningsen P. Provocative testing with prolonged hyperventilation and ergometrine in patients suspected of coronary artery spasm: a comparative study. Int J Cardiol 1987;15:151.
84. Lown B. Mental stress, arrhythmias, and sudden death. Am J Med 1982;72:177.
85. Taylor CB, Ferguson JM, Wermuth BM. Simple techniques to treat medical phobias. Postgrad Med J 1977;53:28.
86. Marks I. Fears and phobias. London: Heinemann, 1969.
87. Marks I. Recent results of behavioral treatments of phobias and obsessions. J Intern Med 1977;5[Suppl 5]:15.
88. Van Ameringen MA, Lane RM, Walker JR, et al. Sertraline treatment of generalized social phobia: a 20-week, double-blind, placebo-controlled study. Am J Psychiatry 2001;158:275.
89. van Vliet IM, den Boer JA, Westernberg HG. Psychopharmacological treatment of social phobia: a double blind placebo controlled study with fluvoxamine. Psychopharmacology 1994; 115:128.
90. Jefferson JW. Benzodiazepines and anticonvulsants for social phobia (social anxiety disorder). J Clin Psychiatry 2001;62[Suppl 1]:50.
91. Altamura AC, Pioli R, Vitto M, et al. Venlafaxine in social phobia: a study in selective serotonin reuptake inhibitor non-responders. Int Clin Psychopharmacol 1999;14:239.
92. Helzer JE, Robins LN, McEvoy L. Post-traumatic stress disorder in the general population: findings of the Epidemiologic Catchment Area Survey. N Engl J Med 1987;317:1630.
93. Acierno R, Resnick H, Kilpatrick D, et al. Risk factors for rape, physical assault, and posttraumatic stress disorder in women: examination of differential multivariate relationships. J Anxiety Disord 1999;13:541.
94. Breslau N, Kessler RC, Chilcoat HD, et al. Trauma and posttraumatic stress disorder in the community: the 1996 Detroit Area Survey of Trauma. Arch Gen Psychiatry 1998;55:626.
95. Kessler RC, Sonnega A, Bromet E, et al. Posttraumatic stress disorder in the National Comorbidity Survey. Arch Gen Psychiatry 1995;52:1048.
96. Kessler RC. Posttraumatic stress disorder: the burden to the individual and to society. J Clin Psychiatry 2000;61[Suppl 5]:4.
97. Kolb LC. A neuropsychological hypothesis explaining posttraumatic stress disorders. Am J Psychiatry 1987;144:989.
98. Ross RJ, Ball WA, Sullivan KA, et al. Sleep disturbance as the hallmark of posttraumatic stress disorder. Am J Psychiatry 1988;146:697.
99. Andreasen NJ, Noyes R, Hartford CE. Factors influencing adjustment of burn patients during hospitalization. Psychosom Med 1972;34: 517.
100. Bisson JI, Shepherd JP, Joy D, et al. Early cognitive-behavioural therapy for post-traumatic stress symptoms after physical injury. Randomised controlled trial. Br J Psychiatry 2004;184:63.
101. Brom D, Kleber RJ, Hofman MC. Victims of traffic accidents: incidence and prevention of post-traumatic stress disorder. J Clin Psychol 1993;49:131.
102. Davidson J, Kudler H, Smith R, et al. Treatment of posttraumatic stress disorder with amitriptyline and placebo. Arch Gen Psychiatry 1990;47:259.
103. Kosten TR, Frank JB, Dan E, et al. Pharmacotherapy for posttraumatic stress disorder using phenelzine or imipramine. J Nerv Ment Dis 1991;179:366.
104. Alarcon RD, Glover S, Boyer W, et al. Proposing an algorithm for the pharmacological management of posttraumatic stress disorder. Ann Clin Psychiatry 2000;12:239.
105. Goldberg RJ. Anxiety reduction by self-regulation: theory, practice, and evaluation. Ann Intern Med 1982;96:483.
106. Benson H. The relaxation response. New York: William Morrow, 1976.
107. Gaarder KR, Montgomery PS. Clinical biofeedback: a procedural manual for behavioral medicine. 2nd ed. Baltimore: Williams & Wilkins, 1981.
108. Benson H, Beary JF, Carol MP. The relaxation response. Psychiatry 1974;37:37.
109. National Institutes of Health. Drugs and insomnia: Consensus Development Conference Summary. Bethesda, MD: National Institutes of Health, 1984;4:1.
110. Giffiths RR, Weerts EM. Benzodiazepine self-administration in humans and laboratory animals: implications for problems of long-term use and abuse. Psychopharmacology 1997; 134:1.
111. Romach M, Busto U, Somer G, et al. Clinical aspects of chronic use of alprazolam and lorazepam. Am J Psychiatry 1995;152:1161.

For annotated ***General References*** *and resources related to this chapter, visit www.hopkinsbayview.org/PAMreferences.*

Chapter 23

Personality and Personality Disorders

Robert P. Roca

CONCEPT OF PERSONALITY AND PERSONALITY DISORDER

Definition and Methods of Classification

The enduring attitudes, behaviors, and capacities that distinguish individuals from each other are collectively called personality. Personality is commonly conceptualized categorically or dimensionally.

Categorical approaches specify qualitatively distinct personality *types* and classify individuals according to the type they most closely resemble. The ancient Greek typology (i.e., phlegmatic, choleric, sanguine, melancholic) is one such example. The American Psychiatric Association uses this approach in the classification of personality disorders published in the most recent *Diagnostic and Statistical Manual of Mental Disorders, 4th Edition, Text Revision* (*DSM-IV-TR*) (see Subtyping of Personality Disorder).

Dimensional approaches view personality as a mosaic of *traits,* each possessed by individuals in differing quantities (1). Intelligence, as defined by the *intelligence quotient* (IQ), is a model of such a trait. IQ scores are normally distributed in the population and are highly correlated with academic and occupational achievement. People with above-average IQ scores tend to be successful in school and work, whereas those with below-average IQs often have difficulty meeting the demands of daily life independently. Knowledge of a person's position on the dimension of intelligence thus illuminates strengths and vulnerabilities and allows one to predict circumstances that the person might find overwhelming.

A 30-year-old man was admitted to the hospital for cellulitis of the feet. His physician discovered that he had only completed the third grade and that he was unable to read, write, or calculate. Further investigation disclosed that he had recently lost his job in a laundromat and that he had been observed walking barefoot in a dumpster looking for items he needed. His physician explained to him, carefully and repeatedly, the relationship between his infection and his behavior. A social worker was called to help him apply for financial assistance and other entitlements.

Dimensions can be translated into categorical terms, sometimes with misleading consequences. "Mental retardation," for example, is said to be present when the IQ is lower than 70. By this definition, a man with an IQ of 68 is categorized as mentally retarded but one with an IQ of 72 is not, despite the fact that their risk of intelligence-related difficulty is essentially identical. In the latter case, a categorical approach may obscure clinically important vulnerability.

While IQ is by far the best-studied dimension of personality, other personality traits may also be described dimensionally. We use dimensional thinking informally when we recognize that some people are more meticulous, more gregarious, or more ambitious than others. Psychologists use this approach technically when they administer standardized tests to describe quantitatively how meticulous, introverted, agreeable, or conscientious someone is. At some arbitrary point, the meticulous person may be categorized as obsessional or the introverted person as schizoid and thus be said to have a categorical personality disorder; however, it is useful to recognize that certain patients are more meticulous or more introverted than others even when they are not categorically obsessional or schizoid. A dimensional view facilitates the recognition of such traits in every patient, and helps health care practitioners adapt assessment, relational, and management strategies to the personalities of their individual patients (see Chapters 3 and 4).

Development of Personality

Personality is believed to evolve out of interactions between constitutional, or inborn, factors and the molding influences of the environment. *Constitutional factors* include capacities, such as intelligence, and aspects of temperament, such as sociability and emotionality, all of which may have neurobiologic correlates and genetic determinants (2). The most important *environmental influences* are interpersonal relationships, particularly with parents. Many theories have been offered to account more specifically for personality development, but none has yet proved fully adequate (3).

Conceptualization of Personality Disorder

Personality disorders are among the most controversial conditions in psychiatry. There is no doubt that some people have enduring patterns of maladaptive attitudes and behaviors that interfere with their ability to work effectively and to develop and sustain gratifying interpersonal relationships. It is also clear that such people are at increased risk for long-term social impairment and for many major psychiatric illnesses (4,5). The controversy lies in how best to conceptualize and subdivide these disorders. This chapter describes three such conceptualizations.

The dominant approach in the United States—that adopted by the American Psychiatric Association in *DSM-IV-TR*—is categorical. In this scheme, the *diagnostic criteria* for the personality disorders are lists of attitudes and behaviors (e.g., self-dramatization) that, in combination, evoke an ideal prototype (e.g., the histrionic personality). Only a person exhibiting the requisite number of such attitudes and behaviors (e.g., at least five of eight, in the case of histrionic personality disorder) is said to have the condition.

Maladaptive personalities can also be conceptualized in terms of quantitative deviations from normal along specific personality dimensions. As mentioned earlier, many clinically important personality traits (e.g., meticulousness, dependency, self-confidence) can be viewed in this way. Extreme deviations from "normal" along any of these dimensions may produce special vulnerability, particularly under certain circumstances. For example, excessive meticulousness may lead to great distress when the environment is out of order, and poor self-confidence may predispose one to demoralization in response to criticism from a superior. Thus dimensional thinking about personality disturbances creates a model for understanding the interaction between environmental stresses and trait-based vulnerabilities.

Finally, personality disorders may be viewed as incomplete or atypical expressions of schizophrenia, mood disorders, or other major psychiatric illnesses.

Subtyping of Personality Disorder

The *DSM-IV-TR* describes ten types of personality disorders and groups them into *three clusters:* the dramatic (histrionic, borderline, narcissistic, and antisocial types), the anxious or fearful (obsessive-compulsive, dependent, and avoidant types), and the odd or eccentric (schizoid, schizotypal, and paranoid types) clusters. In the descriptions of the categorical disorders that follow in this chapter, it is clear that many of the disorders may be viewed as manifestations of extreme positions on dimensions of personality such as emotionality, narcissism, trust, sociability, self-esteem, and assertiveness. It is also seen that the types within each cluster tend to share traits and vulnerabilities and, therefore, implications for management. A few disorders are linked to major psychiatric illnesses. It is important to emphasize that a patient with clinically obvious disturbances involving dimensions of personality may meet criteria for several *DSM-IV-TR* personality disorders or may meet criteria for none.

Personality disorders are listed on axis II of the multiaxial assessment system that is recommended in *DSM-IV-TR*. Table 23.1 shows the estimated population prevalence and sex ratios for the major personality disorders.

TABLE 23.1 Estimated Prevalence and Sex Ratios of the Major Personality Disorders

Personality Disorder	*Prevalence (General Population)*	*Sex Ratio*
Dramatic cluster		
Histrionic	2%–3%	F > M
Narcissistic	<1%	M > F
Borderline	1%–2%	F > M
Antisocial	1%–3%	M(~ 3%) > F(1%)
Anxious cluster		
Avoidant	0.5%–1%	F = M
Dependent	Common	F > M
Obsessive Compulsive	1%	M > F
Odd/Eccentric cluster		
Paranoid	0.5%–2.5%	M > F
Schizotypal	3%	M > F
Schizoid	Uncommon	M > F

Adapted from Diagnostic and statistical manual of mental disorders. 4th ed. Text Revision. Washington, DC: American Psychiatric Association, 2000.

GENERAL APPROACH TO MANAGEMENT OF PERSONALITY TRAITS AND DISORDERS

Several points are useful to bear in mind when dealing with patients with maladaptive traits or categorical personality disorders of any subtype. Because maladaptive traits are generally well established and deeply ingrained, it is doubtful that they will change in response to the health care practitioner's efforts. An exception to this rule is when particular aspects of temperament (e.g., harm avoidance) change in response to pharmacologic treatment of concurrent mood disorders that are making these traits more prominent (6). Otherwise, the general approach to primary care management of personality disorders is to recognize these sources of vulnerability, take them into account when interacting with the patient, and minimize their adverse impact on the provision of medical care.

Patients may become resentful when maladaptive traits are pointed out to them, and this response defeats the practitioner's purposes. Yet it is often important to call patients' attention to ways in which they are undermining their medical care. When such action is necessary, it is usually advisable to avoid personality disorder labels, referring instead to specific problematic behaviors, and to present clinical observations plainly and without criticism (e.g., "It is difficult for us to provide you with the care you need when you curse at us and criticize every effort we make.").

Generally, counseling by the generalist, if undertaken at all, is best when it is symptom-focused and short-term (see Chapter 20). For long-term treatment, patients with seriously disturbed personalities should be referred to a mental health professional.

DRAMATIC CLUSTER

Patients with personality disturbances in this cluster tend to occupy extreme positions on the dimensions of emotionality and self-esteem. They are intensely emotional, sometimes acting impulsively, aggressively, or self-destructively. They are also self-absorbed, lacking in empathy for others, and extreme (unrealistically high or low) in their self-regard. They tend to be demanding of others, and their relationships are unstable, tempestuous, and exploitive, qualities that may characterize their interactions with health care practitioners and complicate the provision of medical care.

Histrionic Personality

The essence of the histrionic type is *excessive emotionality, self-dramatization, and attention-seeking*. Patients meeting criteria for the categoric disorder are self-centered, unusually eager for approval and praise, overly concerned with physical attractiveness, and often inappropriately sexually seductive or flattering ("Of all the doctors I've had, you are the first to really listen to me"). Their style of speech is dramatic, impressionistic, and factually imprecise, and their expression of emotions is often exaggerated, rapidly shifting, and apparently shallow. They may manifest an unusually warm and sometimes seductive manner with the practitioner and present to the office with complaints that are dramatically expressed but vague in medically relevant detail. Histrionic patients may be especially inclined to develop somatization disorder (see Chapter 21).

Narcissistic Personality

The narcissistic personality type is characterized by *an exaggerated sense of self-importance,* intolerance of criticism, and insensitivity to the needs of others. Narcissistic people may exploit others for their own ends, require constant admiration and attention, believe themselves entitled to special treatment, and envy those who are more successful, attractive, intelligent, or otherwise praiseworthy. Such patients are often difficult to care for because they tend to believe that their problems are unique and can be solved only by remarkable health care providers. They may challenge the doctor's knowledge, skill, and judgment and expect that their convenience will be the prime consideration in the scheduling of tests and appointments.

Borderline Personality

Extreme instability—in mood, identity, interpersonal relationships, and self-regard—is the essence of the borderline personality. Although this condition was once believed to lie on the "border" of schizophrenia, recent data more strongly support a link with affective disorders. Substance abuse, sexual impulsiveness, poor self-esteem, self-mutilation, recurrent (often manipulative) suicidal threats, and brief bouts of intense depression and rage, superimposed on chronic feelings of emptiness or boredom, characterize the long-term functioning of these patients. A shifting tendency to view other people as all good or all bad and to react to them with extremes of idealization or devaluation creates difficulties in all interpersonal relationships, including those with health care practitioners and other caretakers, who are seen as either good or bad and are pitted against one another (staff splitting).

Antisocial Personality

The antisocial personality type is characterized by a chronic and *pervasive pattern of irresponsible and socially unacceptable behavior*. Truancy, vandalism, fire setting, lying, and theft in childhood give way to impulsiveness, recklessness, aggressiveness, sexual promiscuity, financial irresponsibility, and outright criminality in adulthood. Often complaining of mistreatment themselves, they shamelessly exploit others in their relationships. In medical settings they may be malingerers (see Chapter 21), consciously feigning disease for obvious gain; and in their dealings with medical staff they may be either demanding and abusive or flattering and ingratiating, depending on which approach they perceive to be most expedient.

Management of Dramatic Subtypes

When dealing with dramatic patients one can expect a show of emotional extremes and pressure to bestow emotional and material favors as well as medical care. It is helpful to maintain equanimity in the face of the patient's emotional excesses, to avoid defensiveness when challenged, and to give special attention to professional boundaries. Socializing or becoming unusually familiar with histrionic or borderline patients is particularly risky. Because patients with these traits lack empathy and exploit others, it is often necessary to spell out, firmly but nonpunitively, the limits of acceptable behavior with medical staff, nurses, and other members of the health care team; such limit-setting is most often needed with narcissistic and antisocial patients.

ANXIOUS OR FEARFUL CLUSTER

Patients with personality disturbances in this cluster tend to be self-doubting, timid, and tense. Lacking confidence in themselves, they may seek to avoid making decisions or taking on responsibility, preferring to have others decide or perform for them; however, they are often dissatisfied with and critical of the efforts of others. They tend to be socially unassertive, submitting to the wishes of others and even avoiding friendships in the first place for fear of ultimate rejection. Levels of generalized anxiety are chronically high.

Avoidant Personality

The avoidant person *craves social contact but avoids it* because of intense social discomfort related to expectations of criticism and rejection. These people often complain of loneliness, but they are too shy to make the social contacts required to solve the problem unless they are certain of acceptance. Major depression and social phobia commonly occur. Because health care practitioners are generally viewed as accepting of their patients, avoidant people may feel particularly comfortable in the presence of their practitioner and may develop symptoms justifying regular visits to alleviate their loneliness.

Dependent Personality

Dependent people *lack self-confidence and go to great lengths to ensure the availability of others* on whom they can depend for advice and reassurance. Because they feel uneasy and helpless when alone, they may endure abuse and perform unpleasant or demeaning tasks to preserve the dependent relationship. They are exceedingly sensitive to criticism and abandonment. Patients of this type may become quite dependent on their health care practitioners, particularly when other relationships are unsatisfactory, and may use vague, chronic complaints as a means of remaining in close touch, especially in times of stress. Such patients may also become ill before a period of planned unavailability on the part of the practitioner (e.g., a vacation).

Obsessive-Compulsive Personality

People with obsessive-compulsive personalities are *rigid, parsimonious, morally scrupulous, and emotionally constricted*. Exceedingly committed to work, they are reluctant to delegate duties, convinced that no one else can do things correctly, yet they are also indecisive and at times are rendered ineffective by perfectionism or preoccupation with trivial details. They tend to describe upsetting emotional experiences in a cool, detached manner (isolation of affect). When ill, they often present their health care providers with extremely detailed accounts of their symptoms and request lengthy explanations of their disease and its treatment, including very precise instructions about medication use and likely side effects. They are usually aware of hospital rules and routines and are intolerant of lateness and inefficiency. People with obsessive-compulsive personalities may be especially prone to developing hypochondriasis (see Chapter 21) and obsessive-compulsive disorder, a condition characterized by recurrent, resisted thoughts and repetitive, senseless actions (see Chapter 22).

Passive-Aggressive Personality

Although not listed in *DSM-IV TR*, passive-aggressive personality disorder warrants brief mention because of its potential impact on the provision of medical care. Passive-aggressive people *do not want to meet the expectations of others but do not want to be held responsible for this decision*. Thus they do not say "no" directly but express hostile resistance in terms of procrastination, intentional inefficiency, and feigned forgetfulness. Usually dependent and lacking in self-confidence, they seek the counsel of others, yet often paradoxically resist following the advice of those whom they consult. In medical settings they insist that they intend to comply with treatment recommendations but then, for example, forget to keep a symptom log required to assess the effectiveness of a new treatment or forget to make it to the laboratory for an important blood test.

Management of Anxious Subtypes

The general guidelines described previously are applicable. Because patients with these types of personality traits tend to develop anxious attachment to their health care practitioners, the management of dependency is a central issue. It may be necessary to allow patients to be excessively dependent, within manageable bounds, during times of unusual stress. It may be helpful to give them regular, brief appointments so that they do not need to develop new symptomatic complaints to gain access to attention (see Chapter 21), and it may be useful to advise them to call weekly at a specified time to provide updates on their status; this may preempt emergency calls at less convenient times. Such patients also generally benefit from advance notice about vacations and may appreciate meeting the covering practitioner ahead of time. Treatment for generalized anxiety disorder, phobias, and major depression may be indicated in selected cases (see Chapters 22 and 24).

ODD OR ECCENTRIC CLUSTER

Patients with disorders in this cluster occupy extreme positions on the dimensions of trust and sociability. They tend to be highly suspicious and to isolate themselves from other people due to anxious mistrust, awkwardness, or indifference.

Paranoid Personality

Patients with paranoid personalities *tend to perceive threats and insults at every turn*. Expecting to be exploited or harmed by others, they hear veiled threats in neutral remarks and readily question the loyalty of friends and the fidelity of spouses. They are guarded, easily slighted, defensive, and unforgiving. Although their suspiciousness does not carry the intensity or conviction of a true delusion, they have family histories of schizophrenia and delusional disorders more often than other people (2). In medical settings these patients may be reluctant to provide a complete history, especially a social history ("What does this have to do with my medical problem?") and may balk at undergoing laboratory tests ("You doctors are just trying to make money off me").

Schizotypal Personality

People with schizotypal personality type exhibit odd behavior, *have peculiar beliefs, and suffer social isolation*—as a result of their own social anxiety as well as the impact of their beliefs and behavior on others. Their affect is often constricted, their talk vague and digressive, and their appearance unkempt. They tend to be suspicious and superstitious. People with this disorder are generally severely impaired, often meeting criteria for other personality disorders simultaneously (5). There are family links with schizophrenia (7,8), and there is evidence that this disorder should be viewed as belonging to the "schizophrenia spectrum" (7). Schizotypal patients may be guarded and suspicious in medical settings but may also present to health care practitioners with unusual symptoms (e.g., "feelings of electricity in my scalp") or idiosyncratic theories of causation ("Could my neighbors be doing this to me?").

Schizoid Personality

The essential features of the schizoid personality are *indifference to the company of others and constricted emotionality.* These people are loners who seldom marry, prefer solitary activities, and appear cold and aloof. Despite its name, this disorder does not appear to be closely linked to schizophrenia. Schizoid people tend to shun contact with health care practitioners and may appear very uncomfortable when hospitalization thrusts them into close and constant proximity to others.

Management of Eccentric Subtypes

The general guidelines described previously apply here as well. The most important specific principle of management is to work gradually toward the establishment of rapport by meticulous honesty, composure in the face of the patient's suspiciousness and reserve, and a consistent demonstration of sincere concern for the patient's well-being and respect for his or her privacy.

SPECIFIC REFERENCES*

1. McHugh PR, Slavney PR. The perspectives of psychiatry. 2nd ed. Baltimore: Johns Hopkins University Press, 1998.
2. Rutter M. Temperament, personality, and personality disorder. Br J Psychiatry 1987; 150:443.
3. Herbst JH, Zonderman AB, McCrae RR, et al. Do the dimensions of the Temperament and Character Inventory map a simple genetic architecture? Evidence from molecular genetics and factor analysis. Am J Psychiatry 2000;157:1285.
4. Rutter M, Quinton D. Parental psychiatric disorder: effects on children. Psychol Med 1984;14:853.
5. Zimmerman M, Coryell W. DSM-III personality disorder diagnoses in a nonpatient sample. Arch Gen Psychiatry 1989;46:682.
6. Hellerstein DJ, Kocsis JH, Chapman D, et al. Double-blind comparison of sertraline, imipramine, and placebo in treatment of dysthymia: effects on personality. Am J Psychiatry 2000;157:1436.
7. Cadenhead KS, Light GA, Geyer MA, et al. Sensory gating deficits assessed by the P50 event-related potential in subjects with schizotypal personality disorder. Am J Psychiatry 2000;157:55.
8. Kendler KS, Gruenberg AM, Strauss JS. An independent analysis of the Danish adoption study of schizophrenia. II. Arch Gen Psychiatry 1981;38:982.

*Bold numerals denote published controlled clinical trials, meta-analyses, or consensus-based recommendations.

For annotated ***General References*** *and resources related to this chapter, visit www.hopkinsbayview.org/PAMreferences.*

Chapter 24

Mood Disorders

Francis M. Mondimore

Clinically significant depressions often go undetected and undiagnosed in the ambulatory medical setting (1). As a consequence, patients with untreated depression may receive costly and misdirected diagnostic procedures and symptomatic therapies instead (2). Undiagnosed depressions exact a substantial toll on patients and families in the form of severe and persistent functional impairments (3). This chapter outlines the public health consequences of depressive conditions, describes the spectrum of mood disorders that afflict patients, and provides an approach to the treatment of these disorders for the generalist.

PUBLIC HEALTH IMPACT OF MOOD DISORDERS

By any measurement, depressive conditions are major public health problems. In one medical outcome study, the *poor functioning uniquely associated with depressive symptoms* was comparable to or worse than that associated with eight major chronic medical conditions: arthritis, current advanced coronary artery disease (CAD) (recent myocardial infarction [MI]), current angina, current back problems, current severe lung problems, current gastrointestinal (GI) disorders (ulcers or inflammatory bowel disorders), diabetes, and hypertension (4). Depressed subjects ranked fourth in impairment in physical functioning, third in impairment in role functioning, second (behind advanced coronary disease) in the number of bed days, and worst in social functioning and sense of well-being about their current health.

Excess deaths attributed to depression are primarily from suicides. Studies of populations of depressed patients show that over 2% eventually die by suicide (5). Suicide was the eleventh leading cause of death in the United States in 2003, and the third leading cause of death among 15- to 24-year-olds. Illicit substance abuse is thought to account for a dramatic rise in suicide rates between the mid-1950s and the mid-1990s among male adolescents. The suicide rate for white males age 15 to 24 years peaked in the mid-1990s and appears now to be dropping, a trend attributed to the passage of laws designed to keep firearms out of the hands of adolescents and also to the increased treatment of adolescent depression with selective serotonin reuptake inhibitors (SSRIs) (6). In the Old Order Amish population, where there is very little if any drug and alcohol abuse, more than 90% of all suicides between 1880 and 1980 were by people with major depression or bipolar disorder (7). Several studies have shown that the *incidence and outcome of other medical disorders are affected adversely by depression.* The incidence of MI is increased about fourfold in subjects with a prior episode of major depression (8). The odds of dying in the 18 months after a MI are three times greater in patients with concurrent depression than in those without depression (9).

In economic terms, the burden of depressive illnesses in the United States in 2000 was 83.1 billion dollars, of which 26.1 billion dollars (31%) were direct medical costs, 5.4 billion dollars (7%) were suicide-related mortality costs, and 51.5 billion dollars (62%) were workplace costs (10). This was despite a dramatic increase in the proportion of depression sufferers who received treatment. In comparison, the estimated burden of diabetes was estimated to be 57.6 billion dollars in 1996 (11).

PREVALENCE OF MOOD DISORDERS

Mood disorders are among the most prevalent forms of mental illness. Serious depression is especially common, with the past-year prevalence rate of clinically significant *major depressive disorder* estimated to be between 4% and 16.6% in epidemiologic studies, affecting more than 9 million Americans in 1999 (12). A national community survey of mental disorders, the Epidemiological Catchment Area Study, estimated that 6% to 12% of women and 2% to 5% of men experience at least one major depressive episode during their adult life, and such an episode may occur at any age (13). Perhaps just as many patients suffer from depressive symptoms that are clinically significant but do not reach a level of severity sufficient to be diagnosed as major depression, so-called *minor depression* (14). The 12-month prevalence of *dysthymic disorder*, characterized by chronic, smoldering depressive symptoms that last for years, has recently been estimated to be 2.5% (15).

Only 0.6% to 1.2% of adults develop bipolar disorder; which is equally common in men and in women (16). Over the past decade the concept of *bipolar spectrum disorders* has developed to describe illnesses, usually with predominantly depressive symptomatology, that also include briefer periods of elation or extreme irritability. The inclusion of these less severe disorders may increase the prevalence of bipolar disorders as much as fivefold, to about 5% of the general population (17).

As this discussion may suggest, the classification of mood disorders continues to be unsatisfactory. Many patients with mood disturbances do not fit neatly into the *Diagnostic and Statistical Manual of Mental Disorders, 4th Edition Text Revision (DSM-IV TR)* categories of major depression, dysthymia, or bipolar disorder, and are classified as *depressive disorder, not otherwise specified*, a subcategory of which is *minor depression*. Sometimes patients meet criteria for different *DSM-IV TR* disorders at different times.

BEREAVEMENT AND ADJUSTMENT DISORDERS

Some disturbances of mood are the normal and expected, perhaps even the inevitable sequelae of personal, medical, or financial setbacks. It is important and appropriate to evaluate and help patients in these situations not only because these symptoms affect the patient's sense of well-being but also because patients with nonpathologic mood disturbances are at risk for development of significant medical conditions. Bereavement, for example, is associated with increased rates of medical visits, heart attacks, and death in the first year after the loss of a spouse (18). Various medical conditions have been noted to have poor medical outcomes in patients with even mild depression (19).

Normal Bereavement

Although grief reactions are individual in their content, they share characteristic features as to course. The intensity of distress reflects the bereaved person's closeness to the deceased. The grief reaction tends to proceed in phases, beginning at the time at which the death is made known. The *first phase* is called the numbness or shock phase. Although painful, this first period of about 1 week is remarkable for the organized or calm way in which many bereaved people appear to go through the societal rituals of mourning, funeral, burial, and the visits with close family and friends. In retrospect, patients often describe themselves as confused and not fully appreciating their loss during this first week. A *second phase* has been called *confrontation* and emerges after completion of the structured rituals of mourning with increasingly intense feelings of sadness, loneliness, and pining for the lost loved one. During this periods of weeks to months, the bereaved becomes more fully aware of his loss and begins to face the changes the loss has brought about in his life. *Wellings* of grief, intense feelings of loss that come in waves, are initially as relentless as ocean surges but usually begin to come less frequently over a period of several weeks. The waves then progressively and substantially diminish in frequency and intensity over a period of 6 to 12 months, although they may recur from time to time for years, perhaps for a lifetime, especially when reminders of the loved one are encountered. Apathy, a diminished sense of organization, disinterest in doing a job that was previously engaging, and an inability to enjoy things are the characteristic signs of this period. The feelings of apathy and disengagement usually remit slowly and incrementally over many months as they are replaced by a sense of re-engagement in old and new activities. As the wellings of grief diminish in frequency, a *third phase,* that of *acceptance,* emerges as the bereaved person returns to his or her normal daily activities such as work, school, and social activities and is able to reclaim the emotional energy that was invested in the relationship with the deceased and re-invest it in other relationships and activities.

Patients may seek out or be brought to primary care clinicians during any of the three phases of bereavement. In the early stages, it is usually because of sleeplessness or agitation. Validating the reasons for distress, normalizing and explaining the grieving process, and instructing family members on how to help are useful responses. Prescribing hypnotic or anxiolytic medications may sometimes be necessary. Patients may come on their own during the later phases of grief because they are concerned about their physical health or about persistent problems in functioning at work or at home. These patients benefit from reassurance and from explanations of the phenomenology of the normal bereavement process, emphasizing that 12 months is usually necessary for the substantial completion of "grief work."

The bereavement process may be more lengthy, complex, and difficult if the loss has been very unexpected, and especially if the death has been violent or the result of a crime. Referral to a grief counselor is often appropriate in such cases. The death of a child is especially difficult. Local chapters of a national organization, *The Compassionate Friends*, provide grief counseling for families who have experienced the death of a child. Local hospices often have grief counselors on staff or can be a source of referrals.

It is important to remember that major depression is often precipitated by the loss of a loved one in susceptible patients. This becomes apparent in the later phases of bereavement when persistent mood symptoms can give way to the full-blown depressive syndrome. Chapter 13 contains additional information about the experience of the family members of dying and deceased patients.

Adjustment Disorder with Depressed Mood

Adjustment disorder with depressed mood is a normal or an exaggerated emotional reaction to a recent or imminent loss or stressful life event that is characterized by predominantly depressive symptomatology. Table 24.1 shows the criteria for the diagnosis of adjustment disorder from the *Diagnostic and Statistical Manual of Mental Disorders, 4th edition (DSM-IV)*, published by the American Psychiatric Association. The diagnosis of adjustment disorder is usually straightforward and depends on identifying the link between emotional or behavioral symptoms and the precipitating stressors.

TABLE 24.1 Diagnostic Criteria for Adjustment Disorder

A. The development of emotional or behavioral symptoms in response to an identifiable stressor occurring within 3 months after the onset of the stressor.
B. These symptoms or behaviors are clinically significant as evidenced by either of the following:
   1. Marked distress that is in excess of what would be expected from exposure to the stressor
   2. Significant impairment in social or occupational (academic) functioning
C. The stress-related disturbance does not meet the criteria for any specific axis I disorder and is not merely an exacerbation of a preexisting axis I or axis II disorder[a]
D. Does not represent bereavement.
E. The symptoms do not persist for more than 6 months after the termination of the stressor (or its consequences).

Acute: if the symptoms have persisted for less than 6 months
Chronic: if the symptoms have persisted for 6 months or longer

[a]See Chapter 19 for definition of axis I and axis II disorders.
Reprinted with permission from the Diagnostic and statistical manual of mental disorders. 4th Ed. Text Revision. American Psychiatric Association, 2000.

A critical and sometimes difficult diagnostic task is the assessment of individuals who present with what seem like unexpected, exaggerated, or prolonged emotional reactions to stressful events. Patients with any form of depression and those with personality disorders are more likely to overreact or to become functionally impaired in the face of a significant stressor. The identification of axis I disorders (e.g., major depression) or of personality disorders becomes a priority in these cases.

Major depressive disorders regularly manifest in the context of an apparent adjustment disorder. At the time of presentation the patient's distress is often focused on the stressor, and the doctor needs to help the patient adapt to the stressor, but this empathic task is distinct from the diagnostic task of identifying a major depression.

If the history does not suggest a coexisting axis I or II disorder, the appropriate intervention for an adjustment disorder is very similar to the approaches described earlier for bereaved patients and to those described in Chapter 20.

IDENTIFYING PATIENTS WITH DEPRESSIVE DISORDERS

Symptoms of Depression

Depressed patients who seek medical attention often do not complain of depressed mood as a primary symptom. Even if they acknowledge depressed feelings, they may do so in relation to other complaints that they see as primary.

Depressed patients usually present to generalists with three types of general complaints: (a) vegetative symptoms of depression (loss of energy, inability to concentrate, poor sleep, poor appetite, weight loss, decreased motivation or interests) and autonomic anxiety symptoms (tachycardia, chest discomfort, light-headedness); (b) aches and pains that may have anatomic bases but are out of proportion to what the patient usually experiences (e.g., worsening of migraine headaches, irritable bowel, or back pains) or what is expected (e.g., postsurgical pain that continues to require narcotic analgesics a month after surgery); and (c) nervous complaints such as increased tension and feelings of anxiety, often expressed in relation to stressful life circumstances such as marital distress or job difficulty. The presence of a mood disturbance should not, however be taken to explain or invalidate physical complaints: coexistence of psychiatric and medical disorders is the rule rather than the exception.

Even when specifically asked about mood, almost half of depressed patients deny depression or sadness as their predominant mood. They may describe their predominant mood as apathetic (e.g., "blah"), anxious, or even "numb" (i.e., unable to experience normal emotions including sadness, love, and grief). If appropriate inquiries are made however, it is likely that typical symptoms of depression can be elicited. Changes in mood (e.g., sadness, anger, irritability), mental sluggishness, decreased physical energy, pessimistic feelings about the future, and negative self-attitude are features central to depressive disorders. Despite the difficulty describing these pathologic states, patients should be asked specifically about them as well as about their sleep, appetite, and libido.

The term *atypical depression* appears in the *DSM-IV* and refers to depressive states in which hypersomnia, overeating, and lethargy are seen rather than insomnia, anorexia, and psychomotor agitation. Patients with atypical depression seem particularly prone to panic and anxiety symptoms and although they have the characteristic depressive changes in self-attitude and vital sense, they often describe their mood as fatigued rather than as sad. The term *atypical* may not be strictly justified, because all three of the "atypical" symptoms are common among depressed patients. However, the concept of atypical depression serves to remind clinicians of the importance of surveying *both* sides of eating and sleeping behaviors. When asked, "How is your appetite?" a depressed patient may respond, "Good," or "Too good," or "No problem." It easy to misinterpret these answers as negative screening responses rather than as clues to the overeating that can be associated with depression.

Family members, if available, should be asked to corroborate and augment the information obtained from the patient. With the patient's agreement, the physician also should share with the family the diagnostic assessment, the plans for treatment, and the prognosis as the depressed patient is often hard pressed to remember what was said by the doctor during the appointment.

Routine Depression Screening in Primary Care

Studies in primary care settings over many years have shown that depressive disorders are under-diagnosed in primary care settings, with between 30% and 50% of depressed patients going unrecognized during usual care by primary care physicians (20). Since 2002, the U.S. Preventive Services Task Force (USPSTF), which conducts rigorous, impartial assessments of the scientific evidence for the effectiveness of a broad range of clinical preventive services, has recommended screening adults for depression as a part of routine clinical practice in primary care settings (21).

A whole variety of screening methods have been suggested, including formal screening instruments such as the Beck Depression Inventory and the PRIME-MD (Primary Care Evaluation of Mental Disorders) (19). All appear to be effective and correlate well with each other (22); clinicians may choose any method that fits their patient population and clinical setting.

A positive response to either of two questions: (a) "Have you had a down, low, or depressed mood in the past month?" or (b) "Have you been bothered by a loss of interest and pleasure in your usual activities?," has been reported to have a 96% sensitivity in the diagnosis of major depression (23).

Positive screening should trigger a more complete diagnostic interview to elicit symptoms of depression as above.

MAJOR DEPRESSIVE DISORDER

Diagnosis

The most common form of clinical depression is major depressive disorder (Table 24.2). The *differential diagnosis* of symptoms that suggest major depression varies depending on the patient's age, the presenting manifestations, and other associated factors. In *younger patients*, the differential is between adjustment disorder and major depression in those with recent onset of symptoms, and between adjustment disorder and dysthymia in those with more chronic presentation. In adolescents, irritability, oppositional behaviors, or substance abuse can predominate, although low mood, anhedonia, and vegetative symptoms can usually be easily elicited upon careful questioning. In *elderly patients* with memory complaints, the differential diagnosis is more complex because memory complaints without substantial memory performance problems are common in the depressed elderly and also because a modest but reversible dementia can result from the depression alone (so-called pseudodementia; see Chapter 26). Additionally, depression and dementia syndromes can both be related to underlying neuropathologic disorders, particularly Parkinson disease and stroke (see Chapters 90 and 91).

Stressful life events are common precipitating factors for major depression, so their presence is not useful for either making or excluding the diagnosis. In patients with panic attacks or obsessive-compulsive symptoms, it is important to remember that both panic disorder and obsessive-compulsive disorder (see Chapter 22) can occur in the context of a major depressive syndrome.

Alcohol abuse and the abuse of other substances commonly cause mood syndromes that may be indistinguishable from those of the major affective disorders. Substance abuse is a comorbidity common in patients with major affective disorders as well. Therefore, screening for substance abuse should be a routine part of the assessment of the depressed patient.

TABLE 24.2 American Psychiatric Association Diagnostic Criteria for Major Depressive Episode[a]

A. At least five of the following symptoms have been present during the same 2-week period and represent a change from previous functioning; at least one of the symptoms is either (1) depressed mood or (2) loss of interest or pleasure.
   1. Depressed mood most of the day, nearly every day, as indicated by either subjective report (e.g., feels sad or empty) or observation made by others (e.g., appears tearful)
   2. Marked diminished interest or pleasure in all, or almost all, activities most of the day, nearly every day (as indicated either by subjective account or observation made by others)
   3. Significant weight loss or weight gain when not dieting (e.g., more than 5% of body weight in a month), or decrease or increase in appetite nearly every day
   4. Insomnia or hypersomnia nearly every day
   5. Psychomotor agitation or retardation nearly every day (observable by others, not merely subjective feelings of restlessness or being slowed down)
   6. Fatigue or loss of energy nearly every day
   7. Feelings of worthlessness or excessive or inappropriate guilt (which may be delusional) nearly every day (not merely self-reproach or guilt about being sick)
   8. Diminished ability to think or concentrate, or indecisiveness, nearly every day (either by subjective account or as observed by others)
   9. Recurrent thoughts of death (not just fear of dying), recurrent suicidal ideation without a specific plan, or a suicide attempt or a specific plan for committing suicide

B. The symptoms cause clinically significant distress or impairment in social, occupational, or other important areas of functioning.

C. Not due to the direct effects of a substance (e.g., drugs of abuse, medication) or a general medical condition (e.g., hypothyroidism).

D. Not occurring within 2 months of the loss of a loved one (except if associated with marked functional impairment, morbid preoccupation with worthlessness, suicidal ideation, psychotic symptoms, or psychomotor retardation).

[a] Criteria for children have been omitted from this table.
Reprinted with permission from the Diagnostic and statistical manual of mental disorders. 4th Ed. Text Revision. American Psychiatric Association, 2000.

A variety of *prescribed medications* have been reported to cause mood syndromes (Table 24.3). Unfortunately, the lengthy lists of pharmaceutical agents reported to be depressogenic that appear in most textbooks are often based on case reports or uncontrolled case series and are of questionable utility for the physician who is trying to decide whether to discontinue an effective medication in a patient who becomes depressed while taking it. A survey of more than 2000 community subjects found that most commonly prescribed medications are not associated with depressive syndromes. In this study, β-blockers, angiotensin-converting enzyme (ACE) inhibitors, lipid-lowering agents, and digoxin—all drugs often reported to cause depression—showed no association with the depressive syndrome (24). An association between β-blockers and depression, touted as a clinical pearl since this class of drugs first became available, remains unproven and controversial despite many years of investigation (25). A more impressive association between depression and treatment with digitalis has been demonstrated, and digitalis intoxication can present as a depressive syndrome (26). Steroid medications have clearly been shown to precipitate both the major depressive syndrome and manic syndrome in some patients (27). Drug-induced depression caused by interferon during treatment for hepatitis C or malignancy, by acute estrogen deficiency during the treatment of breast cancer with tamoxifen, and by naltrexone in the treatment of alcoholism has also been well established. Medication-induced mood syndromes often respond to reduction in dose of the causative agent or to treatment with antidepressant or mood-stabilizing medication (28). The differentiation of affective disorders from drug-induced syndromes and the management of mood symptoms in the medically ill patient who is taking multiple needed medications can be complex and challenging. Close coordination with a psychiatric consultant and thoughtful risk–benefit analysis of various medication approaches is the best course for the generalist in these situations.

TABLE 24.3 Drugs and Substances That May Cause or Precipitate Mood Syndromes

Agents associated with depressed states
- Alcohol
- Benzodiazepines
- Corticosteroids
- Digitalis
- "Ecstasy" and other "club drug" withdrawal
- Interferon
- Naltrexone
- Oral contraceptives
- Stimulant and cocaine withdrawal
- Tamoxifen

Agents associated with hypomanic and manic states
- Amphetamines, cocaine, "ecstasy" and "club drugs"
- Anabolic-androgenic steroids
- Antidepressants (all classes)
- Corticosteroids
- Levodopa
- Thyroid hormones

Modified from: Patten SB, Love EJ. Drug-induced depression. Psychother Psychosom, 1997;66:63, and Peet P, Peters S. Drug-induced mania. Drug Saf 1995;12:1466.

Finally, it is important to differentiate unipolar from bipolar depressive states, because antidepressants can precipitate manic or mixed manic mood swings in patients with bipolar disorder.

The specific criteria of the American Psychiatric Association for major depressive episode (Table 24.2) require the presence of at least five of nine depressive symptoms and related functional impairment for 2 weeks, not caused by the direct effect of a medication or a drug of abuse or of a general medical condition. *Either depressed mood or loss of interest or pleasure in usual activities (anhedonia) are always present;* these symptoms can be considered core symptoms of major depression and should always be sought. A patient with a history of episodic depressive disorder and the fully developed symptom cluster is not difficult to diagnose. However, patients with major depression who present with a dominant somatic complaint or with a clear "reason" to be depressed, guilty, or hopeless may easily be missed if they are not specifically asked about depressive symptoms. When major depression is strongly suspected, probing inquiry about symptoms from both the patient and those close to the patient usually clarifies the diagnosis.

A *fully developed major depression* is characterized by a sustained alteration in mood, self-attitude, and vital sense. The sustained lowering of mood is impervious to environmental influence once the depression becomes severe. Events that are not usually stressful are perceived as overwhelming by a depressed patient as the syndrome develops. The *change in self-attitude* is usually manifested in expressions of guilt, inferiority, uselessness, and hopelessness. The *changes in vital sense* (the subjective assessment of one's physical and mental functioning) result in complaints of confusion or poor memory, inability to concentrate, lack of energy, and easy fatigability. Sometimes patients complain only of a vague sense of ill health. This preoccupation with physical symptoms can occasionally reach delusional intensity, and seriously depressed patients can become convinced that they are dying of cancer or another fatal illness when there is no evidence of these diseases.

Marked psychomotor retardation (i.e., slowed speech and movements), *delusions* with depressive content, and *diurnal mood variation* (worst mood in the morning) occur in a minority of patients but are diagnostically useful when present because they are fairly specific to this disorder.

Treatment

Once the diagnosis of major depression is made, treatment consists of explaining the diagnosis to the patient (and family), prescription and monitoring of antidepressant medication, and supportive counseling for the patient and family.

For the patient with major depression who is in good physical condition and who is neither overwhelmed with depressive delusions nor suicidal, antidepressant medication is the appropriate initial treatment. Any antidepressant drug is effective in approximately 70% of patients with major depression, and no antidepressant approved for use has been shown to be more effective than the others. Depressed patients tolerate side effects (and what they perceive to be side effects) poorly and often stop taking antidepressants without completing a full 8-week trial of the medication. Therefore, the selection of the first antidepressant has more to do with convenience of administration and side effect profile than with the probability of a therapeutic response. The exception to this rule is the patient who has had a prior good (or poor) response to a particular antidepressant.

Depressed patients with delusions, hallucinations, or profound psychomotor retardation tend to be less responsive to drugs. Referral for psychiatric consultation and consideration of electroconvulsive therapy (ECT) are appropriate for such patients. Among patients with suicidal intent (see Suicide Prevention), antidepressants, especially tricyclics, should be dispensed in small amounts to avoid providing enough drug for a lethal overdose.

Characteristics of Available Antidepressants

Table 24.4 lists characteristics of available antidepressant drugs. There are six selective serotonin reuptake inhibitors (SSRIs) available in the United States: citalopram, (Celexa) and its S-enantiomer, escitalopram (Lexapro), fluoxetine (Prozac and Sarafem), fluvoxamine (Luvox), paroxetine (Paxil), and sertraline (Zoloft). They are similar in efficacy and side effect profiles. Fluvoxamine, citalopram, and paroxetine are more sedating than fluoxetine and sertraline. Because of its extremely long half-life (up to 4 days), fluoxetine has been formulated for once-a-week dosing during the maintenance phase of treatment (Prozac Weekly). Although preliminary studies support the efficacy of once-weekly compared with daily dosing of fluoxetine (29), whether it actually improves patient compliance is not known.

Bupropion (Wellbutrin) is an antidepressant of the aminoketone class, unrelated to the tricyclic and SSRI antidepressants that inhibits serotonin, norepinephrine, and dopamine reuptake. At the higher dosages (up to 700 mg) originally approved by the U.S. Food and Drug Administration (FDA), bupropion was associated with a higher rate of seizures; a finding that led to the recommended 450-mg limit on total daily dosage. Several controlled release preparations (Wellbutrin SR, Wellbutrin XL) have become available that now allow for twice daily or even once daily dosing. Bupropion has also been found to be useful in smoking cessation and is marketed under the brand Zyban for this indication.

Venlafaxine (Effexor) and *duloxetine* (Cymbalta) are phenylethylamine antidepressants that have been dubbed selective serotonin and norepinephrine reuptake inhibitors. Both venlafaxine and, to a lesser extent, duloxetine cause diastolic hypertension in a small fraction of patients, particularly at higher dosages, therefore, blood

TABLE 24.4 Characteristics of Antidepressant Drugs

Drug	Strengths of Available Oral Preparations (mg)	Low or Starting Dosage Range	Usual Dosage Range	Common Side Effects	Special Considerations
Selective Serotonin reuptake inhibitors (SSRIs)					
Citalopram[a] (Celexa)	20, 40	20 mg q.d.	20–60 mg q.d.	Insomnia, gastrointestinal discomfort, restlessness, diarrhea, headache, sweating, anxiety, sexual dysfunction	Note: All SSRIs can raise levels of other drugs, including anticonvulsants, tricyclics, theophylline, digoxin, Coumadin, some antiarrhythmics, β-blockers, calcium channel blockers
Escitalopram (Lexapro)	5, 10, 20	10 mg q.d.	10–20 mg q.d.	Same as citalopram (perhaps less severe)	
Fluoxetine[a] (Prozac, Sarafem)	10, 20,40	10–20 mg q.d.	20–40 mg q.d.	Same as citalopram but more activating	Very long half life, available in once-a-week preparation
Sertraline (Zoloft)	25, 50, 100	25–50 mg q.d.	100–200 mg q.d.	Same as citalopram but perhaps more gastrointestinal symptoms	—
Paroxetine[a] (Paxil)	10, 20, 30, 40	10–20 mg q.d.	20–40 mg q.d.	Same as citalopram, sometimes sedation	May be taken at bedtime
Fluvoxamine[a] (Luvox)	50, 100	25–50 mg q.d.	150–200 mg q.d.	Similar to sertraline but more sedating	—
Selective serotonin norepinephrine reuptake inhibitors (SSNRIs)					
Venlafaxine				Nausea, insomnia, sedation, sweating, gastrointestinal discomfort	Can increase blood pressure
(Effexor)	37.5, 75	37.5–75 mg b.i.d.	100–150 mg b.i.d.		
(Effexor XR)	37.5, 75, 150	37.5–75 mg q.d.	100–225 mg q.d.		
Duloxetine (Cymbalta)	20, 30, 60	20 mgs b.i.d.	40–60 mg b.i.d.	Same as venlafaxine	
Tricyclics					
Secondary amines					
Nortriptyline[a] (Pamelor, Aventyl, others)	10, 25, 50, 75, 100	25 mg q.h.s.	50–150 mg q.h.s.	Dry mouth, sedation, orthostasis, constipation, weight gain, sexual dysfunction	Titrate to am, trough serum level 90–150 ng per dL
Desipramine[a] (Norpramin, others)	10, 25, 50	25–50 mg q.h.s.	150–250 mg q.h.s.	Same as other tricyclics	Titrate to level >150 ng per dL upper limit unclear—?250 ng per dL
Tertiary amines					
Amitriptyline[a] (Elavil, others)	10, 25, 50, 75, 100	25–50 mg q.h.s.	150–250 mg q.h.s.	Same as other tricyclics, but more severe	Titrate to combined amitriptyline plus nortriptyline level >150 ng per dL
Doxepin[a] (Sinequan, Adapin, others)	10, 25, 50, 100	25–50 mg h.s.	150–250 mg q.h.s.	Same as amitriptyline	Titrate to level >125–250 ng per dL

(continued)

TABLE 24.4 (Continued) Characteristics of Antidepressant Drugs

Drug	Strengths of Available Oral Preparations (mg)	Low or Starting Dosage Range	Usual Dosage Range	Common Side Effects	Special Considerations
Imipramine[a] (Tofranil, others)	10, 25, 50, 100	25–50 mg h.s.	150–250 mg q.h.s.	Same as amitriptyline	Titrate to level >180 ng per dL
Atypical/others					
Nefazodone[a] (Serzone)	100, 150	37.5–75 mg b.i.d.	100–200 mg b.i.d.	Nausea, dry mouth, headache, sedation, occasional orthostasis, priapism	"Black box" warning of risk of hepatic failure issued in 2002
Trazodone[a] (Desyrel, others)	50, 150, 300	25–100 mg q.h.s.	300–500 mg q.h.s.	Same as nefazodone but more sedation	Useful in low dose (25–100 mg h.s.) as relatively safe hypnotic without dependence or cognitive impairment
Bupropion[a]				Insomnia, gastrointestinal upset, more reduction of seizure threshold than others; less sexual dysfunction than other antidepressants	Incompatible with ritonavir; new sustained-release preparations for b.i.d. and once daily dosing
(Wellbutrin)	75, 100	75 mg q.d. or b.i.d.	100–150 mg b.i.d. or t.i.d.		
(Wellbutrin SR)	100, 150	150 mg q.d.	100–200 mg b.i.d.		
(Wellbutrin XL)	150, 300	150 mg q.d.	300–450 mg q.d.		Once daily preparation
Mirtazapine[a] (Remeron)	15, 30, 45	7.5–15 mg q.h.s.	15–45 mg q.h.s.	Sedation, weight gain, dizziness, rarely granulocytopenia	—

[a]Generic preparation available.

pressure monitoring for 2 weeks after starting the drug and after any dosage elevation is recommended. Duloxetine has also been approved for the treatment of diabetic neuropathy.

Trazodone (Desyrel) and *nefazodone* (Serzone) are closely related agents that have been called atypical antidepressants. Trazodone is usually too sedating at the doses required to treat depression for it to be recommended as such. However, in smaller small doses (50 to 100 mg), it is a reasonably effective alternative to benzodiazepine hypnotics for depressed patients. Cases of life-threatening hepatic failure reported in patients taking nefazodone led the manufacturer of Serzone to discontinue its manufacture, although it is still available as a generic preparation. Both trazodone and nefazodone have been associated with priapism that has required surgical intervention (30). Male patients should be instructed to discontinue these drugs immediately if they experience prolonged or painful erections and seek emergency treatment as necessary.

Mirtazapine (Remeron) is associated with significant sedation but has a sufficiently long half-life to allow bedtime dosing. It is available as an instantly dissolving wafer that can be taken without water (Remeron SolTab), a useful option for patients unable to swallow. An uncommon but serious side effect is granulocytopenia.

Tricyclic antidepressants (TCAs), the oldest class, include two subgroups: secondary and tertiary amines. The side effect burden of these agents is significant and they are usually reserved for use in patients who have failed to respond to newer drugs. *Nortriptyline* has fewer side effects than the other TCAs and has the most clearly established therapeutically effective serum concentration range. *Imipramine, desipramine, amitriptyline,* and *doxepin* blood levels are also available. Starting dosages of TCAs should be reduced by approximately 50% in *older patients* (especially those with medical illnesses). Giving the total daily dosage at bedtime is desirable for most patients to minimize side effects.

The *monoamine oxidase inhibitors* (MAOIs) were the main alternatives to tricyclics before 1990, but are uncommonly used today except by psychiatrists specializing in the treatment of mood disorders because of their substantial side effects and the need for patients to follow a low-tyramine diet while taking them. Nevertheless, some patients are uniquely responsive to these agents. Patients who are taking MAOIs have usually failed all other treatments for depression. For this reason, primary care physicians should become comfortable treating patients for medical problems who are also taking MAOIs for depression, and avoid advising patients to discontinue MAOIs without psychiatric consultation.

Complementary and Alternative Treatments

A number of nutritional supplements and herbs have been claimed by enthusiasts to be safe and effective for depression (see Chapter 5). Patients may ask about alternative treatment because trials with standard antidepressants have failed or because of the misconception that herbal and nutritional preparations must be safer than the FDA-approved medications for which numerous possible adverse reactions are listed. *St. John's wort* gained considerable attention in the late 1990s after several studies seemed to indicate its effectiveness in depressed patients. One meta-analysis of 22 controlled clinical trials found St. John's wort to be as effective as standard antidepressants for the treatment of depression but a Cochrane collaboration report concluded that evidence for superior efficacy was weak in patients who meet diagnostic criteria for major depression or who suffer from "prolonged" depression (31). Several randomized, placebo-controlled studies have found no difference between St. John's wort extract and placebo in the treatment of patients with *DSM-IV* major depression (32,33).

Selection and Dosage Adjustment of Antidepressants

Because of their favorable side effect profile and ease of use, the SSRIs have become the drugs of first choice for most depressed patients. Because almost every patient is more prone to or more intolerant of some side effects than others, selection of an antidepressant for a particular patient depends on the fit between the patient's medical history and the antidepressant's side effect profile. The SSRIs have a significant advantage over the TCAs because of their relative safety in overdose. Both fluoxetine and the tricyclic nortriptyline have been shown to be safe for use during the first trimester of pregnancy. Although both were associated with a small increase in spontaneous abortions, neither was associated with any increase in fetal abnormalities (34).

In the otherwise healthy depressed patient, it is reasonable to initiate antidepressant treatment with 20 mg/day of *fluoxetine* or *paroxetine*. These two SSRIs are administered once a day and require no titration of the daily dosage as studies show that most responders do as well on the usual starting dosage of 20 mg/day as on higher dosages (35). For patients who are very sensitive to medication side effects, initiating treatment at 10 mg/day and advancing to 20 mg/day after 1 week is a reasonable option.

The benefits of pharmaceutical interventions for depression may take several weeks to become apparent and it is important to warn patients that they may notice little or no improvement during the first weeks of treatment. Patients should take a new medication at the starting dosage for 2 to 4 weeks before a dose increase is considered. Dosage increases likewise should occur at intervals of not less than 2 to 4 weeks. Symptoms should not be considered refractory to a particular agent unless the patient has taken it at the top of the recommended dosage range or, if serum determinations are available, at the top of the therapeutic range, for 4 to 8 weeks. Patients may continue to improve for months after starting on a new medication.

Recovery from depression can be slow and characterized by starts and stops in the recuperation process. Even as they are trending toward steady improvement, patients will frequently have good days and bad along the way. Frequent assessment (weekly during the initial stages of treatment, and at least every 2 weeks as long as there are significant symptoms) is necessary to ensure accurate assessment of recovery over time. Cross-sectional assessments at longer intervals may mislead as to the extent of progress. Family members should be encouraged to attend followup appointments in order to report their impressions. Patients can also be encouraged to keep a journal or mood chart and bring the results to appointments.

Antidepressant Side Effects

Mild side effects often occur before the therapeutic effects of antidepressant drugs begin and depressed may patients tolerate even mild side effects poorly and need frequent reassurance that the treatment is safe and likely to be effective (in 3 to 8 weeks). Emphasizing that side effects are not unusual, that they are benign and usually temporary is very helpful in getting patients through this period.

The common side effects of all SSRIs are transient mild nausea, transient insomnia, and transient nervousness and muscular irritability. All SSRIs have good antianxiety properties when taken for 2 weeks or longer at a steady dosage.

The *SSRIs and selective serotonin and norepinephrine reuptake inhibitors can cause sexual dysfunction* in up to one third of patients, usually decreased interest in sex (decreased libido), delayed orgasm or anorgasmia, and, less commonly, diminished sensation in the genital areas. Erectile function usually is not affected by these agents, but impotence can be caused by TCAs. Strategies for managing SSRI-related sexual dysfunction fall into several categories (36). Monitoring and waiting is appropriate for patients with delayed orgasm, because many patients notice improvement in this side effect after several months.

Decreased libido and anorgasmia do not often resolve spontaneously, and other measures are usually necessary to relieve these problems. The section on antidepressant side effects in Chapter 6 provides details about the approaches that can be tried in these patients.

The most common side effects of the *TCAs* are anticholinergic: dry mouth, constipation, and, less often, delayed micturition, blurred vision, and an anticholinergic delirium. Orthostatic hypotension is particularly problematic in elderly patients and in any patient with unsteady gait or balance problems. TCAs may also produce increased appetite with weight gain, granulocytopenia (rarely), hypomania or mania, slowed cardiac conduction, and cardiac arrhythmias.

Because of the *cardiac side effects,* TCAs should be given cautiously to patients with pre-existing conduction abnormalities or any unstable cardiac conditions (e.g., recent MI). Nortriptyline has been studied in cardiac patients and can be safely administered to those with pre-existing stable heart disease (37). SSRIs, venlafaxine, and bupropion have few cardiac effects and therefore offer greater safety for the cardiac patient.

Bupropion is contraindicated in patients with a seizure disorder. The FDA recommends that the dosage not exceed 150 mg/dose or 450 mg/day (400 mg/day of Wellbutrin SR) to minimize the risk of seizures.

Drug Kinetics and Interactions

Among the TCAs and SSRIs, fluoxetine has an unusually long half-life (7 days for its active metabolite, norfluoxetine). This property can be advantageous because this antidepressant is less often associated with a withdrawal syndrome when discontinued, compared with other SSRIs and the selective serotonin and norepinephrine reuptake inhibitors. However, the long half-life increases the time required to achieve washout before changing to another antidepressant.

All SSRIs inhibit one or more of the cytochrome P-450 enzymes, but the clinical impact of this property, first reported in 1991, has proven to be modest. In patients taking paroxetine, fluoxetine, citalopram, or sertraline, blood levels of coadministered benzodiazepines, antipsychotics, TCAs, and flecainide-type antiarrhythmic agents may increase (Table 24.5).

TABLE 24.5 Drugs That May Interact with Antidepressants

Antidepressant Drug Class	*Interaction*
Tricyclics (TCAs)	
Anticholinergic antispasmodics	Enhanced anticholinergic side effects
Anticholinergic antiparkinsonian drugs	Enhanced anticholinergic side effects
Antihypertensive drugs	Enhanced orthostatic hypotension
Selective serotonin reuptake inhibitors (SSRIs)	
TCAs, anxiolytics, hypnotics, neuroleptics	SSRIs block metabolism so blood levels rise; TCA plasma levels may rise twofold or more
Monoamine oxidase inhibitors	Potentially fatal serotonin syndrome

Switching Antidepressants

Almost one third of depressed patients fail to respond to an adequate trial of an antidepressant medication. Switching antidepressants is one reasonable approach to the patient with treatment-resistant depression. Naturalistic studies indicate that switching antidepressants results in a treatment response approximately 50% of the time. Most authorities recommend switching to an antidepressant with a mechanism of action different from that of the failed agent, such as switching from an SSRI to a selective serotonin and norepinephrine reuptake inhibitor, bupropion or mirtazapine, agents that have actions on both serotonin and norepinephrine transport. Open label studies indicate, however, that switching from one SSRI to another can also be effective (38). A medication wash-out period is clearly indicated only with a switch from a MAOI to another antidepressant. Immediate substitution is usually well tolerated when switching within the same medication class (e.g., one SSRI or TCA to another) and has the advantage of avoiding discontinuation symptoms. Immediate substitution of mirtazapine for a SSRI has also been shown to be well tolerated. Gradual introduction of the new agent while gradually tapering the failed one is another well-tolerated strategy (39). The time to treatment response after switching to another agent cannot be estimated with any reliability. Numerous studies indicate that some patients require up to 12 weeks or even longer to have a response to changes in treatment approaches (40).

Treatment-Resistant Depression

The management of treatment-resistant depression is challenging and requires not only experience in managing complex mood disorders, but also a substantial investment of time and considerable patience on the part of both the patient and the clinician. Biweekly or weekly monitoring visits are fairly standard practice in psychiatric settings for such patients during the many weeks, sometime many months, required for adequate new trials of antidepressant agents and for treatment augmentation strategies such as the addition of lithium, anticonvulsant mood stabilizers, atypical antipsychotics, thyroid hormones and dopaminergic and glutamatergic agents. Clinicians should consider psychiatric referral of the patient who has not benefited from even an initial antidepressant trial if these time-intensive interventions are not possible in their own practice and for patients who have failed several adequate trials of antidepressants.

Duration of Drug Treatment

In a patient with persistent and significant depressive symptoms, an adequate therapeutic trial usually requires 2 months at a therapeutically effective dosage. After recovery from a first or from an infrequently recurrent depressive syndrome, the medication that induced the remission should be continued for at least 12 months, the time of highest risk for relapse (41). Most patients with a history of episodes and relapses should be advised to continue their antidepressant for a number of years. The terms "indefinite" and "for the rest of your life" may convey a sense of pessimism to patients. The commitment to long-term treatment should rather be an incremental decision, made after comparing 1 and then 2 years of treatment experience with the period before treatment. The use of a lower dosage of the patient's antidepressant for "maintenance" treatment is not recommended. Patients who took half of the acute antidepressant dosage had no better outcome than the placebo group in one controlled study (42). After electroconvulsive therapy (ECT) (see later section), maintenance treatment with antidepressants is essential for most patients to reduce the risk of relapse.

Drug Discontinuation

Patients who discontinue antidepressant medications can experience a variety of uncomfortable physical symptoms, especially if they stop a medication abruptly. Symptoms including dizziness, light-headedness, headache, insomnia, fatigue, nausea, sensory disturbances, and flu-like malaise have been reported after discontinuation of TCAs, SSRIs, and selective serotonin and norepinephrine reuptake inhibitors (43). Discontinuation symptoms are more common with agents that have a shorter half-life (e.g., paroxetine) and less likely with agents that have a longer half-life (e.g., fluoxetine) (44). The overall incidence of antidepressant withdrawal symptoms is difficult to estimate because of the wide variation among antidepressants and probable variations in patient sensitivity, but discontinuation symptoms have been reported in up to one third of patients within the context of controlled trials of drug efficacy (43). Symptoms can occur within hours or days and may persist for up to several weeks.

When medications must be discontinued, tapering the dosage usually, but not always, prevents discontinuation symptoms from developing. Antidepressants should be tapered over a period of at least 10 days and over a longer period if the drug has been taken at higher dosages. A reasonable approach is to taper by 25% of the patient's dose every 3 to 4 days until the patient has been taking half of the usual *starting* dose for 3 to 4 days, and then discontinuing altogether. Patients taking low doses of antidepressants can be tapered more rapidly. Other than reassurance, treatment of discontinuation symptoms is rarely necessary. However, if necessary, they can usually be aborted by restarting or increasing the dose of the medication being discontinued, followed by a more gradual taper.

Counseling and Psychotherapy

Counseling Visits

For the first 6 to 8 weeks, the patient with major depression should be seen at least every other week for adjustment of medication and for brief supportive psychotherapy as described in Chapter 20. For patients with major depression, the first priority in supportive counseling is consistent repetition of the answers to the three questions most troublesome to depressed patients: "What is wrong with me?"; "Is this treatment going to work?" (this question may be presented as a concern: "I think this pill is making me worse; I want to stop it."); and "What is going to happen to me (if this doesn't work for me)?" Answers to these questions should be prefaced by a reassuring statement, like, "You have clinical depression. We don't understand how it is caused, but it is not your fault. It is a medical disease. You will get better. We are going to continue to care for you and fight the depression with you until you are better." Supportive counseling is important for members of the patient's family as well.

A second focus of counseling is more directive. It is remarkable how many patients resign jobs and separate from spouses based on distorted depressive perceptions about not being able to do their usual work, or not being able to feel love for a spouse. It is important therefore that the physician counsel patients not to attempt any *major life decisions* while they are depressed. Job-related and personal relationship changes should likewise be deferred until the patient's ability to maintain a more objective and positive perspective recovers.

Frank discussion of *suicidal feelings,* plans, and intentions should be a routine part of each visit (see Suicide Prevention). Candid discussion of the level of risk and protective measures available is equally important and may require the participation of a family member or loved one.

The patient should be routinely assessed for the *side effects* that are most typical of the antidepressant being used. The more depressed the patient, the less tolerant he or she will be of minor adverse drug effects and the more likely to give up on the treatment before it has been given an adequate trial. The support of the doctor in encouraging persistence with drug therapy is crucial.

Office Psychotherapy

Traditional or "insight-oriented" psychotherapy has been a two-edged sword for depressed patients. On one hand, it engages depressed patients in an empathic consideration of their feelings and concerns. On the other hand, the theories behind the practice propose that depression results from maladaptive responses to life experiences and can therefore be alleviated through the insights and personal growth that psychotherapy facilitates. Psychodynamic therapy may thus convey the message that, when depressive symptoms persist, the patient rather than the treatment has failed—a distinctly inaccurate and even harmful implication for patients with major depression.

Several specialized types of psychotherapy have been found to be effective in treating depressive disorders. Cognitive therapy (also called cognitive behavior therapy or CBT) challenges the ingrained self-deprecating thoughts and attitudes (called *schemas*) that are common in depressed persons that are thought to lead to self-defeating behaviors that intensify and sustain depressive symptoms. Table 24.6 lists some of the more common *cognitive distortions* that depressed patients experience and express. Even someone who is not trained in cognitive therapy can help patients by gently challenging negative thoughts such as those listed. A supportively offered challenge can help patients access what they already know and what they have experienced, both of which usually argue against the most negative and distorted conclusions of the depressed state. *Interpersonal therapy* (IPT) emphasizes the social contexts and consequences of the patient's depression. It includes skills such as identifying and addressing stressors, pointing out assets, and providing alternative choices. Chapter 20 describes these and other skills useful in interpersonal therapy. A meta-analysis of six trials comparing treatment with CBT or IPT to antidepressant medication and placebo in 883 outpatients found these psychotherapies to be as effective as medication in treating mild to moderate nonpsychotic major depression (45).

A combination of psychotherapy and medication has been shown to be more effective than either intervention alone for some patients. Thase et al. found in a meta-analysis of six clinical trials that CBT or IPT were as effective as medication in milder depression, but that there was a highly significant advantage of combining psychotherapy with medication in patients with more severe, recurrent depressions (46). When 707 patients being treated for dysthymic disorder were randomized to treatment with sertraline, with IPT, or with combination treatment, patients in either medication group had superior and equivalent symptomatic remission compared to patients receiving IPT, but patients on combination therapy had significantly lower health care and social services costs over the 2 years of treatment (47).

Psychotherapy is not indicated during the most acute depressive states however, as it requires that the patient be able to concentrate, recall, and maintain a level of objectivity and hopefulness that is not possible for the severely depressed patient.

TABLE 24.6 Cognitive Distortions in Depression

All-or-nothing thinking: Thinking occurs in black-and-white terms with no recognition of a middle ground. Things are wonderful or awful. One's actions reflect either perfection or total failure.
Overgeneralization: Words such as "always" and "never" may portray a single negative event as a never-ending pattern of defeat.
Selective abstraction: A single negative detail is focused on and ruminated about until it colors everything.
Disqualifying the positive: Positive experiences are often discounted as not relevant, not real, or not deserved.
Arbitrary inferences: It is assumed that things are or will be negative, regardless of the facts.
Magnification or minimization: One's own failures and others' successes are magnified; one's own successes and others' failures are minimized.
Emotional reasoning: Bad feelings are taken as the litmus test of reality.
"Should" statements: Repetitive "I should/should not" or "I must/must not" statements often contribute to depression, resentment, guilt, and hopelessness.
Labeling and mislabeling: Mistakes or shortcomings become sweeping self-condemnations.
Personalization: Depressed people often assume they are the cause of some unfortunate or unpleasant event for which, in actuality, they are not responsible.

Adapted from Burns DD. Feeling good: the new mood therapy. New York: New American Library, 1980.

Referral for Psychiatric Treatment

General physicians should be able to treat many of the patients in whom they diagnose major depression. However, some depressed patients should be referred to a psychiatrist: those in whom the diagnosis is not clear enough to allow confident treatment; those who show no improvement after 8 weeks of treatment with therapeutic dosages of antidepressant medications (about one in three patients); those who cannot or will not take antidepressant medications; those who are overtly suicidal; and those with delusions, hallucinations, or depressive stupor (i.e., mute and unresponsive). Hospitalization, more aggressive drug therapy, or ECT are often appropriate for these patients.

Although many patients initially resist the idea of seeing a psychiatrist, a primary care physician with whom a patient has good rapport can be most persuasive in helping the patient understand the need for and reasons necessitating psychiatric consultation or referral. Because patients may interpret psychiatric referral as an indication that their situation is hopeless, or that they are being shunned by their physician (as many depressed patients fear), it is important to explain the reasons for referral, specifically, that additional treatments, with which the psychiatrist has more experience, are available.

Electroconvulsive Therapy

ECT is an effective and rapid treatment for major depressive disorder. The decision to use ECT should be made in consultation with a psychiatrist, with the informed consent of the patient and, when available, with the informed consent of the patient's family. This treatment was previously given only to hospitalized patients, but outpatient ECT is increasingly available and suitable for medically and behaviorally stable patients. The indications for ECT involve emergency situations mandating a rapid response (such as the malnourished, dehydrated, or suicidal patient); the presence of medical illness that makes drug therapy excessively risky; the presence of delusions or overwhelming severity of the depression; and failure of drug therapy. The likelihood of marked benefit from ECT is higher than with antidepressants: It is approximately 80% in patients with major depression. The benefit is short-term however, lasting anywhere from several weeks to 6 months. Therefore, ECT is an excellent first choice for patients with clearly episodic depressions that are severe but infrequent. The benefit usually requires 6 to 12 treatments given two to three times per week. The procedure involves anesthetization administered with a muscle-relaxing agent.

Aside from the small risk of brief anesthesia, the *adverse effects* that follow ECT primarily involve memory. Retention of new and occasionally old memories is mildly defective for weeks to months after a series of ECT treatments. These memory gaps are usually spotty and involve primarily declarative memories (events, things that were heard or read) as opposed to procedural memories (how to perform a task). Typically, the patient in whom this effect becomes clinically apparent (perhaps 40% of treated patients) has trouble recalling names of recent acquaintances or forgets events that occurred during or just before beginning ECT. Clinically apparent memory defects typically resolve within 2 months. Formal testing has revealed mild defects lasting up to 3 months, but none at 6 months after treatment.

Prognosis

The clinical course of depressive illness varies greatly in individuals. A significant number of patients completely recover from a single major depressive episode and suffer no further recurrences (48). Some patients have recurrent illness, but enjoy sustained periods of virtually complete symptom remission between their illness episodes. But approximately 25% of patients with major depression have a chronic course of illness with long periods of residual symptoms and only incomplete remission over many years (49). These patients have been shown to have worse long-term outcomes than patients without chronic symptoms, having a greater number of relapses into periods of incapacitating depression, and worse occupational and social functioning over the long term (50). A naturalistic, prospective study of 431 patients with unipolar major depressive disorder found that they met diagnostic criteria for major depression or for dysthymic disorder or had subthreshold depressive symptoms during 59% of the weeks of the 12-year study. Twenty-seven percent of these patients had no weeks during which they were completely free of symptoms (49). The term *double depression* has been coined to describe patients with major depressive episodes superimposed on the chronic symptoms of dysthymic disorder.

DYSTHYMIC DISORDER

Dysthymia is a chronic depressive state (lasting 2 years or longer) in which the number of depressive symptoms experienced is fewer than what is required for the diagnosis of major depressive disorder (Table 24.7 versus Table 24.2). Although many dysthymic patients are fairly functional in their occupational life, this chronic illness is often associated with marked impairment in *social* functioning, especially in close personal relationships. Long-term avoidant behavioral patterns and lonely solitary lifestyles are not unusual in dysthymic patients. Superimposed substance abuse problems are not uncommon and can mask the underlying low grade, but debilitating depressive symptoms. Dysthymia not infrequently begins in childhood and, because the low mood is so persistent, patients, their family and friends, and also their physician often judge the problem to be an innate part of a chronically unhappy person's disposition (i.e., a personality disorder) rather than a mood disorder. For this reason, many dysthymic patients do not present for treatment of depression because they do not identify their mood problems as symptoms of illness. In reality, the disposition of dysthymic patients derives to a large degree from their chronic depression. Heightened public awareness of depression brought about by public service campaigns, advertisements for antidepressant medications in the lay media, and celebrity accounts on television may be leading more patients with chronic depression to seek treatment. Pharmacotherapy can be dramatically beneficial for these patients.

Diagnosis

In addition to self-recognition of depressive symptoms, complicating problems associated with depressed mood such as suicide attempts, self-injurious behavior, excessive medical care-seeking behavior, or abnormal illness behavior may prompt dysthymic patients to seek treatment.

TABLE 24.7 American Psychiatric Association Diagnostic Criteria for Dysthymic Disorder[a]

A. Depressed mood for most of the day, for more days than not, as indicated either by subjective account or observation made by others, for at least 2 years.
B. Presence, while depressed, of at least three of the following:
 1. Low self-esteem or self-confidence, or feelings of inadequacy
 2. Feelings of pessimism, despair, or hopelessness
 3. Generalized loss of interest or pleasure
 4. Social withdrawal
 5. Chronic fatigue or tiredness
 6. Feelings of guilt, brooding about the past
 7. Subjective feelings of irritability or excessive anger
 8. Decreased activity, effectiveness, or productivity
 9. Difficulty in thinking reflected by poor concentration, poor memory, or indecisiveness
C. During the 2-year period of the disturbance, the person has never been without the symptoms in criteria A and B for more than 2 months at a time.
D. No major depressive episode during the first 2 years of the disturbance, that is, not better accounted for by chronic major depressive disorder, or major depressive disorder in partial remission.
E. Has never had a manic episode, or an unequivocal hypomanic episode.
F. Does not occur exclusively during the course of a chronic psychotic disorder, such as schizophrenia or delusional disorder.
G. Not due to the direct effects of a substance (e.g., drugs of abuse, medication) or a general medical condition (e.g., hypothyroidism).

[a]Criteria for children have been omitted from this table.
Reprinted with permission from the Diagnostic and statistical manual of mental disorders. 4th Ed. Text Revision. American Psychiatric Association, 2000.

Serious diagnosable medical disorders, alcohol and drug abuse, and worries about family and marital discord or job difficulties may also bring the dysthymic to the attention of primary care physicians.

Patients with dysthymic disorder have the characteristic sustained changes in self-attitude and vital sense seen with major depression. Hypersomnia, increased appetite and weight gain, and loss of energy and libido are common, as are anxiety symptoms.

Table 24.7 shows the criteria of the American Psychiatric Association for making the diagnosis of dysthymic disorder.

Treatment

Studies have revealed strong similarities in treatment response between patients with dysthymia and those with major depression. Also, dysthymic patients have a high likelihood of developing a superimposed major depression (so-called *double depression*). Thus the treatment of dysthymia has increasingly resembled the treatment of major depressive episodes.

SSRIs and TCAs have been shown to be effective in reducing dysthymic symptoms (51). In addition, brief psychotherapies are also known to be helpful (see Chapter 20). The major differences in treatment for the two types of depression relate to the increased rate of comorbid behavioral and social problems associated with this more chronic form of depression (dysthymia), problems usually requiring intensive psychotherapeutic interventions.

Recognizing that depression plays an important part in their life problems can be helpful for dysthymic patients. However, appreciating the difference between accepting medical regimens to treat mood disorders and making the effort required to overcome maladaptive behavior patterns is equally important.

Prognosis

In contrast to the major affective syndromes, discussions of prognosis in dysthymic disorder is problematic. The disorder typically continues beyond a 2-year period, and the time to remission cannot be estimated with much confidence. Superimposed major depressive episodes in dysthymic patients tend to respond well to antidepressants but subsyndromal symptoms are not uncommon. Poor outcomes are most common among patients with severe social maladjustments and personality disorders (see Chapter 23).

BIPOLAR DISORDERS

Diagnosis

The manic syndrome, like major depression, is defined by a sustained change in mood, self-attitude, and vital sense. The manic patient's mood may be euphoric or irritable, or may alternate between or even seem to be a combination of the two. The *self-attitude* is usually one of overconfidence; in more severe cases, it is reflected in an inflated sense of power, position, and importance. *Heightened vital sense* is manifested in the patient's sense of quickened and totally accurate thinking. The patient has an overconfident ease in decision-making and a sense of heightened perception of sounds, colors, and tastes. The patient sees only continued well-being in his or her future. The patient manifests dramatically increased energy and a decreased need for sleep. In the speeded-up and overconfident state, the patient is observed by his or her family to be very distractible in speech (jumping from topic to topic) and behavior (jumping from one new project to another, completing none). Finally, judgment ranges from poor to catastrophic as patients spend impulsively, including giving away money and

TABLE 24.8 American Psychiatric Association Diagnostic Criteria for a Manic Episode

A. A distinct period of abnormally and persistently elevated, expansive, or irritable mood, lasting at least 1 week (or any duration if hospitalization is necessary).
B. During the period of mood disturbance, at least three of the following symptoms have persisted (four if the mood is only irritable) and have been present to a significant degree:
   1. Inflated self-esteem or grandiosity
   2. Decreased need for sleep (e.g., feels rested after only 3 hours of sleep)
   3. More talkative than usual or pressured to keep talking
   4. Flight of ideas or subjective experience that thoughts are racing
   5. Distractibility (i.e., attention too easily drawn to unimportant or irrelevant external stimuli)
   6. Increase in goal-directed activity (either social, at work or school, or sexually) or psychomotor agitation
   7. Excessive involvement in pleasurable activities that have a high potential for painful consequences (e.g., the person engages in unrestrained buying sprees, sexual indiscretions, or foolish business investments)
C. The mood disturbance is sufficiently severe to cause marked impairment in occupational functioning or in usual social activities or relationships with others, or to necessitate hospitalization to prevent harm to self or others.
D. Not due to the direct effects of a substance (e.g., drugs of abuse, medication) or a general medical condition (e.g., hyperthyroidism).

Reprinted with permission from the Diagnostic and statistical manual of mental disorders. 4th Ed. Text Revision. American Psychiatric Association, 2000.

personal belongings on the street, and are uncharacteristically disinhibited and provocative in word and deed.

Delusions and hallucinations, when present, are usually either persecutory or grandiose. Occasionally symptoms characteristic of schizophrenia occur (see Chapter 25), but follow the course of the other manic symptoms, remitting as the mood and behavior normalize. The diagnosis of *schizoaffective disorder–manic type* is reserved for patients in whom the psychotic symptoms persist well beyond the manic syndrome so that the patient is psychotic in the absence of the manic symptoms throughout most of the course of the illness. Whether these patients have an unusually severe form of bipolar disorder or a condition more related to schizophrenia is currently unknown. Table 24.8 shows the specific criteria of the American Psychiatric Association for mania.

Initial Treatment

General Principles

The disruptive and disinhibited symptoms of mania are more difficult to manage in medical terms, and the manic patient's behavior can be quite agitated and out of control. Therefore, manic patients are almost always best referred to psychiatrists, and many will require inpatient psychiatric treatment.

The referral may be difficult, because acceptance by a manic patient of the need for help is the exception rather than the rule. The patient's personal physician can be a crucial—at times the only—clinician involved with the manic patient in the initial presentation, and by virtue of an already established relationship with the patient or the family, this physician may be able to persuade the patient to take some medication and to accept a referral to a psychiatrist, emergency room, or hospital inpatient unit. Basic knowledge about the use of antipsychotic drugs and mood-stabilizing medications is therefore important for primary care physicians.

Hypomania, a milder form of the manic syndrome, can sometimes by treated on an outpatient basis but usually indicates the presence of a complex mood disorder that will require specialized care. Close symptom monitoring, discontinuation of any antidepressant medication that the patient may be taking, and prompt psychiatric evaluation usually are indicated. Hypomania can escalate rapidly and dangerously into full-blown mania, and initiation of antipsychotic medication is often appropriate.

Winning the cooperation of the acutely manic patient can be very difficult. The euphoric or irritable manic patient often will not accept the notion that his or her behavior is disturbed, much less that it requires hospitalization. Explaining the need for medical treatment in a manner that does not inflame the patient and provoke even more disordered behavior is a valuable skill. If possible, consultation with the family about the diagnosis and plan of treatment should be arranged before, not after, confronting the patient with the diagnosis and treatment plan. Despite the uncontrollable behavior of the manic patient, family members may be afraid to support the doctor's resolve to have the patient treated out of fear of being seen by the patient as betraying his or her trust. The clinician's task is to calm the patient and the family, to persuade the manic patient to accept hospitalization voluntarily if needed, and to resort to civil commitment if necessary.

Although *laws on commitment* vary among states, all states currently have legal provisions to allow the involuntary hospitalization of patients with mental disorders who are clearly dangerous to themselves or others and for whom no less restrictive alternative is appropriate. Physicians should make themselves familiar with commitment laws in the community where they practice and know the steps necessary to initiate commitment procedures *before* they are faced with this psychiatric emergency. These procedures often require the teamwork of the clinician, the family, the staff of an emergency room, and sometimes law enforcement officials to be successful.

Medication for Severe Mania

Severe acute mania requires initial treatment with antipsychotic medications and later with mood stabilizers, such as lithium, anticonvulsant mood stabilizers, and/or atypical antipsychotics. For the first week or two, this treatment is usually carried out in the hospital. The generalist's role with such patients many include initial diagnosis, treatment with sufficient medication to get the manic patient to the hospital, and then continued participation in followup care.

For acute manic agitation, the use of parenteral fluphenazine (Prolixin) or another high-potency neuroleptic is usually effective. Modest doses (5 to 10 mg intramuscularly) calm most patients with little or no depression of blood pressure and little sedation. Parenteral preparations of the newer atypical antipsychotic medications are becoming available (olanzapine and ziprasidone as of this writing) and have been shown to be effective in the treatment of acute agitated states including mania (52). Older, more sedating phenothiazines such as chlorpromazine (Thorazine) are more difficult to work with because repeated doses are often necessary to break the agitated manic state and these preparations often produce significant orthostatic hypotension. Within 15 to 20 minutes, intramuscular high-potency neuroleptics usually bring about a calming effect that may last for several hours. This period can be used to get the patient admitted to hospital. Even in this short period, however, patients may develop *extrapyramidal side effects* from the high-potency neuroleptics, most often acute dystonic reactions. This condition is alleviated by 50 mg of intramuscular diphenhydramine (Benadryl) or 1 to 2 mg of trihexyphenidate (Cogentin).

Maintenance Therapy for Bipolar Disorder

Although the management of patients with bipolar disorder on a long-term basis is best thought of as requiring specialty care, primary care physicians will encounter patients on maintenance medications for bipolar disorder in their routine practice and should be knowledgeable about the agents used. Additionally, patients in remission from bipolar symptoms may request that their primary care physician manage their maintenance medications, either on an ongoing basis or during transitions in psychiatric care as might be necessitated by relocation to a new community. This necessarily brief overview summarizes the use of several of the most commonly used agents for maintenance treatment.

Patients recovering from an episode of mania will usually be taking a lithium preparation, an anticonvulsant mood stabilizer and/or an atypical antipsychotic medication. Patients recovering from an episode of depression may be taking an antidepressant in addition to lithium and/or an anticonvulsant. Since many patients can be protected against recurrences of their illness with lithium or an anticonvulsant alone, adjunctive medications are often gradually tapered and discontinued. Substantial numbers of patients with bipolar disorder will, however, need to take a combination of medications to remain well.

Lithium

Lithium continues to be the standard criterion for the maintenance treatment of bipolar disorder despite a fairly substantial side-effect burden and the need for ongoing monitoring of serum lithium levels and other laboratory tests.

Regular serum lithium levels are necessary during lithium maintenance not only because of a narrow therapeutic index but also because of an extensive literature indicating that the prophylactic efficacy of lithium requires that it be taken at a dose sufficient to achieve a threshold level. The American Psychiatric Association's guidelines note that 0.6 to 0.8 meq/L is the range "commonly chosen by patients and their psychiatrists" for lithium monotherapy (53). Serum lithium levels, which should be measured 12 hours after a dose (trough levels), should be obtained whenever there has been a change in dosage and at least every 6 months in stable patients. Elderly and medically frail patients should be tested more often.

Most of lithium's side effects correlate with peak serum levels and can often be ameliorated by changing the dosage schedule or using sustained-release preparations. Gastrointestinal symptoms are not uncommon; polydipsia and polyuria as well as edema that occur early on often resolve with time and can be managed with low doses of loop diuretics (patients who develop polyuria only after months or years should be evaluated for nephrogenic diabetes insipidus, discussed in this section). Diuretics, especially thiazide diuretics, alter lithium excretion, and serum lithium levels must be closely monitored in these patients to avoid toxicity. Nonsteroidal anti-inflammatory drugs (NSAIDs) also alter lithium excretion and should be avoided by patients taking lithium. Table 24.9 lists drugs that interact with lithium.

Side effects associated with long-term lithium treatment include weight gain, cognitive dulling, and fine hand tremor (all dose-related). Dermatologic problems associated with lithium use include acne and hair loss. Lithium can exacerbate pre-existing psoriasis so severely as to preclude lithium therapy in some individuals, although some patients with psoriasis will respond to the agents usually effective for this problem (54). Lithium has been associated with a variety of benign electrocardiogram (EKG) changes but significant cardiac conduction changes or arrhythmias are very uncommon.

TABLE 24.9 Important Drug Interactions with Lithium

Drugs that may enhance lithium toxicity
ACE inhibitors[b]
Amiloride[a]
Ethacrynic acid[a]
Furosemide[a]
Nonsteroidal anti-inflammatory drugs[a]
Spectinamycin[a]
Spironolactone[a]
Tetracycline[a]
Thiazide diuretics[a]
Triamterene[a]
Drugs that may increase lithium excretion
Acetazolamide[c]
Theophylline[c]
Drugs that may aggravate lithium tremor
Caffeine[b]
Neuroleptics[b]
Theophylline[b]
Tricyclic antidepressants[b]
Valproate[b]

[a]Decreased renal excretion.
[b]Mechanism not established.
[c]Increased renal excretion.

As the long-term effects of lithium on the kidney have become clearer, earlier concerns about it as a nephrotoxic substance have eased significantly. Although the risk of reduced glomerular function appears very low, a very small group of patients appear to develop glomerular and tubulointerstitial nephropathy that can progress to renal insufficiency and be irreversible if not detected early enough. In a review of such cases, the reversibility of renal insufficiency after discontinuation of lithium appeared correlated with serum creatinine levels under 2.5 mg/dL, further emphasizing the need for monitoring of renal function in patients taking lithium (55). Creatinine clearance (CrCl) determinations are no longer recommended for routine monitoring and obtaining serum creatinine determinations every 3 to 12 months depending on factors such as age and general medical conditions is reasonable. Patients with serum creatinine levels consistently above 1.6 mg/mL (or when the level has increased by 25% or more) should be referred for specialty evaluation.

The more common lithium associated renal problem is a nephrogenic diabetes insipidus caused by loss of renal concentrating ability. A mild but significant decrease in urine concentrating ability has been demonstrated in most (though not all) longitudinal studies of lithium's effect on the kidney. Patients should be asked about polyuria and a 24-hour urine volume measurement obtained if polyuria is suspected.

Lithium decreases thyroid hormone release and may interfere with other steps in the synthesis of thyroid hormones. Patients may respond to these thyroid suppressing effects with a rise in thyroid-stimulating hormone (TSH) that is usually temporary, but some progress to clinical or subclinical hypothyroidism. Kleiner et al. recommends that both antithyroperoxidase autoantibodies and antithyroid globulin determinations be done on patient at the beginning of lithium therapy to identify patients at greater risk for developing hypothyroidism. They recommend that TSH, the most sensitive and therefore only needed test, be measured every 3 months during the first year of therapy and semi-annually to annually thereafter to detect lithium-induced thyroid dysfunction (56).

Although lithium remains a Class D drug for teratogenic risk, there is some evidence that the risk is much lower than initially thought and that healthy outcomes in patients who become pregnant while taking lithium can be expected (57). However, lithium levels change dramatically during pregnancy and the postpartum period is one of extremely high risk for the development of mania. The management of the pregnant and postpartum patient with bipolar disorder is a complex challenge best left to a psychiatrist skilled in the management of mood disorders.

Lamotrigine

Lamotrigine (Lamictal) is a phenyltriazine anticonvulsant that has been found to be effective for the maintenance treatment of bipolar disorder in a number of open and controlled trials, and its use for this purpose will only continue to grow. It has a very low side-effect burden compared to lithium and does not require any ongoing laboratory monitoring.

Headache and dizziness are the most common side effect complaints. At higher doses, some patients complain of cognitive dulling similar to that seen with lithium and other anticonvulsants.

Early trials with lamotrigine for the treatment of epilepsy were marked with relatively high rates of erythema multiforme, including Stevens-Johnson syndrome and toxic epidermal necrolysis (TEN). It was noted however, that pediatric age range, rapid upward titration of dose, and the combined use with valproate were associated with the highest risk of serious rash. Since the introduction of new dosing guidelines, the incidence of serious rash has dropped to levels similar to that of other anticonvulsant agents.

A few case reports of agranulocytosis have been reported but a causal relationship has not been established.

Valproate

Valproate is another anticonvulsant medication of proven efficacy in the treatment of acute mania (58). Although its efficacy for maintenance treatment is more controversial, it is often used for that purpose, especially in combination with other agents (59).

Serum valproate levels are routinely used to monitor its use in epilepsy but there is substantially less data on the serum levels that are effective in bipolar disorder and essentially no data on effective levels for maintenance treatment. Studies suggest that levels above 45 μg/mL are necessary for antimanic efficacy and side effects become increasingly problematic at levels above 125 μg/mL.

Dose-related side effects of valproate include nausea, vomiting, and other gastrointestinal complaints such as abdominal pain and heartburn. A fine tremor is frequently seen at higher levels. Other reversible adverse effects include weight gain, increased appetite, and hair loss.

Transient minor elevations in hepatic transaminases are common when starting treatment with valproate and usually subside over time and the risk of severe hepatotoxicity in adults appears to be very low. Careful monitoring of liver functions is recommended when starting the drug as the hepatotoxicity is often reversible if the drug is withdrawn. Rare cases of hemorrhagic pancreatitis have been reported that seem related to initiation of the drug or dosage increase in susceptible individuals. Delay of diagnosis has been implicated as a contributing factor to these rare cases, and patients should be warned about the symptoms and potential severity of pancreatitis. Thrombocytopenia is a rare idiosyncratic response to valproate.

There have been reports linking valproate with gynecologic problems including menstrual irregularities, polycystic ovary syndrome, and androgenization in women taking it for the treatment of epilepsy. Other studies have not replicated this work and the topic is intensely controversial (60). Regular monitoring of reproductive function in female patients taking valproate is recommended with questioning during visits regarding menstrual disorders, fertility, weight gain, hirsutism, and galactorrhea.

Epidemiologic studies of valproate suggest an increased incidence of spina bifida in the offspring of women who took the drug during pregnancy. Additionally, an increased incidence of cardiovascular, orofacial, and digital abnormalities has been reported. Women in the childbearing years should practice birth control while taking valproate.

Atypical Antipsychotic Medications

Antipsychotic medications have been used mainly as adjunctive agents in the acute phases of bipolar disorder, especially manic states, for many years but a role for the atypical antipsychotics in maintenance treatment is developing. Although their use as monotherapy agents for prophylaxis is still being evaluated in controlled trials, impressive results have been obtained in studies of olanzapine (Zyprexa), especially for the prevention of mania, leading to FDA approval of olanzapine as maintenance treatment for bipolar disorder (61).

Sedation is the main dose-related side effect of these agents, which usually cause little in the way of extrapyramidal symptoms making adjunctive treatment with anticholinergic agents rarely necessary.

Soon after the introduction of this class of drugs in the mid-1970s, excessive weight gain was reported in some patients taking atypical antipsychotics, especially clozapine and olanzapine. Although weight gain in the short term is usually small, several studies have shown that it can continue for many months after starting on antipsychotic medications making the potential for significant weight gain in patients on long-term treatment substantial (62). The weight gain from these drugs more often results in central or abdominal obesity, a pattern thought to impose more health risks than generalized obesity. Such health risks include type 2 diabetes mellitus, coronary artery disease secondary to hyperlipidemia, osteoarthritis, and other conditions. Body weight, blood glucose, and serum lipid levels should be monitored at the beginning of treatment and regularly thereafter in patients taking antipsychotics for maintenance treatment. Nutritional counseling for patients taking these agents is important, emphasizing portion size, low-fat foods, and regular exercise.

Prognosis

The course of the bipolar disorders is so widely variable as to defy simple description or easy categorization. Some patients enjoy many years of symptom remission with maintenance treatment, and others endure almost unrelenting mood cycling and substantial psychosocial morbidity (63).

Cyclothymic Disorder

An episodic bipolar affective disorder that is sufficiently mild or so brief that the episodes fail to meet the American Psychiatric Association criteria for major depression or mania is categorized as a *cyclothymic disorder.* Patients with cyclothymic disorder must be distinguished from patients with the personality traits of emotional lability and self-dramatization who often report rapid but unsustained mood changes. The family histories of cyclothymic patients are similar to those of patients with bipolar affective disorders. The long-term course is also similar to that of bipolar disorder, and 35% of such patients have been found to experience full-blown manic, hypomanic, or depressive episodes in a 2- to 3-year period of followup (64).

COUNSELING THE FAMILY

Family members of patients with serious affective disorders often experience feelings of confusion, hopelessness, guilt, and recrimination toward the patient. Not only are these feelings painful, but they impede the family's attempts to support their ill relative. Physicians need to address the family's needs directly through meetings with them. Above all, the family must recognize major affective disorders as diseases and realize that these disorders are not caused by the family, the patient, or even the social predicaments affecting the patient. The family also should know that although the pathophysiology of affective disorders is unknown, empiric treatments are effective and the prognosis for complete recovery from an episode is generally good, although relapses occur frequently. These points usually require some repetition and are best repeated in response to questions that the family should be encouraged to raise in such a meeting or consultation. It is equally important to reassure families and patients with dysthymic and transiently demoralized mood states that the patients are not suffering from a major mental illness.

Educational materials on affective disorders are available from the American Psychiatric Association and the National Institutes of Mental Health (NIMH), and a number of accessible and well-written books about the disorders for patients and their families are available (see www.hopkinsbayview.org/PAMreferences). Additionally, patients and families will gain considerable help from patient and family-member support groups (see Sources of Information at www.hopkinsbayview.org/PAMreferences).

HEREDITY OF DEPRESSION

Evidence from many studies of concordance comparing identical and nonidentical twins has established a substantial genetic contribution to major affective disorders, although the relevant genes have not yet been isolated. The modest findings to date support the supposition that genetic heterogeneity underlies these disorders and that the disease genotype comprises an ensemble of genes that act in concert to predispose people to these illnesses. It appears that a sibling or offspring of a patient with a major affective disorder has a 10% chance of developing the disorder. However, in some families this risk may be as high as 50%. The risk is also greater for monozygotic twins. Counseling of patients and their families about the genetic risk should be tailored to the needs and relevant history in each family. The major themes of counseling should be that most cases are genetically influenced, that effective treatment is available, and that treatment is greatly enhanced by early detection of the disorder.

SUICIDE PREVENTION

The rate of suicide in most countries is so low (11 per 100,000 in the United States) that successful prediction of an individual suicide at a given point in time is very unlikely.

Practical strategies in this area are to protect those with high risk in the short term and to reduce the risk in these patients over a longer term. *Risk factors for successful suicide* include depressive disorder (greater severity is associated with greater risk), older age, male gender, alcoholism, living alone, previous suicide attempt, and refusal to accept referral for psychiatric treatment. Retrospective studies of patient groups with major affective disorders in the era before affective drugs were available suggest that approximately 15% of the deaths were caused by suicide. Additionally, clinical observations suggest that the risk of suicide increases when improvement begins (or just after a depressed patient is discharged from the hospital) or when the depressive ruminations become frankly delusional convictions. Retrospective studies also suggest that there are fewer suicides among patients treated with ECT or long-term lithium therapy (65).

When evaluating any patient with depressed mood, direct and open inquiry should be made regarding suicidal ideas (e.g., "Have you at times felt so low that you feel life is not worth living," followed by "Have you had any thoughts of hurting yourself or taking your own life?"), and the patient should be asked about specific plans that he or she may have formulated ("Have you thought about how you might try to harm yourself?"). An assessment of the lethality of the patient's plans and the availability of the means to carry them out should be made. Seriously depressed patients should always be asked about the presence of firearms in the home, and any weapons should be removed, even in the face of a patient's disavowal of plans to use them. A study of adolescent suicide showed that the presence of a firearm in the home increased the risk of completed suicide regardless of whether the weapon was a handgun or a long gun, kept loaded or unloaded, locked up or not (66). Information about the capability and availability of constant family supervision is also helpful in determining whether treatment may be attempted safely on an outpatient basis. Asking patients to *"contract for safety"*—that is, to promise verbally or even in writing to contact a family member or the physician, to call police or to go to an emergency room, if their suicidal impulses should intensify or become difficult to resist—has frequently been recommended in the management of suicidal patients. Obtaining a *"no-harm contract"* helps the physician engage the patient in a discussion of his or her suicidal thinking, emphasizes the physician's concern for the safety of the patient, communicates the physician's assessment of the gravity of the situation, and also requires the development and discussion of an action plan should suicidal thinking worsen. This "contract" does not, however, substitute for a complete assessment of the patient's risk for suicidal behavior, and it is only as effective as the soundness of the underlying therapeutic alliance (67). The suicide risk evaluation should also be guided by the knowledge that delusionally depressed patients have a significantly increased risk of suicide and that patients with prior suicide attempts are more likely than others to attempt it again when depressed.

Short-term protection of patients with suicidal intent by means of hospitalization, including involuntary commitment, is sometimes required. The most crucial activities of physicians in preventing suicides, however, are the diagnosis, treatment, and prophylaxis of major depressive episodes.

Most patients who present to emergency facilities after an *overdose of pills* do not have major depression but rather an adjustment disorder or personality disorder, and they usually do not die by suicide. However, they should be methodically evaluated in the same manner as noted previously because many such patients are prone to take overdoses again when stressed. These patients may benefit from brief hospital admissions when social support for them is lacking and suicidal feelings are intense. All should have outpatient counseling.

SPECIFIC REFERENCES*

1. Wells KB, Hays RD, Burnam MA, et al. Detection of depressive disorder for patients receiving prepaid or fee-for-service care. Results from the Medical Outcomes Study. JAMA 1989;262:3298.
2. Simon GE, VonKorff M, Barlow W. Health care costs of primary care patients with recognized depression. Arch Gen Psychiatry 1995;52:850.
3. Mintz J, Mintz LI, Arruda MJ, et al. Treatments of depression and the functional capacity to work. Arch Gen Psychiatry 1992;49:761.
4. Wells KB, Stewart A, Hays RD, et al. The functioning and well-being of depressed patients. Results from the Medical Outcomes Study. JAMA 1989;262:914.
5. Bostwick JM, Pankratz VS. Affective disorders and suicide risk: a reexamination. Am J Psychiatry 2000;157:1925.
6. Bridge JA, Barbe RP, Brent DA. Datapoints: recent trends in suicide among U.S. adolescent males, 1992–2001. Psychiatr Serv 2005;56:522.
7. Egeland JA Sussex JN. Suicide and family loading for affective disorders. JAMA 1985;254:915.
8. Pratt LA, Ford DE, Crum RM, et al. Depression, dsychotropic dedication, and risk of myocardial infarction: prospective data from the Baltimore ECA Follow-up. Circulation 1996;94:3123.
9. Frasure-Smith N, Lesperance F, Talajic M. Depression and 18-month prognosis after myocardial infarction. Circulation 1995;91:999.
10. Greenberg PE, Kessler RC, Birnbaum HG, et al. The economic burden of depression in the United States: how did it change between 1990 and 2000? J Clin Psychiatry 2003;64:1465.
11. Druss BG, Marcus SC, Olfson M, et al. Comparing the national economic burden of five chronic conditions. Health Aff 2001;20:233.
12. Narrow WE, Rae DS, Robins LN, et al. Revised prevalence estimates of mental disorders in the United States: using a clinical significance criterion to reconcile 2 surveys' estimates. Arch Gen Psychiatry 2002;59:115.
13. Weissman MM, Bruce ML, Leaf PJ, et al. Affective Disorders. In: Robins LN, Regier DA (eds). Psychiatric Disorders in North America, The Epidemiologic Catchment Area Study. New York: Free Press, 1991.
14. **14.** Hermens MLM, van Hout HPJ,Terluin B, et al. The prognosis of minor depression in the general population: a systematic review. Gen Hosp Psychiatry 2004;26:453.
15. Kessler RC, Berglund P, Demler O, et al. Lifetime prevalence and age-of-onset distributions of DSM-IV disorders in the National Comorbidity Survey Replication. Arch Gen Psychiatry 2005;62:593.
16. Robins LN, Helzer JE, Weissman MM, et al. Lifetime prevalence of specific psychiatric disorders in three sites. Arch Gen Psychiatry 1984;41:949.
17. Akiskal HS, Bourgeois ML, Angst J, et al. Re-evaluating the prevalence of and diagnostic composition within the broad clinical spectrum of bipolar disorders. J Affect Disord 2000; 59:S5.
18. Schaefer C, Quesenberry CP, Jr., Wi S. Mortality following conjugal bereavement and the effects of a shared environment. Am J Epidemiol 1995;141:1142.
19. Spitzer RL, Kroenke K, Linzer M, et al. Health-related quality of life in primary care patients with mental disorders. Results from the PRIME-MD 1000 Study. JAMA 1995;274:1511.
20. Simon GE, VonKorff M. Recognition, management, and outcomes of depression in primary care. Arch Fam Med 1995;4:99.
21. **21.** U.S. Preventive Task Force. Screening for depression: recommendations and rationale. Ann Intern Med 2002;136:760.
22. Rogers WH, Adler DA, Bungay KM, et al. Depression screening instruments made good severity measures in a cross-sectional analysis. J Clin Epidemiol 2005;58:370.
23. Whooley MA, Avins AL, Miranda J, et al. Case-finding instruments for depression. Two questions are as good as many. J Gen Intern Med 1997;12:439.
24. Patten SB, Lavorato DH. Medication use and major depressive syndrome in a community population. Compr Psychiatry 2001;42:124.
25. Ried LD, McFarland BH, Johnson RE, et al. Beta-blockers and depression: the more the murkier? Ann Pharmacother 1998;32:699.
26. Seiner SJ, Mallya G. Treating depression in patients with cardiovascular disease. Harv Rev Psychiatry 1999;7:85.
27. Brown ES, Suppes T. Mood symptoms during corticosteroid therapy: a review. Harv Rev Psychiatry 1998;5:239.
28. Gleason OC, Yates WR. Five cases of interferon-alpha-induced depression treated with antidepressant therapy. Psychosomatics 1999;40:510.
29. Schmidt ME, Fava M, Robinson JM, et al. The efficacy and safety of a new enteric-coated formulation of fluoxetine given once weekly during the continuation treatment of major depressive disorder. J Clin Psychiatry 2000;61:851.
30. Pecknold JC, Langer SF. Priapism: trazodone versus nefazodone. J Clin Psychiatry 1996; 57:547.
31. **31.** Linde K, Mulrow CD, Berner M, et al. St John's Wort for depression. Cochrane Database Syst Rev 2005;2:CD000448.
32. **32.** Linde K, Ramirez G, Mulrow CD, et al. St John's wort for depression—an overview and meta-analysis of randomised clinical trials. BMJ 1996;313:253.
33. **33.** Shelton RC, Keller MB, Gelenberg A, et al. Effectiveness of St John's wort in major depression: a randomized controlled trial. JAMA 2001;285:1978.
34. Pastuszak A, Schick-Boschetto B, Zuber C, et al. Pregnancy outcome following first-trimester exposure to fluoxetine (Prozac). JAMA 1993;269:2246.
35. Beasley CM, Jr., Bosomworth JC, Wernicke JF. Fluoxetine: relationships among dose, response, adverse events, and plasma concentrations in the treatment of depression. Psychopharmacol Bull 1990;26:18.
36. Zajecka J. Strategies for the treatment of antidepressant-related sexual dysfunction. J Clin Psychiatry 2001;62 Suppl 3:35.
37. Veith RC, Raskind MA, Caldwell JH, et al. Cardiovascular effects of tricyclic antidepressants in depressed patients with chronic heart disease. N Engl J Med 1982;306:954.
38. Posternak MA, Zimmerman M. Switching versus augmentation: a prospective, naturalistic comparison in depressed, treatment-resistant patients. J Clin Psychiatry 2001;62:135.
39. Thase ME, Blomgren SL, Birkett MA, et al. Fluoxetine treatment of patients with major depressive disorder who failed initial treatment with sertraline. J Clin Psychiatry 1997;58:16.
40. Fava M. Management of nonresponse and intolerance: switching strategies. J Clin Psychiatry 2000;61 Suppl 2:10.
41. Maj M, Veltro F, Pirozzi R, et al. Pattern of recurrence of illness after recovery from an episode of major depression: a prospective study. Am J Psychiatry 1992;149:795.
42. Kupfer DJ, Frank E, Perel JM, et al. Five-year outcome for maintenance therapies in recurrent depression. Arch Gen Psychiatry 1992;49:769.
43. Zajecka J, Tracy KA, Mitchell S. Discontinuation symptoms after treatment with serotonin reuptake inhibitors: a literature review. J Clin Psychiatry 1997;58:291.
44. **44.** Rosenbaum JF, Fava M, Hoog SL, et al. Selective serotonin reuptake inhibitor discontinuation syndrome: a randomized clinical trial. Biol Psychiatry 1998;44:77.
45. **45.** Casacalenda N, Perry JC, Looper K. Remission in major depressive disorder: a comparison of pharmacotherapy, psychotherapy, and control conditions. Am J Psychiatry 2002;159:1354.
46. **46.** Thase ME, Greenhouse JB, Frank E, et al. Treatment of major depression with psychotherapy or psychotherapy-pharmacotherapy combinations. Arch Gen Psychiatry 1997;54:1009.
47. **47.** Browne G, Steiner M, Roberts J, et al. Sertraline and/or interpersonal psychotherapy for patients with dysthymic disorder in primary care: 6-month comparison with longitudinal 2-year follow-up of effectiveness and costs. J Affect Disord 2002;68:317.
48. Brodaty H, Luscombe G, Peisah C, et al. A 25-year longitudinal, comparison study of the outcome of depression. Psychol Med 2001;31:1347.
49. Judd LL, Akiskal HS, Maser JD, et al. A prospective 12-year study of subsyndromal and syndromal depressive symptoms in unipolar major depressive disorders. Arch Gen Psychiatry 1998;55:694.

*Bold numerals denote published controlled clinical trials, meta-analyses, or consensus-based recommendations.

50. Kennedy N, Paykel ES. Residual symptoms at remission from depression: impact on long-term outcome. J Affect Disord 2004;80:135.
51. Williams JW, Jr., Barrett J, Oxman T, et al. Treatment of dysthymia and minor depression in primary care: a randomized controlled trial in older adults. JAMA 2000;284:1519.
52. Battaglia J. Pharmacological management of acute agitation. Drugs 2005;65:1207.
53. American Psychiatric Association. Practice guideline for the treatment of patients with bipolar disorder (revision). Am J Psychiatry 2002;159:1.
54. Tsankov N, Angelova I, Kazandjieva J. Drug-induced psoriasis. Recognition and management. Am J Clin Dermatol 2000;1:159.
55. Bendz H, Aurell M, Lanke J. A historical cohort study of kidney damage in long-term lithium patients: continued surveillance needed. European Psychiatry 2001;16:199.
56. Kleiner J, Altshuler L, Hendrick V, et al. Lithium-induced subclinical hypothyroidism: review of the literature and guidelines for treatment. J Clin Psychiatry 1999;60:249.
57. Viguera AC, Cohen LS, Baldessarini RJ, et al. Managing bipolar disorder during pregnancy: weighing the risks and benefits. Can J Psychiatry 2002;47:426.
58. Pope HG, Jr., McElroy SL, Keck PE, Jr., et al., Valproate in the treatment of acute mania. A placebo-controlled study. Arch Gen Psychiatry 1991;48:62.
59. Gyulai L, Bowden CL, McElroy SL, et al. Maintenance efficacy of divalproex in the prevention of bipolar depression. Neuropsychopharmacology 2003;28:1374.
60. Bauer J, Isojarvi JIT, Herzog AG, et al. Reproductive dysfunction in women with epilepsy: recommendations for evaluation and management. J Neurol Neurosurg Psychiatry 2002;73:121.
61. Tohen M, Ketter TA, Zarate CA, et al. Olanzapine versus divalproex sodium for the treatment of acute mania and maintenance of remission: a 47-week study. Am J Psychiatry 2003;160: 1263.
62. Allison DB, Mentore JL, Heo M, et al. Antipsychotic-Induced Weight Gain: A Comprehensive Research Synthesis. Am J Psychiatry 1999;156:1686.
63. Suppes T, Dennehy EB, Gibbons EW. The longitudinal course of bipolar disorder. J Clin Psychiatry 2000;61 Suppl 9:23.
64. Howland RH Thase ME. A comprehensive review of cyclothymic disorder. J Nerv Ment Dis 1993;181:485.
65. Nierenberg AA, Gray SM, Grandin LD. Mood disorders and suicide. J Clin Psychiatry 2001;62 Suppl 25:27.
66. Brent DA, Perper JA, Allman CJ, et al. The presence and accessibility of firearms in the homes of adolescent suicides. A case-control study. JAMA 1991;266:2989.
67. Simon RI. The suicide prevention contract: clinical, legal, and risk management issues. J Am Acad Psychiatry Law 1999;27:445.

*For annotated **General References** and resources related to this chapter, visit www.hopkinsbayview.org/PAMreferences.*

Chapter 25

Schizophrenia and Related Psychotic Disorders

Andrew F. Angelino and Chester W. Schmidt, Jr.

Schizophrenia is a mental disorder, or group of disorders, for which the etiology is unknown. In the *Diagnostic and Statistical Manual of Mental Disorders, 4th Edition Text Revision (DSM-IV TR)*, the American Psychiatric Association lists the essential features of the disorder as the presence of certain psychotic features for a significant length of time (i.e., a 1-month period, with some signs persisting for at least 6 months); characteristic chronic symptoms involving multiple psychological processes; deterioration from a previous level of functioning; and median age at onset in the mid-twenties for men and late twenties for women. As noted later (see Diagnosis), none of these symptoms is pathognomonic for schizophrenia, and each is seen in other psychotic states.

Familiarity with schizophrenia is important to the generalist for three reasons: In the prodromal stage, the patient often presents first to a general physician; the interested generalist may provide much of the care for a patient with this lifelong disorder; and patients with schizophrenia have significant medical comorbidity as a result of diminished self-care and adverse effects of psychotropic medications.

EPIDEMIOLOGY

Schizophrenia has been found in all societies throughout the world. The distribution is similar throughout all populations. Epidemiologic studies in Western societies have found the lifetime prevalence of schizophrenia to be slightly less than 1 case per 100 persons. Lifetime incidence rates have been reported to range from 0.6% to 1.9% (1). Studies of incidence and prevalence in Europe using strict and somewhat narrow criteria for schizophrenia have produced case numbers and rates lower than similar studies done in the United States, which used broader criteria. In 1943, Lemkau et al. (2) determined that 15% to 25% of patients with schizophrenia never entered the hospital. Developments in psychopharmacology over the past three decades and the wide availability of ambulatory treatment resources have expanded the number of patients who never enter the hospital and greatly reduced the duration of confinement for those who do require hospitalization.

Schizophrenia is equally common in men and women. Onset is usually during young adulthood, with the first hospitalization usually occurring between the ages of 25 and 34 years. Most schizophrenic patients are single and are members of lower socioeconomic groups. The proposed reason for the clustering of patients in the lower socioeconomic groups is a downward social drift resulting from deterioration of social and vocational function.

CAUSES

The cause or causes of schizophrenia remain unknown. Numerous constitutional, genetic, neurologic, anatomic, biochemical, nutritional, psychosocial, and psychoanalytic theories have been offered. Present evidence strongly suggests some genetic transmission, because schizophrenia has long been known to run in families. The increased risk ranges from 3% for second-degree relatives, to 7% to 15% for siblings and children of one schizophrenic parent, to 40% for children of two schizophrenic parents. Concordance rates are 10% to 15% in dizygotic twins and 45% in monozygotic twins (3). Children born of schizophrenic parents but raised in adoptive families also show a higher incidence of the disease. This evidence indicates that transmission of schizophrenia is not explained by simple mendelian inheritance. Current research is seeking a polygenic mechanism, possibly with incomplete penetrance. Further, the study of "biomarkers," subtle neurologic signs and physical features, is emerging to help determine the precise genes involved.

In regard to the pathology of schizophrenia, many autopsy and neuroimaging efforts have played a significant role in the last decade. As the data emerge, it is becoming evident that schizophrenia is not a disease of one specific brain area but rather a functional disorder of brain systems that affects the developing brain of adolescents and young adults, causing several types of symptoms to emerge gradually. A significant research effort is now being directed at the heteromodal association cortex, a group of related brain structures thought to be involved in the higher, executive functions of the neocortex (4).

Neurochemical mechanisms involved in the production of symptoms of schizophrenia are still being investigated. An important clue emerged from studies of the pharmacologic effects of antipsychotic agents on schizophrenia. These medicines antagonize dopamine-mediated neurotransmission, leading to the speculation that excessive activity of the dopamine systems may be part of a biochemical defect in schizophrenic patients (5). Research has now shown that cortical serotoninergic systems modify the activity of the mesocortical and mesolimbic dopamine systems (6) and has led to the development of newer medicines that tend to have reduced rates of certain adverse effects.

NATURAL HISTORY OF SCHIZOPHRENIA

Although the first episode of acute psychosis usually occurs in late adolescence or early adulthood, *prodromal manifestations* of the disease are often present for years before the acute episode. During the prodromal phase, patients gradually withdraw from social relationships. They become indifferent to their grooming, ignore social graces and social rituals, and may develop suspicious attitudes about others. They appear different, peculiar, and sometimes bizarre. Timing of the onset of this phase plays a significant role in the achievement of social, educational, and occupational milestones. In some patients, the deterioration of social and vocational skills may be so striking that the patient seems to have a changed personality. In many cases of early onset schizophrenia, the patient has developed only marginal social and vocational skills, so his or her deterioration appears more insidious.

In one study of the prodromal stage of schizophrenia, many patients had some behavioral concern, most commonly depression or school or work decline, but the majority did not seek any health professional contact. Those patients that did seek out health care visited primary care physicians 35.7% of the time—at least twice as often as any other health care professional. Further, once psychotic symptoms began, the most frequent presentation site for patients became emergency departments, but family physicians were again more than twice as likely to be visited than any mental health care provider (7).

Psychiatrists classify psychotic symptoms into categories of positive, disorganized, and negative symptoms. *Positive symptoms* include delusions (fixed, false, idiosyncratic ideas) and hallucinations (perceptions without stimuli). Thought disorders—including loosening of associations, illogical or magical thinking, and inability to carry on discourse—and bizarre behavior and emotions make up the *disorganized symptoms.* The *negative symptoms* include apathy, preoccupation with fantasies and an inner psychological world (autism), inability to carry out goal-directed behavior because of preoccupation with consequences of alternatives (ambivalence), and anhedonia (loss of pleasure in activities). Occasionally, patients display catatonic symptoms, which include stereotypical movements, mutism, and sometimes rigid posturing.

Acute psychotic episodes are marked by the development or exacerbation of any of the positive or disorganized symptoms and are often brought on by stressful life events. Before antipsychotic medications were available, these episodes could last from weeks to years. Currently, most episodes are brought under pharmacologic control within several weeks. After treatment, positive and disorganized psychotic symptoms subside and in some cases seem to disappear completely. Some patients, however, develop a more chronic course, with persistent positive and disorganized symptoms. Many patients also suffer from prominent negative symptoms, which may be evident only between acute exacerbations. With each subsequent psychotic episode, the patient may slip further into a dependent, regressed state in which he or she is unable to function and becomes entirely dependent on family or society. Scholastic and vocational ability often diminish. Fewer than 20% of patients work full-time; most are financially supported by welfare programs or federal disability programs. Institutionalization is required in some cases because the patients lose all ability to care for themselves.

Schizophrenia is a lifelong disease consisting of psychotic symptoms that periodically become intense and an arrest or deterioration of social and vocational functioning, probably caused by massive withdrawal of interest in the outside world. The devastation of the disease is supported by the fact that 30.6% of suicides by schizophrenics occur within the first 2 years after onset or first hospitalization, and overall lifetime prevalence of suicide in schizophrenic patients is 4.9% (8).

DIAGNOSIS

The diagnosis of schizophrenia, especially during the initial episodes of acute psychosis, is based on clinical judgment and diagnostic criteria that, until recently, were unreliable. No pathognomonic symptoms, signs, or laboratory findings point to the diagnosis. The medical history of the patient does not contribute to the diagnosis, and, as discussed earlier, family history of the disease provides only partial information.

The diagnostic criteria for schizophrenia described in the *DSM-IV TR* are an excellent synthesis of several recognized diagnostic formulations (Table 25.1). Diagnosis rests on the findings of the symptoms of psychosis elicited by a mental status examination (see Chapter 19) and a history that documents the prodromal phase.

DIFFERENTIAL DIAGNOSIS

Any kind of psychotic state may resemble acute schizophrenia. However, differences in symptoms permit differentiation and diagnosis. *Delirium, dementia, and amnestic and other cognitive disorders* (see Chapter 26) are marked by disturbances in consciousness (delirium); by disorientation with respect to time, place, and person; and by

TABLE 25.1 Diagnostic Criteria for Schizophrenia

A. Characteristic symptoms: Two (or more) of the following, each present for a significant portion of time during a 1-month period (or less if successfully treated)
   1. Delusions
   2. Hallucinations
   3. Disorganized speech (e.g., frequent derailment or incoherence)
   4. Grossly disorganized or catatonic behavior
   5. Negative symptoms, i.e., affective flattening, alogia, or avolition (Note: Only one criterion A symptom is required if delusions are bizarre or hallucinations consist of a voice keeping up a running commentary on the person's behavior or thoughts, or two or more voices conversing with each other.)

B. Social/occupational dysfunction: For a significant portion of the time since the onset of the disturbance, one or more major areas of functioning such as work, interpersonal relations, or self-care is markedly below the level achieved before the onset (or when the onset is in childhood or adolescence, failure to achieve expected level of interpersonal, academic, or occupational achievement)

C. Duration: Continuous signs of the disturbance persist for at least 6 months. This 6-month period must include at least 1 month of symptoms (or less if successfully treated) that meet criterion A (i.e., active-phase symptoms), and may include periods of prodromal or residual symptoms. During these prodromal or residual periods, the signs of the disturbance may be manifested by only negative symptoms or two or more symptoms listed in criterion A present in an attenuated form (e.g., odd beliefs, unusual perceptual experiences).

D. Schizoaffective and mood disorder exclusion: Schizoaffective disorder and mood disorder with psychotic features have been ruled out because either (a) no major depressive, manic, or mixed episodes have occurred concurrently with the active-phase symptoms, or (b) if mood episodes have occurred during active-phase symptoms, their total duration has been brief relative to the duration of the active and residual periods.

E. Substance/general medical condition exclusion: The disturbance is not due to the direct psychologic effects of a substance (e.g., a drug of abuse, a medication) or a general medical condition.

F. Relationship to a pervasive developmental disorder: If there is a history of autistic disorder or another pervasive developmental disorder, the additional diagnosis of schizophrenia is made only if prominent delusions or hallucinations are also present for at least a month (or less if successfully treated).

Reprinted with permission from Diagnostic and statistical manual of mental disorders. 4th ed., text revision. Washington, DC: American Psychiatric Association, 2000.

TABLE 25.2 Prescription Drugs That Have Been Reported Occasionally to Cause Hallucinations or Other Manifestations of Psychosis

Angiotensin-converting enzyme inhibitors	Fluoxetine (Prozac)
Acyclovir (Zovirax)	Ganciclovir (Cytovene)
Albuterol (Proventil; Ventolin)	Ethchlorvynol (Placidyl)
Alfa-interferon	Histamine H_2-receptor antagonists
Amantadine (Symmetrel)	Isoniazid (INH, others)
Amiodarone (Cordarone)	Levodopa (Sinemet)
Amphetamine-like drugs	Methyldopa (Aldomet)
Anabolic steroids	Methylphenidate (Ritalin)
Anticonvulsants	Metronidazole (Flagyl)
Antidepressants, tricyclic	Nalidixic acid (NegGram)
Antihistamines	Narcotics
Atropine and anticholinergics	Nonsteroidal anti-inflammatory drugs
Baclofen (Lioresal)	Pentazocine (Talwin)
Benzodiazepines	Pergolide (Permax)
Beta-adrenergic blockers	Phenelzine (Nardil)
Bromocriptine (Parlodel)	Phenylephrine (Neo-Synephrine)
Bupropion (Wellbutrin)	Prazosin (Minipress)
Caffeine	Procainamide (Pronestyl)
Chloroquine (Aralen)	Procaine penicillin G
Ciprofloxacin (Cipro)	Pseudoephedrine
Clonidine (Catapres)	Quinacrine (Atabrine)
Cocaine	Quinidine
Corticosteroids (prednisone, cortisone, adrenocorticotropic hormone, other)	Salicylates
	Selegiline (Eldepryl)
Cyclobenzaprine (Flexeril)	Sulfonamides
Cyclosporine (Sandimmune)	Tamoxifen (Nolvadex)
Deet (Off)	Thyroid hormones
Digitalis glycosides	Trazodone (Desyrel)
Disopyramide (Norpace)	Verapamil
Disulfiram (Antabuse)	Zidovudine (Retrovir)

Adapted from Drugs that cause psychiatric symptoms. Med Lett 1993;35:65 (which includes references to reports).

impairment in intellectual functions (e.g., memory, calculations). Additionally, especially in patients younger than 50 years of age, there is usually evidence from the history, physical examination, and laboratory tests of specific organic findings that are etiologically related to the mental condition. *Single psychotic symptoms,* such as persecutory delusions or auditory hallucinations, may occur *de novo* in elderly patients as symptoms of dementia or paraphrenia (see Chapter 26). Effects of illicit drugs, especially amphetamine and phencyclidine (see Chapter 29), may mimic the acute phase of schizophrenia. Additionally, a number of *prescription drugs* may occasionally produce hallucinations and other manifestations that suggest psychosis (Table 25.2). History of drug use and absence of the prodromal phase help differentiate these conditions from schizophrenia.

The *psychotic symptoms of major affective episodes* (both mania and depression; see Chapter 24) can also be similar to those seen during acute episodes in the course of schizophrenia. Affective disorders differ from schizophrenia in that psychotic symptoms (e.g., delusions, hallucinations) appear after the development of the affective disturbance (depression or mania) and generally remit when the affective disturbance remits. In schizophrenia, marked depression or mania may appear, but the affective disturbance occurs after the onset of the psychotic symptoms, which often exist as well in the complete absence of affective symptoms. These principles of differential diagnosis are far from perfect, and patients with both types of disorder have been mislabeled. Because the prognosis associated with schizophrenia is often worse than of affective disorders, mislabeling has significant consequences, including attitudes toward the patient and actual treatment provided.

Schizoid and schizotypal personality disorders, described in Chapter 23, are personality types that may share some of the features of withdrawal from society, but they are not accompanied by the psychotic features seen in schizophrenia (Table 25.1). There is some evidence that these personality types may comprise part of a spectrum of schizophrenic illness, including data showing higher rates of these personality types in families of patients with schizophrenia.

TREATMENT AND PROGNOSIS

Antipsychotic Drugs

The primary treatment of the acute and chronic psychotic manifestations of schizophrenia in ambulatory or hospitalized patients centers around the antipsychotic agents. There are several classes of antipsychotics, with numerous drugs in each class. Table 25.3 lists the common drugs, together with available strengths and potency equivalents to chlorpromazine.

Although the structures of the various antipsychotics are well known, the pharmacology is not. Dose–response relationships have not yet been worked out for humans. The drugs generally produce effects within 1 hour after oral administration and within 10 to 15 minutes after intramuscular injection. They are lipid soluble with a high affinity for cell membranes. The drugs and their metabolites are distributed generally throughout the central nervous system with no local or regional accumulation. Metabolites are partially excreted each day, with significant portions retained in lipid-rich tissues and connective tissues. As these tissues become saturated, the drugs undergo slow turnover. The drugs are detoxified and inactivated mainly through oxidation by hepatic microsomal enzymes, and they are excreted through both bile and urine.

There is no evidence that these agents are addicting, although tolerance to some of the side effects (sedation, hypotension, anticholinergic effects, parkinsonian

TABLE 25.3 Available Strengths and Equivalent Doses of Commonly Used Neuroleptic Antipsychotic Agents

Generic Name	Trade Name	Available Strengths of Oral Preparations (mg)	Approximate Equivalent Dose of Chlorpromazine (mg)
Phenothiazines			
Aliphatic			
Chlorpromazine[a]	Thorazine	10, 25, 50, 100, 200	100
Triflupromazine	Vesprin	10, 25	30
Piperidines			
Mesoridazine	Serentil	10, 25, 100	50
Thioridazine[a]	Mellaril	10, 15, 25, 50, 100, 150, 200	95
Piperazines			
Fluphenazine[a,b]	Prolixin, Permitil	1, 2.5, 5, 10	2
Perphenazine[a]	Trilafon	2, 4, 8, 16	10
Trifluoperazine[a]	Stelazine	1, 2, 5, 10	5
Thioxanthenes			
Aliphatic			
Chlorprothixene	Taractan	10, 25, 50, 100	65
Piperazine			
Thiothixene[a]	Navane	1, 2, 5, 10, 25	5
Dibenzazepine			
Loxapine	Loxitane, Daxolin	10, 25, 50	15
Butyrophenone			
Haloperidol[a,c]	Haldol	0.5, 1, 2, 5, 10	2
Indolone			
Molindone	Moban	5, 10, 25	10
Diphenylbutyrylpiperidine			
Pimozide	Orap	1, 2	1
Atypicals			
Aripiprazole	Abilify	5, 10, 15, 20, 30	7.5
Clozapine	Clozaril	25, 100	50
Risperidone[d,f]	Risperdal	0.5,1, 2, 3, 4	1–2
Olanzapine[e,f]	Zyprexa	2.5, 5, 7.5, 10, 15	5
Quetiapine	Seroquel	25, 100, 200, 300	75
Ziprasidone[e]	Geodon	20, 40, 80	60

[a]Generic available.
[b]Long-acting fluphenazine decanoate or enanthate, for injection, comes in a concentration of 25 mg per mL; also available for injection as fluphenazine hydrochloride, a short-acting preparation.
[c]Haloperidol for injection comes in a concentration of 2 mg per mL.
[d]Long acting risperidone available as Risperdal Consta.
[e]Also available as short-acting injection.
[f]Also available in oral disintegrating wafers.

symptoms) has been reported. The drugs are fairly safe but may induce delirium if used in great excess. Further, antipsychotic drugs prolong the QTc interval (Q-T interval corrected for heart rate) to a varying degree depending on the specific agent, and care should be exercised when prescribing them to patients with cardiac conduction delays, because cases of sudden cardiac death have been reported. If patients are found to have a prolonged QTc interval (longer than 500 msec), the antipsychotic medicine should be evaluated for discontinuation, and consultation with a cardiologist should be obtained.

The mechanisms of action of the antipsychotics are not fully understood. Although it has been speculated that specific antipsychotic activity may result from the dopamine-antagonist action of these agents, the drugs have a variety of effects on many metabolic processes. Newer, so-called atypical or second-generation, antipsychotics affect neurotransmitters other than dopamine, especially serotonin, and additional dopamine receptor types compared with the older agents. This is the proposed basis for their lower rates of certain side effects, such as extrapyramidal symptoms, and it may be the mechanism of action of their effect on negative symptoms. These atypicals include aripiprazole (Abilify), clozapine (Clozaril), olanzapine (Zyprexa), quetiapine (Seroquel), risperidone (Risperdal), and ziprasidone (Geodon).

Treatment of Acute Psychotic Episodes

All antipsychotics are equally efficacious for controlling positive psychotic symptoms associated with schizophrenia, but only the atypical antipsychotics have been shown to have any efficacy in the treatment of negative symptoms. The choice of one drug over another depends on predicted differences in side effects, the history of a particular patient's response, and the clinician's familiarity with the agent. The treatment of acute psychotic episodes should begin with the equivalent of 300 to 1,000 mg of chlorpromazine (Thorazine) per day, in divided doses (usually three times daily). This dose range is equivalent to 6 to 20 mg of haloperidol (Haldol), which may be given as a single or divided dose. Only one antipsychotic should be given at a time, because administration of more than one agent increases the probability of side effects.

Combativeness, hyperactivity, and agitation are usually controlled within 24 to 48 hours after beginning treatment. If these symptoms are not modified within that period, the dosage should be increased, up to the equivalent of 800 to 2,000 mg of chlorpromazine, or 16 to 40 mg of haloperidol. It may be necessary to administer the drugs intramuscularly during the acute phase of agitation if the patient is unable to take oral medication. Haloperidol 2 to 5 mg is a good choice for intramuscular injection because of its minimal effects on circulatory regulation, but intramuscular preparations of the atypical agents ziprasidone and olanzapine are now available and becoming increasingly used because of lower incidence of acute dystonic reactions. For patients who do not respond to an adequate trial (4 to 6 weeks) of two or more antipsychotics, a trial of clozapine should be considered. Because clozapine causes fatal agranulocytosis in up to 1% of patients, a history of blood dyscrasias and poor compliance are contraindications. Clozapine trials should last at least 3 months at a dosage of 200 to 600 mg/day.

Delusions, hallucinations, associational defects, negativism, and withdrawal begin to subside within 1 to 2 weeks after treatment begins. Continued improvement of these symptoms may take place over an additional 4 to 8 weeks. If very high dosages of antipsychotic agents are initially required, the dosage should be cautiously reduced to the equivalent of 300 to 600 mg of chlorpromazine, because high doses of conventional antipsychotic agents can worsen apathy and negativism. This adjustment in dosage can usually begin 1 to 2 weeks after the peak dosage is reached.

Early Side Effects of Antipsychotics

Antipsychotic drugs with lower potency per milligram, such as chlorpromazine (Table 25.3), produce *sedation,* which can be a useful side effect in treating hyperactive or combative patients but is a disadvantage in regressed, withdrawn patients. The *anticholinergic properties* of all phenothiazines produces annoying symptoms of dry mouth, stuffy nose, blurred vision, and occasional urinary retention in older patients and delirium at high dosages. These side effects often abate or disappear within 2 to 4 weeks. A common worrisome side effect is drug-induced *Parkinson syndrome,* also called *extrapyramidal symptoms.* This occurs with greatest frequency in association with drugs of higher potency per milligram, such as haloperidol, the piperazine class of phenothiazines, thioxanthene, loxapine, and molindone (Table 25.3). The syndrome usually appears within 5 to 30 days after beginning treatment and includes tremor, rigidity, bradykinesia, fixed facies, drooling, and stooped posture. Because this problem commonly causes patients to discontinue antipsychotic treatment, it should be managed properly. In most cases reduction of dosage or addition of small amounts of an antiparkinsonism agent controls these side effects (see Chapter 90). The parkinsonian effects of antipsychotic drugs tend to decrease after 1 or 2 months. Therefore, withdrawal of antiparkinsonism drugs should be attempted after 6 to 12 weeks. Prophylactic treatment of all patients with antiparkinsonism drugs is generally discouraged because of the additional anticholinergic effects of these drugs.

The incidence of extrapyramidal symptoms is lower with the *newer antipsychotic agents* such as aripiprazole, olanzapine, quetiapine, and ziprasidone. Risperidone also shows a lower incidence at lower doses, but the symptoms appear at doses greater than 8 to 10 mg with the same regularity as with haloperidol or other potent agents.

Acute dystonias occur in some patients within 1 to 5 days after initiation of any antipsychotic; these effects are most often seen with haloperidol and the piperazine class of phenothiazines. The symptoms are sudden onset of severe, tonic contractions of the musculature of the neck (torticollis), the spine, the heels (opisthotonos), the extraocular muscles (oculogyric crises), the mouth, and the tongue. These symptoms remit promptly after intravenous or intramuscular injection of diphenhydramine (Benadryl, 25 to 50 mg) or benztropine (Cogentin, 1 to 2 mg). Antipsychotic treatment can be continued in these patients; an antiparkinsonism agent should be added for about 1 month to protect against recurrent dystonia. *Akathisia* may also occur early in treatment. This side effect is marked by motor restlessness with pacing, fidgeting, and restless legs. It does not resolve with treatment as predictably as the acute dystonias do. Treatment is the same as that prescribed for drug-induced parkinsonism. In a small, controlled trial the lipophilic β-blocker, propranolol, in daily doses of 20 to 60 mg, was shown to improve symptoms of akathisia in most patients (9).

A number of *nonneurologic side effects* can result from administration of the antipsychotics. *Cardiovascular toxicity* includes orthostatic hypotension; this problem is most commonly seen with the aliphatic and piperidine classes of phenothiazines and with chlorprothixene. Frank syncope may occur, rarely, after intramuscular administration of low-potency antipsychotics. Many agents have been shown to prolong the QTc to varying degrees. In particular, thioridazine and mesoridazine have been shown to cause significant QTc prolongation, and those drugs contain warnings in their prescription information mandated by the U.S. Food and Drug Administration (FDA). Torsades de pointes and ventricular tachycardia are rare side effects; there are no baseline characteristics that help one recognize patients at risk for this problem (see Chapter 64 for a discussion of cardiac arrhythmias). Reversible *cholestatic jaundice* can occur as an allergic response. *Agranulocytosis* is an exceedingly rare side effect.

The *neuroleptic malignant syndrome* is a rare, and occasionally lethal, idiosyncratic complication. It usually occurs within 1 month after the onset of treatment, when the dosage is increased, or when a second drug is introduced. Over 24 to 72 hours, the patient develops confusion, muscle rigidity, hypertension or severe orthostatic hypotension, and a high temperature (as high as 107.6°F [42°C]). Patients with this syndrome should be hospitalized immediately in an intensive care unit, because hypoventilation occurs as a consequence of the rigidity of the patient's chest wall muscles. The treatment involves discontinuation of all antipsychotic agents, aggressive intravenous hydration, and, in some cases, the administration of dantrolene or bromocriptine. Patients should remain off all antipsychotic drugs for a minimum of 2 weeks before reintroduction. In the interim period, acute exacerbations of symptoms are common, and patients may require inpatient psychiatric hospitalization.

Because *older schizophrenic patients* are more prone to the development of the common side effects, dosages should be lower for these patients, by the equivalent of 100 to 200 mg of chlorpromazine or 2 to 4 mg of haloperidol. The very high dosages described for treatment of combativeness and hyperactivity should be avoided in elderly patients.

Long-Term Drug Treatment of Schizophrenia

Interested generalists can assume responsibility for the long-term care of schizophrenic patients. Pharmacotherapy is the principal mode of long-term treatment. Many studies show that 60% to 70% of schizophrenic patients relapse within 1 year if they do not receive medication (10). A large meta-analysis of relapse demonstrated that patients withdrawn from antipsychotic therapy had a rate of relapse three times higher than those maintained on medication, with a mean follow up time of 9.7 months. However, almost half of the patients for whom antipsychotics were withdrawn remained stable without relapse during the followup period (11). These data support the conclusion that for most patients, antipsychotics should be maintained at the lowest level necessary to control symptoms and relapses, while minimizing risk of long-term side effects. Withdrawal of antipsychotics should be undertaken only in very stable situations, and for patients who have no history of violence, suicide attempts, or other serious consequences of relapse.

The goal of long-term pharmacotherapy is to minimize psychotic symptoms with the lowest dosage of antipsychotic possible. Moderate maintenance dosages appear to be as effective as, and safer than, the larger dosages that have been popular in the United States (12). For most patients a low to moderate dosage is the equivalent of 200 to 400 mg of chlorpromazine (or 4 to 8 mg of haloperidol) daily. Patients receiving this dosage often continue to have psychotic symptoms but do not seem to be disturbed by them (e.g., "I still hear the voices, but they don't bother me").

Compliance Problems

Some patients temporarily have difficulty maintaining a regular medication schedule because of psychotic disorganization, negativism, or fear of medication. Inability to comply with the medication regimen may signal the onset of an acute episode. With the first indication of a disruption in medication schedule, the patient should be evaluated, the frequency of visits increased to at least once a week, and the medication dosage increased if warranted. If the patient remains unable to comply, a long-acting intramuscular agent, such as fluphenazine decanoate (Prolixin Decanoate, available in doses of 25 mg/mL), 1 to 2 mL every 2 weeks, haloperidol decanoate (Haldol Decanoate, available in doses of 50 mg/mL), 2 to 4 mL every 4 weeks, or risperidone (Risperdal Consta, available in doses of 25 mg/mL) 1 to 2 mL every 2 weeks should be used. The patient can be returned to an oral medication when symptom control is reestablished. Long-acting intramuscular agents are also useful for new patients for whom no information is available on compliance in aftercare or ambulatory programs. Evidence suggests that family therapy and cognitive behavioral therapy improve compliance with medication regimens (13). Patients having difficulty with medication compliance should be referred for one of these types of therapy in addition to the previously described measures.

Nonresponders

Between 5% and 25% of schizophrenic patients do not respond to antipsychotics, and a similar number are intolerant of the side effects. Both groups of patients are candidates for treatment with *clozapine* (Clozaril) (14), a tricyclic dibenzodiazepine. The recommended starting dosage is 25 mg once or twice per day, to be increased by 25 mg every other day to 100 mg per dose, then increased by 50 mg every other day to 300 to 450 mg per day by 2 weeks. Clozapine is available in 25- and 100-mg tablets. The risk of agranulocytosis is 1% to 2% and necessitates initial weekly blood monitoring. Because of dose-related incidence of seizures, the dosage should not exceed 600 mg. Common side effects are weight gain, sedation, drooling, and dizziness. There are reports of increased incidence of type 2 diabetes mellitus (DM) in patients treated with clozapine.

Late Side Effects of Antipsychotics

Onset of the early type side effects is uncommon in patients taking maintenance dosages of antipsychotics (see Treatment of Acute Psychotic Episodes discussed earlier). When an increase in medication is necessary, drug-induced parkinsonism may appear. Patients who experience symptoms of parkinsonism over a long period should try other antipsychotic medications until one is found that does not produce the side effect. As noted previously, long-term use of antiparkinsonism medication is to be avoided if possible (see Chapter 90).

Tardive dyskinesia is an extrapyramidal syndrome that occurs in patients after prolonged (months to years) moderate- to high-dosage antipsychotic treatment. The cumulative prevalence is approximately 24% to 27% in women and 22% in men—but is much lower with the newer, atypical antipsychotic agents and is nonexistent for clozapine. The prevalence reaches its peak in men between 50 and 70 years of age but continues to rise after age 70 years in women. Asians have lower prevalence than North Americans, Europeans, or Africans (15). The disorder has been reported in association with long-term treatment with anticonvulsants, and there is a very small incidence among untreated schizophrenic patients. Up to 25% of patients treated with antipsychotics who are evaluated for drug-induced tardive dyskinesia are found to have another disorder causing their dyskinesia. The most common of these is the oral-buccal-lingual dyskinesia that arises in 10% of edentulous patients.

The syndrome of tardive dyskinesia consists of *involuntary or semivoluntary movements* of a choreiform, tic-like nature, sometimes associated with a dystonic component that classically involves the tongue, facial, and neck muscles. Early manifestations include fine, worm-like movements of the tongue at rest, facial tics, and jaw movements. Later symptoms are bucco-lingual-masticatory movements, chewing motions, lip smacking, puffing of cheeks, blinking of eyes, and choreoathetoid movements of the extremities. Younger patients often have significant involvement of the extremities and trunk. Although the syndrome is painless, it can be socially embarrassing and can interfere with patients' ability to feed and care for themselves.

The prognosis for remission of tardive dyskinesia is poor, regardless of treatment, and symptoms last for years if not indefinitely. The emphasis of antipsychotic use should therefore be on prevention of tardive dyskinesia, by careful selection of patients for long-term antipsychotic treatment, trials of atypical agents first, and use of the lowest possible dosage. At the first sign of the disorder, antipsychotics should be tapered and discontinued if possible. Symptoms gradually diminish or disappear over several months in approximately one third of patients who can be taken off drugs early.

Because there is no satisfactory treatment for tardive dyskinesia, understanding support by the physician and family members is especially important in long-term care of the patient. Antiparkinsonism medications usually worsen the symptoms. One short-term effective treatment is the use of more potent antipsychotics to suppress the symptoms, but this usually requires increasing dosages of the suppressing agent, and subsequent withdrawal of antipsychotics often leads to worsening of the symptoms for a period of time. In case reports, benzodiazepines, pure lecithin, lithium, sodium valproate, and vitamin E have been reported to be useful, but there are no well-delineated guidelines for selecting one of these agents. Another strategy is to switch the patient to clozapine, so that antipsychotic therapy is continued with a medication that does not cause tardive dyskinesia; this strategy is best done in consultation with a psychiatrist.

Overall Psychiatric Treatment of the Patient

The schizophrenic patient is sensitive to change or instability in any aspect of his or her life. Whenever possible, a single practitioner should provide continuous care, so that that practitioner becomes a predictable resource for helping the patient to maintain his or her role in the community. Although few schizophrenic patients work full time, patients should be referred for vocational rehabilitation (see Chapter 9) or for sheltered workshops when requested. Most patients determine their own levels of social activity and may not change despite encouragement, but offers and suggestions should be made. The clinician should be available to the patient's family or to foster care providers for periodic review of the patient's progress and expectations. The book, *Surviving Schizophrenia,* should be recommended to the patient's family (see *www.hopkinsbayview.org/PAMreferences*).

Ideally, residential facilities are available when there is no family with whom the patient may live or when the family is a harmful influence. However, in many communities, such facilities do not exist. For some patients, the clinician and the ambulatory center itself become the sources of the few social contacts that the patient has outside his or her home and inner psychological world.

Regular office visits should be scheduled. Frequency of visits should be determined on the basis of current status of the patient, history of the course of the patient's illness, reliability of the patient in taking medication, and the patient's ability to recognize early signs of onset of acute episodes. Routine office visits need last only 15 to 20 minutes and should include an interim history, a brief mental status examination, a review of the effectiveness of medications and of significant side effects, and provision of support or advice regarding the ways in which the patient is dealing with day-to-day matters. In other words, these office visits may be defined as supportive therapy, as described in Chapter 20.

In addition to individual office visits, *a family management approach* may be useful for patients who are having difficulties with their families (16). The method involves a two-step process:

1. Sessions devoted to educating the patient and family about the nature, course, and treatment of schizophrenia.
2. Family sessions aimed at reducing existing family tensions and improving problem-solving skills of the family in coping with causes of stress (see Family Counseling in Chapter 20).

Management is enhanced if the clinician has ready access to social services, emergency mental health services, and psychiatric day care and inpatient services. Social services, especially for financial support (e.g., welfare, food stamps, disability payments), are important in the treatment of schizophrenic patients because of their usual dependent status. Many acute episodes of psychosis are precipitated by threatened or actual withdrawal of welfare and disability payments.

The generalist caring for a schizophrenic patient may need to consult with a psychiatrist for confirmation of the initial diagnosis, decisions regarding hospitalization, or treatment recommendations when symptoms respond poorly to antipsychotics or when side effects are intolerable.

Medical Comorbidity in Patients with Schizophrenia

Patients who suffer from schizophrenia may have little contact with primary care physicians unless they are part of a program that mandates medical visits or have family members dedicated to keeping up with general health issues. The number one cause of death for schizophrenic patients is heart disease, and the patients have several risk factors.

First, there is a growing body of evidence that patients with schizophrenia are frequently comorbid with obesity (17). It is as yet unclear how much of this problem is caused by the lifestyle of the diseased patient and how much by side effects of medications used to treat the disorder. In fact, most antipsychotic agents are associated with weight gain, the notable exceptions being pimozide and molindone, two older typical antipsychotics and ziprasidone, a second-generation agent. The mechanism for this effect is still unclear but may involve several factors, including sedation, rigidity side effects of medications, increased appetite caused by antihistamine properties of some medications, or other metabolic changes resulting in increased fat storage. In general, weight issues and diet should be addressed in all patients with schizophrenia, and attempts should be made to help obese and overweight patients reduce weight. Attention should be given to possible medication effects, and attempts to alleviate sedation and/or rigidity should be actively pursued. If necessary, patients may try switching to antipsychotics associated with less weight gain, under careful supervision for recurrence of psychotic symptoms.

Second, there is a high rate of comorbidity between schizophrenia and nicotine addiction. Although there are theories about the specific effects of nicotine on schizophrenic brains, suggesting a self-medication model for this behavior, the untoward effects of smoking on the cardiopulmonary system run rampant. Generally, although efforts to force schizophrenic patients to quit smoking may be fruitless, all attempts should be made to reduce smoking to the lowest level possible, offering nicotine replacement as necessary and behavioral therapy to address cravings.

Third, there is evidence that diabetes is a more common problem in schizophrenia than in the general population (18). The possible mechanisms are that diabetes and schizophrenia are in some way genetically linked, so that risk genes may be transmitted together because of their proximity on chromosomes, and that antipsychotic medications may cause diabetes by directly impairing glucose handling and by causing obesity, which may impair insulin responsiveness. Diabetes complications arise as the disease takes its toll on the body, and schizophrenics may be poorly compliant with diet and hypoglycemic or insulin regimens. All schizophrenic patients should be regularly screened for diabetes on routine examinations.

In addition to heart, lung, and endocrine diseases, patients with schizophrenia are at increased risk for certain infectious diseases. Tuberculosis is associated with homelessness, a far-too-frequent sad consequence of chronic mental illness. The rates of human immunodeficiency virus infection and viral hepatitis in patients with schizophrenia are frighteningly high. Sexual transmission of these viruses may be related to the smaller sample of the population with whom patients with schizophrenia have the opportunity for intercourse. There are data to suggest that schizophrenic patients choose sexual partners most often from among other patients in the psychiatric clinic. Further, there is a profound comorbidity of substance use disorders in schizophrenia. The possible mechanisms for this are (a) as a method of self-medication for positive or negative symptoms, (b) as a means of increasing social interaction via a fairly scripted set of rules that patients with schizophrenia can follow, and (c) as a result of increased availability in impoverished areas, to which schizophrenic patients tend to "drift" due to social disenfranchisement. In any case, intravenous drug use may lead directly to infection, and because many schizophrenic patients do not see internists or family practitioners regularly, the illnesses may be overlooked until later stages of infection, when treatment is more difficult and possibly less efficacious. Patients with schizophrenia should be routinely asked about sexual practices and intravenous drug use, and appropriate serologic testing should be performed.

Prognosis for the Treated Patient

Schizophrenia is a lifelong disease that requires an open-ended commitment by the clinician. The patient's life is disrupted by periodic psychosis, sometimes necessitating hospitalization, and by an arrest or deterioration of social function. Some patients are able to work and maintain satisfying interpersonal relationships. Many lead lonely, withdrawn, socially marginal existences. Psychopharmacologic treatment is effective for controlling the symptoms of acute psychosis and suppressing the intensity of psychotic symptoms over long periods. Suppression of psychosis may permit the patient to use his or her intellectual and social talents more effectively in developing and maintaining some role in the community. The atypical antipsychotics (Table 25.3) are reported to have efficacy in the treatment of the negative symptoms that may impair social function.

SPECIFIC REFERENCES*

1. Regier DA, Boyd JH, Burke JD, et al. One-month prevalence of mental disorders in the United States. Arch Gen Psychiatry 1988;45:977.
2. Lemkau PU, Tietze C, Cooper M. Survey of statistical studies on prevalence and incidence of mental disorder in sample population. Public Health Rep 1943;58:1909.
3. Mowry BJ, Levinson DF. Genetic linkage and schizophrenia: methods, recent findings and future directions. Aust N Z J Psychiatry 1993;27:200.
4. Pearlson GD. Neurobiology of schizophrenia. Ann Neurol 2000;48:56.
5. Snyder SH. The dopamine hypothesis of schizophrenia: focus on the dopamine receptor. Am J Psychiatry 1976;133:197.
6. Kapur S, Remington G. Serotonin-dopamine interaction and its relevance to schizophrenia Am J Psychiatry 1996;153:466.
7. Addington J, van Mastrigt S, Hutchinson J, et al. Pathways to care: help seeking behavior in first episode psychosis. Acta Psychiatr Scand 2002;106:358–364.
8. Palmer BA, Pankratz VS, Bostwick JM. The lifetime risk of suicide in schizophrenia: a reexmaination. Arch Gen Psychiatry 2005;62:247–257.
9. Lipinski JF, Zubenko GS, Barreira P, et al. Propranolol in the treatment of neuroleptic-induced akathisia [Letter]. Lancet 1983;2:685.
10. Hogarty GE, Goldberg SC, Schooler NR, et al. Drug and sociotherapy in the aftercare of schizophrenic patients: two-year relapse rates. Arch Gen Psychiatry 1974;31:603.
11. Gilbert PL, Harris MJ, McAdams LA, et al. Neuroleptic withdrawal in schizophrenic patients: a review of the literature. Arch Gen Psychiatry 1995;52:173–188.
12. Baldessarini RJ, Cohen BM, Teicher MH. Significance of neuroleptic dose and plasma level in the pharmacologic treatment of psychoses. Arch Gen Psychiatry 1988;45:79.
13. Pilling S, Bebbington P, Kuipers E, et al. Psychological treatments in schizophrenia: I. Meta-analysis of family intervention and cognitive behaviour therapy. Psychol Med 2002;32:763–782.
14. Meltzer HY. Treatment of the neuroleptic-nonresponsive schizophrenic patient. Schizophr Bull 1992;18:515.
15. Yassa R, Jeste DV. Gender differences in tardive dyskinesia: a critical review of the literature. Schizophr Bull 1992;18:701.
16. Falloon IR, Boyd JL, McGill CW, et al. Family management in the prevention of exacerbation of schizophrenia. N Engl J Med 1982;306:1437.
17. Goldman LS. Medical illness in patients with schizophrenia. J Clin Psychiatry 1999;60[Suppl 21]:10.
18. Mukherjee S, Decina P, Bocola V, et al. Diabetes mellitus with schizophrenic patients. Compr Psychiatry 1996;37:68.

*Bold numerals denote published controlled clinical trials, meta-analyses, or consensus-based recommendations.

*For annotated **General References** and resources related to this chapter, visit www.hopkinsbayview.org/PAMreferences.*

Chapter 26

Cognitive Impairment and Mental Illness in the Elderly

Peter V. Rabins

Although overall rates of mental disorders are similar across the adult age span, the elderly are the least likely to seek help for mental illness. Those who do are most likely to receive treatment from a primary care provider during a routine medical visit.

GENERAL PRINCIPLES

Importance of Diagnosis

Making the correct diagnosis is a crucial first step in determining proper treatment. The most common mistakes made in assessing psychiatric symptoms in older patients are ascribing them to normal aging, confusing symptoms with syndromes, and not appreciating the frequent interaction between physical and psychiatric disorders. Asking the appropriate questions and attempting to elicit the classic signs and symptoms should lead to the correct diagnosis even when the presentation is unusual.

Relationship between Physical and Mental States

Physical and psychiatric illnesses commonly coexist in the elderly. A prudent strategy when facing a patient with both physical and psychiatric complaints is to establish a differential diagnosis for each symptom before assuming that either the physical or the psychiatric disorder is primary. The two types of symptoms may be related in a number of ways.

- *Mental distress complicating a primary physical illness.* Demoralization, anxiety, grief, irritability, and frustration are especially common in older patients with significant physical illness. These feelings usually begin after the onset of the physical illness, vary over time, and respond to the techniques for psychotherapy described in Chapter 20.
- *Physical complaints as the primary manifestation of psychiatric disorder.* Particularly in older patients, focused complaints of physical ill health may be the most prominent or only sign of mental illness, especially depression. Although the physical complaint must be appropriately evaluated, a psychiatric cause should be suspected when the somatic complaint is bizarre, seems to be exaggerated, or has been evaluated without a cause being found or when the patient has some symptoms of depression.
- *Psychiatric disorders arising from specific diseases.* Cancer of the pancreas, hypothyroidism, and several structural brain diseases (stroke, Parkinson disease, dementia) are commonly accompanied by a depression. Because the rates of depression are higher in these disorders than in arthritic or orthopedic conditions with similar levels of impairment, it is likely that the medical disorder is the cause of the depression or that the medical and psychiatric disorders share a common etiology. These depressions respond well to antidepressant treatment.
- *Psychiatric syndromes caused by medication and by substance abuse.* Psychiatric syndromes can be precipitated by a variety of medications and by alcohol abuse. Corticosteroids, β-blockers, and other drugs that affect the adrenergic system can induce depressive symptoms. Anticholinergic compounds, dopaminergic agonist compounds, benzodiazepines, and H_2 blockers can induce delirium. Patients with dementia are more vulnerable to developing cognitive side effects from these compounds than are cognitively normal elderly people. Alcoholism, often hard to recognize in elderly patients, can also cause symptoms of depression and anxiety or cognitive defects (see Chapter 28). Abstinence can lead to resolution of the psychiatric symptoms.

Importance of Psychosocial Factors

Psychosocial factors are important to consider in patients of all ages. They become particularly important in the elderly because widowhood, reduced physical mobility, isolation from family and friends, and financial limitations are more common and can directly interfere with the treatment of medical and psychiatric disorders. For elderly patients with mental illness, referring the patient to a social service agency or enlisting the help of the patient's family

TABLE 26.1 Components of a Mental Status Examination

Orientation
- Person [intact patients will know their complete name]
- Date [intact patients should know the date within 3 days]
- Place [intact patients will be fully oriented to place]

Memory, registration
- Give 3–5 words to remember repeat and ask patient to recall them in 2 minutes

Attention/Concentration:
- Days of the week backward, starting with Sunday, or
- Spell a word backwards, e.g. "house", or
- Subtraction of 7 serially from 100 for 5 iterations [intact persons should be able to get all of the days of the week, 4 of 5 of the spelling backwards, or 4 of 5 of the subtractions]

Memory, recall
- Recall the 3–5 words [intact patients should remember 2 of 3 or 4 of 5 words]

Language
- Naming: show two common items (e.g. watch, shoe) and one uncommon item (e.g. lapel, shoelace)
- Repetition: e.g., repeat "Today is a [sunny] day in [March]."
- Reading: e.g., ask "Raise your right hand".
- Writing: ask to write a complete sentence.
- [Intact patients can do all correctly]

Visual–Spatial
- Copy a complex figure, or
- Draw a clock, put in numbers, and put in hands at specific time [intact patients will do correctly]

Executive
- Ask, "What does this proverb mean: 'Don't cry over spilled milk'?" [correct response, "What is done is done" or similar statement: may be missed because of low education or cultural background]

may be especially important in ensuring successful treatment and follow-through. Even when dementia is present, psychosocial interventions provide an important avenue for relieving morbidity.

Importance of Cognitive Assessment

Because dementia and delirium are common disorders of the elderly, it is important to be familiar with the assessment of cognitive function and to perform a cognitive mental status examination on all patients in whom a psychiatric symptom is present. Table 26.1 displays the mental status examination, which allows the clinician to identify the types of cognitive deficits the patient is experiencing and to provide a comparison for future examinations. The Mini-Mental Status Examination is a reliable, brief, widely used screening tool (1) that permits standardized scoring and facilitates following patients over time. However, it may be normal in patients with mild dementia. Formal neuropsychometric testing and/or reevaluation of patients at a later time may be useful in such situations.

SPECIFIC PSYCHOGERIATRIC DISORDERS

Psychiatric disorders in older patients may present with the classic symptoms described in other chapters of this book. The following pages focus on several syndromes that are particularly important in the elderly.

Depression

Depressive Symptoms

Symptoms of depression and sadness become more common in late life even though the syndrome of major depression is less common in the elderly. This dissociation may be caused by both the criteria used to make diagnoses and intrinsic differences between the young and old. The *Diagnostic and Statistical Manual of Mental Disorders, 4th Edition (DSM-IV)*, divides mood disorder into several categories (see Chapter 24). The differences among them depend on both symptom clustering and course. The presentation of these disorders in older patients may differ from the presentation in younger patients in several ways.

An adjustment disorder with depressed mood is characterized by sad or low mood that follows, within 3 months, a clearly identifiable stressor or precipitant. In elderly patients, stressors such as illness, decreases in functional status, isolation, and financial limitations (see Importance of Psychosocial Factors, above) are particularly common. The approaches to office psychotherapy described in Chapter 20 are fully applicable to elderly patients with adjustment disorders.

A dysthymic disorder, conversely, is characterized by the presence of depressive symptoms for more than 2 years. Mood often fluctuates widely but in no discernible pattern. The patient may experience hours, days, or weeks of improved mood, mixed with prolonged periods of unhappiness. In the elderly, a dysthymic disorder should be considered when the patient reports chronic depressive symptoms throughout his or her life and denies the cyclicity and periods of normal mood found in recurrent depressive or bipolar disorder (see Chapter 24). It may require specialty referral because of its chronicity.

Major Depression

The diagnostic criteria of the major affective disorders and their treatment, as described in Chapter 24, are generally applicable to the elderly. Hypochondriacal features, agitation, and suspiciousness or frank paranoia often accompany depression in the elderly and are common sources of diagnostic confusion. A study demonstrated that the elderly with major depressive disorder are less likely to report being sad than the young (2). Therefore, denial of sadness does *not* rule out the diagnosis of major depression.

Elderly patients with a hypochondriacal focus usually deny that their mood is sad but focus on physical symptoms for which there is minimal or no evidence of abnormality on physical examination or laboratory assessment. Depressed hypochondriacal patients often have changes in their vital sense ("something is wrong with me") and a negative self-attitude ("I've done something to deserve this or cause this"). Therefore, the patient should be asked specifically about these cardinal features of major depression when hypochondriasis is present.

Because suspiciousness and paranoia are common in depressed elderly patients, other evidence for a major depression should be sought when these symptoms are present. When paranoia and depression coexist, depression is most commonly the primary disorder.

As in younger patients, major depression in the elderly often requires pharmacotherapy or electroconvulsive therapy. Chapter 24 gives practical details about these modes of treatment. Selective serotonin reuptake inhibitor (SSRI) antidepressants are the treatment of choice for the initiation of antidepressant pharmacotherapy. Sertraline (Zoloft) should be started at a dosage of 25 to 50 mg in the morning; 200 mg is the maximum dosage. Paroxetine (Paxil) should be started at a dosage of 10 mg in the morning; 30 mg is the maximum dosage. Citalopram (Celexa) should be started at a dosage of 15 mg in the morning. The maximum dose is 45 mg. The long half-life of fluoxetine (Prozac) suggests that it should be used in lower dosages in the elderly than in young patients, starting at a dosage of 10 mg in the morning. The maximum dosage is 40 to 60 mg. Tricyclic antidepressants with the most pronounced anticholinergic properties (e.g., amitriptyline and doxepin) should be avoided. The tricyclics with the highest likelihood of causing orthostatic hypotension (e.g., amitriptyline and imipramine) should also be avoided or closely monitored because elderly patients are at higher risk of falls and are more likely to be receiving antihypertensive drugs or other compounds that also can cause orthostasis. Nortriptyline and desipramine are the tricyclic agents that are least likely to cause these side effects. A usual starting dosage in the otherwise healthy elderly person is 10 to 25 mg at bedtime; however, a dosage of 10 mg should be prescribed in the frail elderly or in patients with the potential for medical complications from the drugs.

Electroconvulsive therapy is sometimes safer than pharmacotherapy for older patients with cardiac disease. It is equally effective in all age groups (see details regarding electroconvulsive therapy, Chapter 24). Low-dose antipsychotic drugs (see Table 25.3) are indicated when *delusions* complicate depression, especially when the suspiciousness is significantly interfering with the patient's function, is life threatening (e.g., the patient will not eat because he or she believes that the food is poisoned), or causes distress for the patient or those close to him or her.

Depression-Induced Cognitive Impairment

Patients with the onset of depression in late life can present with the belief that they are becoming demented. Some depressed patients perform poorly on routine tests of cognitive function. Previously this condition was called *pseudodementia,* but this term has fallen into disfavor because patients with this syndrome perform in the demented range on standardized tests of cognitive function and because up to 50% of these patients eventually develop a progressive dementing illness (3). Nonetheless, recognition of the syndrome is important because both the mood disorder and cognitive function can improve with antidepressant treatment. Depression-induced cognitive impairment should be considered when the onset of cognitive impairment has been subacute (less than 6 months and particularly less than 3 months), when the history of an episode of depression earlier in life is elicited, when a dementia is complicated by hypochondriacal or bizarre delusions (4), when the patient constantly emphasizes his or her cognitive disability (a behavior that is uncommon in Alzheimer disease), or when a cognitively impaired patient reports early morning awakening, lack of energy, self-blame, or guilt. At times it is difficult to determine whether the patient has a primary dementing illness with secondary depression or primary depression with reversible dementia. In such cases a therapeutic trial of an antidepressant (e.g., at least 4 weeks at a therapeutic dosage, as described in Chapter 24) may be the best way to determine which disorder is primary.

Depression Coexisting with Brain Disease

Major depression may complicate organic disorders of the central nervous system. Stroke, Parkinson disease, and AD are three common late-life disorders in which major depressive symptoms occur in 20% to 50% of patients. The importance of recognizing these as coexisting disorders is that the physical disorder and the psychiatric disorder may both need to be treated if either problem is to improve. For example, depression has been shown to interfere directly with rehabilitation from *stroke.* Thus, the treatment of depression after stroke improves the degree of recovery from the stroke; at the same time, gains from rehabilitation improve the patient's morale and mood (see details in Chapter 91). In *Parkinson disease,* depressive symptoms and parkinsonian symptoms (e.g., psychomotor retardation) often overlap, and it can be difficult to determine which disorder is causing specific symptoms. In planning treatment, it is best to focus on the depressive or parkinsonian symptoms separately and to treat first the disorder that is causing the worst impairment in function. Chapter 90 describes the treatment of Parkinson disease. The treatment of depression in patients with *Alzheimer disease* or multi-infarct dementia can improve behavior, and mood, although cognitive impairment will persist (5).

Paranoia and Suspiciousness

Suspiciousness is more common among the elderly than in younger people. This becomes clinically relevant when the suspiciousness interferes with the patient's life. Several types of disorders can present with suspiciousness.

Suspiciousness as an Isolated Symptom

Some elderly people become more suspicious as they age but have no accompanying signs or symptoms of other mental illness. It is important to determine whether there is a basis for the patient's suspiciousness because financial abuse of the elderly is not uncommon and concerns about the environment being unsafe can be appropriate. An understandable reaction to difficult circumstances should not be assumed, however, and a review of symptoms that explores other psychiatric conditions is necessary.

Suspiciousness Complicating Depression

As noted above, suspiciousness occurs in some elderly patients with major depression. Depression should be considered primary if the person feels deserving of persecution or punishment or has changes in vital sense and other manifestations of depression (see Chapter 24).

Late-Life Schizophrenia or Paraphrenia

Older patients occasionally develop a syndrome similar to schizophrenia in young people (see Chapter 25). Such patients have *delusions* (fixed, false, idiosyncratic ideas) and *auditory* or *visual hallucinations* and lack symptoms of depression or cognitive impairment.

The treatment of late-life schizophrenia and paranoia is similar to that for younger patients (see Chapter 25) except that significantly lower dosages of antipsychotic drugs are effective. Although no single antipsychotic drug is more efficacious than another, those likely to induce orthostatic hypotension, such as chlorpromazine (Thorazine), should be avoided, if possible. A starting dosage of 0.25 mg of risperidone (Risperdal) two to three times daily, olanzapine (Zyprexa) 2.5 mg at bedtime, quetiapine 12.5 to 25 mg at bedtime or perphenazine 1 mg at bedtime (may be increased to 2 mg twice daily) is recommended. Perphenazine and haloperidol are less expensive than quetiapine, risperidone or olanzapine. So-called second-generation drugs (olanzapine, risperidone and quetiapine) were thought to produce less tardive dyskinesia than first-generation drugs such as haloperidol, but this has been called into question (6). Of note, all antipsychotic drugs, with the possible exception of clozapine, are associated with increased mortality in patients with dementia (7,8). Chapter 25 describes the use of antipsychotic drugs in detail.

Paranoia and Persecutory Delusions as Symptoms of an Organic Disease

Paranoia can be symptomatic of a focal brain disease (e.g., tumor or stroke), a diffuse brain disease such as AD, a systemic condition such as a metabolic disorder (e.g., hyperthyroidism or hypoparathyroidism), or psychoactive substance abuse. Any patient with a persistent suspicious belief should have a clinical assessment for evidence that supports the presence of one of these causes.

Mild Cognitive Impairment

Some older patients complain of memory loss or slower rate of processing information, or members of their families notice these phenomena, but a history from both the patient and family reveals no social or occupational dysfunction and screening cognitive tests reveal minimal impairment in memory. Recent research suggests that 6% to 12% of these individuals develop dementia each year over the next 5 years (9). Those unlikely to have a dementia complain of such things as misplacing keys or having more difficulty remembering names or words than they once did; on questioning they acknowledge that names and words often come to them minutes later and that they have not forgotten important engagements or events. Patients who are especially concerned about memory difficulties and report a decline in function in social, personal, or occupational realms should be referred to a neuropsychologist for *formal neuropsychologic evaluation* to better formulate the problem. Impairments in memory and executive function are the best predictors of subsequent decline (10). Careful attention should be given to the medical status of such patients because they could have a subclinical delirium (see Delerium). When no dysfunction is identified and objective testing makes a progressive dementia unlikely, reassurance and an agreement to reassess the patient in 6 months may help relieve the anxiety associated with this condition.

Dementia

Definition and Epidemiology

Dementia is characterized by a decline in cognitive abilities from a previous level, multiple impairments in cognitive function such as memory (amnesia) or language (aphasia), and the presence of clear consciousness. Dementia can have many etiologies, but fewer than 2% of affected patients have dementia caused by a reversible etiology (10). Moderate to severe dementia affects approximately 8% of people older than 65 years. However, most dementia occurs among the very old; prevalence is 20% to 25% in people 80 years of age and older and approximately 30% to 40% in people older than 90 years. Prevalence rates are similar in European, North American, and

Asian prevalence studies. A study from Africa suggests lower rates in Nigeria (11).

Etiologic Evaluation

The assessment of a person with complaints of cognitive decline has three purposes. The first purpose is to identify the probable cause of the dementia, including the identification of treatable disorders. The three most common causes of treatable dementia in elderly patients are medication toxicity, depression, and thyroid disease. Commonly used medications that have been associated with global cognitive impairment are the benzodiazepines (most common), H_2 blockers, and anticholinergic drugs. The second purpose of assessment is to identify treatable symptoms and comorbidity. Because few patients have a truly reversible dementia, the treatment of medical and behavioral comorbidity is the main focus of both the assessment and the treatment of almost all patients in the ambulatory setting. The third purpose is to identify issues in the caregiver and environment that are amenable to intervention.

Clinical Characteristics

In considering possible etiologies, it is useful to *determine whether the dementia has the clinical characteristics of a subcortical or cortical dementia* (12). Most treatable dementias present as subcortical dementias. *Subcortical dementias* are characterized by memory loss, apathy, slowness, and movement disorder with intact language (i.e., the patient is able to name objects, repeat a phrase, and follow a command) and normal visuospatial function (i.e., the patient is able to copy a diagram) (Table 26.1). Causes of subcortical dementia include hypothyroidism, Parkinson disease, multiple sclerosis, normal pressure hydrocephalus, the dementia syndrome of depression, and most instances of vascular dementia. The *cortical dementias* are characterized by memory loss plus multiple defects in higher cortical functions: *aphasic language* (making paraphasic errors such as substituting a letter, as in "tee" instead of "tie," or saying an incorrect word, such as "paper" instead of "pencil"), *apraxia* (inability to perform skilled movements such as showing how to drink with a cup on command), and *agnosia* (inability to recognize common objects or sensory stimuli). Alzheimer disease is the most common cortical dementia, but frontal dementias, Lewy body dementia (LBD), and rare dementias such as Creutzfeldt-Jakob disease are included in this category.

Screening Tests

The Agency for Health Care Policy and Research (AHCPR) 1996 Consensus Statement (13) on the differential diagnosis of dementia suggests the following inexpensive screening tests, each targeted at potentially treatable causes, for all patients: complete blood count (CBC), serum electrolyte levels, creatinine clearance (CrCl), liver function tests, calcium and phosphate concentrations, thyroid-stimulating hormone (TSH), vitamin B_{12} level, and serologic tests for syphilis. The more recent clinical practice guidelines published by the American Academy of Neurology recommends screening for depression, B_{12} deficiency, and hypothyroidism but, because of its rarity in the United States, recommends against routinely screening for syphilis, except in high prevalence regions or high-risk patients (13). Imaging of the brain is listed as optional by the AHCPR and as appropriate by the American Academy of Neurology. It is reasonable to obtain a noncontrast computed tomography (CT) study on all patients with symptoms of less than 2 years' duration, onset before age 70, or focal findings on neurologic examination. CT or magnetic resonance imaging (MRI) can identify focal lesions such as a tumor, subdural hematoma, or abscess; demonstrate findings compatible with hydrocephalus; or provide confirmatory evidence for vascular etiology of the dementia. However, it is impossible to diagnose AD solely by any imaging study. Overreliance on CT or MRI reports of "white matter hyperintensities" has led to an overdiagnosis of vascular dementia.

Alzheimer disease is diagnosed by inclusion and exclusion criteria. The diagnosis should be made when other specific causes of dementia, including vascular disease, have been excluded, when the condition has been slowly progressive, and when the cognitive disorder includes language impairment, apraxia, or agnosia in addition to memory impairment.

Vascular dementia should be diagnosed when the history suggests distinct episodes of worsening (a stair-step course); when evidence of vascular disease and hypertension are present on examination; when the neurologic examination reveals asymmetries in reflexes, strength, or sensation; and when a lesion on CT or MRI correlates with the abnormalities or neurologic examination. Evidence of prior stroke on neurologic examination or imaging study is necessary because a history of stroke without confirming evidence is an unreliable indicator of vascular dementia.

The *frontotemporal dementias* (FTDs) are a group of slowly progressive diseases that present with pronounced changes in behavior, personality and language early in the disease. They are neuropathologically heterogeneous. On CT or MRI they show disproportionate frontal atrophy. The only Medicare-supported indication for brain PET scan is to distinguish between AD and FTD.

Lewy body dementia presents in a fashion similar to AD but also has extrapyramidal symptoms (rigidity and parkinsonian tremor), hallucinations, delusions, frequent falls, and episodes of worsening early in the course. Antipsychotic medications should be avoided, if possible, because they can cause marked worsening of the parkinsonian symptoms.

Management

The management of irreversible dementia can be divided into six aspects:

1. *The assessment process.* This is the first step in management. The diagnosis has often been suspected by the family or patient, but at times abnormal behavior has been misinterpreted as purposefully irritating. As specific a *diagnosis* as possible should be made and conveyed to the family. The family may ask about long-term *prognosis*. The average patient with AD lives 7 to 10 years after early symptoms, but life span while demented can be as long as 20 years. Generally, a dementia that has progressed slowly will continue to do so, whereas a history of rapid progression predicts rapid decline. Although the patient has the right to know his or her diagnosis, many lack the ability to realize that they have a deficit. Patients who, when asked, deny that they have any problems with their memory usually do not accept that there is a problem when told directly. Some patients, and most families, experience a measure of relief when it is pointed out that the patient's dementia is a medical problem and not just part of getting older or becoming intentionally stubborn.

   The evaluation process should elicit specific *problems in behavior caused by the dementia* (Table 26.2). Difficulty in speaking, dressing, and performing potentially dangerous activities as driving, smoking, and cooking should be inquired about. When present, these problems should be explained as the result of the illness. The family or other caregivers should then try to adapt the environment to the disordered behaviors and should take steps to eliminate dangerous behaviors. Helping caregivers to specifically identify each problem can enable them to institute common-sense solutions they have not otherwise tried. In regard to the patient who continues to drive, the practitioner should instruct the patient to stop driving rather than asking a family member to do so. Most states require periodic relicensure for older people, and some even require health care practitioners to report all patients with dementia. Because these regulations can be helpful, it is important to be aware of them in one's state.

   Families needing legal and financial advice should be advised to seek this out early and not wait for a crisis. Chapter 19 describes guidelines for assessing competence or for obtaining legal guardianship.

2. *Optimizing general medical care.* Medical conditions such as heart failure, urinary tract infection, and chronic obstructive pulmonary disease (COPD) can worsen the functioning of patients with dementia if not optimally treated. Drugs that can affect cognition (e.g., β-blockers, benzodiazepines, methyldopa, digoxin, anticholinergics) should be carefully monitored and all unnecessary medications discontinued. A search for superimposed medical illness should be instituted if there is a sudden deterioration in behavior, cognition, or functional ability.

3. *Addressing environmental problems, behavioral symptoms, and depression.* Not sleeping at night, suspiciousness, easy irritability, and catastrophic reactions (see below) can be more problematic than cognitive impairment. Nonpharmacologic environmental approaches should be tried first. For insomnia, these include keeping the person more active in the daytime (day care centers are a significant help in this regard) and not letting the patient nap during the day. Irritability, suspiciousness, and frustration are usually best managed by eliminating tasks that the patient can no longer do

TABLE 26.2 Behavior Problems of Patients and Problematic Activities of Daily Living Cited by Families of Demented Patients[a]

Behavior	*Percentage of Families Reporting Occurrence*	*Percentage of Families Reporting Behavior as a Problem*
Memory disturbance[b]	100	93
Catastrophic reactions[b,c]	87	89
Demanding/critical behavior	71	73
Night walking	69	59
Hiding things	69	71
Communication difficulties	68	74
Suspiciousness[b]	63	79
Making accusations[b]	60	82
Difficulty eating meals	60	55
Daytime wandering	59	70
Difficulty bathing	53	74
Hallucinations	49	42
Delusions	47	83
Physical violence	47	94
Incontinence[b]	40	86
Difficulty cooking	33	44
Hitting[b]	32	81
Impaired driving	20	73
Smoking	11	67
Inappropriate sexual behavior	2	0

[a]Based on an open-ended interview with the primary caregivers of 55 patients with irreversible dementia.
[b]Cited as most serious problem.
[c]See example in text.
Adapted from Rabins PV, Mace NL, Lucas MJ. The impact of dementia on the family. JAMA 1982;248:333.

and avoiding situations that frustrate the patient. Reminiscence therapy can improve the morale of patients with dementia (15). It is prudent to have the demented patient wear a medical alert bracelet that describes his or her condition.

Antipsychotic medications should be used only when other approaches have failed and a specific target symptom (hallucinations, delusions, aggression) is present that presents a danger to the patient or others or is very distressing to the patient (16). Importantly, these drugs are not indicated for controlling wandering or swearing. The usual dosages for these drugs are listed above (see Late-Life Schizophrenia or Paraphrenia). After target symptoms have been controlled for several months, the dosage can often be lowered, and drugs can be discontinued in about one-fourth of patients. Patients taking these drugs must be monitored for two common side effects, orthostatic hypotension and extrapyramidal symptoms (see details in Chapter 25). If only insomnia is a problem, trazodone, 50 to 100 mg at bedtime, causes the least paradoxical agitation and the least daytime drowsiness.

Aggressive behavior may be treated with antipsychotic drugs or divalproex sodium (Depakote). The starting dosage of the latter is 125 mg daily, in a pill or sprinkles. The dosage can be increased cautiously to 250 mg twice daily. Dosage should be adjusted based on clinical response and blood levels. Ataxia/delirium or gastrointestinal distress can occur. Antipsychotic drugs are associated with increased mortality at 12 weeks in patients with dementia and agitation and psychosis.

Depression is present in at least 20% of patients with dementia (17–18). When it has the characteristics of an adjustment disorder or demoralized state (see above), it is best managed with supportive therapy (see Chapter 20). However, major depressions with symptoms of early morning awakening, anorexia, self-blame, worthlessness, nihilistic attitudes, or morbid hypochondriasis also occur and should be treated with antidepressants. Their treatment is discussed under major depression, above.

In a *catastrophic reaction*, an overwhelming sense of frustration, fear, anger, or anxiety occurs when the patients are brought into a situation in which they are forced to confront their failing aptitudes. These poorly controlled emotions further impair the patient's already limited functional ability, leading to total decompensation of a previously coping patient.

Case Study

A 72-year-old woman with a history of several small strokes experienced moderate forgetfulness and confusion but was generally calm and pleasant. Keeping track of the date with a calendar and making copious notes to herself, she managed to maintain an independent existence at home. At the supermarket checkout counter she could not find her wallet but insisted she had money to pay for her food. The clerk grew impatient, and the patient became increasingly agitated, tearful, and accusatory. When the store manager was called, she picked up grocery items and began throwing them.

These catastrophic reactions can have an adverse impact on both the patient and the patient's family. The explanation of their cause and their prevention through avoidance of provoking circumstances can forestall the need for institutionalization. The use of small dosages of an antipsychotic drug (see Late-Life Schizophrenia or Paraphrenia, above) may be beneficial in patients in whom episodes like this recur despite the caregiver's best efforts.

4. *Family support.* Family distress is common. Its treatment begins with the assessment. The problem-solving approach outlined under step 3 above gives families a sense of control and the hope that most problems can be managed despite the irreversibility and probable progression of the underlying disorder (19). Feelings of guilt, anger, discouragement, and demoralization are common, as are concerns about loss of friends, hobbies, and leisure time; family conflicts; and worry that the principal caregiver will become ill. Allowing families time to express these feelings and concerns and acknowledging that they are common can be helpful. Referring them to support groups can also be helpful. There is evidence from one controlled trial that a combination of counseling that addresses caregivers' needs and support group participation can delay the need for nursing home placement of demented patients, in this study for an average of 329 days (20).

   The *Alzheimer Disease Association* can provide information about nearby resources and has a toll-free telephone number (1-800-272-3900 and website (http://www.alz.org/). It is also helpful to recommend a book, such as *The 36-Hour Day* (see www.hopkinsbayview.org/PAMreferences), which explains dementia and offers practical advice for dealing with the vexing problems created by a demented family member.

5. *Longitudinal care.* Because the dementing illnesses are progressive (new symptoms appear while old symptoms worsen), expected changes should be described to families. It is also prudent to discuss the possibility of eventual nursing home placement soon after the diagnosis is made. Although most families report that they do not want to place their loved one in a nursing home, it is important to urge them not to promise this unconditionally because medical issues or behavioral problems may necessitate placement. The family's emotional needs may change over time. A nonjudgmental

listening approach helps family members to feel supported.

6. *Decisions about limiting therapy.* Chapter 13 describes the processes whereby patients and their families may plan in advance the limitation of therapy (living wills and other forms of advance directives) and the delegation of decision making to others. These processes are especially important in planning the care of a demented patient early in the patient's course of dementia.

Drugs for Dementia

Three cholinesterase inhibitors have been approved for the treatment of cognitive impairment in patients with AD. Their effectiveness is quite modest (about 6 months improvement in some measures of cognitive function on average). All cause GI side effects (nausea, vomiting, and diarrhea), anorexia, and gait disorder. The starting dosage of donepezil (Aricept) is 5 mg at bedtime. If no side effects develop it should be increased to 10 mg at bedtime in 4 to 6 weeks. Rivastigmine (Exelon) is started at 15 mg twice daily and increased monthly to 6 mg twice a day. Galantamine (Razadyne) is started at 4 mg twice a day and increased monthly to a total of 16 or 24 mg daily. Memantine (Namenda) has been approved for the treatment of moderate-severe AD. It is started at 5 mg daily and increased weekly in 5 mg intervals to 10 mg twice daily if tolerated.

Ginkgo biloba, an herbal alternative, has been shown to improve cognitive and social functioning modestly in one study, but this has not been replicated (21,22). Side effects, most commonly gastrointestinal complaints or headaches, are rare (see Chapter 5).

Delirium

Definition and Diagnosis

The essential features of delirium are cognitive impairment, clouding of consciousness, and difficulty sustaining and shifting attention. Delirium usually has rapid onset, brief duration, and marked fluctuation throughout the day. Delirious patients may appear drowsy or hyperalert (hypervigilant), trail off in the middle of sentences, fail to answer questions or ask that questions be repeated, or appear perplexed. Perceptual disturbances such as illusions (misinterpretations of real external stimuli) or hallucinations are common. Delirium is especially common in patients with dementia. Although patients with either dementia or delirium may experience memory impairment, disorientation, hallucinations, delusions, and disturbed thinking, the patient with dementia is alert, whereas the delirious patient is drowsy and fluctuates in alertness over minutes or hours. The abrupt onset of delirium (within hours or days) differs from dementia, which develops over months or years in most instances.

The presence of cognitive impairment and rapid fluctuation distinguishes delirium from schizophrenia and other psychotic disorders. The hallucinations and delusions associated with delirium are often fleeting and poorly systematized in comparison with those of other psychotic disorders, in which they are sustained and well organized. The electroencephalogram (EEG) in the delirious patient often reveals a generalized slowing of background activity, whereas the EEG is generally normal in schizophrenic and depressed patients.

In some patients, the manifestations of delirium may be so subtle that they are not recognized by an examiner who is unfamiliar with the patient's baseline status. At other times the symptoms suggest depression, dementia, or schizophrenia. Older age is a strong risk factor for developing delirium but underlying dementia is the single

TABLE 26.3 Etiologic Classification of Delirium

In a medical or surgical illness (no focal or lateralizing neurologic signs; cerebrospinal fluid usually clear)
Metabolic disorders: hepatic stupor, uremia, hypoxia, hypercapnia, hypoglycemia, porphyria, hyponatremia
Congestive heart failure
Pneumonia, septicemia, typhoid fever, other febrile illnesses (especially in elderly)
Hyperthyroidism and hypothyroidism
Postoperative and posttraumatic states
In neurologic disease that causes focal or lateralizing signs or changes in the cerebrospinal fluid
Cerebrovascular disease
Subarachnoid hemorrhage
Hypertensive encephalopathy
Cerebral contusion
Subdural hematoma
Tumor
Abscess
Meningitis
Encephalitis
Status epilepticus (by electroencephalogram)
The abstinence states and exogenous intoxications (signs of other medical surgical, and neurologic illnesses absent or coincidental)
Withdrawal of alcohol (delirium tremens), barbiturates, and nonbarbiturate sedative drugs, following chronic intoxication
Drug intoxication from benzodiazepines, opiates, neuroleptics, antidepressants, antihistamines, H_2 blockers, centrally acting antihypertensives, anticholinergics, digitalis, illicit drugs (see Chapter 29), etc.
Beclouded dementia
Any dementing or other brain disease in combination with infective fevers, drug reactions, heart failure, or other medical or surgical disease

Adapted from Adams RD. Delirium and other acute confusional states. In: Isselbacher KJ, Adams RD, Braunwald E, et al., eds. Harrison's principles of internal medicine, 9th ed. New York: McGraw-Hill, 1980:126.

strongest risk factor. Delirium can be precipitated by many drugs and acute medical illnesses, drug toxicity, and dehydration.

The key to accurate diagnosis of delirium is a high index of suspicion in any elderly patient with a history of recent or sudden change in mental status and behavior (23). The EEG shows diffuse slowing in both delirium and dementia. In delirium, the EEG slowing is often marked, even when the cognitive and behavioral impairment is minor; conversely, severe cognitive impairment and a mildly abnormal EEG are most common in dementia.

Etiologic Evaluation

Delirium can result from a wide range of organic causes that adversely affect brain metabolism (Table 26.3). Special attention should be given to medications in the elderly because they may produce a delirium at therapeutic dosages. β-Blockers, H_2 blockers, benzodiazepines, and the many compounds with anticholinergic activity are common causes of delirium. Although electrolyte disturbances are the most common metabolic cause of delirium, any disorder of metabolic homeostasis can cause delirium. Withdrawal from alcohol or sedatives is often overlooked in the elderly as a possible cause of delirium. Multiple causes are suspected, and no one specific cause is identified in 30% to 50% of cases. When there is no obvious cause for a patient's apparent delirium, an EEG may be helpful in confirming that delirium is present.

The key to treatment is the identification of the underlying causes when they can be identified. The physical, neurologic, and laboratory examination should focus on causes that are likely in a particular patient. Attention to nutrition, fluid intake, and electrolyte balance is crucial (23).

The treatment of the behavioral and emotional complications of delirium can become as urgent as the identification of the underlying cause. Frequent reorientation and reassurance, a well-lighted environment, and avoidance of overstimulation are important aspects of treatment. If the agitation, hallucinations, or delusions do not respond to environmental intervention and are overwhelming to the patient or adversely affecting the patient's safety, then a low dosage antipsychotic drug given by mouth or intramuscularly (e.g., haloperidol, 0.5 to 1.0 mg every 4 hours) can be ordered.

SPECIFIC REFERENCES*

1. Folstein MF, Folstein SE, McHugh PR. "Mini-mental state": a practical method for grading the cognitive state of patients for the clinician. J Psychiatr Res 1975;12:1975.
2. Gallo JJ, Rabins PV, Lyketsos CG, et al. Depression without sadness: functional outcomes of nondysphoric depression in later life. J Am Geriatr Soc 1997;45:570.
3. Alexopoulos G, Meyer BS, Young, RC, et al. The course of geriatric depression with "reversible dementia." Am J Psychiatry 1993;150:1693.
4. Rabins PV, Merchant A, Nesdadt G. Criteria for diagnosing reversible dementia caused by depression: validation by 2-year follow-up. Br J Psychiatry 1984;144:488.
5. **5.** Lyketsos CG, Sheppard J-ME, Steele CD, et al. Randomized placebo-controlled, double-blind clinical trial of sertraline in the treatment of depression complicating Alzheimer's disease: initial results from the depression in Alzheimer's disease study. Am J Psychiatry 2000;157:1686.
6. Lee PE, Sykora K, Gill SS, et al. Antipsychotic medications and drug-induced movement disorders other than parkinsonism. JAGS 2005;53:374.
7. **7.** Schneider LS, Dagerman KS, Insel P. Risk of death with atypical antipsychotic drug treatment for dementia. JAMA 2005;294:1934.
8. Wang PS, Schneeweiss S, Avorn J, et al. Risk of death elderly users of conventional vs. atypical antipsychotic medications. N Engl J Med. 2005; 353:2335.
9. Petersen RC, Smith GE, Waring SC, et al. Mild cognitive impairment: clinical characterization and outcome. Arch Neurol 1999;56:303.
10. Rabins PV. Does reversible dementia exist and is it reversible?. Arch Intern Med 1988;148:1905.
11. Hendrie HC, Ogunnixi A, Hall KS, et al. Incidence of dementia and Alzheimer disease in 2 communities—Yoruba residing in Ibadan, Nigeria and African Americans residing in Indianapolis, Indiana. JAMA 2001;6:739.
12. Rabins PV, Lyketsos CG, Steele, C. Practical dementia care. Oxford, New York, 2006.
13. **13.** Knopman DS, Dekosky ST, Cummings JL, et al. Practice parameter: diagnosis of dementia (an evidence-based review). Report of the quality standards subcommittee of the American Academy of Neurology. Neurology 2001;56:1143.
14. **14.** Small GW, Rabins PV, Barry PP, et al. Diagnosis and treatment of Alzheimer disease and related disorders: consensus statement of the American Association of Geriatric Psychiatry, the Alzheimer's Association, and the American Geriatrics Society. JAMA 1997;278:1363.
15. **15.** Woods B, Spector A, Jones C, et al. Reminiscence therapy for dementia. Cochrane Database Sys Rev 2004: CD001120. DOI: 10.1002/14651858.CD001120.pub2.
16. Rabins PV, Lyketsos CG. Antipsychotic drugs in dementia: what should be made of the risks? JAMA 2005;294:1963.
17. Burns A, Jacoby R, Levy R. Psychiatric phenomena in Alzheimer's disease. III. Disorders of mood. Br J Psychiatry 1990;157:81.
18. Rovner B, Broadhead J, Spencer M, et al. Depression and Alzheimer's disease. Am J Psychiatry 1989;146:350.
19. **19.** Teri L, Logsdon R, Uomoto J, et al. Behavioral treatment of depression in dementia patients: a controlled clinical trial. J Gerontol Psychol Sci 1997;52B:P159.
20. **20.** Mittelman MS, Ferris SH, Shulman E, et al. A family intervention to delay nursing home placement of patients with Alzheimer disease. JAMA 1996;276:1725.
21. **21.** Lebars PL, Katz MH, Berman N, et al. A placebo-controlled, double-blind, randomized trial of an extract of Ginkgo biloba for dementia. JAMA 1997;340:1136.
22. **22.** Ernst E, Pittler MH. Ginkgo biloba for dementia: a systematic review of double-blind, placebo-controlled trials. Clin Drug Invest 1999;17: 301.
23. **23.** Inouye SK, Bogardus ST, Charpentier PA, et al. A multi-component intervention to prevent delirium in hospitalized older patient. N Engl J Med 1999;340:669.

*Bold numerals denote published controlled clinical trials, meta-analyses, or consensus-based recommendations.

*For annotated **General References** and resources related to this chapter, visit www.hopkinsbayview.org/PAMreferences.*

Chapter 27

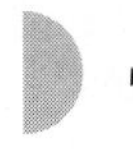

Tobacco Use and Dependence

David W. Blodgett

Tobacco use, primarily in the form of chronic cigarette smoking, is the greatest single cause of illness, disability, and death in the United States. Smoking is estimated to cause more than 440,000 deaths annually—almost 20% of all deaths.

The perniciousness of the habit relates largely to its long history of social acceptability and to the failure by society and by health professionals to recognize and respond to smoking as a health-damaging behavior. This situation has been changing, and it continues to change. Within the United States and many other countries, both society and health professionals are now acting to proscribe, prevent, restrict, and treat smoking. Still, much remains to be done. The prevalence and acceptability of smoking remain high in many subgroups and in many countries. The World Health Organization (WHO) estimates that worldwide tobacco-related deaths will increase from 3 million annually in 1990 to more than 8 million annually in 2020.

PREVALENCE OF TOBACCO USE

The decline of smoking prevalence in the United States in recent decades represents an impressive success of public health and prevention efforts. Beginning in 1965, adult smoking prevalence declined by 0.5% to 1.0% per year, from 42% in 1965 to 25% in 1993. The rate of decline has now slowed; total prevalence fell only two and a half more percentage points over the next 9 years, to 22.5% in 2002. Smoking is becoming concentrated in more resistant individuals. Table 27.1 summarizes the prevalence of adult cigarette smoking in relation to demographic characteristics for the 2002 National Health Interview Survey. There are substantial differences among demographic subgroups. Smoking is more common in poor communities and least common among the highly educated.

Smoking prevalence has been fairly constant in recent years among U.S. adults and adolescents. Prior to 2002, smoking rates had increased among high school students. That trend has since stabilized. Currently 22.9% of high school students in the United States are cigarette smokers.

TABLE 27.1 Percentage of Adults (Age, ≥18 yr) Who Smoke Cigarettes, United States, 2002

Parameter	*Men*	*Women*	*Total*
Race/Ethnicity			
White	25.5	21.8	23.6
African American	27.1	18.7	22.4
Hispanic	22.7	10.8	16.7
Native American	40.5	40.9	40.8
Asian/Pacific	19.0	6.5	13.3
Years of education (for ages ≥25 yr only)			
9–11	38.1	30.9	27.6
12	29.8	22.1	25.6
13–15	24.5	20.6	22.3
≥16	10.7	8.45	9.65
Age (yr)			
18–24	32.4	24.6	28.5
25–44	28.7	22.8	25.7
45–64	24.5	21.1	22.7
≥65	10.1	8.6	9.3
Socioeconomic status			
At or above poverty level	24.8	19.7	22.2
Below poverty level	36.9	30.1	32.9
Total	25.2	20.0	22.5

From Centers for Disease Control. Morb Mortal Wkly Rep May 28, 2004;53:427.

Each day nearly 4,000 young people between the ages of 12 and 17 years initiate cigarette smoking in the United States. Of these 2,000 will become daily cigarette smokers. Adult smoking prevalence is highest among Native Americans, fairly similar among African Americans and whites, somewhat lower among Hispanics (especially Hispanic women), and lowest in Asian/Pacific Americans. In contrast, adolescent prevalence is appreciably lower among African Americans than whites, with Hispanics intermediate; daily smoking prevalence for high school students in 2003 were 25.5% of whites, 20.5% of Hispanics, 14.3% of African Americans, and 12.8% of Asian Americans. Other forms of tobacco use occur predominantly in males: pipe and cigar use in approximately 3% and 5%, respectively, and use of smokeless products (snuff, chewing tobacco) in approximately 6%. However, in some locales and subgroups (e.g., young men in rural or southern areas), the prevalence of smokeless tobacco use may approximate that of smoking.

CAUSES AND RISK FACTORS

The development of tobacco dependence can be viewed as a pediatric disorder. Smoking typically begins in the preteen or teenage years; initiation after 22 years of age is rare. The habit is so widespread that it is not limited to any specific environmental, physiologic, or psychological circumstances. Social influences, such as peer pressures or efforts to display independence and to appear mature and self-confident, are major factors in promoting and sustaining initial smoking experiences. Aversive experiences (e.g., coughing, nausea, dysphoria) are described during the initiation phases of smoking, even by those who proceed to lifelong dependence. Nicotine is the causative pharmacologic agent responsible for establishing and maintaining tobacco use and addiction. The continued easy availability of nicotine-delivering tobacco products, combined with strong learned behavioral habits, memories, and associations, make tobacco use a truly addictive disorder—with characteristic resistance to change (1).

About half of individuals who smoke for 1 month become chronically dependent (2). Certain risk factors are associated with an increased likelihood of becoming a chronic cigarette smoker. Smoking runs in families. An individual with parents and siblings who smoke is four times as likely to become a smoker as is an individual from a nonsmoking family. The familial association results from both genetic and environmental factors. Twin studies indicate an approximately 50% heritability of smoking (3). Other studies suggest that genetic variations in cytochrome P-450, dopamine receptor and transporter, and serotonin transporter genes influence the propensity toward smoking (4). Smoking is also significantly associated with adverse childhood experiences; violence in the family, childhood abuse, and stressful life events are each associated with a two- to fourfold increase in the probability of being a smoker (5,6). In the past, males were more much likely to smoke than females, but this is no longer the case. Alarmingly, it has been well documented that female smokers have a more difficult time quitting smoking than males, perhaps related to differences in reasons for smoking initiation, psychological addiction, and self image (weight gain) (7). There is no distinct personality type that is characteristic of smokers, but on average they tend to be somewhat more extroverted than nonsmokers, more adventuresome or risk taking, and more likely to deviate from social norms or rules. These latter characteristics may, in adolescence, increase the probability of experimentation with smoking, with a consequent increased risk of chronic dependence. Smoking is often referred to as a "gateway drug." Smoking is more prevalent in individuals with other substance use disorders (e.g., 70% to 90% prevalence in alcoholics and other drug abusers). Smoking adolescents are also more likely to have unplanned pregnancies, participate in violent acts, to be involved in automobile accidents or other high-risk activities.

PRIMARY PREVENTION

Primary prevention efforts must be directed to preadolescents and adolescents. An important element is changing societal norms about the acceptability of tobacco use. Formal preventive interventions should begin in elementary grades and continue for several years. Effective interventions are not simple fact-based health education, but instead teach specific skills for resisting social pressure and rejecting enticing tobacco advertising messages. They include explicit instructions and rehearsals with peers in vignettes about resisting offers to use cigarettes, alcohol products, and illegal drugs. Children who receive such training have reduced rates of smoking onset (8). As community health leaders, physicians should encourage and support preventive interventions, including bans on tobacco use in public areas, enforcement of prohibitions on tobacco sales to minors, increasing the price of tobacco, and restrictions on advertising that glamorizes smoking or appeals to youth.

COURSE OF THE HABIT

The health hazards of smoking are now widely recognized, and the social acceptability of smoking has declined. Consequently, most smokers vacillate between defending and justifying their habit and trying to end it. Seventy percent of smokers report wanting to quit, and about half attempt to stop in a given year. Adverse health events and advice from physicians are potent forces in promoting increased cessation efforts by patients. In the United States there are now about twice as many former smokers as there are current smokers.

Patterns of Quitting and Relapse

Approximately 60% to 80% of smokers who attempt to quit achieve at least a minimal period of abstinence. However, the relapse rate is high, most occurring very quickly after quitting (9). Approximately two thirds of quitters resume smoking within 3 to 6 months, many within only a few days. Only 15% to 20% of untreated quitters remain cigarette-free for 6 months or longer. Treatment approximately doubles the long-term success rate, but relapse, repeat quit attempts, and repeat treatments are commonplace. Cessation should not be considered successful until abstinence has been sustained for at least 6 months. The probability of relapse after 6 months of abstinence is reduced but still present.

Approximately 95% of smoking cessation occurs as the result of smokers' self-directed personal efforts, without formal treatment. Abrupt ("cold turkey") cessation is more likely to be successful than is gradual reduction. Most successful quitters require more than one attempt before becoming permanent ex-smokers. Repeated quitting and relapsing are characteristic of the normal, successful cessation process. Success should be applauded with each quit attempt, as each attempt brings a greater likelihood that the next attempt will be successful. The *risk of relapse is increased* when patients are under emotional stress (e.g., anger, frustration, anxiety, depression), when ex-smokers are exposed to cues associated with prior smoking (e.g., after meals, when consuming alcoholic beverages), and in people whose spouse or friends continue to smoke (10).

HEALTH CONSEQUENCES

Risk of Disease

Although smoking dramatically increases overall population morbidity and mortality, its effects on individual smokers are unpredictable, and some smokers escape major health consequences. Age-adjusted mortality rates for smokers are 70% greater than those for nonsmokers. Smoking significantly shortens life expectancy (e.g., 8.1 years less for the 30-year-old two-pack-a-day smoker than for a comparable nonsmoker). Risk is dose related; mortality increases with increasing number of cigarettes smoked, with increasing number of years as a smoker, and with depth of inhalation.

Smoking is associated with an astounding list of health related effects. Most notably, it has been linked to increased risk of cancer (especially of the respiratory tract); cardiovascular disease; chronic obstructive pulmonary disease (COPD); gastric ulcer; breast; prostate and cervix; postmenopausal osteoporosis, diabetes, and macular degeneration. Smoking by pregnant women reduces fetal growth and birth weight and increases the risk of fetal death; smoking interacts with the use of oral contraceptives by women and increases the risk of myocardial infarction (MI), subarachnoid hemorrhage, and thromboembolic disease.

The *risks of cancer and chronic pulmonary disease* in smokers are ten times those in nonsmokers (30% of all cancers have been linked to tobacco use). The percentage of oral, throat, and lung cancer deaths attributable to smoking exceeds 80%. The *risk of atherosclerotic cardiovascular disease* is approximately doubled in smokers. The percentage of cardiovascular disease deaths attributable to smoking is 20%. In sum, tobacco smoking is the single largest underlying cause of death. The morbidity and mortality as well as the economic toll brought on by the use of tobacco present at once a perplexing problem, as well as a golden opportunity to improve health.

Benefits of Cessation

The greatest immediate benefit of smoking cessation is the reduction of cardiovascular risk. Within hours after smoking cessation, both carbon monoxide and nicotine are dissipated from the body, with a consequent reduction in cardiac work requirement and a concurrent increase in oxygenation. There is also prompt reduction in the risk of upper respiratory tract infection (URTI). Slower to accrue are a reduction in the rate of decline of pulmonary function and a reduction in cancer risk; benefits of cessation are measurable in these domains within 3 and 10 years, respectively, after smoking cessation. The risk of coronary artery disease (CAD) and death 15 to 20 years after quitting is similar to that of the nonsmoker.

Health benefits of smoking cessation are greater for smokers who quit before the development of symptoms; however, the benefits of cessation also extend to those who have already experienced symptoms of smoking-related disease. For example, individuals who stop smoking after MI have improved survival rates compared with those who continue smoking. Similarly, there are pulmonary benefits to smoking cessation even late in life (11).

Low-Yield Cigarettes

Because the risks of smoking are dose related, it is tempting to believe that substantial health benefits might be achieved by switching to low-yield cigarettes. This is not the case; the variations in currently marketed tobacco yields have little health impact, and there are negligible correlations between the stated yield values and blood levels of nicotine and its major metabolite, cotinine (12). Biologic yield may differ substantially from stated yield because of behavioral variations in the way the cigarettes are smoked. When nominal yields change, smokers tend to change their behavior so as to keep biologic delivery unchanged (e.g., by smoking more cigarettes, inhaling more smoke). The primary manufacturing technique for producing current low-yield cigarettes is to place ventilation holes in the sides of the filter to dilute the smoke stream with air. With these low-yield brands it is especially likely that biologic delivery will significantly exceed assay delivery, because the smoker's fingers and lips tend to block these ventilation holes (13). Smokers should be cautioned that so-called low-yield cigarettes will not decrease the health-related risks of smoking.

Physical Dependence and Craving

Chronic tobacco use produces physical dependence on nicotine. On cessation of use, an *abstinence syndrome* typically occurs (14–16). The subjective aspects of the syndrome can be very distressing and include irritability, restlessness, sleep disturbances, difficulty in concentrating, anxiety, gastrointestinal (GI) disturbances, hunger, weight gain, and, most important, craving for cigarettes. Most patients feel normal again within approximately 2 weeks of abstinence, except that the craving for tobacco may persist for months or years. Nicotine substitution treatment is effective in reducing the abstinence syndrome. The physiologic aspects of the tobacco abstinence syndrome are generally inconsequential, consisting of a slight and gradual decline in heart rate and blood pressure.

Craving for tobacco is an extraordinarily persistent obstacle to sustained abstinence. Many ex-smokers report cravings years after cessation. The duration of craving is highly variable, but it should be expected to persist for at least 3 to 6 months, with its frequency and urgency diminishing over that interval. Craving may be a learned phenomenon rather than part of an abstinence syndrome, because it is high even among smokers making no attempt to quit or reduce their smoking.

Passive Smoking

Passive smoking exposure of nonsmokers to air contaminated by the smoking of others is not only an irritant to many nonsmokers; it has definite adverse health effects. There are significant health risks associated with passive smoking (17–20). Passive exposure to the smoke of spouses is associated with impaired pulmonary function, increased lung cancer risk, and increased coronary heart disease risk. Children passively exposed to smoke by parents have increased rates of respiratory infections, slower developmental increases in pulmonary function, and an increased incidence of asthma attacks. Maternal smoking contributes to reduced birth weight, and smokers who stop the habit during pregnancy have significantly heavier babies than do those who continue smoking (21).

Physicians should try to protect nonsmokers from cigarette smoke and should recognize that most indoor ventilation systems simply diffuse and redistribute smoke rather than remove it. Smoking (including employee smoking) should be emphatically prohibited in physicians' offices, and physicians should support similar efforts in all public settings, especially in health care facilities. Legal prohibition of indoor smoking in public or commercial facilities is now common.

RECOGNITION AND DIAGNOSIS

Nicotine dependence is a diagnosable substance use disorder in the American Psychiatric Association's *Diagnostic and Statistical Manual of Mental Disorders, 4th Edition* (*DSM-IV*). The diagnostic criteria are identical to those for other substance-related disorders (see Chapter 29), reflecting the growing recognition of extensive commonalities among alcoholism, drug abuse, and tobacco dependence.

There is widespread failure of health professionals to recognize and diagnose tobacco dependence and to maintain it on an active problem list. Tobacco use status should be considered at every visit at the office reception point (22). There should be a clear and prominent chart cue to prompt attention at subsequent visits.

Assessment of smoking status is normally via practitioner questioning and patient self-report. Smoking status can be assessed by measuring carbon monoxide concentrations in expired breath (concentrations greater than 5 to 8 ppm normally indicate smoking). Urine and saliva test-strips for detection of nicotine or its metabolites have been developed.

TREATMENT

Substantial evidence, assistive materials, and pharmacologic modalities are now available for the rational planning and implementation of smoking cessation interventions with patients. They are summarized here.

Role of the Health Care Provider

Concern about health remains the most cited reason smokers quit, and smokers cite physicians as the people most able to influence their decisions to attempt to quit. The optimal role of a physician or other health care practitioner in the treatment of tobacco dependence is to advise and assist all smoking patients to stop. It is a mistake to rely heavily on referral to specialized smoking cessation programs. Results of referral are disappointing when compared with those obtained by devoting equal or less time to brief direct advice.

Brief advice can significantly increase rates of smoking cessation (23,24). A rigorous review of more than 39 studies (with more than 31,000 smokers) found that physician advice resulted in a small but significant increase in the odds of quitting. Although counseling effectiveness is not necessarily related to the intensity of advice, direct comparisons of minimal advice versus intensive counseling found a small advantage for intensive advice; direct comparisons also suggested additional benefit for followup visits. (25). Medical economic analyses have shown that smoking cessation advice is as cost-effective as other common interventions, such as treatment of hypercholesterolemia or mild hypertension. An increase in smoking cessation rates of between 3% and 5% can be expected if practitioners simply caution each smoker to quit during routine office visits for other problems. Addition of pharmacologic treatment further increases success. Among certain patients, advice alone can achieve impressive efficacy. For example, the smoking cessation rate after a first myocardial infarction is as high as 50% for patients given directive smoking cessation advice by their physician, compared with approximately 35% for patients receiving usual care. Similarly high rates of cessation are seen in prenatal care settings, where up to 20% to 30% of smokers may quit during a pregnancy (21).

Consistency of Counseling

Despite its known benefits, the frequency and consistency of physician counseling to quit smoking remain disappointing. Fewer than 50% of smokers report receiving smoking cessation advice from their physician (26,27). Patients who are younger, male, African American, uninsured, healthier, or lighter smokers are less likely to report receiving physician advice to quit smoking. This may be related to frequency of patient health care contacts, or physicians' likelihood to counsel may be influenced by patient characteristics (26,28).

Absolute rates of smoking cessation in response to physician advice are likely to remain frustratingly low. But, it is important to recognize that the overall public health benefit may be very large because of the number of smokers counseled. Routine smoking cessation advice from physicians plays an important role in reducing overall societal smoking rates (29). Further, although patients may not immediately quit smoking as a result of direct physician advice, such counseling may play an important role in increasing readiness to quit smoking in the future (30).

Motivational Communication

The goal of effective doctor–patient communication is to provide advice that maximizes a smoker's motivation and decision to quit. A common error is to rely too much on fact-based health education that implicitly seeks to motivate through fear. Smokers are now well aware of the health risks of smoking and do not respond to that information alone. The five actions described later in this chapter (see Recommended Office Approach) integrate what is known about motivational communication into a practical approach for helping smokers to quit. The approach includes many of the behavioral strategies described in Chapter 4. It focuses on one clear and simple message—"I strongly advise you to quit"—delivered in a manner free of blame or rancor. *The advice should be personally relevant to patients, should describe in a positive way the benefits to be gained, and should prescribe a particular course of action.* These three objectives can be attained by pointing out the association between smoking and the specific symptoms, illnesses, or health risks of the individual patient; by pointing out that smoking cessation can prevent, reverse, or stop the progression of disease (whichever is appropriate); and by stating clearly, simply, and directly the course of action to be taken: stop smoking. A general statement that "Smoking is bad for your health and you can kill yourself if you continue" fails on all three of these points. It is not specifically personal, it describes no benefit, and it is not sufficiently directive. More personalized and directive statements can be more persuasive (e.g., "I strongly advise you to stop smoking; both your coughing and your recurring colds and flus are caused in part by your smoking; I want you to try to quit smoking, and then we should see some improvement").

Patients differ in their readiness and willingness to change their smoking habit. The goal is to move patients along the continuum depicted in Fig. 4.1. When patients are ready to attempt cessation, the goal should be to agree on a cessation date and to provide therapeutic assistance. Patients not yet ready for cessation may become ready in response to repeated nonjudgmental encouragement and motivational advice.

Brochures and Self-Help Materials

Self-help smoking cessation brochures can provide useful motivational advice and specific helpful techniques for smokers. Local health departments have developed excellent resources to help patients quite smoking. Additionally, local offices of the American Cancer Society, the American Heart Association (AHA), or the American Lung Association can be contacted to obtain copies of their smoking cessation self-help brochures. An excellent product, *You Can Quit Smoking,* is available from the Agency for Healthcare Research and Qualtiy (AHRQ) online at http://www.surgeongeneral.gov/tobacco/consorder.pdf, or by calling 1-800-358-9295. Patients with Internet access can also be referred to a wide range of smoking cessation self-help aids, programs, and support groups available on the Internet (see *www.hopkinsbayview.org/PAMreferences*).

TABLE 27.2 Summary of Smoking Cessation Products

Type and Brand Name	Dosage	Package	2005 Retail Cost[a]	Comments
OTC Products				
Nicotine gum				
Nicorette (also as generic)	2 mg × 9–24/day	110 pieces 48 pieces	$47 ($36) $31	Give special instructions on how to "chew-and-park" the gum.
	4 mg × 9–24/day	110 pieces 48 pieces	$56 (42)$33	Absorption is through oral mucosa. Emphasize importance of adequate use. Target is 9–24 per day for 4–6 weeks, then gradual tapering over 2–4 weeks.
Nicotine patch				
NicoDerm CQ	7, 14, 21 mg/24 hr	14 patches	$47 ($38)	Target is maintenance for 4–10 weeks, possibly followed by gradual dosage tapering over 2–6 weeks.
Nicotrol	5, 10, 15 mg/16 hr	14 patches	$47	Step approach step one (15 mg) for weeks 1–6 Step 2 (10 mg) for weeks 7–8 and Step 3 (5 mg) for weeks 9–10
Generic	7, 14, 21 mg/24 hr	14 patches	$26–$38	
Lozenge				
Commit Lozenges	2, 4 mg x 7–25/day	48 pieces 72 pieces	$31 $40	Target is one lozenge every 1–2 hours for first 6 weeks, tapering off by week 12
Prescription Products				
Nicotine nasal spray				
Nicotrol NS	1 mg × 8–40 mg/day 2 sprays = 1 mg	100 mg	$46	Target is maintenance for 6 or more weeks, possibly followed by gradual tapering of use, up to 12 weeks total. Provides most rapid onset of nicotine effects.
Nicotine vapor inhaler				
Nicotrol inhaler	10 mg/cartridge delivers 4 mg	168 cartridges	$168	Absorption is via oral mucosa, not lungs. Similar in appearance to a cigarette; may simulate sensory/manipulation aspects of smoking. 6 to 16 cartridges per day for up to 12 weeks.
Bupropion SR Zyban (also as generic)	150 mg (1/day × 3 days then 2/day)	60 tablets	$149 ($98)	Begin 1 week before quit date No dosage tapering needed. May be combined with NRT for greater total effectiveness.

[a]Based on large pharmacy chain in Baltimore, Maryland region, June 2005.

Pharmacologic Treatments

There have been substantial advances in recent years in the availability of pharmacologic treatments for tobacco dependence. Nicotine chewing gum, lozenge, and transdermal patch products are now available over the counter without prescription. Other types of nicotine replacement treatment products are available by prescription, including nicotine nasal spray and nicotine vapor inhaler. Also, bupropion, the first non-nicotine smoking cessation product, is available by prescription. Table 27.2 summarizes characteristics and 2005 costs of these products. Table 27.3 compares *the costs of smoking and the costs of pharmacologic treatment* with available products.

Mechanism and Indication

Smoking cessation medications are intended to aid patients who are making a serious attempt to stop tobacco use. They will not themselves induce such an attempt. They

TABLE 27.3 Cost of Smoking versus Cost of Treatment

Annual Cost of Smoking	Cigarette Packs Per Day ½	1	2
Price per pack[a]			
$3	$548	$1095	$2190
$4	$730	$1460	$2920
$5	$913	$1825	$3650
Cost of Treatment[b]			
Nicotine gum	$190		
Nicotine Lozenges	$270		
Nicotine patch	$165		
Nicotine nasal spray	$310		
Nicotine inhaler	$525		
Bupropion	$300		

[a]Varies by region and taxation.
[b]Estimates based on current retail prices and typical 8-wk treatment course.

enhance the success of motivated behavior change efforts but do not cause or motivate such behavior change directly. Nicotine replacement products suppress the nicotine abstinence syndrome and reduce subjective desire or craving for tobacco. The mechanism of bupropion's efficacy is uncertain, although it also appears to suppress nicotine withdrawal and craving and to help treat comorbidities that might favor sustained smoking. Medications are to be used in conjunction with a complete cessation of tobacco use. If tobacco use persists beyond the first couple of weeks of treatment, the medication should probably be discontinued until some future renewed effort at total cessation is attempted.

Efficacy

Strong data support the efficacy of all these marketed treatments, but none is clearly superior (31–34). Meta-analyses quantifying their effectiveness are summarized in the recent clinical practice guideline released by the surgeon general (31). All have been shown to increase smoking cessation rates by approximately 50% to 100% over placebo comparison conditions. The absolute rates of smoking cessation depend on many factors: patient motivation and setting, intensity of concurrent behavioral counseling, definition of cessation, and time of assessment. Most clinical efficacy trials described in product labeling are conducted in patients sufficiently motivated to volunteer for smoking cessation treatment and in conjunction with individual or group counseling; success is generally defined as 4 weeks of smoking abstinence during active treatment. Under these conditions cessation success rates of 30% to 50% are often achieved in active medication groups, compared with rates of 10% to 30% in placebo groups. Success rates decline to half of these values when assessed 6 to 12 months after the end of treatment. Despite variations in the absolute rates of success, the relative efficacy of active pharmacologic treatment over placebo is robust and is preserved across different populations, settings, counseling levels, and followup periods.

Nicotine Patch

The nicotine transdermal patch is the treatment of choice at present. This preference relates primarily to its ease of use and relatively good patient compliance. Patches may be worn for either 24 or 16 hours per day with equivalent effectiveness. The rationale for 24-hour use is to minimize nicotine withdrawal on waking. The rationale for 16-hour (daytime only) use is to minimize sleep disturbances that may accompany 24-hour use. The most common side effect is skin irritation at the site of patch application. In a placebo-controlled trial, the nicotine patch was shown to be effective and safe for use in a wide spectrum of patients with chronic cardiac problems (32). While emerging evidence suggests that nicotine contributes to the elevated risk of heart disease among smokers, the benefits to cessation rates from short-term nicotine replacement therapy far outweigh the risks of continued smoking.

Nicotine Chewing Gum

A potential advantage of nicotine gum is the ability to adjust dosage individually and to schedule use as needed in response to situational variations in nicotine withdrawal and craving. Its major disadvantages are the extensive behavioral compliance required for effective use, relatively long periods of time required for onset of action, and the common failure of patients to use enough. Patients must be instructed in proper chewing technique; they must understand that the nicotine is absorbed primarily through the oral mucosa but very poorly if swallowed. Proper use involves a few chews until a peppery taste or tingling is felt, parking the gum inside the cheek to allow absorption, then repeating at intervals of about 1 minute. Nicotine absorption is not rapid, so a regularly timed dosing schedule of 1 gum every 1 to 2 hours is usually more successful than self-selected dosing. Acidic beverages (coffee, juices, soda, and wine) should be avoided before or during gum use because their pH reduces nicotine absorption. The 4-mg dosage form is intended for patients with higher levels of nicotine dependence. Convenient indices of dependence level are number of cigarettes smoked per day (25 or more is considered high dependence) and how soon after waking the first cigarette is smoked (smoking within just a few minutes of waking reflects high dependence).

Nicotine Lozenges

Nicotine lozenges deliver about 25% more nicotine than corresponding doses of the gum (33). The lozenge should be sucked slowly until the taste become strong, then kept between the gum and the cheek and slowly sucked again after the taste has faded. The recommended dose is 7 to 8 up to a maximum of 25 lozenges per day. Lozenges are easier to use than nicotine gum, requiring little instruction to use. Smoking cessation-related weight gain is reduced with 4-mg lozenges as opposed to placebo. Abrupt discontinuation may precipitate withdrawal symptoms.

Nicotine Nasal Spray

The nicotine nasal spray more closely simulates the pharmacokinetics of nicotine delivery via tobacco smoking than the other nicotine substitution medications do. It produces a larger and more rapid increase in blood nicotine levels, although still less than that achieved with smoking. The nasal spray may be especially beneficial to highly dependent smokers, who may need more rapid and more substantial nicotine delivery. The nasal spray's more rapid onset makes as-needed dosing more practical than with gum, but regularly scheduled dosing is still the recommended procedure.

Nicotine Vapor Inhaler

The nicotine vapor inhaler is similar in appearance to a cigarette and may be especially useful to patients who desire the physical manipulation and sensory aspects of smoking. There is no heat or combustion; puffs on the inhaler draw air over an internal nicotine-laden plug. Each puff delivers a very small dose of nicotine vapor (approximately 0.013 mg) to the mouth, where the nicotine is absorbed through the oral mucosa.

Nicotine Vaccine

One potential future approach to smoking cessation is the ongoing development of a nicotine-specific vaccine that removes the rewarding effects of cigarette smoke (34). The vaccine stimulates antibody formation that has a high affinity and specificity for nicotine. These antibodies sequester nicotine in blood, preventing entry into the brain. Theoretically, this would significantly increase cessation success rates. Human studies are in process to elucidate the safety and efficacy of such a vaccine, but initial results are encouraging.

Bupropion

Zyban is a sustained-release tablet formulation containing 150 mg of the antidepressant drug bupropion. The mechanism of action of bupropion in promoting smoking cessation is unknown, but it probably relates to its inhibition of norepinephrine and dopamine uptake. This is the only marketed non-nicotine smoking cessation medication. It is effective as a sole treatment, but its efficacy can perhaps be further enhanced by combination use with a nicotine replacement product (35). In a controlled trial in patients who were not depressed, bupropion, 300 mg (150 mg twice daily), yielded a 1-year cessation rate of 23.1%, compared with 12.4% in patients treated with placebo (36). Treatment was initiated 1 week before each patient's quit date and discontinued after 7 weeks. For the first 3 days, patients took 150 mg/day, then 150 mg twice daily. All patients received simple smoking cessation counseling.

Bupropion is also marketed as an antidepressant under the brand name Wellbutrin (see Chapter 24); patients should not use the two preparations simultaneously.

Chronic Treatment

Current recommendations are for nicotine replacement medications to be used for no longer than 2 to 3 months, during which time they are tapered gradually and discontinued. However, some patients who succeed at stopping smoking continue to use nicotine replacement products for longer periods and may be at risk for smoking relapse if the medication substitution is stopped. There is no consensus on the appropriate response to this circumstance. However, the health risks of chronic nicotine maintenance are certainly much lower than the risks of smoking.

Potential Medication Interactions

Nicotine substitution treatment typically yields nicotine blood levels well below those achieved during tobacco use. Therefore, potential medication interactions relate primarily to the cessation of tobacco use rather than to the administration of smoking cessation medications. After tobacco cessation, a *dosage decrease* may be required for acetaminophen, adrenergic antagonists (e.g., prazosin, labetalol), caffeine, imipramine, insulin, oxazepam, pentazocine, propranolol and other β-blockers, and theophylline. After tobacco cessation a *dosage increase* may be required for adrenergic agonists such as isoproterenol or phenylephrine. Bupropion is contraindicated within 14 days of monoamine oxidase inhibitor (MAOI) use.

Weight Gain

Weight gain is a common, distressing consequence of smoking cessation. Weight gain results both from dietary changes (increased snacking and selection of high-calorie foods) and from discontinuation of the metabolic effects of nicotine (37). Weight gain of patients remaining abstinent for 1 year averages 5 to 15 lb. This magnitude of weight gain is medically insignificant relative to the health benefits of smoking cessation. Unfortunately, the anticipated social, cosmetic, and economic (e.g., wardrobe cost) consequences of weight gain deter some smokers from quitting and contribute to relapse in others. Nicotine replacement treatment and bupropion both significantly attenuate weight gain after smoking cessation (38). Recent research suggests that, among women concerned about weight gain, cognitive behavioral therapy can improve smoking cessation outcomes and decrease weight concerns (39). The goals of the cognitive behavioral therapy were to reduce concerns about, and promote acceptance of, modest weight gain; to discourage dietary restraint, dieting, and active resistance to weight gain; and to encourage moderate consumption of healthy foods in between-meal snacks. The important message for patients concerned about possible postcessation weight gain is perhaps counterintuitive: focusing on weight control concurrent with smoking cessation leads to worse outcomes on both smoking and weight.

Organized Treatment

Health care practitioners often would like to refer smokers to formal cessation programs. For the small minority of smokers who attend them, organized programs at little or no cost are often available through local voluntary service organizations such as the American Lung Association or AHA. There are also available in some communities self-help peer-counseling programs (e.g., Nicotine Anonymous) modeled after the 12-step approaches used with other addictions. Commercial programs offer no clear advantages. Most organized programs incorporate standard behavioral principles of self-monitoring, control of environmental cues, and scheduling of rewards. These principles are also well represented in various self-help guides and in the patient education materials packaged with cessation medications. Patients often express interest in using alternative strategies for smoking cessation, such as acupuncture, hypnosis, or herbal aids. Although research has found no significant benefit of these often costly approaches, patients who are highly motivated to use such alternative strategies may benefit.

Relapse Prevention

As with most addictive disorders, the likelihood of relapse after cessation is high. Most relapses occur within the first few days or weeks of cessation, although patients are at some risk for relapse even after months of abstinence. New quitters face many urges to smoke again. Anticipation and advance planning can prevent relapse. Self-help educational brochures are useful for this purpose. They provide warnings about relapse risk circumstances and suggest coping strategies. Additionally, they help patients recognize the normality of "slips" and the importance of continued commitment to cessation. Slips or brief episodes of relapse are strong predictors of full relapse to smoking; therefore, patients should be carefully counseled that even one cigarette might jeopardize their smoking cessation attempt.

RECOMMENDED OFFICE APPROACH

Most health care practitioners advise smoking cessation for patients with obvious smoking-related illnesses, such as the patient with COPD or the inpatient recovering from a MI. However, too often physicians neglect to give smoking cessation advice in routine office care. Patients with smoking-related diseases obviously require strong smoking cessation interventions, but it is the smoking patient who has not yet experienced negative health consequences of smoking who stands to benefit most from smoking cessation. This section describes the primary care smoking cessation practice developed and recommended in the 2000 *Treating Tobacco Use and Dependence* clinical practice guideline published by the U.S. Public Health Service (http://www.surgeongeneral.gov/tobacco).

Although health care practitioners agree that it is appropriate and important for them to counsel patients to stop smoking, they are inconsistent in providing such advice. Reported barriers to counseling include a belief that such advice is ineffectual, a belief that most smoking patients are uninterested in counseling, a perceived lack of skills, and time constraints. However, studies have repeatedly found that brief, directive smoking interventions delivered during routine care are cost-effective and have the potential for significant public health benefit. A routine office visit for the treatment of eczema, flu, or indigestion can be used successfully to change smoking behavior, in the same way that it may also be used to screen for hypertension. These office-based smoking cessation practices are most effective when the smoking cessation interventions are viewed as essential components of good care. Just as measuring blood pressure at each office visit is now standard practice, so also should smoking status assessment and smoking cessation interventions be systematically integrated into standard office practice (22).

Motivating Smokers to Quit Smoking

Effective motivational counseling for smoking cessation recognizes that smokers cycle through several levels of readiness before attempting smoking cessation (see Fig. 4.1 in Chapter 4). Many factors can influence a smoker's progress through the stages of a change process. Life events, health symptoms, workplace smoking restrictions, and the price of a pack of cigarettes can all move a smoker closer to cessation. Alternatively, stress, weight gain, family problems, and smoking peers can act as barriers to change. The strong, directive advice smokers receive from their health care practitioner regarding the personal importance of quitting smoking is often one of the significant forces that move smokers closer to quitting.

Health concern is one of the most common reasons smokers cite as a motivation for quitting. Physicians and other practitioners can increase overall motivation for cessation by underscoring the personal *relevance* of quitting for that individual patient. The *risks* of smoking to both the smoker and his or her family can be highlighted, as well as the *rewards* of quitting, such as better health, saving money, improved vitality, and fewer wrinkles. And finally, because developing sufficient motivation for change may take a smoker months or years, the effort to motivate patients should be *repeated* at every clinical contact. Practitioners who consistently and repeatedly use these *4 Rs*—Relevance, Risks, Rewards, and Repetition (Fig. 27.1)—and provide smoking patients with advice and encouragement to quit smoking over the course of their medical care are most likely to see success. This *4 Rs* strategy should be used in conjunction with the actions outlined in Figures 27.2 to 27.6.

ACTION	STRATEGIES FOR IMPLEMENTATION
Relevance	Motivational information given to a patient has the greatest impact if it is relevant to a patient's disease status, family or social situation (e.g., having children in the home), health concerns, age, gender, and other important patient characteristics (e.g., prior quitting experience).
Risks	The clinician should *ask the patient to identify the potential negative consequences of smoking.* The clinician may suggest and highlight those that seem most relevant to the patient. The clinician should emphasize that smoking low-tar/low-nicotine cigarettes or use of other forms of tobacco (e.g., smokeless tobacco, cigars, pipes) will not eliminate these risks. Examples of risks follow. • Acute risks: Shortness of breath, exacerbation of asthma, impotence, infertility, increased serum carbon monoxide. • Long-term risks: Heart attacks and strokes, lung and other cancers (larynx, oral cavity, pharynx, esophagus, pancreas, bladder, cervix, leukemia), chronic obstructive pulmonary diseases (chronic bronchitis and emphysema). • Environmental risks: Increased risk of lung cancer in spouse and children; higher rates of smoking by children of smokers; increased risk for SIDS, asthma, middle ear disease, and respiratory infections in children of smokers.
Rewards	The clinician should *ask the patient to identify the potential benefits of quitting smoking.* The clinician may suggest and highlight those that seem most relevant to the patient. Examples of rewards follow. • Improved health • Improved sense of taste • Improved sense of smell • Cost savings • Improved self-esteem • Better-smelling home, car, and breath • No more worrying about quitting • A good example for children • Healthy babies and children • No worrying about exposing others to smoke • Feeling better physically • Freedom from addiction • Better performance in sports
Repetition	The motivational intervention should be repeated every time an unmotivated patient visits the office setting.

FIGURE 27.1. The *4 Rs* Strategy: Components of clinical interventions to enhance motivations to quit smoking. (From the Agency for Health Care Policy and Research. Smoking cessation: clinical practice guideline, no. 18. [USDHHS] AHCPR Publication No. 96-0692. Washington, DC: US Government Printing Office, 1996.)

Action	Strategies for implementation
Implement an office-wide system that ensures that, for EVERY patient at EVERY clinic visit, tobacco-use status is queried and documented. *a*	Expand the vital signs to include tobacco use or use an alternative universal identification system. *b* **Vital Signs** Blood Pressure: ____________ Pulse: ____________ Weight: ____________ Temperature: ____________ Respiratory Rate: ____________ Tobacco Use: Current Former Never (circle one)

a Repeated assessment is not necessary in the case of the adult who has never used tobacco or has not used tobacco for many years, and for whom this information is clearly documented in the medical record.

b Alternatives to expanding the vital signs are to place tobacco-use status stickers on all patient charts or to indicate tobacco use status using electronic medical records or computer reminder systems.

FIGURE 27.2. ASK—Systematically identify all tobacco users at every visit. (From Fiore MC, Bailey WC, Cohen SJ, et al. Treating tobacco use and dependence: clinical practice guideline. Rockville, MD: US Department of Health and Human Services, Public Health Service, June 2000.)

Action	Strategies for Implementation
In a *clear, strong*, and *personalized* manner, urge every tobacco user to quit.	Advice should be: • *Clear*--"I think it is important for you to quit smoking now and I can help you." "Cutting down while you are ill is not enough." • *Strong*--"As your clinician, I need you to know that quitting smoking is the most important thing you can do to protect your health now and in the future. The clinic staff and I will help you." • *Personalized*--Tie tobacco use to current health/ illness, and/or its social and economic costs, motivation level/readiness to quit, and/or the impact of tobacco use on children and others in the household.

FIGURE 27.3. ADVISE—Strongly urge all tobacco users to quit. (From Fiore MC, Bailey WC, Cohen SJ, et al. Treating tobacco use and dependence: clinical practice guideline. Rockville, MD: US Department of Health and Human Services, Public Health Service, June 2000.)

Actions: Ask, Advise, Assess, Assist, and Arrange

The surgeon general's clinical guidelines (see www.hopkinsbayview.org/PAMreferences) for treating tobacco use and dependence were derived from rigorous review of approximately 3,000 scientific reports. Those satisfying scientific quality criteria were analyzed by meta-analytic techniques. This permitted the authors to synthesize outcome data from different smoking cessation treatments and to identify effective treatment elements. Based on this review, the authors concluded that brief interventions are effective in promoting smoking cessation; therefore, "Every patient who uses tobacco should be offered at least brief treatment." The resulting guidelines for brief counseling are based on sound scientific evidence, and they recognize the time constraints on practitioners. These recommended practices are designed to require 3 minutes or less. They consist of five actions that are described more fully in the following paragraphs: Ask, Advise, Assess, Assist, and Arrange.

Office-based practitioners should systematically ***ask*** *about tobacco use* at every visit (Fig. 27.2). Clinicians are more likely to intervene with smoking patients when office procedures are designed to identify smokers and document smoking status. Smoking status should be considered a vital sign that is automatically collected, updated, and integrated into the permanent medical record.

The clinician should next ***advise*** *every smoking patient* in a strong, direct, personalized manner of the importance of quitting smoking (Fig. 27.3). Even brief advice to quit smoking (3 minutes or less) will increase smoking cessation rates.

After advising cessation, the clinician should ***assess*** *the smoker's motivation,* identify those patients who are willing to make a quit attempt, and determine the type of treatment they will accept (Fig. 27.4). For the unmotivated smoker, the clinician can attempt to enhance motivation for future cessation.

For patients interested in quitting smoking, the clinician should ***assist*** *in formalizing a quit* plan by setting a quit date within 2 weeks (Fig. 27.5). Brief counseling can encourage the patient to inform his or her family of the quit date, remove cigarettes from the environment before quitting, review previous quit attempts, identify aids and barriers, and anticipate challenges (e.g., withdrawal symptoms). Nicotine replacement therapy should be encouraged for most patients. Patients should be advised that *total abstinence is essential,* that alcohol should be avoided, and that smoking friends and family members should either join the plan to quit or not smoke around the patient.

Finally, for patients who have set a quit date, a *followup contact should be* ***arranged,*** preferably within 2 weeks after the quit date (Fig. 27.6). This contact can be used to reinforce success, troubleshoot problems, monitor nicotine

Action	Strategies for implementation
Ask every tobacco user if he or she is willing to make a quit attempt at this time (e.g., within the next 30 days).	Assess patient's willingness to quit: • If the patient is willing to make a quit attempt at this time, provide assistance. • If the patient will participate in an intensive treatment, deliver such a treatment or refer to an intensive intervention. • If the patient clearly states he or she is unwilling to make a quit attempt at this time, provide a motivational intervention. • If the patient is a member of a special population (e.g., adolescent, pregnant smoker, racial/ethnic minority), consider providing additional information.

FIGURE 27.4. ASSESS—Determine willingness to make a quit attempt. (From Fiore MC, Bailey WC, Cohen SJ, et al. Treating tobacco use and dependence: clinical practice guideline. Rockville, MD: US Department of Health and Human Services, Public Health Service, June 2000.)

Action	Strategies for implementation
Help the patient with a quit plan.	*A patient's preparations for quitting:* • ***Set** a quit date*--Ideally, the quit date should be within 2 weeks. • ***Tell*** family, friends, and coworkers about quitting and request understanding and support. • ***Anticipate*** challenges to planned quit attempt, particularly during the critical first few weeks. These include nicotine withdrawal symptoms. • ***Remove*** tobacco products from your environment. Prior to quitting, avoid smoking in places where you spend a lot of time (e.g., work, home, and car).
Provide practical counseling (problem solving/training).	• *Abstinence*--Total abstinence is essential. "Not even a single puff after the quit date." • *Past quit experience*--Identify what helped and what hurt in previous quit attempts. • *Anticipate triggers or challenges in upcoming attempt*--Discuss challenges/triggers and how patient will successfully overcome them. • *Alcohol*--Since alcohol can cause relapse, the patient should consider limiting/abstaining from alcohol while quitting. • *Other smokers in the household*--Quitting is more difficult when there is another smoker in the household. Patients should encourage housemates to quit with them or not smoke in their presence.
Provide intra-treatment social support.	• Provide a supportive clinical environment while encouraging the patient in his or her quit attempt. "My office staff and I are available to assist you."
Help patient obtain extra-treatment social support.	• Help patient develop social support for his or her quit attempt in his or her environments outside of treatment. "Ask your spouse/partner, friends, and coworkers to support you in your quit attempt."
Recommend the use of approved pharmacotherapy, except in special circumstances.	• Recommend the use of pharmacotherapies found to be effective. Explain how these medications increase smoking cessation success and reduce withdrawal symptoms. The first-line pharmacotherapy medications include bupropion SR, nicotine gum, nicotine inhaler, nicotine nasal spray, and nicotine patch.
Provide supplementary materials.	• *Sources*--Federal agencies, nonprofit agencies, or local/state health departments (*see website addresses at www.hopkinsbayview.org/ PAMreferences*) • *Type*--Culturally/racially/educationally/age appropriate for the patient. • *Location*--Readily available at every clinician's workstation.

FIGURE 27.5. ASSIST—Aid the patient in quitting. (From Fiore MC, Bailey WC, Cohen SJ, et al. Treating tobacco use and dependence: clinical practice guideline. Rockville, MD: U.S. Department of Health and Human Services, Public Health Service, June 2000.)

Action	Strategies for implementation
Schedule follow-up contact, either in person or via telephone.	*Timing*--Follow-up contact should occur soon after the quit date, preferably during the first week. A second follow-up contact is recommended within the first month. Schedule further follow-up contacts as indicated.
	Actions during follow-up contact--Congratulate success. If tobacco use has occurred, review circumstances, and elicit recommitment to total abstinence. Remind patient that a lapse can be used as a learning experience. Identify problems already encountered and anticipate challenges in the immediate future. Assess pharmacotherapy use and problems. Consider use or referral to more intensive treatment.

FIGURE 27.6. ARRANGE—Schedule followup contact. (From Fiore MC, Bailey WC, Cohen SJ, et al. Treating tobacco use and dependence: clinical practice guideline. Rockville, MD: US Department of Health and Human Services, Public Health Service, June 2000.)

replacement therapy, and recommend more intensive smoking cessation assistance if necessary.

Dealing with Relapse

Risk of relapse is very high for patients who slip and have even one cigarette. Drinking alcohol, socializing with smokers, and high-stress events can all trigger relapse episodes. Patients should be counseled in advance about factors associated with the risk of relapse and reinforced in the continuing challenge of staying abstinent. If relapse occurs, it is important to reassure the patient that relapse is not an indicator that they cannot quit smoking, but instead a common event that most former smokers have experienced before successful quitting. A relapse experience is discouraging for a patient, but it can provide information on the risks and barriers to be addressed in the next cessation effort. Patients should be encouraged to retry cessation as soon as they are ready, and they should be encouraged to use more intensive interventions (e.g., multisession group programs, longer-duration pharmacotherapy) if acceptable (40).

OTHER FORMS OF TOBACCO USE

This chapter focuses on cigarette smoking because it is the most prevalent form of tobacco use and has the greatest health impact. Other forms of tobacco use—cigars, pipes, snuff, and chewing tobacco—also have deleterious health effects (41). Mortality rates associated for these other forms of tobacco use are intermediate between those of cigarette smokers and those of nonusers of tobacco; for example, the total mortality rate of cigar or pipe smokers is approximately 15% to 20% higher than that of comparable nonsmokers. Site-specific cancer rates in the oral-nasal cavity are five times as great as in nonusers of tobacco, and there is increased risk of cardiovascular disease. Treatment approaches for these other varieties of tobacco dependence are the same as for cigarette smoking.

HEALTH CARE PROFESSIONALS AND PUBLIC POLICY

The likelihood of success in overcoming addiction to nicotine is increased not only by the personal motivation and willpower of the cigarette smoker but also by a social and legal environment that encourages nonsmoking, restricts access to tobacco, increases the price of tobacco, and reduces the social acceptability of smoking. An increasing body of evidence supports the value of increased taxation on tobacco, restrictive smoking policies, and anti-tobacco advertising in reducing smoking prevalence in the community. Just as public policies that ensure clean water and adequate sanitation facilities have made dysentery and cholera rare diseases in this country, emerging public policies designed to restrict and control the use of tobacco may someday make smoking-related diseases rare, rather than the leading cause of preventable death. Tobacco use is as much a public health risk as the infectious diseases of the past century, and the primary care clinician should be a vocal member of the anti-tobacco activism within his or her community.

SPECIFIC REFERENCES*

1. Stolerman IP, Jarvis MJ. The scientific case that nicotine is addictive. Psychopharmacology 1995;117:2.
2. Breslau N, Johnson EO, Hiripi E, et al. Nicotine dependence in the United States: prevalence, trends, and smoking persistence. Arch Gen Psychiatry 2001;58:810.
3. Herttema JM, Corey LA, Kendler KS. A multivariate genetic analysis of the use of tobacco, alcohol, and caffeine in a population based sample of male and female twins. Drug Alcohol Depend 1999;57:69.
4. Li MD. The genetics of smoking related behavior: a brief review. Am J Med Sci 2003;326:168.
5. Simantov E, Schoen C, Klein JD. Health-compromising behaviors: why do adolescents smoke or drink? Identifying underlying risk and protective factors. Arch Pediatr Adolesc Med 2000;154:1025.
6. Anda RF, Croft JB, Felitti VJ, et al. Adverse childhood experiences and smoking during adolescence and adulthood. JAMA 1999; 282:1652.
7. Perkins KA. Smoking cessation in women: special considerations. CNS Drugs 2001;15:391.

*Bold numerals denote published controlled clinical trials, meta-analyses, or consensus-based recommendations.

8. Bruvold WH. A meta-analysis of adolescent smoking prevention programs. Am J Public Health 1993;83:872.
9. Ockene JK, Emmons KM, Mermelstein RJ, et al. Relapse and maintenance issues for smoking cessation. Health Psychol 2000;19[1 Suppl]: 17.
10. Shiffman S, Paty JA, Gnys M, et al. First lapses to smoking: within-subjects analysis of real-time reports. J Consult Clin Psychol 1996;64:366.
11. Higgins MW, Enright PL, Kronmal RA, et al. Smoking and lung function in elderly men and women. JAMA 1993;269:2741.
12. Benowitz NL, Jacob P. Nicotine and carbon monoxide intake from high- and low-yield cigarettes. Clin Pharmacol Ther 1984;36:265.
13. Kozlowski LT, Frecker RC, Khouw V, et al. The misuse of less-hazardous cigarettes and its detection: hole-blocking of ventilated filters. Am J Public Health 1980;70:1202.
14. Hughes JR. Tobacco withdrawal in self-quitters. J Consult Clin Psychol 1992;60:689.
15. Hughes JR, Hatsukami D. Signs and symptoms of tobacco withdrawal. Arch Gen Psychiatry 1986;43:289.
16. West R, Shiffman S. Effect of oral nicotine dosing forms on cigarette withdrawal symptoms and craving: a systematic review. Psychopharmacology 2001;155:115.
17. Brownson RC, Alavanja MCR, Hock ET, et al. Passive smoking and lung cancer in nonsmoking women. Am J Public Health 1992;82: 1525.
18. Chilmonczyk BA, Salmun LM, Megathlin KN, et al. Association between exposure to environmental tobacco smoke and exacerbations of asthma in children. N Engl J Med 1993; 328:1665.
19. Fielding JE, Phenow KJ. Health effects of involuntary smoking. N Engl J Med 1988; 319:1452.
20. He J, Vupputuri S, Allen K, et al. Passive smoking and the risk of coronary heart disease: a meta-analysis of epidemiologic studies. N Engl J Med 1999;340:920.
21. Sexton M, Hebel JR. A clinical trial of change in maternal smoking and its effect on birth weight. JAMA 1984;251:911.
22. Ahluwalia JS, Gibson CA, Kenney RE, et al. Smoking status as a vital sign. J Gen Intern Med 1999;14:402.
23. Sippel JM, Osborne ML, Bjornson W, et al. Smoking cessation in primary care clinics. J Gen Intern Med 1999;14:670.
24. Ritvo PG, Irvine MJ, Lindsay EA, et al. A critical review of research related to family physician-assisted smoking cessation interventions. Cancer Prev Control 1997;1:289.

25. Lancaster T, Stead LF. Physician advice for smoking cessation. *Cochrane Database Syst Rev* 2004;4:CD000165.

26. Doescher MP, Saver BG. Physicians' advice to quit smoking: the glass remains half empty. J Fam Pract 2000;49:543.

27. Ellerbeck EF, Ahluwalia JS, Jolicoeur DG, et al. Direct observation of smoking cessation activities in primary care practice. J Fam Pract 2001;50:688.

28. Ossip-Klein DJ, McIntosh S, Utman C, et al. Smokers ages 50+: who gets physician advice to quit? Prev Med 2000;31:364.

29. Orleans CT, Cummings KM. Population-based tobacco control: progress and prospects. Am J Health Promot 1999;14:83.

30. Kreuter MW, Chheda SG, Bull FC. How does physician advice influence patient behavior? Evidence for a priming effect. Arch Fam Med 2000;9:426.

31. Fiore MC, Bailey WC, Cohen SJ, et al. Treating tobacco use and dependence: clinical practice guideline. Rockville, MD: US Department of Health and Human Services, Public Health Service, June 2000.

32. Joseph AM, Norman SM, Ferry LH, et al. The safety of transdermal nicotine as an aid to smoking cessation in patients with cardiac disease. N Engl J Med 1996;335:1792.

33. Shiffman S, Dresler CM, Hajek P, et al. Efficacy of a nicotine lozenge for smoking cessation. Arch Intern Med 2002;162:1267.

34. Hall W. The prospects for immunotherapy in smoking cessation. Lancet. 2002;360:1089.

35. Jorenby DE, Leischow SJ, Nides MA, et al. A controlled trial of sustained-release bupropion, a nicotine patch, or both for smoking cessation. N Engl J Med 1999;340:685.

36. Hurt RD, Sachs DPL, Glover ED, et al. A comparison of sustained-release bupropion and placebo for smoking cessation. N Engl J Med 1997;337:1195.

37. Ferrara CM, Kumar M, Nicklas B, et al. Weight gain and adipose tissue metabolism after smoking cessation in women. Int J Obes Relat Metab Disord 2001;25:1322.

38. Hays JT, Hurt RD, Rigotti NA, et al. Sustained-release bupropion for pharmacologic relapse prevention after smoking cessation: a randomized, controlled trial. Ann Intern Med 2001;135:423.

39. Perkins KA, Marcus MD, Levine MD, et al. Cognitive-behavioral therapy to reduce weight concerns improves smoking cessation outcome in weight-concerned women. J Consult Clin Psychol 2001;69:604.

40. Smith SS, Jorenby DE, Fiore MC, et al. Strike while the iron is hot: can stepped-care treatments resurrect relapsing smokers? J Consult Clin Psychol 2001;69:429.

41. Council on Scientific Affairs. Health effects of smokeless tobacco. JAMA 1986;255:1038.

For annotated ***General References*** *and resources related to this chapter, visit www.hopkinsbayview.org/PAMreferences.*

Chapter 28

Alcoholism and Associated Problems

Michael I. Fingerhood

Along with cardiovascular disease and cancer, alcoholism ranks among the top three causes of death and disability in the United States. However, the majority of alcoholics in the United States do not receive treatment for their alcoholism. Additionally, many people have early alcoholism and could recover successfully if diagnosed and treated.

Until recently, alcoholism was widely regarded as a hopeless condition with a poor prognosis for recovery. Yet alcoholism is one of the most treatable of all medical and psychiatric conditions, with a high long-term success rate when a disease model of alcoholism is used in diagnosis and treatment.

DEFINITION OF ALCOHOLISM

A useful, broad definition of alcoholism is *recurring trouble associated with drinking alcohol.* The trouble may occur in one or more of several domains, including interpersonal (e.g., valued relationships, especially within the family), educational, legal, financial, medical, and occupational. Although there are many exceptions, trouble caused by alcoholism usually occurs in that order of progression, so that one's health and job are last to be affected. The trouble may include the physiologic manifestations of dependence or addiction: *tolerance* (the need for increased amounts of a substance to achieve intoxication or desired effect) and *withdrawal* symptoms. Characteristics of alcoholism include inability to control one's use of alcohol (always present), drinking alone, avoiding situations where alcohol is not available, drinking before going to a party, and continuing to drink alcohol despite occupational, psychosocial, legal or physical problems caused by drinking.

Consensus Definition

In 1992, a multidisciplinary committee of the National Council on Alcoholism and Drug Dependence and the American Society of Addiction Medicine issued its definition of alcoholism: "Alcoholism is a primary, chronic disease with genetic, psychosocial, and environmental factors influencing its development and manifestations. The disease is often progressive and fatal. It is characterized by impaired control over drinking, preoccupation with the drug alcohol despite adverse consequences, and distortions in thinking, most notably denial. Each of these symptoms may be continuous or periodic" (1). Unlike previously issued definitions, this one specifically included denial as a key component of the definition of alcoholism.

Alcoholism is classified by the American Psychiatric Association under the broad rubric *Substance-Related Use Disorders* (2). In its subclassification for these disorders, the American Psychiatric Association has generic criteria for *substance abuse* (abnormal use, with unwanted consequences) and *substance dependence* (more intensive abuse patterns or physiologic manifestations of addiction). Chapter 29 lists the criteria for these two subclassifications. The National Institute on Alcohol Abuse and Alcoholism defines "at-risk drinking" as more than 14 drinks per week or more than 4 drinks per occasion for men and more than 7 drinks per week or more than 3 drinks per occasion for women (3). Recently, the terms "alcohol use disorder," "problem drinking," "hazardous drinking," and "unhealthy alcohol use" have also been used in the literature. These terms aim to include individuals who do not meet *Diagnostic and Statistical Manual of Mental Disorders, 4th Edition (DSM-IV)* criteria for alcohol abuse or dependence, but may be at increased risk for alcohol-related problems or have had problems such as a driving while intoxicated (DWI). Many of these individuals do not need alcohol treatment, but may benefit from primary care intervention to prevent further consequences from drinking.

CAUSES

The causes of alcoholism are multifactorial and poorly understood (4,5). A predisposition to alcoholism appears to be inherited by at least half of all alcoholic patients, and there is some evidence that inherited factors are associated with the inability to control use of alcohol (6). Social conditioning, enabling behavior by others close to the individual (see Co-alcoholism), and being a child in a dysfunctional family are important nongenetic factors. For some alcoholic men, another mental disorder (especially antisocial personality disorder, primary abuse of other substances, or an affective disorder) may play a role. For alcoholic women, preexisting mental illness, especially a phobic disorder or major depression, may play a role. Additionally, for elderly alcoholics whose problem began after 50 years of age, the losses and isolation that accompany aging are often associated with the onset of problem drinking (see Special Populations).

ALCOHOLIC BEVERAGES: CONTENT AND METABOLISM

Alcoholic beverages can be divided into nondistilled (wine and beer) and distilled varieties. The concentration of alcohol (ethanol) in wine ranges from 10% to 22% by volume and is 12% to 14% in most wines. Beer usually contains 4% to 5% alcohol by volume, but beers fermented in the bottle contain a higher percentage of alcohol. The distilled alcoholic beverages—whiskey, brandy, rum, gin, and vodka—contain a higher percentage of alcohol. Alcoholic fermentation ceases when the concentration of alcohol exceeds 15% by volume; consequently, to manufacture more potent beverages, distillation or fortification is necessary. In the United States, *"proof"* is double the percentage of alcohol by volume; for instance, 90 proof whiskeys contain 45% alcohol by volume. One drink of distilled alcohol (1 fluid oz), one glass of wine (4 oz), and one beer (12 oz) all contain approximately 12 grams of alcohol.

In a 154-pound (70-kg) person, on an empty stomach, one drink of distilled alcohol (usually 1 fluid oz or 30 mL) produces a peak blood alcohol level (BAL) of approximately 25 mg/dL within 30 minutes after ingestion. Approximately 15 mg/dL is metabolized per hour. For example, the alcohol in 120 mL of whiskey would take about 6 hours to be metabolized. The rate of metabolism is higher (in the range of 20 to 25 mg/dL/hour) in an individual with alcohol dependence. A BAL of 100 mg/dL is equivalent to 0.08%, in the units commonly used by law enforcement to indicate driving impairment. To reach a BAL of 300 mg/dL, a 70-kg person typically has to consume 14 to 20 drinks over a few hours.

EPIDEMIOLOGY

Prevalence

In 2003, an estimated 119 million Americans (half of all Americans older than age 12 years) were current drinkers, with 16.1 million Americans (6.8% of population) classified as heavy drinkers (5 or more drinks on the same occasion on at least 5 out of the 30 past days) (7). Additionally,

13.6% of the population drove under the influence at least once in the 12 months previous to the survey. Binge drinking (consuming 5 or more drinks on 1 occasion) has steadily increased in the United States with an estimated 1.5 billion episodes in 2001 (8). Rates of binge drinking are highest for young adults (age 18 to 25 years), with resultant high rates of motor vehicle accidents in this population.

Mortality and Morbidity

Prospective studies show that alcoholic patients have two to four times higher death rates and much higher rates of medical and psychosocial morbidity than do matched controls (9). The most common causes of early death in alcoholics are cirrhosis of the liver, cancers of the respiratory and gastrointestinal (GI) tracts, accidents, suicide, and ischemic heart disease. Most alcoholics smoke and, in fact, lung cancer is the most common cancer diagnosed in alcoholics (10). Importantly, alcoholic men who achieve long-term abstinence do not differ from nonalcoholic men in mortality rate (11). However, relapse is significantly related to mortality.

NATURAL HISTORY OF ALCOHOLISM

The natural history of alcoholism in men has been delineated in retrospective and prospective studies. In Jellinek's retrospective study of alcoholic men (4), the majority of subjects identified multiple phases in the progression of their disease: (a) an initial phase, lasting months to years, in which they used alcohol to relieve tension and developed tolerance to alcohol; (b) a phase in which they experienced blackouts (amnesia for drinking-associated events), increasing preoccupation with getting alcohol, and profound loss of control over use of alcohol; (c) a phase in which there were overt psychological and behavioral consequences (rationalization, grandiosity, aggressive behavior, remorse, efforts to abstain); and (d) a stage characterized by chronic intoxication and serious deterioration of health and psychosocial functioning. In Valliant's more recent prospective study (5), this multiphase course of alcoholism characterized three quarters of men who became alcoholic. Most of the remaining men exhibited abnormal drinking patterns, usually rituals to constrain the uncontrolled drinking that they themselves recognized as abnormal, and had less alcohol-related trouble with family, job, and health. Importantly, in these and other studies of the course of alcoholism, it has been found that periodic abstinence or moderation of use is typical. Although anecdotal information suggests that occasionally a person with what appears to be alcoholism can return to normal drinking, this is very uncommon and is not clinically useful to consider.

MANIFESTATIONS OF ALCOHOLISM

Alcoholism is a protean disease, and it is probably the most common great masquerader today. Table 28.1 lists medical, psychosocial, legal, and other manifestations often associated with alcoholism. Manifestations are ranked in the table according to their strength as diagnostic features, ranging from those that are diagnostic of alcoholism to those that should make one at least consider alcoholism. A number of the most important manifestations of alcoholism are discussed here.

Legal Problems

A history or record of DWI highly suggests alcoholism. In one study of 2,358 consecutive people with DWIs, 63.8% of first-time offenders were found to be alcoholic (12). Of those with two DWI arrests, more than 90% were alcoholic, and of those with three, essentially all were alcoholic. A prison record is also strongly suggestive, because most prison inmates have a history of alcoholism or other chemical dependence. Child and spouse or partner abuse is also highly associated with alcoholism.

Behavioral, Psychiatric, and Neurologic Problems

Accidents and trauma, including burns, are often associated with alcoholism; in the majority of patients with severe trauma, alcohol or other psychoactive drug use can be detected. Among patients with symptoms of chronic mental illness, especially symptoms of depression and anxiety, alcoholism is common. Usually alcoholism is the primary problem in these patients, and treatment of mental symptoms is not successful until the alcoholism is treated.

Alcohol Intoxication

The obvious acute consequence of alcoholism is alcohol intoxication, which usually presents no diagnostic problem. Because this condition is so common, diagnostic errors are made when it is forgotten that "drunken" behavior—often with evidence of recent alcohol use—may be caused by a host of conditions, such as infection, metabolic disturbance, neurologic disease, or other drug toxicity. Because alcoholics are especially prone to many disorders that may be manifested as deranged behavior, they should be examined systematically before a diagnosis of simple drunkenness is made.

Alcohol intoxication may be characterized by one or more of the following: relaxation and sedation, euphoria, impaired coordination, loudness, lowered inhibitions, poor memory and judgment, labile mood, slurred speech, nausea, vomiting, and obtundation (Table 28.2). An initial period of excitement and euphoria is often

TABLE 28.1 Medical, Psychiatric, Legal, and Other Findings Suggestive (unmarked to *) to Highly Suggestive (to ***) or Diagnostic (****) of Alcoholism**

Presenting Complaint and History	
****Drinking problem, recurring[a]	*Depression
***Blackouts with drinking	*Suicide attempt
***Spouse/other complains of patient's drinking	*Sexual dysfunction
***Driving while intoxicated (DWI) record	*Legal problem
***Prison record	*Noncompliance in treatment
***Change in alcohol or drug tolerance	*School learning problem
**Frequent requests for mood-changing drugs	*Hypertension
**Gastrointestinal bleeding, especially upper	Headache
**Traumatic injuries, fracture	Palpitations
**Parent, grandparent, or relative alcoholic	Abdominal pain
**Friends alcoholic or other chemical dependence	Amenorrhea
**Family or other violence	Weight loss
**Child abuse or neglect	Vague complaints
**First seizure in an adult	Insomnia
**Job performance problem	Anxiety
*Unexplained syncope	Marital discord
	Financial problem
Alcohol or Other Drug Use History	
****Alcohol use recurring, interfering with health, job, or social functioning[a]	**Other drug misuse or dependence
***Patient says, "I can stop drinking anytime" or the equivalent; or patient gets evasive or angry, or talks glibly during taking of drinking history	*Cigarette smoker
***Patient states that he or she has consciously stopped drinking completely for any length of time	
Physical Examination	
***Odor of beverage alcohol on breath	*Borderline tachycardia
***Parotid gland enlargement, bilateral	*Thin extremities in proportion to trunk
***Spider nevi or angioma	*Splenomegaly
***Tremulousness, hallucinosis	*Hypertension
**Cigarette stains on fingers	Diaphoresis
**Breath mints odor	Alopecia
**Many scars or tattoos	Abdominal tenderness
**Hepatomegaly	Cerebellar signs (e.g., nystagmus)
**Gynecomastia	
**Small testicles	
**Unexplained bruises, abrasions, or cuts	
Laboratory Abnormalities	
****Blood alcohol level >300 mg per 100 mL[a]	**Abnormal liver function tests (especially AST > ALT)
***Blood alcohol level >100 mg per 100 mL without impairment	**Anemia, macrocytic or megaloblastic, microcytic, or mixed
***High serum ammonia	*Hyperuricemia
***Gamma-glutamyl transpeptidase elevation	*Creatine kinase elevation
***Blood alcohol level positive, any amount	*Hypophosphatemia or hypomagnesemia
***High amylase (nonspecific for pancreas)	Electrolyte imbalance (hyponatremia, hypokalemia)
	Low white blood cell or platelet count
	Hyperlipoproteinemia, type 4 or 5

(continued)

TABLE 28.1 (Continued) Medical, Psychiatric, Legal, and Other Findings Suggestive (unmarked to *) to Highly Suggestive (to ***) or Diagnostic (****) of Alcoholism**

Diagnosis	
****Hepatitis, alcoholic[a]	**Attempted suicide
***Pancreatitis, acute or chronic	**Gastritis
***Cirrhosis	**Refractory hypertension
***Portal hypertension	**Cerebellar degeneration
***Wernicke-Korsakoff syndrome	**Peripheral neuropathy
***Frequent trauma	**Aspiration pneumonia
***Cold injury	*Gout
***Nose and throat cancer	*Cardiomyopathy
**Other chemical dependence	*Tuberculosis
**Drownings	*Anxiety
**Burns, especially third degree	*Depression
**Leaves hospital against medical advice	*Marital discord or family problem

ALT, alanine aminotransferase; AST, aspartate aminotransferase.
[a]Major criterian of the National Council on Alcoholism for the diagnosis of alcoholism (see *www.hopkinsbayview.org/PAMreferences*).

followed by depression and sleep, or possibly coma. The duration and magnitude of the intoxication depend on the amount and the rapidity with which the alcohol was drunk and whether the patient drank on an empty stomach (enhancing the rate of absorption). Tolerance is also a significant factor, because an alcoholic may acquire the capacity to increase the rate of alcohol metabolism. Moreover, alcoholics characteristically develop substantial central tolerance, so that they appear fairly sober at BALs of 150 mg/dL or more. Most nonalcoholic people become intoxicated at levels between 100 and 200 mg/dL, and some at levels as low as 30 mg/dL. Levels greater than 400 mg/dL can be lethal, with death usually resulting from depressed respiration or from aspiration of vomitus.

Blackouts

Blackouts—amnesia for events that occurred during a period of intoxication—are common. However, 10% to 25% of alcoholics do not have memory blackouts, and some normal drinkers have experienced blackouts after drinking.

Alcohol Idiosyncratic Intoxication

Alcohol idiosyncratic intoxication (pathologic intoxication) is an uncommon syndrome characterized by an extreme, often aggressive or violent reaction to drinking alcohol, which is often followed by amnesia for the episode. The behavior is atypical of the person when not drinking. The duration of this condition is brief (hours), and the person returns to his or her normal state as the BAL falls. Temporal lobe epilepsy, sedative-hypnotic use, and malingering should be ruled out.

Alcohol Amnestic Disorder (Korsakoff Psychosis)

Alcohol amnestic disorder (Korsakoff psychosis) is characterized chiefly by short-term memory impairment

TABLE 28.2 Expected Effects According to Blood Alcohol Level for a Person without Tolerance to Alcohol

Blood Alcohol Level (mg per dL)	*Expected Effect*	*Approximate Location of Physiologic Disturbance*
25–50	Relaxation, sedation	—
50–100	Coordination impaired; euphoric; loud conversation; apparent reduction of social inhibitions	Cerebral cortex
100–200	Ataxia; depressed fine motor ability, decreased mentation, attention span, and memory; poor judgment; labile mood; beginning of slurred speech	Limbic system and cerebellum
200–300	Marked ataxia and slurred speech, nausea and vomiting, tremor, irritable	Reticular activating system
300–400	Stage 1 anesthesia (unconsciousness), memory lapse	Reticular activating system
>400	Respiratory failure, coma, death	Medulla oblongata

associated with some loss of long-term memory, in the absence of clouded consciousness (or delirium) or general loss of intellectual abilities (dementia). (For definitions and detailed discussions of delirium and dementia, see Chapter 26.) Patients with less advanced forms of this disorder may be substantially impaired, but they may appear superficially to be normal, particularly because they often attempt to minimize their impairment and to confabulate in order to fill in memory gaps.

The amnestic disorder often follows an episode of *Wernicke encephalopathy,* a syndrome of global confusion, ataxia, and impaired eye movement, caused by thiamine deficiency, which may occur suddenly or gradually over several days. Parenteral thiamine given during an acute episode of Wernicke encephalopathy may prevent the amnestic syndrome. With abstention from alcohol and good nutrition for several months, some patients recover entirely from the alcohol amnestic syndrome. However, many remain grossly impaired and require institutional care.

Dementia Associated with Alcoholism

When more generalized intellectual impairment develops after years of heavy drinking, the diagnosis of dementia associated with alcoholism is appropriate. An estimated 70% of actively drinking chronic alcoholics have some cognitive impairment, as measured by psychological testing. Perhaps 10% of these have dementia that is sufficiently apparent and noticeable without psychological testing. Because even detoxified alcoholics are likely to show some cognitive impairment for a period after cessation of drinking, this diagnosis should not be made unless dementia persists for at least 1 month after drinking has stopped. Other causes of dementia must be excluded (see Chapter 26). All alcoholics with any signs of dementia should be treated with high-dosage thiamine (100 mg/day) and long-term multivitamin therapy. Some improve over months to years of abstinence.

Other Medical Complications

The various *deficiency states* involved in a diet composed largely of nutritionally empty alcoholic calories (7 calories per gram), as well as the *direct toxic actions of alcohol* itself, have been implicated in the pathogenesis of many of the medical consequences of alcoholism. These disorders are legion, sparing no body system, and most are related to the quantity and duration of alcohol consumption. Among the more common medical complications of alcoholism are gastritis; fatty liver, hepatitis, or cirrhosis; pancreatitis; cerebellar ataxia; gout; peripheral neuropathy; rhabdomyolysis; hematologic abnormalities (elevated mean corpuscular volume of red blood cells, anemia, thrombocytopenia); hypoglycemia; ketoacidosis; electrolyte abnormalities (hyponatremia, hypokalemia, hypomagnesemia, and hypophosphatemia); pulmonary infections suggesting aspiration or impaired defenses (tuberculosis and pneumonia); cancers of the liver, respiratory, and GI tract; atrial fibrillation; cardiomyopathy; hypertension; and trauma. *Chronic hypertension* is a very common manifestation of alcoholism. Because it often remits within weeks after discontinuation alcohol, it may be the most common reversible cause of hypertension (see Chapter 67).

Because it is both serious and preventable, the *fetal alcohol syndrome* (FAS) deserves special mention. It is manifested by morphologic abnormalities, low birth weight, and developmental and cognitive impairment. This syndrome is a consequence of alcohol ingestion by the mother during pregnancy. The risk of minor abnormalities (e.g., low birth weight) begins with the consumption of one drink per day; this risk increases with increasingly larger amounts of alcohol consumption. It is prudent to advise women not to drink any alcohol during pregnancy.

Medical Consequences: A Summary View

Almost all of the medical consequences of alcoholism tend to have certain common characteristics:

- Drinking alcohol causes them.
- Poor nutrition generally makes most of them worse and makes them occur earlier.
- Harmful habits, such as cigarette smoking and the misuse of other drugs, also tend to compound the medical consequences.

If the patient continues to consume alcohol, damage involving major organs progresses slowly over the course of a few years, often ending in organ failure. The organs affected by alcohol and the rate of decline in function of these organs varies greatly among patients. Severity of damage is loosely correlated with dosage of alcohol. For the liver, damage is more common in women at any level of alcohol consumption (see Special Populations).

Progression of organic damage occurs no matter what medical or psychological intervention the patient receives, as long as drinking continues. If the patient stops drinking, many of the pathophysiologic processes caused by alcohol reverse rapidly, such as those in the blood and bone marrow (cytopenias), those in the small intestine (malabsorption), hypertension, and fluid and electrolyte imbalance. Other processes do not reverse rapidly with abstinence, but they usually do not progress and often improve over weeks and months. Alcoholic hepatitis, chronic pancreatitis, and cognitive deficits are conditions that tend to improve more gradually.

SCREENING FOR AND DIAGNOSING ALCOHOLISM

Overview

Except when a patient presents with overt behavioral or medical evidence of alcoholism (see Table 28.1), the diagnosis of alcoholism requires skillful interviewing and careful evaluation of other information. Such an approach is needed for most alcoholics, whose disease is a private problem experienced by them and those who are close to them. In addition to unwanted psychosocial and physiologic consequences of alcoholism, two cardinal features inevitably emerge when one is obtaining information from an alcoholic or others who know the alcoholic: evidence of inability to control the use of alcohol and denial that a significant problem exists.

Persons who are recognized in the early stages of alcoholism may be helped by *brief interventions* as described in a separate section at the end of this chapter.

Loss of Control

Continuous inability to control the use of alcohol is not always present in alcoholics. Indeed, many can go for periods of a few hours (e.g., at a social gathering) to a few months with apparently normal drinking. Therefore, the absence of overt loss of control for a period of time does not rule out alcoholism. In such patients, the loss of control returns eventually. Additionally, some alcoholic patients describe rituals to constrain their intake because of previous trouble with control (e.g., never having a first drink until after dinner). Nonalcoholic people do not describe drinking in these ways, and such information usually indicates that there is a serious problem. Control of alcohol consumption is always an issue for the alcoholic.

Denial

Denial (i.e., the direct or implied message that there is no problem) is present in almost all actively drinking alcoholics. Denial behavior may be caused by one or more of the following mechanisms: (a) conscious lying (one of the least common mechanisms); (b) classic denial (an adaptive coping response to avoid the shame, lowered self-esteem, and distressing inability to overcome the drinking problem that are experienced by most alcoholics); (c) memory blackout caused by drinking; (d) euphoric recall (the patient remembers only the good times experienced when drinking); (e) the fact that no one points out problems related to drinking; (f) wishful thinking; (g) denial on the part of the family and other close people, including helping professionals; (h) ignorance of what an alcoholic is; (i) toxic effects on information processing and memory; and (j) stigma related to the term *alcoholic.*

Denial presents in some of the following ways: rationalizations (e.g., "I drink because my work is more than anyone should try to do"), glibness and humor, hostility ("I came to you about my blood pressure and I would appreciate it if we could stay out of my personal life"), comparison of oneself with a "real problem drinker" ("Now see here, I have a lovely family, a job that I enjoy...I have nothing in common with those poor guys who have lost it; those are your alcoholics"), reticence to discuss drinking, and the assertion that other physicians or family members do not perceive a problem with alcohol. An alcoholic patient's denial responses are usually the result of years of complex adapting to dependence on alcohol. This helps explain why these responses may seem to be refractory and may cause much frustration during screening and diagnostic interviewing and during efforts to get the patient to accept the diagnosis and agree to treatment.

Screening for Alcoholism

Because alcoholism is common and because the evidence for it is usually private information that patients do not volunteer, all patients should be screened for this problem. The goal of screening, and of further inquiry when there are positive responses to screening, is to be confident that one has ruled out alcoholism, has detected definite alcoholism, or must continue to consider alcoholism as a possible diagnosis.

There are a number of ways to screen for the cardinal features of alcoholism. The approach outlined in Fig. 28.1 incorporates the four so-called CAGE questions into the interview (13). In this approach, exploratory inquiry about the use of alcoholic beverages follows inquiries about less sensitive habit information, and the inquiry begins with an open-ended question that prompts patients to respond with more than a simple *Yes* or *No* or with a quantitative reply (e.g., "a few beers"). In patients who report any current or recent use of alcohol and in those with discomfort, glibness, voluntary reporting of heavy use, or other information suggesting alcoholism (Table 28.1), including that from the patient's medical history, there is increased likelihood that a problem exists (14). In the absence of such clues, all patients who report alcohol use should still complete the followup questions listed in Fig. 28.1 or other questions that focus on similar content.

The approach in Fig. 28.1 is designed to uncover specific data that point to the diagnosis of alcoholism. Lengthier than the CAGE, the Michigan Alcoholism Screening Test (MAST) is a 24-question standardized instrument that has been used extensively for alcoholism screening (Table 28.3) (15). The questions in the MAST may be helpful when one is attempting to uncover occult alcoholism. The questions are best used to gather additional information within the flow of obtaining a history related to drinking, complementing and adding information to positive CAGE answers. Another screening tool, the 10-item Alcohol Use Disorders Identification Test (AUDIT), developed by the World Health Organization (WHO), focuses on alcohol consumption and as such can be regarded as a screening tool for problem drinking (Table 28.4) (16,17). The CAGE questions (Fig. 28.1) have the advantage of being simple to incorporate into an office interview, being phrased in a nonthreatening way, and focusing on several

1. **Integrate alcohol use inquiry into interview** so that it follows inquiry about less sensitive habits.

   Example: "We have talked about your usual diet and your smoking. Can you tell me how you use alcoholic beverages?" (or "How about alcoholic beverages . . .?").

   If the patient says that he/she has never used alcohol and shows no sign of discomfort, inquire about problem use in others (e.g., "Anyone in your family or other close persons who have a drinking problem?"). This helps to identify a risk factor for alcoholism and to identify patients who may suffer because of the alcoholism of another person.[a]

2. **General Questions:** For patients who report present or past use of alcohol, screen for evidence of alcoholism, with a general question such as the following:

   "Has (Did) your use of alcohol caused (cause) any kinds of problems for you?" or "Have you ever been concerned about your drinking?"

3. **CAGE Questions:**[b] If the patient has not disclosed a problem with drinking, use these four focused questions and probe for clarification of positive or ambivalent responses.

   "I'd like to ask you a few more questions about alcohol that I ask all of my patients . . ."

C "Have you ever felt you ought to CUT DOWN on your drinking (use of ___________)?"

A "Have people ANNOYED you by criticizing your drinking (use of ___________)?"

G "Have you ever felt bad or GUILTY about your drinking (use of ___________)?"

E "Have you ever had a drink first thing in the morning (EYE OPENER) to steady your nerves or get rid of a hangover?" (For other substances: "Have you found that you have to take some ___________ most days/some days to feel okay?")

[a]See section on "Co-Alcoholism."
[b]Modifications of questions for substances other than alcohol are shown in parentheses.

FIGURE 28.1. A recommended approach to the use of interviewing to screen all patients for alcoholism and problems with alcohol in the family.

features that are present in most patients with alcoholism:

- Cut Down: *Inability to control* one's drinking, which leads to cutting back or quitting attempts.
- Annoying: *Domestic problems* caused by one's drinking evoke negative responses from other people. The phrasing of this question places the blame on the one criticizing, so that a positive response is not self-incriminating.
- Guilt: *Bad feelings* that one has about drinking-related actions. The phrasing of this question allows the patient to blame the drinking and not himself or herself.
- Eye opener: *Physiologic dependence,* as denoted by the need to drink to suppress withdrawal symptoms.

Studies of the CAGE questions have shown that they are sensitive (70% to 90% of alcoholics respond positively to one or more of the questions, and most have at least two positive responses) and specific (80% to 95% of nonalcoholic people respond negatively to all four questions) (18). An additional tool similar to the CAGE, the TWEAK (Table 28.5) was developed and validated for assessing alcohol misuse in pregnant women and may outperform the CAGE in women (19).

The test characteristics of the CAGE questions are superior to those of laboratory tests—gamma-glutamyl transpeptidase (GGT), other liver function tests, and mean corpuscular volume (MCV)—that are often measured in patients with alcoholism (20). However, abnormalities in these specific tests may be helpful in supporting persistent inquiry and in confrontation of the patient with suspected alcoholism.

Screening questions that focus on one common consequence of alcoholism, *trauma,* may be sensitive—especially the question, "Have you ever been injured after drinking?" A positive response to this question, or a history of unexplained repeated trauma or traffic accidents, may be important in patients whose CAGE responses are equivocal and in those who have few of the social contacts that are implied in the CAGE questions. The latter group includes antisocial younger drinkers, older people, and others who commonly become isolated.

Importantly, the approach in Fig. 28.1 does not include direct inquiry about quantity or frequency of alcohol use. Although *quantitative inquiry* may be helpful for identifying a patient who is ready to discuss problems associated with drinking, its disadvantages are that it does not focus on inability to control use or on adverse consequences of drinking, there is no gold standard for the cutoff quantity below or above which one can confidently exclude or diagnose alcoholism, and problem drinkers usually underreport the amount and frequency of their drinking.

Diagnosis of Alcoholism

The confident diagnosis of alcoholism requires nonjudgmental exploration of any positive information obtained in screening. This may include asking for clarification ("Can you tell me more about the last time you decided to cut back a bit?" or "Exactly what does she say to annoy you?" and gentle confrontation ("That must have made you feel pretty bad—sounds like the drinking had a lot to do with it") (21).

At times, a *planned interview with a family member or close friend,* by telephone or in person, may be needed to make a confident diagnosis of alcoholism. This entails requesting the patient's permission to discuss his or her drinking with another person. Questions to another person regarding the patient's drinking patterns and consequences of the drinking (asking the same questions contained in the CAGE and MAST instruments, such as, "Has your husband ever felt that he ought to cut down on his drinking?") usually yield abundant evidence for alcoholism when the

TABLE 28.3 Michigan Alcoholism Screening Test (MAST)[a]

	Yes	No
0. Do you enjoy having a drink now and then?	0	
1. Do you feel you are a normal drinker? (By normal we mean you drink less than or as much as most other people and you have not gotten into any recurring trouble while drinking.)		2
2. Have you ever awakened the morning after some drinking the night before and found that you could not remember a part of the evening?	2	
3. Does either of your parents, or any other near relative, or your spouse, or any girlfriend or boyfriend ever worry or complain about your drinking?	1	
4. Can you stop drinking without a struggle after one or two drinks?		2
5. Do you feel guilty about your drinking?	1	
6. Do friends or relatives think you are a normal drinker?	2	
7. Are you able to stop drinking when you want to?		2
8. Have you ever attended a meeting of Alcoholics Anonymous (AA)?	5	
9. Have you gotten into physical fights when you have been drinking?	1	
10. Has your drinking ever created problems between you and either of your parents, or another relative, your spouse, or any girlfriend or boyfriend?	2	
11. Has any family member of yours ever gone to anyone for help about your drinking?	2	
12. Have you ever lost friends because of your drinking?	2	
13. Have you ever gotten into trouble at work or at school because of drinking?	2	
14. Have you ever lost a job because of drinking?	2	
15. Have you ever neglected your obligations, your school work, your family, or your job for 2 or more days in a row because you were drinking?	2	
16. Do you drink before noon fairly often?	1	
17. Have you ever been told you have liver trouble? Cirrhosis?	2	
18. After heavy drinking have you ever had severe shaking, or heard voices or seen things that really weren't there?	2 (5 DTs)	
19. Have you ever gone to anyone for help about your drinking?	5	
20. Have you ever been in a hospital because of drinking?	5	
21. Have you ever been a patient in a psychiatric hospital or on a psychiatric ward of a general hospital where drinking was part of the problem that resulted in hospitalization?	2	
22. Have you ever been seen at a psychiatric or mental health clinic or gone to any doctor, social worker, or clergy for help with any emotional problem, where drinking was a part of the problem?	2	
23. Have you ever been arrested for drunk driving, driving while intoxicated, or driving under the influence of alcoholic beverages or any other drug?	2 each	
24. Have you ever been arrested, or taken into custody, even for a few hours, because of other drunk behavior, whether due to alcohol or another drug? (If YES, How many times?)	2 each	

[a]Interpretation of standard MAST: 0 to 3 points, probable normal drinker; 4 points, borderline score; 5 to 9 points, 80% associated with alcoholism/chemical dependence; ≥10 points, 100% associated with alcoholism. The values assigned to each response are shown.

Modified from Seltzer ML: The Michigan alcoholism screening test: The quest for a new diagnostic instrument. Am J Psychiatry 1971;127:89.

problem is present. An exception may be the relatives of an elderly alcoholic who have little contact with the patient or have tacitly agreed to ignore or deny a frustrating, seemingly hopeless situation. In this instance, educating the family about the disease concept of alcoholism may be necessary before they are willing to describe the patterns and consequences of the patient's drinking.

Through contact initiated by one or more family members, information will be produced that supports the diagnosis of alcoholism. Family members should be encouraged to tell the patient that they have contacted his or her doctor to describe these concerns. Ways in which the family can influence the treatment of the patient and can get help for themselves are described in section on Co-Alcoholism.

In summary, except for the presence of the diagnostic manifestations of alcoholism (Table 28.1), there is no simple way to diagnose alcoholism. When the problem is not overt, skillful interviewing of the patient and evaluation of multiple pieces of information are needed to make this diagnosis. This process may be accomplished at one or two visits or over weeks to months.

TABLE 28.4 Alcohol Use Disorders Identification Test (AUDIT) Questionnaire[a]

1. How often do you have a drink containing alcohol?
   (0) Never (1) Monthly or less (2) Two to four times a month (3) Two to three times a week (4) Four more times a week
2. How many drinks containing alcohol do you have on a typical day when you are drinking?
   [Code number of standard drinks.]
   (0) 1 or 2 (1) 3 or 4 (2) 5 or 6 (3) 7 to 9 (4) 10 or more
3. How often do you have six or more drinks on one occasion?
   (0) Never (1) Less than monthly (2) Monthly (3) Weekly (4) Daily or almost daily
4. How often during the last year have you found that you were not able to stop drinking once you had started?
   (0) Never (1) Less than monthly (2) Monthly (3) Weekly (4) Daily or almost daily
5. How often during the last year have you failed to do what was normally expected from you because of drinking?
   (0) Never (1) Less than daily (2) Monthly (3) Weekly (4) Daily or daily
6. How often during the last year have you needed a first drink in the morning to get yourself going after a heaving drinking session?
   (0) Never (1) Less than monthly (2) Monthly (3) Weekly (4) Daily or almost daily
7. How often during the last year have you had a feeling of guilt or remorse after drinking?
   (0) Never (1) Less than monthly (2) Monthly (3) Weekly (4) Daily or almost daily
8. How often during the last year have you been unable to remember what happened the night before because you had been drinking?
   (0) Never (1) Less than monthly (2) Monthly (3) Weekly (4) Daily or almost daily
9. Have you or someone else been injured as a result of your drinking?
   (0) No (2) Yes, but not in the last year (4) Yes, during the last year
10. Has a relative or friend or a doctor or other health worker been concerned about your drinking or suggested you cut down?
    (0) No (2) Yes, but not in the last year (4) Yes, during the last year

[a] A score of 8 or more indicates a strong likelihood of harmful alcohol consumption.
From: Saunders JB, Aasland OG, Babor TF, et al. Development of the Alcohol Use Disorders Identification Test (AUDIT): WHO Collaborative Project on Early Detection of Persons with Harmful Alcohol Consumption-II. Addiction 1993;88:791.

GENERAL PRINCIPLES OF TREATMENT

Definition of Successful Treatment

Alcoholism is a highly treatable disease. Successful treatment depends largely on the skills of those who motivate the alcoholic patient to accept the diagnosis, to undergo detoxification, and to enter and adhere to a long-term treatment process. *Treatment success can be defined as the achievement of abstinence or progressively longer periods of abstinence from alcohol (and other drugs), with improved life functioning for patients and their families.* (A case example is shown in Fig. 28.2.) Factors

TABLE 28.5 The TWEAK Questionnaire

Prior to administering TWEAK, drinkers are identified by a positive response to the question "Do you or have you ever consumed beer, wine, wine coolers, or drinks containing liquor (i.e., whiskey, rum, or vodka)?"

Points

(2) **T**olerance—How many drinks can you hold? ***OR*** How many drinks does it take before begin to feel the first effects of the alcohol, or do you need to feel high?
(2) **W**orried—Have close friends or relatives worried or complained about your drinking in the past year?
(1) **E**ye-openers—Do you sometimes take a drink in the morning when you first get up?
(1) **A**mnesia (blackouts)—Has a friend or family member ever told you about things you said or did while you were drinking that you could not remember?
(1) **K** (C) Cut Down—Do you sometimes feel the need to cut down on your drinking?

- To score the test, a 7-point scale is used
- The Tolerance-hold question scores 2 points if the respondent is able to hold six or more drinks
- The Tolerance-high question scores 2 points if three or more drinks are needed to feel high

A total score or 2 or more indicates that patients are likely to be risk drinkers. A score of 3 or greater identifies harmful drinking or alcoholism.

Adapted from Bradley KA, Boyd-Wickizer BA, Powell SH, et al. Alcohol screening questionnaires in women: a critical review. JAMA 1998;280:166.

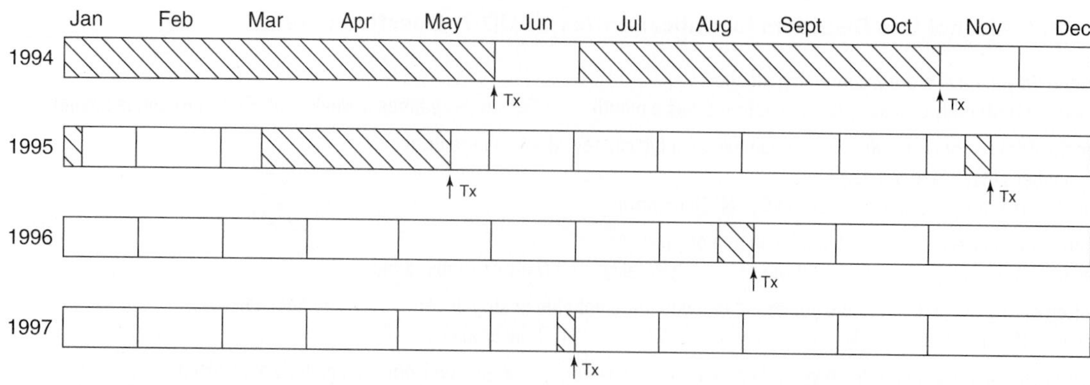

FIGURE 28.2. Drinking–sober profile of a 53-year-old factory supervisor who had been abusing alcohol for 15 years. The achievement of longer and longer periods of abstinence is typical of the process of recovery from alcoholism. *Hatched areas*, drinking; *clear areas*, abstinence; *Tx*, came in for treatment after having dropped out of treatment.

associated with good and poor outcomes after treatment are summarized later (see Prognosis with Treatment). The appropriate terms for describing an alcoholic in recovery are *recovered alcoholic* (a public or polite term) or *recovering alcoholic* (a personal or clinical term). The terms *ex-, reformed, former, or cured alcoholic* are inappropriate. Despite reports that some alcoholics can learn controlled drinking, this goal of treatment has been shown in studies to be unrealistic for most alcoholics and should be avoided.

Avoiding a Psychoanalytic Approach

It has been shown repeatedly that treating alcoholics as though their abnormal drinking behavior is secondary to underlying psychopathology is usually unsuccessful and often counter-therapeutic. Insight-oriented or in-depth psychotherapy early in the treatment of alcoholism is therefore contraindicated. By contrast, supportive and directive psychotherapy, using the treatment methods outlined here and focused on the alcoholism as a primary disease, is usually effective in helping the alcoholic patient reach a successful recovery.

Breaking Down Denial and Motivating the Patient

Denial is the major obstacle to having a patient accept the diagnosis of alcoholism and agree to treatment. Three motivational techniques are fundamental for breaking down denial in patients and, if necessary, in their family members: confrontation, showing empathy, and offering hope. These techniques are equally important in one-on-one interviews and in the other paths to treatment that are described later. *Confrontation* is telling the person what one observes, including that one has diagnosed the disease alcoholism. The patient usually denies the diagnosis and may even get angry. However, with persistent and nonjudgmental confrontation, most patients eventually admit that they have a problem with alcohol. It is important in a confrontation not to argue with the patient but simply to restate the facts.

Statements that convey empathy and offer hope are important in allaying the person's denial, anxiety, anger, and shame. They should be interspersed with confrontational statements. Empathy is conveyed by stating that one recognizes the patient's feelings ("I can see that this is upsetting you") and by conveying concern ("I am very concerned about you"). Offering hope is crucial. The patient must hear, repeatedly, that there is a way out and that there is relief from the misery and bewilderment of the condition. The way out is through abstinence from alcohol and other psychoactive drugs—one day at a time—and regular use of group treatment, which includes self-help groups and group therapy.

Motivation of the patient is an ongoing process. In a model described by Prochaska and DiClemente (Fig. 28.3), one must first facilitate the patient to move from the state of *precontemplation* to *contemplation*. The patient must seriously be ready for change *(determination)*, must *take action* (detoxification and treatment) and, finally, must work toward long-term sobriety (*maintenance*). Unfortunately, because alcoholism is a chronic disease, *relapse* is a likely part of the cycle (22).

After a confident diagnosis of alcoholism has been made, the objectives of care are to have the patient accept the diagnosis and agree to treatment. Specific aspects of this process are described here, beginning with one-on-one confrontation of the patient.

Confrontation

Using the motivational techniques described previously, one can often persuade an alcoholic patient to accept

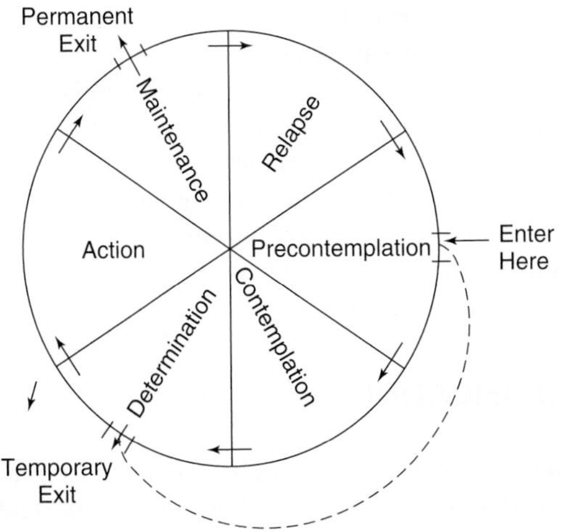

FIGURE 28.3. A stage model of the process of change. (Adapted from Prochaska JO, DiClemente CC. Transtheoretical therapy: toward a more integrative model of change. Psychother Theory Res Pract 1982;19:276. Reprinted with permission from Miller WR, Jackson KA. Practical psychology for pastors. Englewood Cliffs, NJ: Prentice-Hall, 1985:130.)

treatment. Several actions are critical in the confrontation of the patient:

- Stating the diagnosis
- Explaining the disease model
- Making the model specific to the patient
- Telling about treatment
- Getting the patient (and the family) to accept (support) treatment
- Following through

Figure 28.4 summarizes a recommended approach that includes each of these actions. This approach may be incorporated into the interview at a single visit or into interviews at multiple visits. The term *drinking problem* may be used early in the discussion, before the patient's feelings regarding alcoholism are known. Even in the most denying and uncooperative patient, naming the diagnosis is useful because it plants a seed that is likely to grow, given time and motivation. One must be directive in confronting a patient with alcoholism. It is important, however, to include questions that *give the patient some sense of control* during this rather one-sided interaction (see items 3, 5, 7, and 10 in Fig. 28.4). Because most alcoholic patients have negative emotional responses, either overt or private, to being told their diagnosis, it should be assumed that they would not register much of what one says and that *brevity, repetition, and directness* are essential. Repeated *statements of concern, optimism, and support* for the person are as important as statements of fact about the disease. Such statements help patients while they are hearing a diagnosis that inevitably brings shame and help convince them that they have a disease for which they are not to blame. To ensure that patients do not conclude that they cannot avoid further drinking because they have a disease, one should tell them that it is their responsibility to seek treatment.

STATING THE DIAGNOSIS

1. Tell the patient the diagnosis (e.g., "I think that you have the disease alcoholism . . . and I am very concerned about you").
2. Acknowledge the patient's reaction (e.g., "I can see that this is making you pretty uncomfortable . . .").

EXPLAINING THE DISEASE MODEL

3. Ask the patient to tell you his/her idea of what alcoholism is. (Patient usually describes stereotype model of a skidrow alcoholic . . . "and that's not me!". . .)
4. Clarify the patient's model by stating four basic facts:
   a) Alcoholism is a disease ("a disease like other medical diseases . . . for example diabetes").
   b) Like other diseases, alcoholism has an early stage way before what you described.
   c) Like other diseases, alcoholism is not the patient's fault.
   d) Alcoholism can be treated and the chances of recovery are excellent.

MAKING THE MODEL SPECIFIC

5. Ask the patient if he/she knows why you think he/she has alcoholism.
6. Tell the patient the evidence that he/she has alcoholism. (Always restate concern for the patient; if appropriate, stress features of early alcoholism.)

TELLING ABOUT TREATMENT

7. Ask the patient what he/she knows about the treatment of alcoholism.
8. Tell the patient the basic facts about treatment:
   a) Abstinence
   b) Requires the help of other people

GETTING THE PATIENT (AND FAMILY) TO ACCEPT TREATMENT

9. Offer the patient treatment options that you know of (always include a local program that offers detoxification and Alcoholics Anonymous).
10. Get the patient to select a treatment plan and to make contact promptly (e.g., call available detoxification program, call local AA office and let patient speak with AA representative).
11. With the patient's permission, contact his/her spouse or significant person(s) (tell the diagnosis and plan, and initiate plans for family treatment).

FOLLOWING THROUGH

12. Schedule follow-up appointment in 1 or 2 weeks (consider 1 or 2 days if patient has not agreed to make a treatment decision).

FIGURE 28.4. A recommended approach for one-on-one confrontation of the patient in whom alcoholism has been diagnosed.

The first goal of treatment is abstinence from alcohol and other psychoactive drugs. However, it is never sufficient simply to tell the patient to stop drinking. Early in treatment, the patient must accept help in the difficult process of recovery. *This help is multidimensional.* In addition to regular follow-up by a supportive physician who believes the patient can recover, the most important elements are a plan for detoxification, Alcoholics Anonymous or group therapy, and family involvement (see Nonpharmacologic Treatment After Detoxification). Inpatient treatment in a specialized alcoholism treatment facility may be needed. Each of the possible treatment options should be explained to the patient and the family. If the clinician is not familiar with these, an alcoholism counselor should be asked to explain them to the patient. If the patient is in a crisis and not enough time is available during the first visit, a return appointment should be scheduled within a few days or the patient should be immediately referred to a reliable treatment program.

Formal Intervention

All too often, alcoholics with concerned families do not respond to efforts to motivate them to accept treatment. In this situation, the family should be told about the option of using a formal intervention. This consists of a meeting at which people closest to the alcoholic (immediate family members, concerned friends, employer, or other important people) create a crisis that motivates the alcoholic to accept treatment.

The intervention team is composed of as many people as possible who are emotionally important to the alcoholic. Before the actual intervention, this team meets to talk about the alcoholism, to come together in their thinking, and to agree that their purpose is to show the patient in unmistakable terms that there is a problem and that he or she needs treatment. The process is initiated by having each participant put in writing specific dramatic instances of drinking-related incidents that led to anger, fear, disappointment, sadness, embarrassment, or other distress for the team member. The team then rehearses confronting the alcoholic. Each person learns to begin with an expression of concern for the alcoholic, to describe the disturbing event and how it made that person feel, and to name specific measures they will take if the patient does not agree to treatment (e.g., loss of job, no further visits by grandchildren). As part of a formal intervention, arrangements may be made in advance to have the person admitted for alcoholism treatment. Financing of treatment, packing clothes, arranging for absence from work, and other details must all be worked out by the team ahead of time.

Motivating through Employee Assistance Programs

Increasingly, employers have recognized the economic and human costs of alcoholism and have developed employee assistance programs to motivate and assist alcoholics into treatment. Employers threaten to terminate employees who have deteriorating job performance due to alcoholism unless they get treatment and remain in treatment. Physicians asked to write work excuses can often work with employee assistance programs to coerce the denying alcoholic to get appropriate treatment for alcoholism. This approach uses the strong motivation to keep a job as leverage for getting treatment and following through to recovery—leverage the physician alone may not have on the patient. The problem of the impaired professional and the use of measures similar to employee assistance programs are discussed in a later section.

DETOXIFICATION

The majority of alcoholics can be detoxified from alcohol by outpatient procedures (23). With the cost of treatment now a major consideration, the decision between inpatient and outpatient detoxification should be based mostly on medical history and severity of alcohol withdrawal symptoms.

Alcohol Withdrawal Symptoms

The diagnosis of alcohol withdrawal requires a history of recent heavy drinking followed by reduced intake or cessation of use, the absence of other conditions that could cause symptoms mimicking withdrawal, and one or more of the four major manifestations of alcohol withdrawal (tremors, seizures, hallucinosis, and delirium tremens) (24). These occur also in other conditions, ranging from withdrawal from other sedative-hypnotic drugs to meningitis (see list of causes of delirium in Chapter 26).

Tremulousness usually begins 8 to 12 hours after the patient's last drink and peaks in 24 to 36 hours. *Withdrawal seizures* occur within 8 to 24 hours. Withdrawal seizures may occur independent of other manifestations of alcohol withdrawal. Both seizures and tremulousness can occur before the BAL has reached zero.

The *alcohol hallucination* is almost never the mythical pink elephant. Rather, it is usually one of moving insects, small animals, or threatening voices. In a series of 50 consecutive patients, 58% of their hallucinations were purely visual, 16% were purely auditory, and 26% were mixed (25). In certain patients these hallucinations may not be all negative; that is, the patient becomes used to them and is no longer frightened. Hallucinations may begin up to several days after the patient stops or markedly reduces alcohol use (usually in the first 48 hours). Typically, alcoholic hallucinosis lasts from minutes to days (usually less than 1 week) but in a very small percentage of patients hallucinosis continues for weeks to months or, rarely, as a continuous symptom.

Delirium tremens is a late manifestation of withdrawal, occurring from 48 hours (most common interval) to 14 days (uncommon) after cessation of drinking (26). It may begin after the patient has shown signs of improvement from the early manifestations of withdrawal. Any of the symptoms of delirium, described in Chapter 26, may signal the onset of delirium tremens.

At least half of ambulatory alcoholic patients who stop drinking develop none of the four major manifestations of withdrawal. Additional minor symptoms are common. Anorexia, nausea, and sometimes vomiting are present in varying degrees. Tachycardia, systolic hypertension, and paroxysmal diaphoresis also are common. Generalized weakness may be prominent, and tinnitus, hyperacusis, itching, muscle cramps, and mood and sleep disorders are sometimes experienced. The patient often is hyperalert, startles easily, and has difficulty concentrating and usually craves alcohol or other drugs to quiet symptoms.

Selection of Patients for Inpatient versus Outpatient Detoxification

There are a number of indications for referring a withdrawing alcoholic patient for *inpatient detoxification* (Table 28.6). Inpatient detoxification provides careful 24-hour monitoring and treatment of withdrawal symptoms, evaluation of inter-current medical problems, and removal of patients from the environment that has facilitated their drinking. If medically stable, patients participate in groups (usually Alcoholics Anonymous) and receive individual counseling.

For mildly symptomatic patients with a stable home environment and supportive family and friends, *outpatient detoxification* supervised at daily visits to a treatment program or physician's office is as effective as inpatient detoxification. Patients may contract to attend an Alcoholics Anonymous meeting daily with a friend or family member. For moderately sick patients, the choice of outpatient versus inpatient detoxification should be based on what programs are available. Some outpatient detoxification programs are intensive, requiring patients to spend entire days being monitored, with patients receiving medication as needed and participating in group counseling but going home to sleep. Other outpatient detoxification programs consist only of brief daily visits.

TABLE 28.6 Indications for Referring a Withdrawing Alcoholic for Inpatient Detoxification

Evidence of hallucinations, severe tachycardia, severe tremor, fever, extreme agitation, or a history of severe withdrawal symptoms
History of seizure disorder
Presence of ataxia, nystagmus, confusion, or ophthalmoplegia, which may be indicative of Wernicke encephalopathy
Severe nausea and vomiting that would prevent the ingestion of medication
Evidence of acute or chronic liver disease that may alter the metabolism of drugs used in the treatment of withdrawal
Presence of cardiovascular disease such as severe hypertension, ischemic heart disease, or arrhythmia, for which the sympathetic surge of catecholamines during withdrawal poses particular risk
Pregnancy
Presence of associated medical or surgical condition requiring treatment
Lack of medical or social support system to allow outpatient detoxification

Use of Drugs in Detoxification

A useful *tool for making decisions about pharmacologic treatment in the withdrawing alcoholic* is the Clinical Institute Withdrawal Assessment for Alcohol (CIWA-Ar) (Table 28.7) (27). Pharmacologic therapy is not indicated for a score less than 10. For scores of 10 to 20, clinical judgment should determine the need for pharmacologic treatment. For scores greater than 20, treatment with drugs is indicated and should be administered on either an outpatient or an inpatient basis. For scores of 20 to 40, the assessment can be repeated after administration of a dose of medication; patients without improvement need more intensive monitoring as inpatients. Notably, pulse and blood pressure are not part of the CIWA scale. Although elevations of blood pressure and pulse do occur in alcohol withdrawal, the other signs and symptoms are more reliable in the assessment of severity of withdrawal. Therefore, one should not make a decision about whether to prescribe drugs for alcohol withdrawal based solely on blood pressure and pulse measurements.

Detoxification with the use of orally administered psychoactive drugs appears to be most effective when it is combined with the nonpharmacologic techniques described in the next section and when treatment is given early. The safest and most effective drugs for this purpose are the benzodiazepine sedative-hypnotics (28). All of the benzodiazepines are effective. Diazepam has the advantages of having a rapid onset of action, a longer half-life, and a lower cost. Its long half-life permits loading on the first day; that is, 5 to 10 mg every 1 to 4 hours until severe symptoms dissipate, which will reduce or perhaps eliminate the need for further dosing on subsequent days. Lorazepam (Ativan) does not require hepatic metabolism and is safer in patients with severe liver disease (e.g., prolonged prothrombin time [PT]). Patient response to a dose of benzodiazepine is unpredictable and is not necessarily related to the amount of drinking. Ideally, patients should be monitored for response after initial dosing to make an assessment of indicated dosage and dosing interval. Dosing should be titrated to effect. Essential to management is early recognition of withdrawal, early treatment, frequent monitoring, and continual treatment. Given the decision to use sedative drugs in the detoxification process, one can choose low or high dosages (Table 28.8). Low dosages of sedative-hypnotic drugs may be tried first for most patients. The advantage of low-dose treatment is that the

TABLE 28.7 Addiction Research Foundation Clinical Institute Withdrawal Assessment for Alcohol (CIWA-Ar)[a]

Patient ________ Date |___|___|___| (y m d) Time ________ : ________ (24-hour clock, midnight = 00:00)

Pulse or heart rate, taken for 1 min: ________ Blood pressure: ________/ ________

NAUSEA AND VOMITING—Ask "Do you feel sick to your stomach? Have you vomited?" Observation.
0 no nausea and no vomiting
1 mild nausea with no vomiting
2
3
4 intermittent nausea with dry heaves
5
6
7 constant nausea, frequent dry heaves and vomiting

TREMOR—Arms extended and fingers spread apart. Observation.
0 no tremor
1 not visible, but can be felt fingertip to fingertip
2
3
4 moderate, with patient's arms extended
5
6
7 severe, even with arms not extended

PAROXYSMAL SWEATS—Observation.
0 no sweat visible
1 barely perceptible sweating, palms moist
2
3
4 beads of sweat obvious on forehead
5
6
7 drenching sweats

ANXIETY—Ask "Do you feel nervous?" Observation.
0 no anxiety, at ease
1 mildly anxious
2
3
4 moderately anxious, or guarded, so anxiety is inferred
5
6
7 equivalent to acute panic states, as seen in severe delirium, or acute schizophrenic reactions

AGITATION—Observation.
0 normal activity
1 somewhat more than normal activity
2
3
4 moderately fidgety and restless
5
6
7 paces back and forth during most of the interview, or constantly thrashes about

TACTILE DISTURBANCES—Ask "Have you any itching, pins and needles sensations, any burning, any numbness, or do you feel bugs crawling on or under your skin?" Observation.
0 none
1 very mild itching, pins and needles, burning or numbness
2 mild itching, pins and needles, burning or numbness
3 moderate itching, pins and needles, burning or numbness
4 moderately severe hallucinations
5 severe hallucinations
6 extremely severe hallucinations
7 continuous hallucinations

AUDITORY DISTURBANCES—Ask "Are you more aware of sounds around you? Are they harsh? Do they frighten you? Are you hearing anything that is disturbing you? Are you hearing things you know are not there?" Observation.
0 not present
1 very mild harshness or ability to frighten
2 mild harshness or ability to frighten
3 moderate harshness or ability to frighten
4 moderately severe hallucinations
5 severe hallucinations
6 extremely severe hallucinations
7 continuous hallucinations

VISUAL DISTURBANCES—Ask "Does the light appear to be too bright? Is its color different? Does it hurt your eyes? Are you seeing anything that is disturbing to you? Are you seeing things you know are not there?" Observation.
0 not present
1 very mild sensitivity
2 mild sensitivity
3 moderate sensitivity
4 moderately severe hallucinations
5 severe hallucinations
6 extremely severe hallucinations
7 continuous hallucinations

HEADACHE, FULLNESS IN HEAD—Ask "Does your head feel different? Does it feel like there is a band around your head?" Do not rate for dizziness or lightheadedness. Otherwise, rate severity.
0 not present
1 very mild
2 mild
3 moderate
4 moderately severe
5 severe
6 very severe
7 extremely severe

ORIENTATION AND CLOUDING OF SENSORIUM—Ask "What day is this? Where are you? Who am I?"
0 oriented and can do serial additions
1 cannot do serial additions or is uncertain about date
2 disoriented for date by no more than 2 calendar days
3 disoriented for date by more than 2 calendar days
4 disoriented for place and/or person

Total CIWA-A Score to 35________
Rater's Initials to 35________
Maximum Possible Score 67

[a]This scale is not copyrighted and may be used freely.
From: Sullivan JT, Sykora K, Schneiderman J, et al. Assessment of alcohol withdrawal: the revised clinical institute withdrawal assessment for alcohol scale (CIWA-Ar). Br J Addict 1989;84:1353.

TABLE 28.8 Characteristics of Benzodiazepines Used Orally in the Treatment of Alcohol Withdrawal

Drug	*Onset of Action*	*Rate of Metabolism*	*Liver Metabolized*	*Low Dosage (mg per 6 hr)*	*High Dosage (mg per 2–4 hr)*
Chlordiazepoxide	Intermediate	Long	Yes	25	100
Diazepam	Fast	Long	Yes	2–5	10–20
Lorazepam	Intermediate	Intermediate	No	0.5	2
Oxazepam	Slow	Short	No	10–15	30

patient remains more alert. High dosages of these drugs may be indicated when the low dosage does not suppress or prevent symptoms within the first few hours.

The aim of drug treatment is to alleviate the most bothersome symptoms and signs of withdrawal. Symptom-driven therapy, compared to fixed schedule therapy, has been shown to decrease treatment duration and the amount of benzodiazepine used (29). Benzodiazepines should be given in such a manner that withdrawal symptoms are improved without oversedation of the patient. If the patient is being treated as an outpatient, each day's medication should be entrusted to a family member or friend who will be staying with the patient. Most patients need to be medicated for only 24 to 72 hours. Antihypertensive drugs (most notably clonidine and β-blockers) have been used for management of alcohol withdrawal. These drugs effectively alleviate the sympathetic markers of withdrawal (hypertension and tachycardia) but do little for the more severe aspects of withdrawal (seizures and hallucinosis). For this reason, if a patient is so symptomatic that the use of drugs is deemed appropriate, a benzodiazepine should be the drug of choice. Carbamazepine may also be effective in treating patients with mild alcohol withdrawal (30). The prevention of withdrawal seizures is discussed later.

Detoxification without Drugs

Candidates for nonpharmacologic outpatient detoxification should be ambulatory and, except for their chronic alcoholism and acute withdrawal, should be otherwise free from serious chronic illness or acute problems. The primary aim in nonpharmacologic detoxification is to provide a nonthreatening, positive environment for the patient. The patient should be kept ambulatory when possible and given a regular diet. Except when asleep or resting comfortably, the patient should be encouraged to perform purposeful activities, such as carrying out small duties or attending introductory group education and therapy sessions.

Nonpharmacologic therapy can be just as effective as drug therapy in the detoxification of ambulatory patients in uncomplicated cases (31). The advantages of nonpharmacologic detoxification, compared to traditional detoxification with drugs, are that it can be done largely by nonmedical personnel, it is less expensive, and the patient is more likely to remain alert and, consequently, able to participate in treatment. The only routine medication should be vitamins (100 mg of thiamine, 1 mg of folate, and a multivitamin daily). These vitamins should be continued for the first month or more of recovery.

Many communities have established alcoholism facilities that provide a sheltered, supportive environment to care for alcoholics, using a social model for detoxification. Patients are screened and evaluated to detect any obvious medical problems before or shortly after being admitted. Should complications arise, backup hospital/medical support is available. The length of stay varies in each program, from 3 days to more than 30 days. Most social setting programs use Alcoholics Anonymous extensively, and many of the larger programs use techniques used in other alcoholism treatment centers. These centers can be either day treatment or residential facilities.

For detoxification at home without the use of drugs, a reliable family member or other person should be present to observe the patient for at least 2 full days. The physician supervising such detoxification should be in touch with the patient or the family member daily during the 2 to 4 days required for detoxification. The following is a checklist for home detoxification:

1. The patient should be motivated to achieve detoxification at home.
2. A reliable person should stay with or frequently check on the patient.
3. There should be access to a telephone so that the patient can call the physician or counselor daily for reassurance and for monitoring withdrawal.
4. There should be no active medical problems requiring aggressive treatment and no significant chemical dependence to drugs other than alcohol.
5. There should be arrangements to see a supervising physician, nurse, or counselor each day.
6. The patient should be as active as possible (attend Alcoholics Anonymous, take foods and fluids as desired, and take multivitamins daily).
7. The patient should have arrangements to start an outpatient program on completion of detoxification.

Prevention of Withdrawal Seizures

There is no consensus about whether *phenytoin* (Dilantin) should be included in the detoxification of patients with a history of withdrawal seizures. It has been shown that phenytoin at a dosage of 300 mg/day for 5 days can prevent most withdrawal seizures, even though therapeutic plasma levels of phenytoin are not reached (32). However, in another study, when patients received an intravenous load of phenytoin or placebo within 6 hours after a first alcohol withdrawal seizure, phenytoin provided no benefit in preventing further seizures (33).

There is evidence that a *high-dosage benzodiazepine* regimen for withdrawal can prevent seizures (34). Therefore, patients who are significantly symptomatic and are receiving sufficient pharmacologic therapy with a benzodiazepine do not require phenytoin. However, patients who are only mildly symptomatic and have a history of a withdrawal seizure should receive prophylactic phenytoin if they are not going to be treated with a benzodiazepine. This recommendation is based on the fact that a seizure may occur without the presence of any other manifestations of alcohol withdrawal (35).

NONPHARMACOLOGIC TREATMENT AFTER DETOXIFICATION

Overview

Treatment consists of motivating the patient, initiating a treatment plan, and providing regular followup. The clinician who initially motivates an alcoholic to accept treatment may elect not to coordinate the overall treatment but to provide a referral elsewhere. For this important referral, one should select a specialist or a program with demonstrated expertise in helping alcoholics recover.

In selecting skilled help, one should look for several characteristics. Effective programs are abstinence-oriented; use Alcoholics Anonymous or group therapy as a mainstay of treatments; avoid the use of psychoactive drugs in long-term treatment; refer the spouse to Al-Anon or family therapy; provide close followup; and avoid insight-oriented psychotherapy, unless indicated later in the course of recovery. The physician who makes the referral should reinforce participation in the treatment program whenever the patient returns for followup.

Alcoholics Anonymous and Group Therapy

Alcoholics and other chemical-dependent people seem to recover best in group treatment settings. Groups effectively break down the denial process and heal the associated guilt and shame through a combination of identification, nonjudgmental acceptance, confrontation, and support. Every alcoholic should be strongly encouraged to attend Alcoholics Anonymous regularly. Studies show that regular Alcoholics Anonymous attendance is strongly correlated with long-term recovery and improved functioning (36). Patients who continue to attend Alcoholics Anonymous after inpatient treatment have improved outcomes (37).

Many patients are reluctant to attend Alcoholics Anonymous or a therapy group. Therefore, when referring a patient, it is important to convey that one is familiar with these programs and has confidence in them. Immediate action, taken while the patient is in the office, may consist of having the patient contact a family member or friend who is active in Alcoholics Anonymous, telephoning the local Alcoholics Anonymous office and having the patient request a contact to take him or her to a convenient Alcoholics Anonymous meeting, or telephoning an alcoholism treatment program and arranging an intake appointment for the patient. The best way for physicians to learn about these programs is to attend one or more Alcoholics Anonymous meetings and, if available, open group therapy meetings. To locate such meetings, one can call the local Alcoholics Anonymous office or look on the Internet at http://www.alcoholics-anonymous.org. Table 28.9 summarizes the Alcoholics Anonymous process.

Psychotherapy

It is commonly thought that all alcoholic patients have a primary and causative underlying psychological problem. If treatment of this condition is successful, the alcoholism is expected to resolve because it is considered to be chiefly a manifestation of the underlying psychological problem. Although this approach may seem theoretically valid, this therapeutic strategy rarely works unless there happens to be a coexisting psychosis. Patients with alcoholism cannot gain insight into aspects of their lives successfully until they have maintained sobriety. Early psychotherapy may impede maintenance of sobriety and trigger relapse. Even in patients with coexisting psychosis, the alcoholism must also be treated. After rapport is established, therefore, the initial effort in psychotherapy should be to work with the patient toward abstinence and regular participation in group treatment.

Ongoing supportive care by the provider, as described in Chapter 20, is useful for reinforcing the patient's understanding of the disease and the recovery process; for monitoring the patient's functioning in important life areas, such as family, job, and interpersonal relations; and for assisting the patient in change and growth.

Discussions with the Spouse or Closest Family Members

As part of the early treatment of an alcoholic patient, the situation should be discussed with the spouse or person

TABLE 28.9 The Process of Alcoholics Anonymous

Two alcoholics, one a stockbroker and one a physician founded Alcoholics Anonymous in 1935.
Meetings
Alcoholics Anonymous meetings are held frequently in all communities in the United States and in most other countries. Meetings are either open or closed (most are open and most welcome nonalcoholics interested in treating alcoholism). A published directory of meetings, places, times, and information by telephone are available from each local chapter of Alcoholics Anonymous. By contacting Alcoholics Anonymous, an alcoholic can almost always arrange to be taken to a meeting in his or her community; often on the day he or she makes the request. Many Alcoholics Anonymous members attend meetings several times a week. Some attend at least one meeting per day. Lifelong activity in Alcoholics Anonymous is the basis for maintaining health for many recovering alcoholics. Meetings are usually 1 hour in length. Most are held in the evening, although there are many daytime meetings as well. Meetings begin with a recitation by one member of the Twelve Steps and the Twelve Traditions and are devoted to examination and interpretation of these, as illustrated in personal experiences described by a number of members. One member of the group chairs the meeting and calls on speakers. Speakers introduce themselves by their first names (e.g., "I'm Joe-I'm an alcoholic"). Meetings end with group recitation of the Lord's Prayer or the Serenity Prayer "God grant me the Serenity to accept the things I cannot change, Courage to change the things I can, and Wisdom to know the difference." Alcoholics Anonymous on the surface can sometimes look insubstantial and unsophisticated, often turning off newcomers. Often the spiritual overtones of the program are rejected. However, the program is *profound and life changing.* Without an administrative structure, owning no property, and having no dues or fees, it continues to grow because it works and meets human need.
Publications
Alcoholics Anonymous provides printed educational aids in the form of pamphlets (available at meetings) and "the Big Book" (*Alcoholics Anonymous,* a collection of personal stories that illustrate vividly the ways that lives are damaged by alcoholism and the Alcoholics Anonymous path to recovery). One can obtain this book or other literature at meetings, at the local Alcoholics Anonymous office, or at http://www.alcoholics-anonymous.org
The 12 Steps
1. We admitted we were powerless over alcohol, that our lives had become unmanageable. 2. Came to believe that a power greater than ourselves could restore us to sanity. 3. Made a decision to turn our will and our lives over to the care of God, as we understood Him. 4. Made a searching and fearless moral inventory of ourselves. 5. Admitted to God, to ourselves, and to another human being the exact nature of our wrongs. 6. Were entirely ready to have God remove all these defects of character. 7. Humbly asked Him to remove our shortcomings. 8. Made a list of all persons we had harmed, and became willing to make amends to them all. 9. Made direct amends to such people wherever possible, except when to do so would injure them or others. 10. Continued to take personal inventory, and when we were wrong promptly admitted it. 11. Sought through prayer and meditation to improve our conscious contact with God, as we understood Him, praying only for knowledge of His will for us and the power to carry that out. 12. Having had a spiritual awakening as the result of the Steps, we tried to carry this message to alcoholics, and to practice these principles in all our affairs (note: for this step, Altman substitutes "others" for the word "alcoholics"). *Boiled down, these steps mean, simply:* a. Admission of alcoholism. b. Personality analysis and catharsis. c. Adjustment of personal relations. d. Dependence on some higher power. e. Working with other alcoholics.
The 12 Traditions
1. Our common welfare should come first; personal recovery depends upon Alcoholics Anonymous unity. 2. For our group purpose there is but one ultimate authority—a loving God as He may express Himself in our group conscience. Our leaders are but trusted servants; they do not govern. 3. The only requirement for Alcoholics Anonymous membership is a desire to stop drinking. 4. Each group should be autonomous except in matters affecting other groups or Alcoholics Anonymous as a whole. 5. Each group has but one primary purpose—to carry out its message to the alcoholic who still suffers. 6. An Alcoholics Anonymous group ought never endorse, finance, or lend the Alcoholics Anonymous name to any related facility or outside enterprise, lest problems of money, property, and prestige divert us from our primary purpose. 7. Every Alcoholics Anonymous group ought to be fully self-supporting, declining outside contributions. 8. Alcoholics Anonymous should remain forever nonprofessional, but our service centers may employ special workers. 9. Alcoholics Anonymous, as such, ought never to be organized; but we may create service boards or committees directly responsible to those they serve. 10. Alcoholics Anonymous has no opinion on outside issues; hence the Alcoholics Anonymous name ought never be drawn into public controversy. 11. Our public relations policy is based on attraction rather than promotion; we need always maintain personal anonymity at the level of press, radio, and films. 12. Anonymity is the spiritual foundation of our Traditions, ever reminding us to place principles before personalities.

closest to the patient. Such discussions (which should be conducted without breaking the patient's confidentiality) serve to ensure that the family agrees with the goal of abstinence; explore the spouse's own drinking pattern; discern any special problems occurring in any of the close family members, and educate the spouse about the enabling process. *If the family does not change and grow, usually through regular attendance at Al-Anon meetings, it will be more difficult for the patient to recover.* Family treatment and the Al-Anon process are described later (see Co-alcoholism).

PHARMACOLOGIC TREATMENT OF ALCOHOL DEPENDENCE

Disulfiram (Antabuse)

Although disulfiram has not been shown to increase duration of sobriety (38), the use of disulfiram to prevent drinking should be considered for some patients. Patients must be in active recovery, including Alcoholics Anonymous and individual or group therapy. Disulfiram should not be used as the focus of treatment but as an adjunct. Because disulfiram is taken daily, it is a constant reminder that one cannot drink safely. For the patient on disulfiram, the decision not to drink has to be made only once a day.

Alcohol is initially oxidized by the hepatic enzyme alcohol dehydrogenase to acetaldehyde, and disulfiram inhibits acetaldehyde oxidation by interfering with aldehyde dehydrogenase. This effect may persist for up to 2 weeks after cessation of disulfiram. The symptoms of the alcohol–disulfiram reaction are related to *elevated acetaldehyde;* they are usually proportional to the amounts of disulfiram and alcohol ingested. Some people have typical symptoms after drinking as little as 7 mL of alcohol (about half of a drink). A very small percentage of patients seem to be able to drink despite taking disulfiram with no significant symptoms.

The common symptoms of the alcohol–disulfiram reaction usually begins within 10 minutes and includes flushing, throbbing in the head and neck, headaches, anxiety, general discomfort, sweating, and respiratory difficulty. The reaction typically lasts between 30 minutes and several hours.

Patients who are motivated to succeed in recovery and who have experienced relapse or dread the likelihood of relapse are candidates for disulfiram. Table 28.10 summarizes a practical plan that can be used in office practice. This supervised approach is similar in its demands on patients and physicians to the initiation and management of long-term treatment. Patients should carry an identification card that identifies them as taking disulfiram.

Contraindications for the use of disulfiram include a history of hypertension, diabetes, emphysema, seizures, significant liver or renal disease, coronary artery disease (CAD), hypothyroidism, pregnancy, or a history of drinking

TABLE 28.10 The Suggested Approach to Supervised Use of Disulfiram

1. Satisfy the following indications: the patient is willing to take medication several times a week under supervision, the patient can recall making the decision to take the first drink of a relapse, and the patient is actively involved in an organized outpatient treatment program.
2. Rule out contraindications and ask yourself the following question: "Can this patient survive a disulfiram–alcohol reaction?"
3. Ensure sober state before the initiation of treatment.
4. Be sure patient and spouse know how to avoid hidden alcohol in foods, over-the-counter medications, toiletries, etc.
5. Have the patient read, discuss, and sign a consent form before initiating treatment.
6. Begin with a dosage of one tablet (250 mg) daily.
7. *Keep the medication bottle in the office* and have the patient come in three times a week to be dispensed two (or three) doses by the office staff. After 1 month, decrease the visits to twice a week and increase the number of pills dispensed accordingly. After another month, go to weekly visits and continue these for the duration of disulfiram treatment. See the patient at least monthly and repeat laboratory testing every 3 months.
8. If the patient misses more than one or two appointments in a row, have the office staff contact the people on the consent form, and stop administering the medication.

while taking disulfiram. If alcohol-related liver disease is present, prescribing of disulfiram should be delayed until the levels of serum aspartate aminotransferase (AST) and serum alanine aminotransferase (ALT), two serum markers of liver disease, are less than three times the normal range. Cough syrups and foods (e.g., salad dressings) that name alcohol as an ingredient should be avoided.

Naltrexone

Naltrexone (ReVia) is a second drug that is potentially useful as an adjunct to a formal treatment program for individuals with alcohol dependence (39,40). Unlike disulfiram, patients do not get sick if they drink while taking naltrexone. Naltrexone has been shown to *reduce alcohol craving* and as a result may be particularly useful in preventing relapse in motivated patients (38,41). When patients relapse they tend to drink smaller amounts. There is no data supporting naltrexone assisting in long-term abstinence, as most studies have been small and have followed patients for only 3 to 6 months. A large multicenter study of alcoholic veterans did not find a benefit from using naltrexone over 1 year (42). A recent Cochrane review of the use of naltrexone for alcoholism concluded that the evidence supports the use of naltrexone as a "short-term treatment for alcoholism"(43). Long-acting parenteral depot forms of naltrexone for use in alcohol dependence are available in Europe.

Naltrexone is an opiate antagonist and therefore cannot be prescribed to patients who are taking opiate analgesics. Furthermore, patients maintained on naltrexone will not obtain pain relief if prescribed an opiate. Naltrexone is well tolerated, with nausea as its main side effect. Naltrexone can be used in combination with disulfiram. Although there is no clear evidence of hepatotoxicity, the makers of naltrexone advise monitoring of liver function tests (initially at monthly intervals and then less frequently). If naltrexone is tolerated and is successful in aiding abstinence, the recommended initial course of treatment is 3 months. Naltrexone does not cause physical dependence and can be stopped at any time without withdrawal symptoms. If a patient is going to have elective surgery, naltrexone should be stopped at least 72 hours beforehand to allow the use of opiate analgesia.

Acamprosate

Acamprosate (Campral, calcium acetyl homotaurinate), the newest drug approved for treatment of alcoholism, was approved for use in the United States in 2004. Compliance is difficult, as acamprosate must be taken as 666 mg (two pills) three times a day. Most studies of acamprosate examine its effectiveness in individuals who have just completed detoxification. Studies of benefit are mixed, but a recent meta-analysis of acamprosate concluded that it is an effective adjuvant therapy for alcoholism and can significantly improve abstinence (44). A study of the combined use of acamprosate and naltrexone for preventing relapse had a high dropout rate limiting the interpretation of its findings (45).

A decision to stop disulfiram, naltrexone, or acamprosate is best made jointly by the physician, the spouse or other close person, the Alcoholics Anonymous sponsor, and the patient. It should be based on the strength of the patient's recovery. Important guidelines in this decision are active Alcoholics Anonymous or group-therapy participation, coping with crises without recourse to drinking, improved family relationships, dissolution of denial, social ease (diminution in social anxiety), growth in self-esteem, and prolonged abstinence.

Psychoactive Drugs

Although many alcoholics have symptoms such as anxiety, insomnia, and tremors that might be helped by sedatives, in actuality these drugs usually interfere with successful recovery. Anxiolytic drugs may have a role in acute detoxification, and major tranquilizers, antidepressants, and lithium have usefulness in treating, respectively, the schizophrenic, the severe protracted depressive, and the manic-depressive alcoholic (as long as these patients are being treated concomitantly for alcoholism). Apart from these situations, psychoactive drugs should not be prescribed for alcoholics. There are many reasons for this recommendation: (a) all sedatives are cross-tolerant with alcohol and thus have a built-in escalation factor; (b) combining sedatives with alcohol is often dangerously synergistic; (c) inability to control consumption, a cardinal feature of alcoholism, occurs with prescribed sedative drugs; (d) memory blackouts may also occur with other sedatives and minor tranquilizers; (e) patients may alter the prescription to obtain excessive quantities of these drugs; (f) prescribing these drugs reinforces psychoactive substance use as a coping mechanism and impairs development of the patient's own coping mechanisms; and (g) the drugs interfere with learning to relate to others in a healthy manner.

FOLLOWUP: PREVENTION AND MANAGEMENT OF RELAPSE

Next to dealing with denial and motivating the patient, followup is the most difficult part of treatment. One reason is that when an alcoholic recovers there may be an early honeymoon period during which the patient feels and looks so good that one is lulled into believing that regular followup is unnecessary. However, because it takes 2 to 3 years of appropriate treatment before recovery can be secure, regular followup is indicated.

During the first 6 weeks after stopping drinking, patients need much support and direction, for this is the time when they are most likely to relapse. At least weekly patient contacts are indicated for this time, with a gradually decreasing frequency thereafter. Some of these contacts may be by telephone. Other *high-risk times for relapse* include special days and occasions, such as vacations, holidays, business trips, birthdays, and anniversaries, and crises, such as separation, divorce, death of a close person, or illness in the family. Other relapse danger times are when a patient stops taking pharmacologic therapy or stops attending Alcoholics Anonymous or group therapy meetings.

"Dry drunks" are often part of the natural history of recovery. This is the name given by recovering alcoholics to the negative emotions and behaviors reminiscent of those that occurred when the patient was drinking. Dry drunks may last from a few hours to several weeks or even months. Treatment is by recognition, education, and alteration of the diet and other current life habits. Dry drunks are often associated with eating poorly. Regular, well-balanced meals should be recommended, and caffeine intake, including coffee, tea, colas, and chocolate, should be markedly decreased or discontinued. Increased attendance at Alcoholics Anonymous or group therapy meetings at this time is very important. Moderation in the patient's work and recreational activities and rest should be advised.

The *relapse process generally begins long before the person drinks.* It often progresses in the following sequence:

reactivation of denial, progressive isolation and defensiveness, building a crisis to justify symptom progression, immobilization, confusion and overreaction, depression, loss of control over behavior, recognition of loss of control, and finally relapse to drinking.

Although it should not be telegraphed to the patient, relapse is part of the natural history of successful recovery for most alcoholics, and one should not become discouraged if it happens (Fig. 28.3). Instead, one should immediately recruit the patient back into treatment using the same motivational techniques used initially. Relapse is a time for both patient and therapist to learn about their mistakes and to correct them by strengthening treatment.

INPATIENT REHABILITATION

Although controlled studies differ regarding the advantage of inpatient rehabilitation versus outpatient treatment, inpatient rehabilitation for 2 to 6 weeks may be especially helpful for selected patients (46). It is always planned for in advance when a formal intervention is used (see Formal Intervention). Other indications for inpatient rehabilitation are strong denial, especially if it persists in outpatient treatment; unsuccessful or too slow recovery despite adequate outpatient treatment; weak or unavailable support systems; danger to self or others; severe medical, psychiatric, or other problems related to the alcoholism; and patient's desire for inpatient treatment.

Although treatment goals among inpatient rehabilitation programs vary, some of the major goals include breaking down denial, educating about alcoholism, providing an introduction to group treatment (self-help groups and group therapy), learning how to ask for help, learning how to communicate directly and honestly, learning how to enjoy life while abstinent, beginning family restoration, and developing a specific, appropriate, and structured long-term recovery program.

PROGNOSIS WITH TREATMENT

A number of factors, described here, are associated with a good or poor prognosis for recovery. Even factors traditionally thought to be major barriers to treatment success—a skid row lifestyle or being an unattached young adult—do not always preclude successful recovery.

Factors Associated with a Good Prognosis

The first of the factors associated with a good prognosis is *clinician commitment to facilitating patient motivation.* Most patients are only marginally motivated to get well. Patients are ambivalent: A part of them wants to get well, and another part of them wants to continue drinking and stay sick (patients usually do not know what is wrong with them because no one has told them of the diagnosis in an effective way). Such patients have a good chance of getting into recovery if their physician is committed to the treatment of their alcoholism and consistently use the motivational techniques described previously.

The *presence of a crisis situation* is also a positive prognostic factor if the crisis is used as a motivational tool. The crisis may be the threat of a job loss, family separation or divorce, a DWI charge, a health-related crisis, an organized formal intervention or some other dramatic event. The physician actually precipitates a crisis when the confrontation approach is used (Fig. 28.4). As in that approach, it is critical to act promptly if a situational crisis is to be used effectively to motivate the patient to accept treatment. If exploitation of this crisis does not work, at least a seed has been planted that may eventually yield results. A third factor associated with a good prognosis is *appropriate treatment for at least 2 years.* Many alcoholics who begin treatment either believe they can do it on their own or return to drinking and drop out of treatment. To recover effectively, most alcoholics need to be with people who are recovering successfully. This favorable environment is found most easily in self-help groups such as Alcoholics Anonymous and in group therapy. Therefore, if patients show any indication of dropping out of treatment, it is important to promptly persuade them against this move.

The prognosis is also better if *family, job, health, and cognitive function are intact.* The status of family, job, health, and cognitive function usually correlates with how far alcoholism has advanced. Making a diagnosis early in the course of the alcoholism generally portends a better prognosis because each of these aspects of the patient's life tends to be more intact early in the illness. Also, in early illness the patient's and family members' denial systems and other defense systems tend not to be as strong. If one or more members of the patient's family are receiving treatment for co-alcoholism (see Co-Alcoholism), the prognosis for the patient usually is better.

Additional factors that increase the likelihood of long-term success are prompt recognition and intervention when relapse occurs and the acceptance by patient and physician of a recovery model that views alcoholism as a physical, mental, and spiritual illness.

Factors Associated with a Poor Prognosis

If the patient has *no perceived threat of loss* from continued drinking, the prognosis for recovery is generally worse. Factors that may worsen prognosis include: pharmacologic treatment alone, psychoanalytically oriented psychotherapy in the first year of alcoholism treatment, controlled drinking treatment, use of sedatives in long-term management, inpatient or outpatient treatment that does not treat alcoholism as a primary illness, and treatment that is too short in duration.

Although many patients who have a continued self-destructive bent do not tend to recover, some do. Often, intensive inpatient alcoholism treatment for 2 months or longer can be helpful for such patients. However, economic restraints most often limit this option. Cognitive impairment or psychosis often makes treatment difficult. However, the presence of these factors alone does not preclude a full attempt at treatment. With abstinence there is often surprising improvement over time.

Acceptance of a *derelict status* by the patient makes the prognosis virtually hopeless. However, it can be helpful to screen for a potentially reversible derelict status by looking at prior career and duration of dereliction. For example, a person who up until 2 years ago was in a productive profession or trade and is now on skid row has potential for recovery. By contrast, a person who has had no constructive activities for many years usually has less chance for reaching a successful long-term recovery. Patients who have *powerful enablers* to deny, cover up, and protect them from the consequences of drinking or drug using (see Co-alcoholism) are less likely to make a successful recovery.

SPECIAL POPULATIONS

Alcoholism in Older Persons

It is estimated that alcoholism is present in 3 to 4 million Americans older than 60 years of age, with prevalence estimates of 2% to 10%. Most elderly alcoholics have not been diagnosed, and even fewer are in treatment (47). This is true despite the fact that the elderly alcoholic is more likely than a younger alcoholic to have seen a physician recently.

The diagnosis of alcoholism can be more difficult in the elderly because they are less likely to face job loss, legal problems, marital problems, or fear of premature death. However, any change in functional status can be an important clue. The CAGE questionnaire, discussed previously, has been validated in a cohort of 323 elderly patients in an outpatient medical practice of an urban university teaching hospital. The sensitivity and specificity were 86% and 78%, respectively, for a score of 1 and 70% and 91%, respectively, for a score of 2. In this population, scores of 2, 3, and 4 yielded positive predictive values of 79%, 82%, and 94%, respectively (48). The CAGE may not be effective in detecting elderly binge drinkers who are at high risk of falling (49). As an adjunct, a geriatric version of the MAST has been developed (Table 28.11) (50).

TABLE 28.11 Michigan Alcoholism Screening Test—Geriatric Version (MAST-G)

	Yes	No
1. After drinking, have you ever noticed an increase in your heart rate or beating in your chest?	_____	_____
2. When talking with others, do you ever underestimate how much you actually drink?	_____	_____
3. Does alcohol make you sleepy so that you often fall asleep in your chair?	_____	_____
4. After a few drinks, have you sometimes not eaten or been able to skip a meal because you didn't feel hungry?	_____	_____
5. Does having a few drinks help decrease your shakiness or tremors?	_____	_____
6. Does alcohol sometimes make it hard for you to remember parts of the day or night?	_____	_____
7. Do you have rules for yourself that you won't drink before a certain time of the day?	_____	_____
8. Have you lost interest in hobbies or activities you used to enjoy?	_____	_____
9. When you wake up in the morning, do you ever have trouble remembering part of the night before?	_____	_____
10. Does having a drink help you sleep?	_____	_____
11. Do you hide your alcohol bottles from family members?	_____	_____
12. After a social gathering, have you ever felt embarrassed because you drank too much?	_____	_____
13. Have you ever been concerned that drinking might be harmful to your health?	_____	_____
14. Do you like to end an evening with a night cap?	_____	_____
15. Did you find your drinking increased after someone close to you died?	_____	_____
16. In general, would you prefer to have a few drinks at home rather than go out to social events?	_____	_____
17. Are you drinking more now than in the past?	_____	_____
18. Do you usually take a drink to relax or calm your nerves?	_____	_____
19. Do you drink to take your mind off your problems?	_____	_____
20. Have you ever increased your drinking after experiencing a loss in your life?	_____	_____
21. Do you sometimes drive when you have had too much to drink?	_____	_____
22. Has a doctor or nurse ever said they were worried or concerned about your drinking?	_____	_____
23. Have you ever made rules to manage your drinking?	_____	_____
24. When you feel lonely, does having a drink help?	_____	_____
Scoring: 5 or more yes responses indicative of alcohol problem.		

Blow FC, Brower KJ, Schulenberg JE, et al. The Michigan Alcoholism Screening Test - Geriatric Version (MAST-G): A new elderly-specific screening instrument. Alcohol Clin Exp Res 1992;16:372.

Older patients with alcoholism tend to fall into two groups: those with early onset and those with late onset. Two thirds of patients fall into the *early onset group.* These are patients who have had ongoing alcoholism but may have avoided some of the usual sequelae. They are often hidden, functional alcoholics who, as they lose mobility or cognitive abilities, become unable to function normally. The *late-onset patients* are likely to have had a recent stressor (i.e., loss of spouse, retirement, a new impairment in activities of daily living). Occasionally, late-onset alcoholism occurs in a previous teetotaler (51). Compared with younger alcoholic patients, the elderly are more likely to be separated, divorced, or widowed and live alone.

Older people are more sensitive to the acute effects of alcohol, with amplification of preexisting deficits. Dysphoria predominates over euphoria. Additionally, there is more likely to be interaction with prescribed drugs.

Once an older patient is confronted and agrees to treatment, there are some aspects of treatment specific to the elderly. The elderly patient who experiences significant alcohol withdrawal is best monitored in an inpatient setting. For patients with mild withdrawal treated at home, family or friends should stay with the patient for at least the first week of abstinence. In addition, home health care, if available, should be considered (see Chapter 9). Once the patient is medically stable, treatment toward continued abstinence should be initiated. Treatment must be specifically tailored for the elderly. Because of decreased mobility and an inability to drive, patients may find Alcoholics Anonymous meetings more difficult to reach. Meetings during the day must be found for elderly patients who are afraid to go out at night. The elderly tend to be more comfortable in smaller groups. These can often be found in meetings that run in a senior center. The senior center can also be a source of activities to fill the new void of free time formerly spent drinking.

Because older adults are often taking many medications and are more likely to have other chronic medical illnesses, disulfiram should generally be avoided. Many elderly alcoholics would benefit from a 30-day stay at an inpatient treatment center. Some centers have recovery programs specifically for the elderly alcoholic. Access to this type of treatment is usually related to insurance status and cost.

Alcoholism in Women

Alcoholism is more likely to go unrecognized in women than in men, yet suicide, trauma, and liver disease are more common in female than in male alcoholics (52,53). Women are also more likely to develop alcohol dependence after a lesser duration of drinking. An additional concern is the pregnancy-related complication of fetal alcohol syndrome, mentioned previously. Alcoholism decreases a woman's average life expectancy by 15 years (54). More than 50 case-controlled studies and 7 meta-analyses have shown a direct relationship between alcohol consumption and breast cancer (55).

Women tend to drink more subtly and covertly. In part, this is related to society's considering drinking in public, especially in a tavern or bar, less acceptable in women than in men. Women often drink at home and those who are unmarried, divorced, or unemployed drink more. Alcoholic women are also more likely to have alcoholic spouses.

The techniques discussed previously should be used to screen, diagnose, and confront women with alcoholism. There are some particular obstacles to treatment. Women are more likely to need provision of childcare while they are in treatment. In addition, alcoholic women tend to have less spousal support than alcoholic men do. There are treatment programs aimed specifically toward women, including women-only meetings of Alcoholics Anonymous. Alcoholic women, who make up only about 30% of Alcoholics Anonymous participants, should generally seek other women to be their sponsors.

The Impaired Physician or Other Professional

The prevalence among physicians of alcoholism and other chemical dependencies is probably similar to that for the general population (56). Each year, a substantial number of physicians are lost to the profession because of chemical dependence or other treatable illnesses, and many more practice despite being seriously troubled or impaired. Numerous professional organizations have implemented programs to address impairment in colleagues, including organizations of physicians, nurses, dentists, pharmacists, psychologists, social workers, lawyers, and others.

Definitions

Impaired professionals may be defined as those who are troubled by personal difficulties to the extent that they cannot (a) offer reasonable patient care, (b) effectively help others through interpersonal skills, or (c) maintain skills by continuing education. Impairment is also characterized by denial. Intervention with appropriate treatment as soon as alcoholism is recognized is a major goal of the impaired physician movement.

Recognition and Management

The manifestations, symptoms, or signs of impairment from alcoholism or other chemical dependence among professionals are the same as those seen in nonprofessionals. When one is concerned about impairment in a colleague, it is advisable to contact one or more close associates of that colleague to confirm the impairment. Likely reasons for the impairment may be uncovered by this discreet inquiry, and often alcoholism or another chemical dependency is the underlying problem. Persuasion of an impaired physician to accept the existence of a problem and agree to rehabilitation can be attempted by a concerned colleague. Such efforts are likely to be met with intense denial. A second approach is to use the state's physician rehabilitation committee. Each state medical society has a committee and maintains telephone access for confidential reporting of impaired physicians. Subcommittees undertake verification of the problem, followed by confrontation of the troubled physician, similar to the formal intervention technique described earlier in this chapter. The goal of this process is to rehabilitate the physician, usually through intensive treatment in a residential facility.

BRIEF INTERVENTION FOR NONDEPENDENT DRINKERS

Brief interventions are time-limited sessions provided by primary care providers that focus on *reducing alcohol use in the nondependent drinker.* Many targeted people may be in the early stages of alcoholism, having not yet lost control of their drinking. The brief intervention procedures used in studies vary, but none involve more than six contacts. No outside referrals are made, but written materials are often helpful. Typical followup sessions are usually 15 minutes long. Brief interventions have been found to be effective in reducing alcohol consumption (or achieving treatment referral) in problem drinkers in the primary care setting (57,58). Even a single brief 5- to 10-minute intervention may have impact (59). This further illustrates the importance of addressing alcohol use in all patients, even those who are not alcoholic, because problem drinking, independent of alcohol dependence, plays an enormous role in contributing to trauma, especially automobile accidents.

The brief intervention process consists of assessing alcohol use, giving feedback, contracting and goal setting, arriving at a strategy for behavior modification, and providing a plan for followup. There must be an emphasis on personal responsibility for change and clear advice to change. Therapeutic empathy describes the recommended counseling style. Typically, the goal of brief intervention is not abstinence. Therefore, patients must receive followup assessments to confirm that they are problem drinkers and not alcoholics.

The approach to brief intervention parallels the approach previously mentioned for confronting the patient with alcoholism. *Six essential elements* should be included: (a) *feedback* of personal risk (patient-focused review of the evidence for existing or potential risk related to drinking), (b) emphasis on personal *responsibility* for change (empowering the patient to take control of the decision for change), (c) clear *advice* for change ("Based on all we have discussed, you need to make a change"), (d) offering a *menu* of alternative options ("Here's some ways you can make a change"), (e) therapeutic *empathy* as an innate part of the intervention ("I know this may be difficult"), and (f) enhancement of patient *self-efficacy* ("This is not hopeless; with change, things will get better for you"). The mnemonic FRAMES may help remember the six elements. Chapter 4 describes in detail the concepts that underlie these behavior modification techniques.

CO-ALCOHOLISM (CO-DEPENDENCE)

Co-alcoholism can be defined as ill health or maladaptive, problematic, or dysfunctional behavior that is associated with living with, working with, treating, or otherwise being close to a person with alcoholism. Co-alcoholism is a specific example of the more general phenomenon of codependence (i.e., suffering or dysfunction associated with or caused by focusing on the needs or behaviors of others). Children who grow up in a family dominated by alcoholism can experience varied long-term behavioral and psychologic effects, and may benefit from group or individual therapy, either as children or adults (Adult Children of Alcoholics).

Co-alcoholism affects not only individuals and families but also helping professionals, communities, businesses, other institutions, and even whole societies. Its signs and symptoms range from passive acceptance and absence of overt problems to the following range of manifestations:

In People Close to an Alcoholic

- Behaviors to protect the alcoholic (enabling)
- Behavioral or psychological symptoms, such as anxiety disorders, depression, insomnia, hyperactivity, aggression, anorexia nervosa, bulimia, or suicidal gestures
- Functional or psychosomatic illness
- Family violence or neglect
- Alcoholism or another chemical dependence

In Helping Professionals

- Failure to diagnose alcoholism
- Failure to treat alcoholism as a primary illness
- Treating the alcoholic with sedatives or tranquilizers
- Treating the co-alcoholic with sedatives or tranquilizers

In Society at Large

- Not confronting relatives, friends, and colleagues who are inappropriately intoxicated or are chronically abusing alcohol or drugs
- Placing a positive social value on those who drink
- Stigmatizing those who are alcoholics or those who do not drink

TABLE 28.12 Family Drinking Survey[a]

	Yes	No
1. Does someone in your family undergo personality changes when he or she drinks to excess?	1. (1)	(0)
2. Do you feel that drinking is more important to this person than you are?	2. ____	____
3. Do you feel sorry for yourself and frequently indulge in self-pity because of what you feel alcohol is doing to your family?	3. ____	____
4. Has some family member's excessive drinking ruined special occasions?	4. ____	____
5. Do you find yourself covering up for the consequences of someone else's drinking?	5. ____	____
6. Have you ever felt guilty, apologetic, or responsible for the drinking of a member of your family?	6. ____	____
7. Does one of your family member's use of alcohol cause fights and arguments?	7. ____	____
8. Have you ever tried to fight the drinker by joining in the drinking?	8. ____	____
9. Do the drinking habits of some family members make you feel depressed or angry?	9. ____	____
10. Is your family having financial difficulties because of drinking?	10. ____	____
11. Did you ever feel like you had an unhappy home life because of the drinking of some members of your family?	11. ____	____
12. Have you ever tried to control the drinker's behavior by hiding the car keys, pouring liquor down the drain, etc.?	12. ____	____
13. Do you find yourself distracted from your responsibilities because of this person's drinking?	13. ____	____
14. Do you often worry about a family member's drinking?	14. ____	____
15. Are holidays more of a nightmare than a celebration because of a family member's drinking behavior?	15. ____	____
16. Are most of your drinking family member's friends heavy drinkers?	16. ____	____
17. Do you find it necessary to lie to employers, relatives, or friends in order to hide your spouse's drinking?	17. ____	____
18. Do you find yourself responding differently to members of your family when they are using alcohol?	18. ____	____
19. Have you ever been embarrassed or felt the need to apologize for the drinker's actions?	19. ____	____
20. Does some family member's use of alcohol make you fear for your own safety or the safety of other members of your family?	20. ____	____
21. Have you ever thought that one of your family members had a drinking problem?	21. ____	____
22. Have you ever lost sleep because of a family member's drinking?	22. ____	____
23. Have you ever encouraged one of your family members to stop or cut down on his or her drinking?	23. ____	____
24. Have you ever threatened to leave home or to leave a family member because of his or her drinking?	24. ____	____
25. Did a family member ever make promises that he or she did not keep because of drinking?	25. ____	____
26. Did you ever wish that you could talk to someone who could understand and help the alcohol-related problems of a family member?	26. ____	____
27. Have you ever felt sick, cried, or had a "knot" in your stomach after worrying about a family member's drinking?	27. ____	____
28. Has a family member ever failed to remember what occurred during a drinking period?	28. ____	____
29. Does your family member avoid social situations where alcoholic beverages will *not* be served?	29. ____	____
30. Does your family member have periods of remorse after drinking occasions and apologize for his or her behavior?	30. ____	____
31. Please write any symptoms or medical or nervous problems that you have experienced since you have known your heavy drinker. (Write on back if more space is needed.)	31. ____	____

[a]If you answer "Yes" to any two of the above questions, there is a good possibility that someone in your family has a drinking problem.
If you answer "Yes" to four or more of the above questions, there is a definite indication that someone in your family *does* have a drinking problem.
These survey questions are modified or adapted from validated survey instruments such as the Children of Alcoholics Screening Test (CAST) and the Howard Family Questionnaire, and from the Family Alcohol Quiz from Al-Anon.

Co-Alcoholism in the Individual

The following is a typical case history of co-alcoholism in an individual.

A 38-year-old married woman presented with recurring episodes of upper abdominal pain of about 4 years' duration. During that time she had been evaluated by two internists and had been hospitalized once. After extensive evaluations, the working diagnosis was functional abdominal pain. She was treated with antispasmodics and sedatives but there was no substantial improvement. The pain occurred almost every day. On a followup visit 6 months later, the patient said that a friend had suggested that she attend the self-help group Al-Anon because her husband's drinking had been bothering her for at least 5 years. The patient reported that after she attended 12 Al-Anon meetings over 3 months, her abdominal pain gradually abated. On followup 2 years later, she had continued to attend Al-Anon and the symptoms had not recurred. In the meantime, the patient's husband had continued to drink.

This case study illustrates a common manifestation of co-alcoholism: a psychosomatic illness that resolved after the patient recognized an alcohol problem in the family and attended Al-Anon regularly.

Recognition and Treatment of the Co-Alcoholic Patient

When a patient has unexplained somatic or psychological symptoms, it is helpful to ask whether the patient has ever been concerned about the drinking (or drug use) of anyone close to him or her. If the answer is *Yes,* the patient should be asked to describe the problem. If the patient is vague or doubtful, one can administer some or all of the questions in the *Family Drinking Survey* shown in Table 28.12. One can also ask the possible co-alcoholic to answer CAGE questions (Fig. 28.1) or the questions on the MAST (Table 28.3) as though they were addressed to, and answered honestly by, the potentially alcoholic person to whom he or she is close. A positive score on one of these is a strong indication of co-alcoholism.

Initially, the psychological and behavioral adjustments of the co-alcoholic are normal responses to an abnormal situation. However, these adaptive responses eventually lead to the person's becoming dysfunctional. Co-alcoholism, like alcoholism, is chronic and progressive; it is characterized by denial, ill health, and/or maladaptive behavior and by a lack of knowledge about alcoholism.

The major strategies in treating a patient with co-alcoholism are remarkably similar to those for treating the alcoholic:

- Have the patient accept that he or she is a co-alcoholic.
- Motivate the patient to get help (occasionally by using a coercive intervention, such as the formal intervention described previously).
- Refer the patient to Al-Anon or Alateen (as with Alcoholics Anonymous referrals, enthusiasm for and a good understanding of the Al-Anon process [Table 28.13] on the part of the referring physician are critical to successful referral).
- Provide supportive psychotherapy at follow-up visits (see Chapter 20) and refer the patient or the family for additional therapy, especially group therapy for codependents or adult children of dysfunctional families.
- Assist in the process of getting the alcoholics who are the source of the problem into treatment.

Co-Alcoholism in the Helping Professions

Co-alcoholism includes behavior on the part of professionals that enables alcoholics to remain enmeshed in their disease. Enabling behavior often coexists with otherwise excellent clinical skills. Some questions (Table 28.14) are useful for identifying the various ways in which enabling may occur in the context of medical practice. Societal norms (including one's own approach to the use of alcohol or other drugs), plus a lack of awareness of modern

TABLE 28.13 The Al-Anon Process

Al-Anon began in the 1940s as an Alcoholics Anonymous (AA) auxiliary and initially called itself AA Family Groups. In 1952, the wives of the two founders of AA established Al-Anon.

Al-Anon is a fellowship of family members of alcoholics who meet together to share their experiences, strengths, and hopes so that they can achieve health and serenity. The organization is modeled after AA and uses the 12 Steps of AA (see Table 28.8) as its principles for individual recovery. Its focus is not on the alcoholic but on the family members; thus, it powerfully frees families from their dependence on the alcoholic.

Al-Anon meetings are open to the public and often meet at the same time and location as AA meetings. In most communities, Al-Anon has a telephone listing where meeting information, help, and literature can be obtained. Where there is no local Al-Anon office, the AA office can provide Al-Anon information.

Al-Anon meetings generally last 1 hour and follow the format of AA meetings (see Table 28.8), but they are usually smaller and discussion of topics is often freer than in AA.

Al-Anon is the sponsor of Ala-Teen and Ala-Tots, which are organizations for teenage and young children of alcoholics, respectively. These groups follow the Al-Anon discussion format and in general are not open to the nonalcoholic public, but helping professionals are usually welcome if they request to attend ahead of time. In the last several years in some areas, Al-Anon members have begun groups for adult children of alcoholics. These groups offer help to adults who may no longer live with an alcoholic family member, but whose life continues to be adversely affected by the legacy of growing up in an alcoholic home. These are especially powerful, and many patients with this background can be profoundly helped.

Al-Anon publishes a number of pamphlets that are available at meetings for families. *Al-Anon Faces Alcoholism,* Al-Anon's "Big Book," describes the family's plight with alcoholism through a variety of stories that graphically describe how families become sick in response to the alcoholic. Its other major book, *Living with an Alcoholic,* offers practical suggestions for recovery.

More information can be obtained at http://www.alanon.org.za/

TABLE 28.14 Questions to Identify Enabling Behaviors in Health Professionals[a]

	Enabling Response
1. Do you sometimes avoid raising sensitive issues related to drinking because it might offend your patient, or make him or her angry or feel bad?	Yes
2. Do you generally treat the heavy-drinking person's problems without focusing most of the treatment on the drinking behavior?	Yes
3. Do you avoid confronting your heavy-drinking patient when there is good evidence that he or she has misinformed you about his or her drinking?	Yes
4. Do you generally suggest to your alcoholic patients that they cut down on their drinking?	Yes
5. Do you believe what your heavy-drinking patient tells you about his or her drinking without using other sources such as a spouse, employer, screening test, blood alcohol test, or other laboratory test?	Yes
6. Do you generally prescribe a sedative or minor tranquilizer for the nervous conditions or sleep problems of your alcoholic patients?	Yes
7. Do you refer most of your alcoholic patients to attend Alcoholics Anonymous meetings regularly and / or an alcoholism therapy group?	No
8. Do you refer most of the spouses of family members of your alcoholic patients to attend Al-Anon meetings regularly?	No
9. Do you subscribe to the theory that most alcoholics have an underlying psychologic disorder that is the major cause of the alcoholism?	Yes
10. Do you believe that most alcoholics will not respond positively to treatment for their alcoholism?	Yes

[a]The greater the number of enabling responses the greater the enabling behavior.

approaches to diagnosis, motivation, and treatment of the alcoholic, are probably the major reasons for co-alcoholism in helping professionals. Several steps are recommended for the professional who wishes to cease being an enabler:

- Update your knowledge of alcoholism.
- Attend some Alcoholics Anonymous and Al-Anon meetings.
- Start using skills such as those described in this chapter. The best cure for co-alcoholism in the physician is success in getting a number of alcoholics and their families into the recovery process.

DOMESTIC VIOLENCE

Domestic violence is present in all demographic and socioeconomic strata. It is especially prevalent in women whose partners abuse alcohol or other drugs and in women who themselves abuse substances. It is estimated that 75% of wives of alcoholics have been threatened and 45% have been assaulted by their alcoholic partners (60). *Domestic violence has been defined* by the American Medical Association (AMA) (see *www.hopkinsbayview.org/PAMreferences*) as an ongoing debilitating experience of physical, psychological, or sexual abuse in the home, associated with increased isolation from the outside world and limited personal freedom and accessibility to resources.

In the United States, it is estimated that 2 million women are victims of domestic violence each year and that more than 12 million will be abused at some time during their lives. Most of these women never seek help from health care providers for the consequences of domestic violence. However, studies demonstrate a relationship between domestic violence and medical and psychiatric illness.

Brief screening for domestic violence should be incorporated into the medical interview of all women. Because some women may not initially recognize themselves as victims of domestic violence, questioning should be specific (Table 28.15). The issue should be dealt with sensitively, validating the difficulty most women have in discussing the

TABLE 28.15 A Recommended Approach to the Use of Interviewing to Screen Patients for Domestic Violence

Integrating domestic violence inquiry into interview as part of social history:

"Because abuse and violence have unfortunately become a common part of a woman's life, I ask all my patients about it routinely."

We all occasionally fight at home. What happens when you and your partner disagree?

Have you ever been treated badly or threatened by your partner?

Has your partner ever prevented you from leaving the house, seeing friends, getting a job, or continuing your education?

Does your partner ever force you to have sex or force you to engage in sex that is uncomfortable to you?

(if appropriate) You mentioned your partner drinks (uses drugs). How does he (or she) act when he is drinking (using drugs)?

TABLE 28.16 Clinical Signs and Symptoms Suggestive of Domestic Violence

Alcohol or drug abuse
Anxiety
Atypical chest pain
Change in appetite
Chronic headaches
Chronic pain of unclear etiology
Depressed mood
Difficulty concentrating
Dizziness
Fatigue
Frequent evidence of minor trauma
Frequent requests for pain medications or tranquilizers
Frequent visits with vague somatic complaints
Gastrointestinal upset, diarrhea, or dyspepsia
Insomnia
Palpitations
Panic attacks
Paresthesias
Pelvic pain
Suicide attempts or gestures

issue. The patient may be reluctant to disclose information because of shame, humiliation, low self-esteem, or fear of retaliation by the perpetrator. Some women may also believe that they deserve the abuse and do not deserve help or that they need to protect their partner, who is often their only source of affection and support. There may also be a belief on the part of the victim that the medical provider will not understand the problem or will not believe her.

In addition to screening, certain patient problems should alert the practitioner to the possibility of domestic violence (Table 28.16). Problems may range from direct evidence of physical trauma (contusions, abrasions, broken bones) to nonspecific complaints of fatigue and difficulty concentrating. The screening information and medical history related to domestic violence must be well documented in the medical record, because they provide evidence that may be used in a legal case. The record should include detailed descriptions of any injuries and, if possible, photographs of injuries sustained.

Once evidence of abuse is obtained, one must validate the seriousness of the situation to the patient. This must occur even if the patient is not yet ready to leave the abusive spouse. In addition, the immediate safety of the woman should be assessed. Unfortunately, the level of severity of past violence may not be a predictor of the severity of future violence. If safety is in question, the woman (and her children) should be advised to stay with family or friends, or at a shelter that specializes in caring for abused women and their families. Medical attention may also be needed for abused children in the household.

Often, the patient resists taking action. One should continue to show concern and work to motivate the patient toward change. Once the patient has agreed to take action, local community resources that can provide support, safety, and advocacy must be accessed. The *National Domestic Violence Hotline* (1-800-799-7233) is a 24-hour service that helps women find a safe place to stay in their community. At times, psychiatric or substance abuse referral may also be appropriate.

SPECIFIC REFERENCES*

1. Morse RM, Flavin DK. The definition of alcoholism. JAMA 1992;268:1012.
2. American Psychiatric Association. Diagnostic and statistical manual of mental disorders. 4th ed. (DSM-IV). Washington, DC: American Psychiatric Association, 1994.
3. **3.** National Institute on Alcohol Abuse and Alcoholism. The physicians guide to helping patients with alcohol problems. Washington, DC: Government Printing Office, 1995. (NIH publication no. 95-3769)
4. Jellinek EM. Phases of alcohol addiction. Q J Stud Alcohol 1952;13:673.
5. Vaillant GE, ed. The natural history of alcoholism, revisited. Cambridge, MA: Harvard University Press, 1996.
6. Conneally PM. Association between the D2 dopamine receptor gene and alcoholism: a continuing controversy. Arch Gen Psychiatry 1991;48:664.
7. Substance Abuse and Mental Health Services Administration. (2004). Results from the 2003 National Survey on Drug Use and Health: National Findings (Office of Applied Studies, NSDUH Series H-25, DHHS Publication No. SMA 04-3964). Rockville, MD.
8. Naimi TS, Brewer RD, Mokdad A, et al. Binge drinking among US adults. JAMA 2003;289: 70.
9. Klatsky AL, Armstrong MA, Friedman GD. Alcohol and mortality. Ann Intern Med 1992;117:646.
10. Hurt RD, Offord KP, Croghan IT, et al. Mortality following inpatient addictions treatment: role of tobacco use in a community-based cohort. JAMA 1996;275:1097.
11. Bullock KD, Reed RJ, Grant I. Reduced mortality risk in alcoholics who achieve long-term abstinence. JAMA 1992;267:668.
12. Fine EW, Scoles P. Secondary prevention of alcoholism using a population of offenders arrested for driving while intoxicated. Ann N Y Acad Sci 1976;273:637.
13. Ewing JA. Detecting alcoholism: the CAGE questionnaire. JAMA 1984;252:1905.
14. Cyr MG, Wartman SA. The effectiveness of routine screening questions in the detection of alcoholism. JAMA 1988;259:51.
15. Powers JS, Spickard A. Michigan Alcoholism Screening Test to diagnose early alcoholism in a general practice. South Med J 1984;77:852.
16. Bush K, Kivlahan DR, McDonell MB, et al. The AUDIT alcohol consumption questions (AUDIT-C): an effective brief screening test for problem drinking. Arch Intern Med 1998;158:1789.
17. Saunders JB. Development of the Alcohol Use Disorders Identification Test (AUDIT). Addiction 1993;88:791.
18. O'Connor PG, Schottenfeld, et al. Medical progress: patients with alcohol problems. N Engl J Med 1998;338:592.
19. Bradley KA, Boyd-Wickizer BA, Powell SH, Burman ML. Alcohol screening questionnaires in women: a critical review. JAMA 1998;280: 166.
20. Beresford TP, Blow FC, Hill E, et al. Comparison of CAGE questionnaire and computer-assisted laboratory profiles in screening for covert alcoholism. Lancet 1990;336:482.
21. Samet JH, Rollnick S, Barnes H. Beyond CAGE: a brief clinical approach after detection of substance abuse. Arch Intern Med 1996;56:2287.
22. Prochaska JO, DiClemente CC. Toward a comprehensive model of change. In: Miller WR, Heather N, eds. Treating addictive behaviors: process of change. New York: Plenum, 1986.
23. **23.** Hayashida M, Alterman AI, McLellan T, et al. Comparative effectiveness and costs of inpatient and outpatient detoxification of patients with mild-to-moderate alcohol withdrawal syndrome. N Engl J Med 1989;320:358.
24. Turner RC, Lichstein PR, Peden JG Jr, et al. Alcohol withdrawal syndromes: a review of pathophysiology, clinical presentation, and treatment. J Gen Intern Med 1989;4:432.

*Bold numerals denote published controlled clinical trials, meta-analyses, or consensus-based recommendations.

25. Victor M, Hope JM. The phenomenon of auditory hallucinations in chronic alcoholism. J Nerv Ment Dis 1958;126:451.
26. Saunders JB. Delirium tremens: its aetiology, natural history and treatment. Curr Opin Psych 2000;13:629.
27. Sullivan JT, Sykora K, Schneiderman J, et al. Assessment of alcohol withdrawal: the revised clinical institute withdrawal assessment for alcohol scale (CIWA-Ar). Br J Addict 1989;84:1353.
28. Mayo-Smith MF, for the American Society of Addiction Medicine Workshop Group on Pharmacologic Management of Alcohol Withdrawal. Pharmacologic management of alcohol withdrawal: a meta-analysis and evidence-based medicine practice guideline. JAMA 1997;278:144.
29. Saitz R, Mayo-Smith MF, Roberts MS, et al. Individualized treatment for alcohol withdrawal: a randomized double-blind controlled trial. JAMA 1994;272:519.
30. Malcolm R, Myrick H, Roberts J, et al. The effects of carbamazepine and lorazepam on single versus multiple previous alcohol withdrawals in an outpatient randomized trial. J Gen Intern Med 2002;17:349.
31. Whitfield CL, Thompson G, Lamb A, et al. Detoxification of 1,024 alcoholics without psychoactive drugs. JAMA 1978;239: 1409.
32. Sampliner R, Iber F. Diphenylhydantoin control of alcohol withdrawal seizures. JAMA 1974;230:1430.
33. Alldredge BK, Lowenstein DH, Simon RP. Placebo-controlled trial of intravenous diphenylhydantoin for short-term treatment of alcohol withdrawal seizures. Am J Med 1989;87:645.
34. Sellers EM, Naranjo CA, Harrison M, et al. Diazepam loading: simplified treatment of alcohol withdrawal. Clin Pharmacol Ther 1983;34:822.
35. Ng SK, Hauser WA, Brust JC, et al. Alcohol consumption and withdrawal in new-onset seizures. N Engl J Med 1988;319:666.
36. Hoffman NG, Harrison PA, Belille CA. Alcoholics Anonymous after treatment: attendance and abstinence. Int J Addict 1983;18:311.
37. Gossop M, Harris J, Best D, et al. Is attendance at alcoholics anonymous meetings after inpatient treatment related to improved outcomes? A 6-month follow-up study. Alcohol 2003;38:421.
38. Garbutt JC, West SL, Carey TS, et al. Pharmacologic treatment of alcohol dependence. JAMA 1999;281:1318.
39. Fiellin DA, Reid MC, O'Connor PG. New therapies for alcohol problems: application to primary care. Am J Med 2000;108:227.
40. O'Connor PG, Farren CK, Rousanville BJ, et al. A preliminary investigation of the management of alcohol dependence with naltrexone by primary care providers. Am J Med 1997;103:477.
41. Volpicelli JR, Alterman AI, Hayashida M, et al. Naltrexone in the treatment of alcohol dependence. Arch Gen Psychiatry 1992;49: 876.
42. Krystal JH, Cramer JA, Krol WF, et al. Naltrexone in the treatment of alcohol dependence. N Engl J Med 2001;345:1734.
43. Srisurapanont M, Jarusuraisin N. Opioid antagonists for alcohol dependence. The Cochrane Database of Systematic Reviews 2005, Issue 1. Art. No.: CD001867.
44. Bouza C, Angeles M, Munoz A, Amate JM. Efficacy and safety of naltrexone and acamprosate in the treatment of alcohol dependence: a systematic review. Addiction 2004;99:811.
45. Kiefer F, Jahn H, Tarnaske T. Comparing and combining naltrexone and acamprosate in relapse prevention of alcoholism a double-blind, placebo-controlled study. Arch Gen Psychiatry 2003;60:92.
46. Walsh DC, Hingson RW, Merrigan DM, et al. A randomized trial of treatment options for alcohol abusing workers. N Engl J Med 1991;325:775.
47. Reid MC, Tinetti ME, Brown CJ, et al. Physician awareness of alcohol use disorders among older patients. J Gen Intern Med 1998;13:729.
48. Buchsbaum DG, Buchanan RG, Welsh J, et al. Screening for drinking disorders in the elderly using the CAGE questionnaire. J Am Geriatr Soc 1992;40:662.
49. Adams WL, Barry KL, Fleming MF. Screening for problem drinking in older primary care patients. JAMA 1996;276:1964.
50. Blow FC, Brower KJ, Schulenberg JE, et al. The Michigan Alcoholism Screening Test—Geriatric version (MAST-G): a new elderly-specific screening instrument. Alcohol Clin Exp Res 1992;16:372.
51. Atkinson RM, Tolson RL, Turner JA. Late versus early onset problem drinking in older men. Alcohol Clin Exp Res 1990;14:574.
52. Bradley KA, Badrinath S, Bush K, et al. Medical risks for women who drink alcohol. J Gen Intern Med 1998;3:627.
53. Wilsnack SC, Wilsnack RW. Epidemiology of women's drinking. J Subst Abuse Treat 1991;3:133.
54. Roman PM. Biological features of women's alcohol use: a review. Public Health Rep 1988;103:628.
55. Singletary KW, Gapstur SM. Alcohol and breast cancer: review of epidemiologic and experimental evidence and potential mechanisms. JAMA 2001;286:2143.
56. Moore RD, Mead L, Pearson TA. Youthful precursors of alcohol abuse in physicians. Am J Med 1990;88:332.
57. Whitlock EP, Polen MR, Green CA, Orleans T, Klein J; U.S. Preventive Services Task Force. Behavioral counseling interventions in primary care to reduce risky/harmful alcohol use by adults: a summary of the evidence for the U.S. Preventive Services Task Force. Ann Intern Med 2004;140:557.
58. Wilk AI, Jensen NM, Havighurst TC. Meta-analysis of randomized control trials addressing brief interventions in heavy alcohol drinkers. J Gen Intern Med 1997; 12:274.
59. Reiff-Hekking S, Ockene JK, Hurley TG, Reed GW. Brief physician and nurse practitioner-delivered counseling for high risk drinking. Results of a 12-month follow-up. J Gen Intern Med 2005;20:7.
60. Eisenstat SA, Bancroft L. Primary care: domestic violence. N Engl J Med 1999;341: 886.

*For annotated **General References** and resources related to this chapter, visit www.hopkinsbayview.org/PAMreferences.*

Chapter 29

Illicit and Therapeutic Use of Drugs with Abuse Liability

Michael I. Fingerhood

DEFINITIONS

Drugs with abuse liability modify mood, feeling, thinking, and perception. Many are commonly prescribed and are useful therapeutic agents. The use and abuse of such substances date back thousands of years. Plant alkaloids, alcohol, and an ever-increasing array of newly synthesized chemicals have also been used in illicit endeavors. Patterns of use and the social acceptance of use of these agents have differed from time to time and from place to place. Successive generations of the same society have held discordant views about which substance to use, at what age, in what amount, and under which circumstances (e.g., attitudes regarding alcohol use in the pre-Prohibition and post-Prohibition eras in the United States). There are two forms of less problematic use of illicit substances (experimental and social–recreational) and two defined patterns of abnormal use (substance abuse and substance dependence).

Experimental Use

The experimental use of illicit substances is sporadic; the initial trial and experience are usually associated with adolescence. These experiments usually have little impact on mental health. They are potentially dangerous because of possible overdose, because unsterile methods of exposure may occur, because of behaviors that may endanger the user or other people, and because some people may find the drug experience extraordinarily rewarding leading to repeated use. Incorrect labeling of illicit drugs (a common problem) increases the risk of untoward consequences.

Social–Recreational Use

Social and recreational use of illicit substances suggests that they have been used repetitively but that control has been exerted over the dosage and the frequency of use. The risks of unintended overdose and improper exposure are increased by the frequency of use. Recreational use may not be psychologically disabling even though adverse consequences may occur. Adequate social and behavioral function is maintained. Most use of alcohol and marijuana conforms to this pattern of social–recreational use.

Substance Abuse and Substance Dependence

The *Diagnostic and Statistical Manual of the American Psychiatric Association, 4th Edition (DSM-IV)* delineates two diagnostic categories for substance-related disorders (1). The diagnostic criteria are the same for all psychoactive substances, including alcohol.

The Diagnostic and Statistical Manual, 4th Edition, Criteria for Substance Abuse

A. A maladaptive pattern of substance use leading to clinically significant impairment or distress, as manifested by one or more of the following occurring at any time during the same 12-month period:

1. Recurrent substance use resulting in a failure to fulfill major role obligations at work, school, or home (e.g., repeated absences or poor work performance related to substance use; substance-related absences, suspensions, or expulsions from school; neglect of children or household).
2. Recurrent substance use in situations in which it is physically hazardous (e.g., driving an automobile or operating a machine when impaired by substance use).
3. Recurrent substance-related legal problems (e.g., arrests for substance-related disorderly conduct).
4. Continued substance use despite having persistent or recurrent social or interpersonal problems caused or exacerbated by the effects of the substance (e.g., arguments with spouse about consequences of intoxication, physical fights).

B. Has never met the criteria for substance dependence for this class of substance.

The Diagnostic and Statistical Manual, 4th Edition, Criteria for Substance Dependence

A maladaptive pattern of substance use, leading to clinically significant impairment or distress, as manifested by *three or more of the following* occurring at any time in the same 12-month period:

1. Tolerance, as defined by either of the following:
   - **a.** Need for markedly increased amounts of the substance to achieve intoxication or desired effect;
   - **b.** Markedly diminished effect with continued use of the same amount of the substance.
2. Withdrawal, as manifested by either of the following:
   - **a.** The characteristic withdrawal syndrome for substance (refer to the criteria sets for withdrawal from the specific substances);
   - **b.** The same (or closely related) substance is taken to relieve or avoid withdrawal symptoms.
3. The substance is often taken in larger amounts or over a longer period than was intended.
4. There is a persistent desire or unsuccessful efforts to cut down or control substance use.
5. A great deal of time is spent in activities necessary to obtain the substance (e.g., visiting multiple doctors or driving long distances), use the substance (e.g., chain smoking), or recover from its effects.
6. Important social, occupational, or recreational activities are given up or reduced because of substance use.
7. Continued substance use despite knowledge of having had a persistent or recurrent physical or psychological problem that was likely to have been caused or exacerbated by the substance.

Classification by Pharmacologic Effect

Later sections of this chapter describe the manifestations and the principles of management for selected substances of abuse common in the United States (Chapters 27 and 28 describe tobacco and alcohol abuse/dependence, respectively). A list of all drugs that have abuse potential would be extremely long. However, it is possible to group the various substances into broad classes, the members of which share common characteristics and are readily distinguishable from other classes (Table 29.1). Psychoactive substances may be classified as depressants, opioids, stimulants, and drugs that alter perception (including hallucinogens).

Tolerance and Physical Dependence

Most drugs of abuse share the capacity to induce tolerance. *Tolerance* is defined as the phenomenon whereby with repeated use an increased amount of drug is required to

TABLE 29.1 Categories of Psychoactive Drugs

CNS depressants
Alcohol
Sedative-hypnotics
Benzodiazepines
Barbiturates
Other—meprobromate (Equanil or Miltown), eszopiclone (Lunesta), zaleplon (Sonata), zolpidem (Ambien)
Inhalants
Nitrous oxide, toluene, volatile hydrocarbons
Opioids
Morphine, hydromorphone (Dilaudid), heroin, oxycodone, hydrocodone, meperidine (Demerol), codeine, methadone
Stimulants
Cocaine, amphetamine, methamphetamine, methylphenidate (Ritalin), MDMA (Ecstasy), caffeine, nicotine, arecoline
Drugs that alter perception (including hallucinogens)
Marijuana, LSD, psilocybin, mescaline, PCP, MDMA, GHB, belladonna alkaloids (atropine, scopolamine)

CNS, central nervous system; MDMA, methylenedioxymethamphetamine; LSD, lysergic acid diethylamide; PCP, phencyclidine; GHB, gamma hydroxybutyrate.

TABLE 29.2 Characteristics of Dependence on Drugs of Abuse

Drug	*Physiologic Effect*	*Withdrawal Symptoms and Signs (1–7 Days after Last Dose)*	
Opioids	Pupillary constriction Analgesia Constipation Respiratory depression	Pupillary dilation Myalgia Diarrhea Stimulation of respiratory centers ("yawning") Rhinorrhea Gooseflesh Nausea and vomiting Restlessness	
Alcohol, barbiturate, benzodiazepines	Induction of sleep (hypnosis) Sedation Alcohol usually decreases but may increase seizure activity (other sedatives decrease seizure activity)	Insomnia Nausea Tremulousness Anxiety Irritability Autonomic hyperactivity (sweats, tachycardia, hypertension) Delirium Seizures Death (alcohol and barbiturates)	Minor symptoms Onset 24–72 hr after last dose Duration 72–96 hr after last dose Major symptoms Onset 72 hr to 1 wk after last dose Duration up to 2 wk after last dose
Cocaine	Pupillary dilation Tachycardia Hypertension	Bradycardia Hyperphagia Fatigue Hypersomnolence	

produce a given effect. Alternatively, the same amount of drug produces a lesser effect with repeated administration. The time required for the induction of tolerance ranges from days after repeated use of opioids by injection to weeks or months after repeated oral administration of opioids, barbiturates, alcohol, and other sedatives.

Physical dependence is defined as the phenomenon whereby abrupt cessation of a drug results in withdrawal symptoms and signs (the abstinence state). Withdrawal symptoms and signs are often the opposite of the biologic effects exerted by the drug in question (Table 29.2). Physical dependence is not synonymous with addiction. People who are prescribed benzodiazepines may exhibit physical dependence (sometimes called therapeutic dependence) but do not fulfill criteria for substance dependence (see *DSM-IV* criteria above). Similarly, many people exhibit a withdrawal syndrome for caffeine but do not fulfill criteria for substance dependence.

PRIMARY CARE PRACTITIONER'S ROLE

Background

Since the 1920s, with the exception of small numbers of psychiatrists and substance abuse specialists from other disciplines, practitioners in the United States have been reluctant to become involved in problems of substance abuse and dependence. The passage of the Harrison Narcotic Act in 1914, prohibited physicians from prescribing opiates for the treatment of opiate dependence. From 1920 to 1940, health care providers who prescribed or dispensed narcotics in violation of the Harrison Act were prosecuted and imprisoned. This campaign led to avoidance of the problems of addiction by physicians and other health care providers. Providers are still reluctant to become involved in problems with addiction because of a lack of knowledge of how to deal with these patients, their own attitudes toward substance abuse, and the understandable response to the difficult behaviors these patients often exhibit. In recent years, substance abuse has been recognized as a major cause of morbidity seen in medical practice—usually a mix of physical, mental, and social consequences—and the responsibility of primary care practitioners to care for the patient with substance abuse has been emphasized. This role was expanded with recent federal legislation allowing primary care physicians to prescribe buprenorphine as opioid replacement therapy.

Specific Roles

For the patient with substance abuse, the role of the primary care practitioner is recognition of the problem, motivation of the patient to accept treatment, referral to a treatment program, ongoing care for the patient's other medical problems, and continued motivation to help the patient remain in recovery. By prescribing controlled substances wisely, the primary care practitioner can also play an important role in preventing prescription drug abuse.

Recognition/Diagnosis

Discovery of a substance abuse problem starts with a suspicion of the diagnosis if signs, symptoms, and elements of the history suggest the possibility, even in the most unlikely subjects. People from all walks of life abuse drugs. The stereotype of the drug abuser is of a young antisocial male who uses drugs for their euphoric effect. Although this may be true, the abuse of illicit drugs such as marijuana and cocaine also occurs commonly among middle and upper class Americans, and the misuse and abuse of prescription analgesics and sedatives by people who are in the mainstream of American society have been recognized for many years. Patients with chronic anxiety, insomnia, or pain are at risk of abusing medications used to treat those conditions. In some instances, escalated use (and sometimes abuse) develops not because the patient is primarily seeking drug-induced euphoria or intoxication but because the tolerance that develops during continued use leads the patient to increase the dosage to inappropriate levels. Elderly patients are at particular risk because they are more likely to be given medications. Changes in the pharmacokinetics of drugs secondary to the aging process also make the elderly more vulnerable to normally prescribed dosages.

Advice on history taking includes: ask questions about drug use in the context of general medical history, develop a nonjudgmental approach, use direct questions, learn to recognize qualified answers, be persistent and friendly, and do not discuss rationalizations. It is often helpful to obtain information from a family member or close friend, with the patient's consent.

Chapter 28 describes interviewing techniques helpful in screening for alcoholism and motivating the alcoholic to accept treatment. Techniques such as the CAGE questionnaire, as shown in Fig. 28.1, can be adapted to screen patients for the abuse of other drugs and substances.

Urine Testing

Urine testing to establish drug abuse seems a tempting and objective means of cutting through the problems of denial, unreliable histories, and the less than clear-cut signs and symptoms presented to arrive at a diagnosis. In the primary care practitioner's office, however, testing for drug abuse can prove problematic. The patient already knows whether he or she is abusing drugs. The question is whether the patient is willing to share that information with the practitioner.

Drug testing requires informed voluntary consent of any person 18 years of age or older, except in true emergencies. Faced with this requirement, laboratory testing yields no more information than the patient is willing to provide by history. Testing at the request of an employer or school authority, in particular, is fraught with ethical questions. Nevertheless, many employers now require drug testing (which is legal).

TABLE 29.3 Medications That May Give False Positive Results on Drug Screen

False-positive Result	*Drugs*
Opiates	Quinolone antibiotics, rifampin, quinine in tonic water, poppy seeds
Marijuana	Efavirenz (Sustiva), nonsteroidal anti-inflammatory drugs, dronabinol (Marinol)
Benzodiazepines	Sertraline (Zoloft)
Amphetamines	Bupropion (Wellbutrin), selegiline (Eldepryl), over-the-counter decongestants, trazodone, chlorpromazine, desipramine, ranitidine (Zantac), amantadine

There are problems of sensitivity and specificity in using urine-screening tests. False-negative results occur because of deception in collection and insensitive testing. False-positive results occur because of innocent confounding substances (Table 29.3), errors in processing samples, and the normal frequency of testing error. Experimental, social, and recreational use of illicit substances is so widely practiced that a positive test by no means establishes abuse or dependency. It also does not provide evidence of intoxication or impairment.

The testing of minors younger than age 18 years, which theoretically can be authorized by parents and legal guardians regardless of the wishes of the patient, raises issues of patient trust, ethics, and legality if contested. Possible drug use can be explored most productively in the context of the total family relationship, without the referring practitioner appearing to have to take sides.

In most instances, the drug treatment program should perform drug testing. Avoiding urine testing in the primary care setting also helps facilitate the doctor–patient relationship. It is hoped that people who relapse will be open and honest and will be more likely to show up for medical visits if they do not have to worry about urine testing.

Prescribing Controlled Drugs

Prescription drug abuse can be best avoided by careful and thoughtful prescribing of medications. Office-based practitioners prescribe large amounts of controlled drugs. Table 29.4 shows a summary description of the various schedules under the Controlled Substances Act. When prescribing these drugs, it is important to realize that chronic pain, anxiety, and insomnia treated with controlled drugs on a long-term basis will result in physiologic dependence.

TABLE 29.4 Controlled Substances Act

The Controlled Substances Act (Title II of the Federal Comprehensive Drug Abuse Prevention and Control Act of 1970) is designed to improve regulation of the manufacturing, distribution, and dispensing of controlled substances by providing a "closed" system for legitimate handlers of these drugs. If not specifically exempted, every person who manufactures, distributes, *prescribes,* administers, or dispenses any controlled substance must register annually with the Attorney General. Accurate records of drugs purchased, distributed, and dispensed must be maintained and kept on file for 2 years by all persons who regularly dispense and charge for controlled substances in the course of their practice.

Each drug or substance subject to control is assigned to one of five schedules depending on the potential for abuse, medical usefulness, and degree of dependence if abused. The five schedules and the drugs included in them follow:

Schedule I: Drugs and other substances having a high potential for abuse and no current accepted medical usefulness. Included are heroin, methaqualone, MDMA (Ecstasy), marijuana, and lysergic acid diethylamide (LSD).

Schedule II: Drugs having a high potential for abuse and accepted medical usefulness; abuse leads to severe psychologic or physical dependence. Included are most opiates (fentanyl, hydrocodone, hydromorphone, meperidine, methadone, morphine, oxycodone), pentobarbital, and secobarbital.

Schedule III: Drugs having less abuse potential and accepted medical usefulness; abuse leads to moderate dependence. Included in this schedule are buprenorphine, hydrocodone combination tablets, codeine combination tablets, butalbital, anabolic steroids, and dronabinol.

Schedule IV: Drugs having a low abuse potential, accepted medical usefulness, and limited dependence. Included in this schedule are benzodiazepines, phenobarbital, butorphanol, propoxyphene, eszopiclone, zaleplon, zolpidem, modafinil, and phentermine.

Schedule V: Drugs, including a few *over-the-counter preparations,* having a low abuse potential, accepted medical usefulness, and limited dependence. Mixtures containing limited quantities of opioids with nonopioid drugs (e.g., codeine containing cough syrups) and Lomotil (atropine/diphenoxylate) are included in this schedule.

Practitioners must be vigilant to avoid being "duped," acquiescing to patient demands by prescribing inappropriately. To avoid possible abuse, medications with abuse liability should be prescribed on a fixed schedule. This strategy improves control of symptoms, minimizes the development of symptoms (rather than reacting to symptoms after they occur), and avoids patient focus on immediate relief. Medications should be prescribed for short periods during treatment of acute problems. Patients should be seen for reassessment at frequent intervals and telephone refills should be avoided.

There is a definite risk of theft of prescription blanks or alteration of a prescription. All prescription pads should be safeguarded and, ideally, marked "not for scheduled drugs." Prescription blanks for scheduled drugs should

TABLE 29.5 Generally Inappropriate Prescribing Practices

Combinations of scheduled drugs
Two prescriptions for the same scheduled drug filled on the same or consecutive days
Regular prescriptions of "preferred" drugs of abuse
Prescribing for two or more family members of a family the same drug or combination of scheduled drugs
Multiple scheduled drugs for the same purpose
Prescribing scheduled drugs to family members
Prescription of scheduled drugs from two or more practitioners simultaneously

be kept locked separately. Prescriptions should be written clearly, and the number of pills to be dispensed and the number of refills should be written out (not just a number). For some medications, such as sustained release oxycodone, the milligram dose should be spelled out, as a 10 can easily be altered to a 40. If no refills are to be given, "no refill" should be noted. All prescribing of scheduled drugs should be documented clearly in the chart.

Practitioners should be suspicious of patients who: 1) lose prescriptions or medications, 2) obtain prescriptions from multiple practitioners, 3) run out of medication before the time that would be expected, 4) demand one specific drug as the only one that will work, 5) have a sudden deterioration in work, school, or relationships, 6) have a history of substance abuse, 7) have a history of violent behavior, or 8) have slurred speech or unexplained cognitive impairment. Table 29.5 lists prescribing practices that may be illegal, dangerous, or inappropriate or indicate drug abuse.

Two classes of controlled drugs, benzodiazepines and narcotics, are the most commonly abused prescription drugs (2). Long-term use of these drugs is sometimes appropriate (see Chapter 22 and Chronic Pain Management, below). However, intermittent use is required to avoid physical dependence. Nonpharmacologic modalities should always be used to increase the interval between doses, decrease the required dosage, and permit intermittent use of these drugs if possible.

Nonscheduled drugs with abuse liability include muscle relaxants (especially carisoprodol—Soma), clonidine, Phenergan, and amitriptyline. Clonidine, prescribed for hypertension, commonly finds its way onto the streets, where it is sold to opiate addicts to alleviate opiate withdrawal. Muscle relaxants are abused commonly as sleeping pills.

SOCIAL AND EPIDEMIOLOGIC ASPECTS

Social Aspects

Drug abuse has been a dominant public health concern for the past 30 years. Quite apart from toxic effects that may represent specific health threats to the individual abuser (discussed at greater length below under each substance), there are major societal consequences. The loss of impulse control directly associated with drug abuse, especially that caused by depressant intoxication is clearly recognized as conducive to acts of violence (assault, rape, murder, and suicide). Impaired judgment and performance secondary to intoxication are associated with greatly increased rates of vehicular and workplace accidents and trauma, as well as impaired work performance and attendant economic loss.

Finally, not as a result of pharmacologic effects but as an unintended byproduct of illicit status, substances of abuse are closely linked to crime (3). Illegal status raises the cost of such substances and creates an economic stimulus to hook and then supply consumers. Tens of billions of dollars annually in property crime and robberies are committed by addicts to pay the hugely inflated price of their addiction. Thousands of homicides annually are linked to drug abuse, many by dealers to acquire and police their turf. Many more billions of dollars are spent in the criminal justice system in the apprehension, trial, and imprisonment of addicts and dealers.

Epidemiology

Although survey data show changes in the use of some illicit substances among important segments of the U.S. population, drug abuse continues to be one of the most serious problems faced by public health and law enforcement authorities. Overall, in 2003 there were an estimated 19.5 million Americans who were current users of an illicit drug (4). This represents 8.3% of the population older than age 12 years. Marijuana was the most commonly used illicit drug with 14.6 million users, followed by cocaine, with 3.5 million current users. In the past 5 years, there has been a tremendous surge in the use of the so-called "rave" drugs—methamphetamine, 3,4-methylenedioxymethamphetamine (MDMA, Ecstasy), gamma-hydroxybutyrate (GHB, liquid Ecstasy), and Rohypnol. Additionally, in rural areas where heroin is not readily available, illicit OxyContin is commonly snorted or injected.

Drug use and abuse are not evenly distributed throughout various segments of society. The incidence and prevalence of regular use and abuse are greater among inner city populations characterized by low levels of employment and educational achievement. Minorities are overrepresented in this population. *Women* are at lower risk of drug abuse than men but still make up about a third of the treatment population. They also are more likely than men to abuse illicit drugs by smoking or snorting rather than injecting. Particular problems include prostitution and consequent high rates of sexually transmitted diseases (STDs) as well as pregnancy, child care problems, and single-parent status.

The *elderly* are not at high risk for illicit drug use. Addiction to illicit drugs tends to wane over the years in those who survive beyond their fifties or sixties. Most drug problems in the elderly occur with alcohol, tobacco, and prescription drugs (opioids for analgesia and benzodiazepines for insomnia).

Polydrug use, abuse, and dependence are extremely common. For example, more than 80% of alcoholics are cigarette smokers. Many younger alcoholics also abuse cocaine. Alcoholics, in general, are at greater risk of abusing benzodiazepines when compared with non-drug abusing populations. People in methadone maintenance programs often abuse cocaine, benzodiazepines, and alcohol, and more than 90% are cigarette smokers. Heroin and cocaine are frequently injected together as a "speedball." Use of a particular drug can be a function of price and availability, as illustrated by geographic differences in the patterns of drug abuse. Sometimes a drug interaction is desired (e.g., anxiolytic effects of alcohol counteract stimulant effects of cocaine). Generally, people who find one drug of abuse particularly rewarding are likely to find other drugs of abuse also to be rewarding.

Psychiatric disorders are more common among substance abusers than in the population as a whole. These both precede onset of substance abuse and result from substance abuse. Consequences of substance abuse also mimic psychiatric disorders. For example, patients with anxiety disorders may self-medicate with alcohol or benzodiazepines. Withdrawal from these substances produces anxiety regardless of whether the patient has an anxiety disorder. Stimulants acutely produce psychotic reactions, and depression is seen during withdrawal. Substance abusers are often given personality disorder diagnoses (especially the antisocial type).

CAUSES

Predisposing Factors

The causes of substance abuse are clearly complex. Some of the factors involved are:

- *Pharmacologic.* Certain drugs, classes of drugs, and routes of administration are highly rewarding or reinforcing.
- *Genetic.* Certain individuals appear to be biologically predisposed to the rewarding effects of drugs of abuse and to the acquisition of drug dependence. This is most well recognized for alcohol, but is increasingly being recognized for other drugs of abuse.
- *Learning and behavior.* Repeated use of drugs (rewarding stimulus) elicits conditioned responses that perpetuate drug use.
- *Personality and psychiatric disorder.* People who have difficulty in deferring gratification seem to be predisposed

to drug abuse. Those with mood or anxiety disorders may find that certain drugs of abuse normalize these states.

- *Social, environmental, and cultural.* Different societies have different attitudes and customs regarding use of psychoactive substances (e.g., French attitude toward wine). People who have few other rewarding activities (e.g., gainful employment) may be predisposed toward drug abuse as a rewarding activity.

Models for Understanding and Managing Substance Abuse

These causes do not speak to possible legal consequences or to therapeutic maneuvers. Four models, described here, have been proposed to encompass these concerns. The models, although distinct, are not mutually exclusive, and most people fit into more than one model, illustrating the complexity of their disease.

Moral Failure Model

This view attributes substance abuse to a failure by parents or parental surrogates (e.g., religious training, schools, movies, television, and music) to inculcate values, with resultant lack of morality that would prevent the use and abuse of drugs. From a public health viewpoint the model has utility. When applied to the person already dependent on drugs and with a long criminal record, it is not useful unless there is some religious conversion experience or complete acceptance of a 12-step program (e.g., Alcoholics Anonymous or Narcotics Anonymous).

Legal Model

Proponents define behavior as aberrant only when specific acts violate existing law and then recommend existing legal remedies such as trial, fines, and imprisonment to deal with these infractions. This model counters the disease or illness concept of addiction.

Disease Model

The disease model hypothesizes a host susceptibility to drugs of abuse that is lifelong, progressive, and incapable of modification and hence can be coped with only by total abstinence. It takes as its substrate only those meeting the definitions of substance abuse or dependence and does not concern itself with social or experimental use. The disease model partially encompasses research advances in psychopharmacology.

The disease model was originally proposed to counter adverse societal attitudes and judgmental views toward alcohol and drug abuse. This model also offers a nonstigmatizing explanation of substance abuse to organizations such as Alcoholics Anonymous and Narcotics Anonymous. These organizations have helped unleash a vast movement for self-improvement that has helped a significant number of abusers. The disease model is the paradigm for methadone maintenance, developed in the 1960s, for the treatment of heroin dependence. Heroin abuse was seen as a biologic modification of the brain that required supplementation by a narcotic substitute that does not lead to significant dysfunction.

Psychosocial Model

The psychosocial model views chemical dependency as the inadvertent effect of repeated self-medication by a vulnerable individual intent on relieving overwhelming anxiety or psychic pain related to hopelessness, boredom, depression, or fear. Drugs of abuse are potent and effective, albeit short-term, chemical alleviators of these symptoms. Vulnerability in this model is not a function of genetic constitution (although this may define an enhanced susceptibility). Rather it is because of membership in at-risk populations who, because of immaturity, socioeconomic disability, and the lack of responsible familial or peer support systems, have not developed the behaviors that the greater part of society uses to cope with adversity. This model has the virtue of defining an at-risk population from among the young, the dropouts, and the socially and economically disadvantaged that best fits most abusers in our current epidemic. The model helps explain the potential for endemic abuse by people who, although they may be socially and economically advantaged, may also turn to repetitive self-medication in the face of losses or situational anxiety, demoralization, or physical pain. The psychosocial model avoids a simplistic expectation of cure by mere detoxification or by enforced abstinence if release back into the same environment occurs without change in the conditions of vulnerability. The model also relies on support systems and self-help as a condition of remission.

SELECTED DRUGS OF ABUSE

Opioid (Narcotic) Analgesics

Opioids are commonly prescribed drugs and play an essential role in the care of patients. The fear of causing opioid addiction has led some practitioners to under-medicate in the management of acute pain. Less commonly, there has been a tendency in treating patients with chronic pain to continue the use of opioid analgesics when the development of tolerance has rendered them less effective. Patients who have been taking opioid analgesics for long periods may experience little pain relief and may, in fact, confuse incipient withdrawal toward the end of a dosing interval with the onset of pain. An understanding of tolerance, physical dependence, and addiction can ensure more rational prescribing patterns.

The opiate-dependent patient is not generally seen in office practice seeking treatment for drug dependence. Patients often appear in office practice settings attempting to obtain prescription drugs when they experience difficulty in obtaining heroin. Morphine, hydromorphone (Dilaudid), oxycodone, and meperidine (Demerol) are the drugs most preferred by addicts, but they will readily use the whole range of less potent opioid analgesics if preferred drugs are unavailable. The term *opioid* refers both to drugs derived from opium (opiates) and to synthetic drugs with similar actions. Alcohol, benzodiazepines, and promethazine (Phenergan) are often abused by opioid dependent patients because of their tendency to potentiate the effects of opiates.

Usual Effects and Therapeutic Use

Opiates are the prototype for managing patients with pain. To prevent abuse, they should be prescribed on a fixed schedule. For a comparison of the different opioids, see Chapter 13. Used for short intervals after an acute pain syndrome, opioids are safe and effective. Abuse liability increases with potency. Heroin, the most commonly abused illicit opioid, is usually injected intravenously but can also be injected subcutaneously (skin-popping), smoked, or sniffed (snorting). Heroin crosses the blood–brain barrier more effectively than other opioids. The effects after use consist of a brief and intense period of euphoria followed by several hours of a pleasant dreamy state in which the user may slowly nod as if falling asleep. Areas of pain feel numbed. The skin may itch (because of histamine release), which leads to characteristic scratching. Other effects include increased talkativeness (soap boxing), increased activity, and conjunctival suffusion (red eye). Stomach turning and vomiting (pleasant sick) occur. Physiologic effects include miosis and respiratory depression.

Acute Adverse Effects

Depressed consciousness and respiration characterize opioid overdose. Pulmonary edema, a common complication of opioid overdose, contributes to hypoxia and may cause death. Some opioids, such as propoxyphene (Darvon) and meperidine (Demerol), cause convulsions at high dosages. The latter has a proconvulsive metabolite (normeperidine) that accumulates in the setting of renal failure.

Chronic Adverse Effects

The adverse effects of chronic heroin abuse result from use of dirty needles (see Complications of Injecting Drugs, below), the adulterants mixed with the heroin, and the associated life-style (poor nutrition, lack of health care, and criminal activity) rather than from the drug itself. Heroin is usually mixed with lactose and quinine under unsterile conditions. Other more dangerous adulterants may also be included to mask the dilution of the heroin.

Tolerance to heroin develops quickly and can be demonstrated to some degree after only a few days of administration of the drug. The degree of tolerance and the consequent severity of withdrawal symptoms depend primarily on dosage levels and the frequency and duration of use. As outlined in Table 29.2, anxiety, nausea, yawning, diarrhea, sweating, rhinorrhea, dilated pupils, and piloerection (gooseflesh) characterize opioid withdrawal. In the advanced stages of withdrawal, the patient experiences vomiting and muscle spasms. Although the untreated addict experiences significant anxiety and discomfort during withdrawal, the process itself presents no serious medical risks.

Treatment

Opioid overdose must be treated in an emergency room. Emergency treatment requires cardiorespiratory monitoring and support. The opioid antagonist naloxone (Narcan) is safe and effective in countering the central nervous system (CNS) depression caused by opioid overdose but may precipitate withdrawal. The initial dose is 0.4 mg intravenously. This may need to be repeated because naloxone has a shorter duration of action than most opioid agonists.

Any patient who has been abusing heroin or other opioids and is willing to accept help should be referred for treatment. Few addicts voluntarily seek treatment before being faced with the destructive consequences of their drug use.

Detoxification from opiate dependence involves the administration of an opiate agonist (methadone), the nonopiate clonidine, or a partial agonist (buprenorphine). Substitution and slow tapering of methadone effectively reduces the severity of opiate withdrawal (5). It has a long duration of action and is conveniently administered orally. However, federal regulations limit the use of methadone to specially licensed centers. Detoxification may be accomplished by substituting methadone for the opioid previously used by the patient and then gradually reducing the dosage over time (usually at least 7 days). The initial dose should be sufficient to suppress withdrawal symptoms without causing sedation. Methadone detoxification is normally done on an ambulatory basis by specially licensed drug treatment programs.

Clonidine is a nonopioid medication demonstrated effective in suppressing symptoms of opiate withdrawal. A centrally acting α-adrenergic agonist, clonidine reduces sympathetic nervous system related effects of opiate withdrawal. It is more effective in suppressing signs than in relieving symptoms of withdrawal (6). Clonidine is dosed at 0.1 mg every 4 to 6 hours for the first day, followed by 0.1 mg every 8 hours the second day, and 0.1 mg every 12 hours on the third day. Dosages are held for systolic blood pressure less than 100 mm Hg. Transdermal clonidine may be an effective adjunct in outpatient treatment. However, it has a delayed onset of action, not crossing the dermis for at least 24 hours after placement. Recent cases of oral ingestion of the clonidine patch resulting in profound hypotension and bradycardia may limit its use. Outpatient use of clonidine is also impacted by diversion for illicit use. Other pharmacologic aids (dicyclomine for abdominal cramps, ibuprofen for bone pain, and loperamide for diarrhea) provide additional treatment for symptoms of opiate withdrawal.

Buprenorphine is a partial μ-opiate receptor agonist with a long duration of action. It is more effective than clonidine and equally effective to methadone for the management of opiate withdrawal (7). The parenteral formulation has been used to treat opiate withdrawal symptoms in hospitalized medically ill opiate-dependent patients (8). Experimental studies have demonstrated the efficacy of a sublingual preparation of buprenorphine as a maintenance therapy for opiate dependence (9,10). This preparation has recently become available for use in the United States and has become the drug of choice for outpatient treatment of opiate withdrawal. Only physicians who complete an approved eight-hour course and subsequently obtain a special Drug Enforcement Agency (DEA) number may prescribe buprenorphine. For detoxification, sublingual buprenorphine is administered once withdrawal symptoms are present, with typical treatment of 3 to 7 days.

Except for physicians licensed to prescribe buprenorphine, it is illegal for a care provider to prescribe an opiate for the treatment of opiate withdrawal. As with detoxification from any substance, the patient should be engaged in a program of outpatient chemical dependency counseling during and after detoxification (see sections on detoxification and rehabilitation, below). Even short-term detoxification has been shown to impact positively on future outcomes related to opiate dependence (11).

Cocaine and Other Stimulants

Cocaine, the amphetamines (especially methamphetamine), and methylphenidate are the most commonly abused stimulant drugs (nicotine is discussed in Chapter 27). *Cocaine* is used in several forms. The route for cocaine intake depends on the form used. As the natural water-soluble powder, cocaine hydrochloride, it is either sniffed (snorted) and absorbed through the nasal mucosa or injected intravenously. Forms of cocaine that can be smoked (using a water pipe or in cigarette form) are produced by extracting or freeing the cocaine alkaloid from the hydrochloride salt. When ether is used as the reagent in this process, the resulting product is referred to as freebase. When baking soda and water are used as reagents, the resulting product is crack, so named because of the crackling sound that is produced when the drug is smoked. Although they may differ in appearance and concentration, freebase and crack are pharmacologically the same.

Cocaine use appears in variable patterns. In the early stages, sessions of cocaine use typically last 2 to 4 hours, with intervals of days or weeks between sessions. Some users are able to maintain this pattern of use without progressing further. However, many users follow a pattern of rapidly escalating use in which both the length of sessions and the rate of consumption increase; users of freebase and crack may be more likely to succumb to this pattern than users who snort cocaine powder.

Chronic abusers typically engage in runs or periods of intensive cocaine use that can last anywhere from a few hours to several days. A run is terminated when the user runs out of cocaine or money, or is too physically exhausted to continue.

Methamphetamine, a synthetic stimulant, is sold as a white powder that is taken orally, intranasally, or intravenously or as a clear "rock" that is heated and smoked. It is known on the street as ice, speed, crystal meth, crank, tina, or glass. It is easily synthesized from the over-the-counter cold remedy pseudoephedrine by illegal small-time laboratories that quickly change location. Methamphetamine is especially popular in nonurban areas that have less influx of cocaine.

Methylphenidate (Ritalin) mimics the effects of naturally occurring stimulants such as cocaine and can be taken orally or intravenously. Legitimately used for the treatment of attention deficit disorder, methylphenidate is sometimes obtained by diversion from family members with the disorder or by seeking refills for reportedly affected family members from unsuspecting practitioners.

Abusers of stimulants develop some tolerance to the euphoric effects of the drugs but may become more sensitive to other effects such as irritability, restlessness, hypervigilance, and paranoia. Users report that in any given session of cocaine use, the duration and intensity of the euphoric effect seem to recede with successive doses, a phenomenon called "chasing the dragon's tail."

Usual Effects and Therapeutic Use

CNS stimulants produce euphoria, increased confidence and energy, increased heart rate and blood pressure, dilated pupils, constriction of peripheral blood vessels, and increased body temperature. Effects are caused by sympathetic stimulation centrally and peripherally. The duration and intensity of effect depend on the dosage and the route of administration. Single oral doses of amphetamines produce effects lasting 2 to 4 hours. The effects of cocaine, when snorted, are rapid in onset but short in duration. Smoking freebase or crack produces an intense short-duration effect (peak effect in 2 to 3 minutes, duration about 10 minutes) because smoking is an extremely efficient method of drug administration. Intravenous use produces similar (or greater) intensity and longer duration of effects. Smoking and intravenous use of methamphetamine results in a pleasurable rush that lasts a few minutes. Oral use results in a muted longer duration effect.

Its capacity to produce euphoria gives cocaine a high abuse potential. In animals, cocaine produces reinforcing responses that exceed those of other drugs of abuse. The administration of cocaine in humans is associated with an increased desire for more cocaine (i.e., the presence of the drug itself in the body increases desire for cocaine). Users often delay entry into treatment until they are physically and emotionally exhausted or are faced with serious financial, legal, or medical problems.

Acute Adverse Effects

Very large doses of all stimulants may cause hyperpyrexia, arrhythmias, hypertension, and coronary and cerebral artery vasospasm, leading to myocardial infarction, stroke, seizures, cardiovascular collapse, and death (12). Large doses of cocaine may also cause respiratory depression with a fatal outcome. A *reversible organic delusional disorder* that resembles paranoid schizophrenia is occasionally seen. This syndrome may occur in normal subjects with no previous psychiatric history.

Chronic Adverse Effects

The chronic abuser of cocaine, amphetamines, and other long-acting stimulants is typically hyperactive, jittery, and irritable while using and depressed, exhausted, or lethargic afterward. Previously stable individuals may develop unexplained financial problems or uncharacteristic overnight disappearances. With chronic heavy use there is usually a history of sleep disturbance and weight loss. The patient may be emotionally labile, and periods of irritability, depression, and fatigue may alternate with periods of elation and mania. Cases of persistent psychotic disorders have been reported. Intravenous abusers of methylphenidate develop talc lung because talc is contained as filler in the tablet.

Physical examination may reveal needle marks; rhinitis; teeth worn from bruxism (grinding of teeth); ulcers on the lips, tongue, or nose; nasal septum perforation; tremor; flushing; and excessive sweating. Although cocaine may initially enhance sexual functioning, chronic use often interferes with sexual performance. Extremely heavy users may exhibit rapid, repetitious, and ritualistic body movements.

Stimulant withdrawal as outlined in Table 29.3 is characterized by a "crash" with symptoms of fatigue, drowsiness, dysthymia and drug craving. Orthostatic hypotension may accompany amphetamine withdrawal.

Treatment

Stimulant-abusing patients are generally treated in the outpatient setting, except for patients who present a risk of suicide. Treatment preferably involves daily counseling sessions during the first few weeks of abstinence. Necessary external supports include stable employment, a drug-free home environment, and active involvement in Narcotics Anonymous. No specific pharmacologic treatment is indicated for cocaine withdrawal because symptoms are mild. Currently, no drugs have been convincingly demonstrated to be efficacious in maintaining abstinence. A variety of drugs, including fluoxetine, desipramine, topiramate, and ondansetron, has been studied for their effects in reducing the reinforcing responses to cocaine in humans. To date, none has become clinically useful.

Sedative-Hypnotics and Benzodiazepines

The most commonly abused sedatives are alprazolam (Xanax), clonazepam (Klonopin), and diazepam (Valium). Rohypnol (flunitrazepam) has recently gained attention for abuse as "the date rape drug." It is not licensed in the United States but is sold illicitly on the street. Rohypnol may cause paradoxical agitation and is not detectable by routine urine toxicology.

Usual Effects and Therapeutic Use

Sedatives cause intoxication similar to that seen with alcohol. Sufficient amounts are often taken to produce a depression of cortical function and to relax social and personal inhibitions. A high, or a state in which mood is elevated and anxiety is reduced, occurs. Normal individuals and those with anxiety disorders do not necessarily find these effects pleasurable or reinforcing. Because of their safety profile, benzodiazepines have become the only sedative-hypnotics prescribed for anxiolytic or sedating purposes. Chapter 22 discusses the proper prescribing of benzodiazepines for this purpose. This class of medicine should be avoided in all patients with a history of substance abuse. Phenobarbital should be the only prescribed barbiturate, with its indication being a second- to third-line drug for seizure prevention (see Chapter 88). Shorter acting barbiturates are contained in migraine medicines such as Fiorinal. These medications have a high abuse potential and should be avoided.

Acute Adverse Effects

Overdose may lead to slurred speech, impaired judgment, and unsteady gait. Even greater overdose may lead to stupor, coma, respiratory depression, vasomotor collapse, and death. Benzodiazepines (compared with barbiturates) cause less loss of motor coordination and almost never cause death when taken alone in large doses (unless given rapidly intravenously, e.g., midazolam or diazepam). However, the combination of alcohol and benzodiazepines can be lethal.

Chronic Adverse Effects

Benzodiazepine use may increase the risk of accidental injury and in a study of older adults, an elevated rate of automobile accident was found in benzodiazepine users (13). Several epidemiologic studies have shown benzodiazepines increase the risk of falls (14,15) and hip fractures in the elderly (16,17). One study has shown an increased risk of suicide attempt in benzodiazepine users with borderline personality disorder (18).

Almost no organ toxicity is associated with chronic administration of these drugs. From this standpoint, they are safer than alcohol. If prescribed for insomnia, benzodiazepines should be prescribed for short-term treatment (19,20). Otherwise, if patients use the medications on a regular basis, they will induce tolerance and increase the dosage. Chronic use of benzodiazepines may go undetected until confusion, irritability, slurred speech, or ataxia is recognized as a sign of sedative intoxication.

Physical examination may include ecchymoses from injuries sustained during an intoxicated state. Sedative-hypnotics can also produce anterograde amnesia. This is mostly dosage related and has been most often described with flunitrazepam (Rohypnol) and diazepam (Valium).

Physical dependence on benzodiazepines and the potential for major withdrawal symptoms may occur in as little as 2 months if dosages substantially above therapeutic levels are used. Most patients who abuse and have significant physical dependence on benzodiazepines abuse other drugs concurrently. Withdrawal symptoms (outlined in Table 29.2) occur in patients taking therapeutic dosages daily for 6 months or more (21). Tapering the dosage can reduce the risk of withdrawal. Although chronic use may create the risk of withdrawal symptoms, there is evidence that patients may use benzodiazepines on a chronic basis without developing tolerance to the anxiolytic effects of the medication (22,23).

Treatment

Nonbenzodiazepine sedative overdose is a life-threatening occurrence that should be treated in an emergency department. Because of physical dependence, patients who use excessive dosages of sedative drugs are at risk of serious withdrawal reactions, including life-threatening seizures. Outpatient treatment for therapeutic dependence can often be managed by tapering the prescribed benzodiazepine or switching to a benzodiazepine with a longer half-life and tapering it over several weeks (24). Onset time of withdrawal symptoms is inversely related to the half-life of the benzodiazepine of use. Inpatient treatment is often required for high-dose abuse and can be managed using phenobarbital, which has a long half-life (80 to 100 hours) and provides the pharmacokinetic umbrella to prevent withdrawal symptoms (25).

Marijuana and Hashish

Marijuana consists of the dried leaves of the *Cannabis sativa* plant, which are usually smoked in pipes or cigarettes (joints). *Hashish* is a concentrated resin of cannabis and contains approximately 5 to 10 times the concentration of the principal psychoactive ingredient—9-tetrahydrocannabinol—as compared with *marijuana.* The discussion that follows applies to both marijuana and hashish. Cannabis can also be added to foods such as brownies, but when it is eaten, effects appear less rapidly and are less under control of the user.

Usual Effects and Therapeutic Use

The effects of marijuana from usual smoked doses last from 3 to 6 hours. The more common effects are elation or high, an increased tendency to laughter and silliness, tachycardia, reddening of the eyes, and a later stage of relaxation. At higher dosages these effects are enhanced. The user may misjudge the effects of time, and perception of sound, color, and other sensations may be distorted or sharpened. Short-term memory and logical thinking are impaired, as is the ability to drive a car or perform other complex tasks. Additive effects occur with alcohol or other CNS depressants. Dosages three to five times higher than those producing relaxation and mild euphoria can result in effects similar to those of lysergic acid diethylamide (LSD) and other hallucinogenic substances (depersonalization, auditory, and visual hallucinations). Some of the usual effects of marijuana that might be enjoyable to the experienced user, as well as the more alarming effects associated with high dosage, can be frightening to the inexperienced user. The setting is important in determining the effects of the drug. When smoked in a pleasant and familiar setting, marijuana is less likely to produce a negative response than when used in unfamiliar or threatening surroundings.

Cannabis has effects that are *potentially useful for therapeutic purposes* (e.g., decreased intraocular pressure, antiemetic properties). However, other currently approved drugs are of similar or superior efficacy for these indications and have fewer side effects. The principal psychoactive substance in cannabis is marketed in oral preparations; dronabinol (Marinol) is a schedule II drug in the United States and nabilone is available in Canada, where they are approved for use as appetite stimulants.

Acute Adverse Effects

Considering the large number of regular users in the United States, it is clear that adverse reactions to marijuana requiring medical treatment are rare. The most common adverse response is an *acute anxiety reaction,* which may include paranoid ideation. These reactions are most likely to occur in novice users or in users who unexpectedly receive a much larger than usual dose. Most reactions last only the few hours it takes for the effects of the drug to wear off. Some patients experience persistent anxiety for several days after the initial panic subsides.

There have also been reports of delirium induced by marijuana. A dysphoric reaction characterized by disorientation, catatonic immobility, acute panic, and heavy sedation has also been reported. These conditions tend to remit within 2 to 4 hours as the effects of the marijuana diminish. Reports of enduring psychotic reactions after heavy marijuana use have appeared, largely in countries where marijuana is used at much higher dosages than in the United States. Reports of confirmed psychotic reactions to marijuana in this country are rare.

Chronic Adverse Effects

There is substantial evidence that marijuana at dosage levels associated with common social usage results in loss of energy and drive, impaired memory, and apathy. This is sometimes called the amotivational syndrome.

Smoking marijuana alone does not appear to cause a decline in pulmonary function (26). However, heavy cannabis users tend to be heavy tobacco smokers. The tar content of cannabis smoke is 50% higher than that of tobacco. Accordingly, users may develop chronic bronchitis and other respiratory diseases. Marijuana smoke contains 70% more carcinogens than does tobacco smoke (27). There have been conflicting findings concerning possible adverse effects of marijuana on the immune system. Some studies report changes in immunologic responsiveness, but the clinical implications of these changes are currently unknown. There is evidence that marijuana reduces testosterone levels in men, although generally, the testosterone level in users remains within normal limits (28).

Regular use induces moderate *tolerance*. High dosages followed by sudden cessation produces a mild *withdrawal* syndrome in both animals and humans. Regular users of marijuana often exhibit restlessness, sleep disturbance, loss of appetite, and irritability when they stopped using marijuana. For social use, neither tolerance nor physical dependence is a major issue.

Treatment

Because they must be closely observed and may take several hours to recover, patients with panic reactions are best managed in a setting such as a drug abuse program, mental health center, or emergency department where continuing observation and supportive contact can be provided. Generally, these patients require simple reassurance and an explanation that they are experiencing a drug reaction that will dissipate as the drug is eliminated from their bodies.

Delusional or delirious patients should be seen in an emergency department because they present more complicated management problems and may require sedation or hospitalization. Furthermore, other causes of delirium should be ruled out. Restraints should be used only when absolutely necessary for the safety of the patient or others. Medications should not be used unless the patient is extremely agitated and difficult to control.

Treatment for chronic use should involve the support necessary for abstinence: a drug-free environment, active participation in 12-step meetings of Alcoholics Anonymous or Narcotics Anonymous, and, in some circumstances, group counseling.

3,4-Methylenedioxymethamphetamine (Ecstasy)

MDMA is a synthetic drug that is both a stimulant and hallucinogen (LSD-like). It was originally synthesized as a drug to facilitate communication during psychotherapy (29). Street names for MDMA include Ecstasy, Adam, XTC, hug, beans, and love drug. Most MDMA sold on the street has MDMA in combination with other drugs, including LSD, amphetamine, caffeine, heroin, and lactose. Using MDMA with LSD is termed "candyflipping." MDMA comes in the form of a white powder that is usually pressed into pills, but other routes, such as snorting, injecting, and use as a rectal suppository, have been reported.

Usual Effects

When taken on an empty stomach, oral ingestion of MDMA results in a "rush" within minutes. The rush, consisting of euphoria and an intensification of perceptions, lasts 25 to 30 minutes. Individuals crave the effect and take additional doses. However, repeated doses have diminished effect. After the initial intense phase, a plateau phase occurs during which users report a trance-like feeling that lasts a few hours. A down phase, accompanied by feelings of dysphoria and anxiety, occurs 3 to 6 hours after initial ingestion. Despite feelings of exhaustion, users are unable to fall asleep.

Acute and Chronic Adverse Effects

MDMA is neurotoxic, damaging dopamine and serotonin producing neurons in the brain. Acute use of MDMA results in muscle rigidity, involuntary teeth clenching, nausea, blurred vision, faintness, and cold sweats. Cases of acute rhabdomyolysis have been reported. Heart rate and blood pressure increases may be dose dependent. MDMA can cause confusion, depression, sleep problems, severe anxiety, and paranoia. These effects may linger weeks after use. Hepatotoxicity and an acneform rash occur in many individuals after chronic use. Long-term users of MDMA may suffer permanent deficits in thought and memory (30). Motor disturbances may occur resulting in a syndrome resembling Parkinson disease.

Treatment

The acute toxic effects of MDMA are short lived. It is metabolized in the liver and excreted in the urine. Management of overdose is supportive care in a quiet dark setting. For individuals who are agitated and paranoid, treatment with benzodiazepines will ameliorate symptoms. Intravenous hydration is indicated in cases of overdose accompanied by rhabdomyolysis. Dantrolene may be useful if severe persistent muscle spasms occur.

Long-term treatment for abuse of MDMA is similar to other drugs of abuse, consisting of counseling and 12-step groups. Most users of MDMA are young and should seek treatment centers that have programs specific for adolescents and young adults.

γ-Hydroxybutyrate

γ-Hydroxybutyrate (GHB) is a precursor of the neurotransmitter gamma aminobutyric acid. It was developed as an adjunct to anesthesia and is used clinically for narcolepsy. It is sold in small bottles as a salty clear liquid and goes by the street names liquid ecstasy, easy lay, cherry meth, soap, liquid X, liquid G, and liquid E. After ingestion, the onset of action is within 15 to 30 minutes with effects lasting up to 3 hours. The drug's half-life is about 30 minutes with elimination by expiration as carbon dioxide.

Usual Effects

Acting on the central dopaminergic system, GHB produces euphoria and disinhibition without a subsequent dysphoria.

Adverse Effects

Idiosyncratic responses to GHB occur. These include delusions, aggressive behavior, altered mental status, seizures, nausea, vertigo, ataxia, nystagmus, amnesia, somnolence, and coma. Recovery from somnolence and coma is often characterized by myoclonic jerks and confusion. During intoxication, individuals are at risk for aspiration. In severe cases of intoxication, bradycardia and myoclonus may accompany coma. Adverse effects are potentiated by CNS depressants, including alcohol, benzodiazepines, and opiates. Use of GHB with methamphetamine increases the risk of seizures.

Treatment

Management of acute overdose is supportive. Comatose patients may require intubation for airway protection. Atropine should be prescribed in the presence of symptomatic bradycardia. Because many patients ingest GHB with other drugs, a screen for other drugs should be performed with treatment for toxicity from other drugs as indicated.

Long-term treatment for abuse of GHB is similar to other drugs of abuse, consisting of counseling and 12-step groups. GHB users are at high risk of developing dependence to other drugs. Most users of GHB are young and should seek treatment centers that have programs specific for adolescents and young adults.

Phencyclidine

Phencyclidine (PCP) is a barbiturate-like anesthetic and derivative of ketamine. However, PCP exhibits selective action as an anesthetic, appearing to depress sensory tracts—including proprioception, pain, touch, and temperature—to a greater degree than it depresses cortical function. The resultant state of sensory deprivation and relative cortical wakefulness makes for a peculiar sense of detachment, disembodiment, and weightlessness. These sensations are intensely pleasurable for some, whereas for others they induce intense anxiety and even panic. PCP was developed as an anesthetic but was abandoned for this purpose when it was found to cause disturbing side effects. It continues to be used by veterinarians as an animal tranquilizer or immobilizing agent. Pure PCP is a white powder that dissolves in water. It is usually sprinkled on marijuana, dried parsley flakes, or other organic material and smoked. Less often, it is obtained in powder or tablet form and ingested or snorted. Street names for the drug vary considerably from region to region, but it is most commonly known as angel dust, flakes, crystal, greens, hog, or sheets.

Usual Effects

The effects of PCP are dose-related, although both individual responses vary. People who take PCP in the dosages normally associated with street use may experience exhilaration, euphoria, inebriation, tranquilization, and perceptual disturbances. Some unpleasant effects commonly reported include disorientation, hallucinations, anxiety, paranoia, excitability, and irritability. At usual street dosages, most users reach peak intoxication in 5 to 30 minutes and remain high for 4 to 6 hours. It may take 24 hours or more before the user feels completely normal again.

Acute Adverse Effects

Even at low dosages, PCP is capable of occasionally causing severe reactions that may precipitate extreme agitation and acts of violence toward the user and to others. With higher dosages, users are more likely to exhibit delirium, which may include hallucinations. Users may also develop PCP psychosis, a disorder closely resembling schizophrenia that persists for 24 hours or more. Such psychoses may develop out of the original intoxication or may occur days after the intoxication has cleared.

Ataxia, nystagmus, slurred speech, and ptosis are common features of acute PCP toxicity. Very high dosages of PCP, which are normally the result of oral ingestion rather than smoking, can result in coma, severe respiratory depression, seizures, and death.

Chronic Adverse Effects

Chronic use of PCP may produce persistent changes in personal habits (hygiene or dress), problems with memory or speech, sleep disturbances, mood changes (depression, irritability), delusional thinking, and unusual excitability or lethargy. Little is known about long-term physical effects.

Treatment

Consistent correlation has been found between the patient's initial level of consciousness and the time course of improvement. Patients who are delirious at presentation can be treated in an emergency department and do not necessarily require hospitalization. Repeated mental status examinations should be performed to ensure that the patient is in a state of clear consciousness for at least 4 hours before discharge. Members of the family should be cautioned that the patient should stay in the company of family members or reliable friends for several days. Patients can have the onset of severe depression or a PCP psychosis for several days after the acute effects of the drug have subsided. PCP abuse usually occurs in the setting of polysubstance abuse, and long-term treatment should include traditional 12-step meetings.

Lysergic Acid Diethylamide

LSD is the prototype of a number of alkaloid substances of high potency that cause hallucinations. Others include psilocybin, dimethyltryptamine, and mescaline. All are classified as hallucinogens and are CNS depressants at higher dosages. LSD (acid) is sold illicitly in the form of powder, tablets, or capsules. Sugar cubes, small squares of gelatin (window panes), or paper (blotter acid) that have been impregnated with the drug are also available. LSD is usually ingested orally and its effects appear within 30 to 40 minutes, reaching a peak at about 90 minutes, with physiologic effects gone by 6 hours but subjective effects persisting for 8 to 12 hours.

Usual Effects

Subjective effects produced by LSD include depersonalization, altered time perception, labile mood, perceptual distortions (usually visual), body image distortion, and feelings of increased insight. Physiologic effects include slight rises in blood pressure and heart rate, fever, lack of coordination, dilated pupils, increased salivation and lacrimation, hyperreflexia, and occasionally vomiting.

Acute Adverse Effects

Inexperienced users may have an acute panic reaction that occurs because the normal effects of the drug are unfamiliar or unexpected. In more severe reactions, users of LSD may experience hallucinations (usually visual) and delusions that may persist beyond the time when the drug is circulating in the blood.

Flashbacks, spontaneous recurrences of the original LSD experience, occur in some users, often days to years later. They are more likely to occur in chronic users (and can occur after the use of any hallucinogenic drug). There have also been reports of prolonged psychotic reactions after the use of LSD, although these are rare.

Patients with acute LSD toxicity can be differentiated from those with PCP toxicity or schizophrenia in several ways. LSD causes dilation of the pupils, which is absent in PCP toxicity and schizophrenia. PCP toxicity usually is characterized by clouding of consciousness and the patient often exhibits ataxia, nystagmus, and ptosis, which are not features of LSD toxicity or of schizophrenia.

Chronic Adverse Effects

Some degree of tolerance develops with repeated use of LSD, but no chronic effects or withdrawal syndrome has been observed.

Treatment

Adverse reactions to LSD usually remit in 8 to 24 hours, and hospitalization is usually unnecessary. However, the patient should be observed until symptoms clear. Referral to an emergency room or to a drug abuse program that can provide this type of support will usually be necessary. The same supportive measures described earlier for the treatment of adverse reactions to marijuana are appropriate. Extremely agitated patients should be treated with diazepam or lorazepam.

Inhalants: Solvents

The inhalation of solvents is a form of substance abuse that is most commonly found among children and adolescents. Because solvents are easily obtainable and inexpensive, they are likely to be preferred by people who lack the money or other resources needed to obtain more desirable drugs. A partial list of specific substances subject to this type of abuse includes gasoline, ignition spray, airplane glue, paint thinner, spray paint, lighter fluid, nail polish remover, cleaning fluid, and shoe polish. Inhalation is typically accomplished by saturating a rag with the substance and holding it directly over the face or placing it in a bag that is then placed over the nose and the mouth.

Usual Effects

The effects of solvents are immediate and of short duration, usually dissipating in a few hours or less (depending on the dosage). Acute intoxication is similar to alcohol intoxication except for the shorter duration.

Acute Adverse Effects

A hangover, with symptoms of headache and nausea that is similar but perhaps milder than the hangover produced by alcohol has been observed. Some users experience apparent delirium characterized by tactile hallucinations, spatial distortions, and body image distortions. Sudden sniffing deaths have been described when inhalants were used during strenuous activity or under conditions in which blood oxygen is reduced. Such deaths apparently occur as a result of cardiac arrhythmias. Other deaths have been caused by suffocation when the user loses consciousness with the bag containing the solvent covering the nose and mouth.

Chronic Adverse Effects

The effects of solvents on the CNS, liver, kidneys, and bone marrow are not well understood. Cerebellar damage (which is partially reversible with abstinence) and peripheral neuropathy occur with long-term use. Numerous studies have demonstrated organ damage from long-term exposure to low concentrations of industrial solvents, but it is less clear to what extent these findings can be generalized to the short-term high-concentration exposures experienced by inhalant abusers.

There is evidence that tolerance develops with chronic solvent abuse, but withdrawal symptoms and signs are uncommon, probably because the concentration of the substance in neurons is not sustained.

Treatment

Because the acute effects of solvents are usually of short duration, abusers rarely present for medical treatment. On rare occasions, a patient may be brought in for treatment of a solvent-induced delirium. Chronic solvent abuse requires the same type of intense counseling and rehabilitative intervention indicated for other forms of substance abuse.

Anabolic Androgenic Steroids

These drugs are used to enhance athletic performance and improve physique. They are derivatives of testosterone and promote growth of skeletal muscle and may increase lean body mass. Use is widespread but data are limited. Anabolic steroids are mostly used in cycles of weeks or months. Stacking (use of more than one preparation) and pyramiding (dosages gradually increased and then tapered) are common patterns of administration. Dosages used are much greater than those administered for therapeutic purposes.

Usual Effects and Therapeutic Use

Anabolic steroids are prescribed routinely to individuals with hypogonadism. Acute experimental administration of testosterone to eugonadal individuals produces no acute psychoactive effect (31). Total body weight increases in less than a week, partly because of salt and water retention and also because of a true increase in lean body mass. Anabolic steroids contribute to an increase in strength in trained individuals (32).

Anabolic steroids have therapeutic benefit in people with weight loss related to human immunodeficiency virus (HIV) infection. Both oxandrolone, an oral synthetic anabolic steroid, and testosterone are prescribed for involuntary weight loss and wasting related to medical illness. In these settings they are safe to prescribe, with low abuse potential.

Chronic Adverse Effects

Although it is not clear whether there are any acute adverse effects, there are chronic adverse effects if these drugs are taken in excess. Adverse chronic effects include decrease in sperm count, testicular atrophy, masculinization in women (hoarse voice and clitoral hypertrophy), premature fusion of epiphyses in adolescents, decreased glucose tolerance, an unfavorable lipid profile (increased low-density lipoprotein, decreased high-density lipoprotein), acne, alopecia, hirsuteness, hepatitis, and complications of injection drug use (see above). There is a tenuous link with malignancy and case reports of MI and other vascular events. The most reported psychological effect is an increase in aggression. Some users fulfill *DSM-IV* criteria for psychoactive substance abuse and dependence as defined at the beginning of this chapter (33).

Atropinic Drugs

Atropine (the alkaloid produced by nightshade *Atropa belladonna* and by jimsonweed) and scopolamine are acetylcholine antagonists that at high dosages produce hallucinations, delirium, and varying states of excitement, insomnia, or amnesia. CNS depression and coma may follow these effects. The undesired pharmacologic effects of these drugs—dryness of the mouth, blurred vision, anhidrosis, and tachycardia—limit their appeal as psychoactive agents. Thus, the rare instances of abuse are mostly by teenagers experimenting with jimsonweed in rural areas or, in the past, by use of over-the-counter soporifics that contained scopolamine until the Food and Drug Administration (FDA) banned this. Treatment of toxic overdose is a medical emergency requiring gastric lavage and ingestion of activated charcoal to limit intestinal absorption, maintenance of vital signs, administration of physostigmine, and lowering of body temperature.

Arecoline (Betel/Areca Nuts)

Arecoline is a parasympathomimetic alkaloid somewhat similar in structure to nicotine. It is used for its psychoactive effects by about a billion people, mostly in Southeast Asia and the Indian subcontinent. It is the world's fourth most popular psychoactive drug (after caffeine, alcohol, and nicotine). It is a cholinergic drug, exerting effects similar to acetylcholine, including sweating, salivation, and increase in bladder tone. At low dosages it produces general arousal and is usually classified as a stimulant. However, at higher doses there may be sedating effects. The nuts have a bitter taste and produce reddened saliva and stained teeth, and chronic use commonly leads to grinding of the teeth and cancer of the oral cavity. They are usually chewed with lime to enhance absorption. Treatment of arecoline poisoning consists of administration of atropine and cardiorespiratory support.

COMPLICATIONS OF INJECTING DRUGS

Cutaneous complications in injection drug users include needle marks or scars, usually in the antecubital fossae of both arms, on the forearms and wrists, or on the backs of the hands. The presence of old abscess scars and of bluish phlebitis scars from past injections also indicates chronic use. Long-time users are usually forced to seek new injection sites as old sites become unusable because of scarring, and they may exhibit fresh needle marks on the legs and neck.

Skin and soft tissue infections are extremely common. *Staphylococcus aureus* is the most common pathogen (staphylococcal colonization is universal among injecting drug users). Streptococci (groups A and G) are the next most common pathogens. However, almost every common pathogen (as well as some uncommon ones) is seen. The types of infections include cellulitis, abscess, multiple chronic ulcerations, necrotizing fasciitis, pyomyositis, septic phlebitis, and infected aneurysms. Regional lymphangitis and lymphadenitis are common with all of these conditions. Unusual infections introduced at the site of injection include wound botulism, candidiasis, and tetanus.

When needles are shared, there is a high risk of acquiring viral hepatitis. Seroprevalence surveys among injecting drug users reveal positive hepatitis C serology in up to 86% of users (34). Many individuals have chronically elevated aminotransferase levels. Although the natural history of hepatitis C in this population is not yet well described, injecting drug users infected with hepatitis C may be more likely to die from drug overdose or homicide than from hepatitis C (35). Hepatitis B virus (HBV) is also common among injecting drug users with carrier (antigen positive) rates of 4% and previous infection (antibody positive) rates ranging from 30% to 94% (34,36). People who have been infected with HBV are at risk for infection with hepatitis D virus (HDV) (delta virus). Hepatitis B vaccine should be given to seronegative injecting drug users. Chapters 18 and 47 describe hepatitis vaccines and hepatitis in detail.

Approximately 30% of recent cases of acquired immunodeficiency syndrome (AIDS) in the United States relate to injecting drug use (37). Injecting drug users are the main sources of heterosexual, and subsequent perinatal, transmission of HIV. Compared with homosexuals who are HIV-positive, injecting drug users who are HIV-positive are more likely to have morbidity related to bacterial infections (endocarditis, pneumonia, and abscesses). Generally, studies have found that modest behavior change among injecting drug users has occurred as a result of concern about AIDS. This relates mostly to risk reduction rather than to elimination (smoking or snorting rather than injecting drugs). Multiple simultaneous interventions appear to be needed. These include access to drug abuse treatment (including methadone), education, counseling, social support, and needle and syringe exchange/availability (38). Even with these interventions, many individuals (especially those with antisocial personality) do not significantly change their behavior. Chapter 39 describes HIV infection in detail.

Endocarditis usually is caused by bacteria at injection sites and most often affects the tricuspid valve. *S. aureus* is the most common causative organism. Mitral and aortic valves are not uncommonly involved and are more likely to be affected if there is pre-existing pathology. *Streptococci* (enterococcus, viridans, and α-hemolytic) are next most common and are more likely to affect left-sided valves. Other offending organisms include gram-negative organisms (*Pseudomonas*) and fungi (*Candida*). Polymicrobial and culture-negative endocarditis also occur. Prognosis is related to size of vegetations and to complications such as heart failure and embolic events. Treatment should be in a controlled inpatient setting. Chapter 40 describes the posthospital management of endocarditis.

Skeletal infections account for a significant number of admissions of injecting drug abusers. Osteomyelitis and septic arthritis occur, mainly by hematogenous, but occasionally from contiguous, spread. The lumbar spine, sternoarticular structures, and the pelvis and its articular structures are commonly involved. Synovial joints (most commonly the knee) and occasionally the appendicular skeleton can be involved. Tuberculosis and fungal infections are also encountered. Gonococcal arthritis is commonly seen among drug-abusing women who prostitute. Chapter 40 describes the ambulatory aspects of diagnosis and management of osteomyelitis.

Pulmonary complications, other than septic emboli, are mostly related to obtundation and drug intoxication with consequent aspiration pneumonia (or pulmonary edema from opiates), lung abscess, and empyema. Microembolization, talc granulomas, pulmonary fibrosis, and, uncommonly, pulmonary hypertension are sometimes seen. Pneumothorax may occur as a complication of attempted injection in the neck.

Defects in host defense mechanisms (independent of HIV-induced problems) are present in injecting drug users. Cell-mediated immunity is depressed, but the mechanisms involved are not clearly understood. Other factors such as malnutrition and concurrent alcohol abuse complicate the study of this problem. The humoral immune response is not diminished. Polyclonal increases in immunoglobulin, probably related to repeated antigenic exposure, result in elevated total protein levels. Thrombocytopenia commonly occurs as a result of circulating immune complexes reacting with platelets. Up to 25% of drug users have a biological false positive serologic test result for syphilis. Usually, the positive titer is 1:4 or less, and the more specific fluorescent treponemal antibody test is negative.

PHARMACOLOGIC APPROACHES TO THE TREATMENT OF SUBSTANCE ABUSE

As mentioned above, the roles of the primary care practitioner are to recognize substance abuse, discuss the problem nonjudgmentally, motivate patients to accept treatment and to refer patients for treatment. Pharmacologic treatment and rehabilitation are generally managed by specialists in substance abuse in the context of a treatment program.

Detoxification

With the exception of opioid-addicted patients who enter methadone maintenance treatment, rehabilitation usually begins with detoxification. This is the process or set of procedures involved in readjusting the patient to a lower or absent tissue level of the substance of abuse. Where they are available, the specific pharmacologic approaches to detoxification have been described above under descriptions of individual drugs of abuse.

Detoxification is the first and easiest task for the recovering addict. Patients tend to attach too much significance to the task of physiologic withdrawal and too little significance to the behavioral changes that are required to prevent relapse (see Rehabilitation, below).

With proper support, many chemically dependent patients can be detoxified on an outpatient basis. Such patients should be seen on a daily basis throughout the detoxification and should be participating concurrently in an intensive program of counseling and education. Medications should be administered on a daily basis so that the patient has only the dosages needed between visits. Clearly many patients do not have the social support and accessibility to appropriate programs for this to occur. Chapter 28 describes the other conditions needed for successful outpatient detoxification.

In general, *inpatient* detoxification is necessary when (a) the patient is unable to discontinue use of illicit substances on an outpatient basis; (b) the patient has concurrent medical problems that require hospitalization or significant medical problems that would be exacerbated by detoxification (e.g., symptomatic coronary artery disease); (c) the patient has developed an extremely high tolerance and has a history of major withdrawal symptoms such as seizures and delirium tremens; (d) the patient presents a clear risk of suicide or, because of chronic intoxication and impaired judgment, is a danger to self or others; or (e) the patient is dependent on multiple drugs.

For most patients, it is not physical dependence that presents the major obstacle to recovery. Rather, it is the propensity to relapse, and the factors that influence this, that determine the success of the patient's efforts to become drug free.

Methadone Maintenance

Methadone maintenance is the most widely used chemotherapeutic approach to the treatment of opioid addiction. Methadone is a long half-life opioid that is taken orally in a single daily dose. Methadone is substituted for the opioid previously used by the patient at a dosage that prevents withdrawal but causes less sedation or intoxication. The starting dose is usually 30 mg. The methadone dosage is gradually increased, thereby increasing the patient's tolerance for all opioids to a level where the user is less able to experience a significant effect, even from large dosages of illicit narcotics. Although this methadone blockade can be overridden by a sufficiently large dose of another narcotic, the payoff for doing so is small in relation to the cost. Patients taking methadone are partially tolerant to its euphoric–sedative effects and are thus able to function normally in home and work settings.

Numerous studies have shown methadone maintenance to be a cost-effective approach in treating opioid addiction (39). Methadone maintenance reduces heroin use (40). It may reduce crime and increases economic productivity of patients in treatment (41). It has also taken on a new significance because of its potential for reducing the spread of AIDS.

Contingency management treatment has been most often applied to methadone maintenance programs. Attempts are made to change behavior by manipulating consequences. Rewards or punishments are provided as incentives for desirable behavior. For example, take-home privileges are linked to the provision of clean urine tests.

Although cost effective, methadone treatment has limitations. As with other forms of chemical dependency treatment, there is a high turnover and rate of relapse. Patients are required to take methadone under observation at a clinic at least three times a week, and this requirement sometimes conflicts with work and family commitments. Although methadone is effective in suppressing the use of opioids, it has no such effect on alcohol or other drugs, and many methadone-maintained patients develop problems with other substances. Methadone-maintained patients become both physically and psychologically dependent on the drug, and many patients experience considerable difficulty in making the transition from methadone to abstinence. Some treatment professionals believe that opioid addicts have a biochemical abnormality that is corrected by methadone so that it may be necessary for them to remain on methadone for life. No scientific evidence supports this view at this time. However, it is likely that genetic studies will reveal a biologic predisposition to opioid use, as has been demonstrated with alcohol and tobacco. Some patients who make appropriate changes in life-style and develop good social and emotional support systems are able to detoxify successfully from methadone.

Buprenorphine Maintenance

A combination sublingual tablet buprenorphine/naloxone (Suboxone) and a buprenorphine mono-tablet (Subutex) are available in the United States for treatment of opioid dependence in office-based practice. The interaction of buprenorphine at the μ-opioid receptor results in buprenorphine having a good safety profile, low physical dependence, and convenient dosing. The buprenorphine plus naloxone combination product is safer for use than plain buprenorphine with decreased risk of diversion. Only physicians who complete an approved 8-hour course and apply for a special DEA number may prescribe buprenorphine. Courses and information are listed on the Web site at www.buprenorphine.samhsa.gov. Buprenorphine, is as effective as methadone in treating opiate addiction (9,10).

Naltrexone

Naltrexone is an orally administered opioid receptor antagonist that is highly effective in blocking the effects of opioids. It is a long-acting drug that can effectively block the effects of opioids when administered three times a week. Because naltrexone causes an acute withdrawal reaction, candidates for naltrexone treatment must first be detoxified from the opioid to which they are addicted. Unlike methadone, which works by increasing the patient's tolerance for opioids, naltrexone competes with opioids at the receptor site. Another important difference is that naltrexone is not addicting, and patients can discontinue use without difficulty. The major disadvantage of naltrexone is that few patients are willing to use the drug and stay on it for an appropriate length of time. Its effectiveness is thus limited to highly motivated patients or patients who can be required to take the drug. Its effectiveness as maintenance therapy is less certain (42) than is that of methadone (40) or buprenorphine (10). Like methadone, naltrexone is not effective in blocking the use of other substances of abuse. A patch preparation of naltrexone is under development. Equivalents of methadone and naltrexone have not been developed that would allow for the pharmacologic management of other forms of drug abuse, such as cocaine.

REHABILITATION

All forms of drug abuse optimally require both acute and long-term intervention. Acute interventions include the management of overdose, toxicity, and withdrawal under medical supervision (if this is indicated). However, when the immediate physical consequences of drug abuse have been successfully treated, there remains a need to identify and treat, if possible, any underlying conditions that motivated drug misuse in the first place. Many drug abusers have significant problems of psychological and social adjustment and may benefit from counseling and rehabilitation over extended periods. As described above, the primary care practitioner's major role in dealing with long-term rehabilitation is to motivate patients to cease drug abuse and to enter and continue in rehabilitation programs.

Effective rehabilitation programs stress the development of practical social and vocational skills and the avoidance of social environments conducive to drug use. Unfortunately, many employers are reluctant to hire someone with a history of substance abuse. However, employment is a key aspect of recovery. In recent years, there has been an increasing recognition that families may actually enable drug abuse by one or more members. Family therapy has been used successfully with opiate addicts and appears to be the treatment of choice with drug-abusing teenagers who are still living with their parents.

Because many drug abusers have important deficits in education and vocational preparation, lack basic social and recreational skills, and are handicapped by problems of poor impulse control and low self-esteem, the process of rehabilitation often takes considerable time. Some treatment programs serve as therapeutic workplaces, integrating drug treatment and vocational training.

There is evidence that existing treatment modalities improve the course of substance abuse disorders and reduce the amount of injury to both the individual and the community. There is evidence that treatment reduces the economic costs that result from drug abuse and that these cost reductions substantially exceed the actual cost of providing care (43). However, it must also be acknowledged that definitive treatment methods that result in lasting abstinence from drugs in a significant proportion of patients do not currently exist.

Principal Types of Rehabilitation Programs

Residential Treatment Programs

Two types of residential treatment programs are commonly encountered in the United States. *Therapeutic communities* typically require patients to commit themselves to 6 months or more of treatment. Patients are subjected to an intense aggressively confrontational form of group therapy that is intended to facilitate change by stripping away antisocial drug-oriented beliefs and values and replacing them with socially adaptive beliefs and values. Therapeutic communities tend to have high dropout rates in the first few weeks of treatment because many patients are not willing to make the commitment required by this form of treatment. Patients who remain for the duration of treatment, however, often achieve an enduring drug-free adjustment.

A more common form of residential treatment is the *intermediate-term residential program*. These programs are typically 4 weeks in duration and were originally designed to treat alcoholism. Over the last two decades, they have evolved into chemical dependence programs that accept patients with a wide range of substance abuse problems. Intermediate-term residential programs use a more traditional group therapy approach that is less aggressive than the approach used by therapeutic communities. They also place a strong emphasis on education. In most facilities, patients attend lectures and films designed to increase their understanding of the disease of chemical dependency and the nature of the recovery process.

Traditionally, intermediate-term residential programs have been viewed as the treatment of choice for chemical dependency, but in recent years they have come under pressure from a variety of groups concerned about the rising cost of health care benefits. Residential treatment is considerably more expensive than outpatient care, and comparisons of the two approaches for one form of drug abuse—alcoholism—show little difference in outcome for comparable patients (43). There are few data for other drugs of abuse. In response to the demand for more cost-effective treatment approaches, intermediate-term residential facilities now offer flexible lengths of stay rather than admitting all patients for the same 28- or 30-day program.

Intensive Outpatient Treatment Programs

Demands for more cost-effective forms of treatment have led to a greater emphasis on the use of outpatient approaches. Intensive outpatient programs offer a combination of education and group counseling similar to that found in the intermediate-term residential programs, but they provide treatment in the evenings so patients do not have to be absent from home or work. Intensive outpatient programs have patients attend treatment sessions four to six times a week and offer 12 to 20 hours of therapeutic activities each week for 4 to 6 weeks or longer. Traditional individual psychotherapy (rather than counseling) has not proved particularly effective in treating drug dependence.

Self-Help Groups

Self-help groups such as *Alcoholics Anonymous* (see Chapter 28) and *Narcotics Anonymous* (http://www.na.org/) provide another valuable resource for people seeking help for a substance abuse problem. These 12-step programs provide a clearly defined sequence of steps that the addict must take to recover. They also provide immediate access to the emotional support and encouragement of others who have successfully coped with similar problems. Alcoholics Anonymous and Narcotics Anonymous both maintain hotlines that are listed in the telephone directories of every major community in the United States and Canada. Chapter 28 describes the Narcotics Anonymous process, which is identical to the process of Alcoholics Anonymous. Most drug-free treatment programs incorporate the tenets of Narcotics Anonymous into their approach and encourage patients to get actively involved with a 12-step program.

Nar-anon (http://www.naranon.com/home.html) provides support for members of the addict's family using 12 steps modeled on the 12 steps of Al-Anon (see Chapter 28). Even if the patient refuses to accept treatment or try self-help groups, family members (who may be codependents) can be referred to Nar-anon. Codependents may experience a wide range of physical and emotional stresses as a result of another family member's addiction. Codependents often experience guilt, shame, loss of self-esteem, diminished self-confidence, and social isolation. They often believe that they are in some way to blame for the substance abuser's problems, a belief that is often fostered by the substance abuser, who is more than happy to shift responsibility to others. Codependents often engage in enabling behaviors—actions that are intended to help the substance abuser but only shield the substance abuser from the consequences of his or her behavior and therefore delay serious efforts at recovery. Codependents often resort to a variety of strategies intended to control or prevent access to drugs by the substance abuser. Such efforts are usually unsuccessful. Recovery usually occurs when the substance abuser feels the need for change and is willing to accept full responsibility for making change occur. Substance abusers who recover are motivated to change in large part by the unpleasant and painful consequences of their drug use. Nar-anon helps family members recognize and discontinue enabling behaviors and helps them cope with the physical and emotional stresses that result from living with a substance abuser.

Common Obstacles to Recovery

Many patients, particularly those in the early stages of addiction, have difficulty accepting the requirement of total abstinence. Although they might not admit it, many patients enter treatment with the unstated agenda of gaining control of their drug use rather than stopping it. They are reluctant to give up the pleasurable effects of drugs or they doubt their ability to cope with emotional distress without the relief afforded by drugs. They secretly hope to learn how to enjoy the benefits of drugs while avoiding the problems that have accompanied their drug use in the past. This is part of the process of denial. Other patients enter treatment believing that they have a problem with one type of drug but not with others. Cocaine addicts, for example, often believe that they do not have a problem with alcohol or marijuana and see no reason to give up the use of those drugs. Experience has shown, however, that continued use of non–problem drugs tends to predispose patients to relapse with their problem drug. Furthermore, patients who continue to use other drugs are less likely to make the changes in life-style that are important in maintaining recovery over the longer term.

One of the most important tasks for the patient in early recovery is to sever ties with drug users and to develop new relationships with nonusers, or at least with nonabusers. The relationships with other abusers tend to be superficial and based mainly on the shared activity of getting high. In addition to forming new relationships, the recovering addict must learn to form a new type of relationship, one that involves a level of trust, honesty, and intimacy that may seem alien to some. Such relationships are fundamental to recovery because they are the primary source of support for the addict struggling with the physical and emotional demands of recovery. During their addiction, most addicts learn to use drugs as a quick and effective, though ultimately destructive, method of dealing with physical or emotional distress. In recovery, the addict must learn other strategies to cope with distress.

The active abuse of drugs during adolescence and early adulthood seems to interfere with the development of basic social skills. Additionally, addicts are often hampered by diminished self-esteem and self-confidence and by the expectation that they will be rejected by society. Meeting people for the first time and attempting to initiate new relationships generate anxiety for most people under the best circumstances. When normal social anxiety is compounded by the social and emotional deficits that characterize most addicts in early recovery, the task of forming new relationships can become so intimidating that it may be avoided altogether. The recovering addict who feels lonely or isolated is tempted to resume contact with old friends who are still using drugs.

Another important life-style change has to do with the use of leisure time. Drug use is, among other things, a recreational activity. Getting and using drugs provides a daily routine that fills time and provides stimulation and challenge. For some addicts, the enjoyment of certain aspects of the drug-oriented life-style is as important as the reinforcing effects of drug use in maintaining drug involvement. For other users, being high makes it possible to tolerate what would otherwise be a tedious daily routine. It is important for the addict in early recovery to identify new activities that will provide a reasonable amount of stimulation and satisfaction. Boredom greatly increases the risk of relapse, and the recovering addict who fails to find employment that is in some way rewarding or to develop satisfying leisure activities is in danger of relapse.

Self-help groups are an invaluable resource for people in early recovery. In addition to providing emotional support and guidance, they are the best available forums for meeting nonusers and developing new friendships. They also sponsor social and recreational activities and provide opportunities for addicts in early recovery to learn new ways of managing leisure time from people who are further along in recovery.

In summary, recovery from chemical dependency requires a multitude of changes in beliefs, relationships, and life-style. Some of the required changes are difficult to accomplish, and the need for them is not immediately apparent to many addicts. In early episodes of treatment, most addicts make some of the needed changes but not enough to avoid relapse over the long term. As a result, relapse rates among patients successfully completing treatment run as high as 80% in the year after treatment. Of course, results highly depend on how the population is selected. Socially stable higher socioeconomic groups have a better prognosis. With successive treatment episodes, however, one can hope to see a changing pattern in which periods of abstinence grow longer and periods of active drug use grow shorter. Perhaps it is best to view relapse as an indication that the patient has so far failed to make all the necessary changes needed to support an enduring recovery. Instead of regarding relapse as an indication that the patient's case is hopeless, the patient's practitioner can encourage the patient to identify the reasons for the current relapse and to make changes that will help the patient avoid a recurrence. The approach should not be very different from that of other chronic diseases such as hypertension or diabetes, in which complete cure is uncommon.

CHRONIC PAIN MANAGEMENT

Chronic pain of nonmalignant origin is not a single entity. It has a variety of causes and contributing factors. Treatment may vary from behavioral and physical therapy approaches to medications, including opioids. Pain is one of the most common reasons patients consult a practitioner, yet it is often inadequately treated. There is much controversy over the long-term use of opioids for nonmalignant pain. Opioids can clearly be of benefit in some patients with chronic pain who have not responded to other pharmacologic therapies, including nonsteroidal anti-inflammatory drugs (NSAIDs), and have no history of substance abuse. Success or benefit should be measured by improvement in quality of life, as measured by greater ability to perform activities of daily life. Side effects such as respiratory depression and sedation tend to be rare in patients with chronic pain and should not prevent the proper prescribing of opioids.

Evaluation of a patient with chronic pain should include the following: (a) a pain history with specific details of the impact of pain on the patient, (b) an assessment of pain in a typical day (worst score, best score, average score, and response of pain score to pharmacologic and nonpharmacologic interventions—use of a visual analog scale, as illustrated in Chapter 13, Fig. 13.1, can be helpful), (c) a directed physical examination, (d) a review of previous diagnostic studies, (e) a review of previous interventions, (f) an alcohol and drug history, and (g) an assessment of coexisting diseases or conditions. Treatment should be based on the findings in this evaluation and the presenting cause of pain.

Patients with chronic pain require frequent visits and phone calls. Many providers view such patients as time-consuming and frustrating and as a result look to refer them to pain centers. However, referral to pain centers is often limited by insurance as a result of their cost. Most studies of the effectiveness of pain centers focus on patients with chronic back pain. A meta-analytic review of 65 studies of pain centers in the management of chronic back pain tended to show beneficial effects of pain treatment centers, but many studies were poorly designed (44). One randomized controlled study in Denmark of 189 patients with chronic pain of nonmalignant origin showed that the patient group treated at a multidisciplinary pain center had better pain relief and quality of life than the comparison group treated by a general practitioner after initial consultation by a pain specialist (45). No time or cost analysis was performed.

Nonpharmacologic therapies, including acupuncture (see Chapter 5), acupressure, exercise, hydrotherapy, biofeedback, relaxation techniques, massage, and physical therapy, should all be considered and prescribed, if appropriate, as adjuncts to the management of chronic pain (46). They provide an opportunity for patients to be active in their approach to overcoming chronic pain. Psychosocial stress and mood have an impact on pain perception and the ability to cope with pain. Patients should not lose their "identity" to their diagnosis of chronic pain, and these nonpharmacologic modalities often contribute to a better sense of well being.

The relationship between pain and depression is complex because many patients with depression have a history of chronic pain and vice versa. Depression does lower pain tolerance and increase analgesic requirements. There have been a variety of trials using tricyclic antidepressants as adjuncts for pain control (47,48). Additionally, when given at bedtime, they enable sleep, which may have a positive impact on pain during the day. Pain improvement may occur at lower than therapeutic blood levels. Nortriptyline at a dosage of 10 or 25 mg at bedtime is a usual starting point, with gradual increase of dosage depending on effect. Other antidepressants have also been found to be useful as pain management adjuncts, with paroxetine (Paxil) deserving particular mention, especially when coupled with a tricyclic antidepressant (49). Chapter 24 gives details regarding antidepressants.

Other drugs to be considered as adjuncts for pain management include the anticonvulsants gabapentin, phenytoin, and carbamazepine. A recent meta-analysis provides some evidence from randomized controlled trials supporting the efficacy of these agents but recommends that they be withheld until other interventions have been tried (50). Gabapentin in escalating doses up to 3,600 mg/day may be particularly effective for chronic pain of neuropathic origin (51). It may be better tolerated than the other anticonvulsants and can be titrated up in dose with little side effect other than sedation. The above cited meta-analysis, however, found no statistically significant difference in toxicity (numbers needed to harm) among the three agents (50). Capsaicin, a topical substance P inhibitor, is available without prescription and is often useful as an adjunct for treatment of postherpetic neuralgia, arthritis, diabetic neuropathy, and reflex sympathetic dystrophy. Topical lidocaine is also useful for postherpetic neuralgia.

If a trial of opioids is deemed appropriate, the provider should ensure that the patient is informed of the risks and benefits of opioid use. Most patients should have already been tried on a course of NSAIDs. The provider may choose

PAIN CONTRACT

1. I understand that the aim of pain management is to improve my quality of life and increase the amount of activity I can perform.

2. I understand that it is unlikely that all of my pain will be relieved.

3. I agree to pursue any/all non-medication therapies that may improve my pain.

4. I understand that narcotic pain medications used over long periods of time cause dependence and if stopped abruptly may result in withdrawal symptoms.

5. I agree to have only one provider prescribe all of my narcotic pain medications.

6. I agree to always take my pain medication as prescribed. Any changes in dose **must** be made by agreement with my provider.

7. I am responsible for my prescriptions lasting the appropriate amount of time. I understand I will not receive additional medication ahead of time.

____
Patient Signature

____
Provider Signature

FIGURE 29.1. Sample pain contract.

to continue an NSAID while initiating opioid therapy. Specific conditions under which opioids will be prescribed should be agreed upon (e.g., strict adherence with directions, no telephone refills, and patient responsibility for the prescription and all pills). Only one provider should be responsible for all prescriptions related to chronic pain. A written agreement specifying these conditions may be useful (Fig. 29.1).

Generally, long-acting opioids should be used for chronic pain because they reduce the need for frequent dosing, have reduced abuse liability, and alleviate pain while preventing the re-emergence of pain. Both morphine and oxycodone are available as long-acting twice a day preparations for the treatment of pain. Fentanyl is available in a transdermal patch formulation that lasts for 3 days. Transdermal fentanyl should be prescribed only to patients who are already opioid experienced. A recent multicenter controlled study found transdermal fentanyl to be superior to sustain release oral morphine in the treatment of chronic nonmalignant pain (52). Chapter 13 gives details regarding opioid analgesics. In most patients, the effective opiate analgesic dose for chronic pain will stabilize at a set dose, without need for escalation over time and with sustained pain relief.

Review of treatment efficacy should be an ongoing process. Patients should keep a pain diary with a record of daily activity and pain scores during a typical day. Monthly followup visits should include a review of the pain diary, an assessment of functional status, efficacy of analgesia, drug side effects, quality of life, and any sign of medication misuse. All this information should be documented in the patient chart on each visit.

SPECIFIC REFERENCES*

1. American Psychiatric Association. Diagnostic and statistical manual of mental disorders. 4th ed. (DSM-IV).Washington, DC: American Psychiatric Association, 1994.
2. Parran T Jr. Prescription drug abuse. A question of balance. Med Clin North Am 1997;81:967.
3. Deitch D, Koutsenok I, Ruiz A. The relationship between crime and drugs: what we have learned in recent decades. J Psychoactive Drugs 2000;32:391.
4. Substance Abuse and Mental Health Services Administration (2004). Results from the 2003 National Survey on Drug Use and Health: National Findings (Office of Applied Studies, NSDUH Series H-25, DHHS Publication No. SMA 04-3964). Rockville, MD.
5. Amato L, Davoli M, Minozzi S, et al. Methadone at tapered doses for the management of opioid withdrawal. Cochrane Database System Rev 2005;3:CD003409.
6. Jasinski DR, Johnson RE, Kocher TR. Clonidine in morphine withdrawal: differential effects on signs and symptoms. Arch Gen Psychiatry 1985;42:1063.
7. Gowing L, Ali R, White J. Buprenorphine for the management of opioid withdrawal. Cochrane Database System Rev 2004;4:CD002025.
8. Parran TV, Adelman CL, Jasinski DR. Buprenorphine detoxification of medically unstable narcotic dependent patients: a case series. Subst Abuse 1990;11:197.

*Bold numerals denote published controlled clinical trials, meta-analyses, or consensus-based recommendations.

9. Johnson RE, Chutuape MA, Strain EC, et al. A comparison of levomethadyl acetate, buprenorphine, and methadone for opioid dependence. N Engl J Med 2000;343:1290.

10. Mattick RP, Kimber J, Breen C, et al. Buprenorphine maintenance versus placebo or methadone maintenance for opioid dependence. Cochrane Database System Rev 2003;2:CD002207.

11. Chutuape MA, Jasinski DR, Fingerhood MI, et al. One-, three-, and six-month outcomes after brief inpatient opioid detoxification. Am J Drug Alcohol Abuse 2001;27:19.

12. Mouhaffel AH, Madu EC, Satmary WA, et al. Cardiovascular complications of cocaine. Chest 1995;107:1426.

13. Ray WA, Fought RL, Decker MD. Psychoactive drugs and the risk of injurious motor vehicle crashes in elderly drivers. Am J Epidemiol 1992;136:873.

14. Cumming RG, Miller JP, Kelsey JL, et al. Medications and multiple falls in elderly people: the St Louis study. Age Aging 1991;20: 455.

15. Lichtenstein MJ, Griffin MR, Cornell JE, et al. Risk factors for hip fractures occurring in the hospital. Am J Epidemiol 1994;140:830.

16. Wagner AK, Zhang F, Soumerai SB. Benzodiazepine use and hip fractures in the elderly. Arch Intern Med 2004;164:1567.

17. Cummings SR, Nevitt MC, Browner WS, et al. Risk factors for hip fracture in white women. N Engl J Med 1995;332:767.

18. Lekka NP, Paschalis C, Beratis S. Suicide attempts in high-dose benzodiazepine users. Comprehens Psych 2002;43:438.

19. Benzodiazepine dependence, toxicity and abuse. A Task Force Report of the American Psychiatric Association. Washington, DC: American Psychiatric Association, 1990.

20. Kupfer DJ, Reynolds CF 3rd. Management of insomnia. N Engl J Med 1997;336:341.

21. Noyes R Jr.Perry PJ, Crowe RR, et al. Seizures following the withdrawal of alprazolam. J Nerv Mental Dis 1986;174:50.

22. Shader RI, Greenblatt DJ. Use of benzodiazepines in anxiety disorders. N Engl J Med 1993;328:1398.

23. Moller HJ. Effectiveness and safety of benzodiazepines. J Clin Psychopharmacol 1999;19:2S.

24. Sullivan JT, Sellers EM. Detoxification for triazolam physical dependence. J Clin Psychopharmacol 1992;12:124.

25. Sullivan JT, Sellers EM. Treating alcohol, barbiturate and benzodiazepine withdrawal. Ration Drug Ther 1986;20:1.

26. Tashkin DP, Simmons MS, Sherrill DL, et al. Heavy habitual marijuana smoking does not cause an accelerated decline in FEV1 with age. Am J Resp Crit Care Med 1997;155:141.

27. Hollister LE. Health aspects of cannabis: revisited. Int J Neuropsychopharmacol 1998;1:71.

28. Cushman P. Plasma testosterone levels in healthy male marijuana smokers. Am J Drug Alcohol Abuse 1975;2:269.

29. Morton J. Ecstasy: pharmacology and neurotoxicity. Curr Opin Pharmacol. 2005; 5:79.

30. McCann UD, Eligulashvili V, Ricaurte GA. Methylenedioxymethamphetamine ("Ecstasy")-induced serotonin neurotoxicity: clinical studies. Neuropsychobiology 2000;42:11.

31. Fingerhood MI, Sullivan JT, Testa MP, et al. Abuse liability of testosterone. J Psychopharmacol 1997;11:65.

32. Giorgi A, Weatherby RP, Murphy PW. Muscular strength, body composition and health responses to the use of testosterone enanthate: a double blind study. J Sci Med Sport 1999;2:341.

33. Brower KJ, Blow FC, Young JP, et al. Symptoms and correlates of anabolic-androgenic steroid dependence. Br J Addict 1991;86:759.

34. Fingerhood MI, Jasinski DR, Sullivan JT. Prevalence of hepatitis C in a chemical dependence population. Arch Intern Med 1993;153:2025.

35. Thomas DL, Astemborski J, Rai RM, et al. The natural history of hepatitis C virus infection: host, viral, and environmental factors. JAMA 2000;284:450.

36. Lemberg BD, Shaw-Stiffel TA. Hepatic disease in injection drug users. Infect Dis Clin North Am. 2002;16:667.

37. Centers for Disease Control and Prevention. HIV/AIDS Surveillance Report for the year 2003. Available at: www.cdc.gov/hiv/stats.

38. Gostin LO, Lazzarini Z, Jones TS, et al. Prevention of HIV/AIDS and other blood-borne diseases among injection drug users. A national survey on the regulation of syringes and needles. JAMA 1997;277:53.

39. Barnett PG. The cost-effectiveness of methadone maintenance as a health care intervention. Addiction 1999;94:479.

40. Mattick RP, Breen C, Kimber J, Davoli M. Methadone maintenance therapy versus no opioid replacement therapy for opioid dependence. Cochrane Database System Rev 2003:2:CD002209.

41. Gerstein DR, Johnson RA, Harwood H, et al. Evaluating recovery services: the California Drug and Alcohol Treatment Assessment (CALDATA). Sacramento: California Department of Alcohol and Drug Programs, 1994.

42. Kirchmayer U, Davoli M, Verster A. Naltrexone maintenance treatment for opioid dependence. Cochrane Database System Rev 2003; 2:CD001333.

43. Miller WR, Hester RK. Inpatient alcoholism treatment: who benefits? Am Psychol 1986; 41:794.

44. Flor H, Fydrich T, Turk DC. Efficacy of multidisciplinary pain treatment centers: a meta-analytic review. Pain 1992;49:221.

45. Becker N, Sjogren P, Bech P, et al. Treatment outcome of chronic non-malignant pain patients managed in a Danish multidisciplinary pain centre compared to general practice: a randomised controlled trial. Pain 2000;84:203.

46. Allegrante JP. The role of adjunctive therapy in the management of nonmalignant pain. Am J Med 1996;101:33S.

47. Godfrey RG. A guide to the understanding and use of tricycle antidepressants in the overall management of fibromyalgia and other chronic pain syndromes. Arch Intern Med 1996;156: 1047.

48. Sindrup SH, Jensen TS. Efficacy of pharmacological treatments of neuropathic pain: an update and effect related to mechanism of drug action. Pain 1999;83:389.

49. Jung AC, Staiger T, Sullivan M. The efficacy of selective serotonin reuptake inhibitors for the management of chronic pain. J Gen Intern Med 1997;12:384.

50. Wiffen P, Collins S, McQuay H, et al. Anticonvulsant drugs for acute and chronic pain. Cochrane Database System Rev 2005;3: CD001133.

51. Eckhardt K, Ammon S, Hofmann U, et al. Gabapentin enhances the analgesic effect of morphine in healthy volunteers. Anesth Analg 2000;9:1185.

52. Allan L, Hays H, Jensen NH, et al. Randomised crossover trial of transdermal fentanyl and sustained release oral morphine for treating chronic non-cancer pain. BMJ 2001;322:1154.

*For annotated **General References** and resources related to this chapter, visit www.hopkinsbayview.org/PAMreferences.*

SECTION 4

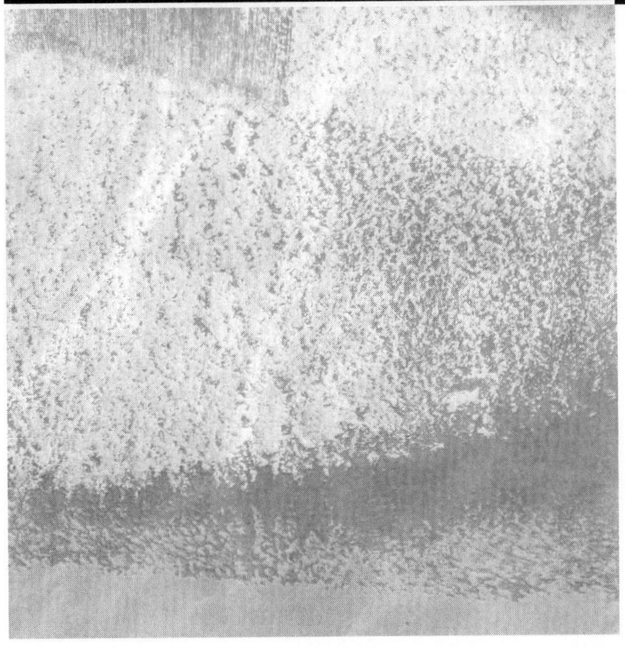

Allergy and Infectious Disease

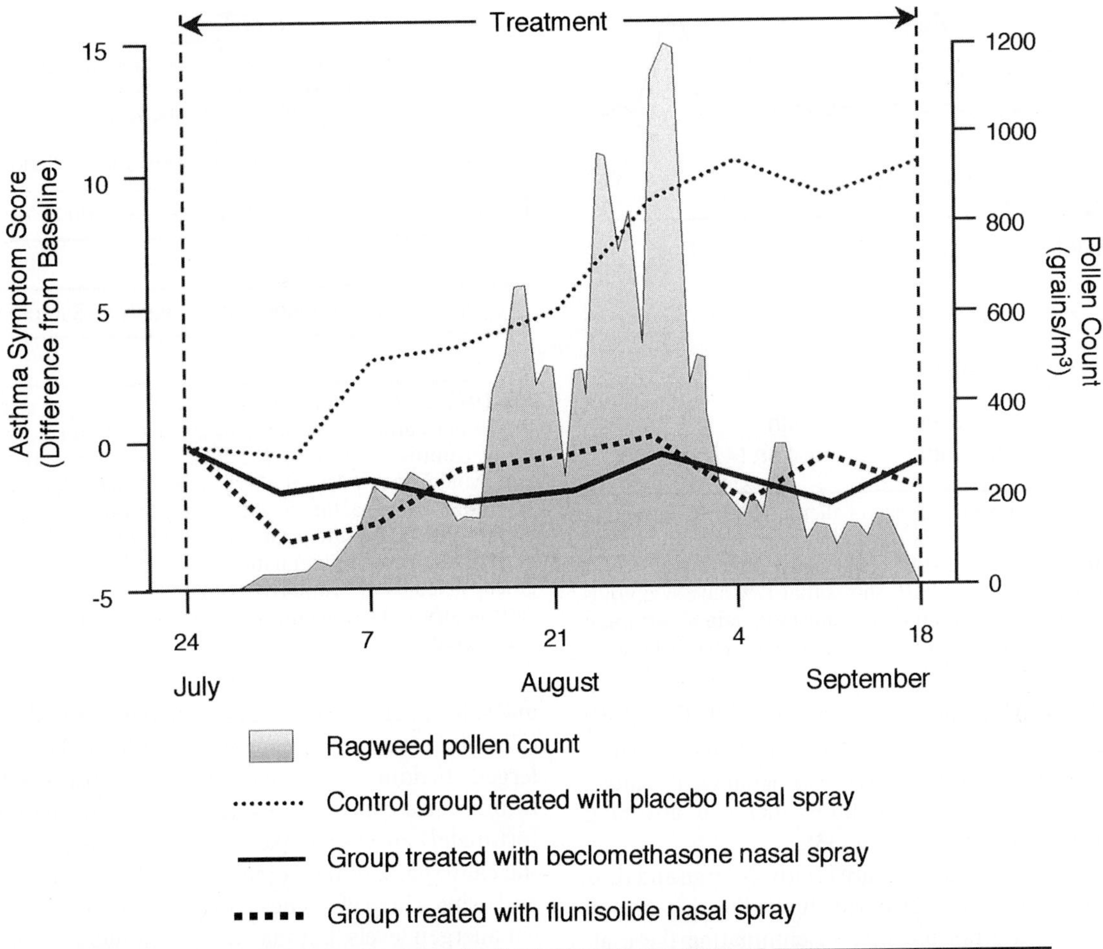

FIGURE 30.3. Improvement in asthma with treatment of allergic rhinitis. Asthma symptom scores of ragweed-sensitive individuals treated with placebo nasal sprays increase as the pollen count rises during the fall season. In contrast, active treatment of allergic rhinitis with beclomethasone or flunisolide nasal sprays not only improves nasal symptoms but also prevents allergen-induced exacerbation of asthma. (Adapted from Welsh P, Stricker W, Chu C, et al. Efficacy of beclomethasone nasal solution, flunisolide, and cromolyn in relieving symptoms of ragweed allergy. Mayo Clin Proc 1987;62:125.)

of the nasal passages and nasopharynx and help to localize polyps, purulent drainage, and other potential pathology (18).

Management

The three main components of the management of allergic rhinitis are allergen avoidance, pharmacotherapy, and immunotherapy. Treatment options are chosen in a stepwise fashion based on the frequency and severity of symptoms (Fig. 30.5). Management of ocular symptoms is described later in this chapter.

Allergen Avoidance

Environmental control measures should be based on a careful assessment of allergen sensitivity. The presence of allergen-specific IgE antibodies may be established through skin testing *in vivo* or *radioallergosorbent testing (RAST)* of blood samples *in vitro*. During skin testing, small concentrations of various allergen extracts are introduced through superficial punctures or through intradermal injections on the arms or back. Skin testing provides immediate results and is generally more cost effective than *in vitro* testing. Results of these tests should be correlated with the patient's history to determine their clinical relevance. The temporal pattern of symptoms and of exposures should be clarified. For example, a positive skin test with dust mite allergen would be more relevant for an individual with perennial, rather than strictly seasonal, symptoms.

Dust Mites

Allergens of dust mites are contained in their fecal matter (30) and are mostly found in bedding. The use of dust mite-proof bedding covers can reduce the level of exposure to dust miteallergens, but as a single avoidance measure may not be enough to reduce symptoms of allergic

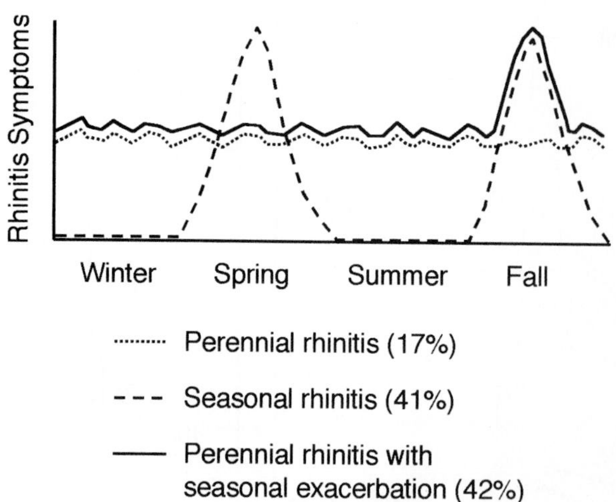

FIGURE 30.4. Temporal patterns of allergic rhinitis. The temporal pattern of rhinitis symptoms may indicate the environmental allergens to which an individual is sensitive. Our survey of 412 individuals with allergic rhinitis shows that 17% have symptoms year-round, 41% have symptoms only during certain seasons, and 42% have year-round symptoms with seasonal exacerbations.

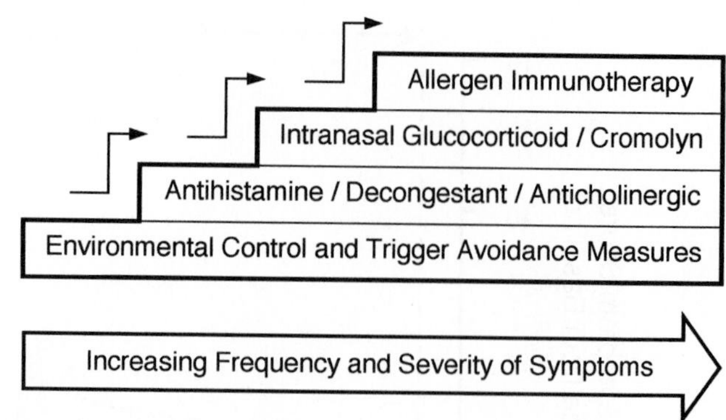

FIGURE 30.5. Stepwise management of allergic rhinitis. The modes of treatment are chosen based on the frequency and severity of rhinitis symptoms. The first step involves identification and avoidance of relevant allergens and other triggers. Relief of symptoms can be achieved with an antihistamine, decongestant, and/or anticholinergic agent as needed. For persistent disease, control of allergic inflammation can be attained with intranasal glucocorticoids or cromolyn. If these measures do not provide satisfactory improvement, allergen immunotherapy should be considered.

rhinitis (31). Washing bedding with hot (>130°F [54.5°C) water every 1 to 2 weeks can kill dust mites on the surface and denature their allergens (32). Maintenance of relative humidity below 50% with a dehumidifier may also help reduce the dust mite population (33).

Because dust mite particles are relatively large and thus do not remain constantly airborne, high efficiency particulate air filters are not effective in eliminating these allergens (34). For the same reason, so-called ion-charging devices would not have any significant impact on the allergen load inside the room (35). Application of so-called acaricides has not been proven to be consistently beneficial on a long-term basis (36).

Pets

Any fur-bearing animal potentially may cause allergic sensitization in a genetically predisposed individual. Cat allergy has been extensively studied in this regard. The allergenic proteins of cats mostly come from their sebaceous and salivary glands and are deposited onto the skin and fur (37). There may be significant variability in the levels of allergen shedding among cats (38). The most effective way to minimize exposure to such allergens in the home unfortunately entails complete removal of the pet. Confining the cat to parts of the home outside the patient's bedroom and using a high efficiency particulate air filter may reduce cat allergen levels, but may not be enough to produce any significant clinical improvement (39). This illustrates that even relatively low levels of allergens are sufficient to cause respiratory symptoms. Washing the cat may reduce levels of airborne allergens, but this effect is not sustained and its clinical benefit has not been proven (40). If and when patients comply with complete removal of the cat, they should be aware that residual allergens may persist for up to 6 months. Elimination of carpeting and thorough cleaning of the walls may facilitate the decline of allergen levels (41). Exposure to animal allergens may also occur outside the home, as shown by findings of significant levels of cat and dog allergens in school buildings (42). Cat allergens in particular tend to adhere to material surfaces and may be transported via clothing (43).

TABLE 30.1 Reported Triggers of Allergic Rhinitis Symptoms

Trigger	*Patients Affected (%)*
Pollens	91
Animals	79
Tobacco smoke	71
Other irritants	69
Cold dry air	57

Adapted from Diemer FB, Sanico AM, Horowitz E, et al. Non-allergenic inhalant triggers in seasonal and perennial allergic rhinitis. J. Allergy Clin Immunol 1999;103:S2.

Pollens

Complete avoidance of outdoor allergens such as pollens is more difficult to achieve. Keeping the windows closed and using air-conditioning while indoors may help minimize exposure to tree, grass, and weed allergens that are typically prevalent during the spring, summer, and fall seasons, respectively. Multiple studies have documented exacerbation of symptoms among untreated patients in parallel with levels of pollen (26,44) (Fig. 30.6). A study on ragweed pollen counts showed that they begin to rise

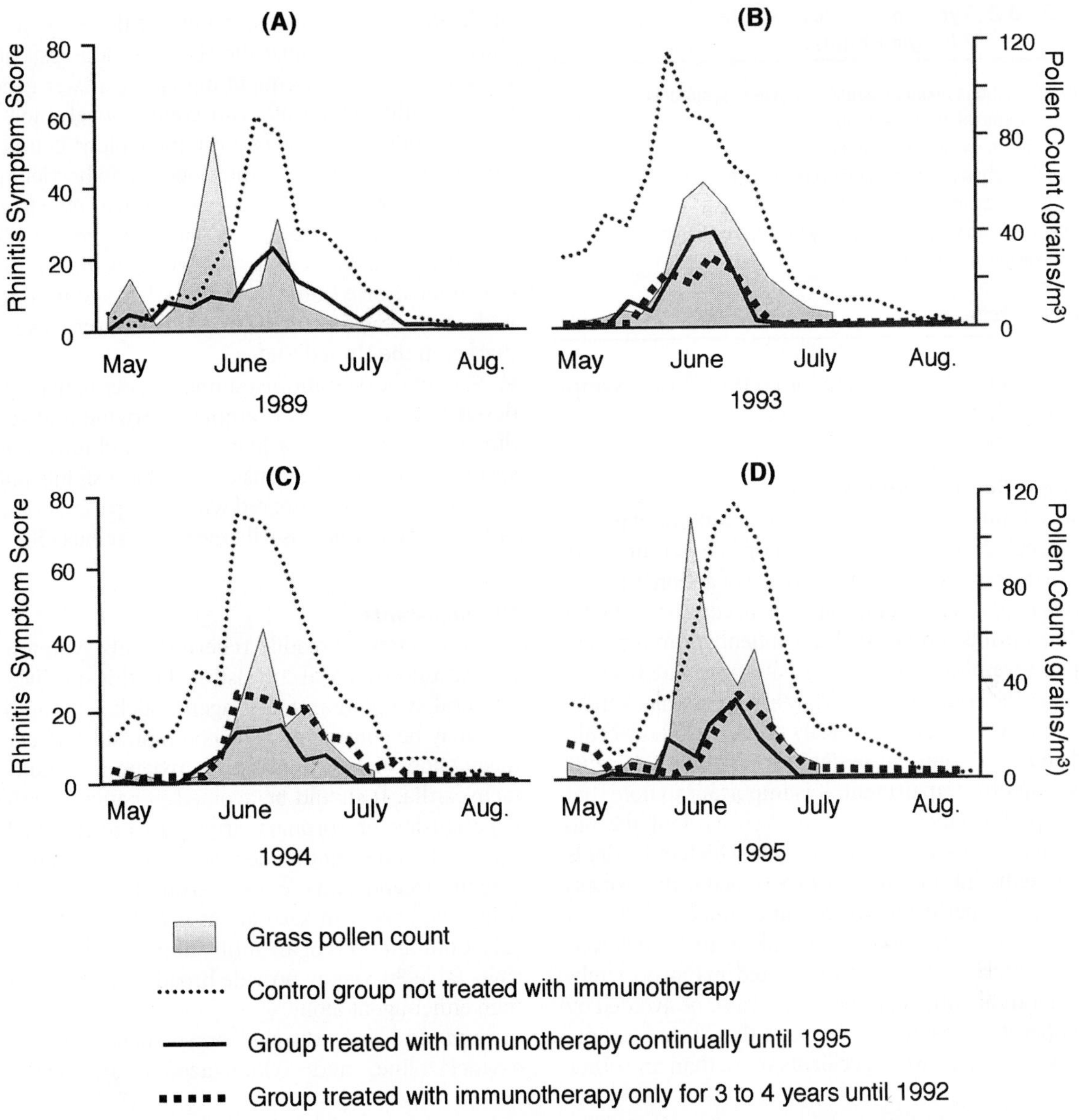

FIGURE 30.6. Long-term improvement of allergic rhinitis with immunotherapy. Symptom scores of control subjects with seasonal allergic rhinitis increased as grass pollen count rose during the summer season (**A to D**). In contrast, those who underwent immunotherapy experienced significantly decreased nasal symptoms within 1 year of treatment (A). Those who received continuous immunotherapy consistently had lower rhinitis symptom scores throughout the study (B to D). Interestingly, even those who stopped receiving immunotherapy after 3 to 4 years of treatment experienced extended relief of symptoms (B to D). (Adapted from Durham S, Walker S, Varga E, et al. Long-term clinical efficacy of grass-pollen immunotherapy. N Engl J Med 1999;341:468.)

at 6:00 a.m. and peak at midday (45). Patients can check prevailing pollen counts that are regularly monitored across the United States and reported by the National Allergy Bureau (www.aaaai.org/nab).

Pharmacotherapy

For most patients with allergic rhinitis, complete allergen avoidance is unattainable or insufficiently effective, necessitating therapeutic intervention. Medications for this disease may be classified into two groups, rescue agents and controller agents (Table 30.2). *Rescue medications* are used as needed to provide immediate but transient relief of symptoms. These include antihistamines, decongestants, and anticholinergic agents. *Controller medications* are optimally used on a regular daily basis to mitigate the underlying pathology of allergic inflammation. These include topical glucocorticoids and cromolyn sodium. Antileukotrienes, which were originally approved for use in

TABLE 30.2 Types of Medications for Allergic Rhinitis

Rescue medications taken as needed to relieve symptoms
- Oral or intranasal antihistamines
- Oral or intranasal decongestants
- Oral antihistamine-decongestant combinations
- Intranasal anticholinergic agent

Controller medications taken regularly to reduce inflammation
- Intranasal glucocorticoids
- Intranasal cromolyn
- Oral antileukotrienes

asthma, are now also indicated for controlling the symptoms of allergic rhinitis.

Histamine-1 Receptor Antagonists

Antihistamines significantly reduce symptoms of paroxysmal sneezing, pruritus, and rhinorrhea within 1 to 3 hours of dosing. Given this rapid onset of action, they are effectively used intermittently on an as-needed basis. Older generation antihistamines such as diphenhydramine were developed several decades ago and are now widely available as over the counter drugs. They are potent blockers of histamine receptors but also easily cross the blood–brain barrier, and commonly cause significant sedation, fatigue, and psychomotor impairment. It is important to note that impaired performance may occur even without the patient's awareness, as shown by a study in which individuals given diphenhydramine denied experiencing drowsiness but nonetheless performed poorly in a simulated driving test (46). These patients are more likely to be involved in motor vehicle accidents if medicated inappropriately. Older generation antihistamines should also be avoided by anyone operating machinery, because they have been associated with serious work accidents more than any other medication (47). The cost benefit of these agents should thus be weighed against the risk of serious psychomotor impairment and consequent injury. The newer generation antihistamines (Table 30.3) are comparatively more expensive but offer advantages over their older counterparts. They do not readily cross the blood–brain barrier and thus cause little or no central nervous system effects at regular doses (48). Two drugs in this class, terfenadine and astemizole which were associated with the development of cardiac dysrhythmias, particularly when used together with erythromycin or ketoconazole (49) were taken off the market in the United States.

Most of the new antihistamines are derivatives of agents developed earlier. For example, cetirizine and fexofenadine are metabolites of hydroxyzine and terfenadine, respectively. The new antihistamines have significantly better safety profiles compared with their parent compounds (49), but are not necessarily more efficacious (50).

Decongestants

Antihistamines readily relieve rhinitis symptoms with the exception of nasal congestion. For this specific indication, oral sympathomimetic agents such as pseudoephedrine may be considered. The common side effects of this medication include insomnia, anxiety, restlessness, and tachycardia. It should be avoided in patients with severe hypertension or coronary artery disease (CAD). Phenylpropanolamine, another decongestant that had been available for decades, was removed from the U.S. market after being implicated in several cases of hemorrhagic stroke (51). Combinations of an antihistamine and pseudoephedrine (Table 30.3) may provide broader symptomatic relief than either agent alone.

Intranasal decongestant sprays such as naphazoline, oxymetazoline, and xylometazoline are available as

TABLE 30.3 Rescue Medications for Rhinitis

Drug	Trade Name	Adult Dosage
New-generation antihistamines		
Azelastine	Astelin	2 sprays each nostril b.i.d.
Cetirizine	Zyrtec	5 to 10 mg qD
Desloratadine	Clarinex	5 mg qD
Fexofenadine	Allegra	60 mg b.i.d. or 180 mg qD
Loratadine	Claritin	10 mg qD
New-generation antihistamine–decongestant combinations		
Cetirizine 5 mg/pseudoephedrine 120 mg	Zyrtec-D	1 tab b.i.d.
Desloratadine 5 mg/pseudoephedrine 240 mg	Clarinex-D 24 Hour	1 tab qD
Fexofenadine 60 mg/pseudoephedrine 120 mg	Allegra-D 12 Hour	1 tab b.i.d.
Fexofenadine 180 mg/pseudoephedrine 240 mg	Allegra-D 24 Hour	1 tab qD
Loratadine 5 mg/pseudoephedrine 120 mg	Claritin-D 12 Hour	1 tab b.i.d.
Loratadine 10 mg/pseudoephedrine 240 mg	Claritin-D 24 Hour	1 tab qD
Anticholinergic agent		
Ipratropium bromide 21 μg	Atrovent 0.03%	2 sprays each nostril b.i.d. to t.i.d.

TABLE 30.4 Controller Medications for Rhinitis

Drug	Trade Name	Dose/Spray (μg)	Initial Adult Dosage[a]
Intranasal glucocorticoids			
Beclomethasone	Beconase AQ[b]	42	1 spray each nostril b.i.d. to q.i.d. q.d.
Budesonide	Rhinocort Aqua[b]	32	1 to 4 sprays each nostril q.d. q.d.
Flunisolide	Nasarel[b]	25	2 sprays each nostril b.i.d. 2 sprays each nostril b.i.d.
Fluticasone	Flonase[b]	50	2 sprays each nostril q.d.
Mometasone	Nasonex[b]	50	2 sprays each nostril q.d.
Triamcinolone	Nasacort AQ[b]	55	2 sprays each nostril q.d. q.d. q.d.
Intranasal Cromolyn			
Cromolyn sodium	NasalCrom	5,200	1 spray each nostril t.i.d. to q.i.d.
Oral Antileukotriene			
Montelukast	Singulair	10 mg	1 tab q.d.

DS, double strength.
[a]The medication should be titrated to the minimum effective dose.
[b]Aqueous sprays; the rest are dry aerosol sprays.

over-the-counter medications. These should not be used for more than 3 to 5 days. Otherwise, rebound nasal congestion (*rhinitis medicamentosa*) may develop.

Intranasal Anticholinergic Agent

For patients with persistent rhinorrhea, ipratropium bromide 0.03% intranasal spray may be beneficial (Table 30.3). It can reduce the production of nasal secretions but does not significantly ameliorate other symptoms of rhinitis (52). Possible side effects include excessive nasal dryness and epistaxis.

Intranasal Glucocorticoids

Topical intranasal glucocorticoids are the most effective medications for persistent allergic rhinitis (53). Used prophylactically, they can attenuate the development of inflammation and of nasal symptoms during the early and late phases of the allergic response (54). Their onset of action may be evident within 1 day of treatment (55–57), and studies have demonstrated favorable results even if they are only used intermittently as needed (58). However, these medications are optimally effective when used on a regular daily basis. Although the various intranasal glucocorticoids are comparable in terms of clinical efficacy, they have significant differences in their bioavailability (53,59). Nonetheless, they do not cause any significant suppression of the hypothalamic–pituitary–adrenal axis when used at recommended doses (59). As in the case for any nasal spray, they may cause local irritation, particularly in the beginning of treatment when ongoing inflammation makes sensory nerves more sensitive to stimuli. To improve compliance, it may be best to give patients a choice of a preparation that they prefer, based on characteristics such as the medication's smell or taste, if any (Table 30.4). Some individuals may find liquid nasal sprays soothing, but others may find it more bothersome than dry sprays. Mild epistaxis may occur, especially when the nasal mucosa becomes too dry, in which case saline nasal sprays may be of benefit. Because anecdotal cases of septal perforation have been reported in association with intranasal sprays, patients should be monitored for the development of any mucosal erosion or incessant bleeding (60). Chronic use of intranasal glucocorticoids itself has not been associated with any detrimental histologic changes such as atrophy (61–63). Intranasal glucocorticoids do not have to be discontinued if the patient incidentally develops an upper respiratory infection, because these medications do not affect the course of such an infection (64).

Chronic or recurrent use of oral or parenteral glucocorticoids for allergic rhinitis is not advisable because of their potential systemic adverse effects.

Intranasal Cromolyn Sodium

Abatement of allergic inflammation may also be achieved with the use of intranasal cromolyn sodium. It typically has to be used up to four times daily to attain optimal benefit (Table 30.4).

Leukotriene Modifiers

Leukotriene receptor antagonists were originally approved for use in asthma but are now used also to treat seasonal and perennial allergic rhinitis (65,66). A study on montelukast showed reduction in allergic rhinitis symptoms by the second day of daily treatment (67).

Immunotherapy

Immunotherapy should be considered for patients who do not satisfactorily respond to environmental control measures and pharmacotherapy, who do not tolerate or consistently comply with the use of medications, or who prefer long-term amelioration of their frequent symptoms of allergic rhinitis. The choice of specific allergens used for this mode of treatment should be tailored according to the individual's clinically relevant skin test or *in vitro* test results. Appropriately dosed allergen immunotherapy may be thoroughly effective alone or in combination with medications. Improvement is typically evident within 1 year of beginning treatment, which should then be continued for 3 to 5 years. Data from a long-term study has shown that clinical benefit may endure several years after discontinuation of immunotherapy (38) (Fig. 30.6). Anaphylactic reactions related to immunotherapy, albeit rare, may occur either during the build-up or maintenance phase. Most such reactions develop within 20 to 30 minutes of the allergen injection (68). This form of treatment should thus be administered only under the supervision of an appropriately trained physician, and patients should remain under observation for at least 20–30 minutes. Personnel, equipment, and medications required for the management of anaphylaxis (see Anaphylaxis and Anaphylactoid Reactions later in this chapter) should be readily available. Immunotherapy should not be administered to patients with ongoing cardiac or pulmonary instability. Alternative forms of treatment should also be considered in patients using β-blockers that may make them less responsive to epinephrine if needed for anaphylaxis. Dosing of allergen extracts should be adjusted accordingly if either systemic or large local reactions develop.

Novel Therapy

Immunomodulation to treat allergic respiratory diseases may also be achieved using novel agents such as omalizumab. This is a humanized monoclonal antibody that links to IgE, thereby preventing the binding of IgE to high-affinity FcεRI receptors on mast cells and basophils. Clinical trials have demonstrated its efficacy in rapidly reducing serum levels of free IgE and subsequently ameliorating symptoms of allergic rhinitis, but presently it is indicated only for moderate to severe allergic asthma that is not well-controlled with other forms of therapy (6).

Consultation with an Allergist

In the assessment and care of patients with allergic rhinitis, consultation with an allergist may be considered for several reasons:

- Identification of specific allergens and other factors that are driving the disease process;
- Insufficient or adverse response of the patient to medications;
- Need for patient education regarding the disease and its treatment;
- Desire for long-term benefit through disease-modifying allergen immunotherapy

Prognosis

A longitudinal study (69) showed that at followup after 23 years, about 23% of individuals with allergic rhinitis reported being symptom free, whereas 32% noted improvement in their disease. The condition was reported to be unchanged in 33%, worse in 9%, and in the remaining 3% of patients the data were not available. The probability of improvement tends to increase with younger age at onset of symptoms. There was improvement in 85% of individuals whose symptoms started at ages 1 to 5 years and in only 39% of those whose symptoms started at age greater than 20 years. The study also showed that patients with allergic rhinitis are about three times more likely to develop subsequent asthma (70). A separate study suggested that immunotherapy in children with allergic rhinitis may reduce the risk for future development of asthma (71).

Allergic Conjunctivitis

Evaluation

Ocular symptoms often accompany allergic rhinitis. Surveys indicate that up to 88% of patients with nasal symptoms also develop itchy, watery, red, teary, and/or swollen eyes. In parallel with rhinitis symptoms, these may occur on a seasonal or perennial basis. Studies in children indicate that it is also possible to have allergic conjunctivitis as the single manifestation of atopy. On physical examination, hyperemia and edema of the conjunctivae, termed chemosis, may be noted bilaterally.

Management

As in rhinitis, the first step in the management of allergic conjunctivitis is the identification and avoidance of offending factors. Cold compresses may provide symptomatic relief. The application of preservative-free artificial tears may help clear the eyes of allergens. For more persistent symptoms, pharmacotherapy with various ophthalmic solutions may provide benefit. These include antihistamines that reduce ocular itching, topical decongestants that reduce redness and swelling, and mast cell stabilizers and other similar agents that ameliorate the underlying inflammation (Table 30.5). As in allergic rhinitis, immunotherapy has likewise been shown to significantly ameliorate symptoms of allergic conjunctivitis (72).

TABLE 30.5 Medications for Allergic Conjunctivitis

Classification *Drug*	*Trade Name*	*Adult Dosage*
Ophthalmic antihistamines		
Emedastine	Emadine	1 drop each eye q.i.d.
Levocabastine	Livostin	1 drop each eye q.i.d.
Oral antihistamines		
See Table 30.3		
Mast cell stabilizers		
Cromolyn	Crolom	1 to 2 drops each eye 4 to 6 times daily
Lodoxamide	Alomide	1 to 2 drops each eye q.i.d.
Pemirolast	Alamast	1 to 2 drops each eye q.i.d.
Nedocromil	Alocril	1 to 2 drops each eye b.i.d.
Ophthalmic antihistamines/Mast cell stabilizers		
Azelastine	Optivar	1 drop each eye b.i.d.
Ketotifen	Zaditor	1 drop each eye b.i.d. to t.i.d.
Olopatadine	Patanol	1 drop each eye b.i.d.
Ophthalmic nonsteroidal anti-inflammatory agents		
Ketorolac	Acular	1 drop each eye q.i.d.
Ophthalmic decongestants		
Naphazoline	Vasocon	1 to 2 drops each eye q.i.d.

Nonallergic Rhinitis

Description

Recurrent nasal symptoms may occur independent of IgE mediation, in which case tests for sensitivity to suspected allergens are negative. Various studies in different clinical settings indicate that 17% to 52% of chronic rhinitis cases have a nonallergic etiology (73). It is difficult to predict whether or not an individual's nasal complaints are IgE mediated simply based on their triggers. Of note, allergic rhinitis symptoms may be triggered not only by allergens but also by nonallergenic irritants such as tobacco smoke and cold dry air (28) (Table 30.1). On the other hand, the age at onset of symptoms may help predict whether a patient has allergic or *nonallergic rhinitis*. The likelihood of obtaining a positive allergy skin test is greater than 90% if the symptoms began before age 10 years but is less than 40% after age 40 (74). Other details in the history may help differentiate allergic rhinitis from nonallergic rhinitis. Symptoms of nonallergic rhinitis typically occur year-round, whereas the pattern for allergic rhinitis may be perennial, seasonal, or perennial with seasonal exacerbation (Fig. 30.4). In contrast to allergic rhinitis, nonallergic rhinitis is less frequently associated with pruritus, ocular symptoms, concomitant asthma, or a family history of atopy. Gender may also be a risk factor for nonallergic rhinitis, as one study showed that 71% of patients with nonallergic rhinitis are female compared with 55% in a group with allergic rhinitis (73).

TABLE 30.6 Possible Causes of Nonallergic Rhinitis Symptoms

Structural
- Septal deformities
- Granulomatous disease
- Nasal polyps
- Nasopharyngeal neoplasms

Hormonal
- Pregnancy
- Hypothyroidism

Infectious
- Bacterial upper respiratory infection
- Viral upper respiratory infection

Medications
- See Table 30.7

In most cases of nonallergic rhinitis, the exact *pathophysiology* is difficult to establish. The commonly used term vasomotor rhinitis may be a misnomer because it suggests an established disease mechanism. Research studies indicate that 15% to 33% of patients with nonallergic rhinitis have more than 10% eosinophilia in nasal smears and/or elevated eosinophil cationic protein in nasal fluids and are thus diagnosed with *nonallergic rhinitis with eosinophilia syndrome* (NARES) (73).

There are several possible *etiologic or contributory factors* for chronic recurrent nasal symptoms in a nonatopic individual (Table 30.6). Rhinorrhea induced by eating spicy foods is termed gustatory rhinitis, which is a reflex response likely involving capsaicin-sensitive and vagal nerve fibers. Nasal obstruction may be related to structural changes due to septal deformities, nasal polyps, granulomatous diseases such as sarcoidosis or Wegener granulomatosis, and benign or malignant tumors of the nasopharynx. Radiographic studies such as sinus computed tomography may be useful in evaluating these possibilities when strongly suspected. Referral to an otorhinolaryngologist is warranted if any of these conditions is discovered. *Pregnancy* may also produce nonallergic rhinitis symptoms, which typically increase during the early and late gestational periods and decline postpartum. These may develop in association with physiologic hormonal or vascular changes. Rhinitis symptoms commonly occur due to *upper respiratory infection,* which may be characterized by mucopurulent discharge and painful sinuses (see Chapter 33). These are usually self-limited if it is viral or otherwise responsive to appropriate antibiotics if it is bacterial in origin.

Recurrent rhinorrhea or nasal congestion may also be associated with over-the-counter and prescription drugs (Table 30.7). For example, prolonged use of intranasal decongestant sprays may lead to rebound congestion and rhinitis medicamentosa. This condition is characterized by a hyperemic and edematous nasal mucosa that becomes

TABLE 30.7 Examples of Medications Reported to Cause Symptoms of Rhinitis

α-Adrenergic antagonists
Prazosin, tamsulosin, terazosin
Angiotensin inhibitors or antagonists
Benazepril, candesartan, lisinopril, losartan, trandolapril, others
β-Adrenergic antagonists
Acebutolol, betaxolol, bisoprolol, carteolol, carvedilol, esmolol, labetalol, nadolol, timolol
Diuretics
Indapamide, torsemide
Other antihypertensive agents
Methyldopa, guanabenz, guanethidine, reserpine
Intranasal decongestants
Naphazoline, oxymetazoline, xylometazoline
Nonsteroidal anti-inflammatory agents
Aspirin, celecoxib, etodolac, felbinac, flurbiprofen, others
Psychoactive agents
Bromperidol, clozapine, femoxetine, fluphenazine, olanzapine, paroxetine, risperidone, trazodone
Other medications
Benzonatate, cilostazol, cisapride, desmopressin, didanosine, nizatadine, pergolide, pilocarpine, sildenafil

progressively unresponsive to vasoconstricting agents. Recalcitrant rhinitis symptoms such as nasal irritation and congestion may also be due to the use of illicit drugs such as snorted cocaine.

Management

The presence of any etiologic or contributory factor for nonallergic rhinitis must be addressed. Avoiding exposure to known triggers, particularly irritants such as tobacco smoke at home and in the workplace, may help ameliorate the patient's condition. Empirical use of intranasal glucocorticoids (Table 30.4), such as those used for allergic rhinitis, is the usual mode of treatment. The efficacy of topical steroids, however, tends to be less consistent in nonallergic rhinitis compared with allergic rhinitis. Patients with NARES tend to respond more favorably to intranasal glucocorticoids compared with those with other forms of nonallergic rhinitis (73). However, the evaluation of nasal smears to detect eosinophilia and diagnose NARES is unnecessary, because patients alternatively may be given a trial of intranasal glucocorticoids. Azelastine nasal spray also has an indication for use in nonallergic rhinitis. For patients with *severe rhinitis medicamentosa*, a short course of oral glucocorticoids (prednisone 30 mg/day for 5 to 7 days) minimizes the rebound phenomenon as the decongestant spray is tapered and discontinued. Oral decongestants and/or anticholinergic agents (Table 30.3) may also be used for symptom-directed treatment of nonallergic rhinitis. Immunotherapy is not a consideration in these cases because they are not IgE mediated.

GENERALIZED ALLERGIC AND PSEUDOALLERGIC CONDITIONS

Anaphylaxis and Anaphylactoid Reactions

Description

Anaphylaxis is a rapidly evolving systemic allergic reaction that may be life threatening. Although most of these reactions develop at home (75), they also occur in the hospital setting. It is estimated to affect 1 of every 3,000 inpatients in the United States with a 1% risk of a fatal outcome (76). A study in Great Britain indicated that approximately half of fatal anaphylactic reactions are iatrogenic (77).

Anaphylaxis involves IgE-mediated release of cellular products such as histamine and leukotrienes from mast cells and basophils upon exposure of a previously sensitized person to a foreign substance. Such products may affect multiple organs, resulting in cutaneous, respiratory, cardiovascular, or gastrointestinal (GI) manifestations. Table 30.8 lists the frequency of occurrence of these signs and symptoms recorded in a case series of anaphylaxis (78). Respiratory distress may be due to upper airway obstruction and/or bronchoconstriction. Hypotension may be due to vasodilatation or increased vascular permeability. These developments typically occur within minutes of exposure to the offending agent but may develop up to an hour later. The more rapid reactions tend to be more severe. Up to one-quarter of affected patients exhibit a biphasic pattern in which signs and symptoms again develop 1 to 8 hours after they initially resolve (75,79). It is thus important to keep affected patients under close observation during this period.

Anaphylactic reactions may be triggered by minute amounts of an allergenic substance. The most commonly

TABLE 30.8 Signs and Symptoms of Anaphylaxis

Signs and Symptoms	*Frequency (%)*
Urticaria, angioedema	90
Dyspnea, wheezing	60
Dizziness, near-syncope	29
Flushed skin	28
Diarrhea, abdominal cramps	26
Upper airway obstruction	24
Nausea, vomiting	20
Hypotension	20
Nasal congestion, rhinorrhea	16
Eye swelling	12
Chest pain	6
Headache	5
Generalized pruritus without rash	4
Blurred vision	2
Seizure	2

Adapted from Kemp SF, Lockey RF, Wolf BL, et al. Anaphylaxis: a review of 266 cases. Arch Intern Med 1995;155:1749.

implicated triggers are certain drugs and foods. Other causes of anaphylaxis include stinging insect venoms and latex. The evaluation and management of allergy to these specific elements are discussed separately later in this chapter. About 6% to 20% of cases have no identifiable cause and are thus termed idiopathic anaphylaxis (75,80).

The term *anaphylactoid* reaction denotes the same clinical picture produced by anaphylaxis but by definition is not mediated by IgE antibodies. Nonetheless, these so-called pseudoallergic reactions may similarly involve bioactive mediators released by mast cells and basophils. These cells can be directly activated, independent of IgE, by opiates (81) or by hyperosmolar agents (82). Other possible mechanisms include activation of the complement cascade and production of anaphylatoxins such as C3a and C5a that trigger mediator release (83). In contrast to anaphylaxis, these pseudoallergic reactions do not require previous exposure.

Depending on the patient's clinical presentation, the *differential diagnosis* may include vasovagal reaction, acute ischemia, asthma exacerbation, hyperventilation syndrome, carcinoid syndrome, and systemic mastocytosis. The diagnosis of anaphylaxis is strongly supported by the demonstration of elevated serum histamine or tryptase. However, this may be difficult to demonstrate because of the short half-lives of these mediators. If possible, histamine should be measured within 10 minutes to 1 hour, and tryptase within 1 to 2 hours, of the anaphylactic reaction (84).

Management

Because acute anaphylactic or anaphylactoid reactions are potentially fatal, the patient's cardiopulmonary status and the need for timely intervention must be quickly addressed. Most anaphylaxis deaths due to food allergy are associated with respiratory arrest, whereas those due to drugs and stinging insect venoms are associated with cardiovascular collapse. The median time to respiratory or cardiac arrest has been found to be 30 minutes for fatal anaphylactic reactions to foods, 15 minutes for insect venom, and 5 minutes for drugs (77).

Epinephrine is the drug of choice for the acute treatment of life-threatening anaphylaxis because of its combined α- and β-agonist properties. The α component increases peripheral vascular resistance and ameliorates hypotension, urticaria, and angioedema, and the β component has inotropic and bronchodilatory effects. The adult dose is 0.2 to 0.5 mL of a 1:1,000 solution (0.2 to 0.5 mg epinephrine) given subcutaneously or intramuscularly (Table 30.9). The recommended route is intramuscular injection into the thigh as it has been shown to produce faster systemic absorption and higher peak levels of the drug (85). Dosing may be repeated every 10 to 15 minutes as needed for up to three doses. A retrospective study has shown that more than one dose of epinephrine is required in 36% of cases of anaphylaxis (86).

TABLE 30.9 Medications for the Acute Management of Anaphylaxis

Drug	*Adult Dose and Administration*
Epinephrine	0.2 to 0.5 mL of 1:1,000 solution i.m. every 10–15 min up to 3 doses
Diphenhydramine	2 mg/kg i.m. or i.v. then 25–50 mg i.v., i.m., or p.o. every 4–6 h
Cimetidine	300 mg i.v. then 300 mg p.o. every 6 h
Methylprednisolone	1–2 mg/kg i.v. every 6–8 h or 60 mg p.o. then 60 mg p.o. per day tapered over several days

Antihistamines help to reduce the effects of histamine released from mast cells and basophils. Diphenhydramine is given intramuscularly or intravenously at an initial dose of 1 to 2 mg/kg, and then 25 to 50 mg intravenously, intramuscularly, or orally every 4 to 6 hours to relieve recurrent signs and symptoms (Table 30.9). Additional treatment with an H_2 blocker such as ranitidine or cimetidine may provide further benefit (87).

Bronchodilator therapy with nebulized albuterol should be given if bronchospasm occurs as part of the anaphylactic reaction, especially in asthmatic patients. Intubation or tracheotomy to allow ventilatory support may be required in severe cases of respiratory distress.

Glucocorticoids are not first-line agents for the treatment of anaphylaxis but are commonly used, putatively to attenuate any late-phase reaction. Methylprednisolone is given at a dose of 1 to 2 mg/kg intravenously (Table 30.9).

A detailed history should be taken to identify any causative agent so preventive measures may be implemented. Referral to an allergist may be considered for further evaluation and management. Skin testing or *in vitro* tests may detect specific IgE against suspected agents. If future re-exposure is anticipated, desensitization against suspect drugs or immunotherapy against insect venom may be indicated, as discussed later in this chapter.

Patient Education

Patients should be educated about the early recognition of anaphylaxis and the need for immediate action. They should always carry epinephrine for self-administration in case of future life-threatening allergic reaction. A survey has shown that a large percentage of patients with a history of anaphylaxis do not carry epinephrine (78). This should be addressed, because failure to promptly administer this drug increases the risk for fatal anaphylaxis (79). *EpiPen* Auto-Injector, a device that delivers 0.3 mL of 1:1,000 epinephrine (0.3 mg) intramuscularly through a spring-activated concealed needle, may be used for this purpose. For small children, the *EpiPen* Jr. Auto-Injector device delivers 0.3 mL of 1:2,000 epinephrine (0.15 mg). The patient should be instructed about the proper use of this device to avoid mistakes that lead to ineffective delivery of the drug (88). Epinephrine should be used only in the event of actual or impending cardiovascular or respiratory compromise. In such cases, the patient should seek emergency medical care because additional treatment could be required. Periodic followup should be made to ensure that unused epinephrine is replaced before its expiration date (89).

Prognosis

A longitudinal study has shown that at followup after an average of 2.5 years, 60% of patients with *recurrent idiopathic anaphylaxis* report resolution of this problem. In 26% of cases, the frequency of anaphylactic episodes decreased, and it increased in 6% (90). The prognosis among patients with allergic reactions to known causes such as foods, drugs, or insect venom is discussed under Specific Allergic and Pseudoallergic Conditions.

Urticaria and Angioedema

It is estimated that 16% to 24% of the U.S. population will develop *urticaria* at least once in a lifetime (91). Affected individuals present with pruritic, erythematous, circumscribed superficial wheals or "hives" that may be coalescent. The individual skin lesions usually resolve within 24 hours, but others may develop at additional sites. The hives, which are largely due to local plasma extravasation, typically appear on the trunk and extremities but may arise anywhere on the body. *Angioedema* is swelling of deeper subcutaneous or submucosal tissue that is less circumscribed than urticaria. Unlike other forms of edema, these are often asymmetrically distributed and have no predilection for dependent areas. Urticaria and angioedema occur together in 49% of cases. About 40% of affected patients develop urticaria alone, whereas 11% develop angioedema without hives (91).

Urticaria and angioedema are arbitrarily classified as *acute* if they occur over a period of less than 6 weeks or *chronic* if they last longer. For acute urticaria and/or angioedema an apparent cause may be found, whereas chronic cases rarely have an identifiable cause.

Evaluation

Acute Urticaria and Angioedema

Possible causes of acute urticaria and/or angioedema that may be gleaned from the history include drugs, foods, insect bites or stings, physical elements, infections, and topical irritants. Of note, only some of these cases have demonstrable involvement of IgE-mediated allergy. It is helpful if a temporal relationship between the onset of symptoms and a particular trigger factor can be established. For example, a history of food ingestion or insect sting minutes before the development of urticaria or angioedema strongly suggests an allergic reaction. Several nonallergic causes may also be identified. A history of exercise or heat exposure preceding the appearance of pinpoint hives suggests *cholinergic urticaria*, a nonallergic state. Other physical elements that can trigger urticaria and/or angioedema include pressure, vibration, and cold temperature (92). Urticaria and angioedema may also be associated with infections, for example, hepatitis viruses or *Helicobacter pylori*, although reports have been conflicting (91,93,94).

If allergen sensitivity is suspected as a cause of recurrent acute urticaria or angioedema, appropriate skin testing or *in vitro* tests by an allergist may be useful. If physical elements are suspected, diagnostic provocation can be performed. For example, an ice cube may be applied for 5 to 10 minutes on the forearm of a patient with a history of cold-induced urticaria to verify such diagnosis (95). If no specific cause can be identified, a limited workup may be considered to screen for any underlying systemic condition based on findings in the history and physical examination.

Chronic Urticaria and/or Angioedema

For patients with chronic urticaria and/or angioedema, differential diagnoses to consider include connective tissue disease or vasculitis, complement-related disorders, presence of autoantibodies, lymphoproliferative diseases, or mastocytosis with urticaria pigmentosa. A thorough review of systems and physical examination should be performed to evaluate the possibility of these conditions.

The cutaneous lesions associated with *urticarial vasculitis* are different from benign urticaria in that they are purpuric, persist longer than 24 hours, are painful rather than pruritic, and typically leave residual skin pigmentation. Cutaneous vasculitis accounts for less than 1% of all cases of chronic urticaria (96).

Angioedema, specifically if it is not accompanied by urticaria, may be due to a *C1 esterase inhibitor deficiency*. This condition may be hereditary or acquired. Laryngeal or gastrointestinal tissue swelling can cause airway obstruction or abdominal discomfort, respectively. Gastrointestinal symptoms may be the sole manifestation of this disease and can lead to unnecessary exploratory laparotomy (97). *Hereditary angioedema* (HAE) is an autosomal dominant disorder due to several possible defects in the C1 esterase inhibitor gene (98). *Acquired angioedema* has been associated with connective tissue diseases, lymphoproliferative disorders, malignancies, or autoantibodies against the C1 esterase inhibitor protein (99). For patients with chronic angioedema without urticaria, complement C4 levels should be measured. These are persistently low during and between attacks of angioedema because of C1 esterase inhibitor deficiency. In contrast, levels of C2 are low only during episodes of active disease, and C3 levels are unaffected. The diagnosis is established by demonstrating low quantitative and/or functional levels of C1 esterase inhibitor. Its quantity is low in type 1 HAE, which accounts for 85% of cases. In the 15% of cases with type 2 HAE, C1 esterase inhibitor is normal in quantity but is functionally impaired (100). To distinguish between hereditary and acquired angioedema, C1q level should be measured. Levels of C1q are normal in HAE but are low in acquired angioedema (99). Resultant elevations in C2 kinin and bradykinin are believed to be the cause of tissue swelling in these patients (99,101). Elevation in bradykinin, which increases vascular permeability, also has been implicated in angioedema associated with angiotensin-converting enzyme (ACE) inhibitors. Angiotensin II receptor blockers (ARBs) can also induce angioedema, especially in patients with a prior history of developing the same problem following treatment with an ACE inhibitor (102).

Some studies suggest that *autoimmunity* may play a role in subgroups of patients with chronic idiopathic urticaria or angioedema. Autoantibodies against thyroid peroxidase or thyroglobulin (103) and against IgE or the α chain of the IgE receptor have been implicated (92,104,105). However, the exact role of autoantibodies in the pathogenesis of chronic urticaria and angioedema remains unclear, and routine measurement of their levels is not recommended. In refractory cases of urticaria or when vasculitis is suspected, skin biopsy should be considered (96).

Management

Management of Urticaria or Angioedema without a Known Cause

Management of *idiopathic* urticaria and angioedema is mainly directed toward amelioration of symptoms. For this purpose, various combinations of antihistamines can provide benefit. Older generation antihistamines are quite effective, but they often cause significant psychomotor impairment in contrast to newer agents (Table 30.3). Addition of H_2 receptor antagonists such as cimetidine or ranitidine to treat persistent cases may provide further benefit (106). Tricyclic antidepressants such as doxepin have potent H_1- and H_2-blocking capabilities and may thus play a therapeutic role. However, their use could be limited by side effects such as sedation and psychomotor impairment (107). Chronic use of oral or parenteral glucocorticoids is not advised in view of their known adverse affects. However, brief courses of oral glucocorticoids may be needed occasionally for severe exacerbations. The use of aspirin and similar nonsteroidal anti-inflammatory drugs (NSAIDs) should be discouraged because they can induce exacerbations of chronic idiopathic urticaria and angioedema (108).

Management of Urticaria or Angioedema with a Known Cause

For *nonidiopathic* cases when a specific cause such as a food or drug has been identified, avoidance measures should be implemented. For patients diagnosed with C1 esterase inhibitor deficiency, prophylactic management with anabolic steroids such as stanozolol or danazol can prevent recurrence of life-threatening angioedema. The dosage should be cautiously reduced to the lowest effective level possible. The patient's liver function, serum cholesterol, and iron profile should be monitored. Adverse effects in women may include signs of virilization such as hoarseness, acne, irregular menses, and changes in hair pattern (109). If available, infusion of vapor-heated C1 esterase inhibitor concentrate can be used to treat acute episodes of angioedema (110).

For patients with chronic urticaria and thyroid autoantibodies, treatment with thyroid hormone has been reported to provide benefit in some individuals (103), but this effect is neither consistent nor predictable.

Prognosis

A study of patients with chronic idiopathic urticaria or angioedema showed that after 1 year, 38% of those with urticaria alone, 20% with angioedema alone, and 60% with combined urticaria and angioedema were symptom free (111). Another study indicated that up to 20% of patients with chronic idiopathic urticaria continue to be affected after 20 years (92).

SPECIFIC ALLERGIC AND PSEUDOALLERGIC CONDITIONS

Drug Allergy

About 10% to 20% of hospitalized patients in the United States experience some form of adverse drug reaction (112), with fatal outcomes in an estimated 100,000 cases a year (113). Although most of these reactions are not IgE-mediated, approximately 6% to 10% may have an allergic or immunologic basis (114). Systematic data about adverse drug reactions in the outpatient setting are lacking, but this problem is nonetheless an important consideration in ambulatory care.

β-Lactam Antibiotics

Penicillin is the most common cause of drug-related fatal anaphylaxis. It is estimated that anaphylactic reactions occur in 0.004% to 0.015% of all courses of penicillin (115). Such reactions tend to occur more frequently when penicillin is given parenterally rather than orally (116).

Although most cases involve middle-aged adults, elderly patients tend to have more fatal outcomes, probably due to underlying cardiovascular insufficiency. The risk of allergic reaction to penicillin may be higher among patients with a history of similar adverse reactions to other drugs such as sulfonamide antibiotics (117).

If patients who give a history of a penicillin-induced allergic reaction require treatment with this drug, *skin testing* should be done first to identify those at risk for anaphylaxis. If the anaphylactic reaction occurred recently, skin testing should be deferred for 1 to 2 weeks; otherwise, the result could be unreliable (118). Skin testing should be performed using major and minor antigenic determinants of this drug. Benzylpenicilloyl polylysine (Pre-Pen) is considered the major determinant because it represents 95% of haptenated penicillin. The minor determinants include benzylpenicillin (penicillin G), which is commercially available, and benzylpenicilloate and benzylpenniloate, which are available only in certain medical centers. It is believed that the minor determinants are responsible for more severe hypersensitivity reactions. Of note, skin testing does not predict adverse effects that are not IgE-mediated such as delayed cutaneous rash, erythema multiforme, Stevens-Johnson syndrome, and toxic epidermal necrolysis. Skin testing is not required if there is no personal history of adverse reaction to this drug, even if there is a family history of penicillin allergy. At present, there is no reliable *in vitro* test for hypersensitivity to this antibiotic.

Only 10% to 20% of patients who give a history of reaction to penicillin are truly allergic to this drug based on skin testing (116). About 97% to 99% of patients with negative skin tests using the major and minor determinants will tolerate penicillin. On the other hand, patients with a positive history and positive skin test have at least a 50% probability of developing an immediate hypersensitivity reaction if they receive penicillin (119). Alternative antibiotics should therefore be used in these cases. If administration of penicillin is mandatory, the patient should first undergo desensitization. This entails administration of incremental doses of the drug in a carefully monitored setting until therapeutic levels are reached to achieve immunologic tolerance.

About 98% of patients with a history of penicillin allergy will tolerate treatment with cephalosporins, especially the second and third generations of this class of antibiotics. However, the 2% who do react will likely have life-threatening anaphylaxis. There is no validated skin test available for cephalosporins, because their antigenic determinants remain to be established. For these reasons, patients with a history of anaphylactic reaction to penicillin and a positive penicillin skin test should either avoid cephalosporins or undergo desensitization (112,120).

Carbapenems such as imipenem can be cross-reactive with penicillin and should be avoided by penicillin-allergic patients (121). In contrast, the monobactam aztreonam rarely cross-reacts with penicillin (122).

Ampicillin and amoxicillin are known to cause *morbilliform rashes*, which are not life threatening, in 5% to 10% of patients. These effects are not IgE mediated, so skin testing is not warranted.

Although some patients maintain their hypersensitivity for long periods of time, in the majority the penicillin skin test becomes negative within 10 years (123). This may partially explain why 80% to 90% of patients who give a past history of allergy to penicillin have no evidence of sensitivity to this drug upon testing. Repeat skin testing before each subsequent course of β-lactam antibiotics is not needed because the risk of resensitization is low (124).

Aspirin and Nonsteroidal Anti-inflammatory Drugs

Aspirin ranks second to penicillin as a frequent cause of adverse drug reactions. Affected patients typically experience exacerbation of their pre-existing rhinoconjunctivitis, asthma, urticaria, and/or angioedema. However, these side effects are largely unrelated to IgE-mediated mechanisms. In addition to aspirin sensitivity, some patients can have concurrent asthma and nasal polyposis. These three conditions constitute the so-called Samter triad.

Patients with sensitivity to aspirin similarly develop adverse reactions to NSAIDs such as those listed in Table 30.10. Furthermore, a study has shown that up to 34%

TABLE 30.10 NSAIDs That Should Be Avoided by Patients with Aspirin Sensitivity

Drug	Trade Name
Diclofenac	Voltaren
Diflunisal	Dolobid
Etodolac	Lodine
Fenoprofen	Nalfon
Flurbiprofen	Ansaid
Ibuprofen	Advil, Motrin
Indomethacin	Indocin
Ketoprofen	Orudis
Ketorolac	Toradol
Meclofenamate	Meclomen
Mefenamic acid	Ponstel
Nabumetone	Relafen
Naproxen	Aleve, Anaprox, Naprosyn
Oxaprozin	Daypro
Piroxicam	Feldene
Sulindac	Clinoril
Tolmetin	Tolectin

NSAIDs, nonsteroidal anti-inflammatory drugs.

of aspirin-sensitive asthmatic patients can have mild reactions to acetaminophen at high doses of 1000 mg or greater (125). As such, patients with aspirin sensitivity should avoid both NSAIDs and high doses of acetaminophen. However, these individuals can tolerate lower doses of acetaminophen.

There is no skin test or *in vitro* test for the diagnosis of aspirin or NSAID intolerance. An oral challenge with aspirin is the only definitive way to establish the presence of sensitivity to this medication.

Desensitization should be considered if the benefit outweighs the risk of an adverse reaction. One example is the use of aspirin in patients with myocardial infarction (MI) (126). Patients who successfully undergo aspirin desensitization are also expected to tolerate NSAIDs. Once tolerance is achieved, administration of therapeutic doses of the drug should be continued on a daily basis. Otherwise, full sensitization may recur if the medication is discontinued for up to 7 days.

Radiographic Contrast Material

The incidence of adverse reactions to radiocontrast material is estimated to be 5% to 8%. These may occur with intravascular administration or during hysterosalpingograms, myelograms, and retrograde pyelograms. Although these effects are believed to be unrelated to IgE-mediated hypersensitivity, the reaction is clinically similar to anaphylaxis. Contrary to common belief, shellfish allergy is not a risk factor for the development of adverse effects from radiocontrast dye. The acute treatment of anaphylactoid reactions to radiocontrast media is similar to the management of anaphylaxis.

Individuals who have a history of reactions to radiocontrast media have a greater risk of experiencing adverse effects upon re-exposure. The reported probability of a recurrent anaphylactoid reaction upon repeat exposure ranges from 16% to 44%. This risk can be lowered to approximately 1% by pretreating the affected patient with glucocorticoids and antihistamines. Prophylaxis can be provided with prednisone given at a dose of 50 mg at 13 hours, 7 hours, and 1 hour before the procedure. An oral antihistamine (Table 30.3) is then given 1 hour before the administration of radiocontrast material (127). The use of radiocontrast media with low osmolality can likewise reduce the risk of anaphylactoid reactions (128).

Food Allergy

Epidemiology

Food allergy affects approximately 2% of the adult population in the United States (129). Anaphylactic reactions to food requiring treatment in the emergency department are estimated to occur about 1,000 times a year, with a number of cases resulting in death (130). More than 90% of fatal cases of food allergy have been attributed to peanuts and tree nuts (131). A significant portion of the population is at risk, as 3 million Americans have been determined to have peanut and/or tree nut allergy. Notably, about half the members of this group have never sought medical evaluation, and only a few have epinephrine available for emergency use (132).

Relatively few foods account for the vast majority of food allergy. Milk, eggs, peanuts, soy, and wheat account for 90% of food hypersensitivity in children, but in adults, peanuts, fish, shellfish, and tree nuts are responsible for 85% of food-related reactions. It is rare for an individual to be allergic to more than three foods (129).

Evaluation

A detailed history is important in evaluating the possibility of IgE-mediated sensitivity to food. When they occur, allergic reactions to food typically develop from a few minutes to an hour after ingestion. The absence of a close temporal relationship between exposure and the development of signs and symptoms should prompt a search for other explanations. The manifestations of allergic reactions to food can range from nausea, vomiting, and abdominal cramping to generalized urticaria and respiratory distress.

Some reported cases of anaphylactic reactions to food have been associated with factors such as exercise after a meal (133). Other case reports suggest that in highly sensitized patients, reactions can be triggered by skin contact or inhalational exposure to food particles (134).

For diagnostic purposes, *tests for food-specific IgE antibodies or food challenges* may be applicable. Although puncture skin testing and *in vitro* assays have low specificity and positive predictive values, they have excellent sensitivity and negative predictive accuracy. Only about 50% of patients with positive skin tests to food will have a reaction to *double-blind placebo-controlled food challenge*. On the other hand, negative skin tests virtually rule out IgE-mediated food sensitivity. For *in vitro* evaluation, cutoff levels of IgE that provide positive and negative predictive values of 95% and 90%, respectively, have been determined for egg, milk, peanuts, and fish (135).

Patient history regarding possible food allergy is not always reliable. Only about 40% of cases can be verified as true food-induced allergic reactions through double-blind placebo-controlled food challenges. This office-based procedure can be considered if no specific item is identified as the cause of an allergic reaction, but certain foods remain strongly suspected. It can be performed under close medical supervision by starting with minute amounts of the suspected food and stopping as soon as symptoms such as oral itching or nausea develop (136).

Management

Once a food item is identified as a possible cause of hypersensitivity reactions, it should be vigilantly eliminated from the patient's diet. Those with a history of severe allergic reaction should be prescribed epinephrine to be self-administered in case of cardiovascular or respiratory compromise due to anaphylaxis (see details in preceding section Anaphylaxis and Anaphylactoid Reactions, Patient Education). Patients and their caregivers can obtain further support and useful updates from the Food Allergy and Anaphylaxis Network (www.foodallergy.org). A study of the use of anti-IgE in patients with peanut allergy had favorable results and opened the possibility of a disease-modifying treatment in the future (137).

Prognosis

About one-third of adults with food allergy will lose their clinical reactivity after 1 to 2 years of allergen avoidance. However, neither skin tests nor *in vitro* tests can predict which patients will experience resolution of their food hypersensitivity (138).

Insect Venom Allergy

Evaluation

Anaphylactic reactions to insect venom account for about 50 deaths annually in the United States (139), and it is possible that additional cases are undiagnosed and unreported. Stinging insects that cause such IgE-mediated reactions include yellow jackets, hornets, wasps, honeybees, and imported fire ants. Yellow jackets dwell in the ground, whereas hornets build nests in trees and shrubs. Both can be quite aggressive and often sting with minimal provocation. Wasps build honeycomb nests in dark areas, whereas honeybees can be wild or domesticated. Imported fire ants dwell in mounds of soil mostly in the southern states, and their habitat is expanding (140).

Most insect stings typically cause localized swelling, erythema, pain, and pruritus, which are largely due to histamine, serotonin, and kinins contained in the venom. Such limited reactions are not life threatening, but potentially fatal anaphylaxis can also develop in susceptible individuals. The signs and symptoms of such serious reactions can include any combination of generalized urticaria, angioedema, and cardiovascular and/or pulmonary distress.

Localized reactions are not associated with increased risk of subsequent anaphylaxis and thus do not require any long-term intervention. Systemic allergic reactions, however, merit further evaluation and management. Skin testing and/or *in vitro* tests should be done to demonstrate the presence of IgE antibodies specific for the suspected insect venom.

Management

Adult patients with a confirmed history of systemic allergic reaction to insect venom have a 30% to 60% risk of developing anaphylaxis again in reaction to subsequent stings. Insect venom immunotherapy is thus indicated because it reduces the risk of a subsequent systemic allergic reaction to approximately 2% (141). In children, immunotherapy reduces the risk of a systemic reaction from about 17% to 3% (142). As in any case of anaphylactic reactions, patients should carry epinephrine that can be self-administered as needed. Unfortunately, this important measure is often overlooked (143).

Prognosis

Prospective studies indicate that insect venom immunotherapy can be discontinued after 5 years of treatment. Data from followup evaluation over the next 5 to 10 years show that the residual risk of a systemic reaction to an insect sting is 5% to 15%. Patients who experienced a life-threatening reaction may opt to continue their treatment indefinitely (141).

Latex Allergy

The prevalence of latex hypersensitivity in the general population is less than 1%. However, certain groups have a significantly higher risk of developing this condition. For example, latex allergy is estimated to affect 24% to 60% of patients with spina bifida and genitourinary abnormalities who have undergone multiple surgeries and to affect 5% to 15% of health care workers (144). This increased risk can be attributed to a higher rate of exposure to latex gloves among these individuals.

Several proteins in the sap of the rubber tree (*Hevea brasiliensis*) have been identified as latex allergens. Exposure can occur by direct contact, parenteral administration, or inhalation of aerosolized particles. Powdered latex gloves are common sources of the latter, because latex allergens are absorbed by cornstarch powder. Individuals with latex allergy may experience similar hypersensitivity reactions to avocado, banana, chestnut, or kiwi because these foods may have cross-reactivity with latex allergens (145). IgE antibodies against latex allergens can be demonstrated by skin testing or by *in vitro* tests.

Avoidance of latex products is the only means of preventing serious allergic reactions in a sensitized individual. Primary prevention of latex allergy through the institution of latex-free environments should be encouraged. In the hospital setting, for example, only nonlatex gloves should be allowed to minimize sensitization of high-risk individuals and to avoid adverse reactions among those who are already sensitized. Affected patients should always carry epinephrine that can be self-administered in case of a life-threatening allergic reaction.

SPECIFIC REFERENCES*

1. Arbes SJ Jr, Gergen PJ, Elliott L, et al. Prevalences of positive skin test responses to 10 common allergens in the US population: results from the third National Health and Nutrition Examination Survey. J Allergy Clin Immunol 2005;116:377.
2. Hopp RJ, Bewtra AK, Watt GD, et al. Genetic analysis of allergic disease in twins. J Allergy Clin Immunol 1984;73:265.
3. Sarafino EP. Connections among parent and child atopic illnesses. Pediatr Allergy Immunol 2000;11:80.
4. Strachan DP. Family size, infection and atopy: the first decade of the "hygiene hypothesis."" Thorax 2000;55:S2.
5. Kay A. Allergy and allergic diseases (First of two parts). N Engl J Med 2001;344:30.
6. Adelroth E, Rak S, Haahtela T, et al. Recombinant humanized mAb-E25, an anti-IgE mAb, in birch pollen-induced seasonal allergic rhinitis. J Allergy Clin Immunol 2000;106:253.
7. Leckie M, Brinke A, Khan J, et al. Effects of an interleukin-5 blocking monoclonal antibody on eosinophils, airway hyper-responsiveness, and the late asthmatic response. Lancet 2000;356:2144.
8. Kinet JP. A new strategy to counter allergy. N Engl J Med 2005;353:310.
9. Durham S, Till S. Immunologic changes associated with allergen immunotherapy. J Allergy Clin Immunol 1998;102:157.
10. Malone DC, Lawson KA, Smith DH, et al. A cost of illness study of allergic rhinitis in the United States. J Allergy Clin Immunol 1997;99:22.
11. Law AW, Reed SD, Sundy JS, et al. Direct costs of allergic rhinitis in the United States: estimates from the 1996 Medical Expenditure Panel Survey. J Allergy Clin Immunol. 2003;111:296.
12. Meltzer EO. Quality of life in adults and children with allergic rhinitis. J Allergy Clin Immunol 2001;108:S45.
13. Blaiss MS. Cognitive, social, and economic costs of allergic rhinitis. Allergy Asthma Proc 2000;21:7.
14. Kay GG, Berman B, Mockoviak SH, et al. Initial and steady-state effects of diphenhydramine and loratadine on sedation, cognition, mood, and psychomotor performance. Arch Intern Med 1997;157:2350.
15. Skoner DP. Complications of allergic rhinitis. J Allergy Clin Immunol 2000;105:S605.
16. Ramadan HH, Fornelli R, Ortiz AO, et al. Correlation of allergy and severity of sinus disease. Am J Rhinol 1999;13:345.
17. Hisamatsu K, Ganbo T, Nakazawa T, et al. Cytotoxicity of human eosinophil granule major basic protein to human nasal sinus mucosa in vitro. J Allergy Clin Immunol 1990;86:52.
18. Meltzer EO, Hamilos DL, Hadley JA, et al. Rhinosinusitis: establishing definitions for clinical research and patient care. J Allergy Clin Immunol 2004;114:155.
19. Alles R, Parikh A, Hawk L, et al. The prevalence of atopic disorders in children with chronic otitis media with effusion. Pediatr Allergy Immunol 2001;12:102.
20. Simons F. Allergic rhinobronchitis: the asthma-allergic rhinitis link. J Allergy Clin Immunol 1999;104:534.
21. Togias A. Rhinitis and asthma: evidence for respiratory system integration. J Allergy Clin Immunol 2003;111:1171.
22. Gaga M, Lambrou P, Papageorgiou N, et al. Eosinophils are a feature of upper and lower airway pathology in non-atopic asthma, irrespective of the presence of rhinitis. Clin Exp Allergy 2000;30:663.
23. Grembiale R, Camporota L, Naty S, et al. Effects of specific immunotherapy in allergic rhinitis individuals with bronchial hyperresponsiveness. Am J Respir Crit Care Med 2000;162:2048.
24. Halpern MT, Schmier JK, Richner R, et al. Allergic rhinitis: a potential cause of increased asthma medication use, costs, and morbidity. J Asthma 2004;41:117.
25. Braunstahl G-J, Overbeek S, Klein JA, et al. Nasal allergen provocation induces adhesion molecules expression and tissue eosinophilia in upper and lower airways. J Allergy Clin Immunol 2001;107:469.
26. Welsh P, Stricker W, Chu C, et al. Efficacy of beclomethasone nasal solution, flunisolide, and cromolyn in relieving symptoms of ragweed allergy. Mayo Clin Proc 1987;62:125.
27. Bousquet J, Cauwenberge P, Khaltaev N, Area Workshop Group, World Health Organization. Allergic rhinitis and its impact on asthma. J Allergy Clin Immunol 2001;108:S147.
28. Diemer FB, Sanico AM, Horowitz E, et al. Non-allergenic inhalant triggers in seasonal and perennial allergic rhinitis (abstr). J Allergy Clin Immunol 1999;103:S2.
29. Sanico AM, Koliatsos VE, Stanisz AM, et al. Neural hyperresponsiveness and nerve growth factor in allergic rhinitis. Int Arch Allergy Immunol 1999;118:153.
30. Tovey ER, Chapman MD, Platts-Mills TA. Mite faeces are a major source of house dust allergens. Nature 1981;289:592.
31. Terreehorst I, Hak E, Oosting AJ, et al. Evaluation of impermeable covers for bedding in patients with allergic rhinitis. N Engl J Med 2003;349:237.
32. Tovey ER, Taylor DJ, Mitakakis TZ, et al. Effectiveness of laundry washing agents and conditions in the removal of cat and dust mite allergen from bedding dust. J Allergy Clin Immunol 2001;108:369.
33. Arlian L, Neal J, Morgan M, et al. Reducing relative humidity is a practical way to control dust mites and their allergens in homes in temperate climates. J Allergy Clin Immunol 2001;107:99.
34. Antonicelli L, Bilo MB, Pucci S, et al. Efficacy of an air-cleaning device equipped with a high efficiency particulate air filter in house dust mite respiratory allergy. Allergy 1991;46:594.
35. Custis NJ, Woodfolk JA, Vaughan JW, et al. Quantitative measurement of airborne allergens from dust mites, dogs, and cats using an ion-charging device. Clin Exp Allergy 2003;33:986.
36. Huss R, Huss K, Squire E, et al. Mite allergen control with acaride fails. J Allergy Clin Immunol 1994;94:27.
37. Bartholome K, Kissler W, Baer H, et al. Where does cat allergen 1 come from? J Allergy Clin Immunol 1985;76:503.
38. Wentz PE, Swanson MC, Reed CE. Variability of cat-allergen shedding. J Allergy Clin Immunol 1990;85:94.
39. Wood R, Johnson E, Van Natta M, et al. A placebo-controlled trial of a HEPA air cleaner in the treatment of cat allergy. Am J Respir Crit Care Med 1998;158:115.
40. Avner DB, Perzanowski MS, Platts-Mills TA, et al. Evaluation of different techniques for washing cats: quantitation of allergen removed from the cat and the effect on airborne Fel d 1. J Allergy Clin Immunol 1997;100:307.
41. Wood R, Chapman M, Adkinson N, et al. The effect of cat removal on allergen content in household dust samples. J Allergy Clin Immunol 1989;83:730.
42. Perzanowski MS, Ronmark E, Nold B, et al. Relevance of allergens from cats and dogs to asthma in the northernmost province of Sweden: schools as a major site of exposure. J Allergy Clin Immunol 1999;103:1018.
43. Almqvist C, Larsson PH, Egmar AC, et al. School as a risk environment for children allergic to cats and a site for transfer of cat allergen to homes. J Allergy Clin Immunol 1999;103:1012.
44. Durham S, Walker S, Varga E, et al. Long-term clinical efficacy of grass-pollen immunotherapy. N Engl J Med 1999;341:468.
45. Barnes C, Pacheco F, Landuyt J, et al. Hourly variation of airborne ragweed pollen in Kansas City. Ann Allergy Asthma Immunol. 2001;86:166.
46. Weiler J, Bloomfield J, Woodworth G, et al. Effects of fexofenadine, diphenhydramine, and alcohol on driving performance. A randomized, placebo-controlled trial in the Iowa driving simulator. Ann Intern Med 2000;132:354.
47. Gilmore TM, Alexander BH, Mueller BA, et al. Occupational injuries and medication use. Am J Ind Med 1996;30:234.
48. Simons FE. Non-cardiac adverse effects of antihistamines (H1-receptor antagonists). Clin Exp Allergy 1999;29:125.
49. Simons FER. H1-receptor antagonists: safety issues. Ann Allergy Asthma Immunol 1999; 83:481.
50. Sanico AM. Latest developments in the management of allergic rhinitis. Clin Rev Allergy Immunol 2004;27:181.
51. Kernan W, Viscoli C, Brass L, et al. Phenylpropanolamine and the risk of hemorrhagic stroke. N Engl J Med 2000;343:1826.
52. Dockhorn R, Aaronson D, Bronsky E, et al. Ipratropium bromide nasal spray 0.03% and beclomethasone nasal spray alone and in combination for the treatment of rhinorrhea in perennial rhinitis. Ann Allergy Asthma Immunol 1999;82:349.
53. Lumry WR. A review of the preclinical and clinical data of newer intranasal steroids used in the treatment of allergic rhinitis. J Allergy Clin Immunol 1999;104:S150.
54. Pipkorn U, Proud D, Lichtenstein L, et al. Inhibition of mediator release in allergic rhinitis by pretreatment with topical glucocorticoids. N Engl J Med 1987;316:1506.
55. Meltzer EO, Rickard KA, Westlund RE, et al. Onset of therapeutic effect of fluticasone propionate aqueous nasal spray. Ann Allergy Asthma Immunol 2001;86:286.
56. Day J, Briscoe M, Rafeiro E, et al. Onset of action of intranasal budesonide (Rhinocort aqua) in seasonal allergic rhinitis studied in a controlled exposure model. J Allergy Clin Immunol 2000;105:489.
57. Berkowitz R, Bernstein D, LaForce C, et al. Onset of action of mometasone furoate nasal spray (NASONEX) in seasonal allergic rhinitis. Allergy 1999;54:64.
58. Jen A, Baroody F, de Tineo M, et al. As-needed use of fluticasone propionate nasal spray reduces symptoms of seasonal allergic rhinitis. J Allergy Clin Immunol 2000;105:732.
59. Allen DB. Systemic effects of intranasal steroids: an endocrinologist's perspective. J Allergy Clin Immunol 2000;106:S179.
60. Schoelzel EP, Menzel ML. Nasal sprays and perforation of the nasal septum. JAMA 1985; 253:2046.
61. Pipkorn U, Pukander J, Suonpaa J, et al. Long-term safety of budesonide nasal aerosol: a 5.5-year follow-up study. Clin Allergy 1988; 18:253.
62. Minshall E, Ghaffar O, Cameron L, et al. Assessment by nasal biopsy of long-term use of mometasone furoate aqueous nasal spray

*Bold numerals denote published controlled clinical trials, meta-analyses, or consensus-based recommendations.

(Nasonex) in the treatment of perennial rhinitis. Otolaryngol Head Neck Surg 1998;118:648.
63. Baroody F, Cheng C-C, Moylan B, et al. Absence of nasal mucosal atrophy with fluticasone aqueous nasal spray. Arch Otolaryngol Head Neck Surg 2001;127:193.
64. Qvarnberg Y, Valtonen H, Laurikainen K. Intranasal beclomethasone dipropionate in the treatment of common cold. Rhinology 2001;39:9.
65. Chervinsky P, Philip G, Malice MP. Montelukast for treating fall allergic rhinitis: effect of pollen exposure in 3 studies. Ann Allergy Asthma Immunol 2004;92:367.
66. Philip G, Malmstrom K, Hampel FC Jr., et al. Montelukast Spring Rhinitis Study Group. Montelukast for treating seasonal allergic rhinitis: a randomized, double-blind, placebo-controlled trial performed in the spring. Clin Exp Allergy 2002;32:1020.
67. Weinstein SF, Philip G, Hampel FC Jr., et al. Onset of efficacy of montelukast in seasonal allergic rhinitis. Allergy Asthma Proc 2005;26:41.
68. Bernstein DI, Wanner M, Borish L, Liss GM, Immunotherapy Committee, American Academy of Allergy, Asthma and Immunology. Twelve-year survey of fatal reactions to allergen injections and skin testing: 1990–2001. J Allergy Clin Immunol 2004;113:1129.
69. Greisner WA 3rd, Settipane RJ, Settipane GA. Natural history of hay fever: a 23-year follow-up of college students. Allergy Asthma Proc 1998; 19:271.
70. Settipane RJ, Hagy GW, Settipane GA. Long-term risk factors for developing asthma and allergic rhinitis: a 23-year follow-up study of college students. Allergy Proc 1994;15:21.
71. Moller C, Dreborg S, Ferdousi HA, et al. Pollen immunotherapy reduces the development of asthma in children with seasonal rhinoconjunctivitis (the PAT-study). J Allergy Clin Immunol 2002;109:251.
72. Bielory L. Allergic and immunologic disorders of the eye. Part II. Ocular allergy. J Allergy Clin Immunol 2000;106:1019.
73. Settipane RA, Lieberman P. Update on nonallergic rhinitis. Ann Allergy Asthma Immunol 2001;86:494.
74. Togias A. Age relationships and clinical features of nonallergic rhinitis. J Allergy Clin Immunol 1990;85:182.
75. Cianferoni A, Novembre E, Mugnaini L, et al. Clinical features of acute anaphylaxis in patients admitted to a university hospital: an 11-year retrospective review (1985–1996). Ann Allergy Asthma Immunol 2001;87:27.
76. Neugut AI, Ghatak AT, Miller RL. Anaphylaxis in the United States: an investigation into its epidemiology. Arch Intern Med 2001;161:15.
77. Pumphrey RS. Lessons for management of anaphylaxis from a study of fatal reactions. Clin Exp Allergy 2000;30:1144.
78. Kemp SF, Lockey RF, Wolf BL, et al. Anaphylaxis: a review of 266 cases. Arch Intern Med 1995;155:1749.
79. Sampson H, Mendelson L, Rosen J. Fatal and near-fatal anaphylactic reactions to food in children and adolescents. N Engl J Med 1992; 327:380.
80. Yocum MW, Khan DA. Assessment of patients who have experienced anaphylaxis: a 3-year survey. Mayo Clin Proc 1994;69:16.
81. Tharp MD, Kagey-Sobotka A, Fox CC, et al. Functional heterogeneity of human mast cells from different anatomic sites: *in vitro* responses to morphine sulfate. J Allergy Clin Immunol 1987;79:646.
82. Silber G, Proud D, Warner J, et al. *In vivo* release of inflammatory mediators by hyperosmolar solutions. Am Rev Respir Dis 1988;137:606.
83. Bochner B, Lichtenstein L. Anaphylaxis. N Engl J Med 1991;324:1785.
84. Laroche D, Vergnaud MC, Sillard B, et al. Biochemical markers of anaphylactoid reactions to drugs. Comparison of plasma histamine and tryptase. Anesthesiology 1991;75:945.
85. Simons FE, Gu X, Simons KJ. Epinephrine absorption in adults: intramuscular versus subcutaneous injection. J Allergy Clin Immunol 2001;108:871.
86. Korenblat P, Lundie MJ, Dankner RE, et al. A retrospective study of epinephrine administration for anaphylaxis: how many doses are needed? Allergy Asthma Proc 1999;20:383.
87. Lin RY, Curry A, Pesola GR, et al. Improved outcomes in patients with acute allergic syndromes who are treated with combined H1 and H2 antagonists. Ann Emerg Med 2000; 36:462.
88. Huang SW. A survey of Epi-PEN use in patients with a history of anaphylaxis. J Allergy Clin Immunol 1998;102:525.
89. Simons FE, Gu X, Simons KJ. Outdated EpiPen and EpiPen Jr autoinjectors: past their prime? J Allergy Clin Immunol 2000;105:1025.
90. Khan DA, Yocum MW. Clinical course of idiopathic anaphylaxis. Ann Allergy 1994;73:370.
91. Mathews K. Urticaria and angioedema. J Allergy Clin Immunol 1983;72:1.
92. Greaves M. Chronic urticaria. J Allergy Clin Immunol 2000;105:664.
93. Cribier BJ, Santinelli F, Schmitt C, et al. Chronic urticaria is not significantly associated with hepatitis C or hepatitis G infection: a case-control study. Arch Dermatol 1999;135:1335.
94. Gala Ortiz G, Cuevas Agustin M, Erias Martinez P, et al. Chronic urticaria and *Helicobacter pylori*. Ann Allergy Asthma Immunol 2001;86:696.
95. Orfan NA, Kolski GB. Physical urticarias. Ann Allergy 1993;71:205.
96. Kaplan AP. Clinical practice. Chronic urticaria and angioedema. N Engl J Med 2002;346:175.
97. Weinstock LB, Kothari T, Sharma RN, et al. Recurrent abdominal pain as the sole manifestation of hereditary angioedema in multiple family members. Gastroenterology 1987;93:1116.
98. Bowen B, Hawk JJ, Sibunka S, et al. A review of the reported defects in the human C1 esterase inhibitor gene producing hereditary angioedema including four new mutations. Clin Immunol 2001;98:157.
99. Markovic SN, Inwards DJ, Frigas EA, et al. Acquired C1 esterase inhibitor deficiency. Ann Intern Med 2000;132:144.
100. Cicardi M, Agostoni A. Hereditary angioedema. N Engl J Med 1996;334:1666.
101. Nussberger J, Cugno M, Cicardi M, et al. Local bradykinin generation in hereditary angio-edema. J Allergy Clin Immunol 1999;104:1321.
102. Warner KK, Visconti JA, Tschampel MM. Angiotensin II receptor blockers in patients with ACE inhibitor-induced angioedema. Ann Pharmacother 2000;34:526.
103. Leznoff A, Sussman GL. Syndrome of idiopathic chronic urticaria and angioedema with thyroid autoimmunity: a study of 90 patients. J Allergy Clin Immunol 1989;84:66.
104. Tong LJ, Balakrishnan G, Kochan JP, et al. Assessment of autoimmunity in patients with chronic urticaria. J Allergy Clin Immunol 1997;99:461.
105. Hide M, Francis DM, Grattan CE, et al. Autoantibodies against the high-affinity IgE receptor as a cause of histamine release in chronic urticaria. N Engl J Med 1993;328:1599.
106. Mansfield LE, Smith JA, Nelson HS. Greater inhibition of dermographia with a combination of H1 and H2 antagonists. Ann Allergy 1983; 50:264.
107. Goldsobel AB, Rohr AS, Siegel SC, et al. Efficacy of doxepin in the treatment of chronic idiopathic urticaria. J Allergy Clin Immunol 1986;78:867.
108. Doeglas HM. Reactions to aspirin and food additives in patients with chronic urticaria, including the physical urticarias. Br J Dermatol 1975;93:135.
109. Cicardi M, Castelli R, Zingale LC, et al. Side effects of long-term prophylaxis with attenuated androgens in hereditary angioedema: comparison of treated and untreated patients. J Allergy Clin Immunol 1997;99:194.
110. Waytes AT, Rosen FS, Frank MM. Treatment of hereditary angioedema with a vapor-heated C1 inihibitor concentrate. N Engl J Med 1996;20:1630.
111. Kozel MM, Mekkes JR, Bossuyt PM, et al. Natural course of physical and chronic urticaria and angioedema in 220 patients. J Am Acad Dermatol 2001;45:387.
112. Gruchalla RS. Drug metabolism, danger signals, and drug-induced hypersensitivity. J Allergy Clin Immunol 2001;108:475.
113. Lazarou J, Pomeranz BH, Corey PN. Incidence of adverse drug reactions in hospitalized patients: a meta-analysis of prospective studies. JAMA 1998;279:1200.
114. Gruchalla R. Understanding drug allergies. J Allergy Clin Immunol 2000;105:S637.
115. Salkind AR, Cuddy PG, Foxworth JW. Is this patient allergic to penicillin? An evidence-based analysis of the likelihood of penicillin allergy. JAMA 2001;285:2498.
116. Adkinson NF Jr. Risk factors for drug allergy. J Allergy Clin Immunol 1984;74:567.
117. Strom BL, Schinnar R, Apter AJ, et al. Absence of cross-reactivity between sulfonamide antibiotics and sulfonamide nonantibiotics. N Engl J Med 2003;349:1628.
118. Gadde J, Spence M, Wheeler B, et al. Clinical experience with penicillin skin testing in a large inner-city STD clinic. JAMA 1993;270:2456.
119. Weiss ME, Adkinson NF. Immediate hypersensitivity reactions to penicillin and related antibiotics. Clin Allergy 1988;18:515.
120. Kelkar PS, Li JT. Cephalosporin allergy. N Engl J Med 2001;345:804.
121. Saxon A, Adelman DC, Patel A, et al. Imipenem cross-reactivity with penicillin in humans. J Allergy Clin Immunol 1988;82:213.
122. Adkinson NF Jr. Immunogenicity and cross-allergenicity of aztreonam. Am J Med 1990;88:12S.
123. Green GR, Rosenblum AH, Sweet LC. Evaluation of penicillin hypersensitivity: value of clinical history and skin testing with penicilloyl-polylysine and penicillin G. A cooperative prospective study of the penicillin study group of the American Academy of Allergy. J Allergy Clin Immunol 1977;60:339.
124. Bittner A, Greenberger PA. Incidence of resensitization after tolerating penicillin treatment in penicillin-allergic patients. Allergy Asthma Proc 2004;25:161.
125. Settipane RA, Schrank PJ, Simon RA, et al. Prevalence of cross-sensitivity with acetaminophen in aspirin-sensitive asthmatic subjects. J Allergy Clin Immunol 1995;96:480.
126. Gollapudi RR, Teirstein PS, Stevenson DD, Simon RA. Aspirin sensitivity: implications for patients with coronary artery disease. JAMA 2004;292:3017.
127. Greenberger PA, Patterson R. The prevention of immediate generalized reactions to radiocontrast media in high-risk patients. J Allergy Clin Immunol 1991;87:867.
128. Barrett BJ, Parfrey PS, McDonald JR, et al. Nonionic low-osmolality versus ionic high-osmolality contrast material for intravenous use in patients perceived to be at high risk: randomized trial. Radiology 1992; 183:105.
129. Sampson HA. Food allergy. Part 1. Immunopathogenesis and clinical disorders. J Allergy Clin Immunol 1999;103:717.

130. Bock SA. The incidence of severe adverse reactions to food in Colorado. J Allergy Clin Immunol 1992;90:683.
131. Bock S, Munoz-Furlong A, Sampson H. Fatalities due to anaphylactic reactions to foods. J Allergy Clin Immunol 2001;107:191.
132. Sicherer SH, Munoz-Furlong A, Burks AW, et al. Prevalence of peanut and tree nut allergy in the US determined by a random digit dial telephone survey. J Allergy Clin Immunol 1999;103:559.
133. Kidd JM 3rd, Cohen SH, Sosman AJ, et al. Food-dependent exercise-induced anaphylaxis. J Allergy Clin Immunol 1983;71:407.
134. Tan BM, Sher MR, Good RA, et al. Severe food allergies by skin contact. Ann Allergy Asthma Immunol 2001;86:583.
135. Sampson HA, Ho DG. Relationship between food-specific IgE concentrations and the risk of positive food challenges in children and adolescents. J Allergy Clin Immunol 1997;100:444.
136. Bock SA, Sampson HA, Atkins FM, et al. Double-blind, placebo-controlled food challenge (DBPCFC) as an office procedure: a manual. J Allergy Clin Immunol 1988;82:986.
137. Leung DY, Sampson HA, Yunginger JW, et al. Effect of anti-IgE therapy in patients with peanut allergy. N Engl J Med. 2003;348:986.
138. Sampson HA. Food allergy. Part 2. Diagnosis and management. J Allergy Clin Immunol 1999;103:981.
139. The discontinuation of Hymenoptera venom immunotherapy. Report from the Committee on Insects. J Allergy Clin Immunol 1998;101:573.
140. Kemp SF, deShazo RD, Moffitt JE, et al. Expanding habitat of the imported fire ant (*Solenopsis invicta*): a public health concern. J Allergy Clin Immunol 2000;105:683.
141. Golden DB, Kagey-Sobotka A, Lichtenstein LM. Survey of patients after discontinuing venom immunotherapy. J Allergy Clin Immunol 2000;105:385.
142. Golden DB, Kagey-Sobotka A, Norman PS, et al. Outcomes of allergy to insect stings in children, with and without venom immunotherapy. N Engl J Med 2004;351:668.
143. Clark S, Long AA, Gaeta TJ, et al. Multicenter study of emergency department visits for insect sting allergies. J Allergy Clin Immunol 2005;116:643.
144. Poley GE Jr, Slater JE. Latex allergy. J Allergy Clin Immunol 2000;105:1054.
145. Rodriguez M, Vega F, Garcia MT, et al. Hypersensitivity to latex, chestnut, and banana. Ann Allergy 1993;70:31.

For annotated ***General References*** *and resources related to this chapter, visit www.hopkinsbayview.org/PAMreferences.*

Chapter 31

Approach to the Patient with Fever

Paul G. Auwaerter

Clinicians may often encounter febrile patients whose initial history and physical examination offer few clues toward achieving a diagnosis. For patients who present with elevated temperatures, the fever may be a secondary concern; for example, when severe headache and meningismus focus attention on meningitis. In other circumstances, a fever with shaking chill may herald an illness soon recognized as pneumonia with the onset of a productive cough and dyspnea, or it may evolve into an apparently self-limiting viral illness. However, for isolated or persisting fevers, achieving a diagnosis often depends on medical sleuthing using a meticulous history, careful physical examination, and judicious application of diagnostic tests.

MEASUREMENT AND DEFINITIONS

Patient temperatures are reported in the United States as either centigrade (C) or Fahrenheit (F). Values may be converted according to the following:

$$°C = 5/9(°F - 32)$$
$$°F = (9/5)°C + 32$$

Defining normal body temperature is an imprecise science, because values obtained from modern studies depend upon the study method used. An individual's normal oral temperature can range between 96°F and 100.7°F (35.6°C to 38.2°C). Normal circadian patterns cause body temperature to vary by 1.8°F (1°C), with the nadir reached typically at 6 a.m. and the peak between 4 and 6 p.m. Individual patient temperatures may differ depending on the recording instrument, because thermometers are often poorly calibrated and differ in design (mercury vs. electronic) and anatomic location of measurement (oral, axillary, rectal, tympanic).

Accurate oral readings depend on whether the probe is properly located in the sublingual pocket. Smokers may have higher than normal readings, whereas recent ingestion of a cold beverage may transiently lower oral readings. In very hot weather or after intense exercise, body temperature may rise 0.9°F to 1.8°F (0.5°C to 1.0°C).

The most commonly recognized "normal" body temperature of 98.6°F (37°C) is based on somewhat antiquated medical lore. Mackowiak et al. (1) described the likely 19th century origin of this criterion; it was derived from the work of a German physician, Carl Wunderlich, who obtained mostly axillary measurements in over 25,000 subjects. In his critical comparative study, Mackowiak et al. found that with modern readings in healthy men and women, the mean oral temperature was 98.2°F ± 0.7°F (36.8°C ± 0.4°C). Rectal thermometry provides measurements with less variation, but patients and health care providers dislike this more accurate form of temperature assessment. To compare temperatures by different methods, consider rectal temperatures as 0.7°F (0.4°C) higher than oral measurements and 1.4°F (0.8°C) higher than those obtained with the convenient and popular aural (tympanic membrane) device (2).

Because defining normal temperature is inexact, it is not surprising that fever terminology is also variable. Surveys of medical textbooks reveal varying proposals for defining fever that range from any temperatures greater than 98.6°F (37.0°C) to only those greater than 100.4°F (38.0°C) (3). Many clinicians define a significant fever as a temperature greater than 101.0°F (38.3°C), which is likely grounded in the classic study on fever of unknown origin (FUO) by Petersdorf and Beeson (4).

FEVER OF ABRUPT ONSET AND LIMITED DURATION

The clinician should first determine whether a fever needs any diagnostic investigation. Many illnesses without localizing signs in otherwise healthy individuals may be due to common viruses, such as rhinovirus infection causing the common cold. These fevers tend to be low grade, with temperatures less than 102.2°F (39°C), and do not last beyond 5 to 7 days. However, some infections that start only with fever and other nonspecific symptoms should be considered in certain situations. Table 31.1 lists selected infections that may first present in the office with fever and require additional attention.

For example, high fevers to 104°F (40°C) associated with chills, myalgia, and cough during wintertime may be due to influenza (see Chapter 33). In contrast, summertime fever with malaise and headache in an active outdoorsman or gardener may be the first sign of a tick-borne infection such as Lyme disease, ehrlichiosis, or Rocky Mountain spotted fever (see Chapter 38). Patients who use intravenous drugs or practice high-risk sex may have acute human immunodeficiency virus (HIV) infection (Chapter 39), viral hepatitis (hepatitis B or C, see Chapter 47), or venereal diseases such as syphilis or gonorrhea (see Chapter 37) as the cause of febrile illness. Teenagers or young adults may have an isolated fever before the development of pharyngitis or lymphadenopathy associated with infectious mononucleosis (see Chapters 33 and 58). Viral exanthems may present first with fever in adolescents or adults who are not naturally immune or who were not adequately vaccinated (see Chapter 18). Nowadays, consideration of bioterrorism agents, such as anthrax and smallpox in the evaluation of fever, may be necessary in certain circumstances.

In the elderly, fever generally indicates the presence of serious infection, most often caused by bacteria from urinary or respiratory sources, even when localizing symptoms are absent (5). Because significant temperature elevation may be absent in 20% to 30% of elderly patients with a serious infection, elderly patients should be considered febrile when they have an elevated body temperature of approximately 2°F (1°C) above baseline values.

DRUG FEVER

Elevation of temperature in response to a drug without the presence of rash is known as a drug fever, though it should be more properly termed "drug hypersensitivity." Although the exact incidence of drug fever is unknown, it may occur in up to 10% of hospitalized patients (6). In ambulatory patients, who are typically on fewer medications, drug fever occurs less frequently.

Contrary to popular conceptions, drug fever usually does not cause a sustained pattern of temperature elevation. There is a variable lag time between initiation of the offending drug and onset of fever, most commonly occurring within 1 or 2 weeks (7). Relative bradycardia is an important clue that may assist the physician in considering drug fever as the cause of an otherwise unexplained temperature elevation, along with a general impression that the patient is not acutely ill. Such a pulse–temperature dissociation can only be determined if a patient has a fever greater than 102°F (38.8°C) and does not have a cardiac conduction disturbance such as sick sinus syndrome or medication effect (e.g., β-blockers). The appropriate pulse for a given temperature is estimated by taking the last digit of the Fahrenheit reading and subtracting 1 and then multiplying by 10 and adding 100 (6). For example, a patient with a temperature of 104°F (40°C) should have a pulse of 130 beats per minutes ($[4 - 1] \times 10 + 100$).

Patients with drug fever will often be unaware of a significant fever, and chills are uncommon. A generalized maculopapular rash may eventually arise in some patients affected by drug fever. There are no diagnostic laboratory features, although the erythrocyte sedimentation rate (ESR) may be elevated to levels exceeding 100 millimeter per hour, and eosinophilia may be found in a small percentage of patients. Fever induced by drugs such as barbiturates, methyldopa, phenytoin, and sulfonamides may herald the development of a serum sickness syndrome with rash, lymphadenopathy, arthritis, and nephritis. Other

TABLE 31.1 Infections That May Present Initially with Fever Alone

Infection	*Clinical Features other than Fever*	*Special Considerations*
Anthrax (*Bacillus anthracis*)	Malaise, mild cough or chest pain; respiratory distress and mediastinitis follow. Bloody pleural effusions are characteristic.	Bioterrorism agent; usually infrequent, sporadic in industrialized areas; occupational hazard of workers exposed to animals or animal products
Chickenpox (varicella)	Pruritic maculopapular rash evolves in hours to vesicles and in days to scabs	Malaise and fever precede or occur simultaneously with rash; highly contagious
Ehrlichia or anaplasma	Headache, chills, myalgia; abnormal liver function tests, leukopenia, thrombocytopenia common	Spring, summer with tick exposure risk
German measles (rubella)	Maculopapular (occasionally confluent) rash begins on forehead and spreads to trunk and extremities	1- to 7-day prodrome of malaise, headache, mild conjunctivitis
Influenza	Headache, myalgia, chills; cough may evolve to pneumonia	Wintertime, may cause epidemics; high mortality among the chronically ill and elderly
Infectious mononucleosis (*Epstein-Barr virus*)	Pharyngitis, lymphadenopathy, splenomegaly	Atypical lymphocytes, Monospot positive 90%; differential diagnosis also includes acute HIV infection, acute viral hepatitis, rubella, acute toxoplasmosis, acute cytomegalovirus infection, adverse drug reaction
Leptospirosis (*Leptospira interrogans*)	Headache, chills, severe myalgia (calves and thighs), conjunctival suffusion, multiple organ involvement	Sudden onset of fever. Acquired from contact with skin, especially if abraded, or mucous membranes of water, moist soil, or vegetation contaminated with urine of infected animals
Lyme disease (*Borrelia burgdorferi*)	Bull's eye rash classic (rash may be not noted ~20%) but homogenous ovoid erythema more common; chills, myalgia, arthralgia, headache	Spring, summer with tick exposure risk; fever usually only with acute disease <4 wks
Malaria (*Plasmodium* species)	Headache, myalgia, back pain, abdominal pain	Any traveler with fever returning from a malarious country should be considered to have malaria until proven otherwise; rare cause of blood transfusion-related infection
Measles (rubeola)	Maculopapular rash spreading from face to neck to trunk, to feet by third day. Koplik's spots on buccal mucosa are characteristic	3- to 4-day prodrome with fever, malaise, hacking cough, rhinitis, subsiding 1–2 days after onset of rash
Parvovirus (B19)	Myalgia, intense arthralgia or arthritis, lacy rash; women more afflicted than men	Exposure to daycare or school-aged children
Q fever (*Rickettsia burnetii*)	Headache, chills, anorexia, myalgias, cough, rales	Spread by airborne rickettsiae in dust contaminated by infected animals (cattle, sheep, goats) or by direct contact with infected animals or their tissue
Rocky Mountain spotted fever (*Rickettsia rickettsii*)	Headache, chills, myalgia; petechial rash; classic, maculopapular rash more commonly, but never present in ~10%	Spring, summer with tick exposure risk; life threatening, early treatment with doxycycline essential
Smallpox (variola major)	Malaise, headache, backache, occasional abdominal pain and vomiting; followed by maculopapular to vesicular to pustular rash beginning on face and extremities	Now only a bioterrorism agent; last naturally acquired case worldwide in 1977

HIV, human immunodeficiency virus.

drugs such as procainamide, quinine, and hydralazine may cause a lupus-like syndrome with arthritis, serositis, and production of antinuclear and antihistone antibodies.

Table 31.2 lists commonly prescribed medications that are most likely to cause drug fever. Drugs that are not known to cause hypersensitivity reactions include aminoglycosides, digitalis preparations, and insulins.

The diagnosis of drug fever requires a high index of suspicion, because the often insidious onset may obscure the cause. Withdrawal of the suspected offending agent should result in defervescence within several days but may take weeks in drugs requiring prolonged periods of elimination (e.g., amiodarone, iodides, isoniazid). Conclusive evidence that a drug has caused a febrile reaction can only be proved

TABLE 31.2 Drugs Commonly Implicated in the Development of Fever due to Hypersensitivity

Allopurinol
Amphotericin B
Anti-thymocyte antibodies
Atropine
Azathioprine
Barbiturates
Bleomycin
Cephalosporins
Heparin
Hydralazine
Interferons
Isoniazid
Iodides (including i.v. contrast media)
Methyldopa
Penicillamine
Penicillins
Phenytoin
Procainamide
Propylthiouracil
Rifampin
Quinidine
Nonsteroidal anti-inflammatory drugs (NSAIDs)
Salicylates
Streptokinase
Sulfonamides

by rechallenge, but this should not be entertained unless that medication is expected to be important for future therapy and no end-organ damage was associated with initial administration.

The most serious febrile reaction to drugs, malignant hyperthermia, occurs as an idiosyncratic response to neuroleptic medications such as haloperidol, thiothixene or phenothiazines (the *neuroleptic malignant syndrome*), or to certain anesthetic agents (8,9). Abrupt fever up to 105.8°F (41°C) is accompanied by altered mentation, muscular rigidity, and labile blood pressure. Few infectious processes cause temperatures elevations beyond 105.8°F (41°C), perhaps with the exception of malaria. The human body usually cannot survive fever greater than 107.6°F (42°C) (10). The differential diagnosis of extreme pyrexia otherwise includes only HIV infection, heat stroke, and central fevers because of hypothalamic injury by stroke, tumor, or infection.

FEVER OF UNKNOWN ORIGIN

Fevers of 101°F (38.3°C) or greater lasting for more than 3 weeks without a diagnosis, despite 1 week of intensive diagnostic investigation in hospital, or fever of unknown origin, has been the traditional definition of FUO (4,11). As a practical matter, this definition has become too restrictive because patients with FUO are less commonly hospitalized and even complex evaluations are now frequently performed on an outpatient basis. Therefore, a patient may be considered to have an FUO if temperature elevations to 101°F (38.3°C) or more persist beyond 3 weeks with negative blood culture studies and no other apparent explanation (12). It has also been proposed that FUO may be diagnosed when fevers remained undiagnosed despite at least three outpatient visits or at least 3 days in the hospital (13).

Diagnostic tests such as computed tomography (CT), magnetic resonance imaging (MRI), and serologic analyses have advanced considerably since the early published literature on FUO. Rheumatologic and infectious etiologies now comprise a smaller proportion of FUOs, although infectious causes remain the leading category, accounting for 25% to 50% of achieved diagnoses in recent series (14–16). Common causes of FUO (Table 31.3) account for up to half of the explanations in published series. Exhaustive lists of potential causes of FUO can be found in several reference sources (12,17).

Some recent demographic trends may be important in the evaluation of FUO. For the category of infection, classic pulmonary tuberculosis rarely leads to FUO because radiographic findings of cavitary disease suggest the proper diagnosis. *Extrapulmonary tuberculosis* such as

TABLE 31.3 Categories and Leading Diseases Causing Fever of Unknown Origin

Infections
Culture-negative endocarditis
Extrapulmonary tuberculosis
Intra-abdominal/hepatic abscess
Chronic osteomyelitis
Cytomegalovirus
Neoplasia
Lymphoma
Metastases to liver or brain
Peritoneal carcinomatosis
Renal cell carcinoma
Myelodysplastic syndrome
Rheumatologic
Temporal (giant cell) arteritis
Still disease (adult-onset, juvenile rheumatoid arthritis)
Vasculitis (polyarteritis nodosa, hypersensitivity vasculitis)
Miscellaneous
Drug fever
Granulomatous hepatitis
Sarcoidosis
Inflammatory bowel disease
Cirrhosis
Alcoholic hepatitis
Factitious fever
Habitual hyperthermia

40. Buysschaert I, Vanderschueren S, Blockmans D, et al. Contribution of (18) fluoro-deoxyglucose positron emission tomography to the work-up of patients with fever of unknown origin. Eur J Med 2004;15:151.
41. Kjaer A, Lebech AM, Eigtved A, et al. Fever of unknown origin: prospective comparison of diagnostic value of 18F-FDG PET and ^{111}In-granulocyte scintigraphy. Eur J Nucl Med Mol Imaging 2004;31:622.
42. Ryan EW, Bolger AF. Transesophageal echocardiography (TEE) in the evaluation of infective endocarditis. Cardiol Clin 2000;18: 773.
43. Volk EE, Miller ML, Kirkley BA, et al. The diagnostic usefulness of bone marrow cultures in patients with fever of unknown origin. Am J Clin Pathol 1998;110:150.
44. Holtz T, Moseley RH, Scheiman JM. Liver biopsy in fever of unknown origin. A reappraisal. J Clin Gastroenterol 1993;17:29.
45. Gleckman R. Fever of unknown origin: the value of abdominal exploration. Postgrad Med 1977; 62:191.
46. Chang JC, Gross HM. Utility of naproxen in the differential diagnosis of fever of undetermined origin in patients with cancer. Am J Med 1984; 76:597.
47. Vanderschueren S, Knockaert D, Peetermans WE, et al. Lack of value of the naproxen test in the differential diagnosis of prolonged febrile illness. Am J Med 2003;115:572.
48. Harris HW, Mentiove S. Miliary tuberculosis. In: Schlossberg D, ed. Tuberculosis. New York: Springer-Verlag, 1994:233.
49. Suzuki A, Ohosone Y, Mita S, et al. Fever of unknown origin responding to steroid therapy. Nihon Rinsho Meneki Gakkai Kaishi 1997;20: 21.
50. Roberts NJ Jr. Temperature and host defense. Microbiol Rev 1979;43:241.
51. Styrt B, Sugarman B. Antipyresis and fever. Arch Intern Med 1990;150:1589.
52. Klein NC, Cunha BA. Treatment of fever. Infect Dis Clin North Am 1996;10:211.
53. Whitcomb DC, Block GD. Association of acetaminophen hepatotoxicity with fasting and ethanol use. JAMA 1994;272:1845.

*For annotated **General References** and resources related to this chapter, visit www.hopkinsbayview.org/PAMreferences.*

Chapter 32

Bacterial Infections of the Skin*

Patrick A. Murphy

*Nathaniel F. Pierce, MD, contributed to earlier versions of this chapter.

Most skin infections are trivial and can be managed at home without medical assistance. Each year, however, approximately 5% of the population develop a skin infection that requires medical attention. The severity of these infections depends on the virulence of the infecting organisms and the state of host defenses. The most common infecting organisms are *Streptococcus pyogenes* and *Staphylococcus aureus*. In otherwise healthy people, these often cause only modest morbidity and respond rapidly to appropriate treatment. They can, however, cause serious infections, especially in diabetic patients, in patients with impaired blood supply to the infected site, impaired lymphatic or venous drainage of the site, and in patients with defects in leukocytic or immunologic defense mechanisms. Serious infection is also more likely when other bacteria, or combinations of bacteria, are involved, as occurs in bites or contaminated wounds.

SUPERFICIAL INFECTIONS CAUSED BY *S. PYOGENES* AND *S. AUREUS*

Impetigo, ecthyma, and erysipelas are superficial infections usually caused by group A hemolytic streptococci (*S. pyogenes*) and *S. aureus* (1). These infections arise from breaks in the skin that are often so minor they are unnoticed.

Impetigo

Impetigo occurs mostly among preschool children, especially in warm, humid climates or when personal hygiene is poor (2). Under these conditions, the disease is highly contagious and outbreaks may occur. Older children and adults are only occasionally affected.

Impetigo begins as a pruritic, focal, superficial eruption of small 1- to 2-mm *vesicles,* often on the face near the nares, chin, or lower extremities. There is usually no history of trauma. In several days, the vesicles change to pustules that break, become crusted, and have an erythematous base. Regional lymphadenopathy is common, but there are no constitutional symptoms. The process may spread because of scratching. Healing occurs without scarring. Impetigo may recur if personal hygiene is not improved.

Bullous impetigo is caused by strains of *S. aureus*that secrete one of the epidermolytic toxins (3). Epidemics of bullous impetigo can occur among newborns, but only sporadic cases are seen in older children, and adult cases are uncommon. The process begins as a macular erythematous rash. The characteristic thin-walled, fluid-filled, superficial bullae appear within 1 to 3 days, range from 1 cm to several centimeters in diameter, and usually involve exposed areas of the body. These bullae rupture, desquamation occurs, and healing without scarring follows in about 7 days. In its most dramatic form, this process causes the scalded skin syndrome, a disease of small children in which there is extensive superficial desquamation.

Ecthyma

Ecthyma occurs under the same conditions of poor hygiene that promote impetigo. It is characterized by 3- to 10-mm *discrete, ulcerating lesions with an adherent necrotic crust and surrounding erythema;* a small amount of pus often underlies the crust. The ulcer is sufficiently deep to cause permanent scarring. Lesions are most common on the anterior tibial surface at sites of minor trauma or insect bites. Left untreated, the lesions tend to spread distally and there may be associated lymphadenopathy; systemic symptoms, however, are lacking. Cultures of pus may yield both *S. pyogenes* and *S. aureus.* There is evidence that *S. aureus* causes a majority of the cases. Lesions with a similar appearance may result from bacteremia with *Pseudomonas aeruginosa.*

Erysipelas

Erysipelas involves progressive, often rapid spread of infection through superficial layers of skin and lymphatics. It may occur after a minor wound in normal skin but is more likely when prior injury or disease has impaired the lymphatic or venous drainage of the skin or left extensive scarring, as, for example, in a patient with chronic venous insufficiency of the lower extremities or lymphedema of the arm after radical mastectomy. Most episodes of erysipelas are caused by *S. pyogenes.* A few are caused by *S. aureus* or other agents, such as *Pasteurella multocida* or *Erysipelothrix rhusiopathiae* (see sections Bites, Cellulitis, Wound Infections, and Table 32.4), and these cannot always be distinguished clinically.

Erysipelas is characterized by a rapidly spreading area of marked erythema with warmth, local pain, an elevated sharp margin between involved and uninvolved skin, and firm edema that gives the skin a typical "orange peel" appearance. There may be seropurulent drainage at the inoculation site, but fluctuation and dermal necrosis are lacking. Erythema often extends centrally along superficial draining lymphatics; regional lymph nodes are often enlarged and tender. Systemic toxicity, chills, and fever are common. If it is untreated, metastatic infection may occur, and there is appreciable mortality. Facial infections are especially dangerous because of possible intracranial spread via draining lymphatics or veins. Extensive involvement of the trunk also carries an increased risk of death.

Management

Bacterial cultures of the lesions of impetigo, bullous impetigo, and ecthyma usually are not helpful. Impetigo and ecthyma may reveal mixed cultures of *S. pyogenes* and *S. aureus,* or either agent alone, whereas lesions of bullous impetigo are often sterile. Blood cultures should be obtained when erysipelas is extensive or is associated with marked systemic toxicity (e.g., temperature greater than 102°F [39°C], shaking chills, severe malaise). Attempts to isolate an organism by culturing sterile saline that has been injected and withdrawn through a fine needle at the edge of the lesion have a low yield and are not useful. If there is seropurulent drainage from the lesions, it should be cultured.

Antimicrobial therapy is required for most of these infections (Tables 32.1 and 32.2). Minor cases of impetigo, with no systemic symptoms and few local symptoms, can be treated with antibacterial ointments such as bacitracin. Topical mupirocin (Bactroban) was recommended previously, but resistance develops very rapidly and it is no longer recommended. If the rash is spreading rapidly, or there are many cases in a school or a village, it is probably wise to use a systemic antibiotic.

Impetigo and ecthyma are treated similarly. Dicloxacillin, cephalexin, and other penicillinase-resistant β-lactams are usually effective oral antimicrobials. Erythromycin is also frequently effective. These simple antibiotics probably work because most of the cases are partially or solely attributable to streptococci. Adjunctive therapy includes careful daily soaking of lesions to remove crusted debris using warm water with an iodophor (a soap that releases iodine in a nontoxic, nonstaining form, such as

TABLE 32.1 Antibiotic Selection for Superficial and Pustular Skin Infections[a]

Infection	Antibiotic	Route
Superficial Infections		
Impetigo	Dicloxacillin or cephalexin	Oral
	Erythromycin	Oral
Ecthyma	As for impetigo	
Erysipelas		
Mild	Penicillin V	Oral
	Erythromycin	Oral
Severe	Penicillin G	Intravenous
Pustular Infections		
Folliculitis	None	
Furunculosis, boils	Dicloxacillin or cephalexin	Oral
	Erythromycin	Oral
Bullous impetigo	As for furunculosis	Oral
Carbuncle	As for furunculosis	Oral
	Nafcillin	Intravenous
	Vancomycin	Intravenous
Cellulitis	As for carbuncle	
Any of the above known or likely to be caused by MRSA infection	Trimethoprim-sulfamethoxazole	Oral
	Linezolid	Oral
	Vancomycin	Intravenous

[a]Dosage recommendations are in Table 32.2. Other penicillinase-resistant oral β-lactams may also be given.

Betadine skin cleanser) or with a soap that contains hexachlorophene (e.g., pHisoHex). Prevention depends primarily on improved personal hygiene; the most important preventive measure is careful frequent skin cleansing with soap and water.

Treatment of *bullous impetigo* should be directed at penicillin-resistant staphylococci. Oral dicloxacillin and cephalexin are the standard initial treatment, but in some communities as many as 50% of *S. aureus* are resistant. If these antibiotics fail, the patient should be treated with a regimen which covers methicillin-resistant *S. aureus* (MRSA, see Pustular Infections Caused by *S. aureus*).

Minor episodes of *erysipelas* may be treated with oral penicillin V or erythromycin. Application of moist heat to the affected area appears to hasten clearing of the infection. Serious episodes are those with marked systemic toxicity, extensive lesions, or facial lesions and those occurring in compromised hosts (e.g., diabetics). Such patients have an appreciable mortality, and they require hospitalization and intravenous treatment with penicillin G (Tables 32.1 and 32.2).

Special attention should also be paid to patients with atherosclerotic peripheral vascular disease who have infections of their lower extremities. Such patients should be put at bed rest, or at least couch rest. The leg should be at approximately the same height as the heart. If the

TABLE 32.2 Antibiotic Dosage and Schedule for Skin Infections Caused by *Streptococcus pyogenes* and *Staphylococcus aureus* in Adults

Antibiotic	Dosage
Ambulatory treatment (mild infection)	
Dicloxacillin	250 mg PO t.i.d.
Cephalexin	500 mg PO q.i.d.
Erythromycin	250–500 mg PO t.i.d.
Penicillin V	500 mg PO t.i.d.
Ambulatory treatment (MRSA)	
Trimethoprim-sulfamethoxazole	1 double-strength tablet q.12h
Linezolid	400 mg q 12h
Parenteral treatment (severe infection)	
Penicillin G	600,000–2,000,000 units IV q6h
Nafcillin or oxacillin	1–2 g IV q4–6h (dose and interval depend on severity)
Vancomycin	1g IV q 12h (less in elderly or in patients with renal failure)

leg is elevated too much, the blood pressure in distal arteries may become so low that blood does not reach the toes. If the leg is too dependent, it may become edematous. Either eventuality will result in difficulty in clearing infection. Sustained pressure on any part of the leg or foot should be avoided because it is likely to result in a decubitus ulcer.

Patients with chronic edema caused by damage to the veins or lymphatics of an extremity may experience repeated episodes of erysipelas or cellulitis that cause further damage. More than 95% of such infections are caused by hemolytic streptococci. While Group A causes some cases, most are due to streptococci of other Lancefield types—B, C, F, or G. Fortunately, hemolytic streptococci have not (yet) developed resistance to penicillin G. Patients who have numerous recurrent infections should receive continuous antibiotic prophylaxis with penicillin V (250 mg twice daily), benzathine penicillin (600,000 units intramuscularly monthly), or erythromycin (250 mg twice daily). Reduction of chronic edema by use of fitted pressure stockings or by administration of diuretics helps reduce susceptibility to this infection.

Superficial skin infections respond rapidly to appropriate therapy. Systemic toxicity and erythema associated with erysipelas usually abate within 3 or 4 days, and discrete skin lesions show marked healing within 10 days. During this period, activity should be restricted in accord with the extent of the infection. Minor lesions require no restrictions. Patients with any form of impetigo should avoid contact with infants and small children until lesions heal.

Complications

Streptococcal skin infections do not cause rheumatic fever, but they may cause *acute glomerulonephritis* if the streptococcal strain is nephritogenic. Nephritis is not prevented by antimicrobial therapy. The average latency period between initial symptoms of a streptococcal skin infection and the onset of glomerulonephritis is 2 weeks. If a nephritogenic strain is known to be in the community, initial and 14-day followup evaluation should include a urinalysis. Most patients who develop poststreptococcal glomerulonephritis are asymptomatic, but in some, glomerulonephritis is first suggested by gross hematuria; acute hypertension; and signs of salt and water retention, such as dependent edema or congestive heart failure (CHF).

Bacteremia with metastatic infection may complicate neglected or severe episodes of erysipelas. Metastatic infection should be considered in patients with severe disease that responds poorly to treatment or if findings develop that are suggestive of distant localized infection. Possible metastatic infections include meningitis, endocarditis, septic arthritis, infection of pre-existing pleural effusions or ascites, and solid organ abscesses (e.g., liver, spleen).

PUSTULAR INFECTIONS CAUSED BY *S. AUREUS*

These include folliculitis, furunculosis, hidradenitis suppurativa, and carbuncles. They represent increasingly severe effects of the infection of hair follicles, sebaceous glands, or sweat glands by *S. aureus,* the result being inflammation and abscess formation.

Folliculitis

Folliculitis involves minor inflammation of individual hair follicles, often with formation of small superficial pustules. There is little pain or surrounding erythema. In some people, lesions recur for months or even years. A common area of involvement is the bearded part of the face, where minor trauma from shaving may be a contributing factor.

Furunculosis

Deeper infection of follicles or cutaneous glands leads to formation of pustular furuncles. *Boils* are large furuncles. They range in diameter from about 5 mm to 2 or 3 cm and occur most commonly on hairy areas exposed to friction, trauma, or maceration (e.g., buttocks, neck, face, axillae, groin, forearms, thighs, upper back). Furunculosis may also complicate the acne of adolescence. Furuncles begin with pruritus, local tenderness, and erythema, followed by swelling and marked local pain. As pus forms in the center of the lesion, the overlying skin becomes thin, the lesion becomes elevated, pain increases, and spontaneous drainage of pus ultimately occurs, usually with prompt relief of pain and rapid healing. Furunculosis may be recurrent in some people, especially diabetics and chronic nasal carriers of *S. aureus*.

Hidradenitis Suppurativa

Hidradenitis suppurativa is a noninfectious skin disease characterized by obstruction of the ducts of apocrine sweat glands in the axilla, perineum, or groin. The process begins at puberty when these glands become active, and it comes to light when staphylococcal infection of one or several of the obstructed glands occurs. Such episodes initially respond well to antimicrobials, but because antimicrobials do nothing for the primary condition, the infections recur. After several years, infection becomes chronic, with multiple scars and numerous draining abscesses and sinus tracts. By this time, the bacterial flora is usually gram negative, with *Proteus* and *Pseudomonas* commonly found.

Carbuncles

A carbuncle is a coalescent mass of deeply infected follicles or sebaceous glands with multiple interconnecting sinus tracts and cutaneous openings that drain pus ineffectively. Carbuncles usually occur in the thick skin on the back of the neck or upper back. Once formed, the lesions steadily worsen, with increasing pain, erythema, swelling, purulent drainage, and lateral enlargement; they vary in diameter from 3 to 10 cm or larger. Fever and systemic toxicity are common, and bacteremia may be present. Carbuncles occur with increased frequency in diabetics and may cause a major increase in the severity of diabetes. Patients who are normally sustained on an oral agent or who were not previously known to be diabetic may present in ketosis.

Management

Bacterial cultures of typical pustular lesions are usually unnecessary because virtually all are caused by *S. aureus* and most isolates prove resistant to penicillin G. Increasingly, these infections are caused by MRSA, and cultures should be done if standard treatment fails.

Minimal lesions, such as *folliculitis,* require little therapy. Careful, twice-daily cleansing with a mild soap, preferably one containing hexachlorophene, and avoidance of minor trauma and irritants, such as cosmetics or abrasive soaps, are usually sufficient.

Furuncles should be managed initially by gentle application of warm moist heat (as moist compresses or baths) for about 30 minutes four times a day. Traditionally, compresses contain hyper-osmotic solutions of substances such as glycerin and magnesium sulfate to "draw the pus out," and they probably work. The patient should be instructed to avoid squeezing or pressing on the furuncle. Lesions less than 1 cm in diameter often drain spontaneously after 1 to 3 days and require no further treatment. Larger lesions, painful lesions, and lesions that do not drain spontaneously should be *drained surgically when they are fluctuant.* This can be done in the office by making a single incision into the abscess with a scalpel, after first infiltrating the incision line with 0.5% or 1.0% lidocaine for local anesthesia. Lifting the anesthetized skin with a forceps when the incision is made helps avoid pain caused by downward pressure from the scalpel. Packing with iodoform gauze for 1 or 2 days may be needed to control oozing of serosanguineous discharge after surgical drainage. Antimicrobial therapy is required only for extensive lesions such as multiple furuncles, carbuncles, or lesions associated with marked surrounding inflammation, or in diabetic patients. In such cases, oral dicloxacillin or cephalexin (Tables 32.1 and 32.2) should be given until signs of inflammation subside completely, which may take 2 weeks or longer. When antibiotics are given, indurated furuncles often resolve without becoming fluctuant. Progression on treatment suggests MRSA infection.

Currently many community-acquired strains of *S. aureus* are methicillin-resistant, and some of them are highly virulent. Such strains can cause epidemic furunculosis in baseball, football, and basketball players, and in athletic locker rooms of high schools and gymnasiums (4). The common factors are minor skin trauma, frequent skin-to-skin contact, and shared towels and clothing. It is difficult to predict which oral agent will be effective in such circumstances, and cultures are, therefore, very helpful. Most MRSA strains are resistant to clindamycin and quinolones, although these drugs are still effective if the organisms are sensitive. Almost all strains are sensitive to linezolid, but this drug is exceedingly expensive ($1,000 or more per course). Most, but not all strains can be treated with trimethoprim/sulfamethoxazole, which is very inexpensive. If all else fails, it may be necessary to install a line, and treat with intravenous vancomycin; in many instances that can be done in an ambulatory setting.

Carbuncles require surgical drainage, which usually can be done in an outpatient facility. Patients with severe systemic toxicity, such as diabetics with carbuncles, require hospital admission and parenteral therapy with a penicillinase-resistant penicillin; vancomycin is an effective alternative for those who are allergic to penicillin, or for MRSA strains.

Recurrent furunculosis may prove a frustrating problem. Management of individual episodes is as described previously, but other steps should also be taken to eliminate colonization with staphylococci. The anterior nares should be cultured. Patients whose nasal cultures contain *S. aureus* should be treated by application of mupirocin ointment to the anterior nares twice daily for 5 days. Alternatively, bacitracin ointment or gentamicin ointment may be applied three or four times daily for 14 days. During topical treatment, bacterial contamination of skin should be meticulously controlled by having the patient bathe and shampoo twice daily with a chlorhexidine soap or lotion, and by changing underclothing and bed and bath linens daily.

Recurrent furunculosis may occur in certain *disorders that impair host defenses.* Tests for diabetes mellitus should be made; if they are positive, control of blood glucose may prove beneficial (see Chapter 79). Defects in polymorphonuclear leukocyte function are a rare cause of recurrent furunculosis but should be considered in young patients who show an increased incidence or severity of infections caused by staphylococci. Gram-negative bacteria and fungi may be cultured from the furuncles of such patients. If an unusual problem, such as a leukocyte defect, is suspected, the patient should be referred to a medical center with the capability to investigate such disorders.

Hidradenitis suppurativa is a difficult problem that requires prolonged, often lifelong treatment by multiple methods. These include selective surgical drainage of abscesses; elimination of irritants such as tight clothing, antiperspirants, and shaving of the axillae; careful, frequent cleansing of skin with antiseptic agents; local application of heat; and intermittent or long-term systemic antimicrobial therapy. The only curative therapy is surgical removal of all involved skin, which is easier said than done. Management of such patients is best supervised by a dermatologist (see Chapter 115).

Complications

Staphylococcal skin infections may spread to other sites. This is especially true in patients with extensive inflammation and systemic toxicity, such as those with carbuncles, in whom bacteremia is common. Even an innocent-appearing furuncle can cause metastatic infection, especially in patients with a focus of increased susceptibility, such as a ventricular septal defect, an artificial heart valve, or an arthritic joint. Patients at risk for bacteremia who have such susceptible foci or whose systemic complaints (fever, focal pain) persist despite antimicrobial treatment, should be carefully examined for possible metastatic infection.

CELLULITIS AND WOUND INFECTIONS

Any break in the skin can become infected. This includes not only obvious trauma, such as lacerations, burns, abrasions, and animal or human bites, but also minor injuries such as scratches and insect bites. The features of the resultant infection vary widely and depend on the nature of the wound, the type of infecting organism, and the defensive responses of the infected person. In many instances, early

TABLE 32.3 Wound Infections: Findings That Necessitate Hospitalization or Surgical Intervention

Finding	*Comment*
Extensive cellulitis or erysipelas with systemic toxicity	Needs parenteral antibiotics, close observation
Diminished arterial pulse in cool, swollen, pale, infected extremity	Possible fasciitis, a surgical emergency
Cellulitis with cutaneous necrosis or subcutaneous gas	Needs parenteral antibiotics and possible surgical drainage/debridement
Closed space infection of the hand	Needs surgical drainage

appropriate management given on an ambulatory basis is sufficient. In others, recognition of serious infection and prompt hospitalization for vigorous medical or surgical treatment are of prime importance. Table 32.3 describes findings that require hospitalization or surgical intervention. Table 32.4 lists organisms that can cause life-threatening forms of cellulitis. The most important are *Vibrio vulnificus*, associated with injuries sustained in brackish water, and *Aeromonas hydrophila*, associated with injuries in fresh water. Both organisms cause severe, rapidly spreading, necrotic cellulitis, with hemorrhagic bulla formation and frequent bacteremia. The most useful treatment is doxycycline, which is not commonly used for cellulitis unless these diagnoses are suspected.

Cellulitis Caused by *S. pyogenes* and *S. aureus*

Acute cellulitis is a spreading infection of subcutaneous tissues. The infection plane is below the epidermis and above the deep fascia, in subcutaneous fat. The involved area, which enlarges steadily, is painful, tender, and intensely erythematous. Chills and fever are common, and bacteremia may occur. The lesion differs from erysipelas in that its margin is not as sharply demarcated, nor is it elevated. There may be purulent or serous drainage at the inoculation site; in severe cases, patches of involved skin may become necrotic.

The most common causes of acute cellulitis are *S. pyogenes* and *S. aureus*. Studies based on full-thickness biopsies of skin and subcutaneous fat show that more than 95% of cases are streptococcal (5). Finding gram-positive cocci in drainage from the wound is presumptive evidence that they are causative. Cellulitis may progress rapidly, especially when it involves an area of chronic edema. Lower extremity infection in patients with peripheral arterial insufficiency can cause tissue necrosis and secondary infection.

TABLE 32.4 Causes of Life-Threatening Bacterial Cellulitis

Cause	*Important Features*
Gram-negative enteric bacilli, especially *Escherichia coli*	Occur in fecally contaminated wounds; gas may be present; surgical drainage required for gas or pus
Mixed anaerobic and enteric aerobic bacteria	Occur in fecally contaminated wounds; gas may be present; symptoms may progress rapidly and may include exquisite pain; surgical drainage required
Bacillus anthracis	Causes anthrax when minor wound is inoculated by spore-contaminated animal products (animal hides and hair, especially from goats); local chancre-like lesion develops, followed by systemic toxicity
Erysipelothrix rhusiopathiae	Erysipelas-like lesion with central clearing; caused by wound contamination with fish or meat products; treated with penicillin V or tetracycline
Pasteurella multocida	Erysipelas-like lesion that follows a dog or cat scratch or bite; treated with penicillin V or tetracycline
Marine vibrios	Necrotizing cellulitis after minor wound is contaminated by sea water or contact with shellfish
Aeromonas hydrophila	Wound contaminated by fresh water swimming

Management of cellulitis should include culture of any wound drainage (as described for erysipelas) and prompt antimicrobial therapy. In mild cases, treatment may be given on an ambulatory basis. Generally, the antimicrobial is designed to cover infections by penicillin-resistant staphylococci as well as penicillin-sensitive streptococci. However, since the overwhelming majority of cellulitis is streptococcal, this is probably unnecessary. Oral dicloxacillin or cephalexin is adequate for infections caused by either type of organism; erythromycin is a suitable alternative for patients who are allergic to penicillin (Tables 32.1 and 32.2). Local application of moist heat is a useful adjunct to antibiotic treatment; care should be taken, however, to avoid causing burns, especially in patients with impaired sensitivity to pain. Improvement is usually apparent in 3 or 4 days; during this period, patients should rest the involved area (with elevation when the cellulitis involves an extremity). Patients should be told to report promptly any worsening of the infection or of constitutional symptoms. Severe infections require hospitalization and parenteral treatment with a penicillinase-resistant β-lactam such as nafcillin, or vancomycin. This includes patients with extensive lesions, lesions of the face, or serious toxicity.

Necrotizing Fasciitis

Most patients with an acutely swollen, painful leg have cellulitis. A very few have a much more serious infection in which the primary infectious process is in the plane of the deep fascia. The infection spreads rapidly and widely in this plane, and a whole limb may be involved in a few hours. Initially, the patient is febrile and toxic out of proportion to the visible changes in the skin, which may be minor or nonexistent. The infection causes thrombosis of small blood vessels as they cross the fascia to supply blood to the skin. The overlying skin becomes dusky blue and edematous, ultimately developing hemorrhagic bullae.

Necrotizing fasciitis is a surgical emergency; the fascia is dead over wide areas, and it must be removed back to normal bleeding tissue. Diagnosis is primarily clinical, although computed tomographic scans may show gas or edema, or both, in the plane of the deep fascia. Treatment involves long incisions with much undermining of skin edges to allow removal of necrotic material. The wounds are drained and left open to heal by secondary intention. Multiple subsequent débridements usually are necessary.

There are two distinct bacterial causes. Group A *S. pyogenes* can cause this syndrome as a single organism (6). Formerly there were epidemics of streptococcal gangrene in hospitals; presently, streptococci are the "flesh-eating bacteria" of the popular media. Streptococci do not form gas, so computed tomography shows only edema. The other kind of necrotizing fasciitis was described by Fournier and is called Fournier gangrene (7). It is caused by a mixed fecal flora involving several bacteria—aerobic gram-negative rods and both gram-positive and gram-negative anaerobes. This flora typically produces abundant gas. Streptococcal fasciitis can start anywhere; Fournier gangrene usually starts near the perineum. These cases are treated in hospital with broad-spectrum antimicrobials as an adjunct to surgery; if a streptococcus is responsible, treatment can be simplified to penicillin.

Secondarily Infected Ulcers

Cutaneous ulcers are caused by a wide variety of conditions (see Chapter 95). By far the most common cause is chronic venous insufficiency, most typically associated with ulceration of the medial side of the leg, just above the ankle.

Management of the ulcer is generally aimed at the underlying cause and seeks to improve blood flow, reduce edema, and avoid pressure and trauma (see Chapter 95).

Control of secondary infection is also important. Superficial colonization with a variety of bacteria is unavoidable and without consequence; however, infection that is deeper or laterally invasive prevents healing and may interfere with other treatments, such as skin grafting. It should be remembered that infection is almost never the primary cause of an ulcer. Ulcers will not respond to antimicrobials if the primary problem is vascular insufficiency. Infection is best controlled by repeated careful cleaning and local debridement. Systemic antimicrobials should be used only after other methods have failed to control surrounding infection. The choice of antimicrobial should be based on cultures of the wound or its purulent drainage. Local antibacterials are sometimes helpful. Those effective against a broad spectrum of bacterial agents include polymyxin–bacitracin–neomycin ointment, topical nitrofurazone (Furacin ointment), and the silver sulfadiazine ointment commonly used to treat burns. These should be applied three times daily until healing occurs or it is apparent that they are ineffective. Soaking with 3% acetic acid three to four times daily is helpful in controlling bacterial growth in ulcers colonized with *P. aeruginosa.*

There is good evidence that local application of fibroblast growth factors speeds healing of ulcers, but the proteins are recombinant and very expensive.

Cutaneous Diphtheria

Cutaneous ulcers and other skin lesions may become secondarily infected with *Corynebacterium diphtheriae,* causing cutaneous diphtheria. Although the cutaneous lesion may appear benign, myocarditis or neuropathy develops in approximately 3% of cases. Outbreaks have occurred in the northwest and southern parts of the United States, primarily among Native Americans or indigent urban residents (8). The presence of cutaneous diphtheria in a community should increase suspicion that skin wounds may harbor this agent. The diagnosis should be suspected when existing wounds develop a *gray-yellow or gray-brown covering membrane* and surrounding erythema. Typically, the membrane can easily be removed to reveal a clean base. Other minor skin lesions may also become infected. Typical organisms can be seen in methylene blue stains of smears from the wound and confirmed by culture on Loeffler or tellurite agar. Presumptive cases should be reported to public health officials and treated with equine diphtheria antitoxin (20,000 to 40,000 units intramuscularly or intravenously after testing for hypersensitivity to horse serum) and either erythromycin (1.5 grams per day, orally) or procaine penicillin (1.2 million units per day, intramuscularly) for 7 to 10 days. Because horse serum is frequently allergenic, attempts are being made to synthesize a human soluble receptor that binds diphtheria toxin.

Cutaneous Anthrax

Until recently, cutaneous anthrax was a curiosity seen occasionally in agricultural areas and in factories where workers handled imported hides or wool. Now that anthrax has been used by bioterrorists, it is not clear how common it may become in the future. The cutaneous form of the disease occurs when anthrax spores become implanted under the skin, germinate, and begin to multiply. The disease is usually found on exposed skin of the hands and arms, sometimes on the face. The anthrax bacilli make two toxins: (a) an edema-forming toxin that poisons capillary endothelium and produces leaky capillaries, and (b) a lethal toxin that poisons most cells by inducing apoptosis (programmed cell death). These two toxins account for the distinctive features of the disease. At the site of initial implantation, the skin rapidly becomes black and necrotic. The lesion is roughly circular, and diameters range from 1 to 3 cm. Although anthrax is described as causing a "malignant pustule," it is more like a vesicle, because the fluid contains bacteria but very few cells. There may be secondary vesicles around the primary one. Spreading from the primary site is an area of pronounced edema that may extend 10 cm or more from the primary lesion. There may be regional lymph node enlargement. Fever and systemic toxicity are rare except in neglected cases.

Cutaneous anthrax must be distinguished primarily from the vastly more common boil (see Pustular Infections Caused by *S. aureus*). Anthrax lesions are curiously painless and may itch. Big boils are very painful, as are the associated nodes. A boil may develop a black or dark red crust of coagulated blood if it has been picked at, but the anthrax lesion is black from the beginning. Edema around boils is less pronounced than that around anthrax lesions. Gram stains from boils show pus, sheets of polymorphonuclear cells, and gram-positive cocci in clusters. Gram stains from anthrax vesicle fluid show big (8 μm) gram-positive rods with few or no cells. The organisms are easily differentiated on culture, but the laboratory should be warned what it may be dealing with.

Without treatment, the mortality rate of cutaneous anthrax is approximately 25%. The most suitable antimicrobials for adults are quinolones (e.g., ciprofloxacin 500 mg orally twice daily) and tetracyclines (e.g., doxycycline 100 mg orally twice daily), given for 60 days. Penicillins, cephalosporins, and vancomycin are commonly used in children. Patients with cutaneous anthrax lesions on the head or neck or with extensive edema or signs of systemic toxicity should be hospitalized for intravenous therapy with a multidrug regimen. With treatment, the mortality rate should be under 5%.

Bites

Bite wounds become infected with the oral, salivary, or dental flora of the biting person or animal and may cause serious local or systemic infections. Initial management before signs of infection appear is of primary importance in preventing certain infections (9). Appropriate prophylaxis for tetanus is required for all bite wounds (see Chapter 18).

Human bites are contaminated with a complex variety of aerobic and anaerobic oral bacteria. Without treatment, a severe necrotizing cellulitis often results. Minor lesions that break the skin should be washed thoroughly and treated with a combination of amoxicillin 875 mg and clavulanic acid (Augmentin) orally twice daily. Oral clindamycin (150 to 300 mg three times a day) is appropriate for patients who are allergic to penicillin. Antimicrobials should be continued for 7 to 10 days. More severe wounds, including wounds of the hands and knuckles, require meticulous debridement and possible tendon repairs. These injuries should be referred for surgical management.

Dog bites carry the risk of local soft tissue infection with various organisms, including *P. multocida*, and raise concern about rabies. Minor abrasions, shallow punctures, and superficial lacerations require no therapy for local infection other than thorough cleansing with soap and water. Puncture wounds should be irrigated vigorously with sterile saline injected through a 20-gauge needle. More extensive or deeper bites require surgical management for debridement. Amoxicillin and clavulanic acid, as described previously, should be given for bites of the hands or face. The same treatment is appropriate for patients who have signs of soft tissue infection when first seen. Patients with hand infection require surgical management and intensive antimicrobial therapy.

Rabies precautions should be taken with all dog bites, including bites by domestic pets, even though the risk of rabies from domestic pets—especially when biting was provoked—is very small. The dog should be quarantined for 10 days. If the dog's owner cannot be identified, the local health department should be called to take charge of the dog. If its owner is known and can prove that the dog was vaccinated against rabies, it may be observed at its home. If it remains well, there is no risk of rabies. If the dog develops neurologic symptoms or dies, its brain should be examined immediately; prophylaxis is required if evidence of rabies is found. If the dog escapes after biting, and especially if the bite was unprovoked, rabies prophylaxis with human rabies immune globulin and human diploid cell rabies vaccine is indicated (see Chapter 18).

Bites by domestic cats should be managed in the same way as dog bites. Cats are not routinely vaccinated against rabies and are now a greater hazard than domestic dogs. *Bites by wild animals* carry a greater risk of rabies, and rabies prophylaxis is usually required unless the animal's brain can be examined. Wild animals with the greatest risk of carrying rabies are raccoons, skunks, foxes, coyotes, and bats. The risk of rabies with rodent bites, including squirrel bites, is very small.

It is recommended that the practitioner seek the help of the local or state health department when dealing with animal bites. Officials with knowledge of disease activity in local animal populations may be able to determine whether a particular exposure is trivial or serious and can also arrange fluorescent antibody testing and viral cultures if the animal is available. Not every animal that appears neurologically impaired has rabies; other causes of animal encephalitis are also found.

Puncture Wounds

Puncture wounds usually involve the feet or hands and may introduce infecting bacteria that cannot be removed by washing or debridement. In all instances, patients should receive appropriate prophylaxis for tetanus (see Chapter 18). *Low-risk wounds* (i.e., those not likely to be contaminated by soil or fecal material and in which the wound site is in healthy, well-vascularized tissue) need only be thoroughly washed and observed for several days for signs of developing infection. Should infection develop, any wound drainage should be cultured and treatment begun with dicloxacillin orally 250 mg three times daily or amoxicillin-clavulanate (see earlier discussion) for presumptive staphylococcal or streptococcal infection. The wound site should also be soaked in warm soapy water for 30 minutes at least four times a day.

Higher-risk wounds (i.e., those likely to be contaminated with fecal material, soil, or foreign debris and those occurring in a diabetic person or in an extremity with an inadequate blood supply) should be treated from the outset with a broad-spectrum antimicrobial. In adults, a quinolone such as ciprofloxacin 750 mg every 12 hours with or without metronidazole 500 mg every 8 hours. In children, probably a third generation cephalosporin or a carbapenem. The wound site should be rested and treated with warm soaks as described for low-risk wounds. The patient should promptly report any evidence of inflammation, swelling, or persisting pain. If purulent drainage develops, it should be cultured. Antimicrobial management should be altered if bacteria resistant to the current treatment are isolated. If pus develops, surgical drainage usually is required.

Felon

A felon is an infection of the pulp of the distal phalanx of a finger; it usually occurs after a recognized local wound. Abscess formation and tissue necrosis are common, and bony or articular involvement may occur. If the felon is neglected or inadequately treated, severe damage, including loss of function, may occur. The most common causative agents are *S. aureus* and *S. pyogenes,* although gram-negative bacilli may also be recovered. Treatment involves surgical drainage by a physician who is familiar with the procedure. Concurrent antibiotic therapy should be guided by Gram staining and culture of infected material. If Gram staining and culture are persistently negative, the diagnosis of herpetic whitlow (Chapter 117) should be considered.

Paronychia

A paronychia is an infection, often chronic or recurrent, that involves tissue immediately adjacent to a fingernail or toenail. The affected tissue is warm, tensely swollen, erythematous, and painful. When infection is chronic, the nail may become ridged or discolored and may be lost. Paronychia occurs most often in people who bite their nails, or whose hands are frequently in water (e.g., dishwashers, mothers of infants). Diabetics also have an increased risk for this infection. *Candida* species appear to play an etiologic role, although a variety of bacteria usually are present. Management involves keeping hands as dry as possible (e.g., using waterproof gloves for dishwashing) and applying an anticandidal medication (e.g., nystatin cream) or a broad-spectrum antifungal agent (clotrimazole or miconazole cream) two times a day for several weeks. If localized swelling does not respond to these measures, drainage may be helpful. This can be done by sliding an 18-gauge needle, bevel down, along the nail into the involved area. Lifting the skin from the nail with the needle usually achieves drainage and relief of pain.

The major cause of paronychia of the toe (usually a great toe) is an ingrown toenail. Chapter 73 describes the diagnosis and management of this problem.

Intertriginous Infections

Chapter 116 describes approaches to diagnosis of infections involving moist intertriginous areas (toe webs, axillae, groin area).

SPECIFIC REFERENCES

1. Bisno AL, Stevens DL. Streptococcal infections of skin and soft tissues. N Engl J Med 1996; 334:240.
2. Esterly NB, Nelson DB, Dunne WM Jr. Impetigo. Am J Dis Child 1991;145:125.
3. Gemmell CG. Staphylococcal scalded skin syndrome. J Med Microbiol 1995;43:318.
4. Kazakova SV, Hageman JC, Matawa M, et al. A clone of methicillin resistant *Staphylococcus aureus* among professional football players. N Engl J Med 2005;352:468.
5. Bernard P, Bedame C, Mounier M. Streptococcal cause of erysipelas and cellulitis in adults. Arch Dermatol 1989;125:779.
6. Barker FG, Leppard BJ, Seal DV. Streptococcal necrotizing fasciitis: comparison between histological and clinical features. J Clin Pathol 1987;40:335.
7. Green RJ, Dafoe DC, Raffin TA. Necrotizing fasciitis. Chest 1996;110:219.
8. Belsey MA, Sinclair M, Roder MR, et al. *Corynebacterium diphtheriae* skin infections in Alabama and Louisiana: a factor in the epidemiology of diphtheria. N Engl J Med 1969;280:135.
9. McDonough JJ, Stern PJ, Alexander JW. Management of animal and human bites and resulting human infections. Curr Clin Top Infect Dis 1987;3:11.

For annotated ***General References*** *and resources related to this chapter, visit www.hopkinsbayview.org/PAMreferences.*

Chapter 33

Respiratory Tract Infections*

Nicholas H. Fiebach and R. Graham Barr

Respiratory tract infections are the most common acute illnesses in the United States and in the industrialized world. These infections are the most frequent causes of absences from school or work. Most upper respiratory infections (URIs) are self-diagnosed and self-treated and do not come to the attention of a clinician. Lower respiratory infections (LRIs) may be minor or amenable to ambulatory treatment, but they also represent one of the leading causes of hospitalization and death in this country. The cost of respiratory tract infections in lost productivity and expenditures for treatments, including over-the-counter (OTC) remedies, is estimated to be billions of dollars.

UPPER RESPIRATORY TRACT INFECTIONS

Common Cold

The common cold, or coryza, is a mild, self-limited syndrome caused usually by viral infection of the upper respiratory tract mucosa and characterized by one or more of the following symptoms: nasal discharge and obstruction, sneezing, sore throat, cough, and hoarseness.

Epidemiology and Transmission

The common cold syndrome is caused by a variety of viruses that are clinically indistinguishable from each other, yet have distinct seasonal peaks (1). *Rhinoviruses* are the etiologic agent in 30% to 50% of colds, with seasonal peaks in fall and spring. *Coronaviruses* account for another 10% to 15% of colds, with a seasonal peak in midwinter. *Influenza, parainfluenza, respiratory syncytial viruses, and adenovirus* are etiologic agents for another 15% to 25%, although this group more commonly causes the typical influenza syndrome. A newly identified virus, metapneumovirus, has been found in children with upper respiratory illnesses, although its role in adult colds is not yet clear. Bacteria associated with pharyngitis can also cause some common cold symptoms.

The incidence of the common cold syndrome decreases with age. On average, adults have two to four colds per year; children have six to eight (1). Because person-to-person spread of colds occurs mainly in the home and at school, schoolchildren often introduce colds into a family (2).

Rhinoviruses may be transmitted from infected persons to others by direct contact with respiratory secretions as well by aerosolization of large or medium droplets of secretions in close quarters (1). Frequent, unconscious touching of virus-laden nasal mucosa contaminates the hands of infected individuals. Infectious material can survive on the hands or on inanimate objects, and hand-to-hand contact or touching these objects transfers the virus to susceptible individuals. Self-inoculation of the nares and conjunctiva (from which the virus is passed along the lacrimal ducts to the nasal passages) then completes the transmission of infection. Exposure to susceptible subjects across short distances of air may also transmit rhinovirus infection. Other viruses, such as adenovirus, respiratory syncytial virus (RSV), and influenza, are spread in similar manners, although adenovirus and influenza can also be spread by tiny droplet nuclei that may be carried by air currents and may cause lower as well as upper respiratory illness. Contagion of viruses that cause the common cold is low in community settings, relatively low from casual contact, but higher in the home and in close living quarters such as dormitories (3). Recirculation of air in an airplane cabin was not associated with an increased risk of URI (4).

Clinical Features

The correct diagnosis of the common cold is readily made by the patient. After an incubation period of 48 to

*In the previous edition, Darius A. Rastegar, MD, contributed to this chapter.

(41°C) in some cases, typically lasts 3 days, although it may persist for 5 to 7 days. Headache and myalgias involving the back, arms, legs, and occasionally the eyes are the predominant symptoms, persisting as long as the fever. Respiratory symptoms, such as nonproductive cough, nasal discharge, hoarseness, and sore throat, appear as systemic symptoms wane. Cough and weakness usually subside after 2 weeks but may persist longer. In the elderly, myalgias and sore throat are less common, whereas dyspnea is a more common symptom (40).

Physical findings include general toxicity, flushed face, hot skin, watery red eyes, clear nasal discharge, tender cervical lymph nodes, and occasionally localized rales in the chest. The white cell count and differential, indicated only if the patient is toxic or pneumonia is suspected, usually demonstrate mild neutropenia and relative lymphocytosis caused by absolute granulocytopenia.

Because specific antimicrobial therapy for influenza infections is available, it is important to determine whether flu syndrome is likely to be caused by this virus. The best clinical predictors of influenza virus as the cause of flu syndrome are fever greater than 100°F (37.8°C), cough, and abrupt onset (44). However, during influenza epidemics, when the prevalence of influenza infection may be 65% or higher among individuals with any respiratory symptoms, this combination is neither sensitive nor specific. Therefore, influenza should be suspected in patients who have respiratory illness during flu season (November through April), and it should be presumed to be the cause of acute respiratory illness with fever and cough when influenza is known to be circulating in the community. Clinicians can obtain information about influenza epidemics from the Centers for Disease Control and Prevention (CDC) website (http://www.cdc.gov/flu/weekly/fluactivity.htm) and Voice Information System (influenza update at 888-232-3228) and from state and local health departments.

Since influenza vaccination is likely to be only 30% to 40% effective in preventing upper respiratory influenza illness in targeted patients (although it is more effective in preventing influenza-associated pneumonia, hospitalization, or death), flu syndrome in vaccinated patients still may be caused by the influenza virus and respond to specific therapy (41,44).

Diagnostic Tests

Influenza virus infection may be diagnosed by viral culture, polymerase chain reaction (PCR) assay, or specific serology (comparing acute and convalescent titers). These tests require specialized techniques, and the results are not available until days to weeks after a patient is evaluated. Immunofluorescence antibody staining and enzyme immunoassay (EIA) tests may be performed on respiratory secretions with results available in several hours, but these tests are not readily available in ambulatory practice. A variety of rapid test kits for point-of-care analysis of nasopharyngeal swabs or nasal aspirates or washes are available to clinicians and provide results within 30 minutes (44). Most of these tests are moderately complex and require CLIA (Clinical Laboratory Improvement Amendments from the Centers for Medicare and Medicaid Services) certification. Some of the rapid diagnostic tests can distinguish between influenza A and B. Reported sensitivity is 70% or more (with no clear advantage for any specific kit), but specificity is better, usually 90% or more. Therefore, a positive test reliably confirms a diagnosis of influenza infection, but a negative test does not exclude influenza or the potential benefit of specific treatment. Testing is not likely to be helpful during an influenza epidemic, when the pretest probability of influenza infection is high in a person with typical symptoms, but it may be most useful when influenza is not known to be circulating widely or when the clinical diagnosis is uncertain (44). Information about diagnostic testing for influenza, including available rapid testing kits, may be found on the CDC website (www.cdc.gov/flu/professionals/labdiagnosis.htm).

Treatment

Options for the specific antimicrobial treatment of influenza include the older, adamantine compounds, *amantadine* and *rimantadine,* and two newer neuraminidase inhibitors, *zanamivir* and *oseltamivir* (Table 33.4). Amantadine and rimantadine are effective only against influenza A, whereas the neuraminidase inhibitors are active against both A and B strains.

All of these drugs attenuate clinical disease by reducing fever by 50% and by shortening the duration of illness by 1 or 2 days. Reductions in illness duration may be somewhat greater when influenza symptoms or fever are more severe, and there is some evidence that viral shedding (and contagion) decreases with treatment. These benefits were observed when the drug was administered within 24 to 48 hours after onset of illness, although some experts suggest treating high-risk patients or severely ill patients who present within 3 to 4 days after symptom onset (45). Evidence for the effectiveness of these drugs in treating influenza illness is based mostly on studies in younger, healthy people with uncomplicated influenza illness, and data in patients at high risk for complications, including the elderly, are limited. There is only limited evidence that neuraminidase drugs are effective in preventing serious complications of influenza (e.g., pneumonia, exacerbations of chronic diseases) (41,46).

Table 33.4 shows dosages, routes of administration, adverse effects, and costs of these drugs. Previously, drug resistance was not a clinically significant problem in treating influenza, but in 2006 the predominant influenza A strain (H3N2) showed widespread resistance to amantadine

TABLE 33.4 Antimicrobial Drugs for the Treatment of Influenza

Generic Name	Trade Name	Active Against Type A	Active Against Type B	Dosage, Route[a]	Cost[b]	Adverse Effects
Amantadine	Symmetrel	Yes	No	100 mg p.o. b.i.d.[c,d]	$	CNS (insomnia, irritability, dizziness, decreased concentration); 10%–15% (higher in elderly); GI, 3%
Rimantadine	Flumadine	Yes	No	100 mg p.o. b.i.d.[c,d,e]	$$	CNS, 2%–6%; GI, 3%
Oseltamivir	Tamiflu	Yes	Yes	75 mg p.o. b.i.d.[d]	$$$	GI, 10%
Zanamivir	Relenza	Yes	Yes	10 mg inhaled b.i.d.	$$$	May cause bronchospasm in patients with obstructive lung disease

CNS, central nervous system; GI, gastrointestinal; p.o., per os.
[a]Amantadine, rimantadine, and oseltamivir are also available as a syrup or suspension. The recommended duration of treatment for amantadine and rimantadine is 3 to 5 days, and for oseltamivir and zanamivir 5 days.
[b]Relative costs.
[c]Reduce dosage in the elderly (= 65 years old) to 100 mg daily or less.
[d]Reduce dosage in patients with renal insufficiency (see package insert for details).
[e]Reduce dosage to 100 mg daily in patients with hepatic disease.

and rimantadine. Resistance to the neuraminidase inhibitors remained rare. If amantadine or rimantadine is used to treat influenza illness, it should be discontinued after 3–5 days, or within 24–48 hours after symptoms have resolved; oseltamivir and zanamivir are given for 5 days (41).

Drug treatment should be considered for patients at high risk for morbidity and mortality who develop an influenza-like illness in a community where local influenza activity has been reported. Groups at high risk include patients with chronic pulmonary, cardiovascular, metabolic, neuromuscular, or immunodeficiency diseases and patients taking immunosuppressive medications. Adults whose activities are vital to community function, including selected hospital personnel, also should be considered for drug treatment of influenza.

Choice of therapy depends on consideration of the type of influenza circulating in the community, the safety, cost, convenience and availability of the drugs, and the concerns about resistance described above. Zanamivir is delivered via an inhalation device that requires assembly, and elderly patients have been shown to have difficulty with its use (47). Some patients with obstructive lung disease have had bronchospasm after using zanamivir, so it is generally not recommended for patients with asthma or chronic obstructive pulmonary diseases (COPD).

Supportive measures are important for symptomatic relief. Rest and adequate fluid intake should be advised. NSAIDs, including aspirin 650 mg every 3 to 4 hours, or acetaminophen 650 to 1,000 mg every 4 to 6 hours (maximum 4 g daily), reduce headache, fever, and myalgia. Aspirin should be avoided in children. Relief of nasal discharge may be obtained by agents discussed previously (see Common Cold). Relief of cough with cough suppressants is discussed later (see Acute Bronchitis).

Complications

Pulmonary complications exhibit a spectrum of severity, from mild airway hyperreactivity without pulmonary infiltrates, to segmental influenza pneumonia or secondary bacterial pneumonia, to fulminant bilateral influenza pneumonia with the acute respiratory distress syndrome (ARDS). Patients should be advised that dyspnea, hemoptysis, wheezing, purulent sputum, fever persisting longer than 7 days, and, rarely, dark urine or severe muscle pain herald complications that demand prompt medical attention and sometimes hospitalization.

Airway hyper-reactivity may occur after some influenza infections and other viral respiratory tract infections manifested clinically by bronchospasm, coughing, or both (48,49). Patients with asthma or chronic bronchitis have even greater bronchoconstrictor responses to influenza infection because of their underlying bronchial smooth muscle hyperreactivity. Airway hyper-reactivity may be demonstrated for 3 to 8 weeks after infection by influenza or other viruses, and occasionally it may last for 4 to 6 months, even in patients who are not atopic. Both cough and wheezing after an otherwise uncomplicated flu syndrome may be treated with a trial of an inhaled bronchodilator (see Chapter 60) as needed and at bedtime. Patients troubled particularly by nighttime cough may obtain additional relief with 15 to 30 mg of codeine at bedtime.

During influenza epidemics, there is an increase in the incidence of pneumonia, although influenza often is not recognized by clinicians as a primary or contributing cause in patients who are admitted to the hospital with community-acquired pneumonia (CAP) (50). The incidence of bronchitis and pneumonia associated with influenza varies with age: it is low in patients younger than 50 years of age and very high in patients older than 70 years of age. The characteristics of pneumonias associated with influenza are described in the section on Lower Respiratory Tract Infections below.

Nonpulmonary complications of influenza are unusual. *Myositis,* with thigh pain and inability to walk, occurs occasionally in children and adolescents. Severe myositis with myoglobinuria and acute renal failure has been observed in adults after both influenza A and B. Guillain-Barré syndrome, encephalitis, and transverse myelitis are *neurologic complications* associated rarely with influenza infection, but no firm causal relationship has been established. *Reye syndrome* (encephalopathy and fatty liver) is a rare but severe complication of influenza, usually type B; patients present with a change in mental status and progress to coma and hepatic failure. The mean age at attack is 6 years, and the incidence has fallen markedly in recent years. The syndrome is rare in adults and, unlike the situation in children, is not associated with aspirin. With the exception of mild myositis, all of the nonpulmonary complications of influenza require hospitalization for differential diagnosis and management.

Prevention

Chapter 18 discusses the use of influenza vaccine and drug prophylaxis in ambulatory practice.

Pharyngitis

Sore throat is among the most common symptoms seen in ambulatory medical practice. Most acute episodes of pharyngitis in adults are self-limited and of short duration, and significant complications are rare. The most important task in the evaluation of patients who complain of sore throat is to identify group A streptococcal and other bacterial infections, for which antibiotic treatment is appropriate, and to recognize less common causes of pharyngitis associated with more serious illnesses. Although many adult patients with sore throat are treated with antibiotics (51), it is increasingly recognized that this practice is often not appropriate.

Epidemiology

Pharyngitis in adults is caused by a variety of viral and bacterial pathogens, with no single etiology predominating (52,53). The majority of cases are caused by common viruses, most often rhinovirus, coronavirus, and adenovirus. Streptococcal bacteria, predominantly group A β-hemolytic *Streptococcus* (GABHS) species, account for only 15% of cases or less. *Mycoplasma pneumoniae,* the TWAR strain of *Chlamydia pneumoniae, Arcanobacterium* (formerly *Corynebacterium*) *haemolyticum, Neisseria gonorrhoeae, H. influenzae* type b, *Corynebacterium diphtheriae, Candida* species, respiratory syncytial virus, influenza types A and B, parainfluenza, herpes simplex virus, adenovirus, and Epstein-Barr virus cause pharyngitis infrequently.

Group A β-Hemolytic Streptococcal Pharyngitis

Clinical Features

Only 5% to 15% of episodes of acute pharyngitis in adults are caused by GABHS (54). It occurs most commonly in the winter and spring. Individuals who have regular contact with children (e.g., parents, teachers), or who have been exposed to others with diagnosed streptococcal pharyngitis, are more likely to have GABHS. The incubation period is 2 to 4 days, followed by the abrupt onset of sore throat, malaise, fever, and headache. Mild neck stiffness and gastrointestinal symptoms are sometimes present (55). All of the features of the classic syndrome, including fever, tender anterior cervical and tonsillar lymph nodes (at the angle of the jaw), and enlarged tonsils with white exudate, occur together infrequently, and each of these features may occur in other types of pharyngitis. Importantly, *cough, hoarseness, and rhinorrhea are not usually present in the patient with strep throat.* A distinctive scarlatiniform rash *(scarlet fever)* occasionally occurs. It is characterized by a diffuse red blush appearing on the trunk early in the disease, spreading centrifugally, blanching with pressure, and acquiring a sandpaper texture; 1 week later the skin desquamates, particularly over the palms and soles. This rash is not seen in most patients with GABHS pharyngitis. A similar rash also occurs in toxic shock syndrome and Kawasaki syndrome and a rash associated with *A. haemolyticum* pharyngitis is localized to the trunk and does not desquamate.

Diagnosis

Because individual clinical findings are nonspecific, the diagnosis of streptococcal pharyngitis relies on clinical prediction rules, rapid antigen tests, or throat culture. Several *clinical prediction rules* for GABHS pharyngitis have been developed (55); the Centor criteria (56) are simple and straightforward, have been validated prospectively, and have emerged as a consensus tool (54,55) (Table 33.5). These criteria include: *tonsillar exudates, tender anterior cervical lymphadenopathy, history of fever* (temperature greater than 100.4°F [38°C]), and *absence of cough.* The presence of three or four of these criteria has a sensitivity of 75% and a specificity of 75% for GABHS pharyngitis, using throat culture as the reference standard. For most

TABLE 33.5 Clinical Features in Patients with Sore Throat That Predict Group A β-Hemolytic Streptococcal (GABHS) Pharyngitis[a]

Tonsillar exudate
Tender anterior cervical lymphadenopathy
History of fever *or* Temperature >100.4°F (38°C)
Absence of cough

[a]Patients with three or four of these features are likely to have group A β-hemolytic *Streptococcus* (GABHS) pharyngitis; patients with zero or one likely do not.

adults, this results in a positive predictive value of 40% to 60% when three or four criteria are present, and a negative predictive value of approximately 80% if none or only one of the criteria is present (54).

Rapid antigen tests, which employ enzyme and optical immunoassay methods to detect GABHS carbohydrate products, are commercially available for point-of-care use in ambulatory practice. The specificity of these tests is reported to be greater than 95%, although the sensitivity is lower, e.g., 80% to 90% (53). For the average prevalence of GABHS in adults with sore throat (i.e., 10%), rapid antigen tests have a positive predictive value of approximately 65% and a negative predictive value of 98%. Therefore, the use of these tests alone (that is, without regard to clinical features) does not reliably establish the diagnosis of strep throat, although they are useful in conjunction with clinical criteria. A negative rapid strep test does accurately confirm the absence of GABHS.

Throat culture has been the gold standard for diagnosing GABHS, although a significant disadvantage is that results are not available for 24 to 48 hours. A small percentage of false negative tests may be caused by inadequate specimen collection or improper handling. False positive tests may occur if the patient is an asymptomatic carrier of GABHS and the acute pharyngitis is caused by another pathogen; this is estimated to occur in only 2% to 4% of adolescents and adults (55). Currently, many physicians prefer to send throat swabs in transport media to commercial laboratories. Inexpensive office throat culture kits are also available and have a high sensitivity (approximately 95%).

The accuracy of rapid antigen tests and throat cultures depends on *proper collection of the throat swab.* The pharynx must be viewed adequately, with elevation of the soft palate and depression of the posterior tongue. Use of a tongue blade and the classic "ahh" phonation by the patient may help; sometimes not having the patient stick out the tongue, or having the patient pant, is useful. The tonsillar tissue and posterior pharynx should be swabbed vigorously; adequate collection often induces the gag reflex.

Diagnostic Approach

Adult patients with sore throat should be screened for the four clinical findings (Centor criteria), as outlined previously. The clinician should also be alert to aspects of the history, symptoms, and signs that suggest other, potentially treatable or serious causes of pharyngitis (see Other Bacterial Causes of Pharyngitis and Noteworthy Viral Causes of Pharyngitis sections). Patients with none or only one of the four clinical criteria should not receive further testing or antibiotic treatment, because they are unlikely to have GABHS. Patients with two or more of the criteria should be tested with a rapid antigen kit or throat culture and treated with antibiotics if the result is positive. One consensus guideline suggests that patients with three or four of the criteria may be treated with antibiotics empirically (54); however up to one half of such patients may not have GABHS and will be treated unnecessarily. *Symptomatic family contacts* of patients with streptococcal pharyngitis should be tested and should be treated with antibiotics if the tests or cultures are positive. Routine testing of *asymptomatic* family members is not indicated.

Acute Rheumatic Fever and the Rationale for Antibiotic Treatment

The benefits of treating sore throat with antibiotics, especially if GABHS can be confirmed, include prevention of acute rheumatic fever and suppurative complications and perhaps more prompt relief of symptoms and interruption of contagious spread of pharyngitis. There is a growing recognition, however, that the magnitude of the benefits of antibiotic treatment may not be as large as previously believed.

Acute rheumatic fever is a clinical syndrome of nonsuppurative inflammatory lesions of the heart, joints, and central nervous system that follows GABHS pharyngitis (57,58). Diagnosis is based on the Jones criteria: two major criteria (carditis, polyarthritis, chorea, subcutaneous nodules, and erythema marginatum), or one major criterion and two minor criteria (fever, arthralgia, heart block, elevated acute-phase reactants including granulocytosis, erythrocyte sedimentation rate, and C-reactive protein). Evidence of recent streptococcal infection must be confirmed by either positive throat culture, streptococcal antigen test, or elevated or rising antistreptococcal antibodies. One third of acute rheumatic fever cases occur after asymptomatic streptococcal infection, but almost all cases are associated with a rise in serum antistreptolysin O (ASO) titers. The latent period between clinical streptococcal pharyngitis and onset of acute rheumatic fever ranges from 1 to 5 weeks, with a mean of 19 days. Clinical trials have confirmed that appropriate antibiotic treatment of GABHS pharyngitis is highly effective in preventing rheumatic fever if administered within approximately 1 week after the onset of illness.

The incidence of acute rheumatic fever declined dramatically in the United States and other industrialized countries during the last century, falling to extremely low levels during the 1960s and 1970s. It continued to be endemic in developing countries, where it accounts for up to 40% of all cardiovascular disease. Outbreaks among school-age children and young adult military recruits in the United States in the 1980s raised fears about a resurgence of rheumatic fever, but since then its occurrence has continued to decrease to only 1 case per 1 million people per year. Although the CDC suspended reporting of acute rheumatic fever in 1995, it has remained endemic at low levels in the region surrounding Salt Lake City, Utah (59).

Because almost all of the recent, very infrequent cases of acute rheumatic fever have been in children or young adults living in close quarters, the risk in most adults after GABHS is likely to be extremely low. The reasons for the overall decline and periodic resurgence of rheumatogenic GABHS infections are not completely understood or predictable, so clinicians should be aware of emerging trends in streptococcal disease.

Suppurative complications, such as peritonsillar or retropharyngeal abscess (see Pharyngeal Abscesses section), are very rare, although a quantitative review demonstrated a further reduction in their occurrence with antibiotic treatment of GABHS pharyngitis (60). However, patients with these infrequent complications often already have them at initial evaluation, or have a negative test initially, or were treated initially with appropriate antibiotics (54). Although antibiotics are often recommended for patients with GABHS pharyngitis to prevent contagion, the utility of this approach for adults in noninstitutionalized settings is not known. There is good evidence from controlled clinical trials and systematic reviews that antibiotic treatment of suspected or confirmed GABHS provides some relief of symptoms; however, therapy must be initiated within 2 to 3 days after the onset of illness, and the benefit is limited to shortening the duration of symptoms by 1 to 2 days (54,60).

Patients in whom GABHS is clinically suspected or confirmed by testing should be treated. In three additional groups of patients who present with sore throat, antibiotic treatment for streptococcal pharyngitis should be started and throat cultures obtained: patients with a history of rheumatic fever not currently taking prophylaxis, young patients with a strong family history of rheumatic fever, and all new cases of pharyngitis in an explosive epidemic of streptococcal disease in close populations such as groups of military personnel or students living in dormitory settings. Local health authorities should be notified promptly in this last situation.

Choice of Antibiotics

The *preferred therapy* for GABHS pharyngitis is parenteral benzathine penicillin, 1.2 million units given once intramuscularly, because it obviates nonadherence and is the only specific treatment proven in clinical trials to prevent rheumatic fever. If oral therapy is given, the recommended regimen is penicillin V, 500 mg twice daily for 10 days (53). Resistance to penicillin has *not* been a problem in GAHBS. For patients who are allergic to penicillin, a 10-day course of erythromycin 250 mg every 6 hours or 500 mg twice daily or a first-generation cephalosporin, is recommended. The use of newer macrolides such as azithromycin to treat GABHS is discouraged because of their increased costs and potentiation of antibiotic resistance. Posttreatment cultures should be performed only if there is a history of rheumatic fever in the patient or in a household contact.

Symptomatic Treatment

In addition to recommending antibiotics only for patients with suspected or confirmed GABHS pharyngitis, clinicians can encourage all patients with sore throat to try antipyretics and systemic and topical analgesics in appropriate doses (see section on Common Cold), along with supportive measures such as gargling.

Other Bacterial Causes of Pharyngitis

Pharyngitis caused by *A. haemolyticum* is characterized by exudative pharyngitis, a scarlatiniform rash, fever, adenopathy, and a negative test for GABHS (52). It may be treated with erythromycin 500 mg orally twice daily for 10 days.

Gonococcal pharyngitis should be considered in patients who complain of sore throat in association with urethritis or vaginitis; it occurs alone without genital symptoms in fewer than 5% of cases and must be diagnosed by throat culture. Special culture techniques (including the use of Thayer-Martin medium, which is available in kits for office cultures, or specific swab kits with appropriate transport media) should be used to detect gonorrhea in specimens from patients practicing orogenital sex. Calcium alginate swabs should be used, because ordinary cotton swabs contain fatty acids inhibitory to gonococcal growth. Gram staining of a direct pharyngeal smear is insensitive and nonspecific. For throat cultures, *N. gonorrhoeae* must be distinguished from *Neisseria meningitidis* and *Neisseria lactamica* by carbohydrate fermentation and serology; therefore, cultures should be sent to state or regional laboratories. Patients with gonococcal infections are often coinfected with chlamydia; although coincident chlamydial pharyngitis is unusual, it is recommended that patients with gonococcal pharyngitis also be treated empirically for possible genital chlamydia infection. Treatment of gonococcal infections, including the oropharynx, are discussed in detail in Chapter 37. Clinicians may also refer to the CDC website (http://www.cdc.gov/STD/treatment/, accessed 3-27-06) for updates.

Diphtheria is exceedingly rare in this country. Pharyngitis and skin infections caused by *C. diphtheriae* have occurred recently only in persons from disadvantaged groups who were inadequately immunized. It should be suspected when there is a grayish membrane in the anterior nares or on the tonsils, uvula, or pharynx. Treatment must begin before bacteriologic confirmation and requires hospitalization for strict isolation, bed rest, close observation, diphtheria antitoxin, and erythromycin or penicillin for 14 days. Chapter 18 discusses vaccination against diphtheria and management of exposed contacts.

Throat cultures sometimes grow *other bacteria*, such as pneumococci, staphylococci, group B, C, or G streptococci, and various gram-negative enterobacteria. These species colonize the pharynx and rarely cause pharyngitis, and patients who harbor them generally should not be treated with antibiotics. Some outbreaks of pharyngitis have been traced to streptococci of groups C and G, and patients with persistent sore throat and throat cultures positive for these organisms may be treated with shorter courses of the antibiotics listed for GABHS (54).

Vincent angina is an anaerobic bacterial infection of the pharynx characterized by fever, tender lymphadenitis, a large grayish-brown pseudomembrane in the pharynx, and very foul odor. It is a complication of acute necrotizing ulcerative gingivitis (see Chapter 112). Hospitalization for antimicrobial treatment with penicillin or tetracycline is the appropriate management plan.

Noteworthy Viral Causes of Pharyngitis

Infectious mononucleosis (see Chapter 58) is characterized by the clinical triad of sore throat, fever, and lymphadenopathy. It can be distinguished on clinical grounds from streptococcal infection only when hepatosplenomegaly and a maculopapular skin rash (similar to a drug eruption or rubella, typically precipitated by ampicillin) are present. Palatal petechiae may be seen in mononucleosis but may also occur with rubella or streptococcal pharyngitis. *Pharyngoconjunctival fever*, caused by several adenovirus strains, is usually accompanied by influenza-like symptoms and can be distinguished by concurrent conjunctivitis in one third of cases and a history of swimming pool exposure 1 week before onset. It has also been reported among military recruits (52). Oropharyngeal infection with *herpes simplex virus or coxsackie A virus* is distinguished by the presence of mucosal vesicles or ulcers (see Chapter 112). The vesicular enanthem in the pharynx caused by coxsackie viruses is sometimes called *herpangina*. The acute retroviral syndrome caused by *HIV infection* may manifest with fever and nonexudative pharyngitis; systemic symptoms and occasionally a rash occur also (see Chapter 39).

Chronic or Relapsing Sore Throat

Some patients describe a sore throat of several weeks' duration at their first visit. Others have either a prolonged course after an illness that began as a typical acute pharyngitis syndrome or frequent recurrence of sore throats. Table 33.6 lists the conditions that can cause prolonged or recurrent pharyngitis. (Most are discussed in more detail elsewhere in this book, as indicated in the table.)

TABLE 33.6 Causes of Chronic or Relapsing Sore Throat

Primary Site of Pain	Condition	See for Details
Pharynx	Chronic tonsillitis	
	Smoking (especially marijuana)	Chapters 27, 29
	Postnasal drip	Chapter 30, 59
	Infectious mononucleosis	Chapter 58
	Chronic fatigue syndrome	Chapter 58
	Agranulocytosis	
	Acute leukemia	
	Pemphigus	
Not the pharynx	Septic thyroiditis	Chapter 80
	Subacute thyroiditis	Chapter 80
	Angina (radiating to neck)	Chapter 62
	Esophageal reflux	Chapter 42
	Psychogenic	Chapter 21

Chronic tonsillitis or *recurrent pharyngitis* is a clinical diagnosis made in patients with frequent sore throats (more than six in 1 year, or three or more episodes in 2 or more years), very large tonsils, and chronically enlarged, periodically tender lymph nodes. The effectiveness of tonsillectomy to alleviate chronic tonsillitis in children has been controversial (61); there have been no controlled trials in adults, and its indications in adults are not well established. Postoperative pain and hemorrhage are the most common complications, the latter occurring in 0.5% to 2% of patients (but perhaps more often in adults) (62).

β-Lactamase–producing organisms in the pharynx, including *S. aureus*, *Haemophilus* species, *Bacteroides* species, and *Branhamella catarrhalis*, can inactivate penicillin and protect mucosal streptococci; these conditions may underlie some cases of chronic or recurrent pharyngitis. Patients who have multiple episodes of GABHS pharyngitis should receive clindamycin 300 mg twice daily or amoxicillin/clavulanate 500 mg twice daily (53).

Pharyngeal Abscesses

Occasionally, after several days of symptoms of a URI, a patient may develop a complicating infection of one of the closed compartments adjacent to the pharynx. The most common of these pharyngeal abscesses are *peritonsillar abscess* (also known as "quinsy") and *retropharyngeal abscess*. If one of these conditions is suspected, the patient should

TABLE 33.7 Differential Diagnosis of Severe Throat Pain, Odynophagia, and Inability to Swallow Saliva

Peritonsillar abscess	Toxic epidermal necrolysis
Retropharyngeal abscess	Stevens–Johnson syndrome
Vincent angina	Botulism
Diphtheria	Tetanus
Pharyngeal zoster	Gastroesophageal reflux
Epiglottitis	Foreign body

be referred immediately for evaluation and management by an otolaryngologist. Table 33.7 lists other conditions to consider when the patient is unable to swallow saliva because of pain.

Patients with *peritonsillar abscess* develop severe odynophagia; they are unable to take liquids and also may be unable to swallow their own saliva, resulting in early dehydration. The voice acquires a muffled quality, and trismus may be present. Fever, malaise, and systemic toxicity are typical. Dramatic relief may occur if the abscess drains spontaneously before the patient seeks medical attention. On physical examination, there is a swelling of the anterior tonsillar pillar at its superior pole. The involved tonsil itself may or may not be enlarged, but it is displaced medially. This condition is almost always unilateral. Half of the cases of peritonsillar abscess are caused by group A *S. pyogenes*.

The symptoms of *retropharyngeal abscess* are similar to those of peritonsillar abscess. In addition, there may be respiratory embarrassment if the process extends inferiorly toward the larynx. Trismus is uncommon. On examination, a swelling in the posterior oropharynx is readily seen. Lateral soft tissue radiographs of the neck may disclose expansion of the soft tissue density in the posterior pharyngeal space.

Management

Unless the airway or swallowing is compromised, needle aspiration and outpatient treatment with oral antibiotics are effective (63). The procedure can be performed by an otolaryngologist, an oral surgeon, or an experienced emergency room physician. Needle aspiration is unsuccessful in a small percentage of patients, necessitating incision and drainage. Non–group A streptococcal peritonsillar abscesses recur in 10% of cases, and abscess tonsillectomy may be required for repeated recurrences (63).

Epiglottitis

Acute epiglottitis is a life-threatening, rare complication of URIs. The epiglottis serves as a valve that closes over the proximal portion of the trachea during swallowing to prevent aspiration. When the epiglottis becomes inflamed, the resultant edema causes it to curl posteriorly and inferiorly, thereby reducing the glottic aperture. Inspiration, which draws the epiglottis down, further reduces the effective airway. Since the introduction of the *H. influenzae* B vaccine, the incidence in children has decreased, and now the incidence in adults is higher than in children (64).

The diagnosis of epiglottitis should be suspected in patients with a sore throat, odynophagia, and muffled voice, all of short duration. Only one half of patients are febrile and show evidence of pharyngitis, and only one third of patients have cervical lymphadenopathy. Sitting erect, complaint of dyspnea, and stridor noted on inspiration are indications of airway obstruction. Soft tissue radiographs of the neck may show edema of the epiglottis and narrowing of the aperture. The diagnosis is confirmed by indirect laryngoscopy, which reveals marked edema of the epiglottis and supraglottic tissue. This procedure must be performed only in circumstances in which emergency intubation can be carried out, because it may induce (rarely in adults) additional respiratory obstruction.

Management

Patients with suspected epiglottitis should be admitted to the hospital for observation; those with signs of airway obstruction should be admitted to an intensive care unit, where close observation and emergency tracheotomy, if necessary, are possible (64). The remainder of the cases can be managed conservatively in a general ward with antibiotic treatment for the most common organisms, including *S. aureus, H. influenzae, S. pneumoniae,* and *S. pyogenes.* Use of topical or systemic corticosteroids does not prevent airway obstruction.

Telephone Assessment and Self-Care for Upper Respiratory Tract Infection

Most clinicians welcome the opportunity to assess URI symptoms initially by telephone. The telephone assessment should accomplish the following:

- Differentiate between infectious and allergic problems
- Among the patients with acute infections, distinguish those with possible bacterial infections or superinfections who should be examined to determine whether antibiotics should be prescribed.
- Identify those who may have complications of a URI that require office evaluation.

The following symptoms and signs should be sought: symptoms lasting longer than 3 weeks; fever lasting longer than 1 week or associated with delirium; purulent nasal discharge with sinus pain; purulent sputum, chest pain, dyspnea, or hemoptysis; ear pain or discharge; sore throat and a history of rheumatic fever; the combination of cough and fever higher than 102°F (39°C); hoarseness for longer than 1 month; pleuritic chest pain; marked odynophagia; and dysphagia, stridor, and difficulty in breathing.

During influenza outbreaks (November through April), it is important to remember that the abrupt onset of fever and cough are fairly sensitive and specific for influenza infection, and that drug treatment for influenza has been shown to be effective only if started within the first 1 to 2 days of illness.

For patients not needing an office visit, simple instructions for self-care can be provided based on the measures described previously.

LOWER RESPIRATORY TRACT INFECTIONS

The cardinal manifestations of lower respiratory tract infections (LRI) are cough and dyspnea, often accompanied by auscultatory evidence of lower respiratory tract inflammation (rhonchi, rales, wheezes, signs of consolidation). Bronchitis and pneumonia are the major infectious syndromes of the lower respiratory tract in adults. A number of noninfectious conditions can also cause a cough that may be confused with a lower respiratory illness. Table 33.8 summarizes the differential diagnosis of acute and persistent cough (see also Chapter 59).

TABLE 33.8 Conditions and Agents That Can Cause Acute or Persistent Cough

Acute (<3 wk)
Acute bronchitis/upper respiratory tract infection
Common: influenza A and B, parainfluenza, respiratory syncytial virus, rhinovirus, adenovirus, coronavirus
Uncommon: *Bordetella pertussis, Mycoplasma pneumoniae, Chlamydia pneumoniae*
Pneumonia
Common: *Streptococcus pneumoniae, Haemophilus influenzae, Mycoplasma pneumoniae, Chlamydia pneumoniae,* respiratory syncytial virus
Uncommon: *Legionella, Mycobacterium tuberculosis, Moraxella catarrhalis,* plague, varicella, tuberculosis, anthrax, hantavirus and others
Persistent (>3 wk)
Noninfectious
Postnasal drip
Gastroesophageal reflux or repeated aspiration
Asthma
Angiotensin converting-enzyme inhibitors
Infectious
Common: *Bordetella pertussis, Mycoplasma pneumoniae, Chlamydia pneumoniae*
Uncommon: Tuberculosis and other mycobacterium, and fungal pneumonias: histoplasmosis, coccidioidomycosis, blastomycosis, aspergillosis

Acute Bronchitis

Acute bronchitis is one of the most common clinical syndromes encountered in outpatient practice. It is defined clinically as an acute illness characterized by a cough, which is usually accompanied by sputum production, and occasionally by fever and pleuritic chest pain. It is differentiated from pneumonia by the absence of dyspnea, a relatively normal chest examination, and lack of abnormalities on chest radiography. Bronchitis appears to be caused by inflammation of the tracheobronchial tree followed by tracheobronchial hypersensitivity that results in a cough of 1 to 3 weeks' duration. A cough that continues for longer than 3 weeks is generally referred to as a "persistent" or "chronic" cough. "Chronic bronchitis" is defined as an illness characterized by daily productive cough for at least 3 months in two or more consecutive years in the absence of any other illness that may account for these symptoms (see also Chapter 60 for a discussion of COPD).

Epidemiology

Acute bronchitis in otherwise healthy adults is generally caused by viral agents, including influenza A and B, parainfluenza, respiratory syncytial virus, rhinovirus, adenovirus, and coronavirus (65). Less commonly, acute bronchitis may be caused by bacterial agents such as *Bordetella pertussis, M. pneumoniae,* or *C. pneumoniae.* Other bacterial pathogens, such as *S. pneumoniae, H. influenzae,* or *M. catarrhalis* generally do not cause bronchitis in persons without underlying lung disease; however, they may be responsible for bacterial superinfections after an acute viral respiratory illness. Bacterial superinfection is rare in otherwise healthy adults and most commonly occurs in elderly persons and those with underlying chronic medical illness, especially chronic heart and lung disease.

Diagnosis

Patients with a cough as the predominant or only respiratory symptom may have pneumonia, bronchitis, or one of a variety of noninfectious conditions associated with persistent cough. Mucoid sputum production develops in many cases and is not helpful in distinguishing etiologic agents. Diagnostic efforts should be directed at identifying patients with pneumonia and those with noninfectious causes of cough, leaving acute bronchitis as a diagnosis of exclusion. For a primary care provider evaluating a patient with an acute illness characterized by cough, the most important question is often whether *chest radiography* is indicated for further evaluation. No single symptom, sign, or constellation of symptoms and signs can predict pneumonia reliably. However, one review suggested that the likelihood of pneumonia is diminished by the absence of signs of focal consolidation on chest examination or of any of the following vital sign abnormalities: heart rate greater than 100 beats/per minute, respiratory rate greater than 24 breaths/per minute, and oral body temperature greater than 100.4°F (38°C) (66). A chest radiograph usually is not necessary if none of these signs are present unless it is indicated for evaluation of dyspnea or an abnormal physical examination of the chest. *Gram stain* and *bacterial cultures of sputum* are not useful in the evaluation of acute bronchitis because most cases are of viral etiology and the sputum is readily contaminated by nasopharyngeal flora.

B. pertussis should be considered in adults with prolonged cough (usually defined as cough lasting longer than 2 weeks), especially if there is a history of exposure to someone with pertussis, since protection from childhood vaccination wanes by late adolescence (67). *B. pertussis* causes less than 1% of episodes of cough lasting more than 5 days but 6% of episodes lasting more than 8 weeks (68). Pertussis initially causes nonspecific symptoms of malaise and rhinorrhea, typically followed by 1 to 14 weeks of severe paroxysms of repetitive coughs terminated by an inspiratory whoop. These classic clinical symptoms are attenuated in previously immunized adults and children, so that it is hard to distinguish clinically from other causes of acute bronchitis. Epidemiologically, pertussis is less frequently associated with fever than are other causes of acute bronchitis, and is more likely to occur in young adults (68). Because of the nonspecific nature of the symptoms, 2 weeks is the duration of cough used as the threshold to initiate investigation of sporadic cases, and 1 week is used during an outbreak. The bacteriologic diagnosis is not easy to confirm. Culture, using a *nasopharyngeal swab* and special medium for *Bordetella*, is the standard diagnostic assay, but it is uncommonly positive, particularly after administration of antibiotics more than 3 weeks after the onset of cough. PCR assays are not yet fully standardized but may be useful also in the first 3 weeks of symptoms. Direct immunofluorescent staining of organisms and PCR on a smear of nasopharyngeal secretions are useful in outbreak investigations. Diagnosis by a single positive antibody test may be helpful to diagnose cases more than 4 weeks after the onset of cough, but repeated measurement of antibody titers to establish a trend is preferred (69).

Treatment

The CDC and the American College of Physicians (ACP) recommend *against* antibiotics for healthy adults with uncomplicated bronchitis (70). A meta-analysis of eight randomized controlled trials of antibiotics (erythromycin, doxycycline, trimethoprim/sulfamethoxazole) for bronchitis found a modest improvement in symptom duration with antibiotics (one-half day, on average) (71), but when side effects, costs, and the increasing problem of antibacterial resistance are taken into account, the risks associated with treatment appear to outweigh the potential benefits. Not surprisingly, antibiotics are more beneficial in patients with suspected acute bronchitis who actually have an underlying pneumonia and less beneficial in patients with only a simple URI (72). The beneficial effects of antibiotics for cigarette smokers appear to be the same or less than for nonsmokers (73). Sputum color is not necessarily an accurate indicator of purulence. *If pertussis is suspected,* appropriate diagnostic studies should be performed rather than using presumptive therapy with antibiotics, unless the patient is in an epidemic area. Treatment for pertussis is either erythromycin 500 mg orally four times daily or a standard course of one of the newer macrolides (azithromycin or clarithromycin). Trimethoprim (160 mg)/sulfamethoxazole (800 mg) orally twice daily for 14 days is an alternative for patients who are allergic to erythromycin. See the section Flu Syndrome earlier in this chapter for treatment for treatment options for influenza.

Treatment of cough and systemic symptoms such as fever, myalgias, malaise, and chest pain is generally symptomatic. Cough suppression may be achieved with dextromethorphan but often requires codeine sulfate, 15 to 30 mg every 4 to 6 hours, especially at bedtime (see Chapter 59). Bronchodilator treatment with a β-agonists is not helpful in patients with acute bronchitis and no underlying lung disease, (74) but is indicated in patients with evidence of bronchospasm (such as wheezing) on examination (65). Inhaled corticosteroids have not been shown to have a role in the treatment of acute bronchitis in patients without underlying lung disease. Chinese herbs may help shorten the duration of episodes of acute bronchitis; however, available trial data are limited in size and quality (75). Conventional wisdom has suggested that antihistamines should be avoided to prevent inspissated secretions, although empiric data are lacking. Encouragement of good oral hydration is appropriate for all patients with respiratory tract infection.

Smokers with acute bronchitis should be strongly encouraged to stop smoking, particularly for the duration of the acute illness. Smokers with a history of chronic cough before their bronchitis may be more motivated to discontinue smoking permanently in the face of the acute illness. In 50% of those who discontinue smoking, the chronic cough resolves completely within 1 month. Chapter 27 describes approaches to smoking cessation. There is no evidence that smokers who have not developed COPD will benefit from antibiotic treatment for acute bronchitis (73). Chapter 60 discusses the treatment of acute exacerbations of COPD.

Prevention

An acellular pertussis vaccine combined with an adult formulation of diphtheria, tetanus toxoid, and acellular pertussis (DTaP) has been shown to be effective and safe (68). It has been proposed that adolescents routinely receive this vaccine in the future, and it may replace the adult tetanus-diphtheria (Td) vaccine for periodic booster immunization in adults.

Pneumonia

More than 3 million episodes of pneumonia occur annually in the United States, and it is responsible for more than 30 million days of disability requiring bed rest and for 600,000 hospitalizations. With influenza, pneumonia ranks seventh among all diseases as a cause of death (76) and first among infectious diseases. Its mortality rate has been rising during the last two decades (77).

Definition and Distinction from Bronchitis

Pneumonia is a LRI usually accompanied by fever, dyspnea, cough, and evidence of consolidation on chest radiography. Cough may be purulent or dry, and associated with malaise, pleuritic chest pain, and constitutional symptoms. Pneumonia is caused by bacterial, fungal, or viral infection of the alveoli, which results in airspace edema and consolidation usually discernable on physical examination and chest radiograph. The resultant arterial-alveolar gradient causes dyspnea. Patients who are early in the disease course of pneumonia or who are dehydrated and patients with emphysema and reduced lung parenchyma may fail to show any infiltrate or may show a patchy infiltrate on their chest film despite the presence of considerable inflammation. Antibiotics are indicated in pneumonia whereas they are not indicated in acute bronchitis, which typically involves a viral infection of the bronchial epithelium.

Pneumonia Syndromes and Causes

Important clues for the etiologic diagnosis of pneumonia may be obtained from knowledge of the seasonal, environmental, and occupational predilections of the various agents that cause pneumonias. Table 33.9 lists pathogens associated with different epidemiologic characteristics of patients.

Bacterial pneumonias make up the majority of all adult pneumonias, and the largest fraction of these are caused by *S. pneumoniae* (78). Pneumococcal pneumonia may occur in a previously healthy adult, or after a URI, usually with the abrupt onset of shaking chills, fever, pleuritic chest pain, and cough productive of purulent or rusty sputum. Patients with compromised pulmonary clearance of secretions (e.g., depressed consciousness, morbid obesity, abdominal surgery, chronic bronchitis, congestive heart failure, alcoholism) are predisposed to pneumococcal and other bacterial pneumonias; the onset of clinical symptoms may be more insidious in these patients.

Drug-resistant *Streptococcus pneumoniae* (DRSP) is increasingly a problem worldwide, with up to one half of isolates showing *in vitro* evidence of resistance (79). Pneumococci resistant to penicillin are often resistant to cephalosporins, macrolides, doxycycline, and trimethoprim/sulfamethoxazole as well. Characteristics of patients at higher risk for DRSP include age older than 65 years, β-lactam therapy in the previous 3 months, alcoholism,

TABLE 33.9 Epidemiologic Characteristics Associated with Specific Community-Acquired Pneumonia Pathogens

Characteristic	*Pathogens*
Alcoholism	*Streptococcus pneumoniae,* anaerobes, gram-negative bacilli, tuberculosis
COPD/smoking	*S. pneumoniae, Haemophilus influenzae, Moraxella catarrhalis, Legionella*
Nursing home residency	*S. pneumoniae,* gram-negative bacilli, *H. influenzae, Staphylococcus aureus,* anaerobes, *Chlamydia pneumoniae,* tuberculosis
Poor dental hygiene	Anaerobes
Exposure to bats	*Histoplasma capsulatum*
Exposure to birds	*Chlamydia psittaci, Cryptococcus neoformans, Histoplasma capsulatum*
Exposure to rabbits	*Francisella tularensis*
Exposure to farm animals or parturient cats	*Coxiella burnetii* (Q fever)
Travel to southwest U.S.	Coccidioidomycosis
Suspected large-volume aspiration	Chemical pneumonitis, anaerobes, or obstruction
Structural lung disease (bronchiectasis, cystic fibrosis, etc.)	*Pseudomonas aeruginosa, Pseudomonas cepacia, S. aureus*
Injection drug use	*S. aureus,* anaerobes, tuberculosis, *Pneumocystis carinii*
Recent antibiotic therapy	Drug-resistant pneumococci, *Pseudomonas aeruginosa*
Endobronchial obstruction	Anaerobes

Adapted from Niederman MS, Mandell LA, et al. Guidelines for the management of adults with community-acquired pneumonia. Am J Respir Crit Care Med 2001;163:1730.

immunosuppressive illness or medication (including corticosteroid therapy), multiple medical comorbidities, and exposure to a child in a day care center (78). The clinical significance of DRSP pneumonia is still not completely understood. There is some evidence of increased morbidity and mortality among patients infected with DRSP with high levels of resistance, but infections with intermediate resistance appear to respond well to β-lactam treatment for pneumonia and may be of clinical significance only in the treatment of otitis media or meningitis (80).

The so-called *atypical pneumonia syndrome,* most common among patients younger than 40 years of age, is characterized by a prodrome of headache and myalgia preceding the onset of respiratory symptoms. Respiratory pathogens commonly causing "atypical pneumonia" include *M. pneumoniae, Legionella pneumophila, C. pneumoniae* (TWAR strain), a number of viruses (influenza A and B, respiratory syncytial virus, parainfluenza, adenovirus), *Chlamydia psittaci, Coxiella burnetii* (Q fever), *Coccidioides immitis,* and *Pneumocystis carinii.* Nonetheless, all of these pathogens may result in a pneumonitis that is clinically and radiographically indistinguishable from pneumococcal pneumonia (81,82); because "typical" bacterial pneumonias are also commonly preceded by a prodrome of headache, myalgias, and malaise, the designation "atypical pneumonia" is of little use in practice.

Pneumonias caused by *Mycoplasma* or *Chlamydia* often manifest with sore throat, as well as fever and cough. *C. pneumoniae* may cause a biphasic illness, with severe pharyngitis and laryngitis in the first phase, followed by pneumonia (83,84).

Complications of *Mycoplasma* pneumonia include sinusitis, otitis media, myringitis (diagnostic if bullae are seen), erythema multiforme or erythema nodosum, intravascular hemolysis, meningoencephalitis, toxic psychosis, myocarditis, and pericarditis. Fulminant infection can occur irrespective of age or host status. Persistent hacking cough, lasting as long as 6 weeks despite therapy, is common and requires symptomatic relief with codeine (see Chapter 59). Relapse of the primary disease occurs in up to 10% of cases, usually 2 to 3 weeks after the initial illness, and is probably related to the fact that mycoplasma persists in bronchial epithelium for up to 14 weeks.

Pseudomonas aeruginosa is an uncommon cause of pneumonia, particularly in the outpatient setting. Risk factors for development of *P. aeruginosa* pneumonia include structural lung disease (e.g., bronchiectasis, cystic fibrosis), corticosteroid therapy, malnutrition, and recent broad-spectrum antibiotic therapy for longer than 7 days. A sputum culture that yields *P. aeruginosa* is not always indicative of true infection and may represent only colonization.

Legionnaire disease (caused by *Legionella pneumophila* and other species), in comparison with other causes of pneumonia, is more likely to be associated with headache, confusion, and diarrhea and is less likely to cause cough, expectoration, and thoracic pain (85). Laboratory abnormalities associated with Legionnaire disease include hyponatremia and elevated serum creatine kinase activity. However, many of these symptoms, signs, and laboratory abnormalities may be seen with other typical and atypical bacterial pneumonias.

Pneumocystis carinii pneumonia (PCP) should be considered if the onset of fever, cough, and dyspnea is insidious over 1 to 4 weeks and the patient is immunocompromised or has risk factors for HIV infection (see Chapter 39). The chest radiograph typically shows diffuse bilateral infiltrates but may show focal infiltrates, cysts, pneumothorax, or no abnormality (86).

Primary influenza viral pneumonia is an *early* complication of influenza illness. It occurs predominantly among the elderly and patients with chronic illnesses and occasionally in healthy young adults. Within the first day or two of illness, the dry cough becomes productive and sometimes bloody, and tachypnea and dyspnea may progress rapidly to hypoxia, cyanosis, and delirium. Diffuse rales are present on examination. The chest radiograph often reveals bilateral interstitial infiltrates, but lobar consolidation may also be seen. ARDS may develop. Immediate hospitalization and intensive care are required, but the mortality rate remains high. Some patients have milder influenza pneumonia, with persistent fever, cough, dyspnea, localized rales, and normal white blood cell (WBC) count, and they subsequently experience a benign course. Although there are no reported studies of antiviral drugs (Table 33.3) for the treatment of influenza pneumonia, their use is reasonable in patients in whom it is suspected.

Influenza may also be complicated by *secondary bacterial pneumonia and bronchitis,* more commonly in the elderly and in patients with chronic pulmonary or cardiac disease. The presentation is typically biphasic; initial respiratory symptoms are followed by several days of clinical improvement, and then there is an exacerbation of fever with production of purulent or bloody sputum. The predominant bacterial pathogens are *S. pneumoniae, H. influenzae,* GABHS species, and *S. aureus*; *S. aureus* pneumonia has a mortality rate of approximately 50% in this setting.

Hantavirus pulmonary syndrome (HPS) is a rare pneumonitis with a high mortality rate (87), now recognized throughout the United States and western Canada. After 1 to 7 days of nonspecific viral prodrome of fever, myalgias, chills, and headache, the respiratory phase is heralded by dry cough and dyspnea, with rapid onset of pulmonary edema caused by a capillary leak syndrome. The most lethal complication is cardiogenic shock.

Severe acute respiratory syndrome (SARS) was transmitted globally by SARS-associated coronavirus between February and July 2003, causing more than 8,000 cases and 800 deaths. SARS was thereafter contained, but it is unclear if or when another outbreak may occur. Continued surveillance is therefore necessary. SARS is characterized by an incubation period of 2 to 10 days; early systemic symptoms followed within 2 to 7 days by dry cough and/or shortness of breath, often without upper respiratory tract symptoms; development of radiographically confirmed pneumonia by day 7 to 10 of illness; lymphopenia in most cases; and recent travel to China or surrounding countries or occupational exposure (88). Further information can be found at http://www.cdc.gov/ncidod/sars/clinicians.htm.

Evaluation

Physical Examination

No specific signs or constellation of signs can confirm the diagnosis of pneumonia (66); however the physical examination is helpful in distinguishing pneumonia from acute bronchitis, from other causes of dyspnea, for evidence of chronic lung disease and for early detection of complications (e.g., pleural effusion). The physical examination cannot reliably distinguish between bacterial and atypical pneumonia syndromes. Crepitant rales that do not clear with cough are suggestive of pneumonia of either type, but signs of consolidation (increased tactile fremitus, dullness to percussion, bronchial breath sounds, and egophony) are more common in typical bacterial pneumonia. In the early stages of pneumonia, the examination may be normal despite an infiltrate on the chest film. Alternatively, rales and rhonchi may indicate pneumonia before the appearance of an infiltrate.

Diagnostic Testing

Every patient with suspected pneumonia should have a chest radiograph to establish the diagnosis and evaluate for possible complications (78). Although chest radiography is essential for the firm diagnosis of pneumonia, a normal film does not necessarily rule out pneumonia, and radiographic patterns are not a specific indication of the cause (89). For patients with underlying heart or lung disease, measurement of oxygenation by pulse oximetry (or arterial blood gas analysis) are recommended to help to determine the need for hospitalization. Routine blood tests, including complete blood counts and serum chemistries, are of little value in determining the cause of the pneumonia but may have prognostic value and can also play a role in determining the need for hospitalization (78).

A sputum Gram stain is generally *not* recommended for the evaluation of outpatients with pneumonia (78). It can be helpful occasionally in directing initial therapy, but discordant results between Gram stain and culture in pneumococcal pneumonia, and the lack of diagnostic data for many other common respiratory pathogens including *Legionella*, *Mycoplasma*, and *Chlamydia*, render the Gram stain of limited utility. *Sputum cultures* likewise have limited utility in the management of ambulatory pneumonias, because sputum samples are often contaminated by oral flora and cultures are often negative if any prior antibiotic therapy has been administered (90).

Serologic testing and *cold agglutinin measurement* are usually *not* useful in the initial evaluation of patients with CAP; consensus guidelines recommend against their use to direct therapy (78). Few pathogens can be diagnosed by serologic study of the acute serum specimen; exceptions include pertussis and hantavirus infection. Rapid test kits are available for the office diagnosis of influenza, but there are limitations to their use (see Flu Syndrome). During an apparent community outbreak of a respiratory illness caused by unculturable agents, it is helpful to the public health authorities for practitioners to collect and save acute and convalescent sera for later study at reference laboratories. Guided by epidemiologic clues (Table 33.8), measurement of acute and convalescent titers for antibodies against selected infectious agents may be considered. Testing for antibodies to *M. pneumoniae,* Q fever, psittacosis, influenza, *Legionella* species, tularemia, *C. immitis,* and *Histoplasma capsulatum* is available at most state diagnostic laboratories and many commercial laboratories.

Management

An etiologic diagnosis of pneumonia would require many different tests and a specific etiology cannot be defined in up to 50% of cases despite extensive diagnostic testing (91). Therefore, antibiotic choices are driven by the epidemiology of host–microbial interaction and treatment decisions focus on the need for hospitalization. The desire to avoid unnecessary hospitalizations has led to studies defining low-risk patients with CAP who can be treated as outpatients (92).

Decision about Hospitalization

The 2003 update to the pneumonia guidelines of the Infectious Disease Society of America suggest a three-step assessment of the need for hospitalization in a patient with pneumonia (93). First, the social setting of the patient should be assessed to determine if it is stable enough to allow reliable oral antibiotic therapy and convalescence. If sufficiently stable, the second step is calculation of the Pneumonia Severity Index (PSI). Third, the PSI should be supplemented as appropriate with clinical judgment.

The PSI originated from a meta-analysis of pneumonia outcomes, which revealed multiple prognostic factors associated with increased mortality: altered mental status, male gender, absence of pleuritic chest pain, hypothermia, systolic hypotension, tachypnea, diabetes mellitus, neoplastic disease, leukopenia, and multilobar pulmonary infiltrates (94). A survey of practitioners making decisions on hospitalization for pneumonia indicated that hypoxemia, inability to maintain oral intake, and lack of patient home care support were almost universal and appropriate criteria for admission. However, practitioners usually overestimated the risk of death from pneumonia, based on examination and comorbidity, resulting in excessive use of hospitalization (95). The large *Patient Outcomes Research Team (PORT) study,* which used data from more than 14,000 patients with CAP, established that *if the answers to all of the following three questions are "No,"* the patient is in the lowest of five risk classes (group I), with a 30-day mortality rate less than 0.4% (92):

- *Is the patient older than 50 years of age?*
- *Is one or more of the following coexisting conditions present:* neoplastic (except skin cancer), cerebrovascular, renal, or liver disease or congestive heart failure?
- *Is one or more of the following abnormalities on physical examination present:* altered mental status, pulse rate faster than 125 beats/per minute, respiratory rate faster than 30 breaths per minute, systolic blood pressure lower than 90 mmHg, temperature lower that 35°C or higher than 40°C?

If the answers to any of these three questions was "Yes," further risk assessment was determined by a point scoring system including the additional characteristics listed in Table 33.10, each of which was independently associated with increased morbidity. Patients in risk class I had a 0.1% to 0.4% risk of mortality within 30 days; class II patients (70 points or less) had a 0.6% to 0.7% risk, and class III patients (71 to 90 points) had a 0.9% to 2.8% risk. (92). Most patients in classes I and II may be safely managed as outpatients; class III patients are potential candidates for outpatient therapy or a brief inpatient observation. In contrast, patients in classes IV (91 to 130 points) and V (more than 130 points) had 30-day mortality rates of 8.2% to 9.3% and 27.0% to 31.1%, respectively, and are usually best treated in hospital settings. The PORT-derived indicators of risk can be used as general guidelines until prospective studies provide even more precise rules, but clinical judgment should supersede such rules. Complications such as concomitant meningitis or septic arthritis, hemoptysis, prior splenectomy, and need for respiratory isolation of potential tuberculosis or pneumonic plague must be considered. Moreover, a patient's social situation and personal preferences should play a role in the decision whether to hospitalize.

TABLE 33.10 Point Scoring System for Step 2 of the Prediction Rule for Assignment to Risk Classes II (=70 Points), III (71–90 Points), IV, and V

Characteristic	*Points Assigned*[a]
Demographic factor	
Age	
Men	Age (yr)
Women	Age (yr) −10
Nursing home resident	+10
Coexisting illness	
Neoplastic disease	+30
Liver disease	+20
Congestive heart failure	+10
Cerebrovascular disease	+10
Renal disease	+10
Physical examination findings	
Altered mental status	+20
Respiratory rate = 30/min	+20
Systolic blood pressure <90 mmHg	+20
Temperature <35°C or = 40°C	+15
Pulse = 125/min	+10
Laboratory and radiographic findings	
Arterial pH <7.35	+30
Blood urea nitrogen = 30 mg/dL (11 mmol/L)	+20
Sodium <130 mmol/L	+20
Glucose = 250 mg/dL (14 mmol/L)	+10
Hematocrit <30%	+10
Partial pressure of arterial oxygen <60 mmHg	+10
Pleural effusion	+10

[a] A total point score for a given patient is obtained by summing the patient's age in years (age minus 10 for women) and the points for each applicable characteristic.

Adapted from Fine MJ, Auble TE, Yealy DM, et al. A prediction rule to identify low-risk patients with community-acquired pneumonia. N Engl J Med 1997;336:243.

Ambulatory Management: Choice and Duration of Antimicrobial Therapy

The treatment of CAP is by necessity empiric and based on a knowledge of epidemiology and estimates of patient risk for different pathogens.

The American Thoracic Society has issued consensus guidelines for the initial treatment of immunocompetent adults with CAP (78); these guidelines are reasonable and practical but require further study to show that adherence improves outcome. The guidelines divide ambulatory patients into two groups, based on the presence or absence of cardiopulmonary disease and modifying factors that increase the risk of infection with drug-resistant pneumococcus, enteric gram-negative bacteria, or *P. aeruginosa* (Table 33.11).

For ambulatory patients with no comorbidity and no risk factors for drug-resistant *S. pneumoniae* or other modifying factors, an advanced-generation macrolide (azithromycin or clarithromycin) is recommended as first-line therapy; doxycycline is an alternative for patients who are allergic to or intolerant of the macrolides (Table 33.12). Clarithromycin and azithromycin provide coverage for pneumococcal, chlamydial, *Legionella,* and mycoplasmal infections. *Azithromycin* has the advantage of once-daily and single dosing. Clarithromycin, but not azithromycin, can raise blood theophylline levels, occasionally into the toxic range, and dosages of the latter drug should be monitored and adjusted.

TABLE 33.11 Modifying Factors That Increase the Risk of Infection with Specific Pneumonia Pathogens

Drug-Resistant *Streptococcus pneumoniae*
Age >65 yr
β-Lactam therapy within the past 3 mo
Alcoholism
Immune-suppressive illness (including corticosteroid therapy)
Multiple medical comorbidities[a]
Exposure to a child in a day care center
Enteric Gram-Negative Bacteria
Nursing home residence
Underlying cardiopulmonary disease
Multiple medical comorbidities[a]
Recent antibiotic therapy
Pseudomonas Aeruginosa
Structural lung disease (bronchiectasis, cystic fibrosis)
Corticosteroid therapy (>10 mg of prednisone per day)
Broad-spectrum antibiotic therapy for >7 days in the past month
Malnutrition

[a]Includes chronic obstructive pulmonary disease, diabetes mellitus, renal insufficiency, congestive heart failure, coronary artery disease, malignancy, chronic neurologic disease, and chronic liver disease.
Adapted from Niederman MS, Mandell LA, et al. Guidelines for the management of adults with community-acquired pneumonia. Am J Respir Crit Care Med 2001;163:1730.

For ambulatory patients with either cardiopulmonary illness (congestive heart failure or COPD), a risk factor for drug resistant *S. pneumoniae,* or another modifying factor, the guidelines recommend treatment with a β-lactam *plus* a macrolide or doxycycline (Table 33.13). The β-lactam options include oral cefpodoxime, cefuroxime, high-dose amoxicillin (1 g every 8 hours), amoxicillin/clavulanate, or parenteral ceftriaxone followed by cefpodoxime. An alternative is an antipneumococcal fluoroquinolone (gatifloxacin, levofloxacin, moxifloxacin) that is active against *S. pneumoniae, M. pneumoniae, Chlamydia trachomatis, Legionella, M. catarrhalis,* and gram-negative aerobes. See Table 33.3 for dosing guidelines for these drugs. The fluoroquinolones are generally effective against DRSP, although resistance has been reported (96) and is increasing due to over-use of these agents. Many experts caution against the indiscriminate use of fluoroquinolones for outpatient treatment of pneumonia, because of concerns about the emerging resistance of pneumococci to this class of antibiotics (80).

TABLE 33.12 Outpatient Treatment of Pneumonia, Group I: Patients with No Cardiopulmonary Disease or Modifying Factors[a]

Possible Pathogens	*Recommended Empiric Therapy*
Streptococcus pneumoniae *Mycoplasma pneumoniae* *Chlamydia pneumoniae* *Haemophilus influenzae* Respiratory viruses *Legionella* species *Mycobacterium tuberculosis* Endemic fungi Miscellaneous	Advanced-generation macrolide: azithromycin or clarithromycin *- or-* Doxycycline

[a]See Table 33.11 for modifying factors. Excludes patients at risk for human immunodeficiency virus infection.
[b]Because many *S. pneumoniae* isolates are resistant to tetracycline, this should only be used if the patient is allergic or intolerant of macrolides.
Adapted from Niederman MS, Mandell LA, et al. Guidelines for the management of adults with community-acquired pneumonia. Am J Respir Crit Care Med 2001;163:1730.

TABLE 33.13 Outpatient Treatment of Pneumonia, Group II: Patients with Cardiopulmonary Disease or Other Modifying Factors[a]

Possible Pathogens	*Recommended Empiric Therapy*
Streptococcus pneumoniae (including DRSP) *Mycoplasma pneumoniae* *Chlamydia pneumoniae* *Haemophilus influenzae* Enteric gram-negatives Respiratory viruses *Legionella* species *Moraxella catarrhalis* *Mycobacterium tuberculosis* Endemic fungi Miscellaneous/mixed infections	β-Lactam (oral cefpodoxime, cefuroxime, high-dose amoxicillin,[b] amoxicillin/clavulanate, or parenteral ceftriaxone followed by cefpodoxime) *plus* Macrolide or doxycycline[c] *- or-* Antipneumococcal fluoroquinolone (gatifloxacin, levofloxacin, moxifloxacin)

DRSP, drug-resistant, *S. pneumoniae.*
[a]See Table 33.11 for modifying factors. Excludes patients at risk for human immunodeficiency virus infection.
[b]One gram every 8 hours.
[c]Erythromycin does not provide coverage against *H. influenzae,* so if amoxicillin is used, it should be with doxycycline or an advanced-generation macrolide (azithromycin or clarithromycin).
Adapted from Niederman MS, Mandell LA, et al. Guidelines for the management of adults with community-acquired pneumonia. Am J Respir Crit Care Med 2001;163:1730.

The duration of therapy for CAP is not precisely defined. The American Thoracic Society guidelines suggest that "typical" bacterial infections, such as pneumococcal pneumonia, should be treated for 7 to 10 days, whereas *Mycoplasma, Chlamydia,* and *Legionella* pneumonias may need longer therapy, ranging from 10 to 14 days. Because an etiologic diagnosis usually is not established in outpatients, clinicians should consider the presence of coexisting illness, the severity of illness at the onset of antibiotic therapy, and the subsequent course in determining the duration of antibiotic therapy. For most infections, a 5-day course of azithromycin is adequate therapy because of its prolonged biologic half-life.

Followup

The patient should be advised to keep in close contact by telephone, maintain good hydration with oral fluids, use aspirin or acetaminophen to control fever and headache, and avoid cigarettes. A telephone contact with the patient 24 hours after the initial visit provides a check on antibiotic adherence and side effects and on the status of symptoms; also it reassures the patient that he or she has access to the clinician should the condition worsen or fail to improve.

A followup visit to the office 3 to 4 days later will help assess response to therapy. Symptoms of pneumococcal pneumonia in the uncompromised host usually abate within 48 to 72 hours after initiation of therapy, and somewhat longer with other pathogens or compromised host defenses. If a substantial clinical response to the initial antibiotic therapy has not occurred in this time, the patient must be reevaluated. Possible reasons for clinical failure include poor adherence to the antibiotic regimen; resistance of the etiologic organism to the empiric antibiotics prescribed; unusual pathogens such as tuberculosis, viral, or fungal pneumonia; and a noninfectious cause such as pulmonary embolus or carcinoma. In any case, hospitalization usually is required to determine the cause of therapeutic failure and to provide additional treatment. Complete resolution of symptoms caused by an episode of pneumonia may not occur for 30 days or longer after diagnosis (96).

After clinical resolution of the pneumonia, a chest radiograph is recommended in 4 to 6 weeks to exclude malignancy or other persistent lung abnormalities, particularly in smokers and in patients older than 40 years of age (78). The rate of radiographic resolution depends on age and extent of pneumonic involvement; although most patients have complete clearance at 4 weeks, elderly patients and those with multilobar pneumonia or underlying lung disease can have delayed resolution (97).

Prevention of Pneumonia

Chapter 18 discusses polyvalent pneumococcal and influenza vaccines in detail. No special precautions need be taken to isolate the ambulatory patient with pneumonia. Household contacts of these patients need no special surveillance, with the exceptions of pneumonic disease caused by tuberculosis (see Chapter 34), tularemia, plague, or meningococci.

Pleuritis and Pleurodynia

Pneumonic infections may cause inflammation or infection of the pleura, resulting in pleuritic chest pain and the appearance of a pleural effusion. Parapneumonic effusions and empyemas are typically caused by bacterial pneumonias, but tuberculosis, atypical bacteria, viruses, fungi, and even parasites may cause pleuritis. Chapter 59 discusses the evaluation of pleural effusions.

Pleurodynia is an uncommon acute illness usually caused by one of the coxsackie viruses. It occurs in summer and early fall. The presenting symptoms may suggest the onset of pneumonia: abrupt onset of *severe paroxysmal pain of the thorax or abdomen,* worse with cough or breathing. Other manifestations of pleurodynia include fever, headache, cough, and anorexia. The physical examination is often normal except that the patient splints to avoid pain, which is commonly felt in the lower rib cage or under the sternum. The chest radiograph is usually normal. Most patients recover within 3 days to 1 week. Rare complications are orchitis, pericarditis, and aseptic meningitis.

APPROPRIATE PRESCRIBING OF ANTIBIOTICS FOR RESPIRATORY TRACT INFECTIONS

Antibiotics for respiratory tract infections account for approximately 50% of antibiotic prescriptions written in physicians' offices in the United States (98). Although there was a decline in the number of antibiotic prescriptions for respiratory tract infections during the last decade, approximately 50% of patients with colds or nonspecific URIs, 60% of patients with acute bronchitis, and 70% of patients with sinusitis still received antibiotics (98–100). More than half of patients who were prescribed an antibiotic for these URIs were treated with a broad-spectrum agent (100). A comparison of these rates with the estimated incidence in adults of acute bacterial sinusitis (15%) and GABHS pharyngitis (10%)—the principal acute URIs for which antibiotics are indicated—strongly suggests that the use of antibiotics for URIs in practice should be reduced.

The overuse of antibiotics for respiratory tract infections exposes patients to unnecessary side effects, especially allergic reactions, diarrhea, and vaginitis (Table 33.3); increases medical care costs both for individual patients and health care payors; and contributes to the increasingly serious problem of antibiotic resistance.

Antibiotic Resistance

The importance of emerging antibiotic resistance in relation to respiratory tract infections is illustrated by the increasing resistance of *S. pneumoniae* to multiple antibiotics. Since the 1990s, the rates of resistant strains of this key respiratory pathogen have increased from 25% to 40% for penicillin, 29% to 35% for trimethoprim/sulfamethoxazole, 8% to 20% for tetracyclines and 20% to 28% for macrolide antibiotics (101–104). Although the most common respiratory bacterial pathogens remain susceptible to the newer fluoroquinolones (Table 33.3), increasing resistance has been reported for older ones such as ofloxacin, with rates of about 5% (105).

The proliferation of day care arrangements for young children and the increase in global travel also contribute to the emergence of antibiotic resistance, but the frequent prescription of antibiotics for respiratory tract infections probably is a major contributor to this problem. There is evidence that individual patients who received multiple or recent courses of antibiotics are more likely to be colonized with resistant strains of bacteria. It is also clear that rising rates of antibiotic resistance for a particular antibiotic parallel increased use of that antibiotic; efforts to decrease the use of certain antibiotics in some countries have resulted in declining rates of resistance to those antibiotics (106). Although the possibility of resistant bacteria in some URIs, such as suspected acute bacterial sinusitis, warrants the consideration of broad-spectrum antibiotics in selected patients, their indiscriminate use will only worsen the problem of resistance.

Successful Approaches to Limiting Antibiotics

Practitioners can use the following principles to limit antibiotic prescriptions for respiratory tract infections to appropriate indications:

- Specific clinical criteria offer reasonable accuracy in the selection of patients who should receive antibiotics for acute bacterial sinusitis (Table 33.2) or GABHS pharyngitis (Table 33.5).
- Nonspecific acute URI generally should not be treated with antibiotics.
- Purulent nasal secretions or productive cough by themselves do not reliably indicate the presence of an acute bacterial infection or the need for antibiotic treatment.
- Symptoms lasting longer than several days do not necessarily indicate bacterial complications or the need for antibiotics; symptoms of most viral URIs and bronchitis typically last for 1 week or longer.
- When antibiotics are indicated for acute sinusitis, GABHS pharyngitis, or pneumonia, treatment should be initiated with the recommended first-line, narrower-spectrum antibiotics; newer, broad-spectrum antibiotics usually should be considered only if there are specific reasons to suspect antibiotic resistance or more serious disease (Table 33.11).

Similar principles have been applied successfully in practice settings (70,107). A multifaceted educational intervention targeted at patients and clinicians successfully reduced antibiotic prescriptions for bronchitis from 74% to 48%, without increasing the duration of illnesses or utilization of medical services or other medications (108). An important component of that intervention was use of the term "chest cold" instead of "bronchitis" in referring to cough illness. This study and others emphasize the importance of providing adequate explanations to patients of the appropriate use of antibiotics.

A successful approach to patients seeking care for respiratory tract infections for whom antibiotics are not indicated should include the following:

- Determining which symptoms are the most bothersome for the patient.
- Recommending or prescribing specific symptomatic treatment (see Table 33.1). Decongestants are often effective for nasal symptoms, systemic and topical analgesics are helpful for sore throat, and cough suppressants and sometimes inhaled bronchodilators may be useful for cough illnesses.
- Explaining to patients the natural history of many viral URIs and bronchitis, which may include the persistence of nasal symptoms or cough for 1 week or longer.
- Emphasizing to patients the personal benefits of foregoing unnecessary antibiotics (decreased exposure to adverse effects, fewer expenditures, lower risk of subsequent infection with antibiotic-resistant bacteria), as well as the importance to society of reducing antibiotic use.

Contrary to the beliefs of many clinicians, patients' expectations for antibiotics may not be insurmountable. Reduced prescribing of antibiotics is not necessarily associated with less-satisfied patients (70). Rather, patient satisfaction with encounters for respiratory complaints may have more to do with the adequacy of explanations for their illness (109). Many governmental, national, and local health care organizations are working to reduce antibiotic use for respiratory tract infections, and clinicians should increasingly be able to find support in this effort. The CDC's Campaign for Appropriate Antibiotic Use in the Community provides some helpful resources and materials for clinicians (www.cdc.gov/drugresistance/community).

SPECIFIC REFERENCES*

1. Heikkinen T, Jarvinen A. The common cold. Lancet 2003;361:51.
2. Monto A. Epidemiology of viral respiratory infections. Am J Med 2002;112:4S.
3. Musher D. Medical progress: how contagious are common respiratory tract infections? N Engl J Med 2003;348:1256.
4. Zitter J, Mazonson P, Miller D, et al. Aircraft cabin air recirculation and symptoms of the common cold. JAMA 2002;288:483.
5. Jepson S, Holbrook JH, Hale D, et al. Management of upper respiratory tract infections by telephone. West J Med 1994;160:529.
6. Graham NMH, Burrell CJ, Douglas RM, et al. Adverse effects of aspirin, acetaminophen, and ibuprofen on immune function, viral shedding, and clinical status in rhinovirus-infected volunteers. J Infect Dis 1990;162:1277.

*Bold numerals denote published controlled clinical trials, meta-analyses, or consensus-based recommendations.

7. Sperber SJ, Hendley JO, Hayden FG, et al. Effects of naproxen on experimental rhinovirus colds: a randomized, double-blind, controlled trial. Ann Intern Med 1992;117:37.
8. Forstall GJ, Macknin ML, Yen-Lieberman BR, et al. Effect of inhaling heated vapor on symptoms of the common cold. JAMA 1994;271:1109.
9. Sakethoo K, Januszkiewicz A, Sackner MA. Effects of drinking hot water and chicken soup on nasal mucus velocity and nasal airflow resistance. Chest 1978;74:408.
10. Jackson J, Peterson C, Lesho E. A meta-analysis of zinc salts lozenges and the common cold. Arch Intern Med 1997;157:2373.
11. Prasad A. Zinc: the biology and therapeutics of an ion. Ann Intern Med 1996;125:142.
12. Smith MBH, Feldman W. Over-the-counter cold medications: a critical review of clinical trials between 1950 and 1991. JAMA 1993;269:2258.
13. Hayden FG, Diamond L, Wood PB, et al. Effectiveness and safety of intranasal ipratropium bromide in common colds: a randomized, double-blind, placebo-controlled trial. Ann Intern Med 1996;125:89.
14. Salerno S, Jackson J, Berbano E. Effect of oral pseudoephedrine on blood pressure and heart rate: a meta-analysis. Arch Intern Med 2005;165:1686.
15. Luks D, Anderson M. Antihistamines and the common cold: a review and critique of the literature. J Gen Intern Med 1996;11:240.
16. Curley FJ, Irwin RS, Pratter MR, et al. Cough and the common cold. Am Rev Respir Dis 1988;138:305.
17. Douglas RM, Chalker EB, Treacy B. Vitamin C for preventing and treating the common cold. Cochrane Database Syst Rev 2001;4.
18. Chalmers T. Effects of ascorbic acid on the common cold: an evaluation of the evidence. Am J Med 1975;58:532.
19. Truswell AS. Ascorbic acid and the common cold [Letter]. N Engl J Med 1986;315:709.
20. Hemila H. Does vitamin C alleviate the symptoms of the common cold? A review of current evidence. Scand J Infect Dis 1994;26:1.
21. Levine M, Rumsey SC, Daruwala R, et al. Criteria and recommendations for vitamin C intake. JAMA 1999;281:1415.
22. Melchart D, Linde K, Fischer P, Kaesmayr J. Echinacea for preventing and treating the common cold. Cochrane Database Syst Rev 2005;4.
23. Gonzales R, Bartlett JG, Besser RE, et al. Principles of appropriate antibiotic use for treatment of nonspecific upper respiratory tract infections in adults: background. Ann Intern Med 2001;134:490.
24. Hendley JO. The host response, not the virus, causes the symptoms of the common cold [Editorial comment]. Clin Infect Dis 1998;26:847.
25. Reuler JB, Lucas LM, Kumar KL. Sinusitis: a review for generalists. West J Med 1995;163:40.
26. Hickner JM, Bartlett JG, Besser RE, et al. Principles of appropriate antibiotic use for acute rhinosinusitis in adults: background. Ann Intern Med 2001;134:498.
27. Sande MA, Gwaltney JM. Acute community-acquired bacterial sinusitis: continuing challenges and current management. Clin Inf Dis 2004;39:S151.
28. Williams JW Jr, Simel DL. Does this patient have sinusitis? Diagnosing acute sinusitis by history and physical examination. JAMA 1993;270:1242.
29. Piccirillo, JF. Acute bacterial sinusitis. N Engl J Med 2004;351:902.
30. Engels EA, Terrin N, Barza M, et al. Meta-analysis of diagnostic tests for acute sinusitis. J Clin Epidemiol 2000;53:852.
31. Williams JW Jr, Roberts L Jr, Distell B, et al. Diagnosing sinusitis by x-ray: is a single Waters view adequate? J Gen Intern Med 1992;7: 481.
32. Gwaltney JM Jr, Phillips CD, Miller RD, et al. Computed tomographic study of the common cold. N Engl J Med 1994;330:25.
33. Williams JW Jr, Aguilar C, Cornell J, et al. Antibiotics for acute maxillary sinusitis. Cochrane Database Syst Rev 2003;2.
34. Balk EM, Zucker DR, Engels EA, et al. Strategies for diagnosing and treating suspected acute bacterial sinusitis: a cost effectiveness analysis. J Gen Intern Med 2001;16:701.
35. Anon JB, Jacobs MR, Poole MD, et al. Sinus and allergy Health partnership. Antimicrobial treatment guidelines for acute bacterial rhinosinusitis. Otolaryngol Head Neck Surg 2004;130:S1.
36. Piccirillo JF, Mager DE, Frisse ME, et al. Impact of first-line vs. second-line antibiotics for the treatment of acute uncomplicated sinusitis. JAMA 2001;286:1849.
37. Williams JW Jr, Holleman DR, Samsa GP, et al. Randomized controlled trial of 3 vs. 10 days of trimethoprim/sulfamethoxazole for acute maxillary sinusitis. JAMA 1995;273:1015.
38. Gross PA, Rodstein M, LaMontagne JR, et al. Epidemiology of acute respiratory illness during an influenza outbreak in a nursing home. Arch Intern Med 1988;148:559.
39. Thompson WW, Shay DK, Weintraub E, et al. Mortality associated with influenza and respiratory syncytial virus in the United States. JAMA 2003;289:179.
40. Cox NJ, Subbarao K. Influenza. Lancet 1999;354:1277.
41. Harper SA, Fukuda K, Uyeki TM, et al. Prevention and control of influenza: recommendations of the advisory committee on immunization practices. MMWR Morb Mortal Wkly Rep 2005;54:1.
42. Thompson WW, Shay DK, Weintraub, E, et al. Influenza-associated hospitalizations in the United States. JAMA 2004;292:1333.
43. Beigel JH, Farrar J, Han AM, et al. Writing Committee of the World Health Organization (WHO) Consultation on Human Influenza A/H5. Avian influenza A (H5N1) infection in humans. N Engl J Med 2005;353:1374.
44. Call SA, Vollenweider MA, Hornung CA, et al. Does this patient have influenza? JAMA 2005;293:987.
45. Couch RB. Prevention and treatment of influenza. N Engl J Med 2000;343:1778.
46. Moscona, A. Neuraminidase inhibitors for influenza. N Engl J Med 2005;353:1363.
47. Diggory P, Fernandez C, Humphrey A, et al. Comparison of elderly people's technique in using two dry powder inhalers to deliver zanamivir: randomised controlled trial. BMJ 2001;322:577.
48. Skoner DP, Doyle WJ, Seroky J, et al. Lower airway responses to influenza A virus in healthy allergic and non allergic subjects. Am J Respir Crit Care Med 1996;154:661.
49. Fraenkel DK, Bardin PG, Sanderson G, et al. Lower airways inflammation during rhinovirus colds in normal and in asthmatic subjects. Am J Respir Crit Care Med 1995;151:879.
50. Oliveira EC, Marik PE, Colice G. Influenza pneumonia: a descriptive study. Chest 2001;119:1717.
51. Linder JA, Stafford RS. Antibiotic treatment of adults with sore throat by community primary care physicians: a national survey, 1989–1999. JAMA 2001;286:1181.
52. Bisno A. Acute pharyngitis. N Engl J Med 2001;344:205.
53. Bisno AL, Gerber MA, Gwaltney JM Jr, et al. Infectious Diseases Society of America. Practice guidelines for the diagnosis and management of group A streptococcal pharyngitis. Clin Infect Dis 2002;35:113.
54. Cooper RJ, Hoffman JR, Bartlett JG, et al. Principles of appropriate use for acute pharyngitis in adults: background. Ann Intern Med 2001;134:509.
55. Ebell MH, Smith MA, Barry HC, et al. Does the patient have strep throat? JAMA 2000;284:2912.
56. Centor RM, Witherspoon JM, Dalton HP, et al. The diagnosis of strep throat in adults in the emergency room. Med Decis Making 1981;1:239.
57. Bisno AL. Group A streptococcal infections and acute rheumatic fever. N Engl J Med 1991;325:783.
58. Stollerman GH. Rheumatic fever. Lancet 1997;349:935.
59. Miner LJ, Petheram SJ, Daly JA, et al. Molecular characterization of *Streptococcus pyogenes* isolates collected during periods of increased acute rheumatic fever activity in Utah. Pediatr Infect Dis J 2004;23:56.
60. Del Mar CB, Glasziou PP, Spinks AB. Antibiotics for sore throat. Cochrane Database Syst Rev 2005;4.
61. Burton MJ, Towler B, Glasziou P. Tonsillectomy versus non-surgical treatment for chronic/recurrent acute tonsillitis. Cochrane Database Syst Rev 2005;4.
62. Richardson MA. Sore throat, tonsillitis, and adenoiditis. Med Clin North Am 1999;83:75.
63. Herzon FS. Peritonsillar abscess: incidence, current management practices, and a proposal for treatment guidelines. Laryngoscope 1995;105[Suppl 74]:1.
64. Rasgon BM, Quesenberry CP Jr. Acute epiglottis in adults: analysis of 129 cases. JAMA 1994;272:1358.
65. Gonzales R, Sande M. Uncomplicated acute bronchitis. Ann Intern Med 2000;133:981.
66. Metlay JP, Kapoor WN, Fine MJ. Does this patient have community-acquired pneumonia? Diagnosing pneumonia by history and physical examination. JAMA 1997;278:1440.
67. Wright SW, Edwards KM, Decker MD, et al. Pertussis infection in adults with persistent cough. JAMA 1995;273:1044.
68. Ward, J. I., et al. Efficacy of an acellular pertussis vaccine among adolescents and adults. New Engl J Med 2005;353:1555.
69. Nenig ME, Shinefield HR, Edwards KM, et al. Prevalence and incidence of adult pertussis in an urban population. JAMA 1996;275:1672.
70. Gonzales R, Bartlett JG, Besser RE, et al. Principles of appropriate antibiotic use for treatment of uncomplicated acute bronchitis: background. Ann Intern Med 2001;134:521.
71. Bent S, Saint S, Vittinghoff E, et al. Antibiotics in acute bronchitis: a meta-analysis. Am J Med 1999;107:62.
72. Fahey T, et al. Antibiotics for acute bronchitis. Cochrane Database Syst Rev 2005;4.
73. Linder JA, Sim I. Antibiotic treatment of acute bronchitis in smokers: a systematic review. J Gen Intern Med 2002;17:230.
74. Smucny J, Flynn C, Becker L, Glazier R. Beta2-agonists for acute bronchitis. Cochrane Database Syst Rev 2004;1.
75. Wei J, et al. Chinese medicinal herbs for acute bronchitis. Cochrane Database Syst Rev 2005;4.
76. Minio AM, Smith BL. Deaths: Preliminary data for 2000. National vital statistics reports, vol. 49, no. 12, Hyattsville, MD: National Center for Health Statistics, 2001: 5.
77. Pinner RW, Teutsch SM, Simonsen L, et al. Trends in infectious disease mortality in the United States. JAMA 1996;275:189.
78. Niederman MS, Mandell LA, Anzueto A, et al. Guidelines for the management of adults with community-acquired pneumonia: diagnosis, assessment of severity, antimicrobial therapy, and prevention. Am J Respir Crit Care Med 2001; 163:1730.
79. Whitney CG, Farley MM, Hadler J, et al. Increasing prevalence of multi-drug resistant

Streptococcus pneumoniae in the United States. N Engl J Med 2000;343:1917.
80. Heffelfinger JD, Dowell SF, Jorgensen JH, et al. Management of community-acquired pneumonia in the era of pneumococcal resistance. Arch Intern Med 2000;160:1399.
81. Fang G-D, Fine M, Orloff J, et al. New and emerging etiologies for community-acquired pneumonia with implications for therapy. Medicine (Baltimore) 1990;69:307.
82. Marrie TJ, Peeling RW, Fine MJ, et al. Ambulatory patients with community-acquired pneumonia: frequency of atypical agents and clinical course. Am J Med 1996;101:508.
83. Steinhoff D, Lode H, Ruckdeschel G, et al. *Chlamydia pneumoniae* as a cause of community acquired pneumonia in hospitalized patients in Berlin. Clin Infect Dis 1996;22:958.
84. Grayston JT. Infections caused by *Chlamydia pneumoniae* strain TWAR. J Infect Dis 1992;15:757.
85. Sopena N, Sabri-Leal, Pedor-Botet ML, et al. Comparative study of the clinical presentation of legionella pneumonia and other community-acquired pneumonias. Chest 1998;113: 1195.
86. Kennedy CA, Goetz MB. Atypical roentgenographic manifestations of *Pneumocystis carinii* pneumonia. Arch Intern Med 1992;152:1390.
87. Duchin J, Koster FT, Peters CJ, et al. Hantavirus pulmonary syndrome: a new illness in the southwestern United States. N Engl J Med 1994;330:949.
88. Centers for Disease Control and Prevention. In the absence of SARS-CoV transmission worldwide: guidance for surveillance, clinical and laboratory evaluation, and reporting. Version 2. 2005 Available at: www.cdc.gov/ncidod/sars/absenceofsars.htm.
89. Bartlett JG, Mundy LM. Community-acquired pneumonia. N Engl J Med 1995;333:1618.
90. Woodhead MA, Arrowsmith J, Chamberlain-Webber R, et al. The value of routine microbial investigation in community-acquired pneumonia. Respir Med 1991;85:313.
91. Ruiz M, Ewig S, Marcos MA, et al. Etiology of community-acquired pneumonia: impact of age, co-morbidity and severity. Am J Respir Crit Care Med 1999;160:397.
92. Fine MJ, Auble TE, Yealy DM, et al. A prediction rule to identify low-risk patients with community-acquired pneumonia. N Engl J Med 1997;336:243.
93. Mandell LA, Bartlett JG, Dowell SF, et al. Update of practice guidelines for the management of community-acquired pneumonia in immunocompetent adults. Clin Inf Dis 2003;37:1405.
94. Fine MJ, Smith MA, Carson CA, et al. Prognosis and outcomes of patients with community-acquired pneumonia. JAMA 1996;275:134.
95. Fine MJ, Hough LJ, Medsger AR, et al. The hospital admission decision for patients with community-acquired pneumonia: results from the Pneumonia Patient Outcomes Research Team Cohort Study. Arch Intern Med 1997;157:36.
96. Metlay JP, Fine MJ, Schulz R, et al. Measuring symptomatic and functional recovery in patients with community-acquired pneumonia. J Gen Intern Med 1997;12:423.
97. Mittl RL Jr, Schwab RJ, Duchin JS, et al. Radiographic resolution of community-acquired pneumonia. Am J Respir Crit Care Med 1994;149:630.
98. Steinman MA, Gonzales R, Lindeer JA, Landefeld CS. Changing use of antibiotics in community-based practice, 1991–1999. Ann Intern Med 2003;138:425.
99. Mainous AG 3rd, Hueston WJ, Davis MP, Pearson WS. Trends in antimicrobial prescribing for bronchitis and upper respiratory infections among adults and children. Am J Public Health 2003;93:1910.
100. Steinman MA, Landefeld CS, Gonzales R. Predictors of broad-spectrum antibiotic prescribing for acute respiratory tract infections in adult primary care. JAMA 2003;289:719.
101. Whitney CG, Farley MM, Hadler J, et al. Increasing prevalence of multidrug-resistant *Streptococcus pneumoniae* in the United States. N Engl J Med 2000;343:1917.
102. Hyde TB, Gay K, Stephens DS, et al. Macrolide resistance among invasive *Streptococcus pneumoniae* isolates. JAMA 2001;286:1857.
103. Ailani RK, Agastya G, Ailani RK, et al. Doxycycline is a cost-effective therapy for hospitalized patients with community-acquired pneumonia. Arch Intern Med 1999;159:266.
104. Jacobs MR. Streptococcus pneumoniae: epidemiology and patterns of resistance. Am J Med 2004;117:3S.
105. Centers for Disease Control and Prevention. Resistance of *Streptococcus pneumoniae* to fluoroquinolones—United States, 1995–1999. MMWR Morb Mortal Wkly Rep 2001;50:800.
106. Spach DH, Black D. Antibiotic resistance in community-acquired respiratory tract infections: current issues. Ann Allergy Asthma Immunol 1998;81:293.
107. Juzych NS, Banerjee M, Essenmacher L, Lerner SA. Improvements in antimicrobial prescribing for treatment of upper respiratory tract infections through provider education. J Gen Intern Med 2005;20:901.
108. Gonzales R, Steiner JF, Lum A, et al. Decreasing antibiotic use in ambulatory practice. JAMA 1999;281:1512.
109. Hamm RM, Hicks RJ, Bemben DA. Antibiotics and respiratory infections: are patients more satisfied when expectations are met? J Fam Pract 1996;43:56.

For annotated ***General References*** *and resources related to this chapter, visit www.hopkinsbayview.org/PAMreferences.*

Chapter 34

Tuberculosis in the Ambulatory Patient

Patrick A. Murphy

EPIDEMIOLOGY

Incidence Trends

In 1990–1992, the United States was experiencing an increase in tuberculosis incidence. The cause was the human immunodeficiency virus (HIV) epidemic, which had created a large number of susceptible hosts. In addition, the number of cases of tuberculosis (TB) caused by bacilli resistant to most or all standard antituberculosis drugs rapidly increased. These multidrug-resistant (MDR) bacilli were highly lethal for patients with HIV infection, and it was feared that they would also produce untreatable infections in the normal population. Because of these problems, there was a resurgence of interest in the disease, medical and hospital practices were changed, and there was intense followup of diagnosed cases by public health officers.

All this activity has paid off, and the current situation looks better (see American Thoracic Society, www.hopkinsbayview.org/PAMreferences). In 2003, there were 14,874 new cases of TB in the United States, well below the 1985 level of 22,201 and the 1992 level of 26,673. Furthermore, 52% of all the cases occurred in people who were born in other countries, and, of those, two-thirds were born in Haiti, Mexico, India, China, Vietnam, or the Philippines. It seems likely that most such cases were acquired abroad and imported. The number of cases in United States natives fell 44% between 1986 and 2003, whereas the incidence in immigrants rose 53%. More than half of all immigrants with TB present within 5 years after entry into the United States. MDR TB is still virtually 100% lethal in the HIV-infected person. However, the incidence of MDR TB nationwide has decreased markedly. In 1993 there were more than 400 cases (2.5% of total) of MDR TB in persons who had never previously been treated for TB. These were presumably primary infections with a resistant organism. In 2003 there were fewer than 120 such cases (0.8%).

This improvement in the national picture can be attributed to many causes. Skin testing for TB has come back as a diagnostic procedure and is mandatory for health care workers. Patients discovered by this method are promptly given isoniazid (INH) preventive therapy. Clinical suspicion for TB by doctors has escalated, and TB is being considered as a possible cause of almost any chest illness and almost any abnormal chest radiograph. Microbiologic methods for diagnosis have improved: polymerase chain reaction (PCR) allows rapid diagnosis of TB from the sputum, and metabolic inhibition tests allow early detection of drug-resistant bacilli. Four-drug therapy for TB has virtually replaced the old two- and three-drug regimens, and therapy is commonly enforced by directly observing the patient take his or her medicines. Finally, hospitals, clinics, and prisons have refined their ventilating systems to reduce airborne transmission of TB. These changes in practice are discussed later in the chapter.

A major improvement in the investigation of cases of TB is the Tuberculosis Genotyping Program funded by the Centers for Disease Control and Prevention (CDC) in 2004. One culture can be submitted for analysis from every case of TB diagnosed in the United States. It used to be thought that most clinical TB in the United States was because of the reactivation of latent TB in persons who were old or ill. Such infections were thought to be an individual, but not a public health problem. Genotyping has shown that 52% of all U.S. cases of TB were associated with at least one other clinical case, and that the average cluster size was six cases. Most of the clusters were in young people, mostly men, with known risk factors for TB such as homelessness, low socioeconomic status, substance abuse, unemployment, and HIV infection. They often lived in places where transmission is known to occur, such as shelters and jails. Genotyping did confirm some of the old teachings. For example, a man with newly diagnosed TB, age older than 60 years, born abroad, with none of the risk factors mentioned above, is likely to have a unique isolate. Also, although it is possible to be reinfected with a new strain of TB, the incidence is very low. A study from Capetown, South Africa, with a very high TB transmission rate, showed that 16 of 698 cases of pulmonary TB who were treated and apparently cured subsequently developed a second episode of clinical TB. Of these, 12 were infected with a new strain, which was clearly different by genotyping when compared with the strain that caused the original infection (1). At least 11 of these patients with exogenous reinfection were HIV negative (the twelfth was not tested). Because of the low TB rate in the United States, it is thought that the incidence of reinfection here must be much less than 1%.

The relatively good news about TB in the United States is not applicable to the worldwide situation. There are approximately 8 million new cases of TB every year, with about 1.8 million deaths. The world incidence is rising at 1.8% per year, and in sub-Saharan Africa, it is rising at 6.4% per year. The main driver of the TB epidemic is HIV infection.

Human Immunodeficiency Virus and Tuberculosis

It is estimated that a normal adult newly infected with TB has approximately a 5% chance of developing clinical illness in the first 5 years after infection, and a total lifetime risk of approximately 10%. The other 90% of normal people infected with TB have a positive skin test but never develop clinical illness. In contrast are people who are tuberculin positive as a result of a long-standing infection and who then acquire HIV infection. Such people have an annual incidence of clinical disease of 8% to 10%, with essentially a 100% lifetime incidence (2). Even more devastating are the consequences of being HIV positive and then becoming infected with TB. Because HIV seropositivity is often unknown to or concealed by the HIV-infected person, precise estimates of annual risk in this situation are not available. However, there are enough epidemics of severe primary TB among HIV-infected people exposed to an index case of TB to make it clear that the risk must be considerably higher than the 8% to 10% noted for the situation in which TB is acquired first. The annual risk is almost certainly greater than 50% and may approach 100% (3).

There are two other reasons why HIV infection amplifies TB rates. The first is based on the intensity of exposure needed to become infected. TB is acquired by inhaling dried droplet nuclei, which typically contain one to three organisms. A normal person usually must inhale several hundred such nuclei before one of them successfully establishes a caseous focus. Most cases of TB in normal people occur after long-standing, intense exposure to an infected person living in the same house or working in daily close contact. By contrast, a person infected with HIV acquires TB after inhaling an average of less than 10 infected nuclei, meaning that HIV-infected people often acquire TB after casual contact with an infected person. The other reason why HIV infection amplifies TB rates is that the clinical disease is often severe, and many bacilli are coughed out. Each case of TB in an HIV-infected person is therefore more infectious for other people than is the average case of TB in an immunocompetent person (3).

No matter how immunosuppressed one is, one cannot develop TB infection unless one is exposed to the organism. HIV infection acquired by a young male homosexual in Iowa is highly unlikely to be complicated by TB because there is little chance that he will ever be exposed to a case of pulmonary TB.

Reactivation and Primary Tuberculosis

There are now two distinct epidemiologic profiles of clinical TB. Most sporadic symptomatic cases still arise as reactivation disease in a patient who was infected many years ago and was never treated or was inadequately treated. When the patient becomes old or develops an immunosuppressive illness, the disease reactivates. Such patients are infectious for others, and TB can develop in people closely exposed to them. The response to primary TB infection depends on the kind of person infected. Children are highly susceptible to TB and tend to have clinical symptoms shortly after primary infection. Primary infection in an adult usually causes no symptoms, but the newly infected person becomes tuberculin positive (4). As discussed earlier, primary TB in an HIV-infected person tends to be severe and progressive (3).

Causes

The cause of TB in an immunologically normal person residing in the United States is almost always *Mycobacterium tuberculosis.* Atypical mycobacteria, such as *Mycobacterium kansasii* and *Mycobacterium avium-intracellulare,* and certain fungi, such as *Cryptococcus neoformans* and *Histoplasma capsulatum,* may produce disease indistinguishable from TB and should be considered in the differential diagnosis. All of these diseases are more common and more severe in immunosuppressed persons. In foreign countries, bovine TB bacilli can be important infectious agents.

Drug Resistance

In populations who have never been treated with antituberculosis drugs, primary resistance of tubercle bacilli to most drugs occurs at a low level (approximately 1% to 3%). Because the mechanisms of resistance are different for every drug, primary resistance to multiple drugs is uncommon. However, during the past 50 years many inner-city patients have been given antituberculosis drugs without close supervision. Such patients are likely to take drugs singly, because of real or perceived side effects from multiple drugs, and to discontinue therapy entirely after symptoms improve. Not only do the bacilli in these patients become resistant to many antituberculosis drugs, but these resistant organisms may then infect other people. In such cases, the TB is "primary" because the infected person has a new infection. Nonetheless, the tubercle bacilli may be resistant to one or more of the standard antituberculosis drugs. Even in 1965, before the HIV epidemic, children in Brooklyn who were younger than 5 years of age and had primary TB had INH-resistant organisms 15% of the time (4).

The HIV epidemic has amplified the problem of drug-resistant tubercle bacilli that already existed in large cities. It is now not uncommon for tubercle bacilli to be resistant to all three standard antituberculosis drugs: INH, rifampin (RIF), and ethambutol (EMB). Some strains have been resistant to all known antituberculosis drugs. Such MDR strains are disastrous for the HIV-infected person because the disease cannot be controlled and is rapidly fatal. MDR strains are also a major public health hazard for immunocompetent people who are exposed to intense concentrations of infectious droplet nuclei. There is no reason to believe that these organisms are any more virulent than average, and presumably a normal person infected with such strains would have a 10% lifetime risk of developing clinical disease. However, if disease developed, it could not be treated with the usual drugs.

DIAGNOSIS

History

When symptomatic, TB almost always presents with signs and symptoms of weeks' to months' duration. Almost the only time it presents as acute disease is in rare cases of acute meningitis or TB pneumonia. These acute episodes occur when a tuberculous focus ruptures into the cerebrospinal fluid (CSF) or a bronchus, and large quantities of tuberculous pus are suddenly discharged. The history should be directed toward both defining the symptom complex and determining possible exposure to known sources of disease.

Because TB has multiple presentations, chronic unexplained symptoms in any patient should be considered suspicious. Weight loss (documented over a defined period), fever (particularly in the late evenings), night sweats (to be differentiated from environmentally induced sweats), decreased appetite, and the loss of a sense of well-being are the most important nonspecific symptoms. Persistent cough (usually with sputum production), hemoptysis, and pleuritic chest pain are more specific findings suggestive of pulmonary involvement.

It is important to know whether the patient has previously had TB, has previously been skin-tested for TB (and if so, when and what the results were), and when the patient has had previous chest films (and where they can be obtained).

Possibly significant history also includes the patient's country of origin, any family member or close friend with known TB, any person in school or at work with known disease, and any recent history of travel to a country where TB is common.

Because extrapulmonary TB can occur in any organ (e.g., pleura, lymph nodes, endometrium, kidneys, ureters, bones and joints, skin, meninges, small intestine, peritoneum) or as a disseminated (miliary) form, chronic symptoms and signs in any organ must raise the consideration of TB.

Physical Examination

The physical examination may be entirely normal, even with obvious evidence of pulmonary disease on the chest radiograph. The following findings, when present, may be of considerable help in suggesting the diagnosis: rales localized to the upper posterior chest or auscultatory evidence of pulmonary cavitation (bronchovesicular breathing and whispered pectoriloquy), evidence of pleural effusion, supraclavicular and infraclavicular retraction, lymphadenopathy, evidence of weight loss, and fever. Although rare in the United States, large, matted, nontender cervical lymph nodes (at times with draining sinuses) are almost diagnostic of scrofula, a form of tuberculous adenitis seen primarily in children (that also may be caused by atypical mycobacteria).

Tuberculin Skin Tests

The standardized skin test (5) for evidence of tuberculous infection uses 5 units of Tween-stabilized intermediate-strength purified protein derivative (PPD), which is injected intradermally on the volar skin of the forearm. The use of control tests with "anergy panel" antigens has been abandoned. The PPD test requires intradermal injection, which is a highly skilled procedure. Tine tests and automated methods of introducing antigen into the skin such as the Heaf gun can be used in population surveys. Positive results elicited with these methods should be confirmed with the standard PPD. The PPD reaction should be read at 48 hours. A practical method for determining the diameter of the indurated area is the *ballpoint pen method:* a line is drawn from a point 1 to 2 cm away from the margin of a positive reaction; when the pen tip reaches the margin of the indurated area, definite resistance is felt; this is repeated on the opposite side, and the diameter of the indurated reaction is measured.

The diameter required for a *positive test* varies according to circumstances.

Cases in which More than 5 mm is Regarded as Positive

- People with HIV infection and people receiving immunosuppressive therapy
- People with recent close contact with a case of pulmonary TB
- People with fibrotic changes on their chest radiograph suggestive of healed TB

Cases in which More than 10 mm is Regarded as Positive

- In general, those with chronic illnesses known to predispose to TB and those from areas with a high incidence of TB
- People with silicosis, malnutrition (including people with gastrectomy or jejunoileal bypass), or diabetes
- Transplant recipients and people being treated with renal dialysis, corticosteroids, or cancer chemotherapy
- Children younger than 4 years of age
- Recent immigrants from high-prevalence areas
- Medical and laboratory personnel with occupational exposure
- The poor, especially injection drug users
- People from prisons, nursing homes, and other group residences

Cases in which More than 15 mm is Regarded as Positive

- People who are generally healthy and not exposed to TB (testing of such persons is discouraged because most positive test results are falsely positive)

A PPD conversion requires an increase of 10 mm within 2 years for patients of any age. Note that a change from 8 to 12 mm is *not* a PPD conversion. The criteria are not foolproof and should be applied with common sense. In particular, it has been suggested that even 2 mm induration may be significant in an HIV-infected patient (6).

The tuberculin skin test is an excellent way of diagnosing recent tuberculous infection in children or young adults. Such people are rarely tuberculin positive in the absence of recently acquired tuberculous infection. The test is also useful for investigating family members or health care personnel who have had known exposure to patients with infectious TB. Because it is neither specific nor sensitive enough to guide a clinical decision, the tuberculin test is not useful for the evaluation of patients with nonspecific symptoms that may be caused by TB. In some populations of elderly patients, up to 50% may be tuberculin positive as a result of long-standing infection that is inactive and has nothing to do with the present illness. Fully 20% of patients who do have active clinical TB are PPD negative. When one adds in other clinical variables such as tumors, steroid therapy, radiation therapy, and organ transplantation, a negative PPD test is often uninterpretable. Also, a negative PPD test may be harmful if it is used to rule out the diagnosis of TB in a patient whose clinical state may be caused by active disease.

A person with a known positive tuberculin skin test should not have it repeated. In such patients, there is a risk of producing a very strong positive reaction characterized by tender induration, axillary adenopathy, temperature elevation, and sloughing of the epidermis after 1 week. If a patient develops this complication, it should be treated with a sterile gauze dressing impregnated with a topical steroid, such as 0.1% triamcinolone.

The CDC recommends that *previous Bacillus Calmette-Guérin*(BCG) *vaccination* be disregarded when interpreting the response to a PPD (5). The reason is that a positive PPD reaction induced by BCG tends to wane with time. There is no reliable way of determining whether a positive PPD reaction is caused by real TB or by the BCG vaccine. There is agreement that when a person is PPD tested for the first time, very pronounced reactions (greater than 20 mm) are unlikely to be a result of BCG vaccination. On the other hand, recall of PPD sensitivity induced by repetitive PPD testing in persons vaccinated with BCG is commonly seen. Necrotic tuberculin reactions are particularly common in people who were vaccinated with BCG in childhood, become health care workers, and must be PPD tested every 6 or 12 months. If the vaccination was done 20 to 30 years earlier, the first tuberculin test is commonly negative. However, with repeated testing the immunologic memory revives and the reaction becomes progressively more intense. Not only does this raise unwarranted fears of tuberculous infection, but the reactions are very painful. The CDC regulations do not cover this situation; however, it is prudent not to do more than one tuberculin test in anyone previously vaccinated with BCG.

M. tuberculosis shares antigens with related mycobacteria, so a positive skin test is not specific. However, most cross-reactions are less than 10 mm in diameter. Skin testing with specific atypical mycobacterial antigens should not be done: The antigens are not available for general use, and the results are difficult to interpret.

Persons with a remote tuberculous or atypical mycobacterial infection who have become skin-test negative may, on repeat annual skin testing, develop a positive response because the repeated exposure to antigen reinvigorates the immune response (*booster effect*) (7). Repeated testing with tuberculin skin test antigen will not induce a positive test in an uninfected person. The booster phenomenon may mimic PPD conversion in persons who are repeatedly tested, such as elderly people, in whom loss of PPD reactivity is common, and people such as hospital employees who may be skin tested frequently. The booster effect is detected by administering a second tuberculin test 2 weeks after the first test in persons who initially have a negative response. If the second response is positive, these individuals can be said to have had past infection but are not considered to have a recently acquired infection.

Current practice in hospitals is that all employees not known to be PPD positive are tested on entry. If they are PPD negative on entry and have contact with patients, they are retested annually, or more often if the hospital is in an area where TB is common.

Laboratory Evaluation

Chest Radiograph

Both posteroanterior and lateral views should be obtained. If the standard radiograph is normal but the patient has strong clinical evidence for TB, an apical lordotic view or a computed tomography scan of the chest should also be obtained. The radiologic findings typical of TB (e.g., apical scarring, hilar adenopathy with peripheral infiltrate, upper lobe cavitation, miliary infiltrate) are not specific; however, a negative chest film rules out pulmonary TB (with the rare exception of early miliary disease), making the chest film a very sensitive test.

Cultures and Smears of Sputum

Sputum for smear and culture should be obtained at least three times. A *positive sputum smear* highly suggests TB (but is not absolutely diagnostic because of the possibility of atypical infection or of contamination), and a *positive culture is diagnostic.* If sputum is difficult to obtain, one can obtain assisted sputum after the patient has inhaled hypertonic saline aerosol. This procedure is obviously dangerous to personnel and should be done only in a special room with proper precautions for infection control. If clinical features suggest infection outside the lung, smears and cultures of other body fluids such as urine and CSF are appropriate.

PCR tests for *M. tuberculosis* are approved by the U.S. Food and Drug Administration (FDA) for direct use on sputum. However, the tests are subject to errors due to the presence of inhibitors, and most clinical laboratories are not able to routinely offer PCR tests directly on sputum.

Cultures usually become positive within 3 or 4 weeks. Any tubercle bacillus isolated from a patient should be tested for sensitivity to standard drugs, because it may be necessary to change treatment if the organism shows resistance. The state laboratory will be glad to do this if necessary. In parts of the world with very limited funds, it may be necessary to confine drug susceptibility tests to tubercle bacilli from patients who have failed standard therapy.

Miscellaneous Laboratory Tests

In patients with active TB, the hematocrit value may be normal or low. The anemia caused by TB is normochromic and normocytic, the so-called anemia of chronic disease (see Chapter 55). The white blood cell (WBC) count and differential count are usually normal; occasionally a monocytosis is seen in patients with severe disease. The urine should be tested routinely; if sterile pyuria is found, it is suggestive of renal TB and cultures should be sent for analysis.

Determinations of serum aminotransferases, alkaline phosphatase, and bilirubin may be helpful if disseminated disease or liver involvement is suspected. Also, these values provide baselines in case the patient develops hepatitis caused by antituberculosis drugs. Other procedures, such as thoracocentesis, lumbar puncture, and liver biopsy, are indicated only when specific organ involvement is suspected.

Presumptive Diagnosis

The presumptive diagnosis of active TB can be made when any of the following is found:

- A typical chest radiograph
- A positive sputum smear
- A biopsy showing caseating granulomas with or without acid-fast organisms
- A recent change (within 1 year) of the tuberculin skin test result from negative to positive, associated with other characteristic systemic symptoms or signs

The diagnosis of active TB is confirmed by a positive culture from any body fluid or biopsy specimen. All patients with a presumptive or confirmed diagnosis of TB must be reported promptly to the appropriate local health department.

Diagnosis of Tuberculosis in HIV-Infected Patients

In 1993, pulmonary TB in an HIV-positive patient was designated as an *acquired immunodeficiency syndrome (AIDS)–defining condition* (see Chapter 39). When clinical TB appears before the development of other AIDS-indicator conditions, presentation occurs in a typical fashion, with pulmonary disease predominantly in the apices and often with cavitation. Fever, sweats, cough, anorexia, and wasting are common complaints. When TB appears after AIDS is already established, many patients have progressive primary disease, with extensive lower lobe involvement, no cavitation, and hilar adenopathy (3). Extrapulmonary TB is more common in patients with AIDS and may involve lymph nodes, liver, brain, meninges, bone marrow, adrenals, and the genitourinary tract. Aspiration or biopsy of the suspected site of infection should be performed for acid-fast stain and culture. If acid-fast bacilli (AFB) are found in one of these specimens, treatment for *M. tuberculosis* should be initiated while awaiting culture results. In most of the world, acid-fast organisms seen on smears or biopsies are likely to be *M. tuberculosis*. In the low-incidence United States, *M. avium-intracellulare* is more common.

The diagnosis of tuberculosis is important because delays have real consequences in the form of clinical infections of contacts. A schoolboy in California developed TB that was not diagnosed for 12 months (8). He exposed 1,293 people. Among these, there were 12 cases of actual clinical tuberculosis, and 292 PPD conversions.

MANAGEMENT AND COURSE

Treatment

When TB is diagnosed in association with systemic signs or symptoms, the patient should be treated for active disease. Patients with positive tuberculin reactions as the only manifestation of disease are more difficult to treat (see Isoniazid Treatment of Latent Tuberculosis Infection).

Isolation

Any patient with symptomatic TB who is hospitalized should be placed at once in respiratory isolation in a negative-pressure room. Isolation must be instituted as soon as the diagnosis is made or even strongly suspected. One can never prevent a patient walking into an emergency room and exposing a doctor, two or three nurses, a clerk, a radiology technician, and other patients to the risk of TB. But an undiagnosed patient who stays on a medical ward for 2 weeks may easily expose 200 people. Isolation should be maintained until the patient is clearly noninfectious (see Respiratory Isolation for Ambulatory Patients).

In some communities, no hospital has the required isolation rooms and MDR tubercle bacilli are uncommon or unknown. In these circumstances, a patient who has a home can be started on treatment and sent home. The logic is that everyone in the home has already been exposed. The patient is instructed not to leave the house for 2 weeks and not to allow any previously unexposed visitors for the same period. Therapy in the home should be directly observed (see Directly Observed Therapy), and the patient should be allowed to leave the house or have visitors only when clearly improving. It should be noted that this exception to the guidelines does not apply to patients who are homeless or are unlikely to follow directions because of alcoholism or drug addiction. It also does not apply in communities where MDR TB is common.

Drug Therapy for Tuberculosis

The imperatives of the MDR TB situation have resulted in a *standard four-drug protocol* for treatment of TB (9). There is little room for individual variation, and attempts to use nonstandard methods usually result in telephone calls from the local health department. The pressure is in favor of *rendering the patient noninfectious in the shortest possible time*. That way, fewer nurses are required to supervise the therapy.

The current standard initial regimen is as follows:

- *Isoniazid* (INH): 300 mg per day (available strengths, 100 and 300 mg)
- *Rifampin* (RIF): 600 mg per day (available strength, 600 mg)
- *Ethambutol* (EMB): 15 mg/kg/day, commonly 1,200 mg per day (available strengths, 100 and 400 mg)
- *Pyrazinamide*(PZA): 2,000 mg per day (available strength, 500 mg)

All four of these drugs are given for 2 months, and then the EMB and PZA are discontinued. INH and RIF are continued for another 4 months, making *6 months of treatment in all*. When patients are treated on a twice-weekly schedule, the daily dose of drugs is larger (Table 34.1).

After a patient's culture results become available, sensitivities should be checked. If the bacilli are susceptible to all four drugs and if directly observed therapy is used, more than 98% of cases of TB are permanently cured (9).

The enthusiasm for four-drug supervised therapy should not obscure the fact that this regimen is not appropriate for everyone. It is possible to cure TB with two or three drugs, but it takes longer. Patients should receive special consideration if they cannot take all of the components of the standard regimen (10).

There are some special situations where the standard therapy for pulmonary tuberculosis should either be prolonged or changed. The recurrence rate after standard therapy is about 2%, and this value appears to be an irreducible minimum, because prolongation of the regimen does not reduce the recurrence rate. However, if a patient either has a pulmonary cavity, or if the sputum culture is positive after 2 months of therapy, the recurrence rate is about 6%. If there is a cavity *and* the sputum culture is positive at 2 months, then the recurrence rate is 22%. There is general agreement that such patients should be treated for longer, perhaps for 9 months.

Drug Toxicity

Patients may develop a number of toxicities from antituberculosis medications (Table 34.1).

TABLE 34.1 Drugs for the Treatment of Mycobacterial Disease in Adults

Commonly Used Agents	Available Strengths of Oral Tablets or Capsules (mg)	Dosage		Most Common Side Effects	Test for Side Effects	Drug Interactions[a]
		Total Once-Daily Dosage	Twice-Weekly Dosage			
Isoniazid[b]	100, 300	5–10 mg/kg up to 300 mg p.o. or IM	15 mg/kg PO up to 900 mg	Peripheral neuritis, hepatitis, hypersensitivity	Aminotransferases (not as a routine)	Carbamazepine: increased toxicity, both drugs Disulfiram: psychosis, ataxia Phenytoin: toxicity increased
Rifampin	150, 300	10 mg/kg up to 600 mg p.o.	10 mg/kg up to 600 mg p.o.	Hepatitis, febrile reaction, purpura (rare)	Aminotransferases (not as a routine)	May reduce the effect of the following drugs due to increased hepatic metabolism: oral contraceptives, quinidine, corticosteroids, anticoagulants, disopyramide, diazepam, barbiturates, methadone, digitoxin, digoxin, oral hypoglycemics; p-aminosalicylic acid may interfere with absorption of rifampin
Streptomycin		15–20 mg/kg up to 1 g IM	25–30 mg/kg up to 1 g IM	Eighth nerve damage, nephrotoxicity	Vestibular function, audiograms; blood urea nitrogen and creatinine	Neuromuscular blocking agents; may be potentiated to cause prolonged paralysis
Pyrazinamide	500	15–30 mg/kg up to 2 g p.o.	50–70 mg/kg up to 4 g	Hyperuricemia, hepatotoxicity	Uric acid, aminotrans-ferases	
Ethambutol	100, 400	15–25 mg/kg p.o.	50 mg/kg p.o. up to 2.5 g	Optic neuritis (reversible with discontinuation of drug; very rare at 15 mg/ kg), skin rash	Red-green color discrim-ination and visual acuity,[c] difficult to test in a child <3 yr	

IM, intramuscularly; p.o., per os.
[a]Reference should be made to current literature, particularly on rifampin, because it induces hepatic microenzymes and therefore interacts with many drugs.
[b]With pyridoxine 25 mg/day for poorly nourished or pregnant patients to prevent peripheral neuropathy.
[c]Initial examination should be done at start of treatment.
Adapted from American Thoracic Society. Treatment of tuberculosis and tuberculosis infection in adults and children. Am Rev Respir Dis 134:355, 1986; and MMWR, Morb Mortal Wkly Rep 1993;42:2.

Isoniazid

Hepatic toxicity is the most common adverse reaction; it occurs at a biochemical level in approximately 20% of patients who take the drug, and the incidence of toxicity increases with age and with excessive alcohol intake (11). Pregnant women are at increased risk for INH toxicity. Laboratory evidence of mild injury to the liver is not in itself a reason to stop the drug, however, because in most subjects the aminotransferase level returns to normal while the drug is being continued. If the patient develops jaundice or develops fever with elevated liver enzymes, the drug should be stopped. The liver injury is usually reversible and heals without further therapy. However, in some patients (elderly men and particularly those with chronic alcohol-related liver disease), the liver injury can be severe and sometimes fatal. INH liver toxicity most often occurs early in therapy, so that the first 2 to 3 months are the most critical in the detection of adverse drug reactions. Specific guidelines for monitoring for INH hepatitis are discussed later (see Monitoring of Patients Taking INH). Sensory peripheral neuropathy is an uncommon complication of INH therapy that occurs only in patients on an inadequate diet; it can be prevented by taking 25 mg of pyridoxine every day.

Ethambutol

The most serious side effect of EMB is *optic neuritis,* which causes decreased visual acuity and inability to distinguish the color green. This problem was seen frequently when the drug was given at a dose of 25 mg/kg. It is extremely uncommon at the current recommended daily dose of 15 mg/kg.

Rifampin

Serious allergic complications of RIF therapy, including thrombocytopenia manifested by purpura, petechiae, and hematuria; acute renal failure; and a flu-like syndrome, occur in approximately 1% of patients and necessitate cessation of therapy. There is a modest increase in hepatic toxicity that may be additive to INH toxicity, so patients taking both drugs should be supervised closely. Patients should be warned that RIF will result in an orange-red color in secretions such as urine and saliva and may irreversibly stain contact lenses. RIF accelerates the metabolism of other drugs (Table 34.1) and may necessitate an increase in the dosage of these drugs. Interaction with HIV protease inhibitors is a major problem and requires expert advice.

Special Situations

Patients with *nonpulmonary TB* can be treated with the 6-month regimen just described. Exceptions are patients with TB meningitis or bone marrow or joint infection. These patients should receive 12 months of treatment (10).

Pregnant women are difficult to treat because of the need to consider the effects of prescribed drugs on the fetus. The standard recommendation, for areas where MDR TB is uncommon, is a three-drug regimen of INH, RIF, and EMB. There is worldwide experience with this regimen, and it is generally regarded as safe. PZA is a category C drug that could be added if necessary; streptomycin is category D (it may cause fetal deafness), and its use is discouraged. For other antituberculosis drugs, one should seek expert advice.

Patients with *renal failure* are difficult to treat because both EMB and PZA are excreted largely by the kidneys. If renal function is only moderately reduced, this situation can be dealt with by dosage reduction. However, if the patient is on hemodialysis, the calculations become a nightmare. Because the toxicity of EMB is blindness and that of PZA is severe hepatitis, errors are serious. Both INH and RIF can be given in full dosage to people with no renal function, and provided the organisms are sensitive to both antimicrobials, INH plus RIF given together for 9 months cures all forms of TB. It seems better to accept the longer treatment. If there is a real possibility of MDR TB, and a four-drug regimen is necessary, INH, RIF, PZA, and streptomycin might be the safest drugs to prescribe. The hepatotoxicity of PZA is generally reversible, and although ototoxicity of streptomycin is irreversible, the blood level of streptomycin can be measured.

Patients who have HIV infection but are infected with drug-sensitive tubercle bacilli have a good prognosis for cure of their TB. It is usual to treat for 9 months rather than 6 and to be meticulous about follow-up. There is good evidence that patients with HIV as well as TB have higher relapse rates than patients with TB who are immunologically normal (12).

Drug Resistance

If the bacilli prove to be resistant to either INH or RIF, treatment should be modified to a three- or four-drug regimen in which the bacilli are susceptible to all components. Such a regimen should be continued for at least 12 months, and perhaps 18 months in a case of extensive disease.

If the bacilli are resistant to both INH and RIF, the organism is by definition MDR. The patient should be referred for treatment to an expert, either at a university or at the state health department. The patient will be kept in isolation as long as bacilli are found on sputum culture. In order to treat MDR cases, one needs to know the sensitivities to all the drugs that might be useful. It is very important not to provide empiric regimens in the absence of such knowledge, because of the probability that the patient will be treated with only one or two effective drugs. Such treatment usually generates even more resistant bacilli. It is best to wait until the information is available, and pick at least three and preferably four drugs that have activity and can be tolerated. Old drugs such as streptomycin, ethionamide, cycloserine, para-amino salicyclic acid (PAS), and capreomycin may be combined with newer ones such as quinolones and linezolid. If the organism is resistant to rifampin, it is usually but not always resistant to rifampin relatives such as rifabutin and rifapentine. It is generally possible to find some regimen that works. Regimens of six to twelve drugs are not uncommon (13). If the response to the best available therapy remains poor, the addition of γ-interferon infusions can be tried (14). If the

Epidemiologic Features				
Source (Reservoir)	***Transmission to Humans***	***Incubation Period***	***Diagnosis***	***Specific Therapy***
Soil	Foodborne	2–16 h	Culture suspected food	None
Animal feces	Foodborne or waterborne[a]	24–48 h	Culture stool, blood	Macrolide (see text)
Animal feces, soil	Foodborne (canned, low pH, anaerobic)	12–36 h	Culture food, identify toxin in food, blood, stool	Polyvalent antitoxin
Ubiquitous, especially in health care environments (spores)	Probably not necessary but occurs via fomites in hospitals	2–10 days after beginning antibiotics (rarely up to 6 wk after antibiotics stopped)	Identify toxin in stool	Metronidazole or vancomycin (see text)
Human feces, animal feces, soil	Foodborne (meats)	12–24 h	Culture suspected food	None
Human feces	Foodborne	24–48 h	Culture stool	Fluoroquinolone, trimethoprim-sulfamethoxazole, rifaximin
Human feces	Foodborne (cheeses)	24–48 h	Culture stool	Same as *Shigella* (see text)
Human feces	Probably foodborne	24–48 h	Culture stool, small bowel	Antibiotics to which organism is sensitive
Animal feces	Foodborne	24–48 h	Culture stool (see text)	None
Dairy cattle, soil, decaying vegetable matter	Foodborne	18 h–21 days	Stool culture; serum antilisterolysin O	Ampicillin or trimethoprim-sulfamethoxazole
Animal feces; eggs	Foodborne (many foods, see text), person-to-person[a]	12–48 h	Culture stool	Fluoroquinolone or trimethoprim-sulfamethoxazole, in selected cases only (see text)
Human feces	Person-to-person, foodborne	4 days–3 wk	Culture blood, stool, antibacterial antibodies	Fluoroquinolone, ceftriaxone for empiric therapy
Human feces	Person-to-person[a]	12–48 h	Culture stool	Trimethoprim-sulfamethoxazole or fluoroquinolone (see text)
Human skin, nares, mouth	Foodborne (many foods, see text)	2–8 h	Culture food, and food handlers	None
Human pharynx, skin lesions	Foodborne	1–3 days	Culture throat, food, skin lesions of food handlers	Penicillin (see Chapter 28)
Human feces	Waterborne and foodborne	12 h–5 days	Culture stools, antibacterial and antitoxin antibody	Tetracycline

(continued)

TABLE 35.1 (Continued) Characteristics of Acute Illness Caused by Ingestion of Infectious Agents

Agent	Pathogenesis	Usual Clinical Features	Frequency in USA	Usual Pattern
Vibrio parahaemolyticus	Probably both invasion and enterotoxin production; exact mechanism unknown	Diarrhea, abdominal cramps	Uncommon	CSO, S
Vibrio vulnificus (51)	Mechanism unknown	Fever, abdominal pain, diarrhea; septicemia, hemorrhagic bullae on skin	Uncommon	S
Yersinia enterocolitica (40)	Invasion of small and large intestine	Fever, abdominal pain, may suggest appendicitis, diarrhea	Uncommon	CSO, S
Viruses				
Norovirus (52)	Invasion of small intestine	Vomiting and diarrhea	Common	CSO, S
Rotavirus (53)	Invasion of small intestine	Severe gastroenteritis in young children, mild in adults	Common	S
Protozoa and helminths				
Entamoeba histolytica (39)	Invasion of large intestine	Diarrhea, often chronic and bloody	Uncommon, except in travelers	CSO, S
Giardia lamblia (54;55)	Colonization and occasional invasion of small intestine	Diarrhea, flatulence with foul-smelling stools	Uncommon	CSO, S
Trichinella spiralis	(a) Encysted trichinae mature, reproduce in small intestine; (b) larvae penetrate intestine, migrate to muscles where they cause inflammation and encyst	Diarrhea, puffy eyes, muscle aching, fever, occasionally severe heart failure; eosinophilia typical	Rare	CSO, S
Cryptosporidium parvum (19;56)	Colonization	Diarrhea, acute in children and healthy adults; chronic in HIV-infected patients	Common, especially in patients with AIDS	CSO, S
Cyclospora cayetanensis (57)	Colonization	Diarrhea, cramping, heartburn, low-grade fever	Uncommon; more common in travelers, patients with AIDS	CSO, S

CSO, common source outbreak; S, sporadic; AIDS, acquired immunodeficiency syndrome.
[a]Anal–oral transmission may occur.

Sources and Modes of Transmission

Tables 35.1 and 35.2 summarize the *sources and modes of transmission* of the etiologic agents causing foodborne illness. The features of four of the most well recognized etiologic agents illustrate the diverse ways that foodborne disease is acquired:

1. Humans whose skin or nasal mucosa is colonized are almost always the source of *Staphylococcus aureus*. Contamination of food with small numbers of staphylococci is undoubtedly very common. Staphylococcal food poisoning occurs when contaminated foods are allowed to stand long enough for organisms to multiply and produce enterotoxin. The principal foods in which this occurs are those high in protein (meats, either cooked or in salads, and cream-filled cakes and pastries) and those with a high salt or sugar content (ham, salads, and custards) (4).
2. Animals are the source of the *Salmonella* serotypes that cause most human disease; only *Salmonella typhi* and *Salmonella paratyphi* are carried by humans. Foodborne transmission from animal to humans occurs chiefly by fecal contamination of equipment and personnel involved in the packaging and preparing of food, most commonly poultry and meats. Foodborne outbreaks of salmonellosis have also been related to use of undercooked eggs (5). Although eggs with visible shell cracks should always be considered suspect, those with

Epidemiologic Features				
Source (Reservoir)	***Transmission to Humans***	***Incubation Period***	***Diagnosis***	***Specific Therapy***
Seawater	Foodborne (various types of seafood from estuary and seawater)	15–24 h	Culture stool	None
Seawater	Foodborne (various types of seafood from estuary and seawater)	24 h–2 days	Culture stool	Minocycline plus 3rd-generation cephalosporin, fluoroquinolone
Animal feces	Foodborne, person-to-person	Probably 3–7 days	Culture stool	Doxycycline or trimethoprim-sulfamethoxazole
Human feces or emesis	Foodborne and waterborne, person-to-person (secondary cases)	1–3 days	Nucleic acid amplification in stool	None
Human feces	Person-to-person (secondary cases)	1–3 days	Virus antigen in stool Rise in antiviral antibody	None
Human feces	Foodborne and waterborne, person-to-person[a]	Few days to months	Examine stool for trophozoites	Metronidazole or tinidazole plus luminal agent (see text)
Human feces	Waterborne, person-to-person[a]	1–4 wk	Stool antigen assays, Examine stool for trophozoites	Metronidazole, tinidazole, or nitazoxamide
Animal muscle (swine, many wild animals)	Foodborne	2–28 days	Skin tests, antibody, muscle biopsy	Mebendazole or albendazole and steroids (see text)
Fresh water (chlorine-resistant); human and animal feces	Waterborne; person-to-person[a]	2–7 days	Examine stool for trophozoites	Antiretroviral therapy +/− paromomycin or nitazoxamide for patients with AIDS
Human feces	Waterborne; person-to-person[a]	12 h–11 days	Examine stool for oocysts	Trimethoprim-sulfamethoxazole

intact shells can also be infected (e.g., from a salmonella abscess in the ovary of a hen). Only hard-cooked eggs and pasteurized eggs are absolutely safe; raw egg dishes (e.g., homemade salad dressings, eggnog, ice cream) and undercooked eggs (e.g., scrambled and soft-cooked eggs) should be avoided, particularly by immunocompromised and elderly people (5,6).

3. *Clostridium perfringens* is a ubiquitous organism found in human and animal feces and in soil. Meats are the most frequently contaminated foods; transmission of enough organisms to produce illness occurs typically with inadequately heated or reheated meats (spores may survive at normal cooking temperatures and then germinate and multiply while foods are being held at warm temperatures or being rewarmed at temperatures that do not inhibit bacterial growth).
4. *Enterohemorrhagic E. coli* are found in the intestines of healthy livestock and can contaminate the surface of whole meat products during slaughter and processing. Most reported outbreaks have been related to *E. coli* O157:H7. Ground meats pose the highest risk because surface contamination is distributed throughout the product. The risk of illness is minimized by cooking ground red meat until it is no longer pink or until juices run clear (internal temperature 155°F [68.3°C]). Ingestion of raw or undercooked contaminated ground meat can lead to infection that can result in bloody

TABLE 35.2 Characteristics of Acute Illness Caused by Ingestion of Chemical Agents

Agent	Pathogenesis	Clinical Features	Frequency in USA	Pattern
Seafood (58)				
Ciguatera fish poisoning	Toxins from algae concentrated in fish, particularly predatory fish; toxins affect human cell sodium channels	Vomiting, diarrhea, paresthesias (warmth, extremities), metallic taste, blurred vision, sharp pains in extremities, respiratory paralysis	Uncommon (Florida)	CSO, S
Domoic acid (amnesic shellfish poisoning)	Neuroexcitatory amino acid produced by phytoplankton and concentrated by mussels	Vomiting, cramps, headache, neurologic symptoms, anterograde amnesia, seizures, coma, death	Rare (surveillance for domoic acid in Canada)	CSO, S
Scombroid fish poisoning	Histamine intoxication	Histamine reaction (flushing, headache, dizziness, burning of mouth and throat; urticaria, pruritus, and bronchospasm)	Uncommon (frozen and fresh fish can be affected)	CSO, S
Paralytic shellfish poisoning	Multiple neurotoxins (saxitoxins) causing motor paralysis	Paresthesias (warmth, extremities), floating sensation, dysphonia, dysphagia, weakness, and respiratory paralysis	Uncommon (surveillance for toxins in shellfish in United States)	CSO, S
Muscarine	Muscarinic cholinergic response	Colicky abdominal pain, nausea, vomiting, diarrhea, salivation, miosis, blurred vision, bradycardia, hypotension	Uncommon	CSO, S
Phalloidin (and other toxins)	Diverse cytotoxin effects, multisystemic	*Stage 1:* Nausea, abdominal pain, vomiting, bloody diarrhea, marked weakness, hypotension (shock) *Stage 2:* Clinical improvement (day 2 or 3) *Stage 3:* Severe hepatic failure, delirium, frequent fatal outcome	Uncommon	CSO, S
Miscellaneous				
Heavy metals (antimony, cadmium, copper, iron, tin, zinc)	Upper GI irritation	Metallic taste to food, nausea, vomiting, or diarrhea	Uncommon	CSO, S
Monosodium glutamate (MSG)	Idiopathic reaction	Burning sensation in chest, neck, abdomen, extremities	Common	S

CSO, common source outbreak; GI, gastrointestinal; S, sporadic; MSG, monosodium glutamate.
Data from Gossalin RE, Hodge HC, Smith RP, et al. Clinical toxicology of commercial products. 5th ed. Baltimore: Williams & Wilkins, 1984; and Morris JG. Natural toxins associated with fish and shellfish. In: Blaser MJ, Smith PD, Randin JI, et al., eds. Infections of the gastrointestinal tract. New York: Raven, 1995, with permission.

diarrhea and hemolytic uremic syndrome (7). The mortality among patients with the latter syndrome can be high. Recently, natural environmental contamination of nonmeat products (e.g., produce and apple juice) has resulted in outbreaks (8,9).

Thus, most episodes of foodborne illness follow the *ingestion of normally safe foods that have been rendered unsafe by one or more of the following factors:* failure to refrigerate foods properly or to heat foods thoroughly, preparing foods a day or more before they are served, allowing

Epidemiologic Features				
Source	**Transmission to Humans**	**Incubation Period**	**Diagnosis**	**Specific Therapy**
Food chain of bottom-dwelling and predatory fish caught in Florida, Hawaii (red snapper, barracuda)	Foodborne	1–6 h	Clinical and epidemiologic features	Mannitol infusion; atropine for bradycardia; dopamine for, hypotension; symptoms may last days to months
Mussels and clams contaminated with domoic acid	Foodborne	Minutes to 48 h	Clinical and epidemiologic features	Supportive care
Bacteria acting on fish flesh (tuna, mackerel, bonito, skipjack, mahi mahi)	Foodborne ("peppery" taste of affected fish reported)	Minutes to 1 h	Clinical and epidemiologic features; elevated urine histamine level	Usually none; Antihistamines (H_1 and H_2), possibly corticosteroids, in severe cases
Toxic dinoflagellates concentrated in filter-feeding bivalves (mussels, clams, oysters, scallops)	Foodborne	<30 min	Clinical and epidemiologic features	Supportive care (lasts few hours to few days)
Amanita muscaria	Foodborne	Few minutes–few hours	Clinical and epidemiologic features	Atropine 0.1–0.5 mg s.c. or i.v.
Amanita phalloides and other Amanita species	Foodborne	6–15 h	Clinical and epidemiologic features	None
Containers made of alloy that includes a heavy metal	Foodborne (food prepared in, stored in, or eaten from a container from which heavy metal leached)	5 min–8 h	Clinical and epidemiologic features	None
Foods prepared with large amounts of MSG	Foodborne (Chinese restaurant foods)	3 min–2 h	Clinical and epidemiologic features	None

foods to remain at warm temperatures, failure to reheat or cook foods at temperatures that kill vegetative bacteria, incorporating raw (contaminated) ingredients into foods that receive no further cooking, failure to clean and disinfect kitchen or processing plant equipment, and contamination by infected food handlers who practice poor personal hygiene. The complexity of the world's food distribution system and the difficulty in controlling food safety even at a national level are exemplified by an outbreak of salmonellosis in Finland and the United States resulting

TABLE 35.3 Burden of Foodborne Illness, United States, 1999

Etiology	*% of Total Foodborne Illness Due to an Identified Pathogen*
Neurovirus	66.6
Campylobacter spp.	14.2
Salmonella spp.	9.7
Clostridium perfringens	1.8
Giardia lamblia	1.4
Staphylococcus aureus	1.3
Shiga-toxigenic *E. coli*	0.7
Shigella spp.	0.6
Yersinia enterocolitica	0.6
Other	3.1

Data from Mead PS, Slutsker L, Dietz V, et al. Food-related illness and death in the United States. Emerging Infect Dis 1999;5:607.

from contaminated alfalfa sprouts grown from seeds supplied by a Dutch shipper (10) and an outbreak of cyclosporiasis in North America related to raspberries from Guatemala (11).

Some foodborne illnesses are caused by the ingestion of *foods that are always unsafe* because of the presence of toxins that cannot be rendered innocuous by cooking or other means (e.g., histamine or scombrotoxin, ciguatoxin, *Amanita* mushroom toxins, paralytic shellfish toxin, and heavy metals) (12). A recent report of histamine poisoning associated with eating tuna burgers highlights the increasing recognition of scombroid poisoning (named for the type of fish most often associated with this illness), which is characterized by flushing, vomiting, and profuse watery diarrhea (13).

Not all gastroenteritis and diarrheal disease is foodborne. Waterborne outbreaks may result from contaminated drinking water or recreational water sources. *Cryptosporidium* is a common cause of waterborne outbreaks because it is chlorine-resistant. A large outbreak of cryptosporidiosis in 1993 resulted from contamination of the public water supply in Milwaukee, Wisconsin, affecting over 400,000 people (14). Recreational water illnesses are on the rise and are caused largely by swallowing contaminated water while swimming. *Cryptosporidium*, *Giardia*, *Shigella*, and *E. coli* are the most common pathogens.

Outbreaks unrelated to contaminated food or water are commonly caused by noroviruses and other viral enteropathogens, especially within institutional settings (e.g., day care centers, nursing homes, and assisted living facilities) and during the winter. A viral cause is more likely when secondary cases develop in a household or institution, a pattern that suggests person-to-person spread rather than one-time exposure to a common food.

More serious forms of diarrheal disease resulting from animal exposures are increasingly recognized. These include infection with *enterohemorrhagic E. coli* while visiting farms or petting zoos (15,16) and salmonellosis associated with pet reptiles or amphibians (17). In both cases, children have borne the brunt of the morbidity and mortality.

Populations at Risk

For many of the conditions listed in Tables 35.1 and 35.2, *people are at risk at all ages*, and a single episode may not confer protective immunity against a later episode. Although most cases of acute diarrhea occur in children, older adults are at increased risk of dying from gastrointestinal illnesses. Of 28,538 diarrhea-related deaths in the United States between 1979 and 1987, 78% occurred in adults aged 55 and older versus 11% in children younger than 5 years old (18). A particularly high rate of diarrheal illness also occurs in people of all ages who travel to developing countries. For older adults who are commonly prescribed cardiovascular medications that can block normal physiologic responses to volume depletion, special counseling is advisable. Patients with cirrhosis are at increased risk for complications of acute hepatitis A infection and infection with *Vibrio vulnificus* and should be counseled to avoid consuming raw or partly cooked shellfish.

Immunocompromised persons are also at greater risk for gastrointestinal (GI) infections and their associated morbidity and mortality. The diagnosis of HIV infection must be considered in patients with unusual diarrheal syndromes. Protracted diarrhea can herald the progression of HIV infection, and a number of enteropathogens can cause not only acute illness but also prolonged symptoms of diarrhea in patients with advanced HIV disease. *Cryptosporidium* infection, usually a benign self-limited diarrheal illness in children and healthy adults, may cause a prolonged and life-threatening illness (19). *Isospora belli*, usually not thought of as a diarrheal pathogen, may also cause diarrheal illness in these patients. Diarrheal illnesses caused by *Salmonella* and *Campylobacter jejuni*, which are usually self-limited normal hosts, may be prolonged in HIV-infected patients. (See Chapter 39 for additional discussion of infection in HIV-infected patients.)

PATHOGENESIS

As indicated in Tables 35.1 and 35.2, most of the etiologic agents produce symptoms by causing inflammation of the GI tract or through the physiologic effects of toxins.

The common bacterial diarrheal syndromes can be separated into invasive and enterotoxigenic syndromes (Table 35.4), and this becomes important when antibiotic

TABLE 35.4 Characteristics Distinguishing Invasive and Enterotoxigenic Diarrhea

Feature	Invasive Diarrhea	Enterotoxigenic Diarrhea
History	Fever, abdominal pain, tenesmus, may have blood in stool	Watery diarrhea with little or no fever or other systemic symptoms
Physical examination	Fever, abdominal tenderness; proctoscopy may be indicated	May be signs of salt and water depletion
Laboratory studies	Stool culture (may be diagnostic) Fecal leukocytes in large numbers[a] White blood cell count may be elevated	Stool culture usually negative unless special culture techniques available No or few fecal leukocytes White count usually normal, but may be elevated
Therapy	Oral fluids and electrolytes (usually only small quantities needed) Antimicrobials often indicated[b]	Oral fluids and electrolytes Bismuth subsalicylate, other symptomatic medications as needed[c] Antimicrobials not indicated
Course	Improvements in 1–2 days, particularly if appropriate antimicrobials used	Duration of 1–2 days usually; may last up to 5 days

[a]Use a drop of methylene blue stain with liquid stool.
[b]See text for recommendations for specific bacterial pathogens.
[c]See text for details.

treatment is considered. In *invasive disease,* the etiologic agent invades the intestinal mucosa and diarrhea results from destruction of mucosal cells that occurs due to inflammation. This usually involves the large bowel and produces systemic symptoms (particularly fever), local symptoms (tenesmus, abdominal discomfort), and frequent small amounts of stool that contain pus cells and often blood. Shigellosis is the prototype of this syndrome. In *enterotoxigenic diarrhea,* the organisms do not invade tissue but colonize and multiply on the small bowel mucosal surface. During this process they produce enterotoxins, which act as chemical mediators and cause net secretion of fluid and electrolytes into the small bowel lumen. Little tissue damage is produced, and inflammation of the mucosa is minimal. Symptoms consist of watery diarrhea (which may be voluminous), accompanied by minimal systemic signs, unless dehydration becomes significant. The prototypes of this syndrome are diarrheas caused by *Vibrio cholerae* and by enterotoxigenic *E. coli* (20).

Unfortunately, not all enteric diseases caused by bacteria fit into this simple dichotomy. Enteroaggregative strains of *E. coli* do not invade mucosal cells, but tightly adhere to the mucosal surface and induce an inflammatory diarrhea, at least in part through the production of one or more enterotoxins. These strains produce diarrhea primarily in small children, HIV-infected patients, and travelers, and many belong to the classic enteropathogenic serotypes (21). In addition, *Clostridium difficile,* a cause of pseudomembranous colitis, produces two toxins: an enterotoxin (toxin A), which causes secretion of fluid into the gut lumen, and a potent cytotoxin (toxin B), which damages the gut epithelium and leads to inflammation (22).

PATIENT EVALUATION

Historical Information

In addition to a history of the specific symptoms, the clinical history should include items that may suggest the most likely pathogens (Table 35.5). The most useful information is as follows:

- A history of *food eaten* within the past 48 hours, particularly noting any deviation from the patient's usual pattern, such as eating an unusual food (e.g., a special fish, raw shellfish, or improperly cooked hamburger), eating at a restaurant, or attending a picnic or potluck dinner.
- A history of a *similar illness in others* (family members or members of a group who ate with the patient). Simultaneous onset of disease among group members suggests a common source outbreak, while sequential onset suggests person-to-person transmission consistent with norovirus gastroenteritis.
- A detailed history of recent *travel.* Chapter 41 discusses the problem of diarrheal illness and other problems related to travel.
- A history of *animal exposures,* including livestock and pet reptiles or amphibians. These exposures increase the risk of illness due to enterohemorrhagic *E. coli* and *Salmonella,* respectively.
- The probable *incubation period.* This may be helpful in suggesting the most likely cause of a patient's illness (Tables 35.1 and 35.2). For example, the onset of symptoms immediately after ingestion always indicates chemical food poisoning, onset of symptoms within a few hours of eating strongly suggests staphylococcal food poisoning,

TABLE 35.5 Evaluation of Acute Gastroenteritis or Diarrhea: Using the Clinical History to Suggest Probable Pathogens

■ Travel to developing world	Enterotoxigenic *Escherichia coli* *Campylobacter* sp *Salmonella* sp (including *S typhi*) *Entamoeba histolytica* *Giardia lamblia* *Cryptosporidium parvum* *Cyclospora cayetanensis*
■ Daycare attendance or employment	*Shigella* sp Norovirus *Giardia lamblia* *Cryptosporidium parvum*
■ Consumption of unsafe food	*Salmonella* sp *Listeria monocytogenes* *Vibrio* sp *Escherichia coli* (including STEC*) *Campylobacter* sp
■ Exposure to untreated water	*Escherichia coli* *Entamoeba histolytica* *Cryptosporidium parvum* *Giardia lamblia*
■ Contact with livestock	*Salmonella* sp *Escherichia coli* (including STEC*) *Campylobacter* sp *Yersinia* sp *Cryptosporidium parvum*
■ Contact with reptiles	*Salmonella* sp
■ Similarly ill contacts suggesting person to person transmission	Norovirus *Salmonella* sp *Shigella* sp
■ HIV/AIDS	*Salmonella* sp *Cryptosporidium parvum* *Giardia lamblia* *Microsporidia* sp *Isospora belli* *Cytomegalovirus*
■ Pregnancy	*Listeria monocytogenes*
■ New medications (especially antibiotics)	*Clostridium difficile* Antibiotic-resistant *Salmonella* sp Antibiotic-resistant *Campylobacter* sp
■ Receptive anal intercourse, oral-anal sex	*Entamoeba histolytica* *Giardia lamblia* *Neisseria gonorrhoeae*
■ Bloody diarrhea	STEC* *Shigella* sp *Salmonella* sp *Campylobacter* sp *Entamoeba histolytica*

*STEC = Shiga-like toxin-producing *E. coli* (a.k.a. enterohemorrhagic *E. coli*)

Table adapted from Nuermberger E. Current issues in the diagnosis, evaluation, and management of gastrointestinal infections. Adv Stud Med 2005;5:90.

onset within 24 to 48 hours suggests *Salmonella* infection, and onset of symptoms 1 week or more after exposure suggests a less common problem, such as giardiasis.

- A *history of taking antimicrobials.* No etiologic agent can be identified in approximately 80% of patients with diarrhea after antibiotic exposure. Although treatment with virtually any antibiotic class has been implicated, receipt of clindamycin, ampicillin, advanced cephalosporins and, more recently, the new methoxy-fluoroquinolones, usually while hospitalized, supports the diagnosis of antibiotic-associated diarrhea caused by *C. difficile.* This agent causes syndromes that range from enterotoxigenic diarrhea to invasive disease and pseudomembranous colitis (23).
- A history of *neurologic symptoms* after ingestion of canned foods should always suggest botulism. Table 35.2 lists other sources of neurotoxins (all rare) and their typical manifestations.
- A history revealing *risk factors for HIV infection* (see Chapter 39) and chronic diarrhea suggests increased risk for infection with *Cryptosporidium* (19,24), *Isospora,* or *Salmonella* among other causes.

Physical Examination

The physical examination is usually of minimal help in establishing a cause. Fever or significant abdominal tenderness in association with diarrhea suggests an invasive organism as the etiologic agent. Poor skin turgor and postural hypotension suggest significant salt and water deficits (uncommon in adults with diarrhea in the United States). Rare conditions in which the physical findings may be helpful are *botulism* and other neurotoxic forms of food poisoning and *trichinosis* (Tables 35.1 and 35.2).

Laboratory Studies

In most outpatients with acute GI illness, no laboratory studies are indicated (25) unless a common source outbreak is suspected. In such cases, the physician should notify local and/or state health authorities since special cultures and assays for viral pathogens, as well as tests for toxins in stools and in food, may be obtained for epidemiologic purposes.

Diarrhea lasting >1 day, especially if accompanied by fever, bloody stools, systemic illness, recent antibiotic use, day care center attendance, recent hospitalization, or dehydration should prompt consideration of the following laboratory studies (25):

- *Stool culture for enterotoxigenic E. coli, Salmonella, Shigella, Campylobacter, and Yersinia.* The clinician should also inquire whether the laboratory routinely seeks to identify enterohemorrhagic *E. coli* or its

correlate well with those obtained by quantitative plate cultures (14).

Culture-Negative Urine

If the patient has not taken an antimicrobial, has symptoms of cystitis with or without pyuria, but the urine does not contain visible or cultured bacteria, the most likely explanation is that the patient has urethritis, prostatitis, or vaginitis. However, adenovirus can cause symptomatic cystitis, and chemical cystitis can be caused by several chemotherapeutic agents. In patients with culture-negative pyuria, tuberculosis of the kidney, bladder stone, bladder tumor, and interstitial cystitis should be considered.

Localizing the Site of Infection

Several techniques may characterize a UTI as either confined to the bladder or involving the kidneys. However, in most cases it is unnecessary to try to decide whether the patient has cystitis, pyelonephritis, or prostatitis. Many patients with pyelonephritis respond to standard 3-day treatment regimens described later in this chapter.

The simplest indication that a patient has pyelonephritis or prostatitis that requires prolonged treatment is that the UTI relapses after a standard 3-day course of antimicrobials that would be expected to clear a simple bladder infection. *Relapse* means that all of the infectious episodes are caused by the same organism, as defined not only by species but also by any other available characteristics such as antimicrobial sensitivity or serotype. Relapsing episodes are not necessarily caused by pyelonephritis: They may be caused by persistent colonization of the introitus and multiple episodes of ascending infection. Most cases of recurrent UTI are managed by prolonged courses of antibiotics, as discussed in section Management of Recurrent Infection, Reinfection Type.

In pyelonephritis, the bacteria in the urine are usually coated with antibody. This can be detected with the use of fluorescent goat antihuman immunoglobulin. In cystitis, bacteria in the urine are generally free of antibody. This test is not absolutely reliable: antibody-coated bacteria may be found in prostatitis, and antibody-negative bacteria may be obtained from some cases of pyelonephritis. For this reason, the test is of limited clinical value and should rarely be performed.

Other techniques are cumbersome because they require urethral or ureteral catheterization. The standard criterion for localization of upper tract infection is bilateral ureteral catheterization with separate collection of the urine from each kidney. There is a less complicated bladder washout technique that detects pyelonephritis but gives no information about the side of the infection. Radiographic abnormalities such as renal cortical scars are not present in most cases of pyelonephritis. Localization of the UTI is so seldom needed in clinical practice that patients who require it should be referred to a urologist.

TABLE 36.1 Indications for Evaluating Patients Who Have Urinary Tract Infections with Ultrasonography

Acute pyelonephritis in male patients
Acute pyelonephritis in women with persistent high fevers or leukocytosis after 2 or 3 days of antimicrobial treatment
Renal colic (see Chapter 51)
Palpable bladder or renal mass
Urea-splitting organism, usually *Proteus* species.
Frequently recurrent urinary tract infections in women (>3–4/yr)
Failure to eradicate infection with appropriate therapy

Imaging

Uncomplicated UTIs that respond to treatment do not require additional workup. However, some clinical situations warrant investigation for anatomic abnormalities (Table 36.1). In office practice, an intravenous pyelogram (IVP) is no longer the most appropriate way to evaluate renal anatomy. *Sonography* is quicker and less dangerous to renal function. It detects kidney size, cortical scars, stones, and hydronephrosis. If sonography is normal, IVP is unlikely to add more information (15). Sonography is particularly useful for detecting and estimating the volume of residual urine in patients who cannot empty the bladder.

Computed tomography (CT) scanning is most useful for the detection of perinephric abscess and as a prelude to operations on the kidneys. *Voiding cystourethrography* is another test that should be delegated to the urologist.

MANAGEMENT OF SYMPTOMATIC URINARY TRACT INFECTIONS IN WOMEN

First Infection, Occasional Infection, or Uncomplicated Infection

Most women with UTIs experience only one or an occasional uncomplicated infection. The diagnosis of a UTI can be confirmed by urinalysis and urine culture; however, as discussed earlier, a therapeutic trial is usually sufficient and is more convenient and far less costly for the patient. Although an uncomplicated infection may clear spontaneously in time, treatment with antimicrobials dramatically shortens the symptomatic period and should be given. Forcing fluids, historically a common practice, is discouraged once antimicrobial therapy has been initiated because it may actually dilute significantly the concentration of antimicrobial in the urine.

TABLE 36.2 Antimicrobial Agents for Uncomplicated Urinary Tract Infections (3-Day Therapy)

Agent	Dosage and Schedule
First choice (effective and inexpensive)	
Trimethoprim-sulfamethoxazole[a] (Bactrim, Septra, generic)	1 double-strength tablet q12h
Second choice (effective)	
A Quinolone[b]	
Ciprofloxacin (Cipro)	250 or 500 mg q12h
Levofloxacin	500 mg q12h
Norfloxacin (Noroxin)	400 mg q12h
Tetracycline[a]	500 mg q12h
Doxycycline[a]	100 mg q12h
Third choice (effective for cystitis but not for pyelonephritis)	
Nitrofurantoin (Furadantin)	50 or 100 mg q12h
Fourth choice (less effective but can be used during pregnancy)	
β-Lactams (e.g., amoxicillin, cephalexin)	250–500 mg q8h

[a]Three-day course costs less than $5.
[b]Three-day course costs $15–$20.

Antimicrobial Treatment

Uncomplicated UTIs should usually be treated with an antimicrobial for 3 days (Table 36.2). Three days of treatment gives the same cure rate as the traditional 7- to 10-day courses, and there is little superinfection with *Candida,* a common occurrence with the longer course. One-dose therapy was popular a number of years ago, but the cure rate is less than that attainable with 3 days of therapy.

There is a randomized controlled trial showing that UTI in presumably healthy young women can be managed effectively over the telephone (16). There is also a controlled trial showing that patients who are given antibiotics in advance can diagnose and treat their own UTIs (17).

For patients who are not pregnant, a wide range of drugs can be used. Probably the best available therapy is trimethoprim–sulfamethoxazole (TMP-SMX). This produces little in the way of allergy, kills most gram-negative rods, tends to sterilize the vaginal introitus, and is inexpensive. Overall, the cure rate is 90% to 95% (18). Patients who are allergic to sulfonamides can be treated with a quinolone, a tetracycline, or nitrofurantoin. Because TMP-SMX has been extensively used in the last 20 years, the incidence of resistance is rising all over the country. Surveys show that resistance to TMP-SMX varies from a minimum of 7% in Pennsylvania to a maximum of 33% in Iowa (19). Resistance reported in the laboratory is not necessarily correlated with clinical failure because of the very high concentrations of antibiotics in the urine. However, at some point TMP-SMX is going to lose its effectiveness (20).

TABLE 36.3 Points to Consider in Educating Women Who Have Had an Uncomplicated Infection

Infections are often recurrent. However, the following measures may decrease the recurrence rate:

- Avoid a full bladder. This is an especially important reminder during travel.
- High fluid intake (1 L in 2–3 hr) may eradicate an infection that has just become symptomatic.
- Irritation to the urethra, as occurs with sexual intercourse, is associated with the movement of bacteria into the bladder. Voiding after intercourse, therefore, helps to prevent recurrent infection.
- Diaphragm use is associated with development of urinary tract infection.

Infections in the absence of structural urologic disorder are rarely, if ever, associated with the development of chronic renal failure.

Prompt recognition and treatment will help to control symptoms.

Even if recurrent infections are frequent, there is much that can be done to control symptoms.

β-Lactams such as ampicillin and cephalosporins are less effective than the four drugs mentioned earlier. However, in pregnant women there is no reasonable alternative to β-lactams because of the risk of harm to the fetus. Therefore, a somewhat increased risk of recurrent UTI must be accepted. In the rare pregnant woman with a serious penicillin allergy, aztreonam should not cause anaphylaxis, and will be effective against most gram-negative rods. One could consider an aminoglycoside, but there is a risk of fetal deafness.

Any of the above treatments usually sterilizes the urine and produces total relief of symptoms in 24 hours or less. In very symptomatic patients, one could add the bladder analgesic *phenazopyridine* (Pyridium), 200 mg three times a day for 1 day or longer. This drug, which requires a prescription, usually alleviates annoying symptoms, especially dysuria and urgency, within hours after the first dose. The patient should be told that phenazopyridine will cause the urine to become dark orange.

If the patient remains asymptomatic after treatment, she may be regarded as cured without the need for any additional followup.

Table 36.3 summarizes the *points to stress to women after a UTI episode*. The behaviors that most often help prevent recurrent UTI are emptying the bladder after sexual intercourse and avoiding a full bladder. If a woman is using a diaphragm for contraception, a change in contraceptive method should be considered (see Chapter 100).

Management of Recurrent Infection, Reinfection Type

Most women with recurrent UTIs have *reinfection* (rather than *relapse,* which is discussed below). Although the infections are symptomatic and occasionally may be associated with pyelonephritis, recurrent reinfections in women with structurally normal urinary tracts rarely, if ever, lead to chronic renal failure.

The approach to women with anatomically normal urinary tracts and the syndrome of reinfection has been vastly improved by the understanding of the pathogenesis of UTI in women. In the past, women often were treated with a variety of painful manipulations such as urethral dilation, urethral incision, transurethral resection of the bladder neck, installation of a variety of intravesical agents, and other inappropriate and ineffective maneuvers. Instead, each episode of bacterial infection should be treated as outlined previously in the section on first infections. If there are three or more recurrences in a year, the urinary tract should be evaluated for anatomic abnormalities (see General Diagnostic Evaluation). Patients with structural problems should be referred to the appropriate specialist (urologist or gynecologist). If the urinary tract is normal, prophylactic antimicrobials should be considered.

Prophylactic Antimicrobial Therapy

A number of studies have confirmed the efficacy of prophylaxis in reducing the frequency of UTI in women, and prophylactic therapy has dramatically improved the lives of many women with multiple UTIs. The agents that have been used are effective when given as a single small dose at bedtime. A dose taken only after sexual intercourse is also effective in patients whose recurrent UTIs are clearly associated with sexual activity. Patient acceptance is good, and side effects are uncommon.

Many agents have been shown to be effective prophylactically, but nitrofurantoin (Furadantin), a 50-mg tablet at bedtime; TMP-SMX, 40/200 mg (half a tablet of regular strength Bactrim, Septra, or generic) at bedtime; and cephalexin (Keflex or generic), a 250-mg capsule at bedtime, are used most commonly and are recommended. In some patients, the antibiotic may be effective when given on 3 days of the week. Prophylactic therapy should be continued for 6 months. If there are still frequent recurrences after the cessation of prophylaxis, prophylaxis for a longer period (e.g., 1 year) should be tried.

Estrogens

In elderly women, the vaginal cells lose glycogen, lactobacilli vanish from the vaginal flora, and the introitus becomes colonized with gram-negative rods. A controlled trial demonstrated that the frequency of recurrent UTIs in elderly women can be greatly reduced (from an average incidence of 5.9 to 0.5 episodes per year) by the use of intravaginal estrogen creams (21). Treated patients used intravaginal cream containing 0.5 mg of estriol on the following schedule: nightly for 2 weeks, then twice weekly for 8 months. Presumably, systemic estrogens would have the same effect.

CLINICAL SYNDROMES THAT MIMIC URINARY TRACT INFECTIONS IN WOMEN

There are two syndromes in women that mimic classic UTI: the urethral syndrome, which is common, and interstitial cystitis, which is rare.

Urethral Syndrome (Dysuria–Pyuria Syndrome)

The urethral syndrome is characterized by bladder irritation, frequency, urgency, and dysuria without significant (greater than 10^5) bacterial colonies per milliliter on culture. *Dysuria–pyuria syndrome* may be the better term, because *dysuria is invariable and most patients have pyuria* (more than eight WBCs per cubic millimeter of clean uncentrifuged urine). Studies show that many women with the syndrome have bacterial infection with a low bacterial colony count (22). These infections respond to the standard therapy for uncomplicated UTI described earlier.

The urethral syndrome can also be caused by any of several sexually transmitted infections. *Chlamydia, gonorrhea, and herpes simplex* are the most common causes. Other agents such as *Mycoplasma hominis* and *Ureaplasma urealyticum* may be found, but their significance is uncertain. Any woman who has acute onset of *dysuria and has urine that is apparently sterile* may have one of these infections. The patient should have a pelvic examination to check for the signs of common STDs, and the appropriate specimens should be obtained for culture and other examinations (see Chapter 37).

If the patient has never been sexually active, or has not been sexually active for years, then the dysuria–pyuria syndrome is occasionally caused by a viral infection. Adenovirus is the most common cause.

Of women who have the urethral syndrome, *5% to 10% do not have a demonstrable infectious agent* even when special culture methods are used; most often these patients do not have pyuria. The cause of the syndrome in these instances is unknown. In this group, treatment with reassurance, sitz baths, and the urinary tract analgesic phenazopyridine (Pyridium), 200 mg three times a day for 5 to 10 days, will provide some relief. The patient should be informed that this medication causes the urine to appear orange. If symptoms persist, referral to a urologist is indicated for cystoscopic evaluation.

Measures to be recommended to patients with this syndrome should be identical to those outlined for UTI (Table 36.3) or, if there is vaginitis or an STD present, as outlined in Chapter 37.

Interstitial Cystitis

Interstitial cystitis is an occasionally seen disorder affecting middle-aged women that, early in its course, may be confused with the urethral syndrome. Interstitial cystitis causes symptoms of suprapubic discomfort, especially when the bladder is full, and symptoms are relieved by voiding. The patient may experience progressive loss of bladder volume and increasing urinary frequency, and eventually may have to void four to six times per hour throughout the night. The urinalysis is often normal, but hematuria may be present. The urine is sterile. This disease is difficult to diagnose. If it is suspected on the basis of the history, referral to a urologist is indicated. The urologist performs cystoscopy and often a biopsy of the bladder to establish the diagnosis (usually a normal-appearing mucosa with a very small vesical capacity is identified; tissue histology may show changes consistent with the diagnosis; mucosal hemorrhage may appear with bladder filling). Also, a cystoscopic evaluation permits the urologist to exclude other causes of the symptoms (e.g., bladder tumor). No definitive therapy has yet been developed for treatment of this condition.

Vaginitis and Cervicitis

For detailed discussion of these conditions, see Chapter 37.

SYMPTOMATIC URINARY TRACT INFECTIONS IN MEN

Bacterial Cystitis

Bacterial cystitis in men is similar in presentation to that in female patients and is diagnosed by the same method, but a urine culture should always be obtained. A UTI in a man suggests the presence of an underlying structural problem or the presence of bacterial prostatitis. In the past, it was felt that the initial evaluation should always include a prostate examination. However, because young men who are either homosexual or uncircumcised can develop UTIs in the absence of a structural abnormality, some easing of this standard is reasonable in men from either of these groups (4,5). If a workup is initiated, sonography is preferable to IVP as a screening tool.

A small number of young boys develop UTI in the apparent absence of a structural abnormality. Most turn out to have a congenital abnormality such as urethral valves. Young men with UTIs most often have stones or hydronephrosis. Older men usually have prostatic enlargement or stones.

Bacterial cystitis in men should always be treated for a minimum of 7 to 10 days (see daily dosages and schedules for antibiotics, Table 36.2). Structural problems are so common that short courses are ineffective. Even if no structural anomaly is found, men should be carefully followed up, because many of the infections relapse. Many men with relapse-type recurrences have bacterial prostatitis; therefore, a followup visit 4 to 6 weeks after the initial infection should be arranged to reculture the urine and, if it is positive, to consider treatment for chronic prostatitis.

Prostatitis

Prostatitis is classified as bacterial prostatitis (acute or chronic), nonbacterial prostatitis (prostatosis), or the much less common prostatic infections caused by a virus, a parasite, tuberculosis, a fungus, or nonspecific granulomatous changes.

Acute Bacterial Prostatitis

Acute bacterial prostatitis is characterized often by the abrupt onset of fever, chills, low back pain, and perineal pain with irritative urinary tract symptoms, although on some occasions, systemic symptoms are not pronounced. Perineal discomfort may be worsened by defecation. In addition, the patient may have initial, terminal, or occasionally total hematuria (see Chapter 49). Rectal examination usually discloses a tender, swollen, and boggy prostate. The urine and the expressed prostatic secretions contain leukocytes, and culture often grows the responsible bacterial pathogen, which most commonly is *E. coli* in older men and *Chlamydia* or *Neisseria gonorrhoeae* in younger men.

When the diagnosis is made, the patient may require hospitalization, although if systemic symptoms are minimal, ambulatory therapy is appropriate. Most antibiotics do not achieve high concentrations in prostatic fluid. The best initial choice for younger patients is *levofloxacin* (500 mg once or twice daily), which penetrates the prostate well and covers the common etiologic organisms. If quinolones cannot be used, a number of other antimicrobials may be tried. *TMP-SMX* does penetrate prostatic epithelium and is an alternative for treating *E. coli.* Penicillins and cephalosporins do not achieve effective concentrations in the prostate and are not useful. Because of the overriding effects of local antimicrobial concentration, antibiotics such as *erythromycin,* which would not normally be used to treat *E. coli,* may also prove effective. Therapy with antimicrobials for acute prostatitis should be continued for 2 weeks. Table 36.2 lists dosages and schedules.

Bed rest and sitz baths for 20 to 30 minutes two or three times a day may provide comfort. Occasionally, prostatitis results in acute urinary retention, which requires hospitalization and urgent urologic consultation. The palpable irregularity of the prostate gland after acute infection may persist for several months. The acute infection is readily controlled, but recurrences may occur, especially in older patients.

Chronic Bacterial Prostatitis

The organisms that cause chronic bacterial prostatitis most often are gram-negative bacilli, *E. coli* being the most common organism, followed by *Enterococcus*, *Proteus*, and *Klebsiella*. Most patients with chronic bacterial prostatitis have mild irritative symptoms (frequency, urgency, and dysuria), and occasionally there is a urethral discharge. Fever is absent. Patients may also have painless hematuria or painful ejaculation with hematospermia. On rectal examination, the prostate gland feels somewhat irregular and may be mildly tender, although the examination is often unremarkable.

Obstructive symptoms are rare. Most often the patients have intermittent symptomatic episodes that have been controlled with short courses of antibiotics. However, recurrent infection is common because of persistence of bacteria within the urinary tract. Chronic prostatitis may also be a reservoir for acute symptomatic cystitis, pyelonephritis, or epididymitis. Therefore, a prolonged course of therapy is indicated when chronic prostatitis is diagnosed clinically. If the infectious organism is sensitive, *ciprofloxacin, 250 mg twice daily for 2 weeks,* has been shown to be effective in eradicating infection in more than 60% of patients with chronic prostatitis (23).

If all efforts to eradicate infection fail, symptoms usually can be controlled with *suppressive therapy* using a low dose of *TMP–SMX,* one-half tablet of regular strength (Bactrim, Septra, or generic) nightly, indefinitely. The only way to effect a cure is by radical prostatectomy, but the morbidity of this procedure precludes its use for benign disease. Repeated prostatic massage has not been shown to be effective. Patients with refractory chronic bacterial prostatitis should be evaluated by an urologist.

Nonbacterial Prostatitis (Prostatosis)

Some patients have all of the symptoms and signs of chronic bacterial infection of the prostate, but no organism can be demonstrated. They have nonbacterial prostatitis (prostatosis), which is the most common form of prostatic inflammation. These patients have mild perineal pain and irritative symptoms on urination with *WBCs in the urine sediment, but negative urine cultures.* Culture of the secretions and urine by special techniques occasionally reveals infectious agents such as *Mycoplasma, Gardnerella vaginalis, U. urealyticum,* or *Chlamydia* species; however, the significance of these findings is unknown. Most patients with this condition cannot be cured; nevertheless, treatment with an antimicrobial such as ciprofloxacin or levofloxacin at the dosage and schedule described for acute prostatitis may control symptoms. An antispasmodic agent such as oxybutynin (Ditropan), 5 mg two to three times a day, may be tried. Therapeutic prostatic massage has not been shown to be of value.

If there is no response to therapy, the patient should be referred to a urologist to exclude conditions such as interstitial cystitis and *in situ* bladder cancer. Both conditions require cystoscopic examination for confirmation.

Prostatodynia

Patients with a syndrome called prostatodynia have symptoms suggesting prostatic inflammation but have no evidence of inflammation on physical examination, have *no WBCs in the urine or in expressed prostatic secretions, and have sterile urine cultures.* There is some evidence that the syndrome may be caused by a neurologic disorder and that muscle relaxants or α-sympathetic blocking agents such as phenoxybenzamine (Dibenzyline) are effective in treating it. If this syndrome is suspected, urologic consultation is suggested to confirm the diagnosis, to rule out interstitial cystitis and bladder cancer, and to initiate therapy.

Epididymitis

In young men, this infection is usually caused by sexually transmitted pathogens. Chapter 37 describes the manifestations, management, and course of sexually transmitted pathogens.

The *older patient* with acute epididymitis should always have a urine culture and should be evaluated for obstruction at the bladder outlet (see Chapter 53) as soon as the acute symptoms are controlled. On rare occasions, continued pain from chronic epididymitis may occur; if it does, a urologist should be consulted, because an epididymectomy may be required.

With great rarity, chronic epididymitis may turn out to be caused by tuberculous or fungal infection of the urinary tract. There is commonly involvement of the kidneys and/or the prostate in such cases, and the urine is generally positive on culture for tubercle bacilli or one of the fungi capable of causing invasive disease.

Urethritis

Urethritis is an acute inflammation of the urethra that may be classified as gonococcal or nongonococcal. All forms of urethritis are assumed to be sexually transmitted. Chapter 37 discusses this topic in detail.

PERSISTENT URINARY TRACT INFECTION IN MEN AND WOMEN

As noted earlier, treatment in the male or female patient of infection in a normal urinary tract with an appropriate antimicrobial should result in the sterilization of the urine within 72 hours. By this time, symptoms should have abated or at least markedly diminished. If symptoms continue, a persistent infection may be present, and the urine culture should be repeated. If the urine culture is still positive despite antimicrobial therapy, further investigation is required. Modern antimicrobials are so effective and the concentrations achieved in urine are so high that persistent infection is unusual.

The possibilities to be considered are that the patient is not taking the antimicrobial or has taken it but vomited subsequently; the organism is totally resistant (unusual but seen with certain pseudomonads and enterococci); the patient's renal function is so poor (e.g., creatinine greater than 3 mg/dL) that little antimicrobial reaches the urine; the antimicrobial does not work at the current urinary pH; there is a gross structural anomaly such as bladder carcinoma, a vesicocolic fistula, or a leaking pyonephrosis; there is a nidus of sequestered bacteria such as a staghorn calculus; or the organism is not a bacterium at all, but a fungus. Once one has decided which of the above applies, the indicated treatment is usually obvious.

RECURRENT INFECTION, RELAPSE TYPE, IN MEN AND WOMEN

Recurrent infection with the same organism is called relapse infection and implies the persistence of bacteria in tissue within the urinary tract. Relapse infection is similar to persistent infection except that in relapse the urine was shown to be sterile while the patient was taking or had completed antimicrobial therapy, whereas sterility is never demonstrated with persistent infection. Relapse occurs most often within 6 weeks after completion of a course of antimicrobial therapy. An underlying structural problem is often present in both men and women with this condition. In women, relapse is much less common than reinfection but is difficult to document because most infections are caused by *E. coli,* which has many serotypes that cannot be differentiated by routine bacteriologic laboratory techniques. Therefore, recurrent UTI caused by *E. coli* may be either relapse (same serotype) or reinfection (different serotype). On the other hand, relapse of infection with organisms other than *E. coli* may be diagnosed by routine bacteriologic culture. In women, if recurrent infection with *E. coli* occurs four times in a 12-month period or if relapse infection with other species occurs, evaluation as described previously (see Persistent Urinary Tract Infection in Men and Women) to exclude the possibility of structural abnormality is appropriate. If a structural abnormality is identified, it should be corrected if possible.

If a woman or man has a structural or functional abnormality of the urinary tract that cannot be corrected, sterilization of the urinary tract usually is not possible. In a patient who has had recurrent infections because of urine stasis caused by an atonic bladder, *intermittent straight catheterization* by the patient or a trained member of the family may help to prevent recurrent infections (see Urinary Incontinence in Chapter 54). In patients with other abnormalities, *suppressive therapy* (see regimens for prophylaxis of recurrent cystitis, discussed previously) may decrease the frequency of symptomatic exacerbations or episodes of sepsis. Relapsing infection may occur in *patients with no evidence of a structural abnormality.* In women, that usually means that the patient has chronic pyelonephritis. In men, the most common cause is chronic bacterial prostatitis. Chronic pyelonephritis is generally treated with a 6-week course of an appropriate antimicrobial, on several occasions if necessary. Some patients may eventually respond to prolonged antimicrobial courses of 6 months or more. These prolonged courses are generally indicated only in young patients where there is some hope of cure.

If the patient has chronic bacteriuria that cannot be eradicated, there is some evidence that the ingestion of large quantities of cranberry juice will reduce the number of symptomatic episodes (24).

INFECTION IN CATHETERIZED PATIENTS

In the ambulatory setting, one often sees patients who were catheterized while acutely ill in the hospital, developed infection, and now have bacteriuria, even though the catheter has been removed. In general, these patients should be treated based on bacterial sensitivities, because otherwise they will probably develop symptomatic episodes of cystitis or pyelonephritis. The usual course of treatment is 10 days, and because recurrence is common, a "cure" urine culture should be done.

ACUTE PYELONEPHRITIS IN MEN AND WOMEN

Pyelonephritis is a bacterial infection of the kidney that most often results from ascending infection. It is suggested by flank pain, fever, and often, abdominal pain in addition to symptoms of bladder irritation. Bacterial infection of the kidney may also be present without any of these signs or symptoms or with only bladder irritation. The urinalysis will show changes as outlined previously, but only

TABLE 37.1 Oral Therapy of Genital Herpes

Drug	Dosage	Frequency	Duration
First Clinical Episode			
Acyclovir	200 mg	5 times a day	7–10 days
Acyclovir	400 mg	3 times a day	7–10 days
Famciclovir	250 mg	3 times a day	7–10 days
Valacyclovir	1 g	Twice a day	7–10 days
Episodic Therapy of Recurrences			
Acyclovir	400 mg	3 times a day	5 days
Acyclovir	800 mg	Twice a day	5 days
Acyclovir	800 mg	3 times a day	2 days
Famciclovir	125 mg	Twice a day	5 days
Famciclovir	1000 mg	Twice a day	1 day
Valacyclovir	500 mg	Twice a day	3 days
Valacyclovir	1 g	Once a day	5 days
Daily Suppressive Therapy			
Acyclovir	400 mg	Twice a day	
Famciclovir	250 mg	Twice a day	
Valacyclovir*	500 mg	Once a day	
Valacyclovir	1 g	Once a day	
Episodic Therapy of Recurrences in HIV-infected Patients			
Acyclovir	400 mg	3 times a day	5–10 days
Famciclovir	500 mg	Twice a day	5–10 days
Valacyclovir	1 g	Twice a day	5–10 days
Daily Suppressive Therapy in HIV-infected Patients			
Acyclovir	400–800 mg	2–3 times a day	
Famciclovir	500 mg	Twice a day	
Valacyclovir	500 mg	Twice a day	

*Valacyclovir 500 mg once a day may be less effective in patients with frequent recurrences (≥10 a year).

and valacyclovir, a valine ester of acyclovir, have better absorption after oral dosing than acyclovir. As a result, they can be taken less frequently, but are more expensive. These drugs have little toxicity. Acyclovir has been safe in patients using it daily for greater than 10 years (2). Topical acyclovir is not recommended for treatment of genital herpes.

In patients with HIV infection, HSV outbreaks may be more prolonged and severe, and they often require higher doses and prolonged courses of treatment for HSV. Severe episodes of HSV in immunocompromised patients, especially when HSV becomes disseminated, may necessitate hospital admission. Acyclovir-resistant HSV is unusual and has been reported almost exclusively in immunosuppressed patients who have had prolonged exposure to the drug. In these patients, valacyclovir will be ineffective, and the virus is often also resistant to famciclovir. These patients usually require therapy with intravenous foscarnet. Patients with refractory HSV infection should have viral cultures and acyclovir drug-sensitivity testing performed at a reference center. Patients with acyclovir-resistant HSV should be managed in consultation with an expert.

Along with antiviral therapy, counseling plays a central role in the care of patients with newly diagnosed HSV. Patients must be educated about the potential for recurrences and the availability of episodic and suppressive therapy. They should be aware that viral shedding occurs not only during the times of active lesions but can also occur during asymptomatic periods. With this in mind, they should be instructed to inform their sexual partners about their HSV status prior to sexual activity, and abstain from sex with uninfected partners when prodromal symptoms or active lesions are present. Patients should be informed that the use of condoms might decrease the risk of transmission of HSV during asymptomatic periods and given the option of suppressive therapy to attempt to decrease transmission to a seronegative partner (31). Men and women should be informed about the risks of neonatal herpes infection. Type-specific serologies for HSV may prove helpful in determining if sexual partners are truly discordant for HSV-2 infection. Patients may obtain more HSV information by accessing informational Internet sites including the CDC site (http://www.cdc.gov/std/Herpes/STDFact-Herpes.htm) and the Planned Parenthood site (http://www.plannedparenthood.org/pp2/portal/files/portal/medicalinfo/sti/pub-sti-herpes.xml). A free patient pamphlet, "Genital Herpes: A Patient Guide to Treatment," can be ordered from the American Medical Association by calling 312-464-2588.

Syphilis (Chancre)

See section on "Syphilis—Primary Syphilis."

Chancroid

Chancroid is caused by the organism *Haemophilus ducreyi*. It is relatively common in Africa, the Caribbean, and Southwest Asia, but is seen infrequently in the United States. Chancroid has been seen in episodic outbreaks especially associated with prostitution and drug use and is endemic in several large cities in the United States (32–34). Its incidence is likely underreported secondary to difficulties in diagnosis. In 1987, almost 5,000 cases were reported to the CDC but in 1996 only 386 were reported (35). Chancroid should be suspected in individuals with a genital ulcer who have recently had sexual exposure in a developing country.

The incubation period for chancroid is 4 to 7 days. Initially a papule forms and over several days erodes into a deep ulcer with irregular undermined borders. The ulcers are generally multiple but can be solitary and are extremely painful. Chancroid ulcers are friable and often have a purulent base. The ulcers are usually found on the coronal sulcus in circumcised men or on the prepuce of uncircumcised men and in women on the labia or perineum (17). After a week, about 50% of patients develop inguinal lymphadenopathy that is most frequently unilateral. Women are less likely to develop lymphadenopathy (36). Lymph nodes may become fluctuant and may spontaneously rupture. The combination of a painful ulcer and suppurative lymphadenopathy is almost pathognomonic for chancroid.

Definitive diagnosis of *H. ducreyi* requires isolation of the organism in special culture media that is not commonly available. The sensitivity of culture is <80% (37). A Gram stain revealing short, wide gram-negative rods in chains or clusters is suggestive of the diagnosis but the sensitivity and specificity of Gram stain is generally felt to be poor (38). There is no FDA-approved PCR test for chancroid. Given these diagnostic limitations, the CDC treatment guidelines suggest that a probable diagnosis of chancroid can be based on the following criteria: one or more painful genital ulcers; *T. pallidum* is not identified on dark-field examination of the ulcer exudates and serologic testing for syphilis is negative at least 7 days after onset of the ulcers; the presentation, ulcer appearance and, if present, lymphadenopathy are typical for chancroid; and, HSV culture of the ulcer exudates is negative.

The recommended treatments for chancroid include: azithromycin 1 g orally as a single dose; ceftriaxone 250 mg intramuscularly in a single dose; ciprofloxacin 500 mg orally twice daily for 3 days; or erythromycin base 500 mg orally 3 times daily for 7 days (2). Little data is available regarding the efficacy of the short-term ceftriaxone and azithromycin regimens in HIV-infected patients. Some experts prefer erythromycin therapy in HIV-infected patients. Pregnant or lactating women and patients less than 18 years of age should avoid ciprofloxacin.

Clinical re-evaluation should be performed between 3 to 7 days after initiation of therapy. Symptoms rapidly improve within 3 days of initiating therapy and clinical improvement of ulcers is usually evident in 7 days. Large ulcers may take over 2 weeks to heal. Healing of lymphadenopathy is slower and large fluctuant lymph nodes may require aspiration or incision and drainage (39). Response to therapy may be slow or inadequate in uncircumcised men or HIV-infected patients and these patients should be followed more closely (40–42). Overall, the cure rate with recommended therapy in HIV-negative patients is ≥92% and in HIV-positive patients is ≥76% (40–43).

Patients should be counseled to notify their recent sexual partners so that they may receive clinical evaluation and therapy if indicated. All persons who have had sexual contact with the patient within 10 days of the development of symptoms of chancroid should be empirically treated for chancroid even if no abnormalities are detected on examination. The patient should be provided HIV and syphilis testing at time of diagnosis and instructed to return for repeat testing in 3 months (2).

Granuloma Inguinale (Donavonosis)

Granuloma inguinale is caused by the intracellular, encapsulated, short gram-negative bacillus, *Klebsiella granulomatis*. The disorder is found most commonly in tropical and subtropical areas, especially in the Western Pacific, and is rare in the United States. The incubation period is between 8 days and 12 weeks. It can present as large ulcerative lesions, erythematous papules with overlying granulation tissue, large papules resembling severe condyloma acuminatum, or expanding plaques of scar tissue (16). Most commonly it is a slowly progressive disorder with large, painless, friable ulcers with heaped up borders and "beefy" vascular bases. Lymphadenopathy is rare. Without treatment, granuloma inguinale is a slowly destructive process that can result in serious sequelae for the genitourinary tract. The organism is difficult to culture and diagnosis relies on histopathology. A sample of tissue from the leading edge of an ulcer is placed between a slide and cover slip, crushed (crush preparation), and stained. The diagnosis of granuloma inguinale is made by identification of rods within cytoplasmic vacuoles of macrophages (Donovan bodies).

The CDC-recommended treatment is doxycycline 100 mg orally twice daily for at least 3 weeks and until the lesions have completely healed (2,44). Alternative regimens include: ciprofloxacin 750 mg twice daily for at least 3 weeks; erythromycin base 500 mg 4 times a day for at least 3 weeks; azithromycin 1 g weekly for at least 3 weeks; or trimethoprim-sulfamethoxazole one double strength tablet twice daily for at least 3 weeks. The 2003 World Health Organization (WHO) Sexually Transmitted Infections Management Guidelines also recommended a 1 g dose of azithromycin followed by azithromycin 500 mg daily until symptoms resolve (44). Therapy should be continued until all lesions have re-epithelialized. In patients with HIV-infection, pregnant patients, or patients with slow improvement, gentamicin 1 mg/kg intravenously every 8 hours can be added. The erythromycin-based regimen is preferred in pregnancy. The benefit of empiric drug therapy for sexual contacts is not clear, but all sexual contacts within 60 days of the patient's symptom onset should be evaluated clinically and offered therapy.

Lymphogranuloma Venereum

Chlamydia trachomatis serovars L1, L2, and L3 are the causative organisms of lymphogranuloma venereum (LGV). Until recently, LGV was infrequently seen in the Western world and was chiefly seen in South and Central America, the Caribbean, Southeast Asia, India, and areas of Africa. In 2003, an outbreak was noted among MSM in the Netherlands in association with proctitis. Investigation revealed 30 cases in 2003 and 62 cases in 2004 (1). Since then cases and case clusters of LGV proctitis have been scrotal abscess, hydrocele, varicocele, viral orchitis, testicular neoplasm, Fournier gangrene, Henoch-Schonlein purpura, renal colic, peritonitis, or intraperitoneal hemorrhage with a patent processus vaginalis and a leaking abdominal aortic aneurysm (143).

Testicular torsion and torsion of the testicular appendage are the most common alternative diagnoses (144). Expeditious diagnosis of testicular torsion is critical. The total time of ischemia determines the viability of the testes. Therefore, when evaluating acute scrotal pain, clinicians must consider the history, risk factors, and clinical examination. A history of previous episodes of scrotal pain that resolved without intervention is compatible with intermittent or recurrent testicular torsion (145–147). Classically the pain of testicular torsion is acute in onset and severe but there is significant overlap in the clinical presentations of the common causes of acute scrotal pain. Physical findings suggestive of testicular torsion include an abnormal axis of the affected testicle, an abnormal position of the epididymis, an abnormal axis of the unaffected testicle, or abnormal elevation of the affected testicle with a palpable twist of the spermatic cord (145). Any findings on history or physical examination that are suggestive of testicular torsion should prompt emergent urosurgical evaluation.

Clinical findings suggestive of epididymitis include: gradual onset of pain; dysuria, urethral discharge, or recent genitourinary instrumentation; a history of UTI, imperforate anus, neurogenic bladder, or genitourinary surgery; fever of $>101°F$ (38.3°C); tenderness and induration at the epididymis; and urinalysis showing ≥ 10 WBCs per high-power field or ≥ 10 red blood cells (RBC) per high-power field (145). Patients with three or more of these findings are likely to have epididymitis.

Evaluation of patients with epididymitis should include Gram stain of a urethral swab for evidence of urethritis or gonorrhea, testing for gonorrhea and chlamydia preferably with NAAT for optimal chlamydia sensitivity, and sampling of first-void urine for leukocyte count, leukocyte esterase measurement, and culture (2). Patients with suspected gonorrhea or chlamydia infection should also be screened for syphilis and HIV infection.

Empiric treatment should be initiated at the time of first evaluation. Treatment in patients with a high risk of sexually transmitted epididymitis should include ceftriaxone 250 mg intramuscularly as a single dose with doxycycline 100 mg orally twice daily for 10 days. Ofloxacin 300 mg orally twice daily or levofloxacin 500 mg orally daily for 10 days are also acceptable regimens if the patient has not traveled abroad, has not recently visited California or Hawaii, and is not a homosexual man (2). In patients with epididymitis more likely caused by gram-negative enteric bacteria or patients intolerant of cephalosporins or tetracyclines, treatment with levofloxacin is recommended with the dose, duration, and caveats specified above. Symptomatic treatment should include bed rest, scrotal elevation, and antipyretics/analgesics. Hospital admission should be considered for patients with fever, testicular abscess, toxic appearance, severe pain, immunocompromise, a history of noncompliance, or intolerance of oral intake.

Patients should have significant improvement within 3 days. Patients who fail to improve appropriately or whose symptoms do not completely resolve with treatment should be reevaluated with consideration of the differential diagnosis outlined above and the possibility of quinolone resistant *N. gonorrhoeae*. Patients may benefit from radiologic imaging and urosurgical evaluation. Treatment failure may indicate error in the initial diagnosis or infection with an antibiotic resistant or atypical organism. Tuberculosis, brucellosis, bacillus Calmette-Guérin (BCG), and fungal infections are rare causes of epididymitis. If gonorrhea or chlamydia infection is suspected or proven, all of the patient's sexual partners in the last 60 days should be referred for medical evaluation and treatment. If the patient's last sexual activity was more than 60 days prior to diagnosis, the patient's last partner should be referred to medical care. The patient and his sexual partners should abstain from sexual activity until symptoms have resolved and treatment has been completed.

SYPHILIS

Syphilis caused significant morbidity and mortality in the first half of the last century, but after the introduction of penicillin in the 1940s, the rates of disease in the United States declined significantly (148,149). The epidemiology has been characterized by epidemics at 7- to 10-year intervals. In the late 1980s, syphilis was associated with crack cocaine use and sex-for-drugs prostitution (149–151). More recently, the focus of outbreaks has been in the gay community. Overall, nonwhite minorities are disproportionately affected (148). In addition to the known sequelae of cardiovascular and neurologic disease and the continued morbidity and mortality from congenital syphilis, syphilis facilitates HIV transmission. The HIV epidemic, the concentration of new syphilis cases in specific geographic locations, the disproportionate impact on minority populations, and the availability of new biomedical and public health tools led the CDC to call for a new drive for syphilis elimination. In order to reach this goal, the reported rates of primary and secondary syphilis will need to fall to 0.4 per 100,000 people nationally per year.

Syphilis control requires the rapid treatment of newly identified cases, aggressive contact tracing, and active screening by primary care providers. In most office settings, asymptomatic sexually active patients should be screened for syphilis at their first visit with a nontreponemal serologic test and should be retested at followup visits if they report risk behaviors or have been diagnosed with another STD.

TABLE 37.3 Outline of the Clinical Stages of Syphilis

Stage	Characteristic Findings	Usual Onset after Exposure	Duration of Stage if Untreated	Dark-Field
Primary	Chancre—may be absent or not visible (e.g., in vagina or mouth)	10–90 days (average 21 days)	2–6 weeks	+ (Chancre, lymph nodes)
Secondary	Rash, condyloma lata, lymphadenopathy	6 weeks to 6 months	2–6 weeks; recurrences in 25% over 4 yrs	+ (Especially moist lesions)
Latent			May be lifelong because only 1/3 of untreated patients develop tertiary syphilis	Negative
Early	None	<1 year after infection		
Late	None	>1 year after infection		
Late (tertiary)				
Benign	Gumma	2–10 yrs	Indolent	Negative
Cardiovascular	Aortic aneurysm, aortic insufficiency, coronary artery disease	10–30 yrs	Progressive; may be fatal	Aorta may be +
Neurosyphilis		2–35 yrs	Progressive; may be fatal	Brain may be +
Asymptomatic	None			
Acute syphilitic meningitis	Headache, cranial nerve lesions, papilledema	6 weeks to 2 yrs	Not applicable	
Meningovascular	Signs of infection depend on area involved	2–10 yrs		
Tabes dorsalis	Signs of posterior column degeneration	5–30 yrs		
Paresis	Minor personality change to frank psychosis	15–35 yrs		

Clinical Classification

Syphilis is caused by *Treponema pallidum*. The clinical manifestations of disease vary during the different stages of disease (Table 37.3).

Primary Syphilis

Primary syphilis is classically characterized by the development of a chancre, a painless ulcer with indurated edges and a clean base. A chancre forms 10 to 90 days (average 21 days) after infection. Lesions begin as painless papules at the sites of sexual contact, most commonly on the genitals. Extragenital chancres are infrequent but primarily occur in the mouth (152). Approximately 30% of cases will have multiple lesions. Chancres are frequently associated with painless regional and generalized lymphadenopathy. This painless, initial stage of disease can easily be missed, and up to 60% of patients diagnosed with syphilis have no history of ulcerative lesions (152). (See Genital Ulcer Disease for differential diagnosis.)

Secondary Syphilis

Approximately 50% of patients with untreated primary syphilis will develop signs of secondary syphilis. The onset of secondary syphilis is generally between 6 weeks and 6 months after infection. In 15% to 20% of patients, the primary chancre is still present. Secondary syphilis is a systemic disorder, the classic manifestation of which is a maculopapular, follicular, or occasionally pustular rash. The rash can be widespread and often affects the palms and soles. Patchy alopecia may result from follicular involvement on the scalp or along the eyelids. Oral lesions known as mucous patches occur in 5% to 22% of patients and present as gray lesions on an erythematous base (153). Flat, waxy, wart-like lesions usually found in the moist intertriginous regions of the genital or anal areas are known as condylomata lata. Both mucous patches and condylomata lata are highly infectious. Dermatologic manifestations of secondary syphilis will generally resolve within 2 to 6 weeks even without treatment. A quarter of patients will have a recurrence of symptoms within 4 years.

Constitutional symptoms of malaise, low-grade fever, headache, and generalized lymphadenopathy are common in patients with secondary syphilis. Asymptomatic meningitis and cranial nerve palsies may also occur (152). Other infrequent manifestations of secondary syphilis include anorexia, nausea, vomiting, jaundice, granulomatous hepatitis, proteinuria, nephrotic syndrome, acute nephritic syndromes, gastric ulcerations or rugal hypertrophy, ocular inflammation, tinnitus, and sensorineural deafness.

Latent Syphilis

Latent syphilis is the period of asymptomatic *T. pallidum* infection that begins with the resolution of secondary symptoms and ends either with treatment or development of signs and symptoms of tertiary disease. The period is divided into two categories: early latent and late latent. The cut-off between these two categories is somewhat arbitrarily set at 1 year. It is within the year of early latent syphilis that 90% of recurrences of secondary symptoms will occur (154). During latent syphilis, recurrences are rare. For this reason persons with early latent syphilis also pose a higher risk of syphilis transmission.

Tertiary Syphilis

Even without appropriate treatment, only one third of patients with syphilis will develop tertiary manifestations. Since the introduction of penicillin, tertiary manifestations have become uncommon and more subtle in their presentation. There are three principal forms of tertiary syphilis: late benign (gummatous) syphilis, cardiovascular syphilis, and neurosyphilis.

1) ***Late Benign Syphilis.*** The classic lesion of late benign syphilis is the gumma, a granulomatous lesion that typically develops 2 to 10 years after infection. Gummas can be several centimeters in size and most commonly affect the skin (nodular or ulcerative lesions), bone, or liver. Significant morbidity and mortality can be associated with lesions in the brain or heart.
2) ***Cardiovascular Syphilis.*** In untreated patients, cardiovascular manifestations generally occur 5 to 30 years after initial infection. The most common manifestation is syphilitic aortitis. *T. pallidum* characteristically causes destruction of the elastic and muscular tissues of the ascending aorta resulting in aneurysm formation, aortic ring dilatation, aortic regurgitation, and progressive heart failure. Stenosis of the coronary ostia may result in angina pectoris but is rarely associated with myocardial infarction (155).
3) ***Neurosyphilis.*** *T. pallidum* infection of the central nervous system (CNS) occurs at all stages of disease. Early infection may proceed to spontaneous resolution, asymptomatic meningitis, or acute aseptic meningitis. Late disease may remain asymptomatic or patients may develop meningovascular syphilis, tabes dorsalis, or general paresis (152).

Neurosyphilis

Asymptomatic neurosyphilis is defined as a reactive Venereal Disease Research Laboratory (VDRL) test for syphilis in cerebrospinal fluid (CSF) or elevations in CSF WBC or protein concentrations in a syphilitic patient without clinical neurologic or psychiatric abnormalities. The diagnosis of asymptomatic neurosyphilis also requires that other causes of these CSF abnormalities are excluded. These abnormalities in CSF parameters are most commonly detected during primary, secondary, and early latent syphilis. Predictors of CSF abnormalities include a nontreponemal test titer $\geq$1:32 (see Diagnosis) and in HIV-infected patients, a CD4 count $<$350 lymphocytes per milliliter (156). Detection of CSF abnormalities in asymptomatic patients is of unclear significance. Use of penicillin in primary and secondary syphilis at doses inadequate for spirochetal eradication in the CNS has nevertheless been associated with remarkably low rates of symptomatic neurosyphilis. Similarly, the presence of CSF abnormalities or mild neurologic complaints in patients with early disease has not been associated with serologic treatment failure after treatment with regimens recommended for early disease (157).

Syphilitic meningitis most commonly occurs during secondary or early latent syphilis and is characterized by severe headache, meningismus, seizures, and cranial nerve involvement. Patients may develop facial palsies, sensorineural deafness, or optic nerve or primary ocular involvement (152).

Meningovascular syphilis can occur after 2 to 10 years of untreated infection. Clinical findings include headache, irritability, confusion, personality changes, emotional lability, seizures, and altered level of consciousness (158). Vasculitis of small end arteries can produce focal findings specific to areas of involvement.

Tabes dorsalis occurs 5 to 30 years after untreated infection. It affects pupillomotor structures and the posterior columns in the CNS. Patients initially develop lightning pains in their lower extremities and paresthesias. Disease progresses with the onset of sensory ataxia, loss of position and vibratory sense, areflexia, broad-based gait, incontinence, and impotence. Joint changes (Charcot joint) and neuropathic ulcers may develop. Another feature of tabes dorsalis is gastric crises with vomiting, and/or abdominal pain. Some patients also develop the classic Argyll Robertson pupil (small, irregular pupil that accommodates but does not react to light).

General paresis occurs in patients with untreated syphilis 15 to 35 years after infection. It is a complication of untreated syphilis that is characterized by progressive personality changes, irritability, poor judgment, memory loss, and psychotic features.

Pregnancy

In addition to the manifestations and complications above, syphilis has been associated with spontaneous abortion, stillbirth, premature delivery, and perinatal death (159). Syphilis can be transmitted vertically to the neonate and result in serious systemic complications.

Diagnosis

There are several tools that are useful in the diagnosis and staging of syphilis. All patients diagnosed with syphilis by dark-field microscopy or serologic testing should be tested for HIV-infection at the time of diagnosis, and in the case of primary and secondary syphilis, at 3 months after diagnosis. Dark-field microscopy and direct fluorescent antibody (DFA-TP) tests are used in early stages of syphilis to identify organisms in primary chancres and condylomata lata. Dark-field microscopy is not available at all centers but is usually available at STD clinics. Patients can usually be referred to one of these clinics for complete evaluation. To obtain a sample, the lesion should be lightly abraded with a gauze pad and then squeezed so that the serous exudate can be collected on a microscope slide or slide cover. Three microscopic samples should be evaluated immediately to avoid drying. Slides should be evaluated at 45X to identify possible organisms. Any suspected organisms should be examined under oil immersion and the 100X objective. Although *T. pallidum* is a corkscrew shape organism with a characteristic motility, it can be difficult to differentiate from the oral spirochete, *T. macrodentium*. For this reason oral lesions should not be evaluated with dark-field microscopy. A negative dark-field examination of a genital lesion does not rule out syphilis.

Two different types of serological tests are available for diagnosis of syphilis and are useful during all stages of disease. Nontreponemal tests include VDRL and rapid plasma reagin (RPR). These tests detect nonspecific antibody to reagin, a cardiolipin-lecithin-cholesterol antigen complex. The titers of these tests usually correlate with disease activity. These tests cannot be used by themselves due to their limited sensitivity in early and late syphilis and the occurrence of false positives. For this reason positive nontreponemal tests must be followed with specific treponemal tests to confirm a diagnosis of syphilis.

A patient is considered to have a *biologic false-positive* test if the nontreponemal test is reactive and a specific treponemal test is consistently nonreactive. The titer of the nontreponemal test is generally less than or equal to 1:8. Biologic false-positive nontreponemal tests are designated as acute if they are present less than 6 months or chronic if present more than 6 months. Conditions associated with a biologic false-positive test include: pneumonia, hepatitis, pregnancy, mononucleosis, measles, malaria, intravenous drug use, rheumatologic disorders, chronic liver disease, Waldenstrom macroglobulinemia, older age, and hereditary biologic false-positive.

Treponemal tests include the fluorescent treponemal antibody absorption (FTA-ABS), *T. pallidum* particle agglutination, and treponemal enzyme immunoassay (EIA) tests. FTA-ABS and *T. pallidum* particle agglutination tests detect specific antibodies to *T. pallidum*. They have higher sensitivity and specificity than nontreponemal tests but are more difficult to perform and are more expensive. False-positive tests are rare but can occur in patients with autoimmune disease, viral infections, and pregnancy (160). There are rare reports of false-negative FTA-ABS tests in HIV-infected patients with syphilis (161). FTA-ABS and *T. pallidum* particle agglutination should generally be used as confirmatory tests except in cases of suspected primary or tertiary syphilis when the nontreponemal tests may be negative and the treponemal test may be more sensitive.

Treponemal EIA tests are used by some large clinical labs and blood banks. In 2000, approximately 13% of public health laboratories used treponemal EIA tests (162). A positive EIA generally should be followed with a titered nontreponemal test. If the RPR or VDRL is negative, the patient may have partially treated syphilis, previously treated disease, untreated late infection, or a false-positive result. These patients need a careful history and laboratory evaluation with FTA-ABS or TP-PA.

The diagnosis of neurosyphilis in a patient with positive serologic tests for syphilis depends on the results of CSF analysis. Any patient with neurologic or ophthalmic signs or symptoms, evidence of tertiary aortitis or gummas, evidence of serologic treatment failure, or patients with HIV infection and late latent syphilis or syphilis of unknown duration should be evaluated for neurosyphilis with CSF evaluation. CSF examination should also be considered for patients with latent syphilis and serologic titers $\geq$1:32 or HIV-infected patients with CD4 counts $\leq$350 lymphocytes per milliliter (156). A positive CSF VDRL is the best laboratory evidence of neurosyphilis. Although its specificity is virtually 100%, its reported sensitivity ranges widely from 10% to 89%. The CSF VDRL is less sensitive in detecting asymptomatic neurosyphilis and tabes dorsalis. However, in patients without other identifiable CNS infections, an elevated protein concentration (>40 mg/dL) or WBC count (>5 mononuclear cells per μL) in the CSF can also indicate CNS syphilis infection. The role of the CSF FTA-ABS test in neurosyphilis diagnosis is controversial. Most studies agree that a nonreactive CSF FTA-ABS is useful for ruling out neurosyphilis, but the significance of a reactive CSF FTA-ABS without other CSF abnormalities is unclear (163–165).

Treatment and Followup

The treatment of choice for all stages of syphilis is parenteral penicillin G (benzathine, aqueous procaine, or aqueous crystalline). Combinations of benzathine penicillin and procaine penicillin or oral penicillin should not be used. Unfortunately, inadvertent syphilis treatment errors continue to occur due to inappropriate use of Bicillin CR (1.2 million units procaine penicillin G and 1.2 million units benzathine penicillin G) instead of Bicillin LA (2.4 mu benzathine penicillin G) (166). The duration of treatment depends on the stage of disease. Therefore, before deciding on a treatment plan every patient should have a thorough physical examination, including speculum examination in women, to evaluate for evidence of chancres, skin rash, ocular changes, or cardiologic or neurologic manifestations. Knowledge of a patient's HIV status is also important.

Primary and Secondary Syphilis

Primary and secondary syphilis should be treated with benzathine penicillin G 2.4 million units intramuscularly (IM) in a single dose (2). Evidence for alternatives to penicillin in nonpregnant, HIV-seronegative patients is limited. Doxycycline 100 mg orally twice daily or tetracycline 500 mg four times daily for 14 days has been used for many years. Less is known about the efficacy of ceftriaxone, but some experts recommend 1 g IM or intravenously (IV) for 8 to 10 days.

Azithromycin 2 g as a single dose has been considered a potential oral option for syphilis treatment (167). Although the potential for directly observed oral therapy makes the use of azithromycin attractive especially in penicillin allergic patients, a considerable rate of *in vitro* resistance has been demonstrated in the United States, and clinical failures have been reported (168). Therefore, azithromycin should be used with caution and only when alternative regimens are impractical.

Followup of patients should include both physical examination and measurement of nontreponemal test titers. Followup should occur at 6 months and 12 months after treatment. Closer followup may be warranted if patients are treated with nonpenicillin regimens or if they are HIV-positive. Nontreponemal test titers should decline fourfold (2 dilutions) within 6 months after therapy. More than 85% of patients treated for primary or secondary syphilis will eventually revert to a nonreactive nontreponemal serologic test. Approximately 10% of patients appropriately treated will also revert to a negative FTA-ABS (169). If serologic titers have not fallen appropriately, the patient is at risk for treatment failure and at a minimum needs close clinical and serologic followup. Persistant or recurrent symptoms or a fourfold increase in nontreponemal test titer suggest reinfection or treatment failure. Patients with treatment failure should have repeat HIV testing and should be retreated with three weekly IM injections of benzathine penicillin G 2.4 million units, unless CSF evaluation suggests the presence of neurosyphilis.

Latent Syphilis

Recommended treatment of early latent syphilis is benzathine penicillin G 2.4 million units intramuscular injection in a single dose (2). Patients who do not have documented seroconversion within the last year, clear signs of primary or secondary syphilis, and do not have a sex partner with documented primary, secondary, or early latent syphilis must be assumed to have late latent syphilis. These patients should be treated with 3 weekly intramuscular injections of benzathine penicillin 2.4 million units. In nonpregnant, HIV-seronegative patients, alternatives to penicillin therapy are poorly studied. Patients with early latent syphilis may be treated with caution with the alternative regimens listed under Treatment and Followup and Primary and Secondary Syphilis. Patients with late latent syphilis can be treated with either doxycycline 100 mg orally twice daily or tetracycline 500 mg orally four times daily for 28 days.

Clinical and serologic followup should be performed at 6, 12, and 24 months. Approximately 75% of patients treated for early latent syphilis and 44% of patients treated for late latent syphilis will have nonreactive nontreponemal serologic tests 5 years after treatment (171). Treatment failure should be considered for patients whose titers increase fourfold, if an initial titer $\geq$1:32 fails to decline at least fourfold within 12 to 24 months, or if signs or symptoms of syphilis develop. These patients should have CSF evaluation for neurosyphilis and if negative should be retreated for latent syphilis.

Tertiary Syphilis

Patients with gummatous or cardiovascular syphilis should be evaluated for neurosyphilis. If CSF evaluation is normal, they should be treated with benzathine penicillin 3 weekly IM injections of 2.4 million units (2). Some experts treat patients with evidence of cardiovascular syphilis with neurosyphilis regimens. Doxycycline or tetracycline for 28 days can be considered for treatment of patients with penicillin allergy and without neurosyphilis. Response to treatment of tertiary syphilis has not been well studied.

Neurosyphilis

Patients with abnormalities on CSF examination or with evidence of ocular syphilis should be treated for neurosyphilis. CDC recommended treatment for neurosyphilis is aqueous crystalline penicillin G 3 to 4 million units IV every 4 hours or as a continuous infusion with a daily dose of 18 to 24 million units IV a day for 10 to 14 days (2). An alternative regimen is daily procaine penicillin 2.4 million units IM with probenecid 500 mg orally four times a day for 10 to 14 days. Some experts give one to three additional weekly IM injections of benzathine penicillin 2.4 million units after the IV treatment to achieve a total duration of therapy that is equivalent to late latent treatment. There is less clinical experience with nonpenicillin containing regimens. Ceftriaxone has been recommended by some experts when penicillin cannot be used (172). Some experts recommend ceftriaxone IV or IM 2 g daily for 10 to 14 days.

Patients with elevated CSF cell counts should have repeat CSF evaluation every 6 months until the cell concentration is normal. The cell count should decrease within 6 months, and patients should be retreated if CSF pleocytosis has not resolved after 2 years (2).

Special Considerations in Pregnancy

Pregnant patients should be treated with penicillin regimens, not with alternative regimens. Pregnant patients with penicillin allergy should be desensitized to penicillin. Some experts recommend 2 weekly doses of intramuscular benzathine penicillin 2.4 million units in pregnant women with primary, secondary, or early latent syphilis. Pregnant patients should be managed with the assistance of an obstetrician.

Jarisch-Herxheimer Reaction

The Jarisch-Herxheimer reaction is an acute febrile reaction that can last several hours and can occur within the first 24 hours of any effective treatment for syphilis. The pathogenesis is unknown but thought to be related to the release of toxin by dying spirochetes. Patients often report headache, myalgias, and worsening cutaneous lesions. Antipyretics may be useful for symptomatic relief. In rare severe reactions patients may develop transient hypotension. In pregnant women, the Jarisch Herxheimer reaction may result in early labor or fetal distress (175). Patients with early stages of syphilis may have a greater risk of developing this reaction and should be informed about this possible side effect of treatment.

HIV-Infected Patients with Syphilis

Although numerous case reports suggest the possibility of a more aggressive course of early syphilis in HIV-infected patients, a recent prospective multicenter, randomized trial comparing manifestations of disease and response to therapy in HIV-infected and uninfected patients with early syphilis found only minor differences in clinical presentation (173). HIV-infected patients had a greater median number of ulcers, and a higher proportion of HIV-infected patients had multiple ulcers. Neurologic signs and symptoms were infrequent in both HIV-infected and uninfected patients.

Although most HIV-infected patients can generally be evaluated and treated with the same diagnostic tests and treatment regimens as HIV-negative patients, clinicians should be aware of several unique considerations. Rarely, false negative serologic tests in the setting of clinical findings suggestive for syphilis in HIV-infected patients may require biopsy of lesions for dark-field examination or direct fluorescent antibody staining. HIV-infected patients with syphilis may also be at somewhat greater risk of developing neurosyphilis even at early stages of disease and may have greater rates of treatment failure with standard treatment regimens (174). A Jarisch-Herxheimer reaction occurs in up to 22% of HIV-infected patients compared to 12% of HIV-negative patients (173).

Current recommendations for treatment do not differ from HIV-negative individuals except that all HIV-infected patients with late latent syphilis or syphilis of unknown duration should have CSF evaluation prior to determination of treatment regimen (2). Recommended followup for HIV-infected patients is at 3, 6, 9, 12, and 24 months after therapy for primary, secondary or early latent syphilis. Patients with late latent syphilis should be re-evaluated serologically at 6, 12, 18, and 24 months after treatment. Patients meeting previously discussed indicators of treatment failure should be reassessed with CSF evaluation and retreated.

Contact Evaluation

Transmission of syphilis occurs through exposure to mucocutaneous syphilitic lesions. Therefore, primary, secondary, and early latent syphilis mark the stages of disease in which sexual partners are at risk of acquiring infection. The CDC STD Treatment Guidelines recommend identifying at-risk sex partners exposed to a patient within 3 months plus the duration of symptoms of primary syphilis, within 6 months plus the duration of symptoms for secondary syphilis, and within 1 year for early latent syphilis (2). Presumptive treatment should be given to all persons regardless of their serology if they have been exposed within 90 days to a case of primary, secondary, or early latent syphilis. If a person has been exposed to primary, secondary, or early latent syphilis greater than 90 days prior to evaluation but serologic tests are not available or followup is in doubt, presumptive treatment should be offered. In cases of syphilis of unknown duration, if the patient has a high titer ($\geq$1:32), partner notification and treatment should follow the guidelines for early syphilis. Persons with a history of exposure to a patient with latent syphilis should be managed based on the results of clinical evaluation and serologic testing.

SPECIFIC REFERENCES

1. Centers for Disease Control and Prevention. Lymphogranuloma venereum among men who have sex with men–Netherlands, 2003–2004. Morb Mortal Wkly Rep 2005;53:985.
2. Centers for Disease Control and Prevention. 2006. Sexually Transmitted Diseases Treatment Guidelines. Morb Mortal Wkly Rep 2006 (in press).
3. Cameron DW, Simonsen JN, D'Costa LJ, et al. Female to male transmission of human immunodeficiency virus type 1: risk factors for seroconversion in men. Lancet 1989;2: 403.
4. Chen CY, Ballard RC, Beck-Sague CM, et al. Human immunodeficiency virus infection and genital ulcer disease in South Africa: the herpetic connection. Sex Transm Dis 2000; 27:21.
5. Greenblatt RM, Lukehart SA, Plummer FA, et al. Genital ulceration as a risk factor for human immunodeficiency virus infection. AIDS 1988;2:47.
6. Schacker T, Ryncarz AJ, Goddard J, et al. Frequent recovery of HIV-1 from genital herpes simplex virus lesions in HIV-1-infected men. JAMA 1998;280:61.
7. Stamm WE, Handsfield HH, Rompalo AM, et al. The association between genital ulcer disease and acquisition of HIV infection in homosexual men. JAMA 1988;260:1429.

8. Chapel TA, Brown WJ, Jeffres C, et al. How reliable is the morphological diagnosis of penile ulcerations? Sex Transm Dis 1977;4:150.
9. O'Farrell N, Hoosen AA, Coetzee KD, et al. Genital ulcer disease: accuracy of clinical diagnosis and strategies to improve control in Durban, South Africa. Genitourin Med 1994;70:7.
10. Zainah S, Cheong YM, Sinniah M, et al. A microbiological study of genital ulcers in Kuala Lumpur. Med J Malaysia 1991;46:274.
11. Ribes JA, Steele AD, Seabolt JP, et al. Six-year study of the incidence of herpes in genital and nongenital cultures in a central Kentucky medical center patient population. J Clin Microbiol 2001;39:3321.
12. Roberts CM, Pfister JR, Spear SJ. Increasing proportion of herpes simplex virus type 1 as a cause of genital herpes infection in college students. Sex Transm Dis 2003;30:797.
13. Fleming DT, McQuillan GM, Johnson RE, et al. Herpes simplex virus type 2 in the United States, 1976 to 1994. N Engl J Med 1997;337:1105.
14. Langenberg AG, Corey L, Ashley RL, et al. A prospective study of new infections with herpes simplex virus type 1 and type 2. Chiron HSV Vaccine Study Group. N Engl J Med 1999;341:1432.
15. Langenberg A, Benedetti J, Jenkins J, et al. Development of clinically recognizable genital lesions among women previously identified as having "asymptomatic" herpes simplex virus type 2 infection. Ann Intern Med 1989;110: 882.
16. Rosen T, Brown TJ. Genital ulcers. Evaluation and treatment. Dermatol Clin 1998;16:673, x.
17. Hoffman IF, Schmitz JL. Genital ulcer disease. Management in the HIV era. Postgrad Med 1995;98:67, 79.
18. Schmid GP. Approach to the patient with genital ulcer disease. Med Clin North Am 1990;74:1559.
19. Benedetti J, Corey L, Ashley R. Recurrence rates in genital herpes after symptomatic first-episode infection. Ann Intern Med 1994;121:847.
20. Koelle DM, Benedetti J, Langenberg A, et al. Asymptomatic reactivation of herpes simplex virus in women after the first episode of genital herpes. Ann Intern Med 1992;116:433.
21. Gupta R, Wald A, Krantz E, et al. Valacyclovir and acyclovir for suppression of shedding of herpes simplex virus in the genital tract. J Infect Dis 2004;190:1374.
22. Cone RW, Swenson PD, Hobson AC, et al. Herpes simplex virus detection from genital lesions: a comparative study using antigen detection (HerpChek) and culture. J Clin Microbiol 1993;31:1774.
23. Slomka MJ, Emery L, Munday PE, et al. A comparison of PCR with virus isolation and direct antigen detection for diagnosis and typing of genital herpes. J Med Virol 1998;55:177.
24. Ashley RL, Wald A, Eagleton M. Premarket evaluation of the POCkit HSV-2 type-specific serologic test in culture-documented cases of genital herpes simplex virus type 2 [see comment]. Sex Transm Dis 2000;27:266.
25. Martins TB, Woolstenhulme RD, Jaskowski TD, et al. Comparison of four enzyme immunoassays with a western blot assay for the determination of type-specific antibodies to herpes simplex virus. Am J Clin Pathol 2001;115:272.
26. Whittington WL, Celum CL, Cent A, et al. Use of a glycoprotein G-based type-specific assay to detect antibodies to herpes simplex virus type 2 among persons attending sexually transmitted disease clinics. Sex Transm Dis 2001;28:99.
27. Prince HE, Ernst CE, Hogrefe WR. Evaluation of an enzyme immunoassay system for measuring herpes simplex virus (HSV) type 1-specific and HSV type 2-specific IgG antibodies. J Clin Lab Anal 2000;14:13.
28. Wald A. New therapies and prevention strategies for genital herpes. Clin Infect Dis 1999;28 Suppl 1:S4.
29. Patel R, Tyring S, Strand A, et al. Impact of suppressive antiviral therapy on the health related quality of life of patients with recurrent genital herpes infection. Sex Transm Infect 1999;75:398.
30. Corey L, Wald A, Patel R, et al. Once-daily valacyclovir to reduce the risk of transmission of genital herpes. N Engl J Med 2004;350:11.
31. Wald A, Langenberg AG, Link K, et al. Effect of condoms on reducing the transmission of herpes simplex virus type 2 from men to women. JAMA 2001;285:3100.
32. Jones C, Rosen T, Clarridge J, et al. Chancroid: results from an outbreak in Houston, Texas. South Med J 1990;83:1384.
33. Dillon SM, Cummings M, Rajagopalan S, et al. Prospective analysis of genital ulcer disease in Brooklyn, New York. Clin Infect Dis 1997;24:945.
34. DiCarlo RP, Armentor BS, Martin DH. Chancroid epidemiology in New Orleans men. J Infect Dis 1995;172:446.
35. Centers for Disease Control and Prevention. STD Surveillance 1996. US Department of Health and Human Services, Public Health Service, Atlanta, September, 1996.
36. Plummer FA, D'Costa LJ, Nsanze H, et al. Clinical and microbiologic studies of genital ulcers in Kenyan women. Sex Transm Dis. 1985;12:193.
37. Orle KA, Gates CA, Martin DH, et al. Simultaneous PCR detection of *Haemophilus ducreyi, Treponema pallidum*, and herpes simplex virus types 1 and 2 from genital ulcers. J Clin Microbiol 1996;34:49.
38. Sturm AW, Stolting GJ, Cormane RH, et al. Clinical and microbiological evaluation of 46 episodes of genital ulceration. Genitourin Med 1987;63:98.
39. Ernst AA, Marvez-Valls E, Martin DH. Incision and drainage versus aspiration of fluctuant buboes in the emergency department during an epidemic of chancroid. Sex Transm Dis 1995;22:217.
40. Ballard RC, Ye H, Matta A, et al. Treatment of chancroid with azithromycin. Int J STD AIDS 1996;7 Suppl 1:9.
41. Kimani J, Bwayo JJ, Anzala AO, et al. Low dose erythromycin regimen for the treatment of chancroid. East Afr Med J 1995;72:645.
42. Tyndall MW, Agoki E, Plummer FA, et al. Single dose azithromycin for the treatment of chancroid: a randomized comparison with erythromycin. Sex Transm Dis 1994;21:231.
43. Malonza IM, Tyndall MW, Ndinya-Achola JO, et al. A randomized, double-blind, placebo-controlled trial of single-dose ciprofloxacin versus erythromycin for the treatment of chancroid in Nairobi, Kenya. J Infect Dis 1999;180:1886.
44. World Health Organization. Guidelines for the management of sexually transmitted infections. Geneva, Switzerland, World Health Organization, 2003;1–89.
45. French P, Ison CA, Macdonald N. Lymphogranuloma venereum in the United Kingdom. Sex Transm Infect 2005;81:97.
46. Kropp RY, Wong T. Emergence of lymphogranuloma venereum in Canada. Cmaj 2005;172:1674.
47. Levine JS, Smith PD, Brugge WR. Chronic proctitis in male homosexuals due to lymphogranuloma venereum. Gastroenterology 1980;79:563.
48. Mostafavi H, O'Donnell KF, Chong FK. Supralevator abscess due to chronic rectal lymphogranuloma venereum. Am J Gastroenterol 1990;85:602.
49. Papagrigoriadis S, Rennie JA. Lymphogranuloma venereum as a cause of rectal strictures. Postgrad Med J 1998;74:168.
50. Quinn TC, Goodell SE, Mkrtichian E, et al. *Chlamydia trachomatis* proctitis. N Engl J Med 1981;305:195.
51. Koutsky LA, Galloway DA, Holmes KK. Epidemiology of genital human papillomavirus infection. Epidemiol Rev 1988;10:122.
52. Meisels A. Cytologic diagnosis of human papillomavirus. Influence of age and pregnancy stage. Acta Cytol 1992;36:480.
53. Syrjanen K, Vayrynen M, Castren O, et al. Sexual behaviour of women with human papillomavirus (HPV) lesions of the uterine cervix. Br J Vener Dis 1984;60:243.
54. Wen LM, Estcourt CS, Simpson JM, et al. Risk factors for the acquisition of genital warts: are condoms protective? Sex Transm Infect 1999; 75:312.
55. Hippelainen M, Syrjanen S, Hippelainen M, et al. Prevalence and risk factors of genital human papillomavirus (HPV) infections in healthy males: a study on Finnish conscripts. Sex Transm Dis 1993;20:321.
56. Kataja V, Syrjanen S, Yliskoski M, et al. Risk factors associated with cervical human papillomavirus infections: a case-control study. Am J Epidemiol 1993;138:735.
57. Negrini BP, Schiffman MH, Kurman RJ, et al. Oral contraceptive use, human papillomavirus infection, and risk of early cytological abnormalities of the cervix. Cancer Res 1990;50:4670.
58. Franceschi S, Doll R, Gallwey J, et al. Genital warts and cervical neoplasia: an epidemiological study. Br J Cancer 1983;48:621.
59. Halpert R, Fruchter RG, Sedlis A, et al. Human papillomavirus and lower genital neoplasia in renal transplant patients. Obstet Gynecol 1986;68:251.
60. Matorras R, Ariceta JM, Rementeria A, et al. Human immunodeficiency virus-induced immunosuppression: a risk factor for human papillomavirus infection. Am J Obstet Gynecol 1991;164(1 Pt 1):42.
61. Durst M, Gissmann L, Ikenberg H, et al. A papillomavirus DNA from a cervical carcinoma and its prevalence in cancer biopsy samples from different geographic regions. Proc Natl Acad Sci U S A 1983;80:3812.
62. Durst M, Kleinheinz A, Hotz M, et al. The physical state of human papillomavirus type 16 DNA in benign and malignant genital tumours. J Gen Virol 1985;66 (Pt 7):1515.
63. Gissmann L, Boshart M, Durst M, et al. Presence of human papillomavirus in genital tumors. J Invest Dermatol 1984;83(1 Suppl): 26S.
64. Koutsky LA, Holmes KK, Critchlow CW, et al. A cohort study of the risk of cervical intraepithelial neoplasia grade 2 or 3 in relation to papillomavirus infection. N Engl J Med 1992;327:1272.
65. Beutner KR, Wiley DJ, Douglas JM, et al. Genital warts and their treatment. Clin Infect Dis 1999;28 Suppl 1:S37.
66. De Panfilis G, Melzani G, Mori G, et al. Relapses after treatment of external genital warts are more frequent in HIV-positive patients than in HIV-negative controls. Sex Transm Dis 2002;29:121.
67. Silverberg MJ, Ahdieh L, Munoz A, et al. The impact of HIV infection and immunodeficiency on human papillomavirus type 6 or 11 infection and on genital warts. Sex Transm Dis 2002;29:427.
68. Handsfield HH. Clinical presentation and natural course of anogenital warts. Am J Med 1997; 102:16.
69. Beutner KR, Reitano MV, Richwald GA, et al. External genital warts: report of the American Medical Association Consensus Conference. AMA Expert Panel on External Genital Warts. Clin Infect Dis 1998;27:796.

70. Carr G, William DC. Anal warts in a population of gay men in New York City. Sex Transm Dis 1977;4:56.
71. Armstrong LR, Preston EJ, Reichert M, et al. Incidence and prevalence of recurrent respiratory papillomatosis among children in Atlanta and Seattle. Clin Infect Dis 2000;31:107.
72. Silverberg MJ, Thorsen P, Lindeberg H, et al. Condyloma in pregnancy is strongly predictive of juvenile-onset recurrent respiratory papillomatosis. Obstet Gynecol 2003;101:645.
73. Wikstrom A, Hedblad MA, Johansson B, et al. The acetic acid test in evaluation of subclinical genital papillomavirus infection: a comparative study on penoscopy, histopathology, virology and scanning electron microscopy findings. Genitourin Med 1992;68:90.
74. Beutner KR, Conant MA, Friedman-Kien AE, et al. Patient-applied podofilox for treatment of genital warts. Lancet 1989;1:831.
75. Duus BR, Philipsen T, Christensen JD, et al. Refractory condylomata acuminata: a controlled clinical trial of carbon dioxide laser versus conventional surgical treatment. Genitourin Med 1985;61:59.
76. Reid R. The management of genital condylomas, intraepithelial neoplasia, and vulvodynia. Obstet Gynecol Clin North Am 1996;23:917.
77. Maw R. Critical appraisal of commonly used treatment for genital warts. Int J STD AIDS 2004;15:357.
78. Beutner KR, Spruance SL, Hougham AJ, et al. Treatment of genital warts with an immune-response modifier (imiquimod). J Am Acad Dermatol 1998;38(2 Pt 1):230.
79. Edwards L, Ferenczy A, Eron L, et al. Self-administered topical 5% imiquimod cream for external anogenital warts. HPV Study Group. Human PapillomaVirus. Arch Dermatol 1998;134:25.
80. Moore RA, Edwards JE, Hopwood J, et al. Imiquimod for the treatment of genital warts: a quantitative systematic review. BMC Infect Dis 2001;1:3.
81. Beutner KR, Ferenczy A. Therapeutic approaches to genital warts. Am J Med 1997;102:28.
82. Schwebke JR, Weiss HL. Interrelationships of bacterial vaginosis and cervical inflammation. Sex Transm Dis 2002;29:59.
83. Geisler WM, Yu S, Venglarik M, et al. Vaginal leucocyte counts in women with bacterial vaginosis relation to vaginal and cervical infections. Sex Transm Infect 2004;80:401.
84. Weinstock H, Berman S, Cates W. Sexually transmitted infections in American youth: incidence and prevalence estimates, 2000. Perspectives on Sexual and Reproductive Health 2004 2004;36:6.
85. Bjekic M, Vlajinac H, Sipetic S, et al. Risk factors for gonorrhoea: case-control study. Genitourin Med 1997;73:518.
86. Cooper DL, Bernstein GS, Ivler D, et al. Gonorrhea screening program in a women's hospital outpatient department: results and analysis of risk factors. J Am Vener Dis Assoc 1976;3(2 Pt 1):71.
87. Evans BA, Tasker T, MacRae KD. Risk profiles for genital infection in women. Genitourin Med 1993;69:257.
88. Gershman KA, Barrow JC. A tale of two sexually transmitted diseases. Prevalences and predictors of chlamydia and gonorrhea in women attending Colorado family planning clinics. Sex Transm Dis 1996;23:481.
89. Hook EW, III, Reichart CA, Upchurch DM, et al. Comparative behavioral epidemiology of gonococcal and chlamydial infections among patients attending a Baltimore, Maryland, sexually transmitted disease clinic. Am J Epidemiol 1992;136:662.
90. Mertz KJ, Finelli L, Levine WC, et al. Gonorrhea in male adolescents and young adults in Newark, New Jersey: implications of risk factors and patient preferences for prevention strategies. Sex Transm Dis 2000;27:201.
91. Upchurch DM, Brady WE, Reichart CA, et al. Behavioral contributions to acquisition of gonorrhea in patients attending an inner city sexually transmitted disease clinic. J Infect Dis 1990;161:938.
92. Holmes KK, Johnson DW, Trostle HJ. An estimate of the risk of men acquiring gonorrhea by sexual contact with infected females. Am J Epidemiol 1970;91:170.
93. Hooper RR, Reynolds GH, Jones OG, et al. Cohort study of venereal disease. I: the risk of gonorrhea transmission from infected women to men. Am J Epidemiol 1978;108:136.
94. Lin JS, Donegan SP, Heeren TC, et al. Transmission of *Chlamydia trachomatis* and *Neisseria gonorrhoeae* among men with urethritis and their female sex partners. J Infect Dis 1998;178:1707.
95. Thin RN, Williams IA, Nicol CS. Direct and delayed methods of immunofluorescent diagnosis of gonorrhoea in women. Br J Vener Dis 1971;47:27.
96. Wiesner PJ, Tronca E, Bonin P, et al. Clinical spectrum of pharyngeal gonococcal infection. N Engl J Med 1973;288:181.
97. Handsfield HH, Lipman TO, Harnisch JP, et al. Asymptomatic gonorrhea in men. Diagnosis, natural course, prevalence and significance. N Engl J Med 1974;290:117.
98. McCormack WM, Stumacher RJ, Johnson K, et al. Clinical spectrum of gonococcal infection in women. Lancet 1977;1:1182.
99. Quinn TC, Stamm WE, Goodell SE, et al. The polymicrobial origin of intestinal infections in homosexual men. N Engl J Med 1983;309: 576.
100. Kerle KK, Mascola JR, Miller TA. Disseminated gonococcal infection. Am Fam Physician 1992;45:209.
101. Bohnhoff M, Morello JA, Lerner SA. Auxotypes, penicillin susceptibility, and serogroups of Neisseria gonorrhoeae from disseminated and uncomplicated infections. J Infect Dis 1986;154:225.
102. Janda WM, Jackson T. Evaluation of Gonodecten for the presumptive diagnosis of gonococcal urethritis in men. J Clin Microbiol 1985;21:143.
103. Juchau SV, Nackman R, Ruppart D. Comparison of Gram stain with DNA probe for detection of *Neisseria gonorrhoeae* in urethras of symptomatic males. J Clin Microbiol 1995;33:3068.
104. Luciano AA, Grubin L. Gonorrhea screening. Comparison of three techniques. JAMA 1980;243:680.
105. Stamm WE, Cole B, Fennell C, et al. Antigen detection for the diagnosis of gonorrhea. J Clin Microbiol 1984;19:399.
106. Koumans EH, Johnson RE, Knapp JS, et al. Laboratory testing for *Neisseria gonorrhoeae* by recently introduced nonculture tests: a performance review with clinical and public health considerations. Clin Infect Dis 1998;27:1171.
107. Carroll KC, Aldeen WE, Morrison M, et al. Evaluation of the Abbott LCx ligase chain reaction assay for detection of *Chlamydia trachomatis* and *Neisseria gonorrhoeae* in urine and genital swab specimens from a sexually transmitted disease clinic population. J Clin Microbiol 1998;36:1630.
108. Hook EW, III, Ching SF, Stephens J, et al. Diagnosis of *Neisseria gonorrhoeae* infections in women by using the ligase chain reaction on patient-obtained vaginal swabs. J Clin Microbiol 1997;35:2129.
109. Centers for Disease Control and Prevention. Increases in Fluoroquinolone-resistant *Neisseria gonorrhoeae* among men who have sex with men—United States, 2003, and revised recommendations for gonorrhea treatment, 2004. Morb Mortal Wkly Rep 2004;53:335.
110. Gaydos CA, Howell MR, Pare B, et al. *Chlamydia trachomatis* infections in female military recruits. N Engl J Med 1998;339:739.
111. Hughes G, Catchpole M, Rogers PA, et al. Comparison of risk factors for four sexually transmitted infections: results from a study of attenders at three genitourinary medicine clinics in England. Sex Transm Infect 2000;76:262.
112. Klausner JD, McFarland W, Bolan G, et al. Knock-knock: a population-based survey of risk behavior, health care access, and *Chlamydia trachomatis* infection among low-income women in the San Francisco Bay area. J Infect Dis 2001;183:1087.
113. Hart G. Factors associated with genital chlamydial and gonococcal infection in males. Genitourin Med 1993;69:393.
114. Magder LS, Harrison HR, Ehret JM, et al. Factors related to genital *Chlamydia trachomatis* and its diagnosis by culture in a sexually transmitted disease clinic. Am J Epidemiol 1988;128:298.
115. Stamm WE, Koutsky LA, Benedetti JK, et al. *Chlamydia trachomatis* urethral infections in men. Prevalence, risk factors, and clinical manifestations. Ann Intern Med 1984;100:47.
116. Laga M, Manoka A, Kivuvu M, et al. Non-ulcerative sexually transmitted diseases as risk factors for HIV-1 transmission in women: results from a cohort study [see comments]. AIDS 1993;7:95.
117. Ghys PD, Fransen K, Diallo MO, et al. The associations between cervicovaginal HIV shedding, sexually transmitted diseases and immunosuppression in female sex workers in Abidjan, Cote d'Ivoire. AIDS 1997;111:F85.
118. Mostad SB, Overbaugh J, DeVange DM, et al. Hormonal contraception, vitamin A deficiency, and other risk factors for shedding of HIV-1 infected cells from the cervix and vagina. Lancet 1997;350:922.
119. Cates W, Jr. , Wasserheit JN. Genital chlamydial infections: epidemiology and reproductive sequelae. Am J Obstet Gynecol 1991;164(6 Pt 2): 1771.
120. Svensson L, Westrom L, Ripa KT, et al. Differences in some clinical and laboratory parameters in acute salpingitis related to culture and serologic findings. Am J Obstet Gynecol 1980;138(7 Pt 2):1017.
121. Nilsen A, Halsos A, Johansen A, et al. A double blind study of single dose azithromycin and doxycycline in the treatment of chlamydial urethritis in males. Genitourin Med 1992;68: 325.
122. Jacobson GF, Autry AM, Kirby RS, et al. A randomized controlled trial comparing amoxicillin and azithromycin for the treatment of *Chlamydia trachomatis* in pregnancy. Am J Obstet Gynecol 2001;184:1352.
123. Kacmar J, Cheh E, Montagno A, et al. A randomized trial of azithromycin versus amoxicillin for the treatment of *Chlamydia trachomatis* in pregnancy. Infect Dis Obstet Gynecol 2001;9:197.
124. Aral SO, Holmes KK. Social and behavioral determinants of the epidemiology of STDs: industrialized and developing countries. In: Holmes KK, Sparling PF, Mardh P-A, et al., eds. Sexually transmitted diseases. 3rd ed. New York: McGraw-Hill,1999;39–76.
125. Burstein GR, Zenilman JM. Nongonococcal urethritis—a new paradigm. Clin Infect Dis 1999;28 Suppl 1:S66.
126. Dixon L, Pearson S, Clutterbuck DJ. Chlamydia trachomatis infection and non-gonococcal urethritis in homosexual and heterosexual men in Edinburgh. Int J STD AIDS 2002;13:425.

127. Dupin N, Bijaoui G, Schwarzinger M, et al. Detection and quantification of Mycoplasma genitalium in male patients with urethritis. Clin Infect Dis 2003;37:602.
128. Falk L, Fredlund H, Jensen JS. Symptomatic urethritis is more prevalent in men infected with *Mycoplasma genitalium* than with *Chlamydia trachomatis*. Sex Transm Infect 2004;80:289.
129. Horner P, Thomas B, Gilroy CB, et al. Role of *Mycoplasma genitalium* and *Ureaplasma urealyticum* in acute and chronic nongonococcal Urethritis. Clin Infect Dis 2001;32:995.
130. McKee KT, Jr. , Jenkins PR, Garner R, et al. Features of urethritis in a cohort of male soldiers. Clin Infect Dis 2000;30:736.
131. Bjornelius E, Lidbrink P, Jensen JS. Mycoplasma genitalium in non-gonococcal urethritis—a study in Swedish male STD patients. Int J STD AIDS 2000;11:292.
132. Mena L, Wang X, Mroczkowski TF, et al. Mycoplasma genitalium infections in asymptomatic men and men with urethritis attending a sexually transmitted diseases clinic in New Orleans. Clin Infect Dis 2002;35:1167.
133. Morency P, Dubois MJ, Gresenguet G, et al. Aetiology of urethral discharge in Bangui, Central African Republic. Sex Transm Infect 2001;77:125.
134. Schwebke JR, Hook EW, III. High rates of *Trichomonas vaginalis* among men attending a sexually transmitted diseases clinic: implications for screening and urethritis management. J Infect Dis 2003;188:465.
135. Leung A, Taylor S, Smith A, et al. Urinary tract infection in patients with acute non-gonococcal urethritis. Int J STD AIDS 2002;13:801.
136. Janier M, Lassau F, Casin I, et al. Male urethritis with and without discharge: a clinical and microbiological study. Sex Transm Dis 1995;22:244.
137. Stamm WE, Hicks CB, Martin DH, et al. Azithromycin for empirical treatment of the nongonococcal urethritis syndrome in men. A randomized double-blind study. JAMA 1995;274:545.
138. Stimson JB, Hale J, Bowie WR, et al. Tetracycline-resistant *Ureaplasma urealyticum*: a cause of persistent nongonococcal urethritis. Ann Intern Med 1981;94:192.
139. Gaydos CA, Crotchfelt KA, Howell MR, et al. Molecular amplification assays to detect chlamydial infections in urine specimens from high school female students and to monitor the persistence of chlamydial DNA after therapy. J Infect Dis 1998;177:417.
140. Berger RE, Alexander ER, Harnisch JP, et al. Etiology, manifestations and therapy of acute epididymitis: prospective study of 50 cases. J Urol 1979;121:750.
141. Grant JB, Costello CB, Sequeira PJ, et al. The role of *Chlamydia trachomatis* in epididymitis. Br J Urol 1987;60:355.
142. Berger RE, Kessler D, Holmes KK. Etiology and manifestations of epididymitis in young men: correlations with sexual orientation. J Infect Dis 1987;155:1341.
143. Burgher SW. Acute scrotal pain. Emerg Med Clin North Am 1998;16:781, vi.
144. Lewis AG, Bukowski TP, Jarvis PD, et al. Evaluation of acute scrotum in the emergency department. J Pediatr Surg 1995;30:277.
145. Knight PJ, Vassy LE. The diagnosis and treatment of the acute scrotum in children and adolescents. Ann Surg 1984;200:664.
146. Melekos MD, Asbach HW, Markou SA. Etiology of acute scrotum in 100 boys with regard to age distribution. J Urol 1988;139:1023.
147. Stillwell TJ, Kramer SA. Intermittent testicular torsion. Pediatrics 1986;77:908.
148. St Louis ME, Wasserheit JN. Elimination of syphilis in the United States. Science 1998;281:353.
149. Nakashima AK, Rolfs RT, Flock ML, et al. Epidemiology of syphilis in the United States, 1941–1993. Sex Transm Dis 1996;23:16.
150. Gunn RA, Montes JM, Toomey KE, et al. Syphilis in San Diego County 1983–1992: crack cocaine, prostitution, and the limitations of partner notification. Sex Transm Dis 1995; 22:60.
151. Rolfs RT, Goldberg M, Sharrar RG. Risk factors for syphilis: cocaine use and prostitution. Am J Public Health 1990;80:853.
152. Singh AE, Romanowski B. Syphilis: review with emphasis on clinical, epidemiologic, and some biologic features. Clin Microbiol Rev 1999;12:187.
153. Mindel A, Tovey SJ, Timmins DJ, Williams P. Primary and secondary syphilis, 20 years' experience. 2. Clinical features. Genitourin Med 1989;65:1.
154. Gjestland T. The Oslo Study of untreated syphilis: an epdiemiologic investigation of the natural course of syphilis infection based upon a restudy of the Boeck-Bruusgaard material. Acta Derm.Venereol 1955;35[Suppl. 34]:1.
155. Burch GE, Winsor T. Syphilitic coronary stenosis, with mycoardial infarction. Am Heart J 1942;24:740.
156. Marra CM, Maxwell CL, Smith SL, et al. Cerebrospinal fluid abnormalities in patients with syphilis: association with clinical and laboratory features. J Infect Dis 2004;189:369.
157. Rolfs RT, Joesoef MR, Hendershot EF, et al. A randomized trial of enhanced therapy for early syphilis in patients with and without human immunodeficiency virus infection. The Syphilis and HIV Study Group. N Engl J Med 1997;337:307.
158. Merritt HH. The early clinical and laboratory manifestations of syphilis of the central nervous system. N Engl J Med 1940;223:446.
159. Wendel GD. Gestational and congenital syphilis. Clin Perinatol 1988;15:287.
160. Sparling PF. Diagnosis and treatment of syphilis. N Engl J Med 1971;284:642.
161. Erbelding EJ, Vlahov D, Nelson KE, et al. Syphilis serology in human immunodeficiency virus infection: evidence for false-negative fluorescent treponemal testing. J Infect Dis 1997;176:1397.
162. Dicker LW, Mosure DJ, Steece R, Stone KM. Laboratory tests used in US public health laboratories for sexually transmitted diseases, 2000. Sex Transm Dis 2004;31:259.
163. Dans PE, Cafferty L, Otter SE, Johnson RJ. Inappropriate use of the cerebrospinal fluid Venereal Disease Research Laboratory (VDRL) test to exclude neurosyphilis. Ann Intern Med 1986;104:86.
164. Hook EW, III, Marra CM. Acquired syphilis in adults. N Engl J Med 1992;326:1060.
165. Jaffe HW, Larsen SA, Peters M, et al. Tests for treponemal antibody in CSF. Arch Intern Med 1978;138:252.
166. Centers for Disease Control and Prevention. Inadvertent use of Bicillin C-R to treat syphilis infection—Los Angeles, California, 1999–2004. Morb Mortal Wkly Rep 2005;54:217.
167. Hook EW, Martin DH, Stephens J, et al. A randomized, comparative pilot study of azithromycin versus benzathine penicillin G for treatment of early syphilis. Sex Transm Dis 2002;29:486.
168. Lukehart SA, Godornes C, Molini BJ, et al. Macrolide resistance in *Treponema pallidum* in the United States and Ireland. N Engl J Med 2004;351:154.
169. Schroeter AL, Lucas JB, Price EV, et al. Treatment for early syphilis and reactivity of serologic tests. JAMA 1972;221:471.
170. Smith NH, Musher DM, Huang DB, et al. Response of HIV-infected patients with asymptomatic syphilis to intensive intramuscular therapy with ceftriaxone or procaine penicillin. Int J STD AIDS 2004;15:328.
171. Fiumara NJ. Serologic responses to treatment of 128 patients with late latent syphilis. Sex Transm Dis 1979;6:243.
172. Marra CM, Boutin P, McArthur JC, et al. A pilot study evaluating ceftriaxone and penicillin G as treatment agents for neurosyphilis in human immunodeficiency virus-infected individuals. Clin Infect Dis 2000;30:540.
173. Rompalo AM, Joesoef MR, O'Donnell JA, et al. Clinical manifestations of early syphilis by HIV status and gender: results of the syphilis and HIV study. Sex Transm Dis 2001;28:158.
174. Berry CD, Hooton TM, Collier AC, et al. Neurologic relapse after benzathine penicillin therapy for secondary syphilis in a patient with HIV infection. N Engl J Med 1987;316:1587.
175. Myles TD, Elam G, Park-Hwang E, et al. The Jarisch-Herxheimer reaction and fetal monitoring changes in pregnant women treated for syphilis. Obstet Gynecol 1998;92:859.

For annotated **General References** *and resources related to this chapter, visit www.hopkinsbayview.org/PAMreferences.*

Chapter 38

Lyme Disease and Other Tick-Borne Illnesses

Paul G. Auwaerter and John A. Flynn

Lyme disease is the most common tick-borne illness in the United States. Although it rarely causes mortality, it can have morbid complications and generates concern among patients. Other arthropod-borne illnesses such as Rocky Mountain spotted fever (RMSF) and ehrlichiosis, although less common than Lyme disease, are among the diseases requiring prompt recognition, because death can occur without proper treatment. The number of recognized tick-borne human diseases other than Lyme disease continues to expand in the United States (Table 38.1).

LYME DISEASE

Epidemiology

Since the original clinical description in 1977 of infection by the spirochete *Borrelia burgdorferi,* Lyme disease has become the most common arthropod-borne illness in the United States (1). It is endemic in more than 15 states and is responsible for an increasing number of cases primarily in Eastern coastal areas and the upper Midwest (Fig. 38.1) (2). This spirochete was originally isolated from the *Ixodes scapularis* tick in the northeastern United States (3). Subsequently, other *Ixodes* species were found to carry this infection in California (*I. pacificus)* and throughout Europe (*I. ricinus*) and Asia (*I. persulcatus*). In addition to the transmitting tick vector, other animal reservoirs are involved in the tick life cycle maintaining *Borrelia* infection. In the United States, the white-footed mouse and the white-tailed deer are the preferred hosts for this very small tick, also known as the black-legged deer tick, which is no larger than 2 by 3 mm in its adult form. Ticks become infected through horizontal transmission among these reservoirs. In endemic areas, up to 50% of ticks may be infected (4). Despite the high carriage rate in ticks, the probability of acquiring Lyme disease from a single tick bite is at most 3.5% in highly endemic areas (5). The disease incidence is greatest in the mid-spring through late fall. This correlates with periods of increased tick populations, especially biting nymphs (less than 2 mm), as well as increased outdoor activities of people in endemic areas. Effective transmission to humans appears to require at least 36 to 48 hours of tick attachment.

Surveillance of this nationally notifiable disease has been conducted by the Centers for Disease Control and Prevention (CDC) since 1982. The following clinical case definition for this surveillance has been established and is discussed later in this chapter:

- Erythema migrans (see below) of 5 cm (2 inches) or greater, or
- At least one late manifestation of neurologic, cardiovascular, or musculoskeletal disease (see below), and laboratory confirmation of infection with *B. burgdorferi*.

The highest number of cases in the United States is reported in the northeastern and mid-Atlantic regions. Endemic pockets also exist in northern California and in regions of Minnesota and Wisconsin. Cases of Lyme disease have been reported in 49 states and the District of Columbia; Connecticut, Rhode Island, New York, and Pennsylvania have reported the highest rates (1). There is no gender predilection, although persons 5 to 19 years of age and 30 years or older appear to have the highest risk of infection. Significant outdoor exposure (e.g., hiking, gardening) in endemic regions increases risk, although cases have occurred without a history of much outdoor activity. In those cases for which the month of illness was identified, June and July were reported most frequently.

Clinical Manifestations and Stages

Patients may develop erythema migrans (EM) and then have no further symptoms even in the absence of antibiotic therapy. Others may present with one of the later manifestations of the infection without any history of EM. Lyme disease is divided into three stages based on its clinical manifestations: 1) early localized disease; 2) early disseminated disease; and, 3) late disease. Approximately 70% to

TABLE 38.1 North American Tick-Borne Infections and Common Characteristics

Disease	*Pathogen*	*Vector*	*Likely U.S. Geography*	*Clinical Hallmarks*
Lyme Disease	*B. burgdorferi*	*I. scapularis* (deer tick) *I. pacificus*	Northeastern, mid-Atlantic, upper Midwest, Pacific coast	Erythema migrans, facial palsy, meningitis, carditis, arthritis
RMSF	*R. rickettsii*	*D. variabilis* (dog tick) *D. andersoni* (wood tick)	Southern, mid-Atlantic	Fever, headache, rash with evolving petechiae
HME	*E. chaffeensis*	*A. americanum* (Lone Star tick)	New York to Texas	Fever, headache, myalgia, leukopenia, thrombocytopenia
HGA	*Anaplasma phagocytophilum*	*I. scapularis* *I. pacificus*	Same as Lyme disease	Fever, headache, myalgia, leukopenia, thrombocytopenia
Relapsing fever	*B. hermsii B. duttonii* and others	*Ornithodoros species* (soft ticks)	Southwest and west, mountainous regions	Intermittent fever, headache, petechial rash
Tularemia	*F. tularensis*	Many hard ticks	South-central	Ulcer, lymphadenitis
Babesiosis	*B. microti*	*I. scapularis*	Same as Lyme disease, especially costal islands	Fever, anemia, malarial-like illness
Colorado tick fever	*Coltivirus*	*D. andersoni*	Rocky Mountains, west	Intermittent fever, headache, myalgia, leukopenia

A, Amblyomma; B, Borrelia; D, Dermacentor; E, Ehrlichia; F, Francisella; HME, human monocytic ehrlichiosis; HGA, human granulocytic anaplasmosis; I, Ixodes; R, Rickettsia; RMSF, Rocky Mountain Spotted Fever.

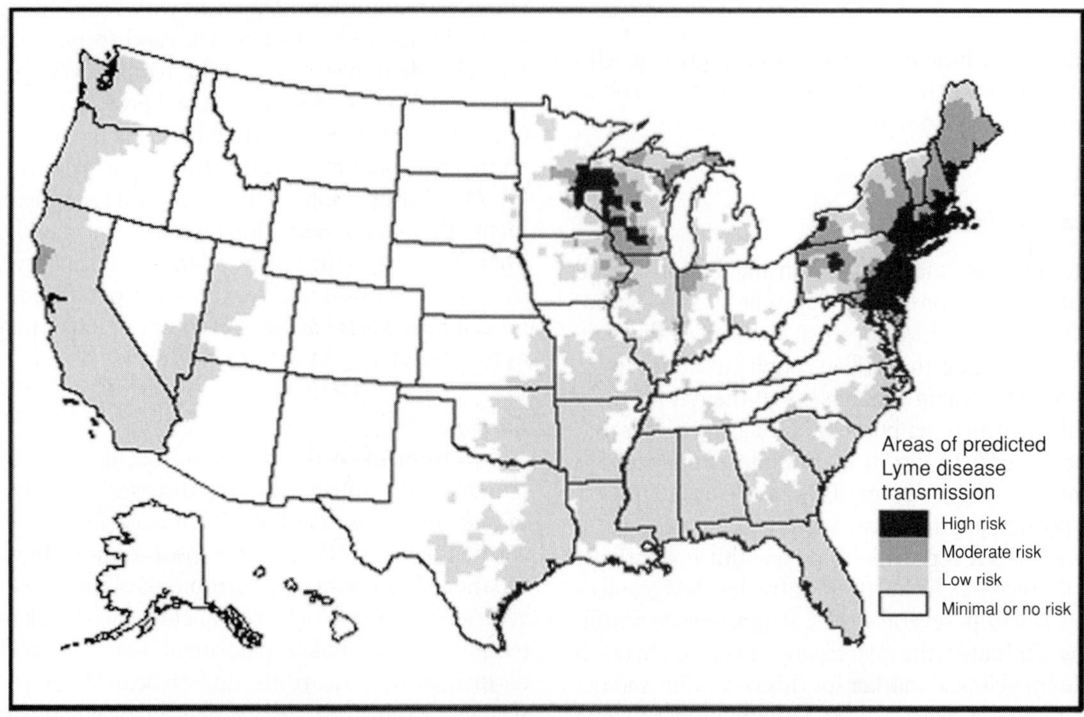

FIGURE 38.1. National Lyme Disease Risk Map. This map demonstrates an approximate distribution of predicted Lyme disease risk in the United States. The true relative risk in any given county compared with other counties might differ from that shown here and might change from year to year. Available at: http://www.cdc.gov/ncidod/dvbid/lyme/riskmap.htm.).

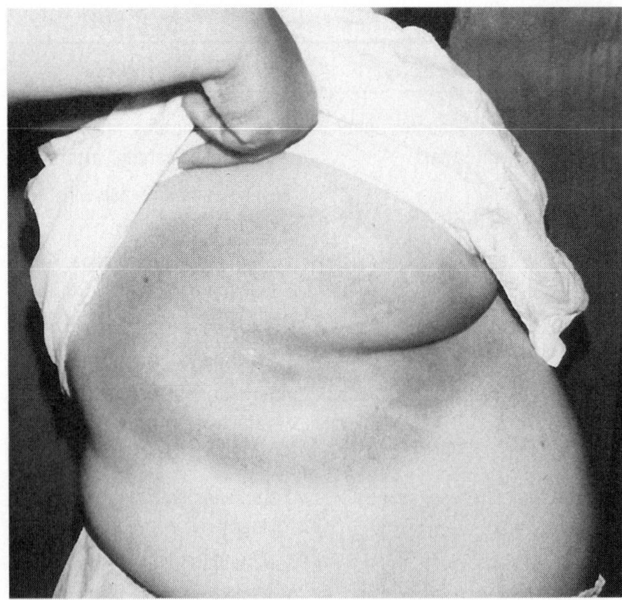

FIGURE 38.2. (See also Color Plate.) Classic erythema migrans rash of early Lyme disease with bright red border and partial central clearing, the so-called "bull's-eye" rash. (Photograph courtesy of Paul Auwaerter, MD)

85% of patients with definite Lyme disease present with early localized disease. In most patients, there is no characteristic progression from one stage to the next.

Early Localized Disease

After a bite from an infected tick, an incubation period of several days to 1 month may elapse before the pathognomonic skin lesion, EM, forms at the site of the bite. Common sites include the axillae, popliteal area, groin, and waistline. This lesion starts as an erythematous macule or papule with an outer border and clearing center that can expand beyond 15 cm in a circumferential manner over several days (Fig. 38.2; see also Color Plate). The border is sharply demarcated, warm to touch, nontender, although sometimes it is pruritic. Only one third of patients are aware of a recent tick bite. If left untreated, EM resolves spontaneously within several weeks. If appropriate antibiotic therapy is initiated, the rash resolves in days. This rash is the single best clinical marker for this condition and occurs in up to 90% of cases (6). Most patients have some nonspecific constitutional symptoms, such as myalgia, fatigue, arthralgia, or headache. Twenty percent of patients have no manifestation other than the rash. Though often described as a "bull's-eye" rash because of central clearing, this feature is frequently not present. In one study of culture-proven Lyme disease less than 40% of rashes had central clearing, and a homogenous or central redness pattern was more common (7).

Early Disseminated Disease

Early localized Lyme disease often progresses to hematogenous dissemination within the first month. During summertime, flu-like illnesses with headache, myalgia, arthralgia, and fever, without EM rash, may also represent Lyme disease. End-organ effects develop within several weeks or up to 1 year after the primary infection in untreated patients. Unusual manifestations include optic neuritis, hepatitis, myositis, and pneumonitis. The section as listed below describes the more common manifestations.

Dermatologic

Multiple secondary annular lesions develop in half of untreated patients because of hematogenous spread (11). These disseminated erythema migrans lesions are smaller than the initial lesion and resolve with appropriate antibiotic therapy.

Neurologic

Ten to fifteen percent of untreated patients develop neurologic involvement including meningitis, cranial neuropathy, or radiculoneuropathy, within 4 to 8 weeks after resolution of EM (8). Patients with meningitis, the most common manifestation, present with fever, meningismus, photophobia, and headache. The cerebrospinal fluid (CSF) typically demonstrates a mild lymphocytic pleocytosis (100 to 500 cells), and an increased protein level. A peripheral seventh nerve palsy (Bell palsy) is the most common cranial neuropathy; it is bilateral in up to a quarter of cases (9). Most cases resolve within 1 month regardless of treatment. Peripheral radiculoneuropathies occur less often. They may involve one or more motor or sensory nerves of the thorax or limbs in an asymmetric pattern, mimicking, for example, spinal nerve root compression or manifesting as focal weakness in the involved areas.

Cardiac

Involvement of the heart can occur in up to 10% of patients with untreated Lyme disease, typically within 3 months of developing EM. The precise incidence of Lyme carditis is unclear because the most common finding when a patient has carditis is asymptomatic first-degree atrioventricular (AV) block. Complete heart block requiring temporary pacemaker placement may occur (10). Cardiomyopathy, pericarditis, and myocarditis have been described but are rare. All cardiac involvement usually resolves within 8 weeks, and complete heart block usually recedes with antimicrobial treatment, making permanent pacemaker placement unnecessary.

Musculoskeletal

Roughly half of untreated patients develop migratory arthralgias, myalgias, tendonitis, bursitis, or bone pain. A self-limited monoarticular or oligoarticular arthritis may develop, primarily in the large joints, most often the knee. Polyarthritis is distinctly unusual. Large synovial effusions contain inflammatory fluid (5,000 to 20,000 white blood cells [WBCs] per cubic millimeter) with neutrophilic predominance.

Late Manifestations

The late manifestations of Lyme disease occur many months to years after the initial infection.

Musculoskeletal

A migratory oligoarthritis develops in up to 60% of patients with untreated disease (12). Recurrent attacks of oligoarthritis chiefly affect weight-bearing joints, most commonly the knee, and persist for weeks to months before resolving. Synovial effusions may be large and inflammatory (up to 100,000 WBCs per cubic millimeter). Even in untreated patients, the arthritis usually improves. A minority of patients go on to develop a chronic arthritis, despite extensive antibiotic therapy and apparent eradication of all spirochetes. In these unresponsive cases, certain human leukocyte antigen (HLA) haplotypes (DR4 and DR2) have been linked to a robust antibody response to outer surface proteins of the spirochete (OspA and OspB), suggesting a perpetuating immune reaction rather than persistence of *Borrelia* spirochetes (13,14).

Neurologic

The most common neurologic manifestation of late Lyme disease is a chronic encephalopathy that occurs years after the initial infection (15). Patients experience memory impairment and mood changes. Additionally, a polyradiculopathy with paresthesia or radicular pain of the extremities may develop with or without encephalopathy. Motor involvement is unusual. Partial improvement may occur in half of those patients who are treated with antibiotics, but the natural history tends toward a chronic progressive course. All forms of chronic neurologic Lyme disease are believed to be uncommon, occurring in fewer than 5% of people with untreated Lyme disease.

Dermatologic

A peculiar cutaneous affliction, *acrodermatitis chronica atrophicans,* is primarily seen in untreated patients in Europe (16). This red to blue nodular plaque develops mostly on the dorsal aspect of the hand, elbow, and extensor surface of the foot and ankle. Over time, the involved skin becomes atrophic or sclerotic. *B. burgdorferi* has been cultured from these lesions.

Diagnosis

The diagnosis of Lyme disease should be based primarily on the presence of characteristic clinical findings, exposure to an endemic area, and response to appropriate antibiotic therapy (17). The clinical presentation of EM is so distinctive that any patient presenting with this rash requires treatment for early Lyme disease with no specific laboratory testing required. In patients with other associated findings (e.g., facial nerve palsy, complete heart block) and no history of EM, serologic testing should be performed if the likelihood of exposure is significant.

With the exception of skin samples from lesions and blood in patients with EM, it is difficult to culture *B. burgdorferi* from any site (4,18). Because this technique is difficult and the skin lesion is pathognomonic, attempts at culturing the organism are limited to research settings.

Routinely available diagnostic testing determines whether there has been an immune response to the spirochete, using an enzyme-linked immunosorbent assay (ELISA) to detect immunoglobulin (Ig)M and IgG antibodies to *B. burgdorferi.* In patients infected with Lyme disease it can take several weeks before detection of an IgM response. This may be completely abrogated with early antibiotic treatment of EM. Once positive, the IgM response can remain present for longer than a year. Although it helps to confirm exposure, it does not establish active infection. After 4 to 8 weeks, the IgG antibody response should develop in untreated patients. False positive results have been noted in a number of situations, including viral infections, rheumatoid arthritis, and other autoimmune diseases as well as in healthy people living in endemic areas (4). In the absence of appropriate clinical and environmental findings, these laboratory studies do not have sufficient sensitivity or specificity to establish or exclude the diagnosis of Lyme disease (19).

Although criteria have been established for the interpretation of Western blot studies of Lyme disease–related antibodies, there is still difficulty with standardization and reliability of this testing (20). The CDC recommends a two-step Lyme diagnostic test strategy in which positive or equivocal ELISA studies are confirmed by Western blot testing for Lyme-specific IgM and IgG bands. These tests are available routinely. The IgM Western blot is often falsely positive and therefore should be obtained only in patients with symptoms of less than 1 month's duration. In these cases, the test is considered positive if two of three Lyme-specific bands are present. The IgG Western blot requires that at least 5 of 10 specific bands be present. Polymerase chain reaction (PCR) testing has detected *B. burgdorferi* deoxyribonucleic acid (DNA) in blood, synovial fluid, spinal fluid, and skin specimens (21). DNA detection with PCR for *B. burgdorferi* continues to be fraught with technical difficulties, risk of contamination, poor sensitivity, and lack of standardization that has prevented wide clinical use (16). Its main role may be in confirming active Lyme infection in synovial fluid.

The CDC has issued a recent warning regarding certain commercial laboratories that present themselves as Lyme specialty centers (22). These labs use assays for which accuracy and clinical utility have not been adequately established, including urine antigen tests, immunofluorescent staining of blood for *B. burgdorferi*, and lymphocyte transformation tests. These laboratories may also use inappropriate specimens such as blood or urine for *B. burgdorferi* DNA PCR tests or interpret Western blots using unvalidated criteria. If unsure, healthcare providers and patients are urged to should ask whether the laboratory offers validated, Food and Drug Administration (FDA)-approved Lyme testing.

Occasionally patients suffering from *B. burgdorferi* may be coinfected with other tick-borne pathogens such as *Ehrlichia* or *Babesia* species. This is an uncommon situation that appears to represent no more than 2% of Lyme disease cases even in highly endemic areas (23).

Treatment

Lyme disease in all stages should respond with clinical improvement to appropriate antibiotic therapy. Recognition and treatment of early Lyme disease prevents development of later manifestations. A Jarisch–Herxheimer reaction with spiking fever, rigor, and rarely hypotension occurs in some patients within several hours after treatment. It peaks in approximately 12 hours and then resolves over 1 to 2 days, and is treated with supportive care.

Early Manifestations

EM can be treated successfully with oral doxycycline in adults, or amoxicillin in pregnant or lactating women (Table 38.2). For people who are allergic to these medications, oral cefuroxime is an effective alternative (24). Although azithromycin has been studied, it is less effective than amoxicillin against EM (25). Most cases of EM resolve within days after initiation of therapy. Although the optimal duration of antibiotic therapy has not been established conclusively, one study suggested that 10 days of doxycycline is sufficient for the treatment of EM (26). A reasonable approach at this time is to treat for 10 to 14 days with doxycycline or 14 to 21 days with amoxicillin (27).

Patients with isolated facial palsy, minor cardiac abnormalities (e.g., first-degree AV block), or disseminated annular lesions at the time of diagnosis should be treated with a 21- to 28-day oral regimen (27). Patient with complete AV block, meningitis, or other early neuroborreliosis syndromes should receive intravenous ceftriaxone therapy for 14 to 28 days (28). Some practitioners use parenteral therapy until acute symptoms have resolved (e.g., in cases of cardiac conduction abnormalities) and then complete the course of antibiotics with oral therapy. Parenteral penicillin is equally efficacious, although ceftriaxone is used more frequently because of dosing simplicity. Patients with significant cardiac involvement may require monitoring and a temporary pacemaker.

TABLE 38.2 Antibiotic Therapy for Lyme Disease[a,b]

Drug	*Dosage and Frequency*	*Duration (days)*
Oral therapy for localized disease (erythema migrans)		
Doxycycline	100 mg b.i.d.	10–14
Amoxicillin	500 mg t.i.d.	14–21
-OR-		
Cefuroxime	500 mg b.i.d.	14–21
Pregnant or lactating women		
Amoxicillin	500 mg t.i.d.	14–21
Oral therapy for early disseminated disease (first-degree atrioventricular block, facial palsy, disseminated annular lesions)		
Doxycycline	100 mg b.i.d.	21–28
-OR-		
Amoxicillin	500 mg t.i.d.	21–28
Intravenous therapy for early disseminated disease (complete atrioventricular block, meningitis, neuritis)		
Ceftriaxone	2 g q.d.	14–28 (some switch to oral therapy with clinical improvement)
-OR-		
Cefotaxime	2 g q8h	
Oral therapy for late disease (arthritis)		
Doxycycline	100 mg b.i.d.	28
-OR-		
Amoxicillin	500 mg q.i.d.	28
Intravenous therapy for late disease (persistent arthritis, late neurologic disease)		
Ceftriaxone	2 g q.d.	14–28
-OR-		
Cefotaxime	2 g q8h	14–28
Penicillin G	18–24 mU IV q.d.	14–28

[a] Preferred choices are listed first, followed (after "-OR-") by alternative choices.
[b] From Wormser GP, Nadelman RB, Dattwyler RJ, et al. IDSA practice guidelines for the treatment of Lyme disease; Clin Infect Dis 2000;31;Suppl 1:1; Wormer GP, Ramanathan R, Nowakowski J, et al. Duration of antibiotic therapy for early Lyme disease. A randomized, double-blind, placebo-controlled trial. Ann Intern Med 2003;138:697.

Late Manifestations

Late manifestations of Lyme disease require longer courses of antibiotics (Table 38.2). Lyme arthritis should be treated with a 28-day course of oral antibiotics. If the patient does not respond, a 14- to 28-day course of intravenous ceftriaxone should be given (29). A small percentage of patients develop a postinfectious immune response with persistent arthritis despite extensive antibiotics (see Late Manifestations, Musculoskeletal). Patients with late neurologic manifestations should be treated with a 28-day course of intravenous ceftriaxone (28). Prolonged treatment with antibiotics, beyond this, is no more effective than placebo in improving persistent symptoms in patients with a

Chapter 39

Human Immunodeficiency Virus Infection

Darius A. Rastegar and Michael I. Fingerhood

In the decades since the onset of the human immunodeficiency virus (HIV) epidemic, the prognosis for patients in the United States has greatly improved (1). Highly active antiretroviral treatment (HAART) and prophylaxis for opportunistic infections have significantly lowered the mortality from acquired immunodeficiency syndrome (AIDS) and have improved the lives of many. These changes have made the care of HIV-infected patient more rewarding yet more complex.

The role of primary care practitioners in caring for HIV-infected individuals is controversial. Some studies have found poorer patient survival and lower adherence with guidelines among physicians who care for small numbers of patients. However, it appears that the care provided by experienced generalists is comparable to that provided by specialists (2). Most would agree that ongoing experience with the care of HIV-infected patients is important and that a physician with only a few HIV-infected patients should consider referring these patients to an expert.

Primary care practitioners certainly do play an important role in identifying those who are infected and counseling those at risk of becoming infected. This chapter reviews the issues involved in the ambulatory care of HIV-infected patients. It does cover all of the details of antiretroviral therapy and HIV-related complications; other resources for obtaining more extensive and updated information are listed at www.hopkinsbayview.org/PAMreferences.

GENERAL CONSIDERATIONS

Causes

HIV is a member of the *lentivirus subfamily of human retroviruses* and was found to be the etiologic agent of AIDS in 1983. These viruses code for an enzyme known as reverse transcriptase, which permits transcription of viral ribonucleic acid (RNA) into proviral deoxyribonucleic acid (DNA) and subsequent integration into the host's cellular genome, leading to a persistent and latent infection. The retroviruses are associated with diseases of long incubation period, involvement with the hematopoietic and central nervous systems, and immune suppression. Other related human retroviruses include HIV-2 and the human T-cell lymphotropic viruses (HTLV-I, and HTLV-II). HIV-2, found primarily in West Africa, has also been associated with AIDS but has a more prolonged incubation period (3). HTLV-1 has been associated with tropical spastic paraparesis and T-cell leukemia/lymphoma, and HTLV-II has not yet been associated definitively with any human disease (4).

TABLE 39.1 Estimated Per-Act Risk of Acquiring HIV, by Exposure*

	Risk per 10,000 Exposures to an HIV-Infected Source
EXPOSURE route	
Blood transfusion	9,000
Needle sharing (injection drug use)	67
Receptive anal intercourse	50
Percutaneous needle stick	30
Receptive penile-vaginal intercourse	10
Insertive anal intercourse	6.5
Insertive penile-vaginal intercourse	5
Receptive oral intercourse	1
Insertive oral intercourse	0.5

*Estimates for sexual transmission assume no condom use.
Source: Centers for Disease Control and Prevention. MMWR 2005;54:7.

Epidemiology

The Centers for Disease Control and Prevention (CDC) estimates that over 1 million Americans are infected with HIV, and 25% of them do not know that they are infected. (5) Worldwide, over 39 million people are HIV infected (6). Most HIV infections occur in adults who belong to the major risk groups for HIV transmission: men who have sex with men (MSM), heterosexual partners of infected persons, injection drug users, and infants of infected women.

Transmission and Prevention of Transmission

Primary care practitioners play an important role in counseling patients at risk of acquiring HIV. However, doing so requires actually evaluating a patient's risk of infection. This involves questions about an individual's sexual practices and drug use; topics that physicians (and patients) are often uncomfortable discussing (7). Primary care practitioners should ask all their patients about their sexual practices, as well as drug and alcohol use, in an open and nonjudgmental fashion, and educate them about the risks they may be taking. Table 39.1 provides estimates of transmission risk associated with different exposures.

HIV-1 occurs in highest concentrations in blood and semen. It also occurs in lower concentrations in cervical and vaginal secretions, saliva, tears, breast milk, and amniotic fluid. HIV transmission is most commonly through blood and semen, but vaginal secretions and breast milk also have been implicated in the transmission process.

Sexual Transmission

HIV infection can be transmitted during sexual intercourse between men and between men and women. The risk of transmission varies depending on a number of factors, including the type of sexual practice, the HIV viral RNA level of the infected person, and likely other factors (yet to be determined) in the immune system of the uninfected person.

The following patterns, practices, and situations carry the greatest risk of infection:

- Unprotected receptive anal intercourse, especially if the mucosal lining has been torn, which may happen with penile insertion itself but is more likely to happen with such sexual practices as fisting. The estimated per-episode risk with anal receptive intercourse is about 0.5%.
- Unprotected vaginal intercourse—the estimated per-episode risk is 0.1% for receptive penile-vaginal intercourse and 0.05% for the insertive partner.
- Unprotected vaginal or rectal intercourse when either partner has genital ulceration (e.g., due to primary syphilis, chancroid, or genital herpes). Genital ulcers can act as conduits for infected blood from, or for infected semen, blood, or vaginal secretions into, the person with the ulcer.

The *prevention of sexual transmission of HIV* requires that sexually active people choose sexual practices that eliminate the high-risk situations listed above, as well as other lower risk practices, including oral–genital contact. In the care of every patient who is sexually active and in public education messages, the fundamentals of safe, possibly safe, and definitely unsafe sex should be clearly communicated (Table 39.2). Specific instructions for the most effective use of condoms (Table 39.3) are particularly important. Postexposure prophylaxis with antiretroviral medication after sexual contact with someone who is infected (similar to postoccupational exposure prophylaxis; see Occupational Exposure, below) may be considered in certain situations (8).

TABLE 39.2 Safe Sex Guidelines

Safe sex practices
Massage
Hugging
Mutual masturbation
Social kissing (dry)
Body-to-body rubbing
Voyeurism, exhibitionism, fantasy
Possibly safe sex practices
French kissing (wet)
Anal intercourse with condom[a]
Vaginal intercourse with condom[a]
Limiting the number of partners with whom one has sex
Unsafe sex practices
Semen, vaginal fluid, menstrual blood, or urine in mouth or in contact with the skin where there is an open cut or sore
Anal intercourse without condom[a]
Vaginal intercourse without condom[a]
Rimming (oral-anal contact)
Fisting (possible percutaneous inoculation with blood from trauma caused by inserting fist into anus)
Having sex when either partner has an open genital sore

[a]See instructions for condom users in Table 39.3.

The risk of sexual transmission also varies depending on the serum level of HIV RNA ("viral load") in the infected person. In a study of 415 HIV infection-discordant heterosexual couples in Uganda, researchers reported an average transmission rate of approximately 12 per 100 person-years. However, there were no instances of transmission when the infected partner's HIV RNA level was below 1,500 (9).

TABLE 39.3 Instructions for Condom Users

Use a condom every time you have intercourse.
Always put the condom on the penis before intercourse begins.
Put the condom on when the penis is erect.
Do not pull the condom tightly against the tip of the penis. Leave a small empty space—about 1 or 2 cm—at the end of the condom to hold semen. Some condoms have a nipple tip that will hold semen.
Unroll the condom all the way to the bottom of the penis.
If the condom breaks during intercourse, withdraw the penis immediately and put on a new condom.
After ejaculation withdraw the penis while it is still erect. Hold onto the rim of the condom as you withdraw so that the condom does not slip off.
Use a new condom each time you have intercourse. Throw used condoms away.
If a lubricant is desired, use water-based lubricants such as contraceptive jelly. Lubricants made with petroleum jelly may damage condoms. Do not use saliva because it may contain virus.
Store condoms in a cool dry place if possible.
Condoms that are sticky or brittle or otherwise damaged should not be used.

Adapted from Population Reports XIV, No. 3, 1986.

Transmission through Transfusion of Blood and Blood Products

HIV can be transmitted only by whole blood, blood cellular components, plasma, and clotting factors. No other blood products (e.g., immune globulin preparations, albumin, plasma protein fraction, hepatitis B vaccine) have been implicated.

The risk of acquiring HIV through a blood transfusion is now infinitesimally small. The estimated risk of HIV infection is 1:153,000 per unit of blood transfused (10). This low risk has been achieved by blood donor education programs (to eliminate donors who belong to high-risk groups), uniform blood product screening since April 1985, HIV-inactivating treatment of clotting factor concentrates, the use of autologous blood transfusions for elective surgery, and efforts to avoid nonessential transfusions.

Needle Transmission

Sharing of needles by injection drug users accounts for a large proportion of patients with AIDS in the United States. HIV-infected patients in this group pose a threat to both needle partners and sexual partners. In developing countries, this mode of transmission may also occur because of reuse of improperly cleaned needles and syringes for the injections of medicines.

Definitive interruption of transmission by injection drug use requires that the user discontinue the practice as part of a recovery program (see Chapter 29). The interruption of transmission by those who continue injection drug use requires that they avoid needle-sharing. Therefore, drug treatment can serve the dual purpose of treating addiction and preventing HIV transmission. Syringe and needle exchange programs have been shown to decrease needle sharing and to decrease spread of HIV infection. Some have advocated that physicians prescribe clean needles to injection drug users who would otherwise not have access to them to prevent transmission of HIV and other blood-borne diseases. Cleaning needles with bleach before reuse (if done properly) may also reduce the risk of transmission (11).

Perinatal Transmission

Although several routes may account for perinatal transmission from an HIV-infected woman to her infant, most infants acquire their infection at or near the time of delivery because of inoculation or ingestion of maternal blood. Intrauterine transmission by cord blood is less common. Transmission also can occur postnatally through breastfeeding. It is estimated that 7% to 39% of infants born to

HIV-infected mothers become infected, with the highest rates occurring in infants born to mothers with high viral loads, late-stage disease, early fetal membrane rupture, and placental inflammation.

Prevention of perinatal transmission requires primary prevention through safer sex practices and secondary prevention through HIV testing and subsequent counseling of HIV-infected women about the risks of pregnancy. Antiretroviral therapy with zidovudine or nevirapine has been shown to reduce transmission of HIV to the fetus. However, the current standard of care in the United States is to treat pregnant women who have an HIV RNA level over 1,000 copies per milliliter with a three-drug regimen with the goal of lowering the HIV RNA level to an undetectable level (12). It has been shown that transmission to the infant is rare if the HIV RNA level is below 500 copies per milliliter at the time of delivery. Additionally, elective cesarean section appears to reduce the risk of transmission but is probably of benefit only if the mother does not receive or respond to antiretroviral treatment or does not achieve on HIV RNA level below 1,000 on therapy.

Casual Contact and the Risk of Human Immunodeficiency Virus Transmission

Casual transmission of HIV does not occur. Thus, household contacts of HIV-infected patients who are not sexual partners are not at risk during ordinary circumstances. Although the virus has been isolated in urine and saliva, there have been no documented cases of transmission through kissing or through exposure to urine, stool, or saliva. Nevertheless, it is generally recommended that the same precautions taken to prevent transmission of hepatitis B in the household setting should be observed by HIV-infected people (see Chapter 47).

Occupational Exposure

Health care workers have an extremely low but finite risk of occupational infection with HIV. The predominant occupational risk is through accidental needlestick exposure. Most cases of HIV transmission by needlestick have occurred via a large-bore needle. Accidental infection is preventable by conscientious use of *universal precautions* (Table 39.4). "Universal" refers to the fact that these precautions should be followed in the direct care and in the handling of the body fluids of *all* patients (not just those known to be infected with HIV).

TABLE 39.4 Health Care Workers' Universal Precautions that Should Be Used in the Care of *All* Patients

Wear gloves for touching blood and body fluids, mucous membranes, or nonintact skin of the patient.
Wash hands immediately before and after patient care.
Wear gown, mask, and goggles if aerosolization or splattering of blood or body fluids is likely.
Handle sharp instruments with great care and discard them immediately in containers designed for this purpose. Used venipuncture needles MUST NOT be recapped.
Clean blood spills promptly with disinfectant such as 1:10 dilution of bleach.
Refrain from direct patient care if you have exudative skin lesions.

If a health care worker has a percutaneous injury (needlestick or cut) or contact of mucous membrane (eye or mouth) or nonintact skin with blood, tissues, or other body fluids, the source patient should be assessed clinically and, tested for HIV infection (if consent is obtained). As soon as possible after exposure, the exposed worker should also be counseled and, if consent is obtained, tested for HIV infection. If the source patient is HIV negative and has no clinical indicators of or risk factors for HIV infection, no further followup of the exposed worker is necessary. The U.S. Public Health Service recommends postexposure prophylaxis with antiretroviral medications for occupational exposures to HIV in certain situations depending on type of exposure and exposure source; these guidelines can be accessed at the AIDSinfo website (AIDSinfo.nih.gov) (13). Postexposure prophylaxis should be initiated within 1 to 2 hours after exposure. The optimal duration of therapy is unknown, but 4 weeks is suggested. Most health care institutions have postexposure protocols and resources for their employees; another resource is the National Clinicians' Postexposure Prophylaxis Hotline run by staff at the University of California-San Francisco and San Francisco General Hospital (phone: 888-448-4911; www.ucsf.edu/hivcntr).

SEROLOGIC DIAGNOSIS AND COUNSELING

Indications for Serologic Testing

Primary care practitioners are the front line of identifying patients infected with HIV and at risk of acquiring the infection. HIV testing and counseling are indicated both to prevent further transmission of disease and to allow people already infected to be identified so that they can seek appropriate medical care. This is especially important now that potent drugs are available to halt the progression of HIV and prevent infection in newborns.

According to the CDC, voluntary testing should be offered to all patients who have sexually transmitted diseases (STDs), are current or former injection drug users, are hemophiliacs, have active tuberculosis (TB), have received blood transfusions or blood products between 1978 and 1985, are prostitutes, are from developing countries with high rates of HIV infection, have regular sexual partners

TABLE 39.5 Factors That Should Trigger Consideration of Testing for Human Immunodeficiency Virus

- Historical factors
  - Alcohol or drug use/detoxification
  - Psychiatric hospitalization
  - Homelessness
  - Unsafe sexual practices
    - Multiple partners
    - Men who have sex with men
    - Sex with prostitutes
- Clinical factors
  - Any sexually transmitted disease, including
    - Herpes
    - Gonorrhea
    - Trichomonas
    - Syphilis
    - Hepatitis B
    - Pelvic inflammatory disease
    - Genital condyloma
    - Abnormal Pap smear
  - Other infections, including
    - Tuberculosis
    - Pneumonia
    - Recurrent vaginal candidiasis
    - Herpes zoster
    - Hepatitis C
  - Skin conditions
    - Psoriasis
    - Seborrhea
    - Molluscum contagiosa
  - Other conditions
    - Unexplained weight loss
    - Bell palsy/other neuropathies
    - Generalized lymphadenopathy/unexplained focal adenopathy
    - Lymphoma
    - Mononucleosis syndrome
    - Pulmonary hypertension
    - Congestive heart failure (unexplained)
    - Renal failure
    - Idiopathic thrombocytopenic purpura (ITP)
    - Thrombotic thrombocytopenic purpura (TTP)

with risk factors or known to be HIV infected, have signs or symptoms suggestive of HIV infection, consider themselves at risk for HIV infection or request testing, or are exposed to blood or other at-risk body fluids (including health care workers who perform invasive procedures); all pregnant women should also be offered voluntary testing. There is a growing list of conditions associated with HIV infection that should also provoke consideration of HIV testing; Table 39.5 lists some of these. There are many HIV-infected persons who do not know that they are infected and who may not have known risk factors; therefore, some have proposed that *all* adults be tested and have argued

TABLE 39.6 HIV Pretest and Posttest Counseling: Points for Discussion

- Pretest counseling
  - Meaning of positive test
    - Positive test means HIV infection
    - Positive test does *not* mean AIDS[a]
    - Positive test means patient is an HIV carrier
  - Confidentiality of test results and medical information
  - Availability of anonymous and confidential counseling and testing sites
  - Potential adverse psychosocial consequences if information becomes known, e.g., possible adverse effects on employment, housing, insurance status
  - Sources of additional AIDS/HIV-related information[b]
  - Means for reducing risk of HIV transmission or exposure (depends on patient's current or likely high-risk behaviors)
    - "Safe sex" practices (see Tables 39.1 and 39.2)
    - Sterilization of intravenous drug equipment
    - Treatment for drug addiction
    - Discontinuation of sharing intravenous needles
- Posttest counseling
  - Interpretation of HIV antibody test results
  - Information about long-term chances of developing symptoms
  - Planning for medical follow-up
  - Referral to psychosocial support services
  - Reinforcement of recommendations for prevention of HIV transmission/exposure
  - Discussion of notification of sexual partners or needle-sharing partners
  - Reproductive issues in women

[a] Most people with a positive test will develop AIDS. Length of time from infection to development of AIDS is variable but averages 10 years.
[b] A single source for information is the National AIDS Information Clearing House. P.O. Box 6003, Rockville, MD 20850 (800-458-5231).
HIV, human immunodeficiency virus; AIDS, acquired immunodeficiency syndrome.

that universal testing (every 3 to 5 years) would be cost effective (14).

Pretest and Posttest Counseling

The most important aspect of HIV testing is pretest and posttest counseling. Because of the ominous meaning of HIV infection, it is important to ensure privacy and to allow sufficient time to respond to the patient's feelings and questions. Many settings require the patient's written informed consent as part of pretest counseling. Table 39.6 shows recommended points of discussion during counseling. Information about behaviors associated with the risk of acquiring HIV infection is important in both stages of counseling.

Information about available printed materials useful in posttest counseling and about regional programs for HIV-infected patients can be obtained by contacting the CDC National Prevention Information Network (www.cdcnpin.org; P.O. Box 6003, Rockville, MD 20850; 1-800-458-5231).

Serologic Tests

Antibody to HIV usually appears 6 to 12 weeks after infection but may take as long as 6 months to appear. However, the immune response to HIV does not lead to elimination of the virus from host tissues. A persistent carrier (and persistent seropositive) state follows infection with this type of virus. The diagnosis of HIV infection is based on detection of *anti-HIV antibodies* by the enzyme-linked immunosorbent assay (ELISA), confirmed by the more specific Western blot (WB) method. In the WB method, several individual HIV proteins are transferred onto nitrocellulose paper and reacted against the patient's serum and known positive and negative sera; HIV antibody is detected by an antihuman immunoglobulin antibody coated with an enzyme that, in the presence of substrate, produces a colored band. A positive WB test (the presence of two of three colored bands representing p24, gp41, and gp120 or gp160) indicates that the patient has been infected with HIV (15).

ELISA tests are reported as positive or negative. WB tests are reported as positive, negative, or indeterminate. The routine processing of a specimen that is positive on initial ELISA testing always includes rerun of the ELISA, to confirm the result, followed by the WB test. The currently used ELISA tests have a sensitivity greater than 99% and a specificity of 99.5%. False-positive ELISA tests (ELISA-positive, WB-negative) may occur when nonspecific serologic reactions are present in patients who have other types of immunologic abnormalities or who have had multiple transfusions or multiple pregnancies. False-positives generally occur in patients from groups at low risk of acquiring HIV infection. False-negative ELISA results may occur in recently infected patients who have not yet made an antibody response.

Patients whose WB tests are reported as indeterminate are those whose sera yield only one of the necessary positive color bands. In most cases, the person is not infected with HIV, especially if the person is at low risk. However, this result may signify that a person is recently infected and will eventually convert to WB-positive. For this reason, the patient should be tested again; if the result remains indeterminate, testing should be repeated in 3 to 6 months. If the WB pattern remains indeterminate for 6 months—in the absence of any known risk factors or clinical findings to suggest HIV infection—the test may be considered negative. Patients who have risk factors or findings compatible with HIV-induced disease should have continued evaluation.

The Food and Drug Administration (FDA) also has licensed a *home HIV test kit* (Home Access Express, Home Access Health Corporation). This system requires the purchaser to pierce his or her skin with the lancet supplied in the kit, place a few drops of blood on a filter paper test card, and then send the sample to a central laboratory. Routine testing with ELISA and, if necessary, WB is then performed. Sensitivity and specificity for this system is reported to be comparable with routine testing on serum. Counseling is provided over the telephone. There are a number of other home testing kits advertised on the Internet that have not been licensed by the FDA and therefore cannot be recommended for use.

In 2004, the FDA approved the first oral rapid HIV antibody test (OraQuick Rapid HIV-1 Antibody Test, Abbott Diagnostics). Individuals have a test device swabbed around the upper and lower outer gums; this is then inserted in a vial containing a developer solution. After 20 minutes, if HIV antibody is present, two purple lines appear. Although the test is over 99% sensitive and specific, it is still recommended that positive tests be confirmed with a blood test.

HIV RNA level ("viral load") should not be used for screening purposes, except when acute HIV infection is suspected. The sensitivity and specificity of this test for diagnosing chronic infection is poorer than the ELISA and WB tests; some chronically infected patients have undetectable viral loads, and false-positive viral loads can also occur (16).

PATHOGENESIS AND NATURAL HISTORY

Pathogenesis of Disease in Human Immunodeficiency Virus-Infected Patients

HIV causes illness by impairing important components of the patient's immune system, making the patient susceptible to a wide variety of infections. This virus also causes illness by its direct effect on other body systems, especially the nervous system (17).

HIV preferentially infects human *T lymphocytes of the helper/inducer subset* (also called *CD4 cells*), resulting in both quantitative and qualitative defects in helper cell function. Because helper T lymphocytes are crucial in cell-mediated immunity, HIV infection impairs this type of immunity, making the patient susceptible to a number of opportunistic infections. Uninfected people usually have more than 800 CD4 cells per cubic millimeter of blood, whereas HIV-infected patients with opportunistic infections usually have less than 200 CD4 cells per cubic millimeter. Thus, monitoring the CD4 cell count has become useful for predicting the degree of suppression of a patient's cell-mediated immunity, guiding the differential diagnosis of new symptoms, and deciding when to initiate antiretroviral treatment and prophylaxis for opportunistic infection (see Prevention of First Episodes of Opportunistic Infections and Antiretroviral Treatment).

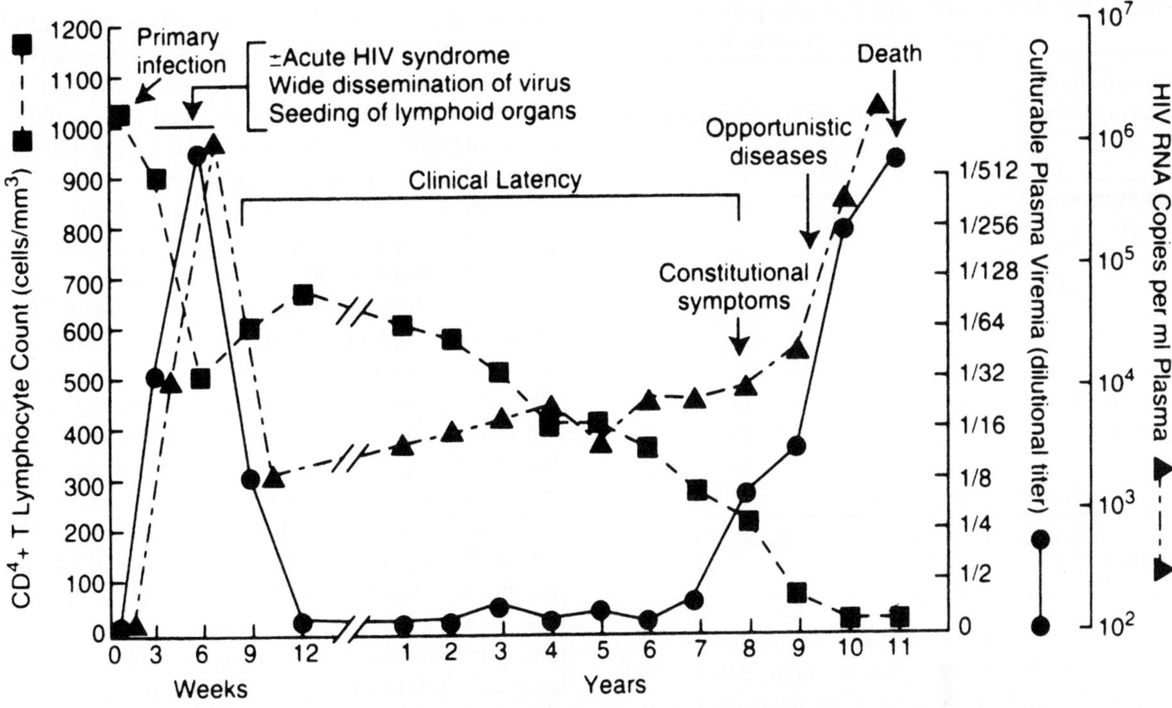

FIGURE 39.1. Natural history of HIV infection, based on CD4 counts and viral load. (From Fauci AS, Pantaleo G, Stanley S, et al. Immunopathogenic mechanisms of HIV infection. Ann Intern Med 1996;124:654, with permission.)

Other abnormalities of immune function are also found in HIV-infected people. HIV can infect and impair the function of macrophages and monocytes and CD4 lymphocytes. HIV infection may also result in B-lymphocyte activation and nonspecific hypergammaglobulinemia, which may impair the *de novo* antibody response to some antigens; this may place the patient at increased risk for infection with encapsulated bacteria. Additionally, some studies suggest that HIV infection may cause derangements in polymorphonuclear neutrophil phagocytosis and intracellular killing.

Although most of the illnesses in patients with HIV infection are caused by impaired resistance to infection, a number of clinical manifestations are direct consequences of HIV infection or the immune response to HIV infection. There is good evidence that the virus plays an etiologic role in some neurologic syndromes. Additionally, the virus, or in some cases the immune response to the virus, may cause disease in the gastrointestinal (GI) tract, heart, lungs, and kidneys.

Natural History and Prognosis in Human Immunodeficiency Virus Infection

The mean length of time from seroconversion to symptomatic AIDS in untreated patients is 10 years. The time from infection to symptoms, however, varies considerably from person to person and probably reflects variations in individuals' immune systems and the virulence of different strains of the virus. Expanded use of antiretroviral therapy, prophylaxis against opportunistic infections, and treatment of AIDS-associated conditions result in delayed progression and longer life expectancies for HIV-infected people. Figure 39.1 shows an overview of the natural history of HIV infection, based on CD4 counts and viral load. Because HIV may remain clinically silent with no demonstrable signs of immunodeficiency or symptoms for many years, asymptomatic patients play a major role in transmitting the virus.

Primary Human Immunodeficiency Virus Infection

Primary HIV infection ("acute retroviral syndrome") is usually symptomatic in the form of a mild to severe flulike illness. The most common signs and symptoms are fever, lymphadenopathy, pharyngitis, and rash (Table 39.7). The syndrome is nonspecific and cannot be differentiated from other acute viral illnesses on the basis of signs or symptoms alone. Patients often do not seek medical attention and even when they do, HIV infection is generally not recognized. There is a wide range of less common presentations of primary HIV infection that have been reported; these include opportunistic infections, acute renal failure, rhabdomyolysis, and vasculitis.

The incubation period (time from exposure to onset of illness) for the acute syndrome may range from 5 days to

TABLE 39.7 Manifestations of Primary Human Immunodeficiency Virus Infection

Common Signs and Symptoms	Expected Frequency (%)
Fever	96
Lymphadenopathy	74
Pharyngitis	70
Rash	70
Myalgia/arthralgia	54
Diarrhea	32
Headache	32
Nausea and vomiting	27
Hepatosplenomegaly	14
Weight loss	13
Thrush	12
Neurologic symptoms	12

Source: Centers for Disease Control and Prevention. MMWR 2005; 54:(RR-02)13.

3 months, but is usually 2 to 4 weeks. During the period of initial infection, blood virus levels are high, HIV is widely disseminated, and there is a transient decrease in circulating CD4 cells. There is an immune response to HIV between 1 week and 3 months after infection, and antibodies are usually detectable 6 to 24 weeks after the initial exposure. The early immune response is associated with a dramatic decrease in viremia, but viral replication is never completely curtailed, particularly in lymphoid tissue.

Because of the nonspecific nature of the illness, primary care practitioners need to maintain a high index of suspicion to identify patients with primary HIV infection. The diagnosis can be made by measuring HIV RNA level (viral load) or HIV p24 antigen; an elevated viral load (usually over 100,000 copies per milliliter) or detectable p24 antigen, in the presence of a negative HIV ELISA, establishes the diagnosis. Viral load is a more sensitive test (100%) than the p24 antigen (89%) but is less specific (97% vs. 100% for p24 antigen); however, specificity for viral load approaches 100% if a cutoff of 10,000 copies per milliliter is used (since false-positive viral load titers are usually below this level) (16). Recognizing primary HIV infection is important because it can help prevent further transmission and gives the opportunity to test for transmission of resistant virus (see Drug Resistance section and Antiretroviral Treatment).

Prognostic Indicators

The marker of disease progression that is most familiar to clinicians and has served the test of time is the *CD4 lymphocyte count*. The absolute number and percentage of CD4 lymphocytes gives the clinician an indication of the degree of immunosuppression and hence can be used to determine to what complications the patient is susceptible. The absolute number of CD4 cells is subject to more variability than the percentage because of normal biologic fluctuations in total lymphocyte counts. Within a year of seroconversion, CD4 cell counts usually drop 200 to 300 per cubic millimeter from the normal range of 800 to 1,200. This decline is followed by an increase to near baseline and then a slow decline of less than 100 cells per year (Fig. 39.1). People with CD4 cell counts greater than 500 are usually asymptomatic and have virtually no risk of developing an AIDS-indicator condition, except for TB, cervical cancer, recurrent bacterial pneumonias, or superficial Kaposi sarcoma (KS), within 18 months. In contrast, those with CD4 cell counts of 100 or less are often symptomatic and have a 60% chance of developing an AIDS-indicator disease (excluding TB, cervical cancer, and recurrent bacterial pneumonias) within 18 months.

A second prognostic indicator of disease progression is *HIV viral load* (measured as circulating HIV RNA). Among patients with equivalent CD4 lymphocyte counts, patients with higher viral loads on average have a more rapid fall in CD4 counts and clinical disease progression (18). Viral loads are an important way to monitor the effectiveness of antiretroviral therapy; a change in viral load usually occurs before a change in CD4 lymphocyte count, so changes in therapy can be made sooner if viral load is used. Nevertheless, changes in viral load should be interpreted with caution because there is wide intrapatient variation and serial changes are significant only when they are greater than 50% (0.3 log). Viral load varies from undetectable, which is currently less than 400 copies/mL (50 copies per milliliter on ultrasensitive assays), to greater than 1 million copies per milliliter. Immediately after infection, plasma viral load begins to rise and peaks at greater than 100,000 copies per milliliter. It then declines and plateaus in about 150 days to a steady state called the viral set point. The viral set point remains constant for months to years and is a good indicator of risk for disease progression. Viral load again rises just before the development of opportunistic diseases and reaches its highest value with end-stage disease.

Guidelines for the use of CD4 count and viral load in clinical decision-making are found below (see the section on antiretroviral therapy).

CLASSIFICATION SYSTEM FOR HUMAN IMMUNODEFICIENCY VIRUS INFECTION AND CASE DEFINITION FOR ACQUIRED IMMUNODEFICIENCY SYNDROME

Since 1993, the CDC has used a revised HIV classification system that emphasizes the importance of the CD4 count. Patients are now classified according to three categories of CD4 cell counts:

1. More than 500 per cubic millimeter;
2. 200 to 499 per cubic millimeter;
3. Less than 200 per cubic millimeter.

They are also classified according to three clinical categories:

A. Asymptomatic, acute HIV, or persistent generalized lymphadenopathy;
B. Symptomatic, not A or C conditions;
C. AIDS-indicator conditions.

Once a person meets criteria for symptomatic HIV or AIDS, that person remains in the same category or advances to a more advanced stage despite interventions that may eliminate symptoms or increase CD4 cell counts. Patients in categories 3 or C meet the case definition of AIDS.

Symptomatic disease in category B includes any condition attributable to immunodeficiency from HIV infection or complicated by HIV infection (except those in categories A and C). Examples of these conditions include bacillary angiomatosis; oropharyngeal candidiasis; vulvovaginal candidiasis that is persistent, frequent, or poorly responsive to therapy; cervical dysplasia (moderate or severe) or cervical carcinoma *in situ*; constitutional symptoms such as fever (38.5°C [101.3°F] or higher) or diarrhea lasting more than 1 month; oral hairy leukoplakia; herpes zoster of more than one dermatome or recurring at least once; idiopathic thrombocytopenic purpura; listeriosis; pelvic inflammatory disease; and peripheral neuropathy.

The CDC has also expanded the list of *AIDS-indicator conditions* (Table 39.8). In addition to the 23 clinical conditions originally used to define AIDS, pulmonary TB, recurrent pneumonia (at least two episodes per year), and invasive cervical cancer are now AIDS-indicator diseases.

TABLE 39.8 AIDS-Indicator Conditions in HIV-Infected Persons

Candidiasis
Bronchi
Trachea
Esophagus
Lungs
Cervical cancer, invasive
Coccidioidomycosis, disseminated or extrapulmonary
Cryptococcosis, extrapulmonary
Cryptosporidiosis, extrapulmonary
Cytomegalovirus disease (other than liver, spleen, or nodes)
Encephalopathy, HIV related (dementia)
Herpes simplex
Chronic ulcer >1 mo duration
Bronchitis
Pneumonitis
Esophagitis
Histoplasmosis, disseminated or extrapulmonary
HIV wasting syndrome (>10% weight loss and either chronic weakness and fever or chronic diarrhea, ≥30 days)
Isosporiasis, intestinal of >1 mo duration
Kaposi sarcoma
Lymphoma
Burkitt
Immunoblastic
Primary of the brain
Mycobacterium
M. avium complex, disseminated or extrapulmonary
M. kansasii, disseminated or extrapulmonary
M. tuberculosis, pulmonary or extrapulmonary
Other species, disseminated or extrapulmonary
Pneumocystis jiroveci (carinii) pneumonia
Pneumonia, two or more episodes within a year
Progressive multifocal leukoencephalopathy
Salmonella septicemia, recurrent
Toxoplasmosis, brain

HIV, human immunodeficiency virus; AIDS, acquired immunodeficiency syndrome.
Adapted from Centers for Disease Control and Prevention. 1993. Revised classification system for HIV infection and expanded surveillance case definition for AIDS among adolescents and adults. MMWR 1992;41 (No. RR-17).

INITIAL EVALUATION AND TREATMENT OF HUMAN IMMUNODEFICIENCY VIRUS-INFECTED PATIENTS

Baseline History, Physical Examination, and Laboratory Studies

The apparently asymptomatic patient with HIV infection requires an initial evaluation and ongoing psychosocial support and medical assessment. This section describes important manifestations to be sought in initial and subsequent evaluations of HIV-positive patients and prophylactic guidelines, as established by the U.S. Public Health Service in collaboration with the Infectious Diseases Society of America (19). Descriptions of symptomatic manifestations are found under Symptomatic Human Immunodeficiency Virus-Infected Patient, below.

In addition to the HIV-oriented review of systems summarized in Table 39.9, seropositive patients should be asked about a history of STDs, TB, or a positive purified protein derivative (PPD) test; exposure to or history of hepatitis B; immunosuppressive therapy (e.g., an asthmatic patient who intermittently requires corticosteroids); and previous immunizations, including pneumococcal and hepatitis B vaccines. Important information to obtain in the social history includes current sexual practices (type and number of sexual partners), types of contraception used, and past or present injection drug use.

The *baseline physical examination* should include all organ systems, with special emphasis on the oral cavity, skin,

TABLE 39.9 HIV-Oriented Review of Symptoms

General: Weight loss, fever, night sweats
Skin: New rashes, pigmented lesions, itching
Lymphoid system: Asymmetric or rapidly growing lymph nodes.
HEENT: Change in vision, unusual headaches, congestion or running nose, oral lesions
Respiratory: Cough, shortness of breath, decrease in exercise tolerance
Gastrointestinal: Pain or difficulty in swallowing, nausea or vomiting, diarrhea, painful defecation
Neuropsychiatric: Difficulty thinking, depression, change in personality, numbness or tingling, muscle weakness, loss of sensation

HIV, human immunodeficiency virus.

lymph nodes, and, in women, the reproductive system. Physical manifestations in these organ systems are particularly important because diseases may be found that are potentially treatable (e.g., seborrheic dermatitis) or that carry prognostic significance (e.g., oral candidiasis).

The *baseline laboratory evaluation* should establish a database that will be useful for identifying already present abnormalities and for comparison when abnormalities are identified at a later time in the care of the patient. This database should include a complete blood count (including a differential and platelet count), hepatitis B surface antigen and antibody, syphilis serology, *Toxoplasma* antibody, HIV viral load, and CD4 lymphocyte count. Injection drug users and their partners should be tested for hepatitis C antibody. Baseline serologic tests for antibody to cytomegalovirus (CMV) are not generally useful because of the high prevalence of positive tests in the normal population. Unless the patient has a history of a positive PPD skin test or TB, the patient should have a PPD. A chest radiograph should be performed in all patients who have a positive PPD (5 mm or more induration) or have respiratory symptoms or a history of respiratory disease. Table 39.10 gives suggested guidelines for periodic monitoring.

Many patients who complain of no symptoms at baseline will have one or more abnormalities found on physical examination or laboratory evaluation, most commonly generalized lymphadenopathy (see Constitutional Manifestations and Lymphadenophy section), reduced CD4 count, elevated HIV viral load, or mild suppression of the elements of the bone marrow. If a history of constitutional symptoms (weight loss, fevers, night sweats) is elicited, this should be evaluated further, as discussed in the next section. Findings in the oral cavity that may not cause symptoms but suggest some degree of immunodeficiency include oral hairy leukoplakia or early *Candida* infection (see Oral Lesions section). A finding of an isolated low platelet count may be indicative of immune thrombocytopenic purpura. Laboratory abnormalities (e.g., anemia) should be evaluated in the same manner as in a non–HIV-infected patient.

Health Maintenance: Monitoring Schedules, Immunizations, and Opportunistic Infection Prophylaxis

Table 39.10 outlines the recommended monitoring schedule for HIV-infected patients according to CD4 cell count. Table 39.11 and this section address immunizations and opportunistic infection prophylaxis to prevent first episodes of preventable diseases. Later sections address the treatment of opportunistic infections (see Symptomatic Human Immunodeficiency Virus-Infected Patient) and the schedule for viral load monitoring and the initiation and long-term use of antiretroviral drugs (Antiretroviral Treatment).

Prevention of First Episodes of Opportunistic Infections

Preventive care for HIV-infected patients should include various vaccinations (Table 39.11). Pneumococcal pneumonia is the leading cause of bacterial pneumonia in HIV-infected patients; *pneumococcal vaccine* is

TABLE 39.10 Health Maintenance in the HIV-Infected Patient: Monitoring Timing and Frequency Based on CD4 Count

CD4 Count (per mm^3)	*>500*	*200–499*	*100–200*	*<100*
CD4 cell count	3–6 mo[a]	3 mo	3 mo	3 mo
HIV viral load	3–6 mo[a]	3 mo	3 mo	3 mo
Syphilis serology	12 mo	12 mo	12 mo	12 mo
Hepatitis B serology	Once	Once	Once	Once
Tuberculosis screening[b]	12 mo	12 mo	12 mo	12 mo
Pap smear	12 mo	6–12 mo	6–12 mo	6–12 mo
Ophthalmologic exam (CMV)	No	No	No	6 mo

[a]A patient on antiretroviral therapy should be monitored every 3 months; a longer interval may be sufficient if not on therapy, especially if the viral load is relatively low.
[b]When positive, do not repeat.
HIV, human immunodeficiency virus; CMV, cytomegalovirus.

TABLE 39.11 Health Maintenance in HIV-infected Individuals: Immunizations and Antimicrobial Prophylaxis to Prevent First Episodes of Opportunistic Disease in Adults

Pathogen	*Indication*	*First Choice*	*Alternative*
Category I: Strongly Recommended as Standard of Care			
Pneumocystis jiroveci (P. carinii)	CD4 count <200 or oropharyngeal candidiasis	TMP/SMZ, 1 SS; or DS daily	Dapsone 50 mg b.i.d. or 100 mg daily; or Aerosolized pentamidine; 9 mo or Atovaquone 1,500 mg daily.
Mycobacterium tuberculosis Isoniazid-sensitive	PPD reaction ≥5 mm or prior positive PPD without treatment or contact with active TB case	Isoniazid 300 mg + pyridoxine 50 mg daily × 9 mo; or Isoniazid 900 mg + pyridoxine 100 mg twice weekly × 9 mo; or rifampin 600 mg + pyrazinamide[a] 20 mg/kg daily× 2 mo	Rifabutin 300 mg + pyrazinamide 20 mg/kg daily. × 2 mo; or rifampin 600 mg daily. × 4 mo.
M. tuberculosis Isoniazid-resistant	Same as above, with high probability of exposure to isoniazid-resistant tuberculosis	Rifampin 600 mg + pyrazinamide[a] 20 mg/kg daily × 2 mo[a]	Rifabutin 300 mg + pyrazinamide[a] 20 mg/kg daily. × 2 mo; or rifampin 600 mg daily. × 4 mo.; or rifabutin 300 mg daily × 4 mo.
M. tuberculosis multidrug-resistant	Same as above, with high probability of exposure to multidrug-resistant tuberculosis	Consult public health authorities.	None
Toxoplasma gondii	IgG antibody to *Toxoplasma* and CD4 count <100	TMP/SMZ, 1 DS daily	TMP-SMZ, 1 SS daily; or dapsone 50 mg daily + pyrimethamine 50 mg weekly + leukovorin 25 mg weekly; or atavoquone 1,500 mg daily ± pyrimethamine 25 mg daily + leukovorin 10 mg daily
Mycobacterium avium complex	CD4 count <50	Azithromycin 1,200 mg weekly; or clarithromycin 500 mg b.i.d.	Rifabutin 300 mg daily or azithromycin 1,200 mg weekly + rifabutin 300 mg daily
Varicella zoster virus (VZV)	Significant exposure to chickenpox or shingles for patients who have no history of either condition or, if available, negative antibody to VZV	Varicella zoster immune globulin (VZIG), 5 vials (1.25 mL each) im administered = 96 h after exposure, ideally within 48 h	None
Category 2: Generally recommended			
Streptococcus pneumoniae	All patients	Pneumococcal vaccine	None
Hepatitis B	All susceptible (anti-HBc-negative) patients	Hepatitis B vaccine (3 doses)	None
Influenza A	All patients (annually, before influenza season)	Influenza vaccine	Rimantadine 100 mg twice daily.; or amantadine 100 mg twice daily

All medications are p.o. unless otherwise noted.
[a]Use with caution; severe cases of hepatotoxicity reported with this combination (see text).
HIV, human immunodeficiency virus.
Source: CDC Guidelines for preventing opportunistic infections among HIV-infected persons—2002. MMWR Recommendations and Reports 2002;51 (RR-08).

recommended for all HIV-infected patients. It should be given early in the course of HIV infection or, if given in later-stage disease, after the patient has responded to antiretroviral therapy. The evidence for the efficacy of the pneumococcal vaccine is mixed: A randomized controlled trial in Uganda unexpectedly showed a trend toward increased pneumococcal disease among vaccine recipients (20), whereas an analysis of a U.S. database of HIV-infected patients suggested a benefit for those with CD4 counts over 500 (21). The *influenza vaccine* has been shown to be effective and safe in HIV-infected adults; however, the intranasal influenza vaccine (FluMist) should not be given to HIV-infected individuals, since it contains attenuated virus (22).

Hepatitis B vaccine should be given in hepatitis B surface antigen and antibody-negative patients who have continued risk factors for hepatitis B because of the increased risk for chronic hepatitis in HIV-infected patients. Although data on the efficacy of *other killed or inactivated vaccines* is not available, it is still recommended that routine vaccines such as tetanus be given to HIV-infected patients.

Live attenuated vaccines such as polio, typhoid, and yellow fever should not be given. Measles vaccine, however, has been shown to be safe in HIV-infected children and can be given according to the recommendations for HIV-negative people. For details regarding dosages and schedules of immunizations, see Chapter 18.

Antimicrobial Prophylaxis

Table 39.11 delineates recommendations for antimicrobial prophylaxis for infections caused by *Pneumocystis jiroveci* (previously known as *P. carinii*), *Mycobacterium avium*, and *Toxoplasma gondii*. These indications for prophylaxis are guided largely by CD4 counts and not symptomatic infection. Recommended prophylaxis regimens for other opportunistic infections, initiated *after episodes of symptomatic infection*, are found below (Symptomatic Human Immunodeficiency Virus-Infected Patient).

P. pneumonia (PCP) prophylaxis should be initiated when the CD4 cell count is less than 200 or if the patient already has had PCP or has oral candidiasis (19). Table 39.12 shows doses and regimens for the oral agents effective for prophylaxis. Oral trimethoprim-sulfamethoxazole (TMP-SMZ) is the preferred agent because it has been shown to be most efficacious and it also has the added benefit of being inexpensive (less than $50 for a year of treatment).

TABLE 39.12 Risks and Benefits of Delayed or Early Initiation of Therapy in the Asymptomatic HIV-Infected Patient

Risks and benefits of delayed initiation of therapy
- Benefits of delayed therapy
  - Avoid negative effects on quality of life (i.e., inconvenience)
  - Avoid drug-related adverse events
  - Delay in development of drug resistance
  - Preserve maximum number of available and future drug options when HIV disease risk is highest
- Risks of delayed therapy
  - Possible risk of irreversible immune system depletion
  - Possible greater difficulty in suppressing viral replication
  - Possible increased risk of HIV transmission

Risks and benefits of early therapy
- Benefits of early therapy
  - Control of viral replication easier to achieve and maintain
  - Delay or prevention of immune system compromise
  - Lower risk of resistance with complete viral suppression
  - Possible decreased risk of HIV transmission
- Risks of early therapy
  - Drug-related reduction in quality of life
  - Greater cumulative drug-related adverse events
  - Earlier development of drug resistance, if viral suppression is suboptimal
  - Limitation of future antiretroviral treatment options

Source: Guidelines for the use of antiretroviral agents in HIV-1 infected adults and adolescents. October 2004.

The most common side effects with TMP-SMZ prophylaxis, in descending order of frequency, include rash, pruritus, nausea and vomiting, fever, anemia, neutropenia, and elevated liver enzymes. These side effects generally occur within the first month of starting therapy, but some, especially cutaneous reactions and fever, may occur later, even years after initiation of therapy. These side effects occasionally necessitate discontinuation of therapy. Often, however, TMP-SMZ can be reintroduced, especially when given in gradually increasing doses using the liquid formulation.

If life-threatening reactions occur, such as Stevens-Johnson syndrome, or if the patient is unwilling to restart TMP-SMZ because of prior side effects, dapsone, aerosolized pentamidine, or atovaquone can be substituted. The major toxicities of dapsone are rash and cytopenias; it is also associated with the uncommon, but serious, complications methemoglobinemia and hemolysis. The side effects of aerosolized pentamidine (300 mg every 4 weeks administered over 20 to 25 minutes with a jet nebulizer) include cough and bronchospasm, most often seen in smokers or in patients with pre-existing asthma. Pretreatment with a metered-dose bronchodilator often prevents this problem. Additionally, because of the risk of aerosolization of a mycobacterial infection not previously suspected, aerosolized pentamidine should be used only in specially designated areas and in patients proven not to have active TB. Atovaquone is another oral alternative to TMP-SMZ but is much more expensive than the other prophylactic agents (~$10,000 a year). Side effects of atovaquone include rash and diarrhea.

All HIV-infected patients with *positive tuberculin tests* (defined as 5 mm or more of induration), regardless of age, should be treated prophylactically with isoniazid 300 mg for at least 9 months or rifampin and pyrazinamide for 2 months (19). The rifampin and pyrazinamide combination has been associated with cases of severe hepatotoxicity and even death; generally it should be avoided, especially for patients receiving other hepatotoxic drugs and those with a history of alcoholism or chronic liver disease. If this combination is used, it is recommended that liver enzymes be checked at baseline and after 2, 4, and 6 weeks of treatment (19a). If the patient is known to have been exposed to a strain that is resistant to isoniazid but sensitive to rifampin, rifampin should be used as preventive therapy (see details in Chapter 34).

Patients with antibodies to *T. gondii* and CD4 cell counts less than 100 cells per cubic millimeter should be given TMP-SMZ (one double-strength dose per day) for prophylaxis (19). Dapsone and pyrimethamine are acceptable alternatives if TMP-SMZ is not tolerated. Folinic acid is also given, with the regimen at 25 mg/week to prevent bone marrow toxicity associated with pyrimethamine.

Prophylaxis is recommended against *M. avium* complex (MAC) when CD4 cell counts are less than 50 cells per cubic millimeter, and has been shown to reduce the risk of disseminated infection and overall mortality (23). Effective regimens include azithromycin 1,200 mg once a week, clarithromycin 500 mg twice daily, or rifabutin 300 mg daily. Azithromycin and clarithromycin are more efficacious than rifabutin, and azithromycin has the added advantage of once-weekly dosing.

Oral ganciclovir has been shown to reduce the risk of *CMV retinitis* in patients with low CD4 cell counts (24), but because of toxicity and difficulty defining which patients are at risk, primary CMV prophylaxis is not routinely recommended (19). However, ophthalmologic screening every 6 months for CMV retinitis is recommended for patients with CD4 cell counts less than 75 cells per cubic millimeter.

Fluconazole has been shown to reduce the risk of invasive fungal infections (esophageal candidiasis and cryptococcosis) for patients with advanced AIDS (CD4 counts <50 per milliliter), but does not reduce overall mortality (25). For this reason, and because of concerns about the development of drug resistance, the routine use of fluconazole as prophylactic agent is not recommended (19).

Since the advent of new antiretroviral agents that can raise CD4 cell counts for prolonged periods (see Antiretroviral Treatment section), there has been increasing evidence that primary (and in some cases secondary) prophylaxis can be discontinued once the CD4 cell count rises above the value used as the threshold for initiation. Discontinuation of primary prophylaxis for *P. jiroveci*, *T. gondii*, and MAC has been shown to be safe when patients have a sustained increase in CD4 counts above the prophylaxis threshold.

Coexisting Medical Problems

HIV-positive patients are as likely as HIV-negative patients to have common acute or chronic diseases. The two groups should be approached in the same way in addressing these problems and in addressing indicated preventive care (see Chapter 14).

Many HIV-infected patients describe minor problems, such as fatigue, night sweats, mild chronic diarrhea, pruritus, and low-grade temperature elevation, for which specific infectious causes cannot be identified. Many of these problems may be manifestations of chronic HIV infection. In addition, for some patients, a focus on somatic concerns is the way in which they present their mental distress (see Chapter 21 for a detailed discussion of somatization). When an identifiable opportunistic infection has been excluded (see Symptomatic HIV-Infected Patients section) and there is no evidence of a conventional infection, simple palliative measures should be recommended. Patients should be encouraged to discuss their mental distress at the same time that they are queried and advised about physical symptoms.

Psychosocial and Ethical Aspects

Dealing with the psychosocial issues accompanying the diagnosis of asymptomatic HIV infection is often more difficult than the medical management. Patients who have learned they have a fatal disease that may have been acquired sexually and is stigmatizing for a variety of reasons usually feel extremely isolated and despondent. Because patients' emotional responses may impair the ability to process information, it is important to check their comprehension of the facts, to be prepared to reiterate points covered in the posttest counseling session (Table 39.6), and to respond to the feelings and questions that these points will evoke. The patient must understand how the virus is and is not transmitted, the usual course of the disease, and available therapeutic interventions.

The HIV-infected patient has an intense need for hope and support. In addition to ensuring the patient of ongoing support and using counseling techniques that are helpful for a patient in crisis (see Chapter 20), it is appropriate to offer psychologic or psychiatric consultation after the diagnosis of HIV infection. Among the possible psychosocial consequences of this diagnosis are the uncovering of homosexuality in men whose gay orientation has been confidential; the threatened loss of family, social, and occupational relationships; an increase in the release of irresponsible promiscuity in antisocial people; and an increased risk of suicide. These problems particularly require expert counseling.

HIV-positive patients should be assured of confidentiality about their condition but at the same time should be instructed to inform others who may have been infected by them. Although asymptomatic HIV infection is not reportable in most jurisdictions, the patient's physician may have a responsibility to inform others who may be infected if the patient will not do so. This raises the difficult conflict between the patient's right to confidentiality and the rights of other people to protect their health. Laws governing physicians' actions and obligations and ethical aspects of caring for an HIV-infected patient are discussed further in a later section (Public Health and Legal Responsibilities of the Physician).

ANTIRETROVIRAL TREATMENT

Multiple clinical trials have shown that HAART dramatically increases CD4 counts, decreases viral load, delays clinical progression, and prolongs life. However, the duration of the efficacious effect and the optimal stage for

TABLE 39.13 Indications for the Initiation of Antiretroviral Therapy in the Chronically HIV-Infected Patient

Clinical Category	*CD4 Cell Count*	*Plasma HIV RNA Level*	*Recommendation*
Symptomatic (AIDS or severe symptoms)	Any value	Any value	Treat
Asymptomatic, AIDS	$CD4^{+}$T cells <200/mm^3	Any value	Treat
Asymptomatic	$CD4^{+}$ T cells >200/mm^3, but >350/mm^3	Any value	Treatment should be offered following full discussion of pros and cons with each patient.
Asymptomatic	$CD4^{+}$T cells >350/mm^3	>100,000	Most clinicians recommend deferring therapy, but some clinicians will treat.
Asymptomatic	$CD4^{+}$T cells >350/mm^3	<100,000	Defer therapy.

HIV, human immunodeficiency virus; AIDS, acquired immunodeficiency virus.
Source: Guidelines for the use of antiretroviral agents in HIV-1 infected adults and adolescents. October 2005. Available at: AIDSinfo.gov.

initiation of therapy are unknown. Development of resistance and long-term side effects of antiretrovirals are concerns in patients on HAART. The long-term side effects include dyslipidemia (dysmorphic changes and hyperlipidemia), hyperglycemia, and peripheral neuropathy. Concerns about these toxicities and uncertainty about the benefits and risks of early versus delayed initiation of HAART (Table 39.12) resulted in extensive revision of consensus recommendations for antiretroviral treatment in 2001. Table 39.13 shows consensus guidelines for antiretroviral treatment that were updated in October of 2004. Most importantly, patients must be willing and able to comply with HAART with the recognition that a very high level of compliance with medication regimen is necessary to prevent viral resistance and treatment failure. Table 39.14 shows strategies for optimizing adherence. Treatment recommendations updated in October 2004 and summarized in Table 39.15 include treatment with at least three agents, usually two nucleoside reverse transcriptase inhibitors (NRTI) with a nonnucleoside reverse transcriptase inhibitor (NNRTI) or protease inhibitor (26). These guidelines are frequently revised; updated recommendations are available from the U.S. government (website: AIDSinfo.nih.gov).

Baseline viral loads and CD4 counts give the most useful information about prognosis without treatment. The CD4 count has increasingly been viewed as the guide for deciding on when to initiate HAART. The viral load is the best guide for monitoring the effectiveness of therapy and deciding when to change antiretroviral therapy. Once HAART is initiated, achieving an undetectable viral load should be the goal. In clinical trials, this is achieved in more than 80% of patients after 1 year of therapy, whereas in most clinical settings it is achieved in only 40% to 60% of patients.

Antiretroviral Drugs

The development of agents that act at different loci in the viral replication cycle has led to the application of principles used with other infectious agents to prevent resistance and promote eradication, such as the principles applied in the treatment of TB. The hallmark of these principles is the use of several agents simultaneously.

There are currently three classes of antiretroviral drugs used for initial treatment: NRTIs; the NNRTIs, which have the same mechanism of action as the NRTIs but a different structure; and the protease inhibitors, which act at a different locus in the process of viral replication than NRTIs or NNRTIs. There is also a fourth class of medications, fusion inhibitors, of which only one drug, enfuvirtide (Fuzeon), is currently available. This agent must be given as a twice-daily subcutaneous injection and currently is only used as a salvage treatment in combination with other

TABLE 39.14 Strategies to Improve Adherence

- Inform patient, anticipate, and treat side effects.
- Avoid adverse drug interactions.
- If possible, reduce dose frequency and number of pills.
- Negotiate a treatment plan, which the patient understands and to which he/she commits.
- Take time, multiple encounters to educate, and explain goals of therapy and need for adherence.
- Establish readiness to take medication *before* first prescription is written.
- Recruit family and friends to support the treatment plan.
- Develop concrete plan for specific regimen, relation to meals, daily schedule, side effects.
- Provide written schedule and pictures of medications, daily or weekly pill boxes, alarm clocks, pagers, other mechanical aids to adherence.
- Develop adherence support groups or add adherence issues to regular agenda of support groups.
- Develop linkages with local community-based organizations around adherence with educational sessions and practical strategies.

Source: Guidelines for the use of antiretroviral agents in HIV-1 infected adults and adolescents. October 2005. Available at: AIDSinfo.gov.

HIV infection is also a financial burden for most patients. The cost of antiretroviral medications alone exceeds $10,000 annually and even those who have private health insurance may be saddled with high co-payments or may exhaust their pharmacy coverage. Patients who are disabled from the complications of this illness may qualify for Social Security disability. This means that the patient receives Social Security income immediately but must wait 24 months before receiving Medicare health insurance. A patient who meets the needs criteria for Supplemental Security Income can obtain health insurance through Medicaid immediately (see Chapter 9 for further information). In the United States, there are a number of other programs that help to provide medical care for HIV-infected patients. The Ryan White Comprehensive AIDS Relief Emergency (CARE) act was first enacted in 1990 and provides funding for HIV care through a number of mechanisms, including grants to states, cities, and health care providers. State-administered AIDS drug assistance programs (ADAPs) provide funding for medications for patients who do not have access through other programs; coverage and access to this program vary from state to state.

A newer and rather unusual problem that has arisen since the advent of HAART is patients having unexpected health restored after years of considering themselves to be terminally ill. This has raised many psychologic and practical issues, including making plans for a future never expected, returning to work after being on disability, and the guilt of surviving when so many did not earlier in the epidemic.

In addressing the social aspects of the patient's disease, the patient's right to privacy and confidentiality should be ensured at the outset, and patients should be asked to specify the people to whom they plan to disclose the nature of their illness. Many AIDS patients require counseling to cope with these decisions and the many changes in their lives caused by their disease. In addition to provider input, the supportive counseling of a social worker or nurse educator and help from community-based support groups should be enlisted.

Death and Dying

Because AIDS is still a fatal disease in many, dealing with the issues of death and dying is extremely important. It is probably not appropriate to begin such discussions when a patient first learns of the HIV diagnosis other than to answer questions about the prognosis frankly. It should be emphasized that HIV infection has a long latency period. Hope is extremely powerful in maintaining the patient's psychological and physical well-being.

The more appropriate time to explore the issues of death and dying is when the patient develops signs and symptoms related to progressive disease. Open discussions should be initiated about financial planning and about advance directives regarding resuscitation and other aspects of care when one may not be competent. These discussions should take place early in the course of AIDS while the patient is still fully competent. Chapter 13 discusses issues of death, dying, and bereavement, and Chapter 12 describes legal considerations in specifying and documenting advance directives.

Public Health and Legal Responsibilities of the Physician

No disease in recent times has emphasized to a greater extent the confrontation between the defense of individual privacy and the protection of public health. Clearly, this remains a major challenge to health care professionals dealing with HIV infection. The physician's primary responsibility is to the patient. The unique trust inherent in the physician–patient relationship allows the physician to guide the patient to protect those who may be at risk because of sexual contact. The physician has the responsibility of emphasizing to the patient, on multiple occasions if necessary, the importance of informing sexual or needle-sharing partners. Guidelines governing the physician's responsibility when the patient refuses to inform others are included in many state laws, and advice regarding these guidelines should be sought from state public health authorities. Many states now have confidential programs for sexual partner notification.

Physicians are required by law to report all newly diagnosed cases of AIDS, using confidential morbidity report forms. In addition, some states now require reporting of most symptomatic HIV-associated diseases.

Information and Support for Household Members

People who live with or care for HIV-infected patients at home have special needs. Most importantly, they need clear information about the transmission of HIV infection, about both the safety of nonintimate contact with the patient and the risks and precautions related to intimate contact. Household caretakers should be advised to follow the universal precautions recommended to health care workers for the care of all patients (Table 39.3).

People close to patients with HIV infection and AIDS invariably have a variety of intense emotional reactions and must also confront distressing social implications of the patient's illness. Thus, taking the time to share information and respond to questions from patients' caretakers is a critical part of caring for patients with HIV and AIDS.

SPECIFIC REFERENCES*

1. Lee LM, Karon JM, Selik R, et al. Survival after AIDS diagnosis in adolescents and adults during the treatment era, United States, 1984–1997. JAMA 2001;285:1308.
2. Landon BE, Wilson IB, Cohn SE, et al. Physician specialization and antiretroviral therapy for HIV. J Gen Intern Med 2003;18:233.
3. Markowitz DM. Infection with the human immunodeficiency virus type 2. Ann Intern Med 1993;118:211.
4. **4.** Centers for Disease Control and Prevention and USPHS Working Group. Guidelines for counseling persons infected with human T-lymphotrophic virus type I (HTLV-1) and type II (HTLV-2). Ann Intern Med 1993;118: 448.
5. Centers for Disease Control and Prevention. HIV/AIDS surveillance report. Cases of HIV infection and AIDS in the United States, 2003. Volume 15. Available at www.cdc.gov/hiv.
6. UNAIDS 2004 report on the global AIDS epidemic. www.unaids.org.
7. Epstein RM, Morse DS, Frankel RM, et al. Awkward moments in patient-physician communication about HIV risk. Ann Intern Med 1998;128:435.
8. **8.** Centers for Disease Control and Prevention. Antiretroviral postexposure prophylaxis after sexual, injection-drug use, or other nonoccupational exposure to HIV in the United States. MMWR 2005;54:(RR-02).
9. Quinn TC, Mawer MJ, Sewankambo N, et al. Viral load and heterosexual transmission of human immunodeficiency virus type 1. N Engl J Med 2000;342:921.
10. Cummings PD, Wallace EL, Schorr JB. Exposure of patients to human immunodeficiency virus through the transfusion of blood components that test antibody-negative. N Engl J Med 1989;321:941.
11. Abdala N, Crowe M, Tolstov Y, et al. Survival of human immunodeficiency virus type 1 after rinsing injection syringes with different cleaning solutions. Subst Use Misuse 2004;39:581.
12. **12.** Perinatal HIV Guidelines Working Group. Recommendations for the use of antiretroviral drugs in pregnant HIV-1 infected women for maternal health and interventions to reduce perinatal HIV-1 transmission in the United States. February 24, 2005. Available at: AIDSinfo.nih.gov.
13. **13.** Centers for Disease Control and Prevention. Updated U.S. Public Health Service guidelines for the management of occupational exposure to HIV and recommendations for postexposure prophylaxis. MMWR 2005;54:(RR-09).
14. Paltiel AD, Weinstein MC, Kimmel AD, et al. Expanded screening for HIV in the United States—an analysis of cost-effectiveness. N Engl J Med 2005;352:586.
15. Centers for Disease Control and Prevention. Interpretation and use of the Western blot assay for serodiagnosis of human immunodeficiency virus type I infections. JAMA 1989;262:3395.
16. Daar ES, Little S, Pitt J, et al. Diagnosis of primary HIV-1 infection. Ann Intern Med 2001;134:25.
17. Panteleo G, Graziosi C, Fauci AS. The immunopathogenesis of human immunodeficiency virus infection. N Engl J Med 1993;328:327.
18. Saksela K, Stevens CE, Rubinstein P, et al. HIV-1 messenger RNA in peripheral blood mononuclear cells as an early marker for risk of progression to AIDS. Ann Intern Med 1995;123:641.
19. **19.** Centers for Disease Control and Prevention. Guidelines for preventing opportunistic infections among HIV-infected persons—2002. MMWR Recommendations and Reports 2002; 51(RR-08).

19a. Centers for Disease Control and Prevention. Update: adverse event data and revised American Thoracic Society/CDC recommendations against the use of rifampin and pyrazinamide for treatment of latent tuberculosis infection—United States, 2003. MMWR 2003;52:735.

20. **20.** French N, Nakiyingi J, Carpenter LM, et al. 23-Valent pneumococcal polysaccharide vaccine in HIV-1-infected Ugandan adults: double-blind, randomised and placebo controlled trial. Lancet 2000;355:2106.
21. Dworkin MS, Ward JW, Hanson DL, et al. Pneumococcal disease among human immunodeficiency virus-infected persons: incidence, risk factors, and impact of vaccination. Clin Infect Dis 2001;32:794.
22. **22.** Tasker SA, Treanor JJ, Paxton WB, et al. Efficacy of influenza vaccination in HIV-infected persons: a randomized double-blind, placebo controlled trial. Ann Intern Med 1999;131:430.
23. **23.** Pierce M, Crampton S, Henry D, et al. A randomized trial of clarithromycin as prophylaxis against disseminated MAC infection in patients with advanced acquired immunodeficiency syndrome. N Engl J Med 1996;335:384.
24. Spector SA, McKinley GF, Lalezari JP, et al. Oral ganciclovir for the prevention of cytomegalovirus disease in persons with AIDS. N Engl J Med 1996;334:1491.
25. Powderly WG, Finklestein DM, Feinberg J, et al. A randomized trial comparing fluconazole with clotrimazole troches for prevention of fungal infections in patients with advanced human immunodeficiency virus infection. N Engl J Med 1995;332:700.
26. **26.** United States Department of Health and Human Services. Guidelines for the use of antiretroviral agents in HIV-infected adults and adolescents. October 2005. Available at: AIDSinfo.gov.
27. **27.** Hirsch MS, Brun-Vezinet F, D'Aquila RT, et al. Antiretroviral drug resistance testing in adult HIV-1 infection: recommendations of an International AIDS Society-USA panel. JAMA 2000;283:2417.
28. McArthur JC, Sacktor N, Selnes O. Human immunodeficiency virus-associated dementia. Semin Neurol 1999;19:129.
29. Sulkowski MS, Thomas DL. Hepatitis C in the HIV-infected person. Ann Intern Med 2003; 138:197.
30. Kartalija M, Sande MA. Diarrhea and AIDS in the era of highly active antiretroviral therapy. Clin Infect Dis 1999;28:701.
31. Nemechek PM, Polsky B, Gottlieb MS. Treatment guidelines for HIV-associated wasting. Mayo Clin Proc 2000;75:386.
32. Dezube BJ. Acquired immunodeficiency syndrome-related Kaposi's sarcoma: clinical features, staging, and treatment. Semin Oncol 2000;27:424.
33. Whitcup SM. Cytomegalovirus retinitis in the era of highly active antiretroviral therapy. JAMA 2000;283:653.
34. Kimmel PL, Barisoni L, Kopp JB. Pathogenesis and treatment of HIV-associated renal diseases: lessons from clinical and animal studies, molecular pathologic correlations, and genetic investigations. Ann Intern Med 2003;139: 214.
35. Rerkpattanapipat P, Wongpraparut N, Jacobs LE, et al. Cardiac manifestations of acquired immunodeficiency syndrome. Arch Intern Med 2000;160:602.
36. Friis-Moller N, Sabin CA, Weber R, et al. Combination antiretroviral therapy and the risk of myocardial infarction. N Engl J Med 2003; 349:1993.

*Bold numerals denote published controlled clinical trials, meta-analyses, or consensus-based recommendations.

*For annotated **General References** and resources related to this chapter, visit www.hopkinsbayview.org/PAMreferences.*

Chapter 40

Ambulatory Care for Selected Infections Including Osteomyelitis, Lung Abscess, and Endocarditis

*Patrick A. Murphy**

Usually, the three types of infections reviewed in detail in this chapter are managed initially with intravenous antibiotics administered in the hospital. Patients with these infections are often seen first in an office setting, and the long courses of antimicrobials used to treat them are then completed after discharge from the hospital. These infections involve diverse bacteria and different anatomic sites but share a propensity for relapse caused by the persistence of bacteria at the infected site. This explains the requirement for prolonged courses of antimicrobial treatment. Antimicrobials may be administered by two different routes out of hospital: the oral route, to complete a course initiated parenterally during hospitalization, and the intravenous route, using the same regimen provided for inpatients and administered by home health agencies (see Gilbert et al., at www.hopkinsbayview.org./PAMreferences.).

*John G. Bartlett, MD, wrote this chapter in previous editions.

EXPANDING ROLE OF ORAL ANTIBIOTICS

In the past, there was reluctance to prescribe oral antimicrobials to be taken at home for most serious infections; however, this approach is gaining acceptance because of a number of studies indicating their efficacy (1–5). The advantages of home use of oral agents are patient convenience, the notable reduction in cost, and a reduction in nosocomial infections. Table 40.1 summarizes these and other considerations. Current estimates of the cost of hospital care that includes intravenous antimicrobials are about $1,000 per day, whereas for intravenous antimicrobials given at home the average charge is 300 to $400 per day and for oral agents the cost is 1 to $6 per day. The benefit of patient convenience is obvious. With regard to nosocomial infections, the cost in terms of morbidity, mortality, hospital lengths of stay, and charges is substantial (6). Of particular concern in recent years has been nosocomial acquisition of tuberculosis (especially the multiply resistant strains); *Clostridium difficile,* associated colitis, which is now recognized largely as a nosocomial complication; and Legionnaires disease. Hospitals also remain the major source of problem pathogens such as *Pseudomonas aeruginosa,* multiply resistant gram-negative bacilli, methicillin-resistant *Staphylococcus aureus* (MRSA), and vancomycin-resistant *Enterococcus.*

Some types of infectious diseases have traditionally been treated with parenteral antimicrobials but may sometimes be treated with oral agents: *P. aeruginosa* urinary

TABLE 40.1 Advantages and Disadvantages of Home Treatment with Oral Antimicrobial Agents

Advantages
Cost reduction
Patient convenience
Reduced nosocomial infections
Demonstrated efficacy
Disadvantages
Bioavailability
Need for supportive care or monitoring
Compliance
Possible legal liability
Selected infections that require parenteral agents
Serious side effects that require immediate care

tract infections (including bacterial prostatitis), pulmonary infections in patients with cystic fibrosis, some forms of osteomyelitis, tricuspid valve endocarditis caused by *S. aureus* in intravenous drug abusers, fever in the patient with neutropenia (see Chapter 10), some cases of pyelonephritis, most cases of pneumonia (see Chapter 33), and selected fungal infections that traditionally have required amphotericin B.

Newer Antimicrobial Agents

Much of the progress in this area has resulted from the development of oral antimicrobial agents in four classes that have an expanded spectrum of activity: cephalosporins, fluoroquinolones, β-lactam–β-lactamase inhibitor combinations, and the triazole antifungal agents. Among the *cephalosporins* and *carbacephams,* the agents with an expanded spectrum of activity for oral administration include cefaclor, cefuroxime axetil, cefprozil, cefpodoxime, loracarbef, and cefixime. All of these agents are active against most strains of Enterobacteriaceae; activity against major gram-positive cocci is variable, and none of these agents is active against *P. aeruginosa,* enterococci, or MRSA. In general, these drugs are advocated for respiratory tract infections, skin and soft tissue infections, and urinary tract infections. The *fluoroquinolones* include norfloxacin, ciprofloxacin, ofloxacin, gatifloxacin, moxifloxacin, and levofloxacin. There are slight differences among these agents in bioavailability, spectrum of activity, pharmacology, and side effects. In general, ciprofloxacin is favored for infections involving *P. aeruginosa*; levofloxacin, gatifloxacin, and moxifloxacin are preferred for infections in which *Streptococcus pneumoniae* is an established or suspected pathogen. *S. aureus* strains are developing resistance to the fluoroquinolones, and resistance to one implies resistance to the entire group. The only available oral *β-lactam–β-lactamase inhibitor* is amoxicillin plus clavulanate (Augmentin), which has effect against the spectrum of amoxicillin plus organisms that are penicillin-resistant because of β-lactamase production: *S. aureus,* many gram-negative bacilli, *Haemophilus influenzae,* and many anaerobes.

For oral treatment of serious anaerobic infections, either of two older drugs, metronidazole and clindamycin, is usually an option.

Newer Antifungal Agents

The triazoles—fluconazole, itraconazole and voricnazole —have supplanted amphotericin B for many fungal infections. All three are effective against most strains of *Candida albicans* and may be used for mucocutaneous candidiasis, but their use for parenchymal and systemic *Candida* infections is limited. Fluconazole has established efficacy for cryptococcosis. Itraconazole now appears to be the preferred agent for most cases of histoplasmosis, blastomycosis, and paracoccidioidomycosis and for many cases of coccidioidomycosis and aspergillosis.

RISKS AND BURDENS OF HOME TREATMENT

The use of oral agents in the home setting for infections traditionally treated with intravenous antibiotics in the hospital is not without some risks and burdens. Supportive care requiring some hospital resources for very sick patients is an example. Although monitoring of drug levels is rarely an issue with oral agents, compliance is always a concern, and physicians have been notoriously unable to predict which patients will take their medications (see Chapter 4). In many communities, this issue is now addressed for tuberculosis by direct observation of pill taking, although here the circumstances are somewhat different because antituberculosis drugs can be given twice weekly and the need is justified on the basis of public health concerns. Certain pathogens are difficult or impossible to treat with currently available oral agents. These include the fluoroquinolone-resistant strains of *P. aeruginosa,* many infections involving methicillin-resistant *S. aureus,* and cytomegalovirus (CMV). An additional concern about outpatient management is the fact that patients are not under direct observation, so emergency care is not immediately available for serious side effects. The major example is immunoglobulin E–mediated hypersensitivity caused by β-lactam agents, which occurs with a frequency of about 1:2,500 to 1:25,000 courses of penicillin G. Finally, there may be concern about legal liability when the use of oral antibiotics is not considered the standard of care, even if efficacy and safety seem well established. Because many third-party payers now mandate home care for stable patients who require long-term antibiotics, the latter concern is unlikely to deter expanded home treatment.

OSTEOMYELITIS

Definition

Osteomyelitis is an infection of bone. There are *four major categories:* osteomyelitis due to hematogenous spread of infection, osteomyelitis secondary to a contiguous focus of infection, infection of prosthetic joints, and osteomyelitis associated with vascular insufficiency. These four categories differ in terms of patient age, bones involved, predisposing conditions, usual bacterial pathogens, and presentation (Table 40.2). Osteomyelitis is also classified as *acute or chronic:* acute osteomyelitis indicates newly recognized bone infection, whereas chronic osteomyelitis indicates prior infection or clinical symptoms exceeding 10 days (3).

TABLE 40.2 Type of Osteomyelitis

	Hematogenous	*Secondary to Contiguous Infection*	*Complications of Vascular Insufficiency*
Approximate proportion of all cases (%)	20	50	30
Most common age groups	1–16 yr, >50 yr	Any age	>50 yr
Bones involved	Long bones (children) Vertebrae (adults)	Hip, femur, tibia, digits	Feet
Predisposing causes	Trauma Bacteremia	Surgery Soft tissue infection	Diabetes mellitus Vascular insufficiency
Usual bacteria	*Staphylococcus aureus* gram-negative bacilli	Often polymicrobial: gram-negative bacilli, *S. aureus*	Usually polymicrobial: gram-negative bacilli, anaerobes, streptococci, *S. aureus*
Presentation			
Initial episode	Fever, local pain swelling, tenderness, limited movement	Fever, local pain swelling, tenderness, limited movement	Ulceration drainage ± pain
Recurrent episode	Sinus drainage ± pain	Sinus drainage ± pain	Drainage ± pain

Clinical Presentation and Bacteriology

Hematogenous

Hematogenous osteomyelitis is classically described as a disease of *children,* usually younger than 16 years of age, which is usually caused by *S. aureus* (3). The tendency for this infection to occur during active growth reflects the enhanced susceptibility of the vascular network of the metaphysis, especially of the femur or tibia. About one third of the patients have a history of preceding nonpenetrating trauma in the area that is subsequently involved. The infection begins in the metaphyseal sinusoidal veins; it is contained by the epiphyseal growth plate and tends to spread laterally, with perforation of the cortex and lifting of the loose periosteum.

Hematogenous osteomyelitis of the long bones in *adults* is rare, different in presentation, and bacteriologically distinct. In these patients, the growth cartilage has been resorbed so that the subarticular space is more vulnerable, and the periosteum is firmly attached so that subperiosteal abscess formation is uncommon. The most common form of hematogenous osteomyelitis in adults involves the vertebrae (Fig. 40.1), and the most common pathogens are gram-negative bacilli and *S. aureus.* The initial site of infection is the richly vascularized bone adjacent to cartilage; there is subsequent involvement of adjacent bone plates and of the intervertebral disc. The infection may extend longitudinally to involve adjacent vertebrae, anteriorly to produce a paraspinal abscess, or posteriorly to form an epidural abscess.

Patients with acute hematogenous osteomyelitis usually present with precipitous onset of pain, swelling, chills, and fever. With vertebral osteomyelitis, there is fever with back pain, stiffness, and often point tenderness over the infected vertebra. Many patients have a more subacute presentation, with vague symptoms of 1 to 2 months' duration before presentation and few constitutional complaints. One well-described variant is the Brodie abscess (also called a cold abscess): subacute staphylococcal osteomyelitis located in the metaphysis of a long bone, which manifests with local pain and fever. Patients with recurrent or chronic osteomyelitis often simply note increased or persistent drainage and pain after an episode involving the same anatomic location.

Contiguous Infection

Osteomyelitis secondary to a contiguous focus of infection accounts for at least half of all cases. The most common precipitating factor is previous surgery, usually involving the lower extremities, such as open reduction of fractures of the femur or tibia. Next in frequency is a soft tissue infection involving the digits of the hands or feet. These infections usually become apparent within 1 month after the precipitating event, although many patients have chronic or recurrent infections that occur intermittently for years or decades.

Prosthetic Joint Infections

Infections that complicate prosthetic joints are classified as acute (within 12 weeks after surgery) or chronic (within 3 to 24 months after surgery) (3). Later infections may result from transient bacteremia in a fashion analogous to the pathogenesis of endocarditis, with the joint serving as a susceptible nidus. The presentation of an infected prosthesis is a painful, unstable joint, often with little or no fever and nonspecific radiographic findings. The diagnosis is best established with semiquantitative culture of an aspirate from the joint space or bone–cement interface.

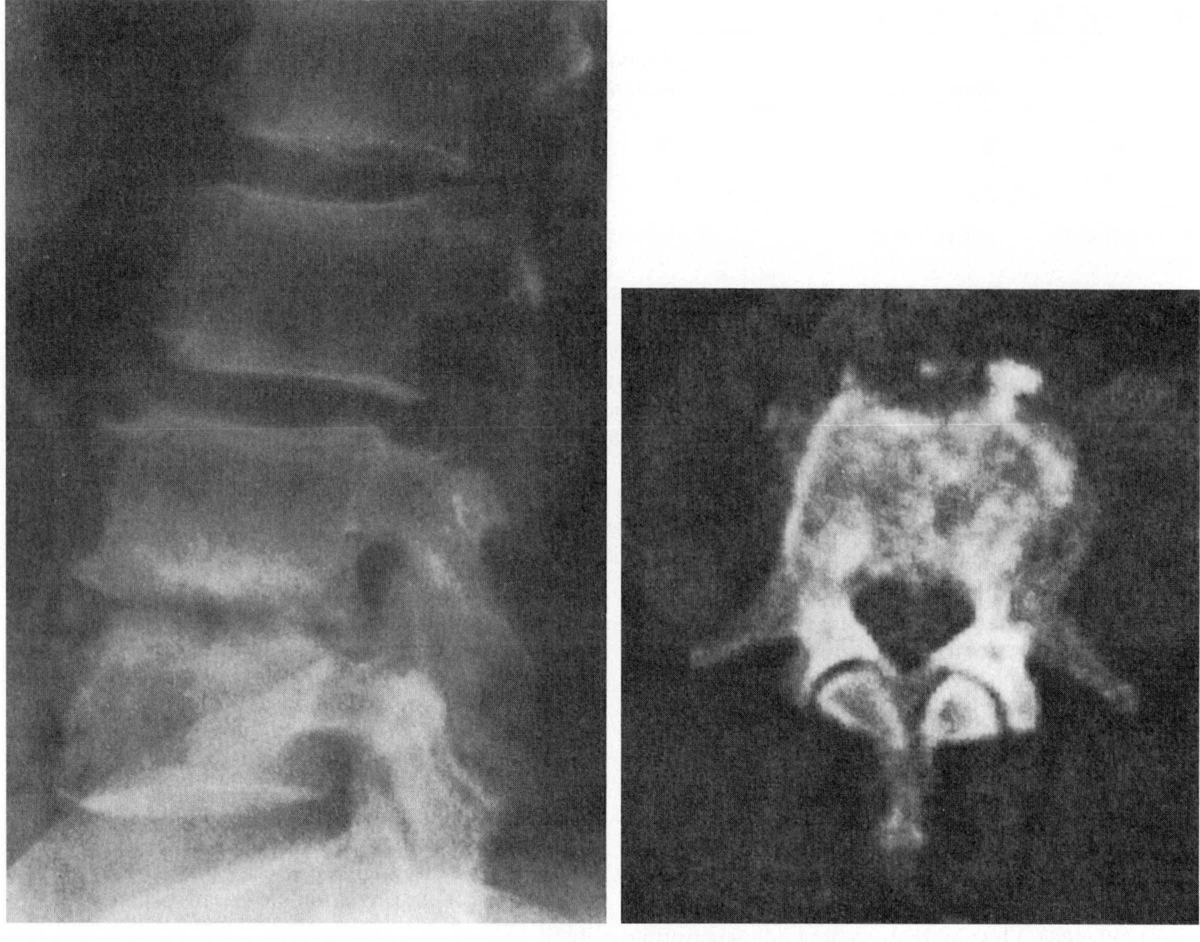

FIGURE 40.1. **A:** L3–4 staphylococcal osteomyelitis of 3 months' duration, with disc narrowing and sclerosis seen on plain film. **B:** Computed tomographic scan in same patient showing small soft tissue abscess and minimal bone destruction. Note hazy bone outline (From Post MJD, ed. Computed tomography of the spine. Baltimore: Williams & Wilkins, 1984:740.)

Staphylococcus epidermidis accounts for 75% of cases; next in frequency are *S. aureus,* streptococci, *Peptococcus magnus,* enteric gram-negative bacilli, and *Candida* species.

Vascular Insufficiency

Osteomyelitis associated with vascular insufficiency is most common in patients with diabetes mellitus or severe atherosclerosis (7,8). The most common sites of infection are the toes and small bones of the feet, usually with overlying soft tissue infections (Fig. 40.2). These infections are often detected on routine radiographs performed to evaluate the chronic draining sinuses or skin ulcers that are so common in the patients at risk. Probing that demonstrates extension of ulcers to bone is essentially diagnostic of osteomyelitis, and this finding supersedes all scanning techniques in terms of specificity (7,8). Both the adjacent soft tissue infection and the osteomyelitis usually involve *polymicrobial flora* that may include anaerobic bacteria, coliforms, pseudomonads, streptococci, and *S. aureus.*

Laboratory Evaluation

Diagnostic studies include radiographs, radionuclide studies, computed tomography (CT), or magnetic resonance imaging (MRI) to demonstrate typical bone changes and cultures to identify the etiologic organism.

The earliest changes on plain radiographs are lytic lesions; other findings may include soft tissue swelling, periosteal reaction, cortical irregularity, demineralization, and sequestrum formation. However, typical changes are not visible on plain films until 30% to 50% of the bone has been resorbed, and this usually requires 10 to 14 days. In a patient with a normal plain film but clinical findings suggesting osteomyelitis, a technetium bone scan or an ^{111}Indium leukocyte scan can be helpful. Both of these

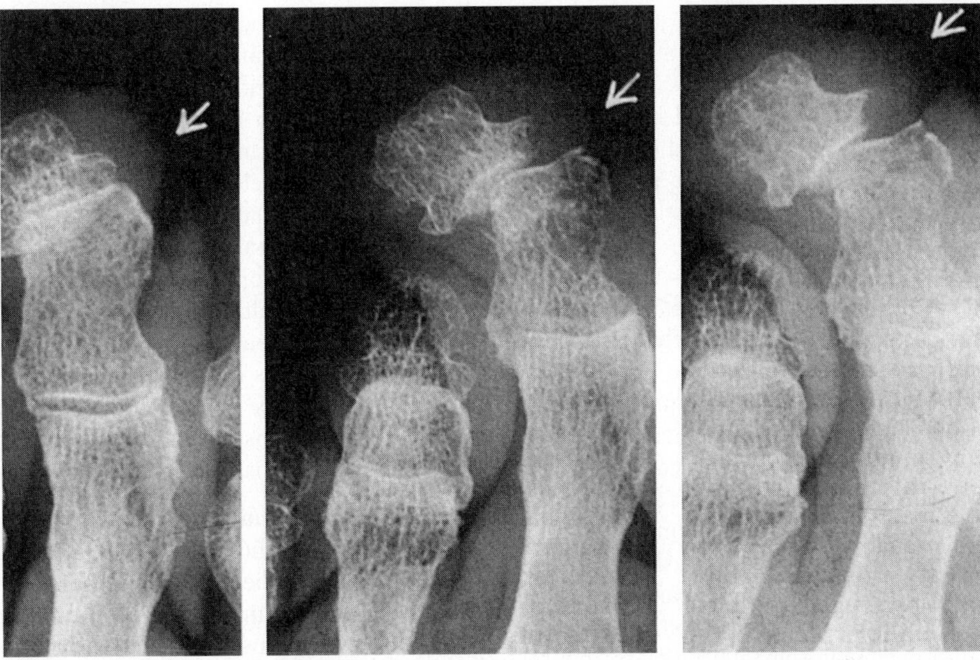

FIGURE 40.2. Arrows indicate, from left to right, infected soft corn, sinus tract, and osteomyelitis in the distal interphalangeal joint. As destruction increases, the joint becomes dislocated. (From Gamble FO, Yale I. Clinical foot roentgenology. Baltimore: Williams & Wilkins, 1966.)

tests are sensitive in early osteomyelitis (70% to 90%), but they lack specificity (50% to 75%) (3,9,10). The bone scan uses technetium ^{99}Tc as a marker bound to diphosphonate, which concentrates in bone because of incorporation at sites of osteoblastic activity. Abnormal studies may occur when there is increased blood flow associated with soft tissue infections or with osteoblastic activity caused by other processes, such as degenerative joint disease. If a three-phase technetium scan (immediate, showing flow; 15-minute, showing blood pooling; and 4-hour showing bone imaging) is used, soft tissue infections give positive images in the first two phases but only bony infection gives positive images in all three phases. Most authorities regard ^{99}Tc scanning as the preferred scintigraphic method (9,11). CT and MRI are also useful in showing osteomyelitis. CT scans are especially helpful for guiding needle biopsy or percutaneous aspirations. MRI is quite sensitive and may show osteomyelitis before changes are evident by scintigraphy (3). Prosthetic material that is ferromagnetic is a contraindication to MRI, but most materials now used in orthopedic surgery do not interfere.

Because antimicrobial treatment, often prolonged, is the mainstay of management, accurate bacteriologic data are helpful for making the diagnosis and planning treatment. The list of possible organisms is long, and sensitivity patterns for these organisms show considerable variation, making empiric selection of antimicrobials hazardous. These considerations may justify an aggressive attempt to identify the responsible organism. Conclusive bacteriologic studies require isolation of the pathogen from bone or blood cultures.

Under ideal circumstances, an orthopedist should perform a *needle aspiration* over the involved bone, either blindly or, preferably, under CT guidance (12). If subperiosteal pus is obtained, surgical drainage is mandatory. If no pus is obtained, the needle is inserted into bone to obtain a specimen. The diagnostic yield with a needle aspirate of bone is approximately 60%, and for a surgical biopsy it is approximately 90% (3). Cultures from draining sinus tracts tend to show poor correlation with cultures obtained directly from bone (12). Needle aspirate specimens should be submitted for Gram stain and for culture of aerobic and anaerobic bacteria. Care must be exercised in the interpretation of culture results, even of bone aspirates, because these are often contaminated, especially if the specimen is obtained by traversing soft-tissue infections (13). Organisms recovered in low concentrations, especially those growing only in the broth culture, must be viewed with skepticism. Common skin contaminants include *S. epidermidis*, diphtheroids, and *Propionibacterium*. These organisms tend to cause osteomyelitis only in the presence of prosthetic devices. Gram staining of exudate or tissue aspirate should verify the culture results and represents an important correlate in determining the etiologic organism. The semiquantitative results of cultures are an important and often overlooked component of interpreting culture results, especially when the organisms detected are common contaminants.

Treatment

General Principles

Immobilization was commonly advocated for the treatment of osteomyelitis in the pre–antimicrobial era. However, it appears to be less important at present, and most authorities conclude that strict immobilization is unnecessary.

Antimicrobial Treatment: Acute Osteomyelitis

For newly diagnosed or acute osteomyelitis, the standard recommendation has been a 3- to 6-week course of parenteral antimicrobials (3). This recommendation is based on several studies noting that patients often developed recurrent or chronic disease when treatment lasted less than 21 days. The standard regimen for acute staphylococcal osteomyelitis in adults is a penicillinase-resistant penicillin such as nafcillin, given intravenously at a dosage of 1.5 to 2 g every 6 hours. Alternative parenteral regimens are cefazolin (1.0 to 1.5 g every 8 hours), vancomycin (1 g every 12 hours), or clindamycin (600 mg every 8 hours) (3). In stable patients, these regimens can be initiated in the hospital and completed at home.

To decrease cost, length of hospitalization, and patient discomfort, a *modified regimen,* consisting of a short course of parenteral antimicrobials followed by a prolonged course of oral agents, has been developed (3). The intravenous antimicrobial is given for at least 3 days, or until the patient is afebrile, or for an arbitrarily defined period such as 1 to 2 weeks. An alternative oral agent selected by *in vitro* sensitivity tests is then taken by mouth, usually at home, to complete a total 3- to 6-week course, usually 4 weeks. The drugs recommended for oral administration are clindamycin (300 mg every 6 hours), an oral antistaphylococcal penicillin such as dicloxacillin or cephalexin (500 mg every 6 hours), or a fluoroquinolone. It should be noted that the importance of bactericidal activity and the relative merits of drugs for bone penetration as factors in drug selection are debated issues that remain unresolved.

Antimicrobial Treatment: Chronic Osteomyelitis

Therapeutic guidelines are less precise for chronic osteomyelitis. Because necrotic bone may serve as a nidus for sequestered bacteria, surgical excision of dead tissue and adequate debridement are often essential components of treatment. Antimicrobial selection should be based on bacteriologic diagnosis using deep aspirates or, preferably, cultures obtained from bone. The daily dosage, route of administration, and duration of treatment are somewhat arbitrary, but most authorities recommend prolonged courses. The initial treatment may consist of parenteral antimicrobials for 1 to 3 months in the hospital or in the home, followed by oral agents for several months. An alternative approach is the use, from the outset of treatment, of oral agents to which the patient's infecting organism is sensitive, for extended periods, such as 6 months or longer (3). Fluoroquinolones such as ofloxacin or ciprofloxacin, alone or in combination with clindamycin or metronidazole, have established efficacy for osteomyelitis with a mixed anaerobic–coliform flora (3). Oral cephalosporins may also be used for infections involving gram negative bacilli; metronidazole by mouth is preferred for oral treatment of deep infections involving anaerobes, although clindamycin and amoxicillin–clavulanate (Augmentin) are probably effective as well. A variety of dosages of these drugs have been proposed; guidelines should be sought in published reports or the most current editions of manuals on the use of antibiotics for specific infections.

Unconfirmed Infections

Many patients who appear to have osteomyelitis or infections of orthopedic devices need a considerable amount of improvised treatment. It is not uncommon to have a patient present with subacute backache, fever, and leukocytosis, and to be unable to establish a bacteriological diagnosis by blood cultures, needle punctures, or cultures of operative specimens, even though the patient may have evidence of bony destruction with local abscess formation. If the patient is an intravenous drug user, it may be assumed that the cause is MRSA, and appropriate treatment should be initiated. In a patient who does not self-inject, *S. aureus* is still the most common cause of spinal osteomyelitis, although most such strains are not MRSA. The effect of therapy may be monitored indirectly by following changes in the evidence of inflammation. Fever, leukocytosis and local pain should improve. Neurologic signs should not develop, nor should they progress if already present. The erythrocyte sedimentation rate (ESR) and C-reactive protein (CRP) should steadily fall; the hematocrit value and the serum albumin should steadily rise. If these changes occur, the diagnosis can be presumed to be correct. If not, other diagnoses should be considered.

Empiric treatment is also commonly required for osteomyelitis of the foot bones in diabetics, chronic osteomyelitis of limb bones (usually old compound fracture sites), and infections of orthopedic hardware such as metal plates and artificial joints. In all of these cases, a bacteriologic diagnosis may not be forthcoming despite the usual investigations including operative exploration. If the patient had an earlier infectious episode in which an organism was isolated, it is usually safe to assume that the same organism has recurred. If there is no information at all, then one must guess at an etiology, and monitor treatment empirically, as above.

Late Complications

The major complication of osteomyelitis is recurrence that may happen months, years, or decades after the initial

Chapter 41

International Medicine: Care of Travelers and Foreign-Born Patients

Stephen D. Sears and Nathaniel W. James, IV

CARE OF TRAVELERS

International travel is increasing in popularity. Americans are visiting exotic locales and trekking to increasingly remote regions of the world. It is now estimated that 25 to 40 million Americans travel by air to foreign countries each year. Many others take boats, cruises, or cars to Canada and Mexico. Of these millions, it is estimated that 4 to 8 million journey to developing areas of the world where they encounter infectious diseases that are uncommon in developed countries. Malaria, schistosomiasis, yellow fever, polio, typhoid fever, and amebiasis are just a few of the diseases that are more prevalent in tropical developing countries. Many travelers make little or no provision for the prevention of illness while traveling. This is unfortunate because the overall attack rate for several infectious diseases is much higher in international travelers than it is in comparable populations that remain at home (1). This fact is well illustrated by the results of a study of Swiss travelers that found that three-fourths had at least one symptom of infectious illness while traveling; of the 16,500 travelers surveyed in this study, more than 30% had at least one episode of a diarrheal illness. In a followup study, not only were travelers found to have illnesses while traveling, but almost one-third became ill within a month of returning home. Another study of 2,000 travelers returning to the United Kingdom found that 43% became ill during or shortly after their journeys (2). In another review, 75% of travelers did not take sufficient basic precautions against infection (3).

These studies offer a small glimpse into the medical problems of travelers. Even so, there is no reliable measurement of the amount or severity of disease encountered by the traveler. Only a portion of the most dramatic cases of illness in travelers, such as malaria, Lassa fever, or African trypanosomiasis, are usually reported to public health authorities. For instance, outbreaks of leptospirosis (4) and coccidiomycosis (5) only came to light well after the travel-related exposures. Additionally, new illnesses such as severe acute respiratory syndrome (SARS) and avian influenza emphasize the need for global surveillance and a continued review of updated reports on emerging infections. At present, there is no mechanism for obtaining accurate surveillance data on the occurrence of illness in American travelers, nor are there data on significant risk factors for acquiring infectious diseases. This lack of data hampers scientific investigation of interventional strategies in travelers. Even so, significant progress has been made in the prevention of malaria, traveler's diarrhea, and diseases for which immunizations exist.

To prevent unnecessary illness, it is imperative that travelers undertake appropriate *pretrip health planning*. When approached by a person about to embark upon an international journey, it is important for the clinician to ascertain several key aspects of the proposed trip. *Where are you going? Where will you stay? What is the purpose of your trip? Where will you be eating? In restaurants or in private homes? Is sex with other travelers or local residents likely?* With this information, one can categorize the types and magnitude of risk. A business person staying for a short time in a first-class hotel in a large city in a developing country has different risks than does a college student who will be living in villages in several developing countries. Most travelers fit somewhere between these two extremes, and a travel consultation must be individualized to fit the traveler's lifestyle, itinerary, medical history, use of medications, allergies, and previous immunizations.

There are several *sources for current recommendations.* Immunizations, malaria prevention, food and water safety, diarrhea, schistosomiasis, and a number of general health hazards are topics that should be discussed with the traveler. Two useful resources that are updated yearly provide practical information on these issues: *Health Information for International Travel,* published by the U.S. Public Health Service (available from the Centers for Disease Control and Prevention, Atlanta, GA 30333) and *Vaccination*

Certificate Requirements for International Travel and Health Advice to Travelers, published by the World Health Organization (WHO) (available from WHO Publication Center, 49 Sheridan Ave., Albany, NY 12210). Other valuable resources include the International Association for Medical Assistance to Travelers (IAMAT, 1623 Military #279, Niagara Falls, NY 14304-1745, telephone 716-754-4883), which provides information on tropical diseases and a list of English-speaking physicians overseas, and the Centers for Disease Control and Prevention (CDC) Traveler's Information Hotline (404-332-4559; will fax current information on all regions).

Additionally, *travel medicine websites* have proliferated. At least 65 websites cover a variety of topics, including consumer advice, professional societies, outbreak updates, traveling with chronic illnesses, epidemiology of infectious diseases, and consumer products. For a partial listing, see Table 41.1.

Immunizations

Vaccines are now available against a number of the major viral and bacterial diseases encountered in developing areas. For patients traveling to these areas, it is necessary to administer travel-specific vaccines and to update primary vaccines (Table 41.2). Immunizations can be broadly separated into those that are legally required and those that are recommended. *Legally required vaccinations* are public health measures that certain countries demand before entry, to benefit the country as a whole, whereas *recommended immunizations* are designed to benefit only the patient. No vaccines are legally required to enter or return to the United States. However, many countries have strict entry requirements, and travelers who arrive without proper vaccination certificates may be denied entry, quarantined, or possibly vaccinated at the point of entry. Therefore, it is important to determine what vaccines are required before beginning a journey (6).

Currently, the only legally required vaccination is for yellow fever, and each country has its own requirements. In the past, smallpox and cholera vaccinations were required by many countries, but in 1980, the WHO declared the global eradication of smallpox, and on January 1, 1982, smallpox was deleted from the list of diseases subject to regulation. Although cholera vaccination is not endorsed by the WHO for entry into any country, some local authorities may still require proof of cholera vaccination, especially if the traveler is arriving from endemic areas.

Yellow Fever

Yellow fever, once almost controlled, has made a dramatic resurgence (7). Although generally rare in travelers, two yellow fever deaths in Americans visiting the Amazon Basin were recently reported. Yellow fever vaccine, containing a live attenuated strain of the yellow fever virus, is one of the most important and effective vaccines. It is required by some countries before travelers are allowed

TABLE 41.1 Travel-Related Websites

	Website
Authoritative travel medicine recommendations	
CDC Yellow Book	http://www.cdc.gov/travel/yb/outline.htm
CDC Travel's Health	http://www.cdc.gov/travel/index.htm
CDC Travel Notices	http://www.cdc.gov/travel/outbreaks.htm
Health Canada Online	www.hc-sc.gc.ca
Pan American Health Organization	www.paho.org/
Databases for travel medicine practitioners	
American Society of Travel Medicine and Hygiene	www.astmh.org
The Medical Letter	www.medicalletter.com
Shoreland's Travel Health Online	www.tripprep.com
Consumer websites	
Medical Advisory Services for Travelers Abroad	www.masta.org
International Society of Travel Medicine	www.istm.org
Travax Pre Travel Advice	www.shoreland.com
Medical assistance for overseas travelers	
International Association for Medical Assistance to Travelers	www.iamat.org
International Federation of Red Cross and Red Crescent Societies	www.ifrc.org
U.S. State Department	www.state.gov
World Health Organization	www.who.int/en/

CDC, Centers for Disease Control and Prevention.

TABLE 41.2 Vaccines and Immune Globulin for International Travel

Vaccine/Immune Globulin	Patient Age	Route	Dose	Booster	Comments
Yellow fever	> 9 mo	s.c.	0.5 mL	0.5 mL q10yr	May be required.
Cholera	6 mo–4 yr	s.c. or i.m	0.2 mL	0.2 mL q6mo	May be required.
	5–10 yr		0.3 mL	0.3 mL q6mo	Limited efficacy.
	>10 yr		0.5 mL	0.5 mL q6mo	
Typhoid parenteral	< 10 yr	s.c.	0.25 mL	0.25 mL q3yr	Local reactions common.
	>10 yr		0.50 mL	0.5 mL q3yr	
Typhoid oral (TY21a)	> 1 yr	Oral	1 dose q.o.d. × 4	Repeat series q5yr	Keep refrigerated, avoid antibiotics.
Typhoid parenteral (ViCPS)	≥2 yr	i.m.	0.5 mL	2 yr	Well tolerated.
Poliomyelitis					
OPV	All ages	Oral	3 doses	1 dose pretravel	IPV is preferable for adults.
IPV	All ages	s.c.	3 doses	1 dose q10yr	
Japanese encephalitis	< 3 yr	s.c.	0.5 mL	1 dose at 1 and 4 yr	Delayed allergic reactions.
	> 3 yr		1.0 mL		
Hepatitis A					
Havrix	2–17 yr	i.m.	0.5 mL × 2	6–12 mo then 10 yr	Consider screening for anti-HAV in frequent travelers.
	> 17 yr	i.m.	1 mL × 2	6–12 mo then 10 yr	
Vaqta	2–17 yr	i.m.	0.5 mL × 2	6–12 mo then 10 yr	
	> 17 yr	i.m.	1 mL × 2	6–12 mo then 10 yr	
Immune globulin (short term <3 mo)	< 23 kg	i.m.	0.5 mL	—	Immune globulin is used for prophylaxis of hepatitis A; consider screening for anti-HAV in frequent travelers.
	23–45 kg		1.0 mL	—	
	> 45 kg		2.0 mL	—	
Tetanus-diphtheria	>7 yr	i.m.	3 doses	1 dose q10yr	Always use combined vaccine.
Mennomune	>2 yr	i.m.	0.5 mL	Unclear	For specific areas of travel.
Menactra	>3 yr	i.m.	0.5 mL	Unclear	For specific areas of travel.
Rabies	All ages	i.m.	1.0 mL (3 doses)	1 dose q2yr	Still requires postexposure treatment.
		i.d.	0.1 mL (3 doses)	1 dose q2yr	i.d. only approved for HDCV.
Hepatitis B	All ages	i.m.	1.0 mL (3 doses)	Unclear	Protection lasts 5–7 yr.

OPV, oral polio vaccine; IPV, inactivated polio vaccine; HDCV, human diploid cell vaccine.

entrance, particularly when areas to be visited are endemic for yellow fever and when travelers have recently left a country endemic for yellow fever. If yellow fever exists in the country of destination, the traveler should be vaccinated regardless of the regulations of the country (Figs. 41.1 and 41.2).

The vaccine is nontoxic and induces long-lasting immunity. Although the yellow fever vaccine is quite safe, there have been recent reports of rare adverse effects. Therefore, the vaccine should only be given to travelers who will be at risk for yellow fever. Mild reactions occur in 1% to 5% of patients. These include mild headache, myalgia, low-grade fever, or other minor symptoms 5 to 10 days after inoculation.

Because yellow fever vaccine is a live attenuated virus, it could pose a risk to pregnant women, although teratogenicity has not been encountered. Pregnant women who must travel to areas endemic for yellow fever should be vaccinated. It is presumed that the unknown but small risk to the fetus is less than the risk to the mother. If at all possible, the trip should be postponed until after delivery. The vaccine is contraindicated in immunocompromised patients, including patients with acquired immunodeficiency syndrome with CD4 counts below 200. Because the vaccine strain is grown in chick embryo culture, it should not be given to travelers with known hypersensitivity to eggs. Yellow fever immunization is also discouraged in children younger than 9 months of age because of neurotoxicity in infants.

Yellow fever vaccine is available only through official yellow fever vaccine centers; locations of these centers can be obtained by calling the local health department. The dose of vaccine is 0.5 mL subcutaneously. It must be given within 1 hour of reconstitution and should be stored at 41°F (5°C) until it is reconstituted. The vaccine gives solid immunity for at least 10 years. If it is contraindicated for a traveler to receive yellow fever vaccine for any of the above reasons, a detailed letter explaining the contraindications should be provided to the traveler.

Cholera

Since January 1991, more than a million cases of cholera have occurred in South and Central America, and cholera occurs in nearly all developing countries. Additionally, a new cholera epidemic erupted in India in 1992 with a

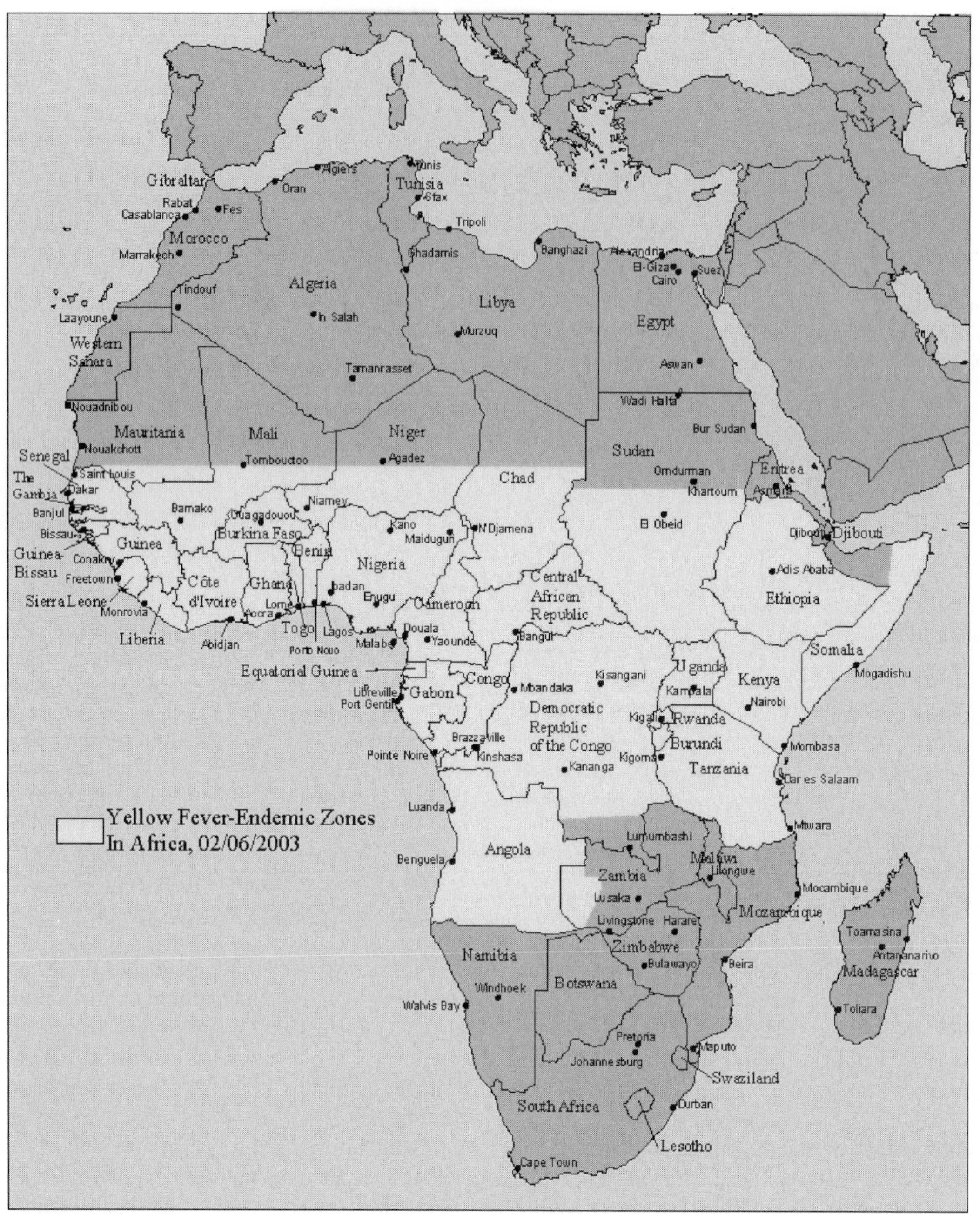

FIGURE 41.1. Yellow fever endemic zone in Africa. (From Centers for Disease Control and Prevention. Health Information for International Travel, 2003–2004, DHHS, Atlanta, GA, with permission.)

non-01 *Vibrio cholerae* strain (0-139) and has spread rapidly (8). Even so, the risk to travelers remains low, especially for those who use caution in food and water acquisition. In 1973, the World Health Assembly recommended discontinuing required vaccination against cholera. By 1992, all countries had officially discontinued this requirement, but a few in Africa still have unofficial requirements at certain border crossings for travelers coming from areas endemic for cholera. Thus, there is still some possibility of difficulty at borders unless a certificate of vaccination is obtained. Unless the vaccine is legally required, the killed whole cell injectable vaccine is discouraged because it causes excessive local inflammation and is not warranted considering the low risk.

Travelers in countries outside the United States may wish to take one of the new safe *oral cholera vaccines* if they travel to high-risk areas. Two recently developed vaccines for cholera are licensed and available in other countries

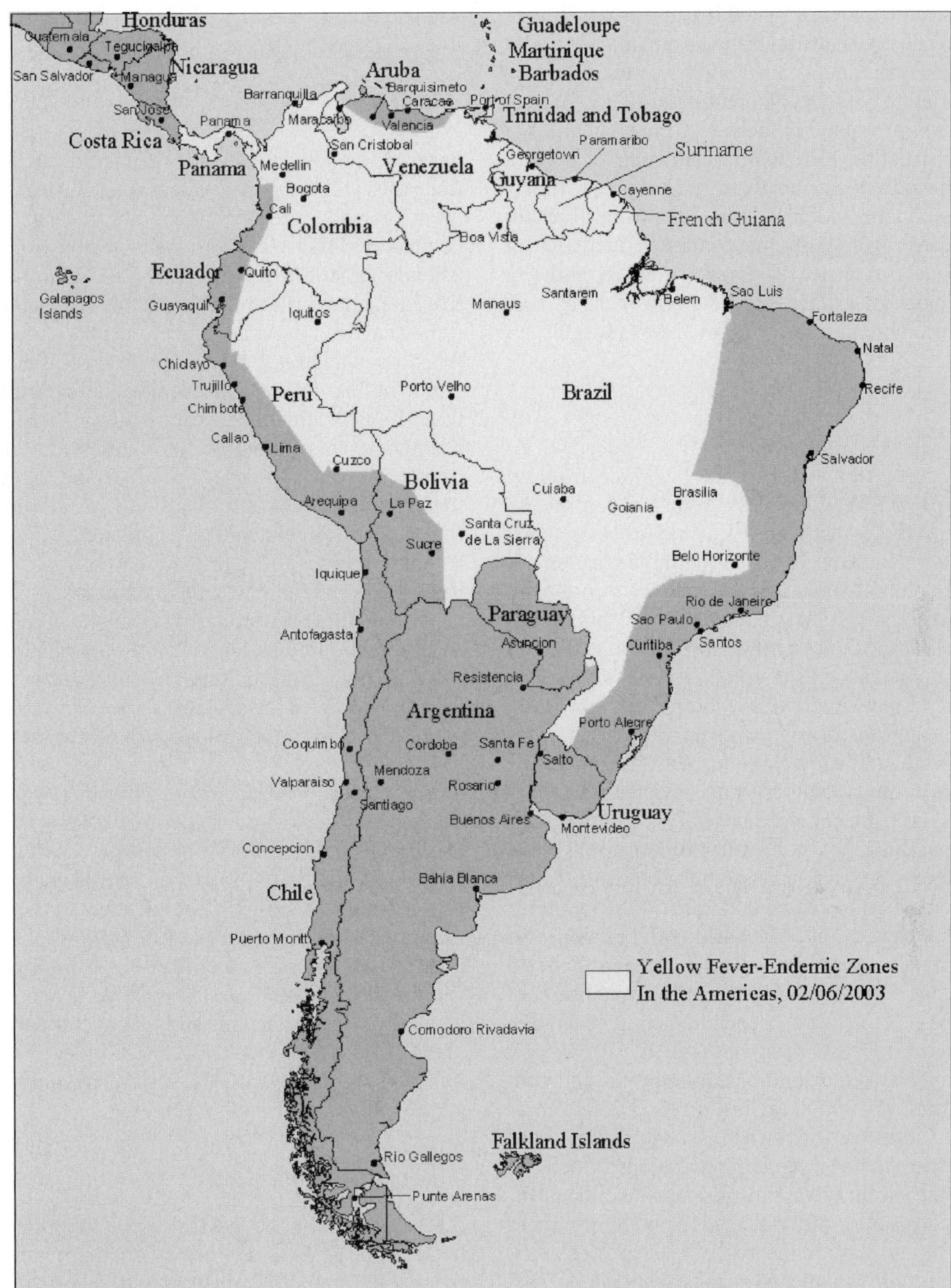

FIGURE 41.2. Yellow fever endemic zone in the Americas. (From Centers for Disease Control and Prevention. Health Information for International Travel, 2003–2004, DHHS, Atlanta, GA, with permission.)

(Dukoral from Biotec AB and Mutacol from Berna). Both vaccines appear to provide somewhat better immunity and have fewer side effects than the parenteral vaccine. Of note, no vaccines presently provide protection against the 0-139 strain. For travelers following usual tourist routes and using standard precautions in countries endemic for cholera, the estimated attack rate is less than 1 per 100,000 returning travelers, but recent studies in Japanese travelers suggest that the rate of cholera infection may be much higher than previously assumed (9). The estimated rates are likely to be significantly underestimated because many cholera episodes may be not be distinguished from other episodes of traveler's diarrhea, and being treated overseas, they may not be reported to the CDC. Nonetheless, rather than recommend immunization routinely, clinicians should emphatically instruct travelers to areas endemic for cholera not to eat uncooked vegetables, to use caution with undercooked seafood, and always to drink boiled water or bottled beverages. With the continued increases in the worldwide prevalence of cholera coupled with reported antibiotic resistance, the new oral vaccines may become a recommended strategy for travelers in the future (10).

Typhoid Fever

Typhoid fever remains a danger for high-risk travelers; more than 70% of the 2,445 cases reported to the CDC in the United States between 1985 and 1994 occurred after international travel (11). Areas with the greatest risk are parts of South America and the Indian subcontinent, although the risk is present in almost all developing countries. *Salmonella typhi* is transmitted by the ingestion of fecally contaminated food and water. Typhoid vaccination, although not legally required, is recommended for travelers who are likely to stray off the usual tourist route, stay in small villages, and eat local food. With the increasing prevalence of antimicrobial resistance to *S. typhi,* vaccination takes on even greater significance.

Typhoid vaccines have been available for over 100 years. Two vaccines currently are licensed for protection against typhoid fever: a live attenuated oral vaccine (Ty21a), and a newly licensed capsular polysaccharide parenteral vaccine (ViCPS, Typhim Vi). The older heat-phenol-inactivated parenteral vaccine has been discontinued. The efficacy of these vaccines is 60% to 70% depending on the degree of subsequent exposure. Ty21a is a mutant of *S. typhi* that produces enough endotoxin to be immunogenic and nonpathogenic and has limited replication. Ty21a is taken as four separate doses over 7 days; it must be refrigerated and is well tolerated, although abdominal cramps sometimes occur with the vaccine. The capsules may be difficult for some to swallow, are contraindicated in children younger than 6 years, and have a theoretical risk in pregnancy, immunocompromised patients, or those with altered gastrointestinal (GI) function. Antibiotics should not be taken during the week that the oral vaccine is being administered.

Typhim Vi is composed of purified Vi (Virulence) antigen, the capsular polysaccharide produced by *S. typhi.* Primary vaccination with ViCPS consists of one 0.5-mL (25-mg) dose given intramuscularly with boosters every 2 to 3 years. It is safe for immunocompromised travelers, is well tolerated, and is not affected by concurrent antibiotics. The vaccine is not recommended for children younger than 2 years of age because of poor immunogenicity at this age.

Polio

Paralytic poliomyelitis had been eradicated from the Americas (12), and in developing countries outside the Americas polio rates are falling, but travelers should still be protected. Travelers who have previously completed a primary series with either the Sabin (oral, live) or Salk (parental, inactivated) vaccine should have a booster dose if they have not previously received a booster as an adult. A history of at least three doses of oral polio vaccine (OPV, Sabin) or four doses of inactivated polio vaccine (IPV, Salk) with IPV boosters each 5 years until age 18 is evidence of adequate primary immunization. Such fully immunized people need only one dose of polio vaccine before traveling to high-risk areas. If a traveler is only partially immunized, the primary series should be completed.

Adults who require a primary series should receive IPV. Recently, a new IPV of enhanced potency has been released (eIPV). IPV is preferred in adults because the risk of OPV-associated paralysis is somewhat higher in adults than in children. If children are not already vaccinated, they should receive a primary series. New guidelines for primary polio immunization with eIPV rather than OPV have just been released. If an unimmunized adult traveler does not have time to complete a primary IPV series before departure, a single dose of OPV may offer reasonable protection. On return, primary immunization with IPV should be completed. Live (OPV) vaccine should not be given routinely to women known to be pregnant, although teratogenicity has not been shown. If the risk of polio is significant and the pregnant woman is unimmunized, primary vaccination with IPV would be prudent. Because OPV is a live virus, immunocompromised patients and their families should not receive OPV; instead they should be immunized with IPV. Table 41.2 summarizes information regarding dosages for polio vaccines.

Tetanus and Diphtheria

Tetanus occurs worldwide but is slightly more common in the tropics. Many adults may not be protected against tetanus (13), so it is important to keep tetanus immunization up to date in travelers. Boosters must be given every 10 years regardless of age. Travelers, if they injure themselves, are less likely to seek medical help, so adequate pretravel immunization becomes more important. Diphtheria is endemic in many developing countries and is currently epidemic in the countries of the former Soviet Union. Most cases occur in unimmunized or partially immunized people. Therefore, routine immunization with tetanus-diphtheria rather than with tetanus toxoid alone should be given. For primary immunization, patients older than 7 years should receive three doses of tetanus-diphtheria. (Before age 7, the primary immunizing agent is the diphtheria-pertussis-tetanus combination.) The first doses are 1 to 2 months apart and the third 6 to 12 months later. Local reactions may occur within 12 to 48 hours after vaccination. Severe local reactions can occur in adults if the booster is given within a short time of the previous vaccine. The only contraindication to tetanus-diphtheria is a history of hypersensitivity reactions after immunization.

Varicella

A live attenuated vaccine against varicella virus (chickenpox) was released in the mid-1990s. Varicella occurs worldwide, is highly contagious, and can be severe in adults. The primary series in childhood is a single dose of vaccine, and in those older than 12 years, it is two doses given 1 month apart. Long-term travelers should be immune; if immune status is not known, serologic testing may be indicated. The vaccine is contraindicated in pregnant women and those with compromised immunity.

Hepatitis A

Hepatitis A (HA) continues to be an important risk for travelers to many areas of the developing world and is the most common vaccine-preventable disease of travelers. Although the risk is less for people who travel on ordinary tourist routes and stay for short periods, it may be considerable for those who bypass the tourist routes and stay for extended periods. HA illness may be asymptomatic but can also be severe, with jaundice and significant morbidity. Protection against HA is strongly recommended for international travelers to developing areas (14). Although immune globulin provides passive protection against HA for a few months and is safe and effective, HA vaccine (active immunization) is generally preferred for most travelers. Two vaccines are licensed, Havrix (SKF) and Vaqta (Merck), and both prevent approximately 90% of expected HA infections. A new combination vaccine for HA and hepatitis B (HB) is also available (see Hepatitis B). Travelers to HA-endemic areas should ideally receive the first dose of vaccine at least 1 month before travel. Recent evidence suggests that vaccine is protective even when given immediately before a trip, although protective antibodies may not be measurable. Immune globulin is less expensive and is still a reasonable choice for travelers making only one trip who need limited (up to 3 months) HA protection. For travelers leaving immediately, administering both immune globulin and HA vaccine is both safe and effective.

The recommended schedules for both Havrix and Vaqta include a primary immunization for all patients and a booster in 6 to 12 months for patients 2 to 18 years of age. A booster for travelers over 18 ensures optimal long-term protection. The dosage of immune globulin may be based on weight, but for adults injection of 2 mL for stays of less than 3 months is adequate in practice. HA vaccines are well tolerated and adverse events are rare. The only side effect of immune globulin is muscle soreness at the injection site. Immune globulins for intramuscular injection prepared in the United States carry no risk of transmission of human immunodeficiency virus (HIV) or other infectious agents, but those produced in developing countries should not be used. Pregnancy is not a contraindication to immune globulin. Screening for anti-HA virus in frequent travelers should also be considered.

Hepatitis B

HB vaccination is now recommended for all infants and adolescents. Although the risk of HB is generally low for the routine traveler, this may be an opportunity to provide this important vaccine. Health care workers who are likely to have contact with blood or secretions from patients in areas endemic for HB should receive the HB vaccine. Travelers who will live for more than 6 months in countries with a high prevalence of HB antigenemia should also be strongly considered for vaccination. The prevalence of HB virus carriers is 5% to 15% in sub-Saharan Africa and Southeast Asia, including China and Indonesia, and 1% to 5% in North Africa, South Central Asia, and Southern Europe. Because HB can be transmitted through sexual contact, travelers should be counseled appropriately when going to endemic areas. Vaccination or HB immune globulin prophylaxis may be appropriate for people who are likely to have sexual contacts. Primary adult vaccination consists of three intramuscular doses of 1 mL of vaccine. The first two doses are given 1 month apart, and the third dose should be given 6 months later. This is often difficult in travelers, and accelerated vaccine schedules have been defined and may be useful for travelers with high exposure risks (see additional details in Chapter 18). A combination vaccine (Twinrix, GlaxoSmithKline) may be given to travelers who need to be protected against HA and HB, as long as there is time to provide two doses (1 month apart) before departure. It is not approved for children.

Rabies

Rabies remains uncontrolled in many areas of the developing world, but the risk to short-term travelers is low (15). Rabies transmission occurs when the rabies virus is introduced into open cuts or wounds, usually through the bite of an infected animal, so counseling on avoidance of animal bites and avoiding street dogs is essential. *Pre-exposure rabies prophylaxis,* which consists of three inoculations of human diploid cell killed virus vaccine (HDCV), purified chick embryo cell vaccine (PCEC), or rabies vaccine adsorbed (RVA) (1 mL intramuscularly on days 0, 7, and 21 or 28) is appropriate for long-term travelers who will live in endemic areas. People who anticipate animal exposure, such as veterinarians, animal handlers, and laboratory workers, should be vaccinated and should also receive a booster dose of vaccine (1 mL) every 2 years. Children are especially at risk because of the increased likelihood of contact with stray dogs. The new vaccines (HDCV, PCEC, and RVA) are more immunogenic and cause fewer reactions than the old duck embryo vaccine. Occasional local reactions and rare systemic reactions such as headaches, myalgias, and dizziness may occur. Vaccine from animal brain tissue is still being used in some developing countries, so if travelers require rabies vaccine, they should be sure to obtain the HDCV, PCEC, or RVA.

The HDCV may also be administered to travelers by the intradermal route (0.1 mL on days 0, 7, and 21 or 28) if the three-dose series is completed 30 days or more before departure. The PCEC and RVA should not be administered intradermally. If there is not sufficient time before departure, one of the intramuscular rabies vaccine should be used. Intradermal rabies vaccine is as immunogenic as intramuscular vaccine, but because the dose is one-tenth of the intramuscular dose, it is less costly. The HDCV should not be administered by the intradermal route when chloroquine or mefloquine, which may interfere with the immune response to the HDCV, is being used.

Pregnancy is not a contraindication to pre-exposure prophylaxis. If the previously vaccinated traveler is exposed to rabies, he or she should still seek medical help for *postexposure immunization* (see Chapter 18). Any animal bite should be thoroughly cleansed with soap and water to help reduce the risk of rabies.

Tuberculosis

Tuberculosis (TB) continues to be a worldwide health problem, but the risk to the short-term traveler is small. *Mycobacterium tuberculosis* is primarily a respiratory pathogen contracted by inhaling droplet nuclei, but unpasteurized milk products can also spread the disease. Travelers who will be spending extended periods in TB endemic areas should have a tuberculin skin test before departure. Bacillus Calmette-Guérin (BCG) vaccine use is controversial, and most U.S. experts do not recommend it. Periodic skin tests in long-term travelers are recommended to detect subclinical infections.

Measles, Mumps, Rubella, and Influenza

In most developing and developed countries other than the United States, measles, mumps, and rubella remain uncontrolled. Therefore, children should receive routine immunizations against these diseases before travel. Adolescents and adults who have neither had these diseases nor been immunized against them are at risk of becoming infected while traveling. People born after 1957 should have a booster dose of vaccine if they have not already received it. Rubella vaccine is indicated for females of childbearing age without serologic evidence of prior rubella infection (see Chapter 18).

Certain travelers may benefit from pretrip vaccination with influenza and pneumococcal vaccine. Influenza causes morbidity and mortality throughout the world and poses a risk to unvaccinated travelers. Influenza vaccination should be considered for high-risk travelers who did not receive influenza vaccine the previous fall if they are traveling to the tropics (where influenza occurs throughout the year), traveling in large tourist groups (which may include persons from areas of the world where influenza viruses are circulating), or traveling to the Southern Hemisphere during April through September. Increasing penicillin resistance in pneumococci throughout the world is also of concern, and pneumococcal vaccine should be given to patients at increased risk. Chapter 18 contains details regarding risk groups, dosages, and schedules for these vaccines.

Japanese Encephalitis

Japanese encephalitis is a mosquito-borne viral encephalitis that occurs in epidemics in much of Asia, including China, and endemically in the tropical areas of Southeast Asia. The risk to short-term travelers and those who confine their travel to urban centers is low. People at greatest risk are those living for prolonged periods in endemic or epidemic areas (Fig. 41.3). A vaccine to protect against Japanese encephalitis is now available in the United States (16). The vaccine (JE-VAX, Japanese encephalitis vaccine, inactivated; distributed by Connaught Laboratories) should be considered for patients planning long-term residence in endemic areas and for travelers visiting rural farming areas or sleeping in unscreened rooms in endemic or epidemic areas. It is especially recommended for people staying more than 1 month in an endemic country. Japanese encephalitis vaccine is associated with a 10% to 20% rate of side effects, including fever, headache, myalgias, and malaise. Serious allergic reactions have also been documented, which may be delayed up to 1 week after immunization. Even so, the vaccine is immunogenic, efficacious, and safe and has been used to vaccinate millions of people. Vaccinees should be observed for 30 minutes after immunization and should be warned about the possibility of delayed allergic reaction. The primary series consists of three subcutaneous injections at weekly intervals, with boosters at 1 and 4 years, and the initial series should be completed at least 3 weeks before departure.

Meningococcal Meningitis

Meningococcal meningitis occurs throughout the developing world, often in devastating epidemics (17). Although

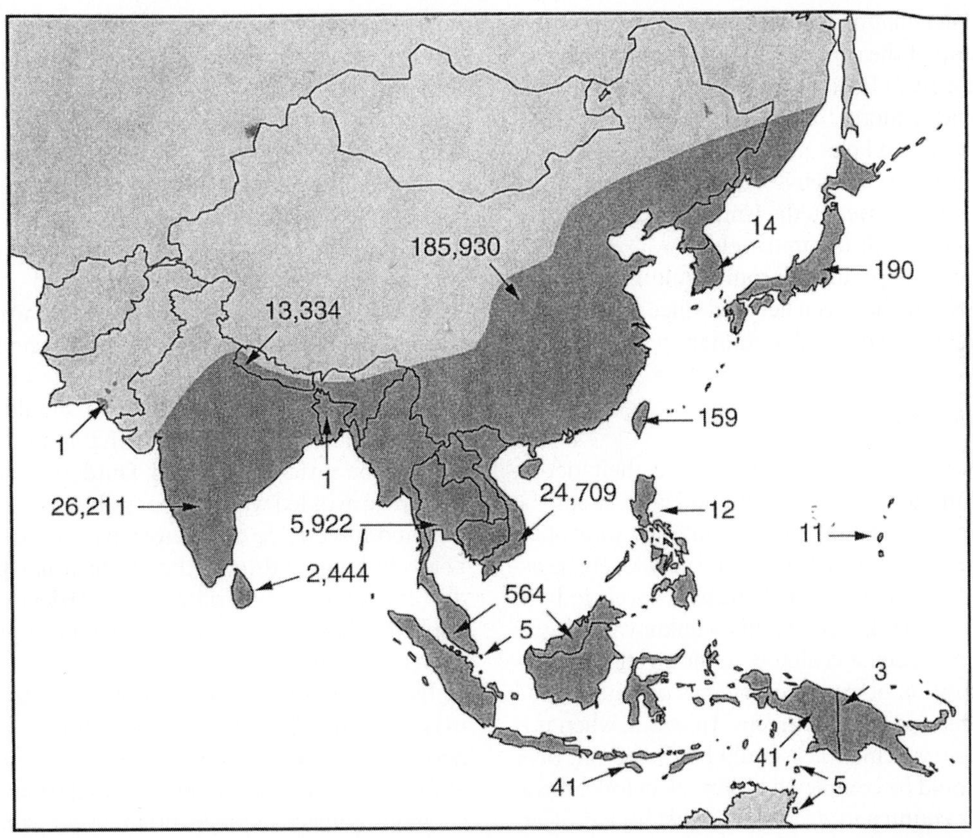

FIGURE 41.3. Reported Japanese encephalitis cases by endemic countries and regions of Southeast Asia where viral transmission is proven or suspected, 1986–2000. (From Halstead SB, Tsai TF. Japanese encephalitis vaccines. In: Plotkin SA, Orenstein WA, eds. Vaccines, 4th ed. Philadelphia: W.B. Saunders, 2004, with permission.)

cases in American travelers are rare, vaccine may be indicated for persons going to countries with high rates of infection. Areas where pretravel immunization has been recommended in the past include Northern India, Nepal, and Kenya. Risk is seasonal in the meningitis belt of Sahel (sub-Saharan Africa), including the dry inland regions of west African countries. Vaccine is required for entry into Saudi Arabia for pilgrims traveling to Mecca for the Hajj. Although meningococcal meningitis epidemics have occurred in Latin America, the prevalent type has been B, a serotype not covered by the vaccine. Two vaccines available for use in the United States are the A, C, Y W-135 Quadrivalent vaccine (Menomune, Connaught) and the newly released conjugated polysaccharide quadrivalent vaccine (Menactra) (18). The dose of vaccine is 0.5 mL given subcutaneously, with boosters recommended between 3 and 5 years.

Miscellaneous Vaccines: Typhus, Plague, Lyme, Anthrax, and Tick-borne Encephalitis

Typhus vaccine is no longer available, and the disease poses little risk except for those working with louse-infected refugees. Anecdotal cases of typhus have been reported in travelers to remote areas and empiric treatment with doxycycline is effective and curative.

Plague exists in certain rural areas in Africa, Asia, and North and South America. Vaccination is not recommended for most travelers, but if the traveler will have direct contact with wild rodents in plague-enzootic areas, vaccination may be considered. Local and systemic reactions after plague vaccine are common. Instead of vaccination, travelers considered to be at high risk for plague due to unavoidable exposures in epidemic areas should consider short-term antibiotic prophylaxis with tetracycline (500 mg twice daily) or doxycycline (100 mg daily). Trimethoprim-sulfamethoxazole (TMP-SMZ) can be substituted in children.

Lyme disease is found in temperate regions of Europe, Asia, and the United States and is generally not transmitted in the tropics (see Chapter 38). A recently licensed vaccine has been withdrawn, but because of genospecies diversity of the infectious agent, *Borrelia burgdorferi*, it was not likely to be efficacious outside North America. Avoiding tick habitats, using repellants, and checking daily for ticks is the recommended strategy to avoid exposure.

Tick-borne encephalitis (spring–summer encephalitis) is a viral infection of the central nervous system occurring in western and central Europe, including the countries of the former Soviet Union. Transmission is from infected ticks, but infection can be acquired by consuming unpasteurized dairy products. Effective vaccines are available in Europe but are not licensed in the United States. Available data do not support their use in travelers.

Anthrax vaccine is produced from a culture filtrate of *Bacillus anthracis* and has been licensed since 1970. Its use is controversial and is confined to military personnel.

Timing of Vaccines

Many travelers see a physician just before their departure. In this situation, all active immunizations can be given concurrently. The simultaneous administration of injectable cholera and yellow fever vaccine may rarely be associated with lower than expected antibody levels to both vaccines. The clinical relevance of this is unknown because injectable cholera vaccine is almost never given. Simultaneous administration of multiple vaccines produces good antibody responses to all the antigens. However, when it is possible, multiple vaccinations should be spread out over time, and all should be completed by 1 week before arrival in a developing country to decrease the likelihood of reactions and to ensure that adequate antibody levels have been attained (19). When vaccines are administered concurrently, they should be given with separate syringes at different body sites. Killed vaccines can be given at the same time as immune globulin. With certain live attenuated vaccines (especially measles, mumps, rubella), passively acquired antibody may interfere with replication of the vaccine virus and poses the possibility of decreasing the efficacy of the vaccine. Therefore, if possible, live virus vaccines should be given at least 14 days before the administration of immune globulin and probably 3 months after administration. Immune globulin does not interfere with yellow fever or OPV, both of which are live.

Malaria Prophylaxis

Malaria is a potentially fatal parasitic disease caused by infection of red blood cells (RBCs) with *Plasmodium* species. It is usually transmitted by *Anopheles mosquitoes* but can be acquired from transfused blood and intravenous drug use. Malaria tends to be more severe in "immunologically virgin" travelers than in residents of endemic areas. The disease is characterized by high fevers, chills, sweats, myalgias, and headache with no obvious focal signs or symptoms of infection. Malaria exists worldwide. The risk of contracting malaria varies from country to country and from season to season depending on local conditions such as rainfall, altitude, and mosquito density. Because malaria is almost totally preventable in travelers, there should be no deaths in travelers caused by malaria. Each year, however, American travelers still die because of inadequate protection against malaria. Prevention of malaria requires minimizing mosquito contact and taking appropriate prophylactic medicine (20).

To avoid mosquito exposure, travelers should sleep in screened rooms and under mosquito nets. *Anopheles* mosquitoes feed predominantly from dusk to dawn. Therefore, travelers who must be out during this time should try to cover the body with clothing and use insect repellent on exposed areas. Long-sleeved shirts, long-legged trousers, and occasionally a face net should be worn if at all possible. Mosquito repellent containing *N,N*-diethyl-*m*-toluamide (DEET, 20% to 40%) should be applied to exposed skin. Use of 100% DEET is not recommended and can be toxic for children. Outdoor nighttime activity should be avoided whenever possible. Permethrin, a repellant and insecticide of low toxicity, can be applied to bed nets, clothing, and tents. Permethrin has been shown to decrease clinical malaria cases in African children when applied to bedding. It is available in most pharmacies and sporting goods stores (21).

Even with appropriate mosquito protection, travelers may get bitten by malarious mosquitoes. It is therefore necessary to take an appropriate *chemoprophylactic* drug (Table 41.3) when traveling to a malarious area. Malaria chemoprophylaxis should preferably begin 1 to 2 weeks before travel and should continue for 4 weeks after leaving the malarious areas. Before deciding on a chemoprophylactic regimen, it is important to obtain recent information regarding country-specific malaria risk. The CDC maintains up to date information that is available by calling 707-488-7788. Regardless of the chemoprophylaxis used, it is still possible to contract malaria. Symptoms of malaria can develop as early as 1 week after initial exposure and as late as several months after departure from a malarious area.

In selecting the appropriate chemoprophylactic agents, several factors must be taken into consideration. The most important consideration is whether the traveler will be at risk of acquiring chloroquine-resistant *Plasmodium falciparum* (CRPF) malaria.

For travel to malarious areas where CRPF has not been reported or is at a very low level (e.g., Central America), once weekly *chloroquine phosphate,* 500 mg of the phosphate salt (300-mg base), should be taken. Chloroquine is usually well tolerated, but a few people may experience mild side effects, including itching, nausea, and disorientation. Side effects can be minimized by taking the drug with meals or in divided twice weekly doses. As an alternative, the related compound *hydroxychloroquine* may be better tolerated. Amodiaquine, another related compound (not available in the United States), should not be used because of associated hepatotoxicity and bone marrow depression. When chloroquine is used for prolonged periods at high dosages, as in the therapy of rheumatoid arthritis, it may be associated with a severe retinopathy.

TABLE 41.3 Drugs Used in the Prophylaxis of Malaria[a]

Drugs	*Adult Dosage*	*Pediatric Dosage*
Chloroquine phosphate (Aralen)	500 mg salt orally, once/wk	5 mg/kg base (8.3 mg/kg salt) orally, once/wk, up to a maximal dose of 300 mg base
Hydroxychloroquine sulfate (Plaquenil)	400 mg salt orally, once/wk	5 mg/kg base (6.5 mg/kg salt) orally, once/wk, up to a maximal adult dose of 310 mg base
Mefloquine	228 mg base (250 mg salt) orally, once/wk	15–19 kg: ¼ tablet/wk 20–30 kg: ½ tablet/wk 31–45 kg: ¾ tablet/wk >45 kg: 1 tablet/wk
Doxycycline	100 mg orally, once/day	> 8 yr of age: 2 mg/kg of body weight orally/day, up to adult dose of 100 mg/day
Atovoquine/Proguanil (Malarone)	250 mg/100 mg daily, 1–2 days, before and for 7 days after entering malaria area	10–20 kg: ¼ tablet 21–30 kg: ½ tablet 31–45 kg: ¾ tablet
Primaquine	30 mg base (52.6 mg salt) orally, daily	0.6 mg/kg base (1.0 mg/kg salt) up to adult dose orally, daily
For presumptive therapy: pyrimethamine-sulfadoxine (Fansidar)	3 tablets (75 mg pyrimethamine and 1500 mg sulfadoxine orally as a single dose)	5–10 kg: ½ tablet 11–20 kg: 1 tablet 21–30 kg: 1.5 tablets 31–45 kg: 2 tablets >45 kg: 3 tablets

[a]See text for indications according to geographic region and *Plasmodium* species.

This serious side effect is extremely rare when chloroquine is used at the low dosages for malaria chemoprophylaxis. The risk of retinopathy appears to increase after a cumulative dosage of 100 g of base, and periodic retinal examinations should be considered in travelers who have taken this much chloroquine. Chloroquine is safe in pregnant and lactating women and should be recommended to pregnant women traveling to malaria endemic zones.

Most malaria endemic areas now have strains of *P. falciparum* that are resistant to chloroquine, and travelers to these areas (Figs. 41.4 and 41.5) are at risk of contracting chloroquine-resistant malaria if chloroquine alone is used for chemoprophylaxis.

Chemoprophylaxis Against Chloroquine-Resistant Malaria

For travel to areas of risk where CRPF exist, three efficacious options exist, which are listed below. Although all three of these regimens are effective, Malarone is becoming increasingly the first choice followed by mefloquine and then doxycycline in special situations. Additionally, there are new recommendations for the use of *Primaquine* for primary prophylaxis in special situations.

Atovaquone/Proguanil (Malarone)

Atovaquone/proguanil is a fixed combination of the two drugs atovoquone and proguanil. Atovaquone/proguanil primary prophylaxis should begin 1 to 2 days before travel to malarious areas and should be taken at the same time each day while in the malarious area and for 7 days after leaving such areas. The most common adverse effects reported in persons using atovaquone/proguanil prophylaxis are abdominal pain, nausea, vomiting and headache. Atovaquone/proguanil should not be used in children weighing less than 11 kg, in pregnant women, in women with breast feeding infants weighing less than 11 kg or in patients with severe renal impairment.

Mefloquine (Lariam and Generic Brands)

Mefloquine primary prophylaxis should begin 1 to 2 weeks before travel to malarious areas. It should be taken once a week on the same day of the week during travel in malarious areas and for 4 weeks after the traveler leaves such areas. Mefloquine has been associated with rare serious adverse reactions such as psychosis or seizures at prophylactic doses. These reactions are more frequent with higher dosages used for treatment. Other side effects that may occur with prophylactic doses include gastrointestinal disturbances, headache, insomnia, abnormal dreams, visual disturbances, depression, anxiety disorder, and dizziness. Mefloquine is contraindicated for frequent use in travelers with active depression or a history of psychosis or seizures. It should be used with caution in persons with psychiatric disturbances if at all. Although it appears that mefloquine is safe for individuals on beta blockers, it should not be recommended for persons with cardiac conduction abnormalities. Mefloquine resistance is increasing and either doxycycline or Malarone can be used by travelers to these areas (the borders of Thailand with Burma and Western Cambodia and Eastern Burma (Fig. 41.6).

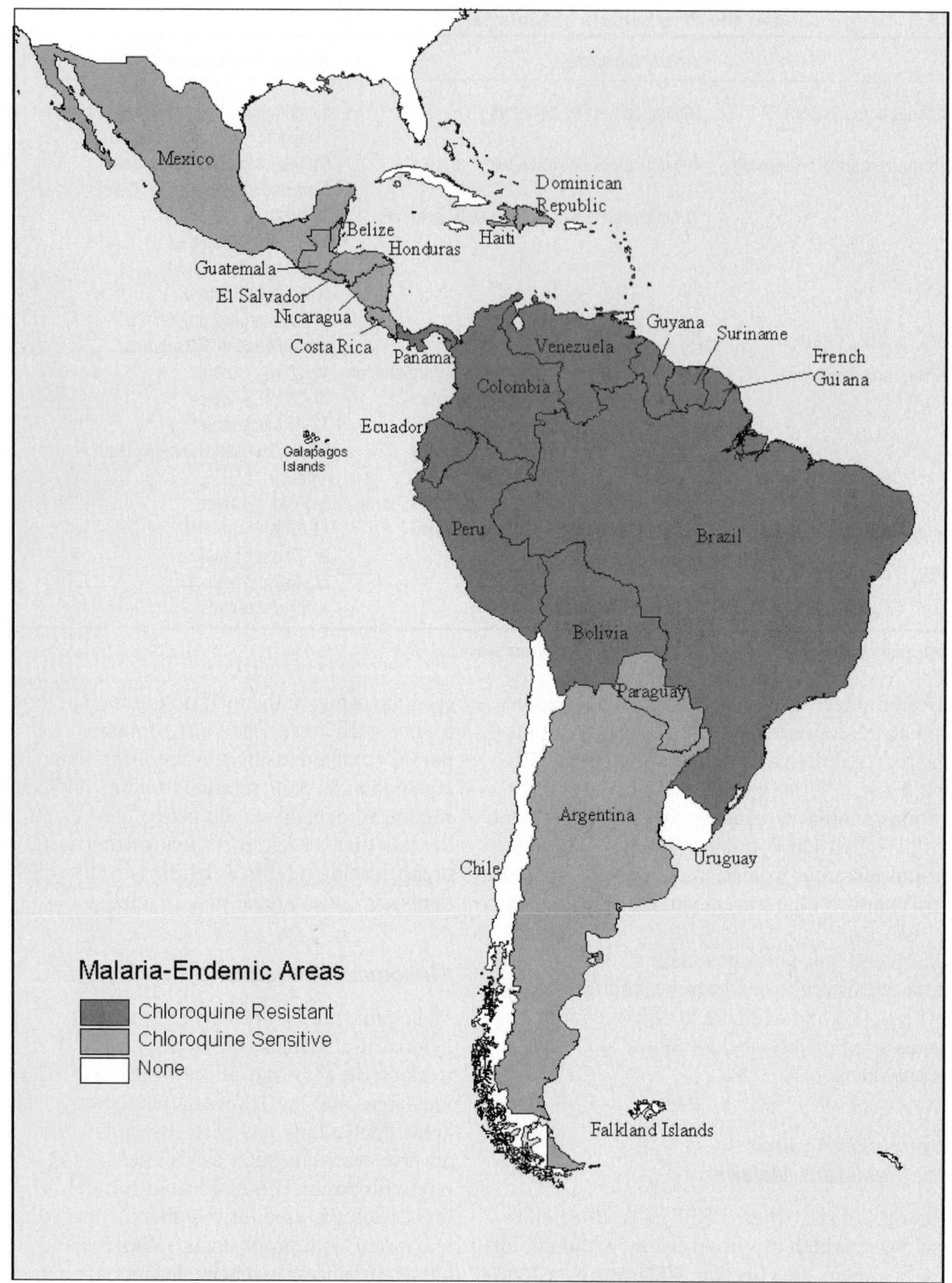

- If risk exists in any area of a country the entire country is shaded accordingly.
- Please refer to specific country information in Chapter 2 for detailed risk and recommended prophylaxis information.

FIGURE 41.4. Malaria endemic countries in the Americas 2002. (From Centers for Disease Control and Prevention. Health Information for International Travel, 2003–2004, DHHS, Atlanta, GA, with permission.)

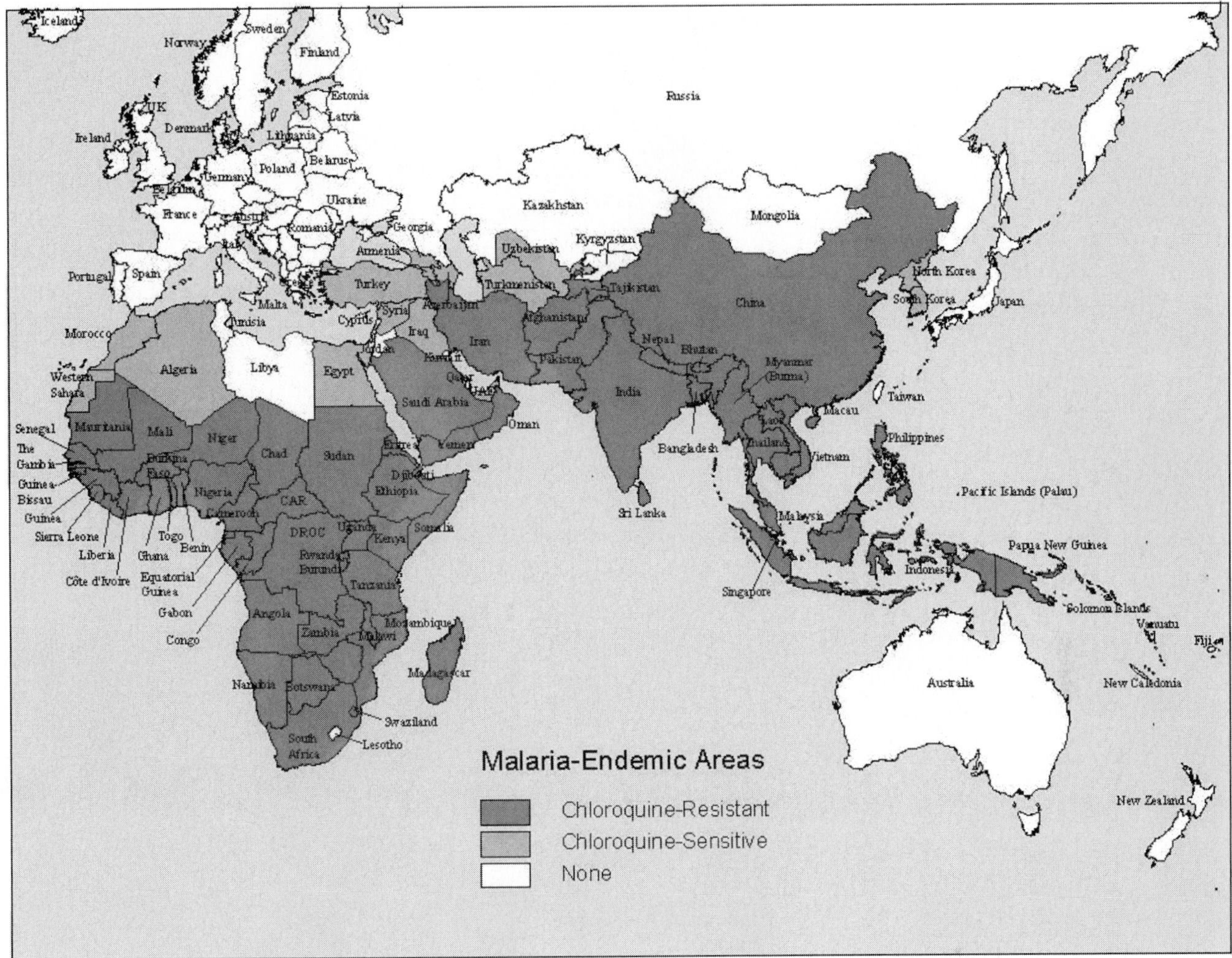

- If risk exists in any area of a country the entire country is shaded accordingly.
- Please refer to specific country information in Chapter 2 for detailed risk and recommended prophylaxis information.

FIGURE 41.5. Malaria endemic countries in Africa, the Middle East, Asia and the South Pacific 2002. (From Centers for Disease Control and Prevention. Health Information for International Travel, 2003–2004, DHHS, Atlanta, GA, with permission.)

Doxycycline (Many Brand Names and Generic)

Primary prophylaxis with doxycycline should begin 1 to 2 days before travel to malarious areas. It should be continued once a day, the same time each day during travel in malarious areas and daily for 4 weeks after leaving such areas. There is insufficient data that related compounds such as *minocycline* and other tetracyclines are effective against malaria. Persons on long term regimens of minocycline for acne should stop taking the minocycline 1 to 2 days prior to travel and start doxycycline instead. Doxycycline can cause photo sensitivity usually manifested as an exaggerated sunburn type reaction. The risk of such a reaction can be minimized by avoiding prolonged direct exposure to sun and by using sunscreens (Chapter 118). Additionally, doxycycline use is associated with an increased frequency of *Candida* vaginitis in women. GI side effects including nausea and vomiting may be minimized by taking the drug with a meal. To reduce the risk of esophagitis, travelers should be advised to not take doxycycline before going to bed.

Primaquine

In rare instances and after consultation with malaria experts such as those available through the CDC malaria hotline, primaquine may be used for primary prophylaxis to

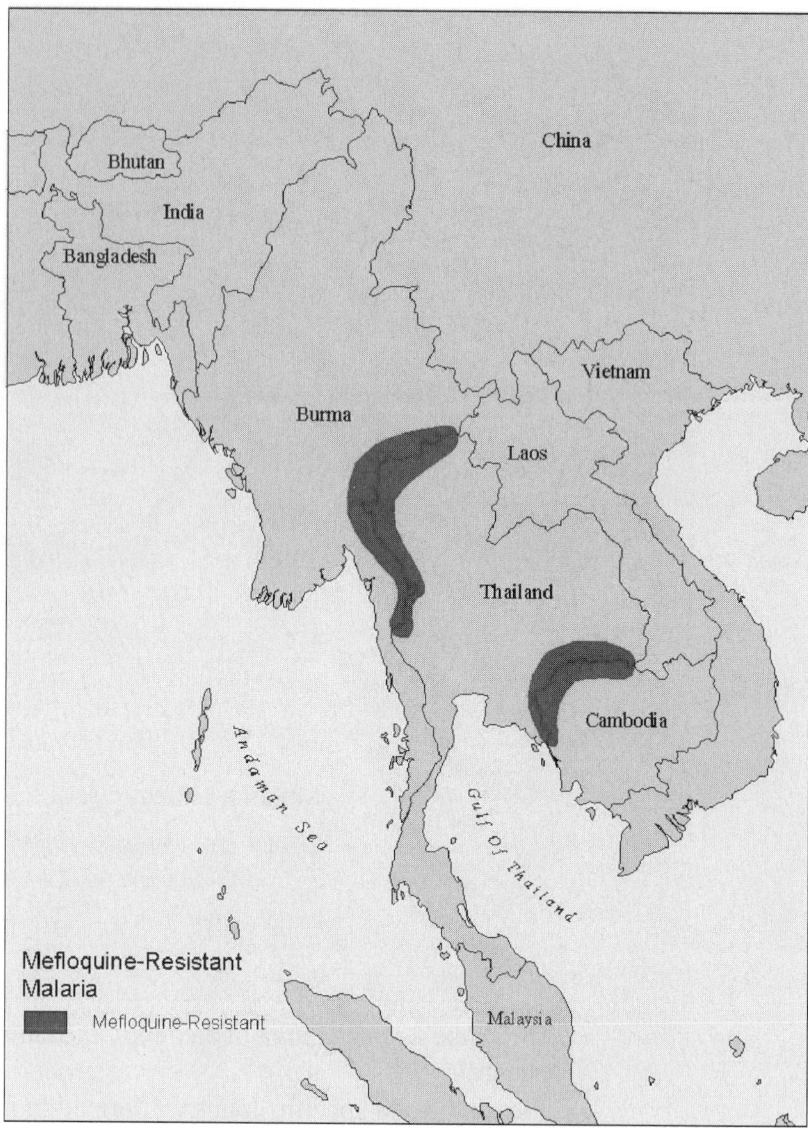

FIGURE 41.6. Mefloquine resistant malaria. (From Centers for Disease Control and Prevention. Health Information for International Travel, 2003–2004, DHHS, Atlanta, GA, with permission.)

Note: Zones with mefloquine-resistant malaria are known to be expanding. Please check the CDC Travelers' Health website: www.cdc.gov/travel, for updates.

travel areas with or without chloroquine resistant *P. falciparum*. This use should generally be reserved for travelers unable to take any of the other *chemoprophylactic regimens* indicated for their region of travel. Prior to taking primaquine the traveler must have a documented level of glucose 6-phosphate dehydrogenase (G6PD) in the normal range. Primaquine primary prophylaxis should begin 1 to 2 days before travel to malarious areas, be taken daily at the same time each day while in the malarious area and daily for 7 days after leaving such areas. Of note, the CDC no longer recommends chloroquine/proguanil (Paludrine) as a preventive option for persons traveling to areas with *chloroquine*-resistant *P. falciparum*. Although not yet approved, recent evidence suggests that azithromycin 250 mg daily may also be an effective and safe agent for *chloroquine* resistant *P. falciparum* prophylaxis (22).

Chemoprophylaxis for Infants, Children, and Adolescents

Infants, children, and adolescents of any age can contract malaria. Therefore, children traveling to malaria risk areas should take an antimalarial drug. In the United States antimalarial drugs are available only in tablet form and may taste quite bitter. Pediatric dosages should be carefully calculated according to body weight and should never exceed adult dosages. Pharmacists can pulverize tablets and prepare gelatin capsules for each measured dose (Table 41.3).

Chemoprophylaxis during Pregnancy

Malaria infection in pregnant women can be more severe than in nonpregnant women. Malaria can increase the risk for adverse pregnancy outcomes including prematurity, abortion, and stillbirth. For these reasons and because no chemoprophylactic regimen is completely effective, women who are pregnant or are likely to become pregnant should be advised to avoid travel to areas with malaria transmission if possible. If travel to malarious areas cannot be deferred, the use of an effective chemoprophylactic regimen is essential.

Changing Prophylactic Medications

The medications recommended for prophylaxis against malaria have different modes of action that affect the parasite at different stages of the life cycle. Thus, if the medication needs to be changed because of side effects prior to the completion of a full course, there are some special considerations. If a traveler starts prophylaxis with a medication such as mefloquine or doxycycline and then changes to atovaquone/proguanil during or after travel, the standard duration of therapy would be insufficient. The atovaquone/proguanil should be continued for 4 weeks after the switch or 1 week after returning, whichever is longer. In situations where malaria chemoprophylaxis is complex or involves pregnant women or small infants, it is best to consider calling the CDC malaria hotline (770-488-7788) for up-to-date guidance.

Travelers who decide to take chloroquine alone in areas of *chloroquine* resistant *P. falciparum* should take with them a treatment supply (three tablets) of pyrimethamine-sulfadoxine (Fansidar). These travelers are at risk of *chloroquine* resistant *P. falciparum* and should be advised to take the Fansidar promptly if they have a febrile illness and can not obtain medical care (Table 41.3). Mefloquine should not be used for self-treatment because of the likelihood of dosage-dependent side effects.

Routine malaria prophylaxis with chloroquine or mefloquine does not prevent delayed attacks of malaria from *Plasmodium vivax* or *Plasmodium ovale* because these species have an extraerythrocytic chronic liver phase that is not eradicated by these two agents. *Primaquine* is an 8-aminoquinolone drug that is effective against the chronic liver forms of vivax and ovale malaria. For travelers with minimal mosquito exposure and short stays in endemic areas, primaquine is not routinely indicated. However, primaquine prophylaxis should be considered in travelers who have had extended stays in areas endemic for either *P. vivax* or *P. ovale* malaria and who have had significant mosquito exposure. Primaquine, 15 mg of base daily for 14 days, is usually given during the last 2 weeks of chloroquine chemoprophylaxis. Primaquine can cause hemolysis in people with G6PD deficiency and has several other potential side effects, such as headache, nausea, vomiting, and gastrointestinal distress. Before treatment with this drug, the patient's G6PD status should be determined.

Food and Water

The traveler should learn the mantra for food and water safety: "boil it, cook it, peel it, or forget it." Food and water are the most common vehicles for the introduction of infectious agents into the body. It is best for the traveler to the developing world to consider any *uncooked* food and any product containing unpasteurized milk as possibly contaminated and therefore not safe to consume. Meats can harbor pathogens such as *Trichinella spiralis* and *Taenia solium* and *Taenia saginata.* Raw or undercooked freshwater fish and crustaceans can transmit liver flukes and tapeworms. Even after foods have been cooked, it is imperative that food is properly stored. Food held at ambient temperatures is a medium in which bacterial pathogens can multiply rapidly. Creamy desserts are often vehicles for *Salmonella* and staphylococcal food poisoning and should be avoided in areas with poor refrigeration (see Chapter 35). Fruits that can be peeled are safe as long as they are peeled by the consumer just before eating. The traveler should be wary of cheese products made from unpasteurized milk as possible sources of *Brucella* and other enteric pathogens. Salads should be avoided because lettuce and leafy vegetables are difficult to clean properly and often harbor infectious parasite eggs, cysts, and bacteria.

Although water may be safe in hotels in large cities, only water that has been adequately boiled or chlorinated should be considered safe to drink. If the traveler is uncertain about the purity of the water, it should be boiled. Routine chlorination may not kill all parasites. In areas where purified water is not available or where hygiene and sanitation are poor, travelers are advised to drink only the following beverages: those that use boiled water, such as hot tea or coffee; canned or bottled carbonated beverages, including carbonated bottled water and soft drinks; and beer or wine.

Boiling is by far the most reliable method of making water safe to drink. If the water contains sediment or floating matter, it should be strained with a cloth before boiling or chemical treatment. The water should be boiled vigorously for at least 10 minutes to kill cysts, viruses, and bacteria and then allowed to cool to room temperature. If boiling is not possible, water can be *chemically disinfected* with tincture of iodine or tetraglycine hydroperiodide tablets. The purification tablets can be purchased from a pharmacy or a sporting goods store. The traveler should follow the manufacturer's instructions. If the water is cloudy, the number of tablets should be doubled. If the water is extremely cold, it should be allowed to warm up before the tablets are added. Tincture of iodine should be used as follows. Per quart or liter of water, for clean water, use 5 drops and let sit

30 minutes. For cloudy or cold water, use 10 drops and let sit several hours.

Water may also be adequately purified by the use of small portable *water filters* that are available in sporting goods stores. These remove all water-borne parasitic and bacterial agents and some remove viruses. The water can be consumed immediately after treatment.

It should be remembered that where water may be contaminated, ice (as well as containers for drinking) should also be considered contaminated. If at all possible, boiled or bottled water should be used for making ice, rinsing drinking vessels, and brushing teeth. If boiled or bottled water is unavailable, the hot water tap can be used as a last resort. Although many infectious agents do not grow at these temperatures, hot tap water is by no means completely safe.

Diarrhea

Diarrhea is the most common illness among travelers to developing countries, occurring in 30% to 60%, and it affects the enjoyment of the trip for many people. Most cases do not pose a serious health threat; however, some episodes are severe and may lead to dehydration. Cases occur when fecally contaminated food or water is ingested, so the precautions mentioned above for food and water should be followed. Even with good personal hygiene and avoidance of suspect food and water, the attack rate for traveler's diarrhea remains high. Approximately 70% of episodes are caused by bacterial agents, with more than 50% caused by enterotoxigenic *Escherichia coli.* Less common etiologies include protozoa and viruses, but no organism is found in 10% to 40% of cases (Table 41.4). Because the causative agents can be assumed to be bacterial three fourths of the time, several strategies to prevent bacterial diarrhea or to treat it early have been studied (23).

Prophylaxis

A consensus conference on traveler's diarrhea held at the National Institutes of Health (NIH) recommended against the routine use of prophylactic antimicrobials (24). The potential risk of adverse reactions to the prophylactic agent was thought to outweigh the benefits. Although routine prophylaxis was not thought to be appropriate, it was also concluded that some travelers may wish to consult with their physician and may elect to use prophylactic antimicrobial agents for travel under special circumstances, once the risks and benefits are clearly understood. The antimicrobials that have been used in this way include ciprofloxacin (250 or 500 mg/day), norfloxacin (400 mg/day), ofloxacin 300 mg/day, levofloxacin 500 mg/day, doxycycline (100 mg/day with meals), and TMP-SMX (one double-strength tablet daily), continued for 2 days after departure from a developing country. Global resistance is increasing and quinolones are generally preferred (25). If prophylaxis is used, it should be limited to less than 3 weeks, and the quinolones listed are preferred in most cases because of the excellent coverage for the enteric pathogens, with consequent high efficacy rates (prevents more than 95% of expected illness) and low rate of adverse reactions. If doxycycline is being used for another indication (e.g., malaria prophylaxis or acne), additional antidiarrheal prophylaxis is not needed; because of possible photosensitivity, people taking doxycycline should wear hats and garments that prevent sun exposure.

Pepto-Bismol, a nonprescription product containing bismuth subsalicylate, can also prevent approximately 65% of diarrhea episodes; the dosage is two tablets four times a day with meals. Pepto-Bismol turns the tongue and stools black, and it may cause tinnitus.

Examples of travelers who would benefit from prophylaxis are those with pre-existing medical conditions (e.g., cardiovascular disease) that would place the person at great risk if diarrhea and even mild dehydration develop. Prophylaxis is also sometimes appropriate for people who will be at high risk for a very limited time (e.g., volunteers in a refugee camp for less than 3 weeks).

TABLE 41.4 Common Causes of Traveler's Diarrhea[a]

Bacteria (50%–70%)	*Protozoa (0%–20%)*	*Viruses (0%–20%)*
Escherichia coli	*Giardia*	Rotavirus
Campylobacter	*Entamoeba*	Calicivirus
Salmonella	*Cryptosporidia*	Enterovirus
Shigella	*Cyclospora*	

[a]No organism found (10%–40%).

Treatment

Most cases of diarrhea are self-limited and may require only rest and replacement of fluids and salts. This can best be accomplished with oral rehydration solution (ORS; e.g., CeraLyte, Cera Products, Inc., Columbia, MD), but certain home-available fluids (e.g., juices, soups) can also be used. Especially when diarrhea is severe, ORS should be used because it contains a complete formulation to replace the needed electrolytes in the appropriate concentrations. The traveler should drink a volume of ORS to approximate the volume of diarrhea losses, although an exact balance of intake and output is not necessary. If no commercial ORS is available, a similar solution can be made by adding one-half teaspoon salt, one-half teaspoon baking soda, and 4 tablespoons sugar to 1 pint (500 mL) water. (If baking soda is not available, 1 teaspoon salt should be used.) The electrolyte concentrations of fluids for sweat replacement

TABLE 41.5 Chemoprophylaxis and Treatment of Traveler's Diarrhea

Drug	Dose
Prophylaxis	
Bismuth subsalicylate	Two 262 mg tablets chewed q.i.d. with meals and at bedtime
Quinolone antibiotics	
Norfloxacin	400 mg/day
Ciprofloxacin	500 mg/day
Ofloxacin	300 mg/day
Levofloxacin	500 mg/day
Doxycycline	100 mg/day
Treatment	
Loperamide	4 mg loading dose, then 2 mg after each loose stool, to a maximum of 16 mg/day
Quinolone antibiotics	
Norfloxacin	400 mg b.i.d. for up to 3 days
Ciprofloxacin	500 mg b.i.d. for up to 3 days
Ofloxacin	300 mg b.i.d. for up to 3 days
Levofloxacin	500 mg/day for up to 3 days
Azithromycin	1,000 mg single dose or 500 mg/day for 3 days
Rifaximin	200 mg t.i.d. for 3 days

(e.g., Gatorade) are not equivalent to ORS. Any ORS remaining after 24 hours should be discarded because there is a chance of bacterial contamination.

Early antimicrobial treatment with ciprofloxacin (250 or 500 mg twice daily), levofloxacin (500 mg daily), norfloxacin (400 mg twice daily), doxycycline (100 mg twice daily), or TMP-SMX (one double-strength tablet twice daily) will shorten the episode caused by susceptible strains of bacteria (Table 41.5). Generally, the drug should be started soon after diarrhea begins and continued for 3 days, although a single dose of ciprofloxacin (500 mg) or levofloxacin (500 mg) has been shown to be effective (26). Recently, campylobacter resistant to quinolones has been increasing in prevalence. Preliminary studies suggest that azithromycin 500 mg daily may be effective therapy for this organism and for traveler's diarrhea in general. If the illness is thought to be *shigellosis* on the basis of signs and symptoms (blood in the stool, fever, and severe cramps), one of the quinolones for 5 days is the regimen of first choice; the second choice would be TMP-SMX for 5 days. Most shigellae are resistant to tetracyclines and sulfa, however. A new approach to the treatment of traveler's diarrhea has been the development of antimicrobial agents that are poorly absorbed. Rifaximin (Xifaxan, 200 mg by mouth twice a day for 3 days) is a nonabsorbable locally active agent effective against enteric pathogens. Early studies with rifaximin look highly promising.

Antimotility drugs such as diphenoxylate/atropine (Lomotil) and loperamide (Imodium) may provide temporary relief when diarrhea is especially inconvenient, such as during a long bus trip or other emergent situations. There continues to be concern that dysentery can be prolonged if antimotility drugs are used, and these agents should be used with care (if at all) with fever or dysentery because of potential clinical deterioration with an invasive bacterial pathogen. They have been used together with antimicrobial agents such as the quinolones to provide more rapid relief than might occur with the antimicrobial alone; however, the improvement is marginal. If loperamide (no prescription needed), which does not cause atropine-like side effects, is used, the dose is two 2-mg tablets after each voluminous watery stool.

Bismuth subsalicylate (Pepto-Bismol) is also helpful, although large amounts are needed to significantly reduce diarrhea. The dosage is 30 mL liquid (or two tablets) every half hour to 1 hour, up to eight doses in 24 hours. Precautions with this drug include complications caused by the salicylates it contains and by the fact that it binds tetracyclines. Kaopectate, Entero Vioform, and Streptotriad are not efficacious and should not be used.

The choices among the modalities described above should be based on the patient's symptoms. Fluid replacement should be encouraged for any episode of diarrhea and is all that is necessary in mild cases. For diarrhea of moderate severity (two to three unformed stools per day, no fever, no symptoms of frank dysentery, e.g., severe crampy pain or bloody stools), nonspecific symptomatic therapy may be all that is needed. Either bismuth subsalicylate or loperamide is useful. Antimicrobial agents should be used only for moderately severe to severe illness (more than four unformed stools per day, mild fever, dysentery). Some travel experts advocate taking antimicrobial agents at the first sign of diarrhea to minimize the length of the illness episode. Balancing adverse drug effects with symptomatic relief is the goal.

For diarrhea that is very severe, is associated with repeated vomiting, or does not improve after several days, the traveler should be advised to consult a physician rather than attempt self-treatment. A doctor should also be consulted if there is blood in the stool; if there is a fever higher than 101°F (38.3°C), especially if accompanied by shaking chills; or if antimicrobial therapy does not provide rapid improvement.

Finally, in preparation for possible diarrhea, the traveler should be reminded that *toilet tissue* is difficult to find in many developing countries and that it is prudent to take a supply. Chapter 35 contains additional information regarding the pathogenesis, epidemiology, and treatment of diarrheal illnesses.

Schistosomiasis

Schistosomiasis is one of the world's major public health problems. Three predominant species exist (*Schistosoma*

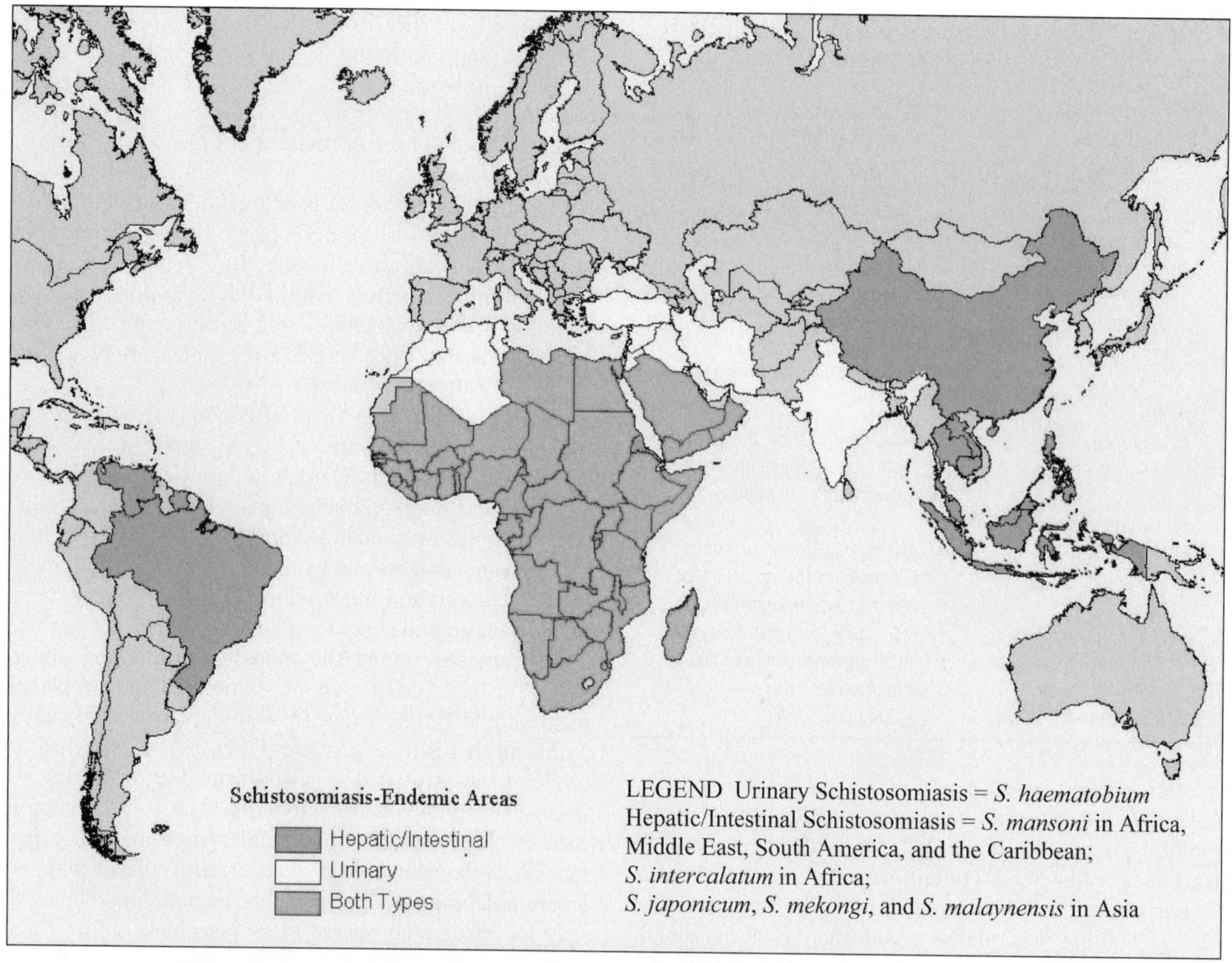

FIGURE 41.7. Geographic distribution of *Schistosomasis*. (From Centers for Disease Control and Prevention. Health Information for International Travel, 2003–2004, DHHS, Atlanta, GA, with permission.)

mansoni, S. japonicum, and *S. haematobium*) and are found worldwide (Fig. 41.7). Although few travelers are aware of schistosomiasis, it is a common disease in much of the developing world (27). After infection, the disease may lie dormant until it causes problems later in life. People contract schistosomiasis by wading or swimming in fresh or estuary water that harbors the snail vector of this trematode parasite. The cercariae (larval stage) can penetrate the skin and pass into the bloodstream without causing any symptoms at the time. Symptoms that may occur with schistosomiasis depend on the stage of the infection. Sometimes, there may be a rash at the site where the cercariae invaded, but this is uncommon. About 4 or 5 weeks after infection, an episode of fever, cough, and general malaise may occur. Still later (6 months to several years), more severe complications may occur, usually related to liver or urinary tract disease.

In recent years, severe cases of schistosomiasis have occurred in Americans after river rafting in Ethiopia and after swimming in fresh water in Kenya. Although treatment has improved with the advent of praziquantel, it is better to advise travelers to avoid fresh water contact in endemic areas and thereby prevent disease acquisition. For a returning traveler who has been exposed to fresh water in a schistosome-endemic area, screening tests, including a complete blood count (CBC) and specific serology, may be useful. This is particularly important in a patient with unexplained systemic symptoms. Eosinophilia in the peripheral blood may be present during the initial stages of the parasitic infection, although it is not a constant finding in late chronic infections. Positive serology indicates likely exposure, especially in the nonimmune traveler. If serology is positive, a further laboratory evaluation including urinalysis and stool examination for ova should be undertaken, recognizing that the acute syndrome described above may occur before there is detectable egg excretion. Proven or strongly suspected acute schistosomal infection requires treatment with *praziquantel* (Biltricide), which

medically relevant, patient categories, based upon similarities in their health care needs or specific vulnerabilities.

Refugees

From a medical perspective there are characteristics that distinguish refugees from other nonrefugee immigrants. These characteristics do not vanish or resolve when their status is adjusted to permanent resident alien or they become a citizen. To the health care professional, refugee patients are special in many ways. They fit into a broad category of patients who share a common refugee experience. Many are victims of physical and psychological trauma. Many have been subjected to systematized abuse or torture. All have experienced forced displacement, loss of their homeland, villages, communities, and personal belongings. Most have been separated from loved ones, have lost family members to war or disease, or have no knowledge of their relatives' condition or whereabouts. Many have experienced the humiliation of life in refugee camps. They are likely to originate from developing parts of the world, disrupted by recent conflict, where modern medicine and public health improvements have never been accessible or have been disrupted. Often the overseas physical examination required for U.S. entry accounts for all of their contact with modern health care. They arrive in the United States with the clothes on their backs, possibly some photographs, and little more.

As a category of patients, refugees have many similar unmet health care needs. Immunization series need to be started and completed. Chronic conditions need to be identified and managed. Many need orientation to the concept of primary health care. Those who have suffered physical trauma need reconstructive surgery and rehabilitation. Posttraumatic stress disorder (PTSD), depression, limited English proficiency, employment requirements, resettlement into substandard housing, and transportation problems can complicate adjustment to life in America. Parents often worry about loss of control over their children who seem to acculturate too quickly into a society often viewed as liberal and devoid of culturally appropriate role modeling.

The U.S. Department of Health and Human Services, Administration for Children and Families, Office of Refugee Resettlement (ORR) oversees services for refugees and disbursement of funds designated for refugee cash assistance (RCA) and refuge medical assistance (RMA). RMA funds reimburse state Medicaid programs for which refugees are automatically eligible for a limited period of time. Federally subsidized, often church-affiliated, refugee resettlement programs, in conjunction with state refugee coordinators, help on the local level with case workers, housing applications, school enrollment, and job acquisition.

The greatest numbers of refugees resettled in the United States in recent years have arrived from Southeast Asia (Cambodia, Vietnam, and Laos) between 1975 and 1990. The Soviet occupation of Afghanistan in 1987 displaced millions of Afghans. Soviet style communism resulted in a trickle of refugees from Hungary, Poland, Bulgaria, Romania, Czechoslovakia, and the former Soviet Union. Serbs, Croats and other refugees from the former Yugoslavia arrived during and following the Balkan conflict. Civil wars in Africa have displaced thousands of people from Ethiopia, Eritrea, Somalia, Sudan, Democratic Republic of Congo (Zaire), Uganda, and Rwanda, among other countries.

Each source of refugees has its own characteristics and, within countries of origin, smaller subsets can be defined. While Cambodian refugees are very homogeneous in culture and experience, other sources of refugees are more ethnically diverse or share other common experience. The Kampuchea (or Khmer) Krom from the south of modern day Vietnam, constitute an ethnically distinct group of people who identify more with Cambodia than Vietnam. Vietnamese "boat people" and re-education camp detainees lived through special circumstances that make them somewhat distinct from other Vietnamese refugees. The Somali Bantu, a more recently resettled subset of Somali refugees are ethnically, physically, and culturally distinct from other Somalis. They were imported as slaves from Mozambique and Zanzibar by Arab slave traders in the 18th century and have remained marginalized within Somali society ever since. Sudanese refugees can be broadly divided into Christians and Muslims and further divided by tribal affiliation.

Secondary Migrant Refugees

Once resettled in the United States, many refugees migrate secondarily, once or more than once, in search of relatives, friends, clan members, ethnic cluster sites, jobs, or better living conditions. This secondary migration disconnects refugees from RCA programs, Medicaid, contact with case workers, housing, schools, and other programs established on their behalf. Health care they receive along the way becomes fragmented. Overseas medical records, carefully guarded in transit to the United States, are often lost. Records of tuberculosis screening and treatment, immunizations, and other care received in the United States are difficult or impossible to reconstruct. These "secondary migrants" must depend upon their own ingenuity to re-enroll in school and jobs. They must find their own way back onto Medicaid rolls and into the health care system. Many become dependent upon local general assistance programs and city shelters. Secondary migrants are refugees with additional issues that can complicate their health care management.

Asylum Seekers and Asylees

People seeking asylum may need medical evidence of injury or torture that can be used to make a case for asylum before a judge. They may also need psychiatric evidence of PTSD or other psychological sequelae of their past or present situation. Clinicians may be asked by lawyers, often working pro bono, to evaluate a person seeking asylum and to render a formal medical or psychiatric opinion. Asylum seekers may or may not be allowed to work legally at the time of their application so the ability to afford a medical evaluation may be a complicating factor. As a general rule, they are not eligible for ORR services and assistance. Financial concerns and preoccupation with satisfying the requirements of their application for asylum may outweigh concerns regarding comorbidities or preventive health care. Addressing unrelated findings such as uncontrolled high blood pressure or suspected diabetes may have to be deferred.

From a health care perspective, asylees are similar to refugees. They are eligible for ORR services and assistance. Access to services, usually available to refugees through refugee resettlement programs, can vary from state to state.

Vietnamese Amerasians

The precipitous collapse of South Vietnam on April 30, 1975 placed many thousands of Vietnamese Amerasian young people under a reunified, communist Vietnam. Their American features, once regarded favorably under the former regime, became reminders of the American occupation. Families with Amerasian children feared reprisals. Many Amerasian children were marginalized and left to fend for themselves on the streets, uneducated and stigmatized as "Dust of Life" or half-breeds. Following implementation of the second Amerasian Homecoming Act, in conjunction with the Orderly Departure Program (ODP), they became "Golden Children," the ticket for safe transit out of Vietnam for America, not just for themselves, but for their immediate family. In many cases the "immediate family" was financially arranged. This became apparent when many Amerasian young people moved away from their "families" shortly after arriving in the United States. Discriminated against in Vietnam and foreign in America, these youth without a country, many in poor health and beyond the age of being able to matriculate easily into schools, have struggled physically and psychologically to survive. Few have been reunited with their biological fathers. Technically, Vietnamese Amerasians are not refugees. Yet, from a health care perspective they share much in common with Vietnamese refugees. Additionally, they have suffered in other ways placing them at additional risk for PTSD, depression, and failure to acculturate and succeed in America.

Lost Boys and Girls of Sudan

Thousands of young boys left their homes in southern Sudan in 1987 to avoid enslavement and conscription. They wandered thousands of miles, becoming known as "The Lost Boys of Sudan," and many died of disease and starvation. In 2001, 4000 of these boys were resettled to the United States. The CDC recommends presumptive treatment for schistosomiasis and strongyloidiasis for this population and for other Sudanese with similar exposure risk (49).

Illegal Immigrants

Illegal immigrants keep a low profile in order to avoid the U.S. immigration justice system. They avoid circumstances where they may be questioned in order to complete forms and applications. Hospital clinics that offer uncompensated care are inaccessible if high barrier patient registration processes or Medicaid denial letters are required. With few exceptions for emergency services, illegal immigrants are not eligible for health benefits under Medicaid. Most work "under the table" and receive no employer-sponsored health benefits.

Migrant Farm Workers

Migrant or seasonal farm workers are a mixture of citizens, permanent resident aliens, non-immigrants working under an H-2A visa, and illegal aliens. Most migrant workers earn wages that are less than 100% of federal poverty guidelines. Eighty-five percent of migrant workers are minorities. Most are Hispanic, while others come from Haiti, Jamaica, Thailand, Laos, and other countries (50,51). Alien migrant workers are generally ineligible for Medicaid. Migrant workers who are eligible for Medicaid may not be able to meet state residency requirements due to high mobility. Few state-sponsored Medicaid programs have reciprocity agreements with other states. Mobility also contributes to the fragmentation of health care and the health care record (52). A Federal, nationwide network of migrant health centers is capable of meeting only approximately 20% of the health needs of this population (50).

Communication across Cultures

As health care practitioners, learning about geographic medicine is relatively easy and an extension of basic training in medicine. Learning effective communication across cultures can be another matter. This requires attention to accurate language interpretation, elimination of knowledge deficits, and sensitivity to cultural differences.

Language

Of all the barriers to communication across cultures, the language barrier is the most obvious and the most important to address. This is accomplished through use of a skilled language interpreter and acquisition of triadic interviewing skills by the practitioner (53). The Joint Commission on Accreditation of Health Care Organizations (JCAHO) identifies a patient's ability to access culturally and linguistically appropriate services as not just a right but a matter of quality and safety (54). The Health Plan Employers Data and Information Set (HEDIS 3.0) now considers availability of an interpreter as a quality measure (55). Standards for interpreters are becoming clearer and go beyond the mere ability to translate (56). Increasingly, interpreters are professionals who are either full-time employees of hospitals or who contract their services through formal vendor agreements. The Health Insurance Portability and Accountability Act (HIPAA) of 1996, has driven expectations around confidentiality. There is an increasing expectation that interpreters will have some training in medical terminology, and that they will be professional in their interactions with patients both inside the examination room and in the community at large. Hospitals and medical offices that accept federal health care reimbursement are required to provide interpreters.

Professional, gender-concordant interpreters present for the medical encounter are generally preferred over other means of providing language interpretation (55). Interpreters who are present in the examination room are better able to engage through eye contact and nonverbal cues, than telephonic translators. Utilization of full-time hospital-employed interpreters may not be associated with longer visit times (57). As a general rule of thumb, young children should not be medical interpreters. They lack sufficient education and sophistication around matters of confidentiality. They may be uncomfortable discussing medical conditions. Their native language and English language development are likely to be imperfect. A patient's own child is likely to be uncomfortable in the examination room and the patient is unlikely to disclose relevant confidential information. On the other hand, a mature adult child may be comfortable accompanying their parent and be the person with whom the patient is most comfortable as an interpreter (55).

The evolution of telephone language lines has helped make interpreters readily available anywhere and at any time of the day or night. Language line services provide trained interpreters for most major languages without prior appointment. Minority dialects may be an exception. With some language lines it may be possible to make prior arrangements for unusual languages or dialects by appointment. In small communities, or under special circumstances involving very private conversations, language lines may be a preferable alternative to having an interpreter in the examination room. If a language line is used, the patient should be introduced to the interpreter using age, sex, and clinical context (examination room, trauma room, etc.) and it should be explained that names are not to be used. If necessary, time should be spent to discuss the patient's concerns about confidentiality and the measures that are in place to protect it. The use of high quality speaker phones with preprogrammed dialing enhances the use of language lines. At registration desks in busy waiting rooms, dual handset telephones may work better. Some of the larger language line services include CyraCom International (http://www.cyracom.net), Language-Line Services (http://www.languageline.com), and Pacific Interpreters (http://www.pacificinterpreters.com).

Being able to access translated written materials such as brochures, educational materials, and informed consents documents can be very helpful but may have some limitations. Translating documents can be complicated and expensive. Back translation is necessary to ensure accuracy. Translated materials have to be kept up to date. Multiple documents are difficult to catalog, access, and keep in stock. Native language illiteracy also may be a factor. The Immunization Action Coalition (http://www.immunize.org/vis/index.htm) has obtained funding for the translation, cataloging, and Internet distribution of vaccine information statements (VIS) in many languages. The continued expansion of high speed Internet access, electronic medical record systems, and computers in examination rooms makes accessing translated materials via the Internet an increasingly practical solution. Computer systems have the flexibility to offer language-appropriate narrated video clips that, in the future, could help explain procedures, disease management, and more (for example, see Healthy Roads Media at http://www.healthyroadsmedia.org/).

Knowledge about Health Care Practices

Foreign-born patients may lack familiarity with Western, scientific approaches to health and illness. Instead, they may adhere to their own, deeply rooted, *culture-bound health beliefs*, *interventions*, and *practices*. Western-trained health care professionals may regard these as curiosities and with skepticism. But, this is a two-way street, as foreign-born patients often regard Western health beliefs, interventions, and practices with equal skepticism.

Depending upon the extent of a patient's exposure to Western, scientific explanations of health and illness, *culture-bound health beliefs* may explain states of wellness or illness in terms of natural or supernatural balance or disturbance. Earth, wind, fire, and water may be viewed as the elements of life. Wellness may be seen as a state of harmony between these elements and the balance of opposing forces such as hot and cold, as in the principle of yin and yang. Illness may be explained on the basis of a "bad wind" that has entered the body, feeling "hot," or as the result of being possessed by a spirit or demon (58,59). Members of many cultures turn to traditional healers who possess special knowledge of these principles to seek cures and remedies based upon them (60,61). Patients may believe that if they feel well or do not have pain that nothing can be wrong. This can complicate explanations of screening tests or interventions for sub-clinical disease. In interactions with Western-trained practitioners, patients may feel a sense of embarrassment if they disclose adherence to a belief system that may be viewed as primitive or unscientific. Nevertheless, adherence to traditional beliefs tends to be strong. Patients are apt to question the ability of Western-trained health care practitioners who are not indoctrinated in their belief system, fearing the practitioner will be incapable of understanding and treating their condition. This perception is likely to be reinforced by the practitioner who resorts to too many questions, questions that are too personal, unfamiliar physical examinations that invade privacy, laboratory testing, and deferral of treatment pending the outcome of testing. Phlebotomy or radiograph imaging may be perceived as injurious within the health belief system of many patients. The patient may expect an injection or have another preconceived notion of appropriate treatment that should be offered at the time of the visit.

Culture-bound health interventions have evolved as traditional or folk remedies that have as their basis the restoration of natural order and the state of well-being. Examples include acupuncture, cupping (Fig. 41.10), coining (Fig. 41.11), pinching, taping, massage, ceremonies to exorcise evil spirits, consumption of herbal tea or alcohol, and inhalation of steam from herbal brews:

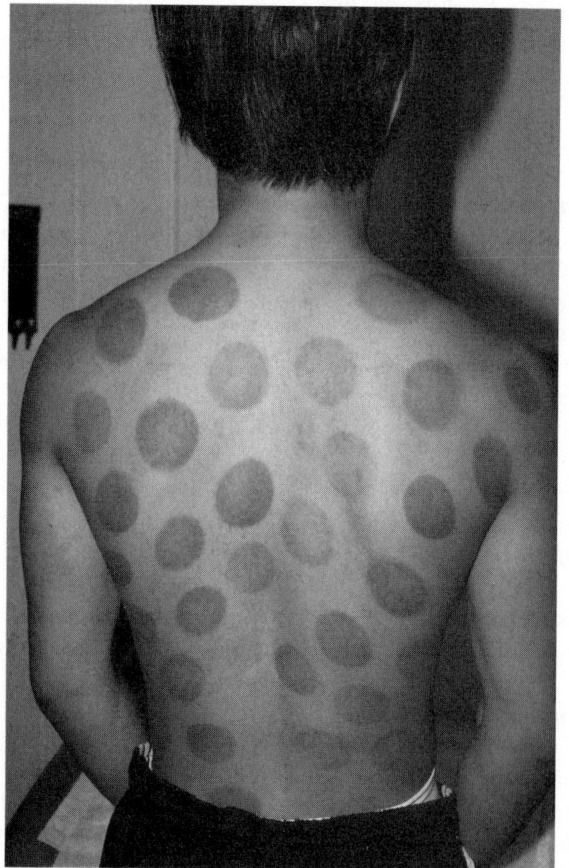

FIGURE 41.10. Cupping. Cambodian refugee adolescent with fever, sore throat, and tonsillar exudate. Portland, Maine 1997. Photographer: Maine Medical Center Audiovisual Department.

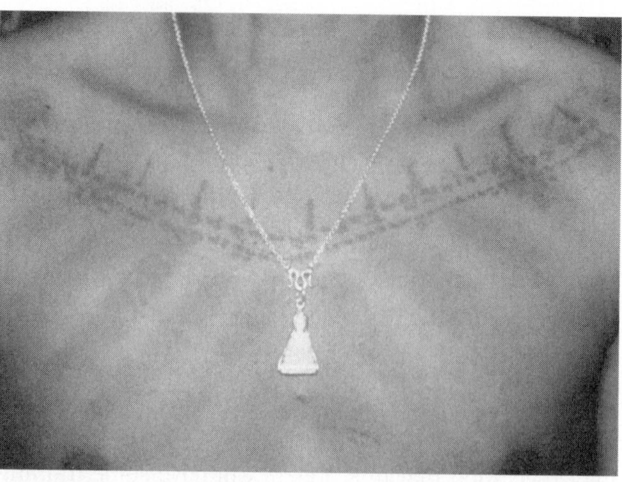

FIGURE 41.11. Coining, tattoo, and amulet. Cambodian adult male. Emergency Department, Maine Medical Center, Portland, Maine ~1994. Photographer: Maine Medical Center Audiovisual Department.

> *Coining* can be a social event usually at the home of the sick person, who is the center of attention. Adult family members and close friends may participate. A small amount of green Tiger Balm oil or other lubricant is applied to skin and rubbed using the edge of a coin until a red bruise is raised. This is repeated until a symmetrical pattern of bruises is created, usually on the neck, trunk, arms, and/or abdomen. The process is thought to help release heat from the body, thereby, reestablishing the harmonic balance of hot and cold. This practice is common in Cambodian culture and is performed on both adults and children.
>
> *Cupping* is performed in much the same way and for the same reasons. The difference is that a small glass cup is pressed over a small lighted candle balanced on the skin until it extinguishes. This creates a perfectly circular suction ecchymosis. This approach might be taken on a level surface such as the forehead of a recumbent patient. An alternative approach employs a preheated cup, sealed to the skin with gentle pressure and allowed to cool.
>
> A Vietnamese patient seen in the office with a red vertical streak in the center of the bridge of the nose between the eyes has been repeatedly *pinching* the skin to relieve headache, "fever" or dizziness. "Fever" in this sense does not necessarily correlate with febrile.
>
> White adhesive *tape* impregnated with aromatic extracts and possibly combined with a salicylate is applied to the temples to relieve headache or to the back or joints to relieve pain in Asian cultures. The practice may extend to other Asian cultures.
>
> Cambodian women traditionally believe it is important to build a *fire under the bed* and to remain on the

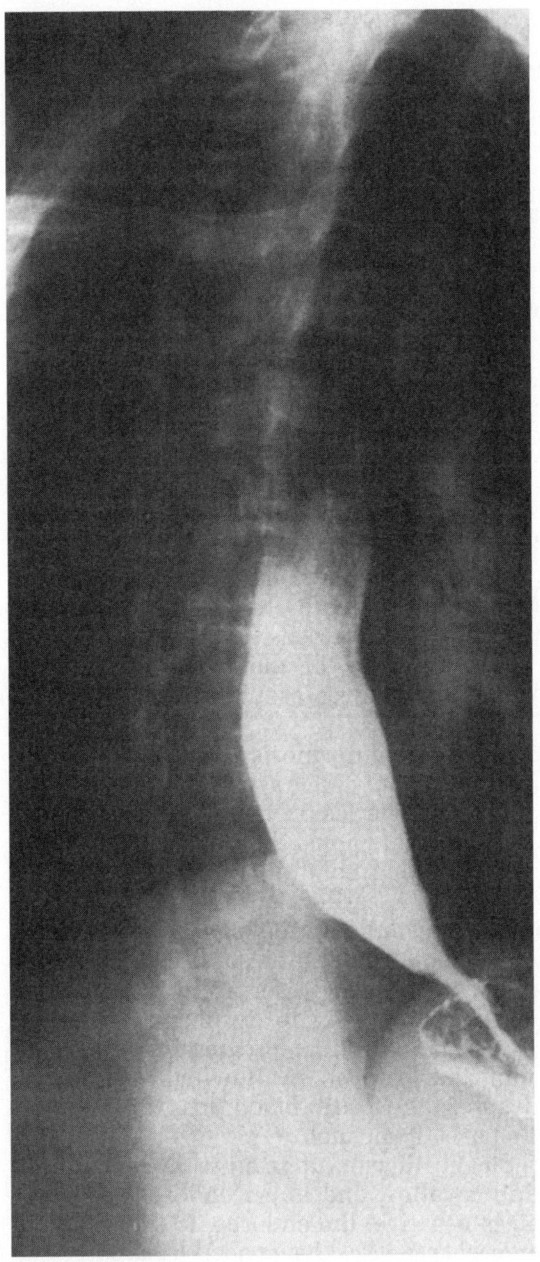

FIGURE 42.1. Barium swallow in a patient with achalasia. The esophagus is dilated and the tapered distal segment never opens normally. Under fluoroscopy, no peristalsis is seen, but simultaneous contractions are noted.

Differential Diagnosis

Achalasia must be differentiated from other disorders that lead to obstruction of the passage of food into the stomach. *Esophageal strictures,* both peptic and neoplastic, and *carcinomas at the esophagogastric junction* may result in symptoms and in a radiographic and manometric picture similar to that of achalasia (8). Thus, all patients with a clinical or radiographic diagnosis of achalasia should be evaluated with endoscopy. Failure to pass the endoscope into the stomach indicates an anatomic obstruction. *Scleroderma,* with its associated esophageal motility disturbance, may result in dysphagia with diminished peristalsis seen on the radiograph. If stricture has not occurred, the patient will demonstrate a wide-open sphincter through which barium passes easily. By the time patients with esophageal scleroderma develop stricture and dilation of the esophagus that may mimic achalasia, they usually have other obvious stigmata of scleroderma (particularly tight skin of the face and hands or Raynaud phenomenon). Furthermore, on esophageal manometry the LES pressure in scleroderma is low rather than high, as it is in achalasia, but like achalasia, the disorder of motility is confined to the smooth muscle portion (distal two-thirds) of the esophagus, with a normally functioning proximal segment. In patients from South America (or individuals who have spent time there), *Chagas disease,* caused by infection of the ganglion cells with *Trypanosoma cruzii,* may cause a megaesophagus with manometric patterns identical to that of achalasia. Some patients with *idiopathic intestinal pseudo-obstruction* may also have a manometric pattern similar to that of achalasia.

Therapy

Two types of definitive therapy exist for achalasia: pneumatic dilation and surgery. Both forms of therapy are aimed at reducing the pressure gradient between the esophagus and the stomach, thus decreasing the severity of the dysphagia. The aperistalsis and impaired sphincter relaxation persist after therapy. *Pneumatic dilation,* an outpatient procedure, is performed by a trained gastroenterologist. The esophagus is aspirated completely before the dilation. After premedication with analgesics and sedatives, a balloon dilator is passed into the stomach. Under fluoroscopic guidance, the balloon portion is positioned across the LES. It is then inflated for 10 to 30 seconds, causing a forceful disruption of the LES muscle. The dilator is then removed and can be blood streaked. The patient usually experiences chest pain during the procedure. The major risk of the procedure is esophageal perforation, which occurs in up to 5% of dilations. Satisfactory results (long-term improvement in dysphagia, weight gain, and decrease in retention of barium) can be expected in approximately 85% of cases. In successful cases, there is immediate relief of symptoms. The patient is observed for 4 to 6 hours and discharged. Dilation can be repeated if symptoms of dysphagia recur or worsen, but most patients have only minimal symptoms for many years after therapy. Repeat esophageal manometry is not necessary unless symptoms recur.

Surgical therapy, the Heller myotomy, involves a transection of the circular muscle of the LES zone to the level of the mucosa. This surgical approach provides results similar to those after pneumatic dilation, with a success rate of 80% to 85%. The procedure may cause significant reflux esophagitis in 10% to 25% of patients. As a result of this complication, some advocate combining a fundoplication

TABLE 42.3 Therapy for Esophageal Motility Abnormalities Associated with Chest Pain

Treatment Modality	Dose	Mode of Administration	Major Complications
Reassurance			
Nitrates[a]			
Nitroglycerin	0.4 mg SL	Usually before meals and PRN	Headache
Isosorbide	10–30 mg p.o.	30 min before meals	
Anticholinergics			
Dicyclomine (Bentyl)	10–20 mg	4 times a day	Dry mouth, blurred vision
Sedatives/antidepressants			
Diazepam (Valium)	2–5 mg	4 times a day	Drowsiness
Trazodone (Desyrel)	50–100 mg	4 times a day	Drowsiness, impotence
Imipramine (Tofranil)	50 mg	At bedtime	Drowsiness
Calcium channel blockers[a]			
Nifedipine (Procardia)	10–30 mg	4 times a day	Dizziness, nausea, dyspepsia
Diltiazem (Cardizem)	90 mg	4 times a day	Headache, edema, nausea
Smooth muscle relaxants[a]			
Hydralazine[a]	20–50 mg	3 times a day	Headache, lupus-like syndrome
Static dilation	50 French	Repeat as needed	None
Pneumatic dilation[b]			Perforation (3%–5%)
Esophagomyotomy[c]			Gastroesophageal reflux (20%)

[a] Orthostatic hypotension is a common complication of this class of drugs.
[b] May be indicated if dysphagia is a prominent symptom.
[c] Rarely indicated (intractability).

with the myotomy. Until recently, the procedure required a thoracotomy, but it can now be performed by either a laparoscopic or thoracoscopic approach. These minimally invasive techniques have made myotomy a better tolerated procedure with shorter hospitalizations, but because pneumatic dilation can be performed on outpatients without general anesthesia, it is usually the procedure of choice. Surgery is reserved for failure of repeated dilations to provide symptomatic relief, esophageal perforation secondary to pneumatic dilation, inability to perform dilation because of the shape of the esophagus or the presence of a large epiphrenic diverticulum, and inability to exclude carcinoma.

Medical therapy with nitrates, calcium channel blockers (Table 42.3), and even mercury bougienage may offer transient improvement in some patients. Pharmacologic therapy should be reserved for patients in whom pneumatic dilation or myotomy is contraindicated or for patients with very mild disease.

Endoscopic injection of botulinum toxin into the LES has been studied as a treatment of achalasia (9). A decrease in LES pressure and improved esophageal emptying are seen immediately after injection. An initial success rate of 70% to 80% has been reported after the first injection, with most patients relapsing (and requiring repeat treatment) in 6 months to 1 year. This procedure can be performed by a trained endoscopist and has no more risk than esophagoscopy alone. The therapy should be considered for patients in whom surgery has high risk and in whom the risk of perforation with pneumatic dilation is also high, but not as a long-term treatment option.

Complications

Many studies suggest that patients with achalasia are at increased risk of developing esophageal cancer. The incidence of this complication ranges from 6% to 29% in various series (8). Tumors in patients with achalasia should not be confused with cancer of the esophagogastric junction presenting with an achalasia-like picture. Cancers in patients with primary achalasia usually occur many years after the diagnosis of achalasia has been established and are usually squamous cell type, occurring in the mid-portion of the esophagus. There is no evidence that successful therapy of achalasia prevents the development of cancer.

Diffuse Esophageal Spasm

Clinical Presentation

Symptomatic diffuse esophageal spasm (DES) (10) is a disorder characterized by intermittent nonperistaltic (simultaneous) esophageal contractions that result in dysphagia and substernal chest pain. The disorder occurs with equal frequency in both sexes and at all ages (although it appears to be rare in children). The dysphagia is intermittent and is experienced for both solids and liquids. The pain is also intermittent and may be provoked by certain foods, particularly hot and cold beverages. At other times, the pain occurs spontaneously and may even awaken the patient at night. The pain is highly variable in quality and is sometimes described as knife-like or as dull and crushing; it may radiate to the neck, back, or arms. It may be brief or last for hours. Because of its location, radiation, and crushing quality, it may be confused with the pain of ischemic heart disease. When no cardiac disease is found, many of these patients are incorrectly believed to have a psychogenic disturbance.

Diagnosis

The procedures for the diagnosis of this condition include radiographic studies and esophageal manometry. A carefully performed *barium swallow,* or *videoesophagogram,* may demonstrate nonperistaltic, spontaneous, and simultaneous contractions (tertiary waves) of the body of the esophagus. However, these abnormal contractions are often encountered during routine barium swallow and by themselves do not make a diagnosis of esophageal spasm without the appropriate clinical history. Furthermore, because DES is an intermittent condition, the barium swallow may be normal or too insensitive to detect the motility disturbance. Because the barium study is not specific, it should be done only on patients with dysphagia. Patients with suspected DES should have *esophageal motility studies* to confirm the diagnosis, even if they have had a barium swallow. Provocative agents (e.g., edrophonium) can be used during the motility studies to identify more clearly patients who experience chest pain of esophageal origin (described later in this chapter) (11).

Therapy

Table 42.3 lists therapy for DES and other motility disorders that cause chest pain, which are discussed in greater detail later in this chapter.

Other Primary Motility Disorders

In addition to achalasia and DES, three distinct primary motility abnormalities of the esophagus have been described that are associated rarely with dysphagia. The *nutcracker esophagus* and the *hypertensive LES* (excessively high LES pressures with normal esophageal peristalsis) are two abnormalities associated primarily with chest pain and, rarely, with dysphagia; they are discussed later in this chapter. Some patients with dysphagia referred for esophageal motility testing demonstrate contractions in the distal esophagus with amplitudes of smooth muscle contraction below 30 mm Hg in more than 30% of swallows. This is called *ineffective esophageal motility* because contractions of this low amplitude are incapable of effective propagation of a bolus. This abnormality is seen commonly with gastroesophageal reflux, and rarely it may be seen with dysphagia alone.

Secondary Motility Disorders

Chronic reflux esophagitis (discussed later) may cause scarring of the distal esophagus, which can result in decreased force of esophageal contractions and/or ineffective esophageal motility, either of which can lead to dysphagia. There is ample evidence that acute acid reflux does not induce esophageal spasm, but chronic reflux may cause symptoms and motility abnormalities that are radiographically similar. Treatment is aggressive antireflux therapy. Improvement in dysphagia and contraction abnormalities is variable, but the pain of chronic reflux usually diminishes with treatment.

Abnormalities of esophageal contractions associated with dysphagia may be seen in patients with hyperthyroidism or hypothyroidism, amyloidosis, and myotonic dystrophy. Diabetes mellitus has been associated with multiple radiographic and manometric abnormalities of the esophagus, but patients are seldom symptomatic. Collagen vascular disease, particularly scleroderma, may affect the esophagus as well. Chronic idiopathic intestinal pseudo-obstruction may produce manometric abnormalities indistinguishable from those of achalasia, as noted earlier in this chapter. Many authorities have used esophageal manometry to help make this diagnosis. Use of the term *presbyesophagus* should be abandoned since normal aging does not produce significant alteration of esophageal motility.

Scleroderma of the Esophagus

The esophagus is affected in up to 80% of patients with scleroderma. At times esophageal symptoms may lead to the diagnosis, since the esophagus may demonstrate the characteristic abnormalities even before skin changes occur. The main symptoms of esophageal scleroderma are heartburn and dysphagia. The cause of these symptoms can be readily appreciated by examining the changes in esophageal motility. In esophageal scleroderma, the LES pressure is very low, resulting in free gastroesophageal reflux. Additionally, the peristaltic waves initially are of reduced amplitude, progressing later to complete aperistalsis in the smooth muscle portion of the esophagus, sparing the skeletal muscle portion. Because peristalsis is impaired, the refluxed acid remains in the esophagus for an abnormally long time, perhaps accounting for the development of an esophageal stricture, commonly seen in this disorder. Thus, the dysphagia may be caused by the primary motor abnormality or may signify the development of a peptic stricture.

The pathogenesis of scleroderma is unknown. In the esophagus, the disorder is not simply secondary to replacement of muscle fibers with collagen because the motility dysfunction can be demonstrated in the absence of histopathologic changes. It has been suggested that there is a neural defect in the esophagus rather than a primary myogenic disorder (12).

Scleroderma is a chronically progressive disease for which no specific treatment exists. Therapy of esophageal

TABLE 42.4 Treatment of Gastroesophageal Reflux

Intervention	Specific Change	Mechanism of Improvement
Lifestyle changes		
Elevate head of bed (6- to 8-inch blocks)		Decreased acid contact time
Avoid drugs that decrease LES pressure	Avoid theophylline, nitrates, calcium channel blockers, benzodiazepines	Avoids decrease of lower sphincter pressure
Avoid irritants	Citrus, coffee	Avoids direct mucosal damage
Stop smoking		Removes inhibition of H_2 blockers, increases lower sphincter pressure
Avoid eating before sleep	3 h	Avoids gastric distension
Antacids	As needed	Decreases gastric acid
Alginic acid (Gaviscon)	As needed	Barrier protectant
H_2 antagonists (OTC)	As needed	Decreases gastric acid
Pharmacologic therapy		
H_2 antagonists[a]		
Cimetidine (Tagamet)	400 mg b.i.d. (nonerosive symptomatic disease) 800 mg b.i.d. (erosive esophagitis)	Decreases acid secretion
Ranitidine (Zantac)	150 mg b.i.d. (nonerosive symptomatic disease) 150 mg q.i.d. (erosive esophagitis)	
Famotidine (Pepcid)	20 mg b.i.d. (nonerosive symptomatic disease) 40 mg b.i.d. (erosive esophagitis)	
Nizatidine (Axid)	150 mg b.i.d. (all forms of reflux disease)	
Metoclopramide (Reglan)	5–10 mg q.i.d.	Metoclopramide increases LES pressure, increases esophageal clearance, and accelerates gastric emptying
Sucralfate (Carafate)	1 g q.i.d.	Mucosal protection (not FDA approved for treatment of reflux)
Proton pump inhibition		
Lansoprazole (Prevacid)	30 mg/day (am) 15 mg/day (am) maintenance	
Omeprazole (Prilosec)	20 mg/day (am)	Decreases acid secretion
Rabeprazole (Aciphex)	20 mg/day (am)	Decreases acid secretion
Pantoprazole (Protonix)	40 mg/day (am)	
Esomeprazole (Nexium)	40 mg/day (am) acute 20 mg/day (am) acute, maintenance	
Surgery	Nissen fundoplication	Creates intra-abdominal esophagus and augments antireflux barrier
	Belsey Mark IV repair	
	Hill procedure	
Endoscopic treatment	Suturing device	Mechanism unknown
	Radiofrequency energy to sphincter	Barrier tightening, decreased sphincter relaxation?

[a] Nocturnal H_2 antagonists are insufficient antireflux therapy.

manifestations is directed at symptomatic relief and prevention of strictures.

Patients with scleroderma who have dysphagia or heartburn should be referred to a gastroenterologist for evaluation of esophageal motility and to rule out reflux esophagitis and stricture formation. If reflux is present, the patient should be treated with intensive antireflux therapy (Table 42.4) to try to prevent stricture formation. Strictures should be dilated by bougienage, followed by long-term medical therapy with proton pump inhibitors (PPIs). In general, patients with scleroderma require a high dosage of a proton pump inhibitor (Table 42.4) for treatment of esophagitis. Antireflux surgery should be avoided because the motility disorder may cause significant dysphagia after fundoplication.

Esophageal Webs and Rings

Dysphagia for solid foods may be caused by esophageal webs or rings. An *esophageal web* is a mucosal structure that protrudes into the lumen, most commonly in the proximal esophagus. The association of iron deficiency anemia with a proximal esophageal web constitutes the *Plummer-Vinson syndrome*. *Esophageal rings* are located in the distal esophagus and may be either mucosal or muscular; rings can be demonstrated in up to 10% of the population but rarely cause symptoms.

The ring that occurs just above the gastroesophageal junction is called a *Schatzki ring*. The origin of these lesions is unclear, but they are probably acquired. They are often found in asymptomatic individuals. There is some evidence that gastroesophageal reflux is associated with the development of a Schatzki ring.

Symptoms arise when the ring narrows the esophageal lumen to less than 13 mm in diameter and are rare if the lumen is more than 20 mm in diameter. A typical presenting symptom of a patient with an esophageal ring is intermittent dysphagia for solid foods. The patient may point to the area of the ring. At times a bolus of food may become impacted; the patient then regurgitates and then may be able to resume eating without further difficulty. The intermittency of the dysphagia, the chronicity of the condition, and the difficulty in making the diagnosis unless specifically suspected often result in misdiagnosis and in inappropriate therapy.

The diagnosis of esophageal ring is best made by barium swallow with a barium-coated marshmallow. The lower esophageal ring is best detected when the lower segment of the esophagus is distended, as it is during a Valsalva maneuver. Endoscopy is sometimes helpful to differentiate rings from annular strictures secondary to either reflux esophagitis or carcinoma. Cervical webs are often missed on conventional radiography but may be detected with cine studies. The webs usually are detected on the anterior surface of the esophagus, and lateral and oblique films are needed to demonstrate these lesions. Endoscopy often fails to visualize cervical webs and may disrupt the lesion during blind passage of the instrument into the esophagus. The endoscope may reveal an esophageal ring during air sufflation of the distal esophagus.

If the webs are associated with iron deficiency, treatment of the anemia causes rapid regression of the web. Otherwise, therapy involves mechanical disruption of the ring or web as well as reassurance, along with the recommendation to chew food well and slowly. Bougienage with a large-caliber dilator often disrupts the lower esophageal ring with complete relief of the dysphagia. The procedure causes transient discomfort but much less pain than does pneumatic dilation. It is ordinarily done by a gastroenterologist. Rarely, symptoms may persist after bougienage, and pneumatic dilation or even surgery may be necessary.

Globus Sensation

Globus sensation is a diagnosis often incorrectly made in patients with dysphagia who have no demonstrable organic disease. However, this condition does not produce dysphagia. Patients with globus describe the sensation of a lump in the throat, but do not have difficulty swallowing. These symptoms may be more pronounced with eating. However, when specifically questioned, patients deny dysphagia or food sticking or being held up in this region and they state that the symptom is present even when they are not eating. The pathogenesis of this condition is unknown, but hypertonicity of the upper esophageal sphincter, as a primary disorder or as a consequence of esophageal reflux, has been suggested. Gastroesophageal reflux should be ruled out (see below) before a psychologic disturbance (see Chapter 21) is diagnosed. Reassurance and an explanation of the problem form the basis for treatment. Recognizing this disorder avoids confusion in patients with true dysphagia.

ESOPHAGEAL CHEST PAIN

Chest pain is a common and difficult diagnostic challenge. Approximately 10% to 30% of patients with chest pain have normal coronary arteries at the time of coronary angiography. Despite reassurance, many of these patients continue to take antianginal medications and are hospitalized on an average of once each year for continuing evaluation (13). Esophageal disorders may account for the symptoms in some of these individuals, but the prevalence of esophageal chest pain is unknown.

Etiology and Pathogenesis

Esophageal chest pain has been attributed to stimulation of esophageal chemoreceptors by acid reflux or of mechanoreceptors by smooth muscle spasm or esophageal distension. Cold or hot liquids may cause severe chest pain, suggesting an alteration in the sensitivity of temperature receptors in the esophagus. Transient esophageal myoischemia may be a cause of pain in patients with spastic motility disorders. Such patients have an increased frequency of psychiatric disorders and have personality profiles similar to those of patients with the irritable bowel syndrome (see Chapter 44), suggesting that chronic stress may play a role in the pathogenesis of their chest pain. Panic disorder has been diagnosed in up to one-third of patients with chest pain and normal coronary angiograms (14).

Two major abnormalities have been associated with esophageal chest pain: esophageal motility disorders and gastroesophageal reflux disease (GERD). Studies using ambulatory pH monitoring have demonstrated clinically significant gastroesophageal reflux in approximately 45% of patients with unexplained chest pain. The typical symptom of gastroesophageal reflux—heartburn—is seen in about half of patients with GERD-related chest pain. Approximately 30% of patients with esophageal chest pain have a demonstrable motility disorder, of which *nutcracker esophagus* (hypertensive esophagus, supersqueezer) is the most common. This manometric abnormality is characterized by peristaltic contractions in the distal esophagus with contraction amplitude greater than two standard deviations above normal (less than 180 mm Hg) associated with chest pain (Table 42.2). Many of these patients have prolonged duration of contractions as well. *DES* (see above) is the motility disorder usually considered the principal cause of esophageal chest pain; however, studies have found it to be uncommon, representing less than 10% of esophageal motility abnormalities in patients with noncardiac chest pain (15). Other disorders, such as an *isolated elevated LES pressure* (hypertensive LES) and *achalasia,* are rarely associated with noncardiac chest pain. A large number of patients (approximately 35%) have contraction abnormalities that do not fit into one of the four categories defined here. These patients have been historically grouped under the general category of *nonspecific esophageal motility disorders;* however, these patients have had their motility abnormalities re-evaluated and are now classified as having ineffective esophageal motility. This abnormality is defined as low amplitude esophageal contractions (<30 mm Hg) in more than 30% of swallows (see Table 42.2) (16). Evaluation requires consultation with a gastroenterologist. Few patients have spontaneous chest pain during stationary esophageal motility testing (even if esophageal motility is abnormal), but chest pain is often reproduced when the esophagus is stimulated with intravenous edrophonium (Tensilon). This cholinergic agonist reproduces chest pain accompanied by high-amplitude esophageal contractions in 20% to 30% of patients with chest pain and normal coronary arteries (13). Edrophonium does not cause narrowing of the coronary arteries nor does it cause chest pain in normal subjects or in patients with irritable bowel syndrome. A positive test indicates that the chest pain is of esophageal origin.

Diagnosis

Unfortunately, the history is not reliable in differentiating esophageal from cardiac pain or in distinguishing among the various esophageal causes of chest pain. Location, exertional onset, and radiation do not distinguish the two entities. Heartburn, dysphagia, or odynophagia suggests an esophageal etiology, but overlap exists. Pain lasting longer than 1 hour or pain that awakens the patient from sleep is more likely to be esophageal but is occasionally seen with cardiac disease. Therapeutic trials with antacids or nitrates do not reliably distinguish between the two diseases. Intraesophageal acid perfusion can cause pain and ST-T wave changes indistinguishable from that due to coronary artery disease, so cardiac disease must be ruled out before the esophagus can be implicated. A musculoskeletal etiology should be sought by careful examination of the chest wall and the costochondral joints. Peptic ulcer disease should be excluded by history, and if biliary tract disease is suspected, it should be excluded by ultrasound. Endoscopy is normal in 80% to 90% of cases and should not be done routinely (17). If heartburn is present, consideration should be given to a short (3- to 4-week) therapeutic trial of antireflux therapy. If this trial is unsuccessful, the patient should be referred for 24-hour ambulatory esophageal pH monitoring to assess the frequency of reflux and to correlate acid reflux with episodes of pain. Esophageal pH can be monitored during exercise to determine whether there is associated acid reflux. If this study is negative, esophageal manometry with provocative testing using edrophonium should be performed. Using this systematic approach, an esophageal etiology can be established in more than 60% of patients with noncardiac chest pain.

Treatment

If gastroesophageal reflux is diagnosed, treatment should proceed as outlined later in this chapter, although most patients require higher dosages of PPIs for pain relief. Treatment of patients who have only positive provocative tests is more difficult and controversial (Table 42.3). Once cardiac disease has been ruled out, reassurance should be given to all patients, specifically indicating that the esophagus, and not the heart, is the cause of their pain. Many experience a decrease in pain with this single intervention. Patients with spastic disorders or with nutcracker esophagus may respond to a nitrate or to a calcium channel blocker. Hydralazine may be tried in patients with symptomatic esophageal spasm if nitrates or calcium blockers are not successful. Trazodone HCl (Desyrel), an antidepressant, has been used successfully to relieve chest pain in these patients and is particularly useful in patients with other symptoms suggestive of depression. Imipramine (50 mg at bedtime) also has been shown to lower the frequency of esophageal chest pain (18). This dosage, lower than that typically used to treat depression, is suspected to have a visceral analgesic effect on smooth muscle. Tranquilizers and anticholinergics have been used successfully in some patients. Patients with symptoms unresponsive to these measures may respond to biofeedback or to other psychologic interventions. Several uncontrolled studies have shown improvement in chest pain caused by esophageal motility disorders after injection with botulinum toxin (19). Rarely surgery with a long esophageal myotomy is required in patients with severe pain in whom pharmacologic therapy has failed. Many patients with esophageal chest pain, whatever the cause, continue to have intermittent symptoms despite therapeutic intervention.

GASTROESOPHAGEAL REFLUX

GERD is common in the United States. Approximately 10% of Americans experience daily heartburn and up to 33%

have symptoms at least monthly. Most patients complain of burning substernal pain that radiates upward, often aggravated by meals and by lying down and relieved by sitting up. Approximately 10% of people have chest pain that is similar to that of angina pectoris as the sole manifestation of reflux. The percentage of people with hoarseness, cough, or wheezing caused by GERD is unknown (20). In most cases the diagnosis and treatment of GERD can be managed successfully by the primary care provider; however, 10% to 15% of patients develop complications and require referral to a gastroenterologist.

Etiology and Pathogenesis

The etiology of GERD is unknown. Several defects contribute to the development and progression of the disease. By far the most significant is an abnormality of the antireflux barrier: the LES. Two major abnormalities of the LES are associated with an increased frequency of reflux: *a low basal LES pressure* and *transient LES relaxation* unassociated with a swallow. The latter abnormality is the most common cause of an episode of reflux. Abnormal esophageal epithelial resistance (increased permeability to hydrogen ions), abnormalities of gastric emptying, gastric distension, and the nature of the gastric refluxate (acid, pepsin, and bile) all contribute to the development of GERD.

Diagnosis

Several diagnostic tests are available to establish the clinical diagnosis. No single test provides complete information about the cause and consequences of reflux, so careful selection among the available modalities is required. In patients with mild heartburn, a therapeutic trial of what has been termed phase I therapy, including antacids or H_2 receptor antagonists in over-the-counter doses, may be an effective diagnostic approach. Studies have evaluated the utility of high dose PPIs (the equivalent of 40 to 60 mg omeprazole daily for 1 to 2 weeks) to determine if symptoms are relieved (21). If successful, no further workup may be needed. Patients with dysphagia and chest pain should be considered for further evaluation to determine the cause of their symptoms. If the diagnosis of reflux disease is established, treatment can proceed as outlined below. Patients with symptoms for more than 10 years, especially if they are 50 years or older, should have endoscopy because of the higher prevalence of Barrett esophagus (see below).

A *barium swallow* may be used to define macroscopic anatomic abnormalities in patients with GERD. However, since hiatal hernia or free reflux may be present in 30% to 40% of the general population, these findings, together or alone, should not be used to make a diagnosis of reflux disease. The presence of mucosal irregularities, stricture, or esophageal ulcer suggests a high likelihood (85% to 95%) that GERD is present.

Endoscopy (esophagoscopy) is the best study for the diagnosis and evaluation of reflux esophagitis or of other complications of GERD such as stricture or Barrett epithelium. If esophagitis is present at endoscopy, the diagnosis of GERD is established with 95% certainty, and no further workup is required. If a stricture is encountered, it should be biopsied to rule out carcinoma (dilation may be done at the same sitting in some patients). If Barrett mucosa is observed, biopsies can be taken to confirm the diagnosis and to rule out dysplasia or *in situ* carcinoma.

The diagnosis of GERD is established in most patients by the combination of history, response to therapy, and endoscopy. If the diagnosis is still in doubt or the patient presents with an atypical symptom, 24-hour *ambulatory pH monitoring* should be performed. Endoscopy may be normal in 40% of patients in whom reflux is subsequently verified by prolonged intraesophageal pH monitoring. The test is performed by placing a 2-mm flexible antimony probe transnasally so that the tip of the probe rests 5 cm above the LES. The probe is connected to a recording box similar to an ambulatory electrocardiographic monitor and worn about the waist. The patient can then be monitored at home eating a normal diet. Ambulatory monitoring is extremely useful in patients with noncardiac chest pain, in patients with wheezing, cough, or hoarseness due to reflux, or in patients with typical symptoms when a diagnosis is elusive. Probes may be placed at multiple levels in the esophagus to evaluate patients with atypical symptoms. All patients who are being considered for surgery should have pH monitoring to confirm the diagnosis before the operation. The study is extremely reproducible and is currently the most sensitive and specific diagnostic test for the presence of abnormal acid reflux.

Figure 42.2 outlines a suggested approach to the diagnosis of GERD.

Treatment

Treatment has traditionally been divided into phases (Table 42.4), implying that each is a distinct step to be followed in all patients. At present it is accepted that therapy should be individualized using a combination of lifestyle modifications (historically *phase I therapy*) and pharmacologic or surgical interventions. The overall goals of treatment are the complete relief of symptoms to improve the quality of life of the patient, the healing of erosive esophagitis if present, and the prevention of symptomatic relapse or complications.

Lifestyle modifications include elevating the head of the bed on 6- to 8-inch blocks or using a wedge designed to be placed in the bed under the shoulders and upper back. The patient should avoid sleeping on more pillows because this might actually increase abdominal pressure

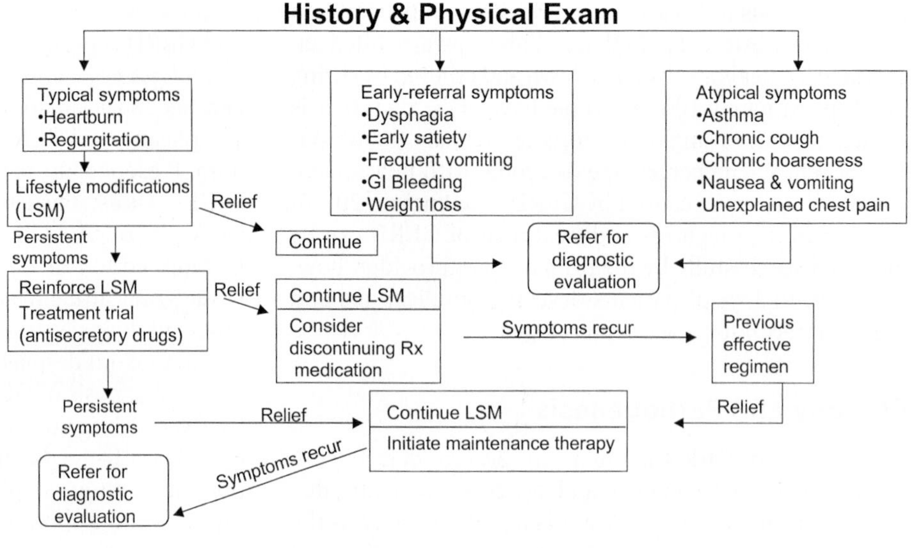

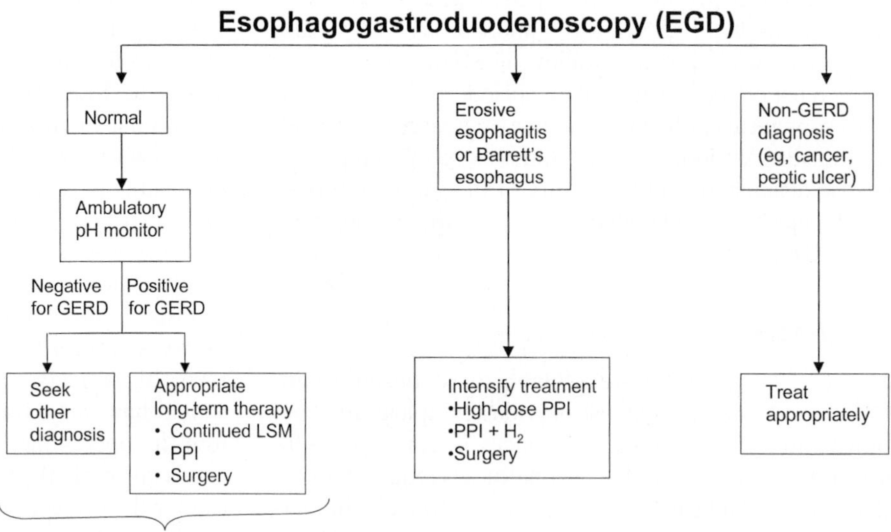

FIGURE 42.2. Approach to patients with gastroesophageal reflux. GERD, gastroesophageal reflux disease; PPI, proton pump inhibitor.

and contribute to more reflux. Certain foods (e.g., coffee, citrus juice, and spices) are direct esophageal irritants and should be avoided. The patient should be instructed not to lie down after a meal because this promotes greater reflux. Avoidance of food 3 hours before going to bed has also been shown to decrease episodes of reflux. Obesity and alcohol use are both risk factors for the development of GERD, and weight loss and avoidance of alcohol may contribute to reducing the severity of reflux. Drugs that decrease LES pressure (e.g., calcium channel blockers, nitrates, sedatives, and theophylline) should be avoided. Antacids and over the counter H_2 antagonists can be considered adjuncts to lifestyle modifications and should be used as needed to relieve daytime symptoms. The current practice of using PPIs as first-line therapy has relegated lifestyle modifications to a minor role in many guidelines, though the American College of Gastroenterology guidelines recommend that such modifications are part of any treatment program for GERD. Few would use behavioral modification as the only therapy for established GERD.

Pharmacologic therapy is aimed at decreasing gastric acid secretion (H_2 antagonists or PPIs). Prokinetic agents that augment LES pressure and improve esophageal clearance are rarely used as primary therapy. Metoclopramide is the only prokinetic agent currently approved for heartburn; however, the high frequency of side effects precludes its widespread use except as a combination agent in patients refractory to antisecretory therapy. Proton pump inhibitors have replaced H_2 antagonists as the initial choice of antisecretory therapy in GERD. If an H_2 receptor antagonist is used, treatment should be given with a twice-daily dose and continued for 6 to 8 weeks. Average acute healing rates are approximately 50% with this regimen. If symptoms do not resolve, a proton pump inhibitor should be started. Although doubling the dose of H_2 receptor antagonists may be mandated by some managed care algorithms, there is no evidence of improved efficacy with this strategy (22).

Current data support PPIs as the most effective therapy for all symptoms of GERD, for both acute and long-term therapy. Healing rates for omeprazole, lansoprazole, rabeprazole, and pantoprazole are equivalent and average 85% after 8 weeks of therapy. Esomeprazole, an optical isomer of omeprazole, is the only proton pump inhibitor to demonstrate superior-healing rates when compared with omeprazole (23). Proton pump inhibitors should be considered in all patients as potential first-line agents for treatment.

Long-Term Treatment

GERD is a chronic disease. Symptomatic and endoscopic relapse of esophagitis occurs in up to 80% of patients initially treated successfully. Therefore, most patients require some form of long-term therapy (24,25), that must be individualized. H_2 receptor antagonists at full dosage are approved for maintenance treatment but are effective in maintaining symptomatic and endoscopic remission in fewer than 50% of patients. The PPIs give the best symptomatic relief, and all five available agents are effective agents in maintaining symptom relief and remission of esophagitis (approximately 85% of patients, on daily therapy) (25). It is now clear that it may be as difficult to maintain remission in patients with nonerosive GERD as it is to treat patients with erosive esophagitis or Barrett esophagus, so PPIs can be considered the most effective agents for long-term therapy regardless of the presence or absence of erosions. Continuous treatment with PPIs for up to 11 years has been demonstrated to be safe without a need for special monitoring, including measurement of serum gastrin (26). It is likely that patients can be treated indefinitely with these agents.

Surgery may be considered in patients who require long-term daily medical therapy. However, there are no absolute indications for surgery, since most patients can be treated effectively with high-dose proton pump inhibitor therapy. The best predictor of a positive outcome from surgery is an initial response to medical therapy with PPIs (25). All patients, prior to surgery, should have esophageal manometry to evaluate LES pressure and esophageal peristalsis and ambulatory pH monitoring to confirm the diagnosis of abnormal acid exposure before surgery. Fundoplication around the distal esophagus provides symptomatic improvement in approximately 90% of patients. Success with the laparoscopic operation is equal to that of the open procedure (27). In experienced hands, hospitalization is reduced to 1 to 2 days, with a marked decrease in pain and an earlier return to normal activity. Simple repair of hiatus hernia, if present, has not been as effective nor have the benefits been as long-lasting. Fundoplication provides an effective barrier to reflux. Several variations of the operation are available, and local surgical expertise generally dictates the specific operation that is performed. Complications include dysphagia, which may require esophageal dilatation, and the gas-bloat syndrome from inability to belch. Studies indicate that over half of the patients treated with antireflux surgery have returned to using medication 10 years or more after the operation, a reminder that the benefit from this intervention may not be permanent (28). Care in selecting an experienced surgeon is critical. Antireflux surgery for patients with scleroderma should be avoided, because it may markedly exacerbate dysphagia. Vagotomy is not indicated in the treatment of GERD. There is no evidence that surgery reduces the risk of esophageal cancer or improves symptoms in patients with Barrett epithelium.

The Food and Drug Administration (FDA) has approved two endoscopic therapies for GERD: radiofrequency ablation of the LES region and an endoscopic sewing device. Each has been evaluated in only a small number of patients in uncontrolled single studies. Further evaluation is needed to determine the role of these procedures in GERD.

Complications

The complications of reflux include hemorrhage, ulcerations, stricture formation, and development of Barrett mucosa. Esophagitis is the cause of 5% to 10% of all cases of upper gastrointestinal hemorrhage. Peptic ulcers and strictures must be differentiated from malignancy and from ingestion of caustic substances. The presence of a midesophageal ulcer or stricture should raise the suspicion of Barrett mucosa (columnar-type mucosa that replaces the squamous mucosa of the tubular esophagus). This type of mucosa has characteristic staining features that differentiate it from normal gastric tissue. This metaplastic intestinal type of epithelium is a premalignant condition. Patients with Barrett mucosa should therefore undergo regular endoscopic surveillance (every 2 to 3 years) for the development of cancer.

HIATUS HERNIA

Herniation of a part of the stomach through the normal diaphragmatic esophageal hiatus into the thorax is called a hiatus hernia. The defect is common, but the precise prevalence is observer dependent. Estimates of prevalence therefore range from 30% to 60% overall. The defect is twice as common in women as in men and is seen in 70–80% of those older than 60 years of age. Hiatus hernia is not synonymous with reflux esophagitis, as a hernia may exist without producing symptomatic reflux and reflux may occur without hernia. If a patient has clear-cut reflux esophagitis, the treatment should not be influenced by the presence of a hiatus hernia. If a patient who does not have reflux is incidentally discovered to have a hiatus hernia, no treatment is indicated. A large hiatus hernia (>5 cm) may predispose to more serious reflux and itself cause symptoms of chest pain or dysphagia.

A *paraesophageal hernia,* herniation of part of the stomach through the diaphragm adjacent to the gastroesophageal junction, is potentially dangerous because of the risk of incarceration or acute obstruction, which is a surgical emergency.

SPECIFIC REFERENCES*

1. Devesa SS, Blot WJ, Fraumeni JF Jr. Changing patterns in the incidence of esophageal and gastric carcinoma in the United States. Cancer 1998;83:2049.
2. McLoughlin RF, Cooperberg PL, Mathieson JR, et al. High resolution endoluminal ultrasonography in the staging of esophageal carcinoma. J Ultrasound Med 1995;14:725.
3. Fleischer DE, Haddad NG. Neoplasms of the esophagus. In: Castell DO, ed. The esophagus. 4th ed. Philadelphia: Lippincott, Williams & Wilkins, 2003:376.
4. Reed C. Surgical management of esophageal cancer. Oncologist 1999;4:95.
5. Jemal A, Murray T, Ward W, et al. Cancer statistics, 2005. CA Cancer J Clin 2005;55:10.
6. Bondi JL, Goodwin DH, Garrett JM. Vigorous achalasia: its clinical interpretation and significance. Am J Gastroenterol 1972;58:145.
7. Katz PO, Richter JE, Cowan R, et al. Apparent complete lower esophageal sphincter relaxation in achalasia. Gastroenterology 1986;90:978.
8. Meijssen MAC, Tilanus HW, van Blankenstein M, et al. Achalasia complicated by oesophageal squamous cell carcinoma. A prospective study in 195 patients. Gut 1992;33:155.
9. Pasricha PJ, Rai R, Ravich WJ, et al. Botulinum toxin for achalasia: long-term outcome and predictors of response. Gastroenterology 1996; 110:1410.
10. Richter JE, Castell DO. Diffuse esophageal spasm: a reappraisal. Ann Intern Med 1984; 100:242.
11. Katz PO, Dalton CB, Richter JE, et al. Esophageal testing of patients with non-cardiac chest pain or dysphagia. Results of three years experience with 1161 patients. Ann Intern Med 1987;106:593.
12. Cohen S, Fisher R, Lipshutz W, et al. The pathogenesis of esophageal dysfunction in scleroderma and Raynaud's disease. J Clin Invest 1972;51:2663.
13. Katz PO. Approach to the patient with non cardiac chest pain. Semin Gastroenterol Dis 2001;12:38.
14. Katon W, Hall ML, Russo J. Chest pain: relationship of psychiatric illness to coronary arteriographic results. Am J Med 1988;84:1.
15. Dalton CB, Castell DO, Hewson EG, et al. Diffuse esophageal spasm. A rare motility disorder not characterized by high-amplitude contractions. Dig Dis Sci 1991;36:1025.
16. Leite LP, Johnston BT, Barrett J, et al. Ineffective esophageal motility: the primary finding in patients with nonspecific esophageal motility disorder. Dig Dis Sci 1997;42:1859.
17. Cherian P, Smith LF, Bardhan KD, et al. Esophageal tests in the evaluation of non-cardiac chest pain. Dis Esoph 1995;8:129.
18. Cannon RO, Quyyumi AA, Mincemoyer R, et al. Imipramine in patients with chest pain despite normal coronary angiograms. N Engl J Med 1994;330:1411.
19. Miller LS, Pullela SV, Parkman HP, et al. Treatment of chest pain in patients with non-cardiac, non-reflux, non-achalasia, spastic esophageal motor disorders using botulinum toxin injection into the gastoesophageal junction. Am J Gastroenterol 2002;97:1640.
20. Locke GR, Talley NJ, Fett SL, et al. Prevalence and clinical spectrum of gastroesophageal reflux: a population-based study in Olmsted County, Minnesota. Gastroenterology 1997;112:1448.
21. Fass R, Fennerty MB, Ofman JJ, et al. The clinical and economic value of a short course of omeprazole in patients with noncardiac chest pain. Gastroenterology 1998;115:42.
22. Kahrilas PJ, Fennerty MB, Joelsson B. High- versus standard-dose ranitidine for control of heartburn in poorly responsive acid reflux disease: a prospective, controlled trial. Am J Gastroenterol 1999;94:92.
23. Kahrilas PJ, Falk GW, Johnson DA, et al. Esomeprazole improves healing and symptom resolution as compared with omeprazole in reflux oesophagitis patients: a randomized controlled trial. Aliment Pharmacol Ther 2000; 14:1249.
24. Howden CS, Castell DO, Cohen S, et al. The rationale for continuous maintenance treatment of reflux esophagitis. Arch Intern Med 1995; 155:1465.
25. Vigneri S, Termini R, Leandro G, et al. A comparison of five maintenance therapies for reflux esophagitis. N Engl J Med 1995;333: 1106.
26. Klinkenberg-Knol EC, Festen HPM, Jansen JBMJ, et al. Long-term treatment with omeprazole for refractory reflux esophagitis. Ann Intern Med 1994;121:161.
27. So JB, Zeitels SM, Rattner DW. Outcomes of atypical symptoms attributed to gastroesophageal reflux treated by laparoscopic fundoplication. Surgery 1998;124:28.
28. Spechler SJ, Lee E, Ahnen D, et al. Long-term outcome of medical and surgical therapies for gastroesophageal reflux disease: follow-up of a randomized controlled trial. JAMA 2001; 285:2331.

*Bold numerals denote published controlled clinical trials, meta-analyses, or consensus-based recommendations.

For annotated ***General References*** *and resources related to this chapter, visit www.hopkinsbayview.org/PAMreferences.*

Chapter 43

Peptic Ulcer Disease

Mack C. Mitchell, Jr. and H. Franklin Herlong

EPIDEMIOLOGY AND NATURAL HISTORY

Peptic ulcer disease remains a common problem, even though the incidence of duodenal ulcers has decreased over the last 40 years (1). The incidence of gastric ulceration has not changed over this time (1) nor has the incidence of complications, such as bleeding, perforation, obstruction, and penetration of peptic ulcers (2). The economic impact of peptic ulceration is over $5 billion a year in the United States (3).

The prevalence of duodenal and gastric ulcer is approximately the same in men and women (2) but the prevalence and incidence of duodenal and gastric ulcers are higher in older compared with younger age groups (4).

Ulcers are usually less than 1 cm in diameter, although giant ulcers (larger than 2.5 cm) occasionally occur. Duodenal ulcers are almost always located in the duodenal bulb or within 3 cm of the pyloric duodenal junction. Ulcers distal to the duodenal bulb should raise the suspicion of the Zollinger-Ellison syndrome (discussed later in this chapter) or Crohn disease of the duodenum. Gastric ulcers are most commonly located on the lesser curvature, at the junction of the body and antrum of the stomach. There is no risk of cancer in a duodenal ulcer, but 1% to 3% of gastric ulcers not attributable to nonsteroidal anti-inflammatory drugs (NSAIDs) are malignant.

Untreated duodenal ulcers can be chronic. Ulcers recur in 50% to 90% of patients within 1 year of diagnosis if curative therapy is not given (5). The rate of recurrence is highest within the first 5 years and then decreases over 10 to 20 years (6,7). The recurrence rate of gastric ulcers appears to be lower (5). Both duodenal and gastric ulcers tend to recur in the same place as the index ulcer. Long-term studies suggest that bleeding or perforation occurs at a rate of 1% to 3% a year, with a lifetime incidence of approximately 20% (8) if the ulcer is not adequately treated. Recurrent hemorrhage occurs in approximately 50% of patients who have had a previous bleed. The complication rate may be reduced by maintenance therapy (9) and can be eliminated if the bacterium *Helicobacter pylori* is eradicated (see below). The major risk of death from ulcer disease is on the initial presentation (10).

PATHOPHYSIOLOGY

Duodenal Ulcer

Duodenal ulcer disease has traditionally been viewed as the result of an imbalance between the amount of acid delivered to the duodenum from the stomach and the normal duodenal defense mechanisms. A number of factors contribute to this imbalance including increased parietal cell mass, increased capacity of parietal cells to secrete acid, increased vagal drive to secrete acid, and defective inhibition of gastrin release and of gastric secretion. Alterations in normal duodenal defense mechanisms such as bicarbonate secretion, mucus production, vascular integrity, and endogenous prostaglandin production also promote ulcer formation. It is now clear that these imbalances can be caused by hypersecretory states, ingestion of NSAIDs, and most importantly by *H. pylori* infection.

Gastric Ulcer

The pathogenesis of gastric ulceration is unclear, although it is generally accepted that a disruption of the gastric mucosal barrier leads to gastric ulcer formation. This barrier can be affected by irritants such as bile, alcohol, and aspirin. These observations help explain the epidemiologic data associating alcohol with acute gastritis and aspirin with gastric ulcers and erosions. Furthermore, in patients with gastric ulcers, radiologic and manometric studies suggest increased duodenal gastric reflux. This reflux of bile across an incompetent pyloric sphincter results in the disruption of the mucosal barrier. Once the barrier is broken, hydrogen ion may diffuse back into the gastric cells, leading to ulceration via local histamine release, vasodilation, and tissue damage. According to this hypothesis, gastric ulcer formation requires injury to the gastric mucosal barrier and the presence of some, but not necessarily an excessive amount of, acid. *H. pylori* infection, bile acids, and NSAIDs may make the mucosa more susceptible to injury and result in a gastric ulcer.

RISK FACTORS

Helicobacter pylori

H. pylori infection is the most common and important risk factor for duodenal ulcer. The risk of gastric ulcer is probably multifactorial, although many gastric ulcers are also associated with *H. pylori.*

H. pylori is a gram-negative spiral organism found exclusively in gastric epithelium, although it may be seen in the duodenal bulb in regions where there is gastric metaplasia. In the United States, the organism is found in 10% of healthy people under 30 years of age and in approximately 60% of healthy people over age 60 (11). The rate of infection varies by country and by region of the United States and is more common in lower socioeconomic areas and in developing countries (11). The organism is probably spread by person to person contact.

H. pylori is the etiologic agent for chronic nonerosive antral gastritis (see below) and is present in the stomach in 70% of patients with a peptic ulcer, making it the most common cause of that disease (12). It is estimated that 15% to 20% of infected patients will develop an ulcer in their lifetime. Other diseases associated with *H. pylori* infection are B-cell mucosa-associated lymphoid tissue (MALT) lymphoma and gastric adenocarcinoma. As such, *H. pylori* has been recently classified as a class I biologic carcinogen.

Eradication of the organism accelerates duodenal ulcer healing (13) and significantly decreases ulcer recurrence 1 and 2 years after treatment (13,14). The rate of reinfection is unknown but appears to be less than 1% up to 5 years after treatment. Eradication of *H. pylori* also reduces recurrent bleeding in patients who have had ulcer-related gastrointestinal (GI) bleeding.

Although *H. pylori* infection is a major risk factor for peptic ulcer disease, 20% to 30% of gastroduodenal ulcers occur in the absence of *H. pylori* infection (15,16) with most of these caused by NSAID use. False-negative *H. pylori* screening tests may, in part, account for these findings, but the availability of more than one reliable test for *H. pylori* should improve detection. Prior use of antibiotics, particularly macrolides, or proton pump inhibitors (PPIs) within 6 weeks of *H. pylori* testing may also result in false-negative tests.

Nonsteroidal Anti-Inflammatory Drugs

There is good evidence that all *NSAIDs* can cause gastric and duodenal ulcers. The greatest risk of NSAID-induced gastric or duodenal injury occurs in people older than 60 years of age (17), in patients with a history of a GI "event" (peptic ulcer or hemorrhage), in patients who are taking corticosteroids or anticoagulant drugs concurrently, and in patients taking a dose of an NSAID that is two or more times the usual prescribed dose (18). Prospective and retrospective studies have concluded that chronic use of corticosteroids by patients who are not taking NSAIDs does not increase the risk of peptic ulcer disease or its complications (19). The cyclooxygenase (COX)-2 specific NSAIDs are associated with a significantly lower risk of gastric ulceration and major complications, including GI bleeding, compared with traditional nonselective NSAIDs (20,21). Until recently, these NSAIDs were often considered for patients who require anti-inflammatory drugs, especially those at risk for GI complications from this class of agents. However, some of the medications in this class have recently been removed from the market (as of this writing, celecoxib is the only product in this class still available) because use of these drugs has been associated with an increased risk of stroke and myocardial infarction. COX-2 inhibitors, if available, should therefore be reserved for patients who require an NSAID for a relatively short time and who have a low cardiovascular risk profile.

Other Factors

Genetic factors were once thought to play an important role in the development of peptic ulcers, but since the identification of *H. pylori* and NSAIDs as major risk factors, it has been recognized that the role of inheritance is minimal (22). The role of emotional stress in the pathogenesis of peptic ulcer disease seems clinically evident but has been difficult to quantitate. In fact, in a case control study, the number of stressors in the lives of patients with duodenal ulcer was no greater than in control subjects (23).

regimen, ranging from 10% to 30%, and may be reduced by the addition of a PPI. A single daily dose of a PPI will increase compliance, which is the key to a successful regimen. Patients who are intolerant of tetracycline can be given amoxicillin (500 mg four times a day) in its place.

If *H. pylori* is successfully eradicated, there is no need for maintenance therapy. If symptoms recur after adequate treatment, the patient should be tested for the presence of the organism (urea breath test, stool antigen testing, or repeat endoscopy, depending on availability and cost). If *H. pylori* is present, it is probably not due to reinfection but to ineffective treatment, and another course of treatment should be prescribed. If *H. pylori* is not found, evaluation for another cause of symptoms should be pursued.

Though the combination of PPIs with antibiotics is the preferred treatment of *H. pylori*-associated ulcers, antisecretory agents such as antacids and H_2 receptor antagonists are effective in relief of symptoms and may still be used in selected patients with intolerance to PPIs or with *H. pylori*-negative ulcers. lists the currently available drugs used in the treatment of peptic ulcer disease.

Antacids are rapidly acting and are effective for transient relief of symptoms. A large selection of calcium carbonate, aluminum, or magnesium-based antacids is available. They should not be used as the sole treatment to heal peptic ulcers, but they may be used as adjunctive agents to control symptoms. *Histamine receptor antagonists* were the mainstay of therapy before the development of combination PPI-antibiotic regimens to treat peptic ulcer disease. Four H_2 receptor antagonists are available: cimetidine, ranitidine, famotidine, and nizatidine (Table 43.3). All are available as generic compounds, and all are available in over-the-counter (OTC) dosage formulations. They are used to treat ulcers in full dose given twice daily or as a nocturnal dose. When used in FDA-approved dosing schedules, H_2 receptor antagonists reduce acid production by 30% to 50%, keep intragastric pH above 3 (the critical value for ulcer healing) for 8 to 12 hours, and effectively heal more than 80% of peptic ulcers after 6 to 8 weeks of therapy (41). Side effects are infrequent (rare abdominal discomfort, nausea, and vomiting). Of the available H_2 receptor antagonists, cimetidine has the greatest potential for interaction with drugs that effect the cytochrome

TABLE 43.3 Drugs Approved for the Treatment of Peptic Ulcer Disease

Drug	*Available Strength*	*OTC*	*Generic*	*Initial Dose*	*Principal Side Effects*[a]
H_2 Receptor Blockers					
Cimetidine (Tagamet)	100, 200, 300, 400, 800 mg	+	+	400 mg b.i.d. or 800 mg at bedtime	Gynecomastia, confusion, impotence, blood dyscrasia, drug interaction
Ranitidine (Zantac)	75, 150, 300 mg	+	+	150 b.i.d. or 300 mg at bedtime	Gynecomastia, impotence, hepatitis (rare)
Famotidine (Pepcid)	10, 20, 40 mg	+	–	20 mg b.i.d. or 40 mg at bedtime	Headache, decreased libido, depression, mild increase in liver enzymes
Nizatidine (Axid)	75, 150, 300 mg	+	–	150 mg b.i.d. or 300 mg at bedtime	Sweating, urticaria (<1%), somnolence, elevated liver enzymes
Proton Pump Inhibitors[b]					
Omeprazole (Prilosec)	10, 20, 40 mg	–	–	20 mg/day (DU) 40 mg/day (GU)	Headache, dizziness, rash, diarrhea, abdominal pain
Lansoprazole (Prevacid)[c]	15, 30 mg	–	–	30 mg/day	Diarrhea, abdominal pain
Rabeprazole (Aciphex)[c]	20 mg	–	–	20 mg/day	Headache
Pantoprazole (Protonix)[c]	40 mg	–	–	40 mg/day	Chest pain, headache, diarrhea
Esomeprazole (Nexium)[c]	20, 40 mg	–	–	20–40 mg/day	Headache, diarrhea, nausea, abdominal pain
Sucralfate (Carafate)	1 g	–	–	1 g q.i.d. or 2 g q.i.d.	Constipation

[a]1%–10% of patients.
[b]For eradication of *H. pylori* infection, all PPIs are given b.i.d. (i.e., twice the initial dose listed in the table) for 10–14 days except esomeprazole, 40 mg, which is given once a day.
[c]Not approved by FDA for treatment of gastric ulcer.
OTC, over-the-counter; DU, duodenal ulcer; GU, gastric ulcer.

P450 system such as diazepam, phenytoin, warfarin, and theophylline.

Sucralfate forms a protective coating on the mucosa of the stomach and duodenum and is as effective as H_2 blockers in the healing of peptic ulcers. It has been replaced by PPIs as initial and maintenance therapy for peptic ulcer disease.

Most *H. pylori*-negative duodenal ulcers are caused by NSAIDs and resolve with discontinuation of the offending agent. A PPI is often added to promote healing. Maintenance therapy is unnecessary unless the patient has had severe GI bleeding. When used, maintenance therapy consists of one-half the daily dose of whatever drug was given for acute healing.

Gastric Ulcer

In general, the same drugs used to treat duodenal ulcers are effective in the treatment of gastric ulcer (Table 43.3). If *H. pylori* is present, it should be eradicated (Table 43.2), regardless of whether NSAIDs are thought to be implicated.

Healing must be documented by endoscopy 4 to 8 weeks after the diagnosis of a gastric ulcer to exclude possible underlying malignancy. No dietary restrictions affect healing, and hospitalization is unnecessary in the absence of complications. NSAIDs, including aspirin, should be discontinued if possible. Smoking cessation should be strongly recommended. Maintenance therapy is necessary if the ulcer was due to *H. pylori*, until the infection is eradicated.

Chapter 77 discusses the prevention and treatment of NSAID-associated gastropathy.

SURGICAL THERAPY

Although surgery is effective therapy for the relief of ulcer symptoms and for the prevention of ulcer recurrence, with current medical therapy it is rarely indicated. At present the only indications for surgical treatment of peptic ulcer disease are perforation, uncontrolled hemorrhage, gastric outlet obstruction, and, rarely, intractability. Because most operations are performed on an emergency basis, the type of surgery is generally decided upon in the operating room after the surgeon has evaluated the gastroduodenal area.

Duodenal Ulcer

Three operations are currently used for duodenal ulcer: *vagotomy with pyloroplasty, vagotomy with antrectomy,* and *parietal cell (or highly selective) vagotomy.* The first two procedures involve a selective vagotomy (gastric vagal fibers only) plus a drainage procedure to facilitate gastric emptying postoperatively. The third procedure involves cutting vagal fibers to the body (acid-secreting cells) of the stomach, preserving antral innervation, and eliminating the need for a drainage procedure. Vagotomy with pyloroplasty has the lowest mortality, shortest operation time, and a recurrence rate of 6% to 8%. Vagotomy with antrectomy is technically more difficult and may predispose patients to more postoperative morbidity (because an anastomosis to the remaining stomach is required) but has the lowest recurrence rate (less than 2%) (42). Postoperative complications (Table 43.4) are significantly more common with either procedure than with parietal cell vagotomy. A parietal cell vagotomy has a recurrence rate of 10% at 10 years (42), approximately four to five times that of vagotomy with antrectomy. Long-term complications (of dumping syndrome and diarrhea) are less than 60% those of vagotomy with antrectomy. In the hands of experienced surgeons, a parietal cell vagotomy is the operation of choice. The higher recurrence rate (which can be managed medically in 80%) is an acceptable trade-off for the decreased complication rate.

Gastric Ulcer

The surgical approach for gastric ulcers is not as well established since the causes of gastric ulceration are more complicated. In contrast to duodenal ulcer disease, a vagotomy may not be indicated in all patients with a gastric ulcer who undergo surgery. However, in patients who have evidence of concomitant duodenal ulcer disease (approximately 10% to 40% of patients with gastric ulcers) and in patients who have pyloric ulcers, which generally behave as duodenal ulcers, a vagotomy is clearly indicated. If the ulcer is within the antrum, an antrectomy or hemigastrectomy that includes the ulcer is often the preferred operation. When the ulcer cannot be included in the gastric resection, a full-thickness biopsy of the ulcer should be taken for frozen section to rule out malignancy. The recurrence rate for gastric ulcers after these types of operation is very low (1% to 2%).

After antrectomy or hemigastrectomy, the stomach may be anastomosed to the duodenum (Billroth I anastomosis) or to the jejunum (Billroth II). The type of anastomosis is determined by the surgeon, based on the degree of duodenal deformity and on technical considerations.

Postgastrectomy Syndromes

Many problems develop after gastrectomy (Table 43.4). In 10% of patients, postgastrectomy complications are severe. Many of these conditions result from the altered physiology created by the surgery.

ZOLLINGER-ELLISON SYNDROME

The Zollinger-Ellison syndrome dramatically demonstrates the relationship between gastrin, acid secretion,

TABLE 43.4 Postgastrectomy Syndromes

Syndrome	Clinical Features	Pathophysiology	Diagnosis and Treatment
Early			
Stomal dysfunction	Vomiting, gastric retention	Edema, inflammation, hypokalemia	Electrolyte repletion, time, no suction
Duodenal stump dehiscence	Pain, fever, signs of abscess, sepsis, death	Billroth II anastomosis: tension and poor closure, adjacent pancreatitis, excessive inflammation in area of surgery	Reoperation
Afferent loop syndrome	Pain, vomiting bile without food, may occur acutely or chronically	Billroth II anastomosis: afferent loop too long, kinked, twisted, herniated etc.; loop fills, then empties	Reoperation
Vagotomy complications			
Transient dysphagia	Dysphagia	Lower esophageal sphincter dysfunction	Usually transient, disappears in 1–2 wk
Diarrhea	Diarrhea transient or slight, 20%–40% of patients; troublesome, 5%; occurs mainly with selective vagotomy and drainage procedure	Most common after truncal vagotomy; appears to be related to increased output of dihydroxy bile salts, the cause of which is uncertain	Cholestyramine, Amphojel
Late or Persistent			
Dumping syndrome	Early phase: with or shortly after meals–nausea, abdominal fullness or pain, cramping, palpations, dizziness, sweating	Distension of gastric pouch and upper jejunum from rapid emptying; peripheral intravascular volume depletion from rapid entry of fluid into jejunum due to osmotic changes in jejunum; vasomotor symptoms related to release of vasoactive substances into circulation, such as serotonin and bradykinin	Small frequent meals, high protein, low carbohydrate, small volume of liquids only
	Late phase: symptoms of hypoglycemia	Early hyperglycemia → insulin production → late hypoglycemia	
Gastric cancer	Increased incidence of 3%–5% in gastric stump 15–20 yr after surgery	Possibly related to chronic gastritis developing after gastrectomy	Endoscopy for diagnosis, surgical resection
Diarrhea	Chronic diarrhea	Rapid gastric emptying, lactose intolerance unmasked by vagotomy, malabsorption, Z-E syndrome, bile acid output increased, bacterial overgrowth	Lactose-free diet; if no response, malabsorption workup (Chapter 45)
Stomal or recurrent ulcer	Recurrent ulcer symptoms; hemorrhage in approximately 50%	Hyperacidity caused by inadequate resection, incomplete vagotomy, retained antrum, unrecognized Z-E syndrome (gastrinoma)	Endoscopy; H_2 antagonists, (successful in 80%), reoperation
Anemia	Iron deficiency	Chronic blood loss; impaired iron absorption	Repletion of deficient nutrient
	Nutritional anemia	Defective vitamin B_{12} absorption because of decreased intrinsic factor production (resection and gastritis); possible blind loop bacterial overgrowth; folate deficiency	
Osteomalacia	Bone pain	Diminished calcium intake, poor vitamin D absorption; duodenal bypass	

Z-E, Zollinger-Ellison.

and ulcer formation. The syndrome results from a *non–β islet cell tumor* of the pancreas that autonomously secretes gastrin and is therefore called a *gastrinoma.* In most cases multiple tumors are present, most commonly found in the head of the pancreas. These tumors vary considerably in size from several millimeters, often undetectable at surgery, to huge masses that may even be palpable through the abdominal wall. Approximately two thirds of gastrinomas are malignant; although they are usually slow growing, they can metastasize and can be a cause of death.

The appreciation of the clinical features of Zollinger-Ellison syndrome changed when measurement of serum gastrin levels became available. The original description of the syndrome focused on the virulent nature of the ulcer diathesis and on the atypical location for the ulcers. It is now recognized, however, that 75% of ulcers in patients with Zollinger-Ellison syndrome occur in the duodenal bulb and appear as routine single lesions. However, the finding of postbulbar and jejunal ulcerations should still alert the clinician to the possibility of the syndrome. More than one fourth of patients undergo ulcer surgery before the diagnosis of the syndrome, which is usually made only when anastomotic ulcers develop.

Diarrhea occurs in approximately one third of patients, and may precede the formation of ulcers by several years. Some patients have diarrhea and never develop an ulcer. Diarrhea is caused principally by the increased secretion of gastric acid that lowers the pH of the normally alkaline duodenal fluid and interferes with absorption of water and electrolytes.

Diagnosis

The diagnosis of Zollinger-Ellison syndrome should be considered when duodenal ulcers do not heal with medical therapy, or when there are giant ulcers multiple ulcers, postbulbar or jejunal ulcers, or anastomotic ulcers. Ulcer disease associated with diarrhea or with radiographic evidence of gastric hypersecretion also suggests Zollinger-Ellison syndrome.

The diagnosis of Zollinger-Ellison syndrome is usually based on the fasting serum gastrin concentration, normally less than 150 mg/mL. Elevations greater than 1,000 mg/mL in association with the typical clinical picture are virtually diagnostic of a gastrinoma. However, in patients with mild elevations of the serum gastrin concentration (between 150 and 300 mg/mL) and in postoperative patients, differentiation between Zollinger-Ellison syndrome and other causes of hypergastrinemia is important. Other conditions that may lead to hypergastrinemia include retained antrum, G-cell hyperplasia, postvagotomy with pyloroplasty, and pernicious anemia. Also, H_2 receptor blockers and PPIs cause a slight increase in the serum gastrin concentration, and therefore should be stopped for at least several weeks before gastrin levels are measured.

Differentiation of the Zollinger-Ellison syndrome from other causes of hypergastrinemia often requires the use of provocative tests, i.e., the secretin and calcium infusion tests, generally performed by a gastroenterologist. The *secretin test* is preferred because it is more reliable and is safer. In both tests, the response of the serum gastrin level to the infusion of a stimulating substance is monitored. In the secretin test, the serum gastrin level rises, usually within the first half hour after the injection of secretin, in patients with Zollinger-Ellison syndrome, whereas in all other disorders the gastrin level falls or is unchanged.

Gastric analysis may provide further supportive data. Marked hypersecretion is found in both the basal state and after pentagastrin stimulation. Because the stomach is being influenced by an autonomous tumor, further stimulation with exogenous pentagastrin provides little additional stimulation to secretion. Thus, the basal acid output to maximal acid output ratio is 0.6 or greater in this syndrome. However, there is considerable overlap with normal values, so gastric secretory data alone cannot be used to make the diagnosis.

Therapy

Because the tumor mass is rarely localized and therefore rarely curable by local resection, therapy is directed at the end organ. Although total gastrectomy historically was the procedure of choice, in recent years it has become clear that medical therapy is successful in controlling both the ulcer disease and the diarrhea, making surgery often unnecessary. The PPIs (Table 43.3) are also extremely successful in controlling acid secretion in these patients, although high doses are often required. Long-term treatment with these agents is safe. Although gastrectomy prevents the consequences of hypersecretion of acid it does not alter the biologic behavior of the gastrinoma. In the past, patients died from this condition, most often because of the virulent nature of the ulcer disease (with frequent recurrences), because of severe diarrhea (with malabsorption), and as a result of multiple operations and their complications.

DYSPEPSIA

The term dyspepsia is often used to describe epigastric discomfort, occasionally related to meals and sometimes associated with nausea, belching, or bloating. It is estimated to be present in 7% of the U.S. population, most of whom rarely seek medical attention. When patients with dyspepsia are evaluated with endoscopy, only 20% to 25% have peptic ulcer disease or gastric cancer. Non-ulcer dyspepsia presents a diagnostic and therapeutic dilemma.

Four major disorders are associated with nonulcer dyspepsia: irritable bowel syndrome, cholelithiasis, gastroesophageal reflux, and chronic pancreatic disease. In irritable bowel syndrome (see Chapter 44) the dyspepsia is associated with diffuse abdominal pain and altered bowel habits. Patients with gastroesophageal reflux disease have associated heartburn (see Chapter 42). Chronic pancreatic disease is less common but is usually associated with more severe pain and steatorrhea. The most difficult diagnostic dilemma, because of the high prevalence of gallstones in the general population, is distinguishing patients with symptomatic gallstones from patients with dyspepsia and asymptomatic (incidental) gallstones (see Chapter 96). It is now well established that patients with dyspepsia do not respond to cholecystectomy unless they have had an identifiable attack of acute cholecystitis or a history of biliary colic. The absence of either should suggest that gallstones are not the cause of dyspepsia.

Patients without one of these identifiable conditions are said to have *essential dyspepsia*. The etiology of this condition is unknown. A small subset of patients has been described with delayed gastric emptying of solid foods; however, correlation of improvement of symptoms with treatment has been poor. Approximately 50% of patients have *H. pylori* gastritis, but symptomatic response to treatment for this infection has been inconsistent. Patients with essential dyspepsia do not have increased basal acid secretion nor has a definite association with emotional stress been documented.

The patient with essential dyspepsia can be difficult to manage. The yield of radiographic and endoscopic procedures is low and may be confusing. Response to empiric therapy with H_2 blockers or PPIs has been disappointing and may be misleading.

Patients younger than 40 years with a short history and no evidence of organic disease by physical examination and appropriate laboratory tests should be treated with reassurance, some modification of their diet, and avoidance of caffeine, alcohol, and tobacco. A 4-week trial of H_2 blockers or PPIs may be used (Table 43.3). If no response occurs after 4 weeks and no evidence of reflux disease or irritable bowel syndrome is present, endoscopy should be performed. If endoscopy is negative, the other diagnoses should be pursued. Patients older than age 50 are candidates for early investigation (within 1 to 2 weeks), particularly if symptoms are severe and have occurred for the first time. In this group the diagnostic yield of endoscopy is 60% (43). Patients who are not responsive to these measures are often treated for *H. pylori* infection if these organisms are demonstrated on gastric biopsy; however, data from placebo-controlled trials suggest that treatment of *H. pylori* does not result in long-term relief of essential or nonulcer dyspepsia (44). An individualized approach is necessary using a combination of antisecretory agents, reassurance, and supportive care. The long-term prognosis is good with or without treatment in patients in whom endoscopy is negative.

GASTRITIS

Gastritis—inflammation of the stomach mucosa—is a nonspecific diagnosis that is made by endoscopic biopsy. It may be variably associated with dyspepsia, although a cause and effect relationship has not been documented. Several types of gastritis are seen in clinical practice.

Acute erosive, or *hemorrhagic, gastritis* is seen most commonly in seriously ill hospitalized patients; in patients taking NSAIDs, including aspirin; after heavy alcohol ingestion; and rarely in patients taking potassium chloride or iron supplements. Symptoms are variable but usually include nausea or vomiting and gastrointestinal bleeding.

Nonerosive or *chronic antral gastritis* is a histologic entity commonly seen in the general population, particularly the elderly and often caused by *H. pylori* infection. However, it is unclear whether the histologic (or endoscopic) entity of gastritis is associated with symptomatic disease. There is no correlation between eradication of *H. pylori,* histologic resolution of gastritis, and relief of dyspepsia, bloating, abdominal pain, or gas. In practice, patients with these syndromes should be treated as having non-ulcer dyspepsia. Symptomatic treatment of patients with nonerosive gastritis is the same as it is for patients with non-ulcer dyspepsia.

SPECIFIC REFERENCES*

1. Munnangi S, Sonnenberg A. Time trends of physician visits and treatment patterns of peptic ulcer disease in the United States. Arch Intern Med 1997;157:1489.
2. Kurata JH. Epidemiology: peptic ulcer risk factors. Semin Gastrointest Dis 1993;4:2.
3. Sonnenberg A, Everhart JE. Health impact of peptic ulcer in the US. Am J Gastroenterol 1997;92:614.
4. Sonnenberg A. Temporal trends and geographic variations of peptic ulcer disease. Aliment Pharmacol Ther 1995;9[Suppl2]:3.
5. The ACG Committee on FDA-Related Matters. Current status of maintenance therapy in peptic ulcer disease. Am J Gastroenterol 1988;83:607.
6. Fry J. Peptic ulcer disease: a profile. Br Med J 1964;2:809.

*Bold numerals denote published controlled clinical trials, meta-analyses, or consensus-based recommendations.

7. Greibe J, Bugge P, Gjorup T, et al. Long-term prognosis of duodenal ulcer: follow-up study and survey of doctors' estimates. Br Med J 1977; 2:1572.
8. Penston JG, Wormsley KG. Review articles: maintenance treatment with H_2 receptor antagonists for peptic-ulcer disease. Aliment Pharmacol Ther 1997;6:3.
9. Bardhan KD, Hinchliffe RFC, Bose K. Low dose maintenance treatment with cimetidine in duodenal ulcer: intermediate term results. Postgrad Med J 1986;62:347.
10. Bonnevie O. Survival in peptic ulcer. Gastroenterology 1978;75:1055.
11. Pounder RE, Ng D. The prevalence of *Helicobacter pylori* infection in different countries. Aliment Pharmacol Ther 1995;9[Suppl 2]:33.
12. National Institutes of Health. *Helicobacter pylori* in peptic ulcer disease. JAMA 1994;272:65.
13. Graham DY, Lew GM, Evans DG, et al. Effect of triple therapy (antibiotics plus bismuth) on duodenal ulcer healing. A randomized controlled trial. Ann Intern Med 1991;115:266.
14. Hentschel E, Brandstatter G, Dragosics B, et al. Effect of ranitidine and amoxicillin plus metronidazole on the eradication of *Helicobacter pylori* and the recurrence of duodenal ulcer. N Engl J Med 1993;328:308.
15. Laine L, Hopkins RJ, Girardi LS. Has the impact of *Helicobacter pylori* therapy on ulcer recurrence in the US been overstated? A meta-analysis of rigorously designed trials. Am J Gastroenterol 1998;93:1409.
16. Gisbert JP, Blanco M, Mateos JM, et al. *H. pylori* negative duodenal ulcer. Prevalence and causes in 774 patients. Dig Dis Sci 1999;44:2295.
17. Fries JF, Miller SR, Spitz PW, et al. Toward an epidemiology of gastropathy associated with nonsteroidal antiinflammatory drug use. Gastroenterology 1989;96:647.
18. Lanza FL. A guideline for the treatment and

prevention of NSAID-induced ulcers. Am J Gastroenterol 1998;93:2037.
19. Conn HO, Poynard T. Corticosteroid therapy does not induce peptic ulcer. J Intern Med 1994;236:619.
20. Chan, FK, Hung, LC, Suen BY, et al. Celecoxib versus diclofenac and omeprazole in reducing the risk of recurrent ulcer bleeding in patients with arthritis. N Engl J Med 2002;347: 2104.
21. Silverstein FE, Faich G, Goldstein JL, et al. Gastrointestinal toxicity with celecoxib vs nonsteroidal anti-inflammatory drugs for osteoarthritis and rheumatoid arthritis: the CLASS study: A randomized controlled trial. JAMA 2000;284:1247.
22. Del Valle J, Cohen H, Laine L, et al. Acid peptic disorders. In: Textbook of Gastroenterology. Vol 1. Philadelphia: Lippincott, Williams & Wilkins, 1999:1370.
23. Piper DW, McIntosh JH, Ariotti DE, et al. Life events and chronic duodenal ulcer: a case control study. Gut 1981;22:1011.
24. McCarthy DM. Smoking and ulcers: time to quit [Editorial]. N Engl J Med 1984;311:726.
25. Kurata JH, Nogawa AW. Meta-analysis of risk factors for peptic ulcer. Nonsteroidal anti-inflammatory drugs, *Helicobacter pylori*, and smoking. J Clin Gastroenterol 1997;24:2.
26. Sontag S, Graham DY, Belsito A, et al. Cimetidine, cigarette smoking, and recurrence of duodenal ulcer. N Engl J Med 1984;311:689.
27. Stemmermann GN, Marcus EB, Buist AS, et al. Relative impact of smoking and reduced pulmonary function in peptic ulcer risk. A prospective study of Japanese men in Hawaii. Gastroenterology 1989;96:1419.
28. Kirk AP, Dooley JS, Hunt RH. Peptic ulceration in patients with chronic liver disease. Dig Dis Sci 1980;25:756.
29. Kang JY, Wu AY, Sutherland IH, et al. Prevalence of peptic ulcer in patients undergoing maintenance dialysis. Dig Dis Sci 1988;33:774.
30. Aspirin Myocardial Infarction Study Research Group. A randomized, controlled trial of aspirin in persons recovered from myocardial infarction. JAMA 1980;243:661.
31. Dooley CP, Larson AW, Stace NH, et al. Double contrast barium meal and upper gastrointestinal endoscopy. A comparative study. Ann Intern Med 1984;101:538.
32. Committee on Endoscopic Utilization. Appropriate use of gastrointestinal endoscopy. Manchester, MA: American Society for Gastrointestinal Endoscopy, June 6, 1986.
33. McCarthy D. The place of surgery in the Zollinger-Ellison syndrome. N Engl J Med 1980;302:1344.
34. Cutler AF, Havstad S, Ma CK, et al. Accuracy of invasive and noninvasive tests to diagnose *Helicobacter pylori* infection. Gastroenterology 1995;109:136.
35. Cutler AF, Prasad VM. Long-term follow-up of *Helicobacter pylori* serology after successful eradication. Am J Gastroenterol 1996;91:85.
36. Fallone CA, Mitchell A, Paterson WG. Determination of the test performance of less costly methods of *Helicobacter pylori* infection. Clin Invest Med 1995;18:177.
37. Faigel DO, Furth EE, Childs M, et al. Histological predictors of active *Helicobacter pylori* infection. Dig Dis Sci 1996;41:937.
38. Graham DY, Evans DJ, Peacock J, et al. Comparison of rapid serological tests (FlexSure HP and QuickVue) with conventional ELISA for detection of *Helicobacter pylori* infection. Am J Gastroenterol 1996;91:942.
39. Chan F, Sung J, Lee YT, et al. Does smoking predispose to peptic ulcer relapse after eradication of *Helicobacter pylori*? Am J Gastroenterol 1997;92:442.
40. Gisbert, JP, Khorrami, S, Carballo, F, et al. Meta-analysis: *Helicobacter pylori* eradication therapy vs. antisecretory non-eradication therapy for the prevention of recurrent bleeding from peptic ulcer. Aliment Pharmacol Ther 2004;19:617.
41. Lanzon-Miller S, Pounder RE, Hamilton MR, et al. Twenty four hour intragastric acidity and plasma gastrin concentration before and during treatment with either ranitidine or omeprazole. Aliment Pharmacol Therap 1987;1:239.
42. Jordan PH Jr., Thornby J. Should it be parietal cell vagotomy or selective vagotomy-antrectomy for treatment of duodenal ulcer? A progress report. Ann Surg 1987;205:572.
43. Talley NJ, Phillips SF. Nonulcer dyspepsia: potential causes and pathophysiology. Ann Intern Med 1988;108:865.
44. Talley NJ, Hunt RH. What role does *Helicobacter pylori* play in dyspepsia and nonulcer dyspepsia? Arguments for and against. *H. pylori* being associated with dyspeptic syndrome. Gastroenterology 1997;113:S67.

For annotated ***General References*** *and resources related to this chapter, visit www.hopkinsbayview.org/PAMreferences.*

Chapter 44

Abdominal Pain and Irritable Bowel Syndrome

Mack C. Mitchell, Jr. and H. Franklin Herlong

ABDOMINAL PAIN

Abdominal pain is one of the most common complaints of ambulatory patients. Acute abdominal pain (onset within 24 hours before the patient seeks help) almost always reflects an organic process. Whether chronic or acute, abdominal pain resulting from an organic cause is more often a symptom of disease of the digestive system than of a process outside the digestive system.

Important characteristics of abdominal pain are the rapidity of onset, apparent severity, location, and accompanying signs and symptoms (e.g., fever, gastrointestinal [GI] bleeding, diarrhea). *Chronic pain,* if associated with an organic process, may be caused by peptic, gallbladder, or diverticular disease, chronic relapsing pancreatitis (primarily in alcoholics), or carcinoma (most commonly pancreatic or colonic). The symptoms and signs that accompany these processes are discussed in a general way in this chapter and more specifically in the chapters devoted to these conditions. Chronic pain that is not associated with a demonstrable organic process is most often caused by the irritable bowel syndrome (see below).

The significance of pain is determined by two major factors: the characteristics of the pain and the characteristics of the patient. The significance of pain to the patient depends on its severity and frequency, the degree to which it interferes with daily life or sleep patterns, and its meaning (both implied and symbolic). Even severe pain can be tolerated for brief periods if it appears infrequently, whereas less severe pain may be less tolerable if it interrupts important activities or disturbs sleep. Pain that has no anticipated end is generally less well tolerated than pain that, even though intense, has a predictable span. The threshold of pain tolerance varies considerably from one individual to another, because of both neurologic and psychological factors. Also, pain that is primarily organic may be reinforced by the secondary psychosocial gains it provides.

Elderly patients with abdominal pain require special attention (1). Even serious underlying conditions may be manifested by minimal subjective complaints and objective signs. For example, cholecystitis, appendicitis, and ruptured appendix are easily missed because pain may not be severe and fever and leukocytosis may be minimal or absent. Therefore, careful evaluation of abdominal pain in the elderly requires repeated abdominal and rectal examinations and serial determinations of body temperature and laboratory tests (e.g., white blood cell and differential counts).

Management of any type of pain can be significantly improved by consideration of certain general principles. For example, reassurance that pain can be relieved by medication or surgery can significantly raise the threshold of tolerance. On the other hand, the existence of severe pain sensitizes patients to additional, less intense pain (e.g., lumbar puncture, venipuncture), and the patient's overreaction to the second pain should not be taken to imply that the primary pain is psychogenic.

Types

Pain involving the digestive system can be visceral, parietal, referred, neurogenic, or psychogenic. Pain caused by metabolic disease is ordinarily visceral or neurogenic.

Visceral Pain

Visceral pain can result from spasm or stretching of the muscle wall of a hollow viscus from inflammation or ischemia or from distention of the capsule of the liver. Tenderness associated with visceral pain (sometimes including rebound tenderness) is often felt directly over the part of the digestive system that is involved, although small bowel tenderness is usually not well localized (except for the terminal ileum). Abdominal viscera are insensitive to cutting, tearing, crushing, and burning.

Parietal Pain

The parietal peritoneum, mesentery, and posterior peritoneal covering are sensitive to forces similar to those that affect the viscera, but the omentum and anterior abdominal wall are less sensitive. Parietal tenderness is more localized than visceral tenderness, and rebound tenderness is experienced over the involved area. Parietal pain that is the result of generalized inflammation (peritonitis) encompasses a large area of the peritoneum. A rigid abdomen, associated with pain, usually implies severe inflammation.

Referred Pain

Both visceral and parietal pain may be referred to a remote site along shared nerve pathways (dermatomes). Gallbladder pain, for example, typically radiates to the infrascapular area; and right diaphragmatic pain, to the right shoulder. Esophageal pain can be confused with the pain of myocardial ischemia because the sites to which the pain radiates may be identical (e.g., the neck and left arm). The more severe the visceral pain, the more likely it is to be referred to the back, as with esophageal spasm or cholecystitis. The skin overlying the dermatome to which the pain is referred may be hypersensitive. Deep palpation of the primary site of the painful organ may intensify the pain, not only locally but also at its referred site. However, the reverse is not true; deep palpation over the referred site does not usually enhance pain over the primary site.

Abdominal Pain Caused by Metabolic Disease

Metabolic disease may produce intestinal pain by a direct effect on the alimentary tract (e.g., when intestinal spasm is induced by porphyria, lead poisoning, or familial Mediterranean fever). In hereditary angioneurotic edema, C1 esterase deficiency may produce intestinal swelling, which can cause pain as a result of partial obstruction or intestinal spasm. On the other hand, metabolic disorders may secondarily produce abdominal pain; for example, hyperparathyroidism can produce a painful peptic ulcer or pancreatitis. Hyperlipidemia also can cause pancreatitis, but it can be associated with abdominal pain in the absence of pancreatic disease.

Neurogenic Pain

Neurogenic abdominal pain (causalgia) is experienced by the patient as a burning sensation along the route of distribution of the nerve and is sometimes associated with hyperesthesia. Usually the spinal root is involved by herpes zoster, carcinoma, or arthritis, but peripheral neuropathies caused by operative trauma or diabetes mellitus may also produce neurogenic abdominal pain. There is no relationship of neurogenic pain to digestive function (e.g., eating, defecating).

Psychogenic Pain

Psychogenic pain may represent a conversion reaction that results in the perception of pain when no organic dysfunction exists, or it may result from psychophysiologic reactions characterized by pathologic or physiologic responses to psychological stress (see Chapter 21). For example, emotional stress can lead to painful intestinal spasm in patients with irritable bowel syndrome (see below). This spasm is a measurable physiologic event. Similarly, stress may lead to peptic symptoms as a result of gastric hypersecretion, which also can be quantitated. Pain or tenderness that represents a conversion reaction (emotions converted into somatic complaints) may disappear during periods of distraction. Such pain may be inconsistent and incompatible with known neuroanatomy and neurophysiology.

Historical Clues to Diagnosis

Although successful diagnosis of conditions that cause abdominal pain depends on meticulous pursuit of leads that are provided by the history and physical examination, familiarity with standard questions and examination techniques assists in ensuring completeness. A history of previous episodes of pain, medications taken (e.g., nonsteroidal anti-inflammatory drugs [NSAIDs], warfarin), and the existence of a chronic disease (e.g., diabetes mellitus, diverticulosis) is important. Questions relating to local features include the nature and quality of the pain; its location, radiation, intensity, timing, duration, and course; and the factors that precipitate, aggravate, and alleviate it. Associated symptoms and signs include tenderness, fever and chills, anorexia, nausea and vomiting, diarrhea and constipation, obstruction, borborygmus, rectal bleeding, passing of mucus, jaundice, and genitourinary symptoms. Although aggravation of pain by emotional tension is seen with functional disorders such as irritable bowel syndrome, the pain of many organic disorders can also be accentuated by emotional stress.

Rapidity of Onset of Pain

The temporal development of abdominal pain is an important factor that guides the clinician in evaluation. In particular, pain that develops abruptly or within minutes and becomes rapidly severe is ominous (Table 44.1). Additionally, situations in which a silent period follows the initial symptoms are notoriously deceptive problems. For example, a perforated viscus or an intestinal infarction may

TABLE 44.1 Causes of Acute Abdominal Pain According to Rapidity of Onset

Intestinal Causes	*Extraintestinal Causes*
Abrupt Onset (Instantaneous)	
Perforated ulcer	Ruptured aneurysm or aortic dissection
Ruptured abscess or hematoma	Ruptured ectopic pregnancy
Intestinal infarct	Pneumothorax
Ruptured esophagus	Myocardial infarct
	Pulmonary infarct
Rapid Onset (Minutes)	
Perforated viscus	Ureteral colic
Strangulated viscus	Renal colic
Volvulus	Ectopic pregnancy
Pancreatitis	Splenic infarct
Biliary colic	
Mesenteric infarct	
Diverticulitis	
Penetrating peptic ulcer	
High intestinal obstruction	
Appendicitis (gradual onset more common)	
Gradual Onset (Hours)	
Appendicitis	Cystitis
Strangulated hernia	Pyelitis
Low small intestinal obstruction	Salpingitis
Cholecystitis	Prostatitis
Pancreatitis	Threatened abortion
Gastritis	Urinary retention
Peptic ulcer	Pneumonitis
Colonic diverticulitis	
Meckel diverticulitis	
Crohn disease	
Ulcerative colitis	
Mesenteric lymphadenitis	
Abscess	
Intestinal infarct	
Mesenteric cyst	

Adapted from Ridge JA, Way LW. Abdominal pain. In: Sleisenger MH, Fordtran JS, eds. Gastrointestinal disease, 5th ed. Philadelphia: WB Saunders, 1993;156.

be characterized by resolution of the intense initial pain hours after perforation or infarction first occurs and by a recurrence of pain several hours later when peritonitis and volume depletion are well established. If the patient complains of an abrupt onset of severe abdominal pain on the day that he or she visits the clinician, a complete blood count, urinalysis, chest radiograph, plain and upright films of the abdomen, and close surveillance over several hours are imperative.

When the onset of pain is more gradual, many more causes are possible, and considerable judgment is necessary in determining the urgency and direction of the evaluation. Newly experienced abdominal pain, even if it is believed to be innocuous, should never be dismissed

TABLE 44.2 Nature and Location of Gastrointestinal Pain

Organ Involved	Nature of Pain	Location of Pain
Esophagus	Burning, constricting	Upper lesions: high substernal Lower lesions: low sternal or referred upward Severe: back
Stomach	Gnawing discomfort, sensation of hunger	Epigastric Left upper quadrant
Duodenum	Gnawing discomfort, sensation of hunger	Epigastric
Small intestine	Aching, cramping, bloating, sharp	Diffuse Periumbilical Terminal ileum: right lower quadrant
Colon	Aching, cramping, bloating, sharp	Lower abdomen Sigmoid: left lower quadrant Rectum: midline and sacrum
Pancreas	Excruciating, constant	Upper abdomen radiating to back
Gallbladder	Severe, later dull ache	Right upper quadrant Radiates to right scapula or interscapular area
Liver	Ache, occasionally sharp	Right lower rib cage Right upper quadrant if liver is enlarged

without followup (at least by telephone) within a few days so that any important new symptoms are not missed. It is best for the clinician to initiate this followup because it obviates the need for the patient to decide whether a change in symptoms is important enough to be of concern.

Nature and Location of Pain

Esophageal pain is usually described as pressing, constricting, or burning (Tables 44.2 and 44.3). It is usually located in the substernal area and, when severe, radiates through to the back. The location of the pain is a good clue to the location of the underlying disease. Although pain from the lower esophageal region may be referred higher, lesions high in the esophagus do not refer to the lower part of the esophagus (see also Chapter 42).

Gastric pain is usually experienced in the subxiphoid area or in the left upper quadrant of the abdomen. Although gastritis is perceived as a true pain (often burning or cramping in quality), the distress caused by both duodenal and gastric ulceration is experienced as a gnawing discomfort or as a hunger sensation rather than as pain. The discomfort caused by peptic ulcer is often precipitated by fasting and is relieved by eating. The pain of peptic ulcer typically awakens the patient between 1 and 3 a.m. In contrast, pain of gastritis may be aggravated by eating or relieved only momentarily and then subsequently intensified over 10 to 15 minutes. A change from ulcer distress to a burning, boring, or knife-like pain (especially when there is radiation through to the back) is an indication of penetration. Pain that is precipitated by meals also suggests gastric outlet obstruction (often caused by a pyloric channel ulcer) or high intestinal obstruction (see also Chapter 43).

Duodenal pain is felt also in the epigastric area or slightly to the right of it, and it may radiate through to the back. When an ulcer has perforated, the pain appears abruptly in the epigastric region and later settles into the right lower quadrant of the abdomen as gastric contents migrate into the right gutter.

Small intestinal pain is generally diffuse and poorly localized. It is felt in the periumbilical area and, when severe, radiates through to the back. Pain from the terminal ileum may be localized to the right lower quadrant. Uncommonly, it may radiate down the leg. Small intestinal pain is generally crampy, sharp, or aching. *Bloating, distention,* and *dull ache* are terms that often are associated with prolonged mechanical obstruction or reflex ileus, whereas more acute forms may be manifested by sharp, steady pain. Associated fever and chills suggest inflammatory bowel disease.

Colonic pain is better localized, often to the lower abdomen. *Sigmoid pain* is felt in the left lower quadrant, and *rectal pain* is often described as being in the lower mid abdomen or posteriorly in the rectum. Distention of the splenic flexure of the colon (seen most commonly in patients with the irritable bowel syndrome) from gas produces left upper quadrant or left chest pain that may be confused with the pain of myocardial ischemia. Temporary relief may be obtained by passing gas (see also below, Irritable Bowel Syndrome). Colonic pain generally is crampy or of an aching quality unless perforation occurs, and then it is often severe and constant. Associated fever and chills suggest diverticulitis, diverticular abscess, or ulcerative colitis.

Pancreatic pain is excruciating and constant and usually located in the upper abdomen with radiation through

TABLE 44.3 Differential Diagnosis of Abdominal Pain Caused by Gastrointestinal Disorders

Disorder	A. Character, Location, Production, or Relief		
	Character	**Location**	**Produced or Relieved by**
Peptic ulcer	Gnawing hunger discomfort, occasionally burning, gastric (within minutes after meals); duodenal (usually several hours after meals)	Subxiphoid, may radiate to back	Produced by empty stomach, relieved by food, antacids, or H_2-receptor blockers
Penetrating ulcer	Severe, boring, constant pain	Subxiphoid radiating to back	May awaken patient in early morning hours, may be relieved by antacids or H_2-receptor blockers
Perforated ulcer	Abrupt, severe pain followed within 6 hr by deceptive refractory period with diminishing of pain	Initially epigastric, then right lower quadrant (right gutter)	Initial pain spontaneous, peritonitis aggravated by movement
Small bowel obstruction	Crampy severe pain with partial obstruction, constant pain develops with complete obstruction or strangulation	Generalized periumbilical or localized over strangulation	Relieved by intubation decompression
Large bowel obstruction	Crampy pain initially, constant pain with subsequent distention or strangulation, onset less sudden than upper intestinal obstruction	May be localized or generalized	Occasionally relieved by intubation decompression
Intestinal infarct	Severe, excruciating, abrupt onset	Generalized	Relieved only by surgery
Intussusception	Sudden onset severe crampy pain	Periumbilical	Temporary relief may occur with emesis
Appendicitis	Initially colic then continuous with varying intensity	Lower quadrant, occasional perineal radiation	Aggravated by extension of right leg
Pancreatitis	Severe, constant pain	Epigastric, radiation to back or lower abdomen	Often initiated by alcoholic binge or eating after binge, by common duct obstruction, penetrating ulcer, or blunt trauma
Cholecystitis	Constant, severe pain preceding nausea and vomiting; subsidence of pain followed by aching	Right upper quadrant radiating to infrascapular region	Precipitated by heavy meal and aggravated by deep inspiration
Biliary colic	Crampy, severe pain	Epigastric, radiating to right upper quadrant and subscapular region	Precipitated by heavy meal within 1–3 hr
Diverticulitis	Crampy or continuous pain	Left lower quadrant, may radiate to back	Relieved by anticholinergics and antibiotics
Crohn disease	Crampy with partial obstruction and continuous pain with inflammatory mass	Periumbilical or right lower quadrant, may radiate to back	May be precipitated by milk, relieved by defecation or intubation decompression
Ulcerative colitis	Crampy pain usually, may be constant with toxic dilation	Often left lower quadrant or any area of colon, generalized with toxic megacolon or perforation	Precipitated by emotional stress or infection; toxic megacolon by opiates or enemas; relieved temporarily by defecation

Disorder	B. Abnormal Physical Findings, Associated Signs, and Laboratory Features		
	Abnormal Physical Findings	**Associated Signs and Symptoms**	**Laboratory Features**
Peptic ulcer	Subxiphoid tenderness	Nausea, vomiting, retrosternal burning; weight gain with duodenal ulcer; weight stable or loss with gastric ulcer	Endoscopic or radiographic demonstration of ulcer, possible occult blood in stool or melena, and iron deficiency anemia
Penetrating ulcer	Marked subxiphoid tenderness	Writhing, clutching abdomen	Amylase may be elevated
Perforated ulcer	Initially rigid with rebound, during refractory stage tenderness disappears to return later, absence of liver dullness with intraperitoneal air	Patient lies rigidly still, pale, perspiring; emesis may be present	Upright film shows free air under diaphragm; leukocytosis

TABLE 44.3 (Continued) Differential Diagnosis of Abdominal Pain Caused by Gastrointestinal Disorders

Small bowel obstruction	Borborygmus, high-pitched sound with rushes initially; later quiet abdomen; tenderness may be mild or rebound tenderness may be present	Emesis (may be feculent with lower obstruction), obstipation, may be weak with shocklike appearance	Plain film of abdomen showing air–fluid levels may show stepladder pattern
Large bowel obstruction	Initially hyperperistalsis with high-pitched rushes, subsequently distention and decrease in bowel signs	Nausea but less vomiting than with high obstruction, obstipation, or marked constipation	Large bowel distention with air–fluid levels and no air demonstrated distal to obstruction
Intestinal infarct	Quiet bowel sounds, tenderness present but not commensurate with pain, later rebound tenderness	Shock, bloody diarrhea, melena, vomiting; history of intestinal angina	Leukocytosis, hemoconcentration; bloody fluid on paracentesis; plain film of abdomen may reveal normal gas pattern or no gas pattern due to fluid-filled loops
Intussusception	Tender mass in abdomen, high-pitched peristaltic rushes	Initially normal stool after onset, then blood, mucus, and constipation; vomiting is late; fever after strangulation	Barium enema demonstrates coiled spring appearance of invagination; with ileocecal intussusception, small bowel loop is in colon
Appendicitis	Localized rebound tenderness, hyperesthesia over area	Initially diarrhea, then constipation; nausea and vomiting may be present; fever, tachycardia; rectal tenderness in right perirectal area	Leukocytosis
Pancreatitis	Marked epigastric tenderness, guarding and upper abdominal distention; the pain of chronic pancreatic disease may be less pronounced	Emesis almost invariable, fever, with hemorrhagic pancreatitis purple color in flank or periumbilical region; emesis is less common in patients with chronic pancreatic disease	Marked leukocytosis, hyperamylasemia; serum calcium depression on days 2 to 4, toxic psychosis on days 2 to 4; radiograph may show calcification, localized ileus, or colon cutoff sign; upper gastrointestinal series demonstrates pancreatic enlargement and spicules in C loop of duodenum; may have left pleural effusion
Cholecystitis	Tenderness over gallbladder area, especially on deep inspiration; Murphy sign may be positive	More common in obese women $\geq$40 yr or older after pregnancy; high incidence among some American Indian populations	Leukocytosis; plain film may show calcified stone; stones seen on ultrasonography; TcHIDA nonvisualized; cholangiograms may show radiopaque stones
Biliary colic	As for cholecystitis	As for cholecystitis; jaundice may be present	Radiopaque stones may be seen on plain film; stones seen on ultrasonography; intravenous cholangiogram may show dilated duct; bilirubin, alkaline phosphatase increase; may have hyperamylasemia
Diverticulitis	Guarding and tenderness in left lower quadrant	Constipation, fever, tachycardia; rectal tenderness on left; may have urinary frequency or dysuria from pericolonic involvement	Leukocytosis, barium enema shows diverticula but may not visualize during acute episode, may show partial obstruction
Crohn disease	Tender mass in right lower quadrant, borborygmus	Nausea, vomiting, diarrhea, fever; may have perirectal fistula; tender mass in right rectal area, occasional clubbing	Anemia, elevated sedimentation rate; small bowel series shows cobblestone appearance or string sign
Ulcerative colitis	Tender over involved area, distended especially over transverse colon with toxic megacolon	Frequent passing of small amounts of bloody liquid stool; tenesmus with rectal involvement; fever, tachycardia, arthralgia, erythema nodosa; proctoscopy reveals bleeding and friability	Anemia; elevated sedimentation rate; barium enema demonstrates ulcerations, shortening, effacement of colon

Modified from Handbook of Differential Diagnosis, vol 2, part 1: The abdomen. Nutley, NJ: Ro Com Press, 1974.

to the back, but it may be felt in almost any area of the abdomen. Chronic pancreatic pain (caused by inflammation, pseudocyst, or carcinoma) is similar in nature and location to acute pancreatic pain but may be less severe. Pancreatitis is almost invariably associated with vomiting. If vomiting is not present, other diagnoses (e.g., pancreatic carcinoma) should be considered.

Appendicitis often begins as diffuse or periumbilical abdominal pain that intensifies over hours as it settles in the right lower quadrant. The pain of appendicitis is often aggravated by extension of the right leg.

Gallbladder pain generally begins in the right upper quadrant or epigastrium and radiates to the interscapular area or to the right infrascapular area. It is excruciatingly severe, may be aggravated by deep inspiration, and is replaced by a dull, aching sensation that persists for hours after the severe pain subsides. Tenderness can often be elicited by deep palpation under the rib in the area of the gallbladder, especially during deep inspiration. Gallbladder pain often appears several hours after a heavy meal. Associated fever and chills suggest ascending cholangitis (see also Chapter 96).

Hepatic pain localizes over the liver, and a tender liver can be demonstrated by palpation of its edge during deep inspiration or by fist percussion over the lower right rib cage anteriorly (or over the right upper quadrant of the abdomen if the liver is enlarged). Chapters 36 and 51 discuss *genitourinary pain* (e.g., renal colic).

Physical Examination

The patient's general appearance provides clues about the severity, the duration, and often the cause of the underlying condition. The cold sweat and pallor of shock along with the marble skin (superficial vessels seen over blanched skin) indicating vasoconstriction are signs of significant hemorrhage. Tachycardia and perspiration are seen in both shock and sepsis, but the skin in shock is cold and clammy, whereas in sepsis it is warm and moist. Signs of sepsis suggest bacterial enteritis, inflammatory bowel disease, intra-abdominal abscess, cholangitis, pancreatitis, peritonitis, or pyelonephritis.

The position assumed by the patient may be characteristic of a particular disorder. A position of truncal flexure often typifies patients with pancreatitis, whereas patients with gallbladder colic tend to pace or writhe about and appear restless in their unsuccessful attempt to find a comfortable position. This is in sharp contrast to the immobile position assumed by patients with peritonitis, who attempt to avoid even the slightest jarring movement.

Inspection of the abdomen is facilitated by using incident lighting to visualize abdominal asymmetry and to outline masses and pulsations. In thin patients with partial obstruction, peristaltic intestinal movement may be seen through the abdominal wall, and churning peristalsis may coincide with reports of crampy abdominal pain. Flank discoloration (*Gray–Turner sign*) or periumbilical discoloration (*Cullen sign*) results from retroperitoneal or intraperitoneal hemorrhage dissecting into the subcutaneous tissues and may indicate hemorrhagic pancreatitis. A strangulated hernia may protrude visibly from ventral defects, from the inguinal area, or into the scrotum, where peristaltic contractions may occasionally be appreciated. Patients with subphrenic abscess or gallbladder disease may have inspiratory pain that results in splinting and avoidance of deep inspiration.

Auscultation should always be performed before palpation so that abdominal sounds may be evaluated before they are altered by palpation. At times borborygmus is audible without the stethoscope. Specifically, one should search for hyperperistaltic or hypoperistaltic sounds, for the high tinkles of obstruction, and for bruits suggesting vascular distortion from aneurysms, atherosclerosis, compression of blood vessels, or invasion of blood vessels (e.g., invasion of the splenic artery in advanced pancreatic carcinoma). Although a silent abdomen implies reflex ileus, bowel sounds may also be quiet or significantly diminished late in the course of mechanical obstruction. Whenever obstruction (especially gastric outlet obstruction) is considered, an attempt should be made to elicit a succussion splash. This is done by placing the stethoscope over the area (e.g., the stomach) and shaking the patient gently but abruptly. A sloshing sound indicates the presence of air and fluid. This finding in the stomach 3 hours or more after eating or drinking indicates delayed gastric emptying or, rarely, marked hypersecretion.

Gentle percussion should precede palpation and is an excellent means for detecting rebound tenderness, masses, and tympany (either generalized or localized) over an area of ileus or obstruction. Because air rises to the space between the liver and the abdominal wall, absence of liver dullness with the patient in a recumbent position is an important finding indicating the presence of free air in the abdominal cavity. Before *palpation*, it is wise to ask the patient to point to the site of maximum pain. Gentle palpation should at first avoid that site to minimize the chances that muscle guarding will interfere with the examination. The patient should be lying perfectly supine with knees flexed to facilitate relaxation of abdominal muscles. Guarding may be localized over specific lesions (often inflammatory), or there may be marked rigidity if pain is severe, as in perforation or penetration. Subxiphoid tenderness suggests an active ulcer. Tenderness over the liver, especially when the liver edge is brought down against the examining finger by deep inspiration, suggests inflammation in this organ. With gallbladder disease, tenderness is localized to the region of the gallbladder, and with cystic or common duct obstruction, a distended viscus can sometimes be felt as well. Right lower quadrant tenderness is found with appendicitis or with Crohn disease involving the ileum or the ileocecal area. A left lower quadrant tender sigmoid cord is felt most commonly with irritable bowel syndrome but can also indicate diverticular disease. A distinct tender mass in the right lower quadrant suggests inflammation (usually Crohn disease) extending beyond the bowel; a similar finding in the left lower quadrant suggests diverticulitis. Board-like rigidity indicates an intra-abdominal catastrophe such as perforation or infarction. Pulsatile masses should be differentiated from laterally expansile masses because the former can represent a mass overlying an artery, whereas the latter implies aneurysmal dilation. When localized perforation has occurred, rebound tenderness may be localized over the area. Hyperesthesia may exist over the segmental distribution of the spinal nerve that innervates the particular area of the viscus. This finding is detected by gently rubbing the fingers over the skin of the associated dermatome.

Rectal examination can be extremely helpful in localizing areas of tenderness as well as in palpating masses through the rectum. Periappendiceal abscesses can sometimes be identified in this manner, as can a perforated diverticulum. On digital examination the finger should complete a circle that includes the entire perirectal area.

Genital and pelvic examination, like the rectal examination, should be performed in all patients with abdominal pain because it can detect hernias as well as genitourinary and other pelvic problems.

If analgesic drugs have been administered, it is useful to re-examine the patient after pain has been relieved to identify masses or localized tenderness that may have been obscured by guarding and rigidity.

Laboratory Tests

A complete blood count, urinalysis, and test for occult blood in the stool are required in every person with serious acute abdominal pain, as are a chest radiograph and plain and upright films of the abdomen. Other laboratory tests should be ordered as indicated by the specific findings.

A low hematocrit value or hemoglobin concentration can call attention to intraperitoneal or retroperitoneal bleeding, whereas hemoconcentration raises consideration of mesenteric vascular occlusion. A high leukocyte count and a high erythrocyte sedimentation rate suggest inflammation or infection. Blood in the urine points to kidney disease as a possible source of pain.

The presence of occult blood in the stool reinforces concern about the GI tract as a source of painful symptoms; it may be an early sign of vascular ischemia or intussusception or a sign of more common lesions such as peptic ulcer, polyp, or inflammatory bowel disease.

Radiology

Plain and upright films of the abdomen are helpful in delineating gas patterns, which may demonstrate displacement of intestine by intra-abdominal masses or may show localized loops of ileus, as with *pancreatitis* or *pyelonephritis*. Air is distributed more widely in the small bowel in *reflex ileus* and in *intestinal obstruction*. In the latter, the typical stepladder pattern is often encountered on the abdominal radiograph, with slight separation of the loops caused by edema of the wall of the small bowel; an upright film demonstrates air–fluid levels in the dilated loops. Absence of air distal to a specific point suggests *obstruction* at that point. *Volvulus* can be diagnosed on the plain film, which demonstrates a sausage-shaped air-filled or air- and fluid-filled viscus coming to an apex. In gastric volvulus, the greater curvature is seen above the lesser curve, and a double air–fluid level is a classic finding, one level being in the lesser curvature of the fundus and the other in the antrum (because of the inverted U-shaped stomach under these conditions). Free air under the diaphragm on the upright film indicates a *perforated viscus* unless the patient has had recent surgery (at which time air was introduced) or has *pneumatosis cystoides intestinalis,* in which case a large amount of air may appear subdiaphragmatically from ruptured pseudocysts. The important clue to pneumatosis cystoides intestinalis is the presence of free air in the absence of signs or symptoms of perforation or peritonitis. A radiopaque gallbladder or kidney stones or pancreatic calcification seen on plain films may help corroborate a suspected diagnosis or point attention toward one of these organs.

Contrast studies have been largely replaced by endoscopic procedures in the evaluation of patients with abdominal pain. Endoscopy is both more sensitive and more specific than contrast radiology of the bowel, although it is considerably more expensive. An *upper GI series* (see Chapter 43) is useful if extrinsic compression on the stomach or duodenum or partial gastric outlet obstruction is suspected at endoscopy. *Barium enema* (see Chapter 45) can be useful in demonstrating a low site of obstruction and reducing an intussusception. A barium enema should always be preceded by digital examination of the rectum and by proctoscopy to be certain that the rectum is normal (e.g., that there is no rectal carcinoma). When pain is thought to result from gallbladder disease (see Chapter 96) and opaque stones are not visible on plain abdominal films, ultrasonography is an excellent means of demonstrating stones in the gallbladder, although it is less sensitive for detecting stones within the common bile duct. A *TcHIDA or PipHIDA radioisotopic study* may demonstrate obstruction of the common or cystic duct. This technique requires injection of an isotope and serial views for 1 hour.

Ultrasonography is also useful in showing pancreatic edema or pseudocysts, evaluating a suspected abdominal aortic aneurysm, and evaluating a patient who is difficult to examine for an intra-abdominal mass; this technique has the advantage of avoiding irradiation. Sonography is often unsatisfactory in obese patients and in those with

TABLE 44.4 Ultrasound, Computed Tomographic (CT) Scanning, and Magnetic Resonance Imaging (MRI): Comparison of the Technique and the Patient Experience

Characteristic	*Ultrasound*	*CT*	*MRI*
Basis of tissue attenuation	Tissue elasticity, acoustic impedance	Electron density; linear attenuation coefficient	Nuclear resonance
Radiation dose or toxic effect	None known at diagnostic energy levels	8–10 R (skin exposure)	None known
Morphologic detail	Good	Excellent	Excellent
Contrast medium useful	No	Iodinated intravascular and oral agents; diatrizoate meglumine (Gastrografin)	No (in abdomen)
Time for examination	½–1 hr	½–1 hr	1 hr
Operator skill	Substantial	Minimal	Minimal
Ease of interpretation	Complex, many artifacts	Straightforward	Moderately straightforward
Preparation	Nothing by mouth after midnight (for pelvis, three glasses of water 1 hr before study and do not void)	Evacuate barium from recent gastrointestinal studies (or wait 1 wk)	None
Cooperation	Lie still, supine, be able to hold breath	Lie still, supine, be able to hold breath	Lie still, supine, breathe quietly

Adapted from Ferrucci JT Jr. Body ultrasonography [first of two parts]. N Engl J Med 1979;300:538.

metal abdominal sutures because adipose tissue and metal reflect sound waves.

Computed tomography (CT) is a sensitive means of demonstrating free air, masses, infarcted tissue, cysts, and evidence of inflammation due to diverticulitis, pancreatitis, colitis, or perforation.

Magnetic resonance imaging (MRI) is not used as an initial imaging study of the abdomen but is used selectively to define mass lesions, especially in the liver, kidneys, or adrenal glands, and vascular abnormalities, such as hemangiomas and renal or hepatic vein thrombosis. It is considerably more expensive than a CT scan. HASTE MRI, a newer technique, can demonstrate viscera without movement artifact. It is also effective in showing flowing fluid and therefore can demonstrate partial or complete vascular occlusion or the bile ducts.

Table 44.4 compares the ultrasound, CT, and MRI techniques and the patient experience during the performance of these procedures.

Selective mesenteric angiography should be performed in patients with suspected mesenteric vascular ischemia (particularly in elderly patients with postprandial abdominal pain) or mesenteric vascular occlusion (e.g., women taking contraceptive medication). This is particularly helpful in older patients, because normal arteriographic findings rule out mesenteric vascular disease; on the other hand, occlusion of even two of the three major aortic branches (celiac, superior mesenteric, and inferior mesenteric arteries) can occur without symptoms of mesenteric vascular disease. It may be prudent to hospitalize the patient for this procedure. The patient experience is similar to that described for renal arteriography (see Chapter 67).

Endoscopy

Upper GI endoscopy should be considered the ambulatory procedure of choice to diagnose upper GI disease. Endoscopy should be performed promptly when individuals have abdominal pain associated with upper GI bleeding (see earlier discussion), but these patients should be hospitalized.

Flexible sigmoidoscopy should be performed in any patient with abdominal pain and rectal bleeding or a change in bowel habits and in any patient in whom inflammatory bowel disease (proctitis, ulcerative colitis, Crohn disease) is suspected. Prior preparation for *flexible sigmoidoscopy* depends on the suspected pathology. Mucosal lesions are best identified after oral cathartics or without preparation. Most enema preparations tend to produce some mucosal edema that may obscure mucosal lesions. Chapter 45 describes the patient's experience during the procedure.

Colonoscopy, like upper endoscopy, requires referral to a gastroenterologist. It should be considered in patients with abdominal pain who have occult rectal bleeding, in those with suspected diffuse colonic inflammatory disease (ulcerative colitis, Crohn disease) or suspected ischemic colitis, and in patients with polypoid lesions on barium enema who require biopsy or, often, resection of the lesion. Colonoscopy cannot be performed within a day or two after a barium radiograph of the lower or upper GI tract. Chapter 45 also describes the patient's experience during the procedure.

Treatment

The treatment of patients with abdominal pain depends on the severity of the pain, its rapidity of onset, and the nature of the underlying condition, if known. Severe pain with an abrupt or rapid onset often reflects a GI disorder that will require surgical intervention (Table 44.1). Hospitalization and consultation with a surgeon should be requested immediately in almost all such cases. Less severe pain should not be treated aggressively with analgesic drugs until an attempt has been made to establish a diagnosis, because the pain may abate spontaneously within minutes or hours and not recur. If the pain recurs or persists and the cause is not obvious, the screening tests described in this chapter should be performed. If these tests do not provide a diagnosis, referral to a gastroenterologist is indicated. As a general rule, analgesic drugs may be prescribed to patients with persistent pain, but opiates should be avoided if possible, because they can aggravate the underlying condition. (For example, morphine may aggravate pancreatitis by producing duodenal and ampullary spasm, thus enhancing pancreatic duct obstruction, and opiates or anticholinergics may produce toxic megacolon in patients with active ulcerative colitis.) Furthermore, there is a risk of narcotic addiction if opiates are inappropriately used.

IRRITABLE BOWEL SYNDROME

Irritable bowel syndrome (IBS), one of the most common medical conditions in primary care practice today, is characterized by chronic abdominal pain and a change in the frequency or character of bowel movements. In Western societies, IBS accounts for nearly 12% of visits to primary caregivers and approximately 28% of all referrals to gastroenterologists (2). For many patients, IBS is a chronic problem that affects many aspects of daily life. The costs of diagnosing and treating patients with IBS are staggering. More than 3 million people visit clinicians each year for the evaluation or treatment of IBS. A study in 1996 reported that the annual cost of IBS-related health care (health care visits, diagnostic tests) in the United States was more than $8 billion (3). That did not include associated indirect costs, such as lost productivity, lost wages, over the counter medications, and copayments for health care, which may be as much as three times as high. Furthermore, IBS is now second only to the common cold as the reason for days missed from work and school (4). Over the last several decades understanding of the pathophysiology of the disorder has improved significantly and provides a basis for establishing diagnosis and treatment.

Definition

In the past IBS was labeled nervous colitis, spastic colitis, mucus colitis, unstable colon, or irritable colon, all of which are inappropriate because they are both imprecise and inaccurate and may cause confusion with more serious disorders like ulcerative colitis. The term "irritable bowel syndrome" may suggest to both patients and clinicians a vague amalgamation of complaints. At times the intestinal tract does seem "irritable" due to underlying abnormalities in gastrointestinal motility and to alterations in visceral sensitivity. However, IBS is actually a fairly specific constellation of findings. For these reasons IBS remains an appropriate and inclusive term.

Criteria for IBS, initially proposed by Manning in 1978, have subsequently been validated in clinical practice (5,6). These criteria were updated and modified by a panel of international experts in Rome in 1998 (7). The Rome criteria define IBS as a chronic disorder of abdominal pain or discomfort present for at least 12 weeks (which need not be consecutive) over the previous 12 months. The pain should have at least two of the following three features: relief by defecation, association with a change in stool frequency, or association with a change in stool consistency. Although the Rome criteria are helpful in identifying patients for clinical trials, they may underestimate the true prevalence of IBS in the general population (8).

Prevalence and Epidemiology

IBS is a worldwide disorder, with a prevalence of 15% to 20% in the United States (2). IBS may present in all age groups, including children. Most patients begin to develop their typical symptoms in the late teenage years or early 20s, although the problem may not be diagnosed for many years. Peak prevalence occurs in the third and fourth decades of life, and then decreases during the sixth and seventh decades of life. Although IBS can be diagnosed at any age, a new diagnosis of IBS should be made cautiously in patients older than 50 years of age, because other diseases (colon cancer, diverticular disease, etc.) may have similar presenting symptoms. For most patients, IBS is a chronic disorder with symptoms persisting to some degree 5 years after diagnosis (9).

The prevalence of IBS is similar in Caucasians and African Americans (10), but is somewhat lower in Hispanics (2). For unknown reasons, women are nearly three times more likely to be diagnosed with IBS than are men (2).

Pathogenesis

Overview

IBS was once thought to represent a nervous disorder of the gut, hence the terms "nervous colitis" or "spastic colitis." However, our concept of IBS has changed considerably over the last 50 years. To label IBS a "colitis" is inappropriate because the disorder affects multiple parts of the GI tract. It is now believed that IBS is a complex disorder in which a number of physiologic processes are involved. These include abnormalities in intestinal motility, alterations in visceral sensory function, and changes in central nervous system (CNS) processing of sensory information. The realization that the gut and the brain are intimately connected now plays a central role in the theory of the pathogenesis of IBS.

Altered Gut Motility

Although a number of different patterns of abnormal intestinal motility have been described in patients with IBS, no one pattern is pathognomonic of the disorder. In general, the signs and symptoms of IBS, and the alterations in GI motility that underlie them, appear to be related predominantly to an exaggeration of normal patterns of intestinal motility.

Enhanced Visceral Sensitivity

Abdominal pain is a critical feature of IBS. A number of studies have demonstrated that patients with IBS have increased sensitivity to pain within the GI tract (11–13). Many of these studies demonstrated heightened sensitivity to during balloon distention of various locations within the intestinal tract (rectum, sigmoid colon, and ileum). Patients with IBS perceive balloon distention at much lower levels of inflation and describe the distention as more painful than do patients without IBS. This increased sensitivity to pain is not a generalized phenomenon, however, because patients with IBS do not have lower thresholds for somatic pain, when measured by the cold water immersion test. These experiments demonstrate that patients with IBS are very sensitive to stimuli within the gut and suggest that they may interpret normal intestinal function as painful in many circumstances.

Central Nervous System Influences

Some authorities suggest that patients with IBS may process sensory information from the intestinal tract differently than do patients without IBS (2). Additionally, other factors, such as stress, anxiety, or depression, may modulate sensory processing and influence the perception of pain. These findings have significant implications for the treatment of IBS. Therapy focused only on the intestinal tract may be less effective than a multisystem approach.

Other Factors

Clinicians and patients commonly question whether there are unique events that produce IBS or increase the likelihood of developing IBS later in life. Two studies demonstrated that infectious gastroenteritis might increase the likelihood of developing IBS later in life (14,15). Many patients recall the persistence of bloating, abdominal pain, and altered bowel habits after an acute infectious illness (e.g., traveler's diarrhea). The precise mechanism is unknown, but several explanations have been offered (15). An infectious process may injure the enteric nervous system, the intrinsic nerve supply responsible for coordinating peristaltic activity within the gastrointestinal tract. Another possibility involves immune hypersensitivity, where recurrent exposure to an otherwise benign substance might induce inflammation and possibly intestinal dysmotility. Some experts believe an infectious agent could induce a cycle of chronic mucosal inflammation, eventually leading to altered gut motility. However, biopsies of colonic mucosa in patients with documented IBS are not different from specimens from control subjects, an observation that is inconsistent with the hypothesis that mucosal inflammation plays a significant role in the pathogenesis of the disease.

Diagnosis

Most patients with IBS are diagnosed after having symptoms for months to years. The average time between the onset of symptoms and the diagnosis of IBS is just over 3 years (16). The diagnosis of IBS does not need to be difficult or expensive. After a careful interview, physical examination, and a few simple tests, the diagnosis should be apparent, often at the first office visit. In most individuals, IBS should not be a diagnosis of exclusion nor should the patient be told or led to believe that "it is all in your head."

When strict diagnostic criteria are met and there are no alarm features like unexplained weight loss or GI bleeding (see below), unnecessary diagnostic tests and procedures can be avoided during evaluation of patients with IBS. Several studies have shown that, because of errors in diagnosis, patients with IBS are three times more likely to undergo unnecessary surgery, such as appendectomy, hysterectomy, or exploratory laparotomy, than are patients without IBS (17–19).

History

The two most common presenting complaints are *abdominal pain* and *altered bowel habits*. The pattern of symptoms varies considerably from person to person but remains fairly consistent for a given individual, with changes for an individual occurring predominantly in intensity or frequency of occurrence. A sudden change in this pattern, from chronic diarrhea to constipation, for example, would warrant further investigation. Typically, symptoms are intermittent, with symptom-free periods lasting days, weeks,

informed about the indications for surgery and the types of operations that are available. Early attention to this issue enables the patient to accept an operation more readily if it is needed. Surgery for ulcerative colitis involves a proctocolectomy with an ileostomy to which a stomal appliance is attached to ensure continence. Construction of a continent ileostomy (Kock pouch) avoids the need for a stomal appliance, but the procedure is technically difficult and often requires revision. Another alternative is construction of an internal pouch from a loop of small bowel anastomosed to the anus (Park procedure). These last two procedures are most successful in motivated young patients who are undergoing elective colectomy.

Cancer of the Colon

The risk of colorectal cancer is increased 5 to 10 times in patients with ulcerative colitis (26). The major risk factors are duration of disease (risk increases significantly after 8 to 10 years of disease), extent of colonic involvement (pancolitis carries the highest risk, whereas the risk in patients with ulcerative proctitis is similar to that of the general population), and age at onset of disease (patients younger than 25 years of age at the time of onset have the highest risk, independent of the extent of disease). The cancer may be found anywhere in the colon, although most commonly it is within the rectum or rectosigmoid. It may be multicentric and does not arise in adenomatous polyps. It is important that the patient know about the risk of cancer because it may influence a decision to undergo colectomy. After they have had the disease for 8 to 10 years, high-risk patients should have yearly evaluations of the colon by colonoscopy. Because dysplastic changes of the colonic mucosa have been shown to correlate closely with the development of cancer elsewhere in the colon, serial colonic and rectal biopsies should be obtained during this yearly colonoscopy in high-risk patients.

Crohn Disease

Crohn disease, or *regional enteritis,* is a chronic inflammatory condition of unknown cause involving all layers of the intestine, as opposed to involvement of only the mucosa (as in ulcerative colitis; see Table 45.6). The condition most commonly affects the terminal ileum, but any area from the esophagus to the anus can be involved. The onset of the disease most commonly occurs in adolescence or young adulthood. The incidence of Crohn disease has been rising in recent years, particularly Crohn disease of the colon.

Presentation

Crohn disease may be localized initially to the small bowel, involve small bowel and colon, or be confined to the colon only. The inflammatory process often remains confined to the initial site of involvement unless surgery is performed. Recurrence is the rule after surgery, and the condition may then involve additional segments of bowel. Spontaneous progression of the disease tends to occur in a proximal (orad) direction. As the inflammatory process persists, the bowel wall becomes thickened and stenotic, leading to bowel obstruction. Fistula formation is characteristic and may involve any contiguous structure. As a result, abscess formation and infection can complicate the clinical course. Diarrhea, abdominal pain, and weight loss are the most common symptoms. Unlike ulcerative colitis, rectal bleeding is not a prominent feature unless the colon is the major site of involvement.

The *differential diagnosis* includes disorders of both the small and the large bowel. Occasionally the patient presents with fever and acute right lower quadrant pain resembling acute appendicitis. When there is involvement of the terminal ileum, Crohn disease must be distinguished from lymphoma and tuberculosis. Colonic involvement may suggest ulcerative colitis, ischemic colitis, or carcinoma. Involvement of the distal small bowel and the right colon, the presence of characteristic skip areas, stricturing of the bowel, perianal disease, and fistula formation are helpful diagnostic features that suggest Crohn disease.

Treatment

Medical therapy for Crohn disease is similar to that for ulcerative colitis, depending heavily on 5-ASA preparations or sulfasalazine and immune suppression. For mild to moderate active Crohn disease, 5-ASA agents or sulfasalazine (see earlier discussion for dosing schedule) should be used as first-line agents. Metronidazole (1 to 2 g/day) or ciprofloxacin (1 g/day) is as effective as mesalamine or sulfasalazine and may be used in patients who are allergic or intolerant to these latter two drugs or in combination with the first-line agents. Long-term metronidazole therapy is, however, associated with development of peripheral neuropathy in some individuals. Patients with severe disease usually require an initial course of prednisone, 40 to 60 mg/day until the symptoms resolve, followed by a slow taper. A monoclonal antibody to tumor necrosis factor alpha (Infliximab), given in a single intravenous dose of 5 mg/kg, may be used as adjunctive therapy in individuals not responding to corticosteroids. Patients with severe or fulminant disease require aggressive treatment, which often includes hospitalization, parenteral hyperalimentation, and either intravenous cyclosporine or oral tacrolimus. Surgery may become necessary if response to medical therapy is not optimal. As in ulcerative colitis, corticosteroids are not effective in preventing relapses and should not be used for maintenance of remission. After the control of acute disease, mesalamine, sulfasalazine, metronidazole, ciprofloxacin, 6-MP, or azathioprine may be used for maintenance therapy. Infliximab is effective in closing fistulas in one third or more of the patients (27). However, some patients require periodic infusions every 8 to 12 weeks to prevent recurrence. Although they are not as effective, antibiotics, 6-MP, and azathioprine may also be useful in the treatment of fistulizing Crohn disease.

Because of the complexity of the disease, management should be accomplished by, or in consultation with, a gastroenterologist.

Surgery for resection of fibrotic obstructing lesions, drainage of abscesses, and resection of complicated fistulas is sometimes necessary. Occasionally the disease is refractory to medical therapy and the diseased bowel must be resected. It must be recognized that surgery is not intended to be curative, so removal of normal bowel to achieve wide, disease-free margins is not indicated. In the rare patient whose disease is extensive and unresponsive to medical and surgical intervention or in whom a short-bowel syndrome has developed secondary to the disease and to repeated surgery, long-term home parenteral hyperalimentation can be beneficial to provide good nutritional support and ameliorate symptoms.

Course

Despite its chronicity and tendency for recurrence, Crohn disease takes a highly variable course. Prolonged asymptomatic periods occur, even after years of disease activity and multiple operations. There is a poor correlation between clinical severity and the radiographic appearance of the disease, so followup radiographs are not indicated unless there is a suspicion of a new development in the disease (e.g., a fistula). The risk of colorectal carcinoma is elevated significantly only in Crohn disease involving the colon. Mortality from the disease is low, but morbidity is high. Because the natural history is so variable, the clinician should approach the patient with Crohn disease in a positive and hopeful fashion, yet be aware of the potential for significant morbidity. All patients should be monitored in close consultation with a gastroenterologist.

Drug-Induced Diarrhea

A variety of commonly used medications can cause diarrhea (Table 45.4). The diarrhea may be a direct result of the pharmacologic activity of the drug (e.g., magnesium-containing antacids, colchicine), or the mechanism for the induction of diarrhea may be unknown (e.g., hydralazine, propranolol). The diarrhea may also signify drug toxicity (e.g., digitalis). Certain drugs have repeatedly been associated with diarrhea (antibiotics, antacids, quinidine, digitalis, and alcohol), whereas in other cases (hydralazine, propranolol), the relationship is rare and not well defined.

Diarrhea Associated with Antibiotics

Diarrhea associated with antibiotics may range from a mild increase in the frequency and volume of stools to a toxic, life-threatening condition. Diarrhea may develop during the course of antibiotic therapy, or after parenteral or oral use, but it may also occur up to months after discontinuation of the drugs. The antibiotics most commonly associated with diarrhea are ampicillin, tetracycline, clindamycin, and the cephalosporins.

In the more severe forms of antibiotic-associated diarrhea, the diarrhea is bloody and is accompanied by abdominal cramps and fever. Endoscopy may reveal pseudomembranes, which appear as raised yellowish plaques on edematous, friable mucosa. Histologically, these pseudomembranes are collections of fibrin, mucin, and leukocytes. Proliferation of *C. difficile* and the elaboration of its toxin cause pseudomembranous colitis. This organism accounts for the vast majority of cases of pseudomembranous colitis and for 20% to 30% of antibiotic-associated diarrhea in general. The toxin elaborated by *C. difficile* can be assayed in stool. The organism can also be cultured, but it is difficult to grow. Because culture is less sensitive than the toxin titer and does not correlate as well with symptoms, it is not recommended.

Therapy involves discontinuation of the antibiotics and, in cases of pseudomembranous colitis, administration of metronidazole (Flagyl), 500 mg four times a day for 7 days (see Chapter 35). This antimicrobial agent is effective against clostridial organisms, and the response is fairly rapid. Relapses after discontinuation of metronidazole are not uncommon. In such cases, a second course of metronidazole should be administered. Vancomycin may be prescribed (125 to 500 mg orally four times a day for 7 days) for cases repeatedly resistant or relapsing after metronidazole. Oral cholestyramine has also been used effectively to bind the toxin. Antidiarrheal medications are contraindicated because they may actually prolong the duration of the disease. It is probably unnecessary to treat patients who are found to have *C. difficile* toxin–positive stools, as is common in nursing homes, unless there are accompanying symptoms or an outbreak is in progress. Symptomatic patients can be treated with bismuth subsalicylate (Pepto-Bismol), 30 mL or 2 tablets every 4 hours, while results of the assay for the toxin are awaited.

Postsurgical Diarrhea

A variety of surgical procedures may result in diarrhea. Predictably, *extensive small-bowel resections* (e.g., for mesenteric vascular occlusions) result in severe diarrhea and steatorrhea (short-bowel syndrome). Management of such cases requires careful attention to nutritional factors and use of narcotics to control the diarrhea. Long-term home hyperalimentation has allowed patients to overcome the severe malabsorption that would accompany massive small-bowel resection.

Resection of the ileum is less well tolerated than resection of the jejunum, because the ileum serves as the only site for absorption of bile acids. When the ileal resection is limited (less than 100 cm), the total bile acid pool remains sufficient to prevent significant steatorrhea. However, there is still an excessive loading of bile acids into the colon, where they stimulate mucosal secretion and result in diarrhea. Therapy for this form of diarrhea is aimed at binding the fecal bile acids with an agent such as cholestyramine. The dosage is 4 g given before meals and at bedtime. When ileal resection is more extensive (more than 100 cm), the total bile acid pool becomes diminished below the critical level needed for proper digestion and absorption of fat, and steatorrhea develops. The use of cholestyramine in this situation further depletes the bile acid pool and worsens the steatorrhea and diarrhea. Therefore, dietary fat should be supplied in the form of medium-chain triglycerides, which do not require bile acids for absorption. Commercial preparations are available (e.g., Portagen), and consultation with a nutritionist as well as a gastroenterologist is recommended.

Diarrhea may also occur after *gastric surgery* with vagotomy. At times the vagotomy causes diarrhea by altering intestinal motility and, for unclear reasons, by increasing the concentration of fecal bile acids. Therapy with cholestyramine has been successful in this postvagotomy syndrome. Gastric surgery may also unmask latent lactase deficiency or, rarely, latent celiac disease. The blind loop syndrome with resultant bacterial overgrowth, dumping syndrome, inadvertent gastroileal anastomosis, and gastrocolic fistula are all complications that can result in diarrhea in patients who have undergone gastrectomy (see Chapter 43).

Diarrhea may occur after cholecystectomy, in association with an increased concentration of fecal bile acids. Therapy with cholestyramine is effective. Subtotal colectomy, with an ileal-rectal anastomosis (e.g., for multiple polyposis), often results in diarrhea that is usually easily controlled by antidiarrheal medication and diminishes with time. Segmental colonic resection usually does not result in diarrhea because of the large functional reserve of the normal colon.

Symptomatic Antidiarrheal Therapy

Diarrhea is merely a symptom, and therapy, if possible, should be directed at the underlying process. However, a wide variety of agents are available for symptomatic control of diarrhea. The efficacy of these agents is highly variable, and the mechanism of action of many is poorly understood. Symptomatic treatment should be avoided in patients with suspected acute infectious diarrhea because of bacteria like *Salmonella* and *Shigella*, because suppression of bowel movements in these conditions may prolong the diarrhea.

Hydrophilic bulk-forming agents, such as psyllium (Metamucil, Konsyl), have been shown to improve the consistency of ileostomy and colostomy effluent (see earlier discussion). These agents, which paradoxically are also used in treating constipation, are particularly useful in patients with irritable bowel syndrome (Chapter 44).

Another group of antidiarrheal medications consists of those classified as *absorbents,* on the premise that these agents bind factors within the intestinal lumen that cause diarrhea. Medications of this group include kaolin and pectin (Kaopectate), bismuth salts (Pepto-Bismol), aluminum hydroxide (Amphojel), and cholestyramine (Questran). Most are available over the counter, but their value is not well established. However, Pepto-Bismol has been shown to be effective in controlling the symptoms of traveler's diarrhea (see Chapter 35). Cholestyramine is effective in treating bile acid–induced diarrhea, as occurs in patients after ileal resection, vagotomy, or cholecystectomy. This drug also may bind other compounds, such as digoxin and warfarin, and thereby decrease their absorption.

Opioid derivatives are probably the most effective antidiarrheal medications. Opiate drugs delay the transit of intraluminal contents through the small and large intestines. A central effect is also likely. In patients with extensive small-bowel resection, codeine may be the only effective form of therapy. The synthetic agents diphenoxylate–atropine (Lomotil) and loperamide (Imodium) are also effective and are generally well tolerated. The atropine in Lomotil contributes little to its antidiarrheal effect and may cause significant toxicity. Imodium has the theoretical advantages of a more favorable ratio of GI effects to central nervous system effects and a longer duration of action. An OTC formulation is now available. Imodium has the practical disadvantage of being expensive. The development of megacolon, prolongation of symptoms, and worsening of pseudomembranous colitis have all been linked to the injudicious use of these agents in patients with bacterial diarrhea. The potential risk for abuse is theoretically less for Imodium.

Another group of drugs that is under investigation is classified as *antisecretory.* Some of these drugs inhibit the synthesis of prostaglandins, which increase intestinal secretion by stimulating adenylate cyclase activity within intestinal cells. (Adenylate cyclase is the enzyme that catalyzes the formation of cyclic adenosine monophosphate [(cAMP)], the concentration of which influences certain transport systems in cell membranes.) Other drugs of this class inhibit adenylate cyclase directly. For example, indomethacin inhibits prostaglandin synthesis and has been shown experimentally to inhibit the effect of enterotoxin. Propranolol, an inhibitor of adenylate cyclase, suppresses bile acid–induced fluid accumulation in intestinal loops. Certain diuretics (e.g., ethacrynic acid) that act on electrolyte transport have also been shown to be effective enterotoxin antagonists. Endorphin-like peptides are also under study as antidiarrheal agents. Investigation into their mechanism of action may lead to the development of new effective forms of therapy against diarrhea. A somatostatin analog (octreotide) is available for the treatment of GI endocrine tumors (e.g., vasoactive intestinal peptide–secreting tumor, gastrinoma, carcinoid). It is not recommended for use in other forms of diarrhea.

Because there are few data to allow an objective comparison of the various antidiarrheal medications, the choice of drug must be based on efficacy, safety, and cost. For acute, self-limited illnesses, drugs such as Kaopectate and bismuth salts are often tried by patients, even before a health care provider is consulted. For such patients, diphenoxylate–atropine (Lomotil) or loperamide (Imodium) is highly effective. Patients should be instructed to use medication after a diarrheal movement and not to exceed 8 tablets per day. Loperamide may provide longer diarrhea-free intervals with fewer side effects (28). Oral rehydration therapy (see Chapters 35 and 41) is important, especially with voluminous diarrhea in the frail elderly and in children. Both glucose-based and rice-based electrolyte solutions are available for rehydration. Commercial rehydration solutions designed for athletes (e.g., Gatorade) have inadequate concentrations of electrolytes and therefore are not satisfactory in the treatment of diarrhea.

For patients with chronic diarrhea, the choice of medication is based on the severity and cause of the diarrhea. In patients with the diarrhea-predominant form of the irritable bowel syndrome (Chapter 44), hydrophilic agents may be useful. The dosage should be titrated to the desired bowel habits, with dosages ranging from 1 teaspoon to 2 tablespoons per day mixed in 8 ounces of juice or water per dose. In patients with diarrhea from other causes, diphenoxylate–atropine or loperamide should be tried. These medications can be given in divided doses throughout the day. Diarrhea can also be prevented by taking one or two tablets before engaging in an event associated with diarrhea (e.g., meals, examinations).

In more severe cases of diarrhea, narcotics are necessary. Tincture of opium is convenient because it can easily be titrated (by the drop) to control diarrhea at the lowest possible dosage. A recommended starting dosage is six drops every 4 to 6 hours, to be adjusted by one or two drops per dose depending on the patient's response. Codeine, at a dose of 15 to 30 mg, may also be used with the same dosage schedule.

SPECIFIC REFERENCES*

1. Connell AM, Hilton C, Irvine G, et al. Variation of bowel habit in two population samples. BMJ 1965;2:1095.
2. Sonnenberg A, Koch TR. Physician visits in the United States for constipation: 1958–1986. Digest Dis Sci 1989;34:606.
3. Loche GR III. The epidemiology of functional gastrointestinal disorders in North America. Gastroenterol Clin North Am 1996;25:1.
4. Nyam DC, Pemberton JH, Ilstrup DM, et al. Long-term results of surgery for chronic constipation. Dis Colon Rectum 1997;40:273.
5. Locke GR III, Pemberton JH, Phillips SF. AGA technical review on constipation. Gastroenterology 2000;119:1766.
6. Wald A. Colonic and anorectal motility testing in clinical practice. Am J Gastroenterol 1994;89:2109.
7. Metcalf AM, Phillips SF, Zinsmeister AR, et al. Simplified assessment of segmental colonic transit. Gastroenterology 1987;92:40.
8. Voderholzer WA, Schatke W, Muhldorfer BE, et al. Clinical response to dietary fiber treatment of chronic constipation. Am J Gastroenterol 1997;92:95.
9. Anti M, Pignataro G, Armuzzi A, et al. Water supplementation enhances the effect of high-fiber diet on stool frequency and laxative consumption in adults with functional constipation. Hepatogastroenterology 1998;45:727.
10. Tramonte SM, Brand MB, Mulrow CD, et al. The treatment of chronic constipation in adults. J Gen Intern Med 1997;12:15.
11. Ramkumar D, Rao SS. Efficacy and safety of traditional medical therapies for chronic constipation: systematic review. Am J Gastroenterol. 2005;100:936.
12. Nyam DC, Pemberton JH, Ilstrup DM, et al. Long-term results of surgery for chronic constipation. Dis Colon Rectum 1997;40: 273.
13. Dupont HL, Hornick RB. Adverse effects of Lomotil therapy in shigellosis. JAMA 1973;226:1525.
14. Cimolai N, Carter JE, Morrison BJ, et al. Risk factors for the progression of *Escherichia coli* O157:H7 enteritis to hemolytic-uremic syndrome. J Pediatr 1990;116:589.
15. Fine KD, Ogunji F, George J, et al. Utility of a rapid fecal latex agglutination test detecting the neutrophil protein, lactoferrin, for diagnosing inflammatory causes of chronic diarrhea. Am J Gastroenterol 1998;93:1300.
16. Garcia LS, Shimizu RY. Evaluation of nine immunoassay kits (enzyme immunoassay and direct fluorescence) for detection of *Giardia lamblia* and *Cryptosporidum parvum* in human fecal specimens. J Clin Microbiol 1997;35: 1526.
17. Vanpoucke H, De Baere T, Claeys G, et al. Evaluation of six commercial assays for rapid detection of *Clostridium difficile* toxin and/or antigen in stool specimens. Clin Microbiol Infect 2001;7:55.
18. Shah RJ, Fenoglio-Preiser C, Bleau BL, et al. Usefulness of colonoscopy with biopsy in the evaluation of patients with chronic diarrhea. Am J Gastroenterol 2001;96:1091.
19. Eherer AJ, Fordtran JS. Fecal osmotic gap and pH in experimental diarrhea of various causes. Gastroenterology 1992;103:545.
20. Lang C, Gyr K, Stalder GA, et al. Assessment of exocrine pancreatic function by oral administration of *N*-benzoyl-L-tyrosyl-p-aminobenzoic acid (Bentiromide): 5 years' clinical experience. Br J Surg 1981;68:771.
21. Carroccio A, Verghi F, Santini B, et al. Diagnostic accuracy of fecal elastase 1 assay in patients with pancreatic maldigestion or intestinal malabsorption: a collaborative study of the Italian Society of Pediatric Gastroenterology and Hepatology. Dig Dis Sci 2001;46:1335.
22. Scrimshaw NS, Murray EB. The acceptability of milk and milk products in populations with a high prevalence of lactose intolerance. Am J Clin Nutr 1988;48:1079.
23. Tramonte SM, Brand MB, Mulrow CD, et al. The treatment of chronic constipation in adults. J Gen Intern Med 1997;12:15.
24. Edwards FC, Truelove SC. The course and prognosis of ulcerative colitis. Part III: complications. Gut 1964;5:7.
25. Pullan RD, Rhodes J, Garresh S, et al. Transdermal nicotine for active ulcerative colitis. N Engl J Med 1994;330:811.
26. Lennard-Jones JE, Morson BC, Ritchie JK, et al. Cancer surveillance in ulcerative colitis. Lancet 1983;2:149.
27. Panaccione R, Canadian Consensus Group on the use of infliximab in Crohn's disease. Infliximab for the treatment of Crohn's disease: review and indication for clinical use in Canada. Can J Gastroenterol 2001;15:371.
28. Palmer KR, Corbett CL, Holdsworth CD. Double blind cross-over study comparing loperamide, codeine, and diphenoxylate in the treatment of chronic diarrhea. Gastroenterology 1980;79:1272.

*Bold numerals denote published controlled clinical trials, meta-analyses, or consensus-based recommendations.

*For annotated **General References** and resources related to this chapter, visit www.hopkinsbayview.org/PAMreferences.*

Chapter 46

Selected Gastrointestinal Problems: Gastrointestinal Bleeding, Colorectal Cancer Screening, and Diverticular Disease

Mack C. Mitchell, Jr. and H. Franklin Herlong

GASTROINTESTINAL BLEEDING

The presence of blood in the stool or in the upper gastrointestinal (GI) tract is a significant finding that requires thorough investigation. GI bleeding may manifest as occult blood, hematemesis, melena (black stool) or intermittent hematochezia (overtly bloody stool). Massive hemorrhage, whatever the source, requires immediate hospitalization and often emergency diagnostic procedures. In hemodynamically stable individuals, the evaluation of GI bleeding can often be performed in an ambulatory setting. Table 46.1 shows the common conditions associated with GI bleeding.

Tests for Detection of Blood in Stool

In normal subjects, the hemoglobin concentration of the stool is less than 2 mg hemoglobin per g of stool, as measured by tagged red cell assay. The most commonly used test for fecal occult blood is the *modified guaiac slide test (Hemoccult)*. This test depends on the pseudoperoxidase activity of hemoglobin to detect blood in the stool. It is not influenced by supplemental iron in the diet, but false-positive tests may result from ingestion of rare red meat and peroxidase-rich foods (uncooked vegetables such as broccoli, turnips, and cauliflower). False negative results are more likely in patients taking large doses of vitamin C. The stool slides can be stored up to 6 days if necessary without a decrease in the sensitivity of the test. Rehydration of the fecal material on the slide also increases the false-positive rate and is not recommended.

In populations screened with Hemoccult testing to detect colon cancer or polyps, 1% to 5% of subjects have positive test results (1). However, the predictive value of a positive test is only 2% to 17% for colon cancer (1) and 9% to 36% for adenomatous polyps. The remainder of positive tests are because of other causes of bleeding (e.g., gastritis, peptic ulcer) or to bleeding without a detectable source. Salicylates and other nonsteroidal anti-inflammatory drugs (NSAIDs) can cause occult GI bleeding, either because of a direct irritant effect on the stomach or duodenum or because of unmasking of an underlying lesion. Because colonic neoplasms may bleed intermittently, sensitivity is improved when multiple stool specimens are evaluated. Although the optimal number and

TABLE 46.1 Common Causes of Gastrointestinal Bleeding

Occult Bleeding
Gastritis, especially caused by nonsteroidal anti-inflammatory agents or ethanol
Peptic ulcer disease
Colonic polyps
Colonic cancer
Gastric cancer
Esophagitis
Melena
Peptic ulcer disease
Hemorrhagic gastritis
Gastric cancer
Hematochezia
Diverticulosis
Angiodysplasia
Rectal outlet disorders (hemorrhoids, cryptitis, fissures)
Inflammatory bowel disease
Colonic polyps
Colonic cancer
Hematemesis
Peptic ulcer disease
Esophageal varices
Mallory–Weiss tear
Hemorrhagic gastritis
Gastric cancer

timing of stool samples have not been determined, checking two samples from three separate daily stool specimens is recommended for colorectal cancer screening (2). Among asymptomatic patients with a positive slide test who have carcinoma, more than 80% have early lesions limited to the bowel. Therefore, a positive test for occult blood in the stool requires further investigation and may favorably influence prognosis.

Evaluation of Patients with Gastrointestinal Bleeding

Choosing Appropriate Tests

The history and physical examination direct the sequence of the various tests used to investigate GI bleeding. The patient's age and medical history; the nature of associated symptoms, and the severity of bleeding are all important factors. For example, patients younger than 50 years of age are less likely to have a colonic lesion than are older patients. Peptic disease and benign rectal lesions are more evenly distributed among adults of all ages.

In asymptomatic patients with occult fecal blood and in patients with hematochezia but no other symptoms, the lower bowel should be investigated first. In patients with hematemesis or melena but no other symptoms, the upper GI tract should be investigated first. A reasonable approach to the evaluation of lower and upper GI bleeding is described in the next two sections.

Lower Gastrointestinal Tract

For patients presenting with hematochezia, flexible sigmoidoscopy or colonoscopy is usually the first test done to evaluate the lower bowel. In patients older than 40 years of age, colonoscopy should be performed as the initial test. However, in patients younger than 40 years of age, if the pattern of bleeding is consistent with rectal disease (see Chapter 98) colonoscopy is not always necessary. Diverticulosis (see below), should not be considered the cause of intermittent mild hematochezia until colonoscopy has failed to provide an alternative explanation. For patients with occult fecal blood and no localizing symptoms, a colonoscopy or a flexible sigmoidoscopy plus barium enema is the minimum recommended workup (1).

Proctosigmoidoscopy

Anorectal lesions are poorly visualized by barium enema. Cryptitis, bleeding hemorrhoids, fissures, and proctitis can be seen only by endoscopy. Even rectal polyps and cancer are much better revealed by proctoscopy than by radiography.

Flexible sigmoidoscopy is used to evaluate the rectum and descending colon. It has replaced rigid proctosigmoidoscopy for evaluation of the rectum and sigmoid colon. It is useful in screening asymptomatic patients for colorectal adenoma or carcinoma (3), but is not recommended for evaluating patients older than the age of 40 years with GI bleeding because colonoscopy is required to exclude more proximal colonic lesions.

Colonoscopy

Colonoscopy is indicated in patients with GI bleeding of suspected colonic origin, either as the initial test or as a followup examination when flexible sigmoidoscopy and/or barium enema have not provided an unequivocal diagnosis. Most gastroenterologists perform colonoscopy instead of a barium enema plus flexible sigmoidoscopy because colonoscopy has a higher positive predictive value in the evaluation of rectal bleeding (4). In patients with polyps, colonoscopy provides a way to remove the polyps without major surgery. An experienced endoscopist can reach the cecum in more than 95% of cases (5). Complications from the procedure are mainly perforation and hemorrhage; the overall complication rate for diagnostic colonoscopy is 0.3% to 0.4%, with a mortality rate of 0.02% (6). If polypectomy is performed, the morbidity increases to 1% to 2%, but the mortality rate remains the same.

The sensitivity of colonoscopy in experienced hands is much higher than that of an air-contrast barium enema: Only 2% of polyps are not diagnosed by the former procedure. In a study of anemic patients with occult GI bleeding, colonoscopy revealed polyps (greater than 5 mm in diameter) or cancer in 15% of patients with negative barium examinations; of patients with rectal bleeding, 34% had a significant lesion (including 11% with cancer) when the barium enema was reported as negative or simply as showing diverticulosis (7).

Patient Experience. Preparation for colonoscopy usually includes a liquid diet for 1 day and laxatives such as *Fleets Phosphosoda*. An alternative preparation is to drink 4 L of a nonabsorbed isosmolar solution of polyethylene glycol and electrolytes (Go-lytely, Colyte, Nu-lytely) the night before the procedure. Elderly patients may have difficulty ingesting the large amount of fluid. Just before the procedure, the patient is given moderate sedation (usually with meperidine or fentanyl plus midazolam). Propofol is becoming more popular for moderate sedation because of more rapid onset and shorter recovery time after sedation. Moderate sedation is used to avoid the discomfort associated with distention of the bowel with air for inspection and with stretching of the mesentery as the colonoscope is maneuvered through the bowel lumen. However, some patients may be able to tolerate the procedure with only reassurance and no sedatives. There is no additional discomfort when a biopsy or polypectomy is performed. The duration of the procedure is variable, depending on the tortuosity of the colon, the presence of disease, and the skill of the endoscopist, but the average is 20 to 45 minutes.

If moderate sedation is administered, someone must accompany the patient home after the procedure because of possible lingering sedation. Antibiotic prophylaxis must be given to patients who are at high risk of endocarditis (see Chapter 65) before and after the procedure (see Chapter 93).

Upper Gastrointestinal Tract

The sequence of tests performed in evaluating the upper GI tract depends on the severity of the bleeding and the suspected diagnosis. *Upper endoscopy,* or *esophagogastroduodenoscopy (EGD),* is the procedure of choice for most patients with upper GI bleeding. In patients with acute bleeding, actively bleeding lesions can often be treated at the time of the procedure, by endoscopic band ligation or sclerotherapy in the case of bleeding esophageal varices or by electrocautery or the placement of hemoclips in the case of bleeding ulcer or angiodysplasia. If an upper GI series has been performed and is negative or reveals a gastric ulcer (Chapter 43) or a tumor, upper endoscopy should be the next procedure. If the upper and lower GI tracts have been evaluated in a patient with GI bleeding and both the studies are negative, a *small-bowel series* should be considered to investigate the possibility of other disorders that affect mainly the small intestine, such as Crohn disease.

Radiologic Studies

The *upper GI series* may detect mass lesions in the esophagus and stomach and gastric and duodenal ulcerations, although it is insensitive for evaluating mucosal detail. It is well tolerated and inexpensive. Chapter 43 describes the patient's experience during the performance of an upper GI series.

The conventional *small bowel series* is very poor at detecting small lesions of the intestine (e.g., cancer, leiomyoma). Disorders such as Crohn disease or lymphoma are more likely to be revealed by radiography (although a definitive diagnosis can be made only by biopsy). These sources of bleeding are uncommon and should be suspected only when the more common conditions (peptic ulcer disease, colonic polyps) have been excluded. The patient should be warned that the small bowel series requires spending 1 to 5 hours in the radiology department, during which time films are taken every 30 minutes.

Endoscopy

Upper endoscopy is the most widely used means of investigating upper GI bleeding. This technique not only is more sensitive than radiography but also provides a direct means of obtaining specimens for histological examination. Because of its greater sensitivity, endoscopy is indicated when barium studies are negative in the evaluation of a suspected upper GI source of bleeding.

Patient Experience. Upper endoscopy is an outpatient procedure that usually takes less than 15 minutes. The patient fasts overnight before the procedure. Just before the procedure, the patient is sedated with intravenous medication (meperidine or fentanyl plus midazolam) and the throat is sprayed with a topical anesthetic. Under direct vision, mucosal biopsies and cytologic brushings can be obtained from suspicious lesions for histologic diagnosis. Biopsies are completely painless. Complications include perforation and bleeding but are extremely rare. Newer, smaller-caliber endoscopes have greatly improved patient tolerance of the procedure. After the procedure, because of the sedation, someone must accompany the patient home. The patient typically has a sore throat for several hours.

Occult and Obscure Gastrointestinal Bleeding

Occult bleeding is defined as chronic slow bleeding occurring from the GI tract, presenting either as iron deficiency anemia or a positive fecal occult blood test. Evaluation of occult bleeding should always start with a lower GI examination, preferably with a colonoscopy, especially in individuals older than 40 years of age, unless the history is strongly suggestive of an upper GI lesion. If the colonoscopy is negative, proceeding to an upper endoscopy is reasonable.

Obscure bleeding is defined as persistent GI bleeding, occult or overt, for which no source is identified by upper and lower endoscopy. Arteriovenous malformations, peptic ulcer disease, erosions in large hiatus hernias, and NSAID use are some of the causes of obscure bleeding. Obscure bleeding does not necessarily correspond to small-volume bleeding: It can range from occult to massive bleeding. Evaluation of obscure bleeding should begin with repeat upper and lower endoscopy. A duodenal or small bowel biopsy should be obtained for celiac disease during upper endoscopy, especially in young white patients with a history of diarrhea and persistent iron deficiency anemia. If these are again unrevealing, evaluation of the entire small bowel is warranted. A small bowel series may be helpful in patients with a negative endoscopic examination. It can detect lesions larger than 1 to 2 cm in size but is not very sensitive for identifying many causes of obscure GI bleeding. If the small-bowel series is negative, then capsule endoscopy or push enteroscopy should be the next step. (Push enteroscopy is performed by passing a longer endoscope than is typically used for upper endoscopy as far as possible beyond the duodenum [8,9]). A radioisotope-labeled red blood cell scan (the so-called "bleeding scan") and mesenteric angiography should be considered in cases of overt bleeding that remain undiagnosed. Bleeding scans and angiography are helpful only when the rate of bleeding exceeds 0.1 to 0.4 mL/minute and 0.5 mL/minute, respectively, at the time of the study (10,11). In the absence of active bleeding, however, angiography may sometimes be helpful if the characteristic vascular pattern of a Dieulafoy lesion (a dilated submucosal blood vessel that has eroded through the overlying mucosa), tumor, or vascular malformation is seen. Exploratory laparotomy with intraoperative enteroscopy is sometimes necessary in patients who require repeated transfusions because of recurrent bleeding and in whom the source of bleeding remains unidentified despite extensive evaluation as described previously. All patients with persistent bleeding should be evaluated for a disorder of hemostasis (e.g., von Willebrand disease) if an anatomic cause of bleeding has not been identified (see Chapter 56).

Wireless Capsule Endoscopy

Wireless capsule endoscopy can be performed using a small digital camera with memory chip that is embedded in a capsule. After the capsule is swallowed, the chip transmits digital images (2 frames per second) to a recording device that is worn on the belt for up to 8 hours. The capsule is propelled through the GI tract by peristalsis and permits recording of images from the esophagus to the ileocecal valve. The images are then replayed at a faster speed allowing the observer to interpret the "video endoscopy." The technique has been useful in detecting obscure causes of bleeding, particularly from small mucosal lesions in the small bowel and is also useful for the diagnosis of Crohn disease of the small bowel (12,13). The major disadvantage is the inability to perform biopsies at the time of the imaging.

Selected Lesions that Bleed

Chapter 43 discusses the most common cause of upper GI bleeding—peptic disease. Common causes of lower GI bleeding include benign anorectal disorders (Chapter 98), inflammatory bowel disease (discussed later in this chapter), angiodysplasia, colonic neoplasms, and diverticulosis (see below).

Colonic Polyps

Colonic polyps or colonic cancer should be suspected in any patient older than 40 years of age who has GI bleeding or a change in bowel habits. Bleeding from colonic polyps may be occult or may occur as intermittent hematochezia, although most patients are asymptomatic. It is believed that most cancers of the colon (except those associated with ulcerative colitis) arise from these benign adenomas, although only a small percentage of premalignant polyps grow into invasive cancers. The removal of polyps before they become malignant has the potential to reduce the occurrence of colonic cancer in predisposed individuals (14).

TABLE 46.2 Polyps: Relationship of Size, Histologic Type, and Risk of Carcinoma

	% That Are Cancerous		
Histologic Type	*<1 cm*	*1–2 cm*	*>2 cm*
Tubular adenoma	1.0	10.2	34.7
Intermediate type	3.9	7.4	45.8
Villous adenoma	9.5	10.3	52.9

From Muto T, Bussey HJ, Morson BC. The evolution of cancer of the colon and rectum. Cancer 1975;36:2251.

Although polyps are most common in the rectosigmoid region, they may be found anywhere in the colon.

The risk of a polyp becoming malignant is related to the histological type and size. *Hyperplastic polyps* make up 10% to 30% of all colorectal polyps. They tend to be small (less than 0.5 cm in diameter) and to be located in the distal colon or rectum, and probably have no malignant potential. *Villous and tubular adenomas* make up almost two thirds of all colorectal polyps, are found in 25% of people by age 50 years (and in 50% by age 80), and carry a definite risk of malignant transformation that increases as they increase in size (15). The risk that a villous adenoma larger than 2 cm in diameter is cancerous is greater than 50% (Table 46.2) (16). Fortunately, if the cancer remains confined to the mucosa of the polyp (*carcinoma in situ*), colonoscopic polypectomy is curative. Because the cancerous change in the polyp may be focal, single biopsies of a polyp are not sufficient to exclude the presence of a malignancy; instead, the entire polyp must be excised.

Once an adenomatous polyp has been detected, surveillance for additional polyps is indicated. In 30% of patients more than one polyp is present at the time of initial investigation, and the risk of recurrence increases with the number and size of polyps that are initially discovered (17). Subsequent development of new polyps occurs in at least 10% of patients. If one or two adenomatous polyps less than 1 cm are detected during colonoscopy, repeat colonoscopy is indicated in 5 years to continue screening for new polyps or colon cancer. If more than 2 adenomatous polyps are found or if a polyp is greater than 1 cm in size, then colonoscopy should be repeated in 3 years. If a followup examination reveals no further polyps, the screening interval may be increased to once every 5 years (18).

Multiple polyposis syndromes are rare inherited abnormalities that are important to recognize because of their malignant potential. *Familial polyposis, Gardner syndrome,* and *Turcot syndrome* all are associated with multiple adenomatous polyps of the colon and therefore carry a high risk for development of carcinoma. Gardner syndrome includes osteomas and soft tissue tumors, and Turcot syndrome includes tumors of the central nervous system. Familial polyposis and Gardner syndrome are inherited as autosomal dominant defects, while Turcot syndrome is an autosomal recessive disorder. The diagnosis of a polyposis syndrome is usually made in patients in their 20s, with cancer developing in virtually all patients within the next 20 years. There is considerable controversy about the therapy for these conditions. Colonic resection is curative, but the timing and extent of resection are subjects of controversy. When rectal polyps are present, a proctocolectomy should be performed to eliminate the risk of cancer. However, because the patients are generally asymptomatic and young, the prospect of an ileostomy is often overwhelming. The results of ileorectal pull-through procedures are encouraging. Cyclooxygenase-2 (COX-2) inhibitors (e.g., celecoxib), have been demonstrated to reduce the number of polyps in patients with familial polyposis syndromes (19). Whether these agents are of use also in patients with sporadic adenomatous polyps and whether they reduce the risk of malignant transformation is currently being evaluated through long-term prospective trials.

Whereas colonic polyposis syndromes involve adenomatous polyps, other conditions are associated with juvenile polyps or hamartomas. The *Peutz–Jeghers syndrome* consists of multiple hamartomas, predominantly of the small intestine, associated with buccal and cutaneous pigmentation. Although the malignant potential of the hamartomas is low, duodenal and ovarian carcinomas have been reported in these patients and the cumulative risk for colon cancer is 39% (20). Rarely, juvenile polyps may occur throughout the GI tract. In the absence of associated extracolonic manifestations, this syndrome is called *generalized juvenile polyposis*; when accompanied by alopecia, nail bed changes, hyperpigmentation, and malabsorption, it is called the *Cronkhite–Canada* syndrome.

Colorectal Cancer

Epidemiology and Etiology

Cancers of the colon and rectum account for 14% of all cancers and are the second leading cause of cancer death overall in the United States. Overall, there is approximately a 5% lifetime chance of developing a colorectal cancer.

Colorectal cancer occurs with increasing frequency in older age groups, with two-thirds occurring in people older than 65 years of age. Geographic differences in the mortality rate from this neoplasm suggest an etiologic role for dietary and environmental factors. In particular, a high-fat, low-fiber diet appears to be associated with an increased risk of colorectal cancer. For unclear reasons, the proportion of cancers in the right side of the colon has increased in recent years, with a commensurate drop in the proportion of rectosigmoid lesions (21). Currently, approximately half of colorectal cancers are within reach of the flexible sigmoidoscope. The remaining half is proximal to the splenic flexure and accessible only with a colonoscope. The three main predisposing conditions for colorectal cancer are colonic polyps, familial polyposis (see previous discussion), and ulcerative colitis (see Chapter 45). The presence of these conditions dictates the need for a strict colonoscopic surveillance program and, at times, even prophylactic surgery to prevent the development of cancer. (See Chapter 45 for the risk of cancer in ulcerative colitis.) Although it is accepted that a family history of colorectal cancer predisposes a person to polyps and colorectal cancer, there is some evidence that the risk does not rise significantly above that of the general population unless more than one first-degree relative has had colorectal cancer (22) or unless the family member has had cancer before age 60 (18). Based on these observations, individuals with one or more first-degree relatives with colon cancer should begin screening at age 40 or 10 years earlier than the onset of cancer in the youngest affected relative (18).

Screening Tests

Because of the high incidence of colon cancer and its precursor, the colon polyp, population screening has been recommended in all patients older than 50 years of age. Patients at high risk should be screened at an earlier age (Table 46.3). A number of large, randomized trials showed that annual or biennial fecal occult blood testing decreases the 8- to 15-year cumulative mortality from colorectal cancer by 16% to 33%, compared with no screening (23–26). Hemoccult cards are convenient for the patient because they can be mailed to the practitioner's office without a significant loss in sensitivity. For asymptomatic patients, it was recommended that such screenings be combined with a yearly rectal examination and with flexible sigmoidoscopy every 5 years (27). A retrospective case-control study of patients 45 years of age and older who had been monitored for 17 years revealed that screening sigmoidoscopy reduced deaths from colon cancer by almost 60% (3).

However, because of the insensitivity of the test for fecal occult blood (see earlier discussion) and because flexible sigmoidoscopy is limited to the descending colon, a substantial number of cancers may be missed (34% of men in a VA cooperative study [28]). In women, 65% of advanced neoplasms (polyps >1 cm and cancers) would have been missed by flexible sigmoidoscopy alone (29). It is reasonable, therefore, to consider whether colonoscopy at age 50 years, repeated (if normal) every 10 years, might not be the best screening test for colon cancer (30).

Computerized tomographic scanning with oral contrast can visualize the bowel as well as the intra-abdominal organs. Computed tomography (CT) colonography has been advocated as a method of population screening for colorectal cancer. A meta-analysis of 33 studies including

TABLE 46.3 Colon Cancer Screening

Risk Category	Recommendation
Average risk	Begin at age 50 yr with annual fecal occult blood testing *plus one of the following:* Flexible sigmoidoscopy every 5 yr, *or* Flexible sigmoidoscopy + double-contrast barium enema every 5–10 yr *or,* Colonoscopy every 10 yr (arguably the best screening method).
Second- or third-degree relative with colorectal cancer	Same as for average risk.
First-degree relative with colon cancer or adenomatous polyps diagnosed before age 60 yr	Same as for average risk but begin at age 40 yr.
Two or more first-degree relatives with colon cancer, or one first-degree relative with colon cancer or adenomatous polyps diagnosed before age 60 yr	Colonoscopy every 5 yr beginning at age 40 yr or 10 yr younger than the earliest diagnosis in family.
Hereditary Nonpolyposis Colon Cancer (HNPCC), defined as three relatives with colon cancer, two of them being first-degree relatives of the third, at least two generations affected, and one with colon cancer diagnosed before age 50 yr	Colonoscopy every 1–2 yr, beginning at age 20–25 yr or 10 yr younger than the earliest colon cancer diagnosis in the family, whichever comes first.
Familial adenomatous polyposis	Flexible sigmoidoscopy annually, beginning at age 10–12 yr

Modified from: Burt RW (2000) and Byers et al. (1997). See www.hopkinsbayview.org/PAMreferences.

6393 patients showed the sensitivity for detection of polyps >9 mm was 85% (95% confidence interval, 79% to 91%) and 70% (95% confidence intervals, 55% to 84%) for polyps 6 to 9 mm in size (31). While this technique shows promise for the future, there are still technical problems that limit its widespread use today.

Diagnosis

History

The chromosomal changes that accompany the progression of normal colonic mucosa to adenoma and then to carcinoma have been elucidated (32) and may provide a means to detect people who are at increased risk for development of colorectal cancer so that surveillance can be focused on them. Currently, most patients with adenocarcinoma of the colon are diagnosed only after symptoms have developed. Fewer than one-third are asymptomatic at the time of diagnosis (33), yet it is in this group that the highest chance for cure exists. The major presenting symptoms (33,34) are abdominal pain (25% to 75%) and a change in bowel habits (20% to 50%), either constipation or diarrhea. Abdominal pain is least common among patients with cancer of the rectum, where even large lesions can be accommodated without producing symptoms. Gross blood in the stool is another common complaint, occurring in 75% of patients with rectal cancer and 30% to 40% of patients with colon cancer above the rectum. This hematochezia, however, is often mistakenly attributed to hemorrhoids. Presentation with anemia or with weight loss is also common.

Physical Examination

The findings on physical examination vary according to the location and extent of the lesion. The primary tumor may be palpable as an abdominal mass, particularly in cancer of the right colon, where lesions can remain asymptomatic for long periods. Metastatic disease may be suggested by the presence of a large, hard, nodular liver; ascites; or peripheral adenopathy or by the palpation of a mass in the cul-de-sac on rectal examination. Signs of anemia may be present, particularly in lesions of the cecum and ascending colon, which can bleed covertly for months or even years before the diagnosis is made. Most patients have a positive test result for occult blood sometime during their course of illness.

Radiographic Studies

The diagnosis of colon cancer is sometimes made by barium enema or by CT scanning. Findings may include a polypoid mass, stenosis (either as a stricture or with an "apple-core" appearance), distortion of the mucosa, and localized rigidity of the bowel wall. At times, distortion or fixation of adjacent structures may be seen. The accuracy of the barium enema for the diagnosis of colon cancer is excellent, except at opposite ends of the large bowel. The cecum is often difficult to evaluate because of the inability to cleanse the region completely or to distinguish a prominent ileocecal valve or sphincter from a mass. The rectum is also difficult to visualize optimally, because often it is obscured by the balloon through which the barium is administered. Proctoscopy or flexible sigmoidoscopy is recommended in addition to a barium enema for patients with suspected colorectal carcinoma (7).

Endoscopy

Endoscopy plays a major role in the diagnosis of colorectal cancer. Some polypoid lesions, even if large or sessile, can be removed via the colonoscope, avoiding surgery in many cases. Additionally, colonoscopy has an important role in the identification of other colonic lesions. The prevalence of coexistent polyps in patients with colon cancer is high, ranging from 10% to 30%. These residual polyps may develop into carcinomas, accounting for the incidence (5% to 10%) of a second colon cancer in patients with cancer of the colon over 25 years (16). Additionally, synchronous colon carcinomas occur in 3% to 5% of patients. Therefore, colonoscopy is helpful in ensuring that the rest of the colon is free of neoplastic lesions. Unless emergent surgery is required for obstruction, colonoscopy should be performed preoperatively. In a very large survey, the sensitivity of colonoscopy for the detection of colorectal carcinoma was 95%, whereas that of barium enema was 83% (7). There is also a significant miss rate for colonoscopy: For precursor polyps, colonoscopy failed to detect 27% of lesions 0.5 cm or smaller and 6% of lesions 1 cm or larger (35).

Carcinoembryonic Antigen

Carcinoembryonic antigen (CEA) is a fetal antigen found in the blood of many patients with colorectal carcinoma (from 30% of patients with local disease to 83% of patients with metastatic disease). CEA levels may be elevated in the blood of patients with other malignancies, in cigarette smokers, and with a variety of benign conditions, including peptic ulcer, pancreatitis, diverticulitis, and inflammatory bowel disease. Therefore, the level of CEA is not a useful screening test for the presence of colorectal cancer.

Although its efficacy and cost effectiveness for this purpose have been questioned (36), the assay may be helpful in the postoperative treatment of patients who have increased blood CEA levels at the time of diagnosis. Persistently elevated CEA concentrations postoperatively suggest metastatic disease; falling levels that then rise on followup evaluation suggest reemergence of the malignancy, usually at a remote site.

Therapy

A detailed discussion of the treatment of colon cancer is beyond the scope of this chapter. Surgery is the most effective therapy for most cases of colon carcinoma. Inoperable tumors (including metastatic tumors) respond 20% to 40% of the time to 5-fluorouracil (5-FU) combined with leucovorin, preferably prescribed by or with the advice of an oncologist. However, there is no clear effect of such therapy on survival. (5-FU is usually well-tolerated but occasionally mucositis, with severe diarrhea, occurs.) Although 5-FU has been the mainstay of therapy for metastatic colon carcinoma for decades, other agents are now available including irinotecan, oxaliplatin, and two humanized monoclonal antibodies that target vascular endothelial growth factor (bevacizumab) and the epidermal growth factor receptor (cetuximab). These drugs are generally administered in combination, usually with 5-FU. Operable tumors at an advanced stage (stage III or IV; Table 46.4) should be treated with adjuvant systemic chemotherapy. Administration of 5-FU with leucovorin postoperatively decreases recurrence and improves survival (37). The addition of levamisole does not seem to add any benefit. Capecitabine is an oral fluoropyrimidine carbamate preferentially converted to 5-FU in tumor cells. The role of oral chemotherapy agents, in particular capecitabine, is still being defined. It is not yet clear whether patients with stage II colon cancer benefit from adjuvant therapy (38).

TABLE 46.4 Colon Carcinoma

Cancer Stage	TNM Staging	5-Year Survival
Stage 0	Tis N0 M0	—
Stage I	T1-2 N0 M0	93.2%
Stage IIA	T3 N0 M0	84.7%
Stage IIB	T4 N0 M0	72.2%
Stage IIIA	T1-2 N1 M0	83.4%
Stage IIIB	T3-4 N1 M0	64.1%
Stage IIIC	Any T N2 M0	44.3%
Stage IV	Any T Any N M1	8.1%

Tis, carcinoma in situ; T1, tumor invades submucosa; T2, invades muscularis propria; T3, invades into subserosa or local tissues; T4, directly invades other organs and/or perforates visceral peritoneum; N0, no nodal metastases; N1, metastasis in 1 to 3 regional nodes; N2, metastasis in 4 or more regional nodes; M0, no distant metastasis; M1 distant metastasis.
Modified from O'Connell JB, Maggard MA, Ko CY. Colon cancer survival rates with the new American Joint Committee on Cancer. 6th ed. J Natl Cancer Inst 2004;96:1420.

Patients with rectal cancer should be evaluated by an oncologist prior to surgery to determine the need for preoperative adjuvant radiation and/or chemotherapy. Preoperative chemoradiotherapy has been shown to reduce local recurrence rates and complications compared with postoperative chemoradiotherapy in patients with clinical stage T3 or T4 or node-positive (i.e., locally advanced) rectal cancer (39).

Preoperative Evaluation

Before surgery, most patients should undergo evaluation for metastases. Liver function tests and computed tomography (CT) or an ultrasound of the liver should be performed routinely. In patients with bowel obstruction or bleeding, surgery may still be needed as palliation, despite the presence of liver metastases. In patients who are asymptomatic from their bowel lesions, the presence of multiple hepatic metastases should deter surgical intervention, although single hepatic metastases are often resectable. Abnormal liver function tests alone should not be considered absolute evidence of metastatic disease, nor should normal test results be considered to exclude hepatic metastases. A histologic diagnosis should be made, if possible. Needle liver biopsy, guided by ultrasound or CT, is a simple way to obtain tissue. A preoperative CEA concentration should also be determined as a baseline.

For patients requiring an ostomy, preoperative evaluation by an enterostomal therapist is helpful, not only to discuss with the patient problems and concerns about the ostomy, but also to mark the proper location of the ostomy preoperatively.

Prognosis

The prognosis of colorectal carcinoma is based on several variables. The major variable is the extent of the tumor, in terms of its invasion through the bowel wall and its lymph node involvement (Table 46.4). Vessel invasion and the degree of differentiation of the tumor histologically also affect survival.

Followup Care

Patients may develop diarrhea early in the course after partial colectomy, but it is usually transient and easily controlled with antidiarrheal medication. The patient with a colostomy needs continued followup care by the surgeon and the enterostomal therapist to ensure proper functioning and handling of the ostomy.

The goals of long-term followup are detection of recurrence or spread of the cancer and surveillance for new colonic lesions. Most commonly, metastases occur in adjacent nodes, with eventual spread to the liver. Physical examinations, liver enzymes, and CEA determinations usually are done at prescribed intervals for 3 to 5 years. Abdominal CT scans are done to assess a confirmed rise in CEA levels or liver enzymes, but whether long-term outcome is improved is unclear, despite earlier detection of recurrent tumor.

Colonoscopy should be performed within the first 6 to 12 months postoperatively, if it has not already been done preoperatively to determine the presence of synchronous lesions. If no lesions are found, colonoscopy should be repeated 3 years later. The interval may then be increased to once every 5 years if no recurrence or adenomatous polyps are detected. Yearly evaluation for occult fecal blood loss should also be performed, with three Hemoccult cards. If any of these are positive, colonoscopy should be repeated.

Arteriovenous Malformations of the Colon

Arteriovenous malformations of the colon are a common source of GI bleeding (40,41), most often in the elderly and in patients with chronic renal failure. A variety of terms have been used to describe these abnormalities, including *angiodysplasia, hemangioma,* and *vascular ectasia.* The etiology of the disorder is unknown. Although the lesions may occur throughout the GI tract, they appear most commonly in the mucosa of the cecum and ascending colon, where multiple lesions are often found, ranging in size from 1 mm to more than 1 cm. An association of angiodysplasia of the colon with aortic stenosis has been observed repeatedly (40).

The prevalence of angiodysplasias and the frequency with which they cause bleeding are uncertain. With increasing use of endoscopy and selective angiography, the disorder is being recognized more often. In one study of patients older than 60 years of age without a history of GI bleeding, submucosal vascular ectasia was detected in 53% and mucosal lesions in 27% (40). Angiodysplasias may be the most common cause of bleeding from the right colon. Together with diverticula, they are the most common causes of major lower intestinal bleeding in the elderly (41).

When these lesions bleed, they often produce hematochezia. The bleeding is sometimes brisk and may be massive, but occult blood loss may also occur and seems to be a common presentation of this disorder (42). Bleeding often stops spontaneously, but it commonly recurs. The lesions cannot be detected by barium enema, are not recognizable from the serosal surface by the surgeon, and are often overlooked by the pathologist. The diagnosis is best made by colonoscopy or selective arteriography (by which a malformation can be visualized even when the bleeding has stopped). However, as with diverticula, the mere presence of angiodysplasias does not incriminate them as the source of bleeding, and other potential sources should be sought. Endoscopic therapy with a heater probe, injection sclerotherapy, argon plasma coagulation, or laser ablation of discrete mucosal lesions can be performed by an experienced endoscopist. Lesions that are resistant to endoscopic therapy and continue to bleed should be treated by surgical resection of the involved segment of colon. However, angiodysplasias may be present diffusely throughout the intestinal tract and therefore not amenable to endoscopic or surgical therapy. Intra-arterial vasopressin or embolization at angiography may be helpful for actively bleeding lesions of the small and/or large bowel. Medical therapy with a combination of mestranol, 0.05 mg, and norethindrone, 1 mg, may be helpful in preventing rebleeding and decreasing transfusion requirements in patients with diffuse intestinal angiodysplasias (43). Combination therapy is associated with significant adverse effects in both men (gynecomastia, testicular atrophy) and women (vaginal bleeding), and bleeding may recur once the therapy is stopped. Nonetheless, medical therapy may be extremely helpful in selected patients.

Clinicians should be aware of this disorder, especially in elderly patients with GI bleeding in whom the initial evaluation is unrevealing, but the diagnosis is made only after consultation with a gastroenterologist or radiologist.

DIVERTICULAR DISEASE OF THE COLON

Definitions

The terminology for conditions subsumed under the phrase *diverticular disease* is widely misunderstood. The phrase refers to a variety of clinical states that may differ in etiology and prognosis. Table 46.5 lists the nomenclature of diverticular disease of the colon. As can be seen from this classification, *diverticulosis* is simply the presence of

TABLE 46.5 Nomenclature of Diverticular Disease of the Colon

Diverticulosis (presence of multiple diverticula)
Asymptomatic
Symptomatic (pain, altered bowel habits)
Complicated by hemorrhage
Diverticulitis (necrotizing inflammation in one or more diverticula)
With microperforation (local inflammation)
With macroperforation, manifested by abscess, fistula, peritonitis, obstruction, or hemorrhage
Prediverticular state: muscular thickening and shortening of colonic wall without recognizable diverticula

colonic diverticula, without presuming that there are accompanying signs and symptoms. *Symptomatic diverticular disease* is diverticulosis associated with pain or altered bowel habits in the absence of evidence of diverticular inflammation. *Diverticulitis* is inflammation of one or more diverticula, generally implying perforation of a diverticulum, and is almost always symptomatic.

Epidemiology and Pathogenesis

The prevalence of diverticular disease in Western countries increases with age. Approximately 20% of men and women older than 40 years of age, 50% of those older than 60 years, and as many as 66% over age 85 have diverticulosis of the colon (44). Vegetarians have a much lower prevalence of diverticular disease than nonvegetarians. In a prospective study of almost 48,000 men, a low-fiber diet increased the risk of diverticular disease by two- to threefold over a 4-year period (45). This evidence led to the hypothesis that a low-fiber diet increases intraluminal pressure and that the increased pressure leads to herniation of the mucosa through weakened or porous parts of the colonic muscle. In support of this hypothesis is the demonstration in some individuals with diverticula of higher resting pressures in the colon and of exaggerated contractile activity in response to meals and cholinergic stimulation (46). Therefore, both a low-fiber diet and disordered colonic motility have been implicated in the pathogenesis of diverticulosis.

Weakness in the colonic wall through which the mucosa herniates to form the diverticulum is hypothesized to play a role in the pathogenesis of diverticulosis. Herniation occurs at the site of least resistance, most often at points of penetration of intramural vessels through the circular muscle layer. The association of colonic diverticula with scleroderma and with Marfan and Ehlers–Danlos syndromes suggests that loss of muscle mass or defects in collagen may be important factors. Changes in collagen synthesis occur with aging and may explain the increased prevalence of diverticula in elderly people. Therefore, the formation of diverticula may also involve a degenerative process of the colonic muscle with a change in tensile strength of the wall of the colon.

Asymptomatic Diverticulosis

A substantial majority of patients with diverticulosis are entirely asymptomatic. The diverticula may be localized to the sigmoid colon or may involve the entire colon diffusely. The sigmoid colon is almost always involved (95% of the time), and sigmoid diverticula account for 75% of all colonic diverticula (44). It is believed that this predilection is explained by the narrow caliber of the sigmoid colon, which results in higher intraluminal pressures and hence a greater risk of herniation. By contrast, rectal diverticula rarely occur. Diverticula are more common in the ascending colon in Asians, but the reasons for this observation are unclear (47,48).

The natural history of diverticulosis is variable. A majority of patients remain asymptomatic or have symptoms that are not severe enough to cause them to seek medical attention. Symptomatic diverticular disease manifests either as painful diverticular disease (75%) or as diverticulitis or hemorrhage (25%) (49). In a minority of cases, however, typical symptoms precede anatomic disease (the "prediverticular" state).

Although a diet high in fiber may be beneficial in preventing the development of diverticula, there is little evidence that therapy for asymptomatic diverticulosis is of any value in preventing or even delaying the occurrence of symptomatic diverticular disease or of such complications as diverticulitis or hemorrhage. Maintenance of regular bowel habits without the use of laxatives is probably the best advice for patients who are asymptomatic. It is also prudent to alert patients to the manifestations of symptomatic diverticular disease and to urge them to seek medical care promptly should such symptoms develop.

Painful Diverticular Disease

Diagnosis

Diverticular disease may at times become symptomatic. When the predominant symptoms are abdominal pain and an alteration in bowel habits, the cause is usually painful diverticular disease. The hallmark of this disease is abdominal pain without evidence of an inflammatory process. The pain may be colicky or steady, is generally in the left lower quadrant, and is usually made worse by meals (presumably because of gastrocolic reflex) and at least partially relieved by having a bowel movement or by passing flatus. Bowel movements, usually during the painful episodes, often become irregular, with development of constipation, diarrhea, or both in an alternating fashion. Constipation is more common than the other alterations in bowel habits. These attacks are usually episodic rather than continuous. Symptoms may also include nausea, heartburn, and flatulence.

Physical examination may reveal tenderness, at times significant, in the left lower quadrant of the abdomen. A tender sigmoid loop, which feels like a sausage, may be palpable. The stool should be negative for occult blood, but rectal bleeding may be found because of coincidental rectal outlet disorders such as fissures or hemorrhoids. The presence of fever, leukocytosis, or peritoneal signs points toward the more serious diagnosis of diverticulitis.

Colonoscopy or *barium enema* (see Chapter 45) is important both for diagnosing diverticulosis and for excluding other reasons for the symptoms. Spasm may be a feature of diverticular disease, but fistulas or a mass suggests diverticulitis, carcinoma, or Crohn disease. Particularly in elderly patients, in whom the prevalence of diverticulosis is high, it is important not to assume that the patient's symptoms have been explained once diverticula are found; carcinoma, for example, may be the real cause.

Therapy

The therapy for symptomatic diverticular disease is based on the assumption that a low-fiber diet and increased colonic pressure are important pathogenetic factors. Diets high in fiber (Chapter 45, Table 45.2) are prescribed and have been shown to be effective in improving bowel transit and relieving symptoms (50). Commercial preparations of hydrophilic colloids made from vegetable fiber are available and convenient, but they are more expensive than dietary sources (Chapter 45, Table 45.3). Patients should be instructed about high-fiber diets and, if necessary, should be given fiber supplements at a dosage of 4 to 10 g (1 tablespoon one to three times a day in a glass of water or juice). Artificial fiber products in tablet form are also available.

In addition to dietary maneuvers, anticholinergic drugs or antispasmodic drugs may be helpful for the relief of abdominal pain. Although these agents are not of proven value for this condition, some patients do respond. Dicyclomine (Bentyl), at a dosage of 10 to 20 mg before meals and at bedtime, or hyoscyamine (e.g., Levsin, also available in sustained-release and sublingual formulations) 0.125 to 0.375 mg every 4 hours as needed may be helpful. Other, more potent anticholinergics may produce adverse side effects and may aggravate the constipation.

The patient should be told that the course of the disease is unpredictable and that attacks will probably be experienced at irregular intervals (months to years) for the rest of his or her life. There is no benefit in continuing to take medication for the condition between attacks, but maintaining a high-fiber diet is prudent.

Diverticulitis

Diverticulitis results from perforation of one or more diverticula, usually in the sigmoid colon. Perforation may result from persistently high colonic pressures, from obstruction by a fecalith, and/or from an inflammatory process that weakens the wall of the diverticulum. It is important to note that the colonic mucosa is not inflamed in diverticulitis, since the inflammation is within the diverticulum or outside the wall of the bowel. Hinchey and colleagues described four stages of diverticulitis (51). In stage I, the perforation is small and confined to the pericolonic tissue. In stage II, the collection is larger, but in stage III, there is generalized purulent peritonitis. Stage IV is reserved for generalized fecal soilage and peritonitis. Stages III and IV are sometimes referred to as "perforated diverticulitis" (52). Diverticulitis increases in incidence with age and with duration of the underlying diverticulosis, and it is more common in patients who have many diverticula. Fistulas may form to the bladder (colovesical fistula is most common), vagina (especially after hysterectomy), small bowel, or skin (53).

Diverticulitis is the most common complication of diverticulosis. The long-term risk for development of diverticulitis among patients with diverticulosis is 10% to 25% (44), but it is probably much lower in patients with asymptomatic diverticulosis.

Diagnosis

The cardinal symptoms of acute diverticulitis are abdominal pain and fever. In classic cases, the pain is severe, abrupt in onset, and persistent, worsening with time and localizing to the left lower quadrant. The pain is often accompanied by anorexia, nausea, and vomiting. Altered bowel habits, both diarrhea and constipation, are common. Urinary tract symptoms and purulent vaginal discharge may occur because of fistula formation or because of inflammation of contiguous structures.

Abdominal tenderness and fever are found on physical examination. Localized peritonitis may be indicated by marked direct and rebound tenderness over the involved area, usually most pronounced in the left lower quadrant. The abdomen may become distended and tympanitic to percussion and the bowel sounds diminished. A mass may be felt at the site of inflammation in the left lower quadrant or on pelvic or rectal examination. Occult rectal bleeding occurs in approximately 25% of patients.

Leukocytosis is almost always present. Pyuria and/or hematuria may be found when there is involvement of the bladder or ureter.

The presentation of acute diverticulitis may be muted in the elderly patient. A high degree of suspicion is required in this population, because there may be no fever, no leukocytosis, and minimal abdominal pain.

The *differential diagnosis* includes painful diverticular disease, carcinoma of the colon, and inflammatory or ischemic bowel disease. The presence of peritonitis, fever, and leukocytosis rules out simple symptomatic diverticular disease. The other conditions are distinguished from diverticulitis by their clinical course and by endoscopy.

The *diagnosis* of acute diverticulitis is made largely on clinical grounds, but some tests may be useful in confirming the clinical impression. Plain abdominal films are useful initially to detect free air caused by perforation, a surgical emergency. Abdominal CT can be very helpful in visualizing diverticular abscesses and other signs of inflammation in the pericolonic tissues, and has largely supplanted other radiographic and endoscopic modalities in the clinical diagnosis of diverticulitis (54). The role of endoscopy is very limited in acute diverticulitis, since there is seldom enough mucosal inflammation to confirm the diagnosis and the risk of perforation is significantly increased. Weeks later, after successful medical therapy, it is safe to perform colonoscopy to exclude other conditions, such as carcinoma or Crohn disease.

Therapy

Most patients with diverticulitis should be hospitalized, placed on bowel and bed rest, and given analgesics, intravenous hydration, and antimicrobial drugs (such as fluoroquinolones and metronidazole, synthetic penicillins, or third-generation cephalosporins to treat both aerobic and anaerobic infection). Selected patients, particularly younger patients who are otherwise healthy and who have only mild tenderness and low-grade fever, may be treated on an ambulatory basis with oral broad-spectrum antibiotics (e.g., ciprofloxacin 500 mg twice daily plus metronidazole, 500 mg every 6 hours for 2 weeks).

Although more than 75% of patients respond to conservative medical management, surgical consultation should be obtained early in the hospital course to facilitate operative intervention if necessary. The patient's condition usually improves markedly in 3 to 10 days if medical therapy is successful. For patients who respond to conservative management, a recurrence rate of 20% to 25%, mostly in the first 5 years, can be expected (55).

Failure to resolve the acute inflammatory process, recurrent attacks of diverticulitis, and obstructive stricture formation are indications for surgical intervention. It seems reasonable that patients be placed on a high-fiber diet after recovery from an acute episode of diverticulitis.

Diverticular Bleeding

Diverticular disease is the most common cause of gross lower GI bleeding in adults, followed closely by bleeding from angiodysplasia (56). Both diverticulosis and angiodysplasia are common in the older population, and both are commonly found in the proximal colon. Diverticular bleeds, in contrast to diverticulitis, occur in the right colon in two thirds of cases (even though diverticula are much more common in the left colon) (57). The average age of patients with diverticular bleeding is approximately 70 years (58). Bleeding is the presenting manifestation of diverticular disease in approximately 16% of patients (59,60). The exact cause of diverticular bleeding is uncertain. Diverticulitis is rarely, if ever, associated with gross bleeding. There is no evidence that dietary therapy reduces the risk of hemorrhage. Most instances of bleeding occur in patients who are otherwise asymptomatic.

Massive hemorrhage is a common mode of presentation for diverticular bleeding, although in other cases the bleeding may be occult. Massive lower GI bleeding in a patient known to have diverticula is not necessarily diverticular in origin. In 30% of cases, colonoscopy detects a second lesion (e.g., cancer or angiodysplasia) (57). Occult bleeding also should be ascribed to diverticulosis only after other causes have been excluded by a thorough evaluation (see above).

Patients with diverticular hemorrhage require hospitalization for hemodynamic stabilization, diagnosis, and therapy. Approximately 70% of patients stop bleeding spontaneously. Colonoscopy can be performed after purging with polyethylene glycol (PEG) solutions. If the site of bleeding can be identified, intervention with bipolar electrocoagulation, injection of epinephrine or placement of hemoclips can be used to control the bleeding. In the subset of patients who continue to bleed, angiography is the initial procedure of choice, if the bleeding is very brisk. During angiography, transcatheter embolization (with autologous blood clot, Gelfoam, or another agent) can be attempted and is sometimes effective in patients who are poor surgical candidates. Angiography usually does not identify a site of bleeding when the bleeding is slow and intermittent, and in such patients a radionuclide bleeding scan, and a colonoscopy after a standard bowel preparation, should be considered. Emergency surgery is indicated when the bleeding is persistent. It involves a segmental colectomy when the bleeding site has been identified but colonoscopic interventions have failed, or subtotal colectomy with ileorectal anastomosis when the bleeding site in the colon has not been identified. The recurrence rate after the first episode of diverticular bleeding is 20% to 25%; it is approximately 50% after the second episode and increases with each subsequent episode of bleeding (61). Patients with two or more episodes of significant diverticular bleeding should be considered for elective surgical resection (62).

SPECIFIC REFERENCES*

1. American College of Physicians. Suggested technique for fecal occult blood testing and interpretation in colorectal cancer screening. Ann Intern Med 1997;126:808.
2. Mandel JS, Bond JH, Church TR, et al. Reducing mortality from colorectal cancer by screening for fecal occult blood. Minnesota Colon Cancer Screening Study. New Engl J Med 1993;328:1365.
3. Selby J-V, Friedman GD, Quesenberry CP Jr, et al. A case-control study of screening sigmoidoscopy and mortality from colorectal cancer. N Engl J Med 1992;326: 653.

*Bold numerals denote published controlled clinical trials, meta-analyses, or consensus-based recommendations.

4. Irvine EJ, O'Connor J, Frost RA, et al. Prospective comparison of double contrast barium enema plus flexible sigmoidoscopy v. colonoscopy in rectal bleeding. Gut 1988; 29:1188.
5. Waye JD, Bashkoff E. Total colonoscopy: is it always possible? Gastrointest Endosc 1991; 37:152.
6. Kavic SM, Basson MD. Complications of endoscopy. Am J Surg 2001;181:319.
7. Rex DK, Rahmani EY, Haseman JH, et al. Relative sensitivity of colonoscopy and barium enema for detection of colorectal cancer in clinical practice. Gastroenterology 1997;112:17.
8. Foutch PG, Sawyer R, Sanowski RA. Push-enteroscopy for diagnosis of patients with gastrointestinal bleeding of obscure origin. Gastrointest Endosc 1990;36:337.
9. Zaman A, Katon RM. Push enteroscopy for obscure gastrointestinal bleeding yields a high incidence of proximal lesions within reach of a standard endoscope. Gastrointest Endosc 1998;47:372.
10. Dusold R.Burke K, Carpentier W, Dyck WP. The accuracy of technetium-99m-labeled red cell scintigraphy in localizing gastrointestinal bleeding. Am J Gastroenterol 1994;98:345.
11. Zuckerman DA, Bocchini TP, Birnbaum EH. Massive hemorrhage in the lower gastrointestinal tract in adults: diagnostic imaging and intervention. AJR Am J Roentgenol 1993;161:703.
12. Keuchel M and Hagenmuller F. Small bowel endoscopy. Endoscopy 2005;37:122.
13. Swain P. Wireless capsule endoscopy and Crohn's disease. Gut 2005;54:323.
14. Winawer SJ, Zauber AG, Ho WN, et al. Prevention of colorectal cancer by colonoscopic polypectomy. New Engl J Med 1993;329:1977.
15. O'Brien MJ, Winawer SJ, Zauber AG, et al. The National Polyp Study: patient and polyp characteristics associated with high-grade dysplasia in colorectal adenomas. Gastroenterology 1990;98:371.
16. Muto T, Bussey HJ, Morson BC. The evolution of cancer of the colon and rectum. Cancer 1975; 36:2251.
17. Bond JH. Polyp guideline: diagnosis, treatment, and surveillance for patients with colorectal polyps. Practice Parameters Committee of the American College of Gastroenterology. Am J Gastroenterol 2000;95:3053.
18. Winawer S, Fletcher R, Rex D, et al. Colorectal cancer screening and surveillance: clinical guidelines and rationale—update based on new evidence. Gastroenterology 2003;124:544.
19. Steinbach G, Lynch PM, Phillips RK, et al. The effect of celecoxib, a cyclooxygenase-2-inhibitor, in familial adenomatous polyposis. N Engl J Med 2000;342:1946.
20. Schreibman IR, Baker M, Amos C, et al. The hamartomatous polyposis syndromes: a clinical and molecular review. Am J Gastroenterol 2005;100:476.
21. Devesa SS, Chow WH. Variation in colorectal cancer incidence in the United States by subsite of origin. Cancer 1993;71:3819.
22. Grossman S, Milos ML. Colonoscopic screening of persons with suspected risk factors for colon cancer. I: family history. Gastroenterology 1988; 94:395.
23. Hardcastle JD, Chamberlain JO, Robinson MH, et al. Randomized controlled trial of fecal occult-blood screening for colorectal cancer. Lancet 1996;348:1472.
24. Kewenter J, Brevinge H, Engaras B, et al. Results of screening, rescreening, and follow-up in a prospective, randomized study for detection of colorectal cancer by fecal occult blood testing: results for 68,308 subjects. Scand J Gastroenterol 1994;29:468.
25. Kronborg O, Fenger C, Olsen J, et al. Randomized study of screening for colorectal cancer with faecal-occult-blood test. Lancet 1996;348:1467.
26. Mandel JS, Bond JH, Church TR, et al. Reducing mortality from colorectal cancer by screening for fecal occult blood. N Engl J Med 1993;328:1365.
27. Rex DK, Johnson DA, Lieberman DA, et al. Colorectal cancer prevention 2000: recommendations of the American College of Gastroenterology. Am J Gastroenterol 2000;95:868.
28. Lieberman DA, Weiss DG, for the Veterans Affairs Cooperative Study Group. One-time screening for colorectal cancer with combined fecal occult-blood testing and examination of the distal colon. N Engl J Med 2001;345:555.
29. Schoenfeld P, Cash B, Flood A, et al. Colonoscopic screening of average risk women for colorectal neoplasia. New Engl J Med 2005;352:2061.
30. Detsky AS. Screening for colon cancer: can we afford colonoscopy? [Editorial]. N Engl J Med 2001;345:607.
31. Mulhall BP, Veerappan GR andJackson JL. Meta-analysis: computed tomographic colonography. Ann Int Med 2005;142:635.
32. Kinzler KW, Nilber TMC, Vogelstein B, et al. Identification of a gene located at chromosome 5q21 that is mutated in colorectal cancers. Science 1991;251:1366.
33. Speights VO, Johnson MW, Stoltenberg PH, et al. Colorectal cancer: current trends in initial clinical manifestations. South Med J 1991; 84:575.
34. Steinberg SM, Barkin JS, Kaplan RS, et al. Prognostic indicators of colon tumors: the Gastrointestinal Tumor Study Group experience. Cancer 1986;57:1866.
35. Rex DK, Cutler CS, Lemmel GT, et al. Colonoscopic miss rates of adenomas determined by back-to-back colonoscopies. Gastroenterology 1997;112:24.
36. Moertel CG, Fleming TR, Macdonald JS, et al. An evaluation of the CEA test for monitoring patients with resected colon cancer. JAMA 1993;270:943.
37. Macdonald JS, Astrow AB. Adjuvant therapy of colon cancer. Semin Oncol 2001;28:30.
38. Buyse M, Piedbois P. Should Dukes' B patients receive adjuvant therapy? A statistical perspective. Semin Oncol 2001;28:20.
39. Sauer R, Becker H, Hohenberger W, et al. Preoperative versus postoperative chemoradiotherapy for rectal cancer. New Engl J Med 2004;351:1731.
40. Boley SJ, Sammartano R, Adams A, et al. Nature and etiology of vascular ectasias of the colon. Gastroenterology 1977;72:650.
41. Cheung PS, Wong SK, Boey J, et al. Frank rectal bleeding: a prospective study of causes in patients over the age of 40. Postgrad Med J 1988; 64:364.
42. Coppell MS, Gupta A. Changing epidemiology of GI angiodysplasia with increasing recognition of clinically milder cases. Am J Gastroenterol 1992; 87:201.
43. Barkin JS, Ross BS. Medical therapy for chronic gastrointestinal bleeding of obscure origin. Am J Gastroenterol 1998;93:1250.
44. Parks TG. Natural history of diverticular disease of the colon. Clin Gastroenterol 1975;4:53.
45. Aldoori WH, Giovannucci EL, Rimm EB, et al. A prospective study of diet and the risk of symptomatic diverticular disease in men. Am J Clin Nutr 1994;60:757.
46. Locke GR III. The epidemiology of functional gastrointestinal disorders in North America. Gastroenterol Clin North Am 1996;25:1.
47. Sugihara K, Muto T, Morioka Y, et al. Diverticular disease of the colon in Japan: a review of 615 cases. Dis Colon Rectum 1984; 27:531.
48. Mimura T. Pathophysiology of diverticular disease. Best Practice Res Clin Gastroenterol 2002;16:563.
49. Hughes LE. Postmortem survey of diverticular disease of the colon: I. Diverticulosis and diverticulitis. Gut 1969;10:336.
50. Hyland JM, Taylor I. Does a high fibre diet prevent the complications of diverticular disease? Br J Surg 1980;67:77.
51. Hinchey EJ, Schaal PGH, Richards GK. Treatment of perforated diverticular disease of the colon. Adv Surg 1978;12:85.
52. Ferzoco LB, Raptopoulos V and Silen W. Acute diverticulitis. New Engl J Med 2005;338:1521.
53. Woods RJ, Lavery IC, Fazio VW, et al. Internal fistulas in diver-ticular disease. Dis Colon Rectum 1988;31:591.
54. Welch CE. Computerized tomography scans for all patients with diverticulitis. Am J Surg 1988;155:366.
55. Larson DM, Masters SS, Spiro HM. Medical and surgical therapy in diverticular disease: a comparative study. Gastroenterology 1976; 71:734.
56. Levien DH, Mazier WP, Surrell JA, et al. Safe resection for diver-ticular disease of the colon. Dis Colon Rectum 1989;32:30.
57. Tedesco F, Waye J, Raskin J, et al. Colonoscopic evaluation of rectal bleeding: a study of 304 patients. Ann Intern Med 1978;89:907.
58. Deckmann RC, Cheskin LJ. Diverticular disease in the elderly. J Am Geriatr Soc 1993;40:986.
59. McGuire HH, Haynes BW. Massive hemorrhage from divertic-ulosis of the colon: guidelines for therapy based on bleeding patterns observed in fifty cases. Ann Surg 1972;175:847.
60. Ramanath HK, Hinshaw JR. Management and mismanagement of bleeding colonic diverticula. Arch Surg 1971;103:311.
61. McGuire HH Jr. Bleeding colonic diverticula: a reappraisal of natural history and management. Ann Surg 1994;220:653.
62. The Standards Task Force, American Society of Colon and Rectal Surgeons. Practice parameters for sigmoid diverticulitis. Dis Colon Rectum 2000;43:289.

For annotated ***General References*** *and resources related to this chapter, visit www.hopkinsbayview.org/PAMreferences.*

Chapter 47

Diseases of the Liver

Esteban Mezey

HEPATITIS

Hepatitis is an inflammatory condition that may be localized in the liver or may be part of a generalized systemic process. Acute hepatitis is usually a self-limited disease. The principal causes of acute hepatitis are viruses, drugs, and alcohol. Chronic hepatitis is unresolved hepatitis that has persisted for longer than 6 months. Cirrhosis is often the principal consequence of chronic hepatitis.

Acute Hepatitis

Viral Hepatitis

Viral hepatitis is a systemic infection whose principal manifestations are hepatic. The four types of viral hepatitis that are well-defined, separate entities are designated type A, B, C, and E. Delta hepatitis (hepatitis D virus [HDV]) is infection by a defective virus-like particle that is dependent on persisting or concomitant infection with type B virus.

Table 47.1 shows the characteristic features of types A, B, C, and E hepatitis. Type A hepatitis, previously known as infectious hepatitis, is more common than the other types. It is usually transmitted by the fecal-oral route and has a particularly high incidence wherever people come in close contact under poor hygienic conditions. A number of epidemics have been described after fecal contamination of the water or food supply. Ingestion of contaminated shellfish has been associated with both sporadic cases and epidemics.

Type B hepatitis, previously called serum hepatitis, is usually transmitted by the parenteral route from blood, blood products, or contaminated needles. It is also commonly transmitted by sexual contact and from the mother to the fetus. HDV is transmitted by the same routes as type B hepatitis (1). Its incubation period ranges from 3 to 13 weeks. Infection with the δ agent may become manifest as a biphasic pattern of hepatitis when there is simultaneous infection with hepatitis B virus (HBV), or as a clinical exacerbation of hepatitis in patients who are carriers of HBC with or without chronic liver disease. HDV has been implicated in cases of fulminant hepatitis and in worsening of chronic liver disease with more rapid progression to cirrhosis. However, the incidence of HDV is unknown.

Hepatitis C virus (HCV) accounts for most cases of hepatitis acquired by blood transfusion, although it is now more commonly transmitted by other routes. In the West, 4% of cases of HCV are acquired by blood transfusion, 38% by parenteral use of illicit drugs, 10% by sexual or household exposure to people who have had hepatitis or multiple partners, 2% by occupational exposure to infected blood, and 1% by dialysis (2). The principal sources of HCV infection in health care workers are accidental needle sticks; the risk of becoming infected with HCV by needle stick from a patient already infected with HCV is approximately 3%. Skin tattoos are also a risk factor. Ear piercing in men and intranasal cocaine use have been found to be more common in blood donors infected with HCV than in noninfected donors (3). The source of infection in approximately 45% of cases is unknown; a large proportion of these patients are in a low socioeconomic level.

Hepatitis E virus (HEV) is a common cause of hepatitis epidemics in developing countries, but it can also occur sporadically in developed countries. The virus is transmitted by the fecal-oral route, usually by ingestion of contaminated water. It is associated with a high mortality rate in pregnant women (4).

Hepatitis G virus (HGV) is a single-stranded ribonucleic acid (RNA) virus that has a genomic sequence similar to HCV. It is present in 1.8% of healthy blood donors and often is found in the blood of patients with HCV infection. In a few cases HGV is the only virus identified in patients with hepatitis, and in most of these cases the hepatitis is mild. However, definitive proof is lacking to implicate HGV as a causative agent of hepatitis.

Clinical Presentation

The symptoms of the various types of hepatitis are similar. However, in contrast to the other types of viral hepatitis, acute viral HCV is usually a mild illness that is very likely to persist and develop into chronic hepatitis. Most cases of hepatitis are anicteric; patients have a few nonspecific symptoms, such as fatigue and nausea, and the disease is often misdiagnosed as a flu-like illness. The correct diagnosis, if suspected, is made by demonstrating bilirubin in

TABLE 47.1 Comparison of Selected Characteristics of Various Types of Viral Hepatitis

Characteristic	Type A	Type B	Type C	Type E
Hepatitis A IgM antibody	Appearance	Absent	Absent	Absent
Hepatitis B surface antigen (HBsAg)	Absent	Present in early stage of illness	Absent	Absent
Hepatitis C antibody (Anti-HCV)	Absent	Absent	Appears 5–15 wk after infection	Absent
Incubation period	15–50 d	50–160 d	15–160 d	20–50 d
Route of infection	Oral and parenteral	Usually parenteral, also oral or sexual	Usually parenteral, also oral or sexual	Oral, usually from contaminated water
Age preference	Children	Any age	Any age	15–40 yr
Seasonal incidence	Autumn–winter, epidemic outbreaks	All year	All year	Epidemic outbreaks
Severity	Usually mild	Often severe	Often mild	Mild, severe in pregnancy
Mortality	0.1%	0.1%–1.0%	0.1%	0.5% (20% in pregnancy)
Prophylactic value of gammaglobulin	Good	Good with hyperimmune hepatitis B globulin	Unclear	Unclear
Hepatitis vaccine	90%–100% efficacy	90% efficacy		

the urine and an increase in the level of serum aminotransferases. In icteric disease, the symptoms that usually precede jaundice are anorexia, fatigue, abdominal discomfort, and nausea. Erythematous skin rashes, urticaria, arthralgias, and low-grade fever may also appear. These initial symptoms are followed within 10 days by the appearance of dark urine, often pruritus, and jaundice. It is at this stage that most patients seek medical attention. On physical examination, a tender, palpable liver is found in approximately 70% of the patients. Posterior cervical lymphadenopathy and splenomegaly may also be present. Jaundice usually increases in intensity during the first few days and then begins to decrease, disappearing completely by 2 to 8 weeks after onset.

Laboratory Features

A mild degree of transient anemia, granulocytopenia, lymphocytosis with the appearance of atypical lymphocytes, and mild hemolytic anemia, with an increase in the reticulocyte count, are commonly found in patients with acute viral hepatitis. Both the direct (conjugated) and the total fraction of serum bilirubin rise; the height reached by the total bilirubin is an indication of the severity of the disease. However, total serum bilirubin concentrations higher than 30 mg/dL are almost invariably caused by complicating hemolysis. The serum aminotransferases usually rise before the onset of detectable jaundice, may reach levels as high as several thousand units, and may remain elevated for several weeks. The height reached by the aminotransferases in the serum provides only a rough estimate of the degree of hepatocellular injury and is of no prognostic value. However, a rapid fall in aminotransferases from a high peak to normal in less than 1 week may be an indication of fulminant hepatitis with massive necrosis and collapse of liver parenchyma. The serum alkaline phosphatase usually rises in the early, cholestatic phase of hepatitis, remains elevated throughout the illness, and is often the last serum enzyme to return to normal levels after clinical recovery. The concentration of serum albumin is normal in acute hepatitis. Serum gammaglobulins often are transiently elevated. The prothrombin time is usually normal and, if prolonged, is usually responsive to the administration of vitamin K, typically 10 to 15 mg given by subcutaneous injection. Prolongation of the prothrombin time with no response to vitamin K administration suggests severe hepatitis; if the prolongation increases, it is indicative of fulminant hepatitis.

Imaging Studies

Imaging of the liver by either ultrasonography or computed tomography (CT) scanning is not useful in the diagnosis or management of acute viral hepatitis. However, ultrasonography is useful to confirm a decrease in liver size in hospitalized patients with severe necrosis and fulminant hepatitis in whom the liver cannot be palpated.

Virologic Features

Hepatitis A is caused by an RNA virus. In acute type A hepatitis, fecal excretion of hepatitis A antigen (HAAg) can be demonstrated a few days before the increase in serum aminotransferases, rises to a peak during maximal serum aminotransferase elevation, and then falls as jaundice appears. Anti hepatitis A (anti-HA, predominantly immunoglobulin M [IgM]), appears in the serum at approximately the same time as HAAg disappears from the stool. Anti-HA then rises rapidly to high levels and gradually becomes undetectable over 10 to 12 months. Anti-HA IgG remains detectable for at least 10 years, indicative of immunity against reinfection. Because HA infection is very common, many healthy people have detectable anti-HA in the serum. The prevalence of positive anti-HA is approximately 30% to 40% in the United States and as high as 90% in certain areas of Latin America and Asia (5). Hence, identification of an acute episode of hepatitis as type A requires a high titer of anti-HA of the IgM class or the appearance of or a rise in anti-HA titer in the serum collected during the convalescent stage compared with the acute stage of hepatitis.

The HBV by electron microscopy appears as a double-shelled, 42-nm spherical particle, originally called the Dane particle. The outer shell of this particle is hepatitis B surface antigen (HBsAg), and the inner core contains an antigen that has been designated the hepatitis B core antigen (HBcAg). The inner core also contains double-stranded deoxyribonucleic acid (DNA) and DNA polymerase activity. In acute type B viral hepatitis, HBsAg first appears in the blood 1 to 2 weeks before and usually disappears by 2 to 3 months after the onset of clinical symptoms (Fig. 47.1). Hepatitis B core antibody (anti-HBc) appears in the serum at the onset of clinical symptoms, reaches a peak soon after the maximal level of serum aminotransferase is reached, and then falls gradually, becoming undetectable 1 to 2 years after the infection. Antibody to the hepatitis B surface antigen (anti-HBs) usually appears during the convalescence, when HBsAg is no longer detectable, and then persists for many years. The presence of HBsAg or IgM anti-HBc during the acute illness is evidence that the hepatitis is caused by the HBV (6). Persistence of HBsAg in the serum beyond 3 months after the infection suggests that the patient has become a chronic carrier of the HBV (7). The presence of high titers of anti-HBc but absent anti-HBs is usually found in association with HBsAg in the carrier state. The presence of anti-HBs indicates that the patient has had a prior infection with type B hepatitis and now is immune to reinfection. Another antigen, the so-called e antigen, is detectable in some HBsAg-positive sera. The hepatits B e antigen (HBeAg), although associated only with type B hepatitis, is immunologically distinct from HBsAg and HBcAg. HBeAg appears transiently in the serum during the early phase of acute type B hepatitis. In chronic carriers of HBsAg, the presence of HBeAg is a marker of active virus replication and correlates with infectivity of the carrier (8) and, some studies suggest, correlates also with the risk of progression of acute HBV to chronic hepatitis or cirrhosis. Appearance of anti-HBe (and disappearance of HBeAg) usually indicates remission of the disease. However, some patients develop chronic anti-HBeAg hepatitis (without detectable HBeAg) because of a HBV precore or core mutation that abolishes the production of HBeAg (9). Hepatitis B DNA detection (HBV DNA) is used to detect the HBV and to obtain information on viral load.

HDV is a defective virus-like particle that is composed of a small RNA genome surrounded by hepatitis D antigen (HDAg) and a coat of HBsAg. Acute HDV infection (1) is associated with a brief rise in HDAg that lasts approximately

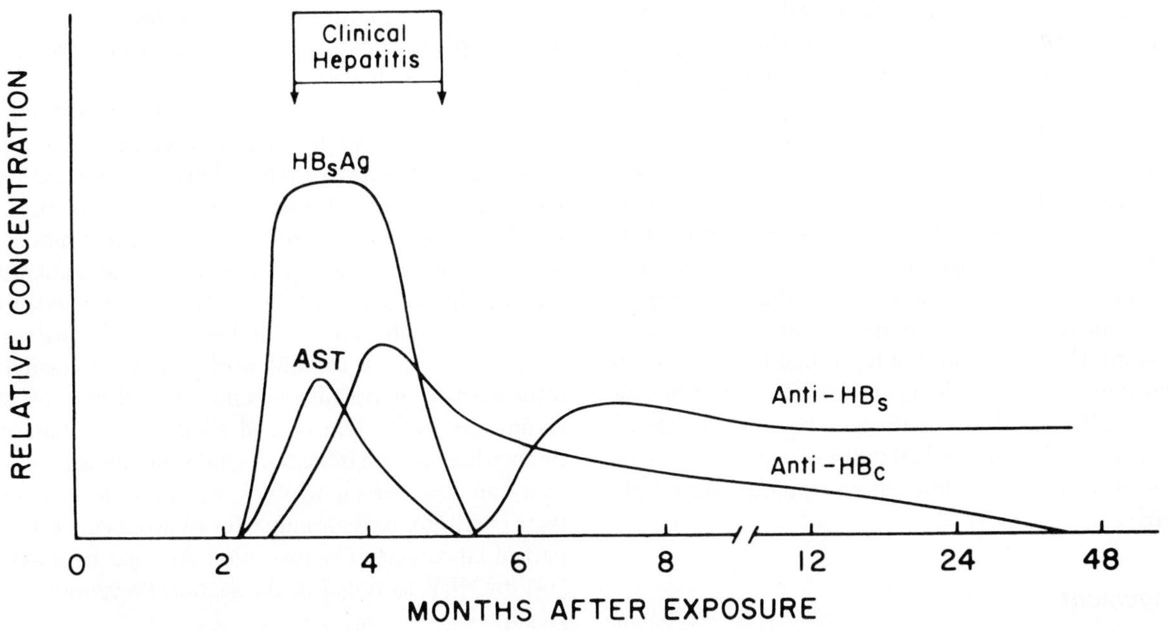

FIGURE 47.1. Pattern of appearance of hepatitis B surface antigen (HbsAg) and antibodies to hepatitis B surface antigen (anti-HBs) and to hepatitis B core antigen (anti-HBc) in acute hepatitis B infection. AST, aspartate aminotransferase. (From Mezey, E. Specific liver diseases. In: Halsted JH, Halsted CH, eds. The laboratory in clinical medicine. 2nd ed. Philadelphia: WB Saunders, 1981.)

10 days and is followed by the appearance of hepatitis D virus antibody (anti-HDV). Initially the antibody is of IgM type, lasting 10 to 20 days; this is followed by the appearance of IgG anti-HD. A characteristic of HDV infection is a lowering of HBsAg titers; probably HDV requires HBV for its replication.

HCV is caused by a single-stranded RNA virus. There are at least six major genotypes of the HCV, which have different geographic distributions and influences on the clinical course of the disease and its response to therapy (10). Hepatitis C virus RNA (HCV RNA) is detectable within 10 days after infection and persists during the development of acute and chronic hepatitis. Anti-HC becomes detectable 5 to 15 weeks after infection. In most cases, it persists in the blood regardless of the outcome of the disease (11).

HEV is also caused by a single-stranded RNA virus. Acute HEV infection is associated with rises of IgM and IgG anti-HEV antibodies. IgM anti-HEV is found in more than 90% of patients 1 week to 2 months after the onset of the illness. IgG anti-HEV appears after the IgM antibody response, and its titer rises after the acute illness, remaining detectable for 1 to 4.5 years. HEV infection in the serum and stool can be detected by reverse transcriptase-polymerase chain reaction (RT-PCR) measurement of HEV RNA (4).

At present, the practical usefulness of the immunologic markers for hepatitis is as follows. Acute HAV infection is confirmed by the demonstration of anti-HA of the IgM class (IgM anti-HAV). Infection with HBV is usually confirmed by the presence of HBsAg, but if the antigen is absent and it is clinically indicated, the diagnosis can be confirmed by demonstrating IgM anti-HBc. The determination of anti-HBs is useful to find out whether a person is immune to HBV or whether that person is a candidate for prophylaxis (see Prevention and Prophylaxis of Viral Hepatitis). HBV DNA is useful in monitoring the virologic response of chronic HBV to treatment. Acute HCV infection is diagnosed by the detection of HCV RNA, whereas chronic HCV is diagnosed by detection of HCV RNA or by anti-HC 6 months or longer after the onset of illness. The false-positive detection of anti-HC is less than 10% and occurs principally in chronic autoimmune hepatitis (see later discussion). HDV, as a cause of fulminant hepatitis or recurrent type B hepatitis, is diagnosed by the presence of HDAg or IgM anti-HD. Hepatitis E is diagnosed by showing initially the presence of IgM anti-HEV in the serum, or later in the course of the infection the appearance of IgG anti-HEV.

Management

Acute viral hepatitis usually resolves completely in 1 to 3 months. There is no specific therapy. Rest often alleviates the symptoms, but there is no evidence that it changes the overall course of the illness (12). As the patient's symptoms improve, a gradual increase in activity is allowed as tolerated by the patient. Intake of a normal-calorie, normal-protein (50 to 70 g protein per day) diet should be encouraged, although it is often difficult for the patient to eat because of nausea and anorexia. However, these symptoms are usually minimal in the morning, so the patient should be encouraged to eat a large breakfast. Strict isolation of the patient to his or her own room and bathroom is often impractical and probably unnecessary. General hygienic measures, such as washing the hands after contact with the patient and careful handling of stool and blood samples, are mandatory (see Prevention and Prophylaxis of Viral Hepatitis).

Hospitalization is indicated for patients in whom the diagnosis is uncertain and for those who have severe symptoms of nausea and vomiting, changes in mental status, or a prothrombin time that is prolonged more than 4 seconds above the control value. Patients with very high levels of serum bilirubin (greater than 30 mg/dL), who most likely have severe hemolysis complicating their hepatitis, should be hospitalized. By contrast, the magnitude of elevation of serum aminotransferase by itself, is not an indication for hospitalization. In addition, it is advisable to admit to the hospital patients who do not have somebody at home who can observe and help them.

Nausea can be controlled with oral diphenhydramine, 25 mg three times a day, or by prochlorperazine, 10 mg two to four times a day, without danger of central nervous system depression. Acetaminophen, 500 mg four times a day, can be safely given for abdominal discomfort (the risk of hepatotoxicity occurs at much higher dosages). No sedatives should be given, because they may precipitate hepatic encephalopathy. Corticosteroids are of no value in the treatment of acute viral hepatitis.

Patients should be monitored at intervals varying from 1 to 3 weeks and should not be discharged from ambulatory care until all symptoms have disappeared and all laboratory tests have returned to normal. Patients are advised not to ingest alcoholic beverages until 1 month after all laboratory tests have returned to normal. Patients who develop chronic hepatitis should avoid alcohol indefinitely.

Patients with acute viral hepatitis who are asymptomatic can return to light work despite abnormal liver tests such as hyperbilirubinemia and elevations of the serum aminotransferases and alkaline phosphatase. Patients whose serum bilirubin is high enough to cause jaundice can also return to work but may need a note of their condition to their employer to avoid concern on the part of coworkers. The exception are food handlers with HAV or HEV, as noted in the section Prevention of Viral Hepatitis.

In patients with HBV, HBsAg should be measured after 6 months. If HBsAg is still detectable at that time, a hepatologist should be consulted for further management. In patients with HCV, chronicity is defined as elevations of serum aminotransferases that persist for longer than 6 months. It is not necessary to continue to measure HCV RNA, except to monitor virologic response to therapy (see later discussion).

Liver Biopsy

A liver biopsy is indicated only if the diagnosis is uncertain or the clinical course of the disease is prolonged beyond 6 months. A specialist in liver disease should be consulted to evaluate the patient and to perform the liver biopsy.

In patients who do not require hospitalization for another reason, liver biopsies are performed as outpatient procedures in a hospital. The patient should have a history of normal hemostasis, a prothrombin time less than 4 seconds above control, and a platelet count greater than 80,000 per cubic millimeter. A liver biopsy is contraindicated if there is an infiltrate in the right lower lung or a right-sided pleural effusion, absent hepatic dullness to percussion, suspected liver hemangioma or abscess, massive ascites, extrahepatic obstruction, severe anemia (hemoglobin less than 10 g/dL), or significantly impaired hemostasis (see above).

Patient Experience. After application of local anesthesia, the liver biopsy is performed by the intercostal right subcutaneous route using suction with a needle 1.6 mm in diameter. It entails minimal risk when done by a skilled operator. The most common complication is pleuritic pain lasting a few hours after the biopsy, which is noted in approximately 5% of the cases. The most serious complications are bleeding and bile peritonitis, which occur in fewer than 1% of cases. The risk of mortality from liver biopsy is 0.2%. After the procedure, patients are observed for approximately 4 hours and then, if no complications have occurred, are sent home accompanied by a friend or relative.

Prognosis

Most patients with acute HAV, HBV, or HEV recover from their illness without any sequelae. The mortality rate from all types of hepatitis is less than 0.1%. The principal cause of death is the development of fulminant hepatitis, which is more common in type B hepatitis. Fulminant hepatitis usually overcomes the patient within 10 days after the onset of the symptoms of hepatitis. Older patients and patients with other medical illnesses, such as diabetes mellitus, are more likely to have a prolonged course and a higher mortality rate. Type E hepatitis, transmitted by the fecal-oral route, results in a high mortality rate in pregnant women. Indications of a poor prognosis are changes in mental status, a nonpalpable liver that is also small on hepatic imaging, a liver that decreases rapidly in size, or a prothrombin time (PT) that is prolonged more than 4 seconds above normal.

Chronic hepatitis occurs in approximately 85% of untreated patients with HCV, and 15% to 20% of those patients eventually develop cirrhosis. Chronic hepatitis occurs in 3% to 5% of patients with type B hepatitis, of whom 6% to 20% develop cirrhosis within 5 years. Chronic hepatitis and cirrhosis do not occur after type A or type E hepatitis. These complications should be suspected in patients with HBV or HCV who continue to have clinical and laboratory evidence of liver disease 6 months after the onset of acute hepatitis (13). Most patients clear the HBsAg from their serum within 3 months of the onset of the illness. Approximately 10% of patients with type B hepatitis become chronic carriers of HBsAg. Chronic carriers of HBsAg with abnormal levels of serum aminotransferases should be evaluated for the development of chronic active hepatitis by liver biopsy. An increased incidence of hepatocellular carcinoma has been found in carriers of HBsAg or HCV RNA.

Differential Diagnosis

A number of other viruses have been reported to cause hepatitis. *Cytomegalovirus (CMV),* usually clinically inapparent in adults, can present with manifestations of hepatitis in patients being administered immunosuppressive therapy, in those who have diseases characterized by immunosuppression (see Chapter 39), or after blood transfusions in healthy subjects. The diagnosis is made by the demonstration of IgM CMV antibody and by examination of biopsy specimens for intranuclear inclusions and detection of the virus in tissue with specific antibodies. *Mononucleosis* (caused by the Epstein-Barr virus, [EBV]) is often associated with hepatocellular dysfunction with mild transient jaundice in 5% to 10% of patients. It is diagnosed by the presence in the serum of a heterophil antibody that is not absorbed by guinea pig kidney or by a positive mononucleosis spot test. Demonstration of IgM EBV antibodies specific for EBV confirms the diagnosis (see Chapter 58).

Hepatitis caused by *leptospirosis* should be suspected in patients who have been in close contact with rodents or with food, water, soil, or other material contaminated with the urine of rodents; the diagnosis is established by recovery of *Leptospira* in culture of the blood or by a rise in antibodies in the course of the disease. *Drug-induced hepatitis* (see later discussion) manifests with clinical features that are indistinguishable from those of viral hepatitis, and a history of drug intake is a most important clue in suspecting the diagnosis. *Alcoholic hepatitis* (discussed later) usually develops after recent heavy alcohol ingestion; the serum aminotransferases are rarely elevated more than 10 times above normal, and the elevation is primarily in the serum aspartate aminotransferase (AST). In patients with marked cholestasis—as evidenced by persistent elevation of the bilirubin, high serum alkaline phosphatase, and pruritus in association with persistently dark urine and light stools—the diagnosis of *extrahepatic biliary obstruction* should be entertained. An abnormal sonogram may provide a clue to extrahepatic obstruction if the biliary ducts are found to be dilated, and the patient should then be referred to a specialist in liver diseases for further evaluation.

Prevention and Prophylaxis of Viral Hepatitis

General hygienic measures, such as washing the hands after contact with the patient, are the most effective means of preventing the spread of hepatitis from the patient to others. In cases of HAV and HEV, which are principally acquired by the oral route, the patient's dishes and eating utensils can be shared by other people only if they have been cleaned and heated to more than 120°F (48.8°C) for 15 to 20 minutes in a dishwasher after the patient has used them. Assignment of the patient to a separate bathroom is ideal but often impractical. The viruses can be present in feces, blood, and other body fluids of the patient; any of these materials should be handled with care. Because the virus appears in the stool during the prodromal period of hepatitis, the precautions mentioned should be taken routinely in environments where there is a high risk of development of hepatitis, such as in institutions for the mentally retarded.

The screening of blood for HBsAg and anti-hepatitis C before transfusion has markedly decreased the risk of posttransfusion infection by HBV and HCV to 1 in 63,000 and 1 in 100,000 units transfused, respectively (14). Other sources of type B and type C hepatitis that can easily be controlled are contaminated needles, pins used to test sensation, and dental and surgical instruments. All used needles or pins should be discarded in specially labeled bottles containing 40% formalin, which is known to inactivate the hepatitis viruses. The preferred method for cleaning surgical and dental instruments is by heat sterilization. The risk that most health care workers who are HBsAg-positive pose to their patients is minimal if high standards of hygiene are maintained. The exceptions are dentists and surgeons (15), who often develop cuts on their hands while operating. Dentists are urged to wear gloves regardless of whether they are HBsAg-positive, to protect themselves and their patients. Patients who have had HBV or HCV and have apparently recovered (clinically and serologically) may still be infectious for many years and therefore should not be allowed to donate blood. Spouses of patients with HBV should receive HBV vaccine. Unvaccinated sexual partners of patients who have recovered from HBV may be at risk. Sexual partners of patients with chronic HCV who are in monogamous relationships have virtually no risk of infection (0% to 0.6%). Therefore, those in long-term monogamous relationships need not change their sexual practices (16). Food handlers with HAV infection should not return to their work with food until 4 months after the onset of symptoms, because HAV can be detected in the stool for that long.

Standard *immune serum globulin* (ISG) is known to prevent the clinical manifestations of HAV in 80% to 90% of persons when administered within 2 weeks after exposure. However, it does not prevent subclinical infection. The recommended dosage of standard ISG is 0.02 mg/kg, given by intramuscular injection. Hepatitis A vaccine is indicated for close personal contacts of patients with known HAV, inmates of institutions during an epidemic of HAV, and travelers to areas where hepatitis is endemic. It is not indicated for casual acquaintances or coworkers of the patient or for people who are known to have anti-HA antibody in their serum. To obtain immediate and long-term protection in people recently exposed to HAV, the vaccine is combined with the administration of ISG. The HAV vaccine results in the development of protective anti-HA antibody 2 weeks after its administration, a protection that lasts approximately 6 months, at which time a booster dose is given to extend the protection for up to 10 years. The vaccination (Havrix or Vaqta) is given as an injection of 0.5 mL to children and adolescents aged 2 to 17 years and as a 1-mL injection to adults (17).

The role of standard ISG in the prevention of type B hepatitis is uncertain. *Hepatitis B immune globulin* (containing a high titer of anti-HBs) prevents approximately 75% of cases of type B hepatitis (if given immediately after exposure) in people who have been stuck with needles contaminated by HBsAg-positive patients, in sexual partners of HBsAg-positive patients, in newborns of HBsAg-positive mothers, and in staff personnel of dialysis units (18). It is not indicated for casual or work contacts of patients with type B hepatitis or for patients who have been demonstrated to have anti-HBs. Testing for anti-HBs should be done routinely before administration of HBV immune globulin, provided that the results of the tests can be obtained within 1 week after exposure to the virus.

Chapter 18 contains details regarding indications, dosages, and schedules for primary prevention of HBV with *hepatitis B vaccine,* postexposure prophylaxis for adults and newborn infants exposed to people who have active HBV or are known HBsAg carriers, and postexposure prophylaxis for adults exposed to people whose HBsAg status is unknown.

There have been insufficient studies to know whether the incidence of posttransfusion HCV or HEV is decreased by the administration of standard ISG. No vaccines are currently available for the prevention of HCV or HEV.

Drug-Induced Hepatitis

The liver is the principal organ concerned with drug metabolism; hence, it is not surprising that it is also a principal target for drug toxicity. Every drug has the potential for producing hepatocellular damage. Drug-induced hepatitis results from either direct hepatotoxicity or from an idiosyncratic reaction (host hypersensitivity). *Hepatotoxic reactions* caused by direct toxins such as carbon tetrachloride and inorganic phosphorus are dose dependent and reproducible with a brief interval after exposure to the drug. *Idiosyncratic reactions* are the more common response to drugs. Characteristically, they are not dose dependent, occur in only a small number of people who are exposed, and are preceded by a sensitizing period of 1 to 4 weeks of exposure or a history of exposure. Drug reactions may be cholestatic, may simulate viral hepatitis, or may combine features of both processes.

Cholestatic Reactions

Cholestasis is caused by a direct dose-related effect of the administration of anabolic steroids and oral contraceptives. Cholestasis occurs in 1% to 2% of patients receiving anabolic steroids but less often after the ingestion of oral contraceptive drugs. Jaundice and pruritus are prominent symptoms. The elevated serum bilirubin is composed principally of the direct conjugated fraction. Serum alkaline phosphatase and cholesterol are elevated, whereas serum aminotransferases are normal or only slightly elevated. Cholestasis disappears soon after withdrawal of the offending drug.

A much larger number of drugs cause cholestasis through *hypersensitivity.* Examples are phenothiazine derivatives such as chlorpromazine, antibiotics such as erythromycin, antithyroid drugs such as propylthiouracil and methimazole, hypoglycemic agents such as tolbutamide and chlorpropamide, immunosuppressant drugs such as azathioprine, and alkylating agents such as chlorambucil. Common clinical features of these drug reactions are fever, right upper quadrant abdominal pain, pruritus, skin rash, and eosinophilia. Serum aminotransferases are moderately elevated (less than 10 times normal). The clinical and laboratory abnormalities usually subside between 2 and 4 weeks after discontinuation of the drug, although on occasion cholestasis persists for months to years. Severe pruritus is treated with cholestyramine (Questran) given in a dosage of 4 g three times a day before meals. Relief of pruritus is obtained in 4 to 7 days after starting this medication. Patients with cholestasis should be hospitalized whenever the jaundice persists unchanged or increases 2 to 4 weeks after discontinuation of the drug, to investigate the possibility of other causes of cholestasis (see Chapter 96).

Hepatocellular Reactions

Most agents that produce direct hepatocellular damage are toxins rather than drugs. Acetaminophen, however, is a drug that produces hepatic necrosis in all people if ingested in a large dose (greater than 10 g), usually in a suicide attempt. Alcoholics and patients taking drugs such as phenobarbital, which are inducers of microsomal enzymes, are at risk for development of hepatic necrosis after the ingestion of lower doses of acetaminophen. Shortly after ingestion the patient develops nausea and vomiting, but evidence of hepatocellular damage often does not become apparent until 48 hours later, when serum aminotransferases rise and the prothrombin time becomes prolonged. The patient's condition then deteriorates; jaundice appears and central nervous system depression may occur. The mortality rate of patients who took an overdose of acetaminophen was found to be 3.5% in one large study (19). Therefore, patients who are known or suspected to have ingested toxic amounts of acetaminophen should be hospitalized for support and treatment (ordinarily with *N*-acetylcysteine).

There has been a marked increase in the use of *herbal medications* in the Western world in recent years (20). Some of these products, the ingredients of which are often poorly defined, are hepatotoxic. A history of taking herbal medicines should be sought in any patient with unexplained liver disease.

Idiosyncratic hepatocellular reactions have been reported after the administration of a number of drugs, the most common of which are isoniazid, α-methyldopa, nitrofurantoin, ketoconazole, sulfonamides, terbinafine (Lamisil), β-hydroxy-beta-methylglutaryl-coenzyme A (HMG-CoA) reductase inhibitors (statins), troglitazone, phenylbutazone, and halothane. Asymptomatic increases in serum aminotransferases, which subside despite continued administration of the drug, have been reported in 5% to 10% of patients taking isoniazid or α-methyldopa. Because of the often transient nature of the serum aminotransferase elevations, there is no need to monitor these tests in asymptomatic patients. However, the development of symptoms of fatigue and anorexia or of nausea and general malaise is an indication for the determination of serum aminotransferase concentrations; if aminotransferase activity is increased, the drug should be discontinued immediately, because this often heralds the onset of severe hepatocellular damage. In some cases rifampin, an occasional cause of hepatotoxicity itself, potentiates the hepatotoxic effects of isoniazid. The incidence of acute hepatitis in patients taking these latter two drugs is 0.1% to 0.3%. Women and older patients are more likely to be affected. The onset of the reaction is between 1 and 10 weeks after the start of therapy. The symptoms, laboratory tests, and findings on liver biopsy are indistinguishable from those of viral hepatitis (see earlier section Acute Hepatitis), so serologic tests to rule out viral hepatitis are often obtained. The hepatitis usually resolves within a few weeks after the drug is discontinued. However, a mortality rate as high as 12% has been reported for severe hepatitis caused by isoniazid. Moreover, chronic active liver disease can develop if the drug responsible for the hepatitis is continued.

Administration of corticosteroids is not indicated in drug-induced hepatitis of any type.

Alcoholic Hepatitis

This condition is seen most often after prolonged heavy alcohol intake. Women are more susceptible to alcoholic liver disease than men are, and it usually does not develop in men who drink less than 40 g of ethanol per day or in women who drink less than 20 g per day (equivalent to 4 and 2 ounces [120 and 60 mL] of 86 proof whiskey, 48 and 24 ounces of beer, and 400 to 200 mL of wine, respectively). Many of the presenting clinical characteristics of patients with alcoholic hepatitis (e.g., anorexia, significant fatigue, jaundice, tender hepatomegaly) are indistinguishable from those of viral hepatitis. However, patients with alcoholic hepatitis are more likely to have fever and leukocytosis. The elevation of the serum aminotransferases is rarely 10 times above normal, and often there is a prolongation of the PT. The elevation of AST is characteristically greater than that of alanine aminotransferase (ALT). Patients with alcoholic hepatitis and jaundice should be admitted to the hospital and have a definite diagnosis established by liver biopsy, if not contraindicated by abnormal hemostatic function. Liver biopsy differentiates alcoholic hepatitis from drug-induced hepatitis and viral hepatitis and gives an indication of any underlying chronic liver disease. The illness is often more severe than in patients with viral hepatitis, and decompensation with hepatic encephalopathy and death can occur. Patients with severe alcoholic hepatitis, manifested by jaundice and prolongation of the PT >4 seconds above control and/or encephalopathy, should be hospitalized and considered for treatment with either corticosteroids or pentoxifylline. Approximately one third of patients with alcoholic hepatitis have been shown to progress to cirrhosis, often within 6 months (21). However, if patients can abstain from further drinking of alcohol (see Chapter 28), approximately one-third recover completely, both clinically and histologically, usually within 1 month.

Chronic Hepatitis

Chronic hepatitis is inflammation of the liver detected by abnormal liver tests or abnormal liver histology that has persisted for longer than 6 months. The spectrum of chronic hepatitis varies from a benign, reversible process to an unrelenting process that often progresses to cirrhosis. Liver biopsy is essential both for the diagnosis and to establish the severity of the disease and the need for treatment. The liver histology is graded semiquantitatively according to the degree of necrosis and inflammation (minimal, mild, moderate, or severe activity) and staged for the amount of fibrosis and the presence of cirrhosis (22).

The principal causes of chronic hepatitis are infection with a hepatitis virus (type B or C), autoimmune disease (formerly called lupoid hepatitis), and drugs such as isoniazid, α-methyldopa, and nitrofurantoin. In addition, patients with Wilson disease, a_1-antitrypsin deficiency, or primary biliary cirrhosis may present with clinical and histologic features of chronic hepatitis.

The onset of chronic hepatitis is usually insidious. The patient may be asymptomatic, with liver disease detected by aminotransferase elevations on routine testing, or there may be symptoms of general malaise, fatigue, abdominal discomfort, anorexia, and jaundice. In approximately one third of the patients, the disease evolves from a clinically overt episode of acute hepatitis. Physical examination in patients with chronic hepatitis often reveals hepatomegaly and sometimes, when the disease is more advanced, splenomegaly, spider angiomas, palmar erythema, and gynecomastia. Elevations of serum aminotransferases may be the only laboratory abnormality, but elevations of bilirubin and globulins are also common. Decreases in serum albumin and prolongation of the PT reflect loss of hepatocellular function and a poor prognosis. Older male patients are more likely to have HBsAg in the serum and to present with an acute onset of illness. Patients with chronic hepatitis caused by HCV may have arthralgias, vasculitis, palpable purpura, and peripheral neuropathy caused by type II cryoglobulinemia. Often these patients have false-negative test results for hepatitis C antibody (anti-HCV) and undetectable HCV RNA because these factors are concentrated in the cryoprecipitates (23).

Patients with *autoimmune hepatitis* are more likely to be women and to present with acne, amenorrhea, arthralgia and arthritis, pleurisy, or intermittent fever (24). Additionally, they may have associated thyroiditis, Sjögren syndrome, ulcerative colitis, glomerulonephritis, or hemolytic anemia. Laboratory tests on these patients show evidence of immunologic hyperactivity: serum γ-globulin is often markedly elevated, and there is elevation in the titers of antinuclear antibodies and smooth muscle antibodies. A small subgroup of patients with chronic autoimmune hepatitis have normal titers of antinuclear antibodies but elevated liver–kidney microsomal (anti-LKM) antibodies. Additionally, antimitochondrial antibodies are found in 15% of these patients.

The diagnosis of *Wilson disease* (which affects approximately 1 in 1 million people) should be considered in all patients, particularly those younger than 25 years of age, who have clinical and laboratory features of otherwise unexplained chronic hepatitis (25). Wilson disease is discussed in more detail in the section Cirrhosis later in this chapter. The diagnosis of chronic hepatitis caused by α_1-antitrypsin *deficiency* (which affects 1 in 1,000 people) is suggested by the finding of an absent or low alpha-1-globulin on serum protein electrophoresis (26). The diagnosis is established by demonstrating a low value of α_1-antitrypsin in the serum by quantitative measurement and by protease inhibitor (Pi) typing (26). The common allele is

PiM; liver disease occurs in approximately 20% of people who are homozygous for the allele PiZ. Liver biopsy reveals periodic acid–Schiff (PAS)–positive cytoplasmic inclusions that are resistant to diastase in both homozygous and heterozygous patients for the allele PiZ. There is no known medical therapy for this deficiency, which is transmitted by codominant inheritance. The diagnostic characteristics of *primary biliary cirrhosis* are discussed later in the section Cirrhosis. The diagnosis of *drug-induced chronic hepatitis* (see Drug-Induced Hepatitis) depends on a careful history and the demonstration of improvement of the patient after discontinuation of drugs that are known to produce this illness. In most cases, chronic active hepatitis caused by drugs reverts to normal after discontinuation of the offending drug.

The clinical course of patients with chronic active hepatitis is variable. Patients can be asymptomatic for a long time, have periods of intermittent worsening and remission, or have a progressive course to cirrhosis and death if untreated. HDV is associated with clinical exacerbation of chronic HBV and more rapid progression to cirrhosis (1).

Therapy

Autoimmune Hepatitis

Corticosteroids are beneficial for symptomatic patients with chronic autoimmune hepatitis. Clinical, biochemical, and histologic improvement and even remission have been observed, and mortality rates have been reduced after therapy with corticosteroids (24). Prednisone or prednisolone, 40 to 60 mg, is given initially to suppress the activity of the disease and then is tapered slowly, usually over 1 to 3 months, to a maintenance dosage of 10 to 20 mg. Symptomatic improvement followed by a fall in serum aminotransferases occurs during the first few weeks. Treatment with corticosteroids is decreased to the smallest dosage possible to maintain normal or minimally increased values of the serum aminotransferases. Discontinuation of the corticosteroid therapy often results in a relapse. *Azathioprine* at an initial dosage of 100 mg/day in combination with prednisone is often effective in maintaining a remission (24). Asymptomatic patients with chronic hepatitis are usually treated only if they have persistent elevations of serum aminotransferases, histologic evidence of at least a mild grade of activity, and evidence of early fibrosis. Administration of corticosteroids to patients with chronic viral hepatitis is contraindicated because it appears to favor replication of hepatitis viruses, resulting in a higher morbidity and mortality (27).

Hepatitis B

Interferon α-2b therapy is effective in eliminating evidence of viral replication (HBeAg) and in normalizing serum aminotransferases in more than one third of patients with type B hepatitis (28). Higher dosages and prolonged administration of interferon α-2b result in improvement in 15% to 25% of patients with chronic HDV (14). *Pegylated interferon α-2a* (Pegasys) in a dose of 180 μg once a week for 6 months was recently found to result in a greater drop in HBV DNA levels than conventional interferon and in HBeAg seroconversion in 37% of patients at 6 months of followup (29).

Lamivudine, a nucleoside analog, in an oral dose of 100 mg/day, results in a decrease in HBV DNA to undetectable levels in 95% of patients after 6 months of treatment, and in a normalization of ALT levels in 52% at 6 months and 70% at 1 year (30). These effects are associated with improvement in liver histology in 75% of patients. After 6 to 8 months of therapy, however, viral mutants that are resistant to the therapy begin to appear; in these cases after discontinuation of the therapy the HBV DNA and ALT return to pretreatment levels as the virus returns to the wild type. Approximately 30% of patients receiving lamivudine for 1 year who experience a loss of HBeAg remain in remission for 6 months after the therapy (31). *Adefovir,* another nucleoside analogue, in an oral dose of 10 mg/day is equally effective in decreasing HBV DNA and normalization of serum aminotransferases, and up to the present time has the advantage of a much lower development of resistant viral mutants (32).

Pegylated interferon α-2a, lamivudine, and adefovir (33) have each been shown to result in biochemical and virological improvement in HBeAg negative chronic HBV; in one comparative study, treatment for 48 weeks with pegylated interferon α-2a was superior to lamivudine in the response during treatment and in the sustained suppression of HBV DNA after 24 weeks of treatment (10). *Entecavir* is the newest nucleoside analogue that shows potent antiviral effect against HBV (34).

Hepatitis C

Pegylated interferons are more effective and have replaced conventional interferon in the treatment of chronic HCV. The two pegylated interferons presently available are *PegInterferon α-2a* (Pegasys) and *PegInterferon α-2b* (Peg Intron). These pegylated interferons are administered by subcutaneous injection once a week (180 μg of *PegInterferon α-2a* or 1.5 μg/kg body weight for *PegInterferon α-2b*) together with ribavirin in a daily oral dose of 1,000 mg (if $<$75 kg body weight) or 1,200 mg (if $>$75 kg body weight). The treatment outcomes and side effects are similar for these two types of pegylated interferons. Patients with genotypes 1 and 4 are treated for 48 weeks, while those with genotypes 2 and 3 are treated for 24 weeks. Early virologic response defined as a decrease in HCV RNA levels by 2 logs at 12 weeks of treatment occurs in approximately 86% of cases (35). The early virologic response is usually associated with a fall or normalization of the serum aminotransferases. The lack of an early virologic response usually predicts a failure to achieve a sustained viral response

(SVR) after treatment. The overall end of treatment viral response (HCV RNA undetectable) is 69%. SVR at 2 years after the end of the treatment are 42% to 46% for genotype 1 and 76% to 82% for genotypes 2 and 3 (35). Decisions about the use of interferon, lamivudine, adefovir, ribavirin, and newer agents should be made in consultation with a hepatologist.

No specific therapy exists for type E hepatitis.

UNEXPLAINED ELEVATIONS OF LIVER ENZYMES IN THE SERUM

Elevations of serum aminotransferases and alkaline phosphatase are occasionally found in normal subjects or in patients without suspected liver disease. In such a situation the abnormality should first be confirmed by repeat testing. Next, it is important to remember that elevated serum aminotransferases and alkaline phosphatase do not necessarily originate from the liver. For example, elevated serum aminotransferases can be caused by injury to the heart and striated muscle; if the source of the serum aminotransferases is muscle, the more specific creatine kinase will also be elevated. Elevation of serum γ-glutamyl transpeptidase (GGTP) is useful to confirm the hepatic origin of elevated serum aminotransferases, because, unlike the latter enzymes, it does not originate from damaged muscle. Elevation of GGPT alone, however, should not be used as an indication of liver damage, because GGPT is a microsomal enzyme and elevations may occur as a result of ingestion of drugs that are microsomal enzyme inducers, such as phenytoin (Dilantin), phenobarbital, and ethanol. An isolated increase of serum alkaline phosphatase can originate from liver or bone. The hepatic origin of alkaline phosphatase can be confirmed by demonstration of an elevated 5′-nucleotidase value; unlike alkaline phosphatase, this enzyme is present only in the liver and in the epithelium of the bile ducts. By contrast, an elevated serum alkaline phosphatase accompanied by a normal serum 5′-nucleotidase value is almost invariably caused by bone disease; a common cause of such an occurrence is Paget disease of bone. A common cause of elevations of serum aminotransferases is nonalcoholic steatohepatitis (see later discussion). Any persistent elevation of serum aminotransferases for longer than 6 months that remains unexplained is an indication for liver biopsy to rule out chronic hepatitis. A persistent elevation of serum alkaline phosphatase in the absence of an elevated serum bilirubin can occur in patients with fatty liver, which is common in diabetic and obese patients, or it can be the result of space-occupying lesions, such as granulomas or metastatic carcinoma. A CT scan with intravenous contrast of the liver, or an magnetic resonance imaging (MRI), if the patient is allergic to the contrast, is recommended in these cases to rule out primary hepatic or metastatic carcinoma. Liver biopsy is indicated if the CT scan or MRI shows a space-occupying lesion or if there is clinical suspicion of diseases such as tuberculosis or sarcoidosis that may result in hepatic granulomas.

ALCOHOLIC FATTY LIVER

Alcoholic fatty liver results from alterations of lipid metabolism caused by alcohol and therefore occurs in all persons who ingest alcohol in excessive amounts. It is manifested mainly by a feeling of abdominal fullness caused by hepatomegaly and mild elevation of the serum aminotransferases (rarely more than twice normal). On occasion, marked fatty infiltration is associated with symptoms of malaise, weakness, anorexia, tender hepatomegaly, and even jaundice. These symptomatic patients require further evaluation, occasionally including liver biopsy, to distinguish fatty liver from alcoholic hepatitis and cirrhosis. The treatment of fatty liver consists of abstinence from alcohol. With abstinence, the abnormal accumulation of fat disappears within 4 to 6 weeks. As the patient's condition improves, the liver decreases in size and becomes nontender. Serum bilirubin and aminotransferase values promptly return to normal. Recurrent episodes of symptomatic fatty liver are common after heavy alcohol ingestion, but there is no evidence that this lesion itself leads to cirrhosis.

NONALCOHOLIC STEATOHEPATITIS

Nonalcoholic steatohepatitis is a chronic disease of unknown origin characterized by fatty infiltration and hepatocellular damage with inflammation in patients who lack a history of significant alcohol ingestion (36). It is a very common cause of elevated serum aminotransferases. It is more common in women. Obesity, defined as a body mass index (the weight in kilograms divided by square of the height in meters) greater than 30, is found in at least 30% of patients, and type 2 diabetes is found in 34% to 75% of patients (36, 37). Hyperlipidemia is also common. Most of the patients are asymptomatic and liver disease is discovered by finding elevated serum aminotransferases. The principal symptoms, when present, are fatigue and right upper abdominal discomfort. Hepatomegaly is a finding in 90% of the patients, but splenomegaly is rare. The serum ALT level is usually higher than the serum AST, which helps in differentiating nonalcoholic from alcoholic steatohepatitis. The serum ferritin and transferrin saturation values are often elevated, but few of these patients are homozygous for the hemochromatosis gene. If the diagnosis is in doubt, fatty infiltration can be confirmed by ultrasonography. Liver biopsy is indicated in symptomatic patients with serum aminotransferase elevations of more than 6 months' duration. Patients with evidence of moderate to severe fibrosis on liver biopsy have at least a 5% risk of

Chapter 48

Proteinuria

Jean Wu and Edward S. Kraus

Normally, 60% of urinary protein is plasma protein that has been filtered by glomeruli and only partially reabsorbed by renal tubules. The remaining 40% is synthesized and secreted into the urine by the renal tubules and by the more distal portions of the urogenital tract. The main plasma protein is albumin, which usually makes up 20% of normal urinary protein excretion.

Proteinuria has been defined traditionally as the urinary excretion of greater than 150 mg per 24 hours. Proteinuria in that range is a common finding in the general population; the prevalence of dipstick-positive proteinuria in adults is approximately 10% (1). It is usually a transient finding without any long-term clinical sequelae. However, persistent proteinuria (see Significance of Proteinuria section) may be a marker of renal disease and merits more aggressive workup and treatment. Additionally, much interest has been focused on low levels of urinary albumin excretion (microalbuminuria), defined as the urinary albumin excretion of 30 to 300 mg/day or as it is commonly reported, 30 to 300 mg of albumin per g creatinine. Microalbuminuria has been well established as a strong predictor of the development of atherosclerotic disease as well as of progressive kidney disease. Also, regardless of the cause, patients with persistent proteinuria have an increase in overall and cardiovascular mortality compared to those without proteinuria. It is therefore important to screen for proteinuria in selected populations at high risk for kidney disease and evaluate and treat the finding of proteinuria in all populations (see Significance of Proteinuria). This chapter discusses the methods of detection of proteinuria, the significance of proteinuria, and an approach to its evaluation and management.

METHODS FOR DETECTING PROTEINURIA

Urinary Dipstick

A dipstick measures protein concentration through a colorimetric change that occurs when protein binds to a pH indicator dye, which ranges from yellow (no protein) to increasing shades of green, representing increasing protein concentration. This test is simple, inexpensive, widely available and highly specific. However, this technique is not very sensitive, as it cannot detect protein excretion of less than 30 mg/dL. Also, as the dipstick is specific for albumin, it may miss positively charged proteins like globulins or parts of globulins (e.g., heavy or light chains and Bence-Jones protein). False-positive results can occur if the urine is alkaline (pH greater than 7.5) and in the presence of leukocytes, gross hematuria, mucus, or semen.

Sulfosalicylic Acid and Limitations of Testing

Other tests are available to detect other urinary proteins. The most commonly used one is the sulfosalicylic acid (SSA) test, which detects the presence of both large and small protein molecules. In this test, a 3% to 10% solution of SSA is added to urine. The results range from "clear" to "flocculent precipitate" suggesting protein levels of 0 to greater than 500 mg/dL respectively. Since this is a turbidimetric test, false positive test results can occur if the urine is already turbid. Also, the SSA test detects proteins of prostatic and vaginal origin. These contaminants can be avoided by not palpating the prostate before collecting urine from men and by obtaining a clean voided urine specimen from women. False-positive results can occur also in the presence of a number of medications, most notably high doses of cephalosporins and penicillins. Additionally, radiocontrast agents can lead to false positive results with both dipstick and SSA testing.

Quantitation of Proteinuria

Quantitation of proteinuria is important to help define the etiology of proteinuria and to follow response to therapy. The "standard criterion" for quantitation has been the measurement of protein in a 24-hour urine collection. However, it has been shown that spot measurement of urinary protein and creatinine is an excellent approximation to the 24-hour collection and is now the preferred method for quantifying urinary protein, as it is simpler, faster, and more readily obtained.

Protein/Creatinine Ratio

There is an excellent correlation between the 24-hour urinary protein excretion and the protein/creatinine concentration ratio (mg/dL of protein divided by mg/dL of creatinine), as determined in a random sample of urine obtained during normal daytime activity (2). The accuracy of this ratio is related to the fortuitous occurrence that daily creatinine excretion is around 1 g/day. Thus, the ratio approximates daily protein excretion. For example, a ratio of 3.5 represents daily protein excretion of around 3.5 g/day and represents nephrotic-range proteinuria. A spot albumin to creatinine ratio is also the preferred method for quantifying albumin excretion.

24-Hour Urine Collection for Protein

Although the spot protein to creatinine ratio is the preferred method for quantifying proteinuria, the ratio may overestimate 24-hour urinary protein excretion in certain circumstances, most notably when urine is collected after strenuous exercise, from patients with diabetes mellitus, or from patients whose daily urinary creatinine excretion is considerably less than 1 g (e.g., frail adults). Conversely, determination of this ratio from a first morning urine specimen may underestimate daily urinary protein losses (see Orthostatic Proteinuria). The first morning urine specimen should therefore not be used for the spot urine protein to creatinine ratio and the spot urine should therefore not be collected after strenuous exercise.

A 24-hour measurement for proteinuria may be required for patients with diabetes mellitus or for frail adults. In this test, a clean container without preservatives, usually a gallon jug, is given to the patient with instructions about the collection process. The 24-hour collection is best done on a day when the patient will be using a single toilet, and it is helpful for the patient to place a note on the toilet on the day of collection, as a reminder to collect all required specimens. On the day of collection, the first voided morning specimen is discarded, and then all urine voided during the next 24 hours, including the next morning's first voided specimen, is collected in the container. Once the urine is collected, it is not critical when protein determination is done. If there is excessive delay, however, bacterial growth can falsely raise protein concentrations. Therefore, it is advisable to refrigerate the urine specimen until it is brought to the laboratory, if it is not brought in on the day the collection is completed. Simultaneous measurement of urinary creatinine and urinary volume is helpful as an index of the adequacy of collection. Most patients who are of average body mass excrete between 800 and 1,500 mg of creatinine per day (21 to 26 mg/kg/day in adult men, 16 to 22 mg/kg/day in adult women).

ASSESSMENT OF PATIENTS WITH PROTEINURIA

Mechanism of Proteinuria

The most common reason for proteinuria is glomerular dysfunction, leading to the presence of increased urinary albumin. Albuminuria (either micro or macro) is thus a potent marker of glomerular disease. However, albuminuria can also occur in states of systemic illness that may lead to changes in renal hemodynamics. In tubulointerstitial disease, tubular reabsorption of proteins is abnormal. This usually leads to the presence of proteins other than albumin in the urine, such as β_2 microglobulins. The other major cause of proteinuria is increased systemic generation of filterable proteins associated with plasma cell dyscrasias.

Approach to Patients with Proteinuria

It is important to determine if proteinuria is transient, intermittent, or persistent (see below). In an otherwise healthy person without any other signs of renal or systemic disease, a positive test for urinary protein should be repeated before pursuing additional workup as the proteinuria is likely to be an inconsequential finding. Transient proteinuria also can occur in a number of circumstances that alter renal hemodynamics such as fever, strenuous exercise, and exposure to cold. Acute illnesses like decompensated congestive heart failure and seizures, and some chronic illnesses like obstructive sleep apnea are also associated with proteinuria. If the proteinuria is a response to the acute event, it usually resolves within several days and is not associated with any other renal abnormalities and may not reflect progressive renal disease. However, testing should be repeated to ensure that persistent proteinuria is not present.

Further laboratory studies to evaluate proteinuria should include microscopic urinalysis to look for other abnormalities that may suggest renal disease. Also, serum creatinine concentration or creatinine clearance should be measured to identify whether renal function is impaired (see Chapter 52). Finally, the amount of protein excreted should be quantitated. Excretion in excess of 3.5 g per 24 hours (protein/creatinine ratio greater than 3.5) defines nephrotic proteinuria.

NONNEPHROTIC PROTEINURIA

Nonnephrotic range proteinuria can be a benign finding or be a marker of underlying renal disease. A variety of primary renal and systemic diseases including hypertensive nephrosclerosis may be associated with nonnephrotic range proteinuria. Also, most patients with nephrotic range proteinuria have had nonnephrotic range protein excretion at some time in the past. Evaluation is best defined by considering patients who have normal physical examinations and laboratory profiles (so called "isolated proteinuria") separately from patients who have other abnormalities in their urinalysis or who have hypertension, diabetes, or signs of systemic illness like rash or arthritis.

Isolated Proteinuria in Apparently Healthy Patients

If the initial evaluation is negative except for the presence of isolated proteinuria, the proteinuria may be further classified as *persistent* (25% to 30% of patients) or *intermittent* (70% to 75% of patients) (3). Making the distinction between these two entities may have some value in that the prognosis of patients with intermittent proteinuria is generally better than the prognosis of patients with persistent proteinuria. However, making this distinction in practice may be challenging because it requires the practitioner to obtain five or six specimens for semiquantitative analysis over several months. The 24-hour urine protein excretion is almost always less than 1 g in patients with isolated proteinuria. If the total protein excretion is greater than 2 g/24 hours, the chance of significant kidney disease is high, and further investigation for nonisolated proteinuria should be considered.

Intermittent Proteinuria

A study of patients with intermittent isolated proteinuria (protein in fewer than 80% of repeat urine dipstick testing) revealed definite abnormalities by light microscopy in the renal tissue of approximately 60% of patients; the remainder had normal or almost normal biopsy findings (4). However, a retrospective study evaluating the prognostic significance of proteinuria in male college students did not find an increased risk of renal disease in this group (5). Although intermittent proteinuria is generally considered to be benign, the prognosis of patients with this finding has not been extensively studied. Thus, it would be prudent to monitor patients with intermittent proteinuria with yearly measurements of urine protein excretion, a urinalysis, and determination of serum creatinine. Should deterioration in renal function, significant increase in protein excretion, or new abnormalities occur, reassessment and possibly a renal biopsy would become necessary.

Persistent Proteinuria

Patients with protein in more than 80% of urine specimens are defined as having persistent proteinuria. The disorder may be further classified by evaluating the effect of posture. *Orthostatic persistent proteinuria* is present when the patient is in the upright position only. *Constant persistent proteinuria* is not influenced by the position of the patient.

Orthostatic Proteinuria

A simple method of determining the presence of this phenomenon is to have the patient collect two urine specimens. The patient rests quietly for 2 hours and then voids just before retiring in the evening to ensure an empty bladder on assuming the recumbent posture. The patient then does not get out of bed for 8 hours. On arising, he or she voids completely into a container labeled *recumbent urine (specimen 1)*. The patient then remains upright but is not vigorously active and collects all subsequent urine over the next 8 hours. This specimen is labeled *ambulatory urine (specimen 2)*. The protein concentrations in the two urine specimens are compared. In patients with orthostatic proteinuria, the recumbent protein excretion is negligible but proteinuria is found when the patient assumes the upright posture.

A renal biopsy is not necessary in the evaluation of a patient with orthostatic proteinuria. When biopsies have been done as part of a research protocol, minor abnormalities have been defined in approximately one half of those patients with orthostatic proteinuria; the others have had a biopsy that appeared normal on light microscopy (3). However, it would be prudent to monitor the patient by measuring urinary protein excretion and serum creatinine on a yearly basis.

Patients with orthostatic proteinuria have an excellent prognosis. Military recruits with this problem have been monitored for 20 years; none developed renal failure, and in approximately 80% proteinuria resolved (6). Not all patients who were free of protein in the urine at 10-year followup remained protein-free after 20 years, but none showed significant deterioration in renal function. A 35-year followup of these same patients did suggest that some developed a decline of renal function greater than expected for normal aging (7).

Constant Isolated Proteinuria

In most patients with constant isolated proteinuria, diverse morphologic changes are identified in kidney biopsy specimens. Few long-term studies of these patients have been made, but the course is likely to be indolent. Renal failure develops very rarely, although most patients develop abnormal urine sediment and 50% develop hypertension (8). It is not necessary to perform a renal biopsy if there are no other findings, but yearly re-evaluation is appropriate and should include blood pressure measurement, urinalysis, and determination of 24-hour protein excretion and serum creatinine and creatinine clearance. If proteinuria exceeds 2 g/day, additional evaluations (such as a renal sonogram or collagen vascular screens, see Proteinuria Nephrotic section) should be pursued.

Nonisolated Proteinuria

Proteinuria associated with impaired renal function, hypertension, or other abnormalities in the urinalysis requires a more aggressive workup. Additionally, the earliest manifestation of diabetic nephropathy is microalbuminuria. Additional workup should follow that outlined for nephrotic proteinuria as discussed below.

TABLE 48.1 Causes of Nephrotic Syndrome in Adults[a]

Most common
Diabetes mellitus
Idiopathic membranous glomerulopathy
Idiopathic lipoid nephrosis (including minimal change disease, mesangial proliferative glomerulonephritis, focal segmental glomerulosclerosis)
Less common
Proliferative glomerulonephritis (crescentic glomerulonephritis)
Membranoproliferative glomerulonephritis
Collagen vascular disease
Amyloidosis

[a] An extensive list of potential causes of nephrotic syndrome can be found in Falk RJ, Jennette JC, Nachman PH. Primary glomerular disease. In: Brenner BM, ed., Brenner and Rector's The Kidney. 7th ed. Philadelphia: WB Saunders, 2004:1293.

NEPHROTIC PROTEINURIA

There are many causes of nephrotic syndrome, but few conditions are seen with significant frequency in general medical practice (Table 48.1). Clinical and laboratory assessments for systemic illness should be performed first in an effort to establish the etiology of the nephrotic syndrome (e.g., detection of Bence Jones proteinuria, collagen vascular screens for SLE). Table 48.2 lists some of the laboratory evaluations that may be helpful in determining

TABLE 48.2 Selected Investigations That May Be Appropriate in the Diagnosis of Proteinuria That Is Not Isolated or Is Nephrotic

Antineutrophil cytoplasmic antibody (ANCA) if vasculitis is suspected
Antinuclear antibody if systemic lupus erythematosus is suspected
Antistreptolysin (ASO) titer if there is a possibility of poststreptococcal glomerulonephritis
Complement (C3, C4) if glomerulonephritis is suspected
Complete blood count to provide a baseline evaluation for subsequent use and to provide a clue to a systemic illness (e.g., leukemia)
Erythrocyte sedimentation rate or C-reactive protein if collagen vascular disease is suspected
Fasting blood sugar to consider the possibility of diabetes mellitus
Hepatitis B surface antigen, hepatitis C antibodies by second- or third-generation enzyme-linked immunosorbent assay (ELISA), if hepatitis-associated vasculitis may be present
Radiologic evaluation: Ultrasound, computed tomography, magnetic resonance imaging or on occasion intravenous pyelogram or voiding cystourethrogram to provide evidence for structural renal disease
Rapid plasma reagin (RPR) with history or risk factors for sexually transmitted disease
Serum albumin if nephrotic range proteinuria is present
Serum electrolytes (Na^+, K^+, Cl^-, HCO_3^-, Ca^{2+}, PO_4^{2-}) to provide a screen for abnormalities as a consequence of renal disease
Serum and urine protein electrophoresis and immunofixation electrophoresis if multiple myeloma is suspected
Uric acid to screen for urate-related renal disease
Urine culture if pyuria is present
Radiograph of chest to provide evidence for systemic disease (e.g., sarcoidosis)

the cause of renal disease. If nephrotic-range proteinuria develops in a patient who has been diabetic for longer than 10 years, the renal lesion is almost always diabetic glomerulosclerosis, particularly if the patient also has diabetic microaneurysms in the retina. In this setting, a renal biopsy usually is unnecessary. On the other hand, a biopsy usually is necessary to diagnose a specific primary renal disease if a diagnosis cannot be made by other tests or it may be needed to guide therapy and to help determine prognosis.

Renal Biopsy

Patient Experience. Generally, in patients without renal failure and normal hemostasis, percutaneous biopsy is performed under local anesthesia with computed tomographic or sonographic guidance. This technique permits the nephrologist to sample the lower portion of the kidney, avoiding the hilar vessels and the renal collecting system. With percutaneous biopsy, the patient usually experiences minimal discomfort and is able to be out of bed in 6 to 12 hours.

The biopsy core is approximately 1 mm in diameter and 10 to 20 mm in length. Usually two such tissue cores are obtained. The risk associated with percutaneous renal biopsy is small if it is performed by an experienced physician.

Microscopic hematuria after the procedure is almost inevitable, and usually there is a small hematoma at the biopsy site on the surface of the kidney. However, it usually is of no clinical consequence. Gross hematuria occurs in 5% to 10% of patients, but less than 5% of this group require a transfusion to replace blood loss. Fewer than 1 in 1,000 patients require nephrectomy because of continued massive bleeding, and death from biopsy is rare. A renal arteriovenous fistula may develop after biopsy, but it usually closes spontaneously. Rarely, this complication may require treatment if bleeding continues or if hypertension develops (see Stiles et al., at www.hopkinsbayview.org/PAMreferences). Even more rarely, there may be perforation of another viscus.

When percutaneous biopsy is not feasible (e.g., obesity, ectopic location, small size of kidney), open transjugular or laparoscopic biopsy can be obtained; some surgeons perform this procedure under local anesthesia in selected patients (see Stiles et al., at www.hopkinsbayview.org/PAMreferences).

Regardless of the technique of obtaining the biopsy, the evaluation of tissue by a pathologist experienced in preparation and interpretation of renal biopsy material includes light, immunofluorescent, and electron microscopy.

The practitioner who has referred to a nephrologist a patient for whom a renal biopsy has been performed should expect communication of the following: the probable diagnosis based on all aspects of the microscopic assessment; whether specific therapy for the condition is indicated; and what prognostic judgment can be made.

SIGNIFICANCE OF PROTEINURIA

It has been well established that the amount or presence of proteinuria is directly correlated with adverse outcomes and with progression of kidney disease, regardless of its underlying etiology. Among diabetic patients, even microalbuminuria is associated with an increased likelihood (up to nine times greater incidence than diabetic patients without microalbuminuria) of developing diabetic nephropathy (9). A recent study also suggests that microalbuminuria may predict future development of renal disease in otherwise healthy patients (10).

Besides its association with adverse renal outcomes, the presence of microalbuminuria is also a powerful predictor of cardiovascular events. In the Framingham study population, overall and cardiovascular mortality rates in men with microalbuminuria were slightly but significantly increased (approximately threefold) compared to the rates of men even with intermittent proteinuria (11). It has also been well established that microalbuminuria is a predictor of cardiovascular risk in diabetic patients (12). The African American Study of Kidney Disease and Hypertension (AASK) trial showed that this relationship is present only in patients with hypertension and that any increase in urinary albumin, even at the current normal range, was associated with adverse cardiovascular outcomes (13). A continuous and graded relationship between urinary albumin excretion and cardiovascular risk has been demonstrated in the general population (14).

Thus, there is strong evidence that even small increases in urinary albumin excretion are associated with increased risks of developing cardiovascular and renal disease. One possible explanation for this relationship is that urinary albumin leakage is a reflection of generalized endothelial dysfunction, which may play a pathophysiological role in accelerated atherosclerosis. Reduction of albuminuria has also been associated with renal protection in both nondiabetic and diabetic renal diseases. Therefore, measuring and reducing urinary protein excretion is key to preventing progression of renal disease and reducing the high cardiovascular mortality in this population.

Currently, screening for proteinuria is not recommended for the general population. In diabetics, clinical practice recommendations (see American Diabetes Association, 2001, at www.hopkinsbayview.org/PAMreferences) recommend that patients with insulin-dependent diabetes for at least 5 years and all non–insulin-dependent diabetic patients be screened annually for the presence of microalbuminuria. The National Kidney Foundation guidelines recommend using a quantitative measurement of microalbuminuria in all patients at risk for kidney disease, particularly patients with hypertension or diabetes mellitus, although the Joint National Committee on Prevention, Detection, Evaluation, and Treatment of High Blood Pressure (JNC) 7 considers testing for proteinuria optional (see NKF/DOQI and JNC 7 guidelines, at www.hopkinsbayview.org/PAMreferences).

TREATMENT OF PATIENTS WITH PROTEINURIA

Patient care is directed at diagnosis, education, surveillance, and treatment of any underlying disease (renal biopsy findings may help target specific interventions). If proteinuria is believed to be caused by a drug, the agent should be discontinued. Proteinuria from drugs may take several months to resolve, and occasionally it is permanent.

Regardless of the cause though, therapy in patients with proteinuria should be directed at reducing urinary protein excretion rate and at modification of cardiovascular risk factors, given the association of proteinuria with both progression of renal disease and cardiovascular mortality.

The mainstay of antiproteinuric therapy is blood pressure control, always including the use of angiotensin-converting enzyme (ACE) inhibitors and/or angiotensin receptor blockers (ARBs). Based on multiple treatment studies, it is clear that lower blood pressure is associated with improved renal outcomes (15). However, the optimal blood pressure target is somewhat controversial. JNC 7 guidelines suggest that the target blood pressure should be 130/80 mm Hg or less while the National Kidney Foundation guidelines recommend decreasing blood pressure to less than 120/75 mm Hg (see NKF/DOQI and JNC 7 guidelines, at www.hopkinsbayview.org/PAMreferences).

In addition, it has now been clearly shown that ACE inhibitors and ARBs can reduce proteinuria and stabilize renal function in both diabetic and nondiabetic renal disease (16–23). Thus, these classes of antihypertensives should be the first line choice in patients with proteinuria and hypertension. Several short-term and few long-term comparative studies have shown these two classes of drugs of have comparative efficacy in slowing progression of renal disease (see Venkat, at www.hopkinsbayview.org/PAMreferences). Thus, it is likely that both have equivalent renoprotective effects and other considerations such as costs and side effects should drive choice of agent.

The goal of treatment is stabilization or fall of at least 30% to 50% in urinary albumin excretion over 3 to 6 months. It has also been advocated that even if blood pressure is at goal, these agents should be titrated until protein excretion is less than 0.5 g/day. Patients should be monitored for a rise in serum creatinine or for the development of hyperkalemia during the first few weeks after initiation of ACE inhibitor or ARB therapy and with each dose increase. Serum creatinine often increases slightly as a result of ACE inhibitor or ARB therapy (usually to less than 15% to 20% above the patient's baseline concentration) and then reaches a plateau. If serum creatinine increases to a more significant extent, the drug usually should be discontinued or the dose decreased to one that was previously well-tolerated. Multiple other therapies such as use of statins, smoking cessation, and weight loss have also been associated with reduction in proteinuria although the data for these therapies are not as strong (see Wilmer et al., at www.hopkinsbayview.org/PAMreferences).

If either edema or hypoalbuminemia is present, special therapy may be indicated. In the absence of renal failure, albumin synthesis is either increased or normal in patients with the nephrotic syndrome. Whereas a high-protein diet was previously recommended to patients with proteinuria, mild to moderate protein restriction is now advised, because it is believed that high protein intake may lead to progressive renal dysfunction by producing hyperfiltration (24). Appropriate standards for protein intake and pharmacologic intervention in this setting remain controversial and are a subject of intense research.

In the presence of edema, salt restriction to a tolerable level, such as a no-added-salt diet (approximately 2 to 3 g/day of sodium; see Chapter 67) is appropriate. If the edema is more severe and is unresponsive to sodium chloride restriction, cautious use of a loop diuretic (furosemide, torsemide, or bumetanide) may be necessary. No attempt should be made to rid the patient entirely of edema, which could risk contraction of the circulating volume, with serious consequences. Potassium-sparing diuretics (spironolactone, triamterene, or amiloride) may be added if renal failure is absent. Metolazone or thiazides may be added if loop diuretics have not been entirely adequate. Monitoring of serum potassium is important for selection and adjustment of the diuretic regimen, especially if ACE inhibitors or ARBs are used in this setting. In many instances, the patient can establish the correct diuretic dosage schedule by keeping a diary of weights and drug intake. If acceptable control is still not achieved, consultation with a nephrologist is appropriate.

Numerous extrarenal complications are associated with nephrotic syndrome. These include alterations in cellular immunity leading to increased infections, hyperlipidemia, and changes in calcium and bone metabolism. Nephrotic syndrome can be associated with a hypercoagulable state with thrombosis of the renal veins as well as other vessels. Clues to the development of renal vein thrombosis include pulmonary embolism, sudden deterioration in renal function, significant increase in the level of proteinuria, back or flank pain, or the development of hematuria. Suspicion of this complication requires hospitalization of the patient for urgent evaluation. Patients with nephrotic syndrome should be counseled about risk factors for deep venous thrombosis, such as long periods of immobilization. This is especially true for patients with membranous glomerulonephritis, although renal vein thrombosis has been reported in all types of glomerulonephritis.

Prediction of the course and selection of specific therapy in patients with nephrotic-range proteinuria depend on the pathologic pattern that is identified in the biopsy. Patients with nephrotic-range proteinuria need regularly scheduled office visits at 1- to 4-month intervals. Usually this followup is done by the primary care provider and the patient sees the nephrologist only once a year. The office visit provides an opportunity to review the patient's symptoms and to perform a physical examination (which, at a minimum, should include weight, volume assessment, and blood pressure) as well as to evaluate the 24-hour urine protein excretion or a protein/creatinine ratio, renal function (creatinine or creatinine clearance), and the serum electrolytes if diuretics are being used. Less often, an assessment of the serum albumin concentration may be necessary.

SPECIFIC REFERENCES*

1. Iseki K, Iseki C, Ikemiya Y, et al. Risk of developing end-stage renal disease in a cohort of mass screening. Kidney Int 1996;49:800.
2. Ginsberg JM, Chang BS, Matarese RA, et al. Use of single voided urine samples to estimate quantitative proteinuria. N Engl J Med 1983; 309:1543.
3. Robinson RR. Isolated proteinuria in asymptomatic patients. Kidney Int 1980;18:395.
4. Muth RG. Asymptomatic mild intermittent proteinuria: a percutaneous renal biopsy study. Arch Intern Med 1965;115:569.
5. Levitt JI. The prognostic significance of proteinuria in young college students. Ann Intern Med 1967;66:685.
6. Springberg PD, Garrett LE Jr., Thompson AL Jr., et al. Fixed and reproducible orthostatic proteinuria: results of a 20-year follow-up study. Ann Intern Med 1982;97:516.
7. Martin-Arevalo DL, Yee J, Pugh J, et al. Fixed and reproducible orthostatic proteinuria: a 35-yr follow-up study [abstract]. J Am Soc Nephrol 1996;7:1323.
8. King SE. Diastolic hypertension and chronic proteinuria. Am J Cardiol 1962;9:669.
9. Nelson RG, Knowler WC, Pettitt DJ, et al. Assessment of risk of overt nephropathy in diabetic patients from albumin excretion in untimed urine specimens. Arch Intern Med 1991;151:1761.
10. Verhave JC, Gansevoort RT, Hillege HL, et al. PREVEND Study Group. An elevated urinary albumin excretion predicts de novo development of renal function impairment in the general population. Kidney Int 2004;66[Suppl 92]:S18.
11. Kannel WB, Stampfer MJ, Castelli WP, et al. The prognostic significance of proteinuria: the Framingham study. Am Heart J 1984;108:1347.
12. Gerstein HC, Mann JF, Yi Q, et al. HOPE Study Investigators. Albuminuria and risk of cardiovascular events, death, and heart failure in diabetic and nondiabetic individuals. JAMA 2001;286:421.
13. Agodoa LY, Appel L, Bakris Gl, et al. African American Study of Kidney Disease and Hypertension (AASK) Study Group. Effect of ramipril vs. amlodipine on renal outcomes in hypertensive nephrosclerosis: a randomized controlled trial. JAMA 2001;285:2719.
14. Hillege HL, Fidler V, Diercks GF, et al. Prevention of Renal and Vascular End Stage Disease (PREVEND) Study Group. Urinary albumin excretion predicts cardiovascular and noncardiovascular mortality in general population. Circulation 2002;106:1777.
15. Jafar TH, Stark PC, Schmid CH, et al. AIPRD Study Group. Progression of chronic kidney disease: the role of blood pressure control, proteinuria, and angiotensin-converting enzyme inhibition: a patient-level meta-analysis. Ann Intern Med 2003;139:244.
16. Lewis EJ, Hunsicker LG, Bain RP, et al. The effect of angiotensin-converting enzyme inhibition on diabetic nephropathy. The Collaborative Study Group. N Engl J Med 1993;329:1456.
17. Mathiesen ER, Hommel E, Giese J, et al. Efficacy of captopril in postponing nephropathy in normotensive insulin dependent diabetic patients with microalbuminuria. BMJ 1991; 303:81.
18. Ravid M, Savin H, Jutrin I, et al. Long-term stabilizing effect of angiotensin-converting enzyme inhibition on plasma creatinine and on proteinuria in normotensive type II diabetic patients. Ann Intern Med 1993;118:577.
19. Sano T, Kawamura T, Matsumae H, et al. Effects of long-term enalapril treatment on persistent micro-albuminuria in well-controlled hypertensive and normotensive NIDDM patients. Diabetes Care 1994;17:420.
20. Heart Outcomes Prevention Evaluation Study Investigators. Effects of ramipril on cardiovascular and microvascular outcomes in people with diabetes mellitus: results of the HOPE study and MICRO-HOPE substudy. Lancet 2000;355:253.
21. The GISEN Group (Gruppo Italiano di Studi Epidemiologici in Nefrologia). Randomised placebo-controlled trial of effect of ramipril on decline in glomerular filtration rate and risk of terminal renal failure in proteinuric, non-diabetic nephropathy. Lancet 1997;349: 1857.
22. Ruggenenti P, Perna A, Gherardi G, et al. Renoprotective properties of ACE-inhibition in non-diabetic nephropathies with non-nephrotic proteinuria. Lancet 1999;354:359.
23. Jafar TH, Schmid CH, Landa M. Angiotensin-converting enzyme inhibitors and progression of nondiabetic renal disease. A meta-analysis of patient-level data. Ann Intern Med 2001: 135:73.
24. Brenner BM, Lawler EV, Mackenzie HS. The hyperfiltration theory: a paradigm shift in nephrology. Kidney Int 1996;49:1774.

*Bold numerals denote published controlled clinical trials, meta-analyses, or consensus-based recommendations.

For annotated **General References** *and resources related to this chapter, visit www.hopkinsbayview.org/PAMreferences.*

Chapter 49

Hematuria

David A. Spector

Normal individuals excrete up to 2 million red blood cells (RBCs) into the urine daily; this is equivalent to one to three RBCs per high-powered microscopic field (HPF) with standard urinalysis techniques. The finding of greater numbers of RBCs in the urine constitutes abnormal hematuria, although the exact level separating normal from abnormal is arbitrary. Benzidine- or orthotolidine-impregnated, hemoglobin-sensitive dipsticks, widely used as screening tests for hemoglobinuria (usually caused by lysis of RBCs in the urine and therefore an indication of hematuria), are less sensitive than microscopy but are usually positive in urine that contains at least three RBCs per HPF. The rate at which RBCs lyse depends on the concentration of the urine in which they are found and the duration of time they are exposed. Usually some lysis occurs within a few minutes, especially when the urine is dilute. There are certain limits to the use of hemoglobin-sensitive dipsticks (Table 49.1).

Microscopic hematuria may or may not indicate serious genitourinary tract disease (1,2). The symptoms, signs, and laboratory findings associated with hematuria and the clinical setting in which it occurs help considerably in predicting the seriousness of the finding. For example, gross hematuria or hematuria associated with proteinuria or pyuria is highly predictive of a significant disease. Conversely, asymptomatic microhematuria in a young adult has little predictive value.

PSEUDOHEMATURIA

A large number of substances can impart a color to urine that may be mistaken for hematuria (3). Table 49.2 lists *exogenous sources* of some of these substances. *Endogenous substances* capable of producing a reddish hue include porphyrins, myoglobin, and hemoglobin. Myoglobin and hemoglobin also cause positive reactions in tests for RBCs. When the urine dipstick is positive and the microscopy is negative for RBCs, myoglobinuria or hemoglobinuria should be suspected. Both are serious findings and warrant further evaluation. Myoglobinuria indicates substantial muscle disease or injury, and hemoglobinuria indicates significant hematuria (with lysis of RBCs) or hemolysis. However, the dipstick reaction will be falsely positive in the presence of oxidizing substances (e.g., if there is heavy hypochlorite [bleach, chlorine] or peroxidase [from bacteria] contamination of the urine specimen or its container). A false-negative dipstick test may also occur when formaldehyde (e.g., present as a breakdown product of the antibacterial agent methenamine) or large amounts of vitamin C are in the urine, because both substances decrease the sensitivity of the test reagent.

INNOCENT HEMATURIA

Microscopic hematuria is sometimes identified after sexual activity or after a genitourinary tract examination such as a pelvic or prostate examination, cystoscopy or bladder catheterization, or biopsy of prostate, bladder, or kidney.

TABLE 49.1 Limits of Dipstick Method for Detection of Blood in the Urine

Reasons for a Positive Test
Hematuria greater than approximately 3 RBCs/HPF
Hematuria with lysis of RBCs
From hypotonic urine (specific gravity <1.008)
From highly alkaline urine (pH >6.5)
Hemoglobinuria from intravascular hemolysis
Myoglobinuria from muscle injury
False-positive reactions
From hypochlorite (bleach) contamination of container
From peroxidase (from heavy growth of bacteria)
Reasons for a False Negative Test
Vitamin C: Ingestion of large amounts of vitamin C (>200 milligrams per day) results in diminished oxidation potential of the test material. The dipstick test may miss trace quantities of blood, although usually there is a quantitative decrease in the estimate of blood (such as 3 + to 2 +). (This is of concern only if RBCs are observed but the dipstick test is negative.)
Formaldehyde: Ingestion of bacterial suppressant agents (such as Mandelamine or Hiprex) that produce formaldehyde in acid urine or contamination of the container with formaldehyde diminishes the oxidizing potential of the reagent strips. This results in a quantitative estimate error or, if hematuria is minimal, a false negative result.

HPF, high-power field; RBCs, red blood cells.

TABLE 49.2 Exogenous Substances That May Cause Pseudohematuria[a]

Type	*Examples*
Medications	
Analgesics	Phenacetin, phenazopyridine (e.g., Pyridium)
Antimicrobials	Nitrofurantoin, rifampin, sulfonamides
Antimalarials	Chloroquine, primaquine
Laxatives	Anthraquinones: cascara, senna, danthron
Anticancer agents	Doxorubicin, daunorubicin
Others	Deferoxamine (an iron-chelating agent), levodopa, phenothiazines, methyldopa (rare)
Vegetable Dyes	
Anthocyanins: beets, blackberries	
Paprika	
Rhubarb	
Fuscin (a reddish dye used in topical agents)	
Others	
Antiseptics	Mercurochrome, phenols, cresols, povidone-iodine (Betadine)
Urate crystals (in acid urine)	

[a]Some of these agents cause hemoglobinuria.

Occasionally, gross hematuria may be seen in this setting. Gross or microscopic hematuria is also sometimes present after vigorous exercise such as swimming, lacrosse, boxing, football, or running. This finding is most common in long-distance runners, and in one study, 18% of athletes were found to have hematuria (mostly microscopic hematuria) after the completion of a marathon (4). Hematuria in all such settings subsides in 24 to 48 hours. It does not signify underlying genitourinary disease if it resolves quickly and does not recur spontaneously. In exercisers (especially runners), proteinuria or cast formation sometimes accompanies the hematuria, and the red cells have been found to be dysmorphic, suggesting that the bleeding site is the glomerulus.

HEMATURIA WITH PYURIA

If a patient is found to have hematuria associated with pyuria (with or without irritative symptoms such as frequency, urgency, or dysuria), an infectious cause is most likely and bacterial cultures of the urine should be obtained. If a specific organism is identified, appropriate antimicrobial therapy should be given (see Chapter 36). After treatment, the patient should be monitored carefully (including urinalysis) in 4 to 6 weeks to ensure that the hematuria has been eradicated and does not recur. If irritative symptoms suggesting infection have been present and the routine culture is sterile, a *sexually transmitted disease* (STD) (especially *Chlamydia* infection or gonorrhea), a viral infection, or genitourinary tuberculosis (now a rare cause of hematuria) should be suspected. In particular, *Chlamydia trachomatis* infection (see Chapters 36 and 102) may be manifested by hematuria and pyuria with minimal irritative symptoms. When a sexually transmitted infection is suspected but cannot be proved, a therapeutic trial of an antimicrobial drug may be given (see Chapters 36 and 102). *Viral cystitis* is a fairly common infection of young women. It has a short natural course (2 to 3 days), and it is nonrecurrent. A diagnosis of *tuberculosis of the urinary tract* requires several weeks to confirm by culture. (An acid-fast stain of a voided specimen of urine is not a reliable indicator because of the regular presence of acid-fast material from smegma bacilli. These bacilli would not be observed in a catheterized urine specimen, but most experts suggest simply waiting for the culture results in the typical patient in whom tuberculosis is a consideration.) Rarely, one may encounter a patient who is from an area endemic for schistosomiasis, and in this situation, the presence of hematuria should raise a question of this infection. Because noninfectious disorders of the bladder (including malignancies) may also present with irritative symptoms (see Chapter 53), one should ensure that those symptoms have abated after treatment, especially in patients older than 50 years of age, and it is probably prudent to confirm that the patient's urinalysis is normal 4 to 6 weeks after completion of treatment for an infection.

HEMATURIA WITH PROTEINURIA, RED BLOOD CELL CASTS, OR DYSMORPHIC RED BLOOD CELLS

Hematuria associated with proteinuria reflects glomerulonephritis or, less often, interstitial nephritis. When proteinuria is greater than 2 g in 24 hours or RBC casts are present, the diagnosis is probably glomerulonephritis (see Chapter 48). The morphologic appearance on microscopy of the RBCs may help differentiate glomerular from nonglomerular bleeding (5). This observation takes advantage of the deformation of RBCs after their passage into the Bowman space. If more than 80% of at least 100 (counted) RBCs appear dysmorphic (abnormal size, shape, and cytoplasmic staining) by Wright stain (or phase contrast microscopy, if available) of the urinary sediment, glomerular bleeding is very likely. In particular, acanthocytes (RBCs with spiny projections), when present, almost always indicate glomerular disease (6). If glomerulonephritis is suspected, estimation of the glomerular filtration rate and measurement of 24-hour urine protein excretion are indicated. Even if proteinuria if not present, when glomerulonephritis is suspected a test for microalbuminuria might also be indicated since, when present in adults with microscopic hematuria, microalbuminuria is predictive of glomerular disease and especially of immunoglobulin A (IgA) nephropathy (Berger disease) (7). Chapter 48 suggests an approach to the patient with suspected glomerulonephritis. Although any form of glomerulonephritis may be present in a patient in whom hematuria is an incidental finding, either IgA nephropathy (8), Alport syndrome (hereditary nephritis, often associated with deafness), or thin basement membrane disease is especially likely. IgA nephropathy and Alport syndrome, in particular, are characterized by recurrent episodes of gross hematuria, dysmorphic red cells, microalbuminuria and/or proteinuria, and a progressive course. A nephrologist should be consulted when these or other forms of glomerulonephritis are suspected. Often the nephrologist will perform a renal biopsy (see Chapter 48) to establish the diagnosis, estimate the prognosis, and determine treatment.

ASYMPTOMATIC ISOLATED MICROHEMATURIA

The prevalence of isolated microscopic hematuria depends on the stringency of the diagnostic criteria (e.g., number of RBCs per HPF, number of "positive" tests required) and the population studied. For example, in each of five studies of young adults, less then 1% of the study population had asymptomatic hematuria (9). In contrast, asymptomatic hematuria was observed in 13% to 21% of older men who were considered to be at high risk for genitourinary carcinoma and other chronic urinary tract diseases (10).

Causes of Asymptomatic Hematuria

Most series describing the causes of microscopic hematuria come from the urology-oriented literature and emphasize diagnoses likely to be made by cystoscopic and radiographic evaluation (Table 49.3). Generally, neoplasia is more commonly reported in series comprising older individuals or patients referred to urologists; conversely, neoplasia is rarely found in population-based series of young patients.

In all series, no specific diagnosis was made for many patients, in part because patient evaluations were usually incomplete. For example, most series did not include a renal biopsy, which may have revealed glomerular or interstitial disease (11,12). The importance of this omission was borne out by one study in which 51 of 65 adult patients with hematuria with minimal or no proteinuria and a negative urologic workup had a specific diagnosis established only after the performance of a renal biopsy (11).

TABLE 49.3 Distribution (%) of Selected Urologic Findings in Asymptomatic Patients with Microhematuria

Finding	*Mariani et al. (14) (694 pts., HMO Urology Referrals[a])*	*Golin and Howard (20) (246 pts., Urology Referral)*	*Khadra et al. (21) (982 pts., Hematuria Clinic[b])*	*Mohr et al. (22) (781 pts., Rochester MN Population[c])*	*Bard (1) (177 Women, Urology Referral)*	*Messing et al. (23) (192 Men >50 Yr Screened for Hematuria)*
Neoplasia	8.5	9.3	5.4	1.0	0.0	8.3
Other disorders						
Renal calculi	3.4	0.0	4.0	3.3	1.6	8.9
Ureteral calculi	0.6	1.0	0.0	0.9	0.6	
Nephritis/renal insufficiency	1.2	2.0	9.4	14.40	0.0	1.0
Benign prostatic hypertrophy	16.50	8.0	—[f]	37.70	—[d]	47.40
Urinary tract infection	4.3	2.0	13.0	0.5	—[d]	2.6
Urethrotrigonitis/prostatitis	37.7	18.0	—[f]	1.8	32.60	—
Any finding[e]	88.30	47.60	31.80	62.50	63.00	84.9

[a]Original series of 1,000 patients included 309 patients with gross hematuria.
[b]Original series of 1,930 patients included 948 with gross hematuria.
[c]Complete urologic workup not performed on all patients.
[d]Women with urinary tract infection excluded from study.
[e]Includes those listed above in addition to other findings that may or may not have been related to the hematuria. These include hydronephrosis, renal cysts, polycystic kidney disease, vesicoureteral reflux, interstitial and radiation cystitis, diverticula, ureteropelvic junction obstruction, ureterocele, cystocele, neurogenic bladder, atrophic vagina, scarred kidney, cystitis cystica, polyps, papillary necrosis, calcified renal mass, and trabeculated bladder. Some patients in all series had more than one disorder.
[f]Unable to determine from data.

TABLE 49.4 Causes of Hematuria

Renal

Glomerular:

IgA nephropathy, hereditary nephritis (Alport syndrome), thin basement membrane disease, **other glomerulonephritis.**

Other:

Renal cell cancer, polycystic kidney disease, pyelonephritis, interstitial nephritis, papillary necrosis, renal infarction, **renal trauma**, crystalluria (usually related to hypercalcemia, hyperuricosuria or drugs), **sickle cell disease, tuberculosis,** medullary sponge kidney, **loin pain hematuria syndrome**, arteriovenous malformation, renal vein thrombosis.

Nonrenal

Cancers (renal pelvis, ureter, bladder, prostate), calculi, benign prostatic hypertrophy, cystitis, prostatitis, urethritis, genitourinary polyps, strictures and diverticula, tuberculosis, schistosomiasis.

Other Site/Uncertain

Exercise, factitious, anticoagulation therapy*, pseudohematuria, contamination from skin

Disorders in bold face commonly cause gross hematuria as well as microscopic hematuria.

*Hematuria in the setting of anticoagulation often has another specific cause.

TABLE 49.5 Examples of Drugs Causing Hematuria

Antimicrobials
Penicillin analogs[a]
Cephalosporin analogs[a]
Sulfa analogs[a]
Polymycin[a]
Rifampin[a]

Analgesics and Anti-Inflammatory Agents
Aspirin[b]
Aminosalicylic acid[b]
Nonsteroidal anti-inflammatory agents[a]

Diuretics
Furosemide[a]
Ethacrynic acid[a]
Thiazides[a]

Anticoagulants
Warfarin (Coumadin)[c]

Other
Cyclophosphamide[d]
Ifosfamide (Isex, an antineoplastic agent)[d]
Danazol[d]

[a]Infrequent bleeding caused by interstitial nephritis, usually occurring within days to weeks of taking drugs; usually reversible.

[b]Infrequent bleeding caused by medullary/papillary necrosis, usually following many months or years of combination analgesic preparations; partially reversible.

[c]An underlying cause of hematuria is often found and a workup should be considered (Cuttino JT Jr, Clark RL, Feaster SH, Zwicke DL. The evaluation of gross hematuria in anticoagulated patients: efficacy of i.v. urography and cystoscopy. AJR Am J Roentgenol 1987;149:527.)

[d]Bleeding caused by hemorrhagic cystitis in 10%–20% of patients; dose-related and usually reversible.

Renal biopsy, when performed, often reveals a glomerular cause of hematuria in younger patients in whom the workup is otherwise unrevealing, and it also may reveal glomerular lesions in up to 40% of cases, even in elderly patients (12). As in patients with combined hematuria and proteinuria, the most likely biopsy findings in patients with asymptomatic hematuria are IgA nephritis, followed by Alport disease and thin basement membrane disease (12).

Additionally, most series did not include quantitation of 24-hour urine calcium and uric acid. Hypercalciuria (more than 300 milligrams per 24 hours) or hyperuricosuria (more than 750 mg/24 hours in women; more than 800 mg/24 hours in men) has been shown to cause hematuria (presumably as a result of irritation of the tubules by microcrystals), and thiazide therapy (which reduces calciuria) or allopurinol stops the bleeding in these circumstances (13). Table 49.4 shows a more complete listing of causes of hematuria.

EVALUATION OF PATIENTS WITH HEMATURIA

Pseudohematuria and drug-induced hematuria (Table 49.5) should be ruled out. The evaluation then depends on associated symptoms, on whether the bleeding is gross or microscopic, and on the results of the complete urinalysis (discussed earlier). Localization of the site of the bleeding in the genitourinary tract is the first priority. The associated symptoms and the history of temporal events often provide diagnostic clues. For example, colicky flank pain suggests that the hematuria is emanating from the ureter, whereas dysuria and urinary frequency suggest that the bleeding is from the bladder. All patients should be asked about the temporal relationship of the hematuria to exercise, to ingestion of medications or food, and to trauma. The urinalysis is helpful also if findings suggest glomerular disease or infection (see earlier discussion). In some studies, the seriousness of the underlying lesion was proportional to the number of RBCs per HPF, and patients with gross hematuria were especially at risk for serious or life-threatening illness (14,15).

A focused history and physical examination should be performed to seek clues to illnesses with which hematuria is associated (e.g., a nodular prostate suggestive of prostate cancer, cutaneous or other abnormalities suggestive of a collagen vascular disease). When the history and physical examination, together with selected laboratory procedures (e.g., urine culture) and treatment (e.g., antimicrobial agents), do not support a working diagnosis, certain laboratory data should be obtained. This evaluation should include a complete blood count (CBC), an estimate of glomerular function (e.g., serum creatinine), a sickle-cell preparation (in the appropriate patient), a 24-hour urine specimen for determination of calcium and uric acid concentrations (see earlier discussion), and a radiologic evaluation. The optimal radiologic procedure(s) for patients presenting with hematuria is not clear. Intravenous pyelography (IVP) has historically been the procedure of choice, with ultrasonography suggested for pregnant women or for those allergic to contrast dye. Although IVP is still recommended as best practice policy by the American Urologic Association (10), multiphasic helical computed tomography (CT) is generally more sensitive than IVP or ultrasonography in detecting small renal calculi (unenhanced CT) (16) and small renal masses (unenhanced CT followed by contrast-enhanced CT), and is specifically more efficacious than IVP in patients presenting with microscopic hematuria (17). Therefore some authors now suggest using helical CT urography without and with contrast as the initial procedure of choice in the evaluation of hematuria (Cohen and Brown; Steele and Michaels, www.hopkinsbayview.org/PAMreferences). In patients with a suspected bleeding disorder, a platelet count and measurement of the prothrombin, partial thromboplastin, and bleeding times should be done. Even if an underlying bleeding diathesis is identified, the search for a pathologic process in the genitourinary tract should continue, because one is usually identified (see Chapter 56). In patients older than 40 to 50 years of age, two or three fresh morning urine specimens should be evaluated by a cytology laboratory for the presence of tumor cells. The sensitivity of cytology in this setting is 30% when an upper tract tumor is present and 50% to 90% when a bladder tumor is present (with higher rates of detection for higher grades of cancer). However, because cystoscopy is the diagnostic procedure of choice when bladder cancer is suspected, many urologists suggest that cytology not be done until after cystoscopy has been performed, and then only when that procedure is negative for cancer but the clinician remains suspicious of the presence of a urinary tract neoplasia. A number of methods of detecting voided protein tumor markers (e.g., BTA, NMP22, Lewis x Antigen, CD44V) have been promoted for use in evaluating recurrence of bladder tumors (10). Although the use of voided tumor markers in the evaluation of patients with hematuria is promising, the available data are insufficient currently to warrant their routine use for that purpose.

Nevertheless, if neoplasia is a consideration (patient older than 40 to 50 years of age or younger but with a risk factor for bladder cancer), a urologist should be consulted and the patient should undergo cystoscopy. Risk factors for bladder cancer include heavy occupational exposure (e.g., to aromatic amines, dyes, benzidine, paint ingredients [see Chapter 8]); a history of smoking; pelvic irradiation; prior use of cyclophosphamide; gross, as opposed to microscopic, hematuria; a history of schistosomiasis; or prolonged daily use of analgesics (phenacetin, acetaminophen, and aspirin combinations have been reported to be associated with genitourinary cancer). If neoplasia is a strong consideration, the urologist might also suggest additional radiologic evaluation of the patient by sonography, CT scanning, magnetic resonance imaging, renal angiography, or retrograde pyelography.

If neoplasia is not strongly suspected and persistent hematuria is present or recurrent, the patient should be referred to a nephrologist for consideration of renal biopsy (see Chapter 48). There is no consensus regarding how long a patient with unexplained microscopic hematuria should be monitored. While in most patients microscopic hematuria is transient and/or benign, in others with persistent hematuria, genitourinary neoplasms or calculi are discovered 1 to 3 years after the onset of hematuria (18,19). It seems reasonable, therefore, to monitor patients with persistent hematuria (in particular older individuals and those with a history of cigarette smoking who are at increased risk of developing genitourinary tract carcinoma) with repeat urinalysis, urine cytology, CT scans, and cystoscopy for at least 3 to 4 years after discovery of hematuria.

Gross Hematuria

If gross hematuria is present, the evaluation should proceed initially in the same manner as for microscopic hematuria, but there are several caveats. Gross hematuria is more likely to reflect genitourinary tract cancer than is microscopic hematuria, and therefore warrants a definitive urologic evaluation regardless of age. In one large prospective study, patients with gross hematuria (even in patients younger than 40 years old), were two to four times more likely to have genitourinary tract cancer than those with microscopic hematuria (21). Patients with gross hematuria should always be referred to a urologist promptly, because the best time to identify the site of bleeding is when the bleeding is active. In patients with gross hematuria, plasma protein is lost into the urine and thereby can be detected by qualitative testing. However, the concentration of urinary protein rarely exceeds 1 g/day when it occurs as a result of blood in the urine alone.

The *three-glass test* is sometimes useful in determining the site of gross bleeding. This test is performed by having the patient void into containers in a sequence: The initial 10 mL of urine represents the urethral specimen, the *middle portion* of urine voided is nondiagnostic of a specific location, and blood in the *terminal portion* (the last few drops of urine) suggests that the site is likely to be the prostate, bladder neck, or proximal urethra. Blood present in all three specimens is not specific for the site of origin.

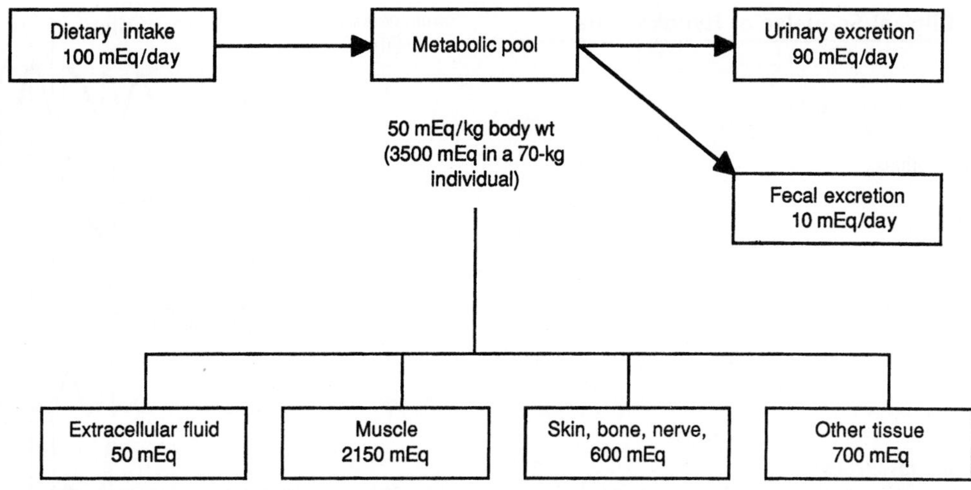

FIGURE 50.1. Balance of potassium (Adapted from Klinger AS, Hayslett JP. Disorders of potassium. In: Brenner BM, Stein JH, eds. Acid-base and potassium homeostasis. New York: Churchilll Livingstone, 1978.)

diarrhea. Severe potassium depletion may, however, have serious symptoms and severe consequences (Table 50.1).

Effects on the Cardiovascular System

Of greatest concern is the effect of hypokalemia on cardiac conduction and rhythm. Severe potassium depletion also rarely causes myocardial necrosis. During hypokalemia, characteristic pathologic electrocardiographic changes may be seen (Fig. 50.3). It is controversial whether mild to moderate hypokalemia per se can cause dangerous ventricular ectopy (4), but it seems certain that hypokalemia may be arrhythmogenic in patients with underlying heart disease (5,6). Hypokalemia also predisposes patients to arrhythmias due to digitalis intoxication. Hypokalemia also reduces the protective effect of diuretics on cardiovascular disease (7,8).

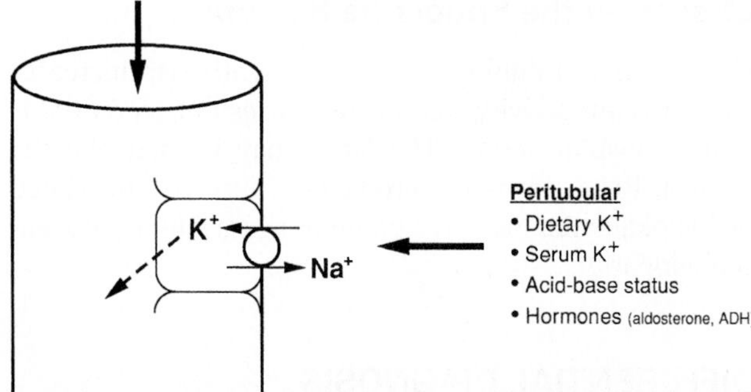

FIGURE 50.2. Factors influencing potassium secretion by the distal tubule. ADH, antidiuretic hormone. (Modified from Giebisch G. Physiology of potassium metabolism. In: Whelton A, Walker WG, eds. Potassium in cardiovascular and renal medicine. New York: Marcel Dekker, 1986.)

Effects on the Neuromuscular System

Potassium depletion alters both smooth and skeletal muscle function. Severe hypokalemia can cause GI tract dysmotility and ileus. Proximal muscle weakness can progress to paralysis. Respiratory muscle involvement can result in respiratory failure. Hypokalemia may also predispose to rhabdomyolysis, at least in part by interfering with exercise-induced vasodilation. Rarely, tetany may be seen even in the absence of changes in serum calcium or pH.

Effects on Blood Pressure

Hypokalemia commonly occurs as a complication of the treatment of hypertension, but potassium balance is also important in the underlying pathophysiology and evolution of hypertension, and of cardiovascular and cerebrovascular diseases. Populations that consume a low-potassium diet, such as African Americans, have very high prevalences of hypertension and cardiovascular disease (9,10). Large studies have shown that blood pressure is partly potassium dependent (11,12). The risk of hypertension increases as the amount of potassium in the diet decreases, independent of sodium intake (13). While the mechanism(s) for the effect of potassium on blood pressure are unclear, simply increasing potassium intake may lower the likelihood of developing hypertension (14,15). Supplementation with 48 to 120 mEq/day of potassium can lower blood pressure (16,17). The correction of hypokalemia by dietary means or by pharmacologic

TABLE 50.1 Clinical Sequelae of Hypokalemia

Cardiovascular
Predisposition to digitalis intoxication
Abnormal electrocardiogram
Ventricular ectopic rhythms
Cardiac necrosis
Increased blood pressure
Neuromuscular
Gastrointestinal
Constipation
Ileus
Skeletal muscle
Weakness, cramps
Tetany
Paralysis (including respiratory)
Rhabdomyolysis
Renal
Decreased renal blood flow
Decreased glomerular filtration rate
Renal hypertrophy
Pathologic alterations (interstitial nephritis)
Predisposition to urinary tract infection
Fluid and Electrolyte
Polyuria and polydipsia
Renal concentrating defect
Stimulation of thirst center
ADH release (?)
Increased renal ammonia production
Predisposition to hepatic coma
Altered urinary acidification
Renal chloride wasting
Metabolic alkalosis
Sodium retention
Hyponatremia (with or without concomitant diuretic)
Endocrine
Decrease in aldosterone
Increase in renin
Altered prostaglandin metabolism
Decrease in insulin secretion (carbohydrate intolerance)

ADH, antidiuretic hormone.
Modified from Tannen RL. Potassium disorders. In: Kokko J Fluids and electrolytes. Philadelphia: WB Saunders, 1986.

supplementation can enhance the treatment of hypertension with minimal risk and expense (18). Increased dietary potassium may have a greater effect than equivalent potassium chloride supplementation, perhaps because dietary potassium is associated with citrate rather than chloride anions (19). In addition, beyond its effect on hypertension, potassium supplementation has been shown to reduce the risk of cerebrovascular disease and stroke (20).

Effects on the Kidney

Hypokalemia impairs urinary concentrating ability. The defect is mild and the associated polyuria is also caused in part by direct stimulation of thirst. Prolonged, severe potassium depletion can produce reversible reductions in glomerular filtration rate and renal blood flow. Hypokalemia increases the risk of nephrotoxic renal failure (21) and rarely causes acute renal injury by itself (22). Hypokalemia-induced chronic tubulointerstitial disease can result in progressive chronic renal failure (23).

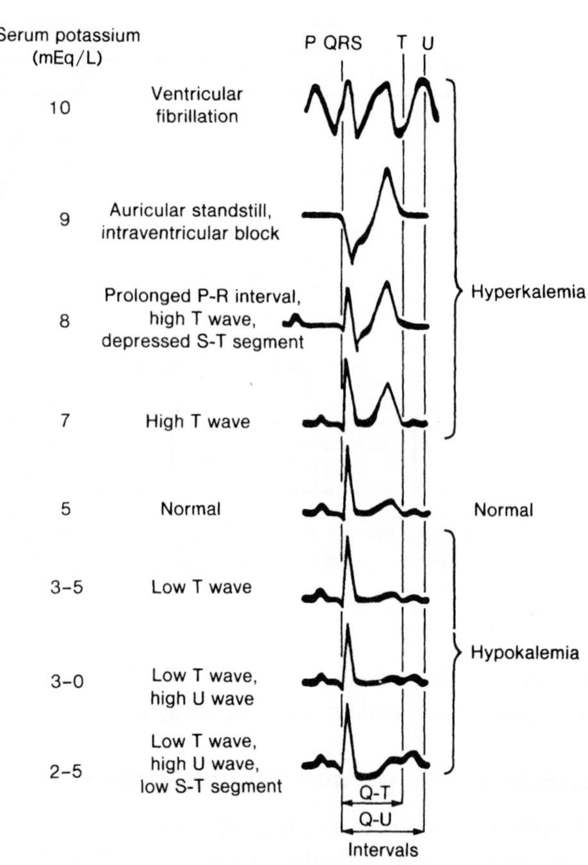

FIGURE 50.3. Electrocardiogram in assessment of potassium. (Adapted from Burch GE, Winsor T. A primer of electrocardiography. 6th ed. Philadelphia: Lea & Febiger, 1972:128.)

Effects on the Endocrine System

Hypokalemia inhibits aldosterone synthesis, increases plasma renin activity, and decreases insulin secretion as well as insulin action. The latter may worsen diabetic control. Renal ammonia production, directly stimulated by hypokalemia, may precipitate or aggravate hepatic encephalopathy.

DIFFERENTIAL DIAGNOSIS AND MANAGEMENT

Diuretic use, vomiting, and diarrhea are the most common causes of hypokalemia. Typically these conditions are evident from the history. Less obvious causes can be diag-

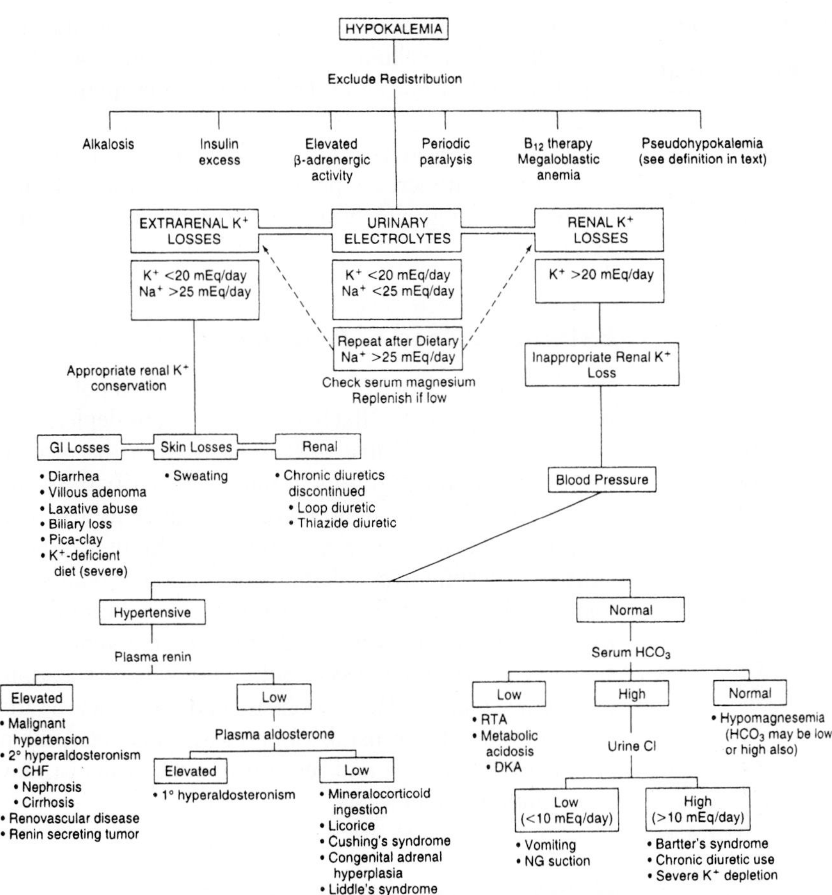

FIGURE 50.4. Diagnostic approach to hypokalemia. RTA, renal tubular acidosis; DKA, diabetic keloacidosis; NG, nasogastric; CHF, congestive heart failure. (Modified from Narins RG, Jones ER, Stom MC, et al. Diagnostic strategies in disorders of fluid, electrolyte and acid-base homeostasis. Am J Med 1982;72:496.)

nosed (Fig. 50.4) (24) by consideration of the fundamental mechanisms of potassium balance: reduced intake, transcellular shift into cells, and excessive loss. Surreptitious vomiting and diuretic abuse, along with Gitelman syndrome (see External Losses of Potassium, Normotensive Hypokalemia, and Bartter and Gitelman Syndromes), are the most common conditions associated with hypokalemia when the cause is difficult to ascertain (25).

Deficient Potassium Intake

Potassium is present in many foods, especially fruits, raw vegetables, fish, and red meat (Table 50.2). Inadequate intake is an unusual cause of hypokalemia except in high-risk situations (dietary fads, pica, alcoholism, cachexia). Hypokalemia can also occur if dietary potassium intake is inadequate during anabolic states such as refeeding of malnourished patients and treatment of megaloblastic anemia. Dietary deficiency of potassium, particularly in the elderly, may also exacerbate diuretic-induced hypokalemia.

Transient Disorders of Internal Potassium Balance

β_2-Adrenergic agonists lower serum potassium concentrations by stimulating cellular uptake of potassium. This is commonly seen when β_2-adrenergic agonists (administered via any route) are used to treat asthma or premature labor. The decrease in potassium is usually mild, but significant hypokalemia can also occur. Resolution occurs within hours of discontinuing the drug. High levels of endogenous catecholamines released during stress may explain transient hypokalemia that resolves with or without supplementation during acute stressful illness (26,27).

Metabolic and respiratory alkalosis are associated with small shifts of potassium from the extracellular to the intracellular space.

Insulin stimulates potassium uptake in liver and skeletal muscle cells independent of effects on glucose transport. This action is the basis for using insulin to treat severe hyperkalemia. Insulin treatment of hyperglycemia may induce hypokalemia even if the serum potassium is normal (28).

Hypokalemic periodic paralysis is a rare familial disorder characterized by spontaneous episodes of paralysis often precipitated by stimuli, including insulin, glucose, and a high-carbohydrate meal (29). A similar syndrome occurs in hyperthyroidism, especially in Asian men (30). Both the serum potassium and urinary potassium excretion decrease dramatically, signifying an intracellular shift of potassium. In the thyrotoxic form, β-blocking agents may be effective in preventing attacks.

TABLE 50.2 Some Common Potassium-Rich Foods

Food Source	Average Portion	Potassium (mEq)
Vegetables		
Artichoke	1 large	22.0
Beans		
Cooked dried	½ cup	10.7
Lima	⅝ cup	10.8
Brussels sprouts	7 medium	7
Corn	1 ear	5.0
Potato		
White	1 boiled	7.3
Sweet	1 boiled	7.7
Tomato		
Fresh	1 medium	9.4
Canned	½ cup	5.6
Squash, winter	½ cup boiled	11.9
Meats		
Hamburger	1 patty	9.8
Rib roast	2 slices	11.2
Fish, haddock	1 medium fillet	8.0
Clams	4 large	6.0
Oysters	6 medium	3.1
Fruits		
Apple	1 medium	2.8
Applesauce	⅓ cup	1.7
Apricots	3 medium	7.2
Avocado	½ pitted	15.5
Banana	1 6-inch	9.5
Cantaloupe	¼ medium	6.4
Dates	10 pitted	16.6
Fruit cocktail	½ cup	4.3
Grapefruit	½ medium	3.5
Melon	¼ small	6.4
Orange	1 small	7.7
Peach	1 medium	5.2
Pear	1 medium	6.7
Plum	2 medium	7.7
Prunes, dried	10 medium	17.8
Raisins	1 tablespoon	2.0
Strawberries	10 large	4.2
Watermelon	1 slice	15.4
Juice		
Grapefruit	1 cup	10.4
Orange	1 cup	12.4
Pineapple	1 cup	9.2
Prune	1 cup	15.0
Tomato	1 cup	13.7
Vegetable	1 cup	14.1
Nuts		
Peanuts, roasted	1 tablespoon	2.0
Peanut butter	2 tablespoon	2.0
Mixed nuts	3.5 oz	2.0
Milk		
Buttermilk	9 oz	8.0
Skim milk	8 oz	8.5
Whole milk	8 oz	9.0

Vitamin B_{12} treatment of megaloblastic anemia may cause large intracellular shifts of potassium. Potassium supplementation and careful monitoring prevent this complication.

Rare causes of transient hypokalemia include hypothermia, which can increase potassium uptake into cells and barium poisoning, which can inhibit potassium potassium exit from cells.

External Losses of Potassium

If there is no evidence of a disorder of internal potassium balance, the patient is likely to be potassium depleted either via renal or GI losses. If unclear from the history, urine potassium measurement may help clarify the route of potassium loss. Potassium greater than 20 mEq/L on a spot urine specimen or greater than 20 mEq in a 24-hour collection despite hypokalemia suggests renal potassium loss is at least partially responsible for potassium depletion. Low urine potassium ($<$20 mEq/L on a spot urine) suggests an extrarenal loss of potassium with appropriate renal conservation. More sophisticated tests such as the calculation of the transtubular potassium concentration gradient (TTKG) (31) and referral to a nephrologist may be required in specific cases.

Gastrointestinal Losses Resulting in Potassium Deficiency

Diarrhea

High concentrations of potassium and bicarbonate are normally present in the stool. Diarrhea can produce significant hypokalemia, often associated with bicarbonate loss that results in a non–anion gap, hyperchloremic metabolic acidosis. While urinary potassium excretion should be low when potassium deficiency results from intestinal losses, this is true only when volume status is maintained. Secondary hyperaldosteronism induced by volume contraction may produce paradoxically high urine potassium losses. Even in the absence of diarrhea, hypokalemia may be a clue to the presence of a villous adenoma of the colon or surreptitious laxative abuse.

Loss of Gastric Fluid

Although gastric fluid contains only small amounts of potassium (approximately 5 to 10 mEq/L), hypokalemia frequently accompanies vomiting or gastric drainage because potassium is lost in the urine (32). The loss of gastric chloride induces metabolic alkalosis, chloride deficiency, extracellular volume depletion, and secondary hyperaldosteronism. The increased distal delivery of bicarbonate and high levels of aldosterone stimulate secretion of potassium. The urine will have high potassium concentrations and very low chloride concentrations.

Correction of potassium depletion and metabolic alkalosis requires provision of adequate amounts of chloride, potassium, and sodium. Potassium administered with anions other than chloride is not retained but is excreted in the urine (33).

Renal Losses Resulting in Potassium Deficiency

Diuretics

Loop and thiazide diuretics accelerate potassium excretion by increasing sodium and water delivery to the potassium secretory sites in the distal nephron and by simultaneously stimulating aldosterone release. The nadir of serum potassium concentration typically is within 7 days after therapy begins (34). Increased sodium intake increases the degree of potassium depletion. At standard dosages, thiazide and thiazide-like diuretics induce an average fall in the serum potassium concentration of 0.6 mEq/L, and 7% to 50% of patients develop a serum potassium less than 3.5 mEq/L. Furosemide causes less potassium depletion, with an average fall in potassium concentration of only 0.3 mEq/L. The use of multiple kaliuretic diuretics acting at different nephron sites (e.g., furosemide and thiazide) is likely to cause hypokalemia that is greater than that produced by a single agent (35).

Levels below 3.0 mEq/L suggest either excessive sodium intake or an unrecognized potassium-wasting state such as primary or secondary hyperaldosteronism (36). Both should be considered when significant hypokalemia develops after the introduction of potassium-wasting diuretics, particularly if the potassium level before treatment was low.

Monitoring Potassium in Patients Receiving Diuretics

The serum potassium should be measured before administration of diuretics and, if normal, it should be measured again 1 and 4 weeks after initiation of, or an increase in the dosage of, a diuretic. Subsequently, semiannual assessment is probably adequate in nonedematous, stable, well-nourished patients. Patients at greater risk of serious consequences of hypokalemia such as those with heart failure on digitalis or with cirrhosis at risk of hepatic coma should have more frequent monitoring.

Prevention and Therapy of Diuretic-Induced Hypokalemia

While the risk of mild diuretic-induced hypokalemia remains controversial (1), simple measures can minimize its occurrence. Both the lowest effective dosage of a diuretic agent, and moderate salt restriction (75 to 100 mEq sodium per day or 2 to 2.5 g sodium or 4 to 6 g sodium chloride) should be used. Increased dietary potassium is easy to achieve, cost-effective, and may be associated with other benefits such as lower blood pressure and decreased risk of stroke, hypertension, and other cerebrovascular diseases.

Even with these measures, approximately 30% of diuretic-treated patients become hypokalemic in the range of 3.0 to 3.5 mEq/L (37). If a diuretic is required, a normal potassium is a prudent goal for those patients listed in Table 50.3. Either potassium supplements or potassium-sparing diuretics can be used. Potassium chloride (Table 50.4) is preferred as potassium with poorly absorbed anions increases potassium loss. Salt substitutes (50 to 65 millmole per teaspoon potassium chloride) are a cheap and effective alternative. Diuretic-induced hypokalemia may seem to be refractory even to large doses of potassium chloride because the renal clearance of potassium remains high during continued diuretic therapy. In one study, potassium chloride at dosages up to 96 millimole per day normalized the serum potassium in only

TABLE 50.3 Indications for Potassium Maintenance Therapy

Digitalis therapy
Predisposition to hepatic coma
Serum potassium concentration <3.0 mEq/L
Development of glucose intolerance
Underlying cardiac disease
Symptoms attributable to hypokalemia

With permission from Tannen RL. Diuretic-induced hypokalemia. Kidney Int 1985;28:988.

TABLE 50.4 Commonly Available Potassium Chloride Supplements

Product	*Amount (mEq)*
Extended-release tablets	
Micro-K Extentabs, Slow K, Klor-Con 8	8
K-Dur, K-Norm, K-Tab, Ten-K, Micro-K 10 Extentabs, Klor-Con 10	10
K-Dur	20
Powders for solution (flavored)[a]	
K-Lor (also 15 mEq), Kato, Klor-Con Klor-Con 125 (25 mEq)	20/packet
Suspension (no taste)	
Micro-K LS	20/packet
Efflorescent granules or tablets (flavored)[a]	
Klorvess, Klor-Con/EF (25 mEq)	20
Solutions (flavored)[a]	
Klorvess 10%, Rum-K 15%	20–30/15 mL

[a]Taste is generally improved by chilling.

8 of 16 hypertensive patients with diuretic-induced hypokalemia (38).

Potassium-sparing diuretics (spironolactone, triamterene, amiloride) reduce urinary potassium losses, minimize development of metabolic alkalosis by reducing acid excretion (spironolactone), and limit renal magnesium wasting. In one study conversion from hydrochlorothiazide (with or without potassium supplements) to hydrochlorothiazide plus amiloride or hydrochlorothiazide plus triamterene without potassium supplements increased the serum potassium by 0.5 to 0.7 mEq/L into the midnormal range (39). Measuring 24-hour urinary potassium excretion and serum potassium may help determine how much supplement to prescribe.

All patients should be assessed for risk of hyperkalemia before potassium supplements or potassium-sparing agents are prescribed. These risks are renal insufficiency (serum creatinine greater than 1.2 mg/dL or glomerular filtration rate less than 60 mL/minute), diabetes mellitus, age 75 or older, and the use of other agents known to interfere with potassium homeostasis such as angiotensin converting enzyme inhibitors, nonsteroidal anti-inflammatory drugs, cyclosporine, and heparin. Even patients with normal renal function generally should not be given potassium supplements and potassium-sparing diuretics together with other drugs that interfere with potassium homeostasis. All patients beginning therapy to raise the serum potassium level should have their serum potassium measured after 1 and 4 weeks and then at least every 6 to 12 months.

Renal Potassium Wasting Unrelated to Diuretics or Gastric Losses

The blood pressure and acid-base status of the patient simplify the complex differential diagnosis of renal potassium wasting (Fig. 50.4) (24), but referral to a specialized center may still be necessary.

Hypokalemia Accompanied by Hypertension

Hypokalemia accompanied by an elevated blood pressure suggests renin/angiotensin, mineralocorticoid/glucocorticoid, or apparent mineralocorticoid excess (Table 50.5). Determination of plasma renin activity is the first step in the evaluation of renal potassium wasting in a hypertensive patient (Fig. 50.4). An elevated renin suggests renovascular disease, malignant hypertension, or a rare renin-producing tumor. A low renin level should be repeated along with a plasma aldosterone level. If both are low, either excess endogenous or exogenous steroids, other than aldosterone, are likely. Licorice, chewing tobacco, carbenoxolone (an agent derived from licorice root), and steroid-containing nasal sprays are rare exogenous causes of this syndrome. Liddle syndrome (hypertension with hypokalemia unresponsive to spironolactone but responsive to amiloride) is caused by an autosomal dominant increased activity of the amiloride-sensitive sodium channel (40). Finally, if the renin level is low but the simultaneous aldosterone level is high, primary aldosteronism is strongly suggested.

TABLE 50.5 Causes of Hypertension with Associated Renal Potassium Wasting

Hyperreninemic Forms
Renovascular
Renin tumor
Malignant or accelerated essential hypertension
Hyporeninemic Steroid-Dependent Forms
Mineralocorticoid
Exogenous
Licorice, desoxycorticosterone, fludrocortisone, chewing tobacco, carbenoxolone
Endogenous
Adrenal adenoma
Adrenal glomerulose hyperplasia
Enzyme deficiency: 17-OHase; 11-OHase
Liddle syndrome
Glucocorticoid
Endogenous
Cushing syndrome, pituitary, ectopic ACTH, adrenal cortical
Exogenous

ACTH, adrenocorticotropic hormone.
With permission from Narins RG, Jones ER, Stom MC, et al. Diagnostic strategies in disorders of fluid, electrolyte and acid-base homeostasis. Am J Med 1982;72:496.

Most patients with primary aldosteronism are asymptomatic. Although once thought to be an extremely rare disorder, the use of the plasma aldosterone to plasma renin activity ratio (41) as a screening test in hypertensive patients has resulted in greater detection of this condition and a higher apparent prevalence than previously believed (42). Clinical manifestations, in addition to hypertension, are related to potassium depletion and occur only when such depletion is severe. These include weakness, paralysis, tetany, arrhythmias, polyuria, and polydipsia. Edema is uncommon because adaptive factors diminish sodium retention. Only a minority of patients with primary hyperaldosteronism have hypokalemia but many of these patients manifest hypokalemia if challenged with potassium-wasting diuretics or with large intakes of sodium chloride (200 millmoles per day, approximately 4 to 5 g of sodium or 10 to 12 g sodium chloride). The development of severe hypokalemia after the initiation of thiazide therapy is sometimes a clue to a hypermineralocorticoid state.

Localization procedures (computerized tomography [CT] or magnetic resonance imaging [MRI]) are needed to distinguish adenomas from bilateral adrenal hyperplasia. Adenomas are usually treated surgically but surgery is seldom curative for bilateral hyperplasia. A spironolactone trial (up to 400 mg daily for several weeks) is useful in almost all patients. Failure of spironolactone to normalize the blood pressure while normalizing hypokalemia strongly suggests that surgery would probably not resolve the hypertension.

Normotensive Hypokalemia

The acid-base status of normotensive, hypokalemia patients with renal potassium wasting should be assessed (Fig. 50.4). Hypokalemia occurs in both renal tubular acidosis and diabetic ketoacidosis. Measuring urine chloride can help distinguish hypokalemic, metabolic alkalosis caused by GI losses from that due to renal losses (43). Upper GI fluid loss is typically associated with low urinary chloride concentration while a high urinary chloride concentration is seen during active diuretic use and with unusual disorders like Bartter syndrome (see Bartter and Gitelman Syndromes). The high urinary chloride concentration that is seen during active or recent diuretic use is typically followed by paradoxically low urine chloride after the drug has been discontinued. Diuretic abuse and self-induced vomiting are commonly concealed causes of hypokalemia and metabolic alkalosis.

Hypomagnesemia is a common finding in up to 40% of hypokalemic patients. Although the mechanism is incompletely understood, enhanced aldosterone secretion is believed to play a role by increasing the urinary excretion of magnesium. Hypomagnesemia of any cause can cause hypokalemia as a result of fecal as well as urinary losses. Serum magnesium therefore should be measured during the evaluation of any refractory hypokalemic patient.

Bartter and Gitelman Syndromes

Bartter syndrome consists of hypokalemic metabolic alkalosis, excessive urinary potassium losses, and normal blood pressure, without edema (40). Plasma renin activity and aldosterone levels are significantly elevated. This presentation is mimicked by diuretic abuse and surreptitious vomiting, from which Bartter syndrome must be differentiated. A urine screening test for surreptitious diuretic use should be done. Urinary chloride is elevated in Bartter syndrome and decreased in surreptitious vomiting. Hypokalemia is usually refractory to potassium supplementation but may be ameliorated by administration of prostaglandin synthesis inhibitors (e.g., nonsteroidal anti-inflammatory drugs [NSAIDs]) or by amiloride 5 to 10 mg/day.

Gitelman syndrome consists of hypokalemic metabolic alkalosis, excessive urinary potassium losses, and normal blood pressure, without edema but also with hypomagnesemia and hypocalciuria. A defect in the thiazide-sensitive sodium chloride transporter causes patients with this condition to appear as if they were taking thiazide diuretics (40).

SPECIFIC REFERENCES*

1. Cohn JN, Kowey PR, Whelton PK, et al. New guidelines for potassium replacement in clinical practice: a contemporary review by the National Council on Potassium in Clinical Practice. Arch Int Med 2000;160:2429.
2. Sterns RH, Cox M, Feig PU, et al. Internal potassium balance and the control of the plasma potassium concentration. Medicine 1981;60:339.
3. McDonough AA, Thompson CB, Youn JH. Skeletal muscle regulates extracellular potassium. Am J Physiol Renal Physiol 2002;282:F967.
4. Siegel D, Hulley SB, Black DM, et al. Diuretics, serum and intracellular electrolyte levels, and ventricular arrhythmias in hypertensive men. JAMA 1992;267:1083.
5. Kuller LH, Hulley SB, Cohen JD, et al. Unexpected effects of treating hypertension in men with electrocardiographic abnormalities: a critical analysis. Circulation 1986;73:114.
6. Caralis PV, Materson BJ, Perez-Stable E. Potassium and diuretic-induced ventricular arrhythmias in ambulatory hypertensive patients. Miner Electrolyte Metab 1984;10:148.
7. Franse LV, Pahor M, Di Bari M, et al. Hypokalemia associated with diuretic use and cardiovascular events in the Systolic Hypertension in the Elderly Program. Hypertension 2000;35:1025.
8. Cohen HW, Madhavan S, Alderman MH. High and low serum potassium associated with cardiovascular events in diuretic-treated patients. J Hypertens 2001;19:1315.
9. Langford HG. Dietary potassium and hypertension: epidemiological data. Ann Intern Med 1983;98(Suppl):770.
10. Linas SL. The role of potassium in the pathogenesis and treatment of hypertension. Kidney Int 1991;39:771.
11. Intersalt: an international study of electrolyte excretion and blood pressure. Results for 24 hour urinary sodium and potassium excretion. Intersalt Cooperative Research Group. BMJ 1988;297:319.
12. McCarron DA, Morris CD, Henry HJ, et al. Blood pressure and nutrient intake in the United States. Science 1984;224:1392.
13. Frisancho AR, Leonard WR, Bollettino LA. Blood pressure in blacks and whites and its relationship to dietary sodium and potassium intake. J Chronic Dis 1984;37:515.
14. Appel LJ, Moore TJ, Obarzanek E, et al. A clinical trial of the effects of dietary patterns on blood pressure. DASH Collaborative Research Group. N Engl J Med 1997;336:1117.
15. Brancati FL, Appel LJ, Seidler AJ, et al. Effect of potassium supplementation on blood pressure in African Americans on a low-potassium diet. A randomized, double-blind, placebo-controlled trial. Arch Intern Med 1996;156:61.
16. Siani A, Strazzullo P, Giacco A, et al. Increasing the dietary potassium intake reduces the need for antihypertensive medication. Ann Intern Med 1991;115:753.
17. Siani A, Strazzullo P, Russo L, et al. Controlled trial of long term oral potassium supplements in patients with mild hypertension. BMJ 1987;294:1453.
18. Svetkey LP, Yarger WE, Feussner JR, et al. Double-blind, placebo-controlled trial of potassium chloride in the treatment of mild hypertension. Hypertension 1987;9:444.
19. Whelton PK, He J, Cutler JA, et al. Effects of oral potassium on blood pressure: metaanalysis of randomized controlled clinical trials. JAMA 1997;277:1624.
20. Khaw KT, Barrett-Connor E. Dietary potassium in stroke-associated mortality: a 12-year prospective population study. N Engl J Med 1987;316:235.
21. Bernardo JF, Murakami S, Branch RA, et al. Potassium depletion potentiates amphotericin-B-induced toxicity to renal tubules. Nephron 1995;70:235.
22. Menahem SA, Perry GJ, Dowling J, et al. Hypokalaemia-induced acute renal failure. Nephrol Dial Transplant 1999;14:2216.
23. Abdel-Rahman EM, Moorthy AV. End-stage renal disease (ESRD) in patients with eating disorders. Clin Nephrol 1997;47:106.
24. Narins RG, Jones ER, Stom MC, et al. Diagnostic strategies in disorders of fluid, electrolyte and acid–base homeostasis. Am J Med 1982;72:496.
25. Reimann D, Gross P. Chronic, diagnosis-resistant hypokalaemia. Nephrol Dial Transplant 1999;14:2957.
26. Sterns RH, Spital A. Disorders of internal potassium balance. Semin Nephrol 1987;7:399.
27. Morgan DB, Young RM. Acute transient hypokalemia: new interpretation of a common event. Lancet 1982;2:751.
28. Heller SR, Robinson RT. Hypoglycemia and associated hypokaelemia in diabetes: Mechanisms, clinical implications and

*Bold numerals denote published controlled clinical trials, meta-analyses, or consensus-based recommendations.

prevention. Diabetes Obes Metab 2000;2:75.
29. Ahlawat SK, Sachdev A. Hypokalaemic paralysis. Postgrad Med J 1999;75:193.
30. McFadzean AJ, Yeung R. Periodic paralysis complicating thyrotoxicosis in Chinese. BMJ 1967;1:451.
31. Ethier JH, Kamel KS, Magner PO, et al. The transtubular potassium concentration in patients with hypokalemia and hyperkalemia. Am J Kidney Dis 1990;15:309.
32. Kassirer JP, Schwartz WB. The response of normal man to selective depletion of hydrochloric acid. Am J Med 1966;40:10.
33. Kassirer JP, Berkman PM, Lawrenz DR, et al. The critical role of chloride in the correction of hypokalemic alkalosis in man. Am J Med 1965;38:172.
34. Morgan DB, Davidson C. Hypokalemia and diuretics: an analysis of publications. BMJ 1980;280:905.
35. Nader PC, Thompson JR, Alpern RJ. Complications of diuretic use. Semin Nephrol 1988;8:365.
36. Tannen RL. Diuretic-induced hypokalemia. Kidney Int 1985;28:988.
37. Gennari FJ. Hypokalemia. N Engl J Med 1998;339:451.
38. Papademetriou V, Burris J, Kukich S, et al. Effectiveness of potassium chloride or triamterene in thiazide hypokalemia. Arch Intern Med 1985;145:1986.
39. Ridgeway NA, Ginn DR, Alley K. Outpatient conversion of treatment to potassium-sparing diuretics. Am J Med 1986;80:785.
40. Scheinman SJ, Guay-Woodford LM, Thakker RV, et al. Genetic disorders of renal electrolyte transport. N Engl J Med 1999;340:1177.
41. Montori VM, Young WF Jr. Use of plasma aldosterone concentration-to-plasma renin activity ratio as a screening test for primary aldosteronism. A systematic review of the literature. Endocrinol Metab Clin North Am 2002;31:619.
42. Mulatero P, Stowasser M, Loh KC, et al. Increased diagnosis of primary aldosteronism, including surgically correctable forms, in centers from five continents. J Clin Endocrinol Metab 2004;89:1045.
43. Kamel KS, Ethier JH, Richardson RM, et al. Urine electrolytes and osmolality: when and how to use them. Am J Nephrol 1990;10:89.

*For annotated **General References** and resources related to this chapter, visit www.hopkinsbayview.org/PAMreferences.*

Chapter 51

Urinary Stones

David A. Spector

Urinary stones are common in the United States. Although urologic intervention or nephrologic consultation may occasionally be required, most patients with stones can be evaluated, treated, and monitored by the primary care provider. This chapter reviews the various manifestations of stone disease, the types of urinary stones, the evaluation of patients with stones, the acute and chronic treatment of patients with urinary stones, and when to obtain consultation for these patients.

PRESENTATION OF URINARY STONE DISEASE

Patients with urinary stone disease may present with acute colic, persistent or recurrent urinary tract infection, isolated hematuria, no symptoms but a stone discovered incidentally on a radiograph taken for other purposes, or a prior history of stones.

Acute Colic

Presentation

Most patients with urinary stones at some time have an acute episode of colic. The stone, if obstructing, causes ureteral spasm, resulting in intermittent paroxysms of pain, which may range from barely noticeable to "the most severe in my life." The location of the pain depends on the location of the stone in the ureter, but it is most often felt in the flank; then, as the stone moves distally, pain radiates in a characteristic pattern around the groin and into the testicles in men or into the labia majora in women. Dysuria and urgency may be present and nausea, vomiting, and other gastrointestinal (GI) symptoms might mistakenly suggest a primary GI problem. Examination reveals an uncomfortable, restless patient. There may be costovertebral tenderness as well as deep tenderness in the abdomen. More importantly, no signs of peritoneal irritation (guarding, rebound, rigidity) are present. Fever is not present unless infection has developed in the obstructed urinary tract. Urinalysis demonstrates microscopic (or gross) hematuria in 91% of cases (1). The presence of pyuria is important because chronic bacterial infection may be associated with the development of urinary stones; however, pyuria may be absent even if infection is present if there is complete urethral obstruction.

A patient with a history strongly suggestive of urinary stone disease may have another cause for the pain. A dissection of the aorta, acute back strain or lumbar disc disease, the passage of blood clots in the ureters (as in sickle cell disease or renal infarct), and, rarely, malingering should be considered. Malingerers are often difficult to identify; these patients may give a classic history of acute renal colic while relating a history of allergy to iodinated contrast dye, prohibiting the performance of an intravenous pyelogram (IVP). These patients may even contaminate the urine specimen they provide for analysis with blood (obtained from a fingerstick or oral injury). (For further information on malingering, see Chapter 21.)

Diagnosis and Management

The aims of management of urinary colic should be confirmation of the diagnosis, relief of discomfort, surveillance for infection, and determination of whether the stones will pass spontaneously or will require surgical removal. For decades, the IVP and abdominal plain film were the standard diagnostic procedures for patients with renal colic, but unenhanced helical computed tomography (CT) is now the imaging technique of choice for the examination of patients with suspected renal calculi (2,3). Although it is more expensive than IVP, unenhanced helical CT is faster, requires no contrast dye exposure, and has greater sensitivity (95%) and specificity (100%) for urinary stones than the IVP (2). Further, CT can give helpful information about other abdominal diseases if urinary stones are not present. On the other hand, IVP gives more information about anatomic urinary tract abnormalities that might predispose to stone formation (e.g., medullary sponge kidney, diverticula). In either case a plain abdominal film should be obtained to assess if the stone(s) is radiolucent (up to 90% of urinary stones are radiopaque) and therefore likely to represent a uric acid or indinavir stone, and as a baseline for future followup radiographs.

Several factors help in the decision whether to hospitalize a patient with renal colic, to obtain urgent urologic consultation, or to treat the patient at home: First, the patient with nausea and vomiting cannot be ensured of an adequate fluid intake or adequate oral analgesia and should be admitted to a hospital. Second, fever suggests infection proximal to an obstructing stone, and urgent urologic consultation should be obtained and hospitalization considered. Third, if the CT scan or IVP reveals a nonfunctioning kidney (completely obstructed ureter), a partially obstructed ureter from a solitary kidney, or urine extravasation, urgent urologic consultation should be obtained. Fourth, the size of the stone helps the clinician to predict whether urologic intervention is likely to be required. In general, stones that are smaller than 5 mm pass spontaneously, those between 5 and 10 mm have a 50% chance of passing spontaneously, and those larger than 10 mm usually require urologic intervention. Of all stones that become symptomatic, 80% are ureteral, and 85% to 90% of these pass spontaneously. Ureteral stones commonly lodge in the ureteropelvic junction, in the ureter at the pelvic brim where the ureter begins to pass over the iliac vessels, in the lower third of the ureter, or at the ureterovesical junction. Only 10% to 15% of ureteral stones require interventional treatment (4).

Once the diagnosis of urinary calculi is confirmed and complications ruled out, most patients can be treated at home. Although the colic associated with urinary calculi has traditionally been treated with narcotics, nonsteroidal anti-inflammatory drugs (NSAIDs) may be more effective. This is so because NSAIDs block prostaglandins, which are known to induce ureteral muscle spasm. In a meta-analysis of randomized controlled trials, NSAIDs provided a greater reduction of pain and less side effects than narcotics (5). Further, NSAID-treated patients were less likely to require "rescue" analgesia. Patients may initially require parenteral administration of either class of analgesics, but rapid conversion to oral medications is usually possible. Indomethacin (Indocin or generic, 50 mg orally or by rectal suppository three to four times per day), ketorolac (Toradol, 10 mg every 4 to 6 hours orally; or 30 mg intravenously or intramuscularly every 6 hours), or diclofenac (Voltaren, 50 mg orally two to three times daily) all provide effective analgesia in renal colic (5). Since NSAIDs may cause GI side effects, simultaneous provision of an H_2 receptor blocker or proton pump inhibitor (PPI) should be considered. Narcotics are a second choice for relief of renal colic. Oxycodone (generic, 5 mg, 1 to 3 tablets) or Tylox, which contains oxycodone and acetaminophen (1 to 3 capsules), every 3 to 4 hours, is a reasonable choice. If needed phenothiazine (e.g., Phenergan, 25 mg), given with the narcotic, provides additional relief by controlling any associated nausea. After pain is relieved, hydration with at least 2 to 3 liters of fluid daily will ensure good urinary flow and will help the stone to pass. All of the urine voided during the period of intermittent colic (usually several days) should be collected and strained through an old stocking, a fine-knit screen, or a filter paper so that the passed stone may be saved and analyzed (see below). Some patients may not realize that a passed "stone" may resemble sand more than a pebble.

If symptoms of colic are intermittent and well controlled at home, the patient should be monitored with a weekly radiograph of the abdomen to determine the progression of the stone. Average expected length of time to stone passage is dependent in part on stone size: for a stone $\leq$2 mm, 8.2 days; between 2 and 4 mm, 12.2 days; $\geq$4 mm, 22.1 days (6). Calcium channel blockers (CCBs) (e.g., nifedipine 30 mg slow release) or tamsulosin (e.g., Flomax 0.4 mg once daily) may significantly shorten the time to stone passage (7). If by 6 weeks the stone has not passed, it is unlikely that spontaneous passage will occur, and urologic consultation should be obtained. For occupational or social reasons, some patients want to consider earlier surgical removal and therefore ask their primary care providers to request urologic consultation sooner.

Stones that pass from the ureter into the bladder usually pass with ease through the urethra. In the event of a bladder outlet obstruction, a stone may be retained in the bladder (*bladder stone*), where it may grow and in time become an infection stone (see Struvite Stones).

Patient Requiring Urologic Referral

When a patient is referred to a urologist for *stone removal,* there are four options: *extracorporeal shock wave lithotripsy (ESWL), percutaneous nephrostolithotomy (PCNL), rigid and flexible ureteroscopy, and open surgery.* During ureteroscopy, lower ureteral stones may be removed with the use of a grasping forceps that is inserted through a cystoscope or ureteroscope or pulverized by ultrasonic, electrohydraulic, or laser lithotripsy. These procedures are similar to cystoscopic examination but require general or spinal anesthesia and hospitalization. These procedures have a success rate greater than 95% and a low rate of complications. Until the early 1980s, stones located more proximally required removal by open ureterolithotomy, open pyelolithotomy, or, in the case of a staghorn calculus, nephrolithotomy. However, PCNL and ESWL have supplanted traditional open stone removal operations. Both techniques give results similar to operative stone removal but are associated with less convalescence time and less morbidity.

PCNL requires that the patient be sedated and an IVP or ultrasound be performed to localize the kidney and the stone. Under fluoroscopy, a percutaneous nephrostomy tube is placed near the posterior axillary line. Subsequently, the tract is dilated and various nephroscopes, buckets, and forceps are used to extract the calculi. For struvite calculi (also called triple phosphate or "infection" stones; see later discussion), *hemiacidrin (Renacidin) irrigation* is sometimes useful to dissolve residual stones. Antegrade radiographs are performed to confirm stone removal and ureteral patency. Successful removal occurs with more than 95% of renal stones and 88% of ureteral stones. On the other hand, PCNL is associated with a significant incidence of complications, including major bleeding (5% to 12%), arteriovenous fistulae (0.6%), perforation/extravasation (5% to 26%), and fever or sepsis (3% to 11%) (8). Typically, a 2- to 3-day hospitalization is needed for a patient to undergo PCNL.

ESWL sometimes requires that the patient have anesthesia (usually spinal), but most often it is performed with only intravenous sedation, after which the stone is located by ultrasound or fluoroscopy. A shock wave, generated by an electrode similar to a spark plug, is focused by the lithotripter for a precise impact on the stone (Fig. 51.1). When the shock wave encounters calculus material that has different acoustic properties from surrounding tissue, a tensile force is produced that shatters that material. This treatment takes an average of 30 to 45 minutes. ESWL usually is done in outpatient settings. After ESWL, fragments of stone usually pass in the urine for a few days and cause mild colic. Retreatment is needed in a few patients, and macroscopic hematuria occurs transiently in most.

The selection of treatment modalities for a given patient depends in part on the characteristics of the stone being treated and in part on local resources and expertise. Where all modalities are available, ESWL used alone is the treatment of choice in 70% of patients. Patients who are suitable for treatment with ESWL are those who have single or multiple renal stones less than 20 mm in diameter, some patients with smaller staghorn stones (those in which the pelvis is not dilated), and some with stones located in the upper third of the ureter. Larger calculi, most staghorn calculi, and calculi composed of cystine (see later discussion) are usually treated by PCNL in combination with ESWL, or by open operation alone.

Results of ESWL are excellent. For patients with stones less than 10 mm in size that are located in the kidney or ureter, 90% become stone free or are left with small, asymptomatic residual fragments. Convalescence from ESWL requires several days. Most patients experience some flank discomfort from the trauma to the kidney. This discomfort often requires use of analgesics for a few days. Immediate complications of ESWL are uncommon, but renal or perirenal tissue injury has been demonstrated in experimental studies and suggested by MRI and tissue enzyme release in up to 85% of patients. Between 1% and 8% of patients develop new hypertension or experience an exacerbation of pre-existing hypertension within 3 years after

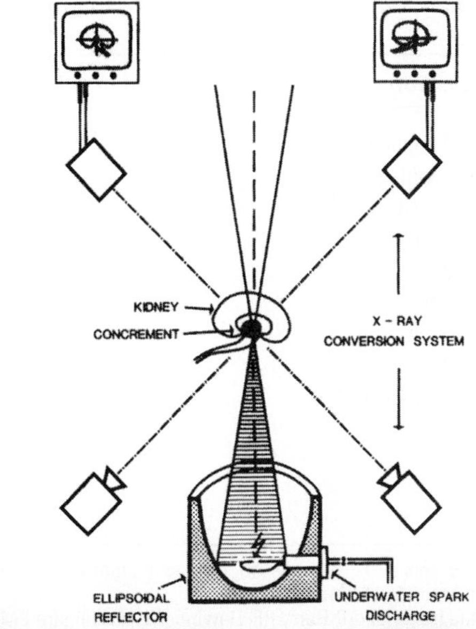

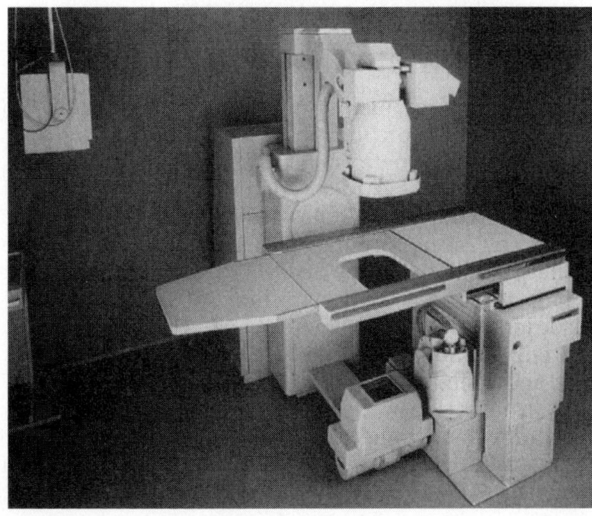

FIGURE 51.1. **Series A:** Schematic drawing of the technical arrangement of a modern lithotripter. (Adapted from Chaussy C, Schmiedt E, Jocham D. Nonsurgical treatment of renal calculi with shock waves. In: Roth RA, Finlayson BF (eds.) Stones Clinical management of Urolithiasis. Baltimore: Williams Wilkins, 1983.) **B:** Photograph of a modern lithotripter. (Courtesy of Domier Medical Systems, Inc, Kennesaw, GA.)

ESWL treatment (9,10). The frequency of this complication may depend on the type of lithotripter.

Other Patterns of Stone Presentation

Urinary stones usually produce symptoms that suggest acute colic, at least at some time in their course. When stones are discovered in patients who do not have colic, the same evaluation and management is indicated as when patients have acute colic (see Diagnostic Workup for Patients with Urinary Stone Disease).

TABLE 51.1 Classification of Stone-Forming Patients by Type of Stone Passed

Type of Stone	*Coe Series (1,431 Patients)*	*Other Series Combined (1,870 Patients)*
Calcium oxalate (with or without phosphate)	69[a]	63.2[a]
Calcium phosphate	2	7.4
Calcium and uric acid	10	
Uric acid	2	5.4
Cystine	1	2.5
Struvite	7	21.5
Unknown	10	

[a] All values expressed as percentages of patients in each series.
From Coe FL. Nephrolithiasis: pathogenesis and treatment. Chicago: Year Book Medical Publishers, 1988.

TYPES OF STONES AND THEIR CAUSES

There are four main types of urinary calculi: calcium oxalate or phosphate, uric acid, struvite–triple phosphate (magnesium ammonium phosphate), and cystine. Calcium stones are by far the most common. Table 51.1 shows the classification of stone-forming patients by the type of stone passed. Not shown in the table are uncommon stones made of xanthine, triamterene, indinavir, or nelfinavir.

It is important to be familiar with the metabolic disorders these patients may have. This understanding is helpful in planning a diagnostic evaluation and specific therapy (see later sections in this chapter). This is particularly true in the evaluation of the patient with the most common stone type, calcium.

Calcium Stones

Table 51.2 shows the metabolic and clinical disorders in calcium stone formers. This table shows that in almost 80% of patients who have had a calcium stone, a specific cause can be identified. In addition to the common disorders shown in the table, other metabolic disorders, such as hypocitraturia, may promote urinary calcium salt precipitation. Hypocitraturia is present as the sole metabolic abnormality in 10% (11) and as one of two or three abnormalities in 19% (12) of calcium stone formers. Urine pH, which affects the prevalence of many types of stones (see Urinalysis), has little influence on the formation of calcium oxalate stones, but formation of calcium phosphate stones

TABLE 51.2 Metabolic and Clinical Disorders in 978 Calcium Oxalate Stone Formers

	No. of Patients (%)	
Disorders	**Men**	**Women**
Systemic Disease		
Primary hyperparathyroidism[a]	26 (4)	24 (10)
Sarcoid	6 (1)	1 (1)
Cushing syndrome	5 (1)	1 (0.4)
Paget disease	1 (0.1)	4 (2)
Renal tubular acidosis, type I	7 (1)	4 (2)
Enteric hyperoxaluria[b]	39 (5)	13 (5)
No Systemic Disease		
Idiopathic (hereditary) hypercalciuria	213 (29)	121 (49)
Hyperuricosuria	126 (17)	9 (4)
Both disorders	120 (16)	22 (9)
No metabolic disorders[c]	186 (26)	52 (11)
Total	**729**	**249**

[a]Seventeen additional patients had primary hyperparathyroidism: either their stones were admixed with uric acid, struvite, or cystine; they had stones with no calcium; or their stone type was unknown.
[b]Includes primary hyperoxaluria (three patients) and hyperoxaluria as a consequence of intestinal bypass for obesity.
[c]Urinary citrate data not available; hypocitraturia has been found alone or in combination with other disorders in 19% of hypercalciurias.
From Coe FL. Nephrolithiasis: pathogenesis and treatment. Chicago: Year Book Medical Publishers, 1988.

is promoted at a pH greater than 6. The approach to these disorders is discussed later in this chapter.

Uric Acid Stones

Uric acid stones are caused by the high insolubility of undissociated uric acid (its pK of 5.7 means that 50% of uric acid is undissociated at pH 5.7 and 90% is undissociated at pH 4.7). Three factors are associated with uric acid stone formation: hyperuricosuria, highly acid urine, and low urinary volume. The lifetime incidence of uric acid stones in the general population is very low (Table 51.3). On the other hand, uric acid stones are very prevalent in patients who have gout, asymptomatic hyperuricemia, and hyperuricosuria, and probably in patients with a history of gout and no hyperuricemia. Many patients have passed uric acid stones long before a gouty attack has occurred. It is known that many patients with gout produce an abnormally high fraction of their daily acid load as titratable acid rather than as ammonium and therefore have an unusually low average urinary pH. Furthermore, patients with chronic diarrhea and those with excessive fluid loss from the skin may have highly concentrated urine, which predisposes them to the formation of uric acid calculi. Patients who have myeloproliferative disease and those with

TABLE 51.3 Prevalence of Urate Stones in Various Populations

Population	Lifetime Incidence (%)
General population	0.01
Patients with gout	22
Hyperuricosuria in primary gout[a] (mg/24 hr)	
<300	11
300–699	21
700–1100	35
>1100	50
Hyperuricemia in men[b] (mg/dL)	
7–8	12.7
8–9	22
>9	40

[a]Adapted from Yu T-F, Gutman AB. Uric acid nephrolithiasis in gout. Ann Intern Med 1967;67:1133.
[b]Adapted from Hall AP, Barry PE, Dawber TR, McNamara PM. Epidemiology of gout and hyperuricemia. Am J Med 1967;42:27.

solid tumors that are undergoing lysis may have excessive uric acid excretion, which may be associated with uric acid stones and tubular plugs of urate. Patients with gout also have more calcium stones than people in the general population (13). The association may result from crystallization of uric acid, which then forms a nidus for calcium deposition.

Struvite Stones (Infection Stones)

It is generally believed that infection stones form primarily as a consequence of the hydrolysis of urea and the production of ammonia by the bacterial enzyme, urease. The production of ammonia leads to a highly alkaline urine, which promotes the precipitation of magnesium, ammonium, and phosphate. These are the components of the infection-induced or struvite stone. Most urea-splitting organisms are *Proteus* species; however, *Pseudomonas, Klebsiella, Staphylococcus,* and some *Escherichia coli* strains are capable of producing urease. Struvite stones usually do not form *de novo* but almost always are a complication of another primary stone disease in which infection has become superimposed, and they are especially likely to grow into staghorn calculi (large stones that cannot pass the ureteropelvic junction and that form a cast of all or a portion of the pelvicaliceal system).

Cystine Stones

Cystine stones are rare and usually are seen in young patients, because the onset is usually in childhood. The stone forms because of crystallization of cystine when the urine is supersaturated with this substance, which occurs when

TABLE 51.4 Urinary Cystine Excretion

Subjects	*Excretion (milligrams per day)*
Normal individuals	<100
Heterozygotes for cystinuria	150–300
Homozygotes for cystinuria	>600

there is an inherited defect in renal tubular resorption of filtered cystine. This is a particularly virulent form of stone disease and may be associated with staghorn calculi. In addition to cystinuria, there is usually urinary loss of other basic amino acids, including ornithine, lysine, and arginine. The disorder is an inherited autosomal recessive trait, although some heterozygous patients have excess cystine excretion, as shown in Table 51.4. Cystine is much less soluble in acid urine than it is in alkaline urine; therefore, cystine stones generally form when urine is acid and cystine excretion is greater than 400 mg/24 hours.

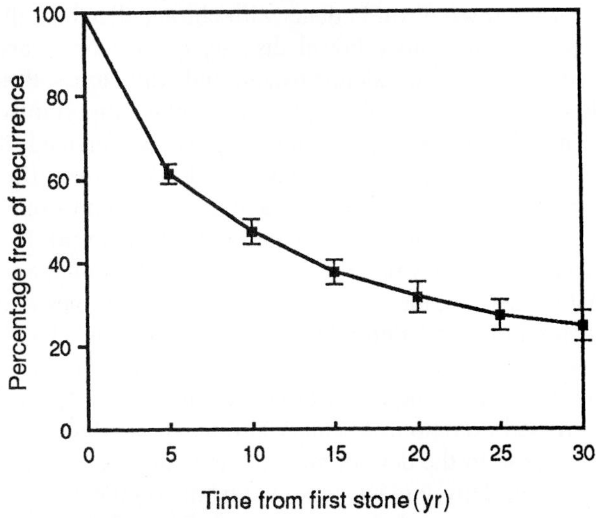

FIGURE 51.2. Life-table calculation of the time course of recurrence after a first renal stone in 515 patients. (From Sutherland JW, Parks JH, Coe FL. Recurrence after a single renal stone in a community practice. Miner Electrolyte Metab 1985;11:267.)

NATURAL HISTORY OF URINARY STONE DISEASE

Urinary calculus disease is a chronic illness. Once a stone has formed there is a tendency for recurrence, and management should be tailored to the stone activity, the type of stone, and any associated metabolic abnormality.

Stone activity—the number of stones formed and the change in size of existing stones—is an important, although at times difficult, determination. It requires a yearly review of stones passed and removed, as well as an evaluation by abdominal radiography of the increase in size of known stones or of the appearance of new stones. The activity of urinary calculi depends on a number of factors: stone type, associated metabolic abnormality, treatment received (both specific and nonspecific), and age. Therefore, precise rates of recurrence cannot be given with accuracy.

Nevertheless, two studies have provided useful and corroborative information regarding the recurrence rate after passage of a first urinary stone. In one retrospective study of 515 patients who were monitored after a single (first) stone and were given no medications to prevent a recurrence, there was a 50% recurrence rate at approximately 9 years and approximately 75% recurrence by 25 years (14). These data are presented as a graph in Fig. 51.2. Another study of patients who passed their first calcium stone showed a recurrence in half of the patients by 5 years and in two-thirds by 9 years (15).

Therefore, it is suggested that evaluation for associated metabolic abnormalities be undertaken in every patient who has formed a new stone, because recurrence is likely, the basic assessment is noninvasive and inexpensive, and a workup may uncover an especially virulent or an important systemic disease or metabolic defect responsible for stone formation.

DIAGNOSTIC WORKUP FOR PATIENTS WITH URINARY STONE DISEASE

Evaluation of patients with stone disease can be accomplished entirely in an ambulatory setting. This evaluation depends on a directed history and physical examination, stone analysis, if the stone is available, and certain laboratory measurements. The extent of the evaluation of patients passing a first stone is somewhat controversial. Some suggest an abbreviated evaluation, because not all patients have recurrent stones and because all treatment modalities have potential side effects; others, citing the likelihood of eventual recurrence, fully evaluate patients after the first stone passage (see Coe et al., at www.hopkinsbayview.org/PAMreferences). The approach outlined in this section is a reasonable and commonly used method for evaluation of patients who have had a urinary calculus (16).

History

A directed medical history is important in determining the activity of stone disease as well as in providing clues to the nature of the stone. The number of passed stones, the frequency of attacks of colic or hematuria, and any history of infection should be obtained. Since most stones are composed of calcium, all conditions that might result in hypercalcemia must be considered, particularly hyperparathyroidism. Patients with chronic diarrheal illnesses, inflammatory bowel disease, or colostomy are predisposed to both calcium oxalate and urate stones. Previous abdominal radiographs and, most importantly, chemical analysis of prior stones should be obtained, if possible. The *family history* may provide a clue to cystine stones, uric acid stones (gout), and many calcium stones (e.g., those associated with idiopathic hypercalciuria). The *dietary history* may reveal excessive intake of sodium, animal protein, purine, or oxalate (see Types of Stones and Their Causes). High-protein meat diets are associated with production of metabolic acids (which leach bone and cause hypercalciuria), increased urine excretion of urate, and decreased excretion of urinary citrate, all of which may predispose to the development of stone disease. The approximate daily *fluid intake* is also an important part of the history. Some people ingest as little as 500 to 700 mL/day and therefore have concentrated urine most of the day. The *medication history* is important. For example, aspirin at high dosages (more than 5 g/day) and probenecid are associated with increased uric acid excretion and may cause a predisposition to uric acid calculi. On the other hand, use of the xanthine oxidase inhibitor allopurinol has led to development of xanthine stones. Use of calcium-containing antacids (e.g., Titralac, Tempo, Tums) as well as vitamins A and D and loop diuretics (e.g., furosemide) may be associated with hypercalciuria and calcium stone formation. Acetazolamide (Diamox) may be associated with the development of chronically alkaline urine and with a higher incidence of calculi made of calcium phosphate. Vitamin C at high dosages can cause hyperoxaluria and increase the risk of stones (17). Triamterene (contained in Dyazide) and its metabolites (18), as well as acyclovir, indinavir (19), and nelfinavir (20) have been found as a nidus in urinary calculi (or as the only constituent). Moreover, certain medications have been shown to decrease calcium excretion (e.g., thiazides) or uric acid excretion (e.g., allopurinol), whereas loop diuretics promote hypercalciuria and interfere with results of testing in a patient who is being evaluated for renal stone disease. The *occupational history* is important because exposure to excessive heat (and therefore fluid losses) and limited accessibility to fluids are factors that influence stone formation by decreasing urine output and by promoting the output of highly concentrated urine.

Physical Examination

Physical examination (when there is no colic) occasionally gives clues to specific problems. For example, band keratopathy (stippled calcification of the perimeter of the cornea, which may require a slit-lamp for visualization) may be seen in hyperparathyroidism, or there may be signs of sarcoidosis, hyperthyroidism, inflammatory bowel disease, neoplasia, or gouty arthritis.

Urinalysis

The urinalysis provides a simple assessment that may give specific direction to the determination of the cause of the urinary calculus. It is important that the urinalysis be complete, including the determination of pH. The pH is usually acid in patients with a uric acid or a cystine stone and is invariably alkaline in patients with struvite stones. Also, the pH may suggest the presence of renal tubular acidosis. Because the first voided morning urine is usually acid, a urine pH greater than 6.0 in such a specimen suggests the possibility of renal tubular acidosis. The microscopic analysis may show hematuria (although this is often absent in the intercritical period), crystals, or evidence of infection. Crystals of cystine have the appearance of a benzene ring and are highly suggestive of cystinuria. Other crystals are more variable and are not diagnostic but may give a clue to the stone composition in patients with lithiasis (see Coe et al., at www.hopkinsbayview.org/PAMreferences for photographs of typical examples). In patients with calcium stones crystalluria, when repeatedly found in early morning urine samples, the finding is highly predictive of stone recurrence (21).

Stone Analysis

If a stone is available, it should be analyzed to determine its composition, because the stone type determines the approach to evaluation and treatment. Stones can be analyzed inexpensively at commercial laboratories and may be mailed without preservative for this purpose.

Laboratory Assessment

A laboratory assessment is important even for patients in whom a stone is available for analysis (Table 51.5). This evaluation is necessary because it is increasingly recognized that many patients have more than one metabolic disorder that predisposes them to stone formation. For example, struvite stones often start as some other primary stone type, most often calcium; patients with a calcium oxalate stone may have hypercalciuria, hyperuricosuria, or hypocitraturia. Patients usually comply with the testing necessary for proper evaluation of a metabolic disorder if they understand the ease with which it can be accomplished, the substantial rate of recurrent calculi, and the effectiveness of specific therapy for metabolic problems (see Preventive Treatment of Urinary Calculus Disease). The 24-hour urine volume and individual constituents provide objective guides about when the most basic interventions, such as increasing fluid intake (if urinary volume is low) or decreasing salt intake (if sodium excretion is high), are useful (see General Measures) and provide baseline data to ascertain the effectiveness of treatment at followup.

TABLE 52.7 Clinical Presentations of Atheromatous Renal Disease

Acute renal failure following reduction in blood pressure (particularly with ACE inhibitors)
Progressive azotemia in a patient with known renovascular disease
Azotemia associated with new-onset hypertension or a change in severity of hypertension
Unexplained azotemia in an elderly patient with peripheral arterial disease
Progressive renal failure with evidence of cholesterol embolization

Adapted from Jacobson HR. Ischemic renal disease: an overlooked entity? Kidney Int 1988;34:729.

which depends on captopril-induced hemodynamic alterations (and is helpful in diagnosing unilateral renal artery stenosis in the absence of significant renal failure), is less valuable in patients with renal insufficiency and suspected bilateral renovascular disease, and often is not diagnostic. *Doppler or duplex sonography* has been used as a screening tool for diagnosing bilateral renal artery stenosis, but these modalities do not provide anatomic detail and are operator dependent. An arteriogram should be obtained if the index of suspicion is high and a therapeutic decision (e.g., balloon dilation, often with stent placement) would be made based on the results. *Gadolinium-enhanced magnetic resonance imaging* has become another less invasive means of assessing the renal arteries in high-risk patients with suspected renal artery stenosis. It avoids the use of potentially nephrotoxic radiographic dyes and the use of intra-arterial catheters and is recommended by many nephrologists as a screening test in patients suspected of having renovascular disease. *Carbon dioxide angiography* provides good definition without the use of traditional dyes. *Intravenous digital subtraction angiography* has been suggested as a lower-risk method of imaging the renal arteries, because the risks of dye-induced acute renal failure (ARF) or atheroembolic disease appear to be reduced, probably because of the lesser amount of dye given and the use of smaller catheters. Finally, *high-speed spiral CT scans* produce excellent images of the renal arteries and veins, but require a large infusion of radiocontrast material. Given the complex decisions encountered when evaluating patients with suspected ischemic renal artery disease, a vascular surgeon, a radiologist, or a nephrologist should be consulted before a modality for imaging the kidneys is selected. The most difficult decisions arise in patients with probable diabetic nephropathy, who often have significant peripheral arterial disease. The decision to perform angiography is usually based on the clinical judgment that the course deviates from what is usually seen in diabetics, or when the vascular component seems prominent (severe hypertension, claudication, bruits).

The incidence of *radiocontrast-induced ARF* seems highest in patients with serum creatinine concentrations greater than 1.6 mg/dL, diabetic patients, and in the elderly. The incidence of ARF ranges from 3% to 50% depending on the presence of risk factors, on the type of radiocontrast agent employed, and on whether prophylactic measures have been used (see below) (11,12). In most cases the rise in serum creatinine after administration of radiocontrast agents is transient and small. The use of a nonionic, iso-osmotic radiocontrast agent like iodixinol, appears to reduce the occurrence of postangiography ARF in patients with pre-existing renal insufficiency (13). The use of the antioxidant acetylcysteine (600 mg orally twice a day, the day before and the day of the study) in combination with intravenous saline has been shown to reduce the frequency of renal function deterioration after the administration of nonionic, iso-osmolar radiocontrast agents in patients with renal insufficiency (14). In one study, the use of sodium bicarbonate given as a 3 mL/kg bolus 1 hour prior to the procedure, followed by a 6-hour infusion, reduced the incidence of ARF as compared to a sodium chloride infusion (15). The benefits of giving mannitol infusions or other pretreatments prophylactically are still unsettled. In summary, the presence of renal insufficiency should not be considered an absolute contraindication to the performance of intravascular dye studies, particularly when the needed information cannot be obtained by alternative means. Because the decline in renal function after use of radiocontrast materials appears to be particularly preventable by avoiding volume depletion, patients should be instructed to maintain sodium intake (6 to 8 g/day) and fluid intake (1.5 to 2 L/day) both before and after the examination, unless this is otherwise not advisable (e.g., in a patient with congestive heart failure [CHF]). Iso-osmotic radiocontrast agents should be used for patients who have pre-existing renal insufficiency.

Renal Biopsy

Once the baseline data have been accumulated, a nephrologist should be consulted to help interpret the information and to decide whether a renal biopsy is indicated. Early consultation with a nephrologist (if the serum creatinine concentration is greater than 1.5 mg/dL or other signs of significant renal disease are present) is advisable. A complete record of past laboratory investigations, a recent urinalysis, and a recent renal ultrasound test should be provided for patients who are being referred for evaluation of chronic renal insufficiency. If the diagnosis remains unknown despite all available information, a renal biopsy provides histologic information and, for many disease entities, is the most specific diagnostic test available. The biopsy should be considered when the diagnosis is uncertain, to estimate prognosis, to help demonstrate renal involvement of a systemic illness, and to help make therapeutic decisions. Most renal biopsies can be performed percutaneously with the use of local anesthesia.

Although overnight observation in the hospital is still common, many nephrologists perform renal biopsies in ambulatory surgery settings with 6 to 8 hours of postprocedure monitoring (see Chapter 48). If the kidneys are very small or if renal failure is advanced, a biopsy is usually not done.

MONITORING THE PATIENT WITH CHRONIC KIDNEY DISEASE

The interval between visits is determined by the stage of renal insufficiency, the rate of progression, and the presence of complicating disorders. Early in the course, patients should have office visits scheduled every 4 to 6 months for monitoring of their symptoms, signs (e.g., weight, blood pressure, edema), and laboratory data (e.g., serum creatinine concentration, SUN, electrolytes, complete blood count [CBC], urinalysis, and possibly CrCl). As renal failure progresses, visits must be spaced more closely, usually at 1-month intervals until dialysis becomes necessary. Drug dosages of prescription, over-the-counter (OTC), and herbal medications should be reviewed at each visit and adjusted according to the degree of renal dysfunction (see Drug Use in Chronic Kidney Disease, below).

COURSE AND PROGNOSIS

The underlying renal disease largely determines prognosis. Many renal diseases have characteristic rates of progression. For example, patients with polycystic kidney disease typically have very indolent courses and some never progress to ESRD. More aggressive courses, with advanced renal failure developing within months to a year, are more likely to occur in patients with diseases such as rapidly progressive glomerulonephritis, systemic sclerosis, or malignant hypertension. However, most renal diseases fall into an intermediate group, with ESRD developing within 1 to 5 years after the initial diagnosis.

Therapy

Goals

The goals of therapy fall into five major categories. The first is to treat the underlying renal disease, if possible, with specific therapies (e.g., corticosteroids or chlorambucil for membranous nephropathy). The second is to slow the progression of renal deterioration by modifying the known or suspected factors that aggravate the primary process. A number of potentially modifiable factors have been identified that if treated have been shown in animal or human studies to slow the progression of established renal disease (Table 52.8). The third goal is to identify and treat comorbidities that can lead to increased cardiovascular complications (e.g. hypertension, diabetes, hyperlipidemia, anemia). The fourth is to treat the specific complications of renal disease (e.g., acidosis) as they occur, and to prevent the long-term complications of uremia before they can become fully established (e.g., secondary hyperparathyroidism). Finally, the patient should be referred to a dialysis and transplantation center well before the need for renal replacement therapy (see Dialysis and Transplantation).

TABLE 52.8 Modifiable Risk Factors for the Progression of Chronic Kidney Disease (CKD)

Modifiable Risk Factors
Systemic hypertension
Intraglomerular hypertension
Proteinuria
Hyperglycemia
Hyperlipidemia
Nephrotoxic drugs
Inflammation
Hyperuricemia
Microcrystal deposition

Specific Treatments

Once a diagnosis is established, a nephrologist should be consulted, if not already accomplished, to determine whether effective therapy is available for the patient's renal disease. In general, the earlier in the course a treatment is started, the more likely it is to be successful in halting or reversing the disease. When the patient's renal disease is advanced or the effectiveness of the treatment is not well established, it is often advisable to forgo potentially toxic therapies, because the hazards often outweigh the benefits.

Many immunologically mediated renal diseases (e.g., membranous nephropathy, Wegener granulomatosis, Goodpasture syndrome, lupus nephritis) may respond to treatment with corticosteroids, cytotoxic agents, or plasmapheresis. For others (e.g., immunoglobulin A nephropathy), there is no proven effective therapy. Patients with immunologically mediated renal disease who require therapy should be under the care of a rheumatologist or nephrologist.

When the renal disease is associated with a metabolic disorder such as occurs in DM, it is critical to treat the underlying abnormality (e.g., hyperglycemia). Treatment directed at metabolic control may slow the course of renal deterioration but is not likely to result in significant reversal of established disease.

When a drug (e.g., methicillin, indomethacin) or other toxic substance (e.g., a heavy metal) is identified as the cause of renal failure, the offending agent should be withheld. A trial of corticosteroids may be given to patients with drug-induced interstitial nephritis, but this treatment is still controversial and the decision should be made in conjunction with a nephrologist.

Vascular lesions in the kidney caused by malignant hypertension may resolve slowly, but usually only partially, with control of blood pressure. In some patients this correlates with significant improvement in the GFR. Patients with renal failure secondary to bilateral renal vascular disease may have significant improvement in their renal function after successful angioplasty or bypass surgery, particularly if intervention occurs before renal insufficiency becomes too far advanced (serum creatinine less than approximately 4 mg/dL).

Obstructing lesions of the urinary tract may require surgical excision (e.g., benign prostatic hypertrophy) or urinary diversion (e.g., retroperitoneal fibrosis) to preserve or improve renal function. Other cases can be managed more conservatively (e.g., intermittent straight catheterization of the bladder) if the lesion is not amenable to surgical therapy (e.g., flaccid neurogenic bladder).

Nonspecific Treatments to Prevent Progression of Renal Disease

There are important treatment options that can reduce the rate of renal deterioration even when no specific therapies can be directed at the primary renal disorder. These therapies are directed at treating the modifiable risk factors listed in Table 52.8. This section will focus on treatment guidelines for hypertension, the use of specific drugs (e.g., the angiotensin-converting enzyme inhibitors [ACEIs] and the angiotensin receptor blockers [ARBs]), reduction of proteinuria and protein-restricted diets. *Systemic hypertension,* which is present in most patients with stages 2 through 5 CKDs (Table 52.2), contributes to the progression of pre-existing kidney failure. Of the 1,795 patients with renal insufficiency admitted to the MDRD study, 83% were hypertensive at study entry (16). The factors that correlated with the prevalence of hypertension included older age, lower GFR, presence of glomerular disease, high body mass index (BMI), male sex, and African American race. The presence of hypertension in the MDRD study predicted a greater probability of progressive renal insufficiency with a faster rate of decline. That long-term control of hypertension slows the progression of renal insufficiency seems to be beyond debate (see Chapter 67), but a number of important clinical questions remain unresolved.

One important question is what levels of blood pressure should be targeted? Few studies have addressed the issue of whether renal function is better preserved by lowering blood pressure to less than the usual target of 140/90 mm Hg. In addition to varying the protein intake, patients in the MDRD study were randomly assigned to receive usual or aggressive antihypertension therapies. Patients in the aggressively treated group (mean arterial pressure [MAP] target, 92 mm Hg) whose GFRs were between 25 and 55 mL/min/1.73 m^2 had a more rapid decline in renal function during the first 4 months than those in the usual care group (MAP target, 107 mm Hg), but a more gradual decline thereafter. It was postulated that the initial rapid decline was hemodynamically mediated and did not reflect actual kidney damage. The beneficial effect of aggressive blood pressure control was greatest in patients with proteinuria (greater than 1 g/day). These findings led to the recommendation that the target blood pressure should be 130/80 to 130/85 mmHg for patients with chronic renal disease without proteinuria, but that patients with proteinuria greater than 1 g/day should have their blood pressure lowered to levels near 125/75 mm Hg. Interestingly, the effectiveness of more aggressive lowering of blood pressure was not confirmed in African Americans with hypertensive nephrosclerosis, a population that seems to be most sensitive to the harmful effects of hypertension (17). The Ramipril Efficacy In Nephropathy 2 (REIN-2) study (18) also did not show an additional benefit when felodipine (a dihydropyridine calcium channel blocker [CCB]) was added to ramipril to see whether reducing blood pressure below 130/80 mm Hg was effective at slowing the rate of renal progression. One meta-analysis raised the possibility that lowering the systolic blood pressure below 110 mmHg could be associated with worse renal outcomes (19). Table 52.9 summarizes recommendations for blood pressure treatment goals. Achieving these goals generally requires multiple antihypertensive medications.

A second important question is whether certain antihypertensive agents offer advantages over others—that is, do some medications have beneficial effects beyond the consequences of lowering of blood pressure? Intraglomerular hypertension leading to hyperfiltration is believed to be

TABLE 52.9 Recommended Target Blood Pressures

Source	*Target Blood Pressure (mm Hg)*	*Notes*
JNC VI	<130/85	<1 gram per day proteinuria
	<125/75	>1 gram per day proteinuria
	<130/80	ACEI or ARB
JNC VII	<130/80	
K/DOQI	<125/75	>1 g/day proteinuria
MDRD	<140/90	Hypertensive nephrosclerosis in blacks
AASK		

AASK, African American Study of Kidney Disease and Hypertension trial; ACEI, angiotensin-converting enzyme inhibitor; ARB, angiotensin receptor blocker; JNC, Joint National Council; KDOQI, Kidney Disease Outcomes Quality Initiative; MDRD, Modification of Diet in Renal Disease.
Adapted from Rosenberg M, Hsu C. Chronic disease and progression. NephSAP 2004;3:204.

an important factor leading to the progression of kidney disease. ACEIs and ARBs have the theoretical advantage of reducing both systemic and intraglomerular pressures. They also have the additional effects of reducing proteinuria, and the cytokine mediated effects of angiotensin, factors associated with renal injury.

Most studies comparing the use of various ACEIs with other antihypertensive medications in humans with nondiabetic renal failure show that ACEIs offer an advantage in slowing the progression of renal insufficiency (20–22). The general recommendations for treating hypertension in patients with renal insufficiency are to use an ACEI as initial therapy unless renal artery stenosis is suspected or the patient has hyperkalemia (serum potassium concentration greater than 5.0 mEq/L). The serum potassium and creatinine levels should be checked 1 to 2 weeks after initiating therapy and periodically thereafter. A small rise in creatinine (below 0.5 mg/dL) or potassium (below 0.5 mEq/L) may occur but does not necessarily mean that therapy should stop. ARBs, as primary therapy, have been shown to be effective in diabetic renal disease (see Diabetes Mellitus), but the data in nondiabetic renal disease is not as well established. Nevertheless, ARBs are recommended by K/DOQI as initial therapy, particularly if there are reasons not to use an ACEI. The COOPERATE study showed that the combination of an ACEI with an ARB resulted in less proteinuria and in fewer patients reaching the primary endpoint (doubling of serum creatinine) than when either therapy was used alone (Fig. 52.6) (23). ACEIs/ARBs can be used in all stages of CKD unless precluded by hyperkalemia. Since proteinuria is an independent risk factor for the progression of renal disease, minimizing proteinuria using combinations of drugs such as ACEIs, ARBs, and CCBs (see below) makes sense. Most studies show that proteinuria can be reduced by 50% to 60% by the use of ACEIs/ARBs.

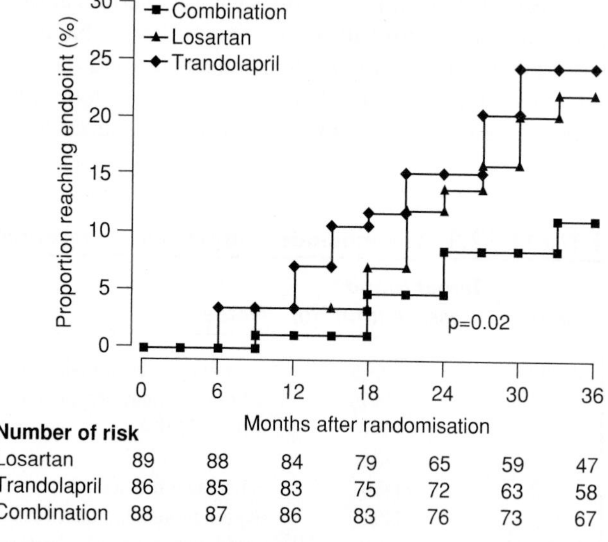

FIGURE 52.6. Effect of combined treatment on the course of CKD. (From Nakao N, Yoshimura A, Morita H, et al. Combination treatment of angiotensin-II receptor blocker and angiotensin-converting-enzyme inhibitor in non-diabetic renal disease (COOPERATE): a randomised controlled trial. Lancet 2003;361: 117.)

CCBs seem to be an adequate alternative to ACEIs when the latter cannot be used or there are other reasons for choosing a CCB. Nondihydropyridine CCBs may also have specific local protective effects on the renal vasculature or glomerular basement membrane that could be advantageous beyond their systemic effects on hypertension. Dihydropyridine CCBs do not seem to offer additional benefit beyond their effects on systemic hypertension since they do not reduce proteinuria. Also, there are some concerns about their use since they cause arteriolar vasodilatation that can lead to intraglomerular hyperperfusion.

Diuretics are almost always needed as part of antihypertensive therapy, particularly as renal function deteriorates. Diuretic therapy in patients with stage 1through 3 CKD (Table 52.2) is similar to that for patients with normal renal function and hypertension. A sodium-restricted diet (e.g., 2 g/day) may be attempted as a first step. Loop diuretics such as furosemide, bumetanide, or torsemide can be added if sodium restriction is insufficient or if nondiuretic drugs (e.g., hydralazine, captopril) lead to secondary sodium retention. Thiazides are generally avoided in patients with GFRs lower than 30 mL/min/1.73 m^2 because they often lose their diuretic effect. Spironolactone, a diuretic whose use is increasing, has been reported frequently (24) to cause hyperkalemia in patients with renal failure, especially if they also have been prescribed an ACEI. Therefore, it and other potassium-sparing diuretics (triamterene, amiloride) should be used only with extreme caution and careful monitoring in patients with significant renal impairment. In patients who have refractory edema or advanced renal failure with severe sodium retention, it may be necessary to use large daily doses of diuretic (furosemide up to 400 mg, bumetanide up to 10 mg, or torsemide up to 200 mg) or to use a combination of loop diuretic and thiazide (e.g., metolazone 2.5 to 5 mg). Patients need to have their body weight and blood chemistries closely monitored when they use combination diuretic therapy, because some patients experience exaggerated responses.

There is often a fine line between effective blood pressure control and hypotension when potent diuretics and antihypertensives are being used; therefore, careful monitoring of blood pressure (both supine and upright) and of serum creatinine concentration is necessary.

Nonpharmacologic therapy to reverse intraglomerular hypertension may involve the use of *protein-restricted diets*. The GFR in healthy animals and humans varies directly with protein intake. Dietary protein restriction has been shown in animal experiments, using various models of partial renal injury, to reduce the degree of compensatory hypertrophy and hyperperfusion (see Pathophysiology of CKD) and to forestall the development of glomerular sclerosis, proteinuria, and progressive renal failure. Dietary treatments have been extensively studied in humans as well.

Despite several small studies that seemed to confirm the benefits of dietary protein restriction in humans, questions remained about its value in the treatment of CKD. Some, but not all, of these questions were resolved by the Modification of Diet in Renal Disease (MDRD) Study (25). Patients with varying degrees of renal insufficiency (GFR, 25 to 55 mL/min/1.73 m^2) were randomly assigned to a usual blood pressure group (mean arterial pressure [MAP], 107 mm Hg) or to a low blood pressure group (MAP, 92 mm Hg). ACEIs were used in a significant proportion of both groups. On the basis of an intention-to-treat analysis, despite the achievement of dietary and blood pressure goals, there were no significant differences between the interventions in rate of decline of GFR (as measured by radioisotope techniques), time until dialysis was required, or mortality. Although the mean protein intake between the groups was different, there was considerable variation and overlap among individual patients. When the data from the group with advanced renal failure were reanalyzed, correlating actual achieved dietary protein intake with GFR (controlling for other factors known to influence the rate of decline in GFR), it was concluded that, within the range 0.5 to 1.0 g/kg daily protein intake, a lower intake was associated with a slower rate of decline in GFR (26).

Based on current literature, a National Institutes of Health Consensus Conference (27) made the following recommendations for nutritional management of nondiabetic patients with renal insufficiency: There is insufficient evidence to warrant protein restriction in patients whose GFR is greater than 25 mL/min/1.73 m^2, who therefore should be maintained on a normal protein intake of more than 0.8 g/kg daily. A diet restricted in protein (0.6 g/kg daily) should be prescribed for patients with a GFR less than 25 mL/min/1.73 m^2, with the understanding that good dietary counseling should be available and that there should be careful monitoring for signs of malnutrition (weight loss, falling albumin concentration, transferrin less than 200 mg/dL). Given the remaining controversy about dietary protein restriction in patients with renal failure, consultation with a nephrologist should be obtained before embarking on such therapy.

Treating Reversible Causes of Deterioration of Renal Function

Before any change in serum creatinine concentration is attributed to natural progression of the underlying renal disease, several alternative possibilities should be considered.

Extracellular volume depletion is probably the most common cause for a fall in GFR. It may be related to an intercurrent illness associated with anorexia, fever, gastrointestinal (GI) losses of sodium and water, excessive sodium restriction, or diuretic use. The usual clinical signs of volume depletion (low jugular venous pressure, orthostatic hypotension, tachycardia, decreased skin turgor, and weight loss) may be absent. Weight loss between office visits is usually the most important diagnostic clue to the presence of volume depletion. The urinary sodium concentration or urine osmolality, usually helpful in establishing the diagnosis of volume depletion in oliguric patients, is of little value in the patient with chronic renal failure because concentrating and sodium-conserving abilities in these patients are often impaired.

Patients with decompensated CHF may also have superimposed prerenal azotemia because of diminished cardiac output and renal perfusion. Optimal treatment of heart failure may improve renal function in these patients (see Chapter 66).

Drugs given for treatment of various other disorders can be related to worsening of renal function (Table 52.5). A careful review of both prescribed and OTC medications is therefore necessary when assessing unexpected changes in kidney function. Of the drugs prescribed in the ambulatory setting, diuretics and NSAIDs are probably the most common offenders. Diuretics can aggravate pre-existing renal failure by inducing intravascular volume depletion and, less commonly, by producing an interstitial nephritis. Careful monitoring of the blood pressure, weight, SUN, and serum creatinine concentration helps detect early signs of prerenal azotemia in patients receiving diuretics. Withholding diuretic therapy for several days usually allows intravascular volume and GFR to return to baseline values. Use of NSAIDs can result in deterioration in kidney function, either by causing a reversible redistribution of renal blood flow or by producing an interstitial nephritis. NSAIDs are most likely to reduce GFR in patients with prerenal states (e.g., volume depletion, CHF, nephrosis). At this time it cannot be said that one nonsteroidal compound is safer to use in the patient with renal insufficiency than another. It is therefore best to avoid them altogether once the GFR is less than 50 mL/min/1.73 m^2.

There are numerous reports of reversible renal dysfunction when ACEIs were administered to patients with bilateral renovascular disease or renal artery stenosis of a solitary kidney.

Obstruction, because of its reversibility, should always be considered in patients with a fall in the GFR. This is particularly true in elderly men who are predisposed to prostatic hypertrophy and in diabetic patients who may have autonomic neuropathy affecting bladder emptying. Drugs that reduce bladder tone (e.g., antidepressants, antispasmodics, antiparkinsonian drugs with anticholinergic properties) should always be considered as causes of urinary retention. If obstruction is a possibility, the postvoid residual volume should be measured (see Chapter 53).

Microcrystal deposition in the kidney has been suggested as a cause of progressive deterioration in patients with azotemia. Serum uric acid concentrations are often elevated in patients with renal insufficiency. However, there is no evidence that reducing the serum uric acid concentration will prevent further deterioration when the original kidney disease was not caused by tophaceous gout. Allopurinol therefore is not used unless it is needed to control symptomatic gout.

Dietary Management

In addition to the possible effects of slowing the progression of kidney disease (see Nonspecific Treatments to Prevent Progression of Renal Disease), the major goals of dietary management in the patient with chronic renal disease are to optimize intravascular volume, correct electrolyte abnormalities, and relieve uremic symptoms. The dietary and general treatment of nephrotic syndrome, occasionally a component of chronic renal failure, is discussed in Chapter 48.

The *volume of the intravascular space* is directly related to sodium balance, which is in turn regulated by the kidney. As renal function declines, the ability of the kidney to maintain sodium balance in response to changes in sodium intake becomes limited, especially when the changes occur abruptly. The intravascular volume may be depleted if the intake of sodium is reduced (e.g., excessive sodium restriction, anorexia) or if there are losses of sodium (e.g., vomiting, diarrhea, diuretics). A reduction in intravascular volume can lead to a further increase in the SUN and to serum creatinine concentrations above the baseline values (prerenal azotemia). Conversely, the intravascular volume will increase if the intake of sodium is suddenly augmented (dietary indiscretion), and the patient can develop hypertension, edema, or heart failure.

Most patients with chronic renal insufficiency maintain sodium balance on a sodium intake of 4 to 6 g/day. Patients with CHF or hypertension may need further limitation of sodium intake (2 g/day of sodium), whereas the rare patient with severe salt-wasting nephropathy may require salt supplements to prevent volume depletion. Most of these latter patients have some form of interstitial renal disease.

Salt intake should be adjusted to maintain intravascular volume at the level that maximizes the GFR for any given degree of renal failure. Assessment of the state of the intravascular volume can be aided by obtaining serial body weights (rapid changes in weight are usually caused by fluid gains or losses), performing a physical examination (e.g., orthostatic change of pulse and blood pressure, jugular venous pressure, skin turgor, edema), and by measuring changes in the SUN and serum creatinine concentrations (increases in the level of SUN are proportionately greater than those of the serum creatinine concentration in states of volume depletion). It is often useful to establish an "ideal weight." This is the weight at which the patient has optimal renal function without overt signs of volume overload. For some patients (e.g., those with CHF or nephrotic syndrome), a small amount of edema is acceptable because worsening of azotemia may develop when further diuresis is attempted. Whenever there is a significant change in the GFR, the intravascular volume and the ideal weight should be re-evaluated.

If volume overload develops or persists despite sodium restriction, diuretics can be used to increase sodium excretion. Because the thiazide diuretics, with the exception of metolazone (Zaroxolyn), lose their effectiveness when the GFR falls below 30 mL/min/1.73 m^2, it is often necessary to use a loop diuretic, such as furosemide (Lasix), torsemide (Demadex), or bumetanide (Bumex). Another loop diuretic, ethacrynic acid (Edecrin), has been associated with an unacceptable level of ototoxicity and should not be used in patients with renal insufficiency. The potassium-sparing diuretics spironolactone (Aldactone), triamterene (Dyrenium), and amiloride (Midamor; also in Moduretic) are also best avoided without consultation from a nephrologist when there is significant renal failure because of the risk of inducing serious hyperkalemia.

Potassium restriction is usually unnecessary until the late stages of renal failure (GFR less than 15 mL/min/1.73 m^2), except in the small number of patients with the syndrome of hyporeninemic hypoaldosteronism (see next paragraph), but careful monitoring of serum potassium levels is indicated nonetheless. If hyperkalemia develops, potassium restriction to between 2 and 2.4 g/day (40 to 50 mEq/day) is necessary. A dietitian should be consulted to help plan a potassium-restricted diet. Foods with high potassium content include dairy products, many greens, beans, potatoes, tomatoes, bananas, dates, prunes, raisins, and citrus fruits. Patients who are on sodium-restricted diets must also be informed that many salt substitutes are unacceptable because they are often composed of potassium salts.

The association of hyperkalemia and hyperchloremic metabolic acidosis in patients with GFR greater than 25 mL/min/1.73 m^2 should lead one to consider the presence of the *hyporenin-hypoaldosterone syndrome* (28). This syndrome occurs most often in azotemic patients with hypertension, DM, or interstitial nephritis. This disorder probably has many causes, but it is caused in part by a suppression of the renin–aldosterone axis. The diagnosis is usually made on clinical grounds, after excluding other reasons for hyperkalemia (e.g., severe renal failure, high potassium intake, drugs that reduce renal excretion of potassium), but it can be more firmly established by the demonstration of a low plasma renin concentration that fails to rise after stimulation with furosemide (Lasix, 40 mg orally) in a patient who has been upright posture for 2 or more hours. The patient should also have no evidence of glucocorticoid deficiency (random cortisol concentration, 15 to 25 mg/mL; see Chapter 81). Because, in the absence of aldosterone, potassium excretion by the kidney depends on an adequate urine flow rate (1.5 to 2 L/day), patients with this syndrome are at risk for development of severe hyperkalemia during periods of sodium restriction or volume depletion. Normotensive patients may be treated with a mineralocorticoid (fluorohydrocortisone [Florinef], 0.1-mg tablets, $\frac{1}{2}$ to 1 tablet per day). Alternatively, if hypertension is present or develops after administration of the mineralocorticoid, the patient may be treated with a combination of furosemide (Lasix, 40 to 80 mg twice a day) plus sodium bicarbonate (600 mg four times a day). The furosemide is used to promote a good urine flow rate, whereas the sodium bicarbonate helps prevent sodium depletion and also is of use in correcting the associated metabolic acidosis. The goal of therapy is to keep the serum potassium concentration within the normal range. Because therapy is often complicated, these cases are best managed with the help of a nephrologist or endocrinologist.

Although diluting and concentrating abilities are impaired in renal failure, most patients can ingest 1 to 3 L of fluid daily without developing hyponatremia. If hyponatremia occurs, fluids should be limited to less than 1.5 L/day to prevent water intoxication.

As GFR falls, patients often consume less protein. Because protein deficient diets are often low in vitamins, calcium, and phosphorus, patients should receive a daily vitamin supplement and 1 to 1.5 g of elemental calcium per day (a single 600-mg calcium carbonate tablet provides 250 mg of elemental calcium). The reduction in dietary phosphorus is desirable (see later discussion), so phosphorus supplements are not given.

Considering the complexity of such diets and the need for individualization of salt, mineral, protein, and potassium intake, consultation with a dietitian or a nephrologist proficient in prescribing renal diets is suggested. Constant encouragement and supervision of dietary therapy are needed. The success of dietary treatment often depends on the involvement of family members as well as an enthusiastic dietitian.

Calcium and Phosphorus

Renal osteodystrophy is a general term that encompasses osteitis fibrosa, osteomalacia, adynamic bone disease, and a variety of other bone lesions that occur in patients with kidney failure. Many aspects of the diagnosis and treatment of renal osteodystrophy remain controversial. However, it is clear that the pathophysiologic factors that lead to osteodystrophy originate in the early stages of renal failure (stages 3 and 4, Table 52.2), although clinical manifestations generally do not develop until the patient is on dialysis.

The pathophysiology of renal osteodystrophy is complex but can be briefly summarized as follows: PTH hypersecretion occurs in response to an absolute or relative deficiency of the active form of vitamin D (see later discussion). The relative deficiency of vitamin D, in turn, leads to diminished calcium absorption, skeletal resistance to the effects of PTH, and resetting of the setpoint of PTH secretion in response to calcium.

The increased rate of PTH secretion keeps serum calcium and phosphorus levels within the normal range until the GFR is less than 30 mL/min/1.73m^2. In more advanced renal failure, hypocalcemia and hyperphosphatemia develop. Hyperphosphatemia further blunts the calcemic response to PTH and diminishes vitamin D secretion. It also predisposes to tissue and vascular calcification. Hyperphosphatemia is linked to increased mortality in the dialysis population (29). A major consequence of prolonged secondary hyperparathyroidism is the development of bone disease (*osteitis fibrosa cystica*).

Osteomalacia, in renal insufficiency, is caused partly by the failure of the diseased kidney to convert 25-hydroxyvitamin D_3 to its more active form, 1,25-dihydroxyvitamin D_3. The active form of vitamin D is necessary for normal bone mineralization. Serum levels of vitamin D can be in the normal range in patients with renal failure, but with GFRs greater than 30 mL/min/1.73m^2 such levels may still represent a relative deficiency of the vitamin, because increased levels of vitamin D would be expected in response to the low calcium concentration in renal failure. Absolute deficiencies of vitamin D are found once the GFR falls below 30 mL/min/1.73 m^2 (Fig. 52.7). Abnormal collagen synthesis, titration of bone buffers, and accumulation of aluminum in the bone matrix have also been implicated in the pathogenesis of osteomalacia. A growing number of patients, mainly with stage 5 CKD (Table 52.2) who have been treated with vitamin D, have relatively low PTH values and show histomorphic evidence of low bone turnover or *adynamic bone disease*. Many will show a combination of histological patterns. The diagnosis of this condition can only reliably be made by bone biopsy.

Much of the current controversy in the diagnosis of renal osteodystrophy centers on the use of PTH measurements. Assays that measure the "intact hormone" have been used for years and were assumed to measure the level of active hormone. These assays only measured the 6–84 fragment and are being replaced by newer "biointact" assays that measure the complete hormone (1–84). In general, very high levels of hormone correlate with the presence of osteitis fibrosa cystica and very low levels are associated with adynamic bone disease. Many patients, unfortunately, have intermediate values that do not predict

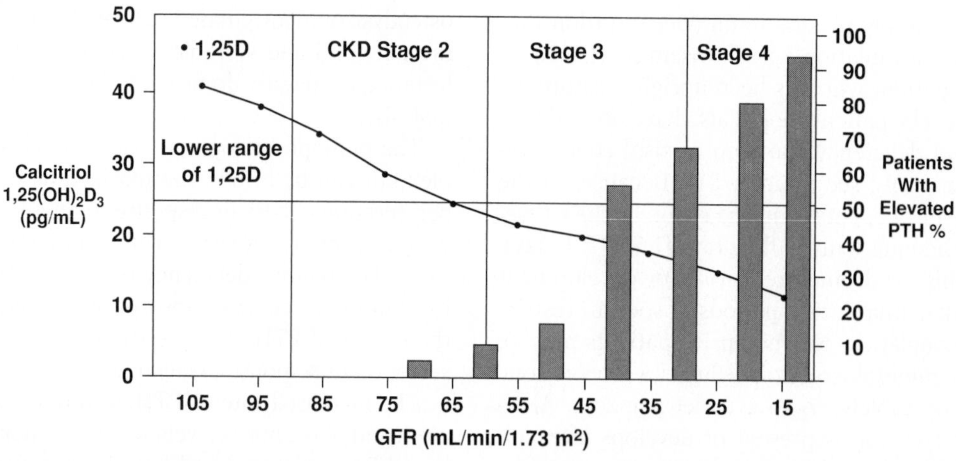

FIGURE 52.7. Vitamin D and PTH in patients with CKD. (Modified from Friedman EA. Consequences and management of hyperphosphatemia in patients with renal insufficiency. Kidney Int 2005;95:S1.)

the bone histology pattern well. Because this is an area of great uncertainty and new information is accumulating rapidly, it would be advisable to discuss interpretation of PTH levels with a nephrologist before initiating therapy.

Patients with CKD should have periodic measurements of calcium, phosphorus, magnesium, and alkaline phosphatase once the GFR falls below 60 mL/min/1.73 m^2 (Table 52.10). The clinical features of deranged calcium and phosphorus metabolism, including bone pain, fractures, and proximal myopathy, are not often seen until after the patient is on dialysis. However, it is generally acknowledged that preventing parathyroid hyperplasia is easier than reversing it once it is established. Therefore, therapy to correct these abnormalities should begin during the early stages of kidney disease.

The goals of therapy are to limit the rise in PTH secretion that usually accompanies renal failure, to prevent the development of osteomalacia, and to maintain normal calcium and phosphorus levels. Maintaining a positive calcium balance, providing vitamin D supplements, and reducing phosphorus intake can achieve these goals.

TABLE 52.10 Frequency of Measurement of PTH and Calcium/Phosphorus by Stage of CKD

CKD Stage	*GFR Range (mL/min/1.73 m^2)*	*Measurement of PTH*	*Measurement of Calcium/Phosphorus*
3	30–59	Every 12 months	Every 12 months
4	15–29	Every 3 months	Every 3 months
5	<15	Every 3 months	Every month

CKD, chronic kidney disease; GFR, glomerular filtration rate; PTH, parathyroid hormone.

Treatment

Because calcium absorption is diminished in patients with CKD, the first step in treatment is to *ensure an adequate intake of calcium*. This is particularly important for patients on protein-restricted diets, which often contain only 300 to 400 mg of calcium per day (normal calcium intake is 800 to 1,000 mg/day). Supplements in the form of calcium carbonate (generic), 600 mg four times per day, provide 1,000 mg of elemental calcium per day. Calcium lactate (generic, 300 mg, in two tablets four times a day) may be substituted if the carbonate is not tolerated because of constipation or bloating.

Restriction of Dietary Phosphorous

Restriction of dietary phosphorus to approximately 800 mg/day (normal intake is 1 to 1.8 g/day) should be initiated when either the PTH begins to rise or when the serum phosphorus level first becomes elevated (stage 4). This degree of phosphorus restriction can be achieved by restricting the intake of protein to 60 g/day (foods such as eggs, meat, and fish contain 15 mg of phosphorus per gram of protein, and dairy products 20 to 30 mg/g). Despite restriction of phosphorus intake, the serum phosphorus level often becomes elevated when the GFR falls below 30 mL/min/1.73m^2. At this juncture, it is necessary to start treatment with phosphate binders. Calcium-containing compounds such as calcium carbonate and calcium acetate, which bind phosphate in the intestine and thereby reduce phosphate absorption, have supplanted the use of oral antacids containing aluminum because aluminum from the antacids is absorbed and can accumulate in the brain and bones of patients with renal failure. This aluminum accumulation has been implicated in the pathogenesis of the dialysis dementia syndrome (myoclonus, seizures, and dementia), and in the development of anemia (see Chapter 55), and of a particular form of osteomalacia (characterized by the appearance of aluminum in the mineralization front of bone studied histochemically) that develop in some patients with ESRD. Nephrologists now recommend the addition of aluminum-containing compounds only in refractory cases of hyperphosphatemia. The initial dosage of calcium carbonate or calcium acetate should be 1 or 2 tablets or capsules given with meals; the dosage should be increased (at 2-week intervals) until the serum phosphorus concentration is reduced to between 4 and 6 mg/dL. Serum phosphorus levels should be monitored every 1 to 2 months to avoid the syndrome of phosphate depletion (low serum phosphorus), which may result in muscle weakness, osteomalacia, and fractures. Many patients report constipation with calcium salts and object to the number of pills they must take.

A serious concern has been raised about the use of calcium-containing phosphate binders in patients with renal failure. A study in which young dialysis patients were screened with electron-beam CT scans revealed significant cardiac calcification (which in the general population is associated with atherosclerosis) in 14 of 16 subjects who were between 20 and 30 years of age. One correlate of cardiac calcification was higher calcium intake (30). Therefore, it is recommended that the total amount of calcium intake in the form of binders be limited to 1,500 mg/day or patients whose serum calcium is greater than 10.2 mg/dL. Fortunately, new options for binding phosphate using calcium free binders are now available. One option is to use a non–calcium-containing, nonabsorbable resin called sevelamer hydrochloride (Renagel). The starting dose should be one 800 mg capsule taken three times per day with meals and titrated to normalize the phosphorus level. Sevelamer hydrochloride also lowers total and low-density lipoprotein (LDL) cholesterol concentrations, but can worsen acidosis. This product is as effective as calcium carbonate, but it is considerably more expensive and some patients complain of gastric bloating. Lanthanum carbonate (Fosrenol) is available in 250 and 500 mg tablets and appears to be as effective as the aluminum-containing binders. Doses are to be given with meals to maximize phosphorus binding and tablets need to be chewed before swallowing.

Vitamin D Therapy

If PTH levels remain elevated despite adequate calcium intake and control of serum phosphorus with diet and binders, consideration should be given to use of *vitamin D therapy*. Vitamin D can reduce PTH secretion by increasing serum calcium, but there is also a direct suppressive effect of vitamin D on the parathyroid gland. The normal kidney is responsible for the conversion of 25-hydroxyvitamin D_3 to 1,25-dihydroxyvitamin D_3 (calcitriol), which is the active form. Low levels of 25-hydroxyvitamin D_3 (<30 ng/mL) are common in patients with stage 3 or 4 CKD and result in low levels of 1,25-dihydroxyvitamin D_3. Correction with ergocalciferol has been shown to ameliorate bone lesions.

Until now, the most commonly used vitamin D preparation that does not require renal activation was 1,25-dihydroxyvitamin D_3 (Rocaltrol). When given orally, Rocaltrol (0.25 to 1.0 μg/day) is effective in improving calcium absorption and raising serum calcium levels in azotemic patients and can reverse some of the biochemical and histologic evidence of osteodystrophy (31). However, Rocaltrol also increases phosphorus absorption through the GI tract and can aggravate hyperphosphatemia. Newer vitamin D analogues have been developed that are effective in reducing PTH secretion, but do not promote calcium and phosphorus absorption to the extent that calcitriol does. Paricalcitol (Zemplar) is available in intravenously administered and oral formulations and is used extensively in patients on hemodialysis. Doxercalciferol or 1 α-hydroxyvitamin D_2 (Hectorol) has been shown to reduce PTH levels in stage 3 or 4 patients (Fig. 52.8) with only minor effects on calcium and phosphorus concentrations (32). The recommended starting dose is 1 mg by mouth daily. If, after consultation with a nephrologist, it is decided to treat, the lowest dosage of the vitamin D preparation should be selected, and the dosage should be raised every 4 weeks until the PTH level is in the desired range (Table 52.11). Vitamin D doses should be reduced if the PTH levels fall below the target range or if serum calcium or phosphorus levels exceed 9.5 or 4.6 mg/dL respectively. Suppression of PTH to "normal" levels with vitamin D therapy leads to a syndrome of adynamic bone disease in dialysis patients who manifest a resistance to PTH.

Vitamin D therapy should not be initiated when serum calcium or phosphorus levels are greater than 10.5 and 6.0 mg/dL, respectively, because of the possibility of inducing metastatic calcification or renal dysfunction. If the serum phosphorus concentration is elevated, as is common in patients whose GFR is less than 30 mL/min/1.73 m^2, it is necessary to first reduce the level of phosphorus to normal before starting vitamin D therapy.

The serum phosphorus concentration may rise after institution of vitamin D therapy because both calcium and phosphorus absorption are increased. If dietary phosphate restriction (approximately 800 mg/day) is not sufficient to maintain serum phosphorus levels within the normal range, phosphate binders must be used (see Restriction of Dietary Phosphorus). Patients who have elevated serum calcium levels or increased calcium X phosphorus products might not be candidates for vitamin D therapy. Cinacalcet (Sensipar), a calcium-sensing receptor antagonist (Fig. 52.9), has been used in both dialysis and

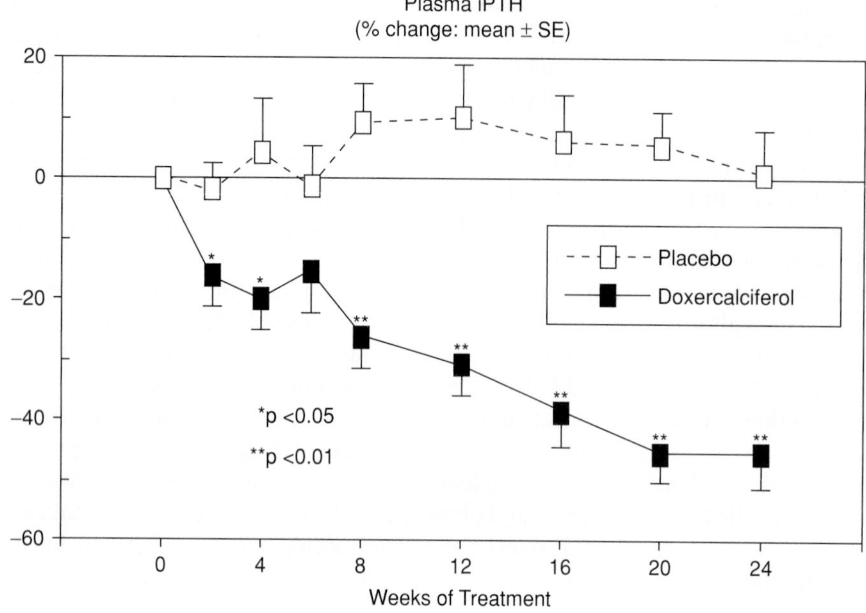

FIGURE 52.8. Reduction in PTH in stages 3 and 4 CKD with doxercalciferol therapy. (From Coburn JW, Maung HM, Elangovan L, et al. Doxercalciferol safely suppresses PTH levels in patients with secondary hyperparathyroidism associated with chronic kidney disease stages 3 and 4. Am J Kidney Dis 2004;43:877.)

pre-dialysis patients to treat hyperparathyroidism (33). This drug "fools" the parathyroid gland into thinking that the calcium level is higher than it actually is. The starting dose is 30 mg by mouth daily. The serum calcium and phosphorus levels typically fall after starting therapy and have to be monitored closely.

Acidosis

A mild hyperchloremic (normal anion gap) metabolic acidosis develops commonly in patients with stage 3 CKD (Fig. 52.10) (34). This occurs because the decrease in production of ammonia by the failing kidney results in inability of the kidney to excrete metabolically produced acids (sulfates and phosphates). The hypochloremic (with an abnormal anion gap) acidosis that is commonly associated with renal failure usually does not appear until the GFR has fallen below 20 mL/min/1.73 m^2.

Chronic metabolic acidosis contributes to the long-term complications of patients who have renal failure by decreasing bone mineralization and suppressing protein synthesis. The goal of treating the acidosis is to maintain a serum bicarbonate level greater than 22 mEq/L. If protein restriction (see Dietary Management), which reduces the exogenous acid load, is insufficient to restore buffering capacity, base in the form of sodium citrate liquid (1 mL liquid = 1 mEq bicarbonate) can be given. Dosages of 30 to 60 mEq/day of base, given in divided doses, are generally sufficient to maintain acid–base balance. Sodium bicarbonate (600 mg = 14 mEq base) can also be used, but it is less well tolerated than citrate because of GI complaints such as belching and bloating. Finally, calcium carbonate, given as a calcium supplement and phosphate binder, may also be effective in correcting the acidosis.

TABLE 52.11 Target Range of Intact Plasma PTH by Stage of CKD

CKD Stage	*GFR (mL/min/1.73 m^2)*	*Target "Intact" PTH (picograms per milliliter)*
3	30–59	35–70
4	15–29	70–110
5	<15	150–300

CKD, chronic kidney disease; GFR, glomerular filtration rate; PTH, parathyroid hormone

Anemia

A normochromic, normocytic anemia typically develops in patients with chronic renal failure, and its severity is proportional to the degree of renal insufficiency (Fig. 52.5). Up to 45% of patients with a serum creatinine concentration of 2 mg/dL or more are anemic (35). The anemia of renal failure results mainly from decreased erythropoietin production. The presence of anemia in patients with CKD affects their quality of life, sexual function, and exercise capacity, and is a major contributor to left ventricular hypertrophy and heart failure. Other causes of anemia (e.g., iron deficiency, GI bleed, vitamin deficiencies) must also be considered.

All patients should be prescribed a multivitamin regimen that includes folate to replace the vitamins lacking

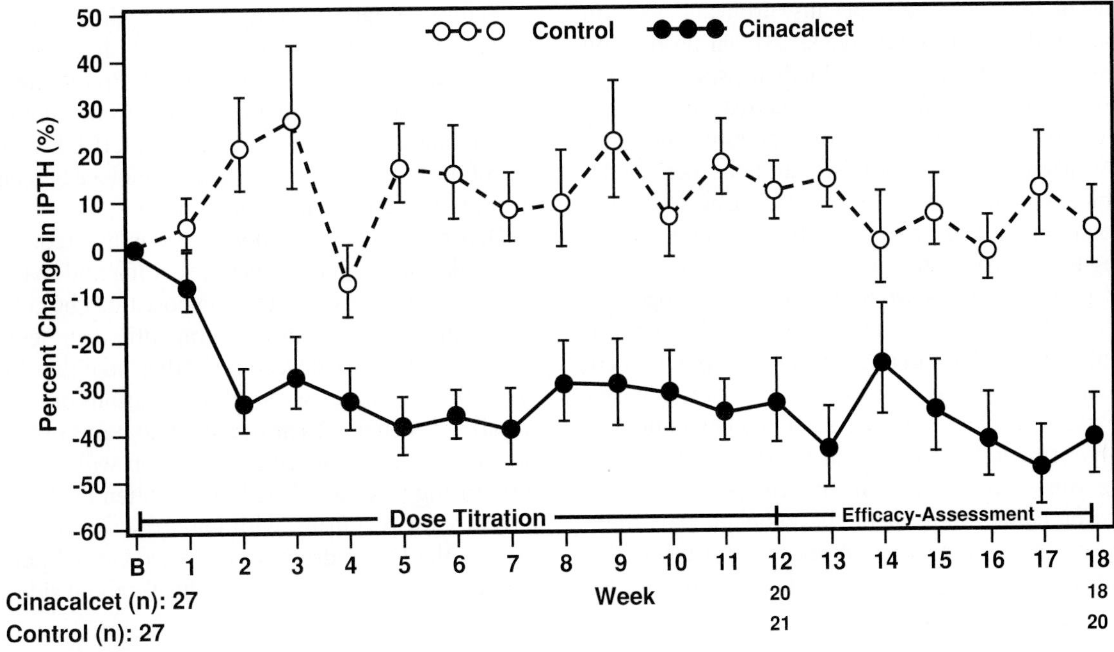

FIGURE 52.9. Reduction in PTH in stages 3 and 4 CKD with cinacalcet. (Modified from Block GA, Martin KJ, de Francisco AL. Cinacalcet for secondary hyperparathyroidism in patients receiving hemodialysis.N Engl J Med 2004;350:1516.)

in the restrictive diets. Iron deficiency is almost universal in patients on hemodialysis, but it may also occur in the predialysis patient, particularly if multiple blood samples have been taken or if there is bleeding. Iron deficiency is best diagnosed in patients with chronic renal failure by measuring the level of serum ferritin and/or iron saturation. The ferritin, serum iron and iron-binding capacity may be "normal" in CKD, but a transferrin saturation less than 20% or ferritin <100 nanograms per milliliter suggest the possibility of iron deficiency. Some CKD patients with "adequate" iron stores who do not respond to erythropoietin and oral iron may respond to intravenously administered iron (Venofer or Ferrlecit) (36) (see Chapter 55).

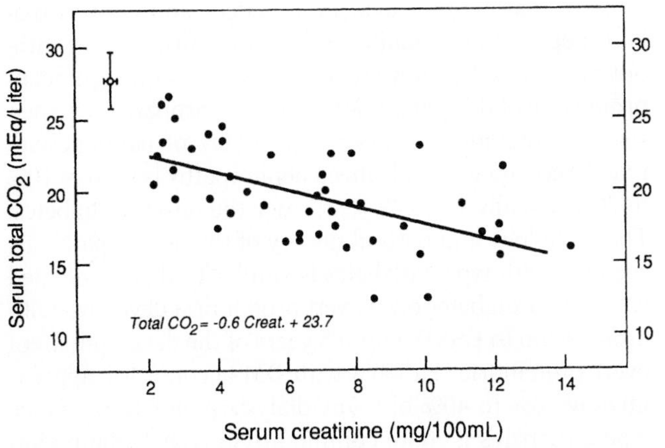

FIGURE 52.10. Relationship between serum bicarbonate and serum creatinine concentrations in patients with chronic renal insufficiency. (From Widmer B, et al. The influence of graded degrees of chronic renal failure. Arch Intern Med 1979;139:1099.)

Patients whose hemoglobin levels fall below 12 g/dL or who have symptoms related to anemia should be treated with recombinant human erythropoietin (Epogen, Procrit, Aranesp). Weekly doses of Procrit/ Epogen starting at 10,000 units given subcutaneously have been shown to be safe and effective (37). Darbepoetin alfa (Aranesp), a glycosylated form of erythropoietin with a longer half-life, can be given less frequently (0.45 μg/kg by subcutaneous injection weekly or 0.75 μg/kg by subcutaneous injection every other week). The hematocrit value or hemoglobin concentration should be measured every other week until stable and monthly thereafter. In general, dose titration should not be done more often than monthly. Most patients become asymptomatic when the hemoglobin level is between 11 and 12 g/dL. The optimal target value for hematocrit or hemoglobin is much debated. There has not been convincing evidence that increasing the hemoglobin above 12 g/dL is beneficial and there is even some evidence that in some patients, higher levels may be harmful (38,39).

Even patients who are not iron-deficient but are taking erythropoietin should be given ferrous sulfate 300 mg and 1 mg of folic acid daily because iron and vitamin stores can be depleted rapidly when red cell production is increased. In some patients, blood pressure may become more difficult to control with this treatment, and it is therefore recommended that blood pressure measurements be taken on a weekly basis until the hematocrit level stabilizes (usually 6 to 8 weeks). Despite evidence that correction of anemia improves quality of life and may reduce long-term cardiovascular complications, only a minority of uremic patients are treated with erythropoietin before starting dialysis treatment. The reasons for suboptimal use of erythropoietin in the predialysis population are not known, but they may be related to lack of familiarity with the use of erythropoietin or to difficulties in obtaining reimbursement. For the treatment to be reimbursable, Medicare rules require that the injections be given in the office or clinic. Many patients complain that there are many obstacles (i.e., large prepayments) to obtaining private insurance coverage for erythropoietin, given its expense.

DRUG USE IN CHRONIC KIDNEY DISEASE

The incidence of adverse drug effects is increased in patients with renal failure, a fact that is attributable largely to the alterations in pharmacokinetics that occur as renal function declines. Adverse drug effects in these patients can be divided into those that are caused by abnormal drug metabolism (e.g., increased incidence of digitalis toxicity) and those that are caused by an effect on renal function that is part of the anticipated pharmacologic action of the drug (e.g., reduction in GFR with diuretics or NSAIDs). In renal failure, drug bioavailability, volume of distribution, and protein binding may be abnormal; however, the most significant derangement is the prolongation of half-life of many drugs or their metabolites. Therefore, it is necessary to have a basic understanding of how a drug's administration should be modified when renal failure is present.

Because even OTC preparations (e.g., aspirin, ibuprofen, magnesium-containing antacids) have the potential for causing toxicity, patients should be reminded to telephone their primary care provider before using nonprescription drugs. Whenever possible, drugs that require no modification of dosage or that do not affect kidney function adversely should be substituted for those with a greater potential for inducing toxicity. The avoidance of drugs with marginal efficacy will help reduce the frequency of adverse effects.

A complete review of drug usage in renal failure may be found in *Drug Prescribing in Renal Failure,* published by the American College of Physicians (40) or by using online resources such as MicroMedix.

Before initiating therapy with a drug that requires dosage modification in renal failure, it is necessary to have an accurate estimation of GFR. Predicting the GFR from the serum creatinine level alone is not recommended; rather, one should either measure the CrCl directly or use one of the formulas for estimating GFR (see Screening and Primary Prevention and equations).

Depending on what modifications are required for a particular drug, an appropriate loading and maintenance dosage can be chosen. A loading dose must be given whenever rapid achievement of therapeutic drug levels is desired. Maintenance dosages are adjusted either by lengthening the interval between administrations or by reducing the size of each dose. The use of nomograms or tables does not guarantee that adverse drug effects will not occur. The monitoring of serum drug levels is often helpful, particularly when using drugs with low toxic/therapeutic ratios. Finally, the list of drugs should be reviewed periodically and the patient questioned specifically about side effects.

CHRONIC KIDNEY DISEASE AND COEXISTING DISORDERS

Nonrenal diseases often occur in patients with kidney disease. In some patients, such as those with SLE or DM, the renal disease is part of a generalized illness that affects many other organ systems. Other patients may have diseases unrelated to the kidneys, such as coronary artery disease (CAD), chronic obstructive pulmonary disease, or malignancy. The coexistence of multiple disorders often complicates management. For example, angina in patients with CAD may be aggravated by the anemia of CKD.

Diabetes Mellitus

Patients with diabetes represent a substantial portion of most primary care providers' practices and clinical diabetic nephropathy, manifested by proteinuria with or without an elevated serum creatinine occurs in a significant proportion of this population. Overt nephropathy with persistent proteinuria occurs in up to 50% of patients with type 1 DM and more advanced nephropathy is seen in 10% to 20%, usually 15 to 20 years after the onset of diabetes. The pathology and natural history of the nephropathy associated with type 2 diabetes is similar to that associated with type 1 diabetes once overt proteinuria develops, with progression to ESRD within 5 years of the development of overt proteinuria. Patients with DM account for approximately 30% to 40% of many dialysis populations. Since type 2 diabetes is more common than type 1, the majority of diabetic patients requiring renal replacement therapy have type 2 diabetes. The pathophysiology of diabetic nephropathy is complex and involves genetic, metabolic, and hemodynamic factors. It is becoming increasingly important for the generalist to recognize and treat these patients, because efforts to prevent the development of advanced renal failure must take place early, usually before the patient is referred to the nephrologist.

Microalbuminuria (30 to 300 mg/24 hours), is the earliest clinical manifestation of diabetic nephropathy and identifies a subpopulation of patients who need more aggressive therapy, including tight glucose and blood pressure control. Without specific interventions, a high proportion of patients (50%) with type 1 disease who have microalbuminuria develop more advanced CKD. The predictive value of microalbuminuria in type 2 diabetes is weaker (20% to 40% who have microalbuminuria develop more advanced CKD). Overt proteinuria (greater than 300 mg/day), as detected by a urine dipstick is seen on average 10 to 15 years after the onset of type 1 DM and sooner in patients with type 2. By this time, pathologic changes of diabetic glomerulosclerosis are well established. The presence of proteinuria is also associated with an increased incidence of cardiovascular disease and death.

The Council on Diabetes Mellitus of the National Kidney Foundation has published guidelines for the screening and treatment of diabetic patients with microalbuminuria (41). Screening for microalbuminuria should be performed annually for all diabetics between the ages of 12 and 70 years. Measurement of a morning spot urine for albumin and creatinine, using a specific assay to detect microalbuminuria, is a practical screening method. Microalbuminuria is present if the albumin/creatinine ratio is between 30 and 300 mg/g on two occasions in a 3-month period. Urine protein may be falsely elevated if the patient is performing strenuous exercise, has a febrile illness, has a urinary tract infection, or is in heart failure. Studies have shown that treatments (usually involving the use of ACEIs or ARBs) that reduce proteinuria have significant renoprotective effects in patients with or without hypertension (42,43).

The prevention of progressive kidney disease and reduction of cardiovascular risks should be the major goals in treating patients with early diabetic nephropathy. Therapeutic strategies include glycemic control, lowering of blood pressure, reduction of proteinuria, use of protein restricted diets, treatment of dyslipidemia and smoking cessation.

Short-term studies of patients with early diabetes showed that tight glycemic control can reverse some of the abnormalities, such as hyperfiltration, which are thought to be important in the development of diabetic nephropathy. Most studies that have looked at the effects of glycemic control in diabetes are relatively short-term and use the development of proteinuria as a surrogate endpoint for nephropathy. There is relatively little information on the effects of tight glycemic control on GFR. The Diabetes Control and Complications Trial (DCCT) (44) showed that the rate of development of microalbuminuria and macroalbuminuria was reduced when intensive therapy (glycated or glycosylated hemoglobin [$HgbA_{1c}$] value <7%) with multiple-dose insulin or an insulin pump was coupled with frequent glucose monitoring in patients with type 1 diabetes. In a study of 102 patients with uncontrolled type 1 diabetes initially without evidence of nephropathy, none of the patients in the intensive treated group developed an abnormal reduction in GFR as opposed to six in the standard treatment group (45). The effects of strict glycemic control on more advanced nephropathy are less certain, but reversal of histologic lesions have been seen after pancreas transplantation. Furthermore, strict glycemic control helps prevent other microvascular complications of diabetes.

Similar data are available for populations of patients with early type 2 diabetes. The Steno study (46), which included a group of patients with type 2 diabetes and microalbuminuria who received intensive therapy aimed at controlling glucose, blood pressure, and dyslipidemia, showed a reduced risk of developing nephropathy (>300 mg protein per day). The United Kingdom Prospective Diabetes Study (UKPDS) (47) also showed a reduced risk of developing proteinuria and of doubling of serum creatinine levels with more intensive glucose control. In a Japanese study of type 2 diabetics, similar in design to the DCCT, the progression of microvascular complications, including nephropathy, was delayed in patients treated with intensive regimens that included multiple doses of insulin as compared to conventional therapy (48). Based on the results of these studies, the American Diabetes Association recommends keeping $HgbA_{1c}$ levels less than 7% to prevent long-term diabetic complications including nephropathy. Attempts at preventing diabetic complications by using drugs that inhibit the formation of advanced glycation end products have only met with limited success and cannot yet be recommended for routine use.

Hypertension is often present in diabetic patients, particularly if they have evidence of nephropathy. A number of studies in both type 1 and type 2 diabetes have demonstrated that the speed of renal deterioration is correlated with the degree of hypertension and that reducing the blood pressure to normal levels slows the rate of deterioration. Animal studies and short-term human studies suggest that ACEIs, ARBs, and nondihydropyridine CCBs provide additional protective effects beyond those afforded by the lowering of blood pressure. These impressions have been confirmed in large-scale, randomized studies (49). Most nephrologists would now recommend the use of an ACEI as first-line antihypertensive therapy in diabetic patients with nephropathy (the earliest sign of which is microalbuminuria). Although hyperkalemia and renal insufficiency (in patients with bilateral renal artery stenosis) are uncommon complications of ACEI therapy, the serum potassium and creatinine levels should be checked approximately

1 week after starting treatment. A decrease in GFR, reflected in a small but measurable increase in serum creatinine level, is expected and should not be a reason for discontinuing the ACEI. Clinical trials have demonstrated that the ARBs can reduce proteinuria and slow the progression of renal insufficiency in hypertensive, nephropathic patients with type 2 diabetes, even in patients with elevated creatinine levels (50,51). In at least one study, the nondihydropyridine CCBs verapamil and diltiazem were as effective as lisinopril in reducing protein excretion and the rate of decline in GFR in patients with type 2 DM, renal insufficiency, and proteinuria (52). The combination of an ACEI and an ARB has been shown to produce a greater reduction in proteinuria and blood pressure than either used alone. It is recommended that diabetic patients with proteinuria be started on an ACEI, since cardioprotective effects have been shown for this class of drug, and that an ARB be added for maximal effect on proteinuria. Regardless of which antihypertensive agent is used, it is important to maintain good control of the blood pressure (130/80 mm Hg or lower).

The renoprotective effect of ACEIs appears to extend to normotensive patients with type 1 diabetes and probably also to those with type 2 as well (53–56). The Heart Outcomes Prevention Evaluation (HOPE) trial (57) demonstrated the value of using ramipril in reducing cardiovascular events in diabetic patients who were considered to be at high risk, including those with microalbuminuria. Therefore, the consensus recommendation is to treat all diabetic patients who have microalbuminuria or macroalbuminuria, regardless of blood pressure, with ACEIs or ARBs unless contraindicated. One study has shown that the use of trandolapril could reduce the incidence of microalbuminuria in type 2 diabetics with hypertension suggesting that an ACEI should be employed as initial antihypertensive therapy in these patients (58).

The burden of implementing the therapies shown to attenuate the course of diabetic nephropathy falls on the primary care provider. A study that compared intensified versus usual treatment for diabetics that focused on glucose, blood pressure, and lipid targets showed that to achieve a significant benefit in renoprotection and a reduction in hospitalization an average of 11 visits per year was required (59).

As in nondiabetic patients, the value of a low-protein diet in retarding the progression of renal damage in diabetic populations remains controversial. If such therapy is attempted, it is important to refer the patient to a dietitian who is familiar with the prescription of the diets and who will work with the patient over time to help with compliance.

Renal disease may reduce the requirement for insulin, an effect related at least in part to decreased hormone degradation in the renal tubules as nephrons are progressively lost. Some oral hypoglycemic agents, notably chlorpropamide and acetohexamide, also have prolonged half-lives in uremic patients. As a consequence of these pharmacologic abnormalities, the first overt manifestation of renal disease in some diabetic patients is the occurrence of hypoglycemia. Therefore, the dosage of insulin or oral hypoglycemic drugs should be assessed regularly in patients with renal impairment.

Diabetes per se is not a contraindication to dialysis or transplantation, although the course of diabetic patients is more complicated than that of patients with isolated renal failure. The form of therapy best suited for those patients with ESRD is uncertain. Hemodialysis, peritoneal dialysis, and transplantation have their proponents. Diabetic patients should be reminded that dialysis and transplantation are supportive therapies for renal dysfunction and will not improve their diabetes (see Dialysis and Transplantation). The vasculopathy that destroys the kidney also affects the retinal and peripheral vessels. Because blindness and peripheral arterial disease are important causes of morbidity and mortality in the dialysis and transplantation population, it is critical for these patients to have appropriate attention to their eyes (see Chapter 79) and feet (see Chapter 73).

Cardiovascular Disease

Cardiovascular complications (e.g. ischemic heart disease, left ventricular hypertrophy, CHF, sudden death) are common in patients with CKD and are a leading cause of morbidity and mortality (Fig. 52.11). A large proportion of patients with CKD die of cardiovascular causes before reaching ESRD. In addition to the usual risk factors (hypertension, hypercholesterolemia, smoking, diabetes), patients with CKD are predisposed to cardiovascular disease through "nontraditional" risk factors (hyperhomocysteinemia, systemic inflammation, calcium and phosphate abnormalities) (Table 52.12). CKD and proteinuria are also independent risk factors for the development of cardiovascular disease (60). Therefore, the primary care provider needs to identify these risk factors and to recognize that patients with CKD are at high risk for cardiovascular disease and must be treated aggressively.

The majority of patients with CKD develop hypertension during the course of their illness (Fig. 52.12). More than 70% of patients starting renal replacement therapy have LVH. Analysis of data from the Third National Health and Nutrition Examination Survey (NHANES III) on the adequacy of drug treatment of hypertension in patients with elevated serum creatinine revealed that only 75% of patients with hypertension and elevated serum creatinine had received treatment (61). Furthermore, only 11% had their blood pressure reduced to below 130/85 mmHg, the level recommended by the Sixth Report of the Joint National Committee (JNC VI) on the Prevention, Detection, Evaluation and Treatment of High Blood Pressure (62)

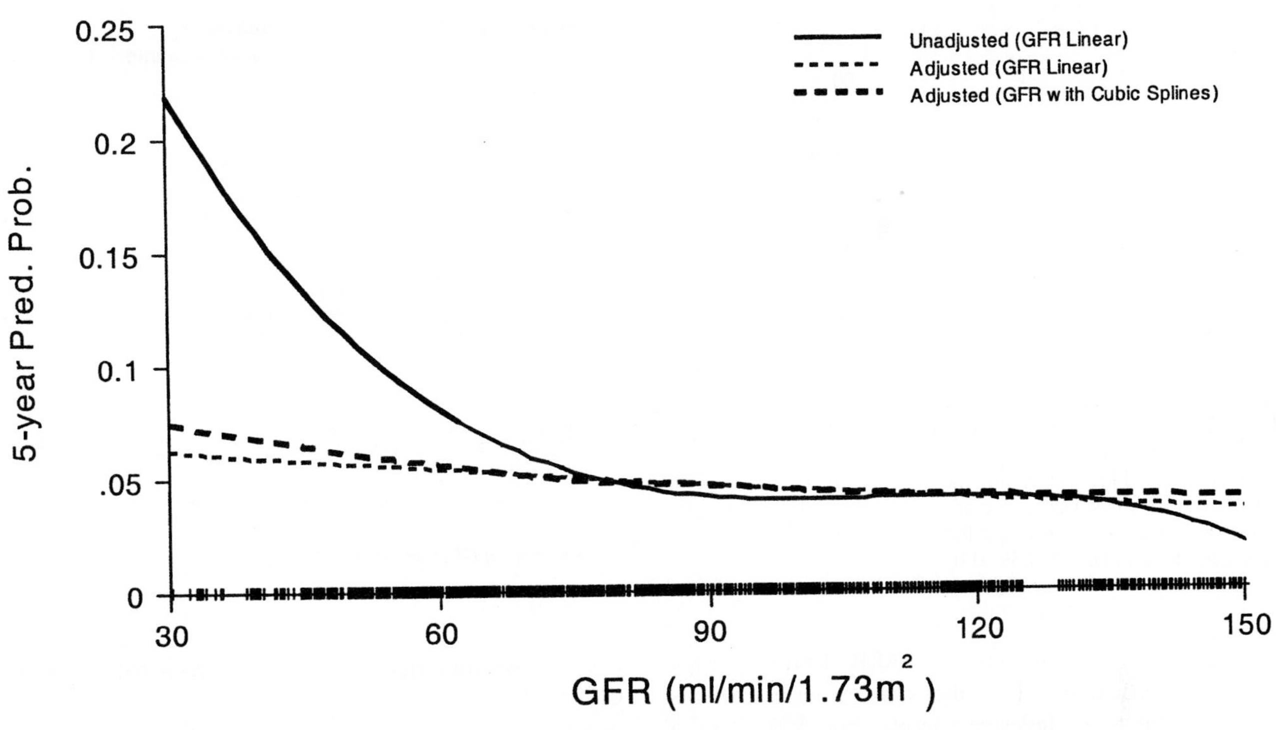

FIGURE 52.11. Probability of cardiovascular mortality versus GFR. (From Manjunath G, Tighiouart H, Ibrahim H, et al. Level of kidney function as a risk factor for atherosclerotic cardiovascular outcomes in the community. J Am Coll Cardiol 2003;41:47.)

and by the NKF to slow the progression of chronic kidney disease. Only 27% had their blood pressure reduced to <140/90 mm Hg, the level recommended by JNC VI to prevent cardiovascular disease in individuals without preexisting target organ damage. Thus, the goals of antihypertensive therapy should be to reduce the risk of cardiovascular disease (as part of an overall risk reduction program), in addition to slowing the progression of renal disease. In addition to lifestyle modifications, most patients will need more than one antihypertensive medication. The goal of therapy should be to lower the systolic pressure to below 130 mm Hg and diastolic pressure to below 80 mm Hg. The type of medication should be tailored to the individual, but most patients, particularly those with proteinuria, would benefit from an ACEI/ARB and a diuretic.

TABLE 52.12 Traditional vs. CKD-Related Factors Potentially Related to an Increased Risk for CVD

Traditional CVD Risk Factors	*CKD Related Nontraditional Risk Factors*
Older age	Decreased GFR
Male gender	Proteinuria
Family history	Renin-angiotensin activity
Hypertension	Volume overload
Elevated LDL cholesterol	Abnormal calcium-phosphorus metabolism
Decreased HDL cholesterol	Dyslipidemia
Diabetes	Anemia
Smoking	Malnutrition
	Inflammation
	Oxidative stress
	Elevated homocysteine
	Infection
	Advanced glycation end-products
	Uremic toxins

LDL, low-density lipoprotein; HDL, high-density lipoprotein; GFR, glomerular filtration rate

Lipid abnormalities are common in patients with CKD, particularly those with diabetes and/or proteinuria. The pattern of dyslipidemia differs depending on the stage of CKD and on associated disorders. Treatment of hypercholesterolemia in the general population has been shown to reduce cardiovascular mortality. Unfortunately, patients with CKD have generally been excluded from these studies; however, a secondary prevention study that included patients with GFRs below 75 mL/min/1.73 m^2 showed a reduction in major coronary events, but not in all cause mortality (63). Therefore, recommendations for treating dyslipidemia in patients with CKD are largely based on extrapolations. Studies in predialysis populations are being done to provide better evidence to guide therapy. The K/DOQI guidelines recommend that all patients with CKD have a fasting lipid panel at least annually. Patients with hyperlipidemia and diabetes should have strict control of blood sugar and patients with nephrotic range proteinuria

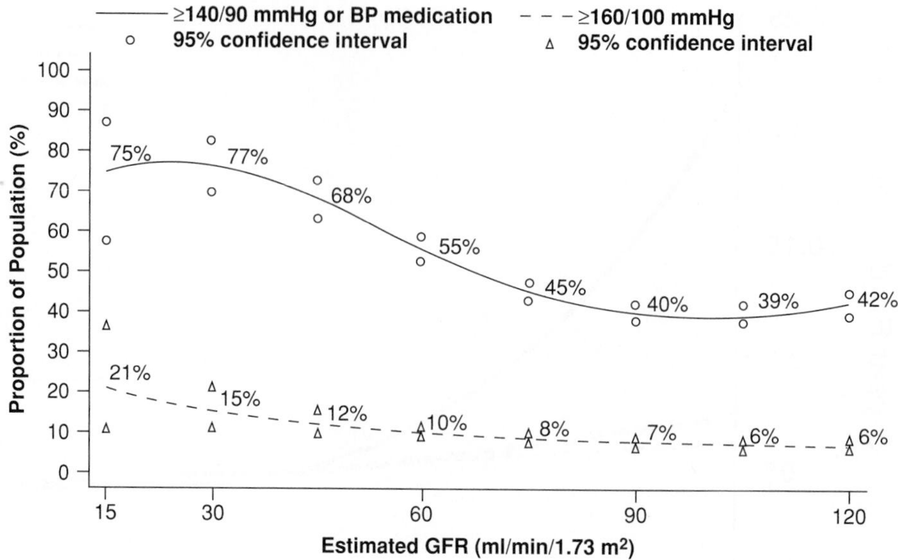

FIGURE 52.12. Prevalence of hypertension relative to GFR. (From K/DOQI Clinical Practice Guidelines for Chronic Kidney Disease: Evaluation, Classification, and Stratification. Am J Kidney Dis 2002;39:S116.)

should be treated with an ACEI/ARB. Initial therapy should include weight loss, diet and exercise. Patients with elevated LDL cholesterol levels should be given a statin (there is some evidence that statin therapy can slow the progression of CKD) and those with triglycerides >500 mg/dL can be treated with a fibrate (gemfibrozil preferred) or with niacin (Fig. 52.13). Patients with stage 5 CKD should be considered at high risk for cardiovascular disease and targeted for LDL cholesterol levels of less than 100 mg/dL. Attention should be paid to adjusting drug dosages and monitoring for side effects (e.g., myopathy) (64). Combining a statin with a fibrate is problematic in patients with reduced GFRs. A pilot study has shown that statins (simvastatin 20 mg/day) and low dose aspirin therapy appear safe and that statins are effective in lowering cholesterol in predialysis patients with CKD (65).

Human Immunodeficiency Virus Infection

A *chronic,* progressive nephropathy, human immunodeficiency virus-associated nephropathy (HIVAN) characterized by heavy proteinuria and renal failure can be seen in patients with the acquired immunodeficiency syndrome (AIDS). Most of these patients have a history of intravenous drug abuse, but AIDS nephropathy has also been found in patients with other HIV exposures. Small studies have reported a beneficial effect of steroids alone or in combination with highly active antiretroviral therapy

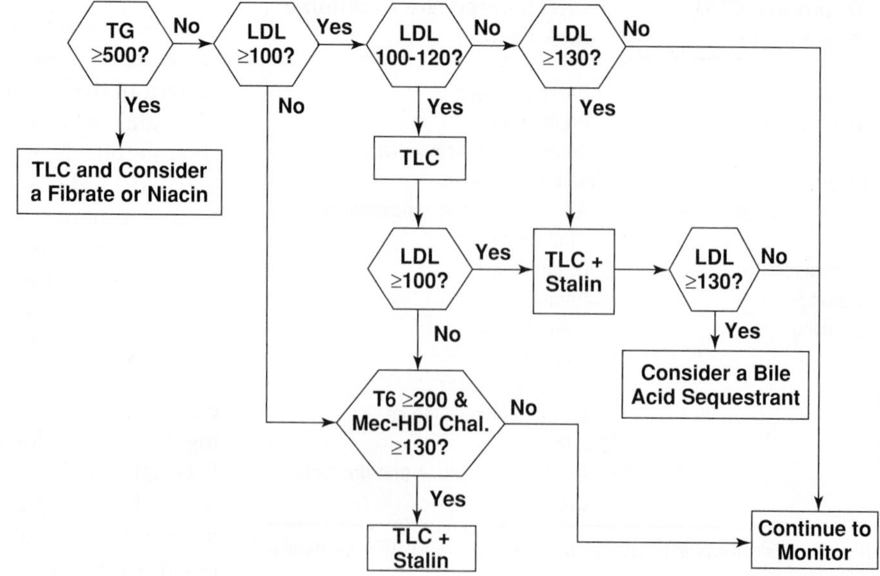

FIGURE 52.13. Treatment algorithm for cholesterol in patients with CKD. (From K/DOQI Clinical Practice Guidelines for Management of Dyslipidemias in Patients with Kidney Disease. Am J Kidney Dis 2003;41;4 Suppl 3:I-IV, S1.)

(HAART) on the course of HIV nephropathy (66,67). The early experience with dialysis in AIDS patients was poor, but more recent reports suggest a more optimistic prognosis, particularly for asymptomatic patients and for those treated with HAART (68). The experience is best for patients who are HIV-positive but have unrelated renal failure. Some centers are performing kidney transplantation in patients with HIVAN who are on HAART and have low viral titers.

Malignancy

Renal failure resulting from hypercalcemia, sepsis, or drug nephrotoxicity is not an uncommon occurrence in patients who are dying with a malignancy. In many of these patients it would be inappropriate to prolong their lives by initiating dialysis. However, patients with neoplasms, such as multiple myeloma, who may have a relatively long survival time, might benefit from dialysis. Dialysis in patients with neoplastic diseases should be recommended only after careful discussion with the patient, the family, an oncologist, and a nephrologist.

Pregnancy and Chronic Kidney Disease

The presence of even mild renal insufficiency has important ramifications for the health of the mother and baby. The frequency of hypertensive complications is increased and proteinuria is exacerbated in women with renal disease who become pregnant. Aside from the increased incidence of hypertension, women who have antepartum serum creatinine levels of 1.4 mg/dL or less do not generally experience a worsening of renal function during the pregnancy. The renal outcome for women with initial serum creatinine levels greater than 1.4 milligrams per deciliter is not as good; almost half experience a decline in renal function during pregnancy, a decline that persists in many (69). Prematurity and low birth weight are much more common in babies born to women with renal insufficiency, but fetal survival is greater than 90% in most series when women get appropriate prenatal attention and high-quality neonatal intensive care is available.

SYMPTOMATIC THERAPY FOR ADVANCED (STAGE 4 OR 5) CHRONIC KIDNEY DISEASE

Initiation of Dialysis

Patients with advanced kidney disease (GFR less than 15 mL/min/1.73 m^2) invariably develop a variety of uremic symptoms. GI disturbances such as nausea, anorexia, and vomiting are common. Although the patient and health care provider should try to minimize the symptoms of uremia with conservative therapy including protein-restricted diets, there is a point when this effort becomes counterproductive and dialysis should be started. There are no absolute laboratory criteria defining the time at which dialysis should be initiated. Delay in starting dialysis can lead to the development of severe peripheral neuropathy, malnutrition, or pericarditis from which complete recovery might not be possible. A falling serum albumin, reflecting malnutrition, has been shown to be a strong predictor for increased mortality in both dialysis and predialysis populations. As patients become uremic, there is a tendency for them to spontaneously decrease their food intake, which predisposes these patients to malnutrition. Most nephrologists would consider any sign of malnutrition, such as weight loss or low serum albumin (not attributable to other causes), to be an indication for starting dialysis (70). A National Kidney Foundation consensus group recommended that dialysis be started when the CrCl falls below that provided by peritoneal dialysis on a weekly basis (less than 9 to 14 mL/min/1.73 m^2), particularly if there is evidence of malnutrition or signs of uremia (71).

The importance of timely referral to a nephrologist for dialysis planning cannot be overemphasized. Late referral, defined as less than 3 months before the actual initiation of dialysis, has been associated with poorer metabolic control, lower likelihood of being treated with erythropoietin for anemia, greater chance of starting hemodialysis with a temporary catheter, starting dialysis as an inpatient, and having higher medical care costs and higher mortality rates (72). If the patient is not already under the care of a nephrologist, referral for dialysis planning should take place when the CrCl is less than 30 mL/min/1.7 m^2. In some instances the primary care provider may question whether referral for dialysis treatments is appropriate. This question most often arises in very old patients, those with severe heart disease, significant cognitive impairment, malignancies, or otherwise short life expectancies. Several sets of guidelines have been developed to help assist in these difficult decisions (73,74).

DIALYSIS AND TRANSPLANTATION

There are now more than 300,000 patients being maintained on dialysis in the United States. Most facilities provide hemodialysis, peritoneal dialysis, and transplantation (or referral to a transplantation center) for patients with ESRD. Either form of dialysis therapy can be performed at a center or at the patient's home. Some patients choose dialysis as a permanent form of treatment, whereas others undergo dialysis temporarily until they receive a kidney transplant. Although dialysis does not correct all of the metabolic abnormalities of chronic renal failure, it has enabled thousands of patients to lead productive lives. The nephrologist often serves as primary care provider for patients who do not have another. For those patients who do, it is important for the nephrologist and the generalist to coordinate care carefully.

Hemodialysis

The hemodialysis procedure involves circulating the patient's blood through a machine that corrects electrolyte abnormalities and can remove excess fluid and toxic metabolic wastes. In the case of slowly progressive renal failure, provisions for dialysis should be made months in advance of need. The goal of dialysis therapy is to maintain health at a level consistent with a normal lifestyle. Therefore, it is not advisable to wait for signs and symptoms of far-advanced uremia (e.g., pericarditis, seizures, coma, bleeding) to appear before initiating dialysis. The patient should be referred to a nephrologist associated with a dialysis center at a point that allows for sufficient time for the patient to become familiar with the various forms of therapy offered at that facility and to become acquainted with the staff.

Before starting dialysis, it is necessary to provide vascular access to allow for the repeated venipunctures required for this form of therapy. It is important that the access be placed well before the patient needs dialysis treatments; otherwise, it is necessary to use temporary access techniques (central vein or femoral vein cannulation), which are associated with both short-term problems (pneumothorax, infection) and long-term complications (subclavian vein stenosis or thrombosis). The preferred access is the arteriovenous fistula, which is usually created at the wrist of the nondominant arm. The creation of a fistula can be performed, in most instances, under local anesthesia and often in an outpatient surgical unit. Fistulas can also be created in the upper arm. An experienced vascular surgeon can almost always find a vein to create a fistula. Because a 2- to 3-month maturation period is often necessary before the fistula can be used, arrangements for the creation of the fistula should be made early, and always before the GFR falls to less than 10 to 15 mL/min/1.73 m^2. If the patient's vessels are inadequate to support the creation of an arteriovenous fistula, an alternative would be to insert a synthetic (Dacron, Gore-Tex) graft under the skin of the forearm. In most cases the synthetic graft can be used within 3 weeks after placement. The most common complications after placement of a fistula or graft are clotting and infection.

Hemodialysis is performed in most centers three times a week, and each session lasts 3 to 4 hours. Except for needle insertion, the procedure is not painful, but some patients do experience muscle cramps, headaches, or nausea during or just after dialysis. Home dialysis is encouraged for patients with good home situations who have willing and able partners. Home dialysis patients have the advantage of more flexible schedules and a greater sense of control than do hospital-based patients; for these reasons, they have a greater chance of maintaining their previous lifestyle. The remainder of the patients can be treated at outpatient dialysis centers. Small, uncontrolled studies suggest that short daily or slow nocturnal hemodialysis offers better metabolic control and sense of well-being, compared with traditional intermittent hemodialysis.

As a group, hemodialysis patients have an 80% survival rate for the first year; by 5 years, the survival rate falls to approximately 55%. The development of long-term complications of chronic renal failure, including progressive neuropathy, osteodystrophy, cardiovascular disease, and an array of endocrine disturbances, reflects the fact that dialysis does not correct all of the metabolic disturbances of uremia.

Peritoneal Dialysis

Peritoneal dialysis procedures involve the instillation of dialysis fluid through a catheter into the abdominal cavity. Fluid and toxic solutes are transferred across the mesenteric capillary bed into the dialysis fluid, which is then removed through the catheter. Improvements in the techniques of peritoneal dialysis have increased its popularity among patients. Its simplicity and freedom from hemodynamic complications make this form of therapy attractive, particularly to the elderly and to those with heart disease. With *continuous ambulatory peritoneal dialysis* (CAPD) the patient constantly carries 2 to 3 L of dialysis solution in the abdomen (75). The fluid is exchanged four to five times a day, every day. However, because fluid movement is determined by gravity and no machine is necessary, the patient is able to perform dialysis at home, at work, or virtually anywhere. This degree of freedom is one of the most attractive aspects of CAPD. Its other attributes, at least theoretically, are that it provides greater removal of higher–molecular-weight substances than hemodialysis does and that the continuous nature of the dialysis eliminates the large swings in concentration of electrolytes and creatinine that occur with the more intermittent forms of therapy. Also, the abdominal catheter for CAPD can be placed at the time of the first dialysis and does not require a maturation period. The major difficulty associated with peritoneal dialysis is the development of peritonitis. The incidence in the typical patient is approximately one infection every 12 to 24 months, but these infections usually respond to antimicrobial therapy and continued peritoneal dialysis, and often treatment of peritonitis does not require hospitalization. However, the peritoneal dialysis catheter may need periodic replacement.

Continuous cyclic peritoneal dialysis (CCPD) is a variant of peritoneal dialysis in which the patient is connected to an automated cycling device that performs the exchanges while the patient is sleeping, further reducing the impact of dialysis on the patient's daytime schedule.

Comparative survival statistics between hemodialysis and peritoneal dialysis are difficult to interpret because of significant population selection biases. An increased risk

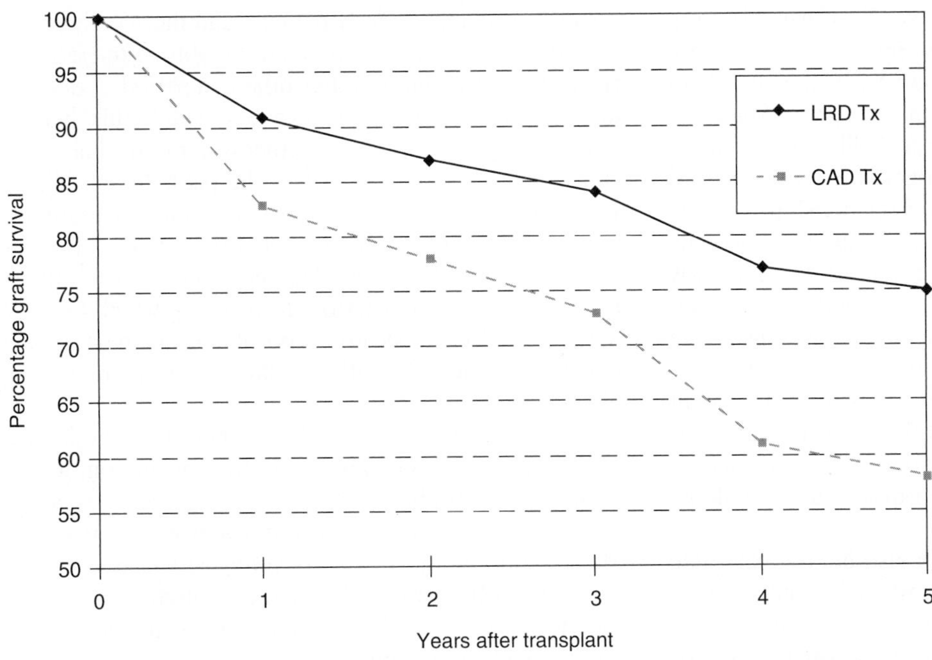

FIGURE 52.14. Two-year kidney graft survival according to donor source in patients treated with cyclosporine. (Modified from Agodoa LYC, Held PJ, Port FK, eds. U.S. Renal Data System: USRDS 1996 annual data report. Bethesda, MD: National Institute of Diabetes and Digestive and Kidney Diseases, 1996.)

of death in peritoneal dialysis as compared to hemodialysis patients after the first year of treatment was reported in a cohort study in which patients were not randomly assigned to their type of dialysis (76). Without a randomized study, however, firm conclusions about the superiority of one treatment over another will remain conjectural. The results of this study (76) should be interpreted in conjunction with previous studies that did not show a difference in survival between the two dialysis modalities. Whether hemodialysis or peritoneal dialysis is used depends on the center to which the patient is referred and on patient preference. Obese patients or those with previous abdominal surgery may not be candidates for peritoneal dialysis. At most dialysis facilities, the patient has a choice and may change dialysis modes if the outcome of one is unsatisfactory.

Renal Transplantation

Of all available therapies, successful renal transplantation provides for the most complete correction of the uremic syndrome. Innovations in antirejection therapy, such as use of the potent immunosuppressant drugs cyclosporine, tacrolimus, sirolimus, mycophenolate mofetil, and monoclonal antibodies (OKT3), have improved the rate of graft survival.

The success of renal transplantation depends partly on the antigenic similarity between donor and recipient. Except in the case of identical twins (in which rejection does not occur), the best results are found with living related donor, human leukocyte antigen (HLA)–identical transplants. In this instance, kidney survival is greater than 90% at 2 years. More commonly performed are HLA-matched (but not identical) sibling-to-sibling or parent-to-child organ transplantations, with a kidney survival of 92% at 1 year and 87% at 2 years (Fig. 52.14). Patient survival for non–HLA-identical living related donor transplants is greater than 90% at both 1 year and 2 years. Living unrelated donor transplants are being done with greater frequency and also have excellent outcomes. Most patients (more than 75%) do not have the possibility of a living donor and must await a cadaveric transplant, which, despite the best tissue typing, has a significantly lower kidney survival of 83% at 1 year and 77% at 2 years. Patient survival rates for cadaveric transplants are 90% at 1 year and 88% at 2 years. Comparison of survival statistics between cadaveric transplants and dialysis patients is complicated because of selection bias. Transplant recipients tend to be younger, have better myocardial function, and have fewer coexisting illnesses than their dialysis counterparts. If these factors are taken into account, no significant difference in survival rate can be found between patients receiving cadaveric kidney transplants and those being treated by dialysis.

Patients with uncomplicated renal transplantation usually require a 3- to 5-day hospitalization. The use of laparoscopic donor nephrectomy has reduced the convalescence of donors and increased the frequency of living related and living unrelated donor transplants (77). After transplantation (except with identical twins), the patient requires lifelong immunosuppression, usually with a combination of cyclosporine (Sandimmune) or tacrolimus (Prograf); prednisone; and sirolimus (Rapamune), or mycophenolate mofetil (CellCept). The patient must understand that there is always the risk of rejection and the possibility of graft failure, with a return to dialysis. Although there is no doubt that a successfully functioning transplant restores health better than any other therapy, patients on immunosuppressive therapy have considerable risks from corticosteroid use and immunosuppressive therapy, including nephrotoxicity, obesity, diabetes, cataracts, osteoporosis, serious infections, and malignancies. Since patients who have received transplants will still need to be seen by their primary care providers for routine medical care, it is important to establish a relationship with the nephrologist caring for the patient in order to coordinate care. Discussion about medication changes is particularly important due to the frequency of potential drug interactions. The primary care provider should also be aware of long-term complications such as obesity, osteoporosis, hyperglycemia, opportunistic infections, post-transplant lymphoproliferative disease and other cancers that occur in higher frequency in this population. These patients are also at high risk for cardiovascular disease and should be treated accordingly (78).

The primary care provider can also be of great value in advising which forms of therapy might coincide best with the patient's expectations. Often, patients have a better understanding of their choices if they visit a dialysis or transplantation unit and talk with patients or staff. The decision to suggest renal transplantation is most clear-cut in adolescents or young adults who wish to pursue an active, vigorous life, have a job, and have intact sexual functions. This is particularly so if a well-matched living donor is available. Elderly patients and those with extensive multisystem disease may not be able to tolerate the rigors of transplantation. For others, a period of dialysis and assessment of the patient's adjustment to this therapy often helps in determining whether to continue dialysis or consider transplantation. Often, the patient who adjusts well to dialysis can be fully rehabilitated and can maintain a job as efficiently as the patient with a successful renal transplantation. At present it appears that quality of life is the most important criterion determining which form of therapy is selected, because survival appears to be similar in patients undergoing either cadaveric transplantation or dialysis.

The personal financial impact of chronic renal failure and the cost of hemodialysis and transplantation, which initially were prohibitively expensive, have been minimized for patients and their families by extension of the Medicare program to patients younger than 65 years of age with ESRD. Nevertheless, patients often have to leave their jobs because of chronic illness or because of the time requirements of therapy.

Despite advances in dialysis and transplantation in recent years, the best hope for patients with chronic renal disease lies in prevention and appropriate therapy in the early stages of renal insufficiency. The patient's primary care provider must accomplish these objectives.

SPECIFIC REFERENCES*

1. Collins AJ, Li S, Gilbertson, DT, et al. Chronic kidney disease and cardiovascular disease in the Medicare population. Kidney Int Suppl 2003: 87:S24.
2. Jones CA, McQuillan GM, Kusek JW, et al. Serum creatinine levels in the US population: Third National Health and Nutrition Examination Survey. Am J Kid Dis 1998; 32:992.
3. U.S. Renal Data System, USRDS 2004 Annual Data Report: Atlas of End-Stage Renal Disease in the United States, National Institutes of Health, National Institute of Diabetes and Digestive and Kidney Disease. Bethesda, MD, 2004.
4. U.S. Renal Data System, USRDS 2001 Annual Data Report: Atlas of End-Stage Renal Disease in the United States, National Institutes of Health, National Institute of Diabetes and Digestive and Kidney Disease. Bethesda, MD, 2001.
5. Brenner BM, Meyer TW, Hostetter TH. Dietary protein intake and the progressive nature of kidney disease: the role of hemodynamically mediated glomerular injury in the pathogenesis of progressive glomerular sclerosis, aging, renal ablation, and intrinsic renal disease. N Engl J Med 1982;307:652.
6. Ohmit SE, Flack JM, Peters RM, et al. Longitudinal study of the National Kidney Foundation's Kidney Early Evaluation Program (KEEP). J Am Soc Nephrol 2003:14:S117.
7. McClellan WM, Ramirez SP, Jurkovitz C. Screening for chronic kidney disease: Unresolved issues. J Am Soc Nephrol 2003;14:S81.
8. Lindeman RD, Tobin J, Shock NW. Longitudinal studies on the rate of decline in renal function with age. J Am Geriatr Soc 1985;33:278.
9. Rowe JW, Andres R, Tobin JD, et al. Age-adjusted standards for creatinine clearance. Ann Intern Med 1976;84:567.
10. Levey AS, Bosch JP, Lewis JB, et al. A more accurate method to estimate glomerular filtration rate from serum creatinine: a new prediction equation. Ann Intern Med 1999;130:461.
11. Rudnick MR, Goldfarb S, Wexler L, et al. Nephrotoxicity of ionic and nonionic contrast media in 1196 patients: a randomized trial. The Iohexol Cooperative Study. Kidney Int 1995;47:254.
12. Manske CL, Sprafka JM, Strony JT, et al. Contrast nephropathy in azotemic diabetic patients undergoing coronary angiography. Am J Med 1990;89:615.
13. Lautin EM, Freeman NJ, Schoenfeld AH, et al. Radiocontrast-associated renal dysfunction: a comparison of lower-osmolarity and conventional high-osmolality contrast media. AJR Am J Roentgenol 1991;157:59.
14. Tepel M, van der Giet M, Schwartzfeld C, et al. Prevention of radiographic-contrast-agent–induced reductions in renal function by acetylcysteine. N Engl J Med 2000;343:180.
15. Merten GJ, Burgess WP, Gray LV, al. Prevention of contrast-induced nephropathy with sodium bicarbonate: a randomized controlled trial. JAMA 2004;291:2328.
16. Levey AS, Adler S, Caggiula AW, et al. Effects of dietary protein restriction on the progression of advanced renal disease in the Modification of Diet in Renal Disease Study. Am J Kidney Dis 1996;27:652.
17. Agodoa LY, Appel L, Bakris GL, et al. Effect of ramipril vs amlodipine on renal outcomes in hypertensive nephrosclerosis: a randomized controlled trial. JAMA 2001;285:2719.
18. Ruggenenti P, Perna A, Loriga G, et al.; REIN-2 Study Group. Blood-pressure control for renoprotection in patients with non-diabetic chronic renal disease (REIN-2): multicentre, randomised controlled trial. Lancet 2005;365: 939.
19. Jafar TH, Stark PC, Schmid CH, et al. Progression of chronic kidney disease: the role of blood pressure control, proteinuria, and angiotensin-converting enzyme inhibition: a patient-level meta-analysis. Ann Intern Med 2003;139:244.
20. Hannedouche T, Landais P, Goldfarb B, et al. Randomized controlled trial of enalapril and beta blockers in non-diabetic chronic renal failure. Br Med J 1994;309:833.
21. Maschio M, Alberti D, Janin G, et al. Effect of angiotensin converting enzyme inhibitor benazepril in the progression of renal insufficiency. N Engl J Med 1996;334:939.
22. Zuccelli P, Zuccla A, Borghi M, et al. Long-term comparison between captopril and nifedipine in the progression of renal insufficiency. Kidney Int 1992;42:452.
23. Nakao N, Yoshimura A, Morita H, et al. Combination treatment of angiotensin-II receptor blocker and angiotensin-converting-enzyme inhibitor in non-diabetic renal disease (COOPERATE): a randomised controlled trial. Lancet 2003;361:117.
24. Juurlink DN, Mamdani MM, Lee DS, et al. Rates of hyperkalemia after publication of the Randomized Aldactone Evaluation Study. N Engl J Med 2004;351:543.

*Bold numerals denote published controlled clinical trials, meta-analyses, or consensus-based recommendations.

25. Klahr S, Levey AS, Beck GH, et al. The effects of dietary protein restriction and blood-pressure control on the progression of chronic renal disease. N Engl J Med 1994;330:877.
26. Levey AS, Adler S, Caggiula AW, et al. Effects of dietary protein restriction on the progression of advanced renal disease in the Modification of Diet in Renal Disease Study. Am J Kidney Dis 1996;27:652.
27. Striker G. Report on a workshop to develop management recommendations for the prevention of progression in chronic renal disease. J Am Soc Nephrol 1995;5:1537.
28. Phelps KR, Lieberman RL, Oh MS, et al. Pathophysiology of the syndrome of hyporeninemic hypoaldosteronism. Metabolism 1980;29:186.
29. Friedman EA. Consequences and management of hyperphosphatemia in patients with renal insufficiency. Kidney Int Suppl 2005;95:S1.
30. Goodman WG, Goldin J, Kuizon BD. Coronary-artery calcification in young adults with end-stage renal disease who are undergoing dialysis. N Engl J Med 2000;342:1478.
31. Barker LRI, Louise Abrams SM, Roe C, et al. 1,25(OH)2 D3 administration in moderate renal failure: a prospective double blind trial. Kidney Int 1989;35:661.
32. Coburn JW, Maung HM, Elangovan L, et al. Doxercalciferol safely suppresses PTH levels in patients with secondary hyperparathyroidism associated with chronic kidney disease stages 3 and 4. Am J Kidney Dis 2004;43:877.
33. Block GA, Martin KJ, de Francisco AL. Cinacalcet for secondary hyperparathyroidism in patients receiving hemodialysis. N Engl J Med 2004;350:1516.
34. Kraut JA, Kurtz I. Metabolic acidosis of CKD: diagnosis, clinical characteristics and treatment. Am J Kidney Dis 2005;45:978.
35. Kazmi WH, Kausz AT, Khan S, et al. Anemia: an early complication of chronic renal insufficiency. Am J Kidney Dis 2001;38:803.
36. Silverberg DS, Iaina A, Peer G, et al. Intravenous iron supplementation for the treatment of the anemia of moderate to severe chronic renal failure patients not receiving dialysis. Am J Kidney Dis 1996;27:234.
37. Provenzano R, Garcia-Mayol L, Suchinda P, et al. Once-weekly epoetin alfa for treating the anemia of chronic kidney disease. Clin Nephrol 2004;61:392.
38. Besarab A, Bolton WK, Browne JK, et al. The effects of normal as compared with low hematocrit values in patients with cardiac disease who are receiving hemodialysis and epoetin. N Engl J Med 1998;339:584.
39. McMahon LP, Roger SD, Levin A; Slimheart Investigator's Group. Development, prevention, and potential reversal of left ventricular hypertrophy in chronic kidney disease. J Am Soc Nephrol 2004;15:1640.
40. Aronoff GR, Bennett WM, Berns JS, et al. Drug prescribing in renal failure. Dosing guidelines for adults. 4th ed. Philadelphia, PA: American College of Physicians, 1999.
41. Bennett PH, Haffner S, Kasiske BL, et al. Screening and management of microalbuminuria in patient with diabetes mellitus: recommendations to the Scientific Advisory Board of the National Kidney Foundation from an ad hoc committee of the Council on Diabetes Mellitus of the National Kidney Foundation. Am J Kidney Dis 1995;25:107.
42. Parving HH, Lehnert H, Brochner-Mortensen J, et al. The effect of irbesartan on the development of diabetic nephropathy in patient with type 2 diabetes. N Engl J Med 2001;345:870.
43. Ravid M, Lang R, Rachmani R, et al. Long-term renoprotective effect of angiotensin-converting enzyme inhibition in non-insulin-dependent diabetes mellitus: a 7-year-follow-up study. Arch Intern Med 1996;156:286.
44. The Diabetes Control and Complications Research Group. The effect of intensive treatment of diabetes of the development and progression of long-term complication in insulin-dependent diabetes mellitus. N Engl J Med 2001;329:997.
45. Rechard P, Nilsson BY, Rosenqvist U. The effect of long-term intensified insulin treatment on the development of microvascular complications of diabetes mellitus. N Engl J Med 1993;329:304.
46. Gaede P, Vedel P, Parving HH, et al. Intensified multifactorial intervention in patients with type 2 diabetes mellitus and microalbuminuria: the STENO type 2 randomized study. Lancet 1999;353:617.
47. UK Prospective Diabetes Study (UKPDS) Group. Intensive blood-glucose control with sulphonylureas or insulin compared with conventional treatment and risk of complications in patients with type 2 diabetes (UKPDS 33). Lancet 1998;352:837.
48. Ohkubo Y, Kishikawa H, Araki E, et al. Intensive insulin therapy prevents the progression of diabetic microvascular complications in Japanese patients with non-insulin-dependent diabetes mellitus: a randomized prospective 6-year study. Diabetes Res Clin Pract 1995; 28:103.
49. Lewis EJ, Hunsicker LG, Bain RP, et al. The effect of angiotensin-converting enzyme inhibition on diabetic nephropathy. N Engl J Med 1993;239:1456.
50. Lewis EJ, Hunsicker LG, Clarke WR, et al. Renoprotective effect of the angiotensin receptor antagonist irbesartan in patients with nephropathy due to type 2 diabetes. N Engl J Med 2001;345:851.
51. Brenner BM, Cooper ME, de Zeeuw D, et al. Effects of losartan on renal and cardiovascular outcomes in patients with nephropathy due to type 2 diabetes. N Engl J Med 2001;345:861.
52. Bakris GL, Copley JB, Vicknair N, et al. Calcium channel blockers versus other antihypertensive therapies on progression of type 2 diabetes and nephropathy. Kidney Int 1996;50:1641.
53. Ravid M, Savin H, Jutrin I, et al. Long-term stabilizing effect of angiotensin-converting enzyme inhibition on plasma creatinine and on proteinuria in normotensive type 2 diabetic patients. Ann Intern Med 1993;118:577.
54. Laffel LM, McGill JB, Gans DJ, et al. The beneficial effect of angiotensin-converting enzyme inhibition with captopril in diabetic nephropathy in normotensive type 1 patients with microalbuminuria. Am J Med 1995;99:497.
55. Jerums G, Allen TJ, Campbell DJ, et al. Long-term comparison between perindopril and nifedipine in normotensive patients with type 1 diabetes and microalbuminuria. Am J Kidney Dis 2001;37:890.
56. Parving HH, Hommel E, Jensen BR, et al. Long-term comparison between perindopril and nifedipine in normotensive patient with type 1 diabetic patients. Kidney Int 2001;60:228.
57. Yusuf S, Sleight P, Pogue J, et al. Effects of an angiotensin-converting-enzyme inhibitor, ramipril, on cardiovascular events in high-risk patients. The Heart Outcomes Prevention Evaluation Study Investigators. N Engl J Med 2000;342:145.
58. Ruggenenti P, Fassi A, Ilieva AP, et al. Preventing microalbuminuria in type 2 diabetes. N Engl J Med 2004;351:1941.
59. Joss N, Ferguson C, Brown C, et al. Intensified treatment of patients with type 2 diabetes mellitus and overt nephropathy. QJM 2004;97:219.
60. Manjunath G, Tighiouart H, Ibrahim H, et al. Level of kidney function as a risk factor for atherosclerotic cardiovascular outcomes in the community. J Am Coll Cardiol 2003;41:47.
61. Coresh J, Wei GL, McQuillan G, et al. Prevalence of high blood pressure and serum creatinine level in the United States. Arch Intern Med 2001;161:1207.
62. Chobanian AV, Bakris GL, Black HR, et al. The Seventh Report of the Joint National Committee on Prevention, Detection, Evaluation, and Treatment of High Blood Pressure: The JNC 7 report. JAMA 2003;289:2560.
63. Tonelli M, Moye L, Sacks FM et al. Pravastatin for secondary prevention of cardiovascular events in persons with mild chronic renal insufficiency. Ann Intern Med 2003;138:98.
64. Weiner DE, Sarnak MJ. Managing dyslipidemia in chronic kidney disease. J Gen Intern Med 2004;19:1045.
65. Baigent C, Landray M, Leaper C, et al. First United Kingdom Heart and Renal Protection (UK-HARP-I) study: biochemical efficacy and safety of simvastatin and safety of low-dose aspirin in chronic kidney disease. Am J Kidney Dis 2005;45:473.
66. Smith MC, Austen JL, Carey JT, et al. Prednisone improves renal function and proteinuria in human immunodeficiency virus-associated nephropathy. Am J Med 1996;101:41.
67. Nacarrete JE, Pastan SO. Effect of highly active antiretroviral treatment and prednisone in biopsy-proven HIV-associated nephropathy [Abstract]. J Am Soc Nephrol 2000;11:93A.
68. Ifudu O, Mayers JD, Mathew JJ, et al. Uremia therapy with end-stage renal disease and human immunodeficiency virus infection: has the outcome changed in the 1990s? Am J Kidney Dis 1997;29:549.
69. Jones DC, Hayslett JP. Outcome of pregnancy in women with moderate or severe renal insufficiency. N Engl J Med 1996;335:226.
70. Hakim RM, Lazarus JM. Initiation of dialysis. J Am Soc Nephrol 1995;6:1319.
71. NKF-DOQI Clinical Practice Guidelines for Peritoneal Dialysis Adequacy: guidelines 1 and 2. Am J Kidney Dis 2001;37:S70.
72. Stack AG. Impact of timing of nephrology referral and pre-ESRD care on mortality risk among new ESRD patients in the United States. Am J Kidney Dis 2003;41:505.
73. Renal Physicians Association and American Society of Nephrology. Clinical practice guidelines on shared decision making in the appropriate initiation and withdrawal from dialysis. Rockville, MD: Renal Physicians Association, 2000.
74. Mendelssohn DC, Barrett BJ, Brownscombe LM, et al. Elevated levels of serum creatinine: recommendations for management and referral. CMAJ 1999;161:414.
75. Levey AS, Harrington JT. Continuous peritoneal dialysis for chronic renal failure. Medicine 1982; 61:330.
76. Jaar BG, Coresh J, Plantinga LC, et al. Comparing the risk for death with peritoneal dialysis and hemodialysis in a national cohort of patients with chronic kidney disease. Ann Internal Med 2005;143:174.
77. Cadeddu JA, Ratner L, Kavoussi LR. Laparoscopic donor nephrectomy. Semin Laparosc Surg 2000;7:195.
78. Olyaei AJ, deMattos A, Bennett W. Cardiovascular disease in kidney transplant patients: Are patients truly stable. Graft 2005;7:136.

For annotated ***General References*** *and resources related to this chapter, visit www.hopkinsbayview.org/PAMreferences.*

Chapter 53

Selected Disorders of the Prostate

E. James Wright

The lower urinary tract (bladder, prostate, and urethra) can be the source of a significant number of disorders, especially in the aging patient. For men, both benign and malignant prostate diseases pose risk for urinary retention, incontinence, and decline in health-related quality of life. This chapter will examine several of the conditions affecting lower urinary tract function commonly seen in the ambulatory setting. The pathophysiology and epidemiology of these conditions will be addressed, as will strategies for diagnosis and therapy.

LOWER URINARY TRACT SYMPTOMS

Taken together, dysfunction in the prostate and bladder accounts for the development of a well-described constellation of lower urinary tract symptoms (LUTS) (Table 53.1). These include urinary hesitancy, urinary urgency, nocturia, decreased force of the urinary stream, and incomplete bladder emptying. The traditional view of urethral compression from an enlarging prostate is recognized as inadequate to fully explain the pathophysiology of LUTS. The origin of LUTS is multifactorial, with both benign prostatic hyperplasia (BPH, see below) as well as age-related changes in bladder function contributing to the problem. The complex interplay between bladder dysfunction and BPH has emerged as an area for exploration with regard to both diagnosis and therapy for LUTS.

Prostatitis and interstitial cystitis (see Chapter 36) are other sources of lower urinary tract dysfunction, accounting for a significant number of visits to primary care providers. The cause and pathophysiology of these conditions are often unclear but the symptoms they elicit negatively impact on quality of life and lead to substantial use of health care resources by affected patients. Advances in diagnosis and in disease stratification have helped to guide therapy and to provide additional understanding of the natural history and epidemiology of these conditions.

In addition to benign conditions of the prostate, malignant change also represents a significant health risk in the aging male. Carcinoma of the prostate is currently the second most common form of cancer in American men. Although significant strides have been made in the diagnosis and management of prostate cancer since the advent of serum prostate-specific antigen (PSA) testing in the early 1990s, it is not clear that overall survival has improved.

EXAMINATION OF THE LOWER URINARY TRACT

Examination of the lower urinary tract begins with palpation of the abdomen and suprapubic region. Although normally confined to the deep portion of the pelvis, the bladder rises into the lower abdomen when distended. With volumes greater than 150 mL, palpation of the bladder becomes possible. Assessment should identify any masses, areas of tenderness, or hernia. The presence of inguinal lymphadenopathy should be noted, as this may indicate either an infectious or malignant condition.

The genital exam in the male begins with visual assessment of the skin, looking for rash or other lesions. Uncircumcised men should have the prepuce retracted to see if they have phimosis or lesions on the glans penis and inner aspect of the foreskin. Carcinoma of the penis is rare in industrialized countries and is extremely unusual in males circumcised in infancy. The testis, epididymis, and spermatic cord should be palpated bilaterally.

TABLE 53.1 Traditional Classification of Lower Urinary Tract Symptoms (LUTS)

Irritative	*Obstructive*
Frequency	Weak stream
Urgency	Intermittency
Nocturia	Hesitancy
Dysuria	Incomplete voiding
	Post-void dribbling
	Straining to void

Any masses, asymmetry, tenderness or atrophy should be noted. Scrotal masses can be transilluminated if there is a suspicion of hydrocele or spermatocele. Varicocele is commonly associated with thickening of the spermatic cord, and the presence of a transmitted impulse with Valsalva is often an associated finding. Varicoceles should decompress when patients are in the supine position and the testicle is elevated. Persistent distension of a left-sided varicocele should prompt evaluation of the kidneys to rule out renal vein occlusion by a mass or a malignancy.

Neurologic assessment is an important part of the examination of the lower urinary tract. This should include sensory evaluation in the sacral dermatomes (perineal, perianal, scrotal, penile). Presence of the bulbocavernosus reflex can verify the integrity of local sacral reflex arcs. This reflex can be elicited by gentle compression of the glans penis during rectal examination. Normally, a contraction of the anal sphincter and bulbocavernosus muscles can be felt, signaling integrity of the sacral reflex arcs S2–S4. Anal sphincter tone, gait, and peripheral reflexes should also be assessed as part of the examination.

Rectal examination of the prostate is an essential part of lower urinary tract assessment in men. The examination is useful for defining the size, shape, contour, and consistency of the prostate gland, and for determining the presence of BPH or prostate carcinoma. It is useful also for assessment of tenderness, hypersensitivity, and the presence of any other rectal masses. The lateral lobes and peripheral zone of the prostate are palpable to the examining finger. The anterior aspect and median lobe cannot be examined. As prostate cancer arises most commonly in the peripheral zone, the rectal examination has significant utility in identifying abnormal areas. The prostate can be felt 2 to 5 cm from the anal verge; its normal consistency is similar to that of the tense thenar eminence or the tip of the nose. A median sulcus can be appreciated, and the lateral lobes are most commonly symmetric. BPH often causes loss of the median sulcus as well as inability to palpate the base portions due to increase in size of the gland. It is important to note, however, that the degree of enlargement of the prostate due to BPH does not necessarily correlate with the degree of bladder outlet obstruction or with the severity of symptoms. In contrast to changes associated with BPH, prostate cancer is most often manifest as a firm nodule or nodules. These can be asymmetrically located and of varying size. In the setting of advanced disease, loss of the lateral sulcus can be appreciated. A variety of other conditions affecting the prostate (prostatic calculi, granulomas, and inflammation) also can lead to nodular changes. Approximately 30% to 40% of such nodules are found to be malignant on biopsy.

The rectal examination can be performed in a number of ways. Some prefer to place the patient in the lateral decubitus position, while others have the patient stand, bend at the waist, and place both elbows on the examining table. Adequate palpation can be obtained from either position. An explanation of the process and of the importance of the examination can reduce anxiety. Sufficient lubrication should be used to reduce discomfort, and asking the patient to bear down slightly as the finger passes through the anus can help minimize spasm and resistance.

As an adjunct to physical examination, urinalysis and urine culture (if pyuria is present) should be included in men with LUTS. Testing for PSA may also be useful for further assessment of prostate cancer (see below).

BENIGN PROSTATIC HYPERPLASIA

BPH is characterized by uncontrolled, nonmalignant growth of the prostate. This growth is generally confined to the centrally located transition zone of the gland. As such, it accounts for a diffuse increase in size, rather than for the peripheral nodularity described above, which is a finding more suggestive of malignancy. The condition has its onset most commonly between the 5th and 8th decade of life. The prevalence of BPH in American men is approximately 40% in those older than 60 years old. This rate increases to more than 90% in men older than 80. It is difficult to accurately assess the incidence of BPH from a symptomatic standpoint, as a unified definition of what constitutes the condition has not been established. For this reason, BPH and LUTS are viewed together, along a continuum of symptom and disease progression.

The development of BPH and LUTS is multifactorial. Androgens, estrogen, interaction between prostate stroma and epithelium, and heredity have all been implicated. Although androgens do not cause the hyperplasia associated with BPH, testosterone and dehydrotestosterone (DHT) metabolism play important roles. With advancing age, testosterone levels decline. In the face of this change, the level of estrogen in the blood proportionate to the level of androgens increases, and this in turn can stimulate androgen receptor production in the prostate. Whereas levels of prostatic DHT are relatively constant in the aging male, this greater availability of androgen receptor likely accounts for some modulation of prostate growth (1).

Although increase in prostate size is associated with a greater risk of acute urinary retention and the need for surgical intervention, bulk enlargement does not fully explain the development of LUTS. Prostate size does not necessarily correlate with the degree of obstruction or with the severity of symptoms, and complex interactions between prostatic, urethral, and bladder smooth muscle must be taken into account. The model most commonly described is one that includes compressive effects on the urethra from hyperplastic prostate tissue, and increased dynamic tone in the smooth muscle components of the bladder. This latter phenomenon may be sympathetically mediated. In the face of these influences on bladder outflow obstruction, changes in bladder function may develop that account for many bothersome BPH-related symptoms (2).

Diagnosis and Evaluation of Benign Prostatic Hyperplasia/Lower Urinary Tract Symptoms

The constellation of LUTS (Table 53.1) is nonspecific, with BPH being one potential source. Other etiologies of LUTS include neurologic dysfunction (e.g., multiple sclerosis, Parkinson disease, Alzheimer), urinary tract infection (UTI), diabetes mellitus (DM), urethral stricture, urolithiasis, and bladder carcinoma. The aim of evaluation is to establish whether BPH or another process accounts for the symptoms.

A comprehensive medical history is essential in the workup of LUTS. Comorbid conditions should be identified for their potential influence on voiding dysfunction. Medications should be examined, as many can influence voiding function (e.g., diuretics, cold medicines). Physical examination as described earlier is also important. A useful tool for stratifying symptoms and for assessing their severity is the International Prostate Symptom Score (IPSS) (3). This instrument is useful to establish a baseline, to determine the need for treatment, and to assess outcome. Additional studies to consider include urine cytology, serum creatinine, and PSA. Table 53.2 includes a summary of these studies.

TABLE 53.2 Studies to Consider in the Evaluation of LUTS/BPH

Study	Comment
Urinalysis	Useful to rule out infection, assess hematuria, glucosuria, proteinuria.
Urine Cytology	Recommended when there is a history of irritative symptoms or cigarette smoking or risk factors for urothelial carcinoma.
PSA	Recommended in men with >10 year life expectancy or in those in whom BPH therapy would be impacted by a diagnosis of prostate cancer. Useful to establish baseline for therapy with 5 α-reductase inhibitor.
Serum Creatinine	Not recommended for initial evaluation. Can be used as screen for renal insufficiency in men with long-standing obstruction or prior to surgery.
IPSS	Not specific for diagnosis of BPH. Helpful to assess type and severity of LUTS. Stratification according to mild, moderate, and severe symptoms.
Cystoscopy	Not necessary in absence of specific indication (i.e., hematuria, stricture, calculi). May be useful prior to surgical intervention.
Renal Ultrasound	Indicated if serum creatinine abnormal.
Other	Post-void residual testing, flow rate assessment, urodynamic testing are optional and may be considered prior to surgical intervention or for evaluation of other etiologies of LUTS.

LUTS, lower urinary tract symptoms; BPH, benign prostatic hyperplasia; PSA, prostate specific antigen; IPSS, International Prostate Symptom Score.

Therapeutic Strategies for Benign Prostatic Hyperplasia/Lower Urinary Tract Symptoms

There is wide variability in symptomatology among patients with BPH and LUTS. As complications from these conditions are relatively rare, the patient's perception of the impact of urinary symptoms on his quality of life is the primary determinant of which therapy is selected. Treatment options are generally stratified into four main categories. These include *watchful waiting, medical therapy, minimally invasive therapy, and surgical therapy.* The majority of symptomatic men pursue nonsurgical therapy in the absence of any of the following conditions: refractory urinary retention, urinary tract infection, persistent gross hematuria, azotemia, or bladder stones because of BPH.

Watchful Waiting

In men who are not greatly bothered by their symptoms or who wish to avoid other intervention, a strategy of watchful waiting can be pursued. This option does not imply therapeutic neglect, but rather a systematic reevaluation of symptoms and of their impact, using the IPSS or another instrument, along with exclusion of any indicators of disease progression. This strategy is sound, as it is unclear whether early intervention in minimally symptomatic men affects the natural history of BPH and LUTS.

Medical Therapy

Medical therapy is very important in the treatment of BPH and resulting LUTS. In keeping with a model that implicates both dynamic smooth muscle tone and bulk enlargement of the prostate in the compressive effects of BPH, two targets emerge for medical therapy. These are the α-adrenergic receptor and the androgen influence of DHT. Table 53.3 includes a summary of the agents used in this regard.

Smooth muscle represents roughly 40% of the cellular constituents of BPH tissue. This smooth muscle is influenced by norepinephrine found in high levels in the prostate. The α_1-adrenergic receptor is the mediator of smooth muscle tone, accounting for bladder outlet

TABLE 53.3 Agents Used for Medical Treatment of BPH/LUTS

Class	Primary Adverse Effects	Medication	Dose
α-Adrenergic Antagonists	■ Orthostatic hypotension ■ Dizziness ■ Asthenia (tiredness) ■ Ejaculatory dysfunction ■ Nasal congestion	Doxazosin (Cardura)	■ Begin at 1 mg daily. ■ Titrate upwards once per week as tolerated (2 mg, 4 mg, 8 mg) to maximum dose of 8 mg daily.
		Terazosin (Hytrin)	■ Begin at 1 mg daily, ■ Titrate upwards once per week as tolerated (2 mg, 5 mg,10 mg) to maximum dose of 10 mg daily.
		Tamsulosin (Flomax)	■ Begin at 0.4 mg daily. ■ May titrate as tolerated to maximum dose of 0.8 mg daily.
		Alfuzosin (Uroxatral)	■ 10 mg daily ■ Titration not required.
5α-Reductase Inhibitors	■ Decreased libido ■ Ejaculatory dysfunction ■ Erectile dysfunction ■ Gynecomastia	Finasteride (Proscar)	■ 5 mg daily
		Dutasteride (Avodart)	■ 0.5 mg daily

LUTS, lower urinary tract symptoms; BPH, benign prostatic hyperplasia.

obstruction secondary to prostatic hyperplasia (4). The density of α-adrenergic receptors is increased in the prostate stroma and bladder neck. Based on this observation, α_1-adrenergic receptor antagonists were found to alter voiding pressure and flow characteristics in men with symptomatic bladder outlet obstruction. As a result of these effects the so-called "α-blockers" remain an essential component of medical therapy for BPH and resulting LUTS.

There are only subtle differences among the various α_1-adrenergic antagonists. No single agent has demonstrated superior efficacy. As a group, they do not alter serum PSA levels. All are associated with up to a 50% reduction in symptom score. Differences can be seen in the adverse effects of these medications, with varying degrees of postural hypotension, drowsiness, asthenia, nasal congestion, and retrograde ejaculation. Generally, though, these medications are well-tolerated; only 10% of men must discontinue α-blocker therapy because of side effects.

The rationale for androgen manipulation to modulate BPH and related symptoms relates to the influence of DHT on prostatic hyperplasia and to the observed decrease in prostate size with androgen deprivation. DHT is formed from testosterone by the enzyme 5-α reductase. DHT is then available to bind to the androgen receptor to stimulate hyperplasia. By blocking formation of DHT, inhibitors of 5-α reductase decrease prostate size. Nearly 30% of men will have a 30% reduction in prostate size within 6 months. As a consequence, the risk of acute urinary retention and the need for invasive therapy are reduced (5). These benefits appear to be most prominent in men with larger prostates (greater than 40 g). Two agents, finasteride (Proscar) and dutasteride (Avodart) are currently available.

The members of the class of 5-α reductase inhibitors reduce serum PSA by roughly 50%, but leave testosterone levels essentially unchanged. They do not exert any specific antiandrogenic effects and they have few side effects. Patients occasionally report gynecomastia, a reduction in ejaculate volume, and decreases in erectile function or in libido.

The potential benefits of combined therapy with α_1-antagonists and 5-α reductase inhibitors have recently been examined. The Medical Therapy of Prostatic Symptoms (MTOPS) trial found that combined therapy with finasteride and doxazosin led to a 66% reduction in symptom score progression, urinary incontinence, UTI, and azotemia (6). Multidrug therapy also reduced the risk of acute urinary retention and the need for invasive therapy. These results were enhanced beyond either agent alone in comparison to placebo.

In addition to prescription medications, a number of supplements have found favor in the treatment of BPH and LUTS. These phytotherapeutic agents are variable in their formulation and are poorly studied. Nevertheless, they continue to engender great enthusiasm as primary therapy or in combination with standard agents (7). *Serenoa repens* (saw palmetto) is perhaps the most widely known, with *Pygeum africanum* (African plum) and *Hypoxis rooperi* (South African star grass, Harzol) also gaining appeal. The mechanism of action of these agents is unknown, although histologic evidence suggests induction of cellular atrophy and epithelial contraction. These changes imply

TABLE 53.4 Summary of Minimally Invasive BPH Therapies

Modality/Device	Description	Clinical Efficacy	Duration of Procedure
Microwave Thermotherapy (TUMT)	Coagulative necrosis of prostate via microwave thermal energy. Office-based. Minimal sedation necessary.	Improvement in IPSS and peak flow by 12 weeks. 67% with durable benefit at 60 months.	40–60 min
Radiofrequency Ablation (TUNA)	Coagulative necrosis via radiofrequency thermal energy. Higher temperature than TUMT. Hospital-based or ambulatory surgical center. Slightly greater anesthetic requirement than TUMT.	77% improvement in symptom score at 12 months.	15–30 min
Prostatic Stents	Minimal anesthetic requirement. Useful for patients with significant comorbidity, advanced age, and urinary retention. Immediate effect.	90% or greater relief of urinary retention. Long-term difficulty with encrustation and stent occlusion limit its appeal.	10–15 min
Laser Ablation	Interstitial therapy with thermal tissue destruction. Outpatient.	Variable	30–60 min

BPH, benign prostatic hyperplasia; TUMT, transurethral microwave thermotherapy; TURP, transurethral resection of the prostate; IPSS, International Prostate Symptom Score.

an effect similar to that of the 5-α reductase inhibitors, although alterations in serum PSA have not been observed.

Minimally Invasive Therapies

A number of minimally invasive therapies have emerged in recent years to compete with traditional surgical approaches. Advances in technology and a greater acceptance of the trade-offs between efficacy, side effects, invasiveness, and recovery have increased the appeal of these treatments. Table 53.4 includes a summary of available options.

Transurethral microwave thermotherapy (TUMT) uses thermal energy to heat the prostate and produce coagulative necrosis in the transition and central zones. A catheter is inserted into the urethra to deliver the heat treatment, which lasts 40 to 60 minutes. The latest generation devices have thermal sensors to monitor rectal temperature and also have elements to provide penile and bulbar urethral cooling to avoid thermal injury. This therapy is office-based and can be performed with local anesthetic or moderate sedation. The tolerance for the procedure in the office setting varies with the device employed and temperature threshold. In sham studies, improvement was seen in symptom scores and flow rate after 12 weeks, suggesting a gradual onset of benefit. This improvement was durable in 67% of men after 5 years in one long-term study (8).

Transurethral needle ablation (TUNA) of the prostate is another minimally invasive therapy using thermal energy to induce coagulative necrosis of prostate tissue. A device similar to a cystoscope is introduced into the urethra to deploy two small needles that pierce the prostate lobes. A series of 3-minute treatments are delivered along the length of the prostate at an average of four to six sites. Intraoperative cooling prevents thermal injury to the urethra. Thermal sensors monitor device impedance based on tissue characteristics to prevent collateral injury and enhance safety. The procedure has a greater anesthetic requirement than TUMT because of a higher final temperature. It is usually done in an ambulatory surgery center or hospital setting. Improvement develops in the 4 to 12 weeks following the procedure. A 77% improvement in symptom score was noted 1 year after therapy in a multicenter study (9). The therapy is additionally useful in men with enlargement of the middle lobe of the prostate.

A number of *laser devices* have been developed to treat BPH. Some of these devices are used for interstitial tissue destruction (similar to TUMT and TUNA) whereas others are designed for more formal tissue ablation and removal. The characteristics of the interstitial devices are similar to microwave and radiofrequency therapies. Lasers with a tissue ablative effect produce results similar to those of transurethral resection of the prostate but have less blood loss.

Expandable wire-mesh stents have been used to relieve bladder outlet obstruction due to BPH. These devices can be placed cystoscopically under moderate sedation and provide immediate relief of prostatic occlusion. Because of side effects of encrustation, stent occlusion, and occasional perineal pain, prostatic stents are generally reserved for men of advanced age with significant comorbid conditions and urinary retention (10).

TABLE 53.5 TNM Classification of Prostate Carcinoma

TNM Stage	Description
T1a	Nonpalpable, with 5% or less of resected tissue with cancer found during TURP or simple prostatectomy
T1b	Nonpalpable, with greater than 5% of resected tissue with cancer found during TURP or simple prostatectomy
T1c	Nonpalpable, with serum elevation of PSA. Diagnosis by TRUS-guided biopsy of prostate.
T2a	Palpable disease in half of 1 lobe or less
T2b	Palpable disease in greater than half of 1 lobe but not both lobes
T2c	Palpable disease involving both lobes
T3a	Palpable disease with unilateral capsular penetration
T3b	Palpable disease with bilateral extracapsular extension
T3c	Palpable disease with invasion of the seminal vesicles
T4	Tumor is fixed or invades adjacent structures (i.e., bladder neck, sphincter, rectum, pelvic sidewall)
N	Regional lymph node metastases
M	Distant metastasis (e.g., bone)

TURP, transurethral resection of the prostate; PSA, prostate specific antigen; TRUS, transrectal ultrasound.

When prostate cancer has progressed locally beyond the capsule of the gland, the stage is T3. Subcategories a, b, and c are assigned based on the location and volume used similarly in stage T2. For T3 disease, therapeutic options include radiation and androgen ablation. With more extensive local advancement, prostate cancer is stage T4. For T4 disease and known metastasis, radiation therapy and androgen ablation therapy are again options.

Treatment of Prostate Cancer

Therapy for prostate cancer therefore may include watchful waiting, surgery, radiation, and/or hormonal manipulation. The selection of therapy is based on many factors including physical examination, PSA level, tumor histology, patient age and comorbidities, and patient preferences. A strategy of *watchful waiting* may have a place in the management of low volume, low Gleason-grade tumors in an older population of men. This protocol involves frequent PSA measurements, clinical evaluation at regular intervals, and annual prostate biopsy (16). It is important to note that watchful waiting is an active process. It is also unclear with current data exactly which men are suited to this course. Research to more accurately stratify such patients is ongoing.

For localized disease, surgery is an effective option. *Radical prostatectomy* involves removal of the entire prostate gland and seminal vesicles and reconnection of the bladder to the urethra. This procedure can be done through a lower abdominal incision (radical retropubic prostatectomy), through an incision in the perineum (radical perineal prostatectomy), and, more recently, via an abdominal laparoscopic approach. These procedures require 2 to 5 hours of operative time and a hospital stay from 1 to 3 days on average. A Foley catheter is left in place for 7 to 10 days postoperatively.

As an alternative to surgery, *radiation therapy* offers an additional curative therapy. This can be delivered with either an external-beam technique or through placement of radioactive seeds into the prostate (*brachytherapy*). External beam radiation therapy requires daily treatments for 6 to 8 weeks. Brachytherapy is done in the operating room with collaboration between a radiation oncologist and urologist. Fine hollow needles containing the radioactive seeds are placed into the prostate through a grid fixed to the perineum. Preplanned dosimetry dictates the location and placement of the small seeds into the prostate to achieve the maximal effective radiation dose. An overnight hospital stay is most common.

The side effects of therapy for localized disease primarily affect urinary control and sexual function. The prostate is contiguous with the bladder neck and external urethral sphincter. Injury to these structures during surgery or as a result of radiation can lead to varying degrees of urinary incontinence or to scarring and occlusion of the bladder outlet. Many men experience some degree of urinary incontinence after the procedure that requires behavior modification (e.g., the timing and amount of fluid intake) and the use of absorptive pads; this typically lasts up to several months. Occasionally other treatment options are required such as pelvic floor exercises, anticholinergic medications, an artificial urinary sphincter or other surgical procedures depending on the cause and severity of the incontinence (17). The cavernous nerves responsible for erectile function are located along the posterolateral aspect of the prostate gland, and injury to one or both of these nerves can lead to impotence. The incidence of impotence after radical prostatectomy is highly variable and is dependent on a number of factors, including whether nerve-sparing surgery is performed. The majority of men with adequate erectile function preoperatively remain potent after bilateral nerve-sparing surgery (18).

For disease that is locally invasive or metastatic, *androgen ablation therapy* is often indicated. Many prostate cancers are androgen-dependent, and shutting down the production of testosterone and of its conversion to DHT can suppress production of PSA and the hormone-sensitive cancer cells. This can be accomplished via surgical or medical castration. Medical options for androgen ablation therapy include estrogens, luteinizing hormone-releasing hormone (LHRH) agonists, and antiandrogens. The classic estrogen therapy for prostate cancer is diethylstilbestrol.

When given in a low dose (1 mg/day), diethylstilbestrol was found to be equivalent to orchiectomy with regard to survival (19). Estrogen therapy, however, can be associated with breast enlargement, water retention, and cardiovascular side effects. Gynecomastia can be avoided by preemptive low-dose radiation to the breast, and much of the cardiovascular risk can be reduced with daily aspirin. Nevertheless, diethylstilbestrol therapy for advanced prostate cancer has fallen out of favor despite its efficacy and low cost.

Another avenue for androgen suppression is through use of LHRH agonists. These agents inhibit production of luteinizing hormone (LH) and follicle-stimulating hormone (FSH), thereby preventing testosterone production. They have been shown to be as effective as surgical castration. LHRH agonists initially lead to an increase in testosterone production prior to a nadir 3 to 4 weeks after initiation of therapy. This "flare" can cause a worsening of bone pain and other symptoms until testosterone levels fall. In order to avoid this side effect an antiandrogen is given for 2 to 3 weeks. Although here might seem to be additional benefit to complete androgen ablation using combination therapy (a LHRH agonist and an antiandrogen), this has not been demonstrated.

As an alternative to medical hormonal ablation, surgical castration (orchiectomy) is an effective option. This procedure can be performed as an outpatient with a light anesthetic. Complications are uncommon, and testosterone levels fall almost immediately.

Medical or surgical castration is generally well-tolerated and are equally effective in reducing PSA and improving performance status in men with advanced prostate cancer. Side effects can sometimes be bothersome, however, and these include osteopenia and osteoporosis, anemia, loss of libido, hot flashes, and asthenia. Hormonal ablation therapy does not prevent or delay progression of prostate cancer, and overall survival is not improved. Roughly 10% of men started on hormonal therapy for metastatic prostate cancer survive less than 6 months. An additional 10% survive longer than 10 years. The remainder fall somewhere between these intervals, with median survival in this group approximately 3 years. The wide range of these numbers is because of great variability in the tumor kinetics and androgen dependence of prostate cancer.

Prostate cancer continues to be an elusive target in terms of diagnosis and cure. The search for improved markers of disease, for more accurate patient stratification, and for effective treatment continues.

PROSTATITIS/PROSTATODYNIA

Prostatitis is the most common urologic diagnosis in men with lower urinary tract symptoms who are younger than age 50 years, and the third most common urologic diagnosis in men older than 50 years old. The general term prostatitis can be subdivided based on etiology and presentation into four categories as defined by the National Institute of Health (NIH) consensus group on prostatitis in 1995 (20). These include acute bacterial prostatitis (category I), chronic bacterial prostatitis (category II), chronic pelvic pain syndrome (category III), and asymptomatic inflammatory prostatitis (category IV). This schema allows for distinction between identifiable bacterial causes of infection and inflammation in the prostate and symptomatic disorders in the absence of an infectious agent. It is helpful in clarifying diagnosis and therapy selection.

Acute bacterial prostatitis is associated with the acute onset of pain in the perineum, pelvis and lower urinary tract as well as of symptoms of urgency, dysuria, and bladder outlet obstruction. Systemic symptoms of fever, malaise, and nausea are typical. Rectal examination reveals a tender, boggy prostate. If fluctuance is present, an abscess should be suspected and urologic consultation obtained. Vigorous manipulation of the prostate should not be done in the setting of acute prostatitis as this may increase bacteremia. Urine culture most commonly reveals gram-negative bacteria with *Escherichia coli* the most common (65% to 85%). *Pseudomonas, Klebsiella,* and *Serratia* species can also be found. Infection with gram-positive bacteria (e.g., *Enterococcus* or *Staphylococcus aureus*) is occasionally seen. Impaired host defense, bacterial virulence, dysfunctional voiding, and reflux into the ejaculatory ducts are some of the presumed mechanisms for development of prostatitis. Antibiotic therapy is indicated for bacterial prostatitis. Trimethoprim-sulfamethoxazole (TMP-SMX) or a fluoroquinolone is preferred. Therapy is continued for 4 to 12 weeks. In the acute setting, adequate urinary drainage should be established with placement of a urethral catheter or suprapubic catheter if significant obstruction or urinary retention is present. An α-blocker is commonly included to minimize bladder outlet obstruction. Hospital admission for intravenous antibiotic therapy is sometimes necessary.

Chronic bacterial prostatitis produces dysuria and urinary frequency or recurrent UTIs, but generally not the systemic symptoms or the acute onset of pain found in acute bacterial prostatitis. Rectal examination may reveal a tender, swollen prostate, but is often normal. The infection is typically caused by gram-negative bacilli, but *Chlamydia* infection is also a cause. Similar antibiotic therapy is used as in acute disease. Persistence of symptoms in the face of negative urine cultures should prompt consideration of a chronic pelvic pain syndrome and alternate therapy. For these men, combination therapy with an α-blocker and a nonsteroidal anti-inflammatory drug (NSAID) is customary.

However, many months of therapy are required for repletion of iron stores (the status of which can be evaluated by repeat measurement of serum ferritin after iron therapy is concluded). Iron absorption is variable and unpredictable. Only a fraction of ingested iron is absorbed, even under optimal conditions. In the menstruating woman with iron-deficiency anemia, treatment for 1 year or longer may be necessary. Iron deficiency is common in menstruating women, especially in those with heavy menstrual periods and a history of multiple pregnancies. Some women may require perpetual iron therapy to maintain a normal Hct level. Standard treatment with oral iron consists of one tablet of iron (e.g., ferrous sulfate 300 mg, which contains 60 mg elemental iron) taken three times daily on an empty stomach (1 hour before meals), separate from H_2 blockers, antacids, and proton pump inhibitors. If patients experience difficulty taking the noontime dose, it reasonably can be omitted. Numerous preparations of iron other than ferrous sulfate are available, but recommendations for their use usually are not justified unless a reduction in the dosage of elemental iron is required (see Side Effects). Generally, time-release capsules and enteric-coated preparations are to be avoided. They are costly, and absorption is variable. Preparations containing iron, including ferrous sulfate, can be obtained without prescription.

Side Effects

Approximately 15% of patients have gastrointestinal side effects from oral iron, most commonly constipation, but nausea, abdominal cramping, and diarrhea also occur. If these side effects develop, the practitioner may elect to administer iron only once per day or may instruct the patient to take iron with meals instead of on an empty stomach (but not with tea or antacids). Taking iron with food decreases iron absorption by approximately 50%, but absorption still is sufficient to replenish the body's iron if treatment is continued long enough. If symptoms continue after these alterations in dosage and schedule, then decreasing the individual dosage of oral iron may be helpful. If the dosage is decreased to <40 mg elemental iron, symptoms often abate. This dosage decrease can be accomplished by using pediatric liquid preparations, which usually are well tolerated.

If these adjustments in the dosage and schedule of oral iron administration are made, parenteral iron is rarely indicated. However, parenteral therapy is indicated in patients with small or large bowel inflammation, rapid gastrointestinal transit, or malabsorption, or if the patient has severe iron deficiency and noncompliance has been repetitively proven. Iron dextran has been the most commonly used form of parenteral iron, but ferric gluconate in sucrose appears to be a safer preparation (6). It now is used preferentially in patients undergoing renal dialysis and may be prescribed to other patients as well. Parenteral iron usually is given in small doses intramuscularly or intravenously. If the intravenous route is chosen, the infusion must be given slowly. Guidelines for the dosage of parenteral iron are provided in the *Physicians' Desk Reference* but can be calculated grossly from the patient's age and Hb value (Table 55.8). A test dose is administered 1 hour before the first therapeutic dose to ensure that the patient is not allergic to the preparation. Injections can be given daily until the calculated required dosage has been administered. Large doses of intravenous iron, appropriately diluted and given over several hours, are not approved by the U.S. Food and Drug Administration (FDA) but are generally safe when supervised by experienced clinicians. Side effects from parenteral iron include pain and rash at the injection site, arthralgias, staining of the skin, fever, and rare anaphylactoid reactions.

TABLE 55.8 Representative Total Body Iron Deficits at Various Body Weights and Hemoglobin Levels

Patient Weight (lb)	*Iron Deficit (mg) at Various Hemoglobin Levels*			
	4 g/dL	*6 g/dL*	*8 g/dL*	*10 g/dL*
100	2,250	1,750	1,400	1,000
120	2,650	2,100	1,650	1,150
140	3,050	2,500	1,950	1,350
160	3,550	2,850	2,200	1,550
180	3,950	3,200	2,500	1,750

Thalassemia

In the normal adult, three types of hemoglobins are present in mature red cells: the major component A and two minor components A_2 and F (fetal). Each hemoglobin molecule consists of four heme groups and four globin chains. The globin chains in each molecule are of two different types. All three hemoglobins have two α-globin chains but differ in their second set of globin chains (β, γ, or δ) (Table 55.9).

Thalassemia is an inherited defect in globin chain production. Anemia is caused by a combination of decreased hemoglobin production and, usually, mild hemolysis.

TABLE 55.9 Globin Chain Composition of Normal Adult Hemoglobins

Hemoglobin Type	*Composition*	*Percentage of Total in Normal Adults*
A	$\alpha_2\beta_2$	97
A_2	$\alpha_2\delta_2$	2
F	$\alpha_2\gamma_2$	1

TABLE 55.10 Heterozygous Thalassemia: Typical Database

Characteristic	Finding
Hematocrit value	37%
MCV	69 fL
MCH	20 pg
MCHC	32 g/dL
Reticulocyte count	2.5%
Red blood cell morphology	Microcytosis, poikilocytosis, stippling
Ferritin	Normal or increased

MCH, mean corpuscular hemoglobin; MCHC, mean corpuscular hemoglobin concentration; MCV, mean corpuscular volume.

β-Thalassemia is seen in the United States primarily in African American patients, patients from Southeast Asia, and patients of Mediterranean (Greek or Italian) origin. The genetics of α-thalassemia are complicated. The disorder appears to have a wider racial distribution than does β-thalassemia, but it is especially common in African Americans (7). Most patients are heterozygous and clinically asymptomatic, but they may have microcytosis. The diagnosis is important because the entity often is confused with iron-deficiency anemia, resulting in lifelong repetitive workups for gastrointestinal bleeding and inappropriate treatment with iron. Except possibly for menstruating women, microcytosis in African American patients is more likely to be caused by α-thalassemia than by iron deficiency.

Diagnosis

Table 55.10 lists the typical database for patients with heterozygous α-thalassemia or β-thalassemia. The combination of low MCV and only very mild anemia should alert the practitioner to the diagnosis because in iron deficiency the degree of microcytosis parallels the severity of the anemia (Table 55.6).

In the forms of β-thalassemia most commonly seen in the United States, production of β chains is decreased, with a compensatory increase in production of δ chains, resulting in decreased production of hemoglobin A and increased production of hemoglobin A_2. This increase can be assessed by electrophoresis of the hemoglobin and is a definitive diagnostic test for β-thalassemia. Increases in hemoglobin F levels are seen less commonly in patients with β-thalassemia in the United States.

The α-thalassemias are more difficult to diagnose because decreased production of α chains affects the relative concentrations of all of the normal adult hemoglobins. A definitive diagnosis of one of the α-thalassemia syndromes may be difficult and may require family studies or techniques available primarily in research laboratories. However, the diagnosis of presumptive α-thalassemia in the setting of an appropriate database (hematologic values consistent with the diagnosis in the absence of iron deficiency and of β-thalassemia) is reasonable even in the absence of laboratory confirmation.

Patient Education

It is important to explain to patients with heterozygous thalassemia that the clinical features of the condition mimic those of iron deficiency. The patient should be put on guard against repetitive diagnostic workups for iron deficiency. The clinician should emphasize the benign nature of the illness and that the anemia, being mild, usually does not cause any symptoms. The patient should be cautioned against taking oral iron because thalassemic patients have increased iron stores. Genetic counseling is important. A couple, both heterozygous for β-thalassemia, has a 25% chance of having a child with homozygous β-thalassemia. Furthermore, the genes for thalassemia and those for hemoglobin S and C are alleles. Hemoglobin S–β-thalassemia is a clinically significant disease.

Miscellaneous

The anemia of chronic disease and the anemia of malignancy may be associated with a low MCV, although MCV usually is normal (see Anemias with Normal Mean Corpuscular Volume and an Inappropriately Low Reticulocyte Index). Sideroblastic anemias (characterized by increased iron stores and ringed sideroblasts in the bone marrow) occasionally are microcytic, and some hemoglobinopathies are associated with a low MCV (hemoglobin E). The former conditions are best treated in consultation with a hematologist. The latter condition is seen primarily in Southeast Asians. Aluminum toxicity, now seen infrequently, sometimes causes a further reduction in red cell mass, with microcytosis (8).

ANEMIA WITH A HIGH MEAN CORPUSCULAR VOLUME

An MCV >100 fL is abnormal, and an attempt should be made to explain the abnormality. Table 55.11 lists conditions associated with an increased MCV (9). For the most part, the diseases associated with an elevated MCV are liver disease, the megaloblastic anemias (including drug-induced megaloblastosis), and the refractory anemias with hypercellular bone marrows (myelodysplastic syndromes). Occasionally an elevated MCV measured by the automatic counter is spurious, caused by red cell antibodies (cold agglutinins). Because young RBCs are large, patients with a marked reticulocytosis may have an increased MCV.

TABLE 55.11 Differential Diagnosis of Mean Corpuscular Volume >100 fL

Spurious
Reticulocytosis (marked)
Liver disease
Alcoholism
Myelodysplastic syndromes
Myelophthisis
Drugs
Megaloblastic anemias
Normal variant

Liver Disease

Chronic hepatocellular and obstructive liver disease results in cholesterol loading in the lipid portion of the red cell membrane so that cell size increases. MCV often is elevated but usually is not >115 fL (Table 55.12). On smears, cells appear to be round and centrally targeted, without significant variation in shape. This morphologic abnormality is not a cause of anemia. However, patients with liver disease often have other reasons for their anemia (bleeding, hemolysis, folic acid deficiency). The severe alcoholic often has an increased MCV even in the absence of overt liver disease or marked megaloblastosis (10). Presumably the elevated MCV results from periodic episodes of alcoholic liver disease, folic acid deficiency, or both. Because of poor diet, the alcoholic often becomes depleted of folic acid. In addition, alcohol interferes with folic acid metabolism.

Megaloblastic Anemia

A megaloblast is a larger than normal hematopoietic precursor with a nucleus that contains characteristic granular chromatin, the result of abnormal deoxyribonucleic acid (DNA) synthesis (11,12). Table 55.13 lists the various etiologies of megaloblastic anemia related to deficiency of vitamin B_{12} (cobalamin) or folic acid (essential cofactors in DNA synthesis). The body's stores of B_{12} are such that a diet without this vitamin (one in which animal protein is completely excluded) would not result in megaloblastosis due to B_{12} deficiency for several years; therefore, dietary B_{12} deficiency is extremely rare. By far the most common cause of B_{12} deficiency is pernicious anemia, an acquired autoimmune defect of the gastric mucosa resulting in deficient formation of intrinsic factor, which binds ingested B_{12} and allows its absorption in the terminal ileum. Patients with pernicious anemia usually are elderly and often complain of sore mouth, indigestion, and constipation or diarrhea. Neurologic problems, including peripheral neuropathy, dorsal column dysfunction (loss of vibratory and position sense in the lower extremities), and changes in affect, are common. If the deficiency is not corrected, lateral column dysfunction (weakness and spasticity) occurs. The anemia develops so slowly that patients often have very low Hcts and yet remarkably good cardiovascular compensation for their anemia. Such patients usually have an expanded total blood volume and are prone to develop heart failure if given transfusions. B_{12} deficiency from other causes (Table 55.13) is less common. Patients who have undergone total gastrectomy or ileal resection

TABLE 55.12 Laboratory Features in Three Conditions Associated with Elevated Mean Corpuscular Volume

Feature	*Liver Disease*	*Megaloblastic Anemia*	*Myelodysplastic Syndrome*
Mean corpuscular volume	Usually <115 fL	Often >115 fL	Usually <115 fL
WBC count	Variable	Often decreased	Often decreased
Platelet count	Variable	Often decreased	Often decreased
RBC morphology	Target cells, no poikilocytosis	Marked anisocytosis and poikilocytosis, macro-ovalocytes	Marked anisocytosis and poikilocytosis, may mimic megaloblastic anemia
Nucleated RBCs	Not common	Common	Common
WBC morphology	Normal	Hypersegmented nuclei of neutrophils	May have abnormal mononuclear cells, no nuclear hypersegmentation of neutrophils
Platelet morphology	Normal	Normal	May be large and degranulated
RBC folate	Depends on diet	Decreased in folate deficiency, normal or slightly decreased in B_{12} deficiency	Normal or elevated
Serum B_{12}	Normal	Decreased in B_{12} deficiency, may be slightly decreased in folate deficiency	Normal or elevated

RBC, red blood cell; WBC, white blood cell.

TABLE 55.13 Causes of Megaloblastosis Due to Vitamin B_{12} or Folic Acid Deficiency

Vitamin B_{12}
Pernicious anemia (acquired or congenital)
Gastrectomy
Ileal resection
Bariatric surgery
Crohn disease and tropical sprue
Fish tapeworm infestation
Blind loop syndrome
Nutritional deficiency (vegan diet, rare)
Metformin
Proton pump inhibitors
Familial selective malabsorption (Imerslund-Grasbeck disease)
Folic Acid
Dietary (old age, alcoholism, chronic disease)
Malabsorption (sprue)
Hemodialysis
Severe exfoliative skin disease (e.g., psoriasis)
Drugs
Interference with absorption or use (phenytoin, alcohol)
Dihydrofolate reductase inhibitors (methotrexate, trimethoprim)
Increased requirements
Pregnancy
Infancy
Hemolysis (e.g., sickle cell anemia)

or who have ileal disease (Crohn disease, tropical sprue) are likely to develop B_{12} deficiency and should receive prophylactic vitamin B_{12}. B_{12} deficiency after partial gastrectomy is less common. Evidence indicates that B_{12} malabsorption may occur and lead to neuropsychiatric sequelae secondary to vitamin B_{12} deficiency despite normal hematologic values and normal Schilling tests (discussed later in this chapter). In such cases, vitamin B_{12} levels usually are low, although often not as low as in pernicious anemia. Diagnosis may require more sensitive (and more expensive) tests of B_{12} metabolism, such as measurement of serum or urine methylmalonic acid and serum homocysteine (13). The mechanism of B_{12} deficiency in such patients is unclear, although it may be caused, at least in some patients, by an inability to absorb food-bound B_{12} even though they secrete normal amounts of intrinsic factor (14). If this problem is suspected, the patient should be referred to a hematologist or neurologist for further evaluation. A therapeutic trial of vitamin B_{12} is often recommended.

In contrast to vitamin B_{12}, the body's stores of folic acid are depleted rapidly when patients eat a diet deficient in folate. The main sources of folate in the diet are leafy vegetables, fruits, nuts, and liver. Therefore, the cause of folic acid deficiency most often is dietary. For example, pregnant women have an increased need for folate and without prenatal supplementation may develop folate deficiency, as may patients whose dietary intake is severely restricted because of chronic disease or multiple surgical procedures. Intestinal malabsorption for any reason is a common cause of folate deficiency. Finally, a number of drugs may be associated with folate deficiency: phenytoin (Dilantin) interferes with folate absorption, alcohol interferes with folate utilization, and methotrexate and trimethoprim–sulfamethoxazole (Bactrim, Septra) interfere with folate metabolism. Some chemotherapeutic agents (e.g., hydroxyurea, cytosine arabinoside, methotrexate, azathioprine) that are used in the treatment of cancer or for immunosuppression induction in patients with a variety of disorders cause megaloblastosis by inhibiting DNA synthesis.

Diagnosis

The morphology of the peripheral blood and bone marrow is the same in patients with folic acid deficiency and in those with vitamin B_{12} deficiency (12). With severe megaloblastic anemia, MCV often is significantly increased. MCV >120 fL almost always is caused by a megaloblastic anemia. The red cells in the peripheral blood are characterized by marked variation in size and shape. The common cell is a macro-ovalocyte (large egg-shaped cell). Howell–Jolly bodies (nuclear fragments), Pappenheimer bodies (iron granules), and nucleated RBCs also may be seen. The nuclei of the neutrophils often are hypersegmented, and commonly neutropenia and thrombocytopenia are present. The bone marrow typically is markedly cellular, revealing characteristic megaloblastic changes of all cell lines. The bone marrow iron stain usually reveals increased numbers of iron-containing nucleated RBCs (sideroblasts).

Folic Acid and Vitamin B_{12} Assay

Classically, in vitamin B_{12} deficiency the serum B_{12} level is quite low (<100 pg/mL) and the serum folate level is high. Spuriously normal B_{12} levels occasionally are seen in B_{12} deficiency (see earlier discussion), and spuriously low levels may be seen without B_{12} deficiency in some patients with folic acid deficiency (Table 55.14). The serum folate assay has little clinical usefulness in the workup of megaloblastic anemia secondary to folic acid deficiency. The red cell folate concentration does reflect chronic folate deficiency, although it may be falsely low in some patients with vitamin B_{12} deficiency (Table 55.14).

Schilling Test

The Schilling test is a measure of B_{12} absorption. It requires the measurement of total radioactivity excreted during a 24-hour period after ingestion of radioactive vitamin B_{12}. This test is useful primarily in cases where the data are confusing and for patients already treated with vitamin B_{12} in whom the serum levels are no longer helpful. The Schilling test requires a cooperative patient who can collect a 24-hour urine sample. The test includes the

TABLE 55.14 Vitamin B_{12} and Folate Concentrations

Serum B_{12} Concentration
Spuriously low in some patients with folate deficiency
Spuriously low in some pregnant patients
May be spuriously low in patients taking large daily doses of vitamin C
May be low in strict vegetarians
May be elevated for weeks after one injection of B_{12}
Increased in myeloproliferative syndromes
Red Blood Cell Folate Concentration
Reflects chronic folate deficiency
Falsely low in some patients with B_{12} deficiency
Falsely high in patients with reticulocytosis
Serum Folate Concentration
Measure of recent dietary intake of folate
May be low, normal, or elevated in B_{12} deficiency

following steps: after voiding, the patient takes 0.5 μCi of cobalt-labeled vitamin B_{12} (cyanocobalamin Co 60 or Co 57) by mouth. A 24-hour urine collection is initiated. At 2 hours, 1 mg B_{12} is given by injection (the flushing dose), and the percentage of radioactive B_{12} excreted in 24 hours is determined. Normally $\geq$7% of the dose is excreted in 24 hours. Incomplete collection may result in a spuriously low Schilling test and a false diagnosis of B_{12} malabsorption. In addition, in the presence of severe megaloblastic anemia, changes in the gastrointestinal mucosa may affect B_{12} absorption. For example, the Schilling test may be abnormal in patients with folic acid deficiency, because of the effect of folate deficiency on the intestinal mucosa, until the megaloblastic process has been treated for 1 or 2 weeks (Table 55.15).

Table 55.16 outlines a stepwise approach to the use of laboratory tests in differentiating between folic acid and vitamin B_{12} deficiency in a patient with megaloblastic anemia.

After a diagnosis of vitamin B_{12} deficiency is established and treatment is initiated (see later discussion), periodic determination of serum vitamin B_{12} is not required.

TABLE 55.15 Causes, Other than Pernicious Anemia, of a Positive Schilling Test

Incomplete urine collection
Renal failure
Some patients with megaloblastic anemia before treatment
Gastric antibodies to intrinsic factor
Defective intrinsic factor
Drugs (alcohol, colchicine, cholestyramine)
Pancreatic insufficiency
Partial gastrectomy

Other Laboratory Features

Megaloblastic anemias essentially are hemolytic in that there is marked destruction of abnormally formed cells within the marrow (ineffective erythropoiesis), which often results in indirect hyperbilirubinemia and an elevated serum lactate dehydrogenase concentration. The SI concentration usually is elevated, and the reticulocyte index is inappropriately low.

Gastric achlorhydria is present in pernicious anemia. Antibodies to gastric mucosal cells and intrinsic factor are often present, as are other autoantibodies, especially antithyroid and antiadrenal antibodies. The most useful test in this regard is the assay of anti-intrinsic factor antibody in serum, which is reasonably specific for pernicious anemia and is present in approximately 70% of cases. Anti-intrinsic factor antibody assay may be helpful in the occasional patient with megaloblastic anemia of uncertain etiology. There is an increased prevalence of thyroid disease (hypothyroidism, hyperthyroidism, and euthyroid goiter) in patients with pernicious anemia.

Treatment

The traditional treatment for B_{12} deficiency is monthly intramuscular administration of 1,000 μg vitamin B_{12} for the rest of the patient's life. Many clinicians treat patients daily while they are in the hospital, particularly if they have neurologic signs; however, there is little evidence that this practice is more efficacious than simply starting maintenance

TABLE 55.16 Differentiating between Folate and B_{12} Megaloblastosis

Etiology by History	*Red Blood Cell Folate*	*Serum B_{12}*	*Interpretation*	*Further Testing*
Suggests folate	↓	Normal or ↑	Folate deficiency	None
Suggests folate	↓	Slightly ↑	Folate deficiency	Recheck B_{12} after folate treatment for 1 wk
Suggests B_{12}	Normal or ↑	↓	B_{12} deficiency	None
Suggests B_{12}	↓	↓	B_{12} deficiency	May confirm with Schilling test
All other combinations → Schilling test				

monthly injections. There is evidence that B_{12} deficiency secondary to pernicious anemia can be treated successfully with oral vitamin B_{12}, 2,000 μg per day (15). Although ingested vitamin B_{12} is primarily absorbed in the terminal ileum as a complex with intrinsic factor (see above), an alternate transport system may exist that allows the absorption of sufficient quantities of vitamin B_{12} when administered orally in high doses (11). Vitamin B_{12} tablets in doses up to 1,000 μg are available over the counter.

Folic acid 1 to 5 mg daily is adequate treatment for patients with folic acid deficiency. Treatment should be given at least until a normal Hct is reached and should be continued if the patient is not eating an adequate diet or if the underlying cause persists (e.g., malabsorption). Patients with a chronic hemolytic state, such as children with sickle cell anemia, patients on hemodialysis (folic acid is dialyzable), and pregnant women, should receive prophylactic treatment.

With appropriate treatment of megaloblastic anemia, rapid reticulocytosis occurs and reaches a peak at approximately 7 to 10 days. Hct begins to rise in approximately 1 week and, in uncomplicated cases, rises at a rate of four to five percentage points per week. The leukopenia and thrombocytopenia respond dramatically, and leukocyte and platelet counts may return to normal in 1 to 2 days. The responses of the neurologic complications of vitamin B_{12} deficiency are variable. Psychiatric symptoms usually abate dramatically. Dorsal column problems and peripheral neuropathies usually improve, but more slowly. Lateral spinal tract signs usually are refractory to treatment.

Myelodysplastic Syndromes

Myelodysplastic syndromes are acquired disorders of bone marrow stem cells that usually are seen in elderly patients and may mimic a megaloblastic anemia at presentation (16). However, the morphologic features of the bone marrow, and usually the peripheral smear, are different (Table 55.12). WBC and platelet morphology may be abnormal, serum vitamin B_{12} and folic acid levels are normal or high, and patients do not respond to folic acid or vitamin B_{12} therapy. In the bone marrow, ringed sideroblasts (red cell precursors containing granules of iron that form a ring around the nuclei) are common, as are "megaloblastoid changes." Approximately 25% of patients develop acute nonlymphocytic leukemia, usually within 1 year but sometimes only after several years. Treatment frequently is supportive (transfusion, erythropoietin) (17), although a randomized controlled trial demonstrated the effectiveness of treatment with 5-azacytidine in selected patients (18). A number of other cytotoxic and immunosuppressive drugs have been tested, but none can yet be recommended for routine use. Patients who require more than supportive treatment should be referred to a hematologist or oncologist.

ANEMIAS WITH NORMAL MEAN CORPUSCULAR VOLUME AND APPROPRIATE RETICULOCYTE INDEX (HEMOLYSIS AND BLEEDING)

Anemias caused by bleeding and hemolysis are associated with an appropriate bone marrow response manifested by an appropriate reticulocyte index (Table 55.3). MCV usually is normal but may be slightly elevated if the reticulocyte count is very high. The diagnosis of hemolysis is suggested by an anemia with a reticulocyte index of at least 3% in the absence of overt bleeding. Bleeding is far more common than hemolysis, and bleeding in certain body sites (e.g., retroperitoneal bleeding in patients taking anticoagulants, bleeding into the site of a hip fracture) may be associated with a marked drop in Hct and a high reticulocyte count without external evidence of blood loss. Furthermore, correction of anemias that are caused by decreased bone marrow production may yield a database that mimics hemolysis, as in patients with an appropriate reticulocyte response after treatment with iron, folic acid, or vitamin B_{12} or after alcohol withdrawal.

Approach to Hemolysis

It is appropriate to attempt to prove the occurrence of hemolysis before obtaining diagnostic tests in a search for specific etiologies. The diagnostic approach to hemolysis varies depending on whether the hemolysis is primarily intravascular or extravascular.

Intravascular Hemolysis

Table 55.17 lists hemolytic mechanisms associated with intravascular destruction of RBCs. Almost all of the conditions require patient hospitalization, and, if possible, diagnostic testing and treatment planned in consultation with

TABLE 55.17 Clinical States Associated with Intravascular Hemolysis

Acute hemolytic transfusion reactions
Severe and extensive burns
Physical trauma (e.g., march hemoglobinuria)
Severe microangiopathic hemolysis (e.g., aortic valve prosthesis, TTP)
G6PD deficiency
Paroxysmal nocturnal hemoglobinuria

G6PD, glucose-6-phosphate dehydrogenase; TTP, thrombotic thrombocytopenic purpura.

TABLE 55.18 Appropriate Database when Intravascular Hemolysis Is Suspected

Observation of the color of the serum/plasma
Observation of the color of the urine
Measurement of free plasma hemoglobin
Heme pigment test of the urine if there are no red cells in the urine sediment
Measurement of serum haptoglobin
Iron stain of urine sediment for hemosiderin several days after a presumed hemolytic event

a hematologist. In intravascular hemolysis, red cell lysis occurs within the vascular space, resulting in hemoglobinemia. The plasma becomes visibly red or brown (methemoglobinemia) at a low hemoglobin concentration (approximately 30 mg/100 mL). Free hemoglobin initially binds to haptoglobin (a binding protein produced in the liver). Once haptoglobin is saturated, free hemoglobin passes through the glomerulus and hemoglobinuria occurs. Some of the hemoglobin in the renal tubules is absorbed by the renal tubular cells, which slough into the urine several days later and stain positively for iron (urine hemosiderin). Therefore, the latter test is helpful in documenting the presence of intravascular hemolysis several days after it has occurred. Table 55.18 suggests an appropriate database when hemolysis is suspected in the clinical states associated with intravascular hemolysis.

Extravascular Hemolysis

Most hemolysis occurs extravascularly within cells of the reticuloendothelial system. A diagnosis of extravascular hemolysis is more difficult to prove than that of intravascular hemolysis. There is no hemoglobinemia, hemoglobinuria, or hemosiderinuria. Haptoglobin is only partially saturated because there is only a slight leakage of free hemoglobin into the circulation. Indirect hyperbilirubinemia may be seen but is an insensitive sign of hemolysis. Fecal and urine urobilinogen levels increase but are difficult to quantitate. Other tests of hemolysis, such as red cell survival, are difficult, and the results are not known for several days. Often the clinician must be satisfied with only a presumptive diagnosis of extravascular hemolysis. Therefore, if extravascular hemolysis is suspected, it may be appropriate to obtain tests diagnostic of specific disease states based on a knowledge of the patient's other problems and on the baseline database (Table 55.19).

TABLE 55.19 Most Common Causes of Extravascular Hemolysis

Autoimmune hemolysis
Delayed hemolytic transfusion reactions
Hemoglobinopathies
Hereditary spherocytic and nonspherocytic anemias
Hypersplenism
Hemolysis with liver disease

Information from the Peripheral Smear

In hemolytic states the peripheral smear often reveals only evidence of the response of the bone marrow to hemolysis (large polychromatophilic or finely stippled red cells). It is a common misconception that hemolysis always causes fragmented red cells on the smear; they are seen only in microangiopathic hemolytic anemias. However, the smear may give further clues about the specific cause of the hemolysis (as indicated below).

Spherocytes

Spherocytes are seen in small numbers in many hemolytic states. When present in large numbers, they suggest hereditary spherocytosis, autoimmune hemolysis, or one of the hemoglobin C hemoglobinopathies.

Elliptocytes

In large numbers, elliptocytes suggest a diagnosis of hereditary elliptocytosis.

Fragmented Cells (Schistocytes)

Sharply pointed, fragmented cells (helmet cells, spiculated cells, triangle cells) are seen in microangiopathic states (see later discussion).

Spiculated Cells

Spiculated cells are sometimes seen in patients with severe liver disease and hemolysis (usually in a terminal stage of liver disease). Spiculated cells are one type of schistocyte found in the blood of patients with microangiopathic hemolysis.

Bite Cells (Blister Cells)

Bite cells are sometimes seen in patients with oxidative hemolysis (e.g., G6PD deficiency). In bite cells, all of the hemoglobin appears to be pushed to one side of the cell.

Poikilocytosis and the Hemoglobinopathies

The peripheral smear often is diagnostic in patients with sickle cell disease or the various other sickle cell syndromes (see later discussion).

Hemolysis with a Positive Coombs Test

Once hemolysis is suspected, the diagnostic testing should be guided by the patient's problem list. Because of the relatively common occurrence of immune hemolysis and the important therapeutic implications of such a diagnosis, it is desirable to obtain a Coombs test at this stage of the workup (19,20).

Positive Direct Coombs Test

The direct Coombs test is done by mixing the patient's cells with Coombs antiserum containing antibody to immunoglobulin G (IgG) and to complement. If the test is positive, the clinician should first ascertain from the laboratory personnel that the positive result is attributable to antibody and/or complement on the red cell surface. If this is the case, it is important to determine whether the antibody is an alloantibody or an autoantibody.

Alloantibodies are antibodies induced by prior transfusion or, in a woman, by placental transfer of fetal red cells. The antibodies are directed against specific minor red cell antigens, and identification of these antibodies is important in case future transfusions are necessary. Ordinarily the antibody is present primarily in the patient's plasma and is identified by an antibody screen (indirect Coombs test). However, a direct Coombs test also would be positive because of the presence of alloantibodies if the patient had been recently transfused with cells that were still circulating and sensitized by the antibody.

In a patient with hemolysis but no history of a recent transfusion, a positive direct Coombs test usually implies the presence of an autoantibody. In this situation, the antibody may be present in the serum as well as on the surface of the red cells. Table 55.20 lists the differences between alloantibodies and autoantibodies. Autoantibodies are classified as either warm antibodies or cold antibodies. Warm antibodies usually are IgG and cannot be identified by direct agglutination of red cells; a Coombs test is required to detect them. Cold antibodies usually are IgM, cause direct agglutination of red cells in the cold, and result in a positive Coombs test because of fixation of complement to the red cell.

Hemolysis Caused by Warm Antibodies

Table 55.21 lists the conditions commonly associated with autoimmune hemolysis resulting from a warm antibody.

TABLE 55.20 Comparison of Alloantibody and Autoantibody

Test	*Alloantibody*	*Autoantibody*
Direct Coombs test	Often negative; may be positive if sensitized foreign red cells are still circulating	Positive
Indirect Coombs test	Positive	Positive or negative
Antibody screen (panel)	Specificity is seen	Panagglutination, no specificity seen

TABLE 55.21 Autoimmune Hemolysis Caused by a Warm Antibody: Differential Diagnosis

- Idiopathic
- Secondary
  - Infection (particularly viral)
  - Drugs
    - α-Methyldopa
    - Penicillin
    - Quinine/quinidine
- Collagen vascular disease (systemic lupus erythematosus)
- Lymphoproliferative disorders
- Miscellaneous (e.g., thyroid disease, malignancy)

Patients may develop such antibodies secondary to use of certain drugs or to any of a number of conditions, including infections (particularly viral), collagen vascular disease (systemic lupus erythematosus [SLE]), lymphoproliferative diseases, and other malignancies. The classic example of a drug that induces a positive Coombs test is α-methyldopa (Aldomet) (21).

Autoimmune hemolysis is a relatively infrequent condition. Sometimes it precedes the development of SLE or lymphoma, but it may occur at any time during the course of the disease. Patients usually have anemia, which may be severe. On physical examination, the spleen is slightly enlarged in 50% of patients, and mild jaundice and fever are not uncommon. The peripheral smear shows marked polychromatophilia, spherocytosis, and often, but not always, an elevated reticulocyte index. Autoimmune hemolysis that is temporary, such as that caused by drug administration or viral infection, usually requires no treatment (although a drug, if implicated, should be discontinued). The process gradually remits over 2 to 3 weeks. Patients with chronic primary autoimmune hemolysis should be referred to a hematologist, who usually prescribes corticosteroids, which are generally effective if first given at a reasonably high dosage and slowly tapered as the anemia improves. Occasionally, splenectomy, cytotoxic drugs, or both are required for refractory cases. In patients with secondary chronic autoimmune hemolysis, treatment of the underlying disease is the most important therapy. Autoimmune hemolysis may present as a fulminant life-threatening anemia, sometimes associated with reticulocytopenia. In such cases, patients should be hospitalized immediately and transfused despite the incompatible cross-match.

Cold Agglutinin Hemolysis

The most common etiology of autoimmune hemolysis caused by a cold antibody is a viral illness or *Mycoplasma* pneumonia (22). Severe hemolysis is rare. Chronic idiopathic cold agglutinin hemolysis or cold agglutinin

TABLE 55.22 Hemolysis with Fragmented Red Cells on Peripheral Smear: Differential Diagnosis

Aortic valve prosthesis
Arteritis (e.g., malignant hypertension, polyarteritis)
Disseminated intravascular coagulation
Thrombotic thrombocytopenic purpura
Hemolytic uremic syndrome
Malignancy
Giant hemangiomas
Renal transplant rejection
Eclampsia
Metastatic cancer (gastric)
Some chemotherapy

hemolysis secondary to a lymphoproliferative disease often is more refractory to treatment with steroids and splenectomy than is the case with warm antibody hemolysis. Transfusion therapy may be a problem in such cases because the antibody is a panagglutinin and reacts with all blood types; therefore, a compatible cross-match may be impossible to obtain. Ordinarily, the IgM antibody in cold agglutinin hemolysis is not significantly hemolytic, and transfusions with warmed washed red cells or plasmapheresis can be attempted when absolutely necessary (23).

Hemolysis with Fragmented Red Cells on Peripheral Smear

Table 55.22 lists the conditions associated with hemolysis and the presence of fragmented red cells on peripheral smear. The peripheral blood contains sharply pointed poikilocytes (schistocytes). Such cells are characteristic and are clearly differentiated from abnormally shaped red cells seen in other conditions (24). The hemolysis may be severe and in such cases usually is intravascular, resulting in hemoglobinemia, hemoglobinuria, haptoglobin saturation, and subsequently hemosiderinuria (see earlier discussion). Red cell fragmentation may occur after insertion of a prosthetic, usually an aortic, valve. Rarely this is associated with clinically significant hemolysis. More often, red cell fragmentation is caused by arteriolar lesions (e.g., fibrin, inflammation) that damage the cells as they pass through the damaged vessel. When fragmented RBCs are accompanied by thrombocytopenia, one should consider the possibility of disseminated intravascular coagulation (see Chapter 56) or thrombotic thrombocytopenic purpura. This latter syndrome often is accompanied by fever and neurologic deficits, which characteristically fluctuate. If this condition is suspected, the patient should be hospitalized immediately and treated in consultation with a hematologist. The hemolytic uremic syndrome is a related (perhaps identical) syndrome, more common in children, that is characterized by the prominence of renal failure over other organ dysfunction.

Hemolysis with Enlarged Spleen (Hypersplenism)

Not all large spleens cause cytopenias, and the degree of cytopenia does not necessarily correlate with the size of the spleen (25). Thrombocytopenia and leukopenia are more common than is anemia. Splenomegaly from almost any cause may result in hypersplenism, but the syndrome is seen most often in patients who have chronic liver disease and congestive splenomegaly. Splenomegaly is sometimes seen in patients with hemolysis from other mechanisms, such as autoimmune hemolysis or hereditary spherocytosis. Rarely, splenectomy is necessary because of severe cytopenias resulting from hypersplenism. Occasionally patients with Felty syndrome (see Chapter 77) benefit from splenectomy, as do some patients with chronic leukemia or lymphoma.

Glucose-6-Phosphate Dehydrogenase Deficiency

G6PD deficiency (26) is seen primarily in African American patients in the United States. Inheritance is sex linked. Ten percent of African American males are affected (hemizygotes), as are 20% of African American females (heterozygotes). In these patients, hemolysis caused by G6PD deficiency is an acute intravascular hemolytic event usually precipitated by infection or an oxidant drug. Drugs known to precipitate hemolysis include sulfonamides, nitrofurantoin, and primaquine. Caucasian-type G6PD deficiency is seen primarily in patients from Mediterranean countries and usually is more severe than the African type. It sometimes causes chronic, persisting, partially compensated hemolysis.

Diagnosis after a hemolytic event may be difficult, especially in female heterozygotes. Screening tests for G6PD deficiency may give a normal result at this time, and even the affected hemizygote African American male may have a normal screening test for several weeks after hemolysis (young cells contain more G6PD activity). Occasionally a characteristic cell (bite cell) is seen in the peripheral blood during a hemolytic event.

Although the frequency of the genetic defect is high, the incidence of severe hemolysis with provocation (infection, drugs) is low. Ordinarily, routine screening before treatment with a known oxidant drug (e.g., sulfonamide) is not recommended. Affected patients should be given a list of drugs to avoid (26).

Sickle Cell Disorders

Approximately 8% of the African American population in the United States carry the sickle cell gene (27). The gene also is present to much less an extent in Greeks, Italians, Arabs, and people from India. Hemoglobin S results from a mutation in the β-globin chain in hemoglobin that, in the presence of reduced oxygen tension, causes the formation of rigid polymers that distort the shape of the RBC and increase its rigidity, leading to tissue ischemia and infarction. A number of common inherited disorders involving hemoglobin S are listed in this section.

Sickle Cell Trait

Most people who are heterozygous for hemoglobin S (sickle cell trait) are completely well and are not anemic. The peripheral smear appears normal, although sickling is seen if the blood is deoxygenated. Hemoglobin electrophoresis reveals approximately 40% hemoglobin S and 60% hemoglobin A. Hemoglobins A_2 and F are present in normal concentrations.

Most patients with the sickle trait lead a normal life. However, rare clinical events attributable to the presence of sickle cell hemoglobin do occur. For example, splenic infarction at high altitudes (above 10,000 feet) has been reported. (Oxygen pressures in commercial aircraft are high enough that people with sickle cell trait may fly safely.) Occasionally, infarctions occur in more vital organs during vigorous exercise. All people with sickle cell trait have renal tubular dysfunction resulting in hyposthenuria. On occasion, severe hematuria occurs from hypertonicity in the renal medulla, resulting in sickling and leading to ischemia and tubular infarction. People with sickle cell trait have a higher incidence of renal infections, especially during pregnancy.

Identification of patients with sickle cell trait is important so that they can be given genetic counseling. A couple, both heterozygous for hemoglobin S, should be informed that they have a 25% chance of having a child with sickle cell anemia.

Sickle Cell Anemia (Hemoglobin SS)

Sickle cell anemia exists in approximately 0.15% of the African American population (27–29). The disease usually is severe and results in significant morbidity as well as a shortened life expectancy. However, survival has improved considerably in the last 30 years. Mean survival of patients with SS disease is approximately 45 years and of persons with hemoglobin SC disease is approximately 64 years (30). One of the most disturbing clinical features of the illness is the occurrence of painful vaso-occlusive episodes: recurrent episodes of severe pain, usually in the limbs and the abdomen, caused by sickling-induced ischemia. Patients have lifelong, often severe anemia, with Hct values that range from the mid-teens to the high twenties. The primary mechanism of the anemia is extravascular hemolysis. Chronic reticulocytosis and chronic indirect hyperbilirubinemia are seen. Patients usually have leukocytosis, with the white cell count occasionally rising as high as 30,000 to 40,000 cells/mm^3 during a painful crisis. A mild thrombocytosis is also common. The peripheral smear shows markedly distorted red cells, including characteristically sickled cells. On electrophoresis, only hemoglobin S with a variable amount of hemoglobin F (no hemoglobin A) is detected.

The multiple and repetitive episodes of organ ischemia caused by sickling result in a host of abnormalities. The bones characteristically appear abnormal on radiography, revealing old infarctions that mimic the changes of osteomyelitis. The medullary spaces usually are widened by the marked compensatory expansion of bone marrow. The spine often takes on a distorted appearance, and aseptic necrosis of the femoral head (and, rarely, of the humeral head) is common, sometimes requiring joint replacement. Puberty often is delayed. Splenomegaly usually disappears by age 8 years because of repeated infarctions of the spleen. An adult with sickle cell anemia essentially is autosplenectomized. This lack of splenic function contributes to the propensity for infections, related especially to a decreased ability to resist pneumococcal infections. Gallstones (pigment stones) are common, and sicklers develop cholecystitis, which may be extremely difficult to differentiate clinically from a syndrome of intrahepatic cholestasis secondary to sickling in the hepatic sinusoids. There is some hazard to surgery, but patients with recurrent abdominal pain consistent with cholecystitis, who have gallstones, probably should have elective cholecystectomy (see Chapter 96). Pregnancy in women with SS disease is complicated by an increased risk for pyelonephritis, pulmonary infarction, antepartum hemorrhage, prematurity, and fetal death. With time, patients develop cardiomegaly and chronic myocardial disease related to repetitive microinfarctions of the heart. Murmurs are common and may suggest rheumatic or congenital heart disease. Patients with sickle cell anemia may develop venous thromboses and pulmonary embolism. They also may develop thromboses in situ in the lungs, followed by chronic scarring and fibrosis after many years. Pulmonary thrombosis/embolism may lead to pulmonary hypertension and right-sided heart failure. Cerebral vascular accidents, including infarction and intracerebral and subarachnoid hemorrhage, are common. Seizures are common as well. Up to 75% of patients with sickle cell anemia develop leg ulcerations that may be chronic and extremely difficult to heal. Patients with sickle cell anemia are prone to serious retinopathy, which in rare cases leads to blindness because of plugging of small retinal capillaries and subsequent neovascularization. It is important that these patients be examined yearly by an ophthalmologist because some of the problems can be prevented by photocoagulation of abnormal new retinal vessels (31).

Hemoglobin SC Disease

The genes that code for hemoglobin S and hemoglobin C are alleles. The C hemoglobin mutation is common in African Americans (approximately 2% prevalence), and patients doubly heterozygous for S and C constitute approximately 0.15% of that population. The syndrome is similar to that of SS disease but usually milder. In contrast to sickle cell anemia, the spleen is palpable in 50% of adult patients.

Hemoglobin S–β-Thalassemia

Patients doubly heterozygous for hemoglobin S and β-thalassemia trait have a syndrome similar to sickle cell anemia but usually more mild. Characteristically the MCV is low. The spleen may be palpable, and hemoglobin electrophoresis reveals 70% to 80% hemoglobin S and smaller amounts of hemoglobin A and F (the reverse of the pattern in sickle cell trait).

Treatment

Vaso-Occlusive Episodes

Painful vaso-occlusive episodes often are severe and may last for a few hours to several days and occasionally for several weeks. They may be associated with high fever and neutrophilia, which makes it difficult but important to differentiate crises from infection. No specific therapy exists. Hospitalization is indicated when pain is persistent. It is important to aggressively treat patients in painful crisis. Relatively large doses of intravenous narcotics frequently are needed. Routine, rather than as-needed (p.r.n.) orders, are appropriate in the hospital. Patients with sickle cell disease metabolize narcotics rapidly, and doses must be repeated every 2 hours. Patient-controlled analgesia has been found to be useful (32). Although narcotic abuse can occur, sickle cell pain, like pain due to cancer, should be treated based on the patient's description and tolerance of the pain. The data suggest that prompt, aggressive treatment of pain decreases hospitalizations and emergency room visits (33).

Infection

Patients with sickle cell anemia are prone to infections, especially with pneumococci. Patients with sickle cell anemia should receive pneumococcal vaccine (see Chapter 18) and should be encouraged to seek medical help at the first evidence of infection or fever.

Hemolytic and Aplastic Crises

Acceleration of hemolysis is unusual in adults. An Hct that drops significantly below baseline probably is the result of decreased marrow production, associated with infection. Hemolytic episodes are much more common in children. If they occur, hospitalization and transfusion often are necessary. Patients with chronic severe hemolysis have an increased requirement for folic acid, and folic acid deficiency may occur, resulting in reticulocytopenia and more severe anemia. Therefore, daily folic acid therapy (1 mg) is reasonable for all patients with sickle cell anemia.

Thromboembolization

Patients with sickle cell disease who develop deep vein thrombosis or pulmonary embolism should be treated with anticoagulants, as should any patient with such problems (see Chapter 57). However, venography should be avoided because of the danger of development of leg ulcers in any patient with SS hemoglobin whose lower extremities are traumatized. It often is difficult to distinguish pulmonary thrombotic/embolic problems from pneumonia. The *acute chest syndrome,* an episode characterized by chest pain, shortness of breath, and cough—often with fever and a pulmonary infiltrate—is common in patients with sickle cell anemia and usually warrants hospitalization to evaluate the diagnostic possibilities and institute appropriate treatment. When it is associated with significant hypoxia, the syndrome can be fatal, and patients may benefit from exchange transfusion. There is evidence that use of incentive spirometry during pain crises may decrease pulmonary complications in sickle cell disease.

Leg Ulcers

Leg ulcers often are large and are particularly refractory to treatment. Skin grafting frequently is only temporarily helpful. It is important to keep the ulcers clean, to elevate the legs frequently, and to use surgical stockings and elastic wraps (see Chapter 95).

Hematuria

Patients with sickle cell trait, sickle cell anemia, SC disease, or sickle cell thalassemia are all prone to bouts of severe hematuria related to sickling and medullary ischemia precipitated by the hypertonicity of the renal medulla. Bleeding can occur for days or even weeks. Maintenance of a high urine flow is important to prevent clots from causing obstruction. Usually the hematuria stops spontaneously.

Priapism

Priapism, an undesired painful penile erection, is common in men with SS and SC disease and often results in permanent impotence once it has resolved. Urologic intervention, if attempted, must be done within a few hours of the onset of the priapism. It often is only temporarily helpful. Once impotence has occurred, penile protheses often are helpful (see Chapter 6).

Preventive Treatment with Hydroxyurea

A large controlled study demonstrated that treatment with hydroxyurea decreases the incidence of painful crises in some patients with sickle cell anemia (34). The mechanism may be partly (but not completely) caused by increased intracellular levels of hemoglobin F. The benefit is modest in most patients, and a therapeutic trial requires close monitoring by a hematologist. The long-term side effects of hydroxyurea must be weighed carefully before a patient is prescribed this therapy. There is a growing experience with stem cell transplantation in children with sickle cell syndromes (35).

Recommendations for Preventive Care

Patients with sickle cell disorders have a lifelong chronic illness and require frequent and recurrent use of the health care system. The patient needs one general practitioner who is familiar with his or her case. The availability of emergency care 24 hours per day is exceedingly important.

Infection

There should be rapid evaluation of fever, chills, or other signs of infection. The patient should be immunized with the pneumococcal, influenza, and *Haemophilus influenzae* type B vaccines (see Chapter 18). Because heart murmurs and cardiomegaly are common, determining whether a patient with sickle cell anemia has valvular heart disease may be difficult based on physical examination alone. Echocardiography is appropriate if valvular disease is suspected.

Folic Acid

It is generally recommended that patients receive 1 mg folic acid daily.

Ophthalmologic Examination

Patients should see an ophthalmologist yearly.

Transfusions

In general, transfusions should be avoided because of the dangers of iron overload, sensitization to minor red cell antigens, infection, and other hazards of transfusion. Exchange transfusion (supervised by a hematologist) may help interrupt a prolonged pain crisis and is indicated in severe, life-threatening acute chest syndrome (discussed earlier). Hypertransfusion is useful in preventing recurrent neurologic vascular events. Alloimmunization occurs much more frequently in patients with sickle cell disease than in other patients with anemia because of minor red cell antigen incompatibilities in racially mismatched blood (36). This occurrence can be minimized by routinely performing extended cross-matches using blood matched for the predominant offending antigens (Duffy, Kidd, Kell, E, C).

The question of prophylactic transfusion for patients with sickle cell disease who are undergoing surgery with a general anesthetic has been long debated. A large multicenter study suggested there is no benefit to aggressive exchange transfusion over simple preoperative transfusion to hemoglobin levels of approximately 10 g/dL (37).

Hydroxyurea

Patients with frequent, severe, life-altering, painful vaso-occlusive episodes should be referred to a hematologist for consideration for hydroxyurea therapy.

ANEMIAS WITH NORMAL MEAN CORPUSCULAR VOLUME AND AN INAPPROPRIATELY LOW RETICULOCYTE INDEX

Mild normocytic anemias without appropriate reticulocyte responses are among the most common problems seen in clinical practice. Before considering possible etiologies and embarking on a diagnostic workup, it is important to be sure that Hct/Hb is reproducibly low. Moreover, the normal values for the testing laboratory should be known. For example, in some laboratories, an Hct of 35% in a woman is normal. One also should consider the variation in normal values related to age, sex, pregnancy, and other factors. Finally, one should be sure that volume overload is not the cause. Volume shifts may result in swings in Hct of six or eight percentage points. Table 55.23 lists

TABLE 55.23 Anemia with a Normal Mean Corpuscular Volume and Low Reticulocyte Index: Differential Diagnosis

Renal failure
Anemia of chronic disease (inflammatory disease and malignancy)
Anemia of hypoendocrine states (hypothyroidism, etc.)
Mild (early) iron deficiency
Combined iron deficiency and megaloblastic anemia
Drug-induced marrow depression
Primary bone marrow disorders
Bone marrow infiltration (myelophthisis)
Bleeding or hemolysis plus one of the above

the differential diagnosis of a normocytic anemia with an inappropriately low reticulocyte count.

Primary Bone Marrow Disorders

A minority of anemic patients with normal MCVs and a low reticulocyte index have primary bone marrow disorders and should be referred to a hematologist/oncologist. They require bone marrow aspiration or biopsy, and it is helpful to talk with them about the procedure before their referral visit.

Patient Experience. The procedure sounds more frightening than it is. Patients should be told that the procedure usually is done in the specialist's office and usually takes only 15 to 30 minutes. The patient lies on the side or abdomen. The usual site is the posterior superior iliac crest. A local anesthetic is used to deaden pain receptors in the dermis and periosteum. The aspirate or biopsy needles are small in diameter, and the procedure is minimally uncomfortable when done by an experienced clinician. Very anxious patients can be given an oral or parenteral analgesic, a mild sedative for anxiety, or both before the procedure if they are accompanied by someone who can drive them home. A gauze adhesive bandage (Band-Aid) is all that is used after the procedure, and acetaminophen is all that is needed for postprocedural discomfort.

Anemia of Renal Failure

Patients with uremia are anemic primarily because of decreased production of erythropoietin (38). The red cell morphology on smear usually is normal, but occasionally spiculated cells (burr cells) are seen. Some patients have a microangiopathic peripheral smear. There may be a mild thrombocytopenia, and the nuclei of the neutrophils may be hypersegmented even in the absence of folic acid deficiency. Hct depends on the degree of renal failure (see Fig. 52.4). Significant anemia is unusual if the creatinine concentration is <2 mg/100 mL. Hct values in patients with renal failure who are undergoing dialysis are extremely variable (ranging from the low teens, requiring transfusion, to the mid-thirties). Recombinant human erythropoietin is helpful for treatment of anemia of renal failure. Responses can be dramatic, and although the preparation is expensive, side effects are few (e.g., hypertension in some patients) (39). Erythropoietin levels are not reliable in predicting response to erythropoietin injections in patients with mild renal insufficiency. Patients in renal failure may be anemic because of iron deficiency (secondary to blood loss) or folate deficiency (because folic acid is dialyzable). Some patients with glomerulonephritis or arteritis have a microangiopathic hemolytic anemia.

Anemia of Chronic Disease

Any chronic inflammatory disease (e.g., rheumatoid arthritis) or malignant disease can cause mild to moderate anemia, unrelated to blood loss or hemolysis (40–42). (If the Hct is <25%, another explanation should be sought.) It is important to note that other chronic illnesses are not associated with this kind of anemia. Red cell morphology usually is normal, but sometimes the MCV is <80 fL, requiring differentiation of the process from other causes of a microcytic anemia (see earlier discussion). SI concentration and TIBC are low; the percentage of saturation may be just as low as it is in iron deficiency (<10%). The serum ferritin level is normal or elevated, and bone marrow iron stores are normal or increased. Treatment with erythropoietin sometimes is helpful in certain patients (e.g., those with cancer, human immunodeficiency infection, rheumatoid arthritis) who have severe, symptomatic anemia if the serum erythropoietin level is <500 IU/mL, and especially if it is <100 IU/mL (43–45).

In addition to chronic infections, acute infection or inflammation causes a decrease in SI, a reticulocytopenia, and a decrease in bone marrow red cell production. If present for 1 week or longer, an acute inflammatory process may result in an Hct fall of several percentage points.

Mild Early Iron Deficiency

Although severe iron deficiency results in microcytic anemia (discussed earlier), in the early stages mild iron deficiency may result in anemia with a normal peripheral smear and a normal MCV. Diagnosis usually can be made by measurement of serum ferritin or by a bone marrow iron stain. In addition, a patient with severe iron deficiency, when it accompanies a macrocytic anemia such as a megaloblastic anemia (e.g., an alcoholic patient with iron deficiency and folic acid deficiency), may have a severe anemia that is normocytic. The reticulocyte count is inappropriately low until (in the alcoholic patient) alcohol is withdrawn and iron and folate are administered.

Anemia in the Elderly

Old age per se is not an explanation for a significant normocytic anemia (46). The Hct in healthy individuals in their seventies is only slightly lower than the normal adult range (Table 55.1). However, it is in elderly patients that frustrating, mild, unexplained, normocytic anemias occur. In such patients, the following possible explanations should be considered: fluid overload, blood loss from phlebotomy if the patient has been hospitalized recently, and any recent inflammatory disease (viral or bacterial infection, inflammatory joint problem) that may depress bone marrow production and, if present for several days, may result in a drop in Hct. If none of these explanations seems appropriate and there is no reason to suspect an underlying problem, it is reasonable to simply monitor the Hct without further diagnostic workup. If the onset of the anemia is known to be recent (e.g., if there is a record of a normal Hct finding 3 months previously), other efforts should be made to explain the anemia. For example, the possibility of occult gastrointestinal bleeding with early iron deficiency or the anemia of chronic disease or malignancy should be entertained. There is evidence that unexplained anemias are more common in elderly poor persons with inadequate access to health care and that anemia in the very old is associated with increased mortality risk (47).

SPECIFIC REFERENCES*

1. Umbreit J. Iron deficiency: a concise review. Am J Hematol 2005;78:225.
2. England JM, Ward S, Down MC. Microcytosis, anisocytosis and the red cell indices in iron deficiency. Br J Haematol 1976;34:589.
3. Suominen P, Punnonen K, Rajamaki A, et al. Serum transferrin receptor and transferrin receptor-ferritin index identify healthy subjects with subclinical iron deficits. Blood 1998; 92:2934.
4. Junca J, Fernandez-Aviles F, Oriol A, et al. The usefulness of serum transferrin receptor in detecting iron deficiency in the anemia of chronic disorders. Haematologica 1998;83: 676.
5. Halliday JW, Powell LW. Serum ferritin and isoferritins in clinical medicine. Prog Hematol 1979;11:229.
6. Faich G, Strobos J. Sodium ferric gluconate complex in sucrose: safer intravenous iron therapy than iron dextrans. Am J Kidney Dis 1999;33:464.
7. Pierce HI, Kurachi S, Sofroniadou K, et al. Frequencies of thalassemia in American blacks. Blood 1977;49:981.
8. Kaiser L, Schwartz KA. Aluminum induced anemia. Am J Kidney Dis 1985;5:348.
9. Davidson RJL, Hamilton PJ. High mean red cell volume: its incidence and significance in routine hematology. J Clin Pathol 1978;31:493.
10. Colman N, Herbert J. Hematologic complications of alcoholism: overview. Semin Hematol 1980;17:164.
11. Oh RC, Brown DL. Vitamin B_{12} deficiency. Am Fam Physician 2003;67:979.
12. Lindenbaum J. Status of laboratory testing in the diagnosis of megaloblastic anemia. Blood 1983;61:624.
13. Lindenbaum J, Healton EB, Savage DG, et al. Neuropsychiatric disorders caused by cobalamin deficiency in the absence of anemia or macrocytosis. N Engl J Med 1988;318: 1720.
14. Carmel R, Sinow RM, Siegel ME, et al. Food cobalamin malabsorption occurs frequently in patients with unexplained low serum cobalamin levels. Arch Intern Med 1988;148:1715.
15. Kuzminski AM, De Giacco EJ, Allen RH, et al. Effective treatment of cobalamin deficiency with oral cobalamin. Blood 1998;92:1191.
16. Ganser A, Haelyer D. Clinical course of myelodysplastic syndromes. Hematol Oncol Clin North Am 1992;6:607.
17. Hellstrom-Lindberg E. Management of anemia associated with myelodysplastic syndrome. Semin Hematol 2005;42(2 Suppl 1):S10.
18. Silverman LR, Demakos EP, Peterson BL, et al. Randomized controlled trial of azacitidine in patients with the myelodysplastic syndrome: a study of the cancer and leukemia group B. J Clin Oncol 2002;20:2429.
19. Collins PW, Newland AC. Treatment modalities of autoimmune blood disorders. Semin Hematol 1992;29:64.
20. Pirofsky G. Clinical aspects of autoimmune hemolytic anemia. Semin Hematol 1976;13:251.
21. Salama A, Mueller-Eckhardt C. Immune-mediated blood cell dyscrasias related to drugs. Semin Hematol 1992;29:54.
22. Jacobson LB, Longstreth GF, Edgington TS. Clinical and immunologic features of transient cold agglutinin hemolytic anemia. Am J Med 1973;54:514.
23. Jefferies LC. Transfusion therapy in autoimmune hemolytic anemias. Hematol Clin North Am 1994;8:1087.
24. Brain MC. Microangiopathic hemolytic anemia. N Engl J Med 1969;281:833.
25. Dameshek W. Hypersplenism. Bull N Y Acad Med 1955;31:113.
26. Beutler E. Glucose-6-phosphate dehydrogenase deficiency. N Engl J Med 1991;324:169.
27. Abramson H, Bertles JF, Wethers DL, eds. Sickle cell disease. St. Louis: Mosby, 1973.
28. Steinberg MH. Management of sickle cell disease. N Engl J Med 1999;340:1021.
29. Vichinsky EP. Comprehensive care in sickle cell disease: its impact on morbidity and mortality. Semin Hematol 1991;28:220.
30. Platt OS, Brambilla DJ, Rosse WF, et al. Mortality in sickle cell disease: life expectancy and risk factors for early death. N Engl J Med 1994;330:1639.
31. King W, Nadel AJ. Ophthalmologic complications in hemoglobinopathies. Hematol Oncol Clin North Am 1991;5:535.
32. McPherson E, Perlin E, Finke H, et al. Patient-controlled analgesia in patients with sickle cell vaso-occlusive crisis. Am J Med Sci 1990;299:10.
33. Brookoff D, Polomano RA. Treating sickle cell pain. Ann Intern Med 1992;116:364.
34. Charache S, Barton FB, Moore RD. Hydroxyurea and sickle cell anemia: clinical utility of a myelosuppressive "switching" agent. The Multicenter Study of Hydroxyurea in Sickle Cell Anemia. Medicine (Baltimore) 1996;75: 300.
35. Walters MC, Storb R, Patience M, et al. Impact of bone marrow transplantation for symptomatic sickle cell disease: an interim report. Blood 2000;95:1918.
36. Vichinsky EP, Earles A, Johnson RA, et al. Alloimmunization in sickle cell anemia and transfusion of racially unmatched blood. N Engl J Med 1990;322:1617.
37. Vichinsky EP, Haberkern CM, Neumayr L, et al. A comparison of conservative and aggressive transfusion regimens in the perioperative management of sickle cell disease: the Preoperative Transfusion in Sickle Cell Disease Study Group. N Engl J Med 1995;333:206.
38. Erslev AJ. Management of anemia of chronic renal failure. Clin Nephrol 1974;2:174.
39. Eschbach JW, Eqrie JC, Downing MR, et al. Correction of the anemia of end-stage renal disease with recombinant human erythropoietin: results of a combined phase I and II clinical trial. N Engl J Med 1987;316:73.
40. Cartwright GE. The anemia of chronic disorders. Semin Hematol 1966;3:351.
41. Cash JM, Sears DA. The anemia of chronic disease: spectrum of associated diseases in a series of unselected hospitalized patients. Am J Med 1989;87:638.
42. Weiss G, Goodnough LT. Anemia of chronic disease. N Engl J Med 2005;352:1011.
43. Henry DH, Beall GN, Benson CFA, et al. Recombinant human erythropoietin in the treatment of anemia associated with human immunodeficiency virus (HIV) infection and zidovudine therapy. Ann Intern Med 1992; 117:739.
44. Ludwig H, Fritz E, Leitgeb C, et al. Prediction of response to erythropoietin treatment in chronic anemia of cancer. Blood 1994;84:1056.
45. Pincus T, Olsen NJ, Russell I, et al. Multicenter study of recombinant human erythropoietin in correction of anemia in rheumatoid arthritis. Am J Med 1990;89:161.
46. Lipschitz DA, Udupa KB, Milton KY, et al. Effects of age on hematopoiesis in man. Blood 1984;63:502.

*Bold numerals denote published controlled clinical trials, meta-analyses, or consensus-based recommendations.

*For annotated **General References** and resources related to this chapter, visit www.hopkinsbayview.org/PAMreferences.*

Chapter 56

Disorders of Hemostasis

Larry Waterbury and Philip D. Zieve

In a healthy person, a number of different processes interact to ensure that blood is maintained in a fluid state until the integrity of a blood vessel wall is compromised. At that point, a plug is rapidly formed to prevent exsanguination. Three major systems are involved in this process: the vasculature itself, the blood platelets, and the coagulation system.

EVALUATION OF PATIENTS

The history is the most important aid in determining whether a patient has a hemorrhagic diathesis (1). Patients with congenital disorders of hemostasis or acquired disorders of long standing almost certainly have a history of unexpectedly excessive bleeding in response to minor trauma or to surgery. The clinician should ask specifically whether the patient has required transfusion after an operative procedure or a seemingly minor trauma.

Bleeding caused by injury to the vasculature is overwhelmingly more common than bleeding caused by defective hemostasis. Therefore, patients with gastrointestinal or genitourinary hemorrhage, for example, are more likely to have a lesion (e.g., peptic ulcer, carcinoma, diverticulum, or tumor of the kidney or bladder) that has bled than a disorder of hemostasis. Similarly, nosebleeds, bleeding gums, or excessive menstrual flow probably reflect local (usually benign) problems. Furthermore, even if patients have hemostatic dysfunction, they are likely to bleed from local lesions, the propensity to bleed of which has been accentuated by the hemostatic abnormality.

Specific disorders of hemostasis may be strongly suspected based on the patient's history and because of characteristic findings on physical examination (Fig. 56.1), but in almost all instances, laboratory tests are required before a specific diagnosis can be made. Screening tests, procedures that are extremely sensitive to alterations in hemostasis, ordinarily are relied on first in a patient with a suspected hemorrhagic diathesis (Table 56.1). More specific tests are indicated if any of these screening test results are abnormal or if a disorder of hemostasis is strongly suspected, even if the test results are not abnormal. These more specific tests are best performed in consultation with a hematologist.

DISORDERS OF BLOOD VESSELS

Vascular disease is diagnosed uncommonly as a cause of a hemorrhagic diathesis, in part because, except for trauma, disorders of the vasculature that result in untoward bleeding are rare (2) and in part because there is no reliable screening test to detect generalized vascular dysfunction. The primary hemorrhagic manifestation of vascular disease is purpura, a confluent purplish discoloration of the skin caused by extravasation of blood from cutaneous and subcutaneous blood vessels. Although patients with an abnormal vasculature occasionally experience bleeding from large blood vessels, most commonly they bleed into the skin or mucous membranes. Because purpura is a common response to minor trauma, it cannot in itself be taken as evidence of an underlying hemorrhagic diathesis.

Cutaneous Lesions

Unexplained bruises, especially on the lower extremities, are common and usually are not associated with an underlying disease process. Therefore, a history of easy bruising is unlikely, by itself, to lead to a diagnosis of a disorder of hemostasis. Similarly, *senile purpura,* which occurs characteristically on the dorsum of the hand and the extensor surfaces of the forearms, does not represent a generalized hemorrhagic diathesis but results from the loss of connective tissue support to intracutaneous blood vessels, which then are easily traumatized and bleed within the substance of the skin. Identical lesions are seen sometimes in patients with Cushing syndrome or in patients who have received corticosteroid therapy.

Allergic purpura is a hypersensitivity reaction to an antigenic stimulus that usually cannot be identified (although sometimes a drug or an infection can be incriminated as a provocative agent) (3,4). Characteristically, patients

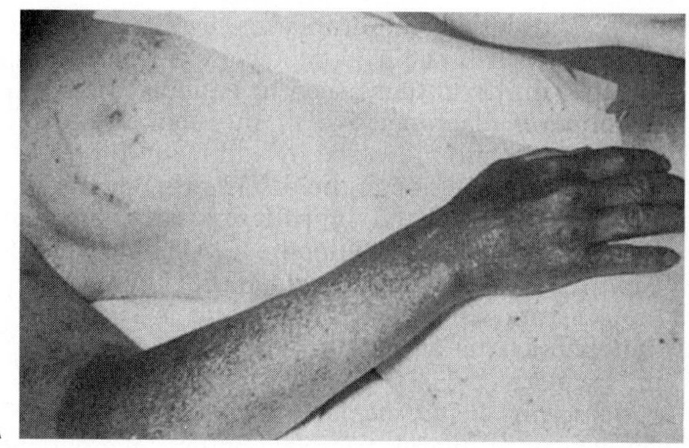

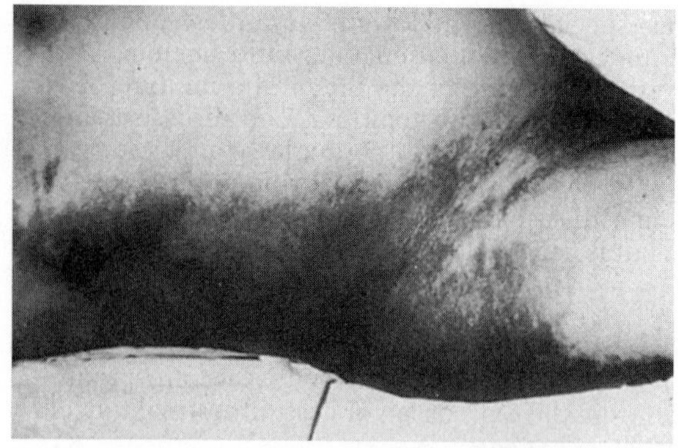

FIGURE 56.1. Bleeding caused by thrombocytopenia compared with bleeding caused by abnormal coagulation. **A:** Immune thrombocytopenic purpura with typical petechial lesions. **B:** Hemophilia A with extensive purpuric bleeding. (From Zieve PD, Levin J. Disorders of hemostasis. Philadelphia: WB Saunders, 1976, with permission.)

develop a symmetrical petechial rash, which is most prominent on the extremities. The lesions are slightly raised, distinguishing them from the petechiae of thrombocytopenia. No hemostatic dysfunction is associated with this condition. The cutaneous manifestations of the disorder are part of a widespread small-vessel vasculitis, the manifestations of which may include arthralgias (sometimes with evidence of joint effusions), fever, malaise, abdominal pain, gastrointestinal bleeding, and renal disease caused by a focal glomerulonephritis that occasionally progresses to chronic renal failure. There is no specific treatment for this condition. If the patient is taking a drug that is suspected of being a sensitizing agent, the drug should be discontinued. In fact, because the offending agent often is not readily identified, all drugs that are not absolutely essential to care should be discontinued. Most patients recover spontaneously within 3 to 4 weeks, but signs and symptoms of the disease may continue or recur for up to 1 year. Patients should be reassured while they are symptomatic that unless they have evidence of progressive renal disease, they ultimately will recover.

TABLE 56.1 Laboratory Evaluation of Hemostatic Function

System	Screening Tests	Specific Tests
Blood vessels	None	Depends on suspected underlying disorder (see text)
Platelets		
Quantitative	Scanning of a stained smear of the peripheral blood	Platelet count
Qualitative	Bleeding time	Platelet aggregation
Coagulation	Partial thromboplastin time, prothrombin time, thrombin time	Factor assays

Autoerythrocyte sensitization (5) is a disorder, predominantly of women, characterized by apparently spontaneous painful ecchymoses, usually on the lower extremities and anterior trunk. The disorder is so named because of a one-time belief that the disorder arose as the result of a hypersensitivity response to patients' red cells or red cell stroma. In fact, the lesions can sometimes be produced by injection of autologous red cells into the skin of these patients. It has become apparent, however, that virtually all patients with the disorder are severely psychoneurotic and, in some instances, frankly psychotic. Many people now believe that the lesions are self-inflicted.

Cryoglobulinemia (6) as a primary abnormality or as a special feature of an underlying disease such as dysproteinemia (see Dysproteinemia), lymphoma, or collagen vascular disease may cause purpuric bleeding, especially on the lower extremities. The cryoglobulins may be isolated monoclonal proteins or may be immune complexes of monoclonal immunoglobulin IgG or IgM and polyclonal IgG or of mixed polyclonal immunoglobulins. There often is an associated glomerulonephritis and, in the patient with immune complex formation, sometimes evidence of hepatitis B or hepatitis C infection.

The diagnosis of cryoglobulinemia can be made by placing a sample of the patient's serum in a refrigerator overnight and then inspecting the serum for the formation of a white gel or precipitate that disappears when the specimen is warmed. The blood for this test should be drawn in a warm syringe and the clot that forms should be allowed to retract in a 37°C water bath. Primary cryoglobulinemia is poorly responsive to treatment. Secondary cryoglobulinemia may respond to treatment of the underlying disease.

Patients with other vasculitides sometimes also present with petechialike lesions and systemic disease (e.g., renal or pulmonary disease) typically much more severe than in patients with allergic purpura. These conditions are sometimes associated with antineutrophilic cytoplasmic antibodies (ANCAs). Such patients are best managed in consultation with a rheumatologist.

Mucocutaneous Lesions

Some patients with vascular disease are prone to bleeding from the oral, nasal, or gastrointestinal mucosa, as well as from the skin. Such patients may present to their providers not only with cutaneous hemorrhage but also with bleeding gums, epistaxis, hematemesis, or melena.

Amyloidosis

Mucocutaneous bleeding may be a symptom of amyloidosis because of the deposition of amyloid within the walls of blood vessels (7). Periorbital bleeding and bleeding in skin folds are especially common. The skin in the areas of hemorrhage sometimes appears thickened because of palpable amyloid deposits within it. Patients suspected of having this disorder should have biopsies with appropriate staining and serum and urine electrophoresis in an attempt to make a specific diagnosis.

Dysproteinemia

Myeloma or macroglobulinemia may be associated with untoward bleeding, either because of increased viscosity of the blood or because the coating of blood vessels and platelets with the abnormal protein interferes with normal hemostatic function (8). Abnormal coagulation is common in patients with these disorders. Patients suspected of having dysproteinemia should have samples of their serum and urine examined by electrophoresis in an attempt to demonstrate a monoclonal protein. If the diagnosis of dysproteinemia seems likely based on the result of this test and the clinical presentation, consultation with a hematologist or oncologist is appropriate.

Vitamin C Deficiency

In the United States, symptomatic vitamin C deficiency (scurvy) might be seen in three specific groups: chronic alcoholics, food faddists, and chronically ill or debilitated patients (9). Because humans, unlike most animals, are unable to synthesize vitamin C, they depend on exogenous sources such as fruits and leafy vegetables. People who cannot, or will not, eat an adequate diet of foods that contain the vitamin are subject to the manifestations of scurvy. The signs and symptoms of scurvy are attributable largely to the formation of defective connective tissue, because of the human body's absolute dependence on vitamin C for the synthesis of normal collagen. Mucocutaneous bleeding is common in patients with vitamin C deficiency who characteristically have large ecchymoses on their extremities, bleeding gums, and, very suggestive of this disorder, perifollicular hemorrhages that commonly appear on the lower extremities and anterior trunk. Sometimes patients with vitamin C deficiency develop hemarthroses similar to those seen in patients with severe coagulation disorders. All manifestations of scurvy are readily reversed by administration of vitamin C, so scurvy should be considered in patients with compatible signs and symptoms even though the disorder is uncommon. Vitamin C deficiency can be confirmed by assay of the blood, but this test usually is unnecessary because, if the diagnosis is suspected, a therapeutic trial of vitamin C (250 mg once per day) is innocuous.

Hereditary Hemorrhagic Telangiectasia

Hereditary hemorrhagic telangiectasia (Osler-Weber-Rendu disease) is an inherited abnormality of blood vessels (an autosomal dominant condition) in which there is dilation of abnormally thin-walled venules and capillaries (10). The dilations result in characteristic telangiectases, which are small, flat, red, or purple lesions that blanch on pressure. They occur throughout the body but most commonly are seen externally on the lips, tongue, hand, and mucous membranes of the nose. Lesions of larger blood vessels also occur in this disease, most commonly pulmonary arteriovenous fistulas, which develop in up to one third of patients and may cause high-output heart failure. Vascular malformations of the liver or the brain may occur. The mucocutaneous lesions may bleed excessively when traumatized. Recurrent epistaxis is the most common symptom of patients with the disorder, but the most troublesome problem is recurrent gastrointestinal bleeding, which is difficult to manage. Accessible lesions ordinarily can be treated by local compression. No pharmacologic agent will alter the course of the condition, but symptoms are variable. Many patients experience little difficulty during the course of their lives.

DISORDERS OF PLATELETS

Platelets provide a cellular defense against the loss of blood from traumatized vessels, especially where blood flow is relatively rapid, as on the arterial side of the circulation and the left side of the heart. Platelets are particularly effective in sealing leaks from small arterioles and capillaries. When platelets are abnormal, either quantitatively or qualitatively, these vessels bleed most prominently. The platelet plug is initiated by contact of platelets with subendothelial collagen, which is exposed by injury to the vascular intima. The absorption of a protein, von Willebrand factor (see below), to specific receptor sites on the platelet surface is important in the mediation of this process. Thereafter, aggregating agents such as thrombin and adenosine diphosphate cause the accretion of platelets at that site, eventually forming an adhesive plug that within minutes prevents the further flow of blood. Eventually, the plug is replaced by fibrin laid down by the activation of the coagulation mechanism, which occurs simultaneously with the initiation of platelet plug formation.

Thrombocytopenia is one of the most common acquired disorders of hemostasis. The normal platelet count is between 150,000 and 400,000/mm^3, but the platelet count ordinarily must be reduced to <50,000/mm^3 before untoward bleeding is observed, and even then bleeding usually does not occur unless the patient is traumatized. So-called *spontaneous bleeding* is unlikely unless the platelet count is reduced to <20,000/mm^3. There is a general impression that there is a higher risk of bleeding when thrombocytopenia is secondary to decreased bone marrow production rather than to decreased survival of platelets. For example, patients with immune thrombocytopenia may not have significant bleeding even with platelet counts as low as 5,000/mm^3. At any given platelet count, the risk of bleeding varies with the cause of thrombocytopenia.

The characteristic lesion of thrombocytopenia is the petechia, a small purpuric hemorrhage occurring on the skin or mucous membranes, especially at sites of elevated capillary pressure, such as the lower extremities, the forearm after inflation of a blood pressure cuff, or the face after prolonged crying or coughing. In fact, if capillary pressure is raised high enough or if capillaries are damaged after sunburn, for example, petechiae may be seen in otherwise normal people. Although cutaneous bleeding may be the first clue to the diagnosis of thrombocytopenia, morbidity from the disorder is more likely to result from gastrointestinal or genitourinary hemorrhage. If bleeding occurs from these sites, the patient should be examined at an appropriate time to determine whether an organic lesion, such as carcinoma of the colon or kidney, has bled in association with defective hemostasis. The most feared complication of thrombocytopenia is intracerebral bleeding that, although it occurs infrequently, is still one of the major causes of death in patients with the disorder.

Evaluation of the Thrombocytopenic Patient

The best screening test for evaluation of the numbers of platelets in the blood is observation of a stained smear of the peripheral blood. With relatively little experience it is easy to determine whether the platelet count is unusually low or high. In unanticoagulated blood (e.g., from a fingerstick), at least one clump of platelets, on the average, should be seen in every oil immersion field. In anticoagulated blood, one platelet should be seen for every 10 to 20 red cells. If a quantitative abnormality is suspected, a precise platelet count can be obtained. The bleeding time is not useful as a screening test for detecting quantitative abnormalities of platelets or for predicting which patients are likely to bleed excessively when traumatized (11). However, despite its limitations, the bleeding time still is used commonly to evaluate qualitative abnormalities of platelet function (described later in this chapter).

Patients with an immune thrombocytopenia (see below) characteristically have increased amounts of γ-globulin adsorbed to their platelets. Tests to detect these proteins are widely available but have proved to be nonspecific and therefore of little value in establishing a precise diagnosis.

In ambulatory practice, many patients with mild thrombocytopenia are encountered. The precise pathophysiology of the condition is not clear. Many patients are found to have thrombocytopenia during the course of routine hematologic studies performed to obtain baseline data or as part of an evaluation of an apparently unrelated condition. The first task for the clinician is to rule out spurious thrombocytopenia secondary to marked platelet clumping affecting the accuracy of the automated platelet count. This artifact usually is secondary to antibodies to the anticoagulant used to obtain blood for a complete blood count. When spurious thrombocytopenia is suspected, blood should be collected using another anticoagulant (usually citrate) and the platelet count repeated. The technician should inspect a smear from anticoagulated blood for increased clumping. Once spurious thrombocytopenia has been ruled out, if the platelet count is >50,000/mm^3 and the history, physical examination, and other hematologic evaluations do not suggest an underlying disease that urgently requires diagnosis and treatment, it probably is justifiable simply to follow the patient with serial platelet counts performed monthly until the stability of the counts are determined.

Symptomatic thrombocytopenia caused by decreased production of platelets usually is observed in conjunction with processes such as aplastic anemia, leukemia, myelodysplasia, disseminated tuberculosis, or metastatic carcinoma that affect other hematologic cell lines. In contrast, severe thrombocytopenia caused by increased destruction of platelets does not necessarily indicate the presence of a disease process that is affecting parts or systems of the body other than the blood platelets or their precursors. To be reasonably certain about the pathophysiology of thrombocytopenia, however, it sometimes is necessary to perform an aspiration of the bone marrow and to evaluate the numbers of megakaryocytes and the appearance of the other blood cell precursors. Patients who have thrombocytopenia because of diseases involving the bone marrow, except in cases of megaloblastic anemia, have reduced numbers of megakaryocytes. If the thrombocytopenia is severe, abnormalities of production of, or qualitative changes in, other cell lines likely will be noted. On the other hand, if the patient is thrombocytopenic because of increased destruction of platelets, the numbers of megakaryocytes will be increased and the marrow will otherwise appear normal (although increased erythroid

TABLE 56.2 Etiology of Thrombocytopenia by Mechanism

Decreased production
- Primary bone marrow disorders (leukemia, myelodysplasia, aplastic anemia, myeloma)
- Replacement (by metastatic cancer, etc.)
- Infection
- Drugs

Ineffective myelopoiesis
- Megaloblastic anemia

Decreased survival/increased sequestration
- Immune thrombocytopenia
- Thrombotic thrombocytopenic purpura/hemolytic-uremic syndrome
- Disseminated intravascular coagulation
- Large spleen syndrome

activity might be seen in those patients who are bleeding). It has been proposed that bone marrow aspiration need not be done routinely in patients with isolated thrombocytopenia (thought to be immune mediated) (12,13). In any case, patients with severe thrombocytopenia (<30,000/mm^3) require consultation with a hematologist.

Decreased Production of Platelets

Decreased production of platelets is a common mechanism for thrombocytopenia in ambulatory patients (Table 56.2). Apparent suppression of thrombopoiesis often is associated with viral infections such as upper respiratory infections, infectious mononucleosis, and childhood exanthems. In most cases, bone marrow aspirates show megakaryocytes in normal or reduced numbers, although they sometimes appear morphologically abnormal. At other times, increased numbers of megakaryocytes are found in patients with thrombocytopenia in association with viral infections, suggestive of a destructive process (perhaps immunologic) to which the marrow has responded with increased production of platelets. In general, patients with benign *viral infections* are not likely to have severe thrombocytopenia and so are not at major risk for bleeding. The process ordinarily dissipates as the infection resolves.

Certain drugs predictably produce thrombocytopenia by affecting thrombopoiesis. Among these drugs, cytotoxic agents are unlikely to be administered by the general practitioner. Although thiazide diuretics have been reported to produce mild to moderate thrombocytopenia commonly, a clear-cut cause-and-effect relationship has not been demonstrated. In the reported studies, platelet counts have fallen several weeks after the beginning of therapy, sometimes associated with morphologically abnormal megakaryocytes. Rarely, however, thiazides have been clearly implicated in immunologically induced destructive thrombocytopenia (see Increased Destruction of Platelets). Thiazide diuretics also are a common cause of allergic purpura (see above), but patients with this condition have normal platelet counts.

A large number of drugs have been implicated, on occasion, in the production of thrombocytopenia by the suppression of thrombopoiesis. Therefore, if patients are symptomatic from thrombocytopenia or have counts <50,000/mm^3 and the cause of thrombocytopenia is unknown, it would be reasonable to discontinue the administration of all drugs that are not considered absolutely essential.

Management

Clearly, the cause of decreased platelet production should be removed, if possible (e.g., discontinuing administration of an offending drug). If there is no evidence of mucous membrane or internal bleeding, treatment of the thrombocytopenia itself usually is unnecessary. Patients with severe bleeding should receive platelet transfusions when thrombocytopenia is due to decreased platelet production and counts are <50,000/mm^3. Some patients with chronic diseases of the bone marrow, such as myelodysplasia or aplastic anemia, require periodic platelet transfusions. Such patients should be followed by a hematologist or oncologist, as well as by a primary caregiver.

Increased Destruction of Platelets

In ambulatory practice, probably the most common cause of thrombocytopenia seen is thrombocytopenia secondary to an immune mechanism (Table 56.3). Patients with *autoimmune thrombocytopenia* characteristically present with petechiae (12–14). Physical examination reveals no other evidence of disease; in particular, the spleen usually is not palpable. It is helpful to look at platelet morphology on a peripheral blood smear. Typically, platelets are large and sometimes elongated in severe destructive thrombocytopenia as opposed to the small platelets seen when the

TABLE 56.3 Immune Thrombocytopenia

Primary (idiopathic thrombocytopenic purpura, autoimmune thrombocytopenia)

Secondary immune thrombocytopenia
- Acute
  - Viral infections
  - Drugs (e.g., quinine, quinidine, sulfa, heparin)
- Posttransfusion purpura
- Chronic
  - Collagen vascular disorders (e.g., lupus, scleroderma)
  - Lymphoproliferative disorders (chronic lymphocytic leukemia, lymphoma, macroglobulinemia, Hodgkin disease)
  - Other autoimmune disorders (e.g., Hashimoto thyroiditis, Graves disease, sarcoidosis, biliary cirrhosis)

thrombocytopenia is due to decreased production. The smear should be made with blood from a fingerstick because anticoagulants cause platelets to swell. Bone marrow aspirates appear normal except for increased numbers of megakaryocytes. An acute disease, often preceded by an otherwise benign viral infection, is seen more commonly in children and, by definition, lasts <6 months. The chronic illness (often still called idiopathic thrombocytopenic purpura) lasts >6 months and is seen more often in women than men (ratio of 3:1 or 4:1). It sometimes is associated with an underlying lymphoproliferative disorder or a collagen vascular disease, especially systemic lupus erythematosus and, more rarely, autoimmune hemolytic anemia. There is an increased incidence of immune thrombocytopenia in association with human immunodeficiency virus (HIV) infection (15) (see Chapter 39). Autoimmune thrombocytopenia is caused by an antibody adsorbed to the surface of circulating platelets that results in their premature destruction by the reticuloendothelial system. The disorder is characterized by ineffective production of platelets as well (16).

Many drugs are associated with thrombocytopenia on an immunologic basis (17). Heparin is the drug most commonly implicated (see Chapter 57). Many other drugs (e.g., quinine, quinidine, sulfa, β-lactam antibiotics, carbamazepine, phenytoin, rifampin, sulfonylureas, ticlopidine, valproic acid) have been less frequently implicated (for a review of drugs associated with thrombocytopenia, see http//moon.ouhsc.edu/jgeorge). If a patient presents to the practitioner with severe thrombocytopenia caused by increased destruction of circulating platelets, it is important to ask what drugs the patient is taking and to consider stopping them if there is any question that the drugs are involved in the process.

It is not unusual for *alcoholics* to develop thrombocytopenia, usually to a moderate degree, after a binge. Alcohol appears to damage platelet membranes, causing their premature destruction, and to inhibit the compensatory increase in platelet production by marrow megakaryocytes. Once the binge is over, the platelet count returns to normal (or transiently higher than normal) in 4 to 5 days. Alcoholics of long standing who have developed cirrhosis of the liver and portal hypertension may have chronic thrombocytopenia because of increased sequestration of platelets in their spleens.

Management

An American Society of Hematology Practice Guidelines Panel has made recommendations for treatment of autoimmune thrombocytopenia (12,13). The panel found no experimental evidence on which to base recommendations, so they resorted to achieving a consensus among experts. The following recommendations are not precisely those of the panel but are consistent with its views. If the platelet count is <20,000/mm^3, treatment should be instituted immediately with the equivalent of 60 to 100 mg (1 mg/kg of body weight) prednisone, even if the patient is asymptomatic or has only a few petechiae. Patients with mucous membrane or internal bleeding should be hospitalized, and patients with severe internal bleeding should receive intravenous γ-globulin (which corrects immune thrombocytopenia more rapidly than do corticosteroids) in the hospital. Such bleeding usually will not occur if the platelet count is >30,000/mm^3. In general, the risk of major bleeding appears greater in elderly patients (18,19).

Most patients with platelet counts of 20,000 to 30,000/mm^3 or less because of chronic immune thrombocytopenia ultimately require splenectomy. Treatment of immune thrombocytopenia in patients with HIV infection is the same as it is for patients who do not have HIV infection.

Although approximately 70% of patients respond within days to corticosteroids with a rise in platelet count sufficient to maintain adequate hemostasis, many relapse as the dosage is tapered. (A reasonable schedule is to reduce the dosage by 10 mg/day each week to half the initial dosage and then by 5 mg/day each week.) If patients do not respond to corticosteroids initially, if mucous membrane or internal bleeding recurs, or if the platelet count falls below 30,000/mm^3 as the dosage of corticosteroids is tapered, splenectomy frequently is indicated. Adequate platelet counts (>50,000/mm^3) are maintained in approximately 80% of splenectomized patients. Patients with symptomatic refractory immune thrombocytopenia may respond to an immunosuppressive drug (other than a corticosteroid) and should be treated by a hematologist.

Increased Sequestration of Platelets

Patients with large spleens often have thrombocytopenia because of redistribution of platelets within a larger splenic pool, most commonly because of congestive splenomegaly associated with portal hypertension. Splenectomy reverses thrombocytopenia but is rarely indicated, because usually the thrombocytopenia is not severe and splenectomy should be considered only if there is a clear-cut hemorrhagic diathesis and the underlying disease responsible for the enlarged spleen permits an operation to be performed.

Increased Use of Platelets

Patients with disseminated intravascular coagulation characteristically have thrombocytopenia, almost always in association with multiple defects in coagulation. Such patients often present acutely ill because of the underlying disease that has incited the hemostatic disorder. For example, in women with various complications of pregnancy, patients with disseminated carcinoma, or in some patients with septicemia, hemostatic mechanisms have been activated because of exposure of the circulating blood to thromboplastic material. The hemorrhagic diathesis is manifest most commonly by widespread bruising, petechiae, and mucous membrane bleeding, occasionally, but not often, associated with venous or arterial thrombosis. In addition to thrombocytopenia, patients have disordered coagulation, which can be identified by measuring the prothrombin time (PT), the partial thromboplastin time (PTT), and the concentration of fibrinogen in the plasma, and by demonstrating increased titers of fibrinogen and fibrin degradation products in the plasma or serum. These products are formed by the lysis of fibrinogen and fibrin by plasmin, the major proteolytic enzyme of the blood. Patients who are strongly suspected of having disseminated intravascular coagulation or in whom the diagnosis has been made should be hospitalized for further treatment and for identification and treatment of the underlying disease.

Qualitative Disorders of Platelets

A number of inherited abnormalities of platelets result in impaired hemostasis even though platelet counts often are within normal limits. In general, the hemorrhagic diathesis associated with these conditions is milder than it is in patients with severe thrombocytopenia. Practitioners are unlikely to see these patients, but if patients have unexplained bleeding, such as purpura, epistaxis, or menorrhagia, with apparently normal coagulation and normal or slightly reduced platelet counts, it is reasonable to perform a bleeding time (see below), which often is abnormal in patients with qualitatively abnormal platelets. Similar abnormalities may be acquired in patients with various disease states, most commonly uremia. In fact, patients with chronic renal failure who have a tendency to bleed often improve after hemodialysis. Perhaps the most common acquired qualitative disorder of blood platelets occurs after the ingestion of aspirin, which often prolongs the bleeding time and irreversibly interferes with platelet aggregation and the release of certain intracellular platelet constituents. Although untoward bleeding is unusual in patients who have taken aspirin, the drug may intensify a pre-existing tendency to bleed. Other nonsteroidal anti-inflammatory drugs may impair platelet function, but, compared with aspirin, the effect is even less predictable and is more quickly reversible when the drug is stopped.

Patient Experience. The bleeding time should be performed using a commercially available, spring-loaded, disposable device (Simplate) that makes a small incision in the forearm. The examiner should puncture the skin with the disposable lancet. A blood pressure cuff should be inflated to 40 mm Hg above the elbow during the test. The time between the instant the puncture is made and the point at which blood from the wound can no longer be adsorbed onto a piece of filter paper is the bleeding time (normally 2–9 minutes). The patient should be warned of the very transient sharp pain that will be experienced when the wound is made and of the small scar, usually inapparent, that may form when the wound heals.

Thrombocytosis

Platelet counts $>400,000/mm^3$, unless associated with a myeloproliferative disorder such as polycythemia vera, myeloid metaplasia, or chronic granulocytic leukemia, are not in themselves associated with an increased risk for morbidity from excessive bleeding or clotting. However, they may signify the presence of an underlying disease that requires attention. If thrombocytosis exists, the most common causes are *inflammatory disease* and *solid tumor malignancies*. Other causes include the postsplenectomy state, acute bleeding, and severe chronic iron deficiency. In secondary thrombocytosis, the platelet count usually (but not always) is $<1,000,000/mm^3$.

Patients with chronic myeloproliferative disorders (polycythemia vera, primary myelofibrosis, essential thrombocythemia), if they have thrombocytosis, usually have large distorted platelets on smear and other hematologic abnormalities typical of the particular disease. Many of these patients also have splenomegaly. The platelet counts may be $>1,000,000/mm^3$. Treatment of thrombocytosis associated with chronic myeloproliferative disease should be planned in consultation with a hematologist.

COAGULATION DISORDERS

The generation of a solid fibrin clot from circulating soluble fibrinogen is the body's major defense against the loss of blood from the vasculature, especially from blood vessels larger than the capillary, arteriole, and venule. Coagulation is initiated by the exposure of proteins to thromboplastic substances (tissue factor) when blood vessels are injured. Thereafter, a series of enzymatic reactions occurs that results in the conversion of fibrinogen by the proteolytic enzyme thrombin to fibrin. The best screening tests for detecting abnormalities of clotting are the activated partial thromboplastin time (aPTT) and PT. The aPTT and the PT measure different phases of the early parts of the coagulation process, but both measure the later phase of the process—the conversion of prothrombin to thrombin and the subsequent conversion of fibrinogen to fibrin.

Enzymatic mechanisms oppose coagulation and prevent unwarranted widespread clotting of the blood when a blood vessel is injured. A number of cases of patients with an increased tendency to thrombosis and low levels of activity of one of the various protease inhibitors that normally circulate in the blood and regulate coagulation have been reported (see Chapter 57). The *fibrinolytic system* generates the proteolytic enzyme plasmin, which adsorbs to the clots and results in their ultimate dissolution. Fibrinolytic therapy is commonly used in the treatment of various thrombotic diseases (e.g., acute myocardial infarction), but such therapy requires hospitalization.

Patients who have a deficiency of one or more of the coagulation proteins are more likely to have extensive soft-tissue bleeding or major hemorrhage in response to trauma than are patients with disorders of the vasculature or of blood platelets (petechiae, discussed earlier in this chapter, are never a sign of abnormal coagulation). Hereditary disorders of coagulation are rare. Ordinarily they are readily diagnosed because of the history of lifelong bleeding and, in the case of hemophilia, because of a history of characteristic hemorrhage into joints and soft tissues. Patients who have a severe hemorrhagic diathesis because of a hereditary abnormality of clotting almost always have markedly low levels of the deficient coagulation protein. Therefore, screening tests such as the aPTT almost always are abnormal and provide clues to the presence of the disorder. The practitioner likely will not encounter such patients because most of them are diagnosed in childhood and are treated by hematologists thereafter. However, if such a patient who is suspected of having a hereditary disorder of coagulation but who has not previously been diagnosed is encountered, referral to an appropriate center is warranted.

Von Willebrand disease is an inherited abnormality of hemostasis (20); the majority of cases are autosomal dominant. The condition is marked by a reduction in the concentration or a change in the structure of the protein von Willebrand factor, which ordinarily binds to platelets and mediates their adhesion to subendothelial collagen in the course of platelet plug formation (see above). Normally, von Willebrand factor forms a complex with antihemophilic globulin (factor VIII:c), the protein that is deficient in the blood of patients with classic hemophilia, so patients with von Willebrand disease often have reduced levels of factor VIII. The qualitative disorder of platelets is reflected in a prolonged bleeding time and decreased platelet adhesiveness. The platelets of these patients characteristically do not aggregate in vitro, as normal platelets do, when exposed to the obsolete antibiotic ristocetin. The course of the disease and the extent of the laboratory abnormalities vary among patients, but in general the hemorrhagic diathesis is milder than it is in hemophilia A. Patients bleed most commonly from the gastrointestinal tract. Symptoms of the disease usually are not apparent until the patient is an adult. The bleeding time and aPTT are useful screening tests. The diagnosis and treatment of patients with von Willebrand disease require the ongoing participation of a hematologist.

TABLE 56.4 Advice To Give Patients with a Disorder of Hemostasis

Take only medicine prescribed by your caregiver. Do not take aspirin or cold remedies.
Take acetaminophen (e.g., Tylenol) instead of aspirin.
Avoid unnecessary trauma.
Wear an identification bracelet identifying your bleeding disorder.
Call your caregiver
- If you experience any abnormal bleeding.
- Before you visit your dentist.
- If you are hospitalized for any reason.

Acquired disorders of coagulation are more common than are congenital disorders. By their nature they are more likely to be associated with multiple defects in hemostasis, such as those seen in patients with disseminated intravascular coagulation (discussed earlier in this chapter) or in patients taking anticoagulant drugs (see Chapter 57). The diagnosis and management of these problems are discussed in those sections.

Rarely, an isolated clotting factor deficiency is acquired, often in association with a lymphoproliferative or collagen vascular disease. Such a deficiency may or may not be revealed by a hemorrhagic diathesis but almost always is associated with an abnormal aPTT or PT. Patients with unexplained prolonged aPTTs or PTs should be referred to a hematologist for evaluation.

ADVICE TO PATIENTS WHO HAVE A DISORDER OF HEMOSTASIS

Table 56.4 lists some rules to give patients who have hemostatic dysfunction. It is important that the patient know the name of his or her disease and its clinical manifestations.

SPECIFIC REFERENCES

1. Collier BS, Schneiderman P. Clinical evaluation of hemorrhagic disorders: the bleeding history and differential diagnosis of purpura. In: Hoffman R, Benz EJ Jr, Shattil SJ, et al., eds. Hematology. Basic principles and practice. 3rd ed. New York: Churchill Livingstone,2000:1252.
2. Bick RL. Vascular disorders associated with thrombohemorrhagic phenomena. Semin Thromb Hemost 1979;5:167.
3. Calabrese LH, Duna GF. Drug-induced vasculitis. Curr Opin Rheumatol 1996;8:34.
4. Blanco R, Martinez-Taboada VM, Rodriguez-Valverde V, et al. Cutaneous vasculitis in children and adults: associated diseases and etiologic factors in 303 patients. Medicine 1998;77:403.
5. Ratnoff OD. The psychogenic purpuras: a review of auto-erythrocyte sensitization, autosensitization to DNA, "hysterical" and factitial bleeding, and the religious stigmata. Semin Hematol 1980;17:192.
6. Monti G, Galli M, Invernizzi F, et al. Cryoglobulinaemias: a multi-centre study of the early clinical and laboratory manifestations of primary and secondary disease. QJM 1995;88: 115.
7. Kyle RA, Greipp RR. Amyloidosis (AL): clinical

and laboratory features in 229 cases. Mayo Clin Proc 1983;58:665.
8. Perkins HA, MacKenzie MR, Fudenberg HH. Hemostatic defects in dysproteinemias. Blood 1970;35:695.
9. Reuler JB, Broudy VC, Cooney TG. Adult scurvy. JAMA 1985;253:805
10. Peery WH. Clinical spectrum of hereditary hemorrhagic telangiectasia (Osler-Weber-Rendu disease). Am J Med 1987;82:989.
11. Rodgers RPC, Levin J. A critical reappraisal of the bleeding time. Semin Thromb Hemost 1990;16:1.
12. George JN, Woolf SH, Raskob GE, et al. Idiopathic thrombocytopenic purpura: a practice guideline developed by explicit methods for the American Society of Hematology. Blood 1996;88:3.
13. The American Society of Hematology ITP Practice Guideline Panel. Diagnosis and treatment of idiopathic thrombocytopenic purpura: recommendations of the American Society of Hematology. Ann Intern Med 1997;126:319.
14. Cines DB, Blanchette VS. Immune thrombocytopenic purpura. N Engl J Med 2002;346:995.
15. Morris L, Distenfeld A, Amorosi E, et al. Autoimmune thrombocytopenic purpura in homosexual men. Ann Intern Med 1982;96:714.
16. McMillan R, Wang L, Tomer A, et al. Suppression of in vitro megakaryocyte production by antiplatelet autoantibodies from adult patients with chronic ITP. Blood 2004; 103:1364.
17. Aster RH. Drug-induced immune thrombocytopenia: an overview of pathogenesis. Semin Hematol 1999;36(1 Suppl 1):2.
18. Guthrie TH Jr, Brannan DP, Prisant LM. Idiopathic thrombocytopenic purpura in the older adult patient. Am J Med Sci 1988;296:17.
19. Cortelazzo S, Finazzi M, Buelli M, et al. High risk of severe bleeding in aged patients with chronic idiopathic thrombocytopenic purpura. Blood 1991;77:31.
20. Cox GJ. Diagnosis and treatment of von Willebrand disease. Hematol Oncol Clin North Am 2004;18:1277.

*For annotated **General References** and resources related to this chapter, visit www.hopkinsbayview.org/PAMreferences.*

Chapter 57

Thromboembolic Disease

Michael B. Streiff

VENOUS THROMBOEMBOLISM

Venous thromboembolism (VTE) is a common cause of morbidity and mortality in the United States, affecting one of every 1,000 Americans each year (1). The most common manifestations of VTE are deep venous thrombosis (DVT) and pulmonary embolism (PE). Two thirds of cases of VTE present as DVT alone; the remainder manifest as PE, with or without a demonstrable DVT (2). The 28-day case fatality rate for an initial DVT is 9.4% compared with 15% for PE (3). Therefore, adequate prevention and treatment of VTE are a priority for ambulatory care providers.

Risk Factors

Venous thrombosis occurs as a consequence of one or more of three different factors (commonly called the Virchow triad): stasis of blood flow, disruptions in the integrity of the vascular wall, and hypercoagulability of the blood. The incidence of VTE is strongly influenced by the presence or absence of risk factors that affect one or more of the Virchow triad. Age has a significant impact on the incidence of VTE. VTE is rare among children younger than 15 years (<5 episodes/100,000 per year). The incidence of VTE gradually increases during adult life up to age 59 years, after which there is a sharp increase from 280 episodes/100,000 per year to 1,800 episodes/100,000 per year among individuals 80 to 84 years old (1). Potential explanations for this dramatic difference in incidence may be the increased prevalence of malignancy and the decreased mobility among older individuals.

Ethnicity influences the risk of VTE. Asian Americans (19 events/100,000 per year) and Latinos (37 events/100,000 per year) have a lower incidence of VTE than Caucasians (86 events/100,000 per year) or African Americans (93 events/100,000 per year) (4). Potential reasons for these ethnic differences may be differences in the prevalence of genetic prothrombotic mutations such as factor V Leiden or the prothrombin gene G20210A mutation. Because these mutations are less common among African Americans than Caucasians, other thrombophilic mutations must be responsible for the higher incidence of VTE among African Americans (5). One report has suggested

TABLE 57.1 Prevalence of Inherited Thrombophilia

	Prevalence		
Thrombophilic State	***General Population***	***Unselected VTE Patients***	***Selected VTE Patients***
Factor V Leiden	Caucasian 5% Latino 2% African American 1% Asian American 0.5%	19%	40%
Prothrombin gene G20210A mutation	Caucasian 2%	7%	16%
Antithrombin III deficiency	0.02%–0.05%	2%	4%
Protein C deficiency	0.2%	2%–4%	4%–5%
Protein S deficiency	0.2%	2%–4%	4%–5%

VTE, venous thromboembolism.
Modified from Ridker PM, Miletich JP, Hennekens CH, et al. Ethnic distribution of factor V Leiden in 4047 men and women. Implications for venous thromboembolism screening. JAMA 1997;277:1305; Seligsohn U, Lubetsky A. Genetic susceptibility to venous thrombosis. N Engl J Med 2001;344:1222.

that elevated levels of factor VIII may be a common risk factor for thrombosis among individuals of African descent (6).

Unlike age and ethnicity, gender does not appear to significantly influence the incidence of VTE (3). However, a higher incidence of recurrent VTE has been noted among males in some studies (7).

Inherited prothrombotic conditions have an important influence on the risk of VTE. Surveys indicate that approximately one third of unselected patients presenting with a DVT or PE will have an inherited form of thrombophilia. Among selected patients (i.e., those who are younger than 50 years; patients who have a family history of VTE; individuals who have a history of recurrent VTE; or those who have idiopathic VTE), the prevalence of an inherited prothrombotic condition increases to 70%. Table 57.1 lists the frequencies of individual inherited prothrombotic conditions among different populations (8). The most common inherited thrombophilic condition is factor V Leiden. Factor V Leiden, a mutation in factor V that impairs the ability of activated protein C to inactivate activated forms of factor V and VIII, affects 5% of healthy Caucasians, 2% of Latinos, 1% of African Americans, and 0.5% of Asian Americans (5). Heterozygosity for factor V Leiden increases the risk of VTE fivefold, whereas homozygosity is associated with a 50-fold increase in risk. The presence of factor V Leiden can be identified using a screening assay, the activated protein C resistance assay, followed by confirmatory testing with polymerase chain reaction (PCR)-based genetic testing. The second most common inherited form of thrombophilia, the prothrombin gene G20210A mutation, is found in approximately 2% of European Americans. This mutation results in a 25% increase in prothrombin levels and a twofold increased risk for VTE. The prothrombin gene mutation can be identified only by PCR-based genetic testing (9).

Elevated levels of factors VIII, IX, and XI appear to increase the risk of VTE. Factor VIII levels >90th percentile are associated with at least a fivefold increased risk for initial and recurrent VTE (10,11). Factors IX and XI raise the risk of initial VTE twofold to threefold (12,13). Although the influence of elevated factor VIII levels on the risk of VTE has been identified in multiple independent studies, studies confirming the influence of elevated levels of factors IX and XI on VTE incidence have not been performed. Laboratory testing for coagulation factor levels is available in many clinical laboratories, but the absence of management trials using this information in therapeutic decision making and the sensitivity of test results to other factors (e.g., infection, inflammation, acute thrombosis) have reduced clinical enthusiasm for using factor level testing as a routine part of the thrombophilia evaluation. Table 57.2 provides information on factor level testing in the evaluation of thrombophilia.

Inherited deficiency of endogenous anticoagulants, such as antithrombin III, protein C, and protein S, are potent risk factors for VTE. A deficiency of antithrombin, which inactivates activated forms of factors II, X, IX, and XI, is present in one of every 5,000 in the general population and increases the risk of thrombosis 25-fold. Protein C inactivates activated forms of factors V and VIII in a complex with its cofactor, protein S. Protein C deficiency is present in one of every 500 in the population and is associated with a 10-fold increase in the risk of VTE. Protein S deficiency has a similar prevalence in the general population and similar potency as a risk factor for VTE (9). Dysfibrinogenemia is a rare inherited coagulation disorder (only 250 reported cases) that can predispose individuals to bleeding, thrombosis, or both, depending upon the site of the mutation in the fibrinogen gene. The thrombin time (usually prolonged, occasionally abnormally shortened) is a useful screening test (14). Although defects in the

TABLE 57.2 Thrombophilia Testing Recommendations

Thrombophilic State	*Recommended Test*	*Recommended Time*	*Factors Affecting Test Results*
Factor V Leiden	APC-R, DNA-based assay	Anytime	APC-R: high heparin concentration (>1.0 U/mL), high titer lupus inhibitors DNA: sample contamination
Prothrombin gene G20210A mutation	DNA-based assay	Anytime	DNA: sample contamination
Antithrombin III deficiency	Antithrombin activity	After acute therapy	Acute thrombosis, DIC, heparin
Protein C deficiency	Protein C activity	After acute and chronic therapy	Acute thrombosis, DIC, warfarin, vitamin K deficiency
Protein S deficiency	Protein S activity	After acute and chronic therapy	Acute thrombosis, DIC, warfarin, vitamin K deficiency, pregnancy, estrogen therapy
Antiphospholipid antibody syndrome	aPTT, dRVVT, anticardiolipin antibodies (ACL), β_2-glycoprotein I antibodies (β_2-GPI)	After acute therapy	aPTT: heparin, dRVVT: high heparin concentrations, warfarin? ACL: infections
Factor VIII	Factor VIII activity	At least 6 mo after thrombosis	Inflammation
Homocysteine	Fasting homocysteine	Anytime	
Dysfibrinogenemia	Thrombin time, fibrinogen activity and antigen, reptilase time	After acute therapy	Thrombin time, fibrinogen activity: heparin

APC-R, activated protein C resistance; aPTT, activated partial thromboplastin time; DIC, disseminated intravascular coagulation; dRVVT, dilute Russell viper venom time.

fibrinolytic system and factor XII deficiency have been suggested to predispose to VTE, strong evidence supporting thrombophilia as a consequence of these abnormalities is lacking (15–17).

Elevated plasma levels of homocysteine are associated with an increased risk for venous and arterial thrombosis. Mild to moderate elevations of homocysteine are present in 5% to 7% of Americans. A common inherited cause of elevated homocysteine levels is a thermolabile mutation in N^5,N^{10}-methylene-tetrahydrofolate reductase, the enzyme responsible for maintaining adequate levels of N^5-methyltetrahydrofolate, a cofactor necessary for the conversion of homocysteine into methionine. In the setting of folate deficiency, this abnormality can result in moderate elevations of homocysteine (15–30 μmol/L) and a twofold to threefold increased risk for venous or arterial thrombosis. Homocysteine is also metabolized by cystathionine β-synthase, which converts cystathionine into cysteine. Homozygous mutations in this enzyme result in homocystinuria, a rare disorder (one in 200,000 live births) associated with severe elevations of homocysteine (as high as 400 μmol/L) and premature atherosclerosis and recurrent VTE (18). Because folate, vitamin B_{12}, and pyridoxine (vitamin B_6) are cofactors required for homocysteine metabolism, deficiencies of these vitamins should be investigated in any patient with elevated homocysteine levels. Supplementation with folate, vitamin B_{12}, and pyridoxine (vitamin B_6) can result in reductions in homocysteine, although whether vitamin supplementation reduces the risk of VTE remains to be demonstrated.

The antiphospholipid antibody syndrome (APS) is an important acquired cause of thrombophilia that increases the risk of both venous and arterial thrombosis. Other clinical manifestations of APS include recurrent miscarriages, immune thrombocytopenia or hemolytic anemia, livedo reticularis, and nonbacterial thrombotic endocarditis. APS can present as a primary autoimmune syndrome or in association with rheumatologic disorders (systemic lupus erythematosus [SLE], rheumatoid arthritis, etc.), infections (syphilis, human immunodeficiency virus, etc.), cancers, or exposure to certain medications. Antiphospholipid antibodies have been identified in 1% to 5% of asymptomatic control subjects and in as many as 30% of SLE patients (19,20).

APS is caused by antibodies directed against antiphospholipid binding proteins, such as β_2-glycoprotein I, annexin V, protein C, protein S, and prothrombin. APS may result in thrombosis by disrupting the anticoagulant function of these proteins, inducing endothelial damage and activation or increasing tissue factor expression by monocytes and/or endothelial cells (19,20). In patients with SLE, APS is associated with an incidence of thromboembolism of two events per 100 person-years (21). APS also increases the risk of recurrent thromboembolism (22).

Diagnostic tests for APS include phospholipid-dependent coagulation assays (e.g., dilute activated partial thromboplastin time [aPTT], dilute prothrombin time [PT], dilute Russell viper venom time, and mixing studies with these assays) and anticardiolipin and β_2-glycoprotein I antibody assays. To meet criteria for APS, patients must have documented clinical events (thrombosis or recurrent miscarriage) and repeatedly positive laboratory tests separated by at least 6 to 8 weeks (19,20).

The clinical utility of diagnostic testing for thrombophilia remains a subject of controversy and of active investigation (23). Possible benefits of testing include identification of the potential etiology of a thrombotic event and increased attention to DVT prophylaxis during future risk periods. However, only selected thrombophilic conditions (e.g., APS, factor V Leiden homozygosity, compound heterozygosity for factor V Leiden and the prothrombin gene mutation, elevated factor VIII levels) have been demonstrated in clinical studies to increase the risk of recurrent VTE and thus potentially to influence the duration of anticoagulant therapy (11,22,24). Furthermore, some studies have not identified an increased risk for recurrent VTE associated with inherited thrombophilia (23). Therefore, clinicians should consider the benefits, risks, and cost of thrombophilia evaluation before testing. Some commonly proposed criteria for identifying high-risk patients, who are most likely to benefit from testing, include age younger than 50 years at the time of the initial event, a family history positive for VTE, recurrent episodes of VTE, idiopathic VTE or VTE in association with minimal provocation, thromboses in unusual locations (e.g., intra-abdominal, cerebral venous sinus thrombosis), and recurrent miscarriages (9). However, clinicians also may consider testing individuals with VTE who do not fulfill one of these criteria if the clinical scenario strongly suggests the presence of a thrombophilic disorder. Table 57.2 lists the recommendations regarding the timing of laboratory testing, the most appropriate assays, and factors that can affect the results of testing.

The Virchow triad is influenced by acquired intrinsic or extrinsic thrombotic stimuli. Major acquired risk factors for VTE (odds ratio for thrombosis >10) include hip or leg fractures, hip or knee replacement surgery, major general surgery, major trauma, and spinal cord injury. Moderate risk factors (odds ratio 2–10) include cancer, chemotherapy, hormone replacement or oral contraceptive therapy, central venous catheters, congestive heart failure, respiratory failure, paralytic stroke, and pregnancy. Weak clinical risk factors (odds ratio <2) include bed rest for >3 days, immobility, laparoscopic surgery, varicose veins, and obesity (25). Although the relative risk of developing VTE that is associated with many of the inherited prothrombotic conditions is greater than the relative risk of acquired thrombotic stimuli, the high prevalence of the latter group of conditions makes their overall impact as risk factors for VTE far greater than that of the inherited disorders.

Diagnosis

The diagnosis of VTE requires consideration of a patient's risk factors for VTE, the symptoms and physical findings, and the results of objective diagnostic testing. Common signs and symptoms of DVT are pain, swelling, and tenderness of the affected extremity. PE is commonly associated with dyspnea, chest pain (often pleuritic), tachypnea, tachycardia, and hypoxia. Because individual physical signs of DVT and PE have low specificity, clinical prediction rules incorporating risk factors and signs and symptoms of DVT and PE have been developed and can be useful guides for assessing the probability of disease (26,27) (Tables 57.3 and 57.4). However, these rules were developed based on data obtained from referred patients attending secondary care outpatient clinics. A prospective study in primary care patients found that clinical prediction rules may be less accurate in the primary care setting (28). Until

TABLE 57.3 DVT Clinical Assessment Tool

Clinical Finding	*Points (If Finding Present)*
Active cancer (under treatment or within 6 mo)	1
Paralysis, paresis, or cast immobilization of the extremity	1
Recent bed rest >3 d or surgery within 4 wk	1
Local tenderness along deep venous system	1
Entire leg swollen	1
Calf swelling 3 cm greater than asymptomatic side (at 10 cm below tibial tuberosity)	1
Pitting edema confined to symptomatic leg	1
Collateral superficial veins (nonvaricose)	1
Alternative diagnosis as likely or greater than DVT	–2

DVT, deep venous thrombosis.
Pretest probability of DVT: low = 0 points, moderate = 1–2 points, high = ≥3 points.
Modified from Wells PS, Anderson DR, Bormanis J, et al. Value of assessment of pretest probability of deep-vein thrombosis in clinical management. Lancet 1997;350:1795.

TABLE 57.4 Wells PE Clinical Assessment Tool

Clinical Finding	*Points (If Finding Present)*
Clinical findings for DVT	3.0
Alternative diagnosis is less likely than PE	3.0
Heart rate >100 bpm	1.5
Immobilization or surgery within previous 4 wk	1.5
Previous DVT/PE	1.5
Hemoptysis	1.0
Active cancer (under treatment or within 6 mo)	1.0

DVT, deep venous thrombosis; PE, pulmonary embolism.
Pretest probability of PE: low = <2 points, moderate = 2–6 points, high = ≥6 points.
Modified from Wells PS, Ginsberg JS, Anderson DR, et al. Use of a clinical model for safe management of patients with suspected pulmonary embolism. Ann Intern Med 1998;129:997.

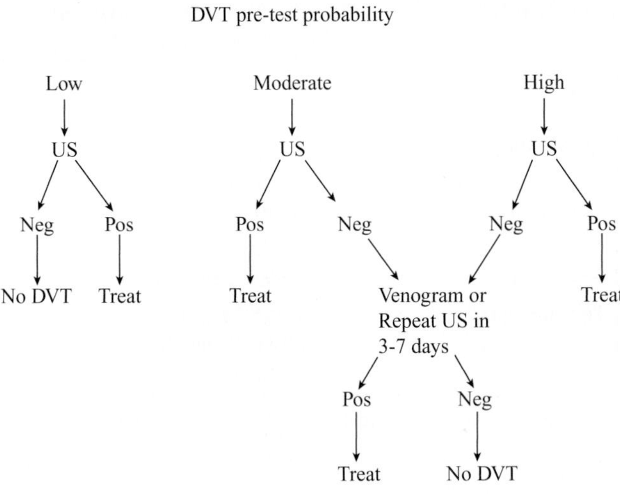

FIGURE 57.1. Algorithm for diagnosis of patients with suspected deep venous thrombosis (DVT). Neg, negative; Pos, positive; US, ultrasound. (Adapted from Wells PS, Anderson DR, Ginsberg J. Assessment of deep vein thrombosis or pulmonary embolism by the combined use of clinical model and noninvasive diagnostic tests. Semin Thromb Hemost 2000;26:643.)

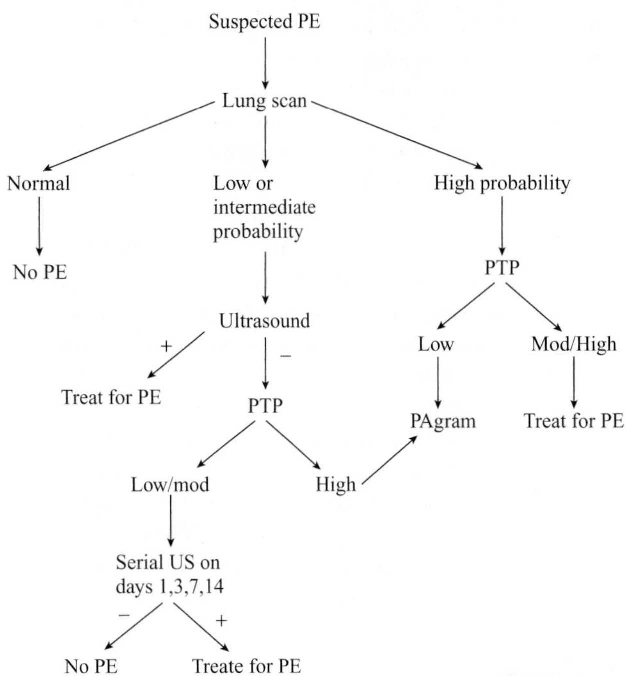

FIGURE 57.3. Ventilation/perfusion scan algorithm for diagnosis of patients with suspected pulmonary embolism (PE). Low/mod, low to moderate clinical probability; PAgram, pulmonary angiogram; PTP, pretest clinical probability. US, ultrasound. (Adapted from Wells PS, Anderson DR, Ginsberg J. Assessment of deep vein thrombosis or pulmonary embolism by the combined use of clinical model and noninvasive diagnostic tests. Semin Thromb Hemost 2000;26:643.)

clinical prediction rules are developed specifically for primary care patients and additional studies are completed, DVT and PE diagnostic algorithms should retain objective radiologic imaging procedures (Figs. 57.1–57.3). The most common diagnostic test for DVT is venous duplex ultrasonography. The sensitivity and specificity of this test both are >95% in patients with symptomatic proximal DVT. However, the sensitivity and specificity of this test for distal DVT (e.g., calf vein DVT) both are only 70%. Contrast venography, once considered the diagnostic gold standard, is rarely used currently because of its invasive nature, the risks of phlebitis and contrast dye reactions, and the limited availability of the procedure.

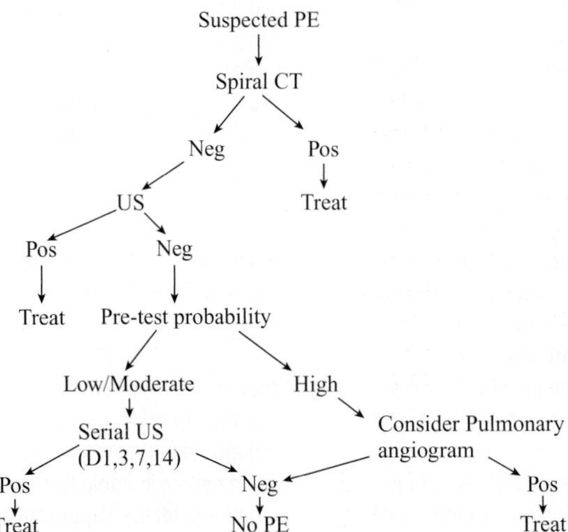

FIGURE 57.2. Algorithm for diagnosis of patients with suspected pulmonary embolism (PE). CT, computed tomography; Neg, negative; Pos, positive; US, ultrasound. (Adapted from Wells PS, Anderson DR, Ginsberg J. Assessment of deep vein thrombosis or pulmonary embolism by the combined use of clinical model and noninvasive diagnostic tests. Semin Thromb Hemost 2000;26:643.)

The most common imaging studies in PE diagnosis are ventilation–perfusion (V/Q) scanning and spiral computer tomography (CT) scanning. V/Q scans are most useful when the results are normal or indicate a high probability of PE. A normal V/Q scan rules out PE, whereas a high probability scan indicates a high likelihood of PE, particularly in patients with a high pretest probability. Unfortunately, more than half of V/Q scans are read as either low (16%) or intermediate probability (41%) (29). Additional studies are necessary to rule out disease in these instances. Helical CT scanning has become an increasingly popular diagnostic tool in the investigation of PE because it is rapidly performed and often identifies alternative diagnoses. The reported sensitivity of helical CT for PE varies greatly (66%–93%), depending upon imaging protocols and technology (30). Clinical outcome studies, however, suggest that subsequent episodes of VTE are infrequent in patients with negative helical CT scans (31). Multidetector row helical CT was demonstrated to have sensitivity of 100% and specificity of 89% in one study that compared this test to digital subtraction pulmonary angiography (32). The greater sensitivity of newer-generation helical CT scanners is likely to make this test the imaging study of choice in PE diagnosis. Figures 57.2 and 57.3 show examples of PE diagnosis algorithms incorporating V/Q and CT scanning. The topic of V/Q and CT scanning in PE diagnosis is discussed in Chapter 59.

In recent years, a large number of studies have documented the utility of D-dimer testing in the diagnosis of VTE. D-Dimers are the cross-linked fragments of fibrin produced by plasmin degradation. When used in conjunction with clinical prediction models, D-dimer assays have been successfully used to exclude the diagnosis of DVT and to reduce the need for additional diagnostic testing (33). Because many D-dimer assays are available for clinical use, only sensitive D-dimer assays validated in the diagnosis of VTE should be used for this purpose. Published thresholds for positive results should be validated in the clinician's laboratory prior to use in diagnosis.

Treatment

Therapeutic alternatives for treatment of VTE include anticoagulation, thrombolytic therapy, and vena caval interruption.

Anticoagulation

Anticoagulation remains the therapeutic option of choice for the vast majority of patients. Either unfractionated heparin (UFH) or low-molecular-weight heparin (LMWH) is used in the acute therapy for VTE. Acute therapy for VTE should be administered for at least 5 to 7 days until therapeutic levels of warfarin are achieved as reflected by an international normalized ratio (INR) of 2.0 to 3.0. The INR is calculated by dividing the patient's PT by the laboratory control PT and raising this result by an exponent, the international sensitivity index (ISI). The ISI reflects the sensitivity of an individual laboratory's PT reagent to reductions in vitamin K-dependent coagulation factors. Because different laboratories may use different reagents to measure the PT, this correction factor helps to normalize PT results for reagent differences and thus reduces variation in PT results between different laboratories. From 7 to 10 days of acute heparin therapy are often given for extensive DVT or PE (34).

Heparin

Most patients with DVT and some with PE can be safely and effectively treated as outpatients using LMWH administered in subcutaneous weight-based doses once or twice daily (for doses, see Table 57.5). UFH ordinarily should not be prescribed to outpatients. Reasons to admit a patient with DVT/PE include the presence of an extensive clot burden at high risk for progression or requiring thrombolytic therapy, significant risk factors for bleeding (e.g., thrombocytopenia or recent surgery or trauma), presence of concomitant medical disorders requiring inpatient management, and medical noncompliance that precludes the safe administration of anticoagulation on an outpatient basis. Although PE previously has been considered an absolute indication for hospital admission, several studies have demonstrated the feasibility and safety of managing hemodynamically stable patients with PE as an outpatient.

TABLE 57.5 Low Molecular Weight Heparin and Fondaparinux Dosing for VTE

Agent	*Dose*
Enoxaparin	1 mg/kg SC q12h or 1.5 mg/kg SC daily
Dalteparin	100 IU/kg SC q12h or 200 IU/kg SC daily
Tinzaparin	175 IU/kg SC daily
Fondaparinux	5 mg SC daily for ≤50 kg 7.5 mg SC daily for 51–99 kg 10 mg SC daily for ≥100 kg

IU, international units; SC, subcutaneously; VTE, venous thromboembolism.

TABLE 57.6 Criteria for Outpatient Management of VTE

Clinical Criteria	
Radiologically confirmed DVT or PE	No recent GI bleeding (within the last 14 d) or Hemoccult (+) stool
Age >18 yr	No history of a bleeding disorder
Medically and hemodynamically stable	No major surgery, trauma, or stroke within 14 d
Willing and able to be discharged to home from the hospital, outpatient setting, or emergency department	No history of hemorrhagic stroke or intracranial hemorrhage
Absence of a massive symptomatic iliofemoral DVT requiring thrombolysis	No history of HIT or current platelet count <100,000 mm^3
Absence of phlegmasia cerulea dolens[a]	No severe liver disease (INR >1.5 in the absence of warfarin therapy)
Absence of symptomatic pulmonary embolism (e.g., hypotension, hypoxia on room air or ambulation)	Must have a suitable home environment to support therapy
	No history of medical noncompliance or unreliable followup

DVT, deep venous thrombosis; GI, gastrointestinal; HIT, heparin-induced thrombocytopenia; INR, international normalized ratio; PE, pulmonary embolism; VTE, venous thromboembolism.
[a]Phlegmasia cerulean dolens is massive thrombosis of the veins of the leg that results in circulatory compromise.

Table 57.6 lists the criteria for outpatient VTE management.

LMWH has predictable pharmacokinetics such that laboratory measurement to evaluate its effect is unnecessary in most patients. Situations in which monitoring can be useful include pregnancy, obesity (body weight >150 kg), and significant renal insufficiency (creatinine <25 mL/min). If monitoring is necessary, the aPTT is not a useful test because it is insensitive to LMWH. The anti–factor Xa assay, which determines the concentration of LMWH by virtue of its inhibitory activity on the activated form of factor X, is used to monitor LMWH therapy when necessary. Samples for anti–factor Xa assays should be drawn 4 hours after subcutaneous administration of LMWH. For twice daily doses of enoxaparin, dalteparin, or tinzaparin, the recommended therapeutic range is 0.6 to 1.0 IU/mL. A therapeutic range of 1.0 to 2.0 IU/mL should be used for once daily doses of enoxaparin, dalteparin, or tinzaparin (34,35). UFH is preferred for treatment of patients with significant renal insufficiency. However, if use of LMWH is necessary in a patient with kidney disease, enoxaparin is the LMWH of choice because Food and Drug Administration (FDA)-approved dosing guidelines for this agent are available (1 mg/kg by subcutaneous injection every 24 hours). When treating patients with body weights >150 kg, actual body weight (i.e., *not* ideal body weight) should be used for dose calculation. Dose capping in obese patients is to be avoided because this practice can result in subtherapeutic drug levels and increase the risk of recurrent thrombotic events.

Fondaparinux

Another alternative for acute therapy of VTE is *fondaparinux,* a synthetic indirect factor Xa inhibitor. Fondaparinux is administered in weight-based subcutaneous injection once daily (Table 57.5). In randomized clinical trials, fondaparinux was found to be as efficacious as enoxaparin and UFH in the treatment of DVT and PE, respectively (36,37). Unlike UFH and LMWH, heparin-induced thrombocytopenia (HIT) (see below) has not been observed during fondaparinux therapy, and case reports suggest that it may be a useful agent for treatment of HIT (38). However, exclusive renal elimination precludes the use of fondaparinux in patients with estimated creatinine clearances <30 mL/min.

Over the next few years, additional options for the acute and chronic treatment of DVT and PE undoubtedly will become available. Idraparinux, a long-acting indirect factor Xa inhibitor similar to fondaparinux that only requires once weekly dosing, currently is in testing for the prevention and treatment of VTE. The long half-life of this agent may limit its popularity until a specific reversal agent is available. Parenteral and oral compounds that directly inhibit factor Xa are in earlier stages of clinical development for VTE treatment (39).

Direct Thrombin Inhibitors

Among investigational antithrombotic agents, oral direct thrombin inhibitors have generated the most interest among clinicians. Ximelagatran, an oral prodrug of the parenteral direct thrombin inhibitor melagatran, has been demonstrated to be noninferior to enoxaparin/warfarin in the acute and chronic treatment of VTE (40). Although ximelagatran has not received FDA approval due to concerns about liver toxicity and rare cardiac events, this drug or another oral direct thrombin inhibitor likely will become available for clinical use in the next 5 to 10 years (41).

Warfarin

Warfarin is the principal agent used for chronic therapy of VTE. Warfarin can be initiated on the first day of acute therapy once therapeutic anticoagulation with UFH, LMWH, or fondaparinux is achieved. Initial warfarin doses should be chosen based upon the expected maintenance dose. Loading doses do not accelerate the pace of warfarin anticoagulation but do increase the likelihood of supratherapeutic INR values. For most patients, 5 mg is an appropriate initial dose. Elderly patients (age >70 years), patients with liver dysfunction, postoperative patients, or patients being treated with medications that reduce warfarin metabolism or disrupt vitamin K absorption or metabolism should start on no more than 2.5 mg warfarin. Use of a warfarin dosing nomogram can help simplify dosing decisions (Table 57.7) (42). The target INR for the majority of VTE patients is 2.5 (range 2.0–3.0). Possible exceptions to this rule include patients with recurrent VTE despite therapeutic anticoagulation and patients with APS and recurrent thromboembolism in whom a higher target range (2.5–3.5 or 3.0–4.0) may be appropriate (34,43).

A number of dietary and medicinal factors can influence warfarin therapy, either enhancing or inhibiting its effect (Table 57.8). Patients need not exclude all vitamin K-containing foods from their diets but should maintain moderate and consistent vitamin K intake to avoid excessive INR fluctuations (a list of the vitamin K content of foods is available at http://www.coumacarenews.com). To reduce the likelihood of drug–drug interactions with warfarin, patients should be instructed to always mention to health care providers that they are taking warfarin when they are prescribed new medications. In light of its effects on warfarin metabolism, alcohol consumption should be minimized (no more than one to two glasses of beer or wine or two ounces of liquor daily). To avoid missed doses, warfarin should be taken at the same time each day.

During the transition from another anticoagulant (e.g., LMWH or UFH) to solo warfarin therapy, the INR should be monitored at least every other day to ensure that therapy with the other anticoagulant is discontinued once the INR reaches the therapeutic range (e.g., 2.0–3.0). Once acute therapy is completed, the INR should be measured initially

TABLE 57.7 Warfarin Initiation Guidelines

Day	INR	Dose (mg)
1		5.0
2	<1.5	5.0
	1.5–1.9	2.5
	2.0–2.5	1.0–2.5
	>2.5	0.0
3	<1.5	5.0–10.0
	1.5–1.9	2.5–5
	2.0–2.5	0.0–2.5
	2.5–3.0	0.0–2.5
	>3.0	0.0
4	<1.5	5–10
	1.5–1.9	5.0–7.5
	2.0–3.0	0.0–5.0
	>3.0	0.0
5	<1.5	10.0
	1.5–1.9	7.5–10.0
	2.0–3.0	0.0–5.0
	>3.0	0.0
6	<1.5	7.5–12.5
	1.5–1.9	5.0–10.0
	2.0–3.0	0.0–7.5
	>3.0	0.0

Modified from Crowther MA, Harrison L, Hirsh J. Warfarin: less may be better. Ann Intern Med 1997;127:332.

TABLE 57.8 Factors That Commonly Influence a Patient's Response to Warfarin

Increase in INR	Decrease in INR
Alcohol	Barbiturates
Amiodarone	**Carbamazepine (Tegretol)**
Anabolic steroids	Chlordiazepoxide
Broad-spectrum antibiotics	Cholestyramine
Cimetidine	Griseofulvin
Clofibrate	Methimazole
Erythromycin	Nafcillin
Fluconazole	Phenytoin
Isoniazid	**Rifampin**
Metronidazole (Flagyl)	Rifabutin
Miconazole	Spironolactone
Omeprazole	Sucralfate
Phenylbutazone	**Vitamin K and vitamin K-rich foods,** including
Piroxicam (Feldene)	**Avocado**
Propafenone	Broccoli
Propranolol	Brussel sprouts
Quinidine	Cabbage
Sulfinpyrazone	Collard greens
Trimethoprim/sulfamethoxazole (Bactrim/Septra)	Cauliflower
	Kale
Omeprazole	Spinach

INR, international normalized ratio.
Especially commonly seen influences on warfarin therapy are indicated in **bold** print.

at least twice weekly. Once patients achieve a stable INR on a stable dose of warfarin, the frequency of INR monitoring can be gradually reduced from weekly to monthly. Because there is a direct correlation between the frequency of INR monitoring and the time spent in the therapeutic range, less frequent monitoring is inadvisable. When dictated by the INR, small graduated dose adjustments (increases or decreases of 5%–20% of the weekly dose) should be made with weekly INR monitoring (Table 57.9). To reduce confusion, a single tablet size (e.g., 5 mg) should be used if possible. Dose schedules should assign specific doses to specific days of the week (avoid every other day or every third day schedules). Dose alterations can be made by splitting tablets (using a tablet splitter that is available from pharmacies and medical equipment stores) and by increasing or decreasing the number of days a patient receives a particular dose (e.g., 5 mg on Monday, Wednesday, and Friday; 2.5 mg on Tuesday, Thursday, Saturday, and Sunday). Dramatic changes in INR should always prompt investigation for the causative factor. Table 57.10 provides guidelines for the management of supratherapeutic INR values in the presence and absence of bleeding (43).

Cancer patients are at higher risk for recurrent VTE and bleeding during treatment. A study of cancer patients demonstrated that dalteparin therapy for 6 months was associated with fewer recurrent VTE without increased bleeding compared with warfarin therapy (44). LMWH should be considered for patients likely to develop complications during warfarin therapy (e.g., cancer patients with liver metastases, poor oral intake, dramatically fluctuating INR values, etc.). Drug cost may be a significant barrier to broader use of LMWH for chronic VTE therapy.

Duration of Anticoagulation

The duration of anticoagulation depends upon the type of VTE, the presence of transient or permanent risk factors, and whether the event prompting treatment represents an initial or recurrent episode. Thrombotic events that occur in association with transient major risk factors require a shorter duration of therapy than do other events or VTE associated with major, long-term risk factors (e.g., malignancy, antithrombin deficiency, APS, etc.). PE is generally treated for a longer duration than DVT because of its higher case fatality rate. Recurrent episodes of VTE generally warrant long-term therapy unless they are associated with transient risk factors. Any decision about the duration of anticoagulation in a given patient should consider the patient's risk for bleeding as well as for recurrent VTE. Validated tools to assess bleeding risk in association with warfarin therapy are available (Table 57.11). Table 57.12 provides guidelines for the duration of VTE therapy (34).

Complications of Anticoagulants

The primary complication of anticoagulation is bleeding. The risk of bleeding associated with UFH or LMWH

TABLE 57.9 Warfarin Management Guidelines

INR	Management
INR >0.3 Below Target Range	
With removable causative factor (e.g., missed dose, drug interaction, more vitamin K consumption)	Remove causative risk factor, then make no change in dose, or increase weekly dose by 10%–20%
Without causative factor	Increase weekly dose by 10%–20%
INR 0.1–0.3 Below Target Range	
With removable causative factor	Remove causative risk factor, but make no change in dose
Without removable causative factor	Take extra 5%–10% of weekly dose × 1 d, and continue weekly dose
2–3 consecutive subtherapeutic INRs, with or without a causative factor	Increase weekly dose by 5%–10%
INR Within Target Range	No change in weekly dose
INR 0.1–0.5 Above Target Range	
With removable causative factor (e.g., extra dose, drug interaction, less vitamin K consumption)	Remove causative factor, continue same dose
Without removable causative factor	No change, or decrease weekly dose by 5%–10%
2–3 consecutive supratherapeutic INRs, *with/without* causative factor	Decrease weekly dose by 5%–10%
INR 0.6 Above Target Range (INR <4.5)	
With removable causative factor	Consider repeat INR If elevation confirmed or test not repeated, remove causative factor, then hold 0–1 dose and continue weekly dose Repeat INR in 1 wk
Without removable causative factor	Consider repeat INR If elevation confirmed or test not repeated, hold 0–1 dose, then decrease weekly dose by 10%–20%
INR >4.5	Repeat INR See Table 57.10

INR, international normalized ratio.
Modified from Ansell J, Hirsh J, Poller L, et al. The pharmacology and management of the vitamin K antagonists. Chest 2004;126:204S; Guidelines on oral anticoagulation: third edition. Br J Haematol 1998;101:374; A guide to oral anticoagulant treatment. Haematologica 2003;88:1.

is influenced by patient age, intensity of anticoagulation, presence of renal insufficiency, and, in some studies, patient gender (female higher risk than male). The frequency of major and fatal bleeding associated with UFH therapy for VTE is 2% and 0.25%, respectively. Major (1.2%) and fatal bleeding (0.1%) are slightly less with LMWH (45). Use of fondaparinux for VTE is associated with a frequency of major bleeding and fatal bleeding of 1.2% and 0.14%, respectively (36,37).

Determinants of bleeding risk associated with warfarin therapy include the intensity of anticoagulation, patient age, previous history of bleeding, comorbidities (hypertension, cerebrovascular disease, renal insufficiency, and cancer), and use of concomitant antithrombotic medications (e.g., aspirin, clopidogrel, nonsteroidal anti-inflammatory drugs). The risk of major bleeding is greatest in the first month of therapy and declines thereafter. Elderly patients are at greater risk of bleeding than younger patients because of their greater number of comorbidities, their use of multiple medications, and their greater vascular fragility and likelihood of falling (45). Clinical trials of chronic warfarin therapy for VTE have estimated the incidence of major bleeding to be one to two episodes per 100 patient-years (34). Given the strict selection criteria for participation in these studies, the incidence of major bleeding derived from a cohort of anticoagulation clinic patients (7.6 events per 100 patient-years) probably is a more realistic estimate for most ambulatory care populations (46). Validated assessment models that allow prediction of a patient's bleeding risk on warfarin therapy have been developed (Table 57.11) (47).

Management of bleeding during warfarin therapy depends on careful assessment by the clinician of the risks associated with anticoagulation during a bleeding episode, as well as the risk of recurrent thromboembolism if anticoagulation is discontinued. The risk of recurrent VTE in the absence of anticoagulation depends on the amount of time that has elapsed since the thrombotic event and on the presence of ongoing risk factors for thrombosis (e.g., malignancy, thrombophilia, idiopathic or recurrent VTE). The risk of recurrent VTE declines as time elapses. During the first month, absence of anticoagulation is associated with a higher risk of recurrence (40% for the 1-month time interval) than during months 2 and 3 after thrombosis (10%

TABLE 57.10 Management of Excessive Warfarin Anticoagulation

INR and Clinical Scenario	*Management*
INR <5.0 without significant bleeding	Review medication list for interacting medications Lower dose or omit one dose, recheck INR in 24–48 hr, resume warfarin at 10%–20% lower weekly dose when INR approaches therapeutic range
INR ≥5 but <9 without significant bleeding	Review medication list for interacting medications Omit next 1–2 doses, recheck INR in 24 hr If at high risk for bleeding or requires invasive procedure (within 48 hr), consider oral vitamin K_1 (1–5 mg × 1) If INR still high at 24 hr, consider additional oral vitamin K_1 (1–2 mg) When INR approaches therapeutic range, resume warfarin at 20% lower weekly dose
INR ≥9 without significant bleeding	Review medication list for interacting medications Hold warfarin, give higher dose vitamin K_1 (5–10 mg PO) and monitor INR daily Use additional vitamin K if needed Resume warfarin at 20% lower weekly dose
Serious bleeding at any INR elevation	Hold warfarin, give vitamin K_1 (10 mg IV over 1 hr) Anaphylaxis kit at bedside Consider use of FFP, NovoSeven 20 μg/kg, or FEIBA 50 IU/kg × 1 Monitor INR closely Vitamin K_1 can be repeated if needed
Life-threatening bleeding	Hold warfarin, Give NovoSeven 20 μg/kg or FEIBA 50 IU/kg IV × 1 Give vitamin K_1 (10 mg IV over 1 hr) Anaphylaxis kit at bedside Monitor INR closely Vitamin K_1 can be repeated if needed, depending upon INR

FEIBA, Factor Eight Inhibitor Bypass Activity (Baxter Healthcare, Round Lake, IL), an activated prothrombin complex concentrate; FFP, fresh-frozen plasma; INR, international normalized ratio; NovoSeven (NovoNordisk, Princeton, NJ), recombinant human factor VIIa.
Modified from Ansell J, Hirsh J, Poller L, et al. The pharmacology and management of the vitamin K antagonists: The Seventh ACCP Conference on Antithrombotic and Thrombolytic Therapy. Chest 2004;126:204S.fresh-frozen plasma.

for the 2-month interval) (48). Potent thrombophilic states (e.g., APS, active cancer, or idiopathic VTE) are associated with a greater risk of recurrence than VTE associated with transient risk factors.

The decision to withhold anticoagulation must consider the clinical severity of bleeding. Minor bleeding (easy bruisability, gum bleeding, etc.) generally does not require a change in therapy (unless associated with a supratherapeutic INR). In contrast, major life-threatening bleeding (e.g. massive hematuria, gastrointestinal bleeding, retroperitoneal bleeding, or intracranial bleeding) generally warrants prompt discontinuation of warfarin and reversal of anticoagulation so that the cause can be identified and treated. Tables 57.9 and 57.10 provide recommendations for warfarin reversal (43). Once the cause of bleeding is identified and hemostasis is achieved, anticoagulation, if still warranted based upon the risk of recurrent VTE, can be reinstituted with close monitoring. Hemorrhage during anticoagulation should not be attributed solely to the presence of anticoagulation, even when the INR is supratherapeutic, as causative lesions are often identified (49,50).

TABLE 57.11 Outpatient Bleeding Risk Index

Risk Factor	*Points (If Factor Present)*
Age ≥65 yr	1
History of stroke	1
History of gastrointestinal bleeding	1
Recent myocardial infarction, hematocrit <30%, serum creatinine >1.5 mg/dL, or diabetes mellitus	1

Bleeding risk index: 0 points = low (2% risk of major bleed in 3 mo); 1–2 points = moderate (5% risk of major bleed in 3 mo); 3–4 points = high (23% risk of major bleed in 3 mo).
Modified from Beyth RJ, Quinn LM, Landefeld CS. Prospective evaluation of an index for predicting the risk of major bleeding in outpatients treated with warfarin. Am J Med 1998;105:91.

Another complication of UFH or LMWH therapy is *osteoporosis* (in patients receiving prolonged therapy, typically for more than a few months). Osteoporotic fractures occurred in 2.2% of patients treated with subcutaneous UFH during pregnancy (51). Osteoporosis appears to be much less common in patients treated with LMWH (52).

A significant complication of heparin therapy is *heparin-induced thrombocytopenia* (HIT). HIT is an

TABLE 57.12 Duration of Anticoagulation for VTE

Diagnosis	*Duration*
DVT	
Transient risk factor, first episode	3 mo
Idiopathic, first episode	At least 6–12 mo
Recurrent DVT	Consider indefinite therapy
Malignancy-associated	Until malignancy in remission
PE	
Transient risk factor, first episode	3–6 mo
Idiopathic, first episode	At least 6–12 mo
Recurrent DVT	Consider indefinite therapy
Malignancy-associated	Until malignancy in remission
Hypercoagulable states	
Antiphospholipid syndrome, two or more thrombophilic mutations (e.g., combined factor V Leiden and prothrombin gene mutations) or homozygous factor V Leiden or prothrombin gene mutation	Consider indefinite therapy
Antithrombin, protein C, or protein S deficiency	At least 6–12 mo, consider indefinite therapy for idiopathic VTE
Factor V Leiden or prothrombin mutation heterozygosity, hyperhomocysteinemia, high factor VIII levels	At least 6–12 mo, consider indefinite therapy for idiopathic VTE

DVT, deep venous thrombosis; PE, pulmonary embolism; VTE, venous thromboembolism.
Modified from Buller HR, Agnelli G, Hull RD, et al. Antithrombotic therapy for venous thromboembolic disease: the Seventh ACCP Conference on Antithrombotic and Thrombolytic Therapy. Chest 2004;126:401S.

immune-mediated prothrombotic state caused by antibodies directed against heparin-bound platelet factor 4 (PF4). It occurs in approximately 1% of patients treated with intravenous UFH and is eightfold to 10-fold less common with LMWH therapy. HIT is characterized by a ≥50% decrease in the platelet count beginning most commonly 4 to 14 days after initiation of heparin therapy. Confirmatory diagnostic tests include the heparin–PF4 assay (HIT antibodies) and the serotonin release assay. Any patient suspected of having HIT should have all heparin products eliminated and should be started on treatment with a direct thrombin inhibitor (e.g., lepirudin or argatroban) because of the increased risk for venous and/or arterial thrombosis in patients with HIT. Upper- and lower-extremity duplex ultrasonography is indicated to identify asymptomatic DVT because studies have demonstrated that 50% of HIT patients have subclinical thrombosis, the presence of which alters the duration of anticoagulation therapy (see above) (53). In the absence of thrombosis, treatment with a direct thrombin inhibitor should continue until the platelet count has returned to baseline. Although fondaparinux therapy for HIT has been used in clinically stable ambulatory patients with adequate renal function, outpatients who develop HIT should be hospitalized for initial therapy. Osteoporosis and HIT have not been seen with fondaparinux.

Warfarin skin necrosis is a rare complication of warfarin therapy (estimated frequency 0.01%–0.1% of warfarin-treated patients). Warfarin skin necrosis is characterized by thrombosis of small dermal vessels that results in skin necrosis, particularly in women, in the areas of the breasts, buttocks, and thighs. Warfarin skin necrosis most commonly occurs when warfarin is used (often in large loading doses) to treat an acute thrombotic disorder in the absence of concomitant UFH or LMWH therapy and in the presence of an underlying thrombophilic state. Although the presence of protein C deficiency has been traditionally linked to warfarin skin necrosis, factor V Leiden, protein S deficiency, antithrombin deficiency, and APS also have been associated with this devastating complication. In patients who develop warfarin skin necrosis and require long-term anticoagulation, warfarin can still be used if therapy is initiated slowly and gradually over a 10-day period (starting with doses of 1–2 mg/day) once therapeutic anticoagulation with heparin is achieved and if heparin therapy is not discontinued until INR ≥2 is achieved with warfarin (54).

Thrombolytic Therapy

Anticoagulation alone rarely results in complete thrombus resolution. Thrombolytic therapy produces substantially greater clot lysis that theoretically may reduce the frequency of postthrombotic syndrome (PTS) (see below for discussion of this syndrome) (55). In a study of patients with submassive PE, systemic thrombolysis reduced the need for treatment escalation compared to anticoagulation alone, although mortality was similar (56). Consequently, despite its therapeutic potential in VTE, thrombolytic therapy is primarily reserved for patients with extensive iliofemoral thrombosis and/or massive life-threatening PE. Randomized clinical trials are needed to determine if the benefits of applying thrombolytic therapy to a broader population are worth the risks of greater bleeding. Thrombolytic drugs should be administered only to inpatients.

Vena Caval Filters

Vena caval filters are sieves generally constructed of nonferromagnetic wire that can be placed percutaneously into the inferior vena cava (IVC) using catheter-directed techniques by an interventional radiologist or vascular surgeon. Numerous case series have demonstrated that vena caval filters are an effective means of PE prevention when anticoagulation is contraindicated or when a patient experiences a PE despite therapeutic anticoagulation. However, permanent vena caval filters are clearly associated with an increased risk for DVT compared to anticoagulation alone. Other complications of permanent filters include IVC thrombosis (2%–10%); penetration of filter components through the IVC wall (0.3%), occasionally involving adjacent anatomic structures; migration from the placement site (0.3%); and tilting (5%) or fracture (3%) of the filter, which theoretically may result in reduced performance. Acute procedure-related complications include misplacement (1.3% of insertions), pneumothorax (0.02%), hematoma (0.6%), air embolism (0.2%), inadvertent carotid artery puncture (0.04%), and arteriovenous fistula (0.02%). Based upon the published case series, fatal complications of placement are rare (0.13% of insertions). Several retrievable vena caval filters are approved for use in the United States. These devices can be removed weeks or, in some cases, months after implantation. Whether retrievable filters will perform as well as permanent filters remains unclear. If retrievable filters are demonstrated to reduce the risk of PE as effectively as permanent filters, retrievable filters should prove to be a very useful treatment option for patients with a transient absolute contraindication to anticoagulation (57).

Management of Venous Thromboembolism during Pregnancy

Pregnancy is associated with a twofold to fourfold increased risk for VTE. Therefore, primary care providers may be involved in the management of patients with VTE during pregnancy. When a pregnant patient is suspected of having DVT or PE, the diagnosis must be confirmed (duplex ultrasonography, V/Q scanning, or helical CT scanning) using fetal shielding when appropriate rather than forgoing diagnostic testing for fear of harming the fetus. A misdiagnosis resulting in inappropriately omitted or prescribed anticoagulation is far more likely to harm the mother and fetus than the effects of diagnostic testing (58). Warfarin therapy during pregnancy is associated with teratogenicity and with an increased risk for bleeding in the fetus. Therefore, UFH or LMWH is generally used for acute and chronic therapy during pregnancy. The lower risk of osteoporosis and HIT and the more favorable pharmacokinetics of LMWH have made it the preferred anticoagulant for VTE during pregnancy. Since maternal weight increases during pregnancy, LMWH doses should be adjusted accordingly as pregnancy progresses. Twice daily dosing is preferred given the shorter half-life of LMWH during pregnancy. LMWH should be discontinued 24 hours prior to the induction of labor. In the postpartum period, either LMWH or warfarin may be used for antithrombotic therapy as maternal warfarin use does not appear to result in an anticoagulant effect in breast-fed infants. Patients with an episode of VTE during pregnancy should be treated for at least 6 weeks post-partum or for the duration of therapy that is appropriate for their thrombotic episode, whichever is longer. Patients with VTE during pregnancy and patients on long-term anticoagulation for previous VTE should receive prophylactic LMWH during subsequent pregnancies (59).

Considerations in Patients with Recurrent Venous Thromboembolism

Recurrent VTE generally indicates persistent abnormalities affecting one or more factors of the Virchow triad. If a patient presents with a recurrence soon after completion of acute VTE therapy, two diagnostic entities should be strongly considered: delayed HIT and Trousseau syndrome. HIT will be apparent by the presence of a reduced platelet count and can be confirmed by laboratory testing. Avoidance of heparin exposure and therapy with a direct thrombin inhibitor are indicated (see above for a discussion of the treatment of HIT). Trousseau syndrome is a prothrombotic disorder associated with solid tumor malignancies that is characterized classically by recurrent migratory thrombophlebitis despite adequate warfarin anticoagulation, laboratory findings consistent with disseminated intravascular coagulation (including thrombocytopenia, hypofibrinogenemia, and elevated D-dimers), and nonbacterial thrombotic endocarditis (60). Anticoagulation with UFH or LWMH is the most effective treatment. Occasional resistance to LMWH therapy has been reported.

APS is another common cause of recurrent VTE despite adequate warfarin anticoagulation. Although most patients with APS can be managed with conventional-intensity warfarin anticoagulation (INR 2.0–3.0), occasional patients require higher INR target ranges (INR 3.0–4.0). Less commonly, other causes of hypercoagulability can trigger recurrent VTE despite adequate anticoagulation and should be investigated as dictated by the clinical circumstances. Recurrent events in the same location should prompt consideration of vascular abnormalities such as May-Thurner syndrome or Paget-Schroetter syndrome (thoracic outlet syndrome, see below), which are underrecognized causes of recurrent VTE. May-Thurner syndrome is characterized by deformation and stenosis of the left iliac vein as a consequence of compression by the overlying right iliac artery. The resulting stenosis precipitates recurrent episodes of left iliofemoral DVT. Thrombolysis and stenting of the affected vein segment can result in long-lasting resolution (61). Management of the Paget-Schroetter syndrome is discussed below.

Calf Vein Thrombosis

Calf vein thrombosis consists of DVT involving the deep vessels of the legs distal to the popliteal vein (when extension into the thigh is not also present). Calf vein DVT is associated with a significant risk of recurrent VTE when treated with short durations of anticoagulation (e.g., 5-day course of UFH); therefore, warfarin anticoagulation in addition to acute therapy with heparin is recommended for 6 to 12 weeks to prevent recurrent DVT or PE (62,63).

Upper-Extremity Deep Venous Thrombosis

Upper-extremity DVT generally consists of thrombosis involving the brachial, axillary, and/or subclavian veins with occasional extension into the superior vena cava. Common risk factors for upper-extremity DVT include central vein catheterization, pacemaker and implantable cardioverter-defibrillator (ICD) placement, cancer, chemotherapy, thrombophilia, and anatomic abnormalities such as the thoracic outlet syndrome (Paget-Schroetter syndrome). Upper-extremity DVT typically is heralded by pain and swelling of the affected extremity and later by the development of superficial venous collaterals. Duplex or color flow ultrasonography is useful to confirm the diagnosis. As in lower-extremity DVT, anticoagulation is indicated, with or without thrombolytic therapy. If the DVT is catheter associated, the catheter often is removed, but it may remain in place if indications for its use remain.

Occurrence of an upper-extremity DVT without clear risk factors should prompt investigation for the Paget-Schroetter syndrome, a venous manifestation of thoracic outlet syndrome. In affected individuals, the subclavian vein is compressed by local anatomic structures (anterior scalene muscle, cervical ribs, etc.). Vascular wall damage and stasis result in thrombosis. Historically, patients may relate a recent history of heavy lifting or exertion involving the affected extremity. Venography of the upper limb vessels in stress position (abduction, external rotation) is useful to demonstrate compression of the subclavian vein (64,65). Therapy for Paget-Schroetter syndrome consists of catheter-directed thrombolysis followed by surgical correction of the anatomic abnormality and anticoagulation (66).

As with lower-extremity DVT, hypercoagulable states may play a role in the pathogenesis of upper-extremity DVT. The risk of PE associated with upper-extremity DVT (10%–15%) appears to be less than that associated with lower-extremity DVT (50%–60%), but the risk is not insignificant (64,67). PTS (see below) can also occur in the affected extremity. Therefore, at least 3 months of anticoagulation with warfarin is recommended (64).

Superficial Venous Thrombophlebitis

Superficial venous thrombophlebitis (SVT) consists of thrombosis of the superficial veins of the legs or arms. Risk factors for SVT are similar to risk factors for DVT and include peripheral venous catheters, thrombophilia, oral contraceptives or hormone replacement therapy, pregnancy, recent surgery or trauma, and a history of previous DVT or SVT. Less common etiologies include Trousseau syndrome, Buerger disease (thromboangiitis obliterans), and Behçet syndrome. SVT traditionally has been managed symptomatically with compression, elevation of the affected extremity, and anti-inflammatory agents, or less commonly with vein ligation. A study indicates that prophylactic or therapeutic doses of LMWH may be a useful option in some patients with SVT (68). Further investigation is needed to define the patient populations likely to benefit from anticoagulation and the appropriate duration of therapy. Until these studies are performed, traditional approaches to SVT probably should remain the first-line therapy with consideration of anticoagulation in patients with progressive disease. Any episode of proximal lower-extremity SVT should prompt duplex ultrasonography to rule out extension into the deep venous system given that PE has occurred in this situation. Conventional anticoagulation for at least 3 months would be appropriate in this instance (68).

Postthrombotic Syndrome (PTS)

PTS is a common cause of chronic morbidity after DVT. PTS is characterized by edema, pain, heaviness, and occasionally skin ulceration of the affected extremity that develop as a consequence of chronic venous obstruction and valvular incompetence. Symptoms worsen with standing and ambulation (69). PTS affects almost 30% of patients within 5 years of an episode of DVT (70). Risk factors for PTS include recurrent ipsilateral DVT, obesity, female gender, and increased age (69). Consistent use of knee-high compression stockings (30–40 mm Hg) has been shown to reduce the incidence of PTS by 50% (71,72). Therefore, all patients should be prescribed knee-high compression stockings after an episode of DVT. Optimally, compression stockings should be worn daily starting within several weeks of completion of acute therapy and then for at least 2 years post-DVT. Whether patients with upper-extremity DVT will benefit from similar treatment remains unclear (73). By reducing the thrombus burden and venous valvular damage, it is possible that catheter-directed thrombolysis may reduce the risk of PTS, but this has not been demonstrated in a randomized clinical trial.

ARTERIAL THROMBOEMBOLISM

Arterial thromboembolism (AT), as manifested by cerebrovascular, cardiovascular, or peripheral vascular disease, remains the most common cause of morbidity and mortality in developed countries. Unlike the venous circulation where coagulation factors play the principal role in the pathogenesis of thromboembolism, arterial thrombosis is primarily the result of platelet-rich thrombi. Consequently, the most important risk factors for arterial thrombosis affect vascular wall and platelet function. Atherosclerosis is an important risk factor for AT, which induces endothelial dysfunction, tissue factor formation, and, ultimately, platelet plug formation that can result in local stenosis and ischemia or embolization. Other risk factors for AT include hypertension, diabetes, smoking, obesity, elevated low-density lipoprotein (LDL) cholesterol and fibrinogen levels, abnormalities of fibrinolysis, hyperhomocysteinemia, APS, and rarely malignancy-associated thrombosis including Trousseau syndrome. Whereas anticoagulation is clearly indicated in the acute treatment of unstable angina, myocardial infarction (see Chapter 62), and cardioembolic stroke (see Chapter 91) and in the prevention of thromboembolism associated with atrial fibrillation (see Chapter 64), left ventricular thrombus, APS, and malignancy-associated thrombosis, inhibiting platelet function remains preeminent in the treatment of AT (74).

Aspirin

Aspirin remains the most commonly used medication for the prevention and treatment of AT. The antithrombotic activity of aspirin is primarily due to its ability to irreversibly acetylate and thus inhibit cyclooxygenase, the enzyme that converts arachidonic acid into prostaglandin H_2. This interferes with the synthesis of thromboxane A_2, a potent vasoconstrictor and platelet aggregating substance (75).

Aspirin has been widely studied in doses ranging from 50 to 1,500 mg/day in the prevention and treatment of AT, including myocardial infarction, stroke, and peripheral vascular disease. The decision to use aspirin in the primary prevention of AT requires an assessment of the individual's risk of AT as well as his or her risk of gastrointestinal toxicity and bleeding associated with aspirin therapy. The risk of a major bleed associated with aspirin in doses of 81 to 325 mg/day is small (approximately one to two major bleeds per 1,000 patient-years, approximately 10-fold less than that associated with warfarin). This risk is not reduced with enteric-coated aspirin or buffered aspirin. However, the benefits of aspirin for healthy individuals at low risk for AT are equally small. Therefore, aspirin should not be used for primary prevention of AT in low-risk healthy adults (75). In contrast, three large studies have demonstrated that low doses of aspirin (75–100 mg/day) significantly reduce (by 15%–23%) vascular events in high-risk patients with one or more risk factors for vascular disease (76–78).

Aspirin has also proven to have activity in the treatment of patients with pre-existing vascular disease. Among patients with stable angina, aspirin therapy results in 10 fewer vascular events per 1,000 patient-years. The benefits of aspirin are even greater among patients with unstable angina or previous myocardial infarction who experienced 50 and 36 fewer vascular events per 1,000 patient-years, respectively. Similar benefits have been seen in patients with transient ischemic attack (TIA) and stroke. It is important to emphasize that although daily doses of aspirin ranging from 50 to 1,500 mg have been demonstrated to be effective in the prevention and treatment of AT, the incidence of gastrointestinal side effects and clinical bleeding increases with high doses, and the clinical benefits of aspirin do not appear to increase at doses >100 mg/day. Therefore, daily doses of aspirin of 75 to 100 mg probably are sufficient for most patients, particularly patients deemed to be at higher risk of bleeding complications (75,79–81).

Thienopyridines

Thienopyridines represent the second class of antiplatelet agents used for AT. Ticlopidine (Ticlid) and clopidogrel (Plavix) belong to this drug class. These agents inhibit platelet aggregation induced by adenosine diphosphate. Ticlopidine has been demonstrated to be superior to aspirin in patients with stroke or TIA and of comparable efficacy in patients with a recent myocardial infarction (82,83). However, hematologic adverse effects, including neutropenia (0.8% of patients), thrombocytopenia, aplastic anemia, and thrombotic thrombocytopenic purpura (TTP; estimated frequency, one case per 1,600–5,000 patients treated) have greatly reduced the use of ticlopidine in clinical practice (75,84).

Clopidogrel has equivalent efficacy to aspirin in prevention of vascular events in patients with myocardial infarction, stroke, and peripheral arterial disease. When added to aspirin, clopidogrel is associated with a reduction in vascular events compared with aspirin alone and has become standard therapy for patients after percutaneous coronary interventions. Clopidogrel is associated with a comparable risk of bleeding and thrombocytopenia compared to aspirin. TTP rarely occurs with clopidogrel, and the incidence may not exceed that seen in the general population. When it occurs, TTP develops within the first 2 weeks of therapy (75,85). Because it does not cause neutropenia and is associated much less often with TTP (86), clopidogrel has become the thienopyridine of choice in clinical practice.

Dipyridamole

Dipyridamole affects platelet function by inhibiting phosphodiesterase that results in increased intraplatelet cyclic adenosine monophosphate levels. The European Stroke Prevention Study 2 demonstrated that the combination of dipyridamole and aspirin was superior to aspirin alone in the prevention of stroke in patients with a previous stroke or TIA (87).

Glycoprotein IIb/IIIa Inhibitors

Glycoprotein IIb/IIIa is the platelet receptor responsible for platelet aggregation. Congenital deficiency of this protein is the cause of the platelet function disorder Glanzmann thrombasthenia. As predicted by its physiologic role, glycoprotein IIb/IIIa inhibitors have proven to be important treatments for coronary artery disease. The currently available glycoprotein IIb/IIIa inhibitors include abciximab, a chimeric mouse–human monoclonal antibody, and two synthetic receptor antagonists, tirofiban and eptifibatide. Development of effective oral glycoprotein IIb/IIIa inhibitors is an active area of clinical investigation that may have a significant impact on the future ambulatory care of patients with AT (75). Currently, none of these drugs is suitable for use in ambulatory patients.

SPECIFIC REFERENCES*

1. Silverstein MD, Heit JA, Mohr DN, et al. Trends in the incidence of deep vein thrombosis and pulmonary embolism: a 25-year population-based study. Arch Intern Med 1998;158:585.
2. Murin S, Romano PS, White RH. Comparison of outcomes after hospitalization for deep venous thrombosis or pulmonary embolism. Thromb Haemost 2002;88:407.
3. White RH. The epidemiology of venous thromboembolism. Circulation 2003;107:I4.
4. White RH, Zhou H, Romano PS. Incidence of idiopathic deep venous thrombosis and secondary thromboembolism among ethnic groups in California. Ann Intern Med 1998; 128:737.
5. Ridker PM, Miletich JP, Hennekens CH, et al. Ethnic distribution of factor V Leiden in 4047 men and women. Implications for venous thromboembolism screening. JAMA 1997; 277:1305.
6. Patel RK, Ford E, Thumpston J, et al. Risk factors for venous thrombosis in the black population. Thromb Haemost 2003;90:835.
7. Kyrle PA, Minar E, Bialonczyk C, et al. The risk of recurrent venous thromboembolism in men and women. N Engl J Med 2004;350:2558.
8. Seligsohn U, Lubetsky A. Genetic susceptibility to venous thrombosis. N Engl J Med 2001; 344:1222.
9. Kearon C, Crowther M, Hirsh J. Management of patients with hereditary hypercoagulable disorders. Annu Rev Med 2000;51:169.
10. Koster T, Blann AD, Briet E, et al. Role of clotting factor VIII in effect of von Willebrand factor on occurrence of deep-vein thrombosis. Lancet 1995;345:152.
11. Kyrle PA, Minar E, Hirschl M, et al. High plasma levels of factor VIII and the risk of recurrent venous thromboembolism. N Engl J Med 2000;343:457.
12. van Hylckama Vlieg, van der Linden IK, Bertina RM, et al. High levels of factor IX increase the risk of venous thrombosis. Blood 2000;95:3678.
13. Meijers JC, Tekelenburg WL, Bouma BN, et al. High levels of coagulation factor XI as a risk factor for venous thrombosis. N Engl J Med 2000;342:696.
14. Roberts HR, Stinchcombe TE, Gabriel DA. The dysfibrinogenaemias. Br J Haematol 2001;114:249.
15. Ridker PM, Vaughan DE, Stampfer MJ, et al. Baseline fibrinolytic state and the risk of future venous thrombosis. A prospective study of endogenous tissue-type plasminogen activator and plasminogen activator inhibitor. Circulation 1992;85:1822.
16. Crowther MA, Roberts J, Roberts R, et al. Fibrinolytic variables in patients with recurrent venous thrombosis: a prospective cohort study. Thromb Haemost 2001;85:390.
17. Koster T, Rosendaal FR, Briet E, et al. John Hageman's factor and deep-vein thrombosis: Leiden thrombophilia Study. Br J Haematol 1994;87:422.
18. Welch GN, Loscalzo J. Homocysteine and atherothrombosis. N Engl J Med 1998;338:1042.
19. Levine JS, Branch DW, Rauch J. The antiphospholipid syndrome. N Engl J Med 2002;346:752.
20. Hanly JG. Antiphospholipid syndrome: an overview. CMAJ 2003;168:1675.
21. Petri M. Thrombosis and systemic lupus erythematosus: the Hopkins Lupus Cohort perspective. Scand J Rheumatol 1996;25:191.
22. Schulman S, Svenungsson E, Granqvist S. Anticardiolipin antibodies predict early recurrence of thromboembolism and death among patients with venous thromboembolism following anticoagulant therapy. Duration of Anticoagulation Study Group. Am J Med 1998;104:332.
23. Christiansen SC, Cannegieter SC, Koster T, et al. Thrombophilia, clinical factors, and recurrent venous thrombotic events. JAMA 2005;293:2352.
24. DeStefano V, Martinelli I, Mannucci PM, et al. The risk of recurrent deep venous thrombosis among heterozygous carriers of both factor V Leiden and the G20210A prothrombin mutation. N Engl J Med 1999;341:801.
25. Anderson FAJr, Spencer FA. Risk factors for venous thromboembolism. Circulation 2003;107:I9.
26. Wells PS, Anderson DR, Bormanis J, et al. Value of assessment of pretest probability of deep-vein thrombosis in clinical management. Lancet 1997;350:1795.
27. Wells PS, Ginsberg JS, Anderson DR, et al. Use of a clinical model for safe management of patients with suspected pulmonary embolism. Ann Intern Med 1998;129:997.
28. Oudega R, Hoes AW, Moons KG. The Wells rule does not accurately rule out deep venous thrombosis in primary care patients. Ann Intern Med 2005;143:100.
29. Value of the ventilation/perfusion scan in acute pulmonary embolism. Results of the prospective investigation of pulmonary embolism diagnosis (PIOPED). The PIOPED Investigators. JAMA 1990;263:2753.
30. Eng J, Krishnan JA, Segal JB, et al. Accuracy of CT in the diagnosis of pulmonary embolism: a systematic literature review. AJR Am J Roentgenol 2004;183:1819.
31. Moores LK, Jackson WL Jr, Shorr AF, et al. Meta-analysis: outcomes in patients with suspected pulmonary embolism managed with computed tomographic pulmonary angiography. Ann Intern Med 2004;141:866.
32. Winer-Muram HT, Rydberg J, Johnson MS, et al. Suspected acute pulmonary embolism: evaluation with multi-detector row CT versus digital subtraction pulmonary arteriography. Radiology 2004;233:806.
33. Wells PS, Anderson DR, Rodger M, et al. Evaluation of D-dimer in the diagnosis of suspected deep-vein thrombosis. N Engl J Med 2003;349:1227.
34. Buller HR, Agnelli G, Hull RD, et al. Antithrombotic therapy for venous thromboembolic disease: the Seventh ACCP Conference on Antithrombotic and Thrombolytic Therapy. Chest 2004;126:401S.
35. Hirsh J, Raschke R. Heparin and low-molecular-weight heparin: the Seventh ACCP Conference on Antithrombotic and Thrombolytic Therapy. Chest 2004;126:188S.
36. Buller HR, Davidson BL, Decousus H, et al. Subcutaneous fondaparinux versus intravenous unfractionated heparin in the initial treatment of pulmonary embolism. N Engl J Med 2003; 349:1695.
37. Buller HR, Davidson BL, Decousus H, et al. Fondaparinux or enoxaparin for the initial treatment of symptomatic deep venous thrombosis: a randomized trial. Ann Intern Med 2004;140:867.
38. Kuo KH, Kovacs MJ. Fondaparinux: a potential new therapy for HIT. Hematology 2005;10:271.
39. Weitz JI, Hirsh J, Samama MM. New anticoagulant drugs: the Seventh ACCP Conference on Antithrombotic and Thrombolytic Therapy. Chest 2004;126:265S.
40. Fiessinger JN, Huisman MV, Davidson BL, et al. Ximelagatran vs low-molecular-weight heparin and warfarin for the treatment of deep vein thrombosis: a randomized trial. JAMA 2005; 293:681.
41. Di Nisio M, Middeldorp S, Buller HR. Direct thrombin inhibitors. N Engl J Med 2005; 353:1028.
42. Harrison L, Johnston M, Massicotte MP, et al. Comparison of 5-mg and 10-mg loading doses in initiation of warfarin therapy. Ann Intern Med 1997;126:133.
43. Ansell J, Hirsh J, Poller L, et al. The pharmacology and management of the vitamin K antagonists: the Seventh ACCP Conference on Antithrombotic and Thrombolytic Therapy. Chest 2004;126:204S.
44. Lee AY, Levine MN, Baker RI, et al. Low-molecular-weight heparin versus a coumarin for the prevention of recurrent venous thromboembolism in patients with cancer. N Engl J Med 2003;349:146.
45. Levine MN, Raskob G, Beyth RJ, et al. Hemorrhagic complications of anticoagulant treatment: the Seventh ACCP Conference on Antithrombotic and Thrombolytic Therapy. Chest 2004;126:287S.
46. Palareti G, Leali N, Coccheri S, et al. Bleeding complications of oral anticoagulant treatment: an inception-cohort, prospective collaborative study (ISCOAT). Italian Study on Complications of Oral Anticoagulant Therapy. Lancet 1996; 348:423.
47. Beyth RJ, Quinn LM, Landefeld CS. Prospective evaluation of an index for predicting the risk of major bleeding in outpatients treated with warfarin. Am J Med 1998;105:91.
48. Kearon C, Hirsh J. Management of anticoagulation before and after elective surgery. N Engl J Med 1997;336:1506.
49. Jaffin BW, Bliss CM, LaMont JT. Significance of occult gastrointestinal bleeding during anticoagulation therapy. Am J Med 1987;83:269.
50. Culclasure TF, Bray VJ, Hasbargen JA. The significance of hematuria in the anticoagulated patient. Arch Intern Med 1994;154:649.
51. Dahlman TC. Osteoporotic fractures and the recurrence of thromboembolism during pregnancy and the puerperium in 184 women undergoing thromboprophylaxis with heparin. Am J Obstet Gynecol 1993;168:1265.
52. Pettila V, Leinonen P, Markkola A, et al. Postpartum bone mineral density in women treated for thromboprophylaxis with

*Bold numerals denote published controlled clinical trials, meta-analyses, or consensus-based recommendations.

unfractionated heparin or LMW heparin. Thromb Haemost 2002;87:182.

53. Warkentin TE, Greinacher A. Heparin-induced thrombocytopenia: recognition, treatment, and prevention: the Seventh ACCP Conference on Antithrombotic and Thrombolytic Therapy. Chest 2004;126:311S.

54. Chan YC, Valenti D, Mansfield AO, et al. Warfarin induced skin necrosis. Br J Surg 2000;87:266.

55. Comerota AJ, Aldridge SC. Thrombolytic therapy for deep venous thrombosis: a clinical review. Can J Surg 1993;36:359.

56. Konstantinides S, Geibel A, Heusel G, et al. Heparin plus alteplase compared with heparin alone in patients with submassive pulmonary embolism. N Engl J Med 2002;347:1143.

57. Hann CL, Streiff MB. The role of vena caval filters in the management of venous thromboembolism. Blood Rev 2005;19:179.

58. Bates SM, Ginsberg JS. How we manage venous thromboembolism during pregnancy. Blood 2002;100:3470.

59. Bates SM, Greer IA, Hirsh J, et al. Use of antithrombotic agents during pregnancy: the Seventh ACCP Conference on Antithrombotic and Thrombolytic Therapy. Chest 2004; 126:627S.

60. Sack GH Jr, Levin J, Bell WR. Trousseau's syndrome and other manifestations of chronic disseminated coagulopathy in patients with neoplasms: clinical, pathophysiological and therapeutic features. Medicine 1977;56:1.

61. O'Sullivan GJ, Semba CP, Bittner CA, et al. Endovascular management of iliac vein compression (May-Thurner) syndrome. J Vasc Interv Radiol 2000;11:823.

62. Lagerstedt CI, Olsson CG, Fagher BO, et al. Need for long-term anticoagulant treatment in symptomatic calf-vein thrombosis. Lancet 1985;2:515.

63. Pinede L, Ninet J, Duhaut P, et al. Comparison of 3 and 6 months of oral anticoagulant therapy after a first episode of proximal deep vein thrombosis or pulmonary embolism and comparison of 6 and 12 weeks of therapy after isolated calf deep vein thrombosis. Circulation 2001;103:2453.

64. Kommareddy A, Zaroukian MH, Hassouna HI. Upper extremity deep venous thrombosis. Semin Thromb Hemost 2002;28:89.

65. Prandoni P, Polistena P, Bernardi E, et al. Upper-extremity deep vein thrombosis. Risk factors, diagnosis, and complications. Arch Intern Med 1997;157:57.

66. Angle N, Gelabert HA, Farooq MM, et al. Safety and efficacy of early surgical decompression of the thoracic outlet for Paget-Schroetter syndrome. Ann Vasc Surg 2001;15:37.

67. Moser KM, Fedullo PF, LitteJohn JK, et al. Frequent asymptomatic pulmonary embolism in patients with deep venous thrombosis. JAMA 1994;271:223.

68. Decousus H, Epinat M, Guillot K, et al. Superficial vein thrombosis: risk factors, diagnosis, and treatment. Curr Opin Pulm Med 2003;9:393.

69. Kahn SR, Ginsberg JS. Relationship between deep venous thrombosis and the postthrombotic syndrome. Arch Intern Med 2004;164:17.

70. Prandoni P, Lensing AW, Cogo A, et al. The long-term clinical course of acute deep venous thrombosis. Ann Intern.Med 1996;125:1.

71. Prandoni P, Lensing AW, Prins MH, et al. Below-knee elastic compression stockings to prevent the post-thrombotic syndrome: a randomized, controlled trial. Ann Intern Med 2004;141:249.

72. Brandjes DP, Buller HR, Heijboer H, et al. Randomised trial of effect of compression stockings in patients with symptomatic proximal-vein thrombosis. Lancet 1997;349:759.

73. Elman EE, Kahn SR. The post-thrombotic syndrome after upper extremity deep venous thrombosis in adults: a systematic review. Thromb Res 2005 Jul 5; [Epub ahead of print].

74. Viles-Gonzalez JF, Fuster V, Badimon JJ. Atherothrombosis: a widespread disease with unpredictable and life-threatening consequences. Eur Heart J 2004;25:1197.

75. Patrono C, Coller B, FitzGerald GA, et al. Platelet-active drugs: the relationships among dose, effectiveness, and side effects: the Seventh ACCP Conference on Antithrombotic and Thrombolytic Therapy. Chest 2004;126:234S.

76. Hansson L, Zanchetti A, Carruthers SG, et al. Effects of intensive blood-pressure lowering and low-dose aspirin in patients with hypertension: principal results of the Hypertension Optimal Treatment (HOT) randomised trial. HOT Study Group. Lancet 1998;351:1755.

77. de Gaetano G. Low-dose aspirin and vitamin E in people at cardiovascular risk: a randomised trial in general practice. Collaborative Group of the Primary Prevention Project. Lancet 2001;357:89.

78. Thrombosis prevention trial: randomised trial of low-intensity oral anticoagulation with warfarin and low-dose aspirin in the primary prevention of ischaemic heart disease in men at increased risk. The Medical Research Council's General Practice Research Framework. Lancet 1998;351:233.

79. Harrington RA, Becker RC, Ezekowitz M, et al. Antithrombotic therapy for coronary artery disease: the Seventh ACCP Conference on Antithrombotic and Thrombolytic Therapy. Chest 2004;126:513S.

80. Albers GW, Amarenco P, Easton JD, et al. Antithrombotic and thrombolytic therapy for ischemic stroke: the Seventh ACCP Conference on Antithrombotic and Thrombolytic Therapy. Chest 2004;126:483S.

81. Singer DE, Albers GW, Dalen JE, et al. Antithrombotic therapy in atrial fibrillation: the Seventh ACCP Conference on Antithrombotic and Thrombolytic Therapy. Chest 2004; 126:429S.

82. Hass WK, Easton JD, Adams HP Jr, et al. A randomized trial comparing ticlopidine hydrochloride with aspirin for the prevention of stroke in high-risk patients. Ticlopidine Aspirin Stroke Study Group. N Engl J Med 1989;321:501.

83. Scrutinio D, Cimminiello C, Marubini E, et al. Ticlopidine versus aspirin after myocardial infarction (STAMI) trial. J Am Coll Cardiol 2001;37:1259.

84. Bennett CL, Davidson CJ, Raisch DW, et al. Thrombotic thrombocytopenic purpura associated with ticlopidine in the setting of coronary artery stents and stroke prevention. Arch Intern Med 1999;159:2524.

85. Allford SL, Hunt BJ, Rose P, et al. Guidelines on the diagnosis and management of the thrombotic microangiopathic haemolytic anaemias. Br J Haematol 2003;120:556.

86. Bennett CL, Connors JM, Carwile JM, et al. Thrombotic thrombocytopenic purpura associated with clopidogrel. N Engl J Med 2000; 342:1773.

87. Diener HC, Cunha L, Forbes C, et al. European Stroke Prevention Study. 2. Dipyridamole and acetylsalicylic acid in the secondary prevention of stroke. J Neurol Sci 1996;143:1.

For annotated ***General References*** *and resources related to this chapter, visit www.hopkinsbayview.org/PAMreferences.*

supportive care. There is no evidence that prolonged bed rest is helpful. It is reasonable for patients to avoid strenuous activities until they feel strong enough to participate. Contact sports should be avoided if the spleen is tender or significantly enlarged. Because splenomegaly may persist for months, however, it seems unreasonable to avoid such sports until the spleen is no longer palpable. Although contacts occasionally develop infectious mononucleosis, there is no evidence that the disease is highly infectious, and patients should not be rigidly restricted from interpersonal contacts (3). Patients continue to shed the virus for up to 18 months after onset of the illness (10), but close personal exposure during this period only occasionally results in transmission of the disease.

Surgery may be needed for splenic rupture, although some cases have been handled with only transfusion support (9). Corticosteroids usually are reserved for patients with severe pharyngitis or impending airway obstruction (11) and other rare life-threatening complications of the illness. Controlled studies have not proved the clinical usefulness of steroids or steroids plus acyclovir (12,13).

Other Causes of the Mononucleosis Syndrome

Cytomegalovirus Infection

Although CMV infections may cause devastating clinical illness in the newborn (in utero) and in the immunocompromised host, infection in the noncompromised adult causes a clinical syndrome essentially indistinguishable from infectious mononucleosis, except that exudative pharyngitis is unusual in CMV infection. Unlike exposure to EBV, which has occurred in most adults in the United States by age 25 years, primary CMV infections usually occur at an older age, making CMV mononucleosis the most common cause of the mononucleosis syndrome in patients older than 30 years. Up to 50% of people older than 40 years have antibodies to CMV, although most do not have a history of infection. Diagnosis can be made by finding an increased titer of serum IgM antibody to CMV.

Toxoplasmosis

Acute toxoplasmosis usually is asymptomatic in people with normal immune responses but may cause a syndrome that resembles infectious mononucleosis. However, pharyngitis does not occur, and splenomegaly and lymphadenopathy usually are not as prominent. In addition, patients usually do not develop hepatitis or the hematologic manifestations of EBV infections. Diagnosis usually depends on serologic findings indicative of recent primary infection (presence of anti-IgM antibodies by an indirect fluorescent antibody test or demonstration of rising titers of IgG antibodies by indirect fluorescent antibody).

Other Infections

Conditions other than EBV, CMV, and toxoplasmosis can cause the mononucleosis syndrome (8). Some of these conditions include viral hepatitis (see Chapter 47), acute human immunodeficiency virus infection (see Chapter 39), and human herpesvirus 6 infection. Sometimes an etiologic agent cannot be identified even after extensive serologic testing. Table 58.3 suggests a stepwise plan for the serologic evaluation of patients with the mononucleosis syndrome. Seronegative patients need further evaluation only if symptoms persist for more than 1 to 2 weeks, if symptoms intensify, or if worrisome adenopathy persists (see The Undiagnosed Patient with Lymphadenopathy).

CHRONIC FATIGUE SYNDROME

Since 1985, there has been an epidemic in the United States, predominantly in young women, of an illness characterized universally by debilitating and persistent fatigue and by a host of other symptoms (sore throat, tender lymph nodes, myalgia, joint pain, headaches, malaise, impaired memory or concentration), many of them suggestive of EBV infection. Initially, people who complained of these symptoms were thought to have chronic mononucleosis because of the demonstration of antibodies to EBV in their blood. It soon became evident, however, that antibody titers to a number of viruses (retroviruses, CMV, human herpesvirus 6, Coxsackie B virus, measles) were elevated in the blood of these patients, casting doubt on the role of EBV as an etiologic agent of the illness. Extensive seroepidemiologic study by the Centers for Disease Control and Prevention has revealed no consistent association with any infectious agent (14). Therefore, the illness was renamed the *chronic fatigue syndrome,* and criteria were formulated for its diagnosis (15). It has become obvious that the prevalence of psychiatric illness (e.g., depression, somatoform disorder, anxiety) is increased considerably in patients with the syndrome, so it is tempting to believe that all the symptoms reflect underlying psychopathology. Studies have failed to identify differences between control subjects and cases in a host of tests of immunologic function (16). In addition to infectious agents, psychiatric illness, and immunologic dysfunction, other potential causes of chronic fatigue syndrome that have been considered include allergies, disturbances of the hypothalamic–pituitary–adrenal axis, neurally mediated hypotension, and nutritional deficiency. Affected patients likely will remain symptomatic indefinitely; they need the understanding and support of their families and their caregiver and specific attention to psychiatric problems when symptoms are manifest (see Chapters 21, 22, and 24). The likelihood of patients returning to totally normal function is low (17). Poor prognostic features include older age, more chronic illness, presence of comorbid psychiatric disease, and a persistent belief by

TABLE 58.3 Stepwise Serologic Testing in the Diagnosis of the Cause of Mononucleosis Syndrome

	Recommendation
1. Typical clinical features with a positive heterophil slide test essentially establishes a diagnosis of infectious mononucleosis, usually caused by EBV	No further testing is needed.
2. Typical clinical features with a negative heterophil slide test at the time the patient first presents to the caregiver	Draw acute serum samples (save frozen in two containers) for pertinent serologic testing for EBV (IgM VCA and IgG EBNA antibodies), toxoplasmosis, CMV, HIV. Repeat heterophil slide test during the third week of clinical illness. If positive, no further testing is necessary. If negative, repeat EBV serology (at least 2 wk after acute sample) and send with one of the acute serologic samples for EBV IgM anti-VCA testing and IgG EBNA antibodies. If the EBV serologies are diagnostic of recent infection, no further testing is necessary.
3. Typical clinical features, negative slide test at week 3 of clinical illness, and negative EBV serology (negative IgM anti-VCA and negative or positive IgG EBNA)	Draw convalescent sera for testing for toxoplasmosis and CMV and send with acute sera for appropriate serologic testing. Consider HIV infection in patients at risk.
4. Typical or atypical clinical features with negative serologies for all of the above. Consider other causes (e.g., leukemia, lymphoproliferative disease, granulomatous disease, collagen vascular disease).	Consider lymph node biopsy and other tests (e.g., bone marrow aspiration and biopsy).

CMV, cytomegalovirus; EBNA, Epstein-Barr nuclear antigen; EBV, Epstein-Barr virus; HIV, human immunodeficiency virus; IgG, immunoglobulin G; IgM, immunoglobulin M; VCA, viral capsid antigen.

the patient that the illness has a physical cause (18). Psychiatric intervention, especially cognitive therapy, may be helpful (19,20).

CHRONIC LYMPHOCYTIC LEUKEMIA

Clinical Features

Chronic lymphocytic leukemia (CLL) is the most common type of leukemia in the United States. It is primarily a disease of older men (21). Two thirds of patients are 60 years or older, and two to three times as many men are afflicted as are women. A mild tendency for the disease to segregate in families suggests that genetic factors play a role in its acquisition (22).

Many patients are asymptomatic when diagnosed (see below), but complaints of malaise and increased fatigability are common. Ultimately, most patients develop generalized lymphadenopathy and splenomegaly.

A persistent absolute lymphocytosis (>10,000/μL for ≥3 months) is the hallmark of the disease. Lymphocyte counts as high as 200,000 to 300,000/μL are seen occasionally. Other tests (bone marrow aspiration, lymph node biopsy) ordinarily are not necessary to establish the diagnosis.

As the disease progresses, hypogammaglobulinemia, anemia, granulocytopenia, and thrombocytopenia may develop. Autoimmune disorders (autoimmune hemolytic anemia, thrombocytopenia, pure red cell aplasia) develop in 10% to 15% of patients.

Treatment and Course

The survival of patients with CLL correlates best with the stage of their disease at diagnosis (23–25). For example, asymptomatic patients with only an absolute lymphocytosis (approximately 25% of the patients) have an essentially normal life expectancy. Patients with lymphadenopathy alone have a median survival of 6 to 8 years (approximately 50% of patients), and patients with significant anemia or thrombocytopenia (approximately 25% of patients) have a median survival of 2 to 3 years. A number of other features, such as age (older, better) and performance status, help predict prognosis. Bone marrow infiltration pattern is prognostically useful (nodular better than diffuse). An elevated β_2-microglobulin level carries a worse prognosis. There are genetic markers, such as chromosome abnormalities and the mutation status of the variable segment of the immunoglobulin heavy chain (mutated better than not), and surrogate markers for these factors, such as ZAP-70 (26).

The evidence on whether or not treatment influences survival is controversial, but treatment can be helpful in decreasing the severity of signs and symptoms in the later stages of the disease. Thus, stable asymptomatic patients with or without lymphadenopathy or splenomegaly may not require treatment. On the other hand, patients with marked constitutional symptoms (weight loss, severe malaise) or with symptomatic anemia or thrombocytopenia should be treated. For years, standard treatment of CLL included alkylating agents (e.g., chlorambucil) and prednisone. Later studies suggest that treatment of CLL with the purine analogue fludarabine results in a higher rate of remission (especially of complete remission) and in more prolonged remissions than does treatment with alkylating agents (although whether or not survival is improved is controversial) (27). Rituximab, a monoclonal antibody against the CD20 lymphocyte antigen, is another drug that may be useful for treatment of CLL. Aggressive treatment (including bone marrow and stem cell transplant) of early-stage disease in younger patients with CLL is under active investigation. Patients with autoimmune hemolysis and thrombocytopenia require more aggressive treatment with corticosteroids, and splenectomy sometimes is necessary in severely anemic or thrombocytopenic patients who are unresponsive to corticosteroids. A hematologist or medical oncologist should be consulted at the time of diagnosis of CLL and should be involved in the care of patients who require treatment.

Differential Diagnosis

A number of neoplastic conditions other than CLL may be associated with a chronic lymphocytosis, such as macroglobulinemia, B- and T-cell lymphomas, hairy cell leukemia, prolymphocytic leukemia, and adult T-cell leukemia. The morphology of the cells, evaluation of peripheral lymphocyte surface markers by flow cytometry, or other manifestations of the disease usually lead to the correct diagnosis. These conditions should be managed in close consultation with an oncologist.

A syndrome has been recognized, most often in older people, characterized by clonal proliferation of large granular T lymphocytes (up to 10,000/μL) and, usually, chronic neutropenia (28). Anemia (rarely, red cell aplasia) and thrombocytopenia are uncommon. Lymphocytic infiltration of the bone marrow and spleen (with splenomegaly) is characteristic; lymph node involvement is rare. Some patients have coexistent seropositive rheumatoid arthritis. Most patients, with or without arthritis, have serologic abnormalities (e.g., in addition to increased titers of rheumatoid factor, antinuclear antibodies, polyclonal hypergammaglobulinemia, and circulating immune complexes). The major morbidity from the disease is caused by recurrent bacterial infections; otherwise, most patients require no treatment, and their mortality rate is low.

THE UNDIAGNOSED PATIENT WITH LYMPHADENOPATHY: WHEN TO RECOMMEND LYMPH NODE BIOPSY

Lymphadenopathy is a common physical finding that is associated with multiple disease processes (29). The decision about when to biopsy an enlarged lymph node is difficult (30). The problem arises most often in younger patients. Older patients with localized lymphadenopathy unexplained by infection or inflammation should be assumed to have cancer until proven otherwise; therefore, the biopsy decision in older patients usually is easy. However, lymphadenopathy in children and young adults usually is caused by inflammation, and biopsy usually is not diagnostic. In such circumstances, the clinician often is concerned about the possible harm from a delayed diagnosis of a malignancy (Hodgkin disease or non-Hodgkin lymphoma most commonly) or a granulomatous condition (e.g., tuberculosis, sarcoidosis) for which specific treatment is indicated. However, harm can result from unnecessary biopsy. The procedure is associated with both psychologic and physical discomfort to the patient, and, most importantly, interpretation of the biopsy of a reactive node can be uncertain. The histology of reactive nodes, especially those encountered in the mononucleosis syndrome, can be difficult to interpret. Reed–Sternberg cells (ordinarily pathognomonic of Hodgkin disease) can be seen in the nodes of patients with infectious mononucleosis, and reactive nodes sometimes look like and are interpreted as diagnostic of Hodgkin disease or of non-Hodgkin lymphoma. Because of these problems, biopsy of a lymph node should be avoided in a patient with the mononucleosis syndrome if possible.

If a specific diagnosis cannot be made based on the clinical features and serologic studies, few reliable criteria are available to assist with the decision as to whether a biopsy is indicated. However, one helpful retrospective study reported that in the age range from 9 to 25 years, three variables were important in determining whether a lymph node biopsy might be diagnostic of an illness requiring specific treatment (31): the size of the node to be tested by biopsy, the presence or absence of ear/nose/throat

TABLE 58.4 When to Recommend Lymph Node Biopsy in the Teenager and Young Adult

Features against early biopsy
- Mononucleosis syndrome, especially when proven serologically.
- Ear/nose/throat symptoms (earache, sore throat, coryza, tonsillar or dental infection)
- Lymph nodes <2 cm in diameter.
- Normal chest radiograph, especially when associated with one of the above

Features for early biopsy
- Systemic illness with atypical features of the mononucleosis syndrome and without serologic proof of a cause of the mononucleosis syndrome (Table 58.3).
- Lymph nodes >2 cm in diameter and an abnormal chest radiograph, absence of ear/nose/throat symptoms, or no proof of a typical mononucleosis syndrome
- Localized supraclavicular lymphadenopathy may be seen in the mononucleosis syndrome but in its absence is suggestive of mediastinal (right supraclavicular) or abdominal (left supraclavicular) granulomatous or neoplastic disease

symptoms, and the presence or absence of an abnormality on chest radiograph. Nodes >2 cm in diameter were more likely to contain important histologic information than were smaller nodes. An abnormal chest radiograph (adenopathy, infiltrate) in a patient with peripheral adenopathy correlated with useful biopsy information. Patients with cervical lymphadenopathy but without any ear/nose/throat symptoms were more likely to have a diagnostic lymph node biopsy. Unfortunately, no validated method differentiates patients with adenopathy whose biopsy would lead to definitive diagnosis and treatment from those whose biopsies would not be clinically useful, and to date no specific clinical factors reliably help practitioners identify those patients with adenopathy who should undergo biopsy. Table 58.4 summarizes some of the features that can be used, especially in the young patient, to help determine the advisability and timing of a lymph node biopsy.

SPECIFIC REFERENCES*

1. Evans AS, Niederman JC, McCollum RW. Seroepidemiologic studies of infectious mononucleosis with EB virus. N Engl J Med 1968;279:1121.
2. Strauss SE, Cohen JI, Tosato G, et al. Epstein-Barr virus infections: biology, pathogenesis, and management. Ann Intern Med 1993;118:45.
3. Sawyer RN, Evans AS, Niederman JC, et al. Prospective studies of a group of Yale University freshmen. I. Occurrence of infectious mononucleosis. J Infect Dis 1971;123:263.
4. Horwitz CA, Henle W, Henle G, et al. Infectious mononucleosis in patients aged 40 to 72 years: report of 27 cases, including 3 without heterophil-antibody responses. Medicine (Baltimore) 1983;62:256.
5. Auwaerter PG. Infectious mononucleosis in middle age. JAMA 1999;281:454.
6. Evans AS, Niederman JC, Cenabre LC, et al. A prospective evaluation of heterophile and Epstein-Barr versus specific IgM antibody tests in clinical and subclinical infectious mononucleosis: specificity and sensitivity of the tests and persistence of antibody. J Infect Dis 1975;132:546.
7. Linderholm M, Borman J, Juto P, et al. A comparative evaluation of nine kits for rapid diagnosis of infectious mononucleosis and Epstein-Barr virus-specific serology. J Clin Microbiol 1994;32:259.
8. Evans AS. Infectious mononucleosis and related syndromes. Am J Med Sci 1978;276:325.
9. Asgari MM, Begos DG. Spontaneous splenic rupture in infectious mononucleosis: a review. Yale J Biol Med 1997;70:175.
10. Miller G, Niederman JC, Andrews LL. Prolonged oropharyngeal excretion of Epstein-Barr virus after infectious mononucleosis. N Engl J Med 1973;288:229.
11. McGowan JE Jr.Chesney PJ, Grossley KB, et al. Guidelines for the use of systemic glucocorticoids in the management of selected infections. Working Group on Steroid Use, Antimicrobial Agents Committee, Infectious Disease Society of America. J Infect Dis 1992;165:1.
12. Tynell E, Aurelius E, Brandell A, et al. Acyclovir and prednisolone treatment of acute infectious mononucleosis: a multicenter, double-blind, placebo-controlled study. J Infect Dis 1996; 174:324.
13. Torre D, Tambini R. Acyclovir for treatment of infectious mononucleosis: a meta-analysis. Scand J Infect Dis 1999;31:543.
14. Mawle AC, Nisenbaum R, Dobbins JG, et al. Seroepidemiology of chronic fatigue syndrome: a case control study. Clin Infect Dis 1995; 21:1386.
15. Fukuda K, Straus SE, Hickie I. The chronic fatigue syndrome: a comprehensive approach to its definition and study. Ann Intern Med 1994;121:953.
16. Mawle AC, Nisenbaum R, Dobbins JG, et al. Immune responses associated with chronic fatigue syndrome: a case control study. J Infect Dis 1997;175:136.
17. Bombardier CH, Buchwald D. Outcome and prognosis of patients with chronic fatigue vs chronic fatigue syndrome. Arch Intern Med 1995;155:2105.
18. Joyce J, Hotopf M, Wessely S. The prognosis of chronic fatigue and chronic fatigue syndrome: a systematic review. Q J Med 1997;90:223.
19. Deale A, Chalder T, Marks I, et al. Cognitive behavior therapy for chronic fatigue syndrome: a randomized controlled trial. Am J Psych 1997; 154:408.
20. Sharpe M, Hawkins K, Simkin S, et al. Cognitive behaviour therapy for the chronic fatigue syndrome: a randomized controlled trial. BMJ 1996;312:22.
21. Skinnider LF, Tan L, Schmidt J, et al. Chronic lymphocytic leukemia. A review of 745 cases and assessment of clinical staging. Cancer (Philadelphia) 1982;50:2951.
22. Conley CL, Misiti J, Laster AJ. Genetic factors predisposing to chronic lymphocytic leukemia. Medicine (Baltimore) 1980;59:323.
23. Kokhaei P, Palma M, Mellstedt H, et al. Biology and treatment of chronic lymphocytic leukemia. Ann Oncol 2005;16 Suppl 2:II113.
24. Rai KR, Han T. Prognostic factors and clinical staging in chronic lymphocytic leukemia. Hematol Oncol Clin North Am 1990;4:447.
25. Rozman C, Montserrat E. Chronic lymphocytic leukemia. N Engl J Med 1995;333:1052.
26. Crespo M, Bosch F, Villamor N, et al. ZAP-70 expression as a surrogate for immunoglobulin-variable-region mutations in chronic lymphocytic leukemia. N Engl J Med 2003;348:1764.
27. Rai KR, Peterson BL, Appelbaum FR, et al. Fludarabine compared with chlorambucil as primary therapy for chronic lymphocytic leukemia. N Engl J Med 2000;343:1750.
28. Loughran TP, Starkebaum G. Large granular lymphocyte leukemia. Report of 38 cases and review of the literature. Medicine (Baltimore) 1987;66:397.
29. Libman H. Generalized lymphadenopathy. J Gen Intern Med 1987;2:48.
30. Greenfield S, Jordan MC. The clinical investigation of lymphadenopathy in primary care practice. JAMA 1978;240:1388.
31. Slap GB, Brooks SJ, Schwartz JS. When to perform biopsies of enlarged peripheral lymph nodes in young patients. JAMA 1984;252:1321.

*Bold numerals denote published controlled clinical trials, meta-analyses, or consensus-based recommendations.

For annotated **General References** *and resources related to this chapter, visit www.hopkinsbayview.org/PAMreferences.*

SECTION 8

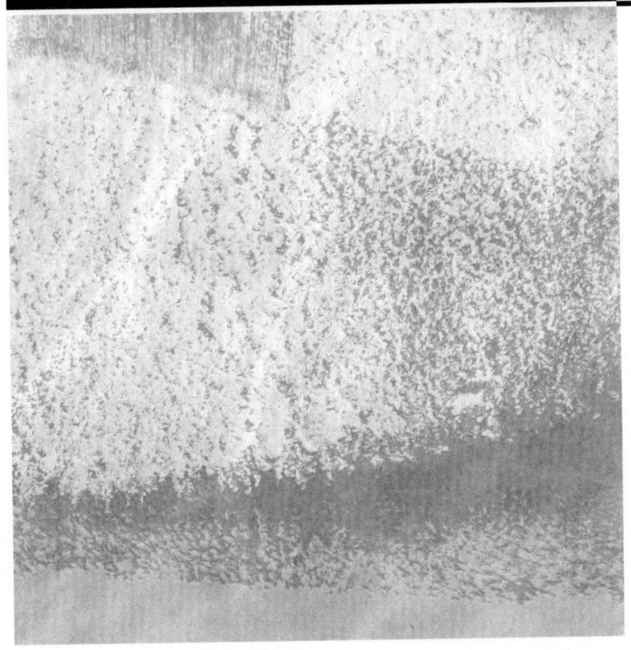

Pulmonary Problems

Chapter 59

Common Pulmonary Problems: Cough, Hemoptysis, Dyspnea, Chest Pain, and Abnormal Chest X-Ray*

Irina Petrache and Steve N. Georas

*Philip L. Smith, E. James Britt, and Peter B. Terry contributed to this chapter in previous editions.

Patients who develop acute respiratory problems usually present with symptoms that result in the rapid diagnosis and treatment of the underlying disorder. On the other hand, chronic diseases of the lung that cause slowly progressive symptoms may go undetected unless incidentally discovered as part of a general medical evaluation. This chapter discusses common pulmonary problems with which the general practitioner is often confronted: cough, hemoptysis, dyspnea, noncardiac chest pain, and the abnormal chest x-ray.

COUGH

Cough is an important defense mechanism that clears the airways of both secretions and inhaled particles (1). Although it often is associated with other respiratory symptoms, cough may be the symptom that prompts a patient to seek medical advice, especially if the cough is associated with complications (e.g., fear of serious disease, exhaustion, insomnia, lifestyle change, pain, hoarseness, urinary incontinence). A cough is composed of three phases: a deep inspiration, closure of the glottis accompanied by a rapid increase in intrathoracic pressure, and a final opening of the glottis with an explosive release of pressure.

Mucosal neural receptors that initiate a *cough reflex* are located throughout the nasopharynx, ears, larynx, trachea, and bronchi down to the level of the terminal bronchioles. They are rapidly adapting receptors with thin myelinated nerve fibers and show varied sensitivities to different stimuli. Stimulation of cough receptors in the nasopharynx also may cause sneezing. In contrast, stimulation of laryngeal receptors may initiate cardiovascular, bronchoconstrictor, and laryngoconstrictor reflexes, whereas stimulation of tracheal and bronchial receptors may also cause bronchospasm and airway mucus secretion. After activation of the receptors, impulses are conducted along afferent pathways in the ninth and tenth cranial nerves to the cough center located diffusely in the medulla. The reflex is completed through efferent pathways that cause forceful contraction of the diaphragm and other expiratory muscles. Although many different stimuli activate these receptors, all initiate cough by some form of mechanical or chemical irritation. The expression of some irritant receptors appears to be increased in the airways of people with chronic cough. Additional factors, such as acute inflammation of the airways,

TABLE 59.1 Causes of Cough

Causes	Examples
Common	
Acute	
Inflammation	Tracheitis, bronchitis, pneumonia
Irritation	Environmental pollutants
Bronchospasm	Infection
Chronic	
Inflammation	Bronchitis, pollution, cigarettes, bronchiectasis, aspirated foreign body, chronic pneumonia (tuberculosis and nontuberculous mycobacterial infection, *Pneumocystis carinii* pneumonia in acquired immunodeficiency syndrome)
Irritation	Cigarettes, cancer, postnasal drip
Bronchospasm	Asthma, heart failure
Less common	
Drug induced	Angiotensin-converting enzyme inhibitor, β-blockers (oral or ophthalmic), inhaled medication
Irritation	Esophageal reflux, chronic aspiration, auditory canal stimulation (cerumen, hair), aortic aneurysm
Inflammation	Sarcoidosis, alveolitis, bronchiolitis obliterans organizing pneumonia (BOOP)

may disrupt the bronchial mucosa, increase its permeability, and expose the receptors. The accompanying increases in respiratory secretions will lead to cough. Environmental pollutants, such as cigarette smoke, can directly stimulate the receptors without necessarily provoking an inflammatory reaction. Finally, although stimulation of irritant receptors may cause reflex bronchoconstriction, the bronchospasm itself, through reflex pathways, induces cough.

Acute Cough Syndromes

Table 59.1 lists the causes of cough. Generally, acute coughs are self-limited (<3 weeks) and are caused by viral *upper respiratory tract infections* (2). In contrast, cough that is triggered by mild bronchospasm may persist for weeks to months after a viral upper respiratory tract infection. Usually, viral infections, atypical pneumonias, and *Pneumocystis carinii* pneumonia are associated with nonproductive coughs, and bacterial infections are associated with significant sputum production. Younger patients tend to have a more productive cough associated with pneumonia, whereas older individuals, especially those with chronic obstructive pulmonary disease (COPD), may retain secretions because of impaired ability to clear them. A productive cough that follows a typical viral syndrome may signal the development of a superimposed bacterial bronchitis or pneumonia. High concentrations of air pollutants, such as insoluble gases (e.g., ozone, SO_3, NO_2), which are not irritating to the upper airway, can cause either a dry or a productive cough secondary to chemical irritation.

Chronic Cough Syndromes

A persistent cough (generally lasting >3 weeks) often is more bothersome than the acute cough syndrome. The most common cause of chronic coughing is *cigarette smoking* (2). The so-called *smokers' cough,* a manifestation of *chronic bronchitis,* is generally described as hacking, worse in the morning, and productive or dry, as sputum often is ignored by cigarette smokers. The number of cigarettes smoked bears little relationship to the development of cough. Perhaps because they inhale more deeply, smokers of marijuana may complain of a persistent cough after smoking only one to two cigarettes daily. Patients with central *bronchogenic and mediastinal tumors* often present with cough, whereas patients with metastatic tumors or peripheral lung cancers that arise outside the airways or beyond irritant receptors seldom do.

In nonsmokers, three entities account for most cases of chronic cough: postnasal drip, asthma, and gastroesophageal reflux disease (GERD). The most common cause of chronic cough is *postnasal drip,* resulting from chronic sinusitis or allergic rhinitis (1,2). It is important to recognize that *bronchospasm* in both smokers and nonsmokers can be associated with a chronic dry cough. Cough may be the only manifestation of mild *asthma* (cough variant asthma) and need not be associated with dyspnea, wheezing, or changes in baseline pulmonary function (3). *GERD* may present with only minimal gastrointestinal symptoms, significant nagging cough, and, occasionally, hoarseness (see Chapter 42). A nocturnal cough that is precipitated or increased by lying flat makes this diagnosis more likely.

A dry hacking cough associated with dyspnea is common in patients in *heart failure* (see Chapter 66). Cough due to congestive heart failure also is often initiated by lying down. Similarly, cough may precede the complaint of dyspnea in patients with pulmonary emboli or bronchiolitis obliterans organizing pneumonia (a patchy pneumonia, probably immunologic, that often responds to treatment with corticosteroids). *Bronchiectasis and chronic pulmonary infections,* such as tuberculosis or nontuberculous mycobacterial pneumonia in immunocompetent patients, and *P. carinii* pneumonia in patients with acquired immunodeficiency syndrome (AIDS) commonly cause coughing. A chronic nonproductive cough occurs in up to 10% of patients taking an *angiotensin-converting enzyme inhibitor* and remits shortly (within 4 weeks) after the drug is discontinued. Because angiotensin-converting enzyme inhibitors are the treatment of choice for many conditions (e.g., congestive heart failure), it may be worth trying to "treat through" the cough in some patients.

Pharmacologic approaches can be used to try to suppress cough in patients who require angiotensin-converting enzyme inhibitors, including cromolyn sodium (e.g., via metered-dose inhalers, two puffs four times per day), baclofen (5 mg three times per day for 1 week, 10 mg three times per day for 3 weeks), low-dose theophylline, or sulindac. However, these regimens have not been evaluated in controlled studies or with large numbers of patients (4). Because the incidence of cough is much lower with angiotensin II receptor antagonists, a trial of these agents also may be reasonable.

There are numerous less common causes of chronic cough. For example, paroxysmal coughing often followed by an inspiratory whoop may indicate infection with *Bordetella pertussis*. A chronic cough may be caused by a process that stimulates the neural receptors in the pleura and pericardium. Even *impacted cerumen* in the external auditory canal can elicit a chronic cough. If the history and physical examination are unrevealing, it often is tempting to attribute chronic cough to a psychogenic cause; however, this is a rare cause of coughing, most often reported in children (1).

Evaluation

The acute and chronic cough syndromes are evaluated in similar ways. Usually, a history and physical examination yield a presumptive diagnosis. Information should be obtained about the development, duration, character, and precipitants of the cough; environmental or occupational exposure; smoking history; and any history of asthma or COPD. A history of constant swallowing or of throat clearing is associated with postnasal drip, even though the patient may deny many other symptoms associated with rhinitis or sinusitis.

Although the physical examination seldom provides a specific diagnosis, it may provide important clues. Careful examination of the ears, nose, throat, and lungs may yield relevant clues to a diagnosis. Cobblestoning in the posterior oropharynx represents lymphoid hyperplasia and is commonly seen in patients with chronic sinusitis. Examination of the chest may reveal rhonchi caused by the loose secretions that result from acute or chronic infection. A localized wheeze suggests a bronchogenic tumor, whereas wheezing at end expiration suggests active bronchospasm. Finally, the physical examination allows observation of the quality and severity of the cough. A harsh cough associated with loose secretions is characteristic of tracheobronchitis resulting from viral upper respiratory tract infection. When little or no coughing occurs in the course of the visit, the patient should be asked to cough to determine whether the cough is productive or is associated with wheezing. This procedure is useful because some patients refuse to admit to expectoration of sputum and often unconsciously swallow their secretions.

If a diagnosis is not obvious after a history and physical examination, a chest x-ray is indicated. It may reveal a tumor, pneumonia, or another chronic inflammatory process involving the lung parenchyma. The x-ray also may demonstrate atelectasis associated with a bronchogenic tumor, aspirated foreign body, or bilateral hilar adenopathy suggesting sarcoidosis. In patients with a normal x-ray, spirometry can be used to look for obstructive airway disease. However, a normal spirogram does not necessarily exclude the diagnosis (see Chapter 60). When the chest x-ray is normal, bronchoscopy seldom provides additional useful information (2). Although a proximal bronchogenic tumor can be hidden on a chest x-ray by the mediastinal shadows, patients with these tumors often have associated hemoptysis. If the history, physical examination, chest x-ray, and spirogram are unrevealing and if the patient's cough persists after stopping new medicines, including angiotensin-converting enzyme inhibitors and β-blockers (including eye drops), referral to a subspecialist may be appropriate. Additional tests might include methacholine challenge (asthma), high-resolution chest computed tomography (CT) (bronchiectasis, interstitial lung disease), sinus x-ray or CT (chronic sinusitis), 24-hour pH probe (GERD), and, rarely, bronchoscopy (endobronchial tumor or aspirated foreign body) or cardiac evaluation (heart failure). Use of an algorithm-based approach that incorporates the clinical assessment of disease probability in evaluating patients with chronic cough has been validated, identifying a cause for cough in 93% of patients (2). Figure 59.1 shows such an algorithm, which was developed by a consensus panel.

Therapy

Specific therapy for the various acute inflammatory and irritating processes likely to cause coughing is discussed in detail in individual chapters dealing with these topics.

In general, viral tracheobronchitis requires only symptomatic therapy because coughing usually subsides spontaneously in 2 to 4 weeks. Patients with persistent coughing and a history or physical examination compatible with bronchospasm may benefit from bronchodilators. Treatment should begin with an inhaled β_2-sympathomimetic agonist. A detailed therapeutic approach to the pharmacologic treatment of bronchospasm is presented in Chapter 60.

Cessation of cigarette smoking and avoidance of a polluted environment may be the most important aspects of the therapy for both acute and chronic cough. It often is difficult to convey to a smoker that smoking as few as one or two cigarettes per day causes airway irritation and inflammation. Ipratropium bromide may improve cough and decrease sputum production in patients with chronic bronchitis (see Chapter 60) (1).

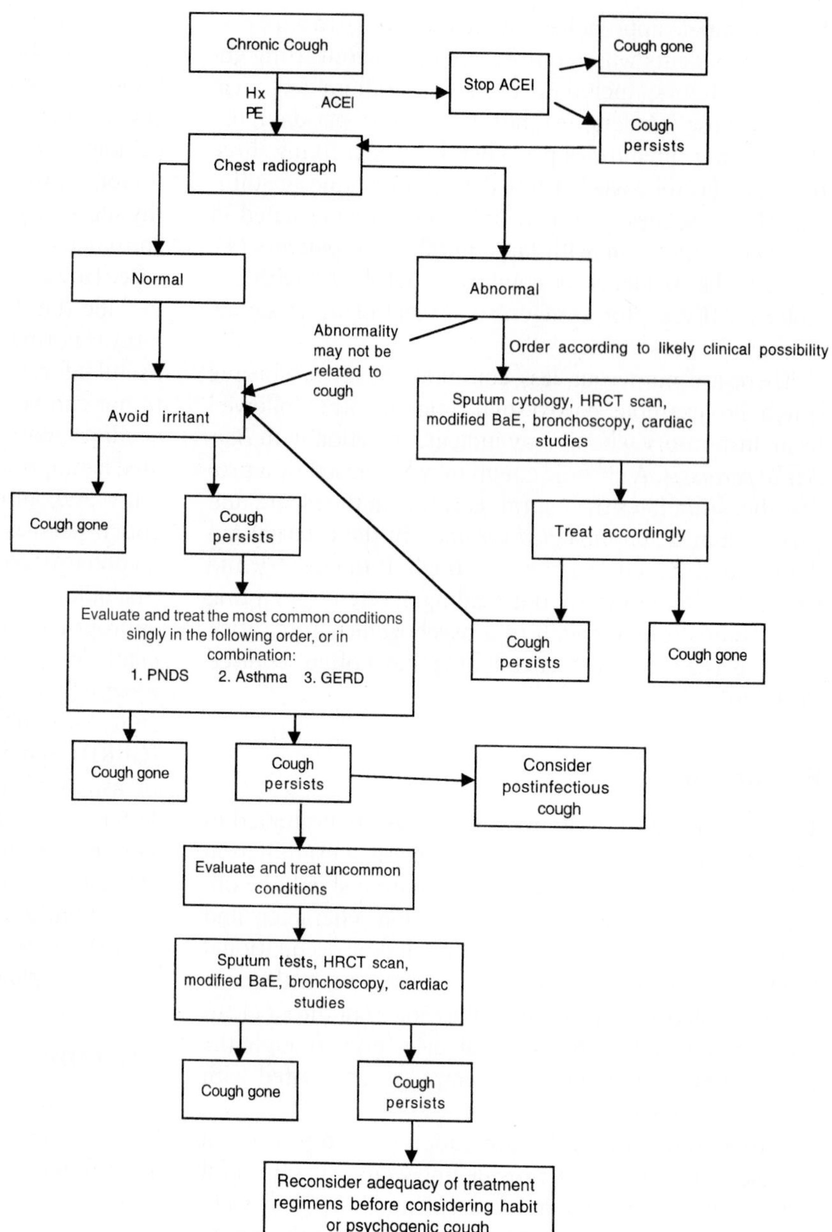

FIGURE 59.1. Guidelines for evaluating chronic cough in immunocompetent adults. ACEI, angiotensin-converting enzyme inhibitor; BaE, barium esophagography; GERD, gastroesophageal reflux disease; HRCT, high-resolution computed tomography; Hx, history; PE, physical examination; PNDS, postnasal drip syndrome. (From Irwin RS, Boulet LP, Cloutier MM, et al. Managing cough as a defense mechanism and as a symptom. A consensus panel report of the American College of Chest Physicians. Chest 1998;114: 133S, with permission.)

The treatment of postnasal drip and GERD is discussed in Chapters 33 and 42, respectively. In most patients, cough improves within 1 week of initiation of therapy for postnasal drip, but GERD may not resolve for months, even with optimal therapy (2). Removal of impacted cerumen in the auditory canal provides immediate relief. Approximately one fourth of patients with chronic cough referred for subspecialty evaluation had more than one cause (2). Thus, if specific therapy does not eliminate the cause, additional testing and treatment should be pursued.

After specific therapy has been initiated, the use of *antitussives* should be considered. Despite the enormous demands for antitussives, these preparations are absolutely necessary in only a few situations. Moreover, the expectoration of sputum is a major goal of therapy for chronic obstructive airway disease. Therefore, when antitussives are needed in patients with productive coughs, it usually is better to attempt cough reduction (not total suppression), primarily to allow patients to sleep and to avoid posttussive syncope, stress incontinence, or straining of the chest wall or abdominal muscles. In the United States, several hundred cough and decongestant preparations, usually sold as combination products, are available. Many of these preparations combine so-called expectorants with antitussives and should be avoided because, insofar as they

TABLE 59.2 Nonnarcotic Antitussives

Drug	Brand Name	Usual Dose	Site of Action	Comment
Dextromethorphan	Many preparations	15–30 mg four times per day	Central	Considered most effective central agent
Benzonatate	Tessalon	100–200 mg four times per day	Peripheral	Considered most effective peripheral agent

have an effect, they work at cross purposes. In prospective double-blinded studies of patients with cough associated with the common cold, the combination of dexbrompheniramine, an antihistamine (contained, for example, in Cheracol and Drixoral), and pseudoephedrine, a vasoconstrictor (6 mg/120 mg twice per day, orally for 1 week), reduced symptoms compared with placebo (5), as did naproxen (500 mg loading dose, then 200–500 mg three times per day orally for 5 days) (6). Another randomized study of 97 patients with cough secondary to upper respiratory tract infections found no difference between guaifenesin alone versus guaifenesin plus codeine or guaifenesin plus dextromethorphan in reducing coughing (7).

Antitussives act on the cough reflex by either anesthetizing the peripheral irritant receptors or increasing the threshold of the cough center. The two most effective nonnarcotic antitussives are *dextromethorphan* and *benzonatate,* although the latter has not been rigorously studied in a placebo-controlled randomized trial (Table 59.2). Dextromethorphan is chemically derived from the opiates; however, it is classified as nonnarcotic because at prescribed dosages it has no sedative or analgesic effects and therefore has little potential for abuse. It is available over the counter in a variety of preparations (e.g., Dimetane DX). Dextromethorphan suppresses cough centrally. Occasionally, the drug causes nausea, dizziness, or vertigo, and overdosage of >200 mg may lead to central nervous system (CNS) depression. Benzonatate is a peripherally acting anesthetic similar to tetracaine. Rarely, it causes headaches, dizziness, and nausea or gastrointestinal upset. The drug should not be chewed or sucked because this action will result in an unpleasant taste and prolonged oral pharyngeal anesthesia. Overdosage has been associated with CNS stimulation and tremors, which may lead to seizures followed by profound CNS depression. It is reasonable to treat patients initially with dextromethorphan and, if intolerable cough persists, to substitute benzonatate.

If nonnarcotic antitussives are ineffective, *codeine* can be tried. Many clinicians prescribe codeine preferentially to patients with persistent cough because it is a more potent cough suppressant than the nonnarcotic agents. Codeine is effective in dosages of 15 to 30 mg administered every 3 to 6 hours. The common side effects—nausea, vomiting, constipation, dry mouth, and sedation—usually are not experienced at these lower dosages.

HEMOPTYSIS

Hemoptysis is defined as the expectoration of blood from below the vocal cords. It can range from flecks of blood in sputum to the coughing of large amounts (>1 L) of blood. Distinguishing between hemoptysis and hematemesis occasionally is difficult. Blood from the lungs usually is bright red and frothy, has an alkaline pH, and usually is mixed with sputum containing macrophages and white blood cells. Often, patients with hemoptysis complain of a tickling or irritation in the chest. On the other hand, hematemesis is characterized by blood that is darker brown, has an acid pH, and is mixed with food particles. Sometimes blood from a lesion in the sinuses or in the upper airway is aspirated and later expectorated, giving the appearance that bleeding occurred in the lower respiratory tract. A careful history and physical examination must be performed to avoid inappropriate evaluation or treatment. The patient should be instructed to collect and save the bloody sputum so that the hemoptysis can be quantified. Nevertheless, a history of hemoptysis should not be ignored if a patient cannot produce a specimen on command, because the symptoms can be intermittent. Table 59.3 summarizes the various pulmonary causes of hemoptysis.

In the typical ambulatory practice, *chronic bronchitis* is by far the most common cause of blood streaking of the sputum, followed less commonly by *lung cancer* (8,9). The likelihood of a particular diagnosis depends on the patient population (e.g., smokers vs. nonsmokers) (8). *Bronchiectasis* is less common today in the industrial world because of mass screening for tuberculosis, childhood vaccinations for measles and whooping cough, and antibiotic treatment of serious respiratory infections. *Active cavitary tuberculosis* is also a less common cause of hemoptysis than it once was, but residual upper lobe bronchiectasis, the result of old tuberculosis infection, is still seen. *Bronchogenic carcinoma* (see Chapter 61) presents with hemoptysis at two stages. Blood-streaked sputum may be a brief manifestation of a small irritative mucosal lesion. This symptom may resolve, only to be replaced by major hemoptysis from a large endobronchial tumor that is friable or necrotic or is eroding central vessels. Usually blood from a *necrotizing pneumonia* or a *lung abscess* is mixed with pus, and the sputum appears red-brown or red-green. Hemoptysis from *pulmonary emboli,* a manifestation of pulmonary

TABLE 59.3 Pulmonary Causes of Hemoptysis

Causes	Examples
Common	
Inflammation	Bronchitis, bronchiectasis (including cystic fibrosis), tuberculosis, pneumonia, lung abscess
Neoplasm	Lung cancer
Less common	
Inflammation	Goodpasture syndrome, idiopathic pulmonary hemosiderosis, Wegener granulomatosis, systemic lupus erythematosus, systemic necrotizing vasculitis
Infection	Parasitic, pre-existing cavitary disease with mycetoma (old tuberculosis or fibrocystic sarcoidosis), broncholithiasis
Neoplasm	Bronchial carcinoid, endobronchial metastasis
Vascular disease	Pulmonary embolus with infarction, arteriovenous malformation, aortic aneurysm, mitral stenosis, tricuspid endocarditis with septic pulmonary emboli, pulmonary hypertension
Iatrogenic cause	Bronchoscopy, transthoracic lung biopsy, transtracheal oxygen catheter, transtracheal suctioning, pulmonary artery catheterization, airway stenting
Drugs	Anticoagulation, aspirin, thrombolytics, crack cocaine, solvents, penicillamine
Chest trauma	
Foreign body	

infarction, is rare because of the lung's dual blood supply, unless patients have significant heart or lung disease. Even with the advent of fiberoptic bronchoscopy, the cause of hemoptysis remains undiagnosed 8% to 15% of the time (10,11). The 5-year survival rate for patients with cryptogenic hemoptysis (hemoptysis with normal chest x-ray and a negative bronchoscopy) is very good (85%–95%) (10).

Table 59.3 also lists less common causes of hemoptysis, but this ranking reflects to some extent the location of a practice. For example, mycetomas and parasitic infections that cause hemoptysis are much more common in areas of the country where those problems are endemic. Hemoptysis is common in *bronchial carcinoids* by virtue of their endobronchial location and marked vascularity. Hemoptysis caused by *pulmonary metastasis* from a solid tumor is rare. Its presence raises the possibility of endobronchial metastases, which are most common in patients with breast, colon, and kidney cancer and those with malignant melanoma. Patients with *mitral stenosis* and pulmonary vascular congestion are prone to hemoptysis with any source of lung irritation. Although certainly less common today, this valvular abnormality often is silent and the history of rheumatic fever forgotten. Patients taking the *anticoagulants* warfarin or heparin may develop hemoptysis, especially if there is an associated inflammation of the airways. Occasionally, *blunt chest trauma* produces hemoptysis in an otherwise healthy individual. Very rarely, hemoptysis is due to intrathoracic endometriosis, in which case it occurs at the time of menstruation.

Evaluation

The diagnostic evaluation of hemoptysis is aimed at determining the cause, localizing the site, and quantifying the amount of bleeding. The history and physical examination are directed at uncovering clues to the causes outlined in Table 59.3. An attempt should be made to quantitate the amount of hemoptysis by history and by collection of expectorated blood. Massive hemoptysis, generally defined as more than a few hundred milliliters of blood during a 24-hour period, is a medical emergency, and survival of the patient depends on rapid diagnosis and treatment (12). The principal risk of massive hemoptysis is asphyxiation, not exsanguination, with the rate of bleeding as the most important prognostic factor. Patients with underlying lung disease are less able to tolerate spillage of blood into other portions of the lung before acute respiratory failure develops.

During the physical examination, extrathoracic sources of bleeding from the nasal passages, sinuses, and pharynx should be sought. Physical findings may be helpful. Digital clubbing may be seen in non–small cell lung cancer, lung abscess, or bronchiectasis. Scattered ecchymoses, multiple petechiae, or gastrointestinal bleeding suggests a defect in hemostasis, and telangiectasia of the skin, lips, or buccal mucosa is consistent with hereditary hemorrhagic telangiectasia (or Osler–Weber–Rendu syndrome). Ulceration and crusting of the nasal septum may represent upper airway involvement of Wegener granulomatosis. The significance of unilateral wheezing or crackles must be interpreted with caution because these sounds may be produced by aspirated blood or secretions rather than by endobronchial tumor.

A chest x-ray is essential because acute inflammatory diseases, such as active tuberculosis, pneumonia, and lung abscess, will produce obvious radiographic abnormalities. Typically, lung cancers associated with hemoptysis are centrally located squamous cell carcinomas, and approximately half are cavitary. However, localization of the bleeding source often is precluded by bilateral aspiration of blood or by the presence of bilateral pulmonary disease. Patients with bronchitis often have normal chest x-rays, and the findings on plain film of focal bronchiectasis may be nonspecific. If the bronchiectasis is a result of old tuberculosis, however, apical scarring may suggest the diagnosis; otherwise, there may be increased or crowded lung markings, thickened dilated bronchi, multiple cystic cavities (1–3 mm in diameter), or infiltrates because of recurrent infection. The chest CT is more sensitive than the chest x-ray in detecting bronchiectasis and generally is sufficient to make the diagnosis (13). Differentiating bronchitis from bronchiectasis by history and chest x-ray sometimes is difficult. This distinction may not be critical, however, because the acute medical management of bronchitis and bronchiectasis in patients with hemoptysis is the same.

When the chest x-ray is normal or nonlocalizing, endobronchial malignancy is the principal diagnosis to exclude, although bronchitis is the most likely diagnosis. Individuals younger than 40 years, including smokers, with hemoptysis that has lasted <1 week are unlikely to have cancer. In such patients, observation is a reasonable initial approach (14).

Persistent or recurrent hemoptysis mandates a thorough evaluation that includes bronchoscopy. Patients with normal chest x-rays who are at increased risk for lung cancer (age >40 years, >20 pack per year cigarette smoker) should undergo bronchoscopy. Still, lung cancer will be discovered at bronchoscopy in only approximately 5% of these patients (see Chapter 61) (14,15). Sputum cytology may provide the diagnosis in as many as half of these patients, but in general bronchoscopy still is required to locate the site of malignancy (lung vs. upper aerodigestive tract) and to plan for therapy. In the evaluation of recurrent or persistent hemoptysis, most clinicians view bronchoscopy and chest CT as complementary, with CT being helpful in guiding the bronchoscopy and/or angiography to the regions of highest yield (13,16).

Therapy

Blood irritates the tracheobronchial tree and triggers constant coughing, which by itself is traumatic. Mild cough suppression may help, but the patient must be able to expectorate blood as it accumulates. Specific treatment depends on the underlying cause of hemoptysis. Chronic bronchitis, with intercurrent hemoptysis, usually is treated on an ambulatory basis with antimicrobial drugs (see Chapter 60) for 10 to 14 days. In such circumstances, blood streaking of the sputum usually stops in 2 to 3 days.

No clinical criteria or radiographic signs predict massive hemoptysis, and the quantity of hemoptysis does not necessarily indicate the seriousness of the patient's underlying disease. Thus, given the tendency for rebleeding and the often unpredictable clinical course, a low threshold for hospitalization is warranted. If massive hemoptysis is present, consideration should be given to early bronchoscopy and interventional angiography with bronchial artery embolization (12,17) or to surgical resection.

DYSPNEA

Breathing is an unconscious act that usually occurs effortlessly, yet even normal people become aware of their breathing during deep sighs or during moderate to severe exercise. Dyspnea, the abnormal uncomfortable sensation of breathlessness, is difficult to define because patients often cannot accurately perceive or quantitate the feeling. Similar to an individual's threshold for pain recognition, the complaint of dyspnea depends on both the individual's limit for discomfort and the specific circumstances that provoke shortness of breath. Thus, dyspnea must be defined in terms of what is abnormal for a particular individual in the context of his or her fitness level and of the amount of activity that is associated with breathlessness. Some patients become dyspneic with relatively small measurable alterations in ventilation, whereas others (e.g., patients who are hyperventilating with Kussmaul breathing) may not complain of dyspnea. Fortunately, a reasonable correlation exists between the degree of dyspnea and objective measurements of physiologic dysfunction.

Often, the actual complaint of dyspnea may not be expressed as such. It may vary depending on the type of precipitating illness and on whether it developed abruptly or over a longer period. Thus, asthmatic patients may complain of tightness in the chest and acute shortness of breath, whereas patients with acute pulmonary embolism (PE) may state that their breath has suddenly "been taken away," and they cannot get enough air even though they ventilate easily. A sensation of air hunger or suffocating is typical for patients with congestive heart failure. In contrast, patients with emphysema or neuromuscular diseases may note an increased effort or work of breathing and may modify their lifestyles and dismiss the sensation of breathlessness as part of their advancing age.

Normal Ventilation

No single mechanism is responsible for dyspnea. Because dyspnea is the result of a variety of diverse influences acting alone or together, a brief discussion of the control of ventilation may help the practitioner understand the complexity of dyspnea and the reason why this sensation often does not immediately respond to correction of obvious physiologic abnormalities. Normally, ventilation is coupled to the individual's metabolic demands as reflected in the oxygen consumption and carbon dioxide elimination necessary to meet a given level of activity. These needs are sensed by peripheral (carotid and aortic bodies) and central (medullary) chemical chemoreceptors that respond to the O_2, CO_2, and pH of blood and cerebrospinal fluid. The acute stimulation of these receptors provokes changes in minute ventilation. In addition, the control and regulation of the rate and pattern of breathing are influenced

TABLE 59.4 Causes of Dyspnea

Causes	*Acute*	*Chronic*
Common		
Pulmonary		
Obstructive airway disease	Asthma, bronchitis	Asthma, chronic obstructive pulmonary disease
Restrictive lung disease	Pneumothorax	Diffuse interstitial lung disease, pleural effusion
Inflammatory	Pneumonia	
Vascular	Pulmonary embolism	
Cardiac	CHF (angina equivalent)	CHF (cardiomyopathy)
Other	Psychogenic	Chronic anemia, obesity
Less common		
Pulmonary		
Upper airway obstruction	Epiglottitis, foreign-body aspiration	Goiter
Restrictive lung disease		Diaphragm paralysis, neuromuscular disease, kyphoscoliosis, pulmonary metastases (lymphangitic)
Vascular		Pulmonary hypertension (thromboembolic, idiopathic), hepatopulmonary syndrome (cirrhosis)
Cardiac		CHF (pericardial disease)
Other	Carbon monoxide intoxication, acute blood loss or hemolysis, thyroid disease	

CHF, congestive heart failure.

by the reflex effects of activation of neural receptors that lie in the lung parenchyma, airways, blood vessels, respiratory muscles, and chest wall. For example, receptors in the chest wall and diaphragm respond to increased stiffness (decreased compliance) in the lung that occurs with fluid accumulation or with interstitial fibrosis. In addition, interstitial edema may activate nerve fibers located in the alveolar interstitium and may cause reflex dyspnea in patients with pulmonary edema. Other receptors located in the airway epithelium cause rapid shallow breathing, coughing, and bronchospasm when irritating substances are inhaled. Finally, the CNS alone can cause large alterations in breathing that lead to hyperventilation in association with anxiety attacks. This discussion should help in understanding, for example, why correction of arterial hypoxemia alone in a patient with an asthmatic attack usually does not relieve the sensation of breathlessness. In this situation, dyspnea results from the complex interaction of both chemical and neural stimuli to breathe, coupled with an individual's response to these signals. Therefore, correction of only one of these problems is not sufficient to abolish dyspnea. A detailed consensus panel report on the pathophysiology and management of dyspnea has been published (18).

Evaluation

The causes of dyspnea are diverse and include essentially all diseases that result in significant functional impairment of either the respiratory system (gas exchange and pulmonary mechanics) or the cardiovascular system (circulatory and cardiac function) and any hematologic abnormality that impairs oxygen delivery. Table 59.4 summarizes the general disease categories likely to cause abnormal breathlessness.

In ambulatory practice, the major causes of dyspnea are obstructive airway disease and atherosclerotic and hypertensive heart disease, either alone or in combination. The prevalence of symptomatic lung disease in a specific geographic region or socioeconomic group is further modified by the prevalence of cigarette use, urban pollution, and occupational exposure to inhaled toxic substances. The clinical circumstances and sequence of events in which dyspnea occurs will aid in its evaluation.

One of the first steps in evaluating a patient who complains of dyspnea is deciding whether the symptoms reflect an acute or a chronic event, because the more serious causes of dyspnea tend to present abruptly. In general, dyspnea of sudden onset is easier to evaluate, but the workup must proceed quickly to determine whether the patient should be admitted to the hospital for more intensive evaluation and therapy. On the other hand, the evaluation of chronic dyspnea usually can be accomplished more slowly in an ambulatory setting.

Acute Dyspnea

The history, physical examination, and chest x-ray form the focal point of the evaluation of a patient with acute dyspnea. In a young patient, the medical history and physical examination alone often suggest the presumptive diagnosis. When necessary, additional distinction of primary cardiac from pulmonary disorders will be aided by the chest x-ray, spirogram, and electrocardiogram.

Acute tracheobronchitis should be considered in the middle-aged smoker with cough, dyspnea, and purulent sputum in association with a clear chest x-ray. When wheezing and rhonchi are present, the term *asthmatic bronchitis* is often used. *Spontaneous pneumothorax* (see below) presents with sudden sharp chest pain and dyspnea. A small but significant pneumothorax on chest x-ray can easily be missed, and diagnostic accuracy will be improved with an expiratory film. Previously undiagnosed *interstitial lung disease, bullous lung disease,* and *cystic fibrosis* also may present with spontaneous *pneumothoraces.* In these cases, the chest film should demonstrate characteristic abnormalities.

Acute dyspnea in association with fever, cough, and purulent sputum with localized infiltrates suggests *pneumonia,* usually bacterial. Diffuse infiltrates and nonproductive cough suggest atypical pneumonia (see Chapter 33).

The patient with acute dyspnea and *heart failure* has usual cardiac symptoms and signs, including paroxysmal nocturnal dyspnea, crackles, cardiomegaly, and a symmetric interstitial pattern with or without pleural effusions (see Chapter 66). *Psychogenic dyspnea,* or the hyperventilation syndrome, has a rapid onset and usually is found in patients with anxiety disorders (see Chapter 22). This syndrome should be considered in young patients in whom dyspnea is unrelated to exertion and is associated with somatic complaints and excessive fearfulness (19).

Less common, but important, causes of acute dyspnea include acute *foreign-body aspiration,* usually evident from the history of aspiration and a physical examination that demonstrates decreased breath sounds over the part of the lung supplied by the occluded bronchus. During the heating season or in certain industrial settings, *carbon monoxide intoxication* should be considered as a cause of headaches and dyspnea. Diagnosis requires a high degree of suspicion and awareness of the problem. Confirmation requires measurement of carboxyhemoglobin with a co-oximeter. The partial pressure of oxygen measured in the arterial blood gas sample will remain normal.

Pulmonary Embolism

PE is a major life-threatening cause of acute dyspnea, but the diagnosis can be difficult. Its evaluation requires a systematic approach with a logical sequence of diagnostic testing. Approximately 75% of patients suspected of having deep venous thrombosis (DVT) or PE do not actually have these conditions (20).

The incidence of PE is high in patients with chronic obstructive lung disease or congestive heart failure and in those with risk factors for venous thromboembolism (e.g., cancer, prolonged immobilization, or a strong family history of DVT; see Chapter 57) (20). In a prospective study of older women (>60 years of age), obesity, heavy cigarette smoking, and high blood pressure were significant risk factors for PE (21). In younger women, use of oral contraceptives substantially increases the risk of PE (21). The physical examination usually is not helpful in the diagnosis, especially because many of the patients have underlying respiratory and cardiovascular diseases that may themselves produce abnormal physical findings, such as tachycardia, tachypnea, distended neck veins, and an accentuated pulmonic component of the second heart sound.

Most laboratory tests are not useful in the diagnosis of PE. Chest x-rays often are abnormal, but the findings are nonspecific (localized infiltrates or oligemia, atelectasis, elevated hemidiaphragm, pleural effusion). Arterial blood gas tensions often are abnormal (reduced Pa_{O_2} and Pa_{CO_2}) but are not helpful diagnostically, in part because of considerable variation and in part because of the high prevalence of cardiopulmonary diseases that alters both Pa_{O_2} and Pa_{CO_2}. An exception is the D-dimer assay. D-Dimer is a breakdown product of fibrinolysis, and its concentration in the blood is increased when clotting occurs. When coupled with a low clinical suspicion of DVT or PE, a negative quantitative D-dimer assay essentially excludes the diagnosis (22–24). For example, if the pretest probability of DVT is <10%, then the posttest probability of DVT after a negative D-dimer rapid enzyme-linked immunosorbent assay (ELISA) is <1% (23). In a 2005 study, none of 232 patients with low or intermediate clinical probability of PE and negative D-dimer assay developed venous thromboembolism after 3 months of followup (24). The diagnostic utility of the D-dimer assays is strongly dependent on how it is measured. ELISAs and quantitative rapid ELISAs have the best sensitivity and negative likelihood ratios (23). Of note, a positive D-dimer assay is not useful in establishing the diagnosis of PE. Furthermore, if the pretest probability of PE is high, then a negative D-dimer assay should not be used to rule out the diagnosis, and additional imaging studies should be obtained. The best way to determine the pretest probability of PE currently not known. In general, the overall impression of an experienced clinician fares about as well as clinical prediction rules for PE, which may be especially valuable for less experienced clinicians (e.g., house staff in training) (25). This is an active area of research where additional prospective studies are needed (see Chapter 57).

If the pretest probability of PE is high (or if the D-dimer assay is positive), then additional imaging studies should be obtained. Three imaging studies of the chest can be performed: pulmonary angiography, ventilation–perfusion (V/Q) scanning, and contrast-enhanced CT. Pulmonary angiography has been considered the "gold standard" for diagnosing pulmonary emboli. However, angiography is uncomfortable for the patient, involves a significant dye load, and requires prolonged breath-holding (up to 30 seconds).

This can be challenging in acutely dyspneic patients and may result in angiograms that are difficult to interpret, especially in subsegmental vessels. V/Q scans or chest CT scans are much less invasive and are the preferred initial tests in the workup of suspected PE. Which of these two scans is the test of choice is a subject of debate. CT scans now are more commonly ordered than V/Q scans in hospitalized patients with suspected PE (26). The choice of V/Q versus CT scan likely will be determined by local institutional expertise in the acquisition and interpretation of these two studies.

Patient Experience. Little discomfort is associated with a lung scan. With a V/Q scan, the patient should be instructed that he or she will inhale a mixture of oxygen and xenon for 3 to 4 minutes, followed by a venous injection of radioactive-labeled technetium. Several different projections are recorded on a scanner while the patient is lying on a table and breathing spontaneously. During a spiral CT scan, as the patient moves through the scanner without stopping, the x-ray tube rotates continuously in the same direction. Acquisition of the scan is carefully timed with an intravenous injection of contrast dye. The patient will have to hold his or her breath, for as little as 10 seconds in newer CT scanners. Patients may experience some mild hot flashes as the dye is injected.

The V/Q scan is a highly sensitive test, but it can be nonspecific depending on the configuration, location, and number of perfusion defects seen. There are well-established criteria for interpreting the results of V/Q scans (27). In general, the greater the perfusion defects without corresponding ventilation defects, the higher the "probability" of the scan. If the V/Q scan is normal, the diagnosis of an acute PE is excluded. Conversely, a high-probability scan is associated with an 85% to 90% chance of PE. As with the D-dimer assay, the predictive value of V/Q scans is highly dependent on the pretest probability of PE (27). Unfortunately, only 10% to 15% of patients with suspected PE will have a high-probability scan, and fewer than 5% of scans will be normal (27). Most patients will have an intermediate-probability (or nondiagnostic) V/Q scan and require further testing to confirm or exclude the diagnosis. Remember that a "low-probability" scan does not exclude the diagnosis of PE. In particular, if there is a high clinical suspicion, up to 40% of patients with low-probability V/Q scans will have documented PE on pulmonary angiography (27). In patients with nondiagnostic V/Q scans, abnormal compression ultrasonography (or impedance plethysmography) may detect a proximal DVT and confirm the need for anticoagulation (22). DVT will be detected by initial testing in approximately 10% of these patients, who should be hospitalized for initiation of anticoagulant therapy (see Chapter 57). Because ultrasonography does not detect calf vein thromboses, some patients with an initially negative test are at risk for propagating a thrombus and having a PE. This occurs 2% to 15% of the time, depending on risk factors for DVT. If there is adequate cardiopulmonary reserve, serial noninvasive testing (e.g., at days 5 and 10) is a reasonable strategy. Alternatively, if clinical suspicion for PE is high or there is limited cardiorespiratory reserve, additional imaging studies should be obtained.

Newer-generation "multislice" CT scanners are becoming widely available and provide exceptional resolution of lung structures and vessels even to the subsegmental level. By injecting a carefully timed bolus of contrast medium, images can be obtained in a single breath-hold, thus allowing visualization of the main, lobar, and segmental pulmonary arteries in most patients. The diagnosis of PE usually is obvious as a low-density filling defect within the vessel lumen, but there is a lack of widely agreed upon standards for diagnosing PE by spiral CT. Therefore, a highly trained interpreter with a knowledge of bronchovascular anatomy (and its variants) is essential. The advantages of a spiral CT include its relatively quick acquisition time and its ability to diagnose abnormalities within the lung parenchyma and mediastinum. In several studies, unsuspected abnormalities (e.g., pneumothorax, cancer) were found in 10% to 30% of subjects undergoing spiral CT to "rule out PE" (28). Studies have shown that multislice CT scanners are very sensitive. For example, a clinical trial that used a D-dimer assay in conjunction with multislice CT scanning found that compression ultrasonography did not improve diagnostic yield in patients with a negative CT scan (24). Therefore, ultrasonography may be unnecessary in patients with negative multislice CT scans. Furthermore, the subsequent rate of venous thromboembolism in patients with negative CT scans is very low (e.g., approximately 1.5% at 3 months), comparable to the rate in patients with negative pulmonary angiography (24,29). This finding has fueled the argument that CT scans should become the new "gold standard." The CT scan versus angiogram debate is unlikely to be resolved by a clinical trial. A definitive study would require randomly assigning patients to CT scan or angiography, withholding anticoagulation in those with negative studies, and observing patients for subsequent venous thromboembolism. Such a study would require thousands of patients in each arm and is unlikely to be performed soon.

The resolution of PE varies and can occur as early as 1 to 2 weeks in patients with small emboli. In patients with larger emboli and in patients with underlying cardiopulmonary disease, angiographic evidence of emboli may persists for 2 to 3 months (30). If chest pain occurs after discharge, a subsequent lung V/Q or chest CT scan is necessary to determine whether embolization has recurred.

Evaluation of Chronic or Progressive Dyspnea

In contrast to acute dyspnea, chronic dyspnea usually is more difficult to diagnose and often requires more extensive diagnostic procedures; therefore, the evaluation should proceed in a logical sequence to avoid expensive and invasive laboratory testing. Because shortness of breath is appropriate to certain levels of activity depending on the fitness of the individual, the clinician must decide whether the patient's symptoms are abnormal and over what period they have developed. Many patients with chronic cardiopulmonary disease or chronic anemia adapt to the insidious onset of dyspnea by subconsciously changing daily habits and avoiding physical activity. The degree of dyspnea should be determined by comparing the patient's abilities to perform work with an appropriate peer group and with his or her baseline performance. Thus, the complaint of dyspnea in a 35-year-old patient who normally runs 5 miles and now becomes short of breath after running only 2 miles should not be ignored.

The most useful initial test is the chest x-ray, which often is abnormal and therefore directs subsequent evaluation. Patients with *COPD* associated with emphysema have hyperinflation, decreased lung markings, and often evidence of bullous formation (see Chapter 60). Large *pleural effusions, lung cancer,* or *heart disease* associated with dyspnea results in obvious changes in the chest roentgenogram with evidence of fluid occupying at least half of one hemithorax, large mass lesions, or cardiomegaly, respectively. *Interstitial lung disease* that has led to fibrosis is revealed by chest x-ray, although early cases of interstitial lung disease will be detectable only by high-resolution CT scan. *Unilateral hemidiaphragm paralysis* results in obvious asymmetry in lung expansion. Patients with this condition often describe orthopnea secondary to difficulty with diaphragmatic excursion in the recumbent position.

Patients with dyspnea and a normal or nonspecific chest x-ray represent a challenging group to diagnose. Table 59.5 provides an approach to the evaluation of these patients. Most of these patients have obstructive lung disease. A spirogram is useful to screen for occult lung disease because a normal spirogram nearly excludes significant parenchymal disease. Although patients with exercise-induced asthma may have a normal spirogram during symptom-free periods, more commonly there is evidence of slight reduction in the baseline forced expiratory volume as a percentage of forced vital capacity. Home peak flow monitoring may confirm the diagnosis in these patients. Chapter 60 discusses additional specialized procedures that aid in the diagnosis of exercise-induced asthma. In one study of 72 patients referred for evaluation of chronic dyspnea not diagnosed by history, physical examination, chest x-ray, or spirometry, the two most common diagnoses were asthma/reactive airway diseases (approximately 17%) and hyperventilation syndrome (approximately 20%). There was a wide spectrum of underlying diseases in the remaining cases. Notably, 20% of patients remained undiagnosed despite extensive evaluation (31).

In general, *obesity* is not associated with dyspnea unless body weight is markedly increased (50%–100% or more, or ≥100 lb over ideal weight). *Primary pulmonary hypertension* may be associated with subtle dilation of the pulmonary arteries on chest x-ray and is most commonly seen in young women. Pulmonary hypertension also can occur in association with collagen vascular diseases and should be suspected especially in patients with dyspnea on exertion in whom the chest X-ray does not show parenchymal lung disease. *Upper airway obstruction* resulting from *goiter,* for example, often is not apparent on a routine posteroanterior and lateral chest x-ray. Anemia usually does not cause dyspnea unless it has developed acutely (blood loss or hemolysis) or is relatively severe (e.g., hematocrit values ≤20%). Some patients with advanced *hepatic cirrhosis* complain of severe dyspnea that is especially worse when they are upright ("platypnea"). These patients experience excess shunting of blood through abnormal vascular channels in the lung (the *hepatopulmonary syndrome*) (32).

In patients in whom the diagnosis is uncertain, laboratory testing should include a hemoglobin determination or hematocrit value to determine whether the patient has severe anemia or erythrocytosis, and thyroid function

TABLE 59.5 Workup of Chronic Dyspnea when the Initial Workup (e.g., Chest X-Ray, Spirometry) Is Unrevealing

Disease Suspected	*Test*
Pulmonary	
Obstructive airway disease	Home peak flow monitoring, bronchoprovocation
Interstitial lung disease	Helium lung volumes, diffusing capacity, high-resolution chest computed tomography
Respiratory muscle weakness	Helium lung volumes, diffusing capacity, inspiratory/expiratory pressures
Pulmonary hypertension (thromboembolic, idiopathic)	Ventilation–perfusion scan, echocardiography, pulmonary angiography
Unclear	Helium lung volumes, diffusing capacity
Cardiac	
Coronary artery disease	Electrocardiography/ multiple-gated acquisition scan: rest ± exercise
Cardiomyopathy	Echocardiography
Other	
Thyroid disease	Thyroid function tests
Anemia	Hemoglobin concentration or hematocrit value
Mixed cardiac/respiratory disease	Cardiopulmonary exercise testing
Deconditioning	Cardiopulmonary exercise testing
Anxiety/hyperventilation	Cardiopulmonary exercise testing

studies if symptoms of thyroid dysfunction (e.g., unexplained weight gain, fatigue) are noted.

Complete pulmonary function tests should be performed. In addition to baseline spirometry (see Chapter 60), other pulmonary function tests include measurements of *total lung capacity* and *functional residual capacity,* which quantitate the degree of hyperinflation or restriction. Categorization of a disorder as obstructive or restrictive will direct the clinician to a narrowed list of causes. The *diffusing capacity* measures the amount of alveolar capillary surface area available for gas exchange. Thus, the diffusing capacity is reduced in patients with PE and other vascular occlusive diseases and in patients with emphysema. In contrast, an elevated diffusing capacity is found in conditions that increase the pulmonary blood volume, for example, erythrocytosis, early congestive heart failure, or obesity. Measurement of inspiratory and expiratory pressures helps characterize neuromuscular problems. *Flow–volume loops* help identify upper airway sources of obstruction. Chapter 60 describes the experience of the patient during the performance of these tests.

Cardiovascular testing should be performed. Chapters 65 and 66 discuss the use of specialized noninvasive cardiovascular evaluation, including *echocardiography* and *nuclear scanning,* to assess right and left ventricular function or the presence of valvular heart disease.

If a patient is dyspneic on exertion and baseline testing of cardiopulmonary function, as described earlier, is normal or only mildly abnormal, *exercise testing* should be considered. In general, two types of exercise tests are available. The first is a standard *cardiac stress test,* during which the patient exercises and is observed for the development of chest pain and for electrocardiographic or radionuclide ischemic changes (see Chapter 62). The second type of exercise test is a *cardiopulmonary stress test* in which cardiac function, pulmonary gas exchange, ventilation, and physical fitness are quantitated at specific workloads. The two types of tests are similar, but the patient should be told that the cardiopulmonary test requires continuous exercise while breathing into a mouthpiece, and measurement of oxygenation is made by either an oximeter or an indwelling arterial line. Such complicated cardiopulmonary stress testing is justified and useful to determine whether dyspnea is caused by cardiac disease; pulmonary disease, including exercise-induced asthma or occult pulmonary vascular disease; deconditioning; or combinations of these conditions. This type of testing is particularly useful in evaluating patients for disability compensation because static pulmonary function and noninvasive cardiac testing may not accurately predict the functional state of a given patient during actual working conditions. The referring clinician usually can determine presumptively the most likely cause of dyspnea and can make the appropriate referral for the specific exercise test. In large hospital centers having combined cardiopulmonary laboratories, simultaneous consultation and exercise testing by cardiologists and pulmonologists may be available. Stress testing also can be useful in deciding whether or not the patient needs supplemental oxygen (see Chapter 60).

This approach to the evaluation of dyspnea almost always answers the questions necessary for diagnosis of the underlying condition and for establishment of a therapeutic regimen.

Therapy

Treatment of dyspnea is primarily aimed at therapy for the underlying cardiac, pulmonary, neuromuscular, or hematologic disorders causing the abnormal breathlessness. In certain patients with underlying irreversible lung disease, specific measures that improve respiratory muscle function may alleviate symptomatic dyspnea. Training programs that increase both muscle strength and endurance are available in selected pulmonary rehabilitation centers, even for patients with advanced lung disease. Pulmonary rehabilitation can result in decreased shortness of breath in many patients. Because anxiety and depression are commonly associated with the development of chronic cardiopulmonary disorders associated with dyspnea, appropriate anxiolytics or antidepressants may be considered. In patients with pulmonary disease, buspirone (20–30 mg/day) may be an effective anxiolytic and does not impair respiratory drive. Selective serotonin reuptake inhibitors may be particularly useful in patients with panic attacks (19). Patients with dyspnea and terminal lung diseases (e.g., cancer, COPD, interstitial pulmonary fibrosis) represent a particularly challenging group to manage. The patient and/or the primary caregiver should make plans early on (and not in the setting of acute decompensation) to deal with progressive dyspnea and end-of-life care. Low-dose narcotics (e.g., morphine sulfate) can be extremely useful as a palliative therapy for terminally ill dyspneic patients. Some subjects obtain marked relief from nebulized morphine, which may act via bronchial opioid receptors. The optimal dosing of nebulized morphine is unknown (typically initially 20 mg morphine sulfate in 5 mL normal saline) and requires further study.

NONCARDIAC CHEST PAIN

Chest pain is a particularly frightening symptom because of the widespread knowledge and concern about heart disease. However, nonspecific musculoskeletal pain is more common than angina, especially in younger patients (<40 years old). Most patients with chest pain can be evaluated and treated in an ambulatory setting; a few patients require referral to a specialist. The common noncardiac causes of chest pain are discussed in this section.

TABLE 59.6 Causes of Chest Pain

Causes	Examples
Common	
Chest wall	Nonspecific musculoskeletal, costochondritis (Tietze syndrome)
Cardiovascular	Angina
Pulmonary	Tracheitis, pleurodynia, pneumonia
Gastrointestinal	Esophageal reflux/spasm
Neurologic	Cervical spine disease (radicular)
Less common	
Chest wall	Herpes zoster, thoracic outlet syndrome, fractured rib, tumor
Cardiovascular	Aortic dissection, pericarditis
Pulmonary	Pneumothorax, pulmonary hypertension, pulmonary infarction
Gastrointestinal	Peptic ulcer disease, abdominal infection/peritonitis

Afferent neural impulses responsible for thoracic pain are carried by the sympathetic chain, vagus, and phrenic nerves. Visceral structures, which include the lung, diaphragm, heart, and esophagus, all lie within the thoracic cage and have overlapping innervation. Chest pain arising from these different organs often has similar referral patterns; thus, irritation of the diaphragmatic pleura, diaphragm, or pericardium from either thoracic or abdominal disease causes chest pain that radiates to the shoulder. In addition, patients may have difficulty localizing pain from the deeper anatomic structures within the chest, whereas diseases involving the superficial structures, muscles, and ribs are more easily localized. Because there is no sensory innervation of the lung parenchyma, alveolar or interstitial disease does not cause chest pain unless the pulmonary vasculature, bronchi, or pleura are involved. One study found that enhanced visceral (esophageal) pain perception underlies many cases of unexplained angina-like chest pain (33). Table 59.6 lists causes of chest pain.

Musculoskeletal pain is common in young individuals who increase their exercise abruptly (including patients who acutely hyperventilate as part of an anxiety state. A history of unusual exertion with increased breathing plus tenderness of intercostal muscles usually suffices to make this diagnosis.

Pain caused by *tracheitis* or *tracheobronchitis* is a distinctive substernal burning sensation that is precipitated by coughing and most often is associated with viral respiratory infections. This is in contrast to the sharp, stabbing, pleuritic chest pain experienced with pneumonia. The latter is clearly localized to the chest wall and arises from stretching the inflamed parietal pleura during breathing or coughing. *Pleurodynia* (or epidemic myalgia), characterized by fever, headache, and sudden onset of intense lower thoracic pleuritic pain, usually results from infection with Coxsackie B viruses.

Other causes of chest pain include *costochondritis* (Tietze syndrome), which is anterior localized pain associated with tenderness over one or more costochondral junctions; *herpes zoster,* which commonly causes unilateral aching or itching, limited to one dermatome, which may precede by several days the eruption of vesicles; *rib fracture* or *bone metastases,* which are more chronic and pleuritic in nature; and *cervical spine disease* with referred pain to the chest (see Chapter 70). Acute stabbing chest pain can occur with a *spontaneous pneumothorax,* which occurs primarily in young men or in older patients with obstructive pulmonary disease. Often, a small (<20%) pneumothorax is not accompanied by significant dyspnea in otherwise healthy individuals. Pleuritic chest pain that follows the abrupt onset of dyspnea should raise the suspicion of a PE. The pain associated with *pulmonary hypertension* is heavy and aching and often similar to that of cardiac ischemia. *Gastrointestinal disorders,* such as GERD or gastric or duodenal ulcer, usually are distinguished from cardiopulmonary chest pain by their association with eating and by their relief with use of antacids (see Chapters 42 and 43).

Evaluation

Many common causes of noncardiac chest pain can be diagnosed by a thorough history and physical examination. Because discrete anatomic structures must be involved to cause noncardiac chest pain, the physical examination is more useful in the diagnosis of noncardiac chest pain than in the diagnosis of dyspnea and hemoptysis. Inspection of the chest wall may reveal the characteristic unilateral eruption of herpes zoster along a dermatome. Light palpation over the chest wall elicits pain and crepitus from fractured ribs. Mild pressure over the costochondral junctions anteriorly reproduces the pain of Tietze syndrome. (In general, cardiac pain is not worsened by pressure over the chest wall.) In pneumonia or pulmonary infarction, a distinct friction rub is sometimes heard directly over the specific area of chest pain. With pericardial involvement, a friction rub that varies with respiration or with the cardiac cycle usually is present. A thorough abdominal examination is important because diseases involving the abdominal visceral organs can cause referred chest pain that is indistinguishable from that produced by involvement of the thoracic structures. Often, laboratory studies and a chest x-ray will not be necessary for the diagnosis of these common causes of chest pain.

Therapy

The treatment of chest pain requires therapy for the underlying disease process, as well as analgesic drugs for the pain itself. Tracheal irritation is limited to the duration of the viral illness but can be treated by cough suppression and bronchodilators (see Cough). Tietze syndrome is treated with standard anti-inflammatory agents and heat. Although the pain of herpes zoster often is severe, it may be controlled with mild narcotics such as codeine 30 to 60 mg every 4 to 6 hours. The chest pain experienced in pulmonary hypertension often does not respond to treatment with nonnarcotic analgesics, and narcotics may be required if the hypertension does not improve with treatment.

Pleuritic pain in patients with pneumonia or PE responds to specific therapy for the inflammatory process. Nevertheless, narcotics may be needed to reduce splinting of the chest wall and thereby prevent atelectasis. Codeine (60 mg every 4 hours) usually is adequate therapy.

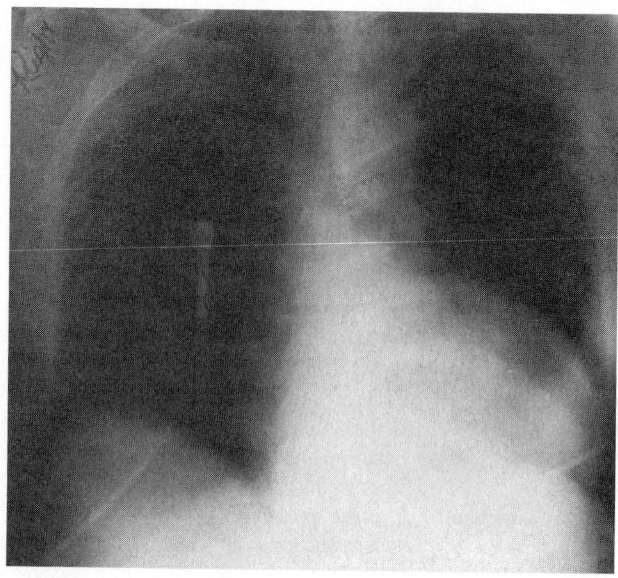

FIGURE 59.2. Air bronchogram. The patient had fever and sputum production. The initial x-ray demonstrates a branching air bronchogram seen behind the heart on the left, which is consistent with a lower-lobe infiltrate.

ABNORMAL CHEST X-RAY

A chest x-ray must always be compared with prior films because an abnormality that has been stable in size for >2 years almost certainly is benign and may not require further evaluation. In addition, depending on the appearance of the abnormality and the patient's age, the most appropriate plan may be observation with serial chest x-rays.

Specific Patterns Indicative of an Abnormal Chest X-Ray

This section reviews common abnormalities that indicate the presence of pulmonary disease requiring further evaluation.

Air Bronchogram

Normally, bronchi beyond the mainstem division cannot be seen. However, when the alveoli surrounding a bronchus are devoid of air because of consolidation or, less commonly, collapse, an air bronchogram can be seen (Fig. 59.2). The presence of an air bronchogram indicates an alveolar filling process and is most commonly seen in pneumonia and pulmonary edema (cardiogenic and noncardiogenic). However, an air bronchogram is not present in every consolidated lung because bronchi may fill with secretions or exudate. Therefore, its absence is less significant than its presence.

Silhouette Sign

Obliteration on a chest x-ray of the margin of a normally opaque structure in the chest by an abnormal pulmonary density is called the *silhouette sign.* If the clinician has knowledge of thoracic anatomy and spatial relations, the silhouette sign can be used to localize abnormalities within the lung parenchyma. Edges of organs that are in contact with parenchymal infiltrates will be obliterated because the normal air interface is eliminated. On the other hand, intrathoracic lesions that are not anatomically contiguous will not interfere with the outlines of nearby structures. For example, obliteration of the right or left cardiac borders, which are anterior, localizes an abnormality to the right middle lobe or to the lingular segment of the left upper lobe, respectively (Fig. 59.3). In contrast, an infiltrate that overlaps, but does not obliterate, the cardiac border is posterior and represents a lower lobe lesion. Lower-lobe abnormalities obliterate diaphragmatic borders and on lateral chest x-ray are seen as an increased density over the vertebrae (spine sign). Obliteration of the left border of the aortic knob, a posterior structure, occurs with lesions in the apical posterior segment of the left upper lobe, whereas obliteration of the border of the ascending aorta, an anterior structure, occurs with lesions in the anterior segment of the right upper lobe.

Collapse

The collapse (Fig. 59.4) or diminution in volume of the whole lung, a lobe, or a segment of one of the lobes can be an important clue to the presence of asymptomatic pulmonary disease, such as bronchogenic carcinoma, or it may be the cause of a symptom, such as dyspnea in an asthmatic patient with mucous plugging. The primary mechanisms that cause pulmonary collapse are *bronchial obstruction* from either an intrinsic bronchial mass or an extrinsic or intrinsic stenosis of the bronchus, *compression of the lung* from a large pleural effusion or from a

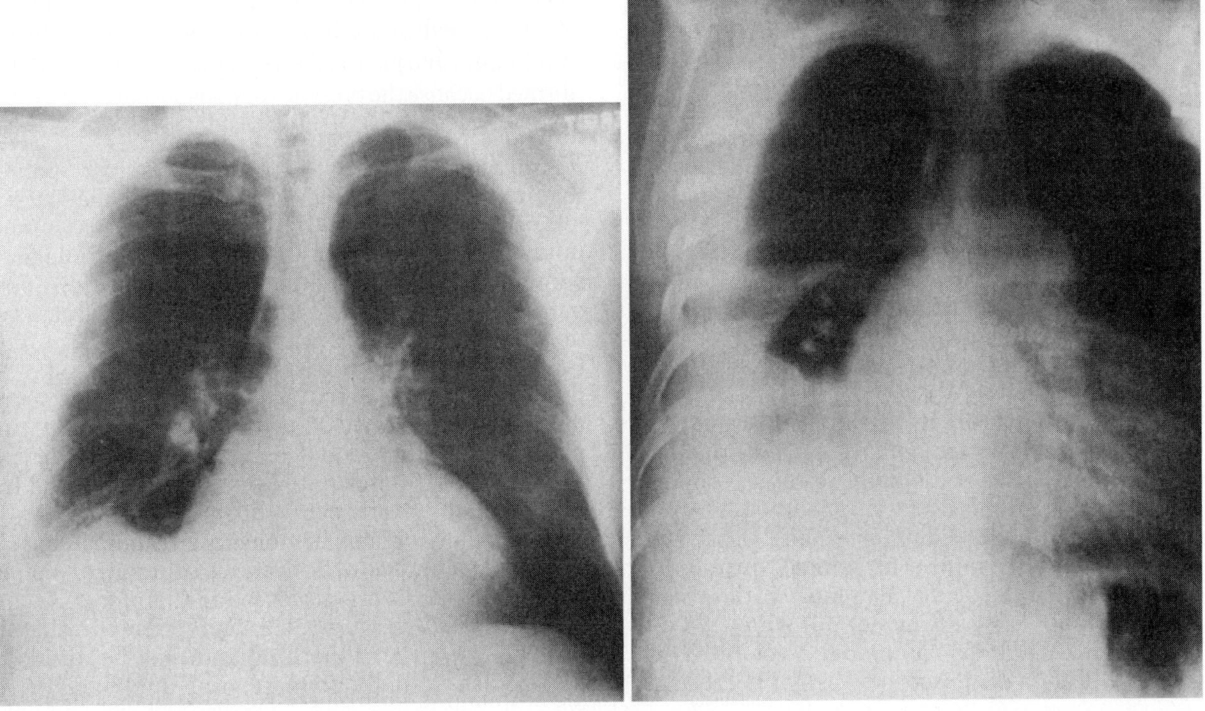

FIGURE 59.7. Subpulmonic effusion. **A:** The diaphragm appears to be elevated on the right, representing subpulmonic fluid. **B:** When the patient is placed in the right lateral decubitus position, fluid layers on the right and tracks in the minor fissure and along the apex and the diaphragm.

from an isolated chest x-ray. If old chest x-rays demonstrate that no change has occurred, further evaluation may be unnecessary. Chapter 34 discusses the evaluation and treatment of patients with tuberculosis.

Superior sulcus tumors, usually squamous cell carcinomas, arise in the extreme apex of the lung and may be difficult to distinguish from pleural thickening or old granulomatous disease. Later in the disease course, x-rays may reveal erosion of adjacent ribs or vertebrae by the tumor (see Chapter 61).

Pleural Effusion

Small amounts of free fluid within the pleural space will obliterate the costophrenic or costocardiac angles. Because the density of pleural fluid is greater than the density of the lung, a subpulmonic collection will laterally displace the crest of the diaphragm (Fig. 59.7A). An increased density between the stomach gas bubble and pulmonary tissue may also indicate the presence of fluid within the pleural space. The diagnosis of a large pleural effusion is not difficult because fluid within the pleural space on an upright chest x-ray will form a concave density across the chest cavity; decubitus x-rays will demonstrate the free flowing pleural fluid in the dependent hemithorax (Fig. 59.7B). If the patient is recumbent, the pleural fluid will layer over the entire hemithorax, causing the lung to appear opaque.

In general, when pleural effusion is seen on a chest x-ray, a sample should be obtained for analysis. The obvious exception is a patient who develops acute pulmonary edema associated with a rapidly developing pleural effusion that resolves with therapy for congestive heart failure (see Chapter 66). Table 59.9 lists the causes of pleural effusion. A diagnostic thoracentesis to determine the cause of the effusion generally can be done when the thickness of the fluid between the inner border of the rib and lung is >1 cm on a lateral decubitus x-ray. The fluid should be sent for white blood cell and differential count, total protein concentration, lactate dehydrogenase (LDH) concentration, glucose concentration, Gram stain, cultures (aerobic and anaerobic bacteria, mycobacterium, fungus), pH (if parapneumonic effusion is present), and cytopathology (if malignancy is suspected). Specialized analysis of pleural fluid can help in cases where the diagnosis is not immediately obvious (e.g., amylase in cases of esophageal rupture or pancreatic disease, or adenosine deaminase in suspected tuberculous pleuritis). Most pleural effusions are clear and straw colored, and deviations from this norm may be diagnostically helpful. For example, a bloody effusion suggests tumor and, less commonly, PE with infarction, tuberculosis, or trauma; a lime-green effusion

TABLE 59.9 Causes of Pleural Effusion

Effusion	Common	Uncommon
Transudate	CHF Cirrhosis, nephrosis	Pericardial disease Myxedema, peritoneal dialysis
Exudate		
Malignancy	Metastatic disease (solid tumors)	Lymphoma, mesothelioma
Infection	Bacterial (parapneumonia and empyema), tuberculosis	Atypical pneumonias, fungal, viral, parasites (amebiasis, paragonimiasis)
Trauma	Hemothorax	Chylothorax
Gastrointestinal		Pancreatitis, esophageal rupture, subphrenic abscess
Collagen vascular disease		Systemic lupus erythematosus, rheumatoid arthritis
Miscellaneous	Postcoronary artery bypass surgery	Pulmonary infarction, benign asbestos effusion, drug hypersensitivity, postmyocardial infarction syndrome, uremia, trapped lung, lymphatic abnormalities

CHF, congestive heart failure.

suggests tuberculosis; a white milky effusion suggests a chylous exudate; and a viscous fluid with feculent odor strongly suggests an anaerobic empyema.

It is important to classify pleural effusion as either transudative or exudative (35,36). *Transudates* caused by increased hydrostatic pressure or decreased plasma oncotic pressure have low protein and LDH concentrations. They generally are caused by congestive heart failure, cirrhosis with ascites, or nephrotic syndrome. They do not require further diagnostic evaluation (with respect to the effusion itself), and treatment is directed at the underlying cause. *Exudates,* as a result of increased protein permeability of the pleural blood vessels, generally are caused by inflammation or tumor infiltration. Exudates are defined by one of the following criteria: pleural fluid protein concentration that is >50% of the concentration of serum protein, pleural fluid LDH concentration that is >60% of the concentration of serum LDH, or pleural fluid LDH concentration that is >67% of the upper limit of normal serum LDH (35,36). Figure 59.8 shows a useful algorithm for working up a pleural effusion. Pleural effusions with protein concentrations >3 g/100 mL nearly always are exudates. If the pleural fluid is defined as exudative but the clinical picture is more consistent with a transudate, the serum–pleural fluid albumin gradient should be measured. If this gradient is >1.2 g/dL, the effusion probably is transudative (36). A cell count and pleural fluid cytologic study should be performed because the presence of polymorphonuclear leukocytes in pleural fluid suggests acute inflammation and infection, whereas >50% lymphocytes suggests tuberculosis or malignancy. Tuberculous pleuritis should be considered in any patient with an exudative pleural effusion and a history of tuberculosis exposure or a positive tuberculin skin reaction. The presence of >5% pleural mesothelial cells makes the diagnosis of tuberculosis unlikely. Low pleural fluid glucose concentration (<50 mg/dL) occurs in infections (parapneumonic effusions, tuberculosis), rheumatoid arthritis, and occasionally in malignancy. Pleural fluid pH determination is important not only in the differential diagnosis (acidic pH is seen with infection, malignancy, severe inflammation, esophageal rupture) but also in the management of parapneumonic pleural effusions. In this setting, pH <7.20 signals the possibility of a complicated parapneumonic effusion, which requires a more aggressive approach (e.g., a drainage procedure) (37). If a pleural effusion is bloody or appears infected, the patient should be hospitalized for further diagnostic studies and therapy (e.g., chest tube drainage, pleural biopsy).

Pneumothorax

The three major types of pneumothorax are spontaneous, iatrogenic, and traumatic. Of the three types, the general practitioner is most commonly faced with a spontaneous pneumothorax either in a young healthy individual or in an older patient with underlying pulmonary disease. In the former, a subpleural apical bleb ruptures into the pleural space, causing collection of varying amounts of air. Patients with spontaneous pneumothoraces tend to be tall, thin, young, male smokers (38). These patients generally are at rest when they first experience symptoms. In the older patient, emphysema with concomitant bullous disease is commonly associated with a pneumothorax. The abrupt onset of pleuritic chest pain or dyspnea is characteristic. Pneumothoraces are diagnosed by demonstrating a visceral pleural line on the chest x-ray.

After the diagnosis of pneumothorax is made, the patient may require observation (ambulatory or inpatient) or insertion of a chest tube. For patients with a pneumothorax >15% of the volume of the hemithorax, needle or catheter aspiration (e.g., using a thoracentesis kit) can obviate the need for hospitalization. This should be performed only by experienced personnel because of the risk for visceral pleural laceration. In general, patients with underlying lung disease should be hospitalized and may require a chest tube because of their limited pulmonary reserve. On the other hand, a healthy patient with a small pneumothorax (<15%) who is not in distress can remain at home and be followed by serial chest x-rays. The rate of reabsorption

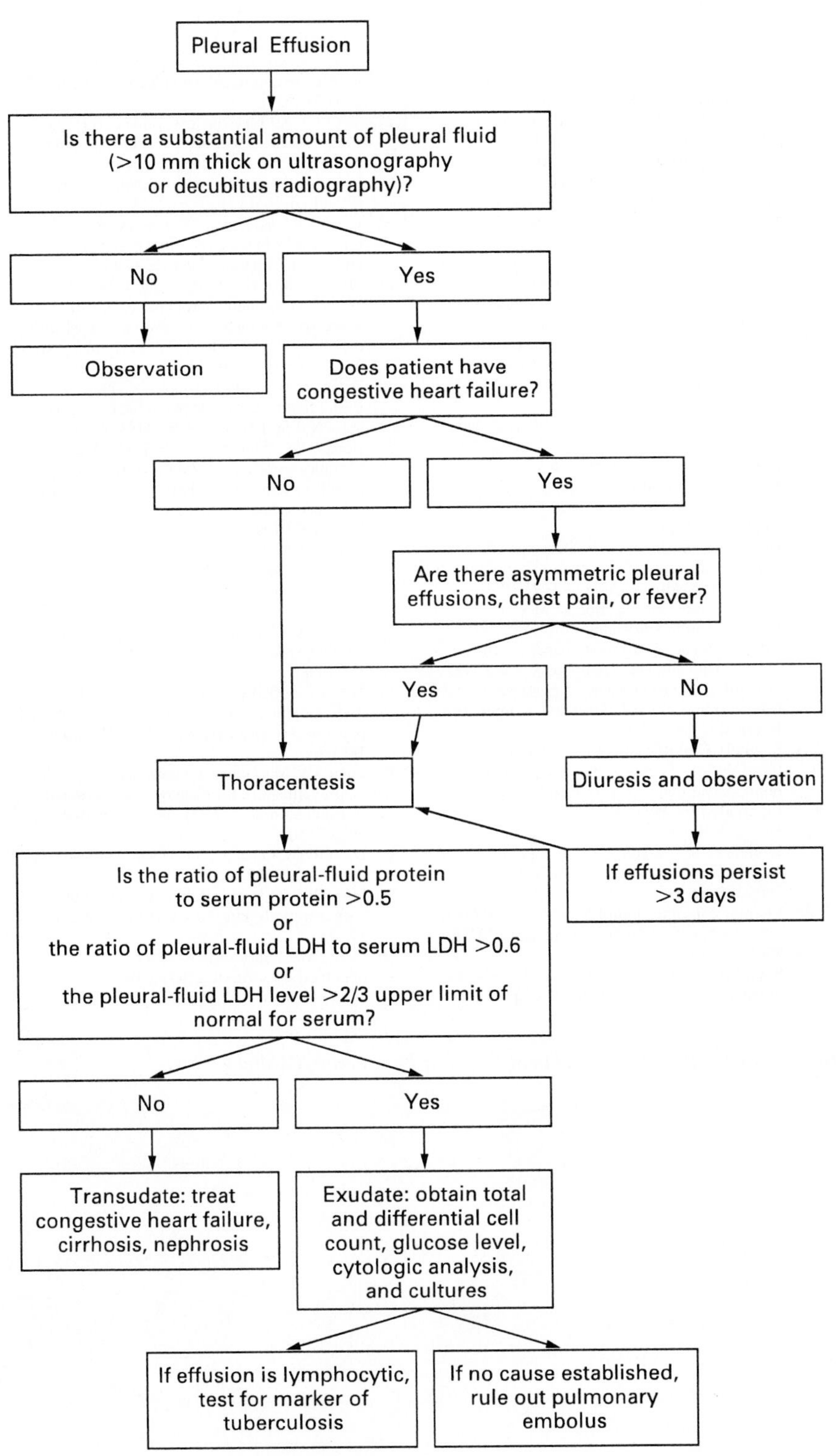

FIGURE 59.8. Algorithm for working up undiagnosed pleural effusions. (From Light RW. Clinical practice. Pleural effusion. N Engl J Med 2002;346:1971, with permission.)

is slow. Assuming approximately 1.25% of the volume is reabsorbed per day (38), a 15% pneumothorax will take approximately 12 days to reabsorb spontaneously. Supplemental oxygen can enhance the rate of reabsorption by increasing the transpulmonary nitrogen gradient.

Solitary Nodule

A solitary nodule is a radiologic finding that always requires evaluation. Chapter 61 provides a detailed discussion of the problem.

SPECIFIC REFERENCES

1. Irwin RS, Madison JM. The diagnosis and treatment of cough. N Engl J Med 2000; 343:1715.
2. Kastelik JA, Aziz I, Ojoo JC, et al. Investigation and management of chronic cough using a probability-based algorithm. Eur Respir J 2005;25:235.
3. Corrao WM, Braman SS, Irwin RS. Chronic cough as the sole presenting manifestation of bronchial asthma. N Engl J Med 1979;300:633.
4. Luque CA, Vazquez Ortiz M. Treatment of ACE inhibitor-induced cough. Pharmacotherapy 1999;19:804.
5. Irwin RS, Madison JM. The persistently troublesome cough. Am J Respir Crit Care Med 2002;165:1469.
6. Sperber SJ, Hendley JO, Hayden FG, et al. Effects of naproxen on experimental rhinovirus colds. A randomized, double-blind, controlled trial. Ann Intern Med 1992;117:37.
7. Croughan-Minihane MS, Petitti DB, Rodnick JE, et al. Clinical trial examining the effectiveness of three cough syrups. J Am Board Fam Pract 1993;6:109.
8. Johnston H, Reisz G. Changing spectrum of hemoptysis. Underlying causes in 148 patients undergoing diagnostic flexible fiberoptic bronchoscopy. Arch Intern Med 1989;149:1666.
9. Santiago S, Tobias J, Williams AJ. A reappraisal of the causes of hemoptysis. Arch Intern Med 1991;151:2449.
10. Adelman M, Haponik EF, Bleecker ER, et al. Cryptogenic hemoptysis. Clinical features, bronchoscopic findings, and natural history in 67 patients. Ann Intern Med 1985;102:829.
11. Hirshberg B, Biran I, Glazer M, et al. Hemoptysis: etiology, evaluation and outcome in a tertiary referral hospital. Chest 1997;112:440.
12. Cahill BC, Ingbar DH. Massive hemoptysis: assessment and management. Clin Chest Med 1994;15:147.
13. Tasker AD, Flower CD. Imaging the airways. Hemoptysis, bronchiectasis, and small airways disease. Clin Chest Med 1999;20:761.
14. O'Neil KM, Lazarus AA. Hemoptysis. Indications for bronchoscopy. Arch Intern Med 1991;151:171.
15. Poe RH, Israel RH, Marin MG, et al. Utility of fiberoptic bronchoscopy in patients with hemoptysis and a nonlocalizing chest roentgenogram. Chest 1988;93:70.
16. McGuinness G, Beacher JR, Harkin TJ, et al. Hemoptysis: prospective high-resolution CT/bronchoscopic correlation. Chest 1994; 105:1155.
17. Mal H, Rullon I, Mellot F, et al. Immediate and long-term results of bronchial artery embolization for life-threatening hemoptysis. Chest 1999;115:996.
18. American Thoracic Society. Dyspnea. Mechanisms, assessment, and management: a consensus statement. Am J Respir Crit Care Med 1999;159:321.
19. Smoller JW, Pollack MH, Otto MW, et al. Panic anxiety, dyspnea, and respiratory disease. Am J Respir Crit Care Med 1996;154:6.
20. Fedullo PF, Tapson VF. Clinical practice. The evaluation of suspected pulmonary embolism. N Engl J Med 2003;349:1247.
21. Goldhaber SZ, Grodstein F, Stampfer MJ, et al. A prospective study of risk factors for pulmonary embolism in women. JAMA 1997;277:642.
22. Wells PS, Anderson DR, Rodger M, et al. Excluding pulmonary embolism at the bedside without diagnostic imaging: management of patients with suspected pulmonary embolism presenting to the emergency department by using a simple clinical model and D-dimer. Ann Intern Med 2001;135:98.
23. Stein PD, Hull RD, Patel KC, et al. D-dimer for the exclusion of acute venous thrombosis and pulmonary embolism: a systematic review. Ann Intern Med 2004;140:602.
24. Perrier A, Roy PM, Sanchez O, et al. Multidetector-row computed tomography in suspected pulmonary embolism. N Engl J Med 2005;352:1760.
25. Chunilal SD, Eikelboom JW, Attia J, et al. Does this patient have pulmonary embolism? JAMA 2003;290:2849.
26. Stein PD, Kayali F, Olson RE. Trends in the use of diagnostic imaging in patients hospitalized with acute pulmonary embolism. Am J Cardiol 2004;93:1316.
27. The PIOPED Investigators. Value of the ventilation/perfusion scan in acute pulmonary embolism. Results of the prospective investigation of pulmonary embolism diagnosis (PIOPED). JAMA 1990;263:2753.
28. Lipchik RJ, Goodman LR. Spiral computed tomography in the evaluation of pulmonary embolism. Clin Chest Med 1999;20:731.
29. Moores LK, Jackson WL Jr, Shorr AF, et al. Meta-analysis: outcomes in patients with suspected pulmonary embolism managed with computed tomographic pulmonary angiography. Ann Intern Med 2004;141:866.
30. Dalen JE, Banas JS Jr, Brooks HL, et al. Resolution rate of acute pulmonary embolism in man. N Engl J Med 1969;280:1194.
31. DePaso WJ, Winterbauer RH, Lusk JA, et al. Chronic dyspnea unexplained by history, physical examination, chest roentgenogram, and spirometry: analysis of a seven-year experience. Chest 1991;100:1293.
32. Hoeper MM, Krowka MJ, Strassburg CP. Portopulmonary hypertension and hepatopulmonary syndrome. Lancet 2004; 363:1461.
33. Goyal RK. Changing focus on unexplained esophageal chest pain. Ann Intern Med 1996; 124:1008.
34. Mittl RL Jr, Schwab RJ, Duchin JS, et al. Radiographic resolution of community-acquired pneumonia. Am J Respir Crit Care Med 1994; 149:630.
35. Light RW, MacGregor I, Luchsinger PC, et al. Pleural effusions: the diagnostic separation of transudates and exudates. Ann Intern Med 1972;77:507.
36. Light RW. Clinical practice. Pleural effusion. N Engl J Med 2002;346:1971.
37. Light RW, Rodriguez RM. Management of parapneumonic effusions. Clin Chest Med 1998; 19:373.
38. Light RW. Management of spontaneous pneumothorax. Am Rev Respir Dis 1993;148:245.

*For annotated **General References** and resources related to this chapter, visit www.hopkinsbayview.org/PAMreferences.*

Chapter 60

Obstructive Airway Diseases: Asthma and Chronic Obstructive Pulmonary Disease

Robert A. Wise and Mark C. Liu

Obstructive lung diseases are the most common chronic pulmonary diseases encountered in ambulatory practice. *Asthma, chronic bronchitis,* and *emphysema* are the most common disorders. Chronic bronchitis and emphysema often coexist. Both are predominantly caused by tobacco smoking, so they both usually are referred to as *chronic obstructive pulmonary disease (COPD)*. Less common conditions that lead to COPD include bronchiectasis, chronic forms of bronchiolitis, and cystic fibrosis. These disorders have different clinical presentations, causes, and prognoses, but all share the same physiologic abnormality, namely, airflow limitation.

EPIDEMIOLOGY

COPD is increasing in prevalence and severity throughout the world and is projected to become the fifth leading cause of disease burden worldwide by 2020 (1). Between 1979 and 1999, the mortality rate of chronic bronchitis and emphysema increased by 40%, which is notable because the all-cause death rate fell by 18% in the same period (2,3). Since then, COPD mortality in men has stabilized, whereas it continues to increase in women. Overall, COPD is the fourth leading cause of death in the United States, accounting for 120,000 deaths per year, equally distributed between men and women. Eleven million Americans alive today have been diagnosed with COPD, including three million with emphysema. The direct health care costs for COPD are $21 billion ($US) per year.

Asthma occurs at some time in approximately 11% of the general population, with 31 million Americans reporting a lifetime history of asthma and 20 million reporting currently active asthma. The disease is more prevalent among African American and Hispanic minorities, who suffer the greatest morbidity and mortality from the disease. Approximately 5,000 deaths per year are caused by asthma, occurring disproportionately in inner-city minorities. Since 1996, there has been a slow downward trend in asthma mortality (4). The direct medical costs from asthma are $9 billion per year, with approximately half resulting from hospitalization. Asthma is the most common chronic condition leading to missed school days in children, costing more than $1.4 billion dollars in indirect health costs (2).

PATHOPHYSIOLOGIC ABNORMALITIES IN OBSTRUCTIVE LUNG DISEASE

The diagnosis, severity, clinical course, and response to treatment can best be established by objective tests of lung function. How these disorders lead to chronic airflow limitation and how this limitation is measured in the ambulatory patient are discussed.

Forced Expiratory Spirometry

Obstructive lung diseases cause the lung to empty slowly during a forced expiratory maneuver. Normal people can forcefully expel all of the air that can leave their lungs (vital capacity) within 4 to 6 seconds. People with established obstructive lung disease may continue to expire during a forced expiratory maneuver for 10 to 20 seconds or more.

Forced Expiratory Vital Capacity and Forced Expiratory Volume in 1 Second

The forced expiratory vital capacity test is used to diagnose and follow the course of obstructive lung diseases.

TABLE 60.1 Indications for Spirometry

Establish diagnosis of obstructive lung disease
Establish prognosis of obstructive lung disease
Evaluate acute bronchodilator response
Evaluate response to treatment
Measure physiologic impairment for disability rating
Evaluate thoracic and nonthoracic surgical risk

The test is performed by having the patient blow forcefully into a device that records the volume of air leaving the lungs as a function of time. The record of the maneuver is called a *spirogram,* and the test itself is called forced *expiratory spirometry.* Devices that record the spirogram may either measure flow directly (a pneumotachometer) and calculate volume electronically or measure volume directly (a spirometer). Many such devices are commercially available and are accurate and reliable, but it is important to ascertain that the devices meet established standards that are promulgated for either screening or diagnostic purposes (5). More common than inaccurate equipment is the inability of the technician to elicit maximum effort from the test subject. A good spirometry technician must be both enthusiastic and demanding. Although diagnostic spirometers require daily calibration, office spirometers do not (5). Anyone caring for patients with obstructive lung diseases should have ready access to spirometry. Table 60.1 lists indications for spirometry.

The *forced expiratory maneuver* is performed by having the patient take a maximal inspiration and then forcefully blow all of the air into the spirometer. A technically satisfactory maneuver is one that has a rapid onset, has a smooth contour without hesitation or coughing, and is prolonged until airflow ceases, with a minimum duration of 6 seconds. The test is repeated until three technically satisfactory maneuvers are obtained, two of which give reproducible measurements. Reproducible measurements are defined as being within 5% of each other or within 150 mL, whichever is greater (Table 60.2).

Many measures can be derived from the forced expiratory spirogram, but the most useful are FVC (forced vital capacity; total amount of air leaving the lung); FEV_1 (forced expiratory volume in the first second; amount of air leaving the lung in the first second); and FEV_1/FVC or FEV_1% (percentage of total air leaving the lung in 1 second). The volume measures are expressed as absolute values adjusted to reflect the volume of gas at body temperature with 100% humidity (BTPS). FEV_1 and FVC are compared to predicted values based on age, gender, race, and height from a healthy reference population, usually as a percent of predicted. Airflow limitation is present when FEV_1/FVC is reduced below the value found in 95% of healthy nonsmokers (Table 60.3), although many people use an operational definition of $FEV_1/FVC < 0.70$. The severity of airflow obstruction is determined by the reduction in FEV_1. Because diseases of airflow limitation also cause increased trapping of gas in the lung at the end of a forced expiration, FVC commonly is reduced as well. This should not, however, be confused with disorders that are associated with small lungs, the *restrictive lung diseases* (see Chapter 59). Despite the low FVC, the maximum gas volume of the lung—the *total lung capacity* (TLC) (see below)—usually is normal or increased in patients with obstructive disease. Typically, restrictive lung diseases cause an increased FEV_1/FVC in combination with reduced FVC (Table 60.4 and Fig. 60.1).

The degree to which airflow limitation can be reversed rapidly is measured by performing spirometry before and after treatment with an inhaled bronchodilator. A positive response of either FEV_1 or FVC to bronchodilators is defined as a >12% increase above baseline and an increment of at least 200 mL. Although this test is helpful in determining the potential for improvement when there is a rapid response to inhaled bronchodilators, many patients without a rapid response show improvement after several weeks or months of treatment with bronchodilators or anti-inflammatory agents.

Patient Experience. Forced expiratory spirometry can be safely and accurately performed on people with normal lung function as well as those with advanced lung disease, even those who are critically ill. After a nose clip is attached, the patient inspires deeply and then forcefully expires for approximately 6 seconds. Because of the high pleural pressures, patients occasionally experience light-headedness during the maneuver. This can be minimized by having the patient sit during the test. Some patients experience soreness of the chest wall or abdomen for 1 to 2 days after the test, although analgesics are rarely needed.

TABLE 60.2 Criteria for Good Spirometry Session

At least three technically acceptable maneuvers
Rapid start of expiration
Continuous effort without hesitation or coughing
Prolonged effort until plateau (at least 6 seconds)
At least two reproducible maneuvers
FEV_1 and FVC within 5% or 150 mL of highest value

FEV_1, forced expiratory volume in the first second; FVC, forced vital capacity.

Flow–Volume Loops

Forced expiratory airflow is high during the initial part of expiration and gradually falls to zero throughout the maneuver. The forced expiratory maneuver can be plotted as flow in relation to volume. If this is also done during a forced inspiration, the resultant display is called a *flow–volume loop.* Flow–volume loops can be readily calculated

specific antigen challenge does give insight into the pathogenesis of chronic asthma. After inhalation of an antigen of sufficient dose, acute bronchoconstriction lasts for 20 to 60 minutes, the *early phase reaction*. Left untreated, this early bronchospasm resolves within 1 to 2 hours, although it may be reversed earlier with inhaled bronchodilators. Approximately 4 to 24 hours later, however, bronchospasm recurs in less than half of allergic people. It is generally thought that the early-phase reaction is the result of bronchial smooth muscle constriction but that the *late-phase reaction* is the consequence of inflammatory cell recruitment with consequent airway mucosal edema and bronchoconstriction.

Exercise-induced bronchospasm is present in nearly all asthmatics if challenged sufficiently. Following cessation of vigorous exercise, normal individuals show a small amount of bronchodilation. In contrast, susceptible asthmatics develop bronchoconstriction 5 to 20 minutes after stopping exercise. Similar responses can be elicited by breathing cold, dry air. Postulated causes for exercise-induced bronchoconstriction include increases in the osmolality of the airway fluid lining layer because of drying of the airways causing release of inflammatory mediators, direct response of the airways to cooling during exercise hyperpnea, and vascular engorgement of the bronchial mucosa (12,13). Exercise-induced bronchospasm can be effectively prevented by pretreatment with an inhaled β_2-adrenergic agonist, a leukotriene inhibitor, or a mast-cell stabilizer such as nedocromil. If a patient does not report improvement of exercise-induced symptoms with β agonists, pretreatment exercise-induced bronchospasm usually is not demonstrated on formal testing (14).

Patient Experience (Exercise Bronchoprovocation). The patient should avoid bronchodilators in the same fashion as for methacholine challenge testing and leukotriene antagonists and mast-cell stabilizing agents such as cromolyn or nedocromil for 24 hours. The patient exercises on a bicycle ergometer or treadmill to tolerance. After stopping exercise, spirometry is performed several times for the following 30 minutes. If bronchospasm occurs, it is reversed with an inhaled bronchodilator (11).

Airway Inflammation and Remodeling

The mechanisms that cause nonspecific airway reactivity are not completely understood; however, it is now recognized that airway inflammation is linked to the presence of airway reactivity. Even mild asymptomatic asthmatics show submucosal infiltration with neutrophils, eosinophils, monocytes, T lymphocytes, and mast cells; edema; vascular engorgement; subepithelial collagen and fibronectin deposition; and epithelial desquamation. Patients with more long-standing asthma show hyperplasia of smooth muscle, goblet cell metaplasia, and mucous gland hypertrophy. It is thought that the chronic changes in airway morphology contribute to the nonreversible changes in lung function found in long-standing asthmatics (15,16).

Numerous theories explaining how airway inflammation leads to airway reactivity and remodeling have been advanced. It is likely that asthma is the common expression of several mechanisms or that one mechanism is predominant in some situations but not others. Whatever the mechanism, there is strong evidence that treatment of the underlying airway inflammation can reduce airway reactivity and improve asthma symptoms (17). There is no evidence, however, that anti-inflammatory treatment can prevent remodeling of the airways and improve long-term lung function (18).

Pathophysiology of the Acute Asthmatic Attack

The acute asthmatic attack may occur suddenly as a consequence of exposure to an allergic or irritant substance producing severe bronchospasm in an individual with previously well-controlled asthma and normal lung function. More commonly, the attack occurs after many days of progressive reductions in lung function, increasing lability of lung function, progressive exertional dyspnea and cough, nocturnal awakening, and increasing requirements for symptomatic use of inhaled bronchodilators.

During the acute attack, bronchospasm, mucosal edema, and mucous plugging lead to narrowing and closure of small peripheral airways. This causes an increase in resistance to inspiratory and expiratory airflow and, more important, trapping of air. The patient must breathe at high volume to keep the airways open. The consequences of this hyperinflation are increased work of breathing, impaired mechanical advantage of the shortened respiratory muscles and of the flattened diaphragm, pulmonary hypertension, and markedly negative inspiratory swings in pleural pressure to initiate airflow. If the attack is severe or prolonged, respiratory muscle fatigue can occur with consequent hypoventilation, carbon dioxide retention, hypoxemia, respiratory failure, and death. Arterial blood gas tensions in nonsevere asthma attacks usually show hypocapnia from hyperventilation. A normal arterial carbon dioxide tension may indicate either resolution of the attack or impending respiratory failure and therefore must be correlated with other clinical features. Ventilation–perfusion mismatch accounts for the hypoxemia that accompanies an asthma attack; however, treatment with β-adrenergic bronchodilators usually worsens ventilation–perfusion matching, causing transient worsening hypoxemia as the asthma attack improves. Resolution of the attack often is preceded by expectoration of copious secretions with small mucous plugs. As the attack resolves, dyspnea and chest tightness disappear before wheezing resolves, whereas abnormalities of lung function can persist for many days or weeks.

Clinical Presentations

Clinical presentations of asthma differ with regard to chronicity and inciting factors. There is broad overlap between these categories of asthma, and they should not necessarily be considered to have differing underlying mechanisms.

Extrinsic or *allergic asthma* is a condition in which worsening of the asthma can be clearly associated with exposure to a specific allergen (Table 60.6). In >80% of cases, allergic asthma is associated with allergic rhinitis. The most common perennial allergens associated with worsening of asthma include molds (particularly *Alternaria*), house dust mite feces, cockroach trailings, cat secretions, and mouse feces (19,20). The most common seasonal allergens are ragweed (autumn), tree pollen (spring), and grass pollens (summer). Diagnosis of a specific allergen triggering asthma requires a history of worsening asthma after exposure, improvement of the asthma when the allergen is removed, and positive wheal and flare reaction to the offending agent on allergy skin testing. Clear association of asthma with a specific allergen is important because control of environmental exposure or specific immunotherapy can be time consuming, expensive, or impractical. When an aeroallergen is clearly associated with asthma symptoms, immunotherapy with weekly allergy injections may lead to mild, although transient, improvement in the disease (21). In most cases, however, asthma is adequately treated in the absence of immunotherapy (22). When allergic asthma is severe and does not respond to usual treatments, maintenance treatment with monoclonal antibodies to immunoglobulin (Ig)E (i.e., omalizumab [Xolair] 150–375 mg by subcutaneous injection every 2–4 weeks based on body weight and IgE level) may be helpful (23,24).

Intrinsic or nonallergic asthma is a condition in which there is no clear association with specific allergen exposure. This form of asthma is more common in adults than in children, and it is more common in women than in men. Typically, the asthma symptoms are perennial. Acute episodes may be triggered by viral illnesses, but often no specific provocative stimulus can be found. In approximately half of the cases, the asthma persists or worsens throughout life, leading to incompletely reversible abnormalities of pulmonary function. When this is associated with chronic cough and sputum production, it often is called *chronic asthmatic bronchitis* and may be difficult to distinguish from smoking-related chronic obstructive lung disease. The cause of this form of asthma is unclear. Many patients show some traits of allergic tendencies with elevation of serum IgE levels and eosinophilic airway inflammation, but allergy skin testing is negative. In some cases, it appears that the onset of disease followed a severe lower respiratory tract viral infection, whereas in others it may be associated with long-term exposure to specific allergens or respiratory irritants.

Occupational asthma (see Chapter 8) is a condition in which a specific occupational exposure leads to cough, wheezing, and chest tightness. If exposure to the offending antigen persists, a chronic asthmatic condition with sensitivity to nonspecific agents may occur. If exposure to the sensitizing agent is stopped soon enough, symptoms and nonspecific airway reactivity often resolve, although it may take up to 2 years. Because the prognosis for remission is better in those who cease exposure early, the treating clinician needs to diagnose occupational asthma early and initiate steps to avoid continued exposure (25). Table 60.7 lists common substances that may cause occupational asthma.

Reactive airways dysfunction syndrome (RADS) is a disorder that follows an intense short-term exposure to a toxic, nonallergenic substance, such as sulfuric acid, nitric acid, chlorine, or hydrochloric acid fumes. After the exposure—often the result of an industrial accident or fire—and resolution of the resultant acute lung injury, the individual is left with chronic airway reactivity to nonspecific physicochemical agents such as tobacco smoke or cold air. The disorder may resolve after several months but can lead to chronic airway reactivity (26).

Exercise-induced bronchospasm is present in most asthmatics, although some children and young adults experience asthma only after exercise. Although this syndrome may be confused with exertional dyspnea or angina, careful questioning will reveal that the dyspnea occurs after a 5- to 20-minute symptom-free interval after the cessation of exercise. Exercise-induced bronchospasm is thought to be caused by airway cooling and drying leading to hyperosmolar airway lining fluids and release of bronchoconstrictor and vasodilator mediators (13). For this reason, exercise-induced bronchospasm often is worse in cold, dry environments whereas warm, humid environments, such as indoor swimming pools, often are well tolerated. The symptoms can be prevented by inhalation of a β-agonist bronchodilator or nedocromil approximately 20 minutes before exercise or by regular use of a leukotriene antagonist (see below for a discussion of these agents).

Triad asthma (Samter syndrome) is a syndrome of nasal polyps, asthma, and aspirin sensitivity. One of three asthmatics with nasal polyps has aspirin sensitivity, in comparison to one in 15 asthmatics without nasal polyps. These individuals often have severe chronic asthma and occasionally experience systemic anaphylactic reactions to aspirin or aspirinlike compounds, including nonsteroidal anti-inflammatory drugs (NSAIDs) (27). Even asthmatics who are aware that they are sensitive to aspirin (10% of asthmatics) may inadvertently use compounded drugs that contain aspirin (see Chapter 30 for a list of common medicines that contain aspirin). The mechanism

TABLE 60.7 Occupational Exposures Causing Asthma

Agent	Specific Examples	Occupation
Birds	Pigeons, chickens	Pigeon breeders, poultry workers
Chemicals	Hexachlorophene, formalin, ethylene diamine, metabisulfite	Hospital workers, photographers, food preparation workers, water purification workers
Crustaceans	Crabs, shrimp	Food processing workers
Drugs	Antibiotics, sulfa derivatives	Workers in pharmaceutical industry, agricultural feed mixing
Enzymes	*Bacillus subtilis,* trypsin, papain	Detergent handlers, pharmaceutical industry workers
Epoxy resins	Anhydride compounds	Workers in manufacturing, auto body repair
Laboratory animals	Rats, mice, rabbits, guinea pigs	Laboratory workers, veterinarians
Metals	Platinum, nickle, chromium, cobalt, vanadium	Workers in metal plating, leather tanning, hard metal industry
Plants	Grain dust, flour	Grain handlers, bakers, millers
Plastics and rubber	TDI (toluene diisocyanate), DDI (diphenylmethane diisocyanate), azodicarbonamide	Polyurethane plastic, paint, varnish, and rubber workers
Soldering fluxes	Colophony, aminoethylethanolamine	Electronics, aluminum fabrication workers
Vegetable products	Gum acacia	Printing workers
Wood dust	Cedar, redwood	Carpenters, construction workers, woodmill workers

Adapted from Chan-Yeung M. Occupational asthma. Chest 1990;98:148S, with permission.

by which this occurs is thought to involve blockade of cyclooxygenase-derived prostaglandins and the induction of lipoxygenase-derived leukotrienes from inflammatory cells. The asthma may improve with surgical removal of the nasal polyps, but the polyps often recur and require long-term topical or systemic corticosteroid treatment. If aspirin is required for treatment of another condition, rapid desensitization can be performed, but daily maintenance doses of aspirin are required to sustain the effect. Aspirin-sensitive asthma is an indication for use of leukotriene antagonists or inhibitors such as montelukast, zafirlukast, or zileuton because increased leukotriene production is a prominent feature of this syndrome. Specific cyclooxygenase-2 inhibitors appear to be well tolerated by patients with aspirin sensitivity, likely because of the lack of effect on the constitutive form of cyclooxygenase (28,29). Some epidemiologic evidence also suggests that acetaminophen use may be associated with asthma. However, in most people with asthma, acetaminophen is a safe analgesic and should be avoided only in individuals who demonstrate an association of its use with worsening asthma symptoms (30).

Cough-variant asthma is a condition in which wheezing, dyspnea, and chest tightness are minimal symptoms, but chronic cough is the major complaint. Approximately 30% of patients with chronic persistent cough for >8 weeks have airway reactivity and respond to treatment with bronchodilators and corticosteroids (31,32).

Allergic bronchopulmonary aspergillosis (ABPA) is an uncommon form of asthma that is difficult to treat and can lead to chronic respiratory failure. The disorder is caused by local allergic reaction to noninvasive *Aspergillus* or to other fungal species colonizing the airway. *Aspergillus fumigatus,* a ubiquitous saprophyte, is the most common organism, but other fungi can cause the syndrome. The chronic inflammatory condition leads to dilation and bronchiectasis of the central airways, recurrent mucous plugging and segmental atelectasis, and eventually fibrotic destruction of lung parenchyma. Criteria for the diagnosis of ABPA include recurrent atelectasis and pulmonary infiltrates; radiographic evidence of proximal bronchiectasis or mucoid impactions, blood, and sputum eosinophilia; immediate skin test reactivity to *Aspergillus;* serum precipitins to *Aspergillus;* elevated serum IgE; and specific IgG and IgE antibodies to *Aspergillus* by radioallergosorbent test (RAST) or enzyme-linked immunosorbent assay (ELISA) testing (see below). Individuals with variants of the cystic fibrosis transmembrane regulator gene and certain HLA-DR genotypes are predisposed to develop ABPA (33,34).

The usual treatment for ABPA consists of systemic corticosteroids with starting dosages of 0.5 to 1.0 mg/kg/day of prednisone or equivalent. At least 6 months of therapy usually is required, but many patients are never able to tolerate permanent steroid cessation. Inhaled or systemic antifungal therapy is not helpful in eradicating the offending agent, although evidence indicates that long-term treatment with oral agents such as itraconazole may permit a reduction in the steroid dose (35,36). Early diagnosis and treatment are necessary to prevent the progressive bronchiectasis and lung fibrosis that can occur. The effectiveness of therapy is monitored with serum IgE levels and chest x-ray films. Because ABPA is found in approximately 10% of cystic fibrosis patients, the clinician should consider screening for cystic fibrosis with sweat chloride concentrations or genetic analysis in patients with ABPA.

Refractory or *severe asthma* is defined as dyspnea, wheezing, and frequent exacerbations despite maximum therapy with bronchodilators and inhaled and systemic corticosteroids (37). When symptoms are intractable, the possibility should be considered that a condition that mimics asthma (see below) is present. Other circumstances that may contribute to intractable asthma include an occult persistent exposure to an allergen or irritant at home or at work, use of β-blockers either systemically or as eye drops, use of aspirin or related drugs, exposure to dietary chemicals such as sulfites, hypothyroidism or hyperthyroidism, gastroesophageal reflux, sinusitis, bronchopulmonary aspergillosis, and mucocutaneous fungal infection. However, the most likely cause of intractable asthma is nonadherence to prescribed treatment, a behavior that often is underestimated (38). When aggravating factors are eliminated, some patients still have episodes of life-threatening asthma. The inflammatory profile in these patients is quite variable; some exhibit persistent airway eosinophilia whereas others show neutrophilia or little cellular inflammation (39).

Catastrophic asthma occurs in individuals who experience rapid deterioration of asthma with fatal or near-fatal consequences. In most cases this occurs in people with severe underlying disease, but it can occur in those without such a history. The severity of the attack often is not recognized by the patient or caregiver, and the ability to predict such events is poor. Approximately one third of fatal asthma attacks are preceded by recurrent hospitalizations, but only one of 20 is preceded by previous near-fatal attacks. The prognosis of patients who had a near-fatal attack of asthma is poor, with 10% dying within 1 year (40).

A wheezing condition not due to asthma may be confused with asthma, often as an intractable case, by the patient or clinician. Such conditions include congestive heart failure, mitral stenosis, cystic fibrosis, immotile cilia syndrome, immunoglobulin deficiency, laryngeal tumors, vocal cord paralysis, laryngospasm, airway foreign body, hypereosinophilic syndromes, endobronchial sarcoidosis, bronchiolitis obliterans, Churg–Strauss vasculitis, multiple pulmonary emboli, reaction to angiotensin-converting enzyme inhibitors, pertussis, and diphtheria. A common disorder mimicking severe episodic asthma is paroxysmal vocal cord dysfunction syndrome, where inspiration is accompanied by paradoxical closure of the vocal cords. Careful examination may allow differentiation of upper airway conditions from asthma. Upper airway obstructions cause monophonic (i.e., single-pitch) inspiratory or inspiratory–expiratory high-pitched sounds (stridor) heard loudest over the central airways. In contrast, asthmatic wheezing causes polyphonic expiratory sounds that are heard loudest over the chest. When there is a question of upper airway obstruction, laryngoscopy and flow–volume loops should be obtained, particularly during a symptomatic episode. A variant of paroxysmal vocal cord dysfunction is the "irritable larynx" syndrome, which is characterized by severe episodes of cough, stridor, and dysphonia. This syndrome may follow exposure to an inhaled irritant or a viral syndrome and often is exacerbated by gastroesophageal reflux and anxiety (41). Another common disorder that is sometimes confused with asthma is the syndrome of "sighing dyspnea" or "functional dyspnea." The characteristic presentation of this syndrome is the episodic sensation that a deep breath is not adequately refreshing or that the lungs cannot expand enough. In contrast to most intrinsic lung disorders, the symptoms are relieved by exercise. In some cases, particularly if it occurs in a background setting of asthma or if the symptoms are described as chest tightness and associated with anxiety, sighing dyspnea can be misdiagnosed as asthma (42).

Evaluation of Chronic Asthma

Medical History and Clinical Interview

A thorough medical history is essential for establishing the diagnosis of asthma and for guiding treatment. The following factors should be evaluated: duration, frequency, and severity of attacks; seasonal variation of disease; specific triggers; occupational and recreational exposures; home conditions; other allergic conditions; and medication use and adherence.

Asthmatics describe their episodic shortness of breath differently than do patients with other forms of lung disease or heart failure. Asthmatics use terms such as *chest tightness* and *wheeziness* rather than *air hunger, suffocation,* or *rapid breathing.* Asthmatics often say the site of obstruction is in their neck. They tend to report more difficulty with inspiration than expiration, in contrast to patients with emphysema, who cannot distinguish inspiratory from expiratory distress (43,44).

Asthma should not be considered well controlled if patients have more than occasional requirement for symptomatic use of inhaled bronchodilators or experience nocturnal awakening with symptoms. The presence of nocturnal symptoms is such a characteristic feature of asthma that the absence of this history should stimulate the investigation of other causes of episodic wheezing and chest tightness. Although pollen seasons and common aeroallergens vary geographically, asthma that is worse in the early fall suggests ragweed allergy; worse in the summer, grass pollen allergy; and worse in the spring, tree pollen allergy. Specific asthma triggers (Table 60.6) should be elicited. Because the symptoms of asthma may follow an allergic exposure by 2 to 24 hours, elicitation of such exposures requires careful questioning or the maintenance of a prospective asthma diary recording exposures, symptoms, and peak flow. Occupational exposures may be obvious (Table 60.7) but also can occur from operations in an adjacent workspace or via ventilation systems. Supportive evidence of an occupational trigger exposure is the absence of symptoms on weekends and during vacations. Occasionally a worksite inspection performed by an expert in occupational medicine is necessary (see Chapter 8).

In cases where the importance of home exposure is unclear, the patient should be questioned about whether the asthma worsened upon moving to a new home and whether it improves during periods away from home. Perennial allergen and irritant exposures at home contribute to the chronic airway inflammation that causes asthma, particularly in children. House dust mites feed on desquamated human skin and produce allergenic feces that are easily respirable. Dust mites thrive in humid, warm environments, particularly feather pillows, comforters, carpets, upholstered furniture, and mattresses. Cockroaches and their excreta are highly allergenic. Pets, particularly cats and dogs, secrete antigen in their saliva that may persist in the home environment many years after the pets are no longer present. Frequent vacuuming, although useful in eliminating home allergens, also disperses antigen into the air for several hours. Smokers in the home also disperse irritant sidestream smoke that worsens asthma. Humidifiers or other causes of high ambient humidity promote the growth of molds as well as of dust mites. Some exposures may be difficult to uncover. Urea–formaldehyde foam insulation can cause low-level irritant exposure that is a potential aggravator of asthma. Newly varnished floors or furniture can give off isocyanate fumes that worsen asthma. Toluene diisocyanate (TDI) exposure can trigger severe asthma in those who use polyurethane paint or varnish (45). Heavy mold exposure occurs in those who engage in water sports or boating. Seminal fluid allergy can rarely occur in those who have coitus (46).

Knowledge of associated allergic conditions is helpful. Histories of allergic rhinitis, eczema, and urticaria can assist in determining specific asthma triggers and would support more specific therapies directed toward those allergens. Chronic allergic or infectious sinusitis can exacerbate asthma, and symptoms or sinus pain or drainage should be elicited (47).

Gastroesophageal reflux, often otherwise asymptomatic, may trigger nocturnal asthma either through reflex distention and irritation of the esophagus or through aspiration of gastric contents into the larynx and lower airways (48–50). *Tartrazine* (yellow dye no. 5) is found in yellow or orange foods, particularly powdered orange juice substitutes. Although tartrazine once was thought to be a common cause of asthma in aspirin-sensitive individuals, true tartrazine sensitivity now is considered to be exceedingly rare (51). *Sulfites,* present in dried fruits, wines, processed potatoes, seafood, and salad greens, can cause acute asthma attacks. The mechanism is thought to be associated with production of sulfur dioxide. Although some patients attribute asthma symptoms to ingestion of *monosodium glutamate,* sometimes found in Asian cooking or snack foods, this trigger rarely can be verified objectively (52). It should not be assumed that asthmatics do not smoke *cigarettes.* As many as 30% of asthmatics are cigarette smokers. Evidence indicates that cigarette-smoking asthmatics receive less benefit from inhaled steroids and leukotriene antagonists. Air pollution (particularly respirable particulates, ozone, SO_2, and NO_2) has been implicated as an exacerbating factor for asthma during atmospheric inversions in the summer (53,54).

Only approximately 50% of asthmatics adhere to their prescribed drug regimen, often without admitting this to the treating practitioner. Adherence worsens as the drug program becomes more complex, and there is less adherence with drugs that prevent but do not relieve symptoms (55). It is important to elicit in a friendly and supportive manner whether the patient actually is following the prescribed program. This can be aided by questions such as, "How often do you have difficulty taking your medications on a routine basis?" or "What problems have you had in taking your medicines?" Barriers to adherence (see Chapter 4) include failure to accept or understand the benefit and purpose of medication and environmental controls, the high cost of drugs and supplies, frequent dosing of multiple drugs, side effects of treatment, and disorganized, stressful living conditions. These elements need to be explored and modified when possible.

Obesity is a risk factor for the development of asthma, particularly in women. The pathophysiologic link between asthma and obesity is not known but may be related to mechanical effects of obesity preventing periodic dilation of airways with tidal breathing, production of inflammatory adducts by adipose cells, or predisposition to gastroesophageal reflux (56).

Physical Examination

Physical examination of the patient with asthma should be directed toward confirming the diagnosis, estimating the severity of disease, evaluating related conditions, and ruling out other disorders that mimic asthma.

During an *acute asthmatic attack,* the patient appears frightened and fatigued. The respiratory pattern is deep and slow with a prolonged expiratory phase but may progress to rapid shallow breathing with expiratory grunting that heralds the onset of respiratory failure. Speech is telegraphic or absent. Coughing is ineffective. The chest appears hyperinflated, with reduced tidal expansion compared to the strong respiratory efforts. The sternomastoid muscles are contracted with each inspiration during severe episodes. Hyperinflation of the lungs causes the lower lateral rib cage to move inward with each inspiratory contraction of the flattened diaphragm rather than outward as normally occurs. Tachycardia is present, with weakening of the pulse during inspiration. An inspiratory fall in systolic blood pressure *(pulsus paradoxus)* of >15 mm Hg is present in severe attacks but may disappear with the onset of respiratory failure (57). The chest has diffuse polyphonic expiratory wheezes, but in the most severe attacks may be silent. Inspiratory wheezing suggests the presence of upper airway obstruction, whereas localized or monophonic wheezing suggests mechanical bronchial obstruction from tumor or foreign body. Absent breath sounds in one hemithorax with wheezing in the other should raise the possibility of *pneumothorax,* a potentially lethal complication.

In chronic asymptomatic asthma, the chest examination often is normal. The presence of mild airflow obstruction can be determined by listening for wheezes during a forced expiration. However, this finding is neither sensitive nor specific for asthma. Associated allergic rhinitis causes the nasal mucosa to be pale and edematous. Nasal polyps appear as tan–gray mucoid lesions that obstruct the nasal aperture.

Examination should be directed at disorders that mimic asthma. Listening over the neck during forced inspiration or with the arm extended over the head can bring out inspiratory stridor with upper airway obstruction. Findings of congestive heart failure, such as chest crackles, cardiomegaly, or mitral regurgitation, should be carefully evaluated. High-pitched monophonic localized inspiratory squeaks suggest the presence of bronchiolitis.

Laboratory Testing

Spirometry (see above) should be performed in all asthmatics in the asymptomatic phase and periodically during the course of therapy to establish a baseline severity and to monitor therapy. Persistent abnormalities of pulmonary function, which form the basis for recurrent attacks of asthma, are present in the asymptomatic phase. The chest x-ray film usually is normal in asymptomatic asthma but shows hyperinflation during acute attacks. ABPA shows characteristic central bronchiectasis and ovoid shadows that are signs of mucus impaction. During severe acute asthma attacks, pneumothorax or pneumonia may require specific treatment. Peripheral blood eosinophilia is common in the patient with asthma, particularly if the patient is not receiving corticosteroids. Microscopic examination of unstained sputum can distinguish eosinophils from neutrophils in the presence of purulence, guiding the need for corticosteroids versus antibiotics. In severe corticosteroid-treated asthma, however, neutrophils may predominate in the absence of bacterial infection (58). Other features characteristic of asthmatic sputum are *Charcot–Leyden crystals,* which are spear-shaped crystals derived from eosinophil granules; *Curschmann spirals,* which are mucous casts of small airways; and *Creola bodies*, which are clumps of desquamated ciliated epithelial cells.

Skin testing for specific allergens is helpful for diagnosing specific allergies, particularly when environmental control procedures are costly or difficult, such as changing occupations or residences or eliminating a beloved pet. However, positive allergy skin tests do not indicate allergy to a particular substance as the cause of asthma unless there is a compatible history. *RASTs* measure allergen-specific IgE in the blood and may be substituted for skin testing. *Total serum IgE* is elevated in asthma but is useful mainly for diagnosis and monitoring of ABPA (see above). *Methacholine challenge* is helpful when the diagnosis of asthma is uncertain. A normal methacholine challenge in a symptomatic person virtually eliminates the diagnosis of active asthma. *Flow–volume loops* and *nasopharyngoscopy* are useful tests for determining whether vocal cord dysfunction is mimicking asthma.

Treatment

The goals of asthma treatment are to keep the patient symptom-free day and night, with full activity levels, normal lung function, absent side effects, and satisfaction with the process of care. For most patients who can adhere to a comprehensive asthma management plan, these goals are realistically attainable.

Treatment in the ambulatory setting has four major components: monitoring of symptoms and lung function, control of environmental triggers, education of the patient and family, and drug therapy (Table 60.8).

Home Monitoring of Lung Function

Monitoring lung function with objective tests is important in asthmatics who must use symptomatic bronchodilator treatments more than twice per week or who have experienced severe attacks. Inexpensive peak flow monitors are commercially available. Recording peak flow gives an indication of maximal lung function, can forecast the worsening of asthma before severe symptoms develop, allows objective identification of harmful environmental or occupational exposures, and facilitates telephone contact between the patient and medical caregivers. A practical regimen is to record the peak flow daily in the morning. If the value is <80% of the patient's personal best level, additional recordings during the day are warranted. The determination of a patient's personal best level can be obtained during a 2- or 3-week period of intensive asthma treatment and should be periodically updated. Asthma diaries are helpful for recording patterns of peak flow variation, symptoms, and use of symptomatic bronchodilators (Fig. 60.3).

TABLE 60.8 Components of Asthma Treatment

Components
Monitor symptoms and lung function
Control adverse environmental exposures
Educate patient and family
Administer drug therapy

ASTHMA SYMPTOM AND PEAK FLOW DIARY

__**My predicted peak flow**
__**My personal best peak flow**
__**My Green (OK) Zone (80-100% of personal best)**
__**My Yellow (Caution) Zone (50-80% of personal best)**
__**My Red (Danger) Zone (below 50% of personal best)**

Date														
	a.m.	p.m.	a.m.	p.m.	a.m.	p.m.	a.m.	p.m.	a.m.	p.m.	a.m.	p.m.	a.m.	p.m.
Peak flow reading														
No asthma symptoms														
Mild asthma symptoms														
Moderate asthma symptoms														
Serious asthma symptoms														
Medicine used to stop														
Urgent visit to the doctor														

1. Take your peak flow reading every morning (a.m.) when you wake up and every night (p.m.) at bedtime. Try to take your peak flow readings at the same time each day. If you take an inhaled beta$_2$-agonist medicine, take your peak flow reading *before* taking that medicine. Write down the highest reading of three tries in the box that says peak flow reading.
2. Look at the box in the upper left of this sheet to see whether your number is in the green, yellow, or red zone.
3. In the space below the date and time, put an "X" in the box that matches the symptoms you have when you record your peak flow reading.
4. Look at your asthma control plan for what to do when your number is in one of the zones and you have asthma symptoms.
5. Put an "X" in the box beside "medicine use" if you took *extra* asthma medicine to stop your symptoms.
6. If you made any visit to your doctor's office, emergency room, or hospital for treatment of an asthma episode, put an "X" in the box marked "urgent visit." Tell your doctor if you went to the emergency room or hospital.

No symptoms = No symptoms (wheeze, cough, chest tightness, or shortness of breath) even with normal physical activity.

Mild symptoms = Symptoms during physical activity, but not at rest. It does not keep you from sleeping or being active.

Moderate symptoms = Symptoms while at rest; symptoms may keep you from sleeping or being active.

Serious symptoms = Serious symptoms at rest (wheeze may be absent); symptoms cause problems walking or talking; muscles in neck or between ribs are pulled in when breathing.

FIGURE 60.3. Asthma symptom and peak flow diary.

Control of Environmental Triggers and Complicating Conditions

Environmental controls for asthma include the identification and removal of nonspecific irritants and the reduction of exposure to specific allergens. Smoking should be discouraged, and *smoking cessation* may require repeated strong personalized messages, referral to smoking cessation group programs, and drug therapy (see Chapter 27). Household members should be discouraged from smoking, or they should be encouraged to smoke outdoors or to confine smoking to parts of the home not occupied by the asthma patient.

Gastroesophageal reflux may worsen asthma, but whether treatment is indicated in the absence of reflux symptoms is controversial. Small, frequent feedings; elevation of the bed; and antacids, histamine-2 receptor blockers, or proton pump blockers may be prescribed (see Chapter 42) (references above). *Allergic or infectious sinusitis* should be aggressively treated with antibiotics, intranasal steroids, or surgical procedures (59).

Common specific perennial *allergen sources* include house dust mites, cockroaches, molds, and pets. *House dust mites* can be controlled by maintaining low humidity and by removing carpeting and stuffed furniture from the bedroom. Impermeable bedding covers have not been found to be an effective treatment for dust-sensitive asthma (60). Asthmatics should avoid vacuuming or entering a freshly vacuumed area for 1 to 2 hours, or they should wear a protective face mask. High-efficiency vacuum cleaners are available but are of unproven value. Bedding should be washed weekly in hot water (>130°F) to eliminate dust mites. *Fur-bearing animals* shed allergenic saliva and urine, and they should be eliminated from the household if they exacerbate asthma. If the patient or family is unwilling to part with the pet, other partially effective measures include washing the pet frequently, excluding the pet from the asthmatic's bedroom, and blocking forced hot air vents in the asthmatic's bedroom (61). *Cockroach infestation* is a particularly important cause of asthma in inner cities and can be controlled with insecticides, although repeat treatment is required. The preferred methods of cockroach control are boric acid powder, poison baits, and traps (62). *Insecticide sprays,* particularly cholinesterase inhibitors, can cause severe asthma exacerbations by themselves. *Molds* can be controlled in the home by using dehumidifiers and providing adequate ventilation in the kitchen and bathroom. *Mouse antigens* are ubiquitous in the inner city. They have an uncertain relationship to asthma, but elimination of mice is a prudent measure. Indoor air cleaning devices using high-efficiency filters or electrostatic filters can diminish suspended particles of tobacco smoke and mold spores, but they have not been found to improve asthma symptoms in controlled studies (63). Therefore, they are not recommended for routine use and do not substitute for other methods of environmental control. Room or house humidifiers should be avoided because they can increase concentrations of mold spores and house dust mites.

During specific pollen allergy seasons or high air pollution days, asthmatics should stay indoors at midday when pollen concentration is highest and air quality is worst. Outdoor exercise during high air pollution periods should be avoided because high levels of ventilation increase the damaging effect of air pollutants. Closing doors and windows and using a recirculating air conditioner minimize indoor pollen and air pollution exposure.

Exposure to occupational allergens should be controlled by ventilation changes in the workplace. If not possible, personal respiratory protection or job reassignment are required to control exposures. Sources of nonspecific respiratory irritants should be avoided. These include unvented gas, kerosene, or wood-burning stoves and heaters. In highly sensitive individuals, aerosol sprays and perfumed cosmetics may worsen asthma and should be eliminated.

Drugs that worsen asthma, such as aspirin, other NSAIDs, and β-adrenergic blockers, should be avoided or should be monitored closely if no alternatives are possible. Many over-the-counter medications for upper respiratory infections, sinusitis, gastroenteritis, musculoskeletal pain, or menstrual pain contain aspirin, which can worsen asthma in susceptible unaware individuals, and use of such drugs should be avoided. β-Adrenergic blockers may inadvertently be used as eye drops for treatment of glaucoma, with the potential for severe asthma exacerbation. Angiotensin-converting enzyme inhibitors may worsen cough in patients with asthma (64).

Although not based on experimental evidence, annual influenza vaccination is recommended for asthmatics of all ages because the infection can precipitate severe and prolonged exacerbations of asthma (65). Influenza immunization does not induce asthma exacerbations (66).

Education of the Asthmatic

Education of the asthmatic patient is an important obligation of the practitioner. Excellent materials to assist in this process are available from volunteer and government agencies (67–69). The specific aims of education should be to teach the patient to recognize the signs and symptoms of asthma, to use the peak flow meter correctly, to take medication properly, to establish and follow treatment plans for exacerbations, to avoid and control asthma triggers, and to make appropriate use of urgent medical care. Table 60.9 lists important specific topics.

TABLE 60.9 Components of Asthma Education

Description of asthma
What asthma medicines do
Community resources for asthma patients and their families
Correct use of metered-dose inhaler and nebulizer
How to use a peak flow meter
How to record an asthma diary
Warning signs of asthma attacks
Asthma trigger control plan
Steps to manage an asthma attack
School, work, and exercise activity plans

TABLE 60.10 Proper Use of Metered-Dose Inhaler

Action	*Reason for Action*
Shake MDI gently.	Disperses drug evenly with vehicle. Check that canister is full.
Hold the MDI two fingerbreadths from the widely opened mouth.	Larger droplets will rain out in the air rather than impact in the mouth. This prevents mouth and throat irritation with some vehicles and thrush with inhaled corticosteroids.
Breathe normally and pause at quiet end expiration.	Inhaling from a low lung volume allows greater peripheral penetration of the drug.
Actuate the MDI at the onset of inspiration and slowly inhale over 4–6 s.	Slow inspiratory flow rates enhance deposition of particles in the peripheral airways and reduce turbulence and impaction in the upper airway.
Hold the breath for 5–10 s at total lung capacity.	Small respirable particles will be allowed to settle in the smaller airways during the breath-hold.
Exhale slowly.	Slow expiration reduces exhalation of drug from the lung.

MDI, metered-dose inhaler.
Adapted from Newhouse MT, Dolovitch MB. Control of asthma by aerosols. N Engl J Med 1986;315:870, with permission.

Asthmatic patients must be instructed on the proper use of *metered-dose inhalers* (MDIs) for delivery of inhaled medications. Patients should be observed using their inhaler during office visits, and proper technique should be repeatedly taught because some studies have shown that 40% of asthmatics do not use their inhalers properly. Proper technique (Table 60.10) involves the following steps: gently shake the MDI; hold the MDI 2 inches away from the open mouth; trigger the device at the onset of inspiration from normal end-tidal lung volume; inhale slowly to TLC over 5 seconds; hold the breath at TLC for 5 to 10 seconds; and exhale slowly. For patients who cannot perform this maneuver properly despite training and practice, the effectiveness of the MDI can be enhanced by use of a spacer or reservoir device. Some drugs are available in single-dose or multiple-dose dry-powder inhalers or breath-triggered MDIs. These devices are breath activated and are effective for people with poor coordination; however, they require good inspiratory flows to work properly. In uncommon cases where use of an MDI is not effective, small electrically powered nebulizers can deliver bronchodilators. However, use of nebulizers is limited by their lack of portability, their expense, and the need for meticulous cleaning and preparation of solutions. Rinsing the mouth after inhalation of drugs effectively reduces local oropharyngeal side effects and minimizes systemic absorption.

Each asthmatic should have a well-understood action plan for treatment of exacerbations and should be able to recognize the signs of worsening asthma and know what action to take. Such a plan should be based on the patient's history of severity of exacerbations, access to health care, and reliability. Table 60.11 gives a typical action plan.

Drug Treatment for Asthma

Drugs should be used in the treatment of asthma in a stepped approach to normalize activity levels and lung function and to minimize exacerbations (Table 60.12). Once control of asthma is achieved, the program can be slowly tapered to maintain the lowest necessary drug dosage. It is important to distinguish between drugs that are used for short-term relief of symptoms and drugs that are used for long-term control of the underlying disease. The patient's failure to understand this distinction often leads to underuse of anti-inflammatory agents and to overreliance on inhaled short-acting bronchodilators, with consequent failure to meet the goals of asthma care.

Inhaled short-acting selective β_2-agonists should be prescribed for patients with mild asthma. Use should be confined to the minimum number of inhalations needed to control symptoms. Table 60.13 lists several selective β_2-agonists available in MDIs. The choice of which β_2-agonist to use initially should be based on symptomatic relief of the patient and cost, because little else distinguishes most of the agents available by prescription in the United States. Nonprescription asthma inhalers should be avoided

TABLE 60.11 Self-Management of Acute Exacerbations

Monitor peak flow and symptoms.
Use inhaled β-adrenergic agonist every 20 min for three doses, then every 3–4 h for 6–12 h as needed.
Contact clinician or visit emergency department if response to initial treatment is incomplete and peak flow is 50%–70% of baseline.
Go to emergency department if response to initial therapy is poor or peak flow is $<$50% of baseline.

TABLE 60.12 Stepwise Approach to Asthma Care

	Symptoms	*Lung Function*	*Quick Relief Drugs*	*Long-Term Control Drugs*
Step 1: mild intermittent	Symptoms less than twice weekly Brief exacerbations Nocturnal symptoms less than two times per month	FEV_1 or PEFR 80% predicted	Short-acting inhaled β-agonists Use of β-agonist more than twice weekly may indicate need to start control treatment	None needed
Step 2: mild persistent	Symptoms more than twice weekly but not daily Limitation of activity during exacerbations Nocturnal symptoms more than two times per month	FEV_1 or PEFR 80% predicted	Short-acting inhaled β-agonists Use of β-agonist more than once daily may indicate need to increase control treatment	Low-dose inhaled corticosteroid, leukotriene antagonist, or sustained-release theophylline
Step 3: moderate persistent	Daily symptoms Daily use of short-acting bronchodilator Nocturnal symptoms more than once weekly	FEV_1 or PEFR 60%–80% predicted	Short-acting inhaled β-agonists Use of β-agonist more than once daily may indicate need to increase control treatment	Medium-dose inhaled corticosteroid or low-dose inhaled corticosteroid with long-acting bronchodilator (e.g., salmeterol or formoterol) or with leukotriene antagonist
Step 4: severe persistent	Continual symptoms Limited physical activity Frequent exacerbations Frequent nocturnal symptoms	FEV_1 or PEFR 60% predicted	Short-acting inhaled β-agonists Use of β-agonist more than once daily may indicate need to increase control treatment	High-dose inhaled corticosteroid and long-acting bronchodilator (e.g., salmeterol or formoterol) or oral corticosteroid as needed to treat and prevent exacerbations

Principles of Stepwise Care of Asthma

Gain control of asthma as quickly as possible, then decrease treatment to the least medication necessary to maintain control.

A short course of oral corticosteroids may be needed at any step to gain control of asthma or treat exacerbations.

Review treatment at 1- to 6-mo intervals for possible stepwise reduction in treatment.

If control is not maintained, review patient inhaler technique, adherence, and control of environmental irritants, allergens, or adverse drug response (e.g., aspirin, β-blockers).

FEV_1, forced expiratory volume in first second; PEFR, peak expiratory flow rate.

Adapted from National Asthma Education and Prevention Program Expert Panel Report II. Guidelines for the Diagnosis and Management of Asthma. Update of Selected Topics 2002. HHS publication 02-5074. Bethesda: National Heart, Lung and Blood Institute, June 2003, with permission.

TABLE 60.13 β-Sympathomimetic Agonists

Generic Name	Trade Name	β_2 Selectivity	Onset of Action (min)	Inhalation Peak Effect (min)	Effect (h)	Dosage Form
Metaproterenol	Bronkometer Alupent	$\beta_2 >>> \beta_1$	1–5	30–60	2–5	Nebulized solution, 1% Metered-dose inhaler, 650 μg/puff
Terbutaline	Brethine	$\beta_2 >>> \beta_1$	1–5	30–60	2–5	Nebulized solution, 5% Metered-dose inhaler, 200 μg/puff
	Bricanyl					Injection, 1 mg/mL
Bitolterol	Brethaire Tornalate	$\beta_2 >>> \beta_1$	3–5	30–60	4–8	Metered-dose inhaler, 370 μg/puff
Pirbuterol	Maxair	$\beta_2 >>> \beta_1$	5	30–60	4–5	Metered-dose inhaler, 200 μg/puff
Albuterol	Proventil Ventolin	$\beta_2 >>>> \beta_1$	5–15	60–90	3–6	Metered-dose inhaler, 90 μg/puff Nebulized solution 0.5%
Salmeterol	Serevent	$\beta_2 >>>> \beta_1$	10–20	180	12	Metered-dose inhaler, 25 μg/puff
Formoterol	Foradil	$\beta_2 >>>> \beta_1$	5–10	180	12	Dry-powder inhaler, 12 μg/capsule

because many contain epinephrine, which has potentially serious cardiovascular side effects from its α- and β_1-adrenergic properties. For this reason, most of these inhalers have been taken off the retail market. Because selective β_2-agonists are so effective in relieving symptoms of bronchospasm but do not treat the underlying airway inflammation, they have the potential for permitting patients to increase exposure to harmful agents and delay more definitive treatment. Because there are neither harmful nor beneficial effects from regular use of short-acting bronchodilators compared to symptomatic use, it is reasonable to limit their use to control of symptoms only (70). There is evidence that certain β-receptor genotypes, which are more prevalent in African Americans, can predispose to deterioration of asthma control with regular β-agonist use in individual patients (71).

Long-acting selective β-agonists may lead to the development of tolerance to their protective effect against nonspecific bronchial challenge while the acute bronchodilating effects of these drugs are unchanged (72). The typical MDI contains 200 to 300 inhalations and therefore should last approximately 3 to 4 weeks or longer. More frequent use of bronchodilator MDIs usually indicates the need for more intensive anti-inflammatory therapy. In general, however, modern selective β agonists are safe and effective drugs, and they should not be withheld from the symptomatic asthmatic. The most common side effects are tremor and cardiac arrhythmias. An often neglected side effect of chronic use of β-agonists is hypokalemia (apparently caused by an intracellular shift of potassium), which can be corrected with supplemental potassium (see Chapter 50). Long-acting β-agonists, such as salmeterol (Serevent) or formoterol (Foradil), which have a slower onset and longer duration of action, are used for long-term control of symptoms. The use of such agents for short-term relief of symptoms may lead to excessive adrenergic stimulation. Therefore, drugs in this class should be prescribed in conjunction with a shorter-acting agent to be used for acute relief of symptoms. Monotherapy with a long-acting β-agonist should not be substituted for inhaled corticosteroids for prevention of asthma symptoms (73,74).

If bronchodilators are used to treat asthma symptoms more than twice weekly (excluding prophylactic use for exercise), an inhaled anti-inflammatory agent should usually be prescribed. *Inhaled nonsteroidal antiallergy drugs* include cromolyn (Intal-2 metered sprays four times per day) and nedocromil (Tilade-2 metered sprays two to four times per day). These agents have few side effects but have limited efficacy for control of asthma. However, these agents are effective in preventing exercise-induced bronchospasm. Their use is limited by the lack of availability of the high-concentration preparations that have been shown to be most effective and by the recommended frequency of dosing. For patients with mild persistent asthma, particularly those who exhibit aspirin sensitivity, *leukotriene inhibitors* and *antagonists* are effective (75–78). However, some patients show little or no response to leukotriene inhibitors, which may reflect genetic polymorphisms of the enzymes that produce leukotrienes (79).

TABLE 60.14 Approximate Comparative Daily Dosages for Inhaled Corticosteroids in Adults

Drug	Low Dose	Medium Dose	High Dose
Beclomethasone	168–504 μg	504–840 μg	>840 μg
42 μg/puff	4–12 puffs	12–20 puffs	>20 puffs
84 μg/puff	2–6 puffs	6–10 puffs	>10 puffs
Budesonide	200–400 μg	400–600 μg	>600 μg
Turbuhaler			
200 μg/dose	1–2 inhalations	2–3 inhalations	>3 inhalations
Flunisolide	500–1,000 μg	1,000–2,000 μg	>2,000 μg
250 μg/puff	2–4 puffs	4–8 puffs	>8 puffs
Fluticasone	88–264 μg	264–660 μg	>660 μg
44 μg/puff	2–6 puffs		
110 μg/puff		2–6 puffs	>6 puffs
220 μg/puff			>3 puffs
Triamcinolone	400–1,000 μg	1,000–2,000 μg	>2,000 μg
100 μg/puff	4–10 puffs	10–20 puffs	>20 puffs

Adapted from National Asthma Education and Prevention Program Expert Panel Report II. Guidelines for the Diagnosis and Management of Asthma. Update of Selected Topics 2002. HHS publication 02-5074. Bethesda: National Heart, Lung and Blood Institute, June 2003, with permission.

Inhaled corticosteroids are important anti-inflammatory agents and have become the mainstay of treatment for patients with persistent asthma symptoms. They reduce airway inflammation and airway reactivity (80). Although daily inhaled corticosteroids improve asthma control, there is no evidence that daily inhaled corticosteroid treatment of mild persistent asthma improves long-term lung function compared to intermittent symptom-based treatment (81). Most of the side effects are caused by local effects such as oral candidiasis and dysphonia, which can be prevented by use of a spacer/reservoir device or by rinsing the mouth with water after each use. Although biochemical evidence of chemical adrenal suppression and increased bone metabolism is found with high-dose inhalation (>1,200 μg/day) of these agents, clinically noteworthy systemic toxicity is rarely observed. However, reports of increased prevalence of cataracts and bone fractures in older people receiving large doses of inhaled steroids and transiently decreased growth in children receiving moderate doses of inhaled steroids emphasize the importance of using the smallest effective dose (82,83). Inhaled corticosteroids available in the United States include beclomethasone, budesonide, flunisolide, fluticasone, and triamcinolone.

Mometasone and ciclesonide likely will be available in the United States in the near future. All have approximately equivalent efficacy and side effects, although some have more convenient dosages and delivery devices. The drug usually is started at a dosage that is adequate to control asthma symptoms and is decreased to the lowest effective dosage (84). The effect of a change in dosage of inhaled corticosteroids may take 3 to 4 weeks to ascertain. Increasing the dose of inhaled steroids during deterioration of asthma control does not seem to be an effective strategy, and often a better strategy is to add a second class of drugs (85). Table 60.14 lists the equivalence of available formulations of inhaled corticosteroids.

If inhaled corticosteroids do not control symptoms and optimize lung function, consideration should be given to adding a second long-acting drug, such as an oral or inhaled long-acting β-agonist, a leukotriene inhibitor, or a long-acting oral theophylline preparation, to control asthma (86–90). Long-acting agents are particularly helpful when symptoms occur at night. Addition of a long-acting β-agonist has become the most widely used and effective combination therapy. A long-acting *theophylline* preparation may be given at a dosage of 400 to 1,200 mg/day in one or two daily doses. Theophylline should be started at a low dosage that is increased at weekly or longer intervals with monitoring of symptoms. Whether monitoring of blood levels is necessary in the absence of side effects is not clear. Theophylline is a mild bronchodilator that also has a modest anti-inflammatory effect (91,92). Side effects of theophylline include anorexia, nausea, gastroesophageal reflux, anxiety, and palpitations. Serious toxic effects at serum levels >20 μg/mL include seizures and atrial and ventricular tachyarrhythmias. Because theophylline is metabolized by the liver, theophylline interacts with numerous other drugs. Erythromycin, ciprofloxacin and other quinolones, and cimetidine decrease theophylline metabolism and elevate serum levels. Cigarette smoking and hyperthyroidism are associated with increased metabolism and decreased theophylline levels. Congestive heart failure and hepatic insufficiency require a dosage reduction or use of an alternative agent.

Albuterol (2- to 4-mg tablets), an oral, long-acting β-agonist, can be given twice daily. Maximal doses of oral β-adrenergic agonists often are limited by tremor and a sensation of nervousness; therefore, they should be titrated upward starting at half to one quarter the maximum recommended dose. Tolerance to this side effect occurs over several weeks, whereas the bronchodilator action is retained. The availability of *inhaled long-acting β-agonists,* such as salmeterol and formoterol, has supplanted the use of oral agents except in circumstances where cost, adherence, or patient preference dictate their use.

Antileukotriene drugs, leukotriene D_4 receptor antagonists (zafirlukast [Accolate], 20 mg twice per day; montelukast [Singulair] 10 mg once daily), are useful in some asthmatics. The 5-lipoxygenase inhibitor zileuton (Zyflo 600 mg four times daily) has a broader leukotriene inhibitory profile but requires monitoring of liver enzymes. Antileukotriene drugs are best reserved for the patient with mild or moderate asthma, the patient with aspirin sensitivity, the athlete who suffers from exercise-induced asthma, and the patient who is unwilling or unable to use adequate doses of inhaled steroids. Rarely, patients treated with leukotriene antagonists develop a syndrome similar to Churg–Strauss vasculitis, which may reflect unmasking of an underlying disease after tapering of systemic steroids (93). Some patients do not respond to these agents, likely because of genetic predisposition; therefore, treatment should be abandoned if there is no apparent benefit.

Inhaled anticholinergic drugs (e.g., ipratropium bromide) are safe and effective bronchodilators in asthma, and they add some marginal benefit when added to β_2-adrenergic agonists, particularly during an acute exacerbation (94).

When these measures are ineffective in controlling asthma or when previously stable asthma is punctuated by an exacerbation, *oral corticosteroids* should be used. They can be prescribed as a 5- to 14-day course starting at 30 to 60 mg/day of prednisone or equivalent prednisolone, either stopping abruptly or tapering gradually. In more severe cases, tapering of the steroids may take several months or require chronic treatment with daily or every-other-day prednisone. In dosages $>$20 mg/day for long periods, serious complications, including diabetes mellitus, posterior subcapsular cataracts, osteoporosis with compression fractures, and hypothalamic–pituitary–adrenal axis suppression, are common. Because of the serious side effects of chronic steroid use, vigorous efforts should be made to optimize adherence with environmental controls and maximum inhalational drug therapy in these patients. Other disorders that mimic asthma should be investigated. If long-term steroids are necessary, tuberculin skin testing should be considered, although the benefit of isoniazid prophylaxis compared with monitoring with chest x-ray films in this setting is controversial. In those receiving long-term corticosteroid therapy, particularly postmenopausal women, prophylaxis of corticosteroid-induced osteoporosis with vitamin D and calcium supplements or bisphosphonates is recommended (see Chapter 103).

For asthmatic patients who cannot taper steroids, treatment with monoclonal antibodies to IgE should be considered for those with underlying allergies (95). Omalizumab (Xolair) is approved for treatment of moderate to severe allergic asthma. It is given by subcutaneous injection every 2 to 4 weeks. Dosing is based on body weight and total IgE level. For those without atopy, several options may be considered, although none is well established at present. These include methotrexate, cyclosporine, troleandomycin, oral gold salts, hydroxychloroquine, dapsone, inhaled lidocaine, and intravenous immunoglobulin infusions (96–98). If gastroesophageal reflux and associated asthma exacerbations can be documented by esophageal pH probe recording and medical treatment is not helpful, surgical treatment of the reflux should be considered (99) (see Chapter 42). Initiation of these treatments should be undertaken by someone familiar with the treatment of steroid-dependent asthmatics because many such patients will have other diagnoses or can be successfully tapered with consistent comprehensive asthma care.

Emergency Treatment of the Acute Asthma Attack

When asthma fails to respond to home management (Table 60.12), the patient should be instructed to receive immediate treatment in a hospital emergency department or a similarly equipped facility. Both patients and practitioners should understand that untreated severe asthma can be fatal and should recognize the individual at risk (100) (Table 60.15). Treatment should be initiated with nebulized treatments of selective β-adrenergic agonists given as three treatments in the first 60 to 90 minutes (Table 60.16). MDI administration of four to eight inhalations using a reservoir device is as effective as nebulizer therapy and can be used when a nebulizer is not available.

Supplemental oxygen should be given to patients who are hypoxemic or to those in whom arterial oxygen saturation is unknown. Because bronchodilators initially can worsen ventilation–perfusion matching, oxygen saturation

TABLE 60.15 Risk Factors for Fatal Asthma

Previous episode of mechanical ventilation for asthma
Hospitalization for asthma in previous year
Steroid-dependent asthma
Nonadherence to medical treatment
Overuse of inhaled β-adrenergic agonists
Recent steroid taper or abrupt withdrawal
Lack of objective measures of asthma severity
Psychiatric disorder
Inner-city residence, poverty

TABLE 60.16 Dosages of Inhaled β-Adrenergic Agonists in Acute Asthma Exacerbations in Adults

Drug	*Dose (Nebulized in 3–5 mL Sterile Saline Solution)*
Albuterol	2.5 mg (0.5 mL of 0.5% solution)
Levalbuterol	0.63 mg (3.0 mL unit-dose vial, premixed)
Metaproterenol	15 mg (0.3 mL of 5% solution)
Isoetharine	5 mg (0.5 mL of 1% solution)

may fall during the early phases of treatment even as lung function is improving. Peak flow measurement or spirometry should be performed on admission and after each nebulizer treatment to determine response. Arterial blood gases should be checked in patients who appear severely ill to determine whether hypercapnia is present and whether mechanical ventilation might be required. A chest x-ray film should be obtained for patients in whom the possibility of pneumonia, pulmonary edema, or pneumothorax is suspected. Serum theophylline levels should be measured in patients taking theophylline to guide possible therapy with this drug. Serum electrolytes may reveal hypokalemia from excess β-agonist use.

If the initial treatment is unsuccessful, systemic corticosteroids at a dosage of 60 to 125 mg prednisolone intravenously every 6 hours should be initiated (101). Hourly treatments with nebulized bronchodilators should be continued and the response measured. If no response to nebulized bronchodilators is observed over the first 2 to 3 hours, subcutaneous epinephrine 0.2 to 0.4 mg or terbutaline 0.25 mg may be administered. In patients with peak flow <50% of baseline, intravenous theophylline may be beneficial in improving lung function and preventing hospital admission, starting with an infusion of 0.6 mg/kg lean body weight (102). The infusion rate should be 0.3 mg/kg for patients with hepatic disease or for those taking drugs that diminish aminophylline metabolism. In patients not previously taking theophylline, a loading dose of 5 to 6 mg/kg should be given. In those who have been taking theophylline, the dosage should be guided by serum levels, with no more than a 3 mg/kg loading dose. Intravenous fluids should be given for dehydration, but excessive administration of intravenous fluids may worsen the asthma by promoting airway edema.

After the initial treatment, if the patient shows peak flow or FEV_1 <25% of baseline, develops altered sensorium, has an arterial oxygen tension <60 mm Hg on supplemental oxygen, or has arterial carbon dioxide tension >40 mm Hg, the patient should be transferred to an intensive care facility for further treatment, monitoring, and possible mechanical ventilation. In some circumstances, noninvasive positive-pressure ventilation or inhalation of a helium–oxygen mixture may prevent the need for intubation (103).

In most circumstances, the response to the first 4 hours of therapy should determine whether the patient requires hospital admission. Considerations favoring hospitalization include peak flow <40% of baseline, continued severe symptoms, recent history of failed emergency treatment, history of respiratory failure, and inadequate home support or access to medications.

Management of the Pregnant Asthma Patient

Pregnancy has an unpredictable effect on asthma; approximately one third of patients experience no change in symptoms, one third improve, and one third worsen. Poorly controlled asthma may pose an increased risk for prematurity, intrauterine growth retardation, and perinatal morbidity (104). Prolonged or severe asthmatic attacks with hypoxemia or acid–base disturbances pose risks to the fetus, which has borderline oxygenation. Thus, prompt and aggressive management of acute asthmatic episodes should take precedence over concerns that the medications used to manage asthma may pose theoretical risks to the fetus.

In pregnant women, initial treatment during an acute asthmatic attack should include supplemental oxygen to maintain an oxygen saturation >95% for prevention of fetal hypoxemia. Fetal monitoring should be instituted for all but mild asthma attacks.

In general, management of pregnant and nonpregnant asthmatics is the same. Control of symptoms should be attempted with minimal use of medications, but no special attempt to discontinue medications is indicated.

β_2-Adrenergic agents and theophylline are smooth muscle relaxants and therefore may inhibit uterine contractions during labor. They have been used for decades and generally are safe for the fetus. Epinephrine causes vasoconstriction because of its α-adrenergic properties and may diminish placental and fetal blood flow; therefore, it should be avoided if possible. Prednisone and prednisolone, the most commonly used systemic corticosteroids, cross the placenta poorly, so steroid production by the fetus is unaffected. Adrenal steroid suppression in the mother, however, may require administration of supplemental corticosteroids during the stresses of labor and delivery. Long-term use of oral steroids in other conditions has been associated with lower-birth-weight infants, so maximizing inhaled forms of therapy before instituting long-term oral steroids is prudent. The benefits of inhaled steroids outweigh any potential risk to the pregnant asthmatic or her fetus. Controlled trials have shown similar perinatal outcomes with theophylline versus inhaled steroids in pregnant women with asthma, although the inhaled corticosteroids result in greater improvement of FEV_1 (105). As a general rule, relying on drugs that have a long record of safe experience in pregnant asthmatics is prudent (see National Heart, Lung, and Blood Institute; National Asthma Education and Prevention Program Asthma and Pregnancy Working Group, at www.hopkinsbayview.org/PAMreferences).

Course and Prognosis

Asthma that begins at an early age generally improves, and rates of prolonged remission from 30% to 70% have been reported. The severity of asthma correlates with the remission rate, so children with mild disease likely will experience remission, whereas those with severe disease often continue to be symptomatic. Some childhood asthmatics experience a remission but then have a recurrence of asthma in adulthood. Such patients tend to develop disease that is persistent and severe and have deficits in pulmonary function (106).

Patients who first develop asthma as adults have more rapid decline of lung function with aging, which may lead to irreversible airway obstruction. Additional risk factors, such as cigarette smoking, environmental exposures, and infection, may influence the progression of asthma to COPD (see below).

Death from asthma or one of its complications is uncommon, with overall death rates in the United States of approximately 1.5 per 100,000 population. However, asthma mortality increased 31% between 1980 and 1990, with the greatest burden of death sustained by inner-city African-American males. Since 1988, the United States death rate from asthma has tended to stabilize or decrease in association with the wider use of inhaled corticosteroids (4). Similar trends have been documented in other countries (107).

CHRONIC OBSTRUCTIVE PULMONARY DISEASE

Definition

The American Thoracic Society and the European Respiratory Society have adopted similar definitions: "Chronic obstructive pulmonary disease (COPD) is a preventable and treatable disease state characterised by airflow limitation that is not fully reversible. The airflow limitation is usually progressive and is associated with an abnormal inflammatory response of the lungs to noxious particles or gases, primarily caused by cigarette smoking. Although COPD affects the lungs, it also produces significant systemic consequences" (108). COPD can be subclassified further into emphysema and chronic bronchitis.

Emphysema is defined by morphologic criteria as abnormal dilation of the terminal airspaces of the lung with destruction of alveolar septa in the absence of interstitial fibrosis (109). Whereas a formal diagnosis of emphysema requires gross anatomic inspection of the lung, a clinical diagnosis can be reasonably based on a compatible history, physical examination, pulmonary function tests, and radiographic studies. *Panacinar emphysema* is a condition in which all of the airspaces in an acinus are equally dilated. Typically, the bases of the lung are more involved than the apices. This is the typical finding in patients with α_1-antitrypsin deficiency and in some elderly nonsmoking individuals. *Centroacinar emphysema* describes the more prevalent condition in which the respiratory bronchiole at the proximal end of the acinus is more dilated than other portions of the acinus. Commonly, the apices of the lung are more involved in this disorder, which occurs predominantly in cigarette smokers. Peripheral airway disease is commonly associated with centroacinar emphysema, manifested by inflammation, fibrosis, and tortuosity of the terminal and respiratory bronchioles. The physiologic abnormality is the consequence of both the emphysema and the small airway narrowing and fibrosis (110).

Chronic bronchitis is a condition of chronic cough and sputum production that excludes other specific disorders such as bronchiectasis, tuberculosis, or cystic fibrosis. The formal epidemiologic definition of this disorder is the presence of cough and sputum production for the majority of days of the week for at least 3 months of the year for at least 2 years in a row. However, nearly everyone with chronic bronchitis has cough and sputum production on a perennial basis. Chronic bronchitis is common in cigarette smokers and often is incorrectly perceived by the patient to be a normal smoker's cough. The morbid anatomy of chronic bronchitis shows hyperplasia and hypertrophy of the mucous glands of the large central airways with central mucous plugging, variable degrees of smooth muscle hyperplasia, and airway wall thickening and inflammation (111). Chronic bronchitis can occur in the absence of major physiologic abnormalities, and the extent to which it contributes to mortality and morbidity in COPD is controversial. In patients with advanced COPD, mortality is best predicted by the postbronchodilator FEV_1, with little additional information provided by other clinical factors (112). Some epidemiologic studies of people with less severe disease have shown some excess mortality associated with cough and phlegm, but the magnitude is not large (113). Approximately 30% of those with abnormal lung function report cough and phlegm, and the magnitude of the physiologic abnormality is worse in those who report more severe cough and phlegm. COPD patients with chronic cough and phlegm are more prone to exacerbations of COPD than are those without. Some smokers with chronic bronchitis develop severe airflow limitation without emphysema. These individuals are best classified as having *chronic obstructive bronchitis* or, when there is prominent reversible airflow obstruction, *chronic asthmatic bronchitis*.

Natural History

COPD is a chronic disease that has its origins in early adulthood, or possibly even childhood, but it does not produce symptoms or impairment of activity until the disease is far advanced, usually in late middle-age or in the elderly. The normal aging process causes slowly progressive degeneration of lung function after the third decade, so a normal person loses approximately 20% of vital capacity and approximately 25% of FEV_1 between the ages of 25 and 75 years. The average decline in FEV_1 is approximately 30 mL/year, with some acceleration after age 65 years. These changes result from the loss of elastic recoil in the lung from degradation of elastin fibers, similar to the changes that occur in the skin and cause wrinkles. In most cigarette smokers, the rate of decline of FEV_1 is normal or only moderately increased. In susceptible smokers, however, degeneration of lung function is accelerated, at 60 to 150 mL/year loss of FEV_1 (114). Over the course of several decades, the degeneration leads to progressive breathlessness and, if unchecked, to disability, respiratory failure, and death. It has been suggested that children who have serious respiratory ailments or exposure to respiratory toxins, such as passive cigarette smoke, will be at increased risk for development of COPD because of impaired lung function when they are young adults and consequently will have less reserve capacity (Fig. 60.4).

Because of the reserve capacity of the lungs, the early stages of COPD do not cause any limitation of activity. When FEV_1 reaches approximately 50% of predicted, there is ventilatory limitation of exercise capacity, but this often is ignored or attributed to deconditioning, and heavy exercise is progressively curtailed. Respiratory infections may cause severe and prolonged symptoms in this phase of the disease, prompting the patient to seek medical care. When FEV_1 reaches approximately 30% to 35% of predicted (approximately 1.2 L in men and 1.0 L in women), symptoms prevent normal execution of daily living and work activities, and approximately half of afflicted individuals stop working. With continued decline in FEV_1, chronic hypoxemia, hypercapnia, and cor pulmonale develop. Viral infections, mucus plugging, or respiratory irritants—including exposure to air pollutants—can precipitate episodes of acute respiratory failure, leading to hospitalization, mechanical ventilation, or death. More than half of patients with COPD compatible with emphysema die within 10 years after initial diagnosis, whereas approximately 15% of those with chronic asthmatic bronchitis die in the first decade after diagnosis (115).

Cigarette smoking is a major risk factor for development of COPD. Both observational studies and clinical trials have shown that cessation of smoking earlier in the course of disease can slow the rate of degeneration of lung function to the normal or near-normal range and can prolong life expectancy (116–118).

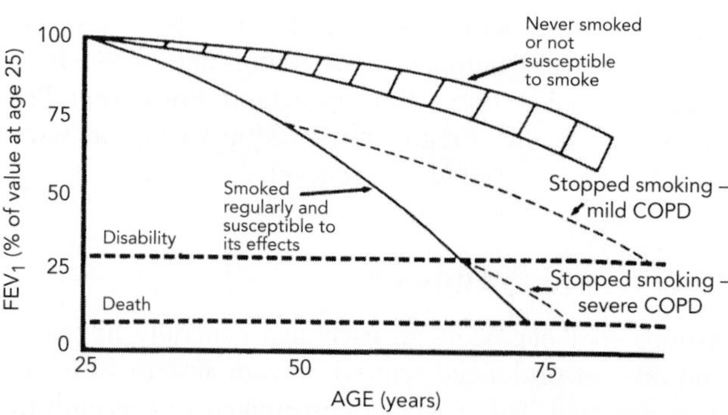

FIGURE 60.4. Effect of risk factors from smoking on loss of lung function (forced expiratory volume in the first second [FEV_1]). *Upper curves* are derived from subjects who do not smoke or are not susceptible to the effects of smoking. They lose lung function gradually throughout adult life (15–30 mL/year). *Lower curves* show accelerated loss of lung function in subjects who are susceptible to the effects of cigarette smoke. At age 65 years there is respiratory disability because FEV_1 has decreased to 25% to 30% of predicted (1–1.2 L), and further functional deterioration eventually will cause death because of complications of respiratory insufficiency. If the subject stops smoking, life may be prolonged but a respiratory death still eventually will result. If intervention is initiated earlier in life (age 40–50 years) when chronic obstructive pulmonary disease (COPD) is mild, accelerated loss of lung function is reversible and a respiratory death will be prevented. Although this figure illustrates theoretical loss of FEV_1 for an adult cigarette smoker, susceptible smokers will lose lung function at different rates, thereby becoming disabled at different ages. (Modified from Fletcher C, Peto R. The natural history of chronic airflow obstruction. BMJ 1977;1:1645, with permission.)

Pathogenesis

It is impossible to predict which individuals are susceptible to COPD. However, several risk factors that increase an individual's risk for developing COPD have been identified (119) (Table 60.17). Among these risk factors, *cigarette smoking* is the most prominent and potentially the most amenable to change. The mechanism by which cigarette smoking leads to COPD is thought to be mediated by proinflammatory components of cigarette smoke, such as the hydrocarbon compound *acrolein*. Fourfold to fivefold increases in the numbers of activated neutrophils are present in the terminal airspaces and the peribronchial regions in smokers. These cells produce elastase, which can destroy the elastin elements in the alveolar walls and induces emphysema in animal models. Normally, the small amount of neutrophil elastase is inactivated by antiproteases present in serum and lung liquid lining layer, with α_1-antitrypsin present in the largest quantities. Increasing evidence indicates that proteases secreted by alveolar macrophages and alveolar lining cells, including the cathepsins and matrix metalloproteinases (MMPs), play a pathobiologic role in the development of emphysema (120,121). These enzymes degrade a range of matrix proteins and inactivate the antiproteases that protect the lung from enzymatic

TABLE 60.17 Risk Factors for Developing Chronic Obstructive Pulmonary Disease

Established Risk Factors
Cigarette smoking
Age
Reduced lung function
Accelerated decline in lung function
Occupational dust exposure
α_1-Antitrypsin deficiency (Pi-ZZ phenotype)
Probable and Possible Risk Factors
Air pollution
Childhood respiratory infections
Allergic diathesis
Airway reactivity
Low socioeconomic status
Poor nutrition
ABO blood type (absence of "B" or presence of "A" in whites)
ABH nonsecretor status
Family members with chronic obstructive pulmonary disease

Adapted from Burrows B. Airways obstructive diseases: pathogenetic mechanisms and natural histories of the disorders. Med Clin North Am 1990;74:547; and Higgins M. Risk factors associated with chronic obstructive lung disease. Ann N Y Acad Sci 1991;624:7, with permission.

destruction. Animals exposed to high levels of cigarette smoke are protected from emphysema if they are genetically unable to produce matrix metalloelastase (MMP-12). Animals that overexpress matrix metallocollagenase (MMP-1) are highly susceptible to development of emphysema, and this enzyme has been found in increased quantities in smokers who develop emphysema (121). Thus, although we are not certain which enzymes are critical to the development of pulmonary emphysema, it seems likely that the balance between free protease activity within the alveolus and alveolar duct and local antiprotease activity determines the rate of destruction of the lung parenchyma. Oxidative lung injury and other pathways that promote apoptosis of endothelial or epithelial cells that form the alveolar structure also may play a role in development of emphysema (122).

α_1-Antitrypsin deficiency is an uncommon genetic disorder (found in approximately one in 2,500 white individuals of European descent) in which the circulating levels of antiproteases are <10% of normal. Normal α_1-antitrypsin activity is produced by the allele Pi-M (protease inhibitor M), for which approximately 90% of the population is homozygous. Pi-S is an allele with intermediate antiprotease activity, and Pi-Z is an allele with marked reduction in antiprotease activity. More than 75 minor alleles of the Pi gene have been identified, although most are rare and are uncommonly associated with disease. Individuals who are homozygous for the Pi-Z phenotype are at greatest risk for developing premature emphysema. Such individuals account for approximately 1% to 2% of cases of emphysema. The Pi-Z phenotype is the result of a single DNA base substitution causing an amino acid substitution that prevents secretion of the material from liver cells (123). Serum levels are <15% of normal despite hepatic intracellular accumulation of the enzyme inhibitor. In addition, the Pi-Z inhibitor has a slower reaction rate in neutralizing proteases, so the material that is secreted is less effective. Most studies have shown little increased risk for emphysema in people with intermediate α_1-antitrypsin levels, that is, the Pi-MS, Pi-MZ, and Pi-SZ phenotypes, suggesting that there is a threshold level of antiprotease activity for development of premature emphysema in deficient patients. Although affected people present for medical care with severe emphysema in the third and fourth decades, many people with α_1-antitrypsin deficiency have normal or only mildly abnormal lung function if they do not smoke (124).

Other *genetic polymorphisms* involved in the inflammatory and antioxidant pathways may play a role in susceptibility to COPD, but they are poorly understood (125).

Occupational exposure to dusts, fumes, and noxious gases has been implicated in the development of COPD (126). In most of these circumstances, however, the offending agents are additive to the effects of cigarette smoking, and it is uncommon to find occupationally related symptomatic COPD in the absence of cigarette smoking. The mechanism is presumed to be the result of nonspecific irritation or activation of alveolar macrophages, enhancing lower respiratory inflammation. Although far-advanced silicosis and asbestosis may be associated with airflow obstruction, the predominant lesion in these disorders is fibrosis with localized compensatory emphysema and honeycombing leading to restrictive ventilatory defects. Occupational exposure to sensitizing agents found in grain, wood, and cotton dust and to polyurethane compounds not only may cause asthma but may lead to fixed airflow obstruction with chronic asthmatic bronchitis if the exposure is prolonged. In nonindustrialized countries, however, intense exposure to particulates from biomass fuels has been implicated as a common cause of COPD in the absence of tobacco smoke exposure.

Nonspecific airway reactivity occurs in approximately 70% of people with COPD, even those with mild abnormalities and minimal symptoms, and is more common in women than in men (127). However, the interpretation of this finding is controversial. One school of thought, the so-called Dutch hypothesis, holds that this is a constitutional state that predisposes the individual to develop accelerated degeneration of pulmonary function when exposed to cigarette smoke or to other environmental agents (128). The alternative viewpoint is that airway reactivity is a marker for inflammatory or geometric changes that have already occurred and therefore is the result, not the cause, of the disease process.

The magnitude of airway reactivity correlates with the rate of decline of lung function (129,130) as well as with markers of inflammation. Whereas inflammatory mediators or airway wall thickening may contribute to increased tendency for airways to narrow, it also is possible that destruction of alveolar septal attachments and thickening of airway walls, which are the result of smoking-induced inflammation and early emphysema, lead to the increased tendency of the airways to constrict. This hypothesis is supported by the findings that airway reactivity is inversely correlated with baseline lung function in smokers, does not disappear with smoking cessation, and is induced in animals with emphysema caused by proteolytic enzymes (131).

Abnormal lung function, particularly FEV_1/FVC during early adulthood, is a predictor of accelerated degeneration in lung function, a phenomenon known as the *horse race effect* (132). People with lower lung function have already experienced some increased decline in lung function. Even individuals within the normal range of lung function who show lower spirometric indices have increased mortality from lung disease and other causes.

Aging is normally associated with changes in lung function, including reduction in vital capacity and FEV_1 and increases in residual volume and FRC. Physiologically, all of these changes can be attributed to a reduction in the elastic recoil of the lung that accompanies the aging process. The mechanism for these changes is unknown but is presumed to be the cumulative effect of endogenous and exogenous factors that degrade the elastin in the lung and the balance of processes that repair or prevent this damage. Emphysema of the panacinar type, which is similar to that occurring with α_1-antitrypsin deficiency, is found in some elderly nonsmoking individuals, particularly women. Development of emphysema in smokers may reflect either the additive effects of toxic exposure that accelerate the normal aging of the lung or interference with the processes that inhibit such degeneration. Most of the increased mortality from COPD over the last 2 decades has been confined to individuals older than 65 years, raising the possibility that the disease is being unmasked as mortality from heart disease, stroke, and infectious diseases is declining (133).

COPD is more common among the poor and poorly educated. Although cigarette smoking is more common in lower socioeconomic groups, the indigent have worse lung function even when adjusted for smoking status. Race is not thought to be a component; some evidence suggests that African Americans are less susceptible to COPD than whites (134). Factors that may contribute include crowded living conditions with exposure to frequent viral respiratory infections, indoor air pollutants from heating or cooking devices in poorly ventilated homes, poor nutrition, exposure to passive cigarette smoke, inadequate access to medical care for childhood respiratory infections, or increased exposure to respiratory irritants and toxins in the workplace. Although COPD mortality rates are highest in white men, women and African Americans have shown disproportionate increases in COPD mortality over the past decade, likely reflecting changing smoking patterns over the past 30 years (133).

The evidence that high levels of *air pollution* are important in the genesis of COPD is suggestive but not definitive. In animal models, high levels of NO_2 and ozone can induce emphysema independently and can potentiate protease-induced emphysema, suggesting that oxidant air pollutants inhibit lung protective mechanisms. There is more convincing evidence that acid aerosols, ozone, and fine particulates contribute to COPD exacerbations, hospitalizations, and death (135–137).

Whereas allergic tendencies are strongly associated with the presence of asthma and symptoms of cough and wheeze in nonsmokers, the effect of atopy on respiratory symptoms and decline in lung function in smokers is less clear, possibly in part because of the tendency of adolescents and young adults with highly reactive airways to avoid cigarette smoking. Some evidence suggests that allergies or nonspecific elevation of serum IgE levels contribute to the development of fixed airway obstruction in smokers.

Evaluation of the Patient with Chronic Obstructive Pulmonary Disease

History

COPD must be considered a diagnostic possibility in all individuals who smoke, even in the absence of respiratory symptoms. The clinician should inquire about smoking habits in every patient encounter. Specific questioning about the age at onset of smoking, average number of packs smoked per day, and number and duration of quit attempts should be elicited. Often patients report being nonsmokers to the practitioner when they have only recently quit smoking. Other respiratory symptoms, such as cough, phlegm, and exertional dyspnea, should be quantified. Morning sputum production often is erroneously considered to be normal by smokers. Shortness of breath can be detected by asking whether the individual has trouble keeping up with peers performing routine activities such as walking, sports, and work functions. More advanced dyspnea is roughly quantified by distance walked or flights of stairs walked before stopping. Sleep disturbance is a common and often overlooked symptom of COPD and may impair quality of life more than exertional dyspnea.

Physical Examination

Although historical and physical findings of COPD (see below) may confirm the diagnosis when they are present, they usually are apparent only with advanced disease (see below for spirometric guidelines). The absence of these findings is not sufficiently sensitive to exclude the diagnosis in the person at risk (Table 60.18) (138,139).

TABLE 60.18 Sensitivity and Specificity of History and Physical Findings for Diagnosis of Moderate Chronic Obstructive Pulmonary Disease

Historical Items			
Historical Finding	***Cutoff***	***Sensitivity (%)***	***Specificity (%)***
Age	75 y	13	99
Previous diagnosis of chronic obstructive pulmonary disease	Yes vs. no	80	74
Smoking history	≥70 pack-years	40	95
Dyspnea severity (five-point scale)	≥4	60	75
Phlegm	≥2 oz in a.m. when present	20	95
Theophylline use	Yes vs. no	60	71
Steroid use	Yes vs. no	40	87
Inhaler use	Yes vs. no	27	94
Home oxygen	Yes vs. no	20	96
Physical Examination Items			
Physical Finding	***Cutoff***	***Sensitivity (%)***	***Specificity (%)***
Initial impression[a]	Yes vs. no	25	95
Diaphragm excursion	<2 cm TLC vs. RV	12	98
Chest percussion	Increased resonance	32	94
Cardiac dullness	Decreased area ≤10 cm	16	99
Blow out a match		53	88
Wheeze	Yes vs. no	9	100
Reduced breath sounds	Yes vs. no	65	96
Forced expiratory time	>10 s	12	99
Cardiac point of maximum Impulse	Abdominal	27	98
Final overall opinion	Yes vs. no	51	93

[a]Based on general inspection.
RV, residual volume; TLC, total lung capacity.
Adapted from Badgett RG, Tanaka DJ, Hunt DK, et al. Can moderate chronic obstructive pulmonary disease be diagnosed by historical and physical findings alone? Am J Med 1993;94:188, with permission.

In advanced COPD, general physical findings include those caused by hyperinflation: increase in resting chest anteroposterior diameter, elevation of the clavicles, widening of the xiphocostal angle, and increase in the intercostal spaces. The distance between the larynx and the sternal notch is reduced to <4 cm (139). With inspiration there is diminished movement of the rib cage and increased movement of the abdominal wall. The patient has hypertrophied and well-defined abdominal and sternomastoid muscles but diminished muscle mass in the arms, thighs, and legs. The characteristic seated posture is leaning forward with both hands on the knees to fix the shoulders, permitting more effective use of the accessory cervical muscles. This may lead to hyperkeratosis of the anterior thighs. Pursed-lip breathing and prolonged time of expiration are spontaneously adopted to diminish the energy expenditure of breathing. The fingers often show tobacco staining. Clubbing of the nails is rare and suggests the presence of bronchiectasis or bronchogenic carcinoma. Chest percussion shows increased resonance and low diaphragms that move poorly with full inspiration and expiration. Auscultation shows diminished transmission of breath sounds over areas of emphysema and is the most reliable physical finding indicative of chronic airflow limitation. Early inspiratory crackles indicate opening of closed airways and are common in COPD, whereas late and pan-inspiratory crackles are more common with interstitial lung diseases (140). Wheezing may be elicited in most COPD patients by forced expiration, but the presence of wheezing during quiet breathing is more common with reversible bronchospasm.

In far-advanced disease with *cor pulmonale,* elevated right atrial pressures cause neck vein distention, peripheral edema, and hepatomegaly. The pulmonary hypertension and distention of the right ventricle cause a pronounced cardiac impulse in the epigastrium. Tricuspid regurgitation from dilation of the right ventricle and pulmonary hypertension causes a systolic murmur over the epigastrium that increases with inspiration. In contrast to other forms of pulmonary hypertension, a ventricular heave and increased intensity of the second heart sound usually are not appreciated because of the interposed emphysematous lung.

Additional Studies

The ability to blow out a paper match from >10 cm away with an open mouth is a rudimentary lung function test that is helpful when abnormal, but the test is not sensitive. Another simple bedside lung function test is to measure the forced expiratory time with a stethoscope over the trachea during an FVC maneuver. However, the test is not sufficiently sensitive in practice to screen for airflow limitation (141).

The *chest x-ray film* is abnormal only in advanced disease. Signs of COPD include hyperinflation with flattening of the diaphragm, increased retrosternal airspace on the lateral view, narrow cardiac silhouette, paucity and tapering of peripheral blood vessels, and bullae. In some smokers with COPD, particularly those with bronchitis symptoms, small rounded opacities or increased linear markings representing thickened airway walls may be seen.

High-resolution computerized tomography of the chest is becoming the standard for evaluation of emphysema in the absence of an anatomic diagnosis. In practice, however, this study rarely is necessary because less expensive tests of lung function—spirometry and diffusing capacity—usually are adequate to distinguish asthma from emphysema and to follow the course of the disease and the response to treatment.

Spirometry (see above) should be performed initially for diagnosis and assessment of severity. Whether spirometry should be performed for COPD screening in asymptomatic smokers is not clear, because the sole effective means of halting disease progression, smoking cessation, should be universally promoted regardless of lung function. After initial diagnosis of COPD, however, spirometry should be repeated to monitor disease progression and response to treatment, particularly when the patient's health status changes (142). As a general rule, FEV_1 measurement >80% predicted indicates mild obstruction, 50% to 80% predicted indicates moderate obstruction, 30% to 50% predicted indicates severe obstruction, and <30% predicted indicates very severe obstruction. Peak flow monitoring, useful in asthma, may be misleading in COPD because the peak flow can be well maintained despite worsening airflow obstruction.

Sensitive tests, such as the *single-breath nitrogen washout test,* measure the function of the small airways. Such tests are abnormal in most smokers and do not predict who will develop symptomatic COPD, so these tests are not routinely recommended. In smokers, forced expiratory spirometry is effective in screening for COPD. With serial measures of spirometry, it is possible to identify individuals who are demonstrating accelerated declines in lung function before symptoms intervene. Of spirometric indices, FEV_1/FVC <70% predicts future decline in lung function (132).

Bronchodilator testing can reveal reversible bronchospasm, and the postbronchodilator measure of FEV_1 is the best overall predictor of life expectancy in COPD. Failure to respond rapidly to a single dose of an inhaled bronchodilator does not indicate that lung function will not improve with more long-term treatment or at different times (143). Approximately one in five patients who do not demonstrate a rapid bronchodilator response will show improvement in lung function after several weeks of treatment with bronchodilators or corticosteroids (144). Abnormal methacholine reactivity is common in COPD but usually does not provide sufficient information to warrant its routine use.

The *carbon monoxide diffusing capacity test* (see above) is helpful for distinguishing emphysema from asthma. Cigarette smokers without emphysema have mild reductions in diffusing capacity because of accumulation of carbon monoxide in the blood, which is only partially reversible with smoking cessation. A diffusing capacity <70% of the predicted value is present with emphysema but also may be found with interstitial fibrosis and pulmonary vascular diseases. In chronic asthmatic bronchitis, the diffusing capacity tends to be preserved (145,146).

Measurements of lung volume (see above) help distinguish obstructive lung diseases from restrictive lung diseases. They are particularly helpful during the initial assessment or when the presence of an interstitial process is unclear, such as that caused by occupational exposure to silica or asbestos. Some patients experience significant improvement in symptoms after bronchodilator treatment as a consequence of reversal of resting or exercise-induced dynamic hyperinflation with little change in FEV_1. However, it often is not necessary to follow response to bronchodilator treatment with lung volume measurements if simple spirometric measures improve. Measurements of airway resistance and lung compliance often are abnormal in COPD but do not add useful clinical information in most circumstances.

Exercise testing is indicated in individuals who demonstrate reduction in diffusing capacity <50% to 60% of predicted and who are not hypoxemic at rest, if supplemental oxygen is being considered for improving exercise capacity. Exercise testing should be performed in a monitored facility. Measurement of oxygen saturation with a pulse oximeter usually suffices to determine whether oxygen should be prescribed. More complex and invasive exercise testing with measurement of arterial blood gas tensions, oxygen consumption, and ventilation are used for evaluation of disability (see Chapter 9) or if the cause of dyspnea is unclear. Maximum exercise capacity on a cycle ergometer before and after an exercise training program is useful in selecting individuals who are good candidates for lung volume reduction surgery (see below). Measurement of the distance that an individual can walk in 6 minutes, the *six-minute walk test,* is used as an indicator of functional ability and is one of several predictors of survival in COPD (147).

Arterial blood gas measurements may reveal disorders of oxygenation or ventilation. *Hypoxemia* occurs in COPD as a consequence of ventilation–perfusion mismatching. In those with advanced disease, particularly obese individuals, hypoventilation also promotes hypoxemia. With exercise, particularly at higher altitude, hypoxemia can worsen because of impaired diffusion of oxygen across the alveolar–capillary membrane. Arterial oxygen saturation should be measured in patients who have moderately advanced disease and FEV_1 <1.5 L, because this group is at risk for chronic hypoxemia and development of cor pulmonale. At higher altitudes, hypoxemia develops with less severe pulmonary involvement, and oxygen tensions should be measured more liberally. When the FEV_1 falls to <1.0 L, chronic *hypercapnia* becomes more common, often in patients with the least dyspnea.

Other blood tests are indicated only as needed for the general care of the patient. An elevated hematocrit value is uncommon in COPD in comparison with similar levels of hypoxemia at altitude, but when it does occur should alert the clinician to the possible presence of chronic hypoxemia. Anemia is not uncommon in COPD patients with comorbidities and is a reversible cause of fatigue and dyspnea in patients with COPD (148). Hypokalemia and hypomagnesemia are common as a consequence of β-adrenergic agonists in conjunction with diuretics and, if severe, may contribute to fatigue or respiratory muscle failure.

Screening for *severe* α_1*-antitrypsin deficiency* can be accomplished with serum protein electrophoresis to evaluate for a marked decrease in α_1-globulin level. Genotyping or measurements of protease inhibitor levels are more specific and can detect intermediate deficiencies. Screening should be done for persons with a family history suggesting α_1-antitrypsin deficiency, for patients with symptomatic airflow limitation at a relatively young age, and for those with unexplained liver disease or necrotizing panniculitis. Although recommended by some, it is not clear that adequate evidence of effective treatment is sufficiently well established to recommend screening in typical older smokers presenting with advanced disease (149).

Cystic fibrosis may present in adulthood with chronic cough and phlegm associated with chronic airflow limitation. It should be suspected if the patient has radiographic evidence of bronchiectasis, has a family history of cystic fibrosis or severe chronic childhood lung disease, has ABPA, or if sputum cultures persistently grow mucoid colonies of *Pseudomonas.* Elevations of chloride in sweat iontophoresis samples confirm the diagnosis, but genetic testing now is widely available to test for polymorphisms of the CFTR gene.

The *electrocardiogram* in COPD shows a vertical or indeterminate heart axis and low voltage. Enlarged P waves, right-axis deviation, or right ventricular hypertrophy is present with cor pulmonale. Echocardiography can confirm right ventricular dilation and tricuspid regurgitation. *Doppler studies* of tricuspid retrograde flow can be used to estimate pulmonary artery pressures but may be inaccurate with severe lung hyperinflation. Transesophageal echocardiography (see Chapter 65) provides better views, but the more invasive nature of the procedure limits its application. In most circumstances, echocardiography should be reserved for patients in whom there is a question of associated left ventricular dysfunction or valve disease.

Sputum examination by Gram stain or wet preparation during exacerbations can help determine whether there is a predominance of neutrophils or eosinophils, guiding the choice between corticosteroids and antibiotics. The presence of green phlegm, a marker for neutrophil myeloperoxidase, is a sensitive finding for the presence of a high bacterial load in phlegm (150). Culture of the sputum is unnecessary unless pneumonia is present or unusual or resistant organisms are suspected. Lower respiratory tract bacterial infections are associated with COPD exacerbations in approximately half of the events, often following colonization of the lower respiratory tract with immunologically new strains of previously colonizing species (151). Common pathogens such as *Streptococcus pneumoniae, Haemophilus influenzae,* or *Moraxella (Branhamella) catarrhalis* can be found in the lower airways in approximately half of COPD flares (152).

Management

The components of care in COPD consist of education about the disease, prevention of disease progression, treatment of complications, drug treatment to maximize lung function, and rehabilitation to optimize activity levels.

Education is important so that the patient can develop an understanding of what COPD is, what causes it, and what possible courses the disorder may take. The patient should be given realistic expectations about the chronic but variable course of the disease, tempered by the understanding that temporary periods of worsening are preventable and treatable. The patient should try to achieve maximum social and physical functioning and to make use of whatever family, social, and medical support is available. Simple measures such as the availability of special parking areas for the disabled, wheelchairs and motorized carts in shopping malls and airports, portable oxygen, and oxygen supplementation during air travel are not always known by patients with advanced COPD, who may unnecessarily confine themselves to home and become socially isolated. Local volunteer health associations commonly sponsor groups in which these issues are discussed, and they often provide instructional materials via the Internet (American Lung Association at http://www.lungusa.org; National Heart, Lung, and Blood Institute at http://www.nhlbi.nih.gov/health/public/lung/index.htm). Patients and their families should understand that the dyspnea that occurs with exertion is not harmful to the lung and that, with appropriate pacing of activities, a certain level of dyspnea actually is desirable to achieve and maintain physical conditioning. Inquiries about sexual functioning should not be avoided. Education of the patient's bed partner on techniques to limit the patient's level of exertion and on the use of prophylactic bronchodilators and oxygen can establish more normal sexual functioning, even with severe disease. Advance directives regarding intensive or long-term medical care should be discussed with patients and their families, and the physician should encourage this communication. Both clinician and patient should understand that episodes of acute respiratory failure in COPD requiring mechanical ventilation often are successfully treated but that the long-term survival is poor, although unpredictable, in those who have incapacitating dyspnea, cor pulmonale, poor nutrition, or persistent hypercapnia (153,154).

Prevention of disease progression and complications is one of the most important goals of treatment. By the time most patients present with advanced disease, they have discontinued smoking, although a sizable minority have not. Many with mild or moderate disease continue to smoke, unaware of their illness and the potential for arresting its progression by smoking cessation. Chapter 27 discusses the practical approaches to smoking cessation. In the patient with lung disease, the physician should deliver a strong personalized smoking cessation message that emphasizes the definite and progressive nature of the disease, the likelihood of early disability with continued smoking, and the potential for arresting the disease when smoking is stopped. Referral to a smoking group program and use of bupropion and nicotine replacement therapy improve smoking cessation rates.

Exposure to respiratory irritants should be avoided in the workplace as well as the home. If the disease is complicated by allergy or overlaps with allergic asthma, environmental control measures should be instituted. Smoking of marijuana and cocaine may cause airway irritation, and although there is little evidence that they contribute to airway reactivity or to development of COPD, their use should be discouraged.

Pneumococcal vaccination (see Chapter 18) is recommended, although evidence of its particular efficacy in COPD is lacking (155). *Influenza vaccination* taken annually (see Chapter 18) or amantadine/rimantadine prophylaxis for unimmunized individuals during an influenza epidemic can prevent or attenuate this potentially fatal infection. During influenza epidemics, the use of neuraminidase inhibitors such as zanamivir and oseltamivir can minimize the severity of infection if taken within 48 hours of onset of illness (156).

Patients with α_1-antitrypsin deficiency are candidates for intravenous replacement therapy with protease inhibitors, although the long-term benefits of this treatment are not proven, particularly in those with mild impairment and those with severe impairment (157–159).

Treatment of Complications

Tracheobronchial infections are common in COPD, heralded by a change in the quantity, viscosity, or color of sputum. Although many infections are initiated by viruses, bacterial contamination or superinfection of the lower respiratory tract is common. Inexpensive broad-spectrum antibiotics, such as doxycycline, erythromycin, amoxicillin, or trimethoprim–sulfamethoxazole, can shorten the duration of these symptoms if they are suggestive of infection (160). When the patient is intolerant of first-line antibiotics, has severe underlying disease, has frequent exacerbations, or manifests evidence of resistant organisms, amoxicillin–clavulanate, ketolide, macrolide, or quinolone antibiotics should be prescribed (161). Antibiotics generally should be given only in exacerbations manifesting the triad of increased cough, worsening dyspnea, and change in sputum color or quantity. The oral route of administration is preferred, if tolerated by the patient.

Chronic hypoxemia causes pulmonary hypertension and cor pulmonale, a condition associated with poor survival if untreated. Oxygen therapy prolongs survival and improves physical and psychologic functioning in hypoxemic patients with COPD (162,163). When indicated (Table 60.19), oxygen can be administered with a nasal cannula. Oxygen concentrators, compressed oxygen tanks, and liquid oxygen storage reservoirs all are suitable for home use. Portable liquid oxygen systems and small compressed oxygen tanks with reservoir devices or demand valves allow mobility out of the home and should be used whenever possible. Oxygen should be prescribed at the lowest level necessary to maintain an arterial oxygen saturation $\geq$90%, usually 1 to 4 L/min. Supplemental oxygen must be used for at least 18 hours/day to have a significant survival benefit. The patient should understand that oxygen is used to prevent cardiac complications and not just to relieve dyspnea. Transtracheal oxygen catheters are used for the

TABLE 60.19 Indications for Continuous Oxygen Therapy

Arterial oxygen tension $\leq$55 mm Hg or sat O_2 $\leq$88% while in usual state of health
Arterial oxygen tension $\leq$60 mm Hg or sat O_2 $\leq$89% with evidence of chronic hypoxemia, such as erythrocytosis, ankle edema, venous engorgement, electrocardiographic P-pulmonale, or psychological impairment

occasional patient who requires high oxygen concentrations or who cannot tolerate a nasal cannula (164).

If desaturation occurs with exercise, increased flows of oxygen during activity can improve exercise tolerance and enhance the ability to engage in an exercise conditioning program. *Nocturnal hypoxemia* in COPD is common and often unsuspected. The importance of screening for nocturnal oxygen desaturation and the benefit of treatment in terms of survival are not known. Preliminary evidence suggests that nocturnal oxygen prevents progression of pulmonary hypertension in COPD patients with nocturnal desaturation (165,166). Nonetheless, testing for nocturnal hypoxemia (in a sleep center or a hospital) in individuals who have erythrocytosis, unexplained peripheral edema without waking abnormalities of blood gases, or daytime hypersomnolence is prudent.

When *pulmonary hypertension* and *cor pulmonale* are present, treatment consists of continuous oxygen to overcome hypoxemia and diuretics to control peripheral edema. Digitalis is not useful unless there is concomitant left ventricular disease or atrial tachyarrhythmias. Calcium channel blockers can vasodilate the pulmonary circulation, but they often worsen hypoxemia, and their benefit is not established. Almitrine, a respiratory stimulant not available in the United States, improves arterial oxygen tension through improved ventilation–perfusion matching but does not reduce pulmonary artery pressure (167,168). Phlebotomy increases exercise capacity when hematocrit is >55%, but persistent erythrocytosis suggests inadequate oxygen supplementation or another cause (169). Anticoagulation, which is considered beneficial in severe pulmonary vascular hypertension (e.g., primary pulmonary hypertension), is of uncertain benefit in patients with pulmonary hypertension caused by COPD.

Supraventricular tachyarrhythmias are common in patients with COPD, as a consequence of right atrial enlargement, increased endogenous adrenergic tone, hypoxemia, and drug treatment, particularly with theophylline. Anticholinergic inhalers also have been implicated as an uncommon cause of supraventricular tachyarrhythmias (170). Treatment is similar to that in nonpulmonary patients (see Chapter 64). However, the presence of COPD should not prevent evaluation for treatable causes of arrhythmias, such as pulmonary embolism, hyperthyroidism, or valvular heart disease, which may be difficult to diagnose in these patients.

Control of *mucus hypersecretion* with use of expectorants and physical means such as high-frequency chest wall oscillation is not of proven benefit in improving lung function, although symptoms sometimes improve (171).

Hypercapnia may be an adaptive response to obstructive lung disease by decreasing the work of breathing, preventing respiratory muscle fatigue, and allowing a diminished sensation of dyspnea. Therefore, respiratory stimulants may be detrimental over long periods. Bronchospasm (see below), obesity (see Chapter 83), and sleep apnea (see Chapter 7) are reversible conditions that can contribute to hypercapnia and therefore should be treated. Narcotics and sedatives with potential for respiratory depression should be avoided.

Malnutrition is present in 50% of patients with advanced COPD, usually when the FEV_1 is <35% of predicted. This is the consequence of increased metabolic demands, insufficient caloric intake, and possibly elaboration of cachexia-producing cytokines such as tumor necrosis factor-α and interleukin-6. Body weight <90% of ideal is associated with increased mortality and decreased exercise capacity in patients with otherwise similar lung function. Muscle wasting and loss of bone mass may be present even in patients who have a normal body mass index (172). Although results of clinical trials of nutritional supplementation have been disappointing, monitoring body weight in COPD patients and prescribing caloric supplementation as needed are prudent because those patients who do gain weight show improved survival (173).

Drug Therapy to Maximize Functional Status

Bronchodilators and anti-inflammatory agents are used in patients with COPD to reverse bronchospasm and prevent bronchoconstriction in response to provocative agents. Small amounts of bronchoconstriction and air trapping can cause marked deterioration in symptoms; conversely, small amounts of bronchodilation can cause considerable improvement in functional capacity. Inhaled corticosteroids do not alter the progression of COPD but do reduce the frequency of exacerbations. Inhaled corticosteroids should be reserved for patients who have an asthmatic component to their disease or those who have frequent exacerbations (174–177).

Stepped drug treatment should use the minimum number of agents and the least frequent dosing schedule possible, starting with the agents having the greatest benefit and least toxicity. Bronchodilators are given to COPD patients on a regular basis to maintain bronchodilation and on an as-needed basis for relief of symptoms. Most breathless patients benefit from regular use of a bronchodilator. Both β-agonist and anticholinergic classes are available in short-acting (4- to 6-hour duration) and long-acting (12- to 24-hour duration) preparations. The choice between class of bronchodilator and duration of effect depends upon the cost of the preparation and the clinician's preference. A combination of different classes of bronchodilators often is more effective than increasing the dose of a single agent. Many patients with advanced COPD require a combination of bronchodilators, including long-acting maintenance anticholinergics and β-agonists as well as symptomatic use of shorter-acting bronchodilators. In individuals who have frequent exacerbations, inhaled corticosteroids or a combination inhaler of inhaled corticosteroids and long-acting bronchodilator may be added. Theophylline in long-acting oral preparations is a useful adjunct to therapy in cases where inhaled medication is too expensive or not acceptable for the patient. Chronic use of systemic corticosteroids should be reserved for individuals with very frequent or life-threatening exacerbations who cannot tolerate their discontinuation. Response to treatment is judged by symptomatic improvement, functional status, and spirometry.

Ipratropium bromide (Atrovent) is an inhaled anticholinergic drug that causes 4 to 8 hours of bronchodilation through inhibition of vagal stimulation of the airways. Although it usually is more expensive than β-agonists, it is the usual choice for first-line therapy. The dosage is started at two MDI inhalations three times daily and can be increased to six inhalations four times daily. Systemic side effects are uncommon, even with relatively high doses (178). Local side effects include mouth irritation and cough, which can be diminished by good inhaler technique or by use of a spacer. Although ipratropium provides sustained benefit in patients with moderate disease, it does not inhibit progression of the disease if smoking is continued (116). *Tiotropium* (Spiriva) is an anticholinergic bronchodilator that has the benefit of once-daily dosing and is more effective than usual doses of ipratropium in bronchodilation, quality of life, and reducing exacerbations (179–181). Tolerance does not develop with prolonged use. It is inhaled once daily from a capsule inserted into a dry-powder inhaler. Proper instruction on use of the inhaler is needed, but the dry-powder inhaler does not require as much coordination as an MDI.

β-Adrenergic agonists are used at dosages comparable to those used for asthma (see above). The dosages of inhaled selective β-agonists should be increased before oral agents are prescribed so that tremor and hypokalemia are minimized. *Long-acting inhaled β-agonists* such as salmeterol (Serevent) and formoterol (Foradil) are useful because of the long duration of action and documented benefit on quality of life (182,183). Both are available in dry-powder inhaler formulations that do not require as much hand-breathing coordination as MDIs. Combination inhaler therapy with a β-agonist and a short-acting anticholinergic provides better bronchodilation than either agent alone, and the simplified treatment regimen may aid compliance (184,185). Combinations of inhaled corticosteroids and long-acting bronchodilators provide more bronchodilation than either alone in patients with chronic bronchitis and airflow obstruction (186).

Theophylline is best taken in a long-acting preparation once or twice daily. Although monitoring of blood levels is possible, there is only a rough correlation between side effects and serum levels. If typical side effects such as nausea, vomiting, tremor, or tachyarrhythmias occur, the dose should be adjusted irrespective of serum levels. Use of theophylline in COPD has diminished because of the availability of long-acting inhaled agents, but it still is an effective and inexpensive second-line drug. Although the bronchodilating effects of theophylline are moderate compared with inhaled drugs, it has other putative pharmacologic actions that improve the well-being of the COPD patient, including improvement in diaphragm function, prevention of respiratory muscle fatigue, increased ventilatory drive, potentiation of catecholamine function, prevention of increased microvascular permeability, increased mucociliary clearance, prevention of late-phase antigen responses, inhibition of mast cell histamine release, and suppression of leukocyte activation (187,188). Clinical trials showing improvement in functional status beyond that gained from the effects of bronchodilation are consistent with improvement in respiratory muscle function (189). New drugs that are more specific inhibitors of phosphodiesterase-4 have not yet been marketed in the United States but hold the promise of similar efficacy with less toxicity.

Oral corticosteroids are effective for treatment of COPD exacerbations (190,191). Among chronic symptomatic patients, 10% to 20% show substantial short-term improvement, defined as $\geq$25% increase in FEV_1. In general, the patients studied had far-advanced disease and did not differ from other COPD patients except with regard to their steroid response. Some have suggested that long-term low-dose oral steroids may slow the progression of the disease, but the evidence is not strong in comparison to the well-defined side effects of such treatment. Most patients with COPD who are on chronic corticosteroid therapy can safely taper the dose at the equivalent of 5 mg prednisone per week and reserve their use exclusively for exacerbations (192). In selected cases, long-term low doses of oral corticosteroids may be prescribed for patients who cannot afford or tolerate inhaled agents.

Inhaled corticosteroids do not alter the progression of COPD in those who continue to smoke (174,176,177). They are most useful in patients who have an overlap between asthma and COPD and those with more advanced disease who have frequent exacerbations. Inhaled corticosteroids can reduce the frequency of exacerbations and improve airway reactivity (174,176). Combined with long-acting bronchodilators, inhaled corticosteroids can reduce symptoms and improve quality of life (186).

Treatment of Chronic Obstructive Pulmonary Disease Exacerbations

COPD exacerbations are characterized by worsening dyspnea, cough, and increased phlegm production. On average, patients with COPD have two to three exacerbations per year, but the number varies widely. Only half of these cases come to the attention of treating practitioners. Precipitating events include respiratory and nonrespiratory infections, exposure to respiratory irritants and air pollution, or comorbid conditions such as heart failure, pulmonary embolism, myocardial ischemia, or pneumothorax. The management of these exacerbations depends upon the severity (193). Patients with severe acute onset of dyspnea; evidence of hypoxemia such as mental confusion, cyanosis or desaturation; new onset of chest pain, edema, or arrhythmias; and those with important comorbidities or inadequate social support should be referred for hospitalization. Arterial blood gas studies and chest radiographs are useful for evaluating etiology and severity of acutely ill patients. Increasing the frequency and intensity of inhaled short-acting bronchodilators for several days is effective in mild exacerbations and usually can be managed by patients at home. A hand-held inhaler and spacer usually is adequate, but a nebulizer may be needed for those who cannot coordinate well. Patients who have increasing dyspnea accompanied by a change in the quantity or color of phlegm should be prescribed an antibiotic, with the choice of antibiotic determined by the severity of the underlying disease and the likelihood of treatment failure. A course of corticosteroids, equivalent to 30 to 60 mg prednisone for 7 to 14 days, will shorten the duration of symptoms for ambulatory patients with exacerbations.

Pulmonary Rehabilitation

In patients lacking the capacity to restore damaged lung parenchyma, efforts should be made to optimize activity levels through rehabilitation programs. The content of such programs varies widely but includes some or all of the following elements: education about COPD and its treatment, nutritional counseling, psychological support, pacing and energy conservation training for daily activities, aerobic exercise conditioning, and upper-extremity strength training. Generally, these programs have demonstrated improved exercise endurance and sense of well-being without changes in lung function. The benefits of some components of these programs are better documented than others (194). If a coordinated rehabilitation program is not accessible, many of these elements can be provided individually to ambulatory patients. For example, a regular daily walk for 15 to 30 minutes at a pace that induces mild to moderate dyspnea can be safely prescribed for most patients with COPD. Even with severe COPD, most patients should be able to achieve a goal of walking at 1 to 1.5 mph for 30 min/day. Ambulatory oxygen may be particularly helpful as an adjunct for those with oxygen desaturation during exercise. Instructional materials and support groups for patients and families are widely available through volunteer agencies and the Internet.

Surgery

Surgical resection of bullae is rarely indicated for treatment of COPD. An individual with a single large bulla that occupies more than one third of the hemithorax with preserved carbon monoxide diffusing capacity is likely to do best after bullectomy. Unilateral or bilateral lung transplantation is indicated in some patients with advanced emphysema, usually in individuals younger than 60 years when FEV_1 is <25% predicted or if severe pulmonary hypertension is present (195). The goal of lung transplantation is to improve quality of life, but whether that goal is achieved is unclear (196). Lung transplantation is limited by the availability of donor organs and accessibility to transplant centers. Lung volume reduction surgery is a useful procedure in highly selected patients. In this operation, lung tissue is resected, increasing elasticity of the remaining lung and improving the contour and function of the diaphragm. The operative mortality from the procedure ranges from 4% to 10%. Patients who have emphysema most severe in the upper lung regions and severe exercise limitation after rehabilitation are most likely to benefit from this operation (197). Patients with very low diffusion capacity or diffuse emphysema and low FEV_1 are at highest surgical risk (198). Chapter 93 discusses the perioperative management of patients with COPD.

Prognosis

In general, the prognosis of patients with chronic airway obstruction (see Natural History) can be estimated from the FEV_1 obtained when the patient is clinically stable. One study showed that in moderate obstruction, when FEV_1 was >1.25 L, the 5-year survival of patients was only slightly decreased from that of matched controls. If FEV_1 was between 0.75 and 1.25 L, 5-year survival decreased to approximately 66% of expected, and if FEV_1 was <0.75 L, 5-year survival decreased to 33% of expected (115). Cardiac disease, resting tachycardia, hypercapnia, hypoxemia, and frequent exacerbations pose additional risks to survival, whereas a significant response to bronchodilator therapy (>10% improvement in FEV_1) is associated with improved survival. Serial tests of lung function intervals help identify patients with excessive rates of decline.

SPECIFIC REFERENCES

1. Murray CJ, Lopez AD. Global mortality, disability, and the contribution of risk factors: Global Burden of Disease Study. Lancet 1997;349:1436.
2. National Heart, Lung, and Blood Institute. Morbidity & Mortality 2004: Chartbook on Cardiovascular, Lung, and Blood Diseases. Bethesda: U.S. Department of Health and Human Services, Public Health Service, National Institutes of Health, 2004. Available at: http://www.nhlbi.nih.gov/resources/docs/04_chtbk.pdf.
3. Mannino DM, Homa DM, Akinbami LJ, et al. Chronic obstructive pulmonary disease surveillance—United States, 1971–2000. MMWR Surveill Summ 2002; 51:1.
4. Sly RM. Decreases in asthma mortality in the United States. Ann Allergy Asthma Immunol 2000;85:121.
5. Ferguson GT, Enright PL, Buist AS, et al. Office spirometry for lung health assessment in adults: a consensus statement from the National Lung Health Education Program. Chest 2000;117:1146.
6. Morrison, NJ, Abboud, RT, Ramadan, F, et al. Comparison of single breath carbon monoxide diffusing capacity and pressure-volume curves in detecting emphysema. Am Rev Respir Dis 1989;139:1179.

7. Owens GR, Rogers RM, Pennock BE, et al. The diffusing capacity as a predictor of arterial oxygen desaturation during exercise in patients with chronic obstructive pulmonary disease. N Engl J Med 1984;310:1218.
8. Busse WW, Lemanske RF Jr. Asthma. N Engl J Med 2001;344:350.
9. Burrows B, Martinez FD, Halonen M, et al. Association of asthma with serum IgE levels and skin-test reactivity to allergens. N Engl J Med 1989;320:271.
10. Tashkin DP, Altose MD, Bleecker ER, et al. The lung health study: airway responsiveness to inhaled methacholine in smokers with mild to moderate airflow limitation. Am Rev Respir Dis 1992;145:301.
11. American Thoracic Society. Guidelines for methacholine and exercise challenge testing—1999. Am J Respir Crit Care Med 2000;161:309.
12. O'Byrne, PM. Leukotriene bronchoconstriction induced by allergen and exercise Am J Respir Crit Care Med 2000;161:S68.
13. Gilbert IA, McFadden ER Jr. Airway cooling and rewarming. The second reaction sequence in exercise-induced asthma. J Clin Invest 1992; 90:699.
14. Abu-Hasan M, Tannous B, Weinberger M. Exercise-induced dyspnea in children and adolescents: if not asthma then what? Ann Allergy Asthma Immunol 2005;94:366.
15. Bousquet J, Jeffery PK, Busse WW, et al. Asthma: from bronchoconstriction to airways inflammation and remodeling. Am J Respir Crit Care Med 2000;161:1720.
16. Chiappara G, Gagliardo R, Siena A, et al. Airway remodelling in the pathogenesis of asthma. Curr Opin Allergy Clin Immunol 2001;1:85.
17. Barnes PJ. Inhaled glucocorticoids for asthma. N Engl J Med 1995;332:868.
18. CAMP Research Group. Long-term effects of budesonide or nedocromil in children with asthma. The Childhood Asthma Management Program Research Group. N Engl J Med 2000; 343:1054.
19. Eggleston PA, Arruda LK. Ecology and elimination of cockroaches and allergens in the home. J Allergy Clin Immunol 2001;107:S422.
20. Weiss ST, Horner A, Shapiro G, et al. The prevalence of environmental exposure to perceived asthma triggers in children with mild-to-moderate asthma: data from the Childhood Asthma Management Program (CAMP). J Allergy Clin Immunol 2001;107:634.
21. Creticos PS, Reed CE, Norman PS, et al. Ragweed immunotherapy in adult asthma. N Engl J Med 1996;334:501.
22. Adkinson NF, Eggleston PA, Eney D, et al. A controlled trial of immunotherapy for asthma in allergic children. N Engl J Med 1997;336:324.
23. Holgate S, Casale T, Wenzel S, et al. The anti-inflammatory effects of omalizumab confirm the central role of IgE in allergic inflammation. J Allergy Clin Immunol 2005; 115:459.
24. Buhl R. Anti-IgE antibodies for the treatment of asthma. Curr Opin Pulm Med 2005;11:27.
25. Mapp CE, Boschetto P, Maestrelli P, et al. Occupational asthma. Am J Respir Crit Care Med 2005;172:280.
26. Alberts WM, do Pico GA. Reactive airways dysfunction syndrome. Chest 1996;109:1618.
27. Szczeklik A. Aspirin-induced asthma: pathogenesis and clinical presentation. Allergy Proc 1992;13:163.
28. Stevenson DD, Simon RA. Lack of cross-reactivity between rofecoxib and aspirin in aspirin-sensitive patients with asthma. J Allergy Clin Immunol 2001;108:47.
29. Hamad AM, Sutcliffe AM, Knox AJ. Aspirin-induced asthma: clinical aspects, pathogenesis and management. Drugs 2004;64:2417.
30. Eneli I, Sadri K, Camargo C Jr, et al. Acetaminophen and the risk of asthma: the epidemiologic and pathophysiologic evidence. Chest 2005;127:604.
31. Irwin RS, Madison JM. The diagnosis and treatment of cough. N Engl J Med 2000; 343:1715.
32. Johnson D, Osborn LM. Cough variant asthma: a review of the clinical literature. J Asthma 1991;28:85.
33. Miller PW, Hamosh A, Macek M Jr, et al. Cystic fibrosis transmembrane conductance regulator (CFTR) gene mutations in allergic bronchopulmonary aspergillosis. Am J Hum Genet 1996;59:45.
34. Slavin RG, Hutcheson PS, Chauhan B, et al. An overview of allergic bronchopulmonary aspergillosis with some new insights. Allergy Asthma Proc 2004;25:395.
35. Wark P, Wilson AW, Gibson PG. Azoles for allergic bronchopulmonary aspergillosis (Cochrane review). Cochrane Database Syst Rev 2000;3:CD001108.
36. Stevens DA, Schwartz HJ, Lee JY, et al. A randomized trial of itraconazole in allergic bronchopulmonary aspergillosis. N Engl J Med 2000;342:756.
37. American Thoracic Society. Proceedings of the ATS workshop on refractory asthma: current understanding, recommendations, and unanswered questions. Am J Respir Crit Care Med 2000;162:2341.
38. Rand CS, Mellins RB, Malveaux F, et al. The role of patient adherence in fatal asthma. In: Sheffer A, ed. Fatal asthma. New York: Marcel Dekker, 1998:429.
39. Wenzel S. Severe asthma in adults. Am J Respir Crit Care Med 2005;172:149.
40. McFadden ER Jr.Warren EL. Observations on asthma mortality. Ann Intern Med 1997;127:142.
41. Andrianopoulos MV, Gallivan GJ, Gallivan KH. PVCM, PVCD, EPL, and irritable larynx syndrome: what are we talking about and how do we treat it? J Voice 2000;14:607.
42. Perin PV, Perin RJ, Rooklin AR. When a sigh is just a sigh . . . and not asthma. Ann Allergy 1993;71:478.
43. Mahler DA, Harver A, Lentine T, et al. Descriptors of breathlessness in cardiorespiratory diseases. Am J Respir Crit Care Med 1996;154:1357.
44. Govindaraj M. What is the cause of dyspnea in asthma and emphysema? Ann Allergy 1987; 59:63.
45. Fabbri LM, Picotti G, Mapp CE. Late asthmatic reactions, airway inflammation and chronic asthma in TDI sensitized subjects. Eur Respir J 1991;13:136s.
46. Shah A, Panjabi C, Singh AB. Asthma caused by human seminal plasma allergy. J Asthma 2003;40:125.
47. Muller BA. Sinusitis and its relationship to asthma. Can treating one airway disease ameliorate another? Postgrad Med 2000;108:55.
48. Gibson PG, Henry RL, Coughlan JL. Gastro-oesophageal reflux treatment for asthma in adults and children. Cochrane Database Syst Rev 2000;2:CD001496.
49. Alexander JA, Hunt LW, Patel AM. Prevalence, pathophysiology, and treatment of patients with asthma and gastroesophageal reflux disease. Mayo Clin Proc 2000;75:1055.
50. Kiljander TO, Laitinen JO. The prevalence of gastroesophageal reflux disease in adult asthmatics. Chest 2004;126:1490.
51. Virchow C, Szczeklik A, Bianco S, et al. Intolerance to tartrazine in aspirin-induced asthma: results of a multicenter study. Respiration 1988;53:20.
52. Woessner KM, Simon RA, Stevenson DD. Monosodium glutamate sensitivity in asthma. J Allergy Clin Immunol 1999;104:305.
53. Koenig JQ. Air pollution and asthma. J Allergy Clin Immunol 1999;104:717.
54. Friedman MS, Powell KE, Hutwagner L, et al. Impact of changes in transportation and commuting behaviors during the 1996 Summer Olympic Games in Atlanta on air quality and childhood asthma. JAMA 2001;285:897.
55. Rand CS, Wise RA. Adherence with asthma therapy in the management of asthma. In: Szefler SJ, Leung DYM, eds. Lung Biology in health and disease. Vol. 86. Severe asthma: pathogenesis and clinical management. New York: Marcel Dekker, 1995:435.
56. Weiss ST, Shore S. Obesity and asthma: directions for research. Am J Respir Crit Care Med 2004;169:963.
57. Shim C, Williams MH Jr. Pulsus paradoxus in asthma. Lancet 1973;1:530.
58. Fukakusa M, Bergeron C, Tulic MK, et al. Oral corticosteroids decrease eosinophil and CC chemokine expression but increase neutrophil, IL-8, and IFN-gamma-inducible protein 10 expression in asthmatic airway mucosa. J Allergy Clin Immunol 2005;115:280.
59. de Benedictis FM, Bush A. Rhinosinusitis and asthma: epiphenomenon or causal association? Chest 1999;115:550.
60. Woodcock A, Forster L, Matthews E, et al. Medical Research Council General Practice Research Framework. Control of exposure to mite allergen and allergen-impermeable bed covers for adults with asthma. N Engl J Med 2003;349:225.
61. de Blay F, Chapman MD, Platts-Mills TA, et al. Airborne cat allergen (Fel d I). Environmental control with the cat *in situ*. Am Rev Respir Dis 1991;143:1334.
62. Gergen PJ, Mortimer KM, Eggleston PA, et al. Results of the National Cooperative Inner-City Asthma Study (NCICAS) environmental intervention to reduce cockroach allergen exposure in inner-city homes. J Allergy Clin Immunol 1999;103:501.
63. Wood RA, Johnson EF, Van Natta ML, et al. A placebo-controlled trial of a HEPA air cleaner in the treatment of cat allergy. Am J Respir Crit Care Med 1998;158:115.
64. Covar RA, Macomber BA, Szefler SJ. Medications as asthma triggers. Immunol Allergy Clin North Am 2005;25:169.
65. Cates CJ, Jefferson TO, Bara AI, et al. Vaccines for preventing influenza in people with asthma. Cochrane Database Syst Rev 2004;2:CD000364.
66. American Lung Association Asthma Clinical Research Centers. The safety of inactivated influenza vaccine in adults and children with asthma. N Engl J Med 2001;345:1529.
67. http://www.nhlbi.nih.gov/health/index.htm
68. http://www.lungusa.org
69. http://www.aanma.org/breatherville.htm
70. Drazen JM, Israel E, Boushey HA, et al. Comparison of regularly scheduled with as-needed use of albuterol in mild asthma. Asthma Clinical Research Network. N Engl J Med 1996;335:841.
71. Israel E, Chinchilli VM, Ford JG, et al. National Heart, Lung, and Blood Institute's Asthma Clinical Research Network. Use of regularly scheduled albuterol treatment in asthma: genotype-stratified, randomised, placebo-controlled cross-over trial. Lancet 2004;364: 1505.
72. Cheung D, Timmers MC, Zwinderman AH, et al. Long-term effects of a long-acting beta 2-adrenoceptor agonist, salmeterol, on airway hyperresponsiveness in patients with mild asthma. N Engl J Med 1992;327:1198.
73. Lemanske RF Jr, Sorkness CA, Mauger EA, et al. Inhaled corticosteroid reduction and elimination in patients with persistent asthma receiving salmeterol: a randomized controlled trial. JAMA 2001;285:2594.

74. Lazarus SC, Boushey HA, Fahy JV, et al. Long-acting beta2-agonist monotherapy vs continued therapy with inhaled corticosteroids in patients with persistent asthma: a randomized controlled trial. JAMA 2001;285:2583.
75. Edelman JM, Turpin JA, Bronsky EA, et al. Oral montelukast compared with inhaled salmeterol to prevent exercise-induced bronchoconstriction. A randomized, double-blind trial. Ann Intern Med 2000;132: 97.
76. Malmstrom K, Rodriguez-Gomez G, Guerra J, et al. Oral montelukast, inhaled beclomethasone, and placebo for chronic asthma. A randomized, controlled trial. Montelukast/Beclomethasone Study Group. Ann Intern Med 1999;130:487.
77. Leff JA, Busse WW, Pearlman D, et al. Montelukast, a leukotriene-receptor antagonist, for the treatment of mild asthma and exercise-induced bronchoconstriction. N Engl J Med 1998;339:147.
78. Drazen JM, Israel E, O'Byrne PM. Treatment of asthma with drugs modifying the leukotriene pathway. N Engl J Med 1999;340:197.
79. Silverman ES, Drazen JM. Genetic variations in the 5-lipoxygenase core promoter. Description and functional implications. Am J Respir Crit Care Med 2000;161:S77.
80. Juniper EF, Kline PA, Vanzieleghem MA, et al. Effect of long-term treatment with an inhaled corticosteroid (budesonide) on airway hyperresponsiveness and clinical asthma in nonsteroid-dependent asthmatics. Am Rev Respir Dis 1990;142:832.
81. Boushey HA, Sorkness CA, King TS, et al. ; National Heart, Lung, and Blood Institute's Asthma Clinical Research Network. Daily versus as-needed corticosteroids for mild persistent asthma. N Engl J Med 2005;352:1519.
82. Lipworth BJ. Systemic adverse effects of inhaled corticosteroid therapy: a systematic review and meta-analysis. Arch Intern Med 1999;159:941.
83. Suissa S, Baltzan M, Kremer R, et al. Inhaled and nasal corticosteroid use and the risk of fracture. Am J Respir Crit Care Med 2004;169:83.
84. Barnes PJ. Inhaled glucocorticoids for asthma. N Engl J Med 1995;332:868.
85. Harrison TW, Oborne J, Newton S, et al. Doubling the dose of inhaled corticosteroid to prevent asthma exacerbations: randomised controlled trial. Lancet 2004;363:271.
86. Evans DJ, Taylor DA, Zetterstrom O, et al. A comparison of low-dose inhaled budesonide plus theophylline and high-dose inhaled budesonide for moderate asthma. N Engl J Med 1997;337:1412.
87. Greening AP, Ind PW, Northfield M, et al. Added salmeterol versus higher-dose corticosteroid in asthma patients with symptoms on existing inhaled corticosteroid. Allen & Hanburys Limited UK Study Group. Lancet 1994;344:219.
88. Laviolette M, Malmstrom K, Lu S, et al. Montelukast added to inhaled beclomethasone in treatment of asthma. Montelukast/Beclomethasone Additivity Group. Am J Respir Crit Care Med 1999;160:1862.
89. Lofdahl CG, Reiss TF, Leff JA, et al. Randomised, placebo controlled trial of effect of a leukotriene receptor antagonist, montelukast, on tapering inhaled corticosteroids in asthmatic patients. BMJ 1999;319:87.
90. Pauwels RA, Lofdahl CG, Postma DS, et al. , for the Formoterol and Corticosteroids Establishing Therapy (FACET) International Study Group. Effect of inhaled formoterol and budesonide on exacerbations of asthma. N Engl J Med 1997;337:1405.
91. Kidney J, Dominguez M, Taylor PM, et al. Immunomodulation by theophylline in asthma. Demonstration by withdrawal of therapy. Am J Respir Crit Care Med 1995;151:1907.
92. Weinberger M, Hendeles L. Theophylline in asthma. N Engl J Med 1996;334:1380.
93. Wechsler ME, Garpestad E, Flier SR, et al. Pulmonary infiltrates, eosinophilia, and cardiomyopathy following corticosteroid withdrawal in patients with asthma receiving zafirlukast. JAMA 1998;279:455.
94. Stoodley RG, Aaron SD, Dales RE. The role of ipratropium bromide in the emergency management of acute asthma exacerbation: a metaanalysis of randomized clinical trials. Ann Emerg Med 1999;34:8.
95. Milgrom H, Fick RB Jr.Su JQ, et al. Treatment of allergic asthma with monoclonal anti-IgE antibody. N Engl J Med 1999;341:1966.
96. Dykewicz MS. Newer and alternative non-steroidal treatments for asthmatic inflammation. Allergy Asthma Proc 2001;22:11.
97. Davies H, Olson L, Gibson P. Methotrexate as a steroid sparing agent for asthma in adults. Cochrane Database Syst Rev 2000;2:CD000391.
98. Aaron SD, Dales RE, Pham B. Management of steroid-dependent asthma with methotrexate: a meta-analysis of randomized clinical trials. Respir Med 1998;92:1059.
99. Larrain A, Carrasco E, Galleguillos F, et al. Medical and surgical treatment of nonallergic asthma associated with gastroesophageal reflux. Chest 1991;99:1330.
100. Strunk RC. Identification of the fatality-prone subject with asthma. J Allergy Clin Immunol 1989;83:477.
101. Littenberg B, Gluck EH. A controlled trial of methylprednisolone in the emergency treatment of acute asthma. N Engl J Med 1986;314:150.
102. Wrenn K, Slovis CM, Murphy F, et al. Aminophylline therapy for acute bronchospastic disease in the emergency room. Ann Intern Med 1991;115:241.
103. Thys F, Roeseler J, Delaere S, et al. Two-level non-invasive positive pressure ventilation in the initial treatment of acute respiratory failure in an emergency department. Eur J Emerg Med 1999;6:207.
104. Namazy JA, Schatz M. Treatment of asthma during pregnancy and perinatal outcomes. Curr Opin Allergy Clin Immunol 2005;5:229.
105. Dombrowski MP, Schatz M, Wise R, et al. National Institute of Child Health and Human Development Maternal-Fetal Medicine Units Network; National Heart, Lung, and Blood Institute. Randomized trial of inhaled beclomethasone dipropionate versus theophylline for moderate asthma during pregnancy. Am J Obstet Gynecol 2004;190:737.
106. Sears MR, Greene JM, Willan AR, et al. A longitudinal, population-based, cohort study of childhood asthma followed to adulthood. N Engl J Med 2003;349:1414.
107. Goldman M, Rachmiel M, Gendler L, et al. Decrease in asthma mortality rate in Israel from 1991–1995: is it related to increased use of inhaled corticosteroids? J Allergy Clin Immunol 2000;105:71.
108. Celli BR, MacNee W; ATS/ERS Task Force. Standards for the diagnosis and treatment of patients with COPD: a summary of the ATS/ERS position paper. Eur Respir J 2004;23:932.
109. National Heart, Lung, and Blood Institute, Division of Lung Diseases. Workshop report: the definition of emphysema. Am Rev Respir Dis 1985;132:182.
110. Hogg JC, Chu F, Utokaparch S, et al. The nature of small-airway obstruction in chronic obstructive pulmonary disease. N Engl J Med 2004;350:2645.
111. Jeffery PK. Structural and inflammatory changes in COPD: a comparison with asthma. Thorax 1998;53:129.
112. Anthonisen NR, Wright EC, Hodgkin JE; IPPB Trial Group. Prognosis in obstructive pulmonary disease. Am Rev Respir Dis 1986;133:14.
113. Peto R, Speizer FE, Cochrane AL, et al. The relevance in adults of air-flow obstruction, but not of mucus hypersecretion, to mortality from chronic lung disease: results from 20 years of prospective observation. Am Rev Respir Dis 1983;128:491.
114. Fletcher C, Peto R. The natural history of chronic airflow obstruction. BMJ 1977;1:1645.
115. Burrows B, Bloom JW, Trayer GA, et al. The course and prognosis of different forms of chronic airways obstruction in a sample from the general population. N Engl J Med 1987;317:1309.
116. Anthonisen NR, Connett JE, Kiley JP, et al. Effects of smoking intervention and the use of an inhaled anticholinergic bronchodilator on the rate of decline of FEV_1. The Lung Health Study. JAMA 1994;272:1497.
117. Scanlon PD, Connett JE, Waller LA, et al. Smoking cessation and lung function in mild-to-moderate chronic obstructive pulmonary disease. The Lung Health Study. Am J Respir Crit Care Med 2000;161:381.
118. Anthonisen NR, Skeans MA, Wise RA, et al. Lung Health Study Research Group. The effects of a smoking cessation intervention on 14.5-year mortality: a randomized clinical trial. Ann Intern Med 2005;142:233.
119. Higgins M. Risk factors associated with chronic obstructive lung disease. Ann N Y Acad Sci 1991;624:7.
120. Imai K, Dalal SS, Chen ES, et al. Human collagenase (matrix metalloproteinase-1) expression in the lungs of patients with emphysema. Am J Respir Crit Care Med 2001;163:786.
121. Finlay GA, O'Driscoll L, Russell KJ, et al. Matrix metalloproteinase expression and production by alveolar macrophages in emphysema. Am J Respir Crit Care Med 1997;156:240.
122. Tuder RM, Petrache I, Elias JA, et al. Apoptosis and emphysema: the missing link. Am J Respir Cell Mol Biol 2003;28:551.
123. Crystal RG, Brantly ML, Hubbard RC, et al. The alpha-1-antitrypsin gene and its mutations: clinical consequences and strategies for therapy. Chest 1989;95:196.
124. Silverman EK, Province MA, Rao DC, et al. A family study of the variability of pulmonary function in a1-antitrypsin deficiency: quantitative phenotypes. Am Rev Respir Dis 1990;142:1015.
125. Sandford AJ, Chagani T, Weir TD, et al. Susceptibility genes for rapid decline of lung function in the lung health study. Am J Respir Crit Care Med 2001;163:469.
126. Meldrum M, Rawbone R, Curran AD, et al. The role of occupation in the development of chronic obstructive pulmonary disease (COPD). Occup Environ Med 2005;62:212.
127. Kanner RE, Connett JE, Altose MD, et al. Gender difference in airway hyperresponsiveness in smokers with mild COPD. The Lung Health Study. Am J Respir Crit Care Med 1994;150: 956.
128. Sluiter HJ, Keoter GH, de Monchy JG, et al. The Dutch hypothesis (chronic non-specific lung disease) revisited. Eur Respir J 1991;4:479.
129. O'Conner GT, Sparrow D, Weiss S. The role of allergy and nonspecific airway hyperresponsiveness in the pathogenesis of chronic obstructive pulmonary disease. State of the art review. Am Rev Respir Dis 1989;140:225.
130. Tashkin DP, Altose MD, Connett JE, et al. Methacholine reactivity predicts changes in lung function over time in smokers with early chronic obstructive pulmonary disease. Am J Respir Crit Care Med 1996;153:1802.
131. Bellofiore S, Eidelman DH, Macklem PT, et al. Effects of elastase-induced emphysema on airway responsiveness to methacholine in rats. J Appl Physiol 1989;66:606.

132. Burrows B, Knudson RJ, Camilli AE, et al. The horse-racing effect and predicting decline in forced expiratory volume in one second from screening spirometry. Am Rev Respir Dis 1987;135:788.
133. Wise RA. Changing smoking patterns and mortality from chronic obstructive pulmonary disease. Prev Med 1997;26:418.
134. Viegi G, Scognamiglio A, Baldacci S, et al. Epidemiology of chronic obstructive pulmonary disease (COPD). Respiration 2001;68:4.
135. American Thoracic Society. Health effects of outdoor air pollution. Am J Respir Crit Care Med 1996;153:3.
136. MacNee W, Donaldson K. Exacerbations of COPD: environmental mechanisms. Chest 2000;117:390S.
137. Samet JM, Dominici F, Curriero FC, et al. Fine particulate air pollution and mortality in 20 U.S. cities, 1987–1994. N Engl J Med 2000;343:1742.
138. Badgett RG, Tanaka DJ, Hunt DK, et al. Can moderate chronic obstructive pulmonary disease be diagnosed by historical and physical findings alone? Am J Med 1993;94:188.
139. Straus SE, McAlister FA, Sackett DL, et al. The accuracy of patient history, wheezing, and laryngeal measurements in diagnosing obstructive airway disease. CARE-COAD1 Group. Clinical Assessment of the Reliability of the Examination-Chronic Obstructive Airways Disease. JAMA 2000;283:1853.
140. Piirila P, Sovijarvi AR, Kaisla T, et al. Crackles in patients with fibrosing alveolitis, bronchiectasis, COPD, and heart failure. Chest 1991;99:1076.
141. Schapira RM, Schapira MM, Funahashi A, et al. The value of the forced expiratory time in the physical diagnosis of obstructive airways disease. JAMA 1993;270:731.
142. Pauwels RA, Buist AS, Calverley PM, et al. Global strategy for the diagnosis, management, and prevention of chronic obstructive pulmonary disease. NHLBI/WHO Global Initiative for Chronic Obstructive Lung Disease (GOLD) Workshop summary. Am J Respir Crit Care Med 2001;163:1256.
143. Calverley PM, Burge PS, Spencer S, et al. Bronchodilator reversibility testing in chronic obstructive pulmonary disease. Thorax 2003;58:659.
144. Eaton ML, Green BA, Church MS, et al. Efficacy of theophylline in irreversible airflow obstruction. Ann Intern Med 1980;92:758.
145. Knudson RJ, Kaltenborn WT, Burrows B. Single breath carbon monoxide transfer factor in different forms of chronic airflow obstruction in a general population sample. Thorax 1990;45:514.
146. ATS Committee on Proficiency Standards for Clinical Pulmonary Function Laboratories. ATS statement: guidelines for the six-minute walk test. Am J Respir Crit Care Med 2002;166:111.
147. Solway S, Brooks D, Lacasse Y, et al. A qualitative systematic overview of the measurement properties of functional walk tests used in the cardiorespiratory domain. Chest 2001;119:256.
148. John M, Hoernig S, Doehner W, et al. Anemia and inflammation in COPD. Chest 2005;127:825.
149. American Thoracic Society/European Respiratory Society Statement: Standards for the Diagnosis and Management of Individuals with Alpha-1 Antitrypsin Deficiency. Am J Respir Crit Care Med 2003;168:818.
150. Stockley RA,O'Brien C, Pye A, et al. Relationship of sputum color to nature and outpatient management of acute exacerbations of COPD. Chest 2000;117:1638.
151. Sethi S, Wrona C, Grant BJ, et al. Strain-specific immune response to Haemophilus influenzae in chronic obstructive pulmonary disease. Am J Respir Crit Care Med 2004;169:448.
152. Sethi S, Murphy TF. Bacterial infection in chronic obstructive pulmonary disease in 2000: a state-of-the-art review. Clin Microbiol Rev 2001;14:336.
153. Menzies R, Gibbons W, Goldberg P. Determinants of weaning and survival among patients with COPD who require mechanical ventilation for acute respiratory failure. Chest 1989;95:398.
154. Rieves RD, Bass D, Carter RR, et al. Severe COPD and acute respiratory failure. Correlates for survival at the time of tracheal intubation. Chest 1993;104:854.
155. Williams JH Jr.Moser KM. Pneumococcal vaccine and patients with chronic lung disease. Ann Intern Med 1986;104:106.
156. Bridges CB, Fukuda K, Cox NJ, et al. Prevention and control of influenza. Recommendations of the Advisory Committee on Immunization Practices (ACIP). MMWR Recomm Rep 2001;50:1.
157. Alkins SA, O'Malley P. Should health-care systems pay for replacement therapy in patients with alpha$_1$-antitrypsin deficiency? A critical review and cost-effectiveness analysis. Chest 2000;117:875.
158. Seersholm N, Wencker M, Banik N, et al. Does α_1-antitrypsin augmentation therapy slow the annual decline in FEV_1 in patients with severe hereditary alpha1-antitrypsin deficiency? Eur Respir J 1997;10:2260.
159. Abboud RT, Ford GT, Chapman KR; Standards Committee of the Canadian Thoracic Society. Alpha$_1$-antitrypsin deficiency: a position statement of the Canadian Thoracic Society. Can Respir J 2001;8:81.
160. Anthonisen NR, Manfreda J, Warren CWP, et al. Antibiotic therapy in exacerbations of chronic obstructive pulmonary disease. Ann Intern Med 1987;106:196.
161. Snow V, Lascher S, Mottur-Pilson C. Evidence base for management of acute exacerbations of chronic obstructive pulmonary disease. Ann Intern Med 2001;134:595.
162. Medical Research Council Working Party. Long-term domiciliary oxygen therapy in chronic hypoxic cor pulmonale complicating chronic bronchitis and emphysema: report of the Medical Research Council Working Party. Lancet 1981;1:681.
163. Nocturnal Oxygen Therapy Trial Group. Continuous or nocturnal oxygen therapy in hypoxemic chronic obstructive lung disease: a clinical trial. Ann Intern Med 1980;3:391.
164. Tarpy SP, Celli BR. Long-term oxygen therapy. N Engl J Med 1995;333:710.
165. Fletcher EC, Luckett RA, Goodnight-White S, et al. A double-blind trial of nocturnal supplemental oxygen for sleep desaturation in patients with chronic obstructive pulmonary disease and a daytime PaO_2 above 60 mm Hg. Am Rev Respir Dis 1992;145:1070.
166. Chaouat A, Weitzenblum E, Kessler R, et al. A randomized trial of nocturnal oxygen therapy in chronic obstructive pulmonary disease patients. Eur Respir J 1999;14:1002.
167. Weitzenblum E, Schrijen F, Apprill M, et al. One year treatment with almitrine improves hypoxaemia but does not increase pulmonary artery pressure in COPD patients. Eur Respir J 1991;4:1215.
168. Winkelmann BR, Kullmer TH, Kneissl DG, et al. Low-dose almitrine bismesylate in the treatment of hypoxemia due to chronic obstructive pulmonary disease. Chest 1994;105:1383.
169. Chetty KG, Light RW, Stansbury DW, et al. Exercise performance of polycythemic chronic obstructive pulmonary disease patients. Effect of phlebotomies. Chest 1990;98:1073.
170. Huerta C, Lanes SF, Garcia Rodriguez LA. Respiratory medications and the risk of cardiac arrhythmias. Epidemiology 2005;16:360.
171. Poole PJ, Black PN. Mucolytic agents for chronic bronchitis or chronic obstructive pulmonary disease. Cochrane Database Syst Rev 2000;CD001287.
172. Bolton CE, Ionescu AA, Shiels KM, et al. Associated loss of fat free mass and bone mineral density in chronic obstructive pulmonary disease. Am J Respir Crit Care Med 2004;170:1286.
173. Ferreira IM, Brooks D, Lacasse Y, et al. Nutritional intervention in COPD: a systematic overview. Chest 2004;119:353.
174. Lung Health Study Research Group. Effect of inhaled triamcinolone on the decline in pulmonary function in chronic obstructive pulmonary disease. N Engl J Med 2000;343:1902.
175. Vestbo J, Sorensen T, Lange P, et al. Long-term effect of inhaled budesonide in mild and moderate chronic obstructive pulmonary disease: a randomised controlled trial. Lancet 1999;353:1819.
176. Pauwels RA, Löfdahl C-G, Laitinen LA, et al. Long-term treatment with inhaled budesonide in persons with mild chronic obstructive pulmonary disease who continue smoking. N Engl J Med 1999;340:1948.
177. Burge PS, Calverley PM, Jones PW, et al. Randomised, double blind, placebo controlled study of fluticasone propionate in patients with moderate to severe chronic obstructive pulmonary disease: the ISOLDE trial. BMJ 2000;320:1297.
178. Gross NJ, Petty TL, Friedman M, et al. Dose response to ipratropium as a nebulized solution in patients with chronic obstructive pulmonary disease. A three-center study. Am Rev Respir Dis 1989;139:1188.
179. Casaburi R, Briggs DD Jr, Donohue JF, et al. The spirometric efficacy of once-daily dosing with tiotropium in stable COPD: a 13-week multicenter trial. Chest 2000;118:1294.
180. van Noord JA, Bantje TA, Eland ME, et al. A randomised controlled comparison of tiotropium and ipratropium in the treatment of chronic obstructive pulmonary disease. Thorax 2000;55:289.
181. Barr R, Bourbeau J, Camargo C, et al. Inhaled tiotropium for stable chronic obstructive pulmonary disease. Cochrane Database Syst Rev 2005;2:CD002876.
182. Rennard SI, Anderson W, ZuWallack R, et al. Use of a long-acting inhaled beta$_2$-adrenergic agonist, salmeterol xinafoate, in patients with chronic obstructive pulmonary disease. Am J Respir Crit Care Med 2001;163:1087.
183. D'Urzo AD, De Salvo MC, Ramirez-Rivera A, et al. In patients with COPD, treatment with a combination of formoterol and ipratropium is more effective than a combination of salbutamol and ipratropium: a 3-week, randomized, double-blind, within-patient, multicenter study. Chest 2001;119:1347.
184. Combivent Inhalation Solution Study Group. Routine nebulized ipratropium and albuterol together are better than either alone in COPD. Chest 1997;112:1514.
185. Friedman M, Serby CW, Menjoge SS, et al. Pharmacoeconomic evaluation of a combination of ipratropium plus albuterol compared with ipratropium alone and albuterol alone in COPD. Chest 1999;115:635.
186. Hanania NA, Darken P, Horstman D, et al. The efficacy and safety of fluticasone propionate (250 microg)/salmeterol (50 microg) combined in the Diskus inhaler for the treatment of COPD. Chest 2003;124:834.
187. Pauwels RA. New aspects of the therapeutic potential of theophylline in asthma. J Allergy Clin Immunol 1989;83:548.
188. Culpitt SV, de Matos C, Russell RE, et al. Effect of theophylline on induced sputum inflammatory indices and neutrophil chemotaxis

in chronic obstructive pulmonary disease. Am J Respir Crit Care Med 2002;165:1371.
189. Murciano D, Auclair MH, Pariente R, et al. M. A randomized, controlled trial of theophylline in patients with severe chronic obstructive pulmonary disease. N Engl J Med 1989; 320:1521.
190. Niewoehner DE, Erbland ML, Deupree RH, et al. Effect of systemic glucocorticoids on exacerbations of chronic obstructive pulmonary disease. N Engl J Med 1999;340:1941.
191. Thompson WH, Nielson CP, Carvalho P, et al. Controlled trial of oral prednisone in outpatients with acute COPD exacerbation. Am J Respir Crit Care Med 1996;154:407.
192. Rice KL, Rubins JB, Lebahn F, et al. Withdrawal of chronic systemic corticosteroids in patients with COPD: a randomized trial. Am J Respir Crit Care Med 2000;162:174.
193. Bach PB, Brown C, Gelfand SE, et al. Management of acute exacerbations of chronic obstructive pulmonary disease: a summary and appraisal of published evidence. Ann Intern Med 2001;134:600.
194. American College of Chest Physicians and American Association of Cardiovascular and Pulmonary Rehabilitation. Pulmonary rehabilitation: joint ACCP/AACVPR evidence-based guidelines. Chest 1997;112:1363.
195. The American Society for Transplant Physicians (ASTP)/American Thoracic Society (ATS)/European Respiratory Society (ERS)/International Society for Heart and Lung Transplantation (ISHLT). International guidelines for the selection of lung transplant candidates. Am J Respir Crit Care Med 1998; 158:335.
196. Trulock EP 3rd. Lung transplantation for COPD. Chest 1998;113:269S.
197. Fishman A, Martinez F, Naunheim K, et al. National Emphysema Treatment Trial Research Group. A randomized trial comparing lung-volume-reduction surgery with medical therapy for severe emphysema. N Engl J Med 2003;348:2059.
198. National Emphysema Treatment Trial Research Group. Patients at high risk of death after lung-volume-reduction surgery. N Engl J Med 2003;345:1075.

*For annotated **General References** and resources related to this chapter, visit www.hopkinsbayview.org/PAMreferences.*

Chapter 61

Lung Cancer

Linda F. Barr

Lung cancer is the leading cause of visceral cancer and cancer-related death in the United States. In 1999 there were an estimated 171,600 new cases of lung cancer and 158,900 deaths from the disease. For each lung cancer patient, an average of 14.7 years of life is lost prematurely (1). The turn of the millennium has seen a small decline in lung cancer mortality for men but a large increase in mortality for women (2). Because of its close association with tobacco smoke, lung cancer is generally a preventable tumor. Unfortunately, the diagnosis usually occurs late in the course of the disease after metastasis has occurred and determined the outcome. New radiographic methods enhance lung cancer detection but remain unproven for benefiting survival. Advances in the management of lung cancer have resulted from both the improved delivery of older chemotherapeutic agents and the addition of new, tumor-specific drugs.

EPIDEMIOLOGY

Tobacco

From 80% to 90% of lung cancers are caused by tobacco smoke, most importantly from cigarettes, but also from pipes and cigars. The increasing death rate from lung cancer in the past 50 years lags 20 years behind a parallel rise in cigarette smoking. Ominously, although the prevalence of current cigarette use declined over >30 years, it significantly increased among high-school students in the United States from 27.5% in 1991 to 36.4% in 1997. Furthermore, cigar smoking has increased by 50% among all age groups (3). When cigarette use has declined, so also has lung cancer incidence. During its first decade, the California tobacco control program led to significant declines in smoking, in association with declines in lung cancer and heart disease mortality (4).

The lifetime lung cancer mortality for the general population is approximately 10% for moderate smokers, 20% for heavy smokers, and 1% for nonsmokers (5), a compelling statistic because 47 million Americans smoke. For smokers, the most important determinant of lung cancer risk is the duration of cigarette smoking, and the number of cigarettes smoked per day has a multiplicative effect (6). The risk of lung cancer increases approximately with the fourth power of the number of years of smoking and the square of the number of cigarettes smoked daily (7). Because of the duration effect, individuals who start smoking before age 15 years are four times more likely to develop lung cancer than those who begin after age 25 years (6). Furthermore, exposure to smoke from other persons' cigarettes ("passive smoking") leads to an increased risk for lung cancer (8–10). The risk of lung cancer declines after 5 years from smoking cessation and continues to decrease with duration of time from quitting; however, some risk remains for former heavy smokers. Indeed, almost half of lung cancers occur in former smokers.

Although those who smoke nonfiltered cigarettes have the highest risk for lung cancer, the amount of tar in each cigarette does not correlate with cancer risk (11). This is because smokers of low-tar and low-nicotine cigarettes typically increase the depth and length of their cigarette inhalation to get their required dose of nicotine (12). Research demonstrates that carcinogen uptake is only modestly and transiently reduced when the number of daily cigarettes is decreased (13). Although the risk of lung cancer is strongly related to the number of cigarettes smoked daily, these results suggest that the only way to decrease lung cancer risk from cigarettes is to stop smoking completely.

Occupational Exposure

Table 61.1 lists other exposures that increase the risk for lung cancer and examples of relevant occupations (14). It is especially important to identify people with asbestos exposure. Not only do asbestos-exposed individuals have an increased incidence of mesothelioma, they also have a sixfold greater risk for developing lung cancer than the general population. Those exposed people who smoke are 60 times more likely to develop bronchogenic carcinoma than are nonsmoking nonexposed people (15).

TABLE 61.1 Occupational Agents Associated with Lung Cancer

Agent	*Occupational Examples*
Arsenic	Copper smelting, pesticide manufacturing, manufacture of "pressure-treated" wood
Asbestos	*Historically:* production, shipfitters *Currently:* maintenance and construction workers exposed to asbestos insulation, mechanics exposed to asbestos brake linings
Beryllium	Mining, refining, manufacture of ceramics, electronic, and aerospace equipment
Bis(chloromethyl)ether	Production, construction
Cadmium	Electroplating, manufacture of plastics and alloys, pigments, battery electrodes
Chromium, hexavalent	Manufacturing of pigments, stainless steel, plating
Mustard gas	Production, warfare
Nickel	Manufacturing of stainless steel, nonferrous alloys, batteries, and electroplating
Polycyclic aromatic compounds	Aluminum production, coal gasification, coke production, soot, and iron and steel founding
Radon	Mining
Vinyl chloride	Production of polyvinyl chloride
Probable Carcinogens	
Acrylonitrile	Manufacture of acrylic fiber for textiles, pipes
Diesel exhaust	Mining, trucking, construction
Formaldehyde	Manufacture, biology
Silica	Mining, masonry, concrete, pottery

Based on classifications of the International Agency for Research on Cancer and the National Institute of Occupational Safety and Health.

Radon

Radon is a pulmonary carcinogen that is a naturally produced radioactive gas found universally in the soil and air. The contribution of radon exposure to excess lung cancer in uranium and other underground miners (including those who mine iron, zinc, tin, and fluorspar) is well established. Of unproven but theoretical concern is the lung cancer risk from exposure to radon in contaminated soil beneath some homes. By extrapolation from miners' data, it is estimated that such exposure may be responsible for a relative risk of 1.14 (95% confidence interval = 1.0–1.3) at 150 Bq/m^3 (the standard measure of radiation exposure) and may account for 6,000 to 36,000 lung cancer deaths each year in the United States. There may be a greater than additive risk for cigarette smoking and home radon exposure (16). Because of uncertainty in the risk estimates, it has been suggested that homes should be tested for radon using commercially available tests and corrective measures taken when the exposure rate approaches 150 Bq/m^3. Whether such measures are effective in reducing the risk of lung cancer is unknown.

Other Risk Factors

It is important to consider other groups with increased risk for bronchogenic carcinoma. First, those with *previous lung cancers* or with other tobacco-associated cancers are at markedly increased risk for developing a second cancer of the respiratory or upper digestive tract (discussed later in Follow-up of Patients Surviving Lung Cancer section). Second, some studies suggest that *genetic predisposition* influences the risk of lung cancer. Stratified case control studies controlled for cigarette smoking have determined that lung cancer patients have an odds ratio of 1.7 to 5.3 for having a first-order relative with lung cancer (17,18). This increased risk may be the result of an inadequacy of DNA repair capacity. Studies of the repair of bleomycin- and benzo[*a*]pyrene diol epoxide–induced chromatid damage (the latter chemical is a carcinogenic derivative of tobacco smoke) show significant differences in the DNA repair ability between lymphocytes derived from lung cancer patients and those derived from age- and ethnicity-matched control subjects (19). Alternatively, genetic differences in lung cancer risk may reflect differences in the functioning of enzymes in the metabolic pathways of carcinogens.

Third, the presence of *chronic lung disease* may increase lung cancer risk. This has been described for both chronic obstructive pulmonary disease (20) and interstitial disease (21). Fourth, *human immunodeficiency virus infection* is associated with a relative risk of lung cancer of 6.5 compared with the general population. As with other acquired immunodeficiency syndrome (AIDS)-associated malignancies, lung cancer is more aggressive and manifests a worse prognosis in the AIDS patient (22).

SCREENING

The diagnosis of lung cancer is generally made in the last quarter of the tumor's life cycle, usually after metastases have occurred and essentially have determined the outcome (23). This observation underlies the dismal survival of patients with the disease. For all stages combined, 5-year survival for patients with non–small cell lung cancer (NSCLC) is 14% and for those with small cell lung cancer (SCLC) is 6%, with only a modest gain over the past 2 decades. However, more than half of patients with disease discovered at a localized stage survive for at least 5 years (24). Thus, there is much interest in detecting lung cancers at an earlier curable stage. As with other adult solid tumors, lung cancers have a long preclinical phase characterized by accumulating genetic changes over a decade or more. This may reflect the relationship between tumor size and doubling time. A 1-mm tumor has already undergone 20 doublings, and a 1-cm tumor has already undergone 30 doublings. Over the extrapolated range of tumor doubling times, this implies a lifespan of 5 to 10 years with accumulating genetic damage, angiogenesis, and metastasis occurring along the way (25).

The presence of a large pool of undiagnosed lung cancer in current and former smokers is supported by the discovery of a 6.4% incidence of unsuspected malignant nodules in the lung specimens of patients undergoing lung volume reduction surgery (26). Earlier large randomized studies at multiple centers showed that screening cigarette smokers with yearly chest x-ray films and sputum cytology improved the detection of cancer and the survival (time from detection to death) but did not lead to a significant reduction in mortality (27). Whether this paradox results from lead time bias (the time of diagnosis moved forward but the date of death unaffected) or overdiagnosis (length) bias (bias toward detection of less aggressive or indolent tumors in a periodically screened sample) (28), or whether the tumors were not detected at a sufficiently early point in their development to have altered outcome is controversial.

The same debates surround the development of low-energy chest computed tomography (CT) as a screening tool for lung cancer (29). This technique is more sensitive than chest radiography and detects nodules <1 cm; however, it has relatively poor specificity. This is exemplified by the findings from a prospective study of annual screening using low-dose helical chest CT at the Mayo Clinic (30). Two years after baseline CT scanning, noncalcified nodules were detected in 69% of 1,520 current and former smokers, with the majority of tumors almost certainly benign. Given the high rate of benign nodule detection, the researchers cautioned that if the annual rate of new indeterminate pulmonary nodules seen in the study remained at 9% to 13%, then "almost all patients will have at least one false-positive CT examination result after several more years of screening." At the 3-year point, 55 participants (3.6%) underwent 60 thoracic operations: benign disease was found in 10 patients (18%) and lung cancer was found in 45 (82%). A 5-year followup study of the Mayo Clinic cohort showed that annual screening chest CT did not lead to a difference in the percentage of patients diagnosed with stage I disease. The authors note, "CT screening for lung cancer offers the possibility of reducing mortality from lung cancer. Our preliminary results do not support this possibility and may raise concerns that false-positive results and overdiagnosis could actually result in more harm than good." In addition to the considerable economic burden of screening and then followup of all these patients, the interventional evaluation carried a significant morbidity: surgical complications occurred in 27% of patients, and operative mortality was 1.7% (31). Larger trials to measure the benefits of screening chest CT in at-risk patients are ongoing.

In addition to improving radiologic methods for lung cancer detection, research has focused on developing lung cancer biomarkers. Candidate abnormalities found in cigarette smokers include mutations in *ras* and *p53* genes and DNA sequence loss at three loci: 3p14 (location of the *FHIT* tumor suppressor gene), 9p21 (location of the *p16* tumor-suppressor gene), and 17p13 (location of the *p53* tumor-suppressor gene). Differences between lung cancer patients and control subjects have also been found for the functional status of members of the family of enzymes responsible for carcinogen activation and degradation and the ability of patients' lymphocytes to repair the genetic damage induced by the cigarette carcinogen benzo[*a*]pyrene (19,32). Analysis of the expression of large numbers of genes and proteins in individual tumors by DNA microarrays and advances in proteomics highlight patterns that may later prove useful for tumor detection and for tumor characterization both by type and by chemotherapeutic responsiveness. Measurement of these markers is not yet clinically useful.

The U.S. Preventive Services Task Force has extensively reviewed the current data and concluded that there is no support for lung cancer screening by any method, although the data also are insufficient to conclude that screening does not work (33).

HISTOLOGY

Lung cancer is classified broadly into two major groups—NSCLC and SCLC—both of which are associated with cigarette smoking. The distribution of these cancers is 80% and 20%, respectively. In the NSCLC category, approximately 36% of patients have *squamous cell carcinomas*, 45% have *adenocarcinomas*, 9% have *large cell carcinomas*, 2% to 4% have *bronchioloalveolar carcinomas*, and 1% to 2% have *carcinoids*. There is significant heterogeneity in the histology: 45% of patients with NSCLC have mixed NSCLC phenotypes, 10% to 20% of NSCLC tumors have SCLC-like neuroendocrine features, and 9% of SCLC have regions of NSCLC tumor cells (34). This heterogeneity supports the hypothesis that all pulmonary cancers arise from a single pluripotent stem cell that has the capacity to differentiate into the major bronchioloalveolar mucosal cell types, including neuroendocrine, glandular, and epithelial.

The past 15 to 20 years have seen a significant shift in NSCLC subtypes in North America, but not in Europe, from a majority squamous cell to a majority that is adenocarcinoma. This has been attributed to the use of "low-tar" cigarettes in the United States and Canada, which lead to a deeper inhalation pattern that allows greater carcinogen exposure to the peripheral lung (where adenocarcinomas generally arise). Another contributor may be the increased proportion of women with lung cancer, a population that is more prone to adenocarcinomas (35,36).

The incidence of bronchioloalveolar carcinoma has doubled over the past 20 years; in one study, this tumor constituted 15% of all lung cancers (37). The reason for this increase is unclear. Patients with this cancer tend to be younger, are more likely to be female, and are less likely to be smokers than are those with other lung cancers. The treatment of bronchioloalveolar carcinoma is similar to that of other non–small cell carcinomas. However, this tumor has a greater propensity to spread locally (or to arise in multiple locations, consistent with a "field" defect) compared with other NSCLC phenotypes, and repeated surgical excisions may be necessary (38).

Malignant mesothelioma is a pleural tumor strongly associated with asbestos exposure. There is a time lag of 25 to 40 years between asbestos exposure and cancer presentation. A proposed relationship between the development of this tumor and infection with the DNA virus SV40 (simian virus) is controversial. Mesothelioma usually is heralded by a pleural effusion. The diagnostic yield of thoracentesis for mesothelioma is <40%, improved by only 10% by repeat thoracentesis and pleural needle biopsy. Thus, thoracoscopic-guided biopsy or open lung biopsy may be required for this diagnosis. A common problem with procedures used to diagnose this tumor is malignant seeding along needle and incisional tracts. A positron emission tomography (PET) scan is useful in the evaluation of tumor extent and prognosis. The histologic differentiation of malignant mesothelioma from adenocarcinoma is an occasional problem and may necessitate electron microscopy or staining for immunohistochemical markers. The treatment of mesothelioma entails debulking surgery, with either intracavitary or external radiation. Platinum-based chemotherapy in conjunction with gemcitabine and other agents may be useful. A promising new treatment for mesothelioma is pemetrexed, which targets folate metabolic enzymes to disrupt nucleotide synthesis. Still, the prognosis is poor, and the median survival time is 12 months (39,40).

HISTORY

The symptoms of lung cancer can be categorized according to those caused by the mass effect of the tumor in the airway, those caused by impingement of the tumor on extrapulmonary mediastinal structures, those of paraneoplastic syndromes, and those of distant metastases.

Pulmonary Symptoms

Ninety percent of patients with lung cancer have symptoms at the time of diagnosis, and most of these symptoms are respiratory. The respiratory manifestations include cough, dyspnea, chest pain, hemoptysis, and symptoms related to postobstructive pneumonia. Cough occurs in almost all patients during the course of lung cancer. *Cough* and sputum production are nonspecific symptoms in smokers, but the appearance of a chronic cough, with or without expectoration, or a change in cough pattern in an older smoker should raise a suspicion of lung cancer.

Hemoptysis (generally blood-streaked sputum) is the initial manifestation of cancer in many patients. Potential extrapulmonary sources of hemoptysis include the mouth, nasopharynx, and gastrointestinal tract. Evaluation includes history and physical examination, including oral pharyngeal and nasal examination, and a chest CT scan, preferably with contrast. Referral for bronchoscopy should be considered for patients who are older than 40 years or who have an abnormal radiograph, a history of hemoptysis for >1 week, a history of tobacco smoking, a chronic cough, anemia, or weight loss. Lung cancer is found at bronchoscopy in one third of patients with hemoptysis and one or more of these risk factors (41). Whether bronchoscopy is indicated in the absence of these risk factors is unclear. With rare exceptions, a negative bronchoscopy is reliable for excluding lung cancer in patients with hemoptysis and negative radiologic studies (42). Because a bronchoscopy is not as good for diagnosing upper airway disease as a nasopharyngoscopy and mirror examination, patients with a negative pulmonary evaluation will require examination by an otolaryngologist and possibly also by a gastroenterologist.

Chest pain is reported by approximately half of patients with lung cancer on presentation, usually as an intermittent dull ache on the side of the tumor. The cause of this pain is unclear. If the tumor appears otherwise resectable, this symptom should not preclude surgery. More severe pain may indicate metastatic disease to the parietal pleura or to bone and may necessitate a bone scan or PET scan. Shoulder pain, sometimes mistaken for arthritis, may be caused by a *Pancoast* (superior sulcus) tumor (see Extrapulmonary Thoracic Symptoms section) or may be caused by a tumor involving the diaphragm.

Dyspnea in a patient with lung cancer may be caused directly by the primary tumor or may result from factors indirectly related to the tumor, from treatment of the cancer, and from other concurrent medical disease. Primary tumor-related etiologies include obstruction of the airway with postobstructive atelectasis or pneumonia, pleural effusion, lymphangitic carcinomatosis, or pericardial metastasis. The tumor can impinge on nerves and lead to recurrent laryngeal or phrenic nerve palsy. Dyspnea indirectly related to the cancer may result from pulmonary embolism, an electrolyte or hormonal disorder from a paraneoplastic syndrome, or inanition. Radiation may result in pneumonitis. Chemotherapeutic agents may cause anemia or other toxicities, such as cardiomyopathy or pneumonitis, which may contribute to this symptom. Finally, because cigarettes are a common risk factor for other medical conditions, patients with lung cancer may have pre-existing lung disease, usually chronic obstructive lung disease or cardiac disease that may produce dyspnea.

Pneumonia resulting from airway obstruction by tumor may be the presenting manifestation of lung cancer. There are no formal recommendations on whether to obtain a followup chest x-ray film in a patient with pneumonia. Whether to obtain a chest x-ray film to document resolution of pneumonia several weeks after the acute illness should therefore be based on (a) whether there were findings suggestive of lung cancer on the patient's initial film; (b) the patient's risk factors for lung cancer, including age and history of cigarette smoking or other exposure; (c) the presence of pre-existing lung disease or other medical comorbidities that increase the risk of pneumonia complications; and (d) the patient's clinical course. A pneumonia that fails to resolve should prompt a consultation with a pulmonologist.

Extrapulmonary Thoracic Symptoms

Intrathoracic extrapulmonary extension may present in a variety of ways, including the superior vena cava syndrome, Pancoast tumor syndrome, Horner syndrome, dysphagia, hoarseness, and symptoms of pericardial disease. Patients with these symptoms should be rapidly evaluated for definitive diagnosis and treatment.

The *superior vena cava syndrome* consists of edema and rubor of the upper trunk and face, sometimes with syncope. It is caused by obstruction of the superior vena cava by involvement of the mediastinum with tumor. The chest x-ray film usually shows a right upper lobe mass and a widened mediastinum. In 25% of cases, a right pleural effusion is noted.

The *Pancoast syndrome* is caused by a tumor that is located at the pulmonary apex and involves adjacent structures such as the chest wall, lymphatics, ribs, vertebrae, vessels, and nerves. The tumor may cause shoulder pain, arm pain, and paresthesia, usually in the ulnar distribution, indicating encroachment of the brachial plexus.

Horner syndrome results from tumor invasion of the lower cervical or upper thoracic sympathetic trunk and consists of miosis, ptosis, enophthalmos, facial flushing, and anhidrosis on the affected side.

Persistent hoarseness may be caused by involvement of the trachea with tumor or by vocal cord paralysis caused by entrapment of the recurrent laryngeal nerve, usually on the left, by a mediastinal mass. This symptom should be evaluated with a flow–volume loop (performed in a pulmonary function laboratory) or by laryngoscopy. Additionally, contrast CT should be performed, starting at the sinuses and down through the chest, to evaluate the upper airway, mediastinum, and pulmonary parenchyma.

Wheezing usually is caused by small airway obstruction but also may be produced by upper airway or bronchial obstruction by an intrinsic or extrinsic mass. Therefore, upper airway involvement should be evaluated in all wheezing patients by auscultation over the neck. The presence of stridor or of monophonic wheezing that localizes to the neck should be emergently evaluated with flow–volume loops and/or laryngoscopy and chest x-ray and neck films.

Mediastinal tumors or enlarged lymph nodes can cause dysphagia by extrinsically impinging on the esophagus. Finally, lung cancers can directly invade, or metastasize to, the pericardium and produce tamponade.

Extrathoracic Symptoms

Anorexia, cachexia, weight loss, and fever are common in patients with lung cancer, particularly as the disease advances. Extrathoracic metastatic disease is found at autopsy in most patients with NSCLC and in almost all patients with SCLC. Metastases may be seen in any organ. Common metastatic sites for lung cancer include the pleura, bone, brain, liver, and adrenal glands. In addition, SCLC frequently invades the bone marrow, leading to hematologic abnormalities.

Paraneoplastic Syndromes

Paraneoplastic syndromes are common in patients with lung cancer. It is important to recognize that the symptoms of paraneoplastic syndromes may precede the other symptoms of lung cancer. Manifestations of these syndromes may mimic metastatic disease and mislead treatment decisions. These symptoms generally improve with successful treatment of the underlying malignancy.

Endocrine syndromes may be seen in 10% to 15% of patients. The most common is *hypercalcemia* secondary to a parathyroid hormone-related protein, with an N-terminus homologous with that of normal parathyroid hormone so that it binds to the parathyroid hormone receptor. This syndrome is usually caused by an NSCLC. The *syndromes of inappropriate antidiuretic hormone release* and of *ectopic adrenocorticotropic hormone secretion* are less common and are more likely to be seen in patients with SCLC. Increased levels of these ectopic hormones can be found in the blood of many more patients with SCLC than in the few percent that have clinical manifestations of the syndromes. The syndrome of inappropriate antidiuretic hormone release is associated with hyponatremia (see Chapter 81). The ectopic adrenocorticotropic hormone syndrome is characterized by mild hypertension, hyperglycemia, hypokalemia, alkalosis, and occasional hyperpigmentation but generally does not have the other manifestations of Cushing syndrome.

Clubbing and *hypertrophic pulmonary osteoarthropathy* are common in, although not limited to, patients with lung cancer. Clubbing is seen in one third of patients with lung cancer. Hypertrophic pulmonary osteoarthropathy with pain, swelling, tenderness, and positive bone scan may be seen in as many as 10% of these patients. Lung cancer is the underlying cause in >80% of adult cases of this osteoarthropathy. The symptoms usually respond to aspirin or other nonsteroidal anti-inflammatory medicines.

Neurologic paraneoplastic processes are rare but dramatic and may be the presenting symptoms of SCLC and occasionally of NSCLC (43). PET scanning may be useful for diagnosis of occult malignancy, whereas magnetic resonance imaging (MRI) seems to have limited value (44). In the *Eaton-Lambert syndrome*, proximal muscle weakness and paresthesias may mimic myasthenia gravis, from which it can be distinguished by electromyography. The diagnosis of other neurologic paraneoplastic syndromes, including peripheral neuropathies, subacute cerebellar degeneration, cortical degeneration, polymyositis, and intestinal dysmotility, may be facilitated by measurement of type I antineuronal nuclear antibody (ANNA-1/Hu-1) (43). Treatment of the tumor may result in improvement of these symptoms.

Hematologic abnormalities may occur in patients with lung cancer and with mesotheliomas. An increased tendency to clot may be manifest as either typical or atypical (*Trousseau syndrome*) venous or arterial thromboembolic disease (see Chapter 57). Anemia and thrombocytosis are common.

PHYSICAL EXAMINATION

The purpose of a careful physical examination of patients with lung cancer is to determine the presence of metastatic disease, to evaluate the patient's candidacy for therapy, and to assess the patient's functional capacity, which is a major contributor to prognosis. Constitutional findings are important; weight loss may be evidence of advanced disease. Attention must be paid to areas of pain or tenderness, which may indicate bony metastasis. The examination should include an evaluation of lymph nodes in the anterior and posterior cervical, supraclavicular, and axillary regions. Suspicious lymph nodes are those >1 cm in diameter, hard in consistency, or fixed. Hoarseness or signs of superior vena cava syndrome or Horner syndrome should be noted. The pulmonary examination may reveal evidence of chronic lung disease and local wheezing or bronchial breath sounds from bronchial obstruction or basilar dullness from a pleural effusion. D'Éspene sign, the inappropriate transmission of whispered pectoriloquy below the level of the T2 vertebral body, suggests mediastinal involvement with tumor. The cardiac examination, including evaluation of the jugular veins, is important in preoperative assessment and when considering the possibility of a malignant pericardial effusion. Hepatomegaly (liver span >13 cm) may suggest hepatic metastases. The extremities may demonstrate clubbing, edema, or cyanosis. A careful neurologic examination is important to look for evidence of brain metastases.

DIAGNOSTIC PROCEDURES

Chest X-Ray Film

A review of old chest x-ray films can demonstrate the rapidity of disease onset and may aid in prognostication. A mass with a doubling time of <2 weeks or >450 days is unlikely to be malignant. (For a more extensive discussion of radiologic characteristics helpful in differentiating benign from malignant pulmonary lesions, see Solitary Pulmonary Nodule.)

Certain chest x-ray patterns are suggestive of particular types of lung cancer. Squamous cell and small cell carcinomas tend to be centrally located. Adenocarcinomas and large cell carcinomas tend to arise peripherally. Centrally located tumors are more likely to present with symptoms of obstruction, such as atelectasis, pneumonia, and dyspnea. SCLC may demonstrate only hilar adenopathy with no visible primary tumor on the initial chest x-ray film. Squamous cell carcinoma is the most likely bronchogenic carcinoma to cavitate, although even this tumor cavitates uncommonly.

Bronchioloalveolar cell carcinoma usually presents peripherally and tends to be multifocal. This cancer has a variety of radiologic manifestations and may appear as a single mass or as multiple nodules, or it may imitate a pneumonia. Malignant mesothelioma is associated with a pleural effusion, and the underlying pleural surface is thickened and lumpy.

Computed Tomography and Magnetic Resonance Imaging of the Chest

A contrast CT of the chest is routine in the evaluation of patients with suspected lung cancer to determine the anatomic extent of the tumor and to guide diagnostic and therapeutic procedures (reviewed in ref. 45). CT may demonstrate lesions that are unseen on chest x-ray film. Furthermore, CT may aid in characterizing the size, shape, and composition of these lesions. For example, CT is better than chest x-ray film in determining calcification of a solitary pulmonary nodule (SPN); a densely calcified nodule is more likely to be benign. CT may demonstrate fat in a nodule, highly suggestive of a hamartoma. In addition, the presence and size of mediastinal or hilar lymph nodes can be evaluated by CT. In patients with lung cancer, nodes >1 cm in diameter have a 60% chance of representing metastatic disease (46). If a surgical cure is contemplated, sampling by transbronchial needle aspiration (TBNA), mediastinoscopy, or mediastinotomy is required (see these specific subsections to follow). Finally, extending CT cuts down through the upper abdomen may demonstrate hepatic or adrenal metastases, although these radiographic findings will require biopsy if therapy would be influenced by the histology of these lesions. CT is neither sensitive nor specific in detecting the invasion of chest wall or mediastinal structures.

MRI is superior to CT for evaluation of possible chest wall or vascular invasion by tumor and for examination of superior sulcus tumors. MRI is more sensitive than contrast CT for diagnosing brain metastases. MRI is not as informative as CT for evaluating pulmonary parenchymal disease, nor is it helpful for evaluating mediastinal lymph nodes.

Positron Emission Tomography

PET, using the glucose analogue fluorodeoxyglucose (FDG), aids in the evaluation of some patients with SPN and in the staging of lung cancer (see Staging). FDG is taken up more avidly by more metabolically active cells and is not easily eliminated. Malignant tissue is enhanced by this method, whereas normal tissue is not. For focal pulmonary densities of all sizes, the sensitivity of PET is 97% and the specificity is 78% (47). Infections, other inflammatory lesions, and granulomatous disease such as sarcoidosis can demonstrate high FDG uptake, leading to false-positive results. Some tumors are falsely identified as benign by this study, especially bronchioloalveolar carcinomas and some adenocarcinomas (see Solitary Pulmonary Nodule). Finally, the PET scan is insensitive for densities <1 cm and in the presence of a high serum glucose level.

Sputum Cytology

The frequency of diagnosis of lung cancer from cytology submitted from spontaneously expectorated sputum depends on the cell type and the tumor location (48). Squamous cell tumors shed cells into the airways, and cytologies are positive approximately 80% of the time. However, patients with a peripheral adenocarcinoma have positive cytologies <5% of the time. Patients should be instructed to produce a forceful cough. Three early morning specimens should be collected in a tightly fitting container. If the specimens cannot be submitted to the laboratory within 2 to 3 hours of collection, a fixative should be added, in which case the specimens can be pooled and submitted together. Saccomanno solution, which contains alcohol and Carbowax, is one of the best fixatives. Submitting more than three samples does not increase the likelihood of a positive diagnosis of cancer. If the patient is not producing sputum, induction by inhalation of an aerosolized solution of saline can be helpful. The patient inhales normal saline or Hanks balanced salt solution that is aerosolized by an ultrasonic nebulizer (DeVilbiss 3583). In general, sputum induction is not a routine office procedure and should be done by experienced personnel. In addition to the sputum collected immediately after induction, good material is produced the following morning. The addition of chest vibration or percussion does not improve the yield from sputum cytology. In cases with obstruction of the bronchus as evidenced by the physical examination or chest x-ray film, it is reasonable to start collecting sputum after therapy, which includes antibiotics and perhaps bronchodilators and may reestablish airway patency and allow sputum production.

Bronchoscopy

Bronchoscopy is used both to diagnose and to stage bronchogenic carcinoma (49). Bronchoscopy is important to search for a second synchronous malignancy and to evaluate vocal cord function. A fixed vocal cord suggests involvement of the recurrent laryngeal nerve in the mediastinum. Furthermore, the bronchoscope visualizes the proximal extent of the tumor, which is helpful in planning surgery (tracheal "sleeve" resections allow resection of tumors close to the carina). Transbronchial biopsy using forceps, brushing for cytology, and bronchoalveolar lavage all can be performed through the bronchoscope. In addition, transbronchial needle aspiration (TBNA) allows sampling of hilar, subcarinal, and other mediastinal lymph nodes. The diagnostic yield for sampling tumors outside of the airway is improved with endoscopic guidance, which is not available in all centers. Fiberoptic bronchoscopy is an outpatient procedure that causes minimal discomfort with use of mild sedation (e.g., midazolam or propofol), a short-acting narcotic (fentanyl), sometimes a drying and vagolytic agent (usually atropine or glycopyrrolate), and topical lidocaine. Occasional circumstances dictate preoperative endotracheal intubation or use of a rigid bronchoscope; these procedures are done with general anesthesia.

The diagnostic yield of bronchoscopy is 60% to 80% for tumors >2 cm in diameter and 20% to 40% for those <2 cm, and it is higher for visualized masses in the central airways. Necrotic tumors, submucosal carcinomas, and large tumors that displace feeding bronchi may be more of a diagnostic challenge and may require more than one bronchoscopic procedure to obtain diagnostic material. Many peripheral tumors are accessible by bronchoscopy using fluoroscopically guided needles, brushes, and biopsy forceps. However, masses <2 cm or in the outer third of the lung usually are better approached from the outside by percutaneous transthoracic needle aspiration (PTNA).

Although bronchoscopy is generally a safe and well-tolerated procedure, potential complications include pulmonary hemorrhage, pneumothorax, laryngospasm or bronchospasm, hypoxemia, and transient cardiac arrhythmias. Patients with primary or secondary coagulation disorders, thrombocytopenia, uremia, pulmonary hypertension, or the superior vena cava syndrome are at increased risk for bleeding. Patients receive supplemental oxygen during the procedure and shortly thereafter, and they are monitored with continuous oximetry. Pneumothorax complicates approximately 5% of transbronchial forceps biopsies and <1% of TBNA procedures, although only half of patients who develop a pneumothorax require a chest tube. Transient atrial and ventricular arrhythmias occur in approximately 5% of elderly patients and may be related to transient hypoxemia or induction of the vagal response by passage of the bronchoscope through the upper airway. However, death is rare and almost always is associated with a transbronchial biopsy that caused significant bleeding (50).

Patients may have a low-grade fever after bronchoscopy, but the occurrence of pneumonia is low. Although the incidence of bacteremia during bronchoscopy is <2%, some advocate prophylactic antibiotics for patients at risk for bacterial endocarditis (50).

The interval between a myocardial infarction and safe performance of fiberoptic bronchoscopy is unknown and must be established on an individual basis, balancing the goals of the procedure and the therapeutic implication of the results.

Patient Experience. Bronchoscopy can be performed on an ambulatory basis by a pulmonologist or a thoracic surgeon. The patient is told to fast (including liquids) for at least 8 hours before bronchoscopy (although generally medicines can be taken with a sip of water) and to not eat for approximately 1 to 2 hours after completion of the procedure until the effects of topical anesthesia wear off. The only discomfort the patient will experience is coughing caused by irritation of the trachea and main bronchi, which is treated with topical 1% to 2% lidocaine. There usually is no pain associated with this procedure. A low-grade fever (<100.5°F oral) or blood-streaked hemoptysis may be present during the first 24 hours after bronchoscopy; however, the patient should call the pulmonologist or go to the emergency room for higher fever, hemoptysis that is more than blood streaking, chest pain, severe shoulder pain (which may indicate a pneumothorax), or exacerbation of shortness of breath.

In the unusual situation where sputum cytology demonstrates malignancy but the chest x-ray film and chest CT scan do not localize a suspicious area ("occult carcinoma"), a long bronchoscopic procedure is undertaken under general anesthesia. In the procedure, a meticulous upper airway evaluation is followed by sequential sampling of each pulmonary segment. Positive findings mandate a confirmatory procedure in which repeat sampling is done of subsegments corresponding to the positive material. The yield of this procedure is 13% to 35%, and up to 15% of these patients have multicentric carcinomas. New metachronous primary lung cancer develops in patients with "occult carcinoma" at the rate of 5% per year. Almost all these patients are heavy smokers and have increased surgical morbidity and mortality; thus, lung-sparing surgery or photodynamic therapies may be indicated (51).

Percutaneous Transthoracic Needle Aspiration

CT-directed PTNA of the lung is most useful when a mass or a nodule is located peripherally near the pleura or in the apex of the lung. It is especially helpful in the diagnosis of metastatic carcinoma because these tumors arise outside of the airway and are difficult to diagnose by bronchoscopy, particularly when they are <2 cm in size. It also may be preferred when the differential diagnosis includes infection because interpretation of the significance of an infectious agent obtained by bronchoscopy is complicated by passage of the scope through the nonsterile nasopharynx or oropharynx. PTNA is performed by either a radiologist or a pulmonologist with fluoroscopic or CT guidance. The technique and experience of the operator and the cytopathologist are of paramount importance in the success of the procedure, and the yield is increased with a repeat procedure. However, the false-negative rate for any fluoroscopically guided procedure is significant. Thus, nondiagnostic or nonspecific findings require followup, the nature of which is determined by the adequacy of the sample and the clinical scenario. PTNA is usually an outpatient procedure, done with local anesthetic, and requires a cooperative patient (52).

Contraindications to the procedure include large blebs or blood vessels that are in the direct path of the needle; a patient with an uncontrollable cough, in which case general anesthesia may be necessary; and contralateral pneumonectomy, in which case the production of a pneumothorax would be devastating. In addition, patients with pulmonary hypertension have an increased risk for bleeding.

Patient Experience. Patients will receive intravenous sedation and local anesthetic. The patient will feel a mild pressure sensation with introduction of the needle. Otherwise, there is no significant pain. Potential complications include a 5% risk of bleeding (usually of minimal amount) and a 10% to 15% risk of pneumothorax (half of these cases require chest tube insertion). Most patients can resume normal activity within 24 hours.

Mediastinoscopy, Mediastinotomy, and Thoracoscopy

Mediastinoscopy and mediastinotomy are indicated when enlarged mediastinal lymph nodes or masses cannot be adequately sampled by less invasive techniques (TBNA or PTNA; see specific sections above). Lymph nodes accessible to cervical mediastinoscopy are those located in the pretracheal area from the thoracic inlet to 1 cm beyond the carina bilaterally. Those anterior to the aortic arch and in the aortic–pulmonary window are not accessible to the cervical mediastinoscope and require anterior mediastinotomy. Potential complications include wound infection, injury to major vascular structures, and recurrent laryngeal nerve paralysis (53). These procedures are done by thoracic surgeons and require general anesthesia and hospitalization.

A biopsy done through a thoracoscope may be better tolerated than one done during a limited thoracotomy. Thoracoscopy may also be helpful, in selected cases, in the removal of peripheral lung masses (54) and in diagnosing the cause of pleural effusions. A medical thoracoscopy can be done under general anesthesia or in the patient sedated with local anesthetic. The visceral and parietal pleuras are examined with either a rigid or fiberoptic endoscope inserted through a chest tube.

A video-assisted thoracic surgical procedure usually requires general anesthesia. The procedure involves inducing a controlled pneumothorax and single lung ventilation, followed by insertion of the instruments through multiple small incisions. The patient generally has 2 to 3 days of hospital observation with a chest tube in place after thoracoscopy. The incidence of complications is similar to that of the closed procedures (55).

STAGING

The staging of the patient with lung cancer has two goals: to determine the anatomic extent of the tumor and to determine the physiologic capacity of the patient to undergo therapy.

Non–Small Cell Lung Cancer

For NSCLC, the anatomic extent of the tumor is defined by the TNM classification system, where T is tumor size, N is nodal involvement, and M is distant metastasis. The TNM categories then are grouped into four stages with therapeutic and prognostic implications (Tables 61.2, 61.3, and 61.4).

Mediastinal nodal involvement can be assessed by chest CT, with sampling of lymph nodes >1 cm in transverse diameter, by bronchoscopy (TBNA), or by mediastinoscopy or surgery. PET is complementary to CT for this examination. For detection of mediastinal node metastases, the

TABLE 61.2 Staging of Non–Small Cell Lung Cancer: TNM Definitions

Primary Tumor (T)	
TX	Primary tumor cannot be assessed or tumor proven by presence of malignant cells in sputum or bronchial washings but not visualized by imaging on bronchoscopy
T0	No evidence of primary tumor
Tis	Carcinoma in situ
T1	Tumor ≤3 cm in greatest dimension, surrounded by lung or visceral pleura, without bronchoscopic evidence of invasion more proximal than lobar bronchus (i.e., not in main bronchus)[a]
T2	Tumor with any of the following features of size or extent: >3 cm in greatest dimension Involves main bronchus, ≥2 cm distal to the carina Invades the visceral pleura Associated with atelectasis or obstructive pneumonitis that extends to the hilar region but does not involve the entire lung
T3	Tumor of any size that directly invades any of the following: chest wall (including superior sulcus tumors), diaphragm, mediastinal pleura, or pericardium; tumor in the main bronchus <2 cm distal to the carina but without involvement of the carina; or associated atelectasis or obstructive pneumonitis
T4	Tumor of any size that invades any of the following: mediastinum, heart, great vessels, trachea, esophagus, vertebral body, or carina; or tumor with a malignant pleural effusion[b] or pericardial effusion, or satellite nodule(s) within the primary bearing lobe
Lymph Node (N)	
NX	Regional lymph nodes cannot be assessed
N0	No regional lymph node metastasis
N1	Metastasis in ipsilateral peribronchial or ipsilateral hilar lymph nodes, including direct extension
N2	Metastasis in ipsilateral mediastinal or subcarinal lymph node(s)
N3	Metastasis in contralateral mediastinal, contralateral hilar, ipsilateral or contralateral scalene, or supraclavicular lymph node(s)
Distant Metastasis (M)	
MX	Presence of distant metastasis cannot be assessed
M0	No distant metastasis
M1	Distant metastasis[c]

[a]The uncommon superficial tumor or any size with its invasive component limited to the bronchial wall, which may extend proximal to the main bronchus, is also classified as T1.

[b]Most pleural effusions associated with lung cancer are caused by tumor. However, in a few patients, multiple cytologic examinations or pleural fluid are negative for cancer. In these cases, the fluid is nonbloody and is not an exudate. When these elements and clinical judgment dictate that the effusion is not related to tumor, the effusion should be excluded as a staging element, and the patient should be staged T1, T2, T3. Pericardial effusion is classified according to the same rules.

[c]Tumor nodule(s) in the ipsilateral lung nonprimary tumor-bearing lobe is classified as M1.

From Mountain CF. Revisions in the international system for staging lung cancer. Chest 1997;111:1710, with permission.

TABLE 61.3 Staging of Non–Small Cell Lung Cancer: New International Revised Stage Grouping

Stage 0	Tis
Stage IA	T1, N0, M0
Stage IB	T2, N0, M0
Stage IIA	T1, N1, M0
Stage IIB	T2, N1, M0
	T3, N0, M0
Stage IIIA	T1-3, N2, M0
	T3, N1, M0
Stage IIIB	T4, Any N, M0
	Any T, N3, M0
Stage IV	Any T, Any N, M1

Modified from Mountain CF. Revisions in the international system for staging lung cancer. Chest 1997;111:1710, with permission.

TABLE 61.4 Five-Year Survival of Non–Small Cell Lung Cancer by Stage at Presentation

Stage	*TNM*	*Frequency (%)*	*5-Year Survival (%)*
IA	T1, N0, M0	~10	67
IB	T2, N0, M0		57
IIA	T1, NI, M0		34
IIB	T2, NI, M0	~13	24
	T3, N0, M0		22
IIIA	T1-3, N2, M0	~22	13
	T3, N1, M0		9
IIIB	T4, Any N, M0	~22	7
	T1-4, N3, M0		3
IV	T1-4, N0-3, M1	~32	1

From Bunn PA Jr, Mault J, Kelly K. Adjuvant and neoadjuvant chemotherapy for non-small cell lung cancer: a time for reassessment? Chest 2000;117: 119S, with permission.

sensitivity and specificity of PET scans are 79% and 91%, respectively, and of CT scans are 60% and 77%, respectively (56,57). However, unlike CT, PET scans cannot adequately distinguish between intrapulmonary lymph nodes and those in the mediastinum, nor can PET differentiate hyperplastic from neoplastic disease, which may require histologic sampling of positive areas.

The major sites of NSCLC metastases are brain, bones, liver, and adrenal glands. The extent of routine pretreatment evaluation of these sites has been controversial. However, two large meta-analyses have demonstrated that the negative predictive value of a good clinical evaluation for metastatic disease is >97% (58,59). This finding led the American Thoracic Society/European Respiratory Society (60) to recommend the NSCLC staging evaluation (Table 61.5). These recommendations may require modification for use in the individual patient. For example, constitutional signs or symptoms of advanced disease or evidence of borderline operability by physiologic criteria may necessitate a more aggressive staging evaluation.

Whole-body PET helps in the preoperative staging of patients with potentially resectable NSCLC. PET has good sensitivity and specificity for detection of distant metastases (56,57). In one prospective study of 102 patients, PET resulted in a change in tumor stage in 62 patients (56). However, because of a 17% false-positive rate for distant metastases, these areas need to be sampled. In addition, PET cannot visualize tumors in the brain. A combined PET–CT scan improves the diagnostic accuracy for diagnosing and staging malignancies (61).

MRI is useful for specific indications, such as examination of paravertebral tumors, or when imaging of vascular and neural structures in the mediastinum or thoracic inlet is required. Gadolinium-enhanced brain MRI scans are superior to CT for detection of brain metastases and should be considered for patients with stage III or IV NSCLC.

Both patients with NSCLC and those with SCLC should undergo evaluation of their performance status. The performance status determines the ability to undergo therapy and is a major contributor to the prognosis (62). Common scales for this measurement are the Eastern Cooperative Oncology Group (ECOG) and Karnofsky performance scales, which measure the patient's physiologic status as a result of the cancer and concurrent medical problems (Table 61.6).

TABLE 61.5 Pretreatment Evaluation of Patients with Lung Cancer

Part A: Recommended Tests for All Patients

Complete blood count
Electrolytes, calcium, alkaline phosphatase, albumin, AST, ALT, T bili, creatinine
Chest roentgenogram
CT of chest through the adrenals[a]
Histologic confirmation of malignancy[b]

Part B: Recommended Tests for Selected Patients

Test	*Indication*
CT of liver with contrast or liver ultrasound	Elevated liver enzymes; abnormal non–contrast-enhanced CT of liver or abnormal clinical evaluation
CT with contrast of brain or MRI brain	CNS symptoms or abnormal clinical evaluation
Radionuclide bone scan	Elevated alkaline phosphatase (bony fraction), elevated calcium, bone pain, or abnormal clinical evaluation
Pulmonary function tests	If lung resection or thoracic radiotherapy planned
Arterial blood gases	Patients with borderline resectability because of limited cardiopulmonary status
Quantitative radionuclide perfusion lung scan or exercise testing to evaluate maximum oxygen consumption	Patients with borderline resectability because of limited cardiopulmonary status

[a]May not be necessary if patient has obvious M1 disease on chest x-ray film or physical examination.
[b]Although optimal in most cases, tissue diagnosis may not be necessary in some cases where the lesion is enlarging and/or the patient will undergo surgical resection regardless of biopsy outcome.
ALT; alanine aminotransferase; AST, aspartate aminotransferase; CNS, central nervous system; CT, computed tomography; MRI, magnetic resonance imaging; T bili, total bilirubin.
Modified from American Thoracic Society/European Respiratory Society. Pretreatment evaluation of non–small-cell lung cancer. Am J Respir Crit Care Med 1997;156:320, with permission.

Small Cell Lung Cancer

SCLC is classified by a two-stage system. In *limited-stage disease*, the cancer is confined to the hemithorax and regional lymph nodes (including mediastinal, ipsilateral hilar, and supraclavicular nodes), which essentially delineate the extent of disease that can be contained within a tolerable radiation port. In *extensive-stage disease*, the cancer lies outside these boundaries. Rarely SCLC presents as a localized nodule, which is the only time curative surgery is possible. SCLC is a more aggressive tumor than NSCLC and metastasizes early and widely. Therefore, the staging on presentation is more extensive than with NSCLC. The staging of SCLC patients generally entails the same recommendations as in Table 61.5, part A, as well as additional studies. Because one third of these patients have bone involvement at presentation, a bone scan or PET scan is indicated. One fourth of patients have liver metastases. Because liver enzymes are not sensitive for metastases, a CT through the liver is necessary. The central nervous system is involved at presentation in one fourth, and eventually in half, of the patients with SCLC. Symptoms are absent in 10% of those with central nervous system

TABLE 61.6 Performance Status Scales

Karnofsky Performance Scale[a]	
Point	**Description**
100	Normal: no complaints; no evidence of disease
90	Able to perform normal activity; minor signs/symptoms of disease
80	Normal activity with effort; some signs/symptoms of disease
70	Cares for self; unable to perform normal activity or do active work
60	Requires occasional assistance but is able to care for most personal needs
50	Requires considerable assistance and frequent medical care
40	Disabled; requires special care and assistance
30	Severely disabled; hospitalization indicated; death not imminent
20	Very sick; hospitalization and active supportive treatment are necessary
10	Moribund; fatal processes progressing rapidly
0	Dead
	ECOG Performance Status Scale[b]
0	Fully active; able to carry on all predisease activities without restriction (Karnofsky 90–100)
1	Restricted in physically strenuous activity but ambulatory and able to carry out work of a light or sedentary nature, e.g., light housework or office work (Karnofsky 70–80)
2	Ambulatory and capable of all self-care but unable to carry out any work activities; up and about ≥50% of waking hours (Karnofsky 50–60)
3	Capable of only limited self-care; confined to bed or chair ≥50% of waking hours (Karnofsky 30–40)
4	Completely disabled; cannot carry on any self-care; totally confined to bed or chair (Karnofsky 10–20)

ECOG, Eastern Cooperative Oncology Group.
[a]From Vaporiciyan AA, Nesbitt JC, Lee JS, et al. Neoplasms of the thorax: cancer of the lung. In: Bast RC, Kufe DW, Pollock RE, et al., eds. Cancer medicine. 5th ed. Hamilton, Ontario: BC Decker Inc., 2000, with permission.
[b]From American Society of Clinical Oncology. Clinical practice guidelines for the treatment of unresectable non–small-cell lung cancer. J Clin Oncol 1997;15:3002, with permission.

involvement. A cranial MRI with gadolinium is superior to head CT for demonstration of metastases. A bone marrow aspirate and biopsy are no longer routine. Performance status must be evaluated, as for NSCLC (Table 61.6).

TREATMENT

Lung cancer therapy has been evolving. Treatment options may be complicated and often require the input of a pulmonologist, oncologist, radiotherapist, and thoracic surgeon. Current therapeutic trends include (a) optimizing the current therapies for benefit and risks; (b) introducing new chemotherapy agents, notably those resulting from improved understanding of cancer biology; (c) targeting therapy to the tumor to spare normal tissue and to be patient specific; and (d) improving supportive care.

The indication for chemotherapy has expanded to include all stages of lung cancer. Alternative radiation strategies are being investigated. Multimodality therapy, including concurrent radiation and chemotherapy, is increasingly being used. *Adjuvant therapy* is the addition of chemotherapy or radiotherapy to surgical treatment. Studies suggest that adjuvant therapy may have a role for some patients with complete surgical resection of NSCLC. *Neoadjuvant therapy* is the use of chemotherapy or radiotherapy prior to surgery, to shrink the tumor and allow for more complete resection.

The current standard treatments for NSCLC and SCLC are reviewed by Spira and Ettinger (63) and outlined in Table 61.7.

Non–Small Cell Lung Cancer

The most important prognostic criterion for NSCLC is the TNM classification because it defines resectable, and thus most of the potentially curable, disease. Surgery is the standard treatment for patients without clinical evidence of mediastinal or metastatic disease and is an option for selected patients with tumor involvement of the mediastinum or chest wall. Chemotherapy and radiotherapy improve survival of most stages (compare the 5-year survival outlined in Table 61.4 with that in Table 61.7).

Stages I, II, and IIIA

Surgical resection results in a 5-year survival of approximately 70% and 50% for patients with clinical stage I and stage II NSCLC, respectively, and is appropriate for selected patients with stage IIIA disease for whom 5-year survival is 15% by presurgical staging (although better for those defined by surgical staging). These results indicate significant mortality even in patients with disease that appears to be local at presentation. Postoperative radiation therapy improves local control and may have a small effect on survival for stage II and IIIA patients. Adjuvant or neoadjuvant platinum-based chemotherapy (e.g., cisplatin or carboplatin), generally in combination with other chemotherapeutic agents and external radiation, improves survival of patients with stage IIIA disease. Cisplatin-based chemotherapy has a small impact on survival of patients with stage I and II disease but is associated with considerable toxicity (64). Recommendations may be changed by newer therapies currently being evaluated, such as the well-tolerated oral agent uracil–tegafur (65,66).

SECTION 9

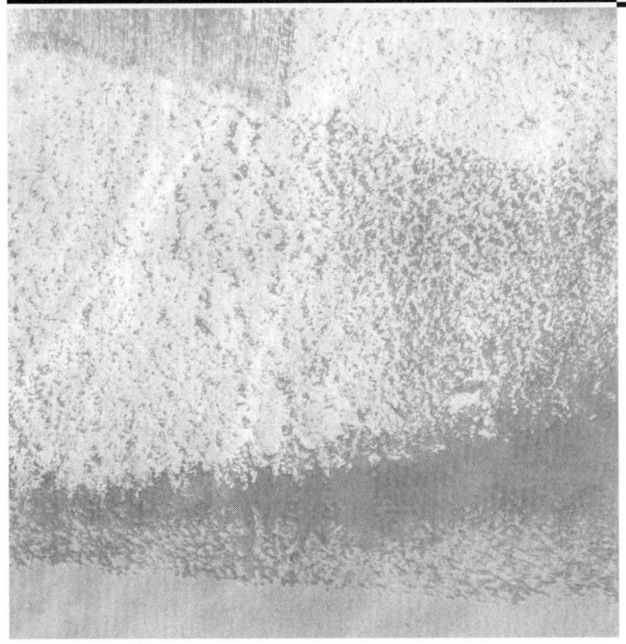

Cardiovascular Problems

Chapter 62

Coronary Artery Disease

Nisha Chandra-Strobos and Glenn A. Hirsch

Chest pain is one of the most common complaints of patients in an ambulatory practice. The major early objective in the diagnosis of patients with chest pain is separating noncardiac from cardiac etiologies. Chapters 42 and 59 describe the various causes of noncardiac chest pain. This chapter describes the pathogenesis of coronary artery disease (CAD) and its most common clinical symptom, angina pectoris. Chapter 63 describes the posthospital medical care and rehabilitation of patients who had a myocardial infarction (MI).

CAD caused by atherosclerosis is one of the most common ailments in the Western world, and it remains the leading nontraumatic cause of disability and death in the United States. Increased public awareness and health education have reduced CAD mortality by >20% in the last 25 years. However, CAD still affects approximately 13,000,000 Americans. Cardiovascular disease accounts for 38% of the total mortality in the United States or approximately the same number of deaths as the next five leading causes combined (cancer, chronic lower respiratory diseases, accidents, diabetes mellitus, and influenza and pneumonia). Of these cardiovascular deaths, coronary heart disease accounts for 53% (1). Chest pain is one of the most common presenting symptoms of patients with CAD who seek medical attention. Health care providers must understand the appropriate diagnostic evaluation and subsequent therapeutic options for patients with chest pain. A detailed history and physical examination are essential when evaluating patients with chest pain. They cannot be replaced by sophisticated procedures; rather, they guide the clinician in selecting the most appropriate diagnostic evaluation.

PATHOGENESIS

CAD presents in a variety of ways, largely related to the underlying pathophysiology of plaque formation and atherosclerosis. The endothelium plays an integral role in defending against atherosclerosis, modulating vascular tone, and preventing intravascular thrombosis. These endothelial functions are adversely affected by CAD risk factors, even before the development of overt atherosclerosis. In the earliest stages of disease, circulating monocytes adhere to vascular endothelial cells (via adhesion molecules) and migrate into the intima of the blood vessel, where they ingest oxidatively modified low-density lipoprotein (LDL) and become trapped as foam cells. Collections of foam cells, known as *fatty streaks,* may be present even in early childhood. Foam cells die, leading to the development of a lipid core. Smooth muscle cells are signaled to migrate from the media, destroying the internal elastic lamina of the vessel in the process. Calcification of the plaque occurs early and can be visualized noninvasively by electron-beam computed tomography (EBCT; see later discussion). The arterial wall progressively thickens and remodels. Encroachment of plaque into the lumen of a coronary artery occurs late in the atherosclerotic process, reflecting advanced disease. Arterial cross-sectional area is reduced by approximately 40% before a lesion is visible as "significant" CAD on catheterization, a finding demonstrated by use of in vivo intravascular ultrasound (2).

Atherosclerotic progression is accelerated by three processes: endothelial dysfunction, inflammation, and thrombosis. Advanced lesions may be calcified and fibrotic, but more concerning are plaques that have a core of lipid and necrotic tissue surrounded by a thin fibrous cap. This cap contains collagen, and its characteristics are closely related to the risk of plaque rupture, the major cause of acute coronary syndromes. Specifically, a thinner fibrous cap is more likely to rupture. A ruptured plaque exposes the highly thrombogenic underlying collagen matrix and leads to rapid thrombus formation. Complete occlusion of a coronary vessel by thrombus on a ruptured plaque typically causes an acute transmural MI characterized by ST-segment elevation on the electrocardiogram (ECG). Nonocclusive thrombus can cause unstable angina or an MI without ST-segment elevation. Nonocclusive thrombus may not cause symptoms but instead may change plaque geometry and lead to rapid plaque growth.

MIs are classified by their appearance on 12-lead ECG during the acute phase as either ST-segment elevation or non–ST-segment elevation and are treated differently (3–6). It is important to recognize that an acute MI often arises from rupture of an atherosclerotic plaque that caused $<50\%$ luminal reduction by angiography prior to plaque rupture (7,8). On the other hand, a coronary artery that is narrowed by $\geq 70\%$ is more likely than is a less severe narrowing to cause exertional angina. The discordance between plaque severity and the development of an acute MI indicates that coronary disease is not simply a mechanical problem but instead occurs as the end result of the interplay between mechanical stresses, inflammation, cholesterol deposition, and thrombosis.

Most patients with classic exertional angina by history have fixed atherosclerotic lesions of $\geq 70\%$ in at least one major coronary artery. Fundamentally, angina is caused by a mismatch between myocardial oxygen supply and demand. Supply is affected by coronary perfusion pressure, coronary vascular resistance, and the oxygen-carrying capacity of blood. Flow is autoregulated over a wide variety of perfusion pressures; therefore, most of the changes in flow result from changes in resistance (i.e., vasodilation). However, the coronary bed beyond a significant flow-limiting stenosis already is maximally vasodilated such that small increases in demand (e.g., increased heart rate and blood pressure during exercise) may result in myocardial ischemia. Oxygen demand is related to heart rate, systolic blood pressure, and wall tension. Wall tension is determined by ventricular pressure, cavity size, and wall thickness. Physical exertion and emotional stress have potent effects on these variables and, not coincidentally, are the common triggers for ischemic chest pain.

RISK FACTORS

Both genetic and environmental risk factors influence the development of atherosclerotic heart disease. The recognition of risk factors is especially important because many of these conditions can be modified to prevent disease. Landmark epidemiologic surveys, such as the Framingham Heart Study, have helped to define levels of risk for individual risk factors. Treatment guidelines have been revised to include the important interactions between individual risk factors and age. Risk calculators (CAD event risk over 10 years) are available on the Internet at http://www.intmed.mcw.edu/clincalc/heartrisk.html. The 27th Bethesda Conference was designed to bring attention to specific patients at high risk for development of CAD events (9). This work has been incorporated into the National Cholesterol Education Program (NCEP) Expert Panel on Detection, Evaluation and Treatment of High Blood Cholesterol in Adults (Adult Treatment Panel III [ATP-III]) (see Chapter 82) (10). The concepts of "risk" and "risk factor" are important in understanding and using the guidelines. The Bethesda Conference outlined four categories of risk based on observational studies and efficacy studies (clinical trials). Table 62.1 summarizes these risk factors.

Category I risk factors are those for which interventions have been proven to reduce the risk of CAD events. They include smoking, elevated LDL cholesterol, diet high in saturated fat, hypertension, left ventricular hypertrophy, and "thrombogenic factors," which are unnamed but have the potential of being reduced by aspirin.

Category II risk factors are those for which interventions are likely to lower CAD risk. They include diabetes mellitus, physical inactivity, low levels of high-density lipoprotein (HDL) cholesterol, increased levels of triglycerides, obesity, and postmenopausal estrogen deficiency. Since the publication of these findings, diabetes has been reclassified as a CAD "risk equivalent" based on data suggesting that diabetic patients without known CAD have survival rates similar to those of nondiabetic patients who have experienced an MI. The ATP-III guidelines focus attention

TABLE 62.1 Risk Factors for Cardiovascular Disease

Category I (Factors for which Interventions Have Been Proved to Lower CVD Risk)
Cigarette smoking
Elevated LDL cholesterol
High-fat/high-cholesterol diet
Hypertension
Left ventricular hypertrophy
Thrombogenic factors (as affected by aspirin)
Category II (Factors for which Interventions Are Likely to Lower CVD Risk)
Diabetes mellitus
Physical inactivity
Low levels of HDL cholesterol[a]
Elevated triglycerides
Small, dense LDL particle size
Obesity
Postmenopausal status (women)
Category III (Factors Associated with Increased CVD Risk That, if Modified, Might Lower Risk)
Psychosocial factors
Elevated lipoprotein (a)
Elevated homocysteine
Oxidative stress
No alcohol consumption
Category IV (Factors Associated with Increased Risk That Cannot Be Modified)
Age
Male gender
Low socioeconomic status
Family history of early-onset coronary artery disease

[a]May now be considered a category I risk factor; see text.
CVD, cardiovascular disease; HDL, high-density lipoprotein LDL; low-density lipoprotein.
Adapted from Pasternak RC, Grundy SM, Levy D, et al. 27th Bethesda Conference: matching the intensity of risk factor management with the hazard for coronary disease events. Task Force 3. Spectrum of risk factors for coronary heart disease. J Am Coll Cardiol 1996;27:978.

on the "metabolic syndrome," which incorporates abdominal obesity, atherogenic dyslipidemia (elevated triglycerides, small LDL particles, low HDL cholesterol), elevated blood pressure, insulin resistance (with or without glucose intolerance), and prothrombotic and proinflammatory states. Patients with this syndrome now are appropriately targeted for intensive risk factor modification. Low HDL cholesterol, with the publication of the Veterans Affairs High-Density Lipoprotein Intervention Trial (VA-HIT) (11), now may be considered a category I risk factor, because an intervention to raise HDL cholesterol (i.e., with gemfibrozil) in this trial reduced the incidence of cardiovascular events (12). Although postmenopausal status correctly identifies a cardiac risk factor, evidence from randomized trials demonstrates that hormone replacement therapy may actually increase the risk of cardiovascular events and therefore is not recommended for treatment or prevention of CAD (13,14).

Category III risk factors are those associated with increased CAD risk that may, if modified, lower risk. These include the "emerging" risk factors such as depression, elevated lipoprotein (a) levels, and hyperhomocysteinemia. This list probably should be expanded to include inflammatory markers (elevated white blood cell count, high-sensitivity C-reactive protein, serum fibrinogen, soluble adhesion molecules), thrombotic risk factors (plasminogen activator inhibitor-1), and sleep apnea. Coronary calcification as measured by EBCT (15) can correctly be considered a category III risk factor for now, but it may need to be reclassified (like diabetes mellitus) as a CAD risk equivalent because it is a measure of the subclinical coronary artery plaque burden.

Category IV risk factors are those that are associated with increased risk but cannot be modified. They include age, male gender, low socioeconomic status, and family history of early-onset CAD. Positive family history has been defined as CAD in a male first-degree relative younger than 55 years or in a female first-degree relative younger than 65 years. These factors usually are taken into consideration with the available risk scoring systems.

DIAGNOSIS

History

Character and Location of Ischemic Pain

The discomfort of myocardial ischemia can be described in a variety of ways. Classically, the term *angina pectoris* describes a "strangulation of the chest," a helpful point to remember because many individuals describe something other than "pain" and instead mention chest tightness or heaviness. Often it is more effective to ask the patient to describe the discomfort. Some patients may simply hold their clenched fist in the middle of their chest (Levine sign).

Angina typically begins and ends gradually over 2 to 5 minutes and usually is steady in character, although occasionally it waxes and wanes. If ischemic pain continues for >20 minutes, myocardial necrosis (i.e., an MI) is more likely to have occurred. The discomfort of angina pectoris usually is midline and substernal, sometimes with radiation to the shoulder, arm, hand, or fingers, usually to the left. Radiation down the inside of the arm into the fingers supplied by the ulnar nerve is classic. Pain also may radiate into the neck, lower jaw, or interscapular region. Occasionally, a patient has pain only in a referred location and experiences no chest discomfort at all. The pain of myocardial ischemia is diffuse and cannot easily be localized. Rarely is the patient able to point with one finger to the location. When pain can be localized in this way, it likely is noncardiac in origin. The elderly, especially the frail elderly, are more likely than are younger patients to experience atypical symptoms such as dyspnea, confusion, or dyspepsia rather than pain.

The Canadian Cardiovascular Society (CCS) Classification System was designed to provide a simple way of grading anginal symptoms (16). *Class I angina* occurs with strenuous, rapid, or prolonged exertion but not with ordinary physical activity. Patients with *class II angina* experience slight limitation of ordinary activity. Class II angina occurs on walking or climbing stairs rapidly; walking uphill; walking or climbing stairs after a meal, in cold, or in wind; or under emotional stress. *Class III angina* produces marked limitations of ordinary physical activity. Angina occurs on walking one or two blocks on level terrain or climbing one flight of stairs under normal conditions and at a normal pace. With *class IV angina*, the most severe type, the patient is unable to carry on any physical activity without discomfort, and anginal symptoms may be present at rest. A higher CCS class is associated with more extensive CAD and a higher risk of CAD events.

Precipitating Factors

The single most important diagnostic feature of the discomfort of myocardial ischemia is its predictable relationship to exertion, emotional stress, or other situations that may either increase myocardial oxygen demand or reduce supply. The cause of atypical pain, pain in an unusual location or of an unusual character, may be clarified by this relationship. Pain that is experienced at rest, if it is caused by ischemia, suggests unstable angina or MI.

Anxiety and mental stress are important and often overlooked provoking factors in many patients. Angina is more likely to occur during cold or windy weather because of increased peripheral vascular resistance and, consequently, increased myocardial work. Other triggers include sexual intercourse or a heavy meal.

Relief of Ischemic Pain

Because angina is fundamentally caused by a discrepancy between oxygen supply and demand, relief of pain is achieved by increasing coronary blood flow or decreasing oxygen demand. Most people must stop or at least slow the activity responsible for precipitating the pain before it is relieved. Angina often is relieved by sublingual nitroglycerin, but the practitioner and the patient both need to realize that relief of chest pain by nitroglycerin is not specific for myocardial ischemia (17). For example, the pain of esophageal spasm can also be relieved by nitroglycerin.

Physical Examination

The physical findings in patients with CAD are nonspecific. A complete cardiovascular examination should focus on identifying markers of hypertension and dyslipidemia, peripheral vascular disease, or diabetes mellitus. Severe aortic valve disease (stenosis or regurgitation) or pulmonary hypertension without CAD can cause angina pectoris either from left or right ventricular wall strain, respectively, leading to myocardial ischemia.

Electrocardiography

A 12-lead ECG should be obtained as soon as possible in a patient with suspected CAD, although in many cases the ECG is completely normal. The most reliable ECG sign of chronic ischemic heart disease is the presence of a prior MI as manifested by two or more pathologic Q waves in a particular myocardial territory (e.g., anterior, lateral, inferior, etc.) (Fig. 62.1A). The differential diagnosis of Q waves on ECG includes prior MI, healed myocarditis, hypertrophic cardiomyopathy, an infiltrative myocardial disorder such as amyloidosis or sarcoidosis, and Wolff-Parkinson-White syndrome (usually with characteristic findings of preexcitation; see Chapter 64). Nonspecific ST-T wave changes, conduction abnormalities (except for left bundle-branch block [LBBB], discussed later), and arrhythmias do not help establish the diagnosis of myocardial ischemia. However, ST-segment depression with a flat or downsloping ST segment is suggestive of subendocardial ischemia (Fig. 62.1B). It is seldom present on the resting ECG of patients with ischemic heart disease unless they are experiencing angina at the time the tracing is recorded. On the other hand, transient ischemic changes are seen commonly when a patient with CAD is exercised to a point at which chest pain develops. Such ECG changes, appearing with exercise or pain and resolving with rest or with the resolution of pain, usually are an indication of myocardial ischemia. Therefore, the necessity of repeating the ECG at rest or after the chest pain has resolved cannot be overemphasized. ST-segment elevation during chest pain (Fig. 62.1C) suggests acute myocardial injury (e.g., MI) or variant angina (discussed later). T-wave inversion on an ECG taken at rest is a nonspecific finding but can occur after infarction or as a specific transient finding in a patient experiencing angina. Therefore, ECG changes noted during episodes of chest pain not only can confirm the diagnosis of myocardial ischemia but also may indicate the extent and location of the ischemic myocardium. As a general rule, the more widespread the changes on ECG, the greater the extent of myocardium that is involved. ST-segment elevation in the absence of chest pain is common on the resting ECG of healthy young adults and is caused by rapid or "early" repolarization of the ventricle. This pattern (Fig. 62.1D) usually is noted in the mid–left chest leads (V_2–V_4) but may be more widespread. ST-segment elevation from pericarditis is diffuse and can be associated with PR-segment depression in the limb leads (except aVR, which may show PR-segment elevation).

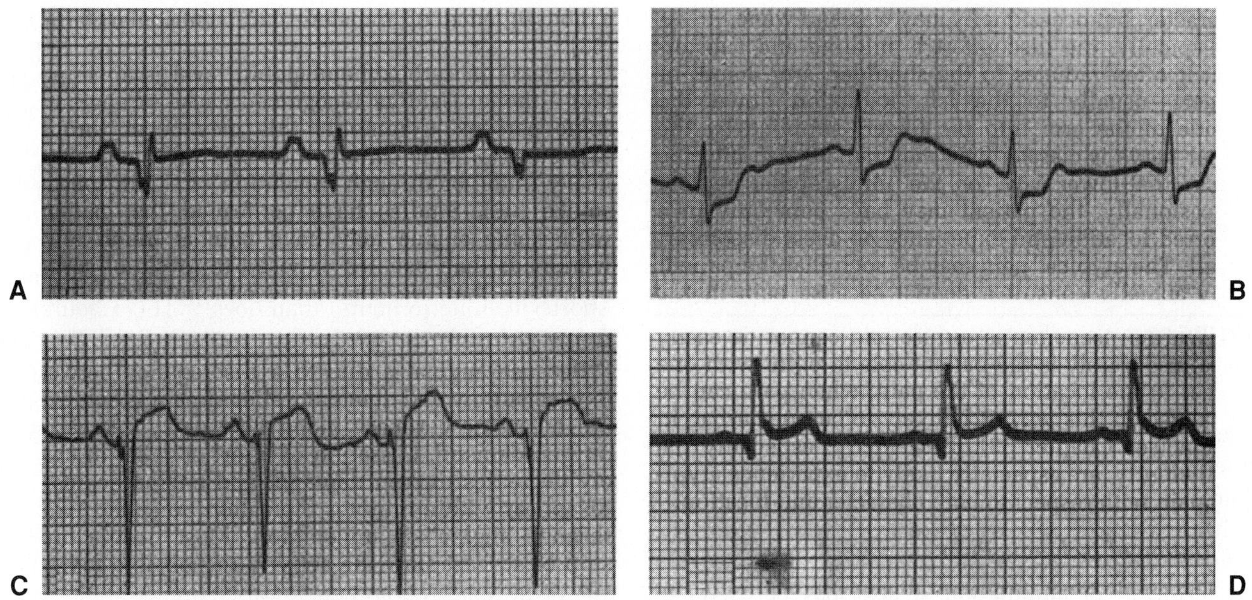

FIGURE 62.1. Electrocardiographic strips from patients with suspected ischemic heart disease. **A:** Q waves suggestive of prior myocardial infarction. **B:** ST-segment depression developing after exertion. **C:** ST-segment elevation during coronary artery spasm (variant angina). **D:** Early repolarization (a normal variant).

The presence of ST-T abnormalities in an otherwise healthy person is a nonspecific finding and should not be considered confirmation of CAD. There is a high association of LBBB with organic heart disease (see Chapter 64), especially CAD. Right bundle-branch block (RBBB), on the other hand, is seen commonly in the absence of other cardiac abnormalities.

Cardiac Stress Testing

Exercise Electrocardiography

The exercise stress test is a means of establishing the diagnosis of myocardial ischemia. It also can be used to assess the efficacy of antianginal therapy, to identify patients who are likely to have more severe CAD and a large area of myocardium at risk, and to assess serially the degree of conditioning or exercise capacity in patients of all age groups. The American College of Cardiology (ACC)/American Heart Association (AHA) exercise testing guidelines outline the recommendations for the use of exercise testing in establishing the diagnosis of CAD, in assessing risk and prognosis in patients with symptoms or a prior history of CAD, and the use of exercise testing after MI (18,19). The usefulness of exercise testing in establishing the diagnosis of CAD is based in part on the likelihood that the patient has this condition (i.e., the "pretest probability" of CAD). This can be determined by the patient's age, gender, and symptoms. For example, exercise testing would not be expected to greatly improve the accuracy of diagnosing CAD in an older patient with typical angina (who has a high pretest probability of CAD) nor in a young, asymptomatic individual (who has a low pretest probability of CAD). The usefulness of stress testing in these situations would be limited by false-negative and false-positive findings, respectively. The ACC/AHA guidelines recommend exercise testing to diagnose CAD in adult patients with an intermediate pretest probability of CAD based on gender, age, and symptoms (18,19). For patients with known CAD, the guidelines recommend stress testing for those with a significant change in clinical status. Patients with unstable angina, decompensated heart failure, severe aortic stenosis, or uncontrolled hypertension should not be referred for stress testing because of an unacceptably high risk for provoking a cardiac event during exercise.

Exercise stress testing is based on the rationale that, as the work performed by the patient increases, cardiac work is increased. The increased cardiac work results in increased myocardial oxygen utilization, with a subsequent increased demand in coronary blood flow. If narrowed or obstructed coronary arteries prevent the required increase in coronary blood flow, myocardial ischemia may occur and be manifested as chest pain and/or ECG changes (20).

The simplest and least expensive exercise stress test is the graded, symptom-limited exercise treadmill test. The test requires 12-lead ECG monitoring of the patient while walking on a treadmill at workloads that can be progressively increased by increasing the speed and inclination of the treadmill. A stationary bicycle ergometer (with hand

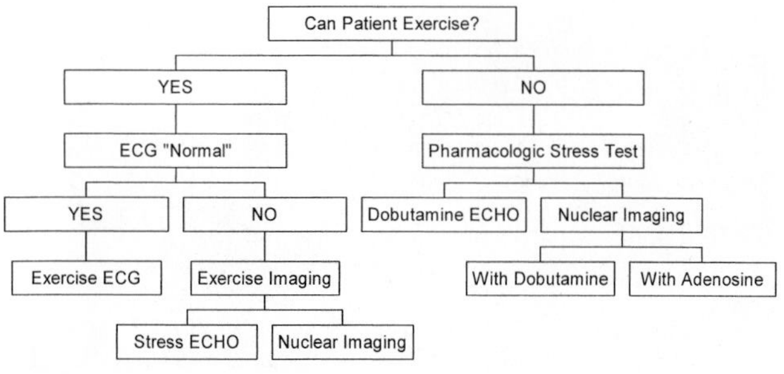

FIGURE 62.2. Algorithm for determining the appropriate stress test. See text for a description of the procedures.

pedals) can be substituted for a treadmill, permitting the patient to exercise with his or her arms instead of legs. Although it is not commonly used, this method of stress testing permits exercise by a patient who may otherwise be unable to do so because of lower-extremity claudication, arthritis, or amputation. It also may be useful in the evaluation of patients who have chest pain predominantly or exclusively with work that involves the arms and shoulders.

A simple algorithm can be used to decide the type of stress test to recommend (Fig. 62.2). First, the patient's ability to exercise should be assessed. If the patient can walk up a flight of stairs carrying laundry or groceries, for example, a treadmill exercise protocol can generally be chosen to allow the patient to achieve a level of cardiac work that permits meaningful information to be obtained from the test. If the patient cannot perform this task, or one that is comparable, a pharmacologic stress test with cardiac imaging (discussed later) should generally be recommended. The patient's baseline ECG should be reviewed to determine the presence of baseline ST-segment abnormalities that might lower the predictive value of exercise-induced changes. False-positive stress tests are often encountered in women, in patients taking medications such as digoxin or amiodarone, and in patients with left ventricular hypertrophy or mitral valve prolapse (21). For these patients and in those with baseline ST-segment abnormalities, intraventricular conduction defects (i.e., LBBB or RBBB), or other conduction system disorders (e.g., Wolff-Parkinson-White syndrome), the diagnostic accuracy of the exercise stress test can be enhanced by concurrent radioisotopic or echocardiographic imaging (see later discussion). The choice between radioisotopic or echocardiographic imaging depends largely on the expertise of local laboratories.

Radioisotope Imaging

Radioisotope imaging can enhance the specificity of stress testing by evaluating myocardial function or flow (22). Radioisotope imaging can be used in conjunction with either treadmill exercise testing or pharmacologic stress testing, using either dobutamine to increase cardiac work or adenosine or dipyridamole to alter coronary blood flow (see later discussion). Commonly used imaging modalities include radioisotope imaging with thallium 201 (^{201}Tl)–and/or technetium 99 (^{99}Tc)–based agents (e.g., ^{99m}Tc-sestamibi). The usefulness of ^{201}Tl as a perfusion tracer is based on its ability to function as an analogue of ionic potassium. It is very efficiently extracted by healthy myocardial cells, and uptake is proportional to regional perfusion and myocardial viability. ^{99m}Tc-sestamibi has a shorter half-life (6 hours) than does ^{201}Tl (73 hours), allowing administration of a larger tracer dose. This and its higher emission energy make it an excellent agent for cardiac imaging. ^{99m}Tc-sestamibi is particularly useful in obese patients and in patients with large breasts (because of possible attenuation of the radioisotopic images in the area of the anterior myocardium).

Both ^{201}Tl and ^{99m}Tc-sestamibi can be used to assess regional myocardial blood flow, either by planar imaging or by single-photon emission computed tomography (SPECT). Imaging usually occurs at two separate times: the stress scan, obtained very shortly after the patient has exercised or received a pharmacologic agent, and the rest scan, obtained either before or several hours after stress. The radioisotope is injected intravenously at the time of peak exercise (or at the time of peak infusion during a pharmacologic stress test), and scintigraphic images are obtained shortly thereafter, depicting regional myocardial perfusion at the time of peak stress. The rest scan typically is obtained several hours later and shows redistribution of the isotope. Ischemia is indicated by the filling in of a cold spot defined on the stress images (i.e., normalization or "redistribution" of a radioisotopic defect), and infarction is indicated by a persisting cold spot or one with only partial redistribution.

Radioisotope imaging with stress gated blood pool scans (multiple-gated acquisition [MUGA]) also can be used to assess myocardial ischemia. To allow for continuous imaging during exercise, stress MUGA is performed with the patient exercising on a semirecumbent bicycle. The rationale for this test is based on the fact that myocardium that becomes ischemic during graded exercise develops regional wall-motion abnormalities that can be detected by sequential image analyses. This type of imaging labels the blood pool with a radioisotope and gates image acquisition to the ECG. Right and left ventricular volumes, regional left ventricular wall motion, and global and regional ejection fractions can be measured, both at rest and with stress.

The cost of stress testing with radioisotope scanning usually is several times that of a standard exercise test.

Stress Echocardiography

Two-dimensional echocardiography can be used instead of radioisotope scanning to detect areas of regional myocardial dysfunction (as evidenced by a wall-motion abnormality) with exercise or pharmacologic stress (23,24). Typically, baseline images are first obtained at rest to determine the adequacy of the echocardiographic images. If these images are technically inadequate (e.g., because of obesity or severe obstructive lung disease), an intravenous ultrasound contrast agent can be used if available; if not, radioisotope images are preferable. If the rest images are technically adequate, the patient undergoes treadmill exercise stress and then images are reacquired immediately, using special software to allow for direct comparison of pre-exercise and postexercise images. If pharmacologic stress testing with dobutamine (see Pharmacologic Stress Testing) is used, the dose of dobutamine is increased in stepwise fashion, and echocardiographic images typically are obtained each time the dose is increased. The safety of dobutamine stress echocardiography is comparable to that of a routine exercise stress test (23,25,26). The sensitivity, specificity, and cost of the test are similar to those of radioisotopic stress testing. Stress echocardiography may be preferred in some cases because additional information is provided that is not obtained with radioisotopic scanning (e.g., presence of pericardial effusion, ventricular hypertrophy, or valvular abnormality). It also avoids exposure to radioactivity.

Pharmacologic Stress Testing

Patients who are unable to exercise because of physical limitations can be evaluated after intravenous administration of dipyridamole, adenosine, or dobutamine in conjunction with an imaging modality. Dipyridamole and adenosine dilate all coronary vessels and generally increase flow to all areas of the heart. Enhanced dilation of normal coronary arteries, compared to that of significantly narrowed vessels, augments differences in flow that usually are not apparent at rest. These agents are suitable for use with radioisotopic imaging modalities that may readily demonstrate this flow heterogeneity. After administration of dipyridamole or adenosine followed by either ^{201}Tl or ^{99m}Tc-sestamibi (i.e., the stress image), myocardium supplied by a narrowed coronary artery typically demonstrates a perfusion defect that "fills in" during the rest image. Because of its ultrashort duration of action, adenosine is preferable to dipyridamole for this test.

Dobutamine is a β_1-receptor agonist that at high dosages (20–40 μg/kg/min intravenously) increases myocardial contractility and heart rate in a similar manner and extent to exercise. Heart rate may not be affected to the same extent as contractility, and atropine often is administered intravenously to increase the heart rate to the maximal predicted heart rate for age. Dobutamine can be used in conjunction with either echocardiography or radioisotopic imaging for diagnosis of CAD.

Mild side effects (e.g., nausea, flushing, and headache) are common with dipyridamole, adenosine, and dobutamine. Dipyridamole and adenosine (but not dobutamine) can produce severe bronchospasm and therefore must be used with caution or not at all in patients with asthma or chronic obstructive pulmonary disease. Adenosine can cause transient heart block, typically lasting several seconds. Because dobutamine increases atrioventricular conduction, it should not be used in patients with atrial flutter and should be used carefully in patients with atrial fibrillation.

Implications of an Abnormal Stress Test

If treadmill exercise stress testing is performed, factors affecting prognosis include the degree of ST-segment depression, time to development of ST-segment depression during exercise, duration of the ST-segment depression in recovery, and speed of heart rate decline during recovery. In addition, an ischemic ECG response that is accompanied by hypotension generally implies a large amount of myocardium at risk. Prognostic information from pharmacologic stress testing-induced ECG abnormalities is less reliable. The number, size, and location of abnormalities evident on stress imaging studies reflect the location and extent of functionally significant coronary stenoses (27). Both radioisotopic and echocardiographic imaging can detect left ventricular dilation with stress, a finding that suggests global, severe ischemia. Lung uptake of a radioisotopic tracer indicates stress-induced left ventricular dysfunction and suggests multivessel CAD. Many studies have shown that high-risk abnormal stress tests are associated with an increased risk for cardiac events. On the other hand, normal radioisotopic or echocardiographic stress tests are associated with a favorable prognosis. In a review of 16 studies involving almost 4,000 patients over 2 years, a negative perfusion scan was associated with a 0.9% rate of cardiac death per year, similar to that of the general population (28).

Ambulatory Electrocardiography

The ambulatory ECG (Holter monitor) may be useful for detecting myocardial ischemia. However, it is not a good tool for screening patients to make the diagnosis of CAD. In patients with CAD who are symptomatic during ambulatory ECG monitoring, ST-segment elevation or depression can be observed during episodes of pain and at other times as well (silent ischemia; see later discussion). In patients with silent ischemia, the ambulatory ECG is particularly useful for quantifying the degree and frequency of ischemia and assessing the efficacy of therapy.

Electron-Beam Computed Tomography

Studies in the 1970s demonstrated that coronary calcification (detected by cardiac fluoroscopy) was useful in identifying patients with angiographically significant CAD (29).

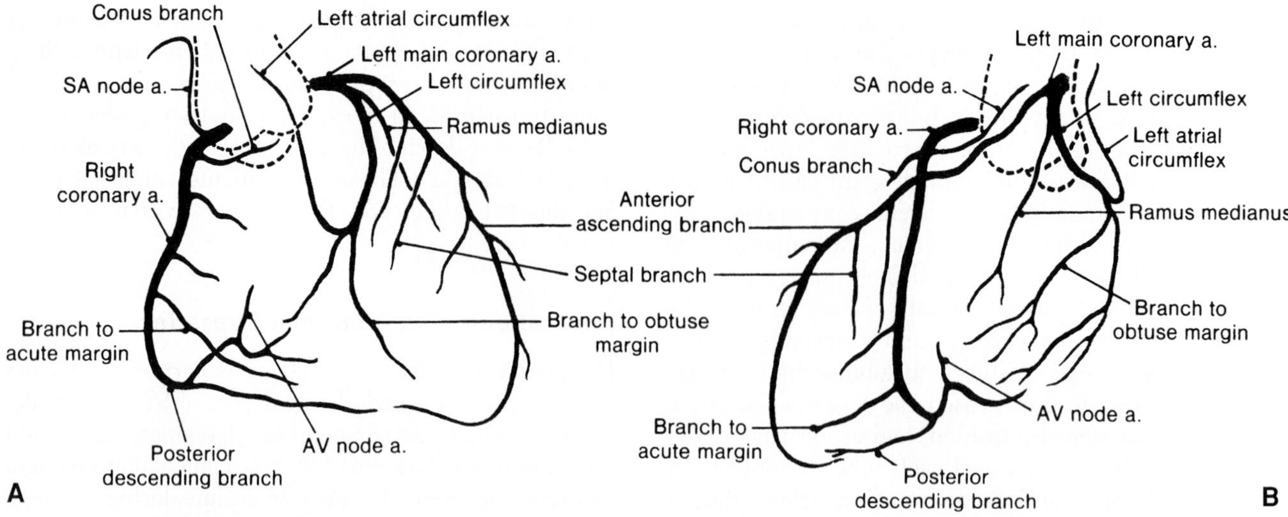

FIGURE 62.3. Anatomic representation of the coronary arteries. These vessels are represented as they would be seen on the angiogram. No attempt has been made to convey the third dimension. Careful study of the changes in position of the various branches with rotation of the heart is essential to intelligent interpretation of arteriograms. **A:** Anteroposterior. **B:** Lateral. (Modified from Abrams HL, Adams DF. The coronary arteriogram: structural and functional aspects [First of two parts]. N Engl J Med 1969;281:1276, with permission.)

EBCT is a highly sensitive technique for detecting coronary artery calcium and may be useful for diagnosing CAD noninvasively (11). ECG gating allows data acquisition within one or two breath-holds, making it a rapid test with limited radiation exposure. The images obtained by this technique allow the determination of a calcium score, which is an index of calcium deposition in multiple arterial segments and is a good approximation for overall plaque burden in the coronary tree. High calcium scores are associated with increased risk for MI (30). The test offers improved discrimination over conventional risk factors in the identification of people with CAD (31). The negative predictive value of EBCT is high. The test is particularly useful for screening asymptomatic individuals with multiple risk factors, in whom an abnormal EBCT should prompt further testing and/or treatment. A very low EBCT score would be reassuring (32).

Cardiac Catheterization and Coronary Angiography

Coronary angiography is defined as the radiographic visualization of the coronary vessels after injection of radiopaque contrast medium (33). This technique provides direct information about the presence of CAD and defines the distribution and severity of obstructive coronary lesions. It is considered the "gold standard" to confirm the diagnosis of CAD. The images obtained are stored as either 35-mm cine film or, more commonly, a digital recording. Percutaneous or cutdown techniques of the femoral or brachial arteries allow insertion of sheaths for the introduction of selective catheters for the right and left coronary ostia, saphenous bypass grafts, or internal mammary arteries. Arteriography is performed as part of cardiac catheterization, which may include left ventriculography and hemodynamic assessment. Figure 62.3 shows diagrammatically the coronary arteries and their branches as they appear on coronary arteriography. The three major coronary arteries are the left anterior descending, left circumflex, and right coronary artery. The coronary tree can be divided into 29 segments, but the extent of disease usually is defined as one-vessel, two-vessel, three-vessel, or left main disease, with significant disease taken to mean the presence of ≥50% reduction in diameter (some operators and texts use ≥70% reduction in diameter).

The 1999 ACC/AHA Guidelines for Coronary Angiography outline the indications and contraindications for the procedure (33). The guidelines recommend arteriography for patients with CCS class III or IV angina while receiving medical treatment (marked limitations of ordinary physical activity because of angina or angina at rest, discussed earlier) and those with high-risk criteria on noninvasive testing regardless of angina severity. It may be reasonable to consider coronary arteriography for patients whose angina has improved with medical treatment but remains present, those in whom noninvasive testing has shown evidence of worsening disease, those who cannot tolerate medical therapy, those with angina who cannot be adequately risk stratified because of disability or illness, and those whose occupation involves the safety of others (e.g., pilots, bus drivers) and who have abnormal, but not high-risk, stress test results.

Inherent in the recommendation for coronary arteriography is the assumption that the patient is a potential candidate for coronary revascularization. If the patient's general medical condition or other medical problems preclude revascularization, or if the patient refuses to consider revascularization regardless of catheterization results, arteriography is ill advised.

Indications for percutaneous coronary intervention ([PCI] including angioplasty and stenting) (34) and coronary artery bypass surgery (35) are reviewed in separate ACC/AHA guidelines and are discussed later in this chapter.

Patient Experience. The patient may undergo cardiac catheterization as part of an evaluation during a hospitalization, but the test itself does not require that the patient be admitted to the hospital. The procedure is not painful, and the patient remains awake throughout the study. Approximately 1 hour before the procedure, the patient is given a sedative, often diazepam (Valium), 5 to 10 mg orally. After the patient is brought to the catheterization laboratory, either the area of the brachial artery or the femoral artery is prepared for sterile procedure. The site of introduction of the catheter usually is selected based on the preference of the operator but also is guided by the presence and extent of peripheral vascular disease. Typically, a catheter is introduced percutaneously through a wire that is threaded through an introducer needle. Under fluoroscopic guidance, the catheter is threaded to the coronary sinuses, and the orifices of the right and left coronary arteries are injected sequentially with contrast medium. The patient is asked to hold his or her breath during the few seconds of the injection. In addition to this part of the test, which visualizes the coronary arteries, studies are typically performed to measure ventricular pressures and to assess left ventricular contraction during injection of dye directly into the left ventricular cavity. During ventriculography, focal wall-motion abnormalities, ventricular aneurysms, and valvular lesions such as mitral regurgitation can be assessed in addition to the measurement of overall left ventricular function and ejection fraction. At the end of the procedure, the catheter is withdrawn, and pressure is applied to the arteriotomy site to achieve hemostasis.

During the procedure, the patient should feel relaxed or even slightly drowsy from the sedation. The patient usually does not feel pain except for the moment when the needle is initially introduced. There is some pressure as the catheter is held in place. The patient may experience a sensation of hot flushing when the dye is injected, particularly when the larger bolus of dye is injected into the left ventricle during ventriculography.

Risks and Relative Contraindications

The major complications of coronary arteriography are MI, stroke, and death. These risks are related to the experience of the laboratory performing the study and to the risk profile of the patient undergoing the test. Risks tend to be lower in young, otherwise healthy patients. Risks tend to be higher in older patients with poor left ventricular function, diabetes mellitus, or peripheral vascular disease, and those who are clinically unstable (e.g., patients with cardiogenic shock, recent acute MI, or decompensated heart failure) at the time of the procedure. In a survey of almost 60,000 patients, mortality from angiography was 0.11%, MI occurred in 0.05%, and stroke occurred in 0.07%. The most common complication was a problem with vascular access, which occurred in 0.43% of patients (36).

There are no absolute contraindications to coronary arteriography. Relative contraindications include renal failure, active gastrointestinal bleeding, acute stroke, severe anemia, coagulopathy, unexplained fever or active untreated infection, severe uncontrolled hypertension, allergic reaction to angiographic contrast agents, and decompensated congestive heart failure (CHF). Renal insufficiency has been the most well-studied complication. It occurs in up to 5% of patients without preexisting renal dysfunction and in 10% to 40% of patients with baseline renal insufficiency. More than 75% of patients who develop renal insufficiency recover normal renal function, although 10% of these patients may require dialysis temporarily. Pretreatment with intravenous hydration (0.9% saline) (37) and limiting the amount of intravenous contrast material used are effective means to avoid contrast-induced renal dysfunction.

For patients with underlying renal dysfunction, pretreatment with *N*-acetylcysteine (38) or intravenous sodium bicarbonate (39) has been shown to reduce contrast-induced acute renal failure following cardiac catheterization. No direct comparison of these prophylactic measures has been performed to date. Patients taking the oral hypoglycemic metformin should be asked to withhold it for 48 hours prior to the procedure, because the use of iodinated contrast dye in patients taking metformin has been associated with development of lactic acidosis (40). The major predictors of contrast allergy are prior contrast allergy (50% risk of subsequent reaction), iodine allergy, and shellfish allergy. These conditions should be discussed with the patient before referral for angiography. The use of nonionic contrast medium along with pretreatment using corticosteroids and antihistamines may reduce allergic complications.

Computed Tomography Coronary Angiography

High-definition rapid CT scanning has evolved as a potent diagnostic tool for identifying CAD noninvasively. Newer CT devices are able to rapidly scan through a patient's chest using many slices for image acquisition (the current state of the art is to use a 64-slice scanner), quickly and accurately identifying unique features of coronary and cardiac anatomy. Multislice cardiac CT scanning is extremely accurate in detecting coronary narrowings in the proximal two thirds of the coronary tree that are demonstrated by conventional coronary angiography, but its resolution of the distal third is less accurate. However, it is superior to conventional coronary angiography in identifying extraluminal vascular abnormalities that result in coronary narrowings but cannot be seen by conventional techniques. Additionally, other noncardiac causes of chest pain, such as aortic dissection, pneumonia, or pulmonary embolus, may be diagnosed by this imaging technique. CT coronary angiography is particularly useful in patients with peripheral vascular disease because it can minimize or avoid catheter-related complications. During CT angiography, the patient receives intravenous radiographic contrast, and the total scanning time usually is $\leq$15 minutes. Image quality is improved at slower heart rates and patients may receive low doses of β-blockers to facilitate this. Because iodinated contrast is used for this procedure, the risks and precautionary treatment associated with such therapy is the same as for cardiac catheterization.

TREATMENT OF ANGINA PECTORIS

General Therapeutic Considerations

In evaluating and treating patients with angina, it is of paramount importance to identify and treat underlying contributing factors and to modify cardiac risk factors that promote CAD progression if possible.

Hypertension often is present in patients with angina. There is a linear relationship between left ventricular work and myocardial oxygen demand. Left ventricular systolic pressure increases in response to an increase in peripheral vascular resistance. Both systolic and diastolic hypertension can increase myocardial oxygen demand. An attempt should always be made to reduce resting blood pressure to normal in patients with chronic hypertension, including those with isolated systolic hypertension. This can be of crucial importance in reducing the frequency and severity of angina pectoris in the hypertensive patient. β-Blockers and calcium channel blockers (see Chapter 67) are excellent choices in such patients because these agents have other antianginal properties as well. Agents such as hydralazine and minoxidil, which cause a reflex tachycardia, are less desirable.

It is important to achieve a maximal level of pulmonary compensation in patients with *angina and coexisting lung disease* (see Chapter 60). Chronic hypoxemia, acidosis, and the increased work of breathing in patients with pulmonary disease increase myocardial oxygen demand, decrease myocardial oxygen delivery, or both. Unfortunately, the treatment of angina in patients with severe lung disease often is limited by a real, or perceived, need to avoid the use of β-blockers (see later discussion).

Abstinence from tobacco products is essential because nicotine in tobacco can cause coronary vasoconstriction. Chapter 27 describes techniques used to achieve this goal. Similarly, passive tobacco smoke should be avoided.

The possibility of *hyperthyroidism* (see Chapter 80) in patients with angina should never be overlooked, particularly in older patients or in those with increasing angina. Often, particularly in the older patient, other obvious signs of hyperthyroidism are not present. For example, hyperthyroidism may be manifested only by an increased frequency or severity of angina, an increase in heart rate in people with atrial fibrillation, or increasing heart failure.

Anemia is important to consider in patients with angina, particularly if the hemoglobin concentration falls to <7 g/dL, when cardiac output must increase to maintain adequate peripheral oxygen delivery at rest. Obviously, this problem is exacerbated in patients with concomitant chronic lung disease and hypoxemia.

Heart failure (see Chapter 66) in patients with angina should always be optimally treated. The real possibility that heart failure is producing angina at rest (see later discussion) or nocturnal angina should be considered. Diuretics, vasodilators, and β-blockers may be useful in patients with rest or nocturnal angina and may reduce the frequency and severity of angina. The calcium channel blocker amlodipine has been shown to be safe in patients with left ventricular dysfunction and may be useful for patients with angina in this setting because it has little negative inotropic effect, reduces preload and afterload, helps decrease left ventricular end-diastolic pressure, and lowers peripheral vascular resistance.

Lipids and Diet

Most of the recent decline in mortality from heart disease is believed to be related to primary and secondary risk factor reductions (41,42). Numerous randomized controlled trials involving cholesterol reduction have been performed and have supported the ability to reduce CAD morbidity and mortality with both primary and secondary prevention strategies. The West of Scotland Coronary Prevention Study demonstrated significant mortality reduction with treatment of hyperlipidemia with pravastatin in asymptomatic people; the greatest benefit occurred in patients with other risk factors for CAD (43). The landmark Heart Protection Study in the United Kingdom randomized subjects with CAD, peripheral vascular disease, or diabetes to 40 mg of simvastatin or placebo and demonstrated reductions in mortality in simvastatin-treated patients regardless of baseline LDL cholesterol levels (44). The value of secondary prevention was established by the Scandinavian Simvastatin Survival Study (45) and the Cholesterol and Recurrent Events (CARE) trial (46). Both trials demonstrated a significant reduction in mortality when LDL cholesterol levels were lowered to approximately 100 to 120 mg/dL. Other trials also have clearly demonstrated that coronary artery lesions did not progress when elevated LDL cholesterol levels were reduced to <100 mg/dL (47,48). More recent trials have compared the effects of more aggressive to less aggressive lipid-lowering strategies, usually by examining the effects of high-dose and lower-dose therapy with a β-hydroxy-β-methylglutaryl-coenzyme A (HMG-CoA) reductase inhibitor or "statin." One of these trials demonstrated that 80 mg of atorvastatin reduced the frequency of cardiovascular events to a greater degree than did 40 mg of pravastatin by more intensive lowering of LDL cholesterol (mean LDL cholesterol lowered to 62 mg/dL) (49). Another study compared the effects of 80 mg and 10 mg of atorvastatin in patients with stable CAD and demonstrated clinical benefit with the more aggressive lipid-lowering approach, achieving mean LDL cholesterol levels of 77 mg/dL and 101 mg/dL in the 80-mg and 10-mg groups, respectively (50).

The NCEP guidelines indicate that the desirable LDL cholesterol level is <100 mg/dL in patients with established CAD or with coronary heart disease risk equivalents including diabetes mellitus, multiple risk factors that confer a 10-year CAD risk >20%, or other clinical forms of atherosclerotic disease (i.e., peripheral arterial disease, abdominal aortic aneurysm, or symptomatic carotid artery disease) (10). Updates recommend considering an LDL cholesterol target <70 mg/dL in very-high-risk patients, defined as those with an acute coronary syndrome or with established CAD and multiple major CAD risk factors (especially diabetes mellitus), severe and poorly controlled risk factors (especially cigarette smoking), or the metabolic syndrome (51). Treatment of patients having low HDL cholesterol levels with the fibrate gemfibrozil was shown to reduce the risk of major cardiovascular events in patients with CAD (12). In addition to pharmacologic options for lipid-lowering drug therapy, the guidelines recommend a multifaceted lifestyle approach to reduce CAD risk. This approach calls for reducing the intake of saturated fats to <7% of total calories and reducing dietary cholesterol to <200 mg/day. Achieving an ideal body weight and increasing physical activity also are advised. These lifestyle recommendations are an essential part of treatment for all patients with coronary disease. Chapter 82 discusses these changes in more detail. Obesity has emerged as a national epidemic, with several studies confirming the increased mortality and morbidity from this condition (52). Chapter 83 discusses in detail the various treatment options for this condition.

Alcohol

Alcohol is an acute pressor agent and may be responsible for as many as 10% of all cases of hypertension (53). However, moderate drinking (1–3 drinks per day) is accompanied by an increase in HDL cholesterol level (54). The extent to which the increase in blood pressure associated with heavy drinking mitigates the beneficial effect on HDL remains to be determined (55). A review of lifestyle recommendations for patients with CAD estimated a 20% reduction in mortality with moderate alcohol use (compared with 24% reduction from physical activity and 36% reduction with smoking cessation) (56).

Antioxidants

Although antioxidants may be important in inhibiting atherosclerosis, clinical trials of antioxidant therapy have not demonstrated conclusive long-term benefit. In the Heart Outcomes Prevention Evaluation (HOPE) study, for example, approximately 9,500 patients at high risk for cardiovascular events were randomly assigned to therapy with either 400 IU of vitamin E or placebo for an average of 4.5 years. There was no apparent effect of treatment with vitamin E on cardiovascular outcomes in this study (57). More recently, a meta-analysis of 19 trials suggested the possibility of increasing mortality with high-dosage vitamin E supplementation for CAD prevention, with risk increasing as the dosage of vitamin E exceeded 150 IU/day (58).

Fish Oil and ω-3 Fatty Acids

Fish oils (ω-3 fatty acids) have demonstrated cardiovascular benefit in people who have taken them by decreasing the risk of potentially fatal arrhythmias, slowing plaque progression, decreasing levels of triglycerides, and mildly decreasing blood pressure. Currently, the AHA recommends two servings of fish per week. Similarly, other foods that contain α-linolenic acid, which can be metabolized into ω-3 fatty acids by the body, such as flaxseed, walnuts, soy products, and tofu, are recommended, but the benefit of ω-3 fatty acid production via α-linolenic acid intake is not well delineated (59).

Postmenopausal Hormone Replacement Therapy

Earlier studies demonstrated improvements in surrogate measures such as endothelial function from hormone replacement therapy (HRT). Observational studies suggested a decreased risk for cardiovascular events in women taking HRT compared to women who did not (60,61). This finding led to two randomized, placebo-controlled studies to definitively evaluate the role of HRT in postmenopausal women with chronic stable CAD. The Heart and Estrogen/

Progestin Replacement Study (HERS) showed that HRT did not result in a reduced risk for cardiovascular death or nonfatal MI (13). The Estrogen Replacement and Atherosclerosis Study (ERAS) failed to show an effect of HRT on the angiographic progression of atherosclerotic heart disease (62). There also is evidence that postmenopausal HRT increases the risk of venous thromboembolic disease (13,63) and gallbladder disease (13) in women with CAD. Therefore, HRT is not recommended for reducing cardiovascular morbidity or mortality in postmenopausal women.

Physical Conditioning

Physical conditioning can improve the exercise tolerance and psychological well-being of patients with stable angina. Additionally, improvements in atherosclerotic risk factors, such as hypertension, glucose intolerance, low HDL cholesterol concentrations, elevated triglyceride levels, and obesity, reduce CAD risk from the perspective of both primary and secondary prevention. The combination of weight reduction and exercise lowers LDL cholesterol concentrations (64). Studies confirm that moderate exercise (20 minutes three times per week) is as effective for weight loss as more vigorous exercise (65). Most large communities have developed supervised exercise programs for patients with CAD. Chapter 63 details the benefits of physical conditioning and exercise programs for patients with heart disease. The AHA-published guidelines for exercise in various patient groups are available on their website (www.americanheart.org). Patients with angina should be counseled to avoid physical activities that are known to provoke their symptoms. Health care providers should specifically discuss the safety of sexual intercourse, a subject that people often are reluctant to broach (see Chapter 63). The appropriate level of sexual activity or participation in any stressful physical activity ideally should be based on the results of an exercise stress test. The energy requirements for a broad range of activities are summarized in Table 63.5.

Medical Treatment

The basic objective in treating patients with angina pectoris is not only to relieve or prevent symptoms but also to prevent disease progression. The former goal may be achieved by medical therapy that improves the relationship between myocardial oxygen demand and supply. The latter goal may be accomplished by preventing platelet aggregation and by decreasing the growth of atherosclerotic plaque and the risk of plaque rupture. The major advance in the medical management of angina has been the demonstration that long-acting antiplatelet and antithrombotic agents and vigorous lipid-lowering therapy can improve outcomes in selected patients with CAD. Table 62.2 lists practical information about the drugs used most often for treatment of angina.

Nitrates

Traditionally, nitroglycerin and related compounds have been an inexpensive mainstay of treatment of patients with angina pectoris. Nitrates increase coronary blood flow in patients with spasm, but the predominant mechanism of action in most patients is not an increase in blood flow but rather a decrease in myocardial oxygen demand and peripheral vascular resistance. These compounds produce dilation of the venous circulation, reduced venous return, decreased ventricular volume, and decreased wall tension. These effects ultimately reduce myocardial oxygen demand. Nitrates also produce arterial dilation to a lesser degree and thereby reduce the resistance to ventricular ejection. Therefore, the beneficial antianginal effect of nitrates is caused primarily by peripheral vasodilation.

Sublingual nitroglycerin is still the drug of choice in most patients for the relief and prevention of discrete episodes of angina pectoris. The initial dose should be small (0.4 mg) to minimize unpleasant side effects (flushing, headache, light-headedness). Patients should be taught the importance of relieving their pain as soon as possible, and they should be instructed to take nitroglycerin whenever such symptoms appear. If pain is not relieved by two to three tablets of nitroglycerin (the patient should wait at least 5 minutes between doses) or if the need for nitroglycerin increases suddenly and dramatically, the patient should be instructed to call his or her health care provider or go to an emergency facility immediately because of the danger of impending MI. Because nitroglycerin may lose potency on storage, patients should be advised not to keep tablets longer than 3 to 4 months after opening the bottle. If the use of nitroglycerin does not result relieve the angina and the usual side effects are not experienced, the problem may be caused by outdated medicine that has lost its potency rather than by a change in cardiac status. Prophylactic use of nitroglycerin is of particular value in patients who have angina in response to specific and reproducible stress despite other therapies. For example, the patient who develops angina after walking from a car to a place of work can be instructed to take nitroglycerin after the car is parked, wait a few minutes, and then walk to work, thereby preventing pain altogether. The most common side effects of nitroglycerin therapy are flushing and headache. A nitroglycerin sublingual spray has been developed that is designed to deliver 0.4 mg of nitroglycerin with each compression of the nebulizer. Some patients find this preparation more acceptable and more reliable than the tablet.

Long-acting nitrates are available in a variety of preparations (Table 62.2). Careful studies confirm the clinical efficacy of both nitroglycerin ointment and isosorbide tablets

28. Brown KA. Prognostic value of thallium-201 myocardial perfusion imaging: a diagnostic tool comes of age. Circulation 1991;83:363.
29. Bartel AG, Chen JTT, Peter RH, et al. The significance of coronary calcification detected by fluoroscopy: a report of 360 patients. Circulation 1974;49:1247.
30. Raggi P, Callister TQ, Cooil B, et al. Identification of patients at increased risk of first unheralded acute myocardial infarction by electron-beam computed tomography. Circulation 2000;101:850.
31. Guerci AD, Arad Y, Agatston A. Predictive value of EBCT scanning. Circulation 1998;97:2583.
32. Budhoff MJ, Georgiou D, Brody A, et al. Ultrafast computed tomography as a diagnostic modality in the detection of coronary artery disease: a multicenter study. Circulation 1996;93:898.
33. Scanlon PJ, Faxon DP, Audet AM, et al. ACC/AHA guidelines for coronary angiography. A report of the American College of Cardiology/American Heart Association Task Force on practice guidelines (Committee on Coronary Angiography). Developed in collaboration with the Society for Cardiac Angiography and Interventions. J Am Coll Cardiol 1999;33:1756.
34. Smith SC Jr, Dove JT, Jacobs AK, et al. ACC/AHA guidelines of percutaneous coronary interventions (revision of the 1993 PTCA guidelines)—executive summary. A report of the American College of Cardiology/American Heart Association Task Force on Practice Guidelines (Committee to Revise the 1993 Guidelines for Percutaneous Transluminal Coronary Angioplasty). J Am Coll Cardiol 2001;37:2215.
35. Eagle KA, Guyton RA, Davidoff R, et al. ACC/AHA guidelines for coronary artery bypass graft surgery: executive summary and recommendations. A report of the American College of Cardiology/American Heart Association Task Force on Practice Guidelines (Committee to Revise the 1991 Guidelines for Coronary Artery Bypass Graft Surgery). Circulation 1999;100:1464.
36. Noto TJ Jr, Johnson LW, Krone R, et al. Cardiac catheterization 1990: a report of the Registry of the Society for Cardiac Angiography and Interventions (SCA&I). Cathet Cardiovasc Diagn 1991;24:75.
37. Trivedi HS, Moore H, Nasr S, et al. A randomized prospective trial to assess the role of saline hydration on the development of contrast nephrotoxicity. Nephron 2003;93:C29.
38. Kay J, Chow WH, Chan TM, et al. Acetylcysteine for prevention of acute deterioration of renal function following elective coronary angiography and intervention: a randomized controlled trial. JAMA 2003;289:553.
39. Merten GJ, Burgess WP, Gray LV, et al. Prevention of contrast induced nephropathy with sodium bicarbonate. JAMA 2003;291:2328.
40. Misbin RI, Green L, Stadel BV, et al. Lactic acidosis in patients with diabetes treated with metformin. N Engl J Med 1998;338:265.
41. Hunink MGM, Goldman L, Tosteson ANA, et al. The recent decline in mortality from coronary heart disease, 1980–1990. The effect of secular trends in risk factors and treatment. JAMA 1997;277:535.
42. Arciero TJ, Jacobsen SJ, Reeder GS, et al. Temporal trends in the incidence of coronary disease. Am J Med 2004;117:228.
43. Shepherd J, Cobbe SM, Ford I, et al. Prevention of coronary heart disease with pravastatin in men with hypercholesterolemia. West of Scotland Coronary Prevention Study Group. N Engl J Med 1995;333:1301.
44. Heart Protection Study Collaborative Group. MRC/BHF Heart Protection Study of cholesterol lowering with simvastatin in 20,536 high-risk individuals: a randomised placebo-controlled trial. Lancet 2002;360:7.
45. Scandinavian Simvastatin Survival Study Group. Baseline serum cholesterol and treatment effect in the Scandinavian Simvastatin Survival Study (4S). Lancet 1995;345:1274.
46. Sacks FM, Pfeffer MA, Moye LA, et al. The effect of pravastatin on coronary events after myocardial infarction in patients with average cholesterol levels. Cholesterol and Recurrent Events Trial Investigators. N Engl J Med 1996;335:1001.
47. Brown G, Albers JJ, Fisher LD, et al. Regression of coronary artery disease as a result of intensive lipid lowering therapy in men with high level of apolipoprotein B. N Engl J Med 1990;323:1289.
48. Nissen SE, Tuzcu EM, Schoenhagen P, et al.; REVERSAL Investigators. Effect of intensive compared with moderate lipid-lowering therapy on progression of coronary atherosclerosis: a randomized controlled trial. JAMA 2004;291: 1071.
49. Cannon CP, Braunwald E, McCabe CH, et al. Intensive versus moderate lipid lowering with statins after acute coronary syndromes. N Engl J Med 2004;350:1495.
50. LaRosa JC, Grundy SM, Waters DD, et al. Treating to New Targets (TNT) Investigators. Intensive lipid lowering with atorvastatin in patients with stable coronary disease. N Engl J Med 2005;352:1425.
51. Grundy SM, Cleeman JI, Merz CN, et al. Implications of recent clinical trials for the National Cholesterol Education Program Adult Treatment Panel III guidelines. Circulation 2004;110:227.
52. Flegal KM, Graubard BI, Williamson DF, et al. Excess deaths associated with underweight, overweight, and obesity. JAMA 2005;293:1861.
53. Randin D, Vollenweider P, Tappy L, et al. Suppression of alcohol-induced hypertension by dexamethasone. N Engl J Med 1995;332:1733.
54. Langer RD, Criqui MH, Reed DM. Lipoproteins and blood pressure as biological pathways for effect of moderate alcohol consumption on coronary heart disease. Circulation 1992;85:910.
55. Victor RG, Hansen J. Alcohol and blood pressure: a drink a day. N Engl J Med 1995; 332:1782.
56. Iestra JA, Kromhout D, van der Schouw YT, et al. Effect size estimates of lifestyle and dietary changes on all-cause mortality in coronary artery disease patients: a systematic review. Circulation 2005;112:924.
57. Yusuf S, Dagenais G, Pogue J, et al. Vitamin E supplementation and cardiovascular events in high-risk patients. The Heart Outcomes Prevention Evaluation Study Investigators. N Engl J Med 2000;342:154.
58. Miller ER 3rd, Pastor-Barriuso R, Dalal D, et al. Meta-analysis: high-dosage vitamin E supplementation may increase all-cause mortality. Ann Intern Med 2005;142:37.
59. AHA Scientific Statement: Fish consumption, fish oil, omega-3 fatty acids and cardiovascular disease, #71-0241 Circulation 2002;106:2747.
60. Grady D, Rubin SM, Petitti DB, et al. Hormone therapy to prevent disease and prolong life in postmenopausal women. Ann Intern Med 1992;117:1016.
61. Sullivan JM, Vander-Zwaag R, Hughes JP, et al. Estrogen replacement and coronary artery disease: effect on survival in postmenopausal women. Arch Intern Med 1990;150:2557.
62. Herrington DM, Reboussin DM, Brosnihan KB, et al. Effects of estrogen replacement on the progression of coronary-artery atherosclerosis. N Engl J Med 2000;343:522.
63. Grady D, Wenger NK, Herrington D, et al. Postmenopausal hormone therapy increases risk for venous thromboembolic disease. The Heart and Estrogen/Progestin Replacement Study. Ann Intern Med 2000;132:689.
64. Stefanick ML, Mackey S, Sheehan M, et al. Effects of diet and exercise in men and postmenopausal women with low levels of HDL cholesterol and high levels of LDL cholesterol. N Engl J Med 1998;339:12.
65. Jakicic JM, Marcus BH, Gallagher KI, et al. Effect of exercise duration and intensity on weight loss in overweight, sedentary women: a randomized trial. JAMA 2003;290:1323.
66. Danahy DT, Aronow WS. Hemodynamics and antianginal effects of high-dose oral isosorbide dinitrate after chronic use. Circulation 1977; 56:205.
67. Thadani U, Fung HL, Darke AC, et al. Oral isosorbide dinitrate in angina pectoris: comparison of duration of action and dose-response relation during acute and sustained therapy. Am J Cardiol 1982;49:411.
68. Elkayam U. Tolerance to organic nitrates: evidence, mechanisms, clinical relevance, and strategies for prevention. Ann Intern Med 1991;114:667.
69. Psaty BM, Smith NL, Siscovick DS, et al. Health outcomes associated with antihypertensive therapies used as first-line agents: a systematic review and meta-analysis. JAMA 1997;277:739.
70. Pahor M, Psaty BM, Alderman MH, et al. Health outcomes associated with calcium antagonists compared with other first-line antihypertensive therapies: a meta-analysis of randomised controlled trials. Lancet 2000;356:1949.
71. Packer M, O'Connor CM, Ghali JK, et al. Effect of amlodipine on morbidity and mortality in severe chronic heart failure. N Engl J Med 1996;335:1107.
72. Gibbons RJ, Chatterjee K, Daley J, et al. ACC/AHA/ACP-ASIM guidelines for the management of patients with chronic stable angina: executive summary and recommendations. A report of the American College of Cardiology/American Heart Association Task Force on Practice Guidelines (Committee on Management of Patients with Chronic Stable Angina). Circulation 1999; 99:2829.
73. Steinhubl SR.Berger PB, Mann JT, et al. Early and sustained dual oral antiplatelet therapy following percutaneous coronary intervention a randomized controlled trial. JAMA 2002; 288:2411.
74. Yusuf S, Zhao F, Mehta SR, et al. Effects of clopidogrel in addition to aspirin in patients with acute coronary syndromes without ST-segment elevation. N Engl J Med 2001;345: 494.
75. Beinart SC, Kolm P, Vedledar E, et al. Long-term cost effectiveness of early and sustained dual oral antiplatelet therapy with clopidogrel given for up to one year after percutaneous coronary intervention results from the Clopidogrel for the Reduction of Events During Observation (CREDO) Trial. J Am Coll Cardiol 2005;46:761.
76. Braunwald E, Domanski MJ, Fowler SE, et al.; PEACE Trial Investigators. Angiotensin-converting-enzyme inhibition in stable coronary artery disease. N Engl J Med 2004;351:2058.
77. Fischman, DL, Leon, MB, Baim, DS, et al. A randomized comparison of coronary stent placement and balloon angioplasty in the treatment of coronary artery disease. N Engl J Med 1994;331:496.
78. Serruys PW, de Jaegere P, Kiemeneij F, et al. A comparison of balloon expandable stent implantation with balloon angioplasty in patients with coronary artery disease. N Engl J Med 1994;331:489.
79. Indolfi C, Pavia M, Angelillo IF. Drug-eluting stents versus bare metal stents in percutaneous coronary interventions (a meta-analysis). Am J Cardiol 2005;95:1146.

80. Chaitman BR, Fisher LD, Bourassa MG, et al. Effect of coronary bypass surgery on survival patterns in subsets of patients with left main coronary artery disease. Report of the Collaborative Study in Coronary Artery Surgery (CASS). Am J Cardiol 1981;48:765.
81. Passamani E, Davis KB, Gillespie MJ, et al. A randomized trial of coronary artery bypass surgery: survival of patients with a low ejection fraction. N Engl J Med 1985;312:1665.
82. Caracciolo EA, Davis KB, Sopko G, et al. Comparison of surgical and medical group survival in patients with left main coronary artery disease: long-term CASS experience. Circulation 1995;91:2325.
83. The Bypass Angioplasty Revascularization Investigation (BARI) Investigators. Comparison of coronary bypass surgery with angioplasty in patients with multivessel disease. The Bypass Angioplasty Revascularization Investigation (BARI) Investigators. N Engl J Med 1996; 335:217.
84. Hultgren HN, Peduzzi P, Detre K, et al. The 5 year effect of bypass surgery on relief of angina and exercise performance. Circulation 1985; 72[Suppl 5]:79.
85. Puskas JD, Winston AD, Wright CE, et al. Stroke after coronary artery operation: incidence, correlates, outcome, and cost. Ann Thorac Surg 2000;69:1053.
86. Roach GW, Kanchuger M, Mangano CM, et al. Adverse cerebral outcomes after coronary bypass surgery. Multicenter Study of Perioperative Ischemia Research Group and the Ischemia Research and Education Foundation Investigators. N Engl J Med 1996;335:1857.
87. McKhann, GM, Goldsborough, MA, Borowics, LM, et al. Predictors of stroke risk in coronary artery bypass patients. Ann Thorac Surg 1997;63:516.
88. Yoon BW, Bae HJ, Kang DW, et al. Intracranial cerebral artery disease as a risk factor for central nervous system complications of coronary artery bypass graft surgery. Stroke 2001;32:94.
89. van der Linden J, Hadjinikolaou L, Bergman P, et al. Postoperative stroke in cardiac surgery is related to the location and extent of atherosclerotic disease in the ascending aorta. J Am Coll Cardiol 2001;38:131.
90. van Dijk D, Keizer AM, Diephuis JC, et al. Neurocognitive dysfunction after coronary artery bypass surgery: a systematic review. J Thorac Cardiovasc Surg 2000;120:632.
91. Newman MF, Kirchner JL, Phillips-Bute B, et al. Longitudinal assessment of neurocognitive function after coronary-artery bypass surgery. N Engl J Med 2001;344:395.
92. Daoud EG, Strickberger A, Man KC, et al. Preoperative amiodarone as prophylaxis against atrial fibrillation after heart surgery. N Engl J Med 1997;337:1785.
93. Guarnieri T, Nolan S, Gottleib SO, et al. Intravenous amiodarone for the prevention of atrial fibrillation after open heart surgery. The Amiodarone Reduction in Coronary Heart (ARCH) trial. J Am Coll Cardiol 1999;34:343.
94. Arora RR, Chou TM, Jain D, et al. The multicenter study of enhanced external counterpulsation (MUSTEECP): effect of EECP on exercise-induced myocardial ischemia and anginal episodes. J Am Coll Cardiol 1999;33:1833.
95. Ernst E. Chelation therapy for coronary heart disease: an overview of all clinical investigations. Am Heart J 2000;140:139.
96. Oesterle SN, Reifart N, Hauptmann E, et al. Percutaneous in situ coronary venous arterialization: report of the first human catheter-based coronary artery bypass. Circulation 2001;103:2539.
97. Proudfit WL, Bruschke AVG, Sones FM. Clinical course of patients with normal or slightly or moderately abnormal coronary arteriograms: 10 year follow-up of 571 patients. Circulation 1980;62:712.
98. Gottlieb SO, Gottlieb SH, Achuff SC, et al. Silent ischemia on Holter monitoring predicts mortality in high-risk postinfarction patients. JAMA 1988;259:1030.
99. Chandra NC, Ziegelstein RC, Rogers WJ, et al. Observations of the treatment of women in the United States with myocardial infarction: a report from the National Registry of Myocardial Infarction–I. Arch Intern Med 1998;158:981.
100. Thompson SG, Kienast J, Pyke SDM, et al. Hemostatic factors and the risk of myocardial infarction or sudden death in patients with angina pectoris. N Engl J Med 1995;332:635.
101. Anderson HV, Cannon CP, Stone PH, et al. One-year results of the thrombolysis in myocardial infarction (TIMI) IIIB clinical trial: a randomized comparison of tissue-type plasminogen activator versus placebo and early invasive versus early conservative strategies in unstable angina and non-Q wave myocardial infarction. J Am Coll Cardiol 1995;26:1643.
102. Califf RM, White HD, Van de Werf F, et al. One-year results from the Global Utilization of Streptokinase and TPA for Occluded Coronary Arteries (GUSTO-I) Trial. Circulation 1996; 94:1233.
103. GUSTO Investigators. An international randomized trial comparing four thrombolytic strategies for acute myocardial infarction. N Engl J Med 1993;329:673.
104. Hennekens CH, Buring JE, Sandercock P, et al. Aspirin and other antiplatelet agents in the secondary and primary prevention of cardiovascular disease. Circulation 1989;80:749.

For annotated **General References** *and resources related to this chapter, visit www.hopkinsbayview.org/PAMreferences.*

Chapter 63

Postmyocardial Infarction Care and Cardiac Rehabilitation

Kerry J. Stewart and Roy C. Ziegelstein

EPIDEMIOLOGY OF MYOCARDIAL INFARCTION

Overview

Cardiovascular diseases are the major cause of mortality in the United States, accounting for more than one million deaths annually. These conditions are responsible for approximately 40% of all deaths in this country (1). Approximately 35% of these deaths are caused by myocardial infarction (MI). Approximately 25% of men and 38% of women will die within 1 year after having an MI (1). Although the overall death rate after MI has decreased, the rate of hospitalizations for MI has been relatively stable. The greater number of patients surviving an MI has increased the number of individuals with chronic heart failure (see Chapter 66) and the number of individuals who should be considered for cardiac rehabilitation and secondary prevention (2). In both older and younger patients, mortality after MI could be reduced still further with more consistent use of interventions known to benefit patients after MI, which is the focus of this chapter (3).

Patients who survive an acute MI are far more likely to suffer recurring illness or death from coronary artery disease (CAD). Approximately 7.1 million people alive today in the United States have a history of heart attack (1). Two of every three survivors of MIs do not make a complete recovery but still have a good long-term prognosis. The longitudinal care of the patient who has survived an MI usually is the responsibility of the patient's primary care provider.

Demographic Subgroups

The average age of a person having a first heart attack is 65.8 years for men and 70.4 years for women (1). Aging of the population undoubtedly will result in greater numbers of individuals with chronic diseases, including CAD, congestive heart failure (CHF), and stroke (4).

Death rates from CAD are highest among African American men and women. Whereas the mortality from cardiovascular disease has declined for men over the last two decades, it has increased for women during this period (1). For *patients hospitalized with an acute MI,* women, particularly African-American women, have higher case mortality than men both during hospitalization and in the 48 months after discharge (5). The higher mortality in women admitted for acute MI has been found in all age groups irrespective of type of treatment (6).

PROGNOSIS OF PATIENTS DISCHARGED FROM CORONARY CARE UNITS

Survivors of Myocardial Infarction

Mortality

Over the last several decades, the in-hospital mortality rate for patients with acute MI has decreased to approximately 10% (1,7). Although the in-hospital mortality rate is higher for patients with Q-wave MI, there is a higher

TABLE 63.1 Characteristics Associated with Increased Mortality after Discharge of Patients Who Have Had an MI

Admission characteristics
History of a previous MI
CHF (chest x-ray or Killip classification)
History of hypertension
Extent of LV ischemia (radionuclide scintigraphy, cardiac enzymes)
Characteristics at discharge
Early (within 10 days) post-MI angina, with transient ST–T changes[a]
LV ejection fraction ≤40% (echocardiography, radionuclide ventriculography, arteriography)
Complex ventricular arrhythmia[b] (Holter monitor)
Left main, proximal left anterior descending, or three-vessel CAD (arteriography)
Positive limited early post-MI ECG stress test (within 2–3 weeks after MI)
Ventricular aneurysm developing in acute stage of MI
Characteristics after discharge
ECG abnormalities, especially ischemic ST-segment depression, 1 month after MI
Decreased heart rate variability
Cigarette smoking
Depression

[a]Mortality risk highest when ECG shows ischemia at a distance (i.e., transient ischemic ST changes in myocardial location that is different from the location of the patient's MI).
[b]Multifocal premature ventricular contractions (PVCs), runs of two or more sequential ectopic ventricular beats, or PVCs with R-on-T pattern. CAD, coronary artery disease; CHF, congestive heart failure; ECG, electrocardiogram; LV, left ventricular; MI, myocardial infarction.

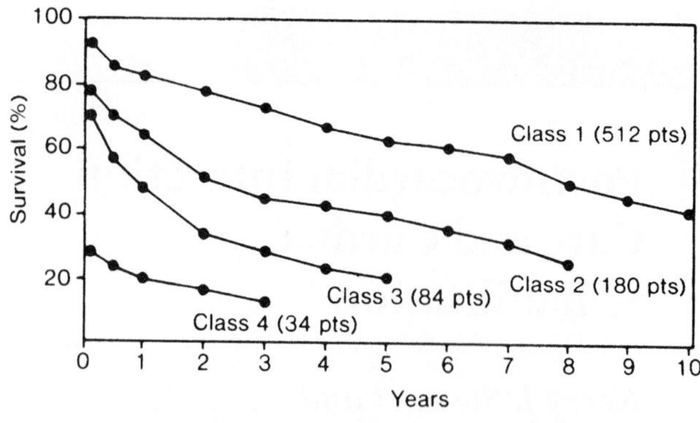

FIGURE 63.1. Survival after acute myocardial infarction based on Killip classification (810 patients admitted to the Duke Medical Center Coronary Care Unit from 1967 to 1978). (From Rosati RA, Harris PJ. Acute myocardial infarction. In: Fries J, Ehrlich GE, eds. Prognosis: contemporary outcomes of disease. Bowie, MD: Charles Press, 1981:275, with permission.)

long-term mortality for those with non–Q-wave MI. The overall first-year mortality for hospital survivors of an MI is approximately 10% to 15% (7,8). Most of the deaths in the first year occur during the 3 months after discharge, and they occur chiefly in patients with one or more of the high-risk characteristics listed in Table 63.1.

The *classification of acute MI developed by Killip* according to the presence and severity of CHF on admission to the hospital is one of the most useful prognostic indices. Class I patients have no evidence of CHF on admission, class II patients have mild CHF, class III patients present with pulmonary edema, and class IV patients have cardiogenic shock. Figure 63.1 shows the strikingly different survival rates among patients in these four classes (9). Improvement in survival rates in each of the Killip classes has been observed, but the classification remains a valid index of morbidity and mortality after MI (10,11).

Table 63.1 lists the *clinical factors predictive of an increased mortality after hospital discharge.* Patients with the greatest risk of mortality during the first year after an MI have one or more of the following factors: previous MI; development of early (within 10 days) post-MI angina accompanied by transient ST-segment or T-wave changes; ejection fraction ≤40%; late hospital phase (predischarge) complex ventricular arrhythmia; left main, proximal left anterior, left anterior descending, or three-vessel CAD; positive stress test at low workload within a few weeks after MI; presence of ischemic ST changes on resting electrocardiogram (ECG) taken ≥1 month after MI; and low heart rate variability (amount of heart rate fluctuation around the mean heart rate) (12). The Gruppo Italiano per lo Studio della Sopravvivenza nell'Infarto Miocardico (GISSI)-2 study also clearly showed that the significantly increased risk of in-hospital mortality with older age persists after discharge (13). Left ventricular (LV) aneurysm developing within 2 days of acute MI also brings a high risk of death during the first year, independent of LV function (14). In addition to these cardiac complications, post-MI depression is strongly associated with post-MI mortality, even after controlling for other known predictors of survival (15).

In patients who are *clinically stable 1 to 6 months after hospitalization* for an acute MI or unstable angina, the presence of ischemic ST-segment depression on the resting ECG is the strongest predictor of morbidity and mortality over the ensuing 3 years. Posthospitalization stress testing is predictive of future coronary events in stable patients only when ischemia (≥1 mm ST-segment depression on exercise ECG) or a reversible perfusion defect (on thallium exercise test) is present at a low workload (5 metabolic equivalents [METs] or less) or when there is evidence of exercise-induced LV dysfunction (LV cavity dilation and/or increased thallium uptake by the lung during exercise) (16). Each of these high-risk subsets has made up <3% of study populations.

Morbidity

Postinfarction angina occurs during the year after an MI in many patients, and cardiac stress testing can help anticipate who will develop this symptom. Stress testing, during the hospitalization, after discharge, or both, is recommended for many patients who have sustained an MI (17,18). The American College of Cardiology (ACC)/American Heart Association (AHA) guidelines list three class I recommendations for stress testing after MI (19): (a) before discharge for prognostic assessment, activity prescription, and evaluation of medical therapy; (b) early after discharge for prognostic assessment, activity prescription, evaluation of medical therapy, and cardiac rehabilitation if the predischarge exercise test was not done; and (c) late after discharge for prognostic assessment, activity prescription, evaluation of medical therapy, and cardiac rehabilitation if the early exercise test was submaximal. Despite these recommendations, only one of every 10 patients hospitalized in this country undergoes a stress test before hospital discharge (20). The limited utilization of stress testing as part of the care of patients with acute MI may relate to the perception that the test is not as useful in patients who have received reperfusion therapy (i.e., percutaneous coronary intervention or thrombolytic therapy) as it was in patients in the pre-reperfusion era. However, exercise testing after contemporary reperfusion therapies for MI still confers important prognostic information (21).

Patients who can exercise to 5 to 6 METs or to 70% to 80% of their age-predicted maximal heart rate without an abnormal ECG or blood pressure response have a low 1-year mortality (22). Patients with a post-MI symptom-limited stress test that shows early ischemic ST-segment changes (≥1 mm exercise-induced ST-segment depression) or limited work capacity (≤5 METs) have two or more times the risk of recurrent MI and of death over the ensuing year (23).

Postinfarction medical complications other than angina include CHF, life-threatening arrhythmias and sudden death, intracavity thrombi with stroke and systemic emboli, and post-MI syndrome (Dressler syndrome).

The *psychologic and social sequelae* during the year after an MI depend on both the severity of the patient's MI and the patient's premorbid psychosocial situation (see later in this chapter for a more detailed discussion of this topic).

Patients with Unstable Angina

Unstable angina is defined as pain caused by cardiac ischemia that is occurring more frequently, is being provoked by less effort, is occurring at rest, or is being relieved less readily by nitroglycerin. Chapter 62 describes other characteristics.

Patients discharged from the cardiac care unit with the diagnosis of unstable angina have 1-year morbidity and mortality rates similar to the rates of patients discharged with the diagnosis of a completed MI (24). Studies show that the resting ECG and the response to exercise stress testing are especially helpful in predicting future events in patients who are clinically stable after admission for unstable angina (16). The lack of ischemic ST-segment changes during exercise testing helps to identify patients at lower risk.

In an individual patient with unstable angina, a more precise prognosis often can be given by defining the coronary anatomy by *cardiac catheterization and coronary angiography.* In studies of patients with unstable angina, coronary angiography has shown CAD in the left main artery is more common in patients discharged with the diagnosis of unstable angina than in patients discharged with the diagnosis of a completed MI (15% vs. 5%, respectively). Another 10% have diffuse CAD, 10% have normal coronary arteries and are presumed to have coronary artery spasm or small-vessel disease as the cause of their chest pain, and the remaining 65% are equally divided among single-vessel, double-vessel, and triple-vessel CAD (25). This information is clinically important because of the demonstrated superiority of surgical over medical treatment of CAD in the left main artery. Chapter 62 describes the prognoses associated with each of the patterns and the management of unstable angina.

Survivors of Cardiac Arrest Who Have Not Had a Myocardial Infarction

The first-year mortality rate of survivors of out-of-hospital cardiac arrest who have not had an MI is approximately three times the mortality rate of survivors of out-of-hospital cardiac arrest who subsequently are shown to have completed an MI. In a study of >200 survivors of out-of-hospital cardiac arrest followed for >4 years, the rate of recurrence of ventricular fibrillation or sudden death in patients without an acute MI was 31%, compared with 5% for out-of-hospital survivors of cardiac arrest who subsequently evolved ECG changes of acute MI. The median time to recurrent circulatory arrest was 20 weeks. More than 70% of the episodes of ventricular fibrillation were unexpected or occurred during sleep or during the usual activities of daily living (26).

Because the survivors of ventricular fibrillation not associated with an MI have a high risk of sudden death, they require aggressive and highly individualized treatment. Advances in electrophysiology, antiarrhythmics, automatic implantable defibrillators, and the many innovative surgical approaches to ventricular dysrhythmias dictate prompt referral of such high-risk patients to a consulting cardiologist. Survivors of ventricular fibrillation not associated with an MI often receive an implantable cardioverter-defibrillator (ICD). The widespread use of ICDs is likely to produce issues for primary care providers who care for patients with these devices. Increased levels of anxiety and depression have been described in patients after ICD placement (27–29). The experience of a shock may

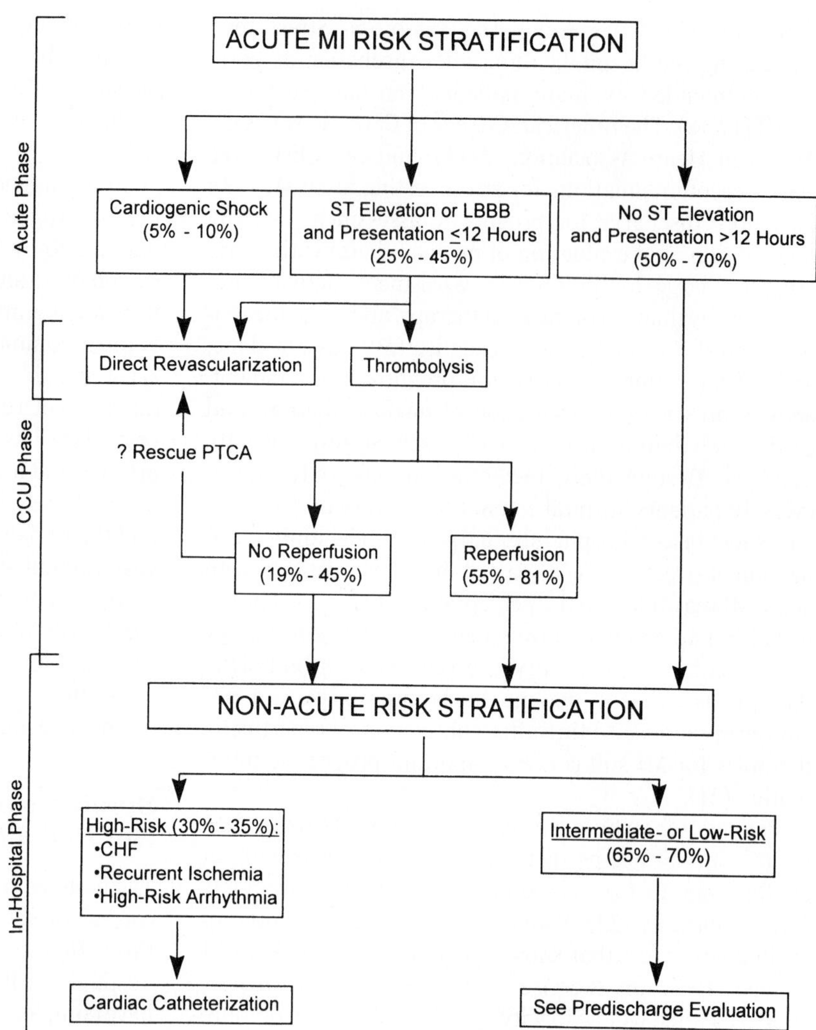

FIGURE 63.2. Flow diagram of risk stratification after myocardial infarction. CCU, coronary care unit; CHF, congestive heart failure; LBBB, left bundle branch block; MI, myocardial infarction; PTCA, percutaneous transluminal coronary angioplasty; ST, ST segment. (From Clinical Guidelines Parts I and II. Guidelines for risk stratification after myocardial infarction [American College of Physicians]. Ann Intern Med 1997;126:561, with permission.)

contribute to psychological distress and diminished quality of life (30,31). Chapter 64 discusses this topic in detail.

RISK STRATIFICATION BEFORE HOSPITAL DISCHARGE

The American College of Physicians has published recommendations for in-hospital risk stratification of MI patients, and the recommendations are summarized in Figs. 63.2 and 63.3 (see American College of Physicians, www.hopkinsbayview.org/PAMreferences). This three-phase scheme delineates decision-making that is supported by outcome data from clinical trials. It was published to guide the care of MI patients before they are discharged from the hospital. It draws on a mix of *baseline characteristics and findings from continuous reevaluation of the patient*. Depending on clinical findings, a patient may have undergone thrombolysis, revascularization, or neither in the acute and nonacute phases of risk stratification. In the *predischarge evaluation,* patients at intermediate or low risk (60%–70% of MI patients) should undergo assessment of LV function and noninvasive stress testing. Often, those patients can be discharged after stays as short as 4 to 5 days. The postdischarge prognosis of MI patients and their appropriate management depend on the predischarge evaluation, postdischarge reevaluations, and the rehabilitation and medical approaches described in this chapter.

REHABILITATION AND MANAGEMENT AFTER MYOCARDIAL INFARCTION

Most patients discharged after MI can expect to return to most of their usual activities within a few weeks to months. For a smaller number of patients, complications of their MI make this outcome impossible. In either situation, an organized plan for care should be followed (Table 63.2). This plan should include the education of the

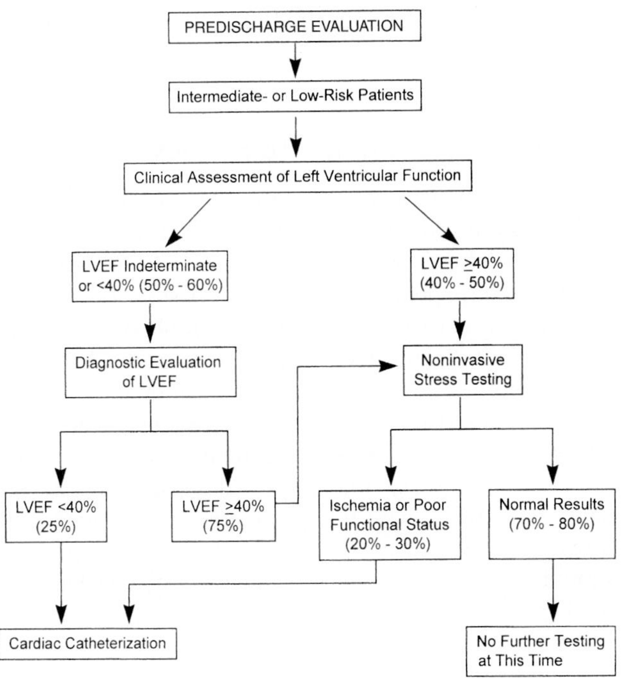

FIGURE 63.3. Flow diagram for predischarge risk stratification after myocardial infarction. LVEF, left ventricular ejection fraction. (From Clinical Guidelines Parts I and II. Guidelines for risk stratification after myocardial infarction [American College of Physicians]. Ann Intern Med 1997;126:561, with permission.)

patient and the patient's family. Because of shorter hospital stays, much of the patient education previously included in inpatient cardiac rehabilitation now is conducted in outpatient programs.

Patient Education

Many hospitals initiate education about MI when the patient is clinically stable. The educational program often is the responsibility of a cardiac rehabilitation professional. Patient education should cover the nature of coronary heart disease, cardiac symptoms, cardiac drugs, modification of major risk factors (smoking, hypertension, hyperlipidemia, obesity, and inactivity), and guidelines for resumption of physical activities (including sexual activity) and return to work. It should be emphasized that MI is a manifestation of a disease process that has been ongoing for many years. Many patients attribute their MI to what they were doing at the moment it actually occurred. Patients must understand that the MI very likely would have occurred regardless of what they were doing that particular day and that the likelihood of a recurrence may best be diminished by following prescribed medical therapy and making lifestyle changes.

Individualized information should be provided in a *predischarge conference* at which the patient and the patient's

TABLE 63.2 Plan of Care for MI Survivors after Hospital Discharge

Patient education (objectives for all patients)[a]
Understands disease process (damage to the heart that heals in a few months, leaves a scar)
Understands likely prognosis
Understands and follows progressive activity schedule[b]
Understands approximate timetable for return to work[b]
Understands importance of controlling major risk factors (smoking, hypercholesterolemia, hypertension) and takes action to control them
Knows how to recognize key cardiac symptoms (angina, tachycardia, heart failure, hypotension) and understands how to use sublingual nitroglycerin
Participates in group classes after discharge[c]
Gets answers to questions specific to his or her lifestyle
Medical management
Review in-hospital course for prognosis characteristics (see Table 63.1) and for medications prescribed at discharge
Assess and reinforce above patient education
Check periodically for complications of infarction (see Table 63.5)
Check for behavioral/psychiatric complications
Check ECG 2–3 months after discharge
Consider β-blocker, ACE inhibitor, statin, and aspirin treatment[d]
Referral for cardiac rehabilitation[d]

[a]Essential to include the patient's partner in all aspects of education.
[b]Serial exercise stress tests can be used to plan progressive activity (see text).
[c]If programs are available in the community.
[d]See text for details.
ACE, angiotensin-converting enzyme; ECG, electrocardiogram; MI, myocardial infarction.

family members are encouraged to ask questions. The conference should include review of any adverse prognostic features identified before discharge (Table 63.1); the medications prescribed at discharge; discussion of specific plans for cardiac rehabilitation, diet, and smoking modification; a chance for ventilation about emotional stress-laden issues; and realistic appraisal of expectations of return to work or usual levels of physical activity. Because of the possibility of postinfarction angina, it is important to describe this symptom to patients who have never experienced it and to point out to all patients that postinfarction angina may occur with the increased activity recommended for the coming weeks. Every patient should be given sublingual nitroglycerin, and the correct use of this drug should be reviewed.

It is important to provide written information and to assess and reinforce patient understanding of the information after discharge. This has perhaps become even more important as length of stay for MI has decreased, resulting in fewer in-hospital opportunities for education and for providing postdischarge recommendations. The patient education booklet *After a Heart Attack* (single copies available without charge from local chapters of the AHA) gives a useful general account of the disease process, prognosis, coronary risk factors, and rehabilitation process.

Many hospitals have developed *group classes for MI survivors and their families.* Typically, they are invited to participate in a number of weekly meetings during the first or second month after discharge. Sessions usually are led by a cardiac rehabilitation professional such as a nurse, social worker, clinical exercise physiologist, or cardiologist, with the objective of having participants raise questions about the recovery period to provide mutual support by sharing experiences with each other. Additional resources available in many communities are patient-run heart clubs and supervised physical conditioning programs (see Physical Conditioning After Myocardial Infarction). The American Association of Cardiovascular and Pulmonary Rehabilitation (401 North Michigan Avenue, Chicago, IL 60611-4267; 312-321-5146; http://www.aacvpr.org) publishes a national directory of cardiac rehabilitation programs and is an excellent source of patient materials and professional publications, such as *Guidelines for Cardiac Rehabilitation and Secondary Prevention Programs* (see American Association of Cardiovascular and Pulmonary Rehabilitation, www.hopkinsbayview.org/PAMreferences). In addition, several resources for patients are available on the Internet, including the sites of the Johns Hopkins Bayview Medical Center and Johns Hopkins Greenspring Station (http://www.hopkinsbayview.org/cardiology) and of the AHA (http://www.americanheart.org). Patients also can be directed to support groups such as The Mended Hearts (http://www.mendedhearts.org/). Many of these sites provide links to other sources of patient information, support, and online newsletters.

Postdischarge Appointments

In general, each patient who has had an MI should be encouraged to contact his or her primary care provider or cardiologist at least once during the first week at home to discuss any questions that arise. An office visit should be scheduled within 2 to 3 weeks. Before this visit, it is important to review the patient's hospital summary to determine whether adverse prognostic features were present (Table 63.1) and to identify the medications prescribed at discharge. The visit should be divided between an assessment of the patient's progress in rehabilitation (physical activity level, diet and smoking modifications, emotional status, understanding of the overall plan of care, expectation about return to work) and an assessment of the patient's medical status (manifestations of ischemia and heart failure, blood pressure status, and review of current medications). Two or more additional office visits, similar to the first visit, should be scheduled during the 3 months after an MI, and the patient should be encouraged to telephone at any time about new symptoms or questions.

Risk Stratification at 3 to 6 Weeks

Approximately 3 to 6 weeks after MI, a *maximal exercise stress test* should be considered, because this test can provide helpful therapeutic and prognostic information regarding the patient's disease (see discussion of stress testing after MI earlier in this chapter). Table 63.3 summarizes the criteria and recommendations of the American College of Physicians, based on stratification into low-risk and moderate-risk findings in this stress test. The stress test is also used to assess functional capacity, to guide the return to work, and to provide goals (e.g., target heart rate, MET level) for an exercise prescription. Approximately 3 months after hospital discharge, an ECG should be obtained and used as the patient's new baseline tracing.

Activity Schedule

Table 63.4 provides a practical summary of symptom recognition for use by the patient and a schedule of progressive physical activities for the first 2 months after MI.

TABLE 63.3 Recommendations According to Stress Test Risk Stratification 3 to 6 Weeks After MI

Low-risk patients
These patients have a peak workload $\geq$5 METs[a] in the absence of exercise-induced angina pectoris or ST-segment depression.
Recommendations: Further diagnostic testing is unlikely to identify patients at an even lower risk and therefore is not indicated. The effect, if any, of medical or surgical therapy on the prognosis of these patients is difficult to demonstrate because of their very low risk. Treatment should emphasize the reduction of risk factors, especially control of hypertension, smoking cessation, diet modification, and exercise training.
Moderate-risk patients
These patients have a peak workload <5 METs, peak systolic pressure <110 mm Hg, or severe myocardial ischemia, defined as angina or ischemic ST-segment depression $\geq$2 mm appearing at a heart rate $\leq$130–140 bpm.
Indication for coronary arteriography: In patients at moderate risk, coronary arteriography is indicated.

[a]MET (metabolic equivalent) is the energy requirement for a certain level of activity. One MET is the energy requirement at rest. METs for common activities are given in Table 16.1.
MI, myocardial infarction.
Data from American College of Physicians. Evaluation of patients after recent acute myocardial infarction (position paper). Ann Intern Med 1989;110:485.

TABLE 63.4 Activity Schedule and Symptom Recognition for Patients Convalescing from MI[a]

General points

All activities, including sitting and lying down, require energy. The amount of energy required to perform a specific activity is expressed as METs. One MET is your resting energy requirement. As activities become more strenuous, the amount of energy required (METs) also increases, as does the workload imposed on your heart.

The schedule recommended in this program is based on the number of METs needed for various activities. Some specific recommendations are given for each of the first 3 months after your return to home. Table 16.1 gives the energy requirements for a wide variety of additional activities. If the table omits your favorite activities, ask your doctor about them.

Warnings: Generally the following activities impose an added strain on your heart and should be avoided, especially during the first 3 months after a heart attack:

- Taking very hot or cold showers or baths
- Extended breath-holding while exercising, lifting, or straining
- Working in a bent or stooped position or with arms held above your head
- Doing work that requires continuous tensing of your muscles
- Working or exercising during very hot, cold, humid, or windy weather (in bad weather, plan your regular exercise at a nearby shopping mall)
- Working or exercising during the first hour after a meal or after consuming alcohol
- Consuming excessive amounts of alcohol (e.g., >1–2 oz of whiskey, 2–3 beers, 1–2 glasses of wine per day)
- Walking or exercising on a hill or an inclined surface
- Engaging in any activity that creates emotional stress or worry for you

Recommended activity schedule[b]

First month (1–3 METs)

From discharge to 1 week

Regular exercise: Walk 5 min at a leisurely pace once per day on a level surface.

Some specific advice: This week, primarily get used to being at home. Occupy yourself with sit-down activities, such as watching television, playing cards, sewing, painting, or sketching. Avoid lifting objects heavier than 5 lb or doing activities that require reaching above your head. You may go up and down the stairs. However, take your time and limit the number of times you need to climb them. Do all of the things you were doing in the hospital. Get up and get dressed each day. You may be surprised at how tired and weak you feel. This is natural. Be sure to take rest periods when you need them, particularly after meals and before you exercise or climb the stairs.

Week 2

Regular exercise: Walk 10 min at a leisurely pace twice per day.

Some specific advice: Continue all of your previous activities and add others, such as taking rides in the car (however, no driving yet), cooking a meal, washing clothes in a machine (have someone else remove them), making your bed, attending a relaxing movie, going out to dinner, going shopping with your family (let others lift things from the shelves to the basket and carry the groceries), shooting pool, playing shuffleboard, throwing a softball underhand, and playing a piano or organ.

Weeks 3 and 4

Regular exercise: Advance gradually to walking 15 min at a leisurely pace twice per day.

Some specific advice: Continue your previous activities and others, such as going to religious services, sweeping floors, polishing furniture, and driving the car (beginning with short drives, avoiding heavy traffic).

Second month (3–5 METs)

Regular physical exercise: Progressively increase leisurely walking from 20 min once per day at a slightly faster pace to 30 min once or twice per day.

Some specific advice: Table 16.1 lists the approximate energy requirements of each activity. You may gradually increase your activities by adding other activities and spending more time at them; see Table 16.1 for activities requiring ≤5 METs or ≥5 METs.

Recognizing heart symptoms

Your heart will give you warning signs if it is not ready for increased activity. Here are some guidelines to use:

Pulse: Locate your pulse and count the number of times it beats for 15 s and multiply that number by 4. This is your heart rate for 1 min. Take your pulse before you begin your walk or any new activity and at the end of the activity. Contact your health care provider before resuming exercise if:

- There is an increase ≥20 bpm in pulse after exercise compared with before exercise pulse
- Your heart rate exceeds 120/min[c]
- You detect abnormal heart action: pulse becomes irregular, fluttering or jumping in chest or throat, very slow pulse rate, sudden burst of rapid heartbeats

Chest pain: Contact your health care provider before resuming exercise if you experience pain or pressure in the chest, arm, or throat precipitated by exercise or following exercise. Remember to take your nitroglycerin and rest if you do experience pain.

Dizziness: Contact your health care provider before resuming exercise if you become dizzy, light-headed, or faint during exercise.

Breathing difficulty: Contact your health care provider before resuming exercise if you become short of breath during or after a new exercise, or if you awaken from sleep short of breath.

[a]Information in Chapter 16, Table 16.1 should be given to patients who receive the instructions in this table.
[b]Pace of these activities may be scaled up or down by results of early post-MI stress test when available.
[c]These figures may be markedly modified by results of early stress test or medication.
MI, myocardial infarction.

In Chapter 16, Table 16.1 lists a broad array of activities corresponding to the recommended energy levels during and after the recuperation period. Resumption of activities with increasing energy requirements should be gradual; in particular, the duration of new activities should be brief at first, with gradual increase, according to how the patient feels. The schedule given in Table 63.4 can be given to most patients. A more aggressive plan can be tailored for the patient if an early physical conditioning program, guided by early stress testing, is available. Similarly, stress test-guided conditioning also can be planned for patients after the first 1 to 2 weeks of convalescence from an MI. Supervised programs that enroll patients soon after MI are widely available. In addition to the American Association of Cardiovascular and Pulmonary Rehabilitation, affiliates of the AHA commonly maintain lists of local exercise programs. A comprehensive discussion of exercise conditioning is found below (see Physical Conditioning After Myocardial Infarction).

Return to Work

Because many patients will have their first MI during their active working years, they are commonly concerned about returning to work. After an MI, 10% to 20% of patients are unable to return to their former occupational and recreational activities. Fortunately, the remaining 80% to 90% of patients are able to do so within 2 to 6 months. In fact, 88% of those younger than 65 years are able to return to their usual work after an MI (1). Patients who do not return to work within 6 months of MI are unlikely ever to return to work (32), and this often is caused by psychological rather than physical factors (see Psychological Problems). Psychological distress is common even in individuals who are able to return to work after an MI (33).

Many factors determine whether an individual returns to work after an MI. Health care providers should be aware that only some of these factors are related to the patient's cardiac or medical condition. An individual's employment history and societal factors are important determinants of the likelihood of returning to work. Local unemployment rates, working conditions, employer attitudes about adjusting workloads, employer return-to-work policies, and medical care benefits are all important determinants (34). Obviously, the type of work is also an essential consideration. Patients whose occupations involve mental stress and hectic schedules should be advised to return to work on a part-time basis at first, leaving plenty of time for rest and relaxation. For patients whose work involves significant physical exertion, the timing of return to work can be based on the information given in Tables 16.1 and 63.4 and guided by the results of exercise stress testing and monitored responses during a supervised rehabilitation program. It is evident from Table 16.1 that most occupations require an energy level of ≤6 METs. Occupational activities classified as heavy work require energy expenditure of ≤7 METs. Certain activities may produce an increased workload on the heart because of psychological stress (e.g., driving a vehicle in heavy traffic) or because they entail significant resistive exercise (e.g., carpentry, plumbing, shoveling, operating pneumatic tools, or carrying objects heavier than 30 lb).

Patients with MIs complicated by poorly controlled angina, CHF, or arrhythmias should be evaluated in conjunction with a consulting cardiologist (see Medical Complications) before a plan for returning to work and other activities is formulated. Some of these patients may qualify for *permanent medical disability* (see Chapter 9) or for job retraining through vocational rehabilitation. The *fundamental difference between impairment and disability* caused by CAD was underscored in the report of the 1989 Bethesda Conference on Insurability and Employability of the Patient with Ischemic Heart Disease (35). Impairment is a medically defined disorder and is a key component of disability, but it is just one of several factors that determine the overall ability of a person to perform meaningful work. Additional factors that affect disability include other medical disorders, age, sex, education, training, and psychosocial support. The main points in the report state that most MI patients can return to work; prognosis can be estimated by clinical examination and noninvasive studies that evaluate LV function (echocardiogram), myocardial jeopardy (thallium stress test), and electrical instability (Holter monitor); cardiac catheterization is not routinely required; special assessment may be needed for jobs requiring sudden or sustained high effort or heat exposure (e.g., firefighters) or for those in whom sudden disability may endanger others (e.g., airline pilots); a trial period of progressively increasing part-time work may be necessary for smooth transition from total disability to full-time work; and maximal functional capacity should be evaluated as soon as the clinical status is stable, usually 3 to 5 weeks after uncomplicated MI, 7 weeks after coronary bypass surgery, and 1 week after coronary angioplasty in patients who have not had an MI.

Although cardiac rehabilitation, including education, counseling, and behavioral intervention, has many benefits, it has not been shown to alter the rates of return to work. This was the conclusion of the 1995 *Cardiac Rehabilitation Clinical Guideline No. 17* of the Agency for Health Care Policy and Research (see Wenger et al., www.hopkinsbayview.org/PAMreferences). The expert panel reported that although education and counseling may improve a patient's potential for return to work, many other factors play a role in return to work, including willingness of the employer to rehire the patient, the patient's level of job satisfaction, economic incentives, and perceived stress of the job.

Sexual Activity

It is safe for patients who are symptom-free during usual activities of daily living to resume sexual intercourse within 4 to 6 weeks of MI. Available data suggest that the energy requirement approximates 3 METs during foreplay and afterplay and 5 METs at climax (36). These are equivalent to the oxygen demands of a brisk walk around the block or climbing one flight of stairs.

The Myocardial Infarction Onset Study provides information about the risk of sexual activity in patients with cardiac disease and is of particular benefit to those counseling individuals about sexual activity after an MI (37). Although this study confirmed that sexual activity can trigger MI, the risk appears to be small and transient. Notably, the relative risk of triggering an MI in individuals with a history of angina or previous MI is not greater than the relative risk in individuals without prior cardiac disease.

The same study indicated that regular exercise appears to reduce, and possibly to eliminate, the small increased risk of MI associated with sexual activity. Thus, health care providers who counsel patients after an MI can reassure them that the risk of triggering an MI during sexual activity is particularly low for those who exercise regularly. When counseling patients about resumption of sexual activity, the health cared provider should *give specific advice* and encourage questions. The pamphlet *Sex and Heart Disease,* available from the AHA (http://www.americanheart.org), is a helpful adjunct to counseling. Frequency of sexual intercourse can be similar to the frequency before the patient's MI. Sexual foreplay without completion of intercourse can be recommended to patients who wish to resume sex cautiously. In general, sexual activity can be resumed in the position that was most gratifying before the MI; however, patients should avoid positions in which they support their weight on their arms because this requires sustained static type of work (see Physical Conditioning After Myocardial Infarction) and may put extra stress on the heart by increasing the blood pressure. Sexual activity should be engaged in when both partners are relaxed. It is best to abstain from intercourse for 2 or 3 hours after eating a large meal because eating increases the work of the heart.

Inability to return to a previous pattern of sexual activity may be caused by angina (precipitated by intercourse), new medications, or psychological stress associated with the recent MI. If an otherwise stable patient develops angina during intercourse, sublingual nitroglycerin can be taken just before sexual activity.

Erectile dysfunction may be particularly common in men with CAD because the two conditions share common risk factors. For this reason, patients recovering from an MI may ask their practitioner about the use of medications to treat erectile dysfunction. Three drugs approved for erectile dysfunction are sildenafil (Viagra), tadalafil (Cialis), and vardenafil (Levitra). These drugs work by inhibiting the action of cyclic guanosine monophosphate (cGMP)-specific phosphodiesterase type 5, thereby blocking the breakdown of cGMP and allowing it to accumulate in the corpus cavernosum of the penis. A study in men with severe coronary stenosis showed that oral sildenafil did not produce any adverse cardiovascular effects, even in coronary flow (38). When patients with CAD were given sildenafil, vardenafil, or tadalafil before exercise stress testing to a level of cardiac work at least as great as that experienced during sexual intercourse, no significant cardiovascular problems were encountered (39–42). Although caution should be used when prescribing sildenafil, tadalafil, and vardenafil to patients with CAD, particularly if the individual is not physically active on a regular basis, these drugs appear safe in the absence of low blood pressure or aortic stenosis. It must be emphasized, however, that these drugs should be used cautiously by men who are taking medicines that contain organic nitrates of any kind, including nitroglycerin. Because nitrates increase cGMP, the concomitant use of an organic nitrate and sildenafil, tadalafil, or vardenafil may result in dramatic, and potentially dangerous, reductions in arterial blood pressure. Chapter 6 discusses the evaluation and management of drug-induced and psychological sexual dysfunction, both of which may occur after MI.

Psychological Problems

It is normal for patients to experience *symptoms of anxiety and depression* during the first few weeks after discharge from the hospital. Some of these symptoms are caused by misconceptions about the nature and prognosis of MI and may respond to simple reassurance and clarification. Most patients do well when they are encouraged to express their concerns and are reassured that their response is normal. A small supply of a minor tranquilizer (see Chapter 22) or a short-acting hypnotic (see Chapter 7) can be prescribed if needed. Participation in group classes and group exercise programs can help patients adjust to changes in their lives after MI (see Patient Education).

Another common psychological complication of MI is an *inappropriate fear of physical activity of any kind* (i.e., the so-called *cardiac cripple* or *ergophobic).* Early participation in supervised physical activity, including the exercise stress test, and exercise conditioning have been shown to enhance the patient's self-confidence and ability to perform physical tasks (43). Having the partner or family member observe an exercise test may help to establish confidence that the patient is not a cardiac cripple. In some medical centers, partners or family members are offered an opportunity to walk on the treadmill. This serves to establish a reference point for estimating ability to engage in activity. Engaging in a wide range of activities in the months after an MI is important because self-confidence is task specific (43,44). Most cardiac exercise programs (see below) initially emphasize activities using the legs, such as walking and jogging. Although these activities increase self-confidence in tasks requiring leg work, they do little for arm self-confidence. To increase arm self-confidence, patients must practice separate arm exercises (44,45). This is especially important for patients who plan to return to work that may require upper-body and arm efforts. The use of resistance training in cardiac rehabilitation now is routinely recommended for physiologic benefits and may help to increase self-confidence (46,47).

Another common problem is *denial of illness persisting beyond the first few days in the hospital.* The behavior associated with persistent denial may create substantial risks. This is especially true of patients who are extremely competitive and are used to controlling most of the circumstances of their lives (48). Typically they are determined to return to work as soon as possible and will refuse cardiac rehabilitation on the basis that they can do it better on their own. This behavior arouses anxiety, fear, and concern in the family and may lead to significant interpersonal conflict. An open discussion with patient and partner, with each acknowledging the other's concerns, often can lead to resolution of these conflicts and more appropriate behavior from each of them.

At times it is useful to teach patients to use *various forms of feedback* to guide their activities. Specifically, patients are taught to use a target heart rate based on an exercise stress test; to observe themselves and how they feel, with the basic instruction to rest if fatigue or any cardiac symptoms occur during exercise; to call their primary care provider or cardiologist if symptoms persist after using nitroglycerin; and to view family members as a source of feedback. In most cases, family members' observation on how the patient looks is remarkably accurate. If a partner says his or her partner looks tired or does not look right, he or she probably is correct (and vice versa). By having the patient agree to consider these comments as well-meaning, the patient usually will comply with the partner's advice. Thereafter, the number of reminding behaviors is reduced progressively, and the rehabilitation process can proceed with greater enthusiasm from both partners. With more difficult patients or with partners having pre-existing interpersonal strife, the consultation of a psychiatrist or psychologist may be helpful in managing adjustment problems.

Some patients have *severe psychological and behavioral problems after MI* that may interfere with their rehabilitation. The most common problem is *persistent depression,* which may have characteristics of a major or minor depressive illness or may present as an adjustment disorder characterized by anxiety, depression, somatization, or a mixture of these responses (49). Chapters 21, 22, and 24 discuss the diagnosis and management of these problems.

Approximately 40% of patients have either minor or major depression soon after an MI (49). *Major depression* occurs in 15% to 20% of patients and is associated with a threefold to fourfold increased cardiovascular mortality at 6 months (13). Individuals with major depression soon after an MI are likely to remain depressed for at least several months and possibly longer (49). Thus, the practitioner who views depression as an expected reaction that is likely to improve and not likely to influence recovery may be missing an opportunity to improve the patient's quality of life and health. Because major depression typically does not resolve spontaneously, the patient who leaves the hospital depressed may continue to experience mood disturbance at the very time when participation in risk-reducing behaviors is critical. It is important for health care providers to recognize that patients with depression after an MI are less likely to adhere to recommended behavior and lifestyle changes intended to reduce the risk of subsequent cardiac events (50).

These findings highlight the importance of recognizing symptoms of depression and offering patients appropriate treatment, which should include a program of cardiac rehabilitation. A study in which depressive symptoms were present in 20% of patients after a major coronary event showed that symptoms resolved in two thirds of these patients after a program of cardiac rehabilitation (51). Unfortunately, patients with depression are more difficult to recruit and retain in these programs than are individuals without depression (52,53). When depression is identified in a patient recovering from an MI, the practitioner should encourage the individual to socialize and to increase interactions with friends and family. Depression resolves more rapidly after an MI when patients have good social support (54). Social support may even buffer the adverse effects of depression on prognosis. The 1-year cardiac mortality of depressed patients with the lowest levels of perceived social support has been observed to be more than five times that of depressed patients with the highest levels of perceived social support (54).

The selective serotonin reuptake inhibitors (SSRIs) can be used safely by patients with ischemic heart disease (55–58). In light of these studies and the general absence of significant cardiovascular side effects of the SSRIs, antidepressants in this class are preferable to tricyclic antidepressants (TCAs) in patients with depression after an MI who require antidepressant therapy. TCAs may increase resting heart rate, produce orthostatic hypotension, and adversely affect intracardiac conduction and, possibly, the susceptibility to ventricular arrhythmias (59). In a study that compared the effects of the SSRI paroxetine to the effects of the TCA nortriptyline in patients with ischemic heart disease and major depression, patients treated with the TCA experienced significantly more adverse cardiac events than patients treated with paroxetine (56). Although concerns about the safety of SSRIs in patients with ischemic heart disease have been allayed, no trial to date has shown that treatment of depression with either an SSRI (58) or with cognitive behavior therapy (60) improves survival. Chapter 24 discusses in detail the treatment of depression.

Medical Therapy

Overview

There is evidence that β-blockers and aspirin reduce the risk of morbidity and mortality after MI. For certain subgroups of patients, long-term treatment with angiotensin-converting enzyme (ACE) inhibitors also improves prognosis. Despite the widespread use of calcium channel blockers after MI, there is no evidence that this class of drug improves prognosis. The evidence for current recommendations regarding each of these classes of drugs is thoroughly reviewed by Hennekens et al. (see www.hopkinsbayview.org/PAMreferences).

β-Adrenoreceptor Blockers

β-Blocker therapy is recommended for all patients who have had an MI. Treatment should begin during the initial hospitalization and should be continued indefinitely. Although the benefits of β-blocker therapy are modest in low-risk patients (i.e., younger patients without a prior MI, those who have not had an anterior MI, or those who do not now have complex ventricular ectopy or significant LV dysfunction) (61), it is generally recommended that unless a clear contraindication exists, even low-risk patients should receive β-blockers indefinitely. When initiated early in the course of an infarction (within 6 hours), β-blockers may limit or reduce infarct size. Later in the postinfarct time period, the mechanism for reduction in mortality is prevention of reinfarction and the antiarrhythmic property of β-blockers. The *overall magnitude of benefit* from the use of β-blockers seems to be an approximately one-third reduction in first-year mortality and about the same magnitude of reduction in reinfarction during the first post-MI year. These benefits may extend beyond 1 year in some subgroups. *Contraindications* or relative contraindications to the use of β-blockers include asthma, bradycardia, and insulin-treated diabetes mellitus. The *recommended dosage* of a β-blocker is the amount required to produce attenuation of heart rate and blood pressure response to exercise without producing side effects. Chapter 67 summarizes the characteristics of the available β-blocking drugs.

Antiplatelet Therapy

Daily aspirin (75–325 mg) is recommended for all patients who have had an MI. Although the efficacy of other types of antiplatelet therapy is less well established, clopidogrel (75 mg/day) may be substituted for aspirin if the patient has an aspirin allergy or aspirin intolerance. Clopidogrel often is recommended in addition to aspirin for patients who have had an MI, particularly if they have been treated with percutaneous coronary intervention (PCI). Clopidogrel is usually given for at least one month, although the optimal duration of clopidogrel therapy is debated. Because many patients have drug-eluting stents placed during PCI, which often require prolonged use of clopidogrel and aspirin, the decision about how long to continue this drug should be made in conjunction with the consulting cardiologist. If the risk is acceptable, warfarin anticoagulation is a reasonable alternative for secondary prevention of MI in patients unable to take aspirin or for those with atrial fibrillation, LV thrombus, or extensive wall-motion abnormality. Multiple randomized trials of antiplatelet therapy for secondary prevention of vascular disease show that prolonged treatment with aspirin has no effect on nonvascular mortality but reduces vascular *mortality* by approximately 15% and nonfatal vascular *events* (stroke or MI) by approximately 30% in patients with pre-existing cardiac or cerebral vascular diseases (62). Post-MI benefits are similar to the benefits in patients after stroke and transient ischemic attack. *In absolute terms,* the benefits of antiplatelet therapy accrued to approximately 40 per 1,000 treated patients during the first month of treatment after an acute MI and to approximately 40 per 1,000 patients with a history of MI who were treated for 3 years. There is no difference in the degree of protection afforded by aspirin alone at a dosage of 325 mg/day and that afforded by higher aspirin dosages or other antiplatelet agents. Aspirin 100 mg/day has been shown to improve coronary artery bypass graft patency at 4 months (90% of grafts patent vs. 68% in the placebo group) (63) and to decrease significantly the frequency of restenosis after percutaneous transluminal coronary angioplasty (64) and thrombolysis (65). Chapter 57 provides additional details on antiplatelet agents.

Angiotensin-Converting Enzyme Inhibitors

All patients who have had an MI and whose LV ejection fraction is <40% should receive an ACE inhibitor in the absence of specific contraindications (see Hennekens, et al., MI management guidelines, www.hopkinsbayview.org/PAMreferences). Although the benefit of ACE inhibitors may be less in those with normal or mildly reduced LV function, even these patients should be considered for treatment with ACE inhibitors, in addition to aspirin and beta blockers. The purpose of using these agents after an MI is to prevent adverse LV remodeling and recurrent ischemic events.

Long-term use of ACE inhibitors by patients with *chronic ischemic congestive cardiomyopathy* is associated with significant improvement in morbidity and mortality irrespective of severity and symptoms of failure. A large placebo-controlled study showed that patients with recent MI and LV dysfunction (ejection fraction ≤40% by radionuclide ventriculography) who were randomized to captopril experienced a modest reduction in cardiovascular and overall mortality, progression to severe heart failure, and recurrent MI during 3 years of treatment (66). Another large study showed that asymptomatic patients with LV ejection fraction ≤35% who were randomized to enalapril also experienced a reduction in mortality or progression to heart failure during 3 years of treatment (67). The benefits accrued chiefly to patients with the lowest ejection fractions. In asymptomatic patients with reduced ejection fractions, ACE inhibitors should be started at low dosages (e.g., enalapril 2.5 mg/day; captopril 6.25 mg three times daily) with gradual increases (e.g., enalapril up to 10 mg/day; captopril up to 25 or 50 mg three times daily) guided by blood pressure response and renal function. An angiotensin II receptor blocker (ARB) is an acceptable alternative for patients who have sustained an MI or who have CHF and who are intolerant of ACE inhibitors. Chapter 67 summarizes the characteristics of ACE inhibitors.

Calcium Channel Blockers

Calcium channel blockers are not recommended for secondary prevention after an MI. Because calcium channel blockers have not been demonstrated to significantly reduce mortality in MI survivors, they should be used only in patients with symptomatic ischemia or hypertension that is not controlled despite treatment with β-blockers and ACE inhibitors or ARBs. Calcium channel blockers may be appropriate for patients with good LV function who have specific contraindications to beta blockers or who tolerate them poorly.

Smoking, Hyperlipidemia, Hypertension, and Exercise

Smoking

All patients who smoke after an MI should be counseled to stop. Post-MI morbidity and mortality are significantly reduced in patients who discontinue smoking. Smokers who have survived an MI usually are motivated to stop. Chapter 27 describes practical ways to assist patients who desire to stop smoking, including the prescription of nicotine substitution products.

Lipid-Lowering Diet and Drugs

A diet low in saturated fat and cholesterol (the AHA Step II diet) should be recommended to all patients after an MI. As noted in the Third Report of the National Cholesterol Education Program (NCEP) Expert Panel on Detection, Evaluation, and Treatment of High Blood Cholesterol in Adults (Adult Treatment Panel III) (see Expert Panel on Detection, Evaluation, and Treatment of High Blood Cholesterol in Adults, www.hopkinsbayview.org/PAMreferences), most patients with CAD require drug therapy to reduce low-density-lipoprotein (LDL) cholesterol. Lipid-lowering therapy should be recommended to reduce LDL cholesterol to <100 mg/dL. In general, treatment should begin with a statin, although whether reducing LDL cholesterol to <100 mg/dL by other means, including the use of other lipid-lowering drugs, produces similar reductions in coronary events in patients who have sustained an MI is not clear. Whereas a target LDL cholesterol of <100 mg/dL has been established by the expert panel, later data suggest that the optimal LDL level may be even lower, perhaps in the 75 to 80 mg/dL range (68). For patients who have normal total and LDL cholesterol levels but whose high-density lipoprotein (HDL) cholesterol is <35 mg/dL, an exercise program should be recommended in an attempt to raise HDL cholesterol. Drug therapy (e.g., with niacin or a fibrate) also may be considered for this purpose.

As pointed out in the American College of Physicians' risk stratification report (see American College of Physicians, www.hopkinsbayview.org/PAMreferences), lipid levels measured within 24 to 48 hours of an MI are accurate and can guide post-MI secondary prevention decisions. Chapter 82 provides detailed information on cholesterol and atherosclerotic disease.

Exercise

The role of formal exercise programs in rehabilitation after MI is described in detail in Physical Conditioning after Myocardial Infarction.

Medical Complications

Table 63.5 lists the principal medical complications of MI, the procedures that may be useful in diagnosing or evaluating them, and potential therapies. As noted earlier (see Risk Stratification Before Hospital Discharge), complications identified early are addressed very aggressively before or shortly after discharge. In general, use of advanced and costly procedures to evaluate the complications listed in Table 63.5 should be coordinated with a consulting cardiologist.

Postinfarction Angina

As discussed in the prognosis, angina is common in survivors of MI. Chapter 62 describes in detail the evaluation and medical management of angina. Because protection of the heart from transient ischemia may be especially important during recovery from an MI, it is advisable to

TABLE 63.5 Medical Complications of MI

Complications	Diagnostic Procedures for Selected Patients[a]	Management Approaches
Angina or other evidence of reversible ischemia	ECG stress testing, echocardiographic or radionuclide stress testing, Holter monitor for silent ischemia, coronary arteriography	Standard antianginal therapy (see Chapter 62), coronary artery bypass or PTCA for selected patients, physical conditioning
CHF	Radionuclide ventriculography or echocardiography (reduced ejection fraction, segmental dysfunction, rupture, ventricular aneurysm)	Afterload reduction, diuretics, ?β-blockers, ?anticoagulants (see Chapter 66 for treatment of heart failure), surgery in a few selected patients
Arrhythmias	Holter monitor, ECG stress testing, electrophysiologic study in selected patients	β-Blockers, other antiarrhythmics (see Chapter 64), surgery or implantable defibrillator in selected patients
Post-MI syndrome (Dressler syndrome)	Echocardiography (pericardial effusion)	Aspirin or other anti-inflammatory agents (see text)
Systemic emboli	Echocardiography (intracardiac thrombus)	Anticoagulant therapy (see Chapter 57), surgery in selected patients

[a]Should be coordinated with and interpreted by consulting cardiologist.
CHF, congestive heart failure; ECG, electrocardiogram; MI, myocardial infarction; PTCA, percutaneous transluminal coronary angioplasty.

prescribe β-blockers in most patients (see above) and to undertake aggressive evaluation and management of patients who develop angina within the first 3 months after MI. Because of the poor prognosis associated with angina that occurs very early after an MI, patients with this problem after hospital discharge should be referred to a cardiologist for consideration of coronary catheterization and possible coronary revascularization.

Postinfarction Symptomatic Congestive Heart Failure

Postinfarction symptomatic CHF usually develops before hospital discharge. Currently, most patients undergo measurement of LV ejection fraction as part of their evaluation before discharge so that those at increased risk for developing symptomatic CHF after discharge are known. As noted above, ACE inhibitors delay deterioration in functional capacity and improve survival in patients with CHF after MI (66). Chapter 66 describes in detail the use of ACE inhibitors and other agents for CHF. Selected patients with persistent CHF may have segmental or global LV dysfunction or mitral regurgitation that may improve after cardiac surgery and may benefit from referral to a cardiologist.

Postinfarction Arrhythmias

A substantial proportion of MI survivors have *complex ventricular arrhythmias* (see criteria in Table 63.1) on 24-hour ambulatory ECG monitoring after the first week of hospitalization. Controlled trials do not show that suppression of ventricular ectopy with drug therapy improves mortality. Therefore, routine testing to determine whether ventricular arrhythmia is present after an MI is not recommended. Studies evaluating the benefits of implantable defibrillators in specific high-risk populations have shown that defibrillators prolong life compared with use of antiarrhythmic drugs (69,70). Chapter 64 provides a comprehensive discussion of the management of symptomatic arrhythmias.

Postmyocardial Infarction (Dressler) Syndrome

An estimated 3% to 4% of patients develop this complication, usually within 1 to 8 weeks after an MI. The syndrome is characterized by the pain of pericarditis (substernal pain relieved by leaning forward and increased with inspiration), presence of a friction rub, pericardial effusion (which can best be demonstrated by echocardiography), malaise, fever, leukocytosis, and often unilateral or bilateral pleural effusion. The principal considerations in the differential diagnosis are pulmonary embolism and recurrence or extension of the recent MI.

A patient with suspected Dressler syndrome should be considered for hospitalization. A possible recurrent MI should be addressed by monitoring, serial ECGs, and measurement of cardiac enzymes. Evaluation for pulmonary embolization requires ventilation–perfusion lung scanning or spiral computed tomography. If these tests do not explain the patient's symptoms, the clinical diagnosis of Dressler syndrome can be made with reasonable assurance. Echocardiographic evidence of a pericardial effusion and an elevated erythrocyte sedimentation rate may be present.

Dressler syndrome usually responds to salicylates or indomethacin. In patients who do not respond to these drugs, prednisone provides prompt relief of symptoms. However, use of steroids within 4 weeks of an MI may interfere with postinfarction healing and may increase the risk of myocardial rupture; therefore, use of steroids should be limited to patients who are >4 weeks postinfarction. Once the diagnosis is secure and symptoms are controlled, the patient can be discharged. The anti-inflammatory drug chosen in the hospital should be administered for a few weeks after discharge. Patients who have recurrent symptoms when anti-inflammatory treatment is discontinued should resume treatment for another month or longer.

Arterial Embolization

Arterial embolization occurs after hospitalization in 5% to 10% of MI survivors. The emboli seem to originate from mural thrombi that typically are seen in the LV apex adjacent to akinetic or dyskinetic wall segments. Approximately 30% to 40% of hearts with akinetic or dyskinetic LV apices show mural thrombi on the echocardiogram. Thus, anticoagulation (see Chapter 57) in patients with mural thrombi is generally recommended, although the impact and appropriate duration of anticoagulation have not been assessed in a prospective trial. However, most cardiologists recommend anticoagulation therapy for 3 to 6 months for MI survivors who have mural thrombi. In patients with LV systolic dysfunction, warfarin use is associated with improved survival and reduced morbidity (71). Patients with atrial fibrillation or a history of embolic events also should be considered for systemic anticoagulation with warfarin.

Referral for Cardiology Consultation

Selected MI survivors may benefit from coronary angioplasty or cardiac surgery by symptom reduction or improved prognosis. Patients in the following groups should be referred promptly to a cardiologist to ensure optimal medical therapy and to obtain an opinion about the advisability and the timing of invasive procedures:

- Patients with *uncontrolled angina* refractory to medical therapy, with a markedly positive exercise stress test at low workload or with evidence of LV dysfunction during exercise (e.g., increased lung uptake of thallium during exercise)
- Patients with a ventricular aneurysm
- Patients with CHF refractory to medical therapy (ACE inhibitors, digitalis, and diuretics)
- Patients with *structural complications,* such as ventricular septal defect (suggested by holosystolic murmur and thrill at the left sternal border), papillary muscle rupture (suggested by refractory CHF and holosystolic apical murmur), segmental akinesis, or ventricular aneurysm
- Patients with *electrical instability* (e.g., symptomatic bradycardia, high-grade atrioventricular blocks, ventricular tachycardia, or other arrhythmias)

Home Care for Acute Myocardial Infarction

Although not generally advisable, management at home may be appropriate for an occasional patient who has a stable acute MI and objects to hospitalization, a patient who is predicted to have a high likelihood of becoming very disoriented and agitated in a cardiac care unit, or a patient who consults a health care provider several days after the onset of symptoms of infarction. The scheme for rehabilitation after MI described in this chapter can be adapted to these situations.

MANAGEMENT OF UNSTABLE ANGINA AFTER DISCHARGE FROM HOSPITAL

Of patients admitted to a hospital with unstable angina but without MI, 15% to 30% continue to have pain despite vigorous medical management. Patients in this group have an estimated 1-year mortality rate of 25%. Therefore, most are evaluated and referred for coronary angioplasty or coronary artery bypass surgery. These interventions relieve or eliminate symptoms in most cases and improve survival for those with left main CAD, three-vessel disease, and two-vessel disease with LV dysfunction.

To date, the rehabilitation of the medically managed patient with unstable angina has not been studied as systematically as the rehabilitation of the patient after MI. These patients should receive education similar to that recommended for patients after MI regarding the nature of CAD, the recognition of symptoms, and the control of risk factors (see above). Because these patients have not sustained an ischemic injury that typically would require ≥2 months to heal, they often return to their usual activities more rapidly than patients who have had an MI. This is true particularly if the angina is well controlled and a stress test shows good effort tolerance (≥9 METs) and minimal or no changes caused by ischemia or LV dysfunction. Chapter 62 provides additional information regarding the management of unstable angina.

PHYSICAL CONDITIONING AFTER MYOCARDIAL INFARCTION

Regular exercise, with the goal of attaining the physiologic adaptation known as the *conditioning effect,* is safe and

50. Ziegelstein RC, Fauerbach JA, Stevens SS, et al. Patients with depression are less likely to follow recommendations to reduce cardiac risk during recovery from a myocardial infarction. Arch Intern Med 2000;160:1818.
51. Milani RV, Lavie CJ, Cassidy MM. Effects of cardiac rehabilitation and exercise training programs on depression in patients after major coronary events. Am Heart J 1996;132:726.
52. Guiry E, Conroy RM, Hickey N, et al. Psychological response to an acute coronary event and its effect on subsequent rehabilitation and lifestyle change. Clin Cardiol 1987;10:256.
53. Blumenthal JA, Williams RS, Wallace AG, et al. Physiological and psychological variables predict compliance to prescribed exercise therapy in patients recovering from myocardial infarction. Psychosomatic Med 1982;44:519.
54. Frasure-Smith N, Lespèrance F, Gravel G, et al. Social support, depression, and mortality during the first year after myocardial infarction. Circulation 2000;101:1919.
55. Shapiro PA, Lesperance F, Frasure-Smith N, et al. An open-label preliminary trial of sertraline for treatment of major depression after acute myocardial infarction (the SADHAT Trial). Sertraline Anti-Depressant Heart Attack Trial. Am Heart J 1999;137:1100.
56. Roose SP, Laghrissi-Thode F, Kennedy JS, et al. Comparison of paroxetine and nortriptyline in depressed patients with ischemic heart disease. JAMA 1998;279:287.
57. Strik JJ, Honig A, Lousberg R, et al. Efficacy and safety of fluoxetine in the treatment of patients with major depression after first myocardial infarction: findings from a double-blind, placebo-controlled trial. Psychosom Med 2000;62:783.
58. Glassman AH, O'Connor CM, Califf RM, et al. Sertraline antidepressant heart attack randomized trial (SADHEART) group. Sertraline treatment of major depression in patients with acute MI or unstable angina. JAMA 2002;288: 701.
59. Roose SP, Glassman AH. Cardiovascular effects of tricyclic antidepressants in depressed patients with and without heart disease. J Clin Psychiatry 1989;50[Suppl]:1.
60. Berkman LF, Blumenthal J, Burg M, et al. Enhancing Recovery in Coronary Heart Disease Patients Investigators (ENRICHD). Effects of treating depression and low perceived social support on clinical events after myocardial infarction: the Enhancing Recovery in Coronary Heart Disease Patients (ENRICHD) Randomized Trial. JAMA 2003;289:3106.
61. Furberg CD, Friedwald WT, Eberlein KA. Proceedings of the workshop on the implications of recent beta-blocker trials for postmyocardial infarction patients. Circulation 1983;67:1.
62. Antiplatelet Trialists' Collaboration. Collaborative overview of randomized trials of antiplatelet therapy. I. Prevention of death, myocardial infarction, and stroke by prolonged antiplatelet therapy in various categories of patients. BMJ 1994;308:81.
63. Lorenz RL, Schacky CV, Weber M, et al. Improved aortocoronary bypass patency by low-dose aspirin (100 mg daily): effects on platelet aggregation and thromboxane formation. Lancet 1984;1:1261.
64. Thornton MA, Greventzig AR, Hollman J, et al. Coumadin and aspirin in prevention of recurrence after transluminal coronary angioplasty: a randomized study. Circulation 1984;69:72.
65. ISIS-2. Randomised trial of intravenous streptokinase, oral aspirin, both or neither among 17,187 cases of suspected acute myocardial infarction. Lancet 1988;2:349.
66. Pfeffer M, Braunwald E, Moye L, et al. Effect of captopril on mortality and morbidity in patients with left ventricular dysfunction after myocardial infarction. N Engl J Med 1992;327: 669.
67. SOLVD Investigators. Effects of enalapril on mortality and development of heart failure in asymptomatic patients with reduced left ventricular ejection fractions. N Engl J Med 1992;32:685.
68. LaRosa JC, Grundy SM, Waters DD, et al. Intensive lipid lowering with atorvastatin in patients with stable coronary disease. N Engl J Med 2005;352:1425.
69. Moss AJ, Hall WJ, Cannom DS, et al. Improved survival with an implanted defibrillator in patients with coronary disease at high risk for ventricular arrhythmias. N Engl J Med 1996; 335:1933.
70. The Antiarrhythmic versus Implantable Defibrillator (AVID) Investigators. A comparison of antiarrhythmic-drug therapy with implantable defibrillator in patients resuscitated form near-fatal ventricular arrhythmias. N Engl J Med 1997;337:1576.
71. Al-Khadra AS, Salem DN, Rand WM, et al. Warfarin anticoagulation and survival: a cohort analysis from the Studies of Left Ventricular Dysfunction. J Am Coll Cardiol 1998;31:749.
72. Ehsani AA, Heath GH, Hagberg JM, et al. Effects of 12 months of intense exercise training on ischemic ST-depression in patients with coronary artery disease. Circulation 1981;64: 1116.
73. Schuler G, Hambrecht R, Schlierf G, et al. Regular exercise and low fat diet: effects on progression of coronary artery disease. Circulation 1992;86:1.
74. Taylor JL, Copeland RB, Cousin AL, et al. The effect of isometric exercise on the graded exercise test in patients with stable angina. J Cardiopulm Rehab 1981;1:450.
75. Coats AJS, Adampoulos S, Meyer TC, et al. Effects of physical training in chronic heart failure. Lancet 1990;335:63.
76. Sullivan MJ, Higgambotham MB, Cobb FR. Exercise training in patients with severe left ventricular dysfunction: hemodynamics and metabolic effects. Circulation 1988;78:506.
77. Gutmann MC, Squires RW, Pollack ML, et al. Perceived exertion–heart rate relationship during exercise testing and training in cardiac patients. J Cardiovasc Rehab 1981;1:52.
78. Taylor RS, Brown A, Ebrahim S, et al. Exercise-based rehabilitation for patients with coronary heart disease: systematic review and meta-analysis of randomized controlled trials. Am J Med 2004;116:682.
79. Council on Scientific Affairs, American Medical Association. Physician-supervised exercise programs in rehabilitation of patients with coronary heart disease. JAMA 1981;245:1463.
80. Stewart KJ, Effron MB, Vaeni SA, et al. Effects of diltiazem or propranolol during exercise training of hypertensive men. Med Sci Sports Exerc 1990;22:171.
81. Kelemen MH, Stewart KJ, Gillilan RE, et al. Circuit weight training in cardiac patients. J Am Coll Cardiol 1986;7:38.
82. Stewart KJ, Mason M, Kelemen MH. Three year participation in circuit weight training improves muscular strength and self-efficacy in cardiac patients. J Cardiopulm Rehab 1988;8:292.
83. Stewart KJ, McFarland LD, Weinhofer JJ, et al. Safety and efficacy of weight training soon after acute myocardial Infarction. J Cardiopulm Rehabil 1998;18:37.

For annotated ***General References*** *and resources related to this chapter, visit www.hopkinsbayview.org/PAMreferences.*

Chapter 64

Cardiac Arrhythmias

Sheldon H. Gottlieb, Joseph E. Marine, and Hugh Calkins

Contraction of the heart normally is the result of a well-orchestrated electromechanical system. The orderly function of the system is maintained by domination of the heart rate by a single biologic pacemaker (the sinoatrial [SA] node), by the relatively fast and uniform conduction of the electrical signal via specialized conduction pathways (His-Purkinje system), and by the relatively long and uniform duration of the electrical signal relative to its velocity of conduction through these pathways, which ensures uniform electrical excitation and contraction of the heart. A *cardiac arrhythmia* is any disturbance in the normal sequence of impulse generation and conduction in the heart.

Arrhythmias may occur in the absence of heart disease, may be symptoms of severe disease, or may themselves cause disease. Their significance and the need for treatment must be evaluated in the context of the clinical situation in which they occur. A precise etiologic diagnosis and an understanding of the pharmacology of the medications used are necessary to treat arrhythmias effectively. In recent years, there have been major advances in nonpharmacologic therapy of arrhythmias with a corresponding de-emphasis on treatment with antiarrhythmic drugs.

PHYSIOLOGY OF IMPULSE GENERATION AND CONDUCTION

Action Potential

Muscle contraction is stimulated by an electrical impulse, the action potential. In skeletal muscle, the action potential lasts several milliseconds, and the electrical activity is dissipated before the beginning of contraction. In cardiac muscle, however, the action potential lasts several hundred milliseconds, almost as long as the mechanical contraction of the myocyte itself (Fig. 64.1). In this way, the action potential not only stimulates contraction of the heart but also determines the duration and intensity of contraction. Furthermore, as long as the action potential is maintained, the heart cannot be stimulated to contract again.

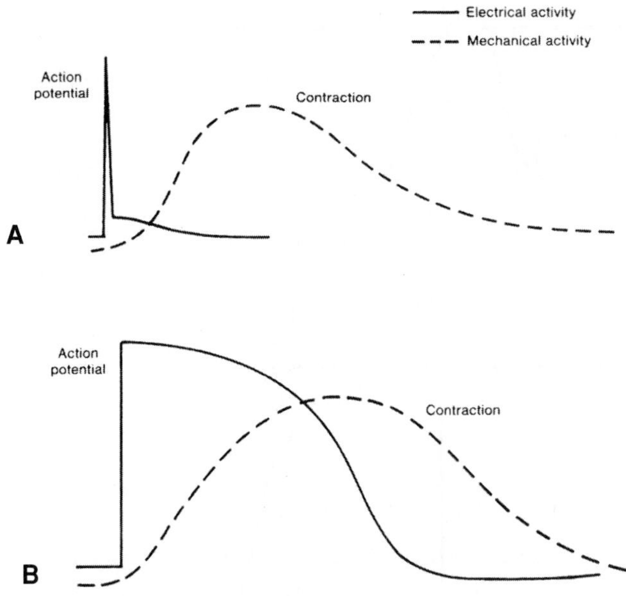

FIGURE 64.1. Comparison between relative time scales of electrical (*solid curve*) and mechanical (*dashed curve*) activity in skeletal (**A**) and cardiac (**B**) muscle. (From Noble D. The initiation of the heart beat. Oxford, England: Clarendon Press, 1975, with permission.)

The action potential is generated by depolarization and repolarization of the cardiomyocyte (Fig. 64.2). In the resting state, the intracellular concentration of potassium is high and that of sodium is low compared with the concentrations in extracellular fluid. The resting gradients of these ions are maintained by metabolic activity within the cell membrane, resulting in the resting membrane potential. This potential is strongly negative (i.e., there is an electrochemical gradient across the membrane so that the inside of the membrane is negatively charged compared with the outside of the membrane). If an electrical stimulus is applied, the membrane becomes highly permeable to sodium ions, which rapidly enter the cell (phase 0). The membrane is thus depolarized (loses its negative charge) and is transiently positively charged (overshoot). Repolarization occurs relatively slowly as chloride (phase 1), calcium (phase 2), and then potassium ions (phase 3) move back into the cell and thereby restore the resting potential (phase 4) (Fig. 64.2) (1).

Relationship to the Electrocardiogram

In the heart, the phases of rapid depolarization and overshoot correspond to the QRS complex of the electrocardiogram (ECG); phase 2 corresponds to the ST segment and phase 3 to the T wave (Fig. 64.2). During phase 2 the membrane is absolutely, and in phase 3 it is relatively, refractory to propagation of another electrical impulse.

Fast and Slow Currents

In most cardiac tissue, excitation is propagated by the rapidly depolarizing sodium current so that the impulses are conducted rapidly. However, in the SA node and the proximal part of the atrioventricular (AV) node, excitation is propagated by a slowly depolarizing current generated by the influx of calcium ions into the cell. Furthermore, in diseased cardiac muscle, the sodium current may be inhibited and depolarization may occur entirely via the slow calcium current; therefore, the action potential may be conducted very slowly. This difference in conduction velocity between cells depolarized by the sodium versus the calcium current has important implications in the generation and treatment of arrhythmias.

Pacemaker Generation

In most cardiac cells, an action potential is not generated until an electrical stimulus is applied. In pacemaker cells, slow spontaneous depolarization occurs during phase 4 until a threshold is reached, whereupon phase 0 rapidly ensues (Fig. 64.2); this process is called *automaticity.* In the absence of heart block, the heart rate is controlled by the pacemaker cells that depolarize most rapidly, because then the action potential is conducted rapidly throughout the heart and initiates rapid depolarization of other cells, even if they already have begun spontaneous slow depolarization. Automaticity is affected by the rate of slow spontaneous depolarization and the threshold potential. Automaticity is enhanced by increased sympathetic tone, decreased vagal tone, increased catecholamine concentration in the blood, thyroxine, and digoxin. It is suppressed by decreased sympathetic tone, increased vagal tone, decreased thyroxine concentration, and numerous drugs, including those used in the treatment of arrhythmias. Antiarrhythmic drugs may increase automaticity under some conditions.

Impulse Generation and Conduction

Sinoatrial Node

The SA node is composed of pacemaker cells and is located at the junction of the right atrium and the superior vena cava (Fig. 64.3). The cells of the SA node spontaneously depolarize more rapidly than any other cells within the heart and thereby control the heart rate under normal conditions.

Atrioventricular Node

The AV node is part of the specialized conduction system that carries the electrical impulse from the atrium to the ventricle. The AV node lies at the junction of the right

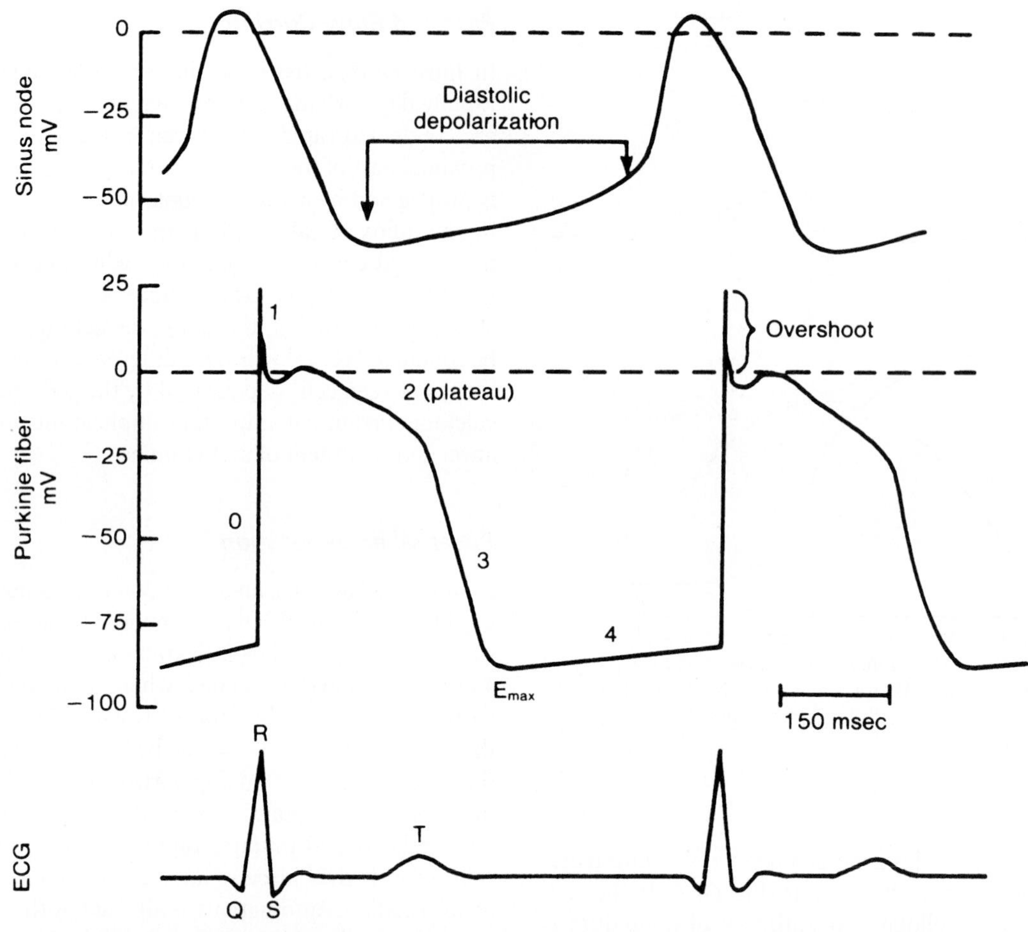

FIGURE 64.2. Transmembrane potentials from the sinus node and a Purkinje fiber. Note the spontaneous diastolic depolarization in the **upper panel,** characteristic of pacemaker fibers. The numbers in the **middle panel** are explained in the text. The **lower panel** shows the correlation of the time sequence of changes in the action potential with the surface electrocardiogram. Alterations in depolarization are reflected in changes in the QRS duration of the surface record; those in repolarization are associated with alterations in the QT interval. (From Singh BN, Collett JT, Chew CYC. New perspectives in the pharmacologic therapy of cardiac arrhythmias. Prog Cardiovasc Dis 1980;22:243, with permission.)

atrium and the interventricular septum, just above the tricuspid valve. Conduction through the AV node, which is mediated by calcium channels, is unique in that it is relatively slow; as a result, there is a 100- to 200-millisecond delay between activation of the atria and ventricles. This delay is important because it ensures that ventricular contraction occurs after atrial contraction is complete, thus maximizing the filling of the ventricles with blood. Another unique property of the AV node is that conduction is decremental; as more impulses arrive at the AV node, fewer get through, and those that do conduct through the AV node travel at a slower rate. The property of decremental conduction allows the AV node to serve as a protective gate, shielding the ventricles from excessively rapid stimulation from the atria, as can occur during atrial fibrillation and atrial flutter. The AV node also has intrinsic pacemaker activity, similar to that of the sinus node but slower (usually at a rate of 40–60 bpm). Because of the slower rate, the AV node may function as a subsidiary pacemaker if the SA node fails or if AV conduction is blocked.

Bundle of His

When the action potential leaves the AV node, it enters the specialized conducting fibers known as the *bundle of His.* The main bundle of His divides into three branches: the right bundle branch, which runs along the right ventricular surface of the septum; the left anterior superior branch, which runs along the left ventricular (LV) surface of the septum; and the left posterior inferior branch, which runs along the posterior wall of the left ventricle. The action

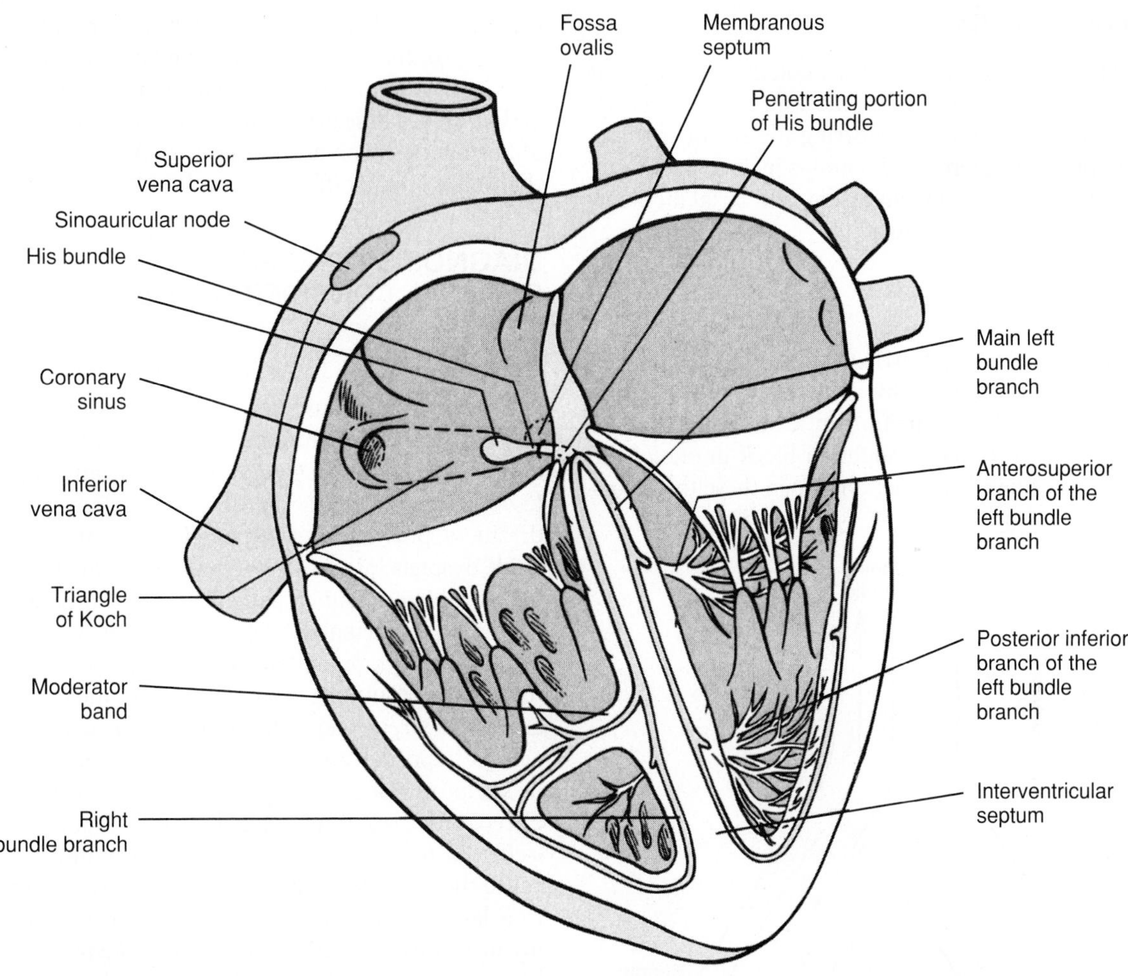

FIGURE 64.3. Anatomy of impulse generation. (From Willerson JT, ed. Treatment of heart diseases. London: Gower Medical Publishers, 1992. By permission of Mosby International.)

potential is conducted through the bundle branches and into the myocardium by a widespread network of smaller fibers known as *Purkinje fibers.*

MECHANISM OF CARDIAC ARRHYTHMIAS

Bradyarrhythmias result from one of two mechanisms: suppression of impulse formation and conduction block. Tachyarrhythmias result from one of three mechanisms: enhanced impulse formation, triggered activity, and reentry of the action potential into a pathway through which it has already passed (1). Multiple mechanisms may coexist in the same patient (e.g., atrial fibrillation with high-degree AV block in a patient with sinus node dysfunction). Furthermore, an arrhythmia may be initiated by one mechanism (enhanced automaticity of pulmonary vein tachycardia) and become sustained by another (reentry), as in the case of paroxysmal atrial fibrillation.

Suppression of Impulse Formation and Conduction Block

A disease process that interferes with pacemaker activity within the SA node or with the movement of the electrical impulse through the normal conduction pathways of the heart results in abnormal slowing of the heart rate (bradyarrhythmia) and/or in one of the various forms of heart block.

Enhanced Impulse Formation

Enhanced automaticity of a part of the cardiac conduction system may result in the initiation of an impulse more rapidly than is normally generated by the SA node. If that happens episodically, occasional premature contractions occur, the nature of which depends on the location of the ectopic pacemaker. On the other hand, if there is rapid sustained firing of the ectopic focus, an ectopic tachycardia ensues.

Triggered Activity

Triggered arrhythmias are the least common; they result from after depolarizations that follow an action potential and that reach threshold for triggering additional impulses (2). Examples of triggered arrhythmias include torsade de pointes, multifocal atrial tachycardia, and atrial tachycardia resulting from digitalis toxicity.

Reentry

Most clinically significant arrhythmias result from reentry (Fig. 64.4). Reentrant arrhythmias occur in the setting of two anatomically or functionally distinct conduction pathways, unidirectional conduction block in one of the pathways, and slowed conduction. When these three conditions are fulfilled, the electrical impulse may travel down one limb of the reentrant circuit and return via the second limb of the circuit, resulting in a "short circuit" or "circus" arrhythmia. These arrhythmias may result from anatomic abnormalities such as an accessory AV connection, as in the case of the Wolff-Parkinson-White (WPW) syndrome.

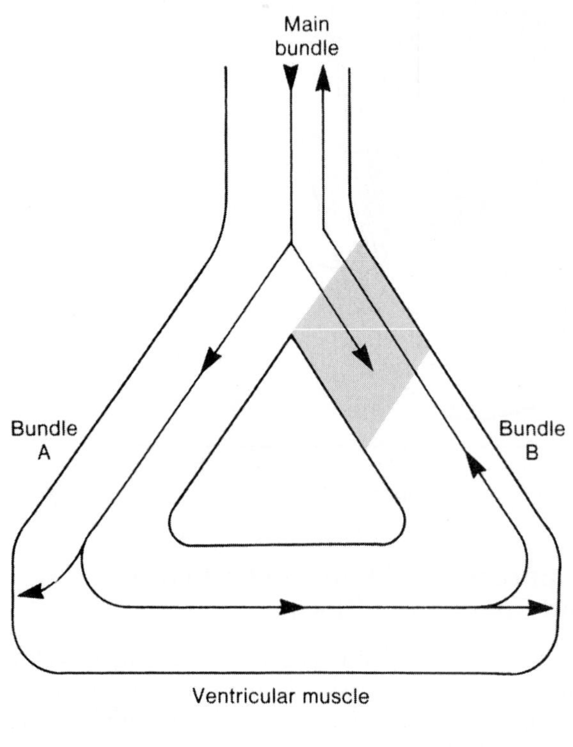

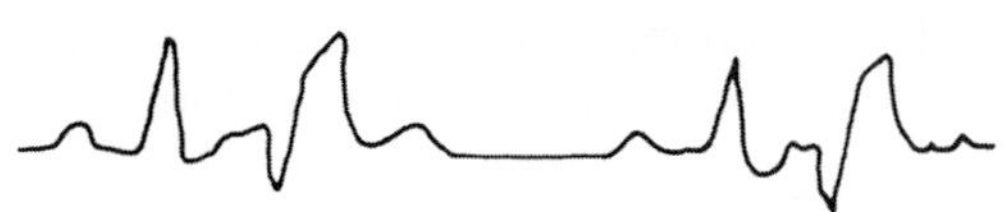

FIGURE 64.4. Sequence of activation of a loop of Purkinje fiber bundles and ventricular muscle during reentry. A region of unidirectional conduction block is indicated by the *dark shaded area* in branch B. Conduction cannot occur through this area in the antegrade direction (from B to ventricular muscle) but only in the retrograde direction (from ventricular muscle to B). Slow conduction is present in the loop. The **bottom** of the figure shows an electrocardiographic pattern that may result from this type of reentry. (From Wit AL, Rosen MR, Hoffman BF. Electrophysiology and pharmacology of cardiac arrhythmias. II: Relationship of normal and abnormal electrical activity of cardiac fibers to the genesis of arrhythmias. B: re-entry, section I. Am Heart J 1974;88:664, with permission.)

DIAGNOSIS OF ARRHYTHMIAS: GENERAL CONSIDERATIONS

History

Arrhythmias may cause a variety of symptoms, or they may be asymptomatic. Symptoms are principally caused by an appreciation of an irregular or rapid rhythm (palpitations) (3,4) or by a reduction in cardiac output (light-headedness, dizziness, presyncope, syncope). Other symptoms may include dyspnea, diaphoresis, chest pain, and anxiety. When taking a history from a patient with a suspected arrhythmia, it is important to define the onset, regularity, and duration of symptoms and whether any factors seem to trigger symptoms (e.g., drinking coffee, smoking, exercise, emotional stress, taking or forgetting to take medications).

It is important to determine whether there is a history or symptoms of an underlying disease that may be associated with arrhythmia (e.g., hypertension, heart failure, ischemic or valvular heart disease, thyrotoxicosis), because the prognosis and recommended treatment depend to a large extent on the nature and severity of underlying heart disease. Patients should be asked about a family history of arrhythmias or sudden death; the taking of stimulant drugs either illicitly (see Chapter 29) or as an attempt to lose weight (see Chapter 83) or to stay awake; and the taking of prescription drugs that can cause arrhythmias (digoxin, theophylline, diuretics, β-blockers, α-agonists, tricyclic antidepressants, and antihypertensives) or even of over-the-counter medicines that might be associated with torsade de pointes (see below for additional discussion).

Palpitations are heartbeats that are sensed, usually because the beats are fast or irregular. However, they do not necessarily imply a significant arrhythmia, and they may represent only sinus tachycardia in an otherwise healthy person (3). In contrast, patients with paroxysmal supraventricular arrhythmias may be misdiagnosed as having a panic disorder (see Chapter 22) (5). Clinical descriptors of palpitations that are predictive of an arrhythmia include "heart fluttering," "heart stopping," and "irregular heartbeat" (1,3). Palpitations often are localized to the area of the apex beat, but paroxysmal supraventricular tachycardias (PSVTs) are commonly sensed in the side of the neck or under the upper sternum. Some people primarily sense the compensatory pause after an extra heartbeat, whereas others sense the extra beat itself. Usually the contraction after an extra beat is more powerful than a normal beat (i.e., postextrasystolic potentiation), and this

less often, and, when they do, nausea and vomiting are more common than diarrhea. Fever and chills or granulocytopenia occurs occasionally.

Within 3 months, 50% of people taking procainamide develop antinuclear antibodies (ANAs), and 90% do so within 12 months (25). From 20% to 30% of patients with ANAs develop a lupus-like syndrome characterized by serositis (pleuritis, pericarditis, synovitis), fever, and hepatomegaly. Unlike classic systemic lupus erythematosus, vasculitis is not a manifestation of drug-induced lupus, so renal disease, for example, does not occur. Most important, the syndrome often abates, usually within days, when the drug is discontinued (ANAs may persist for months). The major threat of the syndrome is hemorrhagic pericarditis, and one must watch for signs and symptoms of pericardial tamponade. For these reasons, procainamide is not recommended for long-term use.

Disopyramide

Disopyramide has direct membrane effects very much like those of quinidine. Like quinidine, disopyramide blocks parasympathetic activity. It is approved by the United States Food and Drug Administration (FDA) for the treatment of specific ventricular arrhythmias: unifocal or multifocal PVCs and VT. Like quinidine and procainamide, disopyramide is not often used in ambulatory practice for treatment of patients with supraventricular or ventricular arrhythmias. One useful niche for this drug is in the treatment of the small subset of patients with vagally mediated atrial fibrillation. Perhaps the most common use of disopyramide today is in the treatment of patients with vasodepressor syncope (see Chapter 89). The effectiveness of disopyramide in the treatment of this condition is related to its vagolytic and negative inotropic effects. Disopyramide has also proved useful in the treatment of hypertrophic cardiomyopathy because of its negative inotropic effects.

The noncardiac toxicity of disopyramide results mainly from its anticholinergic effects, which include dry mouth, blurred vision, urinary hesitancy, and constipation. For these reasons, disopyramide generally is not advised for elderly patients. Nausea, vomiting, and diarrhea are less common than after administration of quinidine or procainamide. The cardiac toxicity of the drug is somewhat similar to that of quinidine in that it can prolong the QT interval and produce torsade de pointes (see later discussion). Disopyramide may cause or intensify heart failure or cause hypotension in patients who have compromised LV function, so it should not be administered to patients with these conditions.

Class IB Drugs

Class IB drugs shorten repolarization and the QT interval and have little effect on the duration of the QRS complex. They are generally not effective for supraventricular arrhythmias. Mexiletine is the principal drug of this class in the United States. This drug has electrophysiologic effects similar to those of lidocaine. Adverse effects include nausea, tremulousness, dizziness, and anxiety. It may be useful in combination with a class IA or III drug (see later discussion), but consultation with a cardiologist is advisable before the drug is prescribed.

Class IC Drugs

Class IC drugs slow conduction and widen the QRS complex but cause only small changes in refractoriness or the QT interval. Flecainide and propafenone, the class IC drugs currently available, both are effective against serious ventricular arrhythmias and may be particularly useful in the treatment of supraventricular arrhythmias, especially atrial fibrillation. Because flecainide has been shown to be associated with an elevated risk of sudden death when used in patients with ventricular dysfunction after MI (19), it should generally not be used in patients with ischemic heart disease, particularly if EF <40%. Common noncardiac side effects are nausea and epigastric pain. These side effects are controlled largely by dosing with meals to reduce peak drug levels. Class IC drugs should be used with caution in patients with a history of atrial flutter, because the anticholinergic effects of these drugs may increase AV conduction and result in 1:1 conduction of atrial flutter at a heart rate of 250 to 300 bpm. These drugs should be used only in consultation with a cardiologist.

Class II Drugs (β-Adrenergic Blocking Agents)

These drugs block the effects of catecholamines (which may potentiate the development of arrhythmias) and slow conduction in the atria, AV node, and ventricular myocardium.

β-Blockers are used to slow the ventricular response in patients with atrial tachyarrhythmia; occasionally, in the process, they convert paroxysmal atrial tachycardia, atrial flutter, or atrial fibrillation to normal sinus rhythm. In addition, ventricular arrhythmias initiated by exercise or ischemia or associated with the congenital long QT syndrome may be prevented by the use of these drugs. Low dosages of a β-blocker (e.g., sustained-release metoprolol) may be effective in controlling heart rate in patients with atrial fibrillation or in maintaining normal sinus rhythm in patients who have been cardioverted. β-Blockers are the only antiarrhythmic medications that have been convincingly shown to reduce the incidence of sudden death after MI (22). Chapter 63 discusses in detail the use of beta blockers in this regard.

A range of *side effects* is associated with β-blocker use. Although they have proved useful in the management of chronic heart failure (see Chapter 66), β-blockers can precipitate heart failure if their dose is not appropriately titrated in patients with poor ventricular function. They are contraindicated in patients with asthma. Most β-blockers occasionally cause hair thinning; this effect appears to be reversible when the dosage is reduced or the drug is discontinued. Many young patients taking β-blockers for supraventricular arrhythmias develop fatigue, malaise, and other symptoms requiring drug discontinuation.

Table 64.3 lists the properties of the currently available β-blocking agents. Propranolol crosses the blood–brain barrier and may cause side effects such as depression and sleep disturbance, although the evidence supporting an association between β-blocker use and depression is not strong (26). Atenolol and metoprolol are long acting, do not cross the blood–brain barrier, and are cardioselective. Because it is largely cleared by renal excretion, atenolol should be dosed carefully in patients with renal insufficiency. The main advantage of the longer-acting agents or sustained-release preparations is the likelihood of better compliance.

Class III (Potassium Channel Blockers)

Sotalol

Sotalol is a racemic mixture of both a class II agent (i.e., a β-blocker, L-sotalol) and a class III agent (i.e., D-sotalol) (27). Although it has few extracardiac side effects, serious ventricular arrhythmias are seen in 3% to 5% of patients. Sotalol should be used with particular caution in patients with heart failure and should not be initiated on an ambulatory basis.

Sotalol, which previously carried an indication only for ventricular arrhythmias, has been repackaged as Betapace-AF and marketed specifically for control of atrial fibrillation in patients with or without structural heart disease. Because of the risk of torsade de pointes, however, a patient beginning sotalol should be monitored as an inpatient for at least several days.

Dofetilide

Dofetilide is approved by the FDA for treatment of atrial arrhythmias. It is used in ambulatory practice for the maintenance of sinus rhythm in patients who have been converted from atrial fibrillation. Initiation of dofetilide requires 72 hours of in-hospital monitoring and careful adjustment based on creatinine clearance and effect on the QT interval.

Amiodarone

Amiodarone is a potent drug that effectively suppresses both supraventricular and ventricular arrhythmias (18). It is unique among the antiarrhythmic drugs in that it has properties of all four classes. Especially at high dosages (>300 mg/day), amiodarone is associated with a number of troublesome side effects, including photosensitivity, hypothyroidism or hyperthyroidism, pulmonary interstitial fibrosis, hepatotoxicity, and a variety of neurologic abnormalities. However, use of the drug is not associated with a high risk of proarrhythmia, and a number of trials of amiodarone in patients with structural heart disease have shown no increased risk of cardiac death. Each 200-mg tablet of amiodarone contains 75 mg of iodine; the likelihood of thyroid dysfunction is high when the drug is taken chronically (28).

Amiodarone interacts with many other drugs. For example, it may potentiate the toxic effects of digoxin and β-blocking agents. It also interferes with the metabolism of warfarin and may markedly prolong the prothrombin time and international normalized ratio (INR) (18). Because of these problems, the risks and benefits of amiodarone must be considered on a patient-by-patient basis. Today amiodarone is one of the most commonly used drugs for treatment of atrial fibrillation (see later discussion). Amiodarone is frequently used in the treatment of patients with sustained ventricular arrhythmias. A cardiologist familiar with the drug should be closely involved in the patient's care. Because of the drug's long mean half-life (almost 2 months), the effects may persist for many weeks after amiodarone is discontinued.

Class IV Drugs (Calcium Channel Blockers)

Calcium channel blockers are effective and useful drugs for controlling supraventricular arrhythmias. Conduction through the AV node is dependent on calcium-mediated currents. By blocking these currents, calcium channel blockers may control the ventricular response in atrial fibrillation and may convert to sinus rhythm those supraventricular arrhythmias that depend on conduction through the AV node. Verapamil may be useful in an ambulatory setting for the conversion of paroxysmal atrioventricular nodal reentrant tachycardia (AVNRT) to sinus rhythm. Doses of 80 to 120 mg orally can be used safely in patients known to have AVNRT; conversion to sinus rhythm usually occurs in 30 to 60 minutes. Alternatively, a dose of 5 to 10 mg intravenously may convert AVNRT in minutes. If the drug is not effective, referral to a hospital emergency room should be considered. Oral verapamil at dosages of 240 to 360 mg/day can be used for prophylaxis against supraventricular arrhythmias. Verapamil also can be used at dosages of 240 to 360 mg/day for ventricular rate control in patients with atrial fibrillation. Diltiazem at dosages of 120 to 300 mg/day also may be effective. The dihydropyridine calcium channel blockers, such as nifedipine and amlodipine, are not useful for control of atrial arrhythmias, nor are calcium channel blockers in general effective for control of ventricular arrhythmias (an unusual exception is idiopathic VT arising from the left ventricle).

Calcium channel blockers such as verapamil and diltiazem, which may be useful in AVNRT, can cause a dangerous acceleration of heart rate in patients with WPW syndrome and atrial fibrillation. If supraventricular tachycardia degenerates to atrial fibrillation in patients with WPW syndrome who are treated with a calcium channel

TABLE 64.3 Characteristics of Currently Available β-Blockers

	Acebutolol (Sectral)	*Labetalol (Normodyne Trandate)*	*Atenolol (Tenormin)*	*Metoprolol (Lopressor)*	*Nadolol (Corgard)*	*Pindolol (Visken)*	*Propranolol (Inderal)*	*Timolol (Blocadren)*	*Carvedilol (Coreg)*[a]
β-Blocking plasma levels	0.2–2.0 μg/mL	0.7–3.0 μg/mL	200–500 ng/mL	50–100 ng/mL	50–100 ng/mL	50–100 ng/mL	50–100 ng/mL	5–10 ng/mL	—
Half-life (h)	3–4	5–6	6–9	3–4[b]	14–24	3–4	3.5–6[b]	4	7–10
Active metabolites	Yes	No	No	No	No	No	Yes	No	No
Predominant route of elimination	HM	HM	RE (mostly unchanged)	HM	RE	RE (40% unchanged) and HM	HM	RE (20% unchanged) and HM	HM (50%) higher plasma levels in elderly and in chronic renal failure)
Relative β_1 selectivity	+	0	+	+	0	0	0	0	0
Available strengths (mg)	200, 400	100, 200, 300	50, 100	50, 100; or 25, 50, 100, 200 XL	40, 80, 120, 160	5, 10	10, 20, 40, 60, 80; and 60, 80, 120, 180 mg long-acting	10	3.125, 6.25, 12.5, 25.0
Usual maintenance dosage	200–600 mg b.i.d.	100–600 mg b.i.d.	50–100 mg q.d.	50–100 mg b.i.d. or 50–200 mg XL q.d.	40–50 mg q.d.	5–20 mg t.i.d.	40–80 mg q.i.d. or 120–160 mg long-acting once per day	20 mg b.i.d.	25 b.i.d.

[a]Has significant α-blocking activity; orthostasis is commonly experienced.
[b]Long-acting preparation also available.
HM, hepatic metabolism; RE, renal excretion.
Modified from Frishman WH. β-Adrenoceptor antagonists: new drugs and new indications. N Engl J Med 1981;305:550, with permission.

blocker, the ventricular rate may suddenly accelerate to >300 bpm. For this reason, calcium channel blockers should generally not be used in patients with WPW syndrome, unless the accessory pathway has been proven to conduct poorly in the anterograde (atrium-to-ventricle) direction.

Verapamil is metabolized by the liver and should be used with caution in patients with impaired hepatic function. Both verapamil and diltiazem are available in extended-release formulations that can be taken once daily. Except perhaps for initial dosage titration, the once-daily formulations are preferred over the short-acting forms. Some elderly patients are very sensitive to diltiazem and require only low dosages of the drug.

The most common *side effects* of calcium channel blockers are headache, light-headedness, dizziness, hypotension, peripheral edema, and constipation. Both verapamil and diltiazem interfere with renal clearance of digoxin and may precipitate digitalis intoxication. All calcium channel blockers are myocardial depressants, and both verapamil and diltiazem may suppress the sinus node, decrease heart rate, and prolong the PR interval. Verapamil should be used with caution in patients with LV dilation and EF ≤40%, although diltiazem can be used with caution in such patients. There is concern that the use of short-acting calcium channel blockers (i.e., nifedipine, verapamil, diltiazem) may be associated with an increased risk of cardiovascular morbidity and mortality, but an increased risk does not appear to be present in patients using long-acting calcium channel blockers (29).

Pacemaker Therapy

Implantable electrical pulse generators (pacemakers) are the treatment of choice for patients with symptomatic bradyarrhythmias and heart block (30,31). The decision to implant a pacemaker and the type of unit to use must be determined in consultation with a cardiologist. In general, patients in atrial fibrillation who require a pacemaker (see later discussion) require ventricular demand pacemakers. Most patients in sinus rhythm are best served by a multiprogrammable AV sequential unit. The modest increases in cost and complexity of the AV sequential units appear to be more than offset by the improved long-term physiologic response of patients. Patients with heart failure, depressed LV systolic function, and interventricular conduction delay have recently been shown to benefit from biventricular pacing, even in the absence of a bradycardia indication (32,33). Pacemaker generators are <0.5 cm thick and may function for up to 10 years. Pacemaker leads are implanted via a percutaneous transvenous technique and rarely become dislodged, even during vigorous activity. Symptoms are relieved in most patients with bradyarrhythmias and conduction block (see later discussion).

Patient Experience. Pacemakers usually are implanted in cardiac catheterization laboratories with fixed fluoroscopy; some operators use surgical operating rooms with portable fluoroscopy. Pacemakers are implanted subcutaneously in the pectoral area with the patient under local anesthesia. The pacemaker lead is inserted via the cephalic vein or directly with the use of a special introducer into the axillary or subclavian vein and lodged in the apex of the right ventricle or in the right atrial appendage. Patients requiring biventricular pacing have a third, specially designed pacemaker lead inserted into a branch of the coronary sinus. The procedure takes approximately 60 to 120 minutes, depending on the number of leads inserted. The patient experiences some discomfort when the anesthetic is injected and, often, an unpleasant sensation when the tissues are manipulated to create a pocket for the pacemaker unit.

After the procedure, patients are discharged from the hospital the next day. Patients with sedentary jobs can return to work within 1 week after pacemaker insertion, but patients with more active jobs should not return to work for up to 4 to 6 weeks to allow the wound to heal completely. After that time, the patient experiences little or no discomfort. The unit feels like part of the chest wall, and no restrictions are placed on the patient's activity. Microwave ovens do not interfere with pacemaker functions, but cellular phones may do so if they are held directly over the pacemaker (34). Magnetic resonance imaging (MRI) currently is contraindicated in patients with permanent pacemakers, but investigation into the compatibility of newer pacemaker models with MRI is ongoing.

Patients with implanted pacemakers require regular long-term followup. The frequency of followup depends on the original indication for the pacemaker. Patients who require constant pacing should be seen more often (approximately every 3–6 months) than patients who require episodic pacing (approximately every 6–12 months). At these followup visits, pacemaker function must be assessed by 12-lead ECG and a computerized pacemaker analyzer, which measures pacemaker data including battery voltage and lead resistance. The pacemaker and its registration number should be entered into the patient's record, and the patient should keep the registration card for the pacemaker on his or her person in the event of device malfunction or an emergency intercurrent problem.

Implantable Cardioverter-Defibrillator Therapy

The implantable cardioverter-defibrillator (ICD) has had a major impact on the clinical approach to prevention of sudden cardiac death from ventricular arrhythmias (35). ICDs are implanted in the same way as are pacemakers, and specific devices can perform all pacemaker functions, including biventricular pacing. They are capable of detecting different forms of ventricular arrhythmias in different rate zones and of treating each with a different sequence of antitachycardia pacing (ATP) and shock therapies. They are capable of storing large amounts of information from each arrhythmia episode that can be retrieved by specialized computers for later analysis.

ICDs detect ventricular arrhythmias from the tip electrode of the lead, which usually is implanted at the right ventricular apex. When a ventricular rate exceeding the programmed detection rate for ventricular fibrillation (usually 150–200 bpm) for the programmed number of beats (usually 10–20) is detected, the ICD begins charging the capacitors. The charging period generally is between 1 and 5 seconds, after which the device confirms continuation of tachycardia before delivering the programmed energy (usually 10–35 J) between the metal shell of the generator and one or more coils on the ICD lead. The ventricular rate then is reanalyzed to determine whether therapy was successful. Further therapies are delivered if needed, up to a maximum of six to eight.

When first released for clinical use in the early 1980s, ICDs were targeted toward patients who had survived multiple cardiac arrests with recurrent ventricular arrhythmias that were refractory to conventional antiarrhythmic drug treatment. As the design of ICDs improved over the next decade and the limitations of antiarrhythmic drugs were exposed through randomized clinical trials, the ICD gained increasing favor for treatment of cardiac arrest survivors and other patients with unstable ventricular arrhythmias. In this setting, several clinical trials were organized to test the efficacy of the ICD in secondary prevention (for patients who had survived a sustained life-threatening ventricular arrhythmia) and primary prevention (for high-risk patients without a history of sustained arrhythmia) of sudden cardiac death.

The Antiarrhythmics Versus Implantable Defibrillators (AVID) trial, published in 1997, established the efficacy of the ICD for patients with prior cardiac arrest or symptomatic sustained VT (36). The Multicenter Automatic Defibrillator Implantation Trial (MADIT) (37) published in 1996 and the Multicenter Unsustained Tachycardia Trial (MUSTT) (38) published in 2000 showed that the ICD improved survival in MI survivors with depressed LV systolic function, nonsustained VT, and inducible sustained VT at electrophysiologic study. MADIT-II, published in 2002, extended the indication for primary prevention ICD therapy to all patients with prior MI and LVEF $\leq$30%, regardless of symptoms or arrhythmia history (39). Most recently, the Sudden Cardiac Death in Heart Failure (SCD-HeFT) investigators demonstrated a significant mortality reduction with primary prevention ICD therapy in patients with depressed LVEF ($\leq$35%) and New York Heart Association (NYHA) class II or III congestive heart failure regardless of etiology (40).

Patient Experience. ICDs are implanted similarly to pacemakers, usually with the patient under local anesthesia. The main differences are that a larger generator is implanted under the skin, and ICD function is tested with the patient under deep sedation. During the latter procedure, known as defibrillation threshold (DFT) testing or noninvasive programmed stimulation (NIPS), VT and/or ventricular fibrillation is induced and then terminated by the device using programmed therapies. External defibrillation is immediately available if the ICD therapy is not successful.

Cardioversion

Electrical conversion of atrial tachyarrhythmias is performed by the application of a short burst of direct current to the chest wall. The shock is synchronized with the QRS complex of the ECG to avoid shock application during the vulnerable period of the cardiac cycle, when VT or ventricular fibrillation might be induced.

Cardioversion is a more reliable technique for conversion of tachyarrhythmias than is administration of antiarrhythmic drugs. It may be required on an emergency basis if a patient has developed severe heart failure, hypotension, or ischemia as a result of an arrhythmia. Otherwise, the procedure should be planned in consultation with a cardiologist. A number of factors must be considered when deciding whether elective cardioversion is appropriate for a patient with atrial fibrillation (41) (see later discussion).

The most cost-effective strategy, in terms of quality-adjusted life years, is to attempt cardioversion before initiation of antiarrhythmic therapy. Typically, patients are anticoagulated for at least 3 weeks before elective cardioversion and for 4 weeks afterward. However, clinical trials have shown that if transesophageal echocardiography (TEE) does not reveal an atrial thrombus, cardioversion may be done without prior anticoagulation (42). (The need for anticoagulation for at least 4 weeks after cardioversion, however, is not obviated.) If atrial fibrillation recurs soon after cardioversion, an antiarrhythmic agent can be started and cardioversion can be repeated (43).

Patient Experience. Cardioversion is performed by a cardiologist in a hospital, either with an anesthesiologist or a nurse experienced in administering conscious sedation, and with resuscitation equipment available. The patient is sedated, usually with intravenous midazolam given to effect. Normally the patient cannot recall afterward any experience of the procedure. For atrial fibrillation, cardioversion is attempted at 200 J; if that attempt is unsuccessful, the energy level is increased and other shocks are administered until conversion occurs or until a level of 360 J is reached. If an initial attempt using anteroposterior patch placement fails, another attempt at cardioversion can be undertaken using an apex–base paddle position. If available, a biphasic defibrillator should be used because of the higher conversion rates with this device. If external cardioversion is unsuccessful, shock delivery through an intracardiac electrode (referred to as *internal cardioversion)* may be successful. Administration of ibutilide, an intravenous class III antiarrhythmic agent, immediately before cardioversion also can lower the amount of energy required for cardioversion (44,45). With the recent availability of biphasic waveforms, this approach is rarely required. Complications, such as embolism or a new arrhythmia, are unusual; however, even with optimal anticoagulation, patients should be aware of a small (0.5%) risk of periprocedural stroke. After cardioversion, the patient is observed for several hours while rhythm is monitored. If the rhythm is stable, then the patient is discharged.

Invasive Electrophysiologic Study

Several categories of patients should be referred for electrophysiologic study; most of these patients already are under the care of a cardiologist. They include patients with a sustained wide-complex tachycardia and those who have survived an episode of sudden cardiac death; patients with nonsustained VT (particularly in the setting of a prior MI) who are thought to be at increased risk for sudden cardiac death; patients with syncope of unknown origin in the setting of structural heart disease; and patients who are considered candidates for a curative catheter ablation procedure for treatment of any of a large variety of supraventricular arrhythmias (including WPW syndrome and PSVT, see below), atrial flutter, atrial tachycardia, atrial fibrillation), and some types of ventricular arrhythmias (frequent PVCs or sustained VT). Although empiric antiarrhythmic drug treatment is appropriate for many patients with PSVT, catheter ablation is also considered appropriate first-line therapy (46,47). Catheter ablation has been shown to be a more cost-effective approach compared with lifelong drug therapy, and it has a much higher success rate in keeping patients free of arrhythmia (48,49).

Patient Experience. The patient's experience during electrophysiologic study is similar in some respects to that during cardiac catheterization (see Chapter 62) in that the patient must lie flat on a table in the cardiac catheterization laboratory. Patients typically receive moderate sedation with midazolam. Catheters usually are advanced, under fluoroscopy, through the femoral vein rather than through the artery, as is done during coronary angiography. The procedure takes longer than does coronary angiography; the average diagnostic procedure takes approximately 1 hour, whereas a radiofrequency catheter ablation procedure can take up to 3 to 5 hours. In a typical diagnostic procedure, intracardiac electrical activity is recorded and the heart is stimulated (either pharmacologically or electrically through a catheter) in an attempt to induce the clinical arrhythmia. If a significant arrhythmia is induced and does not resolve spontaneously, antiarrhythmic drugs or electrical cardioversion is used to restore the patient's intrinsic rhythm. The risks of a diagnostic electrophysiologic study in experienced hands are low and comparable to the risk of diagnostic coronary angiography. The risks associated with catheter ablation vary based on the target arrhythmia. There is a small risk that a permanent pacemaker will be required because of induction of complete heart block during an ablation procedure in no more than 1% of patients (46). The risk of major morbidity (e.g., stroke, MI, significant valve damage) or mortality is generally approximately 0.1%.

SPECIFIC ARRHYTHMIAS

Sinus Tachycardia

Definition and Causes

In adults, the normal resting sinus rate is 50 to 100 bpm. Sinus tachycardia, a sinus rhythm at a rate >100 bpm, usually is a physiologic rhythm in that the rate is ordinarily appropriate to the physiologic state of the patient, a state that requires increased cardiac output to meet increased metabolic demands. The maximal sinus heart rate that can be attained varies with age but usually does not exceed 140 bpm unless demands are excessive (e.g., vigorous exercise). The common factors that stimulate an increase in the rate of sinus rhythm, other than exercise, are fever, emotional stress, intravascular volume depletion, heart failure, hypoxia, and a variety of drugs that affect the autonomic nervous system, including caffeine, aminophylline, amphetamine, alcohol, antidepressants, phenothiazines, and calcium channel blockers of the dihydropyridine class (e.g., nifedipine).

Physical Findings

A regular rapid pulse and heart rate are detected, although there may be a slight variation in rate, called *sinus arrhythmia.* S_1 is normal, and the jugular venous pulsations are normal.

Electrocardiogram

A P wave precedes each QRS complex; the PR interval is normal for the rate (0.16–0.17 second at rates >130 per minute), and the P-wave vector is normal (upright P waves in II, III, and aVF).

Treatment

In most cases, persistent sinus tachycardia need not be treated; it is the underlying condition that requires therapy. In particular, digitalis should not be used to treat a patient with sinus tachycardia unless there is associated heart failure.

In the occasional patient with an unexplained sinus tachycardia for whom a thorough evaluation fails to reveal an underlying cause and in whom tachycardia is symptomatic, use of small dosages of a β-blocker may be justified. Low-dose β-blockers also may be helpful in treating the anxiety and tachycardia associated with anticipated stressful situations.

Sinus Bradycardia

Definition and Causes

Sinus bradycardia is a heart rate <50 bpm (50). Impulse generation in the sinus node often is slow in aerobically well conditioned people (e.g., long-distance runners, heavy laborers) because of high vagal tone. In fact, trained athletes may have asymptomatic sinus bradycardia with resting heart rates as low as 40 bpm. Inappropriately low sinus rates are also commonly caused by increased vagal tone, as is seen in association with pain, vomiting, or vasovagal syncope. A hypersensitive carotid sinus, more common in elderly people, may result in marked bradycardia when the sinus is compressed by a tight collar or by the patient's tensing his or her neck. Parasympathomimetic drugs such as neostigmine, tranquilizers, phenothiazines, digitalis, and sympatholytic drugs such as methyldopa, clonidine, and all β-blockers also may produce sinus bradycardia. Vagally induced bradycardia may be severe and result in asystole (and loss of consciousness) when the stimulus is marked or prolonged or occurs in a hypoxic patient.

Physical Findings

A regular slow pulse and heart rate are detected. S_1 is normal, and the jugular venous pulsations are normal.

Electrocardiogram

A P wave precedes each QRS complex; the PR interval is normal for the rate (up to 0.20–0.21 second), and the P-wave vector is normal (upright P waves in II, III, and aVF).

Treatment

Asymptomatic sinus bradycardia discovered as an incidental finding does not require treatment. If there are no ECG signs of conduction block and structural heart disease is not present, resting heart rates as low as 40 bpm may be well tolerated. However, patients who present with symptoms of light-headedness or syncope and are found to have sinus bradycardia may have underlying sinus node disease or may be subject to paroxysms of tachycardia and bradycardia, the so-called *sick sinus syndrome* (see Sick Sinus Syndrome). Patients with sinus bradycardia and symptoms should be evaluated with an ambulatory ECG to determine whether they have this condition. In any case, patients with symptomatic sinus bradycardia not caused by a drug are best treated with permanent pacemaker implantation.

Sick Sinus Syndrome

Definition and Causes

The term *sick sinus syndrome* refers to a heterogeneous group of arrhythmias involving defective impulse generation by the sinus node or abnormal impulse conduction in the atria and AV node (51). The syndrome is characterized by periods of inappropriate sinus bradycardia (often severe, with rates between 25 and 40 bpm), which may precede or follow supraventricular tachyarrhythmias, and by varying degrees of SA block, sometimes including sinus arrest. The rubrics *bradycardia–tachycardia syndrome* and *tachycardia–bradycardia syndrome* are sometimes used, depending on whether bradycardia precedes or follows a tachyarrhythmia (usually atrial fibrillation), respectively.

The sick sinus syndrome is caused by degenerative fibrotic changes within the sinus node. It often is associated with similar abnormalities in other parts of the cardiac conduction system that result in varying degrees of AV and intraventricular block. These pathologic changes are much more common in patients older than 60 years. Although their precise cause is unknown, they are often associated with hypertensive or ischemic heart disease.

Symptoms and Signs

Many patients are asymptomatic. When symptoms do occur, they are produced either by spontaneous sinus arrest or by the tachyarrhythmia itself (palpitations). If LV dysfunction or coronary artery disease is coexistent, symptoms of heart failure or ischemia may occur as a result of reduced cardiac output or increased cardiac demand.

The results of physical examination often are normal unless the patient is examined during an episode of bradyarrhythmia or tachyarrhythmia, in which case the findings depend on the type of arrhythmia present (see later discussion). Sometimes light carotid sinus massage produces symptomatic bradyarrhythmia in a patient with sick sinus syndrome who is in normal sinus rhythm.

Electrocardiogram

The ECG may be normal or may simply reveal sinus bradycardia. Often, there are varying degrees of SA block, characterized by varying P–P intervals on the ECG. Sometimes sinus arrest occurs, manifested by absent P waves and usually associated with a junctional escape rhythm. Some patients have atrial fibrillation with a slow ventricular response, reflecting a concomitant AV conduction abnormality (see earlier discussion). The ECG changes of the various atrial tachyarrhythmias are described in the discussions of these entities.

If the patient has a history of unexplained syncope or palpitations and the resting ECG is normal, ambulatory

ECG monitoring is indicated (see Diagnosis of Arrhythmias).

Treatment and Course

The treatment of choice for patients with the sick sinus syndrome who are symptomatic from bradyarrhythmias is permanent pacemaker implantation (see Pacemaker Therapy). Otherwise, symptoms are often progressive. Patients with minor symptoms (e.g., light-headedness, dizziness) often feel significantly better after pacemaker therapy.

Tachyarrhythmias associated with the syndrome generally are not prevented by cardiac pacing. However, pacing does allow the use of drugs such as digitalis, calcium channel blockers, amiodarone, and β-blockers that depress the sinus node and increase the likelihood of sinus arrest or asystole. After a pacemaker is implanted, it is reasonable to administer metoprolol 25 mg twice per day and to increase the dosage to 50 mg or 100 mg twice per day in an attempt to prevent tachyarrhythmias. If the β-blocker is not effective, diltiazem or verapamil may be administered in low doses as well, unless the patient has a depressed EF. If tachyarrhythmias continue, then consideration in conjunction with the consulting cardiologist should be given to the use of another antiarrhythmic drug, catheter ablation of the tachyarrhythmia, or ablation of the AV node.

Patients with sick sinus syndrome and atrial fibrillation have an incidence, unaffected by pacemaker therapy, of arterial embolization of approximately 5% to 10% per year. These patients should be anticoagulated with warfarin. The sick sinus syndrome is not itself associated with increased mortality. Life expectancy in these patients is a function of the patient's age and comorbid conditions (51). Patients with chronic atrial fibrillation as a manifestation of sick sinus syndrome should be treated with warfarin (discussed later) or with aspirin if the patient cannot, or will not, take warfarin. Warfarin may generally be restarted within 1 to 2 days after implantation of a permanent pacemaker.

Premature Atrial and Junctional Contractions

Definition and Causes

Premature atrial contractions (PACs) and premature junctional contractions (PJCs) are commonly seen in patients who are otherwise well. They often are induced by the same stimuli that produce sinus tachycardia, especially caffeine or nicotine. However, in patients with congestive heart failure or chronic pulmonary disease, PACs or PJCs may progress to atrial fibrillation or flutter.

Symptoms and Signs

Usually patients are unaware of PACs or PJCs; occasionally they note the PAC or PJC as a palpitation. The clinician, on listening to the heart or palpating the arterial pulse, is aware of a slight irregularity in the cardiac rhythm.

Electrocardiogram

PACs are reflected on the ECG by a premature, morphologically abnormal P wave followed by a premature, morphologically normal QRS complex. Sometimes these impulses are not conducted (Fig. 64.5), in which case, if the P wave is buried in the preceding T wave, a false diagnosis of sinus arrest may be made. At other times the premature impulse is aberrantly conducted, the result of refractoriness of one of the bundle branches (usually a right bundle-branch pattern is seen after the premature atrial beat).

PJCs are reflected on the ECG by a retrograde P wave (negatively deflected in leads II, III, and aVF) that may follow, be hidden in, or precede a morphologically normal but premature QRS complex.

Treatment

Patients with PACs or PJCs who are otherwise well do not require treatment. Rarely, a β-blocker or another antiarrhythmic agent, such as sotalol, flecainide, or amiodarone, is prescribed to reduce the frequency of PACs in patients

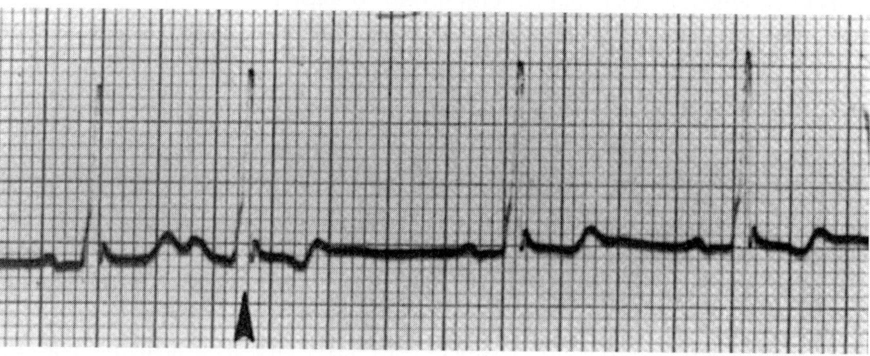

FIGURE 64.5. Premature atrial contraction (*arrowhead*). Note the normal configuration of the premature QRS complex.

who have annoyingly frequent palpitations. Quinidine or procainamide is effective for controlling PACs, but the risk associated with the use of these drugs usually is not warranted (see earlier discussion).

Paroxysmal Supraventricular Tachycardia

Definition and Causes

The term *paroxysmal supraventricular tachycardia* (PSVT) refers to a group of supraventricular arrhythmias that start and terminate abruptly and generally result from reentry (47,52). The most common cause of PSVT is *AVNRT,* which accounts for two thirds of all cases of PSVT (53). AVNRT occurs in the setting of two functionally distinct conduction pathways in the region of the AV node (called the *fast* and *slow pathways).* The second most common cause of PSVT is an accessory pathway-mediated tachycardia called *orthodromic AV reciprocating tachycardia.* This type of tachycardia, which accounts for approximately one third of all cases of PSVT, results when the electrical impulse travels from the atria to the ventricles via the AV node and returns to the atria via an accessory pathway that connects the atrium and ventricle. The third, and least common, cause of PSVT is an *ectopic atrial tachycardia* that is confined to the atrium. This type accounts for <5% of all cases.

The heart rate during episodes of PSVT may vary from 130 to 250 bpm. In general, PSVT involving an accessory pathway tends to be more rapid, and PSVT caused by an atrial tachycardia tends to be slower. However, because of a large degree of overlap, the rate of the tachycardia usually is not helpful in establishing a diagnosis.

Nonparoxysmal atrial tachycardia with block (caused by gradually accelerated automaticity of an ectopic atrial focus) as a manifestation of digitalis toxicity is now rarely seen. If nonparoxysmal atrial tachycardia occurs in association with an AV conduction abnormality (commonly 2:1 block) and the patient is taking digitalis, the drug should be withheld and the serum potassium concentration measured. If the patient is hypokalemic, potassium repletion is in order; usually this can be accomplished by administration of oral potassium salts (i.e., 20 mEq three times per day; see Chapter 50). Patients with refractory arrhythmias with block caused by digitalis toxicity should be hospitalized for more aggressive treatment.

Symptoms and Signs

PSVT usually is suspected or diagnosed based on a careful history. The most important features of PSVT are its abrupt onset and termination and its sustained rapid and regular rate. Patients may complain of dyspnea, diaphoresis, lightheadedness, presyncope, or chest pain. Often the patient is able to terminate the arrhythmia abruptly by performing actions that increase vagal stimulation of the heart, such as a Valsalva maneuver, coughing, or placing a cold wet towel over the face (diving reflex). Occasionally, polyuria is experienced for as long as the arrhythmia lasts; this may be due to atrial dilation and release of atrial natriuretic peptide (54).

Attacks often occur spontaneously but may be precipitated by physical or emotional stress, caffeine, or nicotine. The attacks may be as short as a few seconds or as long as several weeks. The frequency of the attacks is variable: Some people have attacks every day, whereas others have only a few attacks during their lifetime.

On examination, a rapid, regular arterial pulse and heart rate are noted, often faster than those measured in patients with sinus tachycardia and usually not associated with the same stimuli. When the atria and ventricles contract simultaneously, cannon waves are seen in the jugular veins.

Electrocardiogram

PSVT is characterized by a rapid, regular heart rate. There is a fixed relationship of the P wave to the QRS complex. If the impulse is generated in the AV node (as in AVNRT), the P wave may be buried in the QRS complex, but the process can be identified by the normal appearance of the QRS complex and the regularity of the rate. When the P wave is visible, it may follow the QRS complex (in some nodal reentry rhythms and most accessory pathway reentry rhythms). It may also precede the QRS complex and may appear morphologically normal (atrial reentry or ectopic rhythm), in which case the diagnosis can be made (by ECG) only if the rate is sufficiently high to make sinus tachycardia unlikely. The P wave also may be hidden in the T wave, but again the regularity of the rate and the usually normal duration of the QRS complex establish the diagnosis (6,53).

If the ECG recorded from a patient with PSVT demonstrates various degrees of AV block (Fig. 64.6), the most likely cause of the arrhythmia is an atrial tachycardia. The presence of an accessory pathway-mediated tachycardia can be completely eliminated, and the possibility of AVNRT is very unlikely.

Treatment and Course

Therapy for PSVT always starts with attempts to increase vagal tone. As mentioned earlier, the patient often has learned to do this. If the arrhythmia persists despite the patient's efforts, carotid sinus massage should be applied. This must be done after auscultation of the carotid arteries to ensure that there are no bruits; if there are, carotid

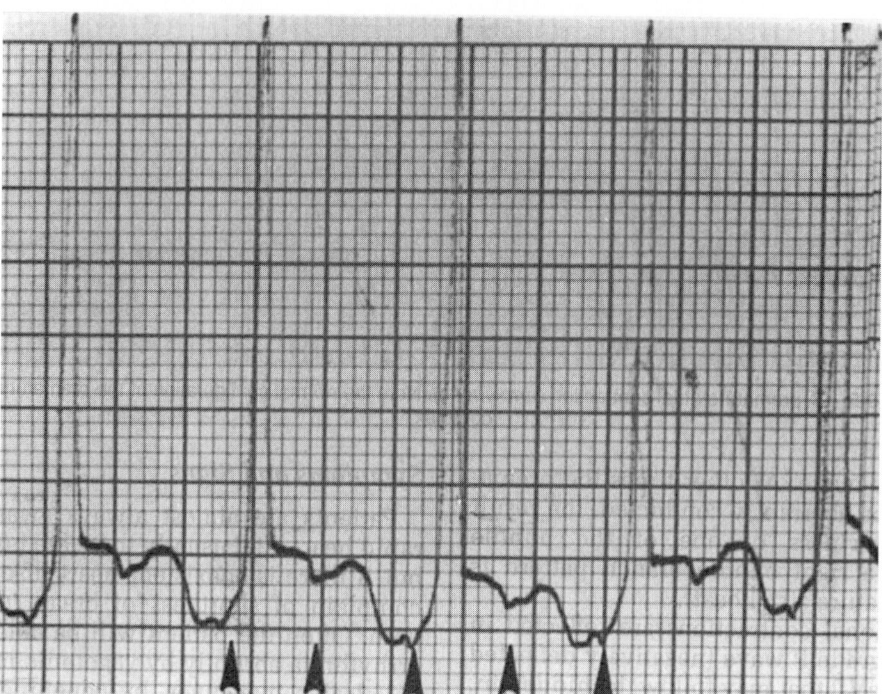

FIGURE 64.6. Supraventricular tachycardia with 2:1 AV block. *Arrowheads* point to consecutive P waves.

sinus massage is contraindicated. The carotid sinus is located at the point of maximal impulse of the carotid artery in the neck. The right sinus should be massaged first for up to 20 seconds; if that has no effect, the left sinus should be massaged. The two sinuses should never be massaged simultaneously. During massage, the patient's ECG should be monitored continuously, and resuscitation equipment should be available.

If carotid sinus massage fails, pharmacologic therapy is indicated. This is best done in an emergency room or a similar facility and always with continuous ECG monitoring. The drug of choice is adenosine (which slows conduction through the AV node), 6 to 18 mg, because the effect of the drug dissipates only 10 to 15 seconds after intravenous administration. Adenosine usually converts the arrhythmia to normal sinus rhythm within 5 to 10 seconds. It is critical that adenosine be administered as a bolus into a rapidly flowing intravenous line. This is best accomplished by using a stopcock and immediately flushing the line with 10 mL of saline after adenosine injection. If PSVT persists after adenosine administration, electrical cardioversion should be considered. Administration of intravenous adenosine should be performed only in a setting where emergency defibrillation can be performed. Alternatives to adenosine include verapamil (80–120 mg orally or 5–10 mg intravenously), diltiazem (60–120 mg orally) (discussed earlier), or metoprolol (25–50 mg orally or 5–10 mg intravenously). As noted previously, calcium channel blockers may increase conduction in the accessory pathway in patients with WPW syndrome. Therefore, calcium channel blockers should not be used to treat PSVT in patients who are known to have an accessory pathway, in order to avoid dangerous acceleration of the ventricular rate if PSVT degenerates to atrial fibrillation.

PSVT can be prevented or the number of episodes reduced by a variety of antiarrhythmic agents. If an initial episode of PSVT terminates spontaneously and is associated with mild symptoms, it would be reasonable to instruct the patient about techniques to terminate the arrhythmia and to delay initiation of antiarrhythmic therapy. On the other hand, if the patient has had multiple episodes of tachycardia, has required emergency room evaluation for termination of tachycardia, or has symptoms of hemodynamic compromise, chronic antiarrhythmic therapy or radiofrequency catheter ablation is indicated.

Digoxin may be used to treat PSVT and perhaps is the most convenient, best tolerated, and least expensive, but it also is the least effective medication for this purpose. β-Blockers and calcium channel blockers are somewhat more effective, are more expensive, and, when given at once-a-day dosing, are equally convenient. On the other end of the spectrum are class IC antiarrhythmic agents such as propafenone and flecainide, which are effective but even more expensive and less convenient. Although amiodarone can be used to treat patients with PSVT, this drug is rarely prescribed because of the benign nature of this arrhythmia, the potential for serious side effects of the drug (see earlier discussion), and the alternative of radiofrequency catheter ablation.

Radiofrequency catheter ablation (described earlier) has evolved from an experimental technique to the preferred therapy for treatment of patients with symptomatic

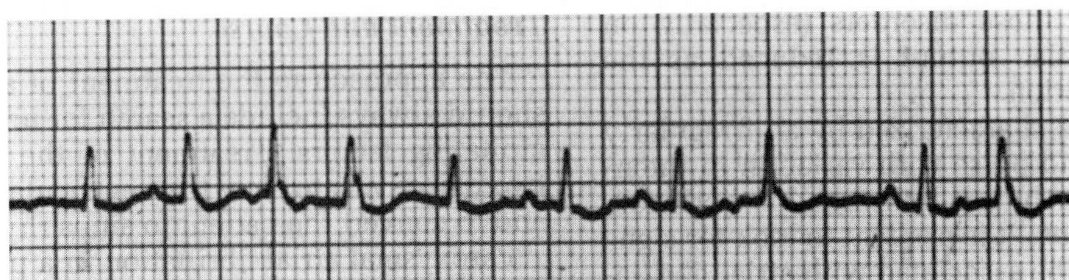

FIGURE 64.7. Multifocal atrial tachycardia. Note the variation in the morphology of the P waves and the duration of the PR intervals.

or frequently recurrent PSVT (47,55). Success rates are >95%, complications are rare (<1%), and the procedure is well tolerated. For this reason, patients with PSVT should be informed about the existence of a curative catheter-based procedure that can be considered as an alternative to lifelong antiarrhythmic therapy or that can be used if antiarrhythmic therapy fails. Electrophysiologic testing and radiofrequency catheter ablation should be recommended as first-line therapy if PSVT occurs in the setting of WPW syndrome (see later discussion). Because of the potentially life-threatening nature of WPW syndrome, these patients should be referred for electrophysiologic testing and radiofrequency catheter ablation (46). Similarly, if a patient with PSVT has symptoms of severe hemodynamic compromise (i.e., syncope), electrophysiologic testing and radiofrequency catheter ablation should be considered early in management.

Although PSVT is generally a benign arrhythmia, it rarely disappears without treatment. Once a patient has had one episode of PSVT, other episodes probably will occur. The frequency of episodes of PSVT increases over time in most patients. In contrast to this generally benign course, the prognosis of patients with PSVT who have WPW syndrome, severe structural heart disease, or symptoms of hemodynamic compromise is not as favorable. For this reason, more aggressive approaches to treatment are used early in these settings.

Multifocal Atrial Tachycardia

Multifocal atrial tachycardia is a chaotic supraventricular arrhythmia characterized on ECG by varying morphology of the P waves, varying PR intervals, and a rapid heart rate, usually 100 to 200 bpm; QRS morphology is normal, and every QRS complex is preceded by a P wave (Fig. 64.7) (56). The arrhythmia usually is seen in patients with serious underlying disease, especially decompensated chronic obstructive pulmonary disease, and is better treated by, for example, improving ventilatory function than by attempting directly to suppress the rhythm. Digitalis does not alter this arrhythmia (which usually is well tolerated) and therefore should not be administered. Either verapamil or diltiazem can be used to control the heart rate in patients with multifocal atrial tachycardia. Oral dosages of verapamil 40 to 80 mg three to four times per day or diltiazem 30 to 60 mg three to four times per day should be tried. If they are effective, a sustained-release preparation of verapamil or diltiazem at the same total daily dosage can be used. Magnesium was effective treatment in one small study (57).

Atrial Fibrillation

Definition and Causes

Atrial fibrillation is defined electrophysiologically as the generation of multiple reentrant wavefronts by the atria. It usually is initiated by one or more PACs (see earlier discussion) that trigger the development of these wavefronts and result in an atrial rate >300 bpm. These impulses enter the AV node randomly. Because of the unique conduction properties of the AV node, including slow conduction and decremental conduction, only a small proportion of the impulses are conducted to the ventricle. This results in a slower (typically 100–180 bpm) and an irregularly irregular ventricular rate.

Atrial fibrillation is classified as *paroxysmal* (starts and stops on its own within 48 hours), *persistent* (continues until/unless converted by drugs, cardioversion, or ablation), or *permanent* (persistent and attempts at conversion either unsuccessful or believed to be futile or medically unnecessary) (58). Studies have shown that *paroxysmal atrial fibrillation* usually is initiated by triggering PACs or bursts of atrial tachycardia arising in the pulmonary veins (59). The causes of *persistent* and *permanent atrial fibrillation* are less clear, but the posterior left atrium and pulmonary veins appear to be important for initiation and/or maintenance of the arrhythmia in a significant percentage of patients.

The prevalence of atrial fibrillation increases with age and with the development of structural heart disease (60). When atrial fibrillation occurs in the absence of any evidence of structural heart disease in patients younger than 50 years, it is called *lone atrial fibrillation.* In some patients, factors that trigger episodes of atrial fibrillation can be identified (e.g., physical or emotional stress, alcohol, nicotine, caffeine). The major noncardiac illness associated with atrial fibrillation is hyperthyroidism. The presence of a fast ventricular response refractory to drugs given to slow the ventricular rate may be a clue to the diagnosis (61).

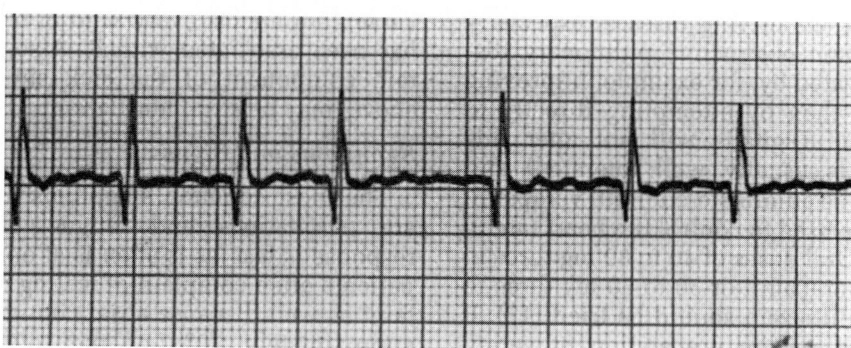

FIGURE 64.8. Atrial fibrillation. The ventricular rate is 90 to 100 bpm, indicative (because digitalis had not been administered) of an associated disorder of atrioventricular conduction.

Hypertensive and rheumatic heart disease (especially if it involves the mitral valve) predisposes to the development of atrial fibrillation, but almost every kind of myocardial disorder has been associated with it. In addition, the tachyarrhythmic component of the sick sinus syndrome (see earlier discussion) usually is atrial fibrillation.

Symptoms and Signs

Atrial fibrillation can be asymptomatic. The most common symptoms of atrial fibrillation are palpitations and fatigue. If the ventricular response is fast, patients often complain of feeling disoriented, light-headed, weak, or faint, especially if they are elderly. Because atrial contraction normally provides approximately 20% of the total cardiac output, patients with incipient heart failure, ischemic heart disease, or valvular heart disease may develop symptoms and signs of those disorders (especially on exertion) when cardiac output is reduced as the result of atrial fibrillation.

Atrial fibrillation is characterized by an irregularly irregular heartbeat and pulse, with variation in intensity of the sounds (including murmurs) on both auscultation and palpation. It is prudent to look for signs of diseases known to be associated with atrial fibrillation (coronary heart disease, heart failure, hypertension, mitral stenosis or regurgitation, and hyperthyroidism), especially because those signs may be subtle or may be altered by the arrhythmia.

Electrocardiogram

The ECG shows rapid irregular fibrillatory atrial activity at rates of 300 to 500 per minute; no P waves are present. The ventricular rhythm is irregularly irregular, at rates that at onset usually are 120 to 180 per minute, unless AV node disease is coexistent or the patient is taking a medication that slows AV conduction, in which case slower rates are likely (Fig. 64.8).

The QRS complex usually is morphologically normal. Occasionally there is aberrant conduction of an impulse in the ventricles, after a beat that has been preceded by a long pause. The aberrant beat usually has a right bundle-branch block (RBBB) configuration. This so-called *Ashman phenomenon* is caused by prolonged refractoriness of (usually) the right bundle branch after the long pause. These aberrant beats must be distinguished from ventricular premature beats (VPBs). Apart from their typical relationship to a preceding long R–R interval, aberrant beats often are triphasic (RSR′) in lead V_1, and their initial vector is the same as that of the normally conducted beats. Neither of these features is characteristic of VPBs.

Other Studies

In addition to ECG and chest x-ray film, all patients presenting for the first time with atrial fibrillation should undergo thyroid function studies and a two-dimensional echocardiogram. Unusual causes of atrial fibrillation, such as atrial myxoma or chronic pericardial effusion, may require echocardiography for diagnosis.

Treatment and Course

The approach to treatment of atrial fibrillation should always include a search for underlying or precipitating factors. Treatment of the arrhythmia has two objectives: to slow the ventricular rate if it is fast and to convert the rhythm to sinus rhythm if symptoms are present.

Paroxysmal atrial fibrillation in a patient who does not have underlying heart disease often reverts to normal sinus rhythm once precipitating factors (e.g., fever, stress, alcohol, nicotine) are controlled or removed. Specific treatment is indicated in the following circumstances: rapid ventricular response associated with symptoms (e.g., extreme fatigue, syncope, angina, shortness of breath); presence of known severe underlying structural heart disease (e.g., aortic stenosis, severe mitral stenosis, ischemic heart disease, chronic congestive heart failure), because such patients are unlikely to revert to normal sinus rhythm spontaneously; and persistent atrial fibrillation, especially if the resting ventricular rate is >110 bpm or the rate after moderate exercise (e.g., climbing a flight of stairs) is >150 bpm.

Symptomatic patients and patients with underlying structural heart disease usually require hospital admission immediately after onset of the arrhythmia for cardioversion (see previous discussion) or for pharmacotherapy.

Cardioversion of atrial fibrillation should be considered in these patients if the arrhythmia has been present for <6 months and significant atrial enlargement (i.e., greater than approximately 5 cm) is not present. Successful cardioversion and maintenance of sinus rhythm are less likely if atrial fibrillation has been present for >6 months or if marked atrial enlargement is noted on echocardiography. Although comparisons of rate control and cardioversion strategies have not shown that patients randomly assigned to cardioversion achieve greater symptomatic improvement or improved quality of life (41) or that cardioversion offers any survival advantage over rate control (62), cardioversion still is typically recommended to highly symptomatic AF patients in whom maintenance of sinus rhythm is believed to be likely and to patients in whom rate control in atrial fibrillation is difficult to achieve. If electrical cardioversion is recommended, the patient should be anticoagulated for at least 3 weeks and then considered for elective cardioversion unless a TEE-guided approach is used (see earlier discussion). In general, cardioversion restores normal sinus rhythm in most patients, but the relapse rate is high (50% in 1 year and 90% in 3 years) unless an underlying disorder can be identified and corrected, the atrial fibrillation has been of short duration, or antiarrhythmic therapy or radiofrequency ablation therapy is used.

Following a second episode of sustained atrial fibrillation, antiarrhythmic therapy is often used, after a repeat successful cardioversion, in an attempt to maintain sinus rhythm. Because no study has demonstrated that antiarrhythmic therapy in patients with atrial fibrillation prolongs survival or reduces the incidence of strokes, the main indication for antiarrhythmic therapy should be symptom reduction.

The selection of an appropriate antiarrhythmic agent for maintaining normal sinus rhythm depends to a large degree on whether structural heart disease is present. For patients with no structural heart disease, almost any antiarrhythmic agent is safe. Class IC antiarrhythmic agents, such as flecainide or propafenone, or the class III antiarrhythmic agent sotalol are often used as first-line antiarrhythmic therapy in this setting. If these drugs are ineffective, low-dose amiodarone can be considered. In contrast, the risk of proarrhythmia is high among patients with impaired ventricular function. Perhaps the most effective and safest antiarrhythmic agent in the setting of structural heart disease is low-dose amiodarone (100–200 mg/day) (63,64). It should be recognized that atrial fibrillation is a difficult arrhythmia to treat and that, even with the most effective antiarrhythmic agents, sinus rhythm can be maintained during long-term followup in <50% to 60% of patients.

If antiarrhythmic therapy fails or is poorly tolerated, the goal of treatment should be to achieve adequate rate control and effective long-term anticoagulation (65). When rate control is attempted, the goal should be to achieve a resting ventricular rate between 70 and 100 bpm and a rate <150 bpm after modest exercise. Digoxin slows the ventricular response in acute atrial fibrillation, but it does not enhance conversion to sinus rhythm (66) and is of limited use in controlling heart rate in paroxysmal atrial fibrillation. The chronic maintenance dose of digoxin is generally 0.125 to 0.25 mg/day.

In contrast to digoxin, calcium channel blockers such as verapamil (120–240 mg/day, sustained-release), diltiazem (120–240 mg/day, sustained-release), or small dosages of a β-blocker (e.g., atenolol 25–50 mg/day, metoprolol 25 mg twice per day, propranolol 10–20 mg four times per day) effectively control heart rate during exercise and are preferred to digoxin (see General Principles in Management of Arrhythmias). Once effectiveness is demonstrated, the drugs can be taken once daily in a sustained-release form at the same total daily dosage.

In patients with permanent atrial fibrillation and a rapid ventricular rate in whom pharmacologic approaches to heart rate control are ineffective or result in intolerable side effects, electrophysiologic modification or ablation of the AV node and permanent pacemaker implantation should be performed (67).

Radiofrequency catheter ablation is emerging as an alternative treatment strategy for selected patients with *paroxysmal* and *persistent* atrial fibrillation that is refractory to pharmacologic therapy (67). Evidence suggests that paroxysmal atrial fibrillation is commonly triggered by rapid bursts of tachycardia arising from muscle sleeves that extend from the left atrium into the pulmonary veins. Radiofrequency catheter ablation targeting these pulmonary vein sleeves may cure atrial fibrillation in up to 70% to 80% of patients (59,68,69). The role of radiofrequency catheter ablation in the management of patients with persistent or chronic atrial fibrillation (other than ablation of the AV node for rate control) is not as well established, but several centers have reported encouraging results using newer ablation techniques (70,71).

A slow ventricular response to atrial fibrillation by untreated patients suggests an associated disorder of AV conduction. Such patients do not require specific therapy for the arrhythmia (other than anticoagulation) unless they are hemodynamically compromised (i.e., in refractory heart failure) and their heart rate is <60 to 70 bpm, in which case implantation of a ventricular pacemaker may be indicated.

Anticoagulation

Patients with chronic atrial fibrillation are at increased risk for arterial embolization. For example, the Framingham study reported that, over a 24-year period, patients with chronic atrial fibrillation with and without rheumatic heart disease had a 17-fold and fivefold increase in the incidence of stroke, respectively (72). Overall, the incidence of arterial embolization in untreated patients with chronic atrial fibrillation is approximately 5% to 10% per year (65). In general, patients should be anticoagulated with warfarin for at least 3 weeks before, and at least 4 weeks after, elective cardioversion (see earlier discussion). An alternative approach is to refer the patient for TEE and, if no intracardiac clots are demonstrated, to perform cardioversion without preliminary anticoagulation but followed by at least 4 weeks of warfarin therapy (42). Prospective randomized trials support the use of anticoagulants in patients with chronic atrial fibrillation if there are no contraindications (73). Anticoagulation with warfarin to obtain an INR of 2.0 to 3.0 is recommended for all patients with atrial fibrillation who are older than 65 years or who have other risk factors for stroke, such as hypertension, diabetes, or a prior transient ischemic episode or stroke. Warfarin should generally be continued indefinitely. The optimal duration of anticoagulation for a patient who is converted to sinus rhythm is unclear, but some clinicians recommend continuing warfarin regardless of whether sinus rhythm is maintained. In patients who cannot, or will not, take warfarin, some studies support the use of aspirin 325 mg/day, particularly in young patients with no risks for embolism (74,75).

Apart from the morbidity and mortality associated with arterial embolization, the prognosis of patients with atrial fibrillation depends on the nature and extent of underlying heart disease.

Atrial Flutter

Definition and Causes

Atrial flutter is a reentrant arrhythmia that usually is confined to the right atrium and results in an atrial rate of approximately 240 to 300 bpm. Usually there is a 2:1 AV conduction block so that the ventricular response is approximately 120 to 150 bpm. In contrast to atrial fibrillation, both atrial and ventricular responses often are regular. Atrial flutter usually is seen in patients who have underlying cardiopulmonary disease—ischemic heart disease, rheumatic heart disease, congestive cardiomyopathy, atrial septal defect, mitral valve disease, chronic obstructive pulmonary disease, or thyrotoxicosis—the same diseases often associated with atrial fibrillation. In contrast to atrial fibrillation, however, atrial flutter is rarely seen in patients who are otherwise healthy.

Symptoms and Signs

Patients usually are aware of a rapid heart rate. Whether other symptoms develop depends on the severity and nature of the underlying heart disease.

A regular, rapid heart rate and arterial pulse are detected. Sometimes the flutter waves are visible in the jugular venous pulse. An S_4 is occasionally audible (in contrast to atrial fibrillation).

Electrocardiogram

In atrial flutter, the ECG commonly shows rapid, regular sawtooth flutter waves at approximately 240 to 300 bpm (Fig. 64.9). The ventricular response may be regular, usually at approximately 120 to 150 bpm, and the QRS complex ordinarily is morphologically normal. If the AV node is diseased or the patient is taking a medication that slows AV conduction, higher degrees of AV block may be seen, usually a multiple of two (e.g., 4:1, 8:1). Aberrant conduction is unusual.

If the diagnosis is unclear, carotid sinus massage may help distinguish atrial flutter from other paroxysmal supraventricular tachyarrhythmias. It usually causes an abrupt temporary slowing of the rate. Flutter waves, which may have been difficult to detect at a higher rate, are visible on the ECG, most commonly in leads II, III, aVF, and V_1 (Fig. 64.9). Diagnostic workup is the same as for atrial fibrillation.

Treatment and Course

Atrial flutter often is a chronic and highly refractory arrhythmia that is difficult to treat with medical therapy. The initial goal of therapy should be to slow the ventricular response, but, in contrast to the situation with atrial fibrillation, it often is difficult to lower the ventricular rate with drugs.

If there is no contraindication, electrical cardioversion (see previous discussion) is the treatment of choice if atrial flutter persists. Most patients can be converted to normal

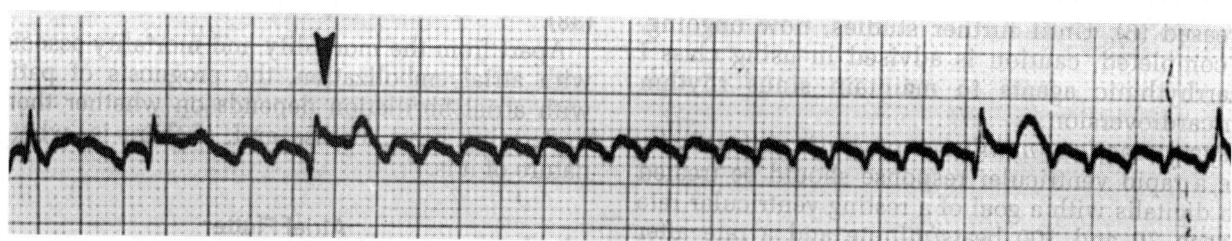

FIGURE 64.9. Atrial flutter. The flutter waves are clearly revealed after carotid sinus massage (*arrowhead*).

sinus rhythm, usually after application of a lower-energy shock than is necessary to convert atrial fibrillation. If atrial flutter recurs after cardioversion, radiofrequency catheter ablation should be considered.

Considerations regarding pharmacologic therapy for atrial flutter are the same as for atrial fibrillation (see previous discussion). Perhaps the only difference is that atrial flutter is even less likely to respond to antiarrhythmic therapy. Patients who have recurrent symptomatic atrial flutter should be considered for electrophysiologic study with possible radiofrequency catheter ablation of the reentrant circuit. Radiofrequency catheter ablation of atrial flutter can be accomplished successfully in >95% of patients, with a very low incidence of complications (76,77). Radiofrequency catheter ablation has been demonstrated to be more effective than antiarrhythmic therapy for treatment of atrial flutter (77).

Ventricular Premature Beats and Ventricular Tachycardia

Definition and Causes

Ventricular premature beats (VPBs) or *premature ventricular contractions (PVCs)* are impulses generated in the ventricles, usually as the result of reentry of an impulse conducted down from the atria through the AV node, but sometimes as the result of the firing of an ectopic (parasystolic) focus. *Ventricular tachycardia (VT)* consists of at least three consecutive PVCs occurring at a rate of at least 100 bpm.

Occasional VPBs occur in many healthy people sporadically during their lives, more often in older people. However, often VPBs are associated with underlying organic heart disease (e.g., hypertensive heart disease, ischemic heart disease, cardiomyopathy). The frequency of VPBs may be increased by caffeine, alcohol, sympathomimetic drugs, tricyclic antidepressants, phenothiazines, hypokalemia, hypomagnesemia, hypoxia, or emotional stress in people both with and without heart disease. VPBs are a common manifestation of digitalis intoxication. Exercise usually abolishes VPBs in people without structural heart disease; conversely, an increase in the number of VPBs after exertion is highly suggestive of structural heart disease.

Symptoms and Signs

Patients may be unaware that they have had a VPB, but often they experience a palpitation. They sense either the premature beat itself or the more forceful normal beat that follows it after a compensatory pause.

Electrocardiogram

The ECG shows a premature ventricular response with a morphologically abnormal, often bizarre, wide QRS complex. No P wave precedes a VPB, but by retrograde conduction a P wave sometimes follows it. The ST segment and T wave have an opposite vector from the QRS complex. Typically, a VPB is followed by a compensatory pause, that is, the R–R interval between two normal beats separated by a VPB is the same as that between two normal beats separated by another normal beat if the patient is in normal sinus rhythm (Fig. 64.10). This occurs because retrograde conduction of the premature beat to the AV node blocks the succeeding sinus beat.

When VPBs are caused by reentry, they have a fixed temporal (coupled) relationship to the preceding normal beats. When they are caused by the firing of an ectopic (parasystolic) focus, they have no fixed relationship to the preceding normal beats but do have a regular pattern (i.e., the ectopic intervals are constant or are multiples of a constant). Ectopic beats occasionally fuse with normal beats, producing a complex that is intermediate between the two (Fig. 64.11).

Treatment and Course

VPBs in patients with otherwise normal hearts are not harmful. However, there is an increased incidence of sudden death and MI in patients with VPBs who have underlying ischemic heart disease (11). Suppression of VPBs has

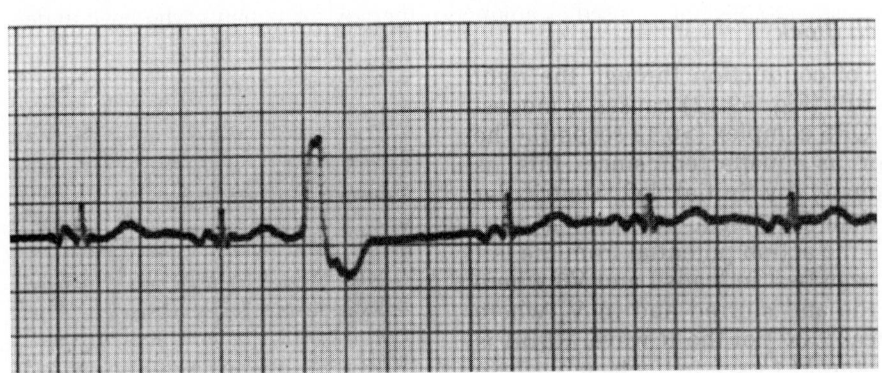

FIGURE 64.10. Premature ventricular beat. Note that the R–R interval between the two normal beats separated by the premature ventricular beat is the same as that between two normal beats separated by another normal beat.

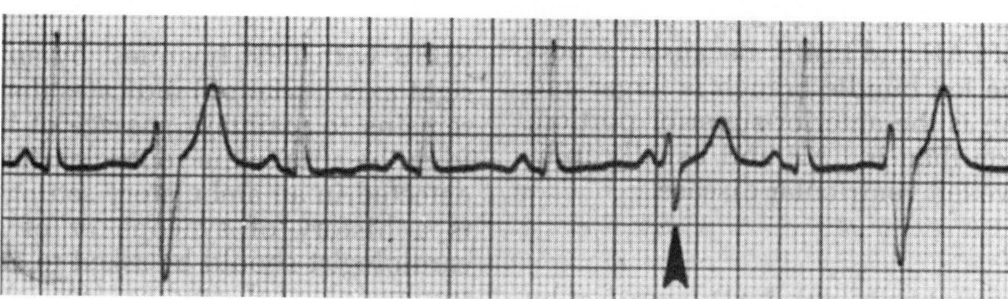

FIGURE 64.11. Premature ventricular beats caused by firing of an ectopic focus. *Arrowhead* points to a fusion beat.

not been demonstrated to alter their course in these latter patients (13). Because all antiarrhythmic agents have potentially serious side effects (Table 64.2), the practitioner must consider for each patient the relative risks of treating versus not treating VPBs. The following generalizations may be useful:

- Apparently healthy young people with asymptomatic VPBs generally do not require treatment (78).
- Apparently healthy young people with VPBs causing symptomatic palpitations do not require pharmacologic treatment. If symptoms interfere with normal lifestyle despite reassurance, a trial of a low-dose β-blocker, such as metoprolol extended-release 25 to 50 mg/day, may abolish VPBs and relieve symptoms. β-blockers can sometimes be discontinued after several weeks; often VPBs do not recur and no further treatment is necessary. Patients with highly symptomatic VPBs who do not respond to β-blocker treatment may benefit from antiarrhythmic drug therapy or catheter ablation.

The management of patients with, or at risk for, VT is evolving rapidly with the more widespread use of catheter ablation and ICD therapy. Patients with significant structural heart disease (evidenced by EF <40%) and symptomatic ventricular arrhythmias, especially symptomatic multifocal premature ventricular beats with a frequency >10 per hour or runs of VT, have an increased risk of sudden death. These patients should be referred to a cardiologist for consideration of electrophysiologic testing and/or ICD therapy. MADIT demonstrated that placement of an implantable defibrillator improves survival among patients with a prior MI and EF <35% who have inducible sustained VT during electrophysiologic testing that is not suppressed with intravenous procainamide (37,79). Sustained VT usually is defined as VT that lasts >30 seconds or requires termination because of hemodynamic compromise, whereas nonsustained VT terminates spontaneously within 30 seconds. MUSTT confirmed these findings and demonstrated that placement of an implantable defibrillator improves survival among patients with a prior MI and EF <40% who have inducible sustained VT during electrophysiologic testing (38). Based on the results of this study, the current recommendation is that patients with nonsustained VT, in the setting of an *ischemic cardiomyopathy,* undergo electrophysiologic testing and that an implantable defibrillator be placed in patients with inducible VT.

The optimal approach to the management of nonsustained VT in the setting of a *nonischemic cardiomyopathy* often also involves ICD therapy, as a result of the findings of the SCD-HeFT trial (40). This trial (see discussion earlier in this chapter) showed that prophylactic placement of an ICD decreased mortality in patients with LVEF ≤35% and NYHA class II or III heart failure, regardless of cause.

When ventricular arrhythmias occur in the setting of congestive heart failure, an attempt should be made to achieve a maximal state of cardiac compensation before antiarrhythmic therapy is instituted. Hemodynamic compensation may decrease or eliminate VPBs so that specific antiarrhythmic therapy is not required. Disopyramide and flecainide are myocardial depressants and are specifically contraindicated in patients whose hearts are enlarged and hypocontractile. Furthermore, patients in severe chronic heart failure, many of whom are taking diuretics, are more likely to experience problems such as hypokalemia, hypomagnesemia, alkalosis, hypoxemia, and digitalis toxicity, thus increasing the risk of serious side effects from antiarrhythmic agents (80). Such patients are best treated in consultation with a cardiologist.

Patients with structural heart disease who have a sustained ventricular arrhythmia (sustained monomorphic VT or ventricular fibrillation) are best managed based on the results of electrophysiologic evaluation. Implantable defibrillators are generally the treatment of choice in this patient population. This approach requires hospitalization and consultation with a cardiologist. Radiofrequency catheter ablation in this patient population is generally used as adjunctive therapy for patients who have undergone placement of an implantable defibrillator and are experiencing frequent shocks because of recurrent slow sustained monomorphic VT (81).

Sustained VT that occurs in the absence of structural heart disease (referred to as *idiopathic VT*) is generally associated with a benign prognosis. Treatment is indicated for relief of symptoms. This type of VT usually responds to treatment with most types of antiarrhythmic agents, including β-blockers, calcium channel blockers, and class IC antiarrhythmic agents. Radiofrequency catheter ablation, which has success rates >90% and a low incidence of complications, is another commonly used treatment option in this patient population (82).

Primary care providers occasionally assume the care of patients who are taking antiarrhythmic agents because of a history of symptomatic ventricular arrhythmias caused by structural heart disease. Consultation with a cardiologist is advisable before therapy is stopped. The possibility that a patient will experience a proarrhythmic effect from an antiarrhythmic agent must always be considered (see earlier discussion).

Preexcitation Syndrome

Definition and Causes

In normal hearts, the atria and ventricles are electrically isolated from each other by the AV groove, and the electrical signal from the atrium is conducted to the ventricle via the AV node and conducting system. If the AV groove is short-circuited by muscle fibers, if muscle fibers from the atria enter the His bundle below the AV node, or if muscle fibers from the His bundle bypass the bundle branches, a variable portion of the right or left ventricle is depolarized early. These short-circuiting fibers are known as accessory AV, nodoventricular, and fasciculoventricular pathways—the atriofascicular bypass tract and the intranodal bypass tract, depending on their location (Fig. 64.12).

The classic example of preexcitation is *WPW syndrome.* This syndrome is characterized electrocardiographically by a short PR interval followed by a wide QRS complex, which is a fusion beat between the ventricular myocardium that is preexcited and that which is excited via normal conduction pathways (Fig. 64.13). The portion of the complex caused by preexcitation is called the *delta wave* because of its resemblance to the Greek capital letter. If the accessory bundle connects the atria with the left ventricle, the ECG pattern resembles RBBB (type A WPW). On the other hand, if the connection is with the right ventricle, the pattern resembles left bundle-branch block (LBBB; type B WPW). The negative delta wave in lead II in this situation may be taken for a Q wave, and the mistaken diagnosis of remote MI may be made.

If the atrial fibers insert into the bundle of His and short-circuit the AV node, the PR interval is short but no delta wave is seen because conduction below the AV node occurs along the usual pathways. This syndrome is known as *Lown-Ganong-Levine syndrome.* A number of other variants of preexcitation syndrome have been described but are much rarer than these two more common disorders (83).

The ECG manifestations of preexcitation may vary from time to time within a given patient because, if conduction occurs through the normal anatomic pathways rather than through accessory fibers, no preexcitation is seen on the ECG. If preexcitation is facilitated because of disease in the AV node or because of drugs that suppress conduction through the AV node (e.g., digitalis, calcium channel blockers, β-blockers), ECG abnormalities are seen.

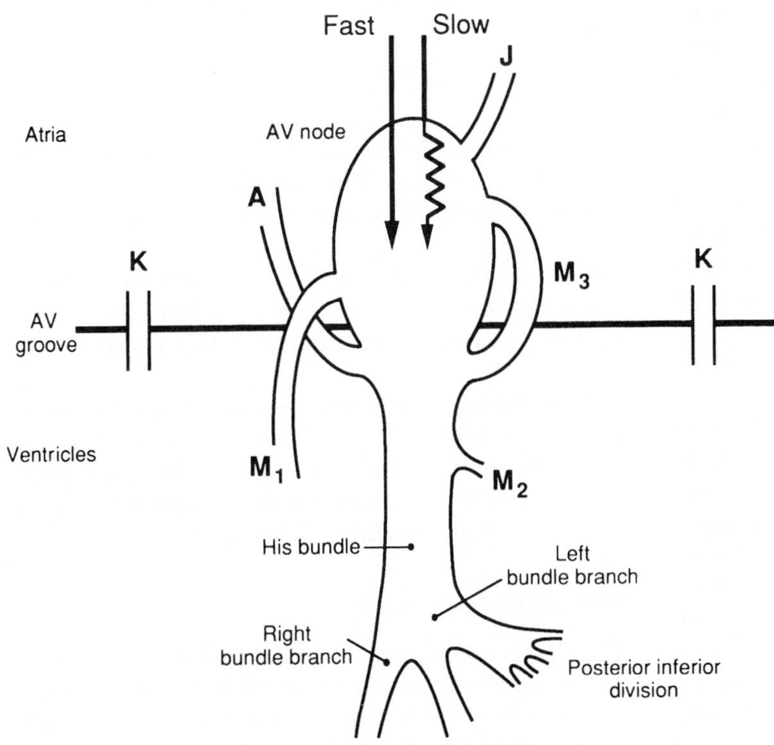

FIGURE 64.12. Schematic diagram of possible accessory conduction pathways (old eponymic nomenclature given in parentheses). A, atriofascicular (atrio-Hisian) bundles; J, intranodal bypass (James) tracts; K, accessory atrioventricular (Kent) bundles; M (Mahaim) fibers—M_1, accessory nodoventricular; M_2, accessory fasciculoventricular; M_3, nodofascicular fibers. Dual atrioventricular node pathways are represented by the *fast* and *slow* labels. (Adapted from Wellens HJJ, Brugada P, Penn OC. The management of preexcitation syndromes. JAMA 1987;257:2325, with permission.)

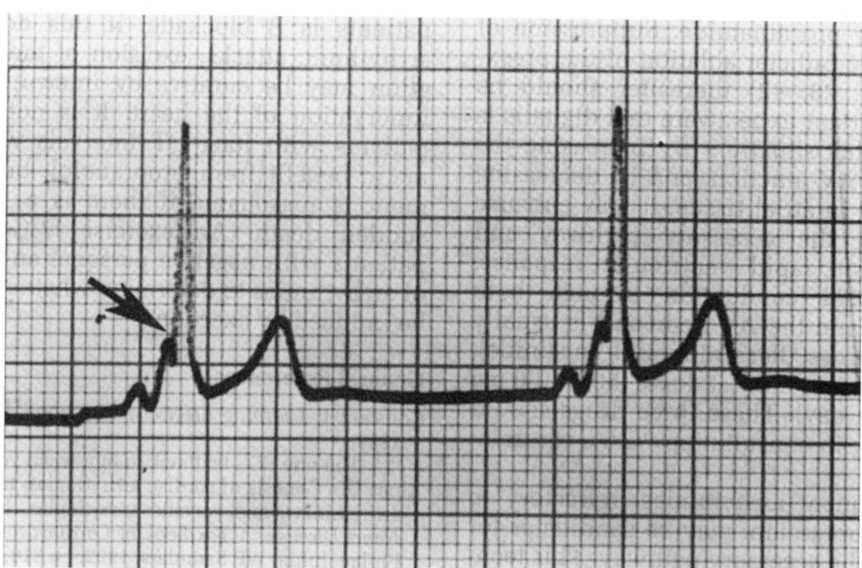

FIGURE 64.13. Wolff-Parkinson-White syndrome. Note the delta wave (*arrowhead*).

Supraventricular arrhythmias are found in 13% to 60% of patients with preexcitation. PSVT is most commonly observed, but atrial fibrillation and flutter also occur (84). Accessory pathways can conduct anterograde (from the atrium to the ventricle), retrograde (from the ventricle to the atrium), or both. The morphology of the QRS complex during the tachyarrhythmia depends on the direction in which the reentrant tachycardia occurs. If reentry occurs with anterograde conduction through the AV conducting system and retrograde conduction through an accessory pathway, then the ventricles are depolarized through the normal AV conduction system, and the QRS duration during the tachyarrhythmia may be normal (i.e., no delta wave is seen during tachycardia). This type of tachycardia, known as *orthodromic atrioventricular reentrant tachycardia (AVRT),* is by far the most common supraventricular tachycardia in patients with WPW syndrome. In a small percentage of patients with WPW syndrome and AVRT, the circuit is established in the opposite direction, with depolarization of the ventricle over the accessory pathway during the tachycardia. In this circumstance, known as *antidromic AVRT,* the QRS complex is wide and the arrhythmia can easily be confused with VT.

It should be noted that the term *preexcitation* refers to evidence of an anterograde-conducting accessory pathway on the ECG. *WPW syndrome* refers to a specific syndrome of supraventricular tachycardia in the setting of preexcitation on the ECG. A patient who has evidence of preexcitation on the ECG but no supraventricular tachycardia is properly described as having *asymptomatic preexcitation.* Accessory pathways that conduct only in the retrograde direction and therefore are not associated with a delta wave on the ECG are referred to as *concealed accessory pathways;* these pathways cannot be identified by a routine 12-lead ECG.

Symptoms and Signs

Preexcitation may be an incidental finding on an ECG, or it may come to the attention of the health care provider because of symptoms of palpitations. Other symptoms of tachyarrhythmia depend on the nature of the arrhythmia and the presence or absence of other structural heart disease.

No physical findings are caused by preexcitation other than an occasional loud S_1, except during periods of tachyarrhythmia, when the findings depend on the type of arrhythmia present.

Prevalence

Preexcitation syndromes are not rare. The prevalence of preexcitation is between one and three per 1,000 people, or approximately 0.15% to 0.3% of the normal population (84). Accurate prevalence rates are difficult to obtain because short PR intervals with normal QRS durations are commonly seen in people without arrhythmias, so no studies are performed to determine whether a bypass tract exists.

Preexcitation syndromes occasionally are associated with certain forms of congenital heart disease. Preexcitation of the WPW type is associated with Ebstein anomaly of the tricuspid valve, corrected transposition of the great vessels, and hypertrophic cardiomyopathy (83).

Treatment and Course

The presence of preexcitation in an asymptomatic patient is associated with an approximately 0.1% annual risk of sudden cardiac death. Because this is not markedly greater than the risk of sudden cardiac death in the general population and because treatment itself is associated with some

32. Abraham WT, Fisher WG, Smith AL, et al. Cardiac resynchronization in chronic heart failure. N Engl J Med 2002;346:1845–1853.
33. Cleland JG, Daubert JC, Erdmann E, et al. The effect of cardiac resynchronization on morbidity and mortality in heart failure. N Engl J Med 2005;352:1539.
34. Hayes DL, Wang PJ, Reynolds DW, et al. Interference with cardiac pacemakers by cellular telephones. N Engl J Med 1997;336:1473.
35. Kadish A, Mehra M. Heart failure devices: implantable cardioverter-defibrillators and biventricular pacing therapy. Circulation 2005;111:3327.
36. The AVID Investigators. A comparison of antiarrhythmic-drug therapy with implantable defibrillators in patients resuscitated from near-fatal ventricular arrhythmias. N Engl J Med 1997;337:1576.
37. Moss AJ, Hall WJ, Cannom DS, et al. Improved survival with an implanted defibrillator in patients with coronary disease at high risk for ventricular arrhythmia. Multicenter Automatic Defibrillator Implantation Trial Investigators. N Engl J Med 1996;335:1933.
38. Buxton AE, Lee KL, DiCarlo L, et al. Electrophysiologic testing to identify patients with coronary artery disease who are at risk for sudden death. Multicenter Unsustained Tachycardia Trial Investigators. N Engl J Med 2000;342:1937.
39. Moss AJ, Zareba W, Hall WJ, et al. Prophylactic implantation of a defibrillator in patients with myocardial infarction and reduced ejection fraction. N Engl J Med 2002;345:877.
40. Bardy GH, Lee KL, Mark DB, et al. Amiodarone or an implantable cardioverter–defibrillator for congestive heart failure. N Engl J Med 2005; 352:225.
41. Hohnloser SH, Kuck KH, Lilienthal J. Rhythm or rate control in atrial fibrillation—Pharmacological Intervention in Atrial Fibrillation (PIAF): a randomised trial. Lancet 2000;356:1789.
42. Klein AL, Grimm RA, Murray RD, et al. Use of transesophageal echocardiography to guide cardioversion in patients with atrial fibrillation. N Engl J Med 2001;344:1411.
43. Catherwood E, Fitzpatrick WD, Greenberg ML, et al. Cost-effectiveness of cardioversion and antiarrhythmic therapy in nonvalvular atrial fibrillation. Ann Intern Med 1999;130:625.
44. Volgman AS, Carberry PA, Stambler B, et al. Conversion efficacy and safety of intravenous ibutilide compared with intravenous procainamide in patients with atrial flutter or fibrillation. J Am Coll Cardiol 1998;31:1414.
45. Oral H, Souza JJ, Michaud GF, et al. Facilitating transthoracic cardioversion of atrial fibrillation with ibutilide pretreatment. N Engl J Med 1999;340:1849.
46. Calkins H, Yong P, Miller JM, et al. Catheter ablation of accessory pathways, atrioventricular nodal reentrant tachycardia, and the atrioventricular junction: final results of a prospective, multicenter clinical trial. Circulation 1999;99:262.
47. Blomstrom-Lundqvist C, Scheinman MM, Aliot EM, et al. European Society of Cardiology Committee, NASPE-Heart Rhythm Society ACC/AHA/ESC guidelines for the management of patients with supraventricular arrhythmias—executive summary. A report of the American college of cardiology/American heart association task force on practice guidelines and the European society of cardiology committee for practice guidelines (writing committee to develop guidelines for the management of patients with supraventricular arrhythmias) developed in collaboration with NASPE-Heart Rhythm Society. J Am Coll Cardiol 2003;42:1493.
48. Cheng CH, Sanders GD, Hlatky MA. Cost-effectiveness of radiofrequency ablation for supraventricular tachycardia. Ann Intern Med. 2000;133:864.
49. Marshall DA, O'Brien BJ, Nichol G. Review of economic evaluations of radiofrequency catheter ablation for cardiac arrhythmias. Can J Cardiol. 2003;19:1285.
50. Mangrum JM, DiMarco JP. The evaluation and management of bradycardia. N Engl J Med 2000;342:703.
51. Andersen HR, Nielsen JC, Thomsen PE, et al. Long-term follow-up of patients from a randomised trial of atrial versus ventricular pacing for sick-sinus syndrome. Lancet 1997;350:1210.
52. Ganz LI, Friedman PL. Supraventricular tachycardia. N Engl J Med 1995;332:162.
53. Kalbfleisch SJ, el Atassi R, Calkins H, et al. Differentiation of paroxysmal narrow QRS complex tachycardias using the 12-lead electrocardiogram. J Am Coll Cardiol 1993;21:85.
54. Levin ER, Gardner DG, Samson WK. Natriuretic peptides. N Engl J Med 1998;339:321.
55. Cheng CH, Sanders GD, Hlatky MA, et al. Cost-effectiveness of radiofrequency ablation for supraventricular tachycardia. Ann Intern Med 2000;133:864.
56. Kastor JA. Multifocal atrial tachycardia. N Engl J Med 1990;322:1713.
57. McCord JK, Borzak S, Davis T, et al. Usefulness of intravenous magnesium for multifocal atrial tachycardia in patients with chronic obstructive pulmonary disease. Am J Cardiol 1998;81:91.
58. Fuster V, Ryden LE, Asinger RW, et al. ACC/AHA/ESC guidelines for the management of patients with atrial fibrillation: executive summary. A report of the American College of Cardiology/American Heart Association Task Force on Practice Guidelines and the European Society of Cardiology Committee for Practice Guidelines and Policy Conferences (Committee to Develop Guidelines for the Management of Patients with Atrial Fibrillation). Developed in Collaboration with the North American Society of Pacing and Electrophysiology. Circulation 2001;104:2118.
59. Haissaguerre M, Jais P, Shah DC, et al. Spontaneous initiation of atrial fibrillation by ectopic beats originating in the pulmonary veins. N Engl J Med 1998;339:659.
60. Allessie MA, Boyden PA, Camm AJ, et al. Pathophysiology and prevention of atrial fibrillation. Circulation 2001;103:769.
61. Klein I, Ojamaa K. Thyroid hormone and the cardiovascular system. N Engl J Med 2001; 344:501.
62. Wyse DG, Waldo AL, DiMarco JP, et al. A comparison of rate control and rhythm control in patients with atrial fibrillation. N Engl J Med 2002;347:1825.
63. Singh BN, Singh SN, Reda DJ, et al. Amiodarone versus sotalol for atrial fibrillation. N Engl J Med 2005;352:1861.
64. Roy D, Talajic M, Dorian P, et al. Amiodarone to prevent recurrence of atrial fibrillation. Canadian Trial of Atrial Fibrillation Investigators. N Engl J Med 2000;342:913.
65. Falk RH. Atrial fibrillation. N Engl J Med 2001;344:1067.
66. Falk RH, Knowlton AA, Bernard SA, et al. Digoxin for converting recent-onset atrial fibrillation to sinus rhythm: a randomized, double-blinded trial. Ann Intern Med 1987;106:503.
67. Scheinman MM, Morady F. Nonpharmacological approaches to atrial fibrillation. Circulation 2001;103:2120.
68. Jais P, Haissaguerre M, Shah DC, et al. A focal source of atrial fibrillation treated by discrete radiofrequency ablation. Circulation 1997; 95:572.
69. Vasamreddy CR, Dalal D, Eldadah Z, et al. Safety and efficacy of circumferential pulmonary vein catheter ablation of atrial fibrillation. Heart Rhythm 2005;2:42.
70. Hsu LF, Jais P, Sanders P, Garrigue S, et al. Catheter ablation for atrial fibrillation in congestive heart failure. N Engl J Med 2004; 351:2373.
71. Pappone C, Oreto G, Rosanio S, et al. Atrial electroanatomic remodeling after circumferential radiofrequency pulmonary vein ablation: efficacy of an anatomic approach in a large cohort of patients with atrial fibrillation. Circulation 2001;104:2539.
72. Wolf PA, Kannel WB, McGee DL, et al. Duration of atrial fibrillation and imminence of stroke: the Framingham study. Stroke 1983;14:664.
73. Matchar DB, McCrory DC, Barnett HJ, et al. Medical treatment for stroke prevention. Ann Intern Med 1994;121:41.
74. Albers GW. Choice of antithrombotic therapy for stroke prevention in atrial fibrillation: warfarin, aspirin, or both? Arch Intern Med 1998; 158:1487.
75. Albers GW, Dalen JE, Laupacis A, et al. Antithrombotic therapy in atrial fibrillation. Chest 2001;119:194S.
76. Natale A, Newby KH, Pisano E, et al. Prospective randomized comparison of antiarrhythmic therapy versus first-line radiofrequency ablation in patients with atrial flutter. J Am Coll Cardiol 2000;35:1898.
77. Nabar A, Rodriguez LM, Timmermans C, et al. Effect of right atrial isthmus ablation on the occurrence of atrial fibrillation: observations in four patient groups having type I atrial flutter with or without associated atrial fibrillation. Circulation 1999;99:1441.
78. Bikkina M, Larson MG, Levy D. Prognostic implications of asymptomatic ventricular arrhythmias: the Framingham Heart Study. Ann Intern Med 1992;117:990.
79. Moss AJ. Implantable cardioverter defibrillator therapy: the sickest patients benefit the most. Circulation 2000;101:1638.
80. Cooper HA, Dries DL, Davis CE, et al. Diuretics and risk of arrhythmic death in patients with left ventricular dysfunction. Circulation 1999; 100:1311.
81. Morady F. Radio-frequency ablation as treatment for cardiac arrhythmias. N Engl J Med 1999;340:534.
82. Coggins DL, Lee RJ, Sweeney J, et al. Radiofrequency catheter ablation as a cure for idiopathic tachycardia of both left and right ventricular origin. J Am Coll Cardiol 1994; 23:1333.
83. Gollob MH, Green MS, Tang AS, et al. Identification of a gene responsible for familial Wolff-Parkinson-White syndrome. N Engl J Med 2001;344:1823.
84. Al Khatib SM, Pritchett EL. Clinical features of Wolff-Parkinson-White syndrome. Am Heart J 1999;138:403.
85. Lerman BB, Basson CT. High-risk patients with ventricular preexcitation—a pendulum in motion. N Engl J Med 2003;349:1787.
86. Makkar RR, Fromm BS, Steinman RT, et al. Female gender as a risk factor for torsades de pointes associated with cardiovascular drugs. JAMA 1993;270:2590.
87. Drici MD, Knollmann BC, Wang WX, et al. Cardiac actions of erythromycin: influence of female sex. JAMA 1998;280:1774.
88. Towbin JA. New revelations about the long-QT syndrome. N Engl J Med 1995;333:384.
89. Schwartz PJ, Moss AJ, Vincent GM, et al. Diagnostic criteria for the long QT syndrome: an update. Circulation 1993;88:782.
90. Page RL. Treatment of arrhythmias during pregnancy. Am Heart J 1995;130:871.
91. Carpenter MW, Sady SP, Hoegsberg B, et al.

Fetal heart rate response to maternal exertion. JAMA 1988;259:3006.
92. Sami M, Kraemer H, Harrison DC, et al. A new method for evaluating antiarrhythmic drug efficacy. Circulation 1980;62:1172.
93. Schneider JF, Thomas HE, Kreger BE, et al. Newly acquired right bundle-branch block: the Framingham Study. Ann Intern Med 1980;92: 37.
94. Schneider JF, Thomas HE Jr, Kreger BE, et al. Newly acquired left bundle-branch block: the Framingham study. Ann Intern Med 1979; 90:303.
95. Kulbertus HE, Demoulin JC. The left hemiblocks: significance, prognosis and treatment. Schweiz Med Wochenschr 1982; 112:1579.
96. Dhingra RC, Wyndham C, Amat-y-Leon F, et al. Incidence and site of atrioventricular block in patients with chronic bifascicular block. Circulation 1979;59:238.
97. Upshaw CB Jr, Silverman ME. The Wenckebach phenomenon: a salute and comment on the centennial of its original description. Ann Intern Med 1999;130:58.

For annotated ***General References*** *and resources related to this chapter, visit www.hopkinsbayview.org/PAMreferences.*

Chapter 65

Common Cardiac Disorders Revealed by Auscultation of the Heart

Susan A. Mayer and Edward P. Shapiro

The past two decades have seen significant changes in the techniques used for the diagnosis of, and the strategies for intervention in, valvular heart disease. For a detailed review and discussion of controversial aspects, the reader is referred to the American College of Cardiology/American Heart Association Guidelines for the Management of Patients with Valvular Disease, published in its full form (1) or executive summary (2). These valuable aids can be accessed on the Internet at www.acc.org and www.americanheart.org, respectively.

HEART SOUNDS

First Heart Sound (S_1)

The first heart sound (S_1) is a high-frequency sound produced by closure of the atrioventricular (AV) valves, that is, M_1 (mitral valve closure) followed closely by T_1 (tricuspid valve closure). Mitral valve closure is louder than tricuspid valve closure.

Abnormally wide splitting of the first heart sound is produced by delays in closure of the tricuspid valve (as in patients with right bundle-branch block), ventricular ectopic beats, idioventricular rhythm, or left ventricular (LV) pacing. In mitral stenosis, mitral valve closure may be so delayed that tricuspid valve closure may actually precede mitral valve closure.

Increased intensity of the first heart sound is associated with a rapid increase in ventricular pressure, which occurs when the ventricles are presented with an increased volume (e.g., ventricular septal defect and atrial septal defect) or with a wide-open AV valve at the end of diastole, which occurs when there is shortening of the AV filling time (e.g., atrial tachycardia and conditions associated with a short PR interval) and when AV filling time is prolonged (e.g., mitral stenosis).

Reduced intensity of the first heart sound may indicate an immobile valve (e.g., severe mitral regurgitation or stenosis) or a long PR interval.

Second Heart Sound (S_2)

The second heart sound (S_2) is produced by closure of the semilunar valves, that is, A_2 (aortic valve closure) followed closely by P_2 (pulmonic valve closure). Normal splitting of the second heart sound occurs at the height of inspiration, when the splitting may be as wide as 0.10 seconds, and is caused by the increase in stroke volume in the right heart with the increase in venous return with inspiration. The two components of the second heart sound normally are synchronous and virtually single during expiration.

Abnormally wide splitting of S_2 without change in expiration is characteristic of an atrial septal defect or anomalous pulmonary venous return. S_2 is widely split but variable in patients with right bundle-branch block or pulmonic stenosis. In the presence of severe aortic stenosis, A_2 is delayed beyond P_2, resulting in wide splitting during expiration with no splitting during inspiration (reversed or paradoxical splitting). Paradoxical splitting of the second heart sound also occurs in the presence of a left bundle-branch block, severe hypertension, or severe LV failure.

Increased intensities of A_2 and P_2 are features of aortic and pulmonary hypertension, respectively. Decreased intensities of A_2 or P_2 are features of an immobile or severely thickened aortic or pulmonic valve.

Gallops

The identification of a gallop sound affords valuable information about diagnosis, prognosis, and treatment. Gallops are diastolic sounds and appear to be related to the two periods of filling of the ventricles: the rapid filling phase (S_3, or ventricular diastolic gallop) and the presystolic filling phase related to atrial systole (S_4, or atrial gallop).

The *atrial gallop sound*, or S_4, is a low-frequency presystolic sound and is found in patients with primary myocardial disease, coronary artery disease, systemic or pulmonary hypertension, or severe aortic or pulmonic stenosis. The atrial gallop indicates severity of the underlying disorder; as the patient's condition improves, the sound may become fainter or disappear. With ventricular hypertrophy, an S_4 is a fixed finding of no prognostic significance. An atrial gallop is commonly heard in people older than 65 years, even in the absence of heart disease or hypertension (see Doppler echocardiography in Clinical Applications of Echocardiography).

The *ventricular gallop sound*, or S_3, is a low-frequency sound (see Chapter 66). It occurs with the same timing as the normal physiologic third sound, approximately 0.14 to 0.16 seconds after the second heart sound. The third sound is a normal finding in children, pregnant women, and young adults up to age 30 years (see Doppler Echocardiography in Clinical Applications of Echocardiography). An S_3 gallop otherwise is a feature of severe cardiac decompensation, whatever the underlying cause (e.g., hypertension, coronary artery disease, rheumatic heart disease), and indicates a poor prognosis.

Ejection Sounds (Clicks)

Ejection sounds are produced at the time of ejection of blood from the left ventricle into the aorta or from the right ventricle into the pulmonary artery. The sound may originate in a thickened valve or dilated great vessel. The *aortic ejection sound* is located in the area of aortic auscultation, namely, from the second right intercostal space in a straight line to the cardiac apex, and occurs 0.05 seconds after M_1. It is a high-frequency sound, often called a *click*. In the presence of systemic hypertension, the aortic ejection sound is an indication of severity. It disappears as hypertension improves. Aortic ejection clicks may also be heard in patients with aortic stenosis, aneurysm of the ascending aorta, and aortic insufficiency.

Pulmonic ejection sounds (or clicks) often are localized to the second left intercostal space and may increase in intensity with expiration. They occur immediately after M_1. Pulmonic clicks are a feature of valvular pulmonic stenosis and pulmonary hypertension.

A *midsystolic clicking sound*, with or without a late systolic murmur, may indicate mitral valve prolapse (see below).

Opening Snaps

An opening snap occurs because of a stenotic, but still mobile, mitral or tricuspid valve. The mitral opening snap is best heard between the pulmonic area and the cardiac apex. It occurs 0.04 to 0.12 seconds after S_2 in early diastole. It is heard in patients with a thickened mitral valve. The earlier the snap, the more severe the stenosis. The tricuspid opening snap is best heard at the lower left or right sternal border and occurs immediately after S_2 in early diastole.

Murmurs

Evaluation of a heart murmur is one of the most common tasks confronting a practitioner conducting a physical examination. Almost all normal people have a systolic murmur at some time in their lives. On the other hand, a murmur may be a sign of serious underlying cardiac or noncardiac disease. It is important to distinguish innocent murmurs from those that reflect an underlying disorder and to appropriately select the tests that will lead to the precise diagnosis and proper management.

General Characteristics of Murmurs

A murmur is a series of audible vibrations produced by turbulence in the circulation. These vibrations can be characterized by intensity, pitch, shape, quality, and timing in the cardiac cycle; precordial location of maximal intensity; and radiation.

The *intensity* or *loudness* of a murmur is, by convention, graded on a scale from 1 to 6. A grade 1 murmur is audible only after concentrated auscultation. A grade 2 murmur is faint but readily audible. A grade 3 murmur is prominent but not loud. Grade 4 murmurs are loud and often, but not always, are associated with a palpable thrill. A grade 5 murmur is very loud and can be heard with only the edge of the stethoscope touching the chest wall. A grade 6 murmur is heard with the stethoscope held 1 cm above, but not actually touching, the chest wall.

The *pitch* of a murmur refers to the frequency of the sound, from high to low. High-frequency murmurs usually reflect high velocity or high pressure.

The *shape* of a murmur refers to the change in intensity throughout the duration of the sound, for example, crescendo (increasing in intensity), decrescendo (decreasing in intensity), or constant.

The *quality* of a murmur refers to the nature of the sound: harsh, blowing, musical, cooing, rumbling, and so forth. Although these terms are not precise, they are useful in identifying various benign and significant conditions, as described below.

The *timing* of a murmur is particularly important in establishing the cause of the sound—first, whether the murmur is systolic, diastolic, or continuous and, second, whether it is heard in early, middle, or late systole or diastole. Murmurs that last throughout systole are called *holosystolic.* Late diastolic murmurs are sometimes called *presystolic.*

The *location* of a murmur refers to the site on the chest wall where the sound is loudest. The *direction of radiation* refers to the other sites where the murmur, although less intense, can still be heard; those sites may be outside the chest (e.g., the back or neck). Aortic murmurs may be heard anywhere in a straight line from the second right interspace to the apex. Pulmonic murmurs are heard best at the second left intercostal space; tricuspid murmurs, at the lower left sternal border; and mitral murmurs, at the cardiac apex radiating into the axilla.

There are two kinds of systolic murmurs: *ejection* and *regurgitant.* The ejection systolic murmur may be an innocent flow murmur, or it may reflect organic heart disease. The regurgitant murmur may be caused by dilation of the annulus of the valve in an otherwise normal heart, or it may represent organic heart disease.

The *ejection murmur* is a crescendo–decrescendo (or diamond-shaped) murmur caused by the turbulence of blood flowing through either the aortic or the pulmonic valve. The murmur is most commonly midsystolic and ends before the second or closing sound (S_2) of the valve from which the murmur was generated, that is, aortic ejection murmurs end before A_2 and pulmonic ejection murmurs end before P_2. The loudness of the murmur depends in part on the pressure gradient across the valve and in part on other factors, such as thickness of the chest and the cardiac output. The shape depends on the acceleration and deceleration of blood flow across the valve as systole proceeds. When diastole is prolonged, for example, by a premature ventricular contraction, ejection murmurs become louder because of the passage of a large volume of blood through the valve. In general, the greater the cardiac output, the louder the murmur. Increases in cardiac output caused by hypermetabolic states, such as anemia, fever, or thyrotoxicosis, increase the loudness of the murmur. Decreases in cardiac output, as in congestive heart failure, decrease the loudness of the murmur.

The *regurgitant murmur* is a murmur produced by backward flow of blood from a high-pressure chamber to a compartment of lower pressure. Intensity may be constant, as in mitral regurgitation, tricuspid regurgitation, or ventricular septal defect, or it may be decrescendo, as in aortic and pulmonary regurgitation.

A number of maneuvers can be performed to alter the intensity of a systolic murmur and to help determine its origin. For example, the strain phase of the Valsalva maneuver reduces intrathoracic venous return and softens the murmur of aortic stenosis while intensifying that of hypertrophic cardiomyopathy (HCM). Squatting, which increases venous return, has the opposite effect. Isometric handgrip, which increases blood pressure and therefore reduces forward flow, softens the murmur of aortic stenosis and intensifies that of mitral regurgitation.

Innocent Murmurs

Innocent murmurs are a series of vibrations that are produced in the absence of significant abnormalities of cardiac anatomy or function (Table 65.1). Innocent murmurs usually can be distinguished from significant murmurs by the absence of other physical, radiologic, or electrocardiographic evidence of disease. Also, innocent murmurs usually are in early systole or midsystole, are grade 1 or 2 in intensity, and vary with respiration and position. Occasionally, echocardiography (see below) is performed to clarify the cause of a murmur, but more elaborate studies, such as stress tests, radionuclide studies, and cardiac catheterization, are used only after a murmur is determined to be not innocent and a more precise diagnosis is necessary.

The most common innocent *systolic murmur of childhood* and young adulthood that is clearly recognizable as benign based on the characteristics of the murmur alone is the *musical* or *vibratory* midsystolic murmur (best heard at the lower left sternal border) caused by the vibration of the leaflets of the pulmonary valve.

The *venous hum* is a continuous murmur, loudest in the neck, caused by altered flow through the jugular veins. It

TABLE 65.1 Benign or Innocent Systolic Murmurs

Vibratory ejection systolic murmur
Continuous murmur of venous hum
Pulmonic ejection systolic murmur
Aortic ejection systolic murmur
Murmur associated with pregnancy

can be eliminated by turning the patient's head, compressing the internal jugular vein on the side where the murmur is heard, or placing the patient in the supine position.

The *pulmonic ejection systolic murmur* is a systolic crescendo–decrescendo murmur generated by the flow of blood through the pulmonary valve. It is loudest in the left second intercostal space or at the midleft sternal border.

Similarly, the *aortic ejection systolic murmur* is an early systolic murmur generated by the flow of blood through the aortic valve. It is loudest in the right second intercostal space or at the apex of the heart. This innocent or flow murmur, caused by sclerosis of the aorta or the aortic valve, is the most common benign systolic murmur in middle-aged or elderly patients and may have a cooing quality. An echocardiogram may be necessary to rule out LV hypertrophy and aortic stenosis.

Benign flow murmurs are commonly heard in *pregnant women*. Because of the normally increased stroke volume at 28 to 30 weeks of gestation, diastolic filling sounds and systolic ejection murmurs of turbulent flow are common. In pregnant women, an S_3 may be prominent enough to be confused with the mid-diastolic murmur of mitral stenosis. The S_3 of pregnancy may be distinguished from the murmur of mitral stenosis, however, by the absence of an opening snap and by the accompanying hyperdynamic apical movement. An echocardiogram is indicated occasionally in some patients to make a precise diagnosis.

In a pregnant woman it is critical to compare the femoral and brachial pulses and the blood pressures in the presence of a heart murmur because coarctation of the aorta may present with a soft heart murmur and, if left untreated, may rarely result in aortic dissection or rupture.

Clinical Applications of Echocardiography

Echocardiography is a valuable adjunct to the clinical assessment of patients suspected of having cardiovascular disease (3). This technique uses high-frequency pulsed sound waves to record echoes of cardiac structures as they move within a beam of sound directed into the chest.

To record a *transthoracic M-mode echocardiogram*, an ultrasound transducer is placed at one point on the chest wall and rocked to inscribe an arc that encompasses several areas of the heart sequentially. The transducer serves as a source of the sound beam and as a receiver of the echoes. A *transthoracic two-dimensional (2D) echocardiogram* is recorded using a pulse transducer that is automatically directed across an arc, providing a simultaneous view of the cardiac structures, which is recorded on videotape. Both modes usually are combined and reported together. These procedures do not cause discomfort, but ideally the patient must be able to lie flat for approximately 30 to 45 minutes for performance of the test.

Echocardiography allows visualization of all four cardiac valves, the aortic root, both atria, the right ventricle, the left ventricle including all individual wall segments (Fig. 65.1), and the pericardium. The size and function of these structures are analyzed and patterns of specific diseases may be recognized.

M-mode echocardiography provides a one-dimensional or "ice pick" view of cardiac structures moving over time. It can be used to measure LV wall thickness and chamber size and to detect some valvular conditions. It has largely been supplanted by 2D echocardiography.

Two-dimensional echocardiography is particularly helpful in assessing LV function in patients with ischemic heart disease, in whom regional structure and function are most important. It should be understood that echo assessment of overall or regional LV function usually is semiquantitative. Wall motion usually is categorized as normal or as mildly, moderately, or severely depressed. An ejection fraction, if reported, often represents a visual estimate by the echocardiographer. Small differences reported in serial studies of the same patient, therefore, may not represent an important change unless the studies have been compared side by side by the same observer. LV systolic function can be quantitated by tracing the endocardial border of the left ventricle at end diastole and end systole in one or more tomographic planes. This technique is limited to patients with adequate endocardial border definition. The Food and Drug Administration has approved two intravenous contrast agents, Definity and Optison, which are microbubbles $<10\ \mu m$ in size with a high acoustic impedance and reflect ultrasonic transmissions better than blood (4). After administration of a contrast agent, the left ventricle is opacified with enhanced endocardial border definition, allowing a more accurate measurement of LV ejection fraction (5).

The noninvasive nature of the test, the lack of associated risks, and its ease of performance make 2D echocardiography extremely important in the evaluation of clinical signs and symptoms in patients with chest pain, palpitations, heart failure, cardiac murmurs, cardiomegaly, hypertension, and a systemic embolic event. The 2D echocardiogram can be diagnostic in cases of valvular heart disease, cardiomyopathy, congenital heart disease, aortic disease, intracardiac masses, pericardial effusion, and pericardial disease. Also, various echocardiographic indices of cardiac function and size add prognostic value to patients with cardiovascular disease. For example, assessments of left atrial size, left and right ventricular size and function, and LV diastolic function provide prognostic information on patients with heart failure (6). The 2D echocardiogram is an important screening tool in first-degree relatives (parents, siblings, and children) of patients with genetic cardiovascular diseases, such as bicuspid aortic valve (7), HCM (8), Marfan syndrome, and other related connective tissue disorders (9).

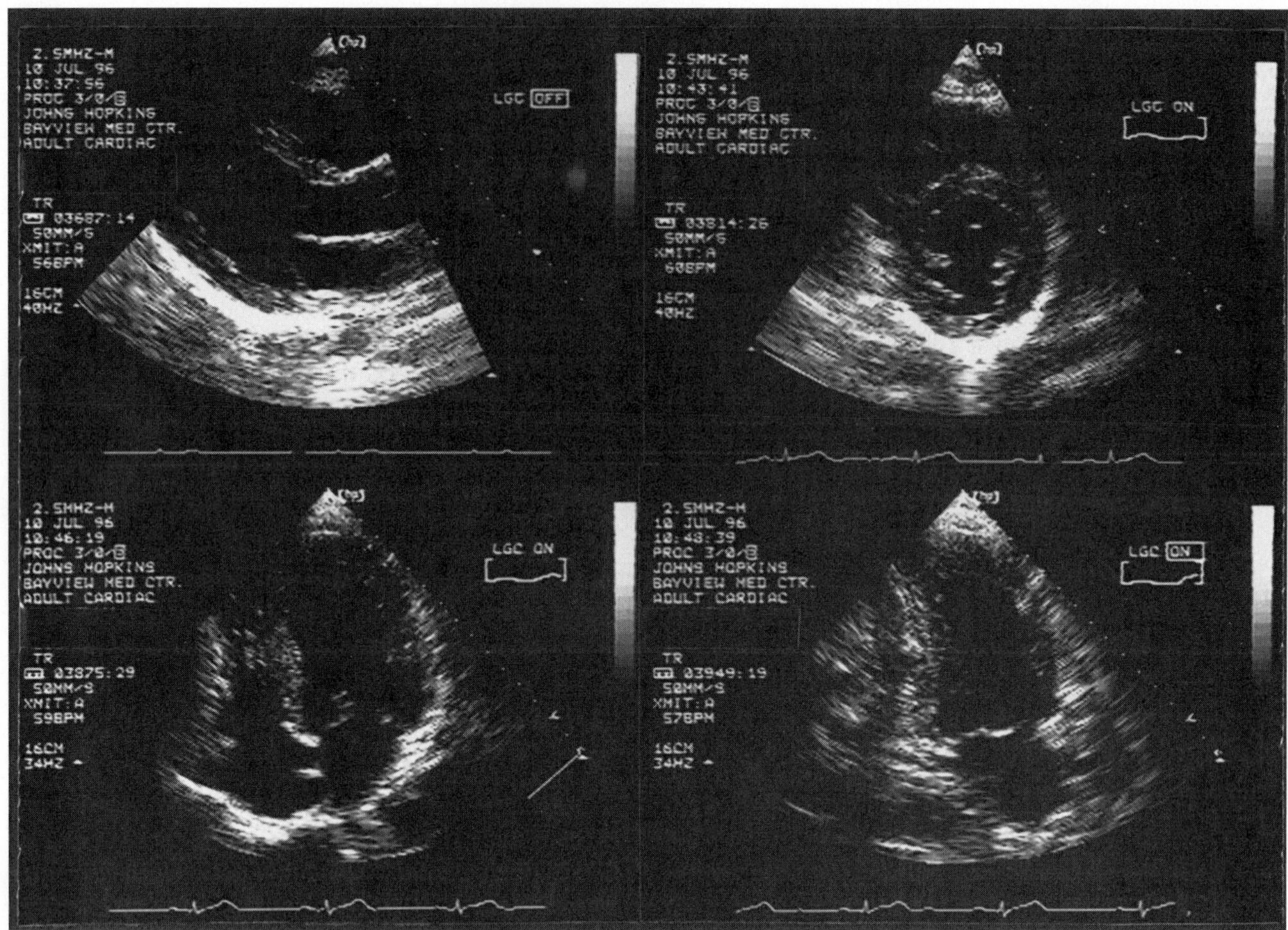

FIGURE 65.1. The four basic views of the two-dimensional echocardiogram. Tomographic slices obtained from different vantage points and angles reveal valvular structure and all left ventricular walls. **Top left:** Parasternal long-axis view demonstrating septum and posterior wall. **Top right:** Parasternal short-axis view displaying a "bread loaf" slice of the left ventricle. **Bottom left:** Apical four-chamber view revealing septum, apex, and lateral wall. **Bottom right:** Apical two-chamber view revealing inferior wall, apex, and lateral wall.

Doppler echocardiography is an extremely useful tool for the detection and quantification of the severity of valvular heart disease. High-frequency sound is directed at a column of moving red blood cells, and the reflected sound is analyzed for changes in frequency, which indicate the direction and velocity of flow. Flow velocity information is color coded and superimposed on the 2D echocardiographic image, providing visual representation of blood flow through the heart and great vessels.

In valvular stenosis, a high-velocity jet of blood is detected distal to the stenosis; the higher the transvalvular gradient, the higher the velocity of the jet. The pressure gradient across a valve and the area of the aortic (10,11) and mitral (12) valves can be calculated, providing precise quantification of the severity of aortic and mitral stenosis.

Valvular regurgitation can be detected by reverse flow and its severity estimated, usually by visualization of the origin, width, direction, and extent of the regurgitant jet in the receiving chamber by color flow Doppler (13). For example, mitral regurgitation is considered severe on a color Doppler study if a central regurgitant jet occupies >40% of the area of the left atrium during systole (14). The qualitative assessment of mitral regurgitation can be difficult, especially with eccentric regurgitant jets. For the severity of aortic and mitral regurgitation, the American Society of Echocardiography has recommended the quantitative assessment of valvular regurgitation (13), and this has been shown to be a powerful predictor of clinical outcomes in patients with asymptomatic mitral regurgitation (15). A small degree of tricuspid regurgitation usually is seen in normal subjects and does not represent disease. The presence of tricuspid regurgitation allows estimation of right ventricular systolic pressure, which is equal to the pulmonary artery systolic pressure in the absence of pulmonic stenosis. This is useful in the detection and followup of patients with pulmonary hypertension of any cause. Small amounts of mitral and pulmonic regurgitation usually are seen in normal people and are not a cause for concern if the echocardiographer comments that the extent is "mild." Small amounts of aortic regurgitation are frequently seen and are considered normal if their extent is graded as "trivial."

Doppler echocardiography often is used to detect *diastolic dysfunction* (16,17), a frequent contributor to the development of congestive heart failure, especially in the elderly (see Chapter 66). The normal diastolic flow pattern consists of two phases: passive filling during early diastole (termed the *E wave*), which is aided by elastic recoil of the ventricle, and filling during late diastole (termed the *A wave*) due to atrial contraction. In young normal people, the left ventricle is pliable, and elastic recoil during diastole is vigorous, resulting in brisk early filling and hence a large E wave. Very little filling then remains to be accomplished during late diastole, hence a small A wave occurs. The ratio of early to late filling (E/A ratio) therefore is high, typically approximately 1.5 to 2.0 in normal people in their thirties or forties. However, the left ventricle loses its pliability in patients with LV hypertrophy, other forms of chronic heart disease, and even during the process of normal aging. Early diastolic elastic recoil then becomes ineffective in aiding filling, and the E wave becomes small. To compensate, a substantial proportion of filling must occur during late diastole, and the A wave enlarges. The E/A ratio thus is reduced. When the ratio falls to <1, "grade I diastolic dysfunction" is said to be present. This pattern is also called "abnormal relaxation." Grade I diastolic dysfunction is a normal finding in people older than 65 years.

However, the E/A ratio is an imperfect index of diastolic function because the velocity of early LV filling depends on several factors in addition to LV relaxation. For instance, a high left atrial pressure, which occurs in congestive heart failure, causes a high AV pressure gradient, which accelerates early filling irrespective of LV stiffness, resulting in a large E wave and a high E/A ratio. This pattern is called *pseudonormalization* of the E/A ratio, or "grade II diastolic dysfunction." Distinguishing pseudonormal from normal may require ancillary Doppler procedures, such as repeating the recording during a Valsalva maneuver, measuring flow through the pulmonary vein, or tissue Doppler imaging of mitral annular motion. However, the presence of grade II diastolic dysfunction should be considered likely in the elderly and in people with LV hypertrophy who are found to have a high E/A ratio, because these individuals are likely to have grade I diastolic dysfunction at baseline. Common causes of grade II diastolic dysfunction include systolic dysfunction, valvular heart disease, fluid overload, and myocardial ischemia. When grade II diastolic dysfunction occurs in the absence of those conditions, "diastolic heart failure" is considered to be present. This latter phenomenon is commonly seen in the elderly in the presence of LV hypertrophy or severe hypertension.

When the E/A ratio is >2.0, "grade III diastolic dysfunction" or a "restrictive pattern" is said to be present. This occurs in restrictive cardiomyopathy and constrictive pericarditis, but also in all conditions that cause grade II diastolic dysfunction, when they are severe.

Several conditions may produce the pattern of grade II or III diastolic dysfunction in the absence of congestive heart failure. For example, in significant mitral regurgitation that is well compensated, the left atrial pressure in *early* diastole may be elevated because of the large "v" wave, increasing the E/A ratio, but the *mean* diastolic pressure may not be high enough to cause pulmonary congestion. Also, in patients who have recently converted from atrial fibrillation to sinus rhythm, a transient atrial myopathy is often present, resulting in a small "A" wave and a high E/A ratio (18).

In patients in whom a large E wave is present, an S_3 is often audible. These patients include normal people younger than 30 years, elderly patients with congestive heart failure, and patients with constrictive cardiomyopathy, in whom the early diastolic sound is called a *pericardial knock*. In patients in whom a large A wave is present, an S_4 is usually audible. These patients include normal elderly people and patients with LV hypertrophy resulting from hypertension or aortic stenosis.

A common limitation of standard transthoracic echocardiography is that ultrasound penetrates lung and bone poorly, and the available acoustic window is limited in many patients, resulting in poor-quality studies. The technique of *transesophageal echocardiography* (TEE) has extended the diagnostic utility of echocardiography by allowing high-quality studies, with markedly increased resolution, in all patients (19,20). Additional structures can be assessed, including the venae cavae, coronary sinus, pulmonary veins, atrial septum, atrial appendages, pulmonary artery, and ascending and descending aorta. Valve leaflets are seen with great clarity. Resolution is adequate to detect atheromas on the walls of the aorta. The method transforms a noninvasive imaging modality into a semi-invasive one; the procedure is similar to esophagoscopy and is often performed in an endoscopy unit, often on an outpatient basis. The patient is asked to fast for 6 to 8 hours and is treated with a pharyngeal topical anesthetic and intravenous sedation. The patient then is assisted in swallowing a small (i.e., 1-cm diameter) echo transducer mounted on a gastroscopelike tube. Visualization of the cardiac structures from the esophagus and stomach usually is accomplished in approximately 20 minutes. The examination may include the intravenous injection of agitated saline, which creates ultrasonic contrast via tiny bubbles, to assess for right-to-left shunting. Complications of TEE are rare and include inability to intubate the esophagus successfully (1.9%), pulmonary difficulties such as laryngospasm (0.14%), cardiac arrhythmias (0.5%), and bleeding (0.2%) (21,22). Esophageal perforation is extremely rare (21). TEE is contraindicated in patients with severe atlantoaxial joint disease with inability to flex the neck, history of radiation to the chest, perforated viscus, and esophageal pathology (e.g., varices, strictures, carcinoma, scleroderma, or diverticula). Respiratory compromise may occur in patients with severe underlying pulmonary disease or obstructive sleep apnea, and an anesthesiologist may need to be consulted for assistance with patient management during the study.

The indications for TEE are evolving. The method allows visualization of almost the entire aorta and is sensitive (97.7%) and specific (76.9%) in the diagnosis of aortic dissection (23). The method is much better than transthoracic echocardiography for visualizing cardiac sources of embolus, such as thrombus in the left atrium or left atrial appendage, sluggish blood flow in the left atrium (spontaneous echo contrast), atrial septal aneurysm, patent foramen ovale, and complex aortic atheromas, sometimes with attached thrombus. Therefore, it often is ordered in patients with cryptogenic strokes (i.e., strokes in patients without evidence of atheroma in the carotid or vertebral systems). Because TEE can detect left atrial thrombi with a high degree of accuracy, TEE can guide treatment of patients with recent-onset atrial fibrillation who are being considered for cardioversion (24). This is the method of choice for assessing the function of prosthetic mitral valves and for visualizing vegetations or intracardiac abscesses caused by endocarditis. TEE is sometimes indicated when transthoracic echo quality is poor and information about cardiac structure or function is deemed crucial.

SELECTED DISORDERS ASSOCIATED WITH ABNORMAL HEART SOUNDS

Aortic Stenosis

Stenosis of the aortic valve obstructs the flow of blood into the aorta and therefore raises the LV pressure above the aortic pressure. The pressure gradient across the valve is related to the severity of the stenosis. The elevated pressure results in a concentric hypertrophy of the left ventricle. Symptoms develop when the left ventricle can no longer compensate for the pressure load; the heart fails and the cardiac output declines.

Aortic stenosis may occur at any one of several levels. The most common obstruction (75% of patients) occurs at the aortic valve, although patients with subvalvular and supravalvular aortic stenosis may have symptoms and signs of severity similar to those of valvular disease. It is particularly important to differentiate fixed aortic outflow obstruction from HCM, in which the obstruction is dynamic in nature (Table 65.2).

Hemodynamically significant stenosis usually is associated with a gradient $\geq$50 mm Hg (unless cardiac output is reduced, in which case the gradient may be much lower even if there is severe stenosis). The effective aortic valve orifice in patients with severe obstruction usually is <0.4 or 0.5 cm^2 per square millimeter of body surface area (compared to 1.6–2.6 cm^2 per square millimeter in normal people). Many laboratories report absolute, rather than normalized, valve areas. At some centers, aortic stenosis is considered severe if the valve area is <0.75 cm^2. At most centers, aortic valve areas of <1.0 cm^2 are considered

TABLE 65.2 Comparison of Valvular Aortic Stenosis and Hypertrophic Cardiomyopathy

	Valvular Aortic Stenosis	*Hypertrophic Cardiomyopathy*
Symptoms and signs	Dyspnea, angina, syncope, or near-syncope. Systolic ejection murmur loudest at aortic area or at apex; louder if patient squats. A_2 may not be audible. S_4 is common. Ejection sounds are common. Carotid upstroke is delayed.	Dyspnea, angina, syncope, or near-syncope. Systolic ejection murmur loudest at left lower sternal border; louder if patient stands or performs a Valsalva maneuver. A_2 usually is audible. S_4 is very common. Ejection sounds are uncommon. Carotid upstroke is brisk.
Electrocardiogram	LVH and strain pattern.	LVH and strain pattern; Q waves in inferior and lateral leads are common.
Chest x-ray film	LVH is a late sign. Aortic valve is always calcified (may be seen only on fluoroscopy). Ascending aorta may be dilated.	LVH may occur but unpredictably. Aortic valve is not calcified. Ascending aorta is not dilated.
Echocardiogram	Characteristic echoes of valvular calcification and valvular stenosis.	Disproportionate septal hypertrophy and systolic anterior displacement of mitral valve may be present.

LVH, left ventricular hypertrophy.

severe, 1.0 to 1.5 cm^2 considered moderate, and >1.5 cm^2 considered mild.

Causes and Epidemiology

In patients younger than 30 years, aortic stenosis most likely is caused by a congenitally stenotic unicuspid valve. Between the ages of 30 and 65 years, a bicuspid aortic valve, which has become calcified and gradually more rigid over the years, is the most common cause of aortic stenosis. A bicuspid aortic valve is found in 1% to 2% of the population, predominantly in men (25). Rheumatic valvular disease accounts for <25% of cases of isolated aortic stenosis in patients between the ages of 30 and 70 years. With the decline of rheumatic fever and the aging of the population, calcific aortic stenosis of an anatomically normal trileaflet valve has become the most common form of the disease encountered, present in 2% to 4% of adults older than 65 years (26). Evidence suggests that calcific aortic stenosis is a chronic, active inflammatory process associated with atherosclerotic risk factors rather than a degenerative process associated with aging (27). Except in the elderly, in whom the prevalence is the same in both sexes, isolated aortic stenosis is three to four times more common in men.

Natural History and Symptoms

Patients with aortic stenosis usually are asymptomatic until late in the course of their disease. Mild to moderate obstruction does not greatly compromise LV function, and even patients with severe stenosis may compensate for years before they develop symptoms. Patients with asymptomatic severe aortic stenosis have a 1% per year risk of sudden death (28). In a series of 622 adults with asymptomatic severe aortic stenosis, most patients became symptomatic within 5 years, and aortic valve area and LV hypertrophy predicted the development of symptoms (28). Once a patient develops symptoms, survival declines precipitously. If the lesion is not corrected, the average patient dies in approximately 4 years.

The earliest symptoms are easy fatigability and excessive dyspnea during or after strenuous exercise. Syncope or near-syncope with effort (see Chapter 89), angina (see Chapter 62), and dyspnea on usual exercise (see Chapter 66) are indicative of severe valvular obstruction. Patients with heart failure do not survive as long (2 years) as do patients with syncope (3 years) or angina (5 years) (29). Sudden death occurs in approximately 15% of symptomatic patients.

Physical Findings

Patients with aortic stenosis usually have a loud (grade 3–4) systolic ejection murmur. The maximal intensity of the murmur is located at the second right intercostal space or at the cardiac apex. The murmur often has a musical cooing quality at the apex. There is often a thrill in the suprasternal notch or the second right intercostal space. However, the loudness of the murmur may not correlate with the severity of stenosis. Also, if cardiac output is reduced, as in congestive heart failure, or if the diameter of the chest is increased, the intensity of the murmur may be less than expected. A late peak to the murmur suggests severe obstruction, but this may be difficult to appreciate with a stethoscope, and absence of the late peak does not mean that obstruction is not severe. Augmentation of the murmur when the patient suddenly squats and diminution of the murmur when the patient stands or performs a Valsalva maneuver are characteristic of aortic stenosis.

The systolic murmur, although it may not be loud, is an invariable sign of aortic stenosis. Other cardiac sounds depend on the nature of the stenotic lesion. An early systolic ejection click is commonly heard when the valve is still mobile. The second aortic sound (A_2) often is not audible when the valve is so rigid that S_2 has only one component (P_2). Paradoxical splitting of the second heart sound, in the absence of left bundle-branch block, is a sign of severity. A small pulse pressure (<30 mm Hg) also indicates severe obstruction (in elderly people, the pulse pressure may be normal despite severe stenosis). A slowly rising pulse—best assessed by palpation of a carotid artery—is characteristic. Under age 40 years, an S_4 is another sign of severe obstruction; over age 40 years, an S_4 is common because of the high prevalence of hypertensive and ischemic heart disease and does not correlate with severity of stenosis.

Based on a review of available evidence of the precision and accuracy of the clinical examination for abnormal systolic murmurs, the likelihood of aortic stenosis is increased by the presence of effort syncope, slowly rising carotid pulse, mid or late systolic peak of murmur, soft or absent S_2, apical to carotid delay, or brachioradial delay (30). The regurgitant early diastolic murmur of aortic insufficiency is heard in 30% to 40% of patients with aortic valve stenosis.

Laboratory Evaluation

An electrocardiogram (ECG), a chest x-ray film, and an echocardiogram should be obtained routinely in a patient suspected of having aortic stenosis.

Electrocardiogram

The ECG usually is normal until stenosis becomes severe, at which point LV hypertrophy (Table 65.3 and Fig. 65.2) and nonspecific ST depression and T-wave inversion are common but not invariable. In older patients particularly, an abnormal ECG cannot be relied upon to reflect severity because there are often other reasons why it might be abnormal.

TABLE 65.3 Principal Electrocardiographic Features of Left Ventricular Hypertrophy

Electrocardiographic Criteria	*Point System for Diagnosis*[a]
Negative components of P in $V_1 \geq 1$ mm and ≥ 0.04 s	3 points
QRS	
Largest limb lead R or S ≥ 20 mm or largest chest lead S before transition or R after transition ≥ 30 mm	3 points
or	
Largest S before transition plus largest R after transition = 45 mm;	
Frontal plane axis ≥ -30 degrees	2 points
Duration in extremity lead ≥ 0.09 s	1 point
Intrinsicoid deflection ≥ 0.05 s	1 point
ST-T	
In general, opposite QRS:	
Without digitalis	3 points
With digitalis	1 point

[a]Interpretation of point score: 6 points, left ventricular hypertrophy; 5 points, probable left ventricular hypertrophy; 4 points, possible left ventricular hypertrophy. If only voltage criteria are met, ECG may be designated as borderline, and left ventricular hypertrophy is suggested only by voltage and should be excluded by other clinical means.

Modified from Horan LG, Flowers NC. Electrocardiography and vectorcardiography. In: Braunwald E, ed. Heart disease: a textbook of cardiovascular medicine. Philadelphia: WB Saunders, 1980:229, with permission.

Chest X-Ray Film

Calcification of the aortic valve is always present in patients older than 40 years with aortic stenosis, but often fluoroscopy is necessary to reveal it. Poststenotic dilation of the ascending aorta is also commonly seen. The heart size and configuration usually are normal until the disease is far advanced.

Echocardiogram

Echocardiography reveals immobile and usually calcified aortic valve leaflets. An increase in ventricular wall thickness on echocardiography implies severe obstruction if there is no other cause for hypertrophy. The severity of aortic stenosis can be accurately assessed in nearly all patients by Doppler echocardiography by measurement of the maximum aortic jet velocity, calculation of the maximum and mean transaortic pressure gradients, and determination of the aortic valve area by the continuity equation (31). Assessment of the aortic valve area by cardiac catheterization is recommended when the echocardiogram is nondiagnostic or when there is a discrepancy between the clinical picture and the echocardiographic data. The valve area is generally considered a better measure of severity of aortic stenosis than the gradient because the gradient may be deceptively low in the presence of reduced cardiac output caused by LV dysfunction, even with severe stenosis (see below). Doppler echocardiography is

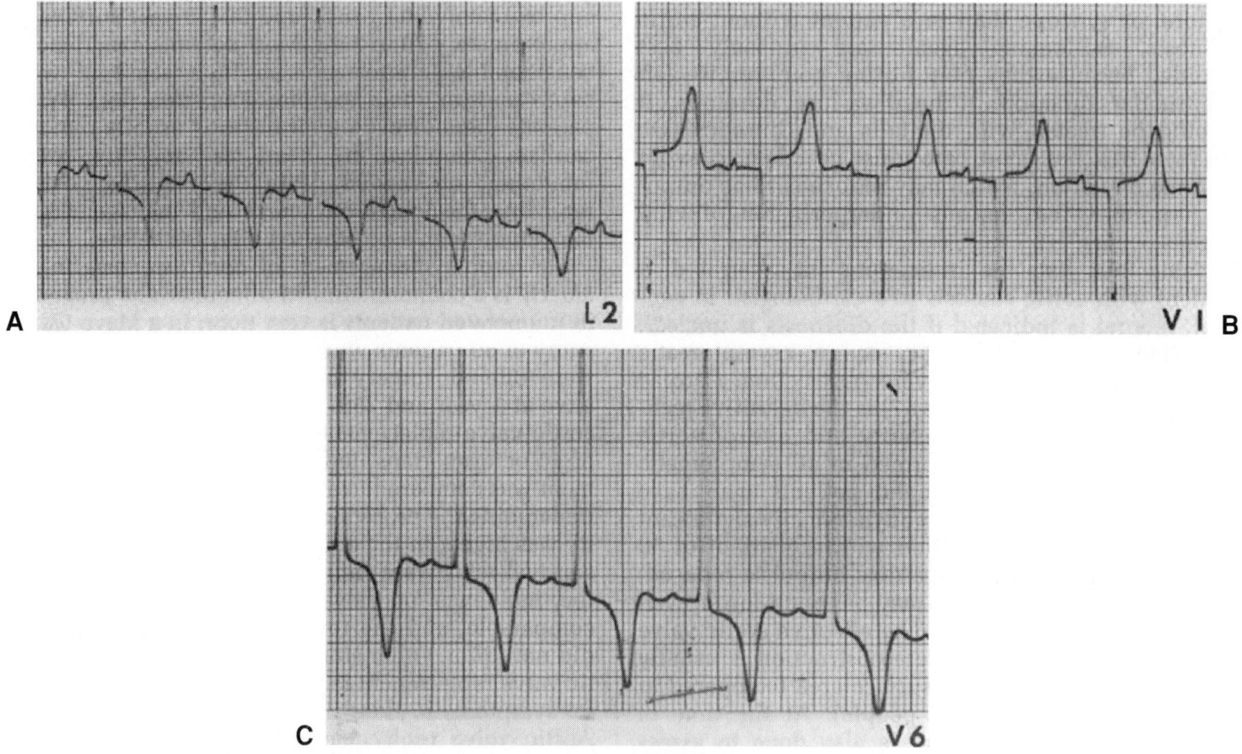

FIGURE 65.2. Electrocardiogram of a patient with left ventricular hypertrophy (Table 65.3).

helpful in distinguishing aortic stenosis from aortic valve sclerosis, in which no significant gradient is present.

Management

Asymptomatic patients with mild or moderate disease should be reassessed every 12 months so that signs of progressive disease can be detected promptly. Reassessment should include interval history, pertinent physical examination, ECG, chest x-ray film, and echocardiogram. Current clinical guidelines recommend a transthoracic echocardiogram annually in severe asymptomatic aortic stenosis, every 2 years in moderate aortic stenosis, and every 5 years in mild aortic stenosis (1). Typically, the rate of progression in the aortic valve area is a decrease of 0.1 cm^2 per year (26).The asymptomatic patient with severe aortic stenosis presents a management dilemma. Although sudden death is extremely rare in asymptomatic patients (approximately 1% per year) (28), symptoms may appear suddenly and progress rapidly to sudden death (as early as 3 months after symptoms appear). There is a 67% probability of remaining asymptomatic at 2 years and a 33% probability at 5 years with severe aortic stenosis (28). Although these factors suggest that prophylactic valve replacement might be indicated in asymptomatic patients with severe disease, this must be weighed against the operative mortality (3%–12%), the risk of prosthetic valve complications (1%–2% per year), and the fact that many patients would be operated on needlessly (32). Patients with moderate to severe asymptomatic aortic stenosis, therefore, should be referred to a cardiologist. However, many cardiologists recommend that asymptomatic patients be followed extremely closely without prophylactic surgery. These issues should be discussed with the patient. It is accepted practice to perform aortic valve replacement in asymptomatic patients with severe (and sometimes moderate) aortic stenosis who require open heart procedures, such as coronary artery bypass grafting or surgery involving the aorta, or in women contemplating pregnancy.

Patients should be cautioned to avoid undue exertion because acute heart failure, arrhythmia, and sudden death are more likely under such circumstances. Patients with mild aortic stenosis do not have to restrict their physical activity. On the other hand, patients with moderate aortic stenosis should not participate in competitive sports, and those with severe aortic stenosis should engage in only low-level activities (1). The risk of subacute bacterial endocarditis is increased in patients with aortic stenosis and is unrelated to the severity of the stenosis (the risk is unchanged after aortic valve surgery; see below). Therefore, antibiotic prophylaxis (see Chapter 93) is necessary before dental and surgical procedures. Because aortic stenosis is an inflammatory process similar to that of atherosclerosis, prospective studies are currently in progress to determine if statin therapy can retard the progression of calcific aortic stenosis. In one small, prospective study, patients with calcific aortic stenosis who did not have an indication for statin therapy were randomized to atorvastatin or placebo, with a median followup period of 25 months (33). Despite the intensive lipid-lowering effect, atorvastatin did not delay the progression nor cause regression of the disease process.

Atrial arrhythmias are uncommon; if they occur, they must be treated aggressively (see Chapter 64) because they are more likely to cause angina, heart failure, or syncope than in a patient without aortic stenosis. β-Blockers are best avoided in patients with severe aortic stenosis because the agents may compromise LV function. Heart failure, if it develops, should be treated with diuretics (see Chapter 66), but great care must be taken to avoid volume depletion, which may reduce cardiac output to a point where serious hypoperfusion of vital organs occurs.

Table 65.4 lists the indications for referral of a patient with aortic stenosis to a cardiologist. In general, referral is indicated if the diagnosis is unclear, if the patient is symptomatic, or if an asymptomatic patient has moderate to severe obstruction.

The cardiologist is likely to recommend replacement of the stenotic aortic valve with a prosthesis in all symptomatic patients and in asymptomatic patients with signs of severe obstruction who are found to have LV dysfunction or other high risk features. Coronary angiography is required in most patients prior to valve surgery to assess the patency of the coronary arteries to determine if concomitant coronary artery bypass graft surgery is needed.

Operative mortality is 1% to 9% in patients without LV failure (26) and 10% to 25% in patients with LV failure (34). The patient's postoperative health and long-term survival depend on a number of factors (including age, general health, and LV function), but overall, the 5-year

TABLE 65.4 Indications for Referral of Patients with Aortic Stenosis

If there is a question about the diagnosis or severity
If the patient is symptomatic
If the asymptomatic patient has signs of severe obstruction
Physical signs
Small pulse pressure (<30 mm Hg)
Late peak of systolic murmur
Diminished A_2
Paradoxical splitting of A_2
Electrocardiogram
Left ventricular hypertrophy (without hypertension)
ST depression and T-wave inversion
Chest x-ray film
Left ventricular hypertrophy (without hypertension)
Echocardiogram
Concentric left ventricular hypertrophy
Doppler-calculated gradient >50 mm Hg or valve area <0.75 cm^2

survival is approximately 80% to 85% and the 10-year survival is approximately 70% to 75%. Most patients experience a considerable improvement in their sense of well-being and exercise tolerance. Death, if it occurs, usually results from a cardiac complication (heart failure, myocardial infarction, or sudden death). (For further details regarding the long-term course and management of the patient with a prosthetic valve, see below.)

The proper management of *aortic stenosis in the elderly* is a common clinical challenge. The prognosis in unoperated patients is very poor. In a study of 50 patients with a mean age of 77 years who were offered surgery but refused, only 57% were alive at 1 year and 25% at 3 years (35). In a study of aortic valve replacement in the elderly (36), a group of 44 octogenarians undergoing aortic valve replacement was compared with a group of 83 younger patients undergoing the procedure. Although the early mortality was higher in the elderly (14% vs. 4%), 2-year survival rates were similar (73% vs. 90%, an insignificant difference), the incidence of valve-related complications was comparable, and the total duration of hospital stay did not differ. Other studies confirm that aortic valve replacement is the most appropriate therapy for symptomatic elderly patients with aortic stenosis. Aortic valve replacement should not be withheld because of age itself, although intercurrent illness, common in the elderly, may complicate decision making.

Percutaneous balloon valvuloplasty is a technique in which one or more balloons are placed across a stenotic aortic valve and are then inflated in an attempt to reduce the severity of stenosis. This method has achieved excellent results in children with congenital aortic stenosis. In adults, it has been applied mainly to elderly patients or to those who are considered to be poor surgical candidates. Although the transaortic gradient usually is reduced and initial clinical improvement is achieved, overall results have not been encouraging because high rates of death (24%) and recurrences of severe symptoms of aortic stenosis (47%) have been reported within 6 months of the procedure (37). Long-term survival after the procedure is dismal and resembles the natural history of untreated aortic stenosis. At present, aortic valvuloplasty for adults has been abandoned at most centers and should be considered only in extraordinary circumstances, for example, for a severely symptomatic and hemodynamically compromised patient who requires urgent management of aortic stenosis as a "bridge" to aortic valve replacement.

Hypertrophic Cardiomyopathy

HCM is a disease of cardiac muscle characterized by severe myocardial hypertrophy in the absence of conditions that cause secondary hypertrophy of the heart muscle, such as hypertension and aortic stenosis. The left ventricle is hypercontractile and, during systole, ejects essentially all of its blood, leaving a "clenched fist" with very high wall stress. HCM has been called by a variety of names, including asymmetrical septal hypertrophy (because of predominant hypertrophy in the septal region) and idiopathic hypertrophic subaortic stenosis (because of the common presence of a dynamic outflow tract gradient) (38). However, some patients with HCM do not have asymmetrical septal hypertrophy and may have either concentric hypertrophy or only apical hypertrophy of the left ventricle. In addition, the majority of patients with HCM do not have a significant resting outflow tract gradient (38). In contrast to the microscopic appearance of secondary LV hypertrophy, in which the fibers are enlarged but are properly oriented, the myofibrils in HCM are characterized by myofibrillary disarray (8).

Causes and Epidemiology

The prevalence of HCM in young adults is thought to be approximately 2 per 1,000 (39) but is higher in the elderly. In fact, HCM is the most common genetic cardiovascular disease. The disease occurs as a familial inherited disease in approximately 60% of cases and as a sporadic disease, without affected first-degree relatives, in the remainder. Men and women are equally likely to be affected. In the familial form, the mode of inheritance is autosomal dominant in approximately 75% of pedigrees. A variety of missense mutations have been identified in patients with HCM, including mutations in the β-myosin heavy chain gene (chromosome 14), the cardiac troponin T gene (chromosome 1), and the α-tropomyosin gene (chromosome 15). All these genes code for sarcomeric proteins. The presence of these mutant components perturbs overall contractile function, and cardiac hypertrophy develops as a compensatory response.

Natural History and Symptoms

As echocardiography has become more widely used for the evaluation of patients with heart murmurs, it has become clear that most patients with HCM are asymptomatic or have only mild symptoms (38). Unless there is a family history of sudden death, the prognosis in this group is excellent. One study of 25 patients showed neither death nor progression of disease over a 4.4-year followup period (40).

The most common symptom of patients with HCM is dyspnea, but patients also often complain of angina (with or without evidence of occlusive coronary artery disease) and syncope or near-syncope. These symptoms are much more likely to be induced by exertion than to occur spontaneously. Once marked symptoms develop, some patients become rapidly worse, with progressive heart failure, angina, or arrhythmias.

The overall mortality for patients with HCM is $<1\%$ per year (8). However, a subset of patients are at high risk for sudden death, primarily from ventricular arrhythmias.

The incidence of sudden death is approximately 3% to 4% per year in symptomatic patients with HCM, but some families have a particularly high incidence, depending on the specific mutation in the pedigree. For example, survival is poor in cardiac troponin T mutations but near normal in α-tropomyosin mutations (41). Some of the major clinical risk factors that are strong predictors of sudden death include a history of cardiac arrest, spontaneous sustained ventricular tachycardia, and a first-degree relative with a history of sudden death. Some of the minor clinical risk factors for sudden death are unexplained syncope, nonsustained ventricular tachycardia, LV wall thickness >30 mm, abnormal blood pressure response with exercise, LV outflow obstruction, and the presence of microvascular obstruction on a nuclear or magnetic resonance imaging study (38).

Physical Findings

Table 65.2 lists the clinical and laboratory features that distinguish aortic stenosis from HCM. The characteristic signs of the disease are a sustained LV apical impulse, a loud S_4, and a harsh systolic ejection murmur, loudest at the left lower border of the sternum and often accompanied by a thrill. The location of the murmur helps to distinguish the condition from valvular aortic stenosis. Other distinguishing features are as follows: the second heart sound (A_2) usually is audible, a diastolic murmur is rare, the pulse pressure is normal, ejection sounds are uncommon, and, most important, the upstroke of the carotid pulse is brisk. In addition, the murmur of HCM is augmented when the patient stands or during the strain phase of a Valsalva maneuver and is diminished when the patient squats—the opposite of the findings in patients with aortic stenosis. The murmur often diminishes rapidly during the release phase of the Valsalva maneuver.

Laboratory Evaluation

An ECG, chest x-ray film, and echocardiogram should be obtained routinely in patients suspected of having HCM. Genetic testing to identify a specific mutation is available at specialized medical centers, although the clinical value of this screening is uncertain.

Electrocardiogram

The ECG is abnormal in most patients and is always abnormal in patients with obstruction. Typically, there is evidence of LV hypertrophy (Fig. 65.2 and Table 65.3), and there is nonspecific ST depression and T-wave inversion. Q waves are often seen in the inferior and lateral leads, reflecting septal hypertrophy.

Chest X-Ray Film

The left ventricle is sometimes enlarged, but unpredictably so. In contrast to aortic valvular stenosis, the aortic valve is not calcified and the ascending aorta is not dilated.

Echocardiogram

Echocardiography is diagnostic; it usually demonstrates a thickened ventricular septum, hypertrophied out of proportion to the posterior wall of the left ventricle, although concentric or apical hypertrophy is sometimes present. Cavity obliteration, or near cavity obliteration, usually occurs during systole. The mitral valve apparatus moves anteriorly during systole (systolic anterior motion), and may contribute to obstruction of the outflow tract and to mitral regurgitation.

Management

The goal of therapy is to relieve symptoms by reducing the hypercontractile state of the left ventricle and the dynamic LV outflow tract obstruction. Currently, this is best accomplished using the calcium channel blocker verapamil (240 mg daily of long-acting formulation, maximum 480 mg daily) (38) unless the patient has signs or symptoms of heart failure or marked LV outflow tract obstruction. Alternatively, a β-blocker may be prescribed (e.g., metoprolol, 25 mg twice daily, with a maximum total dose of 600 mg daily, or an equivalent sustained-release preparation). Angina, especially, is often relieved by treatment, but dyspnea also may be decreased as a result of a slower heart rate and increased LV filling time. Although it is not clear that the risk of sudden death is reduced by therapy, most patients are symptomatically improved or at least stabilized by treatment. Disopyramide (initial dose of 100 mg of sustained-release formulation twice daily, maximum total dose 600 mg daily) (38), a type IA antiarrhythmic agent (see Chapter 64) with negative inotropic properties, has also been used successfully in patients with HCM and does not appear to be proarrhythmic in this patient population (42). However, long-term studies are necessary to assess for the efficacy and side effects of this therapy.

Drugs that increase ventricular contractility or decrease ventricular volume (digitalis, vasodilators, β-adrenergic stimulants, and diuretics) are best avoided, if possible. Patients, even if asymptomatic, should avoid undue exertion (e.g., running) and participation in competitive sports (43).

Patients with HCM have an increased risk for endocarditis and therefore should receive antibiotic prophylaxis before dental and surgical procedures (see Chapter 93).

Many patients with HCM eventually become refractory to beta blockers or verapamil or develop intolerable side effects from those medications. Two other therapies are also sometimes used in patients with HCM, especially when medications are ineffective or are poorly tolerated. First, dual-chamber cardiac pacing, even in the absence of bradyarrhythmias, may reduce the symptoms of angina, dyspnea, and presyncope over 6 to 12 weeks. Some (44,45), but not all (46,47), studies have shown that objective measures of disease, such as exercise treadmill time and outflow tract gradient, also improve with this therapy. Second, studies suggest that alcohol, injected during cardiac catheterization to produce septal ablation, is a helpful procedure in some patients. The alcohol is injected into a septal perforator branch of the left anterior descending coronary artery supplying the proximal septum and results in a controlled and localized myocardial infarction with thinning of the septum and reduction of the LV outflow tract gradient (48). Because of the controlled myocardial infarction and resultant scarring, there may be a potential risk for ventricular arrhythmias and sudden death.

An alternative to alcohol-induced septal ablation in patients who are severely symptomatic and refractory to medical therapy is surgical removal of a portion of the hypertrophied septum (septal myectomy). Improved surgical techniques have reduced the perioperative mortality of this procedure to 1% to 2% (49). However, the elderly are at higher risk for complications. Symptoms of heart failure are relieved through reduction of the LV outflow tract gradient, and long-term mortality is similar to that of the general population (50,51). However, this surgery is not widely available and is performed mainly at tertiary referral centers. Patients with HCM who show progression of symptoms or intolerance of medical treatment should be referred to a cardiologist and, if appropriate, to a cardiac surgeon for consideration of these alternative treatments.

For primary or secondary prevention of sudden cardiac death, an implantable cardiac defibrillator should be placed in patients who have major predictors of sudden cardiac death, such as history of cardiac arrest, sudden death in first-degree relatives with HCM, and sustained ventricular arrhythmias. Patients with three or more minor risk factors for sudden death, as discussed above, also should be considered for an implantable defibrillator. Once the diagnosis of HCM is made, patients should be risk stratified with an exercise treadmill test and a 48-hour Holter monitor.

Screening of first-degree relatives by echocardiography may detect other family members with the syndrome. Because there is a bimodal distribution of the disease process, an echocardiogram should be done approximately every 5 years to assess for the echocardiographic features of HCM. Referral to a center that can perform genetic testing to identify the specific mutation and offer genetic counseling also can be considered.

Atrial Septal Defect

Atrial septal defect of the ostium secundum type (in the midportion of the septum, known as the fossa ovalis) is one of the most common congenital cardiac diseases diagnosed in adults. It causes, until late in the course (see below), a left-to-right atrial shunt with volume overload of the right ventricle and overperfusion of the lungs. Ostium primum atrial septal defect, which occurs as part of the spectrum of endocardial cushion defects, is a less common form of this condition. It is often associated with trisomy 21 (Down syndrome).

Causes and Epidemiology

The defect is more common in females; the reported female/male ratio ranges from 1.5 to 3.5:1. Occasionally the defect is associated with other cardiac abnormalities, including mitral valve prolapse, pulmonic stenosis, and HCM.

Natural History and Symptoms

Patients with atrial septal defect usually are asymptomatic until their third or fourth decade. Thereafter, symptoms almost always develop (usually dyspnea on exertion, fatigue, and palpitations), the result of heart failure and supraventricular arrhythmias. Less commonly, symptoms of pulmonary embolism (see Chapter 59) or paradoxical embolism (e.g., a stroke) occur. Almost all patients are symptomatic by age 60 years. In fact, three fourths of untreated patients are dead by age 50 years and 90% by age 60 years. Increased pulmonary blood flow eventually produces pulmonary vascular disease and, consequently, pulmonary hypertension in approximately 15% of patients (52). When this happens, the left-to-right shunt first decreases and then reverses; at that point, cyanosis develops. Fortunately, this rarely occurs (52). Coexistent atherosclerotic or hypertensive cardiovascular disease may complicate the course of older patients with atrial septal defect and may make diagnosis and treatment more difficult.

Physical Findings

Atrial septal defect usually causes a wide fixed splitting of the second heart sound due to late closure of the pulmonic valve as a result of increased flow into the right atrium and right ventricle. A soft blowing systolic pulmonic ejection murmur and a low to medium frequency middiastolic flow murmur across the tricuspid valve are common. The precordium may be hyperdynamic with a palpable S_3. If pulmonary hypertension has developed (see below), clubbing and cyanosis may be observed, and P_2 is accentuated. Signs of right ventricular failure (edema, distended neck veins, hepatomegaly) are common late in the disease.

Laboratory Evaluation

An ECG, chest x-ray film, and echocardiogram should be obtained routinely in a patient suspected of having an atrial septal defect.

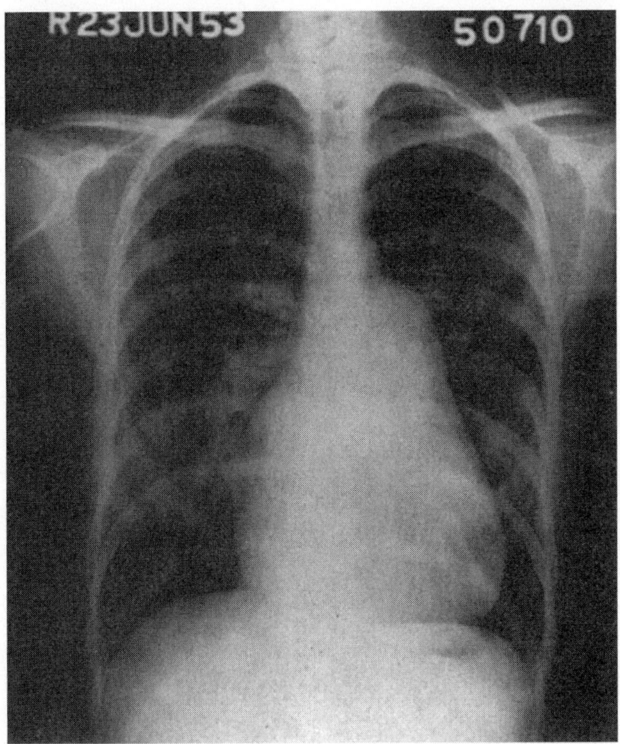

FIGURE 65.3. Chest x-ray film of a patient with atrial septal defect.

Electrocardiogram

The ECG displays an incomplete right bundle-branch block or rSR′ in lead V_1 90% to 95% of the time. If the defect is of the secundum type, a vertical frontal plane axis or right-axis deviation usually is present. The presence of frank right ventricular hypertrophy suggests the development of pulmonary hypertension. Ostium primum atrial septal defect is distinguished by the presence of left-axis deviation. Atrial fibrillation occurs commonly in symptomatic patients; atrial flutter and paroxysmal atrial tachycardia occur less often.

Chest X-Ray Film

The chest x-ray film in this disease is almost always abnormal and shows increased pulmonary vascularity with a prominent main pulmonary artery and increased heart size (Fig. 65.3). The right pulmonary artery usually is more prominent than the left because of differential flow.

Echocardiogram

The echocardiogram demonstrates right ventricular enlargement and paradoxical motion of the ventricular septum with respect to the posterior wall of the left ventricle. These findings are also seen with other lesions that cause volume overload of the right ventricle, such as tricuspid and pulmonic regurgitation, and partial anomalous pulmonary venous return. Flow across the atrial septum often can be visualized by color Doppler echocardiography. Contrast echocardiography, in which agitated saline is injected intravenously and is visualized echocardiographically as bubbles, usually can detect the presence of some right-to-left shunting across the atrial septum, even if the direction of the shunt is predominantly from left to right.

Management

Patients suspected of having an atrial septal defect should be referred to a cardiologist for definitive diagnosis. The cardiologist usually performs TEE and, if the patient is older than 40 years, cardiac catheterization (see Chapter 62 for a description of the patient experience). All patients, even if they are asymptomatic, should undergo repair of their defect if pulmonary blood flow is more than 1.5 times systemic blood flow. The operative mortality is <2%, although some degree of persistent right ventricular or LV dysfunction is common in adults. If severe pulmonary hypertension has developed (pulmonary pressure equal to or greater than the systemic pressure), corrective surgery is generally contraindicated, but patients with lesser degrees of pulmonary hypertension may still benefit from repair of the defect. Survival after corrective surgery is influenced by the age of the patient and the degree of persistent cardiac dysfunction. Patients with otherwise normal hearts have normal survival rates after successful repair of the atrial defect and usually can resume normal activity. An alternative to surgical repair of a secundum atrial septal defect is transcatheter closure with intracardiac or transesophageal echocardiographic guidance. Percutaneous closure using this technique has been successful in >98% of reported cases, with relatively few complications (53,54). After successful transcatheter closure of large atrial septal defects, right atrial area and right ventricular volume are significantly reduced at 6-month followup (55). Percutaneous device closure is now generally preferred over surgical closure if the defect is appropriate for this approach. However, patients who have a large secundum atrial septal defect or a defect with an inadequate tissue rim for deployment of the closure device or patients with atrial septal defects other than the secundum type do not have suitable anatomy for the percutaneous approach and require surgical closure. Unless an associated valvular abnormality is present, endocarditis prophylaxis is not recommended for patients with an atrial septal defect (see Chapter 93).

Mitral Regurgitation

Mitral regurgitation may develop because of an abnormality of any part of the mitral valve apparatus: valve leaflets, chordae tendineae, papillary muscles, or annulus (56). Such abnormalities may result in either acute or chronic signs and symptoms, depending on the nature of the lesion.

An incompetent mitral valve allows regurgitation into the left atrium of blood from the left ventricle. The reduced load on the ventricle reduces the tension in the ventricular muscle and allows it to use more energy in contraction. Therefore, in patients with chronic mitral regurgitation, cardiac output remains normal for years until, because of age or intercurrent disease, the ventricle can no longer compensate and heart failure ensues. In patients with acute mitral regurgitation, ventricular compensation is inadequate and heart failure develops abruptly.

Chronic Mitral Regurgitation

Causes and Epidemiology

Chronic mitral regurgitation in adults may occur in association with a variety of disorders. Mitral valve prolapse appears to be the most common cause of mitral regurgitation today, although the spectrum of this condition is changing as rheumatic heart disease becomes less frequent (rheumatic heart disease is now the cause of only 5%–15% of cases). Other causes of chronic mitral regurgitation include papillary muscle necrosis or dysfunction (the result of ischemic heart disease), an inherited (e.g., Marfan syndrome, see below) or an acquired disorder of connective tissue, idiopathic calcification of the valve (primarily a disorder of the elderly), endocarditis, congenital maldevelopment of the mitral apparatus, or as a consequence of LV remodeling with tethering of the mitral valve leaflets in patients with LV dysfunction (57).

Natural History and Symptoms

The left ventricle characteristically adapts to the increased preload of mitral regurgitation by adding new sarcomeres in series, which returns preload toward normal. The chamber becomes larger and more compliant and fully compensates for the volume overload by increasing the end-diastolic volume and stroke volume. Therefore, patients may remain asymptomatic for many years, even for their entire lives, if the regurgitation is not severe (58). Characteristically, symptoms, when they do develop, appear gradually over years as LV dysfunction slowly develops and the ability to compensate for the loss of more than half of the stroke volume back into the left atrium is lost. Dyspnea and fatigue are the usual symptoms of LV failure. Supraventricular arrhythmias, especially atrial fibrillation, are likely to develop if left atrial enlargement becomes marked, compromising somewhat the ability of the heart to compensate. Acute pulmonary edema occasionally occurs but is uncommon. Sometimes severe pulmonary hypertension develops without much enlargement of the left atrium. Early surgical correction of the lesion in patients with pulmonary hypertension and signs of right ventricular hypertrophy is important.

Patients with symptomatic mitral regurgitation often have adverse health consequences related to their valvular disease. In a series of patients with symptomatic mitral regurgitation, 80% treated medically survived 5 years and 60% survived 10 years (59). Moderately to severely symptomatic patients do less well. In one study, 46% of patients with chronic rheumatic mitral regurgitation survived 5 years (60). Data suggest that even patients with asymptomatic, but severe, mitral regurgitation have adverse health consequences related to their valve disease (61). In asymptomatic patients with severe mitral regurgitation, the 5-year rate of death from any cause was 22%, and there was a 33% incidence of adverse cardiovascular events (death, heart failure, and new-onset atrial fibrillation) (61). Cardiac surgery, especially if mitral valve repair is feasible, is associated with a reduction in the development of heart failure and death. Thus, referral to a cardiologist for discussion of surgical mitral valve repair should be considered for patients with severe mitral regurgitation regardless of the presence of symptoms.

Physical Findings

A high-pitched holosystolic murmur, loudest at the apex, is characteristic of chronic mitral regurgitation (patients with mild regurgitation may have only a late systolic murmur). The holosystolic murmur is constant in intensity and radiates always to the axilla and sometimes to the back and the base of the heart. It is best heard when the patient is in the left lateral decubitus position. The murmur is diminished when the patient stands or performs a Valsalva maneuver and is intensified when the patient squats. Mitral valve prolapse is an exception to this general statement about mitral regurgitation. The onset of the click and murmur in patients with mitral valve prolapse occurs earlier in systole during the strain phase of the Valsalva maneuver or upon standing. Squatting delays the onset of the click and murmur in mitral valve prolapse.

If mitral regurgitation is severe, the precordium usually is hyperdynamic and there is an S_3 gallop. S_1 is soft. If pulmonary hypertension has developed, an S_4 gallop, a loud P_2, and a right ventricular heave may be appreciated. Signs of right ventricular failure—edema, hepatomegaly, distended neck veins, hepatojugular reflux—may be seen late in the course of this disease.

Laboratory Evaluation

An ECG, chest x-ray, and echocardiogram should be obtained routinely if a patient is suspected of having mitral regurgitation.

Electrocardiogram. The ECG shows evidence of left atrial enlargement (Fig. 65.4 and Table 65.5) and, if present, of atrial fibrillation. The pattern of LV hypertrophy (Fig. 65.2 and Table 65.3) is often seen as well, primarily in patients with severe disease. A pattern of right ventricular hypertrophy (Table 65.6), indicating pulmonary hypertension, is less common and, when seen, is cause for great concern.

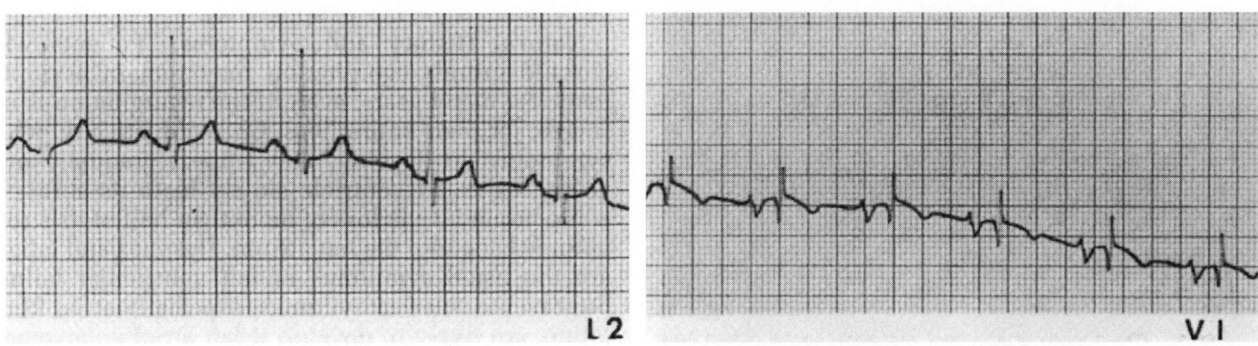

FIGURE 65.4. Electrocardiogram of a patient with left atrial enlargement (Table 65.5).

Chest X-Ray Film. LV and left atrial enlargement are common. On a posteroanterior film, elevation of the left bronchus and prominence of the left atrial appendage are the earliest signs of left atrial enlargement. A double density is seen posteriorly when the left atrium is grossly enlarged (Fig. 65.5).

Echocardiogram. Echocardiography demonstrates left atrial and LV enlargement and hyperdynamic motion of the left ventricle, especially the septum. Two-dimensional echocardiography usually can define the etiology of the valvular disease (i.e., rheumatic, prolapsing, ischemic). Color Doppler echocardiography (see above) is sensitive in detecting mitral regurgitation and can estimate its severity. Occasionally, patients may require TEE for assessment of the mechanism and severity of mitral regurgitation.

Management

Patients who have mild disease (graded by clinical examination and Doppler echocardiography) can be managed medically (see below). Antibiotic prophylaxis against bacterial endocarditis should be administered before all dental and surgical procedures (see Chapter 93). If atrial fibrillation is present, restoration of sinus rhythm may be considered, particularly if the patient is symptomatic. (Chapter 64 gives a detailed discussion of the treatment of atrial fibrillation.) However, the development of atrial fibrillation may represent a marker of severe or progressive disease (management discussed below). Likewise, new-onset heart failure may signal either worsening of mitral regurgitation or the development of secondary LV dysfunction and may constitute an indication for surgical intervention.

The management of moderate and severe mitral regurgitation depends on the severity of symptoms and on LV function. In patients who are symptomatic with fatigue, congestive heart failure, or arrhythmias, mitral valve replacement or repair may be indicated, and referral to a cardiologist should be made (Table 65.7). Cardiac

TABLE 65.5 Principal Electrocardiographic Features of Left Atrial Enlargement

P wave	
Axis	+45 degrees to −30 degrees
Amplitude (II, III, aVF) duration	>0.11 s (broad)
Component (V_1)	
Early	Positive but inside normal
Late	Negative, ≥0.04 area units[a]

[a]Area units = mm·s. One small block on standard ECG paper = 0.04 mm·s.

Modified from Horan LG, Flowers NC. Electrocardiography and vectorcardiography. In: Braunwald E, ed. Heart disease: a textbook of cardiovascular medicine. Philadelphia: WB Saunders, 1980:226, with permission.

TABLE 65.6 Electrocardiographic Criteria of Right Ventricular Hypertrophy in Adults without Conduction Defects Known Not to Have Infarction

Sign	*Points*[a]
Ratio reversal (R/S V_5:R/S V_1 ≤0.4)	5
qR in V_1	5
R/S ratio in V_1 >1	4
S in V_1 <2 mm	4
R in V_1 + S in V_5 or V_6 >10.5 mm	4
Right-axis deviation >100 degrees	4
S in V_5 or V_6 ≥7 mm and each ≥2 mm	3
R/S in V_5 or V_6 ≤1	3
R in V_1 ≥7 mm	3
S_1, S_2, and S_3 each ≥1 mm	2
S_1 and Q_3 each ≥1 mm	2
R′ in V_1 earlier than 0.08 s and ≥2 mm	2
R peak in V_1 or V_2 between 0.04 and 0.07 s	1
S in V_5 or V_6 >2 mm but <7 mm	1
Reduction in V lead R/S ratio between V_1 and V_4	
R in V_5 or V_6 <5 mm	1

[a]Interpretation of point score: 10 points, right ventricular hypertrophy; 7–9 points, probable right ventricular hypertrophy or hemodynamic overload; 5–6 points, possible right ventricular hypertrophy or hemodynamic overload. These criteria do not take into account serial ECG comparisons. Such additional data may alter the interpreter's impression of the likelihood of fixed enlargement or dynamic overload.

Modified from Horan LG, Flowers NC. Electrocardiography and vectorcardiography. In: Braunwald E, ed. Heart disease: a textbook of cardiovascular medicine. Philadelphia: WB Saunders, 1980:226, with permission.

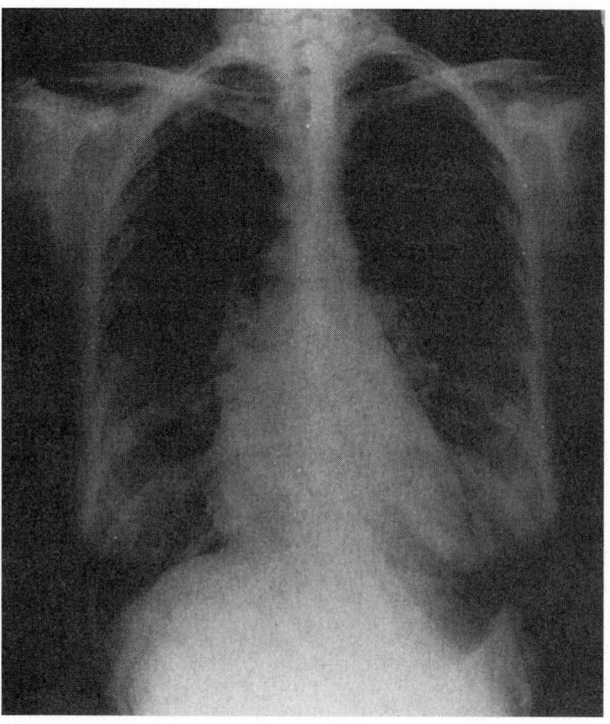

FIGURE 65.5. Chest x-ray film of a patient with left atrial enlargement. Note the straight left heart border and calcification of the left atrial wall.

catheterization and angiography (see Chapter 62) likely will be performed to confirm the severity of the lesion and to determine the patency of the coronary arteries. At this point, a decision is made about the value of operative repair of the lesion. Unless the patient has severe noncardiac disease, replacement or repair of the defective valve is very likely to be recommended.

Surgical reconstruction of the diseased mitral valve has been shown to be an excellent alternative to mitral valve replacement, particularly for valves that are leaking because of myxomatous degeneration (see Mitral Valve Prolapse). Repair most likely is feasible if the etiology of the mitral regurgitation is a flail posterior leaflet. The mitral valve should be repaired whenever possible, but this may not be feasible if the valve has been severely damaged by endocarditis or rheumatic fever. Repaired valves usually maintain their competency and seem not to be as susceptible to infectious endocarditis, and the patient does not require chronic anticoagulation unless another indication is present (1). Valve repair results in better operative mortality, long-term survival, and postoperative ejection fraction than does valve replacement (62,63). Mitral valve repair in severe LV dysfunction is not associated with a reduced mortality rate (64,65), but most patients have improvement of heart failure symptoms, LV systolic function, and LV size (66). The operative mortality is largely dependent on preoperative ejection fraction but averages approximately 2% to 5%.

TABLE 65.7 Indications for Referral of Patients with Mitral Regurgitation

- Dyspnea or fatigue
- Development of supraventricular arrhythmia, particularly atrial fibrillation
- An asymptomatic patient with moderate or severe disease, especially if there is progressive cardiac enlargement or an ejection fraction <60%
- Uncertainty about the diagnosis
- Acute mitral regurgitation
- Patients with mitral valve prolapse who have symptomatic arrhythmias; chronic, moderate, or severe mitral regurgitation; infectious endocarditis; or transient ischemic attacks

The decision about whether to recommend valve repair or replacement depends on the availability of a surgeon who is skilled at this procedure and usually is made in consultation with the cardiologist and the cardiac surgeon. A novel approach for mitral valve repair via a percutaneous route is in early clinical trials and may become available to patients in the future.

Because mitral regurgitation often is well tolerated for years or even decades, many patients are asymptomatic. However, the long-standing chronic volume overload often results in gradual deterioration in LV function, which greatly increases the risk and reduces the benefit of mitral valve repair or replacement when it eventually becomes necessary. Progressive LV dysfunction may be difficult to detect by the usual means of assessment of wall motion (echocardiography and gated blood pool scanning) because regurgitation into the low-pressure left atrium reduces the afterload of the left ventricle during ejection and results in exaggerated wall motion and falsely optimistic estimates of contractility. Many patients develop irreversible LV dysfunction before they note symptoms, even if the ejection fraction has remained within normal limits. In patients with severe mitral regurgitation caused by flail leaflet, this insidious ventricular dysfunction results in a high annual mortality rate (4.1%) even if symptoms are minimal or absent. Early surgery is associated with an improved prognosis (67). In this group, at the end of a followup period of 10 years, 90% of patients have either undergone surgical treatment or died (67). A flail mitral valve leaflet is also associated with an increased risk for sudden cardiac death estimated at 1.8% per year, even in asymptomatic patients (68). As discussed above, patients with asymptomatic, severe mitral regurgitation have a lower survival rate than the general population (61). In the past, surgery has been advised for patients with LV ejection fractions near the low end of normal (55%–60%) or below or with an LV end-systolic dimension ≥4.5 cm (69). The adverse outcomes associated with severe mitral regurgitation and the successes with mitral valve repair (that obviate the need for a prosthetic valve) suggest that patients should be considered for surgery earlier than previously recommended. Therefore, the diagnosis of moderate or severe mitral regurgitation is an indication for referral of the patient to a cardiologist.

Patients with moderate mitral regurgitation should undergo echocardiography annually to assess for worsening mitral regurgitation or the development of LV dysfunction. If there is clinical evidence of worsening mitral regurgitation, an echocardiogram should be requested sooner. Patients with severe mitral regurgitation should undergo echocardiography every 6 to 12 months to exclude asymptomatic LV dysfunction or LV chamber enlargement. Annual echocardiograms are not required in patients with mild mitral regurgitation and can be obtained approximately every 5 years, unless symptoms develop.

Afterload reduction achieved by an arteriolar vasodilator may be particularly useful in this condition; by lowering peripheral resistance, ejection of blood into the aorta, rather than back into the left atrium, is favored. Intravenous vasodilator therapy can result in dramatic hemodynamic improvement in hospitalized patients with congestive heart failure caused by mitral regurgitation. However, the efficacy of vasodilator therapy in asymptomatic patients with preserved LV function has not been studied in multicenter randomized trials. If a beneficial hemodynamic effect could be sustained, it might be possible to delay the development of LV dysfunction or symptoms and postpone the need for surgery. On the other hand, use of vasodilators and β-blocker therapy in patients with congestive heart failure caused by mitral regurgitation is well established.

The health and survival of patients who have undergone successful valve replacement depend on a number of factors (also see below). Advanced age and the preoperative presence of concomitant mitral stenosis, reduced LV function (ejection fraction $<50\%$), and severe symptoms (New York Heart Association class III or IV; see Chapter 66) are adverse factors that reduce long-term postoperative survival (69). In general, patients with mitral regurgitation on the basis of ischemic heart disease do less well than patients with rheumatic heart disease. Nevertheless, even patients with one or more adverse risk factors live longer, on average, with a prosthetic valve than they would without one, and most patients are able to be more active than they were before surgery. The overall 10-year survival for patients who have undergone successful mitral surgery is approximately 70%. Postoperatively, anticoagulation with warfarin is used routinely to prevent thromboembolic complications in patients with mechanical prosthetic valves (see Chapter 57).

Acute Mitral Regurgitation

Causes and Epidemiology

Acute mitral incompetence is most often caused by rupture of the chordae tendineae, the cords that connect the valve cusps to the papillary muscles of the left ventricle. Most often the cause of the rupture is myxomatous degeneration of the valve (see Mitral Valve Prolapse), although occasionally acute mitral regurgitation is caused by papillary muscle rupture or dysfunction (complications of myocardial infarction) or by perforation of a mitral cusp as the result of bacterial endocarditis. The disorder is primarily encountered in middle-aged and elderly patients.

Natural History and Symptoms

Because the left atrium is suddenly presented with a volume load to which it cannot rapidly accommodate, acute pulmonary edema is much more common in patients with acute, compared with chronic, mitral regurgitation.

Physical Findings

A harsh holosystolic murmur of constant intensity, loudest at the apex, is characteristic. If a posterior cord has ruptured, the murmur may radiate to the base of the heart and may mimic the murmur of aortic stenosis. Sometimes an early systolic, midsystolic, or even a crescendo–decrescendo murmur is heard. An S_3 gallop is almost always heard, and an S_4 gallop is common. Unlike the situation in patients with chronic mitral regurgitation, S_1 is normal or even loud. Signs of left-sided heart failure (rales) and right-sided failure (edema, distended neck veins) are common.

Chest X-Ray Film. The chest x-ray film shows marked pulmonary congestion. The left atrium and left ventricle are minimally enlarged.

Echocardiogram. Chamber enlargement usually is not seen, but increased systolic motion of the valve is common. If the chordae have ruptured, the flailing chordae or marked prolapse of the leaflets into the left atrium may be visualized by 2D echocardiography. Doppler echocardiography allows detection of the lesion, but Doppler criteria for estimating the severity of acute mitral regurgitation are not yet established.

Management

Patients suspected of having acute mitral regurgitation should be hospitalized immediately for diagnosis, treatment of acute heart failure, and consideration for early operative repair.

Mitral Valve Prolapse

Causes and Epidemiology

Systolic prolapse of a leaflet of the mitral valve into the left atrium has proved to be a common phenomenon. In the past, the prevalence of mitral valve prolapse was believed to be 5% to 15% of the population. The echocardiographic criteria for the diagnosis of mitral valve prolapse have been refined throughout the years as knowledge has been acquired about how the saddle shape of the mitral annulus influences the diagnosis (70). When strict criteria for mitral valve prolapse were applied to the Framingham Heart Study population, only 2.4% of the patients had the condition (71). Women were slightly more likely to be affected than men in the Framingham Heart Study population (71), although reported sex ratios vary considerably. The exact nature of this abnormality is not entirely clear, but the condition appears to be inherited (autosomal dominant) in some cases, with reduced penetrance in men and children. Most cases are sporadic. Histologic study of prolapsing valves removed at operation shows myxomatous degeneration, a proliferation of the spongiosa layer of mucopolysaccharides into the fibrosa layer and structural alterations of collagen, resulting in weakness in the supporting structure of the valve (72). This abnormality is also seen in a number of known disorders of connective tissue, including Marfan syndrome and Ehlers-Danlos syndrome. However, echocardiographic prolapse has also been reported in patients with ischemic heart disease, HCM, and atrial septal defect. These cases may represent secondary prolapse in which the valve is normal, but changes in ventricular geometry cause prolapsing of the leaflets. In these secondary cases, the click and associated symptoms (see below) usually are not present.

Natural History and Symptoms

Most patients are asymptomatic, and the condition is identified during a routine physical examination. Less often, patients complain of palpitations, chest pain, or dyspnea. The palpitations reflect arrhythmias (see below) or, more commonly, just an awareness of sinus tachycardia. The chest pain often is vague and prolonged and, rather than constituting a true part of the mitral valve prolapse syndrome, its reported association with the condition may represent ascertainment bias (73). That is, patients with nonspecific complaints may be found to have mitral valve prolapse coincidentally and an incorrect association is then made (74). Similarly, dyspnea in the absence of significant mitral regurgitation may be unrelated to the syndrome (75).

The syndrome is benign in most patients. However, significant mitral regurgitation occurs in approximately 15% of patients (76), and patients may complain of dyspnea caused by LV failure. Approximately 3% to 4% of patients require mitral valve surgery during a followup period of approximately 8 years (76).

Some studies have suggested that patients with mitral valve prolapse are at risk for embolic strokes (77), but others have ascribed this association to ascertainment bias (75). The risk of infective endocarditis in patients with mitral valve prolapse is approximately five times that of the general population, and it is the most common condition predisposing patients to infective endocarditis. This risk is highest in patients with mitral regurgitation or thickened mitral leaflets.

Sudden death, the most feared complication of mitral valve prolapse, is extremely rare (78). The risk is higher in patients who have a family history of sudden death or who have a prolonged QT interval on ECG (see below), a flail mitral valve leaflet (68), or LV dysfunction. Sudden death is presumed to be secondary to ventricular arrhythmias. In a small series of seven patients with mitral valve prolapse and malignant ventricular arrhythmias, the patients presented with syncope, out-of-hospital cardiac arrest, palpitations, and near-syncope despite normal LV function and no significant mitral regurgitation (79).

The hemodynamic and infectious complications appear to be more common in men than in women and in patients who have mitral regurgitation at the time of presentation (80). The echocardiographic findings of thickening and redundancy of the mitral leaflet also identify patients with mitral valve prolapse who are at higher risk (81). Patients with the classic form of mitral valve prolapse have mitral leaflet thickening of at least 5 mm, and complications such as infective endocarditis, moderate to severe mitral regurgitation, and mitral valve surgery are more prevalent in this group than in patients with the nonclassic form (leaflet thickening $<$5 mm) (81).

Physical Findings

The characteristic finding in patients with mitral prolapse is a midsystolic click, best heard at the lower left sternal border, caused by sudden tensing of the prolapsed valve. It occurs later than the systolic ejection sound commonly heard in association with systemic hypertension (see above). Very often the click is followed immediately by a crescendo late systolic murmur that continues until A_2.

The physical findings may vary from time to time in any given patient and may vary with the position of the patient. Standing generally augments the click and makes it occur earlier in systole because afterload is reduced and the ventricle becomes smaller with respect to the mitral valve, increasing the prolapse. Squatting and isometric handgrip increase afterload and have the opposite effect. In those instances in which chronic mitral regurgitation has developed, the typical physical findings—including the holosystolic murmur—of this condition will be encountered (see above).

The mitral valve prolapse syndrome is commonly associated with skeletal abnormalities, such as scoliosis and pectus excavatum, suggesting that valve prolapse may be only one component of a generalized disease of connective tissue.

Laboratory Findings

Electrocardiogram

The ECG usually is normal, especially in asymptomatic patients. Symptomatic patients may show nonspecific ST-T wave changes, usually in the inferior leads, and sometimes prolongation of the QT interval. A variety of arrhythmias may occur in patients with mitral valve prolapse. The most common are premature ventricular contractions and paroxysmal supraventricular tachycardia.

Echocardiogram

The echocardiogram usually is diagnostic in this condition. It shows late systolic or holosystolic prolapse of one or both leaflets of the mitral valve of at least 2 mm from the annular plane into the left atrium in the parasternal long-axis or apical long-axis view. Sometimes, however, the echocardiogram shows no abnormalities despite the typical cardiac findings. These patients probably have minor degrees of prolapse. Mitral regurgitation, if present, can be detected by Doppler echocardiography (see above).

Management

Asymptomatic patients require no treatment but should be reassessed by interval history, physical examination, and echocardiogram every few years. Care should be taken to ensure that the diagnosis does not produce unwarranted anxiety. Patients who have a systolic murmur or echocardiographic evidence of thickening or redundancy of the mitral leaflet should receive antibiotic prophylaxis before dental or surgical procedures (see Chapter 93). Other patients probably do not require prophylaxis.

Patients with palpitations should have an ambulatory electrocardiographic monitor or event recorder to determine the nature and severity of their arrhythmia, and therapy should be prescribed based upon the type of arrhythmia present (see Chapter 64). A β-blocking agent is often the drug of choice for the treatment of these patients and for those with mitral prolapse who complain of chest pain or who have persistent palpitations caused by sinus tachycardia (e.g., long-acting propranolol, usual dosage 40–120 mg/day, or atenolol 25–50 mg/day). The drug's mechanism of action in relieving pain is unknown but may be explained by the fact that many untreated patients have increased blood levels of norepinephrine and increased sympathetic tone.

Patients with symptomatic mitral regurgitation should be treated as described above. Referral to a cardiologist is recommended at any time for patients become symptomatic from arrhythmia (other than sinus tachycardia) or develop chronic mitral regurgitation or thromboembolism.

Mitral Stenosis

Stenosis of the mitral valve obstructs the flow of blood out of the left atrium, therefore raising the left atrial pressure above the LV diastolic pressure. The pressure gradient across the valve and the area of the valve orifice are measures of the severity of stenosis. Because of the increase in left atrial pressure, there is an increase in pressure in the pulmonary blood vessels and a tendency to develop atrial fibrillation. Pulmonary congestion and atrial fibrillation account for most of the symptoms of the disease.

Causes and Epidemiology

By far the most common cause of mitral stenosis in adults is rheumatic fever (although a history of rheumatic fever can be elicited in only 50% of patients with pure mitral stenosis). Pure mitral stenosis occurs in 25% of all patients with rheumatic heart disease, and 40% of patients have combined mitral stenosis and regurgitation (82). The remainder of patients with rheumatic heart disease have associated mitral regurgitation, aortic valve disease, and, uncommonly, tricuspid valve disease. Two thirds of patients with rheumatic mitral stenosis are women.

Natural History and Symptoms

On average, there is a latent period of at least 20 years between an attack of acute rheumatic fever and the development of symptomatic mitral stenosis (83). Thus, symptoms usually do not develop before the fourth decade. The severity of symptoms is quite variable. In fact, some people are never symptomatic, some are mildly symptomatic indefinitely, and some develop progressively severe cardiopulmonary decompensation. Of the patients with progressive disease, an estimated average of 7 years elapses between the onset of symptoms and the development of total disability (class IV cardiac status; see Chapter 66).

Pulmonary congestion causes many of the symptoms of mitral stenosis: dyspnea, orthopnea, and paroxysmal nocturnal dyspnea. If left atrial pressure rises acutely because of a sudden stress, frank pulmonary edema may occur. Hemoptysis caused by rupture of small bronchial veins or by pulmonary edema is not unusual.

As the disease progresses, pulmonary hypertension develops and is followed by symptoms of right heart failure: edema, distended neck veins, a tender liver, and ascites. At this point, the flow of blood into the left heart is limited, and the pulmonary arterioles hypertrophy, diminishing the risk of pulmonary edema. Low cardiac output is responsible for the fatigue that is a common complaint of patients at this stage.

Atrial fibrillation (see Chapter 64) complicates the course of 40% to 50% of patients with mitral stenosis (84,85). The 20% reduction in blood flow across the mitral valve by the subsequent loss of left atrial contraction may intensify symptoms of heart failure and fatigue.

At some time in their course, 20% of patients with mitral stenosis experience symptomatic thromboembolism (86), most often to the brain. Eighty percent of these patients have known atrial fibrillation (i.e., atrial fibrillation may be intermittent in some other individuals, so the condition may not be diagnosed).

Physical Findings

A mid-diastolic rumbling murmur with presystolic accentuation is characteristic of mitral stenosis. It is best heard at, and is often limited to, the cardiac apex. To hear it, it may be necessary to turn the patient to the left lateral position and to have the patient expire fully. Sometimes, the patient must be exercised before the murmur is audible. The murmur is best heard with the bell of the stethoscope pressed lightly against the chest. A loud first heart sound and opening snap (see above) usually accompany the murmur when the valve is mobile. Late in the course, signs of pulmonary hypertension (loud P_2 and a right ventricular heave) and right heart failure may be found.

Laboratory Findings

Electrocardiogram

The ECG shows left atrial enlargement (Fig. 65.4 and Table 65.5) in 90% of patients who are in sinus rhythm. With the development of pulmonary hypertension, signs of right ventricular hypertrophy appear (Table 65.6).

Chest X-Ray Film

Left atrial enlargement (see above and Fig. 65.5) is seen in almost all patients with symptomatic mitral stenosis, but left atrial size does not correlate with the severity of stenosis. Late in the course, right ventricular and right atrial hypertrophy are seen as well. Symptomatic patients are likely to show radiologic signs of pulmonary congestion, the severity of which determines the findings (see Chapter 66). Calcification of the mitral valve is not unusual in patients with long-standing mitral stenosis, but it is better visualized by fluoroscopy or echocardiography than by a plain x-ray film.

Echocardiogram

Mitral stenosis can be easily diagnosed by echocardiography. Mitral valve thickening can be seen; there is reduced excursion of the anterior leaflet of the valve with doming during diastole so that the valve leaflet resembles a hockey stick (so-called "hockey stick deformity") and abnormal anterior motion of the posterior leaflet during diastole (it normally moves posteriorly). The severity of the stenosis can be accurately assessed by 2D and Doppler echocardiography (see above). An echocardiographic scoring system has been useful in the selection of patients for percutaneous balloon dilation of the mitral valve (87), a procedure discussed below. This scoring system considers the echocardiographic characteristics of the valve and subvalvular apparatus. The echocardiogram is important in the assessment of mitral regurgitation and of the tricuspid transvalvular gradient for estimation of the pulmonary artery pressure. In selected patients, such as those awaiting balloon mitral valvuloplasty or direct-current cardioversion, a transesophageal echocardiogram is important for excluding left atrial or left atrial appendage thrombus.

Management

Asymptomatic patients in normal sinus rhythm require no treatment except prophylaxis for bacterial endocarditis when they undergo dental or surgical procedures (see Chapter 93). Patients with a history of rheumatic fever with carditis or residual heart disease with valvular abnormalities should receive prophylaxis for β-hemolytic streptococcal infection for at least 10 years or until they reach age 40 years, whichever is longer (1). On occasion, prophylaxis is lifelong in those with relatively high exposure to streptococcal infections, such as day care workers and teachers. For patients without residual heart disease, prophylaxis is recommended for 10 years or well into adulthood, whichever is longer. For those with rheumatic fever without carditis, prophylaxis is given for 5 years or until age 21 years, whichever is longer. When prophylaxis is necessary, one of the easiest regimens is one to two million units of benzathine penicillin G intramuscularly once per month. Alternatively, penicillin V (250 mg) can be taken orally twice daily.

Patients who develop atrial fibrillation should be anticoagulated with warfarin to achieve a target international normalized ratio (INR) of 2.0 to 3.0. Anticoagulation should be continued long term because of the high risk for stroke and venous thrombosis. Patients usually are symptomatic from the atrial fibrillation, and ventricular rate control should be achieved with a β-blocking agent or calcium channel blocker (verapamil or diltiazem). Electrical cardioversion may be necessary and can be performed by a cardiologist if the patient has been adequately anticoagulated for at least 3 weeks; otherwise, a TEE-guided cardioversion is necessary.

Mildly symptomatic patients should be treated with diuretics and sodium restriction (see Chapter 66 for a detailed discussion of the treatment of heart failure). Because it does not affect the hemodynamic abnormality, digitalis is not useful in this situation unless rapid atrial fibrillation or flutter develops. Although the use of β-blockers has been advocated in patients with mitral stenosis in normal sinus rhythm (to reduce heart rate and prolong the diastolic filling period), randomized studies have not demonstrated a clinical benefit (88).

In addition to patients with atrial fibrillation, warfarin anticoagulants should be administered to patients who have a history of a prior embolic event such as venous thromboembolism or pulmonary embolism because of the high risk for recurrent thromboembolism in this patient population (see Chapter 57). The American College of Chest Physicians recommends that patients with severe mitral stenosis and a dilated left atrium (>55 mm by echocardiography) be considered for long-term anticoagulation therapy (89).

The poor prognosis of symptomatic medically treated patients with severe or progressive disease (see Natural History and Symptoms) dictates that such patients be offered a mechanical procedure to improve transmitral flow, either percutaneous balloon valvuloplasty or valve surgery. Percutaneous valvuloplasty can be achieved using a balloon catheter passed through the venous system and then across the atrial septum to the mitral valve. This procedure is generally effective in patients who have low LV end-diastolic pressures, who do not have New York Heart Association class IV symptoms, and in whom the echocardiogram shows good mitral valve mobility and minimal valvular or subvalvular thickening and calcification. It is contraindicated in patients who have moderate to severe mitral regurgitation or a left atrial thrombus by TEE (1). Valvuloplasty should be considered in asymptomatic patients with moderate or severe mitral stenosis who are planning pregnancy, because symptoms are likely to develop late in pregnancy, and pulmonary edema may complicate labor or delivery. Patients with mitral stenosis and moderate to severe tricuspid regurgitation should be referred for surgery because both the mitral and tricuspid valves can be operated on during the same operation. In a prospective randomized trial comparing percutaneous valvuloplasty with open surgical commissurotomy in suitable patients, mitral valve orifice size and functional class after the procedure were better in the percutaneous group than in the surgical group (90). Of the patients who underwent percutaneous valvuloplasty, 72% were asymptomatic after 3 years, compared with 57% of the surgically treated patients. The better hemodynamic results, lower costs, and elimination of the need for thoracotomy suggest that balloon valvuloplasty should be considered for all suitable patients. The procedure is well tolerated and effective, even in elderly frail patients. From the patient's perspective, the procedure is similar to cardiac catheterization. An overnight hospitalization is required for observation after the procedure. In patients with a history of atrial fibrillation, warfarin typically is resumed the day after the procedure and continued long term. In other patients, anticoagulation with warfarin usually is recommended for 4 weeks following balloon valvuloplasty despite the absence of a left atrial thrombus or a history of atrial fibrillation.

TABLE 65.8 Indications for Referral of Patients with Mitral Stenosis

Asymptomatic or symptomatic patients who develop atrial fibrillation or show evidence of pulmonary hypertension
Dyspnea or recurrent attacks of pulmonary edema
Symptomatic disease of the aortic or tricuspid valve
Women, whether symptomatic or not, who wish to become or who are pregnant
Patients with chronic obstructive lung disease
Patients with angina pectoris

Modified from Brandenburg RO, Fuster V, Giuliani ER. Valvular heart disease. When should the patient be referred? Pract Cardiol 1979;5:50, with permission.

In patients requiring mechanical relief of mitral valve obstruction who are not suitable for percutaneous valvuloplasty, the preferred surgical procedure depends on the valve anatomy at the time of operation. If possible, a mitral commissurotomy is performed. The operative mortality of this procedure is low (1%–3%), and the results are excellent for a number of years. However, after commissurotomy, 10% of patients require reoperation within 5 years because of restenosis or because of the development of symptomatic mitral regurgitation or symptomatic aortic stenosis (91,92). If a prosthetic valve is implanted, the operative mortality is 3% to 10%. The course of patients who survive surgery depends on a number of factors (see below) but certainly is better than that of symptomatic patients treated medically. Table 65.8 lists the reasons to refer patients with mitral stenosis to a cardiologist.

Aortic Regurgitation

An incompetent aortic valve allows regurgitation into the left ventricle of blood ejected into the aorta. To compensate for the increased volume load, the left ventricle dilates and hypertrophies, so the effective stroke volume may be normal for a long time. Eventually, however, the left ventricle cannot maintain the workload, and clinical signs and symptoms of heart failure ensue.

Causes and Epidemiology

Aortic regurgitation may be caused by disease of the aortic valve cusps and/or dilation of the aortic root. Rheumatic fever now accounts for <15% of cases of chronic aortic regurgitation in developed countries (93), many fewer than it did 20 to 30 years ago. In developing countries, rheumatic heart disease is still the most common cause of aortic regurgitation. Another cause of chronic aortic regurgitation is a congenitally bicuspid aortic valve. Although aortic stenosis is more common than is aortic regurgitation in patients with a bicuspid aortic valve, aortic regurgitation may occur in isolation or in combination with aortic stenosis, and the majority of patients will require valve surgery during their lifetime (94). Calcific degeneration of the aortic valve is associated with aortic regurgitation, often mild in severity. Less common primary diseases of the aortic valve causing chronic aortic regurgitation include anorectic drugs, systemic lupus erythematosus, and rheumatoid arthritis. Structural degeneration of bioprosthetic aortic valves is becoming an increasingly common cause of chronic aortic regurgitation. Acute valvular incompetence is most often caused by infective endocarditis and, occasionally, by trauma to the aortic valve.

The most common cause of aortic regurgitation requiring aortic valve replacement today is aortic root disease (95). Marked aortic root dilation may be seen in patients with bicuspid aortic valve; connective tissue disorders such as Marfan syndrome, Ehlers-Danlos syndrome, and osteogenesis imperfecta; calcific degeneration of the aortic valve; and in patients with poorly controlled systemic hypertension. When the aortic root is dilated failure of coaptation of the aortic cusps leads to aortic regurgitation. In other diseases, the aortic wall becomes thickened and dilated, such as in ankylosing spondylitis, syphilitic aortitis, and reactive arthritis. Acute aortic regurgitation caused by dilation of the aortic root is most commonly caused by aortic dissection, usually associated with medial necrosis of the aorta. Dissection is associated with systemic hypertension in approximately two thirds of cases (96); occasionally a primary disorder of connective tissue, such as Marfan syndrome, can be incriminated. Aortic regurgitation in general is more common in men than women, but specific exceptions exist (e.g., rheumatoid arthritis).

Natural History and Symptoms

In chronic aortic regurgitation, volume overload usually is tolerated for years or decades because of adaptive dilation and hypertrophy that maintains cardiac performance in or near the normal range. Patients may remain asymptomatic for up to 20 years or have only mild dyspnea on exertion. However, the chronically overloaded heart eventually develops irreversible structural and functional damage, often during the asymptomatic period (97). When symptoms do develop (progressively more severe dyspnea, orthopnea, paroxysmal nocturnal dyspnea, and, less often, angina), they reflect an ominous deterioration in the condition.

Patients with acute aortic regurgitation develop fulminant pulmonary edema because of the inability of the left ventricle to compensate for the sudden volume load and for the abrupt rise in LV end-diastolic pressure. Marked dyspnea and weakness may be experienced virtually overnight and, in most cases, within 2 or 3 months. Other symptoms depend on the underlying cause, for example, fever if the cause is infective endocarditis or severe pain in the chest if the cause is aortic dissection.

Physical Findings

Patients with chronic aortic regurgitation have a characteristic high-frequency early diastolic decrescendo murmur, best heard at the aortic area and at the left sternal border. The duration (but not the intensity) of the murmur correlates with the severity of the lesion, so the murmur is holodiastolic in patients with severe chronic aortic regurgitation. Often an accompanying harsh systolic ejection murmur is heard at the base of the heart. Severe aortic regurgitation may also cause a loud apical diastolic murmur (Austin Flint murmur), simulating the murmur of mitral stenosis. Unlike the situation in true mitral stenosis, however, S_1 in patients with aortic regurgitation is sometimes soft, the result of premature closure of the mitral valve, and there is no opening snap. If aortic regurgitation is moderate or severe, the pulse pressure is ordinarily wide, reflecting peripheral vasodilation. The combination of increased systolic pressure and reduced diastolic pressure (sometimes as low as 30 mm Hg) produces characteristic changes in the peripheral pulse (e.g., the so-called "water-hammer pulse" and pistol-shot sounds heard over the femoral artery) and a typical head bobbing with each heartbeat.

Patients with acute aortic regurgitation often show signs of left- and right-sided heart failure. The regurgitant diastolic murmur is lower pitched and shorter than it is in patients with chronic aortic regurgitation. S_1 often is absent and S_3, uncommon with chronic regurgitation, usually is present. The pulse pressure often is normal, the result of intense peripheral vasoconstriction.

Laboratory Findings

Electrocardiogram

The ECG reflects the severity and duration of aortic regurgitation. Patients with chronic disease show the ECG pattern of LV hypertrophy (Fig. 65.2 and Table 65.3), whereas patients with acute disease do not (although they commonly do show nonspecific ST-T wave changes).

Chest X-Ray Film

The size of the heart in patients with aortic regurgitation depends on the duration and severity of the disease. Patients with chronic severe disease have very large left ventricles, but patients with acute regurgitation may have no cardiac enlargement at all.

Echocardiogram

Echocardiography with Doppler is useful in confirming the diagnosis and assessing LV function and the degree of state of cardiac muscle (see above). The relative position of the curve defines the inotropic state of the muscle. For example, infusing the heart with an inotropic substance such as digitalis causes the ventricular function curve to shift to the left, that is, to perform a higher stroke work at a given preload, assuming that afterload is kept constant. In other words, the contractility of the heart is increased.

Relationship between Preload, Afterload, and Inotropic State (Contractility)

If the end-diastolic pressure–volume relationship (curve) is kept constant, an increase in afterload or a decrease in inotropic state causes a decrease in the volume of the pressure–volume loop (i.e., a depression in ventricular function) as measured clinically by the ejection fraction or stroke volume. Thus, if afterload (end-systolic blood pressure) increases, ventricular function measured by the pressure–volume loop or by the ejection fraction (normally 50%–75%) decreases. A compensatory response is for LVEDP, or preload, to increase, which restores the ventricular function (pressure–volume loop) to baseline. A further increase in afterload leads to a further depression in ventricular function, which again may be restored by an increased preload (i.e., by increasing LVEDP). The *preload reserve* is the LVEDP above which the pulmonary capillary oncotic pressure is exceeded; fluid then passes into the alveoli, and pulmonary congestion, with symptoms of cough and dyspnea, occurs. Any increase in afterload that occurs when the preload reserve is reached causes a decrease in ventricular function and a worsening in symptoms of congestion. The preload reserve varies with the compliance of the ventricle as measured by the position of the LV pressure–volume relationship. If heart muscle is made stiffer or less compliant by a chronic disease process such as hypertension or aortic stenosis or by an acute process such as ischemia or increased heart rate, a higher filling pressure is necessary to set the level of ventricular function by means of the Frank-Starling principle, that is, the pressure–volume loop shifts upward and to the right and the preload reserve is reached at a lower level of stroke work. The only ways to improve ventricular function when the preload reserve is reached are to decrease the afterload or to change the inotropic state of the muscle. The clinical significance of these relationships is discussed at greater length under Management.

Biochemical Basis for Altered Contractility in the Failing Heart

The contractile unit of heart muscle is the sarcomere, which consists of fibers of protein called *actin* and *myosin*. Actin and myosin interact with each other by an interlocking protein, called *troponin*. The interlocking mechanism is facilitated by adenosine triphosphate and magnesium. An inhibitory protein, *tropomyosin*, is present on the myosin fibers. Tropomyosin inhibits the interaction between actin and myosin and allows the muscle to relax. Calcium inhibits the tropomyosin complex, frees the interlocking troponin, and allows actin and myosin to interact and to develop tension. Therefore, calcium is necessary for myocardial contraction to occur. Large amounts of calcium are stored within cardiac myocytes in the *sarcoplasmic reticulum*. Excitation–contraction coupling takes place in heart muscle when an action potential causes a release of calcium from the sarcoplasmic reticulum, thereby initiating contraction.

In classic heart failure, there appears to be decreased energy available for cardiac contraction. This leads to *decreased systolic function* and to slow transport of calcium back into the sarcoplasmic reticulum after contraction, which causes a delay in relaxation (lusitropy) of cardiac muscle. There is a reduction in early diastolic filling and an increased dependence on atrial pumping for ventricular filling. Abnormalities in calcium transport may predispose the failing heart to develop arrhythmias. Embryonic genes for fetal contractile proteins, natriuretic peptides, and inflammatory cytokines are induced by the heart failure state, which may cause profound changes in the structure and function of the heart (8). The pathophysiology of heart failure involves numerous changes in the structure and function of heart muscle cells, including loss of myofilaments, disturbances in calcium handling of the remaining myofilaments, changes in receptor density, and alterations in signal transduction. Processes underlying this condition include the progressive loss of cardiac muscle cells and changes in the extracellular matrix of the myocardium that produce structural changes in the heart. These changes can be produced by the unregulated process of cell *necrosis*, the highly regulated process of cell death called *apoptosis*, and by the expression of *matrix metalloproteinases* that have been shown to play an important role in changing the structure and function of the failing heart (9,10). The changes in ventricular size, shape, and function caused by these processes is called *remodeling*. A normal left ventricle has an ellipsoidal shape. A remodeled left ventricle has a spherical shape that creates mechanical disadvantages. The change in shape results in increased pressure and volume loads that can produce episodic or chronic subendocardial ischemia and in activation of compensatory mechanisms that lead to further malfunction of the heart and worsening symptoms of heart failure. Treatments that may slow or even reverse the remodeling process and thereby improve heart function and decrease symptoms of heart failure are discussed under Management.

In 30% to 50% of patients with the clinical syndrome of heart failure, systolic function as judged by the ejection fraction is normal but diastolic function (relaxation) is impaired. This leads to inadequate LV filling. Any compensatory increase in heart rate shortens diastole disproportionately more than systole, which leads to a further reduction in both LV filling and the time available for calcium uptake, thereby impairing ventricular relaxation (*lusitropy*) and adversely affecting both systolic function and diastolic compliance (11,12). Diastolic dysfunction can be detected and graded by LV filling patterns measured by Doppler echocardiography (13). Diastolic dysfunction is especially prevalent among persons older than 65 years or who have a history of hypertension, coronary heart disease, or diabetes. Both systolic dysfunction and diastolic dysfunction are highly predictive of all-cause mortality (14).

Compensatory Mechanisms

Heart Rate

The neural and hormonal responses to heart failure lead to an increase in heart rate in an attempt to maintain cardiac output. This may lead to rapid deterioration in systolic and diastolic function because of the disproportionate shortening of diastole relative to systole as heart rate increases (see above). The difference between the maximum heart rate during exercise and the resting heart rate (the *heart rate reserve*) is decreased, and the normal vagally mediated resting R–R interval variability is markedly blunted in heart failure. The degree of blunting is highly correlated with plasma norepinephrine levels, which may be very high in advanced heart failure (15).

Hypertrophy and Dilation

Left ventricular hypertrophy (LVH) and dilation may allow compensation of the failing heart to be maintained for many years. The stress in the wall of the heart varies with the radius of the ventricular cavity. If the heart is subjected to a *volume load,* it dilates to accommodate the load and to increase its ability to eject the load (the Frank-Starling principle; see above). However, ventricular dilation causes an increase in ventricular wall stress, which stimulates ventricular hypertrophy. Eventually, the heart becomes both dilated and hypertrophied, and the ratio of wall thickness to cavity size returns to normal, which normalizes wall stress. Therefore, a state of compensated ventricular dilation is achieved. The response to a *pressure overload* is different. An increase in wall stress in the absence of volume overload leads to cellular hypertrophy; wall stress per unit area returns to normal, but the cavity size is unchanged. Although hypertrophy and dilatation initially may be adaptive and beneficial, cardiac remodeling eventually becomes maladaptive and leads to heart failure. The increased myocyte stretch, neurohumoral activation, and myocardial hypoxia associated with cardiac remodeling activate the gene for the precursor of brain natriuretic peptide (prohormone BNP [proBNP]), which results in the synthesis and release of proBNP from ventricular myocytes. ProBNP is cleaved into biologically active BNP and the remaining N-terminal fragment pro-BNP (NT-proBNP, see below for further discussion) (16).

Activation of the Neurohormonal System

The neurohormonal activation triggered by the inability of the failing heart to maintain an effective arterial blood pressure and tissue perfusion is a major cause of the syndrome of heart failure (17). Neurohormonal activation leads to an increase in peripheral vascular resistance, a redistribution of cardiac output (maintaining flow to the heart and brain and reducing it to the kidneys, skin, splanchnic organs, and skeletal muscle), and the retention of salt and water. In less severe heart failure, when the resting cardiac output is normal, redistribution occurs only during exercise. In severe heart failure, when the resting cardiac output is significantly decreased, redistribution occurs at rest. The decrease in blood flow is functionally most important in the kidneys. Decreased renal blood flow causes a release of renin from the juxtaglomerular apparatus, which leads to increased plasma angiotensin activity. *Angiotensin* is a potent vasoconstrictor and acts both directly on smooth muscle and indirectly by increasing norepinephrine release from vascular nerve endings. Norepinephrine and angiotensin may directly damage myocardial cells. Prolonged increased plasma norepinephrine levels lead to a decreased density of β_1-adrenergic receptors on cardiac myocytes and thereby may decrease the normal myocardial response to sympathetic stimulation. The increase in angiotensin activity leads to an increase in aldosterone production, which causes an increase in sodium resorption from the distal nephron, thereby increasing plasma volume.

Increased aldosterone levels contribute to hypokalemia and hypomagnesemia that may make the failing heart more susceptible to ventricular arrhythmias. Aldosterone also appears to stimulate myocardial fibrosis, which in turn may play a role in hypertrophy and dilation of the ventricle (18). The renal resorption of sodium is facilitated by an increased filtration fraction at a given glomerular filtration rate, which causes increased sodium reabsorption in the proximal nephron. Paradoxically, hyponatremia may result from increased thirst and consumption of free water, triggered by increased levels of circulating renin, angiotensin, aldosterone, and antidiuretic hormone and by a decreased renal responsiveness to atrial natriuretic peptide (19). The effect of angiotensin on thirst and on sodium appetite is striking (20). The importance of these compensatory responses to neurohormonal activation in the management of patients with heart failure is discussed below.

Symptoms of *gastrointestinal congestion* may be seen in patients with chronic poorly compensated heart failure. Chronically increased right heart pressure may cause passive congestion of the liver, with swelling and discomfort in the right upper quadrant of the abdomen. Chronic constipation is a common complaint and may be caused by medication, inactivity, and lack of fiber in the diet.

Physical Findings

The physical findings in heart failure depend on its cause, the degree to which neurohormonal compensatory mechanisms are invoked (see above), the degree to which cardiac remodeling has progressed, and whether the heart failure is uncompensated or compensated.

Uncompensated Heart Failure

In chronic uncompensated or poorly compensated heart failure, signs of an attempt at pulmonary and cardiac compensation (increased respiratory and heart rate), signs of cardiac remodeling (increased heart size), and signs of increased renin, angiotensin, and aldosterone activity (vascular redistribution and evidence of cardiac, pulmonary, and peripheral congestion) are seen. Congestion is manifest by a ventricular gallop sound (S_3), pulmonary crackles, jugular venous distention, hepatojugular reflux, and peripheral pitting edema.

Increased heart size may be recognized by inspection, palpation, and percussion of the precordium. The precordium should be palpated with the patient in the supine and the left lateral position. The location, quality, and size of the point of maximal impulse (PMI) should be noted. The PMI of a dilated and enlarged heart is displaced laterally and caudally and is heaving and diffuse. The PMI of a concentrically enlarged heart is not displaced but may be thrusting or sustained.

Sinus tachycardia, defined as a resting heart rate >100 bpm in an adult, is a sensitive but nonspecific sign of heart failure. In patients with poorly compensated heart failure, a relative tachycardia of 85 to 95 bpm may be seen. In patients who have heart failure, tachycardia is a compensatory, but maladaptive, mechanism that attempts to increase cardiac output; the tachycardia shortens diastolic filling time and may lead to further deterioration in function (see above).

The second pulmonic sound (P_2) often is accentuated in patients in LV failure because of increased pulmonary artery pressure. *Paradoxical splitting of the second heart sound,* an indication of prolonged LV ejection time, may be heard in patients with chronic heart failure and often is associated with a left bundle-branch block (see below).

The *ventricular* or *S_3 gallop sound* is the most specific sign of heart failure (27). The sound is heard shortly after the second heart sound (S_2) and is caused by sudden restriction of filling in a noncompliant left ventricle. It usually is heard using the bell of the stethoscope directly over the PMI and may be audible only when the patient is in the left lateral position. The sound is low pitched and often may be sensed by the cadence of the heart sounds rather than specifically heard. The cadence closely approximates that of the word *Kentucky* (pronounced kyn-TUC-ky). The middle syllable is accentuated to represent the loud second heart sound caused by increased pulmonary artery pressure in patients in heart failure. The timing of the last syllable closely approximates the timing of the third heart sound, when the word is repeated at a rate of 85 to 100 times per minute.

Crackles (formally called *rales*) are high-pitched sounds (similar to the sound of a clump of hair rubbed between the fingers) produced by the sudden filling with air of fluid-filled alveoli. They are a sign of moderately to severely decompensated left heart failure.

Neck vein distention and *hepatojugular reflux* are insensitive but specific findings of heart failure (28). In chronic heart failure, right ventricular filling pressure usually increases as LVEDP increases. With time, the right ventricle becomes less compliant. As heart size increases, the pericardium may restrain the heart and thereby limit filling. Neck vein distention is assessed while the patient is semirecumbent, with a small pillow supporting the neck and the head turned slightly away from the examiner. Ideally, the right internal jugular vein is inspected because it is directly in line with the right atrium and accurately reflects right atrial pulsations and pressure. Internal jugular venous distention is seen as a broad-based fullness in the anterior cervical triangle. An arbitrary reference point may be chosen (e.g., the sternal angle; this approximates in many the level of the right atrium), and the column of blood above this point may be measured without regard for the angle of elevation of the thorax. The value of this observation is that accurate serial assessments are possible, permitting the examiner to confirm worsening failure (increasing jugular venous pressure) or to recognize a too vigorous diuretic response (abnormally low jugular venous pressure).

Hepatojugular reflux is assessed by having the patient lie supine and semirecumbent at 45 degrees. The patient is asked to breathe normally and is warned that the examiner will apply pressure over the right upper quadrant of the abdomen. Patients so warned comply and do not hold their breath or perform the Valsalva maneuver, which distends the jugular vein and makes the sign impossible to elicit. The pressure on the vena cava causes right ventricular end-diastolic pressure and right atrial pressure to rise and to remain elevated; this is seen as jugular venous distention.

Peripheral pitting edema is a common but not specific sign of heart failure. It occurs in the dependent portions of the body, which in ambulatory patients are the feet and lower legs. Edema in heart failure is caused by increased resorption of salt and water by the kidney. An increase in weight may precede pitting edema as an early objective manifestation of decompensated heart failure. Patients should be encouraged to weigh themselves daily or at least three times per week, and they should record the values and bring the weight record with them at each visit.

Of note, calcium channel blockers (see below) are a common cause of pitting edema, so if a patient is taking one of these drugs, peripheral edema is not necessarily caused by heart failure. Unilateral pitting edema is also commonly seen in the vein-harvest leg after coronary artery bypass surgery.

Because of low cardiac output and vascular redistribution, patients' extremities may be cool and their nail beds cyanotic. Delayed capillary filling in the skin of the abdomen may be apparent when the examiner's hand is removed after assessing hepatojugular reflux. In patients with decompensated heart failure, hepatic congestion may produce jaundice, hepatomegaly, and abdominal pain that mimic acute hepatitis.

Compensated Heart Failure

In contrast to the findings in patients with acute or chronic uncompensated heart failure, there may be few or no specific physical findings in patients with compensated heart failure at rest other than signs of increased heart size. A presystolic gallop or fourth heart sound (S_4) can be heard in most patients with long-standing high blood pressure or ischemic heart disease who are in normal sinus rhythm. The fourth heart sound is thought to be caused by atrial contraction into a stiff ventricle (see below). A soft systolic murmur, approximately grade 1 to 2/6, is commonly heard at the PMI or along the left sternal border in patients with chronic compensated heart failure. This murmur usually represents a minor degree of mitral or tricuspid insufficiency. A paradoxically split S_2 is often heard in patients who have a left bundle-branch block.

Laboratory Diagnosis

Brain Natriuretic Peptide and N-Terminal Prohormone Brain Natriuretic Peptide

BNP was discovered in porcine brain, but it is produced mainly in the cardiac ventricles. The proBNP gene is activated by myocyte stretch, neurohumoral activation, and hypoxia. These stressors lead to rapid secretion of proBNP from ventricular myocytes. As proBNP is released, it is cleaved into active BNP and inactive NT-proBNP. BNP activates peripheral receptors that cause diuresis, vasodilation, and decreased renin and aldosterone secretion (16). The kidney plays a role in the degradation and clearance of BNP and NT-proBNP, and increased plasma levels of these peptides may be difficult to interpret in the setting of renal dysfunction. However, both tests have a high sensitivity and negative predictive value for the diagnosis of heart failure, allowing their use to "rule out" this condition in the primary care setting (29,30). Thus, the test may be helpful in ambulatory patients in whom the cause of dyspnea is unclear. Diagnostic uncertainty based on routine clinical examination alone is not uncommon in elderly patients with multiple comorbidities, especially when symptoms are mild. Use of BNP and NT-proBNP in this setting may decrease the overdiagnosis of heart failure in primary care (30). BNP also may be very useful in guiding treatment. In one study in which treatment was guided either by BNP levels or by clinical signs and symptoms alone, the number of significant cardiac events in the "BNP group" was reduced by nearly 50% compared with the control group (31).

Chest X-Ray Film

The chest x-ray film is an important diagnostic procedure for evaluation of suspected heart failure. The radiologic signs of heart failure are cardiac enlargement and pulmonary congestion. In advanced or chronic heart failure, pleural effusions are frequently seen.

A number of factors influence heart size on the chest x-ray film, including body build, depth of inspiration when the film is taken, and the chambers that are enlarged. Nevertheless, determination of the ratio of the transverse diameter of the heart to the greatest diameter of the chest, the *cardiothoracic ratio,* is a reliable and valid measurement of heart size and should be part of the database of every patient who is thought to have, or to have had, heart failure. The normal cardiothoracic ratio is <0.5. The pulmonary vasculature should be examined, and signs of vascular redistribution, caused by pulmonary venous hypertension, and of enlarged hilar vessels, caused by acute or chronic pulmonary hypertension, should be noted.

Normally, the lower lobes of the lungs are better perfused than the upper lobes. The earliest radiologic sign of pulmonary congestion is reduction of blood flow to the lower lobes caused by compression of vessels by extravascular fluid that has gravitated to the lung bases. In early heart failure, there is simply an equalization of the size of the vessels to the upper and lower lobes. As congestion increases, the vessels to the upper lobes become more prominent, the so-called *cephalization of flow.* More severe failure is manifest by signs of interstitial edema and ultimately by alveolar edema and a transudative pleural effusion (see Chapter 59). The volume of pleural effusions often is underestimated by routine chest x-ray views. Decubitus films should be obtained if a pleural effusion is present.

Electrocardiogram

No changes on the electrocardiogram (ECG) are diagnostic of heart failure. However, the ECG may reflect an underlying disease (e.g., LVH caused by hypertension; Q waves or ST-T wave changes caused by infarction) or the presence of an unstable rhythm (e.g., atrial fibrillation with rapid ventricular response) that has caused heart failure. Changes reflecting chamber enlargement or hypertrophy (especially LVH or left atrial enlargement), conduction system disease (especially first-degree atrioventricular block and bundle-branch block), or an abnormal rhythm (especially sinus tachycardia, atrial fibrillation, or ventricular ectopy) are common. *A normal ECG is unusual in patients with chronic LV dysfunction.* Because of this finding, use of the ECG as a triage tool has been proposed, which could reduce by 50% the number of echocardiograms ordered for the evaluation of suspected heart failure (32).

Patients with hypertrophy of the heart may show only minor nonspecific ST-T wave changes. Grossly abnormal changes are commonly seen on the ECG of patients who have both dilation and hypertrophy of the left ventricle. The most common manifestations of LVH are *left-axis deviation, increased QRS voltage and QRS duration, and ST-T wave changes.* Evidence of *left atrial enlargement* is frequently seen (see below). Although there are numerous ECG criteria for LVH, a clinically useful criterion is the index of Lewis: net positivity in lead I plus net negativity in lead III $\geq$2.0 mV. Also, an R wave >11 mm in lead aVL is specific for LVH.

Conduction abnormalities are common in patients in heart failure, especially left bundle-branch block. Left bundle-branch block may be an early sign of congestive cardiomyopathy, especially when it occurs in young patients. It nearly always is a sign of organic heart disease. Left bundle-branch block or a nonspecific intraventricular conduction delay with a QRS interval >140 ms is often seen in patients with advanced heart failure. These patients may be candidates for implantation of a biventricular pacemaker resynchronization device (discussed below).

Left atrial enlargement is diagnosed by the presence of a negative P wave with an area >1 mm^2 on lead V_1. It commonly is seen on the ECG of a patient with acute heart failure and may disappear as the patient is treated and the volume of the left atrium decreases.

Right ventricular hypertrophy is most reliably diagnosed in adults by a shift of the QRS axis toward the right >90 degrees in combination with altered precordial R-wave progression.

Certain ECG changes suggest a decreased ejection fraction, especially in patients with heart failure caused by ischemic heart disease. These include Q waves in leads 1, aVL, and V_1 through V_4 with persistently upward coving of the ST segments in the precordial leads (seen in patients with extensive anterior wall infarctions with aneurysms) and deep Q waves in both inferior and precordial leads with QRS duration >0.1 second (suggesting ischemic cardiomyopathy) (32). *Low QRS voltage* (<10 mm in precordial leads and <5 mm in limb leads) is commonly caused by pericardial effusion, hypothyroidism, or infiltrative disease of the heart (e.g., amyloid) but also may be seen in patients with severe emphysema or marked obesity.

Echocardiography

The two-dimensional echocardiogram with Doppler is a reliable technique for determining ventricular size and thickness, the presence of valvular and structural abnormalities, the evaluation of systolic and diastolic function, and the presence or absence of pericardial effusion. If not previously performed, a two-dimensional echocardiogram should be obtained in all patients with a clinical diagnosis of heart failure to assess LV function. This is particularly important because heart failure due to LV systolic dysfunction may be difficult to distinguish from heart failure with normal LV function (i.e., diastolic dysfunction) by history and physical examination alone (see below). Echocardiography should be considered for patients with suspected valvular or pericardial disease or for patients in whom the cause of heart failure is unclear. In the primary care setting, echocardiography is unlikely to be useful in the evaluation of patients with suspected heart failure who have a normal ECG, a normal heart size on chest x-ray film, or a normal BNP or NT-proBNP level. (Use of echocardiography in the diagnosis of valvular heart disease is discussed more fully in Chapter 65.)

Two-dimensional echocardiography with color-flow Doppler is useful in estimating the ejection fraction and detecting valvular stenosis or regurgitation. Pulmonary artery pressures may be estimated accurately but only in patients who have tricuspid regurgitation; this includes most patients with heart failure. Two-dimensional echocardiography with pulsed Doppler evaluation of mitral valve flow velocity also is useful in differentiating between systolic and diastolic dysfunction (13,14).

Radionuclide Angiography and Single-Photon Emission Computed Tomography Scanning

Radionuclide angiography (gated blood pool scan or multigated acquisition study) is a technique for visualizing the cardiac chambers throughout the cardiac cycle. The major advantages of this technique over echocardiography are that good images can be obtained even in patients who are obese or who have severe chronic lung disease, and the ejection fraction can be determined precisely.

Radionuclide angiography is an effective tool for evaluating LV wall-motion abnormalities, including ventricular aneurysm, and for evaluating LV function and diastolic compliance. The primary care provider does not ordinarily consider radionuclide angiography without the advice of a cardiologist. In most institutions, echocardiography has largely replaced radionuclide angiography as a diagnostic tool because it provides much more information regarding systolic and diastolic function, without radiation.

Single-photon emission computed tomography (SPECT) scanning may be used to assess possible ischemia and to determine if viable myocardium is present in patients with heart failure. LV function and wall-motion abnormalities can be assessed. This test usually is ordered after consultation with a cardiologist.

Cardiac Catheterization and Myocardial Biopsy

Cardiac catheterization (see Chapter 62) should be considered in any patient in chronic heart failure in whom an etiologic and anatomic diagnosis has not been made by noninvasive techniques. Sudden onset of heart failure with cardiomegaly in a previously healthy patient is an indication for immediate referral to a cardiologist. Cardiac catheterization may be important in the diagnosis of pericardial disease. Myocardial biopsy may be useful in young patients suspected of having a cardiomyopathy who have sudden onset of heart failure of uncertain cause. Approximately one third of patients with chronic dilated cardiomyopathy are found by cardiac catheterization to have significant coronary disease (33). The procedure should be considered in all patients who have dilated cardiomyopathy of uncertain origin, especially in patients who have diabetes or who may have severe coronary heart disease with mild or no symptoms of chest pain.

Exercise Testing

It often is difficult to determine the functional status of patients with heart failure, and functional limitation often is overestimated or underestimated. Studies show that the most precise determination of functional classification is given by exercise testing with assessment of oxygen consumption (34). The protocol used should be one in which the level of exercise is increased in small increments. The test should be obtained in consultation with a cardiologist or pulmonologist and only if functional classification cannot be satisfactorily determined by clinical means. The 6-minute walk test, in which the distance that the patient is able to walk in 6 minutes is measured, correlates well with function assessed by measurement of oxygen consumption and also with prognosis. It is a useful, inexpensive tool for the assessment of functional status, especially in patients with more advanced heart failure, and changes in performance can be tracked over time (35,36). A carefully taken history is also useful and inexpensive (see above).

Systolic versus Diastolic Dysfunction

The clinical signs and symptoms of heart failure may result from systolic or diastolic dysfunction of the myocardium (see above). It is important to determine whether one or both of these mechanisms are operative in order to prescribe appropriate treatment.

In patients with heart failure caused by *systolic dysfunction,* the heart is typically dilated, often hypertrophied, and the inotropic state of the heart is impaired relative to the afterload so that the ejection fraction, and often the blood pressure, is decreased. A reduced ejection fraction, detected by echocardiography or gated blood pool scan, and an S_4 on auscultation may be the only signs of compensated systolic dysfunction. In uncompensated systolic dysfunction, resting tachycardia usually is present, and an S_3 may be heard. The heart usually is enlarged on chest x-ray film, and Q waves, QRS widening, or left bundle-branch block may be present on the ECG.

In patients with signs and symptoms of heart failure caused by *diastolic dysfunction,* the ventricle is less compliant (i.e., stiffer) and early diastolic passive filling of the left ventricle is decreased. Therefore, immediately before atrial systole, the atrium has a greater than normal volume and pressure and, by the Frank-Starling principle, the force of atrial contraction is increased. Clinically, this may be detected by a palpable presystolic apical filling wave or heard as a loud S_4. On pulsed Doppler echocardiography, diastolic dysfunction may be diagnosed by the increased velocity of the atrial component of diastolic filling relative to the peak velocity of the early diastolic rapid filling phase (see Chapter 65 for a more detailed discussion of this topic) (13).

The diagnosis of diastolic dysfunction should be suspected in patients with evidence of increased filling pressure (jugular venous distention and pulmonary redistribution of blood flow) and concomitant elevation of blood pressure. ECG signs of LVH and elevated levels of natriuretic peptides do not reliably differentiate between systolic and diastolic heart failure. The distinction must be made by echocardiography (13).

MANAGEMENT

The goal of therapy is not merely to control symptoms but to treat specifically the underlying causes of heart failure if possible (Table 66.1). If the underlying disease cannot be effectively treated (Fig. 66.3), an attempt should be made to increase the capacity of the heart to do work or to decrease the amount of work that the heart has to do. Table 66.6 lists the various measures that can be used to accomplish these goals in ambulatory patients. These measures are discussed in detail here.

General Principles

Lifestyle and Nonpharmacologic Therapies

It is not always possible to improve the function of the failing heart, but it usually is possible to decrease the

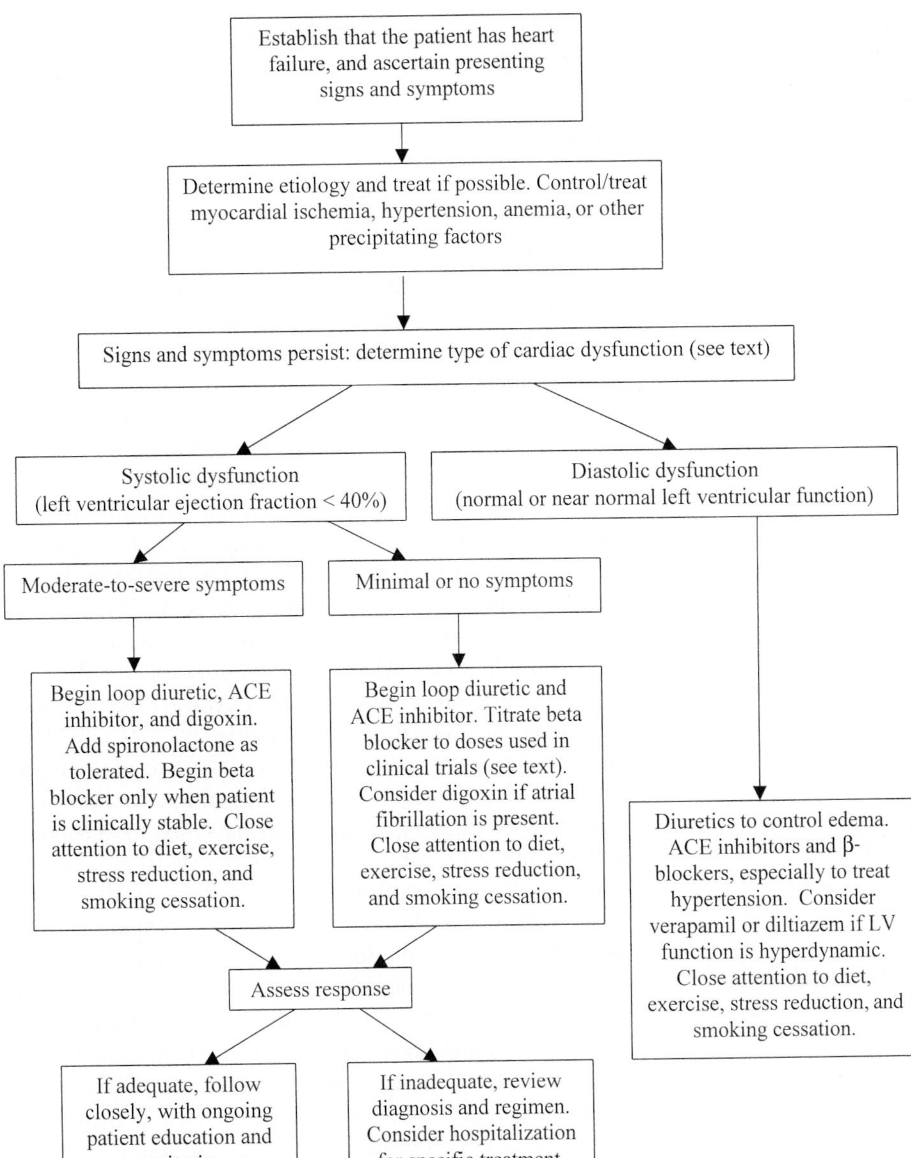

FIGURE 66.3. Algorithm for treatment of heart failure.

TABLE 66.6 Measures Used in Ambulatory Treatment of Heart Failure

Increasing capacity of heart to do work
Appropriate drug regimen (see text)
Control of atrial fibrillation and other arrhythmias (see Chapter 64)
Resynchronization pacemaker and implantable defibrillator therapy (see text)
Decreasing amount of work that heart has to do
Appropriate drug regimen (see text)
Compliance with medication and diet
Adequate rest
Control of other medical illness (e.g., anemia, diabetes, hypertension)
Home oxygen
Exercise training in selected patients
Comprehensive disease management programs

metabolic needs of the body by encouraging a patient to stop smoking (see Chapter 27), to avoid emotional stress, and to get an adequate amount of rest (Table 66.7). Obstructive sleep apnea, if present, must be treated. A thorough understanding of the patient's home and work environments and of the relationship of the patient to his or her supporting family members and caregivers is important. When possible, the recommended treatment regimen should be discussed with both the patient and the patient's family.

The ambulatory patient should be encouraged to exercise (see Chapter 63) but to take care to avoid exertion to the point of causing further symptomatic cardiac decompensation. Sometimes this simply means performing the same activities more slowly.

TABLE 66.7 Suggested Topics for Patient, Family, and Caregiver Education and Counseling

General counseling
Explanation of heart failure and the reason for symptoms
Cause or probable cause of heart failure
Expected symptoms
Symptoms of worsening heart failure
What to do if symptoms worsen—how to obtain help in an emergency
Self-monitoring with daily weight
Explanation of treatment/care plan
Clarification of patient's responsibilities for self-management
Importance of cessation of tobacco use
Role of family members or other caregivers in the treatment/care plan
Availability and value of qualified local support group
Importance of obtaining vaccinations against influenza and pneumococcal disease
Prognosis
Life expectancy
Advance directives
Advice for family members in the event of sudden death
Activity recommendations
Recreation, leisure, and work activity
Exercise
Sex, sexual difficulties, and coping strategies
Dietary recommendations
Sodium restriction
Avoidance of excessive fluid intake
Fluid restriction (if required)
Alcohol restriction (complete abstinence if heart failure is due to alcohol)
Medications
Effects of medications on quality of life and survival
Dosing
Likely side effects and what to do if they occur
Coping mechanisms for complicated medical regimens
Availability of lower cost medications or financial assistance
Importance of compliance with the treatment/care plan

There is a decreased stimulus to renin, angiotensin, and aldosterone production during supine rest, and even severely disabled patients may be able to lead socially useful and satisfying lives if they rest in the afternoon and in the early evening or before social or business engagements. Strict bed rest, which causes muscle weakness and deconditioning, should be strongly discouraged. The best advice for patients with chronic stable heart failure may be to participate in an exercise training regimen in which the exercise is supervised at levels shown to be beneficial in controlled trials (37,38).

The temperature and humidity of the patient's home and work environment must be controlled. Patients should be encouraged to have air conditioners for the summer months to reduce the extra demand placed on the heart by hot humid weather.

Diet

Surprisingly little experimental evidence supports the long-term benefit of a severely salt-restricted diet in controlling heart failure in patients who respond well to moderate dosages of diuretics. However, it is commonly observed that sudden increases in salt intake may precipitate acute pulmonary edema in patients who have moderately well-compensated chronic heart failure. Holiday seasons are particularly dangerous in this regard, probably because of the increased physical activity and emotional stress. The various types of salty food that the patient is likely to eat should be anticipated, based on the patient's cultural background. Examples of frequently eaten salty food include breakfast meats such as sausage, bacon, and scrapple; deli meats including "low-salt" ham; salt pork or fatback in cooking vegetables; and many foods prepared by traditional ethnic cooks. Many patients attempt to substitute condiments in place of salt and are not aware that ketchup, hot sauce, soy sauce, and many other sauces have high sodium concentrations. Homebound patients may eat prepared foods such as frozen pancakes and waffles or frozen convenience dinners, or they may have fast food brought to their home by family and neighbors. Most patients are unaware that the sodium content of these foods often is higher than Atlantic Ocean seawater (1 g sodium/100 g seawater) (39). A no-added-salt diet, which contains approximately 2 to 3 g of sodium, suffices for most patients in compensated heart failure. Patients with poorly compensated heart failure may require a diet that contains 500 mg to 1 g of sodium, along with a restriction of volume intake to no more than 1.5 L. The caregiver must take the time to give specific concrete advice about diet and nutrition.

A high-soluble-fiber diet may help prevent constipation and straining (see Chapter 45). Referral to a dietitian may be essential for patients with frequent episodes of cardiac decompensation caused by noncompliance with salt and fluid restriction. Chapter 67 gives guidelines for planning these diets and a list of foods to be avoided by patients being treated for heart failure.

Patients with heart failure may wish to know whether they can continue to drink alcoholic beverages. More than 2 oz of alcohol per day may increase blood pressure and may impair cardiac function. In any patient with a cardiomyopathy apparently related to prolonged heavy alcohol use, total abstinence from alcohol is essential. However, a published large prospective cohort study suggests that moderate alcohol consumption (approximately 1 oz/day) may decrease the risk of development of heart failure in older persons. This effect may result from the association of moderate alcohol consumption with lower risk of development of coronary artery disease and type

2 diabetes. Moderate alcohol consumption may also decrease blood pressure (40).

Drugs That Promote Positive Sodium Balance

A number of commonly used drugs can promote a positive sodium balance, for example, corticosteroids and estrogens cause renal sodium retention. NSAIDs other than aspirin are strongly associated with the development of heart failure. One study showed an odds ratio of 10.5 for the development of heart failure among patients with known heart disease who took NSAIDs (23). Of note, the effects of cyclooxygenase-2 inhibitors on kidney function may be similar to those of the nonselective NSAIDs (41). Some antacid preparations contain a significant amount of sodium. Patients with heart failure should not take these drugs; however, if the drugs are necessary, the patients should be monitored closely for symptoms of increased heart failure or electrolyte disturbance. There is no convincing evidence that aspirin has a deleterious effect on patients with heart failure; indeed, its use appears to be associated with lower mortality, especially in patients with coronary disease and heart failure (42). Unless patients have a definite history of aspirin allergy or a history of aspirin-induced gastrointestinal or intracerebral bleeding, it seems advisable for patients with heart failure who are not taking warfarin to take daily aspirin, especially if they also have coronary disease or diabetes.

Drugs That May Directly or Indirectly Impair Left Ventricular Function

Calcium channel blockers depress LV function and should be avoided in patients with systolic dysfunction. Second-generation drugs (felodipine and amlodipine; see below) may be exceptions, but they should be considered only if the patient's blood pressure remains poorly controlled despite the careful titration to appropriate doses of ACE inhibitors, β-blockers, and diuretics. The antiarrhythmic agents disopyramide and flecainide should not be used in patients with systolic dysfunction. Use of the insulin sensitizer drugs of the thiazolidinedione class in patients with heart failure (currently pioglitazone and rosiglitazone are available) has been controversial. These drugs are associated with fluid retention in patients with advanced systolic dysfunction. A large observational study, however, showed improved outcomes in patients with type 2 diabetes and heart failure who took insulin sensitizing drugs in the thiazolidinedione class or metformin (43). A consensus panel urges close monitoring of patients with heart failure and diabetes who are taking these drugs (44).

Drug Therapy

The goal of drug therapy for heart failure is to relieve symptoms, improve function, and prolong life. Clinical trials demonstrate that achieving these goals is possible in most patients with chronic heart failure, although in clinical practice appropriate drugs often are not titrated to doses shown to achieve these goals in randomized controlled trials (45).

There may be important differences in the therapeutic approach to patients whose heart failure is caused by systolic dysfunction (dilated left ventricle with decreased ejection fraction) as opposed to patients whose heart failure is caused primarily by diastolic dysfunction (hypertrophied stiff heart with a normal or increased ejection fraction) (see above). Although many patients, especially older patients with chronic hypertension, have heart failure due to diastolic dysfunction, few clinical trials are available to guide therapy for this condition. Control of hypertension, when present, appears to be important in the treatment of diastolic heart failure. Although many antihypertensive drugs may prove beneficial in the treatment of diastolic heart failure, the angiotensin receptor blocker (ARB) candesartan was shown to decrease heart failure hospitalizations in a randomized controlled trial in patients with heart failure and preserved LV function (46).

Diuretic Drugs

Diuretic drugs are used when treatment of the underlying cause of heart failure is not possible or when signs and symptoms of congestion persist despite treatment of the underlying condition. Although diuretic drugs have not been shown to prolong life (with the exception of spironolactone in certain patients with heart failure; see below), they relieve symptoms and improve function in most patients with heart failure. Diuretics reduce symptoms of circulatory congestion by increasing sodium and water excretion.

The goal of diuretic therapy is to reach and maintain the patient's "dry weight." Physiologically, this is the weight at which signs of peripheral congestion are substantially relieved and the LV filling pressure remains near the preload reserve (i.e., function is optimized via the Frank-Starling principle). Clinically, this is the weight at which peripheral edema is no more than a trace, jugular venous distention is absent, hepatojugular reflux, if present, is no more than a few centimeters above the clavicle, the blood urea nitrogen and creatinine determinations are at, or slightly above, baseline, no symptomatic orthostatic blood pressure changes are present, urine output is maintained, and diuretic drug doses do not require adjustment. After diuresis to the dry weight, the decrease in ventricular wall stress (i.e., afterload) and the improvement in ventricular contraction brought about by a decrease in heart size and peripheral vascular resistance often lead to prompt improvement in ventricular function and, in hypertensive patients, a reduction in blood pressure.

TABLE 66.8 Characteristics of Selected Diuretic Drugs

Generic Name	Brand Name	Available Preparations	Usual Daily Dosage (mg/day)	Frequency of Dosing (per day)	Onset of Effect	Peak Effect	Duration
Hydrochlorothiazide	Generic	25-, 50-, 200-mg tablet	25–100	1–2	2 h	4 h	≥12 h
Chlorthalidone	Generic, Hygroton	50-, 100-mg tablet	50–100	1	2 h	6 h	24 h
Metolazone	Zaroxolyn	2.5-, 5-, 10-mg tablet	2.5–10	1	1 h	2 h	12–14 h
Indapamide	Lozol	2.5-mg tablet	2.5–5.0	1	1 h	2 h	28 h
Furosemide	Lasix	20-, 40-, 80-mg tablet	20–160	1–2	1 h	1–2 h	6 h
Ethacrynic acid	Edecrin	50-mg tablet	50–100	1–2	30 min	2 h	6–8 h
Bumetanide	Bumex	0.5-, 1-mg tablet	0.5–2	1–2	30 min to 1 h	1–2 h	4 h
Torsemide	Demadex	20-, 40-mg tablet	20–40	1	30 min to 1 h	3 h	12 h
Triamterene	Dyrenium	100-mg capsule	100–300	1–2	2 h	6–8 h	12–16 h
Spironolactone	Aldactone	25-mg tablet	25–400	1–2	Gradual onset	2–3 days after initiation of therapy	2–3 days after cessation of therapy
Eplerenone	Inspra	25-, 50-, and 100-mg tablets	25–100	1	Several hours	Days-to-weeks after initiation of therapy	At least several days after cessation of therapy
Amiloride	Midamor	5-mg tablet	5–10	1	2 h	6–10 h	24 h

Three classes of diuretics are in common use: thiazides (e.g., hydrochlorothiazide) and thiazidelike agents (e.g., metolazone, chlorthalidone), the so-called loop diuretics (e.g., furosemide, bumetanide, and torsemide), and the potassium-sparing diuretics (spironolactone, eplerenone, triamterene, and amiloride) (Table 66.8).

The *thiazides* and the *thiazidelike diuretics* act on the early portion of the distal convoluted tubule of the nephron. They cause a moderate increase in sodium and chloride excretion. Potassium and hydrogen losses are accentuated because of the increased delivery of solute to the terminal portion of the distal tubule, where potassium secretion occurs and is modulated by aldosterone. Thiazidelike agents such as metolazone act on both the proximal and distal convoluted tubules of the nephron and may be particularly effective in patients with very low renal blood flow.

The *loop diuretics* inhibit tubular resorption of chloride and sodium in the ascending limb of the loop of Henle. These diuretics are potent and result in substantially increased excretion of sodium, chloride, and water. Like the thiazides, the loop diuretics increase the delivery of solute to the more distal portion of the nephron, where potassium and hydrogen secretion is accentuated.

Potassium-sparing diuretics act on the terminal portion of the distal convoluted tubule, where only a small proportion of sodium is reabsorbed. By themselves they are only weak diuretics. However, they may be especially useful in combination with a thiazide or loop diuretic in preventing hypokalemia or when a patient becomes refractory to the more potent diuretics. The effect of thiazides and loop diuretics may be dampened by resorption of sodium in the terminal portion of the distal convoluted tubule because they act proximal to the portion of the distal nephron where aldosterone influences sodium resorption. *Spironolactone* is structurally similar to aldosterone and competitively inhibits aldosterone binding to cellular receptors. It causes gynecomastia or breast pain in approximately 10% of men taking the drug. Eplerenone is a more selective aldosterone blocker that does not appear to cause gynecomastia or breast pain, but it is more expensive than spironolactone (47). *Triamterene* and *amiloride* block sodium resorption and potassium excretion but do not compete with aldosterone or even depend on its presence to be effective. These diuretics may cause life-threatening increases in the serum potassium level. Patients usually should not receive potassium supplementation while taking these diuretics. Patients with renal failure or patients taking an ACE inhibitor are at increased risk for developing hyperkalemia if given these diuretics. Serum potassium levels must be monitored carefully when these agents are used.

Use of Diuretic Drugs

When used for treatment of heart failure, diuretics should always be prescribed with another agent (e.g., ACE inhibitor or β-blocker). In patients with normal renal function, therapy should start with the lowest effective dosage of a thiazide compound (Table 66.8). Generic hydrochlorothiazide is the drug of choice. Many patients with mild heart failure may effectively control symptoms by taking the drug every other day or three times per week, along with an ACE inhibitor and β-blocker. Patients with progressive disease, associated with worsening renal perfusion and albuminuria, should not be treated with a thiazide diuretic, which may decrease renal perfusion. In these cases, a loop diuretic—furosemide, bumetanide, torsemide—should be prescribed (Table 66.8) (ethacrynic acid is no longer widely used). These drugs often are effective in low oral dosages. Furosemide, bumetanide, and torsemide are available in generic forms. Bumetanide and torsemide are less ototoxic than furosemide, and their bioavailability orally is higher than that of furosemide. However, furosemide is still the most popular of these drugs, in part because of cost and custom. Furosemide should be started at a dosage of 20 mg/day and increased as necessary for control of symptoms. Although a single dose of furosemide or bumetanide is commonly administered each day, these drugs are short acting (half-life of 1–1.5 hours), and patients with moderate to severe heart failure may require a second dose in the late afternoon to affect a negative sodium balance. Torsemide has a longer half-life and may be effective given once daily, even in patients with moderately severe heart failure.

Dosages of furosemide higher than 160 to 240 mg/day are rarely required and may cause ototoxicity. Patients who require such large doses of diuretic for control of congestive symptoms probably should be referred to a cardiologist for evaluation. In these cases, substituting bumetanide or torsemide for furosemide or adding a thiazide diuretic in modest dosages (hydrochlorothiazide 12.5–25 mg or metolazone 2.5–5 mg) may be necessary. Combination with a thiazide diuretic may markedly potentiate the effect of loop diuretics, leading to rapid mobilization of fluid, thereby allowing treatment of these patients in an ambulatory setting without the use of intravenous diuretics. Careful monitoring of electrolyte levels is essential (see below). A potassium-sparing diuretic may be appropriate in certain circumstances. In particular, spironolactone or eplerenone should be considered in patients with severe heart failure due to systolic dysfunction because aldosterone blockers have been shown to reduce morbidity and mortality in these patients (48). The diuretic dosage should be reduced when the dry weight is achieved, and the patient should be weighed daily and should keep a written record of the weights to review with the care provider.

Side Effects of Diuretics

Hypokalemia

The thiazides and loop diuretics have marked kaliuretic effects, and hypokalemia is a common complication of the use of diuretic therapy, especially in edematous patients. Hypokalemia may lead to fatigue, muscle cramps, and depression and often precipitates arrhythmias or digitalis toxicity. A high-sodium diet predisposes to hypokalemia in patients taking loop diuretics because of aldosterone-mediated sodium/potassium exchange in the distal tubule. Patients with persistent hypokalemia should be encouraged to adhere to a very-low-sodium diet. The justification for sodium restriction must be explained to the patient in concrete terms. If hypokalemia persists despite a low-sodium diet and treatment with an ACE inhibitor, a potassium-sparing diuretic such as triamterene, spironolactone, or eplerenone should be used in preference to potassium salts. Potassium supplementation should be discontinued before administration of a potassium-sparing diuretic. The patient's electrolyte concentration must be monitored carefully when these medications are started, when the dosage is adjusted, or when there is a change in the severity of heart failure. Patients with diabetes and renal disease, who commonly have some degree of hypoaldosteronism and hyperkalemia (type 4 renal tubular acidosis), may be very sensitive to the potassium-sparing effects of these drugs. The serum potassium level should be measured again 3 days to 1 week later; the goal is to maintain serum potassium concentration in the high–normal range. The usual dosage of triamterene is 50 to 100 mg one to three times per day, spironolactone 12.5 to 100 mg once or twice daily, and eplerenone 25 to 50 mg once daily. The higher dose ranges must be used with caution, especially in diabetics, as noted above. Chapter 50 fully discusses the indications for, and use of, potassium salts in patients taking diuretics.

Hyponatremia

The loop diuretics and the thiazides occasionally are associated with hyponatremia by impairing free water clearance, so caution is especially appropriate in patients who tend to consume large quantities of fluid. These diuretics also may be associated with hyponatremia when the extracellular volume has become contracted (a potent stimulus to release of antidiuretic hormone) and fluid intake has not been restricted. Usually, the hyponatremia can be corrected by restricting water intake to <1 L/day. Finally, the thiazides are associated rarely with hyponatremia in euvolemic patients who also are severely potassium depleted. This situation clinically resembles the syndrome of inappropriate secretion of antidiuretic hormone, although the exact mechanism of the complication is not fully known. The drug must be withdrawn until hyponatremia is corrected.

Contraction of the Extracellular Volume

Diuretics exert their therapeutic effect by causing a net loss of sodium, chloride, and water. If the response is excessive, depletion of the extracellular fluid compartment (the maintenance of which depends on sodium and chloride) occurs. This may have catastrophic consequences, such as postural hypotension, sometimes with loss of consciousness, precipitation of ischemia caused by changes in cerebral, coronary, or renal blood flow, or precipitation of hyperosmolar coma in diabetics. These complications are especially common when loop diuretics are used but may occur after the use of thiazides or combination diuretics, especially in patients also taking an ACE inhibitor. Patients should be monitored carefully for evidence of excessive contraction of extracellular volume by daily self-assessment of weight and for the presence or absence of edema. The caregiver should frequently assess the degree of fullness of the neck veins and evaluate for orthostatic changes in blood pressure and pulse. Glucose levels in diabetics should be checked.

Acid–Base Disturbance

Diuretics have an effect on acid–base balance via their different actions on the nephron. The thiazides and the loop diuretics are often associated with the generation and maintenance of a metabolic alkalosis. This usually requires no therapy. To correct the alkalosis, the associated volume and potassium deficiency would have to be corrected. If the volume were replenished, the effect of the diuretic would be negated. Therefore, usually only potassium-sparing diuretics or potassium chloride supplements are given (see Chapter 50). If the alkalosis is thought to be detrimental, for example, in patients with respiratory failure, the diuretic should be discontinued or the dosage reduced.

Potassium-sparing diuretics may be associated with diminished hydrogen ion excretion and therefore with a mild metabolic acidosis. This usually is of no consequence and requires no treatment.

Hyperuricemia

Thiazides and loop diuretics commonly elevate the concentration of serum urate by blocking urate secretion by the proximal renal tubules or by enhancing resorption through contraction of extracellular volume. However, symptomatic gout is not usual, nor is an elevated uric acid level likely to cause renal injury or stone formation. Therefore, routine measurement of uric acid and treatment are unnecessary unless gout occurs. Chapter 76 discusses treatment of diuretic-induced gout; in general, treatment is the same as for primary gout and does not require discontinuation of the diuretic. If NSAIDs or corticosteroids are used in treatment, the patient should be monitored closely for volume overload and for changes in renal function. Consultation with a rheumatologist may be advisable if gout is severe or recurrent in a patient with heart failure.

Hyperglycemia

Thiazides and, less commonly, loop diuretics may cause glucose intolerance. Hypoglycemic therapy may be required (or changed in diabetic patients already receiving a hypoglycemic agent) if the diuretic is to be continued (see Chapter 79).

Lipid Abnormalities

Thiazides may increase triglyceride concentrations in the blood. In patients with lipid abnormalities, a loop diuretic at low dosages (10–20 mg) may be preferable to a thiazide.

Other Effects

Thiazides occasionally are associated with a hypersensitivity-induced small vessel vasculitis, thrombocytopenia (see Chapter 56), and hypercalcemia and may be associated with impotence. Furosemide at high dosages has been associated with the development of interstitial nephritis and renal failure, especially in patients with marked proteinuria. As noted above, spironolactone, which structurally is closely related to estrogen, may cause gynecomastia, reduce libido in men, or cause impotence. These side effects usually resolve within a few weeks of discontinuing the drug. Eplerenone reportedly has a significantly lower incidence of these side effects. Even when diuretics have substantially relieved the signs and symptoms of CHF, other medications usually are necessary to optimize function and prolong life.

Digitalis

Digitalis may help restore cardiac compensation by increasing the inotropic state, or contractility, of cardiac muscle, thereby increasing the ejection fraction at a given preload and afterload, as described above. It appears to act by increasing calcium delivery to the contractile apparatus of the heart. Digoxin is the only positive inotropic agent that has been convincingly shown both to improve function and quality of life and to not increase mortality in patients with symptomatic heart failure (49). Because digoxin is indicated only for patients with heart failure caused by systolic dysfunction, it is ordinarily used in patients also being treated with a diuretic and an ACE inhibitor (see below).

Chapter 57). There have not been any completed controlled trials of anticoagulation in patients with heart failure. After adjusting for differences in baseline characteristics, warfarin use was associated with improved survival and reduced morbidity in patients with LV systolic dysfunction among patients enrolled in the Studies of Left Ventricular Dysfunction (66). Of note, warfarin use was not assigned in a randomized controlled fashion, and data on compliance with therapy, the intensity of anticoagulation, and complications of therapy were not reported. Warfarin therapy may be hazardous in patients with severe heart failure who may have wide swings in prothrombin time caused by hepatic dysfunction and multiple drug interactions. In such circumstances, the prothrombin time should be checked more frequently, perhaps every few weeks, or within 2 to 4 days after a medication known to interact with warfarin has been introduced or discontinued or if the dosage of warfarin or an interacting medication is changed.

Control of Arrhythmias in Heart Failure and Cardiac Resynchronization Therapy

One of the cardinal features of CHF is a tendency to develop arrhythmias. Between 30% and 50% of patients with chronic heart failure die suddenly, presumably of ventricular tachyarrhythmias, although some studies show bradyarrhythmia is as likely a cause of death. Holter monitoring seldom is useful in evaluating patients without symptomatic arrhythmias.

Patients with heart failure and arrhythmias should be evaluated and treated in consultation with a cardiologist. Consultation also should be considered for patients with severe LV dysfunction and/or advanced symptomatic heart failure. This is especially true because some of these patients, particularly those with an intraventricular conduction delay, might benefit from permanent transvenous biventricular pacing (leads simultaneously pacing both ventricles), "cardiac resynchronization therapy," or placement of an implantable defibrillator (see Chapter 64). Cardiac resynchronization therapy can improve cardiac function by synchronizing ventricular contraction. The rationale for this therapy is that a significant intraventricular conduction delay may adversely affect LV systolic function by producing asynchronous ventricular contraction. Cardiac resynchronization therapy has been shown to significantly improve symptoms and quality of life and to reduce morbidity and mortality in patients with severe heart failure symptoms due to LV systolic dysfunction despite standard pharmacologic therapy (67). The Comparison of Medical Therapy, Pacing, and Defibrillation in Heart Failure (COMPANION) trial studied patients at high risk for death due to advanced heart failure with conduction delays. This trial showed that cardiac resynchronization therapy, with or without a defibrillator, significantly lowered the risk of death from, or hospitalization for, heart failure (68). A pacemaker alone reduces the risk of death from any cause by 24% ($p = 0.059$), and a pacemaker–defibrillator significantly reduced the risk by 36%. In the Sudden Cardiac Death in Heart Failure Trial (SCD-HeFT), patients with LV systolic dysfunction were treated with conventional therapy for CHF plus either placebo, the antiarrhythmic drug amiodarone, or an implantable defibrillator. Whereas amiodarone did not have any significant effect on survival, defibrillator therapy significantly reduced overall mortality (69).

Operative Correction of Problems Causing Heart Failure

The most commonly encountered surgically correctable problems in patients with chronic congestive failure include ischemic heart disease with revascularizable lesions or with resectable ventricular aneurysm, valvular heart disease, and atrial septal defect. Any patient who is in heart failure caused by a surgically correctable cause of myocardial dysfunction should be considered for operative correction, and consultation with a cardiologist should be obtained. Patients whose heart failure is secondary to reversible LV dysfunction may not be easily distinguished by history, physical examination, and echocardiography from those with irreversible ventricular impairment. Noninvasive stress testing may be helpful for detecting ischemia or assessing myocardial viability in patients who are candidates for revascularization. Referral to a cardiologist may help select the appropriate noninvasive test or to determine which patients are appropriate for cardiac catheterization and coronary angiography.

Heart transplants should be considered for patients in severe refractory heart failure. The procedure is being performed in specialized centers throughout the United States. A number of contraindications to transplantation include age $\geq$70 years; irreversible severe renal, hepatic, or pulmonary disease; severe peripheral or cerebral vascular disease; and psychiatric impairment, so the proportion of eligible patients with heart failure is small. Even so, because of the scarcity of donated cadaver organs, the wait for an available compatible heart can be many months, during which time the patient may succumb to his or her disease.

Community Health Services

Many community health services are available to help the caregiver deal with the patient and to help the patient deal with the illness.

Home Visits

In at least two situations, home visits by the patient's health care provider or a visiting nurse should be considered in the management of a patient in heart failure: when the patient has repeatedly returned to the office or has been readmitted to the hospital with heart failure caused by dietary neglect or by failure to use medications correctly (see below) and when the homebound patient's symptoms are so severe (New York Heart Association class IV, Table 66.2) that he or she is unable to come for an office visit without becoming exhausted.

Information Booklets

The American Heart Association has useful free booklets that describe low-salt diets and the management of CHF for the patient and family. These booklets can be obtained from local chapters of the American Heart Association. The American Heart Association website also has excellent information for patients with heart failure (http://www.americanheart.org/chf/working/index.htm). Extensive information that is pertinent and useful is available at other World Wide Web sites, including that of the Heart Failure Society of America (www.hfsa.org).

Exercise Programs

Graduated regular exercise may improve exercise tolerance and increase daily activities and general well-being in some patients with heart failure, even in patients with severe LV dysfunction caused by ischemic heart disease. The improvement in function is thought to be caused by improved efficiency of the skeletal muscles; there is no evidence that myocardial function can be improved by exercise. Patients may also develop a sense of increased confidence in their ability to function.

Patients with class I to III CHF may be trained to exercise to 60% of their maximal heart rate for 20 minutes per day, 3 days per week. Exercise may be contraindicated entirely in patients who have uncompensated heart failure or whose heart failure is caused by valvular heart disease. Isometric exercise should be prescribed with caution in patients in heart failure because of the extra afterload imposed by this form of exercise on the heart. Well-supervised circuit weight training may be safe. Muscle toning exercises using 1-kg hand weights are safe and can be used safely to help maintain function in all but the most frail patients with heart failure.

Management Programs
Comprehensive Disease

Patients with heart failure require the type of coordinated, multidisciplinary care that has been shown to be most efficiently and effectively delivered by a comprehensive disease management program (70). These programs provide frequent contact with trained nurses or pharmacists and close coordination of care between primary care providers and cardiovascular specialists. Patients should be encouraged to participate in these programs if they are available in the community.

PROGNOSIS

The prognosis in heart failure is related clinically to the LV ejection fraction, the functional status of the patient, the initial response to treatment, the patient's compliance with the treatment regimen, the patient's age and comorbidities, and the cause of the heart failure. Physiologically, prognosis is related most importantly to LVEDP and to the degree of neurohumoral activation and LV remodeling. One available measure of these factors is the plasma BNP or NT-proBNP level (see above). Most patients in chronic CHF die suddenly, presumably from ventricular arrhythmia (71). Other common causes of death are progressive heart failure and cerebral and peripheral embolization (65). In the Framingham study reported in 1993, which included heart failure from all causes, the probability of dying within 5 years of onset of heart failure was 62% for men and 42% for women (4,71). The median survival after the onset of heart failure was 1.7 years in men and 3.2 years in women (71). The cause of heart failure in most of these patients was hypertension or ischemic heart disease. Heart failure complicating uncorrected aortic stenosis is particularly ominous, and most of these patients die within 3 years (see Chapter 65) unless aortic valve surgery is performed.

In general, prognosis is related to the patient's functional class (Table 66.2). Patients in functional class I have an annual mortality of approximately 10%. Patients in functional class IV have an annual mortality of nearly 50% (71). The practitioner should avoid discussing prognosis with the patient and family until after the optimal level of response to therapy has been achieved. It has been observed that the median survival in advanced heart failure is similar to that of patients with metastatic breast cancer. Hence, it is appropriate to discuss advance directives and living wills with the patient early in the course of treatment.

Over the 40-year period from 1948 to 1988 (before the widespread use of ACE inhibitors and β-blockers), there was no improvement in survival for patients with heart failure (71). Heart failure remains a lethal disease: age-adjusted 5-year mortality during the period from 1990 to 1999 (the most recent period for which data are available) was approximately 50% (72). However, the treatment of CHF in the ambulatory setting is evolving rapidly. Important advances in nonpharmacologic, pharmacologic, and device therapy for heart failure likely will continue to improve the outlook for patients with this condition.

Hospital Readmission

Patients discharged from the hospital with the diagnosis of heart failure have a high readmission rate. Factors associated with hospitalization include poor adherence to medical therapy and dietary restrictions, inadequate treatment of associated hypertension and ischemic heart disease, and underuse of ACE inhibitors (73). Comprehensive outpatient programs, which include intensive education of the patient and family, social service support, titration of medications, and close followup, have demonstrated reductions in hospitalization rates of up to 87%, associated with clinically significant decreases in sodium intake from 3,400 to 2,100 mg/day and increases in the daily dosages of ACE inhibitors (74,75).

Patients treated successfully for heart failure should be advised to pay attention to even subtle signs and symptoms that may precede overt decompensation. Mild dyspnea or a slight change in weight should not be ignored because these signs may be followed not by a gradual escalation in the severity of the condition but by severe and seemingly abrupt deterioration that requires readmission to the hospital. Decreasing the likelihood of hospital readmission requires (a) patient education about the importance of sodium restriction and careful monitoring of weight, (b) titration of medications to doses shown to be effective in clinical trials, (c) patient compliance with the medical treatment regimen, (d) decreasing the incidence of potentially preventable disease (e.g., influenza or pneumonia), (e) meticulous management of other medical illness (e.g., diabetes and hypertension), (f) constant monitoring of symptoms, and (g) timely reporting of increases in weight or development of symptoms to the patient's health care provider.

End-of-Life Issues

Patients with heart failure have a progressive, complex, costly, and often fatal disease. The primary care provider and/or cardiologist should discuss end-of-life issues with the patient or with friends or family designated by the patient. The clinical course of heart failure is marked by frequent exacerbations with other periods of relative comfort and good function. When symptoms become persistent and are refractory to the maximal medical therapy that can be tolerated by the patient, and when no other options are appropriate for, or desirable to, the patient (e.g., transplantation, cardiac resynchronization therapy), it is appropriate to discuss palliative measures (see Chapter 13) (76). It is important to clarify the patient's health care goals and to identify a person who will make health care decisions when the patient can no longer do so. A useful resource is available on the Internet at www.fivewishes.org.

PREVENTION OF HEART FAILURE

It has been shown in asymptomatic patients that the development of symptomatic heart failure may be predicted by the finding of cardiac enlargement on echocardiography (55). The prognosis of these patients may be improved by treatment with ACE inhibitors, which may delay the development of overt heart failure in patients with LV dysfunction (55).

Although preventing or delaying the development of symptoms in individuals with existent LV dysfunction is important and feasible, the major impact on heart failure prevention will result from a reduction in the prevalence of hypertension, diabetes mellitus, hyperlipidemia, and cigarette smoking and the adoption of a healthier diet and regular exercise programs by a greater proportion of the population. Much time and effort have been expended in identifying the medicines and interventions that will improve and prolong the lives of those with heart failure. The focus now must shift to ensure that patients get those medicines and, more importantly, that a greater number of our population will never need them.

SPECIFIC REFERENCES*

1. Haas GJ. Management of asymptomatic left ventricular dysfunction. Cleve Clin J Med 2001;68:249.
2. Felker GM, Adams KF Jr, Konstam MA, et al. The problem of decompensated heart failure: Nomenclature, classification, and risk stratification. Am Heart J 2003;145 [2 Suppl]: S18.
3. American Heart Association. Heart disease and stroke statistics—2005 update. Dallas, TX: American Heart Association, 2005.
4. Kannel WB. Vital epidemiologic clues in heart failure. J Clin Epidemiol 2000;53:229.
5. Polanczyk CA, Rohde LE, Dec GW, et al. Ten-year trends in hospital care for congestive heart failure: improved outcomes and increased use of resources. Arch Intern Med 2000;160:325.
6. Lakatta EG. Starling's law of the heart is explained by an intimate interaction of muscle length and myofilament calcium activation. J Am Coll Cardiol 1987;10:1157.
7. Katz AM, Lorell BH. Regulation of cardiac contraction and relaxation. Circulation 2000;102:IV69.
8. Hunter JJ, Chien KR. Signaling pathways for cardiac hypertrophy and failure. N Engl J Med 1999;341:1276.
9. Kang PM, Izumo S. Apoptosis and heart failure: a critical review of the literature. Circ Res 2000;86:1107.
10. Libby P, Lee RT. Matrix matters. Circulation 2000;102;1874.
11. Litwin SE, Grossman W. Diastolic dysfunction as a cause of heart failure. J Am Coll Cardiol 1993;22:49A.
12. Kass DA, Bronzwaer JG, Paulus WJ. What mechanisms underlie diastolic dysfunction in heart failure? Circ Res 2004;94:1533.
13. Nishimura RA, Tajik AJ. Evaluation of diastolic filling of left ventricle in health and disease: Doppler echocardiography is the clinician's Rosetta Stone. J Am Coll Cardiol 1997; 30:8.
14. Redfield MM, Jacobsen SJ, Burnett JC Jr, et al. Burden of systolic and diastolic ventricular dysfunction in the community: appreciating the scope of the heart failure epidemic. JAMA 2003;289:194.
15. Porter TR, Eckberg DL, Fritsch JM, et al. Autonomic pathophysiology in heart failure patients. Sympathetic-cholinergic interrelations. J Clin Invest 1990;85:1362.
16. Hall C. NT-proBNP: the mechanism behind the marker. J Card Fail 2005;11[5 Suppl]:81.
17. Schrier RW, Abraham WT. Hormones and hemodynamics in heart failure. N Engl J Med 1999;341:577.
18. Brilla CG. Aldosterone and myocardial fibrosis in heart failure. Herz 2000;25:299.
19. Michell AR. Effective blood volume: an effective concept or a modern myth. Perspect Biol Med 1996;39:471.
20. Fitzsimons JT. Angiotensin, thirst, and sodium appetite. Physiol Rev 1998;78:583.
21. Levy D, Larson MG, Vasan RS, et al. The progression from hypertension to congestive heart failure. JAMA 1996;275:1557.
22. Wittstein IS, Thiemann DR, Lima JA, et al. Neurohumoral features of myocardial stunning due to sudden emotional stress. N Engl J Med 2005;352:539.

*Bold numerals denote published controlled clinical trials, meta-analyses, or consensus-based recommendations.

23. Page J, Henry D. Consumption of NSAIDs and the development of congestive heart failure in elderly patients: an underrecognized public health problem. Arch Intern Med 2000;160:777.
24. Amabile CM, Spencer AP. Keeping your patient with heart failure safe: a review of potentially dangerous medications. Arch Intern Med 2004; 164:709.
25. Green CP, Porter CB, Bresnahan DR, et al. Development and evaluation of the Kansas City Cardiomyopathy Questionnaire: a new health status measure for heart failure. J Am Coll Cardiol 2000;35:1245.
26. Vaccarino V, Kasl SV, Abramson J, et al. Depressive symptoms and risk of functional decline and death in patients with heart failure. J Am Coll Cardiol 2001;38:199.
27. Harlan WR, Oberman A, Grimm R, et al. Chronic congestive heart failure in coronary artery disease: clinical criteria. Ann Intern Med 1977;86:133.
28. Butman SM, Ewy GA, Standen JR, et al. Bedside cardiovascular examination in patients with severe chronic heart failure: importance of rest or inducible jugular venous distension. J Am Coll Cardiol 1993;22:968.
29. Zaphiriou A, Robb S, Murray-Thomas T, et al. The diagnostic accuracy of plasma BNP and NTproBNP in patients referred from primary care with suspected heart failure: results of the UK natriuretic peptide study. Eur J Heart Fail 2005;7:537.
30. Wright SP, Doughty RN, Pearl A, et al. Plasma amino-terminal pro-brain natriuretic peptide and accuracy of heart-failure diagnosis in primary care: a randomized, controlled trial. J Am Coll Cardiol 2003;42:1793.
31. Troughton RW, Frampton CM, Yandle TG, et al. Treatment of heart failure guided by plasma amino terminal brain natriuretic peptide (N-BNP) concentrations. Lancet 2000;355:1126.
32. Davie AP, Francis CM, Love MP, et al. Value of the electrocardiogram in identifying heart failure due to left ventricular systolic dysfunction. BMJ 1996;312:222.
33. Hare JM, Walford GD, Hruban RH, et al. Ischemic cardiomyopathy: endomyocardial biopsy and ventriculographic evaluation of patients with congestive heart failure, dilated cardiomyopathy and coronary artery disease. J Am Coll Cardiol 1992;20:1318.
34. Jennings GL, Esler MD. Circulatory regulation at rest and exercise and the functional assessment of patients with congestive heart failure. Circulation 1990;81:II5.
35. Bittner V, Weiner DH, Yusuf S, et al. Prediction of mortality and morbidity with a 6-minute walk test in patients with left ventricular dysfunction. SOLVD Investigators. JAMA 1993;270:1702.
36. Olsson LG, Swedberg K, Clark AL, et al. Six minute corridor walk test as an outcome measure for the assessment of treatment in randomized, blinded intervention trials of chronic heart failure: a systematic review. Eur Heart J 2005;26:778.
37. Coats AJ. Exercise training for heart failure: coming of age. Circulation 1999;99:1138.
38. Keteyian SJ. How hard should we exercise the failing human heart? J Cardiopulm Rehabil 2001;21:164.
39. MacGregor GA, de Wardener HE. Salt, diet and health: Neptune's poisoned chalice: the origins of high blood pressure. Cambridge: Cambridge University Press, 1998.
40. Abramson JL, Williams SA, Krumholz HM, et al. Moderate alcohol consumption and risk of heart failure among older persons. JAMA 2001;285:1971.
41. Swan SK, Rudy DW, Lasseter KC, et al. Effect of cyclo-oxygenase-2 inhibition on renal function in elderly persons receiving a low-salt diet. A randomized, controlled trial. Ann Intern Med 2000;133:1.
42. Krumholz HM, Chen YT, Radford MJ. Aspirin and the treatment of heart failure in the elderly. Arch Intern Med 2001;161:577.
43. Masoudi FA, Inzucchi SE, Wang Y, et al. Thiazolidinediones, metformin, and outcomes in older patients with diabetes and heart failure: an observational study. Circulation 2005;111:583.
44. Nesto RW, Bell D, Bonow RO, et al. Thiazolidinedione use, fluid retention, and congestive heart failure: a consensus statement from the American Heart Association and American Diabetes Association. Diabetes Care 2004;27:256.
45. Cleland JG, Swedberg K, Poole-Wilson PA. Successes and failures of current treatment of heart failure. Lancet 1998;352[Suppl 1]:SI19.
46. Yusuf S, Pfeffer MA, Swedberg K, et al. Effects of candesartan in patients with chronic heart failure and preserved left-ventricular ejection fraction: the CHARM-Preserved Trial. Lancet 2003;362:777.
47. Pitt B. Aldosterone blockade in patients with systolic left ventricular dysfunction. Circulation 2003;108:1790.
48. Pitt B, Zannad F, Remme WJ, et al. The effect of spironolactone on morbidity and mortality in patients with severe heart failure. Randomized Aldactone Evaluation Study Investigators. N Engl J Med 1999;341:709.
49. The Digitalis Investigation Group. The effect of digoxin on mortality and morbidity in patients with heart failure. N Engl J Med 1997;336:525.
50. Rathore SS, Curtis JP, Wang Y, et al. Association of serum digoxin concentration and outcomes in patients with heart failure. JAMA 2003;289:871.
51. Effect of metoprolol CR/XL in chronic heart failure: Metoprolol CR/XL Randomised Intervention Trial in Congestive Heart Failure (MERIT-HF). Lancet 1999;353:2001.
52. Packer M, Bristow MR, Cohn JN, et al. The effect of carvedilol on morbidity and mortality in patients with chronic heart failure. U.S. Carvedilol Heart Failure Study Group. N Engl J Med 1996;334:1349.
53. Tendera M, Ochala A. Overview of the results of recent beta-blocker trials. Curr Opin Cardiol 2001;16:180.
54. Packer M, Fowler MB, Roecker EB, et al. Effect of carvedilol on the morbidity of patients with severe chronic heart failure: results of the carvedilol prospective randomized cumulative survival (COPERNICUS) study. Circulation 2002;106:2194.
55. Vasan RS, Larson MG, Benjamin EJ, et al. Left ventricular dilatation and the risk of congestive heart failure in people without myocardial infarction. N Engl J Med 1997;336:1350.
56. Brown NJ, Vaughan DE. Angiotensin-converting enzyme inhibitors. Circulation 1998;97:1411.
57. Pitt B, Poole-Wilson PA, Segal R, et al. Effect of losartan compared with captopril on mortality in patients with symptomatic heart failure: randomised trial—the Losartan Heart Failure Survival Study ELITE II. Lancet 2000;355:1582.
58. Granger CB, McMurray JJ, Yusuf S, et al. Effects of candesartan in patients with chronic heart failure and reduced left-ventricular systolic function intolerant to angiotensin-converting-enzyme inhibitors: the CHARM-Alternative trial. Lancet 2003;362:772.
59. Cohn JN, Tognoni G; Valsartan Heart Failure Trial Investigators. A randomized trial of the angiotensin-receptor blocker valsartan in chronic heart failure. N Engl J Med 2001;345:1667.
60. Cohn JN, Archibald DG, Ziesche S, et al. Effect of vasodilator therapy on mortality in chronic congestive heart failure. Results of a Veterans Administration Cooperative Study. N Engl J Med 1986;314:1547.
61. Taylor AL, Ziesche S, Yancy C, et al. Combination of isosorbide dinitrate and hydralazine in blacks with heart failure. N Engl J Med 2004;351:2049.
62. Monane M, Bohn RL, Gurwitz JH, et al. Noncompliance with congestive heart failure therapy in the elderly. Arch Intern Med 1994;154:433.
63. Bennett SJ, Milgrom LB, Champion V, et al. Beliefs about medication and dietary compliance in people with heart failure: an instrument development study. Heart Lung 1997;26:273.
64. DiMatteo MR, Lepper HS, Croghan TW. Depression is a risk factor for noncompliance with medical treatment: meta-analysis of the effects of anxiety and depression on patient adherence. Arch Intern Med 2000;160:2101.
65. Dries DL, Rosenberg YD, Waclawiw MA, et al. Ejection fraction and risk of thromboembolic events in patients with systolic dysfunction and sinus rhythm: evidence for gender differences in the studies of left ventricular dysfunction trials. J Am Coll Cardiol 1997;29:1074.
66. Al Khadra AS, Salem DN, Rand WM, et al. Warfarin anticoagulation and survival: a cohort analysis from the Studies of Left Ventricular Dysfunction. J Am Coll Cardiol 1998;31:749.
67. Cleland JG, Daubert JC, Erdmann E, et al. The effect of cardiac resynchronization on morbidity and mortality in heart failure. N Engl J Med 2005;352:1539.
68. Bristow MR, Saxon LA, Boehmer J, et al. Cardiac-resynchronization therapy with or without an implantable defibrillator in advanced chronic heart failure. N Engl J Med 2004;350: 2140.
69. Bardy GH, Lee KL, Mark DB, et al. Amiodarone or an implantable cardioverter-defibrillator for congestive heart failure. N Engl J Med 2005; 352:225.
70. McAlister FA, Stewart S, Ferrua S, McMurray JJ. Multidisciplinary strategies for the management of heart failure patients at high risk for admission: a systematic review of randomized trials. J Am Coll Cardiol 2004;44:810.
71. Ho KK, Anderson KM, Kannel WB, et al. Survival after the onset of congestive heart failure in Framingham Heart Study subjects. Circulation 1993;88:107.
72. Levy D, Kenchaiah S, Larson MG, et al. Long-term trends in the incidence of and survival with heart failure. N Engl J Med 2002; 347:1397.
73. Chin MH, Goldman L. Factors contributing to the hospitalization of patients with congestive heart failure. Am J Public Health 1997;87:643.
74. Rich MW, Beckham V, Wittenberg C, et al. A multidisciplinary intervention to prevent the readmission of elderly patients with congestive heart failure. N Engl J Med 1995;333:1190.
75. West JA, Miller NH, Parker KM, et al. A comprehensive management system for heart failure improves clinical outcomes and reduces medical resource utilization. Am J Cardiol 1997; 79:58.
76. Gottlieb SH. Palliative care in heart failure. Adv Studies Med 2003;3:456.

For annotated ***General References*** *and resources related to this chapter, visit www.hopkinsbayview.org/PAMreferences.*

Chapter 67

Hypertension

L. Randol Barker

High blood pressure (HBP), or hypertension, is the most common problem addressed in ambulatory care (see Table 1.3). The ambulatory management of this condition is a longitudinal process requiring skill in enlisting the patient's cooperation and in selecting, monitoring, and adjusting treatment. Hypertension has been studied extensively by epidemiologists and clinicians. The recommended care of patients with hypertension is based on findings from numerous clinical and epidemiologic studies.

EPIDEMIOLOGY

Prevalence and Incidence

Prevalence

As shown in data from the 1999–2000 National Health and Nutritional Examination Survey (NHANES) (Fig. 67.1), the prevalence of hypertension increases with age in all gender and race/ethnic subgroups. In this survey, hypertension was defined as a mean systolic blood pressure (SBP) on a single occasion of $\geq$140 mm Hg, a mean diastolic blood pressure (DBP) of $\geq$90 mm Hg, or current treatment for hypertension with prescribed medication.

The *prevalence of isolated systolic hypertension*, seen mainly in the elderly, is approximately 6% in persons 60 to 69 years old and approximately 18% in persons 80 years and older (1).

Of individuals with hypertension, approximately 75% have stage 1 hypertension, which is defined as SBP 140 to 159 mm Hg or DBP 90 to 99 mm Hg (see Clinical Classification). Therefore, in a typical practice, decisions must be made most often for patients with stage 1 hypertension.

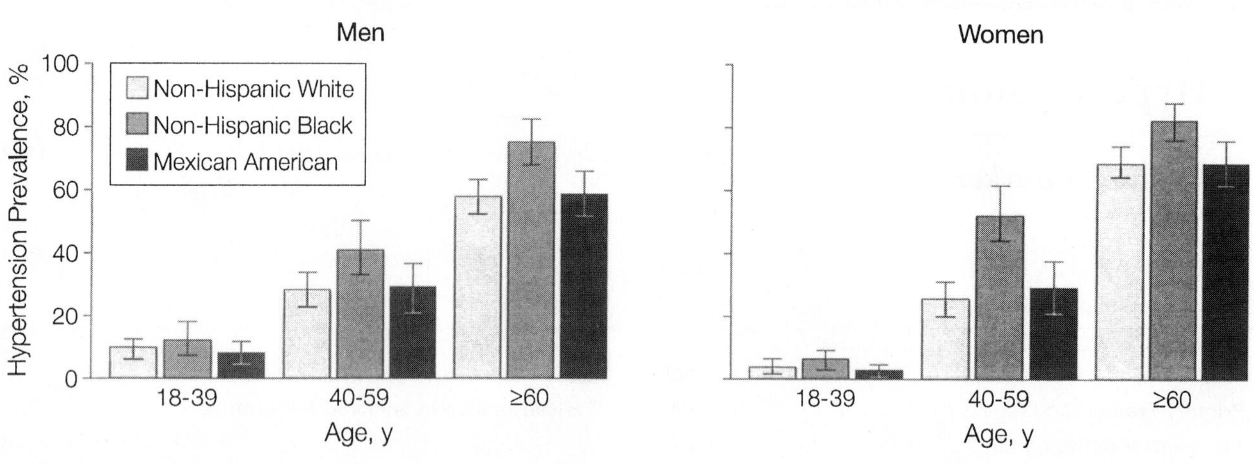

FIGURE 67.1. Hypertension prevalence by age and race/ethnicity in men and women. (From Hajjar I, Kotchen TA. Trends in prevalence, awareness, treatment, and control of hypertension in the United States, 1988–2000. JAMA 2003;290:199, with permission.)

Incidence

An estimated 1.8 million adults in the United States develop hypertension each year (2). An analysis using data from the Framingham Study estimated the 4-year rates of new hypertension in persons with optimal, normal, or high-normal blood pressure (Table 67.1) (3). Four-year incidence varied from 5.3% for persons 35 to 64 years old to 49.5% for those 65 to 94 years old. Increasing age and increasing weight were major predictors of incident hypertension.

Secular Trends in Prevalence, Awareness, Treatment, and Control of High Blood Pressure

The Surgeon General of the United States has named a goal of controlled HBP (<140/<90) for 50% of all persons with hypertension by the year 2010 (4). The record of progress toward that goal has been reported by NHANES for 1988–2002 (5). There has been a gradual increase in the prevalence of HBP and in the proportion of hypertensive persons aware that they have HBP, persons on treatment, and persons with controlled HBP. Table 67.2 summarizes these data for the two major subgroups in the United States: whites and non-Hispanic blacks. Multivariate analysis of the data from 1999–2002 showed that three factors independently predict uncontrolled HBP: being non-Hispanic black, being female, and not completing high school (5).

TABLE 67.1 Adjusted 4-Year Incidence of Hypertension According to Baseline BP Category (Framingham Study)

Baseline BP Category (mm Hg)	*4-Year Rates of Hypertension (95% Confidence Interval)* [a]	
	Age 35–64 y	*Age 65–94 y*
Optimum (<120/<80)	5.3 (4.4–6.3)	16.0 (12.0–20.9)
Normal (120–129/80–84)	17.6 (15.2–20.3)	25.5 (20.4–31.4)
High-normal (130–139/85–89)	37.3 (33.3–41.5)	49.5 (42.6–56.4)

[a] Rates are per 100 and are adjusted for sex, age, body mass index, baseline examinations, and baseline systolic and diastolic blood pressure (BP).
Adapted from Vasan RS, Larson MG, Leip EP, et al. Assessment of frequency of progression in non-hypertensive participants in the Framingham Heart Study: a cohort study. Lancet 2001;358:1682, with permission.

PRIMARY PREVENTION

Many subgroups in the population have an increased risk for development of sustained hypertension, including people who are overweight or sedentary, have high-normal BPs, consume excessive amounts of salt or alcohol, are African American, or have a family history of hypertension. Clinical trials have shown that weight reduction, regular exercise (aerobic and low intensity), reduced salt or alcohol intake, and a diet rich in vegetables and fruits but low in animal fat can prevent the development of hypertension and reduce BP (6–8). Other lifestyle changes evaluated in clinical trials have been found to have inconsistent or unproved efficacy in the prevention or treatment of hypertension. These include stress reduction and increased intake of potassium, fish oil, magnesium, and dietary fiber (7).

The widespread adoption of measures known to help prevent hypertension and of other measures known to protect cardiovascular health (e.g., not smoking, control of

TABLE 67.2 NHANES Data Showing Secular Trends in Prevalence of HBP, Awareness of HBP, Treatment of HBP, and Control of HBP

	Prevalence of HBP[a]		*Awareness of HBP[a]*		*On Treatment for HBP[a]*		*HBP Controlled[a]*	
Racial Group	*1988–1994*	*1999–2002*	*1988–1994*	*1999–2002*	*1988–1994*	*1999–2002*	*1988–1994*	*1999–2002*
White	24	28	70	70	54	60	26	35
Non-Hispanic black	36	41	74	78	58	68	23	32

Data are given as percentages for subjects age ≥20 years in two major racial groups: whites and non-Hispanic blacks.
[a]Age- and sex-adjusted rates.
HBP, high blood pressure; NHANES, National Health and Nutritional Examination Surveys.
Adapted from Hertz RP, Unger AN, Cornell JA, et al. Racial disparities in hypertension prevalence, awareness, and management. Arch Intern Med 2005;165:2098, with permission.

hypercholesterolemia) would reduce significantly the cardiovascular morbidity in the population. Health care professionals can help by recommending these measures to all patients and especially to those who have a family history of hypertension or have prehypertension (see Clinical Classification). A later section of this chapter describes practical details regarding nonpharmacologic measures for controlling or preventing hypertension.

RISKS AND RISK REDUCTION

Risks Attending Untreated Hypertension

Risk Related to Blood Pressure

For the patient and the practitioner, the single most important concept in approaching hypertension is that HBP increases the risk of symptomatic vascular disease (stroke, coronary artery disease, congestive heart failure [CHF], renal insufficiency) during the patient's entire life. This concept was elucidated best by the longitudinal observations on subjects in the Framingham study, which used 140/90 mm Hg as the threshold BP for hypertension (9). A number of other longitudinal studies corroborated the major findings of Framingham study (10). Additional analyses of existing data have shown the following:

- Across the entire BP range (115/75–185/115 mm Hg), the risk of cardiovascular disease doubles with each increment of 20 mm Hg in systolic BP and each 10 mm Hg increment in diastolic BP (11).
- The annual risk is higher for older patients at all BP levels, and incremental increases in SBP and in pulse pressure are the most powerful predictors of cardiovascular events in older hypertensive patients (9,12).
- At all ages and BPs, the annual incidence of events is somewhat higher for men than for women (9).

Coexisting Cardiovascular Risk Factors

Many subjects with hypertension have one or more other treatable risk factors. These risk factors may affect a patient's prognosis far more than does hypertension. This is illustrated by the fact that two hypothetical patients with the following risk-factor profiles have similar long-term cardiovascular risks:

Age	*Cigarettes per Day*	*Total Cholesterol*	*Diastolic Blood Pressure*
50	0	180 mg/day	125 mm Hg
50	30	220 mg/dL	95 mm Hg

Baseline Target Organ Damage

In addition to BP level, age, gender, and other risk factors, *coexisting cardiovascular abnormalities* (target organ damage) increase the degree of risk. This is illustrated in Table 67.3, which summarizes findings in subgroups of

TABLE 67.3 Placebo-Treated Subjects, Veterans Administration Trial: Impact of Blood Pressure and Cardiovascular Abnormalities on Attack Rate

Risk Factor at Entry[a] and Diastolic Blood Pressure (mm Hg)	*No. Patients*	*Attack Rate[b]*
Without Abnormality		
90–104	36	0.145
109–114	51	0.173
With Abnormality		
90–104	48	0.352
105–114	50	0.426

[a]Cardiovascular and renal abnormalities, defined as the presence of any of the following: grade 2 or greater hypertensive retinopathy, cardiomegaly on chest radiograph, left ventricular hypertrophy on electrocardiogram, evidence of renal damage, myocardial infarction, congestive heart failure, cerebrovascular accident.
[b]Rate observed during 3 years.
Adapted from Veterans Administration Cooperative Study Group on Antihypertensive Agents. Effects of treatment on morbidity in hypertension. III: influence of age, diastolic pressure, and prior cardiovascular disease; further analysis of side effects. Circulation 1972;45:991, with permission.

placebo-treated subjects from the Veterans Administration Therapeutic Trial.

Risk Reduction by Treatment of Hypertension

A number of placebo-controlled clinical trials completed between 1970 and 1985 demonstrated that pharmacologic treatment reduces risks in *middle-aged adults with diastolic hypertension* (13–18). In addition, placebo-controlled clinical trials reported between 1985 and 1997 showed convincingly that pharmacologic treatment also reduces morbidity and mortality in *older persons with HBP, including those with isolated systolic hypertension* (19–23).

A network meta-analysis (24) and a standard meta-analysis (25), both published in 2003, assessed the findings of all available placebo-controlled trials and head-to-head drug comparisons. Both of the very large data sets showed that the health benefits of first-line treatment of HBP with low-dose diuretics are equal to or exceed the benefits from first-line treatment with all other classes of antihypertensive drugs. Larger reductions in blood pressure produced larger reductions in risks (25). The health benefits measured were reduction in coronary heart disease, stroke, CHF, major cardiovascular events, cardiovascular disease mortality, and all-cause mortality. The conclusions from these meta-analyses concurred with the findings of the Antihypertensive and Lipid-Lowering Treatment to Prevent Heart Attack Trial (ALLHAT) (26), the very large head-to-head trial of the low-dose diuretic chlorthalidone with the calcium antagonist amlodipine and the angiotensin-converting enzyme (ACE) inhibitor lisinopril.

More than half of subjects in the treatment arms of most clinical trials received *second-line drugs* to achieve treatment goals, and considerable uncertainty exists regarding the optimal regimen for individual patients (see Treatment of Hypertension). In addition, until completion of the placebo-controlled Hypertension in the Very Elderly Trial (HYVET), uncertainty will exist about the health impact of antihypertensive treatment of patients older than 80 years.

Relative Risk Reduction

Aggregate analysis of clinical trial results has shown that antihypertensive treatment is associated with a relative risk reduction of 35% to 40% in stroke incidence, 20% to 25% in myocardial infarction (MI), and >50% in CHF (27). Treatment also prevents the onset or worsening of renal insufficiency, although population-based data suggest that control of HBP among African Americans may not protect renal function as effectively as in whites (2).

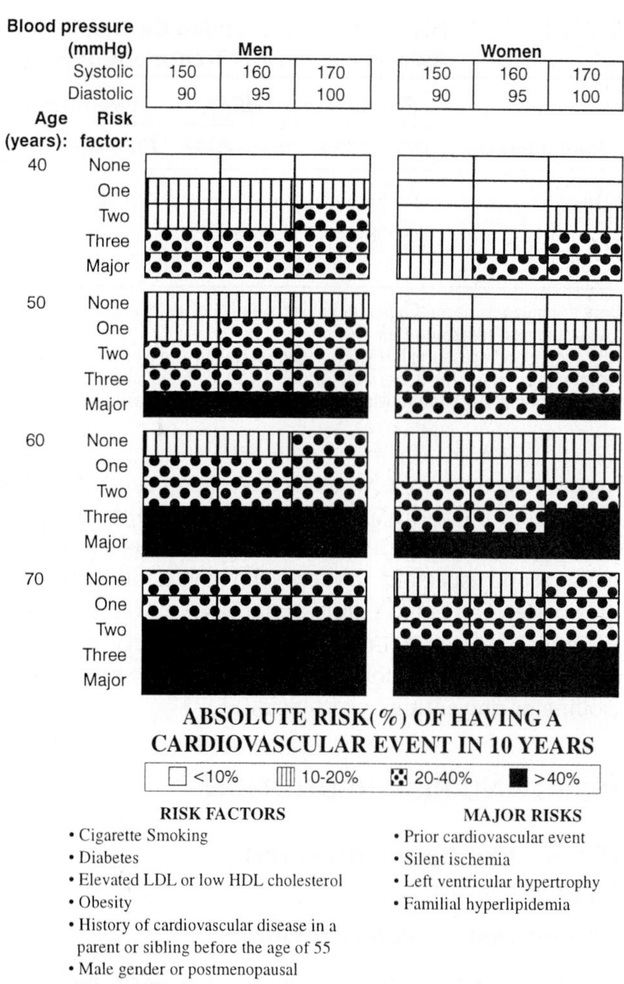

FIGURE 67.2. Matrix developed to help with decisions regarding the active treatment of hypertension based on blood pressure and other risk factors. Note that in 2006, *diabetes* would be regarded as a major risk factor. *Shading patterns* shown in boxes represent absolute risks during 10 years. (Adapted from Jackson R, Barham P, Bills J, et al. Management of raised blood pressure in New Zealand: a discussion document. BMJ 1993;307:107, with permission.)

Gender

Meta-analysis of data from seven clinical trials that included both men and women showed that the relative risk reduction attributable to treatment was *similar for both genders* (28).

Absolute Risk and Risk Reduction

As noted previously, the absolute risk of cardiovascular disease is much higher among patients with hypertension who are elderly and those with target organ damage or multiple risk factors. Figure 67.2 shows the combined impact of these patient characteristics on absolute risk. The absolute benefit of treatment also is higher when patients with these characteristics are treated. Assuming a relative risk reduction of approximately one third for combined cardiovascular events and using the information summarized in Fig. 67.2, it can be seen that the absolute benefits of treatment may differ greatly for patients with similar BPs. For example:

- *In a 70-year-old man with three major risk factors and BP of 160/90 mm Hg,* the 10-year risk of a major cardiovascular event is approximately 45%. A one-third reduction in risk would mean that approximately 15 of an expected 45 events would be prevented in a group of 100 such patients treated for 10 years. Stated another way, the *number needed to treat* for 10 years to prevent one event would be six or seven.
- *In a 40-year-old man with BP of 160/90 mm Hg and no major risk factors,* the 10-year risk of a major cardiovascular event is approximately 10%. A one-third reduction in risk would mean that approximately three of an expected ten events would be prevented in a group of 100 such patients treated for 10 years. In this instance, the *number needed to treat* for 10 years to prevent one event would be approximately 33.

For the following reasons, the findings from randomized controlled trials may underestimate the potential benefits of BP lowering:

- They use intention-to-treat assignment to analyze results.
- Cross-over occurs between treatment groups (no treatment to active treatment or active treatment to discontinuation of treatment).
- The average duration of treatment is 3 to 5 years, so benefits that accrue over longer treatment intervals are not detected.

Gender

Absolute risk reduction differs by type of cardiovascular event in men and women (28). In women, the major benefit is reduction in stroke. This benefit is especially pronounced in African American women, a finding that is partly explained by the greater absolute risk of stroke in these women (29). In men, treatment prevents as many coronary disease events as cerebrovascular events. This difference is thought to reflect the greater absolute risk of coronary events in untreated men.

Nonpharmacologic Measures

In clinical trials, nonpharmacologic measures (weight reduction; salt restriction; physical activity; high-vegetable, low-fat Dietary Approaches to Stop Hypertension [DASH] diet; reduced alcohol consumption) have been shown to reduce BP in hypertensive subjects (30). The approximate impact of each of these measures on blood pressure is summarized later (see Treatment of Hypertension). Although no trial of nonpharmacologic measures has been designed to detect their impact on cardiovascular morbidity and mortality, they likely are efficacious (8,30).

PATHOPHYSIOLOGY AND NATURAL HISTORY OF ESSENTIAL HYPERTENSION

An estimated 95% to 99% of hypertensive patients do not have an identifiable cause for their hypertension. Their problem has been designated *essential hypertension,* a condition whose antecedents probably are a mix of genetic and environmental factors. Several abnormal physiologic characteristics that have been demonstrated in essential hypertension provide a conceptual basis for understanding the clinical consequences of hypertension and the mechanisms of action of antihypertensive drugs.

The patient with established essential hypertension has an increase in peripheral arterial resistance (Fig. 67.3). This condition is hypothesized to be the final consequence of either or both of two mechanisms: inappropriate renal retention of salt and water or increased endogenous pressor activity. Serial studies on small numbers of subjects have suggested that a stage of increased cardiac output may precede the stage of increased peripheral resistance. This earlier stage may be manifested in some young hypertensives as a high resting heart rate. In general, however, evaluation of the individual patient with essential hypertension does not yield much information about the dominant mechanism contributing to that patient's HBP.

Figure 67.3 shows the major complications of untreated HBP. These complications can be seen as the clinical manifestations of two pathophysiologic processes that are

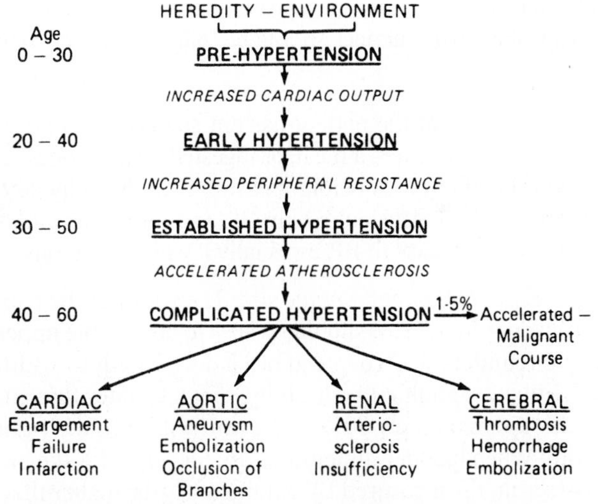

FIGURE 67.3. Representation of the natural history of untreated essential hypertension. (Modified from Kaplan N. Clinical hypertension. 6th ed. Baltimore: Williams & Wilkins, 1994;110, with permission.)

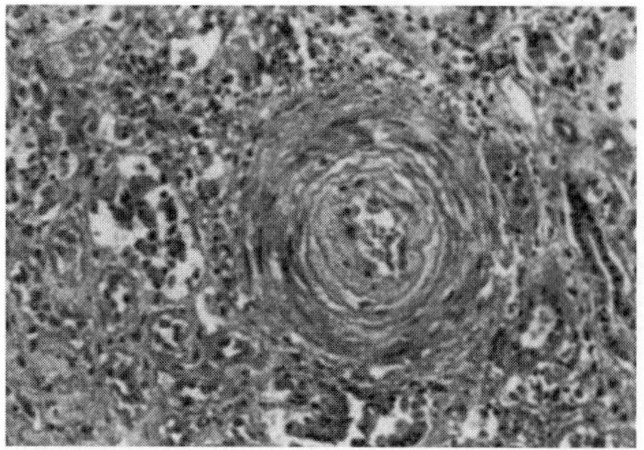

FIGURE 67.4. Hyperplastic arteriosclerosis in renal tissue from a patient with essential hypertension.

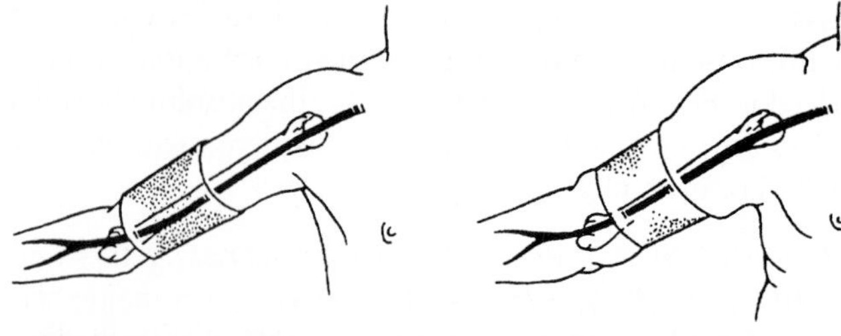

FIGURE 67.5. **Right:** Bladder width is small for arm, and full cuff pressure is never applied to artery. An erroneously high pressure results. **Left:** Bladder width is adequate for arm, and full cuff pressure is applied to brachial artery. (Reproduced with permission from the American Heart Association.)

operating during many silent years of increased peripheral resistance: *trauma to the vessels in the arterial circulation*, leading to accelerated atherosclerosis in large vessels and to obliterative changes (Fig. 67.4) or thinning and rupture in small vessels, and *increase in the workload of the heart*, leading to CHF or angina pectoris.

MEASURING THE BLOOD PRESSURE

Standard Practices

In response to Environmental Protection Agency recommendations, mercury manometers were to be eliminated by the year 2005, and BP measurement was to be accomplished either by auscultation, using aneroid manometry, or by automated electronic manometry. It has been recommended that auscultatory BP measurement be used to diagnose HBP and to verify abnormal BPs obtained electronically (31). A number of factors can affect the level of BP measured by a sphygmomanometer (32). To ensure the validity of the measured BP and to ensure that comparable information is obtained in repeated observations, the following standard practices should be followed at each visit (33,34):

1. Ensure that the patient has not smoked, chewed or snuffed tobacco, eaten a meal, or ingested caffeine or alcohol within 30 minutes before measurement. Nicotine and caffeine cause a transient rise in BP, and eating can cause a transient decrease in BP, especially in elderly persons.

2. *Select cuff of appropriate size.* The width of the rubber bladder in the cuff should be 40% to 50% of the upper arm circumference. The ratio of bladder length to width is 2:1 in most adult cuffs, meaning that a bladder that encircles approximately 80% of the arm will have the right width. When bladder dimensions are too small for the patient's arm, the measured BP obtained may be higher than the actual BP (Fig. 67.5). Overestimation of BP because of small cuff size can be minimized by using large adult cuffs (bladder dimensions approximately 30 × 15 cm) for all adult patients.

3. Apply the cuff to the subject's arm so that the lower margin is 2.5 cm above the antecubital space and the middle of the inflatable bladder is aligned with the brachial artery pulse.

4. Have the patient sit with the back supported in a chair for at least 1 minute. Measure the BP with the arm passively supported across the chest or resting on a table so that the stethoscope head is placed over the brachial artery pulse at the level of the heart (about the level of the junction of the fourth intercostal space with the lower left sternal border). Sitting unsupported or actively holding one's arm across the chest can cause SBP and DBP to increase by 5 to 10 mm Hg. Standing (in the untreated patient) may cause an increase and recumbency a decrease in BP.

5. *In a new patient, measure the pressure in each arm.* If a difference between arms is noted and confirmed on repeated measurement, take all subsequent BPs in the arm with the higher pressure. The most common cause of arm-to-arm difference, which occurs in some patients with atherosclerotic disease, is partial occlusion of blood flow proximal to the brachial artery.

6. *Record the first Korotkoff sound for SBP.* The cuff pressure should be high enough to obliterate the radial pulse; by ensuring that this occurs, one avoids reading a falsely low SBP resulting from the *silent auscultatory gap* that occasionally occurs between the first and second Korotkoff sounds.

7. *Deflate the cuff slowly (approximately 2 mm Hg/s).* This prevents underestimation of SBP and overestimation of DBP. Both may occur with too rapid deflation, especially in a patient with a relatively slow resting heart rate. Underestimation of SBP may occur if the patient has an auscultatory gap.

8. *Record the fifth Korotkoff sound (disappearance) for DBP.*

9. *Wait 30 seconds* before repeating measurement in the same arm to permit the return of the blood that has transiently filled the veins distal to the inflated cuff.

10. *Use the average of two readings* in the same arm to designate the patient's BP. If the two measurements of SBP or DBP differ by >5 mm Hg, repeat measurements until a stable level is reached.

11. To detect orthostatic hypotension before initiating antihypertension treatment, and after starting or increasing therapy with antihypertensive drugs, record the BP with the patient standing for at least 1 minute. In treated patients, consider also measuring the BP after a standard exercise (e.g., ten steps on a footstool or walking a fixed distance) because the orthostatic effect of drugs often is more pronounced after exercise.

12. *Record BP, pulse rate, position, arm, and cuff size* (if a large cuff is used), thereby ensuring that these conditions will be duplicated when BPs are measured at subsequent visits.

Special Situations

Atrial Fibrillation

In patients with atrial fibrillation, whose beat-to-beat stroke volume and BP differ because of varying intervals between ventricular beats, the average of several SBP and DBP values should be recorded.

Pseudohypertension

When the wall of the brachial artery is rigid from calcification, the cuff pressure needed to compress the artery may greatly exceed the intra-arterial pressure, and a very high cuff pressure may be assumed, incorrectly, to be the actual BP. This condition, which has been called *pseudohypertension,* can be tentatively diagnosed by the finding that the (presumably calcified) radial artery does not collapse when the pulse is obliterated during cuff inflation. However, substantial intraobserver and interobserver variability exist in the interpretation of this maneuver (35). Definitive diagnosis of pseudohypertension requires arterial catheterization to directly measure the BP, which then is compared with the cuff pressure. It is important to consider pseudohypertension in the evaluation of patients—usually older patients with widespread atherosclerosis—who describe hypotensive symptoms despite apparently normal or high cuff pressures. A practical approach to management when pseudohypertension is suspected is described later (see Orthostatic Symptoms).

White-Coat Hypertension and White-Coat Effect

Among patients with stage 1 hypertension in the physician's office (see Clinical Classification), ≥20% have normal average daytime BPs if measured at home (36). This pattern is referred to as *white-coat hypertension*. Many patients with apparent white-coat hypertension have normal BPs when the measurement is repeated after the patient has rested quietly in the office. The *white-coat effect* refers to an average office-measured BP that is higher than the average daytime BP. Up to 40% of patients have a white-coat effect of ≥20/10 mm Hg (37). This effect is largest in patients with stage 2 HBP. Although cohort studies have indicated that patients with white-coat hypertension do not have excess cardiovascular risks, cross-sectional studies have found increased risk of left ventricular hypertrophy (LVH) in such patients (38), and evidence indicates that some develop sustained HBP (i.e., elevated home *and* office pressures) (37). Management decisions for patients who demonstrate these patterns are discussed later (see Treatment of Hypertension: General Considerations).

Self-Measurement and Ambulatory Blood Pressure Monitoring

Self-measurement by the patient or someone else and ambulatory blood pressure monitoring (ABPM) are two ways in which the snapshot type of information obtained at office visits can be expanded. Critical assessment of experience with these two methods yields the following conclusions (37,39):

- Neither method was used to classify the subjects in the observational studies and clinical trials described earlier that are the basis for current treatment guidelines. Therefore, neither method is recommended for routine assessment and management of patients.
- The findings from cross-sectional and prospective studies have shown that target organ disease (e.g., LVH) and long-term risks correlate better with BPs from ABPM than with office BPs.
- Both self-measurement and automated ABPM can be helpful when office BPs do not seem to be sufficient for making clinical decisions (Table 67.4) or when patients wish to be more involved in monitoring the status of their BP.
- Based on findings from multiple studies and using a cutoff point of two standard deviations above the mean BP in patients with normal pressure or untreated HBP, it has been recommended that home readings ≥135/85 mm Hg should be considered hypertensive (30,37).
- Self-measurement has a specificity of 85% for identifying white-coat hypertension.
- A large proportion of patients do not adhere to correct technique for self-measurement, and/or they obtain BPs that differ from simultaneous BPs by ABPM.

Home Self-Measurement Devices

Many devices are available, ranging from inexpensive units that require auscultation with a stethoscope to more expensive electronic units that display the BP digitally. These

TABLE 67.4 Situations in Which Self-Measurement Devices or Automated Noninvasive Ambulatory Blood Pressure Monitoring Devices May Be Useful for Clinical Decisions

"Office" or "white-coat" hypertension: blood pressure repeatedly elevated in office setting but repeatedly normal when out of office
Evaluation of apparent drug resistance
Evaluation of nocturnal blood pressure changes
Episodic hypertension
Hypotensive symptoms associated with antihypertensive medications or autonomic dysfunction
Carotid sinus syncope and pacemaker syndromes[a]

[a]Along with electrocardiographic monitoring.
From The sixth report of the Joint National Committee on Prevention, Detection, Evaluation, and Treatment of High Blood Pressure. Arch Intern Med 1997;157:2413, with permission.

devices are reviewed periodically to help consumers select among them. *Finger monitors* are not accurate and should not be recommended (40). When a patient decides to measure BPs at home, it is essential to confirm at periodic office visits that the patient's technique is satisfactory and that similar pressures are obtained with the home monitoring device and the office unit.

Ambulatory Blood Pressure Monitoring Devices

These are portable devices that measure cuff pressures frequently over a 24-hour period. Patients are instructed to hold the arm still during automatic cuff inflation and to keep a diary and report dizziness, headache, or other symptoms of interest. Reports display average daytime, nighttime, and 24-hour pressures; frequencies and temporal distribution of selected pressures; and the *BP load* (e.g., percentage of waking pressures >140/90 mm Hg or sleeping pressures >120/80 mm Hg). The American Society of Hypertension has selected as abnormal an overall average 24-hour SBP >135 mm Hg and DBP >85 mm Hg and has selected the following as *"probable abnormal" awake or asleep BPs* (39):

	Average Systolic BP	Average Diastolic BP	BP Load
Awake	>140	>90	>30% above 140/90
Asleep	>125	>80	>30% above 120/80

Because there are no standard recommendations for the use of these types of aggregate data in decision making, ABPM is mainly useful in selected patients (Table 67.5). The charge for 24-hour monitoring ranges from $150 to $450.

TABLE 67.5 Classification of Blood Pressure for Adults Aged 18 Years or Older (JNC-7)

BP Classification	Systolic BP (mm Hg)	Diastolic BP BP (mm Hg)
Normal	<120 and	<80
Prehypertension	120–139 or	80–89
Stage 1 hypertension	140–159 or	90–99
Stage 2 hypertension	≥160 or	≥100

BP, blood pressure.
Adapted from Chobanian AV, Bakris GL, Black HR, et al. The seventh report of the Joint National Committee on Prevention, Detection, Evaluation, and Treatment of High Blood Pressure: the JNC 7 Report. JAMA 2003;289:2560, with permission.

Clinical trials comparing treatment decisions based on average office BPs to decisions based on average home BPs measured by ABPM (41) or self-monitoring (42) concluded that the latter decisions led to less intensive BP treatment and a better sense of well-being (ABPM) but did not reduce the overall cost of treatment.

Blood Pressure Variability

A number of psychological, biologic, and pharmacologic factors cause BP variability. These factors should be considered when determining the meaning of the measured BP in an individual patient and when following the standard approach to measuring the BP (described earlier).

Normal Patterns

In a 24-hour period, the average person's resting BP fluctuates (SBP 20–40 mm Hg; DBP 10–20 mm Hg) (37). The lowest BPs occur during sleep. These ranges occur in patients with normal BP and in hypertensive patients who are or are not taking antihypertensive drugs. During ordinary activities such as walking, talking on the telephone, attending a meeting, dressing, eating, and working at a desk, slight increases in both SBP (5–20 mm Hg) and DBP (5–10 mm Hg) may occur in untreated subjects. During and after vigorous exercise, SBP may rise as much as 60 mm Hg, and there may be a modest decrease in DBP.

Common causes of transient or short-term high BP are white-coat hypertension (see White-Coat Hypertension and White-Coat Effect); mental stress, both intellectual and psychological; self-medication with excessive amounts of nonprescription sympathomimetic decongestants; nicotine, caffeine, or alcohol use shortly before BP measurement; and alcohol or sedative–hypnotic withdrawal.

Common causes of transient or short-term decrease in a patient's BP are volume contraction during an illness that causes fluid losses or reduced intake; bed rest for several days; hospitalization with or without strict bed rest; and the postprandial state in elderly persons.

Additional findings that increase the prior probability of pheochromocytoma are a marked change in BP or heart rate in response to minor injury, parturition, or general anesthesia; a neurocutaneous syndrome (von Recklinghausen disease or von Hippel–Lindau syndrome); a blood relative with a pheochromocytoma; and type II multiple endocrine neoplasia (medullary carcinoma of the thyroid, parathyroid adenoma, or both, with symptoms suggesting pheochromocytoma).

Screening Tests

Because pheochromocytoma is uncommon, the best practice is to screen only those patients in whom clinical suspicion is high and to refer for consultation or more costly diagnostic evaluation only those patients with positive screening tests. Measurement of 24-hour urinary excretion of one or more of the three markers for increased pressor synthesis (catecholamines, metanephrines, and vanillylmandelic acid) is a screening test that has satisfactory performance characteristics. When used in a patient with an estimated 5% pretest probability of having a pheochromocytoma (e.g., a hypertensive patient with unexplained paroxysms of headache, tachycardia, and/or diaphoresis), excess excretion of any of the three markers would increase to 35% to 45% the probability (positive predictive value) that the patient has pheochromocytoma; normal results would increase from 95% to approximately 99% the probability (negative predictive value) that the patient does not have pheochromocytoma (61). An alternative test, measurement of the plasma level of normetanephrine or metanephrine, may have better performance characteristics but is not yet available for routine screening.

Diagnostic Tests

Patients with positive screening tests should undergo definitive diagnostic testing to localize the presumed tumor. This process has been improved by the availability of radioisotope scanning using labeled iodobenzylguanidine, followed by CT scanning or magnetic resonance imaging of the site that takes up this substance. Almost all pheochromocytomas are located in the adrenal glands; 1% to 3% may be located in the posterior mediastinum. Of these tumors, 90% can be totally removed at surgery. Up to 10% are found to be malignant at surgery.

Sleep Apnea

Sustained hypertension occurs in some patients with obstructive sleep apnea. From one small clinical trial, it appears that the hypertension abates in response to therapeutic but not subtherapeutic treatment with continuous positive airway pressure (62) (see Chapter 7).

Coarctation of the Aorta

Clues to the presence of this condition are hypertension in a relatively young patient (most are recognized in the pediatric age group); decreased BP in the lower extremities as suggested by diminished or absent femoral pulses and corroborated by auscultation over the popliteal artery using a large cuff; and evidence of collateral arterial circulation either on inspection of the trunk or on the plain chest radiograph, which may show poststenotic dilation of the aorta. In a minority of patients, the coarctation occurs proximal to the left subclavian artery, and the BP is high only in the right arm. The patient must undergo aortography to confirm the presence of a coarctation.

Status of Factors Modified by Treatment of Hypertension

Table 67.6 lists factors that should be addressed or documented at baseline because these factors may be modified as part of the treatment plan or as a consequence of treatment. They include information obtained from the history (patient's understanding of hypertension, usual diet, alcohol consumption, current medications), the physical examination (weight, BP, heart rate and rhythm, edema), and laboratory tests (creatinine, electrolytes, fasting glucose, complete blood count, uric acid, cholesterol, and urinalysis).

Status of Other Cardiovascular Risk Factors

Coexisting cardiovascular risk factors are common in patients with hypertension. They greatly affect a patient's long-term probability of morbidity and mortality (Fig. 67.2). Therefore, the baseline evaluation of a hypertensive patient should include checking for other risk factors, which should be considered in planning the overall management. These factors include gender, family history of premature cardiovascular disease, tobacco use (see Chapter 27), high-cholesterol or high-salt diet, hypercholesterolemia (see Chapter 82), sedentary living (see Chapter 16), stressful lifestyle, obesity (see Chapter 83), and diabetes mellitus (see Chapter 79).

TREATMENT OF HYPERTENSION

General Considerations

Goals of Treatment

When sustained hypertension has been confirmed, the goal of treatment is to reduce the patient's risk of future cardiovascular disease by restoring the BP to normal and controlling other risk factors. Normal BP is defined as office SBP <140 mm Hg and DBP <90 mm Hg, or home SBP <135 mm Hg and DBP <85 mm Hg (30). *For diabetic patients and for patients with CHF or chronic renal failure,* a BP <130/80 mm Hg is recommended (30). For patients in whom goal BPs cannot be attained, partial BP control confers some benefit (63).

Timetable

In patients who choose a nonpharmacologic regimen (discussed later), a trial of this approach for 6 to 12 months usually is needed to evaluate its impact on BP. When drug treatment is selected, a goal of satisfactory BP control without significant drug side effects usually can be achieved within 1 to 3 months.

White-Coat Hypertension and White-Coat Effect

The criteria for these two patterns were described earlier (see Measuring the Blood Pressure). The data are not adequate for defining BP goals or treatment recommendations for patients with *white-coat hypertension.* At least one large study showed similar 4-year rates of cardiovascular morbidity in patients with high office BPs (stages 1 or 2) who did or did not manifest a *white-coat effect* (lower, often still high, daytime BPs) and were treated based on their office BPs (64). As noted previously, the current consensus is that home BPs ≥135/85 mm Hg should be considered elevated, meaning that the goal home BPs for these and other patients should be less than these levels (30).

Intensity of Blood Pressure Lowering

Because of the suggestion that an on-treatment DBP <85 mm Hg may increase risk (a "J-curve" effect), particularly in patients with pre-existing coronary artery disease (65), in the early 1990s some authorities recommended that the DBP should not be reduced to <85 mm Hg. However, no J-curve pattern was reported in the Systolic Hypertension in the Elderly Program (SHEP), in which the average on-treatment DBP was 68 mm Hg (21). The subsequent Hypertension Optimal Treatment (HOT) clinical trial, which was designed to compare the effects of on-treatment DBPs ≤90 mm Hg, ≤85 mm Hg, and ≤80 mm Hg, did not find evidence of a J-curve effect (66). A meta-analysis of seven large placebo-controlled clinical trials found an increased mortality risk in patients with the lowest SBPs or DBPs in both treatment and placebo groups. The authors concluded that the increased mortality was the result of poor health but not HBP treatment (67). In two groups of patients (those with diabetes and those with CKD), there is evidence that more intense BP lowering enhances the benefits of treatment (see Pharmacologic Treatment: Specific Considerations).

Initiating and Adjusting Treatment

A recommended approach to initiating and adjusting treatment of HBP is summarized in the algorithm from JNC-7 shown in Fig. 67.6. Despite new data from clinical trials reported since publication of JNC-7, this algorithm, which emphasizes attaining target BPs, remains a valid guide for treatment of most patients.

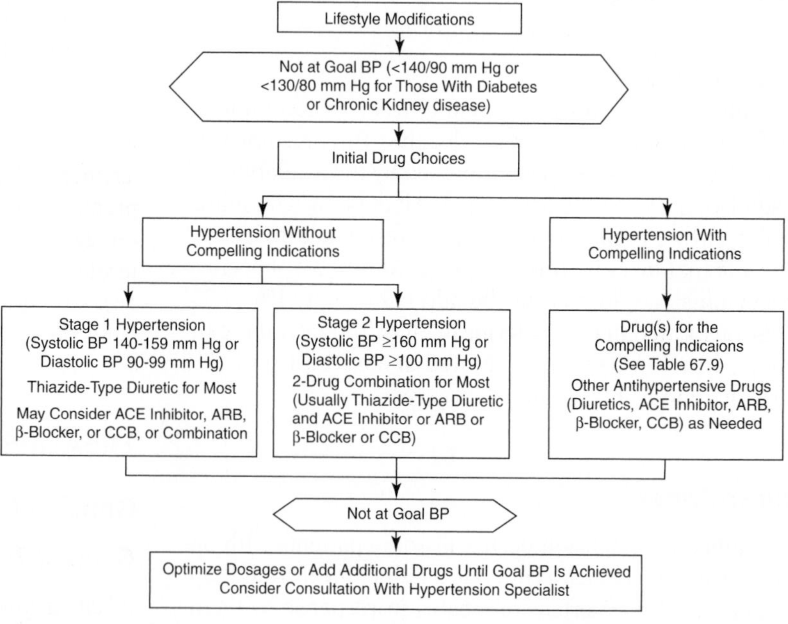

FIGURE 67.6. Algorithm for treatment of hypertension. (Adapted from Chobanian AV, Bakris GL, Black HR, et al. The seventh report of the Joint National Committee on Prevention, Detection, Evaluation, and Treatment of High Blood Pressure: the JNC 7 Report. JAMA 2003;289:2560, with permission.)

Special considerations for the treatment of hypertension in *adolescents, elderly persons, and pregnant women* are discussed in later sections of this chapter.

For stage 1 HBP (sustained SBP 140–159 mm Hg or DBP 90–99 mm Hg), an individualized approach to initial treatment is appropriate. Figure 67.2 shows the graded impact of BP level, other risk factors, and clinical cardiovascular disease on the 10-year prognosis for hypertensive patients. Initial treatment with antihypertensive drugs would be appropriate for stage 1 patients with any *major risk factor* (history of a clinical cardiovascular event, silent ischemia, LVH, diabetes). The presence at baseline of *multiple other cardiovascular risk factors* (smoking, hypercholesterolemia, age older than 60 years, male gender, postmenopausal status, strong family history of cardiovascular morbidity) also favors initial drug treatment. For patients with stage 1 HBP who do not have these associated characteristics, it is reasonable to attempt nonpharmacologic treatment for up to 1 year, especially in those patients who voice a strong preference to try this approach.

For stage 2 HBP (sustained SBP ≥160 mm Hg or DBP ≥100 mm Hg), initial pharmacologic treatment is appropriate. JNC-7 recommends starting drugs from two classes, one of which usually should be a thiazidelike diuretic. This strategy recognizes that (a) two or more drugs have been needed to achieve BP control in more than half of subjects in clinical trials and (b) failure to advance pharmacologic treatment probably explains a substantial proportion of patients who are on treatment but are not controlled (Table 67.2).

Nonpharmacologic Treatment (Lifestyle Modification)

Measures Shown to be Efficacious

A number of nonpharmacologic modalities that require a lifestyle change can either prevent the development of HBP (see Primary Prevention) or lower BP. Although no clinical trials have determined the impact of any these measures on symptomatic cardiovascular disease, there is evidence that nonpharmacologic control of HBP may be as effective as pharmacologic control in preventing LVH (68).

Individual measures for which there is clinical trial evidence for effectiveness in lowering BP include *reducing weight, following a healthy diet (the DASH diet), reducing daily intake of salt, and limiting alcohol intake* (30,68–75). Table 67.7, from JNC-7, shows for each of these lifestyle changes the approximate reduction in SBP reported in clinical trials. Table 67.8, which can be copied for distribution to patients, summarizes what patients need to know in order to follow a low-salt diet. When giving this information to a patient, it is important to point out that approximately 75% of a person's daily intake of salt usually comes from processed foods.

Maintenance of lifestyle modification, and its benefits, requires ongoing motivation of the patient (see Chapter 4). As noted above, for motivated patients with stage 1 HBP and few or no associated risk factors, one or more lifestyle modifications can be tried as primary treatment. Additionally, these measures should be recommended, when pertinent, to all patients who are beginning treatment with

TABLE 67.7 Lifestyle Modifications to Manage Hypertension[a]

Modification	*Recommendation*	*Approximate Systolic BP Reduction, Range*
Weight reduction	Maintain normal body weight (BMI, 18.5–24.9)	5–20 mm Hg/10-kg weight loss
Adopt DASH eating plan	Consume a diet rich in fruits, vegetables, and low-fat dairy products with a reduced content of saturated and total fat	8–14 mm Hg[68,69]
Dietary sodium reduction	Reduce dietary sodium intake to no more than 100 mEq/L (2.4 g sodium or 6 g sodium chloride)	2–8 mm Hg[68,70]
Physical activity	Engage in regular aerobic physical activity such as brisk walking (at least 30 minutes per day, most days of the week)	4–9 mm Hg[71,72]
Moderation of alcohol consumption	Limit consumption to no more than 2 drinks per day (1 oz or 30 mL ethanol [e.g., 24 oz beer, 10 oz wine, or 3 oz 80-proof whiskey]) in most men and no more than 1 drink per day in women and lighter-weight persons	2–4 mm Hg[73]

Abbreviation: BMI, body mass index calculated as weight in kilograms divided by the square of height in meters; BP, blood pressure; DASH, Dietary Approaches to Stop Hypertension.

[a]For overall cardiovascular risk reduction, stop smoking. The effects of implementing these modifications are dose- and time-dependent and could be higher for some individuals.

Adapted from Chobanian AV, Bakris GL, Black HR, et al. The seventh report of the Joint National Committee on Prevention, Detection, Evaluation, and Treatment of High Blood Pressure: the JNC 7 Report. *JAMA* 2003;289:2560.

TABLE 67.8 Information for Patients Who Are Advised to Follow a 2-g Sodium Diet

Americans eat approximately 20 times more sodium than they need, most of which comes from salt, which is one source of sodium.

Sodium[a] is

- found naturally in foods, even those that do not taste salty.
- added to food by manufacturers during food processing.
- added in cooking in the form of salt, baking powder, baking soda, or seasonings such as monosodium glutamate (MSG).
- added as salt to food at the table.

- In the body, sodium acts like a sponge to hold water in the body tissues. Sometimes the body cannot get rid of enough of the sodium. High blood pressure may result. If not controlled, high blood pressure leads to stroke, kidney failure, and heart disease.
- Using no salt in cooking or at the table and eliminating highly salted food cuts down the sodium level of the food you eat to approximately 2,000 mg/day.

Add New Flavors to Your Food!

- Herbs and spices can give new zest to your unsalted cooking.
- A little herb goes a long way. If you are making your own substitution without the benefit of a recipe, try ¼ teaspoon of dried herb or spice to
  - a recipe for four servings,
  - a pound of meat, poultry, fish, or vegetable or two cups of sauce.
    - If you are using red pepper or garlic powder, start with only ⅛ teaspoon. Taste and add a little more, depending on your preference.
- If you use fresh herbs, use four times the amount of dried herb. Instead of ¼ teaspoon of dried herb, use one full teaspoon of fresh herb.
- Add dried herbs to soups and stews during the last hour of cooking.
- Use whole spices in slow-cooking dishes and add them at the beginning of the cooking period.
- When using ground spices, add them 15 minutes before the end of the cooking period. If adding them to uncooked dishes, add them several hours before serving. As a start, try one or a combination of the following popular herbs:

Basil	Rosemary
Celery seed	Sage
Marjoram	Savory
Mint	Thyme

Beware of Hidden Sodium!

Processed Foods

- Salt is added to many packaged, convenience, "fast," and canned foods. Examples are packaged dinners (e.g., macaroni and cheese), packaged coatings and "helpers," combination dinners (e.g., frozen meals and casserole dishes), canned soups, dried soups, canned vegetables, and frozen vegetables with sauces.

"Fast Foods"

- Generally, meals served at "fast-food" places are high in sodium. A typical meal of a hamburger, french fries, and a vanilla shake can total >1,000 mg sodium—more than half of your total daily allowance. Remember that pizza, hot dogs, burgers, fried chicken, fried fish, omelets, and tacos served at fast-food places usually are high in sodium. Just one whole dill pickle contains 1,900 mg sodium, almost the total allowed in this diet.
- Read labels carefully. Foods that list salt or sodium as ingredients should be avoided. Compare different brands of the same product. It is unnecessary to purchase special dietetic foods. Many dietetic foods contain sodium or salt, so read the labels carefully.

Additives

- Sodium may be added to food as a preservative; for quick cooking; to soften or loosen skins of fruits and vegetables; to cure meats, fish, sausage; to stop growth of molds. Additives that contain sodium include
  - MSG
  - Baking soda
  - Disodium phosphate
  - Sodium alginate
  - Sodium benzoate
  - Sodium hydroxide
  - Sodium nitrate
  - Sodium propionate
  - Sodium sulfite

Some Tips on Eating Out

- Select restaurants that offer *á la carte* service.
- For breakfast, order from the allowed cereals. Poached or boiled eggs with toast can be ordered at most restaurants.
- For lunch, try fruit or tossed salads; roast beef, sliced chicken, or turkey breast sandwich; and fruit for dessert.
- When ordering rice, ask if it has been cooked in salted water. Some restaurants cook rice without salt. Rice pilaf usually is prepared with salt.
- You can count on baked potato. For toppings use butter, margarine, or sour cream.
- If in doubt about cooked vegetables, order sliced tomatoes or a salad such as tossed salad, lettuce wedge, or fruit salad. Try lemon or oil and vinegar for the dressing. Ask the waiter to leave off the croutons!

TABLE 67.8 (Continued) Information for Patients Who Are Advised to Follow a 2-g Sodium Diet

- At dinner, try fruit (fresh, canned, or frozen), fruit juice, or fruit cup as an appetizer.
- If you select broiled meats, fresh fish, or chicken, you can request that no salt or other condiments such as garlic salt or onion salt be added before or after broiling.
- Help yourself to the bread basket, but avoid salted breadsticks and crackers with salted tops.
- For dessert select fruit, sherbet, ice cream, or plain yogurt.
- Inside cuts of roast beef, lamb, pork, veal, chicken, and turkey have less sodium than outside cuts. Trim off the edges that would have been salted. Ask that the meat be served without gravy or sauce.
- Most airlines provide "special meals." A low-sodium meal can be ordered at no extra cost when you make your flight reservation.
- Fast-food menu items (except for the salad bar where you can select low-sodium items) usually have been salted. If food can be prepared to order, request that no salted seasonings be added.

To Sum It Up

- Using less salt is advisable for almost everyone, even children, so let the whole family join in.
- Avoid shaking salt on your food. Substitute a blend of herbs for your salt shaker.
- Cook without salt. Try leaving it out of recipes.
- Experiment with new flavors by using herbs and spices. Fine restaurants rely on herbs, spices, and the natural flavor of food, not salt, for good taste.
- Avoid fast foods and other processed foods high in sodium.
- Read the labels of foods and medicines to find "hidden" sodium. Look for the symbol Na; look for the words salt, sodium, soda, brine.
- Become familiar with foods that are high in sodium.
- Low-sodium salt, such as "Lite Salt," is a combination of sodium and potassium. Do not be misled that it is free of sodium. It has about half the sodium content of regular salt.
- Use of low-sodium salt and salt substitutes can be dangerous because of the very high potassium content. It is essential that you ask your doctor if you can use these products. Also ask how much you can use each day.

[a]Useful conversions: 100 mg sodium = 4.35 mEq sodium; 100 mg sodium = 250 mg salt; 1 teaspoon salt = 6 g sodium.
Modified from "Health Is In—Salt Is Out," courtesy of The Maryland High Blood Pressure Coordinating Council.

antihypertensive drugs. As discussed later, when a patient continues to ingest a large amount of salt while taking diuretics, potassium wasting is increased. Therefore, salt restriction may both facilitate BP reduction and prevent excessive potassium loss in patients taking diuretics. Finally, among patients who are taking antihypertensive drugs, the lifestyle modifications listed in Table 67.7 may enable motivated patients to decrease or discontinue drugs and maintain control of their HBP (see Step-Down Therapy).

Physical Activities while Taking Antihypertensive Drug

Most patients want to be informed about the implications of hypertension and antihypertensive drug therapy for ordinary physical activity. Subjects with untreated hypertension have the same patterns of BP fluctuation during exercise as normotensive subjects, only at higher pressures. With vigorous exercise, the SBP rises (as much as 60 mm Hg) while the DBP may rise or fall slightly. Similar patterns usually are found in patients treated with antihypertensive drugs. The effects of a number of antihypertensives and other cardiovascular drugs on BP during exercise are summarized in Table 63.7. In general, it is reasonable to inform patients that their hypertension does not make them different and to reassure them that they can engage in all of their usual activities after beginning treatment for hypertension.

Dietary Potassium

Consuming a diet with substantial potassium content may facilitate the BP-lowering effects of weight reduction, salt restriction, or antihypertensive drugs (76). Increased potassium intake usually occurs as a consequence of changing to a low-sodium diet, which tends to contain more potassium-rich natural foods (e.g., fresh fruits and vegetables) in place of processed food. Because potassium deficiency may cause the BP to increase, maintenance of a normal serum potassium concentration ($\geq$3.5 mEq/L) probably facilitates the BP-lowering effect of diuretics.

Cognitive and Behavioral Techniques

Cognitive and behavioral techniques include biofeedback, stress management, meditation, and muscle relaxation techniques. Critical assessment of clinical trials of these techniques does not support the efficacy of any of the techniques as a primary method for decreasing BP (77). Motivated patients may wish to use one of these techniques as an adjunct to another primary treatment strategy. Chapter 22 describes muscle relaxation techniques useful for stress reduction.

Other Substances and Nutrients

Adequate intake of *calcium and magnesium* or supplemental *garlic* may promote BP reduction, but no evidence

TABLE 67.9 Compelling Indications for Individual Drug Classes

High-Risk Conditions with Compelling Indication*	Recommended Drugs					
	Diuretic	**β-Blocker**	**ACE Inhibitor**	**ARB**	**CCB**	**Aldosterone Antagonist**
Heart failure	•	•	•	•		•
Post-myocardial infarction		•	•			•
High coronary disease risk	•	•	•		•	
Diabeties	•	•	•	•	•	
Chronic kidney disease			•	•		
Recurrent stroke prevention	•		•			

*Compelling Indications for antihypertensive drugs are based on benefits from outcome studies or existing clinical guidelines; the compelling Indication is managed in parallel with the blood pressure. Note: In the JNC-7, this table also designates, with references, the clinical trial basis for each of the compelling indications.
Adapted from Chobanian AV, Bakris GL, Black HR, et al. The seventh report of the joint National Committee on Prevention, Detection, Evaluation, and Treatment of High Blood Pressure: the JNC 7 Report. JAMA 2003;289:2560.

indicates that increased amounts of either of these nutrients should be recommended (37). Although *fish oils* may lower BP, they are associated with adverse effects that counterbalance the small benefit. *Caffeine and nicotine* may transiently raise BP, but their elimination does not lower BP. The amount of nicotine in nicotine substitution products used in smoking cessation aids described in Chapter 27 usually does not raise BP (78).

Pharmacologic Treatment: General Recommendations

To date, objective methods for selecting the most appropriate antihypertensive drug or combination of drugs for an individual patient have not been developed. Therefore, drug treatment for most patients should be initiated and adjusted using the strategies outlined in the algorithm in Fig. 67.6 and those in Table 67.9.

The recommendations shown in Fig. 67.6 for initial choice of antihypertensive drugs are based on clinical trials demonstrating that active drug treatment decreases morbidity and mortality. One or more large placebo-controlled trials or head-to-head equivalence trials have demonstrated this for each of the major classes of drugs: diuretics, β-blockers, ACE inhibitors, calcium antagonists, and ARBs (24,25). The evidence from trials in which a drug from each class was used as first-line treatment was pooled in two meta-analyses published in 2003 (24,25). A major clinical trial published after these meta-analyses, a head-to-head comparison of amlodipine and atenolol, suggested that atenolol may be inferior to other amlodipine HBP drugs. However, critical commentary on the trial concluded that effective BP lowering by any class of drug—or, as is often the case, two or more drugs from different classes—remains the best predictor of health benefit (79).

Table 67.9 lists clinical conditions for which there are *compelling indications, supported by clinical trial results, for choosing individual drug classes.* These indications are based on benefits attributable to BP lowering and/or treatment of a coexisting condition (e.g., β-blockers or ACE inhibitors for a post-MI patient, α-blockers for a patient with benign prostate hypertrophy). These indications and other factors that may guide drug selection are discussed in the next section.

The impact of most antihypertensive drugs on BP occurs within 1 to 7 days. For patients with stage 1 HBP, it is reasonable to evaluate the response to medications within 1 month. Patients with stage 2 hypertension, especially those with SBP $\geq$180 mm Hg or DBP $\geq$110 mm Hg, should be evaluated frequently until there is evidence that the BP is responding to the drugs and dosages prescribed.

PHARMACOLOGIC TREATMENT: SPECIFIC CONSIDERATIONS

Classes of Antihypertensive Drugs

For all available classes of antihypertensive drugs, Table 67.10 provides information about available products, dosages, and common side effects. Table 67.11 summarizes common drug–drug interactions.

Because drugs from each class of antihypertensive agents are available in preparations that are effective for 24 hours or longer, it is prudent to attempt to control a patient's BP with a *once-a-day medication schedule*.

Many proprietary antihypertensive drugs are substantially more expensive than *generic preparations*. Generic preparations are available for drugs from each class except the newest class, the ARBs (Table 67.10).

Monotherapy and Combination Therapy

Overview

Decisions about initiating and adjusting drug treatment of HBP were addressed in a landmark meta-analysis of

TABLE 67.10 Oral Antihypertensive Drugs[a]

Drug Classes and Drugs	Trade Name	Usual Dose Range in Total mg/day (Frequency per Day)	Available Strengths (mg)	Selected Side Effects and Comments[b]
DIURETICS (Partial List)				
Thiazide and Thiazidelike Diuretics				Biochemical abnormalities: ↓ potassium, ↓ sodium, ↑ uric acid Sexual dysfunction: ↑ calcium, ↓ magnesium, short-term ↑ cholesterol, ↑ glucose Rare: blood dyscrasias, photosensitivity, pancreatitis, hyponatremia
Chlorthalidone (G)	Hygroton	12.5–50 (1)	25, 50	
Hydrochlorothiazide (G)	HydroDIURIL, Microzide, Esidrix	12.5–50 (1)	12.5, 25, 50	
Indapamide (G)	Lozol	1.25–5 (1)	2.5	(Less or no hypercholesterolemia)
Metolazone	Mykrox	0.5–1.0 (1)	0.5	
	Zaroxolyn	2.5–10 (1)	2.5, 5	
Loop Diuretics				
Bumetanide (G)	Bumex	0.5–4 (2–3)	0.5, 1	(Short duration of action, no hypercalcemia)
Ethacrynic acid	Edecrin	25–100 (2–3)	50	(Only nonsulfonamide diuretic, ototoxicity)
Furosemide (G)	Lasix	40–240 (2–3)	20, 40, 80	(Short duration of action, no hypercalcemia)
Torsemide (C)	Demadex	5–100 (1–2)	5, 10, 20, 100	(Long duration of action)
Potassium-Sparing Agents				Hyperkalemia
Amiloride (G)	Midamor	5–10 (1)	5	
Spironolactone (G)	Aldactone	25–100 (1)	25, 50, 100	(Gynecomastia)
Triamterene (G)	Dyrenium	25–100 (1)	50, 100	
ADRENERGIC INHIBITORS				
Peripheral-Acting Agents				
Guanadrel	Hylorel	10–75 (2)	10, 25	(Postural hypotension, diarrhea)
Reserpine (G)[c]	Serpasil	0.05–0.25 (1)	0.1, 0.25	(Nasal congestion, sedation, depression, activation of peptic ulcer)
Central-Acting Agents				Sedation, dry mouth, bradycardia, withdrawal hypertension
Clonidine (G)[d]	Catapres	0.2–1.2 (2–3)	0.1, 0.2	(More withdrawal)
Guanabenz (G)	Wytensin	8–32 (2)	4, 8	
Guanfacine (G)	Tenex	1–3 (1)	1, 2	(Less withdrawal)
Methyldopa (G)	Aldomet	500–3000 (2)	250, 500	(Hepatic and "autoimmune" disorders)
Alpha Blockers				Postural hypotension
Doxazosin (G)	Cardura	1–16 (1)	1, 2, 4, 8	
Prazosin (G)	Minipress	2–30 (2–3)	1, 2, 5	
Terazosin (G)	Hytrin	1–20 (1)	1, 2, 5, 10	

(Continued)

TABLE 67.10 (Continued) Oral Antihypertensive Drugs[a]

Drug Classes and Drugs	Trade Name	Usual Dose Range in Total mg/day (Frequency per Day)	Available Strengths (mg)	Selected Side Effects and Comments[b]
***β*-Blockers**				Bronchospasm, bradycardia, heart failure, may mask insulin-induced hypoglycemia Less serious: impaired peripheral circulation, insomnia, fatigue, decreased exercise tolerance, ↓ high-density lipoprotein cholesterol, hypertriglyceridemia (except agents with intrinsic sympathomimetic activity)
Acebutolol (G)[e, f]	Sectral	200–800 (1)	200, 400	
Atenolol (G)[e]	Tenormin	25–100 (1–2)	25, 50, 100	
Betaxolol (G)[e]	Kerlone	5–20 (1)	10, 20	
Bisoprolol (G)[e]	Zebeta	2.5–10 (1)	5, 10	
Carteolol[e, f]	Cartrol	2.5–10 (1)	2.5, 5	
Metoprolol (G)[e]	Lopressor	50–300 (2)	50, 100	
	Toprol-XL	50–300 (1)	50, 100, 200	
Nadolol (G)		20–320 (1)	20, 40, 80, 120, 1, 60	
Penbutol	Levatol	10–80 (1)	20	
Pindolol (G)		10–60 (2)	5,10	
Propranolol (G)	Inderal	40–480 (2)	10, 20, 40, 60, 80	
Timolol (G)	Blocadren	20–60 (2)	5, 10, 20	
Combined α- and β-Blockers				Postural hypotension, bronchospasm
Carvedilol	Coreg	12.5–50 (2)	3.125, 6.25, 12.5, 25	
Labetalol (G)	Normodyne, Trandate	200–1,200 (2)	100, 200, 300	
DIRECT VASODILATORS				Headaches, fluid retention, tachycardia
Hydralazine (G)	Apresoline	50–300 (2)	10, 25, 50, 100	(Lupus syndrome, sensory neuropathy)
Minoxidil (G)	Loniten	15–100 (1)	2.5, 10	(Hirsutism)
CALCIUM ANTAGONISTS				
Nondihydropyridines				Conduction defects, worsening of systolic dysfunction, gingival hyperplasia ankle edema
Diltiazem (G)	Cardizem SR	120–360 (2)	60, 80, 120	(Nausea, headache, lupuslike rash)
	Cardizem CD, Dilacor XR, Tiazac	120–360 (1)	120, 180, 240, 300	
Verapamil (G)	Isoptin, Calan	40, 80, 120 (3)		
	Isoptin SR, Calan SR	90–480 (2)	120, 180, 240	(Constipation)
	Verelan, Covera HS	120–480 (1)	120, 180, 240, 360	

Dihydropyridines				Ankle edema, flushing, headache, gingival hypertrophy
Amlodipine	Norvasc	2.5–10 (1)	2.5, 5, 10	
Felodipine	Plendil	2.5–20 (1)	5, 10	
Isradipine	DynaCirc	5–20 (2)	2.5, 5	
	DynaCirc CR	5–20 (1)	5, 10	
Nicardipine (G)	Cardene SR	60–90 (2)	20, 30	
Nifedipine (G)	Procardia XL, Adalat CC	30–120 (1)	30, 60, 90	
Nisoldipine	Sular	20–60 (1)	10, 20, 30, 40	
ANGIOTENSIN BLOCKERS				
Angiotensin-Converting Enzyme (ACE) Inhibitors				Common: cough Uncommon: angioedema, hyperkalemia, rash, loss of taste, leucopenia, hepatotoxicity, pancreatitis, acute renal failure with bilateral renal artery stenosis, ↑ fetal loss if given in second or third trimester
Benazepril	Lotensin	5–40 (1–2)	5, 10, 20, 40	
Captopril (G)	Capoten	25–150 (2–3)	12.5, 25, 50, 100	
Enalapril (G)	Vasotec	50–40 (1–2)	2.5, 5, 10, 20	
Fosinopril	Monopril	10–40 (1–2)	10, 20	
Lisinopril	Prinivil, Zestril	5–40 (1)	5, 10, 20, 40	
Moexipril (G)	Univasc	7.5–15 (2)	7.5, 15	
Perindopril	Aceon	4–8 (1–2)	2, 4, 8	
Quinapril (G)	Accupril	5–80 (1–2)	5, 10, 20, 40	
Ramipril	Altace	1.25-20 (1–2)	1.25, 2.5, 5, 10	
Trandolapril	Mavik	1–4 (1)	1, 2, 4	
Angiotensin II Receptor Blockers				Similar to ACE Inhibitors, but do not cause cough and rarely cause angioedema, loss of taste, or hepatotoxicity
Candesartan	Atacand	8–32 (1)	4, 8, 16, 32	
Eprosartan	Teveten	400–800 (1–2)	400, 800	
Irbesartan	Avapro	150–300 (1)	150, 300	
Losartan	Cozaar	25–100 (1–2)	25, 50	
Olmesartan	Benicar	20–40 (1)	5, 20, 40	
Perindopril	Aceon	4–8 (1–2)	2, 4, 8	
Telmisartan	Micardis	40–80 (1)	40, 80	
Valsartan	Diovan	80–320 (1)	80, 160	

[a]These dosages may vary from those listed in the *Physicians' Desk Reference,* which can be consulted for additional information. The listing of side effects is not all inclusive; clinicians are urged to refer to the package insert for a more detailed listing.
[b]Parentheses indicate individual drug effect; all others are class effects.
[c]Also acts centrally.
[d]Also available as transdermal therapeutic system (Catapres TTS) in patches that deliver 0.1–0.3 mg/day for 7 days.
[e]Cardioselective.
[f]Has intrinsic sympathomimetic activity.
G, generic available.
Adapted from The sixth report of the Joint National Committee on Prevention, Detection, Evaluation, and Treatment of High Blood Pressure. Arch Intern Med 1997;157:2413, with permission.

TABLE 67.11 Selected Drug Interactions with Antihypertension Therapy

Class of Agent	*Increase Efficacy*	*Decrease Efficacy*	*Effect on Other Drugs*
Diuretics	Diuretics that act at different sites in the nephron (e.g., furosemide + thiazides)	Resin-binding agents NSAIDs Steroids	Diuretics raise serum lithium levels. Potassium-sparing agents may exacerbate hyperkalemia due to ACE inhibitors.
β-blockers	Cimetidine (hepatically metabolized beta blockers) Quinidine (hepatically metabolized β-blockers) Food (hepatically metabolized beta blockers)	NSAIDs Withdrawal of clonidine Agents that induce hepatic enzymes, including rifampin and phenobarbital	Propranolol induces hepatic enzymes to increase clearance of drugs with similar metabolic pathways. β-Blockers may mask and prolong insulin-induced hypoglycemia. Heart block may occur with nondihydropyridine calcium antagonist. Sympathomimetics cause unopposed α-adrenoceptor–mediated vasoconstriction. β-Blockers increase angina-inducing potential of cocaine.
ACE inhibitors	Chlorpromazine or clozapine	NSAIDs Antacids Food decreases absorption (moexipril)	ACE inhibitors may raise serum lithium levels. ACE inhibitors may exacerbate hyperkalemic effect of potassium-sparing diuretics.
Calcium antagonists	Grapefruit juice (some dihydropyridines) Cimetidine or ranitidine (hepatically metabolized calcium antagonists)	Agents that induce hepatic enzymes, including rifampin, phenytoin, and phenobarbital	Cyclosporine levels increase[a] with diltiazem, verapamil, mibefradil, or nicardipine, but not felodipine, isradipine, or nifedipine. Nondihydropyridines increase levels of other drugs metabolized by the same hepatic enzyme system, including carbamazepine, digoxin, quinidine, sulfonylureas, and theophylline.
α-blockers			Verapamil may lower serum lithium levels. Prazosin may decrease clearance of verapamil.
Centrally acting α_2-agonists and peripheral neuronal blockers		Tricyclic antidepressants (and probably phenothiazines) Monoamine oxidase inhibitors Sympathomimetics or phenothiazines antagonize guanethidine or guanadrel Iron salts may reduce methyldopa absorption	Methyldopa may increase serum lithium levels. Severity of clonidine withdrawal may be increased by β-blockers. Many agents used in anesthesiology are potentiated by clonidine.

[a]This is a clinically and economically beneficial drug–drug interaction because it both retards progression of accelerated atherosclerosis in heart transplant recipients and reduces the required daily dosage of cyclosporine.
ACE, angiotensin converting enzyme; NSAIDs, nonsteroidal anti-inflammatory drugs.
From The sixth report of the Joint National Committee on Prevention, Detection, Evaluation, and Treatment of High Blood Pressure. Arch Intern Med 1997;157:2413.

placebo-controlled trials of diuretics, β-blockers, ACE inhibitors, ARBs, and calcium antagonists (80). This study found the following:

- *Monotherapy* with drugs from these five classes caused similar BP reductions at the "usual maintenance doses" listed in reference pharmacopoeias (mean SBP and DBP reductions of 9.1 and 5.5 mm Hg) and lower doses (mean SBP and DBP reductions of 7.1 and 4.4 mm Hg).
- *Lower-dose drug combinations* (from those trials that included this strategy) yielded mean SBP and DBP reductions of 14.6 and 8.6 mm Hg.
- *Adverse effects*: The mean frequency of adverse effects was 5.2% in the monotherapy arms and 7.5% in lower-dose combination drug arms. Adverse effects related to all drugs were strongly dose related, with the exception of ACE inhibitor cough, which was not dose related.

The greater impact of low-dose combination therapy on BP reduction supports the JNC-7 recommendation to consider initiating two drugs for patients with stage 2 hypertension. The fact that side effects were less than additive in two-drug regimens indicates that side effects will only modestly limit the number of patients able to tolerate initial combination therapy.

Monotherapy with drugs from each class, with the exception of vasodilators, can be chosen initially. The vasodilators hydralazine and minoxidil usually require cotreatment with an adrenergic inhibitor to prevent reflex tachycardia. At least 50% of patients with stage 1 HBP reach their BP target with low-dose monotherapy alone. Increasing the dosage of the initial drug or adding another drug makes achievement of the BP target possible in most patients.

Thiazides

Initial monotherapy with a low dose of a thiazide-type diuretic (e.g., 12.5–25 mg hydrochlorothiazide daily) is appropriate for most patients (30). The rationale for this recommendation is that the diuretic arms of multiple clinical trials have shown clinical benefits equal to or better than the benefits in the nondiuretic arms of these trials.

α-Blockers

Because of the increased incidence of heart failure in patients taking the α-blocker doxazosin in a head-to-head comparison of drugs from the major classes, α-blockers should not be selected for initial monotherapy (81). An exception to this is patients prescribed α-blocker treatment to control symptoms from benign prostate hypertrophy (see Chapter 53).

β-Blockers

Although they lower BP, β-blockers, particularly atenolol, the first-line β-blocker in a number of clinical trials, have not been shown to benefit health as much as other BP-lowering drugs (82,83). Because of these findings, beta blockers generally should not be used for monotherapy but do have a role as adjuncts to drugs in other classes.

Fixed-Dose Combination Tablet

Drugs from two or more classes of antihypertensive agents (usually a low-dose thiazide diuretic plus a nondiuretic) are available in a number of fixed-dose combinations. The appropriate combination tablets may provide additional convenience at no extra cost.

Drug Combinations with Beneficial or Risky Synergies

Two antihypertensive drug combinations have been shown to have beneficial synergistic effects:

- An *ACE inhibitor* added to a *thiazide or loop diuretic:* may prevent diuretic-induced hypokalemia
- An *adrenergic inhibitor* (β-blocker or central-acting α-agonist) plus a *vasodilator* (hydralazine or minoxidil): the former prevents reflex tachycardia induced by the latter, enabling the patient to take these potent vasodilations.

Certain two-drug combinations may have potentially harmful synergistic effects:

- An *ACE inhibitor or an ARB* combined with a *potassium-sparing diuretic* and/or potassium supplements: may cause hyperkalemia.
- A *β-blocker* plus a *nondihydropyridine calcium antagonist*: may cause heart block.

Adding a Diuretic

The addition of a diuretic has been shown to enhance the antihypertensive effect of all nondiuretic drugs. Therefore, in a patient who does not achieve control with one of the nondiuretic drugs, the *addition of a low dosage of a thiazide-type diuretic* should be considered. Higher doses of a thiazide, a more potent loop diuretic, or a potassium-sparing diuretic may be needed in some patients who have edema from sodium retention. An especially potent regimen—the combination of a loop diuretic (e.g., furosemide) with a low dosage of a diuretic active at the distal convoluted tubule (e.g., a thiazide or metolazone)—occasionally is needed to control volume overload in a patient whose hypertension is related to this condition.

Demographic Characteristics

African-American subjects respond less often than whites to ACE inhibitor and β-blocker monotherapy and more often to monotherapy with diuretics or calcium antagonists. When their HBP is controlled with combinations of any BP-lowering drugs, the health benefits of treatment appear to be similar (84). In many *older patients with isolated systolic HBP*, low-dose thiazide-type diuretic or long-acting dihydropyridine calcium antagonist monotherapy controls the BP and reduces morbidity and mortality (21,22). *Gender* has not been correlated with selected advantages or disadvantages of any classes of antihypertensive drugs. Because the potent vasodilator minoxidil causes marked hirsutism, it is not an acceptable medication for women. Additional considerations in managing hypertension in *adolescents, older patients*, and *pregnant patients* are discussed in later sections of this chapter.

Miscellaneous Coexisting Medical Conditions

Coexisting medical conditions may influence the selection of antihypertensive drugs. Table 67.9 lists *compelling indications* for each class of drugs, indicating that there is evidence for drug-specific benefits from randomized controlled trials.

Nondiabetic Chronic Kidney Disease

Based on trials that have compared multiple drugs, it appears that ACE inhibitors and ARBs may have a selective renoprotective effect in patients with nondiabetic CKD (30). On the other hand, BP reduction with drugs from all classes has delayed the progression of CKD. A 2004 meta-analysis of clinical trials that used ACE inhibitors and other classes of drugs confirmed that in CKD patients who excrete >1 g/day of protein, (a) an on-treatment SBP of 110 to 129 mm Hg was associated with the lowest risk of CKD progression and (b) an on-treatment SBP <110 mm Hg was associated with an increased risk of progression (85). The on-treatment BP goal of <130/80 mm Hg recommended by JNC-7 (Fig. 67.6) would be appropriate for the majority of CKD patients who excrete <1 g/day of protein. In addition to nondiuretic drugs, large doses of loop *diuretics* may be needed to control volume in patients with advanced CKD.

Diabetes Mellitus

HBP is up to twice as common in diabetic patients as in matched nondiabetic individuals. An association exists between type 2 diabetes, hypertension, and the insulin-resistant state known as the *metabolic syndrome* (hyperinsulinemia, dyslipidemia, and obesity) (86). Nonpharmacologic lifestyle changes that decrease insulin resistance (weight reduction and increased exercise) theoretically may be especially important in treating this subset of hypertensive patients.

The JNC-7 recommendation of an on-treatment goal of ≤130/80 mm Hg for diabetic patients (30) is supported by the findings of the HOT Trial, which showed that more aggressive antihypertensive drug treatment reduces both microvascular (nephropathy, retinopathy) and macrovascular complications of type 2 diabetes (66). Two drug comparison trials showed significantly lower cardiovascular event rates among diabetic patients taking ACE inhibitors versus dihydropyridine calcium antagonists (87,88). Although calcium antagonists were used in the HOT trial, the findings from these two trials suggest that other classes may be more beneficial. In this regard, it is important to recognize that *cotreatment with diuretics* was fundamental to BP control in a large proportion of subjects in the latter trials, and that subsequent analyses of data from many trials have shown that diabetic subjects in low-dose diuretic arms had health outcomes equivalent or superior to outcomes for diabetics in the nondiuretic arms (89,90). Prevention of CKD was not assessed in these trials.

In patients with type 1 diabetes and established nephropathy (urine albumin ≥30 mg/day), ACE inhibitors should be used because they have been shown to reduce proteinuria and delay loss of renal function even in nonhypertensive diabetic patients (91). Cotreatment of type 1 patients with maximum tolerated doses of both ACE inhibitors and ARBs has been shown to reduce proteinuria more than treatment with an ACE inhibitor alone, but the clinical consequences of this aggressive approach are not yet known (92).

In patients with type 2 diabetes and established nephropathy and HBP, ACE inhibitors and ARBs have been studied extensively. Both classes of drugs confer renoprotection that may exceed that conferred by other BP-lowering drugs (30).

A potential unique role for ACE inhibitors in type 2 diabetic patients was found in the Microalbuminuria, Cardiovascular, and Renal Outcomes in Heart Outcomes Prevention Evaluation (MICRO-HOPE) trial. In this placebo-controlled trial, addition of the ACE inhibitor ramipril at a fixed dose (10 mg) to patients' current regimens reduced microvascular and macrovascular end points in diabetic patients (93). The benefit of treatment was at least partly independent of BP lowering, suggesting that ramipril and other ACE inhibitors have a unique vascular protective effect in diabetes.

Pretreatment and posttreatment *standing BPs* should always be measured in diabetic patients. When orthostasis is found, presumably caused by neuropathy, the standing pressure should be monitored and included in treatment decisions.

Left Ventricular Hypertrophy

The finding of LVH on either a baseline ECG or an echocardiogram is a powerful independent predictor of cardiovascular morbidity (94). LVH may regress when BP is reduced by weight reduction, salt restriction, or antihypertensive drugs from all classes except direct vasodilators (95). To date, an ARB (losartan), in a head-to-head comparison with a β-blocker (atenolol), has been shown to have an advantage in reducing LVH (94). A meta-analysis of several small studies has also suggested an advantage for ACE inhibitors (96). It is possible that LVH represents a treatable risk factor independent of HBP. This conclusion is tentatively supported by subgroup analyses of Losartan Intervention for Endpoint Reduction in Hypertension (LIFE) trial data showing that treatment-related lower left ventricular mass is associated with lower rates of end points independent of the degree of BP reduction (94).

In the subset of patients with symptoms of heart failure and echocardiographic evidence for *diastolic dysfunction*, a calcium channel blocker or a β-blocker may provide symptomatic relief as the result of a modest decrease in contractility (47). In the short term, these drugs do not appear to decrease the late-diastolic stiffness present in these patients (97). Over a longer period (3 years), diastolic function does improve in association with regression of LVH in patients treated with ACE inhibitors (98).

Cost of Antihypertensive Drugs

Brand name drugs, especially newer drugs, typically cost the patient more than $1 per dose. Even generic drug prices fluctuate according to what manufacturers choose to charge. The least expensive generic regimens ($10–$40 per month) are monotherapy with a generic product (Table 67.10). When combination therapy is needed, a *combination product* may be less expensive than the component drugs purchased separately.

Drug–Drug Interactions

Table 67.11 provides drug interaction information that may be important in selecting and monitoring both antihypertensive agents and other drugs. This information is not exhaustive. Today, pharmacists usually can provide prompt responses to queries about drug interactions.

Drug Side Effects

Table 67.10 lists the most common side effects for each class or subclass of antihypertensive drugs.

Modification of the regimen may be needed if drugs control the hypertension but cause troublesome side effects. After any drug is initiated, the patient should be encouraged to discuss any drug-associated disturbances, such as reduced mental alertness, mood change, or impairment in physical exercise or sexual activity. From 5% to 20% of enrollees discontinue therapy in the trials of most antihypertensive drugs because of such side effects, and many notice minor side effects as long as they are taking antihypertensive drugs. Even taking a placebo for hypertension is associated commonly with side effects. For many side effects, the frequency is similar in active-drug and placebo patients.

Evidence-based review of the literature (37) and practical experience led to the following conclusions regarding a number of important symptomatic side effects:

- *Cough* is common (up to 30%) in patients taking *ACE inhibitors*. It begins and remits shortly after starting or stopping (or reducing) the drug. ARBs can be substituted.
- *Angioedema* may occur, rarely, >1 month after initiation of *ACE inhibitor* or ARB use and recurs when an ACE inhibitor is inadvertently readministered. It can be life threatening if it affects the upper airway.
- Because they are *teratogenic*, ACE inhibitors, ARBs, and beta blockers are contraindicated during pregnancy.
- *Ankle swelling* is common (up to 25%) in patients taking *calcium antagonists* and can be a reason for reducing the dose or replacing this class of drug. Edema is often present (as part of total-body volume expansion) in patients who require the potent vasodilator *minoxidil*. Loop diuretic treatment, not discontinuation of minoxidil, is appropriate for these patients.
- *Impotence* is common (up to 20%) in men taking *diuretics* and should be addressed before and/or during treatment.
- *Incontinence* is increased in patients with baseline detrusor instability taking *diuretics* and constitutes a reason not to initiate diuretic treatment.
- *Frequent gouty arthritis* may occur after initiation of *diuretic* treatment and constitutes a reason to select an alternative treatment.
- *Peripheral vascular disease* has not been shown to worsen with *β-blocker* treatment. β-Blocker treatment is reasonable in patients with peripheral vascular disease, especially those with coexisting coronary artery disease.
- *Depression* is not increased in patients taking *β-blockers*. Patients taking *reserpine* above the recommended maximum daily dose (0.25 mg) may develop reversible depression at any time during long-term treatment. Reserpine should not be initiated in patients with concurrent or past depression.
- *Hirsutism* predictably occurs, and is pronounced, in patients taking *minoxidil*. For this reason, women do not tolerate this drug.
- *A lupuslike syndrome* can be caused by *hydralazine*. It has the following features in most affected subjects: it occurs after at least 6 months of exposure to ≥200 mg/day, begins as new arthritis or arthralgia, rarely affects the kidneys, stimulates the production of antinuclear antibodies, and remits entirely within a few months after discontinuation of hydralazine (rarely, a patient has persistent rheumatologic symptoms or antinuclear antibodies long after discontinuation of hydralazine).
- *Peripheral sensory neuropathy* may be caused by *hydralazine*. It manifests as paresthesias and numbness and responds to pyridoxine 50 mg/day or to discontinuation of the hydralazine.
- *Orthostatic exaggeration of the BP-lowering effect* can occur with *any antihypertensive drug*. Therefore, patients should be asked about orthostatic symptoms and should have a standing BP measured to check for asymptomatic orthostasis after every change in the regimen. For those with an orthostatic fall in SBP >15 mm Hg, a standing BP should also be measured after exercise (e.g., 10 steps on a footstool or walking a fixed distance) because exercise can exacerbate drug-induced orthostatic hypotension. For patients who report having orthostatic symptoms shortly after they take their daily medication, the

standing BP should be measured when symptoms are present—either at home by the patient or in the office—because profound but transient orthostatic hypotension can occur in some patients (see Problems in the Course of Treatment).

In many clinical trials, *quality-of-life indices* have been used to measure the impact of antihypertensive drugs on patients' energy levels, mental health, physical abilities, and social functioning. In one study, patients taking each of the major classes of drugs or placebo reported modest improvement in most of these measures 4 years after starting treatment (99).

Serum Lipids and Aspirin Use

The clinical approach to two factors that affect cardiovascular risk—serum lipids and aspirin—is related to antihypertensive drug use.

Lipids

Although thiazide diuretics at low dosages can cause a short-term increase in total cholesterol and β-blockers may decrease high-density lipoprotein cholesterol and increase triglyceride levels (100), these unfavorable effects did not persist in a 4-year study of monotherapy that compared a low-dose thiazide diuretic, a β-blocker, an ACE inhibitor, a nondihydropyridine calcium antagonist, and a long-acting α-blocker (101). JNC-7 recommends that any lipid abnormality be addressed according to current guidelines (see Chapter 82) and that antihypertensive drugs, including low-dose diuretics, be used according to the scheme shown in Figure 67.6 (30).

Aspirin

Low-dose aspirin should be considered according to the guidelines summarized in Chapter 62 only when HBP is controlled because of the increased risk for hemorrhagic in patients with uncontrolled HBP (30).

Step-Down Therapy

Patients who are taking one or more antihypertensive drugs may want to take measures that enable them to reduce or discontinue drug treatment. Based on the results of a clinical trial in middle-aged adults, approximately one third of patients who have reduced their weight and restricted their salt intake can maintain control of their HBP without previously administered antihypertensive drugs (102). Similarly, approximately one third of older patients receiving monotherapy for HBP were able to maintain normal BP when drugs were discontinued after 3 months of lifestyle change (salt restriction and/or weight reduction) (103).

Promoting Adherence to Pharmacologic Treatment

Chapter 4 discusses in detail adherence to treatment as a generic feature of ambulatory care. Because poor adherence is common in patients with hypertension, the problem has been studied extensively. Nonjudgmental statements such as the following have been shown to be effective in eliciting accurate information from patients for whom antihypertensive drugs are prescribed: "People often have difficulty taking their medicines for one reason or another, and we are interested in finding out any problems that occur so that we can understand them better." After this statement, patients are asked whether they ever miss taking tablets and are encouraged to discuss any problems they are having with taking medicine.

Certain strategies have been shown to improve adherence to antihypertension treatment. Several of these strategies should be used routinely. More intensive strategies should be used for patients who appear to be especially noncompliant (see Chapter 4).

Strategies recommended for all patients include the following:

- Ensure that the patient knows several critical facts about hypertension: that it increases the risk of disabling illness (stroke, heart disease, kidney failure) or premature death; that it usually is asymptomatic when initially detected; that treatment reduces the risk of illness or premature death by at least one third; and that treatment is continuous for life. This information is covered well in patient information pamphlets available from the American Heart Association.
- Prescribe drugs that can be taken once per day (Table 67.10).
- Have patients state at each visit how they are taking their medication, including when the last dose was taken. Patients taking multiple drugs should be encouraged to bring their bottles of medicine to every visit.
- Ensure that supervision is provided frequently enough. During the first year of treatment, this probably should be at least every 3 months, at scheduled visits.
- Ensure that the practice is planned to maximize convenience for the patient, that is, the waiting time is brief, telephone access to the practice is easy, requests for appointment changes are accommodated, and prescription renewals are easy to obtain.

For patients who admit poor compliance, the reason should be explored and addressed (see Practical Approaches for Detecting and Addressing Noncompliance in Chapter 4).

For patients with uncontrolled hypertension in whom poor compliance is suspected but not admitted, the following strategies have been shown to help:

evaluated for treatable causes of their HBP (see Evaluation for Secondary Hypertension).

Because of the psychological and social stresses associated with adolescence, the care of a chronic condition such as hypertension requires special considerations in this age group (see Chapter 11).

Hypertension in the Elderly

Hypertension is common in older patients (Fig. 67.1), and the risks associated with systolic and diastolic hypertension increase substantially with each decade of life and with the coexistence of other major risk factors (Fig. 67.2). Evidence indicates that SBP and perhaps an elevated pulse pressure (SBP minus DBP) are the strongest predictors of morbidity in older persons with HBP (12,113,114).

Recommendations

The recommendations for older patients in JNC-7 (30) are based on the findings from multiple clinical trials (19–23). One of these trials, the Systolic Hypertension—Europe (Syst-Eur) trial for patients with isolated systolic hypertension, showed that first-line treatment with a long-acting dihydropyridine calcium antagonist had an effect similar in magnitude to that of diuretic-based regimens used in earlier trials (22). The principal JNC-7 recommendations for older patients are the following:

- For older persons with sustained DBPs ≥90 mm Hg, reduction of the pressure to <90 mm Hg is recommended.
- For older persons with SBP >140 mm Hg, reduction of the pressure to <140 mm Hg is recommended.
- A trial of nonpharmacologic measures for up to 1 year before drugs are prescribed is regarded as appropriate initial treatment for older patients with stage 1 hypertension (Table 67.5), particularly those without target organ disease.

Several general points about the published clinical trials in older patients are helpful in making decisions for individual patients:

- *Stage 1 systolic hypertension* (SBP 140–159 mm Hg): Although the JNC-7 recommends BP reduction in older persons with this level of SBP, this recommendation is made in spite of the facts that (a) clinical trials of patients with isolated systolic hypertension enrolled and showed benefits for patients with stage 2, not stage 1, SBP and (b) on-treatment SBPs were not as low as those currently recommended (113).
- *Demographic features:* The older subjects enrolled in clinical trials were relatively healthy men and women whose mean ages ranged from 69 to 75 years. Women, whose hypertension-related morbidity and mortality are similar to those of men after age 60 years, were heavily represented. Notably, African-American subjects were not included in three U.S. trials and were underrepresented in the fourth trial (SHEP). For healthy patients older than 80 years, the impact of HBP treatment is being investigated in the large placebo-controlled trial HYVET, which compares active treatment with a diuretic or a calcium antagonist (115).
- *Antihypertensive medications:* Low-dose diuretic therapy was used as first-step treatment in most of the trials with patients older than 60 years. In at least one trial (British Medical Research Council), benefit accrued to the diuretic-treated subjects but not to subjects treated with a β-blocker (atenolol) (20).
- *Morbidity and mortality:* Treatment reduced morbidity and mortality in subjects with either isolated systolic hypertension or the combination of systolic and diastolic hypertension. The absolute benefit was substantial. During 5 years, stroke, MI, and cardiovascular death are prevented in 50 to 150 of 1,000 subjects.

Caveats Regarding Drug Treatment

Several special characteristics of older persons should be considered when deciding how to treat their hypertension.

Orthostatic hypotension unrelated to drugs is fairly common in elderly patients. The explanation may be an increase in sedentary activity or blunting of autonomic reflexes. Therefore, it is important to obtain baseline and followup standing BPs (including standing after walking) in older patients taking antihypertensive drugs.

Both *pseudohypertension* and *white-coat hypertension* (see Measuring the Blood Pressure) may be more prevalent in older persons, especially those who describe orthostatic symptoms despite apparent high pressures at office visits and in those who have no target organ disease.

Other characteristics of older subjects that increase the risks associated with antihypertensive drugs include the following:

- Salt and fluid intake may vary significantly from week to week.
- Concomitant large-vessel atherosclerosis (kidneys, brain, heart) may increase the risk of ischemic damage resulting from drug-induced hypotension.
- Errors in taking medication may be increased.
- Drug excretion rates are generally reduced as a function of aging.

Chapter 12 discusses these and other characteristics that are important in the care of older persons. *Three precautions* minimize the risks of antihypertensive drugs in older patients: using the lowest recommended dosage and increasing the dosage slowly, keeping the drug schedule simple, and decreasing or discontinuing drugs if signs or symptoms of significant orthostatic hypotension or other annoying side effects develop.

Hypertension in Pregnancy

This section addresses BP and HBP assessment and management in women who are pregnant or lactating. For *nonpregnant women,* longitudinal studies have delineated the risks of HBP, and clinical trials have demonstrated the benefits of treatment. The negligible impact on BP of oral contraceptives and estrogen replacement in most women was addressed earlier (see Evaluation for Secondary Hypertension).

Normally, SBP does not change during pregnancy, but DBP *falls by approximately 10 mm Hg during the first and second trimesters,* then reverts to the prepregnancy level in the third trimester. The maximal fall occurs between weeks 13 and 20. It probably is caused by the general vasodilation that accompanies pregnancy. Increased renin and aldosterone levels also occur in normal pregnancy.

Hypertension (SBP ≥140 mm Hg or DBP ≥90 mm Hg) is present or develops in 6% to 8% of pregnant women in the United States.

Based on previous records or patient history, it should be possible at the first prepartum visit to decide for most women whether they usually are normotensive or have chronic hypertension. This decision is helpful in managing the following *four categories of hypertension,* which have been defined by the National High Blood Pressure Education Program Working Group on High Blood Pressure in Pregnancy (116):

- Chronic hypertension
- Preeclampsia/eclampsia
- Preeclampsia superimposed on chronic hypertension
- Gestational hypertension

This classification, which names gestational hypertension as a distinct category, differs from that issued previously.

Chronic Hypertension in Pregnancy

Chronic hypertension is defined as SBP ≥140 mm Hg or DBP ≥90 mm Hg diagnosed before pregnancy or appearing before week 20 of pregnancy. It is more common in pregnant women who are in their thirties because of the increased prevalence of hypertension with age.

There are two important questions to consider in patients with chronic hypertension:

1. *Should a woman with chronic hypertension avoid pregnancy?* In the woman with uncomplicated stage 1 HBP (Table 67.5), there is only a small increase in the risk to the mother or the infant. However, in women with stage 2 HBP or evidence of target organ disease (cardiomegaly, renal impairment, or eyegrounds changes of accelerated hypertension), infant mortality is greatly increased; these women should be advised to avoid pregnancy.

2. *How should chronic hypertension be treated during pregnancy?* Based on critical assessment of the literature, which contains no high-quality clinical trials, the following approaches are supported (37):

a. A patient who becomes pregnant while taking a nondiuretic antihypertensive medication should substitute methyldopa (labetalol or hydralazine if methyldopa is not tolerated) for her usual medication and should continue treatment unless she becomes hypotensive during the pregnancy.
b. A patient who becomes pregnant while taking a diuretic for hypertension can continue this treatment. In such a patient, it is important to confirm that chronic hypertension was documented before drug treatment was initiated.
c. For patients with chronic hypertension who are not already taking antihypertensives, it is necessary to make a decision about hypertension treatment. Untreated women with uncomplicated stage 1 HBP have pregnancy outcomes similar to those of normotensive women. The evidence favors treatment for women with long-standing stage 2 HBP or already-present target organ disease. Methyldopa (or labetalol or hydralazine) can be recommended, based on the finding of improved fetal survival in a single controlled trial of methyldopa treatment (without diuretics) for women with chronic hypertension and the fact that methyldopa, hydralazine, and labetalol have been found to be safe during pregnancy.
d. ACE inhibitors and ARBs should be avoided because of fetal abnormalities reported with use of these classes of drug.
e. The long-term effects of calcium antagonists on the fetus are unknown.

Preeclampsia/Eclampsia

Preeclampsia is a pregnancy-induced syndrome in which the clinical data must be carefully considered before making the diagnosis, in particular to distinguish it from preexisting chronic hypertension and gestational hypertension. A number of factors increase the risk for developing preeclampsia (Table 67.14). Untreated preeclampsia is associated with a high incidence of fetal mortality and maternal morbidity, especially the convulsive syndrome known as *eclampsia.* The major pathophysiologic derangement in preeclampsia is *placental hypoperfusion* caused by abnormal implantation of the trophoblast. This state leads to endothelial damage, which initiates the release of compounds that cause generalized vasospasm, reduced plasma volume and cardiac output, decreased glomerular filtration rate, and compromised perfusion of the placenta, kidneys, liver, and brain.

SECTION 10

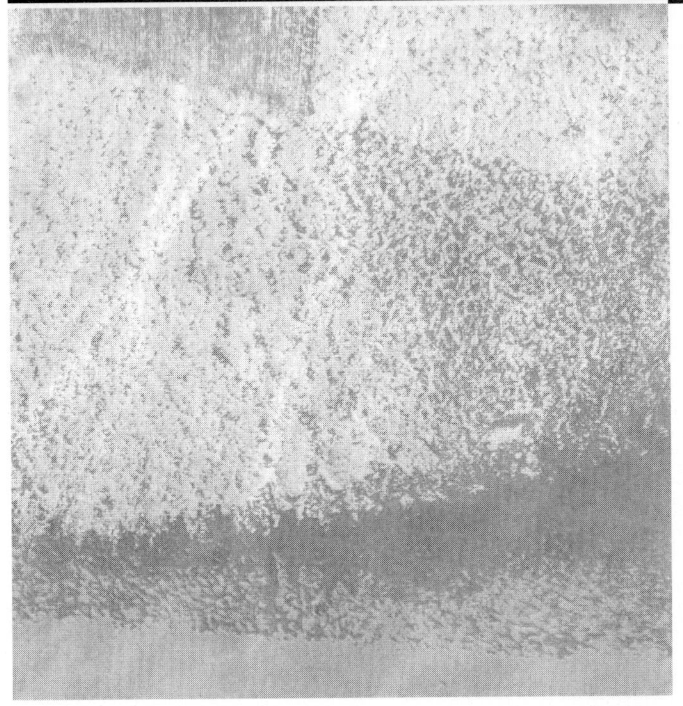

Musculoskeletal Problems

of the ruptured ends of the tendon. Results of tendon repair are favorable, although the joint may lose motion and strength, especially if physical therapy efforts are not followed postoperatively (14,15). Some patients, such as those with rheumatoid arthritis, taking chronic steroids, or who received intratendinous injections of corticosteroids, are vulnerable to tendon tears, and rupture may occur with no inciting traumatic event (16).

Overuse injuries to tendons are common and are thought to result in a condition termed *tendinopathy*. Pathologically, tendinopathy results in fibrotic changes to the tendon fibers. Chronic pain in the tendon can be hard to cure. Initial treatment includes nonoperative measures such as muscle strengthening and stretching. If these efforts fail, surgery to resect the area of altered tendon may be required. Less invasive options, including percutaneous tendinopathy and ultrasound treatments, have been developed (17).

Ligament Injury

Ligaments, fibrous structures around a joint that give it stability, are composed of fibroblasts, type I and type III collagen, elastin, and proteoglycans. Each joint in the body has different requirements for stability and mobility. The shape of the joint and the position and strength of its surrounding ligaments are responsible for the stability and mobility of the particular joint. For example, the sacroiliac joints in the pelvis have little motion and are extremely stable. The sacroiliac joints have a very broad surface and strong constraining ligaments. In contrast, the shoulder is a ball-and-socket joint designed to maximize the motion of the arm. The ligaments of the shoulder provide far less constraint and allow for motion in all directions.

Ligaments are injured when excessive or sudden stress is placed on a joint. Ligament injuries range from a stretching type injury called a *sprain* to full disruption. The amount of force required to injure a ligament depends on the stability of the individual joint. A low-energy twisting motion may have enough force to disrupt the ligaments of a mobile joint, such as the shoulder, but not those in more stable joints, such as the sacroiliac joints of the pelvis. A higher-energy injury, such as that from a car accident, could cause rupture of both the anterior pubis symphysis and the posterior sacroiliac ligaments in the front and back of the sacroiliac joint, resulting in a pelvic ring disruption. As the energy imparted from an injury increases, multiple ligaments around a joint may be injured. The joint may dislocate, and the bones within the joint may sustain fractures.

When a ligament is stretched or sprained, the joint becomes painful and swollen. Point tenderness is present over the sprained ligament, but the joint is stable to examination and is not dislocated. Radiographs reveal no fractures or dislocations. MRI reveals edema in the ligament. Sprains are graded on a three-level continuum (Table 68.2).

TABLE 68.2 Severity of Ligamentous Sprains

Grade	Examination and Underlying Pathology	Recommended Treatment
I	No joint instability or laxity, minor ligamentous stretch without tear	NSAID, RICE protocol (see text), progressive weight-bearing
II	Moderate joint instability, partial ligamentous tear	Immobilization for 4–6 wk
III	Marked joint instability, loss of control of muscle with inability to bear weight Complete rupture of ligament	Immobilize and refer to orthopedist

NSAID, nonsteroidal anti-inflammatory drug; RICE, rest, ice, compression and elevation.

Grade I sprains entail stretching or microscopic tearing of the ligament with no clinical evidence of joint instability or laxity on physical examination. These minor injuries usually resolve in a few days to weeks with minor symptomatic treatment, such as brief periods of immobilization, the RICE protocol, progressive weight-bearing, and use as tolerated.

Grade II sprains are partial tears of the ligament with mild to moderate instability and laxity of the joint. To prevent additional injury in a patient with grade II sprains, the affected area should be immobilized. The best modality for immobilization depends on patient reliability and the extent of injury. Options include prefabricated braces (either soft or hard), moon boots (large ski-boot–like shoes), and a fabricated cast. If the lower extremity is involved, a brief period (usually 1–2 weeks, although the length of time required varies) of no to partial weight-bearing with crutches is followed by gradual, progressive weight-bearing as tolerated. Even when progressive weight-bearing is allowed after 2 weeks, some patients may still require the use of a brace or splint for added protection and stability. Nonsteroidal anti-inflammatory drugs to control pain and inflammation and physical therapy for muscle strengthening and preservation of function can expedite the clinical course.

Grade III sprains are complete ruptures of the ligament(s) and present with obvious signs of joint instability and laxity. If the injury is in the lower extremity, a patient often is unable to bear weight. Radiographs usually show lack of congruency of the articular surfaces of the bones of the joint or opening of the joint with varus or valgus stress (see Imaging Evaluation section). In a patient with such an injury, the area should be immobilized with a splint, and the patient should be referred to an orthopedic surgeon. The orthopedist may consider prolonged immobilization,

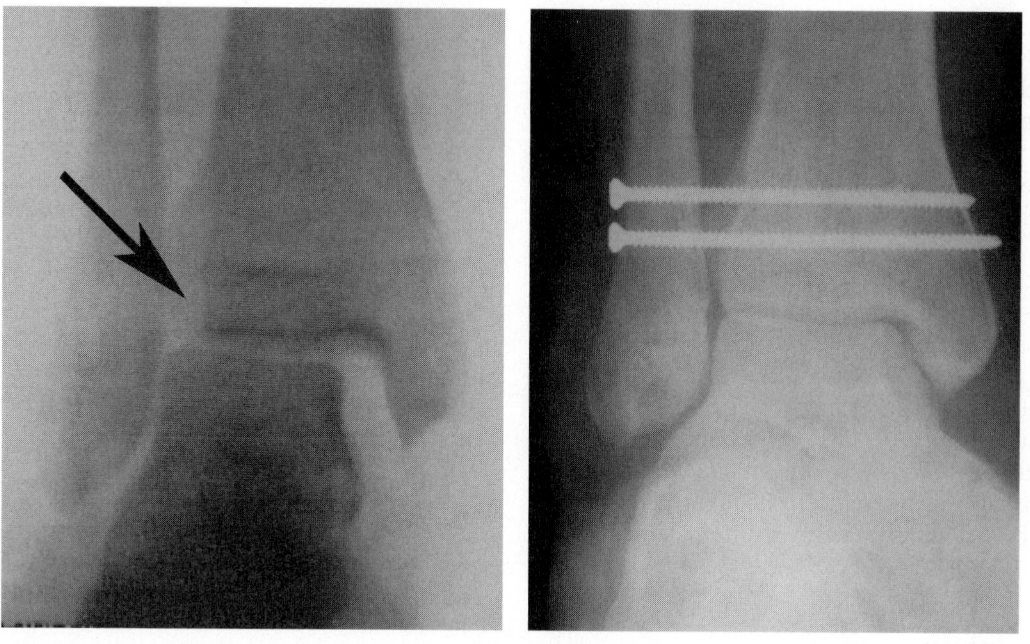

FIGURE 68.2. Ligament injury. **A:** Radiograph showing rupture of the syndesmotic ligament in the ankle. **B:** Screws are used to reduce the syndesmotic injury and allow for healing of the ligaments.

ligament repair, or reconstruction. Occasionally, depending on the severity of the injury and the effect of the problem on the patient's baseline function, these options also may be applicable to patients with severe grade II injuries or those for whom nonoperative methods have failed.

In high-energy injuries, multiple ligaments are disrupted, leading to joint instability and dislocation. Acute dislocations should be referred to an emergency room for treatment. Joint dislocations should be treated emergently by reduction of the joint under local or general anesthesia. Unreduced dislocations may lead to long-term morbidity. A dislocated hip, for example, puts pressure on the blood vessels to the femoral head. The longer the hip remains dislocated, the higher the risk is of femoral head osteonecrosis secondary to disruption of the blood supply.

Reduction of a joint typically requires sedation and an analgesic. Aspiration of the joint to remove the hematoma, combined with intra-articular injection of local anesthetic, may provide enough pain control to allow for joint reduction. However, reduction of a joint with powerful muscles, such as the shoulder or hip, may require a general anesthetic. After joint reduction, radiographs are obtained to assess for joint stability and fracture. MRI or computed tomography scans may be indicated to delineate small fractures, damage to the articular cartilage, or ligaments that may require repair. If a joint is stable after reduction, care includes gentle range of motion of the joint followed by a more formal physical therapy program to regain motion and strength.

In some cases, joint dislocation may lead to chronic joint instability. Chronically unstable joints have damaged ligaments and may dislocate with very little force. Treatment of chronic dislocation involves reconstruction of the weakened or disrupted ligaments to provide a stable joint and allow activity (18). The patterns of injury that lead to chronic joint instability can be identified by an orthopedic surgeon. Injuries such as a syndesmotic ligament rupture in the ankle are best treated with internal fixation to prevent chronic joint instability (Fig. 68.2). In some cases, surgical repair of a ligament may not lead to a good outcome, and reconstruction is required. An example is rupture of the anterior cruciate ligament in the knee. Results of repair are poor, and reconstruction with an autograft or an allograft tendon will provide joint stability.

Cartilage Injury

Injury to the joint may cause damage to the joint's cartilaginous surface of the joint and intra-articular structures such as the labrum or meniscus. All joints have a smooth surface covering made of articular cartilage. Cartilage is attached firmly to the underlying bone and composed of several layers. The upper layers are packed with glycosaminoglycans. This surface is resistant to wear and has slick mechanical properties. Some joints have a rim of cartilaginous tissue that provides support to the joint. In the shoulder and hip, this rim of tissue is called the *labrum,* and it is located around the cup of the joint. In the knee and wrist, this tissue is called the *meniscus.* The labrum and meniscus are important to the joint in terms of shock absorption and articular cartilage protection. Patients present after an injury with pain, tenderness, and joint effusion. Physical examination must rule out ligamentous injury and joint instability. Diagnosis is made with MRI. In the hip and shoulder, enhancement of the MRI with intra-articular injection of gadolinium may be necessary to reveal a labral tear. Nonoperative treatment, including rest, ice, and anti-inflammatory medicines, is the first line of therapy for cartilage injuries. Treatment should be based on MRI findings and on the age and activity of the patient. Operative intervention may be necessary to unlock a joint or to repair or débride the torn cartilage or meniscus (19,20).

Bone Injury

Bones are thought of as inert and lifeless; however, little could be further from the truth. Bones not only provide stability to the body; they also serve as a calcium bank for the body. Bones are made of a stout exterior or cortex and spongy interior or marrow. The cortex is composed of a lamellar structure with precisely aligned type I collagen fibers. Hydroxyapatite crystals deposited within the collagen provide a high tensile strength.

Bone exists in a continual process of breakdown and renewal. In healthy individuals, this balance is established precisely. The collagen structure is permeated with tiny canals that are populated with cells. Osteoclasts are multinucleated cells that function to resorb bone. Osteoblasts are cells of mesenchymal origin that function to produce new bone matrix or osteoid. Because of bone's continued regenerative ability, its healing is unlike that of other tissues. Bones have the ability to heal without the formation of scar tissue (21). If the fine balance between bone breakdown and renewal is disrupted, changes to the bone occur. In osteoporosis, the rate of bone disruption is higher than the rate of renewal, leading to weaker bones. Bones respond by widening their diameter and developing thinner cortices. A wider, thinner bone has some strength but is more brittle and more susceptible to fracture (22) (see Chapter 103).

When an applied load exceeds a bone's mechanical properties, *fracture* occurs. Fractures can be displaced or nondisplaced, and they can occur acutely from an injury or subacutely from continued or repetitive stresses. Repetitive stresses cause microfractures that may lead to a nondisplaced fracture, termed a *stress fracture.*

Stress fractures can occur in young, healthy patients and in older patients with osteoporosis. In the young, healthy patient, a stress fracture occurs as the result of newly applied, sustained loads across the bone, as in the army recruit who must run or march long distances in basic training. In this situation, the bone is not capable of responding to these suddenly applied stresses. The patient notices point tenderness over the area of fracture that worsens with activity. Unchanged activity levels may lead to a displaced fracture. In the osteoporotic patient, the bone becomes so weakened that the simple forces of daily living may lead to progressive microfractures, and stress fractures may develop with no warning signs.

Plain radiographs may not identify stress fractures, and it is important to continue the evaluation to treat a nondisplaced fracture before it becomes displaced. A bone scan can reveal the stress fracture, but it may not do so acutely, that is, within the first 48 hours after injury. An MRI scan shows edema in the bone and is the most sensitive test for stress fracture (23).

Fractures from an acute injury are diagnosed with plain radiographs. Two orthogonal views must be obtained in all cases. Nondisplaced fractures generally are treated with immobilization and reduced weight-bearing. In the acute setting, the joint should be splinted, and the patient should be referred for orthopedic evaluation. The length and amount of restriction is based on the fracture's location and stability or its likelihood for displacement. Some fractures, such as a nondisplaced distal fibula fracture, are stable, and weight-bearing and early motion are safe. Other fractures, such as a nondisplaced femoral neck fracture, may require additional stabilization, such as screws and weight-bearing limitations until healing, to avoid displacement, which could lead to nonunion or osteonecrosis that might require hip replacement (arthroplasty).

Displaced fractures may require immobilization or operative treatment, depending on several factors, including whether the bone has penetrated the skin and the precise location and pattern of the fracture. Fractures are called *open* when the bone pierces the skin. Open fractures may range in severity from a small pinhole through the skin to devastating crush injuries that are massively contaminated. The greater the force to the bone, the more energy must be absorbed by the body, leading to more extensive soft-tissue destruction and more damage to the bone. Patients with displaced fractures should be managed according to Advanced Trauma Life Support guidelines (24).

It is important that the clinician be able to distinguish an open fracture from a closed one. If a wound is present around the area of fracture, a careful examination of the skin must be performed. It is possible for an abrasion of the skin to occur over a broken bone. If, however, a wound around a fractured bone does not stop bleeding or oozing, the fracture should be considered open. Open fractures should be treated initially with removal of gross contamination and gentle washing with sterile saline. A povidone iodine (Betadine) dressing then should be applied and the limb should be splinted. The patient should be transferred emergently to an emergency department for prompt evaluation by an orthopedic surgeon. Open fractures are treated definitively with surgical débridement and fixation. Surgical débridement of the wound allows for decontamination and lessens the risk of infection and osteomyelitis.

In addition to examining for open wounds, the clinician should note the neurologic and vascular condition of the limb. Pulses should be palpated. If pulses cannot be palpated, a Doppler device should be used to check the pulses. A pulseless limb is a true surgical emergency that will lead to loss of limb if not treated within several hours of injury. The physician also should examine the limb for evidence of compartment syndrome. Of note, open fractures are more susceptible than are closed fractures to compartment syndrome because open fractures typically are caused by high-energy trauma, which leads to more muscle injury and swelling. An orthopedic surgeon should evaluate emergently for evidence of massive swelling or decreasing neurologic status.

The position of the fracture and the exact location determine later treatment by the orthopedic surgeon. Displaced fractures that occur in the shaft or diaphysis of the bone may be treated with or without surgery. The goals of fracture treatment are to restore limb length, correct limb rotation, and obtain bony healing. Nonoperative treatment of shaft fractures includes the use of casts and fracture braces. Other displaced fractures require internal or external fixation. Shaft fractures often can be stabilized with minimally invasive techniques and indirect fracture reduction. Intramedullary nailing has been shown to have a >90% chance of healing fractures of the femoral shaft (25).

Fractures that enter the joint or intra-articular fractures require referral to an orthopedic surgeon. Intra-articular fractures cause damage to the articular cartilage, leading to joint incongruity and posttraumatic arthritis (26). The greater the fracture displacement, the higher the rate is of arthritis. Most intra-articular fractures are treated operatively for two reasons: (a) to facilitate joint reduction and maintain of that position for healing, and (b) to allow early motion of within the joint. Without fixation, the joint must be immobilized, which leads to stiffness and dysfunction (27,28).

GENERAL APPROACH TO PATIENT AND REFERRAL GUIDELINES

Most patients with musculoskeletal complaints or injuries can be divided readily into one of two categories: acute or chronic musculoskeletal problems. Acute problems include those related to trauma, recent overuse syndromes, sprains and strains, stress fractures, joint infections, recent peripheral nerve or nerve root impingement, and compartment syndrome. Chronic problems include osteoarthritis, chronic overuse syndromes, bursitis, bony infections, bone and soft-tissue tumors, chronic peripheral nerve or nerve root problems, and claudication. A precise time distinction between acute and chronic problems cannot be made. Nevertheless, it is a common presumption for one to consider any problem that persists for more than 3 months as a chronic condition. There can always be an element of the acute with chronic injury; for example, one may have a recent meniscal injury in the setting of knee osteoarthritis, or an athletic injury may be the presenting complaint that brings attention to a joint affected by rheumatoid arthritis.

TABLE 68.3 Guidelines for Referral of Patients with Musculoskeletal Problems to a Specialist

Fractures
Acute dislocations
Grade III or severe grade II sprains
Suspected joint infections
Suspected compartment syndromes
Suspected cauda equina syndrome or acute myelopathy
Severe or progressive loss of function or work productivity
Problems that do not respond to a reasonable trial of nonoperative treatment

In managed care environments, general clinicians are faced with the challenge of being the "gatekeepers" for referrals to specialists and other allied health professionals. Therefore, knowing when and when not to refer a patient is important. Table 68.3 provides general criteria for referral to an orthopedic surgeon. Problems such as major fractures, open injuries, dislocations, compartment syndromes, and septic joint infections require immediate referral to an orthopedist for evaluation and treatment. Red warning flags of a serious problem in the history and physical examination of a patient include evidence of severe trauma, night pain, fever, chills, joint instability, gross deformity, locked joints, and marked restriction of joint motion. Patients with one or more of these manifestations should be referred urgently to a specialist. On the other hand, the general clinician can comfortably treat, with the nonoperative methods addressed above, most other musculoskeletal injuries. If such measures fail after a reasonable period, then referral to an orthopedist is appropriate.

SPECIFIC REFERENCES*

1. Woodwell DA, Cherry DK. National Ambulatory Medical Care Survey: 2002 summary. Adv Data 2004;346:1.
2. Brinker MR, O'Connor DP. The incidence of fractures and dislocations referred for orthopaedic services in a capitated population. J Bone Joint Surg 2004;86A:290.
3. American College of Rheumatology Ad Hoc Committee on Clinical Guidelines. Guidelines for the initial evaluation of the adult patient with acute musculoskeletal symptoms. Arthritis Rheum 1996;39:1.
4. Institute for Clinical Systems Improvement. Assessment and management of acute pain. 4th ed. Available at: http://www.icsi.org/knowledge/detail.asp?catID=29&itemID.
5. Porter SE, Hanley EN Jr. The musculoskeletal

*Bold numerals denote published controlled clinical trials, meta-analyses, or consensus-based recommendations.

effects of smoking. J Am Acad Orthop Surg 2001;9:9.
6. Senall JA, Kile TA. Stress radiography. Foot Ankle Clin 2000;5:165.
7. Rose NE, Gold SM. A comparison of accuracy between clinical examination and magnetic resonance imaging in the diagnosis of meniscal and anterior cruciate ligament tears. Arthroscopy 1996;12:398.
8. Nerlich ML. Biology of soft tissue injuries. In: Browner BD, Jupiter JB, Levine AM, et al.,eds. Skeletal trauma: basic science, management, and reconstruction. 3rd ed. Philadelphia: WB Saunders, 2003:74.
9. Noonan TJ, Garrett WE, Jr. Muscle strain injury: diagnosis and treatment. J Am Acad Orthop Surg 1999;7:262.
10. Pope RP, Herbert RD, Kirwan JD, et al. A randomized trial of preexercise stretching for prevention of lower-limb injury. Med Sci Sports Exerc 2000;32:271.
11. Kostler W, Strohm PC, Sudkamp NP. Acute compartment syndrome of the limb. Injury 2004;35:1221.
12. Elliott KGB, Johnstone AJ. Diagnosing acute compartment syndrome. J Bone Joint Surg 2003;85B:625.
13. Kaplan FS, Glaser DL, Hebela N, et al. Heterotopic ossification. J Am Acad Orthop Surg 2004;12:116.
14. Ilan DI, Tejwani N, Keschner M, et al. Quadriceps tendon rupture. J Am Acad Orthop Surg 2003;11:192.
15. Maffulli N, Wong J. Rupture of the Achilles and patellar tendons. Clin Sports Med 2003;22:761.
16. Rose PS, Frassica FJ. Atraumatic bilateral patellar tendon rupture: a case report and review of the literature. J Bone Joint Surg 2001;83A:1382.
17. Sharma P, Maffulli N. Tendon injury and tendinopathy: healing and repair. J Bone Joint Surg 2005;87A:187.
18. Robinson CM, Dobson RJ. Anterior instability of the shoulder after trauma. J Bone Joint Surg 2004;86B:469.
19. Alford JW, Cole BJ. Cartilage restoration, part 1: basic science, historical perspective, patient evaluation, and treatment options. Am J Sports Med 2005;33:295.
20. Brittberg M, Lindahl A, Nilsson A, et al. Treatment of deep cartilage defects in the knee with autologous chondrocyte transplantation. N Engl J Med 1994;331:889.
21. Lieberman JR, Daluiski A, Einhorn TA. The role of growth factors in the repair of bone. Biology and clinical applications. J Bone Joint Surg 2002;84A:1032.
22. Lane JM, Cornell CN, Lobo M, et al. Osteoporotic fragility fractures. In: Browner BD, Jupiter JB, Levine AM, et al.,eds. Skeletal trauma: basic science, management, and reconstruction. 3rd ed. Philadelphia: WB Saunders, 2003:427.
23. Lassus J, Tulikoura I, Konttinen YT, et al. Bone stress injuries of the lower extremity: a review. Acta Orthop Scand 2002;73:359.
24. American College of Surgeons Committee on Trauma. Advanced trauma life support program for doctors. 6th ed. Chicago: American College of Surgeons, 1997.
25. Brumback RJ, Uwagie-Ero S, Lakatos R, et al. Intramedullary nailing of femoral shaft fractures. Part II: fracture-healing with static interlocking femoral fixation. J Bone Joint Surg 1988;70A:1453.
26. Buckwalter JA, Brown TD. Joint injury, repair, and remodeling: roles in post-traumatic osteoarthritis. Clin Orthop Relat Res 2004; 423:7.
27. Dirschl DR, Marsh JL, Buckwalter JA, et al. Articular fractures. J Am Acad Orthop Surg 2004;12:416.
28. Hahn DM. Current principles of treatment in the clinical practice of articular fractures. Clin Orthop Relat Res 2004;423:27.

*For annotated **General References** and resources related to this chapter, visit www.hopkinsbayview.org/PAMreferences.*

Chapter 69

Shoulder and Elbow Pain

David E. Kern

SHOULDER PAIN

Shoulder pain is common. Point prevalence ranges from 7% to >26% in the population aged 18 years and older. Lifetime prevalence ranges from 7% to 67%, with the greatest prevalence in individuals of middle and older age (1,2). It is a common reason why patients consult their primary care givers, and often is associated with impairment of function (1,3,4). Persistent and recurrent symptoms are common (4–6).

Usually the primary care practitioner can establish the correct diagnosis and direct appropriate therapy without orthopedic or rheumatologic consultation. This section reviews the major causes of shoulder pain and provides a basis for diagnosis and treatment of these conditions.

ANATOMY AND FUNCTION

To enable accurate diagnosis and treatment of disorders of the shoulder, it is necessary to understand the anatomy and function of the shoulder structures (Figs. 69.1 and 69.2, and Table 69.1). Normal shoulder motion depends on the smooth, integrated movement of the glenohumeral, acromioclavicular, and sternoclavicular joints and the scapulothoracic articulation.

The shoulder structures themselves are organized in four layers (Fig. 69.1).

1. The most superficial layer of the shoulder consists of the deltoid (abducts the shoulder), pectoralis major and minor (adduct the shoulder), and trapezius muscles (elevate and rotate the scapula). The acromion, coracoacromial ligament, and deltoid muscle form a roof overlying the deeper structures.
2. Beneath the superficial layer is the *subacromial* or *subdeltoid bursa,* which assists free movement of underlying structures in relation to the roof.
3. Beneath the bursa lies the *rotator cuff,* a group of muscles and their tendons, which consists of the supraspinatus superiorly, the infraspinatus and teres minor posteriorly, and the subscapularis anteriorly. The rotator cuff muscles stabilize the humeral head in the glenoid fossa. *Abduction* of the shoulder is accomplished by the coordinated action of the deltoid (which initially elevates, or shrugs, the glenohumeral joint, then abducts the arm at the glenohumeral joint) and the rotator cuff muscles, especially the supraspinatus (which hold the humeral head in the glenoid fossa

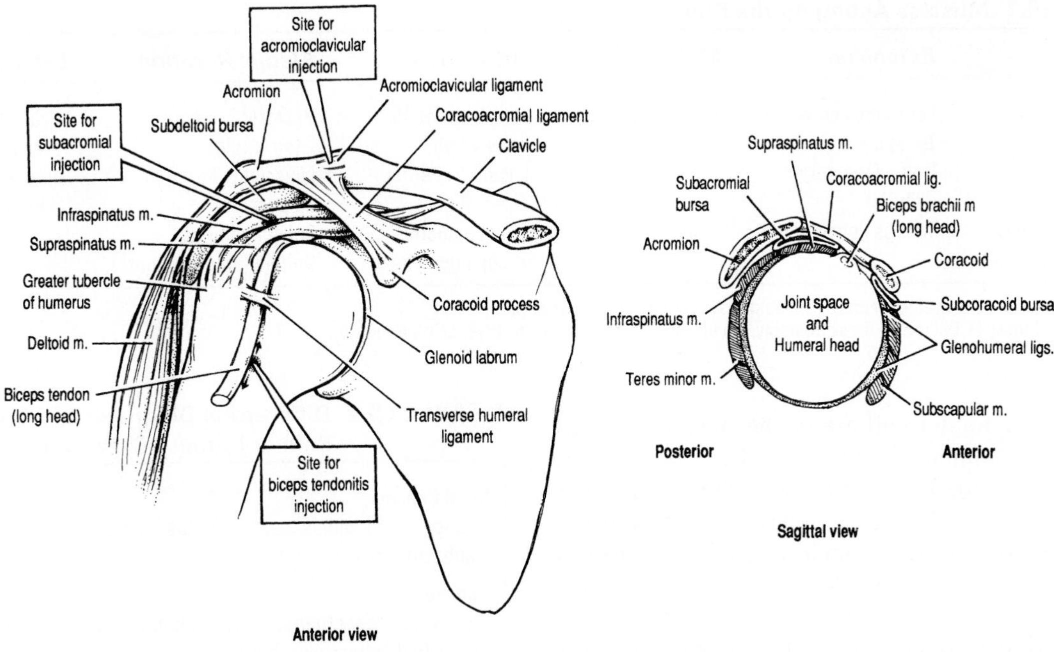

FIGURE 69.1. Structures of the shoulder and their relationships. Note that the subdeltoid or subacromial bursa lies next to the supraspinatus tendon but separate from the shoulder joint. Note the acromion and coracoacromial ligaments, which may impinge on the supraspinatus tendon on abduction of the arm. Note the location for subacromial injection into the bursa and about the rotator cuff tendons. (Sagittal section adapted from Pansky B. Review of gross anatomy. New York: Macmillan, 1979, with permission.)

while abducting). In addition, the rotator cuff muscles assist in internal and external rotation of the shoulder. Repetitive impingement of these structures between the acromion or coracoacromial ligament and the greater tuberosity of the humerus during abduction is thought to lead to inflammatory and degenerative changes within the cuff that are the most common cause of nontraumatic shoulder pain.

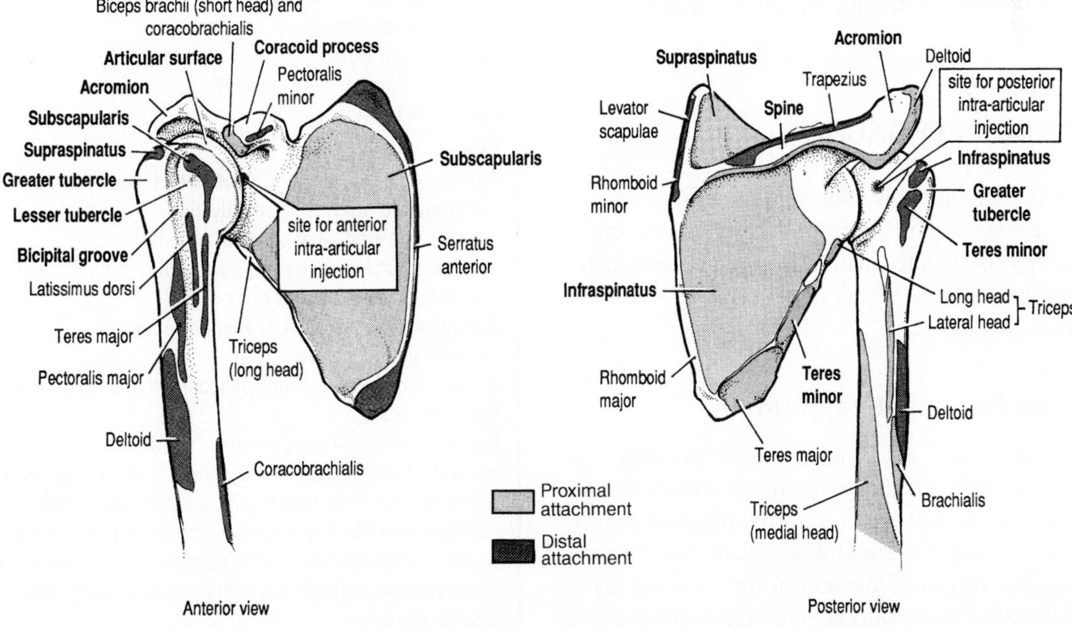

FIGURE 69.2. Humerus and scapula showing attachments of muscles. The distal attachments of the triceps and biceps onto the ulna and radius, respectively, can be seen in Figure 69.5. (Adapted from Agur AMR, Lee MJ, eds. Grant's atlas of anatomy. Baltimore: Williams & Wilkins, 1991, with permission.)

TABLE 69.1 Muscles Acting on the Shoulder Joint

Flexion	*Extension*	*Abduction*	*Adduction*	*Medial Rotation*	*Lateral Rotation*
Pectoralis major (clavicle head) Deltoid (anterior fibers) Coracobrachialis Biceps[a] (long head)	Latissimus dorsi Teres major Deltoid (posterior fibers) Triceps (long head)	Deltoid (as whole) Supraspinatus[a]	Pectoralis major (as whole) Latissimus dorsi Teres major Subscapularis Triceps (long head)	Pectoralis major (as whole) Latissimus dorsi Teres major Subscapularis[a] Deltoid (anterior fibers)	Infraspinatus[a] Teres minor Deltoid (posterior fibers)

[a]Muscles (rotator cuffs and biceps) most commonly associated with shoulder pain.
Modified from Pansky B. Review of gross anatomy. 4th ed. New York: Macmillan, 1979, with permission.

4. Beneath the rotator cuff are the ligamentous capsule and the glenohumeral *joint space*. The tendon of the long head of the biceps runs through the joint capsule and along the bicipital or intertubercular groove of the humerus on its way from its origin on the superior aspect of the glenoid fossa to its muscular attachment on the proximal radius. Its major function is to supinate the flexed forearm and to flex the supinated forearm. Also, it has a modest involvement in flexion of the arm at the shoulder.

The joint is formed by the articulation of the humeral head with the shallow glenoid fossa of the scapula, the diameter and depth of which are increased by the fibrocartilaginous glenoid labrum. The shallowness of the fossa enables nearly hemispheric motion of the arm, but this wide range of motion (ROM) is achieved at the price of joint stability. Stability of the shoulder joint depends primarily not on bony structures but on the integrity of supporting soft-tissue structures, including the labrum, capsule, and rotator cuff.

DIAGNOSTIC APPROACH

Pain about the shoulder usually originates from one of three sites: periarticular structures (e.g., rotator cuff), glenohumeral joint, or sites distant from the shoulder. Table 69.2 lists the causes of shoulder pain arranged by their relative frequencies.

History and Physical Examination

The history and physical examination usually are sufficient to establish a working diagnosis and direct effective treatment. The history is less useful than the physical examination in establishing the anatomic problem, but it is nevertheless helpful. *Perceived location* of the pain usually is not helpful, because most sources of pain (e.g., rotator cuff tendon, subdeltoid bursa, glenohumeral joint space) share a fifth (or sixth) cervical derivation and cause pain in the upper arm only. More severe lesions tend to cause pain

TABLE 69.2 Differential Diagnosis of Shoulder Pain in Primary Care Adult Patients

Most Common
Rotator cuff tendinitis (supraspinatus, infraspinatus-teres minor, subscapularis)

Common
Rotator cuff tears (partial more common than complete)
Subdeltoid/subacromial bursitis

Intermediate
Acromioclavicular arthritis/strain
Adhesive capsulitis/frozen shoulder

Occasional
Arthritis, degenerative or osteoarthritis (often posttraumatic)
Biceps (long head) tendinitis
Cardiac (referred pain)
Carpal tunnel syndrome (referred pain)
Cerebrovascular accident with hemiparesis (see Chapter 91)
Cervical/neck disorders (referred pain)
Dislocation
Fracture (neck of humerus, greater tuberosity)
Glenohumeral instability/subluxation
Glenoid labral tears
Neoplasm (local or referred pain)
Rheumatoid arthritis

Rare
Arthritis, other causes (e.g., gout, pseudogout, psoriasis, neuropathic, ankylosing spondylitis)
Infection (intra-articular or extra-articular)
Nerve entrapment: suprascapular, axillary, long thoracic, or spinal accessory nerves (referred pain)
Osteonecrosis (avascular or aseptic necrosis)
Polymyalgia rheumatica
Reflex sympathetic dystrophy/shoulder–hand syndrome
Sickle cell crisis
Thoracic outlet syndrome (referred pain)
Visceral—referred from sources other than neck or heart (e.g., pleural irritation by lung cancer or other cause; irritation to phrenic nerve or diaphragm by pathologic process such as subdiaphragmatic abscess, ruptured viscus, or disease of the mediastinum, pericardium, liver, spleen, or gallbladder; dissecting aortic aneurysm)
Other traumatic or periarticular soft-tissue problems

Data from references 32, 66, and Cyriax (see www.hopkinsbayview.org/PAMreferences).

radiating down the arm and forearm, usually along the anterolateral aspect. Pain confined to the point of the shoulder suggests a lesion of the acromioclavicular joint, which has a fourth cervical derivation. Involvement of other joints suggests a generalized arthritic process.

Asking about recent trauma and briefly reviewing the patient's problem list, medication list, and past medical history may be helpful in raising the suspicion for less common causes of shoulder pain, such as dislocation (e.g., from trauma), neoplasm (e.g., history of breast or lung cancer), or osteonecrosis (e.g., from corticosteroid use). Dislocation of the glenohumeral joint should be suspected with major injuries to the arm, especially if the shoulder is abducted and externally rotated at impact, whereas injury to, or separation of, the acromioclavicular joint usually results from a direct blow to the acromion. Asking *what precipitates or makes the pain worse* also is helpful. Pain referred to the shoulder from a distant site should not be exacerbated by movement of the shoulder. In contrast, pain with active or passive movement of the shoulder suggests a shoulder or periarticular problem. A history of *occupational* (6) *and sports activities,* such as working with hands elevated, lifting heavy objects, carrying loads supported by the shoulders, hand–arm vibration, pitching baseballs, swimming, or serving tennis balls, can identify exacerbating factors that may both suggest a cause and direct the attention of the clinician to a patient activity that should be modified as part of the treatment plan, especially in a patient with chronic or recurrent shoulder pain.

The physical examination usually is successful in identifying the source of pain. The uninvolved shoulder should be used as a control to confirm any questionable abnormality found on examination of the symptomatic shoulder. *Inspection* is the least helpful part of the examination, but it may reveal evidence of atrophy or displacement of bony landmarks. A popular approach that is most useful and widely accepted for the rest of the examination is given in Cyriax (see www.hopkinsbayview.org/PAMreferences). Excellent interrater reliability has been reported in one study (7). First, the *location of pain origin* is surveyed through a brief examination of the neck, scapula, shoulder, elbow, and wrist, usually involving a combination of active and resisted movements. The suspected abnormal site then is examined in depth. If the shoulder appears normal but another site is abnormal on the survey, the shoulder pain probably is referred from the abnormal site. If the survey reveals no abnormalities, the pain may be referred, or an abnormality in the shoulder may still be present. The shoulder is examined in the following way:

Active motion is studied by having the patient perform a few simple maneuvers. The patient is asked to elevate the arm as far as possible (normal is 180 degrees). External (lateral) and internal (medial) rotation is assessed with the elbow at the patient's side and the forearm held at a right angle in the anteroposterior (AP) plane (normal values are 40–45 degrees and 55–60 degrees, respectively). Internal rotation usually is limited by the patient's body and can be further evaluated by having the patient touch his or her back from below. Alternatively, external and internal rotation can be assessed with the patient's arm in 90-degree abduction. Adduction is assessed by placement of the patient's hands on the opposite shoulders.

Passive ROM then is examined and compared with the active range. Approximately 90 degrees of arm elevation is accomplished through abduction at the glenohumeral joint, 60 degrees by rotation of the scapula by the serratus anterior and upper half of the trapezoid, and 30 degrees by adduction and external rotation, which increases the articulating surface of the humeral head and turns the surgical neck away from the tip of the acromion. Glenohumeral abduction can be isolated by immobilizing the scapula or observing for scapular movement with one's fingers on the inferior angle of the scapula.

Resisted movements are examined next because they help elicit pain from the deep muscles of the rotator cuff. These tests are accomplished without movement of the shoulder joint, with the elbow at the patient's side, and with the forearm at a right angle in the AP plane. Abduction is tested by having the patient press outward at the elbow against the examiner's braced hand so that movement does not occur. Adduction is tested by having the patient press in, flexion forward, and extension backward at the elbow against the examiner's hand. External rotation is tested by having the patient press laterally and internal rotation medially at the wrist against the examiner's braced hand, again without movement and with the elbow kept at the side. Resisted flexion and supination of the elbow are assessed with the arm in the same position in order to test for a lesion of the biceps tendon. Strength and the elicitation of pain are noted.

Palpation is performed last. Palpation is less useful than the combination of active movements, passive ROM, and resisted movements because pain from palpation is common and nonspecific and because some structures are difficult or impossible to palpate. However, differential tenderness, compared with the control side, can help confirm disorders at the acromioclavicular joint, the bursa, or the biceps tendon in the bicipital groove.

Table 69.3 addresses *interpretation of the physical examination.* Both articular and periarticular disorders can cause pain and limitation of active movements. If both active and passive ROMs of the shoulder are limited, a disorder of the glenohumeral joint, adhesive capsulitis, or bursitis should be suspected. Limited ROM with a *capsular pattern* (lateral rotation more impaired than abduction, internal least impaired) suggests adhesive capsulitis or glenohumeral arthritis. A *noncapsular pattern* (abduction limited with little limitation to either rotation) suggests subdeltoid bursitis. If passive ROM is normal or exceeds the active range and passive movements are not painful

TABLE 69.3 Interpretation of the Physical Examination

L = Limited P = Pain W = Weak () = Variably present	Rotator Cuff Lesions: Supraspinatus tendinitis	Supraspinatus tear	Infraspinatus tendinitis	Subscapularis tendinitis	Subacromial/subdeltoid bursitis	Adhesive capsulitis/arthritis	Biceps tendinitis/arthritis	Acromioclavicular joint
Active range of motion	(L)[a]	(L)[a,c]	(L)[a]	(L)[a]	L[d] P	L[e] P		P[f]
Passive range of motion					L[d] P	L[e] P		P[f]
Painful arc	P[b]	P[b]	P[b]	P[b]	P			
Resisted *ab*duction	P	(P)[b,c] W						
Resisted external rotation			P					
Resisted internal rotation				P				
Resisted flexion/ supination of elbow							P	
Full passive *ad*duction								P[f]

[a]Range of motion may be limited by pain.
[b]Pain may be absent in deep or musculotendinous lesions.
[c]When the tear is complete, initiation of abduction may be impossible and pain may be absent.
[d]Limitation is in a noncapsular pattern, with marked limitation of abduction and little restriction of external rotation.
[e]Limitation is in a capsular pattern, with limitation of external rotation greatest, abduction intermediate, and internal rotation least.
[f]Pain usually is felt at acromioclavicular joint or point of shoulder (C4). For all other lesions, pain usually is felt in anterolateral aspect of upper arm (C5), with or without radiation to the forearm.

or are less painful than active movements, a *periarticular cause* is likely. Pain on resisted movements identifies the anatomic location of the disorder (i.e., some element of the muscle or adjacent tissue, such as a bursa, that is being tensed). Weakness on resisted movements suggests a muscle or tendon tear or neurologic compromise. Sometimes strength cannot be accurately assessed because of pain, unless the shoulder is examined after the appropriately placed injection of a local anesthetic.

Additional Diagnostic Tests

Additional diagnostic tests should be used selectively to confirm or further define, for therapeutic purposes, a diagnosis suspected on the basis of history and physical examination. Depending on the circumstances, additional diagnostic tests include a complete blood cell count, erythrocyte sedimentation rate, serologic tests for rheumatologic disorders, diagnostic arthrocentesis, plain radiographs of the shoulder or neck, and other imaging modalities. All have important roles in selected patients. Acute episodes of shoulder pain caused by rotator cuff tendinitis, bursitis, or biceps tendinitis usually should be managed without any additional testing.

Plain shoulder radiographs usually should be ordered in the presence of significant trauma, suspected arthritis (limited ROM in the capsular pattern on physical examination), suspicion of neoplasm, suspicion of osteonecrosis, or chronic, recurrent, or unexplained symptoms. Standard views consist of AP films in external and internal rotation. In external rotation, the humeral head is club shaped and overlaps the glenoid; its greater tuberosity is seen in profile. In internal rotation, the humeral head is rounded. Failure to see this distinction, in the absence of anatomic abnormality, suggests significant limitation in rotational movement. Additional views can be helpful in specific circumstances. An axillary lateral view (which permits accurate evaluation of the glenohumeral articulation but requires that the arm be held in abduction) or a scapular "Y" view (a lateral view that displays the scapula on end) can detect a posterior dislocation, which may not be noticed on routine AP views. A caudal tilt view can help identify subacromial spurs, which may contribute to a chronic impingement or rotator cuff syndrome. A true AP view, in which the patient is turned 40 to 45 degrees toward the symptomatic shoulder, provides a tangential view for evaluation of the glenohumeral joint space in a patient with arthritis. Plain radiographs, although useful in detecting fracture, dislocation, bone destruction, advanced osteonecrosis, calcific tendinitis, and arthritis, are insensitive in the diagnosis of early osteonecrosis and are, at best, only suggestive in the diagnosis of rotator cuff tear and other soft-tissue disorders. For all of these reasons, a detailed explanation of the reason for the radiograph will guide the radiologist to obtain the appropriate views.

Further imaging studies are best ordered in consultation with a specialist when referral or the possibility of surgery is being considered. *Ultrasonography* (approximately 1.2–4 times more expensive than plain radiographs) can be used to evaluate rotator cuff muscles and tendons, the biceps tenon, and the subacromial bursa. Pooled sensitivity and specificity for full thickness rotator cuff tears are 87% and 96%, but ultrasound is less sensitive in detecting partial-thickness tears (sensitivity 67%) (8). Skilled interpretation is required. *Arthrography* (three to eight times more expensive than plain radiographs) is both sensitive (approximately 92%) and specific (approximately 98%) for detecting rotator cuff tears (9), but it causes discomfort and may miss partial tears, particularly those on the bursal side. Communication of dye between the glenohumeral joint and the subacromial space unequivocally confirms a full-thickness tear. Arthrography can also confirm a diagnosis of adhesive capsulitis when clinical findings are equivocal. *Arthrography combined with computed tomography (arthro-CT)* is of value in detecting soft-tissue lesions (e.g., partial tendon tears) and intra-articular pathology (e.g., labral tears, capsular tears, loose bodies, chondral defects), especially in cases of recurrent subluxation/dislocation. *CT* (four to eight times as expensive as plain radiographs) and magnetic resonance imaging (MRI) (seven to 17 times as expensive) are noninvasive but costly techniques for evaluation of soft-tissue lesions. MRI better defines capsule anatomy, supraspinatus tendon integrity, site of impingement, and bursal anatomy than does CT. MRI is equal to arthrography and equal or superior to ultrasonography in detecting rotator cuff tears (sensitivity 75%–100%, specificity 84%–100%) (9,10). A systematic review found a pooled sensitivity and specificity of 89% and 93%, respectively, for full-thickness tears, but 44% and 90%, respectively, for partial-thickness tears (8). MRI is the imaging technique of choice in the diagnosis of early osteonecrosis. MRI arthrography with gadolinium (modestly more expensive than plain MRI) is more sensitive than plain MRI for detecting partial-thickness tears and labral tears (11) and is emerging as the imaging study of choice for glenohumeral instability and labral tears.

MANAGEMENT STRATEGIES

Specific management varies depending on the disorder responsible for the pain. However, some management strategies are broadly applicable.

Physical Activity/Physical Therapy/Acupuncture

In the treatment of acute pain, the patient may benefit from a brief period (2–3 days) of rest with the arm in a sling. Many patients can begin ROM movements immediately to maintain mobility, while avoiding aggressive exercise or overuse. Prolonged immobilization of the shoulder should be avoided whenever possible, because contracture of the shoulder capsule and periarticular structures, known as *adhesive capsulitis* or *frozen shoulder*, may result. When glenohumeral ROM remains restricted after the acute pain has diminished, specific exercises, such as pendular and wall-climbing exercises (Fig. 69.3), should be prescribed for 5 to 10 minutes two to four times per day to maintain joint mobility. Patients with impingement disorders (e.g., rotator cuff lesions, subdeltoid bursitis) should avoid repetitive tasks with their arms overhead or their elbows above midtorso height, especially if the condition is recurrent or chronic. A program of balanced isometric or isotonic exercise of the shoulder abductors, adductors, flexors, extensors, and internal and external rotators, to strengthen the rotator cuff musculature, may help prevent recurrences. Balanced isotonic exercise can be approximated by having the patient loop a long rubber tube around the foot, on the same side as the shoulder being exercised, and do repetitions of shoulder abduction, adduction, flexion, and extension. Repetitions of external rotations can be performed with the tube held in the opposite hand and of internal rotation with the tube looped around an external stationary object. Exercise is beneficial for both short-term recovery and long-term function (12). Manual therapy (manually and/or mechanically applied movement techniques to improve joint motion) may be effective (13).

The efficacy of adjunctive physical therapy measures, such as heat or ultrasound, has not been adequately demonstrated (12,14,15). Nevertheless, on empiric and theoretical grounds, local cooling is generally recommended after acute injury to relieve pain and limit hemorrhage and edema. Similarly, local superficial heat often is recommended to decrease pain and promote tissue extensibility in the subacute and chronic stages, respectively. Some evidence indicates that laser therapy is more effective than placebo for adhesive capsulitis (12).

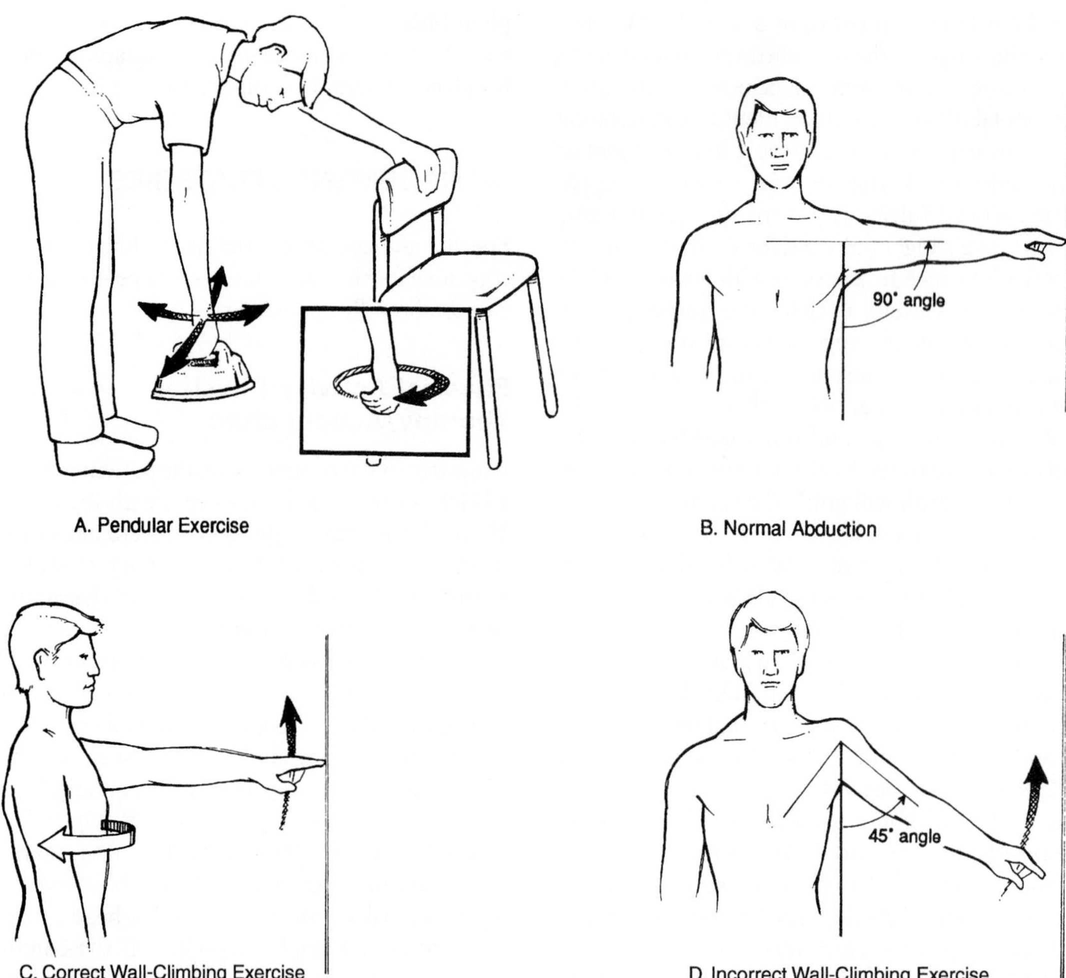

FIGURE 69.3. Range-of-motion exercises of the shoulder. **A:** Pendular exercise can be done with a weight, which facilitates the pendular movement. The arm is moved back and forth in the sagittal and frontal planes, then circumducted in the clockwise and counterclockwise directions in increasingly large circles. **B, C:** Wall-climbing exercise done correctly. The wall climb can be started facing the wall. The body then is turned until the patient is at a right angle to the wall. The shoulder movement is at the glenohumeral joint. **D:** Wall-climbing exercise done incorrectly, with shrugging of the scapula. (Redrawn from Cailliet R. Shoulder pain. Philadelphia: FA Davis, 1981, with permission.)

Referral to a physical therapist is recommended for patients who require a supervised exercise program after surgery or when satisfactory understanding of prescribed exercises or improvements in ROM have not been achieved after counseling by the health care practitioner.

Evidence supporting or refuting the use of acupuncture for shoulder pain is insufficient (16).

Medication

Nonsteroidal anti-inflammatory drugs (NSAIDs) (see Chapter 77) appear to be more effective than placebo but somewhat less effective than steroid injections in decreasing pain and restoring function in periarticular disorders (17–20). Generally, a 2-week course of one of these agents is prescribed for acute disorders (see Chapter 77 for a full discussion of NSAIDs). The effectiveness of NSAIDs for this purpose, compared with analgesics such as acetaminophen, has not been adequately studied (20), although NSAIDs have a theoretical advantage because of their anti-inflammatory properties. Concern has been expressed regarding possible gastrointestinal (peptic disease with bleeding or perforation) or renal (proteinuria and failure) toxicity, particularly in the elderly. The efficacy of topical treatments has been insufficiently studied in patients with shoulder pain.

Injection Therapy

Based on studies using injections of lidocaine only, placebo oral drugs, NSAIDs/analgesics, heat, ultrasound, exercise, and acupuncture, injections of depo corticosteroid appear to reduce pain and speed functional recovery in patients with rotator cuff tendinitis/bursitis and may be more effective than NSAIDs/analgesics (18,19,21,22). A second or even third injection is sometimes required. Based on controlled (22–26) and uncontrolled studies (27), steroid injections (often several), combined with an exercise program designed to increase ROM, may be more effective than analgesic or no therapy (28) in reducing pain and speeding the recovery of patients with adhesive capsulitis. A meta-analysis of the controlled trials of corticosteroid injections for shoulder pain concluded that subacromial steroid injection appears to have a benefit over placebo for rotator cuff tendonitis, but a benefit over NSAIDs could not be demonstrated. It concluded that intra-articular steroid injections may provide early benefit over placebo or physiotherapy alone for adhesive capsulitis (29).

A 60% to 90% success rate can be expected after steroid injections for treatment of bursitis and tendinitis of the shoulder. In one study, after diagnosis by the physical examination strategies described earlier, injection was shown to be much more effective than tender or trigger point injections (20% success rate) (30). Serious complications of treatment (infection, degenerative changes after multiple injections, weakening or rupture of tendons) are rare (<0.1%) (31). They can be minimized by using sterile technique, observing contraindications to intra-articular injection (Table 69.4), following the procedures for injection described in Chapter 74, limiting the number of injections into an area over a given period, and avoiding injection directly into tendons. Instead, the diluted steroid can be injected around the length of the affected tendon. Subcutaneous tissue atrophy occasionally occurs and may be caused by inappropriately superficial injections. Postinjection flares of pain are uncommon (approximately 2% of injections), begin 6 to 12 hours after injection, last up to 72 hours, and can be treated with local cooling and analgesics or NSAIDs. Systemic absorption of locally injected steroid does occur and may cause transient suppression of the hypothalamic–pituitary–adrenal axis. This possibility must be considered in certain situations, as in a diabetic patient in whom the blood sugar concentration could become unusually elevated.

TABLE 69.4 Contraindications to Arthrocentesis or Injection into the Shoulder or Periarticular Structures

Diagnostic and Therapeutic
Overlying soft-tissue infection
Bacteremia
Clotting disorder (relative)
Therapeutic (corticosteroid injection)
Septic arthritis
Unstable joint
Osteonecrosis
Neurotrophic joint
Marked juxta-articular osteoporosis
Intra-articular fracture

Injection Techniques

Because of the frequency of shoulder pain and the apparent efficacy of steroid injections in treating a number of the most common causes, primary care practitioners may want to become proficient in these techniques. Depending on the number and type of sites to be injected, 1 to 5 mL of a short-acting local anesthetic (e.g., 1% lidocaine) is mixed in a syringe with a variable amount (usually 0.5–1.0 mL) of long-acting (depo) corticosteroid preparation (20–40 mg triamcinolone hexacetonide [Aristopan 20 mg/mL] or triamcinolone acetonide [Kenalog 10 or 40 mg/mL], 3–6 mg betamethasone [Celestone 6 mg/mL], or 20–40 mg methylprednisolone acetate [Depo-Medrol 20, 40, and 80 mg/mL]). Injection then is accomplished, observing sterile technique and universal precautions, with a 1.5- to 2-inch, 22- or 25-gauge needle; an 18- or 20-gauge needle is used if joint aspiration is required. For patient comfort, the steroid injection may be preceded by superficial and deep infiltration of a local anesthetic using a 25- to 30-gauge needle. Patients should be told that pain may return 1 to 4 hours after injection, when the effect of the short-acting local anesthetic wears off, but that the pain should improve again as the anti-inflammatory actions of the corticosteroid take effect (several hours or longer after injection).

Rotator cuff lesions and subdeltoid bursitis usually are treated with a *subacromial injection* (Fig. 69.1) of 20 to 40 mg triamcinolone or its equivalent (italics for clarity) in 4 to 6 mL of local anesthetic. The local anesthetic provides an adequate volume for the medication to diffuse through the bursa or along the rotator cuff tendons. The needle is inserted medially along the groove between the midpoint of the lateral acromion and the head of the humerus until grittiness and resistance to depression of the plunger are appreciated as the needle enters the rotator cuff tendon. The needle then is slowly withdrawn while the plunger is depressed lightly, until resistance lessens and some of the solution can be injected. The needle is partially withdrawn and redirected anteriorly and then posteriorly to deposit the remaining solution. This technique probably results in deposition of solution both in the subacromial portion of the bursa and along the rotator cuff tendon. If bursitis is the predominant finding and there is marked tenderness over the lower portion of the bursa, the injection should be directed toward this area as well. Cyriax (see www.hopkinsbayview.org/PAMreferences) has described techniques for injecting around the insertion of the specifically involved tendons, but the therapeutic trials described previously generally used the subacromial fan distribution for injection.

Adhesive capsulitis is treated with *intra-articular injection* of 20 to 40 mg triamcinolone, or its equivalent, in local anesthetic. A posterior or anterior approach can be used (Fig. 69.2). If the *posterior approach* is used, the patient should rotate the shoulder medially, which turns the articular surface posteriorly and presents a larger target. This position can be fixed, if necessary, by having the patient lie prone, with the forearm under the upper abdomen. The practitioner places an index finger on the point of the coracoid process and the thumb on the point where the acromion and spine of the scapula meet at right angles, punctures the skin just inferior to the thumb, and directs the needle along the line joining the fingers, which crosses the glenoid cavity. Once impingement against cartilage and resistance to depression of the plunger are felt, the syringe is minutely withdrawn and the injection accomplished. A 2-inch needle usually is required. If the *anterior approach* is used, the patient is asked to sit with the shoulder externally rotated. The needle is inserted at a point just medial to the head of the humerus and slightly inferiorly and laterally to the coracoid process. It is directed posteriorly and slightly superiorly and laterally. Passage into joint space should be unobstructed. If bone is hit, the needle should be withdrawn and directed at a slightly different angle.

If bicipital tendinitis is the diagnosis, the *bicipital tendon* is identified by palpating it in its groove as the arm is rotated internally and externally with the elbow held in 90 degrees flexion. Then 20 mg triamcinolone or its equivalent in local anesthetic is injected along the length of the affected tendon.

The *acromioclavicular joint* (Fig. 69.1) can be palpated as a groove at the lateral end of the clavicle just medial to the shoulder. A $^5/_8$- to 1-inch needle is directed inferiorly from the superior aspect of the joint. If the needle hits bone at a depth <1 cm or $^3/_8$ inch, the tip probably does not lie intra-articularly, and slightly different spots should be tried until the needle slips in to approximately 2-cm length. Triamcinolone 4 to 10 mg, or its equivalent, in a small volume of local anesthetic is then injected about the joint space. Alternatively, the needle can be inserted from an anterior approach, with the tip of the needle slightly inferior to the joint.

Because the glenohumeral joint capsule juxtaposes the rotator cuff tendons and rotator cuff tendon disorders may accompany adhesive capsulitis, subacromial and intra-articular injections often are combined at the same time. This is particularly true for treatment of adhesive capsulitis. Because intra-articular injections are not consistently successful in entering the joint space, the posterior and anterior approaches are sometimes used sequentially at the same or separate sessions.

Use of a short-acting local anesthetic with or without steroid allows the practitioner to assess immediately after injection the accuracy of the injection by asking the patient whether the pain is gone and by repeating the examination. If the injection was effective, strength and ROM, now uninhibited by pain, can be assessed more accurately.

Because pain may be completely relieved, patients may be tempted to resume full activity of their shoulder immediately after injection. Common sense suggests that the patient should rest the arm for a few days after injection in the case of periarticular disorders, avoid heavy use (or use of the type that may have precipitated the disorder) for several weeks while healing occurs, and take appropriate precautions to prevent recurrence.

Referral

Occasionally, a patient needs to be referred to an orthopedist, rheumatologist, or physical medicine and rehabilitation specialist. Indications for referral include dislocation, fracture, functionally significant rotator cuff tear or rupture, suspected neoplasm, inability to perform indicated steroid injection therapy, nonresponsiveness to therapy, chronic or recurrent symptoms despite appropriate management, and uncertainty regarding the diagnosis or treatment.

PERIARTICULAR DISORDERS

Rotator Cuff Tendinitis

Rotator cuff tendinitis is the most common cause of shoulder pain (30,32,33). The tendinous fibers of the rotator cuff muscles undergo degenerative changes with advancing age. The tendons, particularly the supraspinatus, which is the most superior, are thought to be worn down by repetitive excursion between the greater tuberosity of the humerus and the acromion and acromioclavicular ligament. Edema, hemorrhage, and inflammation associated with repeated trauma cause pain that may lead the patient to seek medical attention. Inflammation of the subacromial bursa also may occur in this manner. The *impingement syndrome* and *pericapsulitis* are less specific terms that are applied to these degenerative and inflammatory disorders of the tendons and bursa. Risk factors for rotator cuff tendinitis include repetitive overhead work or activities and increasing age.

In addition to the history noted previously (see Diagnostic Approach), patients often complain of night pain and difficulty sleeping on the involved side. The physical examination is characterized by pain on resisted abduction (supraspinatus, most common), lateral rotation (infraspinatus), and/or medial rotation (subscapularis, least common). In the most common lesions, which involve the superficial distal end of the tendons, there is a *painful arc*. Pain occurs between 60 and 120 degrees of shoulder abduction (or 60–90 degrees glenohumeral abduction), where the impingement occurs. However, the pain resolves with further elevation as the shoulder is flexed, externally rotated, and adducted, and the impingement is relieved. An impingement sign (pain) also can be elicited by forcibly flexing/elevating the arm to 130 degrees while depressing the scapula *(Neer impingement sign)* or by elevating the shoulder to 90 degrees, flexing the elbow to 90 degrees, and internally rotating the humerus *(Hawkins impingement sign)*. The tests, however, have only modest sensitivity and poor specificity (34). In isolated rotator cuff tendinitis, muscle strength is normal; passive ROM is normal or exceeds active ROM, which may or may not be limited by pain.

The indications for obtaining radiographs were stated (see Additional Diagnostic Tests). If rotator cuff tendinitis is the only problem, the radiographs are normal. However, periarticular calcification in the supraspinatus tendon or subacromial bursa is occasionally seen. Its clinical significance is uncertain because the majority of patients with this radiographic finding do not have symptoms; calcium deposits may disappear spontaneously and usually require no specific treatment (35). In one study, however, ultrasound decreased calcium deposits and relieved pain more effectively than placebo in patients with calcific tendonitis (12). A systematic review found moderate evidence that high-energy extracorporeal shock wave therapy is effective in treating calcific tendinitis (36). If calcium deposits are associated with chronic or recurrent symptoms and do not respond to conservative treatment, removal of the deposit by lavage and aspiration or surgery may be successful. An orthopedist should be consulted in this situation for consideration of the performance of these procedures.

Treatment of most patients with rotator cuff tendinitis was described previously (see Management Strategies). Most patients improve over the course of a few weeks. Relief usually occurs immediately after injection therapy. However, recurrences and eventually the development of chronic symptoms are common (5,37), underscoring the importance of a preventive exercise program and of preventive counseling based on a careful history of occupational and other activities (see History and Physical Examination). Persistent symptoms despite appropriate treatment suggest the possibility of a continued impingement, a tear, or instability (see Rotator Cuff Tear, and Glenohumeral Disorders, Trauma and Instability).

Subdeltoid (Subacromial) Bursitis

Bursitis may involve the subacromial or subdeltoid portion of the bursa and may accompany rotator cuff tendinitis. Its onset often is abrupt. The disorder is characterized by pain, often severe, with a noncapsular limitation (described earlier in History and Physical Examination) of both active and passive ROMs. Active ROM usually is more limited than passive ROM. Abduction is significantly more limited than lateral or medial rotation. The bursa is tender to palpation; the area of tenderness may be used to direct the injection of corticosteroids. A painful arc may not be demonstrable until the patient recovers sufficient ROM. Treatment was described earlier (see Management Strategies).

Rotator Cuff Tear

By the sixth decade, degenerative changes in the rotator cuff are seen almost universally and are thought to be secondary to diminished blood flow. Tears and ruptures of the cuff may then occur even in the absence of significant trauma. In younger patients, trauma (e.g., falling on an outstretched hand), injuries with subluxation or dislocation, and overuse usually are involved.

Most tears occur just proximal to the distal attachment of the supraspinatus tendon. A small tear may be indistinguishable from rotator cuff tendinitis on physical examination. Larger tears are characterized by weakness on resisted abduction. In complete tears (ruptures), the patient may be unable to initiate abduction or to lower the arm to the side smoothly (*drop arm test*) because the supraspinatus is necessary to stabilize the humeral head and to assist the deltoid in the initial phase of abduction. In one study, the drop arm test had low sensitivity but good specificity for complete tears (34).

Radiographs are indicated when symptoms are recurrent or persistent despite treatment (see Diagnostic Approach). An uncommonly seen radiologic sign, narrowing of the space between the acromion and humerus ($\leq$5 mm is abnormal), suggests a tear, as does proximal subluxation of the humeral head and erosive changes in the anterior aspect of the acromion. The techniques of arthrography, CT, ultrasonography, and MRI are more useful than radiography in confirming partial or complete tears (see Diagnostic Approach). An orthopedic surgeon or radiologist may be consulted, to discuss the approach to establishing the diagnosis.

In general, minor tears can be treated conservatively in the manner described for rotator cuff tendinitis. ROM movements, followed by strengthening exercises, usually are part of the rehabilitation program. The decision to treat a patient with a large tear medically or surgically depends on the severity of symptoms, the functional disability, and the functional demands of each patient. Optimally, the patient, the family, the primary care practitioner, and an orthopedist are involved in making decisions. Indications for surgery remain somewhat unclear because of uncertainty about short- and long-term benefits versus risks in the absence of well-designed controlled trials, but they generally include acute posttraumatic weakness, particularly in younger patients and athletes, as well as persistent pain, weakness, and/or dysfunction despite conservative therapy. The traditional surgical approach involves removal of part of the acromion (acromioplasty) and repair of the rotator cuff tendon. The recovery period is more protracted after surgery (6–9 months of painful or restricted movement) than after conservative therapy (typically 8 weeks of painful or restricted movement). Arthroscopic and open repair have similar results; however, with arthroscopic repair, the incision is smaller, there is no need to detach the deltoid for inspection and treatment of intra-articular lesions, the procedure can be performed in the outpatient setting, and return to work and normal activities is shorter (38). One meta-analysis indicated very weak evidence for a long-term superiority of open repair (39). Because immobilization of the shoulder joint after surgery can lead to adhesive capsulitis, early and regular postoperative passive ROM exercises under orthopedic or physical therapy supervision are necessary. Complete pain relief and return to full function are uncommon after surgery.

Bicipital Tendinitis

With aging, the biceps tendon, like the rotator cuff tendons, is subject to inflammation, erosion, and rupture. Because the biceps tendon runs through the joint space and next to the rotator cuff and subacromial bursa, bicipital tendinitis can coexist with inflammation of these structures. However, attrition or chronic subluxation of the tendon in the bicipital groove of the humerus is more often responsible for symptoms.

Pain on resisted supination *(Yergason test or sign)* and flexion of the elbow are the characteristic findings on physical examination. A *Speed test* (pain at the bicipital groove on resisted forward elevation of the humerus with the elbow fully extended and forearm supinated) reportedly is more sensitive but less specific than the Yergason test (34), but it can also be positive in superior labral tears. If the glenoid origin is involved, the pain may be felt purely under the acromion. More often, pain is elicited in the upper arm, and the biceps tendon of the involved arm is tender to palpation in the bicipital groove. If bicipital tendinitis is isolated, active and passive ROM movements of the shoulder are painless and full. Radiographs are not necessary or diagnostic; however, if obtained for other reasons, they may show degenerative changes in the wall of the bicipital groove on tangential views.

Treatment was described earlier (see Management Strategies). Subacromial or intra-articular injection should suffice when this portion of the tendon is involved; otherwise, injection is directed along (but not into) the tendon in the bicipital groove. To reduce the chance of rupture, injections should be repeated no more than once or twice and separated by an interval of at least 4 to 6 weeks. For the same reason, injection usually is followed by a few days to 1 week of resting the tendon and avoidance of fully loading the tendon for a few weeks.

Rupture of the biceps tendon, which occurs rarely, is evident on physical examination as a mass of contracted muscle midway between the shoulder and elbow (*Popeye sign*). Rupture is accompanied by a sudden painful popping sensation, usually during a lifting effort. The upper arm remains painful and tender for several days after the rupture. Surgical repair, if desired (e.g., in an athlete, if an occupation demands maximal biceps function), is best accomplished within 7 days; otherwise, the tendon is likely to be contracted or fibrosed, precluding effective repair. Conservative management is an acceptable alternative. With regular exercise, the strength of forearm flexion and supination gradually returns; however, a 5% to 10% deficit in these movements usually persists.

Acromioclavicular Disorders

The acromioclavicular joint is formed by the articulation of the distal part of the clavicle with the acromion. Osteoarthritis is common in this joint during middle age and later life. Subluxation or dislocation may result from trauma, such as a fall on or a direct blow to the shoulder or acromion, which forces the scapula down and applies stress to the acromioclavicular and coracoclavicular ligaments. Laborers who lift heavy objects overhead or carry weights on their shoulders and athletes who compete in contact sports or weight lifting often sustain repetitive trauma to this joint. Injuries are classified as grade I—injury without subluxation, grade II—subluxation, and grades III to VI—complete dislocation. In grade III separation, there is modest superior displacement of the clavicle relative to the acromion. Types IV through VI are less common; they are characterized by posterior as well as superior, severe superior, and inferior dislocation of the clavicle, respectively.

Pain usually is localized to the exact site of the acromioclavicular joint or to the point of the shoulder (acromial area). There is little or no radiation of pain into the upper deltoid area. On physical examination, active and passive ROM usually are normal. Pain may be felt at the extreme limits of passive motion. *Full passive adduction* of the arm across the front of the upper thorax is often the most painful movement. Local tenderness is present when the superior ligament is involved. In grades III through VI dislocation, the acromion is displaced on palpation. Routine plain radiographs are indicated in situations of severe trauma. A 15-degree caudal tilt view of the acromioclavicular joint at 50% penetrance may be helpful in defining joint anatomy and pathology. Osteoarthritic changes are commonly seen on radiographs, but they also are often present in asymptomatic patients. Osteolysis of the distal clavicle may be seen as a posttraumatic change or in association with diseases such as rheumatoid arthritis, hyperparathyroidism, or sarcoidosis. Alleviation of pain after injection of a short-acting anesthetic directly into the acromioclavicular joint may be helpful in confirming this site as the source of pain. If a severe injury is suspected, the radiologic technician can be asked to obtain AP radiographs with the patient holding weights in both hands to help reveal grade II and grade III separations. However, one study suggested that weighted radiographs may miss acromioclavicular separations (40). Ultrasound, CT, and MRI may also be used when defining acromioclavicular joint pathology is desirable. The choice of methods is best made in consultation with a radiologist, rheumatologist, or orthopedic specialist.

Treatment of pain caused by degenerative arthritis was discussed earlier (see Management Strategies) and includes the use of NSAIDs or nonnarcotic analgesics. Local injection of corticosteroid/anesthetic solution may relieve symptoms in arthritic or low-grade traumatic conditions. If subluxation or complete dislocation is suspected after acute trauma and pain cannot be controlled with conservative measures over a few days, referral to an orthopedist should be obtained for consideration of surgery. However, one caveat should be considered before surgery is contemplated: Several prospective studies of grade III injuries that compared conservative management with strapping or a sling versus open reduction and internal fixation failed to demonstrate improved results from surgical treatment. Therefore, conservative treatment of shoulder separations of grade I, II, or III lesions currently is recommended by most orthopedists (41–43). Conservative management consists of treatment with an analgesic and a sling until the acute pain subsides. The patient should be aware that there will be a permanent prominence of the distal clavicle in grade III separations and a 5% to 10% loss of shoulder strength, which for most people is functionally insignificant. Surgery may be considered in the rare person whose occupation depends on continuous overhead activity (e.g., painters, some athletes) and in whom conservative treatment has failed to control pain. Type IV through VI lesions usually are evaluated for operative repair (42,43).

GLENOHUMERAL DISORDERS

Adhesive Capsulitis

Adhesive capsulitis, or *frozen shoulder,* is a condition of unknown (but likely multiple) causes in which progressive restriction of shoulder motion occurs. It is commonly seen in diabetic patients. Often, an underlying painful condition of the shoulder, such as rotator cuff tendinitis or subdeltoid bursitis, precedes the development of adhesive capsulitis. However, this disorder also may occur in association with a cerebrovascular accident (especially hemiparesis, in which case it affects the paretic side), myocardial infarction, cervical radiculopathy, thyroid disorders, local or lung tumors, or Parkinson disease. A common underlying factor in most of these diverse conditions appears to be immobility of the arm. Eventually, the adhesive capsulitis may represent a greater disability than the initial cause of immobilization. Thickening of the joint capsule and capsular adhesions to the underlying humeral head develop. However, inflammatory findings in the capsule or synovial lining of the joint are not constant findings. Therefore, whether contracture of the shoulder capsule is a passive process related to lack of motion or an active process caused by inflammation remains unclear.

Adhesive capsulitis is somewhat more common in women than in men, and it most frequently occurs between the ages of 40 and 60 years. The patient characteristically complains of the insidious onset of diffuse pain and limitation of motion in the shoulder. In particular, the patient notes difficulty in performing tasks that require overhead arm motion, such as combing the hair and grasping objects from high shelves. Physical examination reveals pain at the extremes of motion and markedly reduced active and passive ROMs of the glenohumeral joint, usually in a *capsular pattern* (see Diagnostic Approach). Injection of an anesthetic agent into the glenohumeral joint may reduce the pain, but it does not result in an improved ROM. If adhesive capsulitis is the only problem, a plain radiograph (see Additional Diagnostic Tests) usually is normal and can help rule out arthritis, osteonecrosis, loose bodies, and other local pathology. Additional studies are rarely indicated. MRI with gadolinium, if done, may reveal thickening of the capsule and synovium. Arthrography, if performed, usually reveals a markedly reduced joint capacity, increased filling pressure, intact tendons, and an absence of inflammatory arthritic changes. If an arthrogram is done, corticosteroid injection and capsular distention by the orthopedist or radiologist can be accomplished at the same time, with accurate placement of solution.

The primary aims of treatment of adhesive capsulitis are pain relief, restoration of motion, and correction of any contributing cause. Treated only with analgesics, most patients recover within 2 to 3 years, but residual slight restriction of movement is common, and severe restriction occasionally is present at 3 to 4 years (28). In controlled (22–26) and uncontrolled (27) trials, intra-articular and periarticular corticosteroid injection, usually combined with a progressive exercise program designed to increase ROM, has been associated with shortened recovery periods of 3 to 8 weeks (22–27). Typically, injections are repeated weekly for several weeks until the patient's pain is controlled and progress in mobility is being made. Capsular distention or rupture with 10 to 90 mL of fluid may actually speed recovery (25,44). An exercise program should be started as soon as the acute pain subsides. This may be limited initially to passive ROM exercises, performed at home with a trained family member. Active ROM often can begin after injection, with pendular and then wall-climbing exercises (Fig. 69.3). Too aggressive mobilization may actually be associated with less satisfactory outcomes. Referral to a physical therapist usually is indicated to increase motivation, to ensure patient understanding of the exercise program, and to train family members. If pain is a limiting factor, consideration may be given to suprascapular nerve block. Two studies have provided some evidence of the effectiveness of suprascapular nerve block in reducing pain in patients with frozen shoulder (45,46). In the past, referral to an orthopedist for manipulation of the shoulder under anesthesia to free capsular adhesions was recommended for patients who did not improve with conservative management. The efficacy of this treatment has not been studied in a controlled fashion. It is no longer generally recommended and should be considered only in recalcitrant cases.

Trauma and Instability

Dislocation

Because of its instability, the shoulder is the joint most commonly dislocated. Dislocation occurs most often in active young to middle-aged adults. *Anterior dislocation* (95% of shoulder dislocations) usually results from a fall on an outstretched hand with forceful abduction, extension, and external rotation of the shoulder. On physical examination, the arm is held in the neutral position, and movement is avoided because of pain. The contour of the shoulder, which normally is convex below the acromion because of the humeral head, is flattened. The tip of the acromion is now the most lateral point of the shoulder region, and a noticeable prominence, caused by the displaced humeral head, is seen and felt inferior to the clavicle. Standard AP radiographs confirm the diagnosis.

Posterior dislocation (5% of shoulder dislocations) is less obvious and more likely to be overlooked on examination and radiography. It results from direct or indirect trauma that forces the humeral head posteriorly out of the glenoid fossa, and it may occur after an electrical shock or convulsion. On physical examination, the arm is held adducted and fixed in internal rotation. Anteriorly, there is flattening of the shoulder contour and prominence of the coracoid process. Posteriorly, there is prominence and rounding of the shoulder. The findings on standard AP radiographs are subtle (slight increase in space between the anterior glenoid rim and the medial humeral head; failure on the external rotation view [see Additional Diagnostic Tests] to see the normal club-shaped humeral head, with its greater tuberosity prominent at the superolateral margin, because the shoulder is locked in internal rotation). An axillary lateral or scapular "Y" view reveals the posterior displacement of the humeral head relative to the glenoid fossa.

Treatment of dislocations requires prompt reduction and usually involves immediate referral to an orthopedist or emergency department. Postreduction management includes a 2- to 6-week period of immobilization in a sling (less time for older patients), with removal a few times per day to extend the elbow, followed by an intensive physical therapy program to restore ROM and strengthen the appropriate anterior or posterior muscle groups in the hope of preventing recurrence. Dislocations may be accompanied by rotator cuff injury, neurovascular compromise (commonly the axillary nerve in anterior dislocation), or fracture, so pretreatment and posttreatment physical examination and radiographic studies should be done to evaluate these complications and to ensure the adequacy of the reduction.

Recurrent dislocation may follow the acute dislocation. It is especially common in younger patients (>50% incidence in patients 25 years of age or younger) (47,48). Each subsequent dislocation may require less force; eventually dislocation may occur even during routine tasks such as combing the hair. A variety of surgical procedures are available to treat this condition. Limited evidence now supports primary surgical intervention for young adults, primarily male, engaged in highly demanding physical activities, who have sustained their first acute traumatic shoulder dislocation (49).

Instability

A syndrome of *glenohumeral instability, with subluxation* with or without recurrent dislocation, is often seen in athletes, particularly in the dominant arm of baseball pitchers, racket sport players, and swimmers. Instability can be anterior, multidirectional, posterior, or inferior; the first two are most common. Patients with multidirectional instability are more likely to have joint laxity, shoulder muscle deconditioning, a history of repetitive injuries, or a previous large rotator cuff tear. *Anterior instability with subluxation* and secondary impingement can be an additional cause of rotator cuff tendinitis.

In addition to pain, patients may describe a sense of instability, weakness, or even radicular symptoms. They may voluntarily reduce their ROM. This syndrome can be difficult to diagnose. Physical examination should include an *apprehension test,* for anterior instability. The arm is placed in 90-degree abduction and full external rotation; patients with a positive test experience apprehension and a sense of impending dislocation. Subsequent application of pressure over the anterior aspect of the proximal humerus may alleviate the apprehension (relocation sign), whereas sudden release of this pressure may cause a return of apprehension, pain, or sense of impending dislocation (anterior release sign). The relocation and anterior release signs have similar sensitivity (~85%) but higher specificity (~87%) than the apprehension test (~50%), giving them better positive predictive values and likelihood ratios (50) (see Chapter 2). Inferior instability may be detected by inferior traction on the patient's arm, revealing a *sulcus sign,* or subacromial indentation, which has low sensitivity (31%) but reasonably high specificity (89%) (50). Posterior instability is tested with a *jerk test.* With the shoulder and elbow in 90 degrees flexion and the shoulder in full internal rotation, the arm is adducted across the body while pushing the humerus posteriorly. A positive test is characterized by posterior subluxation or dislocation. In the case of dislocation, the humeral head can be felt to clunk back into the joint as the arm is abducted. This is not to be confused with the *clunk* test, a test of low sensitivity (35%) and high specificity (98%) used to both assess joint instability and labral tears. With the arm abducted, forward pressure is placed on head of the humerus from behind as the shoulder is externally rotated; a clunk or grinding sensation represents a positive test. *Joint laxity* is tested by having the patient try to touch a thumb to the volar surface of the forearm and by having the patient bend back the fingers at the metacarpophalangeal joints. Plain radiographs usually are normal, but they may show subluxation with the patient holding a weight while relaxing the shoulder musculature.

Special radiographs may demonstrate a *Bankart lesion* (avulsion of the anterior inferior glenoid rim) or a *Hill-Sachs lesion* (compression fracture of the posterior humeral head) apparently caused by recurrent subluxation of the humeral head in front of the anterior glenoid rim. MRI, MRI arthrography, or arthro–CT may demonstrate a glenoid labral tear, laxity of the glenohumeral ligaments, or a Hill-Sachs lesion.

Treatment for anterior instability often requires surgery. The mnemonic *TUBS* applies to anterior instability: *T*rauma, *U*nidirectional, *B*ankart lesion, *S*urgery. Treatment of multidirectional instability involves a program of shoulder strengthening exercises, with a good to excellent response to treatment in approximately 80% of patients (51). The mnemonic *AMBRI* applies to multidirectional instability: *A*traumatic, *M*ultidirectional, *B*ilateral signs of laxity, *R*ehabilitation as the preferred treatment, and *I*nferior capsule tightening if surgery becomes necessary. If conservative treatment fails or if help is needed in making the diagnosis, referral to an orthopedist is appropriate. Surgery is directed toward tightening the capsular structures and stabilizing the joint.

Labral Tears

The labrum is a ring of fibrocartilage that runs around and deepens the glenoid fossa. *Glenoid labral tears* most commonly result from a fall on an outstretched arm with the shoulder in abduction and forward flexion. They also occur in people involved in throwing sports, racket sports, and swimming. The torn labral fragment can catch between the glenoid and humeral head, causing a sensation of catching, locking, and slipping that has been called "functional glenohumeral instability." Tears can be classified as *Bankart* tears, which are anterior and inferior and predispose the shoulder to recurrent dislocation, or *SLAP* (superior labrum anterior and posterior) tears, which commonly occur after a fall on an outstretched arm or in overhead athletes. The diagnosis may be confused with rotator cuff tendinitis or bicipital tendinitis. Physical examination tests for labral tears are being studied. The most common is the *O'Brien test.* With the arm flexed 90 degrees and the elbow extended, downward pressure is applied; pain is felt in full pronation but not full supination. The test, although initially promising, has been found in subsequent studies to have disappointing sensitivity and specificity (50). Labral tears can be confirmed by MRI arthrography, arthro-CT, double-contrast arthrotomography, or arthroscopy. If the diagnosis is suspected, referral to an orthopedist is indicated. Conservative management, usually prior to radiographic confirmation, includes analgesics and/or NSAIDs and a program of stretching and strengthening exercises. Symptomatic tears generally require surgery, which usually is performed arthroscopically.

Fractures

Fractures of the proximal humerus occur most commonly in elderly persons, usually after a fall, although they may accompany traumatic dislocation in patients of any age. The neck and the greater tuberosity are most often involved. Pain, swelling, and deformity are characteristic of displaced fractures. Extensive bruising of the upper and middle arm may appear 1 to 2 days after fracture of the neck. Plain radiography establishes the diagnosis. If fracture is suspected, true AP and axillary lateral (or scapular "Y") views, in addition to standard AP views, are recommended. Because radial nerve injuries are often associated, the practitioner should assess nerve as well as vascular function distal to the fracture site.

Shoulder injuries may result in fractures of the clavicle or of the scapula. *Clavicular fractures* usually result from a fall or direct impact to the clavicle. The patient experiences pain at the fracture site on attempted raising of the arm. *Scapular fractures* usually result from high-impact trauma, such as falls from a height or motor vehicle crashes. They may involve the glenoid, acromion, or coracoid process or the scapula proper. Often there are associated injuries, such as rib fractures, lung contusion, pneumothorax, and brachial plexus or spine injuries. The patient characteristically holds the arm at the side and experiences pain with any attempted movement of the arm. Referral to an emergency department or orthopedist is generally advised for definitive treatment, which varies depending on the type of fracture and the presence or absence of displacement of the segments.

Arthritis and Osteonecrosis

Arthritis

Arthritic conditions are distinguished by pain and limitation in a capsular pattern on active and passive ROM (see Diagnostic Approach). Plain radiographs may show chronic arthritic changes, but they may be normal in early or acute arthritis. Radiologic changes must always be interpreted with the clinical information on hand. Monoarticular arthritis uncommonly is the cause of shoulder pain. *Primary osteoarthritis* of the shoulder is uncommon, although secondary osteoarthritis may occur as a result of recurrent dislocation or instability, complete rotator cuff tear (cuff tear arthropathy), fracture, neuropathy (Charcot joint), osteonecrosis, hemoglobinopathy, or inflammation (see Chapter 75). In chronic *inflammatory arthritides,* such as rheumatoid arthritis, the shoulder usually is involved as part of a constellation of articular complaints (see Chapter 77). A septic (usually gonococcal or staphylococcal, less commonly streptococcal or gram-negative) or microcrystalline (see Chapter 76) process should be suspected if the shoulder is the site of monoarticular arthritis of acute onset. Joint aspiration should be performed promptly to obtain fluid for culture and fluid analysis, including cell count and examination for crystals by polarization microscopy (see Table 74.2, Table 76.1 and Fig. 76.1). The patient with a septic arthritis should be hospitalized and treated with intravenous antibiotics and drainage, usually by percutaneous but occasionally by surgical means.

Osteonecrosis

Osteonecrosis (also called *avascular* or *aseptic necrosis*) of the humeral head should be suspected in the patient with a history of fracture of the humeral head or neck, prolonged corticosteroid therapy, or sickle cell disease. Its incidence is also increased in patients with diabetes, alcohol abuse, or a variety of less common disorders. Diagnosis is confirmed by plain radiography or, if necessary, by bone scan or MRI (most sensitive, see Diagnostic Approach). Patients are staged from 0 to 4: 0—with all imaging studies normal, diagnosis by histology; 1—plain radiographs and CT normal, MRI and biopsy positive; 2—radiographs positive, no collapse; 3—subchondral radiolucency and early flattening of the dome; 4—flattening of the head with joint space narrowing. The disease often is progressive. Treatment includes ROM exercises, analgesics or NSAIDs, and limitation of stress, as discussed previously (see Management Strategies). Evidence from uncontrolled studies indicates that core decompression, which appears to be of benefit in hip osteonecrosis, may be of assistance for grade 1, 2, or 3 disease of the humeral head (52,53); it is a reasonable option in patients with no response after a few months of conservative therapy. Arthroscopic débridement and removal of loose bodies are sometimes used as an alternative or adjunct to core decompression (53). Patients with significant loss of function or severe pain whose condition does not respond to conservative management should be referred to an orthopedist for consideration of core compression, humeral head replacement, or total joint replacement. Total joint replacement is the treatment of choice for stage 4 lesions.

REFERRED PAIN

Occasionally, pain in the shoulder area is referred from other regions of the body. Referred pain should be suspected when (a) the initial physical examination reveals another source for the pain; (b) active, passive, and resisted movements and palpation of the shoulder fail to elicit or exacerbate pain; or (c) the pain is in an atypical distribution (see Diagnostic Approach). The common causes of referred pain are discussed here.

Visceral sources of referred pain may be suggested by a review of the patient's problem list or medical history and the absence of another cause for the referred pain. Irritation of the phrenic nerve or diaphragm may arise from pathologic processes abutting these structures, such as subdiaphragmatic abscess, ruptured viscus, or disease involving the mediastinum, pericardium, liver, spleen, or gallbladder. In addition, ischemic heart disease, apical or superior sulcus tumor of the lung (Pancoast tumor; see Chapter 61), and dissecting aortic aneurysms all may be causes of referred pain (usually acute) to the shoulder.

Reflex sympathetic dystrophy, or *shoulder–hand syndrome,* now designated *complex regional pain syndrome,* is a poorly understood condition that may be a cause of referred shoulder pain. It is characterized by stiffness, swelling without pitting edema, warmth and erythema, vasomotor instability, and patchy bone demineralization of the hand. The syndrome may occur in association with trauma or surgery of the involved extremity, acute myocardial infarction, or cerebrovascular accident (see Chapter 91).

Nerve compression or irritation that is manifested clinically by shoulder pain may originate at the level of the cervical spine, wrist, or shoulder. In addition to pain, the patient may complain of paresthesias, numbness, muscular weakness, or atrophy. Neurologic examination often delineates the nerves or nerve roots affected. *Cervical nerve root* irritation is a common cause of shoulder pain. The pain often is felt above the shoulder, rather than in the upper arm, and it may be accompanied by neck pain. Characteristically the pain is exacerbated by movement of the neck but not of the shoulder. Chapter 70 discusses the diagnosis and management. Compression of the median nerve in the carpal tunnel of the wrist, known as *carpal tunnel syndrome,* occasionally is associated with pain about the shoulder. Usually, the pain originates in the wrist and radiates to the upper arm or shoulder. Chapter 92 discusses this condition. Irritation or compression of the *suprascapular nerve* at the suprascapular or spinoglenoid notch can occur as a result of direct compression from a space-occupying lesion such as a ganglion or lipoma or from nerve entrapment, often seen in athletes involved in excessive overhead activity, often volleyball players (54). Patients experience deep posterior shoulder pain without sensory loss, weakness on external rotation (infraspinatus) with or without weakness on abduction (supraspinatus), and, occasionally, supraspinatus or infraspinatus atrophy. Full adduction of the arm across the chest may increase the pain. MRI, nerve conduction studies, and electromyography can help confirm the diagnosis. Six to 12 months of conservative treatment is recommended, which includes avoidance of repetitive overhead activities, a balanced muscle-strengthening program, and use of NSAIDs and/or gabapentin or a tricyclic antidepressant. Surgery may be required for a space-occupying lesion or to decompress the nerve if conservative treatment fails. Damage to the *axillary nerve,* usually resulting from shoulder dislocation, humeral fracture, or blunt trauma, is characterized predominantly by deltoid weakness but may be accompanied by a patch of sensory loss and pain over the outer shoulder. Other muscles innervated by C5 are not affected. Axillary nerve entrapment, termed the *quadrilateral space syndrome,* can cause similar symptoms. Shoulder pain may result from irritation, compression, or injury of the *long thoracic nerve,* which supplies the serratus anterior and results in winging of the scapula, or of the *spinal accessory nerve,* which supplies the trapezius muscle and results in weakness of shoulder shrugging and abduction, associated with abnormal movement of the scapula.

Thoracic outlet syndrome is an uncommon but serious condition in which pain in the shoulder is a common complaint. Neck pain may be present. The thoracic outlet consists of a series of three narrow, fixed passages within which the neurovascular supply of the upper extremity (brachial plexus and subclavian vessels) can become compressed as it exits the neck and thorax to enter the axilla. These three channels are (a) the space between the scalene muscles and first rib; (b) the costoclavicular space, bordered by the clavicle, first rib, and scapula; and (c) the space under the pectoralis minor where it inserts on the coracoid process (Fig. 69.4). Compression of the neural or vascular structures results most often from mechanical traction caused by muscle weakness, obesity, heavy breasts or arms, poor posture, or the carrying of backpacks or heavy loads on the shoulders. Symptoms may develop from periods of prolonged overhead work or sleeping with the arms hyperabducted. Only a minority of cases are caused by anatomic abnormalities such as a cervical rib (enlargement of the transverse process of C7), anomalies of the clavicle or first rib, cervical bands, hypertrophy of the omohyoid or scalene muscles, or subclavian artery aneurysms. The presenting complaint depends on the predominant structure that is compressed. If it is neural in origin, the patient complains of pain, often extending from the neck or shoulder area to the forearm or hand and accompanied by paresthesias or numbness, usually along

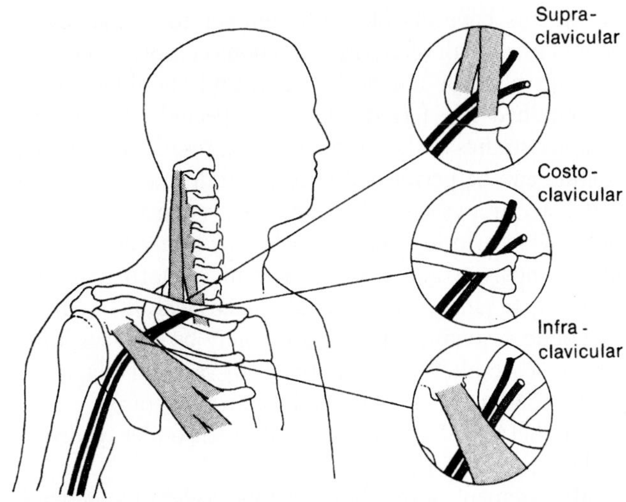

FIGURE 69.4. Points of neurovascular compression in the thoracic outlet syndrome. (From Steinberg GC, Akins CM, Baran DT, eds. Ramamurti's orthopaedics in primary care. Baltimore: Williams & Wilkins, 1992, with permission.)

an ulnar distribution. Muscle weakness and atrophy may be noted on physical examination. If it is vascular in origin, the patient may complain of an alteration in color or temperature, swelling of the affected hand, or a Raynaud-like phenomenon. Neurologic complaints usually predominate.

On physical examination, the force of the patient's radial pulse is palpated during the following maneuvers:

1. The patient holds his or her breath in full inspiration while rotating the extended (posterior) neck toward the side that is being examined (*Adson test*), which constricts the scalene outlet. A modified Adson test includes arm elevation and a Valsalva maneuver.
2. The patient assumes an exaggerated military posture with the shoulder braced posteriorly and inferiorly (*costoclavicular maneuver*), which may constrict the neurovascular bundle in the costoclavicular space.
3. The patient abducts the arm 180 degrees in external rotation (*hyperabduction maneuver*), which constricts the neurovascular bundle beneath the pectoralis minor.
4. The patient repeatedly clenches and unclenches the fists for 3 minutes with the arms abducted to 90 degrees and externally rotated (*Roos test*), which constricts the neurovascular bundle beneath the pectoralis minor.

Unfortunately, the sensitivity and specificity of these tests are low, which seriously limits their usefulness. Because a substantial percentage of normal patients manifest a decrease or obliteration of their radial pulse with these maneuvers (55), reproduction of symptoms in parallel with the change in arterial pulse at the wrist is necessary to properly interpret these physical findings. Only a minority of patients have discoloration, temperature changes, or edema as a result of arterial or venous compression.

Plain films of the neck, chest, and shoulder should be obtained if referred pain is suspected. Noninvasive Doppler studies of the vascular structures of the upper extremity can be performed at rest and during the maneuvers listed if a vascular impingement is considered likely. Subclavian arteriography occasionally is needed to confirm stenosis, to identify an anatomic abnormality such as an aneurysm, or as a prelude to surgical intervention. Magnetic resonance angiography may be an acceptable less invasive alternative approach to vascular diagnosis. Nerve conduction velocity and electromyography can be used to help distinguish between thoracic outlet syndrome and other pathology.

Management of the thoracic outlet syndrome depends on the underlying cause. For most conditions, conservative management is beneficial. This involves the identification and elimination (or reduction) of aggravating factors and the implementation of an appropriate exercise and postural program. Such conservative measures provide relief in 50% to 90% of patients according to Sheon et al. (see www.hopkinsbayview.org/PAMreferences). An occupational therapist (if functional guidance is necessary) or a physical therapist (if exercise guidance is necessary) should be consulted when initiating the exercise program. Occasionally, patients with severe or refractory pain may be helped by surgical intervention, which can involve resection of the first rib, a portion of the scalene muscles, and/or an abnormal constricting structure such as a cervical rib. Consultation with a surgeon should be considered in such situations.

ELBOW PAIN

Elbow pain, although less common than shoulder pain, is a problem not infrequently encountered by the primary care practitioner. It has a prevalence of a few percent in the adult population (1).

ANATOMY AND FUNCTION

The elbow includes the distal humerus, the proximal ulna, and the proximal radius (Fig. 69.5). The *elbow joint* consists of two articulations. The articulation between the trochlea of the humerus and the olecranon of the ulna, sometimes called the *humeroulnar joint,* enables flexion and extension. The articulation between the capitulum of the humerus and the head of the radius, sometimes called the *humeroradial* or *radiocapitellar joint,* enables pronation and supination.

Movements at the elbow joint include flexion, extension, pronation, and supination. *Flexion* at the elbow is powered predominantly by the biceps and brachialis muscles, *extension* primarily by the triceps, *supination* primarily by the supinator and biceps, and *pronation* primarily by the pronators quadratus and teres. Importantly, the *wrist and finger extensors originate from the lateral epicondyle* of the humerus, the most common site of clinical symptoms, and the *wrist and finger flexors originate from the medial epicondyle* of the humerus, the second most common site of clinical symptoms at the elbow. Table 69.5 lists the function and innervation of the major muscles working across the elbow.

The *olecranon bursa,* a common site of bursitis, overlies the olecranon of the ulna and does not connect with the joint space.

Unlike the shoulder, the elbow has considerable articular congruency, and joint instability is much less a problem with the elbow than with the shoulder. Stability is aided by various ligaments shown in Figure 69.5.

DIAGNOSTIC APPROACH

Causes of Elbow Pain

Table 69.6 lists some causes of elbow pain. Lateral epicondylitis (tennis elbow) and medial epicondylitis (golfer's elbow) are discussed in detail in this chapter. General approaches to arthritis and traumatic injuries involving the elbow also are discussed. Chapter 74 discusses olecranon bursitis. Chapter 92 discusses compression and entrapment neuropathies.

History and Physical Examination

History

The history should include questions about the *onset and duration of symptoms; location and radiation of the pain and associated symptoms; precipitating, exacerbating, and relieving factors; and the patient's activities.* Acute onset suggests significant injury, whereas subacute or gradual onset over days to weeks suggests an overuse syndrome. Pain well localized to the lateral or medial epicondyles suggests lateral and medial epicondylitis, respectively, whereas less well-localized pain posterior to the lateral epicondyle is more suggestive of arthritis. Paresthesias or weakness distal to the elbow suggests nerve entrapment. Pain on flexion and extension of the elbow is characteristic of arthritis.

Activities that place individuals at risk include throwing, power gripping, using the elbow as a weight-bearing joint (e.g., gymnasts), and pronation–supination of the forearm, especially with an extended wrist. Particularly important are repetitive movements of these types, such as repetitive wrist turning, hand gripping or shaking, tool use, or twisting movements, and movements that exceed capacity or normal ROM. Individuals at particular risk

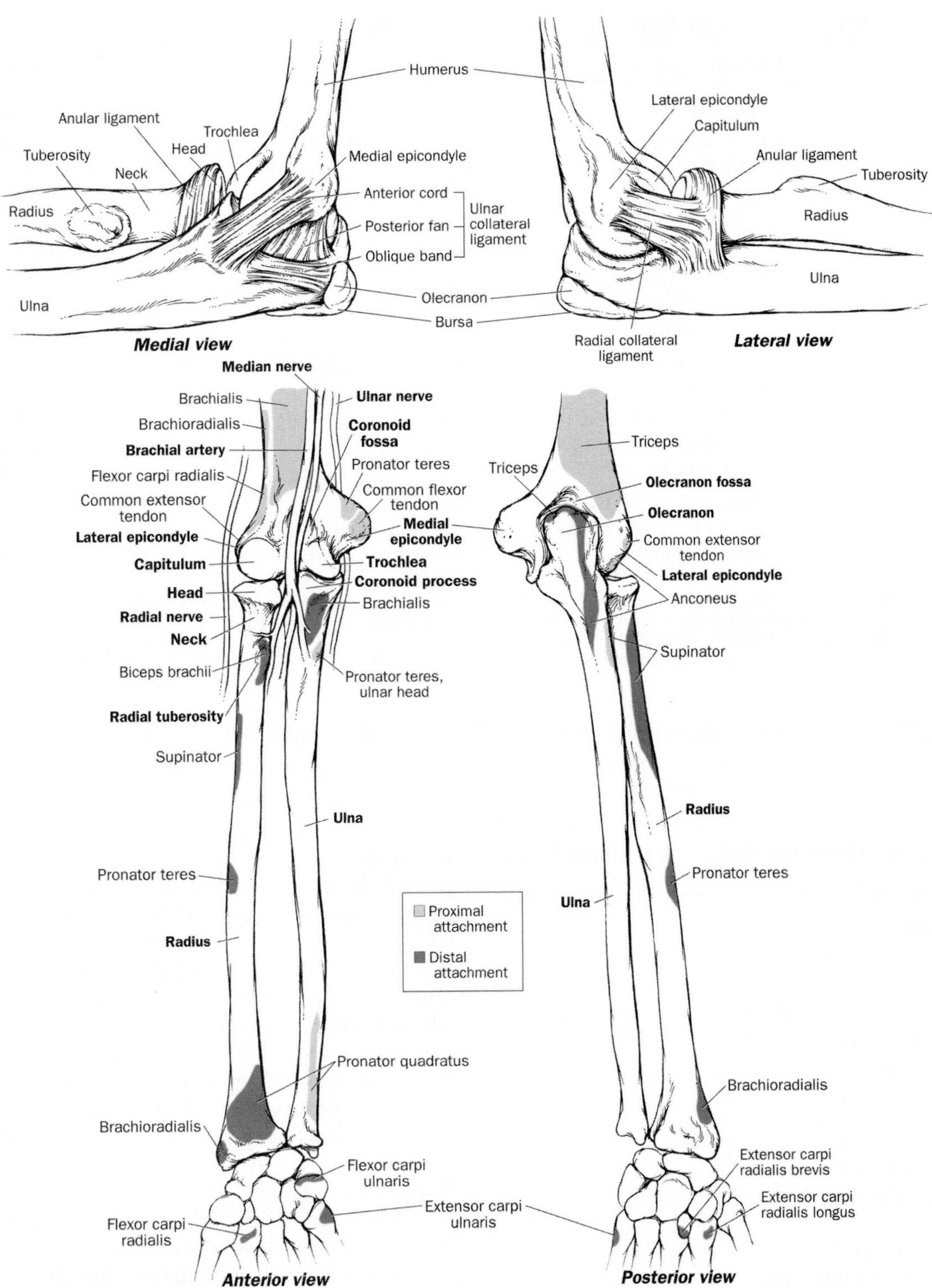

FIGURE 69.5. The elbow: bones, ligaments, arteries, nerves, and attachments of muscles acting on the elbow joint. The proximal attachments of the biceps brachii are shown in Figure 69.2. (Adapted from Agur AMR, Lee MJ, eds. Grant's atlas of anatomy. 9th ed. Baltimore, MD: Williams & Wilkins 1991; and Agur AMR, Lee MJ, eds. Grant's atlas of anatomy. 10th ed. Philadelphia: Lippincott Williams & Wilkins, 1999, with permission.)

TABLE 69.5 Muscles About the Elbow: Actions and Nerve Supply

Action	Muscle	Nerve	Nerve Root[a]
Flexion of elbow	1. Brachialis	Musculocutaneous	C5, **C6**, (C7)
	2. Biceps brachii	Musculocutaneous	C5, **C6**
	3. Brachioradialis	Radial	C5, **C6**, (C7)
	4. Pronator teres	Median	C6, **C7**
	5. Flexor carpi ulnaris	Ulnar	C7, **C8**
Extension of elbow	1. Triceps	Radial	C6, **C7**, C8
	2. Anconeus	Radial	C7, C8, T1
Supination of forearm	1. Supinator	Deep branch of radial nerve	C5, **C6**
	2. Biceps brachii	Musculocutaneous	C5, **C6**
Pronation of forearm	1. Pronator quadratus	Anterior interosseus branch of median nerve	**C8**, T1
	2. Pronator teres	Median	C6, **C7**
	3. Flexor carpi radialis	Median	C6, **C7**
Flexion of wrist	1. Flexor carpi radialis	Median	C6, **C7**
	2. Flexor carpi ulnaris	Ulnar	C7, **C8**
Extension of wrist	1. Extensor carpi radialis longus	Radial	C6, C7
	2. Extensor carpi radialis brevis	Deep branch of radial nerve	**C7**, C8
	3. Extensor carpi ulnaris	Posterior interosseus nerve, branch of radial nerve	**C7**, C8

[a]Boldface type indicates main segmental innervation. From Agur AMR, Lee MJ. Grant's atlas of anatomy. 10th ed. Philadelphia. Lippincott Williams & Wilkins, 1999, with permission.
Modified from Magee DJ. Orthopedic physical assessment. Philadelphia: WB Saunders, 1997, with permission.

include carpenters, gardeners, dentists, politicians, weight lifters, gymnasts, golfers, fly-casting fishers, and racquet and throwing athletes, particularly novices.

TABLE 69.6 Differential Diagnosis of Elbow Pain in Adult Primary Care Patients

Most common
Lateral epicondylitis (tennis elbow)
Second most common
Medial epicondylitis (golfer's elbow)
Common to occasional
Olecranon bursitis
Arthritis
Fracture
Dislocation/subluxation
Median nerve compression
Radial nerve compression
Uncommon
Anterior capsule strain
Biceps tendinitis or tendon rupture
Loose body
Neoplasm
Olecranon impingement
Osteonecrosis
Radiocapitellar chondromalacia
Radial nerve compression
Referred pain, from neck, shoulder, wrist, or visceral organ
Triceps tendinitis
Ulnar collateral ligament sprain

Physical Examination

Physical examination includes inspection and palpation, ROM, and resisted movements.

Inspection

With the patient standing and facing the examiner, the *carrying angle* (the angle made by the axis of the humerus and forearm), which normally is 5 to 10 degrees valgus, can be assessed. An abnormal angle suggests previous or current injury. The presence of *ecchymosis* suggests trauma, whereas *swelling* (using the other elbow for comparison) may be seen in arthritis, bursitis, or trauma. Swelling over the posterior olecranon process is characteristic of olecranon bursitis; associated erythema suggests infection or gout, with overlying cellulitis.

Palpation

In 90 degrees flexion the lateral epicondyle, medial epicondyle, and olecranon form a triangle, which becomes a straight line as the elbow is fully extended. Loss of this relationship suggests dislocation or displaced fracture. Small joint effusions may be detected by noting bulging in the triangular area that connects the lateral epicondyle, radial head, and olecranon in an area posterior and distal to the lateral epicondyle. Lateral and medial epicondylitis are characterized by tenderness over the respective epicondyles. Tenderness 4 to 5 cm distal to the lateral epicondyle suggests radial tunnel syndrome (posterior interosseus compression) (see Chapter 92). A cystic swelling over the olecranon suggests olecranon bursitis; associated warmth and tenderness suggest infection or gout, with overlying cellulitis.

Range of Motion

Normal *ulnohumeral ROM* (flexion–extension) is 0 to 135 or 145 degrees, with at least 30 to 130 degrees required for most normal activities of daily living. *Radiohumeral ROM* (pronation–supination) is tested with the elbow flexed at 90 degrees; findings of 0 to 150 degrees or 180 degrees total motion, and 70 to 90 degrees each of pronation and supination from the sagittal plane, are normal. Most activities of daily living are accomplished with 50 degrees each of pronation and supination. A limitation in ROM suggests arthritis, joint effusion, or previous or current injury involving the joint. Locking suggests a loose body. Bursitis and epicondylitis rarely affect ROM, except when there is overlying cellulitis or the epicondylitis is severe.

Resisted Movements

With the elbow at 90 degrees flexion, the following six isometric movements are tested against counterpressure with no actual movement of the associated joint: elbow flexion, elbow extension, supination, pronation, wrist extension, and wrist flexion. Testing of wrist extension and flexion is indicated because, as noted previously, (see Anatomy and Function) the wrist and finger extensors originate from the lateral epicondyle of the humerus and the wrist and finger flexors originate from the medial epicondyle. Pain on resisted movement that is localized to the tendon or other area of a muscle suggests an injury in the area of pain, such as tendinitis of the common extensor muscles of the wrists and fingers, commonly called lateral *epicondylitis* or *tennis elbow.* True weakness, rather than decreased resistance secondary to pain, suggests muscle or tendon rupture or tear. Soft-tissue injuries (e.g., tendinitis) are characterized by normal, nonpainful ROM with pain, weakness, or both on resisted movements.

Check for Referred Pain

If referred pain is suspected, the physical examination should include the neck (e.g., nerve root impingement, described in Chapter 70), shoulder (discussed previously in this chapter), and/or wrist (e.g., carpal tunnel syndrome, covered in Chapter 92). In the case of referred pain, pain typically is not increased by testing ROM or resisted movements.

Additional Diagnostic Tests

The history and physical examination usually are sufficient to make a diagnosis in the patient with nontraumatic elbow symptoms. *Radiographs* are necessary in the presence of acute trauma to confirm a diagnosis of fracture or dislocation, and they may be useful in confirming and characterizing the type and severity of arthritis. Basic radiologic assessment includes an AP view of the extended elbow and a lateral view with the elbow flexed at 90 degrees and the forearm supinated. Oblique views are used to help diagnose subtle fractures and when the elbow cannot be fully extended. *MRI* can help identify stress fractures; serious ligament, muscle, and tendon injuries; and nerve entrapment. *Neuroelectrodiagnostic studies* are helpful in diagnosing nerve entrapment syndromes (see Chapter 92). *Bursal* or *joint aspiration* is useful in distinguishing traumatic from infectious or other inflammatory etiologies and in diagnosing crystal-induced disease (see Tables 74.2, 76.1, and Fig. 76.1).

LATERAL EPICONDYLITIS (TENNIS ELBOW)

Definition, Epidemiology, and Etiology

The terms *tennis elbow* and *lateral epicondylitis* refer to injury in the region of the lateral epicondyle of the humerus at the origin of the common extensor muscles (see Fig. 69.5). The syndrome is the most common cause of elbow pain. It is associated with activities that involve excessive pronation and supination of the forearm, especially with an extended wrist, or with use of the common extensor muscles that exceeds capacity. Tennis, squash, and badminton players (especially novices), as well as throwers, bowlers, carpenters, gardeners, dentists, and politicians, are at risk. Case reports suggest a relationship with fluoroquinolone use (56). Some studies have shown the pathogenesis of lateral epicondylitis involves collagen degeneration and inflammation and injury (microtearing or microavulsion) of the common extensor muscles and tendons. Whether the anconeus muscle, radial collateral ligament, periosteum, radiohumeral synovium, or bursa is involved is unclear.

Diagnosis

The *history* is characterized by pain and tenderness localized in the *lateral* epicondylar area. It is more likely seen in the dominant arm. Sometimes the pain radiates proximally into the arm or distally into the forearm. The onset usually is gradual but can be acute or subacute. Sometimes the patient complains of intermittent pain or weakness. The pain may be aggravated by lifting (especially with the *palm down)*, by repetitive use of the forearm or wrist, or by shaking hands. On careful questioning, there often is a history of activities that predisposed the patient to this condition.

The *physical examination* characteristically reveals tenderness localized to the region of the *lateral* epicondyle and pain, similarly localized, on *resisted extension* of the wrist. Pain also can be elicited by stretching the wrist extensors through maximal *palmar flexion* of the wrist with the elbow fully extended and the forearm *pronated*. A tight handshake may elicit pain. Sometimes there is pain on resisted radial deviation, supination, or pronation. ROM is normal.

The *differential diagnosis,* which includes arthritis, radial or posterior interosseus nerve entrapment (radial tunnel syndrome), trauma, osteochondral loose body, and referred pain, usually can be distinguished based upon the history and physical examination. In some cases, additional diagnostic tests are required to distinguish among potential causes (see Diagnostic Approach).

Management

A short course of *immobilization* with a sling or long arm splint with the wrist held in dorsiflexion may help to rest the tendons, although evidence supporting this approach is lacking (57). At least *temporary abstention* (usually a few weeks) from the type of overuse that may have precipitated the condition seems wise. *Analgesics, topical or oral NSAIDs, ultrasound, iontophoresis with a steroid gel, acupuncture, or ice* may provide relief, with the current evidence strongest for NSAIDs, ultrasound, and acupuncture (58–60). The weight of current evidence suggests that extracorporeal shock wave therapy is not effective.

Corticosteroid injections are more efficacious than placebo and other conservative treatments in reducing symptoms during the first few weeks after treatment (approximately 80%–90% efficacy, compared with 50%–60% efficacy for placebo or NSAIDs) (61,62). However, long-term outcomes (e.g., at 12 months) are similar; one study suggests that they may be better with physiotherapy (exercises, ultrasound, and deep friction massage) (62). A long-acting corticosteroid preparation (e.g., 10–20 mg triamcinolone) with approximately 1 mL short-acting local anesthetic (e.g., 1% lidocaine) is injected, using a 22- or 25-gauge needle and sterile technique, in the area of maximal tenderness just superficial to the tendon. A painful reaction or resistance to injection suggests that the needle is at bone or within the tendon and should be withdrawn slightly. Contraindications and precautions are similar to those discussed for shoulder disorders (see Injection Therapy). The elbow should be rested for a few days after injection, and consideration should be given to having the patient wear a hook and loop (Velcro) wrist brace for a few weeks.

Recurrence and prolonged minor discomfort that affects some activities are common. *Prevention of recurrence* may be aided by instituting an exercise program after the acute symptoms have subsided. These include grip exercises with a compressible ball or putty and stretch and isometric strengthening/toning exercises of the wrist extensors and flexors. Adjustment in activities that may precipitate or exacerbate symptoms probably is important. For example, changes in technique, racket handle, or frequency of use, combined with an exercise program, may help prevent recurrence in a novice tennis player. Alternating use of the left and right arms may be helpful for others. Referral to a physical therapist may be helpful in motivating patients, teaching them exercises, and analyzing and adjusting precipitating or exacerbating activities. Forearm bands, which theoretically reduce stress on the tendons, appear to help some patients during potentially exacerbating activities, although evidence of their efficacy is lacking (57).

If symptoms fail to respond to conservative treatment, orthopedic consultation should be considered. Surgery occasionally is required, in which case MRI can be helpful in surgical planning by defining the degree of tendon degeneration and tear. No randomized controlled trials have evaluated the efficacy of surgery.

MEDIAL EPICONDYLITIS (GOLFER'S ELBOW)

Definition, Epidemiology, and Etiology

Medial epicondylitis (golfer's elbow) is caused by inflammation of the tissues in the area of the medial epicondyle, where the muscles that flex and pronate the wrist originate (Fig. 69.5). It is caused by overuse of these muscles and is seen most commonly in persons who engage in such activities, including throwing athletes, golfers, swimmers, tennis players who pronate and flex during their serve, and individuals who engage in repetitive lifting, tooling, hammering, or tight gripping. Although medial epicondylitis is not uncommon, it is less common than lateral epicondylitis.

Diagnosis

The *history* is characterized by pain and tenderness localized in the *medial* epicondylar area. It is more likely seen in the dominant arm. Sometimes the pain radiates proximally into the arm or distally into the forearm. The onset usually is gradual but can be acute or subacute. Sometimes the patient complains of intermittent pain or weakness. The pain may be aggravated by lifting (especially with the *palm up),* by repetitive use of the forearm or wrist, or by shaking hands. On careful questioning, there often is a history of activities that predisposed the patient to this condition.

The *physical examination* characteristically reveals tenderness localized to the region of the *medial* epicondyle and pain, similarly localized, on *resisted flexion* of the wrist. Pain may be elicited by stretching the wrist flexors through maximal *extension* of the wrist with the elbow fully extended and the forearm *supinated*. A tight handshake may elicit pain. Sometimes there is pain on resisted radial deviation, supination, or pronation. ROM is normal. The status of the *ulnar nerve,* which runs immediately posterior to the medial epicondyle, should be assessed (see Chapter 92). The *differential diagnosis,* which includes arthritis, ulnar nerve injury or compression (cubital tunnel syndrome), trauma, osteochondral loose body, and referred pain, usually can be distinguished based upon the history and physical examination. In some cases, additional diagnostic tests are required to distinguish among potential causes (see Diagnostic Approach).

Management

Management is similar to management for lateral epicondylitis, except that caution should be taken when injecting corticosteroids to avoid the ulnar nerve (Fig. 69.5). As in lateral epicondylitis, steroid injection appears to have benefit in the short term (several weeks) but not in the long term (3–12 months) (63). Surgical outcomes are worse in patients who have concomitant ulnar neuropathy (64,65).

ARTHRITIS

Definition, Epidemiology, and Etiology

Arthritis refers to disease involving the synovium, cartilage, or bone of the joint space. In the elbow, the most common types are rheumatoid arthritis (see Chapter 77), posttraumatic arthritis, and crystal-induced arthritides (gout, pseudogout, or other; see Chapter 76). Osteoarthritis (see Chapter 75) is relatively uncommon and is seen most often in patients with a history of overuse (e.g., manual laborers, overhead throwing athletes). Infectious causes (e.g., due to local trauma or systemic infection) are seen occasionally.

Diagnosis

On *history,* the pain of arthritis is not as well localized as that of epicondylitis. Early in the course, it often is lateral, but posterior to the epicondyle. Later, it may be more diffuse. On questioning, the practitioner may discover patterns of pain and joint distributions characteristic of rheumatoid, degenerative, or crystal-induced arthritis (see Chapters 75 through 77).

On *physical examination,* there usually is a *limitation in ROM.* Early on, there is a lack of full extension, which maximally reduces joint volume. Extension usually is more limited than flexion. Limitation of pronation and supination usually comes later, unless the arthritis was caused by injury to the radiohumeral area. Often there is *end-point stiffness or pain. Lack of smooth motion, catching, or locking* suggests the presence of a loose body, often seen in osteonecrosis. Soft-tissue swelling or rheumatoid nodules suggest an inflammatory arthritis. Physical examination of *other joints* may reveal findings of degenerative arthritis (see Chapter 75), inflammatory arthritis (see Chapter 77), or crystal-induced arthritis (see Chapter 76).

The *differential diagnosis* includes fracture of the radial head or distal humerus (including stress fractures), loose bodies, and osteonecrosis (avascular or aseptic necrosis or osteochondritis dissecans, most often seen in adolescent athletes with a repetitive overuse history), which often produces loose bodies.

AP and lateral radiographs (see Diagnostic Approach) can demonstrate patterns and characteristics of the various types of arthritides and reveal fractures or loose bodies. *MRI* may be required to reveal subtle fractures or loose bodies. If a septic effusion is suspected, joint aspiration is required for diagnosis. With the elbow resting at 90 degrees flexion, the elbow joint is entered in the center of the triangle connecting the lateral epicondyle, radial head, and olecranon (i.e., inferior and posterior to the lateral epicondyle). Preparation is the same as for shoulder disorders (see Injection Therapy); fluid analysis is described in Tables 74.2 and 76.1.

Management

Chapters 75 through 77 discuss management of the various types of arthritis. Management usually involves a combination of specific medications, joint rest, and physical therapy. Occasionally intra-articular steroid injections are used in the management of rheumatoid arthritis, but this probably is best done in consultation with a rheumatologist. In the presence of disabling deformity or symptoms unresponsive to conservative treatment, the patient can be referred to an orthopedic surgeon for consideration of open or arthroscopic débridement or total joint replacement.

TRAUMATIC DISORDERS OF THE ELBOW

Traumatic injuries to the elbow include dislocation (posterior in >80% of the cases), fracture of the olecranon or coronoid process of the ulna, fracture of the radial head, and distal fracture of the humerus. Although patients usually present to the emergency room, they occasionally present to their primary care practitioner. The practitioner should, therefore, be aware of these injuries and have an approach to diagnosis and referral.

Dislocations and fractures of the radial head commonly result from falls on an outstretched hand with the arm in extension and adduction. Fractures of the olecranon usually result from a direct blow to or fall on the olecranon. Fractures of the coronoid process usually are preceded by sudden, strong resisted contraction of the brachialis muscle or occur in association with dislocation. Humeral fractures are relatively rare. Stress fractures of the olecranon usually are associated with overuse.

The *diagnosis* is suggested by acute and severe pain, swelling, ecchymosis, limited ROM, crepitus, and/or joint deformity. Physical examination should include palpation of the brachial, radial, and ulnar pulses and assessment of the distal vascular supply (warmth, color, and capillary refill). Median, radial, and ulnar nerve function should be assessed distal to the elbow. Radiographs of the elbow are always indicated and usually reveal the diagnosis. Dislocation is not infrequently accompanied by fracture (usually of the radial head or coronoid process of the proximal ulna). Stress fractures, usually of the olecranon, are characterized by a less dramatic history and physical examination and may require a bone scan or MRI for diagnosis.

Once a diagnosis has been made or seriously entertained, *referral* usually is made to an emergency department or orthopedic physician for treatment. In the case of vascular or neurologic compromise, dislocation, or displaced, open, or comminuted fractures, communication and transfer of care are urgent.

SPECIFIC REFERENCES*

1. Walker-Bone K, Palmer KT, Reading I, et al. Prevalence and impact of musculoskeletal disorders of the upper limb in the general population. Arthritis Rheum 2004;5:642.
2. Luime JJ, Koies BW, Hendriksen IJH, et al. Prevalence and incidence of shoulder pain in the general population; a systematic review. Scand J Rheumatol 2004;33:73.
3. Makela M, Heliovaara M, Sainio P, et al. Shoulder joint impairment among Finns aged 30 years or over: prevalence, risk factors and co-morbidity. Rheumatology (Oxford) 1999;38:656.
4. Croft P, Pope D, Silman A. The clinical course of shoulder pain: prospective cohort study in primary care. BMJ 1996;313:601.
5. van der Windt DA, Koes BW, Boeke AJP, et al. Shoulder disorders in general practice: prognostic indicators of outcome. Br J Gen Pract 1996;46:519.
6. Hales TR, Bernard BP. Epidemiology of work-related musculoskeletal disorders. Orthop Clin North Am 1996;27:679.
7. Pellecchia GL, Paolino J, Connell J. Intertester reliability of the Cyriax evaluation in assessing patients with shoulder pain. J Orthop Sports Phys Ther 1996;23:34.
8. Dinnes J, Loveman E, McIntyre L, et al. The effectiveness of diagnostic tests for the assessment of shoulder pain due to soft tissue disorders: a systematic review. Health Technol Assess 2003;7:iii,1.
9. Burk DL, Karasick D, Kurz AB, et al. Rotator cuff tears: prospective comparison of MR imaging with arthrography, sonography, and surgery. AJR Am J Roentgenol 1989;153:87.
10. Boorstein JM, Kneeland JB, Dalinka MK, et al. Magnetic resonance imaging of the shoulder. Curr Probl Diagn Radiol 1992;21:3.
11. Magee T, Williams D, Mani N. Shoulder MR arthrography: which patient group benefits best? AJR Am J Roentgenol 2004;183:969.
12. Green S, Buchbinder R, Hetrick S. Physiotherapy interventions for shoulder pain. Cochrane Database Syst Rev 2003;(2):CD004258.
13. Desmeules F, Cote CH, Fremont P. Therapeutic exercise and orthopedic manual therapy for impingement syndrome: a systematic review. Clin J Sport Med 2003;13:176.
14. van der Heijden GJ, Leffers P, Wolters PJ, et al. No effect of bipolar interferential electrotherapy and pulsed ultrasound for soft tissue shoulder disorders: a randomised controlled trial. Ann Rheum Dis 1999;58:530.
15. van der Windt DA, van der Heijden GJMG, van der Berg SGM, et al. Ultrasound therapy for musculoskeletal disorders: a systematic review. Pain 1999;81:257.
16. Green S, Buchbinder, Hetrick S. Acupuncture for shoulder pain. Cochrane Database Syst Rev 2005;(2):CD005319.
17. Green S, Buchbinder R, Glazier R. Interventions for shoulder pain. Cochrane Database Syst Rev 1999;(2):CD001156.
18. Adebajo AO, Nash P, Hazleman BL. A prospective double blind dummy placebo controlled study comparing triamcinolone hexacetonide injection with oral diclofenac 50 mg TDS in patients with rotator cuff tendinitis. J Rheumatol 1990;17:1207.
19. Petri M, Dobrow R, Neiman R, et al. Randomized, double-blind, placebo-controlled study of the treatment of the painful shoulder. Arthritis Rheum 1987;30:1040.
20. van der Windt DA, van der Heijden GJMG, Scholten RJPM, et al. The efficacy of non-steroidal anti-inflammatory drugs (NSAIDs) for shoulder complaints: a systematic review. J Clin Epidemiol 1995;48:691.
21. Berry H, Fernandes L, Bloom B, et al. Clinical study comparing acupuncture, physiotherapy, injection, and oral anti-inflammatory therapy in shoulder-cuff lesions. Curr Med Res Opin 1980;7:121.
22. Richardson AT. The painful shoulder. Proc R Soc Med 1975;68:731.
23. van der Windt DA, Koes BW, Deville W, et al. Effectiveness of corticosteroid injections versus physiotherapy for treatment of painful stiff shoulder in primary care: randomised trial. BMJ 1998;317:1292.
24. Carette S, Moffet H, Tardif J, et al. Intraarticular corticosteroids, supervised physiotherapy, or a combination of the two in the treatment of adhesive capsulitis of the shoulder: a placebo-controlled trial. Arthritis Rheum 2003;48:829.
25. Buchbinder R, Green S, Forbes A, et al. Arthrographic joint distension with saline and steroid improves function and reduces pain in patients with stiff shoulder: results of a randomized, double blind, placebo controlled trial. Ann Rheum Dis 2004;63:302.
26. Ryans I, Montgomery A, Galway R, et. al. A randomized controlled trial of intra-articular triamcinolone and/or physiotherapy in shoulder capsulitis. Rheumatology (Oxford) 2005;44:529.
27. Rizk TE, Gavant ML, Pinals RS. Treatment of adhesive capsulitis (frozen shoulder) with arthrographic capsular distension and rupture. Arch Phys Med Rehabil 1994;75:803.
28. Grey RG. The natural history of idiopathic frozen shoulder. J Bone Joint Surg Am 1978;60:564.
29. Buchbinder R, Green S, Youd JM. Corticosteroid injections for shoulder pain. Cochrane Database Syst Rev 2003(1):CD0046016.
30. Hollingworth GR, Ellis RM, Hattersley TS. Comparison of injection techniques for shoulder pain: results of a double blind, randomized study. BMJ 1983;287:1339.
31. Gray RG, Gottlieb NL. Intraarticular corticosteroids: an updated assessment. Clin Orthop 1983;177:235.
32. Smith DL, Campbell SM. Painful shoulder syndromes: diagnosis and management. J Gen Intern Med 1992;7:328.
33. Vecchio P, Kavanagh R, Hazleman BL, et al. Shoulder pain in a community-based rheumatology clinic. Br J Rheum 1995;34:440.
34. Calis M, Akgun K, Birtane M, et al. Diagnostic values of clinical diagnostic tests in subacromial impingement syndrome. Ann Rheum Dis 2000;59:44.
35. Faure G, Daculsi G. Calcified tendinitis: a review. Ann Rheum Dis 1983;42[Suppl]:49.
36. Harniman E, Carette S, Kennedy C, et. al. Extracorporeal shock wave therapy for calcific and noncalcific tendonitis of the rotator cuff: a systematic review. J Hand Ther 2004;17:132.
37. Chard MD, Sattelle LM, Hazleman BL. The long-term outcome of rotator cuff tendinitis: a review study. Br J Rheumatol 1988;27:395.
38. Sachs RA, Stone ML, Devine S. Open vs. arthroscopic acromioplasty: a prospective, randomized study. Arthroscopy 1994;10:248.
39. Ejnisman B, Andreoli CV, Soares BGO, et al. Interventions for tears of the rotator cuff in adults. Cochrane Database Syst Rev 2003;(4):CD002758.
40. Bossart PJ, Joyce SM, Manaster BJ, et al. Lack of efficacy of "weighted" radiographs in diagnosing acute acromioclavicular separation. Ann Emerg Med 1988;17:20.
41. Phillips AM, Smart C, Groom AF. Acromioclavicular dislocation: conservative or surgical therapy. Clin Orthop 1998;353:10.
42. Bradley JP, Elkousy H. Decision making: operative versus nonoperative treatment of acromioclavicular joint injuries. Clin Sports Med 2003;22:277.
43. Dumonski M, Mazocca AD, Rios C, et al. Evaluation and management of acromioclavicular joint injuries. Am J Orthop 2004;33:526.
44. Gam AN, Schydlowsky P, Rossel I, et al. Treatment of frozen shoulder with distension and glucocorticoid compared with glucocorticoid alone: a randomised controlled trial. Scand J Rheumatol 1998;27:425.
45. Jones DS, Chattopadhyay C. Suprascapular nerve block for the treatment of frozen shoulder in primary care: a randomized trial. Br J Gen Pract 1999;49:39.

*Bold numerals denote published controlled clinical trials, meta-analyses, or consensus-based recommendations.

46. Dahan TH, Fortin L, Pelletier M, et al. Double blind randomized clinical trial examining the efficacy of bupivacaine suprascapular nerve blocks in frozen shoulder. J Rheumatol 2000;27:1464.
47. Hovelius L, Augustini BG, Fredin H, et al. Primary anterior dislocation of the shoulder in young patients. J Bone Joint Surg Am 1996;78:1677.
48. Yu J. Anterior shoulder dislocations. J Fam Pract 1992;35:567.
49. Handoll HHG, Almaiyah MA, Rangan A. Surgical versus non-surgical treatment for acute anterior shoulder dislocation. Cochrane Database Syst Rev 2004;(1):CD004325.
50. Luime JJ, Verhagen AP, Miedema HS, et al. Does this patient have an instability of the shoulder or a labrum lesion? JAMA 2004;292:1989.
51. Burkhead WZ Jr, Rockwood CA Jr. Treatment of instability of the shoulder with an exercise program. J Bone Joint Surg Am 1992;74:890.
52. Mont MA, Payman RK, Laporte DM, et al. Atraumatic osteonecrosis of the humeral head. J Rheumatol 2000;27:1766.
53. Sarris I, Weiser R, Sotereanos DC. Pathogenesis and treatment of osteonecrosis of the shoulder. Orthop Clin N Am 2004;35:397.
54. Cummins CA, Messer, TM, Nuber GW. Suprascapular nerve entrapment. J Bone Joint Surg Am. 2000;82:415.
55. Rayan GM. Thoracic outlet syndrome. J Shoulder Elbow Surg 1998;7:440.
56. LeHuec JC, Schaeverbeke T, Chauveaus D, et al. Epicondylitis after treatment with fluoroquinolone antibiotics. J Bone Joint Surg Br 1995;77:293.
57. Struijs PAA, Smidt N, Arola, et al. Orthotic devices for tennis elbow. Cochrane Database Syst Rev 2002;(1):CD001821.
58. Green SE, Assendelft WJ, Barnsley L, et al. Non-steroidal anti-inflammatory drugs (NSAIDs) for treating lateral elbow pain in adults. Cochrane Database Syst Rev 2001;(4):CD003686.
59. Smidt N, Assendelft WJ, Arola H, et al. Effectiveness of physiotherapy for lateral epicondylitis: a systematic review. Ann Med 2003;35:51-62.
60. Trinh KV, Phillips SD, Ho E, et al. Acupuncture for the alleviation of lateral epicondyle pain: a systematic review. Rheumatology 2004;43:1085.
61. Smidt N, Assendelft WJ, van der Windt DA, et al. Corticosteroid injections for lateral epicondylitis: a systematic review. Pain 2002;96:23.
62. Smidt N, van der Windt DA, Assendelft WJ, et al. Corticosteroid injections, physiotherapy, or a wait-and-see policy for lateral epicondylitis: a randomised controlled trial. Lancet 2002;359:657.
63. Stahl S, Kaufman T. The efficacy of an injection of steroids for medial epicondylitis: a prospective study of sixty elbows. J Bone Joint Surg Am 1997;79:1648.
64. Kurvers H, Verhaar J. The results of operative treatment of medial epicondylitis. J Bone Joint Surg Am 1995;77:1374.
65. Gabel GT, Morrey GT. Operative treatment of medial epicondylitis: influence of concomitant ulnar neuropathy at the elbow. J Bone Joint Surg Am 1995;77:1065.
66. Vecchio PC, Kavanagh RT, Hazleman BL, et al. Community survey of shoulder disorders in the elderly to assess the natural history and effects of treatment. Ann Rheum Dis 1995;54:152.

For annotated **General References** *and resources related to this chapter, visit www.hopkinsbayview.org/PAMreferences.*

Chapter 70

Neck Pain

Carlos A. Bagley, Ira M. Garonzik, and Frederick A. Lenz

Neck pain is a common problem. Nearly 50% of people older than 50 years experience neck pain at some time. Because of the many structures in the neck that can cause pain when diseased, as well as the multiple sources of referred pain, patients who complain of new or persistent neck pain should be systematically evaluated. This chapter provides a review of the skeletal structures of the neck, the method of evaluation for complaints of neck pain, a description of common problems and their treatment, and guidance for referral of selected patients with neck pain to a physiatrist or a spine specialist.

ANATOMY OF THE NECK AND SOURCES OF PAIN

The cervical spine consists of seven vertebral bodies connected by facet joints, interspinous ligaments, and anterior and posterior longitudinal ligaments (Fig. 70.1). These ligaments provide stability when the neck is flexed and extended. The vertebral bodies are joined by intervertebral disks composed of a gel-like material (the nucleus pulposus) that absorbs increased pressure applied to the spine. The nucleus pulposus is contained within an annulus fibrosus, a fibrous structure ringing the outer margin of the disk. Beginning approximately the fourth decade of life, both the nucleus pulposus and the annulus fibrosus undergo progressive degeneration, seen microscopically as a loss of the fibrous pattern and the collagen alignment. As a result, the ability of the disk to absorb shocks is reduced. Facet joints are found between vertebral elements posteriorly, one on each side of the spine; they are apophyseal (projecting) joints with a synovium-lined capsule and are aligned in an axial plane. It is within these small joints in the posterior spine that osteoarthritis, a breakdown of the articular cartilage within the joints, can occur. The intervertebral neural foramina, located on either side of the vertebral bodies, are the canals through which the nerve roots emerge from the spinal canal. The spinal canal and the

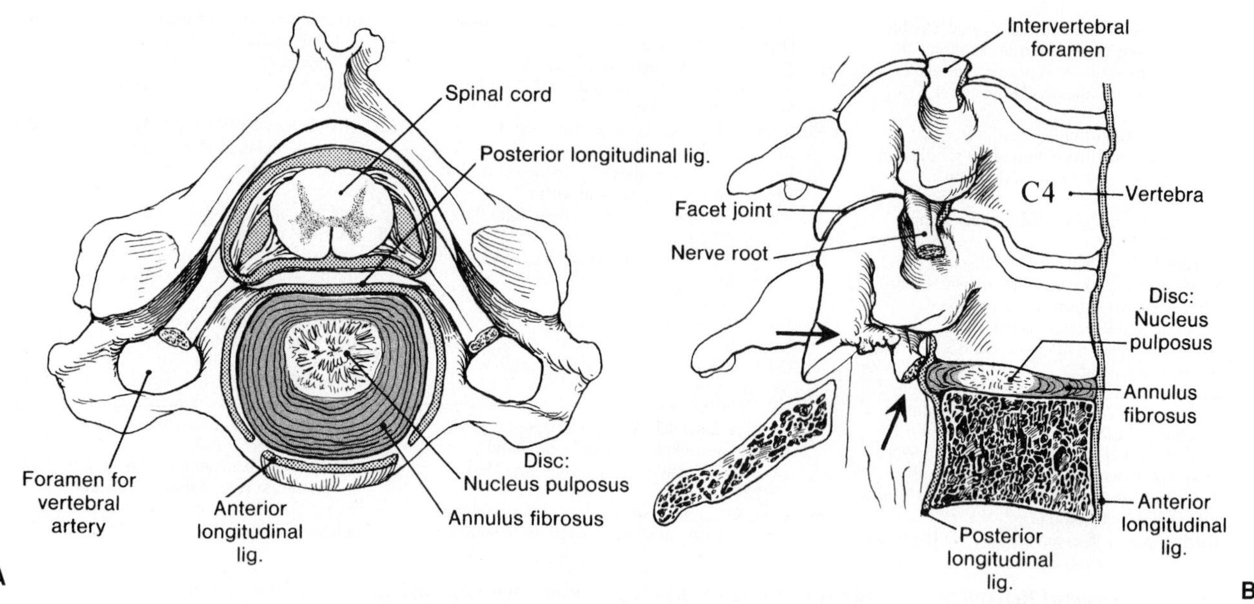

FIGURE 70.1. Anatomy of the disk and ligaments of the cervical spine. **A:** Superior view. Note relationship of anterior and posterior longitudinal ligaments to the intervertebral disk. **B:** Lateral view. Note relationship of the intervertebral foramen to the intervertebral disk and facet joint. Bulging of the intervertebral disk or bone spurs forming from the facet joint may cause compression of the nerve root within the intervertebral foramen (*arrows*).

foramina can be encroached on by a bulging intervertebral disk or an osseous proliferation (bony spur) originating in a vertebral body, by a facet joint, or from the bony margin of a neural foramen (Fig. 70.1). When the encroachment involves a nerve root, pain in the distribution of that root (radicular pain) may occur. The facet joint capsules and the intervertebral disk are innervated by fine nerves that have simple nerve endings (1). When these nerve endings are stimulated by degenerative disease within the disk or joint capsules, the patient may experience pain, which is referred to the posterior aspect of the neck at any level. The pain felt in the neck may not be at the cervical level from which the nerve is arising. In addition, irritation of the nerves can cause pain to be referred to the interscapular area, superiorly and laterally over the shoulders. Spasm of any of the many muscles of the neck region is another common source of pain.

EVALUATION OF THE PATIENT

History

The date of onset of the patient's symptoms and any associated trauma should be ascertained. Often, knowledge of the specific activity the patient was performing at the onset of pain is helpful in establishing potential causes of the pain. Prolonged extension of the neck, as occurs in people doing overhead work, is a common occupational activity that can give rise to pain in the cervical region. Another common occupational cause of neck pain is prolonged sitting with the neck flexed in one position. This occurs commonly in computer operators or typists. The sustained position causes spasm of the neck muscles, which results in pain. Also, patients may sustain minor twisting injuries or trauma to the neck but do not experience neck pain within the first 24 hours, after which pain may begin to appear and progress. Reproduction or exacerbation of pain by neck motion is helpful in localizing the problem to the cervical spine rather than to a referred source (Table 70.1). It is important to know whether the pain is felt outside the neck as well, such as in the head, posteriorly between the scapulae, about the shoulder, down the arm, or in the hand. The patient should be asked about decreased sensation in the arms or hands and, if possible, to specify which fingers are involved. If the pain and numbness are felt in a dermatome distribution (see dermatome map in Chapter 86), this indicates possible nerve compression (Table 70.2).

Muscle weakness in the shoulder, arm, and hand should be elicited to help identify potential nerve compression. Pain associated with motion of the shoulder is not characteristic of cervical spine disease and suggests that the problem is within the shoulder joint (see Chapter 69). Symptoms such as dizziness, visual changes, and ataxia brought on by neck motion (usually rotation) usually are not caused by nerve root compression or degenerative disk disease, but they may be found when bony spurs

TABLE 70.1 Sources of Referred Pain in the Neck[a]

Source	Referred Location
Disorders of the head	
Migraine or tension headache	Anterior or posterior
Sinus infection	Most often anterior but occasionally posterior
Temporomandibular joint problem	Usually anterolateral
Oral problems (see Chapter 112), such as pharyngeal or tonsillar abscess	Middle of the neck
Distant lesions	
Irritation of the surface of the diaphragm innervated by the phrenic nerve (C-3, C-4, C-5)	Often shoulder and low neck pain, but medial diaphragmatic lesion may be associated with neck pain
Shoulder problems (see Chapter 69), such as arthritis or periarticular inflammation	May be referred to the lateral part of the neck
Thoracic outlet syndrome from compression of vascular and neural structures between the rib and the clavicle or between the scalene muscles	May be noted in the lateral aspect of the neck
Lung problems, such as superior sulcus tumor (Pancoast tumor)	Initially may be located in the lateral aspect of the neck and shoulder
Cardiovascular problems, such as a heart attack or thoracic aortic aneurysm	May be localized to the base of the neck

[a]The clue to referred pain is the absence of any tenderness in the neck or of exacerbation of symptoms with manipulation of the neck.

encroach on the vertebral foramina and compress the vertebral arteries. These rare symptoms usually occur when the neck is in a certain position, and they usually are of short duration.

Constitutional signs and symptoms, such as weight loss and fever associated with severe neck pain and hypersensitivity, should raise the concern for an underlying spinal infection or malignancy. Patients with a history of cancer and new-onset neck pain should undergo a workup for metastatic spine disease.

Physical Examination

Examination should begin with inspection of the head, neck, shoulders, and upper extremities from the front and back. Any abnormal posture, such as torticollis (wry neck) or muscle atrophy, should be noted. Next, the patient should be asked to demonstrate active range of motion of the neck, including flexion to touch the chin to the chest, extension by looking up at the ceiling, rotation to touch the chin to the shoulder on both sides, and lateral bending to touch the ear to the shoulder on both sides. Normally, the chin can be placed easily upon the anterior chest, and the neck can be extended so that the patient is looking directly above. Normally, there is almost 90 degrees of rotation of the neck to both sides. Simple hyperextension of the neck commonly exacerbates the pain caused by cervical disk degeneration. The patient should be asked to extend the neck and to maintain this position for 30 seconds to determine whether the pain is made worse. Putting direct compression on top of the head may produce or exacerbate pain in the patient with degenerative disk disease, especially if the head is compressed while the neck is extended (Spurling maneuver). Patients may report an electriclike sensation that travels down the back, arms or legs with neck flexion or extension, known as the Lhermitte sign. The posterior neck muscles are palpated for muscle spasm, which may be asymmetrical and may give the patient the appearance of torticollis. Next, the shoulder should be subjected to a

TABLE 70.2 Characteristic Findings at Individual Cervical Nerve Root Levels

Nerve Root	Disk Level	History	Examination[a]
C3	(C2-3)	Pain into the back of the neck to the pinnae and the angle of the jaw	No reflex changes
C4	(C3-4)	Pain into the back of the neck to the levator scapulae to anterior chest	No reflex changes
C5	(C4-5)	Pain into side of the neck to the superior lateral shoulder, numbness over the deltoid muscle	Deltoid muscle atrophy and weakness of shoulder abduction
C6	(C5-6)	Pain to the lateral aspects of the arm and forearm and into the thumb and index finger, with numbness of thumb and dorsum of hand	Weak biceps and brachioradial muscles and decreased biceps and brachioradial tendon reflexes
C7	(C6-7)	Pain into the midforearm to middle and ring fingers	Triceps muscle weakness with decreased triceps muscle reflex
C8	(C7-T1)	Pain to the medial aspect of the forearm into the ring and small fingers, with numbness of the ulnar border and small finger	Triceps weakness with weakness of intrinsic muscles of the hand

[a]Sensory testing usually shows abnormalities in the dermatome of the affected nerve root (see Chapter 86).

range of motion to determine whether this action elicits pain within the shoulder itself.

Selected neurologic tests (see Chapters 86 and 92) are important in the evaluation of the patient with neck pain whenever there is any suggestion of nerve root involvement or cord compression. These tests for both the upper and lower extremities include reflex testing, muscle strength, and sensory testing. Reflex testing should include the biceps, triceps, brachioradial, quadriceps, and gastrocnemius tendons and the plantar. Muscle strength in the upper extremities should include the biceps (flexion of elbow), triceps (extension of elbow), wrist extensors and flexors, hand and finger flexors, and intrinsic muscles of the hand. Lower extremity motor examinations should include the iliopsoas, quadriceps, hamstrings, gastrocnemius, tibialis anterior, and extensor hallucis longus. A sensory examination should be performed in systemic fashion from the cranial to caudal direction. An objective sensory deficit that conforms to a dermatomal distribution is consistent with nerve root compression (see Chapters 86 and 92).

Cervical spine problems can cause cervical myelopathy. This may result from bone spur formation (spondylosis) posteriorly at the margin of an intervertebral disk, which then impinges on the spinal cord producing signs of cord compression. In addition, degenerative disease of the facet joints may result in hypertrophy and/or synovial cyst formation that also may compress the neural elements. Herniation of the nucleus pulposus of the intervertebral disk may be another source of spinal cord or nerve root compression. Clinical findings consistent with myelopathy include muscle weakness, spasticity, and increased deep tendon reflexes in the upper and lower extremities with Hoffman and/or Babinski signs. Additionally, patients may note subtle changes, such as deterioration in penmanship, difficulty with using buttons or picking up small items such as coins, and worsening gait.

Radiographic Assessment

If the history reveals severe progressive pain or an episode of recent trauma or if the neurologic examination reveals abnormalities, a complete set of cervical spine x-ray films should be obtained (2). These films should include an assessment of levels C1 through C7-T1 with oblique and open-mouth odontoid views. Plain radiographs allow for assessment of the osseous anatomy and spinal alignment and are inexpensive and widely available. These x-ray films will help in assessing the patient for fracture, subluxation, or metastatic disease. However, the correlation between clinical symptoms or signs and degenerative abnormalities on x-ray film is not good. X-ray evidence of cervical degenerative changes (spondylosis) are common and are evident in >90% of people older than 50 years (3). On the other hand, serious cervical disease may demonstrate minimal or no changes on x-ray film. When fracture or subluxation is noted on the initial films, dynamic x-ray films (flexion and extension views) aid in the assessment of the stability of the spinal column. Subluxation of >3.5 mm or of 11 degrees of angulation of the endplates in an adult is considered abnormal and a sign of spinal instability (4).

Computed tomographic (CT) is useful in the evaluation of problems of the cervical spine. CT provides excellent resolution of the bony anatomy and may provide important additional information if a fracture is suspected. Two-dimensional CT reconstructions add information regarding the sagittal and coronal alignment. Magnetic resonance imaging (MRI) is especially useful when evaluating patients suspected of having abnormalities of the soft tissue, such as metastatic cancer or a primary disk problem. CT myelography can be used to assess for neural compression when MRI is contraindicated, inadequate, or inconclusive.

SELECTED SYNDROMES ASSOCIATED WITH NECK PAIN

Many problems of the neck may result in neck pain (Table 70.3). Because the most common surgical problems—herniated cervical disk and cervical spondylosis (degenerative changes)—may have similar manifestations, they are discussed together based on the presence or absence of neurologic findings.

Pain with Neurologic Findings

Diagnosis

Patients with neurologic findings can have signs and symptoms of either nerve root or spinal cord compression (upper motor neuron syndrome, see Chapter 86). The objective signs of nerve root compression include muscle weakness, a decreased or absent deep tendon reflex, and decreased sensation in a dermatomal distribution.

Patients with nerve root compression present with the acute or gradual onset of posterior neck pain that radiates to the shoulder and down one arm. The pain may radiate into the lower arm and often into the hand itself. The pain often radiates into a finger that corresponds to the dermatome of the nerve root involved. The pain may be made worse by movement of the neck and extreme neck positions. In addition, the patient may complain of decreased sensation and paresthesias in the arm and hand. Patients may have nerve root compression in the cervical spine but have little or no neck and arm pain, instead reporting arm weakness and loss of sensation. Nerve root compression can be caused by impingement of the nerve by a cervical disk—most common in younger patients—or by osseous proliferation that can impinge on the nerve as it exits through its foramen—most common in patients

TABLE 70.3 Selected Problems of the Neck That May Result in Neck Pain

Problem	Comment
Arthritis	Especially rheumatoid (see Chapter 77) and degenerative joint disease (see text and Chapter 75)
Disk disease	See text
Fibromyalgia	See Chapter 74
Infection	Osteomyelitis or soft-tissue infection; look for point tenderness (see Chapter 40)
Neoplasia	Myeloma or metastatic disease is associated with point tenderness and abnormalities on x-ray film (or bone scan in the case of metastases).
Neuritis	Any nerve may be involved; a common one is the spinal accessory nerve. Look for tenderness over the nerve and lateral aspects of the upper third of the sternomastoid muscle.
Platybasia	Congenital disorder that may not manifest symptoms before age 40 years or a complication of Paget disease; x-ray films show characteristic changes (i.e., invagination of the base of the skull).
Sprain	Cervical sprain syndrome caused by whiplash and other forms of trauma (see text).
Structures in neck	Any organ or structure located in the neck can become a source of neck pain. Careful examination will detect abnormalities such as thyroiditis, lymphadenitis, pharyngitis, sialadenitis, or tender carotid artery (carotodynia).
Tendinitis	Any tendon can be involved, but occipital and sternomastoid are particularly common. Local tenderness is a clue.
Torticollis (wry neck)	Diagnosis usually is obvious by observation. An underlying structural problem could produce reflex muscle spasm; therefore, with an initial episode an underlying problem (e.g., tumor or infection) should be considered.
Trauma	Because of the danger of cord injury, trauma associated with neck pain should be carefully evaluated.
Vascular	Arteritis or dissection may cause neck pain.

older than 50 years (Fig. 70.1B). Thoracic outlet syndrome may be confused with cervical disease associated with nerve root compression and should be ruled out (see Chapter 69).

Patients with spinal cord compression may have numb clumsy hands or spastic paraparesis. The complaint of neck pain does not need to be prominent, and radicular symptoms may be present. The presence of radicular findings of weakness and fasciculations in addition to long tract findings, such as hyperreflexia, spasticity, and clonus, raises the possibility of motor neuron disease. In younger patients, noncompressive causes of spinal cord dysfunction, such as multiple sclerosis and motor neuron disease, must be considered.

Management

Patients with evidence of *myelopathy* (i.e., involvement of the spinal cord) must be referred to a neurologist or neurosurgeon to establish the cause. Investigation usually includes MRI or CT myelogram. If the myelopathy is secondary to a cervical disk or cervical spondylosis, surgery often is indicated—either laminectomy or anterior cervical fusions. Symptoms of myelopathy, particularly chronic myelopathy, may not remit after decompression, so the goal of surgery is to prevent progression.

Patients with *nerve root compression* leading to muscle weakness and sensory impairment should be referred to a spine specialist for more complete examination and followup. The consultant may further evaluate these patients with CT, MRI, or myelography. Typical surgical criteria include severe, uncontrollable pain; neurologic deficit or myelopathy; and/or bowel or bladder dysfunction. The timing of surgery in these situations remains controversial in the surgical community. Some studies have demonstrated improved outcomes with early surgery, whereas others have not supported this finding (5). If the neurologic deficit would be acceptable should it be permanent, then conservative therapy is an option and has a good chance of success (6).

A period of bedrest may be necessary in rare circumstances. Activity modification and avoidance of exacerbating activities or position are most appropriate during the acute phase. A *cervical collar* may be helpful in providing some relief of the neck pain for short periods. It may be helpful to place a small pillow under the nape of the neck to provide proper positioning. If muscle spasm is present, moist or dry heat applied to the neck may give symptomatic relief. Analgesia using a nonsteroidal anti-inflammatory drug (NSAID) (see Chapter 77) or acetaminophen may help. If a stronger analgesic becomes necessary, a short-acting narcotic may be added. Although not a first-line agent, a muscle relaxant may be helpful (see Chapter 71) if symptoms persist after 3 or 4 days.

The acute phase usually lasts only 1 or 2 weeks. When symptoms become recurrent or chronic (lasting >2–3 weeks), *cervical traction* may provide relief. This procedure is performed initially under the supervision of a physical therapist or physiatrist, after x-ray films of the cervical spine have been obtained to rule out instability. For 30 minutes, 15 to 20 lb of chin halter traction is applied to the neck. The neck must be positioned in slight flexion; extension could worsen symptoms and must be avoided.

After several sessions, the patient can be instructed on the use of a home cervical traction unit, which can be applied for 30 minutes at a time, up to three times per day, for several months. If symptoms persist for more than 2 or 3 weeks, a brief course of steroids, although somewhat controversial, may be clinical benefit (7). Prednisone 60 mg/day is administered for 3 days, followed by a 4-day taper. Even when signs and symptoms subside, the rate of symptom recurrence is high. Therefore, it is important to educate the patient on activities or positions that should be avoided and on exercises that may help relieve muscle spasm (Figs. 70.2 and 70.3).

If the acute symptoms do not subside or if new signs develop, referral to a spine surgeon is necessary for confirmation of the diagnosis and consideration of surgery (most commonly a discectomy and anterior interbody fusion). The surgery should be performed to relieve compression of neural structures as demonstrated by signs, symptoms, and radiologic findings (8). A trial of conservative therapy is indicated in all cases except those with evidence of myelopathy, functionally significant weakness, or spinal instability. In some patients, neurologic deficits can take months to resolve postoperatively and may never resolve, particularly in the case of myelopathy.

Pain without Neurologic Findings

Diagnosis

Most patients with neck pain have no objective neurologic findings. The patient may present with either acute-onset pain or a slowly progressive discomfort (most often from osteoarthritis) that has been building over several months. In the acute disk herniation syndrome, the patient experiences sudden onset of neck pain that is associated with decreased range of motion of the cervical spine, bilateral muscle spasm, or occasionally asymmetrical muscle spasm that produces torticollis (wry neck). The patient may have pain in the shoulder or arm but have no objective weakness or sensory findings on examination. Other patients may have quite debilitating neck pain without evidence of significant disk herniations. MRI of the cervical spine may demonstrate evidence of disk degeneration (i.e., loss of disk height or hydration). This group of patients with axial, "discogenic" neck pain, presumably from disk degeneration, remains one of the most controversial and difficult groups to treat. The surgical outcomes are inferior to those achieved in patients with radiculopathy. Provocative discography may aid in determining the concordance of the imaging findings of disk degeneration and the patient's pain complaints of neck pain (9). Provocation of the patient's pain by injection of saline into the disk space and relief of the pain by injection of local anesthetic is assumed to implicate that particular level in producing the patient's pain. However, the utility of these findings in predicting the ultimate surgical outcomes remains an area of intense controversy, and a great deal of research is needed to more clearly define the role of this technique.

Treatment

Initial treatment is the same as that outlined for patients with neurologic findings. The neck can be "immobilized" with a cervical collar. Several cervical collars are available, but a soft collar often is prescribed first, although it may serve only as a reminder to the patient not to move the neck too quickly or too far. Local heat and analgesics or NSAIDs (see Chapter 77) also may provide symptomatic relief. Muscle relaxants (see Chapter 71) may be tried if symptoms persist after 3 or 4 days of initial treatment. In patients who have a chronic more insidious onset of pain, examining the patient's occupational situation more closely may help determine any exacerbating circumstances (10). Any activity that creates a prolonged extension of the neck, such as overhead work (e.g., painting), or prolonged flexion of the neck, such as sitting at a computer or typewriter, may aggravate a pre-existing problem. If pain lasts for >2 or 3 weeks after initial treatment, x-ray films of the cervical spine should be obtained. The treatment is based on the severity of symptoms. A rapidly acting oral agent, such as ibuprofen 400 mg three times per day, may be tried over a course of 2 or 3 weeks. (Alternative NSAIDs, including aspirin, also can be tried, see Chapter 77.) The patient should be informed that symptoms often may be chronic or recurrent and should be advised about how to avoid recurrences (Fig. 70.2).

If an acute severe episode of neck pain does not respond to treatment within a few weeks, the patient should be referred to a spine specialist. When the symptoms are more mild and chronic, a trial of treatment for several months would be reasonable before referral. Anterior cervical fusions carried out on the basis of positive discograms are sometimes effective in treating patients with neck pain without neurologic symptoms (11).

Cervical Sprain Syndrome

Mechanism

Cervical sprain syndrome is a term given to acute injuries of the neck caused by sudden extension of the cervical spine (*whiplash*). Patients involved in rear-end automobile accidents may have such acute hyperextension injuries to the neck. In experiments, monkeys subjected to acute hyperextension forces can show tearing of sternocleidomastoid and longus colli muscles in the absence of injuries to the anterior longitudinal ligament or disk. Thus, this syndrome may have physical causes (12), although a psychological contribution may be important, particularly in the case of litigation or workman's compensation (13).

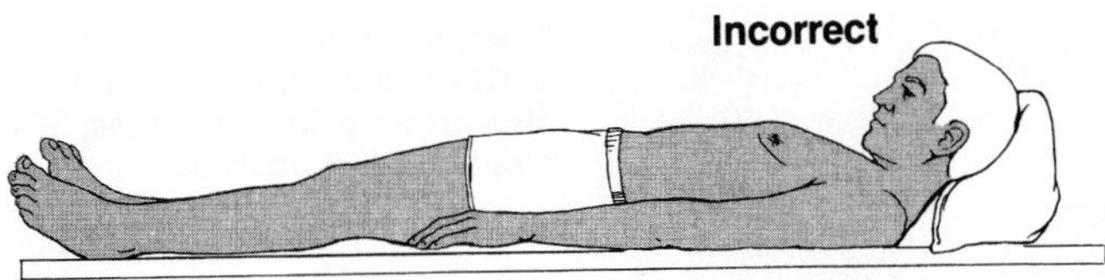

SLEEPING
Maintain normal lordotic curvature.

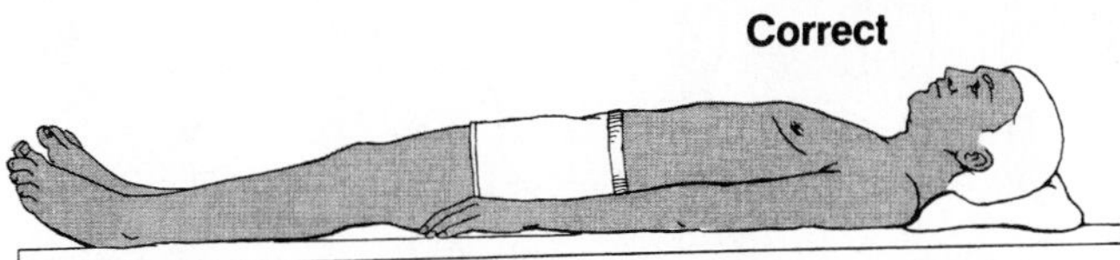

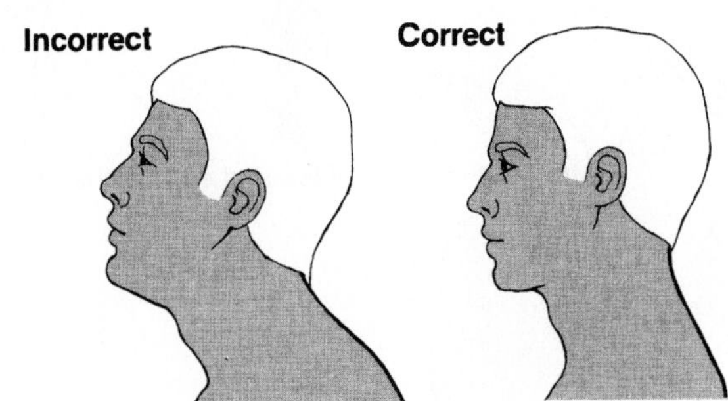

STANDING or SITTING
Maintain normal lordosis. Keep chin in.

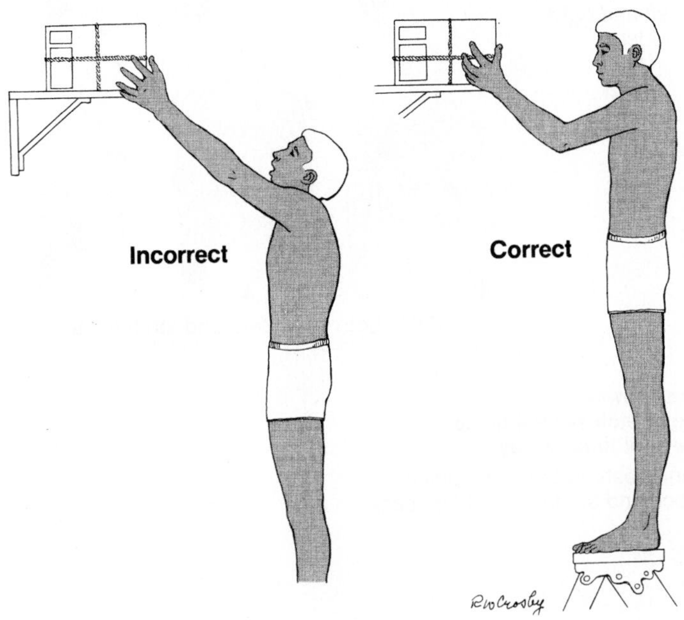

REACHING
Don't reach higher than your head.

FIGURE 70.2. Positions to prevent recurrence of neck pain.

Neck pain from more mild forms of injury that result from repeated hyperextension, such as movements associated with painting a ceiling, usually resolves in 1 to 2 days and is not known to be associated with pathologic changes. The reason why this syndrome can become persistent is unclear. Several clinical studies have found a high initial pain intensity to be an adverse prognostic factor (14), suggesting that psychological variables are important.

Diagnosis

Although patients usually have pain after the accident, patients not uncommonly do not experience discomfort initially. Typically the patient experiences pain in the posterior or anterior region of the neck. It commonly radiates to the occipital aspect of the head and may radiate to the shoulders. Occipital headaches often occur. Disk

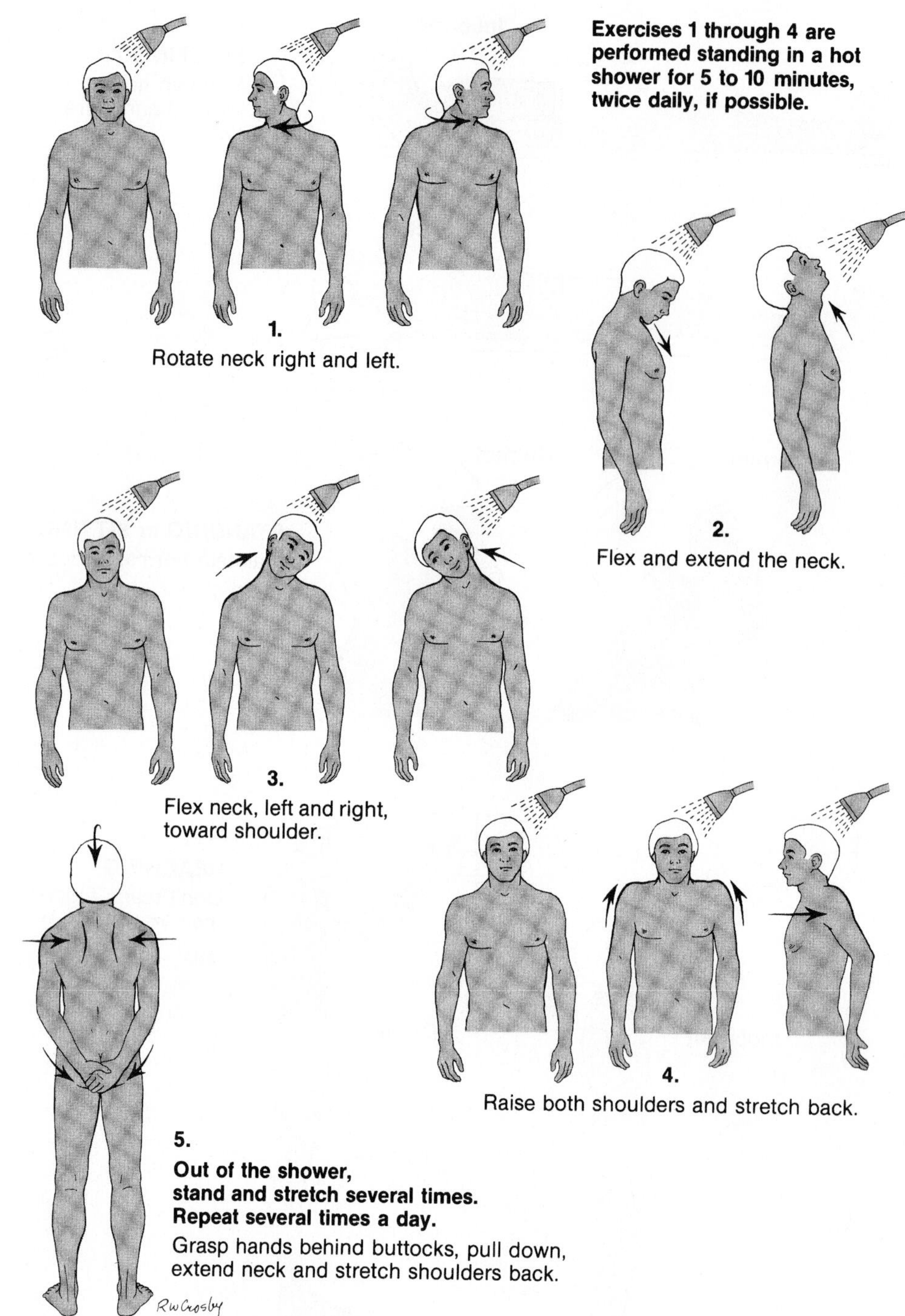

FIGURE 70.3. Exercises to rehabilitate the neck.

herniation, fracture, or subluxation also can occur in this setting. Therefore, it is essential to visualize the cervical spine radiologically from the occipital condyles down to C7–T1 to rule out a fracture or dislocation. If plain x-ray films are normal, flexion–extension x-ray films should be obtained. Any patient with neurologic findings in this setting should be immobilized in a hard collar and seen urgently by a spine surgeon before flexion–extension x-rays are taken.

Treatment

If muscle spasm or limitation of motion is present without neurologic findings, the patient can be placed in a cervical collar. Analgesics such as acetaminophen or NSAIDs (or occasionally a narcotic for short periods), at adequate dosages, should be given. The patient should be warned that extension of the neck will exacerbate the pain. Heat, either moist or dry, applied to the cervical spine may give symptomatic relief but does not speed healing. Patients may seek manipulation for treatment of this condition and should be aware that the value of this modality is uncertain (15). The patient should be encouraged to perform daily work and activities as much as possible. If the patient has severe pain and muscle spasm at the initial injury, the clinical course probably will last 4 to 6 weeks. When the patient's pain subsides and he or she has full range of motion without muscle spasm, the collar can be gradually discontinued, and the patient should be advised of methods for relieving muscle spasm and preventing recurrent symptoms (Figs. 70.2 and 70.3). If no symptoms of nerve root compression are present, the patient with persistent symptoms should be considered for further workup.

SPECIFIC REFERENCES

1. Bogduk N. Zygapophysial joint and anulus fibrosus. Spine 1994;19:1771.
2. Tong C, Barest G. Approach to imaging the patient with neck pain. J Neuroimaging 2003;13:5.
3. Kaiser JA, Holland BA. Imaging of the cervical spine. Spine 1998;23:2701.
4. Panjabi MM, White AA 3rd. Basic biomechanics of the spine. Neurosurgery 1980;7:76.
5. Woertgen C, Rothoerl RD, Henkel J, et al. Long term outcome after cervical foraminotomy. Clin Neurosci 2000;7:312.
6. Wolff MW, Levine LA. Cervical radiculopathies: conservative approaches to management. Phys Med Rehabil Clin N Am 2002;13:589.
7. Ellenberg MR, Honet JC, Treanor WJ. Cervical radiculopathy. Arch Phys Med Rehabil 1994; 75:342.
8. Rothman RH, Simeone FA, eds. The spine. Philadelphia: WB Saunders, 1992.
9. Carragee EJ, Alamin TF. Discography. a review. Spine J 2001;1:364.
10. Dryer SJ, Boden S. Nonoperative treatment of neck and arm pain. Spine 1998;23:2746.
11. Zheng Y, Liew SM, Simmons ED. Value of magnetic resonance imaging and discography in determining the level of cervical discectomy and fusion. Spine 2004;29:2140.
12. Bogduk N. Whiplash: the evidence for a organic etiology. Arch Neurol 2000;57:590.
13. Berry H. Chronic whiplash syndrome as a functional disorder. Arch Neurol 2000;57:592.
14. Scholten-Peeters GG, Verhagen AP, Bekkering GE, et al. Prognostic factors of whiplash-associated disorders: a systematic review of prospective cohort studies. Pain 2003;104: 303.
15. Hurwitz EL, Aker PD, Adams AH, et al. Manipulation and mobilization of the cervical spine. A systematic review of the literature. Spine 1996;21:1746; discussion 1759.

*For annotated **General References** and resources related to this chapter, visit www.hopkinsbayview.org/PAMreferences.*

Chapter 71

Low Back Pain

David G. Borenstein

Low back pain is one of the most common human afflictions. Between 70% and 80% of the population experiences back pain some time during their lives. The prevalence of back pain reported ranges from a low of 10% of adults during a 2-year period to a high of 20% of the population of a Western industrial society during a 2-week period. Although as many as 30% of people with back pain do not seek medical evaluation, the remainder eventually request medical advice. The office is the appropriate setting for the evaluation of these patients. A review of three time periods (1980–1981, 1985, and 1989–1990) studied by the National Ambulatory Medical Care Survey revealed mechanical low back pain (defined below) as the fifth most common reason for all physician office visits. Nonspecific low back pain was the most common diagnosis, accounting for 56.8% of these cases (1). Most patients with low back pain have underlying conditions that can be diagnosed and treated in the ambulatory setting. Most patients do not require expensive imaging tests, hospitalization, or surgery. The task is to separate the few who require more aggressive assessment from those who will recover with only office evaluation and conservative management.

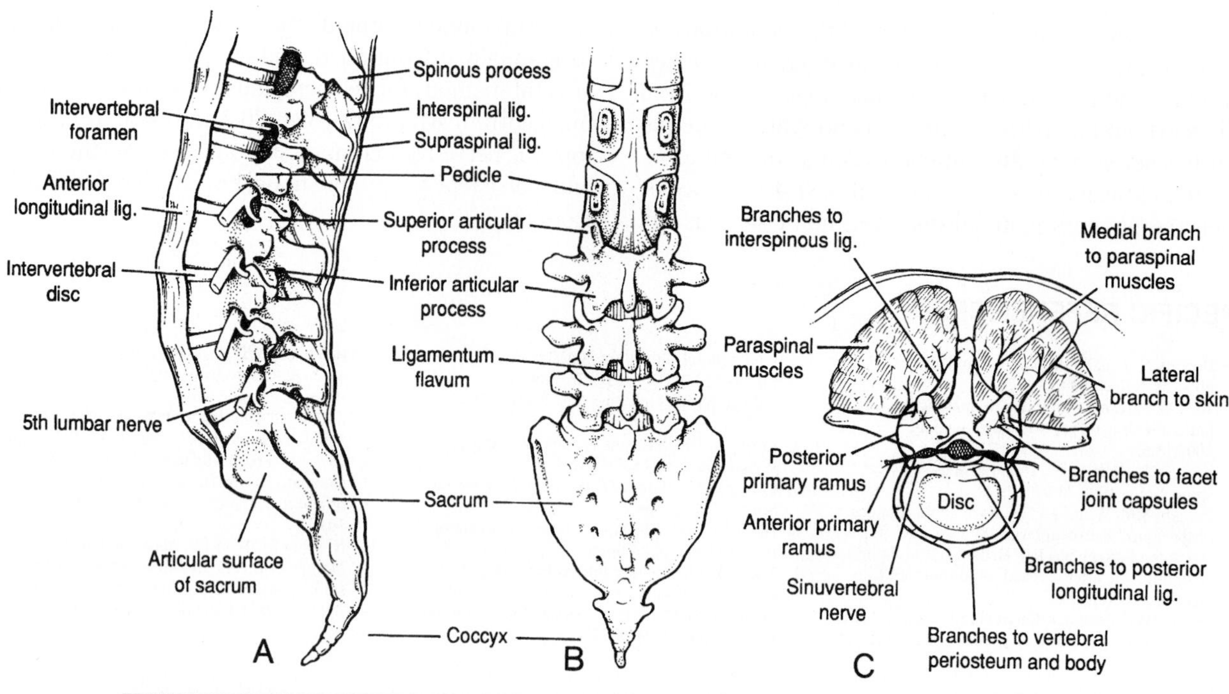

FIGURE 71.1. Anatomic relationships of the lumbosacral spine. **A:** Lateral view. **B:** Posterior view. **C:** Cross-sectional view.

ANATOMY AND BIOMECHANICS OF THE LUMBOSACRAL SPINE AND ASSOCIATED STRUCTURES

The structure of the lumbosacral spine is complex (Fig. 71.1A–C). The lumbar spine is composed of five vertebrae with interposed intervertebral disks that consist of a gelatinous nucleus pulposus and a surrounding annulus fibrosus. The vertebrae and disks are supported by strong ligamentous structures and paraspinous muscles. The posterior aspects of the vertebrae surround the spinal canal, form the neural foramina, and interlock to form apophyseal joints (facet joints) whose main purpose is motion (Fig. 71.1A–B). The sacrum is the part of the spine that interdigitates with the iliac bones to form part of the pelvis.

An understanding of the nerve supply to the lumbosacral spine is essential to recognizing the patterns of pain associated with disease processes that affect components of the back. The *sinuvertebral nerve* (Fig. 71.1C) is the major sensory nerve supplying structures in the lumbar spine. The nerve arises from the corresponding spinal nerve before it divides into anterior and posterior branches. The nerve enters the intervertebral foramen and divides into ascending, descending, and transverse branches that anastomose with the contralateral side and with sensory nerves at adjacent levels above and below. The sinuvertebral nerve supplies the posterior longitudinal ligament, superficial annulus fibrosus, epidural blood vessels, anterior dura mater, dural sleeve, and posterior vertebral periosteum. The posterior rami of the spinal nerves supply the apophyseal joints above and below the nerve and the paraspinous muscles at multiple levels. The complex innervation of lumbar spine structures helps explain the diffuse nature of pain associated with a wide variety of disorders.

A number of organs are situated in the retroperitoneum, anterior to the lumbar spine. The kidneys, ureters, aorta, inferior vena cava, pancreas, and periaortic lymph nodes are retroperitoneal organs. Diseases that affect these organs may result in referred pain that is localized to the lumbar spine.

In the upright position with a normal spinal curvature (lordosis), the ligamentous structures maintain the position of the spine with little need for contraction of the paraspinous muscles or for weight-bearing by the apophyseal (facet) joints (Fig. 71.1A). However, if the normal curve is flattened or accentuated, the paraspinous muscles contract and the apophyseal (facet) joints become weight-bearing. This change in body mechanics results in pain.

The lumbar vertebrae are exposed to tremendous forces. This is caused principally by the magnification of stresses that result from the lever effect of the arm in lifting and by vertical forces associated with the human upright position. Figure 71.2 shows how lifting an object away from the body introduces the lever magnification phenomenon, resulting in a marked increase in forces on

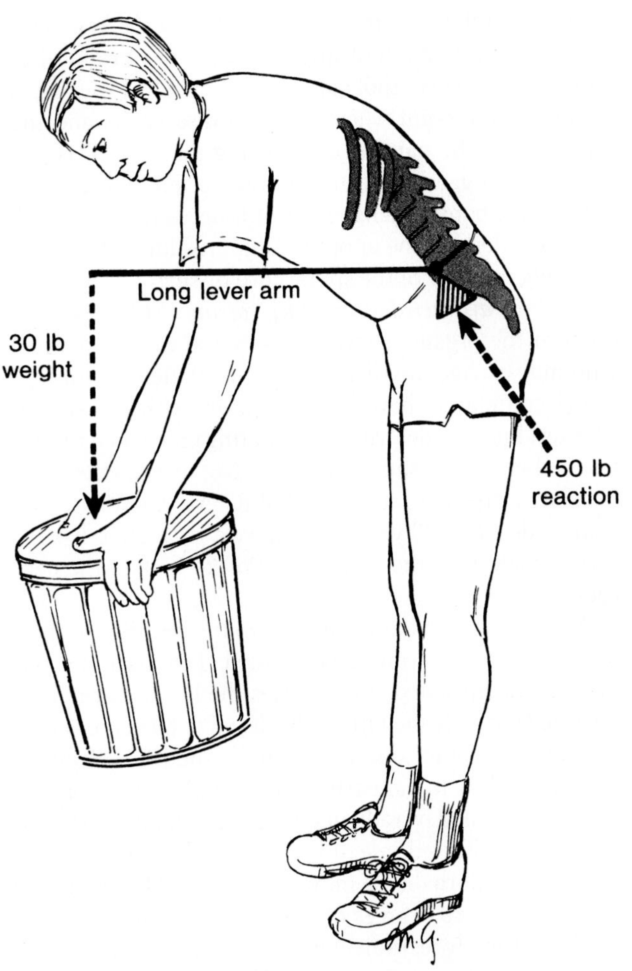

FIGURE 71.2. Forces in the lumbar area.

the vertebral bodies and disks. Because each intervertebral disk is a fluid system, hydraulic pressure is created whenever a load is placed on the axial skeleton. This hydraulic pressure magnifies three to five times the force that occurs on the annulus fibrosus. This force is akin to the hoop stress that occurs in a barrel when pressure is applied to its liquid content. A study using a pressure transducer placed *in vivo* in the nucleus pulposus of an asymptomatic 45-year-old man documented highest intradiscal pressures associated with lifting a 20-kg weight. The lowest intradiscal pressures were associated with the prone position (2). The ability of the annulus fibrosus to withstand stress in any position decreases significantly with age, and by age 60 years many people have only 50% of the strength in these fibers that they had at age 30 years. Alterations in the nucleus pulposus associated with oxidative damage and the appearance of reparative collagen as a manifestation of disk degeneration are observed in pathology specimens obtained from individuals as early as the adolescent years (3).

However, the lumbar spine is not just an isolated structure. Much support is obtained by the muscles and ligaments of the spine and by the muscles of the thoracic and abdominal cavities. These latter structures act as a sort of muscular cylinder that helps decrease the load on the axial skeleton by as much as 30% in the lumbar area and 50% in the thoracic spine.

EVALUATION OF PATIENTS WITH LOW BACK PAIN

Certain facts pertaining to the causes and natural history of back pain influence the evaluation and treatment of patients with this symptom. Back pain is most often associated with a mechanical cause, although it sometimes has a nonmechanical (called *medical* or *systemic* in this text) cause. Mechanical low back pain may be defined as pain secondary to overuse of a normal anatomic structure (e.g., muscle strain) or deformity of an anatomic structure (e.g., herniated nucleus pulposus). Medical back pain syndromes are simply the manifestation, in the area of the lower back, of a systemic disorder. These are defined more fully below (see Approach to Diagnosis and Treatment of Low Back Pain). Most patients with mechanical back pain do not have an associated history of acute trauma, lifting, or strain. Most low back pain problems are self-limited. Of patients evaluated by physicians, 40% to 50% are better in 1 week, 51% to 86% in 1 month, and 92% within 2 months (4). Although most patients have resolution of their episode of back pain within 2 months, as many as 75% may have a relapse within the next 12 months (5). Most patients with low back pain do not require surgery.

History

Questions about back pain should concentrate on a history of episodes and, for the current episode, the onset, duration, frequency, location, radiation, time of day, quality, intensity, and the aggravating and alleviating factors. A history of motor or sensory nerve root irritation or sphincter (bladder or rectal incontinence) or sexual dysfunction is important in identifying patients with *cauda equina compression* (see Physical Examination). Occupational history may reveal predisposing factors associated with recurrent episodes of back injury.

Patients should be questioned about systemic symptoms that are indicative of a medical (systemic) cause of their back pain. Patients with fever, weight loss, pain with recumbency, extended morning stiffness, acute bone pain, or viscerogenic pain should be evaluated for a systemic illness. Patients who are older than 50 years also are at greater risk for a medical (systemic) cause of their pain. A history of cancer is a "red flag" for a medical cause of low back pain (6).

Physical Examination

Physical Examination of the Lumbosacral Spine and Associated Musculoskeletal Areas

Abnormalities of the spine may be discovered while the spine is stationary or in motion. The patient should be examined in an orderly fashion that evaluates the function of musculoskeletal and neurologic structures of the lumbosacral spine.

Initially, the patient is examined in a gown while he or she is *standing* barefoot or wearing only socks. The spinal column is examined from all directions to check for excessive kyphosis, lordosis, or scoliosis. The presence of scoliosis is best determined by having the patient flex at the waist with arms extended in front. Any asymmetry of the height of the shoulders can be appreciated. Any deviation of a spinous process from the midline is noted. Firm palpation of the paravertebral muscles and of each vertebral spine is performed. Isolated tenderness over a bone suggests a localized problem such as tumor, infection, or compression fracture. Firm paraspinous muscles result from spasm secondary to local injury or referred pain.

Mobility of the spine is assessed by having the patient bend forward and attempt to touch the toes (normal is approximately 50–80 degrees). However, the hip joints also participate in the movement. Range of flexion can be determined by quantifying the expansion of a 10-cm line measured from the lumbosacral junction superiorly during maximal flexion (*Schober test,* see Chapter 78) or noting the distance of the fingertips from the floor. During this movement the normally smooth rhythm of the reversal of the lumbar lordosis is noted. If the rhythm is interrupted or hesitant, an abnormality of the apophyseal joints or of paraspinous structures may be present.

Lateral flexion (normal is to approximately 30 degrees) and extension (normal is to approximately 30 degrees) are assessed. Lateral flexion usually is preserved in disk disease but may be limited in patients with a spondyloarthropathy (i.e., joint problem of the spine). Increased discomfort with extension suggests disease of the apophyseal joints or spinal stenosis.

The patient then is examined while he or she is *bent forward* over the examining table. In this position, the inferior portion of the sacroiliac joints, ischial tuberosities, and sciatic notch are more easily palpated.

The *gait of the patient* should be observed. Patients with back pain may walk in a stiff guarded fashion or may favor one leg if a radiculopathy is present.

The patient is next examined *sitting with his or her legs dangling.* The deep tendon reflexes of the knees (L4) and ankles (S1) are elicited to test the integrity of the reflex arcs. An absent reflex may signify nerve root impingement secondary to a herniated nucleus pulposus. The patient extends each knee while seated. Flexion of the hip and extension of the knee stretch the lumbar nerve roots. Radicular pain that radiates from the back to below the knee is associated with nerve root impingement. The origin of the pain from the nerve root can be confirmed by lowering the leg just to the point where the pain disappears and then reproducing the pain by dorsiflexing the foot. This sign, if positive, suggests a herniated intervertebral disk or, less commonly, bony impingement of a nerve root caused by arthritis affecting the apophyseal joints, lumbar stenosis, or, rarely, a tumor of the spinal cord or surrounding structures. This *distracted straight-leg raising* (SLR) test helps confirm the organic source of pain and identify patients who may exaggerate their symptoms. Patients with functional complaints have no discomfort with a distracted SLR test but may describe excruciating pain when the SLR test is done in the supine position. Not all patients with a herniated disk have a positive SLR test. A patient, especially older than 30 years, may have a herniated disk that is too small or in the wrong location to irritate the nerve roots.

Next, the patient assumes the *supine* position so that a *standard* SLR test can be performed. The examiner fully extends the knee and slowly flexes the lower extremity at the hip. Normally the hip can be flexed to 80 degrees without pain, except for discomfort in the thigh or behind the knee secondary to hamstring muscle tightness. A positive test is manifested by radicular pain that radiates below the knee on the affected side or bilaterally. The nerve root and surrounding dura do not move in the neural foramen until an elevation ≥30 degrees of the lower extremity has been reached. Therefore, radicular pain that is elicited at an elevation <30 degrees is suspect. The SLR test is sensitive but nonspecific for the presence of a herniated intervertebral disk causing sciatica (7). After the SLR test, the unaffected lower extremity should be raised, thus performing the *crossed SLR test*. This procedure causes tension and stretch of the nerve roots of the opposite (affected) lower extremity and reproduces the radicular pain caused by SLR in that lower extremity. The test is uncommonly positive, but when so there is a strong but not absolute correlation with disk herniation (8).

Next, *sensory assessment* of the buttock, perineum, and lower extremities should be performed. Chapter 86 shows the relevant sensory dermatomes that can be evaluated by pinprick and touch. Abnormalities help to localize a lesion and to determine the need and urgency of an orthopedic or neurosurgical consultation. An important component of the sensory assessment is the search for signs compatible with a *cauda equina syndrome* (syndrome of neurologic dysfunction from compression of the nerves at the L4–5 level and inferior to the spinal cord proper, often secondary to a central disk herniation). The signs of compression of the cauda equina include saddle anesthesia, loss of anal sphincter tone (assessed by rectal examination), bilateral *sciatica* (pain in the distribution of the sciatic nerve), lower extremity motor weakness, and a history of bowel, bladder, or sexual dysfunction. This syndrome, if present, is an indication for immediate referral to a neurosurgeon or orthopedic surgeon for hospitalization and surgical decompression of the spinal cord. The best neurologic outcome occurs when decompression occurs in the first 48 hours after onset of cauda equina compression signs (9).

A detailed assessment of *motor function* of the lower extremities also helps localize a lesion in the patient in whom neurologic involvement is suspected (see Chapter 92). This assessment can be done while the patient is supine, sitting, or standing. Muscles tested include hip flexors (L2–3) and extensors (L4–5), knee extensors (L3–4), dorsiflexors of the foot (L4–5), knee flexors (L5–S1), and plantar flexors of the foot (S1–2). Subtle weakness may be elicited by having the patient walk on his or her toes (gastrocnemius muscle group, S1–2) and heels (tibialis anterior muscles, L4–5).

The hip, sacroiliac, and knee joints are assessed while the patient is in the supine position. The hip and knee joints are assessed by moving these joints through a normal range of motion when they are unweighted. Pain with motion suggests an articular cause of leg pain. The *sacroiliac joint* is assessed by the Patrick or FABER (flexion, abduction, external rotation) test. The test is done by positioning the lateral malleolus of the tested leg on the patella of the opposite leg. Downward pressure is placed on the medial aspect of the knee while the pelvis is stabilized by placing a hand on the contralateral anterior superior iliac spine. Pain associated with a quick pulse or downward pressure usually is localized to the lateral aspect of the lumbar spine and originates in the sacroiliac joint. Slow pressure may elicit groin pain indicative of hip joint dysfunction.

The sacroiliac joint and muscles of hip abduction (L2–3) are tested while the patient is in the *lateral* position. Pressure is applied to the iliac wing, compressing the sacroiliac joints. Pain felt in the sacroiliac joint suggests an intraarticular process or a strain of the posterior sacroiliac ligaments. The muscles of hip abduction are tested as the patient elevates the upper leg against downward pressure applied below the knee by the examiner.

The symmetry of the buttocks is assessed (gluteus maximus, L5, S1–2) while the patient is in the *prone* position. A femoral stretch test (i.e., extending the hip joint) elicits pain in the anterior thigh (L2–3) or the medial aspect of the leg (L4) in patients with corresponding herniated intervertebral disks.

To evaluate the rare patients suspected of *malingering* or of having a psychiatric origin for their back pain, Waddell et al. (10) identified five physical signs associated with functional disorders. First, overreaction during examination was found to be the single most important sign indicating a nonorganic cause. Overreaction may take the form of collapsing, sweating, tremors, muscle tension, bizarre facial expression, or disproportionate verbalization. Second, simulation testing can be used to elicit nonorganic pain. Two useful examples are axial loading and rotation. In the first example, with the patient standing, low back pain is reported in overreactors (but not in others) on vertical loading by pressing down on the patient's head. Neck pain is common during this examination in all and does not constitute a positive sign. In the hip rotation test, the patient stands with feet together and arms fixed firmly to the lateral sides of the body at the hip level by the examiner's hands. In this manner, the torso (and the spine) is passively rotated on the hips. Because the units of the spine itself are not moved, reports of low back pain are a positive sign of a nonorganic cause. However, in the presence of true radiculopathy, leg pain may be produced because there is movement at the hip joint, and nerve roots may be stretched. Third is the use of distraction testing. This consists of observing the patient during the course of the examination for variable findings when the patient is unaware of being observed or tested, such as during the *distracted SLR* (see Physical Examination of the Lumbosacral Spine and Associated Musculoskeletal Areas). Fourth, superficial, nonanatomic, or variable tenderness is a nonorganic sign. A useful technique is the Magnuson test, in which tender areas are subtly marked and later examined again for reproducibility. Fifth, motor or sensory findings that are not explained by an anatomic lesion provide clues that the problem is psychiatric in origin. Also, sudden giving away or flaccidity of a muscle during strength testing of the symptomatic area supports a nonorganic problem. A finding of at least three of the five types of signs is clinically significant. The presence of positive findings is not correlated absolutely with malingering. These individuals require treatment for physical problems in association with a complete psychological assessment (11).

Examination of Other Regions

Patients with constitutional symptoms or with symptoms not attributed to a local process in the back (e.g., abdominal pain) should undergo a focused physical examination. The physical examination, including pelvic and rectal and breast examinations in women, is particularly important in patients who describe new back pain and are 50 years of age or older.

Common origins of metastatic cancer to the spine are the breast, lung, prostate, thyroid, kidney, and rectum. Referred pain from cancer or other lesions may also be felt in the back. For example, pancreatic tumors or duodenal ulcers cause pain to be referred to the high lumbar or low thoracic vertebral region. Bowel or urinary tract cancer may cause pain to be referred to the mid or low lumbar region, and a disease process located in the pelvis may cause lower lumbar or sacral pain. Neoplasia primarily affecting the bones, especially multiple myeloma, is an important consideration in the elderly.

Assessment of the adequacy of the arteries of the lower extremities is important. Vascular abnormalities may cause pain due to ischemia in the back, buttock, or lower extremities during exertion. In addition to diminished pulses and bruits over arteries, cutaneous signs of ischemia (ulcers, loss of hair or nails) should be sought in the legs or feet (see Chapter 94). Sudden change in a pain pattern associated with an abdominal aneurysm or an episode of hypotension should alert one to the possibility of impending extension or rupture of the aneurysm.

Although the physical examination adds essential information to the evaluation of low back pain, the reproducibility of findings can vary widely among examiners and at different times. In one study of the physical examination of patients with low back pain, McCombe et al. (12) evaluated the reproducibility of a number of signs. They concluded that precise examination, careful measurement of locations of pain and tenderness and degrees of movement of the back and legs, and careful documentation of the findings were most important to accurately reproducing a patient's physical signs. Certain caveats relevant to this examination were developed. The most important among these were as follows:

- Bony tenderness is more reproducible and of greater diagnostic significance than soft-tissue tenderness.
- Pain on hip flexion and external rotation is reproducible and valuable.
- Heel and toe standing are not an accurate method of assessing muscle strength.
- SLR test is reliable and reproducible if measurement and documentation of the extent of pain radiation are precise.
- Measurements of the range of flexion and lateral bend are reliable.

A study by Jensen (13) of the accuracy of certain signs in predicting a precise cause and location of a problem showed a reasonable but imperfect correlation of disturbed sensory and motor function with anatomic abnormalities confirmed at surgery in 52 patients with lumbar disk herniations. The time of day of the examination also may have an effect on physical findings. Ensink et al. (14) measured lumbar spine motion in 29 patients with chronic back pain in the morning and afternoon. Flexion was increased to the greatest degree at the end of the day, and extension was independent of time of measurement. The sum of all these studies is that careful examination and precise measurements of dysfunction and pain location are important in evaluating back pain. However, no sign is absolutely diagnostic or perfectly reproducible, and some signs are frankly unreliable. The entire constellation of findings must be considered in developing a proper approach to a patient.

With information obtained from the history and physical examination, a working diagnosis can be generated based on first defining the pain as mechanical or nonmechanical (medical or systemic) in nature. Patients with mechanical disorders may be treated without additional laboratory or radiographic tests during the initial visit. On the other hand, those believed to have a nonmechanical (medical or systemic) problem should undergo further diagnostic testing.

Laboratory Evaluation

Radiographic Assessment

A *plain x-ray film of the lumbar spine* is not a necessary part of the initial evaluation of patients with back pain unless they have a history of recent major trauma or acute constitutional symptoms. Patients with back pain of a mechanical origin often have normal x-ray films. In addition, many patients with abnormal x-ray films may be entirely asymptomatic. By age 50 years, 67% of normal people have evidence of disk disease characterized by narrowing of one or more disk spaces or disk calcifications; an additional 20% of people have lumbar osteophytes. In fact, only 13% of 50-year-olds have normal x-ray films. Two thirds of patients with roentgenographic evidence of lumbar disk degeneration are asymptomatic. Osteoarthritis of the apophyseal (facet) joints is not correlated with symptoms. In addition, plain films may not be sufficiently sensitive to identify bony lesions unless 50% of the medullary portion of the bone has been destroyed. Therefore, plain x-ray films of the lumbar spine should be obtained only in patients who have not responded to a course of conservative therapy, persist with pain, have reflex asymmetry, have point vertebral tenderness, or are elderly and have new-onset pain (because of the higher incidence of a fracture or a systemic cause of their symptoms) (15). In patients with exacerbation of low back pain with extension of the spine, radiographs of the lumbar spine identify facet joint alterations that are more likely associated with clinical symptoms (16).

Other radiographic techniques that are useful in the evaluation of patients with back pain include *bone scan* (infection, tumor [but multiple myeloma is notoriously missed], arthritis, fracture), *computed tomography* (CT; disk herniation, spinal stenosis, myeloma, retroperitoneal structures), and magnetic resonance imaging (MRI; disk herniation, intraspinal tumors). Each should be highly selected on the basis of the history and physical examination, and often a consultation with a radiologist, rheumatologist, neurosurgeon, or orthopedist is helpful in deciding the approach. *MRI* can detect specific anatomic lesions in the lumbar spine with greater sensitivity than any other radiographic technique (17). MRI detects degenerative intervertebral disk disease and spinal stenosis and is an excellent method for detecting medical disorders affecting the lumbar spine, including primary and metastatic malignancies and osteomyelitis (18). Contrast MRI with gadolinium differentiates scar tissue from recurrent disk herniations in individuals who have undergone surgical discectomies. CT is especially valuable for the definition of trabecular architecture of bone. Benign and malignant tumors and infectious lesions may be differentiated by CT. Radiographic findings become significant only when the history, physical examination, and radiographic findings agree. These more expensive imaging techniques are confirmatory, not diagnostic, tests. Nearly one third of asymptomatic patients have identifiable abnormalities that are of no significance (19). MRI scans have no value in predicting those individuals who will develop back pain over extended periods of time (20).

Other Laboratory Evaluations

Most patients with low back pain do not require laboratory studies with their initial evaluation. Patients who are elderly, have constitutional symptoms, or have not responded to conservative therapy may benefit from a laboratory evaluation (see Radiographic Assessment). The laboratory evaluations that may be useful include complete blood count and erythrocyte sedimentation rate (inflammatory and neoplastic disorders), serum calcium concentration and alkaline phosphatase activity (diffuse bone disease), serum and urine electrophoresis (multiple myeloma), prostate-specific antigen (metastatic prostate cancer), urinalysis (renal disease), and occult blood in the stool (ulcers, gastrointestinal tumors). All such evaluations should be based on distinct diagnostic possibilities based on the history and physical examination.

Electrophysiologic tests are not a substitute for neurologic evaluation of patients with back and leg pain. Electromyographic and nerve conduction tests should be reserved for individuals in whom the spinal nerve root level causing leg pain is unclear (21).

APPROACH TO DIAGNOSIS AND TREATMENT OF LOW BACK PAIN

When describing various conditions that result in back pain, it is useful to place them into two categories: regional (mechanical) and medical (systemic or nonmechanical). Differentiating medical back pain syndromes from a mechanical cause can be difficult when the back is the only anatomic area in which symptoms are manifest. This difficulty is most commonly experienced when evaluating elderly patients. In many patients, a specific causative pathologic entity causing pain is not demonstrable in many individuals (22). Systemic conditions that typically affect the low back region, including infections and tumors, are discussed below.

Most patients with acute onset of low back pain have a regional (mechanical) cause of their symptoms. Up to 90% of these patients respond to a course of conservative medical therapy. Back pain may resolve in as few as 2 weeks in a significant number of patients (23). Serial observation is important in the management of patients with back pain. If symptoms or signs of progression or of incomplete response to treatment are present on reassessment, evaluation for an alternative diagnosis is indicated. The followup contact should occur 3 to 4 weeks after the initial visit for all patients because by this time most patients with nonserious disorders as the cause of their symptoms are markedly improved. The followup visit also is important for patients whose back pain has resolved so that they have an opportunity to be educated with regard to recurrent symptoms and advised regarding prophylactic measures.

COMMON REGIONAL (MECHANICAL) BACK SYNDROMES

Lumbosacral Strain Syndrome

Lumbosacral strain is the most common cause of low back pain. The cause of back strain is not always clear but may be related to muscular, ligamentous, or fascial strain secondary to either a specific traumatic episode or continuous mechanical stress. People between the ages of 20 and 40 years are at greatest risk of developing muscle strain. Predisposing factors include failure to use good techniques in lifting, obesity, abnormal forward pelvic tilt (accentuated lordosis, most usually an acquired posture resulting from abdominal obesity), and leg-length discrepancy.

Diagnosis

The patient complains of pain that may be severe in the back, buttock, or one or both thighs. Usually symptoms follow a recent increase in physical activity, such as gardening, lifting, or participating in an infrequently played sport. Usually the patient experiences no (or minimal) discomfort during or immediately after the activity. Within the next 12 to 36 hours, as the soft tissues swell, pain develops and is associated with a feeling of muscular stiffness. The patient complains of pain that is accentuated by standing and bending and alleviated by lying. Table 71.1 provides information useful in the differential diagnosis of mechanical low back pain.

Examination of the back may show nonspecific signs of muscle spasm and loss of lumbar lordosis, but characteristically no evidence of nerve root impingement is seen. Pain radiating to the low back from an inflamed ischial or trochanteric bursa is occasionally seen, but marked tenderness over the inflamed bursa should reveal the correct diagnosis (see Chapter 74).

TABLE 71.1 Information Useful in the Differential Diagnosis of Mechanical Low Back Pain

Characteristics	Lumbosacral Strain	Herniated Nucleus Pulposus	Osteoarthritis	Spinal Stenosis
Age (yr)	20–40	30–50	>50	>60
Pain characteristics				
Location	Back (unilateral)	Back and leg (unilateral)	Back (bilateral)	Leg (bilateral)
Onset	Acute	Acute (prior episodes)	Insidious	Insidious
Standing[a]	+	−	+	+
Sitting[a]	−	+	−	−
Bending[a]	+	−	−	−
Straight-leg raising test	−	+	−	+ (stress, i.e., after walking)
Plain x-ray film	−	−	+	+

[a]+, Exacerbating; −, alleviating.
Adapted from Borenstein DG, Wiesel SW, Boden SD. Low back and neck pain: medical comprehensive diagnosis and management. Philadelphia: WB Saunders, 2004, with permission.

Management

In December 1994, the Agency for Health Care Policy and Research (AHCPR; now the Agency for Healthcare Research and Quality) published a Clinical Practice Guideline booklet on the diagnosis and management of acute low back pain (24). The booklet included the recommendations of a 23-member panel that critically reviewed 3,918 published scientific articles. Table 71.2 lists the recommendations. The reviewed articles related to management were rated from A to D, ranging from studies with strong research-based evidence to studies in which the design did not meet inclusion criteria. The final recommendations were based on the strength of evidence, risk/benefit ratios, and cost of each intervention. In the absence of controlled trials, the potential benefit of an intervention had to outweigh its possible risks to be considered cost-effective.

In general, the guidelines encourage early return of function. The recommended medications have mild toxicities and little abuse potential. Invasive therapies are limited to patients who do not improve over 4 to 12 weeks. The guidelines do have limitations: the recommendations are options and not the sole method for treating low back pain; they are based on a small number of studies (although many were reviewed), and they are made for patients with acute low back pain and do not apply to patients with chronic low back pain. These guidelines have not been updated since their initial publication. Reviews of the relative value of diagnostic tests and therapies appear in the literature, but no comprehensive revision of recommendations for acute low back pain is extant (25).

Conservative therapy of low back pain from lumbosacral strain includes controlled physical activity (low stress, gradually increasing aerobic and back-strengthening exercises), physical therapy, nonsteroidal anti-inflammatory drugs (NSAIDs), and muscle relaxants. In a study of medical therapy for low back pain with or without leg pain, the combination of an NSAID and a muscle relaxant was associated with the greatest number of individuals with improvement at 1 week (26). To minimize back motion and provide support, the bed should be firm but comfortable. A bed board cut from ⅝-inch plywood placed between the mattress and box spring usually is effective. Avoiding strenuous activity for most patients is appropriate, and even for those with severe pain, a minimal period of strict bed rest as short as 2 days has been shown to be adequate in relieving back pain (27). Controlled physical activity allows injured tissues to rest, permitting a greater opportunity for healing without reinjury. Pushing this concept further, Malmivaara et al. (28) reported on the efficacy of ordinary activity as tolerated in comparison with efficacy of bed rest for 2 days and back-mobilizing exercises. Better recovery, improved function, and fewer missed work days were associated with ordinary activity. Other studies also have reported the benefits of continuation of usual activities for recovery of low back pain (29). Faas et al. (30) showed the absence of significant benefit in the resolution of low back pain from exercise taught and monitored by a physiotherapist. In this study of 473 patients, flexion and stretching exercises were only minimally better at decreasing the duration of low back pain recurrences and had no other benefit compared with placebo interventions, which consisted of ultrasonography by a physiotherapist and usual care. The important lesson is that one should encourage the patient to do gentle activity as tolerated early in the course of acute low back pain when the cause is believed to be secondary to lumbosacral strain.

Physical therapy modalities, in the form of cold (ice massage) initially or heat subsequently, may decrease pain and diminish muscle spasm. Application of dry heat by a heating pad for 20 to 30 minutes several times per day (on low or medium setting with a protective towel between skin and pad to prevent burns) is preferred by some patients.

TABLE 71.2 Agency for Health Care Policy and Research Guidelines for Management of Acute Low Back Pain

I. Patient education
Patients with acute low back problems should be given accurate information about the following (strength of evidence = B):
A. Expectations for both rapid recovery and recurrences of symptoms based on natural history of low back symptoms
B. Safe and effective methods of symptom control
C. Safe and reasonable activity modifications
D. Best means of limiting recurrent low back problems
E. Lack of need for special investigations unless danger signs are present (see text)
F. Effectiveness and risks of commonly available diagnostic and further treatment measures to be considered should symptoms persist

II. Medications
Acetaminophen and NSAIDs
A. Acetaminophen is reasonably safe and is acceptable for treating patients with acute low back problems (strength of evidence = C).
B. NSAIDs, including aspirin, are acceptable for treating patients with acute low back pain (strength of evidence = B).
C. NSAIDs have a number of potential side effects. The most common complication is gastrointestinal irritation. The decision to use these medications can be guided by comorbidity, side effects, cost, and patient and provider preference (strength of evidence = C).

III. Physical treatments
Spinal manipulation
A. Manipulation can be helpful for patients with acute low back problems without radiculopathy when used within the first month of symptoms (strength of evidence = B).
B. A trial of manipulation in patients without radiculopathy with symptoms longer than a month probably is safe, but efficacy is unproven (strength of evidence = C).

IV. Activity modification
Activity recommendations for bed rest and exercise
A. A gradual return to normal activities is more effective than prolonged bed rest for treating acute low back problems (strength of evidence = B).
B. Prolonged bed rest for >4 days may lead to debilitation and is not recommended for treating acute low back problems (strength of evidence = B).
C. Low-stress aerobic exercise can prevent debilitation due to inactivity during the first month of symptoms and thereafter may help to return patients to the highest level of functioning appropriate to their circumstances (strength of evidence = C).

Ratings for strength of evidence: A, strong research-based evidence (multiple relevant and high-quality studies); B, moderate research-based evidence (one relevant high-quality, or multiple adequate studies); C, limited research-based evidence (one adequate scientific study); D, studies did not meet inclusion criteria.
NSAIDs, nonsteroidal anti-inflammatory drugs.

Others prefer moist heat, which is accomplished by using hot towels or a heat pack, which produces sustained heat for up to 30 minutes (available at pharmacies). Application of a continuous low-level heat wrap is as effective as an NSAID for treatment of acute low back pain (31).

Nonnarcotic analgesics such as NSAIDs help make patients comfortable while their injury heals. NSAIDs with rapid onset of action (e.g., aspirin 600 mg four times per day, ibuprofen 400–800 mg three times per day, diflunisal 500 mg twice per day, ketoprofen 25–50 mg three to four times per day, diclofenac 50 mg three times per day, or naproxen 250–500 mg twice per day) are most appropriate. In general, all NSAIDs should be used for a limited time (e.g., 2–6 weeks) when treating patients with acute mechanical back pain. The choice of any of these NSAIDs must be made in consideration of both patient and drug characteristics. For example, some patients prefer twice-per-day drug administration, whereas a few prefer more frequent dosing. In general, NSAIDs are effective for short-term symptomatic relief of low back pain but are less effective for sciatica (32). A systematic review of NSAID studies has confirmed the benefit of the active drugs compared to placebo for acute low back pain (33). Some groups of patients are especially vulnerable to the side effects of these drugs. Particularly important are the gastrointestinal and renal toxicity that occur often in elderly patients, especially women, who take NSAIDs. These drugs must be used with great caution or avoided in this population. Chapter 77 describes NSAID use in detail.

The cytochrome cyclooxygenase-2 (COX-2) inhibitors decrease the risk for gastrointestinal toxicities in older patients. However, COX-2 inhibitors and nonselective NSAIDs have been associated with an increased number of cardiovascular events compared to placebo with variable durations of exposure. Therefore, the benefits and risks of these agents must be determined for each patient. For the older patient who is sensitive to NSAIDs, pain control with acetaminophen alone (or occasionally with small doses of a narcotic for a short time) is generally preferred. Narcotic analgesia may be an appropriate therapy for individuals with comorbid conditions that preclude the use of NSAIDs (34,35).

Muscle relaxants should be considered for the patient with significant muscle spasm on physical examination. Only a small number of clinical trials have defined the benefits of muscle relaxants (36). Clinical trials have reported the benefits of using cyclobenzaprine 5 mg three times per day compared to placebo in patients with acute muscle spasm of the lumbar or cervical spine (37). The 5-mg dose was as effective as the 10-mg dose but was associated with fewer toxicities, including sedation. An interesting finding of the study was the absence of any sedation in 71% of patients who had complete resolution of muscle spasm with the 5-mg dose. Taking the drug at least 2 hours before bedtime may limit early-morning drowsiness. The efficacy of cyclobenzaprine can be judged after a 7- to 10-day trial. If cyclobenzaprine is ineffective, other muscle relaxants that may be useful include methocarbamol 750 mg four times per day, chlorzoxazone 500 mg four times per day, or orphenadrine citrate 100 mg twice per day. Drugs used for muscle spasticity (e.g., tizanidine 1 or 2 mg at night) may be helpful in some patients. Diazepam is no more effective than placebo in improving back spasm.

Biofeedback, transcutaneous electrical nerve stimulation, and acupuncture are not recommended by the AHCPR for the treatment of patients with acute low back pain (24).

During the recovery period, the patient should be advised to avoid activities that greatly increase the forces applied to the lower spine (e.g., lifting, pushing, force on outstretched upper extremity, as when making beds or vacuuming, lurching, or bending). If the patient does not respond or pain recurs, the patient should be reexamined 3 to 4 weeks later to investigate the possibility of a medical (systemic) cause of back pain. If a mechanical cause remains the most likely diagnosis, a modification of drug therapy (prescribing an alternative nonsteroidal and, if needed, muscle relaxant drug) is indicated.

For the patient who is recovering satisfactorily, various exercise programs have been advocated. One simple back-strengthening exercise program combines isometric gluteal and abdominal muscle contractions and pelvic tilt (Fig. 71.3). These exercises, which are performed standing with the back against a wall, should be recommended as soon as tolerated. These exercises strengthen the muscles that support the spine and may relieve current symptoms and help prevent future episodes of back pain. The exercises should be performed for a few minutes four to six times per day. Exercises designed to strengthen the abdominal musculature, such as sit-ups with the knees flexed, increase intradiscal pressure, may exacerbate symptoms, and are not recommended (however, see Management of the Intercritical Period).

Braces are reserved for the occasional patient with persisting back pain who must remain active while healing continues. However, only limited data support their use. Lumbosacral supports theoretically help relieve back pain by increasing intra-abdominal pressure, which results in greater support of the vertebral column, allowing paraspinous muscles to relax. The lumbosacral support may be a cloth corset fitted with metal stays posteriorly or a smaller cloth brace with a molded plastic insert. The patient should be provided a prescription for the corset or brace, which will be fitted by an orthotist or physical therapist. The patient should use the support while working and then remove the appliance. Use of a lumbosacral support weakens supporting back muscles, so patients should be weaned gradually but steadily from their supports. It is important for this group of patients to return gradually to full activity because an abrupt return may cause a recurrence of low back pain. Although use of a prophylactic lumbar brace will not prevent the onset of low back pain, use of such a device seems to decrease the degree of pain workers experience while continuing to work (38).

Patient education is an important component of the healing process. Patient education can be as effective as an exercise program or chiropractic manipulation treatments at a much reduced cost (39). Patients should be informed about the natural history to recovery with low back pain. They should be made aware of the potential for recurrence of low back pain over the next 12 months. Individuals educated about their problem are less likely to be dissatisfied with their care. A number of educational materials with information that removes misconceptions regarding this common disorder are available (40,41).

Herniated Intervertebral Disk

The intervertebral disk is composed of the annulus fibrosus and the nucleus pulposus. The annulus fibrosus maintains pressure on the contents of the nucleus pulposus, allowing the intervertebral disk to cushion the forces placed on the spine. Tears in the annulus fibrosus allow the contents of the nucleus pulposus to herniate beyond their normal confines. Tears in the annulus may be associated with transient episodes of low back pain. Controversy exists regarding the amount of discomfort that is associated with anatomic alterations of intervertebral disks without modifications of surrounding structures. *Discogenic back pain* is the term associated with individuals with disk abnormalities who have pain reproduced by a provocative discogram (a procedure that involves injecting dye into an intervertebral disk). Studies have demonstrated the inability of discography to identify the level of disk disease that is causing an individual's low back pain (42). Considerable disagreement exists regarding the amount of back pain associated with this entity and its appropriate treatment (43).

Herniation of the nucleus may result in sudden severe pain if neural elements are compressed and inflamed by the nuclear contents (Fig. 71.4). A sudden pressure placed on the lumbar spine that may occur with flexion (e.g., bending over to lift a heavy object, lifting with the arms extended away from the body, a sudden lurch, or even a sneeze or cough) can precipitate the rupture. However, many patients who have a herniated disk do not give a history of injury or of a sudden increase in pressure. Lumbar disk disease is most common at the L4–5 and L5–S1 levels and is less common between the other vertebral bodies.

Diagnosis

Patients with herniated intervertebral disks complain of sharp lancinating pain. The pain radiates from the back down the leg in the anatomic distribution of the affected

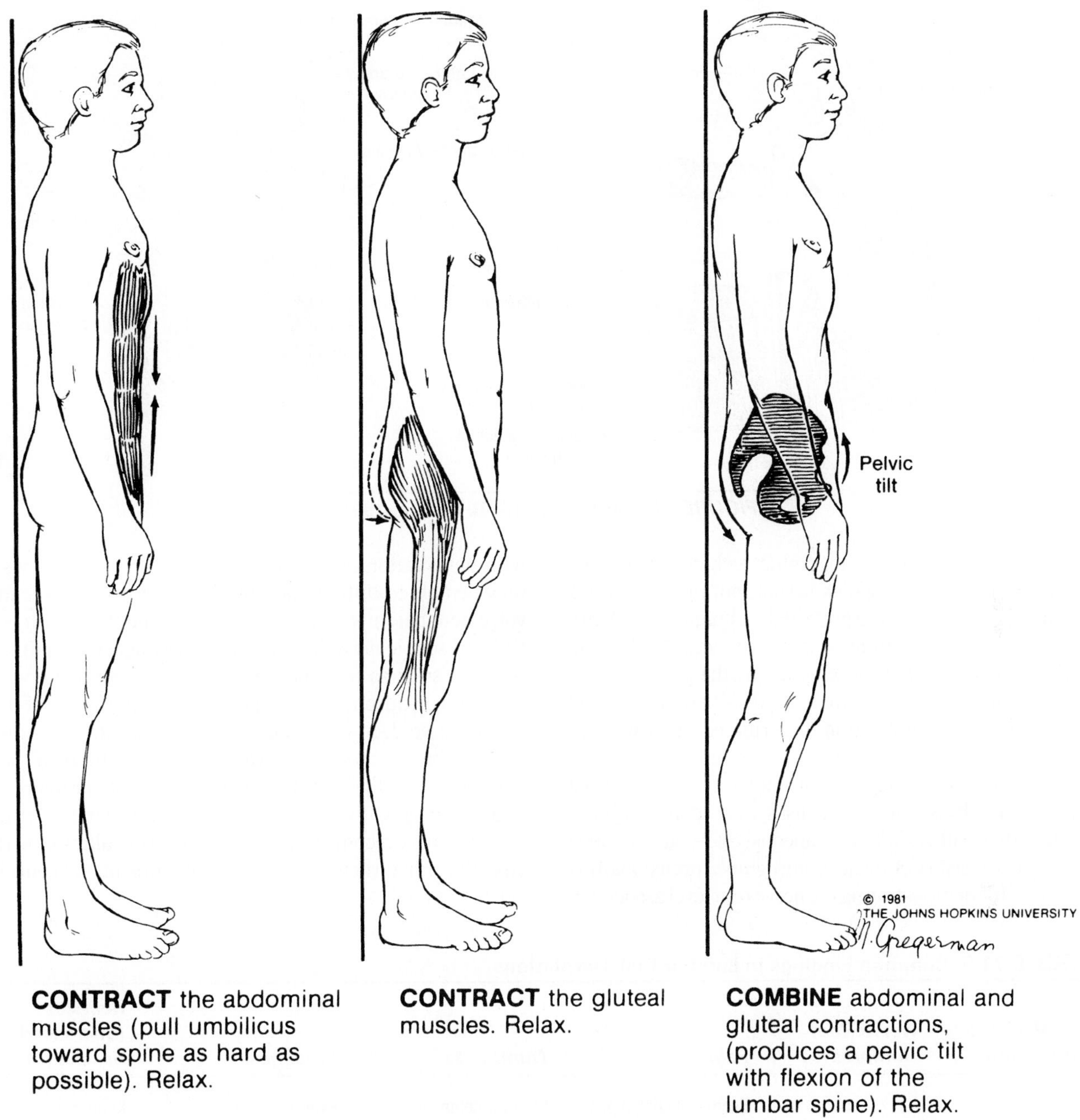

FIGURE 71.3. Exercises: abdominal muscles and pelvic tilt.

nerve root. The pain may be so severe that the patient resists examination and splints the back in an awkward position of lateral lumbar flexion and hip flexion. Patients with bilateral sciatica (pain in the distribution of the sciatic nerve L5–S1 roots [buttocks, posterior thighs, and extending below the knees]), progressive muscle weakness, or bladder or bowel incontinence should be evaluated for cauda equina compression (see Physical Examination). The diagnosis of acute intervertebral disk herniation is most likely when physical examination reveals signs of nerve root compression with loss of motor function, loss of deep tendon reflexes, or localized sensory deficit. Specific disk herniations may result in well-defined motor, sensory, and reflex deficits that aid in their diagnosis (Table 71.3). Patients with progressive neurologic deficits, particularly muscle weakness, should be referred to an orthopedist or neurosurgeon for close observation. These patients may benefit from early surgical intervention.

Documentation of the anatomic abnormality associated with radicular pain is necessary for patients who have continued pain despite a 3- to 4-week course of conservative

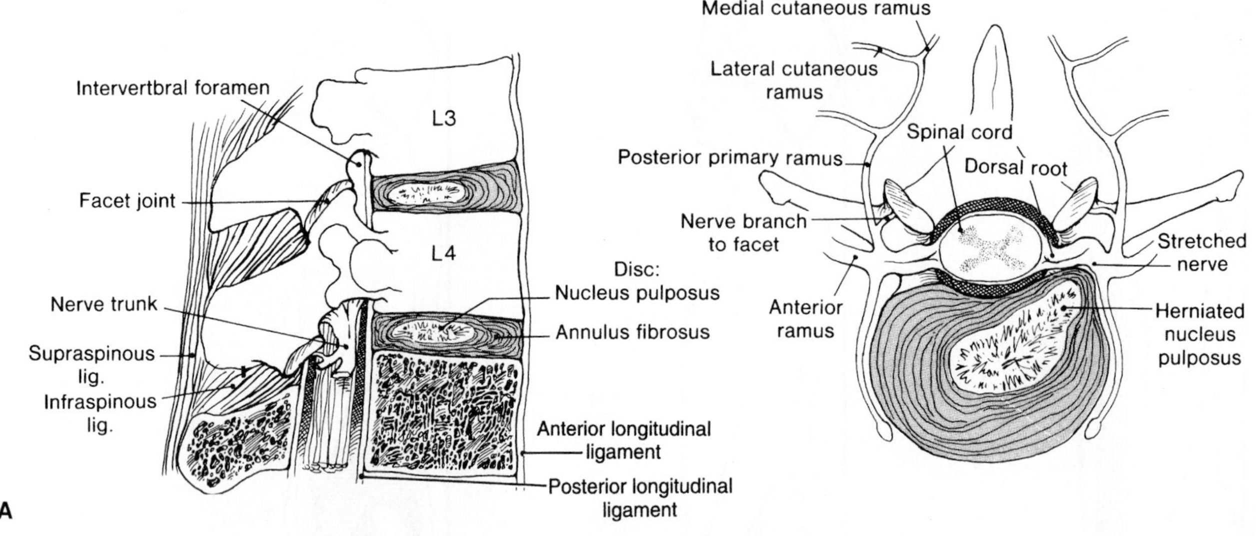

FIGURE 71.4. **A:** Normal disk. **B:** Herniated disk.

therapy. A number of radiographic techniques may be useful for demonstrating disk herniation. In the past, CT and myelography were the preferred techniques for identifying herniated disks. In most circumstances, MRI examination has replaced the myelogram as the preferred test by most surgeons for documenting disk herniation. MRI readily identifies the location of herniated disks without the need for myelographic dye or radiation exposure (44). Preliminary studies suggest that uptake of MRI contrast (gadolinium) by sequestrated disks may identify abnormalities that will resorb spontaneously without the need for surgical excision (45). *Electromyography* occasionally is necessary for demonstrating the nerve root level associated with denervation of leg muscles. Electromyography also may be able to differentiate by the pattern of muscle involvement patients with herniated disk and those with peripheral sciatic nerve abnormalities secondary to another problem such as trauma, tumor, or *piriformis syndrome*. Piriformis syndrome is associated with compression of the sciatic nerve deep in the buttocks by the piriformis muscle. Compression of the nerve results in sciatic pain that may radiate to the foot, following no specific dermatome or association with definitive neurologic deficits. Electromyography is recommended only after consultation with an orthopedist, rheumatologist, neurosurgeon, or neurologist.

TABLE 71.3 Common Findings in Lumbar Disk Herniations

Level of Disk Herniation	*Nerve Root Compressed*	*Pain*	*Numbness*[a]	*Weakness*	*Reflexes (Decreased or Absent)*
L3–4	L4	Sacroiliac joint, hip, posterolateral thigh, anterior aspect of leg	L4 dermatome	Extension of knee (quadriceps)	Knee jerk
L4–5	L5	Sacroiliac joint, hip	L5 dermatome (includes great toe)	Dorsiflexion of great toe (extensor hallucis longus)	
L5–S1	S1	Lateral aspect of leg and foot	S1 dermatome (includes lateral toes)	Unusual (plantar flexion of foot)	Ankle jerk
Massive midline lumbar disk herniation Cauda equina syndrome (usually L4 or L5)	Multiple roots in dural sac	Midline of back, posterior aspect of both thighs and legs	Perineum, posterior thighs, plantar aspect of feet	Paralysis of feet and sphincters	Absent ankle jerk

[a]See Figure 78.2.

Adapted from Vanden Briuk KD, Edmonson AS. The spine. In: Edmonson AS, Crenshaw AH, eds. Campbell's operative orthopaedics. St. Louis: CV Mosby, 1980, with permission.

Management

For most patients with a herniated disk, treatment is nonoperative because 80% of patients respond to conservative therapy (see below) and are completely free of pain within 2 months. In patients whose pain and other neurologic abnormalities remit without surgical reduction of the disk, an adjustment of the annulus and posterior longitudinal ligament relative to the herniated disk fragment is the most likely reason for the diminution of edema, inflammation, back pain, and leg pain. Desiccation of the fragment may play a role in resolution of symptoms.

Conservative therapy consists of limiting physical activity, with the patient at bed rest in the semi-Fowler position (hips and knees flexed, supported by pillows) for 2 days. NSAIDs and muscle relaxants (as described above) and narcotic analgesics (if the pain is severe) should be prescribed. Physical therapy usually is unnecessary for patients with acute disk herniations. Active exercise programs may intensify acute symptoms and should be avoided. Therapy such as ultrasound, short-wave diathermy, heat packs, or cold packs may provide short-term pain relief only (as they do in lumbosacral pain) but do not alter disk lesions or have any long-term effect on symptoms. Lumbar traction has not been shown to be more effective than bed rest for treatment of lumbar disk disease and low back pain and is not indicated (46). Patients should be prescribed such a conservative regimen for 3 to 4 weeks, and if this therapy fails, they should be asked to consider an epidural corticosteroid injection. A series of three injections over 3 to 6 weeks may improve back and leg pain (47). Epidural injections can help reduce pain and improve sensory function early in the course of sciatica secondary to a herniated disk (48). Surgical decompression of the appropriate disk space is indicated for persistent pain resistant to conservative therapy. The size of the disk herniation does not correlate with a lack of response to conservative management. Large herniated disks are more likely to decrease in size as documented by CT and contrast MRI (49). New minimally invasive techniques are being used for the removal of accessible disk fragments. These surgeries are associated with less damage to paraspinous soft tissues. Further investigation is needed to determine the efficacy of these techniques, such as arthroscopic discectomy, in comparison with standard discectomies (50). For management of the intercritical period, see Management of the Intercritical Period.

Osteoarthritis and Spinal Stenosis

The lumbar spine is one of the common locations for osteoarthritis. This joint disease is associated with joint pain, stiffness, deformity, and limitation of motion. Alterations over time secondary to osteoarthritis result in loss of disk volume, increased pressure on apophyseal joints, and hypertrophy of soft tissue and bony structures, resulting in a decrease in the size of the spinal canal. Chapter 75 discusses osteoarthritis in full.

Diagnosis

Initially, patients may complain of pain after repeated episodes of hyperextension that traumatizes the apophyseal (facet) joints, resulting in stretching or tearing of the ligamentous capsule of the apophyseal joint. Typically, back flexion (bending forward) relieves the pain, whereas hyperextension (e.g., a painter working overhead) exacerbates it. Patients also may experience back pain related to gradual degeneration of the intervertebral disk or the development of osteophytes, either of which may impinge on a nerve root. Patients with lumbar osteoarthritis or degenerative disk disease describe back, buttock, or unilateral lower extremity pain. Examination usually reveals evidence of irritation of a specific nerve root, resulting in loss of a localized motor or sensory neurologic function or of an absent deep tendon reflex (L5–S1 disk, ankle or L3–4 disk, knee). The SLR test may be positive. Many of these patients respond to conservative therapy because the anti-inflammatory action of NSAIDs is effective in diminishing the swelling of soft tissues, which causes nerve impingement.

As patients grow older, particularly during the fifth to seventh decade, back symptoms become suggestive of impingement of multiple nerve roots at different levels on both sides of the spinal cord. Spinal stenosis occurs most commonly in men, who complain of chronic low back pain with unilateral or bilateral lower extremity discomfort that is exacerbated by extension of the spine while standing. They also may develop frank hyperesthesia or dysesthesias (Table 71.1). They also may have a history of disk surgery. Many patients with spinal stenosis have symptoms of claudication mimicking those of peripheral vascular insufficiency. These patients develop lower extremity pain while standing or walking or hyperextending the spine in the absence of any evidence of peripheral vascular disease. Painful paresthesias are present in the feet or legs and may radiate to the hip girdle or lower trunk. Patients may experience lower extremity numbness and weakness. These symptoms are relieved by rest or flexion of the spine (the patient may report relief by bending forward as if to tie shoelaces). Physical examination may show no abnormalities until the patient is asked to walk. In this regard, the patient suspected of having spinal stenosis should be walked until pain develops—sometimes this requires many minutes—and then examined in the sitting position; abnormal motor or sensory deficits may be present only after such increased activity. Other physical findings may include the loss of peripheral pulses and atrophic skin (51).

Plain x-ray films show degenerative changes in the apophyseal joints (facet joints) and decreased anteroposterior canal diameter. CT is the best diagnostic radiographic technique for demonstrating spinal stenosis because CT shows the narrowed canal or impingement of osteophytes on the intervertebral foramina.

Management

Most patients with spinal stenosis can be treated nonsurgically. Activities that bring on pain should be discouraged. Patients may respond to NSAIDs or a course of epidural corticosteroid injections (administered by a consulting rheumatologist, neurosurgeon, anesthesiologist, or orthopedist). Operative therapy for spinal stenosis is reserved for patients who are severely incapacitated by their condition. Surgery for spinal stenosis requires decompression of the bony impingement of the spinal cord and nervi erigentes. If vertebral instability is documented before surgery, fusion of the vertebral bodies also is accomplished. Postoperative relief of pain is seen within approximately 1 week and full recovery, when surgery is successful, within 1 month. Patients treated successfully with surgery have a more rapid and greater improvement in neurogenic claudication than medically treated patients. However, only two thirds of patients describe improvement with initial decompressive surgery (52). Also, medically treated patients have no severe deterioration of neurologic function. Therefore, medical treatment for 2 to 3 years before considering surgery seems to be a good approach for most patients with spinal stenosis (53). Another study reported that 80% of individuals experienced immediate postsurgical improvement of neurogenic claudication. At 4-year followup, 70% of the surgical group continued with improved symptoms compared with 52% of patients treated nonsurgically (54).

MEDICAL (SYSTEMIC) BACK PAIN SYNDROMES

Spondyloarthropathies

Patients with spondyloarthropathies (ankylosing spondylitis, reactive arthritis, psoriatic spondylitis, enteropathic spondylitis) often complain of low back, buttock, or leg pain. These patients have morning stiffness as a major component of their symptom complex. Although back pain is the first symptom in a number of young patients, it is often associated with other symptoms and signs of the specific disorder (iritis, conjunctivitis, or skin rash). A clue to the presence of a spondyloarthropathy on physical examination is tenderness with percussion over the axial skeleton or sacroiliac joints. The sacroiliac joints may be painful when stressed while the patient is in the prone or supine position. Early identification of a patient with spondyloarthropathy is important because new therapies are available that prevent progressive calcification of spinous structures (55). Chapter 78 discusses conditions affecting the axial skeleton and sacroiliac joints.

Infections

Although rare, infection of the axial skeleton (osteomyelitis, discitis, or septic arthritis) must be considered in any patient with back pain (56). Osteomyelitis is an infection of the vertebral bodies. Discitis is an infection of the intervertebral disk. Septic arthritis of the back is an infection of the sacroiliac joints. Chapter 40 discusses these conditions in detail.

Vertebral Fractures

Vertebral compression fractures are common, especially among the elderly, and usually result from a flexion injury when the spine is abruptly flexed, for example, during jumping. Fractures conceivably could be classified as a regional (mechanical) cause of back pain. It is arbitrarily classified as a medical (systemic) cause of low back pain because it most typically occurs in the elderly and often is a manifestation of a systemic disorder such as osteoporosis. The thoracic spine is most commonly involved. The force needed to compress a vertebral body in healthy bone is considerable. However, when the bone is diseased, as occurs with osteoporosis, myeloma, metastatic cancer, or hyperparathyroidism, the injury may be insignificant. Pain usually is localized and immediate, although it may be delayed for several days after the fracture. Often tenderness over a single vertebra indicates the presence of a fracture, but an x-ray film is necessary to confirm the diagnosis.

Other radiographic techniques are useful for identifying the locations of fractures that may not be detected by plain x-ray films. A bone scan often is useful in demonstrating whether there are single or multiple fractures. CT or MRI is indicated for patients with compression fractures who also have neurologic deficits. These techniques can localize abnormalities associated with nerve impingement. Not all processes that weaken bone are detected by bone scan (e.g., multiple myeloma). Blood chemistries, including the concentration of serum proteins, and the serum and urine electrophoretic pattern of proteins are helpful in identifying patients with myeloma.

With lumbar or thoracic vertebral compression fractures, management includes rest, adequate analgesia, and gradual ambulation when the patient is free from severe pain. Medical therapy in the form of intranasal calcitonin may be beneficial in controlling fracture pain through the release of endogenous β-endorphin (57). Kyphoplasty is a percutaneous technique for reexpanding collapsed vertebral bodies through the use of an inflatable balloon and injectable bone cement. This technique offers pain relief with the potential for restoration of vertebral body height (58). A lumbosacral support or, for the patient with a thoracic vertebral fracture, a chairback or hyperextension brace may be helpful in alleviating pain. These items can be obtained by prescription from an orthopedic appliance shop.

The pain from a vertebral fracture may persist for several months, although the severe and incapacitating component usually lasts for only 2 to 3 weeks.

Tumors

Tumors of the lumbar spine are unusual causes of back pain; however, these diseases are associated with the highest morbidity, mortality, and dysfunction. Patients with tumors of the lumbar spine usually have back pain as their initial complaint. Commonly, patients with tumor-associated pain have increased discomfort with recumbency. Physical examination demonstrates localized tenderness and neurologic dysfunction if the spinal cord or a nerve root is compressed. Although laboratory evaluation often yields nonspecific results, radiographic evaluation is useful in identifying the location and type of neoplastic lesion. In general, benign tumors are located in the posterior elements of vertebrae (spinous, transverse process), and malignant (both primary and metastatic) tumors are located in the anterior components of vertebrae (body). The most common neoplastic lesion of the lumbar spine is a metastatic tumor. The most common primary tumor located in the lumbar spine is myeloma. The definitive diagnosis of a tumor must be derived from histologic examination of biopsy material obtained from the lesion. The most effective therapy for both benign and malignant tumors is removal of the lesions that are accessible to surgical excision. When excision is impossible, partial resection, radiation therapy, corticosteroids, or chemotherapy may be indicated to control symptoms and compression of the spinal cord and nerve roots.

Referred Pain

Disease processes that affect organs in the retroperitoneum not only may cause pain locally but may refer pain in the distribution of the sensory nerve supplying the diseased tissue. Diseases of the vascular, genitourinary, and gastrointestinal systems may refer pain to the lumbar spine. Characteristically, referred pain is unaffected by the physical position of the patient. Patients usually have symptoms in the affected organ, raising the possibility of a medical cause of the patient's back pain (Tables 71.4 and 71.5).

MANAGEMENT OF CHRONIC BACK PAIN

Although most patients with low back pain have complete remission of symptoms within 3 to 4 weeks, many patients experience a recurrence (5). Patients should return to the caregiver's office even if they have had a resolution of their pain. The purpose of these visits is to discuss ways to prevent recurrent attacks of back pain by focusing education on posture, weight control, exercise, and work activities. In addition, a small but significant number of individuals with low back pain have persistent pain resistant to therapies effective for acute episodes.

Figure 71.5 shows some correct and incorrect postures and practical advice that may be useful to give to patients

TABLE 71.4 Medical Causes of Low Back Pain

Systemic: Constitutional symptoms, severe localized pain, morning stiffness are clues suggestive of generalized disorder.
- Rheumatologic: spondyloarthropathies, polymyalgia rheumatica, fibromyalgia
- Infectious: vertebral osteomyelitis, Pott disease (tuberculosis of spine), discitis, septic arthritis, epidural abscess, herpes zoster
- Neoplastic:
  - Benign: osteoid osteoma, osteochondroma, giant cell tumor
  - Malignant: metastatic, multiple myeloma, chondrosarcoma, chordoma, lymphoma, retroperitoneal sarcoma, neural tumor
- Neurologic-psychiatric: neuropathic (Charcot) joints, femoral neuropathy, depression, hysteria
- Miscellaneous: vertebral sarcoidosis, Paget disease, retroperitoneal fibrosis

Referred pain: Absence of any tenderness, limitation of motion, or aggravation of pain or spasm during the physical examination is suggestive of referred pain (see Table 71.5 for dermatome to which pain from various visceral structures may be referred).
- Lower thoracic and upper lumbar pain from an upper abdominal disease process (e.g., pancreas)
- Low lumbar pain from a lower abdominal disease process (e.g., aortic aneurysm)
- Sacral pain from a pelvic problem (e.g., endometriosis, prostate cancer)

TABLE 71.5 Dermatome to which Pain from Various Visceral Structures May Be Referred

Dermatome[a]	*Viscera*
L1	Kidney, ureter, body of uterus, abdominal aorta, small intestine
L2	Bladder, abdominal aorta, ascending colon
L3	Abdominal aorta
L4	Abdominal aorta
L5, S1, S2	—
S3	Rectum, anus, lower portion of bladder, cervix, upper vagina, prostate
S4	Rectum, anus, base of bladder, cervix, upper vagina, prostate
S5	—

[a] See Figure 86.2 for cutaneous pattern of dermatomes.
Modified from Borenstein DG, Wiesel SW, Boden SD. Low back and neck pain. Philadelphia: WB Saunders, 2004;64, with permission.

Incorrect
Correct
SITTING
Avoid leaning forward.
Support spine with backrest and armrests.
Straight standing is preferable to unsupported sitting.
Incorrect
Correct
STANDING
Eliminate work done at slight flexion.
To avoid this posture, the height of the work area may be raised.
Incorrect
Correct
LIFTING
Avoid back flexion.
Flex knees, keep spine straight.
Hold objects close to the body.
Incorrect
SLEEPING
Avoid the prone position.
Rest on one side, with pillow under head, knees flexed.
Correct
© 1981 THE JOHNS HOPKINS UNIVERSITY

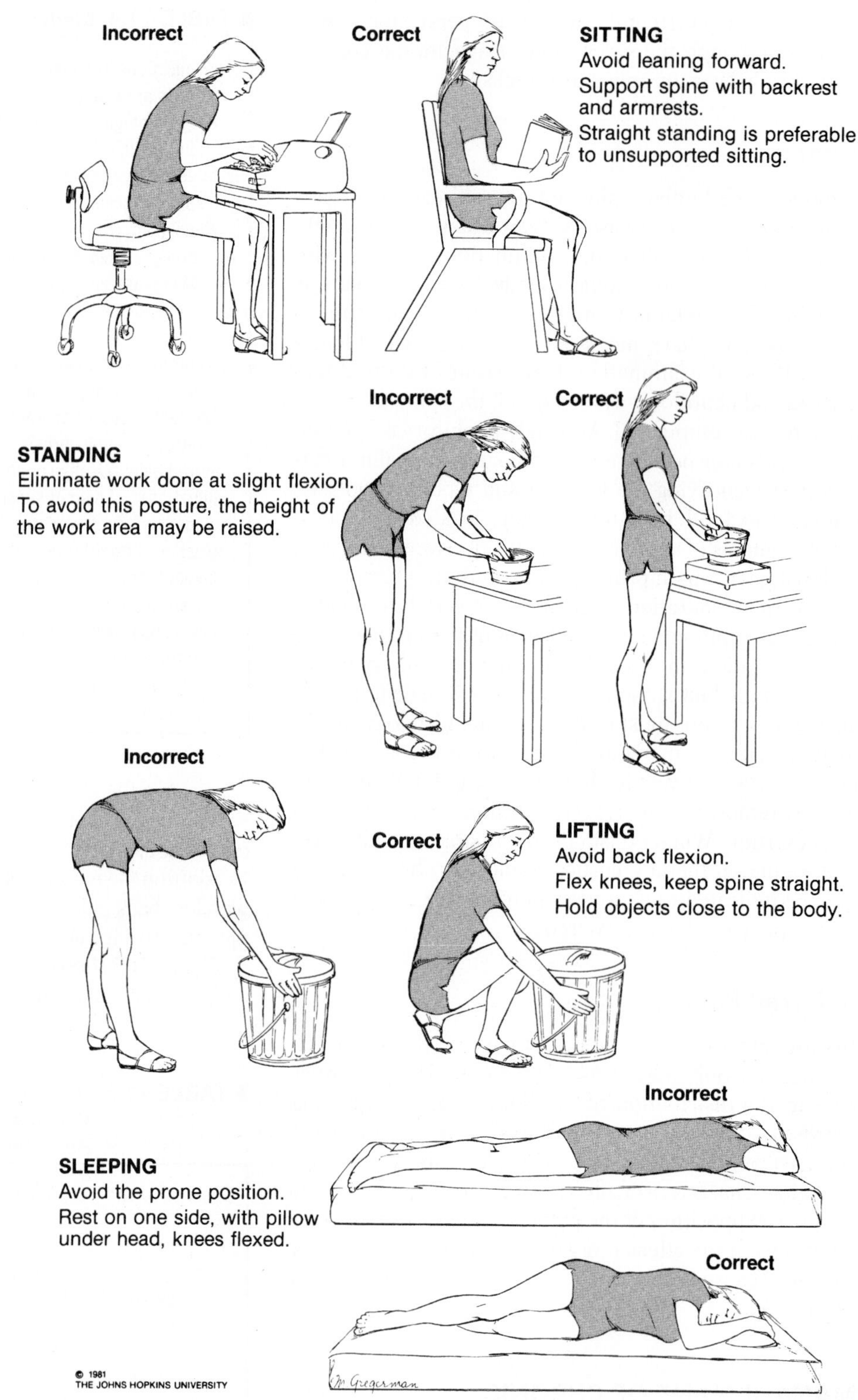

FIGURE 71.5. Incorrect and correct postural attitudes.

who have experienced low back pain. Weight reduction is desirable in the obese patient, because excessive weight directly increases the load on the lower vertebral column and its supporting structures. Exercise initiated as soon as the acute pain subsides (usually 2–4 days after onset) may improve function and decrease pain (59). At a minimum, such exercises alert patients to their back problem, which increases the likelihood of performing daily activities in a way that may allow them to avoid reinjury. Prolonged bed rest weakens back muscles and should be avoided.

Certain advice to the patient regarding lifting is prudent. Sudden loading of the spine when the back is flexed and the knees are straight markedly increases forces placed on the lumbar spine (Fig. 71.2) compared with a position where the knees are bent and the back is straight. Exercises that strengthen the quadriceps (extend knees) are theoretically sound for anyone who may have to lift at all. These exercises include swimming, cycling, or jogging on a flat even surface. The patient should be advised to exercise only if it does not initiate or increase back pain. In addition, because the abdominal muscles are important in supporting the spine when a weight is brought to bear on it, exercises that strengthen the abdominal muscles (Fig. 71.3) are helpful. Patient education is an effective component in the treatment of all patients who have experienced back pain. Education about such matters may improve a patient's lifestyle and the likelihood of returning to work. So-called *back schools,* which generally are conducted by physical therapists, have been organized in many work sites. However, a large controlled trial of an educational program to prevent low back injuries organized as a back school for postal workers failed to prevent work-associated back injury in employees with or without a history of back injury, although the knowledge of safe behavior was increased by the training (60).

Complementary therapies are used frequently for a variety of medical problems, including low back pain (61). A wide variety of therapies has been promoted for the therapy of low back pain, including spinal manipulation, massage, acupuncture, and magnets. Chapter 5 discusses acupuncture and chiropractic.

Spinal manipulation seems to help many patients and has been recommended by the practice guidelines published by the AHCPR (24). These guidelines do not specifically recommend that manipulation be done by a chiropractor. Initial evaluation of low back pain by a *chiropractor* may not include screening evaluation with history and physical examination for systemic disorders. Also, chiropractors generally do not offer additional therapies beyond those offered by an experienced physical therapist. Patient satisfaction with chiropractors seems to be related to the chiropractor's willingness to spend more time with the patient and to listen to his or her concerns (62). Too often physicians and physical therapists do not show such a level of concern and may even minimize the patient's problems. Studies of manipulation of the back do not define precisely what a standard manipulation is or what it accomplishes physiologically, making comparisons of it with other treatments impossible. Concerns also arise between the applicability of manipulation to chronic low back pain versus acute back pain. In general, manipulation may be helpful but is of no greater benefit than conventional therapies (63).

Therapeutic massage has benefited many individuals with chronic low back pain. This therapy given once per week for 10 weeks has demonstrated benefit months after the last treatment. The efficacy of this form of treatment is limited to the availability of experienced massage therapists (64). This same study failed to identify significant benefit of acupuncture for chronic low back pain. Acupuncture techniques can vary, and this may have an effect on the outcome of a clinical trial. Anecdotally, patients have described benefit of additional analgesia associated with acupuncture treatments. Additional trials are warranted to determine the efficacy of this treatment.

Magnets have been suggested as effective for treatment of low back pain. A pilot double-blinded, placebo-controlled trial using magnets for low back pain demonstrated no significant difference between study groups (65).

The patient may need to modify *work or athletic activities* once an episode of back pain occurs. Of note, however, there is no convincing evidence to support the concept that heavy labor or lifting predisposes to the development of the initial episode of back pain. Certain factors do predispose patients to injury, including improper technique in lifting, sitting for prolonged periods or not at all during the workday, and sudden maximal physical activity (e.g., participation in an occasional vigorous game without conditioning). Furthermore, back pain occurs more often in people who consider their occupation to be physically hard and in those who believe their work to be stressful to the spine or who are dissatisfied with their work (66,67).

SPECIFIC REFERENCES*

1. Hart LG, Deyo RA, Cherkin DC. Physician office visits for low back pain: frequency, clinical evaluation, and treatment patterns from a US national survey. Spine 1995;20:11.
2. Wilke H, Need P, Caimi M, et al. New in vivo measurements of pressures in the intervertebral disc in daily life. Spine 1999;24:755.
3. Nerlich AG, Schleicher ED, Boos N. 1997 Volvo award winner in basic science studies: immunologic markers for age-related changes of human lumbar intervertebral discs. Spine 1997;22:2781.
4. Dillane JB, Fry J, Kalton G. Acute back syndrome: study from general practice. BMJ 1966;3:82.
5. Van den Hoogen HJM, Koes BW, van Eijk JTM, et al. The prognosis of low back pain in general practice. Spine 1997;22:1515.
6. Deyo RA, Rainville J, Kent DL. What can the history and physical examination tell us about low back pain? JAMA 1992;268:760.
7. Vroomen PC, de Krom MC, Knottnerus JA. Diagnostic value of history and physical examination in patients suspected of sciatica due to disc herniation: a systematic review. J Neurol 1999;246:899.
8. Vaz M, Wadia RS, Gokhale SD. Another cause of positive crossed-straight-leg-raising test. N Engl J Med 1978;295:779.
9. Shapiro S. Medical realities of cauda equina syndrome secondary to lumbar disc herniation. Spine 2000;25:348.
10. Waddell G, McCulloch JA, Kummel E, et al. Nonorganic physical signs in low-back pain. Spine 1980;5:117.

*Bold numerals denote published controlled clinical trials, meta-analyses, or consensus-based recommendations.

11. Main CJ, Waddell G: Behavioral responses to examination: a reappraisal of the interpretation of "nonorganic signs." Spine 1998;2367.
12. McCombe PF, Fairbank JCT, Cockersole BC, et al. Reproducibility of physical signs in low back pain. Spine 1989;14:908.
13. Jensen OH. The level-diagnosis of a lower lumbar disc herniation: the value of sensitivity and motor testing. Clin Rheumatol 1987;6:564.
14. Ensink F, Saur PMM, Frese K, et al. Lumbar range of motion: influence of time of day and individual factors on measurements. Spine 1996;21:1339.
15. Jarvik JG, Deyo RA. Diagnostic evaluation of low back pain with emphasis on imaging. Ann Intern Med 2002;137:586.
16. Borenstein D. Does osteoarthritis of the lumbar spine cause chronic low back pain? Curr Rheumatol Rep 2004: 6:14.
17. Albeck MJ, Hilden J, Kjaer L, et al. A controlled comparison of myelography, computed tomography, and magnetic resonance imaging in clinically suspected lumbar disc herniation. Spine 1995;20:443.
18. Alexander AR. Magnetic resonance imaging of the spine and spinal cord tumors. Spine State Art Rev 1988;2:499.
19. Weishaupt D, Zanetti M, Hodler J, et al. MR imaging of the lumbar spine: prevalence of intervertebral disk extrusion and sequestration, nerve root compression, end plate abnormalities, and osteoarthritis of the facet joints in asymptomatic volunteers. Radiology 1998;209:661.
20. Borenstein DG, O'Mara JW Jr, Boden SD et al. The value of magnetic resonance imaging of the lumbar spine to predict low-back in asymptomatic subjects: A seven-year follow-up study. J Bone Joint Surg 2001: 83A:1306.
21. Albeck MJ, Taher G, Lauritzen M et al. Diagnostic value of electrophysiological tests in patients with sciatica. Acta Neurol Scand 2000;101:249.
22. Deyo RA. Diagnostic evaluation of LBP: reaching a specific is often impossible. Arch Intern Med 2002;162:1444.
23. Coste J, Delecocuillerie G, Cohen de Lara A, et al. Clinical course and prognostic factors in acute low back pain: an inception cohort study in primary care practice. BMJ 1994;308:577.
24. Bigos SJ, Bowyer O, Braen G, et al. Acute low back problems in adults. Clinical Practice Guideline No. 14. AHCPR Publication No. 95-0642. Rockville, MD: Agency for Health Care Policy and Research, Public Health Service, U.S. Department of Health and Human Services, December 1994.
25. Bouter LM, Pennick V, Bombardier C, et al. Cochrane back review group. Spine 2003;1215.
26. Cherkin DC, Wheeler KJ, Barlow W, et al. Medication use for low back pain in primary care. Spine 1998;23:607.
27. Deyo RA, Diehl AK, Rosenthal M. How many days of bed rest for acute low back pain? N Engl J Med 1986;315:1064.
28. Malmivaara A, Hakkinen U, Aro T, et al. The treatment of acute low back pain: bed rest, exercises, or ordinary activity? N Engl J Med 1995;332:351.
29. Rozenberg S, Delval D, Rezvani Y et al. Bed rest or normal activity for patients with acute low back pain: a randomized controlled trial. Spine 2002;27:1487.
30. Faas A, Chavannes AW, van Eijk JTM, et al. A randomized, placebo-controlled trial of exercise therapy in patients with acute low back pain. Spine 1993;18:1388.
31. Nadler SF, Steiner DJ, Erasala GN, et al. Continuous low-level heat wrap therapy provides more efficacy than ibuprofen and acetaminophen for acute low back pain. Spine 2002;27:1012.
32. Koes BW, Scholten RJPM, Mens JMA, et al. Efficacy of non-steroidal anti-inflammatory drugs for low back: a systematic review of randomized clinical trials. Ann Rheum Dis 1997;56:214.
33. van Tulder MW, Scholten RJPM, Koes BW, et al. Nonsteroidal anti-inflammatory drugs for low back pain: a systematic review within the framework of the Cochrane Collaboration Back Review Group. Spine 2000;25:2501.
34. Mahowald ML, Singh JA, Majeski P. Opioid use by patients in an orthopedics spine clinic. Arthritis Rheum 2005;52:312.
35. Borenstein D. Opioids: to use or not to use? That is the question. Arthritis Rheum 2005;52:6.
36. Bernstein E, Carey TS, Garrett JM. The use of muscle relaxant medications in acute low back pain. Spine 2004;29:1346.
37. Borenstein DG, Korn S. Efficacy of a low-dose regimen of cyclobenzaprine hydrochloride in acute skeletal muscle spasm: results of two placebo-controlled trials. Clin Ther 2003;25: 1056.
38. van Poppel MNM, Koes BW, van der Ploeg T, et al. Lumbar supports and education for the prevention of low back pain in industry: a randomized controlled trial. JAMA 1998;279: 1789.
39. Cherkin DC, Deyo RA, Battie M et al. A comparison of physical therapy, chiropractic manipulation, and provision of an educational booklet in the treatment of patients with low back pain. N Engl J Med 1998;339:1021.
40. Dunkin MA. All you need to know about back pain. Atlanta, GA: Arthritis Foundation, 2002.
41. Borenstein D. Back in control: a conventional and complementary prescription for eliminating back pain. New York: M Evans, 2001.
42. Carragee EJ. Clinical practice. Persistent low back pain. N Engl J Med 2005;352:1891.
43. Carragee EJ, Alamin TF, Miller JL et al. Discographic, MRI and psychological determinants of low back pain disability and remission: a prospective study in subjects with benign persistent back pain. Spine J 2005;5:24.
44. Boden SD. The use of radiographic imaging studies in the evaluation of patients who have degenerative disorders of the lumbar spine. J Bone Joint Surg 1996;78A:114.
45. Komori H, Okawa A, Haro H, et al. Contrast-enhanced magnetic resonance imaging in conservative management of lumbar disc herniation. Spine 1998;22:67.
46. Beurskens AJ, de Vet HC, Koke AJ, et al. Efficacy of traction for nonspecific low back pain: 12-week and 6-month results of a randomized clinical trial. Spine 1997;22:2756.
47. Spaccarelli KC. Lumbar and caudal epidural corticosteroid injections. Mayo Clin Proc 1996; 71:169.
48. Carette S, Leclaire R, Marcoux S, et al. Epidural corticosteroid injections for sciatica due to herniated nucleus pulposus. N Engl J Med 1997;336:1634.
49. Komori H, Okawa A, Haro H, et al. Contrast-enhanced magnetic resonance imaging in conservative management of lumbar disc herniation. Spine 1998;22:67.
50. Hermantin FU, Peters T, Quartararo L, et al. A prospective, randomized study comparing the results of open discectomy with those of video-assisted arthroscopic microdiscectomy. J Bone Joint Surg 1999;81A:958.
51. Bell GR. Office evaluation of patients with spinal stenosis. Semin Spine Surg 1999;11:191.
52. Herno A, Airaksinen O, Saari T, et al. Surgical results of lumbar spinal stenosis: a comparison of patients with or without previous back surgery. Spine 1995;20:964.
53. Johnsson K, Uden A, Rosen I. The effect of decompression on the natural course of spinal stenosis: a comparison of surgically treated and untreated patients. Spine 1991;16:615.
54. Atlas SJ, Keller RB, Robson D, et al. Surgical and nonsurgical management of lumbar spinal stenosis: four-year outcomes from the Maine Lumbar Spine Study. Spine 2000;25:556.
55. Reveille J, Arnett FC. Spondyloarthritis: update on pathogenesis and management. Am J Med 2005;118:592.
56. Alamin TF, Hanley EN. Profiles of patients with spine infections. Semin Spine Surg 2000;12:212.
57. Gennari C. Analgesic effect of calcitonin in osteoporosis. Bone 2002;30[5 Suppl]:67S.
58. Kasperk C, Hillmeier J, Noldge G, et al. Treatment of painful vertebral fractures by kyphoplasty in patients with primary osteoporosis: a prospective nonrandomized controlled study. J Bone Miner Res 2005;20:604.
59. Hayden JA, van Tulder MW, Malmivaara AV, et al. Meta-analysis: exercise therapy for nonspecific low back pain. Ann Intern Med 2005;142:765–775.
60. Daltroy LH, Iversen MD, Larson MG, et al. A controlled trial of an educational program to prevent low back injuries. N Engl J Med 1997; 337:332.
61. Eisenberg DM, Davis RB, Ettner SL, et al. Trends in alternative medicine use in the United States, 1990–1997: results of a follow-up national survey. JAMA 1998;280:1569.
62. Cherkin DC, MacCornack FA. Patient evaluations of low back pain care from family physicians and chiropractors. West J Med 1989;150:351.
63. Cherkin DC, Sherman KJ, Deyo RA et al. A review of the evidence for the effectiveness, safety, and cost of acupuncture, massage therapy, and spinal manipulation for back pain. Ann Intern Med 2003;138;898.
64. Cherkin DC, Eisenberg D, Sherman KJ, et al. Randomized trial comparing traditional Chinese medical acupuncture, therapeutic massage, and self-care education for chronic low back pain. Arch Intern Med 2001;161:1081.
65. Collacott EA, Zimmerman JT, White DW, et al. Bipolar permanent magnets for the treatment of chronic low back pain: a pilot study. JAMA 2000; 283:1322.
66. Bigos SJ, Battie MC, Spengler DM, et al. A prospective study of work perceptions and psychosocial factors affecting the report of back injury. Spine 1991;16:1.
67. Krause N, Ragland DR, Fisher JM, et al. Psychological job factors, physical workload, and incidence of work-related spinal injury: a 5-year prospective study of urban transit operators. Spine 1998;23:2507.

*For annotated **General References** and resources related to this chapter, visit www.hopkinsbayview.org/PAMreferences.*

Chapter 72

Knee, Lower Leg, and Ankle Pain

John H. Wilckens, Simon C. Mears, and Ronald P. Byank

Knee, leg, or ankle pain represents one of the most common reasons patients visit their physicians. Pain can be the result of injury, overuse, or a degenerative, inflammatory, or neoplastic process. Because the knee, lower leg, and ankle are weight-bearing structures, pain located in these anatomic structures greatly affects ambulation, activities of daily living, recreation, and employment. This chapter provides an overview of the anatomy of the knee, lower leg, and ankle and presents a commonsense approach to the diagnosis and treatment of pain in these areas.

THE KNEE

Anatomy

The knee, which is the largest joint in the body, moves along three axes. The principal anatomic components (Fig. 72.1) and their functions are as follows:

- Three articulations between the femur, tibia, and patella: medial tibial femoral compartment, lateral tibial femoral compartment, and patellofemoral compartment. These three separate compartments function as a single cohesive unit.
- Medial and lateral menisci, semilunar-shaped fibrocartilage located in the medial and lateral tibiofemoral compartments, have an important role not only in shock absorption, but also in joint lubrication, weight distribution, and joint stability.
- The extra-articular medial collateral ligament (MCL) and lateral collateral ligament (LCL) provide valgus and varus stability to the knee joint and serve as secondary stabilizers to anteroposterior and rotary knee motion. The MCL has its origin at the medial epicondyle of the femur and inserts distally under the medial hamstrings and pes anserina bursa on the proximal medial tibia, well below the medial joint line. The LCL originates from the lateral epicondyle of the femur and inserts on the proximal fibular head. With the knee in a figure-four position (hip flexed, knee flexed, with the tibia crossing the contralateral tibia), the LCL can be palpated easily.
- The intraarticular cruciate ligaments provide primary anteroposterior and rotary stability to the knee. The anterior cruciate ligament (ACL) arises from the intercondylar eminence located centrally on the tibial plateau and inserts on the posterior aspect of the lateral wall of the intercondylar notch. The posterior cruciate ligament (PCL) arises from the anterior aspect of the medial wall of the intercondylar notch, crosses the ACL, and inserts midline posteriorly on the proximal tibia. The PCL resists posterior tibial translation of the tibia on the femur, whereas the ACL resists anterior translation.
- Several large muscle groups cross the knee joint, providing dynamic stability and motion to the knee. The medial hamstrings consist of the semimembranosus, semitendinosus, and gracilis that fan out to insert over the proximal medial tibia. The lateral hamstrings, the long and short biceps femoris, insert on the proximal fibular head. The gastrocnemius arises from two heads (the lateral head, from the posterior aspect of the lateral femoral condyle; and the medial head, from the posterior aspect of the medial femoral condyle) to insert

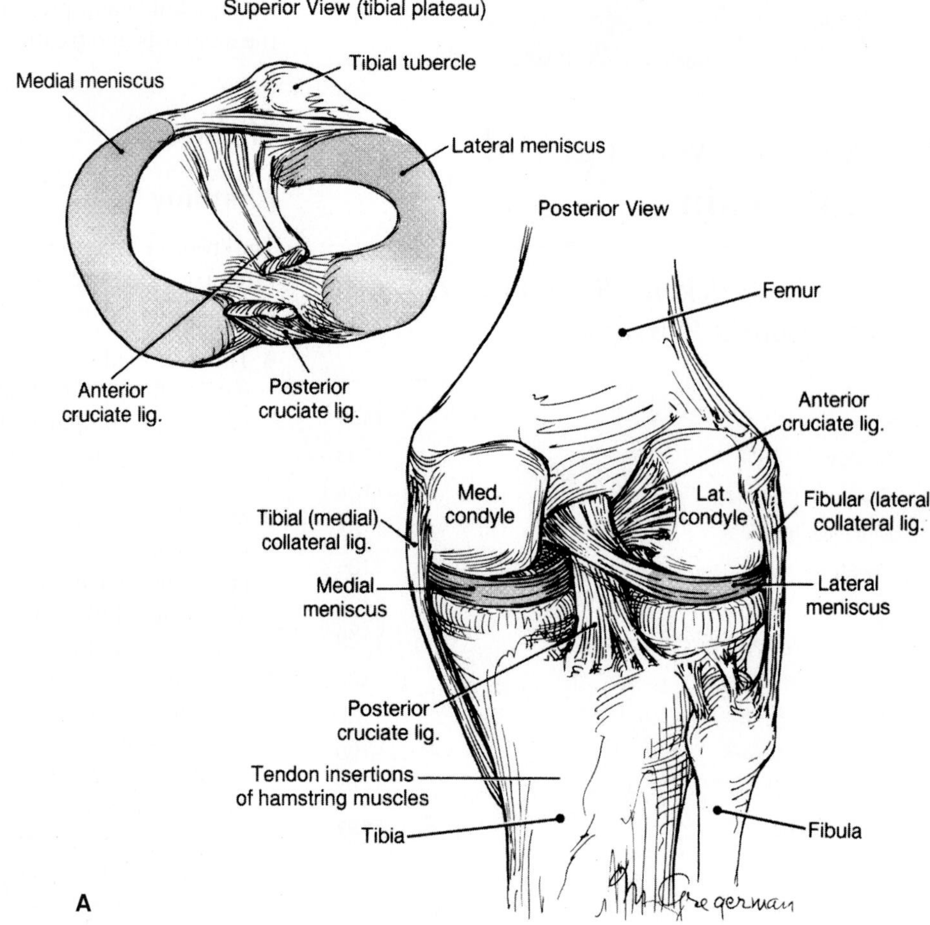

FIGURE 72.1. **A:** Important structures of the knee.

onto the calcaneus as the Achilles tendon. The quadriceps (rectus femoris, vastus medialis, vastus lateralis, and vastus intermedius) forms the extensor mechanism of the knee that inserts onto the patella via the quadriceps tendon and to the tibial tubercle from the patella via the patellar tendon. The patella by its position improves the mechanical advantage of the quadriceps. The patella is stabilized additionally by the medial and lateral retinaculum and the medial patellofemoral ligament (MPFL).

- The suprapatellar, prepatellar superficial patellar, retropatellar, and pes anserinus bursae are located strategically about the knee to reduce friction among its many dynamic components.
- The joint capsule of the knee joint is lined with a synovial membrane.

General Evaluation

A thorough history is essential to evaluation of knee pain. The history should include any episodes of trauma (acute, remote, or chronic), repetitive stress, or overuse; exacerbating factors; location of pain and its radiation; presence of swelling; and mechanical symptoms, such as catching, locking, and giving way.

A systematic, basic knee examination is presented here. Emphasis should be placed on the need to examine the affected knee and to compare it with the contralateral knee.

- The patient should be dressed in a gown or shorts that allow clear visualization and palpation of both knees.
- To visualize alignment, the knee should be inspected from the front, back, and side while the patient is standing. In addition to observing for varus ("bowed leg"), valgus ("knock-knee"), and recurvatum ("hyperextension") alignment of the knee, the overall alignment of the lower limb (e.g., hip anteversion and retroversion, tibial internal and external rotation, and pes planus and cavus) should be noted because it can affect knee function. Alignment of the extensor mechanism can be inspected with the patient supine and with the patient sitting with the knee flexed 90 degrees over the side of the examination table.
- The knee should be examined for swelling. An intra-articular swelling is called an *effusion.* With the patient supine, the suprapatellar pouch is "milked" distally to identify an intra-articular effusion. A large enough effusion can obliterate the dimple along the medial aspect of the knee. A large, tense effusion after an acute injury represents blood in the joint (hemarthrosis).

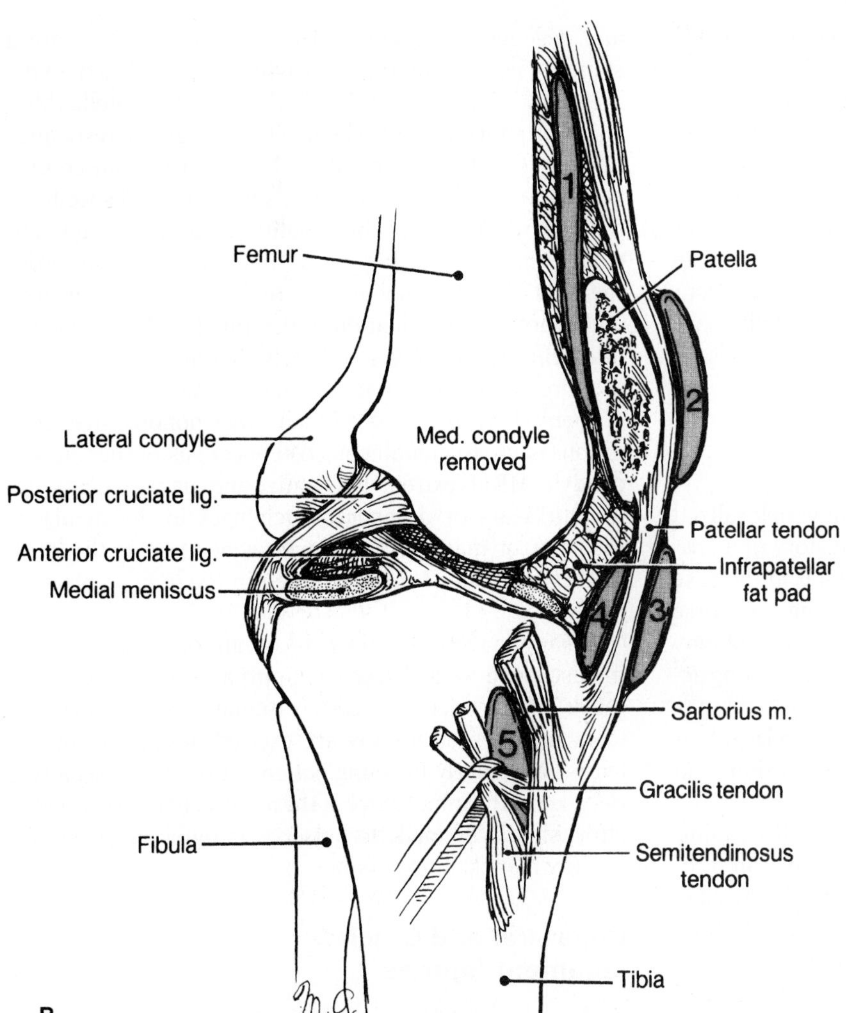

FIGURE 72.1. (Continued) **B:** Five bursae of the knee: suprapatellar, prepatellar, superficial patellar tendon, retropatellar tendon, and pes anserinus.

Varying amounts of chronic effusion represent the synovial membrane's response to inflammation, which may be mechanical or biologic. A large effusion will allow one to ballot or "bob" the patella. Large effusions can result in pain and stimulation of mechanoreceptors in the joint, causing quadriceps mechanism inhibition and weakness. Swelling about the knee can be extra-articular and extensive. Bursae, particularly the prepatellar bursa, can become quite large and mimic an effusion; the discriminating point is that in an effusion the patella can be palpated and balloted, whereas it usually cannot in prepatellar bursitis. With severe injuries to the knee that involve tearing of the capsule, the hemarthrosis may leak out into the surrounding tissues, making the effusion less dramatic, but usually ecchymosis is visible at the area of capsular injury.

- The knee joint's range of motion (ROM) is determined with the patient supine. (Normal range of motion is from 0 degrees full extension to 130 degrees full flexion). First, the knee is examined for hyperextension. Most patients have some degree of hyperextension (0–10 degrees), so the amount of hyperextension in the affected knee should be compared to that of the contralateral knee. Loss of even a small amount of hyperextension can indicate a displaced meniscus tear, arthrofibrosis (i.e., intracapsular and pericapsular scarring), loose body, or impinging osteophytes and soft tissues. Then, flexion in the affected knee is measured and compared with that of the contralateral knee. Intra-articular effusion is the most common cause of lost knee flexion.
- Next, the knee is palpated. Even in obese patients, a careful, systematic palpation can localize an abnormality. Structures to be palpated include the MCL and LCL throughout their courses, the medial and lateral joint lines, the extensor mechanism, the quadriceps tendon, patella, and patellar tendon. Pain elicited along the joint line is very sensitive for meniscal disease and arthritis.

Meniscal Injuries

Definition and Mechanism of Injury

Menisci (see above) frequently are injured, usually as a result of a twisting motion of the knee on a fixed or planted foot. Meniscal tears can occur when an individual performs a deep squat followed by a forceful extension to a standing position. In young patients (<30 years old), meniscal injuries usually occur in concert with an injury to a ligament. A meniscus tear can occur in a knee with normal ligaments, but the tear usually occurs through a degenerated portion of the meniscus. Because the menisci are secondary stabilizers, they are at increased risk for tearing with subsequent giving-way episodes in knees in which the ACLs are defective. Degenerative tears can occur with relatively minor trauma. Such patients usually have a prodrome of joint-line tenderness before the meniscus tear.

Signs and Symptoms

Patients with meniscal tears usually present with localized joint-line tenderness and swelling and a history of a specific twisting injury, which may be incidental in the case of a degenerated meniscus. Pain and swelling are worse with weight-bearing and impact-loading activity and may improve with rest. Patients have difficulty with twisting activities and squatting. If the tear displaces, the patient may complain of the knee catching or giving way. If a large tear displaces, it can lock the knee, block full extension, and cause difficulty with walking.

On examination, patients usually have localized joint-line tenderness and, if the tear is symptomatic, an effusion. The *McMurray* test is a sensitive, but not specific, test for meniscal pathology (1). The test consists of fully flexing the knee of a supine patient, internally rotating the tibia and providing a varus force to pinch the medial meniscus, and then extending the knee. The procedure is repeated with a valgus force to pinch the lateral meniscus. A painful clunk during either part of the test is very suggestive of a displaceable meniscus tear. Some normal mobile menisci may elicit a clear clunk without pain; this finding should be similar in the contralateral knee. Pain alone with the McMurray test is suggestive of a meniscus tear.

Treatment and Prognosis

The overall condition of the knee will dictate the urgency of referral to an orthopedic surgeon. Most symptomatic meniscus tears can be treated with activity modification; rest, ice, compression, and elevation (RICE protocol); and a short course of a nonsteroidal anti-inflammatory medication (NSAID), followed by a referral to an orthopedic surgeon if needed. If the patient's knee is locked (unable to obtain full extension) or the meniscus tear is associated with ligament instability, a more urgent referral to an orthopedic surgeon should be made.

Because meniscus tears usually occur with an injury, radiographs are indicated to rule out a fracture. Radiographs also can provide important information about alignment and degenerative changes. The most useful views are a standing posteroanterior view with the knee flexed 30 degrees and a lateral and tangential view of the patella (Merchant or sunrise view). The need for magnetic resonance imaging (MRI) and who should order it remain controversial. MRI has more than 90% sensitivity and specificity for detecting meniscal abnormality and a strong argument can be made for having the primary care clinician order the MRI. The MRI should not replace a detailed history and thorough examination, but a timely MRI may expedite definitive diagnosis and early treatment. An orthopedic surgeon may order an MRI, not to make the diagnosis of meniscus tear but to rule out other nonoperative conditions such as spontaneous osteonecrosis of the femoral condyle. MRI is extremely sensitive and may detect asymptomatic tears or degenerative changes in the meniscus that may or may not be the pain generators in the knee. MRI findings must be interpreted in the light of physical findings.

Treatment usually consists of an operation on the meniscus via an arthroscopic approach. The central two thirds of the meniscus are avascular, and degenerative tears in this area usually are excised. Large, peripheral tears, particularly in young patients, usually are repaired. Because of the importance of the menisci to the knee, every effort should be made to preserve as much of the stable, healthy meniscus as possible.

Collateral and Cruciate Ligament Injuries

Definition and Mechanism of Injury

Injuries to the ligaments of the knee represent substantial pathology that, if not recognized, can result in instability and additional injury. The MCL is the primary restraint to valgus loading and a secondary restraint to rotational force. The most common mechanism of injury to the MCL is a direct impact on the lateral aspect of the knee, "booking open" the medial compartment. ACL injuries can occur from contact injuries but they occur more commonly from noncontact injuries, as when an individual pivots or changes direction quickly or lands off balance from a jump. PCL injuries usually result from a direct blow to the front of the proximal tibia, such as a dashboard injury in a motor vehicle accident. Isolated LCL injuries are rare (<1% of ligament injuries) because the contralateral leg provides protection against direct contact with the medial aspect of the knee (2). LCL injuries usually occur in concert with ACL and/or PCL injuries.

Signs and Symptoms

ACL injuries usually occur with an audible pop or snap, followed by immediate swelling and pain in the knee and the inability to return to competition. Depending on associated disease, patients may or may not be able to bear weight. They describe a giving-way sensation with any lateral or rotational movement. On examination, a patient has difficulty obtaining full extension and has a large, tense a hemarthrosis. Of all hemarthroses that occur after injury in healthy patients, 75% result from ACL injury (3,4).

Acutely, the knee is very painful and difficult to examine. The most diagnostic test is the *Lachman* test, a gentle, painless, but subtle evaluation. With the knee flexed 15 to 20 degrees, the femur is stabilized with the examiner's opposite hand (for a right-side ACL, the examiner uses the left hand). The tibia is pulled gently forward with the other hand. The observer looks for tibial translation anteriorly and the quality of the termination of motion (end point), that is, does the motion end firmly or softly? The findings are compared with those of the contralateral knee. Other tests with which to diagnose an ACL-deficient knee include the *anterior drawer* and *pivot shift* tests. For the anterior drawer test, the patient is positioned supine with the injured knee flexed 90 degrees and the hamstrings relaxed. The examiner sits on the patient's foot, and the tibia is pulled forward. This test is not very sensitive for an acute ACL injury (5). The pivot shift test is performed with the supine patient's knee fully extended. When the tibia is internally rotated and a valgus force is applied to the knee as it is flexed, the knee "shifts" or reduces from the subluxated position. This test reproduces the giving-way phenomenon the patient experiences. Because this test can be painful and cause apprehension, the patient must be relaxed and cooperative. Typically, the pivot shift cannot be tested in the painful, acutely injured knee. Joint-line tenderness associated with an ACL injury may represent meniscal injury, collateral ligament injury, or bone bruising.

The MCL and LCL are easily palpated, and the site of injury can be localized. The integrity of the collateral ligaments is tested by applying valgus and varus force with the knee in 0 degrees and 15 degrees flexion. In the painful, acutely injured knee, this examination is best accomplished with the patient in the supine position, the affected hip abducted, and the affected thigh resting on the examination table. With the patient in this position, the thigh is supported and the patient is more relaxed. Valgus force is administered to the medial leg to test the MCL, and a varus force is administered to the lateral leg to test the LCL. At 15 degrees flexion, the collateral ligaments are the isolated primary stabilizers. Collateral ligament injury can be categorized in three degrees: *first degree,* varus or valgus force generates pain but does not elicit any joint-line opening; *second degree,* the joint line gaps but has an end point; and *third degree*, the joint opens widely without an end point, indicating complete disruption of the ligament. At 0 degrees flexion, the cruciate ligaments provide additional stability against varus and valgus stress. Medial or lateral joint-line opening at 0 degrees flexion indicates a severe injury involving rupture of at least one collateral and one cruciate ligament.

The PCL is best tested with a posterior drawer test. With the patient in a supine position, the affected knee is flexed 90 degrees, and the examiner sits on the patient's foot to stabilize it. The knee is observed for posterior sagging. The examiner then exerts a posteriorly directed force on the proximal tibia. If the anterior lip of the tibial plateau extends beyond the anterior edge of the femoral condyles, the patient has sustained a severe PCL injury. If the tibia stays anterior or equal to the femoral condyles, the patient has a minor PCL injury (6,7). The quadriceps active drawer test also can demonstrate PCL insufficiency (7). In the same position as for a posterior drawer test (described above), the patient pushes the stabilized foot down on the examination table. In the PCL-injured patient, the quadriceps contraction pulls the proximal tibia anteriorly.

If the examination indicates that two or more ligaments are injured, one must consider that the patient has had a knee dislocation that spontaneously reduced. The clinician should perform a detailed distal neurovascular examination to assess possible injury to the popliteal artery and peroneal nerve.

Treatment and Prognosis

These ligamentous injuries are best treated with the RICE protocol, which reduces pain and swelling. NSAIDs are a useful adjunct. Additionally, the knee should be placed in a knee immobilizer for support. Radiographs should be obtained to rule out fracture. The presence of a Segond fracture, a small avulsion fracture of the proximal lateral tibial plateau, is pathognomonic for an ACL injury. Additionally, each collateral and cruciate ligament can fail by pulling off of its bony insertion. Almost always, MRI is required to assess completely the damage to the knee before a treatment plan is developed.

A patient with an ACL injury should be referred to an orthopedic surgeon for complete evaluation and treatment. Isolated MCL injuries are treated nonoperatively and require protective bracing until healed. If a patient has an MCL injury from a noncontact injury, an ACL injury should be suspected. Treatment of a PCL injury depends on its severity: low-grade PCL injuries are treated nonoperatively, but high-grade PCL injuries may require surgery in high-demand patients. LCL injuries almost always occur in conjunction with a cruciate ligament injury. Isolated or associated LCL injuries almost always are repaired or reconstructed.

Because the natural history of an ACL-deficient knee is not completely understood, there is much discussion and controversy about its treatment. In young, active patients, an ACL-deficient knee is prone to recurrent giving way, with more damage to the knee, particularly to the menisci and articular surfaces, which can lead to posttraumatic arthritis. ACL reconstruction is recommended for these high-risk patients. Many low-demand, typically older patients can function well without an ACL if they observe proper activity modification, such as eliminating pivoting and jumping activities. Some patients without an ACL are disabled, even in terms of activities of daily living, and are candidates for reconstruction. Although an ACL reconstruction is safe, reliable, and predictable, it represents a big decision for the patient and surgeon. An extensive preoperative and postoperative rehabilitation program is essential for an excellent result.

Knee dislocations should be given an urgent referral to an orthopedic surgeon because such injuries almost always require extensive surgery.

Preoperative rehabilitation (improving ROM, obtaining quadriceps function, and reducing swelling) is valuable in preparing patients with ligamentous injury for surgery because it decreases postoperative stiffness and weakness.

Patella Dislocations

Definition and Mechanism of Injury

Dislocation of the patella is a common injury and represents the second most common cause (after ACL injury) of a traumatic knee hemarthrosis. The mechanism is very similar to that of a noncontact ACL injury: a quick, pivoting motion on a planted foot, with the knee relatively extended. The patella dislocates laterally with a pop. It may reduce spontaneously (with another pop) or remain dislocated lateral to the lateral femoral condyle. Medial patellar dislocations are extremely rare and usually are iatrogenic, secondary to overvigorous surgical treatment of lateral patellar instability (8).

There are two distinct types of patella dislocations: (a) traumatic, which results from a severe injury to the knee and has limited increased risk of reinjury after appropriate treatment; and (b) atraumatic, which results from a relatively minor trauma or after a traumatic dislocation and is more likely to recur. Patients at risk for reinjury are those with patellar malalignment, long patellar tendons (patella alta), generalized ligamentous laxity, or a deficient vastus medialis obliquus. Examining the contralateral uninjured knee helps identify patients at risk for reinjury.

Signs and Symptoms

Patients may present acutely to the emergency room with the patella still dislocated. With relaxation and gentle straightening of the knee, the patella can be pushed gently back into place. Many dislocated patellas spontaneously reduce, and the patient presents with large, tense hemarthroses and medial retinacular pain, indicating rupture of the MPFL complex, which courses from the medial epicondyle (just anterior to the proximal MCL attachment) and inserts along the superior medial corner of the patella.

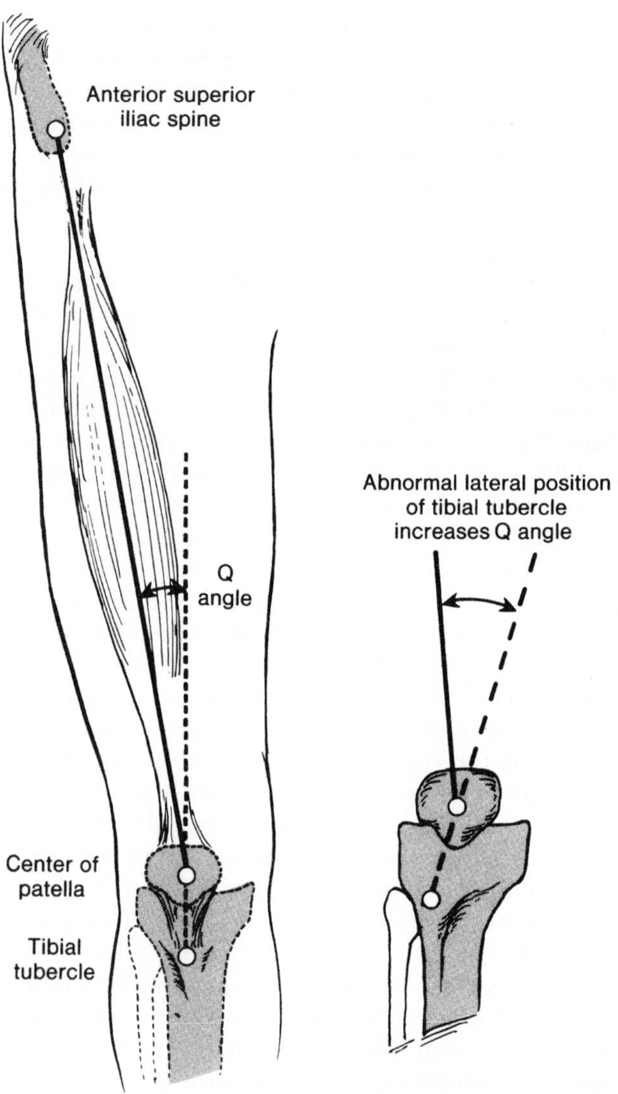

FIGURE 72.2. The Q angle is constructed by a line connecting the anterior superior iliac spine with the center of the patella to a second line connecting the center of the patella with the tibial tubercle **(left).** The normal angle is up to 20 degrees. **Right:** Abnormal Q angle.

In addition to pain over the ligament, blood leaking into the medial patellar retinacular provides a "doughy" feel to the soft tissue in this area. With a laterally directed force on the patella, one can elicit apprehension in the patient. Special attention should be given to overall limb and patellar alignment and tracking. Patients with femoral anteroversion, tibial torsion, patella alta, and a large quadriceps angle (Q angle, Fig. 72.2) are at risk for recurrent dislocation.

Treatment and Prognosis

Patients with a patellar dislocation should be treated with the RICE protocol to reduce pain and swelling. NSAIDs are an appropriate adjunct. Use of a brace or cast is extremely controversial (9). Although knee immobilization is not an unusual treatment for a patellar dislocation, the patella is more unstable in an extended knee than in a flexed knee; therefore, a lateral buttress brace that allows knee flexion and provides a buttress to lateral patellar displacement may be a better choice than immobilization bracing. Additionally, prolonged immobilization leads to quadriceps atrophy and weakness, which is counterproductive; quadriceps strength is the main stabilizer of the patella. Radiographs, including a tangential view of the patella, should be obtained to identify loose fragments that may have occurred with the patellar dislocation or reduction. Use of MRI is helpful but is not indicated for every patellar dislocation. MPFL repair and/or reconstruction is gaining popularity, particularly with patients who have recurrent dislocations. If surgery is contemplated, MRI can identify the area of MPFL injury. MRI can document chondral loose bodies not seen on plain radiographs but which are suspected if the traumatic effusion does not clear in 3 weeks. MRI also should be ordered if an injury in addition to the patellar dislocation, such as an ACL injury, is suspected.

The mainstay of treatment for patella dislocations is physical therapy, which provides most patients with quick resolution of the effusion and improvement in ROM and quadriceps function. Patients with recurrent patella dislocations, atraumatic dislocations, or loose bodies should be referred to an orthopedic surgeon for definitive evaluation and treatment. Surgical treatment may include arthroscopy, open or arthroscopic lateral release, distal patellar realignment, proximal patellar realignment, proximal and distal realignment, and MPFL repair or reconstruction.

Extensor Mechanism Disruption

Definition and Mechanism of Injury

The extensor mechanism, which consists of the quadriceps tendon, patella, and patella tendon, actively extends the knee joint and stabilizes it for locomotion. Rupture of the quadriceps or patellar tendon can result from a forceful quadriceps concentric contraction (such as occurs in jumping) or eccentric contraction (such as occurs when landing from a jump). A direct blow to the patella with the knee in flexion can result in a patella fracture. Tendon rupture also can occur from a corticosteroid injection (e.g., given for tendinitis) in or around the quadriceps or patellar tendon.

Signs and Symptoms

A patient with an extensor mechanism disruption has pain, swelling, inability to extend the knee completely, and difficulty bearing weight. In addition to an effusion and soft-tissue swelling, there is a palpable defect at the site of disruption. With a quadriceps tendon rupture, the patella migrates distally, whereas with a patellar tendon rupture, the patella retracts proximally. A patient with a complete rupture cannot extend the knee, whereas a patient with an incomplete rupture or an intact patellar retinaculum can extend the knee from a partially flexed position.

Treatment and Prognosis

Radiographs should be obtained to document the site of injury to the extensor mechanism. MRI is helpful (but not necessary) for making the diagnosis. The knee should be placed in a knee immobilizer, and the patient should be referred urgently to an orthopedic surgeon. Treatment consists of primary repair of the ruptured tendon or open reduction and internal fixation of a patellar fracture. In rare circumstances, such as a <50% tear in a low-demand patient, partial patellar or quadriceps tendon injuries can be treated with immobilization.

Patellofemoral Pain

Definition and Mechanism of Injury

The extensor mechanism is subjected to magnified forces by many activities, such as ascending/descending stairs, running, squatting, and jumping. Repetitive overuse from such activities can cause pain. In the adolescent, this pain can be localized to the tibial tubercle, the distal insertion of the patellar tendon, causing a traction apophysitis. In adults, such repetitive overactivity may lead to patellar or quadriceps tendinitis. Additionally, patients with malalignment and maltracking have increased patellofemoral pain with repetitive overuse.

Signs and Symptoms

A patient with patellofemoral pain from any of the causes listed has pain around the patella with ascending/descending stairs, running, jumping, squatting, kneeling, or prolonged sitting. Swelling seldom occurs, but there may be crepitus over the patella or quadriceps tendon. Close attention should be paid to patellar stability, alignment, and tracking. A patient with subtle patellar instability has increased patellar mobility, moving more than two quadrants medially or laterally. Patients may have decreased patellar motion and lateral patellar compression. Additionally, patients with chronic patellofemoral pain may have hamstring and hip flexor tightness and core muscle weakness and imbalance. Radiographs should be ordered to rule out rare conditions such as osteochondritis desiccans (osteochondral defect) of the patella, tumor, and bipartite patella, but otherwise they seldom are helpful. Adolescent patients with traction apophysitis may have increased separation or fragmentation of the apophysis. Chronic tendinitis may show tendon calcification. MRI is recommended only for the most recalcitrant cases.

Treatment and Prognosis

Most patellofemoral pain is self-limiting and will respond to the RICE protocol and reduced activity. If symptoms persist, patients should be afforded a trial of physical therapy, consisting of core strengthening, stretching, and quadriceps open and closed concentric and eccentric strengthening. Additionally, a therapist may use a battery of modalities, including ultrasound, cryotherapy, phonophoresis, iontophoresis, electrostimulation, and cross-friction massage. Patellar malalignment, instability, and maltracking can be improved after treatment with McConnell taping (application of tape to the patella) to improve patellofemoral mechanics (10).

Patients with recalcitrant or recurrent patellofemoral pain should be referred to a physiatrist or orthopedic surgeon for additional evaluation. These conditions seldom require surgery.

Bursitis

Definition and Mechanism of Injury

A bursa is a synovial-lined space that separates adjacent moveable structures, such as tendon or skin and bone, to reduce friction. Overuse can create chronic friction and fluid within the bursa. The bursa can collect fluid from direct trauma and inflammatory processes such as gout and infection.

The bursae commonly located about the knee include the prepatellar bursa (anterior to the patella), retropatellar bursa (posterior to the patellar tendon), pes anserinus bursa (between the distal medial hamstrings and the proximal medial tibia), and iliotibial band (ITB) bursa (located between the ITB and the lateral femoral condyle). ITB bursitis usually results from ITB tendinitis, which commonly develops from a change in a running routine, training errors, real or functional limb-length discrepancies, core weakness, and core muscle imbalance. Prepatellar bursitis can arise from chronic irritation to the anterior part of the knee, as occurs with prolonged kneeling by plumbers or commercial carpet installers.

Signs and Symptoms

Prepatellar bursitis usually presents with painful swelling anterior to the patella. Because the fluid is in front of the patella, the patella is not ballotable. Traumatic bursitis may be accompanied by ecchymosis, and the contained fluid is hemorrhagic. Inflammatory bursitis is painful and presents with warmth and redness. Aspiration may be needed to differentiate a septic process. Septic bursitis has marked warmth, cellulitis, and usually a portal of entry (folliculitis or insect bite). Advanced cases may be associated with lymphangitis and fever.

ITB bursitis/tendinitis presents with localized tenderness over the distal ITB at the lateral epicondyle and possibly down to its insertion on the Gerdy tubercle. ITB tightness can be elicited by the *Ober* test (11). The Ober test is performed with the patient lying in the lateral decubitus position with the affected limb up. The examiner uses his/her forearm and hand to cradle the patient's knee, flexes and then abducts the patient's hip, and then extends that hip. If the ITB is tight, the leg will remain suspended above the horizontal. Flexing and extending the knee from 15 to 40 degrees in this position elicits pain, crepitance, or snapping at the lateral femoral epicondyle. (At 30 degrees, the ITB typically lies over the lateral femoral condyle. Extended from this position, it is anterior to the lateral femoral epicondyle; flexed from that position, it is posterior to the femoral epicondyle.)

Pes bursitis presents with pain and swelling along the distal insertion of the medial hamstrings, gracilis, semimembranosus, and semitendinosus along the proximal medial tibial plateau. The hamstrings may be tight. Chapter 74 discusses anserine bursitis and its treatment.

Treatment and Prognosis

Bursitis and tendinitis can be treated effectively with the RICE protocol. A short course of NSAIDs may be a helpful adjunct (see Chapter 74). If tendinitis is associated with the bursitis, a physical therapy evaluation is warranted. In addition to traditional stretching and strengthening, the therapists will assess the patient for underlying alignment problems and imbalances and may use modalities such as cryotherapy, iontophoresis, phonophoresis, cross-friction massage, or electrical stimulation to reduce symptoms and improve healing.

If the bursitis persists despite nonoperative treatment, the fluid can be aspirated and a compression dressing can be applied to prevent reaccumulation of the fluid.

If nonoperative treatment (including a well-documented program of physical therapy) for ITB tendinitis and bursitis has failed, referral to an orthopedic surgeon is indicated. Surgery would include excision of the bursa, with lengthening and/or partial sectioning of the ITB to reduce friction at the lateral femoral epicondyle.

Septic bursitis should be treated with aspiration to obtain fluid for culture and sensitivities, and then appropriate parenteral or intravenous antibiotics should be administered. If the septic bursa is associated with fever or lymphangitis, the bursa should be incised, drained, and packed open. This intervention should be performed in an operating room or procedure room setting, which would necessitate a referral to an orthopedic surgeon.

Baker Cysts

Definition and Mechanism of Injury

A popliteal cyst, commonly called a Baker cyst (see Chapter 74), is a synovial cyst that forms in the popliteal space contiguous to the knee-joint cavity. Typically, it is seen with degenerative meniscal tears. It also can occur with arthritis of the knee and other inflammatory conditions. The knee joint produces fluid in response to mechanical or biologic inflammation and, as the knee is flexed, the fluid is forced posteriorly. Over time, a popliteal cyst may develop.

Signs and Symptoms

Most Baker cysts are asymptomatic and are noted incidentally on physical examination or MRI. As the cyst grows, it produces a sensation of fullness behind the flexed knee. If the Baker cyst becomes extremely large, it can produce compressive symptoms, particularly of the posterior tibial nerve.

Treatment and Prognosis

Most popliteal cysts resolve or reduce with appropriate treatment of the knee effusion. If a cyst accompanies a degenerative meniscus tear, excision of the tear will decompress the cyst. Occasionally, the cyst requires aspiration or, more rarely, excision. Aspiration or excision without addressing the intra-articular problem may result in cyst recurrence.

Popliteal cysts in preadolescent patients usually resolve spontaneously and do not need treatment unless an intra-articular problem is present.

If a large popliteal cyst ruptures, it may be accompanied by intense pain and swelling in the patient's posterior calf. The symptoms mimic deep venous thrombosis, and a vascular study may be required to rule out deep venous thrombosis.

Septic Knee

Definition and Mechanism of Injury

A deep-space knee infection represents an orthopedic emergency. The knee can be seeded from direct inoculation (knee aspiration or penetrating trauma), hematogenous spread (from a distant infection), or local adjacent tissues. Predisposing factors include arthritis, gout, intravenous drug abuse, alcoholism, diabetes, systemic steroids, or immunosuppression.

Signs and Symptoms

Patients present with pain, swelling, warmth, redness, difficulty with weight-bearing, and painful and limited ROM.

Treatment and Prognosis

A knee-joint aspiration is indicated for all painful, nontraumatic knee effusions. It is important to aspirate the knee through noncellulitic skin to avoid inoculating the knee joint. In addition to culture and sensitivity, a cell count of the aspirated fluid is important. Although white blood cell counts >50,000 can be found with gout, such levels are suspicious for infection. White cell counts >100,000 represent a septic process. If the patient is sexually active, a diagnosis of gonorrhea should be investigated. In Lyme-endemic geographic areas, the patient should be assessed for Lyme disease with appropriate cultures and titers.

Treatment almost always requires incision and drainage, historically via arthrotomy followed by inflow/outflow drains. Arthroscopic lavage and synovial resection are adequate for most septic knees. If surgical treatment is delayed, repeat aspirations and intravenous antibiotics are appropriate initial interventions.

THE LOWER LEG

Anatomy

The principal anatomic components of the leg and their function are as follows:

- The bony structures are composed of the tibia medially and the fibula laterally. The tibia is the main weight-bearing bone.
- The leg has four fascial compartments: anterior, lateral, superficial posterior, and deep posterior compartments (Fig. 72.3).
- The anterior compartment contains the tibialis anterior, extensor hallucis longus, extensor digitorum longus, and peroneus tertius muscles. These muscles dorsiflex the ankle, hallux (or great toe), and lesser toes. The neurovascular supply to this compartment is via the deep peroneal nerve and anterior tibial artery.
- The lateral compartment contains the peroneus longus and brevis muscles. These muscles, innervated by the superficial peroneal nerve, primarily evert the foot and are

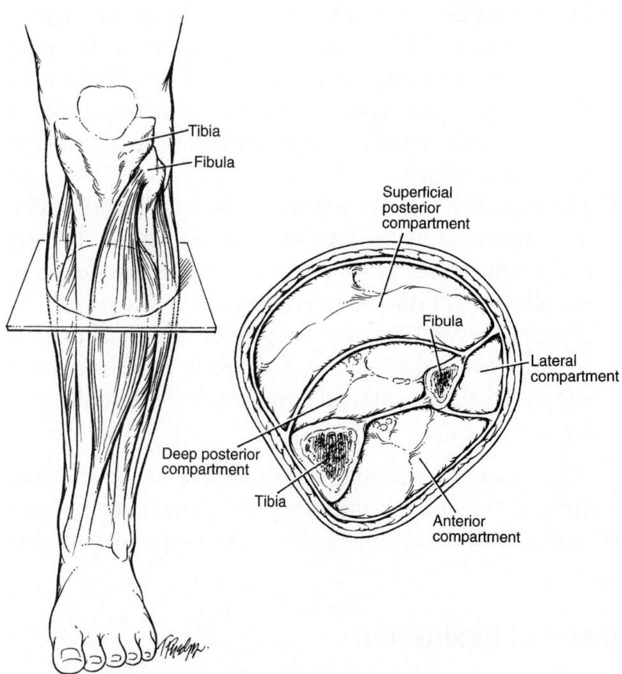

FIGURE 72.3. Leg anatomy. **Left:** Coronal view. **Right:** Cross-sectional view showing compartments.

important dynamic stabilizers for the ankle. This compartment does not contain an artery, but the peroneus muscles receive their blood supply via branches of the peroneal artery, a tributary of the posterior tibial artery.

- The superficial posterior compartment contains the soleus and gastrocnemius muscles and the plantaris tendon. These two muscles merge distally to form the Achilles tendon. These muscles are powerful plantarflexors of the ankle, particularly in the gait cycle. In addition, they act eccentrically at foot strike to control ankle motion. The tibial artery and posterior tibial nerve supply these muscles.
- The deep posterior compartment contains the tibialis posterior, flexor hallucis longus, and the flexor digitorum longus muscles. These muscles are primarily invertors and plantarflexors of the foot, ankle, and lesser toes. The tibialis posterior also is a dynamic ankle stabilizer. This compartment is innervated by the posterior tibial nerve and vascularized by the posterior tibial and peroneal arteries.
- The interosseus membrane, a fibrous connection between the lateral border of the tibia and the medial border of the fibula, runs almost the entire length of each bone, separating the anterior and deep posterior compartments. It also contributes to the syndesmotic stability of the ankle joint.
- The common peroneal nerve courses along the proximal neck of the fibula under the peroneus longus and then branches into its deep and superficial branches. The deep peroneal nerve then enters the anterior compartment, whereas the superficial peroneal nerve stays in the lateral compartment.
- The superficial veins, which include the greater saphenous vein (which lies medial to the crest of the tibia) and the lesser saphenous vein (which lies in the mid-posterior calf and courses around the lateral malleolus), drain the anteromedial and posterolateral aspects of the ankle, respectively.
- The superficial nerves are the saphenous nerve, superficial peroneal nerve, and sural nerve. The saphenous nerve runs along with the greater saphenous vein and supplies the skin on the anteromedial leg. The superficial peroneal nerve innervates the skin on the distal anterolateral leg and the dorsum of the foot. The sural nerve supplies the posterior and posterolateral portions of the leg.

Knowledge of lower-limb neuroanatomy, lumbar root source, nerve course, muscle innervation, and sensory components is invaluable to the evaluation and diagnosis of leg pain.

General Evaluation

As with the knee, injuries to the leg can be caused by a single traumatic event or chronic, repetitive stress. An appropriate history is essential (see Chapter 68). The clinician must define the mechanism of injury. If no acute trauma has occurred, then stress injury from chronic repetitive activity or increase in the frequency or duration of the activity is the likely cause. Pain in the leg may be referred pain from back, pelvis, or hip abnormalities. As with the knee, the general principles of inspection, palpation, and evaluation of ROM and strength are addressed:

- One should *inspect* the leg for any gross deformity or swelling, observe for any superficial abrasion, ecchymosis, or laceration, and compare it with the normal contralateral limb.
- The entire medial crest of the tibia from the plateau to the medial malleolus and the fibular head proximally and its distal extension (the lateral malleolus) should be *palpated*. The common peroneal nerve wraps around the proximal fibula before it branches, and injury to this area can affect both the superficial and the deep peroneal nerves.
- All fascial compartments should feel soft during palpation. If any compartment feels tense or swollen after trauma, a compartment syndrome must be ruled out by physical examination and measurement of compartment pressures (see section Acute Compartment Syndrome). In addition, fascial hernias, or defects in the fascia, may be palpated. These defects occur at normal exit sites for the traversing nerve across the fascia or as a result of direct trauma or exertional compartment syndrome.
- The *strength* of the muscles in each compartment should be tested. Each motion should be graded on a 0- to 5-point muscle strength scale (see Chapter 86).
- *Sensory examination* should be performed over the appropriate dermatomes and superficial nerve distributions.

Differential Diagnosis of Acute Leg Pain

Trauma is a common cause of acute leg pain. Blunt trauma can result in a contusion or, if severe enough, fracture of the tibia and fibula. Because of the superficial nature of the medial border of the tibia, high-energy injuries usually result in an open fracture. Acute pain can result from muscle strain and/or rupture. Rupture (partial or complete) of the proximal medial or lateral head of the gastrocnemius or plantaris can result in severe pain and swelling, mimicking deep venous thrombosis. Delayed-onset muscle soreness and tendinitis are the most common causes of acute pain with a sudden increase in lower leg activity. More rarely, such acute pain can be the result of stress fracture or compartment syndrome. Other etiologies of lower leg pain include sciatica (from a herniated disk or other cause), deep venous thrombosis (see Chapter 57), neurogenic and vascular claudication (see Chapter 94), cellulitis (see Chapter 32), myopathy and neuropathy (see Chapter 92), and acute monoarthritis (see Chapter 76).

Acute Compartment Syndrome

Definition and Mechanism of Injury

Compartment syndrome not only is a cause of acute leg pain; it also is a surgical emergency that requires early recognition for a favorable outcome. It is associated with a high rate and amount of indemnity payments in malpractice suits (12). The lower leg contains four compartments (anterior, lateral, superior posterior, and deep posterior) surrounded by a dense, unifying fascia. Injury to the tissues of the lower extremity causes bleeding and swelling. As this bleeding and swelling increase, the pressure in the compartment(s) rises. This scenario is compounded when the compartment pressure eclipses the venous pressure, stopping flow out of the compartment while arterial flow into the compartment continues, escalating the rise in pressure. When compartment pressure exceeds mean arterial pressure, an ischemic process begins to develop and, with time, can lead to muscle and nerve injury and necrosis.

A common misconception is that a fracture is needed to create a compartment syndrome. A compartment syndrome can develop from seemingly minor trauma (e.g., muscle contusion or ankle sprain) or prolonged pressure (as can occur in an individual, overdosed with drugs or alcohol, lying on the lower leg). It can also be exercise-induced or chronic. (See Exertional or Chronic Compartment Syndrome).

Signs and Symptoms

In the awake patient, the most common sign of compartment syndrome is pain out of proportion to the injury, pain that cannot be managed even with liberal doses of narcotics. The compartment(s) involved is swollen and tense. Passive stretch of the muscles through the compartment causes severe pain. Typically, the skin over the compartment has a red, shiny sheen and could mimic an early cellulitis. As the compartment syndrome develops, the patient experiences paresthesias in the distribution of the nerve traversing the compartment and paresis or weakness of the involved muscles. Pulselessness is a very late clinical finding. In trauma patients with low systolic pressure, compartment syndrome can develop at low pressures. Any diagnosis of compartment syndrome should be confirmed by pressure measurements in all suspected compartments.

If the patient is unconscious or uncooperative, compartment pressures can be measured easily with a commercially available unit. All four compartments should be measured.

Controversy exists regarding what pressure level constitutes a developing compartment syndrome, but most surgeons recommend surgical intervention when pressures are elevated to within 30 mm Hg of the patient's diastolic pressure (13).

Treatment and Prognosis

Acute compartment syndrome necessitates an emergent referral to an orthopedic surgeon for immediate fasciotomy of the involved compartments, which relieves the pressure. Elevated pressures for 6 to 8 hours can lead to irreversible muscle and nerve damage. Because extensive muscle damage can lead to rhabdomyolysis and renal failure, the clinician should monitor the patient for these possible developments and treat them accordingly.

Any injury to the lower leg that could lead to swelling should be treated with the RICE protocol in an effort to prevent the potential development of a compartment syndrome. Once a compartment syndrome develops, the limb should be kept horizontal because elevation can decrease mean arterial pressure.

Exertional Leg Pain

Leg pain with walking, running, or vigorous activity represents exertional leg pain and is a common presenting condition. Differential diagnoses include stress fractures, shin splints, medial tibial periostitis, exertional or chronic compartment syndrome, vascular or neurogenic claudication, and radicular nerve root irritation.

Stress Fractures

Definition and Mechanism of Injury

A stress fracture occurs when a bone undergoes excessive or suddenly increased cyclic loading. This mechanical stress stimulates osteoclastic activity, with eventual osteoblastic bone remodeling in an attempt to meet the increased load. If the bone remodeling cannot keep pace with the mechanical loading, the bone will fail with a microfracture or stress fracture. With continued loading, a stress fracture can progress to a complete fracture.

Stress fractures typically are seen in training athletes and military recruits (14). Although many physiologic and biomechanical factors (e.g., cross-sectional area of the tibia, bone mineral density, pes cavus or valgus, and excessive hip external rotation) have been suggested as etiologies of increased risk for stress fracture, training errors are the most common—and most treatable—causes. Training errors include improper footwear, excessive running mileage, and excessive speed work.

Insufficiency fractures are stress fractures that occur in weakened bones under normal loading stress.

Signs and Symptoms

A patient with a stress fracture typically notes the onset of pain with high-impact activity and abatement of the pain with rest. As the stress fracture evolves, the patient experiences pain with daily activities or even at rest. Detailed questioning usually can identify a training error, and on physical examination the patient usually has well-localized tenderness over the stress fracture site, with or without swelling or periosteal callus.

With excessive repetitive activity, a stress fracture can develop in almost any bone, including the sacrum, pubic rami, femoral neck (hip), femur, tibia, fibula, tarsals, and metatarsals. In the lower leg, stress fractures usually occur distally in the fibula and almost anywhere in the tibia (medial, proximal, and distal): in the tibial plateau (mimicking knee pathology), medial malleolus (mimicking ankle pathology), and anterior cortex of the tibial shaft.

Treatment and Prognosis

Typically, anteroposterior and lateral radiographs of the tibia and fibula do not show a stress fracture within the first 2 to 3 weeks of symptoms. Early radiographic findings actually represent early healing of the stress fracture, including periosteal callus and sclerosis across an invisible fracture line. An advanced stress fracture can display a radiographic fracture line, which indicates a risk for complete fracture and displacement.

A technetium bone scan allows one to identify stress fractures early (24 hours) in most patients; in the elderly, positive identification on bone scan may be delayed for 48 hours or more. MRI is an expensive but sensitive imaging study for identifying stress fractures. Short T1 inversion recovery (STIR) sequences can provide greater prognostic capability for stress fractures, which would be important in a competitive athlete.

Stress fractures should be referred to an orthopedic surgeon or physician who specializes in sports medicine. Most fractures heal uneventfully with "active rest" (i.e., reduction of activity to below-pain level) without immobilization, but some are prone to progression and/or nonunion (15,16). Initial treatment should limit activity to the point at which the pain begins. If the patient experiences pain with walking, crutches are prescribed. If no pain is associated with normal daily activity, some light, low-impact training is permissible as long as it occurs below the threshold of pain. Smoking should be discouraged to promote bone healing (see Chapter 27).

Training errors should be identified and corrected. If the patient with a stress fracture is a young woman, it is important to inquire about eating habits and menstrual irregularities. There is such a high correlation between stress fractures, amenorrhea, and eating disorders that this complex is referred to as the *female triad* (17). These patients may require additional referrals for bone density scanning, gynecologic evaluation, and psychological counseling (see Chapters 11, 101, and 103).

Stress fracture prevention includes proper training methods with cyclic or periodic rest to allow the bone an opportunity to remodel. As a general rule, runners should not increase their mileage by >10% per week. Other methods for reducing the risk of stress fracture include varying the exercise programs (cycling, swimming, elliptical trainers), wearing shock-absorbing shoes and/or insoles, and (especially for an individual in training) paying special attention to proper nutrition to support the increased physical needs.

Shin Splints

Definition and Mechanism of Injury

Shin splints are another common cause of exertional leg pain. They often occur with jogging, running, or sustained walking in poorly conditioned individuals and, as do stress fractures, can occur secondary to training errors, including improper shoe wear. Shin splints have been identified as medial tibial periostitis (18). Pain is thought to result from periostitis at the attachment of the posterior tibial muscle and/or the medial soleus on the midshaft of the medial tibia (Fig. 72.4).

Signs and Symptoms

Patients with shin splints have poorly localized tenderness at the junction of the middle and distal medial tibia. Swelling or crepitus may or may not be present.

Radiographs usually are negative but are obtained (after 2–3 weeks of symptoms) to rule out a stress fracture. MRI or a bone scan can be used to image recalcitrant cases and usually show vertical uptake above the medial tibial cortex.

Treatment and Prognosis

Shin splints respond to the RICE protocol and NSAID medication. As symptoms improve, activity can be advanced to the level of the pain threshold. Training errors should be identified and corrected. Patients will improve with formal physical therapy, which should address limb alignment, eccentric and concentric strengthening of the muscles of the lower leg, core strengthening, and modalities such as electrical stimulation, phonophoresis, iontophoresis, and ultrasound (19,20). If the patient has pes planus or cavus, orthotics should be prescribed (see Chapter 73).

Exertional or Chronic Compartment Syndrome

Definition and Mechanism of Injury

In the lower leg, there are four well-described muscle compartments encapsulated by fascial sheaths. When muscles are exercised, they swell. The fascia adjusts to muscle swelling. However, muscle swelling with activity can result in an exercise-related compartment syndrome, although the direct cause remains elusive. Some patients are unable to exercise vigorously for extended periods because of leg pain; other patients develop symptoms with activities they previously could perform without pain.

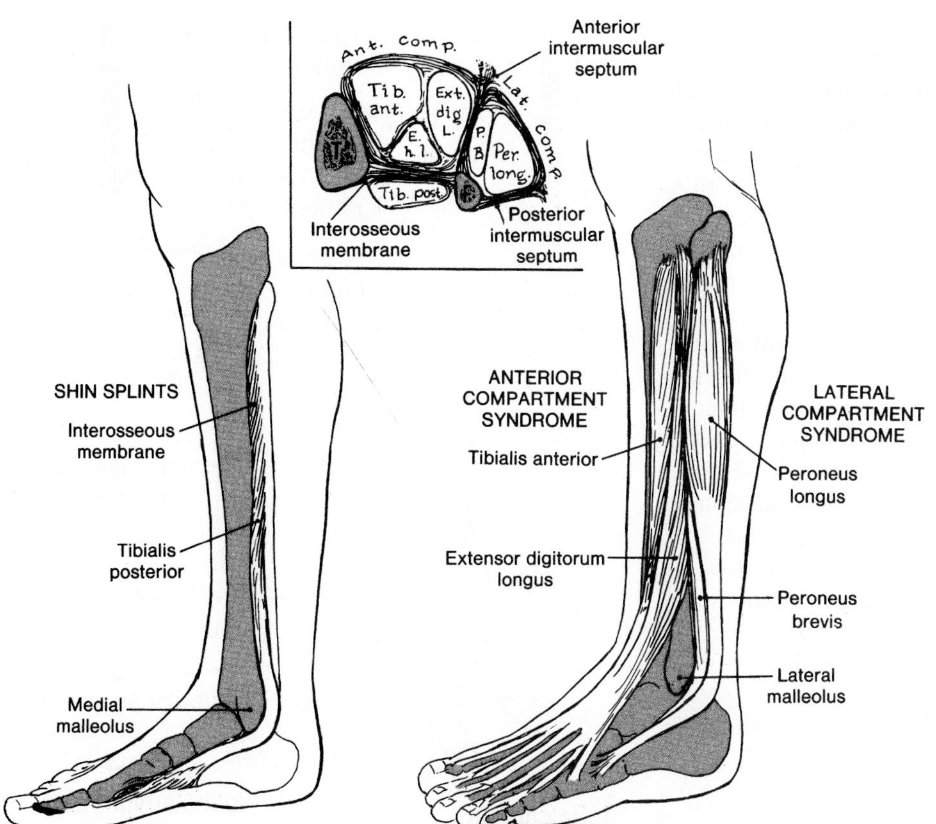

FIGURE 72.4. Sites of pain and relevant anatomy for shin splints, anterior compartment syndrome, and lateral compartment syndrome.

Signs and Symptoms

Patients with exertional compartment syndrome complain of cramping and aching in the affected lower leg with a predictable level of physical activity. For example, a patient may have no symptoms after running 1 mile but may develop pain after running 1.5 miles. As exercise and symptoms persist, the patient may develop lower leg weakness and distal paresthesias. Symptoms gradually resolve over time with rest.

On physical examination, the patient at rest may have no localized pain. Because the anterior compartment is the one most commonly affected, a patient usually describes pain lateral to the crest of the tibia over the anterior or, less commonly, the lateral compartment. Careful palpation of the anterior and lateral compartments may reveal fascial hernias, that is, palpable defects in the fascia that can be associated with exertional compartment syndrome. Examining the patient after exercise to recreate the threshold of symptoms is extremely helpful. The affected compartments are tight and painful, and subtle fascial hernias are more obvious.

The diagnosis of exertional compartment syndrome can be made with a series of compartment pressure readings: before exercise, immediately after exercise, and later after exercise. Normal at-rest compartment pressure usually is <4 mm Hg. A patient with exertional compartment syndrome usually has elevated at-rest compartment pressure (>8 mm Hg). Immediately after exercise that produces the symptoms, the pressure typically is >30 mm Hg and slowly decreases over time.

Treatment and Prognosis

Patients with exertional compartment syndrome should be referred to an orthopedic surgeon or sports medicine specialist. Because the cause of this syndrome is unknown, it is hard to recommend specific treatment. Nonoperative treatment should include reduced activity, eccentric and concentric muscle strengthening, and accommodative shoe inserts. If symptoms continue, an elective fasciotomy of the involved compartment(s) is recommended. If symptoms with activity are neglected, exertional compartment syndrome can evolve into acute compartment syndrome.

Other Causes of Exertional Leg Pain

Vascular and neurologic claudication is a cause of exertional leg pain in the older patient (>50 years). Frequently, the physical examination with the patient at rest is not very helpful. Vascular studies, including Doppler, are indicated (see Chapter 94). In addition, if spinal stenosis is suspected for neurologic claudication, MRI of the lumbar spine is indicated (see Chapter 71).

Bone and Soft-Tissue Tumors

Patients with a primary bone tumor typically complain of constant, deep, aching pain. Night pain is a common feature of malignant tumors. Osteoid osteoma is a benign bony tumor that can cause night pain, which is often relieved by NSAIDs. A sudden increase in pain after mild trauma should raise the possibility of a pathologic fracture and an underlying malignancy. On the other hand, a growing mass, not pain, is the typical presenting complaint of soft-tissue tumors. Constitutional symptoms such as fever, malaise, weakness, and recent weight loss are important symptoms that might be associated with a malignant bone tumor.

The patient should be examined for any local masses, focal tenderness, pain with palpation or weight-bearing, and any peripheral nerve deficit secondary to entrapment. Plain radiographs and other imaging modalities, if needed, should be obtained. Computed tomography is useful for bone tumors, and MRI is useful for soft-tissue tumors. Laboratory studies include a complete blood cell count; calcium, magnesium, and phosphorus levels; alkaline phosphatase activity; and erythrocyte sedimentation rate. Although the results of these tests are nonspecific, they may offer clues regarding bone turnover, an increased inflammatory state, and systemic illness. Patients suspected of having a bone tumor should be referred to an orthopedic surgeon.

Deep Venous Thrombosis

Deep venous thrombosis often presents in a nonspecific manner but is an important potential explanation for lower extremity pain. Chapter 57 provides a full discussion on the management of deep venous thrombosis.

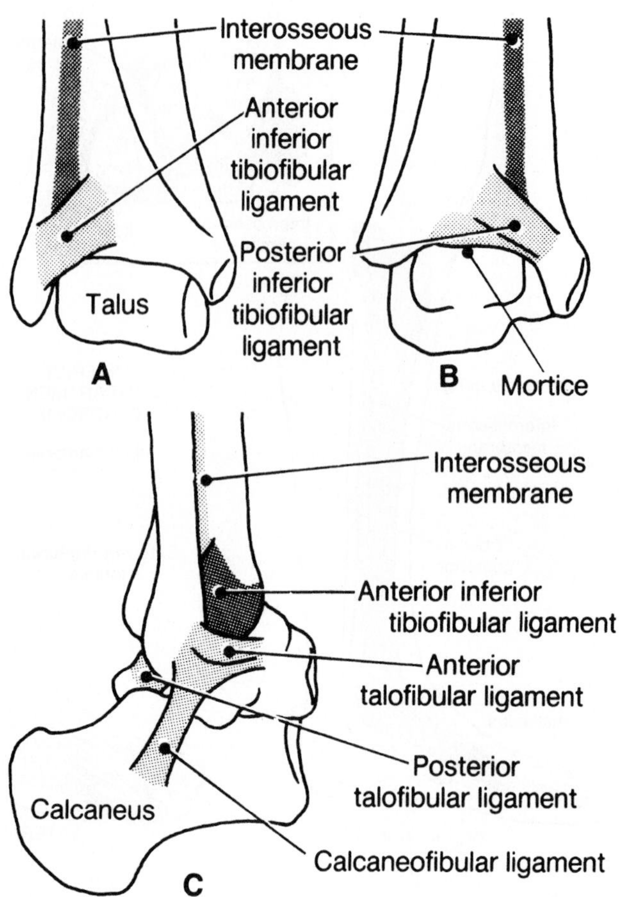

FIGURE 72.5. Ankle joint. **A:** Anterior view. **B:** Posterior view. **C:** Lateral view. (From Ramamurti CP, Tiner RV. Orthopedics in primary care. Baltimore: Williams & Wilkins, 1979:245, with permission.)

THE ANKLE

Anatomy

The ankle joint (Fig. 72.5) consists of articulations of the distal tibia and fibula with the talus. The principal anatomic components and their function are as follows:

- The distal tibia and fibula, with their distal bony extensions, form the medial and lateral malleolus, respectively. The medial and lateral malleolus, along with the distal flat articular surface of the tibia (the tibial plafond), form an arch or mortise that articulates with the dome of the talus.
- The interosseous ligament runs almost completely along the length of the tibia and fibula. This ligament, along with the anterior inferior and posterior inferior tibiofibular ligament, stabilizes the distal tibiofibular joint.
- The talus is stabilized within the mortise by the medial and lateral ligamentous structures. The lateral complex consists of anterior and posterior talofibular ligaments and the calcaneofibular ligament. The medial complex consists of the superficial and deep deltoid ligament connecting the medial malleolus to the talus and calcaneus.

General Evaluation

A focused history is essential (see Chapter 68). As with the knee, ankle injuries can be caused by a single traumatic event or by multiple and chronic stresses. The clinician will need to define the mechanism of injury in order to effect a satisfactory outcome. If no acute trauma has occurred, then stress injury from chronic repetitive activity or increase in the frequency or duration of the activity is the likely cause of injury. As with the knee, the general principles of inspection, palpation, and evaluation of ROM and strength in the ankle are addressed.

- The ankle should be *inspected* for any gross deformity or swelling and for any superficial abrasion, ecchymosis, or laceration. It should be compared with the normal contralateral limb. The resting position of the ankle, the presence of hindfoot varus or valgus (i.e., position of the calcaneus in varus or valgus), and any pronation of the foot or loss of the medial arch should be noted.

- The clinician should palpate the following structures for tenderness or swelling:
  - — Medial and lateral malleolus
  - — Proximal fifth metatarsal
  - — Behind the medial malleolus (tarsal tunnel [tibialis posterior, flexor digitorum longus, or flexor hallucis longus tendon])
  - — Behind the fibula (peroneus brevis or longus tendon)
- The clinician should palpate to determine the presence of tibialis posterior and dorsalis pedis pulses.
- The *strength* of the ankle everters (peroneus brevis and longus), invertors (tibialis posterior), dorsiflexors (tibialis anterior and extensor digitorum longus), and plantarflexors (tibialis posterior, flexor digitorum longus, gastrocnemius, and soleus) should be assessed and graded on a 0- to 5- point muscle strength scale (see Chapter 86).
- *Sensory examination* should be performed over all dermatomes and superficial nerve distributions.
- The *ROM* of dorsiflexion and plantarflexion, including subtalar (side-to-side) motion, should be obtained and compared with that of the normal ankle. (Most ankles have 20 degrees dorsiflexion and 40 degrees plantarflexion.)

Ankle Sprains

Definition and Mechanism of Injury

Ankle sprains are one of the most common conditions that cause a patient to present to a physician or emergency room. The most common mechanism is an inversion injury to the ankle as the foot begins the foot-strike part of the gait cycle. (Once the foot is planted fully, the ankle mortise provides much of the ankle's stability.) The most commonly injured ligament is the lateral anterior talofibular ligament. The calcaneofibular ligament and the posterior talofibular ligament also can be injured, but usually only by high-energy trauma. All sprains are graded with a ligament grading system (Table 72.1). Medial ankle sprains represent severe ankle injuries. Finally, injury to the syndesmosis results in a "high-ankle" or syndesmosis sprain. This injury usually occurs with rotation of the ankle on a planted foot, with the talus acting as a crowbar to pry open the syndesmosis between the tibia and fibula.

Signs and Symptoms

The patient usually can recall the specific mechanism of injury. Pain and swelling usually develop immediately. Depending on the magnitude of the injury, the patient may or may not be able to bear weight. Physical examination reveals swelling, tenderness, and (later) ecchymosis over the injured ligaments. Reproducing the mechanism of injury exacerbates the pain. Increased laxity may be shown by an anterior drawer test. With the patient's knee flexed over the examination table and the ankle plantarflexed by gravity, the clinician stabilizes the patient's anterior tibia with one hand and uses the other hand to apply forward pressure on the back of the patient's heel, drawing the ankle forward. Increased anterior translation represents ligament injury. Pain along the medial deltoid ligament represents a more severe injury.

Special attention should be directed to the ankle syndesmosis. These injuries present with tenderness at the syndesmosis or proximal fibula, which can be elicited with direct palpation, compression of the syndesmosis, or rotation of the talus within the ankle mortise.

To avoid having to obtain radiographs of all sprained ankles, the Ottawa rules (21) present safe and clear indications for radiographically ruling out fracture with an ankle injury. If the patient has tenderness on direct palpation over the lateral or medial malleolus or proximal fifth metatarsal, radiographs should be obtained. If there is no direct tenderness over these bony prominences with an ankle injury, then radiographs for the acute injury are not indicated. Obviously, if ankle pain does not resolve within the next 6 weeks (the usual time frame for an ankle injury), radiographs are then indicated.

Treatment and Prognosis

Most ankle sprains can be treated with the RICE protocol and protected activity. Although compression with an elastic wrap or immobilization in a cast is commonly used, protection can be provided with a removable fracture boot, stirrup, or lace-up ankle splints that will accommodate increases and decreases in ankle swelling. Crutches

TABLE 72.1 Severity of Ligamentous Sprains

Grade	Examination and Underlying Pathology	Recommended Treatment
I	No joint instability or laxity, minor ligamentous stretch without tear	NSAID, RICE protocol (see text), progressive weight-bearing
II	Moderate joint instability, partial ligamentous tear	Immobilization for 4–6 wk
III	Marked joint instability, loss of control of muscle, unable to bear weight, complete rupture of ligament	Immobilize and refer to orthopedist

NSAID, nonsteroidal anti-inflammatory drug; RICE, rest, ice, compression, and elevation.

may be needed to support weight-bearing. Patients with severe, complete, or multiple ankle ligament sprains and syndesmosis sprains (22) should be referred to an orthopedic surgeon or sports medicine specialist.

Most ankle sprains resolve with nonoperative treatment in 2 to 6 weeks. Physical therapy is strongly recommended, particularly for low-energy ankle sprains, to improve not only ROM and strength but also proprioception, or position sense. The therapist can help retrain the ankle and reduce the risk of reinjury.

Medial ankle sprains and syndesmosis ankle sprains represent severe ankle injuries and require prolonged treatment. It may be 2 to 3 months before the patient is symptom-free with full activity. Only chronic, debilitating ankle instability or acute high-grade ankle sprains in the athlete should be considered for surgical repair or reconstruction.

Ankle Fractures

Definition and Mechanism of Injury

Ankle fractures typically occur once the foot is fully planted and the bony mortise is supplying the ankle's stability. Depending on the magnitude and direction of forces, the ankle may fracture. Several systems have been developed for classifying and prognosticating ankle fractures (22).

Signs and Symptoms

The most reliable sign of an ankle fracture is pain with direct palpation over the medial or lateral malleolus. There may or may not be any deformity. Fracture is associated with substantial swelling and ecchymosis. Patients with low-energy ankle fractures may still be able to bear weight.

Treatment and Prognosis

If the patient has pain over the medial or lateral malleoli or proximal fifth metatarsal, anteroposterior, lateral, and mortise (15 degrees internally rotated anteroposterior view) radiographic views of the ankle are indicated. Any fracture of the ankle should be referred to an orthopedic surgeon. If the fracture is nondisplaced and stable, it can be treated with protected immobilization (cast or fracture boot). However, these fractures must be followed closely with serial radiographs to monitor healing and possible displacement. Healing typically takes 8 to 10 weeks in most adult patients; this time frame is twice as long in patients with diabetes. If there is >1-mm fracture displacement or >1-mm mortise widening of the medial joint space, open reduction and internal fixation should be strongly considered because malunion of an ankle fracture predictably leads to posttraumatic arthritis. Open reduction and internal fixation of ankle fractures also provides the patient with early ambulation, reduced immobilization, and a quicker return to full activity. Physical therapy is recommended for improved ROM, strength, and proprioception.

Achilles Tendinitis

Definition and Mechanism of Injury

Achilles tendinitis refers to chronic irritation of the Achilles tendon and its sheath secondary to repetitive use and trauma (23,24). The Achilles tendon is the terminal tendinous attachment of the soleus and gastrocnemius muscles into the calcaneus. Achilles tendinitis commonly is seen in active individuals (adolescents to middle-aged adults) engaging in athletic activities without proper conditioning. However, Achilles tendinitis can occur even in well-conditioned athletes who run on hills or wear shoes with excessively rigid soles. Furthermore, structural abnormalities such as tibia vara (bowed leg deformity), tight hamstrings and calf muscles, cavus foot (high arched foot, often with claw toes), and varus (inverted) heel deformity predispose to Achilles tendinitis. Initially, the peritenon (loose, soft, connective tissue surrounding the tendon) is inflamed, but in chronic cases the tendon itself undergoes mucoid degeneration with formation of longitudinal nodules and fissures in the tendon. This condition can increase the risk of a tendon rupture.

Signs and Symptoms

The patient typically complains of a burning-type pain at the site of tendon insertion onto the calcaneus. The onset of pain usually coincides with the start of the activity; however, it may lessen or disappear completely as the activity continues. The discomfort often recurs at startup or after completion of the activity.

On examination, there is local or diffuse tenderness of the Achilles tendon. A chronic tender nodule may be present in the substance of the tendon with crepitus and swelling. The patient experiences pain with passive stretch of the tendon.

Retrocalcaneal bursitis involving the bursa that lies between the calcaneus and Achilles tendon may produce symptoms similar to those of Achilles tendinitis. On examination a patient with retrocalcaneal bursitis has focal tenderness confined to the calcaneus.

Treatment and Prognosis

The general treatment protocol is like that for any other tendinitis condition. The inciting activity or sport should be stopped initially, and the patient should use the RICE protocol and be placed on a trial of NSAIDs to reduce the inflammation. Runners should not run for several days and should reduce running mileage and avoid hills until symptoms are absent for 10 to 14 days. If symptoms persist after this short rest period, the patient may need to stop the exercises that aggravate the condition for 3 to 4 weeks or longer.

A physical therapy referral is beneficial for refractory cases of Achilles tendinitis because ultrasound and other modalities can be highly effective. A removable heel lift inserted into the shoe may provide some relief. If the syndrome is severe, splinting or casting the ankle joint and using crutches may be necessary to immobilize the Achilles tendon. In mild cases, the prognosis is excellent. Patients with conditions that do not respond in 2 weeks should be referred for an orthopedic consultation. Surgery usually is not necessary, but for some cases, operative options include open débridement and repair of the tendon (25). The patient with retrocalcaneal bursitis is best advised to rest from stressful activity, to obtain properly fitted athletic shoes that are not tight around the Achilles tendon, and to use a heel pad in regular shoes. Corticosteroid injection in and about the Achilles tendon should be avoided because it can lead to rupture of that tendon.

Prevention

Exercises that gently stretch the tendon may help condition runners and prevent recurrences. The use of good shoes is important. Shoes should have flexible soles, a well-molded Achilles pad, and a rigid heel wedge.

Achilles Tendon Rupture

Definition and Mechanism of Injury

An Achilles tendon rupture is a disruption of the tendon, usually 2 to 6 cm proximal to its insertion into the calcaneus. It typically occurs in middle-aged adults, usually during athletic activities that require rapid active plantarflexion of the ankle. Patients with Achilles tendinitis are at risk for tendon ruptures, as are patients with systemic inflammatory diseases (such as lupus and rheumatoid arthritis) or with a history of using systemic steroids (26). Achilles tendinitis and tendon rupture have been associated with fluoroquinolone therapy (27). The rupture can be acute or chronic, complete or incomplete.

Signs and Symptoms

A patient with an acute rupture usually recalls a sudden snap and pain in the area of tendon insertion. A patient with a chronic rupture may not recall a particular event but generally has pain in this area. Depending on how complete the rupture is, the patient may not be able to actively plantarflex the ankle or may be able to do so with weakness and pain. On examination, there is local pain and swelling. A palpable defect may be present in the tendon. The *Thompson test* is positive (28). This test is performed by squeezing the mid to proximal muscular section of the calf. If the tendon is intact or not completely torn, the ankle will plantarflex. If the tendon is completely ruptured, no plantarflexion will occur.

Radiographs should be obtained to rule out an avulsion fracture at the tendon insertion site. If the diagnosis is still not clear, MRI will delineate the degree of the tear and its location. Patients with acute or painful chronic tears or those with avulsion fractures should be referred to an orthopedic surgeon for definitive treatment. For a patient with an acute rupture, referral should be made urgently because delay in treatment beyond a few days may result in retraction of the proximal portion of the tendon.

Treatment and Prognosis

Some controversy exists regarding the management of Achilles tendon ruptures (29,30). Both operative and nonoperative options are available. In the case of operative repair, primary anastomosis at the site of rupture is followed by a period of immobilization to allow for tendon healing. Nonoperative treatment entails immobilizing the ankle joint in plantarflexion to approximate the two ends of the tendon. This position is held for 4 weeks in a below-the-knee cast. Then the foot is brought into more dorsiflexion with another below-the-knee cast, and the process is repeated until the tendon is healed. Most surgeons recommend surgical repair of acute, complete ruptures in young, active patients. The prognosis of Achilles tendon ruptures is varied. Most patients are able to return to routine daily activities, but some may not be able to return to preinjury levels of sporting activities. Generally, compared with nonoperative modalities, surgical repair has a higher success rate of returning patients to preinjury sports levels with a lower chance of recurrence (31).

Prevention

Proper conditioning can prevent a tendon rupture. Appropriate stretching exercises should be performed before and after sporting activities. Appropriate treatment of Achilles tendinitis should be sought to decrease the potential chance of a rupture.

Posterior Tibialis Tendinitis and Rupture

Definition and Mechanism of Injury

Tendinitis of the posterior tibialis tendon is common. This tendon courses posterior to the medial malleolus, inverts the ankle joint, and plantarflexes the foot. Chronic irritation from the malleolus, along with a tenuous blood supply, place this tendon at risk for tendinitis and subsequent rupture. Patients with a history of trauma or previous surgery to the medial aspect of the foot, diabetes, obesity, or local steroid injection are at risk for dysfunction and tearing of this tendon.

Signs and Symptoms

Patients frequently complain of medial foot and ankle pain. The onset of the pain usually is gradual. Examination reveals tenderness along the course of the tendon behind the medial malleolus. Additionally, patients with a torn tendon may have gradual loss of the medial arch of the foot and, eventually, a flatfoot deformity. With complete tendon rupture, the foot abducts and the pain can move laterally into the region of the sinus tarsi or beneath the fibula, where bony impingement can occur secondary to the loss of the medial arch. The hindfoot assumes a valgus position, allowing more of the toes to be visible when viewed from behind the patient ("too-many-toes" sign). In the early stages, when only tenosynovitis is present, the tendon is intact and the patient is able to perform a single-heel rise, that is, stand only on the affected limb and raise the heel from the floor with plantarflexion of the ankle. In more advanced stages of tendon attenuation or tear, however, the patient is unable to perform a heel rise. In advanced stages, radiographs show osteoarthritis in the ankle. MRI is valuable in showing posterior tibial tendon attenuation or tear.

Treatment and Prognosis

In the presence of an intact posterior tibial tendon with tendinitis, the standard RICE protocol with NSAIDs can be followed. The ankle joint should be immobilized for 6 weeks with a rigid below-the-knee cast or boot to allow the inflammation to resolve. Subsequently, the patient can progress to a stiff-soled shoe with a medial heel wedge. Patients for whom such nonoperative measures fail may require surgical débridement of the tendon. For patients with incompetent or torn posterior tibial tendons, nonoperative treatment tends to be less effective and does not prevent progression to flatfoot deformity. Surgical options include reconstruction of the tendon, flexor tendon transfer, medial calcaneal osteotomy to displace the calcaneus medially, lengthening the lateral aspect of the foot, and ankle arthrodesis, or a combination thereof (32,33). The prognosis for this form of tendinitis tends to be good, but it may recur. The prognosis for posterior tibial tendon rupture varies and depends in part on the extent of the acquired flatfoot deformity.

Prevention

The best prevention for posterior tibial tendon rupture is to halt the progression of tibialis posterior tendinitis. Often, early treatment of posterior tibial tendinitis with NSAIDs, immobilization, activity modification, and use of orthotics is successful. Once the tendon is ruptured, the foot can develop a flatfoot deformity, and major surgical reconstruction may be necessary.

SPECIFIC REFERENCES

1. Hardin GT, Farr J, Bach BR Jr. Meniscal tears: diagnosis, evaluation, and treatment. Orthop Rev 1992;21:1311.
2. Hughston JC, Andrews JR, Cross MJ, et al. Classification of knee ligament instabilities. Part II. The lateral compartment. J Bone Joint Surg 1976;58A:173.
3. DeHaven KE. Diagnosis of acute knee injuries with hemarthrosis. Am J Sports Med 1980;8:9.
4. Noyes FR, Bassett RW, Grood ES, et al. Arthroscopy in acute traumatic hemarthrosis of the knee. Incidence of anterior cruciate tears and other injuries. J Bone Joint Surg 1980;62A: 687.
5. Torg JS, Conrad W, Kalen V. Clinical diagnosis of anterior cruciate ligament instability in the athlete. Am J Sports Med 1976;4:84.
6. Shelbourne KD, Davis TJ, Patel DV. The natural history of acute, isolated, nonoperatively treated posterior cruciate ligament injuries. A prospective study. Am J Sports Med 1999;27:276.
7. Miller MD, Bergfeld JA, Fowler PJ, et al. The posterior cruciate ligament injured knee: principles of evaluation and treatment. Instr Course Lect 1999;48:199.
8. Hughston JC, Deese M. Medial subluxation of the patella as a complication of lateral retinacular release. Am J Sports Med 1988;16:383.
9. Diehl LH, Garrett WE Jr.Knee. Section E. Patellofemoral joint. 1. Acute dislocation of the patella in the adult. In: DeLee JC, Drez D Jr, Miller MD, eds. De Lee & Drez's orthopaedic sports medicine: principles and practice. 2nd ed. Philadelphia: WB Saunders, 2003: 1697.
10. McConnell J. The management of chondromalacia patellae: a long term solution. Aust J Physiother 1986;32:215.
11. Safran MR, Fu FH. Uncommon causes of knee pain in the athlete. Orthop Clin North Am 1995;26:547.
12. Bhattacharyya T, Vrahas MS. The medical-legal aspects of compartment syndrome. J Bone Joint Surg 2004;86A:864.
13. McQueen MM, Court-Brown CM. Compartment monitoring in tibial fractures. The pressure threshold for decompression. J Bone Joint Surg 1996;78B:99.
14. Verma RB, Sherman O. Athletic stress fractures: part I. History, epidemiology, physiology, risk factors, radiography, diagnosis, and treatment. Am J Orthop 2001;30:798.
15. Boden BP, Osbahr DC. High-risk stress fractures: evaluation and treatment. J Am Acad Orthop Surg 2000;8:344.
16. Boden BP, Osbahr DC, Jimenez C. Low-risk stress fractures. Am J Sports Med 2001;29:100.
17. Barrow GW, Saha S. Menstrual irregularity and stress fractures in collegiate female distance runners. Am J Sports Med 1988;16:209.
18. Rzonca EC, Baylis WJ. Common sports injuries to the foot and leg. Clin Podiatr Med Surg 1988;5:591.
19. Glorioso JE Jr, Wilckens JH. Exertional leg pain. In: O'Connor FG, Wilder RP, eds. Textbook of running medicine. New York: McGraw-Hill, 2001: 181.
20. James SL, Bates BT, Osternig LR. Injuries to runners. Am J Sports Med 1978;6:40.
21. Stiell IG, McKnight RD, Greenberg GH, et al. Implementation of the Ottawa ankle rules. JAMA 1994;271:827.
22. Marsh JL, Saltzman CL. Ankle fractures. In: Bucholz RW, Heckman JD, eds. Rockwood and Green's fractures in adults. 5th ed. Philadelphia: Lippincott Williams & Wilkins, 2001: 2001.
23. Clain MR, Baxter DE. Achilles tendinitis. Foot Ankle 1992;13:482.
24. Myerson MS, McGarvey W. Disorders of the insertion of the Achilles tendon and Achilles tendinitis. J Bone Joint Surg 1998;80A:1814.
25. Paavola M, Orava S, Leppilahti J, et al. Chronic Achilles tendon overuse injury: complications after surgical treatment. An analysis of 432 consecutive patients. Am J Sports Med 2000;28:77.
26. Kao NL, Moy JN, Richmond GW. Achilles tendon rupture: an underrated complication of corticosteroid treatment [letter]. Thorax 1992;47:484.
27. Ribard P, Audisio F, Kahn MF, et al. Seven Achilles tendinitis including 3 complicated by rupture during fluoroquinolone therapy. J Rheumatol 1992;19:1479.
28. Thompson TC. A test for rupture of the tendo Achilles. Acta Orthop Scand 1962;32:461.
29. Cetti R, Christensen SE, Ejsted R, et al. Operative versus nonoperative treatment of Achilles tendon rupture. A prospective randomized study and review of the literature. Am J Sports Med 1993;21:791.
30. Jarvinen TA, Kannus P, Paavola M, et al. Achilles tendon injuries. Curr Opin Rheumatol 2001;13:150.
31. Jacobs D, Martens M, Van Audekercke R, et al. Comparison of conservative and operative treatment of Achilles tendon rupture. Am J Sports Med 1978;6:107.
32. Weil LS Jr, Benton-Weil W, Borrelli AH, et al. Outcomes for surgical correction for stages 2 and 3 tibialis posterior dysfunction. J Foot Ankle Surg 1998;37:467.
33. Feldman NJ, Oloff LM, Schulhofer SD. In situ tibialis posterior to flexor digitorum longus tendon transfer for tibialis posterior tendon dysfunction: a simplified surgical approach with outcome of 11 patients. J Foot Ankle Surg 2001;40:2.

For annotated ***General References*** *and resources related to this chapter, visit www.hopkinsbayview.org/PAMreferences.*

Chapter 73

Common Problems of the Feet

Bruce S. Lebowitz

The primary care practitioner is often called upon to treat patients who complain of problems with their feet. Although disorders of the feet are not life threatening, they should not be taken lightly. Any patient with a painful foot attests that the pain takes the joy out of living.

STRUCTURE AND FUNCTION

The abnormal foot cannot be understood unless the structure of the foot and its function during gait are understood.

Normal Gait

The bones and joints of the feet facilitate walking and running in an upright position (Fig. 73.1). The foot and leg function together to allow a smooth, even transfer of weight as one extremity moves ahead of the other. During gait, the foot first adjusts to a variable terrain and then acts to propel the body's weight forward.

In the *first stage of gait,* the heel strikes the ground and body weight begins to move distally over the lateral aspect of the foot. The foot is in a pronated position, meaning that the arch is flattened. In effect, the foot resembles a loose bag of bones during this stage, permitting it to adapt to the terrain and to act as a shock absorber when body weight strikes the ground.

In the *second stage of gait,* as weight moves distally to the ball of the foot and the body is propelled forward, the foot must convert to a rigid lever. This conversion, or supination, takes place in the subtalar and midtarsal joints. Supination serves to heighten the arch, pushing the bones and joints of the foot together rigidly enough to propel body weight forward efficiently.

For the lower extremity to function normally, certain structural criteria must be met; if they are not met, compensation occurs. Ideally, the leg should be in a plane perpendicular to the foot and ground, as in a stick figure drawing. The forefoot should be in a plane parallel to the rear foot, but various congenital factors may act to prevent this normal angulation. Varus (toward the midline or inverted) or valgus (away from the midline or everted) positions of the forefoot or hindfoot are the most common of these congenital factors.

Excessive Pronation

Excessive pronation (pronation extended through too much of the gait cycle) is the most common compensating mechanism when structural abnormalities are present. When the foot remains pronated during gait and does not resupinate in time, or at all, the condition known as *flatfoot* exists. The degree of this flatfoot position reflects the degree of pronation that is present. A number of problems may evolve from excessive pronation during gait, including bunions, calluses, and hammertoes. As pointed out in the discussion that follows, assessment of the mechanical basis for the condition is important in planning appropriate treatment for it.

Shoes

Shoes clearly play a role in the way feet function. Shoes protect feet from the elements, cushion the effect of walking on hard flat surfaces, and provide some support to the bones and ligaments. Unfortunately, many people favor short narrow shoes, high heels, and pointed toes. Obviously, squeezing a basically rectangular foot into a

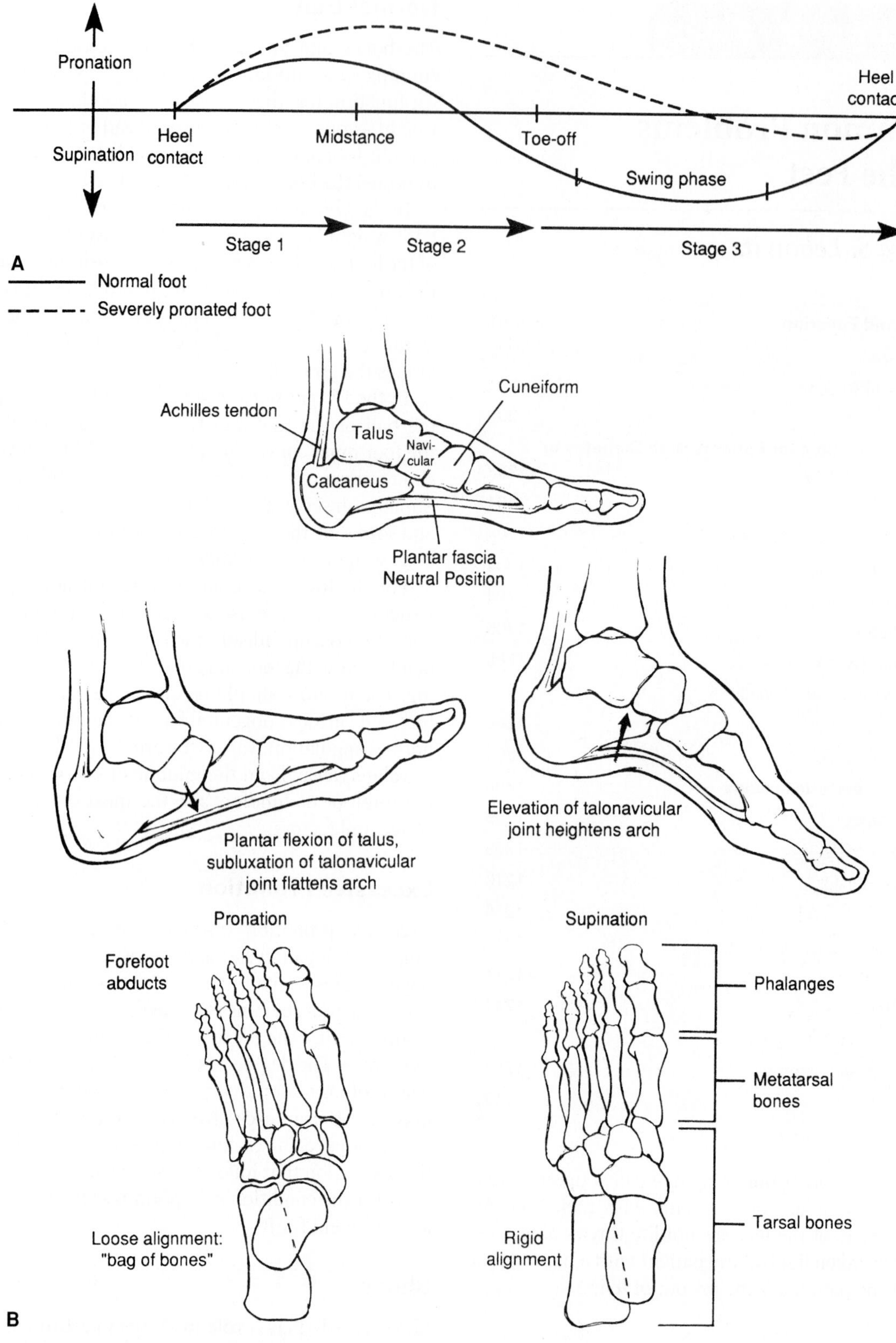

FIGURE 73.1. **A:** Schematic representation of the gait cycle for a normal foot and for a foot with excessive pronation. **B:** Schematic illustration of foot structure during pronation and supination during gait cycle.

triangular shoe with the heels elevated from 2 to 5 inches creates significant stress for the foot. Most of the disorders of the foot discussed in this chapter are intensified by these demands of fashion.

Most people, in fitting themselves for shoes, do not take into account the variations in their foot size throughout the day and the variation in shoe size from manufacturer to manufacturer. Therefore, the following advice often is helpful: buy shoes in the late afternoon when any swelling that might occur is already present; lightweight shoes are preferable to heavy shoes; and leather, because it is more porous, is preferable to synthetic materials in shoe construction.

Interest in shoes appropriate to sports, especially jogging and running, has escalated in recent years. Sneakers or running shoes should be well fitted and firm enough to prevent excessive splaying of the foot during activity. For shock absorption, the shoes should have studded soles, and there should be a raised resilient heel wedge. The midsole should be flexible to help prevent Achilles tendon stress, and there should be a well-molded Achilles pad to prevent irritation of the tendon. The tongue should be well padded to prevent irritation of the dorsum of the foot. Figure 73.2 illustrates these features.

It is a misconception that wearing sneakers excessively harms the feet. Actually, the better running shoes available today are so supportive and so well padded that they can be recommended to patients for numerous painful foot conditions. For example, highly arched feet (which are supinated and may pronate only slightly) lack shock-absorbing qualities; constant impact on the ground can cause severe metatarsal, heel, and arch pain. For patients with this condition, the support and resiliency provided by a modern running shoe are ideal. Likewise, a flat or pronated foot may be very well supported by the built-in arch supports of well-made running shoes.

Running magnifies the problems associated with excessive pronation, and the long-term management of this condition requires the selection of shoes that provide good support. The use of well-designed running shoes is important in preventing most exercise-related injuries of the lower extremity.

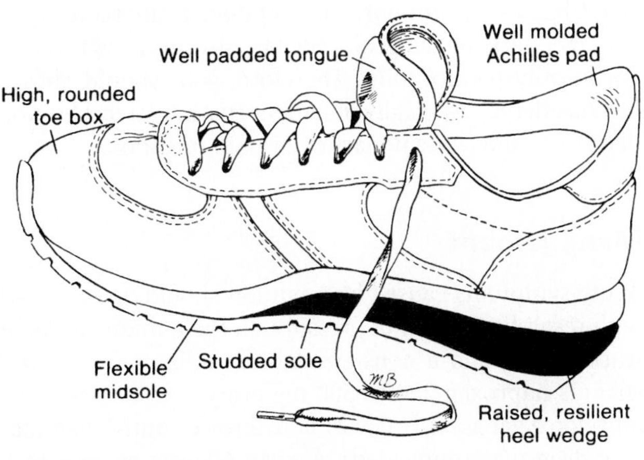

FIGURE 73.2. Features of a well-designed running shoe.

PREVENTIVE FOOT CARE FOR PATIENTS WITH DIABETES OR ARTERIAL INSUFFICIENCY

To understand the need for professional diabetic foot care, one must consider the special devastating effect of diabetes mellitus on the feet. The most important podiatric problem of diabetes is neuropathy (see Chapter 79). Sensory neuropathy may cause burning and sometimes unbearable pain in the feet and legs, especially at night. At the same time, sensory neuropathy lessens the ability of the patient to interpret and respond to painful stimuli. A foreign body that is not felt or a thick corn or callus that is not treated can result in irritation of the tissues with complicating infection.

Motor neuropathy causes wasting of the small muscles of the foot. Without the intrinsic muscles helping to stabilize the motions of the toes and metatarsal phalangeal joints, the tendency to form severe hammertoe and callus is greatly increased. The mechanical forces on the toes and metatarsals are increased as the ability to sense pain is reduced.

Sympathetic neuropathy leads to excessively dry skin, and the feet of a diabetic patient often are anhidrotic and at risk for secondary infection. In addition to neuropathy, the diabetic foot is affected by vascular disease. Vascular disease also occurs in many patients independent of diabetes mellitus, and the same issues apply. Arteriosclerosis is accelerated in the diabetic patient. The changes that are often seen lead to claudication and rest pain. Diabetic small-vessel disease affects the nourishment of tissues, accounting for the finding of normal pedal arterial pulses and yet severely dysvascular digits that sometimes require amputation. Chapters 79, 94, and 95 discuss the management of peripheral vascular disease and lower extremity ulcers and the consequences of diabetic vascular and neuropathic complications.

For all of these reasons, prevention and early detection of problems on the foot's surface are particularly important in patients with diabetes because they can prevent serious foot lesions (1). Prevention and early detection include patient education, routine inspection by the patient, and periodic examination by the practitioner or nurse. Examination is important because symptoms alone are poor indicators for the presence of diabetic neuropathy and because, in the presence of neuropathy, foot lesions may go undetected and progress (2). The single most important advice that can be impressed upon the patient is to look at his or her feet every day. When obesity or lack of visual acuity is a problem, someone else should examine the patient's feet every day. Irritations, abrasions, and calluses that usually produce pain must be identified visually when there are sensory abnormalities in the feet. Advice about selection of shoe gear (see above) should be provided routinely to patients with diabetes and vascular insufficiency. Following these procedures minimizes the risk of serious foot ulcers and infections.

These patients also should be advised not to use over-the-counter remedies for corns and ingrown toenails. Such commercial preparations include acids and tanning agents that can seriously injure the tender skin of these patients. Normal toenails should be allowed to grow past the end of the fleshy part of the toe; thick nails are best trimmed by a podiatrist, as are corns and calluses (see Calluses and Corns). Soft cotton should be worn between toes that tend to rub each other, and talcum powder should be used to prevent interdigital moisture and maceration. Lanolin should be applied to dry and thickened skin to prevent fissuring, especially common in the heels of diabetic patients with anhidrosis from sympathetic neuropathy. Prescription-strength moisturizers such as ammonium lactate cream (Lac-Hydrin 12%) are beneficial in neutralizing the drying effects of neuropathy. Tinea pedis should be treated (see Chapter 117) to prevent breaks in the skin, which could be sources of infection. In-shoe orthotics, which cushion and redistribute pressure, have been shown to be effective in preventing and treating diabetic ulcers (3).

Evaluation and management of diabetic wounds have evolved into a subspecialty of podiatry. Diabetic ulcers are a major source of infections, disability, and loss of limb and life. The costs of treating diabetic foot wounds is enormous and constantly growing (4).

Podiatrists play a special role in débridement, pressure reduction and when necessary, surgical management of diabetic foot wounds. Prevention of wounds is the ultimate goal of all foot care providers. Regular examination of the vascular, neurologic, dermatologic, and biomechanical systems of the foot is essential in identifying risk and addressing pathology. Podiatrists monitor all these systems and provide foot care to the diabetic at-risk population on a constant basis.

A final note on prevention: Patients should be encouraged to shake out their shoes before putting them on as a simple, obvious way to prevent foreign-body penetration. Patients are advised to avoid walking barefoot, to examine their feet daily, and to change shoes frequently.

BUNIONS

Definition and Pathogenesis

Bunion (literally *turnip*) is a term used to describe the collective deformities of the first metatarsophalangeal joint (Fig. 73.3). These deformities include enlargement of the medial, medial–dorsal, or dorsal aspect of the first metatarsophalangeal joint and lateral deviation of the great toe. Enlargement of the joint may consist of bone, soft tissue, or a combination of the two.

For many years, tight-fitting shoes were mistakenly considered to be the cause of bunions. It now is known that, although the pressure of tight shoes on an existing bunion can result in pain that calls attention to the problem, bunions are not caused by poorly fitted shoes. The chief cause of the deformity is a hypermobile first metatarsal bone, most often related to excessive pronation (see Structure Function). The first metatarsal and great toe, which help propel body weight forward, should be stable during the final stage of gait when a tight, rigid, bony structure is needed. The intrinsic and extrinsic musculature should help to hold the metatarsal tight at this point. When there is excessive pronation, the entire foot remains loose and unstable. One result of such laxity in this stage of gait is hypermobility of the first metatarsal and buckling of the first toe; intrinsic and extrinsic muscles cause the first metatarsal to deviate medially and the great toe to deviate laterally. The combined deformity is called *hallux abductovalgus*. Eventually, arthritic hypertrophy of the head of the first metatarsal bone develops.

Symptoms

The presenting complaint of a patient with a bunion is pain localized to the first metatarsophalangeal joint. Pressure of the shoe on the enlarged metatarsal head, with or without pressure on adventitious bursa, can cause pain that is severe and even disabling; pain can also result from the joint motion itself. Often, crepitus can be felt within the joint. Sometimes the patient seeks help not because of pain but because he/she is unable to wear shoes as a result of the deformity.

In evaluating a patient, the practitioner must be certain that the symptoms are a result of the bunion alone. Gout (see Chapter 76) not only may produce acute pain in the first metatarsophalangeal joint but also may aggravate a chronically painful joint. Therefore, gout should always be considered, especially in patients with bilateral bunion deformity and acute nonarticular pain in a foot.

Management

Acute symptoms caused by a bunion should be managed with rest, elimination of pressure on the bunion, soaks in warm water, and a nonsteroidal anti-inflammatory drug such as naproxen 250 to 500 mg every 8 to 12 hours (or a cyclooxygenase-2 [COX-2] nonsteroidal anti-inflammatory drug when indicated). Aspirin 600 mg every 4 to 6 hours also can be used, but the onset of action is slower.

develops as a result of keratin occluding a sweat duct in the skin (Fig. 73.5B). The obstruction and resultant backup create a reaction in the skin similar to a deep large corn. This lesion need not be under a weight-bearing surface. It usually is painful, and after débridement there is characteristically even more distress. Treatment by the dermatologist or podiatrist usually is by local curettage.

Foreign bodies in the plantar surface of the foot can generate a local inflammatory reaction and thus create a hyperkeratotic lesion. One of the most common offending substances is hair (animal or human). For example, a dog hair, trapped in a carpet long enough to have dried out, can penetrate the skin rather easily. This lesion, although grossly resembling a simple callus, has a small aperture (entry wound) near the center, seen upon examination with a magnifying glass. The local reaction may or may not include infection. Treatment is simple excision of the foreign body.

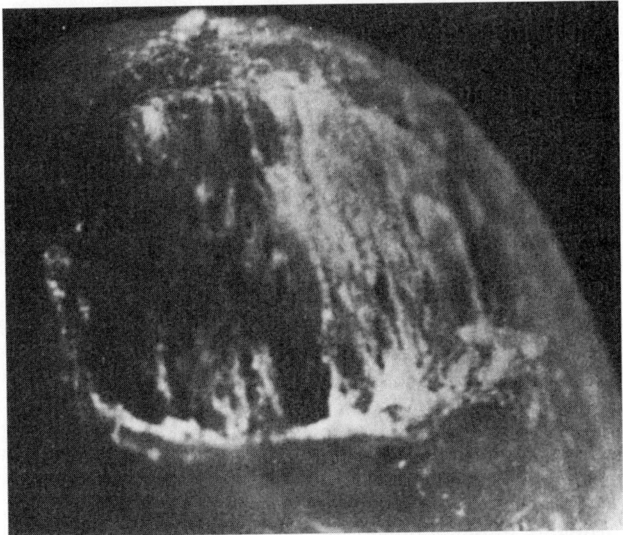

FIGURE 73.6. Mycotic toenail.

NAIL CONDITIONS

Only two nail conditions are commonly brought to medical attention: onychomycosis (fungal infection) and ingrown toenails, with or without concomitant inflammation (paronychia).

Onychomycosis

Causes and Findings

The typical fungal infection of a toenail begins distally at the tip of the toe and moves proximally, subungually, and through the nail plate itself (Fig. 73.6). Etiologic agents are *Trichophyton mentagrophytes, Trichophyton rubrum,* or *Candida albicans*. The fungus produces yellowish discoloration and longitudinal striations in the nails and in the epidermis. The accompanying local inflammatory reaction stimulates hyperkeratosis under the nail. This hyperkeratotic accumulation tends to lift the nail up from the epidermis, facilitating further progression of the fungus. Eventually, the nail becomes mottled brownish yellow, thickened, and powdery. Usually, these infections are asymptomatic; patients are most concerned about the appearance of their nails, the possibility of spread of infection, and sometimes the inability to wear shoes when severe thickening of the nail plate is present.

Treatment

Fungus infections of toenails are difficult to eradicate medically. Oral medications are available to treat and resolve onychomycosis. Itraconazole is effective against dermatophytes such as *T. rubrum* and nondermatophytes such as yeasts and molds. Terbinafine is effective against most dermatophytes. Because not all dystrophic toenails are mycotic, treatment should be based on the results of nail fungal cultures. Both drugs, terbinafine (Lamisil 250 mg) and itraconazole (Sporanox 200 mg), are taken orally once per day for 3 months. Although itraconazole is commonly prescribed as a pulsed dose for fingernail fungus, it is not approved in pulsed form for toenail fungus. (Pulsed doses refer to double dosing for 1 week followed by a 3-week respite.) Potentially serious adverse reactions include congestive heart failure (itraconazole) and hepatic toxicity (both medications). Rare incidents of leukopenia have been reported with terbinafine. White blood cell monitoring with terbinafine and liver function monitoring with both drugs are recommended. Ciclopirox (8% Penlac nail lacquer) is an effective topical antifungal available by prescription. Although it is not as effective as the oral medications, it requires no medical monitoring. Another effective topical agent, amorolfine (5% Loceryl nail lacquer), has not yet been approved for use in the United States.

When nail thickening is regarded as a problem by the patient, the process can be controlled by regular and thorough débridement. The débridement of mycotic or otherwise thickened toenails is a process generally performed by podiatrists. The débridement first involves soaking of the feet and cutting of the nails by heavy-duty cutters. The nails are thoroughly filed down with an electrically powered diamond-studded burr. These drills are fitted with vacuum extraction systems to protect the patient and podiatrist from breathing in the nail dust.

Another treatment is permanent removal of the nail, including matrixectomy. Because toenails serve no useful function, their absence causes no functional impairment. However, surgical correction should be reserved for patients whose nails are painful or for whom the appearance of the feet is a significant factor. The most common type of surgical correction of toenails performed by dermatologists, podiatrists, or surgeons is nail excision, followed by chemical destruction of matrix tissue and nail bed with 88% phenol. After a sterile dressing is applied to the toe, the patient can continue normal activities. The patient needs only to change bandages and soak the feet daily until healing is complete in 2 to 3 weeks. Skin formerly below the nail plate thickens. Anyone can disguise the fact that their nails have been removed by applying nail polish to this thickened skin.

Ingrown Toenails

Causes and Findings

Ingrown toenail, a painful condition in which the medial or lateral border of a toenail penetrates the flesh, is a common problem (Fig. 73.7). Ingrown toenails have been attributed to factors such as improper trimming, heredity, bony pathology, improper shoe fit, tight socks, obesity, and trauma. However, there is no clear-cut cause, and there are probably many contributing causes. The great toe is the one almost always involved, and the problem can be identified by inspection and by finding point tenderness upon pressing the margin of the toenail.

Treatment

There is a popular misconception that cutting a V in the center of a toenail causes the lateral borders to grow toward the center, thereby relieving the ingrown condition. This belief has no basis in fact because the nail plate is merely hornified keratin: nonliving fixed tissue in which growth no longer occurs.

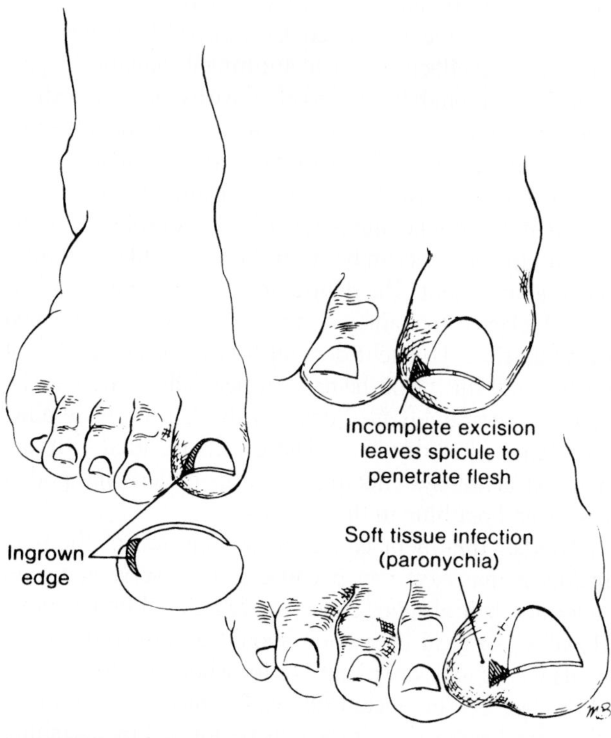

FIGURE 73.7. Schematic illustration of an ingrown toenail and possible complications.

Initial treatment of ingrown toenail depends on whether the patient's toe is infected (paronychia) or is chronically painful but not infected when the patient seeks care. The patient with an ingrown toenail often seeks help after attempting to excise the offending edge of toenail with whatever instruments are available. Most of the nail edge may be removed in this way by the patient, but a small sharp piece of nail usually remains that pierces the skin with each step and promotes infection. The toe becomes red, swollen, and exquisitely tender. The most vigorous soaking and the use of local and systemic antibiotics will not arrest such an infection as long as a nail spicule continues to penetrate the flesh. Therefore, the patient should be referred to a dermatologist, podiatrist, or surgeon for excision of the offending border of the nail; this procedure is done under local anesthesia and is curative. However, approximately 10% of patients have a recurrence, usually within 1 year. Systemic antimicrobials are rarely necessary. Definitive treatment of the ingrown nail itself varies according to the condition and needs of the patient.

For otherwise healthy patients, the procedure described for removal of the entire toenail and for matrix destruction also can be used to eradicate permanently an ingrown border. After local anesthesia (obtained by injecting the base of the toe to create a full block, injecting a field on the medial surface from dorsal to lateral and on the lateral surface from dorsal to lateral), the offending edge of toenail is excised and then phenol and alcohol are applied to cauterize the matrix tissue. This procedure, followed by complete healing in 2 to 3 weeks, usually permanently eliminates this painful and sometimes dangerous condition. Use of phenol dramatically decreases the rate of recurrence of the ingrown nail and increases patient satisfaction but at the cost of an increased postoperative infection rate (7). Even with phenol ablation of the nail matrix, there is still a 20% to 30% chance of recurrence. It is not unusual to rephenolize a nail within 1 year of treatment.

Treatment of diabetic patients and patients with arterial insufficiency must be conservative because wound healing may be poor after surgical removal of the nail. In these patients, frequent and thorough débridement of ingrown borders is effective and safe. Treatment by a podiatrist or other practitioner who is skilled in this procedure may be needed every 3 to 4 weeks to prevent complicating soft-tissue infection.

HEEL PAIN

Diagnosis

Heel pain is a common complaint. The most common pattern is pain that is localized to the medial plantar aspect of

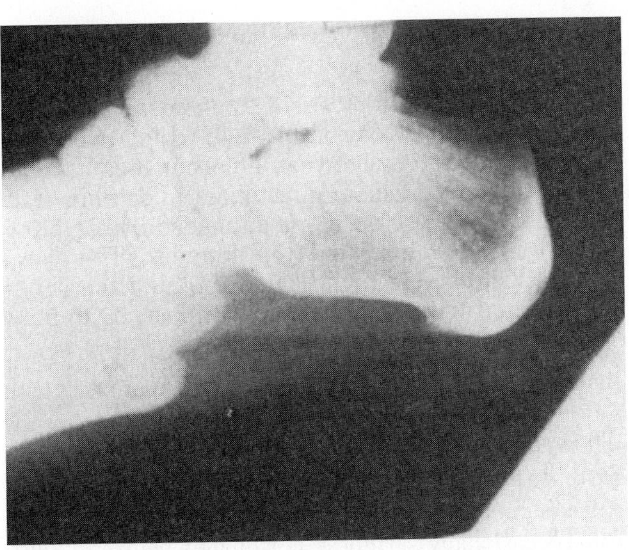

FIGURE 73.8. Radiologic view of a calcaneal exostosis (spur). (Courtesy of Max Weisfeld, DPM.)

the heel. (Chapter 72 discusses heel pain localized to the posterior aspect of the heel, and Chapter 92 discusses heel pain as a manifestation of the tarsal tunnel syndrome.) Characteristically, the first step in the morning is particularly painful. The pain eases after 5 to 10 minutes of walking, but during the course of the day's activities the pain becomes progressively worse. The reason why these symptoms appear, disappear, and reappear is not understood.

Examination of the foot reveals a tender area of the heel approximately 4.5 cm from the posterior margin of the plantar surface, corresponding to the medial condyle of the calcaneus. X-ray films often reveal a calcaneal exostosis or spur at the point of tenderness (Fig. 73.8). These spurs are commonly found on x-ray films of asymptomatic heels, and they are not the cause of pain in symptomatic heels. Because the attachment of the plantar fascia coincides with the point of greatest tenderness, the pain is believed to be caused by *plantar fasciitis*. One can picture the plantar fascia as an extension of the Achilles tendon, with the calcaneus acting as a fulcrum between fascia and tendon (Fig. 73.1B). Any condition that increases stress on the Achilles tendon may also stress the plantar fascia, such as overuse in running or jogging (especially with shoes having inflexible midsoles), excessive pronation (see above), or a sudden change to flat shoes after wearing high heels for prolonged periods. Heel pain may be a manifestation of gout or reactive arthritis, and these diagnoses should always be considered when evaluating such a patient (see Chapters 76 and 78).

Treatment

Treatment should be aimed at both the local inflammatory process and the underlying mechanical problem. Initial treatment includes using an oral anti-inflammatory medication (see Chapter 77), resting, and soaking in warm water. An injection (using a 25-gauge 1-inch needle) of a corticosteroid and lidocaine (approximately 0.5–1 mL of a corticosteroid suspension diluted with 1–2 mL of 1%–2% lidocaine) into the tender area from the medial aspect of the heel usually brings short-term relief from pain that has not responded to other measures (8,9) (see Chapters 69 and 74). Use of high-dose repository steroids should be avoided because of the risk for plantar fascial rupture after injection (9). The potential for fascial rupture may be minimized with the use of a combination solution such as Celestone/Soluspan, which combines a phosphate and acetate in one injection. Topical steroids delivered by iontophoresis may be effective (8). In some cases, stretching of the Achilles tendon brings relief. Spontaneous resolution of symptoms, over the course of months, is common (9).

Recurrent symptoms may be prevented by having the patient obtain a silicone heel pad. These pads are available in sport stores. When this pad is inserted into the shoes, it decreases tension on the Achilles tendon, so tension on the plantar fascia is reduced. The increased angulation of the foot shifts weight away from the heel to the forefoot. When a simple heel pad is not sufficient, consultation with an orthopedist or podiatrist is indicated. The consultant fabricates an appropriate orthotic to minimize pronation, raise the heel, and protect the painful area. Rarely, a painful heel requires surgical fasciotomy and removal of the spur.

Extracorporeal shock wave therapy (administered by a podiatrist) is used in very symptomatic and resistant cases (9). Extracorporeal shock wave therapy uses the same mechanism as lithotripsy but for treatment of plantar fascial pain. Although some studies show symptomatic improvement following extracorporeal shock wave therapy, other studies continue to refute the benefit of this technology. Extracorporeal shock wave therapy can be quite expensive and to date is largely not a covered benefit for many insurance plans, including Medicare (10).

Evidence is conflicting regarding the effectiveness of dorsiflexion night splints, which stretch the Achilles tendon, in patients with chronic pain (>6 months) (8).

METATARSALGIA

Definition and Pathogenesis

Metatarsalgia is pain in the forefoot. The most common condition causing metatarsalgia is *Morton neuroma*. In this condition, two interdigital plantar nerves between adjacent toes become compressed, inflamed, and ultimately painful. Compression of these nerves is enhanced by elevating the heel and compressing the forefoot. Therefore, women's fashionable, high-heeled, pointed-toe shoes are associated with this condition. In fact, 80% to 90% of patients with neuroma are female.

Symptoms and Signs

The symptoms of neuroma are specific and consistent. Typically, the patient describes a shooting, burning, or cramping pain in the foot involving two adjacent toes. The third and fourth toes are involved most commonly. However, the second and third toes often are affected as well. The patient describes spontaneous pain during walking or running. Invariably, the patient instinctively removes the shoe and massages the affected area, thereby relieving the pain. Presumably, the swollen nerve (neuroma) has been pinched by the metatarsal bones, causing the pain that radiates to the toes. Stopping walking eliminates the trauma, and massage may change the position of the neuroma. All of these measures result in alleviation of the pain.

Examination of the foot reveals that the neurovascular status is normal unless another disease is present. Palpation between the metatarsal heads reveals marked tenderness. If the forefoot is compressed while the web space is palpated, the area may be exquisitely tender.

Stress fracture of a metatarsal bone should be suspected in the case of sudden severe pain localized to a metatarsal shaft. X-ray films may be diagnostic but often are negative during the first few weeks of symptoms. Often the fracture will be apparent on repeat x-ray films in 2 to 3 weeks. Bone scans and magnetic resonance images are more sensitive diagnostic tools and often are positive before the radiograph (see Chapter 68).

Treatment

The most effective treatment of metatarsalgia is the wearing of low, flat, wide, soft, leather shoes. Corticosteroid with lidocaine injections into the web space and reaching the plantar surface (0.5 mL depo steroid with 1 mL lidocaine using a 25-gauge 1-inch needle) may provide temporary relief. Nonsteroidal anti-inflammatory drugs are ineffective. Orthotics are helpful; however, if the patient is willing to wear wide enough shoes to accommodate them, the condition usually resolves, even without the orthotic. Surgical excision is successful in 80% to 90% of cases and is indicated if symptoms persist. For patients undergoing surgery, a recovery period of 4 to 6 weeks is necessary before they can return to full activity and wear their usual shoes. Surgical complications are rare. As with most surgery, the possibility of postoperative infection is <3%. Peculiar to neuroma surgery is the possibility of recurrence. Rarely symptoms are not reduced. Because neuroma is entirely a clinical finding, exploration for a neuroma occasionally is fruitless. Fortunately, neuroma is also an uncommon occurrence, but the possibility should always be told to the patient before surgery.

Metatarsalgia not caused by neuroma is more difficult to characterize, evaluate, and treat. Nonneuritic metatarsal pain may occur anywhere in the forefoot with or without radiation and may be exacerbated by high-heeled or, at times, low-heeled shoes. Palpation often reveals pain directly on a metatarsal head rather than between them. Rest, application of ice, and elevation of the foot may help some patients, but most require referral to a podiatrist for padding, orthotics, or other treatment. Metatarsal stress fractures are another cause of metatarsalgia, usually characterized by sudden onset and pain on palpation over the involved metatarsal bone. Often there is no history of trauma. The use of shock-absorbing insoles in footwear has been shown to reduce the incidence of stress fractures in athletes and military personnel (11). Chapter 68 discusses the diagnosis and management of stress fractures.

SPECIFIC REFERENCES*

1. Litzelman DK, Slemenda Cw, Langefeld CD, et al. Reduction of lower extremity clinical abnormalities in patients with non-insulin-dependent diabetes mellitus: a randomized, controlled trial. Ann Intern Med 1993;119:36.
2. Franse LV, Valk GD, Heine RJ, et al. "Numbness of the feet" is a poor indicator for polyneuropathy in type 2 diabetic patients. Diabet Med 2000;17:105.
3. Spencer S. Pressure relieving interventions for preventing and treating diabetic foot ulcers. Cochrane Database Syst Rev 2000;(3):CD002302.
4. Singh N, Lipsky B, Armstrong D. Preventing foot ulcers in patients with diabetes. JAMA 2005;293: 217.
5. Ferrari J, Higgins JPT, Williams RL. Interventions for treating hallux valgus (abductovalgus) and bunions. Cochrane Database Syst Rev 2000;(2):CD000964.
6. Ferrari J. Hallux valgus (bunions). Clin Evid 2000;4:591.
7. Rounding C, Hulm S. Surgical treatments for ingrowing toenails. Cochrane Database Syst Rev 2000;(2):CD001541.
8. Crawford F, Atkins D, Edwards J. Interventions for treating plantar heel pain. Cochrane Database Syst Rev 2003;(3):CD000416.
9. Crawford F. Plantar heel pain (including plantar fasciitis). Clin Evid 2000;4:664.
10. Rompe JD, Decking J, Schoellner C, et al. Shock wave application for chronic plantar fasciitis in running athletes: a prospective, randomized, placebo-controlled trial. Am J Sports Med 2003; 31;268.
11. Gillespie WJ, Grant J. Interventions for preventing and treating stress fractures and stress reactions of bone of the lower limbs in young adults. Cochrane Database Syst Rev 2000;(2):CD000450.

*Bold numerals denote published controlled clinical trials, meta-analyses, or consensus-based recommendations.

For annotated **General References** *and resources related to this chapter, visit www.hopkinsbayview.org/PAMreferences.*

Chapter 74

Nonarticular Rheumatic Disorders

David B. Hellmann

BURSITIS

General Considerations

Bursitis, the inflammation of a bursal sac, is a common problem. Bursal sacs are structures lined with a synovial membrane that secretes and absorbs liquid. The bursae provide a lubricating mechanism between structures such as bones, ligaments, tendons, muscles, and skin. Although they usually are isolated, occasionally they are in communication with a joint space. There are more than 150 such structures in the body, but the number is not fixed. A new bursa may appear whenever there is friction between structures.

Bursitis usually is easy to diagnose and treat in the office. Occasionally, clinicians face the challenge of distinguishing bursitis from arthritis or other conditions. Also, it is important to quickly recognize and treat the few patients who have septic bursitis. When the diagnosis remains uncertain or the usual treatments are unsuccessful, referral to an orthopedist or rheumatologist may be necessary.

Causes

The most common cause of bursitis is minor trauma, as may occur to the subdeltoid bursa from repetitively throwing a baseball or to the prepatellar bursa from prolonged kneeling on a concrete floor. Because the development of bursitis is a function of both physical stresses and the condition of the bursa and surrounding tissues, bursitis is rare before age 20 years; it is particularly common in middle-aged and older people. Less often, bursitis is caused by systemic disorders such as rheumatoid arthritis, polymyalgia rheumatica, or gout. Septic bursitis after trauma is of special concern in patients with superficial bursitis (e.g., olecranon or prepatellar bursitis). Basic calcium phosphate crystals are associated with calcific periarthritis, tendinitis, and bursitis, but little is understood about the exact mechanism of calcium crystal deposition.

Manifestations

Patients with acute bursitis experience abrupt onset of localized pain that is exquisitely tender and usually is aggravated by any movement of the structures adjacent to the bursae. The pain usually is described as a deep aching discomfort. How well the patient can localize the discomfort depends on whether the bursa is superficial or deep to the skin and whether the affected region has extensive or exiguous sensory nerve fibers. Thus, when asked "Where does it hurt?," the patient with anserine bursitis often uses a fingertip to pinpoint the location, whereas a patient with trochanteric bursitis usually waves the entire hand over the general region of pain.

Bursitis near the knee, hip, elbow, or shoulder can mimic arthritis of those structures. Features that suggest bursitis include sudden onset after some repetitive physical activity; swelling, redness, or tenderness localized to the bursa and not the joint (see below); absence of pain on passive motion of the joint; and, if necessary, a normal joint x-ray film or magnetic resonance imaging.

Infection is suggested by fluctuant swelling of the bursa in association with redness and heat of the overlying skin (1). Location is an important consideration because the vast majority of bursal infections involve the olecranon and prepatellar bursae. Some comorbid conditions, notably diabetes, alcoholism, intravenous drug use, and immunosuppression, increase the likelihood of septic bursitis. Fever should always suggest infection, but it also can complicate gouty bursitis. The absence of fever does not exclude infection; only 40% of patients with septic bursitis demonstrate fever (1). A large bursal swelling can compress other structures or even rupture, thus explaining why bursitis around the knee or the hip can present as diffuse leg swelling (mimicking thrombophlebitis), an inguinal hernia, or a pelvic mass (2).

TABLE 74.1 Technique for Aspiration of Superficial Bursae (or Joints) and Analysis of Bursal (or Synovial) Fluid

1. Determine by palpation the area of maximal tenderness or fluctuance and outline with indelible pen.
2. Clean the skin with iodine solution such as povidone (Betadine).
3. Anesthetize the skin with lidocaine in the area of planned aspiration.
4. Use an 18-gauge needle to aspirate.
5. Grossly inspect the fluid and analyze for following:
   A. Cell count and differential; fluid must be in a tube containing heparin or ethylenediamine tetraacetate.
   B. Type of crystals (see Chapter 76).
   C. Gram stain and culture using transport media (even in the absence of a high white cell count).

Aspiration of Bursae

Aspiration usually is easily accomplished by the generalist, especially when the bursa is superficial (Table 74.1). The chief indication for aspirating a bursa is to rule out infection. Analysis of bursa (or joint) fluid can also reveal whether the fluid is inflamed or contains crystals (usually from gout).

The laboratory tests performed on bursal (or joint) fluid depend on the clinical questions (Table 74.2). A bursal or joint fluid white blood cell count >1,000 indicates inflammation; <1,000 white blood cells is characteristic of traumatic fluid (Table 74.2). Bursal infection tends to give very high white blood cell counts, averaging approximately 75,000 for olecranon bursitis (1). Rheumatoid arthritis and gout also occasionally produce markedly elevated bursal fluid white blood cell counts. Gram stains and cultures are the specific tests for infection. Similarly, examining the fluid with a microscope equipped with polarizing lenses is the only way to identify the crystals that are specific for gout (see Chapter 76). Therefore, most bursal fluid can be characterized by the white blood cell count, Gram stain plus culture, and analysis for crystals. Glucose, protein, mucin clot, and other (e.g., enzymes, complement) determinations are not specific and are not needed.

Treatment

Treatment of septic bursitis requires administering antibiotics and draining the bursal sac. Gram stain of the bursal fluid (see below) should guide initial antibiotic choice. More than 75% of cases of septic bursitis are caused by *Staphylococcus aureus,* but Gram stain is positive in only 65%. If the Gram stain shows no bacteria or if gram-positive cocci are found, a penicillinase-resistant antistaphylococcal drug should be used. Vancomycin should be used initially if the patient is acutely ill or has recently been in a facility or lives in a region where methicillin resistant *S. aureus* is prevalent. If gram-negative organisms are found, blood cultures should be obtained and an extrabursal site of infection sought. The antibiotic choice should be based on the organism most likely causing the extrabursal infection. The need for hospitalization depends on both the severity of the infection and the degree of host compromise. Patients with high fever and chills, intense surrounding cellulitis, deep bursal involvement, extrabursal infection, or suspicion of an uncommon organism should be hospitalized for administration of parenteral antibiotics. Hospitalization also should be considered for patients who are compromised by age, alcoholism, diabetes mellitus, or immunosuppression, almost regardless of the intensity of bursal inflammation. Patients who are less ill and less frail can be treated with oral antibiotics on an outpatient basis. Repeat bursal aspiration also is required until the fluid stops accumulating. For example, successful treatment of septic olecranon bursitis requires an average of two to three aspirations over 1 or 2 weeks. The timing of these repeat aspirations is based solely on the clinical response (or absence thereof) of the patient. The duration of antibiotic therapy averages 2 to 4 weeks but should be individualized according to the clinical response and the character of aspirated fluid. In cases requiring repeated bursal aspiration, antibiotics should be continued for at least 5 additional days after the bursal fluid has become sterile or for a total of 2 weeks (whichever is longer).

Gout, pseudogout, or *rheumatoid arthritis* should be treated with anti-inflammatory agents (see Chapters 76 and 77). Usually *traumatic bursitis* resolves spontaneously

TABLE 74.2 Patterns of Bursal (or Joint) Fluid Findings in Common Problems

	Normal	*Trauma*	*Sepsis*	*Rheumatoid Inflammation*	*Microcrystalline Inflammation*
Color of fluid	Clear yellow	Bloody, xanthochromic	Yellow to cloudy	Clear yellow to cloudy	Clear yellow to cloudy
WBC, RBC	0–200/0	<1,000/many	1,000–200,000/few	1,000–20,000[a]/few	1,000–20,000[a]/few
Crystals	~	~	~	~	+[b]
Culture	~	~	+	~	~

[a]Cell count in noninfected inflammatory fluid may be as high as it is with sepsis, thus the need for culture.
[b]Gout, negatively birefringent sodium urate. Pseudogout, positively birefringent sodium pyrophosphate (see Chapter 76).
+, test positive; ~, not applicable or negative; RBC, red blood cell; WBC, white blood cell.

TABLE 74.3 Treatment of Bursitis

1. Avoid repetitive trauma to the bursa; splint where feasible (especially effective in the hand and fingers).
2. Application of heat or cold may be of benefit in some patients.
3. First-line pharmacologic treatment is either injection of lidocaine and a steroid preparation (see Table 74.4) into the bursa or prescription of a nonsteroidal anti-inflammatory agent (see Chapter 77 for a full discussion of these agents).
4. Improvement usually is seen in several days, but the anti-inflammatory agent should be continued an additional 4–5 days to prevent recurrence.
5. If a nonsteroidal anti-inflammatory agent is used first and produces no significant response in 5–7 days and sepsis has been ruled out, the bursa can be injected with lidocaine or a steroid preparation (see Table 74.4).

if the area of inflammation is rested. However, spontaneous resolution requires several weeks, and therapy shortens this period considerably. Therefore, if sepsis and gout are ruled out, the treatment outlined in Table 74.3 is indicated.

First-line therapy for nonseptic bursitis can be either a nonsteroidal anti-inflammatory agent (see Chapter 77) or an injection into the bursa of a mixture of lidocaine and depoglucocorticoid (Table 74.4). Injection usually is the better initial choice when the patient has severe pain (which often intensifies at night) and when the clinician has experience with soft-tissue injections. Cellulitis of skin overlying the bursa contraindicates bursal injection. Systemic anticoagulation with warfarin or heparin is a relative contraindication to bursal injection. Immediate and dramatic but transient relief of pain secondary to lidocaine indicates that the proper site has been injected. The anti-inflammatory effect of the steroid injection is seen in approximately 72 hours. If the response is not satisfactory, the bursa can be reinjected in approximately 2 weeks. Waiting 2 weeks before reinjection provides ample time

TABLE 74.4 Methods of Injection of Bursae or Joints with Lidocaine or Depoglucocorticoid Preparations

1. Be certain sepsis has been ruled out (see Tables 74.1 and 74.2).
2. Prepare the skin carefully with an iodine-containing solution such as povidone (Betadine).
3. Anesthetize the skin with intradermal 1%–2% lidocaine.
4. Mix 2–3 mL of 1%–2% lidocaine with 10–40 mg (depending on size of bursa) of a depo glucocorticoid (e.g., Celestone, Aristocort, or Kenalog), and inject the bursa with 1–3 mL of this mixture using a 22-gauge needle.

Notes of caution: Injection into the skin will cause atrophy and thus should be avoided; the patient should understand there is a possibility of this complication. Injection into tendons themselves may cause degeneration and, in time, rupture; these structures should be avoided by careful palpation.

to rule out iatrogenic sepsis, which occurs rarely after a steroid injection. Depending on the location, other modalities such as ultrasound, heat or cold application, and physical therapy can be used as adjuncts. If a bursitis does not respond to two steroid injections, rheumatologic consultation to rule out associated systemic disease may be necessary. Rarely, definitive treatment by surgical excision of the bursa is necessary.

Specific Forms

Several forms of bursitis are particularly common, and their unique aspects are described.

Olecranon Bursitis

This common form of bursitis—also called student's or miner's elbow—is characterized by a goose egg–like swelling located just behind the olecranon process of the ulna (see Chapter 69). An effusion of the elbow joint itself, in contrast, causes diffuse swelling. Another feature that distinguishes olecranon bursitis from elbow joint inflammation is the near lack of pain with passive extension and flexion of the elbow when olecranon bursitis is the only problem. Important features of olecranon bursitis are that it often is associated with systemic disease, such as rheumatoid arthritis or gout; symptoms often are chronic, in that they have been present for 2 or 3 weeks before a patient sees a physician; and the olecranon is a common site for septic bursitis after trauma and may be associated with surrounding cellulitis. If rheumatoid arthritis or gout is present, it is important to realize that sepsis may coexist. Traumatic olecranon bursitis usually is hemorrhagic, although xanthochromic fluid may be present.

Swelling in the area of the olecranon bursa should be aspirated if symptomatic (Tables 74.1 and 74.2). Gram stain, culture, white blood cell count, and crystal identification with polarizing microscopy should be obtained.

Therapy

Patients with olecranon bursitis should be taught to avoid leaning or resting on their elbows. More specific therapy depends on the characteristics of the fluid (3). If monosodium urate crystals are present, specific therapy for gout is indicated (see Chapter 76). Traumatic bursitis responds to simple removal of fluid; however, if the fluid reaccumulates, a steroid injection (Table 74.4) should be given. If sepsis is identified, the patient should be treated with an antibiotic and bursal aspiration as outlined above.

Prepatellar Bursitis

Prepatellar bursitis (housemaid's or carpenter's knee) is a common form of bursitis, easily recognized by its location overlying the inferior portion of the patella (see Chapter 72). It is particularly common in carpet layers, plumbers, and carpenters and most often is caused by trauma from kneeling. Because it also may be a site of sepsis, usually the bursa should be aspirated.

Anserine Bursitis

The anserine bursa is fan shaped and lies between the confluence of tendons of the sartorius, gracilis, and semitendinosus muscles and the tibia at the anterior medial aspect of the knee just below the joint space (see Chapter 72). Anserine bursitis is seen most in patients with arthritis, especially overweight middle-aged women with osteoarthritis of the knee. It is recognized by its location; the pain typically is produced when the knee is flexed and is particularly troublesome at night. The patient often seeks comfort by sleeping with a pillow between the thighs.

If there is surrounding erythema or if the patient is febrile, aspiration should be attempted because sepsis, although uncommon, may be present. Therapy depends on the findings (Tables 74.2 and 74.3). When injection therapy is used, the solution should be injected in a fan-shaped pattern so that the entire bursa is treated.

Ischial Bursitis

The ischial bursa is located over the ischial tuberosity, close to the sciatic nerve and the posterior femoral cutaneous nerve. When a person is sitting, the ischial bursae are covered only with subcutaneous tissue and skin. When a person is standing, the gluteus maximus also covers the bursa.

The most common reason for inflammation of this bursa is trauma, as may occur in bicycling. It is rarely a site of sepsis. Usually the inflammation results in an abrupt onset of pain, but occasionally the onset is more insidious. The patient often has exquisite pain when sitting or lying. Because of the close proximity of the sciatic nerve to the bursa, there may be an associated neuritis resulting from pressure on the nerve, which causes sciatic pain to radiate into the leg (see Chapter 71). Direct pressure over the ischial tuberosity causes sharp pain, and the patient may hold the painful buttock elevated when sitting. In addition, the pain is intensified when the patient is supine and the hip is passively flexed. The patient has difficulty standing on tiptoe on the affected side.

The differential diagnosis of symptoms suggestive of ischial bursitis includes lumbar spine disease, thrombophlebitis, and inflammatory back disease or sacroiliitis (see Chapter 78). Localization of the pain over the ischial tuberosity and the finding of induration near the ischial tuberosity on rectal examination establish the diagnosis of ischial bursitis.

Aspiration of the bursa, even when it is inflamed, is discouraged because it often is difficult to localize, and the surrounding structures, especially the sciatic nerve, may be injured. If aspiration is indicated because there is associated fever and, therefore, the possibility of septic bursitis, the patient should be referred to an orthopedist for immediate evaluation.

The patient may obtain some comfort when sitting by using a pillow that allows pressure to be eliminated from the ischial tuberosity underlying the inflamed bursa. Standard therapy (Table 74.3) with a nonsteroidal anti-inflammatory agent usually provides dramatic improvement within 2 to 3 days; however, if there has been associated leg pain or weakness from sciatic nerve inflammation, those symptoms may persist for several months. Ultrasound therapy, administered by a physical therapist, may be effective and should be considered if initial therapy has not relieved the symptoms within several days.

If the diagnosis is unclear, there is a question of sepsis, and if the patient does not respond to therapy within 1 week, consultation with a rheumatologist or orthopedist is recommended. If the diagnosis is confirmed, the consultant may aspirate the bursa and, if sepsis is ruled out, inject it with lidocaine and depo glucocorticoid, which often results in dramatic improvement.

Semimembranosus Gastrocnemius Bursitis (Baker Cyst)

The semimembranosus gastrocnemius bursa, commonly called a *cyst,* lies in the posterior medial aspect of the knee behind the femoral condyle and in 50% of patients is continuous with the knee joint (see Chapter 72). The cyst is best seen and palpated when the patient is standing. Swelling of this bursa is commonly associated with other knee problems, such as internal derangements, rheumatoid arthritis, or degenerative arthritis. The bursa is rarely infected. Often, a Baker cyst is asymptomatic. The patient with a large cyst may note a vague discomfort or fullness behind the knee. Many Baker cysts produce symptoms only when they rupture, causing acute swelling, pain, and redness of the calf and lower leg (syndrome of pseudothrombophlebitis). The possibility that a patient with acute calf swelling has pseudothrombophlebitis from a ruptured Baker cyst is strongly suggested by finding swelling of the knee joint. When in doubt, a study to exclude thrombophlebitis should be done (see Chapter 57). Sonography, magnetic resonance imaging, and arthrography can visualize a ruptured cyst but usually are not needed if the clinical picture is consistent and thrombophlebitis has been excluded. Rarely, an unruptured Baker cyst can compress deep veins and cause thrombophlebitis.

The differential diagnosis of a posterior knee fullness includes an aneurysm of the popliteal artery. Therefore, it is important to palpate any fullness for pulsations.

Management of an uncomplicated Baker cyst includes aspiration and instillation of a corticosteroid–anesthetic mixture. Usually, this can be accomplished by aspirating and injecting the joint space. Rarely, the cyst must be aspirated or injected from the posterior approach. Because of the important structures in the popliteal fossa (artery, nerve, and vein), aspiration of the bursa posteriorly should be done by an orthopedist. Weight-bearing should be minimized for several days. The response to this therapy usually is excellent. Management of a ruptured cyst consists of bed rest, heat, and elevation. Although no data confirm this recommendation, an elastic bandage around the knee when treating a Baker cyst is not recommended because it may cause the cyst to compress more severely the venous system, increasing the chance of a thrombophlebitis. Instillation of corticosteroids into the joint that has an effusion may be helpful. Nonsteroidal anti-inflammatory agents may help; after symptoms have started to abate, ambulation can be increased slowly.

Iliopectineal Bursitis

The iliopectineal bursa lies anterior to the hip joint, with which it communicates in approximately 15% of people. It lies between the inguinal ligament and the iliopsoas muscle just lateral to the femoral artery. It may be inflamed from running or other similar trauma. Pain in the anterior pelvis, groin, and thigh is the most common manifestation of iliopectineal bursitis; swelling may result in a bulge resembling a femoral hernia (see Chapter 97) below the inguinal ligament. Bursitis may be present in conjunction with intrinsic inflammatory joint disease such as rheumatoid arthritis. Extension of the hip (e.g., during walking) intensifies the pain, so the patient often limits the stride of the affected side. The anterior crural nerve (the largest branch of the lumbar plexus) lies just below the bursa and may be irritated from bursal inflammation. The resulting neuritis causes pain in the thigh, which often is also intensified by walking. Weakness of anterior muscles of the thigh also may be present. When a bursa is enlarged, it may compress the femoral vein, resulting in edema in the affected leg.

If a hernia can be ruled out (see Chapter 97), the bursa should be aspirated by an orthopedist. Aspiration and injection with lidocaine and usually a corticosteroid result in lasting improvement.

Trochanteric Bursitis

The trochanteric bursa lies in the lateral aspect of the thigh over the greater trochanter of the femur and is closely associated with tendons of the glutei muscles (4). The problem primarily affects older people. Most cases are of unknown cause, although many are thought to result from osteoarthritis. Infection of the bursa is rare. The onset of pain may be abrupt, subacute, or chronic. Patients with trochanteric bursitis often misinterpret their lateral buttock pain to be caused by hip arthritis (which more characteristically produces groin pain). At times, the discomfort mimics that of lumbar spine disease (see Chapter 71). Occasionally, trochanteric bursitis causes pain that radiates to the knee or even to the groin. Discomfort is intensified by movement from the sitting to the standing position, going up and down stairs, or sleeping on the affected side.

On examination, point tenderness over the bursa with reproduction of the pain is observed. The Patrick test (external rotation of the hip combined with abduction) often is painful, whereas internal rotation, flexion, and extension of the hip usually are pain free. Any remaining concern about the knee or lumbar spine causing the pain is eliminated at examination of these structures. X-ray films of the bursa, which sometimes reveal calcifications, usually are not necessary.

Therapy, as outlined in Table 74.3, usually is effective. In addition, the patient should sleep with a small pillow under the involved buttock to keep weight shifted off the bursa.

Subdeltoid Bursitis

Chapter 69 discusses subdeltoid bursitis.

TENOSYNOVITIS

As with bursae, there are many sites of potential tenosynovial inflammation. Tendinitis and tenosynovitis generally occur simultaneously. The synovial-lined tendon sheath usually is the site of maximal inflammation.

Inflammation of a sheath of a tendon is a common problem. For the most part, only long tendons have sheaths. Tenosynovitis most often occurs from exercise, especially when a tendon has been used repetitively in an improperly conditioned person (see Chapter 72). Tenosynovitis also may be part of a generalized inflammatory process. Sometimes tenosynovitis is the first manifestation of this process.

Tenosynovitis often affects the dorsal extensor tendons of the wrist. It manifests most commonly as pain that is intensified with hand extension. In the acute stage, swelling and pain over the dorsal aspect of the wrist or over the dorsal radioulnar joint may occur. Occasionally, a friction rub is felt or heard when the appropriate muscle is contracted.

When tenosynovitis is identified in the absence of trauma, a systemic disease should be suspected and, if present, specific therapy administered. Gonorrhea should be suspected in sexually active people if inflammation involves the tendons of the ankle or wrist in the setting of a monarthritis, fever, and skin rash. Using Transgrow media, culture of the endocervical canal and rectum in women and of the urethra in men is indicated (see Chapter 37).

If the tenosynovitis has developed because of trauma, such as exercise or overuse, or for unknown reasons, nonspecific therapy with a nonsteroidal anti-inflammatory agent, as for bursitis (Table 74.3), is appropriate. The fingers should be splinted in the position of function. If symptoms persist after 3 or 4 days of conservative therapy, the peritenon (loose tissue surrounding the tendon) should be injected with lidocaine and a corticosteroid (e.g., Celestone, Aristocort, or Kenalog) (Table 74.4). To avoid injuring the tendon or causing skin atrophy, only small doses of depo glucocorticoid (i.e., approximately 0.5 mL of steroid mixed with an equal amount of lidocaine depending on the site) should be injected. To avoid injecting directly into the tendon, one should never inject if the syringe plunger cannot be depressed easily. Occasionally, symptoms are recurrent, in which case referral to a rheumatologist or orthopedist is indicated. Chapters 68, 69, 72 and 73 discuss tenosynovitis and tendinitis involving specific tendons.

STENOSING TENOSYNOVITIS

Stenosing tenosynovitis is not a complication of tenosynovitis; rather, it occurs primarily when trauma is severe and localized. In stenosing tenosynovitis, either a nodule forms on a tendon or an actual stenosis of a tendon sheath of a long tendon develops. As a result, the affected part sticks in a fixed position that sometimes is painful. When this condition affects the flexor tendons of the fingers, it is called *trigger finger.* The patient is unable to flex a digit fully or, once it is flexed, the digit locks and literally must be straightened by external force until it suddenly snaps free. When stenosing tenosynovitis is present in the abductor or extensor tendon of the thumb, it is called *de Quervain disease,* the most common form of stenosing tenosynovitis. In this problem, the thumb usually still has motion and does not always lock like a trigger finger. To evaluate for de Quervain tenosynovitis, the patient should make a fist by curling the fingers over the flexed thumb, then passively deviate the fist in an ulnar direction. Exquisite pain over the base of the thumb with this maneuver (*Finkelstein test*) confirms the diagnosis. Stenosing tenosynovitis usually is caused by repeated trauma (e.g., prolonged use of a screwdriver) but occasionally is seen in association with rheumatoid arthritis, amyloidosis, pregnancy, and myxedema.

The treatment is identical to that of bursitis as outlined in Tables 74.3 and 74.4. Splinting is especially helpful in the treatment of stenosing tenosynovitis of the hands and fingers. If the patient does not respond to several weeks of conservative therapy, surgical release may be necessary. When a nodule is palpable, it should be injected with a small amount of corticosteroid (e.g., 10 mg Celestone, Aristocort, or Kenalog) and lidocaine. Often, the condition resolves in several days to weeks.

DUPUYTREN CONTRACTURE

The palmar fascia may undergo nodular hypertrophic fibroplasia of unknown cause. This results over many years in the development of a flexion contracture (Dupuytren contracture). The process causes the skin to be fixed to the underlying fascia by adhesive bands, resulting in a fixed puckered appearance. A Dupuytren contracture almost always is painless but may result in significant functional disability. Although all digits may be involved, the fourth and fifth digits are affected most commonly. The condition affects primarily middle-aged or older men and is bilateral in nearly 40%. It is more common in epileptics and alcoholics, but most affected patients have neither condition. Once the condition is present, passive extension of the fingers does not retard the process and, in fact, may accelerate it. If functional disability is present, the patient should be referred to an orthopedic surgeon for consideration for surgery. Oral anti-inflammatory agents and local cortisone injections are not effective in retarding the process.

GANGLIONS

Ganglions, cystic swellings arising from the synovium of a joint or tendon sheath, are the most common benign tumors of the hand. They tend to occur more often in women from the teens through age 50 years. Onset may be sudden or gradual, and the cyst may change over time, sometimes disappearing and then recurring. The swellings usually are smooth, tense, and fixed to the deep tissues. The most common site is the dorsum of the wrist between the extensor tendon of the thumb and the extensor tendon of the index finger. They also may occur on the volar aspect of the foot (the tarsal area) and ankle. Aching or weakness of the involved area may be associated. Nonoperative treatment in symptomatic patients (generally asymptomatic ganglions are left untreated), consisting of aspiration or cortisone injection, may be successful. Recurrences may require treatment by operative excision.

FIBROMYALGIA

Fibromyalgia (also called *fibrositis*) is a syndrome of widespread chronic musculoskeletal pain, chiefly affecting young women, that is unaccompanied by any objective findings except for increased tenderness at specific anatomic sites, known as *tender points* (5). The diagnosis

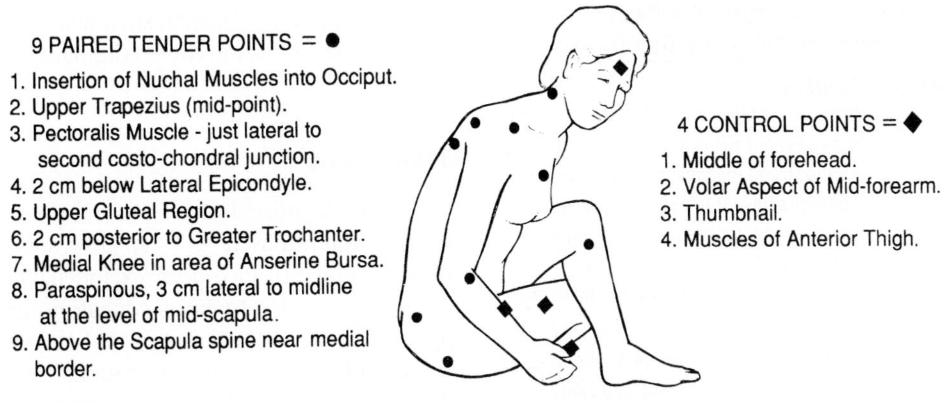

9 PAIRED TENDER POINTS = ●
1. Insertion of Nuchal Muscles into Occiput.
2. Upper Trapezius (mid-point).
3. Pectoralis Muscle - just lateral to second costo-chondral junction.
4. 2 cm below Lateral Epicondyle.
5. Upper Gluteal Region.
6. 2 cm posterior to Greater Trochanter.
7. Medial Knee in area of Anserine Bursa.
8. Paraspinous, 3 cm lateral to midline at the level of mid-scapula.
9. Above the Scapula spine near medial border.

4 CONTROL POINTS = ◆
1. Middle of forehead.
2. Volar Aspect of Mid-forearm.
3. Thumbnail.
4. Muscles of Anterior Thigh.

FIGURE 74.1. The tender point locations in fibromyalgia are remarkably constant from patient to patient. Multiple locations have been described; the nine paired tender points shown represent frequently occurring points in a wide distribution. Most patients with fibrositis usually have 11 or more tender points. Control points are not unduly tender; their examination should be interspersed with that of the tender points. (Modified from Bennett RM. The fibromyalgia syndrome. In: Kelly WN, Harris ED, Ruddy S, et al., eds. Textbook of rheumatology. 5th ed. Philadelphia: WB Saunders, 1997, 2001:513, with permission.)

is purely clinical; no laboratory tests establish the diagnosis of fibromyalgia. The cause of fibromyalgia is unknown, but speculations center on disturbances in rapid eye movement sleep, chronic viral infections, psychological disorders, neuroendocrine abnormalities, and abnormalities of muscle metabolism (5). Usually fibromyalgia is primary, occurring in the absence of other medical conditions. Some patients have secondary fibromyalgia, which is diagnosed when the syndrome accompanies another disorder, most commonly hypothyroidism, rheumatoid arthritis, hepatitis C, or Lyme disease (5).

Fibromyalgia is important to recognize for three reasons. First, fibromyalgia is common, affecting 3% to 10% of the general population and accounting for 20% to 30% of all patients referred to rheumatologists. Second, fibromyalgia responds, albeit imperfectly, to treatment. Third, failure to diagnose and treat fibromyalgia often subjects the patient to multiple consultations and needlessly expensive laboratory testing.

Manifestations

Ninety percent of patients with fibromyalgia are women. Most experience the gradual onset of symptoms between the ages of 20 and 45 years. The cardinal features of fibromyalgia are widespread soft-tissue aching and stiffness that occur essentially daily. The symptoms vary in severity, often involving the axial skeleton, shoulder, and pelvic girdles, with duration of more than 3 months. Typically the pain is chronic, persisting for years. The condition may be aggravated by fatigue, tension, excessive work, immobilization, and weather changes. Although pain is the predominant symptom, most patients with fibromyalgia have many other symptoms, including fatigue, recurrent headaches, sore throat, depression, fitful sleep, difficulty concentrating, alternating constipation and diarrhea, numbness, swollen glands, and subjective sense of fever or joint swelling. In fact, a careful history to rule out depression (see Chapter 24) and somatization (see Chapter 21) is important.

Characteristically in fibromyalgia, the rich history of complaints contrasts starkly with the poverty of physical findings. Objective adenopathy, weakness, and joint inflammation or weakness are notably absent. Indeed, the only physical finding in fibromyalgia is tender points. Although the exact number and location of these tender points are somewhat controversial, the nine paired tender points most commonly found, along with four control points, are illustrated in Fig. 74.1. Nearly 90% of patients with fibromyalgia have tenderness of at least 11 of the 18 (nine paired) tender point sites (5,6).

Laboratory tests in primary fibromyalgia are normal. The purpose of the laboratory tests and physical examination is to exclude other causes of diffuse musculoskeletal pain, which include polymyalgia rheumatica (a condition of elderly people), Parkinson syndrome, polymyositis, endocrine disorders (especially hypothyroidism, but also hyperthyroidism, Addison disease, hyperparathyroidism, and panhypopituitarism), cancer, renal tubular acidosis, and chronic fatigue syndrome (considered by many experts to be a variant of fibromyalgia). Fibromyalgia appears to be slightly more common in patients with hepatitis C and, infrequently, may be triggered by Lyme disease (5). Laboratory testing need not be extensive. Basic laboratory tests should include complete blood cell count, erythrocyte sedimentation rate, thyroid function tests, and

TABLE 74.5 Initial Examination of a Patient with Possible Fibromyalgia Syndrome

Diagnostic Step	*Finding*
Consider diagnosis	In any patient with chronic, poorly defined, generalized musculoskeletal pain; most patients have been studied previously, with normal test results; most often women, aged 20–50 yr; rule out depression and somatization by careful history.
Obtain positive response to most of the following	Chronic fatigue; chronic neck, shoulder, hip, and back pain; disturbed sleep; feeling unrefreshed and stiff in the morning; hypersensitivity to cold, heat; history consistent with tension headaches, irritable bowel syndrome; subjective paresthesias, and swelling of hands and feet without objective abnormalities.
Confirm presumptive diagnosis with physical examination	General physical examination findings normal and no evidence of arthritis or myositis (unless coexistent illness such as rheumatoid arthritis or hypothyroidism is present); tender point examination demonstrates multiple tender points at characteristic locations; associated diffuse muscle spasm and skin hypersensitivity may be present.
Laboratory tests	Complete blood cell count, erythrocyte sedimentation rate, thyroid function tests, and muscle enzyme levels should be normal.

From Goldenberg DL. Fibromyalgia syndrome. An emerging but controversial condition. JAMA 1987;257:2782, with permission.

muscle enzyme levels. Tests for hepatitis C or Lyme disease should be considered in patients with exposures to those infections. By definition, all these studies are normal in patients with primary fibromyalgia, so any abnormalities should warrant a further search for an underlying disorder.

Table 74.5 summarizes the approach to diagnosis of fibromyalgia. The two criteria for diagnosis—widespread pain and mild or greater tenderness in 11 or more of 18 tender point sites—are 88% sensitive and 81% specific. The diagnosis of fibromyalgia should not be made too quickly or too slowly. Because the diagnosis depends on excluding objective abnormalities, rarely is it wise to diagnose primary fibromyalgia on the patient's first visit. Documenting the absence of fever, weight loss, or any other abnormality takes time and increases the certainty of the diagnosis. Because fibromyalgia rarely begins after age 50 years, great caution should be exercised when considering the diagnosis in older patients. On the other hand, there is no benefit to delaying the diagnosis in a typical host with a compatible clinical picture. Indeed, such delays often prompt unnecessary consultations and redundant laboratory investigations.

Treatment

Once the diagnosis of fibromyalgia is confirmed and comorbid conditions (e.g., sleep disorders, depression, or hypothyroidism) have been excluded, the first step and cornerstone of treatment is education. Explaining to the patient that a distinct recognizable syndrome is present significantly reduces the frustrations that may have built up over months, and sometimes years, of previously unproductive medical evaluations. Patients also take solace in learning that fibromyalgia does not shorten life or cause crippling deformities and that the cause and treatment of fibromyalgia are under active investigation.

Step 2 of treatment is to consider initiating both nonpharmacologic and pharmacologic treatment. Although no drug has been specifically approved by the U.S. Food and Drug administration for managing fibromyalgia, controlled trials have demonstrated that several treatments can modestly improve symptoms (5). For example, the tricyclic antidepressants, such as amitriptyline (e.g., Elavil, Endep, or generic, 10–50 mg at bedtime), and cyclobenzaprine compounds, which are structurally related to the tricyclic antidepressants (e.g., Flexeril or generic, 5–30 mg at bedtime), can improve fibromyalgia symptoms (5,7). Fluoxetine (Prozac), a selective serotonin reuptake inhibitor, also has been demonstrated to be effective at 20 mg/day (5,8). Nonsteroidal anti-inflammatory medications are generally not effective. Corticosteroids and narcotics have no role in the treatment of fibromyalgia. Because of the modest efficacy of pharmacologic therapy, treatment often may include other modalities as well, such as cognitive behavioral therapy and an exercise program to maintain a good general level of aerobic fitness (5,9,10). Attempts should be made to modify other aggravating factors, such as mechanical, physical, and psychologic stresses. Should steps 1 and 2 be ineffective, then consideration should be given to referring the patient to specialists (e.g., rheumatologists, psychiatrists, or psychologists) (5).

MYOFASCIAL PAIN SYNDROMES

Related problems, possibly distinct from fibromyalgia, are the myofascial pain syndromes (MPS), which are characterized by the presence of deep tender points. However, in MPS, the tender point is termed a *trigger point* because firm palpation of the point produces pain in a referred distribution. A second feature distinguishing MPS from fibromyalgia is the presence of just one or a regional clustering of points in MPS, in contrast to the widespread distribution of symptoms and tender points in any given patient with fibromyalgia. A wide array of clinical syndromes in many different anatomic areas have been ascribed to MPS.

The pathogenesis of MPS is unknown. Patients with MPS may be helped by passive stretching of involved muscles after injection of the trigger point with a local anesthetic or use of a vapocoolant spray (e.g., ethyl chloride). Attention should be directed to elimination of any possible aggravating factors, such as overuse or repetitive injury to involved muscle areas.

RAYNAUD PHENOMENON

Definition

Raynaud phenomenon is a syndrome characterized by episodic vasospasm of the digital vessels in response to cold or emotional stress. Classically, a triphasic response occurs. First cutaneous pallor extends from the fingertips to the middle of the fingers, followed rapidly by mottling of the skin and cyanosis as venous blood refluxes back into an empty cutaneous capillary bed (this pallor or cyanosis persists until rewarming of the digits). Finally, the recovery phase occurs over 15 to 20 minutes, resulting in intense hyperemia (11,12). Vasospasm usually is triggered by an abrupt change in ambient temperature, so it may occur even in the summer when a patient moves into air-conditioned or refrigerated areas. Attacks may begin in one finger before spreading to other digits in both hands. The feet and other acral parts (e.g., the ears or nose) may be involved. Patients often do not describe spontaneously the classic phases of Raynaud phenomenon but commonly note deep cyanosis associated with numbness, a pins-and-needles sensation, or frank pain on cold exposure.

Causes and Prevalence

Raynaud phenomenon most commonly occurs in an idiopathic or primary form, called Raynaud disease, in which no underlying abnormality can be defined. Raynaud phenomenon also can occur secondary to a defined vascular abnormality or in association with a specific disease process (Table 74.6). Primary Raynaud phenomenon is thought to be common, occurring principally in women aged 20 to 30 years. The true prevalence of Raynaud phenomenon is unknown but is estimated to be 2% to 6% in the general population and up to 20% in the selective population of young women. Patients with primary Raynaud phenomenon are otherwise healthy, generally have infrequent attacks (one to four episodes weekly), and rarely develop local cutaneous complications, such as digital pitting, ulcerations, or loss of hand function. Patients with primary Raynaud phenomenon usually have an uncomplicated course, with gradual decrease in the frequency of episodes over a number of years. Estimates suggest that 8% to 19% of patients believed initially to have the primary form will develop a defined secondary form (usually a connective tissue disease).

TABLE 74.6 Classification of Raynaud Phenomenon

A. Primary: Idiopathic Raynaud, Raynaud disease

B. Secondary: Disorders associated with Raynaud phenomenon

	Percentage of patients with stated disorder who also have Raynaud phenomenon
1. Connective tissue diseases	
A. Systemic sclerosis	90
B. Systemic lupus erythematosus	20
C. "Mixed" connective tissue disease	75
D. Dermatomyositis/polymyositis	20
E. Rheumatoid arthritis	10
2. Neurovascular compression	
A. Thoracic outlet syndrome (e.g., cervical ribs, scalenus anticus syndrome)	
B. Carpal tunnel syndrome	
3. Arterial disease	
A. Arteriosclerosis	
B. Arteritis (e.g., Takayasu arteritis, thromboangiitis obliterans [Buerger disease])	
4. Hematologic disorders	
A. Paraproteinemia	Unknown
B. Cryoglobulinemia	
C. Polycythemia	
D. Hyperviscosity syndrome	
5. Occupational	
A. Vibratory tools (white finger syndrome)	
B. Polyvinyl chloride exposure	
6. Drugs	
A. Ergot-containing drugs (e.g., ergotamine)	
B. β-Adrenergic blockers	
C. Sympathomimetic agents (e.g., Actifed)	
D. Methysergide (Sansert)	
E. Chemotherapy (bleomycin, vinblastine)	
7. Miscellaneous	
A. Primary pulmonary hypertension	30
B. Migraine headache	10

In approximately 40% of patients who present to a general physician with Raynaud phenomenon, the phenomenon is secondary to an underlying condition, the most common being a connective tissue disease (Table 74.6). Raynaud phenomenon occurs in >90% of patients with systemic sclerosis and may be the initial symptom, preceding the other features of the disease by years. Approximately 40% of patients with systemic lupus erythematosus and 10% of patients with rheumatoid arthritis may have associated Raynaud phenomenon. Raynaud phenomenon may be a presenting feature in patients who have a systemic vasculitis. Disturbances of the axillary or cervical neurovascular bundle can lead to Raynaud phenomenon. Patients with neurovascular compression syndromes (cervical rib, scalenus anticus syndrome) and proximal vascular lesions (atherosclerosis) may present with unilateral Raynaud phenomenon. Hematologic abnormalities, such as cryoglobulinemia, paraproteinemia, or cold hemagglutinins, may present as typical Raynaud phenomenon. Ergot-containing drugs, such as ergotamine, and β-blocking agents may be causative or potentiating agents. Occupational injury (vibration white finger syndrome) causing the syndrome occurs in a high proportion of workers who operate vibratory tools (e.g., lumberjacks, shipyard workers, or meat cutters).

Initially, determining whether a patient has a primary or secondary form of Raynaud phenomenon may be difficult. Clues that suggest a secondary form include onset during childhood, male sex, onset in a woman after age 30 years, unilateral Raynaud, Raynaud affecting a single digit, fingertip ulcers, digital gangrene, or symptoms or signs of a systemic disorder.

Evaluation

Patients with Raynaud phenomenon should have a focused history (including a drug review) and physical examination to determine whether their condition is primary or secondary. An extension of the examination, evaluation of the nail bed with an ophthalmoscope (using approximately a 20+ diopter), may reveal small telangiectasias or abnormal cutaneous capillary loops. These small vessel changes may be the earliest findings in an associated underlying connective tissue disease, primarily systemic sclerosis (13). The presence of ulcers on the digits indicates that the Raynaud is very severe and that the patient likely has a secondary form of Raynaud phenomenon. Patients with unilateral Raynaud phenomenon should be carefully evaluated for a local vascular lesion, including bilateral blood pressure determination, auscultation over major vessels to determine the presence or absence of vascular bruits, and assessment of the peripheral pulses. Special testing for possible neurovascular compression syndrome (see Chapter 69) and consideration for chest x-ray film, magnetic resonance angiography, and noninvasive evaluation of the peripheral circulation (Doppler studies or digital plethysmography) are appropriate when only unilateral Raynaud phenomenon is present. Angiography may be necessary in cases where a correctable occlusive vascular lesion is strongly suspected. Carpal tunnel syndrome has been implicated in both unilateral and bilateral Raynaud phenomenon, and nerve conduction studies may be appropriate when the history and physical examination suggest this nerve compression syndrome (see Chapter 92).

If the patient is a woman with onset between the ages of 15 and 30 years who has mild bilateral Raynaud, does not have nail fold capillary changes, has no ulcerations or other ischemic finger tip changes, and exhibits no other manifestations of a connective tissue disease, primary Raynaud is the likely diagnosis (12). For such a patient, laboratory evaluation can be limited to verifying a normal complete blood count, a negative antinuclear antibody test, and ordering renal and liver function tests to screen for collagen disease affecting these organs. If the patient is suspected of having secondary Raynaud, determinations of disease-specific autoantibodies (e.g., anti–double-stranded DNA antibodies for systemic lupus erythematosus, and anti-centromere or anti–SCL-70 antibodies for scleroderma), cryoglobulins, Westergren erythrocyte sedimentation rate, and serum protein electrophoresis are indicated. Referring the patient to a rheumatologist for any additional evaluation is appropriate. Even when a systemic illness is not identified, the patient should be followed expectantly because an underlying illness may emerge several years later.

Treatment

The principal mode of treatment in patients in whom a correctable cause cannot be found is avoiding the cold and staying warm (11). This includes wearing mittens or gloves and avoiding a general chill of the body by wearing a hat and loose-fitting warm clothing in winter months. Smoking aggravates Raynaud phenomenon and should be stopped (see Chapter 27). Drugs that promote vasoconstriction (Table 74.6) should be stopped or avoided. Emotional stress should be assessed and controlled by appropriate measures (see Chapter 20). Patients with mild Raynaud phenomenon often improve with education about the cause and nature of these episodes. Unfortunately, temperature biofeedback therapy is ineffective. Table 74.7 summarizes the nonpharmacologic treatment of patients with Raynaud phenomenon. Most patients, particularly those with primary Raynaud phenomenon, do not need, and should not be treated with, drugs. Rather, pharmacologic treatment should be limited to patients with repeated attacks who limit their daily activities or who have developed digital ulceration or other ischemic changes. There is no evidence that decreasing the number of episodes of Raynaud phenomenon will alter the progressive changes that may occur in patients with scleroderma or another connective tissue disease.

A wide variety of vasoactive agents has been used in patients with Raynaud phenomenon, but few agents have proved to be definite benefit. Many of the patients are young women of child-bearing potential; therefore, unproven treatment that may have a teratogenic effect should be avoided.

TABLE 74.7 Nonpharmacologic Management of Patients with Raynaud Phenomenon

Education and reassurance
- Establish precipitating factors (e.g., refrigerator/freezer, air conditioning, emotional stress).
- Provide emotional support (e.g., assurance of the mild nature of the disease in most patients may reduce some of the stress that can precipitate attacks).

Avoidance of precipitating factors
- Wear gloves before reaching into refrigerator or freezer.
- Wear warm body clothing to avoid cold exposure.
- Keep head covered to prevent heat loss.
- Keep extremities warm and body well covered in cool weather or in air-conditioned environments.
- Be aware that stress can cause Raynaud attacks.

Avoidance of certain drugs that precipitate attacks
- β-blockers (e.g., propranolol)
- Ergot-containing drugs (e.g., ergotamine)
- Sympathomimetic agents (e.g., isoproterenol, Actifed, or other cold remedies)
- Nicotine (smoking)
- Oral contraceptives

Calcium channel blockers are the cornerstone of drug therapy for Raynaud (11,14). Nifedipine has been most extensively used and its efficacy best documented, but other preparations (including amlodipine, isradipine, nicardipine, nisoldipine, and felodipine) also may be effective (11,15). These agents relax smooth muscle, reduce peripheral vascular resistance, and increase peripheral blood flow. Patients with primary Raynaud respond better than patients with Raynaud phenomenon secondary to a connective tissue disease, especially systemic sclerosis. The major side effects of these agents are secondary to their vasodilatory activity and include hypotension, dizziness, headache, and peripheral edema. Approximately 40% to 50% of patients experience some light-headedness caused by hypotension and flushing on initiation of calcium channel blocker therapy. However, these side effects usually are transient, can be minimized by starting with low doses, and do not require discontinuation of the medication. For this reason, the orthostatic blood pressure should be periodically measured. Calcium channel blockers should never be used during pregnancy or in a patient planning to become pregnant because these agents have been shown to be teratogenic in animal models.

The calcium channel blocker that has been most extensively studied, and the drug of first choice, is nifedipine. The initial dosage usually is 30 mg of a sustained-released preparation once daily. The patient should be encouraged to resume usual activities and to keep a diary of the number and intensity of Raynaud attacks. The patient should be monitored for important orthostatic hypotension (symptomatic decrease in systolic pressure $\geq$20 mm Hg below baseline or a fall <90 mm Hg). If needed to improve control of Raynaud phenomenon, the dosage of nifedipine can be increased by 30 mg sustained-release preparation every 2 weeks to a maximum of 90 mg sustained-release preparation daily. Thereafter, monitoring every 2 to 4 months is important because the initial response may be transient, and side effects, such as esophageal reflux, may limit the usefulness of the drug. If the patient does not respond to nifedipine or the drug is not tolerated, amlodipine beginning at 5 mg/day can be initiated (11). Patients generally have resolution or a dramatic reduction in the intensity and number of episodes of Raynaud phenomenon in the summer. For this reason, medication should be discontinued unless repeated cold exposure or active Raynaud phenomenon is documented.

Other drugs have been used for treatment of Raynaud phenomenon. Intravenous iloprost has been shown to be moderately effective for severe Raynaud in patients with scleroderma, but this agent is no longer available in the United States (11,16). Orally administered prostaglandins have not been shown to be effective (14). Losartan, an angiotensin II type 1 receptor antagonist, has shown promise in treating primary and secondary forms of Raynaud phenomenon (17). Topical nitroglycerin paste applied to the digits or nitroglycerin patches have been used with some success, but their indications are not established, and consultation with a rheumatologist is suggested before such agents are prescribed. Prazosin (Minipress) occasionally is of benefit if it is tolerated (2–8 mg/day in two or three divided doses) (18). Nutritional antioxidants have not been shown to be effective.

Surgical sympathectomy once was a popular treatment of Raynaud phenomenon but now is rarely performed, primarily because of the high relapse rate (40%–50%) and frequency of significant postural hypotension. Selective digital sympathectomy may be performed in centers where microsurgery is available; however, long-term controlled studies of this procedure are lacking. Sympathectomy should be considered only for short-term relief from an intractable course complicated by digital ulceration that has failed medical treatment. All patients who have had such a severe course or have ulcers on their digits should be seen by a vascular surgeon or rheumatologist. Local digital block performed by a vascular surgeon or rheumatologist has been used for temporary treatment of significant digital tissue compromise. A good response may predict which patient may have a good effect from digital or cervical sympathectomy. A patient who has severe disease with digital ulcers is susceptible to developing secondary soft-tissue infection. Local débridement and antimicrobial treatment may be necessary if ischemic ulcerations become infected. Whirlpool treatment is the most effective method of ulcer débridement. In cases of secondary complications, consultation with a vascular surgeon or a rheumatologist is advised.

SPECIFIC REFERENCES*

1. Zimmerman B III, Mikolich DJ, Ho G Jr. Septic bursitis. Semin Arthritis Rheum 1995;24:391.
2. Underwood PL, McLeod GA, Ginsburg WW. The varied clinical manifestations of iliopsoas bursitis. J Rheumatol 1988;15:1683.
3. **3.** Smith DL, McAfee JH, Lucas LM, et al. Treatment of nonseptic olecranon bursitis: a controlled, blinded prospective trial. Arch Intern Med 1989;149:2527.
4. Shbeeb MI, Matteson EL. Trochanteric bursitis (greater trochanter pain syndrome). Mayo Clin Proc 1996;71:565.
5. Goldenberg DL, Burckhardt C, Crofford L. Management of fibromyalgia syndrome. JAMA 2004;292:2388.
6. **6.** Wolfe F, Smythe HA, Yunus MB, et al. The American College of Rheumatology 1990 criteria for the classification of fibromyalgia. Arthritis Rheum 1990;33:160.
7. **7.** Carette S, McCain GA, Bell DA, et al. Evaluation of amitriptyline in primary fibrositis: a double-blind, placebo controlled study. Arthritis Rheum 1986;29:655.
8. **8.** Arnold LM, Hess EV, Hudson JI, et al. A randomized, placebo-controlled, double-blind, flexible-dose study of fluoxetine in the treatment of women with fibromyalgia. Am J Med 2002;112:191.
9. **9.** Gowans SE, Dehueck A, Voss S, et al. Six-month and one-year followup of 23 weeks of aerobic exercise for individuals with fibromyalgia. Arthritis Rheum 2004;51:890.
10. Mannerkorpi K. Exercise in fibromyalgia. Curr Opin Rheumatol. 2005;17:190.
11. Wigley FM. Raynaud's phenomenon. N Engl J Med 2002;347:1001.
12. Wigley FM, Flavahan NA. Raynaud's phenomenon. Rheum Dis Clin North Am 1996;22:765.
13. **13.** Fitzgerald O, Hess EV, O'Connor GT, et al. Prospective study of the evaluation of Raynaud's phenomenon. Am J Med 1988;84:718.
14. **14.** Rodeheffer RJ, Rammer JA, Wigley F, et al. Controlled double-blind trial of nifedipine in the treatment of Raynaud's phenomenon. N Engl J Med 1983;303:880.
15. Thompson AE, Shea B, Welch V, et al. Calcium-channel blockers for Raynaud's phenomenon in systemic sclerosis. Arthritis Rheum 2001;44:1841.
16. **16.** Wigley FM, Wise RA, Seibold JR, et al. Intravenous iloprost infusion in patients with Raynaud phenomenon secondary to systemic sclerosis: a multicenter placebo-controlled, double-blind study. Ann Intern Med 1994;120:199.
17. **17.** Dziadzio M, Denton CP, Smith R, et al. Losartan therapy for Raynaud's phenomenon and scleroderma: clinical and biochemical findings in a fifteen-week, randomized, parallel-group, controlled trial. Arthritis Rheum 1999;42:2646.
18. **18.** Wollersheim H, Thien T, Fennis J, et al. Double-blind, placebo-controlled study of prazosin in Raynaud's phenomenon. Clin Pharmacol Ther 1986;40:219.

*Bold numerals denote published controlled clinical trials, meta-analyses, or consensus-based recommendations.

For annotated ***General References*** *and resources related to this chapter, visit www.hopkinsbayview.org/PAMreferences.*

Chapter 75

Osteoarthritis

Shari M. Ling and Joan M. Bathon

Osteoarthritis (OA) is the most common form of arthritis in the United States (1,2). It is projected that OA will affect some 60 million Americans by the year 2020. This estimate reflects the increasing lifespan of Americans but does not account for the astounding rise in obesity that will further boost the prevalence of OA, particularly of weight-bearing joints. OA contributes significantly to limitations in the ability of individuals to ambulate and carry out tasks of daily living (3,4). Treatment of OA remains limited and is focused primarily on modification of behaviors that reduce risk of progression, reduction of pain through medicinal and nonmedicinal approaches, and, in some cases, surgical intervention. The search for clinically relevant biologic markers for early detection of disease has intensified over recent years. Although disease-modifying therapies are being sought, few, if any, interventions have proved to slow the progress of OA. The increasing impact of OA on public health has prompted the National Institutes of Health (NIH) to initiate two collaborative OA research networks: the OA Biomarkers Network and the Osteoarthritis Initiative. These networks will use state-of-the-art immunologic, biochemical, and imaging methods to identify risk factors and biomarkers for the development and progression of OA, with the long-term goal of identifying disease modifying or curative therapies for OA. This chapter highlights the current understanding of the pathophysiology, clinical and diagnostic features, and treatment of OA.

EPIDEMIOLOGY, CAUSES, AND PREDISPOSING FACTORS

OA is the most common form of arthritis in the United States and Europe (1). Given the prolonged life expectancy

TABLE 75.1 Factors Contributing to Development of Osteoarthritis

Aging
Diminished proteoglycan aggregation
Diminished resistance of cartilage to fatigue fracture (?defective collagen network)
Decreased resiliency of soft tissues and bone
Loss of normal anatomic relationship (hip)
Gender
Joint trauma: Excess repetitive stress
Occupational
Sports related
Associated with neuropathy
Abnormal distribution of mechanical stress
Postural or developmental defects
Joint instability or hypermobility
Local incongruity of joint surfaces posttraumatic, after meniscectomy, prolonged immobilization
Obesity
Muscle strength
Heredity/genetics
Heberden nodes
Primary generalized osteoarthritis (female gender)
Postural or developmental defects (e.g., scoliosis, slipped capital femoral epiphyses, Legg-Calvé-Perthes disease)
Procollagen gene (*COL2A1*) defects
Crystalline deposit disease
Calcium pyrophosphate
Hydroxyapatite
Previous inflammatory joint disease
Metabolic abnormalities
Ochronosis
Wilson disease
Acromegaly

in the United States and the aging of the "baby boomer" cohort, the prevalence of OA is expected to increase further. Although the precise cause of OA is unknown, multiple causes and many factors likely influence disease expression. Epidemiologic and observational studies provide important clues to the mechanisms by which OA develops and progresses and thus identify risk factors that might comprise targets for future interventions (5). Table 75.1 lists these risk factors.

The prevalence of OA increases with age and peaks in the 70s. However, OA may begin as early as age 30 years in individuals with multiple risk factors. OA usually is defined in one of two ways in the literature. The diagnosis may be based solely on typical radiographic features ("radiographic OA") or on a combination of pain/stiffness and radiographic findings ("symptomatic OA"). Thus, prevalence estimates vary by the definition used, as well as by the joint that is targeted. Estimates that originate from population-based epidemiologic studies are most commonly based upon radiographic definition.

Age: Advanced age is the strongest risk factor for the development of OA across all anatomic sites (1). Prevalence rates for both radiographic OA and, to a lesser extent, symptomatic OA (moderate or severe) increase with age,with a steep rise after age 50 years in men and age 40 years in women. In the peripheral joints, radiographic OA of the hand is the most prevalent form, followed by the knee and then the hip. Radiographic knee OA has been reported in as many as 44% of individuals aged 80 years or older, although the prevalence of associated painful symptoms was significantly lower (11% in women and 7% in men). This higher rate of radiographic, compared to symptomatic, disease is typical of most studies of OA (5,6). Thus, it is not unusual to find incidental radiographic OA in an otherwise asymptomatic older patient. OA (whether defined radiographically or symptomatically) is uncommon in individuals younger than 35 years. Symptomatic OA of the knee and of the hip are the most prevalent in both sexes, with symptomatic involvement of the hands increasing in women beginning at menopause (1,7). New onset of radiographic and symptomatic OA of the knee continues to develop in older adults at a rate of 1% to 2% per year, again moreso in women than in men (2).

Gender: Until recently, the risk of OA in young adult years had been higher for men than women. This was attributed to the greater risk of sports-related and occupational injuries endured by men (7). However, the recently observed increase in sports-related injuries of the anterior cruciate ligament (ACL) in women (8) may influence the epidemiologic trends in coming years to match the female predominance observed in middle and later life. It has been postulated that the increased prevalence of OA in women may be due to changes in the hormonal milieu (9,10). A reduced risk of incident hip OA has been observed in longitudinal studies of women receiving hormonal therapy, particularly for bilateral radiographic OA and more severe OA (9). However, estrogen/progestin replacement has not been proven to reduce the odds of knee pain or disability in women with knee symptoms (10). Whether estrogen or hormonal therapy is beneficial to patients with OA remains controversial and further emphasizes that symptoms and pathogenesis of OA likely develop by different mechanisms.

Joint Trauma and Nontraumatic Biomechanical Factors: Joint trauma has been shown to increase the risk of OA (11,12). Meniscectomy is associated with a sixfold increase in risk for development of radiographic OA (13–15), even if limited rather than total meniscal resection is used (14,15). Obesity, female sex, and pre-existing early-stage OA further increase the risk of symptomatic OA in patients years after a meniscectomy (13), as does the presence of radiographic hand OA (16). Occupation and sports-related repetitive injury and physical trauma contribute to the development of OA of specific joints (e.g., knees in soccer players, elbows of baseball pitchers, and upper limbs of air hammer operators) (8,17,18) and account for occurrence at sites not usually affected by OA. Although the prevalence of knee

OA is greater in adults who have engaged in occupations that require repetitive bending and strenuous activities, an association with intense exercise or recreational physical activity, such as jogging, has not been proven (19,20).

Malalignment and Laxity: Joint malalignment and laxity are potential causes as well as consequences of OA (21–23). For example, altered alignment, as in the case of acetabular dysplasia, may increase the risk of hip OA (24). Data indicate that cartilage loss in osteoarthritic knees that are malaligned (varus or valgus deformity) progresses at a more rapid rate (as measured radiographically) than cartilage loss in normally aligned knees (25–28). Although laxity and malalignment may coexist, laxity independently increases the risk of OA, as well as attenuating the relationship between strength and physical function (22).

Obesity: Cohort studies have demonstrated a clear association of obesity with the development of radiographic knee OA in older women (11) and a weaker association with hip OA (11). It is estimated that persons in the highest quintile of body weight have up to ten times the risk of knee OA than persons in the lowest quintile. Obesity influences painful symptoms in the knees (11), as indicated by the mild to moderate relief in pain afforded by weight reduction. Malalignment appears to explain some of the risk of knee OA progression attributable to obesity (27–29). Although mechanical factors are assumed to explain the increased risk of knee and hip OA associated with excess weight and obesity (11,29,30), there also is an association of hand OA with weight, which raises the possibility of alternative mechanisms.

Muscle Strength: Weakness of the knee extensor muscles appears to be both a consequence and a risk factor for the development of knee OA (31,32). However, muscle strengthening has not been proven to protect individuals from disease progression (33). In fact, evidence suggests that muscle strengthening may accelerate progression of OA of the knee in individuals whose knees are malaligned (21). Higher hand grip strength is associated with increased risk of proximal interphalangeal and carpometacarpal joint OA in men and of metacarpophalangeal joint OA in men and women (34). However, patients with hand OA often exhibit lower grip and pincer strength (35) than do unaffected individuals.

Genetics: Twin studies have shown that the influence of genetic factors is between 39% and 65% in radiographic OA of the hand and knee in women, approximately 60% in OA of the hip, and approximately 70% in OA of the spine and suggest a heritability of OA of ≥50% (36). Genetic studies of OA to date have focused on identifying polymorphisms of structural components of cartilage. A rare syndrome, inherited as a mendelian dominant, is related to a single base mutation in the type II procollagen gene (*COL2A1*) and results in mild chondrodysplasia and premature OA, often in the fourth decade (37,38). Type II collagen is a major protein component of articular cartilage that contributes structural integrity during mechanical stress. Whether heterogeneity or polymorphisms of alleles of the *COL2A1* gene (37,38) or other molecules such as aggrecan (39) and interleukin (IL)-1 (40,41) play a role in the common forms of OA remains to be determined. One study implicated a defect in the gene for type IX collagen, another collagen important in cartilage structure, as a risk factor for lumbar disk disease and female hip OA (42,43). Other studies have demonstrated an association between early and severe OA with abnormalities in the vitamin D receptor (44–47).

PATHOPHYSIOLOGY OF OSTEOARTHRITIS

The pathogenesis of OA is multifactorial (Fig. 75.1); however, the final common pathway is believed to be progressive depletion of the collagen and proteoglycan matrix and proliferation of underlying bone with osteophyte formation (48,49). Under normal conditions, chondrocytes

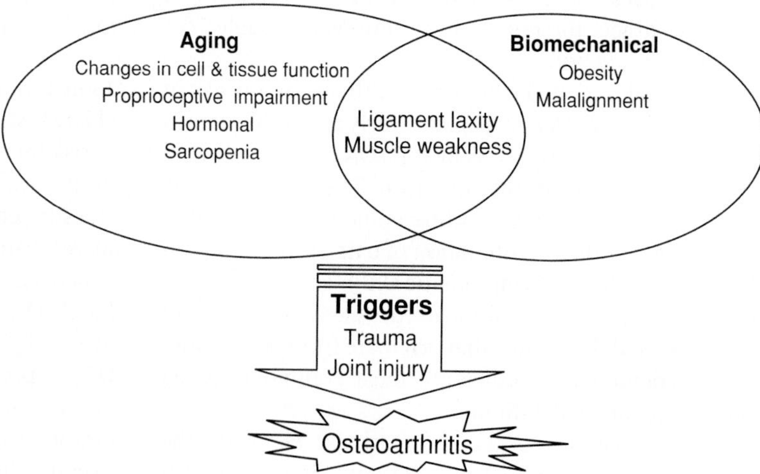

FIGURE 75.1. Predisposing and causative factors implicated in osteoarthritis development. These include cellular, structural, and biomechanical factors associated with aging, biomechanical factors that increase detrimental forces across the joint, and traumatic or repetitive injury.

regulate the amount of extracellular matrix by balancing the synthesis and degradation of its structural components (50,51). In OA, a state of disequilibrium develops in which degradative pathways far outstrip repair processes in a complex milieu of interaction among inflammatory cytokine mediators (51,52), growth factors, degradative enzymes, and chondrocyte apoptosis (53,54). Susceptibility to cartilage damage increases with age and may be the result of abnormal biomechanics that lead to excessive stress or defective matrix components and alteration of the normal structure (55,56). Impact loading and torsional, shear, and repetitive stress are more important than frictional wear (57,58). Changes are most severe in, or may be confined entirely to, areas of maximal stress on the articular cartilage, most striking in weight-bearing areas of the large joints. Synovitis usually is minimal in the early stages but may contribute to joint damage in advanced disease. Changes in the hardness of bone and the cartilage's loss of ability to absorb stress as a primary mechanism in OA also have been proposed. The role of bone pathology in disease progression also has been suggested by observations that higher bone density is positively associated (59), and lower bone density (osteoporosis) negatively associated (60), with OA. The identification of bone marrow lesions in knee OA has contributed significantly to our understanding of the pathogenesis of pain and of the role of bone abnormalities in disease progression (61,62). Finally, deposits of calcium pyrophosphate, hydroxyapatite, or basic calcium salts may play a role in the synovial inflammatory response, pain, or destructive arthropathy in certain patients (63,64).

Because there are no nerve fibers in articular cartilage, early changes in cartilage associated with OA are generally asymptomatic. However, as the disease progresses, pain is thought to evolve from involvement of noncartilaginous structures. Periosteal irritation as a result of proliferating bone, denuded bone, compression of soft tissues by osteophytes in confined spaces, microfractures of subchondral bone, stress on ligaments as a result of loss of cartilage and joint incongruity, low-grade synovitis, effusion, and spasm of surrounding muscles are all potential sources of pain in OA.

GENERAL CLINICAL FEATURES AND DIAGNOSIS

Table 75.2 lists the distribution of joints usually affected by OA. The clinical presentation differs somewhat depending on the particular joint(s) involved, but many of the signs and symptoms are consistent from joint to joint. The American College of Rheumatology (ACR) has developed a set of criteria for the diagnosis of OA. The ACR criteria combine symptoms, physical signs, and x-ray films of the affected joints (65) and are summarized in Table 75.3.

TABLE 75.2 Distribution of Joint Involvement in Primary Osteoarthritis

Commonly affected
Hands
Distal interphalangeal (Heberden nodes)
Proximal interphalangeal (Bouchard nodes)
Carpometacarpal of the thumb (joints between first metacarpal and greater multangular and between greater multangular and navicular)
Knees
Hips
Spine
Cervical
Lumbar
Thoracic
Feet
Metatarsophalangeal (especially first)
Usually spared
Ankles
Hands
Metacarpophalangeal
Carpometacarpal (except first)
Wrists
Elbows
Shoulders

History

Stiffness of the joint after sleep or prolonged inactivity (gel phenomenon) is the most common first symptom. It usually is short in duration (5–30 minutes) and quickly abates with joint movement. This should be distinguished from

TABLE 75.3 Criteria for Diagnosis of Osteoarthritis of the Hand, Knee, and Hip

Hand	*Knee*	*Hip*
Hand pain, aching, or stiffness *and* Hard tissue enlargement of ≥2 joints *and* <3 swollen metacarpophalangeal joints *and* ≥2 DIP joints with hard-tissue enlargement *or* Deformity in ≥2 select joints[a]	Knee pain *and* Radiographic osteophytes *and* ≥1 of the following: Age ≥50 yr Morning stiffness <30 min Crepitus on motion	Hip pain *and* ≥2 of the following: Erythrocyte sedimentation rate <10 mm/h Radiographic femoral or acetabular osteophytes Radiographic joint space narrowing

[a]Select joints = distal interphalangeal, proximal interphalangeal, first carpometacarpal.
From Altman RD. The classification of osteoarthritis. J Rheumatol Suppl 1995;43:42, with permission.

the morning stiffness associated with inflammatory joint diseases that persists beyond 30 minutes.

As the disease progresses, joint pain or aching is the hallmark symptom of OA. The pain is elicited by maneuvers that stress the joint. For example, in patients with patellofemoral OA, knee pain is elicited by squatting and descending stairs. Patients with hip OA often report groin or thigh pain upon weight-bearing pain or with activities that require flexion of the hip, such as the donning of pants. Pain usually begins insidiously but worsens over time in a significant proportion of patients. As the disease advances, pain and aching may persist even when the joint is at rest, often leading to significant sleep interruption. A sensation of "locking" or "giving way" may signal internal derangement of the joint. The patient should be asked about a prior or recent history of joint injury, which may warrant further orthopedic evaluation.

Physical Findings

Physical examination of a joint with early radiographic OA frequently is normal. As the disease becomes more severe and/or symptomatic, however, abnormalities noted on examination are more common. Generally, tenderness can be elicited at the joint margins, and pain may be reproduced by passive range of motion. The examiner can detect crepitus by feeling the joint as it moves through its range of motion. Bony enlargement of the distal interphalangeal joints (*Heberden nodes*), and less commonly of the proximal interphalangeal joints (*Bouchard nodes*), becomes evident as osteophytes and chondrophytes progress. Although less inflammatory than rheumatoid arthritis, mild warmth and/or effusion of the joint may be present, indicating some degree of synovial inflammation. Pain elicited by manual compression of the patella during quadriceps activation usually signals patellofemoral OA. Hip pain is reproduced on passive internal rotation of the hip. Patients with advanced knee OA frequently have varus (or less commonly valgus) malalignment and/or limited extension (flexion contracture). During ambulation, patients with knee or hip OA may exhibit an antalgic gait that limits weight-bearing on the symptomatic side. In addition, patients with advanced hip OA and hip girdle weakness sway toward the affected side during ambulation in the so-called *Trendelenburg lurch.*

Functional Limitations

Numerous cross-sectional and longitudinal studies have clearly established that OA, particularly of the knee and hip, is a major cause of disability in the United States (66–68). Evidence indicates that disability may begin early in the course of the disease (31). Disability is manifested early in the course of hip and knee OA by a slowed and painful gait, often accompanied by a limp (antalgic gait). As the pain worsens, affected individuals curtail their physical activity and avoid difficult or pain-inducing tasks. Muscle weakness accompanies OA in all anatomic locations and may result in difficulty with mobility as well as with self-care tasks. Finally, musculoskeletal pain and OA both predispose older adults to risk of falls, enhancing the possibility of further functional impairment (69,70).

Laboratory Findings

Routine laboratory tests are normal in OA unless the patient has a concomitant disease process(es). Although acute phase reactants, including the erythrocyte sedimentation rate and the C-reactive protein (CRP), are normal in patients with OA compared to patients with more inflammatory arthritides (e.g., rheumatoid arthritis or acute gout), several studies suggest that modestly elevated CRP levels predict the development and/or progression of OA (71–73). However, obesity is common in OA, and obesity itself is associated with elevated levels of inflammatory markers, leading some to call into question the direct association of inflammation with development and progression of OA. Nonetheless, others have demonstrated elevated levels of other inflammatory molecules in OA, including IL-6 and soluble receptors for tumor necrosis factor (74).

Synovial fluid in OA usually is of the noninflammatory type (i.e., white blood cells $<2{,}000/mm^3$, protein content <4 g/dL, and glucose concentration approximately equal to a simultaneous serum glucose concentration; see Chapter 74). A more inflammatory fluid with elevated white cell count may occur when crystals of calcium pyrophosphate or hydroxyapatite are present (see Chapter 76).

Efforts to develop biologic markers for diagnosis, disease activity, or progression of OA have not yet reached a degree of specificity or sensitivity to be clinically useful (49,75–83). Both synthetic and degradative constituents of cartilage and bone can be detected in individuals with OA, illustrating the complexity and delicate balance in degradation and repair processes of cartilage and bone in determining a healthy versus a diseased joint (75–81). Identification of a biomarker(s) is greatly needed because it would facilitate early diagnosis and/or identification of individuals at risk for rapid disease progression (82). It is possible that combinations or clusters of markers may improve the predictive power of identifying OA, rather than relying upon a single marker (83).

Imaging Osteoarthritis

Bony osteophytes at the joint margins, subchondral sclerosis, and joint space narrowing compose the radiographic hallmarks of OA (Fig. 75.2). Conventional radiography remains the definitive procedure in routine clinical care for (a) confirmation of a diagnosis of OA, (b) classification and estimation of disease severity, (c) assessment of disease

nausea and dry mouth. All narcotic preparations can cause constipation and have risk for cross-dependency (130).

Nutritional Supplements

Glucosamine is an amino-monosaccharide component of articular cartilage. Chondroitin sulfate is a proteoglycan component of articular cartilage. The two substances frequently are sold over the counter in combination preparations as dietary supplements. The ACR and European League Against Rheumatism have acknowledged that glucosamine (500 mg three times daily) and chondroitin sulfate (800 mg daily) may be useful for treatment of OA. However, meta-analyses of randomized, placebo-controlled trials have been in conflict about whether or not glucosamine is more effective than placebo (131–133) and do not support the use of chondroitin sulfate for symptom modification in OA (131,134).

Both glucosamine and chondroitin sulfate have been examined for their potential disease-modifying effects. Glucosamine treatment was associated with a slower rate of joint space narrowing over 2 to 3 years compared to placebo in patients with early knee OA in two randomized, controlled studies (135,136). More recently, treatment for 2 years with chondroitin-4 and chondroitin-6 sulfate was associated with less radiographic progression in patients with knee OA compared to patients who received placebo (134). The radiographic methods used in these three studies have been subject to criticism, however, and an NIH-sponsored trial in the United States currently is underway to reexamine these conclusions. Fortunately, all evidence suggests that both agents are well tolerated and safe (131–133). Because glucosamine and chondroitin sulfate are sold in the United States as over-the-counter nutraceuticals, manufacture of these supplements is not as tightly regulated as prescription drugs, and cost is not generally reimbursable by third-party prescription plans. The cost of the two agents combined can be prohibitive.

Intra-Articular Therapies

Judicious use of intra-articular therapies is appropriate for OA patients who are not candidates for, or who have inadequate responses to, oral analgesics or anti-inflammatory agents.

Corticosteroids

Intra-articular injection of corticosteroids has been a time-honored option for treatment of moderate to severe OA. Although not always effective, intra-articular steroids often provide pain relief for several months. Presumably effective because of its anti-inflammatory properties, evidence demonstrating an effect on inflammatory mediators in the joint is lacking. Evidence suggests that repeated injections over time can be effective and do not result in accelerated joint damage (137).

Hyaluronic Acid

Injections of hyaluronic acid derivatives (Synvisc, Hyalgan, Orthovisc) have been demonstrated to relieve pain in some patients with OA of the knee and of the hip (138,139). All preparations are administered over a series of three to five weekly injections and are relatively safe with the exception of occasional flares postinjection. Response has been comparable to that obtained with acetaminophen, NSAIDs, and intra-articular glucocorticoids (140). Although effective, the mechanism of action of this therapy has not been delineated. Furthermore, additional studies are needed to evaluate the long-term effects of these agents (141). Because this mode of therapy is invasive, expensive, and likely, at most, only equally effective as NSAID therapy, it probably should be reserved for patients who have not responded to analgesics and a vigorous nonpharmacologic program or for those in whom NSAIDs are contraindicated. Like NSAIDs, hyaluronic acid injections may be marginally beneficial in patients with very severe disease.

Management of Acute Flare

Some degree of synovial inflammation is common in OA (48). Patients with OA may have occasional acute or subacute painful episodes with swelling and exacerbation of the inflammatory process in the affected joint. These patients may have evidence of inflammation, with pain, swelling, warmth, and some erythema on occasion. When the knee is involved, there usually is an effusion. The episodes, which often are precipitated by minor trauma, may be caused by sudden release into the joint of cartilaginous debris or microcrystalline deposits contained therein, although such crystals are also found in a significant proportion of unselected patients with effusions of the knee due to OA (142). Sepsis occasionally complicates an osteoarthritic joint but is a much less common event than occurs in a rheumatoid arthritic joint.

A patient with established OA who develops an acutely swollen painful joint should have the joint aspirated and the fluid analyzed because of the possibility of a complicating microcrystalline-induced or septic arthritis (see Chapter 74).

Modifying the Disease

At present, no medicinal or nonmedicinal treatments have been proven unequivocally to alter the natural course of OA. This can be accomplished only by altering the underlying pathophysiologic processes that lead to the development and progression of OA. Detection of meaningful differences in radiographic outcomes between study groups over successive visits is fraught with methodologic challenges and requires rigorously standardized imaging methods that are capable of detecting small changes over long periods of time. These requirements have not been met in OA clinical trials to date, and this has tempered acceptance of the results, for example, of published clinical trials of glycosaminoglycan-peptide complex, glycosaminoglycan polysulfate, diacerein, and glucosamine sulfate (143). MRI, as discussed under Imaging Osteoarthritis, offers the potential for more sensitive and accurate measurements of small changes in cartilage volume over time and for assessing the impact of novel therapies on this rate of change (88).

The growing recognition that subchondral bone lesions are associated with pain and more rapid progression of OA of the knee (61) has been strengthened by cross-sectional data suggesting that estrogen and bisphosphonate use reduce the number of bone lesions and overall periarticular bone attrition as measured by MRI (144). The efficacy of antiresorptive therapies for OA depends upon whether the increased bone turnover that occurs in OA results in increased subchondral stiffness (145).

Several pharmacologic agents that target mediators of joint destruction are in various stages of development as potential disease-modifying therapies for OA and are reviewed in detail elsewhere (146,147). These include inhibitors of matrix metalloproteinases that exert their effects by inhibiting the synthesis or activation of an enzyme(s) or as chelators. In a randomized, placebo-controlled trial of patients with unilateral knee OA, treatment with doxycycline (100 mg twice daily) attenuated the rate of loss of joint space width in the index knee but did not reduce pain severity or prevent loss of joint space width in the nonaffected knee (148). Modulation of IL-1 activity with an antagonist of the IL-1 receptor or an inhibitor of IL-1 converting enzyme has been undertaken in clinical trials of rheumatoid arthritis (see Chapter 77) and may hold potential promise as treatment for OA.

Surgical Management

Patients in whom function and mobility are compromised by pain despite maximal medical therapy and in whom there is structural instability may be candidates for surgical intervention.

Arthroscopy, Tidal Irrigation, and Débridement

Although some investigators have argued that these procedures are effective for pain management of OA of the knee, these procedures have come under scrutiny. In a randomized, controlled study, arthroscopy with tidal irrigation of the knee was no more effective in relieving pain or improving function than was sham irrigation (149). Thus, arthroscopic irrigation is no longer justified as a general strategy for pain management in OA (149). Arthroscopy with débridement still is useful principally in patients with meniscal injury and loose bodies that result in knee locking and give-way weakness.

Osteotomy

High tibial osteotomy may be undertaken in patients with painful knee OA who have varus (bowlegged) malalignment due to severe cartilage loss in the medial compartment (150). Surgical realignment is achieved by removing a segment of the proximal tibia. Although osteotomy has been tried in combination with other cartilage-preserving or regenerating procedures, clinical trials have not been undertaken to adequately test the efficacy of specific combinations.

Total joint arthroplasty remains the procedure of choice for patients with severe, deforming OA whose symptoms and disability are unresponsive to maximal nonsurgical therapeutic interventions. Use of unicondylar prosthesis and "minimally invasive" arthroplasty have met with good results, including improved early motion, less blood loss, and shorter hospital stays than standard surgical techniques (151). Despite these advances, consideration must be given first to whether or not a given patient is a surgical candidate, that is, will the patient be able to withstand the risks and stresses of surgery, and will joint replacement restore meaningful function? Patients with OA who have substantial other comorbid conditions face greater perioperative risk (152). Full recovery of mobility and function may not be realistically achieved in the presence of significant cognitive impairment or function-limiting cardiopulmonary disease, because these conditions can impede postoperative rehabilitation. Consideration must be given to timing of joint replacement surgery. That surgical outcomes are best in patients who have not yet developed significant disability, appreciable muscle weakness, or generalized or cardiovascular deconditioning suggests that joint replacement surgery should be considered sooner rather than later. Despite this, preoperative exercise interventions have not improved functional recovery following surgery (153). For patients with severe bilateral OA of the knee or hip, simultaneous replacement of both joints might be contemplated. However, the rate of perioperative complications may be slightly higher with simultaneous bilateral arthroplasties than with staged arthroplasty (154–156). Contraindications to joint arthroplasty include neuromuscular or sensory deficits, severe peripheral vascular disease, and cognitive impairment. Contrary to anecdotal reports, obesity does not appear to independently alter outcomes following total joint arthroplasty (157,158).

Transplantation and Regenerative Interventions

Cartilage is minimally cellular and avascular and thus has limited capacity for self-repair. Numerous attempts have been made to repair cartilage lesions and to re-establish mature cartilage with the biomechanical properties of native tissue. Autologous chondrocyte implantation and osteochondral transplantation have been successful in repairing discrete defects in articular cartilage (159), but no prospective clinical trials support their use over conventional surgical interventions (160,161). Furthermore, these procedures are of limited utility for repairing large defects due to issues of graft viability at the transplantation site, concerns for donor site viability, and limited repair following harvest (161). In contrast, clinical experience with allogeneic osteochondral and chondral grafting has been good. However, enthusiasm for the procedure is tempered by the scarcity of fresh donor tissues.

SPECIFIC REFERENCES*

1. Lawrence RC, Helmick CG, Arnett FC, et al. Estimates of the prevalence of arthritis and selected musculoskeletal disorders in the United States. Arthritis Rheum 1998;41:778.
2. Oliveria SA, Felson DT, Reed JI, et al. Incidence of symptomatic hand, hip, and knee osteoarthritis among patients in a health maintenance organization. Arthritis Rheum 1995;38:1134.
3. Ettinger WH, Davis MA, Neuhaus JM, et al. Long-term physical functioning in persons with knee osteoarthritis from NHANES. I: effects of comorbid medical conditions. J Clin Epidemiol 1994;47:809.
4. Davis MA, Ettinger WH, Neuhaus JM, et al. Knee osteoarthritis and physical functioning: evidence from the NHANES I epidemiologic followup study. J Rheumatol 1991;18:591.
5. Cooper C, Snow S, McAlindon TE, et al. Risk factors for the incidence and progression of radiographic knee osteoarthritis. Arthritis Rheum 2000;43:995.
6. Lethbridge-Cejku M, Scott WW Jr, Reichle R, et al. Association of radiographic features of osteoarthritis of the knee with knee pain: data from the Baltimore Longitudinal Study of Aging. Arthritis Care Res 1995;8:182.
7. Hochberg MC. Epidemiology of osteoarthritis: current concepts and new insights. J Rheumatol Suppl 1991;27:4.
8. Dugan SA. Sports-related knee injuries in female athletes: what gives? Am J Phys Med Rehabil 2005;84:122.
9. Nevitt MC, Cummings SR, Lane NE, et al. Association of estrogen replacement therapy with the risk of osteoarthritis of the hip in elderly white women. Study of Osteoporotic Fractures Research Group. Arch Intern Med 1996;156:2073.
10. Nevitt MC, Felson DT, Williams EN, et al. The effect of estrogen plus progestin on knee symptoms and related disability in postmenopausal women: The Heart and Estrogen/Progestin Replacement Study, a randomized, double-blind, placebo-controlled trial. Arthritis Rheum 2001;44:811.
11. Davis MA, Ettinger WH, Neuhaus JM. Obesity and osteoarthritis of the knee: evidence from the National Health and Nutrition Examination Survey (NHANES I). Semin Arthritis Rheum 1990;20[3 Suppl 1]:34.
12. Davis MA, Ettinger WH, Neuhaus JM, et al. The association of knee injury and obesity with unilateral and bilateral osteoarthritis of the knee. Am J Epidemiol 1989;130:278.
13. Englund M, Lohmander LS. Risk factors for symptomatic knee osteoarthritis fifteen to twenty-two years after meniscectomy. Arthritis Rheum 2004;50:2811.
14. Roos H, Lauren M, Adalberth T, et al. Knee osteoarthritis after meniscectomy: prevalence of radiographic changes after twenty-one years, compared with matched controls. Arthritis Rheum 1998;41:687.
15. Englund M, Roos EM, Lohmander LS. Impact of type of meniscal tear on radiographic and symptomatic knee osteoarthritis: a sixteen-year followup of meniscectomy with matched controls. Arthritis Rheum 2003;48:2178.
16. Englund M, Paradowski PT, Lohmander LS. Association of radiographic hand osteoarthritis with radiographic knee osteoarthritis after meniscectomy. Arthritis Rheum 2004;50:469.
17. Roos EM. Joint injury causes knee osteoarthritis in young adults. Curr Opin Rheumatol 2005; 17:195.
18. Lohmander LS, Ostenberg A, Englund M, et al. High prevalence of knee osteoarthritis, pain, and functional limitations in female soccer players twelve years after anterior cruciate ligament injury. Arthritis Rheum 2004;50:3145.
19. Cheng Y, Macera CA, Davis DR, et al. Physical activity and self-reported, physician-diagnosed osteoarthritis: is physical activity a risk factor? J Clin Epidemiol 2000;53:315.
20. McAlindon TE, Wilson PW, Aliabadi P, et al. Level of physical activity and the risk of radiographic and symptomatic knee osteoarthritis in the elderly: the Framingham study. Am J Med 1999;106:151.
21. Sharma L, Dunlop DD, Cahue S, et al. Quadriceps strength and osteoarthritis progression in malaligned and lax knees. Ann Intern Med 2003;138:613.
22. Sharma L, Hayes KW, Felson DT, et al. Does laxity alter the relationship between strength and physical function in knee osteoarthritis? Arthritis Rheum 1999;42:25.
23. Sharma L, Lou C, Felson DT, et al. Laxity in healthy and osteoarthritic knees. Arthritis Rheum 1999;42:861.
24. Lane NE, Lin P, Christiansen L, et al. Association of mild acetabular dysplasia with an increased risk of incident hip osteoarthritis in elderly white women: the study of osteoporotic fractures. Arthritis Rheum 2000;43:400.
25. Cahue S, Dunlop D, Hayes K, et al. Varus-valgus alignment in the progression of patellofemoral osteoarthritis. Arthritis Rheum 2004;50:2184.
26. Cerejo R, Dunlop DD, Cahue S, et al. The influence of alignment on risk of knee osteoarthritis progression according to baseline stage of disease. Arthritis Rheum 2002;46:2632.
27. Sharma L, Lou C, Cahue S, et al. The mechanism of the effect of obesity in knee osteoarthritis: the mediating role of malalignment. Arthritis Rheum 2000;43:568.
28. Sharma L, Song J, Felson DT, et al. The role of knee alignment in disease progression and functional decline in knee osteoarthritis. JAMA 2001;286:188.
29. Felson DT, Goggins J, Niu J, et al. The effect of body weight on progression of knee osteoarthritis is dependent on alignment. Arthritis Rheum 2004;50:3904.
30. Felson DT, Anderson JJ, Naimark A, et al. Obesity and knee osteoarthritis. The Framingham Study. Ann Intern Med 1988; 109:18.
31. Ling SM, Fried LP, Garrett ES, et al. Knee osteoarthritis compromises early mobility function: The Women's Health and Aging Study II. J Rheumatol 2003;30:114.
32. Slemenda C, Heilman DK, Brandt KD, et al. Reduced quadriceps strength relative to body weight: a risk factor for knee osteoarthritis in women? Arthritis Rheum 1998;41:1951.
33. Brandt KD, Heilman DK, Slemenda C, et al. Quadriceps strength in women with radiographically progressive osteoarthritis of the knee and those with stable radiographic changes. J Rheumatol 1999;26:2431.
34. Chaisson CE, Zhang Y, Sharma L, et al. Higher grip strength increases the risk of incident radiographic osteoarthritis in proximal hand joints. Osteoarthritis Cartilage 2000; 8[Suppl A]:S29.
35. Bagis S, Sahin G, Yapici Y, et al. The effect of hand osteoarthritis on grip and pinch strength and hand function in postmenopausal women. Clin Rheumatol 2003;22:420.
36. Spector TD, MacGregor AJ. Risk factors for osteoarthritis: genetics. Osteoarthritis Cartilage 2004;12[Suppl A]:S39.
37. Vikkula M, Palotie A, Ritvaniemi P, et al. Early-onset osteoarthritis linked to the type II procollagen gene. Detailed clinical phenotype and further analyses of the gene. Arthritis Rheum 1993;36:401.
38. Palotie A, Vaisanen P, Ott J, et al. Predisposition to familial osteoarthrosis linked to type II collagen gene. Lancet 1989;1:924.
39. Horton WE Jr, Lethbridge-Cejku M, Hochberg MC, et al. An association between an aggrecan polymorphic allele and bilateral hand osteoarthritis in elderly white men: data from the Baltimore Longitudinal Study of Aging (BLSA). Osteoarthritis Cartilage 1998;6:245.
40. Frisbie DD, McIlwraith CW. Evaluation of gene therapy as a treatment for equine traumatic arthritis and osteoarthritis. Clin Orthop Relat Res 2000;379[Suppl]:S273.
41. Meulenbelt I, Seymour AB, Nieuwland M, et al. Association of the interleukin-1 gene cluster with radiographic signs of osteoarthritis of the hip. Arthritis Rheum 2004;50:1179.
42. Mustafa Z, Chapman K, Irven C, et al. Linkage analysis of candidate genes as susceptibility loci for osteoarthritis-suggestive linkage of COL9A1 to female hip osteoarthritis. Rheumatology (Oxford) 2000;39:299.
43. Olsen BR. Collagen IX. Int J Biochem Cell Biol 1997;29:555.
44. Huang J, Ushiyama T, Inoue K, et al. Vitamin D receptor gene polymorphisms and osteoarthritis of the hand, hip, and knee: a case-control study in Japan. Rheumatology (Oxford) 2000;39:79.
45. Loughlin J, Sinsheimer JS, Mustafa Z, et al. Association analysis of the vitamin D receptor gene, the type I collagen gene COL1A1, and the estrogen receptor gene in idiopathic osteoarthritis. J Rheumatol 2000;27:779.
46. Uitterlinden AG, Burger H, Huang Q, et al. Vitamin D receptor genotype is associated with radiographic osteoarthritis at the knee. J Clin Invest 1997;100:259.
47. Uitterlinden AG, Burger H, van Duijn CM, et al. Adjacent genes, for COL2A1 and the vitamin D receptor, are associated with separate features of radiographic osteoarthritis of the knee. Arthritis Rheum 2000;43:1456.

*Bold numerals denote published controlled clinical trials, meta-analyses, or consensus-based recommendations.

48. Poole AR. An introduction to the pathophysiology of osteoarthritis. Front Biosci 1999;4:D662.
49. Poole AR. Biochemical/immunochemical biomarkers of osteoarthritis: utility for prediction of incident or progressive osteoarthritis. Rheum Dis Clin North Am 2003;29:803.
50. Goldring MB. The role of the chondrocyte in osteoarthritis. Arthritis Rheum 2000;43:1916.
51. Goldring SR, Goldring MB. The role of cytokines in cartilage matrix degeneration in osteoarthritis. Clin Orthop Relat Res 2004;427[Suppl]:S27.
52. Goldring MB, Berenbaum F. The regulation of chondrocyte function by proinflammatory mediators: prostaglandins and nitric oxide. Clin Orthop Relat Res 2004;427[Suppl]:S37.
53. Kuhn K, D'Lima DD, Hashimoto S, Lotz M. Cell death in cartilage. Osteoarthritis Cartilage 2004;12:1.
54. Lotz M, Hashimoto S, Kuhn K. Mechanisms of chondrocyte apoptosis. Osteoarthritis Cartilage 1999;7:389.
55. D'Lima DD, Hashimoto S, Chen PC, et al. Human chondrocyte apoptosis in response to mechanical injury. Osteoarthritis Cartilage 2001;9:712.
56. D'Lima DD, Hashimoto S, Chen PC, et al. Impact of mechanical trauma on matrix and cells. Clin Orthop Relat Res 2001;391[Suppl]:S90.
57. Setton LA, Elliott DM, Mow VC. Altered mechanics of cartilage with osteoarthritis: human osteoarthritis and an experimental model of joint degeneration. Osteoarthritis Cartilage 1999;7:2.
58. Setton LA, Mow VC, Muller FJ, et al. Altered structure-function relationships for articular cartilage in human osteoarthritis and an experimental canine model. Agents Actions Suppl 1993;39:27.
59. Zhang Y, Hannan MT, Chaisson CE, et al. Bone mineral density and risk of incident and progressive radiographic knee osteoarthritis in women: the Framingham Study. J Rheumatol 2000;27:1032.
60. Dequeker J. Inverse relationship of interface between osteoporosis and osteoarthritis. J Rheumatol 1997;24:795.
61. Felson DT, Chaisson CE, Hill CL, et al. The association of bone marrow lesions with pain in knee osteoarthritis. Ann Intern Med 2001;134: 541.
62. Felson DT, McLaughlin S, Goggins J, et al. Bone marrow edema and its relation to progression of knee osteoarthritis. Ann Intern Med 2003; 139[5 Pt 1]:330.
63. Dieppe PA, Doherty M, Macfarlane DG, et al. Apatite associated destructive arthritis. Br J Rheumatol 1984;23:84.
64. Schumacher HR Jr. Synovial inflammation, crystals, and osteoarthritis. J Rheumatol Suppl 1995;43:101.
65. Altman RD. The classification of osteoarthritis. J Rheumatol Suppl 1995;43:42.
66. Ettinger WH Jr. Physical activity, arthritis, and disability in older people. Clin Geriatr Med 1998;14:633.
67. Fried LP, Young Y, Rubin G, et al. Self-reported preclinical disability identifies older women with early declines in performance and early disease. J Clin Epidemiol 2001;54: 889.
68. Mannoni A, Briganti MP, Di Bari M, et al. Epidemiological profile of symptomatic osteoarthritis in older adults: a population based study in Dicomano, Italy. Ann Rheum Dis 2003;62:576.
69. Leveille SG, Bean J, Bandeen-Roche K, et al. Musculoskeletal pain and risk for falls in older disabled women living in the community. J Am Geriatr Soc 2002;50:671.
70. Ling SM, Bathon JM. Osteoarthritis in older adults. J Am Geriatr Soc 1998;46:216.
71. Sowers M, Jannausch M, Stein E, et al. C-reactive protein as a biomarker of emergent osteoarthritis. Osteoarthritis Cartilage 2002;10:595.
72. Spector TD, Hart DJ, Nandra D, et al. Low-level increases in serum C-reactive protein are present in early osteoarthritis of the knee and predict progressive disease. Arthritis Rheum 1997;40:723.
73. Sharif M, Shepstone L, Elson CJ, et al. Increased serum C reactive protein may reflect events that precede radiographic progression in osteoarthritis of the knee. Ann Rheum Dis 2000;59:71.
74. Penninx BW, Abbas H, Ambrosius W, et al. Inflammatory markers and physical function among older adults with knee osteoarthritis. J Rheumatol 2004;31:2027.
75. Bruyere O, Collette JH, Ethgen O, et al. Biochemical markers of bone and cartilage remodeling in prediction of longterm progression of knee osteoarthritis. J Rheumatol 2003;30:1043.
76. Dragomir AD, Kraus VB, Renner JB, et al. Serum cartilage oligomeric matrix protein and clinical signs and symptoms of potential pre-radiographic hip and knee pathology. Osteoarthritis Cartilage 2002;10:687.
77. Lohmander LS, Ionescu M, Jugessur H, et al. Changes in joint cartilage aggrecan after knee injury and in osteoarthritis. Arthritis Rheum 1999;42:534.
78. Poole AR. Can serum biomarker assays measure the progression of cartilage degeneration in osteoarthritis? Arthritis Rheum 2002;46:2549.
79. Poole AR, Ionescu M, Fitzcharles MA, et al. The assessment of cartilage degradation in vivo: development of an immunoassay for the measurement in body fluids of type II collagen cleaved by collagenases. J Immunol Methods 2004;294:145.
80. Clark AG, Jordan JM, Vilim V, et al. Serum cartilage oligomeric matrix protein reflects osteoarthritis presence and severity: the Johnston County Osteoarthritis Project. Arthritis Rheum 1999;42:2356.
81. Vilim V, Olejarova M, Machacek S, et al. Serum levels of cartilage oligomeric matrix protein (COMP) correlate with radiographic progression of knee osteoarthritis. Osteoarthritis Cartilage 2002;10:707.
82. Garnero P, Delmas PD. Biomarkers in osteoarthritis. Curr Opin Rheumatol 2003;15:641.
83. Otterness IG, Swindell AC, Zimmerer RO, et al. An analysis of 14 molecular markers for monitoring osteoarthritis: segregation of the markers into clusters and distinguishing osteoarthritis at baseline. Osteoarthritis Cartilage 2000;8:180.
84. Kellgren JH, Lawrence JS. Atlas of standard radiographs of arthritis. The epidemiology of chronic rheumatism. Oxford, UK: Blackwell Scientific, 1963.
85. Peterfy CG, Guermazi A, Zaim S, et al. Whole-Organ Magnetic Resonance Imaging Score (WORMS) of the knee in osteoarthritis. Osteoarthritis Cartilage 2004;12:177.
86. McGibbon CA, Trahan CA. Measurement accuracy of focal cartilage defects from MRI and correlation of MRI graded lesions with histology: a preliminary study. Osteoarthritis Cartilage 2003;11:483.
87. Gray ML, Eckstein F, Peterfy C, et al. Toward imaging biomarkers for osteoarthritis. Clin Orthop Relat Res 2004;427[Suppl]:S175.
88. Raynauld JP, Martel-Pelletier J, Berthiaume MJ, et al. Quantitative magnetic resonance imaging evaluation of knee osteoarthritis progression over two years and correlation with clinical symptoms and radiologic changes. Arthritis Rheum 2004;50:476.
89. Ding C, Cicuttini F, Scott F, et al. Association between age and knee structural change: a cross sectional MRI based study. Ann Rheum Dis 2005;64:549.
90. Graichen H, von Eisenhart-Rothe R, Vogl T, et al. Quantitative assessment of cartilage status in osteoarthritis by quantitative magnetic resonance imaging: technical validation for use in analysis of cartilage volume and further morphologic parameters. Arthritis Rheum 2004;50:811.
91. Borenstein DG. Chronic low back pain. Rheum Dis Clin North Am 1996;22:439.
92. Maher M, Hehir DJ, Neary P, et al. Spinal claudication versus arterial claudication. Ir J Med Sci 1996;165:118.
93. Wolfe F. Fibrositis, fibromyalgia, and musculoskeletal disease: the current status of the fibrositis syndrome. Arch Phys Med Rehabil 1988;69:527.
94. Yunus MB, Holt GS, Masi AT, et al. Fibromyalgia syndrome among the elderly. Comparison with younger patients. J Am Geriatr Soc 1988;36:987.
95. Gloth FM 3rd, Tobin JD. Vitamin D deficiency in older people. J Am Geriatr Soc 1995;43:822.
96. Jordan KM, Arden NK, Doherty M, et al. EULAR Recommendations 2003: an evidence based approach to the management of knee osteoarthritis: report of a Task Force of the Standing Committee for International Clinical Studies Including Therapeutic Trials (ESCISIT). Ann Rheum Dis 2003;62:1145.
97. Roddy E, Doherty M. Guidelines for management of osteoarthritis published by the American College of Rheumatology and the European League Against Rheumatism: why are they so different? Rheum Dis Clin North Am 2003;29:717.
98. Zhang W, Doherty M, Arden N, et al. EULAR evidence based recommendations for the management of hip osteoarthritis: report of a task force of the EULAR Standing Committee for International Clinical Studies Including Therapeutics (ESCISIT). Ann Rheum Dis 2005;64:669.
99. Loeser RF Jr. Aging and the etiopathogenesis and treatment of osteoarthritis. Rheum Dis Clin North Am 2000;26:547.
100. Messier SP, Loeser RF, Miller GD, et al. Exercise and dietary weight loss in overweight and obese older adults with knee osteoarthritis: the Arthritis, Diet, and Activity Promotion Trial. Arthritis Rheum 2004;50:1501.
101. Messier SP, DeVita P, Cowan RE, et al. Do older adults with knee osteoarthritis place greater loads on the knee during gait? A preliminary study. Arch Phys Med Rehabil 2005;86:703.
102. Messier SP, Gutekunst DJ, Davis C, Devita P. Weight loss reduces knee-joint loads in overweight and obese older adults with knee osteoarthritis. Arthritis Rheum 2005;52:2026.
103. Fransen M. Dietary weight loss and exercise for obese adults with knee osteoarthritis: modest weight loss targets, mild exercise, modest effects. Arthritis Rheum 2004;50:1366.
104. Ettinger WH Jr, Burns R, Messier SP, et al. A randomized trial comparing aerobic exercise and resistance exercise with a health education program in older adults with knee osteoarthritis. The Fitness Arthritis and Seniors Trial (FAST). JAMA 1997;277:25.
105. Fransen M, McConnell S, Bell M. Therapeutic exercise for people with osteoarthritis of the hip or knee. A systematic review. J Rheumatol 2002; 29:1737.
106. Roddy E, Zhang W, Doherty M, et al. Evidence-based recommendations for the role of exercise in the management of osteoarthritis of the hip or knee—the MOVE consensus. Rheumatology (Oxford) 2005;44:67.

107. Talbot LA, Gaines JM, Huynh TN, et al. A home-based pedometer-driven walking program to increase physical activity in older adults with osteoarthritis of the knee: a preliminary study. J Am Geriatr Soc 2003;51:387.
108. Sharma L, Dunlop DD, Hayes KW. Is a strong quadriceps muscle bad for a patient with knee osteoarthritis? Ann Intern Med 2004;140:150.
109. Gaines JM, Metter EJ, Talbot LA. The effect of neuromuscular electrical stimulation on arthritis knee pain in older adults with osteoarthritis of the knee. Appl Nurs Res 2004;17:201.
110. Talbot LA, Gaines JM, Ling SM, et al. A home-based protocol of electrical muscle stimulation for quadriceps muscle strength in older adults with osteoarthritis of the knee. J Rheumatol 2003;30:1571.
111. Deyle GD, Henderson NE, Matekel RL, et al. Effectiveness of manual physical therapy and exercise in osteoarthritis of the knee. A randomized, controlled trial. Ann Intern Med 2000;132:173.
112. Mayer ME. Physical therapy and exercise in osteoarthritis of the knee. Ann Intern Med 2000;132:923.
113. Fitzgerald GK, Oatis C. Role of physical therapy in management of knee osteoarthritis. Curr Opin Rheumatol 2004;16:143.
114. Rao JK, Kroenke K, Mihaliak KA, et al. Rheumatology patients' use of complementary therapies: results from a one-year longitudinal study. Arthritis Rheum 2003;49:619.
115. Rao JK, Mihaliak K, Kroenke K, et al. Use of complementary therapies for arthritis among patients of rheumatologists. Ann Intern Med 1999;131:409.
116. Berman BM, Lao L, Langenberg P, et al. Effectiveness of acupuncture as adjunctive therapy in osteoarthritis of the knee: a randomized, controlled trial. Ann Intern Med 2004;141:901.
117. Bradley JD, Brandt KD, Katz BP, et al. Comparison of an antiinflammatory dose of ibuprofen, an analgesic dose of ibuprofen, and acetaminophen in the treatment of patients with osteoarthritis of the knee. N Engl J Med 1991;325:87.
118. Pincus T, Koch G, Lei H, et al. Patient Preference for Placebo, Acetaminophen (paracetamol) or Celecoxib Efficacy Studies (PACES): two randomised, double blind, placebo controlled, crossover clinical trials in patients with knee or hip osteoarthritis. Ann Rheum Dis 2004;63:931.
119. Pincus T, Swearingen C, Cummins P, et al. Preference for nonsteroidal antiinflammatory drugs versus acetaminophen and concomitant use of both types of drugs in patients with osteoarthritis. J Rheumatol 2000;27:1020.
120. Felson DT, Lawrence RC, Hochberg MC, et al. Osteoarthritis: new insights. Part 2: treatment approaches. Ann Intern Med 2000;133:726.
121. Zhang W, Jones A, Doherty M. Does paracetamol (acetaminophen) reduce the pain of osteoarthritis? A meta-analysis of randomized controlled trials. Ann Rheum Dis 2004;63:901.
122. Fored CM, Ejerblad E, Lindblad P, et al. Acetaminophen, aspirin, and chronic renal failure. N Engl J Med 2001;345:1801.
123. Adler L, McDonald C, O'Brien C, et al. A comparison of once-daily tramadol with normal release tramadol in the treatment of pain in osteoarthritis. J Rheumatol 2002;29:2196.
124. Babul N, Noveck R, Chipman H, et al. Efficacy and safety of extended-release, once-daily tramadol in chronic pain: a randomized 12-week clinical trial in osteoarthritis of the knee. J Pain Symptom Manage 2004;28:59.
125. Schnitzer T. The new analgesic combination tramadol/acetaminophen. Eur J Anaesthesiol Suppl 2003;28:13.
126. Schnitzer TJ, Kamin M, Olson WH. Tramadol allows reduction of naproxen dose among patients with naproxen-responsive osteoarthritis pain: a randomized, double-blind, placebo-controlled study. Arthritis Rheum 1999;42:1370.
127. Malonne H, Coffiner M, Fontaine D, et al. Long-term tolerability of tramadol LP, a new once-daily formulation, in patients with osteoarthritis or low back pain. J Clin Pharm Ther 2005;30:113.
128. Gibson TP. Pharmacokinetics, efficacy, and safety of analgesia with a focus on tramadol HCl. Am J Med 1996;101:47S.
129. Caldwell JR, Hale ME, Boyd RE, et al. Treatment of osteoarthritis pain with controlled release oxycodone or fixed combination oxycodone plus acetaminophen added to nonsteroidal antiinflammatory drugs: a double blind, randomized, multicenter, placebo controlled trial. J Rheumatol 1999;26:862.
130. Beardsley PM, Aceto MD, Cook CD, et al. Discriminative stimulus, reinforcing, physical dependence, and antinociceptive effects of oxycodone in mice, rats, and rhesus monkeys. Exp Clin Psychopharmacol 2004;12:163.
131. Richy F, Bruyere O, Ethgen O, et al. Structural and symptomatic efficacy of glucosamine and chondroitin in knee osteoarthritis: a comprehensive meta-analysis. Arch Intern Med 2003;163:1514.
132. McAlindon T, Formica M, LaValley M, et al. Effectiveness of glucosamine for symptoms of knee osteoarthritis: results from an internet-based randomized double-blind controlled trial. Am J Med 2004;117:643.
133. Towheed TE, Maxwell L, Anastassiades TP, et al. Glucosamine therapy for treating osteoarthritis. Cochrane Database Syst Rev 2005;(2):CD002946.
134. Michel BA, Stucki G, Frey D, et al. Chondroitins 4 and 6 sulfate in osteoarthritis of the knee: a randomized, controlled trial. Arthritis Rheum 2005;52:779.
135. Reginster JY, Deroisy R, Rovati LC, et al. Long-term effects of glucosamine sulphate on osteoarthritis progression: a randomised, placebo-controlled clinical trial. Lancet 2001;357:251.
136. Pavelka K, Gatterova J, Olejarova M, et al. Glucosamine sulfate use and delay of progression of knee osteoarthritis: a 3-year, randomized, placebo-controlled, double-blind study. Arch Intern Med 2002;162:2113.
137. Raynauld JP, Buckland-Wright C, Ward R, et al. Safety and efficacy of long-term intraarticular steroid injections in osteoarthritis of the knee: a randomized, double-blind, placebo-controlled trial. Arthritis Rheum 2003;48:370.
138. Hochberg MC. Role of intra-articular hyaluronic acid preparations in medical management of osteoarthritis of the knee. Semin Arthritis Rheum 2000;30[2 Suppl 1]:2.
139. Altman RD. Intra-articular sodium hyaluronate in osteoarthritis of the knee. Semin Arthritis Rheum 2000;30[2 Suppl 1]:11.
140. Leopold SS, Redd BB, Warme WJ, et al. Corticosteroid compared with hyaluronic acid injections for the treatment of osteoarthritis of the knee. A prospective, randomized trial. J Bone Joint Surg Am 2003;85-A:1197.
141. Petrella RJ. Hyaluronic acid for the treatment of knee osteoarthritis: long-term outcomes from a naturalistic primary care experience. Am J Phys Med Rehabil 2005;84:278; quiz 84, 93.
142. Huskisson EC, Dieppe PA, Tucker AK, et al. Another look at osteoarthritis. Ann Rheum Dis 1979;38:423.
143. Altman RD. Measurement of structure (disease) modification in osteoarthritis. Osteoarthritis Cartilage 2004;12[Suppl A]:S69.
144. Carbone LD, Nevitt MC, Wildy K, et al. The relationship of antiresorptive drug use to structural findings and symptoms of knee osteoarthritis. Arthritis Rheum 2004;50:3516.
145. Burr DB. Anatomy and physiology of the mineralized tissues: role in the pathogenesis of osteoarthrosis. Osteoarthritis Cartilage 2004;12[Suppl A]:S20.
146. Pelletier JP. Rationale for the use of structure-modifying drugs and agents in the treatment of osteoarthritis. Osteoarthritis Cartilage 2004;12[Suppl A]:S63.
147. Wieland HA, Michaelis M, Kirschbaum BJ, et al. Osteoarthritis—an untreatable disease? Nat Rev Drug Discov 2005;4:331.
148. Brandt KD, Mazzuca SA, Katz BP, et al. Effects of doxycycline on progression of osteoarthritis: results of a randomized, placebo-controlled, double-blind trial. Arthritis Rheum 2005;52: 2015.
149. Moseley JB, O'Malley K, Petersen NJ, et al. A controlled trial of arthroscopic surgery for osteoarthritis of the knee. N Engl J Med 2002; 347:81.
150. Pfahler M, Lutz C, Anetzberger H, et al. Long-term results of high tibial osteotomy for medial osteoarthritis of the knee. Acta Chir Belg 2003;103:603.
151. Tria AJ Jr. Advancements in minimally invasive total knee arthroplasty. Orthopedics 2003; 26[8 Suppl]:S859.
152. Lingard EA, Katz JN, Wright EA, et al. Predicting the outcome of total knee arthroplasty. J Bone Joint Surg Am 2004;86A: 2179.
153. Beaupre LA, Lier D, Davies DM, et al. The effect of a preoperative exercise and education program on functional recovery, health related quality of life, and health service utilization following primary total knee arthroplasty. J Rheumatol 2004;31:1166.
154. Bullock DP, Sporer SM, Shirreffs TG Jr. Comparison of simultaneous bilateral with unilateral total knee arthroplasty in terms of perioperative complications. J Bone Joint Surg Am 2003;85A:1981.
155. Liu TK, Chen SH. Simultaneous bilateral total knee arthroplasty in a single procedure. Int Orthop 1998;22:90.
156. Mangaleshkar SR, Prasad PS, Chugh S, et al. Staged bilateral total knee replacement—a safer approach in older patients. Knee 2001;8:207.
157. Foran JR, Mont MA, Etienne G, et al. The outcome of total knee arthroplasty in obese patients. J Bone Joint Surg Am 2004;86A:1609.
158. Spicer DD, Pomeroy DL, Badenhausen WE, et al. Body mass index as a predictor of outcome in total knee replacement. Int Orthop 2001; 25:246.
159. Brittberg M, Lindahl A, Nilsson A, et al. Treatment of deep cartilage defects in the knee with autologous chondrocyte transplantation. N Engl J Med 1994;331:889.
160. Hunziker EB. Articular cartilage repair: basic science and clinical progress. A review of the current status and prospects. Osteoarthritis Cartilage 2002;10:432.
161. LaPrade RF, Swiontkowski MF. New horizons in the treatment of osteoarthritis of the knee. JAMA 1999;281:876.

For annotated ***General References*** *and resources related to this chapter, visit www.hopkinsbayview.org/PAMreferences.*

Chapter 76

Crystal-Induced Arthritis*

Patricia A. Thomas

Gout was the first form of arthritis that was recognized to be caused by the deposition of (urate) crystals in the joints and periarticular tissues. It now is known that other crystalline substances—most commonly calcium pyrophosphate dihydrate (CPPD), hydroxyapatite, and basic calcium phosphates—also are implicated in the pathogenesis of certain kinds of arthritic disease. Although disorders associated with these various crystals differ in cause and specific characteristics, they have in common the deposition of crystals in and around joints, the propensity to episodes of acute inflammatory arthritis, and sometimes the development of a chronic destructive arthropathy. Therefore, it is appropriate to consider these varied clinical disorders together under the unifying concept of crystal-induced arthritis.

*Alexander S. Townes, MD, wrote this chapter in previous editions.

MECHANISMS OF CRYSTAL-INDUCED ARTHRITIS

When crystals such as monosodium urate and CPPD are experimentally injected into joints, they produce an acute inflammatory response. The mechanisms involved in this response are complex but perhaps are as well studied as any of the stimuli that produce arthritis (1). By virtue of the nature of their electrostatic surface characteristics and mechanical properties, crystals bind to various plasma proteins as well as to cell surface receptors. Binding of crystals to macrophagelike synovial cells results in cellular activation with release of cytokines, which are immunoregulatory proteins that play an important role in the ensuing inflammatory response. Neutrophils are the major inflammatory cells in the synovial fluid during an acute episode of gout or pseudogout. Neutrophils phagocytose crystals and release factors that further intensify the inflammatory response (1). The mechanisms of crystal-induced stimulation and release of inflammatory mediators for the most part are similar with both monosodium urate (in gout) and with CPPD crystals (in pseudogout). Dissemination of cytokines into the circulation probably is responsible for the systemic effects of fever, leukocytosis, and acute phase reactants sometimes observed in acute crystal-induced arthritis (1).

Crystals may be identified in synovial fluid and synovial membrane in the absence of an acute inflammatory response and can be helpful in the diagnosis between acute attacks (2). Usually there is a paucity of neutrophils in this circumstance, with low levels of phagocytosis, mostly by mononuclear cells. The events that then trigger acute inflammation are not entirely clear. Crystals may precipitate from the fluid phase as a result of a change in temperature or pH, or they may be released from soft-tissue deposits. The sudden increase of crystals within the joint space may initiate the cycle of increased phagocytosis and inflammation. In patients with gout, there is an association of acute attacks with rapid changes in serum urate concentration, as may occur with initiation of drugs that lower serum urate, or with alcohol ingestion, dietary indiscretion, or rapid weight loss. In CPPD arthritis, a rapid fall in serum calcium (3) and/or magnesium (4) may precipitate an acute arthritis. The frequent development of acute gout or pseudogout after acute infection, trauma, surgery, or myocardial infarction suggests that the arrival of systemically generated cytokines may alter the balance within the joint toward a proinflammatory response (5). In CPPD deposition disease, release of crystals from tissue deposits in cartilage or soft tissues may result from trauma.

The invariable association between phagocytosis of crystals and the acute inflammatory response is important clinically, because demonstration of *crystals within leukocytes* from synovial fluid (Fig. 76.1A) is a convenient

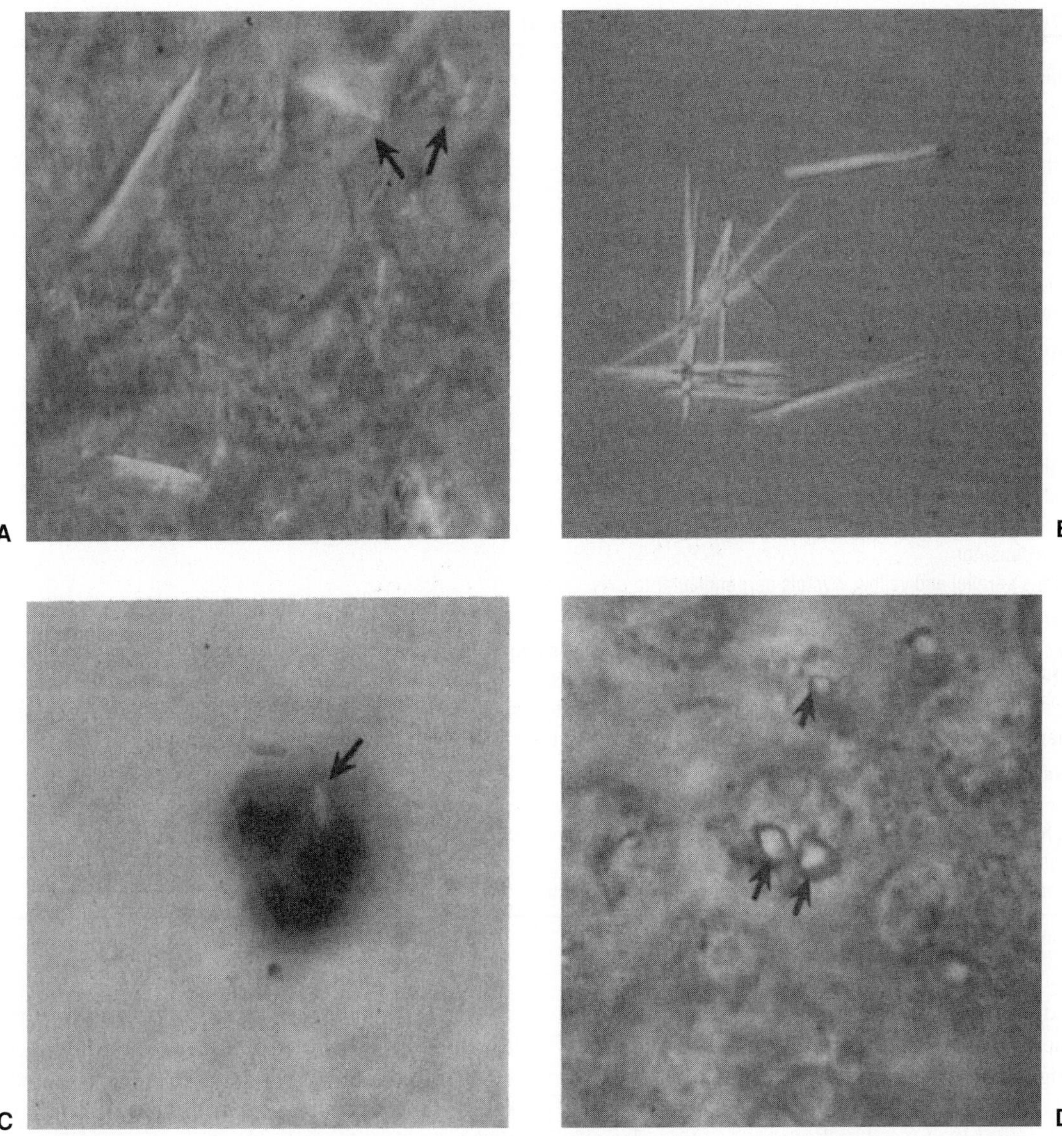

FIGURE 76.1. **A:** Urate crystals in synovial fluid examined by polarized light microscopy. Note the needle shape and variable size (*arrow*), but many have a larger diameter than white blood cells (*arrow*) (100× oil immersion). **B:** Urate crystals from tophus examined by polarized light with red plate compensator (100× oil immersion). **C:** Calcium pyrophosphate dihydrate (CPPD) crystals in white blood cell found on Gram staining (100× oil immersion). Note the shape and size relative to nucleus and cytoplasm. Gram staining is not the usual method of demonstration but occasionally is useful. **D:** Wet preparation of synovial fluid demonstrating variable size and shape of CPPD crystals phagocytized by white blood cells (100× oil immersion lens, polarized light). Size and shape vary from squat rhomboid to rod shaped. Note several crystals in some cells.

method for making a definitive diagnosis in patients with acute inflammatory crystal-induced arthritis.

The acute inflammatory response in crystal-induced arthritis is self-limited. The complex mechanisms that terminate the attack are not well understood but probably involve inactivation of inflammatory mediators by locally elaborated factors. Although gouty arthritis and other crystal-induced diseases usually are characterized by symptoms and signs of acute inflammation, the persistence of crystals in the joint with mild chronic inflammation eventually may contribute to chronic joint damage.

Crystal Identification

The identification of crystals in synovial fluid or periarticular tissue is fundamental to the diagnosis and treatment of patients with crystal-induced arthritis. Crystals of monosodium urate are best identified by placing a drop

TABLE 76.1 Identification of Crystals in Synovial Fluid

Monosodium Urate
Morphology
Rod or needle shape
Length often approaches diameter of PMN leucocyte
Polarized light
Stand out brightly when field is dark
Strongly negative birefringent
Red plate compensator
Yellow crystals parallel and blue crystals perpendicular to axis

Calcium Pyrophosphate Dihydrate
Morphology
Rhomboid, rod, or irregular rhomboid shape
Length variable, often smaller than one lobe of a PMN nucleus
Polarized light
No increase in refractile appearance when field is dark
Weakly positively birefringent (up to 80% nonbirefringent and best seen with ordinary light)
Red plate compensator
Blue crystals parallel and yellow crystals perpendicular to axis

Hydroxyapatite and BCP
Not usually seen with ordinary or polarized light microscopy except as large aggregates that are not birefringent
Aggregates of BCP occasionally seen as "shiny coin" refractile bodies
Stain nonspecifically with alizarin red S (available in histology laboratories) as clusters of crystalline material; useful as a screening test
Requires electron microscopy, x-ray diffraction, or microprobe analysis for more definite identification

Calcium Oxalate
Morphology
Polymorphic, irregular squares, short rods, bipyramidal; may appear in clumps
Polarized light
Variable, most not birefringent, some strongly positively birefringent

BCP, basic calcium phosphates; PMN, polymorphonuclear.

of aspirated tissue fluid directly on a glass slide and examining the wet preparation through a microscope under polarized light. When one lens is rotated so that the field becomes dark, the negatively birefringent urate crystals (i.e., crystals capable of bending light rays in two planes—the notation of negativity is an arbitrary term used by physicists to describe the direction of bend), dimly seen in ordinary light, stand out brightly and can be identified within the cytoplasm of polymorphonuclear leukocytes. The crystals are even more easily identified with a red plate compensator because the field turns red and crystals parallel to the axis of the compensator appear yellow, whereas those perpendicular to the axis appear blue (6). Monosodium urate crystals usually are needle or rod shaped. The size varies, but some large crystals equal to or larger than the diameter of the leukocyte usually are seen. A wet slide of joint fluid prepared in this manner may be kept for a few hours at room temperature; however, once the cells die and lyse, evaluation is less valid. If the aspirated fluid cannot be examined immediately, urate crystals may be preserved overnight by refrigeration in a plain test tube. However, CPPD crystals may dissolve within a few hours even at refrigerator temperatures (7). Methods useful for later examination include Gram-stained smears (Fig. 76.1C) and cytospin-stained smears (8). These methods function well for preservation of specimens for evaluation by light and polarized light microscopy, with sensitivity approximating that of wet mount preparations.

Monosodium urate crystals (which usually are present in abundance) are pathognomonic of gout (Table 76.1 and Fig. 76.1). Absence of crystals in an inflamed joint is strong evidence against the diagnosis. In such cases, especially if leukocytosis is significant, infection or another diagnosis should be considered.

Monosodium urate usually is easily distinguished from CPPD based on the morphology and characteristics of the crystals under polarized light (Table 76.1 and Fig. 76.1). CPPD crystals vary much more in size and shape, from rodlike to rhomboid and irregular forms. They usually are much shorter than monosodium urate crystals, and they are never needlelike. They usually are refractile without polarized light and do not increase appreciably in brilliance when the light is polarized. They are weakly positively birefringent and change color in the opposite direction to urate when the red plate compensator is placed between the polarizing lenses (i.e., blue when parallel to the axis and yellow when perpendicular).

Because CPPD crystals are small and do not stand out in polarized light, they are overlooked more often by the occasional observer. The need to use ordinary light microscopy as well as polarized light has been emphasized by the observation that the majority of CPPD crystals (80% in one study) are not birefringent and could be missed if only polarized light is used (9). Use of 100× oil immersion (difficult for wet preparations) is useful in identifying small CPPD crystals in stained smears. Routine reports from nonspecialized clinical laboratories often are inaccurate. In one review of five quality-control studies, as few as six of 50 CPPD crystals were correctly identified (10). Therefore, it is important to be familiar with the expertise available and the operating characteristics of the particular laboratory called upon for crystal identification (8,11). The clinician needs to alert the pathology laboratory if microcrystals are suspected in a tissue or biopsy specimen, because tissues for microscopy require alcohol fixative rather than formalin to preserve crystals of monosodium urate.

Other crystalline materials that may be seen include those from previously injected corticosteroids (which appear as crystals of varying and unusual configuration) and occasionally cholesterol crystals, which are easily distinguished from all of the others mentioned (they resemble a folded envelope). Contaminating crystalline or refractile substances, such as ethylenediamine tetra-acetic acid (EDTA) anticoagulant and talc, can be prevented by use of careful technique.

GOUT

Pathophysiology

Gout is a word derived from Latin meaning "a drop." It is applied to this form of arthritis because of the false belief, in ancient times, that the disease was caused by drops of bad humor. Gout is caused by an alteration in purine metabolism, the end product of which is uric acid. This alteration results in hyperuricemia and the deposition of urate crystals in various tissues. Periodic attacks of acute inflammatory arthritis, characteristic of gout, are caused by the deposition of urate crystals in and around joints. *Primary gout* is caused by an inborn error in the production or excretion of uric acid. *Secondary gout* is caused by an increased breakdown of nucleic acids in association with one of a variety of acquired diseases or by impaired excretion of urate as a consequence of acquired renal disease (Table 76.2).

Although there is frequently a family history of gout, few specific genetic defects responsible for hyperuricemia

TABLE 76.2 Causes of Hyperuricemia

With Increased Urinary Urate	*With Normal or Low Urinary Urate*
10% of primary gout (defects usually unknown)	90% of primary gout (defects usually unknown)
	Familial juvenile hyperuricemic nephropathy
Specific enzyme defects	
Hypoxanthine-guanine-phosphoribosyltransferase deficiency, partial	
Phosphoribosylpyrophosphate synthetase variants	
Secondary causes	Secondary causes
Myeloproliferative disease	Decreased renal function
	Inhibition of tubular urate excretion (competitive anions)
	Enhanced tubular urate absorption (fasting, dehydration)
	Insulin resistance
	Ethanol abuse
	Hypoxemia and tissue underperfusion
Lymphoproliferative disease	Lead nephropathy
Hemolytic diseases	Drugs
Glycogen storage disease	Diuretics
Psoriasis	Salicylates (low dose)
	Cyclosporine
Severe muscle exertion	Pyrazinamide
	Ethambutol
	Nicotinic acid
	Didanosine
	Others
	Obesity
	Hyperparathyroidism
	Sarcoidosis

Modified from Primer on the Rheumatic Diseases, Edition 11, copyright 1997, the Arthritis Foundation.

have been identified. In a segregation analysis of serum uric acid, the heritability factor was 0.399, supporting the hypothesis that hyperuricemia is a multifactorial trait influenced by complex hereditary and environmental factors (12). Therefore, in patients with primary gout due to overproduction of urate (only approximately 10% of patients), the specific cause usually is not identified. Overproduction of urate in primary gout can occur as a result of an X-linked dominant defect in hypoxanthine-guanine phosphoribosyl transferase, an important enzyme in purine metabolism (13), or from overactivity of 5′-phosphoribosyl-pyrophosphate synthesis (14). An hereditary nephropathy with tubulointerstitial renal damage and early appearance of hyperuricemia and gout is an example of primary gout, with underexcretion of urate caused by an autosomal dominant gene (15,16). A positive family history and onset of gout before age 35 years should suggest the possibility of a primary condition causing overproduction or underexcretion of urate. To assess production and excretion of urate, measurement in a 24-hour sample of urine may be indicated. Normal urinary uric acid excretion is <600 mg/day if the diet for 5 days has been free of purine-rich foods. Because this diet is impractical for most patients, a reasonable estimate can be made on a regular diet. Urinary excretion >1,000 mg/day is clearly abnormal, and 800 to 1,000 mg/day is borderline. An alternative method to screen for increased urate excretion on a regular diet is to measure urate and creatinine in serum and in midmorning urine after a light, low-purine breakfast, calculating the urate excretion normalized to a glomerular filtration rate of 100 mL/min (17). This can be calculated simply by using the formula (Uu × Sc) ÷ Uc, where Uu is urine urate in milligrams per minute, Sc is serum creatinine in milligrams per minute, and Uc is urine creatinine in deciliters per minute. A value >0.6 mg/dL suggests overexcretion. Because overproduction related to a genetic defect is an uncommon cause of primary gout, measurement of urinary urate is unnecessary for the management of most cases of gout unless a secondary cause of hyperuricemia is suspected or uric acid stones have developed.

Normal concentrations of serum urate vary widely in the population (range 3–8 mg/dL); in addition, spontaneous variation may occur within an individual patient. The upper limit of normal for serum urate measured by the uricase method usually is considered 7.0 mg/dL for adult men and 6.0 mg/dL for adult women. Ranges may be higher by ≥1 mg/dL if automated colorimetric methods are used.

Epidemiology

Gout is estimated to occur at a lifetime frequency of three cases per 1,000 population in the United States. The prevalence of gout in the United States has been estimated to be 8.4 per 1,000 persons of all ages and both sexes, corresponding to a total of 2.1 million persons (1.5 million men and 550,000 women) (18). Because this figure is based on self-reported data, it likely is an overestimate. Several population-based studies have indicated that the prevalence of gout has increased recently. One review noted that the prevalence of gout in the United Kingdom increased from 2.6 per 1,000 to 9.5 per 1,000 from the 1970s to 1993 (19). Obesity and excessive weight gain were important risk factors for the development of gout in a prospective study of white men (20). The incidence of gout in African American men was significantly higher than in white men, and gout was associated with systolic blood pressure at baseline and subsequent development of hypertension (21). Gout in all of its forms is ten times more common in men, and it is rare in premenopausal women. Gout is rare before age 30 years and increases in frequency to a plateau at age approximately 60 years. Age at onset probably is related to the duration and severity of preceding hyperuricemia. In a prospective study of 223 men in Taiwan with asymptomatic hyperuricemia, the 5-year cumulative incidence of gout was 19% (22). The only predictor of development of gout at baseline was the concentration of uric acid. Independent risk factors in followup included further increase of serum urate, persistent alcohol consumption, use of diuretics, and increased body mass index. Excessive alcohol consumption was the most important independent risk factor in this group of hyperuricemic men.

Hyperuricemia due to decreased renal clearance of uric acid (23) is a constant feature of a complex cluster of metabolic and clinical abnormalities associated with insulin resistance, the so-called *metabolic syndrome* (24). These abnormalities include hyperinsulinemia, impaired glucose tolerance, dyslipidemia with elevated fasting triglyceride levels and lowered high-density lipoprotein cholesterol levels, hypertension, and central obesity. As a result of long-standing hyperuricemia, gout is often seen in middle-aged men with this syndrome and may be one of the initial clinical presentations (25). Management of gout in such patients may be difficult and requires attention to the other features of the syndrome. Although the etiology involves both genetic and environmental factors, increased visceral fat accumulation (20,26) and alcohol consumption (22,27) are risk factors that contribute to the abnormalities observed and to the development of clinical gout. Alcohol increases the risk of gout in a dose-dependent fashion (27).

Use of thiazide diuretics is a risk factor for gout (28) and complicates the observed association of gout with hypertension. Diuretic use is often a factor in the occurrence of gout in elderly women (29). Gout is often a complication in patients who have undergone renal or cardiac transplantation, in part because of the hyperuricemic effect of cyclosporine (30). In a study of 225 patients after cardiac transplantation, 23 patients developed acute gout that

day for 2 to 3 days, are equally effective (49,50). Moderately high initial dosages of oral corticosteroids (30–60 mg/day prednisone tapered slowly over 7–10 days) usually are required for complete resolution without recrudescence (49).

Drugs administered to lower serum urate concentrations have no place in the treatment of the acute gouty attack. In fact, these agents may exacerbate acute attacks by the associated changes in plasma urate concentration (see Mechanisms of Crystal-Induced Arthritis).

Intercritical Gout

The efficacy of colchicine in dosages of 0.6 mg given one, two, or rarely three times daily (dosage frequency depends on control; most patients tolerate two doses per day without side effects) in reducing the frequency of acute attacks of gout has been well established (30,51). Therefore, prophylactic colchicine is indicated for patients who have had more than one episode of acute gout in a single year or when therapy to lower the concentration urate is initiated (see Chronic Gout). Caution is required in patients with impaired renal function. Reversible myopathy and neuropathy have been observed in some patients whose serum creatinine concentration was >1.6 mg/dL even with two tablets per day (52). Patients with renal insufficiency on colchicine prophylaxis should undergo a complete blood cell count and creatine kinase analysis once every 6 months of therapy to monitor for colchicine-related myopathy and myelosuppression (40). In elderly patients without tophi (nontophaceous gout), with infrequent acute attacks, and only mild hyperuricemia (i.e., <8 mg/dL), prophylactic colchicine may be all that is required. Some patients who have nontophaceous gout with infrequent attacks of arthritis (e.g., fewer than one or two per year) and mild hyperuricemia (<8 mg/dL) may elect not to take regular colchicine prophylaxis. In this instance, episodic use of an NSAID such as indomethacin is appropriate to control acute attacks. However, in most patients with gout and persistent hyperuricemia ≥8 mg/dL, the serum urate concentration should be reduced to prevent recurrent gout and to reverse the accumulation of urate in the tissues. In this instance, colchicine prophylaxis should be continued until the patient has been free of attacks for at least 1 year after the serum urate concentration has returned to normal. As an alternative in patients intolerant of colchicine, NSAIDs can be used for prophylaxis, but they may have more serious toxic effects than colchicine. Omitting prophylactic therapy and treating acute attacks early if they occur is an alternative for some patients with infrequent attacks.

Two classes of drugs that lower serum urate concentration are available: *uricosuric agents* promote urinary excretion of urate by blocking tubular urate resorption, and *allopurinol* decreases urate production through inhibition of purine metabolism. (Oxypurinol, an active metabolite of allopurinol, is not generally available and has few advantages over the parent compound.) Uricosuric agents are most effective in patients with nontophaceous gout who have good renal function (creatinine clearance at least 60–80 mL/min) and normal uric acid excretion (<750 mg/24 hours). The terms *uric acid* and *urate* are sometimes used interchangeably, but the correct terminology uses uric acid where it is the dominant moiety in the uric acid–rate equilibrium. Uric acid is dominant only in very acid situations, as in the distal renal tubule. In blood and at the usual tissue pH, the dominant moiety is urate. In most patients, clinical evidence of impaired urinary excretion rather than overproduction of urate is obvious (Table 76.2). When there is uncertainty, evaluation of urinary uric acid excretion is important not only as a clue to the mechanism of hyperuricemia but also to the choice of therapy (Table 76.2).

Probenecid (Benemid) is the uricosuric agent of choice because of its well-established safety and its long duration of effect. An initial dosage of 250 mg twice daily should be increased to 1.5 g daily or to a maximum of 2 g/day (in two or three divided doses) to achieve a serum urate concentration consistently <6.0 mg/dL, the level required to produce a urate gradient from tissue to plasma and to prevent further deposition of urate. To minimize the chance of precipitating a recurrent arthritic attack, the uricosuric agent should not be initiated until at least 1 week after an acute attack of gout has subsided and only after colchicine prophylaxis (described earlier) has been initiated for 3 or 4 days. The principal side effect of probenecid is gastrointestinal distress (which is uncommon), but there is a risk for formation of uric acid calculi in the renal tubules during the first week of therapy, especially with a large basal uric acid excretion (i.e., 600–800 mg/day). This risk can be minimized by starting at a dosage of 250 mg twice daily and gradually increasing the dosage over 2–3 weeks. The patient may be advised to drink 2 to 3 L of fluid daily and to take an alkalinizing agent such as sodium bicarbonate or citrate salt (polycitrate), 0.5 to 1 mEq/kg of body weight in five or six doses per day, to keep the urine pH (measured occasionally with pH paper) >6.0 or 6.5 for the first few weeks of uricosuric therapy. Small dosages of aspirin (2.4 g/day), but not a single low-dose enteric tablet as used for cardiac prophylaxis (53), block the effect of probenecid on renal excretion of urate and should be avoided. Probenecid may reduce the excretion of other drugs, including NSAIDs and penicillin, and prolong their half-life. Probenecid may cause a false-positive result for glucose in the urine.

Sulfinpyrazone (Anturane) is a more potent uricosuric agent but has more potential for adverse effects, including renal toxicity and nephrolithiasis. It can be given beginning with 50 mg twice daily and increased gradually to 600 mg/day, if required, to achieve the desired serum urate concentration (i.e., <6 mg/dL). Sulfinpyrazone is available in 100- and 200-mg strengths. This agent, which is an analogue of phenylbutazone, can cause gastric ulceration and platelet dysfunction. It can interact with sulfonamides or sulfonylureas to increase their hypoglycemic effect. For these reasons, it should be used principally when probenecid or allopurinol is not tolerated.

Allopurinol (Zyloprim or generic) is a potent agent that reduces the serum urate concentration. Because it blocks urate production by inhibition of xanthine oxidase, it is particularly useful in patients with renal dysfunction or with uric acid calculi and in patients with long-standing gout with tophi or with excessive basal uric acid excretion (>750 mg/24 hours). Serious side effects of rash, fever, leukopenia, hepatitis, and occasionally a generalized vasculitis occur in fewer than 2% of patients. These symptoms are most likely to occur within the first 2 months after initiation of therapy, so patients should be kept under close surveillance during this period. Toxicity is enhanced in patients with severe renal compromise or when the drug is administered concomitantly with ampicillin or thiazide diuretics (54). Allopurinol (available in 100- and 300-mg tablets) should be started at a dosage of 50 to 100 mg/day and increased over 2 or 3 weeks until the serum urate concentration is consistently <6.0 mg/dL; no more than 300 mg should be administered as a single dose. Prolonged use of dosages in excess of 300 mg twice per day increases the risk of toxicity; however, dosages of 400 to 600 mg/day may be required initially for effective control of serum urate concentration and reduction of the tissue urate load. Careful monitoring of the dose in patients with renal insufficiency is mandatory (54). In patients with renal insufficiency and in those who have undergone renal or cardiac transplantation and are receiving cyclosporine, adverse drug reactions are common with allopurinol, as well as with colchicine and NSAIDs (30).

Concomitant use of allopurinol and probenecid has been advocated for patients with chronic tophaceous gout. These agents seem to have an additive effect in lowering the serum uric acid concentration. However, use of a single agent, if possible, is preferred.

Febuxostat, a new nonpurine selective inhibitor of xanthine oxidase, has been submitted for FDA approval. In clinical trials, febuxostat in daily doses of 80 and 120 mg was more effective than allopurinol 300 mg daily in lowering serum urate concentration and similarly Reduced the number of gouty flares (55,56).

Compliance is the major factor in the effective treatment of intercritical gout. Patients feel well between attacks. Continued compliance with medications requires reinforcement in patient education and followup visits to ensure maintenance of normal serum urate concentrations (45). The duration of treatment to lower serum urate is uncertain and depends significantly on the severity of the disease, the presence or absence of tophi, the frequency of acute attacks, and compliance with drug dosage. In one study, patients who were able to achieve a serum concentration ≤6 mg/dL had a reduction in gout attacks and in the finding of crystals on knee joint aspiration compared with patients whose serum urate concentration was higher (57). Continued treatment with drugs to lower the serum urate concentration was estimated to be cost-saving if the patient had two attacks per year and cost-effective if the patient had one attack per year (58).

Dietary advice to patients with gout should be offered, especially to patients who are obese and/or use alcohol (40). High-purine foods (organ meats, seafood, all meats, meat gravies and extracts, lentils, peas, asparagus, yeast, and beer) are common in Western diets, and strict avoidance is neither practical nor necessary in the treatment of most patients with gout. Patients should be aware of these high-purine foods and avoid excesses of intake. More important dietary advice is to avoid alcohol (especially beer because it adds to the purine load) and to avoid fasting beyond 24 hours, because both of these situations may be associated with an acute increase in the serum urate concentration, which may precipitate an attack of gout. Obese patients should practice calorie reduction for weight loss, but a severe restriction may precipitate acute attacks. In a pilot study of patients with gout associated with elevated serum triglyceride concentrations and obesity, weight loss with moderate calorie and carbohydrate restriction and a proportionate increase of unsaturated fat and protein intake resulted in an improved lipid profile, a reduction of serum urate concentration, and a decrease in acute attacks of gout (59). Possibly helpful as a nonpharmacologic management strategy, this diet, which addresses both the complicating factor of dyslipidemia and hyperuricemia, deserves further study with a larger number of patients.

Chronic Gout

Compliance with appropriate therapy should eliminate this phase of gout except in a few patients with severe disease who are intolerant of one or more drugs used in treatment. Continuous or intermittent use of NSAIDs may be required in some of these patients for adequate control of inflammation and chronic symptoms. Effective reduction in serum urate concentration for months or years results in dissolution of tophi and general improvement. However, very large tophi may require surgical removal. After prolonged therapy and resolution of tophi, consideration has been given to discontinuation of therapy with urate-lowering drugs. However, acute attacks and tophi are likely to recur (60), so stopping therapy is generally not recommended.

Patients with chronic tophaceous gout and moderate *renal insufficiency* present a difficult problem in management. Uricosuric drugs usually are not effective. NSAIDs may further impair renal function. Withdrawal of NSAIDs produced a significant improvement in renal function in patients, with an average creatinine clearance of 60 mL/min after control of hyperuricemia was achieved (61). The incidence of adverse reactions to colchicine and allopurinol is increased in patients with renal disease, requiring lower doses and careful monitoring (54). For patients with tophaceous and polyarticular gout whose renal function makes uricosuric drugs ineffective, there are few alternative agents for lowering uric acid when a cutaneous reaction to allopurinol requires withdrawal of this therapy. Success was reported in desensitizing some patients by administering small, gradually increasing doses of allopurinol on a careful protocol beginning with 50 μg/day. A followup study indicated successful continuation of allopurinol and control of hyperuricemia in 78% of patients. Some developed a pruritic skin eruption that responded to withdrawal of allopurinol and dosage adjustment (62). It is important to note that patients with severe reactions, such as toxic epidermal necrolysis, hepatitis, or acute interstitial nephritis, were excluded from this study. Febuxostat (see Intercritical Gout) may prove to be a reasonable alternative in patients who have an adverse reaction to allopurinol.

Asymptomatic Hyperuricemia

Hyperuricemia (>7 mg/dL in men or 6 mg/dL in women) is a common laboratory finding in asymptomatic patients evaluated in a variety of clinical settings. In most patients, clinical findings point to an obvious cause, and no other therapy is required unless gout or nephrolithiasis develops. If the cause is unclear or the serum urate concentration is near 11 mg/dL, further evaluation to estimate urinary excretion and identify secondary causes of excessive urate production (Table 76.2) should be initiated. Although the serum urate concentration often is markedly elevated in patients with end-stage renal disease, clinical gout is rare.

Hyperuricemia Secondary to Diuretics

The renal tubular handling of urate is complex. Complete glomerular filtration is followed by tubular resorption, tubular secretion, and further tubular resorption. Resorption of urate is partly modulated by the volume of extracellular fluid (expansion increases excretion and contraction decreases excretion). Diuretics modify the renal handling of urate and uric acid by their effect on volume, and some diuretics may directly affect urate transport. Thiazides regularly cause a dosage-related rise in the serum urate concentration that is reversed on withdrawal of the agent. The increase in concentration averages 1 to 2 mg/dL but occasionally may be 4 to 5 mg/dL. Furosemide and bumetanide often are associated with a rise in serum urate concentration; less commonly, ethacrynic acid, acetazolamide, and rarely triamterene are associated with hyperuricemia. Spironolactone is not associated with hyperuricemia.

The incidence of gout after initiation of diuretic therapy is a complex issue. Other factors that affect the incidence of gout, such as hypertension and obesity, often are present in patients treated with diuretics. Approximately 10% of hypertensive patients with hyperuricemia secondary to diuretic therapy develop gout. This risk increases in patients with known gout and in patients with diseases associated with elevated serum urate concentration, such as myeloproliferative disorders or psoriasis. With diuretic therapy, uric acid excretion is diminished, and the incidence of urinary calculi does not increase. The risk of developing urate nephropathy is minimal (see Extra-Articular Manifestations). For these reasons, expectant management of patients with asymptomatic hyperuricemia secondary to diuretics is appropriate.

Should acute gout develop, the treatment described previously may be initiated. Intercritical gout is managed similarly to primary gout, and prophylactic colchicine and uricosuric therapy with probenecid (if there is no renal failure) or allopurinol to decrease production of urate may be used. Reducing the dosage or stopping the diuretic usually is associated with a slight fall in the plasma urate concentration, but many patients continue to have attacks of gout. Therefore, if a patient develops gout while taking diuretics and the need for the diuretic continues, it is best to treat the gout as described previously and to continue use of the diuretic at the minimally effective dosage. In the management of hypertension, the use of β-blockers, angiotensin-converting enzyme inhibitors, and long-acting calcium channel-blocking agents, which have no effect on urate excretion, may allow discontinuation of diuretics in some patients. The angiotensin receptor blocking agent losartan 50 mg/day has been shown to decrease serum uric acid concentrations (63).

CALCIUM PYROPHOSPHATE DIHYDRATE-INDUCED ARTHRITIS

Pathophysiology

CPPD deposition disease occurs as a result of altered metabolism of inorganic pyrophosphate (iPP), which causes deposition of CPPD crystals in articular cartilage, fibrocartilage, ligaments, tendons, bursae, and synovia. This may occur as an accompaniment or consequence of aging, often in association with osteoarthritis, or as a result of genetic defects or certain systemic metabolic diseases (Table 76.4). The precise mechanisms by which these deposits develop are not clear and likely are multifactorial. Most of the research toward an understanding of this process has involved alterations of iPP metabolism in articular cartilage. With aging and cartilage degeneration, chondrocytes proliferate, become hypertrophic, and undergo apoptosis (programmed cell death), with increased production

TABLE 76.4 Diseases Associated with Calcium Pyrophosphate Dihydrate Deposition Disease

Osteoarthritis	Hereditary hypophosphatasia
Hemochromatosis–hemosiderosis	Hypothyroidism
Gout	Neurogenic arthropathy
Hyperparathyroidism	Osteochondrodysplasia
Hypomagnesemia	Synovial chondromatosis
	Gitelman syndrome

of iPP and calcification (64). Once formed, calcium crystals may activate processes that enhance degenerative changes in articular cartilage (65). Once released in sufficient quantity into the joint, CPPD crystals induce an acute inflammatory response similar to that of monosodium urate and an acute arthritis, the syndrome of pseudogout.

Epidemiology

Chondrocalcinosis increases in frequency with age. It is present in approximately 5% of the adult population at the time of autopsy and in 20% to 30% of people older than 80 years, most of whom are asymptomatic. The exact prevalence of CPPD deposit disease is unknown. In one series of consecutive patients with newly diagnosed crystal-induced arthritis, CPPD deposit disease accounted for approximately one third of the cases. Men probably are affected more than women, with a male/female ratio of 1.5:1 (66).

Causes

Familial cases with an autosomal dominant inheritance in which chondrocalcinosis appears at an earlier age have been described (67). These families are uncommon, and many of these patients remain asymptomatic for many years. Although genetic defects in the nucleotide pyrophosphohydrolase enzymes have been suspected, the metabolic defect(s) has not been specifically identified. Most cases of CPPD deposit disease are sporadic and idiopathic; a few are associated with one of a variety of metabolic diseases (68). Many of the diseases associated with deposits of CPPD involve metabolic abnormalities in connective tissues, but the precise mechanisms of CPPD crystallization are unknown. Table 76.4 provides a list of these associated diseases. There is a strong association with osteoarthritis (see Chapter 75).

Clinical Features

Patients usually are middle aged to elderly at the time of onset of arthritic symptoms (Table 76.5). Several patterns of presentation are possible. Approximately one fourth of patients have *self-limited, acute, goutlike attacks (pseudogout)* predominantly affecting the knees and wrists, but occasionally involving other joints and rarely the first metatarsophalangeal joint. Monarticular attacks are the rule, but involvement of symmetrical joints and polyarthritis may occur rarely. Symptoms often are less intense than they are in gout, but the presentation is variable, and some attacks may be severe. Systemic symptoms, including fever to 101°F (38°C) or more, may occur as in gout, and patients often are misdiagnosed as having infection. In some elderly patients, fever is the dominant symptom, and the joint abnormalities are subtle and may be overlooked. Attacks often are exacerbated by trauma or acute illness. Long intervals (sometimes years) between attacks are common.

TABLE 76.5 Clinical Features of Calcium Pyrophosphate Dihydrate Deposition Disease

Epidemiology
Age: middle age or elderly

Site
Knee and wrist most common joints involved
Metacarpophalangeal joints, hips, shoulders, elbows, ankles may be affected
Arthritis usually monoarticular

Pattern
Acute goutlike attacks with symptom-free intervals in 25%
Osteoarthritislike disease in 50%, with superimposed acute attacks in half of these patients
Rheumatoidlike polyarthritis in 5%
Neuropathiclike arthritis without neurologic damage (rare)
Asymptomatic chondrocalcinosis in 20% (found on radiography)

Laboratory
Synovial fluid shows leukocytosis and characteristic calcium pyrophosphate dihydrate crystals

In approximately half of patients, and especially in women, the presentation resembles that of osteoarthritis with bilateral involvement, especially of the knees. The wrists, metacarpophalangeal joints, hips, shoulders, elbows, or ankles also may be affected. Acute exacerbations occur in approximately half of these patients, with features that resemble those of osteoarthritis, except that the disease is more progressive and destructive. Varus or valgus knee deformities are common, and extensive calcification around the patella may be seen on radiography. Flexion contractures may occur. The relationship to ordinary osteoarthritis is unclear, except that the involvement of joints not usually affected in osteoarthritis (metacarpophalangeal joints, wrists, shoulders, elbows) suggests a different pathogenesis. In one study, sensitive techniques demonstrated CPPD or basic calcium phosphate crystals in

11 of 12 samples from patients with typical osteoarthritis of the knee when the crystals were too small or too few to be detected by usual methods (see Chapter 75) (69).

In a few patients, persistent subacute inflammation with fatigue, morning stiffness, and synovial swelling in multiple joints lasting weeks or months resembles rheumatoid arthritis.

A few patients with severely *destructive arthritis* that resembles the Charcot joints of neuropathic arthropathy but is associated with a normal neurologic examination have been reported. CPPD deposit disease may be associated with a true neuropathic arthritis caused by tabes dorsalis.

Laboratory Findings

Patients may have peripheral leukocytosis and an elevated erythrocyte sedimentation rate in association with acute or subacute attacks of arthritis. The synovial fluid shows polymorphonuclear leukocytosis that may be >50,000/mm^3 in acute pseudogout but more commonly ranges from 15,000 to 25,000/mm^3. Crystal identification is the key to diagnosis (see earlier discussion). In the absence of acute or subacute inflammation, leukocyte counts may be low (<2,000/mm^3), and crystals may be largely extracellular.

Because of the occasional association with other potentially treatable disorders (Table 76.4), the patient's serum calcium, phosphorus, magnesium, alkaline phosphatase, and uric acid (actually urate, as discussed earlier) concentrations should be measured, although they usually are normal. Chondrocalcinosis is a frequent manifestation of the Gitelman variant of Bartter syndrome, a rare genetic disorder (70). The findings of hypomagnesemia, mild hypokalemic alkalosis, and hypocalciuria lead to the correct diagnosis. The defect is an abnormality in the sodium chloride transporter in the distal convoluted tubule of the kidney. A striking reduction of chondrocalcinosis over a 10-year period and a good prognosis (71) are seen if hypomagnesemia and hypokalemia can be reversed with potassium and magnesium supplementation, sometimes aided with spironolactone. Because pseudogout may be the presenting manifestation of hemochromatosis and because of the importance of early diagnosis in this disorder, measurement of serum ferritin concentration and/or genetic testing are indicated if there is any suspicion of this diagnosis (66).

Radiographic Findings

The typical radiographic findings of CPPD deposit disease are punctate and linear calcifications (chondrocalcinosis), seen most often in the fibrocartilage of the menisci of the knee, usually bilaterally (Fig. 76.3). Other fibrocartilages may show similar changes, including the disc in the distal radioulnar joint, the symphysis pubis, the lip of the acetabulum, the glenoid fossa, and intervertebral discs. Hyaline cartilage may be involved, with similar punctate linear calcifications that may be identified as a dense line parallel to the subchondral bone in the midzone of the articular cartilage. Calcification in the soft tissues of the joint capsule and occasionally in ligaments and

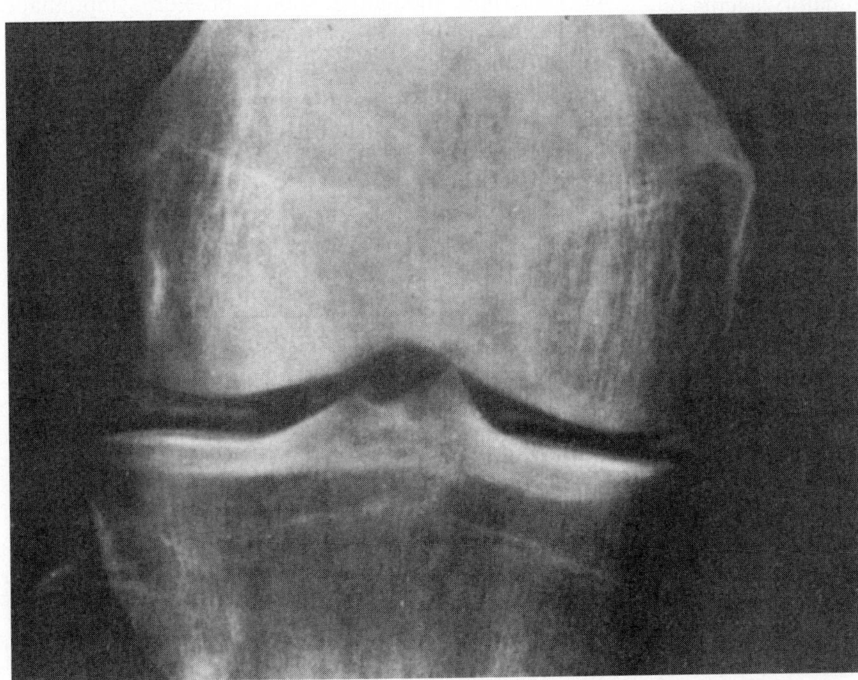

FIGURE 76.3. Radiograph of the knee in a patient with chondrocalcinosis. Stippled calcification of the medial and lateral menisci is easily identified.

tendons may be seen but is less characteristic. In patients with the type of CPPD deposit disease that resembles osteoarthritis, subchondral cyst formation with bony collapse may be prominent. Osteophyte formation is variable and inconsistent.

These radiographic findings may be helpful in suggesting or confirming the diagnosis of CPPD deposit disease (72). However, it may not be possible to visualize the extent of deposits radiographically, and their absence does not exclude the diagnosis if typical crystals can be demonstrated in synovial fluid or in biopsy material.

Management

No therapy influences the deposition or resolution of tissue deposits of CPPD in idiopathic CPPD deposition disease. During the acute attack of pseudogout, diagnostic aspiration of synovial fluid (see Chapter 74) with removal of crystals and leukocytes may provide significant clinical improvement. Local injection of depo corticosteroid (see Chapter 74) often is effective and avoids potential side effects of systemic drug therapy. Efficacy of colchicine has been debated; although it sometimes is effective, use of indomethacin or other NSAIDs as described for acute gout is generally preferred. Because many of these patients are elderly (and therefore may have an impaired glomerular filtration rate), caution regarding renal toxicity of these agents should be exercised (see Chapter 52). As in the treatment of acute gout, a brief course of systemic corticosteroids is an alternative; however, because a single large joint usually is affected, intra-articular steroid administration is preferred. In patients with only recurrent acute attacks, no therapy is indicated between attacks, but early administration of anti-inflammatory agents on exacerbation may minimize or abort attacks. Therapy for patients with more subacute inflammation or for those with osteoarthritislike disease is similar to that described for osteoarthritis (see Chapter 75), except that anti-inflammatory concentrations of drugs may be required for optimal symptomatic control.

HYDROXYAPATITE-INDUCED ARTHRITIS

The capacity of hydroxyapatite crystals to induce an inflammatory response was first appreciated in some patients with acute tendinitis (73). More recently, hydroxyapatite crystals were identified in patients with osteoarthritis, especially in association with acute inflammatory episodes (74), and in patients with destructive arthropathy of the shoulder joint (75). The latter, called *Milwaukee shoulder,* is associated with painful limited shoulder motion, complete disruption of the rotator cuff, and extensive degenerative changes in the bone. In these conditions, crystals of other basic calcium salts, including octacalcium phosphate and tricalcium phosphate in addition to hydroxyapatite, have sometimes been identified. This has prompted the use of the term *basic calcium phosphate (BCP) deposit disease* to describe these syndromes (75). The capacity of the various crystals to induce inflammation varies according to crystal type, surface area, and calcium/phosphate ratio (76). CPPD crystals may be found in addition to BCP crystals in these syndromes and in some familial cases (77). Alizarin red S dye (available from scientific supply houses) may be used to stain wet preparations of synovial fluid to screen for the presence of hydroxyapatite crystals, which appear under ordinary light microscopy as red-stained clumps of crystalline material (78). Because all other calcium-containing crystals and even noncrystalline calcium salts stain with this dye, specific identification of BCP crystals requires techniques that are not usually available, such as electron microscopy, microprobe analysis, or x-ray diffraction. It now is clear that BCP crystals alone or in combination with CPPD are broadly associated with calcinosis in soft tissue, tendons, and bursae as well as in joints. These deposits may be secondary in some instances to trauma, neurologic injury, collagen disease, or chronic renal failure. In any of these locations, an acute goutlike inflammation or a more chronic and sometimes destructive tissue response may ensue. One need only be aware of the potential inflammatory properties of this crystalline material and consider its implication in these various clinical situations. The patient may be treated with aspiration, from a joint or soft tissue, of the crystalline material and subsequent local injection of a lidocaine/corticosteroid solution (see Chapter 74) or with an NSAID (see Chapter 77). These modalities should provide symptomatic relief in patients with acute inflammatory arthritis or tendinitis associated with BCP crystal deposits. If symptoms become chronic or extensive destructive arthropathy is present, rheumatologic or orthopedic referral is indicated.

ARTHRITIS ASSOCIATED WITH CALCIUM OXALATE

Another crystal-associated arthritis has been demonstrated in patients receiving long-term dialysis therapy (usually hemodialysis, but also seen with peritoneal dialysis) for end-stage renal disease. Extensive deposits of calcium oxalate in soft tissues occur in this setting, and these deposits can cause acute arthritis, destructive arthropathy, tenosynovitis, or bursitis (79,80). These patients are difficult to treat because of the presence of extensive and continuing deposits and incomplete response to colchicine, nonsteroidal agents, and corticosteroids.

SPECIFIC REFERENCES*

1. Choi HK, Mount DB, Reginato AM. Pathogenesis of gout. Ann Intern Med 2005;143:499.
2. Pascual E, Batlle-Gualda E, Martinez A, et al. Synovial fluid analysis for diagnosis of intercritical gout. Ann Intern Med 1999;131:756.
3. Malnik SD, Arliel-Romen S, Ervon E, et al. Acute pseudogout as a complication of pamidronate. Ann Pharmacother 1997;31:499.
4. Perez-Ruiz F, Testillano M, Gastoca MA, et al. "Pseudoseptic" pseudogout associated with hypomagnesemia in liver transplant patients. Transplantation 2001;71:696.
5. Terkeltaub RA. Pathogenesis and treatment of crystal-induced inflammation. In: Koopman WJ, ed. Arthritis and allied conditions. Philadelphia: Lippincott Williams & Wilkins, 2001: 23.
6. Fagan TJ, Lidsky MD. Compensated polarized light microscopy using cellophane adhesive tape. Arthritis Rheum 1974;17:256.
7. Kerolous G, Clayburne G, Schumacher HR Jr. Is it mandatory to examine synovial fluids promptly after arthrocentesis. Arthritis Rheum 1989;32:271.
8. Selvi E, Manganelli S.Catenaccio M, et al. Diff Quick staining methods for detection and identification of monosodium urate and calcium pyrophosphate crystals in synovial fluids. Ann Rheum Dis 2001;60:194.
9. Ivorra J, Rosas J, Pascual E. Most calcium pyrophosphate crystals appear as non-birefringent. Ann Rheum Dis 1999;58:582.
10. Swan A, Amer H, Dieppe P. The value of synovial fluid assays in the diagnosis of joint disease: a literature survey. Ann Rheum Dis 2002;61:493.
11. McGill NW, McGill VG. Quality assurance for synovial fluid examination for crystals: an improved method. Ann Rheum Dis 1997;56:504.
12. Wik JB, Djousse L, Boreski I, et al. Segregation analysis of serum uric acid in the NHLBI Family Heart Study. Hum Genet 2000;106:355.
13. Wilson JM, Young AB, Kelley WN. Hypoxanthine-guanine phosphoribosyl transferase deficiency: the molecular basis of the clinical syndrome. N Engl J Med 1983;309:900.
14. Sperling O, Elam G, Pinsky-Brosch S, et al. Accelerated 5′(-phosphoribosyl-pyrophosphate synthesis: a familial abnormality associated with excessive uric acid production and gout. Biochem Med 1992;6:310.
15. Puig JG, Miranda ME, Felicitas A, et al. Hereditary nephropathy associated with hyperuricemia and gout. Arch Intern Med 1993;153:357.
16. Kamatani N, Moritani M, Yamanaka H, et al. Localization of a gene for familial juvenile hyperuricemic nephropathy causing underexcretion-type gout to 16p12 by genome-wide linkage analysis in a large family. Arthritis Rheum 2000;43:925.
17. Simpkin PA. When, why and how should we quantify the excretion rate of urinary uric acid? J Rheumatol 2001;28:1207.
18. Lawrence RC, Helmick CG, Arnett FC, et al. Estimates of the prevalence of arthritis and musculoskeletal disorders in the United States. Arthritis Rheum 1998;41:778.
19. Luk AJ, Simkin PA. Epidemiology of hyperuricemia and gout. Am J Manag Care 2005;11:S435.
20. Roubenoff R, Klag MJ, Mead LA, et al. Incidence and risk factors for gout in white men. JAMA 1991;266:3004.
21. Hochberg MC, Thomas J, Thomas DJ, et al. Racial differences in the incidence of gout: the role of hypertension. Arthritis Rheum 1995;38:628.
22. Lin KC, Lin HY, Chou P. The interaction between uric acid level and other risk factors on the development of gout among hyperuricemic men in a prospective study. J Rheumatol 2001;27:1501.
23. Facchini F, Chen I, Hollenbeck CB, et al. Relationship between resistance to insulin-mediated glucose uptake, urinary uric acid clearance and plasma uric acid concentration. JAMA 1991;166:3008.
24. Kahn R, Buse J, Ferrannini E, et al. The metabolic syndrome: time for a critical appraisal. Diabetes Care 2005;28:2289.
25. Emerson B. Hyperlipidemia in hyperuricemia and gout. Ann Rheum Dis 1998;57:5090.
26. Takahashi S, Moriwaki Y, Tsutsumi Z, et al. Increased visceral fat accumulation further aggravates the risks of insulin resistance in gout. Metabolism 2001;50:393.
27. Choi HK, Atkinson K, Karlson EW, et al. Alcohol intake and risk of incident gout in men: a prospective study. Lancet 2004;363:1277.
28. Scott JT, Higgins CJ. Diuretic induced gout: a multifactorial condition. Ann Rheum Dis 1992;51:259.
29. McFarlane G, Dieppe PA. Diuretic induced gout in elderly females. Br J Rheumatol 1985;24: 155.
30. Lin HY, Rocher LL, McQuillan MA. Cyclosporine-induced hyperuricemia and gout. N Engl J Med 1989;321:287.
31. Wluka AE, Ryan PF, Miller AM, et al. Post cardiac transplantation gout: incidence of therapeutic complications. J Heart Lung Transplant 2000;19:951.
32. Erickson AR, Enzenauer RJ, Nordstrom DM, et al. The prevalence of hypothyroidism in gout. Am J Med 1994;97:231.
33. Gutman AB. The past four decades of progress in the knowledge of gout, with an assessment of the present status. Arthritis Rheum 1972;16: 431.
34. Wall B, Agudelo CA, Tesser JRP, et al. An autopsy study of the prevalence of monosodium urate and calcium pyrophosphate dihydrate crystal deposition in the first metatarsophalangeal joints. Arthritis Rheum 1983;26:1522.
35. Weinberger A, Schumaker HR Jr.Agudelo CA. Urate crystals in asymptomatic metatarsophalangeal joints. Ann Intern Med 1979;91:56.
36. Holland NW, Jost D, Beutler A, et al. Finger pad tophi in gout. J Rheumatol 1996;23:690.
37. Puig JG, Michan AD, Jiminez ML, et al. Female gout: clinical spectrum and uric acid metabolism. Arch Intern Med 1991;151:726.
38. Fam AG, Stein J, Rubenstein J. Gouty arthritis in nodal osteoarthritis. J Rheumatol 1996;23: 684.
39. Schapira D, Stahl S, Izhak OB, et al. Chronic tophaceous gout mimicking rheumatoid arthritis. Semin Arthritis Rheum 1999;29:56.
40. Mikuls TR, MacLean CH, Olivieri J, et al. Quality of care indicators for gout management. Arthritis Rheum 2004;50:937.
41. Hall AP, Barry PE, Dawber TR, et al. Epidemiology of gout and hyperuricemia. Am J Med 1967;42:27.
42. Yu TF, Gutman AB. Uric acid nephrolithiasis in gout: predisposing factors. Ann Intern Med 1967;67:1133.
43. Gerster JL, Landry M, Duvoisin B, et al. Computer tomography of the knee joint as an indication of intra articular tophi in gout. Arthritis Rheum 1996;39:1406.
44. Terkeltaub RA. Gout. N Engl J Med 2003;349:1647.
45. Wortman RL. Effective management of gout: an analogy. Am J Med 1998;105:513.
46. Chin MH, Wang LC, Jin L, et al. Appropriateness of medication selection for older persons in an urban academic emergency department. Acad Emerg Med 1999;6:1232.
47. Ahern MJ, Reid C, Gordon TP, et al. Does colchicine work? The results of the first controlled study in acute gout. Aust N Z J Med. 1987;17:301.
48. Fam AG. Current therapy of acute microcrystalline arthritis and the role of corticosteroids. J Clin Rheumatol 1997;3:35.
49. Groff GO, Frank WA, Raddatz DA. Systemic steroid therapy for acute gout: a clinical trial and review of the literature. Semin Arthritis Rheum 1990;19:329.
50. Alloway JA, Moriarty MJ, Hoogland YT, et al. Comparison of triamcinolone acetonide with indomethacin in the treatment of acute gouty arthritis. J Rheumatol 1993;20:111.
51. Paulus HE, Schlosstein LH, Godfrey RG, et al. Prophylactic colchicine therapy of intercritical gout: a placebo controlled study of probenecid-treated patients. Arthritis Rheum 1974;17:609.
52. Kuncl RW, Duncan G, Watson O, et al. Colchicine myopathy and neuropathy. N Engl J Med 1987;316:1562.
53. Harris M, Bryant LR, Danaker P, et al. Effect of low dose daily aspirin on serum urate levels and urinary excretion in patients receiving probenecid for gouty arthritis. J Rheumatol 2000;27:2873.
54. Hande KR, Noone RM, Stone WJ. Severe allopurinol toxicity: description and guidelines for prevention in patients with renal insufficiency. Am J Med 1984;76:47.
55. Becker MA, Schumacher HR Jr, Wortmann RL, et al. Febuxostat compared with allopurinol in patients with hyperuricemia and gout. N Engl J Med 2005;353:2450.
56. Becker MA, Schumacher HR Jr., Wortmann, RL, et al. Febuxostat, a novel nonpurine selective inhibitor of xanthine oxidase: a twenty-eight day, multicenter, phase II, randomized, double-blind, placebo-controlled, dose-response clinical trial examining safety and efficacy in patients with gout. Arthritis Rheum 2005;52:916.
57. Li-Yu J, Clayburne G, Sieck M, et al. Treatment of chronic gout: can we determine when urate stores are depleted enough to prevent attacks of gout? J Rheumatol 2001;28:577.
58. Ferraz MB, O'Brien B. A cost effective analysis of urate lowering drugs in non-tophaceous recurrent gouty arthritis. J Rheumatol 1995;22:908.
59. Dessein PH, Shipton EA, Stanwix AE, et al. Beneficial effects of weight loss associated with moderate caloric/carbohydrate restriction and increased proportional intake of protein and unsaturated fat on serum uric and lipoprotein levels in gout. Ann Rheum Dis 2000;59: 539.
60. Van Lieshout-Zuidema MF, Breedveld FC. Withdrawal of long term anti-hyperuricemic therapy in tophaceous gout. J Rheumatol 1993;22:1383.
61. Perez-Ruiz F, Calabozo M, Herrero-Beites AM, et al. Improvement of renal function in patients with chronic gout after proper control of hyperuricemia and gouty bouts. Nephron 2000;86:287.
62. Fam AG, Dunne SM, Iazetta J, et al. Efficacy and safety of desensitization to allopurinol following cutaneous reactions. Arthritis Rheum 2001;44:231.
63. Wurzner G, Gerster JC, Chiolero A, et al. Comparative effects of losartan and irbesartan

*Bold numerals denote published controlled clinical trials, meta-analyses, or consensus-based recommendations.

on serum uric acid in hypertensive patients with hyperuricaemia and gout. J Hypertens 2001; 19: 1855.
64. Lotz M, Hashimoto S, Kuhn K. Mechanisms of chondrocyte apoptosis. Osteoarthritis Cartilage 1999;7:389.
65. Cheung HS. Calcium crystals' effects on the cells of the joint: implications for pathogenesis of disease. Curr Opin Rheumatol 2000;12:223.
66. McCarty DJ. Pseudogout and pyrophosphate metabolism. Adv Intern Med 1980;25: 363.
67. Reginato A, Valenzuela F, Martinez V, et al. Polyarticular and familial chondrocalcinosis. Arthritis Rheum 1970;13:197.
68. Jones AC, Chuck AJ, Arie EA, et al. Diseases associated with calcium pyrophosphate dihydrate deposition disease. Semin Arthritis Rheum 1992;22:188.
69. Swan A, Chapman B, Heap P, et al. Submicroscopic crystals in osteoarthritis synovial fluid. Ann Rheum Dis 1994;53:467.
70. Punzi L, Calo L, Schiavon F, et al. Chondrocalcinosis is a feature of Gitelman's variant of Bartter's syndrome: a new look at the hypomagnesemia associated with calcium pyrophosphate dihydrate deposition disease. Rev Rheum Engl Ed 1998;65:571.
71. Barakat AJ, Rennert OM. Gitelman's syndrome (familial hypokalemia-hypomagnesemia). J Nephrol 2001;14:43.
72. Steinbach L, Resnick D. Calcium pyrophosphate dihydrate deposition disease: imaging perspectives. Curr Probl Diagn Radiol 2000; 29:209.
73. Pinals RS, Short CL. Calcific periarthritis involving multiple sites. Arthritis Rheum 1966;9:566.
74. Huskisson EC, Dieppe PA, Tucker AK, et al. Another look at osteoarthritis. Ann Rheum Dis 1979;38:423.
75. Halverson PB, McCarty DJ, Cheung HS, et al. Milwaukee shoulder syndrome: eleven additional cases with involvement of the knee in seven (basic calcium phosphate crystal deposition disease). Semin Arthritis Rheum 1984;14:36.
76. Prudhommeaux F, Schlitz C, Liote F, et al. Variation in the inflammatory properties of basic calcium phosphate crystals according to crystal type. Arthritis Rheum 1996;39: 1319.
77. Pons-Estel BA, Gimenez L, Sacnun M, et al. Familial osteoarthritis and Milwaukee shoulder associated with calcium pyrophosphate and apatite crystal deposition. J Rheumatol 2000;27:471.
78. Paul H, Reginato AJ, Schumacher HR Jr. Alizarin red staining as a screening test for calcium compounds in synovial fluid. Arthritis Rheum 1983;26:191.
79. Reginato AJ, Kurnick BRC. Calcium oxalate and other crystals associated with kidney diseases and arthritis. Semin Arthritis Rheum 1989;18:198.
80. Rosenthal AK, Ryan LM, McCarty DJ. Arthritis associated with calcium oxalate crystals in an anephric patient treated with peritoneal dialysis. JAMA 1988;260:1272.

For annotated ***General References*** *and resources related to this chapter, visit www.hopkinsbayview.org/PAMreferences.*

Chapter 77

Rheumatoid Arthritis

Uzma J. Haque and Joan M. Bathon

Rheumatoid arthritis (RA) is a chronic systemic inflammatory disease of unknown cause that primarily targets the peripheral joints. The articular inflammation has a variable course, but the usual presentation is an additive, progressive, symmetrical polyarthritis that, if inadequately treated, will lead to joint destruction, deformity, and loss of function. Extra-articular features and systemic symptoms are recognized as an integral part of the disease and may antedate the onset of inflammatory arthropathy.

In the last 10 years, a confluence of discoveries from many areas of research has greatly affected our approach to the treatment of RA. Recognition that joint destruction and disability begin early, and that survival in RA is reduced, has led to a much more aggressive approach than in decades past. Advances in immunology and biotechnology have yielded more effective and better-tolerated agents. More than ever, it is imperative for clinicians to make the diagnosis rapidly, identify patients with poor prognosis, and institute an appropriate and effective therapeutic plan.

EPIDEMIOLOGY

The prevalence of RA worldwide is approximately 1% to 2%. However, this figure differs significantly in some populations. For example, Native Americans have a high prevalence of 3.5% to 5.3%, and among rural South African blacks and Japanese the prevalence is only 0.1% (1). The prevalence of RA increases with age, approaching 5% in women older than 55 years. The average annual incidence in the United States is approximately 70 per 100,000 people (1). Both the incidence and the prevalence of RA are two to three times greater in women than in men. Although RA may manifest at any age, it most commonly affects individuals in the fourth to sixth decades.

Genetic influences on disease frequency and severity are suggested by an increased incidence of the human class II histocompatibility antigens human leukocyte antigen (HLA)-DR4 and HLA-DR1 in patients with RA, compared with a matched control population (2). The HLA-DR molecule consists of an α chain and a β chain, with the various HLA-DR specificities determined by heterogeneity at the three hypervariable regions of the HLA-DRβ chain. The molecular basis for the HLA association with RA is defined by a specific sequence of amino acids at positions 70–74 in the third hypervariable region of the DRβ chain. The presence of this shared structural element or "shared epitope" correlates with an increased risk for development of RA and/or greater disease severity (3).

PATHOGENESIS

The normal diarthrodial joint is surrounded by a thin connective tissue structure called the *synovium*. The synovium is the primary site of pathology in RA. Normal synovium is a thin, somewhat amorphous structure consisting of a lining layer one to three cells thick and a sublining layer that is hypocellular but vascularized. Synovial lining cells bear markers of fibroblast and macrophage lineage and secrete joint lubricants such as hyaluronic acid and lubricin. The vascularized sublining area provides nutrients to nearby avascular cartilage. The pathologic hallmark of RA consists of profound hypertrophy of the synovium via increased cellularity in both the lining and sublining areas into a tumorlike structure called the *pannus*. This hypertrophied structure, which consists of lymphocytes, plasma cells, macrophages, and fibroblasts, invades and erodes contiguous cartilage and bone via the elaboration of proinflammatory and degradative enzymes and cytokines (4). The event(s) or factor(s) that triggers the recruitment of inflammatory cells to the joint remains unknown. Local production of rheumatoid factor-containing immune complexes activates complement and attracts inflammatory cells. The predominance and persistence of $CD4^+$ T cells in the rheumatoid synovium suggest an antigen-driven, cell-mediated inflammatory process. The inflammatory process is amplified by a number of macrophage- and fibroblast-derived cytokines found in large quantities in the rheumatoid joint, including tumor necrosis factor (TNF)-α, interleukin (IL)-1, IL-6, IL-8, and granulocyte-macrophage colony-stimulating factor (5). These cytokines drive the recruitment of additional inflammatory cells and subsequent release of destructive enzymes. Enzymes such as collagenase and stromelysin destroy cartilage and bone, leading to loss of normal joint architecture.

HISTORY

RA usually is recognized by its articular manifestations. However, systemic symptoms such as weight loss, fever, and malaise may predate or accompany the onset of joint symptoms, and extraarticular manifestations may occur relatively early. Most commonly, RA presents insidiously over several months with a progressive, additive polyarthritis. Occasionally, patients experience an explosive polyarticular onset over 24 to 48 hours. A relatively uncommon presentation is termed *palindromic rheumatoid arthritis* in which a series of acute, self-limited attacks of inflammatory arthritis occur, usually in a single joint. Regardless of the initial presentation, the usual course is a relentless inflammatory polyarthritis involving small and large joints that is highly destructive and debilitating. The American College of Rheumatology criteria for the diagnosis of RA (6) are outlined in Table 77.1 and are discussed here.

Signs and symptoms of joint inflammation provide the definitive clues to the diagnosis of RA. One of the earliest symptoms is *stiffness* in the joints in the morning upon awakening. The stiffness usually lasts several hours and is accompanied by pain on movement. Patients often volunteer that they warm their hands in warm water or take prolonged showers in order to relieve the debilitating stiffness. Stiffness and pain in the balls of the feet (metatarsalgia) upon arising from bed is another common presenting symptom. Similar stiffness can occur after long periods of sitting or inactivity (gel phenomenon). In contrast, patients with degenerative arthritis complain of stiffness that lasts only 5 to 30 minutes (see Chapter 75). Unlike a patient with gout (see Chapter 76), a patient with RA can bear weight and move the inflamed joint but has a persistent, deep, gnawing discomfort. Severe pain in a patient with established RA, particularly if limited to one joint, should suggest a superimposed infection or an acute structural problem. The number of joints involved initially is highly variable, but almost always the process is eventually polyarticular, involving at least five joints. RA is an additive polyarthritis, with the sequential addition of involved joints, in contrast to the migratory or

TABLE 77.1 1987 American College of Rheumatology Revised Criteria for Classification of Rheumatoid Arthritis

Criterion	Definition
1. Morning stiffness	In and around joints, lasting at least 1 hour before greatest improvement
2. Arthritis of ≥3 joints	Swelling/fluid observed simultaneously by a physician in at least three joint areas
3. Arthritis of hand joints	At least one swollen area in wrist/metacarpophalangeal or proximal interphalangeal joint
4. Symmetrical arthritis	Simultaneous involvement of same joint areas on both sides of the body
5. Rheumatoid nodules	Subcutaneous nodules over bony prominences, extensor surfaces observed by a physician
6. Serum rheumatoid factor	Presence of rheumatoid factor by any method, which has been positive in <5% of normal controls
7. Radiographic changes	Characteristic changes on x-ray films of hands/wrists, including erosions and unequivocal periarticular decalcification

From Arnett FC, Edworthy SM, Bloch DA, et al. The American Rheumatism Association 1987 revised criteria for the classification of rheumatoid arthritis. Arthritis Rheum 1988;31:315, with permission.

self-limited arthritis that can be seen in gout and rheumatic fever.

The other hallmark symptom of RA is *swelling* of the joints as a result of inflammation. Swelling may be accompanied by warmth and mild erythema. Patients complain of inability to remove rings from their fingers and the need to purchase shoes of increased width and size to accommodate their swollen forefeet. The arthritis typically is *symmetrical*, involving the same distribution of joints on the right and left sides of the body. Most typically, the small joints of the hands and feet are affected first. The larger joints also become affected as the disease progresses. The joints involved most often are the proximal interphalangeal (PIP) and metacarpophalangeal (MCP) joints of the hands, the wrists (particularly at the ulnar styloid articulation), shoulders, elbows, knees, ankles, and metatarsophalangeal (MTP) joints. The hips are involved in only approximately 20% of patients with RA. The distal interphalangeal (DIP) joints are nearly always spared, as is the axial skeleton except for the C1–2 articulation (discussed below).

Constitutional symptoms, such as fatigue, weight loss, low-grade fever (37°C–38°C), and malaise, are not uncommon as presenting symptoms and may even precede the arthritis by weeks to months. A higher fever, however, should suggest another illness such as an infection.

It is not unusual for articular symptoms of RA to wax and wane, especially at the beginning of the illness. Furthermore, because patients initially may present only with systemic symptoms and/or transient articular complaints that mimic other musculoskeletal conditions, the diagnosis may be delayed by several months. Atypical presentations include intermittent joint inflammation that can be confused with gout or pseudogout (see Chapter 76), proximal muscle pain and tenderness mimicking polymyalgia rheumatica, and diffuse musculoskeletal pain as seen in fibromyalgia (see Chapter 74).

During the time of diagnostic uncertainty, the physician can best serve the patient by providing reassurance, taking careful interval histories, performing periodic physical examinations (see Physical Examination), and, if appropriate, performing selected tests. Symptomatic treatment with anti-inflammatory drugs can be instituted during this period.

PHYSICAL EXAMINATION

Patients with suspected RA should undergo an initial complete physical examination and then a limited examination every 2 to 4 months. The physical examination is important not only to make the diagnosis but to establish a baseline against which to assess the response to treatment and acceleration of both articular and extra-articular disease. The primary focus of examinations in the physician's office is the joints. Serial joint examinations should be performed with careful records of the status of affected joints, as determined by history and previous examinations (Table 77.2).

Inflammation of the joints, manifested by *swelling* and sometimes warmth and mild erythema, is the signature physical finding of RA. Swelling is usually, but not always, symmetrical in distribution. The swelling is generally confined to the joint capsule, in contrast to gout, for example, in which a tremendous amount of subcutaneous edema is seen as well. In the hands, where the disease often is first manifested, typical fusiform swelling of the PIP joints is often observed (Fig. 77.1). The MCP joints, wrists, and MTP joints often become swollen as well, and involvement of

TABLE 77.2 Components To Be Assessed at Each Clinic Visit

Duration of morning stiffness
Degree of fatigue
Limitations of function
Patient assessment of pain
Number of joints that are painful on passive motion or are tender
Degree of swelling of affected joints

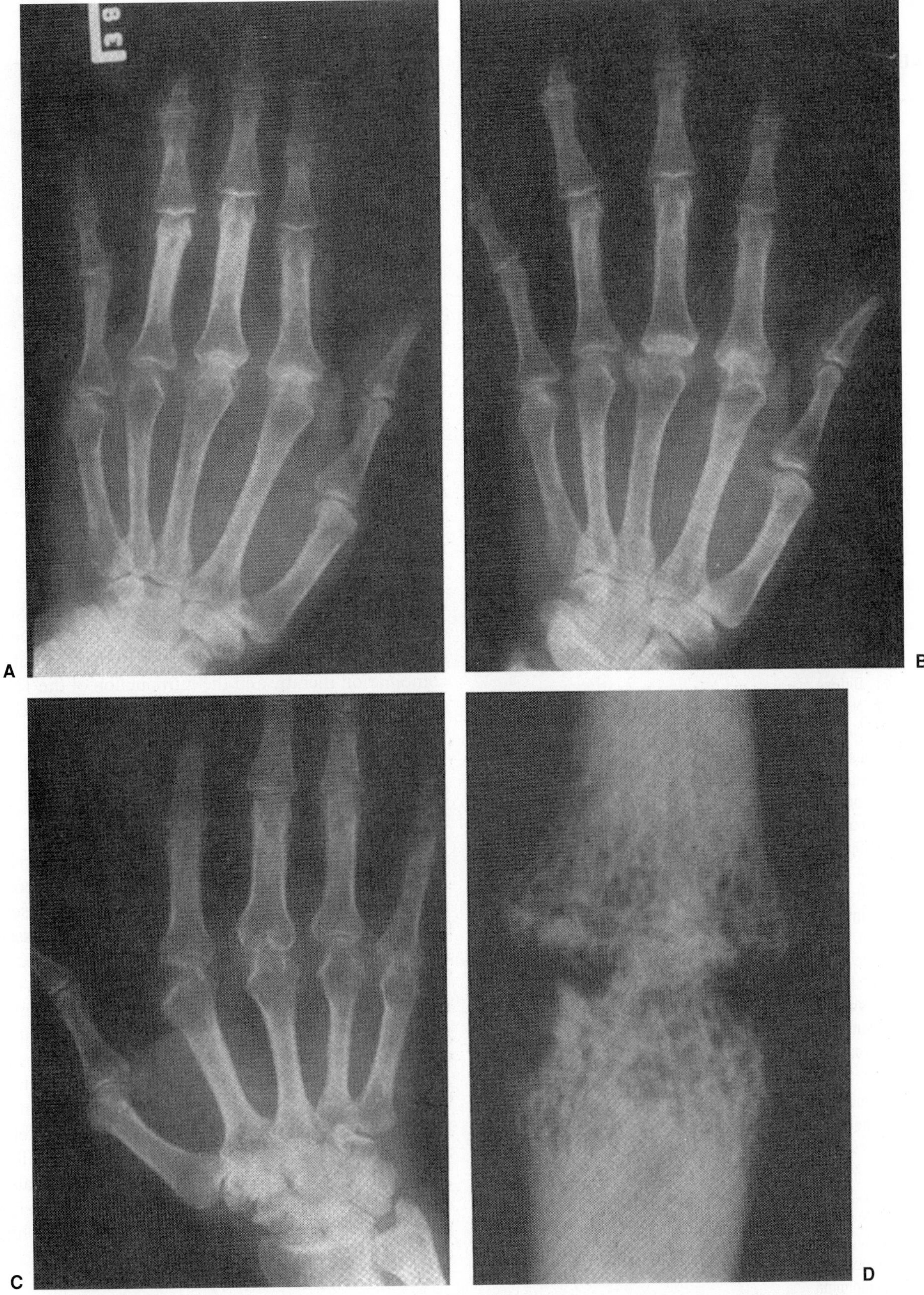

FIGURE 77.3. Radiographic changes in rheumatoid arthritis. **A:** Joint space narrowing in the second and third metacarpophalangeal (MCP) joints. **B:** Cystic changes, erosions, and further bony proliferation in the second and third MCP joints. **C:** Periarticular osteoporosis, most noticeable in the interphalangeal joints, and numerous marginal erosions and cysts in the carpal bones and metacarpal heads. **D:** Juxta-articular erosions in a proximal interphalangeal joint.

TABLE 77.3 Systemic Manifestations of Rheumatoid Arthritis

I. General
   A. Fever
   B. Fatigue, malaise, diffuse stiffness
   C. Adenopathy
   D. Splenomegaly
II. Pulmonary
   A. Pleuritis ($\pm$ effusion)
   B. Intrapulmonary nodules
   C. Interstitial pneumonitis
   D. Rheumatoid pneumoconiosis (Caplan syndrome)
   E. Pulmonary fibrosis
   F. Arteritis (rare)
III. Cardiovascular
   A. Heart
      1. Pericarditis, effusion, tamponade, constriction
      2. Myocarditis
      3. Endocarditis, including valvulitis
      4. Rheumatoid nodule (conduction defects)
   B. Peripheral
      1. Vasculitis or arteritis
IV. Ocular
   A. Keratoconjunctivitis (Sjögren syndrome)
   B. Episcleritis (simple or nodular)
   C. Scleritis
      1. Diffuse
      2. Nodular (scleromalacia perforans)
      3. Necrotizing
V. Nervous system
   A. Peripheral neuropathy (mononeuritis multiplex)—sensory, motor, or both
   B. Central nervous system
      1. Spinal cord lesion
         a. Vascular thrombosis
         b. Rheumatoid nodule
      2. Intracranial
         a. Meningitis (rare)
         b. Rheumatoid nodule (rare)
VI. Hematologic
   A. Anemia (chronic disease)
   B. Neutropenia (Felty syndrome)
   C. Thrombocytosis
VII. Skin
   A. Palmar erythema
   B. Nodules
   C. Vasculitic lesions
   D. Leg ulcers (Felty syndrome)
VIII. Others
   A. Sjögren syndrome
   B. Osteoporosis
   C. Hyperviscosity
   D. Lymphoma
   E. Secondary amyloidosis (controversial)

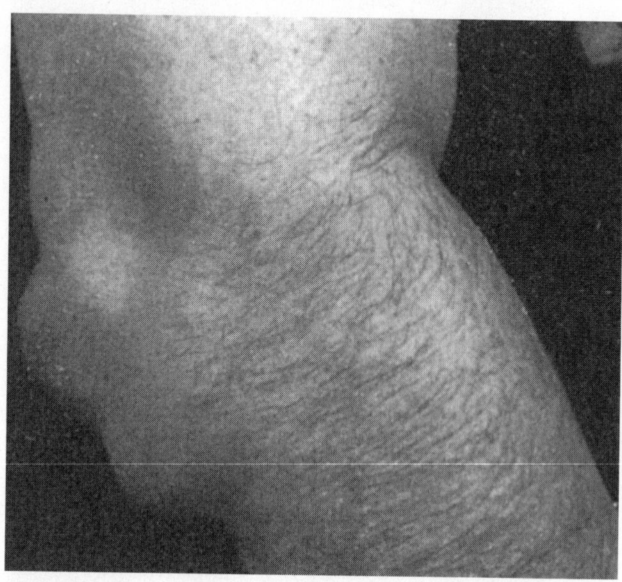

FIGURE 77.4. Rheumatoid nodules along the extensor surface of the forearm.

organ-specific extra-articular disease, the overall incidence of any extra-articular manifestation continues to be high (26). With an emphasis on aggressive management with combination therapy and the introduction of the TNF inhibitors (see Management), this frequency may be reduced over time.

Rheumatoid Nodules

The subcutaneous nodule is the most frequent extra-articular lesion in patients with RA (Fig. 77.4), occurring in 20% to 30% of cases and almost exclusively in seropositive patients. They vary in size from a few millimeters to several centimeters and either are fixed to surrounding tissue or are freely movable beneath the skin. They are located most commonly on the extensor surfaces of the elbows, in the region of the Achilles tendon, and on the fingers. Rheumatoid nodules also may arise within tendons or ligaments and can lead to dysfunction or rupture. Rarely, nodules arise in visceral organs such as lungs, heart, or sclera of the eye. Nodules may regress spontaneously. The course of nodule formation and regression does not seem to parallel that of joint inflammation. Although the nodules usually are asymptomatic, they can be painful and may ulcerate, requiring surgical excision. They frequently recur at sites of resection. Methotrexate has been associated with a higher occurrence of rheumatoid nodules (27).

Pleuropulmonary Disease

The pulmonary manifestations of RA include pleurisy with or without effusion, pleural and parenchymal nodules, rheumatoid pneumoconiosis (Caplan syndrome), diffuse interstitial fibrosis, and, rarely, bronchiolitis obliterans, pneumothorax, or pulmonary arteritis (28). Common findings on pulmonary function testing are a restrictive ventilatory defect with reduced lung volumes and a decreased diffusing capacity for carbon monoxide. Obstructive airways disease (in the absence of a significant smoking history) is described in patients with RA. Extrathoracic upper airway obstruction may occur secondary to involvement of the cricoarytenoid joints of the larynx.

Pulmonary involvement may precede by months the onset of arthritis. Pleurisy, the most common problem, is clinically apparent in 5% of patients, but pleural thickening and inflammation are found in 50% of autopsy cases. Pleural effusions, either unilateral or bilateral, usually are exudates. Even in transudates the glucose concentration of the fluid usually is low (<30 mg/100 mL), a finding otherwise seen only in pleural space infections. The first approach to the management of a pleural effusion includes a diagnostic aspiration and pleural biopsy to exclude infection and malignancy.

Rheumatoid nodules in the lung usually are asymptomatic, but cavitation simulating cancer or infection may occur. Therefore, appropriate diagnostic steps should be taken to ensure that pleural or pulmonary nodules in a patient with RA are not malignant. Interstitial pneumonitis or fibrosing mononuclear alveolitis precedes progressive pulmonary fibrosis, the most severe form of rheumatoid lung disease. Fine dry crackles are heard on auscultation of the lung, and reticulonodular infiltrates are seen on chest radiographs.

Case reports have reported success in treating rheumatoid lung with glucocorticoids and a variety of immunosuppressive regimens, including methotrexate, cyclosporin, cyclophosphamide, and azathioprine. However, no information from controlled clinical trials is available. Patients with symptomatic pleural or pulmonary manifestations of RA should be monitored in consultation with a rheumatologist and a pulmonologist.

Cardiac Disease

Pericarditis is the most common cardiac manifestation of RA (29). In older series, echocardiographic studies demonstrate pericardial effusion in 55% of patients with subcutaneous nodules and 15% of patients without nodules. Patients with symptomatic pericarditis usually present with fever, chest pain, and a pericardial rub that resolve spontaneously. Recurrent or persistent pericardial disease, complicated by tamponade or constriction, is rare. Other unusual cardiac manifestations include nonspecific valvulitis, nodule formation in a valve cusp, myocarditis, and conduction abnormalities secondary to nodule formation in the heart. The treatment of patients with symptomatic cardiac disease is best done in consultation with a rheumatologist and a cardiologist.

Patients with RA now are recognized to have a shorter lifespan than age- and gender-matched controls (30,31). The majority of this increased risk for early mortality results from cardiovascular disease (myocardial infarctions, strokes, and congestive heart failure) (32). Rheumatoid inflammation may initiate or aggravate atherosclerotic lesions and probably constitutes a lifetime independent risk factor (above and beyond conventional cardiovascular risk factors) for the accelerated progression of cardiovascular disease (33). Aggressive control of rheumatoid synovitis and management of conventional cardiovascular risk factors hopefully will reduce cardiovascular morbidity and mortality in patients with RA.

Ocular Disease

Keratoconjunctivitis of Sjögren syndrome is the most common ocular manifestation of RA (see Sjogren Syndrome and Chapter 109). Symptoms include a sensation of dryness and grittiness and can be relieved by artificial tears. Episcleritis occurs occasionally and is manifested by mild pain and intense redness of the affected eye. Ordinarily, episcleritis is a self-limited process of a few weeks' duration. Scleritis and corneal ulcerations are rarer but more serious problems. Unlike episcleritis, scleritis is a slowly progressive, often bilateral process that may lead to perforation and loss of vision. It is characterized by nodularity, intense redness, and often severe pain. The distinction between episcleritis and scleritis is difficult (see Chapter 109), and all patients with a red, painful eye should be referred to an ophthalmologist.

Neurologic Disease

The most common neurologic manifestation of RA is a mild, primarily sensory *peripheral neuropathy* that usually is more marked in the lower extremities. Entrapment neuropathies (e.g., carpal tunnel syndrome, tarsal tunnel syndrome) sometimes occur in patients with RA because of compression of a peripheral nerve by inflamed, swollen tissue (see Chapter 92). Cervical myelopathy secondary to atlantoaxial subluxation is an uncommon but particularly worrisome complication potentially causing permanent, even fatal neurologic damage. Approximately 30% of patients with RA in a referral practice had atlantoaxial subluxation without symptoms, but few of them developed neurologic dysfunction (see Ruddy et al., at www.hopkinsbayview.org/PAMreferences). Imaging of the cervical spine (e.g., MRI) should be performed if neurologic signs and symptoms are present, and neurosurgical consultation should be pursued. A patient with RA who may have sustained cervical injury or is at risk for a neck manipulation (e.g., during general anesthesia) should have flexion/extension cervical spine radiographs so that special caution can be exercised if subluxation, even without symptoms, is present.

Felty Syndrome

Felty syndrome is characterized by RA, splenomegaly, and leukopenia, predominantly granulocytopenia (34). Patients with this syndrome usually are older, and they have high titers of rheumatoid factor and ANA, severe arthritis, and other extra-articular manifestations of the disease. Recurrent bacterial infections and chronic refractory leg ulcers are the major complications. Patients with suspected Felty syndrome should see a rheumatologist urgently because therapy is difficult.

Rheumatoid Vasculitis

Evidence of vasculitis is found in 10% to 25% of autopsy patients with RA. The most common clinical manifestations of vasculitis are small digital infarcts along the nail beds. A syndrome of accelerated vasculitis is seen in fewer than 1% of patients. It is characterized by distal cutaneous ulcerations, gangrene, peripheral polyneuropathy, and visceral (intestinal, renal, cardiac, cerebral) ischemia. The abrupt onset of an ischemic mononeuropathy (mononeuritis multiplex) or progressive scleritis is typical of rheumatoid vasculitis. The syndrome ordinarily emerges after years of seropositive, persistently active RA; however, vasculitis may occur when joints are inactive. Immediate consultation with a rheumatologist and immunosuppressive therapy usually are indicated.

Sjögren Syndrome

Approximately 10% to 15% of patients with RA, mostly women, develop Sjögren syndrome, a chronic inflammatory disorder characterized by lymphocytic infiltration of lacrimal and salivary glands. This leads to impaired secretion of saliva and tears and results in the *sicca complex:* dry mouth (xerostomia) and dry eyes (keratoconjunctivitis sicca). Patients should use lubricating eye drops. They also should be monitored by an ophthalmologist to prevent corneal ulcerations and monitored closely by a dentist to prevent dental caries. Artificial saliva preparations are available, but patients often dislike them because of their taste. Oral pilocarpine derivatives (pilocarpine HCl [Salagen] and cevimeline [Evoxac]) are available for treatment of xerostomia but carry the troublesome side effects of hyperhidrosis and diarrhea.

Other exocrine glands can be affected, manifested clinically as dry skin, decreased perspiration, dry vaginal membranes, or a nonproductive cough. Commonly, a polyclonal lymphoproliferative reaction, characterized by lymphadenopathy and occasionally splenomegaly, is seen. This can mimic and, rarely, transform into a malignant lymphoma. Sjögren syndrome may be associated with a number of other systemic manifestations, including vasculitis, peripheral neuropathy, and thyroiditis.

COURSE

The course of RA, like that of most chronic diseases, cannot be predicted in any individual patient. Several patterns of activity have been described: spontaneous remission, particularly in the seronegative patient; recurrent explosive attacks followed by periods of quiescence, most commonly in the early phases; and the usual pattern of persistent and progressive disease activity that waxes and wanes in intensity.

A self-limited course with spontaneous remission is rare in RA, especially after 6 months of active disease. If long-term remission occurs without disease-modifying antirheumatic drug (DMARD) therapy, the diagnosis should be called into question. Some patients early in the course of the disease, however, will have a course characterized by remissions and exacerbations, each lasting several months. This usually transitions into the typical picture of RA, manifested as sustained joint pain and swelling. Occasionally patients with newly diagnosed RA have severe rapidly progressive disease that leads to early joint destruction and disability. Risk factors for more aggressive disease include high titers of rheumatoid factor and/or anti-CCP antibodies, the presence of radiographic erosions, and markedly elevated inflammatory markers (ESR and/or CRP) at presentation, as well as the presence of the "shared epitope" (35). Patients with one or more of these risk factors should be treated aggressively (see Management) and monitored carefully for signs of advancing joint damage. RA in women may go into remission during pregnancy, but disease activity usually increases again several weeks after childbirth.

Significant morbidity from RA has long been recognized. Approximately 60% of patients with RA were unable to work 10 years after the onset of their disease (36). Only recently, however, have studies demonstrated an increased mortality rate in rheumatoid patients. Median life expectancy was shortened by an average of 7 years for men and 3 years for women, compared with control populations; in >5,000 patients with RA from four centers, the mortality rate was two times greater than in the control population (32). Patients at *higher risk* for shortened survival are those with systemic extra-articular involvement, low functional capacity, low socioeconomic status, low education, and long-term prednisone use. The role of cardiovascular disease in the observed increase in mortality rate in patients with RA was discussed earlier.

TABLE 77.4 Outline of a Diagnostic Approach to Polyarthritis

A. Define the host features
  1. Age, sex, and ethnic background
  2. Family history
  3. Environmental factors
B. Describe the joint involvement
  1. Pattern of joint involvement (symmetrical vs. asymmetrical)
  2. Number of involved joints (monoarthritis vs. oligoarthritis vs. polyarthritis)
  3. Specific joints
  4. Course
C. Extra-articular features
D. Supporting laboratory/radiographic studies
E. Response to therapy

DIFFERENTIAL DIAGNOSIS

The difficulty of diagnosing early RA emphasizes the importance of a systematic approach to patients with arthritis (Table 77.4). The patient's age, sex, ethnic background, and family history influence the likelihood of disease. Therefore, a clear definition of host features forms a framework to begin the evaluation of the patient with arthritis. Table 77.5 outlines examples of the differential diagnosis of polyarthritis based on age and sex. The characteristics of the arthritis itself provide important clues to the differential diagnosis (Tables 77.6 and 77.7).

MANAGEMENT

Overview

RA is a chronic, inflammatory arthritis that can cause joint destruction, significant disability, and increased mortality if adequate treatment is not initiated early and is not appropriately managed throughout the course of the disease (37). Past treatment was based on a pyramid approach beginning with "less potent" NSAIDs, reserving disease-modifying agents only for patients with joint destruction and disability. Thus, institution of appropriate therapeutic intervention often was significantly delayed. We now recognize that articular damage begins early and may progress more rapidly early in the course of the disease (20). Radiologic evidence of bone erosions is apparent in approximately 75% of patients during first 2 years of disease by radiographs (20) and within months if MRI techniques are applied (38).

Several studies have shown that *early initiation of treatment* leads to less joint damage in long-term followup (39,40). In a comparison study of early versus delayed

TABLE 77.5 Differential Diagnosis of Polyarthritis Based on Age and Sex

Age (yr)	*Male*	*Both Sexes*	*Female*
Childhood (1–15)	Juvenile ankylosing spondylitis (see Chapter 78) Kawasaki syndrome[a] Hemophilia (see Chapter 56)	Juvenile rheumatoid arthritis, systemic onset (Still disease)[a] Rheumatic fever[a] Leukemia[a]	Juvenile rheumatoid arthritis, pauciarticular course[a] Juvenile rheumatoid arthritis, polyarticular course
Young adult (15–30)	Ankylosing spondylitis (see Chapter 78) Reiter syndrome (see Chapter 78) "Reactive" arthritis[a] (see Chapter 76) Behçet syndrome[a]	Psoriatic arthritis (see Chapter 116) Lyme disease (see Chapter 38) Inflammatory bowel disease (see Chapter 46)	Systemic lupus erythematosus[a] Gonococcal arthritis (see Chapter 37) Scleroderma[a]
Middle age (30–60)	Gout (see Chapter 76) Whipple disease[a]	Seronegative polyarthritis (see Chapter 77) Hypersensitivity reactions (see Chapter 30) Vasculitic syndromes[a] Relapsing polychondritis[a]	Rheumatoid arthritis Sjögren syndrome Sarcoidosis[a] Polymyositis[a] Erosive osteoarthritis (see Chapter 75)
Elderly (60+)	Diffuse idiopathic skeletal hyperostosis (see Chapter 75) Hypertrophic pulmonary osteoarthropathy (see Chapter 61)	Pseudogout (see Chapter 76) Polymyalgia rheumatica (see Chapter 74) Tumor-related syndromes Secondary osteoarthritis (see Chapter 75) Metabolic disorders	Primary generalized osteoarthritis (see Chapter 75)

[a]These conditions are not discussed in this book. Information about these conditions can be found in the sources listed in the General References.

TABLE 77.6 Assessment of Joint Involvement

Number		
Monoarthritis	**Oligoarthritis (2–4 joints)**	**Polyarthritis (≥5 joints)**
Septic arthritis	Reiter syndrome	Rheumatoid arthritis
Gout	Inflammatory bowel disease	Systemic lupus erythematosus[a]
Pseudogout	Psoriatic arthritis	Serum sickness
Other crystals	Rheumatic fever[a]	Psoriatic arthritis
Local tumor[a]	Rheumatoid arthritis	Tophaceous gout
Patterns		
Symmetrical	**Asymmetrical**	
Rheumatoid arthritis	Psoriatic arthritis	
Serum sickness	Reiter syndrome	
Systemic lupus erythematosus[a]	Gout, pseudogout	
Intensity of Pain		
Severe	**Moderate**	
Septic arthritis	All others, including rheumatoid arthritis	
Microcrystalline arthritis		
Course		
Additive	Rheumatoid arthritis	
Migratory	Rheumatic fever,[a] systemic lupus erythematosus[a]	
Evanescent	Systemic lupus erythematosus,[a] viral[a]	
Episodic	Gout, pseudogout, palindromic rheumatism[a]	

[a]These conditions are not discussed in this book. Information about these conditions can be found in the sources listed in the General References.

therapy in patients with RA, less radiographic damage was noted in the early treatment group after 2 years of followup (40). These and similar data suggest that there is a *"window of opportunity"* during which therapeutic intervention may have greatest impact on disease progression and may potentially "switch" off the disease process if initiated in the first few weeks or months of disease. Thus, in the last 2 decades, there has been a critical shift from the "wait-and-see" paradigm of treatment toward early aggressive intervention to control inflammation and to possibly modify future disease course.

TABLE 77.7 Diagnostic Clues Provided by Arthritis of Specific Joints

Joint Involved	*Diagnosis*
First metatarsal-phalangeal (podagra)	Gout
Knee (acute, episodic)	Pseudogout
Distal Interphalangeal	Psoriatic arthritis, osteoarthritis
Metacarpals, wrist, metatarsals	Rheumatoid arthritis
Sausage digits	Reactive arthritis, psoriatic arthritis, sarcoidosis
Sacroiliac	Ankylosing spondylitis, reactive arthritis, psoriatic arthritis, inflammatory bowel disease
Sternoclavicular	Septic arthritis, polymyalgia rheumatica, rheumatoid arthritis
Heel/ankle	Reactive arthritis, sarcoidosis

The recognition in the 1990s of the safety and efficacy of methotrexate has led to widespread acceptance of this drug as the *"first-line"* treatment of RA and as the "gold standard" against which new therapies are compared. Moreover, *combination* of methotrexate with other DMARDs has been demonstrated to provide cumulative benefit without incurring any unexpected synergistic toxicities (41–43). Thus, one or more DMARDs, conventional or biologic, can be added to methotrexate in a *"step-up"* approach if treatment with methotrexate alone does not achieve adequate control of disease activity. This "step-up" approach is the most commonly used treatment strategy in clinical practice and in clinical trials of RA to date. An alternate approach that has been used primarily in clinical trials, and is also highly effective, is an *"induction"* approach. In this strategy, multiple DMARDs are started simultaneously and then "stepped down" over 6 months to a single DMARD (43,44). Fortunately, the traditional approach of *sequential monotherapy,* in which one DMARD is replaced with another until an effective treatment is found, has been abandoned in favor of step-up and induction approaches.

The advent of biologic agents that block the effects of TNF-α and IL-1 has been a major breakthrough in the treatment of RA and other selected inflammatory disorders. These biologic agents have been shown to be effective in reducing disease activity and improving radiologic outcomes in patients with RA, when used alone or in combination with methotrexate (45–47). Thus, the availability of these new agents, combined with the conceptual advances of early, aggressive treatment and combination therapy, have revolutionized the treatment of RA in the last 10 years.

General Principles

When the diagnosis of inflammatory arthritis is in question, rapid referral of the patient to a rheumatologist is recommended. Delay in therapy can lead to irreversible joint damage and disability. Thus, every effort should be made to prevent delay by referral and access to specialist care. Once the diagnosis is established, the primary goals of treatment of RA are to reduce pain, enhance function and quality of life, and reduce long-term damage to the joints. This is achieved by aggressively suppressing synovitis with pharmacologic therapies and by providing physical and occupational therapy and psychological support to the patient. Treatment usually commences with an NSAID and a DMARD. In cases of very aggressive synovitis and/or disabling systemic symptoms, low-dose prednisone is added. The rapid onset of action of the NSAID and corticosteroid provides some immediate relief while allowing the slower-acting DMARD to exert its effects. Commonly prescribed DMARDs include hydroxychloroquine, sulfasalazine, methotrexate, leflunomide, and TNF inhibitors (etanercept, infliximab, and adalimumab). Older agents, such as gold, penicillamine, and azathioprine, and the newer biologic anakinra (Kineret) are much less commonly prescribed because of their lower rates of efficacy and/or higher rates of toxicity compared to the more commonly prescribed agents.

The choice of the initial DMARD depends to some extent on the cost of the drugs, side-effect profile, comorbidities of the patient, and preferences of the patient and physician. As noted above, however, methotrexate is generally recommended as the initial treatment given its high benefit–risk ratio (48,49). The Early Rheumatoid Arthritis (ERA) trial introduced a dosing schedule for methotrexate that now is widely accepted. The schedule consists of rapid-dose increase over 8 weeks, from 10 mg/week to 20 to 25 mg/week or to maximal tolerated dose (50). If disease activity is not well controlled by 3 to 4 months (allowing for the slow onset of action of methotrexate), a second DMARD should be added. The addition of sulfasalazine and/or hydroxychloroquine to methotrexate is effective and well tolerated. The combination of all three agents, commonly known as "triple therapy," is generally well tolerated (41) but does involve a complicated dosing schedule that may decrease patient adherence over time. Alternatively, an anti-TNF agent may be added to methotrexate, and this combination probably is the most common approach among rheumatologists for patients in whom methotrexate monotherapy is insufficient. The combination of a TNF inhibitor with methotrexate has been demonstrated to be superior to methotrexate monotherapy, for both clinical and radiographic outcomes, for all three available anti-TNF agents (47,51,52). Anakinra, an IL-1 inhibitor, also reduces clinical symptoms and retards radiographic progression when added to methotrexate in patients with RA, but it is a considerably weaker agent than the TNF inhibitors (53). Addition of leflunomide to methotrexate monotherapy is another acceptable combination approach that results in improved clinical outcomes compared to methotrexate alone and is generally well tolerated (54). However, radiographic outcomes comparing this combination to methotrexate alone have not been examined.

Inhibitors of TNF are generally not used as first-line therapy for RA because of their expense and limited data regarding long-term safety. However, first-line treatment with an anti-TNF agent or sulfasalazine is the preferred therapy in certain patients, such as those with chronic liver disease, renal insufficiency, or sulfa allergy, and patients anticipating a pregnancy.

In patients with a mild disease phenotype, seronegativity, and absence of poor prognostic factors, a weaker DMARD such as hydroxychloroquine or minocycline may be sufficient as first-line therapy. However, the disease-modifying potential of these drugs (i.e., to slow or halt joint damage) has not been rigorously proven. Therefore, careful monitoring to evaluate the need to "step-up" the therapy is important.

Despite these significant advances in therapeutics, individual response to treatment is variable, requiring "trial and error" strategy and frequent reassessment of adequacy of response. Even with an aggressive combination approach, therapeutic response may decline over a period of time, making long-term management of this chronic disease a challenge to physicians. Future research in the field of pharmacogenomics may enhance our ability to predict the probability of response to DMARDs and "tailor" treatment to each individual patient.

In addition to aggressive pharmacologic control of synovitis, other important goals of treatment include preservation of joint function, management of pain and disability associated with chronic deformities, and improvement of overall quality of life. To achieve these goals, it is essential that the patient and the patient's family be educated about the nature and course of the disease, the specific causes of the pain, and the goals, problems, and expectations of treatment.

Reduction of joint stress is a critical part of protection of inflamed joints and is accomplished by a number of practical measures that do not depend on the use of drugs. Because obesity stresses the musculoskeletal system, ideal body weight should be achieved and maintained. When the joints are actively inflamed, vigorous activity (heavy work, brisk exercise) should be avoided because of the danger of intensifying joint inflammation or causing traumatic injury to structures weakened by inflammation. On the other hand, patients should be urged to maintain a modest level of activity to prevent joint laxity and muscular atrophy. Splinting of acutely inflamed joints, particularly at night, and the use of walking aids (canes, walkers) are all effective means of reducing stress on specific joints. Specially designed furniture and household utensils can help not only to relieve stress on joints but also to maintain independent function. Such aids are provided on recommendation of the consultant rheumatologist, orthopedist, physiatrist, physical therapist, or occupational therapist and are obtained from an orthotics appliance store.

A consultation with a *physical therapist* and an *occupational therapist* is recommended early in the course of treating a patient with RA. These therapists can effectively design a program of balanced rest and activity that is appropriate for the stage of disease. Passive exercise (moving the joints through a full range of motion) is used when inflammation is active and poorly controlled. An active exercise program, when tolerated, can be designed to prevent contractures and muscular atrophy. The application of local heat, the use of various supporting aids, education on joint protection, and maintenance of good joint function are all part of the therapist's role. The occupational therapies will also assess the patient's need for devices to aid in the performance of activities of daily living, such as buttoning blouses and removing lids from jars.

Specific Pharmacologic Agents

Nonsteroidal Anti-inflammatory Drugs

In the presence of acute or chronic inflammation, it is appropriate to prescribe NSAIDs in patients with RA. The major effect of these agents is to reduce acute inflammation, thereby decreasing pain and improving function. However, NSAIDs are not disease modifying and hence have no role as monotherapy in treatment of RA. They usually are used in conjunction with other DMARDs to reduce pain. All of these drugs have mild to moderate analgesic properties independent of their anti-inflammatory effect.

Aspirin is the oldest drug of the nonsteroidal class. However, because of its higher rate of GI toxicity, the narrow window between toxic and anti-inflammatory serum levels, and the inconvenience of multiple daily doses, aspirin has largely been replaced by NSAIDs. Nonacetylated salicylates (Disalcid, Trilisate) are less potent anti-inflammatory agents but have the advantage of less GI toxicity, lack of inhibition of platelet aggregation, and decreased incidence of NSAID-induced angioedema reactions.

NSAIDs inhibit prostaglandin synthesis by blocking cyclooxygenase enzymes. Prostaglandins are important mediators of pain and inflammation. The two isoforms of cyclooxygenase are COX-1 and COX-2. COX-1 is expressed under basal conditions in the stomach, platelets, and kidney. Because of its tissue localization, COX-1 is thought to play physiologic roles in gastric cytoprotection and platelet aggregation. COX-2 expression is highly restricted under basal conditions and is induced in inflammatory cells by inflammatory or noxious stimuli. Prostaglandins produced by COX-2 mediate symptoms of pain, inflammation, and fever. Conventional NSAIDs inhibit both COX-1 and COX-2, thus putting the patient at higher risk for GI ulcers and bleeding. Selective COX-2 agents are associated with a lower rate of GI ulcers but are associated with a higher rate of acute cardiovascular events presumably mediated by promotion of clotting. A large number of NSAIDs are available from which to choose (Table 77.8), and at full dosage all may be equally effective. However, there is a great deal of variation in tolerance and response to a particular NSAID. Long-acting NSAIDs that allow once- or twice-daily dosing improve compliance. The selective COX-2 inhibitors (celecoxib, rofecoxib, valdecoxib) have been shown to be as efficacious as the older, nonselective NSAIDs, with less GI toxicity and less bleeding (55,56). However, rofecoxib and valdecoxib have now been removed from the market because of the problem with cardiovascular toxicity (see Side Effects).

Dosage

A full dosage of an NSAID should be prescribed for active inflammation (Table 77.8). However, a lower dosage should be used if inflammation is mild and if the patient is elderly or at risk for toxicity (see Side Effects). If a particular NSAID is ineffective after a 4-week trial or is not tolerated, another NSAID can be initiated. An individual patient's response to NSAIDs with respect to both tolerance and effectiveness is unpredictable and varied. Combinations of NSAIDs should be avoided because of the potential for increased toxicity.

Usual Time to Maximal Effect

Although these agents achieve therapeutic blood levels and analgesic effects within hours to days after the first dose, the full anti-inflammatory effect may take several weeks. In the absence of side effects, a reasonable trial period is 1 month.

Side Effects

The most common toxicity of NSAIDs is GI disturbance (57–59) (Table 77.9). The term *NSAID gastropathy* describes a variety of gastric lesions, including mucosal erythema, gastric erosions, and frank ulcerations,

TABLE 77.8 Nonsteroidal Anti-Inflammatory Drugs

Generic Name	Trade Name	Available Strength (mg)	Recommended Dosage and Schedule	Maximal Daily Dosage (mg/day)
Propionic Acid Derivatives				
Ibuprofen[a]	Motrin, Rufen, IBU	300, 400, 600, 800	600–800 mg t.i.d.–q.i.d.	3,200
	Nuprin, Advil	200		
Naproxen[a]	Naprosyn	250, 375, 500	500 mg b.i.d	1,000
	Anaprox, Aleve	275		
Ketoprofen[a]	Orudis	50, 75	50 mg t.i.d.–q.i.d. or 75 mg t.i.d.	300
Flurbiprofen[a]	Ansaid	100	100 mg b.i.d.–t.i.d.	300
Oxaprozin[a]	Daypro	600	600–1,200 mg q.d.	1,200
Oxicams				
Piroxicam[a]	Feldene	10, 20	10–20 mg/day	20
Meloxicam	Mobic	7.5, 15	15–30 mg/day	30
Acetic Acids				
Indomethacin[a]	Indocin	25, 50	50 mg t.i.d.–q.i.d.	150–200
		75 (slow release)	q.d.– b.i.d.	
Sulindac[a]	Clinoril	150, 200	150–200 mg b.i.d.	400
Tolmetin[a]	Tolectin	200, 400	400 mg t.i.d.–q.i.d.	2,000
Diclofenac[a]	Voltaren	25, 50, 75	50 mg b.i.d.–t.i.d. or 75 mg b.i.d.	150
Etodolac[a]	Lodine	200, 300, 400, 500	200–400 mg t.i.d.	1,200
Nabumetone[a]	Relafen	500, 750	1,000–2,000 mg q.d.	2,000
Pyrazoles				
Ketorolac tromethamine	Toradol	10	10 mg q4–6h	Use only for short periods
Nonacetylated Salicylates				
Diflunisal	Dolobid	250, 500	250–500 mg b.i.d.	1,000
Magnesium choline salicylate[a]	Trilisate	500, 750, 1,000	1,500 mg b.i.d.	3,000
Salsalate[a]	Disalcid	500, 750	1,500 mg b.i.d.	3,000
Cyclooxygenase-2 Inhibitors				
Celecoxib	Celebrex	100, 200	100–200 mg b.i.d.	400
Rofecoxib	Vioxx	Removed from market		
Valdecoxib	Bextra	Removed from market		

[a] Approved for use in rheumatoid arthritis.

although NSAID-related lower GI bleeding also has been described (60). Serious complications of NSAID-induced peptic ulcers include obstruction, bleeding, and perforation, which may be life threatening. Risk factors for these serious complications include age over 70 years, RA, concomitant use of steroids or anticoagulants, prior history of ulcer-related GI bleed, and comorbid cardiopulmonary disease (61). NSAID-induced gastropathy is caused by reduced production of gastroprotective prostaglandins by the stomach lining as a result of COX-1 inhibition. Patients should be carefully monitored for GI symptoms and evidence of GI blood loss while receiving NSAIDs. For patients at risk for NSAID-related gastropathy, management strategies may include lower doses of NSAIDs (although this strategy may not provide adequate pain control), coadministration of a gastroprotective agent, or use of an NSAID that selectively inhibits COX-2.

Although the relative efficacies of the latter two strategies have never been compared head to head, independent clinical trials have demonstrated that both reduce the risk of serious NSAID-induced ulcer complications (55,56). Proton pump inhibitors such as omeprazole and the prostaglandin analogue misoprostol, for example, decrease the incidence of new endoscopic and/or symptomatic gastric ulcers and their complications in NSAID users (62,63). Furthermore, healing of pre-existing, endoscopically documented peptic ulcers occurs at a high rate without discontinuing NSAID treatment if a proton pump inhibitor or H_2 blocker is added (64). As for the COX-2 selective NSAIDs, several large clinical trials in arthritis patients have demonstrated a 50% reduction in risk of serious ulcer complications (perforation, bleeding, and obstruction) in patients receiving these agents compared to those receiving nonselective NSAIDs (55,56). It should be noted that the gastropathy is not completely eliminated

TABLE 77.9 Side Effects of Nonsteroidal Anti-Inflammatory Drugs

	Approximate Incidence
Gastrointestinal Effects	10%–20%
Epigastric pain, nausea	
Anorexia, dyspepsia, peptic ulceration	
Overt or occult bleeding	<1%
Hypersensitivity Reactions	1%–5%
Rashes	
Stevens–Johnson syndrome (rare)	
Anaphylactoid reactions (very rare)	
Aggravation of Allergic Rhinitis or Asthma	10% of sufferers
Renal Effects	>5%
Transient renal failure	
Water and salt retention	
Hypokalemia, inhibit diuretic action	
Interstitial nephritis, nephrotic syndrome	>1%
Hepatic Effects	5%–15%
Cholestatic hepatitis	
Central Nervous System Effects	>5%
Tinnitus/deafness	Primarily aspirin
Headache, vertigo, confusion	Higher with indomethacin
Other Effects	
Diarrhea	10%–15% (mefenamic acid, other fenamates)
Aggravation of congestive heart failure, angina	>1%
Toxic amblyopia	<1% (ibuprofen)

with the use of the COX-2 agents, and continued caution is needed in patients at risk for GI bleeding. Furthermore, the protective GI effect of COX-2 selective agents is largely lost if the patient is taking concomitant low-dose aspirin for cardiovascular prophylaxis (65). In these cases, COX-2 selective agents have no apparent advantage over a nonselective NSAID.

Unlike aspirin and nonselective NSAIDs, COX-2 selective NSAIDs do *not* inhibit platelet clotting because the prostanoid product that promotes platelet aggregation (thromboxane B_2) is produced by platelet COX-1. However, COX-2 agents do inhibit production of the anticlotting, vasodilatory prostanoid (prostacyclin) produced by endothelium. An increase in thromboxane/prostacyclin ratio in the vasculature in patients receiving selective COX-2 agents is likely to occur and may be responsible for the increase in acute coronary events and/or cerebrovascular events that were observed in several clinical trials and population studies of patients treated with COX-2 agents compared to nonselective NSAIDs (56,66,67). This serious complication of COX-2 treatment has led to the removal of two of the three Food and Drug Administration (FDA)-approved COX-2 selective NSAIDs (rofecoxib and valdecoxib) from the market, leaving only celecoxib at this time. In adenoma prevention trials, celecoxib showed inconsistent results with regard to cardiovascular toxicity. Although a dose-related increase in acute cardiovascular events was noted with celecoxib use (400 and 200 mg bid) in the Adenoma Prevention with Celecoxib (APC) trial, this effect was not seen in the Prevention of Spontaneous Adenomatous Polyposis (PreSAP) trial (68,69).

Thus, before prescribing celecoxib, the relative benefit (GI protection) versus risk (cardiovascular toxicity) of selective COX-2 inhibition, as well as alternative strategies (e.g., conventional NSAID with proton pump inhibitor), must be weighed carefully for each individual patient (56,66). Celecoxib should be reserved for patients at high risk for recurrent bleeding ulcers, those taking warfarin, and those with significant GI discomfort taking conventional NSAIDs who cannot be managed effectively with gastroprotective agents such as misoprostol or proton pump inhibitors. Celecoxib should be avoided in patients at high risk for new or recurrent cardiovascular events; however, if it is selected as the optimal NSAID, concomitant low-dose aspirin should be continued.

Of note, recent population-based studies have implicated the conventional NSAIDs in promoting acute ischemic events (70). In 2004, the National Institutes of Health (NIH) terminated the Alzheimer's Disease Anti-inflammatory Prevention Trial (ADAPT) because of an apparent increase in cardiovascular events noted in patients taking naproxen compared to placebo. No increased risk was seen with celecoxib in this trial (FDA webcast). This potential adverse effect of nonselective NSAIDs has not been confirmed in any prospective long-term study, and available data are insufficient to draw any definite conclusion. Thus, the long-term cardiovascular safety of both selective and nonselective NSAIDs need to be evaluated in future trials.

Because renal prostaglandins from both COX-1 and COX-2 pathways play a role in the regulation of renal blood flow and maintenance of glomerular filtration, both nonselective and COX-2 selective NSAIDs have the potential to impair renal function (71). Patients at highest risk are those with fluid imbalances or compromised renal function (e.g., heart failure, diuretic use, cirrhosis, dehydration, renal insufficiency) (72). If an NSAID is prescribed for such patients, it should be initiated at low dose, and renal function should be monitored early on and throughout the course of treatment. The drugs should be stopped if there is a rise in serum creatinine concentration or increased edema. Usually, the creatinine concentration returns to normal within 1 or 2 weeks. Rarely, an interstitial nephritis develops in association with a sustained rise in

TABLE 77.10 Nonsteroidal Anti-Inflammatory Drugs and Drug Interactions

Antacids	Reduce rate and extent of absorption of NSAIDs; variable effect.
Anticoagulants	Aspirin, and potentially all NSAIDs, increases the risk of bleeding in a patient taking an anticoagulant.
Oral hypoglycemic drugs	NSAIDs may potentiate the activity of sulfonylurea drugs.
Digoxin	NSAIDs may increase serum concentration.
Antihypertensive/diuretics	NSAIDs may attenuate the effect of diuretics, β-blockers, hydralazine, prazosin, angiotensin-converting enzyme inhibitors.
Lithium	Elevation of plasma lithium concentration level occur, particularly with indomethacin and diclofenac.
Methotrexate	Salicylate inhibits renal clearance of methotrexate, and toxic concentrations may occur.
Phenytoin	NSAIDs may displace phenytoin from albumin and increase the concentration of free drug.
Probenecid	Inhibits renal clearance of several NSAIDs.
Combination of NSAIDs	Should be avoided.

NSAID, nonsteroidal anti-inflammatory drug.

serum creatinine concentration and eosinophiluria. Urinalysis usually is normal.

Fewer than 5% of patients develop a hypersensitivity reaction, usually a rash, to an NSAID. This reaction usually is specific to a particular drug, so another NSAID of a different class can be substituted. Rarely, an anaphylactoid reaction or worsening asthma can occur (see Chapter 30) that can be intrinsic to the mechanism of prostaglandin inhibition. If anaphylaxis or worsening asthma occurs with NSAID therapy, subsequent exposure to all classes of NSAIDs (including aspirin) is contraindicated. If NSAID therapy is deemed essential in the case of anaphylaxis, an allergy consultation is recommended for evaluation and possible desensitization. Although theoretically a selective COX-2 inhibitor might be safe in these instances, this has not been conclusively proven.

Significant drug interactions can occur with any of the NSAIDs (Table 77.10).

Corticosteroids

Glucocorticoids are potent anti-inflammatory agents that inhibit the cascade of inflammatory and immune mechanisms at multiple levels. They have a rapid onset of action and thus are very useful as "bridging therapy" for patients with early debilitating RA. In this context, treatment with low-dose oral prednisone is initiated early on to reduce pain and inflammation while waiting for the delayed action of a coadministered DMARD(s) to take full effect. Once the DMARD effect is evident, prednisone should be tapered slowly to the smallest tolerated dose or, preferably, discontinued entirely. Low-dose prednisone (7.5 mg/day) has been shown to have disease-modifying effects compared to placebo, with retardation of joint damage (73,74), but this effect is relatively modest compared to DMARDs such as methotrexate and the TNF inhibitors. Furthermore, significant side effects associated with chronic steroid use limit their long-term use, and every effort should be made to use the smallest required dose of these agents. Chronic low-dose prednisone as the *sole* disease-modifying therapy is not acceptable treatment. Indications for oral prednisone use in RA therefore include (a) short-term use in early disease until the DMARD effect is realized; (b) short-term use for disease flares; and (c) chronic use only in patients with severe, difficult-to-treat disease.

Corticosteroids can be administered by other systemic routes (intravenously and intramuscularly) or by local route (intra-articularly). Intra-articular steroid injection is indicated when the disease is under excellent control except for one or two joints; however, infection as the cause of the synovitis must be ruled out via arthrocentesis and culture prior to the steroid injection. Intra-articular injections can circumvent the need for systemic glucocorticoids and their side effects. Generally, the same joint should not be injected with a corticosteroid more than three to four times per year because of the risk for deterioration of intra-articular cartilage, although it must be recognized that uncontrolled joint inflammation also can cause rapid deterioration of cartilage.

High doses of intravenous glucocorticoids, or so-called "pulse therapy" (methylprednisolone 100 mg intravenously daily on 3 consecutive days), for management of severe flares usually are reserved for patients for whom most other therapies have failed and who are experiencing a great deal of functional disability. A randomized clinical trial showed equivalent efficacy of 100 versus 1,000 mg of intravenous methylprednisolone daily for 3 days; consequently, the 100-mg dose is preferred (75).

Weight gain and cushingoid appearance are common complaints with high-dose steroids, although their frequency at a chronic low dose of prednisone ($<$10 mg/day) are unclear. Because of the proatherogenic and bone-resorbing effects of steroids, increased cardiovascular risk and accelerated osteoporosis have been described in association with prednisone, particularly at dosages $>$10 mg/day (76). RA itself is a risk factor for osteoporosis (77); consequently, patients receiving corticosteroids should undergo baseline bone densitometry to assess fracture risk. Bisphosphonates are recommended to prevent glucocorticoid-induced osteoporosis in all patients

TABLE 77.11 Toxicities and Monitoring of Commonly Used Disease-Modifying Antirheumatic Drugs

Drug	Common Toxicities	Monitoring
Hydroxychloroquine	Macular damage	Ophthalmology examination every 6 mo
Sulfasalazine	Myelosuppression, hepatotoxicity	CBC, LFTs every month for first 3 mo, then every 3 mo
Methotrexate	Myelosuppression, hepatotoxicity, interstitial pneumonitis, alopecia, oral ulcers	CBC, LFTs, creatinine concentration every 2–3 wk until dosage is stable, then every 4–8 wk
Cyclophosphamide	Myelosuppression, hemorrhagic cystitis, alopecia, secondary malignancy (bladder cancer, myeloproliferative disorders), premature ovarian failure	CBC every 1–2 wk until dosage is stable, then every 1–2 mo; urinalysis every 1–2 mo; urinalysis and urine cytology every 6–12 mo after cessation
Leflunomide	Myelosuppression, hepatotoxicity	CBC, LFTs every mo
Etanercept	Infection, injection site reactions	CBC, chemistries every 3–6 mo
Infliximab	Infection, infusion reactions	CBC, chemistries every 3–6 mo

CBC, complete blood count; LFTs, liver function tests.
From Guidelines for monitoring drug therapy in rheumatoid arthritis. American College of Rheumatology Ad Hoc Committee on Clinical Guidelines. Arthritis Rheum 1996;39:723, with permission.

on chronic glucocorticoid therapy (see Chapters 84 and 103). Other clinically significant side effects include premature cataracts, increased intraocular pressure (78), and glucose intolerance.

Disease-Modifying Antirheumatic Drugs

Table 77.11 lists the toxicities and monitoring of commonly used disease-modifying antirheumatic drugs.

Hydroxychloroquine

An antimalarial agent derived from the bark of the cinchona tree, hydroxychloroquine is rapidly absorbed, safe, well tolerated, and has been used for decades for treatment of RA. In several randomized controlled clinical trials, hydroxychloroquine was shown to be effective in reducing joint pain and swelling, improving physical functioning, however, its effects, particularly on progression of joint damage, are less potent than those of the other DMARDs (48,79). For this reason, hydroxychloroquine as monotherapy usually is reserved for patients with very mild disease. Its greatest use in clinical practice is as adjunctive therapy with other DMARDs, as discussed above.

Mechanism. The mechanism of action of hydroxychloroquine in the treatment of patients with RA is unknown.

Dosage. The usual daily dosage is 400 mg (two tablets). Initial loading with 1,200 mg/day followed by 400 mg/day has been shown to hasten the onset of action (80); however, the long-term safety of this approach is not known. Nonetheless, long-term toxicity is unusual if the chronic daily dose is <6 mg/kg.

Side Effects. The most important toxicity is deposition of hydroxychloroquine in the retina, potentially leading to blindness. This is rare, however, if the drug is used at the recommended doses. Nonetheless, a baseline ophthalmologic examination and a followup examination every 1 to 2 years are recommended during the period of treatment. GI upset, pigmentation changes, leukopenia, and a variety of neurologic side effects are seen rarely.

Methotrexate

Methotrexate is a folic acid antagonist. Its long track record of safety, tolerability and efficacy have made it the first choice for monotherapy of RA and the "anchor" drug for various combinations of DMARDs (48,49). Methotrexate therapy should be considered in all patients who have active disease with one or more risk factors for poor prognosis (see Management).

Mechanism. Although the immunosuppressive and cytotoxic effects of methotrexate are caused by the inhibition of dihydrofolate reductase, the anti-inflammatory effects in RA appear to be unrelated to this mechanism of action. This is evidenced by its continued efficacy in the face of supplementation with folic acid (81). The anti-inflammatory mechanism remains unclear but may be caused by increases in extracellular adenosine, a potent inhibitor of inflammation.

Dosage. Methotrexate (available as a 2.5-mg tablet) is prescribed on a weekly basis. Folic acid (1 mg/day) should be administered with methotrexate. Rapid dose increment to a maximal tolerated dose of 20 to 25 mg/wk was well tolerated in the ERA trial (50), and this regimen has now gained wide acceptance in clinical practice. In this protocol, methotrexate is initiated at a dose of 10 mg/wk and then increased by 5 mg every 4 weeks until a dose of 20 mg/wk is attained. Escalation can be interrupted if a side effect occurs. The total dose can be further escalated to 25 mg/wk if efficacy is not achieved at 20 mg/wk. Because of the slow onset of action, a 4- to 6-week period is required after a dose change before a clinical response is seen. For patients with intolerable GI side effects at higher doses of this medication, substituting intramuscular methotrexate (available as a 25-mg/mL solution) at an equivalent dose may be better tolerated, although this conclusion has been called into question (82).

Contraindications to therapy include renal insufficiency, acute or chronic liver disease, (including chronic hepatitis B and C infection), alcohol abuse, leukopenia, thrombocytopenia, untreated folate deficiency, pregnancy, and breast-feeding. Trimethoprim inhibits folate synthesis and should be avoided or used cautiously in patients receiving methotrexate to avoid cumulative toxicity.

Side Effects. Most side effects of low-dose methotrexate are relatively mild and resolve with a dose adjustment or addition of folic acid; rarely do they require complete discontinuation of the drug. Before starting methotrexate, baseline studies should include a CBC, liver chemistries, serum creatinine concentration, and hepatitis B and C serologies. The need for a baseline chest radiograph is more controversial. American College of Rheumatology (ACR) guidelines call for monitoring of CBC and analysis of concentrations of liver transaminases, serum albumin, and serum creatinine every 8 weeks during therapy (83).

Stomatitis, mild alopecia, and GI upset may occur in 20% to 70% of patients treated with methotrexate, are related to folic acid antagonism, and are improved with folic acid supplementation (81). Folic acid supplementation (1 mg/day by prescription) does not appear to decrease the efficacy of methotrexate (81).

Significant *hepatotoxicity* from methotrexate is rare as long as patients with pre-existing liver disease, alcohol abuse, or hepatic dysfunction are excluded from treatment and as long as liver function tests are periodically checked. Elevated concentrations of liver enzymes (usually transaminases), up to twice the normal value, have been reported in 5% to 9% of patients receiving methotrexate in different clinical trials (84). Transaminitis may be reduced by cotreatment with folic acid (85). Patients are advised to limit alcohol consumption to one to two alcoholic beverages per week while taking methotrexate. Elevated concentrations of liver enzymes often are transient, returning to baseline either spontaneously or with brief discontinuation of the medication. Methotrexate may be restarted at the same dose; however, if the elevation occurs a second time, the dose should be reduced. Persistent elevation of enzyme concentrations have been associated with mild fibrotic changes in the liver (86), but frank progression to cirrhosis is exquisitely rare. Baseline or surveillance liver biopsies are not indicated unless pre-existing liver disease is suspected in a patient who is not a candidate for alternative DMARDs.

The most serious complications of methotrexate therapy (interstitial pneumonitis and severe myelosuppression) are rare (87). *Interstitial pneumonitis* is an idiosyncratic, allergic pneumonitis that is more commonly observed in cancer patients receiving high-dose methotrexate than in patients with RA receiving relatively low doses. Nonetheless, this complication carries a high fatality rate and should be recognized and treated immediately. The patient typically presents with fever, dyspnea, nonproductive cough, hypoxia, and bilateral infiltrates on chest radiograph. Methotrexate pneumonitis can occur at any time during therapy and is not dose related. A baseline chest radiograph may be useful for comparison. Patients with poor pulmonary reserve from other causes, such as emphysema, may be excluded from therapy because of the concern for increased morbidity and/or mortality should methotrexate pneumonitis occur.

Myelosuppression is rare with low dosages of methotrexate. Increased renal insufficiency from other causes, as well as use of trimethoprim (Proloprim, Trimpex), may raise methotrexate concentrations and cause myelosuppression. In general, no conclusive evidence links low-dose methotrexate to an increased risk of infection for either common or opportunistic organisms or for postoperative infections (88). There are case reports of herpes zoster infection with methotrexate use (89). In general, methotrexate is *not* discontinued prior to surgery.

Lymphomas, particularly non-Hodgkin lymphoma, occur at a higher rate in RA populations compared to age- and gender-matched controls, especially in patients with severe disease (90,91). Several cases of Epstein-Barr–associated lymphomas reported in association with methotrexate therapy, interestingly, regressed completely with discontinuation of the drug without the need for chemotherapy (92). However, an overall increase in the occurrence of solid-organ malignancies or lymphomas has not been found in large population-based studies of patients with RA (93).

Based on animal studies, teratogenicity is a potential complication of methotrexate. Consequently, female RA patients of child-bearing potential and male RA patients with partners of child-bearing potential should be advised of this potential for teratogenesis and should be strongly encouraged to practice effective birth control. A washout period of at least 3 months is recommended before conception should be attempted. No detrimental effect of methotrexate on sperm production or ovarian function has been noted (94).

Sulfasalazine

Sulfasalazine is composed of a sulfapyridine moiety linked to 5-amino salicylic acid. Although it has been used for decades for treatment of RA, its ability to slow joint damage was demonstrated only in the last few years (95). Sulfasalazine is effective both as monotherapy and in combination with methotrexate for treatment of moderate to severe RA. A study comparing the efficacy of methotrexate with sulfasalazine showed relative efficacy of the two drugs (96).

Mechanism. Sulfasalazine has antibiotic (sulfapyridine) and anti-inflammatory (5-amino salicylic acid) properties. Yet, its disease-modifying capacity likely is not mediated through either of these mechanisms.

Dosage. Sulfasalazine usually is initiated at a dosage of 500 mg twice daily (available in 500-mg tablets) and increased to 2 to 3 g/day over several months. As with other oral DMARDs, its anti-inflammatory and disease-modifying effects become evident only after several months of treatment.

Side Effects. Like methotrexate, sulfasalazine is generally well tolerated. Although side effects are reported by approximately 30% of patients who receive this drug, most can be reduced or eliminated by dose adjustment and rarely require discontinuation of the drug. Sulfasalazine should be avoided in patients with a known allergy to sulfonamide drugs or with glucose-6-phosphate dehydrogenase deficiency because reactions in these individuals can be severe. Compliance with treatment can be an issue because of the twice-daily dosing.

The most common side effect is nausea, which usually is easily managed by dose reduction or with use of the enteric-coated formulation. Rashes and other cutaneous reactions occur in up to 10% of patients, presumably as an allergic reaction to the sulfa component. In this situation, the drug should be discontinued. Serious side effects, such as myelosuppression and hepatotoxicity, are rare. Sulfasalazine is considered a safe option in patients with chronic hepatitis C infection. Reversible infertility in men treated with sulfasalazine can occur secondary to oligospermia.

Monitoring should include CBC and liver function tests at 4-week intervals for 3 months, then every 6 to 12 weeks for 6 months, and thereafter every 3 months.

Leflunomide

Leflunomide is a reversible inhibitor of pyrimidine synthesis that has disease-modifying and antidestructive effects in RA. It has been shown to have equivalent efficacy to methotrexate (97) and provides additional benefit when combined with methotrexate (54).

Mechanism. Leflunomide selectively inhibits *de novo* pyrimidine ribonucleotide biosynthesis and *in vitro* potently inhibits lymphocyte proliferation. The primary mechanism of action of leflunomide is thought to be cell cycle arrest of pathogenic T cells in the joint by depletion of nucleotide pools and inhibition of DNA synthesis.

Dosage. Leflunomide is a prodrug that is converted in the liver to an active metabolite. It is excreted equally in the kidney and the gut and must be used with caution in patients with hepatic or renal insufficiency. The usual starting dose is 20 mg/day, although a 3-day "loading" dose of 100 mg may be used first to hasten the attainment of therapeutic levels. Four to six weeks are required before the beneficial effects of the drug are seen. The dose should be decreased to 10 mg/day in patients who do not tolerate the higher dose. When necessary, as in the case of serious side effects, the elimination half-life can be decreased to 1 to 2 days by the administration of cholestyramine 8 g three times daily for 11 days. Leflunomide can be added safely to methotrexate, but in this case the starting dose should be 10 mg/day. If 10 mg/day is not efficacious and if the liver enzymes remain normal, the dose can be increased to 20 mg/day (54). Because of the additive potential of methotrexate and leflunomide for hepatotoxicity, regular monitoring of the liver enzymes should continue throughout the course of treatment.

Side Effects. In clinical trials, the most commonly reported adverse events were transaminitis, alopecia, rash, and GI complaints, especially diarrhea. Diarrhea occurs in approximately 25% of patients; it usually is self-limited but may necessitate discontinuation of the drug. As with methotrexate, alanine aminotransferase and aspartate aminotransferase elevation (two to three times the upper limits of normal) occurs in 6% of patients taking leflunomide. Liver enzyme abnormalities normalize with cessation of the drug. Alopecia occurs in approximately 10% of patients (98). Some patients develop loss of appetite and weight loss. Contraindications to drug use include active or chronic liver disease and alcoholism. Like methotrexate, leflunomide is teratogenic in animals and should not be giving during pregnancy. It should be washed out prior to attempts at conception.

Monitoring should include CBC and liver enzyme testing monthly initially, followed by monitoring every 2 months.

Inhibitors of Tumor Necrosis Factor-α

Inhibitors of TNF-α include etanercept (Enbrel), infliximab (Remicade), and adalimumab (Humira). *Etanercept (Enbrel)* was the first TNF inhibitor approved by the FDA. It is a recombinant human TNF receptor that binds both TNF-α and lymphotoxin with high affinity. It is created by linking two molecules of the extracellular portion of TNF receptor II (p75) to the Fc portion of a human IgG1 molecule. Etanercept binds TNF-α in the circulation, thus preventing TNF-mediated activation of inflammatory cells.

TNF-α probably is cleared from the circulation through Fc binding by the reticuloendothelial system. Although the patient may report clinical improvement within the first week or two, the maximal effect generally requires up to 3 months (99). Subcutaneously injected etanercept is slowly absorbed and has a half-life >4 days (100). It is administered as either 25 mg twice weekly or 50 mg once weekly (101).

Infliximab (Remicade) is a chimeric mouse–human anti-TNF monoclonal antibody composed of human IgG1-α coupled to the variable regions of a murine anti–human TNF-α antibody. Infliximab exhibits high affinity for TNF-α and prevents binding to cell-associated receptors (102). Infliximab therapy is initiated at a dose of 3 mg/kg by intravenous infusion at weeks 0, 2, and 6, followed by maintenance therapy at the same dose every 8 weeks. For patients with an incomplete response, dosing may be increased to a maximum of 10 mg/kg every 4 weeks. Patients may report improvement after the first or second dose; however, as with etanercept, maximal improvement usually requires several months. Because a significant portion of the infliximab molecule is of mouse origin, patients may develop human antimouse antibodies with repeat dosing, which limits response duration between doses. Methotrexate decreases the frequency of these human antimouse antibodies, and current recommendations indicate administration of infliximab concomitantly with methotrexate (103).

Adalimumab (Humira) is the latest of the TNF inhibitors to be approved by the FDA. Like infliximab, it is an anti-TNF monoclonal antibody; however, unlike infliximab, it is composed entirely of human sequences. As with the other TNF inhibitors, it binds to TNF with high affinity and specificity, preventing its binding to the cell surface receptors. It has a terminal half-life of 2 weeks (104). Although adalimumab is composed entirely of human sequences, antibodies against the drug can develop and can be suppressed by concomitant methotrexate, although there is no FDA-mandated requirement for methotrexate cotreatment. Adalimumab is initiated at a dose of 40 mg subcutaneously every 2 weeks but can be increased to 40 mg weekly if needed. As with other TNF inhibitors, patients usually experience some improvement within the first two injections, but maximal response takes several months.

Side Effects. *Injection site reactions* occur in approximately 20% to 40% of patients treated with the injectable TNF inhibitors (etanercept and adalimumab) and consist of erythema and induration at the injection site (45,50,105). Reactions occur early after initiation of treatment, are generally mild and self-limited, decrease, and then resolve completely with repeated dosing. The injection site reactions are not associated with other features of hypersensitivity, and no specific therapy is generally required (99). *Infusion reactions* occur in approximately 20% of patients treated with infliximab and consist mainly of mild headache, nausea, and flushing. The reactions are transient and can be controlled by slowing the rate of infusion or by pretreating with antihistamines or acetaminophen. Infusion reactions do not increase over time or after multiple infusions (103). Anaphylactic reactions are rare.

INFECTIONS. TNF-α plays an important role in host defense against infection and in initiation and maintenance of granuloma formation (106–108). Despite concerns, there was no increase in overall frequency of infections, nor in the frequency of serious infections, in clinical trials of TNF antagonists compared to placebo (46,50,99,109). However, postmarketing experience has revealed increased susceptibility of patients treated with TNF inhibitors to opportunistic organisms such as *Mycobacterium tuberculosis*, *Histoplasmosis*, *Listeria monocytogenes*, *Pneumocystis carinii,* and others (110,111). Infection with *M. tuberculosis* appears to result from TNF inhibitor-induced dissolution of pre-existing granulomas (latent infection), resulting in widespread dissemination of the organisms. Thus, patients infected with *M. tuberculosis* following treatment with a TNF inhibitor typically have presented with atypical, extrapulmonary disease usually within the first 2 to 3 months after initiating therapy. Opportunistic infections may occur more commonly with infliximab, but the physician's index of suspicion for infection should be high for all patients treated with TNF inhibitors. Before initiation of a TNF inhibitor, all patients should be tested for latent *M. tuberculosis* infection with a purified peptide derivative (PPD). If the lesional induration is >0.5 cm in diameter at 24 to 48 hours, a decision should be made either to use an alternate (non-TNF inhibitor) DMARD or to begin appropriate antibiotic therapy for *M. tuberculosis* (usually for 1–2 months) before initiating treatment with a TNF inhibitor. Antibiotic treatment should continue for the usual recommended period of time. Most commonly, isoniazid is prescribed at a dose of 300 mg/day for a total of 9 months. Patients with *active M. tuberculosis* infections should *never* receive treatment with a TNF inhibitor until after the active infection is adequately controlled/eradicated. Infections with *Staphylococcus aureus* have been reported in patients treated with TNF inhibitors, both during clinical trials and in postmarketing experience (111). Patients with a history of recurrent Staphylococcal infections should *not* receive a TNF inhibitor. In general, the physician should have a heightened awareness for all potential infections in patients treated with TNF inhibitors.

MALIGNANCY. The immune system plays an important role in the surveillance for malignancy, and increased risk of malignancy is a theoretical concern with chronic long-term TNF-α inhibition. Pooled data from clinical trials and open-label extension do not show an increased incidence of solid-organ tumors in patients treated with anti-TNF agents (46,50,105). However, an increased risk of lymphomas in association with anti-TNF therapy has been suggested by data from clinical trials and observational studies (112–114). Interpretation of these data is confounded, however, by the fact that RA patients, in general, are at an overall higher risk for developing lymphoma whether treated with TNF inhibitors or conventional DMARDs. Furthermore, this risk is related to the severity of RA (114). Because treatment with anti-TNF therapy tends to be reserved for patients with severe disease, it is challenging to extract and differentiate the potential effect of the TNF inhibitors from RA in assessing causality for risk of lymphoma. Until further data are available, patients with lymphomas should not be treated with TNF inhibitors, and all RA patients should be watched carefully for signs and symptoms of lymphoma.

DEMYELINATING DISEASE. TNF appears to be an important cytokine in the pathogenesis of multiple sclerosis; however, a clinical trial using an investigational TNF inhibitor resulted in exacerbation, rather than improvement, in signs and symptoms of multiple sclerosis (115). Furthermore, in non-MS patients treated with TNF inhibitors, a small number of demyelinating syndromes have been reported (116). The most common symptoms were paresthesias, visual disturbance due to optic neuritis, and, less commonly, gait disturbance and facial palsy. Discontinuation of anti-TNF therapy led to partial or complete resolution of symptoms in some cases. However, the causal association of TNF inhibitors with these neurologic events remains unclear. Patients with multiple sclerosis or other demyelinating disease should *not* receive treatment with TNF inhibitors.

AUTOIMMUNITY. Autoantibodies, both antinuclear (ANA) and anti–double-stranded (anti-ds) DNA, have been reported in patients treated with TNF inhibitors. In clinical trials, up to 15% patients receiving etanercept or adalimumab developed new ANA (50,99,105). In the infliximab trials, up to 15% and 50% of patients developed ANA and anti-ds DNA antibodies, respectively, compared to 20% and 0% of controls (109,117). However, reports of lupus or lupuslike syndrome are relatively rare in these patients (118).

HEMATOLOGIC AND BONE MARROW. No serious hematologic events occurred in controlled trials of anti-TNF agents, but rare cases of pancytopenia have been reported in postmarketing experience. Thus, although specific routine monitoring for anti-TNF agents is not required according to FDA guidelines, a CBC and chemistry profile every 3 to 6 months is prudent.

Inhibitor of Interleukin-1. *Anakinra (Kineret)* is a recombinant soluble IL-1 human receptor antagonist (IL-1ra) and is the only FDA-approved IL-1 inhibitor. It has been demonstrated to improve clinical and radiographic outcomes when used alone or in combination with methotrexate (53,119,120). In general, the efficacy of anakinra is considerably more modest effect than that of the TNF inhibitors (119,120).

Anakinra binds to the IL-1 receptor, thereby preventing binding of IL-1β to its cellular receptor. The half-life of anakinra is relatively short. Anakinra is administered once daily at a dose of 100 mg by subcutaneous injection. Injection site reaction, primarily erythema and induration, is the most common side effect of anakinra, reported at a frequency of 73% compared to 33% in placebo-treated patients (119). In the controlled clinical trials as well as open-label extension data, no increase in malignancies, either solid-organ tumors or lymphomas, have been reported in anakinra-treated patients (53,119,120). Similarly, no increase in the rate of infections has been observed with either anakinra monotherapy or anakinra in combination with methotrexate, except in one trial, where a modest increase in bacterial pneumonia and cellulitis was observed in combination with other DMARDs (120). However, no increased risk of TB or other opportunistic infections has been associated with anakinra therapy.

Other Nonbiologic Disease-Modifying Antirheumatic Drugs. *Azathioprine, cyclophosphamide, intramuscular gold, oral gold, cyclosporine, and* D-*penicillamine* are rarely used today to treat RA because of their greater toxicity, inferior efficacy, and slower onset of action in comparison with new DMARDs. Cyclophosphamide continues to be used with caution in patients with severe systemic manifestations of RA (e.g., vasculitis, interstitial lung disease). Serious risks associated with cyclophosphamide therapy include premature ovarian failure, bladder cancer, hemorrhagic cystitis, and secondary hematologic malignancies.

Analgesic Drugs. Inflammatory joint pain is best treated by maximizing the anti-inflammatory drug regimen (see Management). However, short-term or occasional use of opioid therapy is acceptable in some situations. For example, patients in the midst of an acute flare and patients with severe destruction of one or more joints who are awaiting surgery may benefit from short-term opioid use. Patients with severe joint destruction who are not surgical candidates may require long-term opioid use. For the average RA patient, however, opioids should be avoided because they do not treat the underlying disease and have addictive potential. Side effects include diminished mental status, hypersomnolence, and constipation, particularly in the elderly. Dependency and addiction occur infrequently, but the clinician must be alert to these behavior patterns and avoid opioid therapy in patients with a history of substance abuse.

TREATMENT DURING PREGNANCY

RA therapy during pregnancy is complicated by the fact that *no placebo-controlled studies have assessed the risk of specific therapies during pregnancy for any of the drugs discussed*. Although signs and symptoms of RA may remit during pregnancy (121), this effect is not universal. Treatment decisions require careful consideration of the risks and benefits to the mother and fetus and should be made together with obstetric consultation.

If possible, all DMARD therapy should be stopped in women who are planning to conceive and in pregnant and lactating women. Infliximab and etanercept are pregnancy category B, whereas hydroxychloroquine is category C (122). Category B drugs are those for which animal studies have shown no adverse results and controlled human data are unavailable. Category C drugs have known adverse effects on animal fetuses but controlled human data is undocumented. Because of evidence of potential teratogenicity, methotrexate and leflunomide should be stopped in men and women who are planning conception; these drugs are category X. In the case of leflunomide, cholestyramine should be given to speed elimination (see Leflunomide). Although safety has not been proven in controlled trials, no evidence exists for risks to the fetus from low-dose *prednisone* (<20 mg/day) or NSAIDs used in the first and second trimesters. If necessary, joint symptoms are best managed with the lowest possible dosage of prednisone. Potential prednisone complications include worsening of maternal gestational diabetes, hypertension, and intrauterine growth retardation. NSAIDs should be avoided in the third trimester because of the potential for premature closure of the ductus, prolonged labor, and peripartum hemorrhage.

SURGERY

Despite aggressive management of RA, destruction of one or more joints, leading to chronic pain and malalignment, will occur in some patients with RA and will require surgical intervention. The primary physician, the rheumatologist, and the orthopedist together can help the patient understand the risks and benefits of the surgical procedure. The decision to have surgery is complex and must take into consideration the motivation and goals of the patient, the patient's ability to undergo rehabilitation, and the patient's general medical status.

TABLE 77.12 Indications for Referral of Patients with Rheumatoid Arthritis for Consultation

To a Rheumatologist
If there is any question about the validity of the diagnosis
During the early phase of the disease to develop a management program
During the course of disease, to assess the need to change therapy or add a second disease-modifying antirheumatic drug
To assess need for, and safety of, biologic agent
If there are severe manifestations of extra-articular disease
For arthrocentesis/injection if the primary physician is not comfortable performing the procedure (an orthopedist can also do this procedure)
For advice about splinting and corrective surgery (an orthopedist can also provide this advice)
To an Orthopedist
For advice about splinting and corrective surgery
To a Physical or Occupational Therapist
To advise and institute appropriate physical therapy, provide aids for daily activities, to provide ambulatory assistive devices.

Total joint arthroplasties of the knee and hip are highly successful procedures as they restore function and reduce or eliminate pain. Arthroplasty of the elbow and shoulder are done primarily for pain relief, as range of motion may not significantly increase. Arthroplasty of the MCP joints also may reduce pain and improve function. Other operations include release of nerve entrapments (e.g., carpal tunnel syndrome), arthroscopic procedures, and, occasionally, removal of a symptomatic rheumatoid nodule. *Synovectomy* is ordinarily not recommended for patients with RA, primarily because relief is only transient. However, an exception is synovectomy of the wrist and/or extensor tendons of the fingers, which is recommended if intense synovitis persists despite medical treatment over 6 to 12 months, to prevent extensor tendon rupture.

SUMMARY OF INDICATIONS FOR REFERRAL

Table 77.12 lists the indications for referral of patients with rheumatoid arthritis.

SPECIFIC REFERENCES*

1. Hochberg MC, Spector TD. Epidemiology of rheumatoid arthritis: update. Epidemiol Rev 1990;12:247.
2. Ollier W, Thomson W. Population genetics of rheumatoid arthritis. Rheum Dis Clin North Am 1992;18:741.
3. Weyand CM, Hicok KC, Conn DL, et al. The influence of Hla-Drb1 genes on disease severity in rheumatoid-arthritis. Ann Intern Med 1992;117:801.
4. Harris ED Jr. Rheumatoid arthritis. Pathophysiology and implications for therapy. N Engl J Med 1990;322:1277.
5. Firestein GS, Alvaro-Gracia JM, Maki R, et al. Quantitative analysis of cytokine gene

*Bold numerals denote published controlled clinical trials, meta-analyses, or consensus-based recommendations.

expression in rheumatoid arthritis. J Immunol 1990;144:3347.
6. Arnett FC, Edworthy SM, Bloch DA, et al. The American Rheumatism Association 1987 revised criteria for the classification of rheumatoid arthritis. Arthritis Rheum 1988;31:315.
7. Roubenoff R, Roubenoff RA, Cannon JG, et al. Rheumatoid cachexia: cytokine-driven hypermetabolism accompanying reduced body cell mass in chronic inflammation. J Clin Invest 1994;93:2379.
8. Wilson A, Hsing-Ting Y, Goodnough LT, et al. Prevalence and outcomes of anemia in rheumatoid arthritis: a systematic review of the literature. Am J Med 2004;116:50.
9. Bertero MT, Caligaris-Cappio F. Anemia of chronic disorders in systemic autoimmune diseases. Haematologica 1997;82:375.
10. Wolfe F, Cathey MA, Roberts FK. The latex test revisited: rheumatoid-factor testing in 8,287 rheumatic disease patients. Arthritis Rheum 1991;34:951.
11. Eberhardt K, Fex E. Clinical course and remission rate in patients with early rheumatoid arthritis: relationship to outcome after 5 years. Br J Rheumatol 1998;37:1324.
12. Shmerling RH, Delbanco TL. The rheumatoid-factor: an analysis of clinical utility. Am J Med 1991;91:528.
13. Schellekens GA, de Jong BAW, van den Hoogen FHJ, et al. Citrulline is an essential constituent of antigenic determinants recognized by rheumatoid arthritis-specific autoantibodies. J Clin Invest 1998;101:273.
14. Vossenaar ER, Despres N, Lapointe E, et al. Rheumatoid arthritis specific anti-Sa antibodies target citrullinated vimentin. Arthritis Res Ther 2004;6:R142.
15. Masson-Bessiere C, Sebbag M, Girbal-Neuhauser E, et al. The major synovial targets of the rheumatoid arthritis-specific antifilaggrin autoantibodies are deiminated forms of the alpha- and beta-chains of fibrin. J Immunol 2001;166:4177.
16. Schellekens GA, Visser H, de Jong BAW, et al. The diagnostic properties of rheumatoid arthritis antibodies recognizing a cyclic citrullinated peptide. Arthritis Rheum 2000;43:155.
17. Nielen MMJ, van Schaardenburg D, Reesink HW, et al. Specific autoantibodies precede the symptoms of rheumatoid arthritis: a study of serial measurements in blood donors. Arthritis Rheum 2004;50:380.
18. Paulus HE, Wiesner J, Bulpitt KJ, et al. Autoantibodies in early seropositive rheumatoid arthritis, before and during disease modifying antirheumatic drug treatment. J Rheumatol 2002;29:2513.
19. Kaandorp CJ, van Schaardenburg D, Krijnen P, et al. Risk factors for septic arthritis in patients with joint disease. A prospective study. Arthritis Rheum 1995;38:1819.
20. van der Heijde DM. Joint erosions and patients with early rheumatoid arthritis. Br J Rheumatol 1995;34[Suppl 2]:74.
21. Visser H, le Cessie S, Vos K, et al. How to diagnose rheumatoid arthritis early: a prediction model for persistent (erosive) arthritis. Arthritis Rheum 2002;46:357.
22. McQueen FM, Stewart N, Crabbe J, et al. Magnetic resonance imaging of the wrist in early rheumatoid arthritis reveals progression of erosions despite clinical improvement. Ann Rheum Dis 1999;58:156.
23. McQueen FM, Stewart N, Crabbe J, et al. Magnetic resonance imaging of the wrist in early rheumatoid arthritis reveals a high prevalence of erosions at four months after symptom onset. Ann Rheum Dis 1998;57:350.
24. Backhaus M, Kamradt T, Sandrock D, et al. Arthritis of the finger joints: a comprehensive approach comparing conventional radiography, scintigraphy, ultrasound, and contrast-enhanced magnetic resonance imaging. Arthritis Rheum 1999;42:1232.
25. Hurd ER. Extraarticular manifestations of rheumatoid arthritis. Semin Arthritis Rheum 1979;8:151.
26. Turesson C, O'Fallon WM, Crowson CS, et al. Occurrence of extraarticular disease manifestations is associated with excess mortality in a community based cohort of patients with rheumatoid arthritis. J Rheumatol 2002;29:62.
27. Kersten PJ. Accelerated nodulosis during low dose methotrexate therapy for rheumatoid arthritis. An analysis of ten cases. J Rheumatol 1992;19;867.
28. Tanoue LT. Pulmonary manifestations of rheumatoid arthritis. Clin Chest Med 1998;19:667.
29. Lebowitz WB. The heart in rheumatoid arthritis (rheumatoid disease). A clinical and pathological study of sixty-two cases. Ann Intern Med 1963;58:102.
30. Mitchell DM, Spitz PW, Young DY, et al. Survival, prognosis, and causes of death in rheumatoid arthritis. Arthritis Rheum 1986;29:706.
31. Doran MF, Crowson CS, Pond GR, et al. Predictors of infection in rheumatoid arthritis. Arthritis Rheum 2002;46:2294.
32. Wolfe F, Mitchell DM, Sibley JT, et al. The mortality of rheumatoid arthritis. Arthritis Rheum 1994;37:481.
33. Goodson N. Coronary artery disease and rheumatoid arthritis. Curr Opin Rheumatol 2002;14:115.
34. Rosenstein ED, Kramer N. Felty's and pseudo-Felty's syndromes. Semin Arthritis Rheum 1991;21:129.
35. Goronzy JJ, Matteson EL, Fulbright JW, et al. Prognostic markers of radiographic progression in early rheumatoid arthritis. Arthritis Rheum 2004;50:43.
36. Yelin E, Meenan R, Nevitt M, Epstein W. Work disability in rheumatoid arthritis: effects of disease, social, and work factors. Ann Intern Med 1980;93:551.
37. Gabriel SE, Crowson CS, O'Fallon WM. Comorbidity in arthritis. J Rheumatol 1999;26:2475.
38. McQueen FM, Benton N, Crabbe J, et al. What is the fate of erosions in early rheumatoid arthritis? Tracking individual lesions using x-rays and magnetic resonance imaging over the first two years of disease. Ann Rheum Dis 2001;60:859.
39. Egsmose C, Lund B, Borg G, et al. Patients with rheumatoid arthritis benefit from early 2nd line therapy: 5-year follow-up of a prospective double blind placebo controlled study. J Rheumatol 1995;22:2208.
40. Lard LR, Visser H, Speyer I, et al. Early versus delayed treatment in patients with recent-onset rheumatoid arthritis: comparison of two cohorts who received different treatment strategies. Am J Med 2001;111:446.
41. O'Dell JR, Haire CE, Erikson N, et al. Treatment of rheumatoid arthritis with methotrexate alone, sulfasalazine and hydroxychloroquine, or a combination of all three medications. N Engl J Med 1996;334:1287.
42. vanderHeide A, Jacobs JWG, Bijlsma JWJ, et al. The effectiveness of early treatment with "second-line" antirheumatic drugs: a randomized, controlled trial. Ann Intern Med 1996;124:699.
43. Boers M, Verhoeven AC, Markusse HM, et al. Randomised comparison of combined step-down prednisolone, methotrexate and sulphasalazine with sulphasalazine alone in early rheumatoid arthritis. Lancet 1997;350:309.
44. Mottonen T, Hannonen P, Leirisalo-Repo M, et al. Comparison of combination therapy with single-drug therapy in early rheumatoid arthritis: a randomised trial. FIN-RACo trial group. Lancet 1999;353:1568.
45. Moreland LW, Baumgartner SW, Schiff MH, et al. Treatment of rheumatoid arthritis with a recombinant human tumor necrosis factor receptor (p75)-Fc fusion protein. N Engl J Med 1997;337:141.
46. Maini R, St.Clair EW, Breedveld F, et al. Infliximab (chimeric anti-tumour necrosis factor alpha monoclonal antibody) versus placebo in rheumatoid arthritis patients receiving concomitant methotrexate: a randomised phase III trial. Lancet 1999;354:1932.
47. Weinblatt ME, Keystone EC, Furst DE, et al. Adalimumab, a fully human anti-tumor necrosis factor alpha monoclonal antibody, for the treatment of rheumatoid arthritis in patients taking concomitant methotrexate: the ARMADA trial. Arthritis Rheum 2003;48:35.
48. Wolfe F, Hawley DJ, Cathey MA. Termination of slow acting antirheumatic therapy in rheumatoid arthritis: a 14-year prospective evaluation of 1017 consecutive starts. J Rheumatol 1990;17:994.
49. O'Dell JR. Methotrexate use in rheumatoid arthritis. Rheum Dis Clin North Am 1997;23: 779.
50. Bathon JM, Martin RW, Fleischmann RM, et al. A comparison of etanercept and methotrexate in patients with early rheumatoid arthritis. N Engl J Med 2000;343:1586.
51. Klareskog L, van der Heijde D, de Jager JP, et al. Therapeutic effect of the combination of etanercept and methotrexate compared with each treatment alone in patients with rheumatoid arthritis: double-blind randomised controlled trial. Lancet 2004;363:675.
52. St. Clair EW, van der Heijde DM, Smolen JS, et al. Combination of infliximab and methotrexate therapy for early rheumatoid arthritis: a randomized, controlled trial. Arthritis Rheum 2004;50:3432.
53. Cohen S, Hurd E, Cush J, et al. Treatment of rheumatoid arthritis with anakinra, a recombinant human interleukin-1 receptor antagonist, in combination with methotrexate: Results of a twenty-four-week, multicenter, randomized, double-blind, placebo-controlled trial. Arthritis Rheum 2002;46:614.
54. Kremer JM, Genovese MC, Cannon GW, et al. Concomitant leflunomide therapy in patients with active rheumatoid arthritis despite stable doses of methotrexate: a randomized, double-blind, placebo-controlled trial. Ann Intern Med 2002;137:726.
55. Silverstein FE, Faich G, Goldstein JL, et al. Gastrointestinal toxicity with celecoxib vs nonsteroidal anti-inflammatory drugs for osteoarthritis and rheumatoid arthritis: the CLASS study: a randomized controlled trial. Celecoxib Long-term Arthritis Safety Study. JAMA 2000;284:1247.
56. Bombardier C, Laine L, Reicin A, et al. Comparison of upper gastrointestinal toxicity of rofecoxib and naproxen in patients with rheumatoid arthritis. VIGOR Study Group. N Engl J Med 2000;343:1520, 2.
57. Allison MC, Howatson AG, Torrance CJ, et al. Gastrointestinal damage associated with the use of nonsteroidal antiinflammatory drugs. N Engl J Med 1992;327:749.
58. Simm LS. Nonsteroidal anti-inflammatory drug toxicity. Curr Opin Rheumatol 1993;5:265.
59. Soll AH, Weinstein WM, Kurata J, et al. Nonsteroidal anti-inflammatory drugs and peptic ulcer disease. Ann Intern Med 1991;114:307.
60. Saw KC, Higgins AF, Quick CRG. Ileocecal perforation and bleeding: are nonsteroidal

anti-inflammatory drugs (NSAID) responsible. J R Soc Med 1990;83:114.
61. Shorr RI, Ray WA, Daugherty JR, et al. Concurrent use of nonsteroidal antiinflammatory drugs and oral anticoagulants places elderly persons at high-risk for hemorrhagic peptic-ulcer disease. Arch Intern Med 1993;153:1665.
62. Silverstein FE, Graham DY, Senior JR, et al. Misoprostol reduces serious gastrointestinal complications in patients with rheumatoid arthritis receiving nonsteroidal anti-inflammatory drugs. A randomized, double-blind, placebo-controlled trial. Ann Intern Med 1995;123:241.
63. Hawkey CJ, Karrasch JA, Szczepanski L, et al. Omeprazole compared with misoprostol for ulcers associated with nonsteroidal antiinflammatory drugs. Omeprazole versus Misoprostol for NSAID-induced Ulcer Management (OMNIUM) Study Group. N Engl J Med 1998;338:727.
64. Agrawal NM, Campbell DR, Safdi MA, et al. Superiority of lansoprazole vs ranitidine in healing nonsteroidal anti-inflammatory drug-associated gastric ulcers: results of a double-blind, randomized, multicenter study. NSAID-Associated Gastric Ulcer Study Group. Arch Intern Med 2000;160:1455.
65. Laine L, Maller ES, Yu C, et al. Ulcer formation with low-dose enteric-coated aspirin and the effect of COX-2 selective inhibition: a double-blind trial. Gastroenterology 2004;127:395.
66. Mukherjee D, Nissen SE, Topol EJ. Risk of cardiovascular events associated with selective COX-2 inhibitors. JAMA 2001;286:954.
67. Nussmeier NA, Whelton AA, Brown MT, et al. Complications of the COX-2 inhibitors parecoxib and valdecoxib after cardiac surgery. N Engl J Med 2005;352:1081.
68. Solomon SD, McMurray JJ, Pfeffer MA, et al. Cardiovascular risk associated with celecoxib in a clinical trial for colorectal adenoma prevention. N Engl J Med 2005;352:1071.
69. FDA Alert for Practitioners Celecoxib (marketed as Celebrex). April 7, 2005.
70. Graham DJ, Campen D, Hui R, et al. Risk of acute myocardial infarction and sudden cardiac death in patients treated with cyclo-oxygenase 2 selective and non-selective non-steroidal anti-inflammatory drugs: nested case-control study. Lancet 2005;365:475.
71. Breyer MD, Hao C, Qi Z. Cyclooxygenase-2 selective inhibitors and the kidney. Curr Opin Crit Care 2001;7:393.
72. Whelton A, Hamilton CW. Nonsteroidal anti-inflammatory drugs: effects on kidney function. J Clin Pharmacol 1991;31:588.
73. Kirwan JR. The effect of glucocorticoids on joint destruction in rheumatoid arthritis. The Arthritis and Rheumatism Council Low-Dose Glucocorticoid Study Group. N Engl J Med 1995;333:142.
74. van Everdingen AA, Jacobs JW, Siewertsz Van Reesema DR, et al. Low-dose prednisone therapy for patients with early active rheumatoid arthritis: clinical efficacy, disease-modifying properties, and side effects: a randomized, double-blind, placebo-controlled clinical trial. Ann Intern Med 2002;136:1.
75. Iglehart IW III, Sutton JD, Bender JC, et al. Intravenous pulsed steroids in rheumatoid arthritis: a comparative dose study. J Rheumatol 1990;17:159.
76. Saag KG, Koehnke R, Caldwell JR, et al. Low dose long-term corticosteroid therapy in rheumatoid arthritis: an analysis of serious adverse events. Am J Med 1994;96:115.
77. Lodder MC, de Jong Z, Kostense PJ, et al. Bone mineral density in patients with rheumatoid arthritis: relation between disease severity and low bone mineral density. Ann Rheum Dis 2004;63:1576.
78. Garbe E, LeLorier J, Boivin JF, et al. Risk of ocular hypertension or open-angle glaucoma in elderly patients on oral glucocorticoids. Lancet 1997;350:979.
79. A randomized trial of hydroxychloroquine in early rheumatoid arthritis: the HERA Study. Am J Med 1995;98:156.
80. Furst DE, Lindsley H, Baethge B, et al. Dose-loading with hydroxychloroquine improves the rate of response in early, active rheumatoid arthritis: a randomized, double-blind six-week trial with eighteen-week extension. Arthritis Rheum 1999;42:357.
81. Morgan SL, Baggott JE, Vaughn WH, et al. Supplementation with folic acid during methotrexate therapy for rheumatoid arthritis. A double-blind, placebo-controlled trial. Ann Intern Med 1994;121:833.
82. Lambert CM, Sandhu S, Lochhead A, et al. Dose escalation of parenteral methotrexate in active rheumatoid arthritis that has been unresponsive to conventional doses of methotrexate: a randomized, controlled trial. Arthritis Rheum 2004;50:364.
83. Guidelines for monitoring drug therapy in rheumatoid arthritis. American College of Rheumatology Ad Hoc Committee on Clinical Guidelines. Arthritis Rheum 1996;39:723.
84. Kremer JM, Alarcon GS, Lightfoot RW Jr, et al. Methotrexate for rheumatoid arthritis. Suggested guidelines for monitoring liver toxicity. American College of Rheumatology. Arthritis Rheum 1994;37:316.
85. van Ede AE, Laan RF, Rood MJ, et al. Effect of folic or folinic acid supplementation on the toxicity and efficacy of methotrexate in rheumatoid arthritis: a forty-eight week, multicenter, randomized, double-blind, placebo-controlled study. Arthritis Rheum 2001;44:1515.
86. Kremer JM, Lee RG, Tolman KG. Liver histology in rheumatoid arthritis patients receiving long-term methotrexate therapy. A prospective study with baseline and sequential biopsy samples. Arthritis Rheum 1989;32:121.
87. Weinblatt ME, Kaplan H, Germain BF, et al. Methotrexate in rheumatoid arthritis. A five-year prospective multicenter study. Arthritis Rheum 1994;37:1492.
88. Perhala RS, Wilke WS, Clough JD, et al. Local infectious complications following large joint replacement in rheumatoid-arthritis patients treated with methotrexate versus those not treated with methotrexate. Arthritis Rheum 1991;34:146.
89. Shiroky JB, Frost A, Skelton JD, et al. Complications of immunosuppression associated with weekly low dose methotrexate. J Rheumatol 1991;18:1172.
90. Isomaki HA, Hakulinen T, Joutsenlahti U. Excess risk of lymphomas, leukemia and myeloma in patients with rheumatoid arthritis. J Chronic Dis 1978;31:691.
91. Gridley G, Mclaughlin JK, Ekbom A, et al. Incidence of cancer among patients with rheumatoid-arthritis. J Natl Cancer Inst 1993;85:307.
92. Kamel O, Vanderijn M, Weiss L, et al. EBV-associated lymphoproliferative disorders occurring in the setting of methotrexate therapy for rheumatoid-arthritis and dermatomyositis. Lab Invest 1993;68:A93.
93. Moder KG, Tefferi A, Cohen MD, et al. Hematologic malignancies and the use of methotrexate in rheumatoid arthritis: a retrospective study. Am J Med 1995;99:276.
94. Lloyd ME, Carr M, McElhatton P, et al. The effects of methotrexate on pregnancy, fertility and lactation. QJM 1999;92:551.
95. Scott DL, Smolen JS, Kalden JR, et al. Treatment of active rheumatoid arthritis with leflunomide: two year follow up of a double blind, placebo controlled trial versus sulfasalazine. Ann Rheum Dis 2001;60:913.
96. Haagsma CJ, van Riel PL, de Jong AJ, et al. Combination of sulphasalazine and methotrexate versus the single components in early rheumatoid arthritis: a randomized, controlled, double-blind, 52 week clinical trial. Br J Rheumatol 1997;36:1082.
97. Strand V, Cohen S, Schiff M, et al. Treatment of active rheumatoid arthritis with leflunomide compared with placebo and methotrexate. Leflunomide Rheumatoid Arthritis Investigators Group. Arch Intern Med 1999;159:2542.
98. Smolen JS, Kalden JR, Scott DL, et al. Efficacy and safety of leflunomide compared with placebo and sulphasalazine in active rheumatoid arthritis: a double-blind, randomised, multicentre trial. European Leflunomide Study Group. Lancet 1999;353:259.
99. Moreland LW, Schiff MH, Baumgartner SW, et al. Etanercept therapy in rheumatoid arthritis. a randomized, controlled trial. Ann Intern Med 1999;130:478.
100. Korth-Bradley JM, Rubin AS, Hanna RK, et al. The pharmacokinetics of etanercept in healthy volunteers. Ann Pharmacother 2000;34:161.
101. Keystone EC, Schiff MH, Kremer JM, et al. Once-weekly administration of 50 mg etanercept in patients with active rheumatoid arthritis: results of a multicenter, randomized, double-blind, placebo-controlled trial. Arthritis Rheum 2004;50:353.
102. Elliott MJ, Maini RN, Feldmann M, et al. Treatment of rheumatoid arthritis with chimeric monoclonal antibodies to tumor necrosis factor alpha. Arthritis Rheum 1993;36:1681.
103. Lipsky PE, van der Heijde DMFM, St.Clair EW, et al. Infliximab and methotrexate in the treatment of rheumatoid arthritis. N Engl J Med 2000;343:1594.
104. den Broeder A, van de Putte L, Rau R, et al. A single dose, placebo controlled study of the fully human anti-tumor necrosis factor-alpha antibody adalimumab (D2E7) in patients with rheumatoid arthritis. J Rheumatol 2002;29:2288.
105. van de Putte LB, Atkins C, Malaise M, et al. Efficacy and safety of adalimumab as monotherapy in patients with rheumatoid arthritis for whom previous disease modifying antirheumatic drug treatment has failed. Ann Rheum Dis 2004;63:508.
106. Pasparakis M, Alexopoulou L, Episkopou V, et al. Immune and inflammatory responses in TNF alpha-deficient mice: a critical requirement for TNF alpha in the formation of primary B cell follicles, follicular dendritic cell networks and germinal centers, and in the maturation of the humoral immune response. J Exp Med 1996;184:1397.
107. Rothe J, Lesslauer W, Lotscher H, et al. Mice lacking the tumour necrosis factor receptor 1 are resistant to TNF-mediated toxicity but highly susceptible to infection by *Listeria monocytogenes*. Nature 1993;364:798.
108. Gordon S, Keshav S, Stein M. BCG-induced granuloma-formation in murine tissues. Immunobiology 1994;191:369.
109. Elliott MJ, Maini RN, Feldmann M, et al. Randomised double-blind comparison of chimeric monoclonal antibody to tumour necrosis factor alpha (cA2) versus placebo in rheumatoid arthritis. Lancet 1994;344:1105.
110. Keane J, Gershon S, Wise RP, et al. Tuberculosis associated with infliximab, a tumor necrosis factor alpha-neutralizing agent. N Engl J Med 2001;345:1098.
111. Wallis WJ, Burge DJ, Holmdahl R, et al. Infection reports with etanercept (Enbrel) therapy. Arthritis Rheum 2001;44:S154.

112. Brown SL, Greene MH, Gershon SK, et al. Tumor necrosis factor antagonist therapy and lymphoma development: twenty-six cases reported to the Food and Drug Administration. Arthritis Rheum 2002;46:3151.
113. Wolfe F, Michaud K. Lymphoma in rheumatoid arthritis: the effect of methotrexate and anti-tumor necrosis factor therapy in 18,572 patients. Arthritis Rheum 2004;50:1740.
114. Baecklund E, Ekbom A, Sparen P, et al. Disease activity and risk of lymphoma in patients with rheumatoid arthritis: nested case-control study. BMJ 1998;317:180.
115. TNF neutralization in MS: results of a randomized, placebo-controlled multicenter study. The Lenercept Multiple Sclerosis Study Group and The University of British Columbia MS/MRI Analysis Group. Neurology 1999;53:457.
116. Mohan N, Edwards ET, Cupps TR, et al. Demyelination occurring during anti-tumor necrosis factor alpha therapy for inflammatory arthritides. Arthritis Rheum 2001;44:2862.
117. Maini RN, Breedveld FC, Kalden JR, et al. Therapeutic efficacy of multiple intravenous infusions of anti-tumor necrosis factor alpha monoclonal antibody combined with low-dose weekly methotrexate in rheumatoid arthritis. Arthritis Rheum 1998;41:1552.
118. Eriksson C, Engstrand S, Sundqvist KG, et al. Autoantibody formation in patients with rheumatoid arthritis treated with anti-TNF alpha. Ann Rheum Dis 2005;64:403.
119. Bresnihan B, Alvaro-Gracia JM, Cobby M, et al. Treatment of rheumatoid arthritis with recombinant human interleukin-1 receptor antagonist. Arthritis Rheum 1998;41:2196.
120. Fleischmann RM, Schechtman J, Bennett R, et al. Anakinra, a recombinant human interleukin-1 receptor antagonist (r-metHuIL-1ra), in patients with rheumatoid arthritis: a large, international, multicenter, placebo-controlled trial. Arthritis Rheum 2003;48:927.
121. Barrett JH, Brennan P, Fiddler M, et al. Does rheumatoid arthritis remit during pregnancy and relapse postpartum? Results from a nationwide study in the United Kingdom performed prospectively from late pregnancy. Arthritis Rheum 1999;42:1219.
122. Janssen NM, Genta MS. The effects of immunosuppressive and anti-inflammatory medications on fertility, pregnancy, and lactation. Arch Intern Med 2000;160:610.

For annotated ***General References*** *and resources related to this chapter, visit www.hopkinsbayview.org/PAMreferences.*

Chapter 78

Spondyloarthritis, Ankylosing Spondylitis, and Reactive Arthritis

John A. Flynn and Frank C. Arnett, Jr.

SPONDYLOARTHRITIS

Spondyloarthritis is the term used for an overlapping group of diseases that are characterized variably by inflammation of the sacroiliac joints (sacroiliitis), axial spine (spondylitis), tendon, fascia, and ligament insertion sites (enthesitis), and, in some patients, an oligoarthritis, rash, or inflammatory eye disease (uveitis). These diseases also have been grouped under the heading of seronegative spondyloarthritis based on the absence in the blood of affected patients of rheumatoid factor. The diseases include ankylosing spondylitis, psoriatic arthritis, the arthritis of inflammatory bowel disease, and reactive arthritis.

The dominant problems that bring the patient with spondyloarthritis to a clinician and require careful management over many years are pain, limitation of motion, and deformity of the spine. In all forms of spondyloarthritis, the same principles of diagnosis and management of the axial problem apply but must be accompanied by attention to the cutaneous, gastrointestinal (GI), genitourinary, ocular, and peripheral articular manifestations of the primary disorders.

The pathogenesis of spinal inflammation is unknown; however, there is a strong hereditary component marked by the histocompatibility antigen HLA-B27 (1,2). This genetic marker is strongly associated with sacroiliitis and spondylitis regardless of clinical setting (Table 78.1). More than 90% of patients with ankylosing spondylitis have the HLA-B27 antigen. Conversely, if normal subjects with HLA-B27 are carefully assessed, clinical or radiographic evidence of disease can be found in only 2% (3). Transgenic rats possessing the human HLA-B27 gene develop nearly all the clinical features of spondyloarthritis and

TABLE 78.1 Classification of Spondylitis and Frequency of HLA-B27[a]

Classification	*HLA-B27 Positive*
Primary	
Isolated sacroiliitis	70%–90%
Ankylosing spondylitis	>90%
Secondary	
Spondylitis of inflammatory bowel disease	50%
Psoriatic spondylitis	50%
Reactive arthritis with spondylitis	90%

[a]Found in 8% to 10% of normal white subjects and 2% to 4% of normal black subjects.

have confirmed the direct participation of this gene in disease pathogenesis (4). In addition to genetic predisposition, certain environmental agents appear to be associated with these diseases in the B27-positive host. There is evidence that normal bacterial flora in the GI tract participate in the pathogenesis of ankylosing spondylitis and in the disease seen in HLA-B27 transgenic animals (4). Reactive arthritis is known to be triggered by certain specific GI, genitourinary, or other infections (5) (see Reactive Arthritis).

Sacroiliitis

Sacroiliitis may occur as an isolated clinical syndrome or be a component feature of a spondyloarthritis (6,7). Osteoarthritis may affect the sacroiliac joints in older people, but these are radiologic changes that usually are readily differentiated from inflammatory sacroiliitis and typically are unassociated with symptoms. Sacroiliitis is considered the *sine qua non* for *ankylosing spondylitis;* however, this latter diagnosis should be applied only when symptoms or signs indicate progression of inflammation into additional segments of the axial skeleton. *Sacroiliitis* or spondylitis may develop in 10% of patients with inflammatory bowel disease (ulcerative colitis and Crohn disease), 20% of those with psoriatic arthritis, and 20% of those with reactive arthritis.

Enthesitis

The entheses are important sites of inflammation and subsequent pathology in spondyloarthritis. The entheses are locations where tendons, fascia, and ligaments insert into bone. Clinical manifestations include heel pain with involvement of the Achilles tendon, foot pain at the site of insertion of the plantar aponeurosis, or swelling of an entire digit (sausage digit) due to inflammation of the flexor and extensor tendons of the fingers or toes (8).

ANKYLOSING SPONDYLITIS

Prevalence

The prevalence of ankylosing spondylitis parallels the frequency of HLA-B27 in different populations in the United States and in other regions of the world. This gene occurs in 8% to 10% of white Americans, and the disease occurs in 0.1% to 0.2% of the white population (4,5). African Americans have a much lower frequency of both disease and of the HLA-B27 gene. On the other hand, there is a high frequency of ankylosing spondylitis and of HLA-B27 in certain Native American and Eskimo groups. Ankylosing spondylitis is common in Europeans and most Asian groups but is found rarely in African blacks and in Japanese, again reflecting the relative frequency of the B27 marker.

Histopathology

Spondyloarthritis is characterized by chronic inflammation of *synovial* joints, especially those in the axial skeleton; *fibrous* joints such as sacroiliacs and symphysis pubis; and the entheses where tendons, ligaments, and fascia have their insertions (2,9). The chronic inflammatory infiltrates are nonspecific and histologically indistinguishable from those of rheumatoid arthritis. Although erosive bone disease does occur, unlike the rheumatoid process, this inflammatory process also promotes new bone formation across previous articulations. This ossification of the articular and ligamentous structures of the spine results in eventual fusion and gives rise to the characteristic radiographic findings.

History and Examination

The typical patient with ankylosing spondylitis is a young white man younger than 40 years (Table 78.2). Occasionally, the diagnosis is made in older patients, but careful questioning often reveals that symptoms began years earlier. However, the impression that women are affected less often than men (ratio 1:3) may be caused by underrecognition of the disease in women. The initial symptoms of the disorder in women may be peripheral or cervical spine arthritis, and low back involvement may be absent or

TABLE 78.2 Clues to Early Ankylosing Spondylitis

Young man (less often a woman)
Pain/stiffness in buttocks, low back, chest wall
Worse with rest
Better with exercise
Sciaticlike pains
Family history of spondylitis
History of iritis

overshadowed by these complaints. Therefore, one should be mindful of these differences between men and women and must consider an emerging spondylitic process in young women who present with a seronegative arthritis.

The usual presenting symptoms of ankylosing spondylitis are pain and stiffness in the low back or deep within the buttocks. These symptoms begin insidiously, and the patient usually noticed them for at least 3 months before seeking medical advice. Unlike mechanical low back syndromes, the pain and stiffness of inflammatory disease usually are worsened by rest and improved by exercise. The patient is unable to rest at night or sit for prolonged periods and must arise and stretch to obtain relief. As in discogenic disease, however, symptoms of shooting pains into the buttocks and down the posterior or lateral thighs may occur and mimic sciatica. These pains usually are transient, may alternate to the opposite side, and are not associated with any demonstrable neurologic deficits.

With time, the disease progresses into the lumbar and thoracic regions, with enthesitis of costosternal joints. Chest wall pain occurs and may mimic pleuritic, pericardial, or anginal pain syndromes. Progressive limitation of spinal movements ensues, and patients may note more difficulty in bending forward, the development of a stooped posture, and actual loss of height. When the disease process affects the cervical spine, the neck may become fused in a flexed position. Although peripheral joints are uncommonly affected, the root joints (hips and shoulders) eventually become involved in nearly 50% of patients. Occasionally, fusion of the back may be entirely asymptomatic, and the patient develops complaints only when the disease reaches the cervical spine, hips, or shoulders.

Additional important historical facts should be sought during assessment of the patient. In 16% of patients, the family history is positive for a first-degree relative with spondyloarthritis (5). Acute anterior uveitis (iritis) may have been a harbinger of the articular syndrome, and at least 25% of patients will have iritis at some time before or during their course of illness. With the review of systems and family history, one should seek symptoms or diagnoses of psoriasis or inflammatory bowel disease in the patient or in family members. Because of the insidious nature of these symptoms, a delay of up to 8 to 11 years between first symptoms and diagnosis is not unusual (10).

A physical examination initially and every 4 to 6 months is important in patients with suspected spondyloarthritis. Although the primary focus of examinations is the musculoskeletal system, especially the axial skeleton, shoulders, hips, and peripheral joints, additional attention must be directed toward the eyes, heart, skin, and GI tract. This practice ensures the diagnosis and provides the baseline with which the clinician can assess future articular or extra-articular complications or the superimposition of unrelated systemic or musculoskeletal disorders. It must be emphasized that ankylosing spondylitis is a disease that requires management over decades, and each new complaint cannot necessarily be ascribed to the basic disease process.

TABLE 78.3 Physical Examination in Ankylosing Spondylitis

Sacroiliac Joints	Thoracic Spine
Tenderness	Increased kyphosis
Pain with compression/ stress	Tenderness
Lumbar Spine	Pain with rib cage compression
Tenderness	Decreased chest expansion (<3 cm)
Paravertebral muscle spasm	Cervical Spine
Loss of lordosis	Tenderness
Decreased flexion: Schober test (<5 cm) (see text)	Pain on motion
Decreased lateral motion and extension	Muscle spasm
Hips, shoulders	Decreased motion
Pain on motion	Kyphosis, decreased lordosis
Decreased range	Occiput-to-wall distance (see text)

Articular Features

Only a few measurable abnormalities are seen in patients with early disease (Table 78.3). In fact, the patient with sacroiliitis may have an entirely normal physical examination, despite significant symptoms of pain and stiffness in the low back region. At most, tenderness on direct palpation of these joints in the buttocks or upon compression of the pelvis is observed. Stressing the sacroiliac joint to elicit pain (see Chapter 71) may be useful.

Abnormalities that eventually appear in the patient with progressive disease relate to loss of range of motion and deformity in mobile structures. After evaluation of the sacroiliac regions, the clinician should direct attention to the lumbar spine. The patient with lumbar involvement often has lost the normal lordosis, and that segment of the back flattens. In addition, loss in range of motion is seen when the patient attempts to bend forward. Recall that hip motion accounts for 90 degrees of the flexion of the trunk on the lower extremities and that the lumbar spine provides the remaining stretch by reversing its lordosis and becoming kyphotic. An objective measurement of lumbar motion is the *Schober test.* With the patient standing erect, a horizontal line is drawn at the L5–S1 region and another line 10 cm above that in the midline of the back. With forward flexion, the distance between these two ends of the 10-cm line should increase from 10 to 15 cm in the normal lumbar spine. This test is best applied and interpreted in the young patient because lumbar motion normally decreases with age. Lateral bending and extension of the lumbar spine should be assessed at the same time.

Involvement of the *thoracic spine* is determined subjectively by the patient's complaints of pain or stiffness in that region and by demonstrable tenderness along the vertebral column and paravertebral muscles. Compression of the rib cage laterally and over the sternum may elicit pain. Objective determination of fusion of the costovertebral joints is obtained by measuring the chest expansion. A tape measure is placed around the patient's chest wall at the nipple line or fourth intercostal space, and the change in circumference from full expiration to full inspiration is measured. Less than 3 cm is considered abnormal. Chest expansion in normal people decreases with increasing age.

The range of motion of the cervical spine should be determined for extension, right and left rotation, lateral flexion, and forward flexion. Loss of extension usually is the earliest abnormality. As the disease progresses, the patient tends to develop fixed deformity in the forward flexed position. Therefore, another rough estimate of developing cervical kyphosis is the occiput-to-wall measurement. This is obtained with the patient placing both heels against the base of the wall and attempting to extend the neck fully to touch the wall with the back of the head. The horizontal distance from posterior occiput to the wall is a measure of the fixed cervical deformity, as this distance usually is zero.

Examination of the range of motion and elicitation of any pain on motion of both shoulders and hips is important because, as discussed earlier, up to half of patients develop involvement of these joints some time during the course of the disease. Less often, more peripheral joints (e.g., knees, ankles and wrists) become inflamed, but usually only transiently. Approximately 10% of patients with ankylosing spondylitis complain of pain in the heels either at the Achilles tendon insertion or over the attachment of the plantar aponeurosis in the sole of the foot (enthesitis). Swelling is not always apparent in these areas, but tenderness to direct palpation is found.

Extra-Articular Features

Anterior uveitis (iritis) occurs in approximately 25% of patients with ankylosing spondylitis and does not necessarily parallel the course of the articular disease. It occasionally is the sentinel symptom. Its onset usually is abrupt and unilateral, with intense pain, redness, and photophobia as the cardinal symptoms. Immediate ophthalmologic attention is required to prevent serious damage to the anterior chamber of the eye. Local corticosteroids usually are successful in abating an acute episode; however, frequent slit-lamp examinations determine the response and help determine whether systemic steroids are required.

Cardiac abnormalities occur in <5% of patients with ankylosing spondylitis (Table 78.4) (11). The most common cardiac abnormality, first-degree atrioventricular block, can be determined only electrocardiographically. A history of palpitations or syncope and the finding of a slow or irregular pulse on examination should alert one to higher degrees of atrioventricular block. A cardiac pacemaker is required for some cases of serious arrhythmia or complete atrioventricular dissociation. Aortic regurgitation caused by inflammatory thickening of the aortic valve and root is another serious cardiac complication. Once the diastolic murmur becomes apparent, usually cardiac decompensation occurs and requires valve replacement in 1 to 2 years.

TABLE 78.4 Extra-Articular Manifestations and Complications of Ankylosing Spondylitis

Cardiac	5%
First-degree atrioventricular block	
Second- and third-degree atrioventricular block	
Aortic regurgitation	
Ocular	25%
Acute iritis	
Chronic iritis	
Neurologic	Rare
Cauda equina syndrome	
Cord injury caused by fractures	
Renal	Rare
Immunoglobulin A nephropathy	
Amyloidosis	4%
Pulmonary apical fibrosis	Rare

The *cauda equina syndrome* is a rare but serious neurologic complication of ankylosing spondylitis (see Chapter 71). It is believed to be related to entrapment of exiting lumbar and sacral nerves through the inflamed spinal column; however, compressive inflammatory lesions within the spinal column are found in some cases and are surgically remediable. Patients with ankylosing spondylitis should be questioned regularly about paresthesias and pain or weakness in the legs and about symptoms of bladder or bowel sphincter dysfunction. Other neurologic sequelae of the disorder include injuries to the spinal cord from fracture and dislocation of a rigid and brittle spine. The neck is especially prone to fracture, and paraplegia or quadriplegia may result (12).

Secondary amyloidosis can be found in approximately 4% of patients with ankylosing spondylitis, usually after many decades of persistent inflammatory disease. Proteinuria and nephrotic syndrome indicate renal involvement, which usually is the most serious manifestation of amyloidosis. *Immunoglobulin A nephropathy* has been reported as another cause of proteinuria and renal insufficiency in this disease.

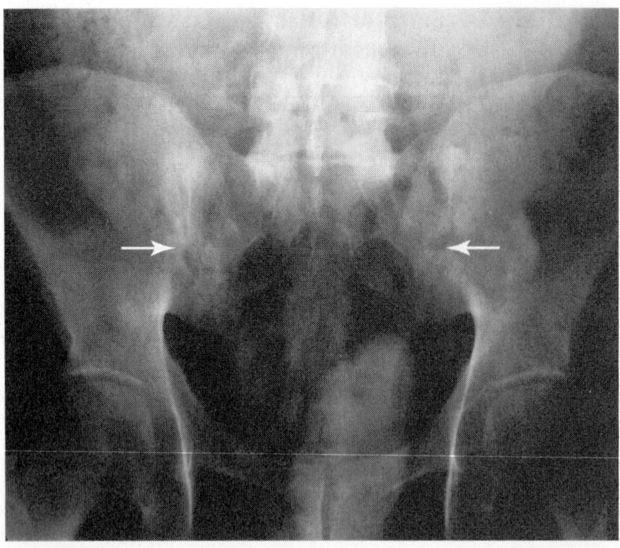

FIGURE 78.1. Radiographic changes of sacroiliitis indicated by bony sclerosis (*small arrow*) with joint space erosions (*large arrow*). (Courtesy John A. Flynn, MD, MBA.)

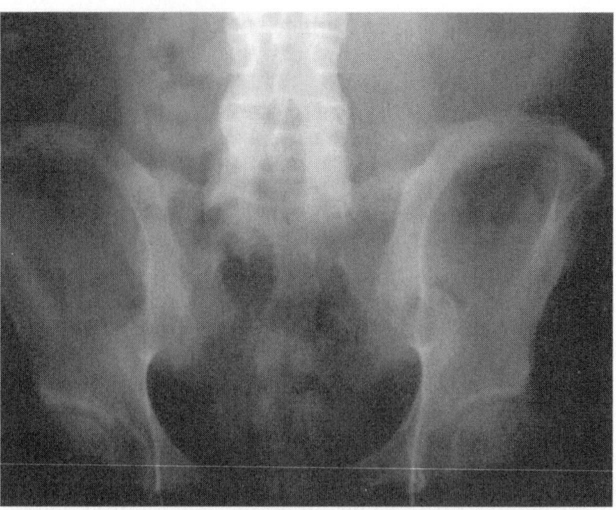

FIGURE 78.2. Late radiographic changes of sacroiliitis showing complete fusion of joint space (*small arrow*). Bridging syndesmophytes are present in the lumbar spine (*large arrow*). (Courtesy John A. Flynn, MD, MBA.)

Apical pulmonary fibrosis, sometimes with cavity formation, is rare and usually of no clinical consequence. This radiographic abnormality may mimic tuberculosis, and vice versa.

Laboratory Evaluation

Radiographic evaluation of the sacroiliac joints is the single most specific test for this disorder. Although a diagnosis of spondyloarthritis can be suspected based on the history and physical examination, definitive diagnosis cannot be established without radiographic findings. A single anteroposterior view of the pelvis may be adequate to define sacroiliitis; however, Ferguson or oblique views may be necessary to evaluate fully the integrity of the sacroiliac joints (2,13). The earliest radiographic change usually is bony sclerosis on the iliac sides of the joint margins. Thereafter, bony erosions occur (Fig. 78.1). There is eventual fusion across the joint space with subsequent loss of the early sclerotic changes (Fig. 78.2). Sacroiliitis often is confused with the radiographic anomaly *osteitis condensans ilii,* a condition in which symmetrical sclerosis occurs on the iliac side of each sacroiliac joint without any erosions. This finding is most common in young women who have borne children.

An early radiographic finding on lateral lumbar spine films is squaring of the vertebral bodies. This phenomenon also may be seen in the thoracic and cervical regions. The apophyseal joints of the spine become fused and, presumably because of surrounding inflammation and resulting immobility, diffuse osteoporosis ensues. Calcification and ossification of the ligamentous structures between vertebral bodies result in the characteristic syndesmophytes seen on radiograph (i.e., the bamboo spine). Large "flowing" syndesmophytes, typically most prominent in the right thoracic spine but also common in the lumbar and cervical areas, are seen in another disease, diffuse idiopathic skeletal hyperostosis (Fig. 78.3), which may clinically and radiographically mimic ankylosing spondylitis. Such patients usually can be discriminated by disease onset in late middle age and the absence of sacroiliitis. Computed tomography and magnetic resonance imaging are more sensitive than conventional x-ray films in early disease but are more expensive (13) (Fig. 78.4). Typing for HLA-B27 may be a more practical diagnostic approach when x-ray films are not definitively abnormal (3) (see below).

Hematologic studies usually are normal. However, a mild normocytic–normochromic anemia reflective of chronic disease may be seen in patients with severe disease. The white blood cell count usually is normal, as is the platelet count, although patients with highly inflammatory disease may demonstrate mild thrombocytosis. The erythrocyte sedimentation rate (ESR) and C-reactive protein (CRP) concentration frequently are elevated. *Serologic studies* for rheumatoid factor and antinuclear antibodies are negative, and serum complement levels are normal.

On tissue typing, HLA-B27 occurs in 85% to 90% of patients with spondyloarthritis. However, this genetic marker also occurs in 8% to 10% of the normal white American population (see Prevalence). It must be emphasized that indiscriminate HLA typing cannot be substituted for a thorough clinical and radiographic evaluation of the patient. In fact, determination of B27 is rarely needed in making the diagnosis of spondyloarthritis. Under unusual circumstances, however, the patient gives a strong history

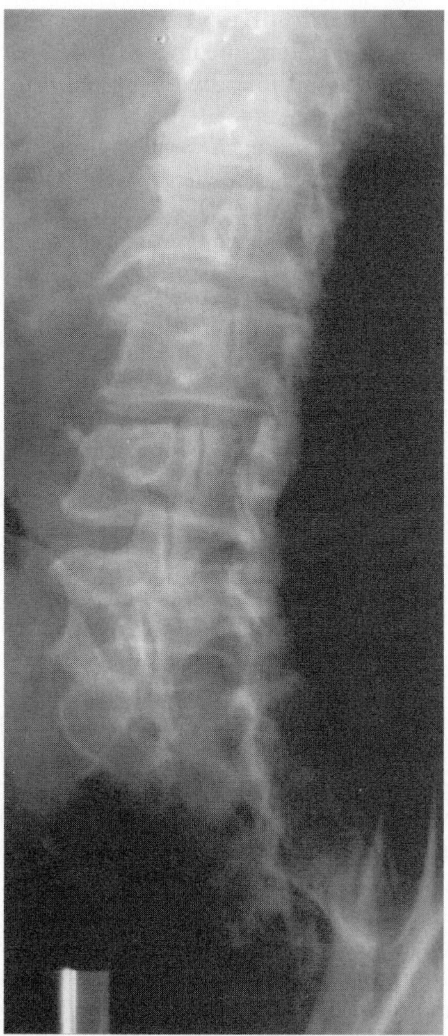

FIGURE 78.3. Diffuse idiopathic skeletal hyperostosis may be misdiagnosed as ankylosing spondylitis. This radiograph shows "flowing" osteophytes (*arrow*). In this condition, sacroiliitis is absent. (Courtesy John A. Flynn, MD, MBA.)

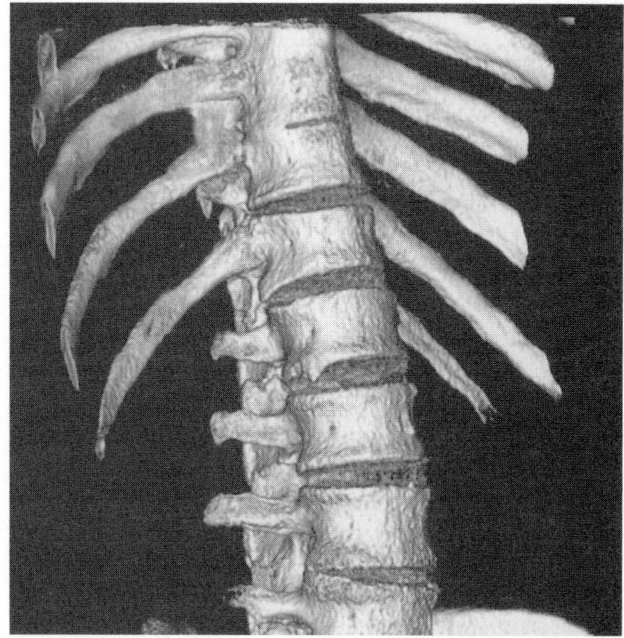

FIGURE 78.4. High-resolution computed tomography of ankylosing spondylitis showing vertebral fusion (*large arrow*) and syndesmophytes (*small arrow*). (From M. Ward, NIAMS, NIH, DHHS. Courtesy John A. Flynn, MD, MBA.)

suggestive of inflammatory axial skeletal disease but the x-ray films are not yet diagnostic of sacroiliitis. In such situations, HLA typing may be helpful, as well as in women with early or atypical disease (14). Even then, a positive B27 does not establish a diagnosis of sacroiliitis but only provides supporting data for the diagnosis when the most specific finding (radiographic sacroiliitis) is not present. In this setting, MRI is being more commonly used to determine any evidence of sacroiliac inflammation.

Many patients already know their B27 status or wish to have the test performed because of the hereditary impact of disease on their family. In these circumstances, one must offer proper genetic counseling. The facts should be simply presented to the patient as they are currently known. It should be emphasized that ankylosing spondylitis usually is not a life-threatening or crippling disorder and that symptoms can be controlled medically in most patients. The likelihood that a family member will develop inflammatory back disease is low. Because HLA antigens, including B27, are inherited in a mendelian dominant fashion, the risk of inheriting this tissue antigen type is 50% for each of a patient's children (this assumes that the patient is heterozygous and the other parent is negative for B27). Even if a child inherits this tissue antigen type, the likelihood of developing arthritis is only approximately 20% (5). Therefore, without any knowledge of HLA status, every child of a patient with B27-positive ankylosing spondylitis has an approximately 10% (50% × 20%) chance of developing ankylosing spondylitis. The 90% probability of never developing this form of arthritis must be emphasized to patients concerned about this hereditary factor.

Diagnostic Criteria

Table 78.5 summarizes the diagnostic criteria for ankylosing spondylitis.

Management

It is impossible to predict the ultimate course of any patient with sacroiliitis. The inflammatory process may remain confined to these isolated joints, or it may involve the lumbar, thoracic, and cervical spinal segments. Likewise, the duration of time from onset of symptoms to fusion of spinal segments is highly variable (15). Thus, each patient

TABLE 78.5 Modified New York Diagnostic Criteria for Ankylosing Spondylitis[a]

Clinical
1. Low back pain of at least 3 month's duration improved by exercise and not relieved by rest
2. Limitation of lumbar spine in sagittal and frontal planes
3. Limitation of chest expansion relative to normal value for age and gender
4. Unilateral sacroiliitis grade 3 (moderate sacroiliitis) or grade 4 (fusion across the joint) or bilateral sacroiliitis grade 2 (minimal sacroiliitis) to 4

[a]Definite ankylosing spondylitis = criteria 4 with at least one other clinical criterion. Modified from van der Linden SM, Valkenburg HA, Cats A. Evaluation of diagnostic criteria for ankylosing spondylitis: a proposal for modification of New York criteria. Arthritis Rheum 1984;27:361.

should understand the nature of the illness and the need for *continued medical surveillance,* as well as the principles of physical and pharmacologic management of the disorder (Table 78.6).

Pharmacologic

Nonsteroidal anti-inflammatory drugs (NSAIDs) are used to relieve the pain and stiffness of the disease and to promote the patient's ability to perform the physical exercises so important to maintaining a good posture. Most often NSAID use is required throughout the patient's life. However, occasionally when symptoms completely remit the NSAID can be tapered over several weeks and reinstituted if symptoms recur. Silent progression of the disease may occur; therefore, the clinician should closely monitor these patients even when they are not taking medication.

Indomethacin (Indocin) is especially effective therapy in many patients in dosages up to 75 to 150 mg/day. A number of side effects are important to consider (discussed in detail in Chapter 77). Other NSAIDs also can be useful in patients intolerant of indomethacin, especially tolmetin in doses of 600 mg three times daily (see Chapter 77). Aspirin usually is ineffective. Low-dose prednisone (≤10 mg/day) occasionally is necessary, especially in patients with peripheral arthritis or enthesitis, but should not be used in the long term.

Sulfasalazine (Azulfidine), a drug used for inflammatory bowel disease, has been found to be effective therapy for ankylosing spondylitis, especially early in the disease and when peripheral joints are involved (16,17). Its mechanism of action is unknown but is presumed to be anti-inflammatory or antimicrobial. An enteric-coated preparation should be given starting at 500 mg/day for 1 week and gradually increased thereafter to total dosages of 2 to 3 g/day (1 g two to three times per day). Adverse reactions are common and include anorexia, headache, nausea, vomiting, gastric distress, and reversible oligospermia in men. Serious blood dyscrasias (aplastic anemia, agranulocytosis, thrombocytopenia), hypersensitivity reactions, hepatic or renal damage, and central nervous system reactions occur occasionally, and complete blood counts and urinalyses should be monitored. Absorption of folic acid and digoxin are both reduced by sulfasalazine. Consultation with a rheumatologist is suggested before using this agent.

A small number of trials have used oral methotrexate in ankylosing spondylitis refractory to NSAIDs and sulfasalazine. A meta-analysis of these trials did not find a significant benefit of methotrexate (18).

Use of tumor necrosis factor (TNF) antagonists in the treatment of ankylosing spondylitis has led to impressive clinical improvement. However, not all patients with ankylosing spondylitis require TNF inhibitors. Guidelines have been developed by international consensus to facilitate the judicious use of this therapy (19). The agents currently approved are the TNF-α receptor protein etanercept (50 mg subcutaneously weekly) and the anti–TNF-α chimeric monoclonal antibody infliximab (eventual dosing of 3–5 mg/kg infusion every 8 weeks). Studies of these agents have demonstrated efficacy in reducing symptoms of ankylosing spondylitis (20,21) as well as markers of inflammation, including CRP and ESR, within several weeks of initiation of therapy.

For patients who have responded to anti-TNF agents, continued therapy usually is necessary and generally well tolerated (22). Discontinuation of therapy may result in reactivation of the disease within several months' time (23). Although these agents have been a remarkable advance in the therapy of ankylosing spondylitis, their use provokes many unanswered questions regarding long-term safety, the proper timing of initiation of therapy, and the potential role of future biologic agents in combination when such agents become available. These medications should be used under the supervision of a rheumatologist.

Radiation therapy to the spine once was an effective means of relieving pain. This form of treatment is no longer recommended because of the risk of subsequent leukemia.

TABLE 78.6 Principles of Management in Ankylosing Spondylitis

Ensure patient understands disease process and objectives of management.
Alleviate pain and stiffness with appropriate medications.
Use physical measures to maintain posture and range of motion in affected areas.
Prevent disease progression?

Physical Measures

Although these drugs relieve the pain and stiffness of ankylosing spondylitis, an equally important function is their promotion of the patient's ability to perform the physical therapy necessary to prevent spinal deformity and loss of motion in the joints. In fact, such a program usually cannot be instituted until symptoms have been brought under control. The natural history of the disease should be explained so that the patient understands the rationale for the exercise program that must be followed (and that the clinician must reinforce) over many years. An erect posture when sitting or standing should be encouraged. The patient's bed should be firm, and the smallest pillow possible should be used to prevent neck flexion. Sleeping in the prone position is most efficacious in promoting spinal extension, but the supine position is adequate if there is good support. The patient should refrain from sleeping on the side in a curled up position.

An active exercise program to promote extension of the back and increase range of motion of the axial and peripheral joints, as well as breathing exercises to maintain chest expansion, should be performed two to three times per day. Referral to a physical therapist who will provide specific instructions and determine that the patient is performing well is a good investment. Swimming is an excellent recreational exercise for the patient with ankylosing spondylitis. If spinal structures undergo complete ankylosis, the danger of spinal fracture after even minor trauma is increased. This is especially true in the neck, where whiplash types of injury occur.

Prognosis

The prognosis for patients with ankylosing spondylitis is excellent. Most patients can be treated successfully by pharmacologic and physical means. Most continue to lead productive lives, and change in vocational plans usually is not indicated. The morbidity from articular and extra-articular complications is low, and lifespan is not reduced significantly, if at all. In many instances, pain in an affected area of the spine disappears after that segment has fused, and often disease halts at a particular segment and does not proceed to others. Although these facts should be optimistically presented to the patient, they are not cause for complacency in following the postural and exercise program and in maintaining close medical surveillance.

REACTIVE ARTHRITIS

Definition

Reactive arthritis is a disorder that occurs after certain genitourinary or GI infections (5). Studies have demonstrated bacterial antigens from the triggering microbe in the synovial fluid and tissue of patients with reactive arthritis. Moreover, there is increasing evidence for persistence of dormant microorganisms known to be associated with reactive arthritis (see Laboratory Evaluation) in the gut, genitourinary tract, and even the joints in patients with this disease (24,25).

TABLE 78.7 Clues to Diagnosis of Reactive Arthritis

Young person with arthritis
Symptoms
Preceding diarrhea, urethritis, or conjunctivitis
Lower extremity oligoarthritis (knee, ankle, foot)
Heel pain or sausaging of digits
Rash on soles, penis; painless oral ulcers; dystrophic nails
Fever, weight loss, leukocytosis
HLA-B27 antigen

Unlike ankylosing spondylitis, reactive arthritis is primarily a peripheral arthritis. However, it shares with ankylosing spondylitis a predisposition to affect young people and a tendency for sacroiliitis, spondylitis, enthesitis, uveitis, the same cardiac complications, and a strong association with HLA-B27 (60%–75% positive). Although it was classically defined as the triad of nongonococcal urethritis, conjunctivitis, and arthritis (Reiter syndrome), it has been found that most patients do not express the classic triad and that approximately 40% of patients have arthritis as the only feature. Diagnosis depends on recognition of the typical pattern of arthritis, the presence of mucocutaneous lesions, and other features that are discriminating (5). The diagnosis and management of the disease focus primarily on symptoms and signs referable to the joints and on nonarticular musculoskeletal structures. The diagnosis is made on clinical grounds based on a constellation of symptoms and signs. Typing for HLA-B27 may be a useful diagnostic aid in the incomplete or atypical case (1).

History and Examination

Table 78.7 summarizes the principal clues to the diagnosis of reactive arthritis. The patient with reactive arthritis usually is a young white person between puberty and age 40 years. It rarely occurs in older patients. African Americans and Japanese (but not other Asians) are affected far less commonly, presumably because of the low frequency of HLA-B27 in these groups.

The disorder occurs in two main settings. First, the disease may follow an episode of diarrhea caused by *Shigella, Salmonella, Yersinia,* or *Campylobacter* (see Chapter 35). Second, the endemic form results primarily from venereal exposure, and *Chlamydia trachomatis* (see Chapters 37 and 102) is the most common causative agent. The sex ratio is equal in the postenteric form, but men appear to acquire the venereal form more often than women, although women with the disease are being recognized more often.

In the classic form, urethritis, usually painless or with mild dysuria and a mucopurulent discharge, is commonly the first symptom. It generally lasts only 1 to 2 weeks. *Conjunctivitis* usually follows shortly. This is most often mild with redness, weeping, and morning crusting. Generally, the conjunctivitis lasts only a few days. Photophobia is unusual, and its presence suggests uveitis (see below). Arthritis usually is the last feature of the triad to appear, usually from several days up to 1 month after the onset of urethritis. The *arthritis* typically is in the lower extremities, involving only one to four joints, most commonly the knees, ankles, and small joints of the feet. The patient notes pain, swelling, heat, and erythema over the joints. In addition to arthritis, >50% of patients have *nonarticular musculoskeletal pain* caused by inflammation of the insertion of tendons or fascia (enthesitis). Heel pain caused by inflammation of the plantar aponeurosis or of the Achilles tendon insertion is one of the most prominent symptoms of the disease and may be one of the most disabling. Diffuse swelling of digits (sausaging), especially the toes, occurs in >50% of patients and indicates involvement not only of the joints but of tendons and periosteal structures.

The *mucocutaneous features* of reactive arthritis often are asymptomatic and must be sought on physical examination. These include painless shallow oral ulcers, usually on the tongue and palate; circinate balanitis (Fig. 78.5; see also Color Plate) manifested by shallow moist painless ulcers on the glans penis in uncircumcised men or a dry scaling eruption on the glans in circumcised men; keratoderma blennorrhagica, a papulosquamous skin eruption usually beginning on the palms or soles (Fig. 78.6; see also Color Plate) and closely resembling pustular psoriasis; and onychodystrophy (Fig. 78.7). These lesions last for a highly variable period (several days to several months).

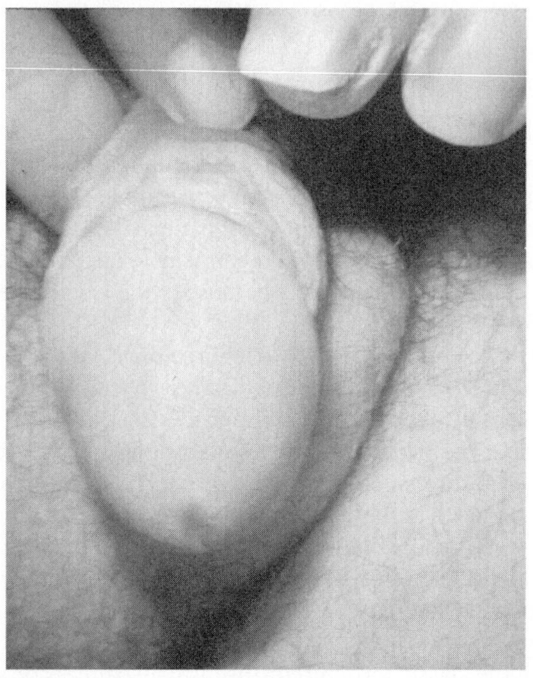

FIGURE 78.5. Moist shallow circular lesions characteristic of circinate balanitis. (Courtesy John A. Flynn, MD, MBA.)

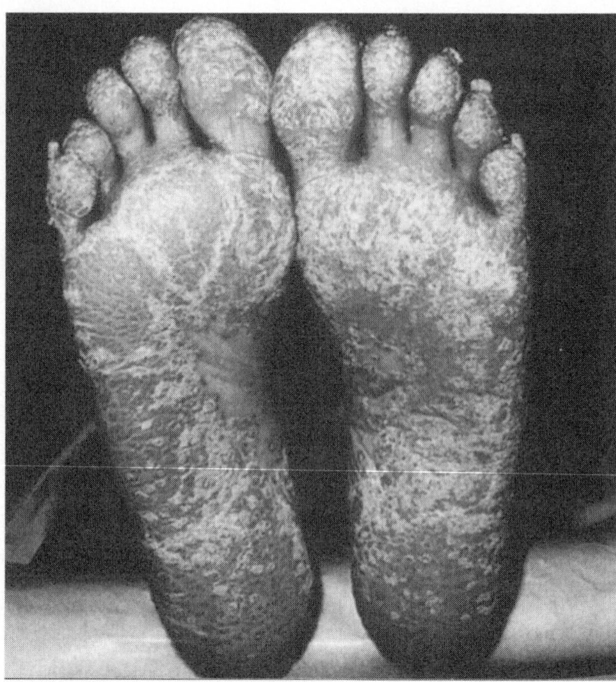

FIGURE 78.6. Extensive keratoderma blennorrhagica involving the soles. (From Provost TT, Flynn JA. Cutaneous medicine: cutaneous manifestations of systemic disease. Hamilton, Ontario: BC Decker, 2001, with permission. Courtesy John A. Flynn, MD, MBA.)

Additional features include fever in approximately one third of patients, weight loss, and uveitis. The disease may begin abruptly and run a toxic course, or begin insidiously and pursue an indolent course. Often, heel pain (see Chapter 73) is the first symptom, and this complaint should raise the question of reactive arthritis.

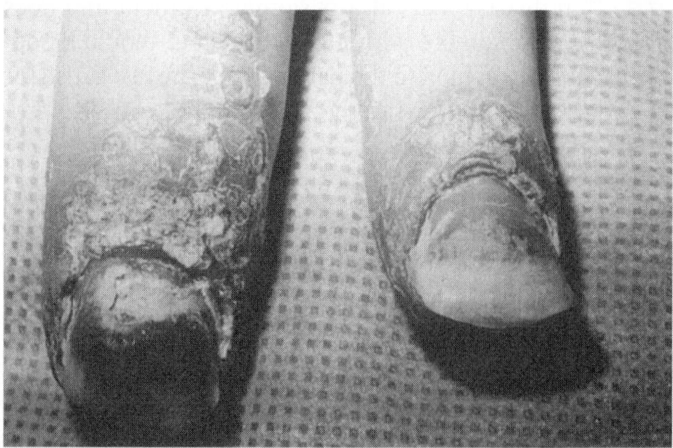

FIGURE 78.7. Onychodystrophy fingernail in reactive arthritis. (From Provost TT, Flynn JA. Cutaneous medicine: cutaneous manifestations of systemic disease. Hamilton, Ontario: BC Decker, 2001, with permission. Courtesy John A. Flynn, MD, MBA.)

offspring of diabetic parents is presently impossible. Even statistical estimates are crude. The prevalence of overt diabetes in offspring of conjugal type 1 diabetic parents is remarkably low, ranging from 3% to 12% in most reports (12). Only 2.5% of siblings of type 1 diabetic patients develop diabetes; when tested initially, these people may show only impaired glucose tolerance (IGT).

If expression of disease in type 1 diabetes was based entirely on genetics, one would expect 100% concordance for diabetes in monozygotic twins. However, this is not the case; both members of pairs develop diabetes only about one-third of the time (13). Thus, environmental factors also must be important (14).

Parents who have a child with insulin-dependent diabetes often wish to know the risk to future offspring. Prenatal histocompatibility leukocyte antigen (HLA) typing of fetal cells obtained at amniocentesis could be compared with that of the sibling with diabetes. A fetus with the same HLA identity would have an increased risk, but the accuracy of the prediction would still be only approximately 50%. The imprecise nature of this assessment is in contrast to the nearly 100% certainty of predicting Tay-Sachs disease or Down syndrome. Thus, even with an accurate family history and pedigree, together with chemical assessment of diabetes (glucose tolerance testing), only crude predictions can be made for a couple who wish to know their own chances of developing diabetes and the risk for their offspring.

At this point, only a few generalities seem safe. Prospective parents should not be told to avoid procreation merely because one parent has diabetes. Even when both parents have diabetes, the risk of having a child likely to develop diabetes is relatively low.

Type 2 Diabetes Mellitus

Type 2 diabetes is often only one component of a complex of abnormalities variously termed the *metabolic syndrome, syndrome X,* the *metabolic syndrome X,* or the *insulin-resistance syndrome* (15). Hyperinsulinemia with or without obvious hyperglycemia is present and denotes the presence of insulin resistance. Other components of the syndrome are obesity (central type), hypertension, fasting and postprandial hyperlipidemia, abnormal concentrations of blood coagulation factors, and premature cardiovascular atherosclerosis. Its pathogenesis remains unclear.

Obesity may be the first manifestation of the metabolic syndrome. Only after some years does an obvious state of diabetes emerge in which all or most of the various features of the metabolic syndrome also become apparent. As the condition evolves, insulin resistance progresses to glucose intolerance and finally to diagnosable type 2 diabetes.

Type 2 diabetes is the most common form of diabetes mellitus and accounts for approximately 80% of patients presenting with an overt abnormality of glucose metabolism. Ordinarily, patients with type 2 disease are neither absolutely dependent on treatment with insulin nor ketosis prone. Nonetheless, some patients being treated with oral hypoglycemic drugs may require insulin to control hyperglycemia or ketoacidosis during stress. Most patients are older than age 40 years at the time of diagnosis, but this type of disease is also seen in young people, which is why older terms such as *maturity-onset diabetes* have been abandoned.

A current concept of the evolution of the common form of type 2 disease is that obesity-related insulin resistance is superimposed on an individual with a limited ability to secrete sufficient insulin (i.e., β-cell dysfunction, presumably genetic) to compensate for the insulin resistance. In this scenario, obesity-related insulin resistance is the immediate cause of the glucose intolerance (hyperglycemia). Without obesity, an overt diabetic state would presumably not develop (16). However, 10% to 15% of type 2 patients are not obese. Some of these individuals are also insulin resistant, presumably secondary to other causes, perhaps genetic as well, but not all of the cases are, in fact, insulin resistant. At this point, the scenario becomes more speculative because longitudinal data on individual patients are not available. Long-standing hyperinsulinemia may eventually diminish, the result of progressive impairment in the patient's ability to secrete insulin, possibly as a result of the accumulation in pancreatic islets of amylin, an amyloid-like protein. The degree of β-cell "exhaustion" is related in part to the duration of the illness. Some patients ultimately develop insulinopenia to the point that they become totally dependent on exogenous insulin and are at risk of developing ketoacidosis if stressed.

Included in the group of type 2 diabetic patients are those who develop the disease before they reach adulthood Maturity Onset Diabetes of the Young (MODY). These young adults (or older children) have what was once considered to be a "variant" of type 2 diabetes shown to be a heterogeneous genetic disorder; usually they are not obese (11). MODY is relatively rare in most populations, accounting for approximately 2% of all cases of type 2 disease (17), but it may be increasing in prevalence. MODY should not be confused with a more common problem: An increasing number of children and young adults are becoming obese and developing "ordinary" type 2 diabetes. This problem is considered to be of epidemic proportions in the United States (18) and is also seen worldwide, mostly in children older than the age of 10 years. When diabetes is diagnosed, most prove to have a strong family history of type 2 diabetes. Nonobese young diabetic individuals should be tested for autoantibodies and C peptide to exclude type 1 diabetes and if these tests are negative or low, respectively, MODY should be considered.

Atypical diabetes is a variant of type 2 diabetes that was first described in adults who seemed to have type 2 but who developed ketoacidosis during stress and required control with insulin. Adult African American patients exhibit this response with some regularity, and it was recently seen in obese African American children. When the ketoacidosis is seen in a child, the issue of type 1 disease is raised, but obesity is the clinical clue that "atypical diabetes" is the correct diagnosis. MODY does not need to be considered in African Americans; to date, it has been described only in whites, Japanese, and, rarely, Chinese persons.

Behavioral, and possibly environmental, factors appear to be involved in the onset of type 2 diabetes. Especially prominent is the role of excessive caloric intake and subsequent obesity in most cases. Although it is clear that obesity somehow aggravates the underlying genetic predisposition for the development of the metabolic abnormalities of the diabetic state and that weight loss often ameliorates them (above), it is also clear that the factors driving the development of obesity are themselves multifactorial. In type 2 diabetes, association with certain HLA subtypes and with antibodies to islet cells has not been found. Blood insulin levels vary depending on the stage of the disease and may be supranormal in the early years and subnormal later in the disease. Insulin resistance is the rule, but measurement of insulin concentration has no clinically diagnostic or therapeutic usefulness. Measurement of insulin C peptide is sometimes useful, along with antibody determinations (see the discussion of LADA under Type 1 Diabetes Mellitus and Its Slowly Progressive Form).

Inheritance

Type 2 diabetes mellitus is genetically and clinically heterogeneous (17,19) with a much more obvious familial pattern of expression than type 1 disease. Impaired first-phase insulin secretion is the earliest detectable abnormality in type 2 disease and is commonly abnormal in the first-degree relatives of patients with type 2 disease, even when their conventionally measured oral glucose tolerance is normal. In contrast to type 1 diabetes mellitus, there is essentially complete concordance for type 2 diabetes in monozygotic twins (20).

Studies of ethnic groups show distinctive patterns of inheritance of type 2 diabetes and superimposed geographic (environmental) effects on these patterns. The most easily apparent correlate is obesity. Certain Native American tribes (e.g., Pima, Navajo) show a remarkably high prevalence of diabetes, with approximately 50% of the adults having the disease; obesity appears to be the major factor in expression of diabetes in these groups. The Hispanic population (Mexican American) of the southwestern United States also shows similar, but less frequent, expressions of obesity and diabetes. In nonnative populations in the United States, no such distinctive ethnic or racial patterns in the pathology of type 2 diabetes have been recognized to date.

TABLE 79.2 Diseases Associated with Diabetes Mellitus

Obesity	Autoimmune disorders
Endocrine disorders	Adrenal insufficiency (Addison disease)
Acromegaly	Thyroid disease
Aldosteronism	Hypoparathyroidism
Glucocorticoid excess (Cushing syndrome; iatrogenic)	Myasthenia gravis
Pheochromocytoma	Pernicious anemia
Thyrotoxicosis from any cause	Polyglandular failure (adrenals, gonads, thyroid)
Somatostatinoma	Primary hypothyroidism
	Graves hyperthyroidism

Other Types of Diabetes

Sometimes diabetes is associated with another disease (Tables 79.1 and 79.2); usually the association is infrequent but more common than in the general population. This heterogeneous group includes some disorders in which there is a clear relationship between the associated disease and the diabetes (e.g., chronic pancreatitis) and many others in which an association has been noted but is not well understood (e.g., primary hyperaldosteronism).

Problems in Classification of Individual Patients

On occasion, classification may be difficult. For example, an adult with ketoacidosis may be erroneously classified as a type 1 diabetic when the diabetes is type 2, with insulin dependence having been precipitated by the temporary stress of infection or trauma (see the discussion of "atypical diabetes" under Type 2 Diabetes Mellitus). Similarly, the process of distinguishing between a patient with type 1 diabetes and a thin patient with type 2 disease for whom insulin has been prescribed may require diagnostic procedures to exclude the possibility that the diabetes is one of the "other types" (Table 79.2).

CLINICAL PRESENTATION

Most diagnoses of diabetes mellitus are now made at an asymptomatic stage of the disease as a result of routine blood tests that reveal elevation of plasma glucose (PG) concentration. When the diagnosis is actively sought, oral glucose tolerance tests (OGTTs) reveal additional cases because up to one-fourth of patients with a diagnostic OGTT have a normal fasting plasma glucose (FPG) concentration. Unless the fasting glucose is elevated, patients do not have enough glucosuria to become symptomatic. Of patients with overt hyperglycemia who are symptomatic at time of diagnosis, most complain of polyuria, which is caused by the osmotic diuresis induced by the glucosuria; polydipsia; and, if the disease is very severe, polyphagia, often associated with weight loss if the increased food intake falls short of full compensation for the caloric loss that results from heavy glucosuria. All these symptoms are manifestations of hyperglycemia and secondary glucosuria. Other symptomatic manifestations include blurred vision (osmolality-related changes in the shape of the lens of the eyes), vaginitis (usually caused by monilial infection), and skin infections. Furuncles and carbuncles, once common, are now rarely seen, but intertriginous candidiasis is common in the obese, and thrush is common in patients with poor oral hygiene or poorly fitting dentures.

Usually, these symptoms are present for weeks or months before medical attention is sought. The onset of symptoms is often insidious and may be attributed by the patient, or even by the clinician, to emotional factors or a common problem such as a urinary tract infection. Indeed, the diagnosis may be missed for a time because the clinician, failing to consider the evolving character of the disease, believes that the patient does not have diabetes on the basis of previous evaluation.

Many patients with type 2 diabetes present with minimal or no symptoms of hyperglycemia and glucosuria but have already developed complications such as neuropathy or, more commonly, vascular disease. Also, it is common to encounter patients who believe that their long-standing diabetes is "mild" only to find themselves with severe complications of the disease. Occasionally, a patient may be completely unaware of having diabetes and yet present with retinopathy or nephropathy.

DIAGNOSIS

Hyperglycemia is the hallmark of diabetes mellitus. Glucosuria alone is not a pathognomonic finding because rare patients may have a renal tubular glucose leak (renal glucosuria) at normal concentrations of blood sugar. Often, patients show diagnostic hyperglycemia (fasting; postglucose load in a glucose tolerance test; or, postprandially) before glucosuria develops.

Criteria for Diagnosis of Diabetes Mellitus

The following revised criteria were established in 2003 by the Expert Committee of the ADA (2): (a) unequivocal elevation of PG concentrations associated with classic symptoms of diabetes mellitus, or (b) elevation of FPG on more than one occasion, or (c) elevation of PG after an oral glucose challenge (standardized OGTT) on more than one occasion. A *single* elevated FPG or a *single* OGTT does not establish the diagnosis (Table 79.3).

The ADA's decision (2) to promote the FPG, with a new and lower cut point rather than the OGTT as the primary basis for a diagnosis of diabetes, was based in part on the practical consideration that few physicians were performing glucose tolerance tests in any event and that the OGTT would best be reserved for research purposes. They further argued that, because of its simplicity, careful attention to the FPG would result overall in a larger number of diagnoses of diabetes than was being made with the OGTT. The diagnostic cut point of 126 mg/dL (7.0 mmol/L) is not arbitrary; it is the level in several studies at which the risk begins for the development of diabetic retinopathy, whereas 110 mg/dL is the point above which acute-phase insulin secretion is lost in response to intravenously administered glucose, the hallmark of early diabetes. The ADA did not completely abandon the OGTT or modify its long-time cut points in the OGTT; a diagnosis of diabetes is established by *either* an elevated FPG *or* the OGTT. Nonetheless, a number of studies of different populations have shown that many fewer diagnoses of diabetes will be made when the ADA's fasting glucose limit is used, even though the new fasting diagnostic level is lower than the old one of 140 mg/dL. These studies clearly show that ADA's criteria for diagnosis are less sensitive than the OGTT (10). There is also poor correlation between the new category of impaired fasting glucose (IFG, see below) and IGT, the latter term applying only to the values obtained using the OGTT (Table 79.3). There is also poor correlation between the new category of impaired fasting glucose (IFG) and impaired glucose tolerance (IGT), the latter term applying only to the values obtained using the OGTT (Table 79.3) (see Impaired Fasting Glucose and Impaired Glucose Tolerance).

TABLE 79.3 Interpretation of Values for Plasma Glucose

Test	*Value (mg/dL)*	*Interpretation*
Fasting PG (no caloric intake for at least 8 h)	<100	Normal
	100–125	Impaired fasting glucose (see text)
	≥126	Provisional diagnosis of diabetes mellitus[a]
Oral glucose tolerance test[b] (OGTT), 2-h PG	<140	Normal
	140–199	Impaired glucose tolerance (see text)
	≥200	Provisional[a] diagnosis of diabetes mellitus

PG, plasma glucose.
[a]The diagnosis must be confirmed on another day according to the criteria described in the text.
[b]OGTT is performed in fasting patients by administration of 75 g of glucose dissolved in water following the standards of the World Health Organization (see text).

In modern laboratories in the United States, glucose is determined in plasma or serum. Plasma and serum values are identical, but both are 5% to 15% higher than those obtained in whole blood from which they are derived. Portable devices for measuring blood glucose are not sufficiently accurate to be used in diagnosis, and abnormal "fingerstick" results should be confirmed with standard tests on venous blood.

Fasting Plasma Glucose

The ADA cut point for making a diagnosis of diabetes is a FPG ≥126 mg/dL (Table 79.3). Two values of 126 mg/dL (7.0 mmol/L) or greater obtained on different days are needed for a definitive diagnosis. Values above 100 mg/dL and less than 126 mg/dL designate *impaired fasting glucose*. It should be remembered that FPG may be elevated transiently by stress or illness.

Oral Glucose Tolerance Test

The OGTT, for many years an accepted diagnostic standard for the diagnosis of type 2 diabetes, is no longer recommended by the ADA for routine clinical use (see Criteria for Diagnosis of Diabetes Mellitus). It is less convenient, more costly, and more variable than the FPG; it is, however, more sensitive for establishing a definitive diagnosis. The test still has a place in diagnosis during pregnancy.

Table 79.3 lists the diagnostic criteria for the OGTT. The test may be falsely abnormal in people who have had a recent stressful illness, have had a reduced food intake (less than 150 g carbohydrate per day), or who have been taking one of a variety of drugs (e.g., glucocorticoids and most diuretics). Even smoking or caffeine or performance of the test in the afternoon can cause an abnormal test result. Also, the values in the OGTT tend to increase with age; that is also true of the FPG, but the latter increase with age is very small.

Measurement of a random 2-hour postprandial blood sugar should never be done for screening purposes; it has low sensitivity, specificity, and reliability.

Previous and Potential Abnormalities of Glucose Tolerance

According to the currently accepted scheme, people with a normal OGTT who previously showed either IGT or overt hyperglycemia should be classified as having a "previous abnormality of glucose tolerance." These people should not be considered diabetic and should not be labeled with the terms *prediabetic* or *latent diabetic*. Terms such as *subclinical, preclinical, chemical,* and *borderline diabetes* should also be avoided.

Impaired Fasting Glucose and Impaired Glucose Tolerance

Patients whose FPG levels or whose glucose levels obtained during an OGTT fall between normal and diabetes (Table 79.3) are now classified by the ADA into a group having *impaired fasting glucose*. The term *impaired glucose tolerance* separates those with glucose intolerance during an OGTT from those who meet the diagnostic criteria for diabetes mellitus.

Significance of Impaired Fasting Glucose or Impaired Glucose Tolerance for Development of Diabetes and Cardiovascular Disease

Both IFG and IGT are risk factors for the development of diabetes. In this combined group, one can expect 1% to 5% per year to develop diagnosable diabetes mellitus. On the other hand, many patients eventually show normalization of glucose tolerance, and still others remain in the IFG or IGT range. The higher the blood sugar within the range of IGT, the greater the tendency to progress to diabetes (21).

Perhaps some of the most convincing evidence on IGT progression has come from long-term studies of Pima Indians (22). The risk of progression to overt diabetes in this group is clearly related to the level of glucose within the range of 160 to 200 mg at 2 hours (three times the risk of that of people with lower values). In this group, however, the rate of decompensation to overt diabetes is still only 3% per year.

Studies of treatment of patients with IFG or IGT with oral antidiabetic (hypoglycemic) agents to prevent or delay the eventual development of diabetes are in progress. Metformin has been shown to have a modest effect (see Prevention of Diabetes Mellitus).

However, IFG and IGT are generally considered to be risk factors for cardiovascular disease (21). Moreover, even the level of fasting blood glucose within the normal range clearly modestly predicts cardiovascular death in nondiabetic men (24). There is no risk of *microvascular* complications (retinopathy or nephropathy) in people with IFG or IGT unless they develop diabetes.

PREVENTION OF DIABETES MELLITUS

Prospective studies show that altering "lifestyle," by modifying diet and increasing physical activity, can prevent or delay the development of diabetes in high-risk patients showing IGT (25). Reduction of progression from IGT to diabetes ranged from 31% to 58% over 3 to 6 years. Whether similar results could be obtained under nonstudy conditions is problematic. Modest weight reduction (mean: about 8.8 lb [4 kg] or 5% to 7% of body weight) and exercise (widely variable but about 2 to 4 hours per week) seem to be the most important contributors to success. Other studies have identified consumption of fiber from cereals and a low glycemic index as contributors to prevention. Total fat intake and type do not seem to relate to the development of diabetes.

A large multicenter randomized prospective study in the United States (Diabetes Prevention Program) included a group who were treated with metformin but who did not receive the other interventions (26). These individuals showed a more modest decrease in the rate at which diabetes developed over the 3 years of study. Metformin is not approved for such preventive use.

TREATMENT OF DIABETES MELLITUS

Patient Education

For all patients with diabetes, the following factors are important: the impact of diet and patterns of eating on diabetes, the implications of having diabetes on ordinary activities and of ordinary activities on diabetes, recognition of the signs of worsening diabetes, the importance of proper foot care and of regular eye examinations, and the clarification of misconceptions about diabetes. For patients receiving insulin, the following additional factors are important: correct administration and timing of insulin injections, the unique constraints that insulin therapy places on dietary management and changes of activity, recognition of the symptoms of hypoglycemia, and adjustment of insulin dosage during intercurrent illness.

Patient responses to being informed of a diagnosis of diabetes varies widely. Many patients already suspected the diagnosis as the result of previous observations of similar symptoms in family members. These patients are often aware of the complications of the disease (loss of vision, amputations) and the use of the needle (insulin self-administration). Transient or even prolonged anxiety or depression is common and should be anticipated by the caregiver. Similar problems at this time are commonly seen in close relatives or friends of the patient. Effective approaches to assisting patients with coping strategies are described in Chapters 4 and 20.

Many patients are reluctant to accept the need for self-injection of insulin, and many clinicians are unwilling to press the issue. The result is poor control, inappropriate use of oral hypoglycemic drugs, or both. Reluctance of both patient and clinician may stem from unfamiliarity with the techniques of insulin injection. In fact, insulin injection is simple and almost without discomfort. A firm attitude on the part of the clinician and input from nurses and, if necessary, other patients can overcome patient reluctance in almost all cases. The use of disposable syringes has eliminated the inconvenience of sterilization, and modern thin, very sharp, plastic-hubbed, or syringe-attached needles render the injections practically painless. Aspects of technique are described under Insulin Therapy.

A substantial proportion of newly diagnosed patients have difficulty making the behavioral changes required for optimal management of their illness. Hence, a multifaceted approach is required, which often involves a diabetes educator, a nutritionist, the primary caregiver, and an endocrinologist. The ADA is a useful resource as well for educational material (see www.hopkinsbayview.org/PAMreferences). General principles and strategies for educating, motivating, and empowering patients and for helping them make desired behavioral changes are discussed in Chapter 4.

Diet Therapy

Different diet strategies guide therapy for diabetes, depending on whether one is dealing with an obese patient with type 2 diabetes or a patient of appropriate weight who has type 1 disease. For the obese patient with type 2 diabetes, the immediate and long-term goal is weight reduction (see Chapter 83). In type 1 patients, timing of meals must be matched to the administration of insulin to prevent excessive postprandial hyperglycemia and to avoid hypoglycemia. In type 2 patients, timing of meals is still important, whether the patient is using insulin or oral hypoglycemic agents. Diet composition is shown in Table 79.4.

Most obese patients with type 2 diabetes are not severely symptomatic and do not require immediate therapy with insulin or oral hypoglycemic agents for control of symptoms; rather, diet therapy is instituted for correction of hyperglycemia and weight. The blood sugar may fall rapidly on initiation of a diet (i.e., within a few days). This effect is caused by caloric restriction and occurs before significant weight loss is seen. Oral agents, if used along with diet, have the advantage that they do not usually produce severe hypoglycemia, but simultaneous institution of a weight-reduction program and treatment with insulin can lead to hypoglycemia and must be done cautiously. No attempt at tight control should be made until active efforts to lose weight have ended. Some, perhaps 10%, of type 2 patients are not overweight. Such patients should not be advised to lose weight.

Population studies indicate that most type 2 diabetes is either made manifest by obesity in genetically predisposed persons or is actually caused by obesity. Overt diabetes in obese patients is potentially preventable or can be ameliorated by weight reduction; sometimes loss of even 5 or 10 pounds (4.5 kg) has a salutary effect. However, most patients are unable to achieve or maintain a weight that will reverse overt diabetes. In one study, a group of patients with IGT were shown to lose weight over a 1-year period using a reduced-fat diet (average weight loss 7.3 lb [3.3 kg]);

TABLE 79.4 Distribution of Major Nutrients in Diabetic Diets (United States)

	Nutrients (Percentage of Total Calories)						
				Fat			
	Starch and Other Complex Polysaccharides	*Sugars and Dextrins*	*Total Carbohydrates*	*Total*	*% Monounsaturated or Polyunsaturated*	*Protein*	*Alcohol*
Typical American diet	25–35	20–30	45–50	35–45	30	12–20	1–10
Current diabetic diets	40	10	50	30	50	20	—
Diet suggested by recent research	30	5	35	50	40 (monounsaturated or polyunsaturated) $\geq$10 (saturated)	15–20	1–10

this reduced the number of patients who progressed to diabetes. Over the following 4 years, however, weight was generally regained to baseline and glucose tolerance deteriorated (27).

A guiding principle for formulating diabetic diets should be the recognition that individual food preferences must be respected whenever possible. The dietitian should obtain the patient's preferred dietary history and then should attempt to construct the diet around these preferences. Such an approach is demanding for the dietitian, but the issuance of a standardized "American" diet to a patient from an ethnic minority who has diabetes is unlikely to be helpful. Chapter 83 on obesity and Chapter 4 on patient education deal with these principles in greater detail.

Prevention of Atherosclerosis

A goal of diet therapy, beyond weight reduction, is the prevention of atherosclerotic disease. This problem is both more prevalent and accelerated in all types of diabetes and accounts for approximately 25% of deaths among patients with type 1 diabetes with onset before age 20 years. Without treatment, adults with type 2 diabetes are two to four times more likely than those in the general population to die from coronary artery disease. A large portion of this excess mortality is undoubtedly caused by the abnormalities of lipids that are so common in diabetes mellitus.

The evidence that atherosclerosis in the patient with diabetes may be preventable is based to a large degree on comparisons of the prevalence of atherosclerotic disease in different populations with widely varying diets (28,29). The diabetic subjects in the United States who followed conventional, widely used, high-fat, low-carbohydrate diabetic diets—at least until about 1970—had the highest rate of coronary disease seen anywhere in the world (three times the rate of the general population). For this reason and because of the evidence from population studies, the ADA recommended that its old standard diabetic diets should be abandoned. Ironically, no strong evidence exists to support the notion that only the high-fat diets used for diabetes were responsible for the high rate of coronary atherosclerosis, although they sometimes contained up to 70% of calories as fat. Type 2 diabetes is now recognized to be part of a syndrome that includes hyperlipidemia and a propensity to the development of atherosclerosis, probably regardless of diet (see the discussion of the metabolic syndrome under Definition and Classification). Currently, the ADA recommends that diet should be individualized to accommodate individual preferences along ethnic lines, but also advocates a diet high in carbohydrates (50% of calories) and relatively low in fat (30%), a diet similar to that recommended by the American Heart Association for people without diabetes (Table 79.4).

The ADA nutritional recommendations are in general, but not completely, followed in this chapter. For details, the reader is referred to the ADA's position paper (30). Although such diets have been successfully used in diabetic patients studied on metabolic wards, their reported beneficial effects on blood lipids may result from other factors: control of caloric intake with concomitant weight reduction, very low cholesterol content, high fiber content, and absence of sucrose. Several studies in which patients with type 2 diabetes received such diets resulted in unchanged low-density lipoprotein (LDL) cholesterol, lowered high-density lipoprotein (HDL) cholesterol, and increased triglyceride levels (31,32), as well as in accentuated postprandial lipemia with accompanying potential for increased atherogenicity. In contrast, another study used a high monounsaturated fat diet (50% of calories) low in carbohydrates (35%) that resulted in improved PG, triglycerides, and HDL cholesterol when compared to the ADA diet (33). A later report comparing a high-carbohydrate (60% of calories) diet to a high-fat diet (40% of calories) rich in monounsaturates saw no differences in lipid profiles between these regimens (34). It is unclear whether seemingly small differences of carbohydrate and monounsaturated fat are critical or whether other factors are involved in this apparent discrepancy. The optimal diet for the control of blood lipids and glucose in the patient with diabetes must still be considered unsettled, but it is reasonable currently to recommend up to 50% of calories from fat, provided that it is high in monounsaturates, and 35% of calories from carbohydrates.

Role of Alcohol (Ethanol)

Objective discussion of the role of moderate amounts of alcohol (ethanol) in the diet is confounded by cultural, social, and religious considerations, and by concern for potential abuse and addiction. Moderate alcohol use in men is associated with decreased development of type 2 diabetes (35) and in women with diabetes, with a reduced risk of atherosclerotic heart disease (36). Therefore, given the high risk of atherosclerosis, it is reasonable, until evidence to the contrary is presented, for clinicians to tolerate moderate amounts of alcohol in the diet, especially if the patient is already a user of alcohol. In people without diabetes, two to three drinks per day for men and one to two per day for women seem to be optimal for reducing cardiovascular risks, although the dose–response is difficult to define (37). On the other hand, alcohol, especially when ingested in the fasting state, can readily produce hypoglycemia in both nondiabetic and diabetic individuals. Diabetics receiving oral agents and/or insulin are probably especially vulnerable to this effect of alcohol. Although alcohol generally increases HDL, which appears to be at least part of its mechanism in preventing cardiovascular disease (see Chapter 82), it induces hypertriglyceridemia. If lipid control proves difficult with ordinary therapy in a particular patient, attention should be paid to a possible contributing role of excessive alcohol consumption, which may be unreported. Alcohol can also induce or worsen hypertension, another major problem in diabetes.

Role of Hyperglycemic Control in Control of Hyperlipidemia

Before hypolipidemic drug therapy is considered, efforts to control hyperlipidemia (especially hypertriglyceridemia) in diabetic patients should include at least an attempt at near normalization of the fasting blood glucose (along with initiation of an appropriate diet [Table 79.4] for at least 3 months). At present, no evidence is available that favors insulin or oral hypoglycemic drugs to achieve this goal in type 2 diabetes, although a theoretical advantage for glipizide has been suggested (38). Treatment of coexisting diseases that can cause hyperlipidemia (e.g., hypothyroidism) is also necessary.

It is inappropriate and usually ineffective to introduce hypolipidemic drug therapy (see Chapter 82) if hyperglycemia is not controlled. However, gross elevations of triglycerides (above 1,000 to 1,500 mg/dL) can predispose to acute pancreatitis. Early institution of drug therapy (gemfibrozil or fenofibrate) is indicated under these circumstances (i.e., even before glucose control is achieved).

Glycemic Index

The magnitude of the increase in blood glucose in the 3 hours after a meal is determined not only by the carbohydrate content of the meal but by the carbohydrate type(s) consumed. By comparing the percent increase of the blood glucose to a reference food, usually white bread or potato with the equivalent carbohydrate content, an index can be calculated to predict the glucose elevating effect of the food. Diets incorporating foods with low glycemic indices do reduce postprandial hyperglycemia. When combined with a high fiber content, which probably acts by slowing absorption, meals with low glycemic indices can be beneficial in terms of the total period of postprandial hyperglycemia. Adopting an optimal diet in terms of the glycemic indices and content of fiber may be quite effective and even comparable with the effect of an oral diabetic drug in a type 2 diabetic, but this approach requires a highly motivated patient and the services of a skillful dietitian (39).

Fiber

It is now recommended that most of the carbohydrate in the diet of both type 1 and type 2 diabetics be in the form of high-fiber foods (fruits and vegetables, especially legumes). The ADA currently recommends 25 g of such foods should be eaten each day, but there is evidence that 40 g per day may be preferable (40). A high-fiber diet results in lower mean blood glucose levels and may allow the administration of lower doses of hypoglycemic agents. There is often a modest reduction in LDL concentrations as well (see Chapter 82). In many patients these diets produce a variety of unpleasant side effects, including increased frequency of stools, diarrhea, abdominal pain, and flatulence. The formulation of fiber-rich diets is difficult, and most patients do not accept the major alterations of diet that are necessary to produce the desired effects on blood glucose levels.

Estimation of Caloric Needs

Caloric requirements for maintenance of weight vary considerably from person to person and are influenced by activity level. Required calories are approximately 40 kcal/kg or 20 kcal/lb per day for an adult with normal activity. Thus, a person weighing 70 kg may require 2,800 kcal, although some lean men performing ordinary activities may require as much as 3,000 to 3,500 kcal per day. Individuals who perform manual labor may need 4,000 or more kcal per day, whereas sedentary people may need only 2,000 kcal, or less, per day.

In prescribing diets, caloric requirements are often underestimated. Clinicians commonly prescribe a 1,800-kcal diet for maintenance even if it is grossly inadequate for a particular patient's caloric needs. Prescription of such a diet leads to frustration and noncompliance. Overzealous decreases of calories for weight reduction may be equally defeating. When maintenance of weight is the goal, a careful dietary history by a skilled dietitian may be a good starting point for establishment of a patient's needs; the prescribed diet should then become simply a modification of that patient's ordinary pattern.

Diet during Conventional Insulin Therapy

Any patient who receives insulin faces a special problem. Unlike patients who are not receiving insulin and whose total intake can vary from day to day, patients who are receiving standard therapy with insulin require fixed patterns of food intake; greater flexibility is possible with intensive therapy (see Insulin Therapy). Total caloric intake must be distributed among the meals of the day, which usually include bedtime snacks. Occasional patients strive to reduce insulin dosage by senseless restriction of intake, incorrectly reasoning that disease severity will somehow be less if they can treat their diabetes with less insulin. Needless to say, they must be dissuaded from such practices.

The exact composition of the diet for the patient with type 1 diabetes is less important for blood sugar control than is the constancy of distribution of the amount of food at each meal from day to day. Insulin effect (duration, intensity), even for a particular type of insulin, varies from patient to patient. Accordingly, avoidance of extremes of blood sugar concentration (hypoglycemia and hyperglycemia) requires some adjustment of food apportionment for each patient. However, one should attempt to simulate as closely as possible the patient's usual and preferred pattern of food intake. The main modification is usually to add between-meal snacks. Once an acceptable food pattern has been established and insulin dosage adjusted to that pattern, the patient must adhere to the program if extremes of blood sugar are to be avoided. Patients learn by trial and error how much latitude they can tolerate. Problems, not easily solved, are encountered in individuals who engage in strenuous sports or work that varies from day to day. Such people may have to eat more on some days than others or make frequent adjustments of their insulin dosage. Intensive therapy (see below) actually allows for better control of blood sugar and greater variation in diet and in the level of physical activity.

Exchange Lists and Special Foods

After a dietitian estimates the constituents that will be acceptable to a patient, joint discussion should be held with the spouse or other involved family members. Cooperation and participation of a spouse in the process may be essential for successful adaptation, which, for practical reasons, may require that both partners participate in the diet modifications.

The intelligent use of diet exchange lists (food equivalents) is helpful for many patients. Such lists are available from the ADA, the American Dietetic Association, and most hospital dietetic units.

Special diabetic or dietetic foods are expensive and usually are unnecessary. Some such foods do contain less simple sugar than is ordinarily the case, but sucrose has no worse a glycemic index than bread or potatoes. The patient must read the labels carefully to avoid deception.

Exercise as Therapy

Historically, exercise was recommended for control of hyperglycemia as part of a basic program of diet and insulin for type 1 patients, but conclusive data indicating such a benefit are not available. Although diabetics, like others, derive health benefits from regular exercise, the complexities of avoiding hypoglycemia during exercise in type 1 patients makes blanket recommendations tenuous (see Exercise During Insulin Therapy). The case for exercise is better in type 2 diabetes. Regular exercise may actually help prevent the emergence of type 2 diabetes (41). The conditioning effect of regular exercise also decreases insulin resistance and can improve hyperglycemia. In patients with type 2 diabetes who receive sulfonylurea drugs, the likelihood of provoking hypoglycemia by an exercise program is not great, but obese patients on low-calorie weight-reduction diets who exercise at high intensity may be severely limited by lack of muscle glycogen unless they consume additional carbohydrates immediately before exercising. Walking or cycling may be the least-threatening form of exercise for these patients; attention to a period of adaptation is vital. All patients must avoid exercise that aggravates latent or existing problems (e.g., foot trauma that can lead to ulceration). It should be assumed that patients with long-standing diabetes who may have occult cardiac disease must be especially cautious when initiating an exercise program. A stress electrocardiogram is a prudent but minimal measure in such patients (see Cardiovascular Problems). The clearest rationale for exercise as therapy is as an adjunct to weight-reduction programs. With weight loss, sensitivity to endogenous insulin may be restored in obese insulin-resistant patients and normoglycemia may ensue, sometimes obviating the need for oral agents or insulin. The blood sugar-lowering effect of exercise often antedates significant weight loss. Approaches to exercise therapy in healthy people and in patients with heart disease are described in Chapters 16 and 63, respectively.

Selection of Patients for Insulin or Oral Therapy

Type 1 Diabetes

Many patients with type 1 diabetes are started on insulin during an episode of ketoacidosis. The insulin dependence has been established by the occurrence of the acute episode. Unless this acute event was precipitated by stress in a type 2 diabetic patient, insulin dependence is usually absolute and permanent. Occasionally in adults (more often in children), the insulin requirement may decrease or even disappear over several months, but relapse is the rule in such cases. Many nonobese adults were in the past considered to have type 2 disease when first diagnosed because they had not developed ketoacidosis on presentation. It is now understood that such patients may have LADA (see Type 1 Diabetes Mellitus and Its Slowly Progressive Form). Conversely, patients presenting with ketoacidosis and thought to have type 1 may prove to have type 2 diabetes. The presence of type 1 diabetes can be suspected from the lack of obesity, lack of response to sulfonylurea, an unequivocally low level of insulin C peptide (a marker for endogenous insulin secretion), and appropriate antibody determinations (anti-islet cell and antiglutamic acid decarboxylase [anti-GAD] antibodies).

Type 2 Diabetes

There is no direct relationship between the level of glycemia and the type of pharmacologic therapy to be used. Although it is true that the magnitude of the hyperglycemia suggests which patients are likely to respond to oral agents, the glycemic goal of therapy should determine the selection of the agent(s) to be used. Obviously, if a single oral agent can achieve the glycemic objective, it is the simplest if not always the least expensive route. Other factors, including age of the patient, life expectancy, and the presence of comorbid disease(s) (such as renal disease or dementia), are important considerations in selecting a therapeutic regimen. As noted, the initial approach to the obese non–insulin-dependent patient should be caloric restriction and weight reduction. Such therapy, if successfully followed, can be expected to reduce if not normalize the blood sugar within a few weeks. However, significant caloric restriction may induce a marked fall in the blood sugar within a few days, well before significant weight loss has occurred. If FPG is less than 200 to 250 mg/dL, hyperglycemia and glucosuria will not ordinarily produce enough symptoms to be troublesome during this period and no additional drug therapy (oral hypoglycemics or insulin) is needed. Even an FPG of 300 mg/dL may be tolerated. These patients are not prone to ketosis; no urgency exists for instituting drug therapy. On the other hand, symptomatic hyperglycemia or glucosuria, persisting for weeks despite efforts at (or actual) weight loss, should not be ignored. In this case, drug therapy is indicated for symptomatic relief of polyuria and thirst and can be discontinued if weight reduction is successful. Most patients with symptomatic type 2 diabetes are treated initially with oral hypoglycemic drugs, although some require insulin or a combination of oral agents or oral agents plus insulin.

The imperative for use of insulin in patients with asymptomatic type 2 diabetes, whose blood sugar cannot be controlled with oral agents is no longer in question. The evidence is clear that modest elevations of blood sugar do indeed relate to at least the microvascular complications of diabetes. The United Kingdom Prospective Diabetes Study (UKPDS) data (42) plus other studies and experimental observations have settled this issue. Patients with type 2 diabetes who do not respond to initial treatment with oral hypoglycemic agents are termed primary failures. Others, adequately controlled by oral hypoglycemic drugs for a time, become unresponsive to these agents (secondary failures). Insulin therapy may become essential in such cases. Other patients with type 2 disease develop grossly uncontrolled hyperglycemia during stress (trauma, infection, surgery, glucocorticoid therapy). Whether or not ketosis ensues, the gross hyperglycemia may produce severe osmotic diuresis and its sequelae. Such patients require control of hyperglycemia with insulin therapy, which may be discontinued as soon as the situation warrants. Occasionally adults, usually not obese and not necessarily exhibiting much glucosuria, may exhibit unexplained weight loss and lack of well-being. Such patients may show dramatic improvement with insulin.

Determination of glycosylated hemoglobin (HbA_{1c}) in cases of modest elevation of blood sugar is an important guide to therapy. Using the best available methodology for measurement, the normal mean HbA_{1c} is approximately 5% and the upper limit of normal is 6.5% (3 standard deviations). A near-normal value (e.g., below 7.0%) might deter a recommendation for drug or insulin therapy, whereas an elevated value would suggest that long-term benefit might outweigh the possible risks or inconvenience of treatment. Recommendations for or against therapy under these circumstances are currently determined not only by the clinical circumstances, including lipid abnormalities, but by the long-term deleterious effect of hyperglycemia.

Special Considerations in the Treatment of the Geriatric Patient

Many elderly patients are best treated with oral agents. Simple symptomatic therapy may be the foremost consideration for these patients. Insulin therapy may present special problems for elderly diabetics (because of poor vision, poor manipulative skill, or cognitive decline) that make self-administration of insulin difficult. On the other hand, many elderly patients can manage insulin therapy, especially of the type that is not excessively aggressive, and age alone should not deter the clinician from instituting insulin therapy. As noted earlier, insulin syringes can be prefilled and stored in the refrigerator for 1 to 2 weeks; this plan is useful for the older person who cannot accurately draw up the correct amount of insulin. The elderly are especially likely to have multiple diseases and to use multiple drugs. The risk of drug interactions in this group is therefore greater than in younger people; insulin therapy avoids this problem. A study of various insulin regimens in the elderly, as well as of insulin–sulfonylurea combinations, concluded that twice-daily insulin administration was the simplest, most effective, and most cost-effective regimen (43).

Normoglycemia as a Goal of Therapy

Type 1 Diabetes Mellitus

The results of a National Institutes of Health-sponsored multicenter study, the Diabetes Control and Complications Trial (DCCT) were released in 1993 (44). The study's definitive results have profoundly altered the goals of clinical practice in patients with type 1 diabetes and have provoked new efforts to control blood glucose in type 2 diabetes. The DCCT enrolled only patients with minimal evidence of complications at entry, and the beneficial results were striking. The results of this trial were summarized in a Position Statement by the ADA (45):

> The Diabetes Control and Complications Trial (DCCT) [was] designed to test the proposition that the complications of diabetes mellitus are related to elevation of the plasma glucose concentration. The study design was simple. Two groups of patients [with Type 1 diabetes mellitus, all younger than 30 years of age] were followed long term, one treated conventionally (goal: clinical well-being; called the standard treatment group) and another treated intensively (goal: normalization of blood glucose; called the intensive treatment group). The intensive treatment group was clearly distinguished from the standard treatment group in terms of glycated hemoglobin levels and capillary blood glucose values throughout the duration of the study. Normalization of glucose values was not achieved in the intensively treated cohort as a group because mean glucose values were ~40% above normal limits. Nonetheless, over the study period, which averaged 7 years, there was an ~60% reduction in risk between the intensive treatment group and the standard treatment group in diabetic retinopathy, nephropathy, and neuropathy. The benefit of intensive therapy resulted in a delay in the onset and a major slowing of the progression of these three complications. Finally, the benefits of intensive therapy were seen in all categories of subjects regardless of age, sex, or duration of diabetes.

A computer model that used the DCCT data projected considerable gains for patients with type 1 diabetes who maintain over their lifetimes a near-normal blood sugar: an extra 5 years of longevity, 8 years of sight, and 6 years' delay of renal failure, amputations, and neuropathy. The costs of the required intensive therapy were two to three times as much as those for conventional therapy. The DCCT is the longest and largest, although not the only, prospective study showing that lowering blood glucose concentration slows or prevents the development of diabetic complications. As such, it has major therapeutic implications for healthcare providers and their patients.

A primary treatment goal in type 1 diabetes should be blood glucose control at least equal to that achieved in the intensively treated cohort of the DCCT. This goal may not apply to all patients with type 1 disease and its pursuit must be based on sound clinical judgment. Of importance, intensively treated patients had a threefold greater risk of hypoglycemia than did patients in the control group. Because serious hypoglycemia is dangerous and is not entirely avoidable, the goal of near normalization of blood sugar may, after an initial effort, have to be abandoned for some patients.

There is no favored form of treatment to achieve tight control of blood glucose levels in type 1 diabetes. However, the goal is certainly not achievable in type 1 diabetic patients by use of a single-dose, or even a two-dose, insulin regimen. The decision to use multiple injections of insulin versus an insulin pump depends on patient preference and the ability of the healthcare team to provide the necessary resources and support, but even with these regimens normoglycemia can be achieved in only about half of the patients. The improvement seen in some of the others may, nonetheless, be worthwhile.

Young patients with type 1 diabetes in the early years of their disease stand to gain the most from normalization of blood sugar (tight control) because prevention of complications is the goal. Patients with type 1 disease who already have advanced complications of diabetes will not benefit at all because such complications are irreversible and probably cannot even be stabilized.

At what point in the course of type 1 diabetes should clinicians consider initiation of intensive therapy? After an initial period of conventional therapy for several months, the issue of intensive therapy should be considered and discussed with patients who are suitable candidates. In those to whom tight control is suggested, the clinician must explain the current view that maintained normoglycemia prevents the long-term complications of diabetes mellitus. The magnitude of the effort that is necessary to maintain normoglycemia must also be explained, including the need for self-monitoring of blood glucose (SMBG). One of the frequent-dose intensive insulin therapy schemes (basal-bolus or multidose) or its alternative, infusion pump delivery of insulin, must also be presented. If the patient understands and accepts the problems and effort required, the clinician may consider a program of tight control. However, serious consideration should be given to referral of the patient to an endocrinologist familiar with such a program because the process is difficult, very demanding of the clinician's time, and usually requires a team approach using a specially trained physician's assistant or nurse. The demands on the patient and the clinician are greatest at onset of intensive therapy. *When is conventional glycemic control rather than intensive therapy appropriate in type 1 diabetes?* Often intensive therapy proves to be less than intensive, regardless of the initial intent. Conventional therapy attempts to achieve near normalization of *fasting* PG, as opposed to near normalization of blood sugar throughout the day. Even this degree of control is simply not possible using conventional therapy. Many clinicians, failing to realize the limitations of one- and two-dose schedules, nonetheless still go through an agonizing trial of conventional therapy with such patients, only to have the effort end in failure and produce frustration for all involved. In such futile efforts, several types and mixtures of insulin are often tried along with both one- and two-dose schedules. At this point, the options include acceptance of a simplified treatment scheme that merely avoids excessive symptomatic glucosuria with resultant symptoms and prevents development of ketoacidosis (minimal therapy) or reconsideration of intensive therapy, perhaps under the direction of a specialist team.

Type 2 Diabetes Mellitus

The major conclusion of the DCCT—that control of hyperglycemia prevents microvascular complications in type 1 diabetics—has since been proven valid for type 2 diabetics as well. The UKPDS, the largest of the studies of type 2 diabetes, reported on 5,102 patients studied for an average of 10 years (42,46,47). The UKPDS produced some clear results. With intensified therapy with insulin, a sulfonylurea, or metformin, a decrease of HbA_{1c} was accompanied by a decrease of microvascular complications (retinopathy, nephropathy, and possibly neuropathy) of 25%. For every percentage point decrease of HbA_{1c} (e.g., from 9% to 8%), there was a 35% decrease in the risk of these complications.

Thus, young or even middle-aged patients with type 2 diabetes stand to gain as much from tight control as do young patients with type 1 disease. On the other hand, in patients whose life expectancy is limited by age, complications of diabetes, or concurrent disease, the problems associated with intensive insulin therapy should temper the clinician's approach to glucose control.

A major problem in type 2 diabetes is *macrovascular (atherosclerotic) disease.* Whereas hyperglycemia per se may directly contribute to the development of atherosclerosis, the clinical evidence is weak. Although the DCCT trial produced a favorable trend for type 1 diabetes, the data were not statistically significant. In fact, DCCT was so small and was conducted in such young patients (younger than age 30 years) that it could not have been expected to yield useful information on slowing atherosclerosis through control of glycemia. The UKPDS did not demonstrate a significant effect on the development of cardiovascular complications except in a subgroup of obese patients treated with metformin (47).

Oral Therapy

Obese type 2 diabetic patients who have not responded to a weight reduction diet within 3 to 4 months or who, having started on a diet, need interim symptomatic relief from hyperglycemia that is producing osmotic diuresis (polyuria, polydipsia) may benefit from an oral hypoglycemic drug. Typically, these patients are older than age 40 years and are more likely to respond if their diabetes has been present for only a few years. Other candidates are those who are unwilling to accept insulin therapy or in whom the risks of insulin-induced hypoglycemia seem unacceptable. The latter might include patients with occupations involving hazardous conditions (vehicle or dangerous equipment operators). Still others include nonobese patients in whom insulin therapy is unacceptable but for whom persistent hyperglycemia is a risk factor for microvascular disease.

Oral agents should not be prescribed for patients with a history of ketoacidosis, unless the latter has developed in relation to stress. Available oral agents may be problematic in patients with severe cardiac, hepatic, or renal disease, although the correct choice of an agent may make such therapy possible.

When selecting oral hypoglycemic agents, consideration should be given to the onset of action of the different medications and the need to ameliorate symptoms. In general, if patients are symptomatic, consideration should be given to using insulin secretogogues (sulfonylureas), which have a shorter onset of action, versus metformin or glitazones, which are slower in onset of action.

Transfer from Insulin to an Oral Agent

Type 2 diabetics receiving insulin can be abruptly switched to an oral agent, provided that they do not need more than 40 units of insulin a day. Patients who require such large dosages are unlikely to respond well to an oral agent. Patients with a history of ketoacidosis are ordinarily not candidates for a transfer from insulin. If the patient has manifested ketosis in the past (e.g., during stress) but is otherwise thought to be a candidate for a switch to an oral agent, the dosage of insulin may be cut in half as the drug is started. Subsequent monitoring over the next few days will show whether the oral agent can control hyperglycemia or must be abandoned. A history of hyperosmolar nonketotic coma does not preclude a successful change from insulin. A patient with no tendency to ketosis but whose diabetes is so severe that it has produced weight loss might not respond to an oral agent given as initial therapy but might respond after hyperglycemia has been controlled for a short time with insulin.

Sulfonylureas

Within a few years after their introduction nearly 50 years ago, sulfonylureas came into wide use for the treatment of type 2 diabetes. The acute hypoglycemic effects of the sulfonylureas appear to be mediated through insulin release. However, in chronic administration, during which blood glucose has been lowered or even normalized, no increase of plasma insulin is apparent. Studies of the mechanisms of action of these drugs show both an increase in the number of insulin receptors and a potentiation of insulin action.

Although the University Group Diabetes Program (UGDP) study, a multicenter study published in 1970 suggested that tolbutamide was no more effective than placebo and might even increase the risk of death from cardiovascular disease, that study is now considered flawed (48). The recent UKPDS followed a much larger number of patients than did the UGDP and established unequivocally the value of sulfonylureas in the treatment of type 2 diabetics (42,44,45).

Effectiveness

In optimally selected patients, about one-half can be expected to experience normalization of fasting blood sugar and about one-third do not respond. In others, some drug effect is evident, perhaps to a degree that permits symptomatic relief. Maximal drug effect can be expected within a few days to a week. Those who do not respond during initial therapy are considered to be primary sulfonylurea failures. In other cases, after a month or more of good response, the drug seems to become ineffective (secondary sulfonylurea failure). The frequency of this response has been estimated at 3% to 10% per year. Some apparent secondary failures are in fact caused by noncompliance. Only rarely in secondary failure is a switch from a maximal dosage of one sulfonylurea to another successful.

Dosing

In initiating therapy, an average dosage is usually appropriate. Hypoglycemia can occur and may be both severe and protracted, especially in the elderly and in patients with decreased hepatic or renal function. A single adjustment upward or downward by a factor of 2 may then be made as indicated by the blood sugar response after a suitable interval. When switching from insulin to an oral agent, initial dosage can usually safely be at the maximum recommended level for the particular oral agent or at least in its mid-dosage range. Before switching from one sulfonylurea to another, or from one type of oral agent to another, the first should have been tried at a maximal recommended dosage for at least 1 week; trials of more than 2 weeks are not indicated. In changing from a first- to a second-generation sulfonylurea, similar time intervals pertain.

Choice of Sulfonylureas

For patients with normal hepatic and renal function, there is little to lead one to choose among the first- or second-generation agents (Table 79.5) except for cost and convenience of dosing in that the longer-acting drugs do not need to be taken as often. The frequency of toxicity with any of these drugs is very low. *Chlorpropamide* is less frequently used than it once was; it should never be taken at a dosage greater than 500 mg per day, above which hepatic toxicity becomes common and additional therapeutic effect is not seen. Because of the ability of chlorpropamide to produce a syndrome of drug-induced water intoxication, this drug should be avoided in the elderly, in whom this effect has been seen almost exclusively. Second-generation sulfonylureas have been in wide use in the United States and abroad for many years. *Glyburide* (Micronase, DiaBeta) and *glipizide* (Glucotrol) are both safe agents. Although all sulfonylureas improve the second phase of insulin secretion, claims have been made that only glipizide, in response to glucose stimulation, improves both first- and second-phase responses. The second-generation sulfonylureas are more potent on a per milligram basis. Slow-release forms of glipizide (Glucotrol-XL) and glyburide (Glynase PresTab) are available and may help with patient compliance. *Glimepiride* (Amaryl) is also available in generic form. Glibenclamide and other sulfonylureas are widely used outside the United States.

Comparative Cost

At present, the approximate monthly retail cost of therapy with these drugs has a wide range, depending on the dosage and the agent used. All the drugs are currently available in their generic forms at one-half to one-third the price of the trade name products.

Instruction to the Patient

The obese patient must realize that weight reduction is the mainstay of therapy and is not simply a general

TABLE 79.5 Oral Agents for Type 2 Diabetes

Drug	Brand Name	Generic	Tablet Size (mg)	Dosage Range (mg/dL)	Doses/day	Route of Inactivation
Sulfonylureas						
First generation						
Acetohexamide	Dymelor	+	250, 500	250–1,500	1–2	Liver, kidneys
Chlorpropamide	Diabinese	+	100, 250	100–500	1	Liver, kidneys
Tolazamide	Tolinase	+	100, 250, 500	250–1,000	1–2	Liver, kidneys
Tolbutamide	Orinase, Tol-Tab	+	500	1,000–3,000	2–3	Liver
Second generation						
Glipizide	Glucotrol; Glucotrol XL	+	5, 10 (tabs) 2.5, 5., 10 (XL)	2.5–40	1–2	Liver
Glyburide	DiaBeta, Micronase	+	1.5, 2.5, 6	1.25–20	1–2	Liver + 50% unmetabolized
	Glynase, PresTab		1.5, 3, 4.5, 6 (micronized)	0.75–12		
Glimepiride	Amaryl	–	1, 2, 4	1–8	1	Liver
Biguanide						
Metformin	Glucophage	–	500, 850, 1,000	1,000–2,500	2 (3 for 2,500 mg)	Kidneys
	Glucophage XR		500	500–2,000	1	
Meglitinides						
Nateglinide	Starlix	–	60, 120	360	3	Liver, kidneys
Repaglinide	Prandin	–	0.5, 1, 2	1.5–16	3–4	Liver
α-Glucosidase inhibitors						
Miglitol	Glyset	–	25, 50, 100	75–300	3	Excreted intact by kidneys
Acarbose	Precose	–	25, 50, 100	75–300	3	Gastrointestinal tract
Thiazolidinediones ("Glitazones")						
Pioglitazone	Actos	–	15, 30, 45	15–45	1	Liver
Rosiglitazone	Avandia	–	2, 4, 8	4–8	1–2	Liver

health measure; weight loss has a specific beneficial effect in diabetes. Drug therapy is an adjunct, not a substitute, for weight reduction. The possible risks and goals of therapy should be clearly outlined. Although hypoglycemia is uncommon with the sulfonylureas, when it does occur, it is likely to be both severe and prolonged. The symptoms of hypoglycemia should be clearly described to the patient and to whomever is in close contact with the patient, usually family or friends, and corrective measures outlined and understood. The possibility of drug interactions should be mentioned lest another clinician prescribe a drug that potentiates or decreases the effectiveness of the sulfonylureas, or vice versa. The sulfonylureas are most effective when administered about 30 minutes before breakfast or dinner.

The elderly are especially prone to development of severe and prolonged hypoglycemia with use of the sulfonylureas, which may be related, in part, to the decrease of renal function that normally accompanies aging and may be worse in the diabetic. Decreased renal function (glomerular filtration rate, creatinine clearance) is often present in the elderly even when the serum creatinine is normal because creatinine production decreases with age as muscle mass decreases.

Drug Interactions

Various drugs enhance the hypoglycemic action of sulfonylureas, and others decrease their effect. Among the more commonly used drugs, salicylates, some sulfonamides, and warfarin all enhance the hypoglycemic action of the sulfonylureas. Nonspecific β-blockers may mask the hypoglycemia-induced release of epinephrine, thus prolonging and intensifying hypoglycemic reactions. β-blockers may also block insulin release. Clonidine (Catapres), like β-blockers, may mask the signs and symptoms of hypoglycemia. Acute ingestion of alcohol can enhance hypoglycemia; chronic alcohol use accelerates metabolic disposal of sulfonylureas and antagonizes their hypoglycemic action. Sulfonylureas interfere with the metabolism of alcohol and may produce a disulfiram (Antabuse)-like effect. Diuretics (the thiazides, chlorthalidone, and loop diuretics) may produce hyperglycemia even in normal people and antagonize the sulfonylureas. The anticonvulsant phenytoin (Dilantin), another commonly used drug, also has an antagonist action. Numerous other drugs may enhance or negate the effect of the sulfonylureas; equally important, the sulfonylureas themselves produce numerous alterations of drug action. These problems should not be overstated, but the clinician should be aware of these possibilities and interactions, especially in the elderly, who may be receiving many drugs.

Biguanides

Metformin (Glucophage), a biguanide, was approved for use in the United States several years ago, after decades of use elsewhere (Table 79.5). The drug's lowering of blood sugar is probably the result of multiple actions; it does not enhance insulin secretion. Another biguanide, *phenformin*, was at one time in wide use in the United States, but was withdrawn because of occasional cases of fatal lactic acidosis and other problems. Metformin causes lactic acidosis much less often. The drug is effective as monotherapy, producing a 50- to 60-mg/dL fall of PG (decrease of HbA_{1c} of 1% to 1.5%). Currently, metformin is preferred by many as the initial oral agent over a sulfonylurea, although no consensus exists on this issue. The main advantages over sulfonylureas are that metformin does not produce hypoglycemia and is less likely to be associated with weight gain. The main disadvantage is that nearly 25% of patients cannot tolerate the gastrointestinal side effects of metformin, whereas sulfonylureas are very well tolerated. Data on overall efficacy are scarce; primary failures occur in 10% to 15% of patients and secondary failures in about 5%. Metformin is often used in combination with a sulfonylurea, as an add-on after failure of the latter. If the combination is effective, an attempt to reduce or withdraw the sulfonylurea can be made after a month. After another month, the need for readministration of the sulfonylurea can be determined. Small decreases of LDL cholesterol and triglycerides are common, as is minimal weight loss (2.2 to 6.6 lb [1 to 3 kg]). Metformin is not well tolerated by all patients: Nausea, anorexia, and diarrhea are fairly common side effects. These symptoms can be minimized by starting at a once-daily dose (500 mg) and increasing the dosage at weekly intervals until a maximum dosage of 2,500 mg in divided doses is reached. Lactic acidosis is very rare in younger patients, but if the patient has renal or cardiopulmonary disease with hypoxia, a significant risk is present. Metformin is not metabolized and is disposed of by renal excretion. It should not be used if renal function is decreased (serum creatinine above 1.5 mg/dL). The drug should be used with great caution in the elderly because their renal function is often compromised even when the serum creatinine is normal, the result of age- or disease-related diminution of muscle mass that causes decreased endogenous creatinine production. It is recommended that metformin be discontinued temporarily before procedures that may result in hypotension or impaired renal function, such as surgery or radiologic studies with iodinated contrast agents.

Thiazolidinediones ("Glitazones")

Pioglitazone (Actos) and *rosiglitazone (Avandia)* are the currently available drugs of this class (Table 79.5). The term *insulin sensitizers* has been applied to these drugs, but the term is misleading in that it implies specificity of action. Although their effect on glucose metabolism is to facilitate insulin's action, they also affect many other cellular processes. These drugs appear to be safe, although the first one marketed, troglitazone (Rezulin), was withdrawn from the market because of hepatic toxicity that resulted in some deaths. At present, the two agents marketed in the United States are probably less effective than sulfonylureas or metformin when used as monotherapy. Side effects include fluid retention and plasma volume expansion, a concern in patients with cardiac disease (49). In patients who are at risk for congestive heart failure (CHF), or who have diagnosed but mild or compensated CHF (class I or II symptoms), these drugs can be prescribed in lower doses with careful monitoring for increased symptoms. Thiazolidinediones should not be given to patients with class III or IV symptoms. Other disadvantages include weight gain, a delayed onset of action (1 to 3 weeks), a prolonged time to reach a full effect (4 to 12 weeks), and increases in LDL cholesterol. The glitazones can be used in combination with other hypoglycemic agents, including insulin. Side effects, such as pedal edema, are more apparent when high doses of the glitazones are used in combination with insulin therapy. This does not necessarily preclude their usage with insulin, but should serve as a reminder to discuss this potential problem with patients.

α-Glucosidase Inhibitors

Acarbose (Precose) is a nonabsorbable α-glucosidase inhibitor that acts by inhibition of the enzymes in the mucosal cells of the small intestine that digest complex carbohydrates. As monotherapy it can be expected to produce only a minimal effect on the FPG (15 to 20 mg/dL) and then only in patients with no more than modest hyperglycemia. A greater effect is seen on postprandial than on fasting glucose (a reduction of 30 to 60 mg/dL). Abdominal fullness, flatulence, and, less commonly, diarrhea are the side effects, all of which tend to abate with time. The drug (50 to 100 mg) is taken at the beginning of each meal.

Meglitinides

Repaglinide (Prandin) and *nateglinide (Starlix)* act by rapidly stimulating the secretion of insulin from pancreatic beta cells by a mechanism different from that of the sulfonylureas (Table 79.5). The drugs are given shortly before meals, have a short duration of action, and are not prone to producing hypoglycemia. Repaglinide and nateglinide have been recommended for treatment of hyperglycemia in the elderly, a group in whom hypoglycemia is especially hazardous. In patients with moderate hyperglycemia, these agents are reported to reduce, on average, FPG by about 60 mg/dL and HbA_{1c} by 1.7%. When substituted for metformin in patients whose response to metformin as monotherapy had become unsatisfactory, repaglinide produced only a minimal response, but when given in combination, the mean decrease in glucose was nearly 40 mg/dL and in HbA_{1c}, 1.4%.

Combinations of Oral Agents

The increasing number of available oral agents and the relative ineffectiveness of monotherapy for control of glycemia have led in the last few years to a proliferation of combination therapies. A significant number of type 2 patients do initially reach glycemic targets with monotherapy but within several years require more than a single drug to maintain satisfactory levels of PG.

Metformin plus a sulfonylurea is probably the most commonly used combination therapy at present. This combination of a "sensitizer" and an insulin secretagogue target the two defects in the pathophysiology of type 2 diabetes mellitus (insulin resistance and defective insulin secretion). Various fixed-dosage combinations of metformin with glyburide (Glucovance) and glipizide (Metaglip) are available. A glitazone plus either a sulfonylurea or metformin (e.g., the rosiglitazone and metformin combination, Avandamet) may also be used. In one study, patients received metformin (2,500 mg) plus 4 or 8 mg of rosiglitazone, all given together once daily. At the end of 26 weeks, patients receiving the combination had a mean FPG of about 180 mg/dL (50). Whereas this was 40 to 50 mg/dL lower than the metformin-only group, only 28% of these patients reached an HbA_{1c} level of 7% or less. These suboptimal results are likely is attributable to the lack of insulin action, and emphasize the need to use a combination of medications that include an insulin secretagogue (a sulfonylurea or either repaglinide or nateglinide) or insulin itself.

Insulin Therapy

Table 79.6 list the insulins sold in the United States today. Until about 10 years ago, insulins were prepared from the pancreas of animals (cattle and pigs). Only a few of these preparations are still available. Most insulin is now made by recombinant methodology and has the amino acid sequence of the human or is modified from that sequence. Thus, so-called human insulin is actually produced in bacteria and purified for clinical use.

Except for the rapid-acting insulins, which are clear solutions, most preparations now in use are suspensions of insulin that have been modified by complexing the insulin with the protein protamine (neutral protamine Hagedorn [NPH]) or precipitated from solution (Lente) to prolong their action by delayed absorption after subcutaneous injection. However, some of the newest preparations have modified sequences so that they are clear solutions with altered durations of action related to their physicochemical properties, which, in turn, has been tailored to ensure delayed absorption (e.g., insulin glargine; see Long-Acting Insulins). The characteristics and uses of these insulins are summarized below.

Rapid-Acting Insulins

Regular Insulin (Crystalline Zinc Insulin)

Regular insulin is a completely dissolved (clear) preparation that has long been used intravenously in hospitalized patients for acute therapy of ketoacidosis. In the treatment of ambulatory patients, regular insulin is used subcutaneously, often in mixtures with other insulins. The onset of action of subcutaneously injected regular insulin is 20 minutes; peak action is at 2 to 4 hours, and the duration of action is 4 to 6 hours. Regular insulin also is used for continuous subcutaneous injection with portable infusion pumps and is increasingly used in combination with Ultralente insulin or insulin glargine in intensive control schemes; the long-acting component provides the equivalent of background activity provided by the basal infusion rate of a pump, whereas additional subcutaneous injections before meals are equivalent to the bolus injections of the pump (Fig. 79.1). Regular insulin is available as mixtures with NPH to provide a more rapid-acting component (Table 79.6).

Insulin Lispro

Insulin lispro, an amino acid-modified recombinant human insulin, when given subcutaneously has a more rapid onset of action (5 to 10 minutes) than ordinary regular insulin and a somewhat shorter duration of action, both resulting from its more rapid absorption. Lispro's main usefulness is in multidose programs involving intensive therapy and in insulin pumps.

TABLE 79.6 Insulins Sold in the United States

Trade Name	Manufacturer	Form
Rapid acting (regular and analogue)		
Humulin-R	Lilly	Human (rDNA)
Humulin-R Regular U-500[a] (concentrated)	Lilly	Human (rDNA)
Humalog (Lispro)	Lilly	Human (rDNA)
Iletin II Regular	Lilly	Pork
NovoLog (Aspart)	Novo-Nordisk	Human (rDNA)
Novolin R	Novo-Nordisk	Human (rDNA)
Novolin R PenFill and Prefilled	Novo-Nordisk	Human (rDNA)
Velosulin BR (for use with pumps)	Novo-Nordisk	Human (rDNA)
Apidra	Sanofi-Aventis	Human (rDNA)
Intermediate acting (NPH, Lente, and analogue)		
Humalog Mix 75/25[b]	Lilly	Analogue (rDNA)
Humulin L (Lente)	Lilly	Human (rDNA)
Humulin N (NPH)	Lilly	Human (rDNA)
Lente Iletin II	Lilly	Pork
Novolin L (Lente)	Novo-Nordisk	Human (rDNA)
Novolin N (NPH)	Novo-Nordisk	Human (rDNA)
Novolin N PenFill and Prefilled	Novo-Nordisk	Human (rDNA)
NPH Iletin II	Lilly	Pork
Long acting (insulin zinc suspension)		
Humulin U (Ultralente)	Lilly	Human (rDNA)
	Novo-Nordisk	Human (rDNA)
Lantus (Glargine)	Aventis	Analogue (rDNA)
Mixtures (NPH/regular and analogue)		
Humulin 70:30	Lilly	Human (rDNA)
Humulin 50:50	Lilly	Human (rDNA)
Novolin 70:30	Novo-Nordisk	Human (rDNA)
Novolin 70:30 PenFill and Prefilled	Novo-Nordisk	Human (rDNA)

NPH, neutral promatine Hagedorn; rDNA, recombinant deoxyribonucleic acid.
[a]All insulins are now marketed in a single strength (100 U/mL, U100) with the exception of Humulin-R Regular (500 U/mL, U500).
[b]Humalog Mix contains 25% or 50% insulin lispro. The remaining 75% or 50% is a protamine-lispro crystalline complex that provides a prolonged effect. Mix 75/25 approximates the action of NPH.
Adapted from Pharm Lett 2003;Aug.

Insulins Aspart and Glulisine

These rapid-acting insulins have a similar mode of action as the other rapid-acting insulin analogues. Aspart (NovoLog, Novo-Nordisk) and glulisine (Apidra, Sanofi-Aventis) insulins should be administered subcutaneously 15 minutes before meals, have an onset of action within 60 minutes and duration of action of approximately 2 hours. They are approved for use in insulin pumps.

Intermediate-Acting Insulins

Neutral Protamine Hagedorn Insulin

NPH insulin is a standardized neutral crystalline suspension prepared from an excess of regular insulin and protamine zinc insulin. NPH is the most commonly used intermediate-acting insulin in the United States. NPH exhibits a relatively rapid onset of action and a duration of action that begins to wane after about 12 hours but may last up to 20 hours. When a single injection of NPH is given in the morning, its onset of action usually occurs in the early afternoon, which essentially provides coverage for the midday meal. NPH can be given in the evenings and in multidose schemes described in Initiation of Insulin Therapy. It should be remembered that if NPH is given early in the evening (around 5 p.m.), some patients may experience nocturnal hypoglycemia (especially if the NPH dose is too high) or, alternatively, they may experience fasting hyperglycemia because the effects of NPH have worn off by the next morning. For most patients the achieved effect of a single dose of NPH is inadequate. Nonetheless, in the United States, many physicians continue to prescribe a single daily injection of NPH, a practice that has long been discontinued in Europe, where NPH is almost always given in two doses. Recently, NPH has been increasingly used in combination with sulfonylureas. Mixtures of NPH and regular insulin (e.g., 70:30; Table 79.6) are now marketed and are useful in some patients in controlling the postprandial increase in blood sugar.

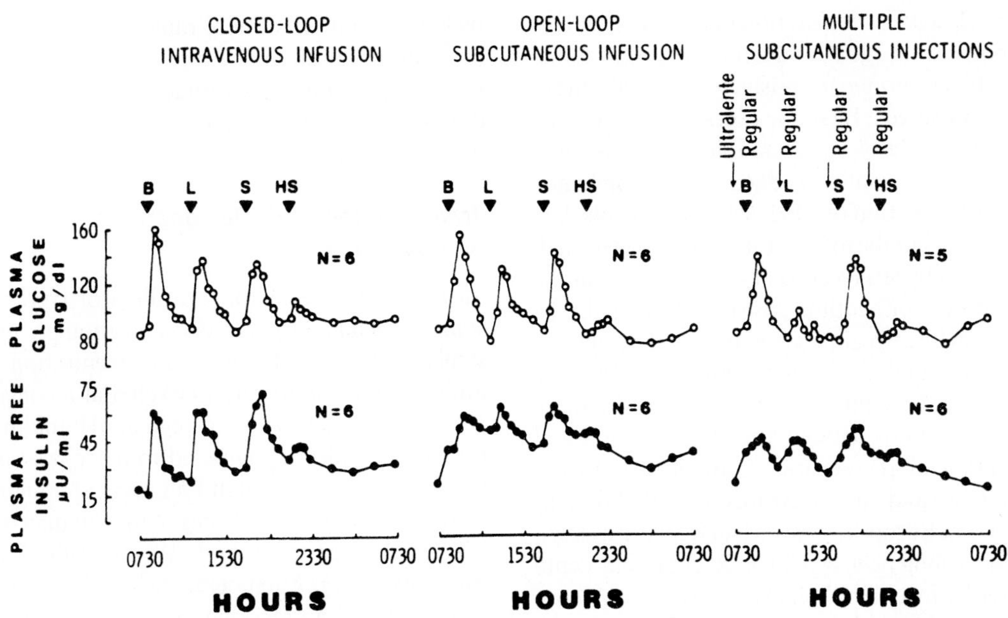

FIGURE 79.1. Plasma glucose and free insulin levels in patients with type 1 diabetes treated by three methods: closed-loop intravenous infusion (plasma glucose sensor-controlled apparatus), open-loop subcutaneous injections (insulin pump), and multiple subcutaneous injections (intensive conventional therapy). *B*, Breakfast; *L*, lunch; *S*, supper; *HS*, bedtime snacks. Note that the results are essentially the same with all methods used. (Modified from Rizza R, Gerich JE, Haymond MD, et al. Control of blood sugar in insulin-dependent diabetes; comparison of an artificial endocrine pancreas, continuous subcutaneous insulin infusion, and intensified conventional insulin therapy. N Engl J Med 1980;303:1313, and Schade DS, Santiago JV, Skyler JS, et al. Intensive insulin therapy. Garden City, NY: Medica Examination Publishing, 1983:138, with permission.)

Lente Insulin

The Lente insulin series was devised to avoid the use of the foreign protein protamine. Controlled addition of zinc is used to prepare Semilente insulin, an amorphous, rapidly absorbed, and rapidly acting material, and Ultralente insulin, a crystalline product with much slower absorption and longer action. Lente insulin is a mixture (30:70) of amorphous (semilente) and crystalline (ultralente) insulins. Although commonly thought to be equivalent to NPH, Lente is slower in onset and its duration of action is significantly longer, usually exceeding 24 hours. If a single daily dose of insulin is the treatment goal, Lente may be appropriate and a better choice than NPH.

Long-Acting Insulins

Ultralente Insulin

Ultralente insulin of beef origin has a duration of action exceeding 24 hours but is no longer marketed in the United States and has been replaced by the human form. It may occasionally be used alone. Until recently, Ultralente insulin (beef or human) was the backbone of intensive therapy by the basal-bolus technique. The prolonged effect of this preparation provides the basal (background) activity equivalent to that of an insulin pump. It is important to note that unlike the beef product, Humulin U (human recombinant Ultralente) has a duration of action shorter than 24 hours and may not be the best choice for use as a source of basal activity in multidose intensive-therapy schemes, although human Ultralente has been successfully used for this purpose.

Insulin Glargine

Glargine insulin (Lantus), a recombinant long-acting insulin analogue, is a completely soluble preparation that lasts approximately 24 hours. Glargine is comparable in its duration of action to beef Ultralente, but it is more predictable in its absorption than either beef or human Ultralente. Glargine is becoming the agent of choice for basal-bolus regimens. However, it is twice as expensive as Ultralente insulin.

Mixtures of Insulins

A frequent goal for patients receiving conventional insulin therapy is a single injection once daily. This goal is inferior to that of a multidose program for control of glycemia and should only be used if the patient cannot take insulin at least twice daily. If a single dose is to be used, insulin effect must be prolonged sufficiently to produce normoglycemia in the morning and at the same time provide adequate daytime control of the increases of blood glucose that occur postprandially. However, the duration of action of NPH is usually too short for this goal, and Lente, although sometimes a better choice, is often unsatisfactory as well. One of two scenarios is observed. First, the excessive daytime hyperglycemia dictates the need for additional rapid-acting insulin. Thus, regular insulin is added to NPH or Lente. Second, the single injection of NPH or Lente controls daytime hyperglycemia but the total duration of action is inadequate, resulting in hyperglycemia at the beginning of the next day. A predinner or bedtime dose of NPH can also be added to a sulfonylurea regimen (see Insulin Therapy for Type 2 Diabetes in Combination with Other Oral Agents).

Regular and NPH insulins can be mixed in the same syringe in all proportions without affecting the onset and duration of action of the separate components. In the United States, 70:30 and 50:50 mixtures of NPH and regular are now sold; in Europe a series of such mixtures (e.g., 90:10, 80:20) have long been available. Regular and Lente insulins cannot be mixed and allowed to stand for more than a few minutes before injection; delay of injection results in blunting of the action of the rapid-acting regular insulin.

Commercial Insulin Preparations

A number of products are available; Table 79.6 lists the various types, species of origin, and the producers. Clearly, no clinician needs to memorize this ever-changing list. However, even though most clinicians write prescriptions for insulin without specifying the brand, it is important to recognize the product that the pharmacist has dispensed. Not all preparations are available in a given region; pharmacies often supply the products of particular manufacturers according to local profit considerations. At present, two companies market most of the insulin used in the United States: Lilly and Novo-Nordisk. Both produce reliable, clinically comparable products within a particular category. A third company, Sanofi-Aventis, introduced insulin glargine and glulisine insulins.

Most problems caused by impurities in insulin in the past disappeared with the introduction of the highly purified animal insulins several decades ago. Allergic reactions and lipoatrophy were the two most troublesome events; both appear to have been related to impurities and now are rarely seen, except that lispro insulin used in a pump was recently reported to produce lipoatrophy. *Purified animal insulin* of pig origin (the only animal insulin available now in the United States) is about as expensive as human insulin and is of a comparable degree of purity.

In the past, insulin resistance was often ascribed to antibody formation, but little evidence exists to document significant immunogenic differences or clinical improvement as the result of switching insulins. Human insulin is certainly immunogenic in humans. Some types of human insulin do differ from the products of animal origin by having somewhat more rapid onset and peak of action and shorter duration of effect. Given the variability of onset and duration shown under clinical conditions, these differences may not be particularly important, especially in multidose programs.

Trade Names, Unit Designations, and Syringes

All insulin (Table 79.6), regardless of type or source, is standardized at a specific concentration per milliliter. The symbol *U* refers to the insulin concentration in units per milliliter. All insulins are marketed at a concentration of 100 U/mL (U100). Human regular (Humulin R, concentrated, Lilly) also is marketed in a preparation that contains 500 U/mL. Although long-term storage is best done by refrigeration, opened vials of insulin may be kept unrefrigerated for up to 1 month. When insulin is used during travel, extremes of temperature should be avoided, as in a sun-exposed automobile or next to a stove or heating element.

Several sizes of syringes are available for use with U100. A 1-mL syringe can be used for all doses up to 100 units, but most accurate dispensing of less than 30 units is made when syringes of 0.5-mL (50-unit) capacity are used. The bores of these syringes are smaller and the scales are consequently expanded. Some patients require more than 100 units for a single injection. For such use, 2-mL syringes (200-unit capacity) are manufactured, but these are in short supply and are difficult to obtain. No syringe is calibrated for use with U500.

The use of disposable plastic syringes with attached needles has greatly simplified use of insulin and is preferred by almost all patients. Many patients reuse disposable syringes without obvious harm, but the practice should be discouraged. Special syringes are available for use by patients with severe impairment of vision that prevents them from accurately measuring a dose. However, a simple solution to this problem is often possible. Disposable syringes can be prefilled with ordinary sterile precautions by an able person (relative, friend, pharmacist) and safely stored in a refrigerator for at least a week.

Insulin Injection Technique

After initial instruction the patient should be observed during self-administration of insulin to be certain that the correct volume is being drawn into the syringe and that the proper injection technique is used. Sterilization of the skin with an alcohol wipe is not necessary, although the injection site should be clean. If the injection is made through skin that is wet with alcohol, unnecessary burning discomfort is produced. Injections with disposable needles are essentially painless. Repeated punctures of the rubber diaphragm of vials of insulin with the same needle dulls the point and leads to painful injections.

In ambulatory patients, insulin preparations should always be given subcutaneously. Most needles in present use are one-half inch in length. Unless the patient is very thin, the best technique involves insertion of the needle at an angle of 90 degrees to the skin surface. If the patient is very thin, the needle is 5/8-inch in length, or if the site is covered by thin skin, the needle may be inserted at an angle of approximately 45 degrees so as to avoid intramuscular injection. After injection, the area should not be massaged because that may accelerate absorption.

The choice of injection region is important because the rate of insulin absorption, and, hence, the duration and magnitude of insulin effect, varies considerably between anatomic locations. Absorption is slowest from the thigh, fastest from the anterior abdominal wall, and intermediate from the arm. In addition, absorption from an exercising extremity is accelerated. The long-used technique of rotation of sites is unwise and may contribute to erratic control. On the other hand, the repeated use of precisely the same spot within a region should be avoided. Because of the variability of insulin absorption, injections in the abdomen should be encouraged. The patient should also avoid injecting insulin prior to showering or entering a hot tub or spa. The heat in these settings can accelerate insulin absorption, which can lead to serious hypoglycemic episodes.

Insulin Injection Devices

A variety of devices are available to facilitate the injection of insulin. Button-like injection ports are devices that can be left in place, usually over the abdomen, all day and decrease the number of skin punctures when multiple injections are being given. Needleless injectors that use a high-pressure jet are used by some patients, but they are not always painless, and absorption may be more rapid than with ordinary injections. Fountain pen-shaped injectors use a cartridge containing insulin; the needle does not need to be changed for several days. Delivery is with a push button or a preset dial. These devices are especially useful for diabetic patients taking more than one injection daily, who are eating meals in a restaurant, or who are traveling. The cost of the insulin in the cartridges used with these devices is high.

Initiation of Insulin Therapy

Type 1 Versus Type 2 Patients

Typical type 1 patients are almost always started on insulin during an initial acute episode of ketoacidosis that was treated during a hospitalization, and when encountered on an ambulatory basis, most will be receiving at least two injections of NPH insulin and a total dose of between 30 and 50 units per day. Adjustments of dosage must be made on knowledge of at least premeal and prebedtime SMBG. Type 2 patients who require insulin will usually have received oral agents that have failed to control the blood sugar. At the time of initiation of therapy with insulin, the clinician should establish clear targets for the degree of control of glycemia. Especially in patients with type 1 diabetes, but also in patients with type 2 diabetes in whom tight control is sought, it should be understood that both basal and bolus insulin will be required (see Intensive Therapy).

Initiation of Insulin

There is not a single, standard approach to initiating insulin therapy. If cost is an issue, the older NPH and regular insulins can achieve excellent glycemic control, but will require more education and intervention by the health care team. For instance, NPH needs to be resuspended before injection and should be given twice daily; regular insulin should be injected 30 minutes prior to each meal. If cost is not a major issue, then newer agents such as glargine and the rapid-acting insulin analogues lispro, aspart or glulisine can be used. Glargine does not require resuspension and the rapid-acting analogues can be injected within 10 minutes of eating a meal. Various algorithms are available to calculate the dose of insulin, but one of the simplest is to begin with glargine 10 units subcutaneously once daily, at any time of day. The patient can increase the dose by 2 to 4 units every 3 days as long as the fasting glucose levels remain above 120 mg/dL. Once the patient achieves blood sugars below 120 mg/dL, without experiencing hypoglycemia, the current dose of glargine is maintained. The patient may be instructed to increase the initial dosage of basal insulin by 2 to 4 units every 3 days until satisfactory control is approached. Usually such a program brings the patient under control within a few weeks. Increments of 10 units every 3 days are also safe as long as the patient is not markedly symptomatic or if no effect is apparent within a week. This aggressive approach can be used in patients with suspected insulin resistance. During this time the patient should monitor blood glucose at least twice daily (prebreakfast and predinner). A telephone call to the physician, nurse, physician's assistant, or diabetes educator should be made every week (more often if the patient is insecure), but at least when a single-dose program is being established, the patient should be encouraged to proceed with the dosage adjustments as planned and should not require or expect a physician's instructions at every dosage increment. Unnecessary dependence is thus discouraged, and the patient's involvement in management is enhanced.

Use of NPH Insulin Regimens

Most patients cannot be controlled with a single morning dose of intermediate-acting insulin (NPH or Lente; see Table 79.5). A single dose in the morning will improve hyperglycemia and glucosuria; the late morning or afternoon glucose measurements are the first to show a tendency to normalize. However, the effect of the morning insulin is insufficient to ensure normoglycemia in the fasting state (i.e., early in the next morning). Several maneuvers can be tried: changing the timing of a single dose to the evening, using twice daily dosing of NPH, changing to another type of insulin with longer action (such as glargine), or adding an oral agent.

In the two-dose approach, a predinner or bedtime dose of the same intermediate-acting insulin can be added, sometimes requiring a concomitant reduction of the morning dose. For example, if such a patient is receiving 60 units of NPH prebreakfast daily, up to 15 units may instead be given in the evening—usually before dinner—and the morning dose can be reduced to 50 to 55 units. Additional increments of 5 units may then be made to either dose, depending on whether the fasting or postprandial glucose is too high. The evening dose will have its greatest effect on the fasting glucose. Patients using such a split-dose schedule often receive 40 units or more daily, with 50% to 70% of total daily dose in the morning and the remainder in the evening. A two-thirds morning–one-third evening split is common.

A number of investigators report improved control of hyperglycemia using intermediate-acting insulin (NPH) given in the evening (before dinner or at bedtime) rather than, as conventionally used, in the morning. The insulin can be given alone or added to a sulfonylurea if insulin alone is inadequate. Part of the rationale includes a need for increased insulin action during the night to suppress the normal tendency for hepatic glucose output to increase during the early morning. Even patients with severe obesity are candidates for this type of therapy. Improved metabolic control has been claimed for this approach (51).

Insulin Therapy for Type 2 Diabetes in Combination with Oral Agents

There is not a standard approach to adding an oral agent to insulin therapy with regard to which drug should be used preferentially in combination with insulin. Because the pathophysiology of type 2 diabetes entails two problems, insulin deficiency and resistance, it is now commonplace to use combination therapy in the early phase of drug treatment. If the patient is insulin naive and is already receiving an oral agent at maximal dose, NPH or glargine is generally given at bedtime with the aim of achieving a normal FPG; improved daytime control will usually follow. In one study, the addition of a once-nightly dose of either NPH or glargine to oral therapy was effective in reducing fasting plasma glucose and HbA_{1c} (52). However, there were fewer episodes of nocturnal hypoglycemia with glargine.

Intensive Therapy

The term *intensive therapy* has had different meanings over the years. At one time, two doses of NPH was considered "intensive." Currently, the intensive approach is an attempt to normalize not only FPG but also preprandial and postprandial levels, using a multiple-dose basal-bolus insulin regimen. Much evidence suggests that the elevation of HbA_{1c} is a function not only of the FPG or the height of postprandial glucose excursions, but also of the mean 24-hour glucose or the integrated glucose concentration ("area under the curve") over the entire 24 hours of the day. Intensive therapy requires a maximal effort by the patient, the caregiver, and a team of support personnel (trained diabetes nurse and dietitian).

Intensive therapy uses an insulin pump or, alternatively, a long-acting form of insulin is given to provide background insulin activity in addition to three or four daily doses of rapid-acting insulin given preprandially (basal-bolus). Approximately 50% to 60% of the total daily dosage of insulin is given as the long-acting depot injection in the morning or before bedtime; the remainder is divided and given before meals as bolus injections of rapid-acting insulin. Regular insulin can be mixed with the long-acting form (except when used with glargine) before breakfast. The term *basal-bolus* is often used to describe multidose intensive therapy.

Other regimens have been developed that use three or four doses of short-acting insulin in combination with one or more doses of intermediate-acting NPH and sometimes an oral agent (sulfonylurea). Regardless of the exact regimen, frequent smaller doses of insulin at equivalent or somewhat lower total daily amounts appear to produce better overall control than single larger doses, as evidenced by HbA_{1c} (44,53).

Lispro (or the other rapid-acting insulins described above), although more expensive than regular insulin, can be taken immediately before eating instead of 20 to 40 minutes before a meal. Also, because of its shorter duration of action, it is less likely to cause postprandial and nocturnal hypoglycemia. Initiation of bolus insulin may be started by asking the patient to administer 1 unit of rapid-acting insulin for every 15 g of carbohydrates ingested (this usually requires education by a nutritionist) or approximately 4 units of insulin before each meal. It is important for the health care provider to review the patient's dietary history to be sure that the patient is consuming some carbohydrates in each meal. If there is no carbohydrate in the meal, the patient should not inject a rapid-acting insulin.

The goal for *pre*prandial sugars should be 70 to 120 mg/dL. Occasional *post*prandial blood sugars are measured and should not exceed 180 mg. Weekly, three morning levels should be determined to detect nocturnal hypoglycemia. Diet must be optimized and contain as close to a constant total of calories from carbohydrate at each meal

Self-Monitoring of Blood Glucose

If glycemic control to a degree that approaches normoglycemia is the goal, SMBG is mandatory. In the patient with type 2 diabetes, complete absence of glucosuria can often be achieved safely (i.e., with avoidance of most episodes of hypoglycemia) even without the need for frequent determinations of fasting blood glucose, but this is not possible in patients with type 1 diabetes or with intensive insulin therapy. Other indications for SMBG include patients with an unusually low or high renal threshold for glucose, many patients with type 1 diabetes treated conventionally, all patients prone to hypoglycemic episodes, pregnant patients, and some patients with type 2 diabetes who, despite an inability to master effective therapy, seem to find SMBG more satisfying.

The basis for all SMBG methods is a paper strip impregnated with an enzyme reagent (glucose oxidase) and suitable dyes. When placed in contact with a drop of capillary blood, the change of color intensity indicates the glucose concentration. Some strips are read only visually, that is, without a reflectance meter (e.g., Chemstrip bG), others are read either visually or with a reflectance photometer (e.g., Glucostix), and still others are read only with a photometer (e.g., Glucofilm). Accuracy of strips properly examined visually is adequate for monitoring control, except when the goal is intensive therapy with normalization of the blood sugar. For many patients a meter is unnecessary, but most feel more secure with machine readings.

In the United States, the meters in widest use are Accu-Check, which uses Chemstrip bG, and LifeScan. All machines are reliable, portable, battery operated, and relatively inexpensive. The manufacturers have reduced the prices to promote sale of the matching strips, the retail cost of which is approximately 60 to 80 cents each. For patients who check their home blood glucoses several times daily, the monthly cost may be considerable. Medicare now pays all costs of monitoring in eligible patients (older than age 65 years), and many companies now provide all necessary paraphernalia through online orders.

Capillary blood is most commonly obtained from the tip of the finger. Disposable lancets are used to produce the puncture. The required drop of blood may be obtained almost painlessly using a spring-triggered device (e.g., Autolet, about $30).

Blood flow from the finger can be enhanced before puncture by holding the hand in warm (not hot) water for 30 seconds. The skin should be quickly dried. Puncturing the thumb is least painful, but the ring finger has the best blood supply. Puncturing the lateral aspect of the fingertip (distal phalanx) is less painful than puncturing the ball. Pain is also less when sufficient pressure to produce erythema is applied to the palmar surface (ball) of the distal phalanx; an opposing digit of the same hand is used to apply the pressure. The first drop of blood produced suffices; the presence of extravascular fluid does not affect the result. The finger is inverted and the drop of a size recommended by the manufacturer is transferred to the strip according to the manufacturer's directions; then timing is begun and the glucose level is read.

Glycosylated Proteins, Hemoglobin A_{1c}

Chronic elevation of blood glucose results in an increase in the concentration of glycosylated hemoglobins, a major component of which is HbA_{1c}. Determination of the level of HbA_{1c} gives an integrated estimate of the degree of hyperglycemia over 5 weeks to 2 months (Fig. 79.2). The normal range of HbA_{1c} is 3.8% to 6.3% of total hemoglobin (normal range of total glycosylated hemoglobin is slightly higher, e.g., 5.3% to 7.9%) and may rise to 15% with chronic hyperglycemia postprandially. Values of less than 7.5% suggest good control with fasting and 1-hour postprandial sugars in the range of 70 to 120 and 100 to 140 mg/100 mL, respectively. With 120 to 140 mg/100 mL fasting and 141 to 160 mg/ 100 mL postprandial, one might see HbA_{1c} at 7.5% to 9%. At 140 to 160 mg/100 mL fasting and 160 to 200 mg/100 mL postprandially, values of 9.1% to 11% are common, whereas minimal control gives values of greater than 11%. Glycosylated hemoglobin levels fall slowly with

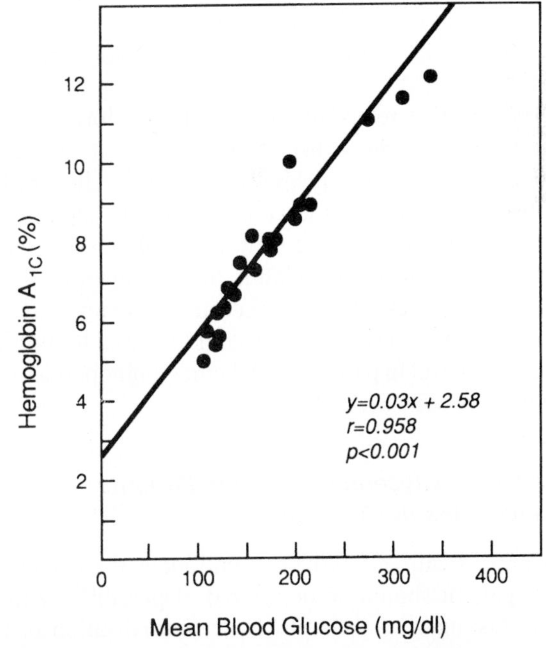

FIGURE 79.2. Relationship between hemoglobin A_{1c} and mean blood glucose. Twenty-one subjects performed self-monitoring of blood glucose four to six times per day for 8 weeks. The arithmetic mean of those values as compared with the hemoglobin A_{1c} value determined at the end of the 8-week period. (Modified from Nathan DM, Singer DE, Hurxthal K, et al. The clinical information value of the glycosylated hemoglobin assay. N Engl J Med 1984;310:341.)

reduction of mean glucose because circulating red blood cells containing high levels of glycosylated hemoglobin disappear normally in approximately 120 days. If euglycemia is established, glycosylated hemoglobins subsequently normalize in 4 to 6 weeks. Conversely, persistent hyperglycemia must be present for 1 to 4 weeks before elevated levels of glycosylated hemoglobins are seen. Short periods of hyperglycemia (6 to 24 hours' duration) may result in disproportionate elevations because some methods include measurement of unstable glycosylated derivatives. Other conditions render interpretations of glycosylated hemoglobin values uncertain, including any in which red cell life span is low (bleeding, hemolysis, sickle diseases) or in which hemoglobin F is increased (some hemoglobinopathies).

HbA_{1c} should, in theory, be usable not only for monitoring glycemic control but in the diagnosis of diabetes (chronic hyperglycemia) and in screening. The objections to such uses have been based on lack of standardization of methodology. Although this is no longer the situation, sensitivity and specificity barriers remain that are population (ethnicity) based. HbA_{1c} has also been found to be remarkably nonreproducible in healthy adults, in contrast to the situation in diabetics. To explain the variability of the HbA_{1c} in normal subjects, it has been postulated that the process of hemoglobin glycation varies from one erythrocyte generation to the next (62). The limitation on the use of HbA_{1c} for diagnosis and screening, therefore, is not technical or analytical but rather biological variability.

Fructosamine refers to the ketoamines formed from glycosylated proteins other than hemoglobin. It can be measured accurately, quickly, and relatively cheaply, but because it varies with the concentration of albumin in the serum and because the turnover of albumin is much shorter than that of hemoglobin, measurement of HbA_{1c} is the preferred test in the evaluation of long-term control of blood glucose. Fructosamine could be used to monitor glycemic control in patients with hemoglobinopathies that lead to erroneous HbA_{1c} levels.

Monitoring Glycemic Control in Patients Receiving Insulin Therapy

Efficacy of treatment in the conventionally treated ambulatory patient should be monitored, if possible, by measuring fasting glucose levels. Near normalization of the fasting (overnight) PG represents the basic or coarse adjustment of insulin dosage. Preprandial and postprandial normalization can be viewed as fine adjustments, both of which are difficult to attain. No useful purpose is served by attempts to adjust preprandial glucose levels before normalization of the fasting level is achieved; only thereafter should blood glucose be monitored at midafternoon or before the evening meal. The availability of techniques for self-monitoring of blood glucose (SMBG) have made blood glucose much easier to track.

The process of SMBG should be initiated as a prelude to tight control because unless the patient is able to master the technique and accept it as an ongoing necessity, the effort at tight control will fail. SMBG does not eliminate the need for dietary compliance. Recent studies indicate that within the wide range of what is grossly considered normal, neither intelligence, socioeconomic status, nor personality type has any predictive value for success with intensive therapy. Patients of limited financial means may be challenged by the high cost of such a program.

Monitoring Glycemic Control with Oral Therapy

The frequency and type of monitoring should be determined by the severity of the diabetes and the goal of treatment. For patients whose FPG becomes normal or reaches an acceptable level, monitoring can be simple because patients receiving oral therapy are not ketosis prone and have fairly stable diabetes. Similar considerations apply to patients being treated with diet alone. These patients must be taught that if they develop symptoms and signs of uncontrolled hyperglycemia (heavy glucosuria, polyuria, polydipsia, blurred vision), prompt advice from a clinician is absolutely necessary. Routine testing for urinary acetone is unnecessary unless the patient has new onset of persistent glucosuria or at some earlier time had an episode of ketoacidosis, perhaps during stress.

FPG should be determined every few months in most patients, but the best means of monitoring patients who respond to oral treatment with normalization of blood sugar is by determination of HbA_{1c}. Development of frank hypoglycemia or excessive lowering of FPG below 70 mg/dL (which may be detected before symptoms develop) is an indication for downward adjustment of drug dosage. When dosages are changed or when drugs are added or removed, monitoring should be done more often, perhaps daily, with SMBG.

Hypoglycemia

When severe, hypoglycemia causes central nervous system symptoms (neuroglycopenic symptoms) ranging from headache or subtle disturbances of mental function, to confusion, visual disturbances, and personality change, or, rarely, to seizures, unconsciousness, and transient hemiparesis. More commonly, when hypoglycemia occurs during waking hours and is accompanied by the usual symptoms of epinephrine release (tremor, sweating, tachycardia, and palpitations), there is no problem in recognizing the condition. However, in some poorly controlled diabetics, as in some normal people, even mild reductions of blood glucose to levels (50 to 70 mg/100 mL) not clearly identifiable as hypoglycemia can sometimes produce epinephrine release with its resulting symptoms (see Chapter 81). Under these circumstances, documentable hypoglycemia is not present and the clinical situation may be confusing.

Diabetic patients often develop defects in mechanisms that normally counterregulate hypoglycemia (63,64). This pathophysiologic state may occur within a few years of onset of the disease. Absolute deficiency of glucagon secretion is common in type 1 diabetes and sometimes occurs in type 2 diabetes as well. Defective endogenous glucagon responsiveness to hypoglycemia in type 1 diabetes is not normalized (reversed) by establishment of tight control (62). Defective counterregulation caused by impaired secretion of epinephrine is also common early in type 1 disease and may become marked in patients with autonomic (adrenergic) neuropathy late in the course of the illness. Other patients may have defective counterregulation caused by impairment of epinephrine action as a result of treatment with β-adrenergic-blocking drugs. In addition, such agents may mask many of the symptoms of epinephrine excess. Regardless of their precise mechanisms, these defective counterregulatory responses undoubtedly contribute in many diabetic patients to their high risk of developing severe hypoglycemia during therapy with insulin.

The most common cause of hypoglycemia in the diabetic patient receiving conventional insulin therapy is failure of the patient to eat at normal times. Skillful questioning usually reveals the problem. Many intensively treated patients appear to develop tolerance to hypoglycemia and remain asymptomatic despite markedly subnormal concentrations of glucose, a state called *hypoglycemia unawareness* (65).

Nocturnal or Early Morning Hypoglycemia in Patients Receiving Insulin

Excessive insulin action often occurs during the night or early morning hours. The hypoglycemia-induced release of epinephrine and other counterregulatory hormones (cortisol, growth hormone, glucagon) then causes rebound hyperglycemia, glucosuria, and ketonuria, an effect known as the *Somogyi phenomenon*. If the clinician notes an elevated blood sugar and prescribes still more insulin, the result is further hypoglycemia, perpetuation of the cycle, and possible serious consequences. Although the existence of the Somogyi phenomenon has been repeatedly challenged, other evidence convincingly points to its contribution to the problem of glucose regulation (66).

To detect this phenomenon, all insulin-receiving patients should be questioned carefully for clues to the presence of nocturnal hypoglycemia (e.g., nightmares, night sweats, and headache during the night or on arising), although these symptoms may not be present and hypoglycemia is revealed only by routine SMBG during the night. The point at which epinephrine release is secreted and produces sweating and other symptoms is quite variable; some diabetic patients trigger secretion at glucose concentrations as high as 50 mg/dL, others do not have counterregulatory release until the blood sugar falls to as low as 30 to 40 mg/dL, and still others have defective counterregulation (see above) and only neuroglycopenic symptoms.

Increasing the intake of carbohydrate in the late evening or reducing insulin dosage by 10% in type 1 diabetes and up to 20% to 30% in type 2 diabetes often corrects the situation. In the latter patients, such a brief and substantial reduction in insulin dosage can be made with impunity.

The classic Somogyi phenomenon must be distinguished from two other possibilities: waning of insulin action and the dawn phenomenon. *Waning of insulin action* occurs when the patient is receiving an insufficient amount of intermediate- or long-acting insulin; either a single morning dose is not carrying into the next day or the second dose, given before dinner or at bedtime, is inadequate. The *dawn phenomenon* is an increase of blood sugar between 3 and 7 a.m. that occurs despite continuous subcutaneous infusion or background insulin action from a long-acting insulin. An increased amount of insulin is necessary to overcome the glucose raising action of growth hormone, which is secreted in pulsatile fashion during the night with considerable interindividual variation and, unfortunately, variation from day to day as well. Because of this variation, an amount of insulin that is sufficient one day may be inadequate or excessive on the next.

Obviously, patients with waning insulin action or the dawn effect need more insulin, whereas the Somogyi effect requires that less be given or dosing times adjusted. The simplest way to distinguish these is by SMBG, often for several nights, with samples at 9 p.m., midnight, 3 a.m., and 7 a.m. More frequent sampling may be needed. Figure 79.3 shows the different patterns. Constantly rising glucose indicates waning insulin. A plateau followed by a rise indicates the dawn phenomenon. A drop during the night to a clearly hypoglycemic level points to the Somogyi effect. If SMBG cannot be done, cautious reduction of the dosage of (evening) insulin should be attempted.

Treatment of Hypoglycemia

The immediate therapy of daytime hypoglycemia in a conscious patient is ingestion of food, preferably sugar. Patients should carry a ready carbohydrate source, such as candy, and must realize that a tiny piece of such material will not suffice. Five or six Life Savers provide the minimum necessary 10 g of carbohydrate, as does a piece of fruit. Glucose tablets (5 to 10 g glucose/tablet) are now available. Also, 4 to 6 oz of sweetened fruit juice or of a nondiet soft drink are satisfactory. A tablespoon of ordinary table sugar (sucrose) may be added to fruit juice

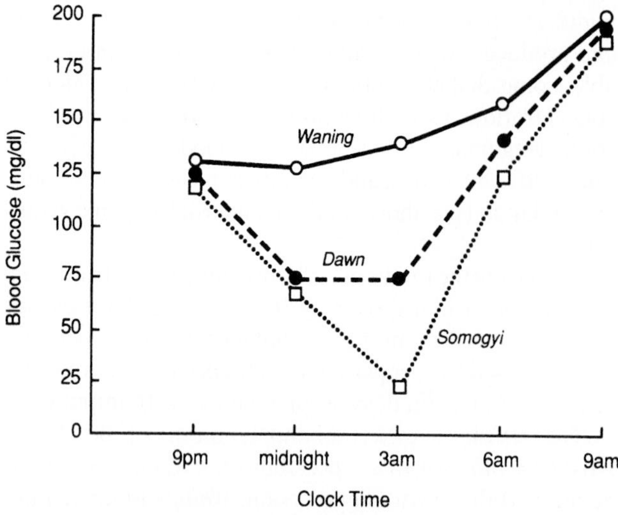

FIGURE 79.3. Idealized patterns of blood glucose concentrations during the night. The three patterns represent waning insulin action, the dawn phenomenon, and the classic Somogyi effect. All result in fasting hyperglycemia but are distinguished by the patterns of blood glucose concentration in the preceding hours.

or dissolved in one-half cup of water. Relief of symptoms should be seen in 10 to 20 minutes. Family members or friends should be instructed in the treatment of such an emergency and should not waste time attempting to reach medical assistance before administering sugar. Emergency medical care may be sought after sugar is given, but the problem is usually resolved by the time medical assistance can be obtained. If no obvious cause is apparent for the episode of hypoglycemia—such as a missed meal that is subsequently eaten—the patient should be on guard for recurrence over the next few hours, during which time repeated ingestion of sugar, at hourly intervals, may be advisable.

Occasional patients cannot be treated by the simple means described. Either because of a hypoglycemia-related alteration of mental status resulting in an uncooperative state or because of unconsciousness, some patients cannot take oral sugar. A safe and effective emergency therapy is administration of 1 mg of glucagon subcutaneously by a person instructed in this technique (glucagon promotes the breakdown of hepatic glycogen to glucose). Glucagon is readily available in single-dose form (1-mg vial) and should be kept available during initiation of insulin therapy and in hypoglycemia-prone patients. About 10 to 15 minutes are required for an obvious effect on the sensorium. As soon as possible, oral sugar should then be given. An effort should always be made to identify the cause of the hypoglycemic episode and to reduce insulin dosage or take other appropriate action to prevent recurrence.

Miscellaneous Factors Contributing to Hypoglycemia

Although defects of counterregulatory responses undoubtedly contribute to recurrent episodes of hypoglycemia in many patients, other factors in their daily lives also contribute. Noncompliance with diet may be deliberate or accidental. The need to consume small snacks can be unappreciated or forgotten. Meals are often taken off schedule, upsetting the effort to adjust insulin dosage to preferred time of meals. Amounts of food, if greatly varied, adversely affect insulin dosage. Emotional upset, difficult to evaluate as a cause of varying control, is nonetheless a significant factor in some circumstances. Injudicious use of alcohol is always a concern. Patients may have trouble measuring their insulin or may reverse the ratio of mixtures. Undocumented hypoglycemic reactions may be improperly treated and unreported. Techniques of blood monitoring are often at fault; patients misread directions or introduce variations that lead to errors of measurements. Not to be ignored is the effect of exercise and accelerated absorption of insulin by factors that raise skin temperature (hot shower, tub or spa).

COMPLICATIONS OF DIABETES MELLITUS

Diabetes mellitus is associated after many years with two distinct types of vascular damage in various organs (Fig. 79.4). Hyperglycemia produces microvascular (capillary) disease that affects the eyes, kidneys, and nerves. The blood lipid abnormalities of diabetes produce accelerated and extensive atherosclerosis of the cardiovascular and peripheral vascular systems. Coronary artery atherosclerosis and renal failure account for most of the deaths attributable to diabetes. Although considerable progress has been made over the past four decades in the understanding and treatment of this disease, diabetes remains a leading and increasing cause of death and enormous morbidity. In the United States and worldwide, the disease is showing a relentless increase.

Cardiovascular Problems

Hypertension and Its Therapy

Hypertension is a common complication of diabetes. Type 1 diabetics have an increasing incidence of hypertension with time (5% by 10 years, 33% by 20 years) (67). In type 2 diabetes, hypertension is often part of the metabolic syndrome at onset.

The risk of microvascular and macrovascular complications is nearly doubled in hypertensive compared with normotensive diabetics (67,68), independent of the risk of

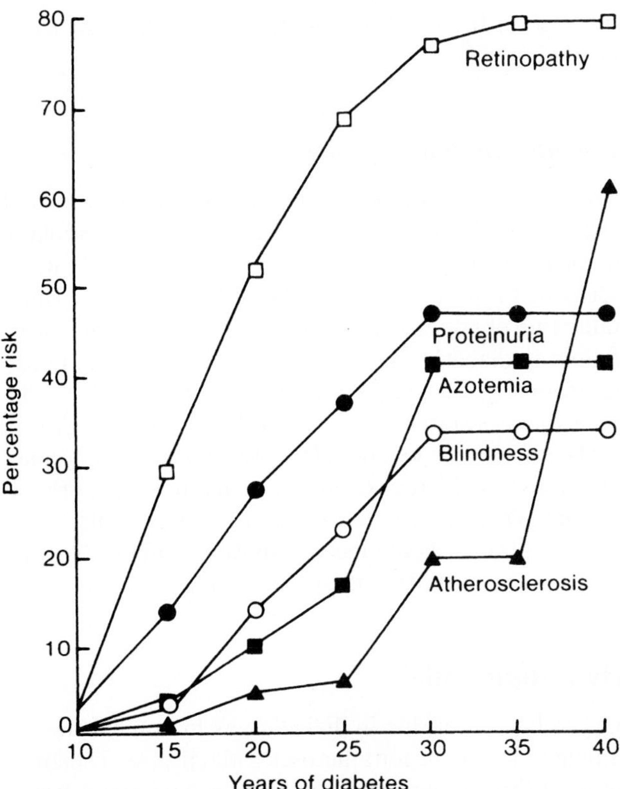

FIGURE 79.4. Complications of diabetes mellitus as a function of duration of the disease. (From Davidson MB. The continually changing "natural history" of diabetes mellitus. J Chronic Dis 1981;34:5, with permission.)

microvascular complications imposed by hyperglycemia. In both type 1 and type 2 diabetics, therefore, control of hypertension is critical. A number of sizable prospective controlled studies support this statement (69,70).

In type 2 diabetes, the same general measures that are important in the treatment of the diabetes itself—exercise and weight reduction—also are important in the control of hypertension. In addition, sodium restriction is important to avoid volume expansion that is part of the syndrome.

If blood pressure cannot be reduced to 130/85 mm Hg or lower, antihypertensive drugs should be prescribed for both type 1 and type 2 diabetics. If patients already have evidence of renal disease, the target blood pressure should probably be 125/80 mm Hg or lower. Detailed recommendations for the pharmacologic treatment of hypertension in diabetic patients are provided in Chapter 67.

There has been concern that previously used, higher doses of thiazide *diuretics* increase morbidity and mortality in this population and decrease glucose tolerance (71). It now seems clear that a low dose of a diuretic (e.g., hydrochlorothiazide 12.5 to 25 mg per day) is as effective as a higher dose in lowering blood pressure and that the development of vascular disease is retarded and the incidence of adverse vascular events is reduced (72).

Although *β-adrenergic blocking agents* provide effective blood pressure control, nonselective agents (propranolol, pindolol, nadolol, timolol) are best avoided because of possible worsening of glucose tolerance (inhibition of insulin release in type 2 diabetes), interference with recovery from hypoglycemia, masking of hypoglycemic symptoms, and occasional promotion of hyperkalemia. However, the selective β_1-blockers (atenolol, metoprolol) can be used because they are unlikely to cause these problems at conventional dosages. Concern over aggravation of hyperlipidemia by selective β-blockers is unwarranted because, unlike the nonspecific propranolol, which gave rise to these concerns, the more selective agents actually have only trivial effects on blood lipids.

As with diuretics there has been concern about the adverse effects of *calcium channel blockers* in the treatment of hypertensive diabetics (73). However, a number of studies have shown that these drugs, too, effectively reduce the risk of macrovascular disease in this population (73,74). Both nondihydropyridine blockers (e.g., verapamil) and dihydropyridine blockers (e.g., nifedipine) appear to be effective. Whether calcium channel inhibitors retard the development of microvascular disease remains to be seen (74).

Angiotensin-converting enzyme (ACE) inhibitors have become the antihypertensive agents of choice in the treatment of hypertensive diabetics. They reduce the risk of macrovascular complications at least as well as other classes of hypotensive drugs (75,76) and have the best risk-to-benefit ratio (see Chapter 67). In type 1 diabetics, ACE inhibitors have the added advantage of retarding the development of renal microvascular disease (77). In type 2 diabetics, the effect of ACE inhibitors on the development of nephropathy has not been as clearly demonstrated, but recent studies show that *angiotensin receptor blockers* do have such an effect (78,79). The accumulated evidence, therefore, supports the preferential use of drugs that inhibit the renin–angiotensin system as primary agents in the treatment of both type 1 and type 2 hypertensive diabetics. As for now, the major difference between ACE inhibitors and angiotensin receptor blockers is cost. (ACE inhibitors are considerably less expensive than receptor blockers and will become even less expensive as the patents on them expire.)

Because of the need to lower blood pressure aggressively in hypertensive diabetics with even early evidence of renal disease, *combinations* of hypotensive agents often need to be prescribed. In such circumstances, adding a diuretic to an ACE inhibitor is probably the first thing to do. If optimum pressures are not reached, a β-blocker and/or a calcium channel blocker can be added sequentially.

Other problems with antihypertensive drugs that may be especially troublesome in diabetic patients are erectile dysfunction (diuretics, α- or β-adrenergic blockers) and hyperkalemia (triamterene, ACE inhibitors), possibly in relation to the subclinical hyporeninemic hypoaldosteronism often present in these patients.

Atherosclerotic Vascular Disease

Diabetics experience two to four times the coronary artery disease of nondiabetics, and when myocardial infarction does occur, the morbidity and mortality in diabetics is twice that of nondiabetics (80). Early attention should be paid to complaints of chest pain and, even in its absence, diaphoresis, dyspnea, or nausea, because these may be anginal equivalents. In addition, diabetics have silent myocardial ischemia more frequently than nondiabetics. These considerations have led to guidelines for screening for cardiac disease in diabetics in the hope of improving outcomes (81). Because coexistent hypertension, diabetic cardiomyopathy, and autonomic neuropathy may alter the sensitivity and specificity of screening tests, more sophisticated studies, such as sestamibi imaging, may be necessary (see Chapter 62).

Because of the prevalence and severity of cardiac disease in diabetics, aggressive management of the risk factors (e.g., smoking cessation, blood pressure control, management of hyperlipidemia) is important (see Hypertension and Its Therapy; Hyperlipidemia; Chapters 67 and 82).

Cardiovascular thrombotic events contribute to the morbidity and mortality of diabetes, no doubt in part because of increased atherosclerosis, but probably also because of a variety of demonstrated alterations of platelet function and of the blood fibrinolytic system. Plasma plasminogen activator inhibitor type 1 and fibrinogenase are often elevated in type 2 patients, especially in the metabolic syndrome, and are correlated with elevated triglycerides and hyperinsulinemia (82). Although diabetes is considered to be a state of hypercoagulability, the relationship of these abnormalities to practical therapy is unclear.

Given the high cardiovascular risk of diabetic patients and the proven usefulness of aspirin therapy in nondiabetic patients, it is unsurprising that antiplatelet therapy is beneficial. The routine use of aspirin in type 2 diabetes is supported by at least six studies that attest to its safety and effectiveness (83). The recommended dose is 81 to 325 mg/day as an enteric-coated preparation, a recommendation sanctioned by the ADA (83). Aspirin does not increase intraocular bleeding in diabetic retinopathy and can be safely used in this condition. Studies of other antiplatelet agents (e.g., clopidogrel [Plavix]) in diabetics are not available, but their use may be considered in aspirin-allergic patients.

Diabetics are also more likely than nondiabetics to develop peripheral vascular disease (up to 30-fold increase in incidence) and cerebrovascular disease (a 2- to 6-fold increase in the incidence of stroke and cerebrovascular deaths).

Diabetic Cardiomyopathy

The Framingham study demonstrated that the risk of heart failure is increased 2.4-fold in diabetic men and 5-fold in diabetic women (84). This risk is associated with an increased mortality rate, even higher than the increased mortality rate of nondiabetics in heart failure. Although heart failure in diabetics is often associated with ischemic cardiomyopathy, a consequence of the accelerated atherosclerosis that is so often associated with diabetes (see above), it also may occur without clear-cut evidence of coronary artery disease. Increased left ventricular mass and primarily diastolic dysfunction are characteristic of this condition. Treatment should include an ACE inhibitor (see Hypertension and Its Therapy, Chapter 66).

Hyperlipidemia

Hypercholesterolemia in diabetics, as in nondiabetics, is a major risk factor for atherosclerotic disease. The kinds of lipid (lipoprotein) abnormalities in type 1 and type 2 diabetic patients differ. The term *diabetic dyslipidemia* embraces both of these patterns, but it is usually used to denote the pattern seen in type 2 diabetes. In patients with type 1 diabetes whose blood sugar is well controlled and who have normal renal function, the serum lipoproteins are not very different from those in normal subjects: LDL is usually normal and HDL may be even higher than normal. Oxidized LDL, the formation of which is facilitated by glycation, is not ordinarily measured but is more atherogenic than normal LDL and is often increased. In contrast, patients with type 2 disease have increased levels of intermediate-density lipoproteins (β-very-low-density lipoprotein, intermediate-density lipoprotein), and HDL is often low. Glycated and oxidized LDL are increased. A direct contribution of hyperinsulinemia to the atherogenic process is also suspected but remains controversial. Current guidelines (see Chapter 82) consider diabetes mellitus equivalent to a cardiac risk factor and recommend treatment should be instituted to lower serum LDL if it exceeds 100 mg/dL, with the goal of achieving levels less than 70 mg/dL.

Management

The hyperlipidemia of type 1 diabetes usually responds to conventional control of hyperglycemia. LDL cholesterol also is usually normalized. Triglycerides are usually not elevated after hyperglycemia is controlled. In patients with type 2 diabetes, as part of the metabolic syndrome, hyperlipidemia may improve somewhat with effective lowering of hyperglycemia, but even euglycemia does not abolish the problem.

The serum lipid abnormalities that persist after the best achievable control of hyperglycemia in both type 1 and type 2 diabetes should be treated aggressively (85,86). At any given level of cholesterol, the type 2 diabetic has two to four times the risk of coronary artery disease of the nondiabetic. It is currently recommended that diabetics with LDL levels above 100 mg/dL should be treated with lipid-lowering agents (see Chapter 82). Using this criterion, 80% of diabetics will be candidates for treatment of hyperlipidemia.

Neuromuscular Disease

Neuropathy

The precise prevalence of neuropathy in diabetic patients is unknown, although it is clear that neuropathy is common and that in most patients the occurrence and severity of involvement are related to duration of the disease. Usually, many years pass before the process becomes obvious, but occasionally even severe neuropathy can have an early onset (see Chapter 92 for a general discussion of peripheral neuropathy).

The most commonly appreciated abnormality is that which affects peripheral sensory nerves. Several types of sensation are involved (pain, proprioception, vibration, light touch) and can lead to unsteadiness, ataxic gait, and such uncommon but striking disorders as neuropathic arthropathy. Less-well appreciated are the autonomic disorders that give rise to disturbances of cardiovascular function (postural hypotension, resting tachycardia), genitourinary function (impotence, bladder dysfunction), and gastrointestinal function (nocturnal diarrhea, fecal incontinence). Motor deficits are much less common but may occur with striking suddenness. Weakness is distal (neuropathic) rather than proximal (myopathic), although a specific type of myopathy also occurs in diabetic patients (see Amyotrophy [Proximal Asymmetric Motor Neuropathy]). Some authors use the term *distal symmetric sensorimotor polyneuropathy* to describe the most common form of diabetic polyneuropathy.

Peripheral Sensory Neuropathy

Classically, the deficit is distal, with the lower extremities affected first, followed by the upper extremities. The term *stocking–glove distribution* is appropriate. The disorder is a symmetric polyneuropathy with a proximal–distal gradient of dysfunction. In severe cases, even the sensory innervation of the trunk is involved; in this instance, the most distal fibers are those of the anterior abdomen and lower thorax. Rarely, even the distal portions of the cranial nerves are affected (e.g., the distal sensory portion of the trigeminal nerve). The patterns of loss are not specific for diabetes mellitus and can be seen in such diverse states as amyloid neuropathy and toxic (e.g., lead) neuropathies.

The nerve damage at first may be asymptomatic, although subtle symptoms may be revealed with careful questioning of the patient. Alternatively, the patient may first complain of hyperesthesia and dysesthesia, including tingling and burning sensations. Later, various symptoms are experienced, including sensations of numbness or heaviness. Patients often complain that their feet feel dead or that they have a sensation of walking on a soft or nonexistent surface. Loss of ability to perceive temperature and firmness gives rise to these complaints. Severe, spontaneous, short-lived, stabbing leg pains and cramps are common. Often, these pains are most troublesome at night.

On neurologic testing, skin hyperesthesia is the most common finding (pinprick, two-point discrimination, light touch). Sensory testing with a standardized (10-gm) monofilament is recommended (information on obtaining monofilaments is found at www.diabetesmonitor.com/footresources.htm). The hyperesthesia and loss of temperature perception lead to unappreciated skin trauma and predispose to infection. Sensory loss in the fingertips can prevent the blind diabetic from learning Braille. Deep tendon reflexes, especially that of the Achilles tendon, are lost, often in the early stages of the neuropathy.

Peripheral Motor Neuropathy

Much less common and less-well recognized are the motor function abnormalities that occur as part of diabetic neuropathy. The intrinsic muscles of the feet are those most commonly involved. Interosseous atrophy produces inability to separate toes but, more important, allows the foot to assume abnormal positions. When claw or hammer toe develops, new pressure points appear at the tips of the toes and along the dorsal aspects; hyperkeratosis, callus formation, and ulceration follow. The interosseous atrophy that may affect the hands does not lead to total loss of function but does result in weakness of grip. Diffuse weakness of the legs and upper extremities may also occur.

Therapy of Painful Peripheral Neuropathies

A recent report from the American Diabetes Association provides an evidence-based algorithm for the management of painful peripheral neuropathy in diabetic patients (87). Nondiabetic etiologies should be considered and excluded when appropriate, and glycemic control stabilized. Drug therapy usually starts with tricyclic drugs, for example, amitriptyline 25 to 150 mg at bedtime. Amitriptyline may have more side effects than desipramine and may be less desirable for use in elderly diabetic patients. Alternative or additional drugs include anticonvulsants (e.g., gabapentin [Neurontin] (88), typically 1,800 mg daily in divided doses) and opioid or opioidlike drugs (e.g., tramadol [Ultram] or oxycodone). Nonpharmacologic therapies, such as acupuncture, and topical treatments, including capsaicin (Zostrix; applied to the skin as a cream three to four times daily) also may be helpful for some patients in the treatment of painful diabetic neuropathy. Referral to a specialized pain clinic should be considered if the patient has bothersome symptoms and does not respond to or tolerate initial therapeutic interventions.

Mononeuropathies

Mononeuropathy (mononeuritis simplex and multiplex) may occur in any superficial nerve (simplex) or asymmetric simultaneous combination (multiplex). The lower extremities are more commonly involved (femoral, lateral femoral cutaneous, sciatic, peroneal) than are the upper (e.g., ulnar, radial). Onset is usually sudden with intense often cramping and lancinating pain (see Chapter 92). Typically, the pain is worse at night and, when the lower extremities are involved, may be relieved by pacing about. When the pain is radicular (trunk or abdomen), intrathoracic or intra-abdominal disease may be misdiagnosed.

At onset, diagnosis can only be surmised, although tenderness along a nerve trunk is suggestive. Herpes zoster may be suspected, especially when hyperesthesia occurs, but when no vesicles appear and muscle weakness and atrophy are eventually evident, the diagnosis becomes obvious. The prognosis is good; complete recovery within a few months is the rule.

Cranial and Oculomotor Neuropathies

Cranial and oculomotor neuropathies are distinguished from other mononeuropathies mainly by their location. Pain and headache may be present. The most common nerves involved are III (palpebral ptosis, pupillary function undisturbed), VI (inward deviation of eye, diplopia), and IV (inward and upward deviations, diplopia). Recovery within 3 months is almost universal. When the facial nerve is involved, distinction from Bell palsy is impossible (see Chapter 92), although the diabetic variety tends to be less severe and recovery is usually complete.

Autonomic Neuropathy

Abnormal Sweat Production

Almost always associated with other evidence of diabetic autonomic neuropathy, this complication in its typical form produces heat intolerance and increased sweating (hyperhidrosis) of the upper half of the body with decreased or absent sweating (anhidrosis) below the midtrunk. In other cases, anhidrosis is generalized, and recognition of the complication may be difficult. In women the condition may be confused with menopausal sweats.

Affected patients have decreased thermoregulatory reserve and are predisposed to hyperthermia and heat stroke. Another consequence of impaired sweating includes failure to recognize hypoglycemia (see Hypoglycemia During Insulin Therapy). This is a serious problem because one of the warning signals of insulin reaction is lost. Many elderly patients, including those without diabetes mellitus, already have impaired sympathetic responses as a result of aging rather than diabetes.

Cardiovascular Autonomic Neuropathies

In addition to abnormalities of innervation that result in abnormal cardiovascular reflexes, diabetic cardiac denervation apparently accounts for the phenomenon of painless myocardial infarction, which is said to occur in more than 30% of diabetic patients who experience an acute event. Diagnosis is difficult unless acute electrocardiographic changes are present. Precipitation of unexplained ketoacidosis or myocardial failure may direct attention to these secondary events.

Resting Tachycardia

Heart rates of 90 to 100 beats/min are common in patients with autonomic neuropathy; occasionally even higher rates are observed. Normal sleep-related bradycardia is absent. Parasympathetic damage is the apparent explanation; the sympathetics appear to be less affected. A β-blocker is useful if therapy is needed. In severe cases, the tachycardia "improves" over the years as denervation becomes more complete and the sympathetics are also lost. Once these abnormal cardiovascular reflexes have developed, there is a marked decrease in 5-year survival. Sudden death, not attributable to myocardial infarction, has been described in many such patients (89).

Postural Hypotension

The most readily recognized troublesome cardiovascular abnormality is postural hypotension (see Chapter 89). The patient may complain merely of dizziness or faintness on standing, or the problem may be more severe, with visual disturbances and syncope. These symptoms may be confused with episodes of hypoglycemia. Remarkably, some patients with fairly marked postural hypotension are asymptomatic.

On initial examination, every diabetic patient should be checked for a postural decrease in blood pressure. In addition, a check for postural hypotension should be made whenever a potentially aggravating condition occurs. The onset or aggravation of postural hypotension is often associated with the beginning of therapy with a variety of drugs often used in diabetic patients, such as antihypertensive drugs, including diuretics, vasodilators such as nitrates, and antidepressants. Occasional diabetic patients may be unable to tolerate effective dosages of these drugs because of this problem.

The mechanism of this disorder is thought to reside in the efferent limb of the baroreceptor arc secondary to damaged sympathetic vasoconstrictor fibers in the splanchnic bed, muscles, and skin. Diminished plasma renin responses to postural change have been noted in such patients, as have abnormalities of plasma norepinephrine, but the role of these defects is unclear.

For patients with severe postural hypotension, the most useful drug has been the mineralocorticoid fludrocortisone (Florinef). In dosages of 0.1 to 1.0 mg/day, the drug is often helpful, but because one of its actions is to expand fluid volume, it can precipitate cardiac failure or produce severe hypertension in the recumbent state. Hypokalemia is common, requiring monitoring of electrolytes and appropriate management (K^+-sparing agents, supplements). Refractoriness may eventually occur. The β-adrenergic agonist midodrine (ProAmatine) has been marketed for the treatment of orthostatic hypotension caused by a variety of causes, including diabetes. The drug requires careful dosing (starting at 2.5 mg twice a day) but seems useful (90). In mild cases, the simple advice that the patient assume upright positions slowly by sitting on the edge of the bed after recumbency may help avoid syncopal episodes; continuing postural hypotension, although readily documented, may not be especially symptomatic and may not warrant therapy (also see Chapter 89).

Amyotrophy (Proximal Asymmetric Motor Neuropathy)

Amyotrophy is a rare, but devastating, complication of diabetes mellitus that is probably a proximal motor neuropathy. Severe asymmetric proximal muscle weakness and pain usually affect the pelvic girdle and thigh muscles, although upper truncal musculature can also be involved. The typical patient is a middle-aged or elderly type 2 diabetic with mild disease. Men are affected more often than women. Onset may be fairly rapid, and a low-grade fever and an elevated erythrocyte sedimentation rate may be present. Cerebrospinal fluid protein concentration may be very high. Muscle biopsy shows fiber degeneration. Electromyography shows a pattern typical of motor denervation. Weight loss of moderate degree is common but may be severe (44 to 66 lb [20 to 30 kg]). Prognosis for spontaneous improvement over 2 to 6 months is good, but complete recovery often requires 24 months or longer and significant residual effects are common.

Infections

Diabetic patients are more prone to infections than are nondiabetics. Clinicians often encounter patients who have experienced repeated bacterial or fungal skin infections (carbuncles, furuncles, external otitis, moniliasis) or gastrointestinal moniliasis at some time before the diagnosis of diabetes was made or in association with uncontrolled hyperglycemia. Once established, infections in the diabetic are difficult to treat and patients are prone to develop complications. Elevated blood glucose appears to be a major cause of this problem. Experimentally, hyperglycemia (blood glucose levels greater than 250 mg/100 mL) inhibits the phagocytic activity of granulocytes and the immune function of lymphocytes, factors that may contribute to lowered host resistance. Consequently, control of blood sugar should be part of any treatment program for an infection. This conclusion is supported by studies of perioperative infections in diabetic patients undergoing coronary artery bypass surgery (91).

Urinary tract infections are an especially troublesome problem in diabetic patients. Although infections are not clearly increased in incidence, a greater prevalence of complications is obvious. Half of all cases of papillary necrosis occur in diabetics. Diabetic patients also seem prone to develop infections with unusual pathogens. However, there is no evidence that treatment of asymptomatic bacteriuria in diabetics is worthwhile. Development of pyelonephritis is an indication for immediate hospitalization and vigorous antibiotic treatment; the risk of a renal abscess is a special hazard for the diabetic.

Skin infections caused by *Candida* are common in diabetics, especially those with type 2 disease who are obese. These infections require therapy with a local antifungal agent (see Chapter 117) and control of hyperglycemia.

Major soft-tissue infections in diabetic patients require prompt hospitalization and treatment with parenteral antibiotics. However, most infections encountered involve the lower extremities, usually the feet, and are not complicated by serious conditions such as osteomyelitis or gangrene (see Neuropathic Foot Ulcers). Until several years ago such uncomplicated infections were treated by hospitalization and a combination of systemic antibiotics, often for several weeks. It is now clear that most of these less-severe infections can be treated with an oral antibiotic and without hospitalization (92).

More than half of *infections of the feet* are acute, with concomitant skin ulceration; others are acute infection of a previously uninfected chronic foot ulcer, whereas a lesser number are abscesses (often paronychias) or cellulitis. Although cultures of such lesions are of limited usefulness, they can be obtained by swab, aspiration, or curettage, the latter being more likely to reveal anaerobes. Aerobic gram-positive organisms are present in more than 50% of lesions, and aerobic gram-negative organisms are present in 15% to 25% of lesions. On average, slightly more than two organisms are isolated, and anaerobes are present in 15% of cases. *Staphylococcus* is the most common organism, followed by *Streptococcus* and the common gram-negative organisms *Klebsiella, Pseudomonas,* and *Proteus*. *Corynebacteria* should not be considered as merely contaminants; they are the only organism present in many cases.

Clindamycin or cephalexin given orally cures 75% of these infections clinically and bacteriologically, even when treatment is without reference to culture results; another 15% to 20% of infections are greatly improved, and some 5% to 15% are treatment failures (92). Other antibiotic regimens yield similar results (93). The value of topical antibiotic preparations (povidone-iodine; silver sulfadiazine) is controversial (94).

It must be emphasized that such results can be expected only in these less-severe infections. Gangrene, severe ischemia, crepitus, and persistent fever are indications for hospitalization. Also to be emphasized is the need for proper adjunctive local care of the foot: elevation of the affected extremity, limitation of ambulation, proper foot hygiene, and, of course, surgical drainage, if appropriate.

Foot Problems

A number of common foot problems (e.g., bunions, calluses, corns, fungal infections, and ingrown toenails) occur in diabetic patients and can lead to devastating complications. Prevention through proper foot care and early recognition and treatment are important considerations in the long-term care of every diabetic patient. These problems are discussed in detail in Chapter 73.

Neuropathic Foot Ulcers

Epidemiology and Etiology

Diabetic foot ulcers and lower extremity amputations occur in 15% of diabetics. The problem is multifactorial. Enormous morbidity and expense are involved. A major technical review of preventive foot care and the ADA position paper that followed have been published (95,96), as have the conclusions of a consensus conference on Diabetic Foot Wound Care (97).

Foot ulcers are typically plantar and occur at the point where weight-bearing is greatest. They are now considered to be primarily the manifestations of diabetic neuropathy, but high plantar pressures and low tissue oxygen tension and blood pressure at the toe are other independent factors (98). Additional risk factors include hammer/claw toe and other acquired foot deformities. Although the diabetic is certainly prone to vascular (arterial) insufficiency and neuropathy and although the presence of vessel disease often contributes, the origin of the problem is primarily the sensory deficit. Neuropathy often is asymptomatic until an ulcer develops. Because the patient does not perceive pain normally, unappreciated trauma occurs, for example, from new or poorly fitting shoes that produce pressure points that go unrelieved and end in penetrating abrasions. Wounds can also result from skin penetration by foreign materials or from accidents during self-trimming of toenails. In addition to the sensory deficit, simultaneous motor weakness of extensor or flexor muscles together with proprioceptive defects can also contribute to anatomic deformity that in turn produces pressure points and ulceration.

Altered motor nerve function leads to muscle atrophy and tendon shortenings, which result in chronic toe flexion and finally hammertoe deformity. This anatomic change shifts weight from the padded ball of the foot to the metatarsal heads, where calluses form and contribute to the formation of new pressure points. The calluses themselves may develop fissures, which further promote ulceration. A contributor to the problem is diabetes or age-related loss of adipose tissue from the submetatarsal "padded" areas of the foot. This adipose padding normally distributes weight of the foot; loss of this tissue is a major anatomic destabilizer.

Management

Prevention is the mainstay of management. A standardized but simple nylon filament touch perception test allows detection of the sensory impairment, which is a major predictor of the risk of foot ulceration. Patients who cannot feel the filament are at about 10 times greater risk of ulceration and 17 times greater risk of amputation. Identification of such patients and institution of preventive measures may be useful in avoiding amputations. When an ulcer is present, decreased weight-bearing ("off loading") is an essential part of treatment. This is best accomplished with a total contact cast, the exact nature of which is best left to the treating practitioner's preference based on experience and technical expertise. Infection is not invariably present but when present is almost always a mixture of aerobic, facultatively anaerobic, and anaerobic organisms (98). In the presence of infection, a total contact cast is contraindicated. Antibiotics of choice and their method of administration are discussed under Infections. Intravenous antibiotics and hospitalization have been standard therapy for many years, but recently oral antibiotics in a home-based setting have been shown to be effective for most patients. Because callus formation aggravates the tendency to increase local pressure and worsens ulceration, regular debridement is essential. Some patients can be taught debridement techniques, which may at least delay the intervals between visits to the caregiver for this purpose, but usually periodic professional assistance is essential. Such care is often best provided by podiatrists (see Chapter 73). Fitting of custom-made molded shoes is helpful and is essential in some cases for prevention of ulceration or its recurrence. Remarkably, with proper treatment the ulcer may heal completely and not recur. However, recurrence is likely as long as the anatomic distortion or continued point pressure is left unmodified. Plantar injection of silicone reduces risk factors for ulceration but has yet to be shown in clinical trials to be effective in preventing actual ulceration (99).

Neuropathic Arthropathy (Diabetic Charcot Foot)

Neuropathic arthropathy, a complication of diabetes, is often unrecognized or misdiagnosed. The disorder, preceded by a sensory neuropathy, is a progressive degenerative change of the bony structure of the foot, most often involving the tarsal and tarsometatarsal joints (60%) but also the metatarsophalangeal joints (30%) and the ankle (10%). The prevalence has been estimated at 1 in 680 cases, but the disorder is probably more common. The patient presents with a swollen foot, often attributed to or associated with recent trauma. The foot may be painful or may be remarkably free of pain, considering the appearance. Examination shows moderate to gross deformity of the foot with rocker-bottom subluxation of the midtarsal region or subluxation of the metatarsophalangeal joints. Usually, the foot is erythematous and warm to the touch. An infected neuropathic ulcer may be present. More often than not, the pulses are intact. Clinicians unfamiliar with this presentation are likely to diagnose some other type of inflammatory arthritis or osteomyelitis, and their impression may be apparently verified by radiographic findings. In these early stages, the radiographs often show severe osteoarthritis, but as the disease progresses, there is complete destruction of the involved joints with resorption of the metatarsal heads and phalangeal diaphyses. Various other bony changes occur, including fractures, joint effusions, and subluxations. When these changes are at the maximal stage (i.e., when soft-tissue involvement is most prominent), the diagnosis of osteomyelitis is often entertained, especially when there is an associated, often infected, ulcer. Synovial biopsy showing a thickened synovium containing osseous debris may provide the correct diagnosis and avoid the necessity of embarking on a prolonged and difficult course of antibiotic therapy for suspected osteomyelitis.

Diabetic Charcot foot may also be confused with the changes associated with osteoarthritis and gouty, rheumatoid, and psoriatic arthritis. Consultation by an orthopedic surgeon, rheumatologist, or podiatrist to confirm the diagnosis and assist with therapy is almost always indicated.

Treatment is based on the cessation of further trauma to the affected area, which is best accomplished by elimination of weight bearing. Hospitalization may be necessary for this purpose. Reduction of edema and signs of inflammation may take several weeks. Immobilization with a cast may be helpful but should not be undertaken in the acute stage, and if used, should be done with great care to ensure the integrity of the areas covered by the cast. Simpler bootlike devices may also be used. Crutches can be used at this point, followed eventually by a walking cast. Up to 4 months of treatment may be required. Thereafter, molded or contoured shoes are essential to proper long-term management. Surgical intervention is inadvisable, although occasionally a stabilization procedure may be required if conservative therapy fails. Amputation is not indicated unless osteomyelitis unequivocally coexists or the entire process fails to respond to prolonged conservative efforts. Despite the discouraging appearance of the foot at its worst stages, sufficient healing and stabilization to produce a useful foot can be anticipated.

Gastrointestinal Dysfunction

Most disorders of the gastrointestinal tract in diabetes are related to disturbances of motility. Esophageal motor dysfunction can be demonstrated on testing but is usually not a clinical problem.

Gastroparesis (atony of the stomach) is often asymptomatic but may be troublesome. Symptoms include anorexia, early satiety, postprandial fullness and bloating, and, occasionally, vomiting. Delayed and unpredictable emptying of the stomach may produce irregular diabetic control in already difficult to manage patients with either type 1 or 2 diabetes. Diagnosis is apparent—sometimes as an incidental finding—on barium radiograph of the upper gastrointestinal tract. Nuclear scintigraphy is the most sensitive method to detect the presence of atony. Gastroparesis has long been thought to be a late complication associated with poor prognosis for survival, but there is no evidence to support this notion (100). Metoclopramide (Reglan) 10 mg three times daily may be helpful (see Chapter 43). In intractable cases, gastrectomy may be needed. Alternatively, insertion of a gastric pacemaker may also ameliorate symptoms and improve quality of life (101).

Small-bowel dysfunction is common and symptomatic, leading to diabetic diarrhea. Typically, the diarrhea is nocturnal. Fecal incontinence, a result of impaired sensation of rectal distention, may occur and is very distressing. The disorder tends to be episodic, with attacks lasting from a few days to weeks or rarely months. Watery brown diarrhea, usually without steatorrhea, is typical. On barium radiograph of the small bowel, the findings are those of disturbed motility. Despite the distressing symptoms, the patient appears well; weight loss is uncommon. When steatorrhea occurs, pancreatic exocrine insufficiency and sprue syndrome, more common in diabetic patients than in the general population, should be considered. Fully developed sprue is associated with gross evidence of malabsorption. A trial of antibiotic therapy (e.g., tetracycline, 250 mg four times a day for 2 weeks) may improve the diarrhea and the malabsorption if the latter is caused by small-bowel stasis and bacterial colonization. Symptomatic treatment with antispasmodics (e.g., loperamide [Imodium]) may be useful, especially when attacks of diarrhea are short lived.

Large-bowel complaints, especially of constipation, are common in the elderly. It does not appear that diabetic patients are especially prone to any additional problems in this regard.

Patients with poorly controlled diabetes may develop *fatty changes of the liver.* Nonalcoholic steatohepatitis, with hepatomegaly or elevations of serum aminotransferases, may occur. Effective control of blood sugar results in disappearance of these abnormalities if diabetes is the cause. However, diabetes and obesity often coexist; fatty liver is also common in uncomplicated obesity.

Genitourinary Problems

Bladder Dysfunction (Neurogenic Bladder)

The symptoms of bladder dysfunction in diabetic patients are often overlooked. Onset is insidious and occurs over many years. Eighty percent of patients have clinical evidence of neuropathy affecting other systems. The first clinical manifestation of bladder dysfunction is an increase in the interval between voiding until urine is passed only twice or even once daily. A need to strain, slow stream, dribbling, and sensation of incomplete voiding may be present. These symptoms should be routinely solicited from diabetic patients, especially when there are symptoms or signs of peripheral neuropathy.

Demonstration of residual urine is the hallmark of clinically symptomatic cystopathy, but many diabetic patients, when studied by cystometric techniques, have objective evidence of neurogenic involvement and a grossly enlarged bladder well before symptoms are evident. At this stage, residual urine is not present and other urinary tract abnormalities (recurrent infections) are not evident. If large volumes of residual urine do develop, patients become prone to infection (see Chapter 36) and incontinence (see Chapter 12). Patients suspected to have cystopathy should be referred to a urologist for evaluation and recommendations about treatment.

Erectile and Sexual Dysfunction

The frequency of erectile dysfunction, formerly termed impotence, is high in diabetic men, perhaps 50% to 60% overall. This complication, like many others in diabetic patients, is related to duration of disease. The problem is usually caused by a type of autonomic neuropathy involving the pelvic parasympathetic nerves, but impaired blood flow is the cause in some cases. Several studies report that sexual function in diabetic women appears to be unaffected by the disease. Others assert that many diabetic women lose the ability to achieve orgasm (102).

The evaluation and management of erectile and sexual dysfunction are described in Chapters 6 and 85. Psychogenic factors probably account for a significant fraction of cases, but there is no evidence that psychogenic problems are more common in diabetic patients. The onset of erectile dysfunction in diabetics usually is slow (6 months to several years), often associated with retrograde ejaculation; impotence eventually becomes complete. Despite this, libido is characteristically retained. Although patients with psychogenic impotence often report nocturnal erections and emissions, these are absent in patients with diabetic impotence. An important point on clinical examination is that testicular sensitivity to pressure and pain is retained in men with psychogenic impotence but is often greatly diminished or lost in the diabetic in whom accompanying sensory neuropathy is common.

A variety of drugs, especially ones that are often used in diabetics, may cause erectile dysfunction. The most common offenders are antihypertensives and antidepressants.

Nephropathy

Progressive renal failure is a major life-threatening complication of diabetes. The relationship between hyperglycemia and the development of microangiopathy with eventual nodular glomerulosclerosis (Kimmelstiel-Wilson disease) is unequivocally established, as strong clinical and experimental evidence has accumulated in favor of such a relationship. One of the earliest indications of incipient diabetic nephropathy is proteinuria, first manifest as microalbuminuria. The detection and significance of proteinuria and of microalbuminuria in diabetic patients are discussed in Chapter 48.

Diabetic patients with even minimal elevations of serum creatinine greater than 1.1 mg/dL, but not those with normal renal function, are at increased risk of acute renal failure from contrast media used in various radiographic procedures. Although the risk is only moderately increased (approximately 10% to 15% in the highest risk patients versus 5% in low-risk patients and less than 2% in those with no renal disease and in nondiabetic subjects), these procedures can often be replaced by others with less risk (magnetic resonance imaging, sonography). If contrast media are to be used, the dosage should be minimal and the patient well hydrated. Diuretics and ACE inhibitors should be reduced or briefly withheld, and metformin should be stopped temporarily. The clinical course of diabetic nephropathy and the impact of failing renal function on insulin requirement and on the dosage of oral hypoglycemic drugs are discussed in Chapter 52.

Skin Lesions

An uncommon abnormality known as *necrobiosis lipoidica diabeticorum* occurs in perhaps 0.3% of all diabetics, seemingly unrelated to glycemic control. Typically, lesions occur on the anterior legs, but also can occur on the arms, trunk, and face. The lesions, described as atrophic plaques, are sharply demarcated, orange or red, and often ulcerate. On biopsy, diagnostic findings include destruction of collagen fibers. Until recently no agent seemed to be useful, but several reports indicate that these lesions respond rapidly to tretinoin-containing creams; pentoxifylline (Trental), 400 mg twice daily, also seems to be effective.

Retinopathy

Diabetic retinopathy has become one of the leading causes of blindness in the United States. In type 1 diabetic patients, some degree of retinopathy can be detected by angiography, the most sensitive technique, after as few as 1 to 2 years in 10% of patients. By 10 years, retinopathy is evident in 50% of cases by ophthalmoscopy, with a 70% prevalence by angiography. At 25 years, nearly all patients can be shown to have some degree of retinopathy. By the time diabetes has been present for 15 to 20 years, approximately 33% of patients have severe disease and another 50% have obvious, but lesser degrees of, progressive retinal involvement. Remarkably, not all cases of early retinopathy are progressive. These figures represent the era prior to the use of intensive therapy to control blood sugar (45).

Type 2 diabetic patients also develop retinopathy, apparently with less frequency, but clearly related to duration and severity of the hyperglycemia. Hyperglycemia, as indirectly measured by glycosylated hemoglobin, clearly predicts the incidence and progression of diabetic retinopathy in type 2 diabetes (103,104).

In patients with retinopathy in whom intensive therapy is initiated, a paradoxical worsening of the retinopathy can be seen. Patients whose retinopathy is mild to moderate usually have no associated visual loss, and long-term intensive treatment of glycemia counterbalances the early worsening (105).

Blindness in Diabetic Retinopathy

The visual loss in diabetic retinopathy is potentially even more severe than is blindness as a result of other causes. Many people who are legally blind (defined as visual acuity less than 20/200 in both eyes) from causes other than diabetes have slow onset of visual loss, thus allowing time for adaptation. In addition, they often retain reasonably full visual fields and visual acuity at or close to the legal limit. Such patients can see well enough to ambulate independently and perform a variety of common activities (self-care, housework). With the aid of special devices they may even be able to read newsprint and to engage in some occupations. In contrast, the visual loss from diabetic retinopathy is often caused by sudden hemorrhage or retinal detachment and often leaves the patient with only light perception. In addition, the diabetic often already has other complications of the disease when blindness develops. Although total blindness afflicts only some diabetic patients, a larger number have some degree of loss of visual acuity caused by macular edema, the most common cause of visual loss in diabetics.

Ocular Symptoms

Diabetic patients who experience symptoms of visual disturbance are not necessarily experiencing a catastrophic complication and deserve reassurance along these lines. Like others, diabetic patients develop changes of visual acuity such as a change in refractive error and astigmatism. In addition, they can experience decreased visual acuity as a result of marked changes in blood sugar (e.g., as the lens swells during acute normalization of blood sugar after prolonged hyperglycemia). However, sudden or persistent change of visual acuity requires examination by an ophthalmologist, especially when advanced retinal disease, proliferative diabetic retinopathy (PDR), is present. A common cause of visual loss in PDR, macular edema, is not readily detectable by the direct ophthalmoscopy available to internists and requires binocular slit lamp or stereoscopic fundus photography by an ophthalmologist.

Sudden painless loss of vision in PDR demands urgent ophthalmologic consultation. This symptom is often caused by hemorrhage from proliferating new vessels or from retinal detachment. Lesser degrees of hemorrhage may cause floaters or cobwebs. Another complication in PDR is outflow obstruction of the aqueous humor produced by fibrous scar tissue extending into the angle of the anterior chamber, causing a marked rise in intraocular pressure and acute (neovascular) glaucoma with severe pain. Loss of vision occurs unless emergency therapy is given.

Types of Retinal Disease in Diabetic Patients

The current classification of diabetic retinal disease is nonproliferative (or background), preproliferative, and PDR. The latter more advanced stage is the point at which sudden and massive visual loss becomes a problem.

Nonproliferative and Preproliferative Retinopathy

The earliest lesions—readily visible with an ordinary ophthalmoscope—are in the region of the macula: microaneurysms, punctate retinal hemorrhages, hard exudates, soft exudates (cotton wool), and so-called intraretinal microvascular anomalies (IRMAs). Both *microaneurysms* and *small-dot intraretinal hemorrhages* appear as red dots, and both tend to fade within months. *Blot hemorrhages* are larger. Distinction can best be made by fluorescein angiograms, in which only microaneurysms light up. This procedure, performed by an ophthalmologist, often identifies extensive intraretinal disease when only a few abnormalities are evident by ophthalmoscopy.

Hard exudates are glistening yellow or white lipid deposits located in the outer retinal layers. If they are greater than 1 disk diameter from the macula, they are not ominous. *Soft exudates* are areas of ischemia or infarction of the nerve fiber layer; they disappear within a few months. *IRMAs* are dilated hypercellular vessels that are thought to represent either dilated capillaries or intraretinal vascular proliferation. These abnormal vessels are identifiable using the green filters of an ordinary ophthalmoscope, but are best seen in the secondary phase of fluorescein angiograms, during which they leak dye into the retina. IRMAs occur adjacent to areas of capillary closure. Their identification is not essential in the routine examination.

Whereas changes of background retinopathy indicate capillary damage and leakage, preproliferative changes (many soft exudates, extensive hemorrhages, IRMAs, and venous bleeding from enlarged dilated [beaded, sausage-link] retinal veins) indicate areas of intraretinal vascular occlusion with resulting nonperfusion. Eyes with retinal ischemia and moderate to severe preproliferative changes have a 50% chance of developing new vessel proliferation (neovascularization) within 1 year.

Macular Edema

It is not usually appreciated by the general clinician that even without proliferative disease, macular edema may result in visual loss as severe as the 20/200 level. Spontaneous improvement is not common but may occur. Visual acuity can also become poor because of lack of proper perfusion of the perifoveal capillaries. In this instance, visual acuity may be as low as 20/200 in the absence of macular edema. Fluorescein angiography reveals the cause of poor visual acuity to be a result of the lack of perfusion of the perifoveal capillaries. In the absence of accompanying proliferative disease, patients at this stage can usually ambulate freely and can engage in some occupations. Ability to read a newspaper, except with a vision aid, is unlikely, and the patient will have to stop driving.

Proliferative Retinopathy

At this stage of retinal disease, new vessels and accompanying fibrous tissue extend from the retinal substance and grow along the inner retinal surface and the posterior surface of the vitreous gel, often causing contraction of the gel and traction on the vessels and the retina. This process creates the conditions for retinal detachment and hemorrhage into the vitreous.

In addition, in advanced PDR, growth of new vessels and scar tissue into the angle of the eye may cause acute glaucoma (see Ocular Symptoms). When the new blood vessels grow out of the surface of the optic nerve heads, they are called new vessels on the disk; elsewhere in the retina, usually extending from large vessels, they are called new vessels elsewhere.

The National Diabetic Retinopathy Study (106) not only established the efficacy of photocoagulation therapy (see Photocoagulation Therapy) but also defined high-risk characteristics as follows: new vessels on the disk greater than 25% of the optic disk area, any new vessels on the disk with preretinal or vitreous hemorrhage, or new vessels elsewhere equal to or exceeding 50% of the disk area with preretinal or vitreous hemorrhage. The presence of high-risk characteristics increases the chance of blindness to 30% to 50% within 3 to 5 years unless appropriate photocoagulation therapy is given.

Treatment of Diabetic Retinopathy

Two forms of surgical therapy are now available for the treatment of proliferative retinopathy and its complications. Photocoagulation is of proven value in the prevention of visual loss caused by proliferative disease, and vitrectomy restores and appears to stabilize vision after hemorrhage and/or retinal detachment.

Photocoagulation Therapy

Argon laser therapy reduces severe visual loss by nearly 60% over 5 years in patients with proliferative disease. Multiple (1,200 to 1,600) 500-μm burns are placed in the retinal periphery. The Early Treatment Diabetic Retinopathy Study (107) evaluated panretinal photocoagulation (and laser photocoagulation using 450- to 650-μm widely spaced burns) to determine whether such therapy affects the course of disease in eyes with high-risk characteristics or preproliferative diabetic retinopathy. Considerable benefit was shown.

Diabetic *macular edema* is also treated with photocoagulation therapy. Leaking microaneurysms and other lesions in the macula are treated with 50- to 100-μm burns. The Early Treatment Diabetic Retinopathy Study showed a reduction of visual loss caused by macular edema of 50% over 3 years.

> *Patient Experience.* Photocoagulation therapy is an office procedure, usually performed in several sessions. Ordinarily only topical (corneal) anesthesia is necessary. Occasionally, some pain is experienced, in which case a local anesthetic is injected into the retro-orbital tissues to allow a completed pain-free procedure.

Vitrectomy

Hemorrhage into the vitreous is the usual indication for vitrectomy, a procedure that removes old blood and opaque vitreous and can be combined with cataract extraction. Retinal detachment resulting from traction bands that are formed in the vitreous is another indication for vitrectomy.

TABLE 79.7 Reasons for Referral of Patients with Diabetes Mellitus to an Ophthalmologist

High-risk patients
Neovascularization covering more than one-third of optic disk
Vitreous or preretinal hemorrhage with any neovascularization, particularly on optic disk
Macular edema (suspect from hard exudates in macula)
Symptomatic patients
Blurry vision persisting for more than 1–2 days or not associated with a change in blood glucose; suspect macular edema
Sudden loss of vision in one or both eyes
Black spots, cobwebs, or flashing lights in field of vision
Asymptomatic patients
Yearly examinations (an optometrist can check pressures if no retinal changes or if only BDR is present)
Hard exudates near macula
Any preproliferative or proliferative characteristics
Pregnancy

BDR, background diabetic retinopathy (see text).
Modified from ADA physician's guide to non–insulin-dependent (type II) diabetes. Diagnosis and treatment, 2nd ed. Alexandria, VA: ADA, 1988.

Other repair procedures can be attempted. The results of vitrectomy can be dramatic in restoring sight after vitreous hemorrhage. Currently, however, vitrectomy is used only in severely diseased eyes. Recovery of near-normal vision is the exception rather than the rule, but the results are definitely worthwhile in many patients.

Every effort should be made to control hypertension in an attempt to prevent retinal hemorrhages. Lifting of heavy objects, jarring exercise, and exposures to high altitudes may also increase the risk of hemorrhages and should be avoided in patients with PDR, but commercial airline travel presents no increased risk. The use of aspirin therapy does not increase the risk or severity of intraocular hemorrhage and is *not* contraindicated in PDR (105).

Role of the Primary Care Physician/Internist Versus That of the Ophthalmologist: Indications for Referral

If there is no evidence of retinal disease, diabetics should have yearly examinations of their eyegrounds, with their pupils dilated. If that cannot be done for any reason or if there is concern about the validity of the examination, referral to an optometrist or ophthalmologist is indicated (Table 79.7). Because most diabetic retinopathy occurs within several disk diameters of the macula, most lesions are visible by examination with the direct ophthalmoscope after dilation of the pupils. Nonophthalmologists often defer this examination out of concern over precipitating acute angle-closure glaucoma. Such reluctance is not warranted because this complication is rare at any age and is hardly ever seen before age 40 years. A drop of dilating solution (2.5% phenylephrine or 1% tropicamide) in each eye is sufficient and causes only sensitivity to bright light (requiring dark glasses) that lasts but a few hours.

If only minimal nonproliferative diabetic retinopathy is present, the patient does not need to be referred immediately if visual acuity is normal. Early preproliferative changes warrant prompt referral to a general ophthalmologist, whereas more extensive changes and proliferative changes should be followed by an ophthalmologist who is also expert in photocoagulation. In addition to examining the retina, the condition of the lens should be evaluated during the examination of the eye because senile cataracts occur prematurely in diabetic patients and metabolic cataracts result from chronic elevation of blood glucose levels.

Periodic checks of intraocular pressure to detect glaucoma, which is more prevalent in diabetics, should also be part of routine health maintenance. These evaluations can be made either by an optometrist or an ophthalmologist (see Chapter 108). Recommendations for followup are given in Table 79.7 and in detail elsewhere (108).

TRACKING AND COORDINATING CARE IN THE DIABETIC PATIENT

Because management of the diabetic patient is complex and multidimensional and because numerous interventions improve healthcare outcomes, it is important for the primary care practitioner to have a systematic approach to monitoring and coordinating the various aspects of longitudinal care of the diabetic patient. A flow sheet or computerized tracking and reminder system that targets treatment and treatment changes, critical laboratory and physical examination parameters, and key referrals is highly recommended (109; and Fig. 1.2). Items that should be tracked include serum glucose and HbA_{1c}; serum lipids; urine protein and renal function; foot examinations; and eye examinations. Prominent display of a *primary care front sheet* that includes a *problem list* (see Fig. 1.1) is particularly important in diabetic patients, because diabetics are likely to have a plethora of associated conditions (see Complications of Diabetes Mellitus). Finally, a preventive care profile and flow sheet (see Fig. 14.3) is as important in care of the diabetic as it is in the care of other patients. Some preventive care recommendations are more specific for diabetic patients, such as recommendations for pneumococcal vaccination and yearly influenza vaccinations at any age and more aggressive lipid management. Knowledge of smoking status and smoking cessation counseling (see Chapter 27) are particularly important in the diabetic patient, whose risk of atherosclerotic disease is very high.

SPECIFIC REFERENCES*

1. National Diabetes Group. Classification and diagnosis of diabetes mellitus and other categories of glucose tolerance. Diabetes 1979;28:1039.

2. Expert Committee on the Diagnosis and Classification of Diabetes Mellitus. Report. Diabetes Care 1997;20:1183.

3. Karjalainen J, Salmela P, Ilonen J, et al. A comparison of childhood and adult type I diabetes mellitus. N Engl J Med 1989;320: 881.

4. Eisenbarth GS. Type I diabetes mellitus. A chronic autoimmune disease. N Engl J Med 1986;314:1360.

5. Yoon JW. Role of viruses in the pathogenesis of IDDM. Ann Med 1991;23:437.

6. Karjalainen J, Martin JM, Knip M, et al. A bovine albumin peptide as a possible trigger of insulin-dependent diabetes mellitus. N Engl J Med 1992;327:302.

7. Niskanen LK, Tuomi T, Karjalainen J, et al. GAD antibodies in NIDDM. Ten-year follow-up from the diagnosis. Diabetes Care 1995;18:1557.

8. Turner R, Stratton I, Horton V, et al. UKPDS 25: autoantibodies to islet-cell cytoplasm and glutamic acid decarboxylase for prediction of insulin requirement in type 2 diabetes. UK Prospective Diabetes Study Group. Lancet 1997;350:1288.

9. Tuomi T, Carlsson A, Li H, et al. Clinical and genetic characteristics of type 2 diabetes with and without GAD antibodies. Diabetes 1999;48:150.

10. Alberti KG, Zimmet PZ. Definition, diagnosis and classification of diabetes mellitus and its complications. Part 1. Diagnosis and classification of diabetes mellitus. Provisional report of a WHO consultation. Diabet Med 1998;15:539.

11. Fajans SS, Bell GI, Polonsky KS. Molecular mechanisms and clinical pathophysiology of maturity-onset diabetes of the young. N Engl J Med 2001: 345:971.

12. Atkinson MA, Maclaren NK. The pathogenesis of insulin-dependent diabetes mellitus. N Engl J Med 1994;331:1428.

13. Olmos P, A'Hern R, Heaton DA, et al. The significance of the concordance rate for type 1 (insulin-dependent) diabetes in identical twins. Diabetologia 1988;31:747.

14. Kumar D, Gemayel NS, Deapen D, et al. North American twins with IDDM. Genetic, etiological, and clinical significance of disease concordance according to age, zygosity, and the interval after diagnosis in first twin. Diabetes 1993;42:1351.

15. Reaven GM. Role of insulin resistance in human disease. Diabetes 1988;37:1595.

16. Gerich JE. Insulin resistance is not necessarily an essential component of type 2 diabetes. J Clin Endocrinol Metab 2000;85:2113.

17. Almind K, Doria A, Kahn CR. Putting the genes for type II on the map. Nat Med 2001;7:277.

18. Rosenbloom AL, Joe JR, Young RS, et al. Emerging epidemic of type 2 diabetes in youth. Diabetes Care 1999;22:345.

19. Kahn CR, Vicent D, Doria A. Genetics of non–insulin-dependent (type II) diabetes mellitus. Annu Rev Med 1996;47:509.

20. Barnett AH, Eff C, Leslie RDG, et al. Diabetes in identical twins: a study of 200 pairs. Diabetologia 1981;20:87.

21. Edelstein S, Knowler WC, Bain RP, et al. Predictors of progression from impaired glucose tolerance to NIDDM. An analysis of six prospective studies. Diabetes 1997;46:701.

*Bold numerals denote published controlled clinical trials, meta-analyses, or consensus-based recommendations.

22. Knowler WC, Saad MF, Pettitt DJ, et al. Determinants of diabetes mellitus in the Pima Indians. Diabetes Care 1993;16:216.

23. Jarrett RJ. The cardiovascular risk associated with impaired glucose tolerance. Diabet Med 1995;13:S15.

24. Bjornholt JV, Erikssen G, Aaser E, et al. Fasting blood glucose: an underestimated risk factor for cardiovascular death. Diabetes Care 1999; 22:45.

25. Tuomilehto J, Lindström J, Eriksson JG, et al. Prevention of type 2 diabetes mellitus by changes in lifestyle among subjects with impaired glucose tolerance. N Engl J Med 2001;344:1343.

26. Tataranni PA, Bogardus C. Changing habits to delay diabetes. N Engl J Med 2001;344:1390.

27. Swinburn BA, Metcalf PA, Ley SJ. Long term (5-year) effects of a reduced-fat diet intervention in individuals with glucose intolerance. Diabetes Care 2001;24:619.

28. West KM. Diet therapy of diabetes: an analysis of failure. Ann Intern Med 1973;79:425.

29. West KM. Diet and diabetes. Postgrad Med 1976;60:209.

30. American Diabetes Association. Nutrition recommendations and principles for people with diabetes mellitus. Diabetes Care 2000;23:543.

31. Chen Y-DI, Swami S, Skowronski R, et al. Effect of variations in dietary fat and carbohydrate intake on postprandial lipemia in patients with noninsulin dependent diabetes mellitus. J Clin Endocrinol Metab 1993;76:347.

32. Coulston AM, Hollenbeck CB, Swislocki ALM, et al. Deleterious metabolic effects of high-carbohydrate, sucrose-containing diets in patients with non–insulin-dependent diabetes mellitus. Am J Med 1987;82:213.

33. Garg A, Bonanome A, Grundy SM, et al. Comparison of a high-carbohydrate diet with a high monounsaturated-fat diet in patients with non–insulin-dependent diabetes mellitus. N Engl J Med 1988;319:829.

34. Bonanome A, Visona A, Lusiani L, et al. Carbohydrate and lipid metabolism in patients with non–insulin-dependent diabetes mellitus: effects of a low-fat, high-carbohydrate diet vs a diet high in monosaturated fatty acids. Am J Clin Nutr 1991;54:586.

35. Ajani UA, Hennekens CH, Spelsberg A, et al. Alcohol consumption and risk of type 2 diabetes mellitus among US male physicians. Arch Intern Med 2000;160:1025.

36. Solomon CG, Hu FB, Stampfer MJ, et al. Moderate alcohol consumption and risk of coronary heart disease among women with type 2 diabetes mellitus. Circulation 2000;102: 494.

37. Gaziano JM, Gaziano TA, Glynn RJ, et al. Light-to-moderate alcohol consumption and mortality in the Physician's Health Study enrollment cohort. J Am Coll Cardiol 2000;35: 96.

38. Stolar MW. Atherosclerosis in diabetes: the role of hyperinsulinemia. Metab Clin Exp 1988;37[Suppl 1]:1.

39. Rendell M. Dietary treatment of diabetes mellitus. N Engl J Med 2000;342:1440.

40. Nuttall FQ. Dietary fiber in the management of diabetes. Diabetes 1993;42:503.

41. Helmrich SP, Ragland DR, Leung RW, et al. Physical activity and reduced occurrence of non–insulin-dependent diabetes mellitus. N Engl J Med 1991;325:147.

42. American Diabetes Association. Implications of the United Kingdom prospective Study. Diabetes Care 1998;21:2180.

43. Wolffenbuttel BH, Sels J-PJE, Rondas-Colbers GJ. Comparison of different insulin regimens in elderly patients with NIDDM. Diabetes Care 1996;19:1326.

44. Diabetes Control and Complications Trial Research Group. The effect of intensive diabetes treatment on the development and progression of long-term complications in insulin-dependent diabetes. N Engl J Med 1993;329:977.

45. American Diabetes Association. Implications of the diabetes control and complications trial. Diabetes Care 2003;26:S25–S27.

46. Intensive blood-glucose control with sulphonylureas or insulin compared with conventional treatment and risk of complications in patients with type 2 diabetes (UKPDS 33). UK Prospective Diabetes Study (UKPDS) Group. Lancet 1998;352:837.

47. Effect of intensive blood-glucose control with metformin on complications in overweight patients with type 2 diabetes (UKPDS 34). UK Prospective Diabetes Study (UKPDS) Group. Lancet 1998;352:854.

48. The University Group Diabetes Program. A study of the effects of hypoglycemic agents on vascular complications in patients with adult onset diabetes. Diabetes 1970;19(Suppl):789.

49. Nesto RW, Bell D, Bonow RO, et al. Thiazolidinedione use, fluid, and congestive heart failure: a consensus statement from the American Heart Association and American Diabetes Association. Diabetes Care 2004; 27:256.

50. Fonesca V, Rosenstock J, Wardham P, et al. Effect of metformin and rosiglitazone combination therapy in patients with type 2 diabetes mellitus. JAMA 2000;283:1695.

51. Garrison CR, Riddle MC. Evening insulin therapy for type II diabetes. Pract Diabetol 1990;9:1.

52. Riddle MC, Rosenstock J, Gerich J et al. The treat-to-target trial: randomized addition of glargine or human NPH insulin to oral therapy of type 2 diabetic patients. Diabetes Care 2003;26:3080.

53. Ohkubo Y, Kishikawa H, Araki E, et al. Intensive insulin therapy prevents the progression of diabetic microvascular complications in Japanese patients with non–insulin-dependent diabetes mellitus: a randomized prospective 6-year study. Diabetes Res Clin Pract 1995;28:103.

54. Bjorntorp P. Visceral obesity: a "civilization syndrome." Obes Res 1993;1:206.

55. Paquot N, Castillo MJ, Lefebvre PJ, et al. No increased insulin sensitivity after a single intravenous administration of a recombinant human tumor necrosis factor receptor: Fc fusion protein in obese insulin-resistant patients. J Clin Endocrinol Metab 2000;85:1316.

56. Rabasa-Lhoret R, Bourque J, Ducros F, et al. Guidelines for premeal insulin dose reduction for postprandial exercise of different durations in type 1 diabetic subjects treated intensively with a basal-bolus insulin regimen. Diabetes Care 2001;24:625.

57. Exenatide (Byetta) for type 2 diabetes. Med Lett Drug Ther 2005;47:45.

58. Pramlintide (Symlin) for diabetes. Med Lett Drug Ther 2005;47:43.

59. American Diabetes Association. Pancreas transplantation in type 1 diabetes. Diabetes Care 2004;27:S105.

60. Sudan D, Sudan R, Stratta R. Long-term outcome of simultaneous kidney-pancreas transplantation: analysis of 61 patients with more than 5 years follow-up. Transplantation 2000;69:550.

61. Shapiro AMJ, Lakey JRT, Ryan EA, et al. Islet transplantation in seven patients with type 1 diabetes mellitus using a glucocorticoid-free

examination is simple, virtually painless, and without complications (see Thyroid Nodules). The procedure is ordinarily performed by an endocrinologist or a pathologist. A few centers use *needle biopsy* (aspiration or cutting), usually performed only if the simpler FNA is not sufficiently informative. In the hands of an appropriate operator, needle biopsy is probably more definitive and, because it is performed with local (cutaneous) anesthesia, is ordinarily painless. The only significant complication is local hemorrhage, but this is an uncommon, usually minor, problem. Ultrasound is often used to guide FNA and may lead to additional information, especially when cystic lesions are present.

Various *imaging techniques* are available to delineate the anatomy of the thyroid and to distinguish functional from nonfunctional nodules, a consideration in the differential diagnosis of thyroid neoplasms. The two commonly used techniques are radioisotopic scanning (scintiscan) and ultrasonography. CT and magnetic resonance imaging are not useful for evaluating nodules, although they have a place in evaluating substernal extension of goiter and in localizing metastatic lesions, as does ^{18}F-fluorodeoxyglucose positron emission tomography (PET) scanning. The isotope most widely used in scintiscans of the thyroid is ^{99m}Tc pertechnetate (TcO_4^-), but ^{123}I is the isotope of choice. However, tumors that can take up ^{123}I but not accumulate pertechnetate in rare circumstances, and thus may give misleading information on the functional state of a nodule. Ultrasonography, now often the initial imaging procedure, is the best technique for determining the size of the thyroid; the number, size, and characteristics of nodules; and whether a nodule is cystic or solid, an important point in differential diagnosis of these lesions. Ultrasonography also provides an objective basis for evaluation of changes in the size of nodules with medical therapy. Both isotopic imaging and ultrasonography can determine whether a nodule is truly single or is in fact one of many in a multinodular gland.

Nonspecificity of Thyroid Function Tests in Nonthyroidal Illness

Thyroid function tests are frequently nonspecifically altered in many nonthyroidal diseases and by drugs and hormones (7–10); that is, these tests are not specific for thyroid disease when severe illness is present (Table 80.3). Moreover, a variety of drugs and hormones affect both thyroid function and tests that assess the hypothalamic–pituitary–thyroid axis (Tables 80.1 and 80.4). T_4, free T_4, FTI, T_3, and TSH may all be affected. Although much of the information on this subject comes from studies of hospitalized patients in whom up to 30% will show one or more abnormalities on admission, ambulatory patients are probably also affected. Some examples are presented below.

Effects of Gonadal and Adrenal Hormones on Thyroid Function Tests

Estrogens (pregnancy, contraceptives) raise and androgens lower T_4, but not free T_4 or FTI, by altering serum TBG. Glucocorticoids inhibit thyroid activity acutely by interfering with TSH secretion, lowering TSH levels, and affecting the pituitary's responsiveness to TRH. The serum T_4 is lowered during chronic glucocorticoid therapy, mainly because of a decrease of TBG.

Liver Disease

Various alterations of thyroid function tests are produced by liver disease. Early in infectious hepatitis, the T_4 level is elevated secondary to an increase of TBG. Chronic liver disease produces many abnormalities in an unpredictable

TABLE 80.3 Nonthyroidal Illness: Effects on T_4, Free T_4, TBG, and TSH in Plasma[a,b]

	T_4	*Free T_4*	*TBG*	*TSH*
Liver disease				
Active hepatitis	↑	↔↑	↑	
Cirrhosis, other chronic diseases	↑↓	↔↑	↑↓	↔↑
Cholangitis	↑	↔↓	↑	
Renal disease				
Nephrotic syndrome	↔↓	↔	↔↓	
Uremia, chronic	↔↓	↔↓	↔↓	
Infections	↓	↑	↔	
Malnutrition	↔↓	↔↑	↔↓	
Severe acute illness[c]	↑↓	↔↑	↔	↑↓

T_4, thyroid hormone thyroxine; TBG, thyroxine-binding globulin; TSH, thyroid-stimulating hormone.
[a]Most illnesses and even such minor alterations of physiologic state as decreased food intake will produce a decrease in plasma T_3.
[b]Changes of TSH levels are unlikely in ambulatory patients.
[c]Not likely to be seen in ambulatory patients.

TABLE 80.4 Drug and Hormone Effects on T_4, Free T_4, TBG, and TSH

Gonadal Hormones	*T_4*	*Free T_4*	*TBG*	*TSH*
Estrogens	↑	↔↓	↑	
Exogenous				↓
Pregnancy				
Androgens	↓	↔		
Testosterone		↑		
Anabolic steroids				
Glucocorticoids	↓	↔	↓	
Cushing syndrome				
Pharmacologic uses				
Psychotropic drugs				
Perphenazine (Trilafon)	↑	↔	↑	
Amphetamines	↑	↑	↔	
Anticonvulsants				
Phenytoin (Dilantin)	↓	↔↓	↔	↔↑
Carbamazepine	↓	↔↓	↔	↔↑
Heparin	↔	↑	↔	
Adrenergic blockers				
Propranolol (Inderal)	↔(↓T_3)	↔	↔	
Antiarrhythmic drugs	↑	↑	↔	
Amiodarone				
Gallbladder dyes				
Iopanoic acid	↑↔(↓T_3)	↔↑	↔↑	↔↑
Ipodate	↑↔(↓T_3)	↔↑	↔	↔↑
Opiates				
Miscellaneous				
Clofibrate	↑		↑	
5-Fluorouracil	↑		↑	

T_4, thyroxine; TBG, thyroxine-binding globulin; TSH, thyroid-stimulating hormone.

fashion. T_4 may be increased or decreased in parallel with TBG and the T_3U. Free T_4 is often elevated with no obvious relationship to the TBG. T_3 is usually low. A frequent and unexplained abnormality is elevation of TSH, although the response to TRH is not exaggerated as it is in hypothyroidism. RaIU is often elevated in acute alcoholic hepatitis with or without cirrhosis and in some cases of cholangitis. These changes have been attributed to both iodide depletion and acceleration of T_4 metabolism.

Renal Disease

The nephrotic syndrome is often associated with depressed T_4 and TBG. The decrease of the T_4 is likely caused by a decrease in TBG and an increase in clearance of both TBG and T_4. In chronic renal disease, the average T_4, free T_4, and TBG, are not significantly different from normal, but the range is greater and values may exceed the usual normal limits. Some patients with severe chronic renal failure receiving long-term dialysis show a progressive decrease of T_4; the mechanism is not known but the prognosis for survival in such patients is poor (see Hypothyroidism versus the Euthyroid Sick Syndrome). As expected in any chronic illness, the serum T_3 is often depressed.

Infections, Malnutrition, and Drugs

The T_4 may drop early in the course of acute infection and free T_4 may rise. Neither change is accounted for by an alteration of TBG. During starvation or severe caloric restriction, serum T_3 falls; free T_4 is often increased without relation to the TBG. Serum T_3 is often decreased in the elderly, a change that has been attributed to aging but may in large part be caused by diminished food intake and nonspecific illness (11). Closely correlated alterations of T_3U and serum TBG have been reported in protein-calorie malnutrition. Some pharmacologic agents affect thyroid hormone levels (Table 80.4). Phenytoin (Dilantin) and carbamazepine promote thyroid hormone metabolism and lower T_4 and free T_4 into the hypothyroid range, but the TSH is normal. The apparently low free T_4 is an artifact of routine methodology and is an excellent example of how misleading this test can be in some circumstances (12). Heparin acutely elevates the free T_4; following heparin administration, the heparin in the specimen can cause stimulation of lipoprotein lipase that liberates free fatty acids that inhibit T_4 binding to serum proteins. β-Adrenergic blockers decrease serum T_3 by inhibition of the normal T_4 deiodination route; rT_3 is increased. A similar decrease of T_3 through reduced hepatic metabolism of

T_4 is produced by propylthiouracil, dexamethasone, amiodarone, and the radiopaque contrast media used for visualization of the gallbladder. In the case of the latter agents, additional mechanisms are operative because these compounds may also elevate T_4 and TSH, an effect attributed to their differential inhibition of conversion of T_4 and T_3 in the pituitary and the periphery. Amphetamine abuse may increase serum T_4, presumably by central stimulation of TSH release (7). In human immunodeficiency virus (HIV) infection, patients have increased T_4 and TBG early in the disease, but no change in T_3 and low rT_3. T_4 and T_3 can be decreased in advanced stages of the disease.

Altered Serum Thyroxine Caused by Inherited and Other Abnormalities of Protein Binding

In addition to those diseases or drugs that alter T_4 levels by affecting binding of the hormone to TBG, altered protein binding also occurs in inherited disorders of TBG excess, TBG deficiency, increased concentration of thyroxine-binding prealbumin, and increases in the number of T_4 binding sites on an albumin variant (familial dysalbuminemic hyperthyroxinemia). The first two conditions are X-linked. The latter two conditions, inherited as autosomal dominants, are rare. In all these conditions, the free T_4 is normal (7).

Alterations of Serum Thyroxine in Nonthyroidal Illness Not Caused by Abnormalities of Protein Binding

Elevations of T_4 that are unexplained by changes in thyroxine binding are common. These situations are difficult to distinguish from hyperthyroidism. Included are the elevation of T_4 seen in acute nonthyroidal illness, in psychiatric disease, and as the effect of some drugs. The stress of serious illness may also lower T_4 and simulate hypothyroidism (see Hypothyroidism versus the Euthyroid Sick Syndrome), but such severe illness is rarely encountered in ambulatory patients. An exception may be seen in patients receiving dialysis for chronic renal failure. Abnormal thyroid hormone levels in these situations and diseases that are regularly associated with such changes (7–9) are described briefly below.

Increase of Serum Thyroxine during Nonspecific Illness: Euthyroid Hyperthyroxinemia

Although the phenomenon of decreased serum T_4 during severe illness is now widely recognized, the frequent occurrence of *increased* T_4 (and free T4) caused by illness is not generally appreciated. The increase of T_4 is modest, and the T_4 generally does not exceed about 15 μg. This problem is commonly seen in severely ill elderly patients in whom it raises the issue of hyperthyroidism (11). Similar findings have been reported in hyperemesis gravidarum.

Acute Psychiatric Disease

Restlessness, hyperactivity, tachycardia, and tremor are often seen as part of severe *acute* psychiatric illness. Clinical suspicion of hyperthyroidism (because of tachycardia, tremor, sweating) leads to thyroid function tests and laboratory results consistent with this diagnosis. Such patients may have elevated T_4, FTI, and T_3. The TSH may not be suppressed (13). In some series, up to one-third of acutely hospitalized psychiatric patients have an elevated T_4. Although the phenomenon is documented only in hospitalized patients, it may be encountered in any severely disturbed person. The T_4 returns to normal within 1 to 2 weeks of clinical improvement of the psychiatric disturbance. This phenomenon may represent a form of centrally driven hyperthyroidism (13).

Increased Serum Thyroxine Caused by Resistance to Thyroid Hormones

Rare but well-recognized cases of increased T_4 unaccompanied by binding protein abnormalities are seen with the syndrome of resistance to thyroid hormone. Originally described as a familial syndrome of increased T_4, goiter, deaf mutism, and some degree of hypothyroidism with delayed bone maturation and epiphyseal stippling, the most common phenotype is actually that of elevated T_4, increased or inappropriately normal TSH, in a person without symptoms of major hypo- or hyperthyroidism. The abnormality occurs both sporadically and in familial form, and is probably part of a heterogeneous group of disorders with variable inheritance (14). Most cases are caused by abnormal (mutant) thyroid hormone receptors.

Statistical Considerations in the Clinical Interpretation of Thyroid Function Tests

No single numerical value divides normal from abnormal in any thyroid function test. The upper and lower limits of normal for serum T_4, FTI, and T_3 are arbitrarily set, as they are for most tests at ± 2 standard deviations from the mean. By definition, therefore, 2.5% of an apparently normal population will have abnormal values at each end of the distribution. To complicate the issue, a small number of hyperthyroid or hypothyroid patients have values that fall clearly within the normal range. In addition to the statistical overlap, both biologic (i.e., day to day) variation and unavoidable analytical error further obscure the dividing line between normal and abnormal. For example, 95% confidence limits for the analytic variation of a single T_4 test are ± 1 μg/dL at the upper and lower limits of the normal range. For all these reasons and because of the occasional instance of laboratory or reporting error, a single laboratory determination should not be relied on to establish or exclude a diagnosis. All abnormal values should be confirmed before therapy is undertaken, and borderline values should be repeated before diagnostic conclusions

TABLE 80.5 Causes of Thyrotoxicosis[a]

Causes
Common
Graves disease
Toxic nodular goiter
Multinodular
Uninodular
Thyrotoxicosis in association with thyroiditis
Postpartum thyrotoxicosis
Iodide induced (iodide, iodine-containing drugs, and contrast media)
Rare to vanishingly rare
Thyrotoxicosis caused by TSH or a TSH-like stimulator
Choriocarcinoma or hydatidiform mole
Embryonal cell carcinoma of testis
Pituitary tumor with TSH excess
Idiopathic TSH excess
Toxic thyroid carcinoma
Thyrotoxicosis caused by exogenous thyroid hormone
Factitia
Medicamentosa (iatrogenic)
Toxic struma ovarii

TSH, thyroid-stimulating hormone.
[a]Listed in approximate decreasing order of frequency.

are drawn. Premature institution of therapy may obscure the diagnosis.

HYPERTHYROIDISM AND THYROTOXICOSIS

Thyrotoxicosis is defined as any condition in which the cells of the body are exposed to excess amounts of circulating thyroid hormone. *Hyperthyroidism* is any condition in which thyrotoxicosis is attributable to hyperfunction of the thyroid gland. Often the terms are used interchangeably, although they do not mean precisely the same thing.

Essentially, the same presentation may result from any of several different pathologic processes (Table 80.5), and selection of proper therapy demands that the correct underlying diagnosis is established. The most common cause of hyperthyroidism is *Graves disease*, an autoimmune process also known as *diffuse toxic goiter*. Only slightly less common is hyperthyroidism caused by a hyperfunctioning multinodular goiter (toxic nodular goiter). Occasionally, hyperthyroidism is caused by a *solitary hyperfunctioning adenoma* ("hot nodule"). Thyrotoxicosis also has been seen with increasing frequency as a transient phenomenon in the evolution of *thyroiditis* (see Thyroiditis) (15,16). In addition, the induction of thyrotoxicosis by iodide and iodide-containing drugs (e.g., amiodarone) and contrast media should be considered for those patients who have had such exposures (see below) (17). The other causes of hyperthyroidism listed in Table 80.5 are rare and are not usually encountered in ordinary practice.

Clinical Presentation and Diagnosis of Thyrotoxicosis

Clinical History

The presentation of patients with thyrotoxicosis is highly variable (Table 80.6). The severity is determined not only by the degree of hormone excess but also by its rapidity of onset, its duration, and the age of the patient. The "typical" thyrotoxic patient has one or more of the following spontaneous complaints: nervousness, weight loss, palpitations (which at first may be intermittent), enlarging neck mass (goiter), change in appearance of the eyes (Graves disease), or symptoms of heart failure. These symptoms usually have been present anywhere from a few weeks to a year or longer. Careful questioning often reveals other symptoms.

TABLE 80.6 Signs and Symptoms of Thyrotoxicosis

Organ or System	*Signs and Symptoms*
Adrenergic manifestations	Excess sweating, heat intolerance, palpitations, tachycardia, tremor, lid lag, stare, nervousness, and excitability
Hypermetabolism and catabolism	Increased appetite, weight loss
One system predominance	
Eyes[a]	Periorbital edema, exophthalmos (proptosis), chemosis, ophthalmoplegia, papilledema
Cardiac	Arrhythmia, congestive heart failure
Muscle	Fatigue and weakness, muscle wasting, proximal myopathy, periodic paralysis
Gastrointestinal	Increased frequency of bowel movements, pernicious vomiting
Bone	Acropachy, osteoporosis, hypercalcemia
Reproductive	Infertility, abortion, scanty menses, testicular atrophy, gynecomastia
Mental	Anxiety, irritability, psychosis, insomnia
Skin	Onycholysis, "pretibial" myxedema, hyperpigmentation

[a]Graves disease only.

The so-called nervousness in thyrotoxicosis is often irritability, inability to concentrate, restlessness, or overt emotional lability, but it is a tremor of the hands that most often leads the patient to express this complaint. Impairment of normal sleep pattern with frequent wakening is common. Some patients with *anxiety* may experience tachycardia, tremor, irritability, and weakness simulating thyrotoxicosis. The "anxiety" of thyrotoxicosis is more likely to appear as irritability and hyperkinesis than as an expressed feeling of being anxious. Primary anxiety disorders are either related to identifiable stresses, coexist with symptoms of depression, or have distinctive characteristics that make them recognizable (see Chapter 22). In depression, weight loss is invariably accompanied by anorexia, a relatively unusual symptom of thyrotoxicosis.

Weight loss classically occurs despite increased appetite, although often no obvious change in appetite is noticed or there may be anorexia, especially in elderly patients. The only prominent gastrointestinal symptom is increased frequency of bowel movements, but actual diarrhea is not seen.

The *heat intolerance* of hyperthyroidism is often apparent only on questioning. Commonly, the patient admits to having reduced the number of covers used on the bed at night or to the development of new and unusual habits, such as sleeping in the nude or with feet extended from under the blankets. Sweating is increased but is not usually a spontaneous complaint and may be denied.

As the disease progresses in severity, *skeletal muscle wasting* occurs, which tends to involve especially the limb girdle musculature, producing a proximal myopathy. This process results in weakness, expressed, for example, as great difficulty in climbing stairs or, on examination, in arising from a squatting position. Exertional dyspnea without evidence of cardiac failure is common and may be related to the myopathy.

Skin changes are hardly ever noticed by the patient, and "silky skin" or hair (a "classic" symptom) is only occasionally seen on examination. Hair loss is common, usually noticed as thinning of the scalp hair by women. Other skin changes include occasional cases in light skinned people of diffuse hyperpigmentation with darkening noted mostly over extensor surfaces of elbows, knees, and small joints. In African American patients, darkening of the skin is common, but its occurrence is discovered only by questioning.

Physical Findings

The thyroid is visibly or palpably enlarged in almost all children and adult patients with hyperthyroidism; however, in the adult population greater than 65 years old, the thyroid may not become enlarged. Asymmetric enlargement is common, especially in patients with toxic nodular goiter. Extreme vascularity of the gland in Graves disease may result in palpable or audible blood flow; a bruit is usually heard over the enlarged lobes but occasionally is best heard more rostrally over the superior thyroidal arteries. A bruit over the thyroid of a hyperthyroid patient is usually diagnostic of Graves disease; this finding is not present in patients with toxic nodular goiter.

Cardiovascular findings include sinus tachycardia, systolic flow murmurs, wide pulse pressure commonly, and atrial fibrillation occasionally. It is a common belief that most patients with hyperthyroidism at least have a tachycardia, but in fact only 50% of patients, regardless of age, have an increased heart rate. The apex impulse is often prominent and forceful. Cardiac failure may develop in severe cases of long duration, especially in the elderly.

The *eye findings* can be separated into those that occur as a result of thyroid hormone excess and those that are part of the ophthalmopathy of Graves disease (see Graves Disease, Opthalmopathy) (18). Excessive thyroid hormone enhances sympathetic tone and the innervation of the eyelids is partially under sympathetic control. Lid retraction with increased scleral visibility above and below the iris (prominent "whites" of the eyes), along with infrequent blinking, leads to the striking "stare" so commonly seen. Failure of the lid to follow movements of the globe ("lid lag") is another manifestation of the same process.

Clubbing of the fingers and toes is rare (thyroid acropachy) and is distinguishable radiographically from that seen in pulmonary disease. A common sign is separation of the distal portion of one or more fingernails from their nail bed (onycholysis; "dirty fingernail" sign). A fine rapid tremor, usually detected in the hands, is a common physical finding.

In some patients, particularly elderly ones, the clinical picture may not suggest thyrotoxicosis. Such patients may have only unexplained weight loss or weakness. Occult neoplasm may first be suspected, and the diagnosis of hyperthyroidism may be missed entirely or considered only after extensive evaluation fails to yield a diagnosis. These are the patients with severe but not clinically obvious disease, termed in the past *apathetic hyperthyroidism*. The term was used to describe patients who did not have obvious activation of the sympathetic nervous system (e.g., tachycardia, lid retraction, tremor). Apathetic hyperthyroidism is only rarely encountered today because of increased awareness on the part of clinician and modern diagnostic techniques that have led to earlier detection of hyperthyroidism.

Congestive heart failure, atrial fibrillation, or new-onset or worsening *angina pectoris* may be the presenting manifestation of thyrotoxicosis.

Laboratory Diagnosis

When prominent symptoms are present, the usual thyroid function tests substantiate the diagnosis in almost all cases: an increase in free T_4 and a suppressed TSH. If these results are borderline or normal, the serum T_3 must be measured, because hyperthyroidism may be caused by elevation of T_3 alone. However, so-called T_3 toxicosis (see Hyperthyroidism Caused by Excessive Secretion of T_3, Triiodothyronine (T_3) Toxicosis) occurs in less than 5% of all cases.

The amount of tracer iodide accumulation (^{131}I, ^{123}I) in the thyroid can be measured using RaIU studies. The uptake of radioactive iodide tracers (RaIU) is increased in Graves disease. RaIU studies are useful when the absence of classical features of Graves disease makes it important to distinguish it from thyroiditis (see Thyroiditis: Thyrotoxicosis Associated with Thyroiditis).

Both antithyroglobulin and antimicrosomal antibodies are elevated in Graves disease but are not useful diagnostically. Assays for TSI are available but usually are not necessary for the diagnosis of Graves disease.

Graves Disease

Graves disease is a complex disorder comprising toxic goiter, ophthalmopathy, and occasionally dermopathy. At any given time during the course of the disease, one of these manifestations may be an isolated finding. Graves ophthalmopathy and Graves dermopathy can occur independently of thyroid hormone excess. It is generally accepted that ophthalmopathy and dermopathy are closely related but separate and overlapping immunologic disorders.

Recognition of Graves disease in a typical case is not difficult. However, its insidious onset and the absence of eye or thyroid findings in early disease may delay the diagnosis for months or years.

Various abnormal immunoglobulins are found in the serum of patients with Graves disease. Some of these immunoglobulins have TSH-like activity and are designated TSIs; they are antibodies to the normal receptor sites for TSH. The reasons for development of abnormal immunoglobulins in Graves disease are not clearly understood. It is currently thought that Graves disease is a failure of T-cell surveillance rather than a response to thyroid antigens released from a thyroid damaged by unknown causes.

Ophthalmopathy

When Graves ophthalmopathy is present, there is forward protrusion of the globe. This process may be unilateral at first and is often asymmetric. The protrusion represents true proptosis and contributes an additional component to the stare produced by increased sympathetic tone. Extraocular muscle weakness may occur and results in limitation of ability to converge and to perform extreme movements of gaze; strabismus and diplopia are its more severe manifestations.

The serum of some patients with Graves ophthalmopathy contains a factor that produces exophthalmos and other abnormalities of orbital tissues in test animals. There is interstitial edema in the extraocular muscles, increased connective tissue, fatty infiltration, and infiltration with lymphocytes (18). Eventually, gross degenerative changes, such as fibrosis, may occur.

The exact frequency of ophthalmopathy in Graves disease is unknown, but most patients have either no obvious infiltrative eye involvement or show only minimal to moderate proptosis, which generally stabilizes at a tolerable level. Severe exophthalmos occurs in no more than a few percent of cases of Graves disease.

Graves ophthalmopathy and thyroid hyperactivity often coincide; in 85% of cases, the two occur within 18 months of each other. However, the ophthalmopathy may occur years before or after the onset of hyperthyroidism. Even if the patient is euthyroid (normal T_4 and T_3), the thyroid can frequently be shown to be autonomous, as demonstrated by a nonsuppressible RaIU and a suppressed TSH. In this phase of the disease, the thyroid's activity is driven by TSIs rather than TSH, but the serum thyroid hormones are within the range of normal. Without evidence of either thyroid hyperfunction, disturbance of the negative feedback system (suppression of TSH), or dermopathy, the diagnosis of Graves ophthalmopathy cannot always be made with absolute assurance. Indeed, other diseases of the orbit or retro-orbital space must be considered. CT of the skull and the orbital contents and/or high-resolution sonography are useful diagnostic tools. These procedures can visualize the enlarged extraocular muscles typical of Graves ophthalmopathy, although such enlargement is also seen in pseudotumor. In cases of Graves ophthalmopathy without overt hyperthyroidism, other aspects of Graves disease usually become apparent eventually, but several years may elapse before that occurs.

Proptosis becomes more than a cosmetic concern when the eyelids fail to close, especially when the patient is sleeping, setting the stage for exposure keratitis or corneal ulceration. This problem may be relieved by the application of liquid tears (available over the counter) and the wearing of eye patches at night and sunglasses in bright sunlight or on windy days. Paresis of the extraocular muscles producing diplopia can also be troublesome and may require use of an eye patch or corrective surgery. The most disturbing, but fortunately uncommon, eye involvement is severe chemosis (marked inflammation and edema) of the conjunctivae and periorbital soft tissues. Ophthalmopathy of this severity is termed malignant or infiltrative exophthalmos. Rarely, optic neuritis leading to blindness occurs.

Treatment of severe ophthalmopathy is best provided by an ophthalmologist who has experience with the problem, working in close collaboration with an endocrinologist. Corticosteroids (e.g., prednisone, 60 mg/day for

1 to 2 weeks, tapered over 6 to 8 weeks) are useful for patients with severe periorbital and conjunctival edema and inflammation. Other therapy, if warranted, includes low-dose orbital radiation, an established and useful therapy (19). Surgical decompression is only rarely needed and is reserved for patients with severe proptosis. There is considerable controversy about which therapy is optimal. It should also be noted that patients with severe Graves ophthalmopathy can have worsened eye symptoms with radioactive iodine therapy, which can be blocked prophylactically by corticosteroids.

Dermopathy

A unique, albeit unusual, finding in Graves disease, consists of somewhat circumscribed areas of mucopolysaccharide deposition, typically over the shins, termed *pretibial myxedema*. This unfortunate designation unjustifiably suggests a relationship between the very different type of generalized mucopolysaccharide deposition in severe hypothyroidism (myxedema) and the localized deposition in Graves disease. No relationship exists between these processes. The lesions usually have sharp raised margins and may have an orange peel-like appearance. The affected area is often intensely pruritic.

Therapy

Hyperthyroidism caused by Graves disease may be a self-limited process that terminates within two years in approximately in one-third of patients. In a few of these individuals, the disease recurs decades later. This natural history strongly influences selection of therapy. Other therapeutic considerations relate to the age of the patient and the presence or absence of complications of the hyperthyroidism, its severity, and the presence of comorbid conditions.

Because there are currently no means of controlling the underlying cause of the disease, presumed to be TSI production, therapy is designed to interfere with thyroid hormone synthesis by drugs or by ablation of thyroid tissue by radioiodide or surgery (20). Antithyroidal therapy and radioablation are the most commonly used treatments, with the latter the preferred choice among endocrinologists in the United States.

Antithyroid Drugs

Antithyroid drugs predictably control excessive production of thyroid hormone in essentially all cases, although in only approximately 20% to 40% of cases will a permanent remission of the hyperthyroidism be seen upon drug withdrawal. Males are much less likely to achieve remission (20%) than females (40%), and younger patients (younger than age 40 years) are less likely (33%) than older patients (older than 40 years) (48%) (21). Relapses may occur early or later (within 6 months to a year) or after apparent remission. Late relapses are uncommon, except in postpartum patients. It is not generally appreciated that about half of the patients who have a permanent remission will become hypothyroid between 15 and 20 years after successful treatment.

In the United States, only two thiocarbamide (thionamide) drugs are available, propylthiouracil (PTU) and methimazole (Tapazole). Other equally effective thiocarbamides are used in other countries. *Propylthiouracil*, unlike methimazole, in addition to its effects in inhibiting thyroid hormone synthesis, also inhibits conversion of T_4 to T_3 in peripheral tissues. On the other hand, *methimazole* is longer acting than propylthiouracil and may be given on a less-frequent dosage schedule, thereby facilitating compliance. In most adults with hyperthyroidism, 100 to 150 mg of propylthiouracil (available in 50-mg tablets) every 8 hours or 15 to 30 mg of methimazole (available in 5- and 10-mg tablets) every 24 hours usually suffice as initial therapy, whereas maintenance is often possible with 50 to 100 mg of propylthiouracil twice daily or 5 to 10 mg of methimazole once a day. The FT_4 level (not the TSH) which can remain suppressed, should be measured after about 2 weeks of treatment, at 1 month and every 2 to 3 months thereafter. If at these relatively low maintenance dosages of antithyroid drug the serum FT_4 falls below normal, efforts to titrate the dosage downward are often tedious and unsuccessful. An euthyroid state can be achieved under these circumstances by the addition of oral T_4, usually at a somewhat-less-than-full replacement dose. Additionally, it should be recalled that antithyroid drug therapy never induces permanent remission in patients with toxic nodular goiter (see below), which is the diagnosis in about half of the thyrotoxic patients older than age 55 years.

Although the recommended dosages of antithyroid drugs control the disease in most cases, some individuals may need higher dosages. Severely ill patients should be given larger doses from the beginning. Although the risk of an adverse drug effect is theoretically increased, this should not be a consideration under such circumstances. To achieve total blockade of hormone synthesis, as much as 400 mg of propylthiouracil every 6 to 8 hours may be necessary. Because methimazole has a longer duration of action, it need not be given so often, but 30 to 40 mg three times daily may be needed in rare cases.

Drug therapy should continue for 12 to 24 months before discontinuation of the drug is considered, although conflicting clinical evidence suggests that lasting remission may not be related to duration of therapy beyond the point at which the patient becomes euthyroid. Patients who have continued to require large doses of drugs are almost certain not to have achieved remission. On the other hand, reduction of thyroid size during therapy is thought by some clinicians to be predictive of lasting clinical remission. Measurement of titers of TSI may be useful in predicting that remission has occurred (22), but such measurements are not widely available and also are not highly accurate predictors. If it appears that remission may have been reached, antithyroid drug therapy is stopped and the patient is observed. Routine determination of serum T_4 every 3 to 4 weeks for 3 to 6 months allows early recognition of the return of thyroid overactivity.

Minor side effects of drug therapy occur in 1% to 5% of patients. Skin rashes, the most common side effect, are usually seen in the first months of therapy and often disappear even if therapy is continued. Antihistamine drugs are useful in controlling these rashes and the associated urticaria and pruritus that sometimes occur. Neutropenia is not uncommon but is usually not severe and is dose related. If the absolute number of polymorphonuclear neutrophils falls below 2,000, the dosage should be reduced, but the drug need not be immediately discontinued. The white blood cell count should be monitored after several weeks of therapy and after increases of drug dosage. If the side effects are not tolerated, a switch to the other thiocarbamide allows continuation of therapy in about half of the cases. Major complications of drug therapy occur in less than 0.1% of cases. *Agranulocytosis* is the most dreaded complication. Unlike neutropenia, thiocarbamide-induced agranulocytosis from antileukocyte antibodies is not dose related and is of such sudden onset that routine blood counts are of no help in prevention. However, the patient should be instructed to contact the physician promptly if severe sore mouth or sore throat and fever occur. Immediate hospitalization is probably indicated. Most patients with agranulocytosis eventually recover, albeit after a stormy course. Other toxic reactions include drug fever, arthralgias, and hepatitis. *Elevations of aminotransferase activity* are commonly seen in patients receiving propylthiouracil. If other liver enzymes are normal, the drug may be continued, but persistent laboratory evidence of hepatocellular damage indicates a need to discontinue therapy. Aminotransferase activity should be measured every 3 to 6 months. Methimazole is rarely a cause of cholestatic jaundice in patients taking the drug; hepatic enzymes (including serum alkaline phosphatase) should be measured at baseline and as indicated thereafter. (However, thyrotoxic patients often have elevations of serum hepatic enzyme activity at onset of their disease, particularly alkaline phosphatase activity.)

Adrenergic Antagonists

Many symptoms and signs of thyrotoxicosis are related to sensitization of the sympathetic nervous system and are in large measure abolished by β-adrenergic-blocking drugs. The indications for use of a beta blocker in hyperthyroidism are severe tachycardia, tremor, sweating, and agitation. Although beta blockers are effective for relief of these manifestations of hyperthyroidism, they do not appreciably affect excessive metabolic rate or reverse the catabolic state of severe cases. β_1-selective agents (e.g., atenolol, nadolol, metoprolol) are probably preferable to avoid unwanted side effects in susceptible individuals (e.g., asthmatics). Other uses for β-blockers are in the prevention of symptoms during a trial of withdrawal of an antithyroid drug when blood hormone levels can be used to assess the progress of therapy and while awaiting the effects of ^{131}I therapy. Most patients require a β-blocker in a dose equivalent to atenolol, 100 mg/day. The drug should be discontinued as soon as the patient is rendered euthyroid (T_4 normal).

Iodide (Nonradioactive)

Nonradioactive (stable) iodide (^{127}I) for the treatment of hyperthyroidism should be reserved for patients with severe illness or for patients with significant comorbidity. Occasionally, iodide therapy produces severe dermatitis. Use of iodide may preclude for many weeks the use of radioactive iodide, the uptake of which by the thyroid will be greatly diminished.

However, iodide is the best agent available for inhibiting hormone release and is useful in patients who need rapid correction of the hyperthyroid state. Iodide also has a time-honored place in preoperative preparation (see Chapter 93) for thyroidectomy to reduce vascularity of the gland. When given for several weeks after radioiodide therapy, iodide seems especially effective in accelerating restoration of euthyroid status. When given in this setting, some endocrinologists advocate initiating antithyroid drug therapy for at least 2 days before starting iodide therapy and continuing combined therapy for 2 months.

The standard dosage of iodide is 1 drop of a saturated solution of potassium iodide (40 mg) diluted in several ounces of water or juice once daily; higher dosages are often given but are unnecessary because a dose of only 5 mg produces a maximal effect. Lugol solution, containing iodine and iodide, is an obsolete pharmacologic concoction and has no virtue over iodide alone.

Iopanoic Acid Therapy

This drug, an oral cholecystogram contrast agent, is a potent inhibitor of the conversion of T_4 to T_3. Some experts believe it is a useful clinical adjunct for the rapid correction of hyperthyroidism (see Thyroid Storm (Thyrotoxic Crisis)).

Radioactive Iodide Therapy

Radioactive iodide (^{131}I) is uniformly effective therapy; it is simple to administer and inexpensive. In the United States, unlike Japan and, to a lesser degree, Europe, it is the preferred form of therapy for most adults with Graves disease. The rapidity of response is dependent on dose and on the size of the gland, but improvement is often apparent in a few weeks and euthyroidism (or hypothyroidism) is achieved usually within a few months. Single-dose radioiodide produces a hypothyroid state in most patients.

Some endocrinologists advocate the use of deliberately ablative doses of ^{131}I. This approach to therapy simplifies patient management, accelerates restoration of the euthyroid state, and is reasonable in view of the high probability of eventual posttherapy hypothyroidism regardless of dose. In the past, elaborate schemes have been used to estimate the required dose of ^{131}I. Unfortunately, none has proven helpful because the variability of the thyroid's sensitivity to radiation, the most important determinant of effect, is not measurable. Ablative doses are typically 12 to 15 mCi. Antithyroid drugs are often used initially to render the patient euthyroid, then interrupted for 96 hours before the ^{131}I is given to maximize iodine uptake, and can be reinstituted 24 to 48 hours afterward. Radioactive iodide can be administered only by an appropriately licensed physician, usually a nuclear medicine physician or an endocrinologist. A few precautions are necessary. In women of child-bearing age, a negative serum test for pregnancy must be obtained by the therapist immediately before the therapy dose is given because exposure of a fetus to radiation is unacceptable. In the United States, women who have a young child at home are given no more than 8 mCi and are instructed to avoid prolonged close contact (e.g., sharing a bed) for a week. Lactating women should not nurse for a month after therapy.

The undocumented notion has long persisted that radiation thyroiditis may produce excessive release of thyroid hormones 7 to 14 days after therapy, with the possibility of consequent worsening of the clinical state. Thus, precarious patients (e.g., those in congestive heart failure) are best brought to euthyroid status or are at least significantly improved by antithyroid drug therapy before ablation with ^{131}I. At 3 months after ^{131}I therapy, when the short-term radiation effect becomes maximal, the antithyroid drug can be discontinued or tapered, provided that the laboratory and clinical evidence indicates return to euthyroid status. Adjunctive therapy with a β-blocker is useful during this period to ameliorate possibly emerging symptoms if the dose of ^{131}I proves to have been inadequate. If the laboratory evidence indicates continuing hyperthyroidism, another dose of ^{131}I is required. Therapy with ^{131}I is always successful if enough ^{131}I is given. "Failure" after one or more doses is never an indication for surgery or indeterminate therapy with antithyroid drug. Rather, additional ^{131}I should be given to complete the process.

Surgical Therapy

For many years surgical ablation of the thyroid (e.g., subtotal thyroidectomy) was the main therapy for hyperthyroidism. Currently, it is rarely used except for patients who cannot, or elect not, to be treated with antithyroid drugs or ^{131}I therapy. In the hands of experienced surgeons, subtotal thyroidectomy is effective therapy, attended by minimal morbidity. However, complications include the small but real risk of anesthetic and operative mortality, recurrent laryngeal nerve damage with vocal cord paralysis, permanent hypoparathyroidism, and most commonly, hypothyroidism.

Hyperthyroidism Associated with Multinodular Goiter (Toxic Nodular Goiter) or with a Solitary ("Hot") Nodule

Toxic nodular goiter is usually seen in adults in midlife or in the elderly. Although the typical patient with Graves disease usually relates symptoms extending over a few months to a year, the history in toxic nodular goiter is often much longer, and many years usually pass before a diagnosis is made. Because of the typical patient's age and the duration of illness, severe cardiac or musculoskeletal involvement is common.

Toxic nodular goiter appears to arise in the evolution of some cases of nodular goiter. Most nodular goiters (see Goiter) are initially TSH dependent (i.e., RaIU is suppressible with exogenous thyroid hormone). Eventually, some of these goiters develop autonomous areas, with other regions of relatively decreased activity. Nodular goiters at this stage of evolution do not secrete enough hormone to produce clinical hyperthyroidism, but 20% of cases nevertheless can be shown to have nonsuppressible function. Some of these autonomously functioning goiters evolve to a stage in which excessive production of hormone and subclinical (see Subclinical Hyperthyroidism) or clinical hyperthyroidism (low TSH, elevated T_4 and T_3, with or without overt clinical symptoms) ensues.

Therapy of toxic nodular goiter is best accomplished with ^{131}I. Large doses, in the range of 15 to 30 mCi, are usually necessary and may have to be repeated more than once. Hypothyroidism occurs much less commonly after ^{131}I therapy for nodular goiter than for Graves disease. If the clinical situation demands prompt relief of the hyperthyroidism, an antithyroid drug can be used after the therapeutic dose of ^{131}I because the response to radioiodide is often slow and/or multiple doses may be needed. Otherwise, ^{131}I given alone is simple therapy, without side effects, and easily monitored by measurements of serum T_4. With ablative therapy (large doses), thyrotoxicosis may be controlled in several weeks or with smaller doses, in several months. Other therapeutic considerations including the use of adjunctive therapy follow those outlined for the therapy of Graves disease with one exception: in hyperthyroidism caused by a solitary toxic nodular goiter, antithyroid drugs alone, although effective while administered, will not produce a lasting remission. The same is true for hyperthyroidism caused by a hot nodule (see Thyroid Nodules).

Hyperthyroidism Caused by Excessive Secretion of T_3

Triiodothyronine (T_3) Toxicosis

In most cases of hyperthyroidism, the thyroid secretes excessive quantities of both T_4 and T_3. However, in perhaps 5% of all cases, T_3 is the predominant hormone secreted. So-called T_3 toxicosis may occur in hyperthyroidism caused by Graves disease, toxic multinodular goiter, or autonomous adenoma. The patient who appears clinically hyperthyroid but whose T_4 is normal or low should have serum T_3 measured. T_3 toxicosis sometimes occurs early in the course of hyperthyroidism caused by Graves disease and can develop during therapy with an antithyroid drug, in which case the dosage should be increased. Continuing clinical findings of hyperthyroidism during such therapy, despite a normal or low T_4, raise the possibility that T_3 toxicosis is now present and that more, rather than less, antithyroid drug is needed. The treatment of T_3 toxicosis is the same as is that of other forms of hyperthyroidism.

Free T_3 Toxicosis

On rare occasions, hyperthyroidism is suspected on clinical grounds and yet the only clue is a low TSH. T_4, free T_4, FTI, and serum T_3 (total) are all normal. Such patients may have the entity of "free T_3 toxicosis" (23). Only a few cases have been reported. These patients may have some anatomic thyroid abnormality or thyroid autonomy (e.g., nodule, multinodular goiter) but the condition can apparently occur without such abnormalities. The only biochemical abnormality of serum hormones in these individuals, aside from a low TSH, is an elevation of their serum free T_3. T_3, like T_4, is mainly protein bound, but T_3 is much less tightly bound than T_4. Free T_3 is measured, like free T_4, by equilibrium dialysis. The metabolic effects of an elevation of free T_3 are clinically identical to that of an increased free T_4.

Factitious Hyperthyroidism

When clinical hyperthyroidism is found in a patient without goiter or true exophthalmos (proptosis), suspicion of *factitious hyperthyroidism* may be warranted. As in true hyperthyroidism, the TSH will be suppressed and the T_4 will be elevated. However, the RaIU test will be very low, and the thyroid will be normal-sized on sonogram. Such findings suggest either the presence of thyroiditis with hyperthyroidism (see Thyroiditis) or ingestion of thyroid hormone. Measurement of thyroglobulin may help differentiate between these two possibilities (thyroglobulin levels will be low if thyroid hormone is being ingested).

Subclinical Hyperthyroidism

The term *subclinical hyperthyroidism* has been applied to the clinical state in which the TSH is suppressed but the free T_4 and free T_3 concentrations are within the normal range (24–26). By definition, the patients are asymptomatic. This condition can occur in the absence of thyroid hormone administration or during treatment with T_4 for replacement or TSH suppression. In one large series, subclinical hyperthyroidism *was* associated with a threefold increased risk in people age 60 years or older of developing atrial fibrillation (but *not* overt hyperthyroidism) over 10 years (25). In that study there were no other adverse outcomes; in fact, the condition may spontaneously abate, that is, the TSH normalizes (26) (see Screening for Thyroid Disease in Healthy Patients). Very few patients with only a low TSH subsequently develop clinical hyperthyroidism with elevation of T_4 or T_3 concentrations. Thus, the term *subclinical hyperthyroidism,* which is based only on a suppressed TSH, may be misleading.

Thyroid Storm (Thyrotoxic Crisis)

Thyroid storm, a severe exacerbation of hyperthyroidism, is rarely encountered. When thyroid storm does occur, it is usually in the setting of severe medical or surgical stress imposed on a patient with uncontrolled or unrecognized hyperthyroidism. Clinical features of full-blown thyroid storm include fever, sometimes to the level of extreme hyperpyrexia; marked tachycardia; great irritability; diarrhea; hypotension; and cardiovascular collapse. Thyroid storm often progresses rapidly to delirium and coma. Any severe exacerbation of hyperthyroidism demands immediate hospitalization and urgent consultation with an endocrinologist.

HYPOTHYROIDISM

Hypothyroidism, the metabolic state resulting from an inadequate level of circulating thyroxine, is common. Most cases can be diagnosed even when symptoms and signs are minimal, provided that the clinician considers the diagnosis and seeks appropriate laboratory confirmation. The manifestations of hypothyroidism are varied and to a large measure age-dependent. *Myxedema* is the term for a severe form of hypothyroidism that results in deposition of mucopolysaccharides in the skin and other tissues, producing a characteristic appearance and a constellation of physical findings. The term *myxedema* is commonly but incorrectly used interchangeably with *hypothyroidism. Primary hypothyroidism* is the term used to indicate that the hormone deficiency results from a disease or other process within the thyroid gland. *Secondary hypothyroidism* or *central hypothyroidism* is much less common and results from lack of thyrotropin (TSH) secretion, a consequence of pituitary or, rarely, hypothalamic disease. The thyroid is usually smaller than normal and is not palpable. Serum TSH, using a second- or third-generation assay, may be low, but TSH assay in this situation can be misleading. Biologically inactive but immunoreactive TSH is often produced so that the measured TSH can be normal or even elevated. Abnormal TSH glycosylation accounts for this phenomenon. Almost invariably the hypothyroidism is part of a decrease in pituitary function involving trophic hormones in addition to TSH with concomitant hypogonadism or adrenal insufficiency. Causes include postpartum necrosis, pituitary tumor, pituitary apoplexy, and granulomatous disease, or sometimes an autoimmune process involving failure of other endocrine glands. Some cases occur without identifiable cause and are termed idiopathic (see also Chapter 81).

Etiology

The most common cause of hypothyroidism worldwide remains dietary *iodide deficiency.* In the United States, iodide deficiency no longer exists because iodide, for more than half a century, has been added to dietary salt to prevent goiter. Most cases of hypothyroidism in this country are a result of *autoimmune destruction* of the thyroid, either with or without goiter (see below). Goitrous autoimmune thyroiditis is also called *Hashimoto thyroiditis*. At a later stage, the gland atrophies and a goiter is no longer palpable. Almost all remaining cases are iatrogenic, the result of therapy of hyperthyroidism, although it should be recalled that hypothyroidism also seems to be a late outcome of Graves disease, regardless of treatment (see Graves Disease). *External radiation of the neck* (e.g., for nonthyroidal neoplastic disease) can also cause thyroid atrophy and subsequent hypothyroidism.

Autoimmune destruction of the thyroid may occur in association with other autoimmune glandular disorders, especially adrenal insufficiency (Schmidt syndrome) and autoimmune ovarian failure (polyglandular failure) and with diseases such as pernicious anemia. High titers of antibodies to thyroid antigens (thyroglobulin, microsomes) are seen in 90% of cases. An easily overlooked form of hypothyroidism is that which occurs *postpartum* (see Postpartum Thyroid Dysfunction). Table 80.7 classifies the causes of hypothyroidism.

Drug-Induced Hypothyroidism

Although a variety of drugs can produce hypothyroidism that is, invariably, associated with goiter formation, only a few in current use have such an effect. Lithium, widely used for the treatment of manic-depressive illness, is one such agent. If goiter occurs, lithium need not be stopped; addition of thyroxine relieves the hypothyroidism and causes regression of the goiter. Overtreatment of hyperthyroidism with an antithyroid drug will, of course, produce hypothyroidism. Iodide in pharmacologic amounts is an antithyroid drug and also occasionally produces goiter and hypothyroidism. However, most adults who are susceptible to the antithyroid action of iodide have an underlying thyroid abnormality, such as Hashimoto thyroiditis or radioiodide-treated Graves disease. Amiodarone, an antiarrhythmic agent, contains iodine and can produce hypothyroidism in up to 13% of patients treated with this drug (see Thyroid Dysfunction Caused by Iodide or Amiodarone).

TABLE 80.7 Clinical Classification of Hypothyroidism[a]

Hypothyroidism without goiter (decrease of thyroid tissue mass)
Postablative for hyperthyroidism (radioiodide therapy or surgery)
Autoimmune atrophy
Postpartum
External radiation
Developmental defect (congenital)
Pituitary or hypothalamic disease
Hypothyroidism with goiter
Autoimmune (Hashimoto disease)
Postpartum
Drug induced (e.g., antithyroid drugs, iodide, lithium[b])
Iodide deficiency (many geographic areas)
Genetic biosynthetic defects

[a]Hypothyroidism in the United States is now most commonly the consequence of therapy for hyperthyroidism. Hypothyroidism from idiopathic atrophy of the thyroid is second in frequency. Developmental defects (e.g., lingual thyroid) are rare. Hypothyroidism with goiter is nearly always caused by Hashimoto thyroiditis, rarely by a drug. Genetic biosynthetic defects are rare and usually become manifest in childhood.
[b]Hypothyroidism from chronic lithium therapy may occur without goiter.

Clinical Features

Hypothyroidism in the adult is highly variable in presentation. Onset is usually insidious, often occurring over many years, with the result that the symptoms go unappreciated by patient and clinician alike. The nonspecificity of the symptoms also contributes to the delayed diagnosis. No predictable progression of symptoms is apparent, but easy fatigability, lethargy, increased sleep requirement (and, sometimes, sleep apnea), cold intolerance, muscle aching, and stiffness are perhaps the most common early symptoms. The skin is dry and may show scaling. Hair loss is common. The eyebrows become sparse, and the face is "puffy" (i.e., full) because of cutaneous deposition of mucopolysaccharides, with edema of the periorbital areas. The voice often becomes low pitched and rough. Constipation is common and may be severe enough to produce megacolon. Diminished hearing, especially in older persons, is easily overlooked or is attributed to aging. Ordinarily, the affected individual becomes abnormally placid, but agitation or frank psychosis may occur. In the elderly, depression is the most common psychiatric accompaniment of hypothyroidism. Despite common medical belief, the few available studies demonstrate that dementia caused by hypothyroidism is rare, if it occurs at all. Coexistence of the two processes in the elderly is, however, not uncommon. Paresthesias and pain in the hands from carpal tunnel syndrome may occur. Diminished sexual function is the rule. Women often experience menorrhagia. Rarely, galactorrhea may be seen in women of child-bearing age. Fertility is diminished, but pregnancy may occur and normal delivery is possible. The newborn is euthyroid, unless the mother's hypothyroidism is drug related or the hypothyroidism is of the rare familial athyrotic variety.

Subclinical Hypothyroidism

The most common stage of hypothyroidism likely to be encountered in ambulatory patients is mild hypothyroidism, commonly termed subclinical hypothyroidism. By definition, such an individual has an elevated TSH but serum thyroid levels that, although within the normal range, are lower, presumably, than they should be for that person (27). This condition is strongly age and gender dependent; it is found in 16% of men and 21% of women older than age 74 years (11,28). It is characterized by nonspecific but suggestive symptoms and few clinical findings. One study suggests that some of these patients improve after therapy with L-thyroxine (29). Many older women have minimal elevations of TSH (6 to 10 μU) despite normal levels of T_4 (see Screening for Thyroid Disease in Healthy Patients). Only those with elevated thyroid autoantibodies are likely to develop overt clinical or laboratory hypothyroidism (50% over 5 years). The significance of minimal TSH elevation in the remainder of this group is unclear. The possibility that the immunoreactive TSH may not reflect its bioactivity has not been excluded in such patients.

Severe Hypothyroidism with Myxedema

In spontaneous cases of hypothyroidism, only with severe long-standing disease does extensive deposition of mucopolysaccharide occur, producing the clinical state of myxedema. Rarely, myxedema may develop rapidly (1 to 2 months) after radioiodide or surgical ablation of the thyroid for hyperthyroidism or after abrupt withdrawal of thyroxine replacement therapy.

In myxedema, a variety of manifestations can be appreciated on physical examination, and of course they vary with the severity and duration of the disease. The skin, in addition to being dry and scaling, is typically cool. The scaling may be extensive, and large flakes may be shed from the elbows and knees. The subcutaneous tissues may be infiltrated by mucopolysaccharides so the skin appears to be "thickened" or "doughy." In the elderly, atrophy of the epidermis may occur simultaneously, producing a stiff, translucent, parchmentlike appearance. Yellow-orange discoloration of the skin from carotene deposition may be evident, especially in the palms. The presence of edema is not obvious because pitting is not noted except in extreme cases complicated by hypoproteinemia. An exception is the collection around the eyes of "bags of water" (lymphedema). This finding is not, however, specific for hypothyroidism. The tongue is sometimes enlarged. The heart rate is usually slow (sinus bradycardia). The heart may appear enlarged, because of either dilation of the myocardium or pericardial effusion. Pleural effusions and ascites may also be present, sometimes even in cases that are otherwise not clinically severe. Indeed, such effusions may be erroneously attributed to malignancy. Hyponatremia, clinically indistinguishable from the syndrome of inappropriate antidiuretic hormone (ADH) excess, may be present (see Chapter 81). Evidence suggests that this phenomenon is not ADH dependent; it disappears slowly as the patient is treated with T_4. The deep tendon reflexes characteristically show a delay in their relaxation phase, the so-called hung-up reflex. This is a highly suggestive finding but may be seen occasionally in other diseases. Mental functioning is slowed, as reflected in characteristically slow speech. The reading speed may be greatly reduced. Hearing loss may be severe or of a degree apparent only on audiometric testing. Cerebellar dysfunction, if present, is usually evident only on extensive neurologic testing, but in rare cases is grossly apparent as ataxia.

Myxedema Coma

Myxedema coma is a severe, often fatal, state that is a rare complication of long-standing disease and is typically seen in an elderly patient. Myxedema coma is often associated with or precipitated by pneumonia, peritonitis, or some other serious infection, the presence of which may not be immediately apparent. Severe respiratory failure is a major feature and can be caused by a variety of factors, ranging from upper airway obstruction to impaired chest wall mechanics. Because elderly patients often become hypothermic on exposure to cold or during sepsis, the diagnosis of myxedema coma is more commonly considered than actually confirmed. However, if myxedema coma is suspected, the patient should be hospitalized in an intensive care setting under the care of an endocrinologist, with administration of intravenous levothyroxine therapy.

Laboratory Findings

In primary hypothyroidism, the combination of low serum T_4, low FTI index (or free T_4), and high TSH is diagnostic. Difficulties in diagnosis are encountered only in occasional cases. The serum T_3 is usually low, but because T_3 decreases in a variety of nonthyroidal illnesses ranging from malnutrition to liver disease, its measurement is not useful for diagnosis of hypothyroidism. Furthermore, the T_3 is normal in many patients with mild hypothyroidism. In hypothyroidism caused by pituitary or hypothalamic disease, the TSH may be "normal," or low (see Chapter 81).

In hypothyroid patients, a common laboratory finding is elevation of serum enzymes that originate in skeletal muscle: creatine kinase and, to lesser extents, serum aspartate aminotransferase, serum alanine aminotransferase, and lactic dehydrogenase. Fractionation studies show that when these enzymes are elevated in hypothyroidism, they do not originate in cardiac muscle. Virtually all phenotypic abnormalities of hyperlipoproteinemia have been observed in hypothyroid patients and are reversible when thyroid hormone is replaced (see Chapter 82). Other abnormalities include electrocardiographic changes (e.g., flattened or inverted T waves, minor ST-segment depressions, and low amplitude QRS complexes) and abnormalities of blood gas measurements caused by hypoventilation. Anemia, usually normocytic and normochromic, may be present, as well as macrocytic anemia of coexistent vitamin B_{12} deficiency (pernicious anemia). An abnormality of red cell shape (spiculation) also has been described in hypothyroidism.

Hypothyroidism versus the Euthyroid Sick Syndrome

Serum thyroid hormone levels drop during starvation and illness. In mild illness, this involves only a decrease in serum T_3 levels. However, as the severity of the illness increases, both serum T_3 and T_4 levels drop. Severely ill patients with these abnormalities of thyroid function are not hypothyroid despite the low hormone levels in blood, and the condition has been called the "euthyroid sick syndrome" or "nonthyroidal illness syndrome." The diagnosis of hypothyroidism in severely ill patients thus may be difficult (8,9). The free T_4 and free T_3 are usually low; however, TSH may be low, normal, or moderately elevated, depending on the stage of the illness. Serum rT_3 is often elevated. In such complicated cases, it generally is best to defer assessment of thyroid dysfunction until the patient is stable, unless there is a compelling reason to think the outcome of the serious illness would be improved. Diagnostic findings of overt hypothyroidism (markedly increased TSH and low T_4) can be relied on, if present, and appropriate treatment can be instituted.

Although the euthyroid sick syndrome has been clearly recognized only in hospitalized, severely ill patients, it probably also occurs in less-dramatic form in chronically ill, nonhospitalized people (9). Many patients with chronic renal failure undergoing hemodialysis appear to fall into this group. The mechanisms underlying this phenomenon appear to involve a combination of factors, including accelerated T_4 metabolism, impairment of TSH secretion (2,9), and impairment of T_4 binding to serum proteins. Most of these pathophysiologic abnormalities probably are due to excessive amounts of circulating cytokines (interleukin-1β, tumor necrosis factor, and others) that are produced during severe illness.

Treatment

T_4 is the best preparation for ordinary use in replacement. T_4 (levothyroxine, sodium L-thyroxine, and the U.S. brand names Synthroid, Levothroid, Levoxyl, and Unithroid) is available in color-coded tablets of 25, 50, 75, 88, 100, 112, 125, 137, 150, 175, 200, and 300 μg. T_3 (liothyronine, Cytomel) is available in 5-, 25-, and 50-μg tablets. Although T_3 is also effective, it has no special advantage for routine therapy of hypothyroidism and has the distinct disadvantage that the serum T_4 or T_3 cannot be monitored to determine adequacy of replacement (because T_4 levels remain low and T_3 levels may fluctuate). Thyroglobulin preparations and desiccated thyroid ("thyroid extract") should no longer be used.

Experts have different opinions concerning the merits of generic versus brand names of T_4 for use in replacement therapy (30). Concern has been expressed over the bioavailability of hormone in certain generic preparations and even lack of standardization of certain brands of T_4, but clinically significant problems are unlikely to be encountered with any of the preparations available in the United States.

Rate of Replacement with Thyroxine

Traditionally, initiation of thyroid hormone replacement therapy has been cautious and has used dosage schedules that ensure slow restoration of the patient to a normal metabolic state. Although this principle is conservative and rational, the practice is often unnecessary. Therapy must be adjusted to the individual case, but with several points kept in mind. If the patient is not elderly and has never had overt cardiac disease, overcautious initiation of therapy will result only in needless prolongation of the hypothyroid state. If the patient has evidence of pre-existing cardiac disease or is frail and elderly, therapy should be started at a low dosage: 12.5 to 25 μg of T_4 a day initially, with 25-μg increases at 4-week intervals, as tolerated. Only rarely will serious heart disease, such as angina pectoris, prevent at least partial replacement therapy sufficient to eliminate myxedema, and most, if not all, unpleasant symptoms of hypothyroidism.

The usual hypothyroid patient, without complicating medical problems, may be started on full daily replacement dosage. Even with this therapeutic approach, the clinical response will be slow. One can expect several months to pass before restoration of a normal metabolic state. The objective of therapy should be to restore the clinically euthyroid state if at all possible. The variability of optimal dosage among individuals is too great to rely on weight-based formulas. Most people need about 125 μg (0.125 mg) per day; and only rarely require as much as 200 μg (0.2 mg). If a larger dose seems to be needed, nonadherence should be suspected (see Chapter 4). Monitoring T_4 dosage changes is best done by measuring TSH and free T_4 levels, initially at 4 weeks after treatment, and then 4 to 6 weeks after any dose changes. TSH measurements alone can be made once the dose is stabilized. If desired, a single weekly dose of T_4 can be used; the dosage is slightly more than seven times the daily dosage (31). The once-weekly dosage has the advantage that it can be more easily supervised, if the circumstances warrant. Because there is decreased clearance of T_4 with aging, elderly patients may require only 100 μg per day or less for maintenance; as little as 50 or 75 μg often suffices. The T_4 requirement during pregnancy is increased by about one-third (32).

Thyroid Hormone Replacement with Thyroxine versus a Combination of Thyroxine and Triiodothyronine

Thyroid hormone replacement therapy has evolved from the use of crude extracts or powdered preparations of thyroid gland (desiccated thyroid) to use of one or two synthetic thyroid hormones, T_4 and T_3. When T_4 is given alone, hypothyroid patients are rendered clinically and biochemically euthyroid (normal) as measured by serum levels of T_4, T_3, and TSH. Serum T_3 is derived from T_4 by deiodination in nonthyroidal (peripheral) tissues. In normal persons, secretion of T_3 from the thyroid amounts to only about 6 μg per day. Nonetheless, for some time clinicians have noted that a significant minority of patients who are receiving only T_4 for replacement report a greater sense of well-being when taking approximately 50 μg of T_4 more than that which restored their TSH to the normal range (3). In a small study, a number of patients were switched from T_4 alone to a combination of T_4 and T_3; they had significantly improved mood and neurologic function on extensive neuropsychological testing (33). However, the available information from several subsequent studies did not support a routine switch from T_4 monotherapy to a combination of T_4 and T_3.

For patients on routine thyroid hormone replacement therapy, judicious use of small amounts of T_3 along with T_4 (10 μg per 100 μg of T_4) may be symptomatically beneficial for occasional patients, but may cause side effects in others (34), and thus it is not generally recommended by this author.

Importance of Avoiding Overtreatment during Thyroxine Replacement Therapy

Considerable concern has been expressed about whether T_4 replacement therapy or overtreatment with T_4 can lead to osteoporosis, because bone demineralization is a known complication of hyperthyroidism. Several studies show that T_4-treated patients, except for those with a history of hyperthyroidism, do not have decreased bone mineral density (35,36). In keeping with those conclusions, a recent study of women 65 years of age and older who were treated with T_4 showed no increase in fracture rate for those whose TSH was maintained in the normal range (0.5 to 5.5 mU/L) or even for those in the "borderline to low" range (0.1 to 0.4 mU/L). However, women whose TSH was suppressed below 0.1 mU/L had a threefold increased risk of hip fracture and a fourfold increased risk of vertebral fracture. Unfortunately, neither measurements of serum T_4 nor the dosages of T_4 were presented. Thus, the possibility exists that only women with overly elevated levels of thyroid hormone were subject to elevated risk of fracture (37), in which case these women may simply have been inadequately monitored. It should also be recalled that the elderly often need substantially less T_4 for replacement than younger persons; failure to appreciate this fact could have contributed to these fractures. Moreover, women older than 65 years with already compromised age-related decreases of bone mineral density, may be an especially high-risk group for the effects of overtreatment. The same concerns could be raised with respect to cardiovascular risk.

THYROID DYSFUNCTION CAUSED BY IODIDE OR AMIODARONE

Excess iodide from a variety of sources can induce hyperthyroidism if the patient ingesting it was previously iodide depleted. In that case, a toxic nodular goiter, or, less often, "latent" Graves disease, may become manifest. This phenomenon is called the Jod-Basedow effect and is more commonly seen in Europe than in the United States. In parts of the world where there is adequate iodine in the diet, excess iodide may cause hypothyroidism, especially if a patient has underlying thyroid disease, such as autoimmune thyroiditis.

Amiodarone (an antiarrhythmic agent; see Chapter 64) contains approximately 40% iodine and, in the United States, is the most likely source of excess iodide, released when the drug is metabolized. The intact drug also can exert a number of effects on the thyroid and on thyroid hormone metabolism; it markedly inhibits peripheral conversion of T_4 to T_3 and coincidentally increases the serum concentration of T_4 and free T_4.

There are two mechanisms by which amiodarone induces thyrotoxicosis (38). The first is by the Jod-Basedow phenomenon (type I amiodarone-induced thyrotoxicosis) in which amiodarone serves as substrate for overproduction of thyroid hormone in a susceptible gland. The second, which is much more common in this country, is from direct drug toxicity that results in thyroid cell destruction with release of preformed thyroid hormones (type II amiodarone-induced thyrotoxicosis) until the gland is depleted of its hormonal stores (1 to 3 months). Potential distinguishing features between the two forms include diffuse or multinodular goiter and increased color Doppler flow in type I; and low RaIU uptake, decreased color Doppler flow and increased serum interleukin 6 in type II. Treatment includes methimazole and perchlorate for type I and glucocorticoids for type II. β-Blockers can be used as an adjunctive treatment for both types of amiodarone-induced thyrotoxicosis. Patients with type I have prolonged hyperthyroidism lasting 6 to 9 months after discontinuation of amiodarone, whereas in type II patients, euthyroidism typically is restored within 3 to 5 months. Type I patients generally return to a normal thyroid state, and type II patients can have transient hypothyroidism, which evolves to permanent hypothyroidism in some cases. Treatment of amiodarone-induced thyrotoxicosis should be supervised by an endocrinologist.

In the United States, hypothyroidism caused by amiodarone (13% of all patients) is more common than thyrotoxicosis (2%). Most of the former cases are presumably a result of iodide-induced effects in persons with subclinical autoimmune thyroiditis.

THYROIDITIS

Thyrotoxicosis Associated with Thyroiditis

Various types of thyroiditis occasionally may be associated with short-lived self-limited thyrotoxicosis. The explanation for this phenomenon has been that the destructive inflammatory process causes release of preformed thyroid hormone. The thyrotoxicosis invariably disappears within a few months.

A RaIU measurement should be obtained in all patients with thyrotoxicosis who do not clearly have Graves disease (i.e., who do not have associated eye findings) or toxic nodular goiter. A very low RaIU establishes the diagnosis of hyperthyroidism associated with thyroiditis and allows the physician to avoid inappropriate therapy (radioiodide or surgery).

Long-term followup studies of these patients show that about half persist in having some degree of thyroid abnormality: antithyroid antibodies or goiter, recurring bouts of thyrotoxicosis, elevation of TSH (decreased thyroid reserve), and, occasionally, hypothyroidism (16).

Lymphocytic Thyroiditis (Silent Thyroiditis)

Lymphocytic thyroiditis is a distinct variant of the thyroiditis–thyrotoxicosis syndrome. Patients have a modestly enlarged nontender thyroid gland. No history of viral illness can be obtained. The RaIU is very low, whereas the T_4 and T_3 levels are high and the TSH level is low. About half of the cases have significant elevations of thyroid antibodies, and about half of these high titers subside within a few months. A propensity of the condition to occur in the postpartum period has been noted, sometimes in successive pregnancies and sometimes followed by the development of hypothyroidism (see Postpartum Thyroid Dysfunction). On biopsy (not ordinarily recommended) the changes that are seen differ from those of the peak phase of classic subacute thyroiditis (see Subacute Thyroiditis), but the latter, in its late stage of evolution, may be indistinguishable from that of lymphocytic thyroiditis. Whether lymphocytic thyroiditis with spontaneously resolving thyrotoxicosis (silent thyroiditis) is a new disease, as has been suggested by some, or is a newly recognized variant of subacute thyroiditis is a matter of debate (16).

Hashimoto Thyroiditis

Hashimoto thyroiditis is common (see Hypothyroidism and Table 80.7). The process is painless and usually produces only modest enlargement of the thyroid. Nodularity is the rule, and the consistency on palpation is classically rubberlike. Distinction from other nontoxic nodular goiters is made by the presence of high titers of thyroid autoantibodies in the serum of approximately 90% of patients with Hashimoto thyroiditis.

Subacute Thyroiditis

Subacute thyroiditis, also known as granulomatous or de Quervain thyroiditis, is common. Many mild cases are probably never diagnosed. The term *subacute* is often deceiving and sometimes inappropriate. Although the onset may be insidious, it is perhaps just as often acute over several days. Many patients give a history of recent antecedent upper respiratory tract infection.

The earliest symptoms may be referred pain, usually to the ear, but pain can appear to originate in the jaw or occiput. This phase may last a few hours or days before tenderness and discomfort in the thyroid area become apparent. Rarely, the patient is concerned only with the referred pain and is unaware of thyroidal tenderness until examination makes it apparent. When the onset is acute, the symptoms and signs are more likely to be severe. Initially, pain and swelling of the thyroid are often unilateral, but the process usually does not remain localized for more than a few days. Systemic symptoms include fever, especially in acute cases, and a sensation of intense fatigue and malaise. The course may be protracted with symptoms persisting for months, although usually they subside within a week or two.

The erythrocyte sedimentation rate is elevated. Early in the disease, the thyroidal RaIU is depressed (but that may be so in many normal people), and serum T_4 may be slightly elevated. Mild cases have no or only borderline abnormalities of these tests. Significant titers of thyroid autoantibodies are not common but can be seen.

Clinical hyperthyroidism can be seen with subacute thyroiditis. Rarely, hypothyroidism occurs and lasts for several months. Permanent hypothyroidism is unusual. A variant of this syndrome has been described in which neither hypothyroidism nor hyperthyroidism is present but symptoms of severe systemic illness with fever and weight loss dominate (39).

Therapy

Therapy of subacute thyroiditis is symptomatic. The patient should be strongly reassured about the benign self-limited character of the disorder. No controlled studies of drug efficacy for symptom relief are available. Widespread practice indicates that thyroid tenderness often responds within several days to aspirin in doses sufficient to maintain therapeutic (anti-inflammatory) blood levels with prompt relapse if the dose is reduced to analgesic levels. There is little published experience with nonsteroidal anti-inflammatory agents, but these agents are probably as effective as aspirin. More potent analgesics, such as codeine, may be necessary if the neck pain is severe. In less than 10% of cases, the process may be severe enough to require glucocorticoid therapy (30 to 60 mg of prednisone daily or equivalent). A glucocorticoid produces prompt relief of pain and tenderness but, if the disease is severe enough to require its use, will usually be necessary for weeks to several months. Relapse is common when glucocorticoid therapy is discontinued, and retreatment may be necessary.

Pyogenic (Suppurative) Thyroiditis

Pyogenic or suppurative thyroiditis, also known as acute thyroiditis, is rare, and most clinicians will never encounter a case. The thyroid infection usually follows bacteremia but can occur as an isolated primary event. The gland shows typical signs of an acute inflammatory process.

Riedel Thyroiditis

Riedel thyroiditis is another rare but indolent and painless form of thyroiditis. The intense induration associated with this process makes the clinical differentiation from infiltrating neoplasm difficult.

THYROID DYSFUNCTION DURING PREGNANCY AND POSTPARTUM

Hyperthyroidism during Pregnancy

Hyperthyroidism complicates about one to two pregnancies per thousand. However, the disease is almost always easily controlled in the mother, and when this is the case, infants are unaffected and there is not any obvious increase in the incidence of congenital anomalies. In contrast, uncontrolled hyperthyroidism leads to preeclampsia, low birth weight, a high percentage of stillbirths, and congestive heart failure in the mothers. If hyperthyroidism is suspected, free T_4 and TSI assays are the preferred tests. Alterations in TBG make total T_4 and T_3 assays difficult to interpret, and TSH levels may be low in euthyroid pregnant women. TSI measurements are useful in the pregnant hyperthyroid patient because high levels are associated with an increased likelihood of neonatal hyperthyroidism caused by placental transfer of the stimulating antibodies. Occasionally, the newborn infant is hyperthyroid at birth as a result of this passive transfer of stimulating antibodies. The clinician who will care for the newborn should always be alerted to this possibility.

Although there have been no prospective clinical trials, consensus opinion is that hyperthyroidism in pregnancy should be treated with an antithyroid drug regardless of whether it is caused by Graves disease or toxic nodular goiter (32,40). Surgery has been used successfully during pregnancy but has no advantage and may be associated with increased fetal loss. Radioactive iodide is contraindicated.

There is little to choose between the two available drugs, although in the United States, propylthiouracil is favored for pregnant women. Methimazole may be associated with an increased incidence of the infrequent congenital skin anomaly, aplasia cutis (1 in 2,000 normal births), a small (up to 3 cm) hairless patch on the head or neck that usually disappears spontaneously after a few years.

Therapy with antithyroid drugs during pregnancy is guided by the consideration that both drugs freely cross the placenta and, in large doses, can produce goiter and hypothyroidism in the infant. The dosage of antithyroid drugs should therefore be the minimal amount adequate to control the hyperthyroidism. A dose of drug that totally blocks hormone synthesis given along with a replacement amount of thyroxine is a scheme that is inappropriate during pregnancy, because it may lead to the use of larger doses of antithyroid drug than are absolutely necessary. When ordinary doses of antithyroid drug are used, the fetus is usually born euthyroid and without a goiter, but as a precaution, some experts reduce the dosage during the last 2 months of pregnancy and, if clinical circumstances permit, discontinue the drug entirely in the last month. This is often possible, because hyperthyroidism during pregnancy tends to ameliorate spontaneously as the pregnancy progresses, although exacerbation in the postpartum period is not unusual. Iodide as an adjunct should not be used during pregnancy because the fetal thyroid is especially susceptible to the goitrogenic effect of iodide.

Conventional thionamide drug therapy (i.e., propylthiouracil and methimazole are used in the United States; see Graves Disease, Antithyroid Drugs) does not preclude nursing. Infants show no effects from the small amounts of the drug that do get into breast milk, at least at daily doses of up to 20 mg of methimazole or 750 mg of propylthiouracil. Intellectual and somatic development is normal in the children of mothers who are receiving an antithyroid drug who are breast-feeding their infants.

Management of Hypothyroidism during Pregnancy

Concern has been expressed over the adverse effects of maternal thyroid hormone deficiency in hypothyroid women receiving T_4 replacement therapy during pregnancy on the subsequent neuropsychological development (intelligence quotient [IQ]) of the child (41). Even a minor degree of maternal hypothyroxinemia may be harmful to the development of the fetal brain. This issue has been carefully reviewed and a strong case made for the avoidance of any T_4 deficiency in the mother during pregnancy, especially in the critical early phase of fetal brain development (41,42). A recent study suggested that the relative T_4 deficiency occurs early, and recommended increasing the replacement T_4 dose by one-third as soon as the patient knows she is pregnant (43). Dependence on a low maternal TSH as an indicator of thyroid hormone adequacy in the first trimester is unreliable, as human chorionic gonadotropin (hCG) levels are high. Free T_4 (or FTI) and not total T_4 is the appropriate measurement for assessing adequacy of thyroxine dosage, given the elevation of TBG in pregnancy. Moreover, free T_4 should be measured by equilibrium dialysis, because in the presence of elevated TBG other methods can yield spuriously high and therefore misleadingly reassuring values (44).

Postpartum Thyroid Dysfunction

Postpartum thyroid dysfunction is common, occurring in some 17% of women in one study (45). Because of its high frequency, a good case has been made for routine screening (46). Both hyperthyroidism and hypothyroidism can occur; in some individuals, one state follows the other. The hypothyroid variation may be transient, lasting only 1 to 4 months, and is most likely to occur in the first 8 months postpartum. However, in 30% of cases the hypothyroidism is permanent. Many cases that are not permanent are caused by the transient occurrence of thyroid-blocking antibodies. Most cases show antimicrosomal (thyroid peroxidase) antibodies; antithyroglobulin antibodies are uncommon. In the United States, the hyperthyroid variety has been associated with postpartum lymphocytic thyroiditis (see Thyrotoxicosis Associated with Thyroiditis). Postpartum hypothyroidism is often misdiagnosed as postpartum depression, and the two conditions are common and can coexist (47). Some women have repeated bouts of postpartum thyroid dysfunction with successive pregnancies. Thyroid abnormalities after pregnancy also have long-term implications as a risk factor for later development of both Graves disease and, especially, permanent hypothyroidism (17% of patients over 5 to 16 years in one series; 23% over 2 to 4 years in another series [48]). Of special interest is the increased incidence (25%) in women with type 1 diabetes, a threefold increase over nondiabetic patients. Because of this high incidence, assessment of TSH and thyroid peroxidase antibodies is recommended 3 months postpartum for all type 1 diabetic patients (49).

SCREENING FOR THYROID DISEASE IN HEALTHY PATIENTS

Because thyroid diseases are common and clinical diagnosis can be difficult (see also Subclinical Hyperthyroidism and Subclinical Hypothyroidism), a rational argument can be made in favor of attempting to detect clinically inapparent thyroid disease by laboratory tests in individuals without overt symptoms (50,51). On the other hand, a recent U.S. Preventative Service Task Report by the U.S. Public Health Service did not find any evidence for or against screening asymptomatic adults for thyroid disease when clinical outcomes of treating identified patients were considered (52). In contrast, the American Thyroid Association recommends screening every 5 years for persons older than age 35 years (53), and the American College of Physicians recommends screening for female patients older than age 50 years with one or more general symptoms that could be associated with thyroid disease (54). Thus, some experts now favor a case-finding approach—that is, testing only patients who are seeing a practitioner for symptoms—although there is not uniform agreement (50,53). In patients who exhibit any clinical findings that could conceivably be attributable to thyroid disease, laboratory testing should be done, but this approach should probably not be termed screening. Some success has been achieved by presenting a list of thyroid-related symptoms at the time of the patient's visit (55).

The results of screening for thyroid disease, using sensitive TSH tests and appropriate followup of abnormal values, are remarkably consistent in various populations

(50,51,56,57). Approximately 1% of apparently healthy individuals, all ages included, are found to be hypothyroid. Many fewer individuals are shown to be hyperthyroid (0.1% to 0.2%). Women older than age 40 years have the most thyroid disease; young men have essentially none. Asymptomatic patients with elevated or depressed levels of TSH may have subclinical hypothyroidism or subclinical hyperthyroidism (see Subclinical Hyperthyroidism), respectively.

Some limitations of screening for thyroid disease with sensitive TSH assays should be kept in mind. For example, in these assays, the TSH is undetectable in patients with hyperthyroidism, a finding that is sensitive but not specific; many sick people and even "normal" elderly patients are found to have low levels of TSH (56,58).

GOITER

A goiter is a thyroid gland that has undergone generalized enlargement. The term goiter should not be applied to a gland that is enlarged by a single nodule, although many physicians continue to do so. The term implies nothing about the functional state of the gland. Goiter is the most common thyroid abnormality. *Diffuse goiter*, also called simple goiter, is a gland that, on gross examination, is uniformly and symmetrically enlarged without apparent irregularities. Most goiters are, in fact, multinodular, as revealed by palpation, sonography, or thyroid scan.

In some areas of the world, thyroid enlargement is so prevalent that it is termed *endemic goiter*. Before the widespread introduction of iodized salt, endemic goiter was common in the United States, but this is no longer the case. Endemic goiter, a term that for practical purposes is synonymous with *iodine deficiency goiter*, is now found principally in geographically isolated areas of the underdeveloped world, but some of these areas are vast, such as much of China, central Asia, and Africa. Moreover, some parts of Europe, such as Germany—which never iodized its salt supply—and parts of Italy, Switzerland, Denmark, and other countries, are still areas of low iodide intake and increased prevalence of goiter. The term *sporadic goiter* refers to thyroid enlargement as now encountered in the United States and other developed areas where iodide intake is adequate. Sporadic goiter is now seen in a small percentage of the U.S. population and increases in frequency with age. Its cause is unknown, but it is clearly not iodide deficiency.

Any process that prevents the synthesis of normal quantities of thyroid hormones, including iodide deficiency, produces goiter. If impairment of hormone synthesis is severe enough, goiter formation is associated with reduction of serum T_4 (but not T_3), eventually to be followed by clinical hypothyroidism. The mechanism of the thyroid enlargement in this situation is increased pituitary TSH secretion via activation of the negative feedback system. The resulting increased thyroid mass is a compensatory mechanism that may allow sufficient hormone synthesis to occur so that the patient remains euthyroid.

Drugs that interfere with thyroid hormone synthesis (e.g., thiocarbamides, lithium, iodides, etc.) can also lead to goiter. Withdrawal of a goitrogenic drug may result in regression of the goiter, as will simultaneous administration of enough T_4 or T_3 to suppress endogenous TSH secretion. The degree of regression depends on how long the goiter has been present. Long-standing goitrous enlargement is associated with the development of multiple large nodules, which are less likely to regress or to do so only incompletely.

Diagnosis

A visible or easily palpable mass in the base of the neck is the usual mode of presentation of goiter. Occasionally, especially in the elderly, an enlarged thyroid is neither visible nor readily palpable but is incidentally found by radiography of the chest or esophagus when either a retrosternal mass is noted or the trachea or esophagus is found to be deviated. The high iodide content of the sporadic goitrous thyroid enhances its radiograph density and identity. Confirmation of the nature of a neck mass as an enlarged thyroid gland and precise determination of its size are now most economically and accurately performed by ultrasonographic examination. CT is accurate in delineating the relationship of a goiter to contiguous structures but is much less useful in defining the thyroid itself.

Except in subacute thyroiditis, pain is not a usual symptom with a goiter but can develop during cyst formation or hemorrhage, a fairly common event, usually accompanied by rapid and sometimes painful enlargement of a portion of the gland. Obstruction of the trachea or esophagus can be produced by goiter, but dysphagia should not be readily attributed to minor degrees of thyroid enlargement. Hoarseness may occur because of involvement of the recurrent laryngeal nerve, but this is rare in patients with benign enlargement and its occurrence is suggestive, although not diagnostic, of thyroid malignancy.

Confronted with a goiter, the clinician's first thought should *not* be cancer. Most goiters (some 95%) represent benign disease (59). The frequency of carcinoma in multinodular goiter has been debated for years. Unwarranted concern has resulted in countless unnecessary operations. The assessment of goiter as a benign condition assumes, however, that malignancy has been excluded. The diagnosis of malignancy in a multinodular goiter is discussed below (see Thyroid Nodules and Thyroid Carcinomas).

Clinical and laboratory assessment of thyroid function should be made in all cases of goiter. Although most goiters are associated with normal serum thyroid hormone levels and a euthyroid state, either hypothyroidism or

Thyroid Carcinomas

General Considerations

Approximately 75% to 85% of thyroid carcinomas are of the papillary variety; 5% to 15% are follicular carcinomas. Anaplastic and medullary carcinomas probably account for no more than 5% of the total. The relative frequency of the various types of thyroid carcinomas is markedly age dependent.

Occult thyroid carcinoma (defined as a lesion with the histologic appearance of carcinoma but less than 1.5 cm in diameter) is found at autopsy in 5% to 10% of U.S. and European populations, and in 30% of Japanese samples. Death from thyroid carcinoma is as rare in Japan as in the United States. Clearly, occult carcinoma behaves as a benign disease and does not warrant aggressive management.

In the United States, more than 10,000 new cases of thyroid carcinoma are seen each year, but only about 1,500 persons die of this disorder. Most of these deaths result from anaplastic tumors (50%) or from unusually aggressive follicular carcinomas. A few deaths are attributable to aggressive papillary tumors and medullary carcinomas.

Papillary Carcinoma

Followup at 10 years indicates a recurrence rate of approximately 20% and a mortality rate of 1.3% after subtotal resection versus 10% and 0.5%, respectively, after total removal of the gland in patients with papillary carcinoma. This small difference was statistically significant in one retrospective study and currently strongly influences the surgical approach. The complication rate for total thyroidectomy (hypoparathyroidism, vocal cord paralysis) is high. As a result, many surgeons have now adopted a modified or near-total thyroidectomy. In this procedure the affected side is completely removed; most of the contralateral lobe is also removed, but the posterior capsule is left, together with the tip of the upper pole. Whether this approach will succeed in reducing complications remains to be established. Conservative surgeons generally support more limited surgery (74). Visibly involved lymph nodes are always removed, but radical neck dissection is not justified even in the presence of obviously involved nodes (65,75). The presence of cervical node metastases at operation or the extent of lymphadenectomy does not seem to influence either recurrence or death rate. The death rate in lesions under 2.5 cm without local invasion and without evident distant metastases at the time of surgery is less than 1% in 10 years and is 4% to 8% in the less-favorable categories (65,75).

Follicular Carcinoma

Well-differentiated follicular carcinomas have been very difficult or impossible to distinguish from benign follicular adenomas on cytopathologic grounds. Thus when the cytology of the FNA of a nodule shows follicular cells, thyroidectomy is often performed. Recently, new immunologic markers such as galectin-3 have shown promise in distinguishing benign follicular neoplasms from malignant ones (6). Additionally, genomic profiling and cluster analysis of ribonucleic acid (RNA) obtained from nodules may be useful in distinguishing benign from malignant follicular lesions and thereby spare some patients needless surgery (76).

Follicular carcinoma can be more aggressive than papillary carcinoma, tends to be angioinvasive, and may metastasize to bones and lungs. The tumor may bypass regional lymph nodes, a marked difference from papillary disease. The most important prognostic feature is invasion of tumor, either through the tumor capsule or into blood vessels. At least one report suggests that, unlike papillary carcinoma, primary tumor size at presentation does not appear to influence prognosis (77). In contrast, in another series not a single patient died who was under 45 and who had an intrathyroidal tumor less than 2.5 cm in diameter (78).

The clinical presentation may be very different from that of papillary disease as the patient may already have metastatic disease involving lungs, bone, brain, or spinal cord at the time of initial diagnosis. In these cases, the primary tumor may be relatively small and initially overlooked. Only rarely do the metastases produce sufficient thyroid hormones to cause thyrotoxicosis.

The surgical approach to follicular carcinoma should be that taken for papillary carcinoma. Suppression therapy with thyroid hormone replacement is routine. Postoperative ablative therapy with radioiodide appears warranted (78), especially for those patients with overtly invasive disease.

Postoperative Therapy for Papillary and Follicular Carcinomas and Its Monitoring

Thyroid-Stimulating Hormone Suppression

Suppression of TSH after surgical treatment of differentiated thyroid cancer is of proven benefit, definitely lowering recurrence and mortality rates. However, supraphysiologic doses of T_4 for long-term TSH suppression can result in iatrogenic hyperthyroidism, usually asymptomatic, but in some instances leading to cardiac hypertrophy, atrial fibrillation, and bone demineralization. Nonetheless, the consensus view is that long-term postthyroidectomy TSH suppression is essential. Unfortunately, the optimal level of suppression is unknown. In practice, a sensitive second- or a third-generation TSH assay should be used to monitor the suppression dose of T_4. During replacement/suppression therapy some experts titrate the T_4 dosage to at least the minimal amount necessary to keep the TSH below the limit of normal (0.4 to

0.5 mU/L) but above 0.1 mU/L. At this level, the development of cardiac complications is avoided and normal bone metabolic parameters are maintained. Others, however, titrate T_4 dosage to the limit of detection of TSH in a third-generation assay (0.01 mU/L) and believe that the minimal effect on cardiac function is not clinically significant (79).

Radioiodide Ablation of Residual Tumor

Postoperative therapy with full replacement doses of T_4 suppresses endogenous TSH, reduces recurrence, and is routine in all cases. In addition, postsurgical ablative therapy with radioactive iodide has a role in those cases of localized disease that need to be treated. Although some have argued that the patient with a minimal papillary lesion may not need such therapy, it is clear that any patient with a large locally invasive lesion or metastases should receive ablative therapy with ^{131}I. In cases with an intermediate-size lesion, without invasion of the thyroid capsule, and without lymph node metastases, the recurrence rate is greatly reduced by treatment with radioiodide, and deaths from recurrent disease may be completely abolished. The hesitation to use radioiodide routinely stems from the fear of radiation-induced leukemia, a problem that is a significant risk only at high (cumulative) dosage of ^{131}I.

Therapy with ^{131}I after surgery requires that the patient's residual tumor is stimulated by TSH to take up a maximal amount of the dose of isotope. This is accomplished by withdrawal of T_4 for 4 weeks. The first course of post-TSH ^{131}I (typically 100 to 150 mCi) therapy is usually given several months after recovery from initial surgery, with additional courses at approximately yearly intervals until posttherapy scans show that no residual functioning tissue in the thyroid bed or metastatic tumor tissue can be detected. A recent study has suggested that recombinant TSH can be used with radioactive iodine to treat low risk thyroid cancer (87).

Monitoring Serum Thyroglobulin

The ideal method for monitoring residual disease is to render the patient hypothyroid, and then measure serum thyroglobulin. Levels below 2 ng/mL suggest no tumor burden. If the level is elevated, an ^{123}I or ^{131}I thyroid scan should be performed to look for focal uptake (80). Typically, these studies are done 6 months after radioablation. Until recently, this was accomplished by withdrawal of T_4 replacement/suppression therapy for 3 to 4 weeks, thus allowing endogenous TSH to rise. However, during the last 1 or 2 weeks of this interval, many individuals experience distressing symptoms of rapidly developing hypothyroidism, which then continue for several weeks even after reinstitution of T_4 therapy. It is no longer necessary to withdraw T_4, and this period of discomfort can now be avoided, because recombinant human TSH has become available for routine use (81). Typically given by injection as two doses over 2 days, the recombinant human TSH primes the residual thyroid tissue and tumor as effectively as endogenous TSH after T_4 withdrawal. Use of recombinant human TSH is a significant advance for reducing morbidity in this situation. In general, at least one evaluation after T_4 withdrawal should be done in low-risk patients, and if there is no evidence of recurrent cancer, the patient can be evaluated annually with recombinant human TSH.

In patients with persistent remission, it may be possible to monitor serum thyroglobulin periodically while the patient is undergoing T_4 suppression. If the thyroglobulin is undetectable with the TSH suppressed, it is likely that no tumor remains.

Medullary Carcinoma

Medullary carcinoma accounts for 1% to 2% of all thyroid cancers. The tumors arise from the parafollicular or C cells and produce thyrocalcitonin. Both sporadic and familial varieties occur. The sporadic case typically presents as a solitary nodule, whereas the familial variety is often multifocal and part of a multiple endocrine adenomatosis syndrome. Diarrhea occurs in some patients. Thyrocalcitonin in serum is elevated in the basal state or after stimulation with calcium or pentagastrin infusion. Some authorities advocate obtaining at least a basal (unstimulated) serum thyrocalcitonin level as part of the initial evaluation of all nonfunctional thyroid nodules (82,83). Although such routine measurement of thyrocalcitonin is not ordinarily done in the United States, it is common practice in Europe. When surgical excision is performed before regional nodes have become involved, 90% of patients survive for 10 years. Once the nodes are involved, only a 40% 10-year survival can be expected. Medullary carcinoma does not appear to respond to suppression therapy with thyroid hormone.

Anaplastic Carcinoma

Fortunately, anaplastic carcinoma is distinctly uncommon; its frequency depends on the age of the population. Anaplastic carcinoma is rare in children and in adults younger than age 35 years. By age 50 years, as many as 10% of cases of thyroid carcinoma are caused by anaplastic disease, and by age 80 years, by which time the overall incidence of thyroid carcinoma has fallen markedly, nearly half of the cases that do occur are of this variety. The disease is locally invasive in a highly aggressive fashion and quickly produces pain, dysphagia, hemoptysis, and hoarseness. Death usually occurs within 6 to 12 months. However, surgically resectable disease without evidence of metastases, even if it has extended outside the thyroid capsule, can be associated with long-term survival (20% to 30%). It is important to distinguish the small cell type of anaplastic carcinoma from lymphoma of the thyroid. This rare disease, unlike anaplastic carcinoma, is radiosensitive and amenable to chemotherapy.

Radiation-Associated Thyroid Carcinoma

Low-dose irradiation of the thyroid is a stimulus to thyroid carcinogenesis, with a latency period of one to several decades (84). The radiation may be from an external source or from radioiodide as has occurred after nuclear bomb fallout or the nuclear reactor accident at Chernobyl. Public health authorities recommend stockpiling stable iodide for distribution to exposed persons in case of a nuclear plant accident. A single dose of 50 mg of sodium iodide would suffice to protect the thyroid in such an event.

In recent years, papillary and follicular thyroid carcinomas have been reported to occur in increased incidence in patients who received radiation therapy years earlier for conditions such as enlarged tonsils or adenoids, or an enlarged thymus, or for acne. A distinction must be made between treatment with penetrating external radiation and local irradiation with point sources (radium rod and plaque treatment). It has not been possible to relate thyroid carcinoma to the limited exposure that occurs with point sources of radiation.

No relationship has been seen between radiation and the development of medullary or anaplastic carcinoma, but radiation-induced cancers appear to present more often with dissemination than those occurring spontaneously, an argument for early detection (82). Accordingly, high-resolution thyroid scintiscans or sonograms should be part of the followup of patients previously exposed to radiation, because nonpalpable lesions can be detected. The only blood test of value is determination of serum thyroglobulin, elevation of which predicts the development of nodules (85).

The approach to the patient with a history of irradiation to the head and neck is not currently standardized. Examination of the patient at 2- to 3-year intervals should suffice. Routine isotopic scintigraphy or sonographic examination of the thyroid to detect patients with nonpalpable lesions is probably indicated. Many nonpalpable lesions (0.5 to 1.0 cm) can be detected by these methods. Thyroid suppression with T_4 is recommended even for patients with nodules detected only by scintigraphy or sonography. If careful followup reveals an increase in the size of the nodule despite suppression, surgery should be performed.

Surgical therapy should involve the same approach as that for nonirradiated patients (i.e., near-total thyroidectomy), although the earlier practice of lobectomy still has its advocates (86). All patients who have had surgery for benign or malignant nodules should receive suppression therapy with thyroid hormone. Recurrence of benign nodules, but not malignant ones, is greatly reduced (84).

Radiation of the head and neck predisposes patients not only to thyroid cancer but to salivary gland tumors with a ratio of benign to malignant lesions similar to that of nodules in the thyroid. The incidence of benign neural tumors (neurilemomas, acoustic neuromas) and parathyroid adenomas is also increased. External radiation can also ablate thyroid tissue and produce hypothyroidism. This has been seen, for example, in mantle irradiation for Hodgkin disease and can occur after combined surgery and irradiation for head and neck cancers.

SPECIFIC REFERENCES*

1. Laurberg P. Iodine intake—what are we aiming at? J Clin Endocrinol Metab 1994;79:17.
2. Dohan O, Carrasco N. Advances in Na(+)/I(−) symporter (NIS) research in the thyroid and beyond. Mol Cell Endocrinol 2003;213:59.
3. Friesema EC, Jansen J, Milici C, Visser TJ. Thyroid hormone transporters. Vitam Horm 2005;70:137.
4. Yen PM. Physiological and molecular basis of thyroid hormone action. Physiol Rev 2001;81:1097.
5. Franklyn JA, Black EG, Betteridge J, et al. Comparison of second and third generation methods for measurement of serum thyrotropin in patients with overt hyperthyroidism, patients receiving thyroxine therapy, and those with nonthyroidal illness. J Clin Endocrinol Metab 1994;78:1368.
6. Bartolazzi A, Gasbarri A, Papotti M, et al. Application of an immunodiagnostic method for improving preoperative diagnosis of nodular thyroid lesions. Lancet 2001;357:1644.
7. Borst GC, Eil C, Burman KD. Euthyroid hyperthyroxinemia. Ann Intern Med 1983;98:366.
8. Wartofsky L, Burman KD. Alterations in thyroid function in patients with systemic illness: the "euthyroid sick syndrome." Endocrinol Rev 1982;3:164.
9. Wehmann RE, Gregerman RI, Burns WH, et al. Suppression of thyrotropin in the low-thyroxine state of severe nonthyroidal illness. N Engl J Med 1985;312:546.
10. Marquesee E, Haden ST, Utiger RD. Subclinical thyrotoxicosis. Endocrinol Metab Clin North Am 1998;27:37.
11. Gregerman RI, Katz MS. Thyroid diseases. In: Hazzard R, Bierman EL, Blass JP, et al., eds. Principles of geriatric medicine. 3rd ed. New York: McGraw-Hill, 1994:807.
12. Surks MI, DeFesi CR. Normal serum free thyroid hormone concentrations in patients treated with phenytoin or carbamazepine. JAMA 1996;275:1495.
13. Roca RP, Blackman MR, Ackerly MB, et al. Nonsuppression of serum TSH during hyperthyroninemia among acute psychiatric inpatients. Endocr Res 1990;16:415.
14. Refetoff S, Weiss RE, Usala SJ. The syndromes of resistance to thyroid hormone. Endocr Rev 1993;14:348.
15. Hamburger JI. Pitfalls in the laboratory diagnosis of atypical hyperthyroidism. Arch Intern Med 1979;139:96.
16. Nikolai TF, Coombs GJ, McKenzie AK. Lymphocytic thyroiditis with spontaneously resolving hyperthyroidism and subacute thyroiditis. Long-term follow-up. Arch Intern Med 1981;141:1455.
17. Daniels GH. Amiodarone-induced thyrotoxicosis. J Clin Endocrinol Metab 2001;86:3.
18. Bahn RS, Heufelder AE. Mechanisms of disease: pathogenesis of Graves ophthalmopathy. N Engl J Med 1993;329:1468.
19. Kahaly GJ, Rosler H-P, Pitz S, et al. Low-versus high-dose radiotherapy for Graves' ophthalmopathy: a randomized, single blind trial. J Clin Endocrinol Metab 2000;85:102.
20. Torring O, Tallstedt L, Wallin G, et al. Graves' hyperthyroidism: treatment with antithyroid drugs, surgery, or radioiodine—a prospective randomized study. J Clin Endocrinol Metab 1996;81:2986.
21. Allahabadia A, Daykin J, Holder RL, et al. Age and gender predict the outcome of treatment for Graves' hyperthyroidism. J Clin Endocrinol Metab 2000;85:1038.
22. Hashizume K, Ichikawa K, Sakurai A, et al. Administration of thyroxine in treated Graves' disease. Effects on the level of antibodies to thyroid-stimulating hormone receptors and on the risk of recurrence of hyperthyroidism. N Engl J Med 1991;324:947.
23. Figge J, Leinung M, Goodman AD, et al. The clinical evaluation of patients with subclinical hyperthyroidism and free triiodothyronine (free T3) toxicosis. Am J Med 1994;96:229.
24. Sawin CT, Geller A, Kaplan MM. Low serum thyrotropin (thyroid-stimulating hormone) in older persons without hyperthyroidism. Arch Intern Med 1991;151:165.
25. Sawin CT, Geller A, Wolf PA, et al. Low serum thyrotropin concentrations as a risk factor for atrial fibrillation in older persons. N Engl J Med 1994;331:1249.
26. Utiger RD. Subclinical hyperthyroidism—just a low serum thyrotropin concentration, or something more? N Engl J Med 1994;331:1302.

*Bold numerals denote published controlled clinical trials, meta-analyses, or consensus-based recommendations.

27. Cooper DS. Subclinical hypothyroidism. N Engl J Med 2001;345:260.
28. Canaris GJ, Manowitz NR, Mayor G, Ridgway EC. The Colorado thyroid disease prevalence study. Arch Intern Med 2000;160:526.
29. Cooper DS, Halpern R, Wood LC, et al. L-Thyroxine therapy in subclinical hypothyroidism. A double-blind, placebo-controlled trial. Ann Intern Med 1984;101:18.
30. Dong BJ, Hauck WW, Gambertoglio JG, Gee L, et al. Bioequivalence of brand name and generic levothyroxine products in the treatment of hypothyroidism. JAMA 1997;277:1205.
31. Grebe SKG, Cooke RR, Ford HC, et al. Treatment of hypothyroidism with once weekly thyroxine. J Clin Endocrinol Metab 1997;82:870.
32. Roti E, Minelli R, Salvi M. Management of hyperthyroidism and hypothyroidism in the pregnant woman. J Clin Endocrinol Metab 1996;81:1679.
33. Bunevicius R, Kazanavicius G, Zalenkevicius R, et al. Effects of thyroxine as compared with thyroxine plus triiodothyronine in patients with hypothyroidism. N Engl J Med 1999;340:424.
34. Escobar-Morreale HF, Botello-Carretero JI, Descobar delRey F, et al. Treatment of hypothyroidism with combinations of levothyroxine plus liothyronine J Clin Endocrinol Metab 2005;90:4940.
35. Baran DT. Detrimental skeletal effects of thyrotropin suppressive doses of thyroxine: fact or fantasy? J Clin Endocrinol Metab 1994;78:816.
36. Marcocci C, Golia F, Bruno-Bossio G, et al. Carefully monitored levothyroxine suppressive therapy is not associated with bone loss in premenopausal women. J Clin Endocrinol Metab 1994;78:818.
37. Bauer DC, Ettinger B, Nevitt MC, et al. Risk for fracture in women with low serum levels of thyroid-stimulating hormone. Ann Intern Med 2001;134:561.
38. Bogazzi F, Bartalena L, Gasperi M, et al. The various effects of amiodarone on thyroid function. Thyroid 2001;11:511.
39. Rotenberg Z, Weinberger I, Fuchs J, et al. Euthyroid atypical subacute thyroiditis simulating systemic or malignant disease. Arch Intern Med 1986;146:105.
40. Mandel SJ, Cooper DS. The use of antithyroid drugs in pregnancy and lactation. J Clin Endocrinol Metab 2001;86:2354.
41. Smallridge RC, Ladenson PW. Hypothyroidism in pregnancy: consequences to neonatal health. J Clin Endocrinol Metab 2001;86:2349.
42. Haddow JE, Palomaki GE, Allan WC, et al. Maternal thyroid deficiency during pregnancy and subsequent neuropsychological development of the child. N Engl J Med 1999;341:549.
43. Alexander EK, Marqusee E, Lawrence J, et al. Timing and magnitude of increases in levothyroxine requirements during pregnancy in women with hypothyroidism. N Engl J Med 2004;351:241.
44. Wang R, Nelson JC, Weiss RM, et al. Accuracy of free thyroxine measurements across natural ranges of thyroxine binding to single proteins. Thyroid 2000;10:31.
45. Fung HYM, Kologlu M, Collison K, et al. Postpartum thyroid dysfunction in Mid Glamorgan. BMJ 1988;296:241.
46. Amino N, Tada H, Hidaka Y, et al. Screening for postpartum thyroiditis. J Clin Endocrinol Metab 1999;84:1813.
47. Kent GN, Stuckey BG, Allen JR, et al. Postpartum thyroid dysfunction: assessment and relationship to psychiatric affective morbidity. Clin Endocrinol 1999;51:429.
48. Premawardhana LDKE, Parkes AB, Ammari F, et al. Postpartum thyroiditis and long-term thyroid status: prognostic influence of thyroid peroxidase antibodies and ultrasound echogenicity. J Clin Endocrinol Metab 2000;85:71.
49. Alvarez-Marfany M, Roman SH, Drexler AJ, et al. Long-term prospective study of postpartum thyroid dysfunction in women with insulin dependent diabetes mellitus. J Clin Endocrinol Metab 1994;79:10.
50. Bagchi N, Brown TR, Parish RF, et al. Thyroid dysfunction in adults over age 55 years: a study in an urban US community. Arch Intern Med 1990;150:785.
51. Danese MD, Powe NR, Sawin CT, Ladenson PW. Screening for mild thyroid failure at the periodic health examination: a decision and cost-effectiveness analysis. JAMA 1996;276:285.
52. U.S. Preventive Services Task Force. Screening Thyroid Disease: Recommendation Statement. January 2004. Rockville, MD: Agency for Healthcare Research and Quality. Available at: www.ahrq.gov/clinic/3rduspstf/thyroid/thyrrs.htm.
53. American College of Physicians. Clinical guideline, part 1. Screening for thyroid disease. Ann Intern Med 1998;129:141.
54. Helfand M, Redfern CC. Screening for thyroid disease: an update. Ann Intern Med 1998;129:144.
55. Parle JV, Franklin JA, Cross KW, et al. Prevalence and follow-up of abnormal thyrotrophin (TSH) concentrations in the elderly in the United Kingdom. Clin Endocrinol 1991;34:77.
56. Finucane P, Rudra T, Church H, et al. Thyroid function tests in elderly patients with and without an acute illness. Age Aging 1989;18:398.
57. Canaris GJ, Manowitz NR, Ridgway EC. The Colorado Thyroid Disease Prevalence Study. Arch Int Med 2000;160:526.
58. Ehrmann DA, Sarne DH. Serum thyrotropin and the assessment of thyroid status. Ann Intern Med 1989;110:179.
59. Samuels MH. Evaluation and treatment of sporadic nontoxic goiter—some answers and more questions. J Clin Endocrinol Metab 2001;86:994.
60. Bistrup C, Nielsen JD, Gregersen G, et al. Preventive effect of levothyroxine in patients operated for non-toxic goitre: a randomized trial of one hundred patients with nine years follow-up. Clin Endocrinol 1994;40:323.
61. Hegedus L, Nygaard B, Hansen JM. Is routine thyroxine treatment to hinder postoperative recurrence of nontoxic goiter justified? J Clin Endocrinol Metab 1999;84:756.
62. Zelmanovitz F, Genro S, Gross JL. Suppressive therapy with levothyroxine for solitary thyroid nodules: a double-blind controlled clinical study and cumulative meta-analyses. J Clin Endocrinol Metab 1998;83:3881.
63. Wesche MT, Tiel-V Buul MM, Lips P, et al. A randomized trial comparing levothyroxine with radioactive iodine in the treatment of sporadic nontoxic goiter. J Clin Endocrinol Metab 2001;86:998.
64. Bonnema SJ, Bertelsen H, Mortensen J, et al. The feasibility of high dose iodine 131 treatment as an alternative to surgery in patients with a very large goiter: effect on thyroid function and size and pulmonary function. J Clin Endocrinol Metab 1999;84:3636.
65. Mazzaferri EL. Management of a solitary thyroid nodule. N Engl J Med 1993;328:553.
66. Vander JB, Gaston EA, Dawber TR. The significance of nontoxic thyroid nodules. Final report of a 15-year study of the incidence of thyroid malignancy. Ann Intern Med 1968;69:537.
67. Aghini-Lombardi F, Antonangeli L, Martino E, et al. The spectrum of thyroid disorders in an iodine-deficient community: the Pescopagano survey. J Clin Endocrinol Metab 1999;84:561.
68. Marqusee E, Benson CB, Frates MC, et al. Usefulness of ultrasound in the management of nodular thyroid disease. Ann Intern Med 2000;133:696.
69. Singer PA, Cooper DS, Daniels GH, et al. Treatment guidelines for patients with thyroid nodules and well-differentiated thyroid cancer. Arch Intern Med 1996;156:2165.
70. Feld S. AACE clinical practice guidelines for the diagnosis and management of thyroid nodules. Endocr Pract 1969;2:78.
71. Hamburger JI. Diagnosis of thyroid nodules by fine needle biopsy: use and abuse. J Clin Endocrinol Metab 1994;79:3.
72. Hamburger JI. The autonomously functioning thyroid nodule: Goetsch's disease. Endocr Rev 1987;8:439.
73. Lippi F, Ferrari C, Manetti L, et al. Treatment of solitary autonomous thyroid nodules by percutaneous ethanol injection: results of an Italian multicenter study. J Clin Endocrinol Metab 1996;81:3261.
74. Baker RR, Hyland J. Papillary carcinoma of the thyroid gland. Surg Gynecol Obstet 1985;161:546.
75. Samaan NA, Schultz PN, Hickey RC, et al. The results of various modalities of treatment of well differentiated thyroid carcinomas: a retrospective review of 1599 patients. J Clin Endocdrinol Metab 1992;75:714.
76. Finley DJ, Lubitz CC, Wei C, et al. Advancing the molecular diagnosis of thyroid nodules: defining benign lesions by molecular profiling. Thyroid 2005;15:562.
77. Young RL, Mazzaferri EL, Rahe AJ, et al. Pure follicular carcinoma: impact of therapy in 214 patients. J Nucl Med 1980;21:733.
78. DeGroot LJ, Kaplan EL, Shukla MS, et al. Morbidity and mortality in follicular thyroid cancer. J Clin Endocrinol Metab 1995;80:2946.
79. Shapiro LE, Sievert R, Ong L, et al. Minimal cardiac effects in asymptomatic athyreotic patients chronically treated with thyrotropin-suppressive doses of L-thyroxine. J Clin Endocrinol Metab 1997;82:2592.
80. Kloos RT. Papillary thyroid cancer: medical management and follow-up. Curr Treat Options Oncol 2005;6:323.
81. Luster M, Lippi F, Jarzab B, et al. rhTSH-aided radioiodine ablation and treatment of differentiated thyroid carcinoma: a comprehensive review. Endocr Relat Cancer 2005;12:49.
82. Dunn JT. When is a thyroid nodule a sporadic medullary carcinoma? J Clin Endocrinol Metab 1994;78:824.
83. Pacini F, Fontanelli M, Fugazzola L, et al. Routine measurement of serum calcitonin in nodular thyroid diseases allows the preoperative diagnosis of unsuspected sporadic medullary thyroid carcinoma. J Clin Endocrinol Metab 1994;78:826.
84. Schneider AB, Recant W, Pinsky SM, et al. Radiation-induced thyroid carcinoma. Clinical course and results of therapy in 296 patients. Ann Intern Med 1986;105:405.
85. Schneider AB, Shore-Freedman E, Ryo UY, et al. Prospective serum thyroglobulin measurements in assessing the risk of developing thyroid nodules in patients exposed to childhood neck irradiation. J Clin Endocrinol Metab 1985;61:547.
86. Fogelfeld L, Wiviott MBT, Shore-Freedman E, et al. Recurrence of thyroid nodules after surgical removal in patients irradiated in childhood for benign conditions. N Engl J Med 1989;320:835.
87. Pacini F, Lodenson PW, Schlumberger M, et al. Radioiodine ablation of thyroid remnants after preparation with recombinant thyrotropin in differentiated thyroid carcinoma: Results of an international randomized controlled study. J Clin Endo Metab 2006;91:878–894.

*For annotated **General References** and resources related to this chapter, visit www.hopkinsbayview.org/PAMreferences.*

Chapter 81

Selected Endocrine Problems: Pituitary and Adrenal Disorders, Therapeutic Use of Steroids, Disorders of Water Metabolism, Hypoglycemia

*Myron Miller**

*In previous editions, Robert I. Gregerman, MD, contributed to this chapter.

PITUITARY DISEASES

Both autopsy studies and the commonly used neuroimaging procedures of computed tomography (CT) and magnetic resonance imaging (MRI) have demonstrated that abnormalities in the region of the pituitary are relatively common findings. The majority of the abnormalities are a result of benign pituitary adenomas, with the remainder caused by pituitary cysts. Unsuspected pituitary adenomas found on CT or MRI are designated as *incidentalomas* (1). Autopsy data indicate that approximately 10% of men and women over the age of 30 years may have such pituitary tumors. A similar incidence has been found in patients who have had CT or MRI scans for nonpituitary-related indications. Pituitary adenomas are commonly classified on the basis of size as microadenomas (<10 mm in diameter) or macroadenomas (>10 mm in diameter).

Clinical Presentation

Clinically, disorders of the pituitary gland are manifest by mass effect with encroachment by a large tumor on adjacent structures, by a disturbance of function (hypersecretion or hyposecretion of trophic hormones), or by a combination of these processes (Table 81.1). The majority of pituitary tumors are benign adenomas that may be nonfunctional. Many of those adenomas that overproduce hormone are clinically inapparent microadenomas. Microadenomas rarely result in hormone hyposecretion. Macroadenomas, however, may either overproduce hormones or may compromise pituitary function and lead to hyposecretion of one or more of the pituitary hormones.

When a patient presents with evidence of decreased endocrine function, routine evaluation must include consideration of whether the process is primary (i.e., in the end organ) or is a result of pituitary disease (i.e., secondary glandular failure). For example, in most patients with hypothyroidism, thyroid-stimulating hormone (TSH) is elevated because of failure of normal inhibition of the negative feedback loop. However, if TSH is low or normal in the face of hypothyroidism, the possibility of pituitary origin of hypothyroidism must be considered. Similarly, in patients with hypogonadism, levels of follicle-stimulating hormone (FSH) and luteinizing hormone (LH) are almost always elevated when there is primary end-organ failure, but are low or normal in hypogonadism caused by pituitary disease.

TABLE 81.1 Presentations of Pituitary Tumors

Mass effect
Erosion of sella: retro-orbital headache
Compression of optic chiasm: visual field defect
Hormone overproduction
Prolactin: galactorrhea, amenorrhea
GH: acromegaly, gigantism
ACTH: Cushing disease
TSH: hyperthyroidism (rare)
Hypopituitarism
GH: short stature, decreased muscle and bone mass
ACTH: secondary adrenal insufficiency
FSH/LH: secondary hypogonadism, amenorrhea, erectile dysfunction
TSH: secondary hypothyroidism
Prolactin: failure of lactation
AVP: diabetes insipidus

ACTH, adrenocorticotropic hormone; AVP, arginine vasopressin; FSH, follicle-stimulating hormone; GH, growth hormone; LH, luteinizing hormone; TSH, thyroid-stimulating hormone.

Mass Effect

When a pituitary tumor is large enough to produce increased pressure within the sella turcica, enlargement and erosion of the bony walls of that structure either produce no symptoms or may cause headache, typically described by the patient as severe and located behind the eyes. Tumor enlargement superiorly leads to encroachment on the adjacent optic chiasm and may produce temporal visual field defects. Pituitary tumors large enough to be anatomically apparent are often associated with failure of hormone secretion (hypopituitarism), a process that results in selective or multiple end-organ failure (hypoadrenalism, hypogonadism, and/or hypothyroidism).

A related problem is that of *craniopharyngioma*. This developmental abnormality may simulate a pituitary tumor. The lesion is usually outside the pituitary and presents as a suprasellar mass lesion readily evident on CT or MRI. Most cases are manifest during childhood.

Radiologic Evaluation of the Sella Turcica

The sella turcica as seen in plain films of the skull may appear deceptively normal when it harbors a pituitary adenoma or may appear abnormal when no tumor is present. MRI has almost totally replaced older techniques for evaluating the sella. MRI is most sensitive when the image is enhanced by gadolinium. CT is less expensive but is less sensitive than MRI in the detection of intrasellar microadenomas. In a few centers, petrosal venous sampling techniques for ACTH can lateralize many of the nonvisualizable adenomas that are the cause of Cushing disease, thus facilitating pituitary hemisectioning at surgery.

Empty Sella Syndrome

An enlarged sella does not always mean that a pituitary tumor is present. Evaluation commonly leads to demonstration of an empty sella turcica (i.e., one not completely filled by the pituitary gland). Empty sellas are often discovered when a head MRI or CT is obtained for reasons other than suspected hypopituitarism, usually headache, and usually are not associated with clinical endocrine disease. The cause of the empty sella syndrome is unknown, but open communication of cerebrospinal fluid through a defect in the diaphragma sellae or a ruptured cyst has been postulated. In most cases, a rim of nonvisualizable normal pituitary tissue remains, and pituitary function, which should be routinely evaluated (e.g., measurement of TSH, FSH, and LH), is normal; in some there is minimal hypopituitarism or a visual field defect for reasons that are not clear, but that could represent effects of a previous cyst. The diagnosis can be made definitively by MRI.

Pituitary Tumors and Disorders of Pituitary Hyperfunction

Chromophobe Adenomas

Chromophobe adenomas, the most common of the pituitary tumors, account for approximately 85% of cases; most occur between the ages of 30 and 60 years, and rarely are associated with parathyroid or pancreatic islet cell adenomas and, sometimes, with the Zollinger-Ellison syndrome (see Chapter 43). These associations constitute the syndrome of multiple endocrine adenomatosis type I.

Chromophobe adenomas are usually noninvasive but may infiltrate local structures and, on rare occasions, even behave as locally malignant lesions. Long thought to be functionless, many are now known to be prolactinomas (see Prolactinomas: Prolactin and Galactorrhea). A few produce growth hormone (GH); even fewer produce gonadotropins. The term *chromophobe adenoma* belongs to the era in which pituitary tumors were classified by their histologic staining characteristics (chromophobe, eosinophile, and basophile). A preferred, more precise contemporary classification is based on the secretory product of the tumor (e.g., somatotrope tumor, GH producing).

Pituitary function remains clinically normal until more than 75% of the normal pituitary has been destroyed by the adenoma. Hypogonadism is usually the earliest evidence of a hormone deficiency state (60% to 80% of cases), but hypothyroidism as an initial manifestation is almost as common. Adrenal insufficiency is usually the last problem to develop and is often inapparent except on laboratory testing. In approximately 10% of cases, diabetes insipidus develops.

The long-term course of nonfunctional microadenomas suggests that most will not undergo further increase in size or become hyperfunctional. Thus, after initial clinical and biochemical screening for hormone overproduction (prolactin, GH, adrenocorticotropic hormone [ACTH]), further followup can be done by obtaining an MRI yearly for 2 years and, if no change has occurred, subsequently lengthening the interval for further MRI (2).

Prolactinomas: Prolactin and Galactorrhea

In women, unilateral or bilateral galactorrhea may be the first clue to the presence of a prolactin-secreting adenoma (prolactinoma). In many cases, discharge from the breast is minimal and may be apparent only on physical examination when a few drops of milk may be expressible. Breast enlargement may occur in the male, but prolactin excess is an uncommon cause of gynecomastia (see Chapter 85). Galactorrhea in men, a rare event, is diagnostic of a prolactinoma. Prolactin secretion appears to inhibit the secretion of gonadotropins and hence may also be associated with evidence of hypogonadism, including impotence and amenorrhea (see Chapters 85 and 101).

Many cases of galactorrhea in women are not caused by tumoral hyperprolactinemia but rather by a functional disturbance of prolactin secretion, which, in turn, is either spontaneous or related to the use of certain drugs. The drugs most commonly incriminated in the production of galactorrhea are estrogens (including oral contraceptives), neuroleptics, tricyclic antidepressants, risperidone, haloperidol, and methadone. In either case, the hallmark of galactorrhea is an increase of the concentration of prolactin in serum. Rarely, galactorrhea occurs secondary to hypothyroidism.

The degree of prolactin elevation is strongly suggestive of the cause of the disorder. Levels of prolactin greater than 200 ng/mL are essentially diagnostic of a pituitary tumor, even in the absence of changes in the sella. Levels of prolactin greater than 250 ng/mL often indicate the presence of a macroadenoma while lesser degrees of elevation are more commonly associated with microadenoma. Elevated levels of prolactin less than 50 ng/mL are more likely to be caused by a functional disorder or a drug, but a pituitary tumor cannot be differentiated from other causes solely by quantification of the prolactin level. If suprasellar extension is present on CT or MRI, the patient should be referred for ophthalmologic examination of the visual fields.

Treatment

Most cases of galactorrhea, whether a result of macro or microadenoma or of another cause, can be treated successfully with the dopamine agonist bromocriptine (Parlodel), which often lowers the prolactin level, abolishes the galactorrhea, and restores normal menses. Bromocriptine not only reduces prolactin secretion, but in many cases caused by macroadenoma, causes the tumor to shrink so dramatically that even visual field defects can be reversed. A favorable response occurs in 80% of cases. The drug is now commonly given preoperatively, even when a large tumor is present, because surgical removal is facilitated. Long-term drug therapy may be an alternative to surgery (3). Treatment with bromocriptine can be undertaken by the nonspecialist if evaluation indicates that tumor is unlikely. The drug is available as 2.5-mg tablets and 5-mg capsules; the initial dosage is 1.25 to 2.50 mg/day. The dosage may be increased by 2.5 mg every 3 to 7 days until an optimal response is achieved—usually 5 to 7.5 mg/day. Adverse effects include nausea, headache, dizziness, and fatigue. If prolactin levels are very high, if radiographic evidence of tumor is present, or if the patient is intolerant of, or unresponsive to, bromocriptine, an endocrinologist should be consulted. An alternative dopamine agonist drug is cabergoline (Dostinex), which has the advantage over bromocriptine of a need for much less frequent dosing, in the range of 0.25 to 1 mg twice weekly (4). The adverse effects of the two drugs are similar.

Prolactin-secreting tumors in men tend to be diagnosed at a much later stage (i.e., as macroadenomas) than in women and to be associated with hypogonadism. Drug therapy is successful in approximately 80% of these cases (5).

Until recently the indications for surgical intervention (transsphenoidal; see Acromegaly) were mainly related to the size of the tumor. In the past, visual field impairment has been the major indication for urgent surgery, but extensive experience indicates that even patients with significant visual loss can be successfully treated with bromocriptine. With transsphenoidal surgery, microadenomas can often be removed successfully and normal pituitary function restored. With marked suprasellar extension, a transfrontal surgical approach may be needed. This is a much more formidable procedure. In many cases, a large tumor cannot be completely removed; postoperative radiation therapy prevents clinical recurrence in these instances.

Acromegaly

Pituitary tumors that produce an excess of GH result in the clinical state termed *acromegaly*. Approximately 75% of pituitary tumors causing acromegaly are macroadenomas, and approximately 25% are mixed tumors that secrete both GH and prolactin.

If GH excess occurs before cessation of growth, gigantism occurs. When GH excess begins in the adult, the most common clinical feature suggesting the presence of acromegaly is insidious alteration of facial appearance over many years. Old photographs may be useful in helping to identify such changes. Physical findings include enlargement (lengthening) of the mandible, sometimes with separation of the teeth; coarsening of facial features because of both overgrowth of frontal, malar, and nasal bones, and of soft tissue producing widening of the nose and protrusion of the lips; enlargement of the hands and feet, often noted by increasing glove and shoe size; and dermatologic changes that include skin thickening and sebaceous gland enlargement (hydradenitis) with accompanying increase in sweating. Patients may present with a nerve entrapment (carpal tunnel) syndrome. Osteoarthritis and diabetes mellitus are often seen in this disorder, but are too common to provide a clue to the presence of acromegaly. Tumors large enough to produce sellar enlargement may lead to headache and suprasellar extension may result in visual field defects.

The laboratory diagnosis is straightforward in overt cases but may be difficult in mild cases. GH varies rapidly during the day in the serum of acromegalic patients, so single measurements may not be helpful. The best test for screening is the determination of serum insulinlike growth factor 1 (IGF-1). The serum concentration of this product of GH action varies little and correlates well with the 24-hour integrated serum GH level, arguably the most definitive test. If GH is measured directly in screening, elevation of serum GH in the fasting basal state to values consistently greater than 10 ng/mL strongly suggests the diagnosis. However, stress, meals and physical activity may also elevate the GH levels. Elevated values must therefore be confirmed with a test of the ability of glucose to suppress the GH. During a standard glucose tolerance test (see Chapter 79), the GH—determined simultaneously with the glucose—should normally fall to a value of less than 1 ng/mL. Most acromegalics show no fall of GH, and a few exhibit a paradoxical rise during the test. Laboratory evidence of elevated IGF-1 or elevated and/or nonsuppressible GH warrants referral to an endocrinologist, as does the presence of equivocal clinical or laboratory findings in a patient with clinical features suggestive of acromegaly (6).

Treatment of Acromegaly

The decision regarding the most appropriate form of therapy should be made by an endocrinologist. Surgery is indicated when there is need for rapid reduction of tumor mass with symptoms of visual field loss or intractable headache. Transsphenoidal hypophysectomy is now standard for most cases and should, if acromegaly is caused by a microadenoma, include an attempt at selective removal of the microadenoma. The transsphenoidal operation involves minimal morbidity, a very low rate of complications, and essentially no mortality. Cure rates for microadenoma vary directly with the experience of the neurosurgeon, reaching approximately 70% in the most experienced hands, but being substantially lower when performed by neurosurgeons who do fewer cases. For macroadenomas, the cure rate even by the most experienced surgeons is only 20% to 50%.

Somatostatin analogues, potent inhibitors of GH secretion, are effective as long-term medical therapy and can be considered as initial therapy in most cases of both macroadenoma and microadenoma. The drugs require subcutaneous injection, but long-acting depot preparations (octreotide acetate [Sandostatin LAR]; lanreotide SR) are now available and can be given every 4 weeks (with usual doses of 20 to 30 mg for octreotide) (7). Tumor shrinkage of up to 40% of original volume is usually evident within 12 to 24 weeks of initiation of therapy and occurs in up to 75% of treated patients. The goals of treatment are to (a) reduce mean GH levels to <2.5 ng/mL and nadir GH after an oral glucose load to <1 ng/mL; (b) reduce IGF-1 to the age-adjusted normal range, a response achieved in approximately 70% of patients; (c) control symptoms of active acromegaly; and (d) reduce tumor mass. Treatment should be directed by an endocrinologist (6).

A second-line drug after somatostatin analogues is pegvisomant (Somavert), a GH receptor antagonist that inhibits the production of IGF-1. Although it normalizes IGF-1 levels in 97% of patients, it does not reduce tumor size and, in some patients, the tumor may actually increase in size. The role of pegvisomant in long-term management of acromegaly appears to be as an additional agent in patients whose GH and IGF-1 levels fail to normalize on a somatostatin analogue alone (8).

Irradiation of the pituitary, usually by external high-voltage techniques, had been standard treatment for years but is no longer considered to be primary therapy. Although it is effective, it may take several years to produce maximal suppression of hormone production and is often accompanied by development of hypopituitarism. The decision about what should be the most appropriate therapy in any individual patient should be determined by an endocrinologist.

Cushing Disease

When there is evidence of overproduction of glucocorticoids and testing suggests the presence of adrenal hyperplasia (see Adrenal Diseases), evaluation of the sella turcica is indicated. Most cases of Cushing disease with adrenal hyperplasia are caused by an ACTH-producing basophilic microadenoma of the pituitary that can be visualized preoperatively, in 80% of cases, with an optimal MRI examination (see Cushing Disease section). Transsphenoidal resection of the microadenoma can be curative.

Other Secretory Pituitary Tumors

Although quite rare, pituitary tumors that secrete thyrotropin (TSH) and produce hyperthyroidism do occur. Even rarer are cases of hypersecretion of TSH without demonstrable tumor. Patients with tumors have been successfully treated with a somatostatin analogue. Tumors that produce excessive amounts of gonadotropins are very rare.

Pituitary Failure (Hypopituitarism)

The most common causes of hypopituitarism are pituitary tumors and surgically induced hypopituitarism following either transsphenoidal or transfrontal resection of a pituitary tumor. Patients who have undergone these procedures will need to have residual pituitary function evaluated, generally at least 2 to 3 weeks after surgery, which is when any deficits will begin to become apparent. The pituitary may also be affected by severe head trauma, as well as by a wide variety of systemic illnesses, including granulomatous, infectious, vascular, and metastatic processes, but all are extremely uncommon causes of hypopituitarism.

Idiopathic Causes

Patients are occasionally encountered in whom pituitary failure occurs without evidence of pituitary tumor or of another demonstrable anatomic defect. Some are eventually found to have infiltrative processes (sarcoidosis, histiocytosis, lymphoma, benign lymphocytic infiltration [hypophysitis]). Hypopituitarism is diagnosed by the demonstration of end-organ failure with concurrent absence of the expected elevation of trophic hormone. Multiple trophic hormone deficiencies are usually present but isolated deficiencies of trophic hormones also rarely occur. Among these, the most likely to be encountered is hypogonadotropic hypogonadism in the male, sometimes associated with anosmia (*Kallmann syndrome*, see Chapter 85). In these patients, no anatomic basis is apparent.

Sheehan Syndrome (Postpartum Pituitary Failure)

Massive uterine hemorrhage occurring at delivery occasionally is accompanied by pituitary infarction and consequent panhypopituitarism. In this syndrome, failure of postpartum lactation and absence of menses are attended by development of debility and other evidence of end-organ failure. Because of improvements in obstetric care (prompt treatment of hemorrhage), such cases are now rare.

Pituitary Hemorrhage and Infarction

Rarely, hemorrhage into the pituitary gland (pituitary apoplexy), usually into an adenoma, leads to severe headache and/or signs of a rapidly expanding intracranial abnormality. Radiographic examination of the sella turcica is abnormal. Hormonal evaluation will demonstrate the presence of hypopituitarism. Another rare phenomenon is that of pituitary infarction occurring during the course of a febrile illness, presumably viral. Intense headache lasts for days and is usually, but not always, severe enough to require hospitalization. The acute febrile illness subsides with symptomatic therapy and without specific clinical or radiographic findings, only to be followed later by the development of hypopituitarism. Both men and women can be affected.

Hypopituitarism Secondary to Head Trauma

Head trauma has long been thought to account for only a tiny fraction of all cases of hypopituitarism, but recent reports indicate that head trauma, usually the result of a motor vehicle accident, can result in hormone deficiencies in as many as 80% of patients early in the period following head trauma. Laboratory findings are highly variable and range from panhypopituitarism to single hormone deficiencies. The most common findings are decreased gonadotropins and growth hormone and increased prolactin. Hormone deficits may resolve over time, but approximately 28% of individuals will be left with permanent deficiencies, most commonly GH, ACTH, and gonadotropins (9). Patients may not recall such an occurrence until helped to remember. Careful questioning of relatives often reveals a positive history that would otherwise remain obscure. The trauma may not have seemed severe; neither skull fracture nor loss of consciousness need occur, although most cases have had both. The typical case is a young male who is found on testing to have evidence of end-organ failure within a year of the traumatic episode, although many years may pass before a diagnosis is made. Pituitary imaging may show an empty sella, pituitary atrophy, and/or areas of hypodensity, cysts, or microcysts. Spontaneous recovery of pituitary function may occur as late as 10 or more years after the event.

Posterior pituitary dysfunction with diabetes insipidus has been found in approximately 22% of patients in the period immediately following traumatic brain injury. When it does occur in the immediate posttrauma period, it often resolves over the next several months with approximately one third of those affected having permanent diabetes insipidus on assessment 6 to 36 months after injury (10).

Disturbances of Pituitary Function Caused by Nonendocrine Disease

Much more common than decreased pituitary function resulting from intrinsic pituitary disease is altered gonadotropin secretion on a functional basis. Many illnesses can affect the functional integrity of the hypothalamic–pituitary–end-organ axis. This phenomenon is most obvious as a disturbance of menstruation in women and, less often, impotence in men (see Chapter 85). Many normal men, generally over the age of 80 years, experience a decline in LH secretion with consequent hypogonadism, a phenomenon sometimes referred to as "andropause." This age-related alteration in hypothalamic/pituitary function of men differs from menopause, which is caused by end-organ failure of the ovary.

Any disease that results in malnutrition can lead to decreased gonadotropins and (secondary) amenorrhea in women or impotence in men. Alcoholism is an outstanding example. Liver disease does not need to be present in alcoholics to produce amenorrhea or impotence, but various liver diseases are themselves associated with loss of menses. The common factor seems to be malnutrition. In recent years, some individuals have undertaken caloric restriction in an attempt to extend their life span. Although such persons maintain that they are not malnourished but rather are undernourished, they share many of the symptomatic features described here.

The classic example of nonendocrine illness that simulates an endocrine disturbance is anorexia nervosa (see Chapter 11). In this psychiatric disturbance, which results in severe malnutrition with resultant weight loss, the most marked disturbance of endocrine function is cessation of menses resulting from a decrease of gonadotropins. Other trophic hormones are not affected. Thyroid function is usually normal. Axillary and pubic hair are retained, giving important clinical evidence for the preservation of adrenal function. Although cortisol secretion is low (urinary glucosteroid excretion is decreased), this results from slow metabolic disposal of cortisol rather than from a decreased ability to increase ACTH secretion appropriately; plasma cortisol is normal. GH concentration may be elevated, a consequence of starvation as a consequence of any cause. The diagnosis of anorexia nervosa should be based on the association of psychiatric abnormalities and obvious decrease in food intake. The tests described serve merely to support the diagnosis.

Women who engage in a high level of physical activity, such as long distance runners or gymnasts, may develop either primary or secondary amenorrhea as a result of hyposecretion of gonadotropins. A number of disorders and diseases may also result in secondary amenorrhea as a consequence of failure of gonadotropin secretion, including such diverse conditions as severe emotional disturbances, marked obesity, poorly controlled diabetes mellitus, and severe chronic infections.

Hormone Replacement Therapy for Hypopituitarism

Pituitary insufficiency, regardless of the cause, is treated with replacement of identified hormone deficiencies, that is, thyroid hormone (thyroxine, see Chapter 80), adrenal glucocorticoid (cortisol, see Glucocorticoid [Steroid] Replacement Therapy section), and gonadal hormone (testosterone [see Chapter 85] or an estrogen [see Chapter 106]). Except for GH, the pituitary trophic hormones themselves are not used routinely (see Growth Hormone Deficiency section). Occasionally, young women may be candidates for therapy with gonadotropins to produce ovulation and restore fertility. Such therapy may be effective but is available at only a few centers. Restoration of fertility in the male is also possible with the use of a combination of gonadotropins, but such therapy is not generally available. In men, normal libido and sexual performance consistent with age can be ensured with testosterone therapy.

Growth Hormone Deficiency

The name "growth hormone" has its historical roots in the period when it was found to be essential for normal growth and development in children. However, GH is a metabolic regulator, even in the adult. Except during aging (see below), GH deficiency in the adult is invariably caused by pituitary disease or pituitary surgery. Although most patients with pituitary disorders do reasonably well when end-organ hormones are replaced (adrenal, thyroid, gonadal), the role of GH replacement only was recognized relatively recently (11).

The clinical state of the adult human with isolated GH deficiency (i.e., patients receiving replacement therapy only with other end-organ hormones) is now considered to be a deficiency "syndrome" (12). The abnormalities attributed to GH deficiency are a reduction in lean body mass, bone mass, and muscle strength, an increase in body fat—especially abdominal fat—and alterations in mood (depression, emotional lability, anxiety) and energy level. Although these features are not specific for GH deficiency, treatment of GH-deficient adults improves psychological well-being, muscle strength, exercise tolerance, and bone mass. Objective evidence validating these changes is available from psychological testing and measurements of lean body mass (body composition studies showing increased muscle, decreased fat), bone mass, and exercise performance testing.

During normal aging, about one-half of the elderly develop a low GH state that is manifest primarily through loss of nocturnal GH secretion with an associated decrease in serum IGF-1. In the past few years, small numbers of such patients have been studied during GH replacement therapy, alone or in combination with sex steroids, in an effort to ameliorate some of the effects of aging, especially the loss of muscle mass (sarcopenia) and strength. Although improvement can be seen in measures of body composition and bone mass, the results of such studies do not suggest that GH will be a panacea for the adverse changes that accompany aging.

The diagnosis of GH deficiency in the adult is not simple. The gold standard is the insulin-tolerance test (ITT), that is, secretion of GH provoked by insulin-induced hypoglycemia. Various stimulatory tests have been proposed, using a variety of agents, alone and in combination. These tests are best left to a consulting endocrinologist, as is the advisability of using GH over the long-term as part of a replacement program. GH is available as a recombinant deoxyribonucleic acid (DNA) product and is administered by daily subcutaneous injection. The potential benefits may be considerable, as is the cost (13).

ADRENAL DISEASES

Adrenocortical Insufficiency (Addison Disease)

Primary adrenal insufficiency is a rare disorder with a prevalence of approximately 100 cases per 1 million people and an incidence of 5 cases per year per 1 million people. In ambulatory patients, the clinical presentation of adrenocortical insufficiency is related to a number of chronic complaints that are nonspecific in character. A high index of suspicion will result in far more tests than positive diagnoses, but detection of this rare problem is important to prevent morbidity culminating in acute hospitalization for full-blown disease (i.e., vascular collapse with addisonian crisis) or death.

Etiology and Association with Other Autoimmune Diseases

Adrenocortical insufficiency is now most commonly the result of autoimmune disease and is associated with the presence of antibodies to adrenal tissue. Most other cases are secondary to pituitary disease.

Many cases of autoimmune adrenocortical insufficiency are associated with autoimmune thyroiditis, although the two problems may develop years apart. The simultaneous occurrence of autoimmune thyroid and adrenal disease is termed *Schmidt syndrome*. Rarely, autoimmune adrenocortical insufficiency, autoimmune hypothyroidism, and autoimmune gonadal failure occur in the syndrome of polyglandular failure. There is also an association of autoimmune adrenocortical insufficiency with pernicious anemia and Sjögren syndrome, and probably with systemic lupus erythematosus. Tuberculosis, once a common cause, now only rarely produces adrenocortical insufficiency in the United States and other developed countries, probably because of a relatively decreased incidence of tuberculosis in the Western world and because of effective therapy. Other rare causes of adrenocortical insufficiency include histoplasmosis, paracoccidiomycosis (in Central and South Americans), and sarcoidosis. Human immunodeficiency virus infection and diseases associated with the acquired immunodeficiency syndrome (e.g., cytomegalovirus, histoplasmosis, mycobacterial infection; see Chapter 39) often cause asymptomatic adrenal dysfunction, but symptomatic adrenal insufficiency is uncommon. Although infectious causes of adrenal insufficiency are unlikely to be encountered in the United States, they should still be excluded, especially in the absence of evidence for coexistent autoimmune disease.

Clinical Presentation

Chronic symptoms include anorexia, weight loss, weakness, and decreased physical endurance. Nausea and vomiting may occur, and abdominal pain, sometimes resembling that of peptic ulcer disease, can be a presenting feature. Other symptoms include mental sluggishness, irritability, and symptoms of either postural hypotension or of hypoglycemia. In primary adrenal insufficiency, increasing pigmentation (white patients) or further darkening of skin (African American patients) may be noted. Loss of axillary and pubic hair—an important finding when present—may occur in women. Such hair loss is commonly overlooked on physical examination and is rarely volunteered as part of the history.

Physical examination often shows postural hypotension. Pigmentation is diffuse but is especially evident in the creases of the hands, the areolae, over pressure areas (knuckles, elbows), and in new scars. Pigmentation of buccal mucous membranes is a pathognomonic finding in white patients but is a normal finding in blacks. Lymphadenopathy is occasionally seen. When the adrenal insufficiency is secondary to pituitary disease, additional findings may relate to the manifestations of a pituitary tumor (headache, visual loss), to hypothyroidism (see Chapter 80), or to hypogonadism.

Laboratory Evaluation

Classically, hyponatremia associated with hyperkalemia and some degree of azotemia provides a clue to the diagnosis. These abnormalities are manifestations of severe disease and are often absent in the less-severe cases that are likely to be encountered in ambulatory practice. Various other nonspecific abnormalities occur occasionally, including anemia, lymphocytosis, and eosinophilia.

Laboratory diagnosis of adrenal insufficiency depends on determination of serum cortisol in the basal state and after adrenal stimulation by injection of the ACTH analogue cosyntropin (Cortrosyn) (14). Both the normal diurnal rhythm of cortisol and the high degree of variability of serum cortisol in normal people must be kept in mind. Serum cortisol can be measured initially at any time of the day, and a robust normal value (15 to 25 μg/dL) will exclude the diagnosis. However, afternoon determinations may be low simply because of the normal diurnal drop, and even the fasting morning cortisol is highly variable. Values lower than 5 μg/dL at any time are highly likely to be a result of adrenal insufficiency. Intermediate values

(5 to 10 μg/dL) may be seen in less-severe cases and may overlap those of normal subjects. Thus, measurement of unstimulated serum cortisol, while useful in excluding the diagnosis, may fail to detect mild cases or may yield indeterminate values.

Further evaluation of low or borderline values of serum cortisol should always be made by administering cosyntropin and then measuring cortisol again. The ease with which such testing is performed—and the common failure of unstimulated serum cortisol values to give definitive information—provides a cogent argument for use of cosyntropin stimulation as the preferred screening procedure for adrenal insufficiency (14). Many variations of cosyntropin stimulation tests have been advocated. The bolus intravenous injection of 0.25 mg of cosyntropin has been used for years as a simple and reliable procedure in the diagnosis of adrenal insufficiency. The serum cortisol is measured at baseline and at 30 and 60 minutes after injection, and will normally rise by at least 7 μg/dL to at least 18 to 20 μg/dL. Patients with adrenocortical insufficiency show a subnormal response. A 1 μg cosyntropin dose has been demonstrated to yield slightly more accurate results and is used in many centers, but requires more frequent blood sampling to detect the peak cortisol response (15). Patients with an abnormal response to cosyntropin should be referred urgently to an endocrinologist for confirmation of the diagnosis and additional testing, including measurement of serum ACTH, in an attempt to distinguish primary from secondary adrenal insufficiency. An elevated ACTH level (>100 pg/mL) is seen in primary adrenal insufficiency.

Other Tests

Tests of adrenal function based on 24-hour urinary steroid excretion (free cortisol) are less useful in screening for adrenal insufficiency. These tests offer no advantage over serum cortisol measurements and will yield artificially low values if urine collection is incomplete. The adrenal response to cosyntropin is slow in secondary adrenal insufficiency and requires stimulation for up to 3 days. In the past, 2- to 3-day infusions were used to discriminate between primary and secondary adrenal insufficiency. However, the presence of low serum ACTH in the setting of low serum cortisol is a more definitive indicator of secondary adrenal insufficiency. The finding of other pituitary hormone deficits, such as follicle-stimulating hormone, LH, and GH, further points to secondary adrenal disease (16).

Although the adrenal mineralocorticoid aldosterone may be low in adrenal insufficiency, the hormone is secreted by the zona glomerulosa rather than the more central portion of the adrenal cortex, and may be relatively unaffected by processes that destroy much of the glucocorticoid-producing zone of the gland. Consequently, measurements of plasma and urinary aldosterone have no place in routine diagnosis of adrenocortical insufficiency. Routine radiographic studies should include a chest radiograph and, if appropriate (e.g., suspicion of adrenal hemorrhage or metastases), CT or MRI of the adrenals.

Functional Adrenal Insufficiency

In recent years, it has been recognized that some patients with critical illness may develop clinical and laboratory features suggestive of adrenal insufficiency, including subnormal serum cortisol response to adrenal stimulation with cosyntropin (17). However, if the individual recovers, the manifestations of adrenal insufficiency will resolve and subsequent assessment of adrenal function will be normal. This condition of transient apparent adrenal insufficiency has been named functional adrenal insufficiency and in the acute setting may be difficult to distinguish from authentic adrenal insufficiency. It can be recognized by the finding in a critically ill person of a serum cortisol less than 15 μg/dL that does not rise by at least 9 μg/dL following stimulation with ACTH (17). These findings warrant prompt treatment with parenteral hydrocortisone at a dose of 50 mg every 6 hours. Complicating making a diagnosis of adrenal insufficiency is the observation that low serum cortisol measured in the presence of severe physiologic stress may be the consequence of altered cortisol binding protein as measurement of serum free cortisol may be normal (18). Functional adrenal insufficiency is unlikely to be diagnosed in an ambulatory setting, but if it is, it warrants immediate hospitalization.

Treatment of Established Adrenal Insufficiency

The addisonian patient should be helped to realize the importance of taking hormone therapy regularly, of self-care (dose adjustment) during situations of stress, and of the necessity of life-long replacement therapy.

Glucocorticoid (Steroid) Replacement Therapy

Replacement dosage for cortisol was established empirically decades ago. Secretion rates determined by stable isotope dilution suggest that 24-hour cortisol secretion is in the range of 8 to 15 mg per day (14), although older studies using radioactive labels gave somewhat higher values. Large or obese persons need more, but too much individual variation exists to make dose-to-weight calculations meaningful. Most patients can be treated with 15 to 25 mg of cortisol or its equivalent daily (20 mg of cortisol is equivalent to 25 mg of cortisone plus 5 mg of prednisone plus 0.5 mg of dexamethasone). The simplest scheme is 10 mg of cortisol (hydrocortisone) given twice daily. Some authorities prefer to simulate the normal diurnal rhythm of cortisol secretion, although no evidence indicates that this scheme is of any special benefit. In this approach, 10 to 15 mg of cortisol is taken on rising and 5 to 10 mg in the evening. Some

TABLE 81.2 Commonly Used Glucocorticoids[a]

Generic Name	Common Trade Name(s)	Equivalent Potency (mg)[b]	Sodium Retention Relative to Cortisol
Cortisol (hydrocortisone)	Cortef	20	—
Cortisone[c]	—	25	1
Prednisone	Deltasone Meticorten Delta Cortef	5	0.1
Prednisolone	Meticortelone Sterane	4	0.1
Methylprednisolone	Medrol	4	0
	Aristocort, Kenacort	4	0
Dexamethasone[d]	Decadron	0.75	0
Betamethasone[d]	Celestone	0.6	0
For parenteral use			
Cortisol	Solu-Cortef		
Methylprednisolone	Solu-Medrol		
Triamcinolone	Aristocort		
Dexamethasone	Decadron		
Betamethasone	Celestone		
For topical use			
Triamcinolone	Aristocort, Kenalog, Triacet		
Fluocinolone	Valisone, Synalar, Capex		
Betamethasone	Betatrex, Betaderm, Luxiq		
For inhalation and intranasal use			
Beclomethasone and others (see Chapters 30 and 60)	Vanceril		

[a]Most of the compounds listed are available in generic forms. All are marketed as ester derivatives or salts of esters (e.g., cortisol sodium hemisuccinate [Solu-Cortef]). For practical purposes, only cortisol and cortisone have significant salt-retaining (mineralocorticoid) action.
[b]Also equivalent to daily physiologic replacement when given in divided doses.
[c]Cortisone acetate has long been given parenterally (intramuscular route) as well as orally; however, this compound is unpredictably absorbed from injection sites and cannot be relied on to produce adequate blood levels.
[d]This compound has a relatively long duration of action and should not be used for alternate-day glucocorticoid therapy.

clinicians still prescribe as much as 30 mg of cortisol (hydrocortisone) per day, an amount that exceeds physiologic replacement for most persons and should be avoided.

Equivalent doses of prednisone or another glucocorticoid (Table 81.2) may be used but have no advantage. Indeed, their use might dictate a requirement for additional mineralocorticoid therapy because glucocorticoids such as prednisone and dexamethasone have much less mineralocorticoid activity than does cortisol (or cortisone).

Overtreatment with glucocorticoids should be avoided. Frequently increasing the dosage for treatment of nonspecific complaints is a common practice but should be avoided because iatrogenic subclinical Cushing syndrome (or, at a minimum, hypertension) is a real hazard to the long-term well-being of patients with Addison disease. The initial response to replacement therapy varies: weakness and lassitude ordinarily abate within hours to days, but other symptoms may diminish somewhat more slowly.

The requirement for glucocorticoids (cortisol) is increased during stress. In the ambulatory patient, minor stress (common "cold" without fever; simple dental extraction under local anesthesia) can be handled by a properly instructed and motivated patient. On such occasions, a modest increase in dosage is often needed, for example, an additional 5 or 10 mg of cortisol. Telephone contact with the caregiver is also useful—or even essential—on many such occasions, especially in the early months of therapy before the patient's ability to deal with these episodes has been demonstrated. The most common stress for the ambulatory patient is an infection, often a febrile viral illness. Ordinarily, a febrile response to approximately 101°F (38°C) that is unaccompanied by vomiting or diarrhea can be handled simply by increasing the cortisol dose to 50 to 75 mg per day in divided doses. A more-severe illness episode may require 100 mg for a few days. The occurrence of vomiting or significant diarrhea requires contact with a physician and may demand the use of parenteral glucocorticoids.

The need for hospitalization during stress must be determined by the caregiver and depends on the circumstances. It is obviously prudent to be cautious, but in this long-term chronic illness, frequent and precipitous hospitalizations should be avoided. Many minor events can be handled by judicious increase of steroid dosage. Perioperative management is described in Chapter 93.

Although not all patients with fully developed adrenal insufficiency require mineralocorticoid therapy in addition to cortisol replacement, such therapy is usually started when the diagnosis is first made. The initial dose is 0.1 mg of fludrocortisone daily (Florinef, 0.1 mg tablets). Aldosterone is not available for therapy of Addison disease. Only rarely will patients require more than 0.1 mg of fludrocortisone. In the early days of replacement therapy, dosages as high as 0.2 mg/day were used, but hypertension and edema were common. A maintenance dosage of 0.05 mg is average, and some individuals require as little as 0.05 mg every other day. Adequacy of therapy can be judged by determinations of serum sodium and potassium levels and clinical observations, including normalization of blood pressure without postural hypotension. During stress, when the dosage of cortisol is increased beyond 50 to 75 mg/day, fludrocortisone therapy becomes unnecessary because the mineralocorticoid activity of cortisol is sufficient to maintain salt balance when taken in greater than basal physiologic amounts.

The patient and members of the patient's household should be educated about the symptoms of addisonian crisis and how to respond in emergencies. In addition, the patient should carry an identification document or wear an inscribed bracelet that identifies the addisonian state and contains instructions for therapy. Appropriate information, in addition to name, address, and telephone number, should read approximately as follows:

> I am a patient with adrenal insufficiency (Addison disease). If I am seriously injured, found unconscious, or am vomiting, I should be given an injection of dexamethasone as emergency treatment for addisonian crisis. A filled syringe is with my belongings. Notify my health care giver (name, telephone number) or other medical authority immediately.

Syringes containing dexamethasone phosphate (4 mg in 1 mL of water) are available for patients and can be carried conveniently.

All patients with Addison disease should consume a liberal quantity of sodium (100 to 150 mEq [6 to 9 g NaCl] per day), regardless of whether mineralocorticoids are used. In the event of intercurrent diarrhea or profuse sweating, additional salt above the normal intake should be consumed. Electrolytes should be checked periodically (every 3 to 4 months during the critical first year of therapy). Mineralocorticoid therapy should be cautiously reduced if edema, hypertension, or hypokalemia is noted, and salt or mineralocorticoid should be increased if postural hypotension, hyponatremia, or hyperkalemia appears. Overtreatment with glucocorticoids should be carefully avoided. Over the long-term, it should be borne in mind that if the Addison disease is idiopathic (i.e., autoimmune), related diseases and their own manifestations may appear at any time (hypothyroidism, hypoparathyroidism, hypogonadism).

Adrenocortical Hyperfunction: Cushing Syndrome

The adrenal glands produce several steroid products: glucocorticoids (chiefly cortisol), mineralocorticoids (chiefly aldosterone), and adrenal androgens. Clinical disorders may affect predominantly the secretion of one or other of these hormones. Table 81.3 lists these disorders of adrenal hyperfunction. Most are rather uncommon or rare, but some essentially functional disorders are commonly encountered. The approach presented here is predominantly oriented to the recognition—or exclusion—and initial evaluation of these diseases in ambulatory patients. Once the practitioner is reasonably certain that a problem exists, detailed evaluation often requires consultation with an endocrinologist and sometimes hospitalization for special procedures. However, many relatively simple tests to assess adrenal function can be performed on an ambulatory basis. The specific steps of this diagnostic workup vary widely even among specialists and are in constant evolution as new hormone assays and tests emerge.

TABLE 81.3 Categories of Adrenocortical Hyperfunction

Glucocorticoid Excess Predominates

Adrenal hyperplasia (60%–70% of all cases)

1. Pituitary microadenoma secreting ACTH (most cases of adrenal hyperplasia)
2. Endocrine tumor (pheochromocytoma, carcinoid, medullary carcinoma of thyroid, others secreting ACTH in addition to other hormones [rare])
3. Nonendocrine tumor secreting ACTH (rare)

Adrenal neoplasm (30%–40% of all cases)

1. Adrenal adenoma
2. Adrenal carcinoma (about equal in frequency)

Adrenal Androgen Excess Predominates (hirsutism/virilism)

Some adrenal adenomas

Some adrenal carcinomas

Partial adrenogenital syndrome[a]

Aldosterone Excess

Primary aldosteronism

1. Adrenal adenoma
2. Adrenal nodular hyperplasia

Secondary aldosteronism

1. Salt and volume depletion, including diuretic use and various disease states causing increased production of renin
2. Juxtaglomerular cell hyperplasia or tumor (rare)

ACTH, adrenocorticotropic hormone.

[a] Complete enzymatic defects in steroid synthesis are rare and are invariably manifest early in life as adrenal insufficiency and abnormalities of genital development. In ambulatory adults, partial defects of synthesis of cortisol lead to compensatory adrenal hyperplasia with production of excessive quantities of adrenal steroids with weak androgenic activity. Hirsutism, with or without virilism, ensues (see Chapters 85 and 101).

A major concern is whether the mass represents a carcinoma. Three considerations are relevant in attempting to make this distinction: biochemical activity, size and appearance of the lesion on CT or MRI, and the very low incidence of adrenal carcinoma. Most carcinomas produce high levels of biochemically measurable products, including glucocorticoids and adrenal androgens. Rarely, only testosterone or aldosterone levels are increased. Benign adenomas may also produce excess quantities of steroids. Nevertheless, tumors producing biochemical products generally should be removed.

If no biochemical abnormality is demonstrable, the size and appearance of the lesion on CT give some indication of whether it is benign or malignant. When discovered, most benign adenomas are small (<6 cm diameter), round and homogeneous, and have a low attenuation value with no enhancement following intravenous contrast. Most carcinomas are large (>6 cm diameter) and the presence of necrosis, hemorrhage, or calcifications on CT or MRI suggest adrenal carcinoma. With tumors larger than 6 cm, approximately three operations would be necessary to remove one carcinoma, and more than 4,000 operations would be needed to remove a single carcinoma if one considers all lesions of diameter greater than 1 cm.

When there is suspicion of malignancy based on the above criteria, adrenal iodocholesterol scanning may be of value in differentiating benign from malignant adenomas as those that take up iodocholesterol are usually benign, whereas those that do not are usually malignant.

Occasionally, the adrenal mass is cystic. Large cystic masses can be aspirated by needle puncture; clear fluid indicates a benign lesion, but bloody fluid is indeterminate and cytology is not helpful. Similarly, needle aspiration biopsy is usually not useful in distinguishing benign from malignant cystic lesions.

In followup of biochemically silent adrenal masses, imaging by CT or MRI at 3, 12, and 18 to 24 months and then yearly are indicated, along with biochemical reassessment at yearly intervals. Lesions that are stable at 18 to 24 months and less than 4 cm in diameter can be considered benign and should not be removed (29). A few cases develop a new contralateral mass; a few others will enlarge and should be surgically removed (30). Subtle hypercortisolism in several standard tests of the hypothalamic–pituitary–adrenal axis may develop in approximately 4% of patients at 1 year and 6% of patients at 5 years of followup. These lesions have come to be termed "subclinical Cushing syndrome" and probably should be removed, as many will progress to overt Cushing syndrome (31).

PHARMACOLOGIC USES OF STEROIDS

Most steroid (glucocorticoid) use is related to treatment of diseases other than adrenal insufficiency. In normal persons, basal cortisol production is approximately 25 mg per 24 hours and under maximal stress can reach approximately 200 mg per 24 hours. Doses of administered glucocorticoid that exceed these values are best termed supraphysiologic or, simply, pharmacologic. The anti-inflammatory and immunosuppressive properties of these drugs constitute an invaluable part of the modern therapeutic armamentarium, but such uses, when prolonged, are invariably associated with side effects. Short-term use, generally for less than 3 weeks, is usually not associated with adverse effects. All available glucocorticoids share these properties to an equal degree, although potency (effectiveness per milligram) varies widely (Table 81.2). Despite this fact, certain glucocorticoid compounds are associated with the treatment of particular conditions (e.g., dexamethasone for treatment of cerebral edema, methylprednisolone for hepatic disease). Often there is no pharmacologic basis to support such exclusive practices. On the other hand, differences between available preparations do exist that include different rates of absorption, metabolic disposal, and solubility and inherent mineralocorticoid activity. Exploitation of such properties is seen in dermatologic use. Triamcinolone and fluocinolone acetonides appear to be much more effective than hydrocortisone for topical use, a phenomenon apparently related to properties of absorption.

Adverse Effects

Table 81.4 lists untoward effects of glucocorticoids. These problems are related to dose and, equally important, to duration of therapy. No contraindication exists to a single dose of glucocorticoid, regardless of the size of that dose. Thus, treatment of an allergic reaction with one or a few doses carries no risk. Long-term therapy, however, should be instituted only after consideration of the risks and benefits.

Adverse effects of steroids are related not only to duration of therapy but also to the dosage used. Obviously, the minimally effective dosage should be used. Nonetheless, some people seem especially vulnerable to unwanted side effects. Poorly nourished, debilitated, and elderly patients are more prone to the muscle-wasting effects of steroids (steroid myopathy). Postmenopausal women (already prone to develop osteoporosis) are especially vulnerable to the demineralization that accompanies steroid use. Bisphosphonate inhibitors of bone resorption (e.g., alendronate) should be considered for such patients (see Chapters 84 and 103). Genetically predisposed individuals or patients in the early phase of the metabolic syndrome may develop overt diabetes mellitus when given glucocorticoids. Peptic ulcer disease may be reactivated, and complications such as bleeding or perforation may be precipitated. Prophylactic use of antiulcer therapy should be considered in patients with a history of peptic ulcer

TABLE 81.4 Untoward Effects of Chronic Glucocorticoid Therapy

Acute
Fluid/electrolyte disturbances
Sodium retention
Fluid retention
Potassium depletion
Hypokalemic alkalosis
Gastrointestinal
Peptic ulcer (hemorrhage, perforation)
Ulcerative esophagitis
Endocrine
Precipitation of diabetes mellitus
Ophthalmic
Glaucoma
Neurologic
Mood swings
Acute psychosis
Convulsions
Chronic
Fluid/electrolyte disturbances
See above, plus hypertension
Musculoskeletal
Muscle weakness
Muscle atrophy
Steroid myopathy
Osteoporosis/pathologic fractures
Aseptic necrosis of femoral or humeral heads
Tendon rupture
Gastrointestinal
Pancreatitis
Dermatologic
Impaired wound healing
Atrophy of skin (fragility)
Ecchymoses
Increased sweating
Neurologic
Convulsions
Increased intracranial pressure
Insomnia
Euphoria
Depression
Endocrine
Menstrual irregularities
Carbohydrate intolerance/diabetes mellitus
Adrenal atrophy/disruption of normal response to stress (iatrogenic Addison disease)
Ophthalmic
Cataracts
Glaucoma
Hematologic
Thromboembolism
Other
Weight gain
Increased susceptibility to infections

disease. Dormant tuberculosis, clinically inapparent except for a positive tuberculin test, may reactivate. The role of isoniazid prophylaxis in this situation is described in Chapter 34. A gamut of psychiatric problems may be seen in patients who receive corticosteroids—emotional lability, depression, euphoria—which may necessitate adjustment of the dosage.

Topical Therapy

When steroids can be used locally, such use is preferred, especially when long-term treatment is involved. Although absorption may be complete from a local site, the amount of steroid required is often far less when use is local. This avoids, to some extent, systemic effects, side effects, and pituitary–adrenal suppression. In addition to dermatologic use of topical steroids, treatments of some ophthalmologic conditions, allergic rhinitis, asthma, and localized joint disease are examples of this principle.

Intermittent Therapy

Usually, severe disease requires initiation of steroid therapy given as multiple daily doses. When the disease intensity has waned (e.g., 1 to 2 weeks), conversion to alternate-day therapy can be made. Intermittent therapy of this type should always be considered when long-term use is contemplated. Such therapy is to be preferred because pituitary–adrenal suppression is less likely, and the adverse effects of glucocorticoids are minimized. When initiating intermittent therapy, the daily dose is given as a single morning dose. After this dose has been shown to be tolerated for several days, the single daily dose may be doubled and given as a single dose every other day. Thereafter, the dose given every other day can be reduced slowly, as clinically indicated. The patient may be symptomatic on the off day, particularly when alternate-day therapy is first started. To handle this situation, small doses of glucocorticoid may be given on this day. Nonsteroidal anti-inflammatory agents may also be helpful in ameliorating symptoms during transition.

Use of Adrenocorticotropic Hormone

The clinical indications for the use of ACTH rather than a glucocorticoid are practically nonexistent. The practice continues, however, because ACTH was available for clinical use even before cortisone was. It is clear that in sufficient amounts (100 units), long-acting preparations (gel or zinc suspensions) given once daily are capable of stimulating adrenal secretion of up to 300 mg of cortisol daily. However, disadvantages are multiple: the route is parenteral, the magnitude of response is unpredictable, the mineralocorticoid effects (salt and fluid retention, potassium wasting) are considerable, and the response in patients previously treated with glucocorticoids is slow and unpredictable. The only advantage is that adrenal responsiveness is maintained during therapy. Combined ACTH–glucocorticoid therapy has been advocated for this reason, as has the occasional injection of ACTH to prevent adrenal atrophy. However, the advantage of such an approach over that of intermittent glucocorticoid therapy is unclear. When ACTH is used alone at high dosages for a prolonged period, pituitary suppression occurs even though adrenal suppression does not. Another disadvantage of ACTH therapy is failure to produce more than the equivalent of 300 mg of cortisol (75 mg of prednisone) despite maximal stimulation of the adrenals. Such a dosage, although considerable, may be insufficient to produce the desired clinical effect.

Withdrawal from Acute or Chronic Glucocorticoid Therapy

Treatment with glucocorticoids (e.g., cortisone, hydrocortisone, prednisone) produces suppression of the hypothalamus–pituitary–adrenal axis; the output of ACTH falls, and there is subsequent adrenal atrophy and an inability to respond to stress with increased cortisol output. The time required for initial suppression is highly variable (see Recovery from Hypothalamus–Pituitary–Adrenal Suppression). Patients receiving daily pharmacologic doses of glucocorticoids (5 mg or more of prednisone or its equivalent daily) for more than 1 week should be presumed to have a suppressed response to stress (32). If stressed by surgery, trauma, or severe infection, these patients should be treated with replacement glucocorticoids as if they had Addison disease. On the other hand, glucocorticoids may be discontinued abruptly after 2 to 4 weeks of pharmacologic steroid therapy provided that the patient is not under stress, because baseline—as opposed to stress-related—adrenal function is almost always adequate. Patients who have been treated with alternate-day steroid therapy are not at risk because pituitary–adrenal function seems well preserved in these individuals.

When it becomes desirable to terminate glucocorticoid therapy, the question arises of how to accomplish this goal while avoiding adrenal insufficiency. In the presence of active underlying disease, for which the glucocorticoids may have been given in the first place, a dilemma quickly becomes apparent. The nonspecific symptoms of adrenal insufficiency may be similar or identical to those of the disease that was under treatment. In addition, the occurrence of the "steroid withdrawal syndrome" (see Steroid Withdrawal Syndrome: Distinction from Acute Adrenal Insufficiency) may further compound the issue.

Withdrawal Schedule

No single scheme can solve this difficult clinical problem, although many have been proposed. However, a few general points can be made. First, even after prolonged therapy, in the absence of active underlying systemic disease, symptoms of true adrenal insufficiency will not occur until the daily dose of glucocorticoid drops below physiologic replacement (20 mg of cortisol, 5 mg of prednisone, or equivalent; see Table 81.2). Symptoms similar to those of adrenal insufficiency may occur as the daily dose is being reduced (see Steroid Withdrawal Syndrome: Distinction from Acute Adrenal Insufficiency), although most patients will not be symptomatic if they take a single 20- to 30-mg daily dose of cortisol (or 5 to 7.5 mg of prednisone). Continuation of 20 mg of cortisol daily for 2 months should ensure some degree of recovery of pituitary–adrenal function. Further withdrawal begins to re-establish the normal pituitary–adrenal relationship. Additional reductions of 5 mg of cortisol can be made every 2 to 3 weeks over the next 2 months or, alternatively, an every-other-day program can be tried over the same period; the glucocorticoid can then usually be stopped without producing symptoms. A laboratory assessment of the functional status of the patient's adrenals at this point is described below (see Recovery from Hypothalamus–Pituitary–Adrenal Suppression: Limitations of Testing with Adrenocorticotropin Hormone).

Steroid Withdrawal Syndrome: Distinction from Acute Adrenal Insufficiency

Abrupt withdrawal of pharmacologic doses of glucocorticoids, even after months of therapy, does not always produce chemical evidence of adrenal insufficiency. Nonetheless, the patient may experience many of the symptoms of adrenal insufficiency (e.g., lethargy, malaise, anorexia, nausea, vomiting, myalgias, fever, and, in severe cases, desquamation of skin in a manner resembling exfoliative dermatitis). Less-than-abrupt withdrawal may result in similar, but not as severe, symptoms. Such patients may be found to have normal or elevated levels of cortisol. This phenomenon is not simply adrenal insufficiency but rather is a pharmacologic withdrawal syndrome. Symptoms subside promptly with reinstitution of glucocorticoid therapy.

Recovery from Hypothalamic–Pituitary–Adrenal Suppression: Limitations of Testing with Adrenocorticotropin Hormone

Recovery of the hypothalamus–pituitary–adrenal axis after 1 week of "steroid burst therapy" (e.g., 40 mg of prednisone for 3 days, followed by a 4-day taper) appears complete within 1 additional week (32), but the rate of recovery is unpredictable after withdrawal from longer courses of therapy. After long-term glucocorticoid therapy (pharmacologic doses for a year or more), recovery of normal pituitary–adrenal responsiveness does not occur for at least several months, even if the patient receives no exogenous steroid therapy during that time. In the first month after withdrawal, both pituitary and adrenal function remain depressed (low plasma ACTH and low plasma cortisol). Over the following 4 months, pituitary function recovers first (plasma ACTH is elevated), but adrenal function remains subnormal (plasma cortisol is lower than normal). Eventually, adrenal function recovers (plasma cortisol levels normalize) and elevated plasma ACTH returns to normal. The entire process may require up to 9 months. During this interval the patient may fare well, provided there is no stress, but replacement therapy with glucocorticoids may become necessary at any time. Accordingly, no patient should be considered to have normal pituitary–adrenal function unless at least 1 year has elapsed after complete withdrawal of chronic glucocorticoid therapy. Occasional patients seem never to recover normal responsiveness. Ideally, therefore, all patients with a history of long-term steroid therapy, if they are to be tested for normality of the axis, should be tested 1 year after withdrawal. It is not clear, however, whether any practical test is available.

Assessment of a glucocorticoid-treated patient's adrenal function under baseline conditions is easy. Both plasma cortisol measurements and urinary excretion of steroid metabolites give a reasonable estimate of baseline function. However, predicting the response to stress is more difficult. Because hypothalamic–pituitary function usually recovers first, followed by adrenal function, a normal response to exogenous ACTH would seem to indicate recovery of the entire axis but in fact does not do so with a reasonable degree of reliability. An accurate assessment of the integrity of the axis can be made by induction of hypoglycemia with insulin (ITT). Hypoglycemia triggers ACTH release and the cortisol secretory response of the adrenal. A normal ITT essentially ensures that if the patient is subjected to stressful circumstances, replacement therapy with steroids will be unnecessary. However, the ITT must be done with careful monitoring and is considered to be dangerous and therefore inappropriate in patients with a history of seizures or who are at risk for or have known cardiac disease. It should be performed only under the direct supervision of an endocrinologist who is experienced in the procedure. An ITT is indicated only in the small number of previously glucocorticoid-treated patients who have experienced symptoms suggestive of adrenal insufficiency when under stress.

Administration of CRH rather than ACTH has been advocated as an alternative to the insulin-induced hypoglycemia test. The end point is the plasma cortisol response. This procedure is easier and is completely safe. However, the correlation between the CRH and ITT is only fair, and the magnitude of the response is only a 1.5-fold mean increase in plasma cortisol, requiring a laboratory with optimal accuracy. Ideally, a CRH stimulation test should be done only by an endocrinologist.

As a practical matter, empirical short-term corticosteroid administration ("coverage") during stress is probably the simplest, safest, and cheapest way to manage patients in whom the status of the adrenal–pituitary axis is uncertain.

DISORDERS OF WATER METABOLISM

Disorders of water metabolism can be divided into two major categories: those associated with impaired ability to conserve water (polyuric disorders) and those associated with impaired ability to excrete water (hyponatremic disorders).

Polyuric Disorders

The combination of excess thirst, increased intake of water, and increased output of urine is a common clinical presentation of a number of conditions (Table 81.5). In most of these, the symptoms are related to some event that results in excessive loss of fluid via the kidney.

Causes

The classical polyuric disorder of water metabolism in ambulatory patients is diabetes insipidus, a deficiency of antidiuretic hormone (ADH) (arginine vasopressin). This condition may be idiopathic, in which case it is unassociated with other evidence of pituitary–hypothalamic disease. More commonly, it is caused by head trauma; neurosurgical procedures in the region of the pituitary; malignancy metastatic to the pituitary; pituitary adenoma or other disease in the hypothalamic–pituitary stalk-pituitary area (craniopharyngioma, aneurysm); hypoxic encephalopathy; a variety of infiltrative diseases (sarcoidosis, tuberculosis); or central nervous system infections.

Less commonly, diabetes insipidus results from nephrogenic diabetes insipidus, an inherited renal tubular resistance to ADH, and usually presents in childhood. Acquired forms of ADH-resistant polyuria are more common in later life and may be less severe than the congenital forms. The most common is the ADH-resistant disorder that results from use of lithium for bipolar affective illness. Other causes of acquired ADH resistance are hypokalemia,

TABLE 81.5 Causes of Polyuria

Disorder	Mechanism
Hypothalamic Diabetes Insipidus	ADH deficiency
Idiopathic and familial	
Head trauma	
Neurosurgical procedures	
Tumor (primary and metastatic)	
Cerebral anoxia	
Granulomatous disease	
Nephrogenic Diabetes Insipidus	ADH unresponsiveness
Familial	
Spontaneous	
Acquired	
Renal disease	
Hypokalemia	
Hypercalcemia	
Drug induced	
Lithium	
Demeclocycline	
Polydipsia	Excess fluid intake
Primary	
Psychogenic	
Hypothalamic disease	
Beer potomania	
Drug induced	
Osmotic Diuresis	Obligatory water loss
Glycosuria (diabetes mellitus)	
Natriuresis	
Chronic renal disease	
Diuretic induced	
Excessive intake	
Mannitol	

ADH, antidiuretic hormone.

hypercalcemia, acute tubular necrosis, chronic pyelonephritis, renal amyloidosis, multiple myeloma and Sjögren syndrome.

A common cause of polyuria is hyperglycemia from poorly controlled diabetes mellitus, which results in a large solute load (glucose) being presented to the renal tubules with an obligatory loss of water (osmotic diuresis). Other causes of osmotic diuresis are increased urinary sodium excretion (diuretic-induced or excessive dietary sodium intake) and mannitol administration.

The ingestion of large quantities of beer, sometimes referred to as beer potomania, can produce polyuria with associated hyponatremia that may be severe enough to produce central nervous system (CNS) symptoms ranging from confusion to stupor to seizures. Patients who present with this disorder are usually binge beer drinkers with poor dietary intake.

Patients with severe psychiatric disorders, especially those with chronic schizophrenia, are at risk of excessive fluid intake that can result in polyuria and dilutional hyponatremia, which may be severe and symptomatic (33). In a study involving a large group of psychiatric inpatients, defects in urinary dilution, osmoregulation of water intake and secretion of ADH were identified. Drugs may play a role in many of the episodes of hyponatremia in these patients as well (34).

A less common cause of polyuria is primary polydipsia, which leads to prolonged, increased fluid intake. The disorder may arise without other evident CNS dysfunction or in response to disease, particularly that affecting the hypothalamic and other regions of the brain associated with control of thirst perception. It is usually accompanied by chronic hyponatremia; symptoms may be few but on occasion can be severe.

Occasionally, people begin excessive water intake in the mistaken impression that drinking large quantities of water is healthful. Regardless of the cause, once such behavior is started, a compulsive pattern tends to persist and is reinforced by a pathophysiologic mechanism. A large urine output, if it persists for a long time, produces a reversible impairment of urine-concentrating ability due to washout of renal medullary solutes. Thus, the behavior pattern, although basically of psychogenic origin, may become self-perpetuating. Attempts to have the patient restrict water intake when urinary concentrating ability is impaired under these conditions lead to continued water loss, and the resulting hyperosmolality leads to intense thirst. Weaning from excessive water intake may be difficult.

Approach to the Patient with Polydipsia and Polyuria

The history should be corroborated by family or friends if possible. Important historical points are rapidity of onset of symptoms, a preference for use of iced water, and nocturnal drinking habits. Sudden onset and preference for iced water are classic features of diabetes insipidus. Numerous spontaneous awakenings at night to drink and urinate also strongly suggest this diagnosis, whereas absence of such events is in favor of functional disease. A careful psychiatric and pharmacologic history is important.

Initial laboratory workup should be straightforward. A morning fasting serum glucose, sodium, and osmolality determination should be made along with serum potassium, calcium, urea nitrogen, and creatinine determinations. Normal serum calcium and potassium concentrations exclude several metabolic problems, whereas abnormalities of calcium, potassium, or renal function make it clear that the problem is caused by altered renal water-conserving ability. If considerable glucosuria and hyperglycemia are present, the cause of the patient's problem is evident and should respond to correction of hyperglycemia.

The patient should collect all urine over one or two 24-hour periods to be examined for volume, osmolality, total urine glucose excretion, and total sodium and creatinine excretion, the latter serving as a marker for completeness of the collection. Measurement of urine specific gravity is inaccurate and obsolete and should be replaced by measurement of urine osmolality. Normal 24-hour urine volume ranges from 1,000 to 2,500 mL. Urine osmolality is decidedly low when the value is well below that of serum (<300 mOsm/kg); the urine is maximally dilute at 50 to 70 mOsm/kg.

The presence of a normal serum sodium or osmolality indicates only that the process is not severe enough to have overwhelmed the ability to excrete water or the homeostatic (thirst) mechanism. Elevated serum osmolality strongly suggests diabetes insipidus while reduced osmolality suggests psychogenic water drinking. In both diabetes insipidus and psychogenic water drinking, urine volume usually exceeds 4 L per day. Values less than 5 to 6 L per day do not distinguish between these possibilities, but do indicate less-than-complete diabetes insipidus, in which urine volumes often approach 10 to 12 L per day, as they may also in cases of severe psychogenic water drinking. If the serum sodium and osmolality are low and the urine volume is large with low osmolality, a diagnosis of psychogenic water drinking is essentially established. If diabetes insipidus is suspected, the next step is to determine the response of urine osmolality to administered antidiuretic hormone (aqueous vasopressin 5 units subcutaneously or 10 μg desmopressin intranasally). Failure of urine osmolality to rise 1 hour after hormone administration indicates the presence of nephrogenic diabetes insipidus.

If there is a large urine volume of low osmolality and normal serum electrolyte concentrations, additional testing is necessary to establish a diagnosis. Referral to an endocrinologist or a nephrologist is appropriate. Hospitalization for testing under metabolic conditions is usually preferred in these cases.

Treatment

The treatment of psychogenic water drinking involves psychiatric counseling. These patients are difficult to manage, especially if they become severely hyponatremic. Weaning such patients from water may also be a slow process, not only because of the profound nature of their psychiatric disturbance but because of their acquired inability to concentrate urine, a process that is only slowly reversible.

The treatment of diabetes insipidus involves use of ADH in some form. For ambulatory patients, ADH is available as the synthetic analogue desmopressin or DDAVP (1-deamino-8-D-arginine vasopressin) and can be administered as a nasal spray, oral tablets, or parenterally. Treatment with nasal spray is begun with 0.05 to 0.1 mL (5 to 10 μg) every 12 to 24 hours with individual titration thereafter. A single dose usually acts for 12 hours or longer. Nasal absorption may be impaired by rhinitis or respiratory tract infections, during which treatment with injectable or oral desmopressin (100 to 400 mg/day) may be necessary. Serum sodium must be monitored closely on initiation of therapy to avoid the development of significant hyponatremia as a consequence of excessive water retention. Patients with partial diabetes insipidus have been managed in the past with chlorpropamide (Diabinese, 250 to 500 mg/day), a drug that potentiates endogenous ADH. However, hypoglycemia is a significant hazard and current preference is for use of desmopressin. Nephrogenic diabetes insipidus, both idiopathic and secondary to lithium, is partially responsive to sodium restriction and thiazide diuretics to induce chronic intravascular volume depletion and consequent increased renal water reabsorption.

Hyponatremic Disorders

Prevalence and Incidence

Hyponatremia is the most common electrolyte disorder, especially among elderly persons. In one study, 7% of healthy subjects older than age 65 years and living at home had a serum sodium of 137 mEq/L or lower. Similarly, hyponatremia was observed in 11% of outpatients from a geriatric medicine clinic (35). Hyponatremia is even more common among hospitalized than nonhospitalized patients, among whom the prevalence increases with age (36). Elderly residents of long-term care institutions appear to be especially susceptible to hyponatremia. In a survey of nursing home residents 60 years of age and older, 18% had a serum sodium less than 136 mEq/L. In a longitudinal analysis of this population, 53% had one or more episodes of hyponatremia during a 12-month period. Persons with CNS and spinal cord disease were at highest risk, and water-load testing indicated that most patients with hyponatremia had features consistent with the syndrome of inappropriate antidiuretic hormone secretion (SIADH) (37).

Causes of Hyponatremia

Medical Diseases

Many diseases can cause SIADH in any population, but the elderly are at highest risk (38). Almost all CNS disorders can lead to dysfunction of the hypothalamic system involved in the normal regulation of arginine vasopressin (AVP) secretion, leading to increased secretion of the hormone and, consequently, to water retention and hyponatremia. Such CNS disorders include vascular injury (thrombosis, embolism, hemorrhage); trauma accompanied by subdural hematoma; vasculitis; tumor; and infection. Cancer can cause SIADH as a result of autonomous release of AVP from malignant tissue, where the hormone is synthesized, stored, and discharged in the absence of known stimuli. The cancer most commonly associated with SIADH is small cell carcinoma of the lung. As many as 68% of patients who have this cancer demonstrate impaired water excretion and elevated blood AVP concentration. Other cancers associated with SIADH include pancreatic carcinoma, thymoma, pharyngeal carcinoma, and lymphoma. Inflammatory lung diseases, such as bronchiectasis, pneumonia, lung abscess, and tuberculosis, can also cause SIADH, perhaps as a result of AVP production by diseased pulmonary tissue.

Many other diseases are associated with an increased risk of hyponatremia, including chronic obstructive pulmonary disease, hypertension, diabetes, heart failure, cirrhosis, nephrotic syndrome, renal failure, and hypothyroidism (39). Approximately 50% of patients hospitalized for acquired immune deficiency syndrome (AIDS) also have hyponatremia. Of these, more than half have symptoms consistent with SIADH (40).

SIADH should be differentiated from another form of hyponatremia mediated by the CNS. Renal sodium excretion from the excessive release of natriuretic factor in the brain can lead to cerebral salt wasting (CSW) (41). CSW and SIADH are both syndromes of hypo-osmotic serum and increased urine sodium. Patients with CSW, however, have a low effective intravascular blood volume as a consequence of marked natriuresis and secondary osmotic diuresis. In contrast, patients with SIADH are usually euvolemic or have mildly increased extracellular fluid volume. CSW can be diagnosed by the clinical and laboratory findings that define diminished extracellular fluid volume, including orthostatic hypotension, tachycardia, and elevated hematocrit, serum urea nitrogen (SUN), and creatinine levels.

Surgery

Although men and women of any age are at risk of hyponatremia after undergoing operative procedures, premenopausal women who undergo surgery, often for elective gynecologic problems, are especially susceptible to severe hyponatremia in the postoperative period. Hyponatremia can appear within 9 days after surgery, but its progress can be rapid enough to produce severe symptoms within a period of hours. Early symptoms include headache, nausea, vomiting, weakness, lethargy, confusion, and slurred speech. Abrupt respiratory arrest may occur and is associated with the development of cerebral edema and hypoxic encephalopathy. Unless the syndrome is recognized and treated promptly, permanent brain damage or death is likely to occur (42).

Drugs

Numerous drugs can cause hyponatremia by increasing the release of AVP from the neurohypophyseal system, by enhancing AVP action on the kidney, or by acting directly on the kidney (43). In particular, many drugs increase the risk of SIADH.

Hyponatremia with the characteristics of SIADH is recognized as an adverse effect of tricyclic antidepressants and of several older antipsychotic agents, such as fluphenazine, thiothixene, and phenothiazine. The selective serotonin reuptake inhibitor (SSRI) antidepressants can also induce SIADH, which occurs in 3.5 to 6.3 per 1,000 patients annually who take these drugs (44). Although fluoxetine is the SSRI most commonly associated with hyponatremia, other SSRIs, including paroxetine, sertraline, and fluvoxamine, are also known to produce the disorder. Patients at highest risk for SSRI-induced hyponatremia are those older than age 65 years, in whom the disorder typically occurs within 2 weeks after the initiation of therapy. In a recent prospective study of depressed elderly patients given paroxetine, approximately 12% had hyponatremia (with a serum sodium as low as 124 mEq/L) within 9 days, on average, after starting SSRI therapy. In all of these patients, the hyponatremia had features consistent with SIADH (45).

Angiotensin-converting enzyme (ACE) inhibitors are also associated with dilutional hyponatremia (46). In most such cases, the hyponatremia has been severe and accompanied by symptoms ranging from confusion to seizures and coma. Although initial reports indicated that the risk was greatest when ACE inhibitors were used in combination with thiazide diuretics, it now appears that the ACE inhibitors alone can precipitate hyponatremia. Hyponatremia induced by ACE inhibitors appears to be dilutional, is accompanied by features of SIADH, and may be mediated by the potentiation of plasma renin activity. This activity subsequently increases angiotensin levels in the brain, which, in turn, stimulate both the release of AVP from the hypothalamus and the thirst response. Discontinuing the ACE inhibitor therapy leads to a resolution of the hyponatremia.

Diuretics, especially thiazides, can decrease renal diluting capacity. In the elderly, generally men over the age of 65 years, this effect becomes especially important when it is superimposed on the already diminished diluting capacity of the aged kidney and thus increases the risk of hyponatremia by impairing the kidney's ability to excrete excess water promptly. In a review of 129 patients with diuretic-induced hyponatremia (serum sodium <115 mEq/L), thiazides were the cause of the disorder in 83% of patients, chlorthalidone in 10%, and furosemide or spirolactone in 7% (47). Loop diuretics appear to have a greater natriuretic effect in older than in younger persons. Hyponatremia can occur when diuretic-induced sodium and water loss is replaced by hypotonic fluid, resulting in a combined depletional and dilutional hyponatremia. Thiazide diuretic-induced sodium loss is often accompanied by the loss of total body potassium, which consequently decreases intracellular solute content and cell volume. This combination can activate hypothalamic volume receptors and thus trigger AVP secretion, water retention, and SIADH, a reaction that occurs almost exclusively in the elderly and can be reversed by correcting the underlying potassium depletion.

Other drugs associated with the development of hyponatremia in the elderly include the sulfonylurea chlorpropamide; the anticonvulsant carbamazepine; the antineoplastic agents vincristine, vinblastine, and cyclophosphamide; calcium channel blockers; nonsteroidal anti-inflammatory drugs; desmopressin acetate; and nicotine. Analgesics, particularly the opioid narcotics, may be responsible for the occurrence of hyponatremia in elderly patients who have undergone surgery.

Of particular concern in the emergency department is the occurrence of acute, severe hyponatremia in young persons who have taken the hallucinogenic drug "ecstasy" (*N*-methyl-3,4-methylenedioxyamphetamine, or MDMA). These patients, who may present with seizures and respiratory arrest caused by cerebral edema, may be resistant to therapy.

Idiopathic Hyponatremia of Aging

Advanced age itself may be a risk factor for hyponatremia. SIADH has been observed in elderly persons, usually older than age 80 years, in whom no identifiable cause for hyponatremia is evident. This finding suggests there is an idiopathic form of SIADH that may occur in response to the physiologic changes that occur in the regulation of water balance during aging. African American patients appear to be at lower risk than whites or Hispanics (35).

Diagnosis

Hyponatremia is often underdiagnosed and undertreated because patients may have only subtle symptoms or remain asymptomatic until the serum sodium drops below 125 mEq/L. The diagnosis of hyponatremia, which can be dilutional, depletional, or of mixed origin, rests on a thorough history of concurrent illness and medication use, physical examination, and an assessment of volume status and readily available laboratory measures (Table 81.6).

Dilutional versus Depletional Hyponatremia

The characteristic features of dilutional hyponatremia, as caused by SIADH, for example, are a low serum sodium and serum hypo-osmolality accompanied by clinical euvolemia without edema. Other features include a failure of the urine to be appropriately dilute, excretion of sodium in the urine at a concentration of greater than 20 mEq/L, and the absence of other disorders that cause hyponatremia, including hypothyroidism, adrenal insufficiency, congestive heart failure, cirrhosis, and renal disease (48).

Depletional hyponatremia typically occurs after a prolonged period of inadequate sodium intake or is caused by increased sodium loss from the gastrointestinal tract or urine. Extracellular fluid volume depletion is often evident

TABLE 81.6 Diagnosis of Dilutional versus Depletional Hyponatremia

Feature	*Dilutional*	*Depletional*
History	Increased fluid intake (oral, IV)	Decreased dietary sodium intake
	Disorders	Sodium loss (vomiting, diarrhea, nasogastric suction)
	Disease (CNS, malignancy)	Renal, adrenal disease
	Drugs	Diuretic use
Physical exam	Euvolemia or edema	Dry mucous membranes
	Evidence of CNS or pulmonary disease, malignancy	Decreased skin turgor
		Hypotension, tachycardia, orthostatic changes
Laboratory	Normal or decreased hematocrit, BUN, creatinine, uric acid,	Increased hematocrit, BUN, creatinine,
	Urinary Na excretion >20 mEq/L	Urinary Na excretion <20 mEq/L

BUN, blood urea nitrogen; CNS, central nervous system; IV, intravenous.
From Miller M. Syndromes of excess antidiuretic hormone release. Crit Care Clin 2001;17:11, adapted.

as well, and the physical findings and laboratory values usually indicate hypovolemia.

Laboratory evaluation plays a critical role in diagnosing hyponatremia. It is important to determine whether the effective serum osmolality reflects true hypo-osmotic hyponatremia, normotonic pseudohyponatremia (caused by hyperproteinemia or hypertriglyceridemia), or elevated tonicity caused by the presence of other osmoles, as may occur in hyperglycemic patients or those undergoing mannitol infusion.

Once serum hypo-osmolality is confirmed, the ability of the kidneys to concentrate urine should be evaluated. Hyponatremia that occurs when the urine is dilute (<100 mOsm/kg) indicates AVP secretion is appropriately suppressed and suggests primary polydipsia as the likely cause of hyponatremia (33,34). Reset osmostat syndrome may underlie hyponatremia that occurs with normal or dilute urine and is caused by a lowered threshold at which osmoreceptors trigger AVP release. This syndrome occurs in patients who have normal adrenal, renal, and thyroid function without cardiac or hepatic disease and whose urine is diluted normally in response to oral water loading (excretion of >80% in 4 hours). Patients who have concentrated urine (>100 mOsm/kg) may have hypovolemic, euvolemic, or hypervolemic hyponatremia. Differentiating hypovolemic from euvolemic hyponatremia by clinical examination alone can be challenging. Decreased effective intravascular blood volume indicates hypovolemia. The serum uric acid concentration may provide insight, as it tends to be elevated in patients with low effective intravascular blood volume and is reduced in volume-expanded states such as SIADH. In most cases, both the urine sodium and volume status will provide clues. An abnormally low urine sodium (<20 mEq/L) in patients with hypovolemia is common and often accompanied by extrarenal volume depletion caused by diarrhea, vomiting, and integumentary losses. In contrast, urine sodium >20 mEq/L in patients with hypovolemia may suggest sodium loss caused by nephropathy, adrenal insufficiency, or CSW. In patients with hypervolemia accompanied by edema, the urinary sodium level will be diminished in the presence of congestive heart failure (CHF), cirrhosis, or nephrotic syndrome, but elevated in the presence of renal failure.

Euvolemic or mildly hypovolemic hyponatremia is often accompanied by hypotonic serum and concentrated urine. Urine sodium of 40 mEq/L or greater in such cases usually indicates SIADH. Hypothyroidism and adrenal insufficiency must be ruled out to confirm the diagnosis of SIADH.

Treatment

The treatment of hyponatremia should not be initiated solely on the evidence of abnormally low serum sodium. The role of management is not only to correct the sodium level, but also to identify and correct the underlying cause of hyponatremia and to restore body-water homeostasis when possible to avoid potentially harmful sequelae. Usually, the most important factors that determine the rapidity of treatment are the absence or presence of symptoms and their severity, whether the disorder is acute or chronic, and, if the hyponatremia is acute, the rapidity of onset of the condition or symptoms.

Asymptomatic Patients

Some patients with hyponatremia may be incorrectly considered asymptomatic if their signs or symptoms are subtle or attributed to another condition. Patients whose hyponatremia is chronic, subacute, or of unknown duration may have few or no overt clinical symptoms. Patients likely to be asymptomatic or mildly symptomatic are those with sodium loss caused by diuretics, digestive losses, or nephrotic syndrome. The treatment of chronic asymptomatic hyponatremia should be conservative, with the initial efforts focused on identifying the cause.

Conservative therapy for asymptomatic euvolemic hyponatremia starts with fluid restriction. The gradual correction of hyponatremia will counteract the stimulus for AVP release and, eventually, sodium balance will be restored. The ability of a patient to produce dilute urine should govern the degree of fluid restriction, but limiting water intake to less than free water loss will increase sodium regardless of the underlying cause of hyponatremia. Fluid restriction should be sufficient to affect serum sodium in euvolemic hyponatremia, whereas in hypervolemic hyponatremia, both salt and fluid intake restrictions may be necessary. Normal saline (0.9%) can be administered to correct extracellular fluid volume deficit in hypovolemic hyponatremia. If thyroid or adrenal insufficiencies are detected, appropriate treatment should be sufficient to correct the hyponatremia. If thiazide diuretics are responsible for hyponatremia, they should be discontinued or replaced with a nonthiazide diuretic. When SIADH is identified as the cause of hyponatremia, treatment of the underlying process causing hormonal imbalance of AVP is the appropriate approach.

The presence of risk factors for neurologic complications should always be considered. The rate of serum sodium correction for asymptomatic and mildly symptomatic hyponatremia should not exceed 0.5 mEq/L per hour on the first day and should not be increased to more than 12 mEq/L in the first 24 hours. After that time, and until symptoms resolve, the rate of correction should be increased no more than 0.25 mEq/L per hour.

Symptomatic Patients

Untreated severe hyponatremia can produce cerebral edema and increased intracranial pressure, both of which lead to neuropathologic sequelae or death. Accordingly, symptomatic or severe hyponatremia justifies prompt treatment. The major risk of correcting sodium too rapidly is the development of central pontine myelinolysis (CPM). Thus, the goal of therapy is to achieve a rate of correction sufficient to resolve the symptoms and to reduce cerebral edema, but not so rapid as to risk CPM. Patients with severe or symptomatic hyponatremia should be hospitalized promptly and correction of the hyponatremia carried out under the guidance of a physician who is experienced with the management of the disorder.

Acute symptomatic hyponatremia is most often associated with polydipsia or postsurgical conditions. The rapid correction of serum sodium levels in cases in which the duration of hyponatremia is known to be short is rarely necessary unless symptoms are severe; however, rapid correction is unlikely, in theory, to increase the risk of neurologic demyelination. When symptoms are present, a prompt initial increase in sodium level is necessary and can be achieved with the intravenous administration of 3.0% NaCl. Such treatment should be carried out in a setting in which serum sodium can be monitored closely, initially at 1- to 2-hour intervals. Most patients are best managed in a hospital intensive care unit.

Chronic hyponatremia may still be symptomatic, even if present for only several days, and there may be a superimposed acute episode. If the duration of hyponatremia is unknown or longer than 48 hours, the clinician must proceed with care because the brain's compensatory mechanisms mandate slow correction. The treatment of chronic hyponatremia accompanied by severe symptoms is similar to that of acute symptomatic hyponatremia, but in this case extreme caution is necessary and is best carried out in an intensive care unit with close laboratory monitoring.

AVP-Receptor Antagonists and Aquaresis

Because hyponatremia associated with water retention is a result of excess AVP, the most rational approach to therapy for this disorder is to either decrease secretion of the AVP hormone or block its effects on the kidney.

The tetracycline antibiotic demeclocycline has been used in doses of 600 to 1,200 mg daily to produce a state of renal AVP resistance through its ability to block AVP-induced activation of the renal adenyl cyclase–cyclic adenosine monophosphate (cAMP) system (49). This drug-induced state of partial nephrogenic diabetes insipidus produces a modest increase in urine volume with a decrease in urine osmolality to near isotonicity and a corresponding rise in serum sodium. Each patient's response to this agent is variable, however, and several days of therapy are necessary before a response does occur. In addition, the treatment may be complicated by renal and hepatotoxicity.

In the treatment of hyponatremia, aquaresis, the excretion of water without electrolyte loss, is preferable to diuresis (50). In recent years, several nonpeptide molecules capable of inhibiting AVP at the level of its tissue receptors have been developed and designated as aquaretics. These compounds are capable of directly inhibiting AVP V_1 vascular and/or V_2 renal receptors located on the distal tubules. By counteracting the effect of AVP V_2 receptors and thus inducing free water excretion, AVP V_2-receptor antagonists can treat hyponatremia directly. Aquaretic agents that target the AVP V_2 receptor or V_{1a} and V_2 receptors have shown promising clinical results, and early trials have demonstrated their ability to normalize sodium levels safely in patients who have euvolemic or hypervolemic hyponatremia with SIADH and CHF (51–53).

Demeclocycline and aquaretics should be considered in patients with chronic hyponatremia when the underlying cause cannot be corrected and when the patient is experiencing symptoms attributable to hyponatremia. The aquaretic agents may play a role in the acute management of symptomatic hyponatremia as their onset of action is within minutes of administration and the dose can be tailored to produce the desired level of water excretion. These agents will be available for clinical use in the near future.

HYPOGLYCEMIA

Because many of the symptoms of hypoglycemia are nonspecific, it is suspected more often than it is present. Chemical hypoglycemia, defined as a serum glucose concentration of less than 40 mg/dL, may not be symptomatic, although levels less than 30 mg/dL are nearly always associated with symptoms. Hypoglycemia produces symptoms by two mechanisms: by triggering the release of epinephrine, one of several homeostatic responses that tend to normalize a low blood sugar, and by depriving the nervous system of glucose, its essential energy source.

Adrenergic versus Neuroglycopenic Symptoms

Many of the symptoms of hypoglycemia relate to stimulation of the release of epinephrine by low blood glucose. These symptoms are termed *adrenergic* or *sympathetic*. Usually, these symptoms are of rapid onset, and more than one is ordinarily present. Typically, they last only 15 to 30 minutes and include sweating, tremor (shakiness), a sensation of hunger, and anxiety. Irritability and palpitations are often mentioned but are rarely spontaneous or prominent complaints.

Symptoms related to glucose deprivation of the central and, to a lesser extent, peripheral nervous systems are termed *neuroglycopenic,* and when severe, mimic those of central nervous system hypoxia. Minimal symptoms are headache, mental dullness, and sudden fatigue. Confusion and visual disturbances (blurring, dimming of vision) are associated with moderate to severe hypoglycemia, whereas unconsciousness and seizures are indications of very severe hypoglycemia.

Causes

The numerous causes of hypoglycemia (Table 81.7) can be divided into two large categories: those mediated by insulin and those caused by impaired glucose production. By far the most common cause is an excess effect of insulin or of sulfonylureas in the treatment of diabetes mellitus, especially in patients who are aggressively managed in an attempt to maintain their blood sugar levels in the normal or near-normal range (see Chapter 79) (54). Of the other conditions that produce hypoglycemia associated with insulin overproduction, the rarest is an insulinoma. So-called postprandial hypoglycemia (within 2 to 4 hours of eating) has been considerably overdiagnosed (55). The attribution of postprandial hypoglycemia to gastrectomy or early diabetes mellitus is not well established and symptomatic hypoglycemia in these conditions is uncommon. Idiopathic postprandial hypoglycemia also appears to be quite rare (55,56). Rarely, some drugs can produce hypoglycemia (Table 81.7). Selected, specific diseases that cause hypoglycemia are discussed below.

Nonhypoglycemia

The frequency with which self-diagnosis of hypoglycemia occurs depends on the patient population (57). The condition has been termed *nonhypoglycemia* and extends the concept of "nondisease," as it originates from misattribution by the clinician, such as misinterpretation of laboratory values, or misattribution of the patient. Identification of such individuals is important, as is their re-education.

The recognition of nonhypoglycemia requires a careful history that fails to demonstrate the legitimate symptoms of hypoglycemia as well as a clear demonstration that glucose metabolism is normal (see below). Exclusion of

TABLE 81.7 Causes of Hypoglycemia in Ambulatory Adults

Postprandial state
- Reactive (idiopathic)
- Early diabetes mellitus
- Ethanol ingestion
- Postgastrectomy state

Fasting state
- Insulin excess
  1. Insulin injection
  2. Sulfonylurea ingestion[a]
  3. Miscellaneous drugs[b]
  4. Insulinoma
  5. Noninsulinoma pancreatogenous hypoglycemia syndrome
  6. Autoimmune hypoglycemia (very rare)
- Alcohol ingestion
- Hormonal deficiencies
  1. Glucocorticoid
  2. Growth hormone
- Fasting in normal young women (24–48 h)
- Malnutrition
- Liver disease
- Extrapancreatic tumors
  1. Mesenchymal tumors
  2. Sarcomas
  3. Hepatocellular tumors
  4. Carcinoid-like tumors
- Renal failure (chronic end stage)
- Congestive heart failure

[a]Many drugs, including such diverse compounds as anti-inflammatory agents, antibiotics, and lipid-lowering agents, potentiate the effects of sulfonylureas and may cause hypoglycemia.
[b]For example, haloperidol, propoxyphene, and salicylates.

other organic disease is important (Table 81.7). Distinction from the rare idiopathic postprandial syndrome must be made. Finally, psychiatric disease must be considered, based on positive findings rather than merely on an exclusion of organic illness.

If the evaluation fails to establish the presence of bona fide hypoglycemia, the issue of the therapy of nonhypoglycemia remains. This difficult problem includes at least three steps that have been termed disattribution, explanation and ventilation, and reattribution (57). Disattribution involves confrontation of the patient with the results of the test procedure. For some patients the mechanics or ritual of the procedure itself is impressive and therefore helpful. If the patient clings to the diagnosis of hypoglycemia despite strong evidence to the contrary, an attempt should be made to explore the reason for the patient's need to do so. During this process, an effort should be made to have the patient fully explain his or her notions about hypoglycemia and verbalize what might happen if those notions are challenged. Finally, an alternate explanation must be provided for the symptoms, that is, reattribution, along with a treatment plan or a willingness to assist the patient in accepting an uncertain and ambiguous situation. Unless grossly apparent psychosocial problems become evident during this process, psychiatric referral may not be necessary. (Chapters 19 and 20 describe in detail interviewing and psychotherapeutic techniques for working with patients such as these.)

Diagnosis

In some patients, the history suggests to the clinician that the patient is experiencing periodic hypoglycemia. Other patients will themselves suggest to their caregiver that hypoglycemia accounts for the symptoms. Verification of the presence of hypoglycemia can be attempted by instructing the patient in the use of a glucometer.

Defining Hypoglycemic Symptoms

Because laboratory confirmation may be difficult in some cases, an extraordinarily careful history is essential. Two issues guide the process. First, what exactly are the symptoms? Second, do the symptoms occur postprandially or in the fasting state?

An accurate history is essential to identify the time at which hypoglycemia occurs. In general, symptoms of true hypoglycemia do not occur within hours of eating a meal unless insulin or sulfonylurea has been prescribed in excess. There are exceptions to this statement, however, both in rare patients with an insuloma and in patients who have a disorder that causes true postprandial hypoglycemia, such as infrequently can occur in persons who have had a gastrectomy.

Inquiry concerning the patient's dietary habits may be revealing. Some patients restrict carbohydrate intake intermittently. When this is done and a large carbohydrate meal follows, hypoglycemia may be precipitated. Moderate to high levels of caffeine intake can cause the development of hypoglycemic symptoms in individuals whose plasma glucose levels are in the low normal range, as can occur in the late postprandial period after ingestion of a large carbohydrate load (58). The amount of alcohol consumed should be noted because ethanol ingestion may precipitate hypoglycemia, even in the nonfasting patient (see Alcohol Abuse section). Often, the patient may recall milder symptomatic episodes experienced over a long period because the intensity of postprandial hypoglycemia tends to wax and wane over the years. A family history of diabetes mellitus should be sought as rarely postprandial hypoglycemia may be an early manifestation of type 2 diabetes mellitus. Although symptoms and signs of anxiety or depression may be present, they have no diagnostic usefulness.

General physical examination can be expected to be negative. Even if early diabetes mellitus is found by glucose tolerance testing to be the cause of the hypoglycemia, complications of diabetes that can be found on physical examination (retinopathy, neuropathy) will not be present.

Laboratory Evaluation

As discussed above, an attempt can be made to determine the presence or absence of hypoglycemia by instructing the patient in the use of a glucometer. If the results are normal or equivocal and the diagnosis is still suspected, determination of serum glucose concentration needs to be done in a controlled setting. Blood sugar should be low at the time symptoms are experienced, and the symptoms should abate when the patient is fed carbohydrate. The glucose tolerance test has been largely abandoned as a diagnostic procedure for postprandial hypoglycemia because of its unreliability in establishing the diagnosis. If it is done, it should be modified to include more frequent sampling (30-minute intervals) and a longer period (5 hours). The patient should be observed during the entire test. Again, correlation of blood sugar values with symptoms is essential.

In patients with a history suggestive of fasting hypoglycemia, evaluation is based on measurement of serum glucose and insulin during a period of closely monitored fasting, which must be done in a hospital setting. An overnight (12-hour) fast followed by determination of serum glucose and insulin is the simplest screening procedure. If hypoglycemia cannot be documented in this time period, the duration of fasting is extended until blood glucose drops to less than 40 mg/dL or the fast has lasted for 72 hours. Frequent blood sampling for glucose level is necessary and blood for simultaneous measurement of glucose, insulin, and C-peptide is drawn at the end of the fasting period. Ninety-five percent of patients with fasting hypoglycemia will be detected by 48 hours (59).

A sex difference in response to fasting is well established. Normal men may fast for up to 72 hours and will not show fasting plasma glucose below 50 mg/dL. In contrast, women often exhibit a progressive fall in the concentration of plasma glucose during prolonged fasting. At 72 hours, many premenopausal women have a concentration of glucose less than 50 mg/dL, with some having a concentration as low as 25 mg/dL. However, these women remain asymptomatic and insulin levels are appropriately suppressed.

Selected Specific Entities Causing Hypoglycemia

Insulinoma

This pancreatic tumor occurs with equal frequency in men and women and at any age. Symptoms of headache on arising, confusion before breakfast, or nocturnal or early morning seizures may be present for years before the diagnosis is suspected. Hyperinsulinism may produce abnormal hunger, weight gain, and obesity (although insulinoma is a very rare cause of obesity). Neuropsychiatric symptoms may lead to neurologic or psychiatric evaluations or to hospitalizations. In some of these cases, permanent neurologic deficits have been seen and are presumably related to long duration of symptomatic hypoglycemia before diagnosis.

Diagnosis

In addition to the demonstration of hypoglycemia, the simultaneous determination of plasma insulin activity remains the most definitive diagnostic test (60). During fasting in normal people, both glucose and insulin levels decline and the ratio of immunoreactive insulin (IRI) to glucose is maintained at less than 0.3 (milliunits of IRI/mg of glucose/dL). In many patients with insulinoma, an abnormally high IRI-to-glucose ratio is apparent after a sufficient period of fasting. These determinations should be made repeatedly because fasting hypoglycemia and an abnormal IRI-to-glucose ratio often occur only intermittently, even in patients with subsequently proven insulinomas. In addition, a single abnormal ratio never establishes the diagnosis. Insulin-to-glucose ratios may be misinterpreted if the glucose concentration is not at hypoglycemic levels. The clinician should be cautious in accepting the accuracy of IRI values obtained from commercial laboratories. Proinsulin levels are elevated in 85% of patients with insulinoma and can be a useful adjunct, especially in those whose insulin levels are low (60).

A variety of other useful procedures should, if deemed necessary, be conducted by an endocrinologist. If fasting for 48 hours fails to provoke hypoglycemia (see above), the fast can be continued to 72 hours or the patient can be exercised as vigorously as tolerable. Up to 2 hours of exercise should be completed with sampling of plasma glucose every 15 to 20 minutes before concluding that hypoglycemia has not developed. An exercise bicycle, jogging, or vigorous calisthenics may be used. Exercise raises glucose levels in normal people but lowers plasma concentration further in patients with insulinoma. Provocative tests of insulin secretion (tolbutamide, leucine, glucagon) can be used with appropriate caution. Suppression of endogenous insulin C-peptide is another useful procedure in difficult cases, but it requires induction of hypoglycemia by infusion of insulin under controlled conditions, a procedure that must be performed by an endocrinologist in a hospital.

The localization procedure of choice is ultrasonography of the pancreas; CT and MRI are less sensitive. Celiac axis arteriography may be useful for localizing lesions smaller than 2 to 3 cm (i.e., those that can be expected to be seen with sonography) (61). These procedures should be performed only after demonstration of abnormal secretion of insulin.

Treatment

The definitive treatment of an insulinoma is surgical, with a cure rate greater than 80%.

Noninsulinoma Pancreatogenous Hypoglycemia Syndrome

An unusually severe form of exclusively postprandial hypoglycemia has been seen in a small number of mostly male adults and in patients who have had gastric bypass surgery for severe obesity (62,63). Their 72-hour fasts were negative for insulinoma and all imaging and angiographic studies of the pancreas failed to identify a pancreatic tumor. Partial pancreatectomy disclosed diffuse islet cell hypertrophy and hyperfunction and was curative in most patients (62,63).

Noninsulinoma Tumoral Hypoglycemia

A number of tumors are associated with severe fasting hypoglycemia, producing a clinical picture identical to insulinoma. However, hyperinsulinemia is absent. Most common are large mesenchymal tumors that can be either benign or malignant. Other neoplasms are sarcomas, hepatocellular tumors, and carcinoidlike tumors. The tumors are usually easily detectable by radiologic or ultrasonograph study because of their large size. Treatment is by surgical resection with followup radiotherapy for residual tumor mass.

Insulin and Sulfonylurea Self-Administration (Factitious Hypoglycemia)

Occasional nondiabetic patients, usually family members of diabetics or people with medically related occupations, engage in surreptitious insulin administration. Examination may reveal needle marks. Other clues can be provided by the presence of antibodies to insulin, which are present only in persons given insulin or by the measurement of insulin C-peptide. In people who are secreting insulin, C-peptide is also produced concomitantly, but C-peptide is not present in commercial insulin and will be present in very low concentrations or will be absent in the serum of patients whose hypoglycemia is induced by exogenous insulin.

Oral hypoglycemic drugs (sulfonylureas; see Chapter 79), like insulin, may occasionally be abused and cause fasting hypoglycemia. In the experience of one group, these agents produce the greatest difficulty in the diagnosis of factitious hypoglycemia (59). Urinary sulfonylurea measurement can be helpful in identifying this problem.

Alcohol Abuse

Alcohol abuse probably produces hypoglycemia more commonly than any other single cause. As stated above, ingestion of ethanol can produce postprandial hypoglycemia in normal well-nourished people who engage in social drinking. However, fasting hypoglycemia related to ethanol ingestion occurs in chronic alcohol abusers and especially in those who are malnourished. The situation most likely to provoke hypoglycemia is cessation of food intake and continued ingestion of ethanol over the ensuing 10 to 20 hours. Under these circumstances, ethanol intoxication (i.e., drunkenness) may mistakenly be thought to be responsible for the symptoms.

Liver Disease, Chronic Congestive Heart Failure, and Renal Disease

Diffuse acquired liver disease can result in impaired hepatic gluconeogenesis. Although hypoglycemia can be seen in severe acute hepatitis or as a result of chronic passive congestion in long-standing congestive heart failure, liver disease does not usually produce hypoglycemia until late in the course. Patients with severe cirrhosis may occasionally have fasting hypoglycemia, but the development of hypoglycemia in such a patient should suggest the presence of a hepatoma. In patients with well-differentiated hepatoma, hypoglycemia may be an early symptom. Diabetic patients with renal insufficiency may become hypoglycemic because of a reduced clearance of insulin (see Chapter 79).

Endocrine Disease

Glucocorticoids and GH are important regulators of glucose metabolism and gluconeogenesis. Thus, either pituitary insufficiency or adrenal insufficiency (primary or secondary to hypopituitarism) can result in hypoglycemia as a presenting manifestation. The diagnosis of these disorders is described elsewhere in this chapter.

Autoimmune Hypoglycemia

There are rare conditions in which autoantibodies develop to insulin receptors. Patients have no history of insulin use. They often have acanthosis nigricans and a variety of clinical features of autoimmune disease. The hypoglycemia is often severe and refractory. These conditions are unlikely to be encountered in a nonspecialty setting.

SPECIFIC REFERENCES*

1. Molitch ME. Evaluation and treatment of the patient with a pituitary incidentaloma. J Clin Endocrinol Metab 1995;80:3.
2. King JT, Justice AC, Aron DC. Management of incidental pituitary microadenomas: a cost-effectiveness analysis. J Clin Endocrinol Metab 1997;82:3625.
3. Molitch ME, Thorner MO, Wilson C. Management of prolactinomas. J Clin Endocrinol Metab 1997;82:996.
4. Verhelst J, Abs R, Maiter D, et al. Cabergoline in the treatment of hyperprolactinemia: a study in 455 patients. J Clin Endocrinol Metab 1999; 84:2518.
5. Pinzone JJ, Katznelson L, Danila DC, et al. Primary medical therapy of micro- and macroprolactinomas in men. J Clin Endocrinol Metab 2000;85:3053.

*Bold numerals denote published controlled clinical trials, meta-analyses, or consensus-based recommendations.

6. AACE Acromegaly Guidelines Task Force. AACE medical guidelines for clinical practice for the diagnosis and treatment of acromegaly. Endocr Pract 2004;10:213.
7. Freda PU. Somatostatin analogs in acromegaly. J Clin Endocrinol Metab 2002;87:3013.
8. Trainer PJ, Drake WM, Katznelson L, et al. Treatment of acromegaly with the growth hormone receptor antagonist pegvisomant. N Engl J Med 2000;342:1171.
9. Agha A, Rogers B, Sherlock M, et al. Anterior pituitary dysfunction in survivors of traumatic brain injury. J Clin Endocrinol Metab 2004;89:4929.
10. Agha A, Thornton E, O'Kelly P, et al. Posterior pituitary dysfunction after traumatic brain injury. J Clin Endocrinol Metab 2004;89:5987.
11. Hoffman AR, Kuntze JE, Baptista J, et al. Growth hormone (GH) replacement therapy in adult-onset GH deficiency: effect on body composition in men and women in a double-blind, randomized, placebo-controlled trial. J Clin Endocrinol Metab 2004;89:2048.
12. Cuneo RC, Salomon F, McGauley GA, et al. The growth hormone deficiency syndrome in adults. Clin Endocrinol 1992;37:387.
13. Bengtsson BA, Johannsson G, Shalet SM, et al. Treatment of growth hormone deficiency in adults. J Clin Endocrinol Metab 2000;85:933.
14. Dorin RI, Qualls CR, Crapo LM. Diagnosis of adrenal insufficiency. Ann Intern Med 2003;139:194.
15. Tordjman K, Jaffe A, Trostanetsky Y, et al. Low-dose (1 microgram) adrenocorticotrophin (ACTH) stimulation as a screening test for impaired hypothalamo-pituitary-adrenal axis function: sensitivity, specificity and accuracy in comparison with the high-dose (250 microgram) test. Clinical Endocrinol 2000;52:633.
16. Grinspoon SK, Biller BM. Laboratory assessment of adrenal insufficiency. J Clin Endocrinol Metab 1994;79:923.
17. Cooper MS, Stewart PM. Corticosteroid insufficiency in acutely ill patients. N Engl J Med 2003;348:727.
18. Hamrahian AH, Oseni TS, Arafah BM. Measurements of serum free cortisol in critically ill patients. N Engl J Med 2004;350:1629.
19. Samuels MH, Brandon DD, Isabelle LM, et al. Cortisol production rates in subjects with suspected Cushing's syndrome: assessment by stable isotope dilution methodology and comparison to other diagnostic methods. J Clin Endocrinol Metab 2000;85:22.
20. Graham KE, Samuels MH, Nesbitt GM, et al. Cavernous sinus sampling is highly accurate in distinguishing Cushing's disease from the ectopic adrenocorticotropin syndrome and in predicting intrapituitary tumor location. J Clin Endocrinol Metab 1999;84:1602.
21. DeHerder WW, Lamberts SW. Tumor localization—the ectopic ACTH syndrome. J Clin Endocrinol Metab 1999;84:1184.
22. Pralong FP, Gomez F, Guillou L, et al. Food-dependent Cushing's syndrome: possible involvement of leptin in cortisol hypersecretion. J Clin Endocrinol Metab 1999;84:3817.
23. Papanicolaou DA, Yanovski JA, Cutler GB Jr, et al. A single midnight serum cortisol measurement distinguishes Cushing's syndrome from pseudo-Cushing states. J Clin Endocrinol Metab 1998;83:1163.
24. Isidori AM, Kaltsas GA, Mohammed S, et al. Discriminatory value of the low-dose dexamethasone suppression test in establishing the diagnosis and differential diagnosis of Cushing's syndrome. J Clin Endocrinol Metab 2003;88:5299.
25. Newell-Price J, Grossman AB. The differential diagnosis of Cushing's syndrome. Ann Endocrinol 2001;62:173.
26. Moro M, Putignano P, Losa M, et al. The desmopressin test in the differential diagnosis between Cushing's disease and pseudo-Cushing states. J Clin Endocrinol Metab 2000;85:3569.
27. Lamberts SW, van der Lely AJ, deHerder WW. Transsphenoidal selective adenomectomy is the treatment of choice in patients with Cushing's disease. Considerations concerning medical treatment and the long-term follow-up. J Clin Endocrinol Metab 1995;80:3111.
28. Nieman LK. Medical therapy of Cushing's disease. Pituitary 2002;5:77.
29. Copeland PM. The incidentally discovered adrenal mass. Ann Intern Med 1983;98:940.
30. Barzon L, Scaroni C, Sonino N, et al. Risk factors and long-term follow-up of adrenal incidentalomas. J Clin Endocrinol Metab 1999;84:520.
31. Rossi R, Tauchmanova L, Luciano A, et al. Subclinical Cushing's syndrome in patients with adrenal incidentaloma: clinical and biochemical features. J Clin Endocrinol Metab 2000;85:1440.
32. Carella MJ, Srivastava LS, Gossain VV, et al. Hypothalamic-pituitary-adrenal function one week after a short burst of steroid therapy. J Clin Endocrinol Metab 1993;76:1188.
33. Goldman MB, Robertson GL, Luchins DJ, et al. The influence of polydipsia on water excretion in hyponatremic, polydipsic, schizophrenic patients. J Clin Endocrinol Metab 1996;81:1465.
34. Goldman MB, Luchins DJ, Robertson GL. Mechanisms of altered water metabolism in psychotic patients with polydipsia and hyponatremia. N Engl J Med 1988;318:397.
35. Miller M, Hecker MS, Friedlander DA, et al. Apparent idiopathic hyponatremia in an ambulatory geriatric population. J Am Geriatr Soc 1996;44:406.
36. Anderson RJ, Chung HM, Kluge R, et al. Hyponatremia: a prospective analysis of its epidemiology and the pathogenetic role of vasopressin. Ann Intern Med 1985;102:164.
37. Miller M, Morley JE, Rubenstein LZ. Hyponatremia in a nursing home population. J Am Geriatr Soc 1995;43:1410.
38. Miller M. Syndromes of excess antidiuretic hormone release. Crit Care Clin 2001;17:11.
39. Wong LL, Verbalis JG. Systemic diseases associated with disorders of water homeostasis. Endocrinol Metab Clin North Am 2002;31:121.
40. Tang WW, Kaptein, EM, Feinstein EI, et al. Hyponatremia in hospitalized patients with the acquired immunodeficiency syndrome (AIDS). Am J Med 1993;94:169.
41. Palmer BF. Hyponatremia in patients with central nervous system disease: SIADH versus CSW. Trends Endocrinol Metab 2003;14:182.
42. Ayus JC, Wheeler JM, Arieff AI. Postoperative hyponatremic encephalopathy in menstruant women. Ann Intern Med 1992;117:891.
43. Miller M, Moses AM. Drug-induced states of impaired water excretion. Kidney Int 1976;10:96.
44. Wilkinson TJ, Begg EJ, Winter AC, Sainsbury R. Incidence and risk factors for hyponatremia following treatment with fluoxetine or paroxetine in elderly people. Br J Clin Pharmacol 1999;47:211.
45. Fabian TJ, Amico JA, Kroboth PD, et al. Paroxetine-induced hyponatremia in older adults. A 12-week prospective study. Arch Intern Med 2004;164:327.
46. Subramanian D, Ayus C. Case report: severe symptomatic hyponatremia associated with lisinopril therapy. Am J Med Sci 1992;303: 177.
47. Sonnenblick M, Friedlander Y, Rosin AJ. Diuretic-induced severe hyponatremia. Review and analysis of 129 reported patients. Chest 1993;103:601.
48. Bartter FC, Schwartz WB. The syndrome of inappropriate secretion of antidiuretic hormone. Am J Med 1967;42:790.
49. Forrest JN Jr, Cox M, Hong C, et al. Superiority of demeclocycline over lithium in the treatment of chronic syndrome of inappropriate secretion of antidiuretic hormone. N Engl J Med 1978; 298:173.
50. Verbalis JG. Vasopressin V2 receptor antagonists. J Mol Endocrinol 2002;29:1.
51. Wong LL, Verbalis JG. Vasopressin V_2 receptor antagonists. Cardiovasc Res 2001;51:391.
52. Costello-Boerrigter LC, Boerrigter G, Burnett JC Jr. Revisiting salt and water retention: new diuretics, aquaretics, and natriuretics. Med Clin North Am 2003;87:475.
53. Martinez-Castelao A. Conivaptan (Yamanouchi). Curr Opin Investig Drugs 2002;3:89.
54. Hart SP, Frier BM. Causes, management and morbidity of acute hypoglycaemia in adults requiring hospital admission. Q J Med 1998; 91:505.
55. Service FJ. Hypoglycemic disorders. N Engl J Med 1995;332:1144.
56. Palardy J, Havrankova J, Lepage R, et al. Blood glucose measurements during symptomatic episodes in patients with suspected postprandial hypoglycemia. N Engl J Med 1989;321:1421.
57. Yager J, Young RT. Non-hypoglycemia is an epidemic condition. N Engl J Med 1974;291: 907.
58. Kerr D, Sherwin RS, Pavalkis F, et al. Effect of caffeine on the recognition of and responses to hypoglycemia in humans. Ann Intern Med 1993; 119:799.
59. Hirshberg B, Livi A, Bartlett DL, et al. Forty-eight-hour fast: the diagnostic test for insulinoma. J Clin Endocrinol Metab 2000; 85:3222.
60. Gordon P, Skarulis MC, Roach P, et al. Plasma proinsulin-like component in insulinoma: a 25-year experience. J Clin Endocrinol Metab 1995;80:2884.
61. Service FJ. Clinical review 42. Hypoglycemias. J Clin Endocrinol Metab 1993;76:269.
62. Service FJ, Natt N, Thompson GB, et al. Noninsulinoma pancreatogenous hypoglycemia: a novel syndrome of hyperinsulinemic hypoglycemia in adults independent of mutations in Kir6. 2 and SUR1 genes. J Clin Endocrinol Metab 1999;84:1582.
63. Service GJ, Thompson GB, Service FJ, et al. Hyperinsulinemic hypoglycemia with nesidioblastosis after gastric-bypass surgery. N Engl J Med 2005;353:249.

*For annotated **General References** and resources related to this chapter, visit www.hopkinsbayview.org/PAMreferences.*

Chapter 82

Disorders of Lipid Metabolism

Annabelle Rodriguez-Oquendo *

*In the previous edition, David E. Kern, MD, and Marc R. Blackman, MD, contributed to this chapter.

Interest in plasma lipids, lipoproteins, and apoproteins stems from their strong relationship to the development of atherosclerosis (1–3). At a time when it is possible to reduce the frequency of premature death and disability from atherosclerotic disease, the clinician should be knowledgeable about and capable of diagnosing and treating the major disorders of lipid metabolism.

LIPID AND LIPOPROTEIN NOMENCLATURE AND COMPOSITION

Lipids are insoluble in the blood. They circulate in plasma as component parts of macromolecules that consist of a nonpolar hydrophobic lipid core of cholesterol esters and triglycerides and a polar hydrophilic monolayer surface coat of protein, phospholipid, and unesterified cholesterol (Fig. 82.1). These macromolecules, which are made miscible in plasma by their surface coat, are called lipoproteins.

Traditionally, lipoproteins have been classified as a family of molecules containing the same basic constituents but in different proportions (Table 82.1). The major classes of lipoproteins can be separated from each other by differences in density (ultracentrifugation), net surface charge (electrophoresis), size, and composition. Ultracentrifugation, which has been the traditional method of classification, separates lipoproteins into five principal classes: *chylomicrons, very-low-density lipoproteins* (VLDLs),

A LIPOPROTEIN PARTICLE

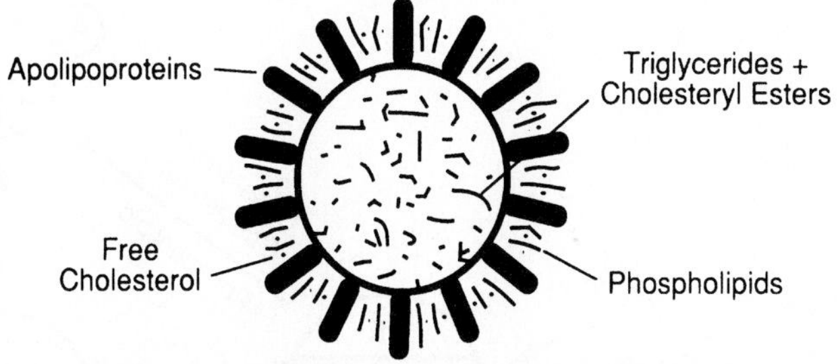

FIGURE 82.1. Structure of the lipoprotein macromolecule with the nonpolar lipids, cholesterol ester, and triglyceride in the lipoprotein core surrounded by a monolayer composed of specific apolipoproteins, proteins, and the polar lipids, unesterified cholesterol and phospholipid. (From The Johns Hopkins Physicians Lipid Education Program. 2nd ed. Baltimore: The Johns Hopkins University, 1988:11, with permission.)

TABLE 82.1 Classification of Plasma Lipoproteins by Physical and Chemical Characteristics

Lipoprotein Fraction (Ultracentrifugation)	Density (g/mL)	Migration (Electrophoresis)	Composition as Percentage of Total Mass			
			Cholesterol	Triglyceride	Apoprotein	Phospholipid
Chylomicron	0.95	Origin	2–7	80–90	2 (A, B-48, C, E)	3
Very low density (VLDL)	<1.006	Pre-β	10–22	50–70	6 (B-100, C, E)	14
β-Very low density (β-VLDL or $VLDL_2$)	<1.006	β	30–40	45	12 (B-100, B-48, C, E)	15
Intermediate density or remnant (IDL)	1.006–1.019	Slow pre-β	30–40	40	18 (B, E)	22
Low density (LDL)	1.019–1.063	β	45–50	5–10	21 (B–100)	22
High density (HDL)	1.063–1.21	α	15–25	3–5	50 (A, C, E)	28

intermediate-density lipoproteins (IDLs), *low-density lipoproteins* (LDLs), and *high-density lipoproteins* (HDLs) (4).

Each lipoprotein contains characteristic proportions of lipids and type-specific apoproteins (apos) such that, with increasing lipoprotein density, the relative amount of lipid decreases and that of apoprotein increases (Table 82.1). For example, triglyceride is the major lipid component in chylomicrons and VLDL, whereas cholesterol is the major component of LDL. Intermediate-density or remnant lipoproteins are catabolic products of chylomicrons and VLDLs, and contain similar amounts of both lipids and apos (see Normal Physiology of Lipoprotein Transport). The HDLs are the most dense lipoproteins; they contain proportionally the most apos and ordinarily consist of 15% to 25% cholesterol with a small amount of triglyceride in the core. HDLs are further subdivided into HDL_2 and HDL_3. The former is more buoyant, as reflected by its higher lipid-to-protein ratio and richer apo A-I and apo C and E content, relative to the more dense HDL_3, which has a lower lipid-to-protein ratio and a higher apo A-II than A-I composition. Some studies have shown an inverse relationship of coronary risk to plasma concentrations of HDL_2 and apo A-I, related to the capacity of the latter molecules to transport cholesterol from cells (this process is termed reverse cholesterol transport) (5).

NORMAL PHYSIOLOGY OF LIPID TRANSPORT

Plasma lipoproteins arise from both exogenous dietary sources and endogenous hepatic sources (Fig. 82.2). They carry lipids in three distinct but interacting pathways: The *exogenous pathway* consists primarily of chylomicrons; the *endogenous pathway* consists mostly of VLDL, IDL, and LDL; and the *reverse cholesterol transport pathway* consists mostly of HDL activity.

After the ingestion of fat, dietary triglycerides are hydrolyzed in the gut and absorbed by intestinal enterocytes. The triglyceride-containing chylomicrons formed in these cells are secreted into lymphatic vessels, and subsequently enter the venous system via the thoracic duct.

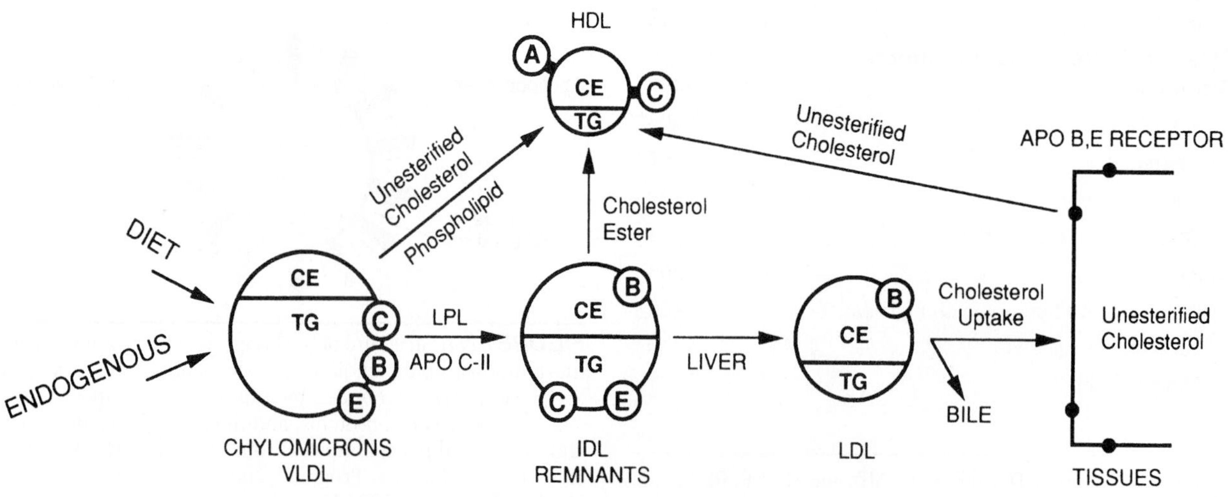

FIGURE 82.2. The normal physiology of lipoprotein transport is illustrated schematically.

Chylomicrons function as a system of high-energy caloric transport, allowing the calories ingested in excess of the immediate needs of the body to be transferred to sites of storage between meals. Absorbed dietary cholesterol is also esterified and transported in chylomicrons.

Other triglyceride-rich lipoproteins are synthesized from endogenous sources by the liver and intestine. Cholesterol synthesis from acetate also occurs in the liver and is regulated by the enzyme hydroxymethylglutaryl coenzyme A (HMG-CoA) reductase. Triglycerides synthesized in the liver combine with cholesterol ester and are enveloped in a lipoprotein monolayer before being secreted into the hepatic venous outflow system as endogenous triglyceride-rich VLDLs.

Chylomicrons and VLDLs are transported to adipose tissue and muscle for storage and use. The uptake and storage of triglyceride are regulated by *lipoprotein lipase* (LPL). LPL hydrolyzes triglyceride and surface components from chylomicrons and VLDL to transform them into *remnant lipoproteins* (Fig. 82.2). The fatty acids released during this reaction migrate to muscle cells for combustion or to adipose cells for resynthesis and storage as triglyceride (6). The remnant lipoproteins are smaller, denser, and relatively enriched in cholesterol, apo B, and apo E, compared with the chylomicrons and VLDL from which they are derived. They are taken up by apo B-E (LDL) receptors in the liver. The chylomicron remnants are further degraded, and the VLDL remnants are processed into IDL and cholesterol-rich LDL (Fig. 82.2). Apo C-II and apo C-III, and the phospholipids and free cholesterol released during the LPL reaction, are transferred to HDL for use. The surface material generated by LPL-mediated removal of core triglyceride from VLDL and chylomicrons is the substrate (apo A-I is the cofactor) for the enzyme *lecithin-cholesterol acyl transferase* (LCAT), which converts nascent HDL to mature spherical HDL and plays a major role in reverse cholesterol transport.

The LDLs are the principal carriers of cholesterol in plasma. Cholesterol is a major structural component of all cell membranes and is a precursor for steroid hormone synthesis by the adrenal glands and gonads. The LDL cholesterol-rich particles are derived mainly from VLDL and their catabolic remnants via the action of LPL and hepatic lipase. The principal removal of LDL occurs in the periphery by cells having a specific cell surface receptor (1) that recognizes all forms of apo B; this is currently referred to as the apo B-E (LDL) receptor (Fig. 82.2). After specific cell receptor binding, LDLs are internalized by receptor-mediated endocytosis and carried to lysosomes, where apo B is irreversibly degraded to amino acids and LDL cholesterol ester is hydrolyzed to free cholesterol. The free cholesterol is transported to an intracellular cholesterol pool, where it regulates, by a cellular feedback pathway, the resynthesis of cholesterol, cholesterol ester, and apo B-E (LDL) receptors (7).

The cholesterol content of the cell is also regulated by a removal system involving HDL as a vehicle for cholesterol transport from peripheral to hepatic cells for catabolism and excretion into bile directly or after conversion to bile acid (7,8). This process, termed *reverse cholesterol transport*, is thought to be one of the mechanisms for the antiatherogenic effect of HDL. It provides an efficient mechanism for the transfer of esterified cholesterol to LDL and VLDL, the absorption of free cholesterol from vascular endothelial cells, and the removal of cholesterol arising from cell membrane turnover and cell death. An apparent antiatherogenic alteration in both the lipoprotein and apoprotein composition of HDL, the formation of HDL_2, occurs during high-cholesterol feeding and represents one pathway by which the body can enhance its capacity to clear excess cholesterol from cells (7). HDL is also thought to be cardioprotective by acting as an antioxidant and endotoxin scavenger. The identification of the HDL receptor SR-BI has shown that the receptor plays a major role in reverse cholesterol transport, with a key role in the selective uptake of cholesteryl esters in hepatocytes and gonadal cells (9,10). Research is currently underway to better define the role of SR-BI in atherosclerosis and to determine whether it might be a useful target for pharmacologic intervention.

Continued LDL catabolism in excess of that performed by hepatic and other parenchymal cells occurs in macrophages via a *scavenger pathway*. The observation that oxidatively modified LDLs are efficiently taken up by the scavenger pathway receptors, and subsequently influence macrophage and monocyte motility, served as the basis for proposing the current oxidative theory of atherogenesis (11). Abnormalities in oxidative metabolism of LDL are considered to account for the dyslipidemia in persons with homozygous familial hypercholesterolemia (11).

Apoproteins occupy specific domains on the three-dimensional structures of the individual lipoproteins. Alterations in lipid–protein interactions occur during the normal metabolism of lipoproteins, resulting in changes in the association of apoproteins with lipoproteins. Abnormalities in lipoprotein transport occur when the domains of apoproteins are altered by substitutions or deletions in amino acids. For example, the abnormal recognition of β-VLDL by the apo B-E receptor on cells occurs because of an abnormality in apo E in dysbetalipoproteinemia (see Pathophysiology of Lipoprotein Disorders), and abnormalities in the apo B-E receptors are responsible for the defect in familial hypercholesterolemia (1,12).

PLASMA LIPOPROTEINS AS RISK FACTORS FOR ATHEROSCLEROSIS

Among the risk factors for atherosclerotic vascular disease (13), the most clearly established ones are plasma total

TABLE 82.2 CAD Risk Factors as Defined by the NCEP Adult Treatment Guidelines[a]

Positive Risk Factors
Age
Male age ≥45 yr
Female age ≥55 yr or premature menopause without estrogen replacement therapy
Family history of premature CAD (definite myocardial infarction or sudden death before 55 yr of age in father or other male first-degree relative, or before 65 yr of age in mother or other female first-degree relative)
Current cigarette smoking
Hypertension (blood pressure ≥140/90 mm Hg or taking antihypertensive medication)
Low HDL cholesterol (<40 mg/dL [1.0 mmol/L] for men, <50 mg/dL [] for women)
Negative Risk Factor
High HDL cholesterol (≥60 mg/dL [1.6 mmol/L])

CAD, coronary artery disease; HDL, high-density lipoprotein.
[a]Diabetes mellitus is now considered a CAD risk equivalent (i.e., equivalent to having CAD) and has been removed from the risk factor table. This designation emphasizes the need to be aggressive in the lipid management of patients with diabetes mellitus.
Expert Panel on Detection, Evaluation, and Treatment of High Blood Cholesterol in Adults. Executive Summary of the Third Report of the National Cholesterol Education Program (NCEP) Expert Panel on Detection, Evaluation, and Treatment of High Blood Cholesterol in Adults (Adult Treatment Panel III). JAMA. 2001 May 16;285(19):2486–97.

cholesterol levels (and plasma LDL and HDL content), hypertension, cigarette smoking, family history of premature coronary artery disease (CAD), and age. Diabetes mellitus is considered a risk equivalent to having CAD (Table 82.2).

Evidence from several large prospective and retrospective epidemiologic studies among diverse populations has demonstrated that variations in plasma levels of certain lipids and lipoproteins are associated with an increased likelihood of developing or having CAD. *Hypercholesterolemia*, for example, is strongly associated with the subsequent development of CAD. The relationship is uniformly consistent, dose related, and independent of gender. The predictive value of the plasma level of total cholesterol is somewhat limited, however, by the fact that it reflects the opposing influences of LDL and HDL cholesterol. Levels of LDL correlate positively, whereas those of HDL, in general, are inversely related to CAD risk. The negative correlation between HDL levels and CAD depends mainly on its subfraction, HDL_2, which may provide, along with its major protein component apo A-I, a better index of risk than the total plasma level of HDL (5). Over the range of total and HDL cholesterol plasma levels found in an average American population, the risk of CAD varies roughly fivefold. Although the impact of cardiovascular risk factors declines after 75 years of age, they are still predictive of CAD in older people. The relative risks of CAD associated with any particular risk factor (e.g., cholesterol levels) decrease with aging because of the increased prevalence of multiple risk factors; however, the absolute risk of morbidity and mortality increases markedly (14). Most, but not all, studies indicate that plasma levels of total cholesterol retain predictive value in the "old old"—that is, in men age 75 to 95 years (15–18). Moreover, HDL cholesterol levels and the ratio of LDL to HDL cholesterol remain useful predictors in this age group.

The relationships of plasma levels of total, LDL, and HDL cholesterol with CAD are independent ones, in that the associations remain significant even after statistical adjustment for other risk factors. A low concentration of HDL cholesterol is a stronger independent risk factor for CAD than is either total cholesterol or LDL cholesterol (3).

Increased fasting levels of plasma *triglyceride* and of its major lipoprotein transporter, VLDL, also correlate with an increased risk of atherosclerotic disease. There has been uncertainty about whether the association is independent of other risk factors (19,20). Recent analyses suggest that plasma triglyceride levels are a risk factor for CAD and are independent of HDL cholesterol levels (21,22). Treatment of hypertriglyceridemia depends on the causes and degree of elevation and on the presence or absence of other risk factors (Table 82.2; see Treatment). Hypertriglyceridemia may be especially important prognostically in patients with diabetes mellitus (23) or end-stage renal disease (24). Not only do these lipoprotein and apoprotein abnormalities increase the risk of CAD, but there also is a parallel increased risk for cerebrovascular disease (13,25), as well as for peripheral vascular disease (25).

A number of lipid fractions are even more strongly related to CAD than are total, LDL, and HDL cholesterol or apo A-I, and measurements of these fractions may become more useful in cardiovascular and cerebrovascular risk factor assessments (3). Elevated plasma concentrations of LDL apo B appear to discriminate between patients with and without atherosclerosis of the coronary and peripheral vasculature, even in the presence of normal total and LDL plasma cholesterol levels (2,26). The determination of the plasma LDL apo B concentration may also prove useful in assessing risk in hypertriglyceridemic patients (2,22). It is known that LDL consists of several lipoprotein subclasses that differ in size and core lipid content, and that LDL subclass pattern B, characterized by small, dense LDL particles, is associated with a threefold increased risk of myocardial infarction (MI), independent of age, gender, and body weight (27).

In addition, MI, the progression of angiographically documented CAD, postangioplasty restenosis, and cerebrovascular disease are strongly associated with the lipoprotein (a) [Lp(a)] blood pattern, particularly in patients with increased levels of LDL cholesterol (28). The evidence (29) suggests that Lp(a) (distinct from apo A) consists of a circulating complex of LDL and apo(a) that is more atherogenic than LDL. Apo(a) exists in more than 30 isoforms and accounts for the substantial variability in the plasma concentrations of Lp(a). Moreover, Lp(a) is structurally similar to plasminogen and inhibits the conversion of plasminogen to plasmin, thus attenuating fibrinolysis. Finally, Lp(a) appears to be directly involved in the formation of atherosclerotic plaques, perhaps because of its susceptibility to oxidative alteration in the arterial wall. However, at present there is no evidence from clinical trials to support routine measurement of Lp(a).

A number of investigations have demonstrated that tissue oxidative damage to LDL, and the subsequent interactions between damaged LDL and vascular endothelium, smooth muscle, macrophages, and monocytes, elicit more atherogenic activity than occurs with native LDL (11). Research in animals indicates that use of exogenous antioxidants retards the progression of experimentally induced atherogenesis by 30% to 80%. Although there have been epidemiologic reports that antioxidants (e.g., vitamin E) protect hyperlipidemic patients from the development or worsening of atherosclerotic heart disease (30,31), several prospective randomized trials have shown no benefit in this regard (32,33).

In *familial dysbetalipoproteinemia*, a genetic disorder characterized by elevated plasma concentrations of IDL and an abnormally migrating β-VLDL (12), there is an increased risk of both peripheral and coronary atherosclerotic disease. In contrast, *fasting chylomicronemia* is associated with recurrent episodes of abdominal pain and pancreatitis, but not with the early development of atherosclerosis.

In several epidemiologic studies, plasma total cholesterol levels lower than 180 to 195 mg/dL were associated with an increased risk of cancer, especially cancer of the colon. The evidence does not, however, suggest a significant causal link because (a) in most studies the association was strongest in the first year of followup, then attenuated and disappeared in subsequent years, suggesting that preclinical cancer might have lowered levels of plasma cholesterol rather than vice versa; (b) studies comparing populations show a positive association between dietary fat intake and risk for major cancers such as breast, prostate, and colon cancer; and (c) the relationship was generally weak, was present in a minority of studies, and demonstrated no consistent relation between cholesterol level and cancer risk (34).

RATIONALE FOR DIAGNOSIS AND TREATMENT

Despite the fact that many risk factors linked with coronary and other atherosclerotic vascular disease have been identified and targeted for intervention, atherosclerotic disease constitutes the leading cause of death and disability in Western industrialized societies. In response, major efforts at risk factor identification and treatment, as well as prevention, primarily targeting hyperlipidemia, hypertension, and smoking, have been undertaken, and mortality from CAD has fallen steadily (35).

The "lipid (or cholesterol) hypothesis," based on the data described, also postulates that favorable alterations of plasma lipoprotein levels by diet, drugs, or other therapy reduce the risk of atherosclerosis in humans. Indeed, randomized primary prevention trials have shown that lowering LDL cholesterol in asymptomatic hyperlipidemic middle-aged men significantly reduces their risk of death from coronary artery disease and of nonfatal MI (36–39). The relative risk reduction over 5 years is approximately 30%, and the absolute risk reduction is approximately 2% (the number needed to treat to avoid an adverse event is 50).

Results from the Air Force/Texas Coronary Atherosclerosis Prevention Study (AFCAPS/TexCAPS) have lent greater support to the rationale for primary prevention treatment (39). A total of 5,608 men and 997 women with average total and LDL cholesterol levels (221 and 150 mg/dL, respectively) and below-average HDL cholesterol levels (36 and 40 mg/dL, respectively) were studied for an average followup period of 5.2 years. This study compared the effects of placebo and lovastatin on the primary end points of unstable angina, fatal and nonfatal MI, and sudden cardiac death in middle-aged patients (men age 45 to 73 years and postmenopausal women age 55 to 73 years). For study subjects receiving lovastatin treatment, the relative risks were significantly reduced for first acute coronary events, MI, unstable angina, coronary revascularization procedures, coronary events, and cardiovascular events. Lovastatin lowered LDL cholesterol levels by 25% (to 115 mg/dL) and increased HDL cholesterol levels by 6% (to 39 mg/dL).

Secondary prevention trials also have shown conclusively that cholesterol-lowering drugs can decrease CAD progression as well as the incidence of new and recurrent CAD-related events in patients with known atherosclerotic vascular disease (40–42). There is a consensus that treatment should be more aggressive in these populations (see Treatment). Relative risk reductions of 20% to 40% have been reported, with absolute risk reductions of 3% to 4% over 5 years of treatment. In these studies, all-cause mortality was also reduced by approximately 20%.

The importance of targeting HDL cholesterol levels, particularly in patients with known CAD, was highlighted in the report from the Veteran's Affairs High-Density Lipoprotein Cholesterol Intervention Study (VA-HIT) (42). In this study, 2,531 men with known CAD, low HDL cholesterol levels (mean: 32 mg/dL), and "desirable" LDL cholesterol levels (mean: 111 mg/dL) were treated with placebo or gemfibrozil 600 mg twice daily for a mean followup period of 5.1 years. Gemfibrozil was chosen as the pharmacologic agent because of its relatively neutral effects on LDL cholesterol levels. The results showed significant relative risk reductions for nonfatal MI, CAD death, transient ischemic attack, angioplasty, carotid endarterectomy, stroke, and hospitalization for congestive heart failure. These beneficial effects of gemfibrozil treatment were associated with significant reduction in plasma triglyceride levels (24%) and increased HDL cholesterol levels (8%).

Results from the Heart Protection Study (HPS) have contributed substantially to the newer guidelines advocating lowering the target LDL cholesterol levels in patients at high risk for CHD (42a). Approximately 20,000 adult men and women, between the ages of 40 and 80 years, with either diabetes mellitus, hypertension, occlusive disease of noncoronary artery disease, or coronary artery disease were enrolled in this double-blind, placebo-controlled, randomized study of statin therapy (simvastatin vs. placebo) of 5 years duration. Overall, the results showed that all participants on statin therapy (regardless of age, gender, baseline LDL cholesterol levels) benefited from statistically significant relative-risk reduction in major coronary events, stroke and revascularization.

HYPERLIPIDEMIA

Definition

The diagnosis of hyperlipidemia historically has been based on plasma levels of lipids or lipoproteins above the 95th percentile of those found in a reference population. The Adult Treatment Panel (ATP) of the National Cholesterol Education Program (NCEP) has established criteria for the diagnosis of hyperlipidemia based on prognostic significance (Table 82.3) (43,44).

TABLE 82.3 Adult Treatment Panel III Criteria for the Classification of LDL, Total, and HDL Cholesterol (mg/dL) Based on Prognostic Significance

LDL Cholesterol	
<100	Optimal
100–129	Near or above optimal
130–159	Borderline high
160–189	High
≥190	Very high
Total Cholesterol	
<200	Desirable
200–239	Borderline high
≥240	High
HDL Cholesterol	
<40	Low
≥60	High

HDL, high-density lipoprotein; LDL, low-density lipoprotein.
Modified from the Executive Summary of the Third Report of the National Cholesterol Education Program (NCEP) Expert Panel on Detection, Evaluation, and Treatment of High Blood Cholesterol in Adults (Adult Treatment Panel III). JAMA 2001;285:2486.

TABLE 82.4 Causes of Secondary Lipoprotein Disorders

Exogenous	Alcohol, oral contraceptives, estrogens, androgens, corticosteroids, diuretics (thiazides, chlorthalidone), β-adrenergic-blocking agents, isotretinoin, obesity, nutrition (diet high in cholesterol/saturated fat)
Endocrine-metabolic	Diabetes mellitus, hypothyroidism, Cushing disease, Addison disease, acromegaly, hypopituitarism, growth hormone deficiency
Hepatic	Obstructive or parenchymal disease, hepatoma
Renal	Nephrotic syndrome, chronic renal failure, hemodialysis
Acute stress situations	Acute myocardial infarction, sepsis, burns
Pregnancy	
Pancreatitis	
Dysgammaglobulinemias	Multiple myeloma, macroglobulinemia
Systemic lupus erythematosus	
Gout	
Viral infections, including acquired immune deficiency syndrome (AIDS)	
Other	Glycogen storage disease, lipodystrophies, progeria, acute intermittent porphyria, anorexia nervosa, Klinefelter syndrome

Classification

Primary versus Secondary

For clinical purposes, hyperlipidemic states should be classified as primary (hereditary or sporadic genetic disorders of metabolism), secondary, or both. Secondary hyperlipidemia is associated with an identifiable disease or condition and is reversible with control or eradication of that disease or condition. Table 82.4 lists the major causes of secondary hyperlipoproteinemia.

Phenotypic versus Genotypic and Pathophysiologic

In the 1960s, it was popular to classify the various hyperlipidemic states *phenotypically*, based on specific concentrations of lipids and lipoproteins and electrophoretic patterns (Table 82.5). Although the phenotypic classification describes in abbreviated fashion the plasma lipoproteins that are present in elevated or low concentrations, it does not reflect the genetic mechanisms or pathophysiology of the lipoprotein disorders. It is desirable to classify patients

TABLE 82.5 Classification of Lipoprotein Disorders by Phenotypes and Genotypes and Corresponding Clinical Manifestations

Phenotype	Lipoprotein in Excess	Plasma Lipid Levels		Plasma Appearance[a]	Genotype	Age at Onset (Primary Form)	Xanthomas[b]	Other Clinical Manifestations
		Cholesterol	Triglyceride					
I	Chylomicrons	Normal or	↑↑↑ Lipemia	Clear plasma, creamy supernatant	Familial lipoprotein lipase deficiency, apo C–II deficiency	Infancy or childhood	Eruptive, tuberoeruptive	Recurrent abdominal pain, other gastrointestinal symptoms, lipemia retinalis, hepatosplenomegaly
IIA	LDL	↑↑↑	Normal	Clear	Familial hyper-cholesterolemia, familial combined hyperlipidemia, polygenic and sporadic hyper-cholesterolemia	Childhood for homozygous FHC, late childhood to middle age for heterozygous FHC, adulthood for others	Tendinous, xanthelasma, tuberous; planar (homozygous)	Premature CAD, arcus corneae, aortic stenosis (homozygous FHC), arthritic symptoms
IIB	LDL + VLDL	↑↑	↑	Clear	Familial combined hyperlipidemia, familial hyper-cholesterolemia			
III	β-VLDL, IDL	↑↑	↑↑	Slightly turbid	Familial dysbeta-lipoproteinemia	Adulthood (occasionally late adolescence)	Planar (especially palmar), tuberous	Premature CAD and peripheral vascular disease, male > female, obesity, abnormal glucose tolerance, hyperuricemia; aggravated by hypothyroidism, good response to therapy
IV	VLDL	Normal or ↑[c]	↑↑	Turbid	Familial hyper-triglyceridemia, familial combined hyperlipidemia, sporadic hyper-triglyceridemia	Early to late adulthood	Usually none; rarely eruptive, or tuberoeruptive	CAD and peripheral vascular disease, obesity, abnormal glucose tolerance, hyperuricemia, arthritic symptoms, gallbladder disease
V	Chylomicrons + VLDL	Normal or ↑	↑↑↑	Turbid plasma, creamy supernatant	Homozygous familial hyper-triglyceridemia	Childhood to middle age, usually adulthood	Eruptive, tuberoeruptive	Recurrent abdominal pain, other gastrointestinal symptoms, lipemia retinalis, hepatosplenomegaly, peripheral paresthesias, abnormal glucose tolerance, hyperuricemia

apo, Apoprotein; CAD, coronary artery disease; FHC, familial hypercholesterolemia; IDL, intermediate-density lipoprotein; LDL, low-density lipoprotein; VLDL, very-low-density lipoprotein.
[a]Plasma obtained after 12 hr of fasting, left undisturbed in refrigerator overnight.
[b]Seen only in a minority of patients, but the frequency increases as plasma lipid levels rise.
[c]Cholesterol normal if triglycerides are less than 400 mg/dL.

pathophysiologically and *genotypically* (Table 82.5) to diagnose and treat lipoprotein disorders accurately. Because apoproteins, enzymes, and cellular receptors are the major regulators of lipoprotein metabolism, it is appropriate to categorize lipoprotein disorders whenever possible in terms of pathophysiologic defects in the structure, function, and metabolism of these molecules, rather than by using a rigidly fixed phenotypic classification. Often, the pathophysiologic and genotypic classification can be surmised from a patient's phenotypic pattern, medical history, family history, and physical examination. Sometimes family members must be studied or more sophisticated laboratory analyses performed, necessitating referral to a specialist in endocrinology and metabolism.

PATHOPHYSIOLOGY OF LIPID DISORDERS

The abnormal accumulation of lipoproteins in plasma results from their excessive production, defective removal, or both. Lipoprotein disorders may be primary (usually genetic); they may be secondary to certain diseases (especially diabetes mellitus, chronic renal disease, hypothyroidism, dysglobulinemia) or drugs (corticosteroids, estrogens, thiazide diuretics); or they may represent an interaction between primary and secondary factors. Abnormalities can occur in triglyceride-rich lipoprotein synthesis, LPL-mediated triglyceride catabolism, remnant lipoprotein catabolism, cholesterol-rich lipoprotein catabolism, or cholesterol-rich lipoprotein (LDL cholesterol) synthesis and absorption.

Increased Triglyceride Synthesis

Most triglyceride input is from the diet in normal individuals. However, abnormalities in the regulation of the endogenous production of triglyceride-rich VLDLs are fairly common and are the most common causes of hypertriglyceridemia. They are associated with an increase in plasma levels of VLDL (type IV) or of VLDL plus chylomicrons (type V). The underlying metabolic cause for endogenous hypertriglyceridemia is usually related to hyperinsulinemia and insulin resistance, most often as a result of obesity, diabetes mellitus, the ingestion of excessive calories or alcohol, or the use of estrogens or corticosteroids.

The primary forms of endogenous hypertriglyceridemia are familial hypertriglyceridemia and primary familial combined hyperlipidemia. *Familial hypertriglyceridemia* results in an increase in the endogenous synthesis of large triglyceride-rich VLDLs. Many such patients are obese and exhibit mild glucose intolerance, hyperinsulinemia, and clinical evidence of diabetes mellitus, conditions that contribute to the excessive hepatic production of VLDL triglyceride.

In contrast, patients with *familial combined hyperlipidemia* (multiple lipoprotein–type hyperlipidemia) exhibit an increase in the production of apo B, which can appear in VLDL, LDL, or both. Various lipoprotein types (IIA, IIB, or IV) are found in patients with familial combined hyperlipidemia, and the presenting sign can be an increase in VLDL triglyceride, LDL cholesterol, or both. The clinical expressions of this disorder vary among individual patients depending on diet, degree of obesity, level of physical activity, and concomitant use of other drugs.

Familial hypertriglyceridemia and familial combined hyperlipidemia are inherited as separate autosomal-dominant disorders, each occurring in approximately 1% of the general population. Familial hypertriglyceridemia is not associated with xanthomas unless hyperchylomicronemia supervenes. Basal concentrations (after a 12-hour fast) of total triglycerides and VLDL triglycerides are characteristically elevated, but plasma levels of total and LDL cholesterol are normal or low unless levels of VLDL cholesterol are also increased. Familial hypertriglyceridemia is not associated with an increased incidence of premature CAD; however, patients with familial combined hyperlipidemia are at high risk, primarily because of their increased plasma levels of apo B as well as abnormalities in the composition of HDL and reduced levels of apo A-I and HDL_2 (2). Familial combined hyperlipidemia may be present in as many as 10% of survivors of MI who are younger than 60 years of age and thus represents a common and important risk factor for atherosclerosis.

The diagnosis of these disorders of lipoprotein metabolism and their exact definition can be established only by family studies. A strongly positive family history of atherosclerosis favors the diagnosis of familial combined hyperlipidemia in hypertriglyceridemic patients in whom secondary causes for hyperlipidemia have been excluded. Differentiating between these two disorders of lipoprotein metabolism is important in the evaluation of a patient with hyperlipidemia, particularly with regard to deciding whether therapeutic intervention is warranted for the prevention of CAD and its complications.

Occasionally, patients have marked *hypertriglyceridemia* and *hyperchylomicronemia* (triglyceride levels greater than 1,000 mg/dL), pancreatitis, eruptive xanthomas, and lipemia retinalis. Coexistence of familial hypertriglyceridemia or familial combined hyperlipidemia with obesity, uremia, untreated diabetes mellitus, chronic alcoholism, or the use of corticosteroids, thiazide diuretics, or estrogens can result in this syndrome. The chylomicronemia syndrome requires immediate treatment with elimination of dietary fat, nasogastric suction when severe, and treatment of the secondary causes. Prevention is the primary means to avoid recurrences, and patients with primary hypertriglyceridemia often receive lipid-lowering agents prophylactically (7).

Decreased Lipoprotein Lipase-Mediated Triglyceride Catabolism

LPL is the rate-limiting enzyme for the uptake and storage of triglyceride by adipose or muscle tissue and for the processing of triglyceride-rich lipoproteins to chylomicrons and VLDL remnants. In patients with the autosomal-recessive trait of *apo C-II deficiency*, LPL activity is normal but marked hypertriglyceridemia is present. In contrast, in the more commonly encountered (yet also rare) autosomal-recessive syndrome of *familial LPL deficiency*, marked hypertriglyceridemia and chylomicronemia are both evident and LPL activity is absent. The type I phenotypic pattern is more likely to occur in patients with the familial form of LPL deficiency, rather than in those with apo C-II deficiency; yet both conditions manifest in childhood with episodes of eruptive xanthomas and with the acute abdominal pain of pancreatitis.

Most adult patients who have an acquired impairment in LPL function have moderately severe type 1 diabetes mellitus, hypothyroidism, end-stage renal disease, or dysgammaglobulinemia or are receiving corticosteroids or thiazide diuretics. The severity of the lipoprotein abnormality seems to be directly related to the decrease in LPL activity in postheparin plasma and adipose tissue.

The hypertriglyceridemia can be controlled by restriction of dietary fat and substitution of carbohydrates or medium-chain triglycerides as energy sources. Effective treatment of diabetes mellitus with diet, insulin, or an oral agent usually normalizes LPL activity and plasma triglyceride levels within several months. Similar beneficial changes are seen after treatment of hypothyroidism or of uremia.

LPL also plays a role in the formation of HDL_2 (see Normal Physiology of Lipoprotein Transport). LPL appears to mediate the increase in HDL_2 seen in endurance-trained athletes (45) and in patients with primary hypercholesterolemia treated with colestipol. Hence, diseases associated with abnormalities in LPL often have concomitant reductions in HDL cholesterol.

Defective Remnant Lipoprotein Catabolism and Dysbetalipoproteinemia

Excessive accumulation of lipoprotein remnants in plasma is usually caused by a defect in their removal as a result of an autosomal-recessive derangement in the structure of apo E (12). *Apo E3*, the predominant form of apo E in the normal population, is absent in patients with the classic form of dysbetalipoproteinemia (type III hyperlipoproteinemia). The mutation causing this syndrome results in the occurrence of an abnormal form of apo E. Of the 1% of people who are homozygous for this condition, only 1% to 2% exhibit hyperlipoproteinemia clinically.

Dysbetalipoproteinemia (remnant removal disease or broad-β disease) has served as a prototype for the study of remnant lipoprotein metabolism. It appears that several defects in lipoprotein metabolism are required before excessive accumulation of IDL and of cholesterol-enriched β-VLDL can occur. The diagnosis is suggested by the initial findings of increased levels of β-VLDL (rather than pre-β-VLDL) and similarly elevated plasma concentrations of cholesterol and triglyceride. It is made more likely by the finding of an abnormally cholesterol-rich VLDL fraction (ratio of VLDL cholesterol to VLDL triglyceride greater than 0.42). The presence of tuberous and planar xanthomas (Fig. 82.3) is highly characteristic of the disorder. Definitive diagnosis, however, requires analysis of VLDL to demonstrate the absence of apo E3. A strong association between this lipoprotein disorder and atherosclerosis of the coronary arteries and peripheral vessels has been reported, and vasculopathy appears to diminish during treatment.

The accumulation of remnants in plasma is also found in certain patients with hypothyroidism, end-stage renal disease, or liver disease. The latter disorders are associated with an increase in the activity of the enzyme hepatic lipase, suggesting that a relationship may exist between this enzyme and the catabolism of remnant lipoproteins by the liver.

Increased Cholesterol Synthesis

The accumulation of cholesterol-rich LDL can occur as a result of an increased input of cholesterol into the plasma from dietary or endogenous sources. The latter occurs because of an increase in HMG-CoA reductase activity and enhanced synthesis of cholesterol, or as a consequence of a primary genetic increase in the hepatic synthesis of apo B and cholesterol. The presence of apo B-enriched VLDL suggests a genetic disorder of overproduction of apo B, compared with the overproduction of VLDL triglyceride in familial hypertriglyceridemia.

The overproduction of apo B-containing LDL and VLDL leads to an increased propensity for the development of atherosclerosis (2). Moreover, the coexistence of obesity promotes the overproduction of apo B-enriched VLDL and cholesterol in these individuals. Finally, the augmented intake of dietary cholesterol usually contributes to the hypercholesterolemia that is characteristic of these patients.

Primary (sporadic) forms of hypercholesterolemia, with a genetic defect in the steps controlling the rate of hepatic synthesis of cholesterol from acetate, lead to an overproduction of cholesterol and resultant hypercholesterolemia. Usually, dietary therapy involving an increase in polyunsaturated fat and a reduction in sucrose and simple carbohydrates is helpful in the treatment of these

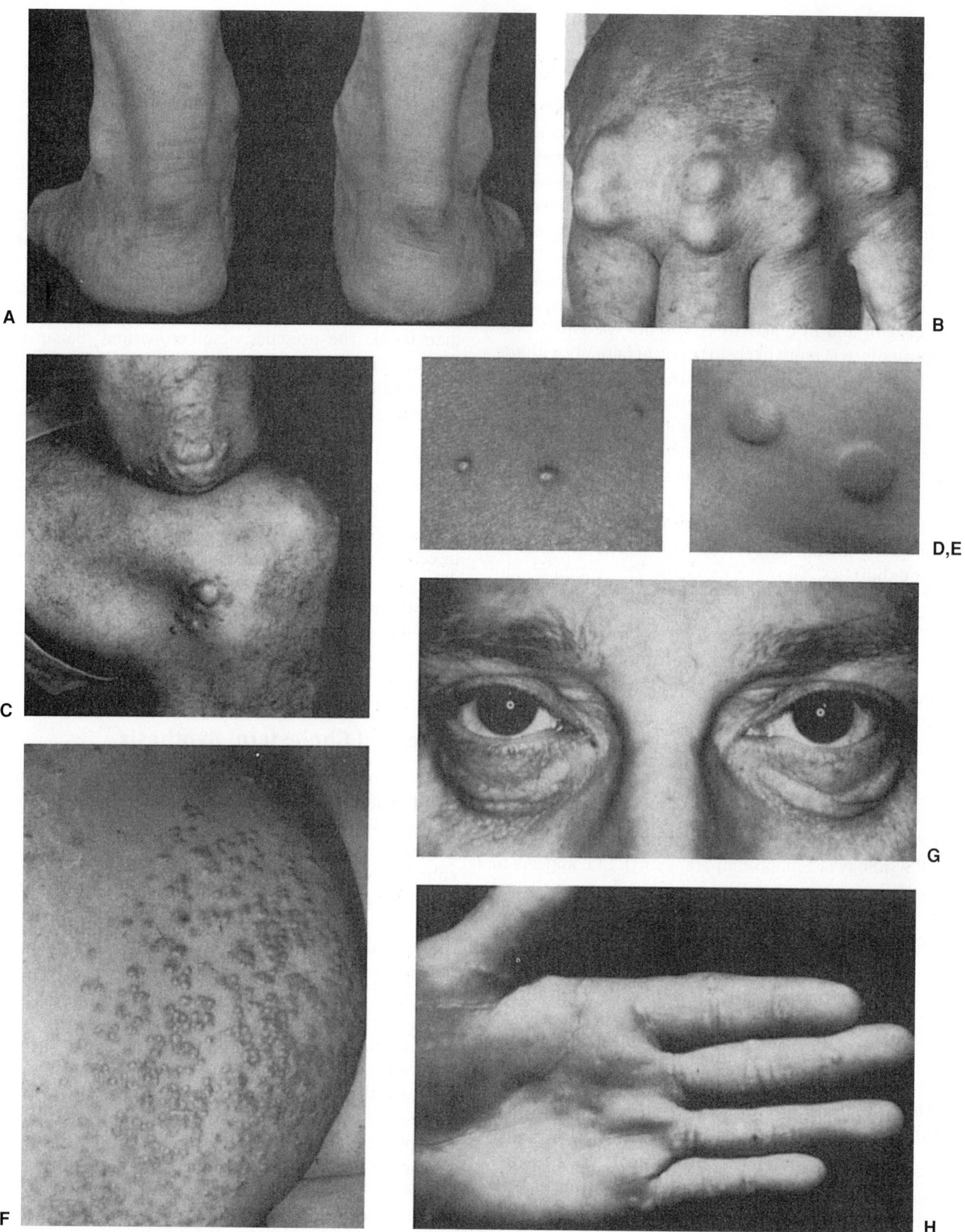

FIGURE 82.3. Dermatologic manifestations of lipid disorders. **A:** Tendinous xanthomas. **B:** Tuberous xanthomas. **C:** Tuberous xanthomas. **D:** Eruptive xanthomas. **E:** Planar xanthomas. **F:** Eruptive xanthomas. **G:** Planar xanthomas on eyelids (xanthelasma). **H:** Planar xanthomas confined to palm creases (xanthoma striata palmaris).

disorders; less often, drugs are required. Hypercholesterolemia in obese hyperinsulinemic patients with type 2 diabetes mellitus is decreased by hypocaloric diets and the return of body weight toward normal. In patients who are noncompliant with dietary measures, therapy with cholestyramine, nicotinic acid, or HMG-CoA reductase inhibitors (commonly known as statins) is usually effective in lowering plasma cholesterol levels.

Defective Removal of Low-Density Lipoproteins

Isolated primary elevations of plasma LDL or combined elevations of LDL and VLDL can be seen in affected members of families with familial hypercholesterolemia (1). Although the cells of some homozygous patients may be totally lacking in identifiable LDL (apo B-E) receptors, in other patients, these receptors are present but functionally defective. Individuals who are heterozygous for familial hypercholesterolemia exhibit more than a 50% reduction in LDL receptor number or a 50% defect in receptor-mediated catabolism; commonly their plasma levels of LDL cholesterol are greater than 400 mg/dL, regardless of their level of cholesterol synthesis. In homozygous patients, plasma levels of LDL cholesterol may reach 1,000 mg/dL (7). Documentation of abnormal receptor binding in cultures of skin fibroblasts is necessary for the precise diagnosis of individuals with familial hypercholesterolemia.

Although primary causes (including familial combined hyperlipoproteinemia) predominate, secondary causes of increased concentrations of LDL cholesterol occur in patients with hypothyroidism, nephrotic syndrome, multiple myeloma, obstructive liver disease, or porphyria, and in patients who have ingested excessive amounts of dietary cholesterol. The primary forms are associated with marked susceptibility to CAD and a high frequency of complications associated with early mortality, such as MI, stroke, and peripheral vascular disease. The hallmark of these disorders is the tendon xanthomas that often affect the Achilles tendon or the extensor tendons of the forearm and hand (Fig. 82.3). Patients with secondary hypercholesterolemia appear not to develop atherosclerosis at as high a rate as people with the primary disorders.

COMMON SECONDARY DISORDERS OF LIPID METABOLISM

Several disease states are commonly associated with increased plasma levels of VLDL, increased levels of both VLDL and LDL, or decreased levels of HDL cholesterol.

Diabetes Mellitus

Abnormalities in fat transport are often noted in patients with diabetes mellitus and are related to abnormalities in insulin action or insulin availability that lead to increased production or decreased removal of plasma lipoproteins. For example, patients with type 2 diabetes mellitus who are often obese, hyperinsulinemic, and insulin resistant exhibit both an enhanced production and reduced plasma clearance of triglycerides. These patients also have abnormalities in HDL cholesterol. In contrast, the hypertriglyceridemia that occurs in patients with insulin-dependent (type 1) diabetes mellitus is caused by markedly reduced levels of LPL activity, because insulin is required for normal synthesis of the enzyme (7). The diabetic lipemia syndrome is characterized by low or absent levels of LPL in the plasma and tissues of these patients. Although the underlying enzyme deficiency can be reversed after insulin repletion, normalization of the lipoprotein abnormalities can take several months.

In the treated diabetic patient, variability in plasma levels of lipoprotein lipids is primarily related to dietary factors, the amount and distribution of body fat, physical activity, and the degree of glycemic control. If glucose tolerance deteriorates because of inadequate insulin administration or increased insulin resistance, severe hypertriglyceridemia may ensue and alter the concentrations of other classes of lipoproteins. In well-treated type 1 diabetic patients, plasma levels of HDL cholesterol are increased; in contrast, even patients with well-treated type 2 diabetes usually have low HDL cholesterol levels. Regardless of the specific treatment or type of diabetes mellitus, women ordinarily exhibit higher plasma levels of VLDL triglyceride and LDL cholesterol, and lower levels of HDL cholesterol, than do diabetic men (23). This may explain the increased prevalence of atherosclerosis in diabetic women and the disappearance of the usual preponderance of atherosclerotic disease in men compared with premenopausal women (13).

Hypercholesterolemia, with increased plasma concentrations of LDL cholesterol and apo B, also can occur in patients with either type 1 or type 2 diabetes mellitus and is usually induced by diet. Intensive therapy with diet, exercise, and insulin usually normalizes lipoprotein levels, unless a genetic lipoprotein disorder coexists.

Hyperlipidemia in the patient with diabetes mellitus increases the risk for the major complications of atherosclerosis, CAD, cerebrovascular disease, and peripheral vascular disease. The severity of peripheral vascular disease is associated with the lipoprotein abnormalities in diabetic women. Whether treatment of the lipid abnormalities in diabetic patients will decrease their risk for CAD and other arteriosclerotic complications remains to be proven, but it can be recommended based on the known efficacy of treatment in other populations.

Chronic Uremia and Treatment with Dialysis

Many patients with chronic uremia have increased plasma levels of VLDL triglycerides and decreased levels of HDL cholesterol (24). These abnormalities persist during maintenance hemodialysis or peritoneal dialysis. The accelerated atherosclerosis observed in white men undergoing long-term hemodialysis, which is not seen in their African American counterparts, appears to be related to the abnormal composition of HDL_2 cholesterol in the plasma of white men. A sedentary lifestyle, obesity, high-fat diets, or treatment with corticosteroids, β-blockers, or androgens worsens the lipoprotein profiles in these patients, and effective reversal of these secondary causes improves the lipid profile (24).

Hypothyroidism

Adequate levels of thyroid hormone appear to be necessary for the homeostatic maintenance of lipoprotein physiology. Decreases in LDL receptor function, abnormalities in LPL and hepatic lipase-mediated metabolism of triglycerides and HDL, and reduced lecithin-cholesterol acyl transferase (LCAT) activity have been demonstrated in some patients with hypothyroidism. Consequently, increased plasma levels of VLDL, IDL, and LDL, and reduced levels of HDL cholesterol have all been reported in patients with this disease. Treatment with thyroid hormone improves LDL receptor function, increases the activity and function of LPL and LCAT, and normalizes lipoprotein profiles.

Other Common Secondary Causes of Hyperlipidemia

Patients with the *nephrotic syndrome* commonly lose apo C-II in the urine, thus decreasing LPL-mediated triglyceride clearance. The hypoalbuminemia that accompanies the nephrotic syndrome increases hepatic VLDL synthesis, thereby elevating plasma levels of VLDL triglyceride and LDL cholesterol. Treatment of the disease that has caused the nephrotic syndrome usually corrects the lipoprotein abnormalities, but drug therapy and a low-fat diet may be required. Reports suggest that statin therapy can ameliorate the nephrosis independently of its benefit in lowering LDL cholesterol levels (46).

Hypercortisolemia of endogenous or exogenous origin increases hepatic synthesis of VLDL, LDL, or both. Kidney transplant recipients treated with high dosages of corticosteroids often exhibit increased plasma levels of both VLDL and LDL as well as reduced levels of HDL cholesterol. The atherosclerosis that develops in such patients is probably related to these lipid abnormalities, which should be treated accordingly.

Obesity, alcohol ingestion, and *androgen administration* tend to increase hepatic lipoprotein synthesis but have different effects on levels of HDL cholesterol and LDL cholesterol. In obese people, plasma levels of VLDL triglyceride and LDL cholesterol are increased, whereas those of HDL are decreased. Mild alcohol ingestion (up to 2 oz/day) increases levels of VLDL triglyceride and HDL cholesterol but lowers levels of LDL cholesterol. Exogenous androgens raise levels of LDL cholesterol and lower HDL cholesterol levels.

Diseases affecting the liver, such as hepatitis or cholelithiasis, alter lipoprotein metabolism. Diseases causing an obstruction in the hepatobiliary system tend to elevate plasma LDL, IDL, and remnant lipoproteins and cause abnormal lipoproteins (Lp X) to accumulate in plasma.

Inflammatory processes usually lower levels of HDL and LDL cholesterol and raise VLDL, depending on the nutritional state of the patient.

Some *drugs* used to treat hypertension, such as thiazide diuretics and β-adrenergic blockers, may cause a modest increase in serum lipids. The benefit of these classes of antihypertensives in reducing the risk of coronary disease is generally greater than their adverse impact on lipids, and in most patients with lipid disorders their use is not contraindicated.

Hyperlipidemia occurs in patients with *systemic lupus erythematosus* or *dysgammaglobulinemia*. This may be related to interactions among amyloid protein, certain immunoglobulin fractions, and various steps in the lipoprotein cascade.

Table 82.6 lists several exogenous and endogenous factors that affect plasma levels of HDL cholesterol.

TABLE 82.6 Factors That Affect High-Density Lipoprotein Cholesterol Levels

Increase	*Decrease*
Exercise	Androgens (male sex, drugs)
Oral estrogens (female sex)	In males, puberty
Alcohol (moderate)	In females, menopause
Familial (hyperalphalipoproteinemia)	Obesity
	Hypertriglyceridemia
Leanness	Type 2 diabetes mellitus
Antihyperlipidemic drugs: nicotinic acid, colestipol, clofibrate, statins, gemfibrozil	Familial hypoalphalipoproteinemia (Tangier disease)
	Cigarettes
Insulin	Sedentary lifestyle
Intravenous heparin	Probucol
	Uremia
	Vegetarian diet
	Progestogens

CLINICAL MANIFESTATIONS OF LIPOPROTEIN DISORDERS

Adverse clinical sequelae of the lipoprotein disorders most commonly manifest as disorders of the vascular, dermatologic, and gastrointestinal systems. Table 82.5 outlines the clinical manifestations associated with each of the major disorders of lipoprotein metabolism.

Vascular

As discussed previously, increased levels of total cholesterol, LDL cholesterol, apo B-enriched lipoproteins, oxidized LDL, and Lp(a) and decreased levels of HDL cholesterol, HDL_2, and apo A-I contribute to the development of atherosclerotic disease. The earlier the onset of symptomatic disease of the coronary, cerebral, or peripheral vasculature, the more likely it is that a lipoprotein abnormality or another major risk factor (cigarette smoking, hypertension, diabetes) is present (13). In the most severe form of hypercholesterolemia, *homozygous familial hypercholesterolemia*, plasma levels of total cholesterol vary from 600 to 1,200 mg/dL, CAD generally develops in childhood, and very few patients survive past 30 years of age. In *heterozygotes*, plasma levels of total cholesterol vary from about 270 to 550 mg/dL and the time of onset of CAD varies between early adulthood and late middle age, with approximately 50% of men becoming symptomatic by age 50 years and 50% of women by age 60 years. Patients with *monogenic familial combined hyperlipoproteinemia* exhibit increased levels of VLDL, LDL, or both, as well as abnormalities in HDL, apo A-I, and apo B; most patients manifest symptoms of CAD by age 60 years. Individuals with *familial dysbetalipoproteinemia* develop premature peripheral vascular disease and CAD at about equal rates, with the mean age at onset in both men and women being about 40 years. Such patients seem to be especially responsive to therapy. Individuals with *monogenic familial hypertriglyceridemia* or with *fasting chylomicronemia* do not appear to be at increased risk for CAD unless other risk factors for atherosclerosis are also present.

Dermatologic

Xanthomas may occur in any of the hyperlipidemias; however, they are present in a minority of hyperlipidemic patients. They occur with increasing frequency as the plasma lipid levels rise. They are present predominantly in the primary forms of hyperlipoproteinemia: familial hypercholesterolemia, familial dysbetalipoproteinemia, and familial LPL deficiency. Xanthomas are cutaneous or subcutaneous papules, plaques, or nodules characterized histopathologically by localized collections of lipid-laden histiocytes (foam cells). The presence or absence of xanthomas should always be noted. If present, their appearance can provide useful information about the nature of the underlying lipid disorder (Table 82.5). Unless tendons (especially the Achilles tendon) are palpated, the tendon thickening that is characteristic of tendon xanthomas may be missed. Xanthomas are divided morphologically into several types:

1. *Tendinous* (Fig. 82.3A)—firm subcutaneous masses that arise in tendons and occasionally in ligaments, fascia, or periosteum. They characteristically move in concert with the associated tendon and can appear as diffuse thickenings of the tendon. They most often occur on the Achilles tendons and the extensor tendons of the hands, knees, and elbows. The overlying skin is normal in color.

2. *Tuberous* (Fig. 82.3B and C)—soft cutaneous and subcutaneous nodules that may harden with age and increasing fibrosis. Occasionally, they occur as superficial extensions of tendinous xanthomas. They can also form from the confluence of eruptive xanthomas, and an intermediate stage is called tuberoeruptive xanthomas. They occur most often on extensor surfaces and areas subjected to trauma, such as the elbows, the knees, the dorsa of the hands, the heels, and the buttocks. The overlying epidermis can be normal in color or have a yellow or orange hue.

3. *Eruptive* (Fig. 82.3D and F)—small (1 to 4 mm) cutaneous papules, that tend to appear in crops, often coincident with an abrupt rise in plasma triglyceride levels. Compared with the other types of xanthomas, they contain more inflammatory cells, free fatty acids, and triglycerides and fewer foam cells and cholesterol esters. They most often occur over pressure areas, such as the buttocks, parts of the trunk, elbows, and knees. They often have a yellow center and red halo. The lesions will disappear in concert with the reduction of triglyceride levels (generally when values are lower than 1,000 mg/dL).

4. *Planar* (Fig. 82.3E, G, and H)—flat, slightly elevated cutaneous lesions that occur most often in skin folds and scars but can be more widely distributed. When present on the eyelids, they are called *xanthelasma*. When located on the palms, they are called palmar xanthomas, and when confined to the palmar creases, *xanthoma striata palmaris*. They tend to be yellow or yellow-brown.

Hypercholesterolemia is associated with tendinous, planar, and tuberous xanthomas. Severe hypertriglyceridemia and chylomicronemia are associated with eruptive and occasionally tuberoeruptive or tuberous xanthomas. Palmar xanthomas are characteristic of familial dysbetalipoproteinemia and florid obstructive liver disease. Planar xanthomas on the body or palms in the presence of a type II lipid profile suggest homozygous monogenic familial hypercholesterolemia. The presence of tendinous or tuberous xanthomas or premature xanthelasma with a type II lipid profile suggests either heterozygous or homozygous monogenic familial hypercholesterolemia, as opposed to the polygenic or nongenetic forms. Tendon xanthomas are found in one-third to one-half of heterozygotes, whereas tuberous xanthomas are seen most often in patients with familial dysbetalipoproteinemia.

Occasionally, xanthomas appear in the absence of a hyperlipidemic state. For example, xanthelasma occur commonly in normolipidemic older individuals and in nonwhites, and planar xanthomas can occur in patients with lymphoma, leukemia, or myeloma. Studies in normolipidemic individuals with xanthelasma have revealed abnormalities in apo B and E suggestive of familial dysbetalipoproteinemia and/or increased levels of LDL apo B (47), suggesting that these individuals may be at an increased risk of developing atherosclerosis.

Differences exist in the responses to treatment of the various hyperlipidemia-associated xanthomas. Tendon xanthomas are the most resistant to treatment and, in practice, seldom disappear. In contrast, eruptive and planar xanthomas can disappear within a few weeks after plasma lipid levels return to normal.

Gastrointestinal

As many as 35% to 55% of patients with fasting chylomicronemia experience episodes of recurrent abdominal pain. Symptoms are ordinarily associated with marked elevations of plasma triglyceride concentrations (>1,000 to 2,000 mg/dL). Abdominal pain may be so severe that it prompts unnecessary surgery, particularly if the lipid disorder is not suspected. The pain is often associated with pancreatitis, although the responsible pathogenetic mechanism is not well understood. Routine serum amylase determinations are often subject to technical artifacts when hyperlipidemia is present because of the presence of an amylase-inhibiting factor that may or may not be triglyceride. In such cases, a more reliable estimate of the serum amylase value can be obtained by determining amylase levels on serial dilutions, until the value obtained no longer changes with further dilution. Another cause of abdominal pain may be rapid hepatic or splenic enlargement with capsular distension from triglyceride deposition in reticuloendothelial cells. Often the cause is unclear. Gastrointestinal symptoms other than abdominal pain, such as nausea, vomiting, borborygmi, and diarrhea, also occur.

Other Clinical Associations

Other clinical concomitants of hyperlipidemia include premature arcus corneae (grayish-white corneal ring caused by lipid droplets) in hypercholesterolemia (elevated LDL); aortic stenosis in homozygous monogenic familial hypercholesterolemia; Achilles tendinitis in heterozygous monogenic familial hypercholesterolemia; obesity, glucose intolerance, hyperinsulinemia, hyperuricemia, and perhaps cholelithiasis in association with hypertriglyceridemia and elevated VLDL; recurrent polyarthralgias, arthritis, tenosynovitis, and siccalike syndromes in hypertriglyceridemia (elevated VLDL) or hypercholesterolemia (elevated LDL); and lipemia retinalis (cream-colored retinal vessels) in chylomicronemia (evident when plasma triglycerides rise above 3,000 mg/dL; obvious when they exceed 10,000 mg/dL).

DIAGNOSIS

Indications for Screening and Evaluation

Over the years there has been disagreement about the optimal, cost-effective approach to the identification of hyperlipidemic patients at high risk for CAD (48–50). Some authorities believe that routine screening of healthy young adults who have no CAD risk factors, family history, or clinical evidence of CAD is unwarranted because the benefits of case finding may be outweighed by the long-term risks of treatment. There is, however, a general consensus that screening is important, although there is some disagreement still about which populations should be targeted. The most widely used guidelines for case findings are those issued by the ATP of the NCEP (44). The NCEP emphasizes LDL as the primary target of cholesterol-lowering therapy, the role of the clinical approach to primary prevention of CAD, and dietary therapy as the initial treatment, with hypolipidemic drug therapy reserved for patients at high risk for CAD. These guidelines, however, emphasize CAD risk status as a major determinant for the type and intensity of treatment, pay more attention to HDL as a risk factor, and underscore the importance of including physical activity and weight loss as components of dietary therapy. With regard to assigning risk factor status, the NCEP report places patients with existing CAD and those with diabetes mellitus or other atherosclerotic disease at highest risk, maintaining lower target levels of LDL cholesterol in these patients. The report uses Framingham projections to predict CAD risk over a 10-year span and targets patients with the metabolic syndrome (see Treatment, General Approach) for aggressive intervention. The panel also continues to recommend that HDL cholesterol greater than 60 mg/dL be considered a negative risk factor and that HDL cholesterol levels be used in the decision making for drug therapy.

The panel continues to recommend that levels of total cholesterol should be measured in all adults 20 years of age or older at least once every 5 years, assuming that blood cholesterol levels are lower than 200 mg/dL, and that HDL should be measured at the same time if accurate results are available (see Laboratory Evaluation). An HDL level of less than 40 mg/dL is considered to be a low value. Measurements of total cholesterol and HDL for screening

TABLE 82.7 LDL Cholesterol Goals and Cutpoints for Therapeutic Lifestyle Changes (TLC)[a] and Drug Therapy in Different Risk Categories

Risk Category	*LDL Goal (mg/dL)*	*Level at which to Initiate TLC (mg/dL)*	*Level at which to Consider Drug Therapy (mg/dL)*
CAD or CAD risk equivalents (10-year risk >20%)	<100 <70 in high-risk patients (optional; see text)	≥100	≥130 (>100 [optional; see text] should consider drug treatment)[b]
2+ Risk factors (10-year risk ≥20%)	<130	≥130	10-year risk 10%–20%: ≥130 10-year risk <10%; ≥160
0–1 Risk factor[c]	<160	≥160	≥190 (160–189: LDL-lowering drug optimal)

CAD, coronary artery disease; LDL, low-density lipoprotein.
[a]Therapeutic lifestyle changes include diet, weight control, increased activity, and smoking cessation.
[b]Some authorities recommend use of LDL-lowering drugs in this category if an LDL cholesterol level of <100 mg/dL cannot be achieved by therapeutic lifestyle changes. Others prefer use of drugs that primarily modify triglycerides and high-density lipoprotein (e.g., nicotinic acid, fibrate). Clinical judgment also may call for deferring drug therapy in this subcategory.
[c]Almost all people with 0–1 risk factor have a 10-year risk of CAD that is <10%; consequently, the 10-year risk assessment in people with 0–1 risk factor is not necessary.
Modified from the Executive Summary of the Third Report of the National Cholesterol Education Program (NCEP) Expert Panel on Detection, Evaluation, and Treatment of High Blood Cholesterol in Adults (Adult Treatment Panel III). JAMA 2001;285:2486.

purposes can be obtained from nonfasting people. However, final classification of abnormal lipid profiles requires lipid determinations in subjects who have fasted overnight. The NCEP classifies individuals by serum levels of total, LDL, and HDL cholesterol (Table 82.7). Serum levels of total cholesterol less than 200 mg/dL are considered *desirable blood cholesterol*; levels between 200 and 239 mg/dL, *borderline-high blood cholesterol*; and levels of 240 mg/dL or higher, *high blood cholesterol*. Data from numerous epidemiologic studies reveal that the relationships between serum levels of total (or LDL) cholesterol and CAD risk are continuous and that CAD risk at a cholesterol value of 240 mg/dL is almost double that at 200 mg/dL and rises rapidly at levels above 240 mg/dL. Total cholesterol levels of 240 mg/dL or more correspond to the uppermost 20% of cholesterol values in the entire population 20 years of age and older. Patients with levels of total serum cholesterol between 200 and 239 mg/dL and either an HDL cholesterol concentration lower than 40 mg/dL, known CAD or diabetes mellitus, or two or more known risk factors for CAD (Table 82.2) are considered to have high blood cholesterol values.

Although there is a consensus on targets for lipid values and intervention in those with the highest CAD risk (e.g., diabetes mellitus) or known CAD, there exists a difference of opinion regarding when to begin screening for lipid disorders in the adult population. The U.S. Preventive Services Task Force (USPSTF) recommends that screening begin at age 35 years for men and at age 45 years for women, and that individuals age 20 years and older be screened only if they have associated risk factors for CAD (50,51). The USPSTF limits screening to measurement of total cholesterol and HDL, and finds no evidence supporting the routine measurement of triglycerides and, by extension, LDL for screening purposes. An older American College of Physicians (ACP) report did not support routine screening in young adult men (age 20 to 35 years), premenopausal women (age 20 to 45 years), or persons older than 65 years of age (52). It should be noted that the NCEP guidelines have been endorsed by more than 40 medical and health care organizations, including the American College of Cardiology, American Academy of Family Physicians, American Medical Association, American College of Preventive Medicine, and American Heart Association (AHA) (53,54).

The practitioner must decide, in consultation with his or her patients, which recommendations to follow. It is clear, however, that screening is indicated and that most patients with hyperlipidemia should be treated.

Evaluation of the Patient with Hypercholesterolemia

Once a patient is found to have a high blood cholesterol level or physical stigmata of hypercholesterolemia (e.g., dermatologic signs), decisions regarding possible diet, drug, or other therapy are made after a more detailed lipoprotein analysis, including measurements of triglyceride levels on a blood specimen obtained after an overnight fast, calculation of the LDL cholesterol level, and determination of other CAD risk factors. The updated NCEP guidelines adjust the classification for LDL cholesterol levels as follows: LDL cholesterol levels greater or equal to 190 mg/dL are considered very high; 160 to 189 mg/dL, high; 130 to 159 mg/dL, borderline high; 100 to 129 mg/dL, near or above optimal; and less than 100 mg/dL, optimal. In patients with known CAD, diabetes mellitus, or two or more major CAD risk factors (Table 82.2), and LDL cholesterol levels between 130 and 159 mg/dL are considered *high risk*. The NCEP considers an HDL level lower than 40 mg/dL to be an independent risk factor for CAD. Therefore, decisions regarding both the implementation and the goals of therapy are based not on ratios of LDL (or total) cholesterol to HDL cholesterol but on absolute levels of LDL and HDL cholesterol. Such decisions are also influenced by the presence or absence of other CAD risk factors.

Triglycerides

The current NCEP guidelines classify fasting triglyceride levels lower than 150 mg/dL as normal levels, those between 150 and 199 mg/dL as *borderline high*, those between 200 and 499 mg/dL as high, and those greater than or equal to 500 mg/dL as very high. There is a complex link between hypertriglyceridemia and CAD, which is explained in part by the association between high triglycerides and low HDL and/or unusually atherogenic forms of LDL. Moreover, elevated triglycerides often reflect increased triglyceride-rich remnant lipoproteins that have atherogenic potential. There is disagreement about the usefulness of measurement of triglyceride levels in the screening of healthy people.

Measurement of plasma levels of total cholesterol, HDL cholesterol, and fasting triglyceride concentrations and calculation of the level of LDL cholesterol are desirable when abnormalities are detected on screening or conditions coexist that could cause secondary abnormalities in lipoprotein metabolism (Table 82.4).

Laboratory Evaluation

Plasma or serum levels of total cholesterol are not appreciably influenced by acute dietary intake and therefore can be obtained from patients in the nonfasting state and at any time of the day. There is considerable biologic variability (6%) and laboratory variability (3%) in repeated measurements of total cholesterol in a given individual (51,55). Therefore, to be within 10% of the true value, two measurements are necessary. It is also important to obtain blood for cholesterol measurements from a nonstressed patient and to send the blood for analysis to a reliable laboratory.

Levels of total (and LDL) cholesterol fall during the first few days after an MI (55), so cholesterol determinations either should be made within 24 hours after a severe acute MI (when they are still valid) or should be postponed until 3 to 4 weeks after recovery. Fasting triglyceride (and VLDL) levels tend to rise slowly after an MI, peaking at 3 to 4 weeks and returning to baseline by 8 to 12 weeks. Therefore, triglyceride levels should be obtained either within 24 hours after the acute event or after 8 to 12 weeks.

The *determination of HDL cholesterol* is the measurement most subject to laboratory error. Again, there is considerable biologic variability (7.5%) and laboratory variability (6%) in repeated measurements of HDL in a given individual (51,55). To be within 10% to 15% of the true value, two to three measurements of HDL are necessary. Such measures to enhance validity are important because there is a relatively narrow range of HDL cholesterol values within which even small differences are prognostically important. For example, a reduction in HDL cholesterol of 5 mg/dL—from 40 to 35 mg/dL—increases the risk for CAD by approximately 25%. HDL levels are unreliable when triglyceride concentrations exceed 400 mg/dL. Under such circumstances, the plasma or serum should be ultrafiltered. If this is required, the clinician should consult the laboratory.

In the nonfasting state, HDL levels are 5% to 10% lower than in the fasting state and therefore may slightly overestimate the risk of CAD. However, for screening purposes, nonfasting levels are acceptable.

Because *triglyceride levels* are 25% to 30% higher in the nonfasting state, it is important that triglyceride measurements be made only in fasting patients.

Calculation of LDL Level

Measurements of HDL and triglyceride levels allow one to calculate the LDL cholesterol level (provided the triglyceride concentration is less than 400 mg/dL) by the following formula: $\text{LDL-C} = \text{TC} - (\text{TG}/5 + \text{HDL-C})$, where LDL-C is the LDL cholesterol level, TC is the plasma level of total cholesterol, TG is the fasting plasma triglyceride level, and HDL-C is the level of HDL cholesterol.

Observation of a fasting plasma sample that has been left undisturbed overnight in a refrigerator at 39.2°F (4°C) is indicated in the presence of a significantly elevated fasting plasma triglyceride level. Increased levels of total (or LDL) cholesterol do not affect the appearance of plasma, whereas hypertriglyceridemia associated with increased levels of VLDL imparts uniform turbidity to plasma, and hypertriglyceridemia associated with chylomicronemia is characterized by a creamy supernatant fraction that floats on the top of plasma.

A marked abnormality in plasma lipid concentrations, especially marked hypertriglyceridemia (greater than 2,000 mg/dL), can affect the validity of other laboratory tests. Marked hypertriglyceridemia has an inhibitory effect on the plasma amylase assay, interferes with the measurement of liver enzymes (aspartate aminotransferase, alanine aminotransferase) and calcium by autoanalyzer, and causes artifactual reductions in the serum concentration of molecules restricted to the aqueous phase (e.g., sodium). Ultracentrifugation of plasma, with the removal of chylomicrons, permits these measurements to be performed accurately; but sometimes serial dilutions of the plasma are necessary, particularly for the measurement of amylase.

Clinical Evaluation

Clinical data contribute substantially to the diagnosis of specific lipoprotein disorders and to decisions about treatment when abnormalities are found. History, physical examination, and indicated laboratory evaluation are required to rule out secondary causes of hyperlipidemia (Table 82.4). A positive family history, the presence of premature atherosclerotic disease, and the presence of specific dermatologic manifestations may permit the diagnosis of a primary form of hyperlipoproteinemia (Table 82.5). Assessment of the patient's family history and cardiovascular status is also important for risk stratification.

If the initial laboratory and clinical evaluations do not clarify an apparent disorder of lipid metabolism, or if the disorder is severe, referral to a lipid disorders clinic or to a specialist in endocrinology and metabolism is indicated. Such specialists can perform (or readily obtain) and interpret more sophisticated tests, such as ultracentrifugal quantification of lipoprotein levels, apoprotein measurement, receptor analysis, and determination of LPL activity. They may also assist in the evaluation of family members, so that the presence of a genetic disorder can be accurately diagnosed. Referral should also be considered for patients who are refractory to lifestyle and pharmacologic management strategies. The Lipid Metabolism Branch of the National Heart, Lung and Blood Institute (National Institutes of Health, Bethesda, MD 20205) can provide the names of research centers in each geographic area where sophisticated evaluation of lipoprotein abnormalities, consultation services, and experimental forms of therapy are offered.

TREATMENT

General Approach

The first step in the management of a lipoprotein disorder is accurate diagnosis. Causes of secondary lipoprotein disorders should be identified (Table 82.4) and treated. If the cause of a secondary disorder is not reversible, or if a primary disorder exists, treatment may be required that is specifically directed at the abnormal lipoprotein pattern.

Such treatment should be part of the comprehensive management of other coexisting CAD risk factors (e.g., cigarette smoking, hypertension, diabetes mellitus, obesity, inactivity). It probably will require behavioral change on the part of the patient and lifelong management, emphasizing the need for a positive patient–clinician relationship, appropriate patient education, and skill on the part of the clinician in promoting patient compliance (see Chapters 3 and 4). Long-term followup and monitoring of such patients are necessary to enhance compliance, to assess the effectiveness of therapy, and to detect drug toxicity or the effect of concomitant therapy (e.g., diuretics, other antihypertensive agents) on plasma lipids.

Patients without CAD who are classified as having a *desirable total cholesterol level* (less than 200 mg/dL) and an HDL cholesterol level higher than 40 mg/dL are usually instructed on the principles of a prudent diet and healthy lifestyle, educated about CAD risk factors (Table 82.2), and advised to have their total cholesterol level rechecked at least once every 5 years.

Patients with CAD, diabetes, secondary causes of lipid disorders, a total cholesterol level higher than 200 mg/dL, an HDL cholesterol level lower than *40 mg/dL, or risk factors* (Table 82.2) should have a fasting lipid panel performed (fasting total cholesterol, triglycerides, and HDL cholesterol, and calculation of LDL; see previous discussion). *Treatment is then based primarily on LDL cholesterol levels* according to guidelines provided by the NCEP (Table 82.7). The guidelines also emphasize the need to assess CAD risk for patients with more than two risk factors and an LDL cholesterol level between 130 and 159 mg/dL (see National Heart, Lung and Blood Institute website in www.hopkinsbayview.org/PAMreferences for instructions on how to calculate risk according to the Framingham scoring system). Drug therapy is suggested for patients who have a 10-year risk of developing ischemic heart disease of more than 10% (Table 82.7).

For patients with a *borderline high total cholesterol* of 200 to 239 mg/dL, HDL cholesterol greater than 40 mg/dL, and fewer than two risk factors, it is also reasonable to provide education about diet, exercise, and other lifestyle modifications and to recheck the total and HDL cholesterol in 1 to 2 years, in the absence of a fasting lipid profile.

Patients with isolated reductions in HDL cholesterol (less than 40 mg/dL) should be instructed in the value of weight loss, aerobic exercise, and discontinuation of cigarette smoking (see Nonpharmacologic Therapy). Although certain drugs used for treatment of increased levels of LDL cholesterol or of triglycerides may also raise HDL levels, at present no data support their use in the healthy patient whose only lipid abnormality is a reduction in the level of HDL.

Management of hypertriglyceridemia must be individualized. When familial combined hyperlipidemia or familial dysbetalipoproteinemia is diagnosed, specific treatment is required. Patients with fasting triglyceride levels greater than 500 mg/dL sometimes accumulate chylomicrons and develop pancreatitis. The risk becomes substantial when triglyceride levels exceed 1,000 mg/dL. The plasma triglyceride level should therefore be lowered in patients whose triglyceride levels exceed 500 mg/dL. For patients with fasting triglyceride levels in the 200- to 499-mg/dL range, control of LDL cholesterol remains the primary goal but control of triglyceride level becomes a secondary goal. Diet, weight control, and regular exercise should be encouraged. Drug therapy should also be considered if treatment goals are not reached through lifestyle change, especially when CAD, diabetes, or coexistent risk factors (see Table 82.2) are present. The presence of the *metabolic syndrome*, which is associated with a very high risk of CAD, should probably also sway the clinician toward the use of drug therapy if treatment goals cannot be achieved by lifestyle change. The metabolic syndrome (also called metabolic syndrome X or insulin resistance syndrome) is characterized by abdominal obesity (see Chapter 83), low HDL cholesterol (less than 40 mg/dL in men, 50 mg/dL in women), hypertension (130/85 mm Hg or higher), fasting plasma glucose concentration 110 mg/dL or higher, and fasting triglycerides 150 mg/dL or higher. *Treatment goals are defined by a non-HDL cholesterol concentration* (i.e., total cholesterol minus HDL cholesterol) that is 30 mg/dL greater than the treatment goals for LDL cholesterol; that is, less than 190 mg/dL for one or no risk factors, 160 mg/dL for two or more risk factors and 10-year risk greater than 20%, and less than 130 mg/dL for CAD or CAD risk equivalent.

Nonpharmacologic Therapy

Diet

It is now well established that plasma lipid levels can be altered by dietary manipulations (Tables 82.8 and 82.9).

TABLE 82.8 Nutrient Composition of the Therapeutic Lifestyle Changes (TLC) Diet

Nutrient	Recommendation
Saturated fat[a]	<7% of total calories
Polyunsaturated fat	Up to 10% of total calories
Monounsaturated fat	Up to 20% of total calories
Total fat	25%–35% of total calories
Carbohydrate[b]	50%–60% of total calories
Fiber	20–30 mg/d
Protein	Approximately 15% of total calories
Cholesterol	<200 mg/d
Total calories[c]	Balance energy intake and expenditure to maintain desirable body weight, prevent weight gain

[a]Trans fatty acids are another low-density lipoprotein-raising fat that should be kept at a low intake.
[b]Carbohydrates should be derived predominantly from foods rich in complex carbohydrates, including grains, especially whole grains, fruits, and vegetables.
[c]Daily energy expenditure should include at least moderate physical activity (contributing approximately 200 kcal/d).
From the Executive Summary of the Third Report of the National Cholesterol Education Program (NCEP) Expert Panel on Detection, Evaluation, and Treatment of High Blood Cholesterol in Adults (Adult Treatment Panel III). JAMA 2001; 285:2486.

Under strictly controlled conditions (e.g., in a metabolic research unit), increased plasma levels of total (or LDL) cholesterol may be reduced by as much as 30% or more, and levels of triglyceride or VLDL (in the presence of marked elevations) by as much as 80% or more. Fasting chylomicronemia can also be eliminated. Under ambulatory conditions, in which diets tend to be less restrictive and noncompliance more common, reductions in lipid levels are less dramatic. For example, among prospective studies of cholesterol-lowering diets, the decrease in plasma cholesterol averaged 15% (range: 8.5% to 22%).

Single-Diet Approach

The ATP of the NCEP (see www.hopkinsbayview.org/PAMreferences) continues to highlight dietary therapy as the first line of treatment of elevated blood cholesterol levels (Table 82.8). In primary prevention trials to date, dietary therapy has not been associated with decreased all-cause mortality. There is insufficient evidence to support treatment of healthy normolipidemic individuals with restrictive diets. Studies have shown little change in the lipid profiles of healthy subjects with intake of either a high- or a low-cholesterol diet (56). Dietary therapy has more impact in those who are dyslipidemic and have risk factors for CAD. It is now appreciated that one diet can be used to treat all of the common forms of hyperlipoproteinemia (Table 82.8). The classification of diets as Step 1 and Step 2 has been eliminated and replaced with the Therapeutic Lifestyle Changes (TLC) diet. Using the principle of graduated regimen implementation (see Chapter 4), the diet can be introduced in a step-wise fashion. If severe chylomicronemia is present, dietary fat must be more severely restricted (see Cholesterol Reduction).

The AHA and other organizations publish useful booklets on this diet for the patient, physician, and nutritionist (see www.hopkinsbayview.org/PAMreferences). Most patients with hyperlipoproteinemia benefit from referral to a suitably trained dietitian. The TLC diet actually incorporates several nutritional strategies, each of which tends to have a selective effect on plasma lipoprotein levels. It is helpful to consider each strategy separately.

Cholesterol Reduction

The TLC diet to lower serum cholesterol levels (Tables 82.8 and 82.9) is characterized by a restriction of dietary cholesterol to less than 200 mg per day and reductions in daily total and saturated fat intake to less than 35% and 7% of caloric intake, respectively. The total fat allowance can range from 25% to 35% as long as the intake of saturated fats and trans fatty acids is low. The other feature of the TLC diet is encouragement of the consumption of plant stanols/sterols (2 g/day) and soluble fiber (10 to 25 g/day). Caloric allowance is adjusted to ensure loss of excess weight or maintenance of ideal body weight (see Chapter 83). Restrictions in dietary cholesterol and

TABLE 82.9 Dietary Guidelines to Lower Blood Cholesterol

Food	Recommended	Avoid or Use Sparingly
Fish, Shellfish, Poultry, Shrimp, Lean Red Meats		
Up to 6 to 7 oz are recommended per day (limit shrimp to 3 oz)	Fish; skinless chicken, turkey, Cornish hen; very lean cuts of beef, lamb, pork and veal; low-fat lunchmeats with 3 g fat or less per oz; dry beans or tofu may be used as a substitute for fish, poultry, and meat	Any fatty cuts of meat; lunchmeats; sausages; scrapple, bacon; hot dogs; caviar, fish roe; deep-fried meats, fish, and poultry; organ meat; duck; goose
Fats and Oils		
Up to 6 to 7 tsp may be used per day, including fat used in cooking	Unsaturated oils: safflower, sunflower, corn, soybean, sesame, rapeseed (canola); soft margarine with first ingredient a liquid unsaturated oil listed above; 4 to 6 nuts or 3 olives count as 1 teaspoon of oil; mayonnaise; salad dressing made with unsaturated oils listed above (2 teaspoons count as 1 teaspoon oil)	Butter; lard; palm kernel oil; meat fat; salt pork; bacon fat; coconut oil; palm oil; hydrogenated or solid shortenings; gravy; cream sauce; salad dressing made with cream, cheese, or sour cream
Milk and Yogurt		
2 or more cups recommended per day	Skim or 1% milk, including evaporated and powdered milk; buttermilk; nonfat and low-fat yogurt	Whole milk, including evaporated and condensed milk; eggnog; yogurt; cream; sour cream; half and half; coconut milk
Cheese		
1 oz of recommended cheese or ¼ cup cottage cheese may be substituted for 1 oz of fish, poultry, or lean red meat	Low-fat cottage cheese; low-fat cheese with 4 g of fat or less per oz	High-fat cheeses containing more than 4 g of fat per oz
Eggs		
Egg yolks should be limited to 2 per week, including those used in cooking	Egg whites (2 egg whites will substitute for 1 whole egg in recipes); cholesterol-free egg substitutes	Egg yolks in excess of 2 per week
Vegetables and Fruits		
5 or more servings are recommended per day; include at least 1 serving of citrus fruit or other source of vitamin C per day	Fresh, frozen, canned, or dried	Vegetables in cream, cheese, or butter sauces, deep-fried vegetables, french fries
Breads and Cereals		
6 or more servings recommended per day	Loaf bread and bagels (except egg); English muffins, pita bread; most sandwich and dinner rolls; Melba toast; water crackers; soda crackers; rice cakes; rye crisp; matzo, pretzels, breadsticks (made without cheese); all cereals except as noted; pasta (except egg); all grains, including rice, barley, buckwheat, bulgur, corn, millet, rye, and oats	Croissants, biscuits, and other rich rolls; pastries; doughnuts; egg breads; commercial baked products; high-fat crackers; cereals with added oils and coconut, such as granola-type; egg pasta
Desserts and Sweets		
Foods high in sugar are best used in small amounts; they should be used infrequently by persons with high triglycerides or excess weight	Fruit; sugar, jelly; cocoa powder, gelatin, Italian ice; frozen fruit bars; frozen low-fat yogurt; pudding made with skim milk; angel food cake; sherbet; sorbet; low-fat cookies; homemade baked products made with skim or low-fat milk, egg whites, and small amounts of unsaturated fat	Chocolate; ice cream; coconut; cream desserts; egg custard; commercial baked products
Miscellaneous	Fat-free broths; air-popped popcorn or popcorn made with small amounts of unsaturated oil; pretzels, nuts (e.g., walnuts) vinegar, spices, herbs, mustard, fat-free salad dressing	Cream or other fatty soups; high-fat snack foods such as potato chips, corn chips, granola bars, microwave popcorn, nondairy creamers, and whipped toppings made with coconut or palm oil

Modified from The Johns Hopkins Physicians Lipid Education Program. 2nd ed. Baltimore: The Johns Hopkins University, 1988.

saturated fats independently contribute to the reduction in plasma cholesterol levels. A modest increase in dietary polyunsaturated fat results in further, although less marked, reduction in plasma cholesterol level.

The two major categories of *polyunsaturated fatty acids* are the omega-6 and omega-3 types. Linoleic acid is the principal *omega-6 fatty acid*; when consumed in large amounts, it can decrease levels of total cholesterol. Lecithin, a phospholipid derived from soybeans, is a widely publicized, popular remedy for hypercholesterolemia and is commonly sold in health food stores. Because it is not absorbed as such from the gastrointestinal tract, any hypocholesterolemic effect probably derives from its high content of linoleic acid. Vegetable oils rich in linoleic acid, such as safflower oil, soybean oil, sunflower oil, and corn oil, are the preferred dietary sources of the omega-6 fatty acids.

The major sources of the *omega-3 fatty acids* are the fish oils. Taken as dietary supplements, high dosages of fish oil lower elevated triglyceride concentrations but do not reduce levels of total or LDL cholesterol. Nevertheless, epidemiologic studies have shown an inverse relationship between the consumption of fish and the risk of adverse cardiac and other cerebrovascular events, in persons with and without ischemic heart disease (57,58). Also, several randomized controlled trials have demonstrated a modest reduction in cardiac events (1% to 3% absolute risk reduction) in patients with documented CAD who were prescribed omega-3 fatty acids (32,59). Side effects are predominantly gastrointestinal (nausea, bloating, flatulence, eructation, diarrhea, fishy aftertaste). Concerns that fish oil supplements may worsen hyperinsulinemia and increase insulin resistance were diminished by a meta-analysis that showed no adverse effects of these supplements on glycosylated hemoglobin levels (60).

The typical North American diet has an unfavorable polyunsaturated-to-saturated fat (P/S) ratio of 0.4. On the other hand, there is no historical precedent that attests to the safety of diets that are very rich in polyunsaturated fats (e.g., P/S ratio of 1.5 or more). It does appear that the latter diets can promote the formation of lithogenic bile and actually increase the incidence of symptomatic biliary tract disease. Although there was a concern that such diets are associated with an increased risk of malignant disease, this finding was not supported when data from several trials were pooled (61). Another disadvantage to substantially increasing dietary intake of polyunsaturated fat is that the resultant high caloric intake might promote obesity. Finally, it should be noted that diets with very high P/S ratios (e.g., 3 or more) may decrease HDL levels and lead to an unfavorable increase in the LDL/HDL ratio. For all of these reasons, a P/S ratio of about 1.0 is recommended in most hypocholesterolemic diets.

Monounsaturated fatty acids, principally oleic acid, found in canola oil, olive oil, and certain forms of safflower and sunflower seed oil, lower levels of LDL cholesterol as effectively as do polyunsaturated fatty acids such as linoleic acid. Therefore, it is now recommended that the TLC diet contain approximately 20% monounsaturated fatty acids, derived mainly from these vegetable oils.

The influence of *dietary fiber* on plasma cholesterol levels is complex, dependent on the type of fiber, and somewhat controversial. Guar, pectin, and unprocessed high-fiber foods, such as legumes and oats, lower plasma total cholesterol levels, whereas other fibers, such as wheat bran, do not. Effects on levels of HDL cholesterol and triglyceride are minimal. In the amounts consumed in a palatable diet, fiber plays a minor role compared with control of dietary fats and cholesterol.

Although *garlic* supplements are effective in reducing total cholesterol, LDL cholesterol, and triglyceride concentrations modestly (approximately 5%) (62), reductions may not persist. The impact on clinical outcomes is unknown. Known side effects are malodorous breath and body odor; there may also be gastrointestinal side effects such as abdominal pain, fullness, anorexia, and flatulence.

Margarines enriched with *plant sterols* (sitostanol and campestanol in Benecol, sitosterol and campesterol in Take Control) have been shown in a few studies to lower total and LDL cholesterol by approximately 10%. They are very poorly absorbed and probably act through the inhibition of cholesterol absorption. Their impact on cardiovascular outcomes is unknown. Although short-term studies have not demonstrated adverse clinical effects, the absorption of fat-soluble vitamins may be affected. A long-term safety profile has not been established. Because of this, the AHA does not recommend their consumption by the general population, but recommends reserving their use for secondary prevention and for patients with moderate to severe hypercholesterolemia (63). Margarines enriched with plant sterols are several times more expensive than ordinary margarines.

Soy proteins, which are found in tofu and soy milk, lower total cholesterol, LDL cholesterol, and triglyceride by approximately 10% (64) and may contribute to the lower risk of heart disease in Asian, as compared to Western, societies. An advisory from the Nutrition Committee of the AHA concluded that 25 to 50 g per day of soy protein is both safe and effective in modestly reducing LDL cholesterol by 4% to 8% (65). The impact of such a diet on health has not been established.

Monitoring and Adjusting Diet

Results of the TLC diet should be monitored after 4 to 6 weeks and again at 3 months, when the effects should be maximal. In general, formal consultation with a dietitian is not required during implementation of the TLC diet, and the physician and other health care providers should serve as the primary sources of education, compliance monitoring, and encouragement for the patient. It is important to emphasize to all patients that dietary treatment of hypercholesterolemia implies permanent, rather than temporary, changes in eating behavior. If the goals of diet therapy are not met after 3 months, it is recommended that the patient continue on the TLC diet and that consideration be given to initiating drug treatment. Patients should also be referred to a dietitian for formal nutritional counseling. For patients with known CAD and for those with diabetes mellitus, it is recommended that pharmacologic and dietary therapy be initiated simultaneously.

Dietary and Drug Therapy

Dietary therapy alone is effective in lowering cholesterol levels in many of the almost 85% of hypercholesterolemic patients with polygenic or nonhereditary forms of hypercholesterolemia. However, numerous studies indicate that dietary therapy alone is less effective in lowering total or LDL cholesterol levels than is the combination of dietary therapy plus drug treatment. For example, in a multicenter trial comparing the separate and combined effects of intensive dietary therapy and low-dose lovastatin in outpatients with moderate hypercholesterolemia, a low-fat diet alone reduced LDL cholesterol by 5%, lovastatin alone lowered LDL by 27%, and lovastatin plus dietary therapy reduced LDL by 32% (66). In elderly patients with hypercholesterolemia, the benefits of diet therapy should be weighed against the possibility of inadequate nutrition.

Triglyceride Reduction

Diets designed to reduce plasma triglyceride and VLDL levels emphasize the loss of excess weight by total caloric restriction. Plasma triglyceride levels usually fall, often to normal, after a few days of caloric restriction. The reduction is maintained as long as weight loss continues at a rate of 1 to 2 lb (0.5 to 1 kg) per week. If normal weight is attained and maintained, further therapy may not be necessary. If hypertriglyceridemia persists or occurs in individuals of normal weight, a cholesterol-lowering diet, as outlined earlier, may be effective. Alcohol intake should be restricted, because it can cause a striking rise in triglyceride levels in some patients with hypertriglyceridemia. Although extreme increases in the carbohydrate content of a diet can cause transient and, rarely, sustained hypertriglyceridemia, there is no firm evidence to suggest that total carbohydrate restriction is helpful in the treatment of hypertriglyceridemia. There are conflicting data regarding the effect on plasma triglyceride level of excessive intake of sucrose (common sugar) and simple sugars. In most studies, especially in patients who are already hypertriglyceridemic, they do raise plasma levels of triglycerides and lower those of HDL cholesterol, but the effect is small. The rationale for dietary restriction of sugar is based more on the need to avoid excessive caloric intake (and to prevent caries) than on any direct effect on plasma lipids. Like alcohol, sucrose provides empty calories in that it contains none of the valuable nutrients (e.g., protein, fiber, minerals, vitamins). Therefore the substitution of complex carbohydrates (e.g., starches) for simple carbohydrates in the diet is recommended. A triglyceride-lowering diet should favorably affect plasma HDL cholesterol levels in most individuals, because obesity and triglyceride concentration are inversely correlated with the level of HDL cholesterol and plasma HDL usually rises during weight reduction. Plasma levels of total (and LDL) cholesterol often fall with loss of excess weight; if they rise, familial combined hyperlipoproteinemia may be present.

Chylomicron Reduction

Treatment of fasting chylomicronemia (type I) involves the restriction of dietary fat intake to 5% to 20% of total calories (0.5 g of fat per kilogram of body weight is a reasonable starting point). The fat deficit should be corrected predominantly by substitution of complex carbohydrates. Because medium-chain triglycerides (available as MCT oil) are transported directly from the intestine to the liver in the portal circulation without incorporation into chylomicrons, they may be added to the diet to provide calories. The recommended dose of MCT oil (available at most pharmacies) is 1 tablespoonful three to four times daily, mixed with foods. Five grams of vegetable fat rich in polyunsaturates should be included to prevent essential fatty acid deficiency.

Dietary fat is severely restricted until fasting chylomicronemia is eliminated and clinical symptoms are prevented or reduced in frequency; dietary fat is then chronically restricted to whatever degree is necessary to prevent fasting chylomicronemia. The efficacy of fat restriction in preventing recurrent abdominal pain is supported by clinical observations in individual patients.

If fasting chylomicronemia is accompanied by increased VLDL triglyceride levels, therapy is initiated with restriction of dietary fat intake and correction of coexistent secondary causes for the disorder. Once chylomicronemia has been eliminated, a triglyceride-lowering diet with a modest reduction in total fat intake (to approximately 30% of total calories) is all that is usually required to prevent recurrence. Total abstinence from alcohol is usually necessary.

Diets to Raise the HDL Level

Some studies have reported that low-fat, low-cholesterol diets have resulted in decreased levels of HDL cholesterol (67), whereas others have found increased HDL values (68). The dietary approach to the patient with an HDL cholesterol level lower than 40 mg/dL should incorporate loss of excess weight with an aerobic exercise program. Although moderate *alcohol* consumption (2 to 3 oz/day) is positively correlated with HDL cholesterol concentration and negatively correlated with CAD, it is discouraged for three reasons: Excessive use (more than two or three drinks per day) increases the overall risk of morbidity and mortality; its use may interfere with attempts to control obesity and hypertriglyceridemia; and evidence is not conclusive that modest intake results in an overall health advantage.

Exercise

During the past decade, evidence has accumulated that regular isotonic exercise enhances fatty acid oxidation and glycogen storage, thus increasing HDL formation, triglyceride clearance, and insulin sensitivity. These metabolic changes favorably affect plasma lipid levels. Most of the exercise programs that have been evaluated, including jogging, rapid walking, swimming, bicycling, cross-country skiing, and mountain climbing, have involved 30 minutes or more of continued effort at 70% to 85% of maximal heart rate at least three times weekly. In most studies, levels of HDL cholesterol have been shown to rise (approximately 20%) and triglyceride levels to fall (approximately 25%) with exercise (45). Although levels of LDL cholesterol usually do not fall in normal subjects, reductions of as much as 10% may occur in individuals with increased concentrations of total and LDL cholesterol.

Resistive training programs conducted in normolipidemic individuals have resulted in increases in HDL cholesterol of 10% to 15% and decreases in LDL cholesterol of 5% to 39% (69). In contrast, in one well-controlled prospective study of resistive training in subjects at risk for CAD (70), no changes in lipid profiles were observed after 20 weeks. Both aerobic and resistive exercise training improve glucose tolerance and insulin sensitivity, reduce blood pressure, and improve body composition (71,72).

To date, most prospective exercise studies have been performed in men. A meta-analysis of the existing longitudinal exercise investigations in women revealed an overall decrease in levels of total cholesterol and triglycerides with little or no change in values of HDL or LDL cholesterol (73). Gender-related differences in the lipoprotein response to exercise may reflect the generally higher endogenous levels of HDL cholesterol in women or differences in metabolic factors such as levels of sex steroids or regulatory enzymes.

It has been demonstrated in both cross-sectional and longitudinal epidemiologic studies that people who exercise regularly have a reduced risk for CAD. Exercise also improves glucose metabolism, assists in weight reduction, and may reduce blood pressure (74,75). Thus exercise counseling (see Chapters 16 and 63) is an important part of the management of patients with abnormalities in lipoprotein metabolism.

Smoking Cessation

Plasma levels of HDL cholesterol have been found to be lower and levels of VLDL triglyceride higher in people who smoke cigarettes than in nonsmokers or ex-smokers. Moreover, an inverse relationship exists between the number of cigarettes smoked daily and the level of HDL cholesterol. Smoking cessation has been associated with a modest rise in plasma HDL concentration. It is not known how much of the increased risk of CAD associated with smoking is mediated through alteration in the plasma lipids and how much via other mechanisms. There is, however, substantial evidence that smoking cessation reduces CAD risk. There is also evidence that counseling of patients increases cessation rates. Therefore, all patients who smoke cigarettes should be counseled to quit, regardless of their lipid profile (see Chapter 27).

Drug Therapy

The recommendations for drug therapy for primary prevention by the ATP (44) are discussed here. Candidates for drug therapy should always continue dietary interventions, because the effects of each mode of treatment are often additive. For all patients, additional lifestyle changes such as weight control, habitual exercise, and cessation of cigarette smoking should be maximized. Table 82.10 provides detailed information on lipid-lowering drugs.

Hypercholesterolemia

In general, the NCEP guidelines suggest a need for drug therapy (Table 82.7) when, despite 3 months of dietary intervention, the LDL level is still higher than the desired range. Patients with marked elevations of LDL cholesterol, in whom dietary therapy alone is unlikely to normalize LDL cholesterol levels, may be considered for drug therapy simultaneously with the initiation of dietary modification. After drugs have been started, LDL cholesterol levels should be checked at 4 to 6 weeks and at 3 months. Once target levels have been achieved, patients should be evaluated with measurement of LDL cholesterol every 4 to 6 months.

For patients at highest risk of adverse cardiovascular events, a recent update from the NCEP suggested that a lower LDL cholesterol target of 70 mg/dL may be appropriate (51). Such patients include those with diagnosed CAD, peripheral arterial disease, or carotid artery disease; diabetes; or 2 or more risk factors for CAD with a calculated 10-year risk more than 20%. In such patients, it is suggested that drug therapy be initiated if the baseline LDL is 100 mg/dL or greater and should even be considered as an option if the LDL is <100 mg/dL but >70 mg/dL. Drug therapy may be delayed in the lowest-risk patients. These include men younger than 35 years of age (with the exception of smokers whose LDL levels are 160 mg/dL or higher and all men whose LDL levels are 190 mg/dL or higher) (44); premenopausal women without other risk factors whose LDL cholesterol levels are less than 220 mg/dL; patients

TABLE 82.10 Commonly Used Lipid-Lowering Drugs[a]

HMG-CoA Reductase Inhibitors (Lovastatin, Pravastatin, Simvastatin, Fluvastatin, Atorvastin, Rosuvastatin)

Efficacy: Decreases total cholesterol (20%–37%), LDL cholesterol (20%–48%), LDL apo B (20%–37%), VLDL cholesterol (27%–40%), and triglycerides (7%–27%). Provides variable and modest increases in HDL cholesterol (4%–12%) and apo A-I and A-II.

Pharmacokinetics: Incompletely absorbed (average 30%); extensive first-pass extraction by liver with <5% reaching systemic circulation; inactive lovastatin converted to several active metabolites; peak plasma concentrations of active metabolites within 2–6 hr; steady-state concentrations of total inhibitors achieved within 2–3 d; 83% of radiolabeled dose eliminated in feces (represents unabsorbed drug and active and inactive metabolites excreted in bile) and 10% in urine (as inactive metabolites).

Side effects: (a) Generally well tolerated, discontinuation required in 1%–2% of patients because of adverse effects; reasonable safety well established; (b) occasional: headache (9% of patients), gastrointestinal (flatulence, abdominal pains or cramps, diarrhea, constipation, nausea, dyspepsia—usually mild and transient [4%–6%]); elevation in liver aminotransferases, and, uncommonly, alkaline phosphatases usually within 3–16 mo (≥3 times increase in 2%), reverses over several weeks after discontinuation of drug; mild increase in creatinine kinase (11%); myalgias (3%); rash and pruritus (5%); (c) uncommon: gastrointestinal (heartburn, dysgeusia), dizziness, insomnia, malaise, fatigue, myopathy (0.5%, but up to 30% in patients taking immunosuppressant drugs or gemfibrozil—also reported in patients taking nicotinic acid or erythromycin), renal failure from rhabdomyolysis.

Administration: Lovastatin (generic, Mevacor)—20–80 mg/d once daily with evening meal or twice daily with meals (administration with food results in 50% higher plasma concentrations of total inhibitors, effectiveness greater when given as evening dose, perhaps because cholesterol synthesis occurs mainly at night). Pravastatin (Pravachol)—10–40 mg once a day at bedtime. Simvastatin (Zocor)—5–40 mg once a day in the evening. Fluvastatin (Lescol)—20–40 mg once a day at bedtime; 40 mg twice daily if no response; absorption not affected by food. Atorvastatin (Lipitor)—10 mg once a day; up to 80 mg once a day if no response. Rosuvastatin (Crestor)—10 mg once a day, up to 40 mg daily.
Obtain baseline creatine kinase and baseline liver function tests, then liver tests at 6, 12 weeks, and semiannually. Discontinue if aminotransferases or creatine kinase rise more than 3 times normal.

Clinical use: First-line effective and well tolerated drugs for the treatment of hypercholesterolemia. When response to a single drug is inadequate, statins are effective in combination with a bile acid sequestering agent or nicotinic acid. Each drug contributes separately to reductions in lipoprotein concentrations.

Cost[b]: $50–130/mo.

Bile Acid Sequestering Resins (Cholestyramine, Colestipol, Colesevelam)

Efficacy: Decreases total and LDL cholesterol up to 25%–40% (onset 4–7 d, maximal effect within 1–3 wk). Mean reductions in total and LDL cholesterol of 13.4% and 20.3% (Lipid Research Clinics trial). Apo B level falls, while HDL level rises slightly. VLDL is unchanged or increased.

Pharmacokinetics: Not absorbed, but may bind other drugs (e.g., thiazides, digitalis preparations, anticoagulants, phenobarbital, thyroxine, phenylbutazone, propranolol, iron).

Side effects: (a) Common: unpleasant sandy/gritty preparations, gastrointestinal (e.g., constipation in 10%–20%, nausea, heartburn, abdominal discomfort, flatulence often resolve with continued therapy or treatment of constipation), lowered serum folate levels; (b) uncommon: gastrointestinal (steatorrhea), hyperchloremic acidosis (small patients on high dosages), fat-soluble vitamin deficiency; increased alkaline phosphatase and amino transferase (usually transient) activity.

Administration: Cholestyramine—12–32 g/d given two to four times daily before or during meals; supplied as Questran 9-g packets each containing 4 g of active drug. Colestipol—15–30 g/d given two to four times daily before or during meals; supplied as Colestid in 5-g packets or 500-g bottles. Colesevelam—3 [WelChol, 625 mg] tablets, twice a day with meals or 6 tablets once a day with a meal. Preparations should be taken with water or juice to prevent esophageal irritation or blockage. Other medicines should be taken 1 hr before or 4 hr after dosage. Monitor serum folate levels and consider supplemental multivitamins with folic acid.

Clinical use: Drugs of first choice in the treatment of hypercholesterolemia, because of their relative safety and efficacy. Well tolerated in combination with niacin or lovastatin. Contraindications include marked hypertriglyceridemia and severe constipation. Poor compliance limits use.

Cost[b]: $50–140/mo.

Cholesterol Absorption Inhibitors (Ezetimibe)

Efficacy: A first-in-class drug that inhibits intestinal cholesterol absorption. In monotherapy it can lower LDL cholesterol approximately 18%. In combination therapy with statins it can lower LDL cholesterol approximately 30%.

Pharmacokinetics: Rapidly absorbed and metabolized to active glucuronide. The half-life of ezetimibe and glucuronide form is approximately 22 hours.

Side effects: No major side effects. Use with caution in patients taking cyclosporine.

Administration: Oral standard dose is 10 mg/d. Can be given with or without food and any time of day.

Clinical use: Indication for hypercholesterolemia either in monotherapy or combination therapy.

Cost: Approximately $70/mo.

(continued)

TABLE 82.10 (Continued) Commonly Used Lipid-Lowering Drugs[a]

Nicotinic Acid (Niacin [generic], and Preparations such as Nicobid [Time-released])

Efficacy: Decreases VLDL triglycerides within 1–4 d (mean: 26% in Coronary Drug Project; range: up to 80% depending on pretreatment levels); decreases LDL cholesterol, onset 5–7 d, maximal effect 3–5 wk (mean decrease of 10% in total cholesterol in Coronary Drug Project; range: up to 30%). Favorable impact on total and LDL cholesterol, triglyceride, VLDL, HDL (increases up to 35%), apos A-I and B.

Pharmacokinetics: Absorbed by mouth; peak concentrations in 20–70 min; at the high dosages used it is partially metabolized in liver and partially excreted unchanged in urine; plasma half-life is about 45 min.

Side effects: (a) Common: cutaneous flushing and pruritus, which diminish after several weeks of therapy; gastrointestinal (nausea, diarrhea, abdominal pain, abnormal liver function); (b) less common: dermatologic disorders (e.g., increased pigmentation); activation of peptic ulcer; arrhythmia; gout; urinary frequency and dysuria; glucose intolerance. Sustained-release forms are associated with irreversible chronic liver disease and fulminant hepatic failure.

Administration: (50-, 100-, 250-, 300-, 400-, and 500-mg tablets). Gradual increase over 1–3 wk from 100–200 mg/d to 2–9 g/d; given two to three times daily; give with meals to diminish side effects. Flushing may be ameliorated by pretreatment with aspirin, one-half to one 325-mg tablet 30 min before each dose. Extended-release forms may pose an increased risk of hepatic toxicity.

Clinical use: First-line (despite side effects) effective drug in the treatment of elevated LDL cholesterol or VLDL triglyceride or low HDL. Well tolerated in combination with bile acid binding resins and statins. Contraindications include peptic ulcer disease, arrhythmia, liver disease, diabetes mellitus, hyperuricemia, and gout.

Cost[b]: $15–50/mo.

Fibric Acid Derivatives (Gemfibrozil, Fenofibrate)

Efficacy: Lowers triglycerides and raises HDL but may raise LDL. In familial combined hyperlipoproteinemia, use of any fibric acid analogue is likely to raise LDL cholesterol.

Pharmacokinetics: Gemfibrozil and fenofibrate: completely absorbed; peak concentration within 2 hr: half-life 1.5 hr; undergoes enterohepatic circulation; metabolized in liver and excreted in urine. May enhance action of oral anticoagulants, phenytoin, and hypoglycemic agents, and of furosemide by displacing them from albumin-binding sites.

Side effects: (a) Usually well tolerated; (b) occasional: (sixfold) increase in the incidence of cholelithiasis (may be less with gemfibrozil and newer analogues); other gastrointestinal (nausea, abdominal pain, diarrhea, weight gain); reduced libido, impotence; unusual flulike syndrome; (c) uncommon: rash, alopecia, breast tenderness, reversible abnormality in liver function, hepatomegaly, myositis, increased plasma glucose, etc; (d) unknown: (?)thromboembolism, (?)intermittent claudication, (?)arrhythmia, (?)neoplasia.

Administration: Gemfibrozil (generic, Lopid)—600 mg twice daily (30 min before meals). Fenofibrate (TriCor)—145 mg/d once daily or 48 mg in three divided doses taken with meals. Dosage reduction required in renal failure patients. Some recommend periodic monitoring of aminotransferase activity and creatinine kinase.

Clinical use: Gemfibrozil is the drug of choice in the treatment of elevated VLDL triglyceride; it can also be used to lower total and LDL cholesterol and to raise HDL cholesterol, of particular utility in type III. Fenofibrate is more effective in lowering LDL. Use with caution in the presence of hepatic or renal insufficiency.

Cost[b]: $35–100/mo.

apo, Apoprotein; HDL, high-density lipoprotein; HMG-CoA, hydroxymethylglutaryl coenzyme A; LDL, low-density lipoprotein; VLDL, very-low-density lipoprotein.
[a]Mechanisms of action are described in the text.
[b]Costs are approximate retail prices as of 2003.

with fewer than two other risk factors and LDL cholesterol levels less than 190 mg/dL; and patients with two other risk factors and LDL cholesterol levels less than 160 mg/dL who have embarked on a trial of adequate diet.

Cholesterol-lowering drugs are categorized into two groups: (a) first-choice agents, such as HMG-CoA reductase inhibitors, bile acid sequestrants, and nicotinic acid, which are effective in lowering total and LDL cholesterol levels, reducing CAD risk, and are generally safe for long-term use; and (b) other drugs, such as gemfibrozil, fenofibrate, and ezetimibe.

HMG-CoA Reductase Inhibitors

The *statins* (lovastatin, simvastatin, pravastatin, fluvastatin, atorvastatin, rosuvastatin) are specific, potent, competitive inhibitors of HMG-CoA reductase, the rate-limiting enzyme in cholesterol biosynthesis. These drugs increase hepatic LDL receptor activity and LDL clearance from the circulation and, in addition, decrease production of LDL (76). More than 15 years of clinical experience with this class of drugs has confirmed their effectiveness in reducing levels of total and LDL cholesterol by 20% to 50%, in decreasing triglyceride levels slightly, and in modestly increasing the levels of HDL cholesterol in some patients (76,77). They appear to be equally effective in individuals with familial and nonfamilial hypercholesterolemia. When compared with bile acid sequestrants and nicotinic acid in the treatment of patients with type IIa hyperlipidemia, statins induce a greater reduction in LDL cholesterol concentrations and better compliance.

A 5-year study demonstrated lovastatin to be comparable in safety to the other major cholesterol-lowering drugs (78). The safety profiles are similar for the other statins, with drug-related adverse events occurring in approximately 2% to 3% of patients. Side effects include increase in aminotransferase activity, myopathy, insomnia, myalgia, arthralgia, and gastrointestinal disturbances. No study has shown a significant increase in the development of lens opacities; consequently, routine ophthalmologic monitoring is not required. Periodic tests of liver function are now suggested before initiation of statin therapy, at weeks 6 and 12, and then semiannually. In general, statin therapy should be reduced or discontinued when aminotransferase levels rise three times above the upper limit of normal. There is no compelling evidence that one statin is superior to another in regard to problems with hepatic toxicity. The same is true for problems with myalgias or myositis. If the patient complains of painful muscles, the serum creatinine kinase (CK) level should be measured. It is prudent to check CK levels before initiating statin therapy as it avoids confusion later if the patient complains of myalgia and then is found to have an elevated CK. Statin therapy should be reduced or discontinued when CK levels rise three times above the upper limit of normal. The incidence of myositis rises when statins are used in combination with gemfibrozil (especially in older females with renal insufficiency), erythromycin, antifungals, or cyclosporine.

Bile Acid Sequestering Resins

The bile acid-binding resins *cholestyramine* and *colestipol* are among the oldest agents used to treat hypercholesterolemia. They are useful for primary prevention therapy in young men and premenopausal women without other risk factors who have moderately increased LDL cholesterol levels. They enhance LDL catabolism and excretion and prevent intestinal absorption by diverting cholesterol and bile acids into the feces. They also increase levels of triglycerides and HDL, particularly HDL_2. At dosages of 20 to 24 g per day, a 20% to 30% reduction in LDL cholesterol may be achieved. Although the resins may be the safest of all of the hypolipidemic drugs, compliance with the older agents was a problem because taste and gastrointestinal side effects prevented many patients from taking a full dose. As many as 30% of clinical trial participants admitted to taking less than half of the prescribed dosage of bile acid-binding resins (36). Gradual increase of dose, continuation of therapy, and concomitant symptomatic management of constipation may diminish side effects. The resins are better tolerated when used at lower dosages in combination with other lipid-lowering agents. They should not be overlooked as adjuvant therapy when other lipid-lowering agents fail to achieve the desired results. Another bile acid resin, now available for prescription, is colesevelam (WelChol), a more palatable preparation and one that has fewer drug interactions than the older bile acid resins. It can be given concurrently with statins and does not interfere with the absorption of vitamins A, D, E, or K (79).

Cholesterol Absorption Inhibitors

Ezetimibe is a relatively new medication that impairs cholesterol absorption in the intestine (80). The standard dose is 10 mg daily and can be prescribed as monotherapy or in combination with other lipid lowering medications. In combination with simvastatin, it is marketed as Vytorin and is available in multiple doses (10 mg of ezetimibe with 10 to 80 mg of simvastatin). It is generally free of major side effects and does not impair absorption of vitamins.

Nicotinic Acid (Niacin)

Nicotinic acid (3 to 6 g/day) significantly lowers plasma levels of LDL and VLDL while raising the level of HDL cholesterol. It is therefore the drug of first choice for patients with concomitant elevations in LDL cholesterol and triglycerides. It is the first lipid-lowering drug shown to lower levels of Lp(a) (26), and it is also one of the most potent agents in elevating HDL cholesterol levels. There is evidence in secondary prevention trials that nicotinic acid may reduce total mortality. Its use is often limited, however, by unpleasant side effects and the frequent presence of coexisting contraindications (see Table 82.10). Therapy should be discontinued if gout, hyperglycemia, or hepatotoxicity develops. By starting at a very low dosage of 100 to 200 mg/day and gradually increasing the dosage of the drug and adding aspirin, increased tolerance often develops to the common side effects of cutaneous flushing, rashes, hives, and pruritus. Sustained-release forms of nicotinic acid were initially thought to produce fewer side effects than immediate-release forms. However, because of reports of irreversible chronic liver disease and fulminant hepatic failure with sustained-release nicotinic acid, immediate-release forms are strongly preferred (81,82).

Fibrates

Gemfibrozil is the most commonly used drug in this class in the United States. *Clofibrate*, rarely used since the World Health Organization Cooperative Trial reported significantly increased all-cause mortality in patients taking the drug (83), and *fenofibrate* are also available in the United States, whereas bezafibrate and ciprofibrate are available in Europe. Although gemfibrozil is approved for the treatment of hypertriglyceridemia, data from the Helsinki Heart and VA-HIT studies (37,42) revealed it to be effective in raising HDL cholesterol and reducing morbidity and mortality from CAD. In general, gemfibrozil is not considered as useful for secondary prevention as other drugs such as the statins, because it does not achieve maximal reductions in LDL cholesterol. Diabetic patients with elevated triglycerides and patients with type III hyperlipoproteinemia are excellent candidates for treatment with this drug. The VA-HIT study showed that gemfibrozil is associated with significant risk reductions for stroke, nonfatal MI, and CAD death in patients with known CAD and low HDL cholesterol levels (42). However, in patients with primary hypertriglyceridemia gemfibrozil may increase LDL cholesterol levels, whereas in patients with elevations of both cholesterol and triglycerides, this drug can cause either an increase or a decrease in LDL cholesterol levels. The newer fibrates may lower LDL cholesterol more effectively than gemfibrozil does (84). A significant side effect of gemfibrozil is its tendency to increase bile lithogenicity.

Combination Drug Therapy

If the response to one of the first-line drugs proves to be inadequate, combined therapy with two drugs with complementary or synergistic mechanisms of action should be considered.. The use of a bile acid sequestrant or ezetimibe in combination with either nicotinic acid or a statin can lower levels of LDL cholesterol by 45% to 60% in patients with hypercholesterolemia and normal triglyceride levels (85). These regimens have been well tolerated, with synergistic effects on LDL cholesterol without an additive effect on drug-related toxicity. Fibrates may also be used in combination with a bile acid-sequestering resin, although these regimens are less effective. The combination of a statin and fibrate causes an increased risk of myopathy, and rhabdomyolysis has been reported with the combination of lovastatin and nicotinic acid (86).

Two placebo-controlled studies of intensive lipid-lowering therapy using combined colestipol and niacin therapy or combined lovastatin and niacin treatment for men with documented CAD showed reduced frequency of progression of coronary lesions, increased frequency of regression, and reduced incidence of cardiovascular events in the active drug groups, without cases of rhabdomyolysis (87,88). Patients with homozygous familial hypercholesterolemia may respond less well to treatment with drugs and diet than patients with heterozygous monogenic, polygenic, or nonhereditary hypercholesterolemia.

Obviously, it is prudent to carefully monitor patients treated with combination therapy. This requires frequent followup visits and advising patients to call the caregiver should they experience excessive muscle aches or weakness. Consultation with a lipid disorders specialist may be helpful in considering and initiating combination drug therapy.

Other Hypocholesterolemic Drugs

The use of *estrogen replacement therapy* (ERT) in postmenopausal women has a number of effects on cholesterol metabolism (see Chapters 103 and 106). Treatment with oral estrogens usually lowers levels of LDL cholesterol and raises those of HDL cholesterol, but the dosages required for these effects probably exceed those for physiologic replacement therapy. In contrast, administration of transdermal estrogens usually results in lower LDL cholesterol levels but unaltered levels of HDL cholesterol. Both oral and transdermal ERT have been shown to significantly lower Lp(a) levels (31% and 16%, respectively) in postmenopausal women. Concomitant use of the progestin medroxyprogesterone acetate (Provera) with either form of ERT appears not to influence either form of ERT adversely. The primary side effect of unopposed estrogen is the increased risk of endometrial cancer, a risk that is greatly attenuated by cotreatment with progestogens (see Chapter 106).

Phytoestrogens, plant-derived estrogens, are substances that have attracted the attention of the American population. These plant derivatives are comprised mainly of three classes: isoflavones, coumestans, and lignans (89). In most studies, phytoestrogens have been reported to exert a favorable effect in improving lipid profiles (89).

The results from the Heart and Estrogen/Progestin Replacement Study (HERS) dampened the enthusiasm for hormone replacement therapy (HRT) in the treatment of women with known CAD. The participants were postmenopausal women younger than 80 years of age with known CAD and an intact uterus. Study participants were treated with either an estrogen/progestin preparation or placebo for an average followup of 4.1 years (90). The results showed no statistically significant difference between the occurrences of nonfatal MI and coronary heart disease death between the two groups. There was an increase in thromboembolic and gallbladder disease among study participants taking the hormone supplements.

In addition, the results from the Women's Health Initiative Study have raised concern that there is an increased risk of invasive breast cancer and of cardiovascular disease associated with hormone replacement therapy (91). The study found excess risk in incident cases of coronary heart disease, stroke, pulmonary embolism, and invasive breast cancer in healthy women using HRT (Premarin 0.625 mg/day plus medroxyprogesterone 2.5 mg/day), but there was also a significant reduction in the risk of colorectal cancer and fracture. It should also be noted that there has been disagreement on whether hormone replacement therapy should be withheld in women at increased risk for coronary disease (92). The most prudent advice for the health care provider is to engage in a candid discussion with the patient regarding the pros and cons of HRT.

Hypertriglyceridemia

Drugs that decrease hepatic production of VLDL and apo B, enhance VLDL clearance by stimulating LPL activity, or both are generally effective in treating hypertriglyceridemia. Fibrates and nicotinic acid do both.

Although *nicotinic acid* may be most efficacious, its use is limited by its side effects and the presence of coexisting contraindications. The fibric acid derivatives *gemfibrozil and fenofibrate* are therefore the drugs most commonly used. Although gemfibrozil is generally well tolerated, an acute myositis, which is occasionally associated with renal failure, may occur, particularly in patients with impaired renal clearance or hypoalbuminemia. Either the drug should not be used or the dosage should be reduced by 70% to 90% in azotemic patients. Periodic monitoring of muscle enzymes (creatine kinase, aldolase) is required to avoid toxicity. If the level of LDL cholesterol rises in a patient taking gemfibrozil, the diagnosis of familial combined hyperlipoproteinemia should be considered.

For compliant patients who remain hypertriglyceridemic with diet and a single drug, combined therapy with a fibric acid drug and nicotinic acid may be useful. Rarely, after consultation with a specialist in lipid disorders, the progestational agent norethindrone acetate or the androgenic anabolic steroid oxandrolone—in women or men, respectively—may be required to treat persistent hypertriglyceridemia plus chylomicronemia.

Dysbetalipoproteinemia

The decreased remnant catabolism characteristic of this clinically uncommon disorder can be corrected or improved by drug therapy. *Gemfibrozil* appears to normalize lipid levels and to enhance remnant clearance in patients with dysbetalipoproteinemia. It is the drug of choice in this disorder. *Ethinyl estradiol* has a similar and even more dramatic effect, but at dosages that greatly exceed those used for postmenopausal replacement therapy. Hence, its use requires careful monitoring for possible adverse estrogenic effects that would necessitate discontinuation of the drug. *Nicotinic acid* is the drug of second choice.

SPECIFIC REFERENCES*

1. Brown MS, Goldstein JL. How LDL receptors influence cholesterol and atherosclerosis. Sci Am 1984;251:58.
2. Brunzell JD, Sniderman AD, Albers JJ, et al. Apoproteins B and A-I and coronary artery disease in humans. Arteriosclerosis 1984;4:79.
3. Lavie CJ. Lipid and lipoprotein fractions and coronary artery disease. Mayo Clin Proc 1993;68:618.
4. Lindgren FT, Jensen LC, Hatch FT. The isolation and quantitative analysis of serum lipoproteins. In: Nelson GJ, ed. Blood lipids and lipoproteins: quantitation, composition, and metabolism. New York: John Wiley, 1972:181.
5. Maciejko JJ, Holmes DR, Kottke BA, et al. Apolipoprotein A-I as a marker of angiographically assessed coronary artery disease. N Engl J Med 1983;309:385.
6. Nilsson-Ehle P. Regulation of lipoprotein lipase: triacylglycerol transport in plasma. In: Carlson LA, Pernow B, eds. Metabolic risk factors in ischemic cardiovascular disease. New York: Raven Press, 1982:49.
7. Havel RJ, ed. Symposium on lipid disorders. Med Clin North Am 1982;66:319.
8. Oram JF, Brenton EA, Bierman EL. Regulation of high density lipoprotein activity in cultured human skin fibroblasts and human arterial smooth muscle cells. J Clin Invest 1983;72:1611.
9. Acton S, Rigotti A, Landschultz KT, et al. Identification of scavenger receptor SR-BI as a high density lipoprotein receptor. Science 1996;271:518.
10. Landschultz KT, Pathak RK, Rigotti A, et al. Regulation of scavenger receptor, class B, type I, a high density lipoprotein receptor, in liver and steroidogenic tissues of the rat. J Clin Invest 1996;98:984.
11. Steinberg D. Antioxidant vitamins and coronary heart disease. N Engl J Med 1993;328:1487.
12. Mahley RW, Angelin B. Type III hyperlipoproteinemia: recent insights into the genetic defect of familial dysbetalipoproteinemia. Adv Intern Med 1984;29:385.
13. Kannel WB, Schatzkin A. Risk factor analysis. Prog Cardiovasc Dis 1983;26:309.

*Bold numerals denote published controlled clinical trials, meta-analyses, or consensus-based recommendations.

14. LaRosa J. Dyslipidemia and coronary artery disease in the elderly. Clin Geriatr Med 1996;12:33.
15. Krumholz HM, Seeman TE, Merrill SS, et al. Lack of association between cholesterol and coronary heart disease mortality and morbidity and all-cause mortality in persons older than 70 years. JAMA 1994;272:1335.
16. Corti M-C, Guralnik JM, Salive ME, et al. Clarifying the direct relation between total cholesterol levels and death from coronary heart disease in older persons. Ann Intern Med 1997;126:753.
17. Sorkin JD, Andres R, Muller DC, et al. Cholesterol as a risk factor for coronary heart disease in elderly men. Ann Epidemiol 1992;2:59.
18. Zimetbaum P, Frishman WH, Ooi WI, et al. Plasma lipids and lipoproteins and the incidence of cardiovascular disease in the very elderly: The Bronx Aging Study. Arterioscler Thromb 1992;12:416.
19. Criqui MH, Heiss G, Cohn R, et al. Plasma triglyceride level and mortality from coronary heart disease. N Engl J Med 1993;328:1220.
20. Castelli WP. The triglyceride issue: a view from Framingham. Am Heart J 1986;112:432.
21. Hokansan JE, Austin MA. Plasma triglyceride level is a risk factor for cardiovascular disease independent of high-density lipoprotein cholesterol level: a meta-analysis of population-based prospective studies. J Cardiovasc Risk 1996;3:213.
22. Ginsberg HN. Hypertriglyceridemia: new insights and new approaches to pharmacologic therapy. Am J Cardiol 2001;87:1174.
23. Walden CE, Knopp RH, Wahl PW, et al. Sex differences in the effect of diabetes mellitus and lipoprotein triglyceride and cholesterol concentrations. N Engl J Med 1984;331:953.
24. Goldberg AP. Lipid abnormalities in hemodialysis: prevalence, implications and treatment. Perspect Lipid Disord 1984;2:17.
25. Heiss G, Johnson NJ, Reiland S, et al. The epidemiology of plasma HDL cholesterol levels. The Lipid Research Clinics Prevalence Study. Summary. Circulation 1980;62(Suppl 4):116.
26. Carlson LA, Hamsten A, Asplund A. Pronounced lowering of serum levels of Lp(a) in hyperlipidemic subjects treated with nicotinic acid. J Intern Med 1989;226:271.
27. Austin MA, Breslow JL, Hennekens CH, et al. Low-density lipoprotein subclass patterns and risk of myocardial infarction. JAMA 1988;260:1917.
28. Rader DJ, Brewer HB Jr. Lipoprotein (a): clinical approach to a unique atherogenic lipoprotein. JAMA 1992;267:1109.
29. Wade DP. Lipoprotein (a). Curr Opin Lipidol 1993;4:244.
30. Rimm EB, Stampfer MJ, Ascherio A, et al. Vitamin E consumption and the risk of coronary disease in men. N Engl J Med 1993;328:1450.
31. Stampfer MJ, Hennekens CH, Manson JE, et al. Vitamin E consumption and the risk of coronary disease in women. N Engl J Med 1993;328:1444.
32. Dietary supplementation with omega-3 polyunsaturated fatty acids and vitamin E after myocardial infarction: results of the GISSI-Prevenzione trial. Gruppo Italiano per lo Studio della Sopravvivenza nell'Infarto miocardico. Lancet 1999;354:447.
33. Collaborative Group of the Primary Prevention Project. Low-dose aspirin and vitamin E in people at cardiovascular risk: a randomized trial in general practice. Lancet 2001;357:89.
34. Levy RI. Consideration of cholesterol and nonvascular mortality. Am Heart J 1982;104:324.
35. Cooper R, Cutler J, Desvigne-Nickens P, et al. Trends and disparities in coronary heart disease, stroke, and other cardiovascular diseases in the United States: findings of the national conference on cardiovascular disease prevention. Circulation 2000;102:3137.
36. Lipid Research Clinics Program. The Lipid Research Clinics Coronary Primary Prevention Trial results: II. The relationship of reduction in incidence of coronary heart disease to cholesterol lowering. JAMA 1984;251:365.
37. Frick MH, Elo O, Haapa K, et al. Helsinki Heart Study: primary prevention trial with gemfibrozil in middle-aged men with dyslipidemia. N Engl J Med 1987;317:1237.
38. Shepherd J, Cobbe SM, Ford I, et al. Prevention of coronary heart disease with pravastatin in men with hypercholesterolemia. West of Scotland Coronary Prevention Study Group. N Engl J Med 1995;333:1301.
39. Downs JR, Clearfield M, Weis S, et al. Primary prevention of acute coronary events with lovastatin in men and women with average cholesterol levels: results of AFCAPS/TexCAPS.

Air Force/Texas Coronary Atherosclerosis Prevention Studies. JAMA 1998;279:1615.

40. Brensike JF, Levy RI, Kelsey SF, et al. Effects of therapy with cholestyramine on progression of coronary arteriosclerosis: results of the NHLBI type II coronary intervention study. Circulation 1984;69:313.

41. Scandinavian Simvastatin Survival Study Group. Randomised trial of cholesterol lowering in 4444 patients with coronary heart disease: The Scandinavian Simvastatin Survival Study (4S). Lancet 1994;344:1383.

42. Robins SJ, Collins D, Wittes JT, et al. Relation of gemfibrozil treatment and lipid levels with major coronary events: VA-HIT: a randomized controlled trial. JAMA 2001;285:1585.

42a. Heart Protection Study Collaborative Group. MRC/BHF Heart Protection Study of cholesterol-lowering with simvastatin in 20,536 high-risk individuals: a randomized, placebo-controlled trial. Lancet 2002;360:7–22.

43. The Expert Panel. Report of the National Cholesterol Education Program Expert Panel on Detection, Evaluation and Treatment of High Blood Cholesterol in Adults. Arch Intern Med 1988;148:36.

44. The Expert Panel. Executive Summary of the Third Report of the National Cholesterol Education Program (NCEP) Expert Panel on Detection, Evaluation, and Treatment of High Blood Cholesterol in Adults (Adult Treatment Panel III). JAMA 2001;285:2486.

45. Dufaux B, Assmann G, Hollman W. Plasma lipoproteins and physical activity: a review. Int J Sports Med 1982;3:123.

46. Fuiano G, Esposito C, Sepe V, et al. Effects of hypercholesterolemia on renal hemodynamics: study in patients with nephrotic syndrome. Nephron 1996;73:430.

47. Bergman R. The pathogenesis and clinical significance of xanthelasma palpebrarum. J Am Acad Dermatol 1994;30:236.

48. Hulley SB, Newman TB, Grady D, et al. Should we be measuring blood cholesterol levels in young adults? JAMA 1993;269:1416.

49. Leaf A. Management of hypercholesterolemia: are preventive interventions advisable? N Engl J Med 1989;321:680.

50. Pignone MP, Phillips CJ, Atkins D, et al. Screening and treating adults for lipid disorders. Am J Prev Med 2001;20:77.

51. NCEP Report. Implications of recent clinical trials for the National Cholesterol Education Program Adult Treatment Panel III Guidelines. Circulation 2004;110:227.

52. American College of Physicians. Guidelines for using serum cholesterol, high-density lipoprotein cholesterol, and triglyceride levels as screening tests for preventing coronary heart disease in adults. Ann Intern Med 1996;124: 515.

53. Cleeman JI, Grundy SM. National Cholesterol Education Program recommendations for cholesterol testing in young adults. Circulation 1997;95:1646.

54. Cleeman JI. Adults aged 20 and older should have their cholesterol measured. Am J Med 1997;102:31.

55. Hegsted DM, Nicolosi RJ. Individual variation in serum cholesterol levels. Proc Natl Acad Sci USA 1987;84:6259.

56. RRamsay LE, Yeo WW, Jackson PR. Dietary reduction of serum cholesterol concentration. BMJ 1991;303:1551.

57. Daviglus ML, Stamler J, Orencia AJ, et al. Fish consumption and the 30-year risk of fatal myocardial infarction. N Engl J Med 1997;336:1046.

58. Oomen CM, Feskens EJ, Rasanen L, et al. Fish consumption and coronary heart disease mortality in Finland, Italy, and The Netherlands. Am J Epidemiol 2000;151:999.

59. Von Schacky C, Angerer P, Kothny W, et al. The effect of dietary omega-3 fatty acids on coronary atherosclerosis: a randomized, double-blind, placebo-controlled trial. Ann Intern Med 1999;130:554.

60. Friedberg CE, Janssen MJ, Heine RJ, et al. Fish oil and glycemic control in diabetes: a meta-analysis. Diabetes Care 1998;21:494.

61. Ederer F, Leren P, Turpeinin O, et al. Cancer among men on cholesterol-lowering diets. Lancet 1971;2:203.

62. Stevinson C, Pittler MH, Ernst E. Garlic for treating hypercholesterolemia: a meta-analysis of randomized clinical trials. Ann Intern Med 2000;133:420.

63. Lichtenstein AH, Deckelbaum RJ. Stanol/sterol ester-containing foods and blood cholesterol levels: a statement for healthcare professionals from the Nutrition Committee of the council on Nutrition, Physical Activity, and Metabolism of the American Heart Association. Circulation 2001;103:1177.

64. Anderson JW, Johnstone BM, Cook-Newell ME. Meta-analysis of the effects of soy protein intake on serum lipids. N Engl J Med 1995;333:276.

65. Erdman JW Jr. Soy protein and cardiovascular disease: a statement for healthcare professionals from the nutrition committee of the AHA. Circulation 2000;102:2555.

66. Hunninghake DB, Stein EA, Dujovne CA, et al. The efficacy of intensive dietary therapy alone or combined with lovastatin in outpatients with hypercholesteremia. N Engl J Med 1993;328:1213.

67. Dattilo AM, Kris-Etherton PM. Effects of weight reduction on blood lipids and lipoproteins: a meta-analysis. Am J Clin Nutr 1991;56:320.

68. Watts GF, Lewis B, Brunt JHN, et al. Effects on coronary artery disease of lipid-lowering diet or diet plus cholestyramine in the St. Thomas Atherosclerosis Regression Study. Lancet 1992;339:563.

69. Hurley BF. Effects of resistive training on lipoprotein-lipid profiles: a comparison to aerobic exercise training. Med Sci Sports Exerc 1989;21:689.

70. Hurley BF, Hagberg JM, Goldberg AP, et al. Resistive training can reduce coronary risk factors without altering VO_2 max or percent body fat. Med Sci Sports Exerc 1988;20:150.

71. Goldberg AP. Aerobic and resistive exercise modify risk factors for coronary heart disease. Med Sci Sports Exerc 1989;21:669.

72. Goldberg LE, Elliot DL, Shutz RW, et al. Changes in lipid and lipoprotein levels after weight training. JAMA 1984;252:504.

73. Tran ZV, Weltman A. Differential effects of exercise on serum lipid and lipoprotein levels seen with changes in body weight: a meta-analysis. JAMA 1985;254:919.

74. Hagberg JM. Exercise, fitness, and hypertension. In: Bouchard C, Shepard RJ, Stephens T, et al, eds. Exercise, fitness and health. Champaign, IL: Human Kinetics, 1990:455.

75. Paffenberger RS, Hyde RT, Wing AL, et al. A natural history of athleticism and cardiovascular health. JAMA 1984;252:491.

76. Grundy S. HMG-CoA reductase inhibitors for treatment of hypercholesterolemia. N Engl J Med 1988;319:24.

77. The Lovastatin Study Group II. Therapeutic response to lovastatin in nonfamilial hypercholesterolemia: a multicenter trial. JAMA 1986;256:2829.

78. Lovastatin Study Group I–IV. Lovastatin 5-year safety and efficacy study. Arch Intern Med 1993;153:1079.

79. Colesevelam (WelChol) for hypercholesterolemia. Med Lett 2000;42:102.

80. Kosoglou T, Statkevich P, Johnson-Levonas AO, et al. Ezetimibe: a review of its metabolism, pharmacokinetics and drug interactions. Clin Pharmacokinet 2005;44:467.

81. Etchason JA, Miller TD, Squires RW, et al. Niacin-induced hepatitis: a potential side effect with low-dose time-release niacin. Mayo Clin Proc 1991;66:23.

82. McKenney JM, Proctor JD, Harris S, et al. A comparison of the efficacy and toxic effects of sustained vs immediate release niacin in hypercholesterolemic patients. JAMA 1994;271:672.

83. World Health Organization Clofibrate Trial. WHO cooperative trial on primary prevention of ischaemic heart disease using clofibrate to lower serum cholesterol: mortality follow-up. Lancet 1980;2:379.

84. Schonfeld G. The effects of fibrates on lipoprotein and hemostatic coronary risk factors. Atherosclerosis 1994;11:161.

85. Illingsworth DR. Mevinolin plus colestipol in therapy for severe heterozygous familial hypercholesterolemia. Ann Intern Med 1984;101:598.

86. Reaven P, Witztum JL. Lovastatin, nicotinic acid and rhabdomyolysis. Ann Intern Med 1988;109:597.

87. Blankenhorn DH, Nessim SA, Johnson RL, et al. Beneficial effects of combined colestipol-niacin therapy on coronary atherosclerosis and coronary venous bypass grafts. JAMA 1987;257:3233.

88. Brown G, Albers JJ, Fisher LD, et al. Regression of coronary artery disease as a result of intensive lipid-lowering therapy in men with high level of apo lipoprotein B. N Engl J Med 1990;323:1289.

89. Murkies AL, Wilcox G, Davis SR. Phytoestrogens. J Clin Endocrinol Metab 1998;83:297.

90. Hulley S, Grady D, Bush T, et al. Randomized trial of estrogen plus progestin for secondary prevention of coronary heart disease in postmenopausal women. Heart and Estrogen/Progestin Replacement Study (HERS) Research Group. JAMA 198;280:605.

91. Writing Group for the Women's Health Initiative Investigators. Risks and benefits of estrogen and progestin in healthy postmenopausal women, principal results from the Women's Health Initiative randomized controlled trial. JAMA 2002;288:321.

92. Machens K, Schmidt-Gollwitzer K. Issues to debate on the Women's Health Initiative (WHI) study. Hormone replacement therapy: an epidemiological dilemma? Hum Reprod 2003; 18:1992.

*For annotated **General References** and resources related to this chapter, visit www.hopkinsbayview.org/PAMreferences.*

Chapter 83

Obesity

Jeanne M. Clark

EPIDEMIOLOGY

Prevalence

Obesity, a state of excess body fat, has reached epidemic proportions in the United States and is increasing throughout the world. During the period 1988 to 1992, 33% of U.S. adults were overweight, 23% were obese, and 3% were extremely obese (1). Despite various efforts to treat and prevent obesity, by 2002, 45% of adults were overweight, and the prevalence of obesity was 30%, with 5% of adults being *extremely* obese (2). No longer just an "American problem," obesity is also becoming common in developed and developing countries throughout the world.

Obesity is not evenly distributed across the U.S. population, but differentially affects groups of different races, ethnicities, and educational and socioeconomic attainment. Overall, women are more likely to be obese than men. Among women, the prevalence of obesity is 31% among non-Hispanic whites, 38% among Mexican Americans, and 49% among non-Hispanic blacks. Obesity is also more common in women with lower educational and economic attainment (3). Men are more likely to be overweight than women, and the prevalence of overweight differs among the different racial/ethnic groups, with Mexican American men (75%) having the highest prevalence, followed by non-Hispanic whites (67%) and non-Hispanic blacks (61%). However, the prevalence of obesity among men is similar across the racial/ethnic groups (27% to 29%).

Etiology

Weight gain, and thus obesity, occurs when caloric intake exceeds caloric expenditure. However, the nuances of energy balance and its regulation are quite complex. Current theories include interplay between genetic predisposition, environment, and social/cultural role of food and activity, as well as the intricate interactions among various hormones, cytokines (e.g., tumor necrosis factor α), and adipokines (e.g., leptin, adiponectin). Currently, these have little or no clinical relevance except as noted below. Although binge-eating disorder is a relatively common problem among people seeking to lose weight, it is not a common cause of obesity. Although most people with this disorder are not obese, they do tend to be overweight.

Genes and the Environment

It has been estimated that 30% to 40% of obesity is attributable to a genetic predisposition, and 60% to 70% is attributable to the environment. Most of the genetic predisposition is polygenic, that is, it is controlled by several different genes, rather than a single gene mutation (monogenic). The one known exception is leptin deficiency, which occurs very rarely and results in severe obesity in childhood. Several mutations in this gene have been described and the patients generally respond to leptin treatment (4). More often, among those genetically predisposed, obesity occurs only under "adverse" conditions, such as high-calorie diets and sedentary lifestyle. These conditions, recently named the "toxic environment," are thought to explain much of the rapid increase in the prevalence of obesity over the past few decades.

Medical Causes of Obesity

There are a number of medical conditions that can lead to weight gain and/or adipose accumulation. Hypercortisolism resulting from Cushing disease can result in adipose accumulation and redistribution. Rarely is this severe enough to cause obesity de novo, and the pattern of fat deposition and associated signs and symptoms are usually recognizable. Similarly, hypothyroidism can cause some weight gain, but is rarely the cause of obesity by itself. Other putative causes of obesity include hyperinsulinemia and polycystic ovary syndrome. However, whether these are causes or consequences of obesity is a matter of some debate. An accurate history and physical examination can distinguish whether such conditions are the underlying cause of weight gain. In general, extensive laboratory testing to identify an underlying cause for obesity is not needed.

A number of medications, including phenothiazines, lithium, glucocorticoids, insulin, insulin secretagogues (i.e., sulfonylureas), and anticonvulsants, can cause weight gain and may exacerbate or cause obesity. An accurate history of the weight trajectory and its relation to new medication can identify the problem. Unfortunately, in some cases, changing the offending medication may not be possible.

Sequelae of Obesity

Increased Mortality

Although mortality directly resulting from obesity can be difficult to separate from that attributable to coexisting conditions (e.g., diabetes, hyperlipidemia, coronary artery disease), the estimated number of deaths attributable to obesity in the United States ranges from 112,000 to 400,000 per year, making obesity an important cause of preventable deaths (5,6). Obese individuals have higher rates of death from all causes (7), and very obese young adults have a life expectancy that is up to 20 years shorter than nonobese adults (8). Furthermore, although generally thought to be associated with deaths from cardiovascular disease and diabetes, obesity is also associated with higher rates of death overall from cancer, and for most specific types of cancer (9).

Medical Consequences

Obesity is also associated with an increased risk of many diseases. Among obese adults, the relative risk of developing hypertension or diabetes is about three times that of people who are not obese; and for hypercholesterolemia it is 1.5 times. Furthermore, obesity independently increases the risk of coronary artery disease, stroke, obstructive sleep apnea, cholelithiasis, osteoarthritis, venous thrombosis, nonalcoholic fatty liver disease, gout, and cancers of the colon, rectum, and prostate in men, and of the uterus and gallbladder in women (10–12). Although there has been a great deal of research into the potential psychiatric consequences of obesity, at this time the bulk of the evidence suggests that obesity does *not* cause psychiatric conditions such as depression or anxiety. Table 83.1 lists the medical consequences of obesity.

In addition to these comorbidities, obesity also increases the morbidity and mortality from unrelated illnesses. For instance, obese persons with liver diseases such as hepatitis C, or alcohol-induced liver disease, have a poorer prognosis than nonobese persons. The impact of

TABLE 83.1 Medical Consequences of Obesity

Cardiovascular
Cerebrovascular disease
Congestive heart failure
Coronary artery disease
Cor pulmonale
Hypertension
Dermatologic
Acanthosis nigricans
Chronic skin infections
Endocrinologic/Metabolic
Decreased growth hormones
Decreased sympathoadrenal activity
Hyperuricemia, gout
Impaired fasting glucose, impaired glucose tolerance, type 2 diabetes
Increased cortisol production
Increased total or free androgens
Insulin resistance, hyperinsulinemia
Lipid abnormalities: increased total cholesterol, LDL, VLDL, and triglycerides; decreased HDL cholesterol
Gastroenterologic
Cholelithiasis
Nonalcoholic fatty liver disease
Genitourinary
Urinary incontinence
Musculoskeletal
Osteoarthritis of weight-bearing joints
Oncologic
Breast cancer (postmenopausal women)
Colon cancer (men)
Endometrial cancer
Esophageal cancer
Gallbladder cancer (women)
Hepatocellular carcinoma
Kidney cancer
Prostate cancer
Pulmonary
Asthma
Obstructive sleep apnea
Pickwickian syndromes (hypoventilation)
Restrictive lung disease
Reproductive
Early menarche
Erectile and other sexual dysfunction, impotence
Gestational diabetes
Oligomenorrhea/amenorrhea
Polycystic ovary syndrome
Surgical
Increased perioperative morbidity and mortality
Incisional hernias
Vascular/Hematologic
Venous stasis
Venous thromboembolism
Thrombophlebitis

HDL, high-density lipoprotein; LDL, low-density lipoprotein; VLDL, very-low-density lipoprotein.

obesity on seemingly unrelated conditions is difficult to measure, but deserves consideration.

Obesity, especially abdominal adiposity (waist circumference >40 inches in men and >35 inches in women), is strongly associated with a number of other adverse health conditions that form the "metabolic syndrome." Widely believed to reflect a state of insulin resistance, this constellation includes elevated blood pressure (>130/85 mm Hg) and triglycerides (≥150 mg/dL), low high-density lipoprotein (HDL) cholesterol (<40 mg/dL for men, <50 mg/dL for women), and impaired glucose tolerance (fasting glucose ≥110 mg/dL). Together these confer a higher cardiovascular risk than each component alone.

Quality of Life

In addition to affecting life expectancy, obesity also reduces quality of life, even in the absence of comorbid diseases (13,14). This is most evident in physical functioning, including activities of daily living, and bodily pain domains. Furthermore, it appears that the morbidly obese and those with predominantly central obesity tend to have the lowest health-related quality-of-life scores.

There are other personal effects of obesity. In the United States and other westernized countries, obese persons experience discrimination that can affect employment opportunities, college acceptance, job earnings, rental availability, and marriage (12). Several studies show that physicians and medical students also harbor negative attitudes toward obese patients, which the patients themselves can sense, and which may negatively affect care.

Health Care Use and Costs

Along with the increased prevalence of obesity, health care use has increased for this disease. In the 1990s, physician visits related to obesity in the United States increased approximately 90% (15). Obese persons, on average, have more physician visits, receive more medical services, and fill more prescriptions than their nonobese counterparts. Given the medical consequences, obesity is also costly to society both directly, in terms of health care dollars, and indirectly, in terms of lost productivity and disability. Although the total economic costs of obesity are difficult to calculate, estimates for the direct health care costs have increased to $78.5 billion per year in the United States, accounting for 9.1% of the overall national health expenditure (3). There is little doubt that patients and society would benefit significantly if obesity were prevented or more successfully treated.

EVALUATION

Despite the known consequences of obesity, both the medical community and society have been reluctant to consider it a disease and to recommend routine screening and treatment. Recently, however, a number of prominent medical organizations, including the U.S. Preventive Services Task Force, the American Medical Association (AMA), the American Association of Family Practice (AAFP), the American Diabetes Association (ADA), and the American Heart Association (AHA) have recommended that all adults be screened for obesity using the body mass index (BMI) and that they be appropriately treated (16–19).

Degree and Distribution of Obesity

Calculating BMI

The first step in assessing obesity is to estimate body fat by calculating the BMI. Other methods, such as bioelectrical impedance, hydrodensitometry, dual-energy x-ray absorptiometry (DEXA), and computerized tomography (CT) scans, are more accurate but are expensive and are impractical in the office setting.

BMI is calculated by dividing weight (in kilograms) by height squared (in meters): BMI = Weight (kg)/Height squared (m^2). If pounds and inches are used, the formula is as follows: BMI = (Weight [lb] × 703)/ Height squared (in^2). For ease of assessment, there are reference tables available, Internet-based online calculators, and programs that can be downloaded into a Personal Data Assistant (PDA), such as from the website of the National Institutes of Health (NIH; www.nhlbi.nih.gov/guidelines/obesity/ob_home.htm). Table 83.2 is an abbreviated BMI table as an example.

Classifying Weight Status by BMI

Based on the risks of mortality, diabetes, hypertension, and atherosclerotic coronary heart disease associated with different BMIs, the NIH and the World Health Organization (WHO) have developed a classification for weight based on BMI (12,20), which is shown in Table 83.3. A BMI ≥30 kg/m^2 is classified as obese, which is further broken down into three subgroups of severity. The term *morbidly*

TABLE 83.2 Body Mass Index Table

BMI	*20*	*25*	*30*	*35*	*40*
Height (in)	Body Weight (lb)				
60	102	128	153	179	204
62	109	136	164	191	218
64	116	145	174	204	232
66	124	155	186	216	247
68	131	164	197	230	262
70	139	174	209	243	278
72	147	184	221	258	294
74	155	194	233	272	328
76	164	205	246	287	328

TABLE 83.3 Classification of Weight Based on BMI

Underweight	<18.5 kg/m^2
Normal weight	18.5–24.9 kg/m^2
Overweight	25–29.9 kg/m^2
Obesity	≥30 kg/m^2
Class I obesity	30–34.9 kg/m^2
Class II obesity	35–39.9 kg/m^2
Class III obesity	≥40 kg/m^2

obese generally refers to a BMI ≥40 kg/m^2, and *superobese* refers to a BMI ≥50 kg/m^2. Although currently the classification is the same for all racial/ethnic groups, it has been proposed that a healthy BMI for people of Asian descent is <23 kg/m^2 and that ≥27 kg/m^2 should be considered obese in this population, based on their risk of morbidity.

Although an increased BMI usually indicates increased body fat in the average person, there are circumstances where this is not the case, such as a professional athlete (who has increased muscle mass) or someone with anasarca (who has increased body fluid). Although such individuals have an elevated BMI, they should not be considered obese.

Measuring Waist Circumference

In addition to the degree of obesity, the *distribution* of body fat is also associated with the risk of complications from obesity. Individuals with more abdominal fat have a greater risk of comorbid conditions (such as diabetes) and mortality (21,22). Abdominal fat can be estimated using the waist circumference. In individuals with a BMI of 25 to 35 kg/m^2, a waist circumference >40 inches (102 cm) in men, or >35 inches (88 cm) in women, portends a higher risk. In individuals with a BMI >35 or 40 kg/m^2, the waist circumference adds little information.

Waist circumference can be measured by placing the tape measure just above the iliac crest in a horizontal plane around the abdomen. The tape should be snug and parallel to the ground, but should not compress the skin. The measurement should be taken at the end of normal respiration.

Another measure of fat distribution is the waist-to-hip ratio. This is calculated by dividing the waist circumference by the hip circumference. The hip circumference is measured similarly to the waist circumference described above, but at the widest part of the hips. A waist-to-hip ratio >1.0 in men or >0.8 in women is associated with higher risk. Either the waist circumference or the waist-to-hip ratio can be used; however, the waist circumference alone provides sufficient information and takes less time to do.

Risk Assessment

Once an individual's BMI and waist circumference have been determined, assessment should turn to whether there is any impact of the weight on other disease states, and whether there are other risk factors for cardiovascular disease. These can be divided into three categories (Table 83.4). The first category comprises diseases associated with a *high risk* of morbidity and mortality such as existing coronary artery disease. The second category comprises the other standard cardiovascular risk factors such as smoking and hypertension. The third category includes other obesity-associated diseases, such as osteoarthritis and stress urinary incontinence, which may be most important to the patient in terms of daily function and quality of life.

TABLE 83.4 Categories of Risk in Obese Patients

High-Risk Conditions
Coronary artery disease
Other vascular diseases (e.g., abdominal aortic aneurysm, carotid artery stenosis, peripheral artery disease)
Diabetes
Obstructive sleep apnea
Standard Cardiovascular Risk Factors
Age >45 for men, >55 (or postmenopausal) for women
Smoking
Hypertension
Hypercholesterolemia (especially high LDL)
Low HDL
High triglycerides
Glucose intolerance
Family history of premature heart disease
Sedentary lifestyle
Abdominal obesity (waist circumference >40 inches in men, >35 inches in women)
Other Obesity-Related Conditions
Oligomenorrhea/reduced fertility
Osteoarthritis
Cholelithiasis
Urinary Incontinence

LDL, low-density lipoprotein.

Putting the entire assessment together, the overall risk associated with obesity can be estimated using the weight classification (or BMI) and the comorbid conditions (Table 83.5). The overall risk will help to determine whether a person needs to be treated, and if so, how aggressively. This is addressed further in the Management section of this chapter.

Assessment of Motivation and Readiness

Because treatment of obesity involves behavioral changes and thus significant patient commitment, the final step in assessment is to determine the patient's current motivation and readiness to lose weight. Reviewing several questions with the patient can help the practitioner decide whether

TABLE 83.5 Estimation of Risk for Obese Patients[a]

		Disease Risk	
Weight Classification	*BMI*	*0 High AND <1 Other Risk Conditions[b]*	*1 High AND/OR 2 or more Other Risk Conditions[b]*
Normal	18.5–24.9	—	Increased
Overweight	25–29.9	Increased	High
Class I obesity	30–34.9	High	Very high
Class II obesity	35–39.9	Very high	Extremely high
Class III obesity	≥40	Extremely high	Extremely high

[a]Relative to people with normal weight and waist circumference.
[b]See Table 83.4.

to counsel the patient to start a weight-loss program now or defer it to another time (Table 83.6).

Whether it is the patient's idea to lose weight or someone else's (family, significant other) affects patient motivation. If the practitioner is the one who raises the issue, then it is helpful to discover whether or not the patient has thought about this, and whether or not the patient thinks losing weight is a good idea. Only if the patient recognizes the importance of weight loss are the efforts likely to be successful.

Understanding what prompted the person to seek help at this time can help the physician understand the underlying motivation and goals. These can be used to reinforce the importance of weight loss, not just for the patient's reasons, but also for appropriate medical reasons. Even if the patient did not seek help for obesity, personalizing the message about weight loss is important. It links the patient's current symptoms, health status, and risk of developing diseases to the benefits they can anticipate by losing even small amounts of weight.

Assessment of stress level and mood can help the physician decide if this is an appropriate time to start a weight-loss program. Although the physician should not postpone treatment indefinitely, it is important to keep in mind that losing weight requires time and effort, so the patient must be able to commit that or the patient will be less successful.

TABLE 83.6 Questions to Ask to Assess Patient Readiness and Motivation to Start a Weight-Loss Program

1. Has the patient sought weight loss on his or her own initiative?
2. What events have led the patient to seek weight loss now?
3. What are the patient's stress level and mood?
4. Does the patient have an eating disorder in addition to obesity?
5. Does the patient understand the requirements of treatment and believe that he or she can fulfill them?
6. How much weight does the patient expect to lose? What other benefits does the patient anticipate?

It is reasonable to assess patients for binge-eating disorder (see Etiology, above). Successful weight loss may be better achieved in combination with or after therapy for this eating disorder. Additionally, a good understanding of the requirements of weight-loss treatment by the patient, *and a belief that he or she can make the needed changes* (good self-efficacy), will increase the likelihood of success.

A careful exploration of *how much* the patient wants to lose and *in what time frame* will help to identify any unrealistic goals in these areas (e.g., trying to lose 30 lb in 2 to 3 months). The physician can then provide feedback on how much weight loss is important for medical reasons (which is often less than the patient desires), and over what time frame (e.g., 1 to 2 lb per week is considered to be the safe and effective rate). Exploring the reasonableness of the weight loss goals and the time frame is essential to setting appropriate short-term goals.

Finally, it is useful to assess the resources (e.g., financial, social, time) available to the patient. The reasonableness and achievability of a patient's goals, as well as the specific approaches to these goals, are often dependent on the resources available to the patient.

The answers to these and similar questions can help determine whether the patient is ready to make the changes needed to lose weight. It is useful, in this regard, to employ a "Stages of Change" Model (23), as in Chapter 4. Depending on the patient's stage, different approaches can be used to get the patient into the action or maintenance stage. For instance, if an obese person is in the precontemplation stage, then the most effective and efficient use of time may be to deliver a concise message about the specific importance of weight loss for the patient and some information for the patient to review. This approach, when followed up over time (or a series of visits), can eventually result in a patient who is ready to lose weight (i.e., is in the action stage) and will reduce the practitioner's frustration related to counseling someone who is not ready to make changes. Furthermore, if weight loss is medically indicated but not discussed, the patient may infer it is not important. Thus a brief discussion about weight management is indicated

TABLE 83.7 Ten Key Steps in Weight Management in the Primary Care Setting

1. Measure height and weight
2. Calculate BMI
3. Measure waist circumference
4. Assess overall disease risk
5. Decide whether the patient should be treated
6. Decide whether the patient is ready and motivated
7. Institute combination therapy: diet, physical activity, and behavior modification
8. Followup and modify or intensify plan as needed
9. Consider pharmacotherapy
10. Consider surgical treatment

for every patient and is discussed further in the Prevention section.

MANAGEMENT

General Approach

Weight management should be approached within the context of a working partnership between the practitioner and patient that takes into account the patient's attitudes and beliefs about weight and weight-loss treatments. More frequent contact during the weight-loss efforts can enhance compliance and produce better results. Such contact need not be limited to office visits with the practitioner, but could include weight checks with a nurse, as well as phone calls or e-mails from physicians or other office personnel. After the initial assessment, the practitioner can turn to weight-loss strategies. Table 83.7 outlines the key steps for weight management in the primary care setting.

The most effective approach to weight loss is a combination of calorie reduction, physical activity, and behavior modification (12,24). These can be added over a series of visits. In addition, similar to the approach to hypercholesterolemia, caregivers should use a stepped approach based on the patient's overall risk (Table 83.8). For instance, in a patient at high risk for complications, the first step should be a trial of caloric reduction, physical activity, and behavior change. These efforts can be intensified over a number of months (6 to 12 months depending on risks). If unsuccessful, pharmacotherapy should be considered. Finally, depending on patient risk, bariatric surgery should be considered.

Patients should be counseled to avoid programs or approaches that are highly restrictive, such as very-low-calorie diets with an intake of <800 kcal per day, or those that exclude or overemphasize entire groups of foods or nutrients. Weight loss can generally be achieved using a balanced diet, and nutritional supplements are not required. Recent public health guidelines nevertheless recommend that adults consider taking one multivitamin per day (25). Even in the absence of weight loss, a balanced diet with fresh fruits, fresh vegetables, low-fat dairy products, chicken and fish (such as the DASH [Dietary Approaches to Stop Hypertension] diet) can significantly impact indices of health such as blood pressure (26).

Weight-Loss Goals

Very few obese patients lose enough weight to be reclassified as "normal." At the same time, a 5% to 10% reduction in weight is achievable and can have a significant impact on comorbidities such as diabetes and blood pressure (27,28). Furthermore, a weight loss of this magnitude also reduces the risk of developing diabetes in people who are at high risk by 50% (29–31). With that in mind, the initial goal should be to lose 10% of current body weight over a 6-month period.

Rate of Weight Loss

Patients can typically lose 0.5 to 1 lb a week by reducing their caloric intake by 300 to 500 kcal per day (1 lb = 3,500

TABLE 83.8 Stepped Obesity Management Recommendations Based on Patient Health Risk[a]

Health Risk	*Best Treatment Options*	*Where to Find*
Minimal or low	Healthy eating habits Increased physical activity Lifestyle change strategies	Self-help resources
Increased or high	All of the above PLUS Reduced-calorie diet	Registered dieticians or community-based programs
Very high	All of the above PLUS Consider pharmacotherapy	Medical office or clinical weight-loss programs
Extremely high	All of the above PLUS Consider surgical intervention	Comprehensive surgery program

[a]Always start with basic treatments and add on components as appropriate given the patient's medical history, medications, and presence/absence of eating or mood disorders.

calories). A reduction in caloric intake by 500 to 1,000 kcal per day can result in the loss of 1 to 2 lb per week. These levels of caloric consumption and rates of weight loss are considered safe without any special monitoring, and faster initial weight loss does not produce better results in the long run (i.e., at 1 year) (32). If the initial caloric reduction does not produce the desired results, calories can be further reduced to about 1,000 kcal per day. Amounts below this require special monitoring.

It is common for weight loss to plateau after 6 months. That should be discussed with patients up front; patients should be reassured that plateauing is normal. If further weight reduction is desired eventually, options include taking a respite of several months (i.e., maintaining weight but not attempting to lose more weight), trying methods that previously worked again, and trying methods they have not previously employed.

Diet

The cornerstone of weight loss is creating a caloric deficit—that is, taking in fewer calories than the number of calories being spent. For most people, this requires a reduction in caloric intake, with or without an increase in expenditure, rather than an increase in caloric expenditure alone. For those with BMIs ranging from 25 to 35 kg/m^2 a reduction in daily caloric intake by 300 to 500 kcal per day is recommended to produce weight loss of 0.5 to 1 lb per week. For men this usually means consuming 1,600 to 1,800 kcal per day, and for women, 1,400 to 1,600 kcal per day. For those with a BMI >35 kg/m^2, reduction in caloric intake by 500 to 1,000 kcal per day is recommended for a weight loss of 1 to 2 lb per week. For men this usually means limiting calories to 1,200 to 1,600 kcal per day, and for women 1,000 to 1,200 kcal per day. Table 83.9 summarizes these recommendations.

Practical suggestions on food shopping and preparation, low-calorie menus, and dining out are available from numerous resources, including the Practical Guidelines from the NIH (available at www.nhlbi.nih.gov/guidelines/obesity/ob_home.htm) (33). For all diet plans, weight regain can occur when the diet is stopped.

Specific Dietary Recommendations

The optimal dietary recommendations for healthy adults are uncertain. The U.S. Department of Agriculture released a revised Food Guide Pyramid in 2005. It recommends a balanced diet that emphasizes grains, fruits, and vegetables, and limits total fat to <30%, saturated fat to <10%, and minimizes sweets (see Chapter 15, Fig. 15.1). The revised Food Guide Pyramid also places greater emphasis on the importance of whole grains that are high in fiber and micronutrients and have less impact on blood sugar (e.g., oatmeal, whole wheat bread, brown rice) (34,35). Consumption of trans fats (e.g., margarine and partially hydrogenated oils found in many packaged foods) have greater negative health consequences than saturated fats and should be kept to a minimum (36–39). Finally, the Food Guide Pyramid encourages consumption of lean proteins, including fish, beans, peas, and nuts, as alternatives for meats.

The "Low Carb" Frenzy

Several proponents of their own diets have argued that diets that emphasize protein intake, minimize carbohydrates, and may or may not ignore fat are more effective at weight reduction than other types of diets. For example, the Atkins diet emphasizes consumption of protein, severe reduction in carbohydrate intake (<20 g per day initially), and pays little attention to fat intake, often resulting in consumption of high-fat foods. Other variations on this theme include the South Beach Diet and the Zone Diet.

Although initially there were few data on the outcomes of low-carbohydrate diets, the results of several controlled clinical trials showed significantly greater weight loss *at 6 months* in the low-carbohydrate groups compared with the low-fat groups (40–44). However, after 1 year, *there was no significant difference* in weight loss between the two groups. The low-carbohydrate diets also increased high-density lipoprotein (HDL) and markedly decreased fasting triglyceride concentrations. Although high dropout rates were seen in all groups, there tended to be fewer dropouts in the low-carbohydrate groups, which may indicate patients are more likely to adhere to this type of diet.

Some studies of low carbohydrate and other very restrictive diets have excluded people with "serious or significant" medical conditions, although people with hypertension, diabetes, and/or the metabolic syndrome have sometimes been included. Thus caution should be used in the face of certain diseases. For example, because the initial weight loss from low-carbohydrate diets is a result

TABLE 83.9 Recommended Initial Caloric Reduction Based on Baseline BMI

BMI Range	*Initial Caloric Reduction*	*Initial Calorie Range*	*Expected Rate of Weight Loss*
25–35 kg/m^2	300–500 kcal/day	Men: 1,600–1,800 kcal/day Women: 1,400–1,600 kcal/day	0.5–1 lb/wk
>35 kg/m^2	500–1,000 kcal/day	Men: 1,200–1,600 kcal/day Women: 1,000–1,200 kcal/day	1–2 lb/wk

of diuresis, persons who are at risk for dehydration should either be discouraged from using the Atkins diet or should be monitored closely.

Finally, it is important to keep in mind that the weight loss from "low-carb" diets is achieved through a reduction in calories eaten, rather than some "magic" with intake of fewer carbohydrates. Just as with any diet plan, a reduction in caloric intake by 500 to 1,000 kcal per day generally results in a weight loss of 1 to 2 lb per week. Overall, the most effective diet is the diet that the patient can "stick with" over time. The decision on which diet to use should be made with the patient's preferences and medical conditions in mind.

Meal Replacements

Another approach to dieting is using meal replacements, such as Slim-Fast, which are widely available to the public. Generally these are used as partial meal replacement (PMR) plans, wherein two meals each day are replaced, and a third is consumed as a balanced low-calorie meal.

Although data are somewhat limited, several trials indicate that PMR plans result in an average 5.5- to 6.6-lb greater weight loss at 3 months and a 5.3- to 7.5-lb greater weight loss at 1 year compared with standard low-calorie diets (45). These also appear to be safe in patients with comorbid conditions including diabetes, and compliance with this approach may be greater for longer time periods. Thus the use of PMR plans should be considered, especially for patients for whom an easy, less-time-consuming way of achieving a low-calorie diet is desirable.

Medically Supervised Programs

Another option for patients is enrolling in a medically supervised program. These generally employ the use of very-low-calorie diets (VLCDs; <800 kcal per day) through the use of liquid supplements (Medifast or Optifast) or other prepackaged meals. Early use of VLCDs was associated with some deaths, with the cause thought to be attributable to a lack of high-quality protein. This was rectified with a change in the formulation of the supplements used and the focus on protein-sparing modified fasts.

Overall, limited available data suggest that the VLCDs used in medically supervised programs may result in faster initial weight loss, but probably do not result in greater long-term (1 year) weight loss (46). Such severe dietary restriction is also associated with more side effects, ranging from dry mouth and constipation to orthostasis, fatigue, hair loss, to increased rates of cholecystitis, which might lower compliance rates over the long-term.

Referral to supervised weight-loss programs that employ VLCDs may be indicated in highly motivated patients interested in faster weight loss. However, these tend to require substantial time commitments (e.g., weekly visits), are often quite costly, and, as with all weight-loss programs, are rarely covered by insurance.

Registered Dieticians

The resources and help of dieticians should not be overlooked. These trained professionals can provide one-on-one counseling that, typically, is based on a balanced, low-calorie diet. As the main focus of their counseling is the diet, the dieticians can spend the extra time needed to explain concepts such as calories and ways to reduce them, different nutrients and their sources, and how to read food labels. They can also develop detailed individual diet plans and provide followup visits to assess compliance and problem solve to overcome barriers. These services are especially useful for the "novice" dieter who knows little about diet and nutrition. Insurance coverage for dietician services varies by type of insurance, state, and presence of other comorbidities. Even without coverage, dietician services are often as affordable as commercial programs and should be considered a useful adjunct.

Community-Based Weight-Loss Programs

There are a variety of commercial weight-loss programs (e.g., Weight Watchers, Jenny Craig) available to patients, including a number of online programs. These typically provide social support and frequent followup, specific dietary information, and information to help identify problematic behaviors and situations and develop different ways to respond. In the face of very little evidence available from randomized controlled trials, these programs (in particular, Weight Watchers) may improve weight loss for periods up to 2 years (47).

Commercial weight-loss programs may be indicated in some patients and can be discussed as an adjunct to their ongoing efforts. However, it is important to keep in mind that not all programs are the same and some may be expensive, ineffective, or even dangerous. Because commercial weight-loss programs change frequently to keep up with consumer demand, it is difficult to provide specific recommendations on programs. Historically, programs such as Weight Watchers (www.weightwatchers.com) and Jenny Craig (www.jennycraig.com) have been developed by registered dieticians and have included physicians and psychologists on their boards. There are also support groups, such as "Take Off Pounds Sensibly" (TOPS, www.tops.org) or Overeaters Anonymous (OA, www.oa.org), which do not offer specific diet information, but simply provide a setting for regular group support and interaction. Other things to consider when helping a patient choose a program are whether the program emphasizes a slow, steady weight loss and includes a program for weight maintenance. Finally, a program should provide detailed information about fees and costs of any additional items (24).

Physical Activity

Regular physical activity is essential to *long-term weight control*. It can help modestly with initial weight loss, but more importantly, it is the best predictor of weight-loss *maintenance* (48). Even in the absence of weight loss, increased physical activity or exercise is associated with redistribution of adiposity away from the abdomen and reduced morbidity and mortality. It is recommended that caregivers regularly monitor and recommend routine physical activity to all patients.

In designing a physical activity plan with a patient, it is important to set appropriate and achievable goals. Setting inappropriately ambitious physical activity goals are likely to result in abandonment of the exercise program (49). In addition, several studies have compared the impact of lifestyle activity (e.g., taking the stairs, parking further away) versus aerobic exercise and demonstrated that they result in similar health benefits (50,51).

As with other behavioral interventions, the physical activity plan should be tailored to the individual. Although some may choose to engage in vigorous physical activity, others should be encouraged to start with low-impact, moderate-intensity physical activity (e.g., walking) of short duration, with a goal of accumulating 30 minutes of physical activity or more on most days of the week. After this goal is met, the practitioner can discuss with the patient if a further increase in activity is realistic. Evidence suggests that physical activity for 60 minutes each day imparts increased benefits and is more likely to help maintain weight loss (52); however, this level of physical activity may be hard to achieve and maintain. Thus, patients should be provided with advice that is realistic and manageable for them.

Whatever plan of physical activity is chosen, it should have the following SMART characteristics: it is *S*pecific (e.g., walking, swimming), *M*easurable (e.g., duration and or distance), *A*ction-oriented (cardiovascular, not weight training or abdominal exercises), *R*ealistic, and *T*imely (start with short-term goals that build in intensity and duration). The following is an example of a SMART goal that a practitioner and patient may negotiate: "I will walk briskly for 20 minutes on Monday, Wednesday, and Friday mornings this coming week. After I reach this goal, I will reward myself by purchasing a new CD. For the following 5 weeks, I will increase my time by 5 minutes per day each week, until I am walking 45 minutes every Monday, Wednesday, and Friday." A followup visit after 6 weeks can assess progress and establish new goals.

Behavior Modification

Behavior modification encompasses a variety of techniques to help people change their behaviors and can be tailored to help achieve weight loss (Table 83.10). Research shows that *the most important behavior change tool* for the majority of people is *self-monitoring* through the use of a food log. Self-monitoring is essential to the process of behavior change. Food and activity logs are frequently the behavioral activities that patients are most resistant to do; the willingness to do them also seems to reflect a readiness to "do what it takes" to change one's lifestyle. In addition, the act of self-monitoring alone may cause people to eat less and/or exercise more.

TABLE 83.10 Examples of Behavior Modification Strategies That May be Useful in Weight Reduction

Behavior Modification Strategy	*Examples*
Self-monitoring	Keeping a daily food and activity log
Stimulus control	Avoiding shopping when hungry
	Keeping high-fat, high-calorie foods out of the house
Meal planning	Planning meals for a week at a time with corresponding shopping list
Reward system	Administering small (nonfood) rewards, such as going to a movie for achieving behavioral goals
Relapse prevention	Avoiding buffets to reduce the likelihood of overeating significantly
Positive social support	Attending weight-loss groups
	Arranging regular physical activity with one or more friends

In addition to self-monitoring, there are a number of other strategies to control portions and reduce caloric intake. S*timulus control* identifies triggers or cues that may encourage unplanned eating and attempts to remove them (53). *Meal planning* can also play a major role in controlling portions and avoiding overeating. These efforts are likely to reinforce dietary adherence by increasing access to appropriate foods and reducing impulsive intake of calorically dense foods.

Relapse prevention is another important behavioral strategy for weight control. Patients are encouraged to identify and limit their exposure to high-risk situations and plan accordingly in an effort to minimize overeating or unplanned eating episodes. Finding ways to overcome predictable dietary or physical activity slips and "get back with the program" is also a key component of relapse prevention. Use of a *reward system* may also enhance compliance with behavior changes. A final behavior modification tool is to seek *positive social support*. For some this can be found in weight-loss groups or can be among friends who may all be trying to lose or maintain their weight actively.

During each office visit the patient and physician can review the weight-loss goals, adherence to the diet and physical activity plans, and any barrier limiting success, and they can problem solve together, identifying behavioral tools that might enhance weight-loss efforts.

Pharmacotherapy

If, after at least 6 months, a regimen of a low-calorie diet, increased physical activity, and behavior modification fails to induce significant weight loss, pharmacotherapy can be considered. Appropriate candidates for pharmacotherapy are patients with (a) a BMI $\geq$30 kg/m^2 or (b) a BMI of 27 to 29.9 kg/m^2 with comorbid conditions (Table 83.8) (12).

Pharmacotherapies can be divided into those that are FDA approved for weight loss (Table 83.11), those that are FDA approved for other indications that also can induce weight loss, and over-the-counter agents promoted for weight loss. No matter which agent is used, weight is often regained after cessation of medication. Medication should only be included along with lifestyle changes as part of a comprehensive weight-loss plan. In addition, the potential side effects and the need to continue drug therapy to maintain weight loss should be discussed with the patient prior to starting medication.

FDA-Approved Drugs for Weight Loss

FDA-approved medications for weight loss can be broadly divided into long-term and short-term agents (Table 83.11). Orlistat (Xenical) reduces dietary fat absorption by approximately 30% and produces an average weight loss of 2.6 kg (5.7 lb) at 6 months and 2.9 kg (6.4 lb) at 1 year when compared with placebo (54). When continued for 2 years, orlistat lessens regain of weight and improves weight-loss maintenance (55). Treatment with orlistat also results in significant decreases in systolic blood pressure, waist circumference, total cholesterol, low-density lipoprotein (LDL) cholesterol, and fasting serum insulin and glucose levels. Orlistat has little systemic absorption, so its side effects are mainly gastrointestinal and include flatus with discharge, steatorrhea, diarrhea, fecal urgency, and incontinence. Reduction of fat intake and the use of psyllium (as found in Metamucil) can decrease these side effects; in

TABLE 83.11 FDA-Approved Weight-Loss Medications

Drug (Generic)	*Brand Name(s)*	*Dose*	*Action*	*Main Adverse Effects*	*Average Cost for 1-Month Supply (2004)*
Long-term use ($\geq$12 Months)					
Sibutramine	Meridia	10 mg PO q.d.	Norepinephrine, serotonin, and dopamine reuptake inhibitor	Increase in heart rate and blood pressure	$170
Orlistat	Xenical	120 mg PO before every meal	Inhibits pancreatic lipase, which reduces dietary fat absorption	Steatorrhea, malabsorption of fat-soluble vitamins	$104
Short-term use (<3 Months)					
Phentermine resin	Ionamin	15–30 mg PO q.d.	Central anorexigenic effects, similar to amphetamines	Palpitations, tachycardia, increased blood pressure, possible pulmonary hypertension with longer use (>3 months); potential for abuse	~$40
Phentermine	Adipex-P	18.75–37.5mg PO q.d.			
Diethylpropion	Tenuate	25 mg PO t.i.d. SR: 75 mg PO q.d.			
Benzphetamine	Didrex	25–50 mg PO q.d.-t.i.d.			
Phendimetrazine	Bontril, X-trozine, X-Trozine LA	17.5–70 mg PO b.i.d.-t.i.d.			

contrast, a high-fat meal after taking orlistat can exacerbate them. Finally, there is the potential for malabsorption of the fat-soluble vitamins (A, D, E, and K), so multivitamin supplementation between meals is recommended, as is careful monitoring of prothrombin time (PT)/international normalized ratio (INR) for patients taking warfarin (see Chapter 57). Orlistat is taken 120 mg by mouth 30 minutes before each meal.

Sibutramine (Meridia) is a serotonin and norepinephrine reuptake inhibitor that acts to enhance satiety. Sibutramine results in an average weight loss of 4.5 kg (9.9 lb) when compared with placebo at 1 year (54). Use of sibutramine has resulted in improvement in blood glucose concentration, but no consistent effect on lipid levels. The effect on blood pressure may vary, but some studies show an increase in diastolic blood pressure when compared to placebo, and a slight increase in average heart rate ($\sim$4 beats/min). Pre-existing hypertension is not an absolute contraindication to the use of sibutramine, but blood pressure should be well-controlled before and during administration of the drug (56). Valvulopathy and pulmonary hypertension have not been seen with sibutramine. Sibutramine is taken orally 10 mg/day.

A number of other prescription medications for weight loss, such as phentermine and diethylpropion, are FDA approved for short-term use, which is defined as less than 12 weeks. On average, phentermine results in 3.6-kg (7.9-lb) greater weight loss than placebo, and diethylpropion results in a 3.0-kg (6.6-lb) greater loss (54). There are some reported cases of pulmonary hypertension and valvulopathies, as well as stroke (phentermine), associated with these drugs after long-term use. Both are thought to work by inhibiting appetite, although there may be separate effects on metabolism or the central nervous system. Similar to amphetamines, these drugs can cause palpitations, tachycardia, increased blood pressure, and tachyphylaxis and tolerance over time. They should be taken in the morning to lessen any sleep disturbance. Several of the short-term agents (benzphetamine and phendimetrazine) have limited potential for abuse and are class IV controlled substances. Several promising new pharmacotherapies for obesity are in testing, including a cannabinoid-1 receptor blocker, rimonabant (57), and a genetically engineered recombinant human variant ciliary neurotrophic factor (rhvCNTF) that signals through leptinlike pathways (58). Clinicians will likely hear more about such approaches in the future.

FDA-Approved Drugs for Other Indications that Can Cause Weight Loss

Several drugs have demonstrated some efficacy for weight loss, but are FDA approved for other indications and not for weight loss. These include metformin, fluoxetine, sertraline, bupropion, topiramate, and zonisamide. It is not appropriate to prescribe these medications primarily for their ability to produce weight loss. However, in patients who have other treatment indications, such as diabetes, it is appropriate and important to consider whether any of the medication options could enhance or promote weight loss (e.g., metformin).

Over-the-Counter Weight-Loss Products

Two over-the-counter agents, phenylpropanolamine (e.g., Acutrim, Dexatrim) and ephedra or ma huang (e.g., Metabolife), have been taken off the market because of concerns of adverse cardiovascular effects (increased risk of stroke). Sale of ephedra-containing products was prohibited by the FDA in April 2004. Because of such safety concerns and limited quality control over dietary supplements, use of over-the-counter products for weight loss should not be recommended.

Bariatric Surgery

If pharmacotherapy is not tolerated or does not achieve the desired weight reduction in combination with diet, physical activity, and behavior modification, bariatric surgery should be considered. Appropriate candidates for weight loss surgery include patients with (a) a BMI $\geq$40 kg/m^2 or (b) a BMI of 35 to 39.9 kg/m^2 with other high-risk comorbid conditions or weight-induced physical problems interfering with performance of daily activities (Table 83.8) (12,59). A discussion of surgical options should include the long-term side effects, such as the possible need for reoperation, gall bladder disease, and malabsorption.

Surgical procedures commonly used today can be classified as predominantly restrictive (vertical-banded gastroplasty, adjustable gastric banding) or malabsorptive (Roux-en-Y gastric bypass, biliopancreatic diversion with duodenal switch), as shown in Figures 83.1 and 83.2. In general, gastric bypass appears to produce more weight loss than gastroplasty, and laparoscopic surgeries tend to have fewer wound complications (e.g., infections).

Numerous case series show marked improvement in most obesity-related comorbidities, including type 2 diabetes (up to 90% resolve), hypertension (up to 66% resolve), and sleep apnea, as well as improvements in lipids, left ventricular wall thickness, mobility, return of fertility, and significant improvement in quality of life. Many patients can be off medications for obesity-related comorbidities 3 years after surgery (60,61). Bariatric surgery has resulted in weight losses between 22 and 37 kg (48 and 81 lb) greater than nonsurgical treatments, which may be maintained for more than 8 years (62).

The risks of bariatric surgery include death, which is reported to be $<$1% in selected patients, and $<$2% in

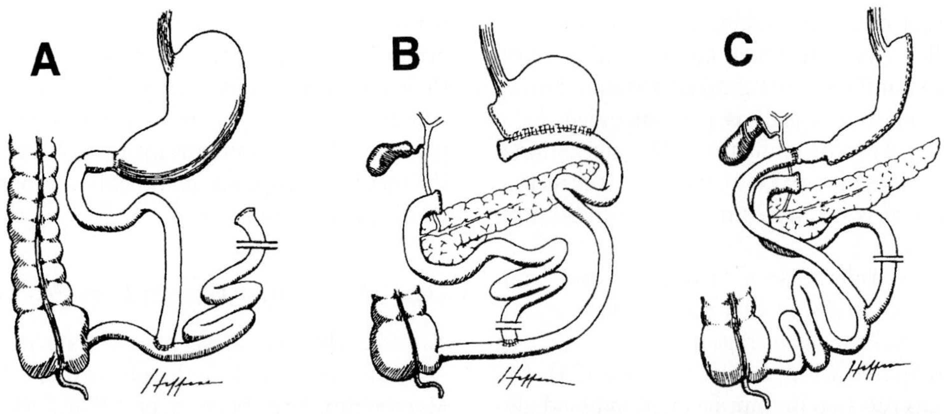

FIGURE 83.1. Bariatric procedures that work predominantly through malabsorption are **(A)** jejunoileal bypass, **(B)** biliopancreatic diversion, and **(C)** duodenal switch. (From Mun EC, Blackburn GL, Matthews JB. Current status of medical and surgical therapy for obesity. Gastroenterology 2001;120:674, with permission.)

studies of administrative data (i.e., unselected patients). Overall rates of complications vary according to the procedure, ranging from 7% to 38% for gastrointestinal symptoms, 3% to 17% for nutrition and electrolyte imbalances, and 2% to 12% for complications requiring reoperation (e.g., stenoses, bleeding). Complication rates are lower in high-volume (>100 procedures per year) centers. Recently, a program to designate Centers of Excellence in Bariatric Surgery was established, which should eventually help providers and patients make informed choices when choosing this option. Finally, as with most surgical referrals, information about the individual surgeon's practice, weight-loss results, and complication rate should be sought prior to making a referral.

Relapse

For most people it is difficult to maintain the lifestyle changes they adopted to achieve weight loss and they face weight regain over the long-term. Efforts to prevent relapse, including informing patients of potential weight regain with the cessation of efforts, are important. Monitoring the patient's weight in the office may also be helpful. Weight regain can be approached in a similar way to a weight-loss plateau—that is, restarting methods that previously worked again or trying methods not previously employed. Motivation frequently wanes over the long-term, so efforts to increase motivation may be needed (e.g., a new reward system) along with increased social support.

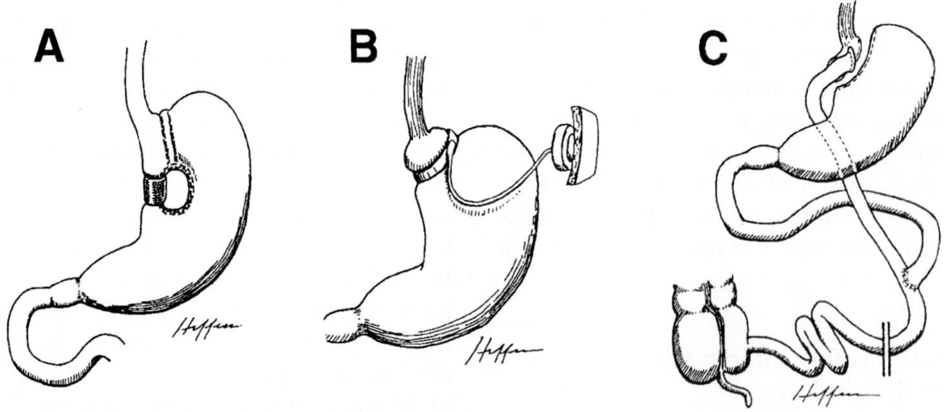

FIGURE 83.2. Bariatric procedures that work predominantly though restriction of food intake are **(A)** vertical-banded gastroplasty, **(B)** adjustable gastric banding, and a combination of restriction and malabsorption **(C)** Roux-en-Y gastric bypass. (From Mun EC, Blackburn GL, Matthews JB. Current status of medical and surgical therapy for obesity. Gastroenterology 2001;120:674, with permission.)

PREVENTION

Overweight and obesity are among the top 10 health priorities established by the U.S. Department of Health and Human Services in *Healthy People 2010*. Given the difficulty of successfully treating obesity, prevention is of paramount importance. Ideally, prevention should begin in childhood and continue through adulthood. Many medical encounters also provide an opportunity for prevention.

Public Health Interventions

Efforts to prevent obesity may be most effective if implemented at the public health level. Like efforts to reduce smoking, efforts to reduce obesity should combine multiple strategies. Information about healthy lifestyles should be taught throughout elementary and high school education, and should continue as much as possible throughout adulthood. Information about foods should be made more available at points of access such as restaurants. Inclusion of portion size and nutrient and calorie information in menus (as is done in some other countries) would help consumers make informed choices.

Access to healthy and affordable foods should be assured for everyone. Furthermore, access to and marketing for unhealthy foods can be limited or eliminated in schools, on billboards, and in media targeted at children (such as cartoons on TV, or kid's magazines). In recent years, policy changes at elementary, middle, and high school levels have attempted to limit access to unhealthy foods at school. Grass-roots movements that encourage people to patronize and support restaurants that offer healthy choices and reasonably sized portions could also make a difference.

To increase physical activity, schools could once again require physical education and include time for active play, especially for young students. City planning could include sidewalks to allow for walking, as well as public parks and recreation sites to encourage regular physical activity. Finally, health policy changes that reimburse for obesity prevention and treatment prior to the onset of significant comorbidities would lessen the burden of obesity on the public. Providers can play a role in effecting such changes at local, state, and national levels, and can encourage their patients to do the same.

Primary Care Interventions

In the practitioner's office, prevention can be approached *very simply,* by measuring height and weight and calculating BMI on all patients and tracking these over time. One or two statements about the patient's weight status each visit (or at annual prevention-oriented visits) can be used. For the patient whose weight is normal, this could include congratulations on having (and maintaining) a normal weight and encouragement to continue. For an overweight patient or a patient who has recently gained some weight, the practitioner should consider a statement that indicates this fact or pattern, and encourages the patient not to gain further weight. In an obese patient, when obesity-related comorbid conditions are diagnosed or suspected, their relation to weight or weight gain can be explained to the patient. Finally, information about BMI, healthy weight, and weight loss can be displayed and/or provided to patients.

SPECIFIC REFERENCES*

1. Flegal KM, Carroll MD, Ogden CL, et al. Prevalence and trends in obesity among US adults, 1999–2000. JAMA 2002;288:1723.
2. Hedley AA, Ogden CL, Johnson CL, et al. Prevalence of overweight and obesity among US children, adolescents, and adults, 1999–2002. JAMA 2004;291:2847.
3. Finkelstein EA, Fiebelkorn IC, Wang G. National medical spending attributable to overweight and obesity: how much, and who's paying? Health Aff 2003;219–226.
4. Clement K, Boutin P, Froguel P. Genetics of obesity. Am J Pharmacogenomics 2002;177–187.
5. Mokdad AH, Marks JS, Stroup DF, et al. Actual causes of death in the United States, 2000. JAMA 2004;291:1238.
6. Flegal KM, Graubard BI, Williamson DF, et al. Excess deaths associated with underweight, overweight, and obesity. JAMA 2005;293:1861.
7. Willett WC, Dietz WH, Colditz GA. Guidelines for healthy weight. N Engl J Med 1999;341:427.
8. Fontaine KR, Redden DT, Wang C, et al. Years of life lost due to obesity. JAMA 2003;289:187.
9. Calle EE, Rodriguez C, Walker-Thurmond K, et al. Overweight, obesity, and mortality from cancer in a prospectively studied cohort of U.S. adults. N Engl J Med 2003;348:1625.
10. Bray GA. Health hazards of obesity. Endocrinol Metab Clin North Am 1996;25:907.
11. Pi-Sunyer FX. Comorbidities of overweight and obesity: current evidence and research issues. Med Sci Sports Exerc 1999;31:S602.
12. U.S. Department of Health and Human Services. Clinical Guidelines on the Identification, Evaluation, and Treatment of Overweight and Obesity in Adults. Washington DC: U.S. Department of Health and Human Services, 1998.
13. Jia H, Lubetkin EI. The impact of obesity on health-related quality-of-life in the general adult US population. J Public Health (Oxf) 2005;27:156.
14. Han TS, Tijhuis MA, Lean ME, et al. Quality of life in relation to overweight and body fat distribution. Am J Public Health 1998;88:1814.
15. Wolf AM, Colditz GA. Social and economic effects of body weight in the United States. Am J Clin Nutr 1996;63:466S.
16. U.S. Preventive Services Task Force. Screening for obesity in adults: recommendations and rationale. Ann Intern Med 2003;139:930.
17. McTigue KM, Harris R, Hemphill B, et al. Screening and interventions for obesity in adults: summary of the evidence for the U.S. Preventive Services Task Force. Ann Intern Med 2003;139:933.
18. Lyznicki JM, Young DC, Riggs JA, et al. Obesity: assessment and management in primary care. Am Fam Physician 2001;63:2185.
19. Eyre H, Kahn R, Robertson RM, et al. Preventing cancer, cardiovascular disease, and diabetes: a common agenda for the American Cancer Society, the American Diabetes Association, and the American Heart Association. Stroke 2004;35:1999.
20. World Health Organization. Obesity epidemic puts millions at risk from related diseases. WHO 1997;6-8-2004.
21. Kuczmarski RJ, Carroll MD, Flegal KM, et al. Varying body mass index cutoff points to describe overweight prevalence among U.S. adults: NHANES III (1988 to 1994). Obes Res 1997;5:542.
22. Chan JM, Rimm EB, Colditz GA, et al. Obesity, fat distribution, and weight gain as risk factors for clinical diabetes in men. Diabetes Care 1994;17:961.
23. Prochaska JO, DiClemente CC, Norcross JC. In search of how people change. Applications to addictive behaviors. Am Psychol 1992;47:1102.

*Bold numerals denote published controlled clinical trials, meta-analyses, or consensus-based recommendations.

24. Stern JS, Hirsch J, Blair SN, et al. Weighing the options: criteria for evaluating weight-management programs. Washington, DC: National Academy Press, 1995.
25. Willett WC. Eat, drink and be healthy: the Harvard Medical School guide to healthy eating. New York: Free Press, 2003.
26. Sacks FM, Appel LJ, Moore TJ, et al. A dietary approach to prevent hypertension: a review of the Dietary Approaches to Stop Hypertension (DASH) study. Clin Cardiol 1999;22:III6–III10.
27. Ross R, Dagnone D, Jones PJ, et al. Reduction in obesity and related comorbid conditions after diet-induced weight loss or exercise-induced weight loss in men. A randomized, controlled trial. Ann Intern Med 2000;133:92.
28. MacMahon S, Cutler J, Brittain E, et al. Obesity and hypertension: epidemiological and clinical issues. Eur Heart J 1987;8S:57.
29. Knowler WC, Barrett-Connor E, Fowler SE, et al. Reduction in the incidence of type 2 diabetes with lifestyle intervention or metformin. N Engl J Med 2002;346:393.
30. Tuomilehto J, Lindstrom J, Eriksson JG, et al. Prevention of type 2 diabetes mellitus by changes in lifestyle among subjects with impaired glucose tolerance. N Engl J Med 2001; 344:1343.
31. Angelo J, Huang J, Carden D. Diabetes prevention: a review of the literature. Adv Stud Med 2005;5:250.
32. Wadden TA, Foster GD, Letizia KA. One-year behavioral treatment of obesity: comparison of moderate and severe caloric restriction and the effects of weight maintenance therapy. J Consult Clin Psychol 1994;165–171.
33. NIH/NHLBI. The Practical Guide: Identification, Evaluation, and Treatment of Overweight and Obesity in Adults. Pub. No. 00-4084. Washington, DC: U.S. Department of Health and Human Services, 2000.
34. Jacobs DR, Pereira MA, Meyer KA, et al. Fiber from whole grains, but not refined grains, is inversely associated with all-cause mortality in older women: the Iowa women's health study. J Am Coll Nutr 2000;19:326S.
35. Liu S, Stampfer MJ, Hu FB, et al. Whole-grain consumption and risk of coronary heart disease: results from the Nurses' Health Study. Am J Clin Nutr 1999;70:412.
36. Dyer AR, Cutter GR, Liu KQ, et al. Alcohol intake and blood pressure in young adults: the CARDIA Study. J Clin Epidemiol 1990;43:1.
37. Mozaffarian D, Pischon T, Hankinson SE, et al. Dietary intake of trans fatty acids and systemic inflammation in women. Am J Clin Nutr 2004;79:606.
38. Stender S, Dyerberg J. Influence of trans fatty acids on health. Ann Nutr Metab 2004;48:61.
39. Oomen CM, Ocke MC, Feskens EJ, et al. Association between trans fatty acid intake and 10-year risk of coronary heart disease in the Zutphen Elderly Study: a prospective population-based study. Lancet 2001;357:746.
40. Brehm BJ, Seeley RJ, Daniels SR, et al. A randomized trial comparing a very low carbohydrate diet and a calorie-restricted low fat diet on body weight and cardiovascular risk factors in healthy women. J Clin Endocrinol Metab 2003;88:1617.
41. Foster GD, Wyatt HR, Hill JO, et al. A randomized trial of a low-carbohydrate diet for obesity. N Engl J Med 2003;348:2082.
42. Yancy WS Jr, Olsen MK, Guyton JR, et al. A low-carbohydrate, ketogenic diet versus a low-fat diet to treat obesity and hyperlipidemia: a randomized, controlled trial. Ann Intern Med 2004;140:769.
43. Stern L, Iqbal N, Seshadri P, et al. The effects of low-carbohydrate versus conventional weight loss diets in severely obese adults: one-year follow-up of a randomized trial. Ann Intern Med 2004;140:778.
44. Dansinger ML, Gleason JA, Griffith JL, et al. Comparison of the Atkins, Ornish, Weight Watchers, and Zone diets for weight loss and heart disease risk reduction: a randomized trial. JAMA 2005;293:43.
45. Heymsfield SB, van Mierlo CA, van der Knaap HC, et al. Weight management using a meal replacement strategy: meta and pooling analysis from six studies. Int J Obes Relat Metab Disord 2003;27:537.
46. Saris WH. Very-low-calorie diets and sustained weight loss. Obes Res 2001;9:295S.
47. Tsai AG, Wadden TA. Systematic review: an evaluation of major commercial weight loss programs in the United States. Ann Intern Med 2005;142:56.
48. Klem ML, Wing RR, McGuire MT, et al. A descriptive study of individuals successful at long-term maintenance of substantial weight loss. Am J Clin Nutr 1997;66:239.
49. American College of Sports Medicine. ACSM's guidelines for exercise testing and prescription. Baltimore: Williams & Wilkins, 1995.
50. Andersen RE, Wadden TA, Bartlett SJ, et al. Effects of lifestyle activity vs structured aerobic exercise in obese women: a randomized trial. JAMA 1999;281:335.
51. Dunn AL, Marcus BH, Kampert JB, et al. Comparison of lifestyle and structured interventions to increase physical activity and cardiorespiratory fitness: a randomized trial. JAMA 1999;281:327.
52. Institute of Medicine. Dietary reference intakes for energy, carbohydrate, fiber, fat, fatty acid, cholesterol, protein and amino acids. Washington DC: National Academies Press, 2002.
53. Ogden CL, Flegal KM, Carroll MD, et al. Prevalence and trends in overweight among US children and adolescents, 1999–2000. JAMA 2002;288:1728.
54. Li Z, Maglione M, Tu W, et al. Meta-analysis: pharmacologic treatment of obesity. Ann Intern Med 2005;142:532.
55. Davidson MH, Hauptman J, DiGirolamo M, et al. Weight control and risk factor reduction in obese subjects treated for 2 years with orlistat: a randomized controlled trial. JAMA 1999;281: 235.
56. McMahon FG, Fujioka K, Singh BN, et al. Efficacy and safety of sibutramine in obese white and African American patients with hypertension: a 1-year, double-blind, placebo-controlled, multicenter trial. Arch Intern Med 2000;160:2185.
57. Van Gaal LF, Rissanen AM, Scheen AJ, et al. Effects of the cannabinoid-1 receptor blocker rimonabant on weight reduction and cardiovascular risk factors in overweight patients: 1-year experience from the RIO-Europe study. Lancet 2005;365:1389.
58. Ettinger MP, Littlejohn TW, Schwartz SL, et al. Recombinant variant of ciliary neurotrophic factor for weight loss in obese adults: a randomized, dose-ranging study. JAMA 2003; 289:1826.
59. Balsiger BM, Luque de Leon E, Sarr MG. Surgical treatment of obesity: who is an appropriate candidate? Mayo Clin Proc 1997; 72:551.
60. Pories WJ, Swanson MS, MacDonald KG, et al. Who would have thought it? An operation proves to be the most effective therapy for adult-onset diabetes mellitus. Ann Surg 1995;222:339.
61. Maggard MA, Shugarman LR, Suttorp M, et al. Meta-analysis: surgical treatment of obesity. Ann Intern Med 2005;142:547.
62. Torgerson JS, Sjostrom L. The Swedish Obese Subjects (SOS) study—rationale and results. Int J Obes Relat Metab Disord 2001;25:S2.

*For annotated **General References** and resources related to this chapter, visit www.hopkinsbayview.org/PAMreferences.*

should be even more diligently sought, as should a family history compatible with osteoporosis. A detailed history of alcohol use and cigarette smoking should be elicited.

Physical Examination

The patient's height and weight should be compared with his previous measurements. An examination of the spine (see Chapter 71) should be done with attention to spinal deformity and spinal tenderness, especially if the patient complains of backache or loss of height. A general examination, including a testicular examination, should be performed to seek secondary causes of osteoporosis.

Radiography

Routine radiographs of the skeleton are often unrevealing, because a loss of 30% or more of bone mass must occur before osteopenia can be appreciated. Thinning of bone is usually seen first in the vertebrae, the pelvis, and the femoral heads.

The diagnosis of osteoporosis is made or confirmed by measurement of bone mineral density by DEXA scan (see Chapter 103). Multiple sites, including hips, lumbar spine, and forearms, are scanned according to standardized protocols.

Laboratory Studies

In contrast to osteomalacia, levels of serum calcium, phosphate, and alkaline phosphatase are typically normal. As there is an identifiable underlying cause in 50% of men with osteoporosis, secondary causes should be considered; therefore, other tests (e.g., measurements of serum testosterone, thyroxine, thyroid-stimulating hormone, cortisol, PTH, 25 hydroxy vitamin D, urine calcium and creatinine, serum and urine protein electrophoresis, urinary free cortisol) may be indicated.

Bone Biopsies

The only reason to do a bone biopsy is if osteoporosis and osteomalacia cannot be distinguished on the basis of the evaluation described above (see also Osteomalacia).

Treatment

There are multiple approaches to treatment. Dietary interventions include calcium supplementation to bring total calcium consumption to 1200 to 1500 mg/day and vitamin D_2 supplementation 800 International Units per day. These interventions are appropriate for all men at risk, including asymptomatic men older than 60 years of age and men taking corticosteroids or other osteoporosis-producing drugs chronically. Physical activity is important in maintaining bone mass. Resistance training and aerobic exercise, alone and in combination, have been effective in stabilizing bone density (48,49).

A number of drugs have been developed to increase bone mass, and one or more of them should be considered for all men with osteoporosis. Men with osteopenia may be treated by diet supplementation and exercise alone and monitored by DEXA scanning.

Bisphosphonates are the primary drugs used in the treatment of men with osteoporosis. They have been shown to be effective in eugonadal and hypogonadal men (50), as well as in men with glucocorticoid-induced bone loss (51,52). Therefore, bisphosphonates are indicated in men with idiopathic osteoporosis, in hypogonadal men with osteoporosis in which testosterone is not indicated or tolerated, and in men with glucocorticoid-induced bone loss. The treatment protocols are similar to those used in the treatment of women with osteoporosis (Chapter 103). A typical regimen is alendronate, 70 mg orally once a week or 10 mg/day. Alternatively, risedronate, a third-generation bisphosphonate, 35 mg a week or 5 mg/day, may be prescribed. Another oral bisphosphonate recently released is ibandronate which is administered 150 mg orally once a month (53).

Bisphosphonates should be taken in the morning, while in the upright position, with a full glass of water, 30 minutes (1 hour for ibandronate) before eating breakfast or taking other medications to avoid esophagitis, the major complication of these drugs. If the oral preparations cannot be tolerated, pamidronate or zoledronic acid, intravenously administered bisphosphonates, can be given (30 mg in saline, once every 3 months or 4 mg yearly respectively); however, these are not Food and Drug Administration (FDA)-approved for osteoporosis in men or women. Intravenous ibandronate has been recently approved by the Food and Drug Administration for treatment of osteoporosis and it is administered 3 mg every 3 months.

Because as many as 30% of men with osteoporosis have been found to be hypogonadal, the use of *testosterone* has been investigated for osteoporosis treatment (54). Many studies have demonstrated that testosterone replacement increases bone mineral density in men with hypogonadism. These studies showed efficacy of testosterone in men with primary and secondary hypogonadism and both congenital and acquired hypogonadism. Testosterone may be administered by injection, patch, gel, or orally (see Chapter 85). Since monitoring for the side effects of testosterone (prostate growth and carcinoma, hyperlipidemia, polycythemia) is critical, referral to an endocrinologist is indicated.

Calcitonin is an alternative for patients who cannot tolerate bisphosphonates. It is administered by nasal spray, one puff (200 IU) daily, alternating nostrils. The major adverse effects are rhinitis and epistaxis. Calcitonin may have an analgesic effect on bone pain. Calcitonin is not as potent as other available agents and is reserved for the patient with intolerance to other medications.

Hydrochlorothiazide has been reported to be effective in increasing bone density, but less so than bisphosphonates or calcitonin (55). It is particularly useful when the underlying reason for the reduced bone mass is hypercalciuria.

Teriparatide (parathyroid hormone) is a potent anabolic agent that builds bone in men and women (56). In a large trial of 437 men with osteoporosis treated with teriparatide (20 or 40 μg) or placebo, after just 11 months, there was a 6% to 9% increase in the bone mineral density in the spine and a 1.5% to 3% increase in the femoral neck compared to placebo (57). Teriparatide has been approved for men who have severe osteoporosis, are at high risk of fracture, or have failed other osteoporosis therapy. The benefits of therapy are weighed against the high cost of the medication (700 dollars per month), the need for daily subcutaneous injection, and concern about the theoretical risks of osteosarcoma.

Followup

The response to treatment of reduced bone density should be assessed by DEXA scan every 12 to 24 months. The use of serum and urine biomarkers of bone metabolism to assess response to therapy is less reliable than DEXA scanning and is not recommended. Patients receiving calcium and vitamin D supplementation should have serum calcium levels measured after 2 to 3 months, and then, if within normal limits, yearly thereafter to be sure that hypercalcemia does not develop. The use of testosterone and teriparatide requires special monitoring, usually by an endocrinologist.

PAGET DISEASE OF BONE

Paget disease is a focal skeletal disorder characterized by rapid absorption and subsequent formation of bone.

Epidemiology

Most commonly, Paget disease is a disorder of older individuals that increases in frequency with increasing age (58). In the United States, it occurs in approximately 3% of Caucasians older than 55 years of age; it appears to be less common among African Americans, although additional data are required to be certain of this impression (59). In the elderly it occurs almost equally often in men and in women. The epidemiology of Paget disease is unusual because of its distinctive geographic distribution throughout the world. Paget disease occurs commonly in England, North America, Australia, New Zealand, France, and Germany. By contrast, it is uncommon in Switzerland and rare in Africa and throughout Asia, including China, India, and the Middle East (60). This information is important because it points to factors, both genetic and environmental, that are essential to the occurrence of the disorder.

Pathogenesis and Etiology

Normal bone remodeling depends on a coupled metabolic response of bone-forming osteoblasts and bone-resorbing osteoclasts. Paget disease is characterized by an initial phase of intense osteoclastic resorption followed by an increase in bone formation. As a result, the rate of bone remodeling is greatly enhanced, leading to the production of excessive, dense, but structurally deficient skeletal tissue. This weakened skeletal tissue is at risk for development of bony deformities and fracture. These changes are responsible for the signs and symptoms of the disease.

Paracrystalline nuclear inclusion bodies have been observed in osteoclasts from patients with Paget disease that are similar to the nuclear inclusions found in subjects with "slow virus" infections such as progressive multifocal leukoencephalopathy and subacute sclerosing panencephalitis (61). The inclusions have been identified, with the use of viral antisera, as nucleocapsids of the paramyxovirus family, with resemblance to both the measles and respiratory syncytial viruses (62). Both measles virus and respiratory syncytial virus nucleocapsids were identified in the same osteoclasts, suggesting the expression of antigen from an altered viral particle (63). However, attempts to isolate or pass an infectious agent from cultured surgical specimens or from cultured bone cells have been unsuccessful. There is also evidence from family studies for a genetic component to Paget disease; 14% to 25% of family members of patients with Paget disease will contract the disease (58,64,65). First-degree relatives of those with Paget disease have a sevenfold to 10-fold increased risk for developing Paget (65,66). In some families with Paget disease, mutations in the SQSTM1 gene have been identified, and in other family studies, genetic susceptibility loci on chromosome 18, 6, and 5 are implicated (66). Taken together, these finding suggest that Paget disease develops in individuals with a latent viral infection in osteoclasts with genetic susceptibility.

Evaluation

History

Early in the disease, patients are asymptomatic and are diagnosed only because a screening blood test has revealed an unexplained elevation of serum alkaline phosphatase activity or when pagetic lesions are incidentally discovered during imaging for another reason (see Radiology).

Chronic pain is the most common complaint of patients with Paget disease of bone. Resulting from either direct pagetic involvement or from osteoarthropathy, pain is the presenting complaint in two thirds of subjects older than 60 years of age (67). Bone pain or limitation of joint function points to the diagnosis in approximately 50% of patients with symptomatic Paget disease. Pagetic pain is typically increased at night and in the limbs with weight bearing (68). Pain in the extremities may result from expansion of bone with involvement of the periosteum. Lumbar spine pain may result from vertebral expansion, collapse, or microfractures. Facet enlargement, cord compression, or impingement of structures in the cauda equina or spinal nerve root may result in pain. The incidence of hip pain in Paget disease ranges from 30% to 50% (69). Pagetic coxopathy refers to involvement of both femur and acetabulum that may be associated with protrusio acetabuli.

Skeletal deformity in Paget disease is most common in the long bones, skull, and clavicle. Deformity of the tibia and femur is typically bowing, caused by enlarging and abnormal contouring of the rapidly remodeling bone. These deformities can result in gait disturbances and abnormal mechanical loads that predispose to pain and fracture. Hyperemia in the vascular pagetic bone results in warmth over the affected area. Involvement of the skull first leads to areas of radiolucency called osteoporosis circumscripta; later, there is skull enlargement in the frontal and occipital area.

Fractures are the most common complication of pagetic lesions. Most frequently seen in the femur, fractures are usually transverse and perpendicular to the cortex. Because of the vascular nature of Paget bone, fractures can be associated with substantial blood loss.

Neurologic symptoms and signs in Paget disease arise from three major sources. First, there can be a reduction in the size of neural foramina, leading to compression of the cranial nerves. Compression of the eighth cranial nerve causes deafness, one of the more common problems in patients with Paget disease, and occurs in more than one third of individuals with the disorder (70). Occasionally, various ocular and facial palsies also develop. Second, brainstem and cerebellar compression and/or hydrocephalus due to basilar invagination (so called platybasia) can occur. Third, spinal cord and nerve root compression occurs occasionally. Rarely, ischemic brain disease may occur secondary to a vascular steal syndrome resulting from increased vascularity of the cranial vault. Myelopathy due to ischemic myelitis has also been reported in the presence of highly vascularized and hypermetabolic bone in the vertebral column or as a consequence of compression of the spinal arteries (71). Spinal stenosis may occur, depending on the level of vertebral involvement; symptoms vary from radicular pain to numbness, paresthesia, and, finally, progressive paraparesis with bladder and bowel involvement.

Physical Examination

Physical examination is normal early in the disease but later may reveal structural deformities of bone (e.g., sabre shins, frontal bossing of the skull), hearing loss, or signs of nerve root compression. Active pagetic areas of bone are warm to palpation on exam.

Laboratory Evaluation

Patients are often diagnosed after a screening blood test has revealed elevated serum alkaline phosphatase activity with normal serum calcium, phosphate, and parathyroid hormone concentrations and normal liver function tests. The alkaline phosphatase can be identified by the laboratory as originating in bone. The level of serum alkaline phosphatase generally correlates with the activity of the disease.

Other biologic markers of bone metabolism may be increased in patients with Paget disease. The high rate of skeletal turnover during the resorptive and mixed stages of the disease has resulted in the development of multiple assays to measure disease activity. Metabolic markers of bone disease, in addition to alkaline phosphatase, include osteocalcin, procollagen type I C-terminal peptide, and newer assays of nonmetabolized collagen peptides, including *N*-telopeptides and pyridinoline crosslinks.

The level of serum osteocalcin, a protein produced by osteoblasts, tends to be increased in states of high bone turnover. Osteocalcin levels are frequently, but not always, increased in Paget disease. Procollagen type I C-terminal peptide, although not specific for bone collagen turnover, is increased when bone turnover is elevated, and a rapid decline in serum levels has been observed after treatment of Paget disease with calcitonin and bisphosphonates (72). Procollagen type I C-terminal peptide, measured in urine, is a highly sensitive assay for the determination of tissue type I collagen breakdown and, consequently, measurement of the rate of bone resorption (72,73). Because pyridinoline crosslink excretion is increased overnight, specimens are collected as second voided urines over a 2-hour period during the morning (e.g., 7 to 9 a.m.). The *N*-telopeptides and procollagen type I C-terminal peptide assays are believed to be the most sensitive markers of bone resorption and are readily available through commercial laboratories (74).

Radiology

The importance of radiologic evaluation in Paget disease cannot be underestimated. Only one third of patients have monostotic disease, with pelvic involvement in 72%, involvement of the lumbar spine in 58%, the thoracic spine in 45%, the femur in 55%, and the skull in 42% (75). The early radiologic lesions of Paget disease reflect severe localized osteolysis. These are typically "flame-shaped" osteolytic lesions that most commonly occur proximal to the distal epiphysis of a long bone. This resorptive lesion gradually progresses to the opposite end of the bone. As the disease evolves, an ingrowth of fibrovascular tissue and a high rate of bone remodeling may lead to deformity of the skull, enlarged dense vertebral bodies, and slowly progressive deformities of weight-bearing bones. Microfractures may occur on the convex side of the femur or tibia, increasing the degree of deformity and leading to the transverse or "banana" fracture that is typical of Paget disease. Pelvic involvement may be limited to the iliac and pubic rami but may involve the acetabulum or both the acetabulum and the femur, resulting in protrusio acetabuli.

For a complete evaluation, each patient should have a *bone scan* at the time of diagnosis to evaluate the extent of disease. Although scintigraphy is diagnostically less specific than radiography, bone scan identifies approximately 15% to 30% of lesions not visualized on radiographs (76). Alternatively, in 5% of cases the radiograph demonstrates diffuse Pagetic involvement (e.g., of the pelvis) whereas the bone scan reveals little uptake of the isotope. In this circumstance, the alkaline phosphatase level may be normal or only slightly elevated, reflecting lesions that are sclerotic, relatively inactive, or "burned out."

Differentiating Paget disease from metastatic cancer may sometimes be difficult. Examination of previous laboratory studies and radiographs may be helpful. If the alkaline phosphatase and bony lesions were not present in the recent past, Paget disease is unlikely. Furthermore, spread of Paget disease to new sites is unusual, therefore, the development of new sites of radiographic involvement should raise suspicion of another process and bone biopsy should be considered.

Bone Biopsy

A bone biopsy is rarely needed to establish the diagnosis of Paget disease. However, a bone biopsy is indicated to rule out malignancy when mixed osteoblastic and osteolytic vertebral lesions are seen. The value of a vertebral needle biopsy is limited. An open biopsy of the involved bone is more likely to be diagnostic.

Complications

In addition to orthopedic and neurologic problems, a few rarer complications may occur.

High-output heart failure may develop if a third or more of the bones are diseased; in addition, *calcific aortic stenosis, heart block, and left bundle branch block* appear to be more common than in the general population (77).

Osteosarcoma is a dreaded but unusual complication, sometimes multicentric; the tumors usually are detected because the patient complains of increased localized pain, sometimes associated with swelling. Radiologically, either osteolytic or osteoblastic lesions may be seen; computed tomography–directed biopsy can often make the definitive diagnosis and distinguish the malignancy from benign giant cell tumor of bone, the incidence of which is also increased in Paget disease.

Increased incidences of *primary hyperparathyroidism* and *hyperuricemia* have been reported in patients with Paget disease (78). *Urinary stones* (see Chapter 51) have been reported in 13% of patients (79).

Treatment

Effective medical therapy for Paget disease has been available for more than 20 years. The availability of newer and more potent agents suggests that treatment should be pursued more aggressively, both to control the disease and to decrease the risk of future complications. Indications for treatment include symptoms of bone pain, headache from skull involvement, hypercalcemia from immobilization, and symptoms of nerve compression. In asymptomatic patients with involvement of the skull, spine, or weight-bearing bones, treatment is also recommended. A general guideline is to treat if the serum alkaline phosphatase concentration is more than two to three times normal. Elevations of alkaline phosphatase indicate either widespread disease or intense activity in a limited area. Such patients are at higher risk for future complications of their disease. Patients with skull involvement or monostotic disease of the tibia or femur should be treated since progression and complications are likely.

Bisphosphonates are the cornerstone of the treatment of Paget disease. Bisphosphonates bind to the surface of the hydroxyapatite crystal and decrease bone resorption by disrupting osteoclast recruitment and cellular activity. The effects of these agents may last several months or produce complete remission. Because it is less potent than newer agents and because it also inhibits bone mineralization, *etidronate,* the first agent widely used to treat Paget disease, is used currently only if subjects have limiting side effects with newer agents (80).

Alendronate, the first of the third-generation oral bisphosphonates, is approved for the treatment of Paget disease at an oral dose of 40 mg/day (5-, 10-, 35-, 40-, 70-mg tablets) for 6 months. In one study, the drug caused a 71% fall in alkaline phosphatase levels, compared with 44% in patients treated with etidronate; osteolytic lesions improved; and no impairment of bone formation was seen on biopsy after 6 months of therapy (80,81). *Tiludronate* (200 to 400 mg/day, available in 200-mg tablets) and risedronate (30 mg/day, available in 5-, 30-, and 35-mg tablets) are newer bisphosphonates approved for the treatment of Paget disease (82,83). They appear comparable to alendronate in potency; however, risedronate requires a shorter course of treatment (2 months) than alendronate (6 months). Treatment of Paget disease should always be accompanied by appropriate calcium and vitamin D supplementation (calcium 1,000 mg/day and vitamin D_2 800 IU/day) to aid in the mineralization of newly formed bone and to prevent the theoretical risk of hypocalcemia related to bisphosphonate therapy. The most common side effects of oral bisphosphonates include epigastric pain, heartburn, and nausea due to esophagitis or gastritis. To avoid these symptoms, oral bisphosphonates must be taken alone on an empty stomach with an 8-ounce glass of water 30 to 60 minutes before breakfast or before taking other medications, and the patient must remain upright for 30 minutes after dosing.

Pamidronate, a potent second-generation bisphosphonate that can be administered intravenously, is useful in refractory disease, producing disease remission for up to 3 years in up to 90% of patients (84–86). After a series of initial infusions, maintenance infusions of pamidronate are then repeated at intervals based on the response of biochemical markers. *Zoledronic acid,* a potent, third-generation IV bisphosphonate administered as a single infusion, is also effective (87). Rare side effects of IV bisphosphonate therapy include a transient flu-like syndrome with leukopenia, anterior uveitis, episcleritis, ototoxicity, and jaw necrosis (88–90). Because the incidence of gastrointestinal (GI) side effects is less with IV bisphosphonates, these agents are an acceptable alternative treatment for patients who are unable to tolerate oral bisphosphonate therapy.

Calcitonin is an alternative treatment to bisphosphonate therapy, although it is less efficacious. The high doses used in subcutaneous administration often result in the development of nausea and transient flushing. Starting subcutaneous doses are in the range of 50 to 100 IU of salmon calcitonin or 50 IU of human calcitonin daily for 1 month; it is then continued three to 4 days per week thereafter (91). It also may be administered by intranasal spray in a dose of 200 to 400 IU daily. Nasal calcitonin causes less nausea, but 11% of patients develop rhinitis (92). Although prolonged remission may occur with calcitonin treatment, a partial or "plateau" response is more common: Biochemical abnormalities wane over a period of months but may not return to normal.

For patients with poor response to bisphosphonate or calcitonin therapy, second-line agents include *gallium nitrate* and *plicamycin (Mithramycin)*. Gallium nitrate, a potent antiresorptive drug, is currently an experimental therapy for Paget disease (93). In a multicenter trial, gallium nitrate was administered in doses of 0.05, 0.25, and 0.5 mg/kg/day by subcutaneous injection in two 14-day cycles; cyclical low-dose subcutaneous administration may be effective for patients with advanced disease that has been resistant to other agents (94).

Surgery

There are several skeletal problems that may require surgical intervention, but only after careful planning with an orthopedist or neurosurgeon. The operations are often complicated by infection and hemorrhage, in part because of the hypervascularity of pagetic bone. For that reason bisphosphonate or calcitonin should be given for approximately 3 months before elective surgery, to decrease the risk of bleeding. To permit unhindered healing, however, it is best to stop treatment at the time of surgery and then resume it 8 weeks postoperatively.

Specific problems that may warrant surgical intervention include *basilar invagination and hydrocephalus* (which may require a ventricular shunt), *nerve compression syndromes* (sometimes reversible by medical therapy), *degenerative disease of joints* that may lead to joint replacement, and *pathologic fractures that require fixation.*

SPECIFIC REFERENCES

1. Jan de Beur SM, Streeten EA, Levine MA. Hypoparathyroidism and other causes of hypocalcemia. In: Becker Bilezikian, Bremner et al., eds. Principles and Practice of Endocrinology and Metabolism. 3rd edition, Philadelphia: JB Lippincott Company, 2001.
2. Zarnegar R, Brunaud L, Clark OH. Prevention, evaluation, and management of complications following thyroidectomy for thyroid carcinoma. Endocrinol Metab Clin North Am 2003;32:483.
3. Pearce SHS, Williamson C, Kifor O, et al. A familial syndrome of hypocalcemia with hypercalciuria due to mutations in the calcium-sensing receptor. N Engl J Med 1996;335:1115.
4. Budarf ML, Collins J, Gong W, et al. Cloning a balanced translocation associated with Di George syndrome and indentification of a disrupted candidate gene. Nat Genet 1995;10:269.
5. Arnold A, Horst Sa, Gardella TJ, et al. Mutation of the signal peptide-encoding region of the preproparathyroid gene in familial isolated hypoparathyroidism. J Clin Invest 1990;86:1084.
6. Ding C, Buckingham B, Levine MA. Familial isolated hyoparathyroidism caused by a mutation in the gene for the transcription factor GCMB. J Clin Invest 2001;108:1215.
7. Suh SM, Tashjian AH Jr., Matsuo N, et al. Pathogenesis of hypocalcemia in primary hypomagnesemia: normal end-organ responsiveness to parathyroid hormone, impaired parathyroid gland function. J Clin Invest 1973;52:153.
8. Cholst IN, Steinberg SF, Tropper PJ, et al. The influence of hypermagnesemia on serum calcium and parathyroid hormone levels in human subjects. N Engl J Med 1984;310:1221.
9. Levine MA, Germain-Lee E, Jan de Beur S. Genetic basis for resistance to parathyroid hormone. Horm Res 2003;60(Suppl 3):87.
10. Lafferty FW. Differential diagnosis of hypercalcemia. J Bone Miner Res 1991;6:S51.
11. Stewart AF. Clinical Practice. Hypercalcemia associated with cancer. N Engl J Med 2005; 352:373.
12. Mundy GR, Guise TA. Hypercalcemia of malignancy. Am J Med 1997;103:134.
13. Silverberg SJ, Bilezekian JP. Evaluation and management of primary hyperparathyroidism. J Clin Endocrinol Metab 1996;81:2036.
14. Silverberg SJ, Gao P, Brown I, et al. Clinical utility of an immunoradiometric assay for parathyroid hormone (1-84) in primary hyperparathyroidism. J Clin Endocrinol Metab 2003;88:4725.
15. Denham DW, Norman J. Cost-effectiveness of pre-operative sestamibi scan for primary hyperparathyroidism is dependent solely on the surgeon's choice of operative procedure. J Am Coll Surg 1998;186:293.
16. Hallfeldt K, Trupka A, Gallwas J, et al. Intraoperative monitoring of intact PTH during

surgery for primary hyperparathyroidism. Zentralbl Chir 2002;127:448.
17. Chan AK, Duh QY, Katz MH, et al. Clinical manifestations of primary hyperparathyroidism before and after parathyroidectomy. A case-control study. Ann Surg 1995;222:402.
18. Bilezikian JP, Potts JT Jr., Fuleihan G el H, et al. Summary statement from a workshop on asymptomatic primary hyperparathyroidism: a perspective for the 21st century. J Clin Endocrinol Metab 2002;87:5353.
19. Rossini M, Gatti D, Isaia G, et al. Effect of oral alendronate in elderly patients with osteoporosis and mild primary hyperparathyroidism. J Bone Miner Res 2001;16:113.
20. Chow CC, Chan WB, Li JK, et al. Oral alendronate increases bone mineral density in post menopausal women with primary hyperparathyroidism. J Clin Endocrinol Metab 2003;88: 581.
21. Khan AA, Bilezikian JP, Kung AW, et al. Alendronate in primary hyperparathyroidism: a double-blind, randomized, placebo-controlled trial. J Clin Endocrinol Metab 2004; 89:3319.
22. Silverberg SJ. Cardiovascular disease in primary hyperparathyroidism. J Clin Endocrinol Metab 2000;85:3513.
23. Silverberg SJ, Bilezikian JP. Asymtpomatic primary hyperparathyroidism: a medical perspective. Surg Clin North Am 2004;84: 787.
24. Silverberg SJ, Bilezikian JP. Therapeutic controversies in primary hyperparathyroidism: to treat or not to treat: conclusions from the NIH consensus conference. J Clin Endocrinol Metab 1999;84:2275.
25. Silverberg SJ, Shane E, Jacobs TP, et al. A 10-year prospective study of primary hyperparathyroidism with or without parathyroid surgery. N Engl J Med 1999;341:1249.
26. Utiger RD. Treatment of primary hyperparathyroidism. N Engl J Med 1999;341:1301.
27. NIH Conference. Diagnosis and management of asymptomatic primary hyperparathyroidism: Consensus Development Conference Statement. Ann Intern Med 1991;114:593.
28. Bone HG, Talpos GB. Therapeutic controversies in primary hyperparathyroidism: who needs parathyroid surgery? The case for parathyroidectomy in nonclassical primary hyperparathyroidism. J Clin Endocrinol Metab 1999;84:2278.
29. Selby PL, Peacock M. Ethinyl estradiol and norethindrone in the treatment of primary hyperparathyroidism in postmenopausal women. N Engl J Med 1986;314:1481.
30. Rubin MR, Lee KH, McMahon DJ, et al. Raloxifene lowers serum calcium and markers of bone turnover in postmenopausal women with primary hyperparathyroidism. J Clin Endocrinol Metab 2003;88:1174.
31. Peacock M, Bilezikian JP, Klassen PS, et al. Cinacalcet hydrochloride maintains long-term normocalcemia in patients with primary hyperparathyroidism. J Clin Endocrinol Metab 2005;90:135.
32. Major P, Lortholary A, Hon J, et al. Zoledronic acid is superior to pamidronate in the treatment of hypercalcemia of malignancy: a pooled analysis of two randomized, controlled clinical trials. J Clin Oncol 2001;19:558.
33. Gloth FM 3rd, Smith CE, Hollis BW, et al. Functional improvement with vitamin D replenishment in a cohort of frail, vitamin D-deficient older people. J Am Geriatr Soc 1995;43:1269.
34. Jan de Beur SM. Tumor-induced osteomalacia. JAMA 2005;294:1260.
35. Jan de Beur SM, Levine MA. Molecular pathogenesis of hypophosphatemic rickets. J Clin Endocrinol Metab 2002;87:2467.
36. Collins N, Maher J, Cole M, et al. A prospective study to evaluate the dose of vitamin D required to correct low 25-hydroxyvitamin D levels, calcium, and alkaline phosphatase in patients at risk of developing antiepileptic drug-induced osteomalacia. Q J Med 1991;78:113.
37. Reginato AJ, Falascia GF, Pappu R, et al. Musculoskeletal manifestations of osteomalacia: report of 26 cases and literature review. Semin Arthritis Rheum 1999;28:287.
38. Bingham CT, Fitzpatrick LA. Noninvasive testing in the diagnosis of osteomalacia. Am J Med 1993;95:519.
39. Seeman E. The dilemma of osteoporosis in men. Am J Med 1995;98(2A):76S.
40. Ringe JD. Hip fractures in men. Osteoporos Int 1996;6[Suppl 3]:48.
41. Nguyen TV, Eisman JA, Kelly PJ, et al. Risk factors for osteoporotic fractures in elderly men. Am J Epidemiol 1996;144:255.
42. Francis RM. Male osteoporosis. Rheumatology (Oxford) 2000;39:1055.
43. Peris P, Guanabens N. Male osteoporosis. Curr Opin Rheumatol 1996;8:357.
44. Wishart JM, Need AG, Horowitz M, et al. Effect of age on bone density and bone turnover in men. Clin Endocrinol 1995;42:141.
45. Kelepouris N, Harper KD, Gannon F, et al. Severe osteoporosis in men. Ann Intern Med 1995;123:452.
46. Bendavid EJ, Shan J, Barrett-Connor E. Factors associated with bone mineral density in middle-aged men. J Bone Miner Res 1996;11:1185.
47. Spencer H, Rubio N, Rubio E, et al. Chronic alcoholism. Frequently overlooked cause of osteoporosis in men. Am J Med 1986;80: 393.
48. Snow-Harter C, Whalen R, Myburgh K, et al. Bone mineral density, muscle strength, and recreational exercise in men. J Bone Miner Res 1992;7:1291.
49. Jackson JA, Kleerekoper M. Osteoporosis in men: diagnosis, pathophysiology, and prevention. Medicine (Baltimore) 1990;69:137.
50. Orwoll E, Ettinget M, Weiss S, et al. Alendronate for the treatment of osteoporosis in men. N Engl J Med 2000;343:604.
51. Cohen S, Levy RM, Keller M, et al. Risedronate therapy prevents corticoid-induced bone loss: a twelve-month, multicenter, randomized, double-blind, placebo-controlled, parallel group study. Arthritis Rheum 1999;42:2309.
52. Saag KG, Emkey R, Schnitzer TJ, et al. Alendronate in the prevention and treatment of glucocorticoid-induced osteoporosis. N Engl J Med 1998;339:292.
53. Miller PD, McClung MR, Macovei L, et al. Monthly oral ibandronate therapy in postmenopausal osteoporosis: 1-year results from the MOBILE study. J Bone Miner Res 2005;20:1315.
54. Medras M, Jankowska EA, Rogucka E. Effects of long-term testosterone substitutive therapy on bone mineral content in men with hypergonadotrophic hypogonadism. Andrologia 2001;33:47.
55. LaCroix AZ, Ott SM, Ichikawa L, et al. Low-dose hydrochlorothiazide and preservation of bone mineral density in older adults: a randomized, double-blind, placebo-controlled trial. Ann Intern Med 2000;133:516.
56. Finkelstein JS, Hayes A, Hunzelman JL, et al. The effects of parathyroid hormone, alendronate or both in men with osteoporosis. N Engl J Med 2003;349:1216.
57. Orwoll ES, Scheele WH, Paul S, et al. The effect of teriparatide therapy on bone density in men with osteoporosis. J Bone Min Res 2003; 18:9.
58. Siris ES. Epidemiological aspects of Paget's disease: family history and relationship to other medical conditions. Semin Arthritis Rheum 1994;23:222.
59. Perry HM III, Kraezle D, Miller DK. Paget's disease in African Americans. Clin Geriatr 1995;3:69.
60. Barker DJ. The epidemiology of Paget's disease of bone. Br Med Bull 1984;40:396.
61. Rebel A, Basle M, Pouplard A, et al. Viral antigens in osteoclasts from Paget's disease of bone. Lancet 1980;2:344.
62. Howatson AF, Fornasier VL. Microfilaments associated with Paget's disease of bone: comparison with nucleocapsids of measles virus and respiratory syncytial virus. Intervirology 1982;18:150.
63. Mills BG, Singer FR, Weiner LP, et al. Evidence for both respiratory syncytial virus and measles virus antigens in the osteoclasts of patients with Paget's disease of bone. Clin Orthop 1984;183:303.
64. Wu RK, Trumble TE, Ruwe PA. Familial incidence of Paget's disease and secondary osteogenic sarcoma. Clin Orthop 1991;265:306.
65. Siris ES, Ottoman R, Flaster F, et al. Familial aggregation of Paget's disease of bone. J Bone Miner Res 1991;6:495.
66. Eekoff EW, Karperien M, Houtsma D, et al. Familial Paget's disease in the Netherlands: occurrence, identification, of new mutations in sequestosome 1 gene, and their clinical associations. Arthritis Rheum 2004;50;1650.
67. Hamdy RC, Moore S, LeRoy J. Clinical presentation of Paget's disease of the bone in older patients. South Med J 1993;8610:1097.
68. Anonymous. Paget's disease and calcitonin. Br Med J 1977;3:505.
69. Altman RD. Articular complications of Paget's disease of bone. Semin Arthritis Rheum 1994;23:248.
70. Gold, DT, Boisture J, Shipp KM, et al. Paget's disease of bone and quality of life. J Bone Miner Res 1996;11:1897.
71. Yost JH, Spencer-Green G, Krant JD. Vascular steal mimicking compression myelopathy in Paget's disease of bone: rapid reversal with calcitonin and systemic steroids. J Rheumatol 1993;20:1064.
72. Ebeling PR, Peterson JM, Riggs BL. Utility of type I procollagen propeptide assays for assessing abnormalities in metabolic bone diseases. J Bone Miner Res 1992;7:1243.
73. Alvarez L, Guanabens N, Peris P, et al. Discriminative value of biochemical markers of bone turnover in assessing the activity of Paget's disease. J Bone Miner Res 1995;10:458.
74. Rosen HN, Dresner-Pollak R, Moses AC, et al. Specificity of urinary excretion of cross-linked N-telopeptides of type I collagen as a marker of bone turnover. Calcif Tissue Int 1994;54:26.
75. Meunier PJ, Salson C, Mathieu L, et al. Skeletal distribution and biochemical parameters of Paget's disease. Clin Orthop 1987;217:37.
76. Fogelman I, Carr D. A comparison of bone scanning and radiology in the assessment of patients with symptomatic Paget's disease. Eur J Nucl Med 1980;5:417.
77. Hultgren HN. Osteitis deformans (Paget's disease) and calcific disease of heart valves. Am J Cardiol 1998;81:1461.
78. Lluberas-Acosta G, Hansell JR, Schumacher HR Jr. Paget's disease of bone in patients with gout. Arch Intern Med 1986;146:2389.
79. Harinck HI, Bijvoet OL, Vellenga CJ, et al. Relation between signs and symptoms in Paget's disease of bone. Q J Med 1986;58:133.
80. Siris E, Weinstein RS, Altman R, et al. Comparative study of alendronate versus etidronate for the treatment of Paget's disease of bone. J Clin Endocrinol Metab 1996;81: 961.

81. Reid IR, Nicholson JC, Weinstein RS et al. Biochemical and radiographic improvement in Paget's disease of bone treated with alendronate: a randomized, placebo-controlled trial. Am J Med 1996;101:341.
82. Reginster JY, Colson F, Morlock G, et al. Evaluation of the efficacy and safety of oral tiludronate in Paget's disease of bone: a double-blind, multiple-dosage, placebo-controlled study. Arthritis Rheum 1992;35:967.
83. Miller PD, Brown JP, Siris ES, et al . A randomized, double-blind comparison of risedronate and etidronate in the treatment of Paget's disease of bone. Am J Med 1999;106:513.
84. DeLaRose RE. Intravenously administered pamidronate for treating refractory Paget's disease of bone. Endocrine Pract 1997;3:214.
85. Wimalawansa SJ, Gunasekera RD. Pamidronate is effective for Paget's disease of bone refractory to conventional therapy. Calcif Tissue Int 1993;53:237.
86. Anderson DC, Richardson PC, Brown JK, et al. Intravenous pamidronate: evolution of an effective treatment strategy. Semin Arthritis Rheum 1994;23:273.
87. Reid IR, Miller P, Lyles K, et al. Comparison of a single infusion of zoledronic acid with risedronate for Paget's's disease. N Engl J Med 2005;353:898.
88. O'Donnell NP, Rao GP, Aguis-Fernandez A. Paget's disease: ocular complications of disodium pamidronate treatment. Br J Clin Pract 1995;49:272.
89. Reid IR, Mills DA, Wattie DJ. Ototoxicity associated with intravenous bisphosphonate administration. Calcif Tissue Int 1995;56:584.
90. Marx RE, Sawatari Y, Fortin M, et al. Bisphosphonate-induced exposed bone (osteonecrosis/osteopetrosis) of the jaws: risk factors, recognition, prevention, and treatment. J Oral Maxillofac Surg 2005;63:1567.
91. Singer FR, Keutman H, Neer RM, et al. Pharmacological effects of salmon calcitonin in man. In: Talmage RV, Munson Pl, eds. Calcium, parathyroid hormone and the calcitonins. Proceedings (Amsterdam) 1972: 89.
92. Silverman SL. Nasal calcitonin. Endocrine 1997;6:199.
93. Bockman RS, Wilhelm F, Siris E, et al. A multicenter trial of low dose gallium nitrate in patients with advanced Paget's disease of bone. J Clin Endocrinol Metab 1995;80:595.
94. Warrell RP Jr., Bosco B, Weinerman S, et al. Gallium nitrate for advanced Paget disease of bone: effectiveness and dose-response analysis. Ann Intern Med 1990;113:847.

*For annotated **General References** and resources related to this chapter, visit www.hopkinsbayview.org/PAMreferences.*

Chapter 85

Male Reproductive and Sexual Disorders

Shehzad Basaria

Disorders of the male reproductive system are common. For example, approximately 1 in 500 males is born with Klinefelter syndrome, a condition associated with low testosterone levels and infertility. More importantly, nearly 50% of men experience some degree of erectile dysfunction between the ages of 20 and 50 years (1). It is important for primary care clinicians to be able to identify and treat (or refer) such patients. Although androgen deficiency is not life threatening, it may have devastating effects on psychological, sexual, and somatic health in men. It is therefore important that clinicians have adequate knowledge about the diagnosis and treatment of reproductive and sexual disorders in men and be able to distinguish patients who only require reassurance from those who need additional evaluation and treatment or who should be referred to a specialist for more complex testing or therapy.

MALE REPRODUCTIVE PHYSIOLOGY

Male Sexual Differentiation

Genetic sex is determined at conception when an egg bearing an X chromosome is fertilized by a sperm bearing either a Y or an X chromosome, resulting in an XY (male) or an XX (female), respectively. The gonadal sex (i.e., the differentiation of testes or ovaries) is determined at the beginning of the 8th week of gestation. The short arm of the Y chromosome contains the "sex-determining region" that causes the gonad to differentiate into a testis. The embryonic testes produce two critical molecules, testosterone and the müllerian-inhibiting factor (MIF). *Testosterone* is the major male sex steroid and is responsible for the development of the undifferentiated external genitalia into a penis and scrotum and of the internal wolffian duct system into epididymis, vas deferens, prostate, and seminal vesicles. Dihydrotestosterone (DHT), a testosterone metabolite, is primarily responsible for the development of external genitalia. Hence, in the absence of the production (or action) of testosterone, female external genitalia (labia and clitoris) form. MIF is a peptide that mediates the regression of the primitive müllerian duct structures in the 6th week of gestation. In the absence of MIF, the müllerian ducts develop into a vagina, uterus, and fallopian tubes. Even in the absence of both ovaries and testes, normal female genitalia can develop. The appearance of the external genitalia identifies an individual's apparent gender at birth. Further sexual development occurs at puberty as a result of greatly increased secretion by the gonads of sex steroid hormones. In males, growth of male pattern body and pubic hair, beard, increase in muscle mass, deepening of voice, and onset of male libido with increased frequency of erections and ejaculations, are characteristic effects of testosterone. In females, rounding of body contours with breast growth and subcutaneous deposition of fat in the hips and buttocks, and also the onset of menses, are effects of cyclic estrogen secretion, whereas growth of pubic and axillary hair (and probably libido) are manifestations of adrenal androgen, and to a lesser extent, ovarian androgen secretion. Both sexes experience a period of accelerated increase in height at puberty (growth spurt), which is followed by closure of the epiphyses and cessation of growth of long bones.

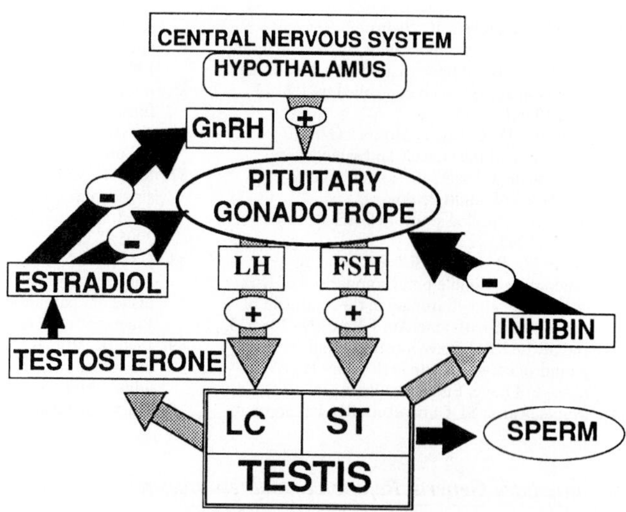

FIGURE 85.1. Reproductive endocrinology in the male. A variety of central nervous system inputs, from both exogenous (e.g., environmental stress) and endogenous (e.g., biorhythms) sources, act via neurotransmitters and neuropeptides to influence the amplitude and frequency of pulsatile hypothalamic neuronal output (*light gray arrows*) of gonadotropin-releasing hormone (GnRH) into the pituitary portal system. GnRH stimulates pituitary gonadotropes to release luteinizing hormone (LH) and follicle-stimulating hormone (FSH). LH induces the Leydig cell (LC) compartment of the testis to secrete testosterone (T). FSH and T act together to stimulate spermatogenesis in the seminiferous tubule compartment (ST). T acts via negative feedback (*dark gray arrows*) to inhibit gonadotropin and GnRH secretion, probably after aromatization locally to estradiol. Inhibin, produced by the ST in response to FSH, also acts by negative feedback to decrease FSH release.

Hypothalamic–Pituitary-Gonadal Axis

The hypothalamus, the pituitary and the testes are the three units forming the hypothalamic–pituitary–gonadal (HPG) axis in men. The neurons in the preoptic area of the hypothalamus secrete a decapeptide, *gonadotropin-releasing hormone* (GnRH). These neurons are also known as the GnRH pulse generator. Axons from these neurons end on capillaries of the median eminence in the pituitary, into which, at intervals of 60 to 120 minutes, they secrete GnRH. These vessels collect into the pituitary portal veins that ramify as sinusoidal capillaries within the pituitary gland. GnRH reaches the pituitary in high concentrations, where it stimulates gonadotropes to secrete luteinizing hormone (LH) and follicle-stimulating hormone (FSH). LH acts on the Leydig (interstitial) cells of the testis to stimulate testosterone secretion (2), which will not only be responsible for maintaining male secondary sexual characteristics, but also spermatogenesis. Testosterone, in turn, acts on both the hypothalamus and the pituitary to inhibit GnRH and LH secretion, respectively (Fig. 85.1). A decline in testosterone production as a result of damage to the Leydig cells results in loss of negative feedback and a rise in LH levels. FSH acts on the seminiferous tubules to initiate and maintain spermatogenesis. Therefore, induction of male fertility depends on the presence of FSH. Another target for FSH is the Sertoli cells (supporting cells), which in turn produce androgen binding protein, and a hormone called *inhibin*. This peptide is responsible for down-regulating pituitary production of FSH, forming a closed-loop negative feedback system (Fig. 85.1). Testosterone secretion follows a diurnal pattern with peak levels occurring around 8 a.m. and nadir around 10 p.m. This rhythm, however, is lost in elderly men (3).

Testosterone Metabolites, Transport, and Secretion

Metabolites

Despite being an active hormone itself, testosterone is also a "pro-hormone" because it is metabolized into two biologically active hormones that play an important role in mediating some of its effects on various tissues. These include *dihydrotestosterone* (DHT) and *estradiol* (E_2) (Fig. 85.2).

DHT

Testosterone is converted to DHT by 5-α reductase. This enzyme has two isoforms (4): type 1, which is expressed in

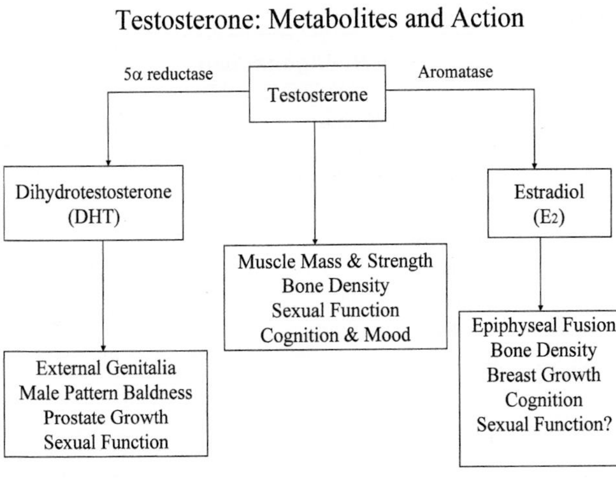

Testosterone: Metabolites and Action

5α reductase	Testosterone	Aromatase
Dihydrotestosterone (DHT)		Estradiol (E_2)
	Muscle Mass & Strength Bone Density Sexual Function Cognition & Mood	
External Genitalia Male Pattern Baldness Prostate Growth Sexual Function		Epiphyseal Fusion Bone Density Breast Growth Cognition Sexual Function?

FIGURE 85.2. Metabolites of testosterone and their actions.

nongenital skin and liver; and, type 2, which is the enzyme of importance since it is expressed in genital skin and the male urogenital tract. It is DHT that is responsible for the development and maturation of the external genitalia and also has a role in male sexual function (5). Congenital deficiency of this enzyme results in children being born with ambiguous genitalia (6). Despite its important role in sexual development, formation of DHT accounts for a fraction of testosterone metabolism. Since there is only one androgen receptor, DHT also acts via this receptor and has a higher affinity for the receptor compared to its parent compound, testosterone.

E_2

Estradiol, or E_2, has long been considered as only a "female" hormone. However, recent studies suggest that it plays an important role in the maintenance of the male skeleton and possibly in male sexual function as well (7,8). Testosterone is converted to E_2 by aromatase, an enzyme that is a product of the CYP19 gene. Though ubiquitous, it is mainly concentrated in adipose tissue, the main site of estrogen formation in men. Approximately 80% to 85% of E_2 is formed in adipose tissue with the remaining 15% directly secreted by the testes. In men, E_2 is responsible for epiphyseal maturation in adolescents (regulating height), regulation of bone mass (in which it is more important than testosterone) (9,10), formation of breast tissue, and for feedback regulation of the HPG axis (E_2 is more potent in suppressing gonadotropins as compared to testosterone).

Transport

Testosterone is mainly transported in the plasma bound to proteins. Approximately 44% of testosterone is bound with very high affinity to the sex hormone-binding globulin (SHBG). About 54% is bound with a low affinity (loosely bound) to albumin. This means that only 2% of testosterone circulates freely and is biologically active (free testosterone). However, when needed, the albumin-bound (loosely bound) testosterone dissociates and is readily available to the tissues. Hence, the combination of free testosterone and albumin-bound testosterone is termed *bioavailable testosterone* (11). SHBG is synthesized in the liver and its levels fluctuate under various circumstances. Estrogen therapy, hyperthyroidism, and male senescence increase SHBG levels while androgen therapy, severe hepatic dysfunction, and hypothyroidism decrease it. Although these changes alter the levels of total testosterone, the HPG unit adjusts to maintain free and bioavailable testosterone levels in the normal range.

Secretion

There are different stages of testosterone secretion.

Stage I

This first stage occurs during fetal life. During the 8th week of gestation, fetal testes begin to secrete testosterone. These levels are maintained until the end of the second trimester and are responsible for fetal androgenization. After that, levels fall at the beginning of the third trimester and remain very low until birth.

Stage II

The second stage of testosterone secretion occurs at birth. Although initial androgen levels are similar in both sexes, shortly after parturition testosterone levels rise in a male infant and remain elevated throughout infancy. Thereafter, levels fall and remain low until the onset of puberty.

Stage III

The third stage of secretion starts at puberty and is responsible for further maturation of sexual organs and development of a male phenotype. Adult levels are achieved by the age of 16 years and are maintained until the fourth decade of life when they begin to decline (see Andropause below). The testes in a normal young man produce 3 to 10 mg of testosterone daily, an amount that translates into normal serum levels of 300 to 1,000 ng/dL (12).

End-Organ Effects of Testosterone

Testosterone acts on many organ systems. It is responsible for anabolic effects on muscle and hypogonadal men have decreased muscle mass and strength, which is improved by testosterone replacement (13). This anabolic effect is directly mediated by testosterone via the androgen receptor, resulting in an increased rate of muscle protein

TABLE 85.1 Causes of Primary and Secondary Hypogonadism

Causes	*Primary Hypogonadism*	*Secondary Hypogonadism*
Genetic	Klinefelter syndrome Y-chromosome microdeletion	Kallmann syndrome PROP-1 mutation Abnormal β subunit of LH and FSH
Infectious	Mumps AIDS-related	Tuberculomas AIDS-related
Infiltrative	Hemachromatosis Sarcoidosis	Sarcoidosis Hemachromatosis
Trauma	Direct trauma Torsion	Deceleration injuries Stalk section
Radiation	External beam	External beam
Drugs	Cyclophosphamide Ketoconazole Glucocorticoids	GnRH agonists Glucocorticoids
Tumors	Varicocele	Prolactinomas Macroadenomas Metastatic disease
Other	Any acute or chronic illness Autoimmune disease	Any acute or chronic illness Idiopathic

AIDS, advanced immune deficiency syndrome; LH, luteinizing hormone; FSH, follicle-stimulating hormone; GnRH, gonadotropin-releasing hormone.

synthesis (14). Similarly, testosterone replacement also reduces fat mass. Hypogonadism of any etiology results in bone loss and predisposes to osteoporosis, a phenomenon that is evident in men with prostate cancer undergoing medical or surgical castration (15). Testosterone replacement results in an improvement in bone mass (16). Estradiol, which is produced by aromatization of testosterone, also has a major role in maintaining bone mass in men. Therefore, the male skeleton benefits from both testosterone and estradiol (7). Testosterone also has a fundamental role in male sexual function. It is responsible for libido (sexual desire), early morning erections, and potency. Patients with hypogonadism present with decreased libido and sexual dysfunction, which are restored by androgen replacement (17). Testosterone also influences cognition. Recent evidence suggests that testosterone replacement in hypogonadal men improves short-term memory, although this effect could be because of its conversion to E_2 (18). In addition to testosterone, DHT also has an independent role in sexual function (5).

MALE HYPOGONADISM

As discussed above, testes have two functional compartments: the Leydig cells, which synthesize and secrete testosterone, and the seminiferous tubules, which are responsible for spermatogenesis. Failure in either compartment (i.e., in testosterone or sperm production) is referred to as male hypogonadism. In certain conditions both compartments are affected simultaneously, whereas in others one is affected predominantly. Hypogonadism can be divided broadly into primary (testicular) or secondary (hypothalamic/pituitary) causes. In the former, pituitary gonadotropins are elevated due to loss of negative feedback whereas in the latter, gonadotropins are low or inappropriately normal despite low testosterone. In some rare cases, hypogonadism occurs due to defects in androgen receptors. In these conditions, serum testosterone levels are normal or elevated; however, the body is unable to respond to its action due to mutant receptors. Table 85.1 summarizes these conditions.

Etiology

Primary Hypogonadism (Hypergonadotropic Hypogonadism)

The most common genetic cause of primary hypogonadism is Klinefelter syndrome, occurring in 1 in 500 live male births (19). In its classic form, it occurs due to chromosomal nondisjunction producing a 47XXY karyotype. These patients have small, firm testes and gynecomastia. They usually enter puberty but fail to progress fully and present with a "eunuchoid habitus" (see later discussion). They typically have erectile dysfunction, a small phallus, and incomplete masculinization. Testosterone levels are generally low, but may be in the low-normal range in patients with mosaicism (47XXY/46XY). Other genetic causes of primary hypogonadism include deficiency of critical enzymes in the sex steroid synthetic pathway and cryptorchidism. Acquired causes include trauma, testicular torsion, cytotoxic agents (alkylating agents like cyclophosphamide and chlorambucil), radiation damage, infection (mumps orchitis) or infiltrative diseases. Certain other drugs, such as ketoconazole and glucocorticoids, inhibit testosterone production. Autoimmune damage to the testis may occur either alone or as part of autoimmune polyglandular syndrome (Hashimoto thyroiditis, Addison disease, vitiligo, primary hypoparathyroidism, or pernicious anemia). Occasionally, a varicocele may also produce hypogonadism (the proposed mechanism being increased scrotal temperature due to pooling of blood).

Secondary Hypogonadism (Hypogonadotropic Hypogonadism)

Among the genetic causes of secondary hypogonadism, Kallmann syndrome is one of the most common. This syndrome is characterized by hypogonadotropic hypogonadism (because of deficient GnRH secretion), anosmia (or hyposmia), red-green color blindness, midline facial abnormalities, and hearing loss (20). The inheritance is X-linked and is due to deletion of the KAL gene on the short arm of the X chromosome. Distinct from Kallman syndrome is another condition called idiopathic isolated hypogonadotropic hypogonadism. This condition is not accompanied by any of the other features of Kallman syndrome and, except for low gonadotropins, the other pituitary axes are normal. The congenital form of idiopathic isolated hypogonadotropic hypogonadism results in micropenis at birth and failure to reach puberty. There is also an acquired variety of idiopathic isolated hypogonadotropic hypogonadism, which occurs in adulthood in men who have undergone normal puberty and have been fertile, but who later develop hypogonadism (21). Acquired central hypogonadism may be infectious (e.g., tuberculosis hypophysitis), infiltrative (sarcoid), traumatic (deceleration injuries leading to interruption of the pituitary stalk), vascular (pituitary apoplexy) or neoplastic (nonsecreting or functioning macroadenomas compressing the gonadotropes) (see Chapter 81). Hyperprolactinemia (of any etiology) also results in central hypogonadism by inhibiting GnRH synthesis. Many drugs (e.g., glucocorticoids, opioids) and many acute or chronic medical conditions may also inhibit GnRH synthesis. Finally, tumors (lung, lymphoma, renal) that metastasize to the hypothalamus or pituitary may also result in central hypogonadism (22).

Androgen Resistance

Hypogonadism because of androgen resistance is always genetic and is caused by absence or dysfunction of the androgen receptor. It is expressed as a continuum, ranging from complete androgen insensitivity (formerly called "testicular feminization syndrome"), in which the phenotype is female and the affected patients have female breasts and external genitalia at birth and normal estrogenization at puberty, but lack a uterus and hence present with primary amenorrhea through varying degrees of partial androgen sensitivity (Reifenstein syndrome), in which the presentation ranges from abnormalities of midline fusion of labioscrotal structures resulting in gender-assignment confusion at birth to minor defects such as hypospadias and cryptorchidism, in which phenotypic gender is still clearly male. In all these cases, the genetic sex is male (i.e., XY).

Diagnosis

The approach to the patient with symptoms suggestive of hypogonadism should be directed first at determining whether hypogonadism truly exists, then at its classification as discussed earlier, next at discovering its specific cause, and finally at providing appropriate therapy and/or referral for the condition diagnosed. Manifestations of hypogonadism vary with the age at which hypogonadism develops.

In Utero

Absolute testosterone deficiency in the first trimester results in female external genitalia at birth; incomplete deficiency results in genital abnormalities such as hypospadias. When testosterone deficiency occurs in the last trimester of pregnancy, the fetus has normal external genitalia but may have a micropenis. These patients are usually identified at birth and referred to an appropriate specialist, so they rarely present as a diagnostic problem for the clinician whose practice is limited to adults.

Prepubertal

Hypogonadism at this stage is expressed as failure of secondary sex characteristics to appear at an appropriate age. It may stem from almost any of the causes cited previously and must be differentiated from constitutional delayed puberty, which is a common, idiopathic, self-limited, familial condition. A strong family history of late blooming and a finding of testicular enlargement are reassuring in this regard. Benchmarks of pubertal development in adolescent boys are available (see Chapter 11). In general, any boy who reaches 16 years of age without signs of pubertal onset (one of the first changes being an increase in testicular size), or who begins but does not complete puberty by age 18 years, deserves further investigation. The index of suspicion should be heightened if the patient has a history of childhood genital abnormalities (e.g., hypospadias, undescended testes) or signs or symptoms of a disease that can produce hypogonadism (e.g., headaches and/or a visual disturbance suggestive of a pituitary tumor).

Postpubertal

The gradual loss of libido, erectile function, and male secondary sex characteristics is a common presentation of hypogonadism at this stage. This may be so insidious that it is taken for granted by the patient, especially in a man progressing from middle age to old age.

History

A proper history should include a chronicle of pubertal progression (i.e., time of pubarche, beard growth, voice change, growth spurts, erections, and ejaculations.) Similarly, loss or diminution of libido, erections or ejaculations, slowing of beard growth, thinning of body and pubic hair, gynecomastia, and loss of aggressive impulse or drive should be evaluated. Severely hypogonadal men may report "hot flashes" similar to those seen in menopausal women. The presence of headaches, double vision, or reduced peripheral vision may give clues to a pituitary tumor. Symptoms of hypothyroidism, adrenal failure, and growth hormone deficiency also indicate pituitary damage. Gynecomastia or galactorrhea indicate hyperprolactinemia. History of urologic problems, cryptorchidism, hypospadias, or orchitis is important. Personal or family history of hemochromatosis suggests iron deposition in the pituitary or testes. Finally, a family history of delayed puberty or of other endocrine abnormalities may suggest either hereditary late blooming or familial autoimmune endocrinopathy.

Physical Examination

The facies should be evaluated first. Does the patient look mature or babyish, masculine or feminine? Secondly, body habitus should be evaluated for "eunuchoid" proportions. This is defined as (a) lower body segment (floor to pubis) more than 2 cm greater than the upper body segment (pubis to crown); and, (b) arm span more than 2 cm greater than the height. These dimensions are equal in normal men. The eunuchoid proportions are seen if hypogonadism occurs before puberty (lack of estrogen results in a delay in fusion of the epiphyses which results in long bones). Appropriate muscle mass, axillary hair, and a palpable prostate on digital rectal examination are evidence against long-standing hypogonadism. Male pattern baldness is also an androgen-dependent process. The presence of acne is also a sign of androgen activity. Eyes should be evaluated for limitation of extraocular movements, papilledema, or restriction of visual fields (especially bitemporal hemianopia); all suggestive of pituitary tumor. Breasts should be evaluated for gynecomastia (see later discussion). Gynecomastia is more common in men with primary hypogonadism, because of the fact that elevated LH levels stimulate synthesis of estradiol by the testes, resulting in increased ductal tissue in the breast. Squeezing of the nipple may elicit galactorrhea, which, although rare in males, is highly suggestive of a prolactinoma.

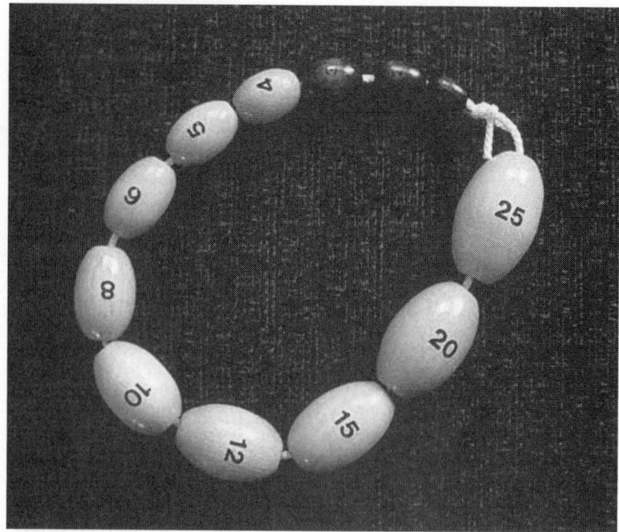

FIGURE 85.3. Prader orchidometer. The beads of various sizes represent testicular volume.

Examination of the genitals is critical. Pubic hair pattern should extend up the linea alba to the umbilicus in a diamond shaped pattern (the so-called male escutcheon). A triangular pattern cut off at the pubis suggests androgen deficiency, as does sparse or excessively fine pubic hair. Penile size and location of the urethral meatus, scrotal rugosity and pigmentation, and size and turgor of the testicles should all be noted. The normal adult testis should be 20 to 25 mL in volume (approximately 7.0 × 4.0 cm). The testicular volume can be measured by use of a Prader Orchidometer (Fig. 85.3). On palpation the testes should have the resistance of a firm plum. An "overripe," softer feeling is a sign of testicular atrophy. Small and firm testes are present in Klinefelter syndrome. Palpation of the left side of the scrotum while the patient performs a Valsalva maneuver may reveal the presence of a varicocele, which is almost always on the left side (venous drainage from the left testis crosses over to the right). Approximately 5% of varicoceles are associated with reduced testosterone production from both testes. Rectal examination should assess prostate size since the prostate shrinks with testosterone deficiency. Careful neurologic examination should include testing the sense of smell to look for Kallmann syndrome.

Laboratory Evaluation

Male hypogonadism is a clinical diagnosis that should be confirmed with laboratory tests. The clinician should measure testosterone only when hypogonadism is suspected based on history and physical examination. Testosterone should not be measured in a hospitalized patient since any acute illness may result in decreased testosterone production (discussed later). Ninety-five percent of healthy young adult men have morning serum testosterone levels of 300 to 1,000 ng/dL (with most between 450 to 700 ng/dL). Since testosterone levels peak in the morning and diurnal variation in testosterone concentration can produce an afternoon or evening decrement of as much as 200 ng/dL, it should be checked at 8 a.m. Early morning values <300 nanograms per deciliter (confirmed twice) in a symptomatic man are considered hypogonadal. Total serum testosterone is generally reliable in most patients and should be the first screening test. If a low total testosterone level is confirmed, the next step is to determine whether it is primary or secondary by measuring LH and FSH. Different assays for LH and FSH have different ranges of normal values. Elevated gonadotropins and low testosterone levels indicate primary gonadal failure. Further workup should be directed to determine the etiology of testicular dysfunction. Karyotyping can be performed to diagnose Klinefelter syndrome. High gonadotropins and normal testosterone levels may also be seen in evolving primary hypogonadism, especially that associated with age, when an increase in pituitary gonadotropin secretion is required to compensate for the testicular failure. To the contrary, low or inappropriately normal gonadotropins in the presence of a subnormal testosterone level indicate secondary hypogonadism. Fasting prolactin should be measured since hyperprolactinemia of any etiology results in secondary hypogonadism by inhibiting GnRH synthesis. All men with tests indicative of secondary hypogonadism should undergo MRI of the pituitary to evaluate for mass lesions. Iron studies should be performed in both forms of hypogonadism since hemochromatosis may involve both the pituitary and the testes.

Although total testosterone measurement is generally accurate, it is affected by variations in plasma SHBG, which may increase with aging and decrease with obesity and liver disease. If the patient is obese and total testosterone levels are repeatedly in the borderline range, it may be helpful to obtain unbound (free) or bioavailable testosterone. Similarly, if an elderly man has borderline normal total testosterone levels but continues to have classic symptoms of hypogonadism, unbound or bioavailable testosterone should be obtained. The unbound testosterone always should be measured by the equilibrium dialysis method and this should be indicated on the request form. Analog and radioimmunoassay methods for direct measurement of unbound testosterone are unreliable and should not be used.

Men with androgen receptor mutations (resistance to testosterone action) present with normal or increased testosterone levels. Gonadotropins may be normal or elevated. Because, as noted earlier, these patients present with ambiguous genitalia at birth, they rarely present as a diagnostic problem for the primary care clinician. Figure 85.4 provides a general algorithm for the evaluation of men with hypogonadism.

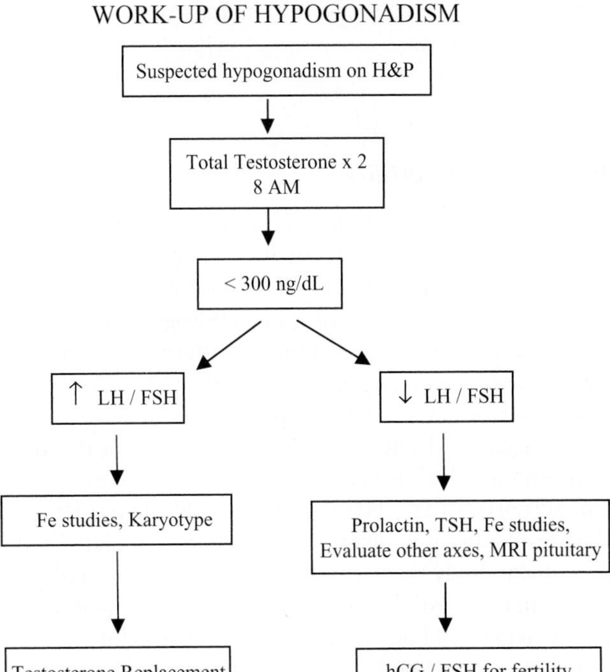

FIGURE 85.4. Algorithm for evaluation of male hypogonadism.

Hypogonadism Associated with Chronic Disease

It is now recognized that a variety of acute and chronic illnesses are often associated with male hypogonadism. A severe acute illness results in a dramatic decline in serum testosterone levels. The etiology is multifactorial and is probably due to a combination of hypothalamic stress, anesthesia (when administered), and starvation. In most situations, the mechanism is central hypogonadism, suggested by the observation that serum gonadotropin levels decline even in postmenopausal women (in whom the levels are elevated) admitted to intensive care units, particularly if there has been weight loss (23).

Before the widespread use of highly active antiretroviral treatment, nearly one third of men infected with the human immunodeficiency virus (HIV) were found to be hypogonadal (24). Similar observations have been made in men with other chronic diseases, such as cancer, heart disease, renal failure, and diabetes mellitus (25,26). Investigations are ongoing to determine whether testosterone therapy would be beneficial in these disease states. There is evidence that HIV-infected men increase their weight, lean body mass, and muscle strength after 3 months of testosterone administration (27,28). It is not clear, however, whether these changes result in increased survival or decreased morbidity.

Treatment

Virilization or Fertility

Once the underlying etiology is addressed, the next question is the specific treatment for hypogonadism. If the patient is interested only in virilization and not in fertility, the aim of therapy is adequate androgen replacement (29). The reasons for replacing testosterone in male hypogonadism are multiple. The most pressing reason is to ameliorate or reverse the symptoms of testosterone deficiency (e.g., hot flashes, decreased libido, erectile dysfunction, emotional lability) and to restore male secondary sex characteristics (e.g., beard growth, pubic hair). Beyond this, testosterone deficiency in adults is associated with loss of lean body mass and muscle strength (30), reduced bone mineral density (i.e., osteoporosis) (15), and an increase in percent body fat with greater central fat distribution. Testosterone replacement can improve or reverse the hypogonadal changes in body composition and function (31,32). Hypogonadism is also accompanied by an adverse lipid profile (increased low-density lipoprotein cholesterol and triglyceride), insulin resistance, and metabolic syndrome (33) (see Chapter 79).

In contrast, an alternative approach is required if fertility induction is desired (see later discussion).

Treatment of Specific Causes

Prolactinomas

The primary therapy of all prolactinomas (micro and macro) is medical. Treatment with the synthetic dopamine agonists bromocriptine or cabergoline normalize (or lower) serum prolactin (34–36), resulting in restoration of testosterone levels, improving libido, shrinking tumor mass, and improving vision. (See Chapter 81 for additional details.)

Hemochromatosis

Hemochromatosis is an underappreciated cause of male hypogonadism, both primary and secondary. Excess iron may be deposited in both the testes and the pituitary (where it has the highest affinity for the gonadotropes). It is important to consider hemochromatosis in the differential diagnosis of male hypogonadism since therapeutic phlebotomy has resulted in normalization of testosterone levels.

Pituitary Adenomas

Central hypogonadism can be caused by a secretory pituitary tumor (prolactinoma or Cushing syndrome) or a nonsecretory adenoma (a macroadenoma that affects production of testosterone by compressing gonadotropes). An imaging procedure, usually magnetic resonance imaging with gadolinium, can detect a mass affecting the hypothalamus, the pituitary stalk, or the pituitary gland. Surgery is performed for functional adenomas (except prolactinomas) and for macroadenomas causing hypopituitarism or visual disturbance. In some cases postoperative radiation therapy is required. (See also Chapter 81.)

Testosterone Replacement Therapy

Options for testosterone replacement include intramuscular esters, transdermal patches or gels, and buccal testosterone. Oral anabolic agents (e.g., oxandrolone, nandrolone, oxymetholone) are not suitable for androgen replacement and should not be used. In Europe and Australia, respectively, oral testosterone undecanoate and testosterone pellets are used. However, these agents are not available in the United States.

Intramuscular Esters

The traditional method of testosterone replacement is injection of testosterone esters such as enanthate, cypionate, or other esters in oil. Esterification of native testosterone makes it more lipophilic. After intramuscular injection, testosterone is gradually released from its oil-based vehicle, prolonging its duration of action. Effective therapy requires injections at regular intervals. Therapy is usually started at a dose of 200 mg every 2 weeks. Although this form of therapy does provide end-organ benefits, injections result in supraphysiological testosterone levels immediately after the dose that may fall to hypogonadal levels before the next injection (depending on the dose and interval). These "roller-coaster" pharmacokinetics result in fluctuation in mood, energy, and libido. Another limitation is that the injections are painful and necessitate regular visits to the caregiver's office or clinic (unless the patient or his family members learn to inject). The advantage of this approach is that it is the cheapest form of testosterone replacement. To judge adequacy of replacement, testosterone levels should be measured at the midpoint between injections (e.g., if injections are administered every 2 weeks, testosterone should be checked at the end of the first week).

Transdermal Testosterone

Testosterone patches are effective at mimicking the normal circadian rhythm (because of slow release of testosterone) and at relieving hypogonadal symptoms. The 5-mg Androderm patch results in peak serum testosterone levels 12 hours after application and can be applied to any skin surface that does not have underlying bony projections (e.g., back, thigh, chest, buttocks). Although the patch adheres fairly well, some men develop skin irritation and, occasionally, severe skin reactions. These reactions are because of permeation-enhancing chemicals in the patch that increase transdermal absorption of testosterone. Such reactions can be prevented by use of 1% triamcinolone ointment before application of Androderm.

A related form of testosterone replacement therapy is transdermal gel. AndroGel 1%, which is available in 2.5- and 5-g packets, was the first gel approved. This clear gel is alcohol-based and is rubbed on the upper arms, back, and abdomen every morning. The gel dries within 10 minutes and the hormone is stored under the skin and slowly diffuses into the circulation over 24 hours. It is advisable not to shower or swim for 4 hours postapplication. Because there can be transference of gel within a few hours of application, direct skin contact with others (including sexual activity) should be avoided for at least 4 hours. The dose of 5 g results in mean serum testosterone levels of approximately 500 to 600 ng/dL. A second gel, Testim, was recently approved in the United States. It is available in 5- and 10-g tubes and has the same pharmacokinetic profile as AndroGel. These gels are well tolerated with little or no skin irritation, but are more expensive than the other forms of replacement.

Buccal Testosterone

Striant, the first buccal testosterone, was recently approved in the United States. Each buccal tablet is 30 mg and is applied twice daily (37). It is applied to the depression in the gum above the upper incisors. Testosterone is absorbed through the buccal mucosa directly into the systemic circulation. Adverse effects include bad taste and problems with adherence. Some subjects have accidentally swallowed the tablet.

Table 85.2 summarizes the various modalities of testosterone replacement.

Fertility

For patients who desire fertility, testosterone replacement alone is not sufficient. Patients with hypogonadism may or may not be infertile, depending on the underlying etiology. Infertility that is primarily testicular is usually resistant to medical intervention and sperm production cannot be induced because of damaged seminiferous tubules. Moreover, testosterone replacement suppresses LH and FSH, causing further reduction in sperm counts and testicular size. Testicular biopsy might be needed in some patients to isolate spermatozoa for procedures such as *in vitro fertilization* and *intra-cytoplasmic sperm insemination*. In contrast, in patients with *central* hypogonadism (i.e., LH or FSH deficiency), infertility as well as deficient testosterone levels may be treated with gonadotropins. Human chorionic gonadotropin (hCG) may be used for its LH-like activity (since human LH is unavailable). Injections of 2000 IU of hCG intramuscularly three times weekly normalize testosterone levels, usually within a few months after initiation of therapy, and may also stimulate spermatogenesis. In patients with a history of cryptorchidism or prepubertal onset of central hypogonadism, both hCG and FSH may be required to initiate spermatogenesis. The dose of FSH is 75 to 150 units intramuscularly three times weekly administered with hCG. Because of the requirement for more frequent injections compared with testosterone, and their expense, use of gonadotropin injections probably should be restricted to those patients with central hypogonadism who are concerned about fertility.

TABLE 85.2 Testosterone Replacement Therapies Available in the United States

Drug	*Route of Delivery*	*Dosage*
Testosterone Esters		
Testosterone propionate	IM	10–25 mg 2–3x per wk
Testosterone enanthate	IM	200–250 mg every 2–4 wks
Cypionate	IM	200 mg every 2–4 wks
Testosterone patch		
Androderm	Topical	5 mg per d
Testosterone gel Androgel		
Androgel, Testim	Topical	5 g per d
Buccal Testosterone		
Striant	Buccal	30 mg twice a day

Adverse Effects of Testosterone Replacement

Generally, testosterone replacement is a safe and effective treatment for male hypogonadism. Although testosterone therapy does not induce prostate cancer, it potentially can promote the growth of a microscopic focus of an existing cancer. The higher prevalence of prostate cancer with older age necessitates that prostate-specific antigen (PSA) be measured and a digital rectal examination (DRE) be done before initiation of therapy in all men older than 50 years of age (see Followup Strategy, below). Testosterone is a known stimulator of erythropoietin and testosterone replacement carries the risk of erythrocytosis. Patients with existing risk factors for erythrocytosis such as hypoxemic lung disease or smoking may be more vulnerable. Hematocrit values should be monitored periodically, initially after 3 months and then annually. There are no definitive data to suggest that physiologic testosterone replacement alters glucose tolerance. A recent study showed that hypogonadism is associated with an adverse lipid profile and that testosterone replacement results in significant lowering of total cholesterol, low-density lipoprotein (LDL) cholesterol, and triglycerides, while causing no significant change in serum high-density liporprotein (HDL) levels (38).

Followup for Men on Testosterone Replacement Therapy

Followup of treated patients should include questions about efficacy and adverse effects. Questions should be asked about sexual function and there should be an assessment of body habitus, beard growth, and in patients with failure of pubertal development, growth in stature, growth of phallus, and depth of voice. Libido and potency usually return within a few weeks after initiation of treatment, whereas secondary sex characteristics improve gradually after 6 to 12 months. The patient should be evaluated for gynecomastia or prostate enlargement (e.g., symptoms of urinary hesitancy and frequency). Hematocrit levels should be measured every 3 to 6 months, and the dose of testosterone should be reduced if the hematocrit rises to more than 54%. PSA should be checked quarterly in the first year and then annually. If PSA increases to >4 ng/mL or rises at a rate of 0.75 ng/ml/year, androgen therapy should be discontinued and a referral to a urologist should be made (39,40).

ANDROPAUSE

Testosterone levels in men begin to decline in the fourth decade of life. This decline is gradual and occurs at the rate of 110 ng/dl/decade (41). At the same time, SHBG levels increase, resulting in a steeper decrease in free and bioavailable testosterone. This decline was observed even in studies in which older men were carefully selected to match younger men in terms of health, obesity, alcohol intake, and social class (42). In the Baltimore Longitudinal Study of Aging, low levels of total testosterone occurred in 19%, 28%, and 49%, respectively, of men in their sixties, seventies, and eighties, whereas the corresponding prevalence of reduced free testosterone levels were 34%, 68%, and 91% (43). Although "male menopause" is a poor choice of words, *andropause* is a more appropriate term, referring to age-related reductions in the production of testosterone. While the timing of menopause in women is usually obvious because it is associated with the cessation of menses, the signs and symptoms of andropause are often subtle and nonspecific, and they do not occur in all men nor do all aging men experience a significant decline in androgen levels (44).

Andropause occurs due to age-related derangements at all levels of the HPG axis. The decline in androgens is generally accompanied by an increase in circulating estrone and estradiol. In the majority of the cases, gonadotropins remain in the normal range. There is a decline in the number of Leydig cells in the testes with aging, and the testes do not respond as robustly to HCG in aging men as they do in young men (45,46). Similarly, there is decreased GnRH production or release from the hypothalamus with aging, suggesting a decrease in activity of the GnRH pulse generator (47).

The clinical significance of andropause remains controversial. Independent of changes in levels of sex steroids, studies in healthy men revealed a steady decrease in sexual interest and ability, with decreases in the frequency of intercourse from an average of two to three events a week to fewer than two a month by age 70 to 75 years (48). This decrease does not appear to be directly related to hypogonadism but probably reflects changes in other systems (i.e., nervous and vascular) that occur with age. Although testosterone treatment may result in improvement in libido in men with hypogonadism, erectile function generally does not improve in elderly men, since they commonly have comorbidities that complicate the mechanism of the sexual function.

Testosterone administration has been shown to improve body composition, with increases in muscle mass and decreases in body fat, in aged andropausal men (49), as it does in frankly hypogonadal young and middle-aged men (32). Whether the increase in muscle mass is associated with improved functional status or with decreased morbidity or mortality remains to be determined. Testosterone supplementation of healthy aged men with low serum testosterone levels also increases lumbosacral spine bone mineral density (50), and improves visuospatial performance and verbal memory (51). Epidemiologic studies suggest that the decline in free testosterone index is associated with an increase in the incidence of Alzheimer disease (52), and that higher bioavailable testosterone concentrations are associated with better long-term verbal memory (53).

There are no data to support a beneficial effect of administration of androgens to aging men whose testosterone levels are normal. Since there are no clear guidelines for routine screening of elderly men, testosterone levels should be checked only if a patient has symptoms suggestive of hypogonadism or has osteopenia or osteoporosis on bone densitometry. Testosterone levels should not be checked simply to know what they are in an asymptomatic, healthy man. The benefits and risks of androgen replacement in andropausal men remain to be determined conclusively. In the meantime, many endocrinologists consider low libido (but not erectile dysfunction) and decreased spinal bone density to be the only indications for androgen replacement in elderly men.

GYNECOMASTIA

Gynecomastia refers to the benign enlargement of the male breast. It occurs as a result of ductal proliferation of the breast tissue and is usually present beneath the areola. It should be distinguished from "pseudogynecomastia," which is simply adipose tissue enlargement seen in obese men. Enlargement of the male breast requires a clinician's attention so that those cases with a serious hormonal or neoplastic cause can be distinguished from the common benign idiopathic forms.

Etiology

There are three physiologic forms of gynecomastia (54). The first occurs after birth and it is due to the influence of maternal estrogens on the fetus. This regresses in a few months. Gynecomastia also occurs during puberty as plasma sex steroid hormone levels rise (occurring in up to 65% of boys at the age of 14 years). This is caused by increased testosterone secretion, resulting in increased formation of estradiol. However, breast enlargement regresses spontaneously in most and is present in fewer than 15% of boys by age 17 years. The prevalence of gynecomastia again increases to approximately 60% in men 50 years of age and older. The reason for this gynecomastia of senescence is an increased estrogen/testosterone ratio (because of declining androgen production and steady levels of estradiol). Mild idiopathic gynecomastia is almost always less than 5 cm in diameter and causes no symptoms. Noticeable gynecomastia of greater than 5 cm in diameter may be the first clue to the presence of a benign or malignant adrenal or testicular neoplasm or a prolactinoma. Hypogonadism, especially primary hypogonadism, may present with gynecomastia. Malignancies of the testis, lung, stomach, and occasionally other cancers may secrete hCG, which may overstimulate testicular androgen production, leading to gynecomastia. Hyperthyroidism also has been associated with breast enlargement. Ingestion of exogenous estrogen (e.g., by individuals with gender dysphoria or prostate carcinoma) or of antiandrogenic drugs such as cimetidine, spironolactone, digoxin, and ketoconazole may cause male breast enlargement. Many other medications have been reported to be associated with gynecomastia, but the causal relationship is less well established. Gynecomastia is also common in liver cirrhosis, in which hepatic metabolism of estrogens is impaired. Approximately 1% of all breast carcinomas occur in men. If a man presents with an eccentric breast mass, nipple retraction, or reddish discharge, one should suspect breast cancer. Table 85.3 summarizes the various causes of gynecomastia.

TABLE 85.3 Causes of Gynecomastia

Physiologic	Infancy Puberty Aging
Benign endocrine disease	Hypogonadism Hyperprolactinemia Hyperthyroidism
Genetic	Androgen receptor mutations (androgen resistance)
Chronic medical conditions	Cirrhosis Chronic renal failure
Nutritional	Refeeding syndrome in malnutrition
Drugs	Spironolactone Ketoconazole Cimetidine Digitalis Verapamil Reserpine Finasteride Cryproterone acetate
Illicit drugs	Heroin Marijuana
Endocrine neoplasms	Testicular (choriocarcinoma, Leydig cell tumor, sex cord tumor) Adrenal (estrogen secreting feminizing tumor)
Non-endocrine neoplasms	Ectopic HCG-producing (lung, hepatoma, renal cell)
Idiopathic	Excessive extraglandular aromatase activity

Diagnosis

History

The duration and age at onset of breast enlargement are important; for example, recent onset of breast swelling in a 30-year-old man would be of more concern than in an adolescent or gradual breast enlargement in a 70-year-old man. The presence of tenderness or discharge and the quality of the discharge (clear, turbid, bloody) should be noted. Any symptoms of hypogonadism (see previous discussion) should be elicited, as should symptoms of hyperthyroidism. A careful medication history and sexual history may reveal an exogenous cause.

Physical Examination

Generally, the examination should be the same as for hypogonadism (described earlier), and signs of thyroid disease should be emphasized. Deep palpation of the upper abdomen may reveal an adrenal tumor or downward displacement of the kidney by such a tumor. Careful bimanual palpation of the testicles may detect a tumor. A system for staging breast development was described by Marshall and Tanner in adolescent girls (see Chapter 11), but it is equally useful for staging gynecomastia. The examiner needs to differentiate between proliferation of glandular breast tissue (firm, slightly lobulated, and symmetrically distributed from the nipple outward with a limited boundary), fat (softer, diffusely distributed, and with no clear separation from surrounding subcutaneous adipose tissue), and tumor (hard, nodular, frequently tender, often fixed to skin or underlying muscle, and eccentrically located with regard to the nipple). Milky nipple discharge on firm squeezing suggests prolactinoma; clear or bloody discharge suggests breast cancer. Unilateral breast enlargement should increase the suspicion of neoplasia, but asymmetry occurs in 10% to 15% of patients with idiopathic gynecomastia. Whether further investigation is required depends on the age of the patient, the rapidity of enlargement of the breast, and the degree of such enlargement. Men between 18 and 45 years of age with recent onset of rapidly enlarging mammary glands, or with glandular breast tissue diameter greater than 5 cm, or with symptoms or signs suggesting hypogonadism or hyperthyroidism should receive further evaluation.

Laboratory Evaluation and Diagnosis

Determinations of serum levels of estradiol, testosterone, gonadotropins (LH and FSH), prolactin, hCG-β, TSH, and free T_4 are indicated. If the serum estradiol is greater than 50 pg/mL and if the testosterone/estradiol ratio is reduced to less than 100:1, the diagnosis of estrogen-secreting testicular tumor is strongly suggested. This should lead a primary care practitioner to obtain a testicular ultrasound. Low or low-normal testosterone levels with increased FSH and LH in late adolescent or young adult males with gynecomastia and testicular atrophy (small, firm testes) suggest the diagnosis of Klinefelter syndrome (47,XXY). Elevated serum hCG should prompt a search for occult malignancy with particular attention to gonads, lungs, and gastrointestinal (GI) tract. Elevated prolactin concentrations may be associated with the use of certain medications (e.g., antipsychotic drugs) or with a prolactinoma (see Chapter 81). Elevated free T_4 and low TSH determinations suggest hyperthyroidism as the cause of gynecomastia. If the above tests are inconclusive, 24-hour urinary 17-ketosteroids should be measured. Elevated levels indicate an adrenal cause of gynecomastia, in which case adrenal hyperfunction should be investigated with the diagnosis of adrenal neoplasm in mind (see Chapter 81).

Imaging

Patients with firm, nodular, unilateral, or notably eccentric breast enlargement should be referred for mammography, ultrasound, or surgical biopsy of the breast.

Treatment

No treatment is needed for physiologic causes of gynecomastia since it remits spontaneously. Similarly, drug-induced gynecomastia remits gradually, in several months, after the drug is discontinued. Treatment of a primary endocrine disease (e.g., prolactinoma, hyperthyroidism, or hypogonadism) should be guided by an endocrinologist. Remission of the accompanying gynecomastia depends on the success of the treatment and the stage of advancement of breast development. Estrogen receptor antagonists such as tamoxifen and aromatase inhibitors have shown some success in the treatment of gynecomastia (55,56). If idiopathic gynecomastia is a cosmetic problem, liposuction or surgical excision of breast tissue may be attempted. Breast development that has progressed to the fibrotic stage will never regress fully, even if the cause is corrected, and therefore will require surgical intervention if complete cosmetic correction is desired.

ERECTILE DYSFUNCTION

In this section, erectile disorder (ED) and loss of libido are considered only as they relate to endocrine disorders. For a more general discussion of sexual dysfunction, see Chapter 6. ED, sometimes referred to as impotence, is the inability to achieve or maintain erection satisfactorily enough to achieve penetration and ejaculation. Transient or occasional ED is common and is not necessarily evidence of a medical problem, but a pattern of repeated episodes (more than 25% of opportunities) lasting longer than 1 month should be investigated. ED may or may not be accompanied by loss of libido, depending on the cause.

Etiology

A disorder of any of the systems that maintain the sexual response may lead to erectile dysfunction. Causes may therefore be of several types: (a) *psychological*; (b) *vascular*, either of the arterial type, with diminished blood supply to the corpora cavernosa (e.g., congenital vascular anomaly, traumatic injury to vessels, large vessel atherosclerosis, disease of smaller peripheral vessels), or as a result of venous incompetence, in which partial erections occur but blood drains off because of "venous leak;" (c) *neuropathic*, involving damage to the peripheral pelvic autonomic nerves (e.g., diabetic neuropathy, heavy metal poisoning, nerve trauma) or disease of the spinal cord or brain (e.g., tumor, multiple sclerosis) that inhibits or obliterates the erectile response; (d) *toxic*, caused by substances of abuse (e.g., alcohol, opiates, sedatives) that can acutely and chronically diminish sexual ability or by a number of medications that affect the autonomic and central nervous system (e.g., antipsychotic drugs, sympatholytic antihypertensives); (e) *debilitative*, related to various severe and chronic medical illnesses (e.g., malignancy, renal failure, cachexia of any etiology) that are accompanied by loss of sex drive; and (f) *endocrine*, including hypogonadism and prolactinoma (see earlier discussions), hyperthyroidism and hypothyroidism, Cushing syndrome, and acromegaly. In one series of patients referred to a major diagnostic center for persistent symptoms, 35% were found to have an endocrine disorder (57).

Diagnosis

History

It is important to differentiate various aspects of sexual dysfunction. These include decreased libido (desire to have sex), erectile dysfunction (inability to attain and maintain erection during intercourse), and premature ejaculation (ejaculation of semen prior to achieving orgasm or intending to achieve it). The duration of symptoms, the frequency with which intercourse is attempted, and the proportion of attempts ending in erectile failure should be ascertained to determine whether the ED is absolute or relative and whether it is progressing. Rapid onset of ED usually indicates psychogenic impotence or genitourinary trauma (e.g., prostate surgery). Partial or nonsustained erections are suggestive of anxiety whereas absolute loss of erections indicates a neurologic or vascular disorder. Erectile dysfunction unaccompanied by loss of libido suggests a neurologic or vascular problem, whereas loss of libido is consistent with either hypogonadism or a psychological cause. The history should include the patient's marital situation, whether there are sex partners other than the spouse, the perceived level of partners' desire, and a social and work history to determine whether there are psychosocial stressors. Situational ED (i.e., experienced with one partner but not another) is also good evidence of a psychological problem. Men are often awakened in the morning with an erection. This is a normal response to a full bladder, with spontaneous detumescence following urination. Preservation of morning erections is good evidence against endocrine, vascular, or neuropathic disease; however, 14% of patients with an endocrine problem maintain morning erections (57). A history of medication use and substance abuse should be sought. Heavy smoking is often associated with a peripheral vascular cause of impotence. The patient should be asked about symptoms of hypothyroidism, hyperthyroidism, Cushing disease, diabetes, peripheral neuropathy (paraesthesia, hyperesthesia), or CNS disease and vascular disease (claudication, angina, cold extremities, skin ulcers). Pain during intercourse or the presence of a curved penile shaft suggests Peyronie disease.

Physical Examination

The physical examination should be conducted with particular attention to the manifestations of hypogonadism described earlier, signs of thyroid or adrenal disease (see Chapters 80 and 81), signs of peripheral vascular disease (peripheral pulses, skin temperature, skin atrophy, hair loss; see Chapter 94) and central or peripheral neuropathy (see Chapter 92). The penile shaft should be palpated to determine whether plaques of Peyronie disease are present. These are fibrous bands within the tunica albuginea that may involve the full length of the penile shaft.

Laboratory Evaluation

Hormone levels should be measured to screen for hypogonadism (serum total testosterone drawn at 8 a.m.) and for a prolactinoma (fasting serum prolactin) (see earlier discussion). If historical or physical findings lead to suspicion of thyroid or adrenal disease, appropriate tests should be done (see Chapters 80 and 81). A fasting blood glucose measurement should always be obtained to screen for diabetes mellitus (see Chapter 79).

Additional Testing

Spontaneous erection during sleep, or *nocturnal penile tumescence*, had been thought to exclude organic etiologies of ED, but that criterion is not completely valid, since some erectile function may be preserved early in organic disease. Many experts and consensus guidelines now emphasize the importance of the history and physical examination in evaluating erectile dysfunction and do not recommend routine testing for nocturnal penile tumescence. If a test is done, it can sometimes be done at home.

The "stamp test" is a simple but unvalidated procedure in which a man fastens a strip of perforated postal stamps around his penis by moistening the overlapping stamp in the usual manner; separation of the stamps at the perforations overnight is considered evidence of erection. Calibrated "snap gauges," which consist of plastic bands of varying strength, and "strain gauges," which include elastic bands that stretch and register changes in circumference, are commercially available.

In selected patients in whom more detailed assessment of the capacity for erection is sought, specialized testing may be undertaken, usually under the direction of a urologist. Electronic monitoring devices are available for home use, and quantitative instrumentation in a sleep laboratory may also be obtained. Definitive diagnosis of vascular disorders may require Doppler studies of penile blood flow or selective angiography, and venous incompetence may be revealed by dynamic cavernosography, procedures used by urologists specializing in ED. If peripheral neuropathy seems a likely cause, it often can be confirmed by referral to a urologist for bladder manometrics and to a neurologist for nerve conduction velocity measurements (see Chapter 92).

Treatment

Therapeutic efforts should be directed at the specific cause of the ED. Psychogenic ED may respond to various therapeutic modalities depending on its severity and associated problems (see Chapter 6). Vascular disease may respond to medication or to surgical revascularization. Caution should be exercised in this regard since, in contrast to young men, results are almost always disappointing in older patients with atherosclerotic disease (perhaps because of the involvement of smaller peripheral vessels). Neuropathic ED is occasionally reversible with removal of an inciting lesion (e.g., spinal cord tumor) or with aggressive diabetic control, but, if irreversible, it may also be treated with other measures (discussed below). Drug-induced ED is usually reversed if the offending agent can be discontinued. Treatment of hypogonadism has been discussed above. If sexual function does not improve within 6 weeks after specific therapy for an organic cause has been instituted, consideration should be given to the possibility that the experience and expectation of sexual failure are inhibiting the response (so-called performance anxiety) even though the primary cause is no longer present. Such secondary psychological ED may respond to psychological or behavioral therapy (see Chapter 6).

Advances in pharmacotherapy have resulted in newer approaches that may succeed in restoring sexual function in a variety of conditions (psychogenic, organic, or multifactorial). Three selective inhibitors of cyclic guanosine monophosphate–specific phosphodiesterase type 5 are currently available. The inhibition of this enzyme leads to increased concentrations of nitric oxide, resulting in vasodilatation and increased genital blood flow. These agents are taken orally. The first drug in this class was sildenafil citrate (Viagra). Doses of 50 to 100 mg are taken 1 hour before planned sexual activity. The second agent that became available was vardenafil (Levitra) that is taken in doses of 10 to 20 mg 1 hour before sexual activity. Both sildenafil and vardenafil are effective for up to 4 hours. The latest drug in this class is tadalafil (Cialis). This drug has the same onset of action, but it has a duration of action of 36 hours. All three drugs have equal efficacy of approximately 60% to 75%. Although these drugs have similar side effects of headaches and dyspepsia, sildenafil results in transient bluish vision in a minority of patients due to cross-reactivity with retinal phosphodiesterase. A few cases of acute loss of vision secondary to ischemic optic neuropathy have been reported among men who took sildenafil. However, this was a rare occurrence and a causal relationship to the phosphodiesterase inhibitors has not been established conclusively (58). The absorption of sildenafil and vardenafil is inhibited by foods with a high fat content, but there are no such interactions with tadalafil. All three drugs are contraindicated in men taking nitroglycerin and nitrate medications.

For patients who cannot take phosphodiesterase type 5 inhibitors, injection of vasoactive agents directly into the corpus cavernosum is the next step. Most effective are prostaglandin E_1 (PGE_1, alprostadil) or papaverine combined with phentolamine. Both treatments are equally effective, but papaverine plus phentolamine use is associated with a lower frequency of priapism and pain (59). These drugs are injected 15 minutes prior to sexual activity and their effects last for 1 hour. Injection therapy should always be supervised by an experienced urologist, because priapism is a potentially serious (2% to 4%) acute complication. A rare long-term complication is gradual fibrosis of the corpora cavernosa with loss of responsiveness. Alprostadil administered as a urethral suppository (available as MUSE or medicated urethral system for erection, provided in doses of 125 μg, 250 μg, 500 μg, and 1,000 μg) is another approach to the treatment of ED. The efficacy and adverse reaction rates of urethral alprostadil appear to be comparable to those of injection therapy (60,61), but experience with this method is still relatively limited. Furthermore, it should not be used if the partner is pregnant.

Still another option is the use of a vacuum device that draws blood into the penis by negative pressure; an occlusive ring applied to the base of the penis maintains the erection. Several different types of suction devices are available. Results with these devices are mixed. For example, one retrospective study found that 81% of men using vacuum devices abandoned them because they "did not work," and the patients' attitudes toward the device were unfavorable overall (62). Another study, however, showed that more than 80% of the men achieved satisfactory erections with vacuum devices (63).

The final option is a penile prosthesis. Implantable penile prostheses have been used extensively but, because of local complications, are no longer as popular as they once were. Implants are available in two basic types: those that are permanently stiff or semiflexible, and more complex devices that inflate by means of a pump and valve mechanism. Complications are related to surgery and wound infections. Implants should be the last modality considered by men with ED, in consultation with a urologist.

SPECIFIC REFERENCES

1. Frank E, Anderson C, Rubinstein D. Frequency of sexual dysfunction in normal couples. N Engl J Med 1978;299:111.
2. Dufau ML, Catt KJ. Gonadotropin receptors and regulation of steroidogenesis in the testis and ovary. Vitam Horm 1978;36:461.
3. Bremner WJ, Vitiello MV, Prinz PN. Loss of circadian rhythmicity in blood testosterone levels with aging in normal men. J Clin Endocrinol Metab 1983;56:1278.
4. Russell DW, Wilson JD. Steroid 5 alpha-reductase: two genes/two enzymes. Annu Rev Biochem 1994;63:25.
5. Mantzoros CS, Georgiadis EI, Trichopoulos D. Contribution of dihydrotestosterone to male sexual behaviour. BMJ 1995;310:1289.
6. Mendonca BB, Inacio M, Costa EMF, et al. Male pseudohermaphroditism due to steroid 5-alpha-reductase 2 deficiency. Medicine 1996; 75:64.
7. Falahati-Nini A, Riggs BL, Atkinson EJ, et al. Relative contributions of testosterone and estrogen in regulating bone resorption and formation in normal elderly men. J Clin Invest 2000;106:1553.
8. Vermeulen A, Kaufman JM, Goemaere S, van Pottelberg I. Estradiol in elderly men. Aging Male 2002;5:98.
9. van den Beld AW, de Jong FH, Grobbee DE, et al. Measures of bioavailable serum testosterone and estradiol and their relationships with muscle strength, bone density, and body composition in elderly men. J Clin Endocrinol Metab 2000;85: 3276.
10. Barrett-Connor E, Mueller JE, von Muhlen DG, et al. Low levels of estradiol are associated with vertebral fractures in older men, but not women: the Rancho Bernardo Study. J Clin Endocrinol Metab 2000;85:219.
11. Manni A, Pardridge WM, Cefalu W, et al. Bioavailability of albumin-bound testosterone. J Clin Endocrinol Metab 1985;61:705.
12. Griffin JE, Wilson JD. Disorders of the testes and the male reproductive tract. In: Wilson, Foster, Kronenberg, Larsen, eds. Williams Textbook of Endocrinology. 9th ed. Philadelphia: W.B. Saunders, 1998;819–875.

13. Bhasin S, Storer TW, Berman N, et al. Testosterone replacement increases fat-free mass and muscle size in hypogonadal men. J Clin Endocrinol Metab 1997;82:407.
14. Basaria S, Wahlstrom JT, Dobs AS. Anabolic-androgenic steroid therapy in the treatment of chronic diseases. J Clin Endocrinol Metab 2001;86:5108.
15. Basaria S, Lieb J 2nd, Tang AM, et al. Long-term effects of androgen deprivation therapy in prostate cancer patients. Clin Endocrinol (Oxf) 2002;56:779.
16. Katznelson L, Finkelstein JS, Schoenfeld DA, et al. Increase in bone density and lean body mass during testosterone administration in men with acquired hypogonadism. J Clin Endocrinol Metab 1996;81:4358.
17. Cunningham GR, Hirshkowitz M, Korenman SG, Karacan I. Testosterone replacement therapy and sleep-related erections in hypogonadal men. J Clin Endocrinol Metab 1990;70:792.
18. Cherrier MM, Matsumoto AM, Amory JK, et al. The role of aromatization in testosterone supplementation: effects on cognition in older men. Neurology 2005, 25;64:290.
19. Amory JK, Anawalt BD, Paulsen CA, Bremner WJ. Klinefelter's syndrome. Lancet. 2000;356:333.
20. Lieblich JM, Rogol AD, White BJ, Rosen SW. Syndrome of anosmia with hypogonadotropic hypogonadism (Kallmann syndrome): clinical and laboratory studies in 23 cases. Am J Med 1982;73:506.
21. Waldstreicher J, Seminara SB, Jameson JL, et al. The genetic and clinical heterogeneity of gonadotropin-releasing hormone deficiency in the human. J Clin Endocrinol Metab 1996;81:4388.
22. Basaria S, Krop JS, Braga-Basaria M. A rare cause of pituitary stalk enlargement and panhypopituitarism. Mt Sinai J Med 2003;70:265.
23. Gebhart SS, Watts NB, Clark RV, et al. Reversible impairment of gonadotropin secretion in critical illness: observations in postmenopausal women. Arch Intern Med 1989;149:1637.
24. Dobs AS, Dempsey MA, Ladenson PW, Polk BF. Endocrine disorders in men infected with human immunodeficiency virus. Am J Med 1988;84:611.
25. Baker HW. Reproductive effects of nontesticular illness. Endocrinol Metab Clin North Am 1998; 27:831.
26. Nierman DM, Mechanick JI. Hypotestosteronemia in chronically critically ill men. Crit Care Med 1999;27:2418.
27. Bhasin S, Woodhouse L, Storer TW. Proof of the effect of testosterone on skeletal muscle. J Endocdrinol 2001;170:27.
28. Fairfield WP, Treat M, Rosenthal DI, et al. Effects of testosterone and exercise on muscle leanness in eugonadal men with AIDS wasting. J Appl Physiol 2001;90:2166.
29. Bhasin S, Bremner WJ. Clinical review 85: emerging issues in androgen replacement therapy. J Clin Endocrinol Metab 1997;82:3.
30. Griggs RC, Kingston W, Jozefowicz RF, et al. Effect of testosterone on muscle mass and muscle protein synthesis. J Appl Physiol 1989;66:498.
31. Muller M, Grobbee DE, den Tonkelaar I, et al. Endogenous sex hormones and metabolic syndrome in aging men. J Clin Endocrinol Metab 2005;90:2618.
32. Bhasin S, Storer TW, Berman N, et al. Testosterone replacement increases fat-free mass and muscle size in hypogonadal men. J Clin Endocrinol Metab 1997;82:407.
33. Brodsky IG, Balagopal P, Nair KS. Effects of testosterone replacement on muscle mass and muscle protein synthesis in hypogonadal men: a clinical research center study. J Clin Endocrinol Metab 1996;81:3469.
34. Biller BM, Molitch ME, Vance ML, et al. Treatment of prolactin-secreting macroadenomas with the once-weekly dopamine agonist cabergoline. J Clin Endocrinol Metab 1996;81:2338.
35. Webster J. A comparative review of the tolerability profiles of dopamine agonists in the treatment of hyperprolactinaemia and inhibition of lactation. Drug Saf 1996;14:228.
36. Colao A, Di Sarno A, Sarnacchiaro F, et al. Prolactinomas resistant to standard dopamine agonists respond to chronic cabergoline treatment. J Clin Endocrinol Metab 1997;82:876.
37. Wang C, Swerdloff R, Kipnes M, et al. New testosterone buccal system (Striant) delivers physiological testosterone levels: pharmacokinetics study in hypogonadal men. J Clin Endocrinol Metab 2004;89:3821.
38. Malkin CJ, Pugh PJ, Jones RD, et al. The effect of testosterone replacement on endogenous inflammatory cytokines and lipid profiles in hypogonadal men. J Clin Endocrinol Metab 2004;89:3313.
39. Catalona WJ, Hudson MA, Scardino PT, et al. Selection of optimal prostate specific antigen cutoffs for early detection of prostate cancer: receiver operating characteristic curves. J Urol 1994;152:2037.
40. Smith DS, Catalona WJ. Rate of change in serum prostate specific antigen levels as a method for prostate cancer detection. J Urol 1994;152:1163.
41. Morley JE, Kaiser FE, Perry HM 3rd, etal. Longitudinal changes in testosterone, luteinizing hormone, and follicle-stimulating hormone in healthy older men. Metabolism. 1997;46:410.
42. Gray A, Feldman HA, McKinlay JB, et al. Age, disease, and changing sex hormone levels in middle-aged men: results of the Massachusetts Male Aging Study. J Clin Endocrinol Metab 1991;73:1016.
43. Harman SM, Metter EJ, Tobin JD, et al. Longitudinal effects of aging on serum total and free testosterone levels in healthy men. Baltimore Longitudinal Study of Aging. J Clin Endocrinol Metab 2001;86:724.
44. Nieschlag E, Lammers U, Freischem CW, et al. Reproductive functions in young fathers and grandfathers. J Clin Endocrinol Metab 1982;55:676.
45. Neaves WB, Johnson L, Porter JC, et al. Leydig cell numbers, daily sperm production, and serum gonadotropin levels in aging men. J Clin Endocrinol Metab 1984;59:756.
46. Rubens R, Dhont M, Vermeulen A. Further studies on Leydig cell function in old age. J Clin Endocrinol Metab 1974;39:40.
47. Basaria S, Dobs AS. Risks versus benefits of testosterone therapy in elderly men. Drugs Aging. 1999;15:131.
48. Martin CE. Sexual activity in the aging male. In: Money J, Musaph N, eds. Handbook of sexology. New York: Elsevier North Holland, 1977: 813.
49. Snyder PJ, Peachey H, Hannoush P, et al. Effect of testosterone on body composition and muscle strength in men over 65 years of age. J Clin Endocrinol Metab 1999;84:2647.
50. Snyder PJ, Peachey H, Hannoush P, et al. Effect of testosterone on bone mineral density in men over 65 years of age. J Clin Endocrinol Metab 1999;84:1966.
51. Cherrier MM, Asthana S, Plymate S, et al. Testosterone supplementatiom improves spatial and verbal memory in healthy older men. Neurology 2001;57:80.
52. Moffat SD, Zonderman AB, Metter EJ, et al. Free testosterone and risk for Alzheimer disease in older men. Neurology 2004;62:188.
53. Barrett-Connor E, Goodman-Gruen D, Patay B. Endogenous sex hormones and cognitive function in older men. J Clin Endocrinol Metab 1999;84:3681.
54. Braunstein GD. Gynecomastia. N Engl J Med 1993;328:490.
55. Braunstein GD. Aromatase and gynecomastia. Endocr Relat Cancer 1999;6:315.
56. Staiman VR, Lowe FC. Tamoxifen for flutamide/finasteride-induced gynecomastia. Urology 1997;50:929.
57. Spark RF, White RA, Connolly PB. Impotence is not always psychogenic: newer insights into hypothalamic-pituitary-gonadal dysfunction. JAMA 1980;243:750.
58. Viagra and loss of vision. Med Lett Drugs Ther 2005;47:49
59. Bechara A, Casabe A, Cheliz G, et al. Comparative study of papaverine plus phentolamine versus prostaglandin E1 in erectile dysfunction. J Urol 1997;157: 2132.
60. Hellstrom WJ, Bennett AH, Gesundheit N, et al. A double-blind, placebo-controlled evaluation of the erectile response to transurethral alprostadil. Urology 1996;48:851.
61. Padma-Nathan H, Hellstrom WJ, Kaiser FE, et al. Treatment of men with erectile dysfunction with transurethral alprostadil. Medicated Urethral System for Erection (MUSE) Study Group. N Engl J Med 1997;336:1.
62. Earle CM, Seah M, Coulden SE, et al. The use of the vacuum erection device in the management of erectile impotence. Int J Impot Res 1996;8: 237.
63. Tay KP, Lim PH. A prospective trial with vacuum-assisted erection devices. Ann Acad Med Singapore 1995;24:705.

For annotated ***General References*** *and resources related to this chapter, visit www.hopkinsbayview.org/PAMreferences.*

SECTION 12

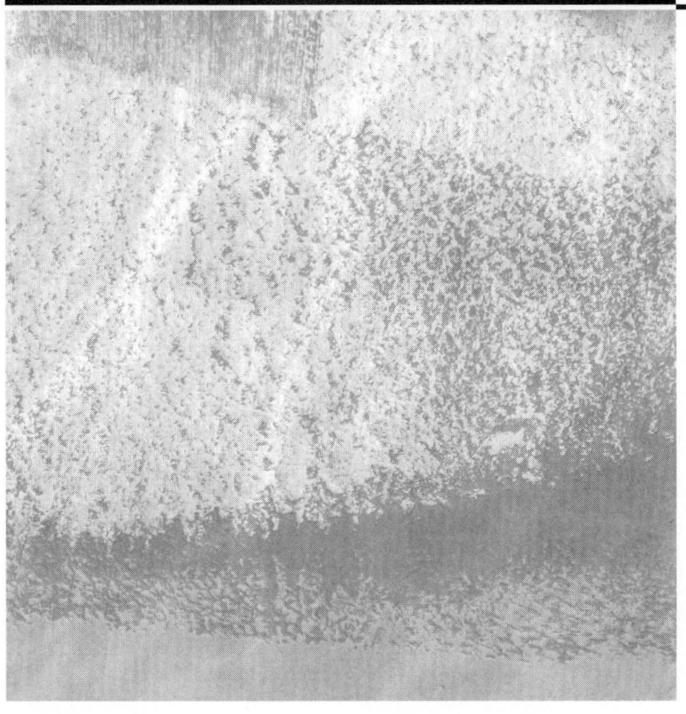

Neurologic Problems

Chapter 86

Evaluation of the Patient with Neurologic Symptoms

Rafael H. Llinas and Constance J. Johnson

This chapter describes the approaches to history taking, physical examination, and laboratory evaluation that are most useful in ambulatory patients with neurologic symptoms. One or more of these approaches is appropriate for patients with each of the neurologic problems discussed in subsequent chapters (headache, seizures, dizziness, vertigo, syncope, tremor, Parkinson disease [PD], cerebrovascular disease [CVD], and peripheral neuropathy).

NEUROLOGIC HISTORY AND PHYSICAL EXAMINATION

General Principles

To proceed with appropriate diagnostic and therapeutic actions, one must localize the lesion in the nervous system and determine the probable cause of the signs and symptoms. This requires knowledge of the presentation, epidemiology, and temporal profile of neurologic diseases. For example, new-onset central paralysis of an arm in a 20-year-old could be caused by multiple sclerosis, whereas in a 60-year-old stroke is far more likely; if the pattern is peripheral, then traumatic nerve injury is likely in the young but tumor is an important consideration in the old. Figures 86.1 and 86.2 summarize facts that are often needed for anatomic localization. Table 70.2 shows additional details regarding the anatomic relationships of peripheral nerves (cervical nerve roots) in Chapter 70, Table 71.3 (lumbar nerve roots) in Chapter 71, and Figs. 92.1 (upper extremity), and 92.2 (lower extremity) in Chapter 92.

Localizing the part of the nervous system affected and then producing a differential diagnosis for a lesion in that area is the best way to address a neurologic sign or symptom. Most individual neurologic symptoms or signs are not specific for a single functional or anatomic disturbance or for a single cause. For example, loss of a reflex is not necessarily caused by motor nerve damage, a hemiparesis is not necessarily a result of cerebrovascular disease, and a resting tremor is not necessarily a symptom of PD. Nevertheless, the constellation of findings from the history and physical examination is often quite specific. Therefore, a thorough history and physical examination are adequate for making a working diagnosis for most neurologic problems encountered in office practice.

Depending on the hypotheses one is entertaining, a brief, general neurologic evaluation may be required; more often, only selected areas of the nervous system require evaluation.

Components of a General History

Higher Functions and Consciousness

Handedness

Is the patient right-handed or left-handed? Regardless of handedness, most people are left-hemisphere dominant

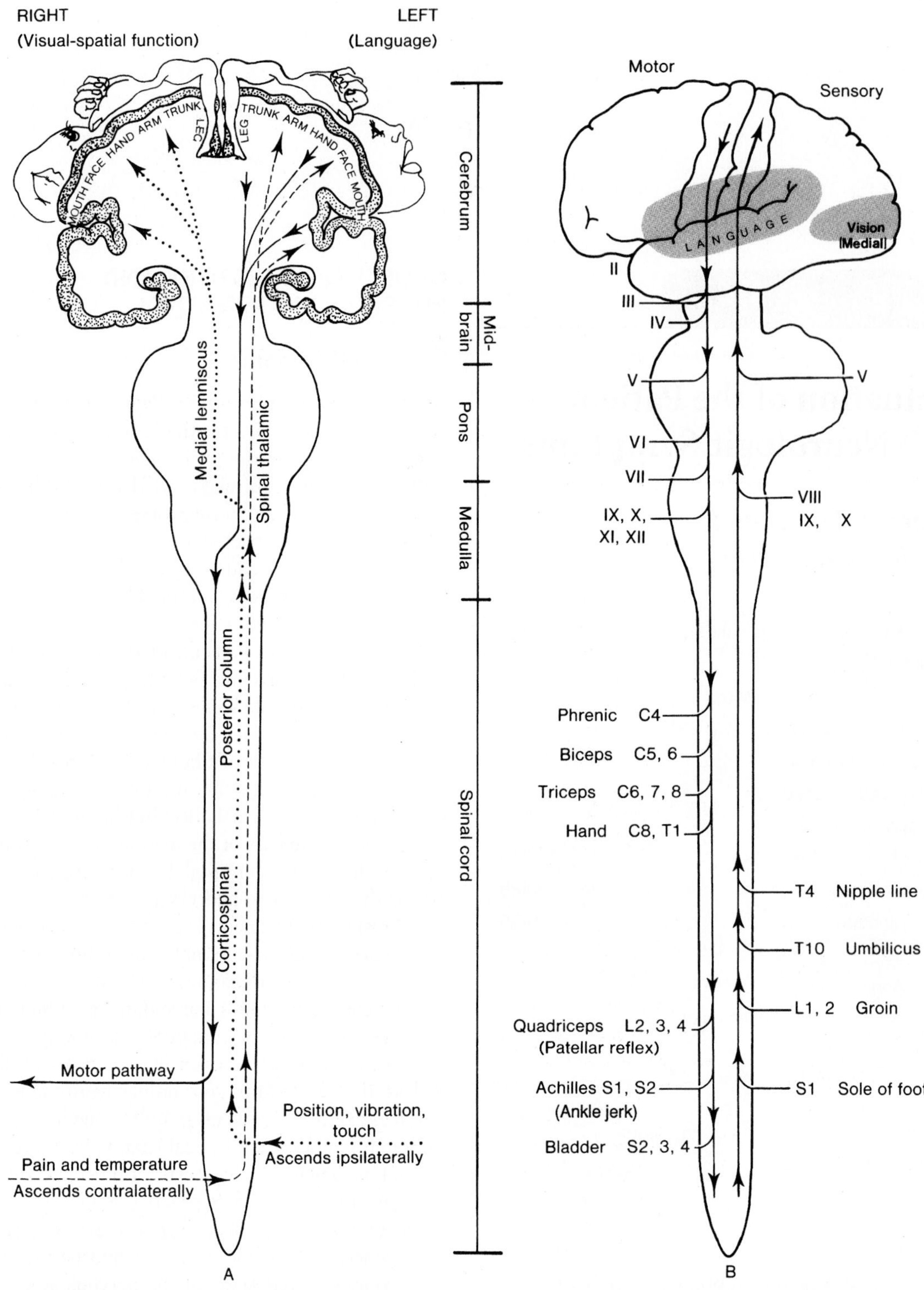

FIGURE 86.1. Schematic diagrams of neurologic localization—anterior **series (A)** and lateral **series (B)** views. Upper motor neuron signs and nonradicular sensory signs can define only the side of the lesion **series (A)**; in general, they do not reveal the level of the lesion. The presence or absence of other neurologic signs or symptoms can help to specify the level of a localized neurologic problem **series (B)**. (Courtesy of Barry Gordon, M.D., Ph.D.)

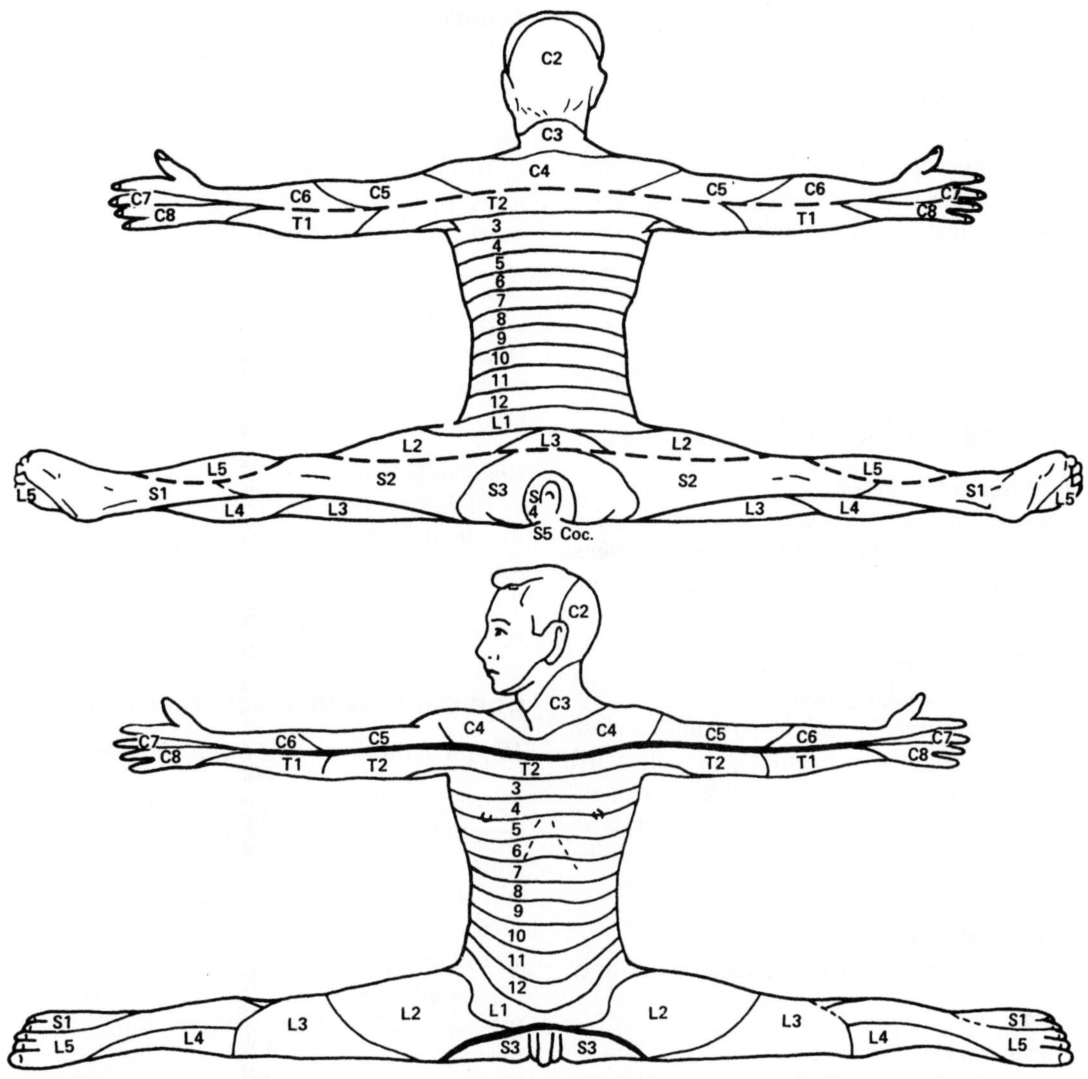

FIGURE 86.2. Cutaneous innervation areas of dermatomes. The numbers correspond to the spinal cord level of the dermatome. C, Cervical; T, thoracic; L, lumbar; S, sacral. (From Haymaker W, Woodhall B. Peripheral nerve injuries. 2nd ed. Philadelphia: WB Saunders, 1953.)

for language; however, some left-handers are right- or mixed-hemisphere dominant. Knowledge of handedness is useful when localizing cortical versus subcortical lesions. A patient with right hemiparesis and intact language who is right-handed has a subcortical lesion. A patient with left hemiparesis and intact language who is left-handed may have a cortical or subcortical lesion.

Language

Has the patient had problems with thinking or speech? Minor difficulty in finding words is common in normal people, as are brief lapses of memory. A basic evaluation for aphasias should include determining whether patients can name, repeat, and comprehend normally.

Memory

How is the patient's memory? What kinds of things are forgotten? (Ask the family whether any problems with the patient's concentration, memory, or general abilities have been noted.) Can the patient work, drive, and do usual chores?

Acute Cerebral Dysfunction

Has the patient ever fainted, lost consciousness, felt dizzy, or had a seizure (fit, convulsion)? Does the patient have frequent or disabling headaches? How often?

Mood

How are the patient's spirits? Does he or she feel depressed? Worry a great deal? How does the patient feel about the future? About self (confident, hopeless, helpless, guilty)?

Hallucinations/Delusions

Has the patient seen or heard things that are unusual or things that are not there? Does the imagination seem to play tricks? What feels wrong? Does he or she perceive being controlled by anything or anybody?

Cranial Nerves

Nerve I (Olfactory)

Not tested in the brief history and physical examination unless the patient specifically mentions a loss of smell or has a history of head trauma with loss of consciousness.

Nerve II (Optic Nerve and Vision)

Is there impaired vision? Do things seem blurred, or are there patches where it is hard to see? Has vision ever been lost in one eye, or has the patient had trouble seeing out of one side or in one direction?

Nerves III, IV, and VI (Extraocular Motions)

Has there ever been double vision?

Double vision during reading or looking at objects close to the patient will often be an oculomotor palsy (III) because of a paresis of eye adduction. Double vision looking far away is often abducens (VI) palsy to paresis of eye abduction). Ask the following questions when doing a quick evaluation.

Nerve V (Trigeminal Nerve)

Has there been numbness over the face or difficulty chewing?

Nerve VII (Facial Nerve)

Has there been any weakness in the face or paralysis of the face?

Nerve VIII (Auditory–Vestibular Nerve)

How is the patient's hearing? Has there been any ringing in the ears or difficulty hearing out of one side? Any loss of balance, spinning sensations, or dizziness?

Nerves IX, X, and XII (Glossopharyngeal, Vagal, and Hypoglossal Nerves)

Have there been any problems swallowing food? Does it seem to get caught anywhere? Where? What kinds of food has the patient had problems with? (Liquids are often the most difficult foods for patients with neurologic problems.)

Other

Motor

Has there been any weakness in the arms or legs? Is it there all the time, or does it come and go? Has there been any twitching or cramps in the muscles? Where? How often? Any wasting of the muscles?

Coordination/Cerebellar

Has there been any shaking or any difficulty in writing, drawing, buttoning, and so on?

Sensation

Has there been any numbness, tingling, or pain in the arms, legs, or feet? Where? Does position change or any other factor seem to bring it on?

Gait

Are there any problems with walking? What kind? Where or when does it happen (e.g., climbing up stairs, walking certain distances)? Is there unsteadiness when erect?

Bladder/Bowel

Have there been any problems in starting to urinate or in urinating? Any difficulty with constipation or diarrhea? Any uncontrolled urination or stool evacuation? If so, was it associated with the urge to urinate/defecate, or was it spontaneous?

Components of a General Examination

Higher Functions and Consciousness

Answers to the questions suggested, together with observations made throughout the history and physical examination, are usually sufficient to determine level of consciousness, language functioning, visual–spatial functioning, mood, level of intelligence, and memory. Chapters 19 and 26, respectively, describe the systematic mental status examinations appropriate for patients with psychiatric problems and for those with suspected cognitive impairments.

Cranial Nerves

Nerve II (Optic Nerve and Vision)

Check vision (make sure that patients wear their glasses, if needed) with the use of the Snellen chart or by having the patient read from a newspaper; test each eye separately. Check fields by confrontation (each eye separately) using finger wiggle. Examine fundi.

Nerves III, IV, and VI (Extraocular Movement and Pupils)

Have the patient move the eyes into all principal positions of gaze (horizontal, vertical, diagonal); observe for dysconjugate movements, and ask, while testing, about diplopia. Look for nystagmus, lid lag, and ptosis, and check pupils for size, symmetry, and reaction to light. The normal pupil size for young adults is 3 to 5 mm. In the elderly, normal pupils are often 2 to 3 mm. A slight degree of pupillary asymmetry, 1 mm or less, is present in about 5% of the normal population; it usually varies from hour to hour and day to day, and it decreases in bright light.

Nerve V (Trigeminal Nerve)

With a pin, check for symmetry of perception over forehead, cheek, and chin. The corneal reflex is not routinely tested in the outpatient setting. There are wide variations in corneal sensitivity among normal individuals; some subjects, particularly those who have worn contact lenses, have virtually no response at all. To test corneal reflexes, touch corresponding points on the cornea of each eye with a cotton swab. Gauze should not be used because it is abrasive. Have the subject look up and away from the testing swab. Asymmetry is the most important clue to disease.

Nerve VII (Facial Nerve)

Inspect for asymmetry of the nasolabial folds when the face is not moving. Have the patient show teeth, close eyes, and frown. Normal people may have a slight degree of resting asymmetry of the face. Normally both sides should move briskly together on showing teeth, smiling, and other facial movements. Lag on one side may be a sign of a slight seventh nerve palsy, central or peripheral.

Nerves IX and X (Glossopharyngeal and Vagus Nerves)

Inspect the uvula for position and for motion when the patient says "Ahh." Test the gag reflex on both sides of the pharynx, looking for asymmetry of response. Some people have asymmetry of the resting uvula. Visualize the palate. If it is unclear if it rises symmetrically, confirm if the uvula is deviated to one side or not. Also, bilaterally hyperactive to bilaterally absent gag responses are within the normal range.

Nerve XI (Accessory Nerve)

Observe shoulder shrug; it should be symmetric.

Nerve XII (Hypoglossal Nerve)

Inspect the tongue at rest in the mouth; have the patient protrude it and move it to both sides. It should protrude in the midline. In cases with a facial droop the lip should be pulled away slightly so the tongue is unimpeded.

Motor Examination

Adventitious Movements

Observe for tremor and other spontaneous movements (see Chapter 90).

Bulk

Examine for asymmetries of muscle mass. Denervation causes loss of muscle bulk, reaching a maximum by 4 months. Disuse over months to years also causes a decrease in muscle bulk (e.g., in the legs of patients who are permanently bedridden).

Muscle Tone (Resistance to Passive Motion)

Test tone by passively flexing and extending the upper and lower extremities. With normal tone there is a slight firmness of muscles and slight resistance to passive motion. In hypotonia the muscles are flaccid, without resistance to passive motion; this may indicate lower motor neuron (LMN) or cerebellar disease.

Hypertonia comprises several subtypes. *Rigidity* is increased resistance to passive motion throughout the whole range of motion around a joint. In *spasticity,* the initial passive motion is easy, but then there is a tightening of the muscle (spastic catch), possibly followed by a sudden release (clasp-knife effect). Spasticity usually affects only one set of muscles around a joint (in the upper extremities, the biceps, forearm pronators, and finger flexors; in the lower extremities, the quadriceps, hamstrings, and plantar flexors). In *gegenhalten or paratonia,* resistance is present in all directions but varies with the examiner's force and speed. It often seems to be voluntary (fighting back). Gegenhalten is seen normally in infants, but it appears pathologically in adults with dementias or with frontal lobe disease.

Voluntary Strength

Test voluntary strength in several major muscle groups. Survey proximal and distal muscles in each extremity. An adequate screen includes testing of shoulder abduction, elbow extension and flexion, wrist and finger extension, grip strength, hip flexion, knee flexion and extension, and foot dorsiflexion. Observe the patient's gait (discussed under Station and Gait).

For precise documentation, the following rating scale for strength can be used: 0: no movement; 1: flicker; 2: able to move with gravity eliminated (e.g., side-to-side movement on the bed.); 3: able to move against gravity; 4: able to move against resistance but less than expected; 5: normal strength.

In conversion reactions and malingering, strength on formal testing is usually jerky or giving. With sudden passive motions in the opposite direction, the examiner may find that the muscles produce normal resistive force. The examiner may find that the subject can do some voluntary activities (e.g., combing hair, reaching for objects, getting up or sitting down) with muscles that he or she states are too weak to use for such motions on formal testing.

Reflexes

The most important reflexes to test can be recalled by simply counting from 1 to 8. These include the achilles tendon (S1–2), patellar (L3–4), biceps (C5–6), and triceps (C7–8). Activity of the reflexes varies widely among patients and can vary depending on a patient's emotional state and ability to relax muscles. As in the rest of the examination, asymmetries between the two sides generally carry more weight than symmetric reflex changes;

comparison must be made with the muscles relaxed to a similar degree and with the two extremities in identical positions. A decrease in the reflex is usually caused by disruption of the sensory or motor nerves of the reflex loop itself. Sometimes decreased reflexes are seen immediately after an acute neurologic injury to be followed later by hyper-reflexia such as in acute cerebrovascular accident or acute spinal cord injury, in which case interpretation does not depend on the reflexes alone. Increased reflexes mean upper motor neuron (UMN) disease located anywhere from just above the anterior horn cell to the cerebral cortex.

A Babinski sign consists of dorsiflexion of the big toe after plantar stimulation; it may be associated with dorsiflexion and spreading of the other toes and dorsiflexion of the foot. The classic Babinski response is slow and deliberate. Nonspecific withdrawal may resemble the Babinski reflex, but it is usually rapid and the patient usually complains of subjective distress; a reliable Babinski sign should occur in the absence of any patient discomfort from the stimulus. A Babinski sign may be found as the sole indicator of UMN disease.

Sensation

The patient should be tested for symmetry and for differences in proximal and distal perception in all four extremities. Light touch (posterior columns) is not a well-delineated modality and can be normal when abnormalities of pinprick (lateral spinothalamic tract) or proprioception/vibration (posterior columns) are present; therefore, it should not be used as the sole screen of sensory function. Sensitivity to pinprick, proprioception, and vibratory sense should be tested. There are normal differences in pinprick perception over different areas of the body (e.g., it is decreased over the beard area), but patients usually ignore these differences. Particularly introspective or anxious patients can give very confusing responses and must be told to ignore small subjective differences. Repeated testing is often important to determine the reliability of a patient's response. Vibration sense should be tested with a 128-Hz tuning fork. Proprioception is tested in the most distal joint of the fingers and toes by moving the digit approximately 30 degrees to 45 degrees and then asking the patient to report the direction in which the digits have moved.

The Romberg test (patient stands with feet together and closed eyes while the ability to maintain balance is assessed) is a test of integrity of proprioception and the posterior columns through which proprioception is conveyed. The ability to stand with eyes closed must be interpreted with caution in patients with cerebellar ataxia. If the patient cannot stand steady with eyes open, the Romberg test may be altered to allow testing of posterior columns by having the patient stand with a wide base (to compensate for cerebellar ataxia) and then close the eyes. If the posterior columns are intact, the patient will not waver more than a slight amount.

Coordination/Cerebellar Function

The patient should be told to touch the thumb sequentially to each of the fingers of each hand separately; speed, effort, and rhythm of the movements should be observed. Finger-to-nose-to-finger movement should be tested (subject must touch examiner's moving finger, then touch his or her own nose, then touch the examiner's finger again) for speed, rhythm, intention tremor, and inaccuracy (dysmetria). The subject should be asked to tap each foot separately, and differences in speed, ease, and rhythm should be observed. In these tests, normal subjects show equal ability with either side or are slightly better on the side of their preferred hand. Slowness and subjective effort on repetitive movements, without a loss of rhythm, are characteristic of UMN lesions. Preserved speed with erratic movements and loss of rhythm may be seen in cerebellar disease. Finger–nose–finger testing may be affected by tremor of various types, as described in Chapter 90.

Station and Gait

Any tendency to list or any need for support while sitting, standing, or walking should be observed. The patient should be asked to walk normally and to walk on the heels and toes (to test strength and balance). Tandem gait testing (walking heel-to-toe) requires the patient to narrow the base of support and reveals abnormalities of balance in patients with ataxia not detected on normal walking.

In *cerebellar disease,* the patient exhibits a wide base (legs widely separated), unsteadiness, and lateral reeling. Lateral reeling can be evaluated by having the patient walk around a chair in both directions; the patient will tend to walk into the chair when it is on the affected side and to veer away from the chair when it is on the unaffected side. Because of fundamental abnormality of motor coordination, the patient with cerebellar disease affecting the lower extremities cannot participate in a standard Romberg test, which requires standing with the two feet together; a modified Romberg test for such patients was described earlier.

In *sensory ataxia* (loss of proprioception), there is uncertainty, slapping or stamping of the feet, and a positive Romberg test (the patient loses balance with eyes closed but can avoid falling when the eyes are open because of visually mediated vestibular or cerebellar compensation).

In a *spastic gait* (in UMN disease), the leg does not flex but circumducts, and there is foot dragging (the toe of the sole of the patient's shoe becomes disproportionately worn); there is also loss of arm swinging on the spastic side.

In a *parkinsonian gait,* there is unilateral or bilateral loss of arm swinging, the patient is bent forward, and there is rigidity, shuffling, and festination (the upper part of the body advances ahead of the lower extremities; gait becomes faster, as if to catch up).

In *LMN paralysis* of the pretibial and peroneal muscles, foot-drop is seen; hip flexion is preserved, and the patient lifts the foot very high, advances it by swinging it forward, then slaps it down.

In *frontal lobe disease,* gait may be wide-based, shuffling, and slow, and turning is slow, but there is no weakness or loss of sensation.

Special Considerations in the Evaluation of Neurologic Symptoms and Signs

Neurologic signs are often subtle in ambulatory patients, compared with patients hospitalized for neurologic disease, and may be related to prior acute neurologic events. Two important considerations in the evaluation of ambulatory patients with neurologic symptoms and signs are the variability in performance over time and the difference between the manifestations of UMN and LMN lesions.

Variability over Time

In patients who have abnormalities of the peripheral nerves, spinal cord, and brainstem, symptoms and signs remain about the same after the basic problem has stabilized; later alterations of the findings usually reflect a change in the patient's disease. On the other hand, cognitive and language impairment can vary greatly from minute to minute, hour to hour, or day to day. The variability affects the psychomotor domain (e.g., performance of everyday tasks, memory, speech and language, and mood). For example,

- The patient may be able to dress, fix breakfast, and bring in the mail one morning, be incapable of these tasks the next morning, and perform them correctly on the third morning.
- The patient may remember his or her spouse's name in the morning but not in the evening of the same day.
- The aphasic patient may be able to say something one minute and unable to say it several minutes later.
- The stroke survivor's affect may vary from depressed to euphoric from hour to hour or day to day.

As a result of this type of variability, members of the patient's family may become confused and angry; they may inquire whether a change in behavior means that the disease is getting worse, or they may conclude that the patient is capable of doing certain tasks but is just not trying sometimes. When the pattern is clearly one of waxing and waning, the family should be reassured that, just as they have their good days and bad days, the patient does also, but in exaggerated and different ways. Chapters 26 (dementia) and 91 (stroke) discuss the evaluation and management of behavioral changes of patients with cerebral damage.

Differences between Upper Motor Neuron and Lower Motor Neuron Symptoms

The manifestations and the course of UMN and LMN damage differ fundamentally. UMN lesions affect the pathways that bring a command from the cortex to the anterior horn cell. UMN function depends on integrity of the cortex and of the corticospinal and corticobulbar tracts. LMN lesions affect the final common pathway for muscle movements. LMN function depends on the integrity of the anterior horn cell in the spinal cord and its nerve fiber for carrying impulses to the muscle cell. A number of points are helpful in recognizing or distinguishing these two patterns of motor abnormality when they are not overt, which is often the case in patients seen in office practice.

Upper Motor Neuron Lesion Syndrome

If a UMN lesion is total, movements are absent. However, there may be preservation of involuntary movements, such as those associated with yawning, laughing, crying, or anger. Classically a patient may have a dense facial weakness with volitional movements but with an emotional smile the face seems to move almost symterically. When there is weakness (paresis) rather than paralysis caused by UMN damage, the following patterns of weakness are seen.

In the face, the lower muscles are usually involved. There is variable but often some involvement of the orbicularis oculi, producing a widened palpebral fissure and weakness of eye closure, but the forehead may be completely spared. This is in contrast to LMN (peripheral) seventh nerve damage, in which both the upper and lower facial muscles are involved, although sometimes mild peripheral seventh nerve weakness (e.g., early Bell palsy, a LMN lesion) can mimic a UMN pattern. One additional differential point is that the LMN lesion produces the same amount of weakness with both a voluntary and an involuntary movement (e.g., laughing). A UMN seventh nerve paresis (e.g., from stroke) may not be apparent when the patient is laughing or crying involuntarily and may be present only when the patient is asked to smile voluntarily.

In the arm, extensors muscles are more affected by UMN lesions and flexor muscles are more affected in the lower extremities. This gives rise to the classic hemiplegic stance with the arm in hyperflexion and leg in hyperextension. Whether or not the muscles are weak in a UMN lesion, voluntary movements are typically slowed and require greater effort than usual, and the ability to make fine movements with the affected limb is lost. A patient with a very mild hemiparesis may be able to squeeze the examiner's hand with normal strength, but movements are slower and clumsier than usual; the patient may be unable to easily use fingers individually. They are likely to have weaker finger extensors and weakness of grip. Also, when the patient is asked to extend both arms with the eyes closed, there may be downward and inward drift of the weak arm (pronator sign). In the lower extremity, a patient with such a mild defect may be able to dorsiflex the foot voluntarily. However, the same patient may not be able to do this very rapidly (as revealed on attempted foot tapping), and the movement may not be automatically coordinated with walking, resulting in a foot-drop.

Typically (but not invariably), UMN lesions are accompanied by spasticity and hyperreflexia.

Lower Motor Neuron Lesion Syndrome

Weakness resulting from a permanent LMN lesion is fixed and unchanging. Only the muscles served by the involved spinal cord segment or peripheral nerve are weak. There are none of the widespread effects characteristic of a UMN lesion. Atrophy is usually apparent within several weeks after a LMN lesion, in contrast to UMN lesions, where atrophy is slight and late (many months). Pathologic fasciculations may be present in affected muscle groups, distinguishable from benign occasional muscle twitching by the fact that they are frequent and occur only in the denervated muscles. Muscles are usually flaccid and hyporeflexic or areflexic. If a peripheral nerve has been involved, there may be associated hypesthesia or anesthesia. In muscle disease (e.g., polymyositis, drug-induced myopathy), muscle tone, reflexes, and sensory function are normal. Weakness is typically proximal in the deltoids, iliopsoas, quadriceps, and neck flexor muscles. The patient complains of difficulty climbing steps or using the arms over the head.

In some situations, UMN and LMN lesions occur together. For instance, spinal cord injury typically gives signs of a LMN lesion at the level of the injury, caused by localized destruction of the anterior horn cells and their nerve roots; below the level of the injury, there may be a partial or complete UMN syndrome, with spasticity, hyperreflexia, and preserved involuntary reflexes. Likewise, amyotrophic lateral sclerosis, an idiopathic degenerative disease, affects both pyramidal tract cells and anterior horn cells. Along with LMN-type weakness, fasciculations, and wasting, these patients have hyperreflexia and may have Babinski signs.

Neurovascular Examination

This examination is especially important in patients in whom cerebrovascular disease or an increased risk of cerebrovascular disease is the problem (see Chapter 91). The examination includes an assessment of the heart and peripheral vasculature, with emphasis on the vessels of the head and neck.

Heart and Peripheral Vessels

The radial arteries should be simultaneously palpated at the wrists to determine any asymmetry in pulse amplitude or timing (pulse delay). The brachial arterial blood pressure should be measured in the supine, sitting, and standing positions. Blood pressure should be measured in both arms to check for asymmetry. Unequal blood pressure in the two arms (20 mm Hg or more difference in systolic pressure, more than 10 mm Hg in diastolic pressure) suggests a stenotic lesion of the subclavian or innominate artery on the side with the lower pressure. Orthostatic hypotension, defined as a fall in systolic pressure of more than 15 mm Hg on moving from a supine to an upright position, is common in autonomic neuropathy and may be important in explaining symptoms in patients with severe stenotic lesions of carotid or vertebral–basilar arteries.

A detailed cardiac examination can provide evidence of cardiomegaly, valvular disease, or arrhythmia, each of which may predispose a patient to a stroke. Finally, a complete assessment of the peripheral vasculature, for evidence of widespread atherosclerosis, should include palpation and auscultation of the femoral arteries and palpation of the arterial pulses in the feet.

Vessels of Head and Neck

Evaluation of the vessels of the head and neck may include inspection, palpation, and auscultation.

Inspection

Prominence of the superficial temporal artery with erythema and, occasionally, ulceration of the overlying skin in a patient with persistent malaise is suggestive of giant cell arteritis, an inflammatory process that can lead to retinal or cerebral infarction (see Chapter 87).

Dilation of the *episcleral arteries* of an eye can result from occlusion of the ipsilateral internal carotid artery; in this instance, the hemisphere on the side of the occlusion is being supplied in a retrograde fashion by the external carotid artery through dilated ophthalmic arteries. The funduscopic examination allows direct visualization of the retinal vessels, and changes resulting from atherosclerosis, hypertension, or diabetes mellitus can be detected. Moreover, the absence of an expected change can be informative, as in the case of the hypertensive patient with normal retinal vessels on the side of a severely stenosed carotid artery; in this instance, occlusive disease of the ipsilateral carotid artery protects the retina from the effects of chronic hypertension. A detailed funduscopic examination may also demonstrate emboli, seen as white or refractile elements in the retinal arterioles (see Fig. 91.1 in

Chapter 91). These emboli may be composed of cholesterol, platelets and fibrin, or calcium and are suggestive of atherosclerotic carotid occlusive disease or cardiac valve disease.

Palpation

Reports of embolic stroke after firm palpation of a diseased carotid artery have left some clinicians with a sense of trepidation regarding manipulation of this vessel. The current consensus, however, is that gentle palpation of the carotid artery can be performed with limited risk and occasionally provides useful information about the status of the vessel. Perhaps more valuable, and without risk, is palpation of the superficial temporal and facial arteries, which are branches of the external carotid artery. A weak or absent pulse in these arteries on one side of the head is suggestive of ipsilateral occlusive disease of the external or common carotid artery. In contrast, an increase in pulsation in these vessels may result from stenosis or occlusion of the ipsilateral internal carotid artery that causes collateral flow through the external system. Finally, the finding of a tender superficial temporal artery with decreased pulsation may support other data consistent with the diagnosis of giant cell arteritis (see Chapter 87).

Auscultation

After auscultation of the heart to check for transmitted cardiac murmur, the examiner should proceed to the supraclavicular regions over the subclavian arteries and to the carotid arteries up to their bifurcation at the angle of the jaw; a cervical bruit is suggestive, but not diagnostic, of atherosclerotic occlusive disease. Auscultation may at times be useful over the occipital, temporal, and parietal regions of the cranium, and over the orbits. The finding of a cephalic bruit in an adult raises the possibility of an arteriovenous malformation; an orbital bruit suggests intracranial internal carotid artery disease.

USE OF DIAGNOSTIC PROCEDURES

Patients may be referred for any of a number of diagnostic procedures in the evaluation of a neurologic problem. The principles described in Chapter 2 are especially important in deciding which of these procedures to select. Costs of neurodiagnostic tests vary widely from region to region and within a region because fee profiles are individually determined. Charges for many of these tests are in the range of $200 to $2,000; however, practitioners should become aware of costs in their own regions. For most of the procedures currently available for ambulatory application, the definition, principal indications, limitations, and a description of the patient experience are provided here. Chapter 92 provides this information for nerve conduction tests and electromyography.

Radiography of the Skull

Definition of Procedure

The term *routine skull radiographs* refers to a set of films that include three standard views: lateral, anteroposterior (AP), and inclined AP. Many other views are possible and may be indicated in specific conditions (e.g., basal skull views for a patient with atypical trigeminal neuralgia).

Principal Indications

The principal indications are suspected skull fracture and problems involving the bones, such as metastatic tumor (osteoblastic or osteolytic), myeloma, or Paget disease.

Limitations

The skull radiograph has little value as a screening or diagnostic test for intracranial disease because few intracranial neurologic conditions are associated with bony changes. It has been almost entirely replaced by computed tomography (CT) imaging of the head.

Patient Experience. The patient will be asked to keep his or her head in several uncomfortable positions for short periods of time; accurate positioning might be impossible for elderly patients or for those who have neck problems.

Radiography of the Spine

Definition of Procedure

Standard spine films are usually AP and lateral views; oblique and flexion–extension views usually must be ordered specifically.

Principal Indications

The principal indications are suspected cervical spondylitic radiculopathy (in which case, oblique films are necessary to examine the intervertebral foramina through which the roots pass); suspected cervical or lumbar stenosis, spondylolisthesis, luxation, or subluxation; suspected vertebral fracture; and suspected metastatic tumor.

Limitations

Asymptomatic cervical spondylosis and interspace narrowing caused by disc degeneration are so common after 40 years of age (see Chapters 70 and 71) that their presence has limited usefulness in the absence of more specific findings from the history and physical examination. Negative films provide good evidence against spondylosis as the cause of radicular symptoms.

Radiographs do not show soft tissue, brain, spinal cord, or nerve roots. In patients with herniated intervertebral discs, films are usually normal or show only nonspecific intervertebral narrowing. However, patients with congenitally small bony canals (cervical or lumbar stenosis) are at risk for neurologic problems occurring secondary to degenerative changes in the disc and ligaments; the radiologist should be asked specifically about these possibilities if they are important diagnostic considerations.

Patient Experience. The patient must cooperate for several views. Patients with neck problems and those who are elderly may be unable to position themselves for adequate cervical spine films.

Electroencephalography

Definition of Procedure

The electroencephalogram (EEG) is a record of the (1- to 50-mV) electrical rhythms of the brain.

Principal Indications

One principal indication is known or suspected seizure disorder (see Chapter 88). Recording during sleep or after sleep deprivation significantly increases the chances of a useful diagnostic examination; for complex partial seizure, sleep deprivation or extended EEG can increase the yield of the study.

The procedure is also used for confirmation of focal brain lesions in the absence of other evidence (e.g., in the diagnosis and localization of stroke) and for confirmation of diffuse brain disease, such as dementia, delirium, cerebral vasculitis, or drug effect or withdrawal. The EEG may at times be helpful in differentiation of the dementia syndrome of depression from organic dementia (see Chapter 26). For sleep disorders (see Chapter 7), routine and special EEG recording techniques are often indicated.

Limitations

The EEG records cortical activity and, although it is sensitive for processes affecting the cortex, it is not useful for delineation of subcortical processes. However, this property can be useful in investigating vascular lesions when a cortical lesion is not identified on CT or magnetic resonance imaging (MRI).

Negative Electroencephalogram

A single negative EEG is not evidence for the absence of a seizure disorder. For example, up to 50% of patients with known epilepsy have normal interictal records. Serial or repeated negative EEGs may be far more significant (see Chapter 88). A normal EEG in a patient with suspected delirium suggests psychiatric illness.

"Mildly Abnormal" Electroencephalogram

Depending on the reader and the classification scheme, some adult EEGs (5% to 30% or more) can be classified as minimally or mildly but nonspecifically abnormal. The relevance of these interpretations must be judged in the context of the patients' problems but should not be given undue weight because of the broad range of normal findings. This is particularly true in infancy, childhood, adolescence, and old age. For instance, temporal slow activity is present after 40 years of age in as many as 30% to 40% of subjects.

Patient Experience. Subjects are asked to lie down or recline while surface electrodes are attached with electrode paste. The total procedure takes an average of 40 to 60 minutes, with 20 to 30 minutes of actual recording time. For most of the actual recording, the patient is simply asked to lie calmly with eyes closed. Additional studies that most laboratories routinely perform include recording during hyperventilation (for 3 to 5 minutes) and during photic simulation with a repetitive flash. For many tracings, subjects are encouraged to fall asleep. Some laboratories induce sleep with oral chloral hydrate if permitted by the referring physician; if this is planned in advance, the patient should be told to bring someone who can drive the patient home.

The EEG is extremely sensitive to patient movement, sweating, and muscle tension, any of which can make a tracing uninterpretable.

For sleep-deprived EEGs, the patient is asked to stay up the night before, and the EEG is done in the laboratory first thing in the morning.

Lumbar Puncture

Definition of Procedure

Lumbar puncture is performed to obtain cerebrospinal fluid (CSF) for analysis and to measure intracranial pressure. A normal opening pressure does not exceed 200 mm. Normal CSF is crystal clear and contains no more than five mononuclear cells; the normal glucose concentration is two thirds that of a simultaneously determined serum glucose level, and the protein concentration is less than 45 mg/dL. Xanthochromia is a yellowish discoloration of the spinal fluid that is present in red cell breakdown (indicating previous subarachnoid hemorrhage), in hyperbilirubinemia, and with extreme elevations of protein.

Principal Indications

Elevated intracranial pressure must be documented to diagnose idiopathic intracranial hypertension (see Chapter 87). The low-pressure headache syndrome (see Chapter 87) can be documented by lumbar puncture but may be exacerbated by the procedure.

Lumbar puncture is used in the evaluation of patients with suspected meningitis; those with suspected or known chronic infection of the CNS, such as syphilis, acquired immunodeficiency syndrome (AIDS), Lyme disease, cryptococcus, or tuberculosis; those with subarachnoid hemorrhage; those with suspected demyelinating or inflammatory disease, such as multiple sclerosis or inflammatory neuropathy (e.g., Guillain–Barre syndrome); and those with undiagnosed CNS disease.

Limitations

The opening pressure depends on the intracranial pressure, which can be elevated by measures that increase venous pressure, such as straining and tightening of the abdominal musculature. A tense patient with an elevated opening pressure should be encouraged to relax, and pressure should be remeasured before fluid is removed. The closing pressure depends on the pressure/volume dynamics, which are influenced by the amount of fluid removed and the intracranial compliance. Abnormalities of CSF are nonspecific; however, when they are interpreted in the context of the clinical presentation and further evaluation in the laboratory, diagnostic accuracy can be increased.

The procedure is completely safe if infection of the skin overlying the puncture site, an intracranial mass lesion, and bilateral brain edema are ruled out. Neurologic consultation and CT or MRI of the brain before the lumbar puncture will eliminate the potential for complications caused by the latter two problems. If papilledema is present, an imaging study to rule out a mass lesion before lumbar puncture is always mandatory in an outpatient.

Patient Experience. Patients are often reluctant to undergo lumbar puncture, based on widespread belief that it is dangerous and very painful. The patient should be reassured that, after neurologic evaluation or an imaging study, the procedure is safe. Under adequate local anesthesia, the discomfort is mild. When lumbar puncture is done properly under aseptic conditions, the most common complication is a postprocedure headache (see Chapter 87). The probability of postprocedure headache can be decreased by using the smallest-gauge needle that is practical (20-gauge in most adults). Newer, blunt-tipped "atraumatic" lumbar puncture needles are postulated to result in a smaller dural hole and have been demonstrated to reduce headache after the procedure. The flow rate through the needle may be compromised with a needle of 22 gauge or higher, but it is adequate with the 20-gauge needle. For most patients, a 20-gauge atraumatic needle is ideal. Performing the tap with the patient in a sitting position also increases the likelihood of a first-pass nontraumatic tap; however, the lateral decubitus position is necessary to obtain a precise opening pressure measurement. After the lumbar puncture, the patient is instructed to lie flat for 5 to 60 minutes and to drink copious amounts of fluid over the ensuing 6 hours. A minority of patients complain of pain at the puncture site, which may be treated with nonnarcotic analgesics.

Duplex Scan

Definition of Procedure

Duplex scanning combines B-mode ultrasonic scanning of the carotid bifurcation with spectral analysis of a Doppler signal to assess plaque disease. The extent of plaque is classified into categories that vary among laboratories but usually approximate the following categories: 0% to 15%, 16% to 40%, 41% to 60%, 61% to 80%, 81% to 99%, and occluded. The percentage of stenosis approximates angiographic measurements; however, some discrepancy occurs because duplex scanning approximates area, whereas angiography is usually a linear measurement. Plaque characteristics such as calcification, hemorrhage, and ulceration can be determined. Plaque distribution in common, internal, and external carotid arteries is delineated.

Principal Indications

This noninvasive screening technique may be used in the evaluation of patients with asymptomatic carotid bruits, transient ischemic attacks (TIAs), or stroke. Duplex ultrasonography compares favorably with MRI angiography (see Cerebral Angiography) in predicting 100% carotid artery occlusion and 70% carotid artery stenosis (1,2). With use of this procedure, stroke-prone patients may be selected for arteriography (see Chapter 91).

Limitations

No more than 3 cm of the internal carotid artery can be imaged above the bifurcation. The proximal common carotid is imaged for a variable distance, depending on its tortuousity. This technique cannot distinguish complete occlusion from a very-high-grade stenosis. No information about intracranial disease is obtained.

Patient Experience. A comprehensive duplex examination of the carotid arteries takes approximately 45 minutes. The transducer head is held over the carotid bifurcation at the angle of the mandible. There is no appreciable discomfort or risk.

Cerebral Angiography

Definition of Procedure

Cerebral angiography provides imaging by intra-arterial injection of a contrast agent, by magnetic resonance technique (magnetic resonance angiography [MRA]), or by helical CT (see Computed Tomography).

For intra-arterial angiography a flexible catheter is placed in an artery, usually the femoral artery, and passed to the aortic arch, where it is selectively advanced into the arteries of interest, including the common carotid or vertebral arteries, which are then injected with a contrast agent. Serial radiographs are taken.

MRA is a noninvasive procedure that uses radiofrequency signals to construct images of the cerebral vessels.

Principal Indications

Cerebral angiography can be used in the delineation of a number of intracranial processes. Since the advent of CT and MRI, the principal indication for angiography has been the definitive diagnosis of cerebrovascular diseases including extracranial and intracranial arterial stenosis, vascular malformations, aneurysms, and vasculitis.

Limitations

Intra-arterial Angiography

Adequate renal function is a prerequisite. Serious complications (approximately 1% to 2% of patients) occur related to femoral puncture, manipulation of the catheter, and reactions to the contrast agent. Serious complications include femoral artery clot with embolization, stroke, and anaphylactic reaction to the contrast agent. The ionic load of the contrast agent may precipitate heart failure in susceptible patients.

Magnetic Resonance Angiography

Resolution with MRA is not yet as acute as with intra-arterial angiography; this limitation is related to disturbances of laminar flow and to the multiplanar course of cerebral vessels. This can lead to intracranial and extracranial arteries appearing more stenotic or artifactually occluded on MRA. The hazards associated with MRA are the same as those listed later for MRI. MRA may be used to noninvasively image the intracranial vessels and the carotid and vertebral arteries in the neck.

Patient Experience. For intra-arterial angiography, the patient lies on a radiography table and a femoral artery puncture is made after local anesthesia with lidocaine. The major discomfort is a burning sensation, which can be intense, that is felt with the injection of contrast material. Less stressful reactions are a metallic taste in the mouth, itching, and occasionally hives. Mild or severe bronchospasm, although uncommon, can occur. The patient must be able to lie still for the radiographs. After the procedure, patients are instructed to drink a large amount of fluid, limit activity, and monitor for signs of bleeding or obstruction at or distal to the site of arterial puncture. Instructions usually include limiting ambulation, no lifting or other strenuous activity for 24 hours, and no bathing for at least 12 hours. For MRA, the patient experience is the same as for MRI (see Magnetic Resonance Imaging).

Computed Tomography Scanning of the Head

Definition of Procedure

CT uses narrow x-ray beams to exploit differences in x-ray absorption between different kinds of intracranial tissues. Without contrast, the CT scanner can distinguish the densities of bone, calcified tissue, blood, gray matter, white matter, CSF, and air. Its resolving power is proportional to the differences in the densities of these tissues. Although CT scanning results are typically presented as horizontal slices through the brain, present technology allows slices to be reconstructed in the vertical plane or in any other plane to give a better perspective on abnormal findings. Helical CT reduces scanning time with some loss of resolution. It is useful for CT angiography.

Intravenous injection of contrast material is used to enhance the x-ray contrast of vascular lesions such as tumors and abscesses; contrast material diffuses into an area where the blood–brain barrier has broken down to increase the x-ray absorption density.

CT scanning is highly sensitive and often diagnostic; therefore, it has a place in both screening and specific investigations. Use of a contrast agent is not necessary for screening studies. CT angiography is becoming a very quick and efficient method for evaluating intracerebral and extracerebral arteries. It does not appear to lead to "over call" stenosis the way MRA can.

Principal Indications

CT is used in the evaluation of patients with intracranial problems when structural alteration is known or suspected, such as tumor, cerebrovascular disease, degenerative disease (e.g., Alzheimer disease, Huntington disease), hydrocephalus, subdural hematoma, or unexplained headache. CT is superior to MRI in identifying calcification and hemorrhage. CT is safe for patients with aneurysm clips, pacemakers, and implanted defibrillators. The imaging time and noise are much less than with MRI, which makes CT useful for uncooperative or confused patients. Many conditions can be assessed without the use of a radiographic contrast agent; this should be strongly considered for patients who have conditions for which the most common causes do not require contrast for visualization (i.e., dementia, remote stroke) and for elderly persons, in whom the risks associated with contrast studies are somewhat greater. CTA can quickly evaluate vascular stenosis with a high degree of accuracy.

Limitations

A negative CT scan does not exclude a structural lesion or damage. The damage may not have caused enough change in local absorption density to produce contrast with its surroundings. This is not uncommon in cases of cerebral infarction within 1 week after the initial insult, when the original edema has cleared and new vessel formation and phagocytosis have not yet begun to affect brain density. A CT scan can also be negative because the damage is in an area of the brain that is poorly visualized, such as the brainstem or spinal cord. Additionally, a CT scan is typically negative after transient ischemia, but this finding does not detract from the significance of the event and the need for further study. CT is less sensitive than MRI for stroke, vascular malformation, tumor, abscess, and demyelinating lesions.

When it is performed without contrast injection, CT scanning is essentially free of risk. When contrast material is used, the risk is that of the contrast agent itself—often a warm flush in the face, nausea, or sometimes vomiting. In approximately 1 case in 100,000 there is the possibility of death from anaphylaxis. The serum creatinine concentration should be measured before the infusion of contrast material. If it is abnormal, the risks and precautions related to renal insult from contrast media must be considered (see Chapter 52).

Patient Experience. The patient is asked to lie down with his or her head inside what looks somewhat like a large doughnut. Straps are usually applied over the forehead to prevent motion. The procedure takes 5 to 20 minutes, depending on the scanner. Contrast material may be given intravenously, by single bolus, or by intravenous drip.

Computed Tomography Scanning of the Spine

The definition of the procedure and the patient experience are the same as for CT scanning of the head.

Principal Indications

CT of the spine is the preferred technique for evaluation of acute fractures and bony impingement on the central canal. It does not visualize the spinal cord or nerve roots and has therefore been replaced by MRI for visualization of the spinal cord and disc disease. CT of the spine can be used for patients with aneurysm clips, pacemakers, and debrillators.

Limitations

If the spinal region to be studied spans three or more vertebrae, MRI is more practical than CT because MRI can visualize an entire region of the spine. Diagnostic accuracy of CT presupposes use of a localizer image for accurate selection of the plane and angle of the slice, as well as a thin slice for optimal resolution.

Magnetic Resonance Imaging of the Central Nervous System

Definition of Procedure

MRI is a noninvasive imaging technique that yields better contrast and sensitivity for most CNS lesions than does radiographic CT. It uses radio waves of a specific (resonance) frequency. No ionizing radiation is required. MRI studies usually are substantially more expensive than CT studies.

Principal Indications

The high tissue contrast achieved with MRI makes it the imaging technique of choice for most CNS diseases, including tumors (especially posterior fossa tumors), cerebral infarctions, vascular malformations, abscesses, white matter disease (e.g., multiple sclerosis), and spinal cord abnormalities including herniated nucleus pulposus.

In several aspects of brain imaging, MRI has been shown to be superior to CT. MRI provides better imaging of the posterior fossa than does CT because the surrounding bone causes no streak artifacts. Tissue contrast with MRI is superior to that obtained with CT. As a result, gray matter and white matter are better delineated and the extent of certain diseases is better appreciated. For example, MRI can reveal many more of the lesions of multiple sclerosis than can CT. Major blood vessels can be identified with MRI without the need for contrast media because the flowing blood, as a result of its velocity, appears dark. The common carotid, internal carotid, external carotid, and vertebral and basilar arteries are easily seen. Aneurysms of the internal carotid artery have been detected, and a thrombus in the lumen of the artery can be identified. Disc disease is easily evaluated without injection of contrast material, as is required for myelography. Diffusion weighted MRI can show strokes within minutes where conventional CT and MRI may not show acute strokes for 6 to 24 hours.

Limitations

MRI has high sensitivity for disease detection in the CNS but is limited and may be less useful than CT in the evaluation of acute hemorrhages, calcified lesions, and bony structures, each of which is easily detected by CT. Because the scanning time is longer than that for CT studies, MRI studies are more subject to artifact caused by patient motion. Some claustrophobic patients cannot undergo the procedure without sedation.

The known hazards of MRI result from the force and torque exerted by the field on ferromagnetic objects brought into the vicinity of the magnet and on patients' prostheses, such as surgical clips, pacemakers, cochlear implants, metal in the eye, and joint replacements. Cardiac pacemaker and implanted defibrillator function can be disrupted and false signals produced. Ferromagnetic metal clips, such as those on cerebral aneurysms, may be dislodged.

Patient Experience. The patient lies supine on a table identical to the CT scanner, but the head holder consists of a plastic coil that passes very close to the patient's face. The entire table is then moved into a larger tunnel. The patient may experience claustrophobia. A loud knocking sound is heard during data collection, during which time the patient must remain absolutely still. The test lasts about 45 minutes.

SPECIFIC REFERENCES*

1. Blakely DD, Oddone EZ, Hasselblad V, et al. Noninvasive carotid artery testing. A meta-analytic review. Ann Intern Med 1995;122:360.
2. Nederkoorn PG, van der Graaf Y, Hunink MG. Duplex ultrasound and magnetic resonance antiography compared with digital subtraction angiography in carotid artery stenosis: a systematic review. Stroke 2003;34:1324.

*Bold numerals denote published controlled clinical trials, meta-analyses, or consensus-based recommendations.

For annotated ***General References*** *and resources related to this chapter, visit www.hopkinsbayview.org/PAMreferences.*

Chapter 87

Headaches and Facial Pain

Constance J. Johnson

EPIDEMIOLOGY

Headache is a common complaint with most adults reporting a history of recurrent headache. In *surveys of visits to physicians*, headache was named by patients as the principal reason for approximately 2% to 4% of all visits to internists, general practitioners, and family practitioners (1). Most patients have a primary headache disorder that meets the criteria for tension-type headache, migraine, or cluster headache. In primary care, a patient with a stable pattern of moderate to severe episodic headache with a normal examination is most likely to have migraine. The Landmark Study of 1,203 patients consulting for headache in the office revealed that 94% of patients had migraine or probable migraine and 25% did not receive a diagnosis of migraine (2). Most headache sufferers depend on self-care with over-the-counter (OTC) remedies rather than on visits to their doctors to deal with their headache problems. Fewer than half of active migraine sufferers consult a physician for headache each year (3).

Less commonly, patients have a secondary headache disorder such as giant cell arteritis, acute sinusitis, or intracranial infection, tumor, and hemorrhage. These patients often have focal neurologic signs or symptoms, systemic disease, and/or abnormal examinations.

of scientific evidence, and side effects. The antiepileptic drug (AED) divalproex sodium is among the drugs receiving the best rating for migraine prevention. Of patients taking divalproex sodium in dosages to achieve levels of 70 to 120 mg/L (500 to 1500), 48% reported headache frequency reduced by 50%, compared to 14% of patients taking placebo (32). Despite this efficacy profile, serious side effects are more likely with divalproex sodium than with other drugs that received this rating. A second AED, topiramate, was approved by the Food and Drug Administration (FDA) for migraine prevention in 2004. In a randomized controlled trial (RCT), topiramate reduced monthly migraine frequency by $\geq$50% at 100 mg/day (33), which is comparable to the effect of divalproex. Patients who are not helped by the standard preventative medications should be referred to a neurologist or other specialist in migraine.

The following general conclusions can be drawn about migraine preventative medication therapy:

- About 50% of treated patients report improvement in their migraine syndrome during initial therapy.
- Most of the improvement consists of a decrease in frequency and severity of headaches and an increased responsiveness to acute/abortive therapies; complete freedom from headaches occurs in only a minority of patients.
- Failure of a drug from one class does not predict response to another from that class or to a drug from another class. Therefore, a sequential trial of different drugs is reasonable.
- Comorbid conditions should be considered when selecting an agent. Patients with asthma or with athletic demands should not be given β-blockers.
- Failure to give an adequate dosage is a common reason for failure of migraine preventative therapy. Each class of drugs listed can be administered in the schedules and dose ranges found elsewhere in this book (antidepressants, Chapter 24; β-blockers and calcium antagonists, Chapter 67; NSAIDs, Chapter 77).
- To facilitate compliance, it is helpful to select agents that can be taken once per day.
- Each patient who chooses preventative therapy should be asked to keep a log in which to record the frequency and severity of headaches and the nature of any associated factors.

Alternative/Complementary Measures to Prevent Migraine. The herbal remedy feverfew has not been shown convincingly superior to placebo (34). Acupuncture has been shown possibly superior to sham treatment (35). Homeopathic remedies have not been shown to be efficacious in the limited clinical trials available for review (36). Magnesium (37) and vitamin B_2 (riboflavin) (38) have been used based in small trials and have low side-effect profiles, but evidence for efficacy is limited. *Petasites hybridus* root (butterbur) was studied in a randomized controlled trial in 245 patients with migraine. After 4 months of treatment the dose of 75 mg b.i.d. was superior to both placebo and to a lower dose and side effects were minimal, primarily burping (39). Chapter 5 contains additional information about nontraditional remedies.

Pregnancy and Migraine

From 50% to 80% of patients with migraine will experience remission of their headaches during pregnancy, especially after the first trimester (40,41). A small number may experience onset of migraine or worsening of headache during pregnancy. Nonpharmacologic measures to reduce or treat attacks in pregnancy include stress reduction, relaxation techniques, cognitive behavioral therapy, and avoidance of triggers. Acetaminophen and prochlorperazine are of low risk and can be used throughout pregnancy for acute attacks. Narcotics can be used judiciously, but should not be used in high doses at term in order to avoid respiratory depression in the newborn. Codeine with acetaminophen is often used. Current recommendations are to avoid ergotamines and triptans during pregnancy (41). Two systematic reviews (42,43) examining the use of sumatriptan in pregnancy have failed to show any impact of sumatriptan on pregnancy outcomes, but there are no RCTs to date, and the evidence is deemed insufficient to rule out a small increase in risk for birth defects. Avoidance of triptans during pregnancy is currently recommended unless the benefit to the mother outweighs the risks to the fetus. Aspirin and NSAIDs are relatively safe, but should be avoided in the last trimester. For women with intractable and frequent migraines, particularly with vomiting, preventative therapy may be necessary. β-Blockers are considered safe, however, intrauterine growth retardation and newborn bradycardia may occur if used in the last trimester. Some of the conventional preventative therapies are absolutely contraindicated, i.e., valproic acid (18).

Patients with Intractable Migraine Headaches

A small number of migraine sufferers have intractable and disabling headaches for which no effective regimen can be found despite trials of all available pharmacologic regimens. For a further assessment and consideration of other therapeutic options, these patients should be referred to a neurologist or headache specialist.

Cluster Headache

Classification and Diagnostic Criteria

Cluster headache is classified separately from migraine because of its distinct clinical characteristics and different therapy. Some of the most common previous names include *Horton headache, histamine headache, Sluder neuralgia*, and *migrainous cranial neuralgia*. Criteria for the diagnosis of cluster headache (4) include the following:

1. The patient has had at least five attacks fulfilling criteria 2 through 4
2. Severe or very severe unilateral orbital, supraorbital, and/or temporal pain lasting 15 to 180 minutes if untreated
3. Headache is accompanied by at least one of the following signs:
   a. Ipsilateral conjunctival injection and/or lacrimation
   b. Ipsilateral nasal congestion and/or rhinorrhea
   c. Ipsilateral eyelid edema
   d. Ipsilateral forehead and facial sweating
   e. Ipsilateral miosis and/or ptosis
   f. A sense of restlessness or agitation
4. Frequency of attacks: from one every other day to eight per day
5. Not attributed to another disorder

Attacks occur in *clusters* extending over days to weeks, giving the syndrome its name. Most cluster episodes last 4 to 6 weeks and are followed by long pain-free intervals. The intervals between episodes range from 3 months to 5 years, and occasionally longer. Most patients have one or two episodes per year; permanent remission occurs in a minority of patients. In a small proportion of patients, the pattern converts from episodic to chronic or from chronic to episodic (44).

The attacks are *stereotyped*. A typical attack begins with sudden unilateral stabbing or burning pain in the eye, orbit, and cheek. The pain is excruciating and *strictly unilateral*. Unlike patients with migraine, patients with cluster headaches are usually agitated and often pace the floor during the attack. The autonomic features are usually prominent, but may be absent. The same side is always involved during a cluster period, and almost always the same side as in previous attacks. If attacks switch sides, the diagnosis of cluster headache should be reconsidered. Attacks may last from 15 minutes to 3 hours (most often 30 to 40 minutes), and they tend to occur at the same time each day, commonly at night after the patient has gone to bed. As alcohol, nitrates, and vasodilator drugs may induce attacks, patients should be asked about concurrent use of alcohol and drugs.

Except during an attack, when the unilateral findings described are present, the physical examination in patients with cluster headache is normal.

Differential Diagnosis

Cluster headache must be distinguished from trigeminal neuralgia (discussed under Facial Pain Syndromes), acute glaucoma (by the presence of miosis, normal tonometry, and no visual impairment), rhinosinusitis (by lack of history of upper respiratory infection, lack of purulent rhinorrhea or sinus tenderness, and negative findings on CT), peripheral dental abscess (by the absence of tenderness on tooth percussion), and atypical facial neuralgia (see Facial Pain Syndromes).

Epidemiology

Cluster headache is much less common than migraine. It occurs predominantly in middle-age men and is associated with smoking cigarettes. The male-to-female gender ratio has been reported as 2.1 to 6.7:1 with an increase in women in more recent studies. Onset usually occurs between the ages of 20 and 50 years of age. Cluster has not been considered an inherited condition; however, studies have revealed a family history in 4% to 7% of patients (45).

Treatment

Acute (Abortive) Treatment

Attacks are short, lasting 15 to 180 minutes and, therefore, oral drug treatment may be ineffective in ameliorating an acute episode (46). When available, *100% oxygen,* administered for approximately 15 minutes at a flow rate of 7 L/minute, may abort an attack. In a double-blind trial, about half of the subjects responded within 10 minutes to 100% oxygen but not to placebo (room air) given through a non-rebreathing face mask (47). The therapeutic effect of oxygen may result from its vasoconstrictor action. Injectable sumatriptan provides the most rapid onset of action of the triptans. *Subcutaneous sumatriptan,* used as described previously for migraine, was shown to decrease the severity of headache in approximately 75% of cluster attacks as compared with placebo (48). A triptan nasal spray (sumatriptan or zolmitriptan) is a reasonable choice in patients who cannot self-inject sumatriptan. *Ergotamine,* administered sublingually, may also be effective abortive therapy for cluster headaches. A sublingual preparation of ergotamine containing 2 mg (Table 87.3) may be given at the beginning of the attack and repeated twice at 30-minute intervals. No more than 6 mg should be taken in a 24-hour period, or more than 10 mg per week.

Preventative Treatment

Cluster attacks consist of frequent, excruciating headache and require preventative medication. These drugs include verapamil, lithium, divalproex sodium, and topiramate in dosages described for migraine prevention. Verapamil is well tolerated and considered by many as first line therapy. Lithium carbonate appears uniquely effective in cluster headache at doses of 300 to 900 mg/day, which results in serum levels lower than usually required for bipolar disease (45). Chapter 24 describes the use of this drug in detail.

Prednisone, beginning at 60 to 80 mg/day and tapering over 2 weeks, may shorten the duration of a cluster episode and decreases the severity and frequency of the attacks (46). A maximal effect occurs within 2 or 3 days after initiation of therapy. (See additional information on prescribing and tapering of corticosteroids in Chapter 81.) Cluster is a very painful condition. If the patient does not respond to initial treatment, prompt referral to a headache specialist is recommended.

Sinus Headache

Chapter 33 discusses diagnosis and management of rhinosinusitis in detail, which is classified as acute, subacute, and chronic. Headache is a minor criterion in the American Academy of Otolaryngology–Head and Neck Surgery diagnostic criteria for rhinosinusitis. The major criteria, of which two or more (or one major plus two minor criteria) must be present to diagnose rhinosinusitis include: purulence in the nasal cavity, facial pain/pressure (must be accompanied by another major criteria), nasal obstruction, fever (acute only), and anosmia/hyposmia (49). Further confounding the problem of diagnosis is the high rate of incidental abnormalities on CT scanning of the sinuses in asymptomatic individuals (50).

The International Classification of Headache Disorders II diagnostic criteria for headache attributed to rhinosinusitis (4) include:

1. Frontal headache accompanied by pain in one or more regions of the face, ears or teeth and fulfilling criteria 3 and 4.
2. Clinical, nasal endoscopic, CT and/or MRI and/or laboratory evidence of acute or acute-on-chronic rhinosinusitis.
3. Headache/facial pain develops simultaneously with onset or acute exacerbation of rhinosinusitis.
4. Headache/facial pain resolves within 7 days after remission or successful treatment of the rhinosinusitis.

Sphenoid sinusitis, although an uncommon cause of sinusitis, is unique in that it is associated with significant morbidity if not diagnosed. Headache is usually unremitting, unchanging in location, and moderately severe, aggravated by activities such as stooping or coughing (51). (See Chapter 33 for further discussion/treatment.)

Chronic sinusitis is often cited as the reason for their headaches by patients requesting repeated courses of antibiotics for episodic headaches. This belief occurs as pain is located over the sinus regions. In a group of self-identified sinus headache patients, 70% met all the criteria for migraine and 28% met all but one criterion and were considered to have migrainous headaches (probable migraine). These patients reported nasal stuffiness (74%), runny nose, and weather change-related onset (45%); all of these symptoms/triggers are associated with migraine (52). Therefore, patients who have recurrent headaches with facial pain and nasal congestion and who do not have purulent nasal discharge or other features of rhinosinusitis most likely have migraine.

Exertional Headache (Cough, Sneeze, Orgasm)

The distinguishing feature of exertional headache is sudden, almost instantaneous, onset of headache related to exertion including coughing, sneezing, straining, bending, running, lifting, and sexual orgasm. It may last from seconds to hours to days. Exertional headaches are usually benign, but may be related to intracranial disease. Exertional headache is associated with Arnold-Chiari malformations in about 40% of cases (4).

Exertional headache must be differentiated from the sentinel headache of *subarachnoid hemorrhage (SAH)*. The latter is usually, but not always, persistent and associated with fever, stiff neck, syncope, and focal neurologic signs. Exertional headaches can be quite severe, but are usually brief and recur with the trigger activity. Distinguishing a first episode of exertional headache from the sentinel headache of SAH is not usually possible on clinical grounds. Brain imaging with CT or MRI scan (see Chapter 86) should be considered at first presentation of exertional headache. For a patient with a negative scan but a clinical presentation strongly suggestive of SAH a lumbar puncture is required.

If imaging findings and lumbar puncture results are normal, the benign nature of the condition should be explained to the patient. The patient may avoid the activity or treat with an NSAID (Table 87.3) prior to the headache-provoking activity.

Sudden-Onset Unprovoked Severe Headache

Sudden-onset, unprovoked severe headache (thunderclap headache) is uncommon but alarming. The headache reaches it peak in seconds. In a large prospective study based in general practice, 37% of patients with this presentation had serious central nervous system disease (25% had subarachnoid hemorrhage). Fewer than 10% of those with subarachnoid hemorrhage had a history of sentinel headaches. In 1 year of followup, none of those with undiagnosed (imaging and lumbar puncture [LP] negative) sudden headache experienced subarachnoid hemorrhage (53). Patients with sudden-onset, severe headache should be referred immediately to a hospital emergency room for prompt evaluation.

Headache Caused by Medications

Headache is a side effect of many drugs, usually occurring in a predictable temporal relationship to ingestion of the substance. It is important to routinely ask about new drugs when evaluating a headache of recent onset. Migraine patients have a more severe immediate headache and reliably develop a delayed migraine type headache with some drugs/substances such as nitric oxide donors (nitroglycerin) or phosphodiesterase (PDE) inhibitors (sildenafil, dipyridamole) (54). Headache may occur with *vasodilator* drugs, but the effect is not predictable.

Management depends on the indications for the drug and severity of the headache. Some patients, if informed of the possibility of headache, choose to take the drug anyway; this is particularly true of administration of nitrates for angina. For the long-acting nitrates, dosage reduction may effectively reduce headache for some patients, whereas alternative antianginal treatment is needed for others (see Chapter 62).

Headache in Acute Febrile Illnesses

Acute febrile illnesses may cause headaches that remit when the illness resolves. A febrile patient in whom the headache is the major symptom and in whom nuchal rigidity or other manifestation of meningeal irritation is present requires a cerebrospinal fluid (CSF) examination to exclude meningitis (see Chapter 86).

Giant Cell Arteritis and Polymyalgia Rheumatica

Giant cell arteritis (GCA) is a chronic vasculitis affecting large and medium arteries throughout the body. Clinical manifestations are usually caused by involvement of the aorta and extracranial branches of the carotid artery, and the most common symptom is headache. GCA has also been called *temporal arteritis (TA),* because temporal headaches and a positive superficial temporal artery biopsy are the findings that are most typical of the disease. The cause of GCA is unknown.

Polymyalgia rheumatica (PMR) is a debilitating condition of older people that manifests with morning stiffness and aching of the neck and proximal musculature. It precedes, accompanies, or follows the onset of GCA in approximately 50% of patients with GCA. In approximately 75% to 80% of patients with PMR in the United States and Europe, GCA does not occur (55). In patients who develop both GCA and PMR, the two syndromes may occur at the same time or GCA may begin months to years after the onset of PMR symptoms. PMR and GCA may be different manifestations of the same vasculitic disorder (56).

Epidemiology

GCA and PMR are almost exclusively diseases of people older than 50 years of age; the average age at onset is 65 to 70 years. Both are uncommon among African Americans, Hispanics, and Asians. They are most common in people of northern European descent, and they are more common in women than in men. It is estimated that the prevalence of GCA is about 200 per 100,000 Americans older than 50 years of age (57). There are no population-based studies of frequency of PMR in the United States; however, it is estimated that the incidence and prevalence rates for PMR are about two or three times higher than the rates for GCA.

TABLE 87.5 Clinical Features of Giant Cell Arteritis

Common Features	%[a]	Less Common but Characteristic Features
Headache	85	Raynaud phenomenon of limbs or tongue
Temporal artery tenderness	70	Tender scalp nodules
Jaw claudication	65	Thick, tender occipital arteries
Lingual, limb, or swallowing claudication	20	Necrotic lesions of scalp, tongue
Brachiocephalic bruits	50	Carotid artery tenderness
Thickened or nodular temporal artery	45	Swelling of the hands
Pulseless temporal artery	40	Taste, smell disturbances
Visual symptoms	40	Distended, beaded retinal veins
Fixed blindness, partial or complete	15	Diminished or absent radial artery pulses
Polymyalgia rheumatica	50	Mononeuropathy (median, peroneal, cervical root)
Weight loss >6 kg	40	
Erythrocyte sedimentation rate		
>50 mm per h	95	
>100 mm per h	60	
Fever (>37.7°C)	20	
Abnormal liver function	50	
Anemia (hematocrit <35%)	50	

TA, temporal arteritis.
[a]Approximate percentage of patients with common feature at initial evaluation.
From Raskin NH, Appenzeller O. Headache. Philadelphia: WB Saunders, 1988.

Manifestations

GCA presents with nonspecific symptoms of fever, anorexia, weight loss, myalgias, and headache. The headache is often temporal; however, it can be frontal, occipital, parietal, or holocephalic. It may be made worse by hair brushing, resting the head on a pillow, or exposure to cold. Table 87.5 lists the most important factors suggesting the diagnosis of GCA. It is important to inquire specifically about pain (claudication) associated with chewing, swallowing, and arm or tongue motion, because these symptoms are highly suggestive of GCA. The combination of one or more of the findings listed in Table 87.5 in a patient older than 50 years of age with a new headache is sufficient to suspect GCA.

PMR is insidious in onset. The chief complaints are aching and stiffness of the shoulder girdle and, less commonly, of the thigh muscles. These symptoms can make it particularly hard for the patient to get up in the morning. Associated low-grade fever, weight loss, and anorexia are common. On physical examination, there may be some tenderness of the shoulder and neck muscles, but there is no significant loss of muscle strength.

Diagnosis

If GCA or PMR is suspected, the erythrocyte sedimentation rate (ESR) measured by the Westergren method is the most useful screening test. The majority of patients have a markedly elevated ESR (often 100 mL/hr or greater). Because the upper limit of normal for people older than 60 years of age may be as high as 40 mL/hr, an ESR of 40 to 60 mL/hr is less informative than a very high ESR. Unlike other chronic inflammatory diseases, GCA and PMR are not associated with autoantibody production or abnormalities in complement factors or immunoglobulin levels.

Definitive diagnosis of GCA is made with a superficial temporal arteritis (TA) biopsy. Examination of serial sections of a long specimen is essential as the typical histologic changes (inflammatory cells, edema, giant cells) are patchy in distribution. In addition to a positive TA biopsy, the American College of Rheumatology has designated four other features that support the diagnosis of GCA: onset after 50 years of age, new localized headache, Westergren ESR greater than 50 mL/hr, and TA tenderness or decreased TA pulse. The presence of three of the five features is considered sufficient evidence to make the clinical diagnosis of GCA (58). One retrospective study reported the feature most predictive of a diagnostic TA biopsy was the presence of either visual symptoms, a TA that is abnormal on examination, or constitutional symptoms (59).

> *Patient Experience.* TA biopsy can be done in an ambulatory surgery facility by a general surgeon, ophthalmologist, vascular surgeon, plastic surgeon, or neurosurgeon. The local scalp hair is shaved, the skin is anesthetized, and a large segment of artery (>2 cm) is excised. The procedure requires about one-half hour and there are no serious sequelae.

The *diagnosis of PMR* is based on the combination of the typical symptoms, a high ESR, and exclusion of other explanations for the patient's symptoms. Normocytic anemia is common. Muscle enzyme levels, electromyography, and muscle histology are all normal. If a patient with typical PMR has manifestations suggesting GCA (Table 87.5), TA biopsy is indicated, because the recommended dosages of corticosteroids for the two conditions are different.

Course and Treatment

Treatment recommendations are based on comparisons of untreated patients with patients treated with corticosteroids. The most serious complication of GCA is unilateral or bilateral vision loss caused by ischemic optic neuropathy. Treatment with corticosteroids appears to prevent vision loss which occurs in 20% to 30% of untreated patients. Although the symptoms of GCA and PMR may respond to aspirin and other NSAIDs, these agents have not been shown to prevent the progressive vasculitis in GCA that can lead to vision loss.

Giant Cell Arteritis

If the diagnosis of GCA is suspected, corticosteroid treatment should be initiated immediately and the TA biopsy should be obtained within 3 to 4 days. If the patient has vision loss that is thought to be from GCA, it is recommended that treatment with steroids should be initiated intravenously (60). The initial oral treatment is prednisone (40 to 60 mg once per day) for 4 to 6 weeks. Within 1 to 3 days, symptoms usually remit entirely and there is a significant decrease in the ESR. After 2 to 3 weeks, the prednisone should be slowly tapered until a dosage of 7.5 to 10 mg daily has been reached (56). Further tapering and duration of treatment depend on the clinical response and ESR. A 2-year course of prednisone is usually recommended. Some authors, who have documented GCA relapse after discontinuation of treatment, recommend lifelong maintenance treatment with low-dose prednisone, especially for patients who have no intolerable side effects from treatment (61). One controlled trial found that combined prednisone and methotrexate treatment for 2 years reduced the frequency of relapse after discontinuation when compared to standard prednisone-only treatment (62).

Polymyalgia Rheumatica

Treatment is begun with prednisone 10 to 20 mg daily, tapered to a daily maintenance dosage of 5 to 7.5 mg after several weeks. Treatment is continued for approximately 2 years, with gradual discontinuation at the end of that time. The symptoms of PMR, as well as the ESR, respond to this regimen dramatically, often within the first 24 hours. PMR recurs in some patients, within months to years after discontinuing prednisone; these patients usually respond to a second course of treatment.

Idiopathic Intracranial Hypertension (Pseudotumor Cerebri)

Idiopathic intracranial hypertension (IIH) is a condition of unknown cause characterized by the following: signs and symptoms of increased intracranial pressure (headache, papilledema, nausea, vomiting, and transient visual obscurations); elevated CSF pressure >25 cm of water;

normal CSF analysis; and the *absence* of a mass lesion, hydrocephalus, or venous sinus thrombosis on brain imaging (63). This condition has had several names including pseudotumor and benign increased intracranial pressure. The signs and symptoms are due to increased intracranial pressure (ICP). Focal neurologic signs are absent with the exception of sixth nerve palsy, which produces diplopia.

Several factors have been associated with IIH including obesity, menstrual irregularity, steroid therapy or withdrawal, oral contraceptives, and a variety of medications and substances, including tetracycline, and vitamin A.

Manifestations

This is an uncommon condition with an incidence of 3.5 per 100,000 in women 15 to 44 years old and 19.3 per 100,000 in women 20 to 44 years old who are *obese*. It is nine times more frequent in women than men although before puberty boys and girls are equally affected (63). The typical patient is an obese young woman who develops progressively more severe headaches, nausea, vomiting, dizziness, and transiently blurred vision. Vision loss lasting seconds at a time can be monocular or binocular and is thought to be because of disc edema. Pulsatile tinnitus described as "hearing my heartbeat," or whooshing sounds is present in 60% of patients (64). The onset may be abrupt or gradual. Headache is usually bilateral, retroocular, constant, and often more severe in the morning, aggravated by coughing, straining, or changing position, and by eye movement. The diagnosis is suggested strongly by daily headache in an obese woman with transient visual obscurations, pulsatile tinnitus, and papilledema without focal neurologic signs. Visual fields may be constricted and the blind spot enlarged. If untreated, vision loss may result.

Differential Diagnosis

The diagnosis of IIH is always one of exclusion. Important considerations in the *differential diagnosis* are intracranial mass, hydrocephalus, and cerebral venous sinus thrombosis. To exclude an intracranial mass or hydrocephalus, a contrast brain MRI scan (see Chapter 86) should be obtained. For women at increased risk of cerebral venous thrombosis (taking oral contraceptives, are postpartum, or, have hypercoagulopathy), brain magnetic resonance venography (MRV) should also be obtained. In IIH, the MRI/MRV is normal. After a negative MRI, a lumbar puncture should be performed (see Chapter 86). The lumbar puncture is *essential* in the diagnosis. The opening pressure is high (250 mm H_2O or more); the analysis of the fluid is normal (include cell count, glucose, protein, cytology, fungal and tuberculosis cultures, and some recommend bacterial cultures) (63). In a very obese woman with a history of amenorrhea for many months, it is also important to consider pregnancy-induced hypertension (toxemia), which is ruled out by a negative pregnancy test.

Treatment and Course

With treatment most patients recover completely from IIH within several weeks or months; however, some patients require ongoing therapy to control headaches and prevent vision loss. Referral to a neurologist and ophthalmologist is almost always necessary as the treatment is specialized and visual fields will need to be formally monitored. In obese patients, weight reduction is recommended.

The goal of therapy is to relieve symptoms by reducing intracranial pressure. At the time of the diagnostic lumbar puncture, enough fluid can be removed to reduce the closing pressure to normal, usually about 25 to 35 mL of fluid. The carbonic anhydrase inhibitor, acetazolamide (500-mg sustained-release capsule up to effect or side effects) has been the traditional therapy as CSF production is believed to be directly inhibited. If the patient remains asymptomatic and the papilledema resolves, acetazolamide can be tapered and discontinued. The use of corticosteroids to treat IIH is controversial. For patients with continued headache, visual impairment, and papilledema, surgical procedures (CSF shunting via a lumboperitoneal shunt or surgical incision of the optic nerve sheath) are sometimes necessary (63). Treatment of these patients is difficult and requires the consultation of neurologists, ophthalmologists, and neurosurgeons experienced in handling this disorder.

Posttraumatic (Postconcussive) Headache

Manifestations

Headache is a common symptom after head and neck trauma and usually occurs within a close temporal relationship to the injury. A number of symptoms, collectively termed the *postconcussion syndrome (PCS)*, occur after traumatic brain injury (TBI): headache, vertigo (often positional; see Chapter 89), light-headedness or giddiness, poor concentration and memory, lack of energy, irritability, anxiety, light and sound sensitivity, change in taste or smell, and insomnia (65). When no structural injury has occurred, the causal mechanism responsible for these symptoms remains unknown.

Headache is common and, typically begins within 24 hours as a dull, constant ache that may wax and wane throughout the day or become concentrated in one location. It may be worsened by sneezing, coughing, stooping, straining, or rapid head motions and changes in body position. Typically, postconcussive symptoms resolve over weeks or months, however, some patients remain symptomatic at 1 year. When persistent, headache may take on migrainous features.

Differential Diagnosis

Subdural Hematoma and Other Expanding Mass Lesions

Headache and nonspecific complaints can occur with chronic subdural hematomas and other slowly expanding mass lesions. Brain imaging either with CT or MRI (see Chapter 86) can be used to evaluate persistent headache after trauma.

Carotid or Vertebral Artery Dissection

Headache occurs on the side of the dissection. Carotid dissections are associated with partial Horner syndrome (miosis, ptosis). Both carotid and vertebral dissections may be accompanied by delayed focal cerebral ischemic symptoms (stroke or TIA, see Chapter 91).

Pre-existing Migraine or Tension Headaches

Head trauma may worsen a pre-existing primary headache disorder such as migraine or tension-type headache.

Objective Tests

A literature search for guidelines for imaging in mild TBI/concussion did not produce guidelines for decision making for patients presenting to the office. Emergency room guidelines for imaging in mild TBI (66) advise *against* skull film radiographs, and do not recommend which patients *should* have a noncontrast CT scan. The guidelines advised that CT is *not indicated in patients who do not have headache.* It can therefore be reasonably recommended to obtain noncontrast CT in patients with mild TBI and headache. Guidelines from the American Academy of Neurology in mild TBI (PCS) because of sports injury recommend brain CT or MRI when headache or other symptoms persist for longer than 7 days or if the symptoms worsen (67). In the absence of other guidelines, it would be reasonable to extrapolate this recommendation to posttraumatic headache due to other injuries.

Treatment

Most patients with posttraumatic headaches recover without specific treatment. There are no randomized controlled trials for posttraumatic headache treatment. Agents used to treat tension-type headache or migraine can reasonably be tried (Table 87.4).

Low Cerebrospinal Fluid Pressure Headache

Low-pressure headache from persistent leakage of CSF occurs most commonly after lumbar puncture. It may occur spontaneously or after trauma and is believed to result from dural tears (68). The headache is markedly positional, brought on by sitting or standing, and relieved almost entirely by lying down. The headache is usually generalized and nausea and dizziness are common nonspecific accompaniments. There are no focal neurologic symptoms or signs, and the patient is afebrile. Brain imaging with MRI may be normal, or positive for diffuse meningeal enhancement, descent of the cerebellar tonsils, decrease in basal cisterns, and for hygromas or chronic subdural hematomas.

The majority of post–lumbar puncture and posttraumatic CSF leaks close spontaneously. Simple medical management includes bedrest, hydration, and ingestion of caffeine. Patients with persistent low pressure headaches can be referred to an anesthesiologist for epidural blood patch. Because of the risk of meningitis, any patient with a suspected persistent CSF leak should be referred to a neurologist or neurosurgeon for further evaluation.

Characteristics of Headache Caused by a Mass Lesion

For both the headache sufferer and the physician, concern about the possibility of a brain tumor often dominates the situation. Important clues to the presence of an intracranial mass lesion are: focal neurologic signs/symptoms, change in mental status, or a seizure. A new headache disorder in a patient older than 50 years of age is suggestive of a secondary headache disorder.

A number of nonspecific features may be clues to the presence of an intracranial mass lesion:

- Although the headache associated with a mass lesion can initially be intermittent, mild, and responsive to mild analgesics, typically it becomes more continuous and less responsive to analgesics.
- The headache awakens the patient from sleep or is present on awakening every day, decreasing after the patient has been up for several hours.
- Coughing, sneezing, and straining aggravate the headache (by transiently increasing intracranial pressure and accentuating the stretching of pain-sensitive structures).
- Nausea and vomiting are prominent features of posterior fossa masses.

When one or more of these historical features are present or focal neurologic signs are found on examination, the patient should be evaluated with brain MRI with contrast (see Chapter 86). If MRI is positive for intracranial disease, the patient should be referred to a neurologist or neurosurgeon for definitive care.

FACIAL PAIN SYNDROMES

Trigeminal Neuralgia (Tic Douloureux)

Manifestations

Trigeminal neuralgia is an idiopathic disorder seen most commonly in patients older than 40 years of age, most of them elderly. It has several distinguishing features: The pain occurs in a branch of the trigeminal nerve, is *severe*, shooting, electric-like, and lasts a *few seconds* to a minute. The patient's face usually contorts with the pain, and the patient may find it impossible to control his/her emotional response. Between attacks the patient is usually pain free, although some patients have a dull ache in the affected area. The interval between paroxysms is usually at least 2 or 3 minutes. The frequency of paroxysms is highly variable; some patients have hundreds each day.

The pain is usually felt in the structures innervated by the second and third divisions of the trigeminal nerve (lips, gums, cheek, chin). *The pain is unilateral, does not cross the midline, and never involves both sides of the face simultaneously*. The patient often can identify trigger points on the face or in the mouth that, when touched (even by contact with a gust of cold air) precipitate pain (69).

Some patients with trigeminal neuralgia have areas of slightly decreased sensation that may be difficult to distinguish from normal; however, there is no objective decrease in sensation.

Other, less common syndromes with paroxysms of lancinating pain include glossopharyngeal neuralgia (pharynx pain) and occipital neuralgia (posterior head pain).

Differential Diagnosis

A syndrome identical or similar to idiopathic trigeminal neuralgia, i.e., secondary trigeminal neuralgia, can be produced by a number of conditions such as multiple sclerosis, acoustic or trigeminal neuroma, aneurysm, meningioma, brainstem infarction or syrinx, and arterial compression. These conditions should be considered, particularly if the patient is younger than 40 years of age, the pain is in the upper division of the trigeminal nerve (forehead and eye), pain is bilateral, or there are abnormalities on neurologic examination.

Treatment

In a patient with a typical clinical presentation and a normal neurologic examination, medical therapy can be initiated without further workup. Patients are in excruciating pain and should be evaluated and treated promptly. If medical therapy is ineffective, or if there are any atypical features, referral to a neurologist is appropriate.

Carbamazepine, widely recognized as the best initial treatment, is usually started at a low dose (100 mg) twice daily. Increases of 100 to 200 mg a day can be made every 3 days until pain relief is obtained. The usual daily dosage is between 400 to 800 mg. Some patients need higher (1500 mg/day) dosages; in these cases, blood levels may be necessary to monitor compliance (69). Most patients can expect excellent to satisfactory relief with carbamazepine. The pharmacokinetics of carbamazepine are complex because of autoinduction with subsequent change in the half life which is complete at 3 to 5 weeks. This may account for apparent loss of efficacy, which can be reversed with an increase in dosage or an increase in dosing frequency. Side effects of the drug include nausea, vomiting, ataxia, vertigo, and transient leukopenia. The most serious side effects are persistent leukopenia and aplastic anemia. A complete blood count and liver function tests are recommended at baseline and at periodic intervals dependent on the clinical course. Trigeminal neuralgia can remit spontaneously. Patients who remain pain free can have their medication slowly tapered periodically to determine if they are in remission

If the patient fails to improve with carbamazepine or fails to tolerate the drug, the muscle relaxant *baclofen* in doses of 30 to 80 mg/day can be tried. A patient whose symptoms cannot be controlled with these medications should be referred for neurologic consultation.

Atypical Facial Pain

Atypical facial pain is a collective term for a variety of painful facial symptoms that do not meet the diagnostic criteria for a recognized entity. These patients should be referred for neurologic consultation to be evaluated for more obscure syndromes.

Temporomandibular Joint Syndrome

Some patients complaining of headache have pain brought on by motion of the jaw and tenderness of the temporomandibular joint. Chapter 112 describes the epidemiology, course, and management of this syndrome.

SPECIFIC REFERENCES*

1. Office visits to internists: National Ambulatory Medical Care Survey, United States, 1975. Advance Data, No. 16, February 7, 1978.
2. Tepper SJ, Dahlof CG, Dowson A, et al. Prevalence and diagnosis of migraine in patients consulting their physician with a complaint of headache: data from the landmark study. Headache 2004;44:856.
3. Lipton RB, Stewart WF, Simon D. Medical consultation for migraine: results from the American Migraine Study. Headache 1998; 38:87.
4. Headache Classification Committee of the International Headache Society. The International Classification of Headache Disorders, 2nd ed. Cephalalgia 2004; 24:1.
5. Frishberg BM, Rosenberg JH, Matchar DB, et al. Evidence-based guidelines in the primary care setting: neuroimaging in patients with nonacute headache. 2001 Am Acad Neurol. Available at: www.aan.com.
6. Scher AL, Stewart WF, Liberman J, et al. Prevalence of frequent headache in a population sample. Headache 1998,38:497.
7. Young WB. Drug-induced headache. Neurolog Clin 2004;22:173.
8. Solomon S, Newman LC. Episodic tension-type headache. In: Silberstein SD, Lipton RB, Dalessio DJ, eds. Wolff's headache and other head pain. 7th ed. New York: Oxford University Press, 2001.

*Bold numerals denote published controlled clinical trials, meta-analyses, or consensus-based recommendations.

9. Tomkins GE, Jackson JL, O'Malley PG, et al. Treatment of chronic headache with antidepressants: a meta-analysis. Am J Med 2001;111:54.

10. Holroyd KA, O'Donnell FJ, Stensland M, et al. Management of chronic tension-type headache with tricyclic antidepressant medication, stress management therapy, and their combination: a randomized controlled trial. JAMA 2001;285: 2208.

11. Launer LJ, Terwindt GM, Ferrari MD. The prevalence and characteristics of migraine in a population-based cohort: the GEM study. Neurology 1999;53:537.

12. Goadsby PJ, Lipton RB, Ferrari MD. Migraine—current understanding and treatment. N Engl J Med 2002;346:257.

13. Edvinsson L. Correlation between CGRP and migraine attacks. Cephalalgia 2005;25:163.

14. Goadsby P. Pathophysiology of headache. In: Silberstein SD, Lipton RB, Dalessio DJ, eds. Wolff's headache and other head pain. 7th ed. New York: Oxford University Press, 2001.

15. Lipton RB, Stewart WF, Diamond S, et al. Prevalence and burden of migraine in the United States: Data from the American Migraine Study II. Headache 2001;41:7.

16. Silberstein SD, Lipton RB, Dalessio DJ. Overview, diagnosis, and classification of headache. In: Silberstein SD, Lipton RB, Dalessio DJ, eds. Wolff's headache and other head pain. 7th ed. New York: Oxford University Press, 2001.

17. Radat F, Swendsen J. Psychiatric comorbidity in migraine: a review. Cephalalgia 2005;25:165.

18. Johnson CJ. Headache in women. Primary care clinics in office practice 2004;31:417.

19. Silberstein SD. Practice parameter: evidence-based guidelines for migraine headache (an evidence based review). A report of the Quality Standards Subcommittee of the American Academy of Neurology. Neurology 2000;55:754.

20. Snow V, Weiss K, Wall EM, Mottur-Pilson C. Pharmacologic management of acute attacks of migraine and prevention of migraine headaches. Ann Intern Med 2002;137:840.

21. Silberstein SD, Saper JR, Freitage FG. Migraine: diagnosis and treatment In: Silberstein SD, Lipton RB, Dalessio DJ, eds. Wolff's headache and other head pain. 7th edition. New York: Oxford University Press, 2001.

22. Mathew NT, Loder EW. Evaluating the triptans. Am J Med 2005;118:285.

23. Pfaffenrath VG, Cunin G, Sjonell G, et al. Efficacy and safety of sumatriptan tablets (25 mg, 50 mg, and 100 mg) in the acute treatment of migraine: defining the optimum doses of oral sumatriptan. Headache 1998;38: 184.

24. Ryan RA, Elkind CC, Baker, et al. Sumatriptan nasal spray for the acute treatment of migraine: results of two clinical studies. Neurology 1997;49:1225.

25. Welch KMA. Drug therapy of migraine. N Engl J Med 1993;329:1476.

26. Ferrari MD, Roon KI, Lipton RB, et al. Oral triptans in acute migraine treatment: a meta-analysis of 53 trials. Lancet 2001;358:1668.

27. Lipton RB, Stewart WF, Cady R, et al. Sumatriptan for the range of headaches in migraine sufferers: results of the spectrum study. Headache 2000;40:783.

28. Dodick D, Lipton RB, Martin V, et al. Consensus statement: cardiovascular safety profile of triptans (5-HT 1B/D agonists) in the acute treatment of migraine. Headache 2004;44:414.

29. Hall GC, Brown MM, Mo J, et al. Triptans in migraine: the risk of stroke, cardiovascular disease, and death in practice. Neurology 2004: 62;563.

30. Colman I, Brown MD, Innes GD, et al. Parenteral dihydroergotamine for acute migraine headache: a systematic review of the literature. Ann Emerg Med 2005;45:393.

31. Colman I, Brown MD, Innes GD, et. al. Parenteral metoclopramide for acute migraine: meta-analysis of randomised controlled trials. BMJ 2004;329:1369.

32. Mathew NT, Saper JR, Silberstein SD, et al. Migraine prophylaxis with divalproex. Arch Neurol 1995;52:281.

33. Silberstein SD, Neto W, Schmitt J, et al. Topiramate in Migraine Prevention. Arch Neurol. 2004;61:490.

34. Pittler MH. Feverfew for preventing migraine. Cochrane Database Syst Rev 2004;1:CD002286.

35. Melchart D, Linde K, Fischer P, et al. Acupuncture for idiopathic headache. Cochrane Database Syst Rev 2001;1:CD001218.

36. Ernst E. Homeopathic prophylaxis of headaches and migraine? A systematic review. J Pain Symptom Manage 1999;118:353.

37. Pfaffenrath V, Wessely P, Meyer C, et al. Magnesium in the prophylaxis of migraine: a double-blind, placebo-controlled study. Cephalalgia 1996;16:436.

38. Schoenen J, Jacquy J, Lenaerts M. Effectiveness of high-dose riboflavin in migraine prophylaxis. Neurology 1998;50:466.

39. Lipton RB, Gobel H, Einhaupl KM, et al. *Petasites hybridus* root (butterbur) is an effective preventive treatment for migraine. Neurology 2004;63:2240.

40. Maggioni F, Alessi C, Maggino T, et al. Headache during pregnancy. Cephalalgia 1997;17:765.

41. Aube M. Migraine in pregnancy. Neurology 1999;53:S26.

42. Loder E. Safety of sumatriptan in pregnancy: a review of the data so far. CNS Drugs 2003;17:1.

43. Hilaire ML, Cross LB, Eicher SF. Treatment of migraine headaches with sumatriptan in pregnancy. Ann Pharmacother 2004;38:1726.

44. Pearce JM. Natural history of cluster headache. Headache 1993;33:253.

45. Dodick DW, Campbell JK. Cluster headache: diagnosis, management, and treatment. In: Silberstein SD, Lipton RB, Dalessio DJ eds. Wolff's headache and other head pain. 7th ed. New York: Oxford University Press, 2001.

46. Dodick DW, Capobianco DJ. Treatment and management of cluster headache. Curr Pain Headache Rep 2001;5:83.

47. Fogan L. Treatment of cluster headache. Arch Neurol 1985;42:362.

48. Sumatriptan Cluster Headache Study Group. Treatment of acute cluster headache with sumatriptan. N Engl J Med 1991;325:322.

49. Lanza DC, Kennedy DW. Adult rhinosinusitis defined. Otolaryngol head neck surg 1997; 117:S1.

50. Bhattacharyya N. Test-retest reliability of computed tomography in the assessment of chronic rhinosinusitis. Laryngoscope 1999;109: 1055.

51. Silberstein SD. Headaches due to nasal and paranasal sinus disease. Neurol Clin N Am 2004; 22:1.

52. Cady RK, Schreiber CP. Sinus headache or migraine? Considerations in making a differential diagnosis. Neurology 2002;58:S10.

53. Linn FH, Mijdicks EF, Graaf Y, et al. Prospective study of sentinel headache in aneurysmal subarachnoid haemorrhage. Lancet 1994;344:590.

54. Young WB. Drug-induced headache. Neurol Clin N Am 2004;22:173.

55. Hunder GG, Allen GL. Giant cell arteritis: a review. Bull Rheum Dis 1978–1979;29:980.

56. Nordborg E, Nordborg C. Giant cell arteritis: strategies in diagnosis and treatment. Curr Opin Rheumatol 2004;16:25.

57. Lawrence RC, Helmick CG, Arnett FC, et al. Estimates of the prevalence of arthritis and selected musculoskeletal disorders in the United States. Arthritis Rheum 1998;41:778.

58. Hunder CG, Bloch DA, Michel BA, et al. The American College of Rheumatology 1990 criteria for the classification of giant cell arteritis. Arthritis Rheum 1990;33:1122.

59. Gonzalez-Gay MA, Garcia-Porrua C, Llorca J, et al. Biopsy-negative giant cell arteritis: clinical spectrum and predictive factors for positive temporal artery biopsy. Semin Arthritis Rheum 2001;30:249.

60. Neff AG, Greifenstein EM. Giant cell arteritis update. Semin Ophthalmol 1999;14:109.

61. Andersson R, Malmvall BE.Bengtsson BA. Long-term cortico-steroid treatment in giant cell arteritis. Acta Med Scand 1986;220:465.

62. Jover JA, Hernandez-Garcia C, Morado IC, et al. Combined treatment of giant-cell arteritis with methotrexate and prednisone: a randomized, double-blind, placebo-controlled trial. Ann Intern Med 2001;134:106.

63. Friedman DI. Pseudotumor cerebri. Neurol Clin N Am 2004;22:99.

64. Giuseffi V, Wall M, Spiegel PZ, et al. Symptoms and disease associations in idiopathic intracranial hypertension (pseudotumor cerebri): a case-control study. Neurology 1991; 41:239.

65. Evans RW. Post-traumatic headaches. Neurol Clin N Am 2004;22:237.

66. Jagoda AS, Cantrill SV, Wears RL. Clinical policy: neuroimaging and decision making in adult mild traumatic brain injury in the acute setting. Ann of Emerg Med 2002;40:231.

67. Practice Parameter: The management of concussion in sports. Neurology 1997; 48:581.

68. Mokri B. Low cerebrospinal fluid pressure syndromes. Neurol Clin N Am 2004;22:55.

69. Rozen TD. Trigeminal neuralgia and glossopharyngeal neuralgia. Neurol Clin N Am 2004;22:185.

For annotated ***General References*** *and resources related to this chapter, visit www.hopkinsbayview.org/PAMreferences.*

Chapter 88

Seizure Disorders

Peter W. Kaplan

About 2 million people in the United States may have epilepsy. An even larger number seek medical advice for treatment of seizures, generating approximately 5% of visits to physicians and 20% of visits to neurologists (1). This chapter addresses the basic principles that should guide the diagnosis and management of seizures in office practice.

DEFINITION AND CLASSIFICATION OF EPILEPTIC SEIZURES

Any paroxysmal disturbance in consciousness, behavior, or motor activity may be called a spell, fit, or seizure, but this chapter addresses primarily *epileptic seizures.* These may be defined as the clinical manifestations of an abnormal, usually brief, excessive, or hypersynchronous neuronal discharge in the cerebral cortex or deep limbic structures. A seizure has a definite start and finish. Seizures are associated with characteristic electrical abnormalities of the brain. Most patients are normal, and their electroencephalograms (EEGs) are often normal, between seizures (the interictal period).

The term *epilepsy* refers to a chronic neurologic condition that causes spontaneous, recurrent seizures. Therefore, single or even multiple seizures arising during transient systemic insult such as fever, infection, toxic causes (e.g., alcohol), or metabolic disturbances should not be labeled as epilepsy and are called *reactive seizures.*

The basic mechanisms underlying epileptic seizures are still uncertain, although much is known about predisposing conditions. The most widely accepted classification is based on behavioral and EEG aspects (Table 88.1) (2).

CLINICAL MANIFESTATIONS OF SEIZURE TYPES

The clinical manifestations of seizures vary according to the degree of maturity of the nervous system, the initial seizure focus, and the pattern of ictal spread. A seizure focus in the motor cortex produces jerking of the corresponding contralateral parts of the body; seizures in sensory regions result in abnormal sensations; and seizures in areas of higher cortical function may produce complex cognitive and behavioral manifestations (Fig. 88.1). Certain types of seizures manifest with sudden changes in vigilance or consciousness rather than with focal motor or sensory signs or symptoms.

Generalized Tonic–Clonic Seizures (Grand Mal)

Generalized tonic–clonic seizures (GTCSs) occur when ictal discharges involve most of the cortex. They may arise

TABLE 88.1 Classification of the Epilepsies

Primary Generalized Epilepsy (Idiopathic Generalized Epilepsy)
Tonic–clonic (grand mal) (GTC)
Absence (petit mal)
Myoclonic
Atonic, others
Secondarily Generalized Seizures
Partial (Focal) Epilepsy
With elementary symptomatology
Focal motor
Focal sensory
Vegetative
Psychic
Mixed
With complex symptomatology
Complex partial (psychomotor) (CPS)
Unclassifiable Seizures

From Dreifuss FE. Proposal for revised clinical and electroencephalographic classification of epileptic seizures. Epilepsia 1981;22:489.

in the context of primary, *idiopathic generalized (genetic) epilepsies*, in which seizure activity appears synchronously over both hemispheres, or they may result from *secondarily generalized seizure* discharges arising from a unilateral focus. GTCSs may be called *major motor seizures,* although the now-disused term *grand mal* referred to bilateral generalization of seizure activity.

Idiopathic generalized epilepsies may appear at any age, although onset is rare after 35 years of age. Frequency may range from two seizures in an entire lifetime to several seizures a day. Symptomatic epilepsies giving rise to focal and secondarily generalized tonic–clonic seizures may occur throughout life, caused by developmental abnormalities, perinatal insults, infection and head trauma, and strokes, particularly in the elderly.

GTCSs typically begin with an arrest of activity and sudden loss of consciousness, followed by trembling, tonic extension of the arms and legs, and then clonic rhythmic but progressively slower limb jerking, followed by flaccidity, stupor, and labored, deep breathing. Seizures usually last less than 2 minutes and are followed by lethargy lasting minutes to hours. During the seizures, consciousness is always lost, so a history of the utterance of meaningful speech, the presence of purposeful eye movements, or a memory of the seizure itself excludes the diagnosis. Although malaise may precede GTCSs, a definite sensory, autonomic, psychic, or motor prelude suggests a *focal onset with subsequent generalization* (secondarily generalized tonic–clonic seizures). Tonic–clonic seizures may be accompanied by incontinence, sweating, tachycardia, elevated blood pressure, minor cardiac arrhythmias, and biting of the lip, cheek, and lateral aspect rather than the tip of the tongue.

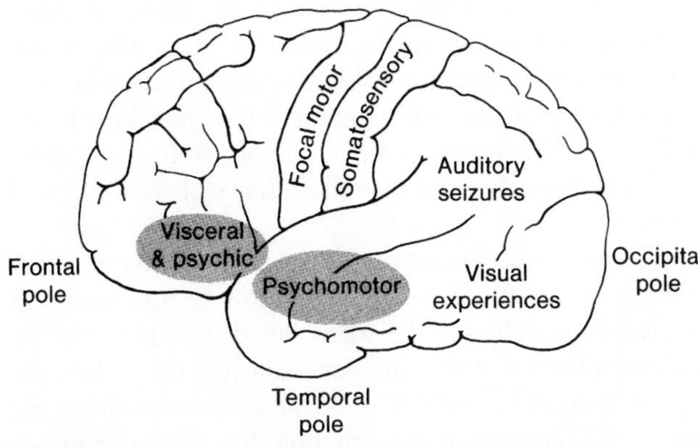

FIGURE 88.1. Relationship of local seizure phenomena to brain topography.

The EEG that is typical in idiopathic generalized epilepsies shows a pattern of bilateral synchronous spike-and-wave discharges, whereas patients with generalized seizures that arise from a lateralized focus may show focal epileptiform discharges over the affected cortical zone.

Generalized Absence Seizures (Petit Mal)

Typical absence seizures are also generalized seizures; they occur in *childhood absence epilepsy* (CAE), a type of idiopathic generalized epilepsy (3). Absence seizures may also occur in Lennox–Gastaut syndrome and in juvenile myoclonic epilepsy. Childhood absence epilepsy constitutes approximately 5% of childhood epilepsy. The onset is usually between 4 and 12 years of age. Most affected children (75%) have absence seizures that remit by the age of 20 years, although about half (especially those with atypical absence) may later develop tonic–clonic seizures.

Because of the previous classification of generalized seizures into "petit mal" and "grand mal" types, some patients incorrectly believe that these two entities represent different severities of the same seizure type (although both can occur with idiopathic generalized epilepsy). There is often confusion also between the staring component of absence seizures and the initial staring phase of partial complex seizures (see Complex Partial Seizures). Finally, the term "petit mal" was often incorrectly used by patients to refer to partial seizures with a motor component or to minor motor seizures. Such confusions in classification may lead to incorrect diagnosis, prognosis, and antiepileptic drug (AED) therapy.

Typical absence seizures in childhood absence epilepsy, consisting of lapses of vigilance or awareness, usually last about 3 to 20 seconds. There is no tonic–clonic phase or loss of posture. Slight rhythmic twitching of the mouth and periorbital musculature or upgaze may be observed. With atypical absence seizures, duration may be prolonged, leading to confusion with complex partial seizures arising from the temporal or other lobes. In childhood absence epilepsy, there is a rapid recovery of awareness after an absence seizure, but amnesia for events occurring during the seizure persists. Absence seizures typically occur up to 100 times per day. Children who have such frequent seizures may be labeled as being inattentive, daydreamers, or slow learners until the correct diagnosis is made.

Both clinical and EEG findings should be used to secure a diagnosis of childhood absence epilepsy; neither alone is diagnostic. The EEG during an absence seizure shows a characteristic bilateral synchronous three-per-second spike-and-wave pattern; between seizures, the EEG may be normal, but brief 3-second bursts usually persist in the absence of AED therapy. Often, hyperventilation or stimulation with regularly flashing lights (intermittent photic stimulation) induces an absence seizure. Three-per-second spike-and-wave patterns on EEG may be seen in asymptomatic close relatives of patients with childhood absence epilepsy as well as other seizure types (e.g., tonic–clonic seizures).

Myoclonus and Myoclonic Seizures

Myoclonus is the predominantly synchronous, involuntary, nonrhythmic jerking of limbs, trunk, or head. Epileptic myoclonus arises from paroxysmal discharges of the central nervous system (CNS) above the brainstem. Conditions in which nonepileptic myoclonus (segmental myoclonus) may occur are conditions affecting the brainstem and the spinal cord.

Myoclonic seizures are most often seen after severe, diffuse cortical injury resulting from cerebral ischemia and anoxia; these seizures are difficult to suppress and carry a poor prognosis. When myoclonic seizures arise from hypoglycemia, severe renal or hepatic failure, or drug toxicity, they are often self-limited and resolve with correction of the underlying disturbance. Primary neurologic diseases, such as viral encephalitis, Jakob–Creutzfeldt disease, Huntington chorea, Wilson disease, and ceroid lipofuscinoses, may also include myoclonic seizures. Myoclonic seizures are also seen in idiopathic generalized epilepsies, benign myoclonic epilepsy of childhood, juvenile myoclonic epilepsy, the Lennox–Gastaut syndrome (triad of multiple seizure types, psychomotor retardation, and a characteristic EEG pattern, seen mainly in children), progressive myoclonic epilepsies, and a wide variety of seizures from toxic and metabolic causes.

Myoclonic seizures consist of brief and violent muscle contractions, usually bilateral, that do not affect consciousness. Myoclonic contractions may be single or multiple, lasting for seconds to hours. Contractions may be rhythmic or irregular. When the upper limbs are involved, patients may drop or toss objects. When the legs or trunk are involved, the patient may suddenly fall. Myoclonic seizures may be spontaneous, or they may be induced by flashes of light, or more rarely by other triggering stimuli.

The usual EEG correlate of myoclonic seizures is generalized or multifocal spikes, polyspikes, and slow waves. Scalp-recorded EEG discharges may be seen in the case of cortical myoclonus but may not be seen in the case of subcortical myoclonus.

Localization-Related or Partial (Focal) Seizures without Impairment of Consciousness

Focal motor or sensory seizures may manifest at any age. The clinical manifestations depend on the brain region involved in the seizure.

The *motor cortex* is a common site of origin for focal seizures. Because the seizure discharges spread across the motor strip, clonus (alternating contraction and relaxation) may march up or down a limb and into the trunk or into another limb. Spread into a sensory area of the brain may cause numbness in the face, trunk, or limbs. *Sensory seizures* can also involve areas of special sensation such as sight or hearing. A focus in or near the visual cortex or its association areas may cause the patient to see spots, lights, or geometric shapes, similar to the experience of patients with classic migraine. Perception of buzzing, clicking, or ringing sounds may be generated from a focus in the superior and mesial temporal lobe. Gustatory and olfactory sensations, usually unpleasant, are components of partial seizures involving mesial temporal lobe structures. Seizures dominated by vestibular symptoms (e.g., dizziness, vertigo) are rare.

Retention of some degree of consciousness is characteristic of focal seizures, so that patients may, for example, walk and talk during a seizure—activities that would be impossible during a generalized seizure. However, a large focus in the dominant hemisphere may generate seizures that blunt awareness.

After a focal motor seizure, there may be *focal weakness of a limb, or Todd paralysis,* which usually resolves within a few hours or, rarely, after a few days. Distinction between cerebrovascular ischemic events with associated seizures and seizures with Todd paralysis may be difficult without clues from the patient's history. A Todd paralysis has localizing value and is good evidence of the focality of a seizure.

EEG does not necessarily reveal a seizure focus, especially if the seizure is small (e.g., motor seizure involving the leg, in which case the focus lies deep within the interhemispheric fissure), and particularly if the EEG is obtained between seizures. With focal seizures involving the leg, the EEG may be normal in more than 88% of patients even during a seizure.

Complex Partial Seizures

The category of complex partial seizures (CPSs) is important for several reasons: The condition is common in the adult population, the seizures are often misdiagnosed, and correct diagnosis leads to a search for potentially correctable lesions and effective AED therapy. CPSs are classified with focal or localization-related seizures because of clinical evidence linking these seizures with focal as opposed to generalized epileptiform discharges. CPSs are largely synonymous with the older term *psychomotor seizures,* but they are not synonymous with temporal lobe seizures because they can arise from any brain region. Although CPSs may begin at any age, the majority begin before age 20 years. An adult onset of CPS carries the same significance as does a new onset of any focal seizure; a treatable structural lesion should be sought. Patients with CPS who come to surgery or to postmortem examination may show either no histologic abnormality of the brain or tumor, infarct, granuloma, or infection; often with temporal lobe origin there is gliosis of the mesial temporal lobe. It is not known whether gliosis causes temporal lobe CPSs or results from them.

CPSs impair attention or consciousness through focal seizure activity. This is why they are called complex. The presentation of these seizures is more varied than that of the other seizure types and may include autonomic, psychic, visceral, sensory, or motor symptoms. Seizures often begin with an aura, which is, in fact, a simple partial seizure. The classic aura, usually consisting of an unpleasant olfactory or gustatory hallucination, is less common than is an aura of poorly described, unpleasant visceral sensations or malaise. Generally, there is no clear boundary between the aura and the seizure itself, particularly when seizures feature distorted visual or auditory sensations, or vertigo or unsteadiness. Arrest of motor activity, rigid posturing of the head and eyes, and slow, repetitive limb movements may occur and are easily distinguished in most cases from the tonic–clonic sequence of convulsive attacks. Autonomic instability, including fluctuating heart rate or blood pressure, flushing, sweating, salivation, or changes in pupillary reactions, may occur in patients with CPSs. Patients often say that they feel strange or as if in a dream, or they experience inappropriate emotions such as intense dread or strange serenity. If they can talk during a CPS, patients may portray what appears to be a psychiatric disturbance. The distinction between CPSs and psychosis may be further obscured in patients who have psychological or psychiatric problems between seizures. Such patients can be misdiagnosed as schizophrenic.

In a condition whose presentation may range from apparent appendicitis to apparent schizophrenia, special efforts should be made to elicit a detailed history of a spell and, if possible, to observe one. CPSs should have a definite start and finish; they should be associated with some impairment in ability to register and process information during the seizure; and they should be stereotyped from episode to episode. Observations of automatic behavior, such as repetitive lip licking or smacking, raising and lowering of the arm, fidgeting or buttoning and unbuttoning of clothing, stroking or rubbing movements, or pacing in circles, may secure the diagnosis of a CPS, because such automatisms are common in CPS but uncommon in other seizure types.

The routine EEG is abnormal in fewer than half of patients with partial seizures, but positive tracings may be found in 80% to 90% of patients by recording multiple EEGs that should include sleep and, in the case of temporal lobe origin, by using special electrodes positioned closer to temporal lobe structures.

Complex electrophysiologic mechanisms determine whether seizure discharges remain localized, spread along particular anatomic pathways, or involve much of the brain. AEDs can limit the spread of a focal seizure and prevent generalization, but generally do not obscure the EEG diagnosis of focal epilepsies. It is unknown how often tonic–clonic seizures are caused by spread from occult primary foci.

Unclassifiable Seizures

With an adequate history, most seizures should be classifiable by the scheme described. Often, however, the history is lacking. The event may not have been witnessed, or observers may report the patient's falling down and shaking but be unable to describe the full sequence of events. In these instances, it is best to list the seizure as unclassifiable or to use descriptive terms that are not otherwise used to classify seizure types, such as *jerks, convulsions,* or *staring spells,* until a specific seizure type can be identified.

CLASSIFICATIONS OF EPILEPSY SYNDROMES

Seizures are observable phenomena with symptoms or signs that last a finite time. An *epilepsy syndrome* is a cluster of signs and symptoms that occur together and constitute a chronic condition of recurrent seizures. There is no single known cause or pathology for epilepsy. Features of a particular epilepsy syndrome include cause, family history, age at onset, seizure frequency, typical course, precipitating factors, imaging studies, and the EEG. For example, damage to the temporal lobe may result in a condition of recurrent seizures characterized by an aura, unresponsiveness with automatisms, and tonic–clonic movements. This would represent a syndrome in which there is a progression of seizure types from simple partial to complex partial to secondarily generalized tonic–clonic seizures. If clinical data point to damage in the temporal lobe (EEG focus, imaging findings), the epilepsy syndrome is that of symptomatic temporal lobe epilepsy. This is also true with idiopathic generalized epilepsies (previously called primary generalized epilepsies). For example, absence seizures may be seen in a number of epilepsy syndromes (e.g., childhood absence epilepsy), each of which may have a different constellation of signs and symptoms and carry a different prognosis.

The importance of establishing a syndromic classification of epilepsy is that the particular prognosis in this chronic condition is tied to the epilepsy syndrome rather than the seizure type. Furthermore, success in the use of AEDs or even seizure surgery is also predicated more on the epilepsy syndrome classification than just on the seizure type (4).

EPIDEMIOLOGY

The annual incidence rate of epilepsy is approximately 40 to 70 per 100,000 population, and the reported prevalence rates are between 1.5 and 57 per 1,000 (5). Partial epilepsies constitute about two thirds of the cases, one fifth are generalized, and the remainder are unclassified (6). In adults, CPSs constitute approximately 40%; GTCSs, about 40%; and simple partial (focal motor or sensory) seizures, approximately 15% (6). For younger age groups, partial seizures are less prevalent and generalized absence seizures are correspondingly more common.

NATURAL HISTORY AND PROGNOSIS

The natural course of epilepsy is difficult to determine because modern studies include a mixture of treated and untreated patients. Comparison of prevalence and incidence ratios suggests a crude mean for the duration of epilepsy of approximately 12 to 13 years (7), not taking into consideration the age at onset of epilepsy, the clinical type, or the response to treatment. *After a first unprovoked seizure, the cumulative risk of recurrence* at 3 to 5 years has been estimated to be 40% (8,9). Until further data are available, a 40% crude risk for recurrence within a few years after a spontaneous tonic–clonic seizure is a reasonable estimate. Of adults who have a recurrence of tonic–clonic seizures, approximately 60% have recurrence in the first year and 70% by 3 years (10). Risk factors that increase the risk of recurrence and decisions about treatment are discussed in a later section (see The Patient with a First Seizure). If a person has a second, unprovoked seizure, the risk for further seizures is higher, and after several unprovoked seizures it exceeds 75%.

Once two spontaneous seizures have occurred, epilepsy is considered to exist, and the epidemiologic focus switches to the possibility for remission. Before the development of AEDs, the spontaneous remission rate for all types of epilepsy was approximately 10% to 32%. Reported remission rates for epilepsy with or without treatment vary between 10% and 82% (11,12), according to when the study was done, retrospective versus prospective methodology, and the length of followup. Studies on prognosis have not yet clarified the role of treatment in the long-term outcome. The probability of going 5 years without a seizure is approximately 40% at 1 year and 50% at 2 years after diagnosis of epilepsy (11). From 50% to 82% of patients are in remission after 2 to 5 years (13,14). The probability of remission at 20 years is 80% to 85% for idiopathic generalized epilepsies but only 65% for localization-related epilepsies. After being free from seizures for 5 years, almost 50% of patients relapse after tapering AEDs, usually in the first year and particularly in the first 6 months (15).

Prognostic factors include age at onset, severity of epilepsy, number of seizures before treatment, number of types of seizures, history of status epilepticus, number of medications required to control the disease, and length of time before attainment of seizure control. CPSs without secondary generalization are the most difficult seizure type to control (16,17).

Epilepsy that has not been controlled after 2 years of treatment represents a significant risk for chronic epilepsy. Some authorities believe that the long-term risk may be decreased by early treatment of seizures; however, this concept remains controversial. An abnormal EEG during AED withdrawal increases the chance of relapse in patients with CPSs (18), but a normal EEG does not exclude a relapse (83% versus 54%) (19). The presence of neurologic or psychiatric problems worsens the prognosis.

It is generally possible to reassure a person with epilepsy that the long-term prognosis for remission is good; however, except for childhood absence epilepsy, which usually remits before young adulthood, the attainment of remission can be expected to require many years.

CAUSES OF SEIZURES

Classification of seizures requires clinical observation, and classification of an epilepsy syndrome often requires clinical, EEG, and imaging data. Because a seizure represents a symptom of cerebral dysfunction, a primary cause should be sought.

Epilepsy that arises from *definable causes* has also been called symptomatic, as opposed to essential or idiopathic. Symptomatic epilepsies often arise from identifiable brain lesions, as from infection, trauma, tumor, or stroke. With idiopathic generalized epilepsies, however, patients have a normal examination, normal screening laboratory tests

TABLE 88.2 Causes of Seizures with Onset at Various Ages

Adolescent (12–21 yr)	*Adult (21–65 yr)*	*Elderly (65+ yr)*
	Common Causes	
Genetic (g or f)	Alcohol withdrawal (g)	Cerebrovascular (m)
Mesial temporal sclerosis (f)	Toxins or drugs (g)[a]	Thrombotic
Infection (m)	Drug withdrawal (g)	Embolic
Meningitis	Tumor (f)	Hemorrhagic
Viral encephalitis	Trauma (f)	Cardiac arrhythmia
Abscess	Scar	Trauma (m)
TORCHS[a]	Subdural hematoma	Scar
Parasites	Mesial temporal sclerosis (f)	Subdural hematoma
Psychogenic (m, usually g)	Genetic (g)	Tumor (m)
Toxins or drugs (g)[a]	Psychogenic (m)	Degenerative CNS disorders (e.g., Alzheimer disease)
Drug withdrawal (g)	Infection (m)	Systemic infection
	Meningitis	
	Viral encephalitis	
	Abscess	
	Syphilis	
	Cerebrovascular (m)	
	Thrombotic	
	Embolic	
	Hemorrhagic	
	Cardiac arrhythmia	
	Occasional Causes	
Metabolic	Metabolic (g)	Alcohol withdrawal (g)
Hypoglycemia	Hypoglycemia	Toxins or drugs (g)[a]
Hyponatremia	Hyponatremia	Drug withdrawal (g)
Hypocalcemia	Hypoxia (g)	Hypoxia (g)
Porphyria	Renal failure (g)	Metabolic (g)
Trauma (f)	Eclampsia (m)	Hypoglycemia
Scar	Parasites	Hyponatremia
Subdural hematoma		Hypocalcemia
Tumor (f)		Infection (m)
Arteriovenous malformation (f)		Meningitis
Subarachnoid hemorrhage (m)		Viral encephalitis
Eclampsia (m)		Abscess
Renal failure (g)		
	Rare Causes	
Collagen disease (m)	Hypocalcemia	Syphilis
Hepatic failure (g)	Hypomagnesemia	Parasites
Multiple sclerosis (f)	Collagen disease (m)	Hypertensive encephalopathy (m)
	Hypertensive encephalopathy (m)	Hyperosmolar (m)
	Hyperosmolar (m)	Renal failure (g)
	Multiple sclerosis (f)	Hepatic failure (g)
	Degenerative (m)	Degenerative (g)
	Abscess	Factitious (m)
	Syphilis	

CNS, central nervous system.
f, Usually focal; g, usually generalized; m, often mixed; TORCHS, toxoplasmosis, rubella, cytomegalovirus, herpes, syphilis.
[a] See list of occupational exposures that may cause seizures, Table 8.2.

(see Laboratory Tests), an EEG often showing a generalized spike-and-wave pattern, and a family history of similar seizures. Such patients would not be exhaustively studied for underlying causes.

Table 88.2 lists *specific causes* that should be considered for different types of seizures at various ages; the causes are listed from top to bottom in approximate order of frequency. It is worth emphasizing that many of the partial epilepsies display secondarily generalized seizures and that the focal onset may be obscured. Therefore, causes of focal seizures should be sought even in apparently generalized seizures.

Special issues are raised by *seizures that are manifested for the first time in the elderly.* First, most seizure disorders have onset in the first three decades of life, and onset of the idiopathic generalized epilepsy is unusual after this age. Second, cerebrovascular disease accounts for 30% to 60% of all new seizures in the elderly population. Tumors, the major cause of focal seizures in middle-age persons, have been found to be the cause of 2% to 30% of seizures in elderly patients (20); brain tumors in this age group are likely to be malignant. No cause is found in about half of elderly patients with seizures. When an elderly patient presents with seizures, a special effort should be made to find treatable conditions such as carotid artery stenosis, cardiac arrhythmias, infection, and toxic–metabolic derangements.

Posttraumatic Seizures

New-onset seizures after head trauma are usually partial (focal) in onset, and often secondarily generalized seizures occur after serious head injuries. There is little risk of seizures after mild head trauma with brief unconsciousness or amnesia, whereas severe injuries with intracranial hematomas, focal neurologic signs, and unconsciousness for longer than 24 hours result in epilepsy in about 10% of patients. Moderately severe injuries (skull fractures or unconsciousness for 30 minutes to 24 hours) impose an intermediate risk. Injuries over the vertex are more epileptogenic.

The value of *prophylactic therapy* to prevent the onset of posttraumatic seizures has not been firmly established. Until more data are available, the following approaches are recommended. Patients with minor scalp lacerations or brief loss of consciousness should not be considered to have a significantly increased risk of epilepsy. A single seizure occurring early (during the first 2 weeks after head injury), or while the patient is still experiencing the acute effects of injury, should not be an indication for long-term therapy; a second seizure in this setting might be grounds for treatment. Some patients with brain injuries might be considered for a 2- to 4-year course of prophylactic AED, especially with severe, penetrating, or vertex injuries. A patient with a seizure occurring more than 2 weeks after a head injury should be evaluated and managed as one would any other patient with new-onset seizures, and the seizure should not be attributed to a recent or remote episode of head trauma until other treatable causes have been excluded.

Alcohol-Related Seizures

Alcohol withdrawal is a common cause of seizures; almost all of them occur within the first 48 hours of abstinence or after marked reduction in alcohol intake, and most of them are generalized. In some series, up to 25% of withdrawal seizures have been focal, presumably because of an old cortical scar from trauma, infection, or vascular disease. The risk of epilepsy in the alcohol abuser is related to the amount of alcohol that was consumed (no longer being consumed at time of seizure) (21), but it may be increased by the higher likelihood of head trauma and intracranial infection in this population. If a known alcohol abuser has had a prior withdrawal seizure, presents a typical picture of a generalized seizure without focal features, and has a normal examination and no complications, then investigations may be limited. More often, the history is imprecise and findings are equivocal, or the patient has a fever or an elevated leukocyte count. In these instances, lumbar puncture, EEG, and continued observation are indicated. A computed tomography (CT) scan may be indicated with new-onset focal seizures, focal neurologic deficits, fever, neck stiffness, or signs of acute head trauma.

The use of AEDs to prevent alcohol withdrawal seizures is controversial. Some investigators recommend the use of AEDs for recent seizures or clusters of seizures during alcohol withdrawal (22), but others argue that alcohol withdrawal seizures are self-limited (23), and some studies show that treatment is usually ineffective (24). Long-term therapy with AEDs is not recommended.

Alcohol abusers may abuse other drugs. Concurrent benzodiazepine or barbiturate withdrawal can cause fulminant seizures. Occasionally, seizures occur during periods of alcohol consumption, as distinct from the period of alcohol withdrawal (25).

Seizures and Brain Tumors

Brain tumor is an uncommon cause of epilepsy, but epilepsy is a common symptom of brain tumors. About one third of intracranial and one half of intrahemispheric tumors are associated with seizures. Our present understanding of epilepsy secondary to tumor has been completely changed with the advent of CT and magnetic resonance imaging (MRI) head scanning (26). More and more often, tumors manifest with a single seizure, leading to early investigation and diagnosis with CT head scan or MRI. Between 1% and 16% of patients with epilepsy are found to have tumors. The probability varies according to age group: In adolescents it is approximately 1%; in young adults, 12% to 16%; and in older people, approximately 10% (27,28). *Young and middle-age adults with new onset of focal seizures* have the greatest chance of having a tumor (35%) (6). Nonetheless, CT or MRI scanning is not indicated in the investigation of patients with idiopathic generalized epilepsies who have diagnostic EEG patterns and in previously investigated patients who present with repeated seizures of unchanged character.

Seizures may be generalized tonic–clonic or partial. Diverse and changing clinical features are highly indicative of neoplasia. The following features suggest that seizures may be associated with a brain tumor: onset after 20 years of age, presence of persistent focal neurologic signs, signs of increased intracranial pressure, and focal unilateral slow waves on the EEG. Seizure frequency varies according to tumor location and histology: Frequent seizures are seen with supratentorial tumors, especially in the rolandic, temporal, or parietal cortical regions. Slow-growing tumors appear to be more epileptogenic.

Seizures and Cerebrovascular Disease

Cerebrovascular disease and epilepsy are the two most common causes of serious neurologic illnesses, and they often occur in the same patient. Ischemia damages brain and can lead to an epileptic focus. The incidence of early seizures (within the first 2 weeks after stroke onset) is approximately 5% in patients with nonembolic stroke (29). The seizures are more likely to be focal (80%) than generalized, and the distribution depends on stroke location. Only a small proportion of stroke patients develop recurrent seizures, i.e., epilepsy: 2.5% of those with intracranial hemorrhage and 3% of those with ischemic stroke (29). In ischemic stroke, although the highest incidence of seizures is shortly after stroke onset (30), epilepsy is most common (90%) in patients with late-onset seizures (more than 2 weeks after stroke) than in those with early-onset seizures (35%). Consequently, early seizures after stroke do not mandate AEDs; late recurrent seizures should be treated as epilepsy.

As previously mentioned, seizures in the elderly should raise the suspicion of cerebrovascular disease and may herald transient ischemia or impending stroke (31). In young patients, cerebral vascular disease is uncommon, but a seizure may lead to a diagnosis of an arteriovenous malformation, an aneurysm, collagen vascular disease, or a rare case of cortical thrombophlebitis.

Seizures and Infections

A seizure may be an early sign of bacterial meningitis, particularly in the very young and in the very old patient in whom the classic signs of meningitis may be lacking. Less fulminant forms of meningitis, such as cryptococcal or tuberculous meningitis, produce seizures that recur over weeks or months. Viral encephalitides, including herpes simplex encephalitis, the childhood exanthems, and the equine viruses, may also produce seizures. Human immunodeficiency virus (HIV) infection (see Chapter 39) is increasingly of concern as a cause of neurologic and systemic disease; most seizures associated with acquired immunodeficiency syndrome (AIDS) result from secondary complications such as cerebral toxoplasmosis, other atypical infections, or CNS lymphoma (32). Any meningoencephalitis can scar the cerebral cortex, resulting in an epileptic focus that can persist after resolution of the infection.

For reasons that are poorly understood, *systemic infections* may trigger seizures in susceptible patients, even if the infection does not directly involve the CNS (CNS). However, when a patient presents with a seizure and signs of infection, especially if the seizure is focal or if focal signs are detected on neurologic examination, the possibility of brain abscess must be explored with the use of head CT scanning or MRI, often with contrast.

EVALUATION OF A PATIENT WITH SEIZURES

In the evaluation of a patient with a history of one or more episodes of self-limited disturbance of consciousness or behavior, three questions must be addressed: First, were the events epileptic seizures? Second, if so, what type of seizures were they (Table 88.1)? Third, are there clues in the history, physical examination, or laboratory tests that point to a cause for the epileptic seizures (Table 88.2) or toward another cause?

Differential Diagnosis of Seizure-Like Behavior

Determination of the nature of a seizure-like episode is often difficult (Table 88.3). Unless the physician has observed an attack, the patient or witnesses must be asked for information about the sequence of behavioral events with attention to specific signs of neurologic dysfunction. Inquiry should be directed at establishing whether there were tonic–clonic features, with or without biting of tongue, lip, or cheek; head and eye deviation; urinary or fecal incontinence; rhythmic face or limb jerking; or speech and motor arrest followed by automatisms. *Syncope* not caused by a seizure is characteristically associated with prodromal

TABLE 88.3 Differential Diagnosis of Seizure-Like Behavior

Condition	*See Chapters*
Syncope	89
Cerebrovascular disease	91
Migraine	87
Narcolepsy	7
Fluctuating delirium	26
Paroxysmal dizziness or vertigo	89
Episodic movement disorders	90
Malingering, factitious illness	21
Conversion disorder	21
Hyperventilation	89
Panic attack	22

malaise, dizziness, and light-headedness, often with pallor, sweating, palpitations, and upright posture (see Chapter 89); if an observer notes sudden loss of consciousness and tone without convulsions and with brief postictal confusion, syncope is a much more likely diagnosis than is seizure. However, syncopal events can include some arrhythmic limb jerking, occasionally accompanied by incontinence and brief confusion. Transient numbness, weakness, speech or vision problems, or dizziness may occur with *cerebrovascular events* (see Chapter 91), including transient ischemic attacks, stroke, bleeding from an arteriovenous malformation or from an aneurysm, or a classic migraine (see Chapter 87). Precipitating factors such as postural changes, changes in antihypertensive medication, and the sequence of seizure characteristics may help distinguish epileptic seizures from cerebrovascular insufficiency. Particularly in the elderly, where the two conditions may be linked, a firm diagnosis may have to be deferred.

Hypoglycemia (see Chapter 81) is most commonly seen in alcoholics, diabetics, and patients who have had gastrointestinal (GI) surgery and often manifests with presyncopal symptoms.

Narcolepsy (see Chapter 7) is a rare disorder characterized by the sudden lapse into rapid eye movement (REM) sleep by episodes, when alert, of brief inhibition of muscle tone (cataplexy). These patients can be aroused from their sleep, often report that they dreamed during the attack, and deny postictal confusion.

In the elderly, a waxing and waning delirium with fluctuating agitation, lethargy, and occasional motor manifestations (see Chapter 26) occurring with intercurrent illness (e.g., renal failure, drug intoxication, infection) may superficially resemble a seizure but usually lacks both the stereotypical aspects of a seizure and a clear start and finish.

Vertigo, caused by disease of the inner ear, can present paroxysmally and may be confused with epilepsy (see Chapter 89).

Certain adults have *face or limb tics,* which, unlike most epileptic seizures, can be partially controlled by volition and often occur at predictable times.

Psychogenic Nonepileptic Seizures

In some patients, the greatest challenge is to distinguish between epileptic and psychogenic nonepileptic events. Misdiagnosis of an epileptic seizure may result in incorrect treatment of the actual underlying condition and the possible social stigma and consequences of being labeled an epileptic. *Panic attacks* can produce recurrent, fulminant, and moderately stereotyped symptoms, all of which may be seen in patients with partial complex seizures (see Chapter 22). Because epileptic seizures may have emotional concomitants (e.g., an aura of extreme fear) and may be triggered by stressful situations, the distinction can be difficult. If a diagnosis of psychogenic illness can be supported on other grounds, if the attacks are strongly linked to preceding anxiety, and if automatisms are lacking, a panic attack becomes a more likely diagnosis.

Patients with seizures caused by a *conversion disorder* may exhibit inattention, staring, deep unresponsiveness, and tonic and clonic movements that closely resemble epileptic events. These psychogenic seizures are involuntary events and must be differentiated from *malingering* and *factitious seizures,* which are produced deliberately by the patient. However, patients with nonepileptic events often also have epilepsy, and the management of epileptic events may be complicated by nonepileptic ones. Thrashing, asynchronous limb movements, crying, screaming, pelvic thrusting, and rapid side-to-side head turning have traditionally been ascribed to nonepileptic events but may also be seen with epileptic seizures. Observation of a generalized attack may reveal features that are atypical of an epileptic event, such as retention of protective reflexes (e.g., the blink reflex), a breathing effort when the airway is briefly occluded, coherent speech, or directed eye movements. Other features include the variability and nonstereotypy of each event, emotional precipitants, the usual presence of witnesses, recall after the event, biting of the tip of the tongue, forced eye closure, and the absence of postictal confusion (33). The motor activity may lack the organized tonic–clonic stages seen with generalized seizures, unless the patient is sophisticated and has observed seizures before. Psychogenic partial complex seizures may be the most difficult to diagnose.

As a general rule, purposeful, goal-directed behavior such as driving, shopping, talking in full sentences, or coordinated acts of violence should not be considered to be part of an epileptic seizure unless there is strong supporting evidence. Some of these features may be seen in the postictal state. Other features typical of a conversion disorder—presence of secondary gain, *la belle indifference,* inappropriate reactions to stress—may contribute to a correct diagnosis. Consultation among primary physician, neurologist, and psychiatrist may be required for proper diagnosis and management (see also Chapter 21).

Initial Determination of Seizure Type and Cause

The identification of seizure type (Table 88.1) should be made at the time of diagnosis of epilepsy. Features of the clinical onset should be especially addressed, because a brief focal onset or an aura may be the only indication that a seizure was secondarily rather than primarily generalized.

The history usually provides the main clues to the cause of the seizure. Contributory factors may include birth trauma or perinatal illness, head trauma, previous cerebral infarction or intracranial hemorrhage, encephalitis or meningitis, malignancies, and prior seizures. A family history of seizures may be pertinent because there is increased risk, particularly with idiopathic generalized epilepsies, for seizures in relatives of people with epilepsy. There should be inquiry into the use of alcohol, benzodiazepines, barbiturates, and other proconvulsants such as cocaine, amphetamine, neuroleptic medications, tricyclic antidepressants, bupropion, and theophylline. Patients may volunteer accounts of precipitating events such as flashing lights or hyperventilation. In some epilepsies, patients identify particular stimuli such as games, music, eating, laughing, or the touching of certain regions of skin. These *reflex seizures* may be avoided by avoiding the offending stimulus.

A general physical examination and neurologic examination (see Chapter 86) may reveal asymmetries or provide evidence for a structural, metabolic, or other cause of the seizure disorder. Some findings (e.g., focal paralysis) may be postictal, indicating focal onset (Todd paralysis), or they conversely may be suppressed, warranting reexamination in a few hours or days.

Investigations in a Patient with Seizures

Laboratory tests are usually not very helpful in determining whether a seizure has taken place, but they may be useful in establishing an underlying cause, in epilepsy classification, and in patient management.

Laboratory Tests

Depending on one's diagnostic hypotheses, investigations may include a full blood count, blood urea nitrogen or serum creatinine concentration, serum glucose, and serum electrolytes. In evaluating test results, it should be remembered that *striking abnormalities may appear transiently immediately after a seizure* (e.g., metabolic acidosis, marked leukocytosis). If clinically indicated, blood gases, liver function tests, and a screen for proconvulsive drugs should be obtained. A baseline electrocardiogram (ECG) may show arrhythmias or ischemia, although immediately after a seizure, these changes also may be results, rather than causes, of the seizure.

At times, measurement of a *serum prolactin level* helps in the evaluation of a patient with a suspected psychogenic seizure (see Kaplan, www.hopkinsbayview.org/PAMreferences). Commonly, the prolactin level rises two- to threefold after an epileptic but not after a psychogenic tonic–clonic event. In a lesser percentage of patients (45%), CPSs may cause serum prolactin increases, as may syncope (34), but 85% of simple partial (epileptic) seizures cause no rise (35). Partial complex seizures of temporal lobe origin are more likely to cause prolactin increases than those from the frontal lobe (36). Because this transient rise is present for 10 to 60 minutes after the event, positive findings are helpful, but negative findings, especially if measured more than 1 hour after the event, are inconclusive.

Electroencephalography

The electroencephalography (EEG) is the most useful laboratory study in the diagnosis of seizure disorders. An EEG may show generalized or focal epileptiform activity, or, even in the absence of such activity, it may demonstrate asymmetries of basic rhythms, focal slow waves, or diffuse slowing, all of which may give direction to further investigation. The appearance of epileptiform discharges on an EEG performed within 1 week after a *first seizure* predicts an 83% recurrence rate within 2 years, compared with a 41% recurrence rate in patients without such findings (37). Usually, the EEG is obtained more than 48 hours after the seizure. About 50% of patients with epilepsy have a normal EEG first. In about 10% of patients with epileptic seizures, multiple EEGs are all normal (38). Generally, the EEG should be relied on not to make a diagnosis of a seizure but to confirm a clinical impression derived from the history. When the history and EEG results are at variance, primacy should go to the history. Patients should not be treated for epilepsy because of an abnormal EEG alone, because interictal epileptiform discharges may be seen in 0.4% of the healthy population, in 2.2% of patients with nonepileptic neurologic disease, and in 3.5% of asymptomatic relatives of people with epilepsy (39). Conversely, one should not be dissuaded from a clinical impression of a seizure disorder just because of a normal EEG.

If EEG confirmation of seizure activity is needed (e.g., the history is equivocal, seizures occur during sleep or drowsiness), a repeat study with sleep deprivation or sleep induction, hyperventilation or intermittent photic stimulation, use of other scalp or semi-invasive electrodes (nasopharyngeal or sphenoidal leads), or eventually the use of prolonged video monitoring with EEG recording may be indicated. Many hospitals have epilepsy monitoring units specializing in the diagnosis and treatment of epilepsy. Referral to such units is sometimes the most effective way to elucidate the nature of spells not delineated by more routine maneuvers.

Epileptiform EEG discharges can usually be observed in the presence of AEDs, although some generalized discharges may be suppressed. Therefore, medications should not be altered for the first EEG. If tracings are repeatedly negative and the diagnosis of epilepsy is suspect, then the patient can be admitted to a hospital for rapid tapering of AEDs and concurrent EEG and video monitoring to look for epileptic activity. However, abrupt withdrawal of barbiturates or benzodiazepines may precipitate seizures even in normal subjects. Among patients with epilepsy, the pattern of generalized EEG slowing without seizure discharges is fairly common, usually resulting from underlying diffuse cortical dysfunction, medication effects, or a postictal state.

Because EEGs can stay abnormal for several weeks after a tonic–clonic seizure, any findings should be re-evaluated with repeated studies. An EEG is without risk (see Chapter 86), barring an injudicious interpretation.

Cerebrospinal Fluid Examination

Certain illnesses that lead to seizures may require examination of cerebrospinal fluid (CSF) to secure a diagnosis; examples are suspected acute or chronic meningitis or subarachnoid hemorrhage. The yield of CSF studies in patients with various seizure types is unknown, and the indication for these studies should be considered on a case-by-case basis. The CSF examination is not indicated in a normal child with classic absence epilepsy or with EEG evidence of focal rolandic spikes, and it is contraindicated in a patient in whom a mass lesion is strongly suspected. Most other patients with focal or generalized seizures of uncertain cause should undergo spinal fluid analysis (see Chapter 86).

After prolonged generalized seizures, the CSF may show a pleocytosis of up to 100 cells, presumably from a transient breakdown of the blood–brain barrier. Clearly, however, infection must be excluded or temporarily considered in this setting.

Cerebral Imaging

CT head scans (see Chapter 86) of patients with primary generalized seizures are abnormal (excluding nonspecific atrophy) in approximately 10% of instances. Scans of patients with focal motor or secondarily generalized seizures show a focal abnormality in 65%. Patients with CPSs show abnormalities about one third of the time. An abnormal and asymmetric neurologic examination has a high correlation with focal abnormalities on the head CT scan. Studies of patients with seizures show that MRI of the head (see Chapter 86) has a higher diagnostic yield than CT scanning and may show specific changes of mesial temporal sclerosis, various angiomas, neuronal migration disorders, or perisylvian polymicrogyria but is not a procedure needed for all patients (40).

Adults with new-onset focal or secondarily generalized seizures should have an MRI or CT scan with contrast if possible, unless the EEG shows a pattern of a genetic disorder. Patients with an abnormal neurologic examination should also be imaged. In patients with a normal examination and in children, this decision should be individualized. Subsequent imaging may also be indicated if there is a change in seizure pattern or neurologic examination.

Other Diagnostic Tests

Skull radiographs, radionuclide brain scans, pneumoencephalography, and arteriography have largely been replaced by newer imaging studies. Several techniques show promise for definition of seizure foci: imaging of brain metabolism and chemistry by positron emission tomographic (PET) scanning; single-photon emission computed tomography (SPECT), which examines cerebral blood flow at particular time points; functional magnetic resonance imaging (fMRI); and magnetoencephalography (MEG), which records brain activity.

TREATMENT OF EPILEPSY

Except in unusual instances, epilepsy cannot be cured. In about three of four patients, it can be controlled so that the patient experiences few or no seizures. Much attention has been focused on the pharmacologic management of seizures, but the importance of a comprehensive approach cannot be overemphasized: A patient who is seizure free but so intoxicated by medicines that employment is impossible represents at best a dubious success. Employment problems and other social aspects of the management of epilepsy are considered in the following sections. General measures of therapy should not be neglected. Removal of precipitating factors for seizures, reduction of stress, and provision for adequate amounts of rest can all be important in the control of epilepsy and are also discussed here. Patients should be advised to wear *medical alert bracelets or medallions.*

The Patient with a First Seizure

In deciding whether to treat a first seizure, one should recall that a single seizure does not constitute epilepsy nor necessarily require treatment. In patients with *"provoked"* or acute symptomatic seizures such as those that occur after alcohol withdrawal, cocaine intake, or overdose of tricyclics, identification and removal of the precipitating cause usually prevents further seizures, and AEDs are rarely indicated. Additionally, single or early seizures, i.e., within 2 weeks after closed head trauma or stroke do not require chronic AED therapy.

In about one third of patients with first seizures, the seizures are *unprovoked.* Such patients may be so frightened by the possibility of having another seizure, with potential repercussions on employment, social relations, and license to drive, that they are willing to accept the inconvenience and morbidity of chronic medication. Most patients first present to a physician after having had several unprovoked seizures. Of this group, more than three-fourths may be expected to have further seizures. This contrasts with the finding from prospective studies that approximately 16% to 36% of patients who present after their first unprovoked seizure have a recurrence within 1 year, and that in the aggregate 27% to 50% have recurrent seizures within 3 years (8,9). Retrospective studies suggest higher recurrence rates.

Because for a given patient the probability of further seizures over a 5-year period may vary from 30% to 80%, it is important to consider the following *risk factors that increase the probability of additional seizures:* an identifiable cause for the first seizure, such as CNS infection or recent stroke or head injury; the presence of EEG epileptiform abnormalities; occurrence of the initial seizure at night; previous febrile seizures; status epilepticus or multiple seizures in the same day; Todd paralysis; and partial seizures (9,16). With genetic epilepsies, typically with childhood onset, in which the EEG shows epileptiform activity, there is an increased risk of seizure recurrence in the short term. Many of these epilepsy syndromes are age dependent and remit after several years.

In one prospective study, addressing the issue of treatment after a first unprovoked tonic–clonic seizure, the rate of recurrence at 1 year in patients randomly assigned to AED treatment was 18%, compared with 38% for those who were not started immediately on treatment (41). Depending on the AED used, the incidence of side effects severe enough to warrant discontinuation of treatment ranges from less than 1% to approximately 6%. These figures usually are not used in deciding whether a patient should be offered a specific AED. Rather, the efficacy profile, the overall side effect profile, and the frequency with which the medication must be taken govern the institution of the drug.

General Principles of Drug Therapy

Patients who have monthly or more frequent generalized seizures are usually undertreated; and the goal of therapy is zero seizures. In contrast, other patients may be taking an unnecessary polypharmacy or incorrect regimens of AEDs. Table 88.4 summarizes general principles for the planning of drug therapy. Prospective observations show that, with adequate AED treatment, the prognosis for seizure control during the first 12 months varies according to seizure type: GTCS, 60% to 70%; mixed (predominately GTCS), 50% to 53%; CPS, 21% to 28% (16).

TABLE 88.4 Principles of Antiepileptic Drug Therapy

Decide whether to treat.
Select the proper drug for the particular form of seizure and epilepsy and for a woman of childbearing age.
Start drugs slowly and build up levels gradually to avoid toxicity or idiosyncratic adverse effects.
Start with one drug, and use it to effect or toxicity before adding another.
Choose the simplest regimen possible.
Suspect compliance problems in treatment failures.
Monitor blood levels in problem cases such as with polypharmacy, toxicity, or questions of compliance.
Withdraw medications gradually and sequentially.
Decide how long to treat considering severity of epilepsy, probability of relapse, social circumstances, driving issues, and professional issues.

Selection of Drugs

To select the appropriate AED, it is important to know the type of epilepsy under consideration. Table 88.5 represents a general but not unanimous consensus on drugs of choice and alternatives for the principal types of seizures and epilepsy (42). Selection of preferred drugs takes into consideration efficacy in suppressing seizures, tolerability, and favorable side effect profiles. Two large controlled clinical trials compared the effectiveness of several AEDs (carbamazepine, phenobarbital, phenytoin, and primidone) and valproic acid versus carbamazepine for the treatment of *partial seizures* or *secondarily generalized tonic–clonic seizures* (43,44). Both carbamazepine and phenytoin were highly effective and were recommended as drugs of choice for these two common types of seizures (44). For complex partial seizures with or without secondarily generalized tonic-clonic seizures, carbamazepine, phenytoin, oxcarbazepine, lamotrigine, and valproate are recommended as first line. Levetiracetam, topiramate, zonisamide, or gabapentin are recommended as second line (42). For efficacy, valproate has been generally recommended as the drug of first choice for idiopathic generalized epilepsies. Newer drugs such as lamotrigine, topiramate, zonisamide, and levetiracetam as well as phenytoin have been favored by an expert consensus committee. *Childhood absence epilepsy* may be treated with either ethosuximide or valproate or lamotrigine, although the former does not always prevent concurrent myoclonic seizures. *Myoclonic seizures* are best treated with valproate, lamotrigine, topiramate, zonisamide, clonazepam, or levetiracetam. A certain percentage of idiopathic generalized epilepsies with GTCSs respond to monotherapy with carbamazepine (although absence seizures may worsen), and a certain percentage of partial seizures respond to valproic acid monotherapy. In several instances, more than one drug may be considered the drug of choice in terms of efficacy, in which case the selection can be made on the basis of personal familiarity with the drug, convenience of dose scheduling, or the relative risk and spectrum of side effects. For example, some practitioners prefer carbamazepine to phenytoin to avoid possible gum hyperplasia and hirsutism, even though these side effects are seen in only approximately 10% of patients.

TABLE 88.5 Drugs of Choice[a] According to Seizure Type

Seizure Category or Epilepsy Syndrome	Drugs of Choice	Alternatives (Preference)	Third Choice
Idiopathic generalized tonic–clonic seizures	Valproate Lamotrigine	Levetiracetam Phenytoin Topiramate Zonisamide	Vagus nerve stimulation Carbamazepine Oxcarbazepine Ketogenic diet Phenobarbital Topiramate Zonisamide
Idiopathic (primary) generalized absence seizures	Ethosuximide Valproate Lamotrigine	Topiramate Clonazepam Levetiracetam	Phenobarbital Phenytoin Ketogenic diet
Idiopathic generalized epilepsy with myoclonic seizures	Valproate Topiramate Lamotrigine	Levetiracetam Clonazepam Zonisamide	Phenobarbital Phenytoin Ketogenic diet Ethosuxmide Vagus nerve stimulation
Partial simple and complex and secondarily generalized epilepsy	Carbamazepine Oxcarbazepine Phenytoin Valproate Lamotrigine	Gabapentin Levetiracetam Topiramate Gabapentin Zonisamide	Phenobarbital Phenytoin Vagus nerve stimulation Ketogenic diet

[a]Not necessarily according to U.S. Food and Drug Administration (FDA)-approved indications.

With phenytoin, the convenience of a simpler dosage regimen, lower cost, and availability of a parenteral preparation may offset these considerations. Several reviews and meta-analyses compared controlled trials of AEDs and revealed no significant differences in efficacy among AEDs in current use (45). Table 88.6 gives dosages, half-lives, serum levels, and principal side effects of the drugs.

Dose Adjustment

The AED dosage should be increased over several weeks to avoid early side effects that might discourage the patient from continuing with treatment. Because some AEDs remain in the blood for some time, it may take several days to weeks before the effects of a dosage adjustment are manifested.

Although initial treatment *with more than one AED,* typically phenytoin and phenobarbital, was once common, there is little evidence that two drugs at subtherapeutic dosages are better tolerated or more effective than one drug at higher dosages. In fact, 90% of new-onset seizures that are controlled can be controlled with one drug. If one drug is unsuccessful, addition of a second helps in only approximately 36% of patients (46).

Compliance is a major factor in the success of drug therapy for epilepsy (see Chapter 4). Every effort should be made to simplify the dosage regimen and choose the best-tolerated drug. Phenobarbital and zonisamide can be given in a once-daily dose. The complexity of providing carbamazepine, valproate, Trileptal, lamotrigine, or levetiracetam which must be given in divided doses, should be offset by a better-suited profile of side effects for the individual patient. At each visit the patient (or other responsible person) should be asked to report on the exact medication regimen and encouraged to bring the most recent medicine bottles with them. All too often, inquiry indicates a need for clearer oral and written communication with the patient. If necessary, the drug regimen should be written out for the patient's use.

Familiarity with cost of medicines is important, because patients may be hesitant to buy an expensive medicine unless the need is clearly explained. *Generic brands* are less expensive, but for several AEDs, such as carbamazepine, primidone, phenytoin, and valproic acid, bioavailability is variable (47). Generally, generic brands should be avoided in patients with seizures that are difficult to control. If generic brands are prescribed, use of the same brand should be encouraged; drug levels may have to be checked more often if toxicity or seizures appear.

The optimal dosage of an AED may vary several-fold among different patients. Determination of serum levels (Table 88.6) is a reliable way to measure how much medication is circulating, but such measurements should not be ordered routinely. If a patient's seizures are controlled on the regimen that is initiated and there is no toxicity from that drug regimen, measurement of a drug serum level might lead one to alter a successful regimen inappropriately. If control is not optimal, drug levels can help

TABLE 88.6 Major Antiepileptic Drugs

Medication[a] *(Brand Name)*	*Available Preparations and Strengths (mg)*	*Typical Adult Dose, Schedule, Range*	*Half-Life (hr)*	*Enzyme Induced*	*Renal Clearance*	*Reference-Target Levels (mg per L)*[b]	*Major Side Effects*
Carbamazepine[c] (Carbatrol)	200-mg, 300-mg capsules	Daily dose 200–800 mg, b.i.d.	10–25	+	<1%	4–12	Same as below
Carbamazepine (Tegretol)	200-mg tablets (100-mg chewable) 100 mg per 5 mL suspension	200 mg t.i.d. or q.i.d. (400–1,600 mg)	10–25	+	<1%	4–12	GI distress Ataxia Blurred vision Blood changes Hepatotoxicity
Carbamazepine extended release (Tegretol XR)	100-, 200-, 400-mg tablets	200–800 mg in two divided doses		+	<1%		Same as above
Clonazepam[c] (Klonopin)	0.5-, 1-, 2-mg tablets	2 mg t.i.d. (2–20 mg)	20–40			0.05–0.7	Drowsiness Ataxia Behavior changes Dizziness
Ethosuximide (Zarontin)	250-mg capsules 250 mg per 5 mL solution	250 mg b.i.d. to q.i.d. (500–1,500 mg)	30	–	20%–25%	50–100	GI distress Sedation Headache Dizziness
Felbamate (Felbatol)	400-mg, 600-mg tablets 600 mg per 5 mL suspension	1,200–3,600 mg per d in 3 or 4 divided doses	20–23	+	45%–55%	30–50	Nausea Vomiting Aplastic anemia Acute liver failure ↑ ALT Insomnia Headache Dizziness Weight loss
Fosphenytoin IV sodium (Cerebyx)	IV preparation 2 mL (100 mg phenytoin equivalent) and 10 mL (500 mg phenytoin equivalent)	150 mg phenytoin equivalent per min diluted in 0.9% saline or 5% dextrose before infusion	15 min Converts to phenytoin with half-life of 22 h			10–20	Pruritis Paresthesia Dizziness Headache Somnolence Ataxia Nystagmus
Gabapentin (Neurontin)	100-mg, 300-mg, 400-mg, 600-mg, 800-mg capsules 250 mg per 5 mL solution	600–1,200 t.i.d.	5–7	–	>95%	>4	Somnolence Ataxia Dizziness Fatigue Nystagmus Tremor Weight gain

(continued)

TABLE 88.6 (Continued) Major Antiepileptic Drugs

Medication[a] (Brand Name)	*Available Preparations and Strengths (mg)*	*Typical Adult Dose, Schedule, Range*	*Half-Life (hr)*	*Enzyme Induced*	*Renal Clearance*	*Reference-Target Levels (mg per L)[b]*	*Major Side Effects*
Lamotrigine (Lamictal)	25-mg, 100-mg, 150-mg and 200-mg tablets 2-mg, 5-mg, 25-mg chewable tablets	75–250 mg b.i.d.	12–14 when added to enzyme-inducing AEDs 25–33 as monotherapy	+	10%	4–18	Rash Dizziness Ataxia Somnolence Headache Blurred vision Nausea Vomiting
Levetiracetam (Keppra)	250-mg, 500-mg, 750-mg scored tablets 100 mg per mL solution	500–1,500 b.i.d.	6–8	–	66%	3–37	Somnolence Asthenias Dizziness
Oxcarbazepine (Trileptal)	150-mg, 300-mg, 600-mg scored tablets 300 mg per 5 mL (60 mg per mL) oral suspension	Starting dose 150–300 mg/d Total: 900–2,400 mg per day, given in two daily doses;	MHD 9.3 ± 1.8	+	27%	Monohydroxy derivative (MHD) 50–200 mmol per L or 10–35 mg per L	Fatigue Dizziness Headache Sedation Ataxia Hypersensitivity reactions Hyponatremia
Phenobarbital[c] (Luminal)	15-mg, 30-mg, 60-mg, 100-mg tablets 15 mg per 5 mL elixir 20 mg per 5 mL elixir	100–200 mg q.d.	72	+	20%–25%	15–40	Sedation Hyperactivity Confusion Mood change
Phenytoin[c] (Dilantin)[c]	30-, 100-mg capsules 50-mg chewable "Infatabs" 125 mg per 5 mL suspension	300 mg q.d.[d,e] (200–500 mg)	22[e]	+	<5%	10–20	Ataxia Cosmetic changes (gum hyperplasia, hirsutism) Sedation Osteoporosis
(Phenytek)	200-mg, 300-mg extended-release capsule 100-mg prompt-release capsule						
Primidone[c] (Mysoline)	50-, 250-mg scored tablets and suspension 250 mg per 5 mL	250 mg t.i.d. or q.i.d. (500–1,500 mg)	3–12[f] 72[g]			6–12[f] 15-40[g]	Sedation Hyperactivity Mood change
Tiagabine (Gabitril)	2-mg, 4-mg, 12-mg, 16-mg, 20-mg tablets	32–56 mg in two to four divided doses	12–15 with other AED 21–24 as monotherapy	–	2%	Unknown	Dizziness Confusion Tiredness GI upset Headache Depression Tremor

Topiramate (Topamax)	25-mg, 100-mg, 200-mg tablets 15-mg, 25-mg sprinkles	100–400 mg per day in two divided doses	12–15 with other AED, 21–24 as monotherapy	+	60%–70%	6.5–30	Somnolence Dizziness Ataxia Psychomotor slowing Paresthesias Weight loss Anorexia Fatigue Kidney stones Glaucoma
Valproate IV (Depacon)	IV preparation 5 mL single-dose vials equal to 100 mg per mL	60-min infusion but not >20 mg per min	16 ± 3			50–100	Same as valproic acid
Valproic acid[c] (Depakene)	250-mg capsules 250 mg per 5 mL syrup	250 mg b.i.d. to q.i.d. (500–4000 mg) per d	8–12	–	<3%	50–100	GI distress Drowsiness Ataxia
Valproic acid; divalproex sodium (Depakote)	125-mg, 350-mg, 500-mg delayed-release tablets 125-mg sprinkles 500-mg extended-release tablet 250 mg per 5 mL syrup	Same as above	8–12	–	<3%	50–100	Alopecia Tremor Blood changes Rare liver toxicity Rare pancreatitis
Zonisamide (Zonegran)	25-mg, 50-mg, 100-mg capsules	Starting dose 100 mg per d; increase by 100 mg per 2 wk as tolerated	63	–	35%	10–40	Fatigue Headache Somnolence Ataxia Agitation Anorexia Nausea Confusion Paresthesias Kidney stone (1%–2%) Mental slowing Hypersensitivity reaction Oligohidrosis

detect inadequate compliance or absorption. They may also provide guidance for patients with symptoms that might be caused by drug intoxication. Ideally, blood specimens obtained to monitor side effects should be taken at times of peak serum concentrations, and specimens obtained to monitor drug efficacy should be taken at times of trough serum levels. It is important to know that for some AEDs, particularly phenytoin, drug dosage and drug level are not linearly related: A saturation point is reached above which small increments in daily dosage (e.g., increasing from 400 to 500 mg of phenytoin per day) may lead to marked increases in serum level and side effects. A serum level is most informative if measured in the steady state (Table 88.6), which requires a stable dosage for approximately five half-lives or longer before measurement.

Many patients with severe and long-standing epilepsy have endured a gradual increase in AED dosage. Excessive polypharmacy may be ineffective, may produce marked side effects, and may even limit the ability to increase a single potentially effective AED to the maximum dosage. In this circumstance, one should consider reduction in AED dosage or number of medications over several months. Other side effects may prompt discontinuation of AEDs.

Although several AEDs can cause modest rises in *liver enzyme levels,* only moderate to marked abnormalities (more than two to three times baseline) necessitate stopping the drug. Conversely, serious hepatotoxicity may not be heralded by changes in liver function tests. Symptoms may include anorexia, malaise, tiredness, and jaundice, usually appearing 2 to 16 weeks after starting treatment. Carbamazepine can cause mild *leukopenia and thrombocytopenia,* but a rapid, progressive leukocyte decline, typically to lower than 3,000 cells/mm^3 with a total neutrophil count of less than 1,000 cells/mm^3, would warrant concern (33). *Nystagmus* should not be used as an indication of toxicity but rather as a marker of AED therapy. Conversely, ataxia, unacceptable somnolence, cognitive impairment, and malaise may indicate the need for modification of therapy.

Duration of Treatment

The determination of how long to maintain treatment with AEDs may be difficult, because seizures remit over time, and therefore freedom from seizures may not be the result of medication. About one half to two thirds of patients are entirely seizure free for 2 years with therapy. If an adult patient is seizure free for about 5 years on medication and then stops treatment by gradual taper, there is a 30% to 50% chance of relapse during the next 5 years (45,15). Approximately 80% of relapses occur within 4 months after starting the taper, and 90% within the first year (48,49).

As with the decision to initiate therapy, the decision to terminate AED therapy must be individualized. A patient with seizures that were initially very difficult to control who has an underlying structural lesion or a persistently abnormal EEG may benefit from lifelong therapy. In contrast, a patient with idiopathic epilepsy who has been seizure free for 2 to 5 years and is willing to accept an increased risk of having a seizure may be a candidate for drug withdrawal. Certain patients who have attained seizure control over a long period do not wish to stop treatment. In these instances, potential benefits and risks of medication reduction should be discussed, but patients should not be forced off medications for the sake of principle. If more than one drug has been prescribed, the medications should be tapered one at a time, each over a period of several months, and reinstated rapidly if seizures recur. The least effective medication or the most toxic may be chosen as the candidate for initial reduction.

An example of a cautious tapering schedule for a patient who has been taking carbamazepine 400 mg (two 200-mg tablets) three times daily would be reduction by one tablet per day every 2 weeks. During tapering and in the first few months after the tapering of all AEDs, it is prudent for the patient to refrain from driving.

Ambulatory Followup

Seizure frequency, medication side effects, and social factors determine the pattern for outpatient followup. Patients who are free from seizures for longer than 1 year and who have no intercurrent problems may be seen yearly. Conversely, patients with frequent seizures, significant side effects, or social problems may need to be seen every few weeks during problem periods. Visits may be necessary every 2 to 4 weeks during adjustment of the drug regimen. For appropriate management and monitoring of therapeutic changes, a patient should be evaluated no sooner than five AED half-lives after the change is initiated.

Specific Antiepileptic Drugs

Carbamazepine (Tegretol, Carbatrol)

Carbamazepine has been used for more than two decades for the treatment of seizures and chronic neuropathic pains. Carbamazepine is one of the drugs of choice for CPSs, but it may worsen absence seizures. Studies comparing carbamazepine with other AEDs for the treatment of partial seizures showed that carbamazepine resulted in the highest rate of complete remission (although mean seizure frequency was similar for patients taking carbamazepine, phenytoin, or phenobarbital) (43). Table 88.6 gives the adult dosage of carbamazepine, which is 400 to 1,600 mg/day, along with dosing guidelines for Carbatrol and Tegretol. It is advisable to initiate therapy with no more than 200 to 400 milligrams per day, increasing to the full dosage over 1 or 2 weeks. The half-life is about

10 to 25 hours. A newer long-acting preparation, Tegretol XR, is available in 100-mg, 200-mg, and 400-mg tablets, with ports that allow slow release. There is also a suspension of 100 mg/5 mL. This form can be taken twice daily. Total daily dosage remains the same, meaning that conversion to the more convenient form is simple, but more even blood levels are obtained. Patients should be warned that the tablet shell may appear in the stool, but this does not represent inadequate release of contents. Patients must be instructed not to chew XR tablets but to swallow them whole. Another long-acting preparation, Carbatrol, also has a long half-life and produces more constant blood levels. Recommended target serum levels with all preparations of carbamazepine are around 4 to 12 mg/dL. Because of erratic absorption of the generic preparation, it should not be continued in any patient who takes it and continues to have seizures.

Because carbamazepine in tablet form may lose one third or more of its effectiveness if stored in humid conditions, patients should be advised to keep their tablet containers in a dry location, away from the bathroom. Recently, manufacturers have been asked by the U.S. Food and Drug Administration (FDA) to package carbamazepine in moisture-proof containers.

The *side effects* of carbamazepine include fatigue, nystagmus, diplopia, dizziness, ataxia, dysarthria, rash (including, rarely, Stevens–Johnson syndrome), inappropriate secretion of antidiuretic hormone, occasionally abnormal liver function tests, and an infrequent lupus-like syndrome. Gastrointestinal distress is the most common side effect, particularly if the medication is initiated too rapidly. Reversible leukopenia or thrombocytopenia is seen in 5% to 10% of patients, so blood counts may be monitored weekly for the first few weeks after the start of therapy. This drug has had a reputation for causing aplastic anemia, based largely on six cases of this complication that were reported in the 1960s (even though a causal relationship to carbamazepine was not established). The actual incidence of aplastic anemia is unknown, but it is thought to be very small (the warning provided by the manufacturer reports a general population incidence of potentially fatal blood dyscrasia of 8 per 1,000,000 and an incidence associated with carbamazepine of about 40 per 1,000,000). Carbamazepine along with phenytoin and the barbiturates are cytochrome-P450 hepatic enzyme inducers and may decrease the efficacy of oral contraceptive pills (OCPs), cholesterol-lowering agents, and Coumadin, among others.

Phenytoin (Diphenylhydantoin, DPH, PHT, Dilantin)

Since its introduction in 1938, phenytoin has been one of the major drugs used to treat seizures. It is most useful in epilepsies with simple and complex partial seizures, with or without secondary generalization. Phenytoin may make absence seizures worse.

Without a loading dose, a full week is required to reach therapeutic levels, but a load given on the first day, achieves immediate therapeutic levels. This rapid dosing scheme is likely to induce transient side effects and is useful chiefly for initiating treatment in a patient who has seized repeatedly (e.g., in an emergency department) and remains unconscious.

The mean half-life of phenytoin is 22 hours, with a range from 7 to 42 hours. It is 90% protein bound, so *low serum albumin* can lead to an increased concentration of the free agent and consequently to increased toxicity. The drug is metabolized in the liver and is not excreted by the kidney. In renal failure, drug-binding proteins may be deficient, resulting in a low measured total serum level with an adequate free drug serum level. Dosage should be lowered only in renal failure to compensate for a decrease in serum protein, and then a reduction of approximately 25% usually suffices. Phenytoin is partially removed by hemodialysis.

The usual starting dosage of phenytoin is 100 mg/day for 3 to 5 days, increasing by 100 mg at similar intervals to 300 mg/day. If seizures are not controlled at this dosage, it is prudent to increase by increments of 50 mg/day, because small increases in dosage may cause large increases in serum levels. Phenytoin (as Dilantin) comes in 30- and 100-mg capsules, suspension (300 mg and 125 mg/5 mL), and chewable 50-mg tablets. This medication can be given once a day if it is given as Dilantin Kapseals, because this preparation is manufactured as a slow-release form. Other forms of phenytoin preparations (e.g., Phenytek) may be less expensive and comes in a 200-mg or 300-mg dosage (Phenytek). A parenteral formulation of phenytoin is fosphenytoin sodium injection (Cerebyx), which can be given intramuscularly or intravenously. It is dosed in phenytoin equivalents and can be given more rapidly intravenously at up to 150 mg/minute. A target range for phenytoin is generally between 10 and 20 mg/L (toxicity usually occurs at levels greater than 20 mg/L, but patients show fairly wide individual susceptibility to side effects). The lethal dose may range from 2 to 20 g.

A number of drugs elevate phenytoin plasma levels—disulfiram and isoniazid commonly. Amiodarone increases phenytoin 1.5 times, while fluconazole and miconazole increase phenytoin 2 to 4 times. Warfarin, chloramphenicol, methylphenidate, phenothiazines, benzodiazepines, propoxyphene, fluoxetine, omeprazole, propoxyphene, thioridazine, haloperidol, cimetidine, and erythromycin less often increase phenytoin plasma levels and OCPs leading to decreased efficacy. Other drugs may lead to *decreased phenytoin* levels: alcohol, folic acid, pyridoxine, theophylline, and occasionally carbamazepine, oral contraceptives, sulfonamides, ticlopidine, trazodone, ciprofloxacin, and antacids. Phenytoin may decrease cyclosporin levels and OCPs, leading to decreased efficacy. These potential drug interactions may be managed best by patient and physician awareness and by observation of serum drug levels during times of medication changes.

There are many potential *undesirable effects of phenytoin.* Dose-related *acute effects* include ataxia (usually beyond 25 to 30 mg/L), lethargy, depression, paradoxical tendency to increase seizures at higher toxic levels (usually greater than 10 mg/L), and allergic reactions. *Chronic side effects* of phenytoin are generally manifested after a few months to several years of daily ingestion. Chronically progressive cosmetic changes can be vexing in young women. Gum hyperplasia occurs in approximately 10%; it may in some be forestalled by good oral hygiene, but once established it may regress only partially. Hirsutism is seen in 5% overall but in 30% of young women. Even more disconcerting are facial changes caused by thickening of subcutaneous tissue about the nose and eyes, the so-called leonine facies. Skin rash occurs in 2% to 10% of users of phenytoin, with a peak incidence about 2 to 8 weeks into the course. Stevens–Johnson syndrome occurs rarely. Lymphadenopathy develops in 2% to 5%, sometimes in association with fever, arthralgia, eosinophilia, and hepatosplenomegaly, presenting a picture of pseudolymphoma and, rarely, true lymphoma. Hepatitis and a variety of blood dyscrasias have been reported. Megaloblastic anemia may occur, which responds to folate. Many patients develop measurable antinuclear antibodies in the serum; a tiny minority of this group progress to symptomatic systemic lupus erythematosus, which remits entirely within days to weeks after discontinuation of phenytoin. The rare instances of pulmonary infiltrates and fibrosis have given rise to the term, *Dilantin lung.* Phenytoin can induce liver enzymes, thereby secondarily affecting metabolism of numerous hormones and drugs. Induced inactivation of vitamin D leads to radiologic or biochemical evidence of bone disease in one of every three chronically treated patients. Teratogenic effects of phenytoin are strongly suspected (see Juvenile Absence Epilepsy section).

Sodium Valproate (Depakote)

The antiseizure effect of valproic acid was discovered in 1963. Its effectiveness is broad, but it is thought to be particularly valuable for absence seizures and childhood absence epilepsy, for idiopathic (JAE and juvenile myoclonic epilepsy [JME]) and symptomatic generalized epilepsies (e.g., Lennox-Gastaut Syndrome), and as a first- or second-line agent for partial epilepsies (49).

Valproic acid is a fatty acid, structurally dissimilar from all other common AEDs. It is usually prescribed as sodium valproate/valproic acid (Depakote), purported by the manufacturer to cause less GI upset than pure valproic acid (Depakene). It is available in 125-mg, 250-mg, and 500-mg tablets delayed release and in 125-mg sprinkle capsules; also available in 250-mg extended-release tablets. Valproic acid is also available in generic form (Depakene), which comes in 250-mg capsules and 250 mg/5 mL syrup. Peak serum levels are reached in 1 to 4 hours after ingestion, and the half-life is about 8 to 12 hours. The drug is metabolized in the liver and excreted in the urine in modified form. The approximate target range is 50 to 100 mg/L. The manufacturer suggests initiation of therapy with a dosage of about 10 to 15 mg/kg/day, to be increased at weekly intervals by about 5 to 10 mg/kg per day to a maximal dosage of 60 mg/kg/day. A common final regimen is 250 to 500 mg orally, two to four times per day.

About one in five patients taking valproate has significant side effects, commonly GI upset, drowsiness, rash, reversible hair loss, weight loss (or more frequently gain), ataxia, tremor, or hyperactivity. A limited number of studies suggest that valproate inhibits platelet aggregation and may prolong the bleeding time, but this effect is poorly documented. There may be a dose-dependent fall in platelets. The health risk from use of valproate that has received the greatest attention is *hepatic toxicity*. Thirty-seven fatalities from hepatic failure associated with use of valproate were reported in the United States between 1978 and 1984 (50). Among patients receiving valproate as monotherapy, the calculated rate of fatality from hepatic injury was 1 per 37,000. This rate was much higher for children younger than 2 years of age and for children receiving polytherapy. These two risk factors together resulted in a fatality rate from hepatic injury of 1 per 500 children. In contrast, no fatalities from hepatic injury were reported in patients older than 10 years of age who were receiving monotherapy. Several patients have developed serious episodes of pancreatitis while taking valproate. Valproate has not yet replaced ethosuximide as the drug of choice for absence epilepsy unless there are concurrent atypical absence attacks or tonic–clonic seizures. There may be drug interactions with aspirin, warfarin, cimetidine, phenothiazines, antacids, the benzodiazepines, and other AEDs such as phenytoin, carbamazepine, and lamotrigine.

Phenobarbital

In past decades, phenobarbital was a drug of choice for GTCSs. It is now a drug of last resort for a variety of seizure types. Phenobarbital has been used in the pediatric age group, where it may be better tolerated than phenytoin because it does not cause cosmetic side effects; however, it can cause significant behavioral side effects (hyperactivity in up to 40% of children).

Phenobarbital is a long-lasting drug. The GI absorption is slow, so it takes 10 to 12 hours for levels to reach their peak after an oral dose, compared with 20 minutes after an intravenous dose. The drug is detoxified by the liver and excreted by the kidney, but the dosage need be only slightly reduced in renal failure. The serum half-life is about 72 hours, ranging from 37 to 96 hours. Therapeutic levels are 15 to 40 mg/L. Phenobarbital is a potent inducer of liver enzymes and leads to rapid tolerance, as well as to alteration of kinetics of numerous other medications. The dosage of phenobarbital is 1 to 3 mg/kg/day, or about 100 mg/day for the average adult. Little justification can be made for giving it in divided doses. Available tablet strengths are 15, 30, 60, and 100 mg; elixir of 15 mg/5 mL and 20 mg/5 mL.

The main *acute side effect* of phenobarbital in adults is sedation. After a few weeks, partial tolerance to the sedation usually develops. In elderly patients, phenobarbital can cause confusion and respiratory depression. Subtle or overt personality changes caused by phenobarbital probably occur more often than is generally recognized, especially in the elderly. Ataxia and nystagmus are common in all patients at high dosages. Occasionally, there is idiosyncratic allergy, with accompanying dermatitis or GI symptoms. Connective tissue problems may occur. Phenobarbital must be administered with caution to potential drug or alcohol abusers or to unreliable patients who might precipitously discontinue their medicine. There are drug interactions with warfarin, β-blockers, and corticosteroids, and possible interactions with acetaminophen, chloramphenicol, chlorpromazine, cimetidine, cyclosporine, desipramine, furosemide, haloperidol, meperidine, methadone, methyldopa, phenacemide, prochlorperazine, propoxyphene, rifampicin, thioridazine, tricyclic antidepressants, verapamil, and other AEDs.

Primidone (Mysoline)

Primidone is a barbiturate used for treatment of CPSs and other partial epilepsies (usually as a drug of last resort). It has also been used in place of phenobarbital for treatment of GTCSs or focal seizures and epilepsies, when the latter drug has failed, but it should not be a drug of first choice for these conditions. Primidone is in part excreted unchanged and in part metabolized to phenobarbital and to phenylethylmalonamide (PEMA). Serum levels of primidone and PEMA can be ascertained, but it often suffices just to confirm that a therapeutic steady-state level of phenobarbital is present. To benefit from the short-lived primidone and PEMA, each of which has some antiepileptic action, primidone must be given in three or four divided doses. A therapeutic dosage is usually about 250 mg orally three or four times a day, but the initial dosages should be much lower to avoid inducing extreme sedation. It is reasonable to start with 125 to 250 mg daily, with increments each week, until therapeutic effect, therapeutic levels, unacceptable sedation, or the maximal dosage of 2 grams per day is reached. If patients are taking other AEDs, it is better to start with a dosage of 100 to 125 milligrams per day. The dosage should be reduced by about half in patients with significant renal failure. Strengths available are 50- and 250-mg tablets and suspension.

Side effects and drug interactions of primidone parallel those of phenobarbital, except that primidone tends to be more sedating.

Ethosuximide (Zarontin)

Ethosuximide is the drug of choice for treatment of absence epilepsy in children when there are concerns for potential hepatotoxicity from valproic acid, and absence seizures are the only seizure type. It is as effective as valproate in controlling absence seizures. It has little efficacy in other types of seizures, and patients with mixed seizure types may respond better to valproate. Peak plasma levels are reached 3 to 7 hours after oral ingestion in children and 2 to 4 hours after ingestion in adults. It is only minimally protein bound, with a volume of distribution of 70% of body weight; it has minimal interaction with other AEDs. The half-life is about 30 hours in children, rising to 60 hours in adults, and 6 to 12 days, respectively, is required to reach steady state. Elimination is primarily by metabolism, with urinary excretion of the metabolites. Absence seizures appear to be controlled by blood levels of about 25 to 165 milligrams per liter, with an average of about 60 mg/L. Levels of 150 mg/L may be needed and tolerated. Dose-related side effects include anxiety, depression, behavioral and psychiatric disturbances, nausea, vomiting, anorexia, fatigue, headache, lethargy, and dizziness. Liver function tests and complete blood counts are recommended monthly for 6 months by the manufacturer and occasionally thereafter. Ethosuximide is supplied as syrup (250 mg/5 mL) and as capsules (250 mg).

Clonazepam (Klonopin)

Clonazepam is a benzodiazepine, closely related to diazepam, that is used principally for treatment of myoclonus. It is not approved for treatment of partial seizures but has been used effectively for these conditions in Europe. Clonazepam is an oral medicine, with a serum half-life of 20 to 40 hours. Serum levels vary from 0.05 to 0.7 mg/L and correlate only very roughly with clinical effect. Because of the sedative effect of the medicine, therapy is usually initiated very gradually, beginning with 0.01 to 0.15 mg/kg, and increased every third day to clinical effect or to maintenance at 0.1 to 0.2 mg/kg/day. In adults the daily maximal dosage is 20 mg. Clonazepam commonly produces drowsiness, ataxia, and behavioral changes and can also cause dizziness and decreased muscle tone. Strengths available are 0.5-, 1-, and 2-mg tablets.

AED Formulations for Rapid Administration

In the acute treatment of seizures, fosphenytoin (Cerebyx) and intravenous valproate (Depakon) (both mentioned previously) are used when rapid intravenous AED supplementation is indicated or a patient cannot take oral preparations. A new rectal diazepam gel (Diastat) has been formulated in prefilled, unit-dose, rectal delivery systems containing 2.5, 5, 10, 15, or 20 mg of diazepam with specialized applicators for children and adults. This product overcomes many of the problems associated with rectal administration by non–health professional caregivers. Rapid plasma concentrations are reached within 15 minutes, and multicenter studies have shown the safety and efficacy of this formulation for reducing seizure frequency in children and adults with acute repetitive seizures, thus forestalling the otherwise necessary admission of the patient to an emergency department.

Newer Antiepileptic Drugs

Newer agents are becoming increasingly available in the United States. Experience with these medications has been gained predominantly in European and American trials. These drugs are often FDA approved for add-on therapy, but they are gaining popularity for use earlier in the treatment of epilepsy because of their *lower side-effect profiles*. They are usually more expensive.

Felbamate (Felbatol)

Felbamate (FDA-approved in 1993) is a drug that has been tested as add-on therapy for drug-resistant CPSs with or without secondary generalization and in patients with Lennox–Gastaut syndrome in several European and American trials.

An oral dose has a half-life of about 20 hours as monotherapy, or 14 hours in patients receiving poly pharmacy, and a volume of distribution of 0.8 L/kg.

Typical dosing regimens vary from 2,400 to 3,600 mg/day. Felbamate may increase phenytoin levels but decrease carbamazepine levels. Little effect has been noted on valproate levels. Felbamate (Felbatol) is available in 400-mg and 600-mg tablets and in suspension.

Side effects include mild problems such as weight loss, nausea, blurred vision, diplopia, headache, and ataxia, as well as severe problems including aplastic anemia (more than 30 reported cases, with 10 deaths) and primary hepatotoxicity (liver failure reported in about 20 cases, with some deaths). At present the drug is largely restricted to use for patients who have epilepsy that cannot be controlled by other AEDs, and in whom the morbidity from epilepsy is believed to outweigh the morbidity risk from felbamate. The patient must sign an informed consent form.

Gabapentin (Neurontin)

This GABA analog (FDA-approved in 1994) was developed and used as an AED based on the GABAergic theory of epileptogenesis; however, it probably does not directly enhance GABA, although whole-brain GABA levels may be increased. Gabapentin is not protein bound, does not alter other AED levels, and is not metabolized. The half-life is 5 to 7 hours. Capsules of 100, 300, and 400 mg as well as tablets of 600 and 800 mg are made.

Clinical trials so far have been as an add-on AED in refractory partial epilepsies with or without secondary generalization. There are usually few if any side effects (Table 88.6), although limb edema has been reported. It is now available in generic form (gabapentin) with dosing at 100-mg, 300-mg, and 400-mg capsules.

Lamotrigine (Lamictal)

Lamotrigine is structurally unrelated to any other AED in current use. Its antiepileptic action is probably related to its inhibitory effect on glutamate release and stabilization of neuronal membrane voltage-sensitive sodium channels. There are over 4.8 million patient exposures.

It appears to be effective in patients with intractable CPSs with or without secondary generalization; patients with primary GTCSs, atypical absences, or nonconvulsive status epilepticus; and some patients with Lennox–Gastaut syndrome. It has also been approved for monotherapy when a patient who is already on an enzyme-inducing AED such as phenytoin or carbamazepine or an enzyme-inhabiting drug such as valproate is then weaned off that medication and maintained on lamotrigine.

The pharmacokinetics in normal human subjects show complete bioavailability, a very long plasma half-life (24 ± 5 to 7 hours), linear kinetics, and approximately 60% protein binding when used as monotherapy.

Enzyme-inducing AEDs reduce its half-life, necessitating b.i.d. dosing while valproate increases it, often to 24 hours. Lamotrigine does not appear to alter other AED levels, but will decrease OCP levels. The drug is well tolerated and side effects are few particularly modest or minimal lethargy in many. Skin rashes, sometimes severe but reversible, occur in about the same percentage of patients as for those starting phenytoin or carbamazepine, if drug escalation is gradual, following new labeling guidelines. The incidence of skin rashes falls the more gradually the drug is started. Diplopia, dizziness, nausea and vomiting, drowsiness, and headache also occur in a small percentage of users.

The drug may be started at 50 mg each night for 2 weeks, 50 mg twice daily for 2 weeks, then 100 mg twice daily, increasing in steps of 50 mg every 2 weeks until seizure control, clinical toxicity, or a maximum dosage of 600 to 700 mg/day is encountered. It may be started as low as 15 mg/day. Initial target levels may be 150 to 200 mg/day on monotherapy or 300 mg to 500 mg as adjunctive therapy. In patients who are also taking valproate, lamotrigine should be started at 25 mg every other day, increasing by 25 mg every 2 weeks so as to minimize the incidence of rash. Lamotrigine serum levels may be used as markers of patient compliance. Lamictal is available in 25-mg, 100-mg, 150-mg and 200-mg tablets with 2-mg, 5-mg, and 25-mg chewable (dispersible tablets).

Topiramate (Topamax)

Topiramate was approved in early 1997 for use as *adjunctive therapy* in adults with partial seizures. It probably has multiple mechanisms of action, including modulating sodium channels, enhancing the effect of gamma-aminobutyric acid (GABA), and decreasing the excitability of brain cells. More than 3 million patients have taken it, with a greater than 50% reduction in seizures in 35% to 44% of patients taking 400 mg/day in early clinical trials. Topiramate has a time to maximum concentration of about 2 hours, a bioavailability of approximately 88% unaffected by food, and little plasma protein binding (13% to 17%). It has linear pharmacokinetics, is not extensively metabolized, and is predominantly excreted by the kidneys. It has limited pharmacokinetic interactions, and its half-life makes it suitable for twice-daily dosing. Clinical studies show that it has no effect on carbamazepine but may increase phenytoin levels in some patients. The side-effect profile is similar to those of most other AEDs, and most side effects are not serious. They occur in the first weeks of therapy and usually resolve by the fourth month. Side effects are predominantly CNS related, including dizziness, drowsiness, and problems with coordination. There is a 1.5% incidence of kidney stones and rare reports in patients with acute myopia of angle closure glaucoma under 40 years of age. Tingling of the tongue, mouth, and digits is frequent. Word finding and other cognitive problems are reported in 10% to 20%, some of which can be moderated by lower ascension rates and lower target levels. Oral contraceptive effectiveness may be affected. The medication is available in 25-mg, 100-mg, and 200-mg tablets with 15-mg and 25-mg sprinkle capsules. Therapy should be initiated at a dosage of 25 mg/day and gradually increased over several weeks to a recommended dosage of 200 mg to 400 mg/day in two divided doses. At doses greater than 200 mg, liver enzyme induction can occur and affect, among others, OCPs.

Tiagabine (Gabitril)

Tiagabine was approved in late 1997 for adjunctive therapy for partial-onset seizures in adults and children 12 years and older. Tiagabine was specifically designed to inhibit the uptake of GABA and prolong its action after synaptic release. Clinical trials have shown it to be effective as an *add-on drug* for patients with intractable focal seizures; 26% of patients have a 50% or greater reduction in focal seizures (51). A reduction of 50% or more of CPSs was seen in 20% to 30% of patients. Tiagabine should be started at 4 mg once daily and increased by 4 mg the first week and 8 mg weekly thereafter to 32 to 56 mg/day. It should be taken with food, in divided doses (two to four times per day), with the largest dose at bedtime. Tablets are available in 2-mg, 4-mg, 12-mg, 16-mg, and 20-mg strengths; side effects include dizziness, confusion, tiredness, GI upset, encephalopathy, and nonconvulsive status epilepticus.

Oxcarbazepine (Trileptal)

Oxcarbazepine is a 10-keto analog of carbamazepine and is active as a prodrug, having similar efficacy but purportedly lower side effects than carbamazepine. It is effective against partial seizures.

Oxcarbazepine is metabolized to the pharmacologically active 10-monohydroxy metabolite. Protein binding is relatively low. The drug does not autoinduce and does not produce an epoxide that normally accounts for most side effects seen with carbamazepine. It is a less potent cytochrome P-450 enzyme inducer, and when patients are switched from carbamazepine to oxcarbazepine, levels of phenytoin, lamotrigine, and topiramate may rise.

In trials at the highest dose of 2,400 mg/day, 50% of patients had a 50% reduction in seizures, compared with 13% in the placebo group. Lower does may be better tolerated as adjunctive therapy. There are more than 1.8 million patient exposures.

Oxcarbazepine has been approved for initial monotherapy in adults and children with partial seizures. The side-effect profile is the same as for carbamazepine, but side effects reportedly occur less frequently and neutropenia is not seen. However, hyponatremia not infrequently occurs. Hypersensitivity and rash reactions are less common than with carbamazepine.

Initial doses are 150 to 300 mg/day in monotherapy, increasing to clinical effect, usually at about 900 to 2,400 mg/day. As adjunctive therapy, initiation is recommended at 150 mg twice daily, with weekly increments of 600 mg/day or less for better tolerability. Serum levels of monohydroxy derivative are available with a target range of 50 to 200 mmol/mL. Oxcarbazepine is available in 150-mg, 300-mg, and 600-mg tablets with a 300-mg/5 mL suspension.

Levetiracetam (Keppra)

This drug has a unique preclinical profile with an efficacy in various animal models of seizures. Mechanic levetiracetam absorption is not affected by food. It has very low protein binding and is not hepatically metabolized. Two thirds of the drug is excreted renally, unchanged. There are no known drug interactions, and levetiracetam is neither an inducer nor an inhibitor of cytochrome P-450 enzymes. It has no effect on oral contraceptives, digoxin, warfarin, or other AEDs. No dosage adjustment is needed for hepatic impairment, but adjustments are needed for renal impairment with creatinine clearance less than 50 mL/minute. Therefore, the dosage may need to be adjusted in elderly patients. Trials have shown a 50% reduction in 23% to 42% of patients with levetiracetam dosages of 1,000 to 3,000 mg/day, compared with 10% to 17% for placebo. At the higher dosage, 8% of patients became seizure free.

The drug is well-tolerated with few adverse events, including somnolence, dizziness, anorexia, which are usually mild to moderate. Of the about one million individuals exposed to date, few serious hepatic, renal, or cardiovascular adverse events have been found. Rash is rare, but fatigue, irritability or personality changes are not.

Levetiracetam is started at 500 mg twice daily, or more gradually, and increased as tolerated to 1,000 mg or 1,500 mg orally twice daily. Levetiracetam is available in 250-mg, 500-mg, and 750-mg tablets and 100 mg/mL oral solution. Target levels typically are 3 mg/L to 20 mg/L.

Zonisamide (Zonegran)

Preclinical studies have suggested a similar profile to phenytoin, but with some action at other channels. The drug is reduced via a cytochrome P-450 (CYP 3A4) and by *N*-acetylene, with about one third excreted unchanged in the urine. The half-life is about 60 hours, and therefore steady state is reached in about 2 weeks. Hepatic metabolism of zonisamide is increased by enzyme-inducing drugs, but protein binding is relatively moderate (40%). Zonisamide neither induces nor inhibits hepatic enzymes; does not affect levels of phenytoin, carbamazepine, or valproate; and does not autoinduce. However, phenytoin and carbamazepine decrease the half-life of zonisamide to about 27 and 38 hours, respectively. Therefore, after enzyme-inducing AEDs are withdrawn, zonisamide levels may increase. Because of its renal excretion, adjustments should be made in renally compromised and elderly patients. With dosages between 100 and 600 mg/day, seizure reductions in up to about one third of patients were seen after exclusion of a placebo response. Zonisamide may be particularly effective in progressive myoclonus epilepsies. Side effects include dizziness, somnolence, headache, anorexia, nausea, and irritability, particularly with more rapid up titration.

Zonisamide is a sulfonamide and may exhibit similar hypersensitivity reactions, occasionally with Stevens–Johnson syndrome. Rash may occur early in treatment. Aplastic anemia and agranulocytosis have been reported. About 1% of patients have renal stones, possibly because of the drug's effect as a carbonic anhydrase inhibitor. Similarly, mouth and digit tingling are not rare. Initial dosing is 100 mg/day, with up titration by 100 mg/day every 2 weeks as tolerated. Treatment may be once or twice daily, and dosages as low as 100 mg/day have been reported to be effective. Optimal plasma zonisamide levels for seizure therapy are reported to be 10 to 40 mg/mL, but evidence is scant. Zonegran is available in 25-mg, 50-mg, and 100-mg capsules.

Other Antiepileptic Drugs

Practitioners often use diazepam, clorazepate, or chlordiazepoxide to treat seizures under certain circumstances. Benzodiazepines (other than clonazepam and clorazepate) have drawbacks for long-term therapy; AED effects tend to diminish as sedative effects accumulate.

Vagal Nerve Stimulation for Refractory Seizures

Vagus nerve stimulation (VNS) is a recent treatment for refractory seizures; it provides a programmed, regular stimulus via coiled electrodes from a chest-implanted generator to the left cervical vagal nerve. The pulse generator is powered by a lithium battery connected to a helical bipolar lead, which is, in turn, attached to the midcervical portion of the left vagal nerve, delivering a biphasic current continuously cycling between on and off periods. Animal data suggest that VNS stimulates small unmyelinated C fibers, with the locus ceruleus playing a crucial role in the mechanism of VNS, because chemical lesioning reduces the anticonvulsant effect of stimulation. VNS inhibits seizures in multiple animal models, including maximum electroshock, penicillin, and pentylenetetrazol models. It also measurably alters cerebral blood flow in the thalamus, cerebellum, and cortex and activates inhibitory structures in the brain.

Several clinical studies using active-control, parallel-blinded formats revealed a substantial reduction in seizure frequency. Long-term studies have shown a sustained reduction of 50% or more in 37% of patients, with a 43% responder rate at 2 and 3 years. Common side effects include voice change and hoarseness. Reductions compared to baseline were about 35% at 1 year, increasing to 44% at 2 and 3 years. Other side effects included paresthesias, headache, and shortness of breath.

Careful patient selection and evaluation by epilepsy centers are optimal techniques for the choice of VNS for refractory epilepsy.

REFERRAL TO A NEUROLOGIST

The role of a consulting neurologist to help with the evaluation and management of epilepsy depends on the experience of the primary physician. Table 88.7 lists common problems for which referral may be helpful.

TABLE 88.7 When to Refer or Hospitalize the Patient with Seizures

Diagnostic Issues for Referral
Question about whether a seizure took place
New abnormality or neurological examination
Focal seizures
Focality on the EEG
Uncertainty about cause
Therapeutic Issues for Referral
Complex medication adjustments
Patient does not respond to appropriate AED
Patient has significant medication side effects
Patient wishes to become pregnant
Patient wishes to taper off medication
Significant change in the pattern of seizures
When to Hospitalize
Most new-onset seizures
New focal signs on examination
Obtunded or prolonged postictal patients
Febrile patients
Crescendo pattern of seizures
All cases of status epilepticus
Barbiturate and benzodiazepine withdrawal seizures
Possibility of rapidly expanding mass lesion
Seizures after recent head trauma
Need for special inpatient studies
Consideration for neurosurgery

AED, antiepileptic drug, CT, computed tomography; EEG, electroencephalogram; MRI, magnetic resonance imaging.

HOSPITALIZATION

Few general statements can be made about the need for hospital admission for seizure patients, because the availability of monitoring systems, emergency room holding rooms, and inpatient beds varies from locale to locale. Table 88.7 shows a set of reasonable guidelines. Patients brought to offices or emergency rooms after a first seizure are usually admitted to facilitate the diagnostic workup and to observe the patient in case a serious underlying cause (e.g., meningitis, subdural hematoma) is present. This principle has exceptions. A young patient with a normal examination and a reliable family may be evaluated in an ambulatory setting. Any patient with new focal signs on examination should be admitted, as should obtunded patients, febrile patients, and those whose postictal lethargy persists for longer than 30 minutes. A patient with a crescendo pattern of seizures, with several in one day, especially if they are tonic–clonic seizures, should be admitted to a hospital immediately. *Status epilepticus,* a condition in which continuous or back-to-back seizures occur without intervening return of consciousness for at least 30 minutes, is a medical emergency and requires immediate hospitalization. Barbiturate withdrawal seizures may become fulminant; therefore, patients having seizures in this setting should be admitted. If the possibility exists of a rapidly expanding mass lesion, such as tumor, abscess, or possible hematoma after head trauma, then admission should not be delayed. Reasons for elective admission include a need for special inpatient studies (arteriography, continuous monitoring), evaluation for possible neurosurgical procedures for intractable epilepsy, and, lastly, trials of supervised drug management to check for noncompliance as a factor in treatment failure.

Admission usually is not needed for patients who are known to have chronically recurrent seizures, whose pattern of seizures is stable, whose cause is established or is thought to be idiopathic on the basis of a prior thorough workup, who have fully recovered from recent seizures, who have normal examinations (or static documented old deficits), and who are reliable enough to return for followup.

SOCIAL ISSUES AND PATIENT EDUCATION

Once a serious underlying cause has been ruled out, there is a tendency for physicians to view epilepsy as a benign disease. From the viewpoint of the patient, this is often far from the case. Seizures are distressing for every patient and for the patient's family. Fear of having a seizure can cause people with epilepsy to withdraw from society, and those who are willing to compete may be faced with nearly insurmountable discrimination.

The Commission for the Control of Epilepsy and Its Consequences (1977) found that the unemployment rate among people with epilepsy is twice the national average, and the underemployment rate is even higher. Suspension of a driver's license (discussed later) may make it almost impossible to get to work. Children may be denied participation in sports or moved unnecessarily to special sections in school. Persons with epilepsy marry less often than matched subjects without epilepsy. A significant fraction of the public believe that people with epilepsy are likely to be physically unattractive. Because of these and other social stigmata associated with epilepsy, it is important to focus on the patient's overall functioning rather than simply on seizure control. The patient and family should be counseled regularly to help them address the concerns that limit full participation in society.

Patients should be told that epilepsy is a medical illness, because too many believe that it is a punishment for some past abuse. Whereas a single or even multiple reactive seizures (e.g., to alcohol) should not be labeled as epilepsy, definite epilepsy should not be mislabeled as something else in an attempt to avoid facing the diagnosis. The patient should know that individual seizures usually do not cause measurable brain damage and that the condition does not lead to mental deterioration. Unfortunately, sudden unexpected death in epilepsy does occur. The prognosis for most patients with epilepsy is good.

Restrictions of Activity

Patients often ask for guidelines about what they can and cannot do. Clearly, if identifiable precipitants such as sleep deprivation, flashing lights, alcohol, or particular medicines can be avoided, the patient should be so advised. Maximal activity consistent with avoidance of risk of personal injury should be the goal. The specifics must be formulated by a physician familiar with the individual patient and the patient's pattern of seizures. Patients with nocturnal seizures need not be restricted during the day. Contact sports are safe for people with infrequent seizures. Common sense dictates limits on activities during which a seizure could be fatal—for example, piloting an airplane, rock climbing, or scuba diving. Some potentially hazardous activities, such as swimming, may be acceptable if provisions can be made for proper supervision. Seizures are not contraindications to strenuous activities, including sex. Alcohol consumption (in moderation) can be enjoyed by most patients with impunity (5,19,52).

Driving a Motor Vehicle

Overall, motor vehicle accident rates for people with epilepsy are about twice the rates in control subjects. The actual proportion of all traffic accidents caused by people with epilepsy has been estimated at 1/10,000 accidents (5,19,53). It is estimated that 6/10,000 of all deaths at the wheel are from natural causes, including epilepsy, and that 5,000/10,000 are caused by alcohol use. Approximately 12% to 20% of accidents involving people with epilepsy occur with the patient's first seizure. As indicated by these statistics, seizures at the wheel do occur and can represent both personal and public dangers. The key element of increased risk is blunting or loss of consciousness. Seizures without this element (e.g., partial simple motor seizures) do not affect the risk of driving, and affected patients are usually exempted from restrictions, although in some, determining momentary loss of consciousness is problematic.

Some states require that physicians directly report occurrence of seizures to the Department of Motor Vehicles (DMV); others require only documentation in the medical record that the patient has been informed of the risks for traffic accidents and has been instructed to contact the DMV for a hearing (see Epilepsy Foundation, www.hopkinsbayview.org/PAMreferences). Patients and physicians should be honest in their communications; both are potentially liable for consequences of inaccurate or incomplete information. Generally, the physician should address the medical facts of a case and leave the final determination of licensing to the state authorities. Often, if an applicant has regular lapses of consciousness, the license will be suspended until a period of 3 months to 2 years without seizures has elapsed (depending on the state); the recent national trend has been to consider shorter periods of suspension.

Employment

It is illegal to discriminate against handicapped people, including people with epilepsy, in the job market. If a person with seizures is unemployed or dissatisfied with work, one should consider prompt referral to a vocational rehabilitation agency for possible retraining, patient and employer education, or advice on legal action. *The Epilepsy Foundation* (4351 Garden City Drive #500, Landover, MD 20774, telephone 301-459-3700; www.efa.org) is a central nonprofit organization that can serve as a source for information and action on social and occupational aspects of epilepsy; at least one chapter exists in each state. Their training and placement service has been effective in training people with epilepsy for work and in finding them employment, either in the general work pool or in sheltered workshops. The same local organizations may further aid patients with regular group counseling for those who cannot live independently, or by providing for regular home visits by visiting nurses and other medical personnel.

Some patients with difficult-to-control seizures should be advised to apply for *Social Security medical disability compensation* (see criteria in Chapter 9).

Pregnancy

Special problems are raised by a woman with epilepsy who is, or wishes to become, pregnant (54). Approximately 0.4% of all pregnancies occur in mothers with seizures. In women with epilepsy, child-bearing carries an above-average risk for eclampsia, vaginal hemorrhage, and complicated labor. The rates of premature birth and perinatal death are increased. Seizures become more difficult to control during pregnancy in approximately 30% to 50% of cases, easier to control in approximately 10% to 30%, and unchanged in the rest. Rarely, pregnancy can induce a new onset of recurring idiopathic seizures. AEDs—phenytoin, carbamazepine, valproate, and, to a lesser extent, most of the other agents—are *teratogenic*. The teratogenic effects of most of the newer AEDs are unknown. Studies suggest that the incidence of congenital abnormalities, particularly cleft lip, cleft palate, and cardiac defects, is two to six times higher in offspring of drug-treated mothers with epilepsy. Valproate has specifically been associated with a 1% to 2% risk of neural tube closure defects and 6% to 9% of major malformations. A minimum of almost 400 first trimester monotherapy exposures is needed to establish with 80%

power, twofold increase in major malformation rate, assuming an expected 3% background incidence. A number of pregnancy registries has provided data, in aggregate, to suggest that the background rate of major malformations in women with epilepsy is 2.1%. For the older AEDs, the North American Registry has shown a major malformation rate of 6.5% (5/77) for phenobarbital and 8.8% for valproate. The UK Registry revealed 2.4% for women with epilepsy on no AED; 2.3% major malformation rate of 700 pregnancies for carbamazepine, and 2.1% in 390 pregnancies for lamotrigine.

Authorities agree that tonic–clonic seizures can produce anoxic, ischemic, or traumatic damage to a fetus and that this risk must be balanced against the teratogenic potential of medication. The best solution to this dilemma is *careful planning*. Physicians should ask their patients not only to plan pregnancies but also to alert the physician to the plan months in advance. Before pregnancy, special efforts can be made to taper medications or to switch to phenobarbital or carbamazepine, which may be less teratogenic than phenytoin or valproate. However, most authorities agree that the AED to be used in pregnancy should be the one best suited for the patient and her epilepsy. Switching drugs after conception, i.e., when the patient discovers that she is pregnant, usually is not recommended, partly because the greatest vulnerability of the developing fetus is early in the pregnancy. Brief CPSs or absence seizures pose no known risk to a fetus, and a decision may be made by the patient to tolerate them during pregnancy rather than take medication. If pregnancy is unexpected, an ongoing successful regimen of AEDs should probably be continued, to avoid the possibility of fulminant withdrawal seizures during a critical obstetric stage. Ultimately, all of these relative risks must be discussed among primary and specialist physicians, the patient, and her partner, so that a mutually satisfactory plan can be derived. The problems of child-bearing are increased for mothers with epilepsy, but not greatly, and only the severely disabled epileptic woman should be flatly discouraged from having children.

Counseling should also include advice on prenatal vitamins, folate, postnatal help with the baby, and further followup in case AEDs need to be adjusted in the postpartum period. No clearly established optimal dosage of folate acid or folate has been established, but dosages recommended usually range between 1 and 4 mg/day, the latter if there is a history of neural tube defects.

Mothers taking AEDs who wish to breast-feed may do so, because the amount of AEDs excreted in breast milk is generally relatively low, and the developing baby was exposed often to even higher doses while *in utero*. Data on the newer AEDs are scarce, but breast milk exposure would be low for topiramate and medium to high for clonazepam, oxcarbazepine, zonisamide, levetiracetam, and tiagabine.

Potential parents wonder about the *likelihood that their child will have epilepsy* if they or one of their children have epilepsy. Although there are methodologic problems in performing studies to answer this question, it can generally be said that there is a risk of about 1 in 40 of transmitting idiopathic generalized epilepsy from the mother. When seizures result from head trauma, tumor, drug withdrawal, or other identified causes, then the risk of heritability is not increased.

There is an increasing body of evidence of long-term effects of antiepileptic drugs. Several studies on enzyme-inducing AEDs, have suggested that chronic usage extending beyond 5 years (in both men and women), particularly after the age of 50, an increasing incidence of osteopenia and osteoporosis. These latter conditions predispose to fractures and their consequent morbidity. With prolonged, chronic enzyme-inducing AED usage and particularly with an unexpected fracture, dual-energy x-ray absorptiometry (DEXA) scans are recommended. Optimal calcium and vitamin D therapy has not been determined, but many practitioners advocate 500 mg twice daily of calcium and 600 international units (IUs) of vitamin D for patients at risk. Higher dosages, or the use of bisphosphonates may be recommended for worse bone disease.

Valproate has been implicated in increase in body mass index often carrying with it, a tendency toward insulin resistance, hyperandrogenism, hirsutism, and a polycystic ovarian syndrome (PCOS) (see Chapter 101). Initial studies showed a high prevalence of PCOS in valproate-treated women when valproate is started before or after the age of 20 years. Further studies to investigate these findings are ongoing in the United States and the United Kingdom. Characteristically, women with PCOS have anovulatory cycles. In affected patients, improvement in anovulatory cycles and other aspects of this syndrome has been obtained by choosing an alternate AED.

Family Education

Families must be told how to *behave during a seizure*; too often, frantic efforts to treat the seizure result in extreme anxiety and broken teeth. Seizures should be allowed to run their course; unless convulsions become continuous or nearly continuous (status epilepticus) they are not dangerous, and no first aid can shorten them. The mouth should not be forced open so that spoons, fingers, towels, pencils, or other objects can be pushed in. The family should be informed that it is impossible to "swallow the tongue." The person undergoing a seizure should be moved away from sharp corners and heights and turned on his or her side to decrease the risk of aspiration. Forcible restraint during a tonic–clonic phase is of no value, and during the automatisms of CPSs restraints may increase agitation. There is little need to fear behavior during automatisms, because directed violence is extremely rare.

Concerned family members may be very helpful in *promoting improved seizure control.* They should be encouraged to discuss compliance, the cost of a pharmaceutical regimen, and how the seizures or drug toxicities affect school, work, and social relations. Patients should be encouraged to keep a log of their seizures, medication times, side effects, and possible precipitating stresses. Perfect control of epilepsy with no toxicity is an ideal attained in only a minority of cases; in the remainder, patient, family, and physician can decide in concert how to balance the inconvenience of seizures against the unpleasant side effects of medication and thereby achieve the best possible results.

Medicolegal Issues

In addition to conducting discussions of the diagnosis, management, prognosis of epilepsy, and potential adverse effects of treatment, it is important to document in the patient's record the principal points that have been addressed with the patient and the family. One should offer patients written information advising them of driving laws, notify them of their obligation to alert the DMV, and warning them to avoid dangerous activities and occupations. They should also have full written records of medications and their side effects, in lay terms, and instructions to contact the physician for any worrisome side effects. In addition, all women of child-bearing age should be counseled regarding fetal teratogenicity effects on fetal and subsequent postnatal cognitive development, possible change in maternal seizure frequency, and the need or lack of need for AED therapy (see Pregnancy). Many of these essential facts are covered well in patient education literature available from the Epilepsy Foundation (see Employment).

Attention to these aspects of patient and family education and a close, compassionate, and open doctor–patient relationship are sound ways to limit malpractice exposure.

SPECIFIC REFERENCES*

1. Annegers JF. Epidemiology of epilepsy. In: Wyllie E, ed. The treatment of epilepsy: principles and practice. 2nd ed. Baltimore: Williams & Wilkins, 1997:165.
2. Commission on classification and terminology of the International League Against Epilepsy. Proposal for revised classification of epilepsies and epileptic syndromes. Epilepsia 1989;30:389.
3. Berkovic SF. Generalized absence seizures. In: Wyllie E, ed. The treatment of epilepsy: principles and practice. 3rd ed. Baltimore: Williams & Wilkins, 1997:451.
4. Benbadis SR, Lüders HO. Epileptic syndromes: an underutilized concept. Epilepsia 1996;37:1029.
5. Sander JWAS, Shorvon SD. Epidemiology of the epilepsies. J Neurol Neurosurg Psychiatry 1996;61:433.
6. Treiman DM. Seizure types and causes of epilepsy. Semin Neurol 1981;1:65.
7. Anderson DW, McLaurin RL. The national head and spinal cord injury survey. J Neurosurg 1980;53[Suppl S]:S1.
8. Annegers JF, Shirts SB, Hauser WA, et al. Risk of recurrence after an initial unprovoked seizure. Epilepsia 1986;27:43.
9. Hauser WA, Rich SS, Annegers YF, et al. Seizure recurrence after a first unprovoked seizure: an extended follow-up. Neurology 1990;40:1163.
10. Hopkins A, Garman A, Clarke C. The first seizure in adult life: value of clinical features, electroencephalography, and computerized tomographic scanning in prediction of seizure recurrence. Lancet 1988;1:721.
11. Annegers JF, Hauser WA, Elveback LR. Remission of seizures and relapse in patients with epilepsy. Epilepsia 1979;20:729.
12. Shorvon SD. The temporal aspects and prognosis in epilepsy. J Neurol Neurosurg Psychiatry 1984;47:1157.
13. Delgado-Escueta AV, Treiman DM, Wahs GO. The treatable epilepsies (second of two parts). N Engl J Med 1983;308:1508.
14. Goodridge DMG, Shorvon SD. Epileptic seizures in a population of 6,000: 1. Demography, diagnosis, and classification, and role of the hospital services. BMJ 1983;287:641.
15. MRC Antiepileptic Drug Withdrawal Study Group. Randomised study of antiepileptic drug withdrawal in patients in remission. Lancet 1991;337:1175.
16. Mattson RH, Cramer JA, Collins JF, et al. Prognosis for total control of complex partial and secondarily generalized tonic clonic seizures. Neurology 1996;47:68.
17. Reynolds EH, Elwes RCD, Shorvon SD. Why does epilepsy become intractable: prevention of chronic epilepsy. Lancet 1983;2:952.
18. Schmidt D. Prognosis of chronic epilepsy with complex partial seizures. J Neurol Neurosurg Psychiatry 1984;47:1274.
19. Tinuper P, Avoni P, Riva R, et al. The prognostic value of the electroencephalogram in antiepileptic drug withdrawal in partial epilepsies. Neurology 1996;47:76.
20. Schold C, Yarnell PR, Earnest MP. Origin of seizures in elderly patients. JAMA 1977;238:1177.
21. Hauser WA, Ng SKC, Brust JCM. Alcohol, seizures and epilepsy. Epilepsia 1988;29[Suppl 2]:S66.
22. Sampliner R, Iber FL. Diphenylhydantoin control of alcohol withdrawal seizures: results of a controlled study. JAMA 1974;230:1430.
23. Victor M, Brausch V. The role of abstinence in the genesis of alcoholic epilepsy. Epilepsia 1967;8:1.
24. Alldredge BK, Lowenstein DH, Simon RP. Placebo-controlled trial of intravenous diphenylhydantoin for short-term treatment of alcohol withdrawal seizures. Am J Med 1989;87:645.
25. Ng SK, Hauser WA, Brust JC, et al. Alcohol consumption and withdrawal in new-onset seizures. N Engl J Med 1988;319:666.
26. Morris HH, Estes ML, Gilmore R, et al. Chronic intractable epilepsy as the only symptom of primary brain tumor. Epilepsia 1993;34:1038.
27. Aicardi J. (ed.). Epilepsies as a presenting manifestation of brain tumors. In: Epilepsy in children. New York: Raven Press, 1986.
28. Luhdorf K, Jensen LK, Plesner AM. Epilepsy in the elderly: etiology of seizures in elderly. Epilepsia 1986;27:458.
29. Sung CY, Chu NS. Epileptic seizures in thrombotic stroke. J Neurol 1990;237:166.
30. Gupta SR, Naheedy MH, Elias D, et al. Postinfarction seizures: a clinical study. Stroke 1988;19:1477.
31. Shorvon CP, Shorvon S, Tallis R. Epilepsy as a warning sign for stroke. Lancet 2004;363:1184.
32. McArthur JC. Neurologic manifestations of AIDS. Medicine (Baltimore) 1987;66:407.
33. Engel JE Jr. Seizures and epilepsy. Philadelphia: FA Davis, 1989.
34. Oribe E, Rohullah A, Nissenbaum E, et al. Serum prolactin concentrations are elevated after syncope. Neurology 1996;47:60.
35. H, MacMillan JP, et al. Serum prolactin levels after epileptic seizures. Neurology 1984;34:1601.
36. Meierkord H, Shorvon S, Lightman S, et al. Comparison of the effects of frontal and temporal lobe partial seizures on prolactin levels. Arch Neurol 1992;49:225.
37. van Donselaar CA, Schimsheimer R-J, Geerts AT, et al. Value of the electroencephalogram in adult patients with untreated idiopathic first seizures. Arch Neurol 1992;49:231.
38. Browne TR, Holmes GL. Epilepsy. N Engl J Med 2001;344:1145.
39. Gastaut H, Tassinari CA. Epilepsies. In: Remand A, ed. Handbook of EEG and clinical neurophysiology, vol. 13, part A. Amsterdam: Elsevier, 1975.
40. Garcia-Herrero D, Fernádez-Torre, Barrasa J, et al. Abdominal epilepsy in an adolescent with bilateral perisylvian polymicrogyria. Epilepsia 1998;39:1370.
41. Bleck TP. Recurrence of tonic–clonic seizures after antiepileptic drugs. Neurology 1993;43:478.
42. Karceski S, Morrell M, Carpenter M. The expert consensus guidelines series: treatment of epilepsy. Epilep Behav 2001;2:A1.
43. Mattson RH, Cramer JA, Collins JF, et al. Comparison of carbamazepine, phenobarbital, phenytoin, and primidone in partial and secondarily generalized tonic-clonic seizures. N Engl J Med 1985;313:145.
44. Mattson RH, Cramer JA, Collins JF. Department

*Bold numerals denote published controlled clinical trials, meta-analyses, or consensus-based recommendations.

of Veterans Affairs Epilepsy Study No. 264 Group. A comparison of valproate with carbamazepine for the treatment of complex partial seizures and secondarily generalized tonic-clonic seizures in adults. N Engl J Med 1992;327:765.
45. Marson AG, Kadir ZA, Chadwick DW. New antiepileptic drugs: a systematic review of their efficacy and tolerability. BMJ 1996;313:1169.
46. Shorvon SD, Chadwick D, Galbraith AW, et al. One drug for epilepsy. BMJ 1978;1:474.
47. Browne TR, Le Duc B. Phenytoin: chemistry and bioinformation. In: Levy RH, Mattson RH, Meldrum BS, eds. Antiepileptic drugs. 4th ed. New York: Raven Press, 1995:235.
48. Buna DK. Antiepileptic drug withdrawal—a good idea! Pharmacotherapy 1998;18:235.
49. Practice parameter: a guideline for discontinuing antiepileptic drugs in seizure-free patients. Summary statement report of the Quality Standards Subcommittee of the American Academy of Neurology. Neurology 1996;47:600.
50. Dreifuss FE, Santilli N, Langer DJ, et al. Valproic acid hepatic fatalities: a retrospective review. Neurology 1987;37:379.
51. Richens A. Chadwick DW, Duncan JS, et al. Adjunctive treatment of partial seizures with Tiagabine: a placebo-controlled trial. Epilepsy Res 1995;21:37.
52. Mattson RH, Sturman JK, Gronowski ML, et al. Effects of alcohol intake in non-alcoholic epileptics. Neurology 1975;25:361.
53. van der Lugt PJ. Traffic accidents caused by epilepsy. Epilepsia 1975;16:747.
54. Morrell MI. Seizures and epilepsy in women. In: Neurologic disease in women, chap. 14. Kaplan PW (ed). New York: Demos Medical Publishing, Inc., 1998:189.

For annotated ***General References*** *and resources related to this chapter, visit www.hopkinsbayview.org/PAMreferences.*

Chapter 89

Dizziness, Vertigo, Motion Sickness, Syncope and Near Syncope, and Disequilibrium

Jeffrey L. Magaziner and Mark F. Walker

DIZZINESS

Dizziness is the ninth most common chief complaint in ambulatory settings (1). The word *dizzy*, however, is a very inexact term. It can refer to impending loss of consciousness, a feeling of motion or spatial disorientation, or imbalance. On the other hand, some patients use "dizziness" to refer to less specific subjective states such as fatigue or anxiety. Occasionally, patients use the word *dizzy* to mean sick. A correct diagnosis for a patient's complaint of dizziness is often possible on the basis of the history and physical examination. A limited number of diagnostic studies can aid the evaluation of selected patients, but these can be interpreted properly only in the light of information gained from the patient.

Categorizing a Patient's Dizziness

Evaluation of the dizzy patient starts with categorizing the exact nature of the symptoms. Categorization of symptoms can help determine what system is involved and give focus to the differential diagnosis. The major categories of dizziness are *vertigo,* the illusion that the patient or the environment is moving; *near syncope or syncope,* a sensation of impending faint or actual loss of consciousness; and *disequilibrium,* a sensation of impaired balance. Finally, some patients' symptoms simply cannot fit into a specific category and are termed nonspecific dizziness. When a patient has ill-defined dizziness that cannot be readily classified, the patient should be asked to *use words more specific*

TABLE 89.1 Categorization of Terms Used by Patients to Describe Dizziness

Vertigo	*Syncope or Presyncope*	*Disequilibrium*
Spinning of self	Fainting	Imbalance
Spinning of environment	Light-headedness	Tilting
Swaying	Woozy	Poor equilibrium
Twisting	Blackout	Impeding fall
Moving	Pass out	Unsteady
Weaving	Spells	Staggering
Rocking	Fall-out	Drunk
Rolling		Listing
Tilting spells		

than dizziness and should be asked to *describe a discrete recent episode.* It is important to ask the patient to describe what they mean by dizzy, rather than asking closed-ended questions like "do you sense the room spinning" in the beginning. Table 89.1 lists typical words they may use and potential categories. If the patient's initial account is too vague, the following questions may help:

- Is there actually the sensation of movement or rotation of you or the environment? (Positive response favors vertigo.)
- Is it a sensation that you might black out? (Positive response favors near syncope.)
- Is it a sensation of unsteadiness on your feet rather than in your head? (Positive response favors disequilibrium.)

Questions about associated auditory, neurologic, or cardiac symptoms may help classify the patient's problem more specifically. Additional important information includes how many episodes of dizziness the patient has had, how long they lasted, and whether there are any specific factors that can provoke episodes.

The patient who claims to be dizzy "right now" while sitting before the physician should be checked for hypotension, first while seated and then while standing, and examined for nystagmus (see Physical Examination).

As part of the preliminary inquiry, it is important to ask the patient whether dizziness has interfered with usual activities, especially driving a motor vehicle. This information will be important in management regardless of the cause of dizziness.

DISORDERS OF THE VESTIBULAR SYSTEM

The purpose of the vestibular system is to sense movement of the head and, through the vestibulo-ocular and vestibulospinal reflexes, to maintain stable vision and posture during movement. Thus, the symptoms of vestibular dysfunction include an inappropriate sense of motion (vertigo), imbalance, and the appearance that the visual world is moving (oscillopsia).

Basic Principles of Vestibular Function

To understand disorders of the vestibular system and their symptoms and signs, it is helpful to keep in mind basic vestibular anatomy and function. The peripheral organs of the vestibular system are the labyrinths. The cochlea is the portion of the labyrinth responsible for hearing (see Chapter 110). The vestibular labyrinth consists of the three semicircular canals (horizontal or lateral, anterior or superior, and posterior) and two gravity-sensitive structures (utricle and saccule) (see Fig. 110.1). Attached to the utricle and saccule are calcium carbonate crystals termed otoconia; these are important in the pathophysiology of benign paroxysmal positional vertigo (BPPV) (see Recurrent Vertigo). The semicircular canals sense angular rotations of the head, and the otoconia in the utricle and saccule sense linear (e.g., side-to-side) motion and the orientation of the head relative to gravity.

When the head is not moving, each vestibular nerve has an equal resting discharge rate, such that there is no net difference in the inputs from the two sides. Rotation of the head excites one labyrinth and inhibits the other, disturbing this balance. This signals the brain that the head is moving and generates the appropriate compensatory eye movement (in the direction opposite to head motion) to maintain steady gaze (*vestibuloocular reflex [VOR]*). For example, when the head rotates to the right, there is an increase in firing from the right horizontal canal. This causes the eyes to rotate to the left in the orbits, so that they remain fixed in space. This compensatory eye movement is called the slow phase of the VOR. If the head continues to rotate, these slow phases will be interrupted by rapid saccade-like movements in the opposite direction, termed quick phases. The combination of slow and quick phases is called *nystagmus. The direction of nystagmus is usually given by the direction of its quick phases,* even though it is the slow phases that reflect vestibular activity. Thus, prolonged rotation of the head to the right generates a right-beating nystagmus. This physiologic nystagmus maintains clear vision during head rotations.

Pathologic vestibular nystagmus results when one labyrinth or vestibular nerve is lesioned, removing the spontaneous discharge from that side and leaving the tonic input from the other side unopposed. The resulting imbalance creates the sensation of spinning and generates a nystagmus, in which *slow phases are directed toward the side of the lesion and quick phases toward the intact side*. Thus, an acute left vestibular lesion causes unopposed input from the right vestibular nerve and a right-beating nystagmus. With time, the brain readjusts central vestibular tone to compensate for the peripheral imbalance, sometimes leaving only minimal residual symptoms and signs.

VERTIGO

Vertigo is a sense of illusory movement, either of oneself or of the surrounding environment. Patients may report feelings of spinning, tilting, or tumbling. Vertigo generally indicates an imbalance in the vestibular system. This may result either from a peripheral lesion, involving one of the labyrinths or vestibular nerves (e.g., vestibular neuritis), or from a central lesion (e.g., infarction) within the vestibular pathways of the brainstem and cerebellum. It is important to keep in mind that bilateral labyrinthine lesions, such as from aminoglycoside ototoxicity, often do not cause vertigo because the lesion is symmetric, thus creating no net imbalance. Vestibular schwannomas (acoustic neuromas) and other slowly growing tumors affecting the vestibular nerve also do not commonly produce vertigo, because the resulting vestibular imbalance is compensated centrally as it develops. The most severe vertigo occurs with an acute unilateral peripheral vestibular lesion.

Evaluation of the Undiagnosed Patient

While most patients who present with vertigo have a benign etiology for their symptoms, a subset can have a potentially life-threatening cause. For the most part, the life-threatening causes of vertigo occur in the central nervous system and are termed central vertigo. Not all causes of central vertigo, however, are life threatening (e.g., vestibular migraine). Lesions of the vestibular apparatus are most often not life-threatening. These disorders are called peripheral vertigo. Differentiation of peripheral and central vertigo is one of the primary goals in evaluating the undiagnosed patient.

History

In taking a history from a patient with vertigo, there are several questions that are particularly helpful:

- Is the vertigo episodic or has it occurred only once?
- How long does each episode last? Episodes of BPPV last less than 1 minute, whereas transient ischemic attacks (TIAs) commonly last at least several minutes. Vertigo from migraine, Ménière disease, vestibular neuritis, or infarcts often lasts longer (hours to days).
- Is there anything that consistently provokes vertigo? BPPV is provoked by head movement. Other possible provoking factors include loud noise and Valsalva maneuvers (coughing, sneezing, and straining during defecation).
- Are there any accompanying symptoms? Auditory symptoms (such as hearing loss or ear pain, pressure, or fullness) suggest a peripheral lesion, whereas symptoms such as double vision, slurred speech, facial numbness, weakness, or limb incoordination should raise the suspicion of a brainstem or cerebellar lesion.

Physical Examination

When examining patients with vertigo, the goals are to look for signs of vestibular hypofunction and to distinguish peripheral from central lesions. It is always important to perform a basic neurologic examination, with particular attention to the cranial nerves, cerebellar function, and walking and balance (see Chapter 86) and to do a basic office assessment of hearing (see Chapter 110). Specific tests of the vestibular system involve looking for vestibular imbalance and impairment of the VOR and testing for positional nystagmus.

As explained above, the hallmark of a static vestibular imbalance is a *spontaneous nystagmus*. However, it is important to remember that *peripheral vestibular nystagmus is suppressed by vision*. Thus, except in the most acute stage of a peripheral lesion, nystagmus is not commonly seen during bedside examination. Techniques must be used to remove the subject's visual fixation while still allowing the examiner to view the eyes. In the vestibular clinic, this is done using specialized goggles with high magnification lenses (Frenzel lenses). An alternative method is to observe the optic disk carefully during direct ophthalmoscopy, while occluding the opposite eye with the hand. A nystagmus can be seen as alternating slow and quick movements of the optic disk. When doing this, it is important to remember that the apparent direction of nystagmus is reversed. This is because the optic disk is at the posterior pole of the eye. Thus, a right-beating movement of the optic disk is really a left-beating nystagmus. *A spontaneous nystagmus that is easily seen in the light is more often a sign of central disease*. Other features indicating a central lesion are a purely vertical (e.g., downbeat) nystagmus and a direction-changing (gaze-evoked) nystagmus.

Often more helpful in identifying a vestibular deficit are tests of dynamic vestibular function, that is, of the VOR. The most important of these is the *head thrust test*. The patient is asked to fixate a target (usually the examiner's nose) during rapid, low-amplitude, horizontal rotations of the head. If the VOR is working normally, gaze will remain stable and the patient will still be looking at the examiner at the end of the rotation. If the function of one or both labyrinths is impaired, rotation toward the affected ear(s) will fail to produce a normal excitatory stimulus, leading to a deficient VOR. The eyes will move with the head, and after the rotation, there will be a corrective rapid eye movement (saccade) to bring the eyes back to the point of original fixation. For example, in the case of a right vestibular lesion, when the head is turned to the left, the response will be normal and the eyes will remain stable in space. However, when the head is turned to the right, the eyes will move to the right with the head and a leftward corrective saccade will be seen. The head thrust test is the best bedside test to identify a peripheral vestibular lesion.

Another useful test of the VOR is *dynamic visual acuity* (2). This is based on the fact that a normal compensatory VOR is required to maintain clear vision when the head is moving. Thus, patients with an impaired VOR (particularly if bilateral as with bilateral vestibular injury) will have reduced visual acuity during head movement. To test dynamic acuity, first determine the patient's baseline visual acuity, using an eye chart or near vision card with appropriate correction (including reading glasses, if the near card is used). This is compared with the best acuity when the head is rotated back and forth (by the examiner) at a frequency of about once per second. A loss of more than one line of acuity is abnormal.

Patients with recurrent episodes of vertigo should undergo *Dix-Hallpike positional testing* to look for evidence of BPPV. This is discussed below in the section on BPPV and Figure 89.1.

Formal Vestibular Testing

Several ancillary tests are helpful in the evaluation of patients who are referred for problematic vestibular disorders. Formal *audiometry* is used to identify evidence of hearing loss, particularly asymmetric (see Chapter 110). *Electronystagmography* consists of a battery of tests of eye movements and vestibular function. The electronystagmography typically includes a recording in the dark to look for spontaneous nystagmus, recordings of saccades and smooth pursuit, recordings of positional nystagmus, Dix-Hallpike testing, and caloric testing. Caloric testing measures the nystagmus generated when one of the external ear canals is irrigated with warm or cold water (or air). Warm water provides an excitatory stimulus to the horizontal canal of the irrigated ear, and cold water provides an inhibitory stimulus. A comparison of responses to irrigation of each ear is used to determine if there is a relative reduction of vestibular function on one side.

Rotatory chair testing uses the natural vestibular stimulus (head rotation) to test the functions of the labyrinths and VOR pathways. The patient is seated in a chair that is rotated in the dark, either at constant velocity or sinusoidally. Unlike caloric testing, rotational testing does not stimulate each labyrinth independently: Rotation in each direction affects both sides, exciting one and inhibiting the other simultaneously. Thus, it is more difficult to identify and localize a unilateral lesion using rotational testing. However, rotational testing is of particular benefit in identifying bilateral vestibular loss.

TABLE 89.2 Causes of Vertigo According to Temporal Pattern

Temporal Pattern of Vertigo	*Cause*
Acute Prolonged (Hours to Days) Vertigo	
Peripheral	Vestibular neuritis/labyrinthitis (if hearing loss present)
	Labyrinthine infarction (usually includes hearing loss)
	Syphilis
	Autoimmune disease
	Bacterial labyrinthitis
	Ramsay-Hunt syndrome (herpes zoster oticus)
	Posttraumatic
Central	Infarct (brainstem, cerebellum)
	Cerebellar hemorrhage
	Multiple sclerosis
	Other inflammatory/autoimmune disorders
Recurrent Vertigo	
Seconds	Benign paroxysmal positional vertigo (provoked by changes in head position)
	Perilymph fistula/superior canal dehiscence (provoked by loud noise/Valsalva)
Minutes	Transient ischemic attack
	Migraine (aura)
	Anxiety/panic
Hours	Migraine
	Ménière disease
	Otosyphilis
	Autoimmune

DISORDERS CAUSING VERTIGO

Table 89.2 lists common causes of vertigo and they are also discussed in this section. Causes are categorized according to the temporal pattern that emerges when the patient gives the history: acute-onset prolonged vertigo, or recurrent vertigo.

Acute Prolonged (Hours to Days) Vertigo

A single episode of prolonged (hours to days) vertigo may be because of either a peripheral or a central lesion. The primary questions to be answered are whether the lesion is in the vestibular periphery or in the brain and whether it is a stroke. It is important to remember that a peripheral lesion can be a stroke.

The symptoms of an acute unilateral vestibular lesion are severe vertigo (from the sudden imbalance of tonic vestibular input), nausea, and vomiting. Some patients will also have a loss of hearing in the affected ear, if the cochlea or auditory nerve is affected. Patients prefer to lie still with the eyes closed, because any head movement makes the symptoms worse. They will have difficulty walking, and on Romberg testing they may fall toward the affected side.

Vestibular neuritis is a common cause of acute unilateral vestibulopathy. When hearing loss is present, the term *labyrinthitis* is often used, although the exact localization is not always certain. The hearing loss is sensorineural, not conductive (see Chapter 110). Vestibular neuritis is generally thought to result from a viral infection of the labyrinth or vestibular nerve or a postinfectious inflammatory process. Bacterial labyrinthitis is rarer but may be a complication of mastoiditis or bacterial meningitis.

The acute severe symptoms of vestibular neuritis usually subside over the first several days with gradual continued improvement over the next several weeks to months, as the brain compensates for the peripheral lesion. If compensation is incomplete, there may be a lingering (usually mild) imbalance that never fully recovers. Once the acute stage has passed, examination findings may be minimal, with no spontaneous nystagmus in the light. The most consistent finding is a head thrust sign when the head is rotated toward the affected side (see Physical Examination). A reduced caloric response confirms the unilateral pathology.

A *labyrinthine infarct* may be difficult to distinguish clinically from labyrinthitis. Thus, older individuals, particularly those with vascular risk factors, should be evaluated for cerebrovascular disease (CVD) affecting the posterior circulation (see Chapter 91). The main concern is that a patient with vertebrobasilar disease could go on to have a second, and potentially more life-threatening, infarct in the brainstem or cerebellum. Other important diagnoses to consider are otosyphilis, vasculitis, and autoimmune inner ear disease, either isolated or as part of a systemic autoimmune process. Thus, patients should have serologic testing for syphilis (rapid plasma reagent [RPR]/fluorescent treponemal antibody [FTA]; see Chapter 37), sedimentation rate, and specific tests for connective tissue disease or vasculitis, when suspected.

Symptoms that should raise suspicion of a central (brainstem or cerebellar) lesion include double vision, facial or limb numbness or weakness, slurred speech, and limb incoordination. A direction changing (gaze-evoked) or vertical (e.g., downbeat) nystagmus indicates central disease, as generally do other cranial nerve or cerebellar signs. Infarction in the territory of the anterior inferior cerebellar artery may produce a combination of both central and peripheral signs (3). A cerebellar or brainstem stroke is a medical emergency.

Some patients with peripheral disease will have ipsilateral facial weakness when there is a combined lesion of cranial nerves VII and VIII. In these cases, the facial weakness should have a peripheral pattern (the forehead is not spared). Ramsey-Hunt syndrome is a reactivation of herpes zoster virus that produces facial paresis, hearing loss, vertigo, and ear pain, with vesicular lesions in the external auditory canal. Early treatment with acyclovir is important.

Although many individuals improve spontaneously from vestibular neuritis, if the patient is seen within the first 3 days after onset, a course of oral steroids may further facilitate recovery (4). Otherwise, treatment of acute peripheral vertigo is largely aimed at explaining the cause and likely course to the patient and ameliorating the symptoms. Vestibular suppressants include antihistamines (e.g., promethazine, meclizine) and benzodiazepines (e.g., diazepam, lorazepam, or clonazepam). Table 89.3 summarizes practical information about these drugs. These should be used only in the acute stage (the first several days), when vertigo is severe, because they may impede the process of central vestibular compensation. Antiemetics may be helpful when nausea and vomiting are present. Ondansetron may have fewer side effects than antidopaminergic agents (e.g., prochlorperazine, chlorpromazine, metoclopramide). Patients should be encouraged to resume activity when possible, because this may facilitate the compensation process. For patients with troublesome persistent symptoms, formal vestibular rehabilitation therapy may also help recovery.

TABLE 89.3 Drugs for Symptomatic Treatment of Vertigo

Type of Action	*Generic (Trade Name)*	*Available Preparations*	*Dosage and Schedule*
Labyrinthine Suppressants			
Antihistamines	Meclizine (Antivert, Bonine)	12.5 and 25 mg	12.5–25 mg b.i.d.–q.i.d.
Benzodiazepines	Clonazepam (Klonopin)	0.5 mg	0.25–0.5 mg q.d.–t.i.d
Antiemetic	Prochlorperazine (Compazine)	5-, 10-mg tablets	5–10 mg q4h p.r.n.
		10-, 25-mg suppositories	10 mg q.i.d., 25 mg b.i.d.
	Odansetron (Zofran)	4-, 8-mg tablets	8 mg b.i.d.

TABLE 89.4 Characteristic Features of Benign Paroxysmal Positional Vertigo

Predisposing factors
Head trauma
Labyrinthine lesion (e.g., labyrinthitis, Ménière disease)
Migraine
Prolonged supine or head back positioning (e.g., dental work)
Age
Vertigo provoked by
Lying down
Rolling to affected side in bed
Putting the head back to look up
Bending over and standing back up
Onset
Latency of several seconds from head movement before vertigo and nystagmus begin
Duration
Seconds (<1 min)
Other
Most common in the morning, after prolonged supine positioning
Symptoms (and nystagmus) fatigue with repeated positioning

Recurrent Vertigo

Recurrent attacks of vertigo can be distinguished by several features, including their duration, provoking factors, and associated symptoms. There are many underlying etiologies (Table 89.2); some common causes include BPPV, migraine, and TIAs.

Benign Paroxysmal Positional Vertigo

BPPV is a common cause of episodic vertigo. It consists of brief attacks of vertigo, provoked by changes in head position relative to gravity. Table 89.4 lists the typical features of BPPV.

BPPV results from the accumulation of otoconial debris in one of the semicircular canals. Otoconia are particles consisting of calcium carbonate crystals that are normally adherent to the membrane of the utricle (see Basic Principles of Vestibular Function). If these particles are dispersed, either spontaneously or by trauma or inner ear injury, they may coalesce into a small clot and become free floating in the endolymph fluid. This clot of particles may fall into one of the semicircular canals, most commonly the posterior canal, because of its orientation. Then, when the head moves, this clot may move within the canal, causing pressure changes in the endolymph and deflecting the cupula. This leads to excitation of the canal, as if the head were rotating.

BPPV is diagnosed by the Dix-Hallpike positioning maneuver, illustrated in Figure 89.1. The head is first turned 45 degrees to one side. This will place the posterior canal on that side in the plane of rotation. Then, the subject is brought quickly from a sitting to a head-hanging position.

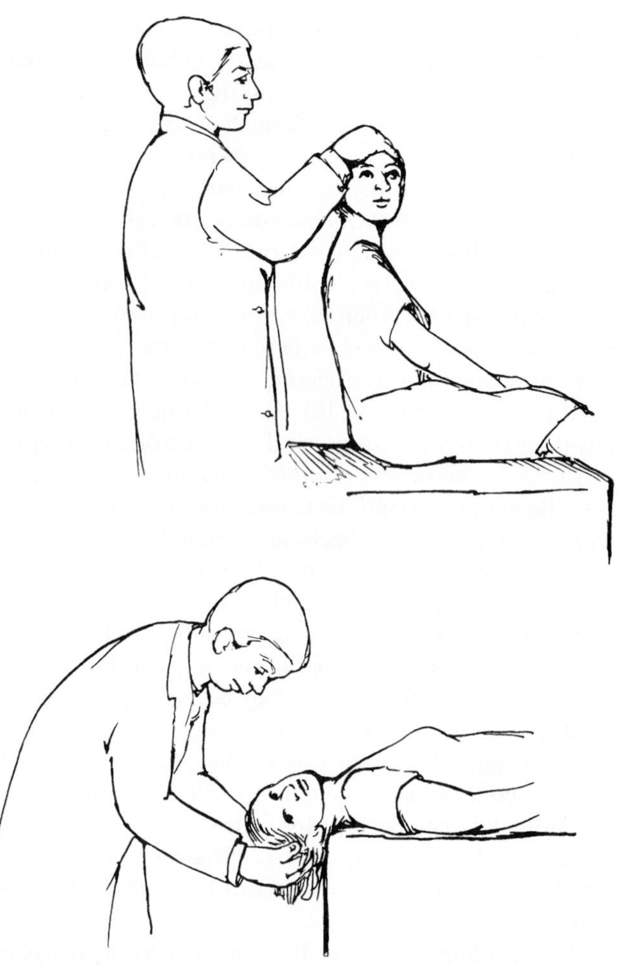

FIGURE 89.1. Dix-Hallpike maneuver for testing a patient for positional vertigo and nystagmus.

A patient with BPPV will describe vertigo when the affected ear is stimulated by bringing the patient to the lying position with the head turned to that side. While supporting the head, the examiner watches the eyes for any nystagmus to indicate excitation of the posterior canal. The expected nystagmus has both vertical and torsional (rotatory) components: *The eyes beat upward and the upper poles of the eyes beat toward the affected (down) ear* (Fig. 89.2). There is usually a latency of several seconds from the initial positioning

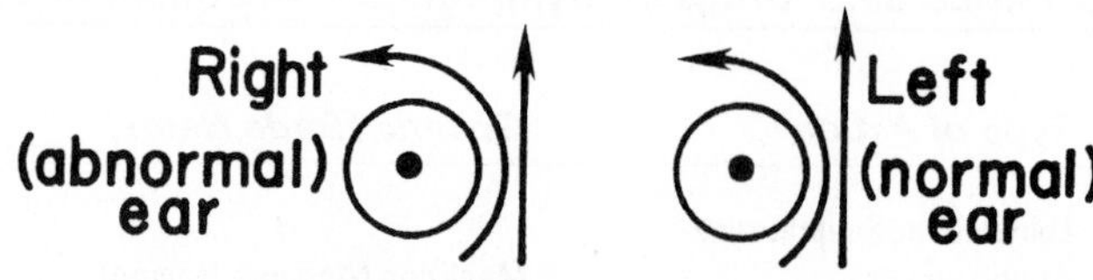

FIGURE 89.2. Pathognomonic nystagmus of benign paroxysmal positional vertigo. The pathognomonic nystagmus consists of quick phases directed upward (with respect to the head) and torsionally toward the abnormal ear. In this example, the torsional element is counterclockwise toward the abnormal right ear.

until the vertigo and nystagmus begin, and the duration is less than 1 minute (commonly about 15 to 30 seconds). It is important to keep in mind that not all positional vertigo and nystagmus is because of BPPV. For example, patients with cerebellar disease or craniocervical junction abnormalities (e.g., Chiari malformation) may have positional nystagmus. In these cases, the nystagmus is usually sustained rather than transient.

Treatment of BPPV consists of the canalith repositioning (Epley) procedure shown in Figure 89.3, which begins with the Dix-Hallpike maneuver, with the head turned to the affected ear (5). The purpose of the maneuver is to relocate the free-floating particles to the utricle. The four-step maneuver is repeated until no nystagmus is observed. This approach to treating BPPV is effective after one session in most patients (6). Contraindications to the Epley maneuver are severe disease of the neck and high-grade carotid artery stenosis. In refractory or recurrent cases, patients can be taught to perform a modification of the maneuver at home, in which the head rests on the bed but with pillows under the shoulders to simulate a head-hanging position (7). Brandt-Daroff physical therapy exercises may also be helpful (8). Making the diagnosis of BPPV quickly and accurately is important, because of the effectiveness of treatment and to avoid an unnecessary and expensive diagnostic workup for other causes (e.g., TIAs). Because BPPV may be a complication of labyrinthine injury, it may coexist with other inner ear diseases (9). Vestibular suppressant drugs (Table 89.3) may reduce the intensity of a patient's symptoms, but they do not reduce the frequency of attacks.

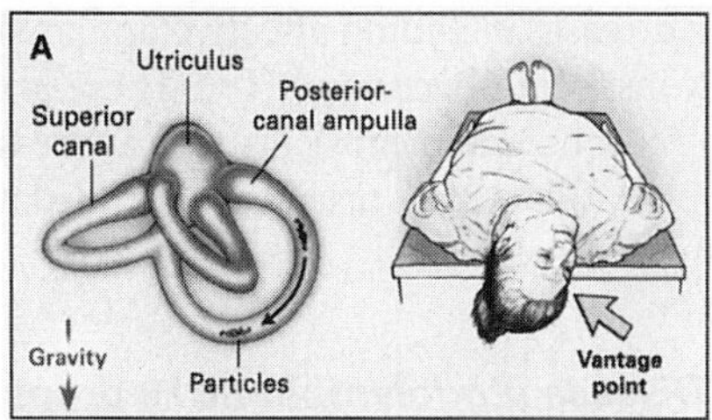

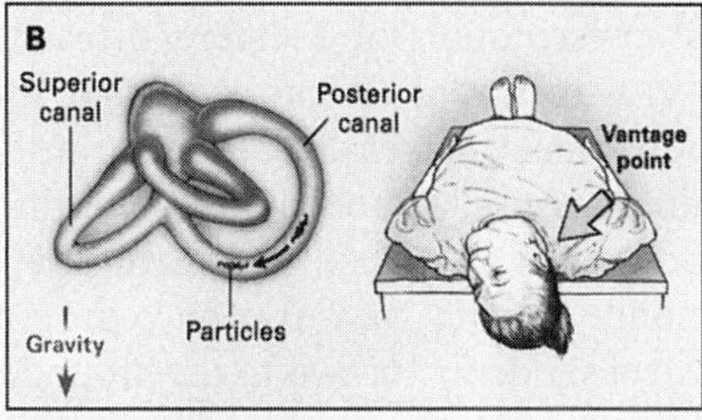

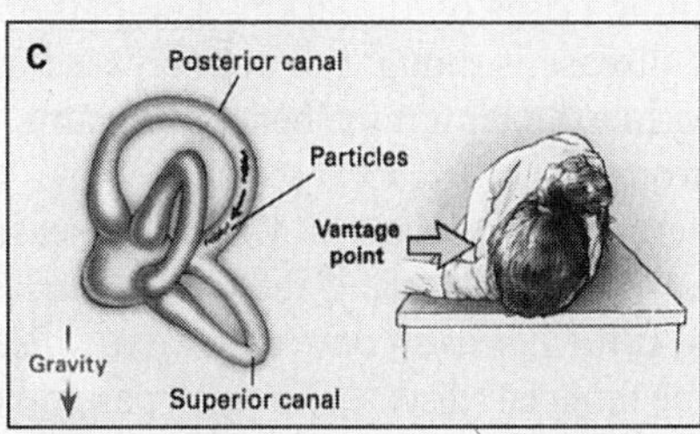

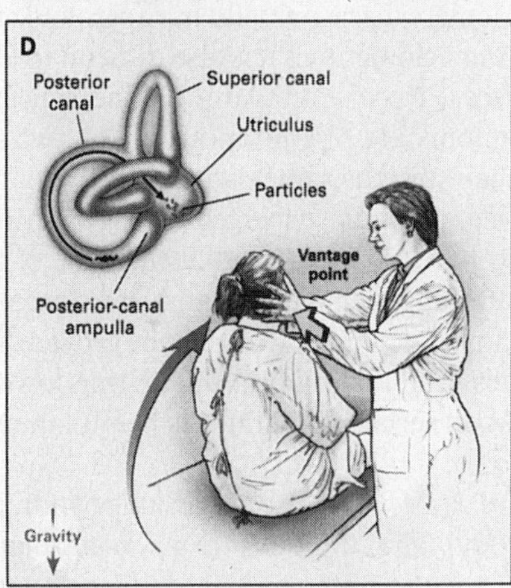

FIGURE 89.3. Bedside maneuver for the treatment of a patient with benign paroxysmal positional vertigo affecting the right ear (Epley maneuver). The presumed position of the debris within the labyrinth during the maneuver is shown in each panel. The maneuver is a four-step procedure. First, a Dix-Hallpike test is performed with the patient's head rotated 45 degrees toward the right ear and the neck slightly extended with the chin pointed slightly upward. This position results in the patient's head hanging to the right **(A)**. Once the vertigo and nystagmus provoked by the Dix-Hallpike test cease, the patient's head is rotated about the rostral-caudal body axis until the left ear is down **(B)**. Then the head and body are further rotated until the head is face down **(C)**. The vertex of the head is kept tilted downward throughout the rotation. The maneuver usually provokes brief vertigo. The patient should be kept in the final face-down position for about 10 to 16 seconds. With the head kept turned toward the left shoulder, the patient is brought into the seated position **(D)**. Once the patient is upright, the head is titled so that the chin is pointed slightly downward. (From Furman JM, Cass SP. Benign paroxysmal positional vertigo. N Engl J Med 1999;341:1590, with permission.)

Vestibular Migraine

Migraine is another common cause of recurrent dizziness (10). Patients with migraine may have a variety of symptoms that include both discrete attacks of vertigo and prolonged episodes of disequilibrium and motion sensitivity. Migrainous vertigo typically lasts minutes to hours. It may occur as an aura, preceding headache, or it may be present simultaneously with headache. In many cases, headache and vertigo occur independently, and occasional patients thought to have vestibular migraine only rarely have headache. Thus, the absence of headache does not rule out migraine as a cause of dizziness, although it should raise suspicion for other causes. Only a small fraction of patients with migrainous vertigo meet criteria for *basilar migraine*; in these patients, vertigo occurs as part of the aura, and there must be at least one other posterior circulation symptom.

The treatment of vestibular migraine is similar to that of migraine headaches. Patients with rare episodes can be given antiemetics and vestibular suppressants (Table 89.4) to be taken at the time of an attack. Patients with chronic refractory migraine are more likely to have comorbid psychiatric disease, including affective and anxiety disorders (see Nonspecific Dizziness) (11). These are very important to recognize and must also be addressed in the treatment plan. Chapter 87 provides a detailed account of migraine management.

Ménière Disease (Endolymphatic Hydrops)

The classic presentation of Ménière disease (see also Chapter 110) is recurrent attacks of vertigo, nausea, and vomiting; a transient decrease in hearing in the affected ear; ear pain, pressure, and/or fullness; and tinnitus, usually low pitched and described as "roaring" or "rushing." Less commonly, patients may also have drop attacks, in which they feel suddenly thrown to the ground. These are called otolithic crises of Tumarkin. The pathophysiology of Ménière disease is thought to be increased endolymph pressure within the labyrinth (hence the name, endolymphatic hydrops).

The differential diagnosis of Ménière disease includes a variety of inflammatory and infectious causes, such as otosyphilis, Lyme disease, connective tissue diseases, and autoimmune inner ear disease. Thus, all patients suspected of having Ménière disease should have serologic testing for these disorders. Sometimes it is also difficult to distinguish Ménière disease from vestibular migraine, especially if auditory symptoms are less prominent. The two diagnoses may also coexist in the same patient (12).

If possible, patients suspected of having Ménière disease should have an audiogram at the time of an attack. The classic finding is a predominantly low-frequency hearing loss in the affected ear that may improve when the attack resolves. The finding of a fluctuating low-frequency hearing loss on serial audiograms is helpful in making the diagnosis.

Treatment of Ménière disease includes sodium restriction (1 g/day) and diuretics (e.g., acetazolamide, hydrochlorthiazide/triamterene). In cases refractory to diuretics, intratympanic steroid or gentamicin injections may be helpful. The goal of gentamicin therapy is to ablate vestibular function partially to eliminate attacks of vertigo with minimal effects on balance. Surgical ablation (labyrinthectomy or vestibular nerve section) is reserved only for the most severe cases, after all other treatments have failed.

Transient Ischemic Attacks

Vertigo may be a symptom of TIAs involving the posterior circulation. Vertigo because of TIAs usually lasts for minutes. Repeated episodes of vertigo on an ischemic basis are unusual in the absence of other posterior circulation symptoms, such as visual field disturbances, double vision, slurred speech, or facial or limb weakness or numbness. However, occasional patients will have isolated vertigo (13). Patients suspected of having TIAs should be evaluated as described in Chapter 91.

Perilymph Fistula

A perilymph fistula is a relatively uncommon cause of recurrent vertigo and is sometimes difficult to diagnose (14). However, it is helpful to keep in mind because it may be amenable to surgical treatment. It results from a defect in the bony labyrinth or the round or oval window, creating a communication between the inner ear and either the middle ear or the intracranial space. Causes include barotrauma, erosion by a tumor (e.g., cholesteatoma), or head trauma. Vertigo is provoked by loud noises, tragal pressure, or Valsalva, with transmission of middle ear or intracranial pressure into the labyrinth through the communicating defect. Surgical exploration and repair may be necessary. Again, this is an uncommon cause of vertigo, but if a patient presents with the above history it is prudent to refer to an otolaryngologist for further evaluation.

Bilateral Loss of Vestibular Function

Patients with bilateral loss of vestibular function have a feeling of imbalance when standing or walking. They do not have dizziness at rest, although they may have a sense of instability or oscillopsia when turning the head quickly. Because several components of the peripheral and central systems are involved in the maintenance of posture and balance, there are many causes of disequilibrium in addition to vestibular disease (see Disequilibrium). Thus, patients with disequilibrium require a thorough neurologic and vestibular examination looking for signs of parkinsonism (e.g., cogwheel rigidity, tremor), myelopathy (spasticity in the legs, increased reflexes), cerebellar disease (limb ataxia, slurred speech, cerebellar eye signs), or neuropathy (loss of vibration sense and proprioception). The diagnosis of bilateral vestibular loss may be missed if vestibular function is not explicitly tested, because there may be few other signs other than gait ataxia, a Romberg sign, and an abnormal VOR.

The chief symptoms of bilateral vestibular loss are imbalance and oscillopsia with head movement (such as when walking or riding in a car, particularly on a bumpy road). These are due to the loss of the vestibulospinal reflex and VOR, respectively. Patients do not have vertigo because the lesion is symmetric, yielding no net imbalance in the inputs from the two labyrinths. Typical findings on examination include a marked loss of dynamic visual acuity (see Physical Examination), bilateral head thrust signs, and a Romberg sign. Reduced rotatory chair responses confirm the diagnosis. The degree of disability depends both on the severity of vestibular loss and the extent of compensation. Some younger patients who are otherwise healthy may compensate well, with limited disability.

Others, particularly those with superimposed neuropathy (causing proprioceptive loss) or poor vision, may be left with more substantial disability.

The most common identified cause of bilateral vestibular loss is *ototoxic drugs*, such as aminoglycosides and cisplatin (15). Gentamicin ototoxicity may occur even in the absence of "toxic" levels. If recognized early, stopping the drug may theoretically limit the damage and allow for some recovery of function. In many cases, however, the vestibular loss is not discovered until the course of treatment has been completed. Early symptoms of disequilibrium may be attributed to a general weakness arising from the patient's underlying systemic illness. Only after recovery from the acute illness, when the patient is more active, is the true balance impairment noted. For this reason, it is important to monitor vestibular function during gentamicin treatment, when possible. This can be done by measuring dynamic acuity with a near card, looking for head thrust signs, and checking for a Romberg sign, if the patient can stand. Because gentamicin is much more toxic to the vestibular organs than to the cochlea, assessing hearing is not a good way to detect ototoxicity. In fact, patients may have little or no change in hearing even with profound loss of vestibular function.

Many cases of bilateral vestibular loss are idiopathic. Other causes include hereditary vestibular loss (16), bilateral sequential vestibular neuritis, combined cerebellar and vestibular degeneration, autoimmune disease, meningitis, sarcoidosis, metabolic disease (e.g., vitamin B_{12} deficiency), bilateral vestibular nerve tumors (e.g., schwannomas), and bilateral Ménière disease (17).

MOTION SICKNESS

Motion sickness is a feeling of nausea and dizziness evoked by excessive or prolonged vestibular or optokinetic stimulation (18). Other symptoms include diaphoresis, yawning, light-headedness, and malaise. Susceptibility to motion sickness varies among individuals; migraineurs are particularly motion sensitive. Most individuals adapt to continued motion (e.g., cruise), although some remain persistently motion sick. Individuals with bilateral vestibular paresis are insensitive to motion.

Several medications may assist in the prevention or reduction of motion sickness, when used occasionally during exposure to a provocative stimulus. Antihistamines such as meclizine (25 to 50 mg), dimenhydrinate (50 to 100 mg), or promethazine (25 mg) may be taken orally about 1 hour before travel. The major adverse effect is sedation, most prominently with promethazine. Transdermal scopolamine is an anticholinergic agent that is effective in preventing motion sickness. The 1.5-mg patch is designed to deliver 0.5 mg of scopolamine over 3 days. It should be applied at least 4 hours before travel. Adverse effects include dry mouth and sedation. Older individuals may be more sensitive to central nervous anticholinergic effects such as confusion and hallucinations. Occasionally, withdrawal symptoms occur, particularly after prolonged use.

After prolonged exposure to motion, such as returning to land after a cruise, many individuals have a feeling of continued motion ("landsickness") that usually resolves within 1 to 2 days. However, in some individuals these symptoms persist for months to years. This has been termed *mal de debarquement syndrome* (19). Typical features are a constant feeling of rocking or swaying when still. In contrast to motion sickness, these individuals feel best when moving and worse when motion stops. Mal de debarquement syndrome has been reported much more commonly in women, usually in their 40s. A history of migraine or other headaches is common.

SYNCOPE AND NEAR SYNCOPE

Definitions and Pathophysiology

Syncope is "a sudden and brief loss of consciousness associated with a loss of postural tone, from which recovery is spontaneous" (20). Syncope typically lasts from seconds to minutes; longer episodes are classified as stupor or coma. *Unconsciousness* implies that both cerebral hemispheres have become impaired or that certain critical structures in the brainstem have failed. Generally, unilateral diseases of the cerebral hemispheres do not lead to unconsciousness (and therefore syncope) unless the brain becomes more generally affected. It is important to note that syncope is a symptom and not a disease.

There are three major pathophysiologic mechanisms of syncope (21):

- *Acute decrease in cerebral blood flow*. This may be caused by cardiac disorders, pulmonary vascular disorders, failure of venous return, CVD, loss of peripheral vascular tone, and vasodepressor syncope, commonly referred to as neurocardiogenic, reflex-mediated, or vasovagal syncope. This last mechanism is thought to result from a triggering of a neural reflex resulting in an episode of hypotension in the setting of bradycardia and peripheral vasodilation. It is the most common diagnosed cause of syncope and carries a good prognosis (see Neurocardiogenic Syncope).
- *Chemical aberration of blood flowing to the brain*. Examples include hypoglycemia, hypocapnia, and hypoxia.
- *Neural or psychologic causes*. These include nonconvulsive seizures and psychogenic syncope.

Syncope must be differentiated from other disorders that may, on initial history taking, sound similar to syncope. *Many types of "spells" are not syncope;* a spell is "a sudden onset of a symptom or symptoms that are recurrent, self-limited, and stereotypic in nature" (22). Such spells are not necessarily syncope and may be caused by endocrine, cardiovascular, psychologic, pharmacologic, neurologic, or other miscellaneous disorders. Carcinoid syndrome and pheochromocytoma are classic examples of disorders in which patients describe spells that are distinct from syncope.

Presyncope, or near syncope, is the sense of imminent loss of consciousness without frank syncope. It may be a prelude to true syncope or it may be related to a spell or to unexplained dizziness.

Incidence and Mortality

In a large epidemiologic study using the Framingham cohort following 7,814 patients for 17 years, a total of 822 patients experienced syncope. The 10-year cumulative incidence was 6%. There was a sharp increase in incidence of syncope in patients over 70 years of age (23). Syncope accounts for 3% to 5% of all emergency room visits and 1% of all admissions (24); however, in the Framingham study only 56% of participants who experienced a syncopal episode sought medical attention (23).

Morbidity and mortality in patients with syncope differ according to the underlying cause of the syncopal event. Studies of patients with syncope report a 1-year mortality of 18% to 33% for patients with a cardiovascular cause of syncope, 0% to 12% for patients with a known noncardiovascular cause, and 6% for patients with an unknown cause of syncope (25). The higher mortality of patients with a cardiovascular cause of syncope appears to be because of the underlying cardiovascular disease, and not the cardiac syncope per se. Four factors, available at the time of presentation, have been shown to predict cardiac arrhythmias or death in the year after presentation with syncope: (a) age older than 45 years, (b) a history of heart failure, (c) a history of ventricular arrhythmias, and (d) an abnormal electrocardiogram. Arrhythmias or death occurred in 4.4% of patients with without any of these factors, and in 58% of patients with three or four risk factors (26).

Syncope also causes significant morbidity. Up to 35% of patients who experience a syncopal episode suffer an injury as a result. Additionally, patients who experience recurrent episodes of syncope can suffer severe functional impairment comparable to other chronic diseases (24).

Differential Diagnosis

The differential diagnosis of disorders presenting as syncope is broad. Table 89.5 lists causes, classified as hypotension, cardiac disease, metabolic conditions, intracranial conditions, or psychiatric disorders. Neurocardiogenic (or reflex-mediated) syncope is thought to be the most common cause of syncope, especially if there is no evidence of a cardiovascular cause. Neurocardiogenic syncope may account for up to 40% of all syncopal events evaluated in the ambulatory setting. The list of medications that may cause syncope continues to expand. Any patient with dizziness or syncope should have all medications, including over-the-counter (OTC) medications, reviewed in light of the patient's presenting complaint. Polypharmacy is a particularly common cause of syncope in the elderly. Depending on the diagnostic criteria used, an underlying cause will not be found for approximately 39% of patients evaluated for syncope, although more recent algorithms have reported lower percentages of unexplained syncope at 14% to 17% (27,28,29).

In a classic prospective evaluation of 204 patients presenting with syncope, 25% had the cause diagnosed on the basis of the history and physical examination. In this study population, in which approximately 50% of patients eventually received a diagnosis, the importance of the history and physical examination was well illustrated. Table 89.6 lists the diagnostic studies (including history and physical) that demonstrated the cause in patients for whom a cause was identified. This study was done before the widespread use of tilt-table testing (see Tilt-Table Testing); recent studies suggest that tilt-table testing will demonstrate neurocardiogenic syncope in one half to two thirds of patients with undiagnosed syncope (20).

Syncope from Hypotension or Circulatory Failure

Because of autoregulation, cerebral blood flow is protected over a wide range of systemic blood pressure. In normal people, a critical decrease in central nervous system (CNS) blood flow (producing near syncope or syncope) does not occur until the mean blood pressure is below 50 mm Hg. Under a number of circumstances (e.g., sympatholytic drug treatment, CVD), however, the minimal tolerated blood pressure may not be this low. Thus, symptomatic failure of the systemic circulation may occur over a wide range of blood pressures.

Neurocardiogenic (Reflex-Mediated, Vasovagal, Vasodepressor, or the Simple Faint) Syncope

Neurocardiogenic syncope has long been known to afflict young people; it is apt to occur in the setting of anxiety, fatigue, or pain and especially during venipuncture or other painful procedures. Additionally, the act of urinating (micturition syncope) and coughing (tussive syncope) can induce symptoms indistinguishable from neurocardiogenic syncope, though some believe that the underlying pathophysiology may be slightly different. Neurocardiogenic syncope is not just a disease of the young but can occur in older patients in identical settings. Episodes are believed

TABLE 89.5 Differential Diagnosis of Syncope/Near Syncope

Hypotension	Cardiac Disease	Hypotension	Cardiac Disease
Vasovagal or neurocardiogenic syncope	Arrhythmia (heart block, bradyarrhythmias, and tachyarrhythmias)	Adrenal insufficiency	Airway obstruction
Vasodilating drugs	Drugs associated with torsade de pointes	Hypoalbuminemia	Carbon monoxide
Angiotensin-converting enzyme inhibitors	Quinidine	Diuretics	Change to moderate/high altitude
Angiotensin receptor blockers	Procainamide	Venous pooling	Hyperviscosity
α-Blockers	Disopyramide	Prolonged Immobility while standing	Drug overdose (sedatives and ethanol)
Calcium channel blockers	Flecainide	Severe varicose veins	**Intracranial Conditions**
Nitroglycerine preparations	Encainide	Late pregnancy	Seizure disorder
Vasodilator antihypertensives	Amiodarone	After exercise	Subarachnoid hemorrhage
Drugs affecting autonomic function	Sotalol	Mobilization after bed rest	Cerebral embolism or thrombosis
Sympatholytic antihypertensives	Terfenadine	Orthostasis of aging	Migraine
Neuroleptics	Astemizole	Valsalva maneuver	Acutely increased intracranial pressure
Tricyclics and monoamine oxidase inhibitors	Outflow obstruction	Tussive	Tumor
Levodopa	Aortic stenosis	Micturition	Trauma
Cholinergic agents	Idiopathic hypertrophic subaortic stenosis	Defecation (with straining)	Ventricular obstruction
Antihistamines	Aortic dissection	Intermittent positive-pressure breathing	Arrhythmia (heart block, bradyarrhythmias, and tachyarrhythmias)
Autonomic neuropathy	Myxoma	Compromise of cerebral blood flow caused by cervical osteoarthritis or subclavian steal	Hypertensive encephalopathy
Peripheral neuropathy	Acute myocardial infarction	Carotid sinus hypersensitivity	Brainstem compression
Postsympathectomy	Mitral valve prolapse	Pulmonary embolism	Cervical or odontoid fractures
Tabes dorsalis and diabetic pseudotabes	Cyanotic congenital heart disease		Metastasis
Idiopathic Parkinsonism (Shy-Drager syndrome)	Cardiac tamponade		Cysts or anomalies of the posterior fossa
Parkinsonism with dysautonomia (multiple system atrophy)	**Metabolic Conditions**		Platybasia
Decreased blood volume	Hypoglycemia or hyperglycemia (consider drugs causing hypo- or hyperglycemia)		**Psychiatric Disorders**
Hemorrhage	Hyponatremia, hypokalemia, or hypocalcemia		Panic disorder
Salt and water deficit	Hypocapnia (hyperventilation)		Generalized anxiety disorder
Fasting	Hypoxia		Major depression
	Anemia		Somatization disorder
			Conversion disorder
			Alcoholism

From Lee JE, Killip T, Plum F. Episodic unconsciousness. In: Baron JA, ed. Diagnostic approaches to presenting syndromes. Baltimore: Williams & Wilkins, 1971, with permission.

to be triggered when venous pooling or catecholamine release leads to increased ventricular contractions and activation of cardiac mechanoreceptors; this causes a reflex increase in parasympathetic and decrease in sympathetic nervous system activity, resulting in symptomatic bradycardia or hypotension, termed the Bezold-Jarisch reflex. Neurocardiogenic syncope nearly always occurs while the patient is upright, but it may occur while seated; consciousness is nearly always regained promptly when the patient lies down. Typically, there is a prodromal warning period, lasting up to 5 minutes, when the patient feels dizzy or flushed, with mild nausea and occasionally palpitations or throat tightness. If the subject lies down during this stage, loss of consciousness may be avoided. An observer will note cold hands, pale skin, and tachycardia just before the patient loses consciousness. A prodrome may be absent in up to 30% of patients (particularly in the elderly), so its absence does not exclude the diagnosis of neurocardiogenic syncope. Additionally, sudden loss of consciousness does not exclude the diagnosis of neurocardiogenic syncope in any patient. After the faint, a flush replaces the pallor. If the patient is unable to lie flat, recovery may be prolonged; an occasional death has been noted if the person is held upright during the spell. Confusion can persist for up to 10 minutes particularly in elderly patients, and bradycardia may persist for up to 30 minutes after neurocardiogenic syncope. During this time the patient should remain lying down. The examination is otherwise normal unless there has been trauma or aspiration.

Neurocardiogenic syncope is often selected as a diagnosis of exclusion because the history and physical examination are often nondiagnostic. As noted above (see Differential Diagnosis), standardized *tilt-table testing* can be used to confirm susceptibility to neurocardiogenic

TABLE 89.6 Diagnostic Studies that Demonstrated the Cause of Syncope in 107 of 204 Patients in Whom Exhaustive Study Established a Cause

Study	No. of Patients
History and physical	52
Electrocardiography	12
Electrocardiographic monitoring	29
Electrophysiologic studies	3
Cardiac catheterization	7
Cerebral angiography	2
Electroencephalography	1
Total	106[a]

[a] In one additional patient a diagnosis of aortic dissection was made at autopsy, 7 days after the patient presented with syncope.
From Kapoor WN, Karpf M, Wieand S, et al. A prospective evaluation and follow-up of patients with syncope. N Engl J Med 1983;309:197, with permission.

syncope in patients for whom this information is needed to make a clinical decision.

In the *treatment of neurocardiogenic syncope*, education plays an important role. Merely lying down when a prodrome develops may abort a syncopal event. There is recent evidence that crossing one's arms or legs tightly during the prodrome of an event can reduce the likelihood of syncope as well (30). Increasing salt intake may also prevent recurrence. A high-salt diet with liberal fluid intake is commonly suggested, occasionally with the addition of compression stockings. Pharmacologic agents, including disopyramide, theophylline, angiotension-converting enzyme (ACE) inhibitors, fludrocortisone, a-agonists, β-blockers, and selective serotonin reuptake inhibitors (SSRIs), have all been used to treat neurocardiogenic syncope. The best studied class of drugs is β-blockers (atenolol 50 mg daily or metoprolol 50 mg twice a day) (31,32). Despite concerns about worsening bradycardia with the addition of β-blockers, these drugs have been well tolerated when used to treat patients with neurocardiogenic syncope. In one study, β-blocker treatment prevented recurrent syncope in 90% of patients for 2 years or longer (33). However, there is also data that shows no benefit from β-blockers. Part of the difficulty in studying drug effects in neurocardiogenic syncope is that there is a very high placebo response rate in this condition (33). Paroxetine (20 mg daily) is also well tolerated in patients with vasodepressor syncope and, in one small controlled study, decreased the recurrence of syncope over 25 months of treatment as compared with those receiving placebo by two-thirds (34). For patients with vasodepressor syncope and significant bradycardia, cardiac pacing showed promise in a preliminary study, however several subsequent studies did not show benefit (35–39). The role of cardiac pacing in neurocardiogenic syncope remains controversial, but it can be considered in patients when their syncope appears to be due predominantly to a cardioinhibitory response and in whom other noninvasive therapies have failed. Even if pacing does not prevent syncopal episodes, it may delay the time from onset of prodromal symptoms to the actual syncope and therefore may provide more time to take evasive action (40).

Carotid Sinus Hypersensitivity

Hypersensitivity of the carotid sinus is common in older men with coronary artery disease (CAD) or hypertension and may be exacerbated by tight collars, cumbersome necklaces, head turning, shaving, or large neck masses; however, this is an uncommon cause of syncope. Syncope may result when stimulation of the baroreceptors in the carotid sinus leads to an increase in vagal activity with resulting bradycardia or may lead to sympathetic relaxation with resulting hypotension. If carotid sinus syncope is suspected, one should consider performing a carotid massage (see Carotid Massage). Patients diagnosed as having carotid sinus syncope should be referred to a cardiologist for consideration of pharmacologic treatment or pacemaker insertion, if the symptoms are recurrent or severe.

Orthostatic Hypotension

There are many causes of orthostatic hypotension that can contribute to syncope. Medications are the most common cause, although autonomic impairment, volume depletion, venous pooling, as well as changes with aging or bedrest can be causes.

Medications

The most common cause of this problem is *antihypertensive drug use*; most syncope caused by these drugs is preventable if the drugs are prescribed cautiously and the standing blood pressure, after exercise, is monitored routinely. Other drugs may also produce orthostatic hypotension (Table 89.5). The management of drug-induced orthostasis requires discontinuation or reduced dosage of the drug.

Autonomic Impairment

Syncope/near syncope caused by autonomic impairment is always associated with orthostatic hypotension. To document this problem, blood pressure must be taken while the patient is supine and again while standing. In some patients, exercise while standing (e.g., walking for a few minutes) may be required for a significant orthostatic drop (20 mm Hg systolic) to occur.

Orthostatic hypotension can also be caused by *autonomic neuropathy*. In patients suspected of having this problem, the integrity of the autonomic nervous system can be assessed by noting the size and reaction of the pupils, the distribution of sweating, and asking about symptoms of gastrointestinal dysmotility. *Sympathetic failure* commonly occurs late in diabetic peripheral neuropathy (see Chapter 79) and may be the presenting feature of amyloidosis or the neuropathy associated with various neoplasms.

Multiple system atrophy (sometimes known as *Shy-Drager syndrome*), which occurs in late life, is caused by failure of central autonomic neurons and causes orthostatic hypotension, parkinsonism, cerebellar ataxia, and other autonomic symptoms in varying combinations. Sympathectomy, particularly when done bilaterally or in the lumbar segments, may be followed immediately by orthostatic hypotension and syncope, although usually venous tone recovers several weeks after the operation. Tabes dorsalis and more commonly diabetic pseudotabes may present with lightning pains and autonomic failure. Chapter 92 summarizes the management of orthostasis caused by autonomic neuropathy, which is symptomatic.

Decreased Intravascular Volume

Decreased intravascular volume caused by hemorrhage or volume loss (e.g., from gastroenteritis, heat exposure, or diuretics) is recognized by the combination of orthostatic hypotension and an associated basis for the volume deficit. Volume expansion, either by increased salt and water ingestion or by intravenous fluids, is the initial treatment.

Venous Pooling

Venous pooling prevents return of blood to the heart, lowering cardiac output, at times sufficiently to produce near syncope or syncope. Symptoms may occur after prolonged standing in one position, particularly after exercise, as in recruits standing at attention. Severe dependent varicose veins or the compression of pelvic veins by a fetus or a large abdominal mass may produce symptoms through a similar mechanism. Syncope 15 to 30 minutes after exercise has been attributed to dilation of the splanchnic circulation before blood flow to the skeletal muscles has completely returned to normal. Management of these conditions involves chiefly avoidance of the precipitating factors. Supportive elastic stockings may be helpful for patients with marked pooling in varicose veins (see Chapter 95).

Orthostatic Syncope/Near Syncope after Bed Rest

This problem is caused by the combined effects of venous pooling, relative hypovolemia, and probably to some degree lowered sensitivity of the baroreceptor system. It is very common at all ages but is especially common among the elderly and should be anticipated in any person who has been at bed rest for more than a few days; moreover, it may persist for 1 or 2 weeks or longer after mobilization begins. Orthostatic symptoms may be minimized or prevented by having the patient gradually stand only after several minutes of sitting on the bed with the legs dependent. Figure 89.4 illustrates practical exercises that may help convalescing or deconditioned patients in overcoming postural weakness and hypotension. These patients should be encouraged to be out of bed for at least 2 hours a day, including morning, afternoon, and evening.

Orthostasis of Aging

Transient orthostatic dizziness and hypotension occur in many healthy older people. A significant fall in systolic blood pressure also is common in elderly patients immediately after eating, even in a seated position, which may make them especially susceptible to syncope when standing up after a meal. The physiologic basis for orthostatic symptoms in the elderly is often multifactorial and may be related not only to postural hypotension but also cerebral ischemia, vestibular dysfunction, visual impairment, and abnormal proprioception. The orthostasis of aging is important because it increases the risk associated with drugs that may cause orthostatic hypotension. Clearly, older patients should have their standing blood pressure checked whenever they complain of even mild orthostatic symptoms, and they should be monitored similarly whenever a drug in one of the groups listed in Table 89.5 is prescribed. Those who are troubled by orthostatic symptoms should be advised to follow the steps recommended above for patients rising after bed rest. Dizziness in the elderly is commonly multifactorial and should prompt consideration of a combination of cardiovascular, neurologic, sensory, pharmacologic, and psychologic causes (41). Mineralocorticoid agents can be used to assist in volume expansion, but patients must be monitored for volume overload, hypokalemia, and peripheral edema. Unfortunately, elderly patients are often unable to tolerate mineralocorticoid agents over a sustained period of time (42).

Other Forms of Syncope Related to Systemic Circulation

Pulmonary embolism may cause sudden loss of consciousness in up to 10% of cases. The diagnosis of pulmonary embolism is suggested by the presence of dyspnea, hypotension, tachycardia, or acute cor pulmonale by electrocardiogram (ECG) or physical examination (see Chapter 57).

Vertebrobasilar insufficiency, due to decreased blood flow to the posterior circulation of the brain, can lead to the sudden onset of loss of postural tone, termed "drop attacks," although loss of consciousness is not necessarily seen. These attacks may also be associated with the abrupt onset of visual loss, diplopia, and dysarthria. Besides the typical history, the diagnosis should be suspected in patients with multiple risk factors for vascular disease.

Leg Exercises

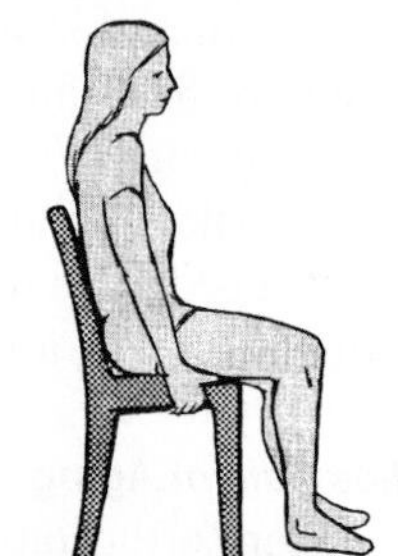

Starting position: Sitting in chair, exercise one leg at a time.

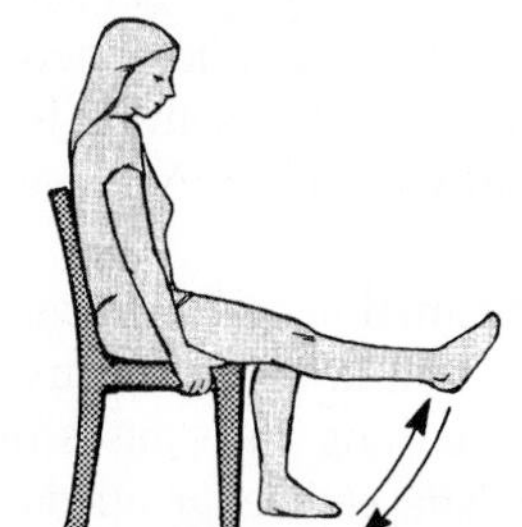

Raise leg up and down. Repeat 10 times.

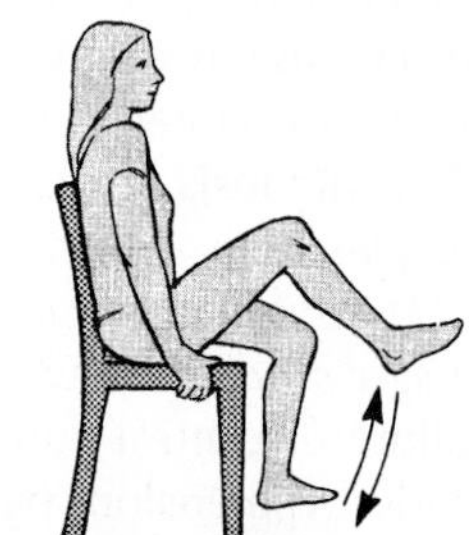

Keeping knee bent, raise leg up and down.

Arm Exercises: To increase effectiveness, hold a soup can in each hand for weight.

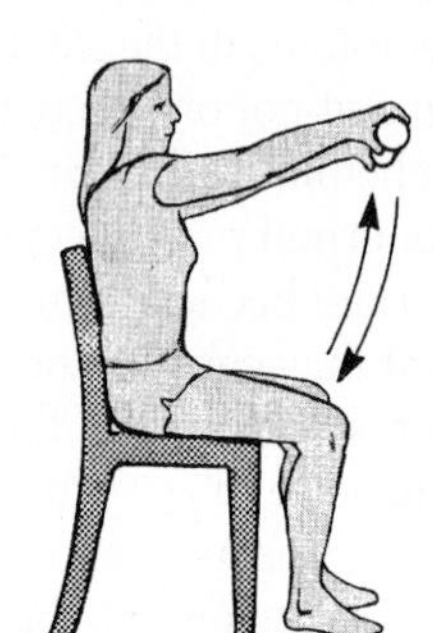

Start with arms straight out in front. Raise arms up and down, only to chin level. Repeat 10 times.

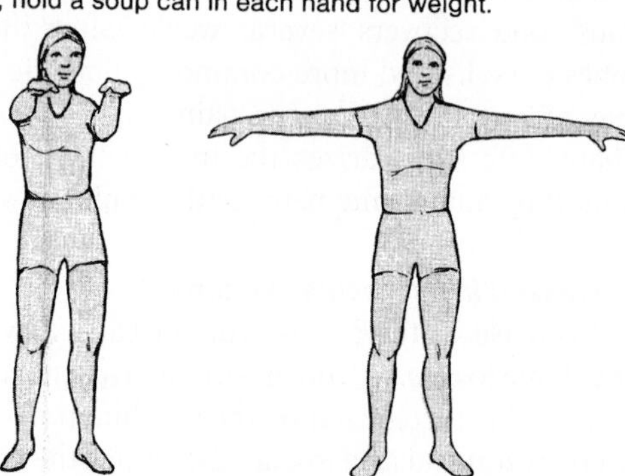

Start with arms straight out in front. Swing arms out to sides and return to front. Repeat 10 times.

Rising Exercise

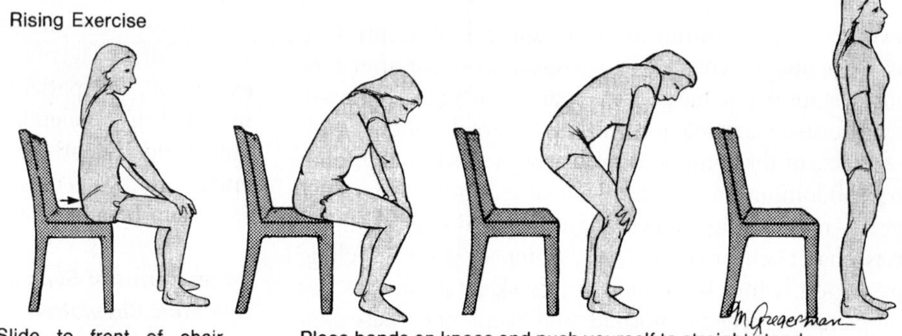

Slide to front of chair, keeping legs apart.

Place hands on knees and push yourself to straight stand. Sit down, using hands on knees to help.

Repeat 3–5 times using hands less and legs more each time. Repeat exercise without using hands to help.

FIGURE 89.4. Exercise for weakness and orthostatic hypotension after prolonged bed rest. Patient must be out of bed 2 hours a day, morning, afternoon, and evening. Exercises are done three times a day. (Courtesy of Karen Ryder, Registered Occupational Therapist.)

Syncope from Cardiac Abnormalities

Rhythm Disturbances

Arrhythmias should always be considered in patients with syncope or near syncope that are older, have known heart disease, describe palpitations, or have syncope while seated or recumbent. Suspicion should also be raised in patients taking medications that may cause arrhythmias, including antiarrhythmics themselves (Table 89.5). Premonitory symptoms such as palpitations, grayouts, sweating, nausea, and fear may be recalled, but the presence or absence of these symptoms is not sufficient to confirm or refute the diagnosis of an arrhythmia. Most patients with cerebral symptoms of arrhythmias have normal resting ECGs. In general, at least 24 hours of ECG monitoring should be performed to identify potentially important arrhythmias in patients with syncope that is not explained by the initial history, physical examination, and 12-lead ECG (see above) and some should have electrophysiology (EP) testing (see Diagnostic Tests).

Outflow Obstruction

An obstruction to ventricular outflow caused by aortic stenosis may lead to syncope. It nearly always follows exertion and is often associated with chest pain. Unconsciousness may be prolonged and may be followed by neurologic abnormalities. Similarly, up to 30% of patients with hypertrophic cardiomyopathy experience syncope by outlet obstruction after exercise or by an arrhythmia (43). Chapter 65 describes the diagnostic approach to patients thought to have outflow obstruction. A left-atrial myxoma (rare) may cause syncope by obstruction of blood flow when a patient leans over or undergoes exertion. Cyanotic congenital heart disease also leads to syncope after exercise or, rarely, during an airplane flight. Hypoxia and increased blood viscosity are contributing factors.

Myocardial Infarction

Acute myocardial infarction (MI) may present with syncope, which may result from an arrhythmia, low cardiac output, or severe pain. However, overall, MI is a rare cause of syncope (44). Embolization from a mural thrombus should be considered when syncope occurs during recovery from MI.

Exercise-Induced Syncope

While exercise can be a trigger of neurocardiogenic syncope, syncope that is brought on with exercise suggests cardiac or vascular causes particularly in older patients. Aortic stenosis and hypertrophic cardiomyopathy may limit cardiac output in response to increased demand (e.g., exercise) leading to syncope. Ischemia-induced arrhythmias may also be unmasked by exercise. An echocardiogram followed by exercise tolerance testing is the appropriate evaluation of patients with exercise-induced syncope (45).

An uncommon cause of exercise-induced ischemia is *subclavian steal*. If the subclavian artery is occluded proximal to the origin of the vertebral artery, increased oxygen demand by the distal subclavian artery territory may result in retrograde blood flow ("steal") from the vertebral artery to the subclavian artery. Exercise involving the arm is the typical activity that unmasks subclavian steal. Much more common on the left than on the right, subclavian steal should be associated with a decreased blood pressure on the affected side.

Syncope from Metabolic Abnormalities

The initial history and physical examination should seek to identify any symptoms or signs of metabolic derangement, especially because some derangements may lead to lasting damage.

Hypoglycemia

Loss of consciousness may occur in hypoglycemic adults, although rarely in older patients, when the blood glucose level is below 40 mg/100 mL. Hunger, palpitations, sweating, and anxiety nearly always occur 5 to 15 minutes before the patient loses consciousness. Because the brain can survive for only about 10 minutes with a blood glucose of 20 mg/100 mL or less, the prophylactic administration of glucose is warranted in anyone who remains unconscious long enough for the physician to prepare the solution. Convulsions and incontinence commonly accompany hypoglycemic coma. Chapter 79 describes the evaluation and management of hypoglycemia caused by exogenous insulin. Reactive hypoglycemia and fasting hypoglycemia (which may be caused by insulinoma) may produce near syncope but only rarely unconsciousness. Chapter 81 describes these problems.

Hypocapnia (Hyperventilation)

Hypocapnia caused by hyperventilation leads to syncope, near syncope, or ill-defined dizziness by decreasing cerebral blood flow through vasoconstriction of small arterioles throughout the brain. A PCO_2 of 25 mm Hg is sufficient to lower cerebral blood flow to levels at which symptoms may occur; such a value may be produced in some people by a few very deep breaths. Athletes preparing to race, musicians playing wind instruments, or anyone who is fearful or anxious may develop transient symptoms in this way. Tetany or carpopedal spasm may or may not precede the cerebral symptoms. Recovery is prompt if ventilation is slowed. Chapter 22 describes the diagnosis and management of hyperventilation related to anxiety, the most common cause of this problem.

Hypoxemia

Hypoxemia caused by any primary cause may predispose to syncope/near syncope. Severe anemia (see Chapter 55) may sufficiently deprive the brain of oxygen to lead to syncope after exercise; it may also predispose to syncope from any other cause. Asphyxiation caused by obstruction of the upper airway should be considered in small children, patients with poor dentition, or patients with masses in the neck. Short-term exposure to moderate or *high altitude*, even in healthy young adults, may lead to syncope, possibly mediated by a decrease in arterial oxygen saturation.

Seizures are common in patients with acute hypoxemia, and neurologic sequelae are the rule after unconsciousness lasting more than 1 or 2 minutes. The management of hypoxemic syncope depends entirely on prompt and accurate diagnosis to prevent recurrence or worsening of the hypoxemia.

Drug Overdose

Overdose of some drugs may cause syncope/near syncope due to orthostatic hypotension. These drugs include sedatives, which may produce venous pooling (particularly chloral hydrate, paraldehyde, and ethanol and less often benzodiazepines and barbiturates), and all the drugs listed as potential causes of autonomic impairment in Table 89.5. However, overdose of most drugs is more likely to cause stupor or coma from their sedating effects than to cause syncope or near syncope from orthostatic hypotension.

Syncope from Intracranial Abnormalities

Seizure

Seizure as a cause of syncope is a diagnosis that is thought to be made easily from historical details. However, as noted above, brief clonic movements are seen in some patients who have syncope unrelated to seizure. In the prospective evaluation of patients presenting with syncope mentioned above, 50% of patients underwent electroencephalographic (EEG) testing, and this confirmed an underlying seizure disorder in only 1.5% (20). It has been demonstrated that the best discriminating finding distinguishing seizure from syncope was orientation immediately after the event, as reported by an eyewitness. A seizure was found to be five times more likely if the patient was reported to be disoriented after the event. In the absence of an eyewitness, the age of the patient was the most useful discriminator; a seizure was three times more likely if the patient was younger than 45 years. Incontinence and trauma were not discriminative findings (46). Chapter 88 describes the diagnosis and management of seizure disorders.

Subarachnoid Hemorrhage

A brief period of unconsciousness at the beginning of subarachnoid hemorrhage is very common. This diagnosis is strongly suggested when the constellation of severe headache, confusion, and neck stiffness follows shortly after a syncopal episode. Any patient who is confused and develops headache during initial evaluation should be admitted for observation and evaluation, even if meningismus has not yet developed.

Cerebral Embolism or Thrombosis

Cerebral embolism or thrombosis may cause brief (TIA) or prolonged (cerebrovascular accident) unconsciousness if the basilar artery is affected; however, more commonly, disease of the posterior circulation leads to loss of postural tone without loss of consciousness. Very rarely, a carotid occlusion may cause unconsciousness initially, even if the remaining vessels are patent. A carotid occlusion likewise may cause loss of consciousness if the contralateral carotid is already occluded. In this instance, the period of unconsciousness is usually prolonged and seizures may occur; neurologic symptoms and signs are nearly always present. Chapter 91 describes the diagnosis and management of CVD.

Migraine

Migraine (see Chapter 87) may produce syncope or near syncope by spasm of the basilar artery or of the posterior cerebral arteries. Syncope that occurs with migraine is more often caused by hyperventilation or a neurocardiogenic mechanism rather than by a central abnormality.

Increased Intracranial Pressure

Increased intracranial pressure, whether caused by a brain tumor, trauma, or an obstruction to the ventricular system, may result in syncope when a Valsalva maneuver is performed such as during straining at defecation or bending over. The hallmarks are pre-existing symptoms, papilledema, and neurologic signs.

General Approach to the Patient (47)

Most patients who come to a physician after an episode of syncope or near syncope do so after their symptoms have resolved. The history should be obtained both from the patient and from anyone who observed the episode. The inquiry should focus on the events immediately before and after the attack, associated problems that may have been present for days to weeks before the episode, and evidence of trauma, neurologic deficit, or aspiration complicating the current episode of syncope. The objectives of these initial steps are to reach a working diagnosis or decide what further evaluation and management is needed for the patient. However, the most important focus during the evaluation of the patient who presents with syncope is to determine if the patient has evidence of intrinsic heart disease (20). As discussed above, the presence of preexisting heart disease significantly increases the risk for a cardiogenic etiology for syncope, which carries a far worse prognosis than a noncardiogenic cause.

Appropriate management may range from reassurance (e.g., the patient with neurocardiogenic syncope), to volume expansion (e.g., the patient with a diarrheal illness), to hospital admission for observation, prompt diagnostic testing, and necessary treatment (e.g., the patient with a history suggesting life-threatening arrhythmias or the patient with a major fracture complicating syncope). Details regarding the critical features of many of the causes of syncope listed in Table 89.5 are discussed in the following section.

History

Current Episode

The patient should always be questioned about his or her situation and body position immediately before the attack. Many patients with a cardiac etiology for syncope have no prodromal symptoms. On the contrary, neurocardiogenic syncope is often preceded by autonomic symptoms (e.g., nausea, pallor, and diaphoresis). If there was psychologic stress (e.g., an argument or fear about a medical procedure), one should consider neurocardiogenic syncope. If exercise preceded the attack, both neurocardiogenic syncope and a number of primary cardiopulmonary abnormalities are possible (including aortic stenosis, hypertrophic cardiomyopathy, arrhythmia, and pulmonary hypertension). (See discussion above of exercise-induced syncope.) If syncope was associated with micturition, coughing, or defecation, the episode may have been caused by an associated Valsalva-induced decrease in venous return as an initiating mechanism for neurocardiogenic syncope.

Syncope from most causes does not occur unless the patient is in the upright position. If the attack occurred when the patient first stood up, orthostatic hypotension should be considered.

Syncope that occurs when the patient is seated or recumbent suggests hypoglycemia, carotid sinus hypersensitivity, cardiac arrhythmia, hyperventilation, seizure, or a psychiatric disorder.

The patient also should be asked *whether consciousness was lost completely* and whether a fall or any injury occurred. Although patients with many different causes of syncope may recall feelings of dizziness, heaviness of the limbs, or dimming of vision before loss of consciousness, other associated symptoms may suggest a diagnosis. Nausea is characteristic of neurocardiogenic syncope but may also occur with bradyarrhythmias, myocardial ischemia, and loss of intravascular volume. Palpitations may suggest an arrhythmia, whereas chest pain and diaphoresis suggest myocardial ischemia. Headache and characteristic visual changes suggest a migraine. Incontinence and tonic–clonic movements of the extremities suggest a seizure; a seizure may be the primary problem or may be secondary to another event, such as cerebral ischemia or cardiac arrhythmia (see Seizure).

Observations made by others who witnessed the period of unconsciousness. Particular attention should be paid to the duration of the spell, whether a convulsion occurred, the sequence of events, and how the patient seemed during the period of recovery. Generally, recovery of consciousness is swift when the cause is from decreased cerebral blood flow. If recovery of clear consciousness takes more than 5 minutes, one should suspect a seizure, hypoglycemia, or stroke.

History preceding the current episode should be sought. Information about the patient during the hours, days, or weeks preceding syncope/near syncope is often helpful in the differential diagnosis. In particular, one should determine the frequency of any previous episodes of syncope or near syncope, as the frequency of episodes influences decisions regarding the urgency of obtaining diagnostic studies. Frequent episodes without injury, especially if the syncope typically is preceded by nonspecific prodromal symptoms, should raise suspicion of a psychiatric disorder. A history of dizziness in addition to syncope is a marker for a greater prevalence of psychiatric disorders, although cardiac arrhythmias may have a similar presentation. Other circumstances surrounding previous episodes of dizziness or syncope may help develop a working diagnosis for the current episode of syncope. For example, a patient may report that previous episodes of dizziness or near syncope occurred after taking a new antihypertensive or psychotropic medication. A patient convalescing from recent illness may relate the symptoms to being up and around after bed rest.

A patient with known organic heart disease, especially a patient with depressed left ventricular function or a history of ischemic heart disease, is at high risk of syncope caused by an arrhythmia. Although uncommon, a family history of cardiomyopathy or arrhythmia (such as prolonged QT syndrome) should be sought while taking the history from the patient.

Physical Examination

General Examination

The physical examination should include a search for abnormalities that may confirm a diagnosis suggested in the history or may reveal an unexpected cause. As patients with organic heart disease may have life-threatening causes of syncope, the cardiovascular examination is particularly important in all patients who present for the evaluation of a syncopal event. The heart rate and blood pressure should be measured after the patient has been recumbent for a few minutes and again after standing for 1 to 2 minutes. Very different blood pressures in the two arms would raise the possibility of aortic dissection or subclavian steal. The strength and upstroke of the carotid pulses should be appraised, and any bruits should be noted. The pulse should be palpated for 1 to 2 minutes to look for irregularities. The heart should be examined for murmurs (particularly the murmurs of aortic stenosis and hypertrophic cardiomyopathy), clicks, or gallops. Abdominal examination may reveal a large bladder or signs of a visceral catastrophe. If orthostatic hypotension has been found, a rectal examination should be performed to check the stool for occult or gross blood.

Carotid Massage

For patients with episodes suggestive of carotid sinus hypersensitivity (see Carotid Sinus Hypersensitivity) or older patients with recurrent syncope and a nondiagnostic evaluation, carotid massage can be performed. However, it should be performed only if there are no carotid bruits and when there is intravenous access and electrocardiographic and blood pressure monitoring, with atropine at hand. Additionally, it should not be performed in patients with a history of TIA or stroke unless recent imaging has shown no carotid disease (48). When performed, carotid massage involves application of digital pressure over each carotid sinus separately, for up to 5 seconds. A resulting carotid asystole of more than 3 seconds or a systolic blood pressure drop of more than 50 mm Hg is considered abnormal.

Neurologic Examination

A brief examination of the major components of the nervous system (see Chapter 86) may reveal evidence of pre-existing neurologic disease or of an acute insult. One should note the patient's orientation, speech, memory (for general information and the episode itself), and judgment. The fundi may reveal microemboli (see Chapter 91, Fig. 91.1) or subhyaloid hemorrhages (a sign of subarachnoid hemorrhage). Involvement of the midbrain, pons, or medulla is suggested by nystagmus, ophthalmoplegia, and other abnormalities of the cranial nerves. Weakness, sensory abnormalities, and pathologic reflexes may indicate a lesion elsewhere in the CNS. Any neurologic abnormalities should raise the suspicion of CVD, intracranial mass, subarachnoid hemorrhage, seizure, or CNS infection. If trauma has occurred in the recent past or if a fall was sustained during the syncopal episode, subdural or epidural hemorrhage should be considered. A nonfocal neurologic examination makes an intracranial cause of syncope unlikely, whereas a focal neurologic examination should prompt imaging of the CNS.

Significance of Seizures and Neurologic Deficits

Seizure activity may occur after syncope with a variety of causes, including neurocardiogenic syncope, cardiac arrhythmias, hyperventilation, orthostatic hypotension, or venous pooling. This is not surprising because unconsciousness signifies a major disruption in normal brain function. A single tonic convulsion is the most common type of postsyncopal seizure; less often a focal seizure may occur. In these instances, the patient's evaluation should include routine tests for a seizure focus (see Chapter 88). However, it should be emphasized that the presence of seizure-like activity in association with a syncopal event does not diagnose a primary neurologic cause for syncope. It makes it more likely and should prompt further neurologic evaluation, but other etiologies for syncope need to be considered.

Minor neurologic signs, such as slight focal weakness, reflex asymmetries, or pathologic reflexes, may be found after syncope from any cause, particularly if the patient is examined immediately after recovering consciousness. Such findings rarely persist for more than a few minutes. If such signs persist, are more profound, or occur in a constellation that suggests a particular anatomic lesion, they warrant further pursuit. However, one should not be surprised if a source is not found because minor neurologic signs are not uncommon after general ischemic or metabolic insults to the brain.

Diagnostic Tests

The history and physical examination lead to a diagnosis in 25% of patients with syncope (47). For these patients, no additional diagnostic tests are necessary. For the remaining patients, however, several diagnostic tests should be considered.

Electrocardiogram

An ECG, with a rhythm strip, *is indicated in all patients with syncope* if the cause is not obvious from the history and physical examination. Although the ECG shows some abnormality in a large proportion of patients with syncope, it confirms a diagnosis in a much smaller number (Table 89.6). Specific diagnostic workups may be prompted by certain ECG abnormalities. For instance, sinus bradycardia in the absence of a β-blocker should prompt concern for sick sinus syndrome or sinus arrest. Sinus tachycardia may be present in patients with volume depletion, congestive heart failure, or pulmonary embolus. Left ventricular hypertrophy may be caused by aortic stenosis or hypertrophic cardiomyopathy, and a prolonged QT interval increases susceptibility to ventricular tachycardia. Left bundle branch block could be caused by cardiomyopathies or MI, and bifascicular block is associated with increased risk for complete heart block (see details in Chapter 64). The noninvasive nature of the test and its low cost, with the potential to uncover a possibly life-threatening disorder, make the ECG a cornerstone of the evaluation of nearly all patients with syncope (47).

Electrocardiographic Monitoring

The *Holter monitor* is one of the most commonly used diagnostic tests in patients with syncope, but the correlation of symptoms and arrhythmia in patients with syncope can be as low as 4% (49). In a prospective study of 140 patients with unexplained syncope, serious diagnostic arrhythmias found with Holter monitoring occurred exclusively in patients with a positive cardiac history and an abnormal electrocardiogram (50), suggesting that the initial evaluation described above can be used in making decisions about Holter monitoring.

There are other methods to monitor patients for arrhythmias for longer periods such as a *loop recorder (event monitor)*, which saves several minutes of rhythm retroactively when activated by a patient while symptoms are experienced. Surprisingly, loop monitors are generally less expensive than Holter monitoring. In a comparison of Holter monitoring and loop recorders in patients with syncope, the diagnostic yield for symptom-rhythm correlations was 56% for loop recorders versus 22% for Holter monitors (51). Unfortunately, while event recorders have many appealing qualities, one major limitation is the dependency on the patient to trigger the device. In one study, 23% of patients who experienced syncope failed to trigger the device at the time of symptoms despite being trained how to use the device (51). This type of testing may be useful in patients in whom arrhythmia is believed to be likely, who have a negative Holter monitor, and who have mild enough symptoms so that they can activate the recorder. Loop recorders may be of particular use in patients without organic heart disease who have frequent episodes of syncope (20).

A relatively new modality is an implantable subcutaneous recorder that can be left in place for more than a year. Some experts recommend using these devices in patients with cardiac disease who have recurrent unexplained syncope or falls with a completely negative evaluation (52). It is reported that a diagnosis is made in up to 55% of patients with implantable recorders versus 19% with traditional external recorders with a distinct advantage in detecting bradyarrhythmias (53). Given the invasive nature of this diagnostic technique, however, its role in the evaluation of syncope is yet to be determined.

Arrhythmias detected during electrocardiographic monitoring but not accompanied by symptoms are difficult to interpret. Although some believe that these arrhythmias, even if unaccompanied by symptoms, may provide a working diagnosis, others disagree. Some arrhythmias, such as sinus arrest and nonsustained ventricular tachycardia, can be seen in normal people. Therefore, the results must be interpreted with caution, with consideration paid to the severity of the detected arrhythmia and the presence of any underlying heart disease. The exception may be nonsustained ventricular tachycardia in a patient with a history of MI or depressed left ventricular function, since this has been shown to increase the risk for sudden death.

Electrophysiologic Testing

EP studies are considered the final step in the evaluation when arrhythmia is strongly suspected and noninvasive testing is nondiagnostic (e.g., in patients with organic heart disease and unexplained syncope). *Indications* for EP testing in patients with syncope include (52):

- Abnormal ECG and/or
- Structureal heart disease or
- Syncope associated with palpitations or a family history of sudden death.
- To evaluate the nature of an arrhythmia which as already been identified
- In persons with high-risk occupations

EP testing is most likely to produce abnormal findings in patients with underlying heart disease. In a study of 111 patients with *unexplained syncope* referred for EP testing, 50% of those with underlying heart disease had positive findings on EP testing, whereas 16% of those without underlying heart disease had positive findings (54). Because other studies have failed to identify clinical predictors that correlate with positive findings on EP studies (55) and because EP findings may lead to treatment that decreases episodes of syncope, there are no clear-cut guidelines for excluding EP testing for patients with unexplained syncope, although the European Society of Cardiology guidelines suggest that EP testing is generally not indicated in persons with no heart disease, no palpitations, and normal ECGs (52).

The most common abnormal finding in patients undergoing EP testing is ventricular tachycardia, followed by conduction disturbances and supraventricular tachycardia, with the percentage of patients with abnormal findings depending on the population studied. As with Holter monitoring, certain abnormalities detected, especially conduction abnormalities and even certain tachyarrhythmias, have questionable clinical significance. It should be noted that EP testing has a lower diagnostic yield in identifying bradyarrhythmias compared to tachyarrhythmias.

Echocardiogram

Transthoracic echocardiography is utilized in up to 60% of patients admitted to hospital for syncope. However, in a recent study, echocardiography proved useful only if the patient had a history of cardiac disease, an abnormal cardiac physical examination, or an abnormal ECG; the echocardiogram showed a significantly reduced ejection fraction in 27% of these patients. However, in patients without cardiac disease and a normal ECG, echocardiography added no useful information (56).

Tilt-Table Testing

In the past 20 years, tilt-table testing has played an increasingly important role in the diagnosis and management of syncope. The most significant impact of tilt-table testing has been in patients without organic heart disease who have unexplained syncope. However, patients with organic heart disease and a negative evaluation for syncope (including EP testing) may also be evaluated with tilt-table testing (57). Tilt-table testing has dramatically reduced the proportion of patients with unexplained syncope.

The tilt-table test is a provocative test used to *document susceptibility to neurocardiogenic syncope* (see Patient Experience). In neurocardiogenic syncope that can be demonstrated by tilt-table testing, blood pooling in the lower extremities leads to central hypovolemia, which ultimately is associated with bradycardia in some individuals (the exact mechanism is a matter of debate). Resultant hypotension leads to decreased CNS perfusion, which leads to syncope. The degree to which bradycardia by the cardioinhibitory response versus hypotension by the vasodepressor response causes syncope varies between individuals and can help predict the efficacy of treatment.

Patient Experience. The tilt-table test is performed by securing a patient to the tilt table in the supine position. The patient is kept in the supine position for 15 to 30 minutes (58) before they are tilted, and then the patient is tilted to a 60- to 80-degree angle within 10 to 15 seconds. (Many patients find this experience unpleasant, because it replicates the syncopal event. It is therefore important to discuss the test with the patient beforehand.) The patient is maintained at the tilted angle for up to 60 minutes, during which time blood pressure and heart rate are monitored. The mean time to syncope in patients with a positive test is 25 minutes (59).

A tilt-table test is deemed positive if syncope or presyncope with hypotension develops. If no event occurs, provocation with either isoproterenol or nitroglycerine may be tried, increasing sensitivity but losing specificity. Even without resorting to provocative testing, establishing susceptibility to neurocardiogenic syncope does not guarantee this as the cause of the patient's event.

Although tilt-table testing is most commonly used to establish susceptibility to neurocardiogenic syncope, other abnormal cardiovascular responses may be uncovered with the test. In the neurocardiogenic response, both heart rate and blood pressure decline. However, in some patients, blood pressure may drop without significant changes in heart rate (termed the *dysautonomic response*). In others, heart rate may increase while blood pressure drops, termed the *postural orthostatic tachycardia syndrome* (60).

The most recent guidelines for the use of tilt table testing in patients with syncope were published by the European Society of Cardiology in 2001, and updated in 2004 (Table 89.7) (52). This consensus document, along with other studies on the evaluation of the patient with syncope, can be summarized as five indications for tilt-table testing:

1. Syncope presumed to be vasovagal, but the history or physical are inconclusive
2. Recurrent syncope in a patient in whom cardiac etiologies have been excluded
3. Syncope resulting in an accident or injury
4. Syncope occurring in a high-risk setting

TABLE 89.7 Summary of Principal Indications for Tilt-Table Testing for Evaluation of Syncope

Tilt-table testing is warranted
Recurrent syncope or single syncopal episode in a high-risk patient, whether or not the medical history is suggestive of neurally mediated (vasovagal) origin, and
No evidence of structural cardiovascular disease, or
Structural cardiovascular disease is present but cardiac causes of syncope have been excluded by appropriate testing
Further evaluation of patients in whom an apparent cause has been established (e.g., asystole, atrioventricular block) but in whom demonstration of susceptibility to neurally mediated syncope would affect treatment plans
Part of the evaluation of exercise-induced or exercise-associated syncope
Conditions for which reasonable differences of opinion exist regarding utility of tilt-table testing
Differentiating convulsive syncope from seizures
Evaluating patients (especially the elderly) with recurrent unexplained falls
Assessing recurrent dizziness or presyncope
Evaluating unexplained syncope in the setting of peripheral neuropathies or dysautonomias
Tilt-table testing not warranted
Single syncopal episode, without injury and not in a high-risk setting with clear-cut vasovagal clinical features
Syncope in which an alternative specific cause has been established and in which additional demonstration of a neurally mediated susceptibility would not alter treatment plans
Assessment of response to treatment
Potential emerging indications
Recurrent idiopathic vertigo
Recurrent transient ischemic attacks
Sudden infant death syndrome

5. When the establishment of a diagnosis of neurocardiogenic syncope will impact management of syncope of another etiology

Tilt table testing can be useful not only for suggesting a diagnosis of neurocardiogenic syncope, but may also allow an opportunity for patient education and reassurance. Patients can learn what their premonitory symptoms are so they can better learn when to take evasive action at the onset of symptoms. Additionally, it is often reassuring for patients to have their symptoms observed by a physician. However, it needs to be emphasized that a positive tilt-table test only suggests a diagnosis of neurocardiogenic syncope but does not prove the diagnosis. Patients with risk factors for cardiac syncope still require evaluation for that even if they have a positive tilt-table test (58).

Guidelines for Admission to a Hospital

Patients should be considered for admission to a hospital for initial evaluation and treatment if there is a high risk of injury from a recurrent event or a high risk of a life-threatening arrhythmia. Assessment of the risk of injury should be based on the degree of injury sustained in the current episode, the frequency of episodes, and the fragility of the patient. Assessment of the risk of an arrhythmia should be based on the status of any underlying heart disease and the presence of any current or previous ECG abnormalities. Unfortunately, there are no studies that specifically look at this issue, but in general if a patient has a good history for neurocardiogenic syncope (or other low-risk etiologies of syncope) and have no evidence of heart disease and a normal ECG, they can be evaluated as an outpatient (20).

Selected Conditions that May Mimic Syncope

Hysterical Faint

Fainting caused by conversion disorder or other forms of somatization occurs in a manner to avoid injury, an important distinguishing feature from true syncope. The patient crumples to the ground with a limp body and shallow respirations. Recovery is usually immediate. Often, the faint may be embellished with movements that resemble seizures, but more often voluntary movements are the rule. Hyperventilation or coaxing may reproduce the spell. Chapter 21 provides additional detail regarding the evaluation and management of such patients. It should be emphasized that in the past up to 30% of patients with syncope were labeled as being psychiatric in origin. However, the improvement in diagnostic evaluation (in particular tilt-table testing) has dramatically reduced this as a diagnostic category.

Drop Attack

Older patients, especially men, may report sudden and unprovoked falls to the ground. Consciousness is not lost, and the patients can usually remember the entire episode. The history of maintenance of consciousness distinguishes drop attacks from syncope. Ischemia of the lower brainstem is one possible cause of drop attacks, and occasionally patients report other concurrent symptoms that suggest vertebrobasilar ischemia. Management is identical to that of TIAs occurring in the posterior circulation (see Chapter 91).

Cataplexy

Cataplexy is a special kind of drop attack, not caused by ischemia, that occurs as part of the syndrome of narcolepsy. The patient falls suddenly to the ground because of a loss of extensor muscle tone but without loss of consciousness. These spells are usually provoked by a sudden startle, a joke, laughing, or sneezing. *Sleep paralysis* (paralysis of the limbs for a minute or 2 upon awakening) and peculiar visual hallucinations on awakening or before falling asleep may also accompany narcolepsy. (See Chapter 7 for additional details.)

DISEQUILIBRIUM OF MISCELLANEOUS ORIGINS

Some patients with persistent dizziness do not have manifestations that make it possible to classify their problem as vertigo or near syncope. Many of these patients have disequilibrium, or a sense of imbalance, that may be caused by multiple sensory deficits (e.g., partial hearing, visual, proprioceptive impairment, or vestibular impairment); lower extremity weakness (e.g., from an old stroke or from disuse after a period of bed rest); pain in a weight-bearing joint (e.g., degenerative arthritis of the hips, knees, or ankles), cerebellar ataxia (see Chapter 86); recently initiated drugs (especially anxiolytics, hypnotics, or neuroleptics); or the onset of a progressive CNS disease (e.g., parkinsonism, normal pressure hydrocephalus, or subcortical small-vessel ischemic disease) (61). These problems often occur in older patients, debilitated patients (particularly chronic alcoholics), or patients with long-standing diabetes mellitus, hypertension, and other vascular risk factors. Cervical myelopathy, either metabolic (e.g., vitamin B_{12} deficiency), infectious (e.g., neurosyphilis), or because of cervical stenosis, should also be considered. In some patients, CVD or autonomic neuropathy may cause periodic vertigo and near syncope to be superimposed on their day-to-day problem with imbalance.

The evaluation of patients describing imbalance consists chiefly of obtaining a history of the duration, progression, and day-to-day characteristics of the problem, focusing on the limitations imposed on their usual activities and on any falls or near accidents that may have occurred. Often, patients with disequilibrium will describe the dizziness as originating in their feet rather than their head (62). Patients with disequilibrium may also report their symptoms are worse in the dark when they lose visual cues that may help them compensate for some of their deficits. In the physical examination, it is important to determine which of the many problems listed above may be contributing to the patient's symptoms focusing on the patient's ophthalmologic examination, sensory examination of the feet, and musculoskeletal examination. When disequilibrium is suspected, it is crucial to observe the patient's gait.

Depending on the individual patient, management by the generalist may include referring the patient for correction of any impairment in hearing or vision (see Chapters 107 and 110), consulting a neurologist if unexplained progressive symptoms are found (e.g., cerebellar ataxia in an otherwise healthy person), consulting a physical therapist if weakness or the need for selecting a cane or walker is apparent, and discontinuing drugs that may be contributing to the patient's symptoms and avoiding drugs that may worsen symptoms (Tables 89.2 and 89.5).

NONSPECIFIC DIZZINESS

A subset of patients who present to primary care physicians will be categorized as having nonspecific dizziness. Up to 15% of dizzy patients in some series fall into this category (1). These patients can be the most challenging of all dizzy patients. Often, patients with nonspecific dizziness are simply incapable of explaining their symptoms beyond general terms of "I just feel dizzy." Invariably, their physical examination is normal. Most patients with nonspecific dizziness are young. Commonly, they have concomitant psychiatric disease including depression, anxiety disorders, and somatization. The role of having the patient hyperventilate to reproduce symptoms is controversial. Some authors advocate this approach. However, as discussed above, hypocarbia can induce dizziness through near syncope in many normal patients. Therefore, the specificity of this technique is highly questionable (63).

The therapeutic approach to patients with nonspecific dizziness is similar to that of patients with somatization disorder (63). Patients require reassurance that their symptoms do not represent life-threatening pathology, but also require recognition of the impact their symptoms have on their life. In a recent study, patients with nonspecific dizziness were shown to benefit from treatment with SSRIs (64).

CHRONIC DIZZINESS: GENERAL MEASURES HELPFUL IN MANAGEMENT

Patients with chronic dizziness, vertigo, syncope, or disequilibrium have a far better prognosis if their home environments are safe and others in their households are aware of risks that should be avoided and devices that may be helpful. A number of general measures to recommend include using night-lights, tacking down loose carpeting and floorboards, installing special railings in the bathroom, selecting proper footwear, and learning to assume an upright posture gradually. These measures can be accomplished most effectively if the physician or a visiting nurse evaluates the patient's home. If vertigo is a contributing factor to chronic dizziness, vestibular rehabilitation can be helpful regardless of the underlying cause (65). In some patients with unsteady gait, a cane or a walker may be helpful; a physical therapist can be very helpful in selecting the best assistive device.

SPECIFIC REFERENCES*

1. Kroenke K, Mangelsdorff AD. Common symptoms in ambulatory care: incidence, evaluation, therapy and outcome. Am J Med 1989;86:262.
2. Demer JL, Honrubia V, Baloh RW. Dynamic visual acuity: a test for oscillopsia and vestibulo-ocular reflex function. Am J Otol 1994;15:340.
3. Oas JG, Baloh RW. Vertigo and the anterior inferior cerebellar artery syndrome. Neurology 1992;42:2274.
4. Strupp M, Zingler VC, Arbusow V, et al. Methylprednisolone, valacyclovir, or the combination for vestibular neuritis. N Engl J Med 2004;351:354.
5. Epley JM. The canalith repositioning procedure: for treatment of benign paroxysmal positional vertigo. Otolaryngol Head Neck Surg 1992;107:399.
6. Lynn S, Pool A, Rose D, et al. Randomized trial of the canalith repositioning procedure. Otolaryngol Head Neck Surg 1995;113:712.
7. Radtke A, Neuhauser H, von Brevern N, et al. A modified Epley's procedure for self-treatment of benign paroxysmal positional vertigo. Neurology 1999;53:1358.
8. Brandt T, Daroff RB. Physical therapy for benign paroxysmal positional vertigo. Arch Otolaryngol 1980;106:484.
9. Karlberg M, Hall K, Quickert N, et al. What inner ear diseases cause benign paroxysmal positional vertigo? Acta Otolaryngol 2000;120:380.
10. Neuhauser H, Leopold M, von Brevern M, et al. The interrelations of migraine, vertigo, and migrainous vertigo. Neurology 2001;56:436.
11. Swartz KL, Pratt LA, Armenian HK, et al. Mental disorders and the incidence of migraine headaches in a community sample: results from the Baltimore Epidemiologic Catchment area follow-up study. Arch Gen Psychiatry 2000; 57:945.
12. Radtke A, Lempert T, Gresty MA, et al. Migraine and Ménière's disease: Is there a link? Neurology 2002;59:1700.
13. Gomez CR, Cruz-Flores S, Malkoff MD, et al. Isolated vertigo as a manifestation of vertebrobasilar ischemia. Neurology 1996;47:94.
14. Friedland DR, Wackym PA. A critical appraisal of spontaneous perilymphatic fistulas of the inner ear. Am J Otol 1999;20:261.
15. Minor LB. Gentamicin-induced bilateral vestibular hypofunction. JAMA 1998;279:541.
16. Baloh RW, Jacobson K, Fife T. Familial vestibulopathy: a new dominantly inherited syndrome. Neurology 1994;44:20.
17. Rinne T, Bronstein AM, Rudge P, et al. Bilateral loss of vestibular function: clinical findings in 53 patients. J Neurol 1998;245:314.

*Bold numerals denote published controlled clinical trials, meta-analyses, or consensus-based recommendations.

18. Takeda N, Matsunaga T. Neurochemical basis of motion sickness and its treatment and prevention. In: Baloh RW, Halmagyi GM, eds. Disorders of the vestibular system. New York: Oxford University Press, 1996: 529.
19. Hain TC. Mal de debarquement. Arch Otolaryngol Head Neck Surg 1999;125:615.
20. Kapoor WN. Syncope. N Engl J Med 2000; 343:1856.
21. Savage DD, Corwin L, McGee DL, et al. Epidemiologic features of isolated syncope: the Framingham Study. Stroke 1985;16:626.
22. Young WF, Maddox DE. Spells: in search of a cause. Mayo Clin Proc 1995;70:757.
23. Soteriades ES, Evans JC, Larson MG, et al. Incidence and prognosis of syncope. N Engl J Med 2002;347:878.
24. Goldschlager N, Epstein AE, Grubb BP, et al. Etiologic considerations in the patient with syncope and an apparently normal heart. Arch Intern Med 2003;163:151.
25. Kapoor WN. Current evaluation and management of syncope. Circulation 2002;106: 1606.
26. Martin TP, Hanusa BH, Kappor WN. Risk stratification of patients with syncope. Ann Emerg Med 1997;29:459.
27. Schnipper JL, Kappor WK. Diagnostic evaluation and management of patients with syncope. Med Clin North Am 2001;84:423.
28. Ammirati F, Colvicchi F, Santini M. Diagnosing syncope in clinical practice: implementation of a simplified diagnostic algorithm in a multicentre proposepctive trial. Eur Heart J 2000;21: 935.
29. Sarasin FP, Louis-Smionet M, Carballo D, et al. Prospective evaluation of patients with syncope: a population-based study. Am J Med 2001;111: 177.
30. Van Dijk N, de Bruin IG, Grisolf J, et al. Hemodynamic effects of leg crossing and skeletal muscle testing during free standing in patients with vasovagal syncope. J Appl Physiol 2005;98:584.
31. Mahanonda N, Bhuripanyo K, Kangkagate C, et al. Randomized double blind, placebo-controlled trial of oral atenolol in patients with unexplained syncope and positive upright tilt table test results. Am Heart J 1995; 130:1250.
32. Cox MM, Perlman BA, Mayor MR, et al. Acute and long-term beta-adrenergic blockade for patients with neurocardiogenic syncope. J Am Coll Cardiol 1995;26:1293.
33. Ventura R, Maas R, Ziedler D, et al. A randomized and controlled pilot trial of beta blockers for the treatment of recurrent syncope in patients with a positive or negative response to head-up tilt testing. Pacing Clin Electrophysiol 2002;25:816.
34. DiGirolamo E, DiIorio C, Sabatini P, et al. Effects of paroxetine hydrochloride, a selective serotonin reuptake inhibitor, on refractory vasovagal syncope: a randomized, double-blind, placebo-controlled study. J Am Coll Cardiol 1999;33:1227.
35. Connolly SJ, Sheldon R, Roberts RS, et al. The North American Vasovagal Pacemaker Study (VPS): a randomized trial of permanent cardiac pacing for the prevention of vasovagal syncope. J Am Coll Cardiol 1999;33:16.
36. Sutton R, Brignole M, Enozi C, et al. Dual-chamber pacing in the treatment of neurally mediated tilt-positive cardioinhibitory syncope: pacemaker vs. no therapy: a multicenter randomized study. Circulation 2000;102:294.
37. Ammirati F, Colivicchi F, Santini M. Permanent Cardiac pacing versus medical treatment for the prevention of recurrent vasovagal syncope: a multicenter, randomized controlled trial. Circulation 2001;104:52.
38. Connolly SJ, Sheldon R, Thorpe TE, et al. Pacemaker Therapy for Prevention of Syncope in Patients with recurrent Severe Vasovagal Syncope: Second Vasovagal Pacemaker Study (VPSII): A Randomized Trial. JAMA 2003; 289:2224.
39. Raviele A, Giada F, Menozzi C, et al. A randomized, doubl-blind, placebo-controlled study of permanent cardiac pacing for the treatment of recurrent tilt-induced vasovagal syncope. The vasovagal syncope and pacing trial (SYNPACE). Eur Heart J 2004;25:1741.
40. Gregoratos G, Abrams J, Epstein AE, et al. ACC/AHA/NASPE 2002 Guidelines Update for implantation of cardiac pacemakers and antiarrhythmia devices: summary article. A Report of the American College of Cardiology/American Heart Association Task Force on Practice Guidelines (ACC/AHA/NASPE Committee to Update the 1998 Pacemaker Guidelines). Circulation 2002;106:2145.
41. Tinetti ME, Williams CS, Gill TM. Dizziness among older adults: a possible geriatric syndrome. Ann Intern Med 2000;132:337.
42. Hussain RM, McIntosh SJ, Lawson J, et al. Fludrocortisone in the treatment of hypotensive disorders in the elderly. Heart 1996;76:507.
43. Nienabe CA, Hiller S, Spielmann RP, et al. Syncope in hypertrophic cardiomyopathy: multivariate analysis of prognostic determinants. J Am Coll Cardiol 1990;15:448.
44. Brieger D, Eagle KA, Goodman SG, et al. Acute Coronary Syndrome without chest pain, an underdiagnosed and undertreated high-risk group: insights from the Global Registry of Acute Coronary Events. Chest 2004;126:461.
45. Linzer M, Yang EH, Estes M III, et al. Clinical guideline—diagnosing syncope. Part 2. Unexplained syncope. Ann Intern Med 1997; 127:76.
46. Hoefnagels WAJ, Padberg GW, Overweg J, et al. Transient loss of consciousness: the value of the history for distinguishing seizure from syncope. J Neurol 1991;238:39.
47. Linzer M, Yang EH, Estes M III, et al. Clinical guideline—diagnosing syncope. Part 1. Value of history, physical examination, and electrocardiography. Ann Intern Med 1997;126:989.
48. Davies AJ, Kenny RA. Frequency of neurologic complications following carotid sinus massage. Am J Cardiol 1998;81:1256.
49. Sarasin FP, Carballo D, Slama S, et. al. Usefulness of 24-h Holter monitoring in patients with unexplained syncope and a high likelihood of arrhythmias. Int J Cardiol 2005;101:203.
50. DiMarco JP, Philbrick JT. Use of ambulatory electrocardiographic (Holter) monitoring. Ann Intern Med 1990;113:53.
51. Sirakumaran S, Krahn AD, Klein GJ, et al. A prospective randomized comparison of loop recorders versus Holter monitors in patients with syncope and presyncope. Am J Med 2003; 115:1.
52. Brignole M, Alboni P, Benditt D, et al. Guidelines on management (diagnosis and treatment) of syncope—Update 2004. Eur Heart J 2004;25:2054.
53. Krahn AD, Klein GJ, Yee R, et al. Randomized Assessment of Syncope Trial. Circulation 2001;1004:46.
54. Denniss AR, Ross DL, Richards DA, et al. Electrophysiologic studies in patients with unexplained syncope. Int J Cardiol 1995;35: 211.
55. Denes P, Uretz E, Ezri MD, et al. Clinical predictors of electrophysiologic findings in patients with syncope of unknown origin. Arch Intern Med 1988;148:1922.
56. Sarasin FP, Junod AF, Carballo D, et al. Role of echocardiography in the evaluation of syncope: a prospective study. Heart 2002;88:363.
57. Sutton R, Bloomfield DM. Indications, methodology, and classification of results of tilt-table testing. Am J Cardiol 1999;84:10Q.
58. Benditt DG, Sutton R. Tilt-table testing in the evaluation of syncope. J Cardiovasc Electrophysiol 2005;16:356.
59. Fitzpatric AP, Theodorakis G, Vardas P, et al. Methodology of head-up tilt testing in patients with unexplained syncope. J Am Coll Cardiol 1991;17:125.
60. Grubb BP. Pathophysiology and differential diagnosis of neurocardiogenic syncope. Am J Cardiol 1999;84:3Q.
61. Whitman GT, Tang Y, Lin A, et al. A prospective study of cerebral white matter abnormalities in older people with gait dysfunction. Neurology 2001;57:990.
62. Tusa RJ. Dizziness. Med Clin N Am 2003;87:609.
63. Furman JM, Jacob RG. Psychiatric Dizziness. Neurology 1997;48:1161.
64. Staab JP, Ruckenstein MJ, Amsterdam JD. A prospective trial of sertraline for chronic subjective dizziness. Laryngoscope 2004;114: 1637.
65. Yardley L, Donovan-Hall M, Smith HE, et al. Effectiveness of primary care-based vestibular rehabilitation for chronic dizziness. Ann Intern Med 2004;141:548.

For annotated ***General References*** *and resources related to this chapter, visit www.hopkinsbayview.org/PAMreferences.*

Chapter 90

Common Disorders of Movement: Tremor and Parkinson Disease

Paul S. Fishman

TREMOR AND OTHER ABNORMAL MOVEMENTS

Definition and Classification of Tremor

Tremor is defined as the involuntary rhythmic or oscillatory movement of a body part, resulting from alternating contractions of antagonistic muscle groups. Tremor is conveniently classified by its relationship to the conditions of rest, postural maintenance, and movement (kinetic or intention tremor). Accurate classification of tremor type is important because each points to a group of specific underlying conditions (Table 90.1), with specific therapy. Several conditions will have tremor that is related to more than one state (resting/action) so that it is useful to note the state where the tremor is most prominent.

Other Abnormal Movements

Tremor can usually be distinguished by its rhythmicity, but can be confused with other abnormal movements. The most basic abnormal movement is *myoclonus*. This is a brief twitch or jerk of a single muscle or muscle group. Such a movement can be normal, such as the myoclonic jerk associated with the early stages of sleep. When occurring repetitively throughout many muscle groups, they are frequently a sign of an underlying metabolic encephalopathy. In this setting myoclonus usually coexists with asterixis (sometimes referred to as negative myoclonus). During *asterixis*, there is a sudden pause in muscle activity with a brief loss of posture. Myoclonus may be repetitive but is usually not rhythmic. The rare forms of repetitive

TABLE 90.1 Conditions Associated with the Three Major Types of Tremor

Resting Tremor
Parkinson disease
Secondary parkinsonism: postencephalitic, toxic (neuroleptics, reserpine, carbon monoxide, manganese, carbon disulfide, MPTP)
Multisystem degenerative diseases with parkinsonian features
Postural tremor
Exaggerated physiological tremor
Anxiety, fright, fatigue, exercise
Endocrine: thyrotoxicosis, hypoglycemia, pheochromocytoma
Drugs: any sympathomimetics, amiodarone, caffeine, theophylline, L-DOPA, lithium, tricyclic antidepressants, neuroleptics, thyroid hormone, hypoglycemic agents, withdrawal from alcohol and sedative-hypnotic drugs
Essential tremor
Familial (autosomal dominant)
Sporadic
With other neurologic disorders: parkinsonism, torsion dystonia, spasmodic torticollis, neuropathy
Kinetic or intention tremor (cerebellar dysfunction)
Cerebellar degeneration: inherited diseases (spinocerebellar atrophies), alcohol-abuse related, paraneoplastic syndromes
Cerebellar lesions due to stroke, hemorrhage, multiple sclerosis, or tumor
Drugs and toxins: phenytoin, barbiturates, lithium, alcohol, mercury, 5-fluorouracil, cyclosporin

MPTP, 1-methyl-4-phenyl-1,2,3,6-tetradhdropyridine.

myoclonus are more commonly confused with focal motor seizures than tremor because of their twitch-like quality. Patients who survive hypoxic/ischemic brain injury can later develop myoclonic jerks with action or intention movements of the limb. This form of action, myoclonus, can be confused with an intention type tremor (1). In patients with metabolic encephalopathy or degenerative diseases of the brain myoclonus and tremor can coexist.

Chorea refers to brief rapid distal movements. These jerky movements are more complex than myoclonus, usually involving a small group of muscles in rapid succession rather than simultaneous activation. The speed and duration of chorea is variable, and these movements usually coexist with slower proximal writhing movements called *athetosis*. The best descriptions of choreoathetosis come from patients with Huntington disease, but these movements can occur with injury to the basal ganglia associated with other conditions such as stroke, acquired immunodeficiency syndrome, systemic lupus erythematosus (SLE), after streptococcal infection (Sydenham chorea) and chronic neuroleptic exposure (tardive dyskinesia). Dramatic, vigorous, flinging movements are termed *ballism* and can be viewed as an extreme form of chorea and are seen particularly after injury to a small basal ganglia center called the subthalamic nucleus (2).

Sustained abnormal posture is referred to as *dystonia*. Dystonia can occur throughout the body (generalized) commonly on an inherited basis, but is usually restricted to a specific body part (focal dystonia). *Cervical dystonia,* also called *spasmodic torticollis* or wry neck, is the most common focal dystonia characterized by intermittent or constant abnormal twisting of the neck (3). Tremor is commonly observed superimposed on a dystonic posture. Focal dystonia can also be provoked by specific movements (*action dystonia*). The involuntary muscle contraction of *writer's cramp* is the most common action dystonia (4). Other common focal dystonias include blepharospasm (involuntary spasm of the eyelids), hemifacial spasm, and spasmodic dysphonia with involuntary laryngeal spasms that interrupt speech (5–7).

Tics are repetitive rapid movements distinguished from chorea by their stereotyped pattern. They can be distinguished from tremor by their lack of rhythmicity, erratic appearance in different body parts, complexity of movement, and onset in childhood or adolescence. Persistent multiple tics with vocalizations are the features of *Tourette syndrome* (8). Tics are often preceded by a buildup of inner tension that subsides after the tic. Patients may be able to temporarily suppress a tic, whereas most other abnormal movements usually lack such a degree of voluntary control. Complex repetitive movements that can be clearly voluntarily suppressed or interrupted are referred to as mannerisms.

EVALUATION OF THE PATIENT WITH TREMOR

The history and physical examination are fundamental in the diagnosis of tremor (Table 90.2), and in almost all cases no further workup is necessary. The differential diagnosis, in general practice, is almost always between Parkinson disease (PD) and essential tremor (ET). Most patients with tremor and other movement disorders do not have any specific abnormality on laboratory investigation (including imaging).

History

Important historical information includes the temporal onset of the tremor, associated neurologic symptoms, family history, a survey of medications and other medical illnesses, and whether the tremor is suppressed by alcohol. Almost all varieties of tremor increase in amplitude under stress, diminish with relaxation, and disappear during

TABLE 90.2 Principal Features of Different Tremor Types

	Resting (Parkinsonian)	*Postural (Essential)*	*Kinetic or Intention (Cerebellar)*
History			
Age at onset	60 yr and older	All ages, more common after age 60	All ages
Family history	Negative	Often positive (autosomal dominant)	Occasionally positive
Response to alcohol	No effect	Often suppresses tremor	No effect or worsening
Physical examination			
Frequency	3–6 Hz[a]	6–12 Hz	3–5 Hz
Symmetry	Almost always begins unilaterally	Symmetric	Either symmetric or asymmetric
Body part(s) affected	Arms > legs	Hand > head > voice	Arms > legs > trunk/head
Associated signs	Bradykinesia, rigidity, postural instability	None	Dysarthria, nystagmus, broad-based gait

[a]Hz (Hertz), cycles per second.

sleep. The impact of the tremor on the patient determines whether treatment is indicated. Some patients do not find their tremor disabling and seek medical attention only for diagnostic purposes. Young patients with ET may need only reassurance that they do not have PD or another degenerative disorder. However, most patients find the tremor physically or emotionally problematic.

Emphasis should be placed on the *activities of daily living* (ADLs). Patients with tremor typically have trouble with tasks requiring fine motor control such as buttoning, feeding, shaving, brushing their teeth, writing, and cooking. Embarrassment is often an unvoiced source of disability, and patients should be questioned about social isolation caused by the tremor. The ADLs also provide objective parameters for judging the effectiveness of therapy.

Physical Examination

The objectives of the physical examination are to determine the frequency, severity, and conditions of maximal activation of the tremor and to search for associated neurologic signs. Patients should be examined with their hands resting on their laps, with their arms held outstretched, and while performing finger-to-nose maneuvers. Samples of handwriting and a drawing of a spiral should also be obtained as an objective means of following response to therapy. Observations while the patient is drinking from a cup or using a fork or spoon are also helpful in assessing functional impairment.

The *resting tremor of parkinsonism* is characterized by 3- to 6-Hz flexion–extension at the metacarpophalangeal joints, abduction–adduction of the thumb, and pronation–supination of the forearm; these produce the so-called pill-rolling tremor. Resting tremor is often brought out by having the patient walk or by distracting the patient with conversation or mental arithmetic. Early in its course, the parkinsonian tremor is almost always unilateral, which is one of the most helpful signs distinguishing it from ET. ET almost always begins bilaterally, although it may be asymmetric.

Postural tremor is characteristic of ET and consists of 6- to 12-Hz symmetric flexion–extension at the wrists and shoulders. It is brought on by having the patient assume an antigravity posture of the upper extremities (e.g., outstretched arms), and it is not present when the arms are resting against the body or on a surface. ET may persist during finger-to-nose testing, leading to the misdiagnosis of a cerebellar tremor.

Kinetic tremor (also called *intention tremor*) is encountered most commonly in cerebellar disease and is characterized by 3- to 5-Hz irregular oscillations as the limb approaches a target. This type of tremor is often accompanied by inaccuracies in direction (dysmetria). In acquired cerebellar diseases, such as stroke and multiple sclerosis, kinetic tremors are often asymmetric, whereas degenerative diseases involving the cerebellum usually produce bilateral symmetric tremor. Conditions that may mimic this aspect of cerebellar disease include severe ET (which may impair purposeful movements) and conditions producing severe proprioceptive loss. Unlike patients with PD or ET, patients with cerebellar impairment rarely present complaining only of tremor. Additional signs pointing toward the cerebellum include gait ataxia, dysarthria, and nystagmus (9).

Generally, it is difficult to estimate the rhythmic frequency of a tremor in a clinical setting. Tremors are commonly described as "fine" or "coarse"—a nonuseful composite of frequency and amplitude. Particularly for ET, it is useful to attempt to rate the severity of tremor by its peak to peak amplitude (severe, greater than 1 to 2 cm). This aspect is most clearly related to both disability and response to treatment. Tremor frequency can be accurately assessed using electromyography (EMG), but can also be assessed with an office form of accelerometry. Using an electrocardiogram solely as a calibrated paper recorder, the patient attempts to make a straight line with a marker pen on the moving paper. The number of oscillations drawn in each marked second gives the tremor frequency.

PHYSIOLOGIC AND EXAGGERATED PHYSIOLOGIC TREMOR

Most people have a barely perceptible postural tremor, so-called physiologic tremor, that may be best appreciated by placing a piece of paper over the outstretched hands. Although asymptomatic, this tremor may be transiently exacerbated during systemic illness, metabolic derangements, stress, and by the use or withdrawal of certain drugs or alcohol (Table 90.1). The most important step in management is identification and removal of the offending cause; resolution of the tremor confirms the diagnosis of exaggerated physiologic tremor. Although discontinuation of tremorogenic drugs usually leads to prompt resolution of the tremor, it may take 1 to 2 weeks for the tremor to resolve after resolution of a systemic illness or a severe metabolic abnormality. It is difficult to distinguish an enhanced physiologic tremor from mild ET. The proof of this diagnosis rests on the resolution of the tremor. If the underlying condition cannot be eliminated (e.g., in patients requiring lithium for manic-depressive illness), the tremor can often be suppressed using medications for ET. For patients subject to situational anxiety manifested by exaggerated physiologic tremor, prophylactic treatment with propranolol (20 to 40 mg) taken 1 hour before an anxiety-producing situation (e.g., public speaking) may be helpful (10).

ESSENTIAL TREMOR

Characteristics

ET is the most common form of postural or kinetic tremor with prevalence of 4% to 6% (11). Estimates of the prevalence of ET are limited by the fact that most patients do not seek treatment for their condition and remain undiagnosed. Although it has been assumed that these undiagnosed patients are only mildly affected, there is recent evidence that the majority of these patients suffer both distress and disability from ET (12). ET is synonymous with familial tremor, benign ET, and senile tremor when it occurs in the elderly. No neuropathologic abnormalities have been identified in ET, but physiologic evidence suggests that both the central and peripheral nervous systems are involved. The onset is insidious and may begin as early as childhood, but ET characteristically presents in adulthood, usually after age 50 years with both incidence and prevalence rising with age. Unlike the tremor of PD, which typically makes the patient seek medical attention within months of its onset, patients with ET often give a history of tremor going back many years. At least 50% of patients with ET give a positive family history; the inheritance is autosomal dominant. Patients with a positive family history are more likely to have a younger age at onset. Genetic linkage studies have identified at least two susceptibility loci with recent identification of a mutation in a neuronal protein (13).

In its prototypical form, ET is characterized by a bilateral and symmetric tremor of the hands, but it may also affect other body parts either in isolation (commonly the head or voice) or combined with a hand tremor. At least half of patients with ET notice a beneficial effect from small amounts of alcohol (14). Although its regular use to suppress tremor should be discouraged, when used sparingly alcohol is an effective treatment for ET, particularly when exacerbated by situational stress. There does not seem to be an increased prevalence of alcoholism among patients with ET (15). ET is a progressively worsening disorder with the tremor gradually increasing in severity, spreading to other body regions (usually hands to head) and occurring at rest along with movement.

Treatment

When ET begins to interfere with the ADLs or causes significant embarrassment, treatment is indicated. Before starting medication, patients should be told that the goal of treatment is not to abolish the tremor, which is rarely possible, but instead to reduce its severity and allow them to function better. The patient's ADLs should be used as a gauge to determine the effectiveness of treatment. As with exaggerated physiologic tremor, treatment begins with elimination of potentially exacerbating factors, including stimulant drugs and medication. ET also has a consistent relationship to exercise where education may help in its control (16). The tremor is worsened directly after vigorous physical exercise of the involved limb due to fatigue, but is also more problematic if exercise is entirely avoided and the involved muscles become deconditioned. Some prosthetic devices, such as handwriting aids, are useful in reducing the disability of ET, particularly for patients who tolerate medications poorly (17).

The two medications most effective for ET are propranolol and primidone. The drugs are equally effective and may be synergistic, but only propranolol is U.S. Food and Drug Administration (FDA)-approved for this indication (18).

Propranolol is started at 10 mg twice per day in elderly patients and gradually increased, depending on the beneficial response and appearance of side effects, to a maximum of 320 mg/day. Once a stable dosage has been reached, patients can be converted to a long-acting form. In younger patients, treatment can be started with the controlled release form (60 mg) with a gradual escalation of the dosage. Although other β-blockers have also been shown to be effective for ET, none is superior to propranolol (19,20). Newer β-blockers have the advantage of being β_1 selective and therefore safer to use in patients with ET and asthma, but at the higher dosages usually needed, β_1 selectivity is diminished. In general, β-blockers should be avoided in the presence of bronchospastic disease, second- or third-degree heart block, or insulin-dependent diabetes.

Primidone, a barbiturate-like anticonvulsant, was found by serendipity to improve ET. The mechanism of action of primidone is unknown, but its effect does not appear to result from either of its metabolites, phenylethylmalonamide and phenobarbital (21). Primidone is available as scored tablets in two strengths, 50 and 250 mg. The starting dosage must be very low (e.g., 25 milligrams per day) because occasional patients (5% to 10%, especially the elderly) develop severe side effects after even a single small dose, known as the first-dose phenomenon. Symptoms include dizziness, lethargy, confusion, nausea, sedation, and ataxia, which usually diminish with continued use. The dose is initially given at bedtime and then gradually escalated to a maximum of 250 mg three times per day as tolerated. In general, if patients show no response to low dosages (250 mg/day), it is rare for higher dosages to be effective. If patients tolerate primidone initially, long-term use is well tolerated and may be superior to propanolol (22).

If there is a beneficial but suboptimal response to either propranolol or primidone used alone, the two should be combined beginning at low dosages and increasing in small increments, watching carefully for side effects, particularly in elderly patients. Blood levels of primidone or phenobarbital are not helpful (unless toxicity or noncompliance is suspected) because they do not correlate with its tremor-suppressing effect.

Generally, patients who fail to respond to propanolol or primidone have a poor chance of success with other drugs. Although benzodiazepines have been widely prescribed for ET, the clinical trial experience with these drugs has been mixed at best. It has been difficult to assign an anti-tremor affect to these agents independent of their anxiolytic effect (23).

The most useful of the benzodiazepines is alprazolam, which has been shown to be effective in the treatment of ET (24). The maintenance dosage is 0.75 to 3.0 mg/day, in divided doses. Its rapid onset of action and intermediate half-life, in comparison with other benzodiazepines, allow for its intermittent use when situational stress temporarily exacerbates ET. Several of the newer anticonvulsant medications have been evaluated for ET and can be viewed as second-line medical therapy. Although gabapentin has been most extensively studied, the experience has been mixed (25,26). Topiramate has shown efficacy in small placebo controlled trials, while there is some promising open-label data using levetiracetam, an anticonvulsant that is useful to suppress some forms of myoclonus (27–29).

Intramuscular injection of *botulinum toxin,* the standard treatment of focal dystonia, has been used to treat ET as well. Treatment of ET involving the hands is difficult to achieve without causing perceptible weakness (30,31). Botulinum neurotoxin has been of greatest use in suppression of tremor of the head, a condition that is both socially distressing and frequently medication resistant (32).

Stereotactic ablation of the ventralis intermedius (VIM) nucleus of the thalamus has long been accepted as the most effective treatment of severe or disabling ET (33). Effective to dramatic reduction of ET (80% to 90% decrease in amplitude) has also been demonstrated after VIM implantation of a high-frequency stimulation device (34). These devices, which cause deep brain stimulation (DBS), are FDA-approved for implantation into the thalamus for control of tremor associated with either ET or PD. Implantation of a thalamic deep brain stimulator has a slightly lower risk of neurologic deficit than thalamotomy but is a more extensive procedure requiring surgical placement of the pacemaker-like device in the chest and a continuing risk of device or lead malfunction (35,36). Deep brain stimulator placement is generally preferred over standard thalamotomy, although the older procedure may be more suitable for specific patients. Although the risk of serious morbidity is relatively low (less than 5%), patients referred for stereotactic surgery should first have an adequate trial of medication to control ET.

The atypical neuroleptic clozapine has also shown efficacy in refractory cases of ET. This drug is worth considering despite its potential to cause agranulocytosis, because its risk is lower than that of surgery for treatment of ET (37,38).

TREMOR CAUSED BY CEREBELLAR DYSFUNCTION (KINETIC OR INTENTION TREMOR)

Tremor is rarely the sole presenting sign of cerebellar dysfunction, and most often the underlying disease is already known or readily apparent (multiple sclerosis, stroke, drug intoxication, long-standing alcoholism, head trauma, inherited disease, or paraneoplastic syndrome). Paraneoplastic syndromes involving the cerebellum are of particular concern with the presentation of tremor and ataxia over a few weeks or months, since brain imaging is frequently unremarkable and these systemic malignancies (usually breast, ovarian, small cell, or lymphoma) are usually occult (39). Occasionally, severe ET may be exacerbated with action, giving the impression of cerebellar disease, but the faster frequency, prominent postural component, and lack of associated cerebellar signs usually suffice to distinguish the ET from cerebellar dysfunction (40).

With the exception of drug-induced cerebellar tremor (Table 90.1), which should be managed by discontinuation or reduction of the dosage of the offending drug, a patient with newly diagnosed cerebellar tremor should be referred to a neurologist. Cerebellar tremors in general respond poorly to medication, which may also reflect the fact the tremor is intimately related to poor control of ballistic movements. Relatively small trials of clonazepam, carbamazepine, and isoniazid have shown some efficacy for cerebellar tremor (41). As with severe ET, there is a role for an occupational therapist. Weighted bracelets have had some benefit in dampening the tremor, and specialized devices to aid in writing and feeding are useful. Computer-controlled tremor damping gloves are under investigation to control severe ataxic tremor. As is the case with severe ET, stereotactic thalamotomy is a viable option for disabling cerebellar tremor (42).

PRIMARY WRITING TREMOR AND ORTHOSTATIC TREMOR

Two uncommon but distinct types of tremor are primary writing tremor (43) and orthostatic tremor (44). *Primary writing tremor* is one variant of a group of task-specific tremors. These are characterized by maximal activation during a specific task. Primary writing tremor occurs exclusively when patients attempt to write. It probably is related to ET but may share some features in common with focal action dystonias, such as writer's cramp. Writing tremor may respond to drugs used to treat ET (see

Essential Tremor, Treatment) or treatments of action dystonias such as anticholinergics, clonazepam, or botulinum therapy. *Primary orthostatic tremor* is characterized by rapid shaking of the legs, only with standing, and may respond to clonazepam (0.5 to 3.0 mg/day). Recent studies suggest that many patients with this syndrome have other extrapyramidal findings as well.

PARKINSON DISEASE AND "PARKINSONISM"

Epidemiology

PD is one of the most common neurologic diseases in the ambulatory setting. Approximately 1 million persons are affected in the United States, with an annual incidence of 18 per 100,000. In general, PD increases in incidence with age, with an average age at onset of 60. The incidence of PD appears to decline in the very old. This observation, along with the increasing incidence of essential (senile) tremor and other extrapyramidal symptoms in the elderly, makes the diagnosis of new-onset PD older than age 80 both difficult and somewhat suspect. Recently, there has been heightened awareness of young-onset PD; up to 5% of PD patients have an age at onset younger than 40 (45).

Pathogenesis

Premature dysfunction and death of *dopamine*-producing (and *neuromelanin*-containing) neurons of the substantia nigra is the basis for both the major motor symptoms of PD and its treatment. Along with neuronal loss, the pathologic hallmark of PD is an eosinophilic cytoplasmic inclusion called a Lewy body. Although the cause of PD in most cases is unknown, PD is emerging as the proving ground for theories of the interaction of environmental and genetic factors in neuronal aging and death. The evidence for an environmental basis of PD comes from two sources. In 1983, it was discovered that an impurity in the illegal production of meperidine, called MPTP (methyl-phenyl-tetrahydropyridine), was capable of causing irreversible Parkinson symptoms in abusers who injected the drug (46). MPTP injection can cause similar symptoms in animals along with the death of dopaminergic nigral neurons. The final steps in MPTP toxicity involve impairment of mitochondrial energy generation, suggesting a role for oxidative injury. Epidemiologic studies also support a role for environmental factors in PD. An increased incidence of PD is found in farm workers with long-standing exposure to herbicides and pesticides (47).

Genetic factors also play a role in the development of PD. Five to ten percent of PD patients have an affected first-degree relative. In the last 10 years the first five genes have been identified that are clearly associated with inherited forms of PD. Mutations in the gene for the protein *α-synuclein* lead to a form of PD, inherited on an autosomal dominant basis (48). Although families carrying these mutations are extremely rare, the role of α-synuclein in both inherited and sporadic PD is first suggested by the observation that α-synuclein is the major component of Lewy bodies (49). Up to 50% of patients with inherited young-onset PD have recessively inherited mutations in the gene for the enzyme *parkin* involved in the ubiquitin-proteasome pathway for degradation of aberrant cellular proteins (50). DJ1 is a multifunctional protein where mutations also cause recessively inherited young onset PD (51). PINK-1 is a mitochondrial protein mutated in inherited PD, while LRRK2 (Dardarin) mutations are the most common cause of inherited, typical late adult onset PD discovered at this time (52,53). Animal model and cellular studies suggest that cell death in PD is the result of interactions of production of abnormal toxic proteins, proteasomal dysfunction and inadequate elimination of these proteins, and mitochondrial dysfunction with resulting oxidative injury (54).

Differential Diagnosis

The cardinal signs of PD include tremor at rest, bradykinesia, muscular rigidity, and postural instability. Common symptoms along with tremor include impaired handwriting (micrographia); difficulty walking; falling; poor coordination; difficulty arising from a deep chair, couch, or the toilet; drooling; and difficulty turning in bed. When the syndrome is fully developed, the diagnosis is straightforward. Patients where tremor dominates the clinical picture can be confused with ET, whereas patients without a resting tremor are difficult to distinguish from the other atypical parkinsonian syndromes described below.

Four of the parkinsonian syndromes in Table 90.3 deserve special mention because their treatment and prognosis differ. Other clinical clues to these syndromes include the following: early onset dementia, rapid progress, early onset dysarthria or dysphagia, prominent and early dysautonomia, early falling, impaired ocular motility, lower motor neuron, cerebellar or pyramidal signs, and bilaterally symmetrical involvement. A positive family history and little or no response to L-dopa are also suggestive of a parkinsonian syndrome rather than Parkinson disease. *Neuroleptic-induced parkinsonism,* may be clinically indistinguishable from idiopathic PD and can be diagnosed only retrospectively when parkinsonian signs resolve after discontinuation of the offending drug. In some patients signs may take as long as 1 year to resolve completely, emphasizing the periodic need to reassess antiparkinsonian therapy. In patients whose signs never resolve, it is likely that the neuroleptic simply uncovered a case of latent PD (55).

Progressive supranuclear palsy (PSP) is the most common nonpharmacologic mimic of PD. It is distinguished by impaired vertical eye movements, although early in its

TABLE 90.3 Differential Diagnosis of Parkinsonism

Toxins
Manganese
Carbon monoxide
Carbon disulfide
Cyanide
Methanol
MPTP
Drug induced
Neuroleptics
Metoclopramide (Reglan), Compazine
Multisystem degenerations
Progressive supranuclear palsy
Multisystem atrophy (includes the Shy-Drager syndrome)
Corticobasal ganglionic degeneration
Primary dementing illnesses
Alzheimer disease
Creutzfeldt-Jakob syndrome
Dementia with Lewy bodies
Heredofamilial diseases
Wilson disease
Juvenile Huntington disease
Pantothenate kinase associated neurodegeneration (formerly Hallervorden-Spatz syndrome)
Vascular parkinsonism
Trauma: dementia parkinsonism pugilistica
Senile gait disorder
Normal pressure hydrocephalus
Other structural lesions of the basal ganglia (tumor, arteriovenous malformation)

course ocular motility may be full with the only clinical clue being slow vertical saccades. Other distinguishing features include neck extension as opposed to the flexion seen in PD, early dysarthria and dysphagia, early and prominent balance and gait impairment with associated falls, greater axial than appendicular rigidity (axial dystonia), progression to severe disability in 5 to 10 years, and limited response to antiparkinsonian medications (56,57).

Multiple system atrophy (MSA) is another more widespread neurodegenerative disease with autonomic, cerebellar, and cortical pathology that can mimic PD. A common form of MSA is parkinsonism signs associated with significant autonomic dysfunction (formerly referred to as the Shy-Drager syndrome). Early identification of these patients is important since treatment of their motor features with dopaminergic drugs will commonly worsen their prominent and symptomatic orthostatic hypotension (58).

Wilson disease (hepatolenticular degeneration) is an autosomal-recessive condition characterized by copper accumulation throughout the body. Parkinsonian features in a young patient should prompt an investigation for this condition. Liver disease may be present at the onset of neurologic disease, but normal liver studies should not deter one from pursuing the diagnosis. The diagnosis is confirmed by demonstrating Kayser-Fleischer rings (green or golden deposits of copper in the Descemet membrane of the cornea), low blood ceruloplasmin, and elevated urinary copper excretion. Although a rare cause of abnormal movements, Wilson disease is noteworthy as a potentially reversible cause of parkinsonism. Timely diagnosis and treatment with copper chelating agents such as penicillamine (1 to 2 g/day) can prevent progression and to some extent reverse neurologic signs and symptoms (59).

Manifestations

Resting Tremor

Tremor is the presenting complaint in at least 70% of patients with PD. The tremor is maximal when the limb is at rest and has a frequency of 3 to 6 Hz. It consists of flexion–extension at the metacarpophalangeal joints, abduction–adduction of the thumb, and pronation–supination of the forearm, producing the typical pill-rolling appearance. The tremor may affect the legs, lips, tongue, or chin but virtually never affects the head (a tremor of the head suggests ET). The parkinsonian tremor is accentuated by stress and distraction, diminishes with relaxation, and disappears during sleep. Although there may be an associated postural tremor in PD, typically the resting tremor suppresses with posture and movement, which helps to distinguish it from ET. Classic resting tremor, which abates transiently with movement, is almost never seen with structural damage to the brain such as stroke (60).

Rigidity

Rigidity is a form of abnormal muscular tone or resistance to passive movement. This feeling of resistance is present and unchanged when moving a patient's limb in flexion or extension, regardless of the speed of the movement, and is described as having a "lead pipe" quality. In this manner, rigidity can be distinguished from spasticity, the other major form of abnormal muscle tone. In spasticity, resistance is greater to extension than flexion and is particularly prominent at the onset of a rapid attempt to flex the arm or leg. This quality gives rise to descriptions of spasticity as "clasp knife" or having a "catch." When the limb of a PD patient is moved passively, there is also a regular ratchet-like quality to the resistance, which gives rise to the term cogwheel rigidity. Deep tendon reflexes are increased in patients with spasticity while they are normal or decreased in parkinsonism rigidity. Patients rarely complain of rigidity per se and instead notice stiffness or describe the abnormal tone as weakness. Cogwheel rigidity is best felt at the elbow, wrist, or neck and may be demonstrated or enhanced by having the patient perform a maneuver with the contralateral limb such as opening and closing the fist or drawing a circle in the air. The cogwheeling phenomenon can also be misleading, since patients with nonparkinsonian tremor such as ET may have a similar ratchet-like quality to passive movement, but without the increased resistance in rigidity.

Bradykinesia and Akinesia

Patients with PD have difficulty initiating movements, and their movements are slow and performed with much greater conscious effort. Speech gradually becomes soft, slow, and monotonal (hypophonia). The blink rate is diminished, as is facial expression (hypomimia), producing the so-called masked face. Movements of PD patients are not only slowed but are reduced in amplitude. This is most prominent with repeated activity, where the movements appear to collapse into a barely visible quiver.

Gait and Postural Abnormalities

Patients with moderate to severe PD are flexed at multiple joints (neck, hips, knees, elbows, and fingers), producing the typical stooped posture. Arising from a chair is often accomplished only with difficulty; patients may need to rock back and forth several times and eventually push off from arm rests. Early changes in gait include a reduction in stride length and diminished associated movements such as arm swing changes usually associated with the very old. The gait later becomes slow and shuffling. Turning is done *en bloc*, with the entire body moving as the feet slowly rotate. There is a tendency to progress involuntarily from walking to running (festination), seemingly in an attempt to catch up with the body's center of gravity thrown forward by the flexed posture. A patient may describe festination as like chasing your shadow. Patients have difficulty maintaining balance and are often unable to correct for a rapid postural displacement, particularly backward. The combination of the flexed posture, bradykinesia, freezing, festination, and impaired postural righting reflexes leads to one of the major problems in the latter stages of PD—falling.

Other Associated Symptoms or Signs

Seborrhea and excessive perspiration and facial oiliness are both common, and although often attributed to inadequate hygiene caused by physical impairment, they are an intrinsic part of the disease process.

Dysphagia often surfaces in the latter stages of the disease where it contributes significantly to morbidity and mortality caused by inanition and aspiration pneumonia. Although not completely understood, swallowing abnormalities have been demonstrated at various levels, including the voluntary muscles of the oral cavity and the involuntary muscles of the pharynx and esophagus. Solids are usually more of a problem than liquids. If patients with advanced PD are unable to maintain sufficient caloric intake, a discussion of the pros and cons of tube feeding should be held with the patient and family.

Sialorrhea is probably the result of decreased initiation of swallowing rather than overproduction of saliva. This can be treated with a low dosage of an anticholinergic, but there is growing experience in the use of injection of the salivary glands with botulinum toxin in the treatment of sialorrhea (61).

Autonomic dysfunction may occur in PD itself and as a side effect of antiparkinsonian medication. Orthostatic hypotension and constipation are the most common autonomic signs in PD, but bladder dysfunction and impotence are also encountered. In each case, medications may be at fault, and a search for other causes should be carried out before the defects are ascribed to PD.

Natural History

PD patients can be viewed as having one of three forms of the disease with implications for both natural history and treatment:

- *Tremor predominant:* These patients have prominent tremor but little other signs and symptoms of PD. They have an earlier average age at onset but a more benign course. They may have little functional disability from bradykinesia or rigidity even years after the onset of tremor. The prominent tremor not only is cosmetically unacceptable and can lead to social isolation as in essential tremor, but can also give a patient a misimpression of a poor prognosis. Frequently medications other than L-dopa are more useful in treatment. Such patients illustrate a poorly understood aspect of parkinsonian tremor. Although a true rest tremor (seen only at rest and suppressed with movement) is the most reliable diagnostic sign of PD, it does not correlate well with bradykinesia and rigidity. These other signs rather than tremor also more closely correlate with overall disease disability and dopaminergic cell loss on radionuclide scans (62). These patients account for approximately 20% of PD.
- *Classic PD:* These patients account for most cases (approximately 60% to 70%) and have all three of the cardinal features (tremor, bradykinesia, rigidity) at the time of diagnosis, frequently in the same body distribution. They generally have a good response to therapy for years after diagnosis, and dominate most clinical trials of medications for PD.
- *Akinetic–rigid*: These patients lack a resting tremor, with stiffness and reduced movement dominating their clinical picture. Akinetic–rigid patients are usually poorly responsive to therapy. It is likely that the poor response of this group is due to its heterogenous nature, with many of these patients having more widespread

neurodegenerative diseases than PD. Expert consultation is essential in evaluation in this group, looking for ocular movement abnormalities, behavioral and cognitive abnormalities, and autonomic and cerebellar dysfunction seen in the atypical parkinsonian syndromes. Not only do these conditions have these other abnormalities, they have more rapidly progressive and disabling disease. Difficulties with speech, swallowing, and posture (with frequent falling) as well as dementia are seen relatively early in the course for many of these patients.

Treatment Overview

The problems facing PD patients vary throughout the course of this disease, which progresses over many years. Treatment strategies that consider both short- and long-term aspects of PD are useful in helping patients, families, and physicians in anticipating and preparing for new problems and maximizing functionality and quality of life.

Treatment of Early Parkinson Disease

Nonmedication Strategies

Education and counseling play a major role in newly diagnosed patients. Fear of disability and death are common but frequently are not voiced. Reassurance is needed that disease progression is in general slow and disability can be forestalled for many years. Patients also need to be reminded that both understanding and treatment of PD are among the most rapidly changing aspects of all of neurology. There is not only reason to be optimistic regarding treatment with current therapy, but therapy will clearly be improving over the patient's lifetime. Patient-oriented books and support groups are often helpful for both patient and families. However, support groups should not be allowed to become the sole source of information for newly diagnosed patients, because they tend to focus on the most severely affected patients. Exercise programs are useful both to reduce physical signs of PD but also in encouraging an active lifestyle (63). Restrictions in activity are only appropriate when activities pose a safety hazard (e.g., working at a height, with heavy machinery, bicycle riding, rollerblading) in early PD.

For tremor predominant patients, declining symptomatic medications remains a viable option. A resting tremor can be quite pronounced and still cause little or no functional impairment. Frequently, embarrassment caused by tremor is the major drive for seeking treatment.

Depression is common in PD (40% to 50% of patients) and frequently is present at the time of diagnosis (64). In general it is not closely related to physical disability (or fear of it), because the incidence of depression in PD is higher than in other disabling conditions. The diagnosis of depression is made more difficult by the presence of facial masking where outward expression of emotion may not be an accurate reflection of mood state. Treatment of depression is accomplished with standard antidepressants (such as the selective serotonin reuptake inhibitor [SSRI] group; see Chapter 24) rather than with purely anti-Parkinson drugs.

Medications

Table 90.4 lists the medications used for the treatment of early PD.

Anticholinergics

Patients with early PD, in whom tremor is the major aspect, can benefit from anticholinergics. Generally, poor patient tolerance limits their use. Dry mouth (which may help sialorrhea), dry eyes, and mild visual blurring are common and dose related. Urinary retention, constipation, memory loss, and confusion are more serious problems, particularly in the elderly with a high prevalence of pre-existing dementia. Narrow angle glaucoma is a contraindication to these agents. Trihexyphenidyl and benztropine are the two most widely used of this class. Trihexyphenidyl is sometimes preferred because of its short duration of action (3 to 5 hours), because it allows a patient to target tremor control to desired situations. The recommended dose for trihexyphenidyl is 2 to 12 mg/day.

Amantadine

Although originally developed as an anti-influenzal drug, amantadine is an FDA-approved antiparkinsonian agent. Its effects are in general modest, but it is better tolerated than anticholinergic drugs. It is useful for mild bradykinesia and rigidity as well as tremor. It has a stimulant effect in many patients, which may account for its use in the treatment of fatigue in multiple sclerosis and chronic fatigue syndrome (65). Dry mouth and insomnia are usually mild. Livedo reticularis on the legs with associated edema occurs in 5% to 10% of patients, leading to discontinuation of amantadine. Exacerbation of congestive heart failure has also been reported with amantadine use. A dose of 100 mg twice daily is usual in early PD.

Carbidopa/Levodopa (L-dopa)

Although the introduction of L-dopa for PD is one of the therapeutic highlights of neurology, its use in early PD remains controversial. Despite the introduction of new medications, L-dopa remains the most effective drug for overall relief of motor symptoms of PD. The controversy surrounding L-dopa use has both theoretical and clinical basis. As mentioned earlier, there is evidence that metabolism of dopamine generates oxidative injury, which may play a role in the progressive cell death in PD. This evidence comes mostly from cell culture studies with relatively

TABLE 90.4 Drugs Used for Parkinson Disease

Drug	Available Preparation (mg)	Schedule	Starting Dose (mg)	Maintenance Dose (mg)
Anticholinergic agents				
Trihexyphenidyl (Artane, generic)	Tablets: 2, 5 Elixir: 2 mg per 5 mL	3–4 times daily	2	2–12
Benztropine mesylate (Cogentin, generic)	Tablets: 0.5, 1, 2	Once or twice daily	1	0.5–6
Dopaminergic agents				
carbidopa/L-dopa	Tablets: 10/100, 25/100, 25/250, 25/100 CR, 50/200 CR	2–4 times daily	50/200 in 2 divided doses	300–1,000 L-dopa
Rapid dissolving carbidopa/L-dopa (Parcopa)	10/100, 25/100, 25/2,500			
Bromocriptine (Parlodel)	Tablets: 2.5 Capsules: 5.0	2–3 times daily	1.25 daily	7.5–30
Pergolide (Permax)	Scored tablets: 0.05, 0.25, 1.0	3 times daily	0.05 daily	1–6
Pramipexole (Mirapex)	Tablets: 0.125, 0.25, 0.5, 1, 1.5	3 times daily	0.375 daily	4.5
Ropinirole (Requip)	Tablets: 0.25, 1, 2, 5	3 times daily	0.75 daily	3–15
Selegiline[a] (Eldepryl)	Tablets: 5.0	2 times daily	5 daily	10
Entacapone (Comtan) Also available in combination with carbidopa/L-dopa combinations of 12.5/50, 25/100 as Stalevo	Tablets: 200	Up to 8 times a day (along with carbidopa/L-dopa)	200	600–1,600
Apomorphine (Apokyn)	Subcutaneous injection	As needed	2 mg per 0.2 mL	2–6 mg per dose total daily dose up to 20 mg
Anticholinergic or dopaminergic activity				
Amantadine (Symmetrel, generic)	Capsules: 100	2 times daily	200 daily	200–400

[a]Alternative generic name: deprenyl.

little animal data, and no clinical studies support the concept that levels of L-dopa used in treatment of PD are toxic. Results of an early clinical study are in direct conflict with the belief that L-dopa treatment accelerates neuronal death in PD. Patients who had L-dopa treatment begun early in the course of their disease had less overall morbidity and mortality than patients where therapy was initiated at a later stage (66). A recent clinical study of initial L-dopa treatment of PD which attempted to resolve the issue of L-dopa's potential neurotoxicity, gave a puzzling result. Patients initiated on L-dopa showed greater signs of degeneration of dopaminergic neurons on imaging studies than placebo treated patients after one year. However, the L-dopa initiated patients not only had greater relief of their PD symptoms than placebo patients, but remained the more improved group even after the placebo patients began on L-dopa. This suggests that early initiation with L-dopa had long lasting benefits in spite of enhanced brain imaging signs of neurodegeneration (67). L-Dopa therapy is however, associated with a major complication of moderate to severe PD—fluctuating motor response (68). Dose fluctuations take two forms:

- Loss of efficacy before the next dose of L-dopa (so-called wearing off).
- Involuntary choreiform movements called dyskinesias that usually occur at the peak effect of each dose. Dyskinesias in particular are associated with duration (in years) of L-dopa treatment.

A practical approach is to defer initiating L-dopa until the patient's motor symptoms interfere with daily activities or cannot be adequately treated with another drug. L-Dopa therapy in early PD is initiated as carbidopa/L-dopa at a dose one 25/100 tablet twice a day, although half of this dose is suggested for elderly patients.

The addition of carbidopa to L-dopa as a combination medication (formerly marketed as Sinemet) dramatically improves its tolerability. Carbidopa inhibits the enzyme dopa-decarboxylase, preventing the conversion of L-dopa to dopamine outside of brain. This leads to marked reduction (10-fold) of the effective L-dopa dose with reduction in so-called peripheral side effects of nausea, gastrointestinal (GI) intolerance (cramps/diarrhea), and hypotension. Patients with refractory nausea on 25/100 combination tablets may benefit from additional carbidopa, available as 25-mg tablets (Lodosyn). Although L-dopa is absorbed best on an empty stomach, this also usually leads to an increased incidence of nausea, so that it is initially prescribed with meals and, once tolerated, can be taken half an hour earlier. Although some patients have an immediate beneficial effect, it may take several weeks before a change is noticed. After that time, if there is no improvement, the dosage is gradually increased every few days to three to four times daily, using full or half-tablet increments, until the patient has shown significant improvement or a total daily dosage of 400 to 600 mg of L-dopa per day has been reached.

Although most patients tolerate carbidopa/L-dopa well, side effects are common, particularly in the elderly or in patients with dementia (see Dementia subsection). These include confusion, hallucinations, hypersexuality, and fluid retention. Orthostatic hypotension is common particularly in patients with autonomic dysfunction related to their untreated PD. Standing and supine blood pressure measurements should be checked before and after initiating treatment.

Dopamine Agonists: Bromocriptine (Parlodel), Pergolide (Permax), Pramipexole (Mirapex), and Ropinirole (Requip)

Medications from this group have been used as adjuvants to L-dopa for patients in the later stages of PD for many years. Recently there has been growing clinical experience with these agents as *initial therapy* of PD, particularly as an alternatives to L-dopa. All four dopamine agonists have been shown to be safe and effective as monotherapy for PD. The three newer agents appear to be somewhat more effective than bromocriptine, the first dopamine agonist introduced. The two newest agonists (pramipexole and ropinirole) have been shown to be virtually as effective as L-dopa in the treatment of mild PD patients (69,70). The major rationale for their use as initial therapy of PD is the significantly lower level of dose fluctuations—particularly dyskinesias—compared to L-dopa over at least the first 5 years of treatment (71,72). As many as half of PD patients can be adequately treated with an agonist without L-dopa for 3 to 5 years. The metabolism of these agents does not produce oxidative injury, so that it has been suggested that they may be less likely to accelerate the underlying neurodegeneration of PD. Both ropinirole and pramipexole initiated patients show fewer signs of dopaminergic degeneration compared to L-dopa–initiated patients with dopamine terminal imaging studies mentioned earlier. Unlike L-dopa, dopamine agonists are not available as a combination pill with an agent to prevent dopamine-related side effects. Dopamine agonists have a higher incidence of nausea and GI disturbances than carbidopa/L-dopa combinations. These side effects can be minimized by a very gradual titration schedule, allowing for tolerance to the drug to occur. The mantra for use of dopamine agonists is "start low, go slow, aim high," because starting doses are typically one tenth of the therapeutic dose (Table 90.4). Patients need to understand both the schedule of dose escalation and its rationale. Overly slow escalation can lead to discontinuation by the patient because of a perceived lack of efficacy, whereas overly rapid escalation leads to discontinuation because of side effects (usually nausea). However, the cost of dopamine agonists is significantly higher than equivalent amounts of carbidopa/L-dopa, particularly in its immediate release generic form.

Domperidone is a useful medication to relieve nausea caused by dopamine agonists (or levodopa) (73). Domperidone is a dopamine antagonist that does not cross the blood–brain barrier and, in contrast to the typical neuroleptics and related antinausea drugs, does not worsen symptoms of PD. It is currently available through Canadian pharmacies as a stimulant for GI motility (its indication worldwide). The two newer agonists ropinirole and pramipexole differ from bromocriptine and pergolide chemically as nonergot derivatives. Fibrotic complications of ergot-based drugs, although rare, are well described. There have been recent reports of valvular abnormalities with long-term pergolide treatment, leading to the recommendation of transthoracic echocardiographic evaluation for patients remaining on this medication (74).

There are no proven neuroprotectants for Parkinson disease. Current data supports the use of either L-dopa or a dopamine agonist as initial therapy for symptomatic PD. Although initial studies suggested that the selective monoamine oxidase type B (MAO-B) inhibitor selegiline may have neuroprotective qualities, it remains uncertain to what extent its unanticipated symptomatic effects contributed to this conclusion (75).

Treatment of Moderate Parkinson Disease

Patients usually experience worsening motor symptoms of PD, requiring increasing amounts of medications (particular L-dopa) within the first 5 years after diagnosis. The most common new problem for patients with moderate stage PD is a reduction in the duration of benefit of each dose of L-dopa, known as wearing off. Although patients with early PD may have uninterrupted benefit from taking L-dopa twice a day, patients with moderate PD may find that their symptoms may worsen at the end of a dose taken three or four times a day. Disease severity plays a major role in this change. L-Dopa has a very short serum half-life (90 minutes), but early PD patients appear to have a capacity for a sustained benefit well beyond its pharmacokinetic effect. As PD worsens, the duration of action of L-dopa approaches its short serum lifetime.

Addressing "Wearing Off" of L-Dopa

Several useful strategies reduce the wearing off of L-dopa. L-Dopa is available in a controlled-release form extending its duration of action by approximately 10% (76). Selegiline inhibits the degradation of dopamine and extends the duration of action of L-dopa by approximately 10% to 15% (77). Selegiline is a virtually irreversible MAO inhibitor and is dosed twice a day regardless of a patient's L-dopa dose schedule. Selegiline is so long acting that when signs of dopamine excess occur with its use, L-dopa dose must be reduced along with discontinuation of selegiline. Inhibitors of the major dopamine degrading enzyme, catechol-O-methyltransferase (COMT), are also available. Tolcapone (Tasmar) was the first COMT inhibitor released, and it remains the most potent drug to prolong the duration of action of carbidopa/L-dopa. Mild elevations of liver function tests were observed in its pivotal clinical trials. After its release, reports of fatal hepatotoxicity mandated regular assessment of alanine aminotransferase (ALT) levels, which has greatly limited its use. Entacapone (Comtan) has not been associated with hepatotoxicity. This COMT inhibitor is more effective than selegiline in prolonging the duration of action of L-dopa and is used in a very different fashion (78). Entacapone is a short-acting medication that is given as a fixed dose (200 mg) along with each dose of L-dopa. Entacapone is available in a preparation combined with carbidopa and L-dopa (Stalevo) (79). For patients requiring frequent doses, L-dopa is also available as a rapidly dissolving tablet that can be taken without water (Parcopa) (80).

Use of the longer acting *dopamine agonists* along with L-dopa is another proven strategy to reduce wearing off and improve the duration of daily "on" time. All the dopamine agonists have shown significant improvement of PD symptoms when used along with L-dopa (81,82). For patients with severe wearing off, a combination of strategies to increase L-dopa action as well as the addition of agonist therapy is commonly used.

Management of dose fluctuations becomes more problematic when patients develop *both wearing off and clinically significant dyskinesias*. The overall strategy is to reduce the total amount of short-acting L-dopa and supplement therapy with a longer acting agent, usually a dopamine agonist. This strategy is based on the observation that most dyskinesias occur at the time of peak action of L-dopa (peak dose dyskinesia), although some dyskinesias may occur during rapid drop in L-dopa levels (wearing off dyskinesias). All forms of L-dopa extension therapy and agonist adjuvant therapy are associated with an increase in dyskinesias, particularly when these treatments are initiated. It is only through the reduction of the daily L-dopa dose that these dyskinesias can be controlled while maintaining an improved duration of "on" time.

Treatment of Severe Parkinson Disease

Drug Treatment of Motor Fluctuations

As PD worsens (usually at least 10 years after diagnosis), patients develop both wearing off and dyskinesias with increasing frequency and severity. The regimens of L-dopa extension drugs and dopamine agonists frequently make such motor fluctuations more unpredictable. Conflict between patients and their physicians over therapy are common in this period. Physicians view dyskinesias as the most medically refractory symptom and aim to reduce them by reducing total daily L-dopa. However, most PD patients do not view dyskinesias as their most significant problem and may even be unaware of mild dyskinesias. Patients usually view the intrusion of PD symptoms during a sudden "off period" as more distressing and functionally more important and may seek increases in their L-dopa daily dose. Direct discussions about both short- and long-term goals of therapy are needed to maximize both patient satisfaction and medication compliance.

Bioavailability of L-dopa is influenced by dietary protein so that a *protein restriction/redistribution* diet is appropriate for patients with severe fluctuation in motor function (83). Consultation with a nutritionist is needed, because weight loss can occur in this population of patients that is already below their ideal weight. Although daytime wearing off usually improves, evening dyskinesias may develop with protein redistribution. Attempts at controlling daytime wearing off with drug therapy may also increase evening dyskinesias as L-dopa levels gradually rise over the day. For sudden unexpected wearing off, injectable apomorphine (Apokyn) has been shown to be effective (84). This short-acting dopamine agonist is self-administered using a subcutaneous injector system. Relief of PD "off" symptoms begins within minutes, much more rapidly attained than with the use of an additional dose of oral L-dopa as a rescue medication. The short half-life of apomorphine allows it to be used along with the patient's usual schedule of medication. Because of the risk of hypotension and the high incidence of nausea and vomiting, initial test use of subcutaneous apomorphine should be done in a physician's office.

Long-term prevention of dyskinesias, as well as optimal dosing to reduce dyskinesia are particularly important since the medical treatment of dyskinesias is extremely limited. The only agent that can be practically used is amantadine. At doses of up to 400 mg/day, this drug has been shown to significantly reduce L-dopa–induced dyskinesias (85).

Surgery

Severe motor fluctuations despite optimal medical therapy is the strongest indication for surgical treatment of PD. Stereotactic thalamotomy and thalamic DBS are effective for parkinsonian tremor, but are now infrequently performed in PD patients (86). Since thalamotomy has little effect on PD signs other than tremor, if a PD patient with thalamotomy develops other PD symptoms years later, he may require a second surgical procedure at a different brain location.

Two other brain regions are targets of stereotactic surgery for relief of not only tremor, but rigidity and bradykinesia as well. The subthalamic nucleus (STN) is currently the most popular target for PD surgery. This small deep brain nucleus was only rarely targeted prior to the introduction of the adjustable/programmable DBS systems. The major benefit of STN DBS is a significant reduction in severity and duration of L-dopa "off" motor symptoms. Many of these patients are able to achieve substantial (30%) reduction in dopaminergic medications with resulting reduction in dyskinesia (87). The globus pallidus interna is also targeted for relief of motor symptoms of PD. Stereotactic lesioning of the globus pallidus interna has been extensively studied and still remains an option for patients who wish to avoid an implanted device and its potential complications. DBS of the globus pallidus interna appears to provide slightly less symptomatic relief than STN DBS. However, like pallidotomy and in contrast to STN surgery, globus pallidus interna DBS directly reduces dyskinesias and can improve patient benefit from medication (88). Careful patient selection is a key to attaining good outcome from DBS surgery. Good surgical candidates have severe motor fluctuation on optimal medical management, but still have good quality (but not duration) L-dopa "on" states.

There is a window of opportunity for PD surgery that cannot be reclaimed once it has passed. Stereotactic surgery for PD is very demanding on patients. For most of the hours of surgery the patient is awake and is an active participant as the target brain region is identified physiologically and test stimulation of the DBS unit is performed. Transient confusion can occur after surgery even in cognitively intact patients. Dementia (see Dementia subsection), a common problem in severe PD, is a clear contraindication to this form of surgery. Poor postural stability, another problem of advanced PD, usually does not improve with surgery. Generally, younger patients (younger than 65 years of age) tolerate PD surgery better and have better outcomes (89). Complications of DBS include not only perioperative bleeding and infection associated with brain lesioning, but device specific problems. A second surgical procedure is needed to implant the pacemaker-like pulse generator in the chest. The generator's battery must be changed on average every 3 years and complications such as device failure, lead fracture, or infection need surgical intervention. After implantation the device must be programmed to attain maximal relief of PD systems without stimulation-related side effects, which include unpleasant sensations, dysarthria, emotional changes, and diplopia. DBS currently is the standard of care for surgical approaches to PD. Fetal brain tissue transplantation has not shown significant benefit in a placebo controlled trial with a patient population resembling optimal DBS candidates (90). These relatively young, L-dopa–responsive PD patients are also the target population for experimental surgical therapies including growth factor infusion, gene therapy, and stem cell transplantation (91,92).

Psychosis

Psychosis, including hallucinosis, can occur in any PD patient receiving dopaminergic therapy. Psychotic symptoms become more prevalent and serious in advanced cases. Age, presence of dementia, and dose of antiparkinsonian drugs are the major risk factors for psychosis in PD patients. Although all forms of PD therapy can cause psychotic symptoms, L-dopa appears to have a superior ratio of relief of motor symptoms of PD to induction of psychosis compared with the dopamine agonists, adjunctive therapy with amantadine or anticholinergics. Psychosis is particularly problematic in demented patients with severe PD. The most common useful strategy to combat psychosis is to lower or simplify the dose of PD therapy. However, many advanced PD patients may not be able to tolerate lowering the dose of their PD medications. In the past, little could be done for these patients because the use of typical neuroleptics worsened motor symptoms to the same extent as reducing a PD medication. The introduction of clozapine (Clozaril) has significantly improved the treatment of these patients. Relatively low doses (12.5 to 50 mg) of clozapine can successfully suppress hallucinations and delusions without worsening motor symptoms (93). Unfortunately, the most common serious side effect of clozapine (agranulocytosis) is an idiosyncratic event, so that regular monitoring of leukocyte count is needed even at these low doses. The newer atypical neuroleptics are also useful to treat psychotic symptoms in PD. At this time quetiapine (Seroquel) appears to be the most useful (25 to 75 mg/day) (94). Risperidone (Risperdal) appears to have a greater propensity to worsen motor symptoms in PD than other atypical neuroleptics.

Dementia

Dementia eventually occurs in at least 30% of PD patients. It is most strongly associated with age (as with virtually all dementing illnesses) but is also associated with duration and severity of motor signs of PD (95). Because dementia is not an invariable part of PD, an evaluation for a reversible cause is needed. The underlying basis for dementia in PD is controversial. Some of these patients have concomitant Alzheimer disease (see Chapter 26). Another group of demented PD patients may have predominantly frontal lobe related abnormalities with loss of spontaneity, poor decision making and planning with less prominent loss of short-term memory (96). A third group of patients have another of the more widespread neurodegenerative diseases known as dementia with Lewy bodies (DLB) or diffuse Lewy body disease. This form of atypical parkinsonism not only shows motor signs, but patients have psychosis and hallucinosis early in the course of their disease even without PD drug therapy. Significant day-to-day fluctuation in behavior, cognition, and motor symptoms are also commonly observed in this condition (97). Clinical and pathologic criteria for DLB have been established relatively recently, but it is clear that it has been underdiagnosed in the past and represents a major form of non-Alzheimer type dementia (98). The anticholinesterase (AchE) that are FDA-approved for Alzheimer disease do provide comparable benefit for patients with PD and dementia (99,100). Worsening of motor signs of PD usually does not occur, and is generally restricted to worsening of resting tremor. Improvement in psychiatric symptoms has also been shown with these medications in patients with DLB, where extremely low levels of acetylcholine synthetic capacity as well as dramatic improvement with AchE treatment has been reported (101,102). Although the antidementia drug memantine has been investigated as an anti-PD medication, it has not been studied in PD with dementia (103,104). Because of its structural similarity to amantadine (contraindicated in PD dementia) this *N*-methyl-D-aspartate (NMDA) antagonist should be avoided in these patients until further information is available.

Autonomic Dysfunction

The most common serious form of autonomic dysfunction in PD is orthostatic hypotension, and it is usually worsened by dopaminergic therapy. Added dietary salt along with the mineralocorticoid fludrocortisone (Florinef) are useful to expand plasma volume. The limitations to this therapy are worsening of congestive heart failure and supine hypertension. Midodrine (ProAmatine) is an α-adrenergic agonist that is FDA-approved for orthostatic hypotension because of autonomic failure (105). This short-acting agent can be dosed during the day (2.5 to 5 mg) every 4 hours to minimize recumbent hypertension. Poor esophageal and intestinal motility are also seen in advanced PD. Domperidone (see Dopamine Agonists) may also be used in this setting since metoclopramide (Reglan) is relatively contraindicated in PD because of its tendency to worsen motor symptoms.

PATIENT SUPPORT ORGANIZATIONS

American Parkinson Disease Association (APDA)
1250 Hylan Avenue
Suite 4B
Staten Island, NY 10305
1-800-223-2732
Website: www.apdaparkinson.org

Dystonia Medical Research Foundation
One East Wacker Drive
Suite 2430
Chicago, IL 60601-1905
1-312-755-0198
Lewy Body Dementia Association
Website: www.dystonia-foundation.org

National Ataxia Foundation
2600 Fenbrook Lane, Suite 119
Minneapolis, MN 55447
1-763-553-0020
Website: www.ataxia.org

International Essential Tremor Foundation (ITF)
P.O. Box 14005
Lenexa, KS 66285-4005
1-888-387-3667
Website: www.essentialtremor.org

National Parkinson Foundation (NPF)
1501 NW 9th Avenue, Bob Hope Road
Miami, FL 33136-1494
Website: www.parkinson.org

Parkinson's Disease Foundation (PDF)
1359 Broadway, Suite 1509
New York, NY 10018
1-800-457-6676
website: www.parkinson.org

Society for Progressive Supranuclear Palsy
Executive Plaza III
11350 McCormick Road
Suite 906
Baltimore, MD 21231
1-800-457-4777
Website: www.psp.org

WE MOVE
204 West 84th Street
New York, NY 10024
Telephone: 1-800-437-MOV2 (in USA)
Website: www.wemove.org

SPECIFIC REFERENCES*

1. Caviness JN, Brown P. Myoclonus: current concepts and recent advances. Lancet Neurol 2004;3:598.
2. Postuma RB, Lang AE. Hemiballism: revisiting a classic disorder. Lancet Neurol 2003;2:661.
3. Jankovic J, Leder S, Warner D, et al. Cervical dystonia: clinical findings and associated movement disorders. Neurology 1991;41:1088.
4. Jedynak PC, Tranchant C, de Beyl DZ. Prospective clinical study of writer's cramp. Mov Disord 2001;16:494.
5. Costa J, Espirito-Santo C, Borges A, et al. Botulinum toxin type A therapy for blepharospasm. Cochrane Database Syst Rev 2005;(1):CD004900.
6. Tan NC, Chan LL, Tan EK. Hemifacial spasm

*Bold numerals denote published controlled clinical trials, meta-analyses, or consensus-based recommendations.

and involuntary facial movements. QJM 2002;95:493.
7. Sulica L. Contemporary management of spasmodic dysphonia. Curr Opin Otolaryngol Head Neck Surg 2004;12:543.
8. Singer HS. Tourette's syndrome: from behaviour to biology. Lancet Neurol 2005;4:149.
9. Diener HC, Dichgans J. Pathophysiology of cerebellar ataxia. Mov Disord 1992;7:95.
10. Hallett M. Overview of human tremor physiology. Mov Disord 1998;13 Suppl 3:43.
11. Bergareche A, De La Puente E, Lopez De, et al. Prevalence of essential tremor: a door-to-door survey in Bidasoa, Spain. Neuroepidemiology 2001;20:125.
12. Louis ED, Barnes L, Albert SM, et al. Correlates of functional disability in essential tremor. Mov Disord 2001;16:914.
13. Higgins JJ, Lombardi RQ, Pucilowska J, et al. A variant in the HS1-BP3 gene is associated with familial essential tremor. Neurology 2005;64: 417.
14. Growdon JH, Shahani BT, Young RR. The effect of alcohol on essential tremor. Neurology 1975;25:259.
15. Koller WC. Alcoholism in essential tremor. Neurology 1983;33:1074.
16. Bilodeau M, Keen DA, Sweeney PJ, et al. Strength training can improve steadiness in persons with essential tremor. Muscle Nerve 2000;23:771.
17. Espay AJ, Hung SW, Sanger TD, et al. A writing device improves writing in primary writing tremor. Neurology 2005;64:1648.
18. Koller WC, Biary N, Cone S. Disability in essential tremor: effect of treatment. Neurology 1986;36:1001.
19. Larsen TA, Terlvainene H, Calne DB. Atenolol vs propanolol in essential tremor. A controlled, quantitative study. Acta Neurol Scan 1982;66:547.
20. Ogawa N, Takayama H, Yamamoto M. Comparative studies on the effects of beta-adrenergic blockers in essential tremor. J Neurol 1987;235:31.
21. Koller WC, Royce JL. Efficacy of primidone in essential tremor. Neurology 1986;36:121.
22. Koller WC, Vetere-Overfield B. Acute and chronic effects of propranolol and primidone in essential tremor. Neurology 1989;39:1587.
23. Thompson C, Lang A, Parkes DJ, et al. A double-blind trial of clonazepam in benign essential tremor. Clin Neuropharmacol 1988;7:83.
24. Huber SJ, Paulson GW. Efficacy of alprazolam for essential tremor. Neurology 1988;38:241.
25. Ondo W, Hunter C, Vuong KD, et al. Gabapentin for essential tremor: a multiple-dose, double-blind, placebo-controlled trial. Mov Disord 2000;15:678.
26. Gironell A, Kulisevsky J, Barbanoj M, et al. A randomized placebo-controlled comparative trial of gabapentin and propranolol in essential tremor. Arch Neurol 1999;56:475.
27. Connor GS. A double-blind placebo-controlled trial of topiramate treatment for essential tremor. Neurology 2002 9;59:132.
28. Bushara KO, Malik T, Exconde RE. The effect of levetiracetam on essential tremor. Neurology 200522;64:1078.
29. Krauss GL, Bergin A, Kramer RE, et al. Suppression of post-hypoxic and post-encephalitic myoclonus with levetiracetam. Neurology 2001;56:411.
30. Jankovic J, Schwartz K, Clemence W, et al. A randomized, double-blind, placebo controlled study to evaluate botulinum toxin type A in essential hand tremor. Mov Disord 1996;11:250.
31. Wissel J, Kabus C, Wenzel R, et al. Botulinum toxin in writer's cramp: objective response evaluation inpatients. J Neurol Neurosurg Psychiatry 1996;61:172.
32. Wissel J, Masuhr F, Schelosky L. Quantitative assessment of botulinum toxin treatment in 43 patients with head tremor. Mov Disord 1997;12:722.
33. Mohadjer M, Goerke H, Milios E, et al. Long-term results of stereotaxy in the treatment of essential tremor. Stereotact Funct Neurosurg 1990;55:125.
34. Pahwa R, Lyons KL, Wilkinson SB, et al. Bilateral thalamic stimulation for the treatment of essential tremor. Neurology 1999;53:1147.
35. Pahwa R, Lyons KE, Wilkinson SB, et al. Comparison of thalamotomy to deep brain stimulation of the thalamus in essential tremor. Mov Disord 2001;16:140.
36. Schuurman PR, Bosch DA, Bossuyt PM, et al. A comparison of continuous thalamic stimulation and thalamotomy for tremor. N Engl J Med 2000;342:461.
37. Ceravolo R, Salvetti S, Piccini P. Acute and chronic effects of clozapine in essential tremor. Mov Disord 1999;14:468.
38. Alvir JM, Lieberman JA. Agranulocytosis: incidence and risk factors. J Clin Psychiatry. 1994;55 Suppl B:137.
39. Darnell RB, Posner JB. Paraneoplastic syndromes involving the nervous system. N Engl J Med 2003;349:1543.
40. Koster B, Deuschl G, Lauk M, et al. Essential tremor and cerebellar dysfunction: abnormal ballistic movements. J Neurol Neurosurg Psychiatry 2002;73:400.
41. Koller WC. Pharmacologic trials in the treatment of cerebellar tremor. Arch Neurol 1984;41:280.
42. Shazadi S, Tasker RR, Lozano A. Thalamotomy for essential and cerebellar tremor. Stereotact Funct Neurosurg 1996;65:11.
43. Bain PG, Findley LJ, Britton TC, et al. Primary writing tremor. Brain 1995;118(Pt 6):1461.
44. Gerschlager W, Munchau A, Katzenschlager R, et al. Natural history and syndromic associations of orthostatic tremor: a review of 41 patients. Mov Disord 2004;19:788.
45. Schrag A, Ben-Shlomo Y, Brown R, et al. Young-onset Parkinson's disease revisited—clinical features, natural history, and mortality. Mov Disord 1998;13:885.
46. Langston JW. The etiology of Parkinson's disease with emphasis on the MPTP story. Neurology 1996;47[Suppl 3]:S153.
47. Lockwood AH. Pesticides and parkinsonism: is there an etiological link? Curr Opin Neurol 2000;13:687.
48. Polymeropoulos MH, Lavedan C, Leroy E, et al. Mutation in the alpha-synuclein gene identified in families with Parkinson's disease. Science 1997;276:2045.
49. Spillantini MG, Schmidt ML, Lee VM, et al. Alpha-synuclein in Lewy bodies. Nature 1997;388:839.
50. Hattori N, Mizuno Y. Pathogenetic mechanisms of parkin in Parkinson's disease. Lancet 2004;364:722.
51. Abou-Sleiman PM, Healy DG, Wood NW. Causes of Parkinson's disease: genetics of DJ-1. Cell Tissue Res 2004;318:185. Epub 2004 26.
52. Hatano Y, Li Y, Sato K, et al. Novel PINK1 mutations in early-onset parkinsonism. Ann Neurol 2004;56:424.
53. Brice A. How much does dardarin contribute to Parkinson's disease? Lancet 2005;365:363.
54. Vila M, Przedborski S. Genetic clues to the pathogenesis of Parkinson's disease. Nat Med 2004;10 Suppl:S58.
55. Sachdev PS. Neuroleptic-induced movement disorders: an overview. Psychiatr Clin North Am 2005;28:255.
56. Rajput A, Rajput AH. Progressive supranuclear palsy: clinical features, pathophysiology and management. Drugs Aging 2001;18:913.
57. Burn DJ, Lees AJ. Progressive supranuclear palsy: where are we now? Lancet Neurol 2002;1:359.
58. Wenning GK, Colosimo C, Geser F, et al. Multiple system atrophy. Lancet Neurol 2004;3:93.
59. Brewer GJ, Askari FK. Wilson's disease: clinical management and therapy. J Hepatol 2005;42 Suppl(1):S13.
60. Bower JH, Dickson DW, Taylor L, et al. Clinical correlates of the pathology underlying parkinsonism: a population perspective. Mov Disord 2002;17:910.
61. Lipp A, Trottenberg T, Schink T, et al. A randomized trial of botulinum toxin A for treatment of drooling. Neurology 2003;61:1279.
62. Pirker W. Correlation of dopamine transporter imaging with parkinsonian motor handicap: how close is it? Mov Disord 2003;18 Suppl 7:S43.
63. Scandalis TA, Bosak A, Berliner JC, et al. Resistance training and gait function in patients with Parkinson's disease. Am J Phys Med Rehabil 2001;80:38.
64. Rojo A, Aguilar M, Garolera MT, et al. Depression in Parkinson's disease: clinical correlates and outcome. Parkinsonism Relat Disord 2003;10:23.
65. Taus C, Giuliani G, Pucci E, et al. Amantadine for fatigue in multiple sclerosis. Cochrane Database Syst Rev 2003;(2):CD002818.
66. Markham CH, Diamond SG. Modification of Parkinson's disease by long-term levodopa treatment. Arch Neurol 1986;43:405.
67. Fahn S, Oakes D, Shoulson I, et al; Parkinson Study Group. Levodopa and the progression of Parkinson's disease. N Engl J Med 2004;351:2498.
68. Ahlskog JE, Muenter MD. Frequency of levodopa-related dyskinesias and motor fluctuation as estimated from the cumulative literature. Mov Disord 2001;16:448.
69. Parkinson Study Group. Pramipexole vs levodopa as initial treatment for Parkinson disease: a randomized controlled trial. JAMA 2000;284:1931.
70. Rascol O, Brooks DJ, Brunt ER, et al. Ropinirole in the treatment of early Parkinson's disease: a 6-month interim report of a 5-year levodopa-controlled study. 056 Study Group. Mov Disord 1998;13:39.
71. Rascol O, Brookes DJ, Korczyn AD, et al. A five-year study of the incidence of dyskinesia in patients with early Parkinson's disease who were treated with ropinirole or levodopa. N Engl J Med 2000;342:1484.
72. Holloway RG, Shoulson I, Fahn S, et al. ; Parkinson Study Group. Pramipexole vs levodopa as initial treatment for Parkinson disease: a 4-year randomized controlled trial. Arch Neurol 2004;61:1044.
73. Jansen PA, Herings RM, Samson MM, et al. Quick titration of pergolide in cotreatment with domperidone is effective. Clin Neuropharmacol 2001;24:177.
74. Van Camp G, Flamez A, Cosyns B, et al. Treatment of Parkinson's disease with pergolide and relation to restrictive valvular heart disease. Lancet 2004;363:1179.
75. Calne DB. Selegiline in Parkinson's disease. BMJ 1995;311:1583.
76. Linazasoro G, Grandas F, Martinez Martin P, et al. Controlled release levodopa in Parkinson's disease: influence of selection criteria and conversion recommendations in the clinical outcome of 450 patients. Clin Neuropharmacol 1999;22:74.
77. Golbe LI, Lieberman AN, Meunter MD, et al. Deprenyl in the treatment of symptom fluctuations in advanced Parkinson's disease. Clin Neuropharmacol 1988;11:45.
78. Schrag A. Entacapone in the treatment of Parkinson's disease. Lancet Neurol 2005;4:366.
79. Brooks DJ, Agid Y, Eggert K, et al. Treatment of

end-of-dose wearing-off in Parkinson's disease: Stalevo (Levodopa/Carbidopa/Entacapone) and Levodopa/DDCI Given in Combination with Comtess((R))/Comtan((R)) (Entacapone) Provide Equivalent Improvements in Symptom Control Superior to That of Traditional Levodopa/DDCI Treatment. Eur Neurol 2005; 53:197.
80. Parcopa: a rapidly dissolving formulation of carbidopa/levodopa. Med Lett Drugs Ther 2005;47:12.
81. Poewe W. Adjuncts to levodopa therapy: dopamine agonists. Neurology 1998;50(6 Suppl 6):S23-6; discussion S44-8.
82. Pahwa R, Koller WC. Dopamine agonists in the treatment of Parkinson's disease. Cleve Clin J Med 1995;62:212.
83. Pincus JH, Barry K. Protein redistribution diet restores motor function in patients dopa-resistant "off" periods. Neurology 1988; 38:481.
84. Factor SA. Literature review: intermittent subcutaneous apomorphine therapy in Parkinson's disease. Neurology 2004;62 (6 Suppl 4):S12.
85. Metman LV, Del Dotto P, LePoole K, et al. Amantadine for levodopa-induced dyskinesias: a 1-year follow up study. Arch Neurol 1999;56: 1383.
86. Fox MW, Ahlsko JE, Kelly PJ. Stereotactic ventrolateralis thalamotomy for medically refractory tremor in post-levodopa era Parkinson's disease patients. J Neurosurg 1991;75:723.
87. Krack P, Batir A, Van Blercom N, et al. Five-year follow-up of bilateral stimulation of the subthalamic nucleus in advanced Parkinson's disease. N Engl J Med 2003;349:1925.
88. Rodriguez-Oroz MC, Obeso JA, Lang AE, et al. Bilateral deep brain stimulation in Parkinson's disease: a multicentre study with 4 years follow-up. Brain 2005; (in press).
89. Russmann H, Ghika J, Villemure JG, et al. Subthalamic nucleus deep brain stimulation in Parkinson disease patients over age 70 years. Neurology 2004;63:1952.
90. Freed CR, Greene PE, Breeze RE, et al. Transplantation of embryonic dopamine neurons for severe Parkinson's disease. N Engl J Med 2001;344:710.
91. Levy YS, Stroomza M, Melamed E, et al. Embryonic and adult stem cells as a source for cell therapy in Parkinson's disease. J Mol Neurosci 2004;24:353.
92. Slevin JT, Gerhardt GA, Smith CD, et al. Improvement of bilateral motor functions in patients with Parkinson disease through the unilateral intraputaminal infusion of glial cell line-derived neurotrophic factor. J Neurosurg 2005;102:216.
93. Parkinson Study Group. Low-dose clozapine for the treatment of drug-induced psycho Parkinson's disease. The Parkinson Study Group. N Engl J Med 1999;340:801.
94. Juncos JL, Roberts VJ, Evatt ML, et al. Quetiapine improves psychotic symptoms and cognition in Parkinson's disease. Mov Disord 2004;19:29.
95. Aarsland D, Andersen K, Larsen JP, et al. Risk of dementia in Parkinson's disease: a community-based, prospective study. Neurology 2001;56: 730.
96. Aarsland D, Andersen K, Larsen JP, et al. The rate of cognitive decline in Parkinson disease. Arch Neurol 2004;61:1906.
97. Barber R, Panikkar A, McKeith IG. Dementia with Lewy bodies: diagnosis and management. Int J Geriatr Psychiatry 2001;16 Suppl 1:S12.
98. Merdes AR, Hansen LA, Jeste DV, et al. Influence of Alzheimer pathology on clinical diagnostic accuracy in dementia with Lewy bodies. Neurology 2003;60:1586.
99. Leroi I, Brandt J, Reich SG, et al. Randomized placebo-controlled trial of donepezil in cognitive impairment in Parkinson's disease. Int J Geriatr Psychiatry 2004;19:1.
100. Emre M, Aarsland D, Albanese A, et al. Rivastigmine for dementia associated with Parkinson's disease. N Engl J Med 2004;351: 2509.
101. Tiraboschi P, Hansen LA, Alford M, et al. Early and widespread cholinergic losses differentiate dementia with Lewy bodies from Alzheimer disease. Arch Gen Psychiatry 2002;59:946.
102. McKeith I, Del Ser T, Spano P, et al. Efficacy of rivastigmine in dementia with Lewy bodies: a randomized, double-blind, placebo-controlled international study. Lancet 2000;356:2031.
103. Reisberg B, Doody R, Stoffler A, et al. Memantine Study Group. Memantine in moderate-to-severe Alzheimer's disease. N Engl J Med 2003;348:1333.
104. Merello M, Nouzeilles MI, Cammarota A, et al. Effect of memantine (NMDA antagonist) on Parkinson's disease: a double-blind crossover randomized study. Clin Neuropharmacol 1999; 22:273.
105. Low PA, Gilden JL, Freeman R, et al. Efficacy of midodrine vs placebo in neurogenic orthostatic hypotension. A randomized, double-blind multicenter study. Midodrine Study Group. JAMA 1997;277:1046.

*For annotated **General References** and resources related to this chapter, visit www.hopkinsbayview.org/PAMreferences.*

Chapter 91

Cerebrovascular Disease

Rafael H. Llinas and Constance J. Johnson

OVERVIEW

Epidemiology

Cerebrovascular disease (CVD) is a major cause of disability and the third leading cause of death in the United States. According to 2005 American Heart Association (AHA) estimates, the annual cost is more than $393.5 billion in direct and indirect costs and there are 4.7 million stroke survivors (2.3 million men, 2.4 million women) (1). Approximately 28% of strokes occur in people younger than age 65 years; men have a 26% greater odds of sustaining a first stroke than women (2). The annual death rate from stroke is higher in African Americans; compared with whites, young African Americans have a two- to threefold greater risk of ischemic stroke, and African American men and women are more likely to die of stroke (1).

Stroke incidence and death rate from stroke have decreased in recent years. This epidemiology of stroke reflects changing risk and demographics as well as more universal application of preventive measures. From 1992 to 2002 death rates from CVD (International Classification of Diseases (and Related Health Problems), 10th edition [ICD-10]) declined 18.0%, while actual CVD deaths increased 0.8% in the same period, (probably reflecting the aging population). Studies in the 1980s showed that stroke incidence had decreased nationwide and worldwide, but this decline stabilized after 1990 (3). Factors that may have contributed to the initial decline include more aggressive treatment of hypertension, more effective and early delivery of health care, and better management and recognition of the cardiogenic sources of cerebral embolization. This is supported by the finding of a community-based study that found a 40% reduction in the incidence of stroke in the past 20 years, as well as significant reductions in smokers, mean total cholesterol, mean systolic and diastolic blood pressures, and increases in preventive treatments (4). Unfortunately, among adults age 18 years and older, the prevalence of two or more risk factors increased from 23.6% in 1991 to 27.9% in 2002 (1).

Ischemic CVD presents two major challenges in ambulatory practice: the prevention of stroke in the large number of people with risk factors that make them prone to stroke and the optimal care of the many stroke survivors in each community. Brain hemorrhage is an acute problem usually presenting to the emergency room and requiring hospitalization and is not covered in this chapter.

Risk Factors and Prevention

A major goal of patient evaluation in ambulatory practice is the identification of the patient with an increased risk of stroke. Stroke risk factors identified in the Framingham study are age, systolic blood pressure, use of antihypertensive therapy, diabetes mellitus (DM), smoking, prior cardiovascular disease, atrial fibrillation, and left ventricular hypertrophy by echocardiogram (5). Subsequent observational data indicated the importance of blood cholesterol, especially for those younger than the age of 45 years (6). In the United States, ethnicity is an important risk factor; blacks have the highest stroke mortality rates, followed by non-Hispanic whites and Asians; Native Amricans and Hispanics have the lowest stroke mortality rates (3).

Patients who have previously had a stroke or transient ischemic attack (TIA) are an important subgroup of this high-risk population. A population-based study found that the risk of stroke after TIA was 9.5% at 90 days, and 14.5% at 1 year (7). The risk of combined stroke, myocardial infarction (MI), or death in this population was 21.8% at 1 year. One in six survivors of a first-ever stroke experience a recurrent stroke over the next 5 years, of which 25% are fatal. The greatest risk of recurrence is in the first 6 months after first stroke (8).

Prevention of stroke includes attention to modifiable risk factors as discussed below, and can be separated into primary prevention and secondary prevention (Table 91.1) (9,10).

Hypertension

Data accumulated during the Framingham study indicate that the risk of stroke is strongly related to hypertension. Atherothrombotic brain infarction occurred in hypertensive subjects (blood pressure greater than 160/95 mm Hg) four times more often than in normotensive subjects (5). Evidence from large controlled trials shows that stroke risk and other cardiovascular disease risk is significantly reduced by the treatment of hypertension in all patients, including those with a history of CVD (11–16). The risk reduction for first stroke with treatment of hypertension was 35% to 47% in these trials. Reduction in stroke risk with treatment of hypertension occurs rapidly, and the lower the blood pressure, the lower the risk of stroke, with no apparent threshold below which there is no further reduction in risk (17). A meta-analysis of nine randomized trials (62,605 hypertensive patients) revealed that calcium channel blockers (CCBs) and angiotensin-converting enzyme inhibitors (ACEIs) reduced cardiovascular events including stroke with reduction in systolic blood pressure. Although all antihypertensive agents were believed to have similar long-term efficacy and safety, a combination of ACEIs and diuretics have been shown very effective in preventing stroke (18). The Antihypertensive and Lipid-Lowering Treatment to Prevent Heart Attack (ALLHAT) trial indicated that blacks may derive greater blood pressure reduction and stroke risk reduction from chorthalidone than lisinopril (19). Chapter 67 discussses the evaluation and long-term management of hypertension.

Lipids

There have been many trials studying β-hydroxy-β-methylglutaryl-coenzyme A (HMG-CoA) reductase inhibitors (see Chapter 82), all of which have shown benefit in lowering chances of having first or recurrent stroke. A meta-analysis of three placebo-controlled randomized

TABLE 91.1 Effectiveness of Stroke Prevention Strategies

Strategy	Relative Risk (RR) Reduction, % (95% Confidence Interval)	Number Needed to Treat to Prevent 1 Stroke a Year[a]
	Primary Prevention Strategies	
Antihypertensive therapy if blood pressure elevated	42 (35–50)	7,937
Statins if cholesterol levels elevated	25 (14–35)	13,333
Antiplatelet therapy		
Aspirin	RR increase, 7 (RR reduction of 5% to RR increase of 22%)	Not significant
Aspirin after myocardial infarction	36 (15–51)	400[b]
Angiotensin-converting enzyme inhibitor	30 (15–43)	11,111
Carotid endarterectomy for asymptomatic stenosis	RR increase, 423(127–1107)	Not significant
	Secondary Prevention Strategies[c]	
Antihypertensive therapy if blood pressure elevated	28 (15–39)	51 (16.5)[d]
Statins if cholesterol levels elevated	25 (14–35)	57 (10.2)[d]
Warfarin for nonrheumatic atrial fibrillation	62 (48–72)	13 (10.5)[d]
Smoking cessation	33 (29–38)	43 (10.5)[d]
Antiplatelet therapy		
Aspirin	28 (19–36)	77 (9.9)[d]
Thienopyridines (vs aspirin)	13 (3–22)	64 (15.9)
Carotid endarterectomy for symptomatic moderate/severe stenosis[f]	44 (21–60)	26 (3.9)[d]

[a]Calculated by assuming that the annual risk of stroke is 0.03% (except where otherwise indicated) and using the best estimates of RR reduction from the literature, assuming constant RR reduction overtime.[††] Note that the baseline risk us variable (ranging from 1%–80%), and therefore the number needed to treat could vary by more than a thousandsfold, depending on this risk.

[b]Calculated by assuming that the risk of stroke is 0.01% over 2 years.

[c]Calculated by assuming that the annual risk of stroke is 7% (except where otherwise indicated) and using the best estimates of RR reduction from the literature, assuming constant RR reduction overtime.[11]

[d]Number in parentheses are the percentage of all recurrent stroke avoided a year, assuming that all eligible patients receive the intervention. The percentage was calculated by factoring the absolute risk reduction from the intervention by the prevalence of the underlying risk factor in the population that has already experienced a stroke or transient isschemic attack.

[e]Calculated by assuming that the annual risk of recurrent stroke in a patient with nonrheumatic atrial fibrillation is 12%.

[f]Calculated by assuming that the annual risk of recurrent stroke in a patient with moderate to severe carotid stenosis is 8.8%.

From Straus SE, Majumdar SR, McAlister FA. New evidence for stroke prevention: scientific review. JAMA 2002;288:1388.

trials (19,768 patients) concluded that pravastatin 40 mg/day reduced ischemic stroke risk 23% across a range of lipid levels with no evidence for benefit in hemorrhagic stroke or stroke of unknown type (6,20). Unfortunately, control of lipids through diet or bile acid sequestering agents have not been found to reduce stroke rates. Target levels of low-density lipoprotein (LDL) cholesterol have not been specified for stroke risk reduction, but should follow similar guidelines to those for cardiac risk reduction (see Chapter 82).

Diabetes Mellitus

Although the presence of DM confers additional risk of stroke, there are no randomized controlled trials (RCTs) demonstrating that tight glucose control in itself reduces risk of stroke. The UK Prospective Diabetes Study found that tight blood sugar control improves microvascular but not macrovascular endpoints in diabetes (21). This same cohort has found that diabetic patients with fatal stroke had higher glycosylated hemoglobin (HbA_{1c}) levels, than those with nonfatal stroke (odds ratio 1.37 per 1% HbA_{1c}) (22). Tight control of glucose with metformin in overweight and obese patients is the only regimen that has been shown to reduce the incidence of macrovascular complications in diabetes (23,24).

Smoking

Cigarette smoking is a predictor of the presence of significant intracranial and extracranial vascular stenosis (25). The duration of cigarette smoking is predictive of extracranial carotid artery stenosis detected by duplex scanning (26). In the Heart Outcomes Prevention Evaluation (HOPE) trial, the risk of stroke among smokers was 1.42 (95% confidence interval [CI] 1.00–2.04) compared with nonsmokers (27). Importantly, the risks for former smokers were the same as for those who had never smoked, suggesting the importance of smoking cessation in this population. As noted below, the major risk to survival in stroke patients is cardiac morbidity, so the implementation of smoking cessation counseling is indicated for this reason alone (see Chapter 27).

Cardiac Impairment

Patients with previous MI and/or cardiac impairment are predisposed to stroke, either directly because of emboli from the heart that lodge in cerebral arteries and lead to cerebral infarction, or indirectly because chronic atherosclerotic cardiac disease is associated with atherothrombotic cerebral disease. Cardioembolic stroke accounts for 15% to 30% of all ischemic strokes and is highly associated with cardiac arrhythmias, particularly atrial fibrillation with or without valvular disease, valvular disease, recent MI, and dilated cardiomyopathy (25). Data from the Framingham study identified cardiac impairment as a significant risk factor in the occurrence of the more common nonembolic atherothrombotic brain infarction. Subjects with electrocardiographic evidence of left ventricular hypertrophy were nine times more likely to develop atherothrombotic brain infarction than those without this abnormality. Patients with coronary artery disease (CAD) had five times the risk of atherothrombotic brain infarction, and those with radiographic evidence of cardiomegaly had three times the risk. When the contribution of concomitant hypertension was eliminated, left ventricular hypertrophy and CAD were each associated with a threefold increase in the risk of atherothrombotic brain infarction; the contribution of cardiomegaly on radiograph was not found to be significant when other variables were controlled. On the basis of these findings it was concluded that cardiac impairment, especially if associated with hypertension, significantly heightens the risk of stroke occurrence.

One of the most important modifiable risk factors is the presence of nonvalvular atrial fibrillation. A meta-analysis of five randomized trials of warfarin or aspirin in nonrheumatic atrial fibriallation concluded that the use of warfarin resulted in a 68% reduction in the risk of stroke (28). The annual rate of stroke in the control group was 4.5%, which was similar to the Framingham study, which found an annual stroke rate of 5%. Risk factors that predicted stroke were age, hypertension, previous history of stroke or TIA, and diabetes. Patients younger than age 65 years with none of these risk factors had an annual stroke rate of 1%. Risk reduction for aspirin in this population was not as consistent, averaging 36%. The current recommendations are to use long-term anticoagulation in all patients with chronic atrial fibrillation, with the exception of those at low risk, targeting an international normalized ratio (INR) = 2.0 to 3.0 (29,30). Patients younger than age 60 years with no risk factors may be treated with aspirin 325 mg daily (29,30).

Other Factors

Elevated blood hemoglobin and hematocrit levels have been implicated as possible risk factors, but a cause-and-effect relationship has not been established. Oral contraceptive use is associated with a five- to 10-fold increase in the risk of vascular diseases, including stroke (see details in Chapter 100). Observational studies initially indicated a decreased risk of ischemic stroke for postmenopausal hormone replacement therapy users (31). The Women's Health Initiative study, however, which studied 10,739 postmenopausal women, age 50 to 79 years of age, found a significant increased effect on the risk for stroke (32). Finally, it is generally accepted that the presence of an asymptomatic cervical bruit correlates with an increased incidence of subsequent stroke, but there is controversy regarding the approach to patients with this finding (see Asymptomatic Carotid Stenosis).

ASYMPTOMATIC CAROTID STENOSIS

Asymptomatic carotid stenosis is detected by the presence of a cervical bruit or because a vascular screening test was performed (see Chapter 86). Bruits occur in 4.5% of the population older than 45 years of age (33). A bruit is not pathognomonic of underlying stenosis (Table 91.2). A duplex scan (see description in Chapter 86) can define which patients with bruits have carotid stenosis and require further evaluation. Stenosis exceeding 75% to 80% of the lumen is associated with an annual risk of ipsilateral stroke of 2% to 3%. A large controlled trial (Asymptomatic Carotid Atherosclerosis Study [ACAS]) demonstrated that, for asymptomatic patients with more than 60% stenosis of the carotid artery, the combination of medical management (risk factor reduction and 325 mg aspirin per day) and carotid endarterectomy was superior to medical management alone (34). Over 5 years, the projected

TABLE 91.2 Possible Causes of Cervical Bruit

Physiologic murmur
Venous hum
Transmitted cardiac murmur
Atherosclerosis and stenosis of carotid, vertebral, subclavian, or innominate artery
Loops, kinks, inflammation, fibromuscular dysplasia of carotid artery
Arteriovenous fistula
Angiomatous malformation
Intracranial neoplasm
Paget disease of the skull

incidence of morbid events (perioperative death or stroke) was 5.1% for carotid endarterectomy patients, and the incidence of ipsilateral stroke was 11.0% for patients treated medically (an aggregate risk reduction of 53%). Patients to whom carotid endarterectomy is offered should be told that in ACAS there was approximately a 3% risk of perioperative stroke or death with carotid endarterectomy and that the benefit found in the ACAS trial accrued over 5 years.

Patients with excess cardiac risk were excluded from the ACAS trial. Medical management alone would probably benefit the latter group. Information about the symptoms of TIA should be given to any patient with a cervical bruit so that the patient does not ignore warning symptoms. The American Heart Association (AHA) has excellent patient education materials on TIA.

TABLE 91.3 Clinical Features of Ischemia Involving the Major Vascular Territories

Carotid artery disease
Paresis (mono- or hemi-)
Sensory loss or paresthesias (mono- or hemi-)
Speech or language disturbances
Loss of vision in one eye or part of one eye (amaurosis fugax)
Homonymous hemianopsia
Cognitive impairment
Vertebrobasilar arterial disease
Vertigo, diplopia, dysphagia, or dysarthria when two occur together or when one occurs with any of the following:
Paresis (any combination of the extremities)
Sensory loss or paresthesias (any combination of the extremities)
Ataxia
Homonymous hemianopsia (unilateral or bilateral)

CLASSIFICATION OF CEREBROVASCULAR EVENTS

Type of Event

Symptoms and signs of vascular origin are characterized by the rapid onset of deficits in a vascular distribution. The following classification has been developed based on duration:

- A *TIA* is defined as a transient episode of focal cerebral dysfunction, rapid in onset (from none to maximal symptoms in less than 5 minutes), that usually lasts from 2 to 15 minutes but always resolves completely within 24 hours.
- A *completed stroke* is defined as an episode of focal cerebral dysfunction that has stabilized and may have improved but has not resolved completely after 3 weeks. The most characteristic pattern is the abrupt occurrence of a neurologic deficit that improves or worsens, sometimes repeatedly, over minutes to hours to days and then becomes a fixed deficit.
- The term *stroke in evolution* is used to describe a vascular syndrome that is acute in onset and progressively worsens during the period of observation.

Vascular Territory

Cerebrovascular events are also classified on the basis of the vascular territory involved. Table 91.3 lists symptoms and signs referable to the two major vascular territories. There is overlap in the symptoms that may make the distinction between carotid and vertebrobasilar disease difficult. The history alone often provides the evidence necessary to identify the arterial territory involved.

A subgroup of ischemic events, called *lacunar syndromes*, is caused by occlusion of penetrating nonanastomosing branches of the major cerebral arteries. The pathology of the involved vessels has been characterized: occlusion is caused either by miniature atherosclerotic plaques at the origin of vessels 400 to 1000 μm in diameter or, more commonly, by a degenerative process called lipohyalinosis affecting vessels 200 μm or less in diameter. These changes correlate strongly with the presence of hypertension. At least 20 clinical lacunar syndromes have been described (35); lacunar infarctions may also be silent, identified only by computed tomography (CT) or magnetic resonance imaging (MRI). The common syndromes include the following:

- *Pure motor hemiparesis* (internal capsule or pons): hemiplegia or hemiparesis involving the face, arm, and leg without sensory deficit, dysphasia, or hemianopsia;
- *Pure sensory stroke* (thalamus): numbness of the face, arm, and leg on one side without weakness or hemianopsia;
- *Ataxic hemiparesis* (internal capsule or pons): cerebellar ataxia, weakness, and pyramidal signs involving the limbs on the same side, the lower extremity more than the arm;
- *The dysarthria or clumsy hand syndrome* (internal capsule or pons): dysarthria, facial weakness, clumsiness of the hand with little or no weakness, a slight imbalance, and a Babinski sign on the affected side;
- *Multi-infarct dementia*: a dementia syndrome characterized by stepwise progression (see description of dementia in Chapter 26).

SYMPTOMATIC PATIENTS

Transient Ischemic Attack and Stroke

Most TIAs and strokes are caused by artery-to-artery embolization, cardiogenic embolus, or small vessel (lacunar) disease. The distinction between TIA and stroke is becoming less important because a rigorous search for cause is indicated in both and many patients with TIA have evidence of brain infarction on imaging. Treatment is based on cause of the event regardless of whether the patient has had a TIA or stroke. Both events signal brain ischemia; stroke occurs when blood supply from collateral vessels is insufficient or the occluding thrombus is too large to be rapidly cleared.

For patients with TIA, other transient neurologic events described elsewhere, such as seizure (see Chapter 88), hypoglycemia (see Chapter 81), syncope (see Chapter 89), and migraine (see Chapter 87) must be considered. A Todd paralysis (transient focal weakness after a focal motor seizure or secondarily generalized tonic–clonic seizure) is diagnosed when the primary event is a seizure. Transient episodes with altered consciousness are almost never vascular in nature. Migraine occurs primarily in younger patients, is associated with headache, and must conform to defined criteria (see Chapter 87). A mass lesion such as a tumor or subdural hematoma may present with transient neurologic symptoms; however, these patients usually have persistent signs and symptoms. CT or MRI (see Chapter 86) is diagnostic. Occasionally, an acute exacerbation of multiple sclerosis may mimic TIA; however, these patients are usually younger and have had multiple episodes with nonvascular localization (e.g., optic neuritis).

Evaluation

Initial evaluation of the patient with TIA or stroke may be in the hospital (the patient who presents within hours or days of the event) or in the ambulatory setting (the patient who presents within weeks of the event). A detailed history is essential to identify risk factors for CVD and to delineate and classify the focal symptoms. The physical examination should include assessment for hypotension, hypertension, cardiac disease, CVD, and peripheral vascular disease, and any persisting neurologic abnormality. The patient should also have a careful funduscopic evaluation to assess the status of the retinal vessels and to detect emboli that suggest atherothrombotic carotid occlusive disease or cardiac disease. A brain MRI or CT (see Chapter 86) can localize the event, demonstrate previous silent events, and rule out other causes of neurologic symptoms that mimic CVD.

If there is clinical evidence of *heart disease*, in particular a murmur, atrial fibrillation, or left ventricular dysfunction, a transesophageal echocardiogram should be obtained to look for a cardiac source of arterial emboli. Transesophageal echocardiogram can also evaluate the aortic arch as a source of embolism. In patients with heart disease, ambulatory cardiac monitoring to check for arrhythmias may be beneficial when the cause of the stroke remains unknown after duplex and transesophageal echocardiogram.

Screening tests to check for *treatable causes* of occlusive CVD include a serologic test for syphilis, hematocrit measurement (polycythemia), and erythrocyte sedimentation rate (vasculitis). If a hypercoagulable state is suspected, anticardiolipin antibodies, anti-nuclear antibodies (AN) and homocysteine levels should be obtained (36).

Patients with carotid territory events should have a *noninvasive carotid evaluation*, using the available technique with the best performance characteristics. A meta-analysis of the various available procedures shows that the preferred noninvasive technique is duplex ultrasonography (37). Chapter 86 describes the characteristics of duplex ultrasonography and the patient experiences associated with it and other noninvasive diagnostic tests.

Cerebral angiography (see description in Chapter 86) should be considered in patients who do not have a definite source of brain embolus identified in the heart, aortic arch, or carotid arteries. Although a duplex scan can rule out carotid stenosis, intracranial vascular disease cannot be identified conclusively by duplex. A limited (noninvasive) evaluation can be justified if the patient's event was so devastating that further evaluation and treatment are precluded.

Early Management

Atherothrombotic Events

Patients with atherothrombotic events, either cortical or lacunar, may be treated medically or surgically.

Medical Therapy

This aspect of management includes risk factor modification and anticoagulant and antiplatelet drugs.

Antihypertensive therapy after an acute ischemic stroke is usually deferred until the patient's neurologic deficit is stable. In a small controlled study of hypertensive patients who had sustained a nonembolic ischemic stroke, 44% of the untreated patients, compared with 20% of the treated patients, suffered another major stroke, and at the end of a 2- to 5-year followup period, 46% of the untreated patients and 26% of the treated patients had died (38). Although the number of recurrent strokes was small, the difference in mortality was statistically significant in favor of the treated group. A meta-analysis of nine trials of blood pressure–lowering agents in hypertensive and nonhypertensive stroke survivors revealed a 28% reduction in stroke recurrence with treatment of hypertension (39). The Preventing Strokes by Lowering Blood Pressure in Patients with Cerebral Ischemia (PROGRESS) trial, a large, randomized, placebo-controlled trial of the ACEI perindopril with and without the diuretic indapamide demonstrated a 43% decrease in recurrent stroke risk in both hypertensive and nonhypertensive stroke and TIA survivors who received both drugs. Perindopril alone lowered blood pressure without affecting stroke recurrence (40). A subsequent meta-analysis found similar reductions in risk of stroke (21% to 24%) with antihypertensive treatment, with ACEIs and diuretics being the most effective (41). Although questions remain about subgroups and specific medications, treatment of hypertension in stroke survivors appears beneficial. (See Chapter 67 for details on the treatment of hypertension.)

The *antiplatelet drugs* aspirin, aspirin and dipyridamole (42), ticlopidine (43), and clopidogrel (44,45) are effective in reducing the recurrence of TIA or stroke. Aspirin is the most widely studied and cheapest agent, with effectiveness in doses of 50 to 1,500 mg (46). Ticlopidine's side-effect profile (fatal neutropenia, diarrhea) outweighs its modest statistical advantage. Clopidogrel's efficacy in secondary stroke prevention was only evident as a combined reduction in MI, stroke, or vascular death (44). The combination of aspirin and clopidogrel has been shown not only not to be more protective but to lead to higher rates of intracerebral and extracerebral hemorrhages (45). In the European Stroke Prevention Study II (ESPS II) trial, aspirin plus dipyridamole (25 mg plus 200 mg twice daily) was compared with aspirin alone (25 mg twice daily), extended-release dipyridamole alone (200 mg twice daily), or placebo. There was a 23.1% reduction of stroke in those on combination therapy compared with aspirin alone. Side effects were minor: headache and gastrointestinal (GI) events with dipyridamole and bleeding and GI events with aspirin, with the combination not significantly affecting side-effect incidence (42). Chapter 57 lists additional details regarding the use of and efficacy of antiplatelet drugs.

Anticoagulant therapy with warfarin (INR 1.4 to 2.8) was compared with aspirin (325 mg/day) in a large, double-blind, randomized trial (Warfarin-Aspirin Recurrent Stroke Study [WARSS]) in patients with prior noncardioembolic stroke, most with lacunar (55% in warfarin group, 56% in aspirin group) or cryptogenic (25% in warfarin group, 26% in aspirin group) stroke. Over 2 years of followup there was no difference in the rates of ischemic stroke, death, or major hemorrhage (approximately 17% in both groups) (47). Warfarin has been recommended for symptomatic patients (TIA or stroke) with known high-grade intracranial stenosis or preocclusive extracranial carotid bifurcation disease that cannot be addressed surgically (e.g., in patients who have cardiac disease precluding surgery). The prospective trial (Warfarin-Aspirin Symptomatic Intracranial Disease [WASID]) trial, however, showed no benefit of warfarin over aspirin and indeed found that there were more fatal events on warfarin than aspirin (48). Ongoing trials of higher on-treatment INRs and of warfarin in subgroups of patients will determine whether warfarin should be recommended for some patients. Based on all available data, aspirin appears superior in most patients with noncardioembolic strokes. Patients with significant intracranial disease probably should not be treated with warfarin unless recurrent events occur without remission; intracranial angioplasty is probably indicated in these patients. A role for *cholesterol lowering* in secondary stroke prevention was examined in a meta-analysis that included patients with stroke. Risk was reduced by 25% (49).

Surgical Therapy

Carotid endarterectomy can be recommended to patients with hemispheric or retinal TIAs or nondisabling stroke with ipsilateral severe (70% or greater) stenosis at the carotid bifurcation. This recommendation is supported by a large clinical trial (North American Symptomatic Carotid Endarterectomy Trial [NASCET]) in which 9% of carotid endarterectomy patients versus 26% of patients receiving antiplatelet treatment experienced an ipsilateral stroke during the 2 years after initiation of treatment (50). For symptomatic patients with moderate (50% to 69%) stenosis, the rate of stroke (average followup of 5 years) was 15.7% in the surgical group compared with 22.2% in the medical group ($p = 0.045$), a modest benefit compared with the benefit in patients with more severe stenosis. For stenosis less than 50%, there was no benefit (51). Patients who have undergone carotid endarterectomy are usually continued on long-term antiplatelet therapy.

In patients with recurrent TIAs or strokes and arteriographic evidence of *severe vertebral or basilar artery stenosis*, bypass procedures, angioplasty, and stenting have been undertaken. The efficacy of these procedures has not yet been established. Because the guidelines for the treatment of patients with TIAs and survivors of stroke are still evolving, the advice of a neurologist who specializes in CVD should be sought.

Cardioembolic Events

Patients with cardioembolic events who benefit from anticoagulation with warfarin include those with atrial fibrillation (both valvular and nonvalvular disease), recent MI, dilated cardiomyopathy, and rheumatic and prosthetic valves. Clinical trials consistently show a reduction in expected events in anticoagulated patients with atrial fibrillation; for those who have had a TIA or minor stroke the annual incidence of a new event is reduced from 12% to 4% and for those with no history of TIA or stroke, the annual incidence is reduced from approximately 5% to 2% (52). Chapter 57 describes specific aspects of anticoagulant therapy to prevent cerebrovascular accident; other chapters cover postinfarct mural thrombi (see Chapter 63), atrial fibrillation (see Chapter 64), and valvular heart disease (see Chapter 65). For patients with both a cardiac source and high-grade carotid stenosis (70% or higher) proximal to the territory of a TIA or stroke, carotid endarterectomy should be considered.

STROKE PROGNOSIS

Morbidity in Stroke Survivors

A number of studies have evaluated stroke survivors on the basis of the degree of neurologic, functional, and psychosocial impairment. In a 1975 study of stroke survivors, half of the patients (63 of 123) had no motor defecit when examined 6 months to 33 years (mean, 7 years) after the event (53). Right and left hempiparesis were equally represented; dysarthria and dysphasia were associated with right hemiparesis in 13 and 9 of 27 survivors respectively. These findings are probably representative of the situation in other communities.

In a classic study of overall function, Katz et al. (54) found that of patients who survive a stroke, approximately 50% are independent 2 years later and can ambulate and perform activities of daily living with minimal or no assistance. Spontaneous improvement is most rapid in the first few months after the stroke and is rarely noted after 2 years. Only a small percentage of stroke survivors remain bedridden and completely dependent. These findings were corroborated by results from the Mayo Clinic, where only 4% of the community-dwelling survivors of a stroke required total care at 6 months, 36% had some degree of neurologic deficit yet were able to work, and 29% were functioning normally (55). On the basis of the authors' assessment, 54% of their patients may have benefited from rehabilitative care, including the 10% who were aphasic.

The Framingham study provided information on the equally important *social and psychologic sequelae* of stroke (53). A significant decrease in the levels of vocational function and socialization outside the home was noted among stroke survivors (compared with age- and sex-matched control subjects), and the decrease exceeded that anticipated based on the levels of neurologic deficit. In a prospective study, the social and psychologic difficulties facing the stroke survivor were evaluated in more detail (56). Within the first 6 months after hospital discharge, 37% of the patients demonstrated moderate or severe depression, 32% anger or anxiety, 56% social isolation, 43% reduction in community involvement, 46% economic strain causing life-style alteration, and 52% disruption of normal family functions. Additional studies have confirmed the high incidence of moderate or severe depression in the first year after stroke and have shown that the risk of depression is particularly high in patients with damage in the left frontal hemisphere. Longitudinal studies show that poststroke depression lasts up to 2 years (57). Patients with poststroke depression respond well to antidepressant therapy (see Management of Psychologic and Behavioral Sequelae). Recognition and treatment of the psychosocial problems of the stroke patient and family are discussed in more detail below.

Mortality in Stroke Survivors

The *death rate among stroke survivors* is significantly greater than that expected for the general population matched for age and sex. The 5-year cumulative mortality is approximately 50% to 60%, with the greatest number of deaths occurring in the first year. With time, however, the mortality rate approaches that of the general population, and in at least one study, the increased rate of death after a stroke subsided completely after 24 to 30 months (54).

Studies that classified strokes on the basis of *type of vascular pathology* indicate that the early prognosis is much better for thrombotic or embolic disease than for hemorrhage (55). There is evidence that the type of pathology is a less reliable predictor of late prognosis. Eisenberg et al. (58) reported that patients with cerebral hemorrhage who lived 1 month had a 5-year survival equal to or better than patients with cerebral thrombosis.

The leading cause of death in stroke survivors is cardiovascular disease, with cardiac-related deaths exceeding deaths attributed to CVD by a factor of 2 to 1. Because cardiac disease is a major contributor to the cause of the stroke, stroke recurrence, and the survival from stroke, thorough evaluation and management of cardiac disease are of great importance in the care of stroke survivors.

LONG-TERM MANAGEMENT

Management of the patient who has survived a stroke involves the evaluation and treatment of physical and psychosocial sequelae and the selection of appropriate therapy to lessen the risk of recurrence. Once the patient has been discharged from the hospital, the patient's personal physician plays a critical role in coordinating care. Reduction in a patient's disability and dependency often requires the concerted efforts of the patient's family, physical, occupational, and speech therapists, and occasionally a psychiatrist. Patients with significant deficits persisting for 3 months or longer may qualify for *disability insurance under Social Security* (see Chapter 9).

Role of the Family

At the time of discharge from the hospital, appropriate education is especially important for the stroke survivor and the patient's family. At this juncture, patients are confronted with the full extent of their functional loss. By dispelling myths regarding stroke and supplanting them with accurate information, physicians and therapists can ensure that the actions of well-meaning family members do not foster the patients' feelings of inadequacy.

The following general suggestions can be helpful for the family of a stroke patient with residual disability:

- Divide duties so that the full burden of care does not fall on one person.
- Help the patient take responsibility for exercising regularly.
- Allow the patient to take on responsibilities for self-care and other activities gradually and by easy steps. It calls for fine judgment to encourage independence and not to frustrate a patient with overly difficult tasks and to stimulate progress without encouraging unrealistic expectations.
- Praise any successful efforts that are made; do not be discouraged by failures. Recovery from stroke is a slow process.
- Have the patient participate in as many family activities and as much family planning as possible. Feeling useful is a tremendous morale builder.
- Help him or her keep in contact with the world.
- Do not relegate the patient to the sidelines and leave him or her with only television and radio. Encourage the patient to develop a hobby. Spend time with him or her and encourage visitors if warranted. Make him or her feel wanted and a part of the social picture.
- Get in touch with the doctor if things are not going as you believe they should.

Role of Rehabilitation

Success in stroke rehabilitation often depends on the extent of permanent damage and the patient's ability to use *alternative methods of function* to compensate for fixed deficits. As noted above, spontaneous improvement in the stroke survivor may continue to occur for the first 6 to 12 months after the stroke, yet the mechanisms underlying such gains remain obscure. In studies to determine whether intensive rehabilitation results in functional gains after the period of spontaneous improvement, it has been found that even significantly impaired patients admitted to a rehabilitation program 12 months after a stroke may show marked improvement in dressing skills, bladder and bowel function, and walking. These findings form the basis for the conclusion that a program of rehabilitation does improve the outcome of the stroke survivor. It is estimated that the savings derived in returning a patient to the family or to independent living more than equals the costs of rehabilitation.

It is clear that not all patients in a rehabilitation program show significant functional improvement. A number of patient characteristics correlate with poor rehabilitation results, including bowel and bladder incontinence, low self-care status on admission, right hemispheric involvement, intellectual and perceptual deficits, heart failure, signs of generalized arteriosclerosis, and lower educational levels. However, because none of these factors correlates strongly with poor outcome, the best approach is to offer rehabilitation services when possible to each stroke survivor with significant functional impairments.

It is generally agreed that, except for patients with evidence of subarachnoid bleeding, for whom bed rest and mild sedation are indicated, a *program of functional rehabilitation* should begin as soon as possible after a stroke occurs and the patient is stable. There are several reasons for the early initiation of a program of rehabilitation. First, it is generally accepted that patients who are provided with rehabilitation services early are likely to experience greater long-term functional improvement. Second, early transfer from bed to chair coupled with physical therapy reduces the complications that can develop in the immobile bedridden patient and that can subsequently limit the extent of functional recovery. Stretching of tight muscles, passive range of motion, and active or resistive exercises minimize the degree of muscle atrophy and prevent the development of contractures. Additionally, even limited mobility of the patient reduces the risk of circulatory complications such as thrombophlebitis, postural hypotension, and pressure sores. Third, early rehabilitation is of particular benefit to the patient who demonstrates an impaired ability to communicate because of either aphasia or dysarthria. Approximately one third of stroke patients exhibit some form of communication disorder, and many of these remain severely impaired beyond the period of spontaneous recovery. Such patients may feel desperately isolated because of their loss of ability to communicate. Therapists who specialize in speech and hearing are skilled in the evaluation and management of these problems and play an integral role in daily interactions with the patient and in recommending appropriate strategies to the patient's family and physician.

Everyone involved in the rehabilitation process must appreciate the significance of the functional losses sustained by the patient, so the losses must be viewed from the patient's perspective. This requires an awareness of the patient's usual activities before the stroke; this essential information should be obtained in conjunction with a social worker who can evaluate the patient's role at home before the stroke and can project how the stroke will alter that role when the patient returns home.

The rehabilitation initiated in the hospital can be continued after discharge. Most communities have physical, occupational, and speech therapists available for both home and ambulatory followup. For patients meeting eligibility criteria, these services are covered by third-party payers. The patient and family should be acquainted with the goals and plans for continued rehabilitation before discharge. Chapter 9 provides information about home health services. The comprehensive text of Brandstater and Basmajian (www.hopkinsbayview.org/PAMreferences) provides details about the many individualized approaches available for rehabilitation.

Management of Psychologic and Behavioral Sequelae

The high incidence of psychologic and behavioral problems among stroke survivors has been noted above. These problems often hinder rehabilitation efforts. Fear of a second stroke and depression caused by loss of functional ability are readily understandable in the context of the patient's predicament. Appropriate counseling of the patient and family (as outlined in Role of Rehabilitation), coupled with participation in an active rehabilitation program, are the best ways to minimize the adverse psychologic reactions to a stroke.

A number of stroke survivors experience *mood disturbances* that do not correlate with the level of functional disability, and there is evidence that for many patients the mood disorder is a specific complication of cerebral damage rather than a reaction to functional loss (57). This mood disorder may augment the cognitive impairment of the patient or on occasion may be expressed as an apparent cognitive impairment (pseudodementia of depression, described in Chapter 26). Response in such patients to antidepressant treatment may be dramatic. Earlier observations suggested that the type of mood disorder depends on the side of the brain affected by the stroke. Gainotti (59) reported that behavior denoting a catastrophic reaction (see Chapter 26) and anxious depressive orientation of mood (anxiety reactions, bursts of tears, provocative utterances, depressed renouncements, or sharp refusals to go on with the examinations) are more common among patients with *left* (dominant) hemisphere damage. Symptoms denoting an opposite emotional reaction (denial of illness, minimization, indifference reactions, and tendency to joke) and expressions of hate toward the paralyzed limbs are more common among patients suffering from a lesion of the *right* (nondominant) hemisphere. Most authorities agree, however, that both psychological and physiologic factors contribute to the development of mood disorders after strokes. Tricyclic antidepressants have been shown to benefit patients with poststroke depression (57). Chapter 24 lists practical information about these and other antidepressant drugs.

The AHA booklet, *How Stroke Affects Behavior,* is particularly helpful for the family and for health care professionals caring for the patient who has survived a stroke.

Management of Late Complications

A number of complications may occur during the months to years after a stroke.

Shoulder Problems

The painful shoulder is one of the most disturbing complications encountered in the patient with a residual hemiparesis. Shoulder pain is often caused by increased traction on the shoulder capsule secondary to abnormal positioning of the paralyzed arm. The normal alignment of the joint can be restored through the use of a sling and proper positioning of the arm at night. Physical therapy, after initial symptomatic treatment with analgesics and the application of heat, can limit the extent of permanent structural damage (see Chapter 69 for additional details).

The *shoulder–hand syndrome* occurs in approximately 5% of stroke patients. It is characterized by the occurrence of a painful shoulder associated with stiffness and swelling of the hand and fingers. Onset is acute or subacute (developing over 3 to 6 months) and may involve the hand and shoulder simultaneously or one followed by the other. Although a number of conditions can result in shoulder discomfort, the dystrophic changes in the hand are characteristic of the development of a complex regional pain syndrome. There is swelling below the wrist, and the intrinsic muscles of the hand atrophy with extension deformities in the metacarpophalangeal joints. At this stage radiographic examination of the hand often shows spotty demineralization of the carpal bones. The severe pain associated with this condition greatly hinders rehabilitation efforts. Therefore, early recognition and treatment are important. A nonsteroidal anti-inflammatory drug (NSAID), local heat, and medications for chronic pain may be helpful.

Complications of Inactivity

The partially paralyzed stroke survivor often leads a sedentary existence, conducive to the development of vascular complications such as thrombophlebitis and pressure sores. Use of elastic stockings and frequent repositioning of the immobile patient by an informed family member minimizes these problems.

Neurologic Complications

Prolonged pressure on a paralyzed limb may lead to a peripheral nerve lesion, which may be difficult to recognize when superimposed on brain damage resulting from the stroke. An awareness of this potential complication can expedite its recognition, and electrodiagnostic studies can confirm the lower motor neuron damage (see Chapter 92). Once a diagnosis is made, prompt initiation of physical therapy limits the degree of functional loss resulting from this potentially reversible lesion.

Approximately 3% to 10% of stroke survivors develop *seizures* (epilepsy) as a late complication (60). Patients with damage to their sensorimotor cortex are the most likely to develop epilepsy, with the first seizure usually occurring 6 to 12 months after the stroke. Transient neurologic dysfunction after a seizure in a stroke survivor is often attributed to a second stroke. The rapid resolution of symptoms and electroencephalographic evidence of an epileptogenic focus point to seizure activity rather than ischemia as the cause. Recurrent seizures in the stroke survivor confirm the diagnosis of epilepsy. Seizure control can usually be achieved through the use of anticonvulsant medication (see Chapter 88).

Finally, *stroke-related deficits may transiently worsen* when the patient develops a major intercurrent illness such as pneumonia or myocardial infarction. In this instance, neurologic status returns to baseline after resolution of the intercurrent illness. (See discussion of upper motor neuron symptoms in Chapter 86.)

General Surgery

Chapter 93 addresses the approach to general surgery in patients who have a history of stroke.

SPECIFIC REFERENCES*

1. American Heart Association. Heart Disease and Stroke Statistics—2005 Update. Dallas: American Heart Association, 2005.
2. Bamford J, Sandercock P, Dennis M, et al. A prospective study of acute cerebrovascular disease in the community: The Oxfordshire community stroke project 1981–86. 1. Methodology, demography and incident cases of first-ever stroke. J Neurol Neurosurg Psychiatry 2988;51:1373.
3. Cooper R, Cutler J, Desvigne-Nickens, et al. Trends and disparities in coronary heart disease, stroke and other cardiovascular diseases in the United States: findings of the National Conference on Cardiovascular Disease Prevention. Circulation 2000;102:3137.
4. Rothwell PM, Coull AJ, Giles MF, et al. Change in stroke incidence, mortality, case-fatality, severity, and risk factors in Oxfordshire, UK from 1981 to 2004 (Oxford Vascular Study). Lancet 2004;363:1925.
5. Wolf PA, D'Agostino RB, Belanger AJ, et al. Probability of stroke: a risk profile from the Framingham Study. Stroke 1991;22:312.
6. Cholesterol, diastolic blood pressure, and stroke: 13,000 strokes in 450,000 people in 45 prospective cohorts. Prospective studies collaboration. Lancet 1995;346:1647.
7. Hill MD, Yiannakoulias N, Jeerakathil T, et al. The high risk of stroke immediately after transient ischemic attack: a population-based study. Neurology 2004;62:2015.
8. Hankey GJ, Jamrozik K, Broadhurst RJ, et al. Long-term risk of first recurrent stroke in the Perth community stroke study. Stroke 1998;29:2491.
9. Gorelick PB, Sacco RL, Smight DB, et al. Prevention of a first stroke: a review of the guidelines and a muldisciplinary consensus statement from the National Stroke Association. JAMA 1999;281:1112.
10. Straus SE, Majumdar SR, McAlister FA. New evidence for stroke prevention: scientific review. JAMA 2002;288:1388.
11. Hypertension Detection and Follow-Up Program Cooperative Group: five-year findings of the Hypertension Detection and Follow-up Program. III. Reduction in stroke incidence among persons with high blood pressure. JAMA 1982;247:633.
12. Dohlof B, Lindholm LH, Hansson L, et al. Morbidity and mortality in the Swedish Trial in Old Patients with Hypertension (STOP-Hypertension). Lancet 1991;338:1281.
13. SHEP Cooperative Research Group. Prevention of stroke by antihypertensive drug treatment in older persons with isolated systolic hypertension: final results of the Systolic Hypertension in the Elderly Program (SHEP). JAMA 1991;265:3255.
14. Randomized double-blind comparison of placebo and active treatment for older patients with isolated systolic hypertension: the Systolic Hypertension in Europe Investigators. Lancet 1997;350;757.
15. PROGRESS Collaborative Group. Randomised trial of perinopril-based blood pressure lowering regiment among 6,105 indivuduals with previous stroke or transient ischemic attack. Lancet 2001;358:1033.
16. Heart Outcomes Prevention Evaluation Study Investigators. Effects of ramipril on cardiovascular and microvascular outcomes in people with diabetes mellitus: results of the HOPE study and MICRO-HOPE substudy. Lancet 2000;355:253.
17. MacMahon S, Peto R, Cutler J, et al. Blood pressure, stroke, and coronary heart disease, I: prolonged differences in blood pressure: prospective observational studies corrected for the regression dilution bias. Lancet 1990;335:765.
18. Aram V. Chobanian MD, George L. Bakris et al. The seventh report of the Joint National Committee on Prevention Detection and Evaluation of High Blood Pressure. JNC 7 report. JAMA 2003;289:2560.
19. Wright JT Jr., Dunn JK, Cutler JA, et al. Outcomes in hypertensive black and nonblack patients treated with chlorthalidone, amlodipine, and lisinopril. JAMA 2005;293:1595.
20. Byington RP, Davis BR, White HD, et al. Reduction of stroke events with pravastatin: the Prospective Pravastatin Poolin (PPP) Project. Circulation 2001;103:387.
21. UK Prospective Diabetes Study (UKPDS) Group. Intensive blood-glucose control with sulphonylureas or insulin compared with conventional treatment and risk of complications in patients with type 2 diabetes (UKPDS 33). Lancet 1998;352:837.
22. Stevens RJ, Coleman RL, Adler AI, et al. Risk factors for myocardial infarction case fatality and stroke case fatality in type 2 diabetes: UKPDS 66. Diabetes Care 2004;27:201.
23. UK Prospective Diabetes Study (UKPDS) Group. Effect of intensive blood-glucose control with metformin on complications in overweight patients with type 2 diabetes (UKPDS 34). Lancet 1998;352:854.
24. Saenz A, Fernandez-Esteban I, Mataix A, et al. Metformin monotherapy for type 2 diabetes mellitus. Cochrane Database System Rev 2005;3:CD002966.
25. Caplan LR. Stroke: a clinical approach. Boston: Butterworth-Heinemann, 1993.
26. Whisnant JP, Homer D, Ingall TJ. Duration of cigarette smoking is the strongest predictor of severe extracranial carotid artery atherosclerosis. Stroke 1990;21:707.
27. Dagenais GE, Yi Q, Lonn E, et al. HOPE Trial Investigators. Impact of cigarette smoking in high-risk patients participating in a clinical trial. A substudy from the Heart Outcomes Prevention Evaluation (HOPE) trial. Eur J Cardiovasc Prev Rehabil 2005;12:75.
28. (No authors listed). Risk factors for stroke and efficacy of antithrombotic therapy in atrial fibrillation. Analysis of pooled data from five randomized controlled trials. Arch Int Med 1994;154:1449.
29. Fuster V, Ryden LE, Asinger RW, et al. ACC/AHA/ESC guidelines for the management of patients with atrial fibrillation. A report of the American College of Cardiology/American Heart Association Task Force on Practice Guidelines and the ESC Committee for Practice Guidelines and Policy [trunc]. Eur Heart J 2001;22:1852.
30. Singer DE, Albers GW, Dalen JE, et al. Antithrombotic therapy in atrial fibrillation: the Seventh ACCP Conference on Antithrombotic and Thrombolytic Therapy. Chest 2004;126:429S.
31. Paganini-Hill A. Estrogen replacement therapy and stroke. Prog Cardiovasc Dis 1995;38:223.
32. The Women's Health Initiative Steering Committee. Effects of conjugated equine estrogen in postmenopausal women with hysterectomy: the Women's Health Initiative randomized controlled trial. JAMA 2004;291:1701.
33. Heyman A, Wilkinson WE, Heyden S, et al. Risk of stroke in asymptomatic persons with cervical arterial bruits: a population study in Evans County, Georgia. N Engl J Med 1980;302:838.
34. Executive Committee for the Asymptomatic Carotid Atherosclerosis Study. Endarterectomy for asymptomatic carotid artery stenosis. JAMA 1995;273:1421.
35. Fisher CM. Lacunar strokes and infarcts: a review. Neurology 1982;32:871.
36. Feinberg W, Coull B. Coagulopathies and stroke. In: Welch KMA, Caplan LR, Reis DJ, et al., eds. Primer on cerebrovascular diseases. New York: Academic Press, 1997.
37. Blakely DD, Oddone EZ, Hasselblad V, et al. Noninvasive carotid artery testing. A meta-analytic review. Ann Intern Med 1995;122:360.
38. Carter AB. Hypertensive therapy in stroke survivors. Lancet 1970;1:485.
39. Gueyffier F, Boissel JP, Boutitie F, et al. Effect of antihypertensive treatment in patients already suffered from stroke. Gathering the evidence. The Indana (Individual Data Analysis of Antihypertensive Intervention trials) Project Collaborators. Stroke 1997;28:2557.
40. Progress Collaborative Group. Randomized trial of a perin- dopril-based blood-pressure-lowering regimen among 6105 individuals with previous stroke or transient ischemic attack. Lancet 2001;358:1033.
41. Rashid P, Leonardi-Bee J, Bath P. Blood pressure reduction and secondary prevention of stroke and other vascular events: a systematic review. Stroke 2003;34:2741.
42. Diener HC, Cunha L, Forbes C, et al. European Stroke Prevention Study. 2. Dipyridamole and

*Bold numerals denote published controlled clinical trials, meta-analyses, or consensus-based recommendations.

acetylsalicylic acid in the secondary prevention of stroke. J Neurol Sci 1996;143:1.
43. Hass WK, Easton JD, Adams HP. A randomized trial comparing ticlopidine hydrochloride with aspirin for the prevention of stroke in high-risk patients. N Engl J Med 1989;321: 501.
44. CAPRIE Steering Committee. A randomized, blinded, trial of clopidogrel versus aspirin in patients at risk of ischemic events (CAPRIE). Lancet 1996;348:1329.
45. MATCH Investigators. Aspirin and clopidogrel compared with clopidogrel alone after recent ischaemic stroke or transient ischaemic attack in high-risk patients (MATCH): randomised, double-blind, placebo-controlled trial. Lancet 2004;364:331.
46. Johnson ES, Lanes SF, Wentworth CE 3rd, et al. A meta-regression analysis of the dose-response effect of aspirin on stroke. Arch Intern Med 1999;159:1248.
47. Mohr JP, Thompson JL, Lazar RM, et al. A comparison of Warfarin and aspirin for the prevention of recurrent ischemic stroke. N Engl J Med 2001;345:1444.
48. Warfarin-Aspirin Symptomatic Intracranial Disease Trial Investigators. WASID Comparison of Warfarin and Aspirin for Symptomatic Intracranial Arterial Stenosis. N Engl J Med 2005;352:1305.
49. Sirol M, Bouzamondo A, Sanchez P, et al. Does statin therapy reduce the risk of stroke? A meta-analysis. Ann Med Intern 2001;152:188.
50. North American Symptomatic Carotid Endarterectomy Trial Collaborators (NASCET). Beneficial effect of carotid endarter- ectomy in symptomatic patients with high-grade carotid stenosis. N Engl J Med 1991;325:445.
51. Barnett HJ, Taylor DW, Eliasziw M, et al. Benefit of carotid endarterectomy in patients with symptomatic moderate or severe stenosis. North American Symptomatic Carotid Endarterectomy Trial Collaborators. N Engl J Med 1998;339:1415.
52. Anticoagulants for atrial fibrillation [Commentary]. Lancet 1993;342:1251.
53. Gresham GE, Fitzpatrick TE, Wolf PA, et al. Residual disability in survivors of stroke: the Framingham study. N Engl J Med 1975;293: 954.
54. Katz S, Ford AB, Chinn AB, et al. Prognosis after strokes. II. Long-term course of 159 patients. Medicine 1966;45:236.
55. Matsumoto N, Whisnant JP, Kurland LT, et al. Natural history of stroke in Rochester, Minnensota, 1955 through 1969: an extension of a previous study, 1945 through 1954. Stroke 1973;4:20.
56. Feibel JH, Berk S, Joynt RJ. The unmet needs of stroke survivors. Neurology 1979;29:592.
57. Robinson RG, Starr LB, Lipsey JR, et al. A two-year longitudinal study of post-stroke mood disorders: dynamic changes in associated variables over the first six months of follow-up. Stroke 1984;15:510.
58. Eisenberg H, Morrison JT, Sullivan P, et al. Cerebrovascular accidents: incidence and survival rates in a defined population. Middlesex County, Connecticut. JAMA 1964;189:883.
59. Gainotti G. Emotional behavior and hemispheric side of the lesion. Cortex 1972;8:41.
60. Lesser RP, Lauders H, Dinner DS, et al. Epileptic seizures due to thrombotic and embolic cerebrovascular disease in older patients. Epilepsia 1985;26:622.

For annotated ***General References*** *and resources related to this chapter, visit www.hopkinsbayview.org/PAMreferences.*

Chapter 92

Peripheral Neuropathy

*Michael J. Polydefkis**

*In previous editions, Gary J. Romano, MD, PhD, and Ralph Kuncl, MD, PhD, contributed to this chapter.

DEFINITIONS AND PATHOPHYSIOLOGY

Peripheral neuropathies result from disease processes that involve the peripheral nervous system. The peripheral nervous system includes cranial nerves III through XII, dorsal and ventral spinal roots, dorsal root ganglia, spinal nerves, and most autonomic ganglia and nerves.

Peripheral nerves consist of a bundle of fibers called *axons;* the large- and medium-sized axons are normally covered with a layer of myelin. Most peripheral nerves are mixed nerves that carry both incoming sensory information (afferent fibers) and outgoing motor and autonomic impulses (efferent fibers). Large-diameter afferent fibers convey information about position and vibration; large-diameter efferent fibers innervate the muscles themselves. Small-diameter, often unmyelinated fibers convey pain and temperature sensation and autonomic information.

Based on the primary site of involvement of the peripheral nerves, peripheral neuropathies can be classified into three categories: neuronopathies, axonopathies, and melanopathies. *Neuronopathies* result from processes affecting primarily the sensory cell bodies in the dorsal root ganglia or motor neuron cell bodies in the spinal cord. By convention, because motor neuron cell bodies are in the central nervous system (CNS), motor neuronopathies are not usually classified among the peripheral neuropathies. *Axonal neuropathies* result from processes affecting primarily the axon, whereas *myelinopathies* (also called demyelinating neuropathies) result from processes affecting primarily the myelin sheath. In some chronic disorders such as diabetes mellitus (DM), irrespective of the primary pathologic process, the interdependence between axon and myelin produces secondary changes that, on biopsy, reveal a mixed pathologic picture. The etiologic diagnosis of peripheral neuropathies, therefore, depends on both the clinical features and the supportive laboratory and pathologic findings.

Three major anatomic patterns of peripheral nerve disease may be distinguished by clinical presentation: mononeuropathy, mononeuropathy multiplex (multifocal neuropathies), and polyneuropathy. *Mononeuropathies* are lesions of individual nerve roots or peripheral nerves; they usually are because of local causes such as trauma or entrapment (compression of a nerve by adjacent structures). *Mononeuropathy multiplex* refers to involvement of two or more named nerves, usually asymmetrically and not contiguously, either at the same time or sequentially. This less common pattern is usually caused by systemic diseases such as the necrotizing vasculitides (e.g., polyarteritis nodosa) or DM, which may affect several nerves focally. *Polyneuropathy* is the result of a generalized disease process affecting many peripheral nerves, often in a symmetric distribution.

In both axonal and demyelinating diseases, the longer larger nerves are generally involved earlier and more severely than the shorter nerves. In demyelinating neuropathies, this vulnerability of the longer axons may reflect the increased number of potential sites for demyelination; in axonal neuropathies, the longer axons require more metabolic support and therefore may be more susceptible to disruption of this support. In axonal neuropathies, the distal ends of the nerve fibers—those that project to the feet—tend to be affected first producing a stocking pattern of involvement. Subsequently, the distal upper extremities become involved in a "glove" pattern. Demyelinating neuropathies generally begin in the lower extremities but can have a more patchy pattern of involvement. Most polyneuropathies indiscriminately affect both the sensory and the motor nerve fibers (mixed polyneuropathies or sensorimotor neuropathies); some affect peripheral autonomic nerves. However, clinically (and occasionally pathologically) in some patients there is a predilection for the sensory nerves (sensory neuropathies), motor nerves (motor neuropathies), or autonomic nerves.

APPROACH TO THE PATIENT

History and Physical Examination

Symptoms of peripheral neuropathy include reduced sensitivity to stimuli (hypesthesia); spontaneous unusual sensations such as tingling, burning, or pain (paresthesias or dysesthesias); weakness; and muscle cramps. If autonomic nerves are involved, impotence, urinary retention or overflow incontinence, constipation or diarrhea, diminished sweating, and orthostatic hypotension are common symptoms. In patients with polyneuropathy, paresthesias in the feet are the most common presenting complaint. Often, patients are bothered by nonnoxious sensory stimuli such as light touch perceived as pain (allodynia) and may report that symptoms of restless legs syndrome that are relieved by pacing the floor or by firm massage. Complaints of heaviness or coldness of the extremities are also common. Diminished joint position sense (proprioception) may be reported as unsteady gait, particularly on uneven surfaces or in the dark.

The *major signs of peripheral neuropathy* are sensory loss, weakness, muscle atrophy, diminished or absent tendon reflexes, and, if autonomic nerves are involved, trophic changes in the skin. The most common sensory modalities affected in polyneuropathy are pain and vibration, in a symmetric stocking–glove distribution. Thermal sensation is usually affected, but this is harder to document in the clinical setting. In polyneuropathies the weakness is most often distal, affecting the intrinsic muscles of the feet (e.g., inability to spread or extend the toes). In long-standing and inherited neuropathies the muscle imbalance causes high arched feet and hammer toes. Eventually, the shin may appear prominent because of atrophy of the tibialis anterior muscle (sharp shin sign), and there may be striking wasting of the small muscles of the hand. Marked loss of proprioception in the feet may be manifest as unsteadiness, ataxia, or a positive Romberg test (see Chapter 86 for additional details about neurologic signs).

Causes and Distinctive Features

Whereas a limited number of conditions produce mononeuropathy and mononeuropathy multiplex (Table 92.1), there are many causes of polyneuropathy (Table 92.2). Diagnosis often depends on obtaining a thorough history (e.g., of alcoholism or of occupational exposure to toxins) or finding a relevant systemic condition (e.g., DM). Table 92.3 lists the three features most useful in the differential diagnosis of a polyneuropathy—time course, selective functional involvement, and distribution—and the causes associated with these features.

Time Course

Mononeuropathies are often acute in onset; that is, the patient remembers the time of onset. The most common of the acute polyneuropathies, the Guillain-Barré syndrome, and other processes—metabolic, vasculitic, or toxic—may cause rapid onset of severe neurologic dysfunction, sometimes within hours. Most toxic neuropathies (e.g., lead poisoning) develop more slowly (within weeks), as do neuropathies associated with malnutrition (e.g., thiamine deficiency). The most common of the chronic neuropathies

TABLE 92.1 Common Causes of Mononeuropathy and Mononeuropathy Multiplex

Mononeuropathy
Trauma: direct (occupational, recreational, e.g., ulnar or peroneal nerve), compression, and entrapment (e.g., carpal tunnel, root compression)
Infection: herpes zoster
Vascular: vasculitis, DM
Neoplasm: neurofibroma, lymphoma
Mononeuropathy multiplex
DM
Vasculitis

DM, diabetes mellitus.

TABLE 92.2 Polyneuropathy: Causes and Modes of Predominant Involvement

	Predominant Nerve Type Involvement
Metabolic	
Diabetes mellitus	
Polyneuropathy	S, SM, A
Mononeuropathy	SM
Lumbar plexopathy (diabetic amyotrophy)	M > S
Alcohol with vitamin deficiency	SM
Uremia	SM
Porphyria	M > S
B_{12} deficiency	S > M
Toxic (see Table 92.5)	
Lead	M > S
Pyridoxine	S
cis-Platinum	S
Most other drugs and toxic agents	SM
Infectious	
Diphtheria	M
Leprosy	S
Lyme disease	SM
Human immunodeficiency virus	S, SM, M
Inflammatory and collagen–vascular	
Guillain-Barré syndrome	M
Chronic inflammatory demyelinating polyneuropathy	M
Noncarcinomatous sensory neuropathy (e.g., Sjögren)	S
Systemic lupus erythematosus	SM
Polyarteritis nodosa	SM
Sjögren syndrome	SM, S
Rheumatoid arthritis	SM
Neoplastic	
Carcinomatous	S, SM
Paraproteinemia, plasma cell dyscrasias	S, SM, A
Benign monoclonal gammopathy	S, SM
Waldenstrom macroglobulinemia	SM, M
Cryoglobulinemia	SM
Hereditary	
Hereditary motor and sensory neuropathies	M > S
Amyloidosis	S > M, A
Dysautonomia (Riley-Day)	S, A
Tomaculous neuropathy	SM
Tangier (Bassen-Kornzweig)	S
Fabry	S

A, autonomic; M, motor; S, sensory.

in the United States (gradual progression over months to years) are associated with DM (see Chapter 79) and alcoholism (see below). Neuropathies related to infections such as leprosy or HIV also tend to be chronic in nature.

Patients with *hereditary neuropathies* sometimes may be unaware that they have a long-standing progressive disorder. A history of a lack of athletic ability in school or problems fitting shoes may be useful clues. Irreducibly high-arched feet and hammer toes reflect long-standing disease occurring during foot development and may therefore suggest a hereditary process.

Selective Functional Involvement

Mononeuropathy usually produces both motor and sensory involvement in the distribution of the affected nerve root or peripheral nerve. Most *polyneuropathies* produce both sensory and motor disturbances. Polyneuropathy with *predominantly sensory involvement* suggests DM, carcinoma, amyloidosis, and dysproteinemia. Occasionally, sensory losses are dissociated, that is, the patient has diminished pain and temperature sensation but preserved vibration and joint position sense; this pattern is typical of small fiber neuropathies. In diabetes, it is not unusual for the neuropathy to start as a small fiber predominant process that then progresses to involve large fiber sensory and then motor nerves. When position and vibratory sense are lost but pain sense is preserved, vitamin B_{12} deficiency (usually pernicious anemia) or, much more rarely, Friedreich ataxia should be considered. In polyneuropathy, *predominantly motor involvement* suggests inflammatory demyelinating neuropathy, hereditary neuropathies, lead intoxication, or acute intermittent porphyria. *Predominantly autonomic involvement* suggests DM, amyloidosis, familial dysautonomia, or dysproteinemia.

INVESTIGATIONS

Clinical Laboratory

The cause of a peripheral neuropathy must be identified because often neurologic dysfunction persists unless the underlying disease can be treated. The common causes of polyneuropathy (shown in italics in Table 92.3) may be obvious to a patient's physician, but sometimes even these require direct questioning (e.g., concerning alcoholism) or specific laboratory tests (e.g., oral glucose tolerance testing) before they are appreciated. If the cause of the neuropathy is not obvious, one should consider the following *screening tests* that may point to a cause: erythrocyte sedimentation rate, fasting blood glucose level, oral glucose tolerance testing, serum creatinine concentration, a complete blood count, serum B_{12} level, a chest radiograph, and a serum and urine immunofixation electrophoresis. Many unusual conditions may be associated with neuropathy,

TABLE 92.3 Polyneuropathy: Differential Diagnosis

- Time course
  - Acute (days)
    - *Guillain-Barré syndrome*
    - Porphyric neuropathy
    - Vasculitic neuropathy
    - Some toxins (e.g., triorthocresyl phosphate)
  - Subacute (weeks)
    - *Many toxins and drugs* (see Table 92.5)
    - *Nutritional neuropathies*
    - Carcinomatous neuropathies
    - Diabetic amyotrophy
    - Uremic neuropathy
  - Relapsing
    - Chronic inflammatory demyelinating polyneuropathy
    - Refsum disease
    - Porphyria
  - Chronic (many months or years)
    - *Diabetic motor and sensory neuropathy*
    - *Alcoholic neuropathy*
    - Chronic inflammatory demyelinating polyneuropathy
  - Very chronic (childhood onset)
    - Hereditary, motor and sensory neuropathies (e.g., Charcot-Marie-Tooth disease)
- Selective functional involvement[a]
  - Predominantly motor
    - Guillain-Barré syndrome
    - Chronic inflammatory demyelinating polyneuropathy
    - Acute intermittent porphyria
    - Lead neuropathy
    - Hereditary motor and sensory neuropathies (e.g., Charcot-Marie-Tooth)
    - Diphtheritic neuropathy
  - Predominately sensory
    - Global sensory loss
      - *Diabetes mellitus*
      - Carcinomatous sensory neuropathy (ganglioradiculitis)
      - Paraproteinemic and cryoglobulinemic neuropathy
      - Tabes dorsalis
  - Dissociated loss of pain and thermal sensibility
    - Diabetes, Impaired Glucose Tolerance (small fiber type)
    - Amyloidosis
    - Hereditary sensory neuropathies
    - Lepromatous leprosy
  - Dissociated loss of joint position and vibration sensibility
    - Subacute combined degeneration
    - Friedreich ataxia
  - Autonomic neuropathy
    - *Diabetes*
    - *Amyloid*
    - Acute, chronic, and relapsing pandysautonomia
    - Dysautonomia (Riley-Day)
- Distribution[b]
  - Proximal weakness
    - Guillain-Barré syndrome
    - Porphyria
    - Diabetic amyotrophy
    - Carcinomatous neuropathy with proximal weakness ("carcinomatous neuromyopathy")
  - Proximal sensory loss
    - Porphyria
    - Tangier disease (analphalipoproteinemia)
  - Temperature-related distribution
    - Lepromatous leprosy

The most common causes are set in Italic.
[a]Most polyneuropathies produce sensory and motor disturbances.
[b]Most polyneuropathies produce distal involvement.
Modified from Griffin JW, Cornblath DR. Peripheral neuropathies. In: Harvey AM, et al., eds. Principles and practice of medicine. 22nd ed. New York: Appleton & Lange, 1988.

but an extensive screening program to rule out all these processes would be expensive and almost always unrewarding unless there is some clue in the history or physical examination to warrant a particular test (e.g., measurement of blood lead levels in a patient with a possible history of occupational exposure). If no cause of the process is identified on evaluation, consultation with a neurologist should be considered.

Nerve Conduction Studies

The measurement of nerve conduction is useful as an *initial diagnostic screen* because it can distinguish major categories of disease (axonal versus demyelinating) and can localize entrapments and other mononeuropathies. A baseline measurement makes it possible to differentiate progression of the peripheral neuropathy from other clinical conditions in the future.

Nerve conduction measurements involve stimulating a nerve at one point and recording the response, either at the muscle (motor nerve) or at some distance along the nerve (sensory nerve). The results of nerve conduction studies usually include latency of response, conduction velocity, and amplitude of response. The *latency of response* refers to the time elapsed between the start of the stimulus and the muscle response (muscle fiber depolarization) or nerve response (sensory nerve action potential). The *conduction velocity* between two points along the nerve is expressed in meters per second.

Conduction disturbances of the peripheral nerve may be localized, as in an entrapment syndrome, or may involve nerves more diffusely, as in polyneuropathies. Generally, early axonal degenerations are associated with normal conduction and the presence of denervation on electromyography (see Electromyography), whereas early demyelination is characterized by slowing of nerve conduction and normal EMG studies. Nerve conduction velocities are normal, and sensory nerve action potentials are spared in cervical or lumbar disk disease with radiculopathy, because the potential site of nerve root compression at the neural foramina is proximal to the sensory cell body in the ganglion and therefore does not cause degeneration of the distal sensory nerve fiber. This is an important point because spondylitic radiculopathy is common and may mimic polyneuropathy (see Chapters 70 and 71).

The procedure has several *limitations*. First, nerve conduction studies test directly only the portion of the nerve between the stimulating and recording electrodes; they generally do not detect damage more distal than (e.g., intramuscular nerve) or more proximal to (e.g., nerve root) the segment tested. Long latency responses such as F waves or H reflexes can provide information about conduction over long segments of nerve, including proximal nerve segments. Second, electrophysiologic studies reflect the function of a subset of peripheral nerve fibers, namely the largest and fastest conducting fibers. Therefore, a patient with a selective small fiber neuropathy can test normally on nerve conduction studies.

Patient Experience. With the patient comfortably positioned, surface electrodes are placed over the nerves and muscles to be tested. Nerves are stimulated with shocks applied to the skin. The shocks are mildly unpleasant. Nerves on both sides of the body may be compared. Testing takes approximately 20 to 60 minutes.

Electromyography

EMG involves the insertion of a needle electrode into a muscle to record muscle electrical activity. By observing muscle activity at rest (spontaneous discharges) and during muscle contraction (volitional activity), much can be inferred about the integrity of motor nerves and the muscle itself.

Spontaneous *fibrillation potentials* are the action potentials of single myofibers that are twitching spontaneously. Fibrillation potentials and positive waves are usually, but not invariably, a good indication of denervation (they also occur in polymyositis and more rarely in other myopathic processes). *Fasciculations* are the spontaneous firings of whole motor units (all the muscle fibers innervated by a single motor neuron and its branches). Fasciculations may be seen in normal subjects, although they are more frequent and likely to be more polyphasic in states of denervation.

Voluntary motor unit potentials are examined individually by asking the patient to contract a given muscle slightly. Long-duration, large-amplitude, polyphasic potentials suggest a denervating process with subsequent reinnervation through axonal sprouting. Brief, small-amplitude, polyphasic potentials are associated with myopathic processes. Graded increasing effort is used to analyze the orderly recruitment of motor unit potentials, including their number and firing rates. Recruitment of a reduced repertoire of large-amplitude motor unit potentials firing at rapid rates is indicative of denervation and reinnervation. Early recruitment of numerous brief small-amplitude motor unit potentials indicates a myopathic process.

One important use of EMG is to detect denervation in muscles that are clinically of normal strength. Because of the process of collateral reinnervation, significant numbers of motor axons may be lost before clinical muscle weakness is detectable. For example, in a slowly progressive chronic entrapment neuropathy such as carpal tunnel syndrome (CTS), more than 50% of the motor axons may be lost before thenar muscles become weak. By revealing such denervation changes, EMG studies help the clinician to determine the severity of the lesion and make informed decisions about prognosis and management. The EMG can also recognize denervation in muscles that are difficult to assess on physical examination. Another use of EMG is to help define entrapment neuropathies (e.g., radial nerve entrapment) and differentiate these from more proximal radicular compression (e.g., apparent carpal tunnel syndrome that is actually caused by C6 radiculopathy: normal nerve conduction velocity [NCV] for the median nerve with abnormal EMG reflecting nerve root pathology). EMG can also help differentiate the muscle wasting of neuropathic or myopathic disorders from disuse atrophy. Table 92.4 summarizes the changes found in denervation and myopathic conditions.

TABLE 92.4 Electromyography: Patterns Typical of Nerve and Muscle Disorders

Disorder	Insertional Activity	Complete Rest (Spontaneous Activity)	Motor Unit Potentials	Recruitment
Neuropathic[a]	Increased	Fibrillations, positive sharp waves, fasciculations	Long duration, high amplitude, polyphasic	Reduced
Myopathic				
Myopathy	Normal	Normal or rare fibrillations	Brief duration, small amplitude, polyphasic	Early
Myositis	Increased	Fibrillations, positive sharp waves	Brief duration, small amplitude, polyphasic	Early

[a]Neuropathy or radiculopathy.

The EMG electrodes mildly inflame the muscles into which they have been inserted though the serum creatine phosphokinase activity is rarely altered by this procedure. Thus, if a muscle biopsy is being considered, EMG should not be performed in the muscle to be biopsied.

Patient Experience. There is usually discomfort with the initial insertion of the recording needles and during movement of the muscles when the needles are in place. Because the needles are very thin and penetrate only skin and muscle, the risks of infection or hemorrhage are almost nil. The procedure takes 30 to 60 minutes.

Nerve Biopsy

Nerve biopsy is a useful last step that should be reserved for patients in whom a specific histologic diagnosis and a management decision that may help the patient are possible (e.g., amyloidosis, demyelination, inflammation, or necrotizing vasculitis). Its use should be guided by the history and electrophysiology. The nerve studied by biopsy is almost always a sensory nerve (the sural) and sometimes may not reflect a disease process that appears to affect only the motor nerves. The biopsy always leads to a fixed numbness in the distribution of the excised nerve (usually the sural distribution on the lateral heel and ankle) but rarely may lead to painful sequelae such as neuroma formation. If a nerve biopsy is done, it should be done at a center where it is performed frequently, where plastic embedded nerve histopathology and electron microscopy are routinely available, and where a pathologist with special expertise in nerve morphology can interpret it, so that maximum information can result from this invasive procedure. Consultation with a neurologist is helpful in determining whether a nerve biopsy is indicated.

Skin Biopsy

The advent of skin biopsy as a diagnostic and research tool has provided an attractive option to the assessment of small caliber unmyelinated sensory nerve fibers. These fibers have historically been difficult to measure as they are not assessed by conventional nerve conduction testing (1). Skin biopsies are well tolerated, relatively noninvasive and can be used to pathologically sample nerve at different locations repeatedly over time. Epidermal nerve fibers are unmyelinated C fiber nociceptors and are typically affected early in the course of sensory neuropathies before large fiber involvement is apparent (2,3). As a result, the skin biopsy technique has become a useful diagnostic tool for small fiber neuropathies in patients who present with distal dysesthesias and normal nerve conduction test results (4). The technique has recently also been adapted to investigate the myelinated nerve fibers within the deep dermis providing insight into demyelinating and inherited neuropathies (5).

Patient Experience. Biopsy sites are numbed with subcutaneous 2% lidocaine producing transient burning. 3 mm punch skin biopsies are performed under sterile conditions using a circular knife identical to ones used for routine dermatologic biopsies. Hemostasis is achieved through local pressure without the need for suture placement—the exception being patients with international normalized ratio (INR) values greater than 2.5. The sites heal by a process of granulation most often with little or no scar formation. People with darkly pigmented skin or those with a predilection to keloid formation can have more prominent scarring. The procedure takes 15 minutes.

SPECIFIC CAUSES

Diabetic Neuropathy

Diabetic neuropathy is one of the most common neuropathies seen in primary care settings (6,7). The diabetic polyneuropathies have protean manifestations. They may present as a symmetric polyneuropathy or as a focal neuropathy. The former include sensory or sensorimotor polyneuropathy and autonomic polyneuropathy. The focal neuropathic syndromes include asymmetric lower limb mononeuropathy (diabetic amyotrophy), mononeuropathy multiplex, cranial neuropathy, entrapment neuropathies, and isolated trunk radiculopathies. Chapter 79 discusses the problem in detail (see Femoral Neuropathy).

Alcoholic Neuropathy

The neuropathy associated with alcoholism and related vitamin deficiencies is a sensorimotor axonal polyneuropathy (8). The presenting symptoms are often pain and paresthesias in the feet and legs though many patients are asymptomatic. Examination often shows diminished ankle jerks and a stocking–glove pattern of decreased sensation to all modalities. Autonomic features, including impotence, bladder dysfunction, and orthostatic hypotension, may rarely be seen. Electrodiagnostic studies commonly reveal reduced amplitudes of the sural sensory nerve action potentials and abnormal H reflexes. Sural nerve sections show primary axonal degeneration. Malnutrition and vitamin deficiencies (particularly thiamine deficiency) probably make a major contribution to the neuropathy, although there is evidence that alcohol has a direct toxic effect on peripheral nerves.

Treatment is aimed toward improved nutrition and vitamin replacement and effective treatment for the alcoholism (see Chapter 28). The paresthesias can improve with treatment in the setting of mild disease but often persist in cases with moderate to severe neuropathy.

Carcinomatous Neuropathies

The most common form of neuropathy associated with malignancies is a distal sensorimotor polyneuropathy. Compression or infiltration of nerves by tumor or a pure sensory neuronopathy occurs less commonly. Both the distal sensorimotor neuropathy and pure sensory neuronopathy are most often associated with carcinoma of the lung, and the onset of the neuropathic symptoms can either precede, follow, or coincide with the diagnosis of the malignancy (9,10).

Distal Sensorimotor Neuropathy

Distal sensorimotor neuropathy is primarily an axonal process with sensory loss and weakness appearing initially in the feet. It is more common in men, develops over weeks or months, and is generally progressive in its course. If the underlying cancer responds to treatment, the neuropathy may improve.

Carcinomatous Sensory Neuropathy

Carcinomatous sensory neuropathy has a distinctive pattern beginning subacutely, often with pain and paresthesias involving legs, arms, or, rarely, the face. Over many weeks a profound proprioceptive sensory loss develops, accompanied by pseudoathetosis (seemingly purposeless movements caused by loss of position sense). Areflexia is common. The patient may be unable to stand or walk unassisted despite normal strength. Nerve conduction studies may show reduced or unobtainable sensory potentials. It occurs more typically in women (9). The underlying tumor is most often small cell carcinoma of the lung, but this neuropathy also may accompany breast, ovarian, uterine, and gastrointestinal tract tumors. The neuropathy is usually progressive. Common chemotherapeutic agents including *cis*-platinum and oxaliplatin can produce a similar picture.

Paraneoplastic Vasculitis of Nerve and Muscle

This disorder is a nonsystemic vasculitic neuropathy that usually affects older men, has a subacute onset, and is progressive. It may present as a painful symmetric or asymmetric sensorimotor polyneuropathy or, less commonly, as a mononeuritis multiplex. The tumors most frequently involved are lymphoma and small-cell lung cancer. Electrodiagnostic studies reveal axonal degeneration affecting motor and sensory fibers. The erythrocyte sedimentation rate may be elevated, and the cerebrospinal fluid protein content is increased. Nerve biopsy reveals intramural and perivascular infiltrates without a necrotizing vasculitis. Muscle is often involved as well. It may respond to treatment of the tumor or to immunosuppression (11,12).

Paraproteinemic Neuropathies

An association between peripheral neuropathies and monoclonal gammopathies has been increasingly recognized. In patients with idiopathic peripheral neuropathy, a monoclonal gammopathy can be identified in nearly 10%. In half of these a plasma cell dyscrasia is diagnosed, whereas in the other half the monoclonal gammopathy is of undetermined significance and the relevance of the association with the neuropathy is unclear (13). In the event of a plasma cell dyscrasia, the treatment of the neuropathy is superceded by treatment of the tumor. The malignancies associated with monoclonal gammopathies include multiple myeloma, osteosclerotic myeloma, Waldenström macroglobulinemia, B-cell lymphoma, and chronic B-cell lymphocytic leukemia. Peripheral neuropathy may be the presenting symptom in plasma cell dyscrasias, such as in primary amyloidosis or the rare osteosclerotic form of myeloma. Patients with multiple myeloma may develop a mild distal sensorimotor neuropathy, a pure sensory neuropathy, or a subacute monophasic or relapsing and remitting neuropathy. Amyloid deposition may occur in these patients, usually causing a distal sensorimotor neuropathy, but may also present as CTS, multiple mononeuropathies, or autonomic dysfunction. Neuropathic symptoms typical in primary amyloidosis are prominent burning dysesthesias and autonomic dysfunction. Like the amyloidosis, the neuropathy generally does not respond to treatment.

Nearly 50% of patients with osteosclerotic myeloma have a neuropathy characterized as a symmetric, demyelinating, primarily motor neuropathy. All or some of the features of the POEMS (polyneuropathy, organomegaly, endocrinopathy, M protein, and skin changes) syndrome may be present (14). Although the course is usually one of steady progression, improvement in the neuropathy occurred in nearly 50% of patients in one series in response to successful treatment of osteosclerotic myeloma.

Five to ten percent of patients with Waldenström macroglobulinemia have a demyelinating sensorimotor polyneuropathy that predominantly affects large sensory fibers. Postural tremor and pseudoathetosis are common. Those patients with demyelinating neuropathy and immunoglobulin (Ig)M to myelin-associated protein (MAG) may respond to therapy with plasma exchange or intravenous Ig, but most require chemotherapy. In patients that are refractory to these treatments, high-dose Cytoxan therapy has provided encouraging results and is a growing focus of research protocols (15).

TABLE 92.5 Toxins and Drugs Associated with Peripheral Neuropathies

Industrial[a]
Pesticides: organophosphates, dichlorophenyoxyacetate (2,4-D), Vacor rodenticide
Metal work: lead, arsenic, mercury, thallium, methyl bromide
Plastics, synthetic fabrics: *n*-hexane, methyl, *n*-butyl ketone, acrylamide, carbon disulfide, perchloroethylene, trichloroethylene,dimethylaminoproprionitrile
Gases: carbon monoxide, ethylene oxide
Euphoriants
Glue sniffing: *n*-hexane, solvents
Nitrous oxide inhalation: whipped cream dispensers, dental offices
Pharmacotherapeutic agents
Antimicrobial: isoniazid, nitrofurantoin, metronidazole
Cardiovascular: hydralazine, procainamide, amiodarone
Other: phenytoin, colchicine, disulfiram, pyridoxine, vincristine, cis-platinum, taxol, thalidomide, pyridoxine (vitamin B_6)

[a]See also Chapter 8, Table 8.2.

Neuropathy Caused by Toxins and Drugs

Toxic neuropathies, including those caused by drugs, are becoming increasingly recognized. Toxic neuropathies are potentially reversible if the toxin can be identified and the exposure to the toxin eliminated. The diagnosis may be made easily if there is a history of drug exposure (e.g., colchicine, isoniazid, hydralazine, vincristine) or industrial exposure (Table 92.5). Because these neuropathies have no distinguishing features on routine history or physical examination, a detailed history of exposure to drugs and the patient's occupation and recreational habits is important. Axonal involvement in the spinal cord may also occur and be masked by the toxic neuropathy. In these cases, a residual spastic paraparesis becomes apparent when the peripheral neuropathy has resolved. Toxic neuropathies are classically associated with chronic low-dose exposure (months to years), although they may appear within days to weeks with high-level exposure. The syndrome of proximal muscle weakness and axonal polyneuropathy caused by colchicine may appear after the patient has taken this drug for years, usually because of elevated drug levels caused by altered renal function. A delayed neuropathy associated with organophosphates develops 10 to 14 days after exposure, whereas Vacor, a rodenticide, produces an acute toxic neuropathy within 2 to 3 days.

Toxicity caused by megadose pyridoxine (vitamin B_6) consumption produces a gradually progressive sensory ataxia with profound distal limb impairment of position and vibratory sense (16). General public acceptance of vitamin B_6 therapy makes direct questioning about vitamin habits necessary. Neuropathy has been reported in patients consuming dosages as low as 200 mg/day.

Patients with familial neuropathy, pre-existing peripheral neuropathy or prominent risk factors such as diabetes or uremia represent a vulnerable population and can experience rapid neuropathy progression in the setting of toxin exposure. This underscores the importance of investigating potential toxic exposures in patients with rapid neuropathy disease courses and not attributing it to a known diagnosis.

Human Immunodeficiency Virus Infection

There are many peripheral nervous system manifestations of human immunodeficiency virus (HIV) infection (17). A *painful sensory neuropathy*, usually confined to the feet, is the most common neurologic complication, affecting 30% of patients with the acquired immunodeficiency syndrome, and typically occurs in the setting of advanced infection. Often reduction in unmyelinated nerve fiber density is the most sensitive pathologic marker, though nerve conduction studies can show reduced or absent sensory potentials. Treatment is currently limited to symptomatic relief using tricyclic antidepressants such as amitriptyline (Elavil) or antiepileptic agents such as lamotrigene (Lamictal), gabapentin (Neurontin), or carbamazepine (Tegretol), described below.

Multiple *mononeuropathies* have been described, most often in HIV-infected patients who have not yet developed AIDS. Both acute Guillain-Barré syndrome (GBS) and chronic inflammatory demyelinating polyneuropathy (CIDP) have been seen, usually in the early stages of HIV infection, in otherwise asymptomatic seropositive patients. Treatment for these demyelinating conditions is generally identical to seronegative patients.

Progressive polyradiculopathy is a cytomegalovirus (CMV) infection-related syndrome that usually occurs late in the course of HIV disease and causes radiating pain and numbness in the low back and buttocks. This is typically followed by progressive flaccid paraparesis, lower extremity areflexia, sphincter dysfunction and occasionally, a thoracic sensory level. Urinary retention occurs in most patients. Cranial nerves and the upper extremities are rarely involved, though many patients have a history of CMV retinitis. The mortality rate is nearly 100% if untreated, with a very rapid and progressive course (measured in days). Cerebrospinal fluid (CSF) findings include a marked polymorphonuclear pleocytosis, and polymerase chain reaction (PCR) for CMV deoxyribonucleic acid (DNA) is highly sensitive and specific. Treatment with ganciclovir is effective if initiated early (18,19).

COMPRESSION AND ENTRAPMENT NEUROPATHIES

When a peripheral neurologic abnormality occurs in one upper or lower extremity, the abnormality is usually caused by nerve entrapment or compression caused by anatomic abnormalities or trauma, although polyneuropathy and

TABLE 92.6 Comparative Data on Root and Nerve Lesions in the Upper Extremity

Roots→	*C5*	*C6*	*C7*	*C8*	*T1*
Sensory loss[a,b]	Lateral upper arm	Dorsolateral forearm and thumb	Mid-dorsal forearm and middle finger	Medial forearm, ring and small fingers	Medial arm, axilla
Motor loss[b]	Deltoid, some biceps, infraspinatus and supraspinatus	Biceps, brachioradialis, some deltoid	Triceps, wrist and finger extensors	Thenar eminence and interossei of hand	Thenar eminence and interossei of hand
Tendon reflex	Biceps, brachioradialis	Biceps, brachioradialis	Triceps	Triceps, finger jerk	Finger jerk
Peripheral Nerves→	***Axillary***	***Musculocutaneous***	***Radial***	***Median (Carpal Tunnel)***	***Ulnar (Cubital Tunnel)***
Sensory loss	Over deltoid	Radial forearm	Dorsal lateral hand	First 3½ digits	4th and 5th digits
Motor loss	Deltoid	Biceps, brachialis	Triceps, wrist and finger extensors	Thenar: abductor pollicis brevis, opponens	Hypothenar: abductor digiti minimi, first dorsal interosseus
Tendon reflex	None	Biceps	Triceps, brachioradialis	Finger jerk	Finger jerk
Pain	Over deltoid	Lateral forearm	Dorsal lateral forearm and hand	Nocturnal in forearm, lateral hand, and first 3½ digits	4th and 5th digits and tenderness at elbow

[a]See dermatomal pattern, Fig. 86.2.
[b]Pain usually radiates from the neck to the distal area of sensory loss.

mononeuropathy multiplex may present initially as a focal deficit in one extremity. With clinical evaluation, it is usually possible to determine whether the patient's problem is caused by nerve root damage or damage to a peripheral nerve or one of its branches. Tables 92.6, 92.7, and 92.8 and Figures 92.1 and 92.2 summarize the information needed to make this distinction: distribution of sensory, motor, and reflex deficits; common causative factors; and critical anatomic relationships.

Several common compression and entrapment neuropathies and specific approaches to treatment are discussed here. Nerve conduction testing is needed to confirm the diagnosis, and distinguish between several possible conditions as well as to support the decision to recommend

TABLE 92.7 Comparative Data on Root and Nerve Lesions in the Lower Extremity

Roots→	*L2*	*L3*	*L4*	*L5*	*S1*
Sensory loss[a]	Upper and medial thigh	Anterior thigh	Lateral thigh to medial leg	Lateral leg to dorsum of foot	Posterior leg to plantar foot
Motor loss	Iliopsoas (hip flexion)	Quadriceps (knee extension), adductor	Quadriceps, tibialis anterior (dorsiflexion of foot)	Great toe extensor, tibialis anterior, tibialis posterior	Gastrocnemius, gluteus maximus (hip extension)
Tendon reflex	Adductor	Adductor, knee jerk	Knee jerk	Medial hamstring	Achilles
Peripheral Nerves→	***Obturator***	***Femoral***	***Lateral Femoral Cutaneous (Meralgia Paresthetica)***	***Sciatic Peroneal Division***	***Sciatic Tibial Division***
Sensory loss, pain area	Medial thigh	Anterior medial thigh	Upper lateral thigh usually to 10–12 inches below the iliac crest	Dorsum of foot and lateral leg	Plantar foot (with burning pain), tips of toes
Motor loss	Adductors	Quadriceps (knee extension)	N/A	Tibialis anterior (dorsiflexion of ankle), extensor digitorum brevis (toe extension)	Gastrocnemius
Tendon reflex	Adductor	Knee jerk	N/A	None	Achilles

[a]See dermatomal pattern, Fig. 86.2.

TABLE 92.8 Entrapment Neuropathies: Common Causative Factors

Nerve, Location	Causative Factors
Median	
At wrist	Meat processing, upholstering, knitting, painting, weight lifting, using vibrating tools, pregnancy, musical instruments
At forearm	Repeated pronation (e.g., screwdriver), weight lifting
Ulnar	
At wrist	Bicycling, leaning on a walker, using pliers, using palm as a hammer
At elbow	Injury to elbow, chronic flexion of elbow (e.g., sitting in wheelchair or lying in bed), leaning on elbow on tables and desks
Radial	
At forearm	Lipoma, tennis, trauma
At arm	Saturday night palsy, bridegroom's palsy, crutches, pneumatic tourniquets
Axillary	Fracture/dislocation of shoulder, deep injections into deltoid muscle
Musculocutaneous	Weight lifting, shoulder dislocations
Tibial	
At knee	Chronic, standing
At ankle	Trauma, weight gain, or edema
Peroneal	
At knee	Ankle sprains, crossed legs, after weight loss, squatting, kneeling
At ankle	Tight shoes, trauma
Femoral	Inguinal surgery, childbirth, psoas hemorrhage, dorsal lithotomy position
Lateral femoral cutaneous	Ascites, overweight, pregnancy, utility belts, blunt sports injury to anterior iliac spine
Obturator	Pelvic fracture, hip surgery, childbirth, retroperitoneal hematoma, malignancy
Sciatic	Hip surgery, pelvic fracture, injections, endometriosis, retroperitoneal hematoma, lipoma

surgery. People with diabetes are at increased risk of developing entrapment neuropathies and generally do not recover axonal loss to the degree that nondiabetic counterparts do. This has prompted some to argue for aggressive early diagnosis and treatment of entrapment neuropathies in people with diabetes—before significant axon loss occurs. Additional general aspects of prognosis and treatment are described in a later section (see Therapeutic Principles). Chapters 70 and 71 discuss root compression symptoms caused by cervical and lumbar spine disease.

Median Nerve (Carpal Tunnel Syndrome)

Causes

CTS is the most common of all the entrapment neuropathies. In CTS, symptoms and signs result from compression by neighboring anatomic structures on the median nerve as it passes from the forearm to the palm (Fig. 92.1). The median nerve and nine digital flexor tendons pass through the carpal tunnel, a rigid compartment formed by the concave arch of the carpal bones and roofed by the transverse carpal ligament. Conditions that cause a decrease in the size of the carpal tunnel (e.g., Colles fracture, rheumatoid arthritis, congenital carpal tunnel stenosis), enlargement of the median nerve (e.g., amyloid, neuroma, endoneural edema in DM), or increase in the volume of other structures within the tunnel (e.g., tenosynovitis, ganglion, lipoma, urate deposits in gout, hematoma, fluid retention in pregnancy) may all result in compression of the median nerve. CTS in the workplace is associated with occupations requiring wrist extension/flexion or hand force in all wrist positions (e.g., meat processing, fruit packing, upholstering, and waiting on tables). Median nerve compression can also be caused by sustained or repeated stress over the base of the palm, such as that caused by the use of hand-tools. Vibration exposure (low frequency, 10 to 40 Hz) is another well-recognized risk factor for CTS (typically from air-powered tools). Repetitive wrist and hand movements in activities such as knitting, crocheting, hooking rugs, playing a musical instrument, painting, woodworking, gardening, lifting weights, or typing when the keyboard is too high may also lead to CTS.

Manifestations and Evaluation

The onset of symptoms of CTS is usually insidious and nocturnal because of sustained posture of wrist flexion during sleep. Symptoms in the hand may initially be described as episodic tingling and numbness with gradual progression to more severe symptoms, such as burning, aching, or a painful numbness in the fingers and deep in the palm. The fingers are sometimes described as feeling swollen, even though little swelling is apparent on inspection. Many patients have accompanying dull aching pain in the forearm, sometimes reaching the shoulder, which can be confused with a C6 radiculopathy.

As CTS progresses, the nocturnal pain and tingling may wake the patient. Relief may be obtained by hanging the arm or shaking or rubbing the hand. Episodic tingling may develop during the day, but the associated pain in the arm occurs less often during the day than at night. Additionally, there can be a subjective feeling of weakness and clumsiness in the fingers with difficulty performing tasks such as unscrewing bottle tops, turning a key, or crocheting.

Objective changes in sensation and strength may appear in the hand, but some patients may have severe attacks of pain for years without developing neurologic signs. Sensory signs within the median nerve distribution (Table 92.6) precede motor signs and are most pronounced in the fingertips. Rarely, instead of decreased sensation, hyperesthesia in the median distribution may occur. Isolated

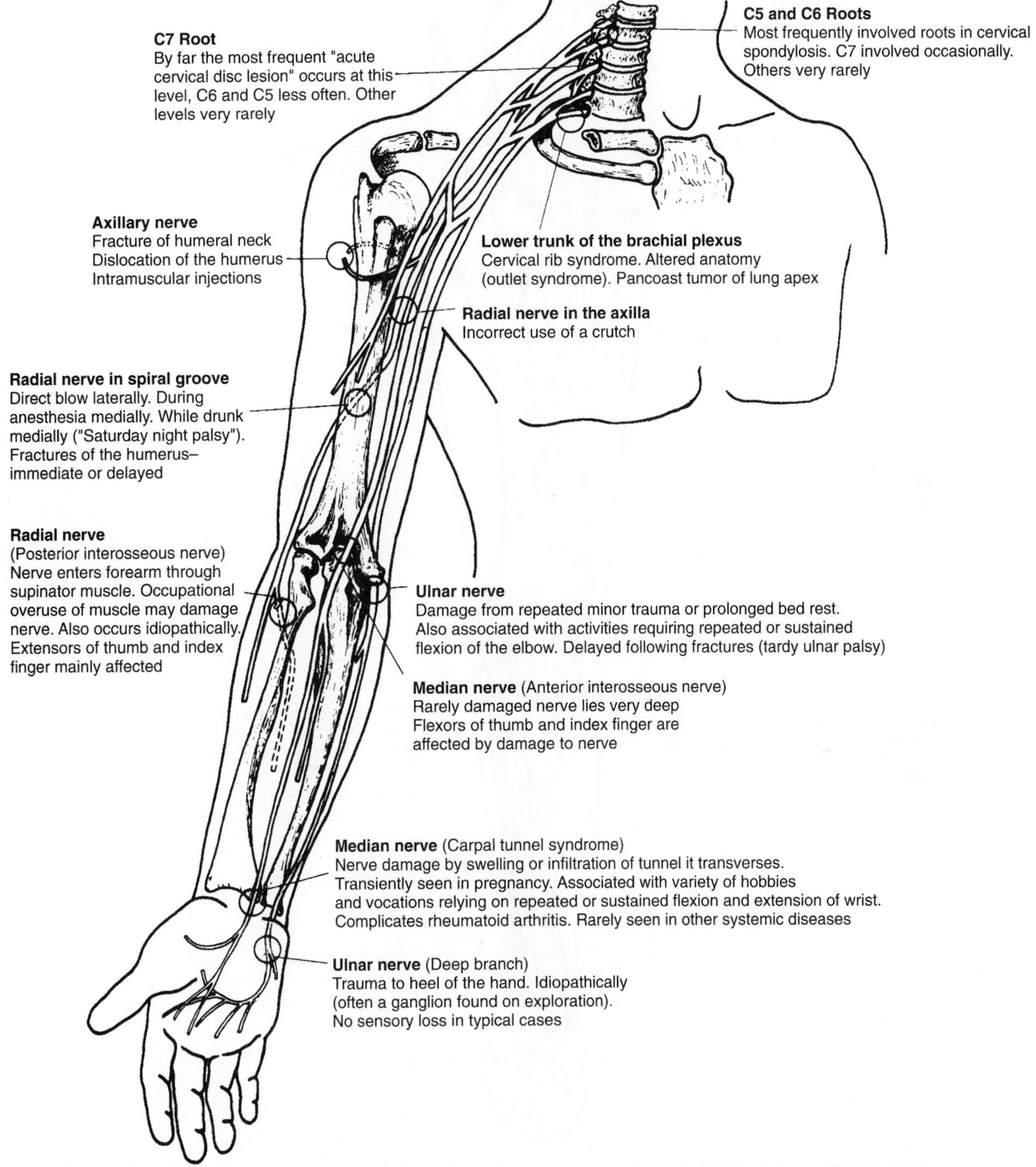

FIGURE 92.1. Anatomic relationships of nerves to the upper extremity. (Modified from Patten J. Neurological differential diagnosis. 2nd ed. New York: Springer-Verlag, 1995.)

sensory impairment in the distribution of one of the lateral three digital (thumb and digits 2, 3, lateral half of 4) nerves may be unusual presenting features of median nerve lesions at the wrist. Mild weakness of the abductor pollicis brevis (to test, patient abducts thumb at right angle to palm, against resistance) or of the opponens pollicis muscle (to test, patient touches base of little finger with thumb, against resistance) is often present with no visually apparent atrophy. Prolonged hyperflexion of the wrist may reproduce sensory symptoms (*Phalen sign*). *Tinel sign,*

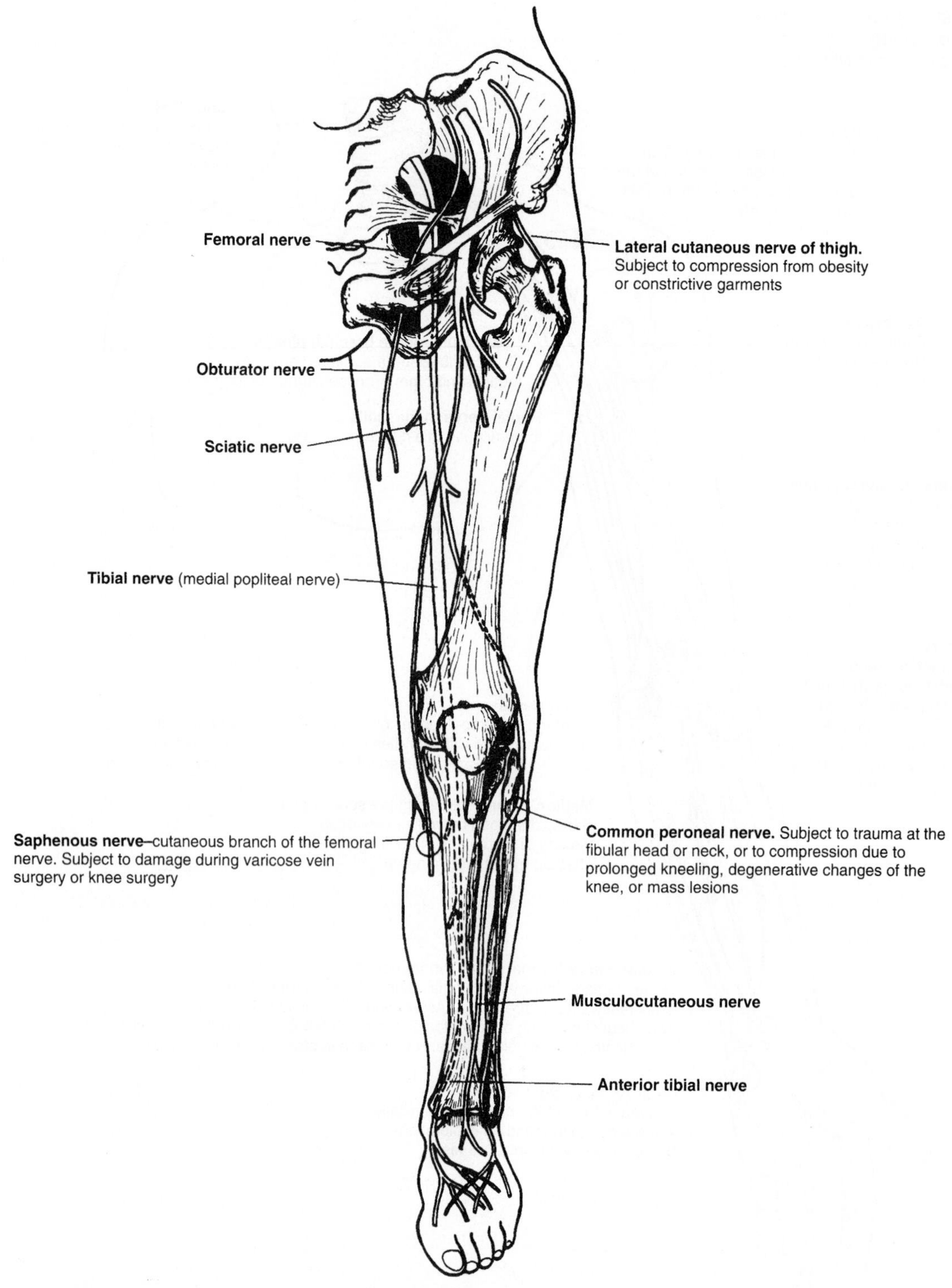

FIGURE 92.2. Anatomic relationships of nerves to the lower extremity. (Modified from Patten J. Neurological differential diagnosis. 2nd ed. New York: Springer-Verlag, 1995.)

consisting of shock-like pain and tingling elicited by percussion of the median nerve at the wrist, is a less specific finding. In a systematic review of the accuracy of the physical examination to diagnose CTS, hypalgesia in the median nerve territory, a classic pattern of pain with hand symptom diagrams, and weak thumb abduction were the strongest predictors of electrodiagnostic CTS (20).

Nerve conduction studies in CTS are invaluable in confirming the diagnosis and qualifying the degree of axon loss if any. In addition, because central nervous system or root lesions can occasionally result in similar sensory symptoms, confirmation of a peripheral nerve lesion by electrophysiologic testing is important. Typically changes in the sensory axons of the median nerve, including segmental reduction in conduction velocity across the wrist segment and axon loss, are the most sensitive measures. Motor axon changes, such as prolonged distal latencies, occur later in the course of entrapment. EMG is important to confirm localization of median nerve entrapment, to look for evidence of associated axonal degeneration and to rule out possible coexistent cervical radiculopathy (double crush syndrome).

Treatment

Immobilization of the wrist with a close-fitting *anterior splint* (extends from the upper part of the forearm to the metacarpophalangeal joints), which is worn by the patient at night or when resting, holds the wrist immobilized in a neutral position. This is often sufficient, but if symptoms persist after a few weeks, additional therapy is indicated. Medications such as NSAIDS, pyridoxine, or diuretics are commonly prescribed but the efficacy of such treatments has not been supported by clinical trials. Steroid injection beneath the transverse carpal ligament has been used for over 60 years to treat CTS though care must be taken not to directly inject the nerve which can result in axonal injury. Several, randomized clinical trials demonstrated that injection with steroids was superior to placebo injection in patients with CTS refractory to splinting. The benefit was frequently short-lived and required repeat injections in many patients (21,22). Two recent RCTs comparing surgical therapy to steroid injection found surgery to be superior for both symptomatic and electrophysiologic improvement (23,24). Steroid injection has an important role as a predictor of treatment success as patients responding transiently to local injection were much more likely to experience relief following surgery (25,26), but likely carries increased risk when used repeatedly in the chronic management of CTS.

Indications for carpal tunnel release include the failure of nonoperative treatment or clinical evidence of thenar atrophy. A relative indication is constant sensory loss, especially if it is long standing. Surgery for CTS is one of the most successful operations that can be performed on the hand. The operation demands care and skill by an orthopedic, plastic, or neurologic surgeon who performs hand surgery regularly. Complications of the operation or poor results such as reflex sympathetic dystrophy, injury to median nerve branches, hypertrophic scar or adherent flexor tendons are almost always related to poor surgical technique. The usual postoperative recovery time is 6 to 8 weeks. An additional month may be needed for occupational rehabilitation. Most patients with jobs that involve repetitive wrist motion such as typing are able to return to their preoperative activities after a work-hardening program.

Ulnar Nerve

Causes

Ulnar nerve compression occurs most often at the elbow (Fig. 92.1). The *cubital tunnel* refers to the area of potential entrapment of the ulnar nerve at the elbow as it runs beneath the aponeurosis of the flexor carpi ulnaris muscle just distal to the medial epicondyle. Minor pressure directly over the cubital tunnel during anesthesia, intoxication, stupor, coma, or by trauma may subsequently cause symptoms.

Compression of the ulnar nerve at the elbow may occur with activities requiring repeated or sustained flexion of the elbow because the cubital tunnel is at its smallest when the elbow is at 90% flexion. Hypermobility of the ulnar nerve can result in subluxation over the medial epicondyle and repeated trauma.

Manifestations and Evaluation

Patients may awaken at night with elbow pain, shooting pain in the hand or fifth digit, and paresthesias and hypesthesia in the ulnar nerve distribution. These symptoms usually improve with elbow extension. The amount of pain and paresthesia varies.

Ulnar sensory loss (Table 92.6) is easiest to establish with two-point discrimination over the distal two phalanges of the little finger. Transition between the ulnar territory over the hypothenar eminence and the medial antebrachial cutaneous nerve (branch from the brachial plexus) of the forearm is often detected at the skin crease at the wrist. Motor disability is usually manifested as decreased grip and pinch strength, which is related to the degree of atrophy of the involved intrinsic muscles, especially the palmar and dorsal interossei and flexor digitorum profundus to the fourth and fifth digits. One of the earliest signs of ulnar nerve entrapment is weakness of fifth finger adduction with a tendency to catch the finger on a pants pocket.

Ulnar neuropathy distal to the elbow occurs at the wrist or in the hand and must be considered if there is no weakness in the flexor digitorum profundus. This is most often caused by a ganglion, rheumatoid arthritis, or trauma (e.g., long-distance bicycling). Often lesions in the wrist or hand produce no paresthesias or sensory loss. Depending on the level of entrapment at the wrist, either all of the ulnar innervated muscles may be weak or there may be selective preservation of hypothenar function, i.e., abductor digiti minimi.

Electrodiagnostic study involves focal slowing of the ulnar motor or sensory nerve conduction across the elbow to localize the nerve damage, depending on the severity. False-positive findings may be obtained, so close correlation with the clinical findings is mandatory. Increased distal latencies are found with entrapment at the wrist but must be correlated with needle electrode examination (see Nerve Conduction Studies) to determine the actual site of the lesion.

Treatment

Nonsurgical treatment is indicated for the patient with intermittent symptoms, acute or chronic mild neuropathy, or mild neuropathy associated with an occupational cause. For a mild ulnar neuropathy, wearing elbow pads during the day and *splinting the elbow* at night in an extended position may be helpful. An easy way to splint the elbow during sleep is to strap a pillow around it. Elbow protection should be continued for 2 to 3 months, especially if the symptoms are intermittent or show improvement. For ulnar compression at the wrist, whether caused by a single traumatic event or by chronic trauma, conservative treatment with a wrist splint (see Median Nerve [Carpal Tunnel Syndrome], above) is generally adequate.

Surgical intervention is generally not necessary. If symptoms progress or if motor involvement develops, surgery can be considered. Surgical approaches to lesions of the ulnar nerve at the elbow depend on the cause and the surgeon. These include simple release of the cubital tunnel, medial epicondylectomy, and anterior transposition of the nerve. Complications from any of the surgical approaches include persistent or recurrent symptoms caused by inadequate surgery or recurrent scarring around the nerve.

Radial Nerve

Causes

Radial nerve lesions are the least common of the major upper extremity nontraumatic compression neuropathies and usually involve the nerve at or proximal to the elbow (Fig. 92.1). Besides traumatic conditions such as humeral fractures, more proximal radial nerve injuries can occur when the arm has been held in a hyperabducted position that causes traction to the nerve, as in surgery or sleep. Proximal nerve injury may also follow axillary pressure caused by incorrect use of a crutch. The middle third of the nerve is compressed against the humerus in the so-called Saturday night palsy, as when an intoxicated person sleeps with the arm draped over a chair. Compression of the posterior interosseous nerve (a motor branch of radial nerve in the forearm) can result from a variety of masses, such as lipomas, fibromas, or calluses from old fractures.

Manifestations and Evaluation

The radial nerve is predominantly a motor nerve. Depending on the location of a high radial compression, the triceps function (elbow extension) may or may not be affected. Elbow flexion and supination may be slightly affected by brachioradialis weakness. The most obvious finding in a radial palsy is wrist drop and digital extensor paralysis (finger drop). A lesion of the posterior interosseous nerve results in finger drop alone.

High radial nerve lesions may produce sensory loss over the dorsum of the hand. Pain and tenderness in the area of nerve damage may be present. Nerve conduction studies and electromyography (see Nerve Conduction Studies) are helpful in localizing and quantifying radial nerve compression. For example, acutely, a Saturday night palsy can cause focal slowing of conduction at the site of pressure injury but normal motor and sensory conduction below this lesion.

Treatment

The treatment of traumatic radial nerve compression is generally conservative and recovery of function occurs within a few weeks to months. To prevent flexor contractures, a *cock-up splint for the wrist joint* should be accompanied by a *spring-loaded extensor brace for the fingers* if the weakness is severe and long lasting. Individually constructed splints made by an occupational therapist are superior to those obtained from a surgical supply house. For compression of the posterior interosseus nerve with no obvious cause, imaging of the nerve should be performed to investigate for possible masses. If no mass is identified, surgical exploration is indicated if there has not been spontaneous recovery within 2 to 3 months.

Peroneal Nerve

Causes

The most common site of compression of the peroneal nerve is at the fibular head (Fig. 92.2). Such compression may result from improperly applied plaster casts or tight stockings and garters or from falling asleep with the side of the leg resting against a protruding object, as in a drug- or alcohol-induced stupor or in the weakened bedridden patient. Prolonged leg crossing, squatting, or kneeling may also result in peroneal compression. Entrapment of the peroneal nerve can also occur in the *fibular tunnel* formed by the peroneus longus muscle.

Manifestations and Evaluation

Symptoms of peroneal palsy consist of painless weakness of ankle dorsiflexion (foot drop) and foot eversion and sensory loss over the lateral calf and dorsum of the foot. *Electrodiagnostic studies* and nerve conduction studies can detect focal slowing or conduction block in the peroneal nerve segment across the fibular head. The superficial peroneal sensory potential may be absent. Needle electrode examination may demonstrate denervation in peroneal innervated muscles with sparing of the short head of the biceps femoris muscle, the most distal of the peroneal innervated muscles above the fibular head. Peroneal palsy with loss of motor function and no clear history of trauma or external compression should be investigated with appropriate physical examination and imaging of the popliteal fossa to rule out a mass lesion.

Treatment

Mild compressive peroneal lesions can be treated conservatively. Patients should be advised to avoid potentially injurious positions for the nerve (e.g., leg crossing, squatting). A custom-fitted *ankle–foot orthotic* is recommended for increased ankle stability and prevention of plantar flexion contractures. Most patients with a transient compressive insult recover peroneal function within weeks to months. Surgical exploration should be considered in severe cases with no clear cause.

Tibial Nerve (Tarsal Tunnel Syndrome)

Causes

The *tarsal tunnel* is located at the inferoposterior margin of the medial malleolus (Fig. 92.2) and is formed by bones of the ankle and the flexor retinaculum (fibrous sheath from medial malleolus posteroinferior to the medial side of the calcaneus) (see Chapter 72). In addition to the posterior tibial nerve, the tunnel contains the posterior tibial artery and three long flexor tendons (27).

Enlarged tortuous veins within the tarsal tunnel, fracture or dislocation at the ankle, and tenosynovitis may lead to compression of the tibial nerve trunk. Prolonged standing and walking often aggravate the pain, indicating that stasis or engorgement within the tunnel is likely to play some role. Also, sensory symptoms are made worse by the venous stasis and engorgement that occur at night during sleep. Except for a high prevalence in jockeys, no common occupational factors have been identified.

Manifestations and Evaluation

The primary symptom of tarsal tunnel syndrome is pain and dysesthesia in the sole of the foot. The burning pain (descriptions by patients may vary, e.g., walking on knives or pins, sole feels very thick) worsens with rest after a day of activity. Nocturnal pain is characteristic. Any or all the three terminal divisions of the tibial nerve (medial plantar, lateral plantar, and calcaneal) may be affected, resulting in sensory disturbance over the entire plantar surface or only one portion of it.

Tinel sign, consisting of shooting pain to the plantar surface produced by gentle percussion over the tarsal tunnel, may be present. Sensory loss, if present, is localized to the plantar surface of the foot and over the tips of the toes (the sural and peroneal territories on the dorsum of the foot do not include the tips of the toes). Weakness in the intrinsic muscles of the foot may lead to a change in configuration of the foot and to instability of the phalanges, which impairs the pushing-off phase of walking. Tarsal tunnel syndrome is usually unilateral.

In the tarsal tunnel syndrome, sensory nerve conduction studies of medial and lateral plantar nerves are the most sensitive electrodiagnostic measures, showing reduced sensory nerve action potential amplitudes or absent responses. Reduced motor or sensory conduction velocities across the flexor retinaculum are found less commonly. Electromyography demonstrates chronic partial denervation in the tibial innervated intrinsic muscles of the feet (e.g., abductor hallucis and abductor digiti quinti). Symptoms of tarsal tunnel syndrome may mimic those of a small fiber neuropathy and often require electrodiagnostic and skin biopsies to distinguish the two.

Treatment

It is important to identify and remove any source of external pressure at the flexor retinaculum. Definitive treatment of tarsal tunnel syndrome is surgical release of the flexor retinaculum, which can result in dramatic relief of symptoms.

Femoral Nerve

Causes

The femoral nerve may be injured by stab wounds to the groin or hip, pelvic fractures, inguinal surgery (inguinal hernia, vascular repair, node resection), angiography, or retraction during pelvic surgery (Fig. 92.2). Stretch injuries can occur with prolonged lithotomy position, during child birth, or with hyperextension during gymnastics or dance. Pressure on the femoral nerve can also be produced at the psoas muscle by hematoma or abscess.

Manifestations and Evaluation

The patient often complains about buckling of the knee (quadriceps weakness), and falls are common. Pain in the groin radiating into the thigh may be severe. Sensory loss is present in the anterior medial thigh and medial leg. Weakness of the quadriceps (knee extension) and loss of the knee jerk are noted on examination. Weakness of hip flexors indicates a more proximal lumbar plexus or root lesion. Electromyography helps differentiate these problems.

Femoral neuropathy is to be distinguished from *diabetic lumbar plexopathy* (diabetic amyotrophy). The latter disorder, seen most commonly in people with diabetes over 50 years of age, begins abruptly with severe pain in the thigh and buttocks, and progresses to produce proximal weakness which can be severe and require the use of a wheelchair. Classically, these patients have significant concomitant weight loss. With electromyography a wider distribution of involvement can be appreciated.

Sensory signs are mild. The prognosis for recovery over 2 to 6 months is variable but generally good (see Chapter 79).

Treatment

Treatment depends on accurate diagnosis (e.g., discontinuation of anticoagulants when a psoas hematoma has been identified as the cause of the neuropathy). Physiotherapy may be required to maintain the mobility of the hip joint. The outcome and extent of rehabilitation measures are determined by the cause and extent of injury.

Saphenous Nerve

The saphenous nerve is one of three sensory branches of the femoral nerve (Fig. 92.2). It is most often injured at Hunter canal (10 cm proximal to the medial condyle of the femur). Vein stripping and knee surgery are common causes. A small medial nerve branch can be injured by knee surgery. The patient has pain and numbness at the medial aspect of the knee and leg. The pain may worsen with walking and climbing. Manual pressure over the Hunter canal produces pain that radiates. If the pain becomes chronic, local anesthetic can be injected to the area of injury.

Sciatic Nerve

Causes

The sciatic nerve is often injured as a complication of trauma (Fig. 92.2), including hip fractures, dislocations, and arthroplastic surgery. Compression of the nerve can occur in comatose or chronically bedridden patients or after sitting on a hard edge. Hematoma, endometriosis, lipoma, and aneurysms of the gluteal artery are other causes of compression. Injections into the buttock are now less common causes of sciatic nerve injury. Injections usually cause immediate dysfunction with poor recovery.

Manifestations and Evaluation

Symptoms of sciatic nerve compression may mimic L5–S1 radiculopathy caused by disk disease (see Chapter 71). The lateral trunk or peroneal division of the sciatic nerve is often affected more severely than the tibial division. Therefore, the distinction between a proximal sciatic injury and a more distal peroneal injury (e.g., after awakening from hip surgery) may be difficult clinically and require electromyography evaluation in order to distinguish the two.

Lateral Femoral Cutaneous Nerve (Meralgia Paresthetica)

The lateral femoral cutaneous nerve may be compressed or stretched at the anterior superior iliac spine at the lateral end of the inguinal canal (see lateral cutaneous nerve of the thigh; Fig. 92.2), causing burning pain, paresthesia, and decreased sensation over the lateral thigh in a distribution that roughly corresponds to the pockets of pants. There is no motor involvement or loss of patellar reflex. Point tenderness can usually be elicited at the passage of the nerve at the ipsilateral anterior iliac crest. Common causes include obesity, acute abdominal enlargement (ascites, pregnancy), external mechanical trauma (girdle, utility belt, climbing with body against utility pole), and DM. The nerve compression may be relieved by weight loss or correction of the aggravating condition. Pain may respond to medical management (see Therapeutic Principles), but generally resolves spontaneously over months. If the pain is severe, local injection of an anesthetic may provide relief for long periods; sectioning of the ligament over the canal or sectioning of the nerve is rarely needed. Paresthesias and pain usually disappear gradually, but a painless sensory loss in the lateral thigh may persist.

Bell Palsy

Paralysis of the facial muscles caused by inflammation and swelling of the seventh (the facial) cranial nerve (Bell palsy) is seen occasionally in a general medical practice. One large series reported an incidence of 23 cases per 100,000 population per year (28). There is no predilection for a particular sex, age group, or race. In most patients, the cause of the condition is unknown. Two specific causes for seventh nerve neuropathy that have been recognized in recent years are Lyme disease (29,30) (see Chapter 38) and HIV infection (see Chapter 39). Bilateral involvement also raises the possibility of sarcoidosis or carcinomatous meningitis. Several small studies have suggested that asymptomatic reactivation of varicella zoster virus is responsible for a substantial proportion of cases of Bell palsy (31).

Manifestations

Usually, patients note the sudden onset, within hours, of a unilateral facial weakness: the eyebrow sags, the eyelid cannot be closed, the nasolabial fold disappears, and the mouth is drawn to the unaffected side. Less commonly, there is loss of taste on the anterior two thirds of the tongue and there is hyperacusis (an accentuation of sounds) in the affected ear. There may be pain behind the ear. Most patients recover spontaneously within weeks to a few months; approximately 15% recover incompletely, but severe residual weakness is rare (28). Patching of the unclosed eye should be performed to avoid corneal injury. Rarely, synkinesis (a contraction of all the facial muscles on the affected side when the patient attempts to move just one or a few of them) caused by aberrant reinnervation can complicate recovery.

Management

Therapeutic trials of treatment for Bell palsy have lacked sufficient power to be conclusive, but meta-analysis of several trials show that corticosteroid therapy early in the course improves facial outcomes (32,33). Combined acyclovir–prednisone was found to improve recovery over prednisone alone in one trial (34). The current standard of treatment when the palsy has been present less than 4 days is prednisone 60 to 80 mg/day for 1 week, and valacyclovir (because of improved oral absorption) 1 g three times a day for 1 week (35).

LESS COMMON PROBLEMS

Hereditary Motor and Sensory Neuropathies

Of the heritable disorders affecting the peripheral nervous system, the hereditary motorsensory neuropathies (HMSN) or Charcot-Marie-Tooth (CMT) disease are the most common. As a group, the HMSN are a heterogeneous group of neuropathy syndromes affecting an estimated 1 per 2,500 people (see www.hopkinsbayview.org/PAMreferences). The nomenclature of these disorders has historically been confusing, though the identification of individual gene mutations has greatly clarified the situation. Patients are now generally classified into four types: CMT 1 refers to patients with reduced conduction velocities and a dominant pattern of inheritance; CMT II if there is a dominant pattern of inheritance and normal nerve conduction velocities but reduced motor or sensory amplitudes; CMTX if they have an X-linked inheritance pattern; and CMT 4 if the inheritance pattern is autosomal recessive. Past eponyms such as Dejerine Sottas disease and the Roussy-Levy syndrome are now appreciated to be phenotypic variants of CMT 1 rather than distinct disease entities.

The most common type, CMT I, is characterized by slowly progressive distal weakness, muscle wasting; foot abnormalities that can include pes cavus and hammer toe, and mildly diminished distal sensation. Symptoms are usually manifest by the fourth decade; however, many patients have few or no symptoms. Sensory symptoms are rarely the presenting complaint and when present suggest an acquired rather than inherited neuropathy.

Physical examination demonstrates a wide range of clinical severity and may include distal weakness, thin peroneal muscles, diminished deep tendon reflexes in the legs, characteristic abnormalities of the feet (see above), and mildly reduced distal sensation. Occasionally, enlarged nerves can be palpated. Electrophysiologic studies of sensory and motor nerves show diffuse involvement, with severely reduced conduction velocities uniformly along the nerve segment. Nerve pathology shows onion bulb formation composed of redundant Schwann cell processes resulting from recurrent demyelination and remyelination. Diagnosis is established by identifying a history of childhood onset and by physical examination, characteristic electrophysiologic findings, electrodiagnostic evaluation of family members, and genetic testing. Genetic mutations have been identified on chromosomes 1, 10, and 17. The most common treatment required is the use of custom-fitted ankle–foot orthotics.

Guillain-Barré Syndrome

GBS or acute inflammatory polyradiculoneuropathy is a rapidly progressive paralytic syndrome affecting all ages. Evidence is strong for an immune-mediated pathogenesis. Most cases of GBS follow a mild viral illness (by 10 to 12 days) (36). The syndrome also may be associated with pregnancy, the postoperative period, recent influenza immunization, and HIV infection. A link between preceding *Campylobacter jejuni* infection and GBS is particularly strong, involving approximately 20% of cases. Molecular mimicry has been implicated as the mechanism and might explain why such cases tend to be more severe. Other prognostic indicators for severe disease are older than 60 years, ventilator dependence, and a rapid progression from initial symptoms to respiratory insufficiency. Diagnosis of *C. jejuni* infection is based on isolation of *C. jejuni* from stool. The *differential diagnosis* for GBS includes acute intermittent porphyria, botulism, diphtheria, poliomyelitis, Lyme disease, and toxic neuropathies (arsenic, thallium).

Manifestations

There is rapid progression of ascending symmetric weakness (usually moving from the lower extremities to the upper extremities) accompanied by loss of deep tendon reflexes. Although acute pain or paresthesias in the back and proximal limbs may be prominent early symptoms, objective evidence of sensory loss is generally limited to mild impairment of distal joint position sense and vibratory sensation. Cranial muscle weakness may be present, with bilateral facial nerve palsy in 40% of patients. Nerve conduction studies show changes of demyelination (prolonged distal motor and F-wave latencies and reduced motor conduction velocities). The CSF may show an increased protein concentration with normal cell counts (cytoalbumin dissociation).

Management and Course

Because of rapid progression of the disease, patients suspected of having this disorder should be admitted to the hospital for close monitoring for potential respiratory failure and autonomic instability (hypotension, hypertension, cardiac arrhythmias, or hyperpyrexia occur in two thirds of patients with GBS). Treatment with either plasmapheresis or intravenous human immunoglobulin early in the course shortens the period of disability, and the combination is no better than either treatment alone (37). Recovery is complete in approximately 50% of patients (although it may take 6 to 18 months); most of the remainder have only mild residual deficits, but 10% have severe permanent disability. Splints (to prevent contractures) and physiotherapy should be used until the recovery period is complete.

Chronic Inflammatory Demyelinating Polyneuropathy

CIDP is an acquired motor and sensory neuropathy of unknown cause but with strong evidence for an immune-mediated pathogenesis. CIDP can occur in the absence of systemic disease or, less commonly, in association with such disorders as systemic lupus erythematosus (SLE), HIV infection, or dysproteinemias. Clinically, CIDP is a predominantly *motor polyneuropathy*. It may affect all ages and may have either a chronic progressive or relapsing course. Weakness typically develops over at least 2 months (distinguishing CIDP from acute inflammatory demyelinating neuropathy or GBS) and generally begins in the legs. Sensory involvement is variable. Most patients experience some degree of numbness or paresthesia; occasionally, there may be painful dysesthesias. On examination, weakness may be both proximal and distal, and the tendon reflexes are reduced or absent in all four limbs.

Electrodiagnostic studies demonstrate features of demyelination, including prolonged distal and F-wave latencies, reduced conduction velocities variably along nerve segments, abnormal temporal dispersion, and conduction block. CSF protein is often elevated. Sural nerve pathology may show evidence of demyelination and remyelination with onion bulb formation, subperineurial and endoneurial edema, and mononuclear cell infiltration.

Management

Common practice is to begin treatment with prednisone 1 mg/kg/day (38) and to use either plasmapheresis or intravenous human Ig as adjuvants (39). Each of these immunomodulating therapies has been demonstrated to be effective in randomized placebo-controlled trials, and most patients respond. Long-term corticosteroid therapy usually is effective but is limited by side effects. Steroid-sparing therapy with azathioprine or mycophenolate are also effective but have a long latency period. The effect of either plasmapheresis or human immunoglobulin is large and of equal likelihood, but for most patients is short-lived and requires continued intermittent treatment (39). For plasmapheresis, improved motor conduction velocities and reversal of conduction block predict improvement in motor function (40). Plasma exchange treatments should be given two to three times per week until improvement is established, then tapered in frequency; concurrent immunosuppressive drug treatment is usually required (40). Human immunoglobulin treatment is effective in about two thirds of patients, most often in patients with acute relapse or disease duration less than 1 year (41). Improvement after a dose of 2 g/kg lasts a median 6 weeks and is reproducible, so that followup pulses of 1 g/kg as single infusions can maintain a stable benefit (41). Of the two adjuvants, both are extraordinarily expensive, but intravenous Ig infusion may be preferable because it does not require expensive medical devices and can be given at home (39).

Multifocal Motor Neuropathy

Patients with multifocal motor neuropathy have progressive, predominantly distal, asymmetric weakness that usually begins in the arms. Early in the disease course, multifocal motor neuropathy can mimic CIDP or the lower motor neuron presentation of amyotrophic lateral sclerosis. Nerve conduction studies show multiple areas of persistent partial motor conduction block, and many patients have high IgM anti-GM 1 ganglioside antibody titers. Most patients with multifocal motor neuropathy respond variably to immunomodulatory therapy with human immune globulin (42). Recently, therapy with rituximab has also been demonstrated to be effective in some patients that became refractory to human immune globulin (43). Corticosteroids are ineffective.

THERAPEUTIC PRINCIPLES

General Measures that Improve Nerve Function

Treatment of peripheral neuropathies first requires identifying and treating any underlying cause, if possible. For type 1 DM, for example, it is now known that intense efforts at tight glucose control dramatically reduce the incidence of neuropathy (see Chapter 79). Efforts should be made also to prevent further damage; for example, patients with an underlying generalized polyneuropathy are more prone to pressure palsies, and it is important to educate them about habits that could be injurious (e.g., leaning on elbows or crossing legs). The daily administration of multivitamins is necessary only in patients whose nutrition may be poor. For entrapment and compression neuropathies, eliminating pressure on the affected nerve is the primary mode of treatment. Pain and paresthesias may be relieved rapidly within hours or days. The prognosis for recovery depends on the pathophysiology of the nerve injury. When little or no denervation is demonstrated by electromyography, which suggests that the predominant pathophysiology is edema or demyelination, recovery of function over weeks is expected. In more severe cases with marked denervation indicating axonal injury, recovery is more prolonged (months).

The most important *prognostic indicators for traumatic nerve injuries* are the site, mechanism, and completeness of the injury. Traumatic injuries can occur at the level of the root, plexus, or peripheral nerve. Root avulsion has the worst prognosis. Electrodiagnostic studies are helpful in localizing the site of injury; however, because denervation may not be evident for at least 14 days, electromyography studies should be done approximately 3 to 4 weeks after injury. Complete nerve transections caused by sharp penetrating injury, although rare, more often benefit from early primary anastomosis than do complicated nerve injuries such as gunshot wounds. Physical therapy, particularly range-of-motion exercises, should be initiated early after injury to prevent contractures. The onset of spontaneous recovery can vary from weeks to 6 months or more after injury. In cases of persistent loss of function or severe pain, surgical exploration should be considered.

Symptomatic Treatment for Irreversible Damage

Polyneuropathy is often irreversible and progressive. Symptomatic therapy and rehabilitative measures are therefore fundamental in helping these patients.

Motor Neuropathies

In most polyneuropathies, weakness usually affects ankle dorsiflexors early (causing foot drop); ambulation can be greatly improved by a custom-fitted ankle–foot orthotic, such as a rigid plastic splint worn in the shoe or a spring-loaded brace attached to the shoe. Fine motor weakness in the hands can be aided by special tools, such as large-handled utensils and other devices, provided by occupational therapists.

Sensory Neuropathies

Small hard objects (keys, faucet handles) can be built up with soft materials. Occupational therapists can make useful suggestions in this regard. Anesthetic limbs are vulnerable to repeated unrecognized trauma. The patient should always check the temperature of bath water, pot handles, and so on with parts of the body that have normal sensation. Meticulous care should be given to feet and toenails to prevent ulceration or infection. Moisturizing cream for dry insensitive skin will reduce serious abrasions.

Pain associated with sensory neuropathies is usually chronic though rewarding to treat. Simple analgesics (aspirin, acetaminophen, or NSAIDS), whirlpool, and massage may help relieve mild pain but are generally of limited benefit. Effective agents generally are from three classes of drugs: anticonvulsants, antidepressants and opiate or opiate-like medications. Gabapentin (Neurontin) was initially developed as an anticonvulsant but its membrane stabilizing properties also renders it quite effective at reducing neuropathic pain and dysesthesias (44). It is generally well tolerated but may be sedating in elderly patients. Therefore, it is usually best to begin gabapentin therapy with a small dose in the evenings (100 to 300 mg) and gradually titrate the dose upwards to the *lowest* effective dose or a maximum of 3,600 mg/day. Similar approaches can be used for other anticonvulsant medications with efficacy in neuropathic pain such as lamotrigene (Lamictal) and pregabalin (Lyrica). Tricyclic antidepressants (e.g., amitriptyline or nortriptyline, 25 to 75 mg at bedtime) are often effective. The selective serotonin reuptake inhibitor (SSRI)/NERI drugs duloxetine and fluoxetine are also effective and have the advantage of being dosed once per day and not requiring a titration period. Duloxetine doses greater than 60 mg/day are generally not associated with improved symptom relief and are complicated by higher side effect rates (45). Tramadol (Ultram), a non-addictive synthetic analgesic structurally related to opiates, or a combination of tramadol and acetaminophen (Ultracet), both have demonstrated efficacy for treatment of neuropathic pain (46). These agents have the advantage that they can be dosed on an as-needed basis while the other agents discussed above generally require constant blood levels for optimum effect. Long-acting opiate preparations such as the fentanyl patch are another attractive option and have the advantage of being dosed every three days. Topical agents such as the Lidoderm patch is another option and is not associated with systemic absorption (47). It most helpful for focal, well-circumscribed neuropathic pain. Another topical agent worth mention is capsaicin cream. While effective (48), the mechanism of action may be associated with epidermal nerve fiber injury (49) from which patients may not fully recover (50). The newer antidepressant and anticonvulsant compounds are so efficacious that their use has supplanted that of the more historical drugs carbamazepine and phenytoin for treatment of neuropathic pain. These historical agents have similar degrees of symptom relief but are associated with much higher rates of side effects.

Autonomic Neuropathies

Autonomic dysfunctions should also be approached symptomatically (51). The *hypotonic bladder* may be treated by drugs that increase bladder tone (Urecholine, 10 to 25 mg every 8 hours), by self-catheterization, or occasionally with surgery to decrease resistance to bladder emptying. For *male sexual impotence,* penile prostheses and pharmacologic erections produced by intracavernous injection or intraurethral suppositories have represented significant advances. The knowledge that sexual dysfunction has a neurologic basis may relieve the anxiety that often accompanies the problem. A check for medications that may be contributing to impotence is important.

TABLE 92.9 Measures that May Help Patients with Orthostatic Hypotension Caused by Autonomic Neuropathy

Avoid sudden changes in position
Avoid excessive intake of alcohol
Avoid diuresis
Correct hypovolemia
Discontinue or reduce the dosage of drugs known to cause orthostatic hypotension:
Antihypertensive drugs
Nitroglycerin
Diuretics
Neuroleptics
Tricyclic antidepressants
CNS depressants (opiates, alcohol)
Levodopa
Prescribe mineralocorticoid (if no congestive heart failure or hypertension)
Supplement diet with salt
Tilt up the head of the bed (may stimulate renin release)
Use elastic support stockings

CNS, central nervous system.

Orthostatic hypotension may be treated with salt supplementation and a volume-expanding mineralocorticoid (fludrocortisone 0.1 to 0.2 mg/day) in patients without congestive heart failure or hypertension. A recently released expensive α_1-adrenergic agonist, midodrine (ProAmatine), has been shown to help patients with orthostatic hypotension. The dosage is 10 mg three times per day. Contraindications are the same as those for fludrocortisone (52). Support stockings with pressure gradients may be helpful to prevent venous pooling, but many patients do not tolerate these stockings well. Arising slowly from recumbent or sitting positions, maintaining active ambulation, and sleeping with the head of the bed elevated on blocks (to stimulate renin release) are other measures that may help. Table 92.9 summarizes the practical ways to manage orthostatic hypotension caused by autonomic dysfunction.

OTHER PROBLEMS

Restless Legs Syndrome

Restless legs syndrome is common, affecting perhaps 5% of the general population. It is an important cause of insomnia (see Chapter 7). Patients complain of an aching or painful crawling sensation deep inside the legs at rest, especially in the evening or in bed. Walking provides some relief, but the dysesthesias often return quickly upon resting (53,54).

The exact pathophysiology has not been elucidated; both peripheral and central mechanisms have been proposed. The syndrome has been related in some patients to the peripheral neuropathies of DM and uremia. An association has also been found with iron and folate deficiency anemias, calcium and potassium deficiency, pregnancy, postgastric surgery state, excessive caffeine, sedative drug withdrawal, and exposure to neuroleptic medication. An idiopathic form is associated with periodic movements during sleep and a positive family history.

These patients should be evaluated for associated conditions for specific treatment. Restricting caffeine use and performing regular exercise before bedtime may be helpful recommendations. Simple analgesics (aspirin, acetaminophen) at bedtime may help early symptoms. In other patients, nonsedating dosages of clonazepam (Klonopin, 0.5 to 2 mg) or triazolam (Halcion, 0.125 mg) may relieve nocturnal symptoms. The drug of choice for people with severe restless leg syndrome is Sinemet (a combination of L-dopa and carbidopa) at dosages of one-half to two 25-/100-mg tablets at bedtime. If the patient is typically awakened later during the night, the controlled-release form of Sinemet is preferable. Sinemet is generally well tolerated (see details in Chapter 90). Dopamine agonists such as ropinirole and pramipexole have also been reported to be useful in treating this disorder (54).

Muscle Cramps

Cramps are localized involuntary painful contractions of skeletal muscles that produce a visible, palpable, hard, and bulging muscle. They must be distinguished from the sensation of cramp such as that described with intermittent claudication; the latter is not associated with a palpable hard and bulging muscle.

Ordinary muscle cramps are common and may be stopped by stretching the affected muscles. Frequent cramps are most often associated with denervating diseases, fatiguing exercises, salt depletion, dehydration, pregnancy, hypothyroidism, alcoholism, uremia, or hypomagnesemia. Patients with frequent daytime cramps related to exercise or fasting should be referred to a neurologist for evaluation for one of the rare muscle enzymatic defects (e.g., myophosphorylase, phosphofructokinase, or carnitine palmitoyltransferase deficiency). If no correctable associated condition exists, these patients may be given a therapeutic trial of phenytoin, carbamazepine, or amitriptyline (see Sensory Neuropathies).

Nocturnal cramps occur in 15% of healthy young adults and are even more common in the elderly. Regular passive stretching of leg muscles often prevents nocturnal cramps. If this is not effective, empiric trial of medicine can be considered. Meta-analysis of published and unpublished controlled trials showed that quinine, which requires a prescription (usual dose 325 mg at bedtime), reduced by about 21% the frequency of night cramps (55). Another drug reported to be effective is single-dose clonazepam, 0.25 to 0.5 mg at bedtime.

SPECIFIC REFERENCES*

1. McArthur JC, Stocks EA, Hauer P, et al. Epidermal nerve fiber density: normative reference range and diagnostic efficiency. Arch Neurol 1998;55:1513.
2. Herrmann DN, Griffin JW, Hauer P, et al. Epidermal nerve fiber density and sural nerve morphometry in peripheral neuropathies. Neurology 1999;53:1634.
3. Sumner CJ, Sheth S, Griffin JW, et al. The spectrum of neuropathy in diabetes and impaired glucose tolerance. Neurology 2003;60:108.
4. Holland NR, Crawford TO, Hauer P, et al. Small-fiber sensory neuropathies: clinical course and neuropathology of idiopathic cases. Ann Neurol 1998;44:47.
5. Lombardi R, Erne B, Lauria G, et al. IgM deposits on skin nerves in anti-myelin-associated glycoprotein neuropathy. Ann Neurol 2005;57:180.
6. Ewing DJ, Clarke BF. Diabetic autonomic neuropathy: present insights and future prospects. Diabetes Care 1986;9:648.
7. Vinik A, Mitchell B. Clinical aspects of diabetic neuropathies. Diabetes Metab Rev 1988;4:223.
8. Behse F, Buchthal F. Alcoholic neuropathy: clinical, electrophysiological and biopsy findings. Ann Neurol 1977;2:95.
9. Horwich MS, Cho L, Porro RS, et al. Subacute sensory neuropathy: a remote effect of cancer. Ann Neurol 1977;2:7.
10. Wilkinson M, Croft PB, Urich H. The remote effects of cancer on the nervous system. Proc R Soc Med 1967;60:683.
11. Oh SJ. Paraneoplastic vasculitis of the peripheral nervous system. Neurol Clin 1997;15:849.
12. Oh SJ, Slaughter R, Harrell L. Paraneoplastic vasculitic neuropathy: a treatable neuropathy. Muscle Nerve 1991;14:152.
13. Kissel J, Mendell JR. Neuropathies associated with monoclonal gammopathies. Neuromusc Disord 1996;6:3.
14. Miralles GD, O'Fallon JR, Talley NJ. Plasma-cell dyscrasia with polyneuropathy. The spectrum of POEMS syndrome. N Engl J Med 1992;327:1919.
15. Drachman DB, Brodsky RA. High-dose therapy for autoimmune neurologic diseases. Curr Opin Oncol 2005;17:83-8816.
16. Schaumberg H, Kaplan J, Windebank A, et al. Sensory neuropathy from pyridoxine abuse, a new megavitamin syndrome. N Engl J Med 1983;309:445.
17. Cornblath DR. Treatment of the neuromuscular complications of human immunodeficiency virus infection. Ann Neurol 1988;2:S88.
18. Eidelberg D, Sotrel A, Vogel H, et al. Progressive polyradiculopathy in acquired immuno-deficiency syndrome. Neurology 1986;36:912.
19. De Gans JH, Portugies P, Tiessens G, et al. Treatment for cytomegalovirus polyradiculomyelitis in patients with AIDS: treatment with ganciclovir. AIDS 1990;4:421.

*Bold numerals denote published controlled clinical trials, meta-analyses, or consensus-based recommendations.

20. D'Arcy CA, McGee S. Does this patient have carpal tunnel syndrome? JAMA 2000;283:3110.
21. Armstrong T, Devor W, Borschel L, Contreras R. Intracarpal steroid injection is safe and effective for short-term management of carpal tunnel syndrome. Muscle Nerve 2004;29:82.
22. Dammers JW, Veering MM, Vermeulen M. Injection with methylprednisolone proximal to the carpal tunnel: randomised double blind trial. BMJ 1999;319:884.
23. Hui AC, Wong S, Leung CH, et al. A randomized controlled trial of surgery vs steroid injection for carpal tunnel syndrome. Neurology. 2005;64:2074.
24. Ly-Pen D, Andreu JL, de Blas G, et al. Surgical decompression versus local steroid injection in carpal tunnel syndrome: a one-year, prospective, randomized, open, controlled clinical trial. Arthritis Rheum 2005;52:612.
25. Green DP. Diagnostic and therapeutic value of carpal tunnel injection. J Hand Surg 1984;9:850.
26. Edgell SE, McCabe SJ, Breidenbach WC, et al. Predicting the outcome of carpal tunnel release. J Hand Surg 2003;28:255.
27. Goodgold J, Kopell HP, Spielholz NI. The tarsal tunnel syndrome. N Engl J Med 1965;273:742.
28. Hauser WA, Karnes WE, Annis J, et al. Incidence and prognosis of Bell's palsy in the population of Rochester, Minnesota. Mayo Clin Proc 1971;46:258.
29. Finkel M. Lyme disease and its neurologic complications. Arch Neurol 1988;45:99.
30. Halperin JJ, Little BW, Coyle PK, et al. Lyme disease: cause of treatable peripheral neuropathy. Neurology 1987;37:1700.
31. Furuta Y, Ohtani F, Kawabata H, et al. High prevalence of varicella zoster virus reactivation in herpes simplex virus-seronegative patients with acute facial palsy. Clin Infect Dis 2000;30:529.
32. Williamson IG, Whelan TR. The clinical problem of Bell's palsy: is treatment with steroids effective? Br J Gen Pract 1996;46:743.
33. Ramsey MJ, DerSimonian R, Holtel MR, et al. Corticosteroid treatment for idiopathic facial nerve paralysis: a meta-analysis. Laryngoscope 2000;110:335.
34. Adour KK, Ruboyianes JM, Von Doersten PG, et al. Bell's palsy treatment with acyclovir and prednisone compared with prednisone alone: a double-blind, randomized, controlled trial. Ann Otol Rhinol Laryngol 1996;105:371.
35. Grogan PM, Gronseth GS. Practice parameter: steroids, acyclovir, and surgery for Bell's palsy (an evidence-based review): report of the Quality Standards Subcommittee of the American Academy of Neurology. Neurology 2001;56:830.
36. Ropper AH, Wijdicks EFM, Truax BT. Guillain-Barré syndrome. Philadelphia: FA Davis, 1991.
37. Plasma Exchange/Sandoglobulin Guillain-Barré Syndrome Trial Group. Randomized trial of plasma exchange, intravenous immunoglobulin, and combined treatments in Guillain-Barré syndrome. Lancet 1997;349:225.
38. Dyck PJ, O'Brien PC, Oviatt KF, et al. Prednisone improves chronic inflammatory demyelinating polyradiculoneuropathy more than no treatment. Ann Neurol 1982;11:136.
39. Dyck PJ, Litchy WJ, Kratz KM, et al. A plasma exchange versus immune globulin infusion trial in chronic inflammatory demyelinating polyradiculoneuropathy. Ann Neurol 1994;36: 838.
40. Hahn AF, Bolton CF, Pillay N, et al. Plasma-exchange therapy in chronic inflammatory demyelinating polyneuropathy: a double-blind, sham-controlled, cross-over study. Brain 1996;119:1055.
41. Hahn AF, Bolton CF, Zochodne D, et al. Intravenous immunoglobulin treatment in chronic inflammatory demyelinating polyneuropathy: a double-blind, placebo-controlled, cross-over study. Brain 1996; 119:1067.
42. Azulay JP, Rihet P, Pouget J, et al. Long term follow up of multifocal motor neuropathy with conduction block under treatment. J Neurol Neurosurg Psychiatry 1997;62:391.
43. Pestronk A, Florence J, Miller T, et al. Treatment of IgM antibody associated polyneuropathies using rituximab. J Neurol Neurosurg Psychiatry 2003;74:485.
44. Backonja MM. Use of anticonvulsants for treatment of neuropathic pain. Neurology 2002; 59:S14.
45. Goldstein DJ, Lu Y, Detke MJ, et al. Duloxetine vs. placebo in patients with painful diabetic neuropathy. Pain 2005;116:109.
46. Harati Y, Gooch C, Swenson M, et al. Double-blind randomized trial of tramadol for the treatment of the pain of diabetic neuropathy. Neurology 1998;50:1842.
47. Meier T, Wasner G, et al. Efficacy of lidocaine patch 5% in the treatment of focal peripheral neuropathic pain syndromes: a randomized, double-blind, placebo-controlled study. Pain 2003;106:151.
48. Treatment of painful diabetic neuropathy with topical capsaicin. A multicenter, double-blind, vehicle-controlled study. The Capsaicin Study Group. Arch Intern Med 1991;151:2225.
49. Nolano M, Simone DA, Wendelschafer-Crabb G, et al. Topical capsaicin in humans: parallel loss of epidermal nerve fibers and pain sensation. Pain 1999;81:135.
50. The time course of epidermal nerve fiber regeneration: studies in normal controls and in people with diabetes, with and without neuropathy. Brain 2004;127:1606.
51. McCleod JG, Tuck RR. Disorders of the autonomic nervous system. II. Investigation and treatment. Ann Neurol 1987;21:519.
52. Low PA, Gilden JL, Freeman R, et al. Efficacy of Midodrine vs placebo in neurogenic orthostatic hypotension: a randomized, double-blind multicenter study. JAMA 1997;277:1046.
53. Earley, CJ. Clinical practice. Restless legs syndrome. N Engl J Med 2003;21:2103.
54. Walters A, Hening W. Clinical presentation and neuropharmacology of restless legs syndrome. Clin Pharmacol 1987;10:225.
55. Man-Son-Hing M, Wells G, Lau A. Quinine for nocturnal leg cramps: a meta-analysis including unpublished data. J Gen Intern Med 1998;13: 600.

For annotated ***General References*** *and resources related to this chapter, visit www.hopkinsbayview.org/PAMreferences.*

SECTION 13

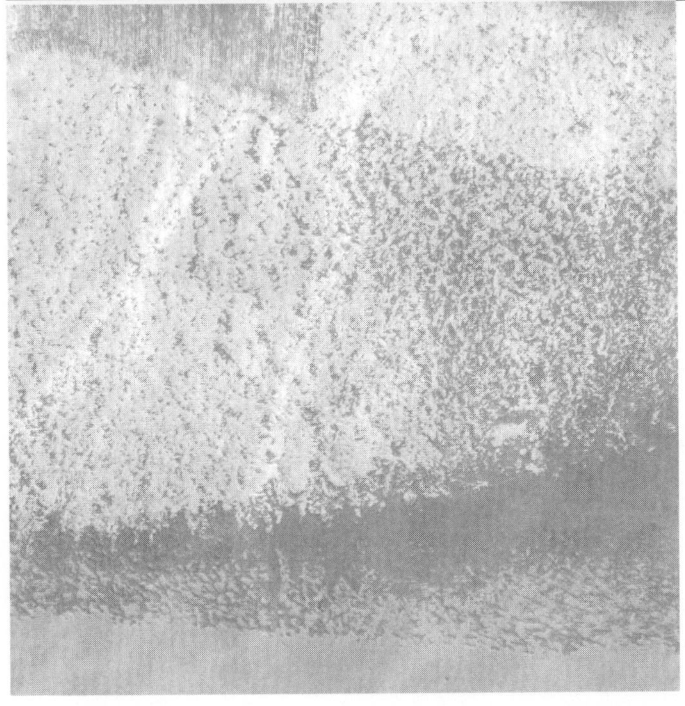

Selected General Surgical Problems

Chapter 93

Preoperative Planning for Ambulatory Patients

Richard J. Gross

PREOPERATIVE PLANNING: OVERVIEW

Preoperative evaluation for elective surgery is now done almost entirely in the ambulatory setting, because most surgery is now performed in outpatient surgical units. For inpatient surgery, most patients are admitted on the day of surgery. The primary care practitioner invests substantial time in establishing a diagnosis for the initial complaint, arriving at the decision to recommend surgery, and discussing the findings with the patient and family. The practitioner then evaluates the medical risks of surgery from factors unrelated to the primary surgical problem and consults on the care of the patient's medical problems in the perioperative period.

The principal reasons for office-based preoperative assessment are that health care insurers reimburse only for same-day surgery for many procedures, insurers do not reimburse for admission the day before surgery for preoperative assessment, office assessment eliminates the costs and inconvenience associated with unanticipated cancellation of surgery after the patient has been admitted, and better planning of care and higher patient satisfaction are often achieved.

Generally, the surgeon expects the referring clinician to have made an independent assessment of the need for surgery and of the medical acceptability of the patient for surgery. Although the surgeon obtains the actual consent for the surgical procedure, the patient's decision is based in part on the counseling provided by the referring practitioner. The referral itself is usually assumed by a patient and the family to be an endorsement of the consulting surgeon and of the surgeon's opinion. For these reasons, it is important for referring practitioners to know the place of surgery in the management of a broad array of conditions.

Table 93.1 summarizes *general guidelines on eligibility for same-day ambulatory surgery,* based on the patient's medical status (1,2).

TABLE 93.1 General Guidelines on Patient Eligibility for Ambulatory Surgery Based on Medical Condition (Not Considering Type of Surgery)

American Society of Anesthesiologists (ASA) class[a] 1 or 2 (some class 3 for minor procedures):
- *Class 1:* There is no physiologic, biochemical, or psychiatric disturbance. The pathologic process for which operation is to be performed is localized and not conducive to systemic disturbance. *Examples:* A fit patient with inguinal hernia; fibroid uterus in an otherwise healthy woman.
- *Class 2:* Mild to moderate systemic disturbance caused either by the condition to be treated surgically or by other pathophysiologic processes. *Examples:* Presence of mild diabetes mellitus, essential hypertension, or anemia.
- *Class 3:* Severe systemic disturbance from whatever cause, even though it may not be possible to define the degree of disability with finality. *Examples:* Severe diabetes mellitus with vascular complications, moderate to severe degrees of pulmonary insufficiency, angina pectoris or healed myocardial infarction.

Stable chronic medical problems well controlled by medicines; absence of acute medical problems.
No recent myocardial infarction or unstable cardiac disease.
No decompensated lung disease.
If diabetic, not taking insulin; if taking insulin; stable and capable of self-monitoring (diabetics should be operated upon in the morning).

[a]For explanation of ASA class see Grossman L. Anesthesia: risks, techniques and agents, organ effects and specific concerns. In: Gross RJ, Caputo GM, eds. Medical consultation: the internist on surgical, obstetric, and psychiatric services. 3rd ed. Baltimore: Williams & Wilkins, 1998:55.
Adapted from Gross RJ, Babbott SF. Evaluation of healthy patients and ambulatory surgical patients. In: Gross RJ, Caputo GM, eds. Medical consultation: the internist on surgical, obstetric, and psychiatric services. 3rd ed. Baltimore: Williams & Wilkins, 1998:37.

Laparoscopic techniques, though more comfortable to the patient, do not necessarily carry a lower medical, anesthetic, or surgical risk. General, spinal, and epidural anesthesia carry similar mortality risks in terms of medical problems. Local and regional anesthesia (usually a block, such as an axillary block) presumably carry lower risk, although data to prove this impression are lacking. Surgery involving the thoracic and abdominal cavities and vascular surgery carry higher medical risks than other types of surgery, with certain exceptions, such as radical head and neck surgery and hip replacement.

In counseling the patient and family, the patient's primary care practitioner and the consulting surgeon should explain clearly the diagnosis; natural history (prognosis) of the disease; and the objective, expected outcome, limitations, potential complications, and alternatives for the operation. This is especially important for surgical procedures that are undertaken for asymptomatic conditions (e.g., elective cholecystectomy) and for procedures that may be disfiguring (e.g., mastectomy or amputation). Preoperative counseling should be documented in the patient's record, including any special issues raised by the patient and how they were resolved (e.g., obtaining additional consultations or providing supportive counseling).

Approximately 50% of adults who undergo surgery are ostensibly in good general health; the other 50% have various medical problems (the percentages vary depending on the age of the population). In perhaps 5% to 10% of patients, new medical problems are identified during preoperative evaluation; a small proportion of these problems have implications for the planning of surgery.

The role of the primary care practitioner in relation to the surgeon and anesthesiologist will vary depending on the setting. In many university hospitals, the anesthesiologist will be more involved in the preoperative evaluation and postoperative care and the surgeon more involved in the postoperative care of medical problems than in community hospitals, but there is wide variation in practices, even among physicians within one institution. The primary care practitioner should be sensitive to the roles of the anesthesiologist and surgeon, usually making recommendations as a consultant rather than mandating management. Perioperative management works best when the primary practitioner, surgeon, and anesthesiologist agree on their individual roles, coordinate care, and work cooperatively. Changes to preoperative medical management before admission will usually be made directly by the primary care practitioner. These changes should be communicated to the anesthesiologist and surgeon before the day of surgery.

Whenever surgery is planned, the patient's referring practitioner should complete an appropriate preoperative evaluation (see General Preoperative Evaluation) to ensure optimal control of existing medical conditions that may affect the outcome of surgery and should communicate specific recommendations to the surgeon and anesthesiologist regarding the care of the patient's medical problems during the perioperative period, including recommendations for office or telephone followup. This chapter provides guidelines for these steps in the management of patients with common medical problems.

GENERAL PREOPERATIVE EVALUATION

There is no consensus on the makeup of a general preoperative evaluation. The recommendations below are based on current clinical practices at several institutions and the literature on preoperative testing. For adult patients undergoing general or spinal anesthesia, the "comprehensive" history and physical examination has mostly been replaced by an examination focused on medical risk factors for anesthesia and surgery. Similarly, ordering an extensive number of routine preoperative tests has been replaced by fewer tests, with additional testing guided by specific risk factors identified for the individual patient.

The previously used comprehensive workup has been criticized for having a low yield and being unnecessarily costly (1). The large number of factors that influence the preoperative evaluation make a consensus unlikely. The patient's age, the nature of the planned surgery (major or minor), the type of anesthesia to be used (general, spinal, regional, or local), and the interval since the patient's last comprehensive evaluation are relevant in the preoperative evaluation of every patient. Additionally, one or more of the following considerations are often pertinent: estimating operative risk, establishing a baseline for expected postoperative changes or possible complications, avoiding harm to other patients or medical personnel (e.g., hepatitis, tuberculosis, or human immunodeficiency virus [HIV] infection), documenting selected information for medicolegal reasons, determining drug dosages, detecting rare but potentially catastrophic circumstances (e.g., thrombocytopenia in a patient scheduled for a craniotomy), evaluating further the surgical problem, and establishing a database in a new patient.

Tables 93.2 and 93.3 summarize a practical approach for the individual patient including history and examination and tests, respectively. The history and examination focus on those items that are important in preoperative evaluation, rather than a "comprehensive" evaluation as

TABLE 93.2 General Preoperative Evaluation[a]

History	HPI, past medical history, allergies, medications, brief ROS (heart, lungs, hemostasis/bleeding problems, endocrine, and new symptoms, especially upper respiratory infection), family history (of surgical/anesthesia problems, bleeding disorders, thromboembolic disease, transfusion reactions)
Physical examination	Vital signs, oral cavity, chest, heart, and abdomen
Laboratory[a]	Hematocrit, urinalysis (dipstick only), ECG (some cases >age 35), serum potassium concentration in some cases, pregnancy test[b]

[a]Basic evaluation for screening and baseline data. Other tests may be added to evaluate risk factors, known disease in a patient or to follow up findings in the preoperative history and physical examination; see also Table 93.3.
[b]Women in child-bearing age group.
HPI, history of present illness; ROS, review of symptoms; ECG, electrocardiogram.

TABLE 93.3 Additional Preoperative Screening Tests for Common High-Risk Situations

High-risk Situation	*Screening Tests*
Patient undergoing neurosurgical, cardiac, vascular, or major abdominal procedure	Tests of hemostasis: platelet count, prothrombin time, partial thromboplastin time
Patient taking diuretics, with vomiting/diarrhea, other abnormal fluid loss, cardiac disease, renal disease	Electrolytes, SUN, creatinine
Patient with increased risk of active liver disease (e.g., alcoholism, drug addiction, homosexuality, dialysis, high-risk medications) who is undergoing general or spinal anesthesia	Liver function tests: serum aminotransferases, alkaline phosphatase, bilirubin, serology for hepatitis B, C
Patient where presence or severity of pulmonary disease not certain; high risk surgery for pulmonary complications	Pulmonary function tests (spirometry)
Patient with increased risk of tuberculosis (e.g., known exposure, HIV positive, underprivileged population)	Chest radiograph, purified protein derivative skin test for TB
Patient with increased risk of coronary artery disease (i.e., smoker, hypertensive, strong family history, diabetic, hyperlipidemia)	ECG
Malnourished patient or prolonged inability to eat	Nutritional assessment

SUN, serum urea nitrogen; HIV, human immunodeficiency virus; TB; tuberculosis; ECG; electrocardiogram.

in the past. Additional items in the history or examination should be asked or done based on the patient's history, risk factors, and type of surgery. Additional tests are added as indicated by the individual patient's medical and surgical problems or risk factors. Selected screening tests should also be added to the workup to avoid potential catastrophes associated with certain high-risk situations (Table 93.3). Routine HIV screening of preoperative patients is currently not recommended; instead, the universal precautions described in Chapter 39 are recommended.

A common approach is to use a grid to select tests based on individual patient characteristics and type of surgery (3). A number of such grids have been published, but recommendations are not uniform (1). Most hospitals or surgical centers have their own grids, which either are sent by the surgical center with the request for preoperative evaluation or may be requested by the referring practitioner. Because of nonuniformity of recommendations, the primary care practitioner should review the grid.

Table 93.4 lists *commonly overlooked aspects of evaluation* and planning in the assessment of the outpatient presurgical patient.

TABLE 93.4 Commonly Forgotten or Underestimated Items in the Office Evaluation and Management of the Surgical Patient

Evaluation
One disease (review the problem list)
The generally sick patient (patient sicker than any one disease alone)
Inquiry about current medications (e.g. aspirin, other over-the-counter [OTC] medications, herbal supplements)
Blood tests indicated by specific medical disease or medications (e.g., drug levels, potassium for diuretics)
Inquiry about abnormal bleeding problems or disorders
Inquiry about history of transfusion or transfusion reactions
Inquiry about current use of alcohol or illicit drugs
Pregnancy test (serum qualitative human chorionic gonadotropin)
Spirometry (indications given under chronic obstructive lung disease)
Echocardiogram (to clarify the need for subacute bacterial endocarditis prophylaxis)
Management
Telling patient to report even minor intercurrent illnesses between physical and day of surgery
Telling patient to stop smoking, drinking alcohol, taking illicit drugs, OTC medications (and no new OTC medications)(see Table 93.6 for medications; smoking should stop 8 weeks before admission; alcohol and illicit drugs 1 or more weeks preoperatively)
Perioperative management of medications (see Table 93.6): whether to take medications the morning of surgery and when to restart postoperatively. Discontinue certain medications (such as aspirin, warfarin). Coverage for corticosteroids if indicated.
Subacute bacterial endocarditis prophylaxis
Informing patient (briefly) what to expect preoperatively and postoperatively; whom to call if unexpected problems arise
Informing patient about, and planning several weeks in advance for, autologous transfusion

Adapted from Gross RJ, Caputo GM, eds. Medical consultation: the internist on surgical, obstetric, and psychiatric services. 3rd ed. Baltimore: Williams & Wilkins, 1998:38.

CURRENT MEDICATIONS AND KNOWN ALLERGIES

Any known drug allergies or adverse drug reactions, reactions to latex, radiocontrast, and prior local or general anesthesia should be included in the preoperative report. All prescribed and nonprescribed drugs that a patient is taking should be communicated to the responsible anesthesiologist, surgeon, or preoperative unit at the surgical center. Over-the-counter (OTC) medications and certain herbal supplements are particularly important. This information is critical for optimal perioperative management (Table 93.5). Some drugs may have to be discontinued days to weeks in advance of surgery. Some are withheld immediately before surgery, whereas others are taken immediately preoperatively. Withholding of important medications may increase the postoperative medical complication rate, especially for cardiovascular medications (4). For most patients it is appropriate to give a dose of medication, with a small amount of water (1 ounce or less), in the early morning before the induction of anesthesia; there is little risk of aspiration as long as there is normal gastric emptying. Many patients can resume their oral medication 6 to 12 hours later. When important oral medications cannot be continued throughout the perioperative period, alternate medications or routes of administration are used.

In addition to the patient's list of current prescribed medications, the referring practitioner should remember to communicate important related information to the anesthesiologist, surgeon, or surgical center. The patient should be asked specifically about nonprescription drug use that, although common, is often not mentioned spontaneously (e.g., aspirin-containing compounds and nonsteroidal anti-inflammatory drugs [NSAIDs], which may potentiate postoperative bleeding, and sedatives, which may interact with anesthetic drugs); and herbal supplements. The use of recreational substances that may affect the patient's course during or after surgery (alcohol, tobacco, illicit drugs) should be documented. The following should also be noted: prior allergic reactions to local and general anesthetic agents (e.g., halothane) and to drugs used for medical conditions, prior reactions to blood products, and a family history of reactions to anesthesia or blood transfusions. Finally, chronic corticosteroid use at any time within the past year should be reported, because perioperative steroids may be required to cover the stresses of surgery.

TABLE 93.5 Recommended Perioperative Management of Medications[a]

Drug Class	Anticipated Problems	Recommended Perioperative Management
Analgesics		
Narcotics	Decreased cough reflex, increased CNS depression by anesthesia, hypotension	Inform anesthesiologist of use.
Aspirin compounds[b]	Increased bleeding	Discontinue 1–2 weeks before surgery.
NSAIDs	Gastrointestinal tract bleeding	Discontinue 1–2 weeks preoperatively.
Antibiotics		
Tetracycline	Risk of renal failure if given with methoxyflurane	Use alternative antibiotic or anesthetic.
Anticoagulants, antiplatelet drugs		
Warfarin[b]	Increased bleeding	Discontinue 4–7 days before surgery, vitamin K_1 if needed, check prothrombin time before operation.
Aspirin, other NSAIDs, clopidogrel[b]		Discontinue aspirin and other NSAIDs 1 week before surgery; clopidogrel 2 weeks before surgery.
Bronchodilators		
Theophylline[b]	Inability to give orally	Switch to intravenous aminophylline.
β_2-Sympathomimetics[b]	Inability to give orally	Switch to aerosolized or subcutaneous beta-2 agent.
Cardiovascular		
Antihypertensives[b]	Interaction with anesthetics, hypotension	Inform anesthesiologist of use.
	Inability to give orally	Plan postoperative regimen with alternative agents if needed.
Antiarrhythmics[b]	Inability to give orally	ECG monitor in operating room and postoperatively, use alternative parenteral agents.
β-Blockers[b]	Myocardial depression, bradycardia	Continue intravenously, taper to lower dosage, or discontinue depending on circumstances.
Digoxin[b]	Toxicity	Obtain serum levels preoperatively.
	Inability to give orally	Give 75% of daily oral dosage of digoxin intravenously each day.
Long-acting oral nitrates[b]	Inability to give orally	Substitute transdermal nitroglycerine.
Corticosteroids[b]	Adrenal insufficiency	Plan coverage (with intravenous corticosteroids) adequate for the stress of surgery.
	Poor wound healing	Discuss with surgeon.
Diabetes		
Oral hypoglycemics[b]	Inability to give orally	Withhold a.m. of surgery; switch to insulin preoperatively in selected patients.
Sulfonylureas		
Thiazolidinediones		
Metformin[b]	Risk of lactic acidosis	Withhold 48 h pre- and postoperatively
Insulin[b]	Risk of hyperglycemia or hypoglycemia	Give one third to one half of usual dosage preoperatively.
Diuretics		
	Electrolyte abnormalities, hypotension, inability to give orally	Obtain electrolytes and check blood pressure (lying, standing) within 24 h preoperatively, use intravenous furosemide if needed.
Gastrointestinal		
Antacids[b]	Inability to give orally	Intravenous H_2 blockers, nasogastric suction (if patient has active peptic ulcer disease).
Gout		
Benemid, allopurinol	Inability to give orally	Observe, treat acute gout with intravenous colchicine.
Lipid lowering		
Lovastatin, other hydroxymethylglutaryl CoA reductase inhibitors	Rhabdomyolysis	? Discontinue preoperatively.
Gemfibrozil	Rhabdomyolysis	? Discontinue preoperatively.

(continued)

TABLE 93.5 (Continued) Recommended Perioperative Management of Medications[a]

Drug Class	*Anticipated Problems*	*Recommended Perioperative Management*
Neurologic		
Levodopa/carbidopa[b]	Interaction with anesthetics (hypertension or hypotension), inability to give orally	Inform anesthesiologist of use; check with anesthesiologist on whether can be given preoperatively, resume orally as soon as possible after surgery.
Barbiturates	Increased CNS depression by anesthesia, inability to give orally	Inform anesthesiologist of use; give daily dosage intramuscularly.
Dilantin	Inability to give orally	Give daily dosage slowly intravenously (or substitute phenobarbital before admitting patient for surgery).
Psychiatric		
Antidepressants[b]	Hypotension or hypertension, arrhythmias	Inform anesthesiologist of use; withhold monoamine oxidase inhibitors 2 weeks preoperatively; selectively withhold other agents 24 h preoperatively.
Neuroleptics (e.g., phenothiazines and haloperidol)[b]	Arrhythmias, enhancement of neuromuscular blocking agents, hypotension	Inform anesthesiologist of use; withhold 24 h preoperatively in some cases.
Benzodiazepines	Increased CNS depression by anesthesia	Inform anesthesiologist of use.
Lithium[b]	Myocardial depression, hypernatremia	Inform anesthesiologist of use: determine blood levels; withhold 24 h preoperatively; avoid diuretics and NSAIDs; follow electrolytes closely.
Recreational drugs		
Alcohol Illicit drugs Tobacco[b]	Affect drug metabolism, drug interactions, withdrawal syndrome, impaired respiratory function Increased bronchospasm, secretions	If possible, have patient discontinue use 1 or more weeks before admission for surgery; inform anesthesiologist and surgeon of recent use.
Thyroid therapy		
Thyroid hormone[b]	Inability to give orally	Usually can be discontinued for up to 7–10 days.
Antithyroid drugs[b]	Inability to give orally	Use parenteral iodides or propranolol if necessary.
Topical drugs for glaucoma		
Timolol	Systemic β-blockage	Notify anesthesiologist preoperatively.
Phospholine iodide	Prolonged muscle relaxant activity	Discontinued 7–10 days preoperatively.

[a]Most maintenance medications should be given with a small amount of water early in the A.M. (e.g., 6 A.M.) before anesthesia. If unable to take orally on the day of surgery, options are intravenous medication or to give orally within 12 h postoperatively.
[b]See additional details in subsequent sections of this chapter.
CNS, central nervous system; NSAIDs, nonsteroidal anti-inflammatory drugs; ECG, electrocardiogram.

PREOPERATIVE DONATION FOR AUTOLOGOUS TRANSFUSION

Donation of one or more units of autologous blood for transfusion for elective surgery is now widely practiced. The risks of autologous transfusion are lower than the risks with bank blood, but bacterial contamination and transfusion of the wrong unit remain small possibilities.

Current blood preservation methods limit autologous donation to about three units. Single units are donated beginning about 4 weeks before surgery, at weekly intervals. In preoperative planning, it is important to leave sufficient time for donation of the required units but not so much time that the units expire if there is a minor delay in the scheduled surgery. Usually this is arranged by the surgeon, but the patient's primary care practitioner may want to discuss this option with the patient, including the time necessary (depending on the number of units needed) and any medical contraindications or limitations to autologous donations.

Medical problems that are potential contraindications or that limit the number of units donated (depending on the severity of the situation) include anemia, cardiovascular disease, hypertension and antihypertensive medication, lung disease with significant hypoxia, orthostatic hypotension, certain infectious diseases (including hepatitis and HIV infection), very frail or debilitated patients, and far advanced age. Despite this list of limitations, most patients, including most elderly patients with chronic diseases, are able to donate blood for autologous transfusion. The patient's practitioner may want to plan for partial volume repletion with saline at the time of donation for some patients who may be very sensitive to the volume loss. Most patients are prescribed iron (see Chapter 55) beginning about 1 week before the first donation and continuing for 2 to 3 months after donation (depending on the number of units donated). Some surgeons administer erythropoietin preoperatively to limit the degree of postoperative anemia, although the utility of this approach is not yet well established.

SURGERY IN THE ELDERLY PATIENT

Risk

The mortality risk associated with anesthesia and surgery is increased in the elderly. However, the risk in elderly patients has fallen substantially over the past 10 to 20 years. The overall mortality risk for major surgery in patients younger than 65 is approximately 1%; the risk is approximately 5% between ages 65 and 80. Patients older than the age of 80 years have a 10% risk, although mortality rates as low as 6% to 8% have been reported (1,6,7).

Several factors are more important than age itself in increasing surgical risk in older patients (7). The most important of these factors are general overall health, nutrition, type of surgery (body cavity versus non–body cavity; emergency versus elective), type of anesthesia, coexisting conditions (cardiac, infectious, renal, pulmonary, central nervous system [CNS]), and psychosocial status (attitude toward surgery, will to live, cognitive level, social situation). Common perioperative causes of death include uncorrectable surgical lesions such as infarcted bowel or ruptured aneurysm, coexisting cardiac disease, infections (especially pneumonia), renal disease, and pulmonary disease. In the preoperative evaluation, attention should be focused on managing or preventing these conditions.

Certain common procedures can be performed at low risk in the elderly, often without general anesthesia. These low-risk operations include cataract surgery, simple hernia repair, and transurethral prostate resection. The risks of some major surgical procedures in the elderly have fallen greatly over the past few years; examples include elective abdominal aortic aneurysm repair and repair of hip fractures. Laparoscopic surgery, such as for cholecystectomy, produces fewer medical complications but has not yet been shown to be associated with a lower mortality rate than does open surgery in the elderly.

Perioperative Management

The elderly patient undergoing major surgery may require a more extensive preoperative evaluation than given in Table 93.2 because of the wide variety of coexisting, often unrecognized, medical conditions found in older patients. The workup should be reviewed specifically for the risk factors listed above. Any major preoperative risks must be weighed against the benefits of the operation, with attention to the fact that quality of life may be as important as longevity in this age group. An accurate estimation of average future longevity for the patient's age group is important; this is often underestimated (see Chapter 12, Table 12.1).

Preoperative cardiac evaluation is discussed in Patients with Cardiovascular Disease. Manifestations of infection (including simple upper respiratory infections) should be carefully sought because classic signs may not be present in the elderly. Spirometry should be performed in patients older than age 65 if there is pulmonary disease, because of the increased incidence of pulmonary complications in older patients. It should be remembered that serum creatinine may be falsely low in elderly patients because of their reduced muscle mass; therefore, a calculated or measured creatinine clearance should be obtained if the state of the patient's renal function is not certain, because of the importance in determining drug dosages. If there is hearing impairment caused by cerumen impaction preoperatively, this problem should be corrected.

Elderly patients often have limitations of understanding because of memory deficits and hearing problems. Because these are often known to the primary care practitioner, informing the surgeon, anesthesiologist, and surgical center of these limitations can improve communication and management at each of these levels. A baseline mental status examination (see Chapter 26) should be completed because postoperative changes in mental status are common in the elderly. Explanation of what to expect during hospitalization and surgery is especially important in the elderly not only because of the above factors, but because elderly patients may be less likely to ask questions of the surgeon and may have outdated conceptions of the nature of surgery.

Simple measures planned before admission may help reduce the high incidence of *postoperative confusion* in older patients, including correction of reversible hearing or vision deficits, planning to allow family members to stay beyond visiting hours, avoiding placing the patient unnecessarily in an intensive care unit, returning the patient to the same room postoperatively, allowing the presence of familiar objects, leaving a night-light on, and avoiding unnecessary instrumentation. Early mobilization, uninterrupted sleep, and frequent orientation to time, place, and current events are also important. Tranquilizers, sedatives, hypnotics, and pain medications should be used in reduced dosages and for appropriate indications, not routinely.

Postoperative mobilization of the elderly patient should be planned and anticipated by the patient, preoperatively. Generally, the patient should expect to resume ambulation as early as possible.

SURGERY IN THE PREGNANT PATIENT

Risk

Up to 2% of women require nonobstetric surgery during pregnancy. Risks posed to the mother and fetus include complications from the surgical problem, effects of anesthesia and medication (including teratogenicity), risks of radiographs and other diagnostic procedures, precipitation of premature labor, and fetal death. Because of these problems, women of child-bearing age who are not known to be pregnant should be screened for pregnancy before surgery. History and sensitive serum human chorionic gonadotropin pregnancy tests usually suffice, but very early pregnancy may still be missed. If it is uncertain whether a woman is pregnant, nonurgent surgery should be postponed for 2 to 3 weeks until the situation is clarified; more urgent surgery requires judgment on an individual basis.

Table 93.6 lists physiologic alterations in pregnancy that may complicate anesthetic and surgical management. Two common changes of pregnancy should be taken into account when evaluating the patient preoperatively: The normal serum creatinine concentration is lower in pregnancy and an S3 gallop, systolic murmur, or edema is commonly present in the pregnant patient without cardiac disease.

Perioperative Management

Preoperative planning and perioperative management for the pregnant surgical patient involves a number of complex issues, considered below.

Urgency

Can the surgery be postponed until after delivery or is it urgent (e.g., acute appendicitis), when delay will increase fetal–maternal mortality? Generally, emergency surgery should not be delayed because of pregnancy, but totally elective surgery should be postponed until the postpartum period. In intermediate situations, the duration and risk to the mother of waiting must be balanced against the risk of immediate surgery.

Testing

Tests should be carefully planned to allow a precise diagnosis with minimal risk, especially risk from radiograph exposure. Whenever possible, other tests should be substituted for radiologic procedures (e.g., renal sonogram instead of computed tomography [CT] scan in suspected renal disease). Routine radiographs, such as chest films or flat abdominal films, should be avoided. When these radiographs are unavoidable, use of lead screening, collimated equipment with minimal exposure, and few films can minimize fetal exposure.

TABLE 93.6 Physiologic Alterations in Pregnancy and Their Relevance to the Surgical Patient

System	Change	Clinical Implications
Cardiovascular	Uterine compression of vena cava and aorta in supine position	Decreased cardiac output and uterine perfusion; avoid supine recumbency; tilt hips 15 degrees in perioperative period.
	Decrease in blood pressure in early to midgestation	Altered criteria for diagnosis of hypotension.
	Presence of dyspnea, third heart sound, and edema	No known increased risk, and such findings are not an indication for diuretic therapy or delay of surgery.
Respiratory	Decreased arterial PO_2 when patient is in the supine position	Avoid supine recumbency.
	Decreased pulmonary functional residual capacity and increased O_2 consumption	Increased risk of hypoxia perioperatively; avoid hypoventilation and increase inspired O_2 content before procedures inducing apnea (intubation or tracheal suctioning).
	Arterial PCO_2 and serum HCO_3 decrease to 30 mm Hg and 20 mmol per L, respectively	Maternal and fetal acidosis may occur in patient ventilated to "normal," nonpregnant values of arterial PCO_2; normal values for pregnancy should be used to guide diagnosis and therapy of acid-base disturbances.
Hematologic	Decreased venous flow in legs and increased levels of clotting factors	Increased risk of thromboembolism; avoid supine position and consider use of support stockings or pneumatic compression device.
	Proximity of fetal and maternal circulations	Risk of isoimmunization; Rh0(D) immune globulin should be considered when uterine trauma is likely.
Gastrointestinal	Decreased gastric motility and reduced competency of gastroesophageal sphincter	Increased risk of aspiration; preoperative antacids should be considered.
Renal	Dilation of urinary collecting system	Increased risk of urinary infection, so catheterization should be avoided when possible.
	30% to 50% increase in glomerular filtration rate and renal plasma flow with a concomitant decrease in serum creatinine and urea nitrogen to 0.5 and 9 mg per dL, respectively	Serum creatinine above 0.8 mg per dL may reflect impaired renal function; the clearance of many drugs is increased, and dosage schedules may require alteration.

From Barron WM. The pregnant surgical patient: medical evaluation and management. Ann Intern Med 1984;101:683.

Medications

Drugs required during the perioperative period should be anticipated. The potential effects on the fetus should be ascertained from obstetric colleagues or available reference sources, and the least toxic alternative should be used. Postoperative medications should be avoided unless they are deemed to be necessary and risk to the fetus has been assessed.

Anesthesia

A decision on the type of anesthesia must be left to the anesthesiologist and obstetrician. Local or regional anesthesia would presumably be safer than general or spinal anesthesia, but no data exist to support this impression.

Monitoring of Fetal Status

Monitoring of fetal status by the obstetrician should be planned throughout the perioperative period.

PROBLEMS AFTER DISCHARGE

During the weeks and months after surgery, patients often have questions about incisional pain, various symptoms in the system that was operated on, restrictions of activity, and return to work. These questions are best answered by the surgeon. Additionally, patients who have major surgery often complain of postoperative fatigue, a problem that can usually be handled by the patient's primary care practitioner.

Postoperative Fatigue

Patients with postoperative fatigue may describe a number of symptoms, including the need for increased sleep, weakness of the arms and legs when resuming usual activity, symptoms of orthostatic hypotension, and loss of interest in resuming usual activities (8). The symptoms of postoperative fatigue often last for 1 or more months. The physiologic changes responsible for these symptoms have not been well defined.

The primary care practitioner should also be aware of specific, often treatable, conditions that may contribute to or cause postoperative fatigue. Sleepiness may be related to sedatives, tranquilizers, or analgesics prescribed at the time of discharge and may improve with discontinuation of these drugs. The patient with orthostatic symptoms may have had a drug prescribed that can produce this problem (diuretics, antihypertensives, long-acting nitrates, antidepressants). Because bed rest alone may cause orthostasis, such drugs should be resumed cautiously in a patient who has had recent major surgery, and blood pressure should be checked in the lying and standing positions. Dosage reduction or discontinuation of the drug should be considered when orthostatic hypotension is documented or orthostatic symptoms persist. Loss of interest may also be secondary to drugs prescribed after surgery (see Chapter 24 for a list of drugs that may cause a depressed mood). Alternatively, this symptom may represent a minor mood disturbance in a patient who has had similar problems at previous times of stress (see Chapter 21), or it may represent a reactive depression, similar to a grief reaction (see Chapter 24), that is related to disfiguring surgery. Because other medical problems related to surgery may occasionally cause postoperative fatigue, a hematocrit value, serum urea nitrogen or creatinine, electrolytes, glucose, liver enzymes, and other tests indicated by clinical findings should be checked if fatigue persists.

When evaluation of postoperative fatigue does not disclose contributing factors that can be treated, patients should be reassured that the problem will gradually resolve; they should also be given a rough timetable for a return to regular activities that is realistic in terms of both the surgical procedure and the fact that postoperative fatigue may take a number of months to resolve entirely. Chapter 89 illustrates simple exercises for patients convalescing from bed rest. For selected patients, these or similar exercises can be recommended during the period of recovery from postoperative fatigue.

PATIENTS WITH CARDIOVASCULAR DISEASE

Most forms of general anesthesia can cause cardiovascular stresses (decreased myocardial contractility, peripheral vasodilatation, arrhythmias, hypotension), and spinal or epidural anesthesia can cause hypotension. These factors and the stresses associated with surgery itself probably account for the greatly increased risk of surgery for patients with underlying cardiovascular disease (9).

Ischemic Heart Disease

Risk

Ischemic heart disease poses four major risks perioperatively in the patient undergoing general anesthesia: myocardial infarction (MI), ischemic pulmonary edema, life-threatening arrhythmias, and cardiac death. These risks depend on the patient's preoperative status. Overall, the risks for patients with arteriosclerotic heart disease are two or three times those of patients of the same age without cardiac disease; patients who have had a prior MI may be at particularly increased risk.

The increased risk posed by ischemic heart disease is partially dependent on the patient's preoperative cardiac status. Stable mild to moderate angina pectoris alone represents only a small increase in risk. The risk attending severe or unstable angina cannot be estimated accurately because of varying definitions and the small number of patients reported in the medical literature, but there is a significantly increased risk. An MI during the 6 months preceding surgery represents a high risk, particularly an MI 3 months or less before surgery. There is some evidence (9,10) that aggressive perioperative management may significantly lower cardiovascular risk (e.g., reduce recurrent MI risk from 30% to 4%). By 6 months after an infarction, the risk of a perioperative MI has plateaued but remains larger than the risk in a control population.

In addition to a recent MI, a number of factors contribute to the risk of perioperative cardiac complications or mortality. The most important of these factors are age older than 70, decompensated congestive heart failure (CHF), arrhythmias, and other organ system disease (11–16). These and other factors were incorporated in 1977 into a Cardiac Risk Index; in 1986 into a Modified Cardiac Risk Index; and in 1999 into a Revised (Simple) Cardiac Risk Index (Table 93.7), all of which have been validated (11–14). The Revised Cardiac Risk Index is used here because it performed slightly to moderately better than the other indices in a single prospective study (14).

The joint American College of Cardiology/American Heart Association (ACC/AHA) Task Force on perioperative cardiovascular evaluation also provided a qualitative index of cardiac risk ("Clinical Predictors") (Table 93.8) (15).

Two algorithms are available (15,16) that provide guidelines on diagnostic and therapeutic approaches (7) based on a patient's level of cardiac risk established by one of the indices. The algorithms were established by expert consensus; neither has been validated. The ACC/AHA algorithm (Fig. 93.1) (15) is used here since it has been updated more recently than the other algorithm from the American College of Physicians (ACP).

Clinical assessment of the cardiac patient is approximately 75% sensitive for detecting high-risk patients. In intermediate- or high-risk *vascular surgery patients,* dipyridamole–thallium or other types of stress tests can accurately identify those with ischemia who have an increased operative risk. In nonvascular surgery patients, the usefulness of preoperative stress testing for risk assessment has not been definitely demonstrated (15). Detailed discussion of the use of noninvasive testing for preoperative decision-making is contained in the ACC/AHA guidelines and in other publications (9,15,16).

TABLE 93.7 Revised (Simple) Cardiac Risk Index[a]

Risk Factors	*Points*
History of ischemic heart disease	1
History of congestive heart failure	1
History of cerebrovascular disease	1
High risk type of surgery	1
Preoperative treatment with insulin	1
Preoperative serum creatinine >2.0 mg/dL	1

[a]Class I, 0 points; class II, 1 point; class III, 2 points; class IV, 3 or more points.

From Lee TH, Marcantonio ER, Mangione CM, et al. Derivation and prospective validation of a simple index for prediction of cardiac risk of major noncardiac surgery. Circulation 1999;100:1043.

TABLE 93.8 Clinical Predictors of Cardiac Risk (from ACC/AHA Guidelines)

Major

Unstable coronary syndrome
—Acute or recent myocardial infarction with evidence of important ischemic risk by clinical symptoms or noninvasive study.
—Unstable or severe angina (Canadian class III or IV)*
Decompensated heart failure
Significant arrhythmias (high grade atrioventricular block; symptomatic ventricular arrhythmias with underlying heart disease; supraventricular arrhythmias with uncontrolled ventricular rate)
Severe valvular heart disease

Intermediate

Mild angina pectoris (Canadian class I or II)
Previous myocardial infarction by history or pathological Q waves
Compensated or prior heart failure
Diabetes mellitus (particularly insulin dependent)
Renal insufficiency

Minor

Advanced age
Abnormal ECG (left ventricular hypertrophy, LBBB, ST-T abnormalities)
Rhythm other than sinus
Low functional capacity (e.g. inability to climb 1 flight stairs with a bag of groceries)
History of stroke
Uncontrolled systemic hypertension

*Severe angina may include "stable" angina in unusually sedentary patients.

Adapted from ACC/AHA Task Force. Guidelines for perioperative cardiovascular evaluation for noncardiac surgery. J Am Coll Cardiol 2002;39:546.

Perioperative Management

Patients with established ischemic heart disease should have a preoperative evaluation (Table 93.2) with emphasis on established cardiac risks for surgery. A *baseline electrocardiogram (ECG)* should be obtained before surgery for all patients with known coronary artery disease (CAD) and for all patients older than 40 to 50 years of age. Noninvasive tests of cardiac function, including echocardiography, nuclear scanning, and stress tests, should generally be reserved for situations where the evidence for the presence or severity of cardiovascular disease is questioned or in certain high-risk situations, such as vascular surgery, where precise information about the degree of severity is desired (see above).

Based on the preoperative evaluation, the risk of general anesthesia and surgery should be estimated for each patient. For patients with an MI within the last 6 months, unstable angina, or less severe CAD and multiple other risk factors (Fig. 93.1 and Tables 93.7 and 93.8), only urgent life-saving surgery should be undertaken until the risk is lowered. Surgery may be done 3 months after infarction when the risk of waiting the additional 3 months is thought to be significant (e.g., recurrent cholecystitis). Patients with stable angina or uncomplicated recovery from MI more than 6 months previously have a small increase in risk that does not decline further with time; thus, there is no need to postpone necessary operations.

Coronary artery bypass surgery or angioplasty should be considered before elective noncardiac surgery, in consultation with a cardiologist, in patients who have other indications for coronary revascularization (see Chapter 62). Although guidelines do not generally recommend bypass surgery or angioplasty prophylactically before noncardiac surgery without other indications, these interventions may need to be considered in an occasional high risk patient. Coronary revascularization in stable non–high-risk patients with CAD undergoing vascular surgery has not been shown to lower cardiac morbidity and mortality (17). Assessing the benefit of coronary angioplasty and stenting before noncardiac surgery is complicated by the need for anticoagulation with antiplatelet agents for 1 month to 1 year or more depending on the type of procedure (18).

Postoperative ECGs should be obtained in high-risk patients, (e.g., those with known CAD or who develop hypotension during surgery.) The yield of useful information from postoperative ECGs is low in low and intermediate risk patients.

For patients taking a long-acting oral nitrate for angina, the drug should be administered on the morning of surgery with a sip of water. If the patient is unable to take medications orally, nitroglycerin paste or a transdermal patch can be substituted at a dosage equivalent to the oral nitrate (or by using an intermediate dose equivalent to 1 to 2 inches of paste every 4 to 6 hours).

For patients taking a β-blocking agent for CAD, small intravenous dosages of an intermediate duration β-blocker (such as propranolol or metoprolol titrated to maintain a pulse of ≤80) can be substituted, while the patient is unable to take medications by mouth. This requires cardiac monitoring, usually in an intensive care unit. This should protect the patient from the risk of acute cardiac ischemia, which occasionally follows abrupt cessation of β-blocking agents. Patients able to resume oral intake within 12 to 24 hours and not at high cardiac risk usually can be observed without intravenous β-blockers, particularly if a long acting β-blocker was administered preoperatively.

For patients who are not already taking a β-blocking agent, who have CAD, who are intermediate to high risk, and who are undergoing major surgery, a β-blocker should be started preoperatively and continued during the perioperative period, based on a randomized controlled trial (RCT) (19). Although only patients undergoing vascular surgery were studied, it is reasonable to extend the use of β-blockers to other major surgery until data are available. The authors recommended a β-blocker dose sufficient preoperatively to lower the heart rate to less than 70 beats per minute in the immediate postoperative period and to less than 80 beats per minute (19); this degree of β-blockade may not be achievable in some patients. β-Blockers should be initiated 1 to 2 weeks preoperatively and the patient's response evaluated in the office before surgery. Consideration should be given to chronic β-blockers after surgery because of their efficacy in coronary disease (see Chapters 62 and 63). If β-blockers are not going to be continued indefinitely for chronic indications, they should be continued for a minimum of 2 to 4 weeks postoperatively, longer if there are ongoing cardiac stresses, and then tapered.

Calcium-blocking agents can usually be given on the morning of surgery. Another type of antianginal medication can be used postoperatively until the patient can resume oral intake. Diltiazem and verapamil are available in intravenous form, but maintenance regimens are not established and the cost is high.

Intensive intraoperative monitoring using pulmonary artery and radial artery catheters should be planned in consultation with the anesthesiologist and surgeon for patients who are very sensitive to volume changes, such as those in CHF (see Congestive Heart Failure); for operations when loss and replacement of large volumes of fluid are expected (e.g., aneurysm repair); and for patients with a recent MI (less than 6 months), severe unstable coronary disease, or at very high risk. Routine invasive monitoring of unselected high-risk patients has not been shown to lower perioperative risk.

Hypertension

Risk

Controversy still exists about whether mild to moderate hypertension (diastolic blood pressures less than 110 mm Hg) increases anesthetic and surgical risks. The only prospective study showed no correlation between uncontrolled diastolic pressures in this range and the risk of perioperative cardiac, renal, or cerebrovascular events (20). Patients in this study often had other cardiac risk factors that did correlate with the incidence of perioperative cardiac morbidity (Table 93.10).

Too few patients have been studied to define adequately the risk for patients operated on when their diastolic pressure exceeds 110 mm Hg, but there is probably an increased risk (20). Likewise, risk is probably increased in selected patients with hypertension who also have significant cardiac, renal, or cerebrovascular disease (CBV).

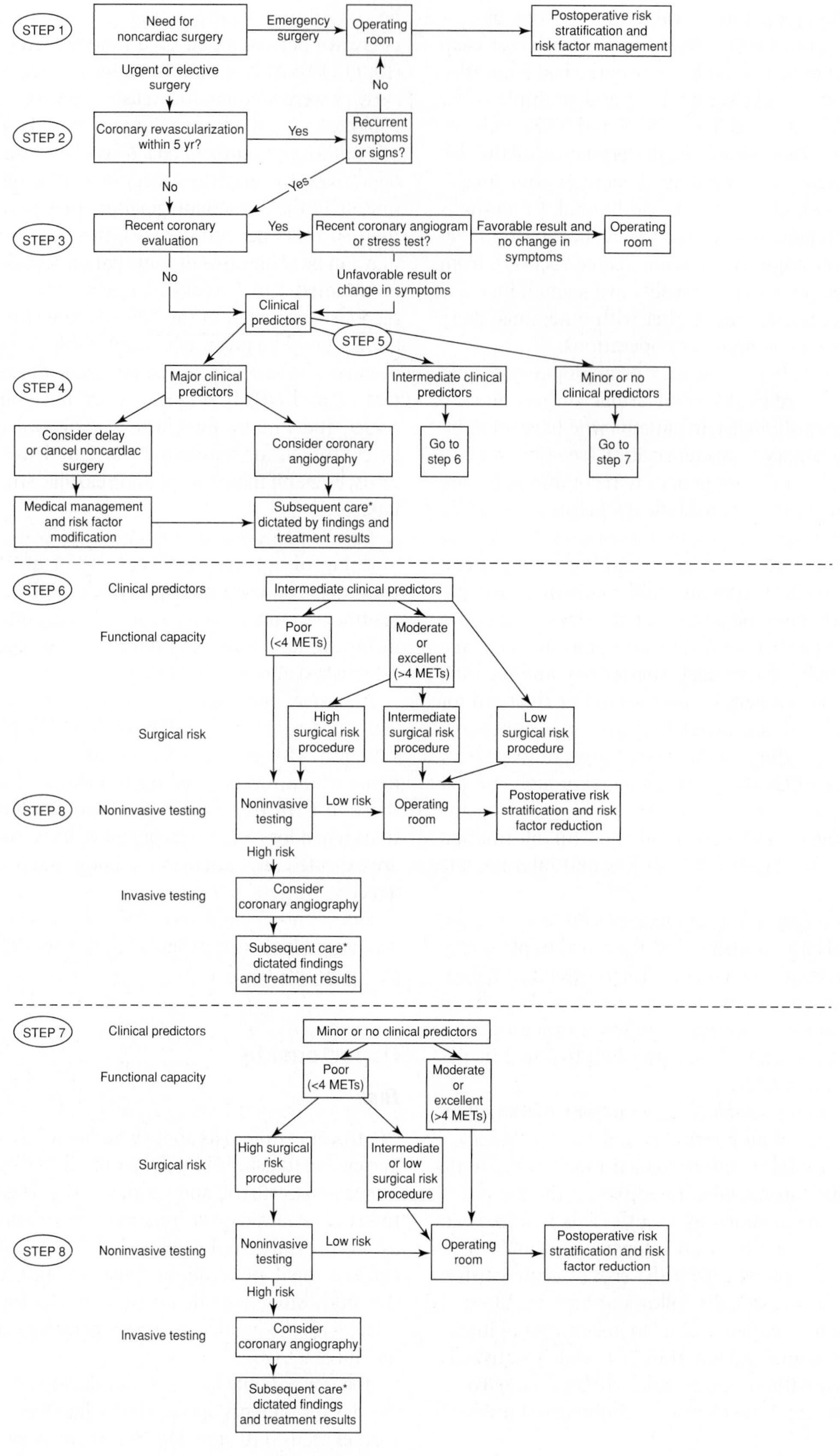
STEP 1
Need for noncardiac surgery
Emergency surgery
Operating room
Postoperative risk stratification and risk factor management
Urgent or elective surgery
No
STEP 2
Coronary revascularization within 5 yr?
Yes
Recurrent symptoms or signs?
No
Yes
STEP 3
Recent coronary evaluation
Yes
Recent coronary angiogram or stress test?
Favorable result and no change in symptoms
Operating room
No
Unfavorable result or change in symptoms
Clinical predictors
STEP 5
STEP 4
Major clinical predictors
Intermediate clinical predictors
Minor or no clinical predictors
Consider delay or cancel noncardiac surgery
Consider coronary angiography
Go to step 6
Go to step 7
Medical management and risk factor modification
Subsequent care* dictated by findings and treatment results
STEP 6
Clinical predictors
Intermediate clinical predictors
Functional capacity
Poor (<4 METs)
Moderate or excellent (>4 METs)
Surgical risk
High surgical risk procedure
Intermediate surgical risk procedure
Low surgical risk procedure
STEP 8
Noninvasive testing
Noninvasive testing
Low risk
Operating room
Postoperative risk stratification and risk factor reduction
High risk
Invasive testing
Consider coronary angiography
Subsequent care* dictated findings and treatment results
STEP 7
Clinical predictors
Minor or no clinical predictors
Functional capacity
Poor (<4 METs)
Moderate or excellent (>4 METs)
Surgical risk
High surgical risk procedure
Intermediate or low surgical risk procedure
STEP 8
Noninvasive testing
Noninvasive testing
Low risk
Operating room
Postoperative risk stratification and risk factor reduction
High risk
Invasive testing
Consider coronary angiography
Subsequent care* dictated findings and treatment results

TABLE 93.9 Cardiac Risk[a] Stratification of Noncardiac Surgical Procedures

High (reported cardiac risk often >5%)
Emergent major operations, particularly in the elderly
Aortic and other major vascular
Peripheral vascular
Anticipated prolonged surgical procedures associated with large fluid shifts or blood loss
Intermediate (reported cardiac risk generally <5%)
Carotid endarterectomy
Head and neck
Intraperitoneal and intrathoracic
Orthopedic
Prostate
Low[b] (reported cardiac risk generally <1%)
Endoscopic procedures
Superficial procedure
Cataract
Breast

[a]Combined incidence of cardiac death and nonfatal myocardial infarction.
[b]Do not generally require further preoperative cardiac testing.
From ACC/AHA Task Force. Guidelines for perioperative cardiovascular evaluation for noncardiac surgery. J Am Coll Cardiol 2002;39:547.

Perioperative Management

The basic preoperative evaluation in the hypertensive patient should establish whether there is end-organ damage (renal: serum creatinine concentration and urinalysis; cerebrovascular: history, neurologic, and neurovascular examination; cardiovascular: history, cardiac examination, chest radigoraph, and ECG). Blood pressure and pulse measurements should be made with the patient lying, sitting, and standing (and after brief exercise, to identify the maximal orthostatic fall in patients taking antihypertensive drugs); the preoperative status of blood pressure control may then be classified as untreated, hypertensive despite therapy, or controlled. The antihypertensive medications being given should be reviewed and evaluated for side effects, particularly orthostatic hypotension, electrolyte disturbances, and changes in renal function (especially with diuretics, angiotensin-converting enzyme [ACE] inhibitors, and angiotensin receptor blockers [ARBs]).

Patients whose hypertension is controlled or partially controlled with diastolic pressures 110 mm Hg or lower should be continued on their prescribed antihypertensive and other medications. Three exceptions to this rule are reserpine, guanethidine, and monoamine oxidase inhibitors (MAOI). A patient taking any of these infrequently used drugs should be switched to different drugs during the 2 weeks preceding surgery, because each of these drugs may cause markedly labile blood pressure during anesthesia.

Untreated patients with diastolic pressures 110 mm Hg or lower may undergo surgery, with institution of antihypertensive therapy after convalescence from surgery, if there are no other complicating cardiovascular risks. Alternatively, as long as adequate time is allowed to measure full effects of antihypertensive medication, there is no reason not to treat hypertension preoperatively. Because for most antihypertensive medications this requires several weeks, a decision may need to be made about delaying surgery versus instituting antihypertensives postoperatively.

Individual judgments must be made about patients with *diastolic pressures that are repeatedly above 110 mm Hg*, depending on the severity and duration of hypertension, the presence of end-organ damage, and the extent of planned surgery. Most patients with diastolic blood pressure above 110 mm Hg should have their blood pressure at least partly controlled before admission for nonurgent surgery, although there are no randomized studies proving that such control modifies risks. Attempts to control blood pressure too rapidly (e.g., with addition of or increases in doses of diuretics, ACE inhibitors, or ARBs over several days) may result in volume depletion, hypotension, or disturbances in electrolytes or renal function at the time of surgery. Therefore, these patients should have their blood pressure stabilized during the 1 to 2 weeks before admission for surgery. There are no data on the perioperative risk of isolated systolic hypertension, but it seems reasonable to aim for a systolic pressure of 160 mm Hg or below (see Chapter 67).

For all hypertensive patients, significant intravascular volume expansion or contraction should be avoided, because these conditions may either cause a significant rise in blood pressure (volume expansion) or fall in blood pressure (volume contraction, especially in the patient who is taking antihypertensive drugs).

Current antihypertensive medications should be continued through the morning of surgery (diuretics are usually withheld the morning of surgery) and resumed

FIGURE 93.1. ACC/AHA algorithm for diagnostic and therapeutic management based on patient cardiac risk. The ACC/AHA algorithm (Fig. 93.1) first addresses three factors (Steps 1–3): need for noncardiac surgery (emergency versus urgent/elective), coronary revascularization within 5 years, and recent coronary evaluation, any of which can lead directly to a cardiac work-up or surgery. If none of these factors is present, the algorithm divides depending on whether major, intermediate, or minor/no clinical predictors are present (Steps 4 and 5). Decision points for Steps 6–8 include functional status (less or more than 4 METS) and cardiac risk of the surgical procedure. The ACC/AHA algorithm gives an estimated cardiac risk for surgery (Table 93.9). From ACC/AHA Task Force. Guidelines for perioperative cardiovascular evaluation for noncardiac surgery. J Am Coll Cardiol 2002;39:545.
*Subsequent care may include cancellation or delay in surgery, coronary revascularization followed by noncardiac surgery, or intensified care.

TABLE 93.10 Risk of Perioperative Cardiac Complications in Patients with Mild to Moderate Hypertension

Preoperative Characteristics	*Mean Point Total[a] (± SEM)*	*Patients with No Cardiac Complication (%)*	*Patients with Minor Complications Only[b] (%)*	*Patients with Major Nonfatal Complications[c] (%)*	*Patients with Cardiac Death[c] (%)*
Normal blood pressure, no history of hypertension	4.3 ± (0.3)	89	9	2	0.2
Hypertension controlled, taking antihypertensive drug(s)	6.9 ± (0.6)	76	15	8	1
Hypertensive					
Taking antihypertensive drug(s)	4.4 ± (0.5)	93	8		1
Not taking antihypertensive drug(s)	5.5 ± (0.6)	88	9	1	1

[a]See reference 11.
[b]New or worse heart failure, supraventricular tachycardia, or intraoperative or postoperative ischemia (typical chest pain or electrocardiogram changes).
[c]Fatal events or life-threatening events (pulmonary edema, myocardial infarction, ventricular tachycardia).
Adapted from Goldman L, Caldera DL. Risks of general anesthesia and elective operation in the hypertensive patient. Anesthesiology 1979;50:285.

postoperatively when the patient is stable and can take oral medications. Because bed rest and inactivity during convalescence can lower blood pressure, some patients require less antihypertensive medication postoperatively and during the first few weeks after major surgery. Because antihypertensive effects may be amplified when a postoperative patient changes position from recumbent to standing, blood pressure should be measured in these positions postoperatively and after antihypertensive treatment has been instituted or resumed.

In some patients, the diastolic pressure exceeds 110 mm Hg postoperatively before oral medication can be resumed. When patients remain severely hypertensive despite control of secondary causes, such as pain, and the hypertension poses immediate health risks, the blood pressure can be controlled by the careful use of parenteral or transcutaneous agents. These include intravenous propranolol, labetalol, hydralazine, enalapril, diuretics, methyldopa, nitroprusside, intravenous or transcutaneous nitroglycerin, and transcutaneous clonidine (especially for patients who were taking clonidine before surgery who are at risk of rebound hypertension and tachycardia if clonidine is withdrawn).

Valvular Heart Disease

Risk

The risk of surgery in the patient with valvular heart disease varies with the valve affected (aortic versus mitral) and the nature (stenosis versus insufficiency) and severity of the lesion (9,12). The severity of valvular lesions as judged clinically by New York Heart Association classification (see Chapter 66) provides a reasonable indication of surgical risk except in patients with aortic stenosis.

Valvular heart disease poses *two major surgical risks: cardiac death and CHF*. The presence of aortic stenosis of any degree of hemodynamic significance poses a high risk of surgical mortality. Mild to moderate mitral lesions or aortic insufficiency pose only slightly increased risk of cardiac death; however, hemodynamically severe valvular disease (New York Heart Association class 3 or 4) caused by these lesions creates major risks. In addition to increasing the risk of perioperative mortality, significant valvular disease poses an increased risk of decompensated heart failure.

Little specific information exists regarding the risks associated with *prolapsed mitral valve* or *hypertrophic cardiomyopathy*. It is reasonable to assume that the risk in patients with prolapsed mitral valve depends on the degree of mitral regurgitation. Patients with hypertrophic cardiomyopathy may be very sensitive to volume contraction and are probably best managed with a pulmonary artery catheter in place during major procedures associated with rapid volume changes.

Patients with artificial heart valves, patients with any evidence of valvular heart disease (including mitral prolapse and hypertrophic cardiomyopathy), and patients with congenital structural defects (e.g., patent ductus arteriosus, ventricular septal defect) have a small but definite risk of acquiring *bacterial endocarditis* when they undergo procedures in the oral cavity and upper respiratory, gastrointestinal (GI), or genitourinary tracts (21).

Perioperative Management

The basic cardiac evaluation should delineate the nature and severity of the valvular disease and should identify any associated cardiac conditions. Chapter 65 describes the uses of echocardiography and cardiac catheterization to evaluate valvular heart disease. Patients with severe valvular disease should have corrective cardiac surgery followed by a period of convalescence before they undergo major elective noncardiac operations. The preoperative management of CHF, arrhythmia, or anticoagulant therapy (in patients with artificial valves) is described in subsequent sections of this chapter.

Patients with valvular disease undergoing procedures attended by a risk of *endocarditis* (Table 93.11) should receive *antimicrobial prophylaxis* (as summarized in Tables 93.11 and 93.12). The information in Table 93.12 is available from the AHA in a wallet-sized card for patients. These recommendations are not based on randomized controlled trials and should not be substituted for clinical judgment (21).

Congestive Heart Failure

Risk

Information on the risk of developing CHF perioperatively is limited because there have been few prospective studies (12–15). The most significant risk factors for postoperative CHF are decompensated failure preoperatively and, to a lesser extent, prior CHF that is clinically stable preoperatively (Table 93.13) (12–15). However, only 40% of patients who develop perioperative CHF have had prior failure. The best predictors for the other 60% of patients are older than 60 years of age, major surgery (especially abdominal aortic aneurysm repair or major abdominal surgery), and nonspecific ECG abnormalities.

Patients with postoperative pulmonary edema have a high total mortality (20% to 57%), most of which is cardiac. Patients who develop less severe postoperative CHF do not have an increased risk of postoperative cardiac death, although the overall mortality from all causes is increased. Most postoperative CHF occurs during or within several hours of surgery.

Perioperative Management

Patients with compensated CHF should have a preoperative evaluation (Table 93.2) with an emphasis on established cardiac risk factors for surgery. This evaluation should include an assessment of volume status (lying and standing blood pressures, inspection of neck veins, determination of whether edema is present) and examination for cardiac gallops and rales. Laboratory data should include blood urea nitrogen (BUN), creatinine, electrolytes, and a digoxin level if that drug is being administered. Noninvasive methods for assessing left ventricular function (see Chapter 66) may be useful when the degree of cardiac dysfunction is uncertain.

Although there are no definitive perioperative studies in this regard, it is prudent to administer digoxin to patients with a confirmed history of moderate or severe dilated congestive cardiomyopathy, ideally during the week before admission. Most controversy about preoperative digitalization has concerned the patient who has a history of no or minimal CHF, yet has a risk of developing CHF because of an enlarged heart or because the surgery will involve major volume shifts. Most experts do not recommend digoxin in

TABLE 93.11 Subacute Bacterial Endocarditis Prophylaxis: Recommendations for Procedures in the Respiratory, Gastrointestinal, and Genitourinary Tracts (See Recommended Antibiotic Regimens, Table 93.12)

Endocarditis prophylaxis recommended
Respiratory tract
Tonsillectomy or adenoidectomy
Surgical operations that involve respiratory mucosa
Bronchoscopy with a rigid bronchoscope
Gastrointestinal tract[a]
Sclerotherapy for esophageal varices
Esophageal stricture dilation
Endoscopic retrograde cholangiography with biliary obstruction
Biliary tract surgery
Surgical operations that involve intestinal mucosa
Genitourinary tract
Prostate surgery
Cytoscopy
Urethral dilation
Endocarditis prophylaxis not recommended
Respiratory tract
Endotracheal intubation
Bronchoscopy with a flexible bronchoscope, with or without biopsy[b]
Tympanostomy tube insertion
Gastrointestinal tract
Transesophageal echocardiography[b]
Endoscopy with or without gastrointestinal biopsy[b]
Genitourinary tract
Vaginal hysterectomy[b]
Vaginal delivery[b]
Cesarean section
In uninfected tissue
Urethral catheterization
Uterine dilation and curettage
Therapeutic abortion
Sterilization procedures
Insertion or removal of intrauterine devices
Other
Cardiac catheterization, including balloon angioplasty
Implanted cardiac pacemakers, implanted defibrillators, and coronary stents
Incision or biopsy of surgically scrubbed skin
Circumcision

[a]Prophylaxis is recommended for high-risk patients; optional for medium-risk patients.
[b]Prophylaxis is optional for high-risk patients.
From Dajani AS, Taubert KA, Wilson W, et al. Prevention of bacterial endocarditis. Recommendations by the American Heart Association. JAMA 1997;277:1794.

TABLE 93.12 Prevention of Bacterial Endocarditis in Patients with Valvular Heart Disease, Prosthetic Heart Valves, and Other Abnormalities of the Cardiovascular System

Situation	Antibiotic	Regimen[a]
	Dental, Oral, Respiratory Tract, or Esophageal Procedures	
Standard general prophylaxis	Amoxicillin	2.0 g 1 h before procedure
Unable to take oral medications	Ampicillin	2.0 g i.m. or i.v.. within 30 min before procedure
Allergic to penicillin	Clindamycin	600 mg orally 1 h before procedure
	or	
	Cephalexin or cefadroxil[b]	2.0 g orally 1 h before procedure
	or	
	Azithromycin or clarithromycin	500 mg orally 1 h before procedure
Allergic to penicillin and unable to take oral medications	Clindamycin	600 mg i.v. within 30 min before procedure
	or	
	Cefazolin[b]	1.0 g i.m. or i.v. within 30 min before procedure
	Genitourinary, Gastrointestinal (Excluding Esophageal) Procedures	
High-risk patients[c]	Ampicillin plus Gentamicin[d]	Ampicillin 2.0 g i.m. or i.v. plus gentamicin 1.5 mg/kg (not to exceed 120 mg) within 30 min of starting the procedure; 6 h later, ampicillin 1 g i.m./i.v. or amoxicillin 1 g orally
High-risk patients allergic to ampicillin/amoxicillin[c]	Vancomycin plus Gentamicin[d]	Vancomycin 1.0 g i.v. over 1–2 h plus gentamicin 1.5 mg/kg i.v./i.m. (not to exceed 120 mg); complete injection/infusion within 30 min of starting the procedure
Moderate-risk patients[c]	Amoxicillin or ampicillin	Amoxicillin 2.0 g orally 1 h before procedure, or ampicillin 2.0 g i.m./i.v. within 30 min of starting the procedure
Moderate-risk patients allergic to ampicillin/amoxicillin[c]	Vancomycin[c]	1.0 g i.v. over 1–2 h; complete infusion within 30 min of starting the procedure

[a]Regimens and dosages are for adults. For children's dosages see reference below.
[b]Cephalosporins should not be used in individuals with immediate-type hypersensitivity reaction (urticaria, angioedema, or anaphylaxis) to penicillins.
[c]High risk: prothestic heart valve, history of endocarditis, complex cyanotic congenital heart disease. Moderate risk: Uncorrected congenital conditions (patent ductus, ventricular septal defect, coarctation, bicuspid aortic valve); rheumatic valve disease; hypertrophic cardiomyopathy; prolapsing or leaking mitral valve (i.e., audible click and murmurs or Doppler-confirmed mitral insufficiency).
[d]No second dose of vancomycin or gentamicin is recommended.
Modified from Dajani AS, Taubert KA, Wilson W, et al. Prevention of bacterial endocarditis. Recommendations by the American Heart Association. JAMA 1997;277:1794.

this situation (15). In patients undergoing major surgery, spironolactone probably should be held the day the operation is performed because of the risk of hyperkalemia; it can be continued for those who undergo minor procedures that do not require general anesthesia. β-Blockers should be continued perioperatively, including a dose the morning of surgery and postoperatively. If the patient cannot take an oral β-blocker postoperatively, one should be given intravenously if CAD is present (see Ischemic Heart Disease); in patients without CAD the decision on intravenous β-blockers should be individualized.

Patients with decompensated CHF should have all but life-saving surgery postponed until the failure is controlled, either in the practitioner's office or in the hospital. Patients with controlled CHF should be maintained on their usual oral regimen until midnight before surgery and maintained with intravenous diuretics and digoxin (75% of the oral dosage) during the immediate postoperative period. Perioperative monitoring with a pulmonary artery catheter should be considered in advance in situations where large volume shifts are anticipated during surgery or the heart failure is severe or decompensated.

Arrhythmias

Chapter 64 describes in detail arrhythmias that are most common in ambulatory patients.

Risk

Patients with arrhythmias before surgery have significantly increased risks of cardiac morbidity and death. These risks have not been quantified for subgroups of patients with specific arrhythmias, except for the broad category of rhythms other than sinus or >5 premature

TABLE 93.13 Risks of Developing CHF in the Perioperative Period

	Size of Risk	
Patient Characteristics	**All CHF (%)**	**Pulmonary Edema (%)**
No prior CHF	4	2
Past CHF		
All–now compensated	16	6
Past pulmonary edema (regardless of current status)	32	23
Decompensated CHF preoperatively	21	16
Preoperative physical findings:		
S3 gallop	47	35
Jugular venous distension	35	30
NYHA class preoperatively (see Table 66.2)		
Class 1	5	3
Class 2	7	7
Class 3	18	6
Class 4	31	25

Table based on 1,001 consecutive patients undergoing general surgery, orthopedic surgery, or urologic surgery (transurethral resection of the prostate omitted because of existing evidence of its safety even in elderly patients).
CHF, congestive heart failure; NYHA, New York Heart Association.
Adapted from Goldman L, Caldera DL, Southwick FS, et al. Cardiac risk factors and complications in non-cardiac surgery. Medicine (Baltimore) 1978;57:357.

ventricular contractions (PVCs) on ECG (10,12). Patients with complete heart block, Mobitz type II second-degree block, and a few patients with sick sinus syndrome (see Chapter 64) have a significant risk of complications during anesthesia if a pacemaker is not inserted. On the other hand, there is little or no increased risk associated with bifascicular or trifascicular block on ECG in patients who are asymptomatic.

Arrhythmias do occur in approximately 20% or more of adult patients during general anesthesia; however, most of these patients do not have preoperative arrhythmias. Most intraoperative arrhythmias are supraventricular, transient, and related to anesthetic or surgical manipulations and do not require specific therapies. The number of arrhythmias that are detected clinically, without the use of continuous monitoring, is lower; supraventricular arrhythmias are detected clinically in 4% of patients and other arrhythmias in 11% (12,22).

Perioperative Management

Patients with arrhythmias should have a preoperative evaluation (Table 93.2) expanded in several ways. The probable cause of the arrhythmia should be delineated (see Chapter 64). If the arrhythmia is intermittent or control is uncertain, 24-hour Holter monitoring should be done. Levels of antiarrhythmic drugs that are being administered should be obtained. This evaluation should be accomplished before admission for surgery.

Patients with *supraventricular arrhythmias* should have their ventricular rates controlled or should be converted to more stable rhythms. Except for atrial fibrillation, this usually means conversion either to normal sinus rhythm or atrial fibrillation because other supraventricular arrhythmias are hemodynamically unstable or give an unpredictable ventricular response even with appropriate drug therapy. Patients with atrial fibrillation should have their rates slowed but should be able to accelerate their heart rate under stress as indicated by their ability to raise their pulse rate more than 10 points by mild exercise.

Established indications for *preoperative digoxin administration* in patients with arrhythmias are control of rate in atrial fibrillation and prophylaxis of supraventricular arrhythmias in selected patients (e.g., some patients with past histories of supraventricular arrhythmias who remain at high risk for recurrence). Patients with *ventricular arrhythmias* should be treated according to the criteria outlined in Chapter 64.

Antiarrhythmic drugs should be continued orally through the morning before surgery, after which the following intravenous treatment should be substituted until the patient can take oral medications again: intravenous digoxin (75% of the oral dosage) for patients taking digoxin and intravenous lidocaine or procainamide for patients taking quinidine, procainamide, or disopyramide for ventricular arrhythmias. Amiodarone is available in an intravenous preparation; its use may be considered in patients maintained on it, a decision best made with the assistance of a cardiologist.

There is general agreement that patients undergoing general anesthesia should have a *prophylactic or therapeutic pacemaker* inserted for the following conditions:

- Symptomatic or significant dysfunction of the sinoatrial node
- Idioventricular rhythm
- Current or past history of third-degree or Mobitz type II second-degree atrioventricular (AV) block
- Occasional instances of Mobitz type I (Wenckebach) second-degree AV block
- Occasional patients with trifascicular block (right bundle branch block plus left anterior hemiblock plus first-degree AV block; alternating left and right bundle branch block; or left bundle branch block and first-degree AV block), especially in the presence of severe valvular disease, ischemic disease, CHF, or syncope
- A history of Stokes-Adams attacks

Patients with a history suggesting symptomatic bradyarrhythmias (especially a history of syncope or near syncope and an underlying ECG abnormality) probably should have a temporary pacemaker recommended if a full workup to evaluate the cause of the symptoms cannot be performed preoperatively. Isolated conditions for which a pacemaker is more controversial, but generally not indicated, include bifascicular block, bundle branch block, first-degree AV block, and asymptomatic sinus bradycardia.

PATIENTS WITH PULMONARY DISEASE

Patients with significant pulmonary disease have increased mortality and morbidity during surgery. The increased risks are caused chiefly by the following physiologic changes produced by the effects of anesthesia, sedatives, and analgesics: abnormalities of pulmonary gas exchange, causing hypoxemia; depression of the cough reflex and decrease in clearance of respiratory tract secretions; respiratory depression; and loss of sighing and normal lung inflation. Each of these changes increases the risk of atelectasis and pneumonia. Additionally, normal breathing and voluntary coughing are decreased after surgery because of pain and discomfort, especially after upper abdominal and thoracic surgery. Optimal preoperative treatment of pulmonary disease can reduce perioperative morbidity and mortality.

Chronic Obstructive Pulmonary Disease

Risk

The precise risk of perioperative death from pulmonary causes for patients with chronic obstructive pulmonary disease (COPD) is not known because of the lack of information regarding patients with mild lung disease. In patients with moderate to severe COPD, pulmonary deaths occur in approximately 4% (versus 0% to 2% of unselected patients), postoperative respiratory failure requiring mechanical ventilation in 3%, and total pulmonary complications in 36% (versus 9% of unselected patients) (23–26).

A *smoking history, dyspnea, cough, or abnormal spirometry* increases the risk of minor postoperative pulmonary complications (i.e., atelectasis or infection without significant respiratory compromise). The risk of respiratory failure requiring vigorous postoperative respiratory therapy is increased in patients with a forced expiratory volume in 1 second (FEV_1) less than 1.5 L. An FEV_1 less than 1.0 L or a carbon dioxide pressure (PCO_2) greater than 45 mm Hg predicts a substantial increase in perioperative pulmonary mortality and in the incidence of postoperative respiratory failure requiring prolonged mechanical ventilation. However, no study has definitively shown that any pulmonary function test, including FEV_1 or arterial blood gases, predicts major pulmonary complications (respiratory failure, need for mechanical ventilation, or death) with enough precision to establish a prohibitive criterion for surgery. The decision for surgery in the presence of pulmonary disease requires consideration of all clinical and laboratory data (23–26).

TABLE 93.14 Nonpulmonary Factors that Increase Pulmonary Risks During General Surgery

Most Important	*Other*
Age older than 60	General anesthesia lasting more than 3 h
Upper abdominal or thoracic operation	Obesity
Repeat operations within 1 yr	Abnormal electrocardiogram
	Poor patient effort/cooperation
	Narcotic analgesics
	Upper respiratory infection

A number of *nonpulmonary factors* are helpful in predicting postoperative pulmonary complications in patients with COPD (Table 93.14). The greatest risks are in patients who are older than 60 years of age, who undergo upper abdominal and thoracic operations or operations under general anesthesia lasting more than 3 hours, or who have repeated operations within 1 year. A much lower risk is posed by operations on the extremities, back, breast, and central nervous system. Lower abdominal surgery represents an intermediate risk. Combining these factors with the pulmonary factors listed above increases the practitioner's ability to predict operative morbidity.

The *type of anesthesia* may affect the risk of pulmonary complications. Local anesthesia creates very little risk; if the patient is also sedated ("moderate sedation"), however, there may be temporary deterioration in respiratory control and there may be a suppression of the cough reflex. Spinal anesthesia has been reported to be associated with a low mortality rate in patients with COPD in some studies (25), but not others (24). However, because of the simultaneous use of sedation, lack of control of the airway, less ability to monitor (especially PCO_2), and because the patient must ventilate in the supine position, spinal anesthesia creates a significant risk of intraoperative and postoperative respiratory complications; this is especially true of obese patients with chronic pulmonary disease. Because of these problems, general anesthesia, which permits control of ventilation and clearance of secretions, is often preferable to spinal anesthesia in patients with moderate or severe COPD.

A respiratory failure risk index (analogous to the cardiac risk indices) has been developed and validated in a Veteran's Administration Hospital (VA) setting (Table 93.15) (24). This index provides useful guidance for clinical decision making, but should not be used solely until it is validated in other settings.

Perioperative Management

Patients with known COPD should have a preoperative evaluation (Table 93.2) with additional evaluation focused

TABLE 93.15 Respiratory Failure Risk Index

Preoperative Predictor	*Points*
Type of surgery	
Abdominal aortic aneurysm	27
Thoracic	21
Neurosurgery, upper abdominal, peripheral vascular	14
Neck	11
Emergency surgery	11
Albumin (<3.0 g/L)	9
SUN (>30 mg/dL)	8
Partially or fully dependent ADLs	7
History of chronic obstructive pulmonary disease	6
Age (years): ≥70	6
60–69	4

Class 1, < 10 points (0.5%); class 2, 11–19 points (2.2%); class 3, 20–27 points (5%); class 4, 28–40 points (11.6%), class 5, >40 points (30.5%). (risk of postoperative respiratory failure parenthesis).
From Arozullah AM, Daley J, Henderson WG, et al. Multifactorial risk index for predicting postoperative respiratory failure in men after major noncardiac surgery. Ann Surgery 2000;232:242.

on established risk factors described above and the status of their pulmonary disease. If they are taking theophylline, they should have measurement of the serum theophylline concentration and adjustment of the dosage if it is above or below the therapeutic range. Any history of smoking, chronic or intermittent sputum production, recent upper respiratory infection (URI), dyspnea on effort, or concomitant cardiovascular disease is particularly pertinent. Ideally, smokers should stop smoking 8 weeks before admission for surgery to be performed under general or spinal anesthesia, and patients with URIs should have surgery postponed at least 2 weeks, regardless of how minor the episode.

For patients undergoing general or spinal anesthesia the principal indications for preadmission spirometry alone (forced vital capacity and FEV_1) or for spirometry plus lung volumes and arterial blood gases have not been firmly established.

Pulmonary function testing is indicated when the presence or severity of lung disease is uncertain clinically, for surgery with a high risk of pulmonary complications, and probably in patients with high risk scores on the respiratory failure risk index. Even experienced clinicians can sometimes misjudge the severity of obstructive lung disease. Spirometry is indicated to clarify the presence and severity of lung disease in questionable cases, including patients without a prior diagnosis of pulmonary disease. However, the ability of pulmonary function testing to predict adverse outcomes for high-risk patients has not been clearly established (26). Pulmonary consultation should be obtained for patients whose FEV_1 is less than 1.0 L or whose PCO_2 is above 45 mm Hg, and for those with less severe pulmonary disease who are being evaluated for thoracic or upper abdominal surgery.

Preoperatively, the patient should be instructed on coughing and deep breathing exercises, as well as on the use of devices such as an incentive spirometer that will be used postoperatively. Patients already taking inhaled or oral bronchodilators and inhaled steroids should continue their regimen through the morning of surgery. Patients who have a history of intermittent airway obstruction should be started on an inhaled bronchodilator before surgery. To prevent bronchospasm, especially in the immediate postoperative period, inhaled (β_2-sympathomimetics) and occasionally intravenous aminophylline should be administered (the serum theophylline level should be kept in the therapeutic range [10 to 20 mg/mL]) while the patient cannot take oral medications. Patients who have received corticosteroids for more than 2 weeks during the year before surgery should be appropriately covered for stress with parenteral steroids (see Adrenal Insufficiency and Chronic Steroid Therapy); occasionally steroids may need to be reinstituted or the dose increased to control the pulmonary disease. Patients with chronic purulent sputum production should receive a 5-to 7-day course of a broad-spectrum antibiotic (tetracycline, amoxicillin, trimethoprim–sulfamethoxazole [TMP-SMX], azithromycin, or clarithromycin) to decrease the quantity and purulence of secretions. Finally, arterial blood gases should be checked in patients with moderate to severe COPD before and, as needed, after surgery. Pulse oximetry is usually obtained pre- and postoperatively but does not measure PCO_2. There is some dispute about the efficacy of most of these individual measures. However, controlled trials show that the combination, preoperatively, of bronchodilators, antibiotics, lung expansion, and mobilization of secretions decreases the number of perioperative complications (25,26).

Lung Resection and Chronic Obstructive Pulmonary Disease

Overall mortality rates for lung resection are about 5% for lobectomy and approximately 15% for total pneumonectomy. The mortality and morbidity rates for lung surgery vary widely depending on patient factors (particularly age and pulmonary function), type of operation (pneumonectomy, lobectomy, segmental resection), and the experience and skill of the surgical team.

Assessment of pulmonary function in the patient with COPD who has an indication for lung resection (usually a tumor) should be performed in the ambulatory setting. Use of the following criteria to select candidates for lung resection has reduced mortality for patients with COPD: *For pneumonectomy,* the major criteria for operability are FEV_1 of 2 L or more and forced vital capacity 50% of predicted or more. Patients with an FEV_1 below 2 L should have quantitative perfusion lung scanning to determine the FEV_1 that can be expected after pneumonectomy (e.g., if 30% of perfusion and ventilation goes to the affected lung, the patient's pulmonary function will be decreased by approximately 30% postoperatively). Those with a predicted postoperative FEV_1 as low as 0.8 to 1 L can undergo pneumonectomy, although their mortality risk is probably increased.

Patients not meeting the criteria for pneumonectomy may tolerate lobectomy or segmental resection. Most patients with a preoperative FEV_1 of 1.5 L or more can tolerate a lobectomy. The patient may undergo resection of the segment or lobe if the predicted postoperative FEV_1 is greater than 0.8 to 1 L by quantitative perfusion lung scanning. Other measures in preoperative planning for the patient with COPD undergoing pulmonary resection are similar to those described for such patients in the preceding section.

Asthma

Risk

Asthma affects approximately 3% of Americans, which makes it one of the most common pulmonary diseases (see Chapter 60). It is difficult to give a firm estimate of the operative risks posed by asthma, because in most reports data on asthma are pooled with results for other types of obstructive airway disease. The most dangerous period for the asthmatic patient is not usually the period during general anesthesia, because the anesthetic may be an effective bronchodilator, but is the immediate postoperative period. The major risks are severe bronchospasm and inspissation of thick secretions.

Perioperative Management

Asthmatic patients should have a preoperative evaluation (Table 93.2) with an emphasis on the severity, stability, and current status of their asthma. The evaluation should be done in the practitioner's office prior to admission to allow adequate time for changes in management. The patient should stop smoking 8 weeks before surgery. Spirometry (FEV_1 and forced vital capacity) should be performed on asthmatic patients before operation; peak flows (if normal) are adequate in mild stable asthmatics undergoing minor surgery. Arterial blood gases should be measured in decompensated or severe asthmatics, in asthmatics with substantial abnormalities of spirometry, and when there is clinical concern about hypoxia or hypercarbia. Pulse oximetry is useful when carbon dioxide (CO_2) retention is not a concern. Serum theophylline levels should be measured in patients on this medication, because levels on standard doses are frequently subtherapeutic or toxic.

β_2-Sympathomimetics and inhaled steroids can be continued as inhaled aerosols until the induction of anesthesia and can be resumed in the recovery room. Planning for the immediate preoperative period should include administration of oral and inhaled bronchodilators on the morning of surgery and scheduling of surgery early in the day. In very severe asthmatic patients who are taking theophylline, a constant infusion of aminophylline may be used in the perioperative period when the patient cannot take medicine by mouth; most patients are adequately treated with intravenous aminophylline or by resuming theophylline orally, in the recovery room. Patients who have taken systemic corticosteroids for more than 2 weeks during the previous year should receive dosages of parenteral steroids sufficient to cover the stress of surgery (see Adrenal Insufficiency and Chronic Steroid Therapy) (27). Some patients will require reinstitution of or an increase in their oral corticosteroid dose to control asthma before surgery.

PATIENTS WITH RENAL DISEASE

Risk

The size of the operative risk for patients with chronic renal disease depends on the severity of their disease (see Chapter 52). The type of surgery also influences risk; high-risk surgery includes trauma, vascular, and some GI surgery (e.g., when bleeding, jaundice, or infection is present preoperatively) (28). Other risk factors include advanced age, volume depletion, hypotension, sepsis, exposure to nephrotoxins, and CHF (28). Overall, the mortality after major surgery in patients with severe renal disease (i.e., creatinine clearance [CrCl] less than 10 to 15 mL/minute, including patients on dialysis) is approximately 2% to 4% when these cases are managed carefully. In patients not requiring dialysis, postoperative acute renal failure is the gravest complication (28).

The major complications associated with surgery in the patient with moderate to severe renal disease are worsened renal failure, electrolyte disturbances (especially acidosis and hyperkalemia), volume contraction, volume overload, toxicity caused by agents that are nephrotoxic or are excreted by the kidneys, anemia, and bleeding. Volume contraction, with the risk of ischemic cerebral, cardiac, or renal damage, is a particular risk in patients with the nephrotic syndrome; these patients usually have a slightly contracted intravascular volume at baseline and are at risk of hypovolemia if an effort is made to decrease their edema with potent diuretics preoperatively. Toxic renal damage may follow the use of two classes of agents that are often used in the perioperative period: radiocontrast materials and aminoglycoside antibiotics.

Perioperative Management

Before admission for surgery, patients with chronic renal failure should have an evaluation as outlined in

Table 93.2, and their intravascular volume status should be documented. Weight and orthostatic blood pressure are important in assessing preoperative volume status. Baseline creatinine clearance should be documented by calculation or actual measurement. Radiocontrast studies should be avoided, if at all possible, in the preoperative workup of patients with significantly elevated serum creatinine concentrations or with other risk factors because of the risk of acute renal failure (28). If radiocontrast studies are required, the use of intravenous hydration with 0.45 (half-normal) saline combined with oral acetylcysteine or an intravenous infusion of sodium bicarbonate may reduce this risk (29,30).

The most important consideration in perioperative management of patients who do not require dialysis is avoidance of fluid imbalance. When the surgery carries a risk of significant volume shifts, pulmonary artery catheterization may be considered to ensure close monitoring of the intravascular volume. Administration of antihypertensives should follow the guidelines stated earlier in this chapter. The dosages of some drugs may need to be adjusted for the patient's degree of renal insufficiency as outlined in Chapter 52 (31). BUN, serum creatinine, and electrolytes should be monitored before and after surgery to detect hyperkalemia and deterioration of renal function. Patients with renal failure often have a metabolic acidosis compensated by hyperventilation; postoperatively, continued appropriate hyperventilation is necessary to avoid a potentially precipitous fall in arterial pH. Preoperative prophylactic dialysis is not generally recommended in the patient not already on chronic dialysis. Patients with chronic anemia secondary to renal failure usually are well compensated and do not require preoperative transfusion unless they are symptomatic from the anemia or a large blood loss is expected during surgery; preoperative use of erythropoietin is a consideration to avoid transfusion.

Generally, the nephrologist caring for patients on chronic dialysis should coordinate the medical management of these patients throughout the surgical episode. Although these patients have a very high postoperative complication rate (caused by hyperkalemia, bleeding, arteriovenous fistula thrombosis, pneumonia, wound infection, and arrhythmias), their risk of dying from surgery remains in the 2% to 4% range if complications are carefully managed (28).

PATIENTS WITH ENDOCRINE DISEASE

Diabetes Mellitus

Risk

Total surgical mortality for all diabetic patients is approximately 2% to 4%; less than 0.3% die as a result of poor control of their diabetes. Approximately 15% of diabetic patients have postoperative complications that may be related to diabetes, particularly wound infection.

Two recent consensus statements have concluded that tight glycemic control during the perioperative period (premeal glucoses $\leq$110 to 126) reduces surgical morbidity and mortality (32,33). Clear guidelines on how to achieve this difficult goal were not offered, except that sliding scale insulin alone is not considered sufficient.

Perioperative Management

Each diabetic patient should have a preoperative evaluation as outlined in Table 93.2, with particular attention to determining diabetes control and the presence of cardiovascular disease. Patients who are responsible can monitor their own glucose, and patients who are compliant are good candidates for outpatient surgery. Relative contraindications to outpatient surgery include significantly uncontrolled diabetes, extremely labile diabetes, and noncompliant diabetic patients requiring insulin.

Measurement of fasting glucose, electrolytes, serum urea nitrogen, and creatinine should be obtained at the time of the preoperative office evaluation. If the patient is monitoring glucose at home, these values should be reviewed, as well as any recent hemoglobin A_{1C} measurements. The patient should be told to call if his or her home glucose measurements are higher or lower than predetermined values (specific values should be given to the patient in writing) between the time of the office medical evaluation and surgery and also postoperatively. The patient or nurse should do a bedside glucose determination on arrival at the hospital. The state of hydration should be determined to ensure that the diabetic is not significantly volume contracted. Elective surgery should not be undertaken if diabetes is uncontrolled (fasting blood glucoses more than 200 to 250 mg/100 mL); better control may decrease perioperative risks, and tight control with pre-meal glucoses less than 110 to 126 are optimal. Table 93.16 summarizes the appropriate perioperative treatment of diabetes, which depends on the type of surgical procedure planned and the preadmission regimen. *Diabetic patients who are controlled by diet* can be monitored with daily fasting blood glucose levels throughout the operative episode and treated with insulin if unacceptable rises in glucose occur.

Treatment of patients taking oral agents varies because they represent a heterogeneous group. Patients with mild elevations of glucose who are undergoing minor procedures that will allow them to eat the same day can take their oral hypoglycemic drug on the day *before* surgery and resume it when they begin eating after surgery. If the patient is to undergo a major procedure, oral agents (including thiazolidinediones) should be discontinued beginning on the morning of surgery and not continued postoperatively

TABLE 93.16 Management of Diabetes on Day of Surgery

	Treatment Required to Control Glucose Preoperatively		
Surgical Procedure	***Diet Only***	***Oral Hypoglycemic Agent***	***Insulin***
Minor	Observe	Withhold until after procedure	Withhold until after procedure or use "major" protocol
Major	Observe	Change to long-acting insulin (achieve control with insulin before operation)	*Preferred regimen:* One half to two thirds of total long-acting insulin dosage preoperatively; regular insulin only if needed *or* One third of total long-acting insulin dosage preoperatively; one third postoperatively; regular insulin only if needed *or* Continuous low-dose infusion of regular insulin *or* Regular insulin in each liter of 5% dextrose in water (D5W)

because they have relatively long half-lives, control is less predictable, and because the drugs cannot be given parenterally postoperatively. Therefore, such patients should be switched to management by diet only or to insulin. Human insulin is preferred for the patient who has not taken insulin previously. An exception is the patient taking *chlorpropamide* (Diabinese), which should be withheld 2 to 3 days before surgery because of its particularly long half-life. *Metformin* (Glucophage) should be withheld at least 48 hours before elective surgery. It should not be restarted (except for minor procedures) until 48 hours postoperatively, and when the patient is stable and eating, and for major procedures, until a postoperative serum creatinine has been measured. Metformin should also be withheld for 48 hours before and after any preoperative imaging procedure involving administration of radiocontrast. It is especially important to withhold metformin in major procedures that carry a risk of hypotension or renal failure (e.g., vascular surgery) because of the risk of lactic acidosis.

For the patient who is taking insulin before surgery, one of several strategies is recommended for the preoperative period (Table 93.16). Because of its simplicity and the small risk of hypoglycemia, the first regimen (giving one half to two thirds of the usual total daily dosage of long-acting insulin preoperatively) is preferred. Postoperative inpatient management of diabetes is beyond the scope of this text (32,33).

Adrenal Insufficiency and Chronic Steroid Therapy

Risk

It is generally agreed that patients who are currently taking a pharmacologic dosage of corticosteroids (more than the equivalent of 20 to 30 mg of hydrocortisone daily), who have taken corticosteroids at a pharmacologic dosage for 2 or more weeks in the past year, or who are receiving replacement dosages for adrenal insufficiency, are at risk of developing perioperative adrenal insufficiency because of the stress of surgery. Patients in each of these groups should therefore receive extra corticosteroids in the perioperative period (see Chapter 81 for additional details) (34).

Perioperative Management

These patients should have an evaluation before admission (Table 93.2) with an emphasis on signs of adrenal insufficiency. For patients with adrenal insufficiency, the evaluation should include particular attention to factors that may reflect the adequacy of corticosteroid replacement (i.e., lying and standing blood pressure, concentration of serum urea nitrogen or serum creatinine, glucose, and electrolytes). Adrenocorticotropic hormone stimulation or insulin-hypoglycemia testing to determine the need for steroid coverage in patients previously on steroids is not recommended for routine use because there is not adequate evidence that a normal response precludes the need for steroid coverage during surgery.

Patients on chronic steroid therapy may receive the usual steroid dosage by mouth the day before surgery. On the day of surgery, hydrocortisone 100 mg should be administered intravenously at 6 a.m. A second 100-mg dose should be given intravenously during surgery and then a 100-mg dose should be given intravenously every 6 hours for the first 24 hours after surgery, followed by 50 mg every 6 hours for the second 24 hours after surgery, and 25 mg every 6 hours for the third 24-hour period. Alternatively, a continuous infusion of hydrocortisone after an initial bolus dose preoperatively may be given (34). The patient may then return to the preoperative medical regimen.

There are two exceptions to these guidelines. First, the regimen is based on the assumption that there is no prolonged stress after surgery; if this occurs, higher dosages of corticosteroids must be continued for a longer time postoperatively. Second, for minor procedures, patients may return to their usual dosage within 24 to 48 hours postoperatively. For outpatient surgery, equivalent dosages of oral prednisone may be given as an outpatient for the postoperative care (preoperative dosage should still be given intravenously).

Hypothyroidism

Risk

The major potential complications of surgery in hypothyroid patients are increased sensitivity to and prolonged half-life of anesthetic agents, hypoventilation and respiratory arrest in the immediate postoperative period, hyponatremia caused by decreased free water clearance, and myxedema coma. The risks of surgery in patients with mild to moderate hypothyroidism are probably not as high as once thought (35). Nonetheless, hypothyroid patients should delay elective surgery for 4 to 6 weeks and should be treated with thyroxine (see Chapter 80).

Perioperative Management

Hypothyroid patients should be evaluated carefully before admission for surgery. The patient should have the evaluation outlined in Table 93.2, and the serum thyroid-stimulating hormone concentration should be checked (unless a value from the past 2 months is available; see Chapter 80 for details).

Specific recommendations for preoperative management depend on the status of the patient's hypothyroidism. Patients with previously known and adequately treated hypothyroidism can undergo surgery. The half-life of administered thyroxine is about 7 days. Therefore, oral thyroxine can usually be omitted on the day of surgery and resumed when the patient is able to take oral medication. The stress of major surgery or severe infection may accelerate the turnover of thyroxine, occasionally necessitating daily treatment with intravenous thyroxine (50% of the oral dosage) in patients in either of these situations.

If the hypothyroidism has been effectively treated for a long period (as indicated by no or only minor symptoms or a normal or only a slightly increased thyroid-stimulating hormone), the patient can usually tolerate surgery and thyroid replacement can be adjusted postoperatively. For hypothyroid patients who have not been treated or who remain significantly hypothyroid because of inadequate replacement therapy, elective surgery should be postponed because of the risks listed above. Such patients should receive adequate thyroid replacement for a minimum of 1 to 2 months before elective surgery (4 to 6 months for patients with profound myxedema). Surgery required before this period in mild to moderately hypothyroid patients may be considered, especially if minor surgery under local anesthesia is being performed, if the patient can be started on a total replacement dosage immediately, and if there is prompt improvement in signs and symptoms of hypothyroidism (see Chapter 80). When a patient with previously undiagnosed hypothyroidism requires immediate major surgery, an endocrinologist should be consulted regarding perioperative treatment and monitoring.

Hyperthyroidism

Risk

The major risk of operation in patients with uncontrolled hyperthyroidism is *thyroid storm* (see Chapter 80). In an old series, there were only 25 episodes of thyroid storm after 1,383 operations on thyrotoxic patients (36). However, surgery accounts for up to one third of the cases of thyroid storm reported, probably in patients with unrecognized hyperthyroidism.

Perioperative Management

The patient with known hyperthyroidism should be reassessed clinically and with thyroid function tests before admission for surgery. In previously undiagnosed patients, the usual approach should be used in evaluation and management (see Chapter 80).

The treatment of the hyperthyroid patient during surgery depends on the patient's current thyroid status. Patients previously diagnosed and adequately treated should take their current treatment until midnight the night before surgery and should resume treatment when they can take medications by mouth again. Patients with new, known, or recurrent hyperthyroidism who are not euthyroid should be brought to an euthyroid state with thyroid-blocking agents or iodides (see Chapter 80). Ideally, surgery should be postponed for several months in these patients until a consistent euthyroid state is attained. An endocrinologist should be consulted regarding the treatment and monitoring of any patient with uncontrolled hyperthyroidism who requires urgent surgery.

Obese Patients

Risk

Massive obesity significantly increases the risk of mortality associated with surgery. In one study, for example, women undergoing surgery for adenocarcinoma of the uterus had a 20% operative mortality if they weighed more than 300 pounds (136 kg), compared with a 1.5% mortality for obese women weighing between 200 and 240 pounds (91 and 110 kg) (37). Less severe obesity probably does not increase mortality risks.

Moderate or massive obesity also increases the risk of a number of perioperative problems, including difficult intubation, difficulty in ventilating the patient during anesthesia, the need for a large amount of anesthesia during induction, potential delay in anesthesia washout because of slow release of anesthetic agents from adipose tissue, postoperative atelectasis and pneumonia, thromboembolism, difficult postoperative mobilization, nosocomial wound infection (particularly when there is increased moisture caused by pannus adjacent to the surgical incision), wound dehiscence, and late incisional hernia.

Perioperative Management

For massively obese patients, a program of gradual weight reduction (see Chapter 83) should be planned, if the patient is amenable, before any elective operation; this may require up to 6 months. When prompt surgery is needed, these patients should have an evaluation (Table 93.2) with the addition of assessment for complications of obesity, particularly cardiopulmonary complications. Particularly, these patients should be checked for uncontrolled diabetes mellitus and significant hypoventilation (sleep apnea), two common complications of obesity that increase the risk of surgery. Either of these two problems should be managed preoperatively, as discussed above.

Massively obese patients should be given preoperative instruction in deep breathing and in the use of the incentive spirometer or other devices designed to prevent pulmonary complications postoperatively. Prophylaxis of thromboembolic disease should be given (see Chapter 57). Other recommendations for perioperative management depend on obesity-associated conditions, such as diabetes, that the patient may have.

PATIENTS WITH GASTROINTESTINAL OR HEPATIC DISEASE

Peptic Ulcer Disease

Risk

Data are lacking on the risk and the management of surgery in patients with active peptic ulcer disease.

Perioperative Management

Patients with active ulcer disease should have elective nonulcer surgery postponed until the ulcer heals. The average time required for the healing of uncomplicated ulcers is 4 to 6 weeks for duodenal ulcer and 6 weeks for gastric ulcer (see Chapter 43). There is no consistent relationship between disappearance of ulcer symptoms, ulcer healing, and recurrence. Therefore, it is best to wait several weeks after all symptoms have disappeared and 6 weeks to 3 months from the beginning of an episode before admission for elective nonulcer surgery. If surgery cannot be deferred this long or if ulcer recurrence is suspected, endoscopy should be considered preoperatively. Before surgery, these patients should also have the medical evaluation summarized in Table 93.2, and multiple stool samples should be checked to exclude active bleeding.

No empiric data confirm these guidelines or indicate whether surgery can be done safely as soon as an ulcer has healed (as shown by endoscopy). If urgent abdominal surgery must be performed in a patient with active ulcer disease, consideration should be given to whether surgical treatment is needed for the ulcer as well (see Chapter 43 for detailed discussion of indications for and types of surgery). Patients with remote or inactive ulcer disease require no special therapy preoperatively or postoperatively.

Patients with recently active ulcer disease should continue their current therapy until midnight the day before surgery. Both H_2 blockers (cimetidine, ranitidine, famotidine) and proton pump inhibitors (lansoprazole, pantoprazole) can be given intravenously or via nasogastric tube. One of these should be used throughout the period when the patient cannot take medications by mouth; nasogastric suctioning may also be recommended during this period.

Hepatitis

Risk

General anesthesia and surgery during acute hepatitis are associated with high rates of mortality and morbidity (38). The major problem accounting for these risks is postoperative hepatic encephalopathy and its complications. The catabolic effects of surgery, hypotension during anesthesia,

TABLE 93.17 Child's Classification of Operative Mortality Risk in the Cirrhotic Patient

	Risk Group by Severity of Liver Disease		
	A (Minimal)	B (Moderate)	C (Advanced)
Bilirubin (mg per 100 mL)	<2.0	2.0–3.0	>3.0
Serum albumin (g per 100 mL)	>3.5	3.0–3.5	<3.0
Ascites	None	Controlled	Poorly controlled
Encephalopathy	None	Minimal	Coma
Nutrition	Excellent	Good	Poor ("wasted")
Operative mortality (%)	0	9	53

From Siefkin AD, Bolt RJ. Preoperative evaluation of the patient with gastrointestinal or liver disease. Med Clin North Am 1979;63:1309.

and hepatic toxicity from anesthetic agents are the principal factors that may precipitate hepatic encephalopathy.

Perioperative Management

Patients with a history of acute hepatitis should have an evaluation (Table 93.2) with the addition of assessment of the severity and complications of the liver disease. Liver function tests (serum aminotransferases, bilirubin, alkaline phosphatase, albumin, and prothrombin time [PT]) should be obtained before admission for surgery. Serologic tests for hepatitis B and hepatitis C should also be performed (see Chapter 47), if they have not been done previously.

Ideally, surgery should be postponed for a minimum of 6 to 12 months after all laboratory evidence of active liver disease has returned to normal. This cautious approach is advised because there is a risk of exacerbating hepatic injury if surgery is performed earlier. Only urgent life-saving surgery should be performed during the acute phase of hepatitis, whatever its cause.

Anticipation of postoperative complications (particularly bleeding and encephalopathy) is important in the patient with active hepatitis who must undergo surgery. For the patient with an abnormal PT, fresh frozen plasma can be given throughout the immediate perioperative period. When immunologic tests or epidemiologic information indicates infectious hepatitis (see Chapter 47), the surgical team should be notified in order to minimize the risk of spreading infection.

Cirrhosis

Risk

Data regarding the risks of surgery in the cirrhotic patient are available from trials of portal–systemic shunts and from more recent studies in general surgical patients (39). The most widely used measure of the mortality risk is the Child index, which incorporates measurements of serum bilirubin, albumin, ascites, encephalopathy, and nutrition (Table 93.17). Elevated PT is also a predictor of bad outcome (39). The perioperative complications encountered in these patients are those associated with chronic cirrhosis: encephalopathy, jaundice, gastrointestinal hemorrhage, infection, and hepatorenal syndrome.

Regional and spinal anesthesia do not entirely eliminate the risks of complications in cirrhotic patients. For example, increased morbidity and mortality caused by liver disease have been associated even with hernia repair under local anesthesia in some patients. The stress of the procedure itself, decreased hepatic blood flow, and complications such as hypotension and wound infection may worsen hepatic function, even in the absence of toxic general anesthetics.

Perioperative Management

In addition to the preoperative evaluation (Table 93.2), patients with cirrhosis should have an assessment of the severity and complications of their liver disease and liver function tests (serum amino transferase, bilirubin, alkaline phosphatase, albumin, and PT). Liver biopsy is indicated in selected patients to establish the presence of cirrhosis, provide an additional indicator of the severity of liver damage, or exclude active hepatitis. CT or sonogram is only occasionally needed to evaluate hepatomegaly. In the history and physical examination, a search should be made for complications of cirrhosis, especially encephalopathy, bleeding, varices, and ascites.

The expected benefits of surgery must be weighed carefully against the risks in patients with cirrhosis. Generally, risks are higher and only essential surgery should be performed. Stable patients with mild cirrhosis, however, who have no ongoing injury (e.g., due to removal of a toxin or discontinuation of alcohol) may tolerate surgery without significant complications.

A number of precautions should be emphasized in the cirrhotic patient who does require surgery. Local (or, as a second choice, spinal) anesthesia may be safer than general anesthesia, although data are lacking. Therapy to prevent complications of liver disease, such as postoperative bleeding (fresh frozen plasma for the patient with an abnormal PT or partial thromboplastin time) and encephalopathy (see Chapter 47), should be established and maintained throughout the operative period, and the patient should be repeatedly checked for evidence of these two problems. The occasional patient who is taking chronic corticosteroid therapy for liver disease should have the steroid dosage increased during the perioperative period as described in Adrenal Insufficiency and Chronic Steroid Therapy.

PATIENTS WITH IATROGENIC IMPAIRMENT OF HEMOSTASIS

All anticoagulants and platelet inhibitors increase the risk of intraoperative and postoperative bleeding and should be discontinued before any type of surgery. Patients receiving drugs in these classes should have a preoperative evaluation (Table 93.2) before admission for surgery, and an appropriate plan for perioperative management of anticoagulation should be communicated to the surgeon, anesthesiologist, or surgical center.

Anticoagulants

On the basis of critical assessment of risks and benefits, recommendations for the perioperative management of patients taking oral anticoagulants have been revised (40). *Warfarin* (Coumadin) should be stopped 4 to 7 days before surgery, depending on the patient's current international normalized ratio (INR). In patients maintained at a high INR, warfarin should be discontinued earlier. The INR should be measured the day before surgery. If the INR remains elevated, 1 mg of vitamin K_1 should be administered subcutaneously. Within 12 hours, this dose will usually normalize the INR of a patient who has been off warfarin for 4 to 7 days. The larger doses of oral vitamin K_1 previously recommended (e.g., 10 mg) are believed not to be necessary and to increase, possibly, the risk of thromboembolism (40).

Preoperative use of intravenous heparin, while the INR is subtherapeutic, is recommended only for patients at very high risk of thromboembolism, such as those with recent (within 1 month) venous thromboembolism or arterial embolism (40). Postoperatively, intravenous heparin is also recommended in these high-risk patients and in patients who have had venous thromboembolism within the 3 months preceding surgery. An alternative to intravenous unfractionated heparin preoperatively is subcutaneous low-molecular-weight heparin (LMWH) in therapeutic or prophylactic doses depending on the underlying diagnosis. Intravenous heparin should be stopped about 6 hours before surgery; the last dose of low-molecular-weight heparin should be given at least 24 hours before surgery. An INR and, if the patient is taking unfractionated heparin, a partial thromboplastin time and a platelet count should be checked before surgery (40). A number of new anticoagulants (e.g., direct thrombin inhibitors and factor X inhibitors) have been developed in recent years. In general, they should not be prescribed perioperatively until more experience is gained with their use.

These recommendations for use of preoperative and postoperative heparin are much more limited than previous recommendations. Other authors recommend preoperative or postoperative intravenous or LMWH for other high-risk patients, such as those with mechanical valves and multiple risks (e.g., mechanical valve, atrial fibrillation, or history of embolization).

Preoperative placement of a vena caval filter is an option in patients with recent venous thromboembolism or patients for whom the risk of bleeding because of heparin is unacceptably high (40). Warfarin ordinarily can be resumed 24 to 72 hours after surgery, at the preoperative dosage, if all surgical bleeding is controlled; the INR usually reaches 2.0 after 3 days. Patients who have undergone intracranial, spinal, or ophthalmologic operations probably should not be anticoagulated for 48 hours to several weeks after surgery. For patients with a high risk of thromboembolism (see above), continuous-infusion heparin can be reinstituted 12 to 24 hours postoperatively without a bolus, if the surgeon is confident that hemostasis is ensured, and continued until full anticoagulation with warfarin has been re-established (40).

Antiplatelet Agents

Aspirin prolongs the bleeding time and may increase blood loss during and after operation in some patients. Generally, if aspirin is not being used as a critical therapy, it should be discontinued 7 or more days before surgery because the effect of aspirin on platelets continues for this period of time. Discontinuation of aspirin is particularly important before procedures for which hemostasis is critical, such as neurosurgical operations or some ophthalmologic surgery. Aspirin may be continued when its indication is important (e.g., CAD) and the risk of bleeding is low (e.g., breast biopsy, some peripheral vascular surgery). Because *some NSAIDs other than aspirin* also may impair platelet function, it is prudent to advise patients to discontinue NSAID use 1 week before surgery, especially surgery for which increased bleeding would be especially harmful (Table 93.4). *Ticlopidine* (Ticlid) and *clopidogrel* (Plavix), platelet aggregation inhibitors, should be discontinued at least 2 weeks before surgery to ensure that the bleeding time is not prolonged in the perioperative period.

PATIENTS WITH A CHRONIC INFECTION

Two types of chronic bacterial infection pose risks to the patient and to others in the operating room: staphylococcal skin infections and pulmonary tuberculosis. They require appropriate management before surgery.

Skin Infections

Chronic bacterial skin infections (usually caused by staphylococci) pose a high risk for wound sepsis and may be the source of infections in other patients. Therefore, they should be suppressed or eradicated before admission of the patient for an elective operation. Chapter 32 describes strategies for accomplishing this.

Tuberculosis

Active pulmonary tuberculosis poses a problem for the surgical patient because of the general debilitation it causes. It also creates the risk of infection for others in the operating room. Therefore, adult patients with a history of unexplained chronic cough or a history of tuberculosis should be evaluated for active tuberculosis before admission for surgery. Patients with active pulmonary tuberculosis should be stable and have negative sputum cultures before admission for elective surgery. Chapter 34 describes the ambulatory treatment of tuberculosis.

Human Immunodeficiency Virus Infection

Acquired immunodeficiency syndrome (AIDS) poses many problems in preoperative evaluation that are beyond the scope of this chapter but are addressed elsewhere (see www.hopkinsbayview.org/PAMreferences and Chapter 39). Several important issues are summarized here.

The risk of transmission to health care workers is very small, but it does exist. Universal precautions are recommended in the care of all patients, not just known HIV-positive patients (see Chapter 39). Screening of all surgical patients for HIV infection is not currently recommended by expert consensus, but this issue continues to be controversial.

HIV-infected patients pose challenges in addition to the usual preoperative evaluation. Decision-making is complicated by the wide spectrum of morbidity in HIV infection, ranging from the lack of symptoms in the recently infected patient to the debilitation in the preterminal patient. Decision-making should balance the status and prognosis of the patient's HIV infection (asymptomatic, symptomatic), mean life expectancy, the patient's wishes, the increased risk for the specific operation posed by the HIV infection, and the indications for and expected benefit of the surgery during the patient's expected length of survival.

PATIENTS WITH NEUROPSYCHIATRIC DISEASE

Neuropsychiatric problems present ill-defined risks during surgery and the postsurgical period. The major concerns are worsening of mental status caused by both metabolic changes and psychologic stresses. The patient with psychiatric disease may decompensate postoperatively, making care difficult and jeopardizing wound healing.

Cerebrovascular Disease

Risk

Patients with recent strokes have a significant risk of worsening focal deficits during carotid artery surgery, but this risk cannot necessarily be extrapolated to other types of surgery. Patients with recent strokes (less than 6 weeks preoperatively) also have a risk of deterioration in their general mental status, regardless of the status of their focal deficits, if they undergo major surgery; however, firm data are lacking on the size of this risk.

Perioperative Management

Patients with recent strokes should have a preoperative evaluation (Table 93.2), emphasizing documentation of the preoperative neurologic impairment and the detection of treatable underlying causes of the stroke. The data regarding the course of the patient's stroke should be reviewed, and additional testing (see Chapter 91) should be performed if necessary to exclude a treatable cause.

No specific perioperative therapy for the patient with a stable completed stroke is needed. In general, it is prudent to delay elective noncarotid surgery for at least 6 weeks after a completed stroke, although no firm data are available to support this practice.

Asymptomatic Cervical Bruit

Risk

Cervical bruits are present in approximately 4% of people older than the age of 45 years. These bruits may be caused by a number of processes (see Chapter 91), including common or internal carotid stenosis. In the patient with an asymptomatic cervical bruit, there is slight or no increased risk of stroke during surgery (41).

Perioperative Management

Apart from a careful history and physical examination to exclude evidence of a prior stroke or transient ischemic attack related to the cervical bruit, no special approach is needed for these patients. Duplex carotid ultrasound can help establish whether the cervical bruit is caused by carotid stenosis and the degree of stenosis; its value has not been established for estimating risk of postoperative stroke. Hypotension and excessive neck manipulation should be avoided during surgery in patients known to have carotid bruits. The patient with a history of symptoms possibly related to the bruit should be evaluated as described in Chapter 91.

Data summarized in Chapter 91 show that patients with high-grade asymptomatic and symptomatic carotid stenosis have a lower long-term stroke rate if carotid endarterectomy is performed. When patients such as these require elective surgery for another condition, a decision must be made on which of the two surgeries to do first. Whether prophylactic carotid endarterectomy should be done before vascular surgery is controversial, but few patients require prophylactic carotid endarterectomy before general surgery who would not require it anyway.

Parkinson Disease

Risk

The perioperative risks in patients with Parkinson disease (PD) are caused by musculoskeletal rigidity, which may impair voluntary postoperative ventilation, mobilization, and swallowing. These patients are also subject to postoperative delirium. The rigidity of patients taking antiparkinson medication may worsen after the patient has missed one or more doses (see Chapter 90). Despite this potential problem, most patients with PD tolerate anesthesia and temporary omission of medications.

Perioperative Management

The patient should have a preoperative evaluation (Table 93.2), and the antiparkinsonian regimen should be tailored to provide the best possible relief of symptoms (see Chapter 90). For patients taking an anticholinergic agent, the drug may be continued until midnight before surgery and resumed when the patient is able to take oral medications. L-Dopa or Sinemet (L-dopa/carbidopa) should be continued until induction of anesthesia, and the drug should be resumed as soon as possible after surgery. Postoperative physical therapy to maintain range of motion may help these patients until they are able to take oral medication. Parkinsonian patients should be observed for postoperative delirium and aspiration.

Dementia and Organic Brain Syndrome

Risk

Patients with dementia have an increased risk of mortality and morbidity during surgery. The increase in mortality is caused largely by lack of cooperation (e.g., with postoperative respiratory care). Much of the morbidity is related to the development of delirium caused by anesthesia, perioperative medications, and surgical stress. Because surgery is always a difficult process for a demented patient and because the degree of increased risk is ill defined, the potential benefits of surgery should be carefully reviewed before a final decision to operate is made.

Perioperative Management

The patient should have an evaluation (Table 93.2) before admission for surgery. Formal mental status testing should be done (see Mini-Mental Status Examination, Chapter 26) so that a baseline is established for postoperative comparison. The patient should be checked for metabolic abnormalities that may worsen cerebral function before admission, just before surgery, and throughout the postoperative period. Emphasis should be placed on detecting and correcting hypovolemia, electrolyte abnormalities, and hypoxia. See Surgery in the Elderly Patient, above, for simple measures to decrease the incidence of postoperative delirium. When demented patients undergo major procedures, constant observation is recommended for the first 24 to 48 hours after surgery.

Other Psychiatric Problems

Risk

The major problems associated with general surgery in psychiatric patients are lack of cooperation with postoperative care, postoperative psychosis, and interactions between psychotropic medications and anesthetic agents. The degree of cooperation that can be expected postoperatively can generally, but not always, be predicted on the basis of the patient's past behavior and preoperative mental status. Obtaining informed consent is also an issue.

Perioperative Management

A careful history of the patient's past psychiatric illness should be obtained. The patient's *mental status* should be documented preoperatively (see Chapter 26) so that it can be compared with postoperative changes. The patient's *ability to give informed consent* should be evaluated (see Chapter 26); involvement of a designated decision-maker other than the patient may be required. A psychiatric consultation should be obtained in all patients with psychosis or other severe psychiatric problems. An additional issue that must be dealt with by the patient's primary care practitioner and surgeon is the likely effect of the patient's psychiatric state on the surgical evaluation and outcomes (e.g., evaluating symptoms in a patient with one of the somatoform disorders, described in Chapter 21, or evaluating the need for cosmetic surgery).

Careful explanation of the operation is especially crucial to management of patients with psychiatric disorders or with anticipated stress reactions to surgery. The procedure should be explained in language the patient can understand. After the explanation, the patient should be asked to express any concerns about the planned surgery, and the patient's comprehension of the planned surgery should be assessed and documented. The need to ventilate about anxiety associated with disfiguring surgery (e.g., mastectomy, amputation) and with the fear of not waking up is particularly common in both anxiety-prone patients and those who are usually free of anxiety.

Patients with severe *psychosis* should be in a stable manageable state before admission for elective surgery. This should be accomplished through close collaboration between the patient's primary care practitioner, the surgeon, and psychiatrist.

Patients with mild to moderate *anxiety or depression* can be managed by supportive counseling, use of support by family members, selective use of antidepressants or minor tranquilizers, and careful explanation of the procedure to the patient. These interventions should be initiated before hospital admission, not at the last minute before surgery.

The patient's use of *psychotropic drugs* should be communicated to the anesthesiologist. Neuroleptics and tricyclic antidepressants can interact with anesthetics to cause increased sedation, hypotension or hypertension, and arrhythmias. Small to moderate dosages of phenothiazines, haloperidol, and tricyclic antidepressants should be continued until about 12 hours before surgery. In the occasional patient taking a very high dosage of these agents, it is recommended that the drug is stopped about 24 hours before surgery, except in patients who have severely decompensated in the past when their medication has been changed. The dosage of benzodiazepines does not need to be changed unless it is very high.

Lithium carbonate may prolong the action of muscle relaxants and cause myocardial depression and hypernatremia. Lithium should be discontinued 24 hours preoperatively; however, the anesthesiologist should be aware that it has been administered recently. A blood lithium level and electrolyte measurements should be obtained before surgery as a guideline. Chapter 24 provides additional information about lithium.

MAOI antidepressants can enhance the effect of sympathomimetic agents and sympathetic responses to anesthesia and can decrease the rate of elimination of certain anesthetic agents. Because of these problems, MAOIs should be discontinued at least 2 weeks before surgery, and the anesthesiologist must be informed of their recent administration.

SPECIFIC REFERENCES*

1. Babbott S, Gross RJ. Evaluation of the healthy patient and the ambulatory surgery patient. In: Gross RJ, Caputo GC, eds. Medical consultation: the internist on surgical, obstetric, and psychiatric services. 3rd ed. Baltimore: Williams & Wilkins, 1998:25.
2. Gold BS, Kitz DS, Lecky JH, et al. Unanticipated admission to the hospital following ambulatory surgery. JAMA 1989;262:3008.
3. Roizen MF. Preoperative evaluation. In: Miller RD, ed. Anesthesia. 4th ed. New York: Churchill-Livingstone, 1994:827.
4. Kennedy JM, van Rij AM, Spears GF, et al. Polypharmacy in a general surgical unit and consequences of drug withdrawal. Br J Clinc Pharmacol 2000;49:353.
5. Djokovic JL, Hedley-White J. Prediction of outcome of surgery and anesthesia in patients over 80. JAMA 1979;242:2301.
6. Hosking MP, Warner MA, Lobdell CM, et al. Outcomes of surgery in patients 90 years of age and older. JAMA 1989;261:1909.
7. Gross RJ. Special topics. In: Gross RJ, Caputo GC, eds. Medical consultation: the internist on surgical, obstetric, and psychiatric services. 3rd ed. Baltimore: Williams & Wilkins, 1998:615.
8. Rose EA, King TC. Understanding postoperative fatigue. Surg Gynecol Obstet 1978;147:97.
9. Falcone RA, Ziegelstein RC. Cardiovascular disease and hypertension. In: Gross RJ, Caputo GC, eds. Medical consultation: the internist on surgical, obstetric, and psychiatric services. 3rd ed. Baltimore: Williams & Wilkins, 1998:149.
10. Rao Tadikonda LK, Jacobs K, El-Etr A. Reinfarction following anesthesia in patients with myocardial infarction. Anesthesiology 1983;59:499.
11. Goldman L, Caldera DL, Nussbaum SR, et al. Multifactorial index of cardiac risk in noncardiac surgical procedures. N Engl J Med 1977;297:845.
12. Goldman L, Caldera DL, Southwick FS, et al. Cardiac risk factors and complications in non-cardiac surgery. Medicine (Baltimore) 1978;57:357.
13. Detsky AS, Abrams HB, McLaughlin JR, et al. Predicting cardiac complications in patients undergoing non-cardiac surgery. J Gen Intern Med 1986;1:211.
14. Lee TH, Marcantonio ER, Mangione CM, et al. Derivation and prospective validation of a simple index for prediction of cardiac risk of major noncardiac surgery. Circulation 1999;100:1043.
15. ACC/AHA Task Force. Guidelines for perioperative cardiovascular evaluation for noncardiac surgery. J Am Coll Cardiol 1996;27:910. (Updated: J Am Coll Cardiol 2002;39:542) (Available at: http://www.acc.org/clinical/guidelines/periobetablocker.pdf. Last accessed April 19, 2006.)
16. American College of Physicians. Guidelines for assessing and managing the perioperative risk from coronary artery disease associated with major noncardiac surgery. Ann Intern Med 1997;127:309.
17. McFalls EO, Ward HB, Moritz TE, et al. Coronary-artery revascularization before elective major vascular surgery. New Engl J Med 2004;351:2795.
18. Brilakis ES, Orford JL, Fasseas P, et al. Outcome of patients undergoing balloon angioplasty in the two months prior to noncardiac surgery. Am J Cardiol 2005;96:512.
19. Poldermans, D, Boersma, E, Bax, JJ, et al. The effect of bisoprolol on perioperative mortality and myocardial infarction in high-risk patients undergoing vascular surgery. N Engl J Med 1999; 341:1789.
20. Goldman L, Caldera DL. Risks of general anesthesia and elective operation in the hypertensive patient. Anesthesiology 1979;50: 285.
21. Dajani AS, Taubert KA, Wilson W, et al. Prevention of bacterial endocarditis. Recommendations by the American Heart Association. JAMA 1997;277:1794.
22. Goldman L. Supraventricular tachyarrhythmias in hospitalized adults after surgery. Chest 1978; 73:450.
23. Kroenke K, Lawrence VA, Theroux JF, et al. Operative risk in patients with severe obstructive pulmonary disease. Arch Intern Med 1992;152:967.
24. Arozullah AM, Daley J, Henderson WG, et al. Multifactorial risk index for predicting postoperative respiratory failure in men after major noncardiac surgery. Ann Surg 2000;232:242.
25. Tarhan S, Moffitt ED, Sessler AD, et al. Risk of anesthesia and surgery in patients with chronic bronchitis and chronic obstructive pulmonary disease. Surgery 1973;74:720.
26. Smetana GW. Preoperative pulmonary evaluation. N Engl J Med 1999;340:937.
27. Oh SH, Patterson R. Surgery in corticosteroid-dependent asthmatics. J Allergy Clin Immunol 1974;53:345.

*Bold numerals denote published controlled clinical trials, meta-analyses, or consensus-based recommendations.

28. Briefel G, Turer P. Renal disease. In: Gross RJ, Caputo GC, eds. Medical consultation: the internist on surgical, obstetric, and psychiatric services. 3rd ed. Baltimore: Williams & Wilkins, 1998:207.
29. Tepel M, van der Giet M, Schwarzfeld C, et al. Prevention of radiographic-contrast-agent-induced reductions in renal function by acetylcysteine. N Engl J Med 2000;343:180.
30. Merten GJ, Burgess WP, Gray LV, et al. Prevention of contrast-induced nephropathy with sodium bicarbonate: a randomized controlled trial. JAMA 2004;291:2328.
31. Bennett WM, Aronoff GR, Golper TA, et al. Drug prescribing in renal failure. Philadelphia: American College of Physicians, 1994.
32. American College of Endocrinology. Position statement on inpatient diabetes and metabolic control. 2004. Available at: http://www.aace.com/pub/positionstatements.
33. Clement S, Braithwaite SS, Magee MF, et al. Management of diabetes and hyperglycemia in hospitals. Diabetes Care 2004;27:553.
34. Lamberts SWJ, Bruining HA, DeJong FH. Corticosteroid therapy in severe illness. N Engl J Med 1997;337:1285.
35. Ladenson PW, Levin AA, Ridgway EC, et al. Complications of surgery in hypothyroid patients. Am J Med 1984;77:261.
36. McArthur JW, Rawson RW, Means JH, et al. Thyrotoxic crisis: an analysis of the thirty-six cases seen at the Massachusetts General Hospital during the past twenty-five years. JAMA 1947;134:868.
37. Strauss RJ, Wise L. Operative risks of obesity. Surg Gynecol Obstet 1978;146:286.
38. Harville DD, Summerskill WHJ. Surgery in acute hepatitis. JAMA 1963;184:257.
39. Mansour A, Watson W, Shayani V, et al. Abdominal operations in patients with cirrhosis: still a major surgical challenge. Surgery 1997;122:730.
40. Kearon C, Hirsh J. Management of anticoagulation before and after elective surgery. N Engl J Med 1997;336:1506.
41. Ropper AH, Wechsler LR, Wilson LS. Carotid bruit and the risk of stroke in elective surgery. N Engl J Med 1982;307:1388.

For annotated ***General References*** *and resources related to this chapter, visit www.hopkinsbayview.org/PAMreferences.*

Chapter 94

Peripheral Arterial Disease, Abdominal Aortic Aneurysms, and Peripheral Aneurysms

James H. Black, III

The aging process is associated with the development of variable degrees of degenerative arterial disease. Longevity and quality of life may be improved by recognition, evaluation, and appropriate therapy of diseases that affect blood vessels (see also Chapters 62 and 91). The purpose of this chapter is to provide guidelines for recognition and management of the more commonly encountered problems of acute and chronic occlusive peripheral arterial disease (PAD) and of abdominal and peripheral arterial aneurysms.

ACUTE PERIPHERAL ARTERIAL OCCLUSION

Acute ischemia occurs when there is a sudden decrease in arterial perfusion of the lower extremities. It demands immediate recognition and management in an effort to minimize morbidity, including limb loss and death, because irreversible changes such as muscle necrosis, extensive arterial thrombosis, and neurologic deficits may occur in the affected extremity as early as 4 to 6 hours after acute arterial occlusion.

Causes

The two major causes of acute arterial occlusion are *cardioarterial embolism* and *in situ thrombosis*. Most large arterial emboli originate in the heart. Arrhythmias and mural thrombi are the major risk factors for embolization. Rare sources of emboli include proximal arterial lesions

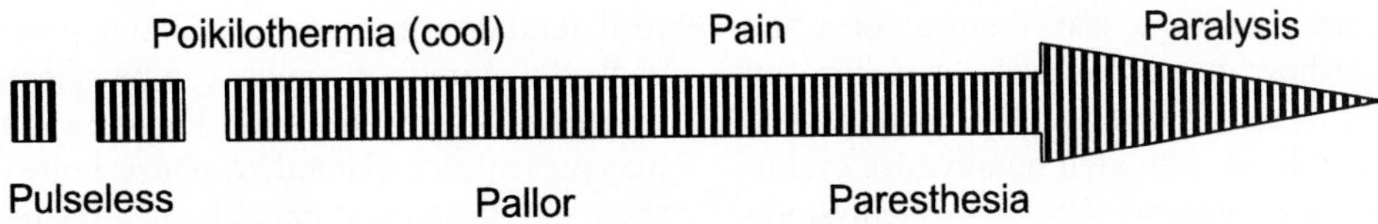

FIGURE 94.1. Stages of acute ischemia and clinical manifestations. Overlap of symptoms is common, especially early in the clinical course. Those patients with underlying chronic peripheral arterial disease (PAD) may progress more slowly than those patients suffering acute limb ischemia without antecedent disease.

such as aortic aneurysms or large ulcerative aortic plaques, which are commonly associated with arterial *cholesterol microemboli.* These microemboli may cause the "blue toe syndrome" (the acute development of cyanosis and pain of the toes or the distal feet, often in association with strong posterior tibial or dorsalis pedis pulses) (1). Left atrial myxomas, debris from prosthetic heart valves, paradoxical emboli (venous clots passing through a congenital cardiac defect into the arterial circulation), and foreign body emboli have also infrequently been associated with sudden arterial occlusion.

In situ thrombosis of a chronic preocclusive arteriosclerotic lesion accounts for approximately 85% of acute occlusive events (2). Such thrombotic complications are most likely to occur in segments of severe stenosis such as the aortic bifurcation, the iliac bifurcation, the common femoral bifurcation, and the superficial femoral artery just above the knee.

Upper extremity ischemia is usually secondary to arterial embolism. Acute thrombosis virtually never causes ischemia in the upper extremity because chronic arteriosclerotic lesions are uncommon and collateralization is excellent. Thoracic outlet compression may rarely give rise to subclavian or axillary arterial thrombosis. Concomitant problems such as hypovolemia from volume depletion or hemorrhage, congestive heart failure (CHF), erythrocytosis, or trauma all have profound influences on management.

Clinical Manifestations

More than 90% of the time, acute embolic occlusion may be distinguished from acute thrombotic occlusion on clinical grounds alone. In instances in which doubt exists about the cause, especially in the absence of atrial fibrillation and recent myocardial infarction (MI), arteriography is essential to distinguish embolus from thrombosis (see Laboratory and Radiographic Studies, below).

Emboli lodge at arterial bifurcations, most often in the lower extremities. Multiple emboli can result from a "shower discharge" of clots from the heart. Therefore, although the legs are affected most often, there may also be symptoms and signs of ischemia elsewhere. The development of new abdominal pain, limb pain, or neurologic deficit in a patient with a recent embolic event should invoke an expeditious diagnostic study, if needed, and prompt therapy.

Clinical manifestations vary depending on the adequacy of pre-existing collateral circulation and the site of occlusion (Fig. 94.1). If pre-existing collateral vessels, stimulated by underlying occlusive arterial disease, are present, acute ischemic symptoms may be mild. Total arterial occlusion of a previously normal arterial tree causes severe symptoms. The cardinal features of acute ischemia include the six *P*s of arterial occlusion: Pulselessness, pallor, poikilothermia ("coolness"), pain, paresthesias, and paralysis. The latter three *P*s reflect neurophysiologic sequelae of ischemia, and the former three result from mechanical occlusion of an artery. Three fourths of patients complain of pain, but 20% note numbness as the first manifestation of sudden arterial occlusion. Initially, the pain may be mild, but as the ischemia progresses, pain worsens, only to subside later as anesthesia and paralysis develop.

Additional findings include absent or faint distal pulses, poor capillary filling, and collapsed or severely sunken veins on the dorsum of the foot. Pedal edema, if present, is not a result of arterial occlusion, but it may be secondary to heart failure or pooling of blood in the extremities of patients who attempt to relieve ischemic pain by maintaining their legs in a dependent position for long periods.

Cardiac examination may reveal atrial fibrillation, a diastolic rumble or the opening snap of mitral stenosis, the click of a prosthetic heart valve, or a third heart sound associated with congestive heart failure. A recent history of chest pain, dysrythymia, or electrocardiographic evidence of MI also suggests a cardiac origin of acute leg ischemia.

Laboratory and Radiographic Studies

Laboratory studies usually are not helpful in making the diagnosis of acute arterial ischemia of the lower extremities. Arterial blood gas measurements and pH should be obtained to serve as baseline studies for subsequent comparative measurement and to identify metabolic acidosis secondary to muscle ischemia. Hyperkalemia may be noted, particularly if prolonged limb ischemia has occurred. A radiograph of the chest may document cardiac enlargement or congestive heart failure. An electrocardiogram

(ECG) and, *if time permits*, a transthoracic or transesophageal echocardiogram may be useful in delineating cardiac disease. All these studies should be obtained after the patient is hospitalized. Although noninvasive evaluation by Doppler ultrasonography (US) or by plethysmography is often superfluous, the inability to obtain any arterial Doppler signal in the foot in a patient with an acute occlusion supports the decision for urgent revascularization.

Contrast arteriography is not performed routinely in patients with acute ischemia except in occasional instances of modest ischemia when it is needed to distinguish between thrombosis and embolus (see Differential Diagnosis). Magnetic resonance angiography is being done in some centers as a less invasive alternative technique, especially when there are contraindications to contrast angiography. It is a key management paradigm that arteriographic investigation should not prolong the treatment interval, especially once neurologic sequelae have occurred. Such delays often lead to permanent nerve and muscle damage that may render a limb functionally useless. Evidence of generalized and severe arteriosclerosis, a tapered arterial occlusion, and well-developed collateral vessels suggest acute thrombosis. Normal-appearing arteries with scanty collateral circulation and an occlusion with an inverted meniscus configuration indicate embolic occlusion. However, embolization can occur in patients who also have chronic occlusive disease, and the diagnosis is occasionally still in question after angiography. In any case, the decision for immediate surgery is based on the clinical status of the extremity, not on the arteriogram.

Differential Diagnosis

Every effort should be made to differentiate embolism from thrombosis because the therapy of the two conditions is different. History is often helpful in separating these two entities. A history of intermittent claudication or of rest pain suggests the acute ischemic event is thrombosis. Absence of a history of intermittent claudication usually indicates embolism. However, a minority of patients who suffer acute superficial femoral arterial occlusion secondary to thrombosis have never had symptoms of intermittent claudication before the sudden occlusive event. On physical examination, classic findings of chronic ischemia such as loss of hair on the toes and dorsum of the foot and the leg, along with nail, skin, and muscle atrophy, suggest arterial thrombosis rather than embolism. A laterally pulsatile abdominal mass suggesting an abdominal aortic aneurysm (AAA) from which a mural thrombus may have embolized to the distal arterial tree might be evident. Finally, if the acute ischemic episode involves only one leg, palpating the popliteal and femoral arteries may detect an aneurysm. If the contralateral vessel is vigorously pulsating and aneurysmal, a thrombosis of an aneurysm on the ipsilateral or symptomatic side may have occurred, especially if a nonpulsatile mass can be palpated.

An acute dissection of the thoracic and abdominal aorta may present as unilateral lower extremity ischemia. Under these circumstances, patients may relate a history of severe, searing, ripping thoracic back pain and may provide a history of long-standing hypertension. Concomitant renal hypoperfusion may be noted, and malperfusion to the visceral vessels may cause vague abdominal pain. Chest radiograph may reveal a widened mediastinal silhouette, and a murmur of aortic insufficiency may be present if the dissection originates in the ascending aorta. Computed tomography (CT) scanning (with IV contrast) can usually demonstrate the septum of the dissection within the main aortic channel, and, often, asymmetric enhancement of the renal arteries or iliac arteries may be present and should heighten the suspicion for hemodynamic compromise of the affected territory.

Treatment

Evaluation and therapy must proceed simultaneously in the management of acute arterial ischemia of the extremities (Fig. 94.2). The cornerstone of early management is the immediate intravenous administration (in the clinician's office or emergency department) of 100 to 150 units heparin sodium per kilogram of body weight (3) (although no prospective controlled studies have established its efficacy) and then urgent vascular surgery consultation.

There may be a role for the interventional radiologist or endovascular surgeon to perform intra-arterial infusion of *fibrinolytic* agents directly into the site of the acute arterial occlusion (2–4). If that is the case, a multiple purpose polyethylene catheter is imbedded into the occluding clot after the arteriographic study is performed. Protocols may vary, but typically urokinase or tissue plasminogen activator is infused for 30 to 60 minutes and a second arteriogram is performed. Therapy is continued for 24 to 48 hours with clinical and angiographic re-evaluation at 8- to 12-hour intervals. Such therapy is contraindicated when the extremity is in dire jeopardy because the time required for lysis to occur may be longer than the safe interval before necrosis occurs. In patients whose limbs are not immediately threatened, this therapeutic approach can be efficacious, particularly for high-risk patients in whom operation may be contraindicated and in those patients with a diagnosis of a thrombosed surgical bypass graft. Results for thrombolysis in regard to restoration of perfusion or salvage of a thrombosed graft are best if the event is recent (<2 weeks). Untoward bleeding is the major complication of fibrinolytic therapy and may result in significant morbidity. The duration of the infusion and the optimal dosage to be administered to restore circulation are not yet firmly established. Therefore, until further experience is gained with this modality, it should be reserved for highly selected

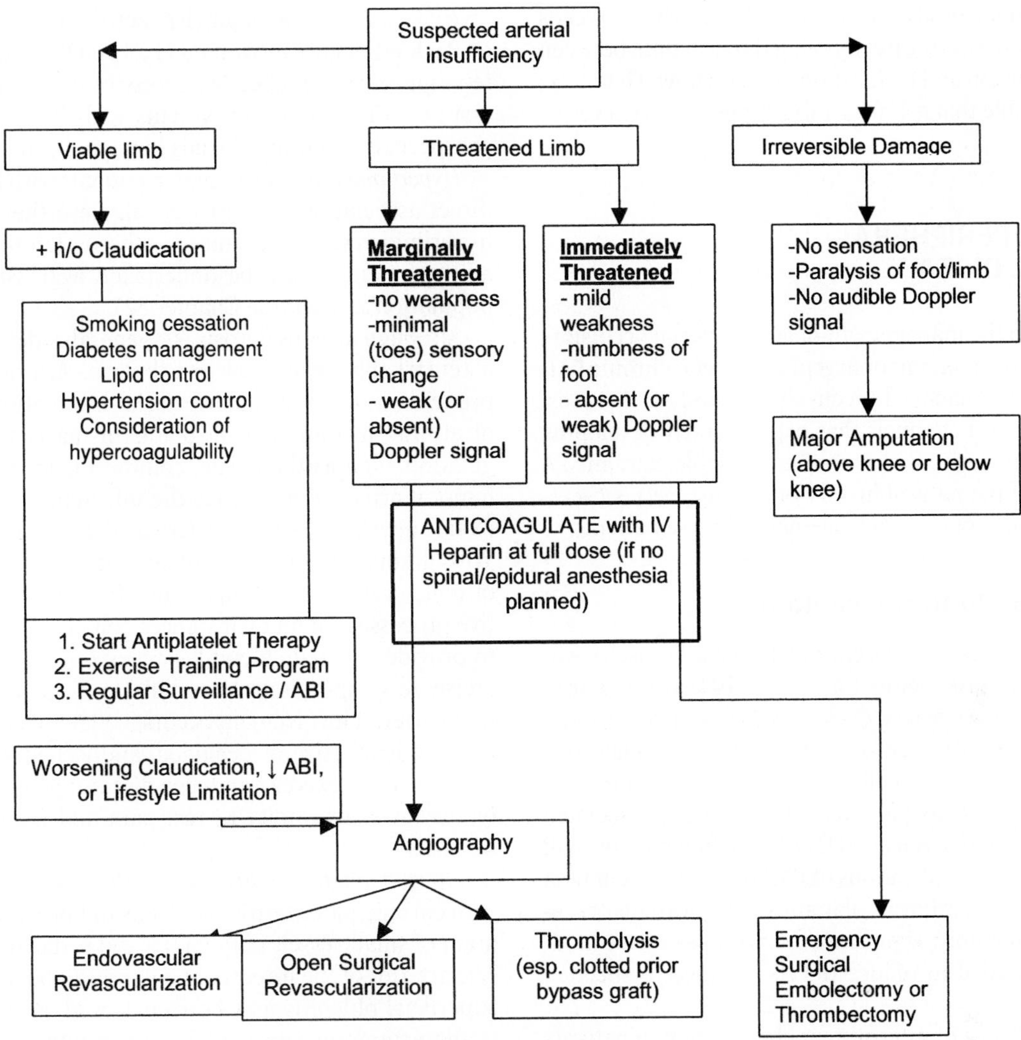

FIGURE 94.2. Overview of treatment of limb ischemia. There may be substantial overlap in those patients who present with threatened limbs. It is not uncommon for IV heparinization to improve the clinical examination of patients with immediately threatened limbs such that investigation (usually by angiography) may be performed; however, it is not acceptable for treatment delay to occur while awaiting investigations. ABI, ankle-brachial index.

patients who are cared for in centers specializing in management of vascular disease.

Surgical revascularization, can then be performed, if necessary, after blood flow to the ischemic extremity is restored. The introduction of the balloon-tipped embolectomy catheter by Fogarty et al. in 1963 revolutionized the management of acute embolic occlusion and converted a previously complex undertaking into a simple operative procedure that invariably can be performed under local anesthesia with improved survival and limb salvage rates.

After discharge from the hospital, patients are almost always maintained on therapeutic levels of oral anticoagulants for the rest of their lives, although only in patients with embolism associated with atrial fibrillation has efficacy been established (see Chapter 57). Furthermore, they must be evaluated several times a year to ensure that optimal cardiac function is maintained and for continued evaluation of their peripheral circulation.

Results

Despite improved diagnosis, preoperative care, operative management, and postoperative support, mortality from acute lower extremity ischemia continues to be discouraging and is likely related to associated cardiovascular disease. Early operative mortality rates still average 15% or more (2). Virtually all deaths are related to complications of cardiovascular disease, which reinforces the contention that recognition and correction of cardiovascular risk factors for arterial embolism or thrombosis are critical in the acute and long-term management of such patients (5).

The likelihood of successful limb salvage, which exceeds 95% in most series, is directly related to the time between arterial occlusion and restoration of blood flow. Therefore, it is improbable that a 100% limb salvage rate will ever be achieved.

CHRONIC PERIPHERAL ARTERIAL DISEASE

In contrast to the management of acute arterial occlusion, which requires emergent or urgent treatment, chronic PAD can usually be managed electively because of the presence of collateral channels that bypass slowly developing atherosclerotic lesions and maintain a viable extremity. A knowledge of the natural history of chronic PAD is necessary for the appropriate management of these patients.

Causes and Pathophysiology

The most common cause of chronic PAD is atherosclerosis. Atherosclerotic risk factors for chronic PAD are similar to those for coronary artery disease (CAD) and cerebrovascular disease (CVD): age older than 50 years, male sex, tobacco use, diabetes mellitus (DM), hypertension, and hyperlipidemia. Many patients with PAD have associated CAD and 10% have associated CVD (6). Often patients will not succumb to complications of PAD but will present with fatal or nonfatal cardiovascular and cerebrovascular complications. Therefore, significant focus on risk factor modification is needed to reduce the risk of these associated events.

The prevalence of intermittent claudication in patients with PAD is 1% to 2% for those younger than the age of 50 years and increases to 5% for those 50 to 70 years of age (6,7). Men are affected 1.5 to 2 times more often than women until age 70 years, when prevalence rates for intermittent claudication for men and women are nearly equal (6).

Smoking is the single most important modifiable risk factor for the development of PAD. Smokers develop PAD a decade earlier than age-matched nonsmokers, are at increased risk of amputation, and have less successful outcomes after lower extremity revascularization surgery (8). Tobacco use is synergistic with other risk factors for the development and progression of arterial disease (9).

Diabetic patients (see Chapter 79) manifest PAD a decade earlier than nondiabetic patients. In diabetics, PAD often develops in the more distal arteries of the leg earlier than it does in nondiabetics, and options for revascularization are therefore often limited. If a limb neuropathy is present, paresthesias and undetected infections and ulcerations can occur. Diabetics have a sevenfold higher rate of amputation than do nondiabetics (10,11).

Hypertension is a major risk factor for the development of PAD, especially in women (10,12). Observational studies support the practice of aggressive blood pressure control (see Chapter 67) in patients with PAD, although no prospective randomized trials have yet been done.

Hyperlipidemia is prevalent in patients with PAD, but the direct association is controversial. Nevertheless, treating hyperlipidemia is important in atherosclerotic patients in any case and should be undertaken aggressively in this population as well (see Chapter 82).

Although atherosclerosis is a generalized disease, it has a remarkably segmental distribution. Arteriosclerosis is prone to develop at major arterial bifurcations, in areas of arterial fixation, and at points of marked arterial angulation such as the aortic, common iliac, and common femoral artery bifurcations; the infrarenal aorta; and the distal superficial femoral artery as it enters Hunter canal. With gradual development of such lesions, the formation of collateral vessels compensates for segmental obstructive processes. In many instances collaterals are sufficient to provide adequate blood flow even during moderate exercise, so symptoms are minimal. However, as progressive main arterial involvement occurs, collateral channels may become ineffective or occluded, and ischemic symptoms progress from exercise-induced discomfort in the muscles of the lower extremity to rest pain and finally to tissue necrosis.

Thromboangiitis obliterans, or *Buerger disease,* is a severe chronic panarteritis that leads to fibrosis and obliteration of small vessels at the tibial and pedal arterial levels. The arteries of the forearm and hand can be involved, and superficial phlebitis may be seen as well. Buerger disease is an uncommon cause of lower extremity arterial insufficiency in the United States. This entity affects young men in their 20s and 30s and is almost always associated with severe tobacco addiction. Successful management hinges on cessation of all forms of tobacco usage.

Natural History

Intermittent claudication reflects a relatively benign condition (13–15). Approximately one third of patients improve, one third remain stable and tolerate their symptoms, and one third deteriorate and require revascularization. Relentless progression of the peripheral atherosclerotic process is unlikely in most nondiabetic patients, particularly if use of all tobacco products is discontinued. Less than 4% of patients will ultimately require amputation, although diabetics are at increased risk (8). On the other hand, patients with ischemic rest pain or gangrene are at very high risk for amputation if revascularization is not undertaken.

The overall 5- and 10-year survival rates among patients with intermittent claudication are approximately 70% and

40%, respectively, and the most common cause of death (in 75%) is CAD (16).

Clinical Manifestations

Symptoms

Many patients with PAD are asymptomatic. When symptoms begin, they are often described as pain or discomfort that develops in the affected limb with exercise and is relieved within several minutes with rest (claudication). The discomfort is often localized to the calf, although it can also affect the buttocks and thigh as well. The distance a patient walks before developing claudication should be documented. When symptoms advance to pain or discomfort at rest or when supine, it may be assumed that blood flow to the lower extremity is marginal. Gravity can increase blood flow slightly, and patients often learn to alleviate the symptoms by dangling the affected leg over the side of a bed or by standing up.

Physical Examination

A complete vascular examination should routinely be performed, noting the status of all peripheral pulses, the presence or absence of bruits and peripheral aneurysms, and the blood pressure measurements in both upper extremities. In patients with mild intermittent claudication, the skin, hair growth, feet, and toenails may appear normal, and faintly palpable dorsalis pedis and posterior tibial pulses may be present. However, with progressive arterial involvement trophic changes may occur with hair loss and the development of thin parchment-like skin. Lack of pulses below the inguinal ligaments, blanching and pallor with elevation of the extremity, and dependent rubor all indicate advanced ischemia. Gangrenous areas may be evident on the toes. The typical locations of ischemic ulcers are the calcaneus, the lateral malleolus, and the dorsum of the foot.

Laboratory and Radiographic Studies

The distribution and severity of PAD can be determined objectively by noninvasive Doppler flow studies. Doppler signals from the dorsalis pedis, posterior tibial, peroneal, or lateral tarsal arteries are located, and a sphygmomanometer cuff is placed immediately above the malleoli and inflated to above systolic pressure to obliterate the Doppler signal. As the cuff is slowly deflated, Doppler signals return at the systolic opening pressure. The highest pressure recorded is compared with the brachial arterial systolic pressure. A resting ankle-brachial index (ABI) of 1 or greater is normal. For patients with intermittent claudication the mean index is 0.59; for those with rest pain, 0.26; and for those with impending gangrene, 0.05 (17). The accuracy of the measurement is quite high (18). The ABI may be artifactually elevated in diabetic patients and those with advanced PAD because of calcific changes in the arterial wall. In this group, the cuff may not be able to occlude the stiffened vessel, and the ABI may be greater than 1.0. Further corroborative examination, usually by Doppler waveform analysis or pulse volume recording will demonstrate the problem if it is present. In normal patients, a triphasic waveform and pulse volume recording tracing are noted, however, as the PAD worsens, the waveform will progress to biphasic ("sine-wave") then monophasic ("flat-line") tracing. A monophasic waveform at any level indicates critical ischemia.

A Doppler study of lower extremity blood flow, although important, is not necessarily required in evaluating all patients with lower extremity arterial occlusive disease. However, noninvasive testing may be helpful in distinguishing vascular insufficiency from other causes of leg pain such as neurogenic claudication secondary to cauda equina compression from spinal stenosis. In the latter condition, Doppler ABI indices are normal at rest and after exercise. Doppler flow studies, with the patient at rest, are almost always sufficient to make the diagnosis of peripheral arterial occlusive disease (19). Rarely, the studies need to be repeated after exercise on a treadmill or even after simply walking the patient to the point of claudication. Noninvasive studies can also document the efficacy of nonoperative therapy and determine whether deterioration of the circulation is progressive (20). Also, comparison of preoperative and postoperative noninvasive data is useful in documenting the effectiveness of operative therapy.

The gold standard study, if it is determined the patient is a candidate for operation, is arteriography. Although risks are very small in experienced hands, arteriography is used only when operation is indicated and agreed to by the patient. Finally, laboratory studies may also reveal hyperglycemia or hyperlipidemia that requires appropriate management.

Treatment and Results

Treatment for arterial insufficiency of the legs may be either operative or nonoperative. Table 94.1 shows indications for operation. Patients should usually be managed nonoperatively unless one of these indications is present

TABLE 94.1 Indications for Operation for Arterial Insufficiency of the Legs

Claudication that is intolerable in a patient at low surgical risk
Ischemic rest pain
Impending gangrene
Nonhealing ulceration

TABLE 94.2 Advice That Should Be Given to Patients with Arterial Insufficiency

Quit smoking. Use *no* tobacco in *any* form[a]
If overweight, lose weight.
Walk to the point of claudication at least 30 minutes a day.
Keep feet very clean. Bathe at least daily in lukewarm water.
Gently apply lanolin or mild hand cream to feet after bathing.
Wear clean, preferably cotton, socks daily (cotton does not retain moisture).
Avoid injury to feet. Wear properly fitting shoes to prevent calluses, corns, blisters.
Avoid shoes made of synthetic material that does not "breathe." Wear slippers at night and use a night light after going to bed.
Place lamb's wool (available from pharmacies) between overriding toes.
Avoid extremes of temperature. Do no put feet in hot water or use heating pads on lower extremities. In cold weather, wear socks to bed to warm feet. Do not get feet cold or wet.
If feet hurt at night, raise head of bed 6–10 in. (15–25 cm) on blocks.
For any sudden change in symptoms such as prolonged pain, numbness or tingling, or inability to move foot or leg, consult your health care provider *immediately*.

[a]See Chapter 27 for ways to help patients to stop smoking.

and medical management has failed. Knowing the natural history of the occlusive process aids significantly in determining whether the patient's symptoms warrant operative intervention in view of associated risk factors and life expectancy. Except for patients who are not considered operative candidates, ischemic rest pain, nonhealing ulcers, pregangrenous changes, and gangrene are unequivocal indications for expeditious revascularization.

General Measures

An itemized list of recommendations written in nontechnical language should be given to and carefully reviewed with the patient (Table 94.2). Meticulous skin hygiene and avoidance of injury to the foot, however slight, cannot be overemphasized. An otherwise asymptomatic ischemic foot becomes symptomatic when trauma leads to a nonhealing ulcer that may require revascularization. If the patient's feet are cold, particularly at night, a warm pair of socks or a muffler is advised but not the use of heating pads or hot water bottles, which may cause tissue breakdown and ulceration. Patients should inspect their feet every day and should bathe them at least once a day in lukewarm water and thereafter apply lanolin or hand cream to the skin to keep it soft and pliable and to avoid cracking and fissuring and subsequent skin breakdown.

Exercise is the cornerstone of therapy for symptomatic PAD. Supervised exercise rehabilitation programs (e.g., in cardiac rehabilitation centers) using a treadmill have been found to be the most successful at relieving intermittent claudication (10,18). Significant improvement in walking times before onset of intermittent claudication can occur when the program includes up to 30-minute sessions of intermittent treadmill exercise three times a week for 3 to 6 months. These programs require a motivated and compliant patient. During sessions, trained personnel may also reinforce the need for risk factor modification. Patients are also encouraged to continue a walking exercise program at home. Other measures that significantly affect outcome include maintaining satisfactory cardiac function.

Smoking cessation (see Chapter 27) is especially critical for patients with chronic PAD, and the decrease in mortality rates for patients who stop smoking is significant (18,20). Smoking cessation improves symptoms of intermittent claudication in up to 85% of patients and improves exercise tolerance by up to 300%. Patients must clearly understand that nicotine absorption occurs through the buccal mucosa with the use of chewing tobacco, pipes, cigars, and cigarettes and does not require inhalation of smoke.

Diabetic patients with PAD have a high risk of eventual amputation, and the general principles of foot care are especially important for them. Additionally, diabetics should be seen by a podiatrist every 3 months for trimming of their nails and calluses and for close inspection for early signs of infection or ulceration. Intensive hypoglycemic therapy, of value in many diabetics, has not yet been demonstrated to affect the course of atherosclerotic peripheral vascular disease (10) (see Chapter 79).

Management of coexistent hypertension (see Chapter 67) is sometimes challenging, and blood pressure control may be less than ideal because the symptoms of the arteriosclerotic occlusive process may worsen if the patient is returned to a normotensive state. It now seems clear that β-blockers, previously thought to be harmful to patients with PAD, may be used in the treatment of hypertension in this population unless the occlusive disease is severe (21). Angiotensin-converting enzyme inhibitors (ACEIs), may, however, be the antihypertensive agents of choice (22). In patients taking antihypertensive drugs, it is important to check at each visit for orthostatic drops in blood pressure and to adjust the treatment regimen accordingly if orthostatic hypotension occurs.

In order to manage hyperlipidemia (see Chapter 82), a fasting lipid profile should be obtained for all patients with PAD. In PAD, the major risk factors for arteriosclerosis are elevated low-density lipoprotein (LDL) cholesterol and triglyceride levels and low high-density lipoprotein (HDL) cholesterol levels. Appropriate diet (and exercise, if possible) are important but lipid-lowering agents are often required. With respect to LDL cholesterol, the goal is to achieve a level less than 100 mg/dL. Several retrospective trials have demonstrated improved patency of vascular reconstructions (carotid endarterectomy, leg bypass grafts) in those patients taking statin medications (23,24).

Pharmacologic Management

Antiplatelet Drugs

Aspirin, 81 to 325 mg/day, has been demonstrated to reduce the risk of vascular events in patients with atherosclerotic disease. It has not, however, been shown unequivocally to alter the progress of PAD (25). Nevertheless, its use in patients with PAD is reasonable, especially considering that most of these patients have systemic atherosclerosis. Ticlopidine and clopidogrel, two other drugs that inhibit platelet plug formation, are approved for treatment of patients with PAD. Ticlopidine is prescribed less often because of hematologic side effects. Clopidogrel has fewer side effects (although rare instances of thrombotic thrombocytopenic purpura have been reported [26]) and has been shown to be slightly more effective than aspirin in preventing progression of PAD (27). Nevertheless, aspirin at present is the more cost-effective drug.

Vasodilator Drugs

There is no objective evidence to suggest that vasodilating drugs are beneficial to patients with PAD. Blood vessels in ischemic tissue beds are already maximally dilated. When systemic vessels are dilated by these drugs, blood flow to the compromised extremity may actually decrease. Therefore, these drugs are not recommended for treatment of patients with PAD.

Pentoxifylline

This drug is a xanthine derivative that has been used for many years to treat patients with PAD. It decreases blood viscosity by a direct effect on the red blood cell membrane. Enough data have now accumulated to show that pentoxifylline (typically one 400-mg tablet three times a day) has little, if any, effect in reducing symptoms in patients with PAD and probably should not be prescribed (10).

Cilostazol

This drug is a phosphodiesterase inhibitor that has been approved relatively recently for treatment of PAD. Its mechanism of action is unknown, although it does affect platelet and endothelial function. A number of controlled trials have shown the drug to be effective in improving exercise tolerance (e.g., walking distance improvement of 45% to 100%) in patients with PAD (10,28). A standard dosing schedule is 100 mg (50- and 100-mg tablets are available) twice a day. Because cilostazol inhibits several hepatic drug-metabolizing enzymes, its daily dosage should be lowered if drugs metabolized by those enzymes (e.g., erythromycin or omeprazole) are prescribed concomitantly. The major side effects reported by the manufacturer are headache (up to 34% of patients), diarrhea (up to 19% of patients), and palpitations (up to 10% of patients). Cilostazol is contraindicated in patients with CHF of any severity.

Anticoagulant Drugs

There is no evidence that heparin or warfarin has any beneficial effect in patients with PAD (29) except in reducing the incidence of embolization in patients with atrial fibrillation.

Operative Intervention

It is only upon failure of nonoperative therapy and among patients with clear indications for surgery that arteriographic studies are obtained. It must be understood that arteriography serves as a roadmap for the vascular surgeon when reconstructing the vascular tree. No characteristic arteriographic findings distinguish between patients with intermittent claudication, those with ischemic rest pain, and those with gangrene and ulceration. As a generalization, however, patients who have intermittent claudication usually have hemodynamically significant proximal arterial occlusive lesions affecting the iliofemoral or the femoral–popliteal system. Characteristically, such patients have reasonably good outflow with two or more tibial vessels patent. Patients with advanced ischemic changes are found to have diffuse multisegment involvement and none or only one patent tibial vessel in the lower leg or foot. However, there is considerable overlap between groups, and no single arteriographic finding consistently characterizes any one symptom complex.

Arteriography occasionally demonstrates a distribution of advanced arterial involvement without reasonable runoff vessels for bypass. Under these circumstances, nonoperative therapy is all that may be offered, and there is a significant risk of subsequent amputation. Indications for operation among patients with intermittent claudication relate mainly to significant limitation of activities of daily living. Nonlimiting claudication and mild ischemic rest pain that is controlled by non-narcotic analgesics are not indications for operation, particularly in high-risk patients. A trial of conservative management is especially important if other risk factors, such as recent MI, are present.

When it is determined that the condition of the patient warrants operative intervention and when arteriography documents adequate outflow vessels, a number of options for arterial reconstruction are open to the vascular surgeon, including autogenous vein or prosthetic graft bypass and endarterectomy. There is a definite preference for bypass surgery rather than endarterectomy. Direct reconstructive procedures include aortofemoral bypass, femoral–popliteal bypass, and femoral–tibial bypass. Extra-anatomic reconstruction includes axillounifemoral bypass, axillobifemoral bypass, and femoral–femoral bypass.

The operative mortality rate for aortofemoral bypass grafting is less than 5% with a patency rate of 80% to 90% at 5 years (8). Operative mortality for extra-anatomic reconstructions is slightly less than for aortofemoral bypass,

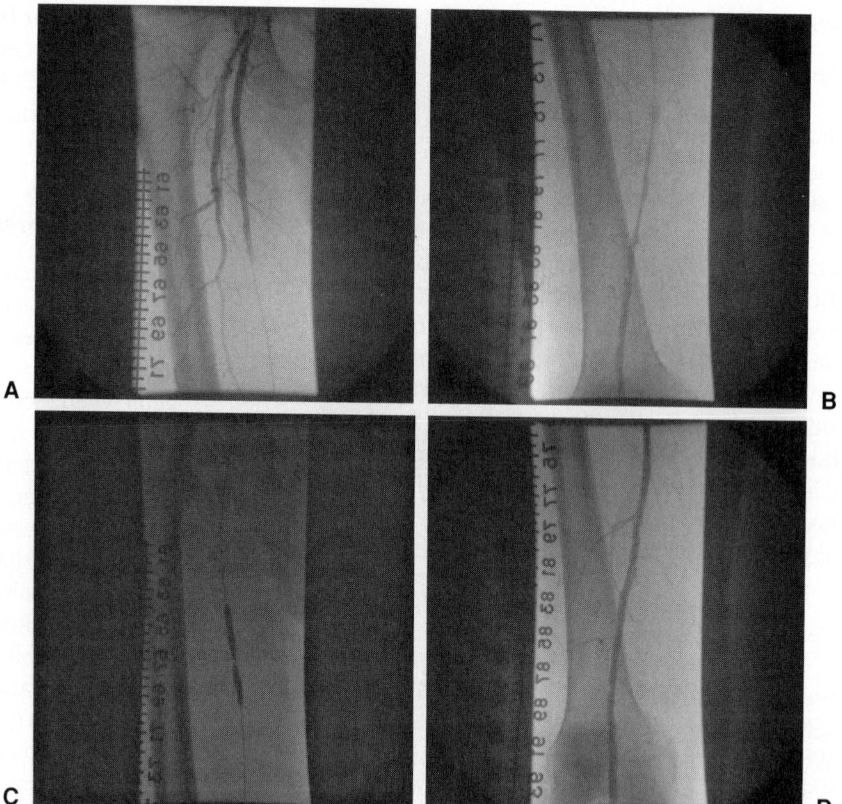

FIGURE 94.3. Percutaneous transluminal angioplasty (PTA) of superficial femoral artery (SFA) atherosclerotic disease in a patient with severe claudication. **A,B:** Diagnostic study reveals diffuse severe disease of the SFA with serial severe stenoses. **C:** PTA balloon demonstrating recalcitrant lesion with tight "waisting" of the balloon. **D:** Final angiographic result with minimal residual stenosis (<20%) and no flow-limiting dissection. The patient had a significant clinical improvement. (James Black, MD)

but the outlook for graft patency is not as good. Operative mortality for autogenous vein femoral–popliteal and femoral–tibial bypass procedures ranges from 0.5% to 1% depending on the general condition of the patient; 5-year patency rates for such procedures vary between 60% and 70% (8,30). It should be emphasized that patency varies directly with adequacy of the vein used and the extent of the disease in the vessel being reconstructed.

Generally, in contrast to aneurysmal disease, arterial reconstruction for occlusive disease is palliative and does not significantly increase the patient's life expectancy because most patients have significant coincident CAD. However, the quality of life may be vastly improved by surgery, particularly for those who would have undergone amputation if successful arterial reconstruction had not been feasible.

Patients with aortofemoral arterial occlusive disease who do not have CAD or DM have survival rates that equal those of the normal age- and sex-adjusted population. It appears that the presence of CAD reduces life expectancy by approximately 10 years, and the presence of DM reduces life expectancy by an additional 15 years (31).

Angioplasty

Percutaneous transluminal arterial dilation (angioplasty) is used as an alternative to surgical reconstruction for highly selected patients with arterial occlusive disease or those with significant surgical risk. It is a technique that uses a catheter with an attached balloon to dilate the stenosed artery. Advantages include lower morbidity, lower mortality, and possibly lower cost compared with arterial reconstruction. Patients who are not candidates for surgery, if subjected to percutaneous transluminal angioplasty (PTA), could conceivably require operation if complications occur after the percutaneous procedure. Therefore, a cooperative approach between the interventional radiologist and the vascular surgeon is mandatory (Fig. 94.3).

The best results with PTA are obtained typically in patients with short segment stenoses of the iliac arteries, in which success rates range from 76% to 93% at 1 year and from 66% to 92% at 2 years. The reported results of angioplasty for femoropopliteal disease range from 51% to 80% at 1 year and from 46% to 75% at 2 years. There is general agreement that results are less satisfactory if the arteriographic runoff is poor. In the properly selected patient, the probability of early success of PTA is high if the involved vessel is the iliac artery, there is a short segment of stenosis and not occlusion, and the runoff is good (32). Results are less satisfactory when multiple dilations are required. Unsatisfactory results of a peripheral angioplasty may require placement of *metallic stents* to improve the technical result if restenosis or dissection is noted.

Patients with longer stenoses and total occlusions have less favorable outcomes, but in very poor-risk patients, angioplasty may be the only alternative to operative reconstruction. In particular, if an adequate length of autogenous vein cannot be harvested (because of prior coronary or leg bypass), a long segment angioplasty may be the only viable therapeutic option. Occlusions more than 5 cm long and stenoses more than 10 cm long appear to be associated with significant restenosis rates (10% to 30% per year) and a regular surveillance program is indicated for such interventions.

Amputation

In debilitated patients with frank gangrene or unremitting ischemic rest pain in whom arterial reconstruction or transluminal angioplasty is not indicated or feasible, amputation is the only alternative. The goal of amputation is to relieve the patient of disabling pain, remove nonviable and potentially infected tissue, and select a level that will provide the greatest chance of healing with maximal prosthetic rehabilitation.

If the gangrenous process is dry and does not involve the great toe, autoamputation may be allowed to occur or formal surgical amputation may be performed. If pulses are palpable in the foot and the ischemic process affects the tips of the digits, primary healing usually occurs after toe amputation. Nonischemic neurotrophic ulcers on the plantar aspects of the foot in diabetic patients often heal if the head of the metatarsal is removed to relieve the pressure necrosis that occurs as a result of the diabetic neuropathy.

Mortality for amputation is directly related to the preoperative condition of the patient and to other complicating diseases. Mortality rates for amputations performed for occlusive arterial disease have been reported to be as high as 30%, with higher mortality rates recorded in the more proximal amputations.

After successful amputation, which includes primary healing that results in a stump amenable to prosthetic fitting, the most important aspect of therapy is rehabilitation. Prosthetic mobility requires almost twice as much energy with an above-knee amputation than with a below-knee amputation, and mobility is further inhibited by increased age, infirmity, obesity, and a poorly fitting prosthesis. Population studies demonstrate that only 50% of patients undergoing below knee amputation because of PAD will be fully ambulatory on a prosthesis; only 10% to 20% of patients with an above-knee amputation become ambulatory. It is difficult to predict successful rehabilitation in the atherosclerotic population, but cooperation between the surgeon and the rehabilitation team is pivotal to a satisfactory outcome.

ABDOMINAL AORTIC ANEURYSMS

An aneurysm, a blood-filled dilatation of a blood vessel, is generally defined as a 50% increase in diameter of a blood vessel. In the infrarenal abdominal aorta, a diameter of greater than 4 cm is also considered diagnostic of an aneurysm. The recognized incidence of AAAs has increased with the advent of sensitive and specific diagnostic noninvasive tests such as US, CT, and magnetic resonance imaging (MRI).

The most common site of an arterial aneurysm is the abdominal aorta. AAA is encountered two to three times more often than the second most common type, the popliteal artery aneurysm, and has been found in almost 2% of consecutive postmortem studies (33).

Etiology and Natural History

An AAA results from disease of the media characterized by degeneration of extracellular matrix proteins, which maintain the integrity of the vessel wall. AAAs are most often infrarenal (75%). Only 5% involve the suprarenal aorta, and 25% involve the iliac arteries (34).

The highest prevalence of such aneurysms is in white males older than 65 years of age (35). Age-adjusted incidence is fourfold to sixfold higher in men than in women for both asymptomatic and ruptured AAAs. Tobacco use is the risk factor most strongly associated with AAA (36). Smokers with small AAAs (4 to 5.5 cm) have been found to have an increased risk of rupture (1.9% per year versus 0.5% per year for nonsmokers) and poorer long-term survival.

The relationship between AAA and atherosclerosis is not clear. It is not known why some patients develop atherosclerosis and calcification of the abdominal aorta and some develop aneurysmal dilatation. Recently, genetic factors have been found to play a role (37). The prevalence of AAA is 1% in elderly siblings of subjects without AAA and increases fourfold in siblings of subjects who have AAA (38).

Our understanding of the *natural history* of AAA is clouded by early studies (39) that documented high risks of rupture but included more patients with large aneurysms than patients with smaller ones. This is important, because the risk of rupture is related to the size of the aneurysm (40). The advent of noninvasive screening techniques has allowed the detection of small asymptomatic aneurysms and improved our understanding of the rate of growth and risk of rupture of AAAs. Studies that have prospectively followed AAA size indicate that the average rate of expansion is 0.3 to 0.4 cm per year, with a range of 0.24 to 0.9 cm per year (41–43). The risk of rupture is negligible for AAAs less than 4.0 cm but increases significantly when the aneurysm reaches a size of 5.0 cm or more or when the rate of expansion is more than 0.5 to 1.0 cm in 6 to 12 months (44) (Fig. 94.4). Thus, whereas early studies demonstrated improved life expectancy with surgical treatment of AAA (45), more recent studies have suggested that early surgery may not offer a long-term survival advantage for patients with small

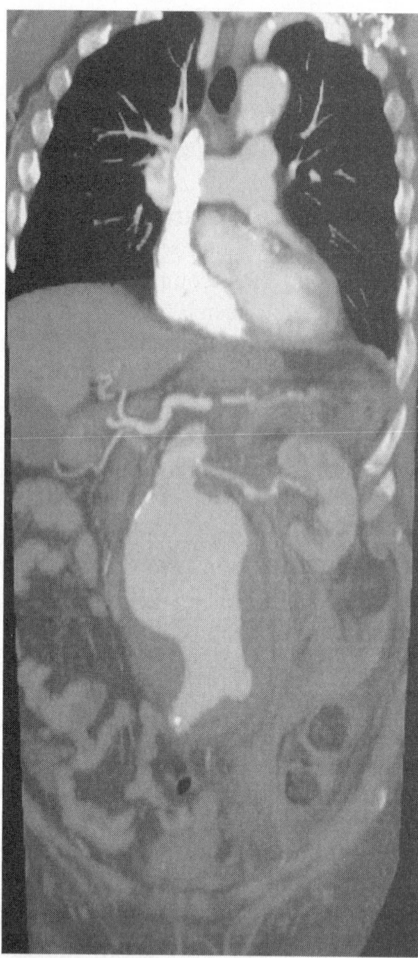

FIGURE 94.4. Sagittal reconstruction of a CT scan demonstrating a ruptured 10 cm abdominal aortic aneurysm. Note the fat stranding created by retroperitoneal blood apparent immediately inferior to left kidney. The patient was hemodynamically stable and underwent endovascular AAA repair (James Black, MD).

asymptomatic aneurysms, who can be followed with serial ultrasound examinations (41) (see Treatment and Results, below).

Screening

The U.S. Preventive Services Task Force (USPSTF) recommends one-time screening for AAA by US in men age 65 to 75 years who have ever smoked (46). Although the USPSTF makes no recommendation for or against screening in men 65 to 75 years old who have never smoked, it acknowledges evidence that an invitation to such men to participate in screening reduces aneurysm-associated mortality (47). Screening for women and for men younger than 65 or older than 75 years is not recommended. Other expert groups have recommended screening all men age 60 to 85 years, women in the same age group with risk factors for atherosclerotic disease, and all patients older than 50 years of age with a family history of AAA. The Center for Medicare and Medicaid Services and the U.S. Congress are considering whether to provide Medicare coverage for screening for AAA by abdominal ultrasound.

Clinical Manifestations

History

The presentation of an AAA depends on whether complications have occurred. More than 50% are asymptomatic when first discovered during routine examination by a caregiver, by the patient who complains of a second heart in the abdomen upon palpating a pulsatile epigastric mass, or serendipitously during radiographic or ultrasonographic abdominal studies in the pursuit of another diagnosis. The patient may complain of abdominal, flank, or back pain as the aneurysm expands and becomes symptomatic, a harbinger of rupture. The most common misdiagnosis of a ruptured AAA is renal colic, thus, a patient suspected to have renal colic should be examined for a pulsatile mass or a confirmatory study should be performed (CT or ultrasound).

Most aneurysms that *rupture* bleed into the retroperitoneal space, affording life-saving tamponade. Under these circumstances, the patient presents with a history of syncope or of flank or back pain in a hypovolemic, but not necessarily a hypotensive, state. On the other hand, the patient with an uncontained intraperitoneal rupture of an AAA typically presents in shock secondary to blood loss and requires immediate operative intervention. Aneurysms may rupture into adjacent structures and cause large arteriovenous fistulas, such as an aortocaval or aortorenal fistula with high-output cardiac failure, or into the gastrointestinal tract, usually the duodenum, causing an aortoenteric fistula with massive hematemesis or hematochezia.

Other Complications

If aneurysms are large enough, they may produce symptoms due to compression of adjacent structures such as the ureter, duodenum, vena cava, or vertebral column. Dislodgment of laminated clots from the wall of the aneurysm occasionally may cause peripheral embolization to femoral, popliteal, or distal vessels. When emboli occur, patients may complain of symptoms of sudden leg ischemia as the first indication of AAA (see Examination section). If emboli are small and distal vessels are patent, small areas of tissue necrosis in the toes or skin of the lower extremities are seen.

After seeking specific historical information regarding the aneurysm, the patient should be questioned about other symptoms so that an estimate of the extent of atherosclerotic involvement is obtained. This information often influences recommendations for or against surgical therapy. Symptoms of transient cerebral ischemia or previous stroke, angina pectoris or previous MI, or cardiac decompensation such as significant shortness of breath, dependent edema, orthopnea, and paroxysmal nocturnal dyspnea are especially important in determining the risks in this group of patients.

Physical Examination

Abdominal palpation is only moderately sensitive and specific in the diagnosis of an AAA (48). As previously noted, most patients with asymptomatic AAAs are discovered on routine physical examination to have an epigastric or left upper quadrant pulsatile mass. However, a pulsatile mass may not be palpable in obese patients or in those with very small aneurysms.

It is important to palpate the epigastrium because the bifurcation of the abdominal aorta is at the level of the umbilicus. Only rarely when palpating inferior to the umbilicus will one identify an AAA unless both common iliac arteries are also aneurysmal. The laterally pulsatile nature of an aneurysm is a clue in differentiating it from the anteriorly transmitted aortic pulsation through viscera or from a mass overlying the aorta. Conditions confused with aneurysms include pancreatic pseudocyst, horseshoe kidneys, neoplasms of the stomach or transverse colon, and retroperitoneal soft tissue tumors. Often, a normal but prominently pulsatile abdominal aorta in a healthy person and an undilated but tortuous aorta in an elderly person may simulate an AAA. In this circumstance, the pulsatile mass is felt to the left of the midline but not to the right. One should palpate the abdomen by approaching the midline both from the right and from the left to identify the laterally pulsatile characteristic of an aneurysm. Risk of rupture correlates best with the size of the aneurysm as determined by US and not by physical examination alone (see Fig. 94.5).

One fourth to one third of patients have significant associated occlusive arterial disease as well as the AAA, so a systematic evaluation should be performed. Systemic blood pressure should be measured in both arms. Carotid bruits can be detected by listening with the bell of the stethoscope over the carotid bifurcations at the angle of the mandible with the patient supine and holding his or her breath. Examination of the lower extremities should be directed to the character of the femoral, popliteal, and pedal pulses and to the presence or absence of femoral and popliteal bruits and aneurysms. In less than 10% of patients with AAA, there may be coexistent peripheral aneurysms involving the popliteal or femoral arteries.

Laboratory and Radiographic Studies

The presence or absence of an AAA must be confirmed by US. The accuracy of sonographic diagnosis of AAAs approaches 100% (49). Anteroposterior and cross-table lateral plain radiographs of the abdomen also document AAAs in 70% to 80% of cases because the aneurysm wall is often calcified. Ultrasonography is simple, safe, and cost-effective and is recommended as the method of choice for verifying or excluding an AAA and for serial followup every 6 months to assess aneurysmal size for patients being treated nonoperatively.

CT and MRI are more expensive and should be used only as an adjunct to US for confirming unusual situations, such as a suspected leak in an otherwise stable patient, extent of visceral artery involvement, inflammatory change, or the presence and characteristics of horseshoe kidney. Generally, the cost of a CT is about double that of a sonogram. The MRI costs twice as much as the CT and rarely provides additional information.

Objective measurement of peripheral pulses in the lower extremities and baseline Doppler blood flow studies are of value during long-term followup. Because atherosclerotic disease may be progressive, the patient should be followed on a yearly basis after convalescence from surgery.

Treatment and Results

Whereas patients with symptomatic AAAs require operative intervention, it is not clear that early surgery improves mortality in patients with small asymptomatic aneurysms in whom a strategy of "watchful waiting" may be reasonable. In one study, 1090 patients age 60 to 76 years with asymptomatic AAA between 4.0 and 5.5 cm in diameter were randomly assigned to undergo elective surgery or serial ultrasonographic surveillance every 6 months. Surgery was recommended to patients randomized to the surveillance strategy if the AAA diameter exceeded 5.5 cm. After an average of 4.6 years, there was no difference in mortality between the groups (41). The decision about when, and if, to recommend surgery to patients with asymptomatic AAA depends on the assessment of the risk of rupture compared with the risk of elective operative repair (50). The risk of rupture, in turn, is most closely related to AAA size and rate of expansion. Patients with an AAA less than 5.5 cm in diameter may be followed by serial ultrasound examinations performed at 6-month intervals. If the aneurysm exceeds 5.5 cm or if the rate of expansion exceeds 0.5 cm in a 6-month interval, the risk of rupture should be considered high and elective surgery should be strongly considered. When surgery is not recommended, therapy with β-blockers should be considered in an effort to reduce the rate of AAA expansion. This recommendation is based largely on a single study of 121 patients with AAA (approximately two thirds of whom received β-blockers) who were monitored with serial ultrasound examinations approximately every 8 months for an average of 43 months. Among patients with AAA 5 cm or greater, β-blockers

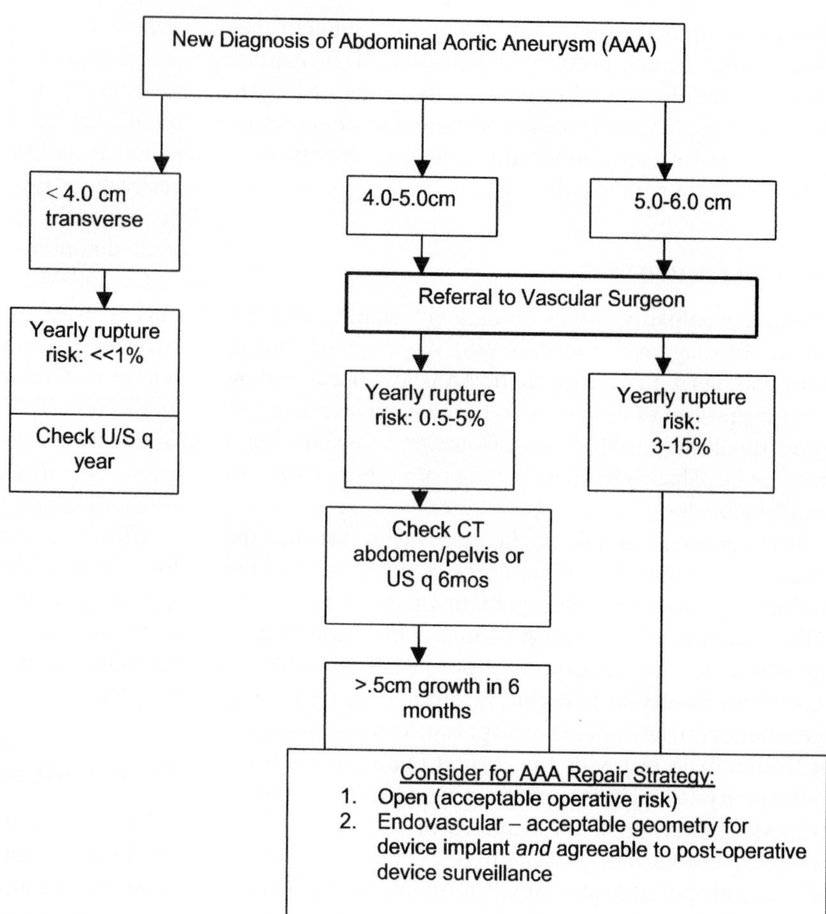

FIGURE 94.5. An approach to AAA. The risk of rupture is weighed against the mortality associated with AAA repair (by both endovascular and open means).

significantly reduced the expansion rate from 0.68 to 0.36 cm per year (42). Figure 94.5 shows an approach to the management of AAA.

Routine use of preoperative aortography among patients with AAAs is very rare. With the advent of multislice CT, outstanding definition can be achieved. A standard protocol CT angiogram with three-dimensional reconstruction can provide all necessary information on the size of the aneurysm as well as anatomic features and suitability for stent-grafting. The procedure requires the administration of 100 to 120 mL of iodinated contrast material. For patients with renal insufficiency, magnetic resonance angiography (MRA) may provide an alternative diagnostic modality. Although surgeons rarely recommend aortography, and most use aortographic studies selectively, under certain circumstances abdominal aortography is helpful and even mandatory. Indications for aortography include the possibility of anomalous renal or visceral vasculature or occlusive disease involving these same vessels that would alter the operative approach. It is important to determine the extent of reconstruction necessary so that the anomalous vessels are not violated and the occlusive lesions are addressed. Drug-resistant renovascular hypertension is an indication for aortography to document renal artery stenosis that can be corrected at the time of abdominal aortic aneurysmectomy. Aortography is essential for delineation of the anomalous circulation of the rare horseshoe kidney initially detected by US.

It is essential to inform the patient of various risks of operative versus nonoperative treatment. Equally important is explaining complications that may occur in the postoperative period. Although this is primarily the responsibility of the operating surgeon, it is appropriate for the primary clinician to discuss with the patient what is likely to occur. The patient should know that a Dacron or polytetrafluoroethylene prosthesis will be used to replace the abdominal aorta and that such arterial grafts are very durable. Fortunately, complications are rare and include (but are not limited to), renal failure, amputation, graft infection, ischemic colitis, paraplegia from spinal cord ischemia, and aortoenteric fistula. It should be stressed to the patient that postoperative complications of abdominal aortic aneurysmectomy are magnified by the urgency of the operative procedure. Proper cardiac risk stratification by noninvasive evaluation (that is, but are not limited to, exercise or nuclear stress test or stress echocardiogram), prior to open AAA repair may identify those patients who may benefit from preoperative coronary angioplasty.

Endovascular stent-grafting of AAAs is gaining favor as the preferred approach for repair of AAA, especially in those patients of advanced age or with significant comorbidity. This technique uses an endoprosthesis that is delivered percutaneously through the femoral artery and deployed in the area of the aneurysm. The endograft is secured with metallic expandable stents and thrombosis of the external surrounding aneurysm, in theory, reduces the risk of rupture. Three Food and Drug Administration (FDA)-approved devices are available for implantation.

Results with each are largely equivalent, with only minor technical differences in device insertion. Randomized trials have demonstrated that endovascular stent-grafting of AAAs is equivalent to open AAA repair for prevention of aneurysm-associated mortality (51).

To date, the most common adverse long-term problem with the current devices is "endoleak," which represents persistent filling of the AAA from either the anastomotic site or through other collateral blood vessels (44). Endoleaks may occur at the interface of the device and the aorta or iliacs, between device junctions, or most commonly from lumbar vessels that back-bleed into the aneurysm sac via collaterals. These endoleaks occur in 10% to 20% of patients per year who have undergone endovascular stent-grafting of AAAs. If associated with expansion of aortic diameter, such endoleaks may require additional procedures to investigate their source.

Patient Experience with Endovascular AAA Repair

Patients are often enticed by the minimally invasive nature of endovascular stent-grafting of AAAs. A standard expected course of endovascular stent-grafting of AAAs is admission on the same day of surgery (if no preoperative overnight hydration for prevention of contrast nephropathy). Patients may have epidural anesthesia (and be kept awake) or general anesthesia. Using bilateral groin incisions, the endovascular implant is introduced via the femoral arteries into the aorta and sealed below the renal arteries to shield the aneurysm sac from the aortic blood flow/pressure. Separate pieces are introduced from either groin to complete the bifurcated device, seal the device at the common iliac arteries bilaterally, and provide passage of blood to pelvis and legs. Transfusion of red blood cells is uncommonly required unless preoperative anemia is present. Patients are monitored in the recovery room or intensive care unit and then convalesce in the hospital for 1 to 2 days prior to discharge. Oral analgesics easily control the pain of the groin incisions, and most patients return to work 2 weeks after endovascular stent-grafting of AAAs. Standard surveillance using CT angiograms of the abdomen and pelvis are required at 1, 6, 12, 18, and 24 months and then yearly to monitor for "endoleaks." Although recovery time is clearly less with EVAR, patients are often frustrated by the intense postoperative surveillance and the potential necessity for additional procedures to eliminate any endoleak. Nonetheless, even with the trade-off of the imposition of regular surveillance versus the extensive incision and recovery of open AAA repair, endovascular stent-grafting of AAAs is often preferred by patients.

If operation is not recommended or accepted, the patient should be evaluated every 3 to 6 months by interval history, physical examination, and US. The warning signs of a rupturing or symptomatic aneurysm, especially steady dull abdominal, flank, or back pain, should be described to the patient. If such pain occurs or if a change in existing symptoms is noted in a patient being followed with an AAA, the patient should be instructed to seek surgical attention promptly.

PERIPHERAL ARTERIAL ANEURYSMS

Peripheral arterial aneurysms may involve the carotid, subclavian, brachial, iliac, femoral, and popliteal arteries. More than 90% of peripheral aneurysms involve either popliteal or femoral arteries. Popliteal arterial aneurysms predominate. Tortuous vessels presenting as serpiginous pulsations under the skin may be mistaken for peripheral aneurysms. The most noted example of this is a tortuous subclavian or common carotid artery in an elderly hypertensive patient that may be confused with a carotid or subclavian artery aneurysm. The pathogenesis of peripheral aneurysms is unknown. There is a male predominance (30:1 ratio, men versus women) and up to 50% are bilateral (52).

Most peripheral arterial aneurysms are arteriosclerotic in origin; mycotic, traumatic, and syphilitic aneurysms are rare. Peripheral arteriosclerotic aneurysms are localized manifestations of a generalized disease process. This is underscored by noting that among a group of 37 patients with common femoral aneurysms, 95% had another aneurysm elsewhere, and 92% had associated aortoiliac aneurysms (53). Femoral aneurysms can be bilateral in up to 60% of cases. Similarly, among 36 patients with popliteal arterial aneurysms, almost 80% had an aneurysm elsewhere, two thirds had aortoiliac aneurysms, and bilateral popliteal aneurysms occurred in 50% of these patients (53). Therefore, when a peripheral aneurysm is found, the clinician should be aware that multiple and bilateral aneurysms can occur, and that the popliteal, femoral, and aortoiliac areas should be carefully assessed by physical examination and US.

Femoral and, particularly, popliteal arterial aneurysms are associated with a high incidence of distal thromboembolism and eventual limb loss. Approximately 75% of untreated peripheral aneurysms may eventuate in limb loss from either distal embolization or acute thrombosis.

On the other hand, rupture with exsanguinating hemorrhage is not a major risk with femoral or popliteal arterial aneurysms, as it is for AAAs.

Clinical Manifestations

Most patients with peripheral arterial aneurysms are elderly, and many are asymptomatic. Femoral arterial aneurysms are usually evident, particularly when they measure 4 or 5 cm in diameter. Similarly, popliteal aneurysms, if they are large, are easily identified. However, popliteal aneurysms may be overlooked because many clinicians do not routinely palpate the popliteal fossa during a physical examination. Approximately 50% of femoral and popliteal aneurysms present with limb-threatening complications of thrombosis, embolization, or rupture. Hence, the discovery of an asymptomatic aneurysm in these anatomic areas is a clear indication for timely repair. Once complications of peripheral aneurysms develop, there is a 25% risk of limb amputation.

An enlarged artery with a very prominent femoral or popliteal pulse to physical examination is characteristic of a femoral or popliteal aneurysm and should be confirmed by US. Diagnosis of femoral aneurysm is easily made on clinical examination alone, but the diagnosis of popliteal aneurysm may be more difficult. When the popliteal fossa is palpated, the patient's leg should be relaxed while the examiner passively flexes the knee with the fingers, compressing the popliteal artery in the fossa, with the thumbs on the patella providing counter-compression. If an unusually prominent popliteal pulsatile mass is palpated and the examiner suspects aneurysm, the patient may be placed in the prone position and the lower leg supported by the examiner's arm to facilitate popliteal arterial palpation. US should be obtained if there is any suspicion of an aneurysm, because diagnosis and treatment before the occurrence of complications are exceedingly important. Occasionally, the only manifestations of a popliteal aneurysm are small punctate necrotic areas of skin over the anterior tibial region or small gangrenous areas of the tips of toes. This "blue toe syndrome" is a result of microemboli from the aneurysm that have showered to the periphery.

Once the diagnosis of a peripheral arterial aneurysm is made, the patient should be referred to a vascular surgeon. Arteriography is mandatory to confirm the anatomy and patency of the femoral–popliteal and tibial arteries when planning operative intervention.

Treatment and Results

Treatment of symptomatic peripheral aneurysms is indicated in all instances. Because the natural history is eventual limb loss, it is important to offer surgical therapy in most cases to maintain or improve quality of life by avoiding amputation. Surgical correction includes replacement of femoral aneurysms with prosthetic or reversed autogenous saphenous vein grafts (SVGs). Similarly, popliteal aneurysms are managed by bypassing the diseased segment with autogenous saphenous vein.

Operative mortality for management of peripheral aneurysms is approximately 1% to 3%. Limb salvage is obtained in more than 90% of cases and is related to the degree of arterial involvement peripheral to the aneurysm. In almost all series of repair of popliteal arterial aneurysms, amputations in the postoperative period have been associated with severe occlusive arterial disease manifested preoperatively by gangrene and rest pain.

SPECIFIC REFERENCES*

1. Kempczinski RF. Lower extremity arterial emboli from ulcerating atherosclerotic plaques. JAMA 1979;241:807.
2. Ouriel K, Veith FJ, Sasahara AA. A comparison of recombinant urokinase with vascular surgery as initial treatment for acute arterial occlusion of the legs. Thrombolysis or Peripheral Arterial Surgery (TOPAS) Investigators. N Engl J Med 1998;338:1105.
3. Jackson MR, Clagett GP. Antithrombotic therapy in peripheral arterial occlusive disease. Chest 2001;119:2835.
4. Results of a prospective randomized trial evaluating surgery versus thrombolysis for ischemia of the lower extremity. The STILE trial. Ann Surg 1994;220:251.
5. Braithwaite BD, Davies B, Birch PA, et al. Management of acute leg ischaemia in the elderly. Br J Surg 1998;85:217.
6. Vogt MT, Wolfson SK, Kuller LH. Lower extremity arterial disease and the aging process: a review. J Clin Epidemiol 1992;45:529.
7. Dormandy J, Mahir M, Ascady G, et al. Fate of the patient with chronic leg ischaemia: a review article. J Cardiovasc Surg 1989;30:50.
8. Weitz JI, Byrne J, Clagett GP, et al. Diagnosis and treatment of chronic arterial insufficiency of the lower extremities: a critical review. Circulation 1996;94:3026.
9. Kannel WB, McGee DL. Update on some epidemiologic features of intermittent claudication: the Framingham Study. J Am Geriatr Soc 1985;33:13.
10. Hiatt WR. Medical treatment of peripheral arterial disease and claudication. N Engl J Med 2001;344:1608.
11. Jonason T, Ringqvist I. Factors of prognostic importance for subsequent rest pain in patients with intermittent claudication. Act Med Scand 1985;218:27.
12. Hughson WG, Mann JI, Garrod A. Intermittent claudication: prevalence and risk factors. Br Med J 1978;1:1379.
13. Boyd AM. The natural course of arteriosclerosis of the lower extremities. Angiology 1960;11:10.
14. Imparato AM, Kim G-E, Davidson T, et al. Intermittent claudication: its natural course. Surgery 1975;78:795.
15. Juergens JC, Barker NW, Hines EA. Arteriosclerosis obliterans. Review of 520 cases with special reference to pathogenic and prognostic factors. Circulation 1960;21:188.
16. Criqui MH, Denenberg JO, Langer RD, et al. The epidemiology of peripheral arterial disease: importance of identifying the population at risk. Vasc Med 1997;2:221.
17. Yao JST. Hemodynamic studies in peripheral arterial disease. Br J Surg 1970;57:561.
18. Dormandy JA, Rutherford RB. Management of peripheral arterial disease (PAD). TransAtlantic Inter-Society consensus (TASC) Working Group. J Vasc Surg 2000;31[Suppl 1]:S1.
19. Pallerito JS, Taylor KJ. Doppler color imaging. Peripheral arteries. Clin Diagn Ultrasound 1992;27:97.
20. Quick CR, Cotton LT. The measured effect of stopping smoking on intermittent claudication. Br J Surg 1982;69:S24.
21. Radack K, Deck C. Beta-adrenergic blocker therapy does not worsen intermittent claudication in subjects with peripheral arterial

*Bold numerals denote published controlled clinical trials, meta-analyses, or consensus-based recommendations.

disease: a meta-analysis of randomized controlled trials. Arch Intern Med 1991;151:1769.
22. Joint National Committee. The Sixth Report of the Joint National Committee on Detection, Evaluation, and Treatment of High Blood Pressure (JNC-VI). Arch Intern Med 1997;157:2413.
23. Abbruzzese TA, Havens J, Belkin M, et al. Statin therapy is associated with improved patency of autogenous infrainquinal grafts. J Vasc Surg. 2004;39:1178.
24. LaMuraglia GM, Stoner MC, Brewster DC, et al. Determinants of carotid endarterectomy anatomic durability: effects of lipids and lipid-lowering drugs. J Vasc Surg. 2005;41:762.
25. Food and Drug Administration. Internal analgesic, antipyretic, and antirheumatic drug products for over-the-counter human use: final rule for professional labeling of aspirin, buffered aspirin, and aspirin in combination with antacid drug products. Federal Register 1998;63: 56802.
26. Bennett CL, Connors JM, Cariwile JM, et al. Thrombotic thrombocytopenic purpura associated with clopidogrel. N Engl J Med 2000;342:1773.
27. CAPRIE Steering Committee. A randomized, blinded, trial of clopidogrel versus aspirin in patients at risk of ischaemic events (CAPRIE). Lancet 1996;348:1329.
28. Dawson DL, Cutler BS, Hiatt WR, et al. A comparison of cilostazol and pentoxifylline for treating intermittent claudication. Am J Med 2000;109:523.
29. Clagett GP, Graor RA, Salzman EW. Antithrombotic therapy in peripheral arterial occlusive disease. Chest 1992;102[Suppl 4]:516S.
30. Taylor LM Jr, Edwards JM, Porter JM. Present status of reversed vein bypass grafting: five-year results of a modern series. J Vasc Surg 1990;11:193.
31. Malone JM, Moore WS, Goldstone J. Life expectancy following aortofemoral arterial grafting. Surgery 1977;81:551.
32. Lally ME, Johnston KW, Andrews D. Percutaneous transluminal dilatation of peripheral arteries: an analysis of factors predicting early success. J Vasc Surg 1984;1: 704.
33. Carlsson J, Sternby NH. Aortic aneurysms. Acta Clin Scand 1964;127:466.
34. Olsen PS, Schroeder T, Agerskov K, et al. Surgery for abdominal aortic aneurysms: a survey of 656 patients. J Cardiovasc Surg 1991;32:636.
35. Hallett JW Jr. Abdominal aortic aneurysm: natural history and treatment. Heart Dis Stroke 1992;1:303.
36. The UK Small Aneurysm Trial Participants. Smoking, lung function and the prognosis of abdominal aortic aneurysm. Eur J Vasc Endovasc Surg 2000;19:626.
37. Marian AJ. On genetics, inflammation and abdominal aortic aneurysm. Circulation 2001;103:2222.
38. Baird PA, Sadovnick AD, Yee IM, et al. Sibling risks of abdominal aortic aneurysm. Lancet 1995;346:601.
39. Estes JE. Abdominal aortic aneurysm. A study of 102 cases. Circulation 1950;2:258.
40. Szilagyi DE, Smith R, DeRusso FJ, et al. Contribution of abdominal aortic aneurysmectomy to prolongation of life. Ann Surg 1966;164:678.
41. The UK Small Aneurysm Trial Participants. Mortality results for randomised controlled trial of early elective surgery of ultrasonographic surveillance for small abdominal aortic aneurysms. Lancet 1998;352:1649.
42. Gadowski GR, Pilcher DB, Ricci MA. Abdominal aortic aneurysm expansion rate: effect of size and beta-adrenergic blockade. J Vasc Surg 1994;19:727.
43. Nevitt MP, Ballard DJ, Hallett JW Jr. Prognosis of abdominal aortic aneurysm: a population-based study. N Engl J Med 1989;321:1009.
44. Hallett JW Jr. Management of abdominal aortic aneurysm. Mayo Clin Proc 2000;75:395.
45. Szilagyi DE, Elliott JP, Smith RF. Clinical fate of the patient with asymptomatic abdominal aortic aneurysm and unfit for surgical treatment. Arch Surg 1972;104:600.
46. U.S. Preventive Services Task Force. Screening for Abdominal Aortic Aneurysm: Recommendation Statement. AHRQ Publication No. 05-0569-A, February 2005. Agency for Healthcare Research and Quality, Rockville, MD. Available at: http://www.ahrq.gov/clinic/uspstf05/aaascr/aaars.htm.
47. Fleming C, Whitlock EP, Beil TL, et al. Screening for abdominal aortic aneurysm: a best-evidence systematic review for the U.S. Preventive Services Task Force. Ann Intern Med 2005;142:203.
48. Fink HA, Lederle FA, Roth CS, et al. The accuracy of physical examination to detect abdominal aortic aneurysm. Arch Intern Med 2000;160:833.
49. La Roy LL, Cormier PJ, Matalon TA, et al. Imaging of abdominal aortic aneurysms. AJR Am J Roentgenol 1989;152:785.
50. Katz DA, Littenberg B, Cronenwett JL. Management of small abdominal aortic aneurysms. Early surgery vs watchful waiting. JAMA 1992;268:2678.
51. Blankensteijn JD, Sjors EC, Prinssen M, et al. for Dutch Randomized Endovascular Aneurysm Management (DREAM) Trial Group. Two year outcomes after conventional or endovascular repair of abdominal aortic aneurysms. N Engl J Med 2005;352:2398.
52. Dawson I, Sie RB, Van Bockel JH. Atherosclerotic popliteal aneurysm. Br J Surg 1997;84:293.
53. Dent TL, Lindenauer SM, Ernst CB, et al. Multiple arteriosclerotic arterial aneurysms. Arch Surg 1972;105;338.

*For annotated **General References** and resources related to this chapter, visit www.hopkinsbayview.org/PAMreferences.*

Chapter 95

Lower Extremity Ulcers and Varicose Veins*

Robert J. Spence and Glen S. Roseborough

*Calvin E. Jones, Jr., MD and James M. Wong, MD, contributed to this chapter in previous editions.

LOWER EXTREMITY ULCERS

Ulceration of the lower extremity, most often caused by either macrovascular or microvascular disease, is a common and important problem in ambulatory medical practice.

As a result of the aging population, the incidence of leg ulcers is rising (1). The ambulatory setting frequently is the best place to treat lower extremity ulcerations to maintain mobility and avoid the complications of hospital bedrest (2).

Accurate diagnosis is based mainly on history and physical examination and is essential for appropriate treatment. Inappropriate therapy can lead to the loss of a toe or even a limb. Generally, it is necessary to give detailed instructions to the patient and to have a great deal of patience. Patient compliance with treatment has been shown to be critical in the success of therapy and the prevention of recurrent ulceration (3).

History

The medical history is important. Illnesses such as arteriosclerotic vascular disease or hypertension, diabetes mellitus, renal failure and dialysis, sickle cell disease, and collagen-vascular disease may be associated with ulcers of the lower extremities. A history of corticosteroid therapy may explain failure of ulcers to heal. Drug abuse or a psychiatric history may be pertinent in the explanation of factitious ulcers. Furthermore, aspects of the patient's lifestyle, particularly mobility and lower extremity dependency, are important.

Specific attention should be paid to duration of ulceration and previous attempts at therapy; symptoms of peripheral arterial vascular disease, such as intermittent calf claudication, intermittent thigh or gluteal claudication, impotence, calf pain at rest, and feelings of coldness and tingling in the legs; a history of deep vein thrombosis, ulceration, or injury to the lower extremities; and a history of discomfort associated with footwear or of chronic swelling, and, if swelling has occurred, whether it has been alleviated by lying down.

Ischemic pain in the calf at rest is usually a symptom of advanced peripheral arterial disease (PAD), and it is characteristically alleviated if the patient dangles his or her feet over the edge of the bed or sits in a chair when awakened at night by ischemic pain. These symptoms must be differentiated from *nocturnal leg cramps* that occur in many people who have no evidence of peripheral vascular disease. Leg cramps are usually accompanied by palpable hardening of the calf muscles and involuntary muscle contraction of the flexor muscles of the toes. The cramps usually are relieved if the patient gets out of bed and walks around. Examination of the extremities in these patients (see below) is usually normal.

Physical Examination

A general physical examination of the patient is undertaken in conjunction with the examination of the lower extremities. The general examination should include a documentation of weight and, ideally, body mass index (BMI). Abdominal aortic aneurysm and other intra-abdominal masses, lymphatic masses in the groin, and signs of long-standing hypertension and cardiac disease should be sought. Needle tracks and brawny indurated hands may indicate a history of drug abuse, as may skin ulcers in areas other than the lower extremities.

Examination of the Lower Extremities

Both lower extremities should be bared. Initial examination is performed while the patient is supine. Both legs are examined and compared. Particular points to be noted include the following:

1. The presence of pitting or nonpitting edema. Pitting edema is a sign of chronic venous obstruction or of an acute inflammatory process. Nonpitting edema is a sign of lymphatic obstruction. If edema is present, it is important to note whether it is unilateral, and if it is bilateral, whether it is asymmetric or symmetric. Very firm brawny edema suggests a long-standing process.
2. The presence of hemosiderin, a brown pigment containing iron, deposited in the skin of the ankles (a sign of venous insufficiency).
3. The general appearance and quality of the skin, including hair growth (hair loss may signify arterial insufficiency).
4. Evidence of fungal infection (scaling, apparently pruritic lesions).
5. The status of the nails (deformity and hypertrophy are associated with arterial insufficiency).

After inspection of the feet and legs, a vascular examination of the lower extremities is conducted. Femoral, popliteal, dorsalis pedis, and posterior tibial *pulses* are palpated and graded. Ideally, an ankle-brachial index (ABI) is obtained, particularly if compression dressings are contemplated as therapy. The *capillary refill time* is observed after placing pressure on the toes with the legs elevated 45 degrees (normally less than 5 seconds). *Auscultation* from the mid-abdomen down to the popliteal regions is performed to detect bruits that are produced by narrowed atherosclerotic arteries. The *temperature* of the legs is felt with the dorsum of the hand, both descending from the thigh to the foot and comparing one side with the other. The patient is asked to sit up and to dangle his or her legs so that *venous filling time* and dependent rubor can be assessed. Evidence of *varicose veins* is best sought with the patient standing.

Inspection and Palpation of Ulcer or Ulcers

Ulcerated areas on the legs are often very tender; palpation, although necessary, should be done gently, with the gloved hand.

more extensive disease and become more symptomatic (23).

The disorder is aggravated, and indeed may be caused, by conditions that elevate intra-abdominal pressure (pregnancy, large intra-abdominal tumors) or chronic straining (prostatic obstruction, carcinoma of the sigmoid colon), and occasionally by mechanical interference with venous return in the venous system itself (thrombosis of the pelvic veins).

Symptoms

The symptoms of uncomplicated varicose veins usually consist of heaviness and aching in the area of the veins or in the calves. The patient may complain of mild edema at the end of the day. Occasionally, patients complain of varicose veins for cosmetic reasons and desire treatment. Patients with uncomplicated varicose veins do not complain of intermittent claudication or severe pain; these symptoms suggest coexistent arterial disease or significant outflow obstruction to the venous system ("venous claudication"). Varicose veins can be complicated by superficial thrombophlebitis, bleeding, and venous stasis ulcers, although these complications occur in only a small minority of patients. Superficial thrombophlebitis is usually associated with an intense inflammatory reaction around a tender palpable subcutaneous cord, and is often mistaken for an infectious process. However, antibiotics usually have no role in the treatment of this problem. After rest, elevation, application of local heat, and appropriate anti-inflammatory therapy (e.g., aspirin), the varix in the thrombosed vein disappears. Bleeding varicose veins may require direct suturing. and the treatment of venous stasis ulcers is discussed earlier in this chapter.

Physical Examination

It is useful to have some idea of the anatomy of the venous system of the leg (Fig. 95.1). This makes it possible to judge the patient's symptoms on the basis of an anatomic abnormality detected by physical examination. There are several types of varicose veins, which conform to the underlying anatomic arrangement of these veins. It is important to classify varicose veins on the basis of the anatomic involvement, since appropriate treatment depends on this information.

Telangiectasia (Sunburst Varices)

These are not, in the true sense of the word, varicose veins but rather dilations of subcutaneous venous plexuses that have a spider-like arrangement and an unsightly purple color. These veins are generally less than a millimeter in diameter and are often the object of cosmetic complaints by patients. Otherwise, they are essentially asymptomatic.

Superficial Varicosities

All varicosities result from dilated subcutaneous veins. Simple (primary) superficial varicosities develop in the absence of involvement of more extensive venous structures. Often, however, superficial varicosities develop secondarily as a consequence of reflux in the saphenous, perforator, or in the deep venous systems. It is important to determine whether varicosities are primary or secondary, since this will influence treatment.

Varicosities of Long Saphenous System

Incompetence of the long saphenous system is the most common cause of varicose veins. The long saphenous vein begins anterior to the medial malleolus at the ankle, courses superficially to the medial side of the knee posterior to the medial femoral condyle, and then passes up the medial side of the thigh to the groin where it joins the common femoral vein just below the inguinal ligament. The vein has several tributaries in the calf and in the thigh that are superficial, and it is also joined by several perforating veins from the deep venous system; the valves at these junctions can become incompetent and lead to focal varicosities (Fig. 95.1). There are several consistent perforators: Dodd vein, located just above the knee, Boyd vein, located just below the tibial plateau, and a group of three veins above the medial malleolus at a distance separated by approximately 3 cm, known as Cockett veins. Incompetence of the long saphenous vein is often clearly visible with the patient standing but may not be evident on visual inspection alone. In these instances it may be evident on palpation or diagnosed with additional noninvasive testing (see Noninvasive Vascular Testing).

Varicosities of Short Saphenous System

The short saphenous vein arises behind the lateral malleolus and courses upward behind the calf to join the popliteal vein in the popliteal space (Fig. 95.1). Varicosities of this system are best seen with the patient standing with his or her back to the examiner.

Perforator Varicosities

Perforator incompetence is usually noticed in the long saphenous vein where the ankle perforators and the perigeniculate perforators join the vein; however, perforators join other superficial veins that, in turn, join the long and short saphenous system. Examination may reveal that there is no incompetence of the short or long saphenous veins, only of the perforators. The location of an incompetent perforator vein may often be determined clinically by palpating a divot in the patient's leg, where the muscular fascia has dilated around a dilated perforator vein. There may not always be a superficial varicose vein visible overlying this area so the examiner must perform a thorough physical examination of the lower leg. Incompetent perforator veins may cause varicose veins in regions other than the saphenous system.

Clinical Testing to Determine Level of Incompetence

One or two easy clinical tests can be performed in the office that will aid in determination of the severity of the problem and selection of appropriate treatment.

Trendelenburg Test

The patient lies supine and raises the affected leg to empty the veins. A venous tourniquet is applied just below the saphenous opening about 3 inches (7 to 8 cm) below the inguinal ligament. The patient then stands up, and constriction is released. If the saphenofemoral valve is incompetent, the veins will fill immediately from above; if not, the veins fill slowly from below. If the veins fill rapidly before the release of the tourniquet, this indicates the presence of incompetent perforator veins allowing reflux from the deep system. This test is then repeated at successively lower levels in the leg so the location of incompetence may be mapped.

Perthes Test

The Perthes test is a test for DVT in association with varicose veins. A tourniquet is lightly applied below the inguinal ligament, as in the Trendelenburg test, and the patient is instructed to walk in place. If varicose veins are accompanied by a thrombosed deep femoral system, the varicose veins become prominent after this exercise.

Noninvasive Vascular Testing

The advent of the modern vascular laboratory has revolutionized the evaluation of varicose veins. Any patient who, by physical examination, is suspected of having venous incompetence at the saphenous femoral junction should be referred to a noninvasive vascular laboratory for evaluation before treatment is planned.

Effective treatment of lower extremity venous insufficiency is predicated on accurate localization of the problem. Various noninvasive vascular examinations and radiologic studies can be successfully used to define the anatomic extent of venous reflux (24). The utility and limitations of these modalities are based on the concept of systolic and diastolic closure of lower extremity venous valves. Venous valves close in response to two distinct physiologic actions. Coaptation of valve cusps occurs during muscular contraction and subsequent forward (toward the heart) flow of blood (systolic closure). These valves include side branches and perforator veins. Diastolic closure occurs immediately after relaxation of muscular contraction when valves proximal to that contraction close to prevent reflux of blood.

The simplest noninvasive test for lower extremity venous reflux is *continuous wave Doppler*. The examiner insolates the venous system with a Doppler probe and listens for venous reflux after provocative maneuvers, such as Valsalva maneuver or manual compression proximal to the transducer. The Valsalva maneuver and proximal compression normally result in the cessation of venous flow. The presence of venous signals during these maneuvers is indicative of venous reflux. Continuous wave Doppler samples any structure in the path of the emitted ultrasound and does not allow for discrimination of the vein being tested. Similarly, anatomic variations such as bifid veins will be unrecognized. Analysis with continuous wave Doppler is qualitative, and may be used at the bedside as an initial test. For the definitive assessment of venous anatomy and abnormalities in the vascular laboratory, plethysmography (photoplethysmography or air plethysmography) has been superseded by duplex ultrasound.

Vascular duplex scanning combines high-resolution ultrasonic imaging with pulsed-wave Doppler. This allows real-time visualization of vascular structures and analysis of physiologic and pathologic flow through valves and vessels. The spectral waveforms and color coding obtained by Doppler depicts the velocity of the blood flow as defined by the Doppler equation. The Doppler-derived velocity is a vector that processes both magnitude and direction. Analysis of the Doppler data can therefore demonstrate the direction of blood flow relative to the transducer (26). The saphenofemoral and saphenopopliteal junctions can be imaged in the groin and popliteal space, respectively, and venous flow recorded by spectral analysis or color Doppler. Venous reflux in response to Valsalva maneuver or proximal limb compression can be observed as either waveforms that are inverted to the normal antegrade flow or with color coding indicating retrograde flow. Duplex ultrasonography offers selective sampling of venous structures and precise localization of disease. Valves can be observed directly and valve incompetence is defined by a prolonged valve closure time. The time to valve closure can be measured after a Valsalva maneuver with the patient in 10 degrees reversed Trendelenburg position, or after a cuff on the thigh is released when the patient is standing. Normal valve closure time is less than 2 seconds with the former method and less than 1 second with the latter method. The entire length of the deep and superficial systems can be evaluated. Careful duplex examination of the medial calf and thigh can demonstrate incompetent perforator veins. Not only is this diagnostic, but it can also be used to localize and mark perforators for surgical ligation. DVT can also be readily identified by this modality.

Venous duplex scanning must be performed by a skilled operator and requires expensive ultrasound equipment (26). However, its noninvasive nature makes it acceptable to patients. Duplex scanning can be used to quantitate the volume of reflux, which correlates with the degree of venous stasis skin changes (24).

Ambulatory venous pressure (AVP) measurement is an invasive technique performed by cannulating a vein on the dorsum of the foot with a small gauge butterfly needle connected to a pressure transducer, amplifier, and recorder. With the use of a pneumatic cuff or elastic tourniquet, it can differentiate between superficial and deep vein or perforator vein incompetence. Elevated AVP correlates with the presence of venous stasis ulcers. AVP measurement is highly sensitive in the detection of venous reflux and is a direct measure of venous pressure. Limitations of this test include inconsistent reproducibility, patient discomfort from its invasive nature, and lack of efficacy as a screening test. It is rarely performed in most vascular labs today.

Descending phlebography is sometimes performed in patients with advanced venous insufficiency who are being considered for repair or autotransplantation of damaged deep venous valves. A catheter is placed in the ipsilateral external iliac vein and the patient is tilted 60 degrees on a fluoroscopy table. As contrast is injected it falls in the leg due to its relative density compared to blood, documenting the extent of reflux. This study defines valvular anatomy well, can identify specific refluxing valves, and can differentiate between primarily insufficient valves that may be repaired and postphlebitic valves that must be replaced.

Treatment

The goals of treatment are to control symptoms and prevent complications. When an intervention is performed, it should be done with full knowledge of the extent of the patient's reflux so that treatment can be aimed at the highest point of reflux. Several options are available.

Observation

Observation is an acceptable option in patients with mild to moderate asymptomatic subcutaneous varices with no history of postural edema, superficial phlebitis, stasis dermatitis, or pain. If the offending telangiectatic venous plexus is large enough to accommodate a 25-gauge needle, a sclerosing solution may be injected. The technique is described below in the section Sclerotherapy. Other treatments such as freezing with carbon dioxide snow, cautery under local anesthesia, and even laser therapy have been advocated, but their use requires a great deal of skill, and unnecessary skin scarring may result that is, in the end, more unsightly than the original vein. Probably the safest treatment of this kind of vein is the use of masking cosmetic creams, together with reassurance.

Support Hose

Support hose maintain compression of subcutaneous varicose veins and prevent edema. Graduated compression hose in the 30- to 40-mm Hg range are available in most pharmacies in various ready-to-fit sizes, including knee, thigh, and panty hose configurations. The patient should be measured and fitted early in the morning before any edema has developed to obtain maximal therapeutic benefit from the compression hose. They should be worn continuously, removed at bedtime, and reapplied immediately upon arising in the morning.

Transcutaneous Laser Ablation

Spider telangiectasias and small varicosities less than 1 to 1.5 mm may be treated with transcutaneous laser ablation. Several lasers have been used for this purpose, including the Nd-to-YAG laser, tunable pulsed-dye laser, copper bromide laser, and the alexandrite laser (27). The procedure is completely noninvasive and is therefore the preferred approach to treating small lesions of this kind. Complications include temporary ulceration and permanent hyperpigmentation or hypopigmentation. Multiple treatments and adjunctive sclerotherapy may be required for optimal results. The lasers are expensive and treatments are typically performed by dermatologists and cosmetic surgeons who use lasers for multiple purposes. Patients are often charged directly for a cosmetic procedure and are not reimbursed by medical insurers, decreasing patient satisfaction with this procedure.

Sclerotherapy

Sclerotherapy is efficacious for segmental subcutaneous varicose veins up to 5 mm in diameter that are not associated with significant greater or lesser saphenous valvular incompetence, and for cosmetically unacceptable telangiectasia (28). The procedure is performed in the office; however, the patient should be told that several treatments may be required for complete elimination of the veins.

The patient stands with a tight tourniquet around the thigh, just enough to make the vein prominent. The area of the vein is lightly prepared with a suitable antiseptic, and 0.5 mL of sclerosing solution is injected by use of a 2-mL syringe, after initial aspiration to make sure the needle is in the vein. Immediately after the end of the injection, the needle is withdrawn and the vein is gently compressed with a 2 × 2-inch gauze for 3 minutes, after which the tourniquet is released and compression is continued for 2 minutes more. The patient wears an elastic bandage on the area for approximately 4 hours. The sclerosant produces an inflammatory reaction in the intima, which obliterates the vein. Failure to use a tourniquet may release an unnecessarily large amount of sclerosant into the major veins of the leg and cause undesirable thrombosis at distant sites. The patient should be warned that extravasation of the sclerosant is a possibility and may cause skin necrosis. Several commercially available sclerosant solutions, including sodium morrhuate, sodium tetradecylsulfate (STS), ethanolamine, polidocanol, and hypertonic saline are suitable for injection. Larger varicose veins, up to 10 mm or more, including the saphenous vein and perforator veins, are being treated with a new technique in which a foam is created by mixing the sclerosant (usually STS or polidocanol) with air and then injecting it (29,30). Perforator and saphenous vein sclerotherapy should be done under ultrasound guidance, whereas superficial varicosities are injected blindly.

Surgical Therapy

Surgical therapy for varicose veins depends on the degree of involvement of perforator veins, the saphenous system, and the deep system. The goal is to control the highest point of reflux. Simple superficial varicosities that are too large for sclerotherapy can be treated with stab phlebectomy. This can be done under local anesthesia in an outpatient setting. Incisions are generally 2 to 3 mm long and phlebectomy is facilitated by specialized hooked instruments. General anesthesia may be required if multiple incisions are anticipated.

Direct ligation of incompetent perforator veins can result in ablation of large clusters of varicose veins, and prevent recurrence of stasis ulcers. It is also performed under local anesthesia but incisions are larger, usually 1 to 2 cm. Multiple incompetent perforator veins were previously controlled by the Linton procedure, a radical operation where the medial leg is opened longitudinally and all perforators are ligated through one continuous incision. This procedure has significant morbidity and has now been abandoned. It has been replaced by subfascial endoscopic perforator vein surgery (SEPS). An operating port and an observation port are placed through two incisions in the medial lower leg and perforators are identified and ligated with clips in the subfascial plane. This procedure requires general anesthesia and can be complicated by significant degloving of the medial skin of the lower leg. Clinical trials have confirmed its effectiveness at healing and preventing stasis ulcers (31,32).

If varicosities are associated with incompetent greater or lessor saphenous systems, these systems should be ablated. Until recently therapy consisted of surgical stripping. The greater saphenous vein is stripped between the groin and just below the knee—stripping more distally may result in injury to the saphenous nerve. The saphenofemoral junction is divided and all branches is this area are ligated. The lesser saphenous vein is stripped from the popliteal fossa from where it inserts on the popliteal vein. Stripping requires general anesthesia and is typically associated with significant postoperative pain and swelling. It can be complicated by significant wound hematomas and infections.

Percutaneous endovenous ablation of the saphenous vein has recently been introduced and has been shown to effectively ablate both the greater and lesser saphenous veins. The vein is cannulated with a wire, a sheath is advanced over the wire and then a probe is advanced through the sheath. The tissues surrounding the saphenous vein are infused with a dilute solution of local anesthetic using tumescent technique, to compress the vein around the probe for more effective ablation and to create a heat sink that protects adjacent tissues from thermal injury. Laser or radiofrequency energy is delivered to the endothelium as the probe is withdrawn from the vein (33,34). The procedure is performed under ultrasound guidance and requires intravenous sedation only.

For varicosities accompanied by valvular incompetence in the iliac, femoral, and popliteal deep veins, reconstructive approaches may include various methods of direct and indirect valvuloplasty (35–37). Postphlebitic valves can be replaced by autotransplanting a valve from the axillary vein. These operations are not practiced widely and results are mixed. They should be performed only after reflux in the perforator and saphenous systems has been addressed, and are usually performed only to control recurrent ulceration.

Varicose veins should not be treated in patients who have an underlying cause associated with increased intra-abdominal pressure until the primary cause has been removed. However, the wearing of elastic stockings may give comfort during this time. Such stockings may be advisable for support in any patient with varicose veins in whom other treatment is undesirable or contraindicated. A further consideration in the selection of therapy is whether the patient has coronary artery disease; although veins that are severely varicose are not suitable for use in coronary bypass surgery, if patients have minimal varicose veins and may become candidates for a coronary artery bypass, these veins should be preserved, if possible, for potential future use (38). Weight reduction in overweight patients is advisable for anyone with varicose veins, regardless of other modes of treatment.

SPECIFIC REFERENCES

1. Margolis DJ, Bilker W, Santanna J, et al. Venous leg ulcer: incidence and prevalence in the elderly. J Am Acad Dermatol 2002;46:381.
2. Simon DA, Dix FP, McCollum CN. Management of venous leg ulcers. BMJ 2004;328:1358.
3. Erickson CA, Lanza DJ, Karp DL, et al. Healing of venous ulcers in an ambulatory care program: the roles of chronic venous insufficiency and patient compliance. J Vasc Surg 1995;22:629.
4. Mekkes JR, Loots MA, Van Der Wal AC, et al. Causes, investigation and treatment of leg ulceration. Br J Dermatol 2003;148:388.
5. Browse NL, Burnand KG. The cause of venous ulceration. Lancet 1982;2:243.
6. Dormandy JA. Pharmacologic treatment of

venous leg ulcers. J Cardiovasc Pharmacol 1995;25:S61.
7. Smith PD. The microcirculation in venous hypertension. Cardiovasc Res 1996;32:789.
8. Mani R, White JE, Barrett DF, et al. Tissue oxygenation, venous ulcers and fibrin cuffs. J R Soc Med 1989;82:345.
9. Graves JW, Morris JC, Sheps SG. Martorell's hypertensive leg ulcer: case report and concise review of the literature. J Hum Hypertens 2001;15:279.
10. Hafner J, Trueb RM. Management of vasculitic leg ulcers and pyoderma gangrenosum. Curr Probl Dermatol 1999;27:277.
11. McClave SA, Finney LS. Nutritional issues in the patient with diabetes and foot ulcers. In: Bowker JH, Pfeifer MA, eds. Levin and O'Neal's the diabetic foot. 6th ed. St. Louis: Mosby, 2001.
12. Thawer HA, Houghton PE. Effects of ultrasound delivered through a mist of saline to wounds in mice with diabetes mellitus. J Wound Care 2004;13:171.
13. Jull A, Waters J, Arroll B. Pentoxifylline for treatment of venous leg ulcers: a systematic review. Lancet 2002;359:1550.
14. van Rijswijk L, Brown D, Friedman S, et al. Multicenter clinical evaluation of a hydrocolloid dressing for leg ulcers. Cutis 1985;35:173.
15. Eginton MT, Brown KR, Seabrook GR, et al. A prospective randomized evaluation of negative-pressure wound dressings for diabetic foot wounds. Ann Vasc Surg 2003;17:645.
16. LoGerfo FW, Coffman JD. Current concepts. Vascular and microvascular disease of the foot in diabetes. Implications for foot care. N Engl J Med 1984;311:1615.
17. Singer AJ, Clark RA. Cutaneous wound healing. N Engl J Med 1999;341:738.
18. Lipsky BA. Osteomyelitis of the foot in diabetic patients. Clin Infect Dis 1997;25:1318.
19. [Anonymous]. Consensus Development Conference on Diabetic Foot Wound Care: 7–8 April 1999, Boston, MA. American Diabetes Association. Diabetes Care 1999;22:1354.
20. Diehm C. Effects of beta-adrenergic blocking drugs on arterial blood flow. Vasa 1984;13:201.
21. Spence RJ, Wong L. The enhancement of wound healing with human skin allograft. Surg Clin North Am 1997;77:731.
22. Nelzen O, Bergqvist D, Lindhagen A. Long-term Prognosis for Patients with Chronic Leg Ulcers: a Prospective Cohort Study. Eur J Vasc Endovasc Surg 1997;13:500.
23. Goldman MP, Fronek A. Anatomy and pathophysiology of varicose veins. J Dermatol Surg Oncol 1989;15:138.
24. Vasdekis SN, Clarke GH, Nicolaides AN. Quantification of venous reflux by means of duplex scanning. J Vasc Surg 1989;10:670.
25. Nicolaides AN, Miles C. Photoplethysmography in the assessment of venous insufficiency. J Vasc Surg 1987;5:405.
26. van Bemmelen PS, Bedford G, Beach K, et al. Quantitative segmental evaluation of venous valvular reflux with duplex ultrasound scanning. J Vasc Surg 1989;10:425.
27. Eremia S, Li C, Umar SH. A side-by-side comparative study of 1064 nm Nd:YAG, 810 nm Diode and 755 nm alexandrite lasers for treatment of 0.3-3 mm leg veins. Dermatol Surg 2002;28:224.
28. Weiss RA, Weiss MA, Goldman MP. Physicians' negative perception of sclerotherapy for venous disorders: review of a 7 year experience with modern sclerotherapy. South Med J 1992; 85:1101.
29. Frullini A, Cavezzi A. Sclerosing foam in the treatment of varicose veins and telangiectases: history and analysis of safety and complications. Dermatol Surg 2002;28:11.
30. Barrett JM, Allen B, Ockelford A, et al. Microfoam ultrasound-guided sclerotherapy treatment for varicose veins in a subgroup with diameters at the junction of 10 mm or greater compared with a subgroup of less than 10 mm. Dermatol Surg 2004;30:1386.
31. Pierik EG, van Urk H, Hop WC, et al. Endoscopic versus open subfascial division of incompetent perforating veins in the treatment of venous leg ulceration: a randomized trial. J Vasc Surg 1997;26:1049.
32. Gloviczki P, Bergan JJ, Rhodes JM, et al. Mid-term results of endoscopic perforator vein interruption for chronic venous insufficiency: lessons learned from the North American Subfascial Endoscopic Perforator Surgery Registry. J Vasc Surg 1999;29:489.
33. Nicolini P, Closure Group. Treatment of primary varicose veins by endovenous obliteration with the VNUS Closure System: results of a prospective multicentre study. Eur J Vasc Endovasc Surg 2005;29:433.
34. Min RJ, Khilnani N, Zimmet SE. Endovenous laser treatment of saphenous vein reflux: long-term results. J Vasc Interv Radiol 2003;14: 991.
35. O'Donnell TF, Mackey WC, Shepard AD, et al. Clinical, hemodynamic, and anatomic follow-up of direct venous reconstruction. Arch Surg 1987; 122:474.
36. Raju S, Fredericks R. Valve reconstruction procedures for nonobstructive venous insufficiency: rationale, techniques, and results in 107 procedures with two to eight-year follow-up. J Vasc Surg 1988;7:301.
37. Wilson NM, Rutt DL, Browse NL. Repair and replacement of deep vein valves in the treatment of venous insufficiency. Br J Surg 1991;78:388.
38. Friedell ML, Samson RH, Cohen MJ, et al. High ligation of the greater saphenous vein for treatment of lower extremity varicosities: the fate of the vein and therapeutic results. Ann Vasc Surg 1992;6:5.

For annotated ***General References*** *and resources related to this chapter, visit www.hopkinsbayview.org/PAMreferences.*

Chapter 96

Diseases of the Biliary Tract

Esteban Mezey and John W. Harmon

Diseases of the biliary tract are commonly encountered in ambulatory practice. Many patients are discovered to have asymptomatic gallstones during the course of evaluation of another condition; others are found to have symptomatic chronic cholecystitis. Less commonly, patients present with an acute illness caused by acute cholecystitis or common bile duct obstruction. This chapter describes the cause, diagnosis, and treatment of these various conditions.

CHOLELITHIASIS

Epidemiology

Approximately 10% of the U.S. population has gallstones. In their lifetime, only 50% will ever be symptomatic, with 80% of them having chronic symptoms and 20% presenting with an acute illness. About 500,000 cholecystectomies are performed each year in the United States.

Ninety percent of gallstones found in patients in the United States are cholesterol gallstones; 10% are pigment (bilirubinate) stones. The prevalence of gallstones is greater in women than in men and increases with age. In the United States, 10% to 15% of men and 20% to 40% of women older than age 60 years are affected (1). The prevalence of cholesterol gallstones is particularly high in the Native Americans of the southwestern United States; for example, 70% of Pima women older than age 25 years have cholelithiasis (2).

Gallstone Formation

Bile is produced in the liver and excreted into the duodenum and contains bile acids (primarily cholic, deoxycholic, and chenodeoxycholic acid), phospholipids (primarily lecithin), and cholesterol. The solubility of cholesterol depends on its incorporation with bile and phospholipids into a micelle. In the intestinal tract, bile salts are necessary for the absorption of dietary fats; they solubilize fatty acids and monoglycerides into micellar solutions. The fatty acids are absorbed in the jejunum, whereas the bile salts are absorbed in the ileum and enter the enterohepatic circulation.

Three major types of gallstones form in human bile: cholesterol stones (more than 70% cholesterol), mixed stones (50% to 70% cholesterol), and pigment stones (12% cholesterol). These stones probably develop in three stages: first, the formation of a supersaturated bile; second, the crystallization or initiation of stone formation; and third, the growth of the stone to a certain detectable size before crystals in the bile are expelled into the intestine. It is likely, but not clearly established, that one of these stages is more important in the formation of certain types of stones than in others.

Cholesterol Stones

The hypersecretion of biliary cholesterol appears to be the real culprit in the pathogenesis of cholesterol stones, but this might not be true in all patients. Several mechanisms of increased cholesterol secretion have been identified (1). Cholesterol crystals form when the amount of cholesterol in bile exceeds the solubilizing properties of bile salts and phospholipid (supersaturated bile). The cholesterol crystals are caught in a film of mucin gel that lines the gallbladder and provides a nucleus for the formation of gallstones. Growth of these stones occurs, especially in a dyskinetic gallbladder, one in which contraction is impaired, as in diabetes mellitus and pregnancy. The mucin gel itself might decrease gallbladder motility and emptying.

Pigment Stones

Formation of pigment stones is probably initiated by supersaturation of unconjugated bilirubin in the gallbladder and common bile duct. Unconjugated bilirubin, like cholesterol, is insoluble in water. An increased concentration of unconjugated bilirubin in bile results either from its formation from conjugated bilirubin in the biliary tree through the action of a glucuronidase (perhaps of bacterial origin, in patients with infected bile; see Signs and Symptoms section) or from increased production of unconjugated bilirubin by the liver (e.g., in patients with hemolytic anemia). A diseased gallbladder is probably not a factor in the formation of pigment stones.

Risk Factors

Because most patients with cholelithiasis are asymptomatic, it is difficult to evaluate risk factors precisely. Table 96.1 lists known risk factors for the development of cholesterol and pigment stones (3).

TABLE 96.1 Risk Factors for Gallstones

Cholesterol stones
Demography: Northern Europe, North and South America more than Asia; Native Americans; probably familial predisposition
Obesity
High-calorie diet
Drugs used in the treatment of hyperlipidemia; clofibrate, cholestyramine, gemfibrozil, colestipol
Gastrointestinal disorders involving major malabsorption of bile acids; ileal disease, resection or bypass; cystic fibrosis, with pancreatic insufficiency
Female sex hormones: women more at risk than men, use of oral contraceptives and other estrogenic medications
Age, especially among men
Probable but not well established: pregnancy, diabetes mellitus, and polyunsaturated fats
Pigment stones
Demography: oriental more than occidental; rural more than urban
Chronic hemolysis
Alcoholic cirrhosis
Biliary infection
Age

From Bennion LJ, Grundy SM. Risk factors for the development of cholelithiasis in man (second of two parts). N Engl J Med 1978;299(22):1221.

Cholesterol Stones

The demography of cholesterol stones probably reflects both genetic predisposition and nongenetic ethnic characteristics. For example, it is known that obese people and nonobese people who eat a high-calorie diet secrete more cholesterol into their bile than the average person. Therefore, populations in whom obesity is common (e.g., the Native Americans of the American southwest) or who consume high-calorie diets (occidental societies in general) are more susceptible to cholelithiasis.

The reasons for the increasing incidence of gallstones in middle-aged and elderly people are unknown but may be related to the time that elapses between formation of supersaturated bile and formation of stones and between formation of stones and recognition of them. The enhancement by estrogens of the secretion of cholesterol in bile is reflected in the higher prevalence of gallstones in women (between puberty and menopause) than in men (see above) and in women who take estrogenic preparations compared with women who do not (see Chapters 100 and 106).

Finally, there are a number of ways by which the concentration of bile acids in bile is reduced, favoring the formation of gallstones: Drugs used to treat hyperlipidemia, such as clofibrate, cholestyramine, gemfibrozil, and colestipol (see Chapter 82), decrease bile acid secretion, and certain disorders of the gastrointestinal (GI) tract (ileal resection, Crohn disease of the ileum) reduce bile acid resorption.

Pigment Stones

The demography of pigment stones is entirely different from that of cholesterol stones. The propensity of Asian people to develop pigment stones is not entirely understood, but it may be attributable to the higher prevalence of bacterial infection of the bile (usually *Escherichia coli* infections) and of *Ascaris* infestation in the Orient compared with the Occident. In the United States, patients with pigment gallstones do not usually have infected or infested bile. The recognized risk factors in the United States are hemolysis and alcoholic cirrhosis. Like cholesterol stones, pigment stones are more common with advancing age, but endogenous and exogenous estrogens and obesity have no influence on their development.

Natural History

Many attempts have been made to study the natural history of gallstones among the 2 to 3 million people in the United States known to have them. Of these people, 50% are asymptomatic, having had gallstones discovered incidentally on abdominal radiography (10% to 15% are radiopaque) or another imaging study or during celiotomy for treatment of another condition. The other 50% are symptomatic and gallstones are discovered during evaluation of the typical or atypical abdominal pain of acute or chronic cholecystitis.

Approximately 18% of people with silent gallstones develop symptoms in 15 to 20 years, and 3% develop complications of biliary tract disease, namely acute cholecystitis, pancreatitis, or obstructive jaundice (4). The risk of developing complications is unrelated to the severity of symptoms but does increase with the length of time symptoms have been present. Most complications occur only among symptomatic patients. However, 20% of the time acute cholecystitis is the first indication of cholelithiasis. Complications, if they occur, are usually experienced within 5 years of the discovery of gallstones.

Causes of death related to cholelithiasis among patients not having cholecystectomy are acute cholecystitis, cholangitis with liver abscess, necrotizing pancreatitis, gallbladder carcinoma, and gallstone ileus with mechanical small bowel obstruction. In Lund's study of the natural history of cholelithiasis, 2.7% of the deaths among patients not operated on were attributed to gallbladder disease (5).

Asymptomatic Patients

It cannot be predicted on the basis of the size or number of stones or the sex or age of the patient which asymptomatic patients are likely to become symptomatic. Whether asymptomatic patients should undergo elective cholecystectomy, therefore, depends largely on the bias of the primary clinician and the consulting surgeon. Approximately 18% of patients become symptomatic some time at a point in their lives when operation is more dangerous because of age, intercurrent illness, or the presence of acute cholecystitis. The risk of complications of cholelithiasis, other than acute cholecystitis, is negligible in the asymptomatic patient. Carcinoma of the gallbladder is more common among people with gallstones and the risk—0.3% to 1% over a lifetime—is approximately the same as the historic operative mortality from cholecystectomy. However, recent technologic changes have decreased the operative risk considerably. If the gallbladder is calcified, the risk of cancer is nearly 50%, however, and cholecystectomy should be performed. Likewise, prophylactic cholecystectomy is recommended for Native Americans with cholelithiasis, because they have a 3% to 5% risk of developing gallbladder cancer (6). Prophylactic cholecystectomy has also been recommended for children with gallstones, in whom symptoms almost always develop (7), and in patients with sickle cell anemia and cholelithiasis because the symptoms of either condition can easily be confused with the other. Otherwise, the current consensus at this point is not to recommend elective cholecystectomy in the asymptomatic patient. The legitimacy of this same approach in the diabetic patient has been endorsed (8). This recommendation is unchanged even with the emergence of laparoscopic cholecystectomy and its attendant lower morbidity and shortened convalescence (see below).

CHOLECYSTITIS

The hallmark of cholecystitis is abdominal pain (9), often epigastric at onset, but localizing within a few hours to the right upper quadrant. The pain is characteristically, but not always, severe and unremitting, with only slight variations in intensity. Use of the term *biliary colic*, therefore, is not precise because colic is defined as pain that waxes and wanes. Some patients describe the pain as heavy and aching and others as knife-like. Occasionally, it radiates into the right side of the back or, less often, into other parts of the abdomen. The pain, often accompanied by slight nausea, usually begins abruptly, within 1 to 3 hours of eating a meal. (The historical association of the pain with fatty food intolerance is unfounded [10].) Patients may also complain of being awakened in the middle of the night. A typical attack subsides spontaneously within 2 to 3 hours. The frequency of such attacks is extremely variable, from every day to only once or twice a year.

A patient who presents with this history is very likely to have gallstones. However, the degree of inflammation of the gallbladder cannot be determined from the history. There may be gallstones without any inflammation at all, there may be acute inflammation, or there may be chronic inflammation with fibrosis. However, an attack lasting more than 6 hours generally heralds the onset of acute cholecystitis (acute inflammation). The severity of the symptoms and the presence or absence of signs of inflammation or biliary obstruction determine the clinician's response (see Cholecystostomy section).

Acute Cholecystitis

Pathophysiology

More than 90% of the time, acute cholecystitis is caused by a gallstone that obstructs the cystic duct. Acute acalculous cholecystitis occurs primarily in patients who have sustained major trauma, including major operations. Inflammation of the gallbladder in early acute cholecystitis is probably caused by irritation by concentrated static bile. As the process progresses, the bile often becomes infected; bile cultures are positive in only 20% to 30% of patients during the first few days of an attack, but by 7 to 10 days, almost 80% of biliary cultures are positive. In certain patients, such as diabetics and patients with acalculous cholecystitis, mural ischemia might also play a role. The difference between the presentation of acute and chronic cholecystitis (see below) is probably caused by the length of time the cystic duct has been totally obstructed and by the intensity of the inflammation.

Signs and Symptoms

The pain of classic acute cholecystitis is severe and persistent. It is usually accompanied by nausea and fever (99°F to 102°F [37°C to 39°C]) and, less often, by vomiting. Unless treated, the symptoms are likely to persist for up to a week.

The severity and persistence of the pain usually cause the patient to see his or her caregiver (see Chapter 45 for a general discussion of abdominal pain). On examination, the patient is restless. There is considerable right upper quadrant abdominal tenderness, associated with involuntary guarding of the abdominal wall. This guarding, indicative of early peritoneal inflammation, is particularly important to recognize. It is not a feature of less acute disease (see Chronic Cholecystitis section). *Murphy sign,* the sudden involuntary arrest of inspiration (because of pain) when the examiner palpates the right upper quadrant during inspiration, is caused by the abutment of the inflamed gallbladder against the examiner's fingers as it moves downward with expansion of the chest cavity. This sign is more often elicited after several days of inflammation. In one third of patients, the gallbladder is palpable during an attack of acute cholecystitis if the right upper quadrant is probed very gently. Occasionally, patients are mildly jaundiced.

Laboratory Tests

Leukocytosis (12,000 to 15,000 white blood cells per cubic millimeter) caused by a neutrophilic granulocytosis is common. Serum amylase activity may be increased in the absence of other evidence of acute pancreatitis. Often, the activity of serum aminotransferases (aspartate aminotransferase and alanine aminotransferase) is increased as well. Twenty percent of patients have mild hyperbilirubinemia (less than 4 mL/100 mL).

Biliary scintigraphy is the test of choice in the diagnosis of acute cholecystitis. The imaging compounds are ^{99m}Technicium (^{99m}Tc)-labeled derivatives of iminodiacetic acid (technetium hepatoiminodiacetic acid [TcHIDA], paraisopropyliminodiacetic acid [PIPIDA], or diisopropyl iminodiacetic acid [DISIDA]), which are concentrated in bile. The study requires injection of isotope intravenously and evaluation of uptake of the isotope by the gallbladder. If the cystic duct is obstructed, because of acute inflammation or because of a stone, uptake does not occur. The test takes 1 to 4 hours to complete. A positive study shows isotope in the biliary tree and in the duodenum but not in the gallbladder. A negative study shows isotope in the gallbladder as well. If isotope is not excreted, the test is uninterpretable, but if it is excreted, the sensitivity of the test is extremely high (essentially 100%). Specificity is also high (95%), but false positive results may occur in patients with chronic cholecystitis or acute biliary obstruction caused by pancreatitis.

Ultrasonography (US) may also be used to diagnose acute cholecystitis in a patient with characteristic symptoms. If there are stones in the gallbladder, thickening or edema of the wall, or an "ultrasonic Murphy sign" (produced by the pressure of the transducer on the inflamed gallbladder), the positive and negative predictive value of the test is greater than 92% (11).

Differential Diagnosis

The differential diagnosis must include disorders that might cause severe right upper quadrant abdominal pain and, usually, leukocytosis and slightly abnormal hepaticT tests: acute pancreatitis, appendicitis, hepatitis, hepatic abscess, a perforated or penetrated peptic ulcer, acute pyelonephritis, myocardial infarction (MI), and right lower lobe pneumonia or pleuritis. Because of the severity of the illness, these distinctions should be made in the hospital.

Treatment

The patient suspected of having acute cholecystitis should be hospitalized for observation, hydration, and further diagnostic procedures (see below and Chapter 45 for a discussion of these procedures as they pertain to ambulatory patients). If the pain is intolerable, the caregiver can administer a narcotic parenterally while arranging admission. The patient should be told that in the hospital intravenous rather than oral feeding will be given, that if there is vomiting a nasogastric tube will be passed, and that antibiotics will be administered. Because 30% to 40% of patients develop gangrenous or perforated gallbladders if cholecystectomy is delayed, urgent operation is generally indicated once the diagnosis is made, especially in diabetics and in the elderly (12,13), among whom rapid development of complications is more likely. A randomized prospective study that compared early and delayed cholecystectomy for acute cholecystitis concluded that the duration of hospitalization and the duration of disability were significantly reduced by early operation (14). The presence of emphysematous cholecystitis caused by gas-forming bacterial infection dictates emergency operation (air bubbles in the right upper quadrant on a plain film of the abdomen indicate the diagnosis). Laparoscopic cholecystectomy is ordinarily the operative procedure of choice (15). A discussion of surgery of the biliary tract and of the results and complications of operations is provided below.

Chronic Cholecystitis

Pathophysiology

Symptomatic chronic cholecystitis is associated with gallstones more than 95% of the time; the remaining cases are caused by other diseases of the gallbladder, such as cholesterolosis (the appearance of macrophages laden with cholesterol crystals in the wall of the gallbladder, often without stones). Recurring attacks of mild acute cholecystitis cause eventual fibrosis, so the gallbladder empties poorly. The symptoms of chronic disease, like those of acute cholecystitis, are caused by obstruction by a gallstone of the cystic duct. In chronic recurrent cholecystitis, obstruction of the cystic duct is of short duration (probably no more than a few hours) compared with the length of time of obstruction in acute cholecystitis, so inflammation is less intense. Chronicity of symptoms may also be related to gallbladder dyskinesia secondary to mural fibrosis.

Signs and Symptoms

Many patients who complain of biliary pain for the first time probably already have chronic gallbladder inflammation. The character and location of the pain are identical to those of acute cholecystitis. Pain is variably associated with nausea and, occasionally, vomiting. Unlike classic acute cholecystitis, fever is unusual with chronic disease. Typically, pain occurs after eating, begins 1 to 6 hours after a meal (see above), and lasts for 2 to 3 hours. Nonspecific symptoms—postprandial pain, bloating, belching, flatulence, so-called fatty food intolerance—thought by many to suggest gallbladder disease, are extremely common in the general population and therefore are not helpful diagnostically.

The patient with chronic cholecystitis usually seeks care less urgently than does the patient with acute cholecystitis. On examination during the attack, although there is tenderness to deep palpation in the right upper quadrant of the abdomen, there is no muscle guarding, as there is in patients with acute inflammation. Murphy sign (see above) is absent, the gallbladder is rarely palpable, and jaundice usually is not present. Between attacks, there is no abdominal tenderness.

Laboratory Tests

The white blood count, serum amylase, serum aminotransferases, and serum bilirubin are usually normal. Unlike patients with acute cholecystitis, patients with symptoms of chronic cholecystitis can be evaluated further in an ambulatory setting, but some are hospitalized early in an attack because of an inability to distinguish it from an episode of acute cholecystitis. If a TcHIDA scan is obtained to help in making that distinction, it may be positive, even in patients with chronic cholecystitis, because of transient obstruction of the cystic duct.

Abdominal Ultrasound

Ultrasound has replaced oral cholecystography (at approximately the same cost) as the principal test for the detection of gallstones. The advantages of ultrasound are that it exposes the patient to no radiation, it is much quicker (5 to 10 minutes), and it has no side effects. It is not influenced by associated GI or hepatic disease. The detection rate for gallstones 3 mm or greater in diameter is 89% to 96% by ultrasound with 93% to 97% specificity (3% to 7% false-positive) (16).

Oral Cholecystogram

The oral cholecystogram documents whether the gallbladder is functioning and whether radiolucent stones are present. Currently, it is obtained only if ultrasound is equivocal. Approximately 75% of gallbladders are visible on the first dose, and another 15% become visible on the second dose. The oral cholecystogram is reliable only if the Telepaque is ingested at the proper time, retained in the GI tract, absorbed from the small bowel, transported to the liver, esterified to glucuronide, and excreted by the liver into the bile. Therefore, GI or hepatic disease may cause a false-positive study. However, the specificity of the test is high (4% false positive) if radiolucent stones are present in an opacified gallbladder or if the gallbladder fails to concentrate contrast material after the second Telepaque dose. The sensitivity of the test is lower (10% false-negative), one of the reasons it has been replaced by ultrasonography.

Computed Tomography

Computed tomography (CT) accurately identifies gallstones 80% of the time. Currently, it has no advantages over (and costs about twice as much as) oral cholecystogram and ultrasonography in the diagnosis of gallbladder disease. However, CT might be useful occasionally if both the oral cholecystogram and ultrasound are equivocal.

Treatment

The treatment of choice for symptomatic chronic cholecystitis is elective cholecystectomy in patients who can tolerate an operation (see Cholecystostomy section). Medical therapies for cholelithiasis such as gallstone dissolution with ursodeoxycholic acid (Actigall) or gallstone lithotripsy are no longer used because of low effectiveness and high recurrence rates. These medical therapies became obsolete with the advent of laparoscopic cholecystectomy. Risks of not treating patients with chronic cholecystitis include gangrene and perforation of the gallbladder, choledocholithiasis (see Choledocholithiasis section), pancreatitis, and, rarely, gallstone ileus (the obstruction of the small bowel by a large gallstone passed through an acute fistula that has formed between the gallbladder and the duodenum).

SYMPTOMATIC PATIENTS WHO HAVE NO DETECTABLE GALLSTONES

Adenomyomatosis of the Gallbladder

Adenomyomatosis of the gallbladder is often asymptomatic, but some patients have symptoms indistinguishable from those with chronic cholecystitis (18). The disease is caused by thickening of the gallbladder wall because of hyperplasia of the epithelium with the formation of glands and diverticula through the muscular wall. The diagnosis is often suspected during ultrasonography or cholecystography, but many cases are revealed by the pathologist after removal of the gallbladder. Adenomyomatosis is found in approximately 20% of patients who undergo cholecystectomy for biliary symptoms. It has been considered not to predispose to gallbladder cancer, but a report of a large number of cases from Japan shows a higher prevalence of gallbladder cancer in segmental adenomyomatosis, which is characterized by a concentric narrowing dividing the gallbladder into two segments (18). Cholecystectomy relieves the symptoms in most patients with symptomatic adenomyomatosis.

Carcinoma of the Gallbladder

Carcinoma of the gallbladder is often asymptomatic, but can present with abdominal pain and, when advanced, with jaundice. It is the most common tumor of the biliary tract with an incidence of approximately 1 in 10,000. It is more common in women than in men. Risk factors for carcinoma of the gallbladder are cholelithiasis, calcification of the gallbladder wall (porcelain gallbladder), and gallbladder polyps (19).

Endoscopic ultrasound (EUS) with fine-needle aspiration (FNA) is a new technique that has greatly improved the ability to diagnose carcinoma of the gallbladder. It facilitates cytological diagnosis by FNA of cholangiocarcinoma and adenocarcinoma of the gallbladder and allows differentiation of these tumors from gallbladder polyps (17). Furthermore EUS can define the extent of a tumor and the involvement of regional lymph nodes providing assistance in determining tumor resectability. The patient's experience is essentially the same as it is with endoscopy alone and the complication rate is low (17).

Surgical resection remains the only potential cure for gall bladder cancer, but unfortunately most tumors, about 90%, are not resectable at the time of diagnosis.

Biliary Dyskinesia

Some patients with symptoms suggestive of gallstones have a normal abdominal sonogram, a normal oral cholecystogram, and a normal abdominal CT. These patients may have *biliary dyskinesia,* a term used to denote abnormally decreased emptying of the gallbladder. The diagnosis is best made by cholecystokinin (Kinevac)-stimulated cholecystography with a TcHIDA. Often, the patient's pain is reproduced after the Kinevac injection (it stimulates gallbladder contraction), and abnormally decreased emptying of the gallbladder can be documented as a markedly decreased ejection fraction (percentage of the isotope excreted) of less than 30% compared with a group of normal subjects. Such patients, if severely symptomatic, should be offered elective cholecystectomy, after which symptoms usually abate. At operation, many of these patients prove to have stones too small to identify by ultrasonography or they have biliary sludge.

Biliary Sludge

In some symptomatic patients who have no gallstones detectable by the standard techniques, the gallbladder reflects, on US, echoes now recognized to be characteristic of biliary sludge. Of note is that EUS is more sensitive in the detection of biliary sludge than is abdominal ultrasound (20). Hence EUS is indicated in patients with symptoms of biliary-type pain who had a negative abdominal ultrasound. In some patients *biliary sludge* is a term applied to excessively viscous bile that contains cholesterol crystals, calcium bilirubinate granules, and mucin. In such patients duodenal drainage, ordinarily done by a consulting gastroenterologist, may prove useful in identifying the cholesterol crystals or the bilirubinate granules.

Patient Experience. The test is performed by having the patient swallow a plastic double-lumen tube, weighted at the end by a mercury-filled bag. There are holes in the tube above the bag. When the bag has passed into the second portion of the duodenum (documented by fluoroscopy), magnesium sulfate is injected into one lumen of the tube to stimulate contraction of the gallbladder. Duodenal contents are then aspirated and the sediment is separated by centrifugation and examined under a microscope. The patient's experience during this procedure is similar to that of patients undergoing upper endoscopy (see Chapter 45).

Biliary sludge may be a precursor of gallstones and of pancreatitis (21), but in a given patient the course is entirely unpredictable. Nevertheless, as with biliary dyskinesia, severely symptomatic patients with biliary sludge should be offered elective cholecystectomy.

CHOLEDOCHOLITHIASIS

Epidemiology

Common duct stones occur in approximately 15% of patients with chronic cholecystitis, either before or after cholecystectomy. The incidence increases with age and the length of time symptoms of gallbladder disease have been present. There are three categories of common duct stones: concomitant gallbladder stones and common duct stones, retained stones found in the common duct soon after cholecystectomy or common duct exploration, and common duct stones identified long after cholecystectomy or common duct exploration. The latter group are thought to develop in the common bile duct, and have a different consistency from stones that form in the gallbladder. They are called "earth stones" because they are soft, and not rocky hard as gallbladder stones usually are. The incidence of common duct stones decreases exponentially in the first year after cholecystectomy only to rise again, reaching a peak at 3 years. In one study, 26% of symptomatic common duct stones occurred 10 or more years after cholecystectomy (22). Also, patients with congenital agenesis of the gallbladder have a 20% incidence of common duct stones. These observations support the concept that common duct stones originate in the gallbladder or in the intrahepatic or common bile ducts.

Signs and Symptoms

Approximately 6% of patients with common duct stones are asymptomatic. More typically, patients develop severe colicky right upper quadrant pain, often associated with jaundice, mild fever, and nausea and vomiting. The pain usually begins abruptly and lasts up to an hour. If nothing is done, attacks recur at variable periods. Eventually cholangitis develops, manifested by persistent malaise and anorexia and intermittent fever, chills, and jaundice, associated with persistently high serum alkaline phosphatase activity. Suppurative ascending cholangitis characterized by right upper quadrant pain, high fever, shaking chills, and jaundice (Charcot triad) is life threatening and constitutes an emergency.

Rarely, painless jaundice is the only presenting complaint of a patient with choledocholithiasis. In such a circumstance the diagnostic studies should be the same ones performed on the patient with more typical signs and symptoms.

On physical examination, if the patient is asymptomatic, no abnormal signs are elicited. If the patient is symptomatic, right upper quadrant abdominal tenderness and muscle guarding are usually present, similar to the findings in patients with acute cholecystitis. The patient is usually mildly to moderately jaundiced.

Laboratory Tests

Because of the acute onset of symptoms and the severity of pain in patients with choledocholithiasis, laboratory studies in the ambulatory setting are usually not appropriate. If such studies are done, leukocytosis and increases in serum alkaline phosphatase, serum aminotransferase, and serum amylase activities and serum bilirubin concentration are likely to be observed. The first diagnostic test is ordinarily *US* (or CT—equally useful, but more expensive). If the common duct is dilated, the next step is visualization of the biliary tree.

The preferred procedure is *magnetic resonance cholangiopancreatography (MRCP).* It has the advantage that it is not invasive and does not carry the small but real risks of pancreatitis and cholangitis associated with *endoscopic retrograde cholangiopancreatography (ERCP).* If there is a normal duct on MRCP then other sources of sepsis can be evaluated, and ERCP may be avoided. If a stone is seen then ERCP is necessary for sphincterotomy and removal of the stone or stones. The initial MRCP can greatly reduce the need for purely diagnostic ERCPs (24). Diagnostic ERCP is still occasionally useful when suspicion of a stone is high, even if the MRCP is apparently normal, and ERCP remains the "standard criterion" for evaluating the biliary tree. (23). The patient's experience during the procedure is essentially the same as it is during other kinds of endoscopy (see Chapter 45) except that ERCP lasts for 30 to 90 minutes and the complication rate is higher (see above).

Percutaneous transhepatic cholangiography (PTC) is most useful in visualizing obstruction of the intrahepatic bile ducts, which can be relieved by stenting in the case of strictures or removal of stones from the small bile ducts. Additionally, PTC is used to visualize the bile ducts in patients who have had a gastrojejunostomy where the sphincter of Oddi is not accessible for ERCP.

Treatment

Therapeutic

Common duct stones should be removed, usually at the time of ERCP by endoscopic sphincterotomy. ERCP is performed in a center where fluoroscopy of the cannulated duct is available. The patient experience during the procedure is essentially the same as it is during other kinds of upper endoscopy (see Chapter 45), except that ERCP usually lasts for 30 to 60 minutes, and may be complicated 5% to 10% of the time by postendoscopic cholangitis, especially if the common duct is manipulated, and by pancreatitis. In an 8-year followup of patients after endoscopic sphincterotomy, papillary stenosis or recurrent bile duct stones occurred in less than 5% of the cases (25).

Although ERCP is the preferred method for removing common bile duct stones, although other approaches are available. Common bile duct exploration and stone removal is possible at either open or laparoscopic cholecystectomy. It is also possible to clear the common bile duct of stones using a percutaneous transhepatic catheter. In special situations these alternative approaches have a place, but generally the most expeditious and effective approach is by ERCP.

Cholangitis

Bacterial infection of the biliary tree generally occurs in association with bile duct obstruction caused by choledocholithiasis, tumor, or biliary strictures. The principal symptoms are fever, chills, and abdominal pain. Jaundice is often but not invariably present. On examination, there is abdominal tenderness and often rebound tenderness. Abnormal laboratory tests include leukocytosis and elevations of the serum bilirubin and alkaline phosphatase. Serum aminotransferases may also be moderately elevated. Blood cultures are often positive. The patient may deteriorate rapidly and develop hypotension and changes in mental status. Hospitalization is mandatory for therapy with antibiotics, followed by appropriate relief of biliary obstruction either surgically, by endoscopic sphincterotomy, or by placement of a biliary stent.

Primary sclerosing cholangitis (26) is a chronic inflammation of unknown cause of intrahepatic and extrahepatic bile ducts that leads ultimately to fibrosis and cholestatic liver disease. Most patients are men. There is a very high correlation with concomitant inflammatory bowel disease, most commonly ulcerative colitis. The course of the cholangitis is unpredictable, but patients with advanced disease develop jaundice, right upper quadrant abdominal pain, fever, pruritus, and weight loss and ultimately die of hepatic failure. Diagnosis is made most easily by the demonstration of typical cholangiographic changes during ERCP or MRCP. Adenocarcinoma of the bile ducts is a common complication that occurs in at least 9% to 15% of patients (27). Patients with ulcerative colitis and primary sclerosing cholangitis are also at increased risk of colon cancer, beyond the risk imposed by ulcerative colitis alone (28,29). High doses of ursodeoxycholic acid (20 to 25 mg/kg/day), but not the lower doses commonly used in the treatment of primary biliary cirrhosis (10 to 15 mg/kg/day), improve liver tests and survival in patients with primary sclerosing cholangitis (30). Patients with advanced cirrhosis and jaundice due to primary sclerosing cholangitis should be referred to a transplant center for liver transplantation (see Chapter 47).

BILIARY TRACT OPERATIONS

Primary caregivers should be aware of the mechanics of biliary surgical procedures so that they can inform and reassure patients who are to be referred to a surgeon.

Cholecystectomy

Laparoscopic cholecystectomy has replaced open cholecystectomy as the procedure of choice for the removal of the gallbladder for cholelithiasis and for acute and chronic cholecystitis. Laparoscopic cholecystectomy is performed under general anesthesia. A pneumoperitoneum is established, and a laparoscope and three additional cannulas are inserted through which instruments are placed to remove the gallbladder. Relative contraindications to laparoscopic cholecystectomy include a gangrenous or perforated gallbladder, peritonitis, cholangitis, previous upper abdominal surgery, and cirrhosis (31). Common duct stones are also a contraindication unless they can be extracted by endoscopic sphincterotomy before the cholecystectomy or unless the surgeon is experienced in laparoscopic common duct exploration. Laparoscopic cholecystectomy has the advantage over open cholecystectomy of a shorter hospital stay. In elective cases, the stay is approximately 24 hours, with a return to normal activity in 10 to 14 days. In one study, laparoscopic cholecystectomy needed to be converted to open cholecystectomy in only 4.7% of cases (32). The common reasons for conversion are severe scarring or acute inflammation that obscures the anatomy, adhesions related to prior surgery, aberrant anatomic features that make dissection difficult, and bile duct, bowel, or vascular injuries that occur during surgery. Common duct stones encountered during the procedure can sometimes be removed by laparoscopic choledochoscopy, but otherwise require open common duct exploration or postoperative ERCP. In a reported series, complications occurred in 5.1% of cases (32). The most common complication is wound infection in 1.1% of cases, followed by bile duct injury in 0.5% of cases. Other complications are prolonged ileus, bowel injury, and operative bleeding. Mortality in elective cases is less than 0.1%.

Elective open cholecystectomy has a mortality rate of 0.3% or less. Urgent or emergency operation for acute cholecystitis has a mortality rate of up to 10% depending on whether common duct stones are present. The morbidity of open cholecystectomy is primarily related to superficial wound infection (less than 5% to 7%). Wound infection is more common if the operation lasts longer than 2 hours, the patient is obese or diabetic, and the patient has acute rather than chronic cholecystitis. Other possible but rare (less than 1%) immediate complications of cholecystectomy are postoperative bleeding, postoperative bile leak, injury to biliary ducts (0.1%), and retained common duct stones.

Cholecystostomy

Cholecystostomy may be required in the patient who is critically ill from acute cholecystitis and who has associated severe cardiac, pulmonary, or renal disease that contraindicates the use of general anesthesia or of a prolonged operation. Another less often cited indication for cholecystostomy is inability to detect normal biliary anatomy because of a severe inflammatory process near the main bile ducts. Rather than risk possible injury to structures in the porta hepatis, a cholecystostomy may be performed.

A cholecystostomy can be done through a small incision in the right upper quadrant. A large drainage tube is inserted into the gallbladder through a stab wound in the fundus. An attempt is made to remove stones. The tube is brought through the abdominal wall and allowed to drain freely. An attempt should be made to empty the gallbladder of stones before placing the tube. If a stone is impacted at the cystic duct, future cholecystectomy will be necessary or a mucous fistula will persist after the tube is removed. However, if all stones are removed, only 30% to 50% of patients will develop recurrent symptoms of cholelithiasis within 2 years after the tube is removed. The operative mortality is very high from cholecystostomy, not because of the operation but because the patient is critically ill.

Choledochotomy

Common duct exploration or choledochotomy, whether combined with cholecystectomy or as an isolated operation, has a higher morbidity and mortality rate than does simple cholecystectomy. The operation takes longer than cholecystectomy and patients are generally older, two factors important in determining morbidity and mortality. Generally the patient is hospitalized 3 to 5 days longer for common duct exploration than for cholecystectomy alone. A drain (called a T-tube) is generally placed in the common duct at the time of operation. This is done to stent the repair and to allow postoperative imaging to rule out retained stones or other technical problems.

COURSE AFTER OPEN BILIARY SURGERY

Normal Course

The patient is usually discharged 5 to 7 days after an uncomplicated open biliary tract operation. Skin sutures or staples will have been removed, and the patient will be allowed to bathe. Usually patients are requested to avoid driving and sexual relations for 1 week from the day of discharge. Patients are generally advised to avoid heavy (approximately 15 pounds [7 kg] or more) lifting for 4 to 6 weeks. The incidence of incisional hernia (see Chapter 97) is low after a right subcostal oblique incision and slightly higher with a vertical midline or paramedian incision. The patient returns to the surgeon's office for evaluation at 1 and 6 weeks after operation. The wound and the drain sites, if present, should be healed unless there has been wound infection. If a common duct exploration was performed, the T tube is removed in 4 to 6 weeks, assuming the postoperative cholangiogram is normal. The patient should be able to resume an unrestricted regular diet within a few days of operation without difficulty. Stools should be at preoperative frequency and of normal color. Immediate weight loss of 10 to 20 pounds is normal, even in uncomplicated cases. Ten percent of patients have diarrhea for up to 6 weeks but rarely longer than that.

The patient should be expected to complain about pulling sensations in the area of the incision because the right rectus muscle has been divided and resutured. If the subcostal incision was made close to the costal margin, the patient often complains also about discomfort on bending or sitting. The area just below a right subcostal incision is apt to be numb for several months because of interruption of a cutaneous sensory nerve to this area. Sensitivity does return, however, in most cases. It is not surprising to find patients gaining weight after cholecystectomy, especially if they had lost weight preoperatively.

Postcholecystectomy Syndrome

Approximately 90% of patients operated on for symptomatic biliary tract disease become asymptomatic or have trivial symptoms (e.g., occasional dyspepsia). The other 10% may continue to be symptomatic, either because they were treated for the wrong disease or because they have developed a postoperative complication. In the former category are patients who had gallstones but whose symptoms actually emanated from another disease (e.g., chronic pancreatitis, peptic ulcer disease, angina, reflux esophagitis, or irritable bowel syndrome).

Postoperative problems associated with the operation itself include retained common duct stones, and common duct injury with eventual bile duct stricture and recurrent cholangitis. Sphincter of Oddi dysfunction occasionally may be a treatable cause of postcholecystectomy syndrome. The diagnosis is made by showing a decrease in the emptying of the biliary tree by cholecystokinin cholecystography with ^{99m}Tc-iminodiacetic derivatives (see Biliary Dyskinesia section) and by demonstrating an elevated sphincter pressure by manometry during ERCP. Sphincterotomy in patients with elevated sphincter pressure results in pain relief in more than 90% of cases (33).

Postcholecystectomy symptoms are occasionally attributed to the cystic duct stump. In the absence of a stone in the stump, this is rarely or ever the cause of the symptoms.

SPECIFIC REFERENCES

1. Johnston DE, Kaplan MM. Pathogenesis and treatment of gallstones. N Engl J Med 1993;328:412.
2. Thistle JL, Schoenfield LJ. Lithogenic bile among young Indian women: lithogenic potential decreased with chenodeoxycholic acid. N Engl J Med 1971;284:177.
3. Bennion LJ, Grundy SM. Risk factors for the development of cholelithiasis in man. N Engl J Med 1978;299:1161.
4. Gracie WA, Ransohoff DF. The natural history of silent gallstones. The innocent gallstone is not a myth. N Engl J Med 1982;307:798.
5. Lund J. Surgical indications in cholelithiasis; prophylactic cholecystectomy elucidated on the basis of long-term follow-up on 526 nonoperated cases. Ann Surg 1960;151:153.
6. Lowenfels AB, Lindstrom CG, Conway MJ, et al. Gallstones and risk of gallbladder cancer. J Natl Cancer Inst 1985;75:77.
7. Pokorny WJ, Saleem M, O'Gorman RB, et al. Cholelithiasis and cholecystitis in childhood. Am J Surg 1984;148:742.
8. Friedman LS, Roberts MS, Brett AS, et al. Management of asymptomatic gallstones in the diabetic patient. A decision analysis. Ann Intern Med 1988;109:913.
9. Diehl AK, Sugarek NJ, Todd KH. Clinical evaluation for gallstone disease: usefulness of symptoms and signs in diagnosis. Am J Med 1990;89:29.
10. Mogadam M, Albarelli J, Ahmed SW, et al. Gallbladder dynamics in response to various meals: is dietary fat restriction necessary in the management of gallstones? Am J Gastroenterol 1984;79:745.
11. Ralls PW, Coletti PM, Lapin SA, et al. Real-time sonography in suspected acute cholecystitis. Prospective evaluation of primary and secondary signs. Radiology 1985;155:767.
12. Mundth ED. Cholecystitis and diabetes mellitus. N Engl J Med 1962;267:642.
13. Morrow DJ, Thompson J, Wilson SE. Acute cholecystitis in the elderly, a surgical emergency. Arch Surg 1978;113:1149.
14. Jarvinen HJ, Hastbacka J. Early cholecystectomy for acute cholecystitis: a prospective randomized study. Ann Surg 1980;191:501.
15. Bender JS, Zenilman ME. Immediate laparoscopic cholecystectomy as definitive therapy for acute cholecystitis. Surg Endosc 1995;9:1081.
16. Ferruci TJ. Body ultrasonography. N Engl J Med 1979;300: 538.
17. Yusuf TE, Bhutani MS. Role of endoscopic ultrasonography in diseases of the extrahepatic biliary system. J. Gastroenterol Hepatol 2004;19:243.
18. Ram MD, Midha D. Adenomyomatosis of the gallbladder. Surgery 1975;78:224.
19. Misra S, Chaturvedi A, Misra NC, et al. Carcinoma of the gallbladder. Lancet Oncol 2003;4:167.
20. Dill JE, Hill S, Callis J, et al. Combined endoscopic ultrasound and stimulated biliary drainage in cholecystitis and microlithiasis—diagnoses and outcomes. Endoscopy 1995;27:424.
21. Lee SP, Nicholls JF, Park HZ. Biliary sludge as a cause of acute pancreatitis. N Engl J Med 1992;326:589.
22. Thurston OG, McDougall RM. The effect of hepatic bile on retained common duct stones. Surg Gynecol Obstet 1976;143:625.
23. Schofl R. Diagnostic endoscopic retrograde cholangiopancreatography. Endoscopy 2001;33:147.
24. Magnuson TH, Bender JS, Duncan MD, et al. Utility of magnetic resonance cholangiography in the evaluation of biliary obstruction. J Am Coll Surg 1999;189:63.
25. Prat F, Malak NA, Pelletier G. Biliary symptoms and complications more than 8 years after endoscopic sphincterotomy. Gastroenterology 1996;110:894.
26. Angulo P, Lindor KD. Primary sclerosing cholangitis. Hepatology 1999;30:325.
27. Rosen CB, Nagorney DM, Wiesner RH, et al. Cholangiocarcinoma complicating primary sclerosing cholangitis. Ann Surg 1991;213:21.
28. Brentnall TA, Haggitt RC, Rabinovitch PS, et al. Risk and natural history of colonic neoplasia in patients with primary sclerosing cholangitis and ulcerative colitis. Gastroenterology 1996;110:331.
29. Shetty K, Rybicki L, Brezezinski A, et al. The risk for cancer or dysplasia in ulcerative colitis patients with primary sclerosing cholangitis. Am J Gastroenterol 1999;94:1643.
30. Harnois DM, Angulo P, Jorgensen RA et al. High-dose ursodeoxycholic acid as a therapy for patients with primary sclerosing cholangitis. Amer J Gastroenterol 2001;96:1598.
31. Gadacz TR. Laparoscopy cholecystectomy. In: Cameron JL, ed. Current surgical therapy. 4th ed. St. Louis: CV Mosby, 1992: 330.
32. Southern Surgeons Club. A prospective analysis of 1518 laparoscopic cholecystectomies. N Engl J Med 1991;324:1073.
33. Greenen JE, Hogan WJ, Dodds WJ, et al. The efficacy of endoscopic sphincterotomy after cholecystectomy in patients with sphincter-of-Oddi dysfunction. N Engl J Med 1989;320:82.

*For annotated **General References** and resources related to this chapter, visit www.hopkinsbayview.org/PAMreferences.*

Chapter 97

Hernias of the Groin and Abdominal Wall*

John W. Harmon and Christopher L. Wolfgang

*In previous editions, Mark D. Duncan, MD, and Jeffrey S. Bender, MD, contributed to this chapter.

DEFINITIONS

A hernia is a protrusion of a viscus or part of a viscus from its normal location in the body. Clinically common hernias involve anatomic defects in the abdominal wall, typically in the inguinal, femoral, or umbilical regions or at the site of a previous surgical incision. The term *ventral hernia,* referring to an anterior abdominal wall hernia, is often used to denote an incisional hernia. A hernia is *reducible* if its contents can be pushed back into the abdominal cavity, and *incarcerated* if they cannot be pushed back. *Strangulation* of a hernia occurs when the blood supply to the herniated tissue is compromised. All strangulated hernias are incarcerated, but incarcerated hernias may not be strangulated.

This chapter describes the more common types of abdominal hernias and discusses the role of the ambulatory practitioner in their diagnosis and treatment.

HERNIAS OF THE GROIN

Inguinal Hernias

Inguinal hernias are classified as direct or indirect; about two thirds are indirect (1). *Direct hernias* are portions of the bowel or omentum that protrude directly through the floor of the inguinal canal to emerge through the external inguinal ring above the inguinal ligament (Fig. 97.1). *Indirect hernias* enter the inguinal canal through its internal ring, lateral to the inferior epigastric vessels, traverse the canal, and emerge also through the external inguinal ring (Fig. 97.1). Indirect hernias, as they get larger, have a propensity to extend into the scrotum.

Epidemiology and Causes

Inguinal hernia is a common problem in ambulatory practice and accounts for approximately 75% of all abdominal wall hernias. Inguinal hernia repair is one of the most common general surgical procedures performed in the United States (1). The majority of inguinal hernias occur in men (1); 5% to 10% of men in the United States develop an inguinal hernia during their lifetime. Although femoral hernias (discussed later) are much more common in women than in men, the most common groin hernia in women is an indirect inguinal hernia. Less than 10% of inguinal hernias in adults are bilateral when the patient is first seen, but a hernia may occur on the opposite side at some time in the future. The chance of developing a contralateral inguinal hernia is the same regardless of which side is affected first.

All *indirect inguinal hernias* are caused by a congenital defect in which the processus vaginalis remains patent. The processus vaginalis is a tract lined with peritoneum that extends from the peritoneal cavity into the scrotum in the male. With time this tract may enlarge, and abdominal contents may herniate into it. The combination of this congenital abnormality and a predisposing acquired condition that increases intra-abdominal pressure (e.g., obesity, chronic obstructive airway disease, ascites, chronic constipation with straining at stool, prostatism with straining at urination, hard physical labor) determines when an inguinal hernia develops. Occasionally, only intra-abdominal fluid gravitates into the scrotum, causing scrotal swelling when the patient is upright but draining back into the abdominal cavity when the patient is supine. Such a lesion is called a *communicating hydrocele*; it is more commonly seen in children than in adults. Indirect hernias, because they are associated with a congenital defect, develop in younger people but increase in incidence with advancing age; they are about four to five times more common after 50 years of age than before.

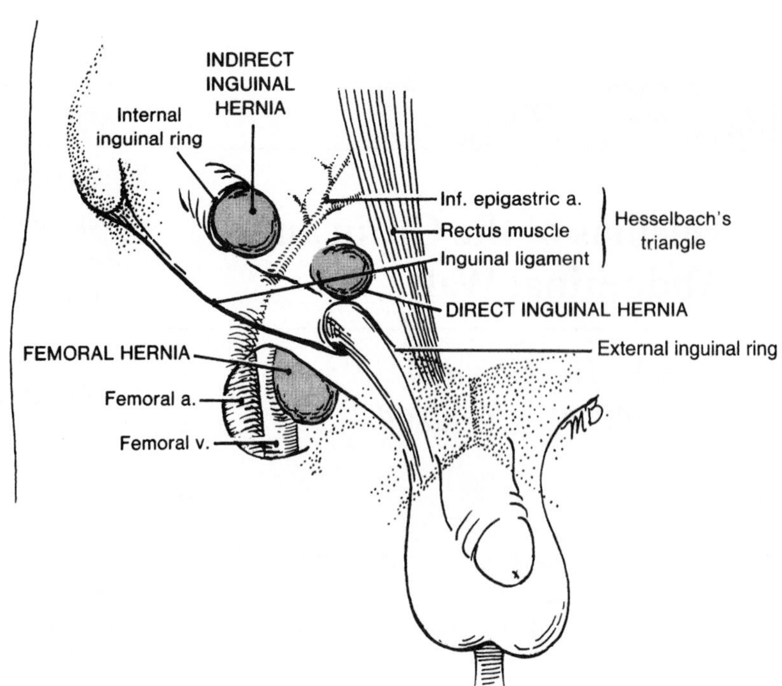

FIGURE 97.1. Artist's rendition of groin region, illustrating indirect and direct inguinal hernias and femoral hernia. (Modified from Dunphy JE, Botsford TW. Physical examination of the surgical patient. 3rd ed. Philadelphia: WB Saunders, 1964:118.)

Direct inguinal hernias are acquired lesions and are influenced not only by changes in intra-abdominal pressure but also by progressive attenuation of the inguinal structures as part of the normal aging process. Rarely, inherited defects in collagen synthesis (e.g., Marfan syndrome) provide an obvious explanation for accelerated weakening of these structures. Direct hernias are predominantly problems of middle-aged and elderly people.

History

Most patients complain of a dull ache in the groin and a bulge, either localized to the groin or at times extending into the scrotum in men or the labia in women. Sometimes pain precedes discovery of the mass by some months (perhaps because, in early stages of herniation, the internal canal is stretched before omentum or bowel manifests as a bulge at the external inguinal ring). Occasionally, the patient recalls a sharp pain during a strenuous event, which represents the initial herniation. Often the patient or the clinician notices a herniated mass in the absence of pain or symptoms. Small reducible hernias may be noticed intermittently, at times of increased intra-abdominal pressure.

If a hernia incarcerates, it may become more painful, although many patients with chronically incarcerated hernias are pain free. Indirect hernias have an approximately 10% chance of incarcerating; direct hernias incarcerate only rarely. Essentially all strangulated hernias are symptomatic; with strangulation, the hernia becomes extremely painful and tender, and nausea, vomiting, abdominal distention, constipation, and fever (with leukocytosis) are common.

Physical Examination

The examination should be performed with the patient standing and then again with the patient recumbent. An indirect hernia sometimes can be distinguished from a direct hernia by inspection. An indirect hernia, once it has entered the inguinal canal, manifests as an elliptical swelling descending toward or even into the scrotum (Fig. 97.2). A direct hernia manifests as an isolated oval swelling near the pubis; it is rarely found in the scrotum (Fig. 97.3). If the hernia is visible, an attempt should be made to push it back the abdominal cavity. If the hernia cannot be reduced, the patient should be asked to lie down and another attempt should be made to reduce it. Approximately 10% of inguinal hernias are incarcerated when they are first diagnosed.

If the hernia is not visible, the physician's finger should be placed at the base of the scrotum and then gently advanced cephalad and laterally into the inguinal canal (Fig. 97.4). The external ring can be examined without causing the patient a great deal of discomfort. The size of the ring, in itself, does not predict the presence of a hernia or the propensity to develop one, because the external ring is an opening in the aponeurosis of the external oblique muscle that does not contribute to the integrity of the floor of the inguinal canal. When the examining finger has been directed through the external ring, having the patient increase intra-abdominal pressure by coughing or straining causes a hernia to protrude and to be felt as an impulse or bulge at the tip of the examining finger.

An attempt should be made to reduce an incarcerated hernia; however, if strangulation is suspected, as when a patient presents with severe pain associated with a preexisting hernia, one should not attempt to reduce the hernia forcefully, because this maneuver carries the risk of

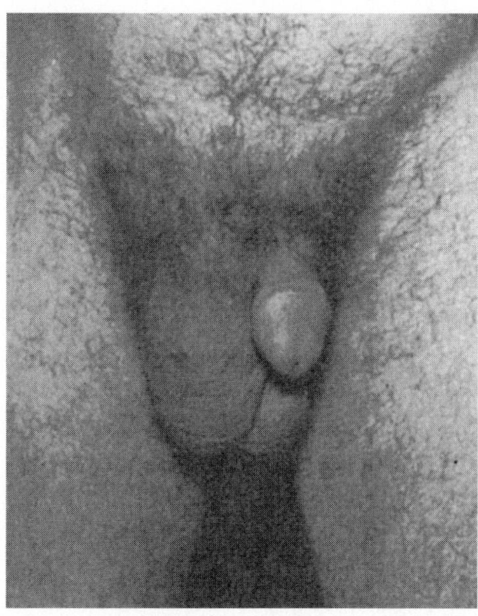

FIGURE 97.2. Indirect inguinal hernia. Swelling is oblique and cylindrical and extends into the scrotum. (From Zimmerman LM, Anson BJ. Anatomy and surgery of hernia. 2nd ed. Baltimore: Williams & Wilkins, 1967:155.)

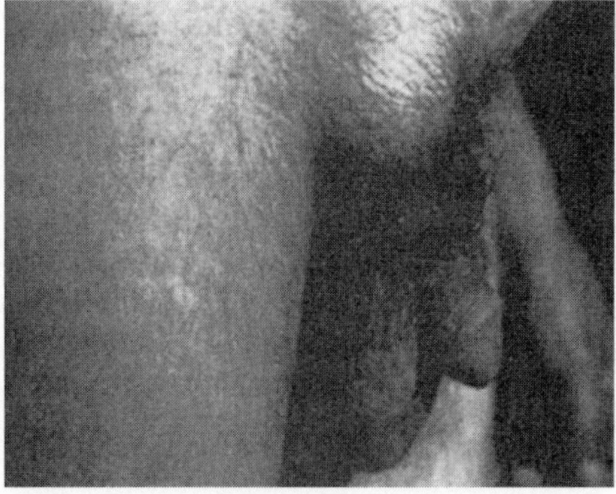

FIGURE 97.3. Direct inguinal hernia. Note medially situated globular swelling. (From Zimmerman LM, Anson BJ. Anatomy and surgery of hernia. 2nd ed. Baltimore: Williams & Wilkins, 1967:154.)

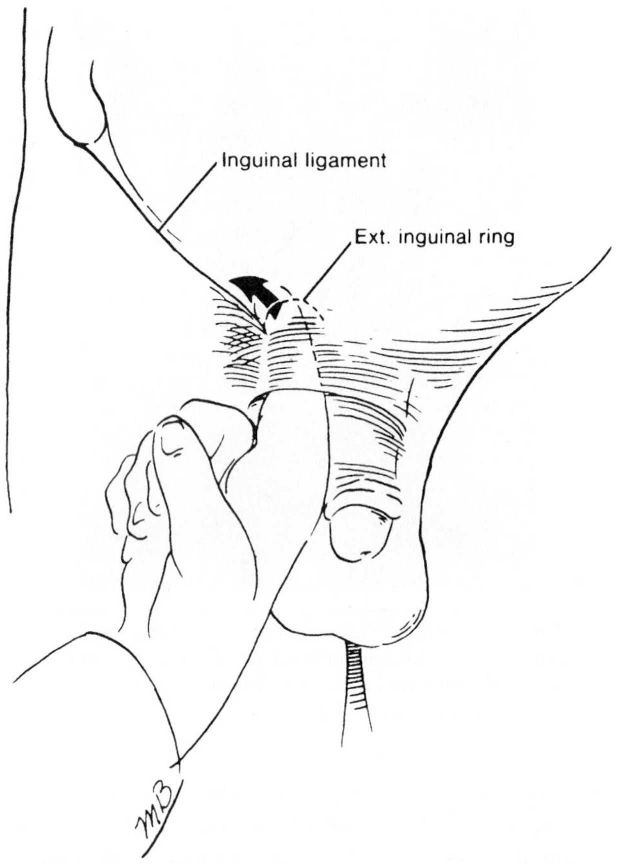

FIGURE 97.4. Examination of the inguinal canal. The examining finger gently invaginates the scrotum into the inguinal canal. (Modified from Dunphy JE, Botsford TW. Physical examination of the surgical patient. 3rd ed. Philadelphia: WB Saunders, 1964:116.)

reducing gangrenous bowel from within the hernia sac into the general peritoneal cavity. A strangulated hernia must be repaired promptly. An incarcerated hernia that is symptomatic should also be repaired on presentation, whereas the hernia of an asymptomatic patient presenting with a chronic incarceration can be fixed electively.

Differential Diagnosis

The most common cause of groin pain that is mistaken for a hernia is *strain of the adductor muscles* of the thigh at their attachment to the pelvis. Because, like groin hernia, the onset of this symptom is related to physical labor, both the patient and the clinician are convinced that a hernia must be present. In the absence of appropriate physical findings, the temptation to surgically explore the groin must be firmly resisted. As with other muscular injuries, groin strain can take months to resolve.

An incarcerated scrotal hernia must be distinguished from other scrotal lesions (Fig. 97.5). One of the most common of these is a *hydrocele*—a tense, slightly fluctuant mass that can be distinguished from a hernia or a solid mass by transillumination. Another common scrotal mass is a *varicocele*—an enlarged venous plexus that on palpation feels soft and worm-like and extends from the testicle up toward the spermatic cord. It does not transilluminate and, when the patient lies down, it collapses. If a varicocele is of recent onset in an adult, occurs on the left, and does not disappear in the supine position, one must consider obstruction of the left spermatic vein (which enters the left renal vein) by a retroperitoneal neoplasm. A *spermatocele* is a localized but vaguely circumscribed mass that also does not transilluminate and that persists when the patient lies down.

Apart from distinguishing a hernia from another kind of scrotal mass, an important component of the physical examination is the examination of the testicle and its surrounding structures. In that way, epididymal cysts, epididymitis, orchitis, testicular torsion, and testicular tumors can be detected. *Epididymal cysts* can occur in any portion of the epididymis and may be smooth or lobulated; some of them transilluminate; they are innocuous and require no treatment. *Epididymitis* manifests as a tender, swollen epididymis (see Chapter 37). Often, elevation and immobilization of the scrotum relieve the pain associated with an inflammatory process. In contrast, the pain produced by *torsion of the testicle* is unremitting. Sudden onset of testicular pain in an otherwise healthy person is characteristic of this problem. On examination, the testicle is enlarged and exquisitely tender. The patient should be referred immediately to a general surgeon or urologist. *Testicular tumors* can involve the entire testicle or simply protrude as a small nodule from the testicular surface. These masses are more indurated than the common benign scrotal masses, and they usually lack the slight tenderness of the normal testicle. Patients with suspected tumors should be referred as soon as possible to a urologist.

Preoperative Evaluation of the Patient with a Hernia

When evaluating a patient with a hernia, it is important to consider whether coexistent disease has allowed the hernia to manifest at that point in time. Focused questions in the medical history should include a specific inquiry about smoking, a history of cough, difficulty urinating, or difficulty with bowel movements, including straining and constipation. A rectal examination, to assess for the presence of prostatic hypertrophy or a rectal mass, is an important part of the preoperative evaluation. The examiner should also ascertain whether ascites is present. Anything that increases intra-abdominal pressure will place tension on the endoabdominal fascia and may contribute to the development or presentation of a hernia. A practitioner would not want to miss a diagnosis of lung cancer, prostate cancer, or colorectal cancer when referring a patient for

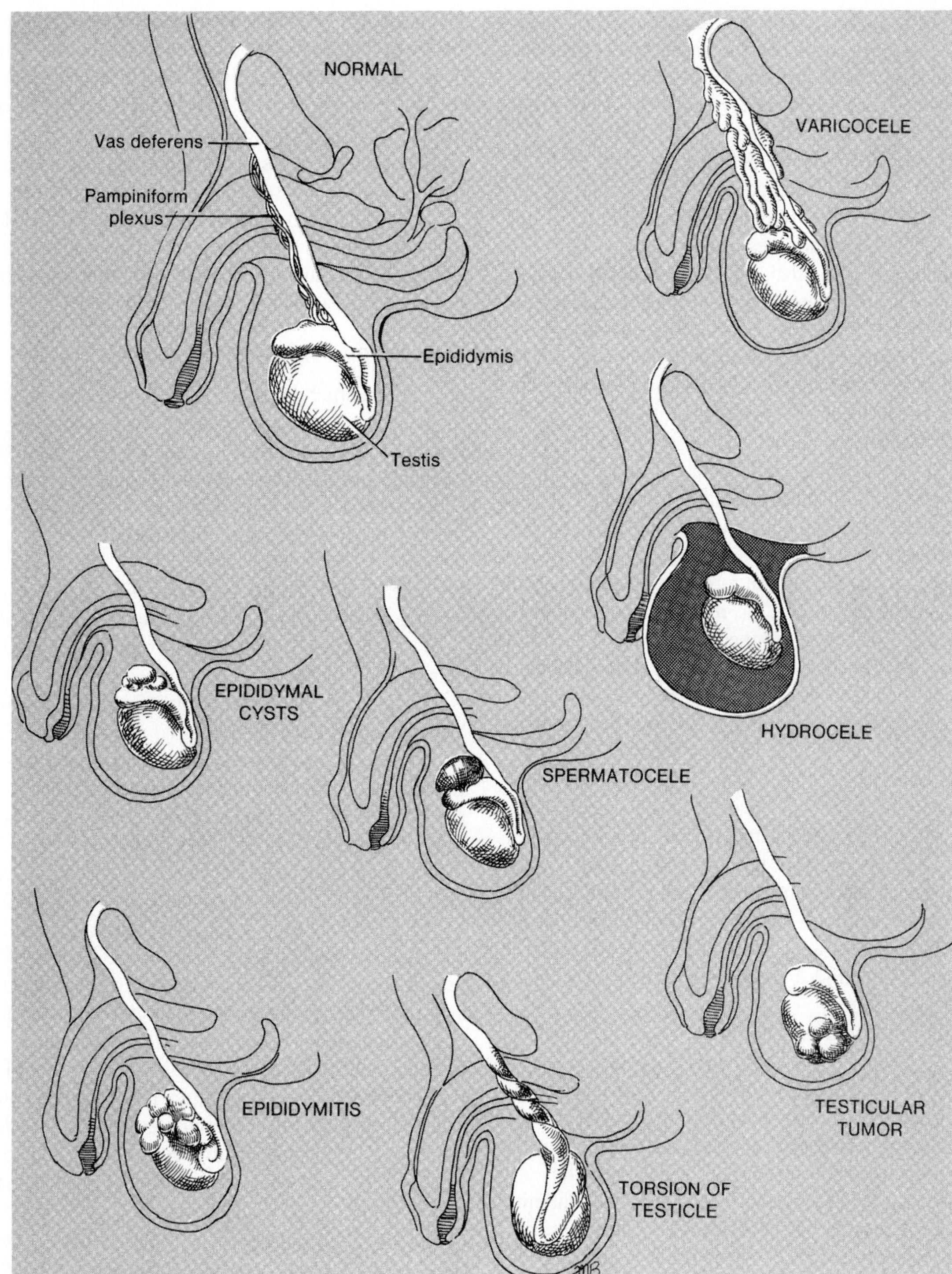

FIGURE 97.5. Lesions palpable in the scrotum. A correct diagnosis can usually be made if the normal anatomic relationships of the contents of the scrotum are borne in mind. (Modified from Dunphy JE, Botsford TW. Physical examination of the surgical patient. 3rd ed. Philadelphia: WB Saunders, 1964:111.)

hernia repair. Furthermore, attention to any predisposing causes of increased intra-abdominal pressure may limit the effect these conditions have on hernia recurrence rates.

Management

Almost all inguinal hernias should be repaired. Severe coexistent illness is the only real contraindication to herniorrhaphy (see Chapter 93 for a discussion of anesthesia and surgery risks in patients with coexistent medical conditions). Although no sense of urgency is associated with elective repair, it should be recognized that the risk of incarceration or of strangulation is greater with indirect than with direct hernia. Accordingly, the repair of a direct hernia may be more confidently deferred, or even declined, in the face of a significant medical illness. Nonoperative therapy should be discouraged; the wearing of a truss is potentially dangerous and does not guarantee that a hernia will remain reduced. Also, the pressure of the truss on the margin of a large defect eventually leads to atrophy of the fascial and aponeurotic (broad tendinous) layers, causing the hernia to enlarge. Subsequent repair is more difficult and therefore carries a greater risk of recurrence.

Elective herniorrhaphy prevents acute incarceration (and strangulation) and the need to perform an emergency operation. If the hernia is chronically incarcerated and there are no symptoms of strangulation (strangulation is primarily a risk in acutely incarcerated, small, indirect hernias), repair may be scheduled electively. If the hernia has incarcerated acutely, the patient must be hospitalized and attempts made to reduce the hernia before operation. A short period of bed rest, combined with an analgesic and an ice pack will often result in reduction of a hernia. Strangulated hernia is a true surgical emergency, because delay in treatment can lead to gangrene of the intestine or omentum. Suspected strangulated hernias require immediate operative intervention.

Bilateral hernias may be repaired at one operation or as staged procedures, depending on their size, the type of repair required, the age of the patient, and coexistent medical conditions. If the patient is elderly and the hernias are large and require complex repair, herniorrhaphies should be staged 4 to 6 weeks apart. Bilateral repairs of indirect inguinal hernias in children or young adults are routinely done at one operation.

Currently, most unilateral inguinal hernias are repaired through a 6- to 8-cm incision under local or regional anesthesia as an outpatient procedure. Many surgeons routinely use prosthetic mesh during the repair. The patient is rarely uncomfortable during the operation. Epidural, spinal, or general anesthesia is used for patients who cannot tolerate the procedure under local anesthesia, patients with large hernias requiring complex repair, and obese patients, in whom repair of the hernia under local anesthesia is technically difficult. Bilateral inguinal herniorrhaphy may also require epidural, spinal, or general anesthesia. Repair of hernias in children is usually done with the patient under general anesthesia.

Laparoscopic Herniorrhaphy

Laparoscopic (or minimally invasive) surgery has lost popularity in the treatment of groin hernias based on poor results in a large Veterans Administration multicenter trial (2). General anesthesia is required for laparoscopic repair, but is often not necessary with an open technique. A laparoscope and two or three instruments are introduced into the peritoneal cavity, usually through separate 0.5- to 1.0-cm incisions rather than one long incision. Under direct visualization, indirect hernia sacs can be dissected and even large defects can be repaired with the use of prosthetic mesh. The cost of laparoscopic repair at this time is significantly higher than that of open repair. Although laparoscopic repair is an accepted technique particularly for bilateral inguinal hernias, the predominant approach still remains the traditional open anterior repair.

Course and Recovery

No matter which anesthesia or technique is used, certain *complications of herniorrhaphy* are possible (in approximately 7% of patients): recurrence (the most common complication), urinary retention, wound infection, hydrocele formation, femoral or ilioinguinal neuralgia, scrotal hematoma, and, rarely, unilateral testicular atrophy. The primary caregiver and the surgeon should discuss these complications with the patient before the operation and provide assurance that, except for recurrence of hernia (and uncommonly testicular atrophy), they are usually transient problems.

When patients are discharged from the hospital, they are ambulatory but typically require narcotic analgesics for relief of pain. For the first week, the patient is advised to avoid lifting or straining and to use a stool softener and a mild laxative. The patient can return to light work (and light activity such as long walks) within another 2 weeks, but an occupation that requires heavy lifting or considerable exertion requires a total convalescence of 6 weeks.

Driving a car during the first 2 weeks should be discouraged, not because it is a form of strenuous activity, but because the patient, fearing pain or injury, may not step on the brake vigorously enough or soon enough in a crisis to avoid a collision. Sexual activity should be avoided for the first 3 weeks after surgery. Resumption of normal recreational and work activities requires common sense. Most patients are fully rehabilitated and working less than 1 month after herniorrhaphy. Because recurrence may be related to premature untoward exertion, patients must be cautioned to avoid strenuous activity for 6 weeks.

Approximately 1% to 7% of indirect and 4% to 10% of direct inguinal hernias recur. More than 50% of the recurrences occur within 5 years after the initial repair. The recurrence rate after repair of a recurrent hernia is even higher, ranging from 5% to 35%. Most surgeons use mesh in the repair of recurrent hernias.

Femoral Hernias

Epidemiology and Causes

A femoral hernia is a protrusion of omentum or bowel through the femoral canal (Fig. 97.1). It is much more common in women than in men, although the indirect inguinal hernia is still the most common hernia in women. The incidence increases with increasing age, presumably because of the degradation of collagen and attenuation of tissue that accompanies aging. It is likely, however, that a contributing cause of a femoral hernia is a congenitally large femoral ring. Preperitoneal fat, forced through the large ring, enlarges it further. Increased pressure produced by straining or pregnancy undoubtedly contributes to femoral herniation. Femoral hernias are bilateral in at least 15% of cases. The risk of incarceration, and particularly of strangulation, is especially high with this type of hernia.

History

The primary symptom of a femoral hernia is a bulge in the groin. A dull pain may be experienced, but less commonly than in patients with an inguinal hernia. Approximately 20% of femoral hernias incarcerate (twice the rate of indirect inguinal hernias). The symptoms of incarceration and strangulation are the same as in patients with inguinal hernias.

Physical Examination

A mass is often palpable, medial to the femoral vessels and inferior to the inguinal ligament. The mass is usually reducible, and occasionally it is tender. Despite careful examination, the hernia often is difficult to detect, especially in obese women, even if it is incarcerated or strangulated. Therefore, women with signs and symptoms of unexplained intestinal obstruction should be examined carefully for evidence of a strangulated femoral hernia.

Differential Diagnosis

A femoral hernia must be distinguished from an enlarged lymph node, a lipoma, a saphenous varix, and a direct inguinal hernia. The first three of these possibilities are not reducible. A *lymph node* or *lipoma* may not transmit an impulse to the examiner's finger when the patient coughs. A *saphenous varix* may simulate a hernia impulse, however, because increased venous pressure induced by the Valsalva maneuver is transmitted to the varix. A lymph node or lipoma is more movable than a hernia, and a varix can be collapsed by compression of the saphenous vein. The distinction between a femoral and other groin hernias sometimes can be made only at operation.

Management and Course

Femoral hernias should be repaired unless the patient is unable to tolerate an operation. The increased risk of incarceration and strangulation adds to the urgency of the recommendation. The operative and postoperative considerations for inguinal hernias (discussed earlier) apply to femoral hernias as well, except that, for technical reasons, a larger proportion of femoral hernias may have to be performed under spinal or general anesthesia, usually as outpatient procedures. Laparoscopy (see earlier discussion) can also be used in femoral hernia repair. Between 1% and 7% of femoral hernias recur and, as with inguinal hernias, 5% to 35% of repaired recurrent hernias also recur.

UMBILICAL HERNIAS

An umbilical hernia is a protrusion of omentum or bowel through the umbilical ring. These hernias are probably caused by congenital defects. Among adults, they appear most often in middle-age multiparous women, in patients with cirrhosis of the liver and ascites, and in frail elderly people. They are also common in infants. Most umbilical hernias are obvious as an enlargement of the umbilical ring with protrusion of intra-abdominal contents through it. However, a few patients complain only of vague intermittent pain and tenderness in the region of the umbilicus. On examination, a small defect is usually found that contains a small piece of omentum, preperitoneal fat, or a knuckle of bowel. If patients are placed in the supine position and then asked to raise their head and cough, the hernia can be palpated.

The most common complication of umbilical hernia is incarceration with or without strangulation. Incarceration is more common with umbilical hernias than with groin hernias. For that reason, unless the patient cannot tolerate an operation, all umbilical hernias in adults should be repaired. Morbidity and mortality from such an operation are much lower if it is performed electively rather than in response to acute incarceration or strangulation. The only exception to this recommendation is umbilical hernias in infants. These tend to close spontaneously as the child gets older, and repair should be deferred until school age.

The repair may be done under local anesthesia if the hernia is small; otherwise, general or spinal anesthesia is preferred. The use of mesh to reinforce the repair is being tried as a strategy to reduce recurrence rates. Laparoscopic repair is also an option, but it is not of proven benefit.

EPIGASTRIC HERNIAS

An epigastric hernia is a protrusion of fat or omentum through the linea alba between the umbilicus and the xiphoid cartilage. These hernias almost never contain a viscus. A congenital defect in the linea alba is probably the major disposing factor. Epigastric hernias most commonly appear between the ages of 20 and 50 years and are three times more common in men than in women. Most patients complain of a small, painless, subcutaneous mass, most often just to the left of the midline. Usually the hernia consists of preperitoneal fat or fat of the falciform ligament.

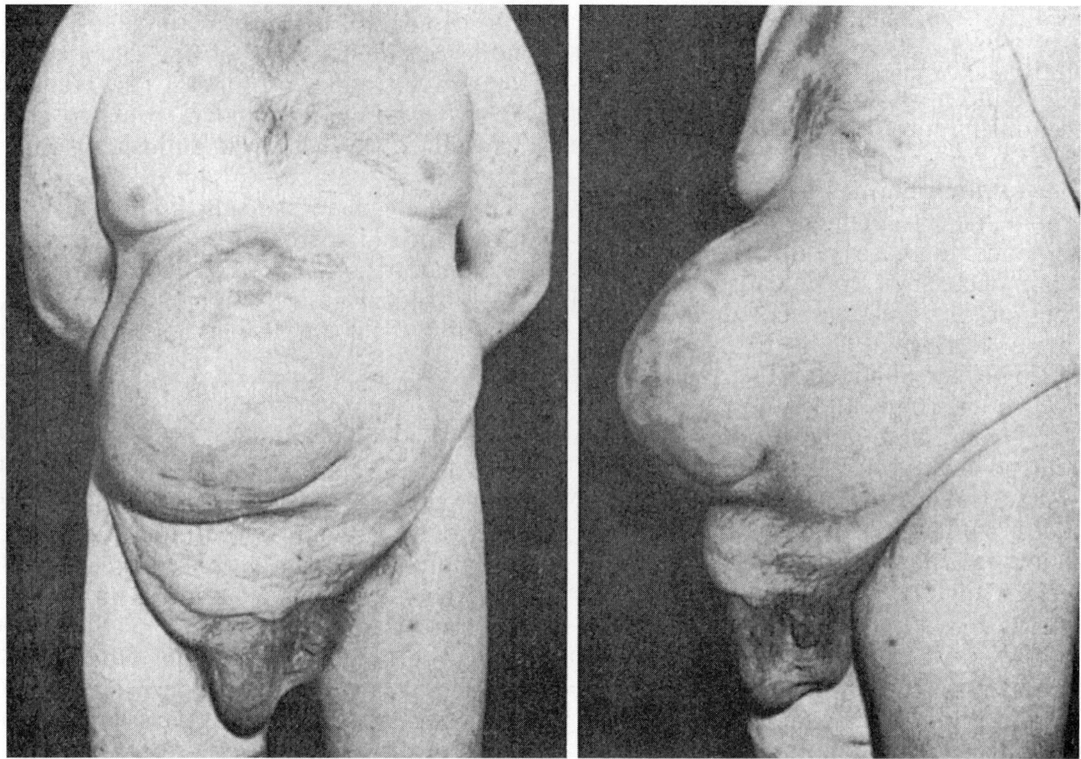

FIGURE 97.6. Large postoperative (ventral) hernia after cholecystectomy. (From Zimmerman LM, Anson BJ. Anatomy and surgery of hernia. 2nd ed. Baltimore: Williams & Wilkins, 1967:287.)

Larger defects also contain omentum. Complications are more common in patients with small hernias because these are more likely to incarcerate. When this happens, there is usually local pain and tenderness and, less often, deep epigastric pain, abdominal distention, and nausea and vomiting. All epigastric hernias should be repaired, usually as outpatient procedures. The recurrence rate after epigastric herniorrhaphy is approximately 10% and usually can be attributed to failure to appreciate multiple defects in the linea alba at the time of the initial operation.

INCISIONAL HERNIAS

An incisional hernia is the protrusion of omentum or bowel through a fascial defect at the site of a prior surgical incision. Unlike the other types of abdominal hernia, a congenital weakness of the abdominal wall does not contribute to the development of the hernia. Any abdominal incision may be the site of a hernia. The major risk factors leading to the development of an incisional hernia are wound infection and obesity. With the increasing use of chronic ambulatory peritoneal dialysis to treat patients in chronic renal failure (see Chapter 52), it has become apparent that incisional hernias (as well as inguinal hernias) are particularly common in this group of patients.

The hernia usually manifests as a bulge through the incision that may enlarge if neglected (Fig. 97.6) and may even lead to intestinal obstruction. It should be repaired electively once the diagnosis is made in order to avoid the development of a larger defect that will complicate repair and be more likely to recur. If possible, an obese patient should lose weight before the operation (see Chapter 83). Laparoscopic repair for these hernias is used in some centers but it is not of proven benefit. The long term recurrence rates are unknown. Prosthetic mesh is commonly employed to repair incisional hernias. In using mesh, effort is taken to avoid exposure of the viscera to coarse textured mesh, which may lead to bowel obstruction or fistula. Instead, the surgeon interposes peritoneum or biodegradable mesh between permanent mesh and underlying viscera. Repaired incisional hernias have a much higher recurrence rate than do other kinds of abdominal hernias. Many patients with incisional hernia have significant comorbidity from underlying medical conditions, which must be taken into account when considering surgery.

For repair of recurrent hernias, advanced techniques include component separation to transfer muscle and fascia to close large defects, and allogeneic keratinocyte grafts (Apligraf) from unrelated donors that may resist infection better than traditional mesh materials (Marlex or Gore-Tex).

DIASTASIS RECTI

Diastasis recti refers to wide separation of the rectus abdominus muscles in the midline, with attenuation of the linea alba. It is not a true hernia. Patients may present with an asymptomatic midline linear bulge that protrudes when the patient strains and is more predominant in the epigastrium. This is usually mistaken for a hernia and can be quite large. On examination, however, there is no scar indicating a prior incision, and there is no palpable fascial defect. Surgical correction of diastasis recti is not required, because this condition is rarely symptomatic and carries no risk of visceral incarceration because the fascia remains intact. Patients who are concerned about the appearance of the abdominal wall can be counseled or referred for cosmetic surgery.

SPECIFIC REFERENCES

1. Rutkow IM, Robbins AW. Demographic, classificatory, and socioeconomic aspects of hernia repair in the United States. Surg Clin North Am 1993;73:413.
2. Neumayer L, Giobbie-Hurder A, Jonasson O, et al. Open mesh versus laparoscopic mesh repair of inguinal hernia. N Engl J Med 2004;350:1819.

For annotated **General References** *and resources related to this chapter, visit www.hopkinsbayview.org/PAMreferences.*

Chapter 98

Benign Conditions of the Anus and Rectum*

John W. Harmon and Christopher L. Wolfgang

*In previous editions, Mark D. Duncan, MD, and Jeffrey S. Bender, MD, contributed to this chapter.

Anorectal disorders are often encountered in an ambulatory practice. The four most common—pruritus ani, anal fissure, hemorrhoids, and perirectal abscess/fistula—are discussed in some detail in this chapter. Also included, because of their importance to the primary care provider, are less common disorders such as proctalgia fugax and rectal prolapse. The final section addresses sexually transmitted and other infectious diseases of the anus and rectum. Chapter 102 and Section 17 discuss cutaneous disorders that involve the perianal area and perineum. Chapters 35 and 45 discuss other conditions that may affect the rectum.

PRURITUS ANI

Pruritus ani, a distressing perianal itch, is more common in men than in women. It varies in intensity but usually is greatest at night. The itching often abates spontaneously, only to recur after variable asymptomatic periods.

Pruritus ani is a symptom, not a disease. Although 50% to 75% of the time the cause is unknown, the symptom may be a manifestation of a myriad of anorectal disorders (Table 98.1). Of these, anal neoplasia is the most serious cause that must be ruled out, especially in older adults. The itching is most often associated with macerated skin,

TABLE 98.1 Causes of Pruritis Ani

Diet
Milk
Caffeine
Chocolate
Tomatoes
Spices
Drugs
Oral antibiotics (e.g., tetracycline)
Colchicine
Laxatives
Dermatologic disorders
Psoriasis
Atopic dermatitis
Contact dermatitis
Lichen planus
Diarrhea
Fissures
Fistulas
Infections and Infestations
Fungi and yeast (especially in diabetic patients) (see Chapter 79)
Erythrasma
Scabies (see Chapter 117)
Pinworm (*Enterobius vermicularis*) infestation, more common in children
Vaginal infections (see Chapter 102)
Viral (condylomata, venereal warts, herpes simplex)
Obesity and excessive sweating
Poor anal hygiene
Rectal prolapse
Prolapsed hemorrhoids
Neoplasia

often complicated by excoriation and secondary infection. These changes may be caused by fecal contamination or excessive cleansing efforts, exacerbated by scratching.

Diagnosis

When a patient complains of perianal itching, several specific historical points should be obtained and several observations should be made to aid in establishing a diagnosis.

History

Dietary history should include information on intake of milk, caffeine (coffee, tea, colas), chocolate, tomatoes, and spices; excessive consumption of any of these can lead to pruritus ani. Medications that cause gastrointestinal (GI) irritation (e.g., laxatives, colchicine) and certain antibiotics (especially tetracycline) can also cause perianal itching, as can chronic diarrhea from any cause. Any history of tissue protrusion or incontinence should be noted. Lastly, personal stress is a major contributing factor, and a careful personal history should be elicited.

Physical Examination

The patient's skin should be examined for signs of a dermatologic problem, such as psoriasis or contact or atopic dermatitis, or a fungal infection (Table 98.1).

With the patient in the lateral decubitus or knee-chest position and the buttocks separated, the perianal area is inspected. During the inspection, the patient should be asked to strain or bear down. This maneuver may demonstrate prolapse or incontinence.

If skin lesions are identified, appropriate evaluation (e.g., a potassium hydroxide preparation) to establish a diagnosis (e.g., *Tinea, Candida*) should be done to initiate definitive therapy (see Chapter 117). In children up to age 14 years, and in adults who live in households with infected children, the evaluation should include several cellophane tape preparations in an attempt to demonstrate the ova of pinworms (see later discussion).

Digital rectal examination should always be performed using a well-lubricated, gloved finger. At initiation of the examination, the patient should be asked to bear down, which minimizes discomfort. Excessive pain localized to a specific area should alert the practitioner to the possible presence of an anal fissure (discussed later). All structures within reach of the finger should be assessed (anus, sphincter, distal rectum, prostate gland, and cervix).

Anoscopy

After rectal examination an anoscopy should be performed. No enema or laxative is required. A well-lubricated anoscope should be inserted gently. The addition of a local anesthetic ointment does little if anything to decrease any discomfort. After removal of the obturator, the rectum should be inspected under adequate light. Visualization of the more distal anal structures is possible only through the side aspect of the instrument as it is slowly withdrawn.

Cellophane Tape Examination for Pinworms

Cellophane tape examination is easily accomplished by the patient at home or by the practitioner in the office. Swabs are commercially available (Pinworm Diagnostic Tapes, Parke-Davis), but they are also easily made by folding clear cellophane tape, sticky side out, over a tongue blade. At night pinworms migrate from the anal canal to the perianal area, where they deposit eggs. Therefore the swab should be obtained on arising, before a bowel movement and before the perianal area is cleansed. The swab is pressed on the anal verge and then afterward the tape is mounted onto a glass microscopic slide. A specimen obtained in this way keeps for several days. The slides should

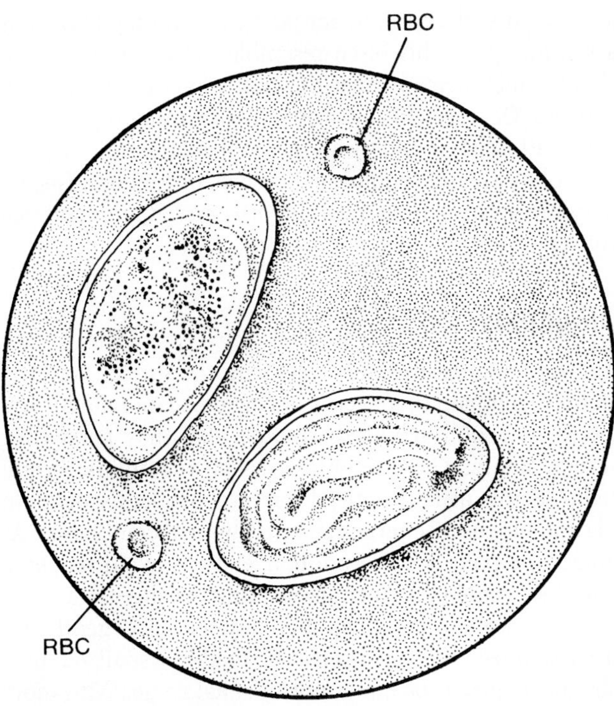

FIGURE 98.1. Appearance of the eggs of shape *Enterobius vermicularis* (pinworm). The egg is approximately 20 to 50 mm and typically has one flattened side.

be examined under the low-power (10×) objective of the microscope, searching for the typical ova of pinworm (Fig. 98.1).

Treatment

Most patients with pruritus ani can be diagnosed and treated adequately by the general practitioner. Even if the evaluation is inconclusive except for the identification of excoriation, symptoms can be controlled by simple measures.

Counseling about the factors responsible for pruritus ani should ensure a clear understanding of the potential roles of stress, lifestyle, and diet.

Dietary change should eliminate potentially causative foods and beverages. It may take 2 weeks for the symptom to resolve after diet modification. It will then recur within 48 hours after resumption of the offending food.

Warm sitz baths for 15 to 20 minutes provide excellent temporary relief (e.g., at bedtime). If possible, these should be used several times daily at the outset of symptoms.

Anal cleanliness and dryness are mandatory and must be gentle. Once or twice daily, and after each bowel movement, the perineal area should be cleansed with a plain mild soap such as Ivory and then rinsed with cotton swabs moistened with warm water. Glycerin–witch hazel wipes (Tucks) or diaper wipes may be used unless they cause irritation or burning. After cleansing, the area should be thoroughly dried by blotting, not rubbing, with soft, white, nonperfumed toilet paper (colored or perfumed tissues, which are potentially allergenic or irritating, should be avoided). A handheld blow dryer is a useful alternative.

The perianal area must be kept dry at all times. This is best accomplished by the application of cornstarch powder or plain talc (Johnson's Baby Powder). A thick layer of zinc oxide or A and D Ointment may be substituted but must be thoroughly and gently removed at the time of each cleaning.

Diarrhea or constipation should be controlled (see Chapters 45 and 46). Bulk laxatives such as psyllium preparations (e.g., Metamucil) and stool softeners such as docusate (e.g., Colace) are preferred. They are not irritating, and they tend to absorb mucus, a possible irritant to the sensitive perianal tissue.

The patient should wear cotton underwear to provide better ventilation and should avoid polyester clothing. Prolonged sitting, especially on synthetic materials (e.g., vinyl seats), which prevent proper ventilation, should be avoided. In general, the use of all other creams, ointments, and medications should be discontinued.

For the occasional patient with symptoms severe enough to cause insomnia, an antihistamine with antipruritic and sedative effects such as diphenhydramine (Benadryl), taken before bedtime, may be helpful. On rare occasions it may be necessary to use minimal amounts of 0.5% or 1.0% hydrocortisone cream to control nocturnal itching. This should be viewed as a temporary measure, and the prolonged use of any topical steroid should be avoided.

A patient with idiopathic pruritus ani that is not responsive to these therapies may be referred to a dermatologist or a gastroenterologist. Further evaluation, especially in the older age group, should include the rectum and colon.

Enterobius vermicularis (Pinworm)

If *E. vermicularis* is identified, all members of the household should be evaluated with the cellophane tape test. The ova are easily disseminated and survive in the environment for up to 3 weeks.

The preferred drugs to eradicate this infestation are mebendazole (Vermox) given as a single dose of 100 mg or albendazole (Albenza) given as a single dose of 400 mg in adults. These drugs should not be used in infants or pregnant women. An alternative is pyrantel pamoate (available over-the-counter in an oral suspension as Pamix, Pin-X, or Reese's Pinworm Medicine), which is also given as a single dose. All of these treatments should be repeated 2 weeks following the initial dose. They are generally well tolerated but can cause mild GI distress. Pyrantel pamoate has been associated with transitory elevation of liver enzymes, and its use should be avoided in patients with known liver disease.

These agents approach 100% effectiveness in killing the worms, and symptoms usually subside within 48 hours. The patient is no longer infective once the deposited eggs are removed from the perianal area and clothing by cleaning. Clothing and bed linens should be laundered with detergent and hot water on the same day that oral treatment is given. It is important that all infected members of the household be treated simultaneously. Reinfestation is common and retreatment may be necessary.

ANAL FISSURE

An anal fissure is an acutely painful, elliptical, mucosal tear, often extending from the anal verge to the pectinate line (Fig. 98.2). It is most often located in the posterior midline of the anal canal, less commonly anteriorly. The inciting factor is usually trauma secondary to the passage of a large, hard stool or anal intercourse. The underlying pathophysiology is thought to be diminished anodermal blood supply abetted by increased anal sphincter tone (1). This leads to an unremitting cycle of pain, reluctance to have a bowel movement, and then further tearing once the bowel movement occurs. The problem is a common one, occurring with equal frequency in men and women (it is uncommon in children). Most patients, and many clinicians, attribute the pain to hemorrhoids, especially when streaking of the stool with blood occurs. It is important to remember that hemorrhoids, unless acutely thrombosed, are not a cause of anal pain.

As an anal fissure becomes chronic it looks more like an ulcer crater, with raised edges, scarring, and the exposed external sphincter at the base. These changes are usually associated with a prominent posterior skin tag known as a sentinel pile. This often resembles an external hemorrhoid, which helps further the confusion of these two diagnoses. Occasionally a chronic fissure, often in an atypical location, is caused by an inflammatory condition such as Crohn disease, syphilis, gonorrhea, or tuberculosis; iatrogenic scarring from local surgery or irradiation; or anal cancer.

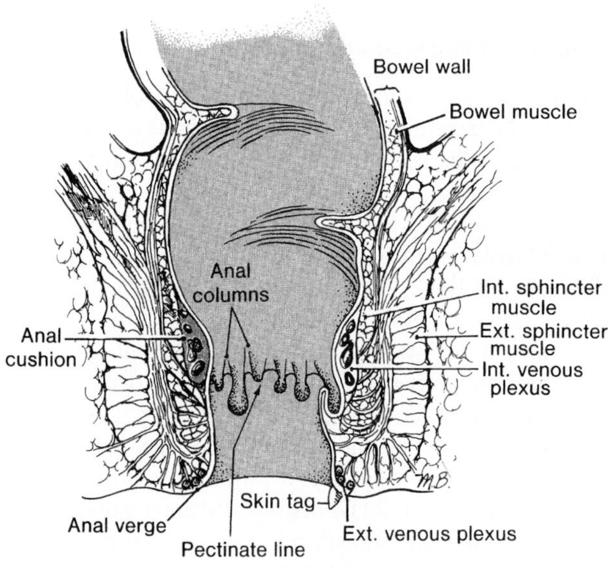

FIGURE 98.2. Important structures of the anal area.

Diagnosis

An acute anal fissure manifests with the sudden onset of sharp rectal pain that occurs during defecation and is followed by a dull aching discomfort that may persist for several hours. There may be associated minimal bright red bleeding, usually noticed just on the toilet tissue. Itching and mucus discharge can be additional complaints. As noted, the pain is so severe that patients avoid having a bowel movement, further aggravating the situation.

On examination, when the buttocks are gently retracted, most anal fissures can be readily visualized, usually at the posterior margin of the anal verge. With more chronic fissures, a posterior sentinel pile may be appreciated. Once an anal fissure has been identified by inspection, usually no attempt should be made to perform a digital examination or anoscopy until treatment has alleviated the symptoms.

Treatment

Many patients with acute anal fissure can be made comfortable within a day or two, and cured within 3 weeks, by the use of conservative therapy. Stool softeners such as docusate or bulk laxatives such as psyllium preparations should be taken, and cathartics should be avoided. A high-fiber diet is recommended, along with the consumption of eight glasses of water daily.

Anal discomfort is relieved by the use of warm baths for 15 to 20 minutes two to three times per day and after each bowel movement (2). Local anesthetic creams (e.g., Nupercainal Cream, Anusol) or suppositories are also useful in providing temporary relief of symptoms.

Nitric oxide (NO) mediates relaxation of the internal anal sphincter. Therapeutic NO donors, such as nitroglycerin (glyceryl trinitrate), may be effective in the treatment of anal fissures. Most (3–5) but not all (6) studies have shown that the topical application of nitrates to the distal anal canal results in early symptomatic relief and in cure of up to 80% of both acute and chronic anal fissures after 6 weeks of treatment. Recurrence rates are unknown. The major side effect has been headache. The topical nitroglycerin preparations used in the reported studies (0.2%, twice daily) were much less concentrated than commercially available preparations (nitroglycerin ointment 2%, e.g., Nitro-Bid or Nitrol); a trial of this approach will require compounding by a pharmacist. Topical calcium channel blocker drugs have been reported to provide similar results, but are not available presently. Healing of anal fissures has been achieved also by the local injection of botulin toxin (7), which should be done only by a surgeon or a gastroenterologist. These approaches obviate operation for at least some chronic fissures (8).

Once a fissure becomes chronic or if 6 weeks of conservative therapy has failed, the next step is surgical referral for a lateral anal sphincterotomy. This procedure is usually done on an ambulatory basis, often under local anesthesia. Postoperative complications (e.g., bleeding, abscess formation) occur in fewer than 5% of cases. There may be early problems with some degree of anal incontinence in up to 8% of cases, but this is a long-term problem in fewer than 1% of patients and is usually confined to difficulty controlling flatus or liquid.

Pain relief is noted within 48 hours, and the fissure is usually healed in 2 to 3 weeks. The recurrence rate is 1% to 8%, and 96% of patients have a lasting excellent or satisfactory result. Transient postoperative incontinence is common.

HEMORRHOIDS

A precise characterization of hemorrhoidal disease is impossible because, despite centuries of medical speculation, neither the pathogenesis nor the cause has ever been elucidated. Hemorrhoids are not varicosities of the rectal venous plexus. There are no certain data to prove any of the popular theories of causation, such as a low-fiber diet, constipation, straining at stool, venous hypertension, obesity, certain occupations, genetic predisposition, and many others.

The currently popular theory associates hemorrhoids with distal displacement of the anal cushions. Anal cushions are part of the normal anatomy of the anal canal (Fig. 98.2). These cushions, which consist of hemorrhoidal venous and arterial plexuses, smooth muscle, and connective tissue, lie under the mucosa. The cushions apparently permit the passage of variable-sized stools without disruption of the rectal mucosa. Three cushions are usually found, in the right anterolateral, right posterolateral, and left lateral portions of the anal canal (Fig. 98.3), the common locations of internal hemorrhoids. This theory is consistent with an observed increase in hemorrhoidal disease in association with aging, groin hernias, and urogenital prolapse, all potentially caused by connective tissue degeneration.

Asymptomatic hemorrhoids are said to be present in half of the population older than 50 years of age, but this figure is suspect because the definition of the diagnosis is uncertain. The prevalence of self-reported hemorrhoidal complaints was 4.4% (equivalent to about 10 million people) in a national health survey, but patients tend to attribute all anorectal symptoms to hemorrhoids (9). The prevalence is the same in both sexes, but women develop hemorrhoids earlier, often in association with pregnancy, and men more commonly seek treatment (9).

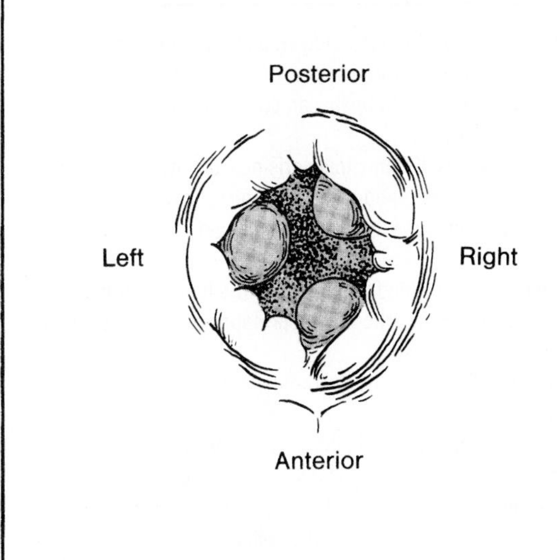

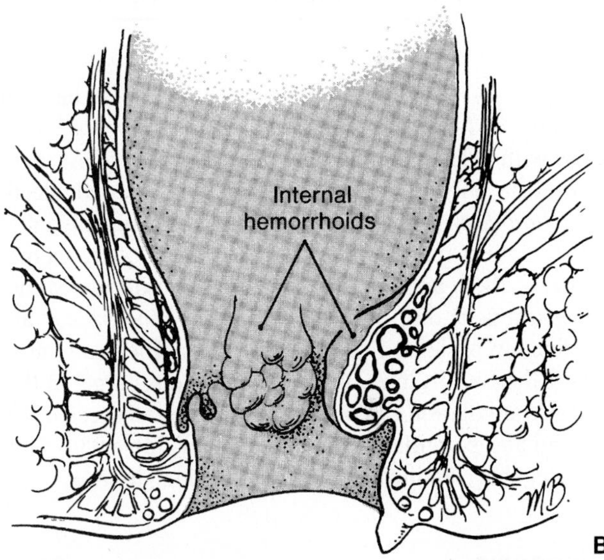

FIGURE 98.3. **A:** Common sites of hemorrhoids. **B:** Protrusion of anal cushions.

Classification

Hemorrhoids are described as internal or external depending on whether they originate above or below the pectinate (dentate) line. External skin tags are commonly, and erroneously, referred to as hemorrhoids as well (Fig 98.2). Internal hemorrhoids are graded based on the degree of

TABLE 98.2 Classification of Hemorrhoids

External hemorrhoids: Hemorrhoids arising from the inferior hemorrhoidal plexus exterior to the anal verge, covered by pain-sensitive skin. Thrombosis can cause acute and sometimes severe discomfort.

Internal hemorrhoids: Hemorrhoids arising from the anal cushions, normal structures lying above the anal verge, covered by pain-insensitive mucosa. Internal hemorrhoids may be classified further.

- *First-degree:* Hemorrhoids bulging into the lumen of the anal canal
- *Second-degree:* Hemorrhoids that prolapse during defecation but reduce spontaneously
- *Third-degree:* Prolapsed hemorrhoids that require manual reduction
- *Fourth-degree:* Hemorrhoids that are irreducibly prolapsed

Thrombosed internal hemorrhoids: An internal hemorrhoid may prolapse and strangulate, which leads to thrombosis, an excruciatingly painful condition. If swelling progresses, gangrene of the hemorrhoids with ulceration, local infection, or pylephlebitis (septic phlebitis of the portal venous system) may result.

prolapse. *First-degree hemorrhoids* project into the anal canal but do not prolapse. *Second-degree hemorrhoids* prolapse with defecation and spontaneously reduce. At these stages the only symptom is painless, bright red bleeding. *Third-degree hemorrhoids* protrude with straining and often require manual reduction. In addition to hematochezia, these are associated with discomfort and sometimes a mucus discharge. *Fourth-degree hemorrhoids* are irreducibly prolapsed through the anus. They can cause severe discomfort, bleeding, and mucus discharge. At this stage strangulation can occur, constituting an exceedingly painful and potentially lethal emergency. Table 98.2 summarizes this classification of hemorrhoidal disease.

Diagnosis

Symptoms

External hemorrhoids manifest with pain, often exquisite, as a result of thrombosis in the external venous plexus. There is a tender lump, and the pain is exacerbated by defecation.

Asymptomatic hemorrhoids noticed incidentally during an examination should not be considered a problem and should not be treated. The symptoms associated with internal hemorrhoids include.

Bleeding

Characteristically, the bleeding from hemorrhoids is mild, intermittent, and bright red. Occasionally it may drip into the commode or be sustained. Massive hemorrhage is rare. Rectal bleeding should never be attributed to hemorrhoids unless all other causes can be ruled out.

Prolapse

Prolapse of internal hemorrhoids produces the sensation of fullness in the anal canal, especially after defecation. This discomfort affects 80% of patients with symptomatic hemorrhoids, but it is not true pain.

Pain

The acute pain attributed to internal hemorrhoids usually is caused by a fissure (see earlier discussion). Pain caused by internal hemorrhoids indicates thrombosis or strangulation and if unresponsive to conservative management (see below), mandates referral to a surgeon. Thrombosis and strangulation occur when fourth-degree hemorrhoids are trapped by congestion and spasm of the anal canal. If ulceration ensues, localized infection may result, which rarely may spread to the portal venous plexus, leading to potentially lethal pylephlebitis.

Physical Examination

The patient is placed in the lateral decubitus or knee-chest position and the buttocks are gently separated. Skin tags are seen as soft, painless excrescences just beyond the anal verge. A thrombosed external hemorrhoid manifests in the anal canal as a firm, tender mass with a bluish discoloration. Internal hemorrhoids can sometimes be visualized as well, especially if the patient strains.

Digital rectal examination is performed principally to rule out other anal and distal rectal disease. Nonvisible internal hemorrhoids are rarely palpable.

Anoscopy is the definitive diagnostic procedure for internal hemorrhoids. It should be performed thoroughly and carefully, as described previously for the diagnosis of pruritus ani, with the use of a good side-viewing anoscope.

Endoscopy, using the flexible fiberoptic sigmoidoscope or colonoscope, should be performed for any patient older than 40 years of age with the recent onset of bleeding thought to be from internal hemorrhoids. This is a part of the assessment of GI bleeding, as discussed more fully in Chapter 45.

Differential Diagnosis

Several other problems may be confused with hemorrhoidal disease. *Hypertrophied anal papillae* occur along the pectinate (dentate) line (Fig. 98.2) in association with an anal fissure (see earlier discussion), with Crohn disease, or without obvious cause. These papillae usually are asymptomatic and require no therapy unless they have become particularly large, eroded, or infected or unless they bleed. Hypertrophied anal papillae often have the appearance of a fibrous polyp and are easily differentiated from hemorrhoids by their location and consistency.

Rectal prolapse is identified by the circumferential abnormal downward displacement, or herniation, of rectal mucosa or of the full thickness of the rectal wall. When mild, it is commonly mistaken for hemorrhoidal disease and may respond to similar methods of treatment (see later discussion in this chapter on its specific diagnosis and treatment).

Protruding tumors such as rectal polyps, anal carcinoma, and even low-lying rectal carcinoma can be confused with hemorrhoids. If there is suspicion about the diagnosis, referral to a surgeon or gastroenterologist for evaluation and biopsy is appropriate.

Treatment

Without treatment, symptoms of hemorrhoids usually resolve spontaneously or in response to self-treatment within several days to several weeks, even when thrombosis is present. However, most patients develop recurrent symptoms, although the asymptomatic intervals may be long.

The aim of treatment (10) is to relieve symptoms, and only symptomatic hemorrhoids need treatment. Therapy does not necessarily reduce venous bulges, although often they do regress, most patients respond to conservative therapy.

Skin tags rarely need treatment. If they are sufficiently prominent to cause true discomfort, the patient can be referred for surgical excision.

Thrombosed external hemorrhoids are often acutely and severely painful and may require surgical referral for management. If the patient presents more than 72 hours after the onset of pain and as the acute symptom is subsiding, conservative measures usually resolve the problem. These consist of the approach used for conservative treatment of symptomatic internal hemorrhoids. In addition, topical analgesics such as Nupercainal or 5% lidocaine ointment should be applied. If prolonged sitting is necessary, an inflatable ring is helpful.

Symptomatic internal hemorrhoids, even fourth-degree ones, in the absence of severe symptoms, deserve a trial of conservative management. The first step is to avoid constipation and straining by giving of a bulk laxative and stool softeners. The patient should eat a high-fiber diet and drink at least eight glasses of water daily. Swelling and prolapse often respond to warm sitz baths taken twice daily and after each bowel movement.

Topical preparations may relieve discomfort, and putatively reduce swelling as well. Corticosteroid-containing preparations such as Anusol-HC and ProctoFoam-HC may be used initially, but their use should be discontinued after 2 to 3 weeks and the non–steroid-containing versions substituted. These preparations come as creams, foams, and suppositories. All three forms are beneficial, and their use depends on patient and clinician preference.

Surgical Management

Patients should be referred to a surgeon for evaluation whenever there is doubt about the diagnosis, if there is no response within 3 or 4 weeks to conservative therapy, if pain is severe (as may occur with thrombosis); or if there is evidence of strangulation, ulceration, perianal infection, or neoplasm. When uncomplicated hemorrhoids are recurrently symptomatic, the patient should be referred to a surgeon for definitive treatment.

The surgeon evaluates the patient, confirms the diagnosis, and then considers several therapeutic options that are not normally provided by general practitioners.

External Hemorrhoids

The usual indication for the surgical treatment of external hemorrhoids is painful acute thrombosis, especially within 48 to 72 hours after onset. The procedure is surgical excision under local anesthesia on an ambulatory basis. Incision and evacuation of the thrombus is a satisfactory maneuver for pain relief in the early stages of thrombosis. A definitive hemorrhoidectomy may be required later. Sometimes external skin tags are sufficiently troublesome to warrant excision. This can be done as an office procedure under local anesthesia.

Internal Hemorrhoids

Injection of Sclerosing Agents

Submucosal injection of a symptomatic hemorrhoid with several milliliters of a sclerosing solution causes fibrosis and retraction of the hemorrhoid. This procedure is excellent therapy for small bleeding internal hemorrhoids (first-or second-degree; Table 98.2); it is simple, requires no anesthesia, and can easily be performed in the office in a few minutes. After this procedure the patient usually requires no recovery period and can return to work immediately. There may be a period of several days when the patient experiences a sensation of anal fullness. This symptom is usually well tolerated or is easily controlled by the use of sitz baths three to four times a day and by mild analgesics such as acetaminophen.

The clinician performing this procedure must be experienced with its use. With the proper technique there are essentially no complications. If the solution is improperly injected, severe pain, necrosis, and rectal stenosis can occur. Injection of sclerosing agents usually provides temporary relief, but recurrence is common. The procedure may be repeated several times, but persistent recurrence should lead to the consideration of another mode of therapy. This approach is most useful for symptomatic first-degree hemorrhoids that are so small that there is insufficient tissue for rubber band ligation.

Rubber Band Ligation

Rubber band ligation of hemorrhoids is a simple office procedure that can be utilized for internal hemorrhoids of all degrees except the fourth (Table 98.2) (11,12). The patient requires no special preparation, and no anesthesia is necessary. Using an anoscope and a special instrument, one or two rubber bands are applied near the base of the hemorrhoid and at least 0.5 cm above the pectinate line. No more than two hemorrhoids should be treated at a single session, but all of the hemorrhoids should be banded ultimately. Constriction by the rubber band results in ischemic necrosis of the hemorrhoid, which sloughs and is passed in the stool 5 to 10 days later, usually along with a small amount of blood. Complications are rare, but delayed massive bleeding and pelvic sepsis have occurred.

Usually, after rubber band ligation of hemorrhoids, the patient is not disabled and has only minimal discomfort characterized by a sensation of rectal fullness, a symptom that is usually well controlled by the use of sitz baths and a mild oral analgesic such as acetaminophen. Aspirin and nonsteroidal anti-inflammatory analgesics should not be used because of the risk of prolonged bleeding. If the discomfort is more severe, a mild relaxant such as diazepam (Valium) is helpful to relieve anal sphincter spasm. If the rubber band is improperly placed below the pectinate line, the patient will experience severe pain and the rubber band must be removed.

After rubber band ligation, the usual conservative measures for internal hemorrhoids should be practiced for 2 to 3 weeks until healing is complete. Further ligation is then performed if necessary. Banding provides good relief of hemorrhoidal disease approximately 70% to 90% of the time. Symptoms recur in 15% to 45% of patients after 18 months to 5 years.

Laser Therapy and Infrared Photocoagulation

Laser therapy and infrared photocoagulation are available as treatment modalities for first-, second-, and third-degree hemorrhoids (Table 98.2). Both require expensive equipment, and the carbon dioxide laser demands special expertise. Therefore neither modality is widely available.

Hemorrhoidectomy

Hemorrhoidectomy is indicated for large internal hemorrhoids after other forms of therapy have failed; for strangulated, ulcerated, or gangrenous third- or fourth-degree hemorrhoids; and when symptomatic hemorrhoids are present in conjunction with other benign anorectal conditions (e.g., fistulas, fissures) that require surgery (1). The procedure is usually done under general or regional anesthesia, although local anesthesia is possible. Patient preparation consists of a Fleet enema the morning prior to surgery. The purpose of the operation is to remove hemorrhoidal tissue and to appose the skin and mucous membrane. The operation has a deserved reputation for severe postoperative pain. Despite newer techniques and the most careful surgical approach the likelihood of postoperative discomfort remains. Postoperative discomfort is best controlled by sitz baths, stool softeners, oral analgesics, and a muscle relaxant such as diazepam (Valium). Topical nitroglycerin may also be beneficial. Postoperative complications are urinary retention and bleeding. The former can be averted by adequate control of pain and muscle spasm. The incidence of significant bleeding is 1% to 2%, and infection is rare. Late complications of incontinence or anal stenosis should occur in fewer than 1% of patients. The late recurrence rate is less than 5%.

Special Considerations

Because of an increased risk of complications associated with operative procedures in patients with severe congestive heart failure (CHF) or debilitating disease, the treatment of hemorrhoids in these patients should be as conservative as possible. Patients who have cirrhosis present a special risk because of the frequent association of hemostatic dysfunction. Hemorrhoidectomy should not be done in patients with Crohn disease and should be done in patients with ulcerative colitis only when they are in remission. Immunocompromised patients should not undergo anorectal surgery.

Hemorrhoids are common in pregnancy and are best managed conservatively. They often resolve spontaneously after delivery. Occasionally, development of strangulated hemorrhoids requires surgical intervention during the pregnancy.

ANORECTAL ABSCESSES AND ANORECTAL FISTULAS

Definition

An *anorectal abscess* is an abscess involving the perineum and perianal structures. Abscesses are classified by their anatomic location (Fig. 98.4). Low intramuscular or perianal abscesses are located in the subcutaneous tissue immediately surrounding the anus, which is the site of 40% to 50% of all anorectal abscesses. *Ischiorectal abscesses* are located in the ischiorectal fossa, a fat-filled space between the distal levator ani (external anal sphincter) and the ischial tuberosity, and account for 20% to 40% of anorectal abscesses. *Intersphincteric, high intermuscular (postanal), and pelvirectal (supralevator) abscesses* are far less common and account for approximately 10% of all abscesses. Anorectal abscesses are common, and the general physician should be familiar with their presentation, so if this problem is suspected, the patient can be promptly referred to a surgeon.

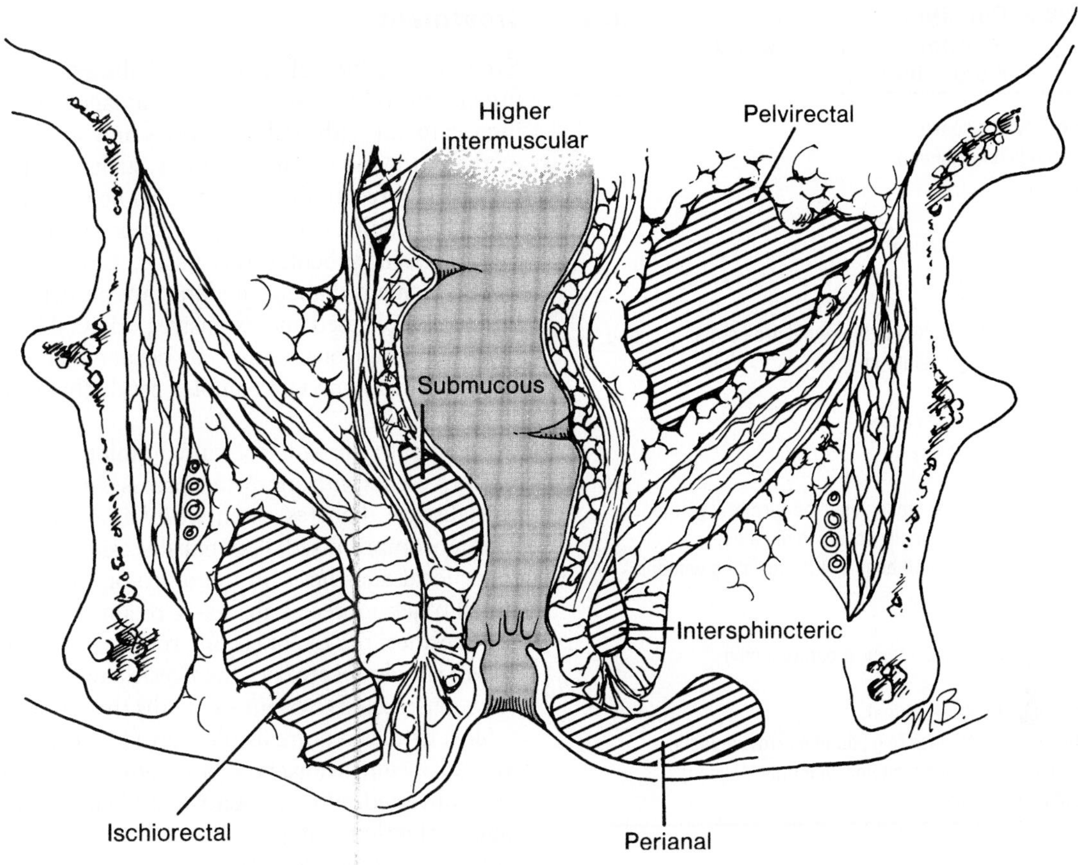

FIGURE 98.4. Anatomic classification of common anorectal abscesses.

An *anorectal fistula (fistula-in-ano)* is a tract lined by granulation tissue that has an internal opening in the anal canal and an external opening in the perianal skin. The internal opening is usually located in one of the anal crypts at the upper end of the anal canal just above the pectinate line (Fig. 98.2).

Anorectal abscesses are more common in men. Most are associated with cryptoglandular infection. Occasionally, anorectal abscesses occur in association with other anal and perianal disorders (Table 98.3). Anal glands, thought to be diverticula of the anal canal mucosa, are located circumferentially around the anus at the level of the pectinate line. Many of these glands pass through the internal sphincter into the intersphincteric space. They normally drain into the anal crypts. Infection and abscess formation result when drainage of these glands is blocked. Bacterial cultures from the abscesses usually grow a mixed flora.

Most anorectal fistulas result from abscess formation in the anal glands and drainage through the perianal skin. Unless this is recognized and treated at the same time, the incidence of fistula formation after drainage of anorectal abscesses is about 50%. Some fistulas are not pyogenic in origin and are associated with inflammatory bowel disease or tuberculosis. Fistulas that do not originate in anal glands may result from diverticular disease, neoplastic disease, or trauma.

Diagnosis

History

Most commonly, a patient with an anorectal abscess describes throbbing perianal pain intensified by sitting, walking, coughing, or defecating (13). Systemic symptoms may be present and include malaise, chills, and fever. These symptoms are more common with ischiorectal than with perianal abscesses. If the abscess has spontaneously drained, the patient may complain of a mucopurulent or bloody discharge.

An uncomplicated anal fistula may create only minor complaints. The most common complaint is painful perianal swelling, but the most common symptom is discharge and soiling. The swelling is often intermittent, and the intensity of the discomfort is variable. Often the patient complains of a purulent anal discharge that, when it ceases, leads to recurrent painful swelling relieved by resumption of the discharge.

TABLE 98.3 Conditions That May Be Complicated by Anorectal Abscess and Fistula-in-Ano

Inflammatory bowel disease
Chronic infections (uncommon)
Actinomycosis
Tuberculosis
Lymphogranuloma venereum
Schistosomiasis (rare)
Amebiasis (rare)
Infection anatomically adjacent to the rectal area and presenting as anorectal abscess or fistula-in-ano
In women
Pelvic inflammatory disease
Bartholin gland abscess
In men
Infections of a Cowper gland (small periurethral glands)
Pilonidal sinus (occasionally occurs in females)
Foreign body (e.g., an ingested bone or a penetrating wooden splinter)
Trauma
Surgery (e.g., hemorrhoidectomy, prostatectomy)
Radiation
Laceration (e.g., from an enema)
Abnormalities of host defense (e.g., bone marrow aplasia, neutropenia, leukemia or lymphoma, diabetes mellitus)
Carcinoma of anus or rectum

Physical Examination

A perianal abscess is easily recognized as a warm, tender, subcutaneous swelling located adjacent to the anus. With an ischiorectal abscess there is often only tenderness and induration detected by pressure on the skin overlying the ischiorectal fossa or the lateral wall of the anal canal during rectal examination. The high anorectal abscesses may present few or no findings on perianal inspection or even on rectal examination. However, these patients complain of severe rectal pain and pyrexia and exhibit a marked leukocytosis.

The diagnosis of an anorectal fistula is established by inspection and palpation of the perianal area and performance of a digital rectal examination. Often the external opening of the fistula in the perianal area can be seen. Digital examination of the rectum may enable identification of the indurated tract of the fistula as it passes to its internal opening at the pectinate line. Often the location of the internal opening is facilitated by anoscopy. Gentle passage of a probe may be attempted, but care must be taken not to create a false passage. Occasionally, accurate localization must await surgical exploration. When complex perineal infection is present, especially if no internal opening is found, the possibility of hydradenitis suppurativa must be considered (see Chapter 115).

Treatment

Even the suspicion of an anorectal abscess should lead to urgent referral to a surgeon for drainage (13). Temporizing treatment with oral antibiotics and sitz baths simply increases the risk of complications, such as systemic infection. An anorectal abscess may also be associated with a rapidly spreading necrotizing infection that destroys large areas of skin, subcutaneous tissue, and fascia. Patients with coincident diabetes mellitus are particularly vulnerable to complicated and extensive perirectal involvement. Finally, spontaneous rupture can occur either externally or internally, resulting in a complex fistula that is difficult to manage.

Preoperative broad-spectrum antibiotics need be given only to patients with anorectal abscesses who have valvular heart disease, diabetes, extensive inflammation or who are immunocompromised. Perianal abscesses may be drained under local anesthesia in the office or emergency room, but all other anorectal abscesses require regional or general anesthesia in the operating room. After drainage, the patient should receive oral analgesics and stool softeners and be instructed to begin sitz baths three times a day.

Most fistulas require fistulotomy (13). The internal and external openings must both be carefully identified and the tract converted into an open wound, which heals by secondary intention. Complex chronic fistulas can present difficult technical problems, and other surgical options may have to be considered. The wounds that result from any of these options commonly take 6 to 12 weeks to heal. The most serious postoperative complication is anal incontinence, which occurs in 3% to 7% of cases. The recurrence rate even for simple fistulas is approximately 5%, and it is higher for complex ones. Injection of fibrin glue to close the fistula appears to be effective in up to 60% of cases, especially for complex or recurrent fistulas (14).

Some patients with fistula-in-ano may be treated nonsurgically, either because of a lack of symptoms or because of complicating factors such as acquired immunodeficiency syndrome (AIDS). If there is a history of inflammatory bowel disease, a gastroenterologist should also be consulted.

PROCTALGIA FUGAX

Occasionally, healthy young adults develop the sudden onset of severe rectal pain, variably intermittent and usually lasting from less than 30 minutes to 1 hour, known as proctalgia fugax. It often awakens the patient at night. It is significantly more common in women than in men, and it can occur after sexual intercourse. The pain is described usually as a spasm or a cramp. The problem is not associated with systemic illness or other GI diseases such as irritable bowel syndrome, and the cause is uncertain. There is often an association with psychiatric disturbances. Proctalgia fugax was long thought to result from spasm of a portion of the levator ani muscle, but it is now thought to be caused by paroxysmal hyperkinesis of the smooth muscle of the internal anal sphincter (15). Patients with proctalgia fugax may obtain relief by taking a hot sitz bath or applying pressure in the perianal area near the site of the discomfort. There are no proven pharmacologic remedies for this affliction. However, if the attacks are severe and frequent, some patients may find relief from the use of sublingual or cutaneous nitrates. There is also the possibility that nifedipine, a calcium channel blocker, decreases the frequency and intensity of attacks, and that the inhalation of albuterol shortens the duration of pain. The problem usually persists for many years but then disappears in later life.

RECTAL PROLAPSE

Prolapse is a protrusion of the rectum through the anus. The protrusion may contain only mucosa (a mucosal prolapse), or it may contain all layers of the bowel wall (a full-thickness prolapse, or procidentia). There can also be an internal prolapse, or internal rectal intussusception, which produces typical symptoms without any external protrusion. This is often associated with the solitary rectal ulcer syndrome.

Prolapse is more prevalent in women (approximately 80% of the cases), with a peak incidence between the age of 60 and 80 years. In men the peak incidence occurs at about 40 years of age. The exact pathogenic mechanism in not known. Multiple factors are associated with this disease. Weakening of the fascial attachments of the rectum, attenuated muscles in the perirectal area and pelvic diaphragm, straining caused by chronic constipation, and even congenital fascial defects all lead to the development of rectal prolapse. Prolapse is often observed after severe chronic diarrhea. Mucosal prolapse also occurs commonly in children, usually before 2 years of age.

Diagnosis

History

Patients have variable symptoms, depending on the degree of prolapse. Initially, the protrusion occurs only with defecation, and the patient can easily reduce it manually. At this stage there may be no associated incontinence and the condition is sometimes mistaken for symptomatic internal hemorrhoids. The patient may complain of a sensation of displaced tissue at the time of a bowel movement, and there is often a feeling of incomplete evacuation. With progression of the problem, prolapse occurs with any straining and, eventually, simply with walking or even standing. At this stage incontinence is almost invariably a problem. With more profound prolapse, the patient may complain of tenesmus and also may develop a continuous mucous discharge. The prolapsed rectum may become excoriated and ulcerated, leading many patients to complain of bleeding. In association with an advanced degree of prolapse, the patient may also have urinary incontinence, and in women there may be associated uterine prolapse. Patients with increasing degrees of prolapse experience considerable embarrassment and consequently may avoid social contact.

Physical Examination

The clinician can best recognize rectal prolapse by inspecting the anus when the patient strains in a squatting position or sits on a commode. It is wise to anticipate incontinence with this maneuver. If the prolapse is full-thickness (procidentia), concentric folds of the rectal mucosa are seen; in mucosal prolapse, only radial folds are seen. Digital examination almost always reveals a patulous and relaxed anal sphincter that often admits two to four fingers. Palpation of the protruding tissue between the examiner's finger provides the sensation of only mucosa in mucosal prolapse or of a double layer of bowel wall in full-thickness prolapse. The rectal examination in patients with prolapse is usually associated with minimal or no discomfort.

Occasionally, prolapsed hemorrhoids are confused with rectal prolapse, but the absence of concentric or radial folds of mucosa and the prominent location of prolapsed hemorrhoids in the left lateral, right anterior, or right posterior edges of the anus suggest the proper diagnosis (Fig. 98.3). On occasion, a prolapse is associated with a rectal tumor. For that reason, a flexible fiberoptic sigmoidoscopic examination should be performed for any patient with rectal prolapse. Other diagnostic studies are not usually required, but a defecatory videoproctogram (available in only a few centers) is useful, especially for identifying an associated rectocele or internal prolapse.

Treatment

If the prolapse is small and limited to the mucosa, the patient may benefit from taking stool softeners and using a stimulant laxative suppository (see Chapter 46) to initiate defecation and thereby avoid straining at stool. If prolapse progresses despite this treatment, or if extensive mucosal prolapse is noted, it is appropriate to refer the patient to a surgeon. Redundant tissue may be treated by rubber band ligation, as for internal hemorrhoids. The procedure can usually be performed in the surgeon's office without anesthesia and is usually successful in preventing progressive degrees of rectal mucosal prolapse.

If procidentia (full-thickness prolapse) is present, only operative treatment is effective. Several procedures are available for the restoration of anal continence and reduction of prolapse. All of these operations require hospitalization, and most require general anesthesia. One important factor to consider before operation is whether incontinence will be improved. If a full preoperative assessment of anorectal function leads the gastroenterologist and surgeon to believe that incontinence is likely to persist, the alternative of providing the patient with a permanent diverting colostomy must be considered.

Both abdominal and perineal operations are available for the treatment of complete procidentia. The perineal approaches have usually been reserved for very elderly or high-risk patients because of perceived less-than-perfect results. However, published studies indicate that these operations may be satisfactory (16). Nonetheless, the most successful operative procedures for full-thickness rectal prolapse require an abdominal proctopexy, in which the rectum is secured to presacral fascia either by primary suture or by the use of synthetic mesh. This may or may not be accompanied by anterior resection of redundant sigmoid colon. Complications associated with the transabdominal surgical repair of prolapse are fecal impaction, presacral hemorrhage, stricture, infection, fistula formation, pelvic abscess, and intestinal obstruction. The complication rate is about 5%. However, fecal impaction can occur in up to 10% of patients after abdominal proctopexy. The complication rate for perineal repairs is low, and fecal impaction is rare. However, anastomotic leak with pelvic abscess, pelvic hematoma, and anastomotic stricture can occur. The operative mortality rate for abdominal operations is less than 3%, and for perineal procedures it is less than 1%.

Recurrence rates are in the range of 2% for the abdominal approaches and up to 30% for the perineal ones. However, of patients with preoperative fecal incontinence, 15% to 30% continue to have some degree of postoperative incontinence. This problem sometimes responds to biofeedback, which ordinarily is available only in specialized gastroenterology laboratories.

SEXUALLY TRANSMITTED DISEASES AND INFECTIOUS PROCTITIS

Anal and rectal problems may be caused by sexually transmitted diseases and infectious proctitis in persons who engage in anal sexual practices. Infection with human immunodeficiency virus (HIV) is also common in such situations (17). In addition to more widespread sexually transmitted diseases such as gonorrhea and syphilis, less common venereal infections may also be the cause of anal lesions.

Although anorectal symptoms may also be a result of nonspecific inflammation caused by trauma, rectal pain, tenesmus, and anal discharge should raise suspicion of infectious proctitis.

Diagnosis

Perianal lesions are seen in association with condylomata acuminata, herpes simplex virus type 2 (HSV-2), syphilis, chancroid, granuloma inguinale, and molluscum contagiosum. Perianal lesions in the form of abscesses, strictures, and fistulas are a late manifestation of lymphogranuloma venereum (LGV) and granuloma inguinale.

Condylomata acuminata are recognized as a typical collection of venereal warts, often extending within the anal canal. There is no specific diagnostic test. Condylomata acuminata associated with certain human papillomavirus (HPV) types are particularly prone to result in high-grade anal dysplasia, or even invasive squamous carcinoma. This is a particular risk for patients with HIV infection.

HSV-2 infection manifests initially as perianal or anal canal vesicles, but these have usually ruptured and coalesced into ulcerations before the patient is seen. Precise diagnosis requires either a direct fluorescent monoclonal antibody technique or culture of the virus. A *perianal chancre* may suggest the diagnosis of primary syphilis, and the typical verrucous excrescence of a *condyloma latum*, although rare, is pathognomonic of primary or secondary syphilis. The diagnosis must be confirmed by dark-field examination for spirochetes. *Chancroid* is associated with anorectal ulcers and abscesses, and the diagnosis is confirmed by culture. *Granuloma inguinale* is a chronic granuloma that eventually causes red, hard, perianal masses; biopsy is necessary for diagnosis. *Molluscum contagiosum* causes self-limited, painless, round, umbilicated lesions that can be confused with cutaneous cryptococcosis in patients with AIDS.

LGV, which is caused by specific immunotypes of *Chlamydia*, may present initially as an ulcer or inflammatory mass, and also causes proctitis. LGV may progress to abscess, fistula, and stricture formation and may require surgical management, occasionally necessitating a colostomy.

Proctitis is a manifestation of gonorrhea, *Chlamydia* infection, HSV-2, amebiasis, shigellosis, or occasionally rectal syphilis. All of these infections cause essentially similar and nonspecific symptoms of rectal discharge, pruritus, tenesmus, hematochezia, and constipation or diarrhea. Pain (odynophagia) is especially typical of HSV-2, *Chlamydia* infection, and chancroid and may also accompany syphilis. The proctitis of amebiasis has a rather typical appearance on sigmoidoscopy, but the symptoms are principally those of colitis, as is also true of shigellosis. Constitutional symptoms accompany HSV-2 infection and consist of urinary retention, impotence, and unexplained but disabling dysesthesias of the perineum, buttocks, and posterior thighs. Inguinal adenopathy is a common finding in conjunction with syphilis, LGV, or HSV-2 infection.

Diagnosis of all of these lesions requires anoscopy and flexible sigmoidoscopy. Gonorrhea causes a nonspecific mucosal inflammation with erythema, friability, and an exudate. Gram staining of the exudate reveals gram-negative intracellular diplococci, and a culture is confirmatory. Syphilitic proctitis is also nonspecific, and the diagnosis is made by dark-field examination of the exudate and serologic tests for syphilis (see Chapter 37). *Chlamydia* causes only a nonspecific proctitis, but LGV causes linear and aphthous ulcers extending from the rectum to the distal colon as well. Histologically as well as clinically, these findings resemble Crohn disease, and the diagnosis of LGV requires culture of the organism, which commonly necessitates tissue culture inoculation. Rising acute convalescent antichlamydial serum antibody titers are confirmatory but usually are not manifested for 1 month. Although the warts of condylomata acuminata usually appear in the perianal area, anoscopy is necessary to look for involvement of the anal canal. HSV-2 also causes predominantly perianal lesions, but anoscopy and sigmoidoscopy should be performed, because the anal canal can contain vesicular lesions or ulcers and the distal rectum may reveal proctitis with or without ulcers as well. Amebiasis often manifests with a characteristic sigmoidoscopic appearance of punched-out ulcers with a yellow base in addition to diffuse inflammation. The diagnosis is confirmed by stool examination for ova and parasites, as is that of giardiasis. A positive stool culture makes the diagnosis of shigellosis; proctitis with ulcerations are shown on proctoscopy.

Since these lesions may not be recognized unless an appropriate history is obtained, it is important that the clinician ask about sexual practices.

Information about the *treatment* of specific anorectal infections can be found in Chapters 35 (amebiasis and shigellosis), 37 (Sexually Transmitted Diseases), 102 (condyloma acuminata in women), and 102 (condyloma acuminata and molluscum contagiosum).

SPECIFIC REFERENCES

1. Schouten WR, Briel JW, Auwerda JJ, et al. Anal fissure: new concepts in pathogenesis and treatment. Scand J Gastroenterol Suppl 1996;218:78.
2. Dodi G, Bogoni F, Infantino A, et al. Hot or cold in anal pain? A study of the changes in internal sphincter pressure profiles. Dis Colon Rectum 1986;29:248.
3. Lund JN, Scholefield JH. A randomised, prospective, double-blind, placebo-controlled trial of glyceryl trinitrate ointment in treatment of anal fissure. Lancet 1997;349:11.
4. Kennedy ML, Sowter S, Nguyen H, et al. Glyceryl trinitrate ointment for the treatment of chronic anal fissure: results of a placebo-controlled trial and long-term follow-up. Dis Colon Rectum 1999;42:1000.
5. Zuberi BF, Rajput MR, Abro H, et al. A randomized trial of glyceryl trinitrate ointment and nitroglycerin patch in healing of anal fissures. Int J Colorectal Dis 2000;15:243.
6. Altomare DF, Rinaldi M, Milito G, et al. Glyceryl trinitrate for chronic anal fissure: healing or headache? Results of a multicenter, randomized, placebo-controlled, double-blind trial. Dis Colon Rectum 2000;43:174.
7. Maria G, Cassetta E, Gui D, et al. A comparison of botulinum toxin and saline for the treatment of chronic anal fissure. N Engl J Med 1998;338:217.
8. Americal Gastroenterological Association. American Gastroenterological Association medical position statement: diagnosis and care of patients with anal fissure. Gastroenterology 2003;124:233.
9. Johanson JF, Sonnenberg A. The prevalence of hemorrhoids and chronic constipation: an epidemiologic study. Gastroenterology 1990;98:380.
10. Standards Practice Task Force, American Society of Colon and Rectal Surgeons. Practice parameters for the treatment of hemorrhoids. Dis Colon Rectum 1993;36:1118.
11. Murie JA, Sim AJW, Mackenzie I. Rubber band ligation versus haemorrhoidectomy for prolapsing haemorrhoids: a long term prospective clinical trial. Br J Surg 1982;69:536.
12. Nivatvongs S, Goldberg SM. An improved technique of rubber band ligation of hemorrhoids. Am J Surg 1982;144:379.
13. Standards Practice Task Force, American Society of Colon and Rectal Surgeons. Practice parameters for treatment of fistula-in-ano: supporting documentation. Dis Colon Rectum 1996;39:1363.
14. Venkatesh KS, Ramanujam P. Fibrin glue application in the treatment of recurrent anorectal fistulas. Dis Colon Rectum 1999;42:1136.
15. Rao SS, Hatfield RA. Paroxysmal anal hyperkinesis: a characteristic feature of proctalgia fugax. Gut 1996;39:609.
16. Agachan F, Pfiefer J, Joo JS, et al. Results of perineal procedures for the treatment of rectal prolapse. Am Surg 1997;63:9.
17. Goldberg GS, Orkin BA, Smith LE. Microbiology of human immunodeficiency virus anorectal disease. Dis Colon Rectum 1994;37:439.

For annotated **General References** *and resources related to this chapter, visit www.hopkinsbayview.org/PAMreferences.*

SECTION 14

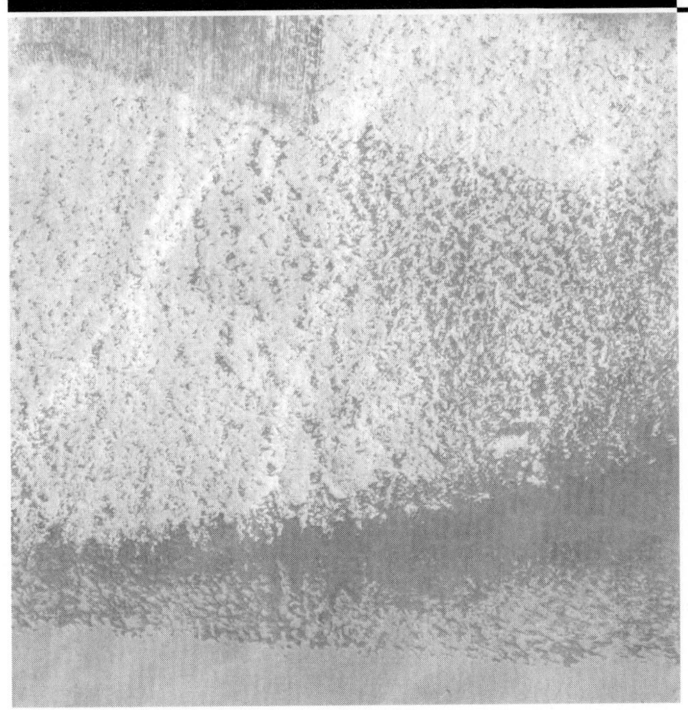

Gynecology and Women's Health

Chapter 99

Approach to Women's Health

Patricia A. Thomas

Women's health is currently conceptualized as a holistic, multidisciplinary approach to the health care of women throughout the life span and, as such, is much evolved from its narrow origins in the biomedical approach to reproductive health (1). On a global scale, women's health embodies a variety of social and economic concerns that affect the lives of girls and women worldwide. Many forces converged to promote the development of this field, but perhaps the most compelling for clinicians was the evidence that previous models failed to deliver quality health care to a substantial proportion of women.

The Council on Graduate Medical Education's *1995 Report on the Status of Women* made several observations about the need for new clinical competencies in women's health (2). First, women have important health needs throughout their life spans, not just during the reproductive years. More than men, the health status of women appears to be impacted by a complex interplay of psychologic, social, and economic factors. For example, women living in states with low scores on women's political and economic indicators are more likely to report poor health (3). Women traditionally earn less than men and are twice as likely to be uninsured. Women report higher rates of depression and chronic illness across all ages, and higher rates of physical disability (Fig. 99.1). Women who become disabled are more likely to have lower employment status and income than men (4). Since women live longer than men, attention to prevention of chronic illness and disability is especially important. Second, demographic shifts, including changes in family structure and aging of the population, which currently affect health trends, relate especially to women's health. As the population ages, a greater percentage of older adults are women. Minority women, whose numbers will increase as the population becomes more diverse, have poorer health outcomes by several measures. The number of single-parent households headed by women, who traditionally have a greater chance of living in poverty, is increasing. A third observation is that inadequate health insurance and fragmented delivery of primary care services have led to poorly coordinated care for many routine and comprehensive health concerns of women. Although community surveys indicate improving trends in cervical and breast cancer screening, colon cancer screening and counseling issues are still underutilized (Fig. 99.2). For women patients more than men, rates of screening seem to relate to characteristics of the physician-patient relationship (5). For a number of chronic illnesses, there appears to be a bias in the provision of care that women receive, compared with men. Men are more likely to undergo noninvasive investigations for coronary artery disease, to undergo renal transplantation, and to receive antiretroviral therapy for human immunodeficiency virus infection (6). The reasons for these gender inequalities are not entirely clear and call for further research.

Although women receive more health services than men, women are less satisfied with their care and are more likely to change caregivers because of dissatisfaction with care (7). This may relate to the traditionally fragmented health care received, since women frequently see more than one clinician for routine care (8). Dissatisfaction has also been traced to gender differences in communication and lack of a sense of partnership with one's physician. In one report, women's overall satisfaction with care was more dependent than men's on informational content, continuity, and multidisciplinarity (9). The rising number of women in medical careers, as well as the lay women's health movement, have advanced the standard toward a woman-centered approach to communication and shared decision-making.

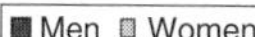

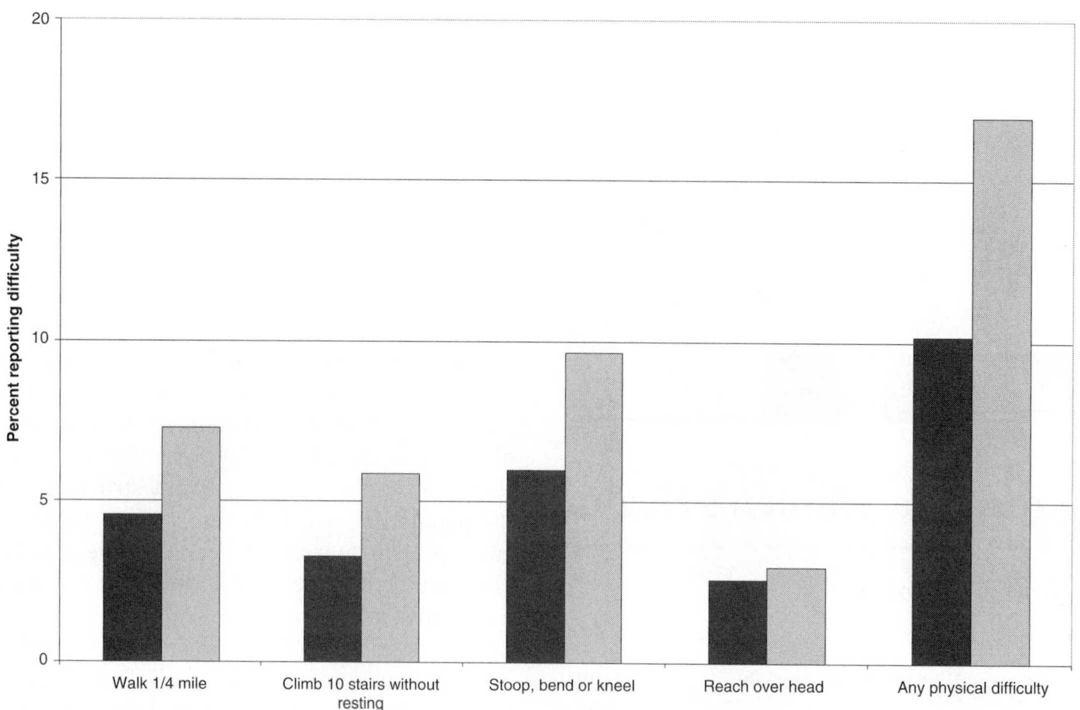

FIGURE 99.1. Frequencies in difficulty of physical functioning among persons 18 years of age and older, United States, 2002. (From Lethbridge-Cejku M, Schiller JS, Bernadel L. Summary Health Statistics for U.S. Adults, National Health Interview Survey, 2002. National Center for Heath Statistics Vital Health Statistics, 2004.)

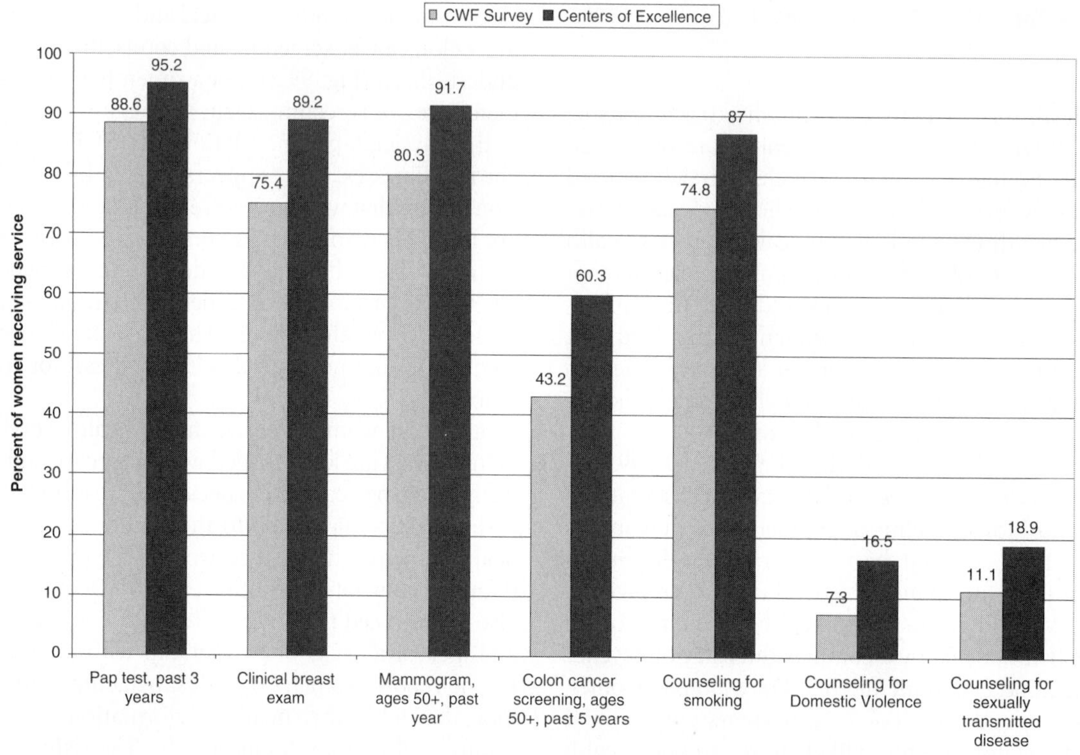

FIGURE 99.2. Provision of screening and counseling services comparing the 1998 Commonwealth Fund Survey of Women's Health (CWF: $n = 3{,}111$) with 15 National Centers of Excellence in Women's Health (COE: $n = 2{,}075$). (Adapted or modified from Anderson RT, Weismna CS, Scholle SH, et al. Evaluation of the quality of care in the Clinical Care Centers of the National Centers of Excellence in Women's Health. Women's Health Issues 2002;12(6):309–325.)

What constitutes effective clinical practice of women's health? In 2001, an interdisciplinary group published core competencies in women's health for medical students, which can be used as a starting point (10). Focus groups of women patients have described the ideal health care experience as holistic, incorporating not only reproductive health, but also attention to psychologic health, social functioning, sexual health, family, and other relationships (11). Women patients want their physicians to offer not only traditional pharmacotherapy, but also lifestyle interventions, alternative medicines, counseling, and education.

The field is still evolving, but a common approach is to consider prevention, risk assessment, and illness by stages of life. Many of the diseases that must be considered in the care of women are common to both men and women. Often the prevalence is higher in women (e.g., eating disorders, autoimmune disease), or the clinical presentation is different in women (e.g., coronary artery disease). A recurrent theme in women's health is that female patients may fail to respond to narrow biomedical approaches to illness, perhaps because of sex-specific biologic and gender-specific psychosocial factors. Throughout this textbook, authors have attempted to highlight these differences in their discussions, and readers are encouraged to use those chapters referred to here for more in-depth discussion of these topics.

A LIFE SPAN APPROACH TO WOMEN'S HEALTH

Most clinicians understand well that health and illness are the result not only of physiologic changes but also of social, cultural, and economic changes in the patient's life. In the field of women's health, newer competencies call for the clinician to possess the knowledge and attitudes necessary to integrate biologic and psychosocial factors in the provision of comprehensive care of women. The following discussion provides some examples of how this integration could be applied over life stages.

Adolescence

Clinicians who care for adult women often care for adolescents. In addition to issues of puberty and sexual differentiation, issues of gender identity and body image become manifest in these years (Chapter 6). Major causes of death in this age group are trauma and suicide. Many chronic adult diseases, such as autoimmune disease, first manifest at puberty. Eating disorders are becoming increasingly prevalent in this age group. The foundation of counseling for health risk behaviors begins in these years. Adolescent women are as likely as men to smoke, drink, and use other drugs, but suffer increased health risks as a result of these behaviors. They are twice as likely to be sexually abused than men (12).

Young Adulthood: Age 18 to 29 Years

In early adulthood, women may be juggling career, social relationships, and family life. Although this age group has the best equity with men's wages, 25% of women in this age group report no health insurance and 30% no usual source of health care (13). Many of the health concerns of women during these years, often referred to as the reproductive years, relate to reproduction, menstrual disorders, and contraception (see Chapters 100, 101, and 102). Counseling issues include avoidance of unintended pregnancy and sexually transmitted diseases (STDs), weight management, and smoking cessation (see Chapter 4). Risk behaviors remain important. As with men, significant mortality and morbidity during these years is related to violence and injury; domestic violence is especially prevalent in this age group (see Chapter 28) (14).

Adult Women: Ages 30 to 44 Years

Economically, women often lose wage equity with men just as family burdens increase; women in this age group earn 75% of men's wages. In the United States, 52% of married women contribute half or more of their household income; 61% of mothers with children under the age of 3 were in the workforce in 2002. Forty-one percent of women head their own households, and 28% of these have dependent children (15). Single mothers living in poverty often must make choices between health care and other commodities. Among low-income single mothers, for instance, childcare consumes almost 20% of the household income. Reproductive and lifestyle counseling issues remain important for this age group. By the close of this period, cancer of the breast and reproductive tract have assumed importance as leading causes of death (see Chapters 104 and 105). Screening and risk assessment for cancer as well as screening for sexually transmitted diseases should be incorporated into routine health care visits.

Midlife: Age 45 to 64 Years

Persons of this age group are sometimes referred to as the sandwich generation, and women during these years often function both as mother to teenage children and daughter to aging parents. More than 60% work outside the home. Transitional issues at this time of life are often accompanied by depression (see Chapter 24). Sixty percent of women in this age group report one or more chronic conditions, such as diabetes, hypertension, and arthritis. Prevalence of cardiovascular disease rises sharply, and cardiovascular risk assessment assumes importance (see Chapter 62). Cancer screening continues to be important,

TABLE 99.1 Suggested Measures of Quality for Women's Health

Process Variables
Adherence to guidelines for screening and preventive care (examples include screening for cervical and breast cancer, sexually transmitted diseases, depression, violence, and osteoporosis; counseling at menopause; and assessment of risk for diabetes and heart disease)
Adherence to guidelines for management of conditions such as cervical dysplasia, osteopenia, diabetes, breast complaints, and chlamydial infection, including timely followup of positive screening tests
Access to Care
Interpersonal aspects of care, such as the amount of information exchanged during an office visit and the active involvement of the patient in the decision-making process
Utilization of health care resources in the ambulatory setting, including number of office visits, use of diagnostic tests, time spent with providers, and changes in source of care over time
Outcome Variables
Functional status, including general health, mental health, and social functioning
Clinical status, including condition-specific measures when available
Changes in patient behavior, such as smoking cessation or initiation of exercise
Patient satisfaction
Professional satisfaction

From Carlson KJ. Multidisciplinary women's health care and quality of care. Women's Health Issues 2000;10(5):219, with permission.

and colorectal cancer screening is added at age 50 years. Menopausal health concerns are also important, beginning with perimenopausal symptoms and culminating with decisions regarding hormone therapy (see Chapter 106).

Late Life: Age 65 Years and Older

At the age of 65 years, the average U.S. woman has 21 years of life ahead. More women than men will assume caregiver roles to sick spouses and, unfortunately, caregivers are more likely to be in poor health themselves and experience difficulty accessing health care (16). In 2002, 41% of women older than 65 years of age lived alone, compared with 18% of men, accounting for the importance of social isolation in this group (17). The frequency of severe depression is 18% to 22% for women in this age group. After life-long lower wages compared with men, the retirement years for women are also often years of economic deprivation. Older women have a higher poverty rate than older men (12.4% versus 7.7% in 2002) (18). Osteoporosis occurs earlier in women (see Chapter 103), and the socially disabling problem of urinary incontinence is more frequent (see Chapter 54). Other health concerns parallel those of men during this phase of life (see Chapter 12).

A SYSTEMS APPROACH TO WOMEN'S HEALTH

Another approach to meeting the complex needs of women has been the development of interdisciplinary women's health centers. These centers are designed to promote coordinated clinical care in one geographic location and to facilitate the comprehensive delivery of that care, which is implied by the suggested quality measures listed in Table 99.1. Disciplines that are frequently represented in such centers include physicians, nurses, nurse practitioners, mental health professionals, physician assistants, health educators, and alternative health care practitioners. Access to care, ease of referral, increased communication, and coordination of care among clinicians can be facilitated with such an integrated center. Many centers are hospital sponsored. Reviews of the experience of these centers note that preventive services are delivered at higher rates and women report higher patient satisfaction (19,20). In addition, the U.S. Department of Health and Human Services has funded National Centers of Excellence in Women's Health in 18 academic medical centers. These Centers of Excellence deliver services to a more diverse population and serve not only as models of integrated clinical care but also as research and training centers (21).

The growth of women's health centers, coupled with the founding of the Office of Research on Women's Health at the National Institutes of Health (NIH) and expanded funding of research initiatives, promises to continue the development of knowledge that will inform clinicians and patients about the delivery of health services to women in the decades ahead.

SPECIFIC REFERENCES

1. Hoffman E, Magrane D, Donoghue GD. Changing perspectives on sex and gender in medical education. Acad Med 2000;75:1051.
2. Council on Graduate Medical Education. Fifth report: women and medicine. Washington, DC: US Department of Health and Human Services, 1995.
3. Jun HJ. A multilevel analysis of women's status and self-rated health in the United States. J Am Med Womens Assoc 2004;59(3):172–80.
4. Randolph DS. Predicting the effect of disability on employment status and income. Work 2004;23(3):257–66.
5. Lemon SC, Zaphka JG, Puleo E. Comprehensive cancer screening in a primary care population: gender differences in the impact of ambulatory care system factors. J Ambulatory Care Manage 2005;28(1):86–97.
6. Raine R. Does gender bias exist in the use of specialist health care? J Health Serv Res Policy 2000;5:237.
7. Falik MM, Collins KS, eds. Women's health: the Commonwealth Fund survey. Baltimore: Johns Hopkins University Press, 1996.
8. Clancy CM, Maisson CT. American women's health care: a patchwork quilt with gaps. JAMA 1992;268:1918.
9. Weisman CS, Rich DE, Rogers J, et al. Gender and patient satisfaction with primary care: tuning in to women in quality measurement. J Womens Health Gend Based Med 2000;9:657.
10. Cain J, Donoghue G, Magrane D, et al., eds. Women's health core competencies for medical

students. Washington, DC: Association of Professors of Gynecology and Obstetrics, 2001.
11. Anderson RT, Barbara AM, Weisman C, et. al. A qualitative analysis of women's satisfaction with primary care from a panel of focus groups in the National Centers of Excellence in Women's Health. J Women's Health 2001;10(7):637–647.
12. Sarigiani PA, Ryan L, Petersen AC. Prevention of high-risk behaviors in adolescent women. J Adoles Health 1999;25(2):109–119.
13. Wyn R, Solis B. Women's health issues across the lifespan. Women's Health Issues 2001;11(3):148–159.
14. Tjaden P, Thoennes N. Prevalence, incidence and consequences of violence against women: findings from the National Violence Against Women Survey. National Institute of Justice, Centers for Disease Control and Prevention. Washington, DC: US Government Printing Office, November 1998.
15. U.S. Department of Labor, Womens Bureau. Available at: http://www.dol.gov/dol/wb.
16. Donelan K, Falik M, DesRoches CM. Caregiving: challenges and implications for women's health. Women's Health Issues 2001; 11(3):185–200.
17. Federal Interagency Forum on Aging-Related Statistics. Older Americans 2000: key indicators of well-being. National Institute of Aging, National Center for Health Statistics. Washington, DC: US Government Printing Office, August 2000. Available at: http://www.agingstats.gov. Accessed February 15, 2002.
18. Current Population Reports. Poverty in the United States: 2002. Publication no. P60-229 Washington, DC: US Bureau of the Census, September 2003.
19. Carlson KJ. Multidisciplinary women's health care and quality of care. Women's Health Issues 2000;10:219.
20. Anderson RT, Weiseman CS, Scholle SH, et al. Evaluation of the quality of care in the Clinical Care Centers of the National Centers of Excellence in Women's Health. Women's Health Issues 2002;12(6):309–325.
21. Weisman CS, Squires GL. Women's health centers: are the National Centers of Excellence in Women's Health a new model? Women's Health Issues 2000;10:248.

*For annotated **General References** and resources related to this chapter, visit www.hopkinsbayview.org/PAMreferences.*

Chapter 100

Contraception and Preconception Counseling

Roxanne M. Jamshidi

Contraception provides a woman and her partner with the ability to determine the number and timing of pregnancies. Generally, avoidance of unwanted pregnancies and continued consistent use of a contraceptive method are issues that require ongoing management and consultation rather than an isolated decision.

There are many contraceptive methods. It is important to understand the benefits and limitations of all of them to be able to educate the patient fully about her options. The caregiver should be prepared to deal with women who have varying knowledge and experience about contraception. Table 100.1 lists the most recent data regarding the percentage distribution of use of contraceptive methods by women in the United States (1).

Table 100.2 shows the failure rates of various methods of contraception. Perfect use refers to the annual percentage of unexpected pregnancy among couples who use the method correctly and consistently, whereas typical use

TABLE 100.1 Contraceptive Use among U.S. Women 15–44 Years of Age, 2002

Contraceptive	*% U.S. Women Age 15–44 Yr in 2002*
Female sterilization	16.7
Oral contraceptive	18.9
Male condom	11.1
Male sterilization	5.7
3-month injectable (Depo Provera)	3.3
Withdrawal	2.9
Intrauterine device	1.3
Periodic abstinence or natural family planning	0.9
Diaphragm	0.2
Implant, Lunelle, or patch	0.8
Others methods[a]	0.6

[a]Includes Today sponge, cervical cap, female condom, and other methods.
From Mosher WD, Gladys MM, Chandra A, et al. Use of contraception and use of family planning services in the United States: 1982–2002. Adv Dat 2004;350:1.

reflects common irregularities in use other than voluntary termination of the method. Clearly there is very little difference between the two failure rates with some methods, whereas others show a considerable difference. This information should be used in helping to educate the patient.

Once it is established that a woman desires fertility regulation, a focused medical history should be obtained, including information about past pregnancies, menstruation, smoking, and medical problems that may affect selection of one method over another. A blood pressure measurement should be made, and if history alone cannot rule out pregnancy, a urine pregnancy test performed. A pelvic examination is not immediately necessary for the initiation or continuation of birth control with the exception of placement of an intrauterine device (IUD) or fitting for a diaphragm or cervical cap. Although an annual pelvic examination, breast examination, Pap smear, and screening for sexually transmitted diseases (STDs) are seen as necessary steps in preventive health care for women of reproductive age, and their deferral should not preclude prescription of a safe contraceptive method and risk an unsafe or unwanted pregnancy (2). After the evaluation, the physician and patient (and, sometimes, her partner) are ready to discuss the various contraceptive methods and develop a satisfactory plan.

SYSTEMIC HORMONAL CONTRACEPTION

Combined Oral Contraceptive Pills

Mechanism of Action

The primary contraceptive action of combined oral contraceptives (COCs) is suppression of ovulation by inhibition of gonadotropin-releasing factors in the hypothalamus. This action is primarily mediated by the progestin component. The principal effect of this inhibition appears to be suppression of the surge in activity of luteinizing hormone at midcycle, thereby removing a major stimulus to ovulation. Additionally, COCs make cervical mucus more viscous and therefore less easily traversed by sperm. They also have a direct effect on endometrial development in high doses, making the uterus less receptive to ovum implantation (3).

Preparations and Dosage Schedules

The COC was first introduced for use in the United States in 1960. In the ensuing years, significant changes were made in steroid dosages and some new steroids were introduced. Since 1970, all new COCs introduced in the United States have contained ethinyl estradiol as their estrogen. As their progestin, many COCs in current use contain levonorgestrel or norethindrone. In 1992, however, two new progestins, norgestimate and desogestrel, were introduced in the United States in an effort to decrease unwanted side effects of oral contraception. A more recently introduced progestin, drospirenone, which is derived from 17 α-spirolactone, has both progestogenic and antimineral corticoid activity.

There are three different preparations of oral contraceptive pills:

- Monophasic—contains the same dosage of estrogen and progestin for 21 days each cycle.
- Multiphasic—contains one to two levels of estrogen and two to three levels of progestin, which vary through the cycle.
- Progestin only (mini-pill)—contains progestin only in a steady, continuous dosage.

Table 100.3 lists conditions requiring precautions for the use of COCs. If a woman chooses oral contraception and has no clinical contraindications, then the first choice should be a combination preparation containing between 20 and 35 μg of estrogen. Use of pills containing 50 μg of estrogen should be avoided, and the few women who may need them should be evaluated by an obstetrician-gynecologist if the clinician is not fully familiar with their use. The choice of progestin is less critical, and no progestin is clearly superior to another. The newer progestins have structural modifications that lower their androgenic activity, and therefore may cause less hirsutism, acne, and weight gain, as well as a more favorable lipid profile. Because of the potassium-sparing effects of drospirenone, caution should be used for women at risk for hyperkalemia.

To suppress ovulation and yet allow periodic bleeding, the combination tablet is taken every day for 3 weeks. COCs are generally packaged in 21-day or 28-day cycles.

TABLE 100.4 Selected Drugs That May Interact with Oral Contraceptive Preparations (OCs)

Drugs That May Decrease the Effectiveness of OCs, Resulting in Breakthrough Bleeding, Pregnancy, or Both
- Well-established, commonly occurring drug reactions
  - Anticonvulsants: barbiturates, phenytoin (Dilantin), primidone (Mysoline)
  - Antimicrobial: rifampin

Reported Instances of Possible Drug Interactions
- Antimicrobials
  - Breakthrough bleeding only: neomycin, nitrofurantoin, phenoxymethylpenicillin (penicillin V)
  - Breakthrough bleeding and pregnancy: ampicillin, chloramphenicol, sulfamethoxypyridazine (Kynex, Midicel)
- Others: chlordiazepoxide (Librium), meprobamate, phenacetin (no longer available in the U.S.), and phenylbutazone (Butazolidin, not longer available in the United States)

Drugs Whose Effectiveness May Be Altered by OCs
- Anticoagulants: effect may be reduced by simultaneous administration of OCs
- Clofibrate (Atromid-S): control of cholesterol and triglyceride levels may be lost when OCs are simultaneously administered
- Thyroid hormone in patients without a functioning thyroid gland: mostly a theoretical concern; however, increased dosage of thyroid hormone may be needed
- Tricyclic antidepressants: higher dosages of estrogen may inhibit the effect of antidepressants, and tricyclic toxicity may be increased
- Caffeine: metabolism of caffeine may be decreased; patients who take large amounts of caffeine (e.g., 4–8 cups of coffee per day) should be cautioned regarding symptoms of caffeinism

prescription. Screening for STDs (see Chapter 102) may need to be done if the woman is at risk. COCs may be discontinued at any time if pregnancy is desired or another method of contraception is planned. The first few menstrual periods after withdrawal may be heavier than during the time COCs were used. There is no change in fertility after a course of COCs, regardless of duration of use. A pill-free or rest period is not advocated when switching to another method or in anticipation of becoming pregnant.

Contraceptive Patch

An alternative method of delivering combined hormonal contraception is in the form of a transdermal patch (Ortho Evra). This thin medicated adhesive is applied to the buttocks, abdomen, upper outer arm, or upper torso (excluding the breast area), and delivers 20 μg of ethinyl estradiol and 150 μg of norelgestromin per day (39). The patch is changed weekly for three weeks, followed by a patch-free week for a withdrawal bleed.

The same side effects and cautions that apply to traditional COCs also apply to the contraceptive patch, with the exception of a higher incidence of application site reactions (20.2%), breast symptoms during the first 2 months (18%), and dysmenorrhea (13%) (40). Because the medication in the transdermal patch is in the adhesive itself, excellent attachment is required. Data on patch adhesion show that approximately 4.7% of patches need to be replaced because of either partial or full detachment (40). The efficacy of the patch is comparable to COCs, with a failure rate of less than 1% (40,41). Clinical data indicate that contraceptive efficacy may decrease in women weighing more than 90 kg (198 lb) (42), however, even low-dose COCs may have decreased efficacy among heavy women (43).

Vaginal Ring

The combined contraceptive vaginal ring (Nuva Ring) is another novel method of delivering the same hormones as those used in COCs. The vaginal ring is a flexible transparent copolymer ring that is placed in the vagina continuously for three weeks, and then removed for a week to allow for a withdrawal bleed. The vaginal ring delivers 15 μg of ethinyl estradiol and 120 μg of etonogestrel daily (44). Although the ring is designed to be worn continuously for 3 weeks, it can be removed for up to 3 hours at a time, without decreasing effectiveness. Additionally, serum concentrations of the hormones remain at contraceptive levels through 5 weeks of continuous use if the ring is left in the vagina. The ring does not have to be fitted or placed in a specific location in the vagina, can be worn during intercourse, and is comfortable for both the patient and her partner. In fact, the vaginal ring can be used concomitantly with tampons, spermicide, or antimycotic comedication without adverse effects or decreased efficacy (45,46,47).

Again, as a combined hormonal method of birth control, the same side effects and cautions which apply to traditional COCs also apply to the vaginal ring. Initial trials showed excellent cycle control with a low incidence (fewer than 5% of women) of irregular bleeding when initiating the vaginal ring. Some side effects are unique to the ring, including an approximate 5% incidence in increased vaginal discharge, 5% incidence of vaginitis, and 2% incidence of vaginal discomfort. Overall, however, acceptability for the ring is quite high for both patients and their partners, with over 90% of users recommending the method to others (48).

Progestin-Only Pill

Because the progestin-only pills are associated with decreased effectiveness and increased breakthrough bleeding compared to COCs, they are rarely prescribed. However, progestin-only contraceptive pills offer an option for women who have medical conditions contraindicating estrogen (such as thrombophilia), are intolerant to estrogenic side effects, or who are lactating.

Injectable Contraception

Depot medroxyprogesterone acetate (DMPA) (Depo-Provera), a synthetic progestogen that is similar to natural progesterone, has been in use in the United States since 1992. DMPA is administered as an intramuscular injection of 150 mg that provides contraceptive efficacy for at least 14 weeks. Administration every 12 weeks provides a margin of error should the woman fail to return at the exact appointed time. In this dosage, the failure rate is comparable to that of sterilization. DMPA acts by inhibiting ovulation, thickening cervical mucus, and altering the composition of the endometrium secondary to the progestin effects.

The most common side effect associated with DMPA is a disruption in the menstrual pattern. This disruption is unpredictable and can range from prolonged periods of amenorrhea (common) to episodes of heavy bleeding (rare). Approximately 50% of women using DMPA for 1 year develop amenorrhea (49). Other reported side effects include skin changes such as acne, breast tenderness, headache, and psychological effects such as decreased libido, depression, nervousness, and fatigue. Variable effects of DMPA IM on body weight have been reported, ranging from nonsignificant changes, to gains of approximately 3 kg to 4 kg at 1 year. However, the only placebo-controlled prospective trial evaluating this issue showed no relationship between DMPA use and weight changes (50).

DMPA is associated with increased bone resorption and, in some studies, a small but statistically significant decrease in bone density when used for more than 2 years. Although this effect appears to be transient and largely reversible (51), the U.S. Food and Drug Administration (FDA) issued a "black box" warning regarding the possible effects of DMPA on bone mineral density (52). In contrast to the FDA, the World Health Organization (WHO) does not believe there should be any restrictions on the use of DMPA (53). Nevertheless, patients should be counseled regarding the recommendation for adequate calcium intake, especially among adolescents. Additionally, women who may be planning to try to conceive in the future should be counseled regarding the delay in ovulation of up to 18 months after cessation of DMPA, although most women have return of fertility 6 to 9 months after the time the next injection would have been given.

A new lower dose (104 mg) DMPA formulation that can be given subcutaneously is undergoing clinical trials. This method of administration offers the advantage of potential self-administration.

A monthly injectable contraceptive combining 25 mg of medroxyprogesterone acetate and 5 mg of estradiol cypionate was approved by the FDA in 2000, and marketed under the name Lunelle. Its mode of action is similar to that of COCs, as are the precautions for prescribing the method (54). The side effect of irregular bleeding is decreased compared to DMPA, and there is a rapid return to fertility within 2 months after the last injection. Unfortunately, Lunelle was recalled by the manufacturer in October 2002, with no known plan for re-introduction to the U.S. market.

Subdermal Contraceptive

Implantable, subdermal capsules that release progestins for several years provide long-acting, reversible contraception. Implants offer the advantage of extremely high effectiveness without maintenance of the user. Like other progestin contraception, the mechanism of action is through a combination of suppression of ovulation, changes in the cervical mucus that make it impenetrable to sperm, and changes to the endometrium that make it thin and atrophic. Implants offer rapid onset of action, with cervical mucus changes seen within hours of placement (55). In general, implants can be placed during any time of the menstrual cycle, with use of backup contraception for the first week of use only. After removal of implants, former patterns of ovulation and menses return rapidly (56). Former use of implants does not alter subsequent rates of fertility, miscarriage, stillbirth, prematurity, or congenital malformations (57).

Like other progestin methods of birth control, the most common side effect with implants are menstrual changes, occurring in almost three quarters of users in the first year (58). Bleeding patterns often become irregular, with an overall decrease in blood loss. Amenorrhea is not uncommon as well. Less common side effects of implants include headaches, weight gain, acne, and psychiatric or mood changes. Local skin irritation occurs in approximately 5% of implant users, but actual infection or inflammation is much less common (59).

In the United States, no implantable methods of birth control have been available since the six-rod implant (Norplant) was removed from the market in 2001. Containing 216 mg of levonorgestrel in six rods, Norplant was approved for use for 5 years in the United States, but two large studies have shown cumulative 7-year pregnancy rates comparable to surgical sterilization, with some decreased efficacy in women weighing more than 80 kg (60,61). Experience with Norplant has led to improvements in the contraceptive implant system, primarily by decreasing the number of implants from six to one or two. Systems with fewer implants can be inserted and removed faster and more easily. Norplant II (Jadelle) is a two-rod system containing 150 mg of levonorgestrel that is left in place for 3 to 5 years. FDA approval was obtained in 1996; but no plans exist to market this system in the United States. However, pending FDA approval, a new single rod system implant should be available in the United States in 2006. This system, Implanon, contains the progestin etonogestrel, which has less androgenic and more progestational activity then levonorgestrel. The single rod comes in a disposable trocar/inserter, which aids subdermal placement. The duration of use is designed for 3 years. With initial studies showing only one pregnancy in over 70,000 cycles, Implanon has extremely high contraceptive efficacy (62).

INTRAUTERINE CONTRACEPTIVES

Intrauterine contraceptives are one of the most effective methods of contraception. Pregnancy rates range from 0.14 to 3 per 100 women per year. The first modern IUDs appeared in the early 1960s and were made of a biologically inert plastic. The second-generation copper and progesterone-containing devices have been available since the early 1970s (63,64).

During the late 1970s, serious concerns were raised regarding the safety of all IUDs. Studies showed a strong relationship between IUD use and the development of PID. The Dalkon Shield specifically was removed from the market because of its link to spontaneous septic abortions and PID. The clearly increased risk for infection with this particular product has been attributed to the multifilament tail (the string that hangs into the vagina), which seemed to act as a wick for bacteria. (Other IUDs used a monofilament tail.) Because of the publicity from the Dalkon Shield, distribution of other devices was discontinued by manufacturers because of low sales volume or concern regarding litigation costs. However, the concern regarding an increased risk of infertility from PID associated with modern IUD use appears to be unfounded. Epidemiologic studies in the 1970s tended to overstate the risk of pelvic infection from IUD use, for the following reasons:

- In most early studies, the control group included women who were using diaphragms and COCs. These modalities are protective against PID.
- The risks for specific IUDs were not analyzed separately. Dalkon Shield wearers, with substantially higher risk for infection, were included in most analyses.
- Most studies did not analyze for factors that significantly affect the risk of PID, such as multiple sexual partners and previous history of pelvic infection.
- Recent epidemiologic studies adjusted the relative risks of tubal infertility by type of IUD used and number of sexual partners. They showed that women who had had only one sexual partner in their lifetime had no significantly increased risk of tubal infertility. However, women who had more than one sexual partner had a three to four times higher risk (65). Also, a case-control study found that tubal infertility in nulliparous women was not linked to a history of IUD use, but rather was associated with the presence of antibodies to chlamydia (66).

Types

Two types of IUDs are available in the United States: progesterone-releasing and copper-bearing. All of the devices have a *monofilament string* attached, which allows for surveillance and removal (see Followup Care). Return to fertility is rapid for both types of IUD.

The copper IUD (ParaGard T380A), which contains no hormone, has a body of polyethylene wound with copper wire and a copper collar on each of its transverse arms. The copper inhibits sperm motility and capacitation, making them unable to penetrate the ovum. There is no evidence that IUDs work after fertilization as an abortifacient. Currently the ParaGard is approved by the FDA for at least 10 years of continuous use. It has a cumulative 10-year failure rate of 2.1% to 2.8%.

The hormone-releasing intrauterine contraceptive the Mirena intrauterine system, was approved by the FDA in 2001. The Mirena has a small, T-shaped frame with a steroid reservoir that releases levonorgestrel at the rate of 20 μg per day. It is currently approved for 5 years of continuous use and has an overall failure rate of 0.14 per 100 woman-years, comparable to that of sterilization. The levonorgestrel thickens cervical mucus and suppresses endometrial proliferation to inhibit passage of sperm, in addition to altering sperm transport as a result of the presence of the IUD in the uterine cavity. The progestin exerts a predominantly local effect; therefore, plasma concentrations of levonorgestrel are lower for Mirena users than for women using oral pills or implants.

Use and Insertion

If the clinician is not experienced in IUD insertion, the woman should be referred to a gynecologist. Traditionally, the IUD is inserted at the time of menstruation, to assure that the woman is not pregnant. However, as long as the provider can be reasonably certain that the woman is not pregnant, the IUD can be inserted at any time of a menstrual period. Prophylactic antibiotics given at the time of insertion do not provide any benefit (67).

Women typically experience some cramps when the IUD is inserted; these can be limited by the administration of nonsteroidal analgesics before the insertion (e.g., ibuprofen 400 mg). If significant cramps persist beyond a few hours, this may be an indication that the device is not inserted properly and should be removed.

After insertion, the woman should feel the string of the IUD. She repeats this monthly, after each menstrual period, to ensure that the device is in place.

Bleeding Patterns

Copper IUD users typically note increased menstrual bleeding, and some experience cramping, which usually subsides within 3 months. Conversely, levonorgestrel IUD users experience a substantial decrease in their menstrual bleeding and cramping. The average number of bleeding days decreases from 5 in the first month to 1 in the sixth month; between 15% and 20% of women are amenorrheic by the end of the first year of use (68,69). This bleeding pattern has prompted the noncontraceptive use of this method for women with irregular bleeding.

Adverse Effects

The most common adverse effects of the IUD are cramping, abnormal uterine bleeding, and expulsion. Expulsion occurs in approximately 5% of users, and is the most common reason for IUD failure (70). Uterine perforation, a rare complication, is most likely to occur at the time of insertion. Although the risk of PID does not increase with prolonged IUD use, the first 20 days after insertion is associated with a small increased risk of infection, presumably from endometrial contamination at the time of insertion (71). After IUD insertion, the woman must be instructed to report any fever, pelvic pain, or discomfort promptly. Copper IUD users must also report any missed menstrual periods and be evaluated for pregnancy (including ectopic pregnancy); however, this does not hold true for levonorgestrel IUD users.

Followup Care

A followup visit should be scheduled after the patient's next menstrual period to check IUD placement and evaluate for signs of infection. Thereafter, the woman can return to annual well-women visits. The followup is best done by a gynecologist if the clinician is not experienced in examining women with an IUD.

If the IUD strings are not visualized on speculum examination, the first step in evaluation is to perform a pregnancy test. Those users found to be pregnant should be promptly referred to a gynecologist for evaluation. If the woman is not pregnant, a cytobrush can be inserted in the endocervical canal to draw out the strings. If this is not successful, the endocervical canal can be examined using a uterine sound or an endocervical speculum. It the IUD is present in the cervix, it should be removed. If the IUD is not in the cervix, radiography or ultrasonography (US) should be used to localize the IUD.

Generally, the IUD is easily removed by gentle traction on the string. As with other methods, if the woman terminates this form of contraception other than to attempt pregnancy, she will need help in choosing another form of contraception.

BARRIER METHODS

Diaphragm

The diaphragm is a low-cost patient-dependent contraceptive device. It is a dome-shaped rubber device that is held open by a metallic band or spring. It is filled with a spermicidal cream or jelly before each use and placed in the vagina over the cervix to prevent sperm deposited during ejaculation from reaching the cervical os. As seen in Table 100.2, with typical use the failure rate is high, whereas correct or ideal use results in a lower failure rate, as is true of all barrier methods.

The diaphragm is fitted by the medical provider. The device fits between the posterior fornix and the symphysis. The largest device that is comfortable is the proper one to use. For better effectiveness, the woman should be asked to insert the diaphragm in the office and have the provider check its placement. Manufacturers of diaphragms have excellent booklets that are useful in helping a woman acquire the skill necessary for comfortable use of this form of contraception.

The woman applies spermicidal jelly to the inside of the dome and inserts the diaphragm in the vagina as long as 4 hours before intercourse. She should check for position with her finger and allow the device to remain in place for at least 6 hours after coitus. If repeated intercourse occurs within 6 to 8 hours, additional jelly should be placed in the vagina first, without removal of the diaphragm.

With care a diaphragm should last 2 years. The woman will need a new fitting if she gains or loses significant weight, has a baby, or has pelvic surgery. Some women report discomfort while the diaphragm is in place. This discomfort is most often related to a wrong design or to improper fitting, and re-evaluation usually identifies the problem. A few women develop recurrent cystitis with frequent diaphragm use; this should lead to a discussion of alternative methods of contraception.

Cervical Cap

The latex Prentif cervical cap is about as effective as the diaphragm (in nulliparous women), offers the advantage of being able to be left in place for a longer time (up to 48 hours), and does not need to be used with spermicide. However, the addition of a tablespoon of spermicide placed in the cap prior to insertion can improve efficacy and decrease the incidence of foul-smelling discharge common after 24 hours of use. The cervical cap comes in several sizes, and must be fitted by a health professional to go over the cervix. Proper fitting can be accomplished in approximately 80% of women. Compared to the diaphragm, the Prentif cervical cap is somewhat harder to fit and is more difficult to insert. Two newer cervical caps have been developed and approved by the FDA: the FemCap and Leas Shield. Both are made from silicone rubber, can be left in place for up to 48 hours, and are designed to be used in conjunction with a spermicide. Unlike the other cervical caps and diaphragms, Leas Shield is "one-size-fits-all."

Condom

The *male condom* is a latex rubber sheath that is placed over the erect penis. It is the only reversible effective male method of contraception except for coitus interruptus. Condoms, when properly used, are an effective form of contraception, and their failure rate with experienced and strongly motivated couples is as low as 1 or 2 per 100 couple-years of exposure. However, rates during the first year of use or in less motivated couples may be considerably higher. Its effectiveness can be enhanced if it is combined with application of a spermicidal jelly or foam in the vagina. Some condoms are being manufactured in containers with a spermicidal lubricant. The condom, when used properly, provides considerable protection against STDs, including gonorrhea, herpes, chlamydia, and human immunodeficiency virus (HIV) infection. Its only side effects are rare instances of sensitivity to the lubricating material or to latex and skin irritation from friction.

The *female condom* is a disposable, prelubricated polyurethane sheath between two rings of differing sizes. One ring is placed in the vagina, as with the diaphragm, and the larger ring rests exteriorly on the vulva. Studies show that it is impenetrable to the passage of HIV as well as other common STD agents. Expected pregnancy rates are comparable to those seen with male condom use (72).

Sponge

The Today sponge is made of a soft, disposable polyurethane foam which contains the spermicide nonoxynol-9. After it is moistened with water and inserted in the vagina, it becomes effective immediately and remains effective for the next 24 hours without the need to add spermicidal cream, even with repeated acts of intercourse. It does not require fitting and was available in the United States as an over-the-counter (OTC) product until 1995 when it was taken off the market because of manufacturing problems. The Today sponge is again available in the United States as of 2005.

VAGINAL SUPPOSITORIES, FOAM, AND JELLY

Vaginal suppositories, foam, and jelly contain a spermicidal material combined with cream, jelly, or foam. The material is inserted in the vagina at least 10 to 15 minutes before intercourse. The spermicidal material is dispersed in the vagina and over the cervix. This creates a barrier around the cervical os to prevent sperm from entering the intrauterine cavity. All of these forms of contraception may be obtained without prescription. They are especially useful when additional protection is desired at midcycle with the condom or to increase the effectiveness of the diaphragm when repeated intercourse occurs. The side effects are minor and are related to sensitivity to the spermicidal material.

NATURAL FAMILY PLANNING

The *rhythm method* or *periodic abstinence* requires avoidance of intercourse during a calculated fertile period. The human ovum probably is viable for only 12 to 24 hours after ovulation, whereas sperm retain the capability for fertilization for 48 hours to 5 days. It is probable that conception is most likely during a 6-day interval ending on the day of ovulation (73). The development of a method of contraception that avoids intercourse at the fertile time is logical; however, the risk of pregnancy in women who use this method of contraception is high (Table 100.2). Three methods have been developed to calculate the fertile period:

1. The *calendar method* attempts to establish the portion of the cycle when intercourse is safe. The woman keeps a careful record for several months of the duration of each menstrual cycle beginning with the first day of bleeding. She then subtracts 14 days from the end of the cycle, which represent the days of ovulation. Intercourse is avoided during this fertile period. Obviously, the woman's cycles need to be extremely regular and predictable in order for this method to work.
2. The *basal body temperature method* takes advantage of the slight drop in body temperature that is associated with ovulation and is followed by a rise in temperature of approximately 1°F (0.5°C). The woman takes her temperature each morning beginning at day 3 of the cycle. The couple avoids intercourse from the onset of menses until 3 days after the woman's basal body temperature has risen.
3. The *cervical mucus method* requires the woman to learn, over a number of cycles, the changes that indicate ovulation. She is taught to examine her cervical mucus for clarity. She learns to identify abdominal discomfort associated with ovulation and to use this information to avoid intercourse when conception is possible. This method requires effort and regular cycles, but it has been used effectively by many women.

STERILIZATION

In the United States, sterilization is the most popular method of contraception, with elective sterilization higher for women than for men (1). Because sterilization is meant to be permanent and nonreversible, individuals and couples considering sterilization need very careful education so that they understand the nature and risks of the procedure and the availability of other contraceptive options.

Vasectomy

Vasectomy, when properly performed, has a very low failure rate. The complication rate is approximately 4 in 1,000, and, for the most part, complications are minor. They include infection, hematoma, epididymitis, and granuloma formation. Long-term serious side effects have not been reported among the very large numbers of men who have had the procedure performed. There was a transient concern, now known to be unwarranted (74), that antibodies to sperm that develop in some men after vasectomy predispose them to atherosclerosis. Additionally, although there had been a concern that the risk of testicular and prostate cancer may be increased in men after vasectomy, data do not support this association (75,76).

Patient Experience

This procedure is done under local anesthesia in the physician's office or outpatient surgical suite. There is minimal operative discomfort. Postoperatively, mild discomfort is common but is usually controlled with a mild analgesic, such as acetaminophen. Vigorous physical activity and sexual activity are restricted for 5 to 7 days until the wound has healed. Followup visits are necessary so that sperm counts can be performed. Usually, 6 to 12 weeks or approximately 20 ejaculations are required for the ejaculate to become free of sperm. Therefore, use of another contraceptive method is necessary until azoospermia is confirmed.

Tubal Ligation

Despite some sterilization failures with tubal ligation, it remains among the best methods of long-term contraception. Overall failure rates are 0.5% at 1 year and approximately 1.8% at 10 years (77). The major complication rate is approximately 4 per 1,000. The complications are bleeding, infection, and bowel, bladder, or uterine trauma.

Patient Experience. Laparoscopy or minilaparotomy in the United States is usually performed with the use of general anesthesia. Uncomplicated tubal ligation is usually performed as an outpatient procedure and is very well tolerated. Mild abdominal discomfort, when present, usually lasts for only a few days, or rarely for a few weeks. Mild analgesics (e.g., acetaminophen) provide relief. The woman typically is able to return to her usual activities in 48 to 72 hours. Sterilization is immediate, and intercourse is permitted as soon as the wound is no longer painful. More recently, a transcervical sterilization technique (Essure) in which tiny nickel-titanium metal coils with polyethylene fibers are inserted into the fallopian tubes hysteroscopically, has become available. Over the next several months after insertion, subsequent growth of local tissue allows scar formation that causes tubal occlusion. Currently, the FDA recommends that women who undergo the Essure method of sterilization continue an alternate form of birth control for the first 3 months after coil placement, at which time a hysterosalpingogram should be performed to confirm tubal occlusion.

Tubal ligation is ideally performed in the first half of the menstrual cycle before ovulation has occurred. This avoids the possibility of fertilization of an ovum occurring a day or two before the surgical procedure. If the woman is using effective contraception, tubal ligation may be performed at any time.

The existence of a posttubal syndrome, characterized by heavier menstrual bleeding and more pelvic pain than in the unsterilized population, has been questioned. After sterilization, most women notice no significant change in symptoms associated with their menstrual periods.

EMERGENCY CONTRACEPTION

Emergency contraception describes the use of a contraceptive method after intercourse to prevent pregnancy. This name is preferred to "morning-after pill," which suggests a very brief window of potential use after unprotected intercourse. Emergency contraception is indicated after intercourse without a method, current method failure (e.g., condom rupture), or rape. Access to emergency contraception can be increased by providing a patient with instructions and a prescription during a routine office visit or by making patients aware of how to access it urgently (1-888-NOT-2-LATE or www.not-2-late.com). Emergency contraception should *not* be used if a pregnancy test is positive.

Insertion of a copper IUD, possible up to 5 days following unprotected intercourse, is the most effective form of emergency contraception, with a pregnancy rate of approximately 0.1 per 100 women. Oral contraceptives are also highly effective as emergency contraceptive measures and are used up to 72 hours following unprotected sex. Progestin-only methods are better tolerated and more effective than combination pills, with pregnancy rates of 1.1% and 3.2%, respectively (78). Emergency contraception is ineffective at disrupting an already established pregnancy.

Method Use

Currently available methods of emergency contraception include COC pills or the copper IUD. There are many possible combinations of oral contraceptives that have been shown to be effective. Plan B, a progestin-only dedicated product contains two tablets of 0.75 mg levonorgestrel. Product labeling instructs that the first dose is taken within 72 hours (earlier administration increases effectiveness), and then repeated (second dose) 12 hours later. However, a large randomized trial shows that a single dose of 1.5 mg is as effective as two separate doses of 0.75 mg (79). Additionally, emergency oral contraception has been shown to have efficacy up to 120 hours after intercourse, although the efficacy is reduced the longer the time delay (79). Neither a pelvic examination nor blood pressure measurement (asymptomatic women) is necessary before providing the method. The IUD can be inserted up to 5 days after unprotected intercourse.

Pregnancy testing is unnecessary before emergency contraception unless there is information to suggest that conception already occurred in a previous cycle. A woman should return for pregnancy testing if she does not get her menses within 3 to 4 weeks after taking emergency contraception. Women given emergency contraception should also receive counseling to help them choose an appropriate method for ongoing contraception.

CONTRACEPTION IN SPECIAL CIRCUMSTANCES

During the time leading up to the menopause, a woman's concern regarding unplanned pregnancy is heightened by abnormal menstrual cycles and episodes of amenorrhea. Although fertility declines with age, missing a period is disturbing to a woman in the perimenopause unless a very reliable method of contraception is being used. Some methods are particularly advantageous to women in the perimenopause.

The postpartum woman needs help in getting back on a contraceptive program, and usually her obstetrician has given her advice in this regard. Also, the woman wishing to use an IUD needs to wait for involution of the uterus—which usually occurs 4 to 6 weeks after delivery—and therefore is at risk for pregnancy until the IUD is inserted. The physiology of the female reproductive cycle, important to an understanding of the many contraceptive methods, is discussed in Chapter 101.

DIAGNOSING PREGNANCY

Human chorionic gonadotropin (hCG) is a glycoprotein hormone that is produced by the blastocyst and the placenta. Its secretion begins very early and can be detected in the maternal blood as early as 6 days after fertilization. Its concentration in serum approximately doubles every 48 hours during the first 10 weeks of a normal pregnancy. In the past, a number of conditions could give rise to a false positive result, such as the presence of foreign protein or cross-reaction with the luteinizing hormone (LH), follicle-stimulating hormone (FSH), and thyroid-stimulating hormone (TSH). The α-subunit for hCG is common to all of these hormones. However, the β-subunit for hCG is unique, and the currently available pregnancy tests that use the monoclonal antibody methodology test only for the β-subunit. A false-positive reaction, even with home pregnancy detection kits, is extremely rare. There are four major types of pregnancy tests, each with its own characteristics; all are very accurate. The Icon, an enzyme-linked immunoassay, is the most commonly used test because of its simplicity, accuracy, and availability. Any clinician who may be asked to diagnose pregnancy should have a rapid pregnancy diagnosing kit in the office. There is no clinical situation in which one of these tests has a distinct advantage over another.

Radioimmunoassay

The radioimmunoassays are performed on serum samples. Tests include Chorion Quant, Beta Tec, and HCG Beta III. Their features are as follows:

- Accurate (almost 100% accuracy for positive result in normal pregnancy) when used at least 7 days after conception
- No LH cross-reaction
- Specific for hCG (detects the β-subunit)
- Used for assessing abnormal pregnancy (ectopic, molar, threatened abortion)
- Requires that the specimen be sent to a laboratory, and the typical turnaround time is 1 day

Enzyme-Linked Immunoassay

The enzyme-linked immunoassay tests (Icon, Confidot, Quest) are performed on urine or serum. Their features are as follows:

- Accurate when used at least 12 days after conception
- No LH cross-reaction
- Specific for hCG (detects the β-subunit)
- Used for routine pregnancy confirmation
- Easy to use, and results are available in a few minutes

Radioreceptor Assay

The radioreceptor assay pregnancy test (Biocept-G) is performed on serum. It has the following features:

- Accurate when used at least 14 days after conception
- LH cross-reaction possible
- Used for early confirmation of normal pregnancy
- Specimen usually is sent to a laboratory, and the turnaround time is typically 1 day

Immunoassay

The immunoassays (Neocept, Pregnosis) are performed on urine or serum. Their features are as follows:

- Accurate when used at least 28 days after conception
- LH cross-reaction possible
- Used for routine pregnancy confirmation
- Serum assay usually is sent to a laboratory, but urine assay can be done in the office

The biological half-life of hCG is approximately 1.5 days. The serum hCG result becomes negative approximately 9 to 13 days after spontaneous abortion, if all trophoblastic tissue is expelled (80). The hCG test may remain positive for weeks to months if small foci of functioning trophoblastic tissue remain. This could be seen after incomplete abortion, persistent hydatidiform mole, or choriocarcinoma.

UNPLANNED PREGNANCY

All contraceptive methods are associated with some failures, which may result in an *unplanned pregnancy*. Women with such a pregnancy are faced with the difficult decision of whether to carry or to terminate the pregnancy. Estimates are that almost 50% of the approximately 4 million births in the United States in 1992 were unplanned.

Currently, about 1.5 million *therapeutic abortions* are performed each year in the United States. The usual method of early termination of pregnancy in the United States is a surgical suction dilation and curettage performed in an outpatient center, free-standing clinic, or obstetrician's office, usually with the patient under local anesthesia. The *antiprogesterone compound*, mifepristone, was approved in 2000 for use in conjunction with misoprostol for the medical termination of early pregnancy. The current FDA-approved regimen provides 600 mg of mifepristone orally on day 1, followed on day 3 by 400 μg of misoprostol given orally in the provider's office.

PRECONCEPTION CARE

A variety of medical conditions, occupational situations, and social practices have consequences on early pregnancy. Because organogenesis begins about 17 days after conception, whereas traditional prenatal care may not commence for several weeks thereafter, there is ample reason to provide preconception care in an effort to optimize a woman's medical, social, and emotional readiness for pregnancy.

Preconception care should include a thorough history, a targeted physical examination, focused laboratory investigations, and specified counseling. The couple should be interviewed regarding family and genetic history, with appropriate carrier screening for inheritable conditions such as hemoglobinopathies, Tay-Sachs disease, or cystic fibrosis, among others. Existing medical conditions should be reviewed and medical therapy optimized, especially for patients with diabetes mellitus or hypertension. Women should discontinue, or be offered alternatives to, drugs known to be contraindicated in pregnancy, such as isotretinoin or Coumadin. Infectious disease risks should be assessed (e.g., rubella, hepatitis B, HIV), and, if appropriate, vaccines should be offered for rubella varicella, and hepatitis B. Additionally, screening should be offered for sexually transmitted diseases such as chlamydia, gonorrhea, and syphilis. Nutrition and eating habits should be evaluated. Although a multivitamin may be suggested, megavitamin supplementation should be avoided. Evidence suggests that daily intake of 0.4 mg of folic acid before conception significantly reduces the risk of neural tube defects.

Finally, a review of a couple's social readiness for pregnancy can help them focus on the upcoming responsibilities of pregnancy and childcare. Social habits of smoking and alcohol intake should be curtailed, and providers should take the opportunity to motivate substance abusers to seek counseling. Patients should consider domestic and economic readiness for pregnancy, and they should know their employer's policy regarding leave benefits for complicated and uncomplicated pregnancies (81).

SPECIFIC REFERENCES*

1. Mosher WD, Gladys MM, Chandra A, et al. Use of contraception and use of family planning services in the United States: 1982–2002. Adv Dat 2004;350:1.
2. Stewart FH, Harper CC, Ellertson CE, et al. Clinical breast and pelvic examination requirements for hormonal contraception: current practice vs evidence. JAMA 2001;285:2232.
3. Durand JL, Bressler R. Clinical pharmacology of the steroidal oral contraceptives. Adv Intern Med 1979;24:97.
4. Westhoff C, Kerns J, Morroni C, et al. Quick Start: a novel oral contraceptive initiation method. Contraception 2002;66:141.
5. Layde PM, McCarthy PS, Lord JAH, Smith CFC. Incidence of arterial disease among oral contraceptive users: Royal College of General Practitioners Oral Contraceptive Study. J R Coll Gen Pract 1983;33:75.
6. Stadel BV. Oral contraceptives and cardiovascular disease (two parts). N Engl J Med 1981;305:612, 672.
7. Vandenbroucke JP, Helmerhorst FM, Bloemenkamp KWM, et al. Third-generation oral contraceptive and deep venous thrombosis: from epidemiologic controversy to new insight in coagulation. Am J Obstet Gynecol 1997;177:887.
8. World Health Organization. Cardiovascular Disease and steroid hormone contraception: Report of a WHO Scientific group. Technical Report Series 877,1998:i-89.
9. Hannaford PC, Croft PR, Kay CR. Oral contraception and stroke: evidence from the Royal College of General Practitioners' Oral Contraception Study. Stroke 1994;25:935.

*Bold numerals denote published controlled clinical trials, meta-analyses, or consensus-based recommendations.

10. Lowe GDO, Greer IA, Cooke TG, et al. Risk of and prophylaxis for venous thromboembolism in hospital patients. BMJ 1992;305:567.
11. World Health Organization. Medical eligibility criteria for contraceptive use. 3rd ed. Geneva: WHO, 2004.
12. Vandenbroucke JP, Koster T, Briet E, et al. Increased risk of venous thrombosis in oral-contraceptive users who are carriers of factor V Leiden mutation. Lancet 1994;334:1453.
13. Vandenbroucke JP, van der Meer FJ, Helmerhorst FM, et al. Factor V Leiden: should we screen oral contraceptive users and pregnant women? BMJ 1996;33:1127.
14. Robinson GE, Burren T, Mackie IJ, et al. Changes in haemostasis after stopping the combined contraceptive pill: implications for major surgery. BMJ (Clin Res Ed) 1986;292:526.
15. Bonnar J. Can more be done in obstetrics and gynecologic practice to reduce morbidity and mortality associated with venous thromboembolism? Am J Obstet Gynecol 1999;180:784.
16. Coagulation and thrombosis with OC use: physiology and clinical relevance. Dialogues in Contraception. Little Falls, NJ: Health Learning Systems, 1996.
17. Edmondson HA, Henderson B, Benton B. Liver-cell adenomas associated with use of oral contraceptives. N Engl J Med 1976;294:470.
18. Centers for Disease Control. Cancer and steroid hormone study: oral contraceptive use and ovarian cancer. JAMA 1983;249:1596.
19. Hankinson SE, Colditz GA, Hunter DJ, et al. A quantitative assessment of oral contraceptive use and risk of ovarian cancer. Obstet Gynecol 1992;80:708.
20. The Cancer and Steroid Hormone Study of the Centers for Disease Control and the National Institute of Child Health and Human Development. The reduction in risk of ovarian cancer associated with oral-contraceptive use. N Engl J Med 1987;316:650.
21. Narod SA, Risch H, Moslehi R, et al. Oral contraceptive use and the risk of hereditary ovarian cancer. Hereditary Ovarian Cancer Clinical Study Group. N Engl J Med 1998;339:424.
22. Combination oral contraceptive use and the risk of endometrial cancer. The Cancer and Steroid Hormone Study of the Centers for Disease Control and the National Institute of Child Health and Human Development JAMA 1987;257:796.
23. Schlesselman JJ. Risk of endometrial cancer in relation to use of combined oral contraceptives: a practitioner's guide to meta-analysis. Hum Reprod 1997;12:1851.
24. Brinton LA, Huggins GR, Lehman HF, et al. Long term use of oral contraceptives and risk of invasive cervical cancer. Int J Cancer 1986;38:339.
25. Moreno V, Bosch FX, Munoz N, et al. Effect of oral contraceptives on risk of cervical cancer in women with human papillomavirus infection: the IARC multicentric case-control study. Lancet 2002;359:1093.
26. Smith JS, Green J, Berrington de Gonzalez A, et al. Cervical cancer and use of hormonal contraceptives: a systematic review. Lancet 2003;361:1159.
27. Skegg DC. Oral contraceptives, parity, and cervical cancer. Lancet 2002;359:1080.
28. Rosenberg L, Palmer JR, Clarke EA, et al. A case-control study of the risk of breast cancer in relation to oral contraceptive use. Am J Epidemiol 1992;136:1437.
29. Collaborative Group on Hormonal Factors in Breast Cancer. Breast cancer and hormonal contraceptives: collaborative reanalysis of individual data on 53,297 women with breast cancer and 100,239 women without breast cancer from 54 epidemiological studies. Lancet 1996;347:1713.
30. Dumeaux V, Alsaker E, Lunde E. Breast cancer and specific types of oral contraceptives: a large Norwegian cohort study. Int J Cancer 2003;105:844.
31. Krauss RM, Burkman RT. The metabolic impact of oral contraceptives. Am J Obstet Gynecol 1992;167:1177.
32. Petitti DB, Sidney S, Bernstein A, et al. Stroke in users of low-dose oral contraceptives. N Engl J Med 1996;335:8.
33. Allais G, DeLorenzo C, Mana O, et al. Oral contraceptives in women with migraines: balancing risks and benefits. Neurol Sci 2004;Suppl 3:S211.
34. Committee on Gynecologic Practice. Contraceptives and congenital anomalies: ACOG committee opinion no. 124, July 1993. Int J Gynecol Obstet 1993;42:316.
35. Linn S, Schoenbaum SC, Monson RR, et al. Lack of association between contraceptive usage and congenital malformation of offspring. Am J Obstet Gynecol 1983;147:923.
36. Galo MF, Grimes DA, Schulz KF, et al. Combination estrogen-progestin contraceptives and body weight: systematic review of randomized controlled trials. Obstet Gynecol 2004;103:359.
37. Effect of oral contraceptives in laboratory test results. Med Lett Drugs Ther 1979;21:54.
38. Dickinson BD, Altman RD, Nielsen NH, et al. Drug interactions between oral contraceptives and antibiotics. Obstet Gynecol 2001;98: 853.
39. Abrams LS, Skee DM, Natarajan J, et al. Multiple-dose pharmacokinetics of a contraceptive patch in healthy women participants. Contraception. 2001;64:287.
40. Audet MC, Moreau M, Koltun WD, et al. Evaluation of contraceptive efficacy and cycle control of a transdermal contraceptive patch vs an oral contraceptive: a randomized controlled trial. JAMA 2001;285:2347.
41. Smallwood GH, Meador ML, Lenihan JP, et al. Efficacy and safety of a transdermal contraceptive system. Obstet Gynecol 2001;98: 799.
42. Zieman M, Guillebaud J, Weisberg G, et al. Contraceptive efficacy and cycle control with the Ortho Evra/Evra transdermal system: the analysis of pooled data. Fertil Steril 2002;77:S13.
43. Holt VL, Cushing-Haugen KL, Daling JR. Body weight and risk of oral contraceptive failure. Obstet Gynecol 2002;99:820.
44. Timmer CJ, Mulders TM. Pharmacokinetics of etonogestrel and ethinylestradiol released from a combined contraceptive vaginal ring. Clin Pharmacokinet 2000;39:233.
45. Verhoeven CH, Dieben TO. The combined contraceptive vaginal ring, NuvaRing, and tampon co-usage. Contraception 2004;69:197.
46. Verhoeven CH, van den Heuvel MW, Mulders TM, et al. The contraceptive vaginal ring, NuvaRing, and antimycotic co-medication. Contraception 2004;69:129.
47. Haring T, Mulders TM. The combined contraceptive ring NuvaRing and spermicide co-medication. Contraception 2003;67:271.
48. Dieben TO, Roumen FJ, Apter D. Efficacy, cycle control, and user acceptability of a novel combined contraceptive vaginal ring. Obstet Gynecol 2002;100:585.
49. Belsey EM. Vaginal bleeding patterns among women using one natural and eight hormonal methods of contraception. Contraception 1988;38:181.
50. Pelkman CL, Chow M, Heinbach RA, et al. Short-term effects of a progestational contraceptive drug on food intake, resting energy expenditure, and body weight in young women. Am J Clin Nutr 2001;73:19.
51. Kaunitz AM. Depo-provera's black box: time to reconsider? Contraception 2005;72:165.
52. "Black box" warning added to contraceptive injection. FDA Consum 2005;39:3.
53. WHO statement on hormonal contraception and bone health. WHO Epidemiologic record No. 35, September 2005.
54. Hall PE. New once a month injectable contraceptives, with particular reference to Cyclofem/Cyclo-provera. Int J Gynaecol Obstet 1998;62[Suppl 1]:S43.
55. Dunson TR, Blumental PD, Alvarez F, et al. Timing of onset of contraceptive effectiveness in Norplant implant users. Part I. Changes in cervical mucus. Fertil Steril 1998;69:258.
56. Huber J. Pharmacokinetics of Implanon: An integrated analysis. Contraception 1998:58; 85S.
57. Buckshee K, Chatterjee P, Dhall GI, et al. Return of fertility following discontinuation of Norplant-II subdermal implants. ICMR Task Force on Hormonal Contraception. Contraception 1995: 51;237.
58. Shoupe D, Mishell DR Jr, Bopp BL, et al. The significance of bleeding patterns in Norplant implant users. Obstet Gynecol 1991: 77;256.
59. Klavon SL, Grubb GS. Insertion site complications during the first year of Norplant use. Contraception 1990: 41;27.
60. Gu S, Sivin I, Du M, et al. Effectiveness of Norplant implants through seven years: A large-scale study in China. Contraception 1995: 52;99.
61. Sivin I, Mishell DR, Diaz S, et al. Prolonged effectiveness of Norplant capsule implants: a 7-year study. Contraception 2000: 61;187.
62. Herjan JT, Bennink HC. Introduction. Presentation of clinical data on Implanon. Contraception 1998: 58;75S.
63. Population Information Program. Population reports: intrauterine devices. IUDs: a new look. Series B, No. 5. Baltimore: Johns Hopkins University, 1988.
64. Luukkainen T, Toivonen J. Levonorgestrel-releasing IUD as a method of contraception with therapeutic properties. Contraception 1995;52:269.
65. Burkman RT. The Woman's Health Study: association between intrauterine device and pelvic inflammatory disease. Obstet Gynecol 1981;57:269.
66. Hubacher D, Lara-Ricalde R, Taylor DJ, et al. Use of copper intrauterine devices and the risk of tubal infertility among nulligravid women. N Engl J Med 2001;345:561.
67. Grimes DA, Schulz KF. Prophylactic antibiotics for intrauterine device insertion: a metaanalysis of the randomized controlled trials. Contraception 1999;68:57.
68. Pakarinen PI, Suvisaari J, Luukkainen T, et al. Intracervical and fundal administration of levonorgestrel for contraception: endometrial thickness, patterns of bleeding and persisting ovarian follicles. Fertil Steril 1997;68:59.
69. Luukkainen T, Allonen H, Haukkamaa M, et al. Effective contraception with the levonorgestrel-releasing intrauterine device: 12-month report of a European multicenter study. Contraception 1987;36:169.
70. Association of Reproductive Health Professionals. New Developments in Intrauterine Contraception. ARHP Clinical Proceedings: September 2004.
71. Farley TM, Rosenberg MJ, Rowe PJ, et al. Intrauterine devices and pelvic inflammatory disease: an international perspective. Lancet 1992;339:785.
72. The female condom. Med Lett Drugs Ther 1993; 35:123.
73. Wilcox AJ, Weinberg CR, Baird DD. Timing of sexual intercourse in relation to ovulation. N Engl J Med 1995;333:1517.

74. Massey FJ Jr, Bernstein GS, O'Fallon WN, et al. Vasectomy and health: results from a large cohort study. JAMA 1984;252:1023.
75. Moller H, Knudsen LB, Lynge E. Risk of testicular cancer after vasectomy: cohort study of over 73,000 men. BMJ 1994;309:295.
76. Cox B, Sneyd MJ, Paul C, et al. Vasectomy and risk of prostate cancer. JAMA 2002;287:3110.
77. Peterson HB, Xia Z, Hughes JM, et al. The risk of pregnancy after tubal sterilization: findings from the U.S. Collaborative Review of Sterilization. Am J Obstet Gynecol 1996;174:1161.
78. Task Force on Postovulatory Methods of Fertility Regulation. Randomised controlled trial of levonorgestrel versus the Yuzpe regimen of combined oral contraceptives for emergency contraception. Lancet 1998;352:428.
79. von Hertzen H, Piaggio G, Ding J, et al. Low dose mifepristone and two regimens of levonorgestrel for emergency contraception; a WHO multicentre randomized trial. Lancet 2002;360:1803.
80. Steier JA, Bergsjo P, Myking OL. Human chorionic gonadotropin in maternal plasma after induced abortion, spontaneous abortion, and removed ectopic pregnancy. Obstet Gynecol 1984;64:391.
81. American College of Obstetrics and Gynecology. The importance of preconception care in the continuum of women's health care. ACOG Committee Opinion no. 212. Washington, DC: ACOG, September 2005.

*For annotated **General References** and resources related to this chapter, visit www.hopkinsbayview.org/PAMreferences.*

Chapter 101

Menstrual Disorders and Other Disorders of Female Reproductive Endocrinology

Meredith B. Loveless and Shehzad Basaria

A normal menstrual cycle in a woman of reproductive age is an indicator of health. Absent or abnormal menses is not only a source of discomfort and anxiety but may also signify pathology in a wide variety of organ systems. Because there are a myriad of causes of abnormal vaginal bleeding, it is helpful to think of relevant etiologies during the various stages of a woman's reproductive life. This chapter reviews the evaluation and management of common menstrual disorders by age group to guide clinical care.

FEMALE REPRODUCTIVE PHYSIOLOGY

The female menstrual cycle is a complex milieu of hormonal functions that establish the normal menstrual pattern. Maturation of the hypothalamic–pituitary axis is required for normal menstrual function. The pulsatile release of gonadotropin releasing hormone (GnRH) from the hypothalamus causes the gonadotropins, luteinizing hormone (LH) and follicle-stimulating hormone (FSH), to be secreted from the pituitary. Under the influence of FSH multiple follicles in the ovary are stimulated. This stimulation causes follicular granulosa cells to increase the number of FSH receptors, and release estrogen and convert

lowers free testosterone and SHBG levels in patients with insulin-resistant PCOS suggests that the insulin resistance may be the underlying cause of the gonadal dysregulation (23). Indeed, a unique insulin receptor defect has been identified in approximately 50% of women with PCOS (18).

The clinical concerns with this process are anovulation and the effects of chronic androgen stimulation. Women with this disorder are classically obese with some degree of hirsutism and acne, although this is not always true. The usual presentation is a complaint of oligomenorrhea or amenorrhea (80%), primary infertility or hirsutism. The most consistent endocrine feature is ovarian hyperandrogenism. Increased LH/FSH secretion and mild hyperprolactinemia may also be present. Diagnostic evaluation should include a detailed history and physical examination with particular attention paid to the degree and distribution of hair, signs of virilization, and presence of acanthosis nigricans (a marker of insulin resistance). A history of sleep apnea should be sought since its prevalence is much higher in women with PCOS compared to age and body mass index (BMI)-matched controls (20).

Studies of patients with PCOS suggest that there are two etiologically distinct subpopulations (24). In approximately 50% of patients, hyperandrogenism is accompanied by carbohydrate intolerance and increased levels of insulin and insulin-like growth factor-1 (IGF-1) (25). These insulin-resistant patients tend to be more obese, have a greater waist-to-hip ratio, are more hirsute, and have higher levels of plasma testosterone and lower levels of SHBG. In contrast, the non–insulin resistant patients have higher LH/FSH ratios than insulin-resistant patients, suggesting that the primary problem in this group involves GnRH regulation.

Laboratory Evaluation

The goals of laboratory evaluation are to assess hyperandrogenism and insulin resistance. Screening tests should include testosterone, free testosterone, SHBG, DHEAS, prolactin, and TSH. Tests to exclude other causes of anovulation and hirsutism should include measuring 24-hour urine free cortisol, 17-OH progesterone, and serum IGF-1. These tests are performed by most commercial laboratories (see Chapter 81). To screen for metabolic complications, fasting levels of glucose, insulin, and lipid profile should be checked. In patients with a history of sleep apnea, polysomnography should be performed. These women should also be referred to gynecologists for evaluation of endometrial thickness, since both endometrial hyperplasia and carcinoma are more common in women with PCOS.

Treatment

Therapeutic options depend on the patient's symptoms and her desire for fertility.

Hirsutism

If hirsutism is mild, mechanical methods of shaving and plucking should be encouraged. For women with moderate to severe hirsutism, the choices include oral contraceptives and anti-androgens. Oral contraceptives suppress LH levels, hence reducing stimulation of theca cells. Furthermore, they also increase SHBG production in the liver, resulting in decreased free testosterone levels. Among anti-androgens, cyproterone acetate has been very effective. It suppresses LH levels due to its progestin component and also prevents the binding of testosterone to its receptor. Cyproterone acetate, however, is not available in the United States. In a recent study, a novel estrogen-progestin combination was used in the treatment of hirsutism in women with PCOS (26). The combination included ethinyl estradiol (30 μg) and drospirenone (3 mg) (Yasmin). Drospirenone is a progestin with a strong antimineralocorticoid activity. There was a significant decrease in the levels of both ovarian and adrenal androgens and the subjects showed a significant improvement in hirsutism scores. Spironolactone in doses of 100 to 200 mg daily also antagonizes the binding of testosterone to the androgen receptor and is commonly used in the United States. It should not be given to women with PCOS who desire fertility (because of its anti-androgen effect on the fetus). Recently, finasteride (Proscar) (a 5α-reductase inhibitor) has also shown some promise. By inhibiting this enzyme, finasteride decreases the formation of dihydrotestosterone (DHT), the active metabolite of testosterone.

Anovulation and Infertility

Life-style modification with diet and exercise is fundamental since weight loss itself may lead to spontaneous ovulation. This should always be attempted first for at least 3 to 6 months. Treatment with insulin sensitizers like metformin (Glucophage) and thiazolidinediones (Avandia, Actos) have resulted in resumption of ovulation and improvement in hirsutism scores by improving insulin sensitivity. In addition to improving insulin sensitivity, metformin also directly inhibits ovarian steroidogenesis (27). Metformin dose is gradually maximized to 1000 mg twice daily to avoid GI side effects. The patients should be counseled that at least 6 months of therapy may be needed before any benefits are noticed. If the patient remains anovulatory, clomiphene (alone or in combination with metformin) or gonadotropins may be useful to induce ovulation. Referral to a reproductive endocrinologist is indicated if the patient desires pregnancy.

Even if fertility is not immediately desired, the danger of unopposed estrogen secretion must be addressed. Women who have had an abnormal bleeding pattern for longer than 1 year should be referred to a gynecologist for endometrial biopsy to rule out endometrial hyperplasia or malignancy. Patients diagnosed in adolescence or in their early twenties with this disorder and those who have had 6 months or less of amenorrhea may benefit from a course of MPA (Provera), 10 mg daily for 10 to 12 days, to induce a withdrawal bleed and restore secretory endometrium. After this initial treatment, maintenance is best achieved with the use of combined OCs with low estrogen analog content for continuous ovarian suppression and also for contraception, since ovulatory cycles may occur after progesterone withdrawal (see Chapter 100).

As noted, these patients tend to have impaired glucose metabolism, increased lipid levels, and a tendency to be overweight, which puts them at increased risk for diabetes and cardiovascular disease. Combination OCs may improve lipid profile, although weight control has been demonstrated to be the most beneficial factor for preventing chronic disease. Therefore, patients should be counseled on lifestyle and cardiac risk reduction for the rest of their lives (see Chapter 79).

Secondary Amenorrhea

Secondary amenorrhea is diagnosed in women with previously normal cycles who have had no menses for a total of 6 months or have missed the equivalent of three previous cycle intervals. There are many causes for this condition, although one of the most prevalent and most easily diagnosed is pregnancy, which must be ruled out before proceeding with the workup (Fig. 101.1). Feminized patients with *central secondary amenorrhea* may have a brain tumor or anorexia nervosa, but most commonly they have hypothalamic amenorrhea. Although this can have an *exogenous* cause (see later discussion), it is often idiopathic with no explanation even after thorough examination. Pituitary amenorrhea is usually *acquired* and is often accompanied by deficiencies in other hormone axes (adrenal, thyroid).

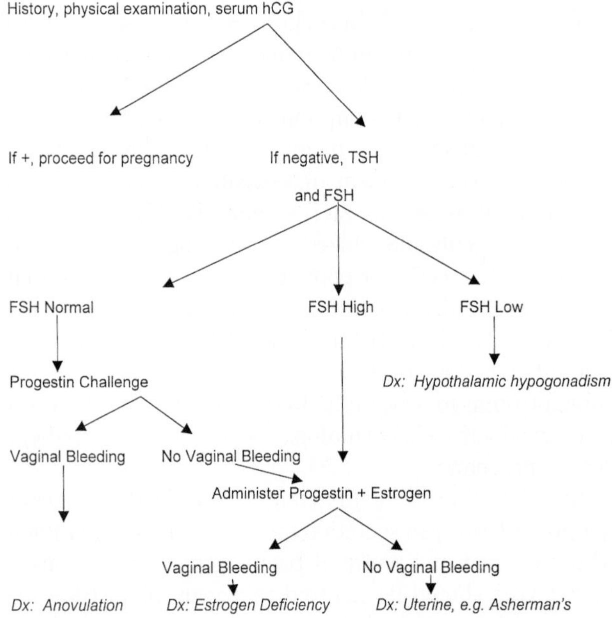

FIGURE 101.1. Approach to secondary amenorrhea.

The term *gonadal secondary amenorrhea* refers to loss of function of the ovary itself after puberty. This can be caused by infection (e.g., tuberculosis), neoplasm (e.g., Krukenberg tumor—metastasis of a GI neoplasm to an ovary), trauma, surgery, or an autoimmune disorder. The latter category is often associated with a syndrome of polyglandular failure that may include disorders of the thyroid (Hashimoto thyroiditis) and adrenal (primary Addison disease), type 1 DM, and, rarely, autoimmune hypophysitis (28). Autoimmune ovarian failure is the most common cause of idiopathic premature menopause.

Exogenous amenorrhea can be caused by other systemic disease, such as hyperthyroidism or hypothyroidism, liver failure, renal failure, or other nonendocrine illness. *Hypothalamic (secondary, central, acquired) amenorrhea* is also often *exogenous* in that there is a proximate cause, such as weight loss (especially in anorexia nervosa), pathologic obesity, vigorous exercise (e.g., runners, ballet dancers), or severe stress, as in grief reactions or mental illness. Another form of *exogenous* interruption of menses may result from consumption of substances of abuse (opiates, alcohol) or prescribed medications (major tranquilizers, estrogens).

Serum or urinary gonadotropins are used to classify hypogonadism as *gonadal* (LH and FSH elevated) or *central* (LH and FSH low or normal). The investigation of central hypogonadism should include a serum prolactin level, especially if galactorrhea is present. Prolactin values between 30 and 100 ng/mL are elevated and are consistent with a prolactinoma, but they may be related to other causes such as hypothalamic (idiopathic) galactorrhea or drug effects. Values greater than 100 ng/mL almost always mean that a prolactinoma is present. Appropriate specialists should undertake further testing which is similar to that outlined for patients with male hypogonadism (see Chapter 85). If hirsutism is present, the serum testosterone and 17-hydroxyprogesterone (17-OHP) levels should be checked (see Hirsutism).

If TSH, FSH, and prolactin levels are normal, a *progestin challenge* should be done to evaluate estrogen production. A progestin challenge is done by prescribing oral MPA (Provera), 10 mg once a day for 7 days. Patients usually bleed 2 to 7 days after the last pill, although sometimes ovulation is triggered and they do not bleed until 14 days later. If the patient bleeds in response to progestin, then the diagnosis is anovulation. The underlying cause of anovulation should then be sought (e.g., stress, weight loss, anorexia, PCOS).

Patients who do not respond to progesterone challenge should be assessed for cessation of estrogen production with a combined estrogen plus progestin challenge (OCs). If the patient bleeds, then the problem is that she does not produce estrogen (as seen in gonadal secondary amenorrhea). The history is important in making the differential diagnosis and will implicate possible underlying causes as well as identify women in whom early menopause follows a clearly familial pattern. When the diagnosis is made in women who are younger than 30 years of age, a karyotype should be performed to exclude gonadal dysgenesis. Among the remainder, precise distinction between autoimmune and idiopathic causes is difficult. All patients with premenopausal estrogen deficiency should be screened periodically for evidence of associated autoimmune endocrinopathy affecting the adrenal, parathyroid, and thyroid glands and the gastric parietal cells (28). These patients are essentially menopausal and must be given hormone replacement therapy for bone protective effects (see Chapter 106). Future fertility is not possible from a native oocyte, although the patient may be referred to a reproductive endocrinologist to explore options of oocyte donation.

If the FSH is low or normal, then the diagnosis is hypothalamic amenorrhea. This is not common but is easily treated. Usually it is caused by stress or weight loss, although a head CT should be obtained to rule out a brain tumor, and the diagnosis of other rare central nervous system disorders should be entertained. This group is characterized by deficient gonadotropin secretion and mimics the endocrine state of the prepubertal girl. The low gonadotropin levels are not necessarily lower than those seen during parts of the normal cycle (particularly the luteal phase) and are of significance only in the context of concurrent diminished ovarian function. When fully expressed, these disorders are markedly hypoestrogenic: withdrawal bleeding does not occur after challenge with a progestational agent. Vasomotor symptoms such as hot flushes and night sweats may be present.

The differential diagnosis of hypothalamic amenorrhea includes conditions associated with destruction of hypothalamic and pituitary tissue such as ischemic necrosis (Sheehan syndrome), head trauma, and neoplasms such as craniopharyngioma and pituitary adenoma. Evaluation should consider both destructive and functional origins of hypogonadotropism through a careful history, physical examination, and, if a functional or nutritional cause is not evident, imaging of the pituitary and juxtapituitary structures. One of the more common intracranial lesions in women is a pituitary microadenoma or macroadenoma, which may be treated with bromocriptine and monitored with prolactin levels and imaging (see Chapter 81). Imaging of the sella turcica and determination of the prolactin level should be repeated annually to rule out or monitor pituitary adenoma, with the possibility of increasing this interval to every 2 to 3 years if results are stable for several years. Because all of these patients are hypoestrogenic and anovulatory, estrogen replacement must be prescribed (either combined OCs or hormone replacement therapy) and the patient reassured that ovulation induction is possible with GnRH analog injections when conception is desired. Treatment is given to remove the cause, restore normal menstrual function, or replace hormones. Patients desiring fertility will not respond to clomiphene and must be treated with gonadotropins for ovulation induction.

A history of dilatation and curettage suggests a uterine cause for secondary amenorrhea. If no bleeding occurred with the combined estrogen/progesterone challenge, a uterine problem such as Asherman syndrome is indicated. A hysterosalpingogram or hysteroscopy will show intrauterine adhesions (Asherman syndrome). This diagnosis is usually suspected with a history of postpartum hemorrhage or menorrhagia that required a dilatation and curettage. The treatment consists of resection of the adhesions, treatment with estrogens for several weeks postoperatively, and re-evaluation with a hysterosalpingogram. Successful pregnancies are achieved in 60% to 85% of patients, although they are at higher risk of abnormal placentation.

Menorrhagia or Intermenstrual Bleeding

Abnormal uterine bleeding (AUB) is a diagnosis of exclusion. Women presenting with menorrhagia or metrorrhagia need to be evaluated for organic, systemic, and iatrogenic causes for their abnormal bleeding (Table 101.2).

TABLE 101.2 Causes of Abnormal Vaginal Bleeding in a Woman of Reproductive Age

Pregnancy
Local pathology
Leiomyoma
Endometrial polyp
Cervical polyp
Cervicitis
Endometritis
Malignancy
Foreign body
Systemic causes
Hypothyroidism
Hyperprolactinemia
Polycystic ovary syndrome
Coagulopathy
Medications
Phenothiazines
Isoniazid
Opiates
Tricyclic antidepressants
Metoclopramide
α-Adrenergic antihypertensives

Organic Causes

The most common causes for abnormal bleeding in the reproductive age group are accidents of pregnancy. Miscarriage and ectopic pregnancy should be evaluated by performing a β-hCG assay, as well as a pelvic ultrasound examination if indicated.

Prolonged excessive bleeding (menorrhagia) as a feature of otherwise normal cycles requires evaluation to exclude pathology affecting the endometrium. The most common reason is leiomyomas or "fibroids," which are a benign overgrowth of the smooth muscle that makes up the myometrium. Leiomyomas are present in up to 40% of women at the time of death (based on autopsy studies), are stimulated by estrogen, and typically become symptomatic in the age range of 30 to 40 years. A history of heavy, prolonged menses with possible clot passage and an enlarged, irregularly shaped uterus on pelvic examination suggests leiomyomas. In this circumstance, evaluation by an experienced examiner, endometrial biopsy in every patient older than 40 years of age, and imaging (pelvic ultrasound) are warranted to exclude another neoplasm masquerading as leiomyoma. Any patient with presumed leiomyomas exhibiting rapid uterine growth should be referred to a gynecologist for evaluation and hysterectomy, because leiomyomas do rarely undergo malignant degeneration (less than 1%). Leiomyomas may also undergo other types of degeneration (cystic, hemorrhagic), typically when blood supply is outgrown, and this may result in a significant amount of abdominal and pelvic pain. Additionally, large leiomyomas may cause other symptoms such as urinary frequency, constipation, and fullness in the lower abdomen.

Abnormal bleeding caused by leiomyomas may respond to hormonal management. Options include high-dose progestins (Depo-Provera, 150 mg or more, by intramuscular injection as frequently as monthly to control symptoms), OCs, or a GnRH agonist. GnRH agonists (leuprolide, goserelin, nafarelin) provide irreversible blockade of estrogen receptors and effectively induce a temporary menopausal state. The GnRH agonists are not options for long-term therapy and may only be used for 6 months because of risks of bone depletion and adversely affected lipid profiles that result from estrogen depletion. However, these medications are useful for decreasing the size of the uterus or allowing the resolution of anemia before surgery. Surgical options are hysterectomy or myomectomy, depending on the patient's preferences for future fertility. Uterine artery embolization through interventional radiology is a nonsurgical option in select patients. Patients who are asymptomatic or who are not anemic and refuse hormonal or surgical therapy may be observed, because these tumors usually decrease in size when the menopause is reached. Leiomyomas should not be considered a contraindication to hormone replacement therapy.

The cause of menorrhagia accompanying otherwise normal cycles in the presence of a normal pelvic examination can be submucous leiomyomas or endometrial polyps, which usually are revealed by ultrasound, especially if it is performed with fluid contrast in the endometrial canal (sonohysterography) (10). The etiology of endometrial polyps is unknown. Because polyps are often associated with endometrial hyperplasia, unopposed estrogen may be the cause. These polyps rarely bleed enough to cause a clinically significant anemia. Occasionally a pedunculated endometrial polyp protrudes through the external cervical os and can cause intermenstrual or postcoital bleeding. The rate of malignant transformation in an endometrial polyp has been estimated to be as high as 0.5%. However, a case-controlled study from Sweden estimated that the increased risk of endometrial cancer in women with endometrial polyps is only twofold (29). Malignant change in an endometrial polyp, when found, is often of a low stage and grade and usually curable. The management of endometrial polyps consists of resection via the hysteroscope and examination of the endometrial lining.

Cervical lesions such as cervical polyps or cervicitis may cause irregular bleeding, particularly postcoital spotting. These lesions can be diagnosed by visualization of the cervix. In addition, traumatic vaginal lesions, severe vaginal infections, and foreign bodies have been associated with abnormal bleeding. Similarly, infections of the upper genital tract, such as endometritis, have been associated with intermenstrual spotting and may even manifest as prolonged menses. Malignancies of any portion of the genital tract may manifest as abnormal bleeding, particularly cervical and endometrial cancer. Less commonly, vaginal, fallopian tube, and ovarian cancer may produce abnormal bleeding. Careful physical examination and evaluation with cervical cytology, endometrial sampling, and ultrasound, when indicated, help to establish the diagnosis.

Systemic Causes

Hypothyroidism is frequently associated with menorrhagia as well as with intermenstrual bleeding. The incidence of this disorder among women with menorrhagia is estimated to range between 0.3% to 2.5%. TSH should be measured and, if abnormal, appropriately treated (see Chapter 80). Although hyperthyroidism is not usually associated with menstrual abnormalities, hypomenorrhea, oligomenorrhea, and amenorrhea have been reported. Similarly, hyperprolactinemia and PCOS are most often associated with amenorrhea but can sometimes manifest as irregular menses.

Systemic disorders that produce abnormalities in coagulation or platelet abnormalities, such as von Willebrand disease, leukemia, severe sepsis, immune thrombocytopenic purpura, cirrhosis, and chronic renal disease, may all be associated with excessive or irregular bleeding (see Chapter 56).

Iatrogenic Causes

Foreign bodies in the uterus, such as an IUD, frequently produce abnormal uterine bleeding. Several medications may interfere with the neurotransmitters responsible for releasing and inhibiting hypothalamic hormones, resulting in anovulation and abnormal bleeding. Medications typically implicated are phenothiazines, isoniazid, opiates, metoclopramide, tricyclic antidepressants, and α-blockade antihypertensives. Exogenous hormones such as danazocrine and OCs or MPA can cause irregular bleeding.

Abnormal Uterine Bleeding

After organic, systemic, and iatrogenic causes for the abnormal bleeding are ruled out, the diagnosis of AUB can be made. Treatment is age dependent and should be tailored to the patient, after reviewing all of her options. For adolescents, either expectant management or OCs may be appropriate. AUB during the reproductive years can usually be well managed with OCs, including the 20-μg pill, or with cyclic progestins (see Chapter 100). OCs offer several advantages, including ease of use, predictable menses and contraceptive benefit. Cyclic progestins are a good option for women who cannot tolerate OCs and those in whom OCs are contraindicated. A low-dose progestin, such as MPA (Provera) 2.5 mg, may be given 12 days during every second or every third month. Another option for some patients is the use of a progestin IUD. AUB in women of late reproductive age to postmenopause can be treated with cyclic progestin, low-dose OCs, or cyclic combination hormone replacement. Treatment choice depends on the patient's symptoms and her need for contraception. Medical management generally offers excellent results for AUB management and should be the first line of treatment in the majority of cases. If medical management fails, surgical options include endometrial ablation, through a variety of techniques, or hysterectomy for definitive management.

Late Reproductive Age through Postmenopause: Greater than 45 Years

Perimenopause usually commences in the fifth decade, heralded by alterations in menstrual rhythm. Although the transition to the postmenopausal state can be brief and uncomplicated, the normal perimenopause is characterized in many women by the unpredictable occurrence of both shortened and lengthened ovulatory cycles as well as anovulatory episodes commencing well before menopause (30,31). The resulting menstrual chaos is a cause for inconvenience, frustration, and fear among affected women. It is in this age group that the term AUB is most commonly applied to the menstrual history. The clinician's focus must be to distinguish those patients whose symptoms are a result of the normal dysfunction of this transition from those who harbor gynecologic pathology. The perimenopausal woman is at increased risk for endometrial hyperplasia, endometrial polyps, and leiomyomas.

Patients approaching the end of the reproductive years often exhibit symptoms long before the manifestation of menopausal symptoms. Patients note bleeding patterns consistent with an anovulatory state, resulting from the decreased number of remaining oocytes. There is also an increased perception of premenstrual symptoms, which is probably secondary to increased levels of hormones resulting from elevated GnRH concentrations required to induce ovulation with limited numbers of recruitable oocytes. In addition to exclusion of pregnancy, patients older than age 40 years with abnormal patterns require endometrial biopsy and ultrasound examination. These patients must undergo workup to exclude other causes of disordered bleeding, especially endometrial neoplasia as the incidence of endometrial carcinoma increases in this age group.

Bleeding after the menopause is the only symptom of many women with endometrial neoplasia, which must be ruled out first. In addition to endometrial hyperplasia and malignancy, there are several benign causes of bleeding that should be considered in the differential diagnosis. Unexpected bleeding is common during hormone replacement therapy, with either cyclic regimens or continuous combined estrogen–progestin regimens, but it requires the same attention given to postmenopausal bleeding in a woman not receiving hormones (8,32) (see Chapter 106). Vaginal bleeding may also occur secondary to atrophic changes occurring after the menopause, in which the mucosal tissue has thinned due to lack of estrogen. This bleeding may occur after examination or coitus, and a tear will be clinically evident. Unless bleeding occurs regularly as a result of hormonal replacement therapy, vaginal bleeding in the postmenopausal woman should be regarded as a result of genital tract malignancy until proven otherwise. Careful clinical examination and endometrial biopsy are mandatory.

Endometrial Neoplasia

Endometrial carcinoma is the most common of the gynecologic malignancies and also one of the most treatable, because it is typically diagnosed at an early stage because of the symptom of postmenopausal bleeding. Because of the possibility of carcinoma, such bleeding must be investigated further immediately. Chapter 104 fully discusses the approach to diagnosis of endometrial carcinoma.

DYSMENORRHEA

Dysmenorrhea (painful menstruation) is a common problem. It is considered primary when no pathologic condition is present. The condition usually presents within 1 to

2 years after the menarche. *Secondary* dysmenorrhea is a result of a specific pathologic process such as uterine myomas, endometriosis, pelvic inflammatory disease, or an intrauterine contraceptive device that causes pelvic pain in conjunction with menses. Therefore, in secondary dysmenorrhea, one should seek an initiating cause. Patients with secondary dysmenorrhea usually should be referred to a gynecologist. Typical primary dysmenorrhea consists of the development within 1 or 2 days after the onset of menstruation of either crampy or sustained lower abdominal and pelvic pain that may radiate into the legs and that can be associated with nausea, vomiting, irritability, diarrhea, back pain, or abdominal distention. In a few patients, symptoms may be so severe that performance of usual daily activities is impaired or prevented. Usually the discomfort is most severe during the initial several hours of menstrual flow, fades gradually, and disappears within 2 or 3 days. The episodes tend to become less severe with increasing age and often disappear spontaneously within 5 or 10 years after the menarche or after the first pregnancy. Occasionally, idiopathic dysmenorrhea reappears (or makes its first appearance) during the perimenopausal period. There is evidence that dysmenorrhea is caused by excess production of prostaglandins from the uterine endometrium, which results in prolonged and sustained uterine contraction during menses. The concentration of prostaglandins found in the endometrium correlates with the severity of dysmenorrhea (33). Further support for this hypothesis is found by the excellent response to nonsteroidal anti-inflammatory drugs (NSAIDs), which act to inhibit prostaglandin synthetase, in treating dysmenorrhea (34).

Mild forms of dysmenorrhea require only analgesic therapy and reassurance from the physician. First-line therapy for dysmenorrhea is NSAIDs, which have been shown to be effective for approximately 70% to 90% or patients (35). They should be taken with food to minimize GI side effects.

Ibuprofen (e.g., Motrin 400 mg four times daily for 5 to 6 days, naproxen (Naprosyn 500 mg two times daily for five doses), and mefenamic acid (Ponstel 250 mg four times daily for 5 to 6 days) have been approved by the U.S. FDA for use in dysmenorrhea. Ibuprofen has the best risk–benefit ratio in this population (36). NSAIDs are most effective if given just before menstrual flow begins and continued for 2 to 3 days thereafter. However, because of the uncertainty of the effects of these agents in early pregnancy, it is suggested that their use be delayed until the beginning of menstrual flow in those patients who are sexually active and who are not using effective means of birth control. The patient should use one agent as a trial for three cycles, then discontinue the agent if there has been inadequate control of the symptoms.

Steroidal contraceptive agents, either oral or injectable, suppress ovarian hormone production and therefore usually control dysmenorrhea; these agents occasionally may be necessary for management of the problem when it is severe. OCs should be considered first line therapy in young women who also desire contraception (see Chapter 100). The unusual patient who does not respond to any of these therapies should be seen by a gynecologist for evaluation for an undetected problem causing secondary dysmenorrhea (such as endometriosis) or to provide more experienced guidance in drug therapy for primary dysmenorrhea.

PREMENSTRUAL DYSPHORIC DISORDER

Premenstrual dysphoric disorder (PMDD) is an ill-defined complex of signs and symptoms that occurs to some degree in approximately 20% to 50% of women of reproductive age. Symptoms include irritability and increased aggressiveness, cravings for sweet or salty foods, nervousness, depression, tearfulness, mood swings, difficulty concentrating, headaches, fullness and tenderness of the breasts, fatigue, and abdominal bloating. Any or all of the symptoms may be present, and the characteristic complaints vary among patients, but the hallmark of the syndrome is that these problems appear during the latter half (luteal phase) of the menstrual cycle, disappear with the onset of menstruation, and are absent during the first part (follicular phase) of the cycle. Approximately 1% to 9% of affected women find such symptoms severely disruptive to their lives and meet the criteria for PMDD (37). To meet the criteria for PMDD as described in the *Diagnostic and Statistical Manual of Mental Disorders, 4th Edition (DSM-IV)* at least five of 11 possible symptoms must be present during the premenstrual phase with resolution within the first few days of menses. Symptoms must be charted over at least two cycles to conform to luteal pattern before the diagnosis can be confirmed.

Investigations of the cause of this entity have not been rewarding. Most studies have found no typical pattern of hormone or electrolyte changes that distinguishes symptomatic from asymptomatic women. Nonetheless, although progesterone supplementation does not eliminate symptoms, the suppression of ovarian activity cyclically medically (e.g., with GnRH analogs) or surgically effectively eliminates premenstrual syndrome, and sex steroid hormone replacement in suppressed patients does not restore symptoms. It therefore seems most likely that the symptoms stem from an "abnormal" physical response to a more or less normal pattern of steroid hormone fluctuations during the menstrual cycle. Serotonin dysregulation has also been implicated in several studies (37).

Randomized controlled trails have demonstrated that treatment with selective serotonin reuptake inhibitors (SSRIs) and other serotonin modulators are effective and can be considered the first line of treatment for PMDD (38). Treatments with SSRIs have shown a significant improvement in premenstrual symptoms compared to placebo. Fluoxetine (Prozac) 20 mg/day has been approved by the FDA for treatment of emotional and physical symptoms of PMDD (37). A meta-analysis found that various SSRIs show equal effectiveness, ranging from 60% to 70%, compared to placebo, given in both the continuous and luteal phase dosing (7 days before menses) (38).

GALACTORRHEA

Galactorrhea refers to the production of milk (confirmed by demonstration of fat after staining of the fluid with Sudan stain) in a woman who is not recently postpartum or nursing a baby. *Secondary central amenorrhea* is often accompanied by galactorrhea (15% of cases). In approximately 40% of cases, galactorrhea/amenorrhea is caused by a prolactin-secreting pituitary adenoma that may or may not be readily detectable by imaging procedures (macroadenoma versus microadenoma). In patients with macroprolactinoma, the serum prolactin levels are generally greater than 200 ng/mL. Other causes of galactorrheic amenorrhea include medication, (phenothiazines, butyrophenones, metoclopramide, resperidol, verapamil), recent pregnancy, hypothyroidism, and idiopathic hypothalamic dysfunction. Occasionally, a woman who has nursed has mild persistent galactorrhea (without amenorrhea) for up to 5 years after weaning. In these cases, prolactin levels are usually normal (less than 30 ng/mL).

HIRSUTISM AND VIRILIZATION

Growth of coarse dark hair (terminal hairs) in various body areas (besides the scalp and eyebrows) depends on the action of androgens. The pattern of hair growth reflects the relative sensitivity of various zones of the skin to androgen effect. Whereas pubic and axillary hair appears in both sexes, further hair growth diverges because of differing androgen levels. Although male patterns vary, maximum expression of androgen effect includes terminal hair development over the face, limbs, chest, superior pubic triangle, linea alba, and back. In those carrying genes for male-pattern baldness, high levels of androgens are also associated with loss of scalp hair, with hair receding first at the temporal hairline ("widow's peak") and later at the crown.

Hirsutism with Virilization

Most women (80%) develop some degree of dark hair growth over the legs and forearms but not much facial hair. About one third have small amounts of hair on the chest and abdomen (extending along the linea alba). Abnormally high levels of plasma androgens can result in male distribution of hair growth, the state of hirsutism. Over time, very high levels of androgen production also lead to virilization, defined as increased muscle mass, redistribution of fat from subcutaneous depots in hips and breasts to abdominal and intra-abdominal areas ("male habitus"), clitoral enlargement (greater than 2.0 cm), deepening of the voice, male-pattern baldness, development of acne, and increased perspiration odor from activation of sebaceous glands.

Excess body hair without signs of virilization is termed "simple hirsutism." Hirsutism with virilization is rare and is usually a result of diagnosable causes, the most common of which are adrenal or ovarian tumor, congenital adrenal hyperplasia, male pseudohermaphroditism, and use of exogenous androgen (e.g., female athletes and body builders). Truly virilized women usually should be referred directly to an endocrinologist for detailed diagnostic investigation.

Hirsutism without Virilization

Although simple hirsutism may be an early manifestation of Cushing syndrome or of an adrenal or ovarian neoplasm, most cases fall into a group termed "idiopathic" hirsutism. The prevalence of simple hirsutism has been estimated to be as high as 10% in adult North American women. It typically develops during the late teens, although progression may be so slow that troublesome amounts of hair do not appear for 10 or more years after onset of menses.

In one half to two thirds of hirsute women, excessive ovarian production of androgens (testosterone or androstenedione) is demonstrable and is often associated with oligomenorrhea and decreased fertility. Ovarian structure may show hyperthecosis (overgrowth of interstitial tissue) or multiple cyst formation (PCOS; see Reproductive Adult: Up to 45 Years).

In about half of all patients with simple hirsutism, elevated serum testosterone levels are not demonstrable. However, approximately half of patients with normal total testosterone have been shown to have increased plasma "free" (or unbound) testosterone due to reduced SHBG. Increased hair follicle conversion of testosterone to the more potent dihydrotestosterone has been demonstrated in some of the remaining cases, and other causes of increased sensitivity of hair follicles to androgens have been reported.

Racial and ethnic factors are also important determinants of hair growth. Women of Asian ancestry and Caucasian women of northern European origin usually have relatively little terminal hair on face, torso, or extremities. In contrast, Caucasian women of Mediterranean origin often develop mustache, beard, or sideburns and have dark hair on legs and arms. Constitutional hirsutism also tends to run in families. Therefore, a patient with moderate hirsutism who is of Mediterranean origin, who has a mother or other close family members with excessive facial hair, and who has normal menses is unlikely to have identifiable endocrine disease. The timing of onset of hirsutism is also important. For example, sudden development of hirsutism many years after menarche is likely to be caused by a tumor of the ovary or adrenal rather than a functional cause.

Transitory hirsutism may occur during pregnancy and occasionally during menopause. A number of pharmacologic agents, including glucocorticoids, phenytoin (Dilantin), minoxidil, diazoxide, and phenothiazines, can result in hirsutism. Drug-induced hirsutism is characterized by increased hair growth that is not limited to the androgen-sensitive areas of the skin. Rare causes include chronic local skin trauma and porphyria cutanea tarda.

Besides PCOS, the other major cause of adult-onset simple hirsutism, sometimes with disturbance of menstrual pattern, is *congenital adrenal hyperplasia (CAH)*. CAH is produced by a deficiency of one of the several enzymes in the steroid synthetic pathway. Although such defects are usually manifested in childhood as ambiguous genitalia with salt loss (21-hydroxylase deficiency) or non–salt losing simple virilization (11-hydroxylase deficiency), patients with partial 21- or 11-hydroxylase defects can manifest hirsutism with onset in puberty or in adult life without symptomatic disturbances of salt and water balance.

Approach to the Patient

A careful ethnic and family history is essential. The temporal evolution of the problem should be noted, including the menstrual history. On physical examination, one should carefully note the distribution and density of terminal hairs in the sideburn and mustache areas, the periareolar and midsternal regions, and over the back and buttocks. Particular attention should be paid to the pattern of pubic hair. In the female, the pubic hair forms an inverted triangle in the inferior pubic region only. The male escutcheon is a rhomboid space with terminal hairs filling the superior pubic triangle and extending up the linea alba to the umbilicus. A male type escutcheon in a female is a good presumptive sign of hyperandrogenism. Physical signs of virilization (discussed earlier) should be sought. Patients with virilism require urgent referral to an endocrinologist, whereas those with severe ovarian dysfunction may require the attention of a gynecologist for treatment of abnormal menstruation or impaired fertility. Finally, symptoms and signs of Cushing syndrome (in which hirsutism and even virilization may occasionally be more prominent than the classic "cushingoid" changes) should also be sought. Obesity with acanthosis nigricans is highly suggestive of the insulin-resistant variant of PCOS.

The decision to proceed with laboratory testing depends on the history and severity of the hirsutism. Laboratory studies can be performed sequentially if financial considerations are dominant or simultaneously if speed is of the essence. Serum testosterone, which is of ovarian and rarely of adrenal origin, is measured first. A normal serum testosterone level suggests idiopathic hirsutism and excludes major ovarian disorders. Not excluded are mild cases of ovarian hyperthecosis/polycystic ovaries with abnormal androstenedione production or cases with decreased SHBG resulting in falsely normal total testosterone (these women have increased free or bioavailable androgen). The uncovering of such borderline cases usually is not worthwhile because management would be unaffected. If the testosterone level is increased to between 85 and 200 ng/dL, a diagnosis of ovarian hyperthecosis or PCOS is most likely. Increased LH and low-normal or reduced FSH are highly suggestive of PCOS but does not occur in all patients. Pelvic sonography usually reveals multiple cysts or thickening of the cortex and enlargement of the ovaries. Levels of testosterone greater than 200 ng/dL suggest a diagnosis of ovarian neoplasm, and specialists should direct further diagnostic evaluation. This may include transvaginal sonography, computerized tomography of the abdomen and pelvis, laparoscopy with ovarian biopsy, or ovarian vein catheterization. It is important to appreciate that the ranges of testosterone elevation mentioned above are a rough guide and should not be considered absolute in terms of making decisions. Hence, each patient should be treated on an individual basis.

If testosterone levels are normal, excess production of weak androgens (e.g., androstenedione, DHEAS) by the adrenal remains a consideration and can be confirmed by appropriate assays. In 21-hydroxylase deficiency, the most common type of CAH resulting in hirsutism in adults, serum 17α-OH progesterone and urinary pregnanetriol may be elevated. However, in about half the patients with this syndrome, these steroid levels are normal at baseline and increase only after stimulation with exogenous adrenocorticotropic hormone (ACTH). Therefore, if CAH is suspected, endocrine specialty referral is appropriate. Large increases in serum DHEAS or 24-hour urinary excretion of 17-ketosteroids suggests adrenal neoplasia (adenoma or carcinoma) and also should be evaluated by an endocrinologist.

Therapy

Treatment of hyperandrogenism and hirsutism includes both local and systemic measures (39). Therapy for simple hirsutism usually is local and essentially cosmetic, even if there is a hormonal abnormality, since medical reduction of androgen excess does not rapidly affect the presence of existing hair and is often incomplete.

Local measures include bleaching, wax stripping, shaving, plucking (tweezing), using hair removal creams (depilatories), and performing electrolysis. Contrary to popular belief, such measures do not accelerate the growth rate of remaining hair. Plucking can occasionally cause local infection. Wax applications and hair removal creams are effective but may be irritating and must be used with care. All of these procedures must be repeated at intervals. Electrolysis and thermolysis are effective procedures for permanent removal of hair, but they are expensive and uncomfortable. Effectiveness and safety (avoidance of burns, scarring, and infection) depend on the technique of the operator. Referral of the patient requires that the clinician be familiar with the electrologist's skill. Under the best of circumstances, electrolysis is generally successful in destroying approximately 50% of the follicles treated at one time. Invariably, therefore, many repetitions are required.

Patients with hyperandrogenic hirsutism (PCOS or CAH) often respond to medical therapy. Such patients should be cautioned not to expect rapid results, because dedifferentiation of androgenized follicles may require 6 to 18 months, even if androgen excess is totally eliminated. The immediate benefit to be expected is prevention of progression of the hirsutism, with variable degrees of reversal occurring only as therapy is continued. Medical therapy is directed toward suppressing androgen production, blocking peripheral androgen action, or both. Although such therapy appears more rational when androgen excess is demonstrable, patients with idiopathic hirsutism may occasionally respond. Adrenal suppression with low dosages of dexamethasone, although introduced on the erroneous assumption that adrenal androgens were responsible for most cases of hirsutism, is nonetheless effective in about one third of cases. This seems to be so because of an accompanying reduction of ovarian androgen secretion, which is either directly dependent on ACTH or indirectly dependent via ovarian conversion of circulating adrenal steroids. Adrenal suppression is, as expected, effective in cases of CAH. This form of therapy is simple and usually free from side effects. Dexamethasone can be given as a single dose of 0.1 to 0.3 mg (as a pediatric solution) orally at bedtime. At these low dosages, neither glucocorticoid excess (iatrogenic Cushing syndrome) nor chronic adrenal suppression with adrenal insufficiency is likely to occur, but levels of both plasma or urinary cortisol and adrenal androgen should be monitored, and the dosage of dexamethasone should be adjusted to keep both in the normal range. Side effects of dexamethasone therapy include occasional insomnia and appetite stimulation.

The most appropriate treatment for ovarian hyperandrogenism is suppression of ovarian androgen production. The first line of treatment is use of a cyclically administered estrogen-progestin combination (OC). This is effective in about half of the cases. Estrogens, especially when given orally, also increase the concentration of plasma SHBG, reducing the concentration of circulating free androgens. Because progestins have some intrinsic androgen-like activity on hair follicles, a combination that minimizes the content of progestational agent may be most appropriate. Agents containing 2 mg or less of norethindrone or 0.5 mg or less of norgestrel are acceptable. Recently, a novel estrogen-progestin combination pill (containing ethinyl estradiol and drospirenone (Yasmin) has also shown good results in the treatment of hirsutism in women with PCOs (26). When used, OCs should be given on the usual schedule recommended for fertility control for the particular preparation (see Chapter 100).

Disadvantages of OCs include their potential for cardiovascular, thrombogenic, and other undesirable effects. These disadvantages have probably been overstated and are less often seen with the low-dose contraceptives of today than with their high-dose predecessors; nonetheless, possible adverse effects must be weighed carefully when they are to be prescribed for an essentially benign problem. Combined adrenal–ovarian suppression may be used if neither alone is effective.

Suppression of ovarian androgen production by OCs precludes pregnancy. Therefore, therapy must be interrupted when fertility is desired and the drug withheld during pregnancy. Spironolactone (Aldactone), at a generally well-tolerated dosage of 25 to 50 mg twice daily, suppresses ovarian androgen production and antagonizes androgen action at the hair follicle. Spironolactone is a well-accepted and relatively safe drug, and the combination of spironolactone with an OC is often effective in more severe cases of hirsutism and in those that are unresponsive to ovarian and/or adrenal suppression alone. Contraindications to spironolactone include concomitant use of potassium supplements or renal insufficiency, either of which may predispose to hyperkalemia.

Cyproterone acetate and flutamide are competitive inhibitors of androgen that block peripheral androgen receptors and have been used successfully in the treatment of hirsutism. Finasteride, which inhibits the enzyme 5-α-reductase that mediates the conversion of testosterone to its active form, dihydrotestosterone (DHT), also appears to be effective in skin and hair follicles (40). Studies of finasteride in the treatment of idiopathic hirsutism (39) and PCOS (41) have shown mixed results. Although none of the latter agents is currently approved by the FDA for the treatment of hirsutism in women, it is not unreasonable to try one of them alone or in combination with ovarian or adrenal suppression in resistant cases.

Suppression of the reproductive system with the use of a GnRH antagonist such as buserelin has also been found to be effective in reducing severe ovarian hyperandrogenism with hirsutism (42). However, because of their attendant risks of osteoporosis or hot flushes, the usefulness of these agents is limited.

Finally, severe hirsutism and virilization can result from benign highly functional ovarian tumors such as luteomas and thecomas (43). These tumors should be removed surgically. Similarly, localized malignant ovarian and adrenal tumors also require surgical excision followed by adjuvant therapy (if needed).

FEMALE SEXUAL DYSFUNCTION (FRIGIDITY AND DYSPAREUNIA)

Definition

As in the male, female hyposexuality can be divided into reduced sexual interest or appetite (hypoactive sexual desire), failure of arousal (inhibition of excitement), and anorgasmia. For a more complete discussion, see Chapter 6. The discussion here is limited to physical and especially to endocrine etiologies.

Etiologies

Organic causes of female hyposexuality include DM with peripheral neuropathy, hyperprolactinemia, hypogonadism with estrogen deficiency, and organic disease of the vagina, uterus, fallopian tubes, or ovaries with resultant dyspareunia. Various endocrine (e.g., hyperthyroidism, hypothyroidism) and other systemic debilitating diseases can also cause loss of interest in sexual activity. Menopausal changes by both surgical oophorectomy or natural menopause often are associated with sexual dysfunction and 40% to 80% of women report experiencing some sexual problems during this time. The loss of ovarian function results in low levels of estrogen and subsequent menopausal symptoms including vaginal dryness. Androgen levels fall with aging and studies have shown that a decrease in testosterone levels is associated with loss of libido (2).

History

Approaching sexual dysfunction requires consideration of medical, sexual, and psychological sources of the problem. Careful history will aid the provider in narrowing this broad spectrum of causes. Questions should be the same as those asked of a woman with hypogonadism (see Secondary Amenorrhea). Additional questions should be asked about dyspareunia. If there is pain or discomfort on intercourse, it is important to know whether it occurs with attempts at penetration (suggesting local vaginal or vulvar problems) or only after deep penetration (suggesting pelvic disease, such as leiomyoma, endometriosis, or salpingitis). The physician should determine whether there was a previous history of satisfactory sexual activity and, if so, the time and circumstances of onset of its deterioration. Careful questioning should reveal to what extent the problem is one of loss of interest, excitation (lubrication and heightened pelvic blood flow), or orgasm. A history of symptoms of DM, peripheral neuropathy, or thyroid, adrenal, or other serious systemic disorders should be obtained. Knowledge of medication use (tranquilizers, OCs, antidepressants) and substance abuse (opiates, alcohol) is also important.

Physical Examination

The physical examination should be conducted in the same way as for patients with female hypogonadism (see Evaluation of Abnormal Bleeding, Physical Examination). Careful attention should be given to the genitalia, uterus, and adnexa for evidence of infection, atrophy, or neoplasia. Endometriosis, a common cause of dyspareunia, is sometimes detected on rectovaginal examination by palpation of nodules in the space between the rectum and vagina (pouch of Douglas). Postmenopausal patients often have significant vaginal atrophy leading to dyspareunia. Neurologic examination should include testing of peripheral sensation, position sense, and deep tendon reflexes.

Diagnostic Procedures

If evidence of hypogonadism exists, appropriate tests should be made (see Secondary Amenorrhea) to classify the syndrome and diagnose the underlying condition. Measurement of the serum prolactin concentration may be helpful even in patients without apparent galactorrhea or amenorrhea (see earlier discussion). Thyroid function with TSH should be considered. To evaluate for androgen deficiency serum total testosterone level can be checked. Levels are altered by SHBG so patients taking a medication that alter SHBG should have a free testosterone level. Patients with pelvic disease should be referred to a gynecologist for further evaluation and therapy.

Therapy

Therapeutic efforts should be directed at the specific organic cause whenever possible. Estrogen deficiency should be corrected, and hyperprolactinemia should be treated surgically or medically (see Secondary Amenorrhea). Vaginal atrophy frequently responds to topical estrogen (Chapter 106). There are no FDA-approved testosterone therapies for women. Testosterone is often used off label in oral, intramuscular and transdermal forms in women with low testosterone levels and hypoactive sexual desire and have shown promise in reports (44,45). Concerns about testosterone treatment in women include virilization, male pattern hair loss, and adverse affects in the lipid panel.

Another non–FDA-approved treatment is use of sildenafil citrate in treatment of physiologic female sexual disfunction. Sildenafil 50 mg given 1 hour before intercourse and not more then once per day was shown to improve sexual arousal and lubrication in a double-blinded trail (46). If no organic cause is evident after careful examination, consideration of various modes of psychological diagnosis and treatment is appropriate (see Chapter 19). Referral to a provider with interest and expertise in sexual dysfunction should be made. A multidisciplinary approach including marital counseling, sex therapy, and mental health care all play a role in successful treatment of sexual dysfunction.

SPECIFIC REFERENCES*

1. Lenton EA, Landren B, Sexton L, et al. Normal variation in the length of the follicular phase of the menstrual cycle: effect of chronologic age. Br J Obstet Gynecol 1984;91:681.
2. Lobo RA, Bachmann GA, Cerey JC, et al. Considerations in evaluating, diagnosing and treating HSDD in postmenopausal women. Cont Ob/Gyn 2005;April supp:4.
3. Kadir RA, Economides DL, Sabin CA, et al. Frequency of inherited bleeding disorders in women with menorrhagia. Lancet 1998;351:485.
4. Shankar M, Lee CA, Sabin CA, et al. von Willebrand disease in women with menorrhagia: a systematic review. BJOG 2004;111:734.
5. Woo YL, White B, Corbally R, et al. von Willebrand's disease: an important cause of dysfunctional uterine bleeding. Blood Coagul Fibrinolysis 2002;13:89.
6. Amesse LS, Pfaff-Amesse T, Leonardi R, et al. Oral contraceptives and DDAVP nasal spray: patterns of use in managing vWD-associated menorrhagia: a single-institution study. J Pediatr Hematol Oncol 2005;27:357.
7. Gay JD, Donaldson LD, Grellner JR. False negative results on cervical cytologic studies. Acta Cytol 1985;29:1043.
8. Ash SJ, Farrell SA, Flowerdew G. Endometrial biopsy in DUB. J Reprod Med 1996;41:892.
9. Langer RD, Pierce JJ, O'Hanlan KA, et al. Transvaginal ultrasonography compared with endometrial biopsy for the detection of endometrial disease. Postmenopausal Estrogen/Progestin Interventions Trial. N Engl J Med 1997;337:1792.
10. O'Connell LP, Fries MH, Zeringue E, et al. Triage of abnormal postmenopausal bleeding: a comparison of endometrial biopsy and transvaginal sonohysterography versus fractional curettage with hysteroscopy. Am J Obstet Gynecol 1998;178:956.
11. Goldstein SR, Zeltser I, Horan CK, et al. Ultrasonography-based triage for perimenopausal patients with abnormal uterine bleeding. Am J Obstet Gynecol 1997;177:102.
12. Meuwissen JH, Oddens BJ, Klinkhamer PJ. Endometrial thickness assessed by transvaginal ultrasound insufficiently predicts occurrence of hyperplasia during unopposed oestrogen use. Maturitas 1996;24:21.
13. Weber AM, Belinson JL, Bradley LD, et al. Vaginal ultrasonography versus endometrial biopsy in women with postmenopausal bleeding. Am J Obstet Gynecol 1997;177:924.
14. James AH, Lukes AS, Brancazio LR, et al. Use of a new platelet function analayzer to detect von Willebrand disease in women with menorrhagia. Am J Obstet Gynecol 2004;191:449.
15. Speroff L, Glass R, Kase N. Anovulation and polycystic ovary syndrome. In: Clinical gynecologic endocrinology and infertility. 6th ed. Philadelphia: Lippincott, Williams & Wilkins, 1999: Chapter 12.
16. Hetland ML, Harbo J, Christiansen C, et al. Running induces menstrual disturbances but bone mass is unaffected except in amenorrheic female athletes. Am J Med 1993;95:53.
17. Prior JC, Vigne YM, Barr LS, et al. Cyclic medroxyprogesterone treatment increases bone density: a controlled trial in active women with menstrual cycle disturbances. Am J Med 1994;96:521.
18. Dunaif A. Hyperandrogenic anovulation (PCOS): a unique disorder of insulin action associated with an increased risk of non-insulin-dependent diabetes mellitus. Am J Med 1995;98:335.
19. Zawadski JK, Dunaif A. Diagnostic criteria for polycystic ovary syndrome: towards a rational approach. In: Dunaif A, Givens JR, Haseltine F, eds. Polycystic ovary syndrome. Boston: Blackwell Scientific, Boston, 1992:377.
20. Ehrmann DA. Polycystic ovary syndrome. New Engl J Med 2005;352:1223.
21. Polson DW, Wadsworth J, Adams J, et al. Polycystic ovaries: a common finding in normal women. Lancet 1988;2:870.
22. Rotterdam ESHRE/ASRM-Sponsored PCOS consensus workshop group, Revised 2003 consensus on diagnostic criteria and long-term health risks related to polycystic ovary syndrome. Fertil Steril 2004;81:19.
23. Dunaif A, Scott D, Finegood D, et al. The insulin-sensitizing agent troglitazone improves metabolic and reproductive abnormalities in the polycystic ovary syndrome. J Clin Endocrinol Metab 1996;81:3299.
24. Meirow D, Yossepowitch O, Rosler A, et al. Insulin resistant and non-resistant polycystic ovary syndrome represent two clinical and endocrinological subgroups. Hum Reprod 1995;10:1951.
25. Falsetti L, Eleftheriou G. Hyperinsulinemia in the polycystic ovary syndrome: a clinical, endocrine and echographic study in 240 patients. Gynecol Endocrinol 1996;10:319.
26. Guido M, Romualdi D, Giuliani M, et al. Drospirenone for the treatment of hirsute women with polycystic ovary syndrome: a clinical, endocrinological, metabolic pilot study. J Clin Endocrinol Metab 2004;89:2817.
27. Mansfield R, Galea R, Brincat M, et al. Metformin has direct effects on human ovarian steroidogenesis. Fertil Steril 2003;79:956.
28. Eisenbarth GS, Gottlieb PA. Autoimmune polyendocrine syndromes. N Engl J Med 2004;350:2068.
29. Pettersson B, Adami HO. Endometrial polyps and hyperplasia as risk factors for endometrial carcinoma. Acta Obstet Gynecol Scand 1985;64:653.
30. Santoro N, Brown JR, Adel T, et al. Characterization of reproductive hormonal dynamics in the perimenopause. J Clin Endocrinol Metab 1996;81:1495.
31. Prior JC. Perimenopause: the complex endocrinology of the menopausal transition. Endocr Rev 1998;19:397.
32. Ettinger B, Li DK, Klein R. Unexpected vaginal bleeding and associated gynecologic care in postmenopausal women using hormone replacement therapy: comparison of cyclic versus continuous combined schedules. Fertil Steril 1998;79:865.
33. Willman EA, Collin WP, Clayton SG. Studies in the involvement of prostaglandin in uterine symptomatology and pathology. B J Obstet Gynacol 1976;83:337.
34. Chan WY, Dawood MF, Fuchs F. Relief of dysmenorrhea with the prostaglandin synthetase inhibitor ibuprofen: effect on prostaglandin levels in menstrual fluid. Am J Obstet Gynecol 1979;135:102.
35. Majorbanks J, Proctor ML, Farquhar C. Nonsteroidal anti-inflammatory drugs for primary dysmenorrhoea. Cochrane Database Syst Rev 20003;4:CD001751.
36. Zhang WY, Li Wan Po A. Efficacy of minor analgesics in primary dysmenorrhoea: a systematic review. Br J Obstet Gyneaecol 1998; 105:780.
37. Pearlstein T. Selective serotonin reuptake inhibitors for premenstrual dysphoria disorder the emerging gold standard? Drugs 2000;62: 1869.
38. Dimmock PW, Wyatt KM, Jones PW, et al. Efficacy of selective serotonin reuptake inhibitors in premenstrual syndrome: a systemic review. Lancet 2000;356:1131.
39. Knochenhauer ES, Azziz R. Advances in the diagnosis and treatment of the hirsute patient. Curr Opin Obstet Gynecol 1995;7:344.
40. Castello R, Tosi F, Perrone F, et al. Outcome of long-term treatment with the 5 alpha-reductase inhibitor finasteride in idiopathic hirsutism: clinical and hormonal effects during a 1-year course of therapy and 1-year follow-up. Fertil Steril 1996;66:734.
41. Tolino A, Petrone A, Sarnacchiaro F, et al. Finasteride in the treatment of hirsutism: new therapeutic perspectives. Fertil Steril 1996;66: 61.
42. Bertoli A, Fusco A, Magnani A, et al. Efficacy of low-dose GnRH analogue (Buserelin) in the treatment of hirsutism. Exp Clin Endocrinol Diabetes 1995;103:15.
43. Klopouh L, Altman K, Nicol T et al. Diabetes in a bearded woman. J Androl 2005;26:455.
44. Speroff L, Glass R, Kase N. Amenorrhea. In: Editors, eds. Clinical gynecologic endocrinology and infertility. 5th ed. Baltimore: Williams & Wilkins, 1994.
45. Shifren JL, Braunstein GD, Simon JA, et al. Transdermal testosterone treatment in women with impaired sexual function after oophorectomy. N Engl J Med 2000;343:682.
46. Berman JR, Berman LA, Toler SM, et al. Safety and efficacy of sildenafil citrate for the treatment of female sexual arousal disorder: a double-blind, placebo controlled study. J Urol 2003;170: 2333.

*Bold numerals denote published controlled clinical trials, meta-analyses, or consensus-based recommendations.

*For annotated **General References** and resources related to this chapter, visit www.hopkinsbayview.org/PAMreferences.*

Chapter 102

Nonmalignant Vulvovaginal Disorders, Pelvic Inflammatory Disease, and Chronic Pelvic Pain

Anne E. Burke and Linda C. Rogers

Vulvovaginal symptoms constitute a significant proportion of problems seen by primary care providers. The diagnosis and treatment of these disorders can be both satisfying and exasperating. Most diagnoses are readily made in one office visit. Treatment is usually easily rendered. However, the patient with recurrent or persistent symptoms presents special problems. Appropriate evaluation and treatment of both the easily treated patient and the patient with persistent symptoms require knowledge of the anatomy, physiology, and pathology of the vulva and vagina.

ANATOMY AND PHYSIOLOGY

Vulva

The external genitalia of the female human is called the vulva (Fig. 102.1). The vulva consists of the labia majora, labia minora, vestibule, clitoris, prepuce, and mons pubis.

The mons pubis (mons veneris) is a cushion of fat covered by stratified squamous skin and its appendages (hair follicles, sebaceous and apocrine sweat glands). The mons is located superior to the clitoris and encompasses the triangular-shaped hair-bearing tissue situated in front of the symphysis pubis. The labia majora are composed of

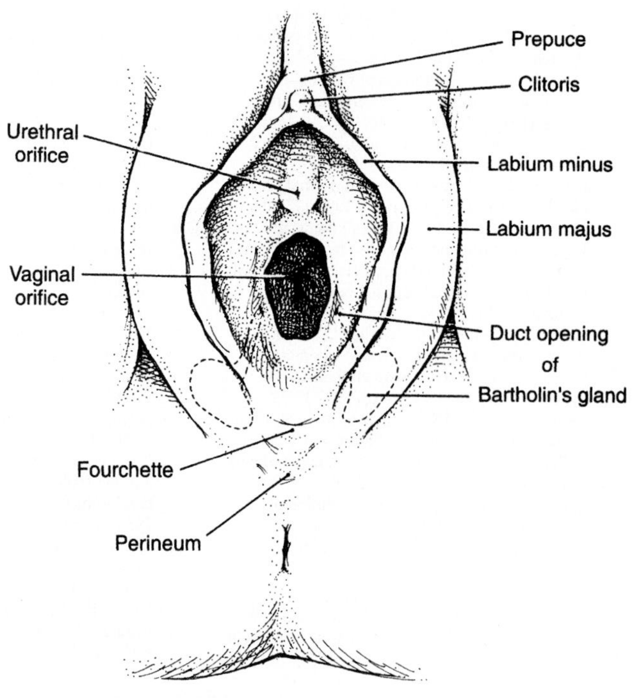

FIGURE 102.1. Anatomy of the vulva.

women who have never been sexually active. Additionally, recurrence rates for the infection are the same for women whose partners do or do not harbor *G. vaginalis* (29). Because of the possible role of sexual transmission, condoms should be used during therapy. However, because there is no clear evidence that treatment of the partner improves recurrence rates, routine treatment of male partners is not currently recommended (11,30).

BV has been associated with preterm birth, and treatment of BV may reduce the risk of preterm complications in high-risk women (31,32,33). However, treatment of asymptomatic BV in all pregnant women has not been shown to affect pregnancy outcome (34). Because of the association between BV and posthysterectomy vaginal cuff cellulitis, preoperative treatment should be given to affected women (35).

Trichomonas

Trichomonas infection (Table 102.1) is the third most common cause of vaginitis, with a prevalence of 4% to 35% (36). It is a sexually transmitted disease (STD) caused by the motile, flagellated protozoan, *Trichomonas vaginalis*. Symptomatic patients classically have a copious, malodorous vaginal discharge accompanied by vulvar pruritus. Additional symptoms include vaginal burning, vaginal spotting, dysuria, frequency, and urgency. Pelvic discomfort may be experienced by some patients. Dyspareunia is common. On physical examination, variable amounts of vulvovaginal erythema may be seen. The vaginal mucosa or cervix may exhibit a characteristic strawberry appearance (reddish color with punctate hemorrhages).

The diagnosis is established by assessing vaginal pH and examining the saline wet slide preparation (see earlier discussion). The vaginal pH is greater than 4.5. On the saline preparation (Fig. 102.3), a multitude of polymorphonuclear leukocytes are seen. Among the white blood cells, trichomonads can be identified by the movement of their flagellae. Sensitivity of the wet mount for the trichomonads is relatively low, at 50% to 70% (37). Culture on a Diamond medium, which has a sensitivity and specificity greater than 95%, can be considered.

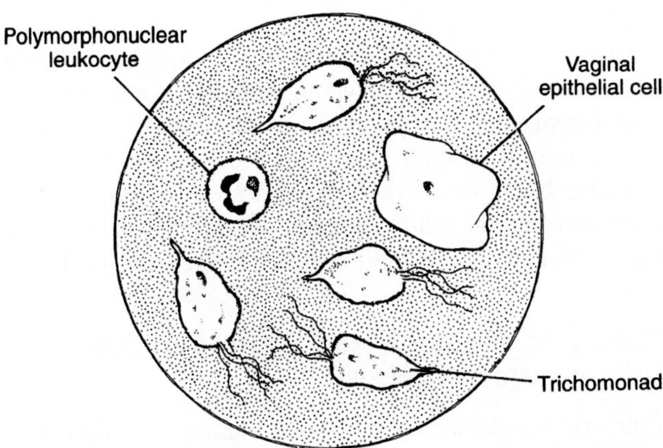

FIGURE 102.3. Saline preparation showing trichomonads.

Liquid-based Pap smears are more sensitive than conventional Pap smears in the diagnosis of trichomoniasis, with sensitivity and specificity of 61% and 99%, respectively (38). Conventional Pap smears, by contrast, have a high false-positive rate (37).

Treatment

Treatment consists of a single 2-g dose of oral metronidazole (11). An alternative regimen is metronidazole 500 mg, twice a day for 7 days. Patients who do not respond to initial therapy may be treated with metronidazole 500 mg, two times per day for 7 days, or tinidazole 500 mg three times daily for 7 days. If treatment failure occurs again, the patient should be treated with a single, 2-g dose of metronidazole once a day for 3 to 5 days (11). Metronidazole should be used cautiously in patients with severe hepatic disease. Some practitioners hesitate to administer metronidazole in the first trimester of pregnancy, although studies have failed to show adverse pregnancy outcomes (39,40). Therefore, current recommendations are that use of metronidazole to treat symptomatic patients is acceptable, even in the first trimester of pregnancy (11).

When taken within 24 hours of alcohol consumption, metronidazole causes severe reactions similar to those that occur when alcohol and disulfiram are consumed together. In these situations or when there is an intolerance to systemic metronidazole, metronidazole gel twice a day for 7 days may be tried as an alternative, although this regimen is less effective (41). Sexual partners should be treated, and there is no need to attempt to recover the organism from the partner. Intercourse should be avoided or a condom used during treatment.

Vaginal Atrophy and Atrophic Vaginitis

Vaginal atrophy occurs in to some degree in nearly all menopausal women, and more than half become symptomatic with vaginal dryness, irritation, and dyspareunia. Women who are breast-feeding or perimenopausal may also be sufficiently estrogen deficient to become symptomatic. Estrogen deficiency results in thinning and fragility of the vaginal and vulvar epithelium, which comes to be comprised primarily of parabasal and intermediate cells. This altered vaginal environment is associated with an elevation of pH to as high as 7.0. In this milieu, pathogenic bacteria may flourish, causing atrophic vaginitis, which affects 10% to 40% of postmenopausal women (42). Because symptoms may appear 10 years or longer after menopause, the condition is often underdiagnosed and undertreated (42). Rarely, atrophic vaginitis develops in girls who are premenarchal (i.e., have unestrogenized tissues) when an additional precipitant, such as wearing of occlusive clothing made of synthetic materials, is encountered.

Atrophy without superimposed infection can cause significant discomfort, especially during coitus, because the atrophic vagina does not lubricate well and is more easily injured. Visual examination of the normal atrophic vagina reveals a pale vaginal mucosa with decreased or absent rugal folds. Vulvar examination demonstrates thin, often shiny skin with decreased subcutaneous tissue and variable loss of hair. In atrophic vaginitis, erythema and petechial hemorrhages may be superimposed on these findings. The patient may complain of a thin, blood-tinged vaginal discharge and vulvar and vaginal dryness.

Examination of a saline wet slide preparation of the discharge of women with atrophic vaginitis typically shows numerous leukocytes mixed with immature, intermediate, and parabasal epithelial cells. Microorganisms seen on the slide are usually secondary invaders of the inflamed mucosa. Often, in the past, diagnosis was made by taking a smear of the vaginal wall and determining the maturation index; however, this test is no longer recommended because it has not proved to be reliable.

Both symptomatic vaginal atrophy and atrophic vaginitis are treated most effectively with vaginally applied estrogen. Vaginal symptoms are relieved in only 55% of women using the estrogen patch, and in 73% of women on oral estrogen, but in 80% to 95% of women on vaginal estrogens (43). Many women on oral or transdermal estrogens may need the addition of vaginally applied estrogen to fully relieve symptoms.

Options for vaginally applied estrogens include creams, tablets, and rings. Creams are most commonly used, and allow for considerable dosing flexibility. As an example, one-half to one applicator of estrogen cream every night for 1 to 2 weeks can be followed by application every other night for 1 to 2 weeks. The medication can then generally be discontinued, and most patients have only infrequent symptoms (e.g., every 1 to 2 months), for which an applicator full on 1 or 2 days when there are symptoms usually provides adequate control. Some patients, however, require up to 24 months of therapy, and the response may still be incomplete (44).

Rings and tablets have been shown to be better accepted by patients, and there is data to support greater safety because of significantly less systemic absorption (45). Most studies find that the low-dose ring and estradiol tablets relieve vaginal dryness and dyspareunia as well as estrogen creams. A reduced risk for urinary tract infections (UTIs) has been demonstrated with vaginal estrogens and some studies have found a decrease in urge incontinence (45). However, recent large studies have demonstrated worsening incontinence of all types with any estrogen therapy (46,47).

The estradiol ring releases 7.5 μgs of estradiol daily. It can remain in the vagina for up to 3 months (48,49). The vaginal tablet contains 25 μg of estradiol and is usually inserted twice a week, but also may be used once a week. Studies have shown an initial increase in serum estradiol levels in the first 2 weeks of therapy because estrogen is well absorbed by an atrophic mucosa. After 2 weeks however, there is no significant effect on serum levels (45). Women with high intake of alcohol or impaired liver function may have higher serum levels of estradiol. Most women maintain an atrophic endometrium with low-dose preparations, but some women do have endometrial effects. There is some evidence that there may be a uterine "first-pass" effect with vaginal estrogen, causing higher uterine levels of estrogen than with the equivalent dose of oral or transdermal estrogen (50). There are currently no evidence-based guidelines on management of unopposed low-dose vaginal estrogen for women with a uterus, but one suggested approach is to do a "progestin challenge" either after 3 months of therapy, or yearly, to assess the amount of endometrial stimulation. Those with any significant bleeding would merit closer monitoring of their endometrium (51).

The clinician should be certain that none of the contraindications for estrogens (e.g., breast cancer) is present and that the same precautionary surveillance (e.g., for hypertension) is provided to the patient using long-term topical estrogen preparations.

Some patients cannot or will not use topical vaginal preparations and prefer to avoid long-term systemic hormonal replacement therapy. In this instance, oral conjugated estrogen 0.625 mg/day may be prescribed for 1 month. Occasionally a repeated course is necessary if symptoms persist. If retreatment courses become frequent, it is necessary to provide close surveillance for the complications of estrogen therapy (see Chapter 106). Generally a gynecologist should be consulted to participate in the care of the patient with frequently recurrent attacks of atrophic vaginitis.

Water soluble vaginal lubricants have also been shown to have some efficacy in relieving vaginal dryness, pruritus, and dyspareunia. These can be recommended to women who cannot or do not want to use estrogens (52). They can also be informed that sexual activity will help them maintain vaginal health. Women who are sexually active have lower vaginal pH and better cell maturation (51).

Cytolytic Vaginosis and Desquamative Inflammatory Vaginitis

Cytolytic vaginosis and desquamative inflammatory vaginitis are uncommonly recognized *vulvovaginitides* that are often confused with other vaginal inflammatory conditions. Cytolytic vaginosis is caused by an overgrowth of lactobacilli, which results in an acidic environment and causes shedding and cytolysis of vaginal epithelial cells. The vaginal discharge of cytolytic vaginosis usually increases during the luteal phase of the menstrual cycle and grossly resembles a candidal discharge; the discharge is thick and white, with an acidic pH. The patient usually experiences severe vulvar burning, dysuria, and dyspareunia (53). KOH preparation reveals an absence of fungi. The saline wet slide preparation reveals an abundance of lactobacilli, fragmented epithelial cells, and naked nuclei. Therapy has not been well established. Currently an intravaginal douche two to three times a week of 30 to 60 mg sodium bicarbonate in 1 L of warm water is recommended. Alternatively, the patient can take amoxicillin clavulanate 500 mg, three times a day for 7 days (53,54).

Desquamative inflammatory vaginitis is a disorder of unknown cause that usually is characterized by copious sterile vaginal discharge and epithelial cell exfoliation (55). Patients experience intense vulvar pain and burning, severe dyspareunia, and dysuria. Conditions such as lichen planus and pemphigus vulgaris have been associated with desquamative inflammatory vaginitis (56,57). The vulva and vagina are usually very inflamed, with various stages of denudation. The discharge is seropurulent, with a pH as high as 7.4 (57). The characteristic violaceous papules and gingival and buccal mucosal lesions of lichen planus may be seen if the patient has the form of desquamative inflammatory vaginitis that is associated with lichen planus (58). Saline wet slide preparation reveals parabasal cells, an absence of lactobacilli, a predominance of inflammatory cells, and fragmented epithelial cells. This entity is distinguished from atrophic vaginitis by the lack of response to topical estrogen, and by a clinical history consistent with normal ovarian function (58). A biopsy of the affected area of the vagina should be taken in order to rule out another cause. Treatment options for desquamative inflammatory vaginitis are not well-established. One study found a 95% improvement rate with use of 2% clindamycin suppositories, although the relapse rate was as high as 30% (55). There may also be a role for topical corticosteroids, with or without clindamycin (57). One half of a 25-mg rectal steroid suppository or one applicator of rectal hydrocortisone foam intravaginally should be used twice daily for 1 to 2 months; the dosage can then be reduced to once a day for an additional 2 months, followed by one- to three-times-a-week maintenance therapy. Estrogen therapy may also help in women with estrogen deficiency (57). If there is no response, a gynecologist or dermatologist should be consulted for confirmation of the diagnosis and consideration of additional treatments, including systemic corticosteroids or antibiotics.

Foreign Body

An occasional cause of vaginal discharge in adults is a foreign body. Lost tampons, forgotten diaphragms, and other smaller objects are easily found by examination. Symptoms improve after removal of the foreign body. Because secondary bacterial infection is also present, use of metronidazole, or clindamycin as prescribed for BV, or a povidone douche once daily for 3 to 4 days may accelerate healing.

GONOCOCCAL AND CHLAMYDIAL INFECTIONS

In the United States, gonococcal and chlamydial infections are the most common STDs of the upper genital tract. These infections may initially manifest as an abnormal discharge that is the result of an associated cervicitis. However, the patient usually considers the discharge a sign of vaginal infection. Although a purulent discharge is classically associated with gonorrhea, a mucopurulent discharge is also seen with chlamydia. Both infections may be asymptomatic. Chapter 37 presents a full discussion of diagnosis and treatment of gonococcal and chlamydial infections.

PELVIC INFLAMMATORY DISEASE

PID is a clinical diagnosis. It refers to upper genital tract inflammation caused by ascending pelvic infection and can include endometritis, salpingitis, tubo-ovarian abscess, and/or peritonitis. Most cases are believed to be attributable to initial infection with gonorrhea or chlamydia, but vaginal flora (e.g. *G. vaginalis, Haemophilus influenzae,* anaerobes, and enteric gram-negative rods) have also been implicated. *Mycoplasma hominis* and *Ureaplasma urealyticum* are also recent suspects (11). The sequelae of PID can be severe: a single episode of acute salpingitis causes infertility in approximately 8% of patients, and this complication rate can increase to 40% after three or more bouts with PID (59).

PID usually begins shortly after a menstrual period, and is typically characterized by fever, nausea, abdominal pain, and marked pelvic tenderness. Nonspecific symptoms such as dyspareunia, abnormal vaginal bleeding, and discharge may also be indicative of PID. The mildness and lack of specificity of symptoms in many cases may delay diagnosis (11). One recent study suggested that one fourth of women presenting to an ambulatory clinic with either gonorrhea or chlamydia actually had subclinical PID (60). The CDC recommends empiric treatment for PID if the following minimum diagnostic criteria are met (11):

- Uterine/adnexal tenderness
- Cervical motion tenderness

Additional criteria that increase the specificity of the diagnosis include

- Fever greater than 101°F (38.3°C)
- Abnormal cervical or vaginal mucopurulent discharge
- Presence of white blood cells (WBCs) on saline microscopy of vaginal secretions
- Documentation of infection with *Neisseria gonorrhoeae* or *C. trachomatis*
- Increased erythrocyte sedimentation rate
- Increase in C-reactive protein

The majority of affected women will have either mucopurulent discharge or WBCs noted on saline wet preparation.

There are additional, highly specific criteria for the diagnosis of PID. While not necessary to confirm in all cases, they may sometimes be useful. These include

- Endometrial biopsy with histopathologic evidence of endometritis
- Transvaginal sonography or magnetic resonance imaging showing thickened, fluid-filled tubes with or without free pelvic fluid or tubo-ovarian complex
- Laparoscopic abnormalities consistent with PID

Treatment

Because PID is usually polymicrobial, broad-spectrum antibiotic coverage must be effective against chlamydia, gonorrhea, and anaerobes, the common organisms involved. Because the male sexual partner is often infected as well, he should be treated (see Chapter 37). Women receiving treatment for PID should either abstain from intercourse or ensure that their partners use condoms until completion of therapy.

Table 102.3 includes indications for hospitalization are included with treatment recommendations. PID during pregnancy is rare. An obstetrician-gynecologist should be consulted promptly if this diagnosis is entertained during pregnancy. Erythromycin, amoxicillin, or azithromycin should be used in pregnant patients.

The presence of a pelvic or tubo-ovarian abscess, poor compliance, immunocompromise, severe illness with nausea, vomiting, or high fever; or failure of outpatient treatment should also prompt hospital admission (11,61). The switch from intravenous to oral antimicrobial therapy should be based on clinical assessment and can be done 24 hours after the patient has shown clinical improvement.

All regimens used to treat PID should cover gonorrhea and chlamydia even if cultures are negative. Anaerobic coverage is also currently recommended. Table 102.3 shows intravenous treatment regimens. A review of the literature suggests that these regimens have clinical cure rates greater than 90% (61). After patients have demonstrated significant clinical improvement, oral therapy should be continued with doxycycline 100 mg orally twice daily or clindamycin 450 mg four times a day to complete a 14-day course. Adequate anaerobic coverage is likely of greater importance in patients with tubo-ovarian abscesses, concurrent BV, or HIV infection (61). If tubo-ovarian abscess is present, the use of clindamycin, clindamycin with doxycycline, or metronidazole with doxycycline should be considered.

Outpatient cefoxitin- and ofloxacin-based regimens, listed in Table 102.3, have cure rates of at least 89%. Outpatient therapy should incorporate followup within 72 hours to assess response to treatment, and to expedite admission, intravenous therapy, and further evaluation if no significant improvement has occurred.

Any sexual partners of the patient within the 60 days preceding the diagnosis of PID should be treated

TABLE 102.3 Management of Pelvic Inflammatory Disease

1. Ambulatory treatment
    a. Ofloxacin 400 mg PO b.i.d. or levofloxacin 500 mg orally once daily for 14 days *with or without* metronidazole 500 mg PO b.i.d. for 14 d *or*
    b. Ceftriaxone 250 mg IM once or cefoxitin 2 g IM once with probenecid 1 g PO *plus* doxycycline 100 mg PO b.i.d. for 14 d, *with or without* metronidazole 500 mg PO b.i.d.
    c. Contact or observation within 72 hr to ensure improvement
2. Criteria for hospitalization
    a. Surgical emergency cannot be excluded;
    b. Diagnosis is certain but patient is toxic or unable to follow or tolerate an outpatient oral regimen
    c. The patient is severely ill, or has nausea, vomiting, or high fever (>100.4°F [38.3°C]),
    d. The patient has a tubo-ovarian abscess
    e. The patient does not respond clinically to oral antimicrobial therapy;
    f. The patient is pregnant
4. Inpatient treatment or ambulatory parenteral treatment
    a. Cefoxitin 2 g IV q6hr or cefotetan 2 g IV q12hr *and* doxycycline 100 mg IV q12hr *or*
    b. Gentamicin 2.0 mg per kg as an initial dose followed by 1.5 mg per kg q8hr (or single daily dosing) *and* clindamycin 900 mg IV q8hr *or*
    c. Ofloxacin 400 mg IV q12hr or levofloxacin 500 mg IV q day with or without metronidazole 500 mg IV q8hr *or*
    d. Ampicillin/sulbactam 3 g IV q6hr and doxycycline 100 mg PO q12hr
    e. After hospital discharge or adequate clinical response from parenteral antibiotics, continue oral therapy with either doxycycline 100 mg b.i.d. or clindamycin 450 mg PO q.i.d. for at least 14 d total therapy

[a] *Note:* Of the antibiotics listed use gentamicin, clindamycin, or cephalosporins in pregnant women. Ceftriaxone is effective against penicillinase-producing *Neisseria gonorrhoeae* (as well as many other organisms).

From Centers for Disease Control and Prevention. 2002 Sexually transmitted diseases treatment guidelines. Available at www.cdc.gov/mmwr/preview/mmwrhtml/rr5106a1.htm.

empirically for gonorrhea and chlamydia even if the patient's cultures are negative. Some experts also recommend rescreening women for gonorrhea and chlamydia 4 to 6 weeks after diagnosis and treatment of PID (11). Future use of condoms should be recommended: consistent condom use following an episode of PID has been associated with significantly reduced risks of recurrence and infertility (62).

VULVAR ULCERATIONS

Herpes Simplex Virus

Herpes simplex virus is a common cause of painful vulvar ulcerations. Chapter 37 discusses HSV and the evaluation of genital ulcers.

Syphilis

Syphilis is an STD caused by the spirochete *Treponema pallidum*. Vulvar ulcerations can be seen in all stages of syphilis. Chapter 37 discusses diagnosis and treatment of syphilis.

Chancroid

Chapter 37 discusses chancroid.

Tampon-Related Ulceration and Toxic Shock Syndrome

Repetitive tampon use during periods of diminished or absent menstrual flow may result in vaginal ulceration. Typically, patients with this problem develop intermenstrual bleeding or abnormal vaginal discharge. The ulcers are usually located in one of the vaginal fornices. They are superficial, erythematous, and 1 or 2 mm in diameter (often they are mistaken for herpes). The ulcers heal spontaneously in a few days if tampon use is discontinued.

Toxic shock syndrome (TSS) is a multisystem illness associated with fever greater than 102°F (39°C), hypotension, rash, skin desquamation, vomiting, and diarrhea (63). Shock may develop within 48 hours after the onset of the disorder. Other manifestations include palmar erythema, myalgias, and multi-organ system involvement. TSS is caused by strains of *Staphylococcus aureus* that produce superantigens, which exert toxic systemic effects (64). Increased incidence of TSS in the 1980s was associated with use of higher-absorbency tampons during menstruation (63). Since then, the incidence has decreased, although there has been concern for a recent increase in incidence since 2002 (11,63).

Pelvic examination typically reveals a purulent vaginal discharge. The vaginal walls are usually inflamed and may be ulcerated. Bimanual examination does not usually reveal any abnormal tenderness. If a tampon is present at the time of the examination, it should be removed and cultured. Testing for gonorrhea and chlamydia should be done to rule out either infection, which may occasionally be associated with symptoms that mimic the toxic shock syndrome.

Treatment of TSS consists of hospitalization for aggressive fluid resuscitation and hemodynamic monitoring. The vagina should be swabbed with Betadine, and any visible abscesses drained. Broad-spectrum antibiotics should be initiated, and continued for 10 to 15 days. First-line agents include β-lactamase-resistant antibiotics, nafcillin, oxacillin, or cephalosporins (65). Vancomycin can be used in case of penicillin allergy.

Cases of TSS must be reported to the state health department and to the CDC. The patient should not use tampons for several subsequent menstrual cycles. Generally, all patients using tampons should be encouraged to change them at least every 6 hours, and to avoid tampons made of superabsorbent material.

Other Causes of Vulvar Ulcerations

Less common causes of vulvar ulceration include granuloma inguinale, lymphogranuloma venereum, chancroid, hidradenitis suppurativa (Chapter 37), Behçet disease, Crohn disease, and tuberculosis. Table 102.4 shows a synopsis of common findings, diagnosis, and treatment of vulvar ulcerations. Any patient with an ulcer that is nonhealing, recurrent, or not easily diagnosed should be referred to a gynecologist or dermatologist.

MISCELLANEOUS LESIONS

Bartholin Gland Cyst or Abscess

Obstruction of the major duct of the Bartholin gland caused, for example, by inflammation, results in a Bartholin cyst (Fig. 102.1; Table 102.5). Infection of the duct can lead to a Bartholin abscess. Most Bartholin cysts occur because of mechanical blockage of the outflow of normal mucus secreted by the gland. If the cyst causes no symptoms and is only 1 to 3 cm in diameter, no treatment is necessary. Large cyst size, associated pain, or dyspareunia may indicate the need for intervention. Antibiotic therapy is not indicated for an uninfected cyst. If the patient is older than 40 years of age, a biopsy or excision to rule out carcinoma should be considered.

When treatment is indicated for a Bartholin cyst, the goal is to create a pathway from the cyst to the vaginal vestibule. This can be accomplished by incision and drainage, marsupialization, or, rarely, excision (66). These procedures should be done by a gynecologist. Infection of

TABLE 102.4 Causes of Vulvar Ulcerations

Disease Entity	*Cause*	*Appearance*	*Transmission*	*Symptoms: Other Manifestations*	*Diagnosis*	*Treatment*
Herpes simplex (see text)	Herpes simplex type 2 or 1	Vulvar vesicle(s) Vulvar ulceration	Sexual	Fever, malaise, lymphadenopathy, burning, paresthesia, dysuria, urinary retention, painful ulcer	Viral culture or direct fluorescent antibody test	Acyclovir Palliative treatment of lesions
Herpes zoster	Varicella zoster	Ulceration following the distribution of dermatome	Previous varicella zoster infection	Fever, malaise, lymphadenopathy, painful ulcer	Distribution of lesions Viral culture or direct fluorescent antibody test	Acyclovir, valacyclovir, or famciclovir Palliative treatment of symptoms
Syphilis (see text and Chapter 37)	*Treponema pallidum*	*Primary:* Chancre (hard, painless lesions with central ulceration, lymphadenopathy) *Secondary:* Condyloma latum (multiple flat plaques, often confluent); rash (especially palm and soles, lymphadenopathy) *Tertiary:* Gummatous tumors or ulceration	Sexual	*Secondary:* Malaise, flu-like syndrome, arthralgias, lymphadenopathy *Tertiary:* Central nervous system signs and symptoms	Positive flurescent treponemal antibody test Rising VDRL or rapid plasma reagin titers	Benzathine penicillin G, tetracycline, or doxycycline
Granuloma inguinale	*Calymmatobacterium granulomatis*	Painless, erythematous nodule that ulcerates (ulcers have irregular borders with a granulation base); lymphadenopathy in latter stages (scarring and lymphedema)	Sexual	Nonhealing ulcer that becomes painful after secondary bacterial infection	Donovan bodies (macrophages containing intracytoplasmic pleomorphic rods) on tissue crush preparation or biopsy	Trimethoprim/ sulfamethoxazole (Bactrim, Septra) or doxycycline, alternatively ciprofloxacin or erythromycin with addition of gentamicin if improvement is inadequate with either in a few days

Lymphogranuloma venereum (LGV)	*Chlamydia trachomatis* serotype L1, L2, or L3	Vulvar papule that ulcerates in 4–6 wk; hallmark inguinal adenitis; nodes are unilateral and edematous; later bubo formation (enlarged, matted nodes held together by inflammatory reaction); fistula formation, vulvar fenestration	Sexual	Fever, malaise, initially painless	Titer of at least 1:64 on LGV complement fixation test	Aspiration of fluctuant buboes Doxycycline Erythromycin Surgical reconstruction
Chancroid	*Haemophilus ducreyi*	Soft, painful, chancre-like ulcer	Sexual	Painful ulcer Inguinal adenopathy	Culturing is difficult; diagnosis of exclusion	Azithromycin Ceftriaxone Erythromycin Ciprofloxacin
Hidradenitis suppurativa (see Chapters 32 and 115)	Inflammation/infection of apocrine sweat glands	Vulvar abscess formation with draining sinuses, scarring, and induration; fistula formation	Nontransmittable	Pruritus, burning	Appearance Biopsy	Surgical excision Occasionally systemic antibiotics Rarely systemic or intralesional corticosteroids
Behçet disease	? Autoimmune	Vulvar ulcerations with associated oral ulcerations and ocular inflammation		Arthritis, erythema nodosum, pyoderma, thrombophlebitis, acne, ulcerative colitis, neurologic symptoms	Diagnosis of exclusion	No definitive treatment High-dose oral contraceptives Intralesional corticosteroids Chlorambucil
Crohn disease	Unknown	Linear ulcerations similar to a knife cut; draining sinuses; fistulous tracts		Oral ulcerations Gastrointestinal symptoms	Biopsy	Corticosteroids Sulfones Metronidazole Surgical reconstruction
Tuberculosis (see Chapter 34)	*Mycobacterium tuberculosis*	Painless ulceration	Airborne Primary inoculation		Biopsy, acid-fast cultures	Antituberculous therapy

TABLE 102.5 Common Nonmalignant Vulvar Lesions

Disease Entity	*Cause*	*Appearance*	*Symptoms*	*Complications*	*Diagnosis*	*Treatment*	*Other*
Bartholin cyst	Obstruction of the duct of the gland	Discrete swelling of the inferior aspect of labium majorum	None or vulvar pain caused by enlargement	Infection, hemorrhage into the cyst; carcinoma, if age ≥40 yr	Visual inspection	None, unless symptomatic, infected, or hemorrhagic—then incision and drainage	
Bartholin abscess	Infection and obstruction of the duct of the gland	Discrete swelling of the inferior aspect of the labium majorum	Pain	Hemorrhage; carcinoma, if age ≥40 yr	Visual inspection	Incision and drainage Marsupialization; rarely, excision	Culture for gonorrhea
Condylomata acuminata	Human papillomavirus	Single or multiple, 2–3 mm in diameter and 10–15 mm high, fine, finger-like projections or flat-topped lesions; lesions may become confluent	Itching, vaginal discharge	Secondary ulceration and infection	Visual inspection, biopsy	Podophyllum 10%–25%; trichloroacetic acid; liquid nitrogen or nitrous oxide or interferon injection	5-Fluorourucil for intravaginal lesions; laser surgery, excision, or electrodesiccation; treat partner
Sebaceous cyst	Unknown	Discrete swelling, often 1 cm in diameter; firm, solid with a yellow color	Vulvar irritation caused by enlargement; pain, if infected	Infection	Visual appearance, biopsy	None; excision, if infected or bothersome	

the Bartholin gland or duct is referred to as a Bartholin abscess. A Bartholin abscess harbors *N. gonorrhoeae* in approximately 10% of cases. Therefore, testing for gonorrhea and chlamydia is indicated. Other common causative organisms include *E. coli* and *Bacteroides* (67). The infection is often polymicrobial. Adequate drainage may obviate the need for systemic antibiotics. Sitz baths provide temporary symptomatic relief until drainage can be performed.

To drain a Bartholin abscess, one should perform the following:

1. Inject lidocaine in a vertical line over the most fluctuant area of the abscess at the medial aspect of the labia majora.
2. With a scalpel, incise the anesthetized area to the abscess cavity.
3. Drain all purulent material.
4. Break up loculation within the abscess cavity with a clamp.
5. Irrigate copiously with a 1:1 solution of physiologic saline and hydrogen peroxide.
6. Pack the cavity with Nu-Gauze packing material or place a small catheter in the cavity.
7. Instruct the patient to take sitz baths three or four times a day.
8. Repeat irrigation and packing one or two times a week until the cavity has healed.

Abscesses can also be treated by placement by a gynecologist of a Word catheter or marsupialization. Broad-spectrum antibiotics (which provide coverage for the likely etiologic agents) can be considered. Options include cephalosporins, clindamycin, or azithromycin (68).

Condylomata Acuminata (Genital Warts)

Condylomata acuminata are caused by human papillomavirus (HPV) and are transmitted sexually. Chapter 37 discusses these lesions.

Vulvar Papules

Folliculitis

Overgrowth of skin staphylococci and streptococci can result in vulvar folliculitis. Predisposing factors for this disorder include immunosuppressive therapy, local trauma, poor hygiene, and occlusive (synthetic) clothing. Infection of the hair follicle is identified by erythematous papules or pustules with a central hair shaft. Treatment consists of cleansing the area with a germicidal soap. Warm sitz baths or compresses help relieve the discomfort. Gentamicin or bacitracin ointment may be prescribed to accelerate healing. If the lesions do not heal within 1 week, systemic dicloxacillin, cephalexin, or erythromycin should be prescribed. In a diabetic patient, the infection could become worse more rapidly; therefore, a systemic and a topical antimicrobial agent are usually prescribed at the time of diagnosis.

Acrochordon

Acrochordons, commonly known as skin tags, are sessile or pedunculated fibroepithelial polyps. Acrochordons are benign and need be removed only if they are large or annoying to the patient. A gynecologist or dermatologist should be consulted or a biopsy performed if there is doubt regarding the diagnosis.

Molluscum Contagiosum

Molluscum contagiosum (see Chapter 117) is a pox virus that causes a benign, uncommon infection that is transmitted by close contact, including sexual intercourse. The adult patient characteristically sees a physician because of a painless new growth in the vulva, perineal area, or thighs. The lesions have a typical appearance, permitting diagnosis by inspection in most instances (Fig. 102.4). The individual lesions are wart-like papules varying from 1 to

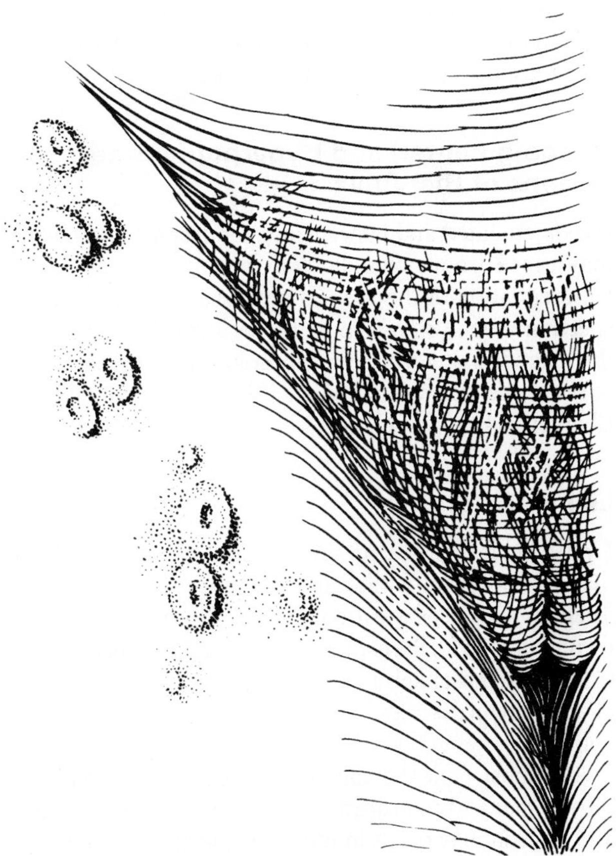

FIGURE 102.4. Molluscum contagiosum.

10 mm in diameter. They have a smooth surface and a central umbilical depression containing keratin. There may be multiple separate lesions or one large, coalesced lesion. If there is any doubt about the diagnosis, the central cheese-like core may be expressed onto a slide and examined under a microscope using the low-power objective. Characteristic large inclusion bodies, which occupy most of the cytoplasm of the cells, are identified. Occasionally, the lesion resembles bacterial infection, such as folliculitis or furunculosis, but in these instances, the expression of pus (rather than a cheesy material) from the lesion permits differentiation. If doubt remains regarding the diagnosis, the patient should be referred to a dermatologist or gynecologist for confirmation.

Most lesions will regress within 9 to 12 months (69). Therapy consists of scraping open the papule (with a scalpel blade), evacuating its contents, and curetting or cauterizing the base. Large lesions may need to be anesthetized with lidocaine injection before they are opened or curetted. The patient should be seen approximately 1 week after the initial treatment for retreatment of any resistant or new lesions. Other treatment options include cryotherapy and imiquimod (69). Also, the patient should be evaluated for the presence of another STD that may have been acquired simultaneously. Tests for chlamydia, gonorrhea, and syphilis should be obtained. The patient's sexual partner should be evaluated for lesions of molluscum contagiosum or evidence of another STD. A condom should be used until the patient's lesions have healed.

Hypopigmented and Hyperpigmented Lesions of the Vulva

Hypopigmented and hyperpigmented lesions of the vulva may range from nonmalignant to malignant disorders. Differentiation of the various processes is difficult by inspection alone. Biopsy must be performed to determine the diagnosis. Referral to a gynecologist or dermatologist is recommended when any such lesion is identified (see Chapter 104).

Lichen Sclerosus

Lichen sclerosus is a progressive and chronic condition marked by inflammation and thinning of the vulvar epithelium (70). It is most commonly seen in the anogenital region (71,72). Premenarchal girls and postmenopausal women are most likely to be affected (73), although women of any age can experience the condition. The etiology is unknown.

The most typical symptoms are itching and pain, although many women are asymptomatic (73). Dyspareunia and dysuria may occur in more advanced cases, in which the labia may become fused and the vulvar architecture is distorted. Classically, lichen sclerosus appears as thin, white skin in the affected area (70). Lesions can appear wrinkled or "parchment-like" (73). Fissuring, excoriations, or petechiae may be seen. The diagnosis must be established with a biopsy.

Vulvar lichen sclerosus carries a risk of malignancy: squamous cell carcinoma of the vulva can occur in approximately 5% of cases (74). Therefore, patients should be examined at least annually.

The mainstay of treatment is a potent topical corticosteroid. Options include clobetasol or halobetasol propionate ointment (0.05%), daily for 6 to 12 weeks, then one to three times weekly for maintenance therapy. Clinical improvement is likely (75). However, symptom recurrence is likely in the absence of maintenance therapy (76). There may also be a role for retinoids or immune system modulators such as pimecrolimus, although these medications should be used with caution, due to potential for skin irritation and unknown long-term effects. There is no role for topical hormones (other than corticosteroids), including testosterone, in the treatment of lichen sclerosus (70,74). Consultations with a dermatologist and a gynecologist may be useful.

Lichen Planus

As with vulvar lichen sclerosus, vulvar lichen planus is a chronic condition. Lichen planus may also involve the skin, oral mucous membranes, scalp, or nails (77). The etiology is unknown, but it is probably immunologically mediated (78).

There are three main subtypes of vulvar lichen planus: papulosquamous, erosive, and hypertrophic (rare). The papulosquamous type is associated with pruritic papules on the vulva or perianal area. The erosive type is associated with erythematous, painful erosions with a white border (Wickham striae) (79). As opposed to lichen sclerosus, vaginal involvement is commonly seen with the erosive form of lichen planus (79). Typical symptoms include vulvar pain or pruritus, vaginal discharge, and dyspareunia. There can be loss or distortion of the vulvar and vaginal architecture. Vaginal narrowing may develop, making intercourse extremely difficult and painful. Diagnosis of lichen planus must be confirmed with a biopsy.

Treatment of lichen planus can be difficult, as genital lesions may not respond well to therapy (80). Ultrapotent topical steroids, such as clobetasol propionate ointment 0.05%, can be applied nightly for 3 to 6 weeks, then twice a week for maintenance. Lower dose topical steroids can also be used for maintenance; regimens may vary. Vaginal suppositories (25 mg hydrocortisone twice a day for 2 months) have been used with success (77). Short courses (up to 4 weeks) of oral steroids may benefit women who have severe cases of lichen planus.

There may also be a role for immune system modulators such as tacrolimus. Some small studies have shown benefit

(81,82), although there is concern about the effects of long-term use of these medications. Vaginal dilator therapy may be helpful in cases of vaginal narrowing. Surgical options are available for severe or non-responsive cases. Consultations with appropriate specialists—dermatologist, gynecologist, or otolaryngologist—may be indicated.

Psoriasis and Seborrheic Dermatitis

Chapter 116 discusses psoriasis and seborrheic dermatitis. The classic appearance of psoriasis is usually altered on the vulva. Because the vulva is moist, the psoriatic scale often is not present, and psoriasis may appear as a nonspecific dermatitis. It is rare for a patient to have psoriasis only on the vulva, so a general dermatologic examination should be performed. Patients with suspected psoriasis on the vulva should be referred to a dermatologist or gynecologist for confirmation of the diagnosis.

Sebaceous Cyst (Epidermal, Keratinous, or Inclusion Cyst)

Sebaceous cysts present as firm, superficial spherical lesions, fixed in the dermis (Chapter 113). No treatment is necessary unless the cyst is infected (Chapter 32), or otherwise bothersome because of its size. Treatment then is excision.

Intertrigo

Chapter 116 discusses intertrigo.

Contact Dermatitis (Reactive Dermatitis)

Chapter 116 discusses contact dermatitis.

VULVODYNIA

Vulvodynia is a syndrome of unexplained vulvar pain. The syndrome is often accompanied by sexual dysfunction and psychological disability. Symptoms must be present for at least three months. The two localized types are clitorodynia and vestibulodynia (83). The most common type of vulvodynia is vestibulodynia. Vulvodynia is still not well understood, and patients often go to many different providers before being diagnosed. A recent population based survey found that 12% of women have had symptoms consistent with vulvodynia at some point in their lives (84).

There are many theories regarding the etiology of vulvodynia, but the most accepted theory is that it is a syndrome of neurologically mediated pain. Many patients identify a history of frequent candidal infections, treatments for condyloma, or other injury that preceded the onset of pain. Tissue injury causes the release of inflammatory neuropeptides, and nociceptors in the region become sensitized, leading to hyperesthesia or allodynia (pain in response to a stimulus that does not ordinarily provoke pain) (85).

Vulvodynia can negatively impact a woman's self esteem and relationship with her partner. Most studies have not found more frequent histories of sexual abuse, but a recent study found there may be higher rates of physical abuse in a subset of patients with vulvodynia (84). Other pain syndromes are also common in patients with vulvodynia, such as irritable bowel syndrome (IBS), interstitial cystitis, and fibromyalgia (86). An increased sensitivity to touch in nongenital sites in the body has also been documented (87). The muscles of the pelvic floor frequently play an important role in the perpetuation of pain in vulvodynia. Muscle hypertonicity may be primary and lead to vulvar pain, or muscle splinting may begin as a response to localized vulvar pain, but then become chronic.

Evaluation

The evaluation of a patient with vulvar pain begins with a careful pelvic examination. Any suspicious areas on the vulva should be biopsied. The vaginal discharge should be assessed, and any vaginitis treated. It is critical to make sure the vagina is well estrogenized. Mild degrees of atrophic vaginitis in perimenopausal women are frequently missed, but can have a large impact on vaginal symptoms. All patients should have vaginal fungal cultures sent because there is significant overlap in symptomatology between fungal infections and vulvodynia. A careful history must be taken to identify potential irritants. Antibacterial and perfumed soaps are frequent culprits, but other possibilities are over-the-counter vaginal products, sanitary pads, fabric softener sheets, and laundry detergents.

Urinary tract symptoms are also common in patients with introital dyspareunia. The presence of interstitial cystitis or urethritis may explain a patient's symptoms, or be an important contributing factor. Any patient with persistent urinary symptoms, especially in the presence of a negative urine culture, should be referred for cystoscopy.

The level of tenderness around the introitus can be assessed at each visit by lightly touching a cotton-tipped swab to various locations around the vulva and recording the patient's rating of the level of pain (Figure 102.5). Assessment of the pelvic floor muscles for hypertonicity or tenderness is equally important.

Treatment

Treatment of vulvodynia is aimed at breaking the cycle of pain, inflammation, sensitization, muscle tension, and maladaptive behaviors. A combination of therapies is usually necessary, frequently requiring a multidisciplinary approach, especially if the pain is long-standing.

Medications that are used to treat neuropathic pain in other areas of the body are used to treat vulvodynia as well (e.g., tricyclic antidepressants, anticonvulsants). Table

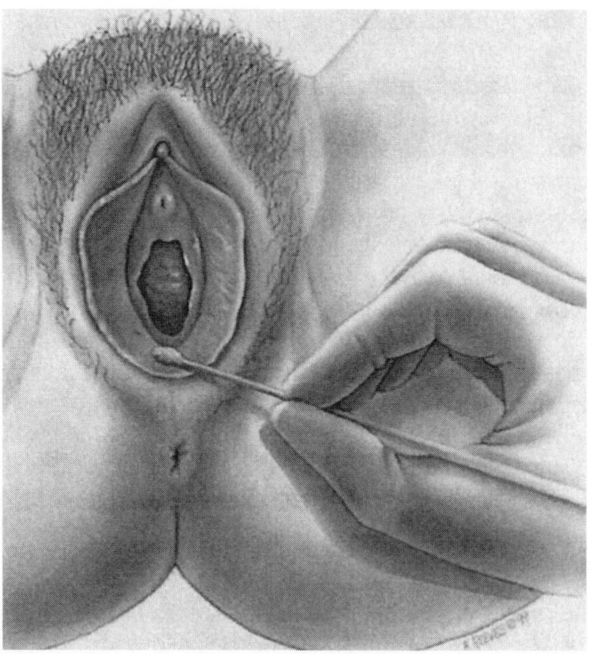

FIGURE 102.5. Vulvar examination for vulvodynia. (From Haefner HK. Critique of new gynecologic surgical procedures: surgery for vulvar vestibulitis. Clin Obstet Gynecol 2000;43:689.)

102.6 summarizes some of these medications (88–93). It may be helpful to explain to the patient that these drugs are used for their effects on the pain pathways rather than for depression.

There are also many topical medications that have been used in the treatment of vulvodynia (Table 102.6) (88,90). Evidence for the efficacy of most is either anecdotal or based on limited evidence. Many of the medications can be prepared by a compounding pharmacist. Many patients receive topical steroids, but there is no evidence of efficacy, and care must be taken to avoid steroid rebound dermatitis and genital atrophy. One small trial supports the use of submucosal infiltrations into the vulva of methylprednisolone and lidocaine (92). Many patients prefer to use a topical medication to avoid the risks and side effects associated with centrally acting drugs. A combination of a peripherally acting and a centrally acting medication is often beneficial.

Physical therapists with specialized training in pelvic floor therapy are invaluable in the treatment of vulvodynia, and should be consulted whenever there is tightness, weakness, or tenderness in the pelvic floor muscles. Biofeedback may be effective for some patients with vulvodynia (93).

Finally, the patient can be referred to a gynecologist for a surgical procedure, such as local excision, vestibulectomy, or perineoplasty, if more conservative techniques are ineffective. Most patients prefer to avoid an invasive procedure if possible, but success rates of 80% or greater are usually reported for surgical treatments. One randomized study comparing cognitive behavioral therapy, biofeedback, and surgical vestibulectomy found that all treatments significantly reduced pain, but that vestibulectomy was the most effective (94).

It is important to treat any muscle hypertonicity prior to surgery to maximize chances of a good outcome. Patients with primary vulvodynia, or pain beginning with their partner's first attempt at vaginal penetration, have poorer responses to surgery (95).

TABLE 102.6 Medications Used for the Treatment of Vulvodynia

Drug	*Usual Dose*	*Comments*
Amitriptyline (91)	10–100 mg by mouth night each night	Side effects common with higher doses: drowsiness, dry mouth, weight gain, dizziness, constipation
Gabapentin (90)	900–3600 mg by mouth daily, divided into three doses	Fewer side effects than amitriptyline Drowsiness, tremor, blurred vision, weight gain
Venlafaxine	37.5 mg–150 mg by mouth, daily	Fewer side effects than either amitriptyline or gabapentin, less evidence for efficacy Discontinuation syndrome common
Lidocaine gel or ointment (88)	2%–5% applied topically (Zolnoun study used saturated cotton ball applied to the fourchette nightly for 6 to 7 weeks)	Can cause burning in some patients Do not exceed 20 gm daily of 5% preparation
Nitroglycerine cream	0.2% applied topically at least three times per week	Headache is a common side effect
Capsaicin cream (89)	0.025% in acid mantle cream applied to the vulva for 20 minutes daily	Patients needed to be pretreated with lidocaine
Estrogen cream	2 g or less intravaginally or topically to the vulva, daily	Use small amounts to minimize risks associated with any estrogens. Endometrial effects are possible with an intact uterus
Amitriptyline 2%/Baclofen 2% in water washable base (93)	Apply 0.5 ml to affected area one to three times daily	Anecdotal evidence only

Postfracture Treatment Program

An osteoporosis treatment program can often be implemented in the setting of new fracture, a time when many patients who were previously unwilling to consider osteoporosis management become interested. Calcium supplementation should be prescribed, although 1500 mg daily may not be tolerated initially because of constipation from narcotics prescribed for fracture pain. Vitamin D, 800 to 1000 units, is recommended. Bisphosphonate therapy in this setting has been difficult to implement because of the high prevalence of gastroesophageal reflux and constipation, although once-weekly and once-monthly dosing may be tolerated. Calcitonin therapy has less adverse effects and is used routinely in the management of acute vertebral fractures.

SPECIFIC REFERENCES

1. Melton LJ III, Chrischilles EA, Cooper C, et al. Perspective: how many women have osteoporosis? J Bone Miner Res 1992;7:1005.
2. Melton LJ III, Atkinson EJ, O'Fallon WM, et al. Long-term fracture prediction by bone mineral assessed at different skeletal sites. J Bone Miner Res 1993;8:1227.
3. Miller PD. Management of osteoporosis. Adv Intern Med 1999;44:175.
4. Riggs BL, Melton LJ 3rd. The prevention and treatment of osteoporosis. N Engl J Med 1992;327:620.
5. National Institutes of Health. Osteoporosis prevention, diagnosis, and therapy. NIH Consensus Statement 2001;285:785.
6. Luckey MM, Wallenstein S, Lapinski R, et al. A prospective study of bone loss in African-American and white women: a clinical research center study. J Clin Endocrinol Metab 1996;81:2948.
7. Cummings SR, Black DM, Nevitt MC, et al. Bone density at various sites for prediction of hip fractures: The Study of Osteoporotic Fractures Research Group. Lancet 1993;341:72.
8. Anonymous. Consensus Development Conference: diagnosis, prophylaxis, and treatment of osteoporosis. Am J Med 1993; 94:646.
9. Stenson WF, Newberry R, Lorenz R, et al. Increased prevalence of celiac disease and need for routine screening among patients with osteoporosis. Arch Intern Med 2005;165:393.
10. The WHO Study Group. Assessment of fracture risk and its application to screening for postmenopausal osteoporosis. Geneva: World Health Organization, 1994.
11. Preventive Services Task Force. Screening for osteoporosis in postmenopausal women: recommendations and rationale. Ann Intern Med 2002;137:526.
12. Raisz, LG. Screening for osteoporosis. N Engl J Med 2005;353:164.
13. Health Care Financing Administration. Medicare Program. Medicare coverage and payment for bone mass measurements. Federal Register 1998;63:34320.
14. Frost ML, Blake GM, Fogelman I. Can the WHO criteria for diagnosing osteoporosis be applied to calcaneal quantitative ultrasound? Osteoporos Int 2000;11:321.
15. Garnero P, Hausherr E, Chapuy MC, et al. Markers of bone resorption predict hip fracture in elderly women: The EPIDOS prospective study. J Bone Miner Res 1996;11:1531.
16. Hamwi A, Ganem AH, Grebe C, et al. Markers of bone turnover in postmenopausal women receiving hormone replacement therapy. Clin Chem Lab Med 2001;39:414.
17. Ross PD, Davis JW, Epstein RS, et al. Pre-existing fractures and bone mass predict vertebral fracture incidence in women. Ann Intern Med 1991;114:919.
18. Cummings SR, Nevitt MC, for the Study of Osteoporotic Fractures Research Group. Non-skeletal determinants of fractures: the potential importance of the mechanics of falls. Osteoporos Int 1994;1[Suppl]:657:67.
19. Rosen, CJ. Postmenopausal osteoporosis. N Engl J Med 2005;353:595.
20. Rossouw JE, Anderson GL, Prentice RL, et al. Risks and benefits of estrogen plus progestin in healthy postmenopausal women: principal results from the Women's Health Initiative randomized controlled trial. JAMA 2002;288: 321.
21. Ettinger B, Black DM, Mitlak BH, et al. Reduction of vertebral fracture risk in postmenopausal women with osteoporosis treated with raloxifene: results of a 3-year randomized clinical trial. JAMA 1999;282:637.
22. Breuer B, Wallenstein S, Anderson R. Effect of tamoxifen on bone fractures in older nursing home residents. J Am Geriatr Soc 1998;46:968.
23. Kreijkamp-Kaspers S, Koh L, Grobbee DE, et al. Effect of soy protein containing isoflavones. JAMA 2004;292:65.
24. McClung M, Clemmesen B, Daifotis A, et al. Alendronate prevents postmenopausal bone loss in women without osteoporosis. Ann Intern Med 1998;128:253.
25. Dawson-Hughes B, Harris SS, Krall EA, et al. Effect of calcium and vitamin D supplementation on bone density in men and women 65 years of age or older. N Engl J Med 1997;337:670.
26. Schousboe JT, Nyman JA, Kane RL, et al. Cost-effectiveness of alendronate therapy for osteopenic postmenopausal women. Ann Intern Med 2005;142:734.
27. Cummings SR, Black DM, Thompson DE, et al. Effect of alendronate on risk of fracture in women with low bone density but without vertebral fractures: results from the Fracture Intervention Trial. JAMA 1998;280:2077.
28. Harris ST, Watts NB, Genant HK, et al. Effects of risedronate treatment on vertebral and nonvertebral fractures in women with postmenopausal osteoporosis. JAMA 1999;282: 1344.
29. Reginster JY, Wilson KM, Dumont E, et al. Monthly oral ibandronate is well tolerated and efficacious in postmenopausal women: results from the monthly oral pilot study. Clin Endocrinol Metab 2005;90:5018.
30. Odvina CV, Zerwekh JE, Rao DS, et al. Severely suppressed bone turnover: a potential complication of alendronate therapy. J Clin Endocrinol Metab. 2005;90:1294.
31. Saag KG, Emkey R, Schnitzer TJ, et al. Alendronate for the prevention and treatment of glucocorticoid-induced osteoporosis. N Engl J Med 1998;339:292.
32. Orwoll E, Ettinger M, Weiss S, et al. Alendronate for the treatment of osteoporosis in men. N Engl J Med 2000;343:604.
33. Reid IR, Brown JP, Burckhardt P, et al. Intravenous zoledronic acid in postmenopausal women with low bone mineral density. N Engl J Med 2002;346:653.
34. Gennari C, Camporeale A. Calcitonin in the treatment of osteoporosis. Osteoporos Int 1997; 7[Suppl 3]:S159.
35. Neer RM, Arnaud CD, Zanchetta JR, et al. Effect of parathyroid hormone (1–34) on fractures and bone mineral density in postmenopausal women with osteoporosis. N Engl J Med 2001;344:1434.
36. Reginster JY, Meurmans L, Zegels B, et al. The effect of sodium monofluorophosphate plus calcium on vertebral fracture rate in postmenopausal women with moderate osteoporosis. Ann Intern Med 1998;129:1.
37. Meunier PJ, Roux C, Seeman E, et al. The effects of strontium ranelate on the risk of vertebral fracture in women with postmenopausal osteoporosis. N Engl J Med 2004;50:459.

*For annotated **General References** and resources related to this chapter, visit www.hopkinsbayview.org/PAMreferences.*

Chapter 104

Early Detection of Gynecologic Malignancy

Robert L. Giuntoli, II, George R. Huggins, and Robert E. Bristow

Malignancies commonly develop in the female reproductive organs. In the United States, cancers of the genital tract account for approximately 12% of cancers in women and results in about 11% of cancer-related deaths (1). Many of the invasive lesions at these sites are preceded by preinvasive lesions. Treatment of lesions during the preinvasive phase results in prevention of malignant sequelae. If a cancer remains confined to the primary organ at the time of treatment, 5-year survival rates are typically in the 80% to 90% range (1). Unfortunately once distant spread has occurred, outcome is significantly worse with 5 year survival rates of approximately 20% to 30% (1). With these findings in mind, the goal of surveillance is the prevention of invasive disease. If a malignancy does develop, surveillance may allow for diagnosis early in the course of the disease, resulting in improved survival.

Both patient and practitioner actively participate in cancer surveillance. Self examination is an important component of early cancer detection. Both the breasts and external genitalia can be evaluated by the patient on a regular basis. Although symptoms such as abnormal vaginal bleeding or vulvar itching are not pathognomonic for malignancy, prompt and appropriate evaluation of these symptoms may result in the diagnosis of a premalignant process or cancer at an early stage. Annual screening of a female patient by a practitioner should include a pelvic exam which allows for inspection and palpation of the pelvic organs and screening with a Papanicolaou smear. Practitioner-initiated screening is vital for women at risk for gynecologic malignancies.

VULVAR LESIONS

The vulva is subject to similar disease processes of the skin seen elsewhere on the body. Malignant conditions of the vulva represent approximately 2% of cancers of the female genital tract (1). Although the area does not typically receive direct sun exposure, malignant conditions associated with ultraviolet radiation such as melanoma involve the vulva and vagina not infrequently. The vast majority of cancers involving the vulva (almost 85%) are squamous cell carcinomas. The second most common vulvar malignancy is melanoma, approximately 5%. Other tumors include adenocarcinomas (such as Bartholin gland tumors, Paget disease), basal cell carcinomas, and sarcomas. The remainder of this section will focus on the more common squamous cell carcinomas. The interested reader is referred to one of several gynecologic oncology texts listed below for more information on the less common vulvar malignancies.

Preinvasive lesions of the vulva are described as vulvar intraepithelial neoplasia (VIN). Over the last 20 years, the rate of VIN has doubled. Although the average age of women with preinvasive lesions is between 40 and 50 years, VIN can and often does develop in young women. In older patients, VIN has a tendency to be unifocal, while in younger patients, the process is typically multifocal (2). Lesions often arise in the labia minora, the anus, and introitus with less common involvement of the clitoris and urethra (3). Evidence of human papillomavirus (HPV) infection is noted in the majority of VIN lesions (4).

Invasive squamous cell carcinomas of the vulva include keratinizing squamous carcinoma and basaloid and warty carcinomas. Most women with invasive vulvar cancer are diagnosed in the seventh decade of life. Occasionally, women younger than 40 may develop a vulvar malignancy. An increased risk of vulvar cancer is associated with a history of condyloma acuminata, increasing number of lifetime sexual partners, immunosuppression, and smoking. The basaloid and warty carcinomas appear to be associated with HPV infection, while keratinizing squamous carcinomas are not (4,5).

VIN and vulvar cancer typically presents as papular or maculopapular lesions with a roughened surface. However, these lesions can have many different appearances, and often appear to be well defined and innocent. The lesions may vary from white to hyperpigmented. They may be sharply demarcated or generalized over the vulva and may even spread to adjacent regions. Some may resemble seborrheic keratoses, nevi, lentigo, intertrigo, condylomata acuminata, or condylomata lata. Biopsy is required to make the diagnosis and to identify invasion.

Several factors unfortunately contribute to the common delay in the diagnosis of VIN and vulvar cancer. First, no vulvar equivalent of the cervical Papanicolaou smear is available. Lesions must be diagnosed by biopsy. Additionally, both patients and practitioners play a role in deferring diagnosis. These lesions typically cause symptoms. Itching occurs in 70% of patients. Other complaints include ulceration, bleeding, pain, or the presence of a mass. Despite these symptoms, most women delay enlisting the care of a medical practitioner. Once a patient does decide to seek medical care however, diagnosis is usually further delayed by the institution of medicinal treatments such as steroid creams. A high index of suspicion is required for all vulvar lesions and symptoms with a low threshold for biopsy or referral to a specialist for biopsy.

The treatment of VIN depends on the extent of the lesion. If the vulvar lesions grossly appear to be *condyloma acuminata* and are not extensive, they may be treated empirically with compounds such as imiquimod (Aldara) cream without biopsy (see Chapter 102). If no decrease in size is apparent within 2 to 4 weeks, the suspected condylomata acuminata should be biopsied to confirm the diagnosis. The pathologist should be made aware of prior treatment of the lesion as several agents can cause histologic changes that would be otherwise concerning. Lesions may be excised or ablated. Prior to use of ablative techniques such as laser, thorough evaluation with the liberal use of biopsy must be performed to rule out invasive disease.

Lichen sclerosus is a common vulvar condition associated with intense itching in postmenopausal females. After the diagnosis is confirmed by biopsy, treatment utilizes steroid creams such as clobetasol (Temovate). If therapy is not successful in improving the lesion and associated symptoms, biopsy should once again be performed to exclude an occult neoplastic lesion.

Prevention of advanced disease requires that the patient be taught to examine her vulva periodically with the use of a mirror and to report any changes in the external genitalia. It is important that one examine the patient promptly if a change is noted and that a periodic examination, usually in conjunction with a routine gynecologic examination, be performed even when there are no complaints. Special sensitivity must be used in older women, who often are reluctant to complain of a vaginal or vulvar problem.

CERVICAL LESIONS

Epidemiology and Etiologic Factors

With the introduction and vigorous promotion of the Papanicolaou smear, an exponential decline in both the incidence of cervical cancer and deaths from this disease has occurred in the United States. Carcinoma of the cervix is the third most common malignancy of the genital tract in the United States after endometrial and ovarian carcinoma. Current estimates predict 10,370 new cases of cervical cancer and 3,710 deaths from this disease in the United States in 2005 (1).

HPV deoxyribonucleic acid (DNA) is found in more than 99% of all cervical cancers (6). Transmission of the virus is primarily through sexual contact. However nonveneral transmission most likely also occurs. More than 100 strains of HPV have been identified, at least 30 of which are tropic for the genital tract. HPV 6 and HPV 11 are most often found in cervical condylomata and low-grade dysplasia. HPV 16 and HPV 18 account for the majority of cervical cancers. HPV 45, HPV 31, and HPV 33 infection are also associated with invasive carcinomas of the cervix (7).

HPV infection is considered necessary but not sufficient for the development of cervical cancer. The incidence of HPV infection appears to be an order of magnitude higher than the incidence of preinvasive or squamous intraepithelial lesions. Only a small minority of women with HPV infections go on to develop a high grade squamous intraepithelial lesion or cervical cancer. The majority of HPV infections appear to resolve over time (8). The causes for the variation in clinical course associated with HPV infection have not been fully elucidated. Given the self-limited nature of most HPV infections and low-grade squamous intraepithelial lesions, conservative management with close followup should be pursued. Intervention, however, is required for progression of disease.

Invasive cervical cancer is considered an acquired immunodeficiency syndrome (AIDS) defining illness. Human immunodeficiency virus (HIV)-infected patients have an approximately 10-fold increase in cervical dysplasia on cytologic screening. Recurrence rates for dysplasia are increased in women with HIV infection. As the prevalence of dysplasia and the risk of recurrence increases with worsening immunodeficiency, cervical pathology in HIV-infected women appears to result from suppression of the immune system (9). Although squamous intraepithelial lesions are precursors for invasive cervical cancer, epidemiologic investigations have reported conflicting data as to the influence of HIV infection on the incidence of carcinoma of the cervix (10,11).

Papanicolaou Smear

The mainstay of cervical cancer control is regular screening by means of Papanicolaou smear, with abnormal results prompting referral for colposcopy and possible biopsy. As mentioned above, the widespread introduction of Papanicolaou smears has been associated with a substantial reduction in the incidence of cervical cancer. There has also been a corresponding increase in the detection of

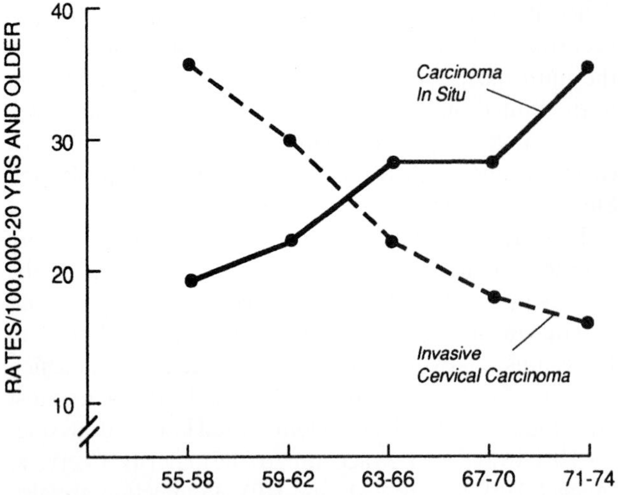

FIGURE 104.1. Average annual age-adjusted incidence rate trends for invasive carcinoma and carcinoma *in situ* of the cervix from the Toledo, Ohio, area. (Redrawn from Kim K, Rigal RD, Patrick JR, et al. The changing trends of uterine cancer and cytology: a study of morbidity and mortality trends over a twenty year period. Cancer 1978;42:2439.)

preinvasive lesions. An investigation of invasive carcinoma and carcinoma in situ of the cervix over a 20-year period during which Papanicolaou smears became widespread clearly demonstrates this association (Fig. 104.1). Despite these results, the efficacy of the Papanicolaou smear as a screening tool has never been tested in a prospective, blinded study. The sensitivity for the Papanicolaou smear is approximately 70% with a specificity of about 75% (12). The effectiveness of the Papanicolaou smear arises not from the accuracy of an individual test but from the use of regular screening. Given the real possibility of a false-negative result, all suspicious cervical lesions require biopsy regardless of the presence of a negative Papanicolaou smear.

The technique for Papanicolaou smear is straightforward. A speculum is inserted. Once the cervix is visualized, the cervical spatula should be placed firmly against the cervix and rotated at least 360 degrees, preferably 720 degrees, in a continuous unidirectional sweep. A plastic brush (Endo-C, Milex, Chicago, IL) should be used to sample the endocervical canal. This increases the recovery of endocervical cells and decreases the number of inadequate Papanicolaou smears. The most important area to be sampled is the squamocolumnar junction, because most cervical neoplastic processes arise at this site. The anatomic relationships of this junction are different in the adolescent, the sexually active woman, and the postmenopausal woman (Fig. 104.2). For a traditional slide Papanicolaou smear, both specimens should then be smeared together onto a clean microscopic slide and immediately sprayed or immersed in fixative to prevent an air-drying artifact. For the newer liquid-based cytology methods, the sample is collected in the usual fashion, but is placed in transport medium rather than on a slide.

A screening Papanicolaou smear should not be obtained if a woman has douched or used vaginal medication or a tampon in the previous 24 hours. These activities may alter or remove cells completely and yield an erroneous interpretation. Lubricants may also interfere with cytologic interpretation. The speculum used in the examination should be unlubricated or, if necessary, lubricated only with water.

New cervical cancer screening methods have recently been introduced: most notably, liquid suspension Pap test techniques. Liquid-based cytology holds several advantages over the traditional Papanicolaou smear. There is an increased detection of high-grade squamous intraepithelial lesions (13). There is a decrease in the presence of obscuring blood and inflammation resulting in an improvement in specimen adequacy (14). Finally, residual cellular material is available for molecular analysis such as HPV DNA testing. The main disadvantage of liquid-based cytology is price. The cost of liquid-based cytology is significantly greater than the traditional, successful slide-based traditional Papanicolaou smear.

In 2003, the American College of Obstetricians and Gynecologists (ACOG) updated their recommendations for cervical cancer screening (15). These recommendations include: Annual cervical cytology screening should begin 3 years after initiation of sexual intercourse, but no later than age 21. Prior to age 30, women should undergo annual cervical cytology screening. Over age 30, women who have had three consecutive negative cervical cytology screening test results and who have no history of HSIL or worse, are not immunocompromised or HIV infected, and were not exposed to diethylstilbestrol in utero may undergo cervical cytology examinations every 2 to 3 years. Both traditional slide-based and liquid-based cervical cytology are acceptable for screening. After hysterectomy with removal of the cervix, women who have no prior history of HSIL or worse may discontinue routine cytology testing. After age 30, the use of a combination of cervical cytology and HPV DNA screening is appropriate. If this combination is used and both tests are negative, rescreening should be performed no more frequently than every 3 years (15).

The Bethesda 2001 Workshop updated the Bethesda System terminology for reporting the results of cervical cytology (16). All Papanicolaou smear require three components. First, the report must contain a comment on the specimen adequacy: satisfactory or unsatisfactory. Second, the report must contain a general categorization: negative for intraepithelial lesion or malignancy, epithelial cell abnormality, or other. Finally, the report must include a description of any epithelial abnormalities. The 2001 Bethesda System places squamous epithelial cell abnormalities include four categories: (a) atypical squamous cells further divided into atypical squamous cells of

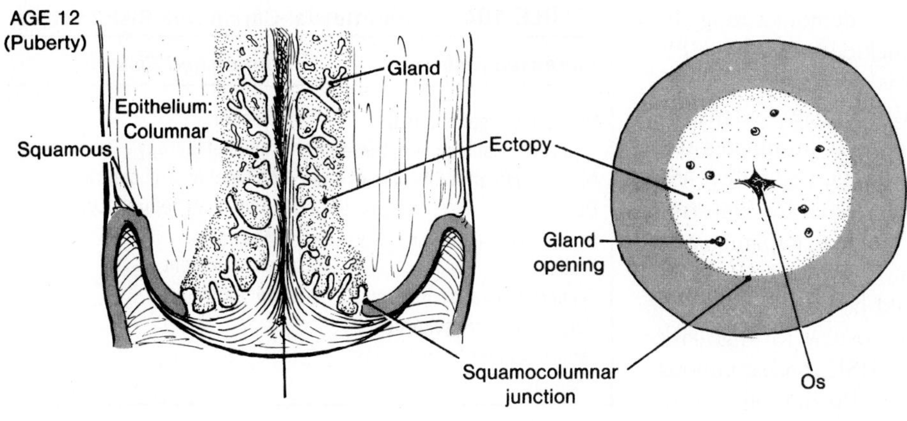

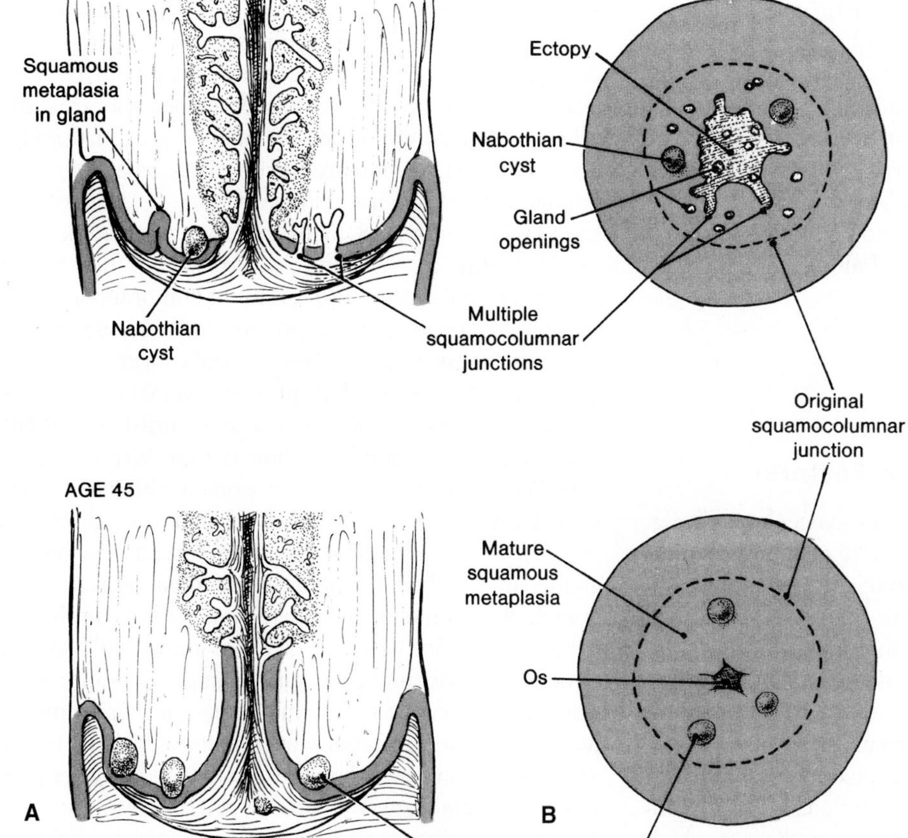

FIGURE 104.2. The uterine cervix in women of various ages. **A:** Coronal section of the cervix and vaginal vault. **B:** Vaginal view of the cervix. (Redrawn from Briggs RM. Dysplasia and early neoplasia of the uterine cervix: a review. Obstet Gynecol Surv 1980;34:70.)

undetermined significance (ASCUS) and cannot exclude high grade, (b) low-grade squamous intraepithelial lesion (LSIL), (c) high-grade squamous intraepithelial lesion (HSIL), and (d) squamous cell carcinoma. Glandular cell abnormalities include three categories: (a) atypical glandular cells, (b) endocervical adenocarcinoma in situ (AIS), and (c) adenocarcinoma.

All glandular cell abnormalities require further evaluation for possible cervical lesions and for possible lesions higher in the genital tract. High-risk HPV testing does not alter the workup process for glandular lesions. All patients with Papanicolaou smears demonstrating abnormal glandular cells should be referred to a specialist for further evaluation and management.

Evaluation of Papanicolaou smears demonstrating abnormal squamous cells typically includes selective HPV testing and colposcopy. *Colposcopy* is an office procedure, done during a pelvic examination with the use of an instrument similar to a dissecting microscope. It illuminates and magnifies (8× to 10×) the cervix, vagina, and vulva. ASCUS Papanicolaou smears should be tested for high-risk HPV DNA. If testing is negative, a repeat Papanicolaou smear should be performed in 6 to 12 months. Referral to a specialist for colposcopy should be obtained for patients with ASCUS smears that test positive for high risk HPV DNA and for patients with LSIL, HSIL, and squamous cell carcinoma on Papanicolaou smear. During colposcopy, biopsies are usually obtained of the ectocervix and the endocervix. Women with biopsy confirmed LSIL may be followed conservatively. Patients with higher grade lesions most often require excisional procedures such as loop electrosurgical excisional procedure (LEEP) or cold-knife cone (CKC). After appropriate workup and treatment, women with a history of a squamous cell abnormality require Papanicolaou smears every 4 to 6 months for several years. If repeat Pap smears show persistent abnormalities, the patient should be once again referred for colposcopy and biopsy. The interested reader is referred to one of several gynecologic oncology texts listed below for more information the evaluation and treatment of abnormal Papanicolaou smears.

TABLE 104.1 Endometrial Carcinoma Risk Factors

Increased Risk	*Diminished Risk*
Unopposed menopausal estrogen replacement therapy	Ovulation
Menopause after 52 years of age	Progestin therapy
Obesity	Combination oral contraceptives
Nulliparity	Menopause before 49 years of age
Diabetes	Normal weight
Feminizing ovarian tumors	Multiparity
Polycystic ovary syndrome	
Tamoxifen therapy for breast cancer	

UTERINE CARCINOMA

Epidemiology and Etiologic Factors

Uterine cancer is the most common gynecologic malignancy. Current estimates predict 40,880 new cases of uterine cancer in the United States in 2005. An estimated 7,310 deaths will occur during the same period in the United States secondary to cancer of the uterus (1). The majority of uterine cancers arise from the endometrium and present with vaginal bleeding.

Endometrial cancer results from exposure to unopposed estrogen stimulation. The exposure may either be endogenous or exogenous. Examples of endogenous stimulation include obesity and polycystic ovary disease, which results in chronic anovulation. Obesity results in increased endogenous exposure secondary to the peripheral conversion of androgens to estrogen in adipose tissue. With chronic anovulation, a woman is exposed to the unopposed estrogen of the follicular phase without the protective progestin component of the luteal phase. An example of exogenous stimulation is unopposed estrogen-only hormone replacement therapy. Table 104.1 lists factors that affect endometrial cancer risk.

Long-term use of unopposed estrogen in postmenopausal women significantly increases the risk of endometrial carcinoma. In the Postmenopausal Estrogen/Progestin Interventions (PEPI) trial, a longitudinal study looking at postmenopausal hormone replacement, 62.2% of women taking continuous unopposed estrogen developed abnormal endometrial histology during the 3 years of the trial. Of those who developed abnormal histology, one third did so during the first year of use (17). There is a 14-fold increase in risk of endometrial cancer among women who use unopposed estrogen replacement therapy for 7 years (18). This increased risk can be nullified by adding a progestin (e.g., Provera) to the estrogen regimen (see Chapter 106). Combination oral contraceptive pills and pregnancy also provide progestin support and result in a reduced risk of endometrial cancer.

Currently, screening asymptomatic women for endometrial cancer is not recommended. In contrast, all patients with abnormal vaginal bleeding require further evaluation. While the vast majority of women with endometrial cancer are postmenopausal or perimenopausal, 5% are younger than 40 years of age. Therefore, as a small but significant number of patients with endometrial adenocarcinoma are premenopausal, irregular bleeding in this age group should not be ignored. Evaluation should include a focused history and physical with a pelvic examination. Additional investigation including endometrial sampling and ultrasound are often warranted. Women at risk for endometrial cancer such as those with hereditary nonpolyposis colorectal cancer should be referred to a specialist. Women ingesting tamoxifen are also at increased risk for endometrial cancer and require thorough evaluation. The significance of a rapidly enlarging uterus is unclear. Historically, this finding was felt to be concerning for smooth muscle tumors of the myometrium.

Diagnostic Techniques

Several methods are available for the evaluation of patients with signs or symptoms suspicious for endometrial cancer. Sampling of the endometrial cavity for histologic examination is commonly deemed the most accurate approach. Dilation and curettage is still considered the gold standard, but is best performed in the operating room. Methods for office evaluation are available. The Pipelle endometrial suction curette (United International Marketing Resources, Wilton, CT) is often used to obtain a pathologic sample. The Pipelle is a flexible plastic tube 3.4 mm in external diameter with a small opening of 2.6 mm near the blunt tip. Suction is applied with an integral movable plastic plunger. This instrument produces minimal pain, and the specimen obtained is equivalent to that obtained with the Novak curette, but with less patient discomfort. However secondary to its flexibility, the Pipelle will occasionally fail to pass through a stenotic cervical os. The Pipelle biopsy is both sensitive and specific, although there have been reports of neoplasms residing solely in a polyp or covering less than 5% of the endometrial surface and not recovered by this method (19,20). If a sample cannot be obtained or if the pathologic findings do not correlate with patient symptoms, further evaluation should be performed.

Transvaginal ultrasound may help determine the need for endometrial sampling. Symptomatic postmenopausal women with an endometrial thickness greater than or equal to 5 mm should undergo endometrial sampling (21). Evaluation of postmenopausal bleeding or irregular bleeding in a patient at risk for endometrial carcinoma is typically managed by referral to a gynecologist.

The Papanicolaou smear is not a screening tool for endometrial cancer. A normal Papanicolaou smear does not exclude a uterine lesion. Symptomatic patients despite a normal cervical cytology still require evaluation. However, the discovery of endometrial cells on Papanicolaou smear is concerning in a woman at risk for endometrial cancer. The presence of normal endometrial cells on cervical cytology in a postmenopausal patient is associated with a 6% risk of endometrial adenocarcinoma. Abnormal endometrial cells are associated with a 25% of cancer in this group.

OVARIAN CARCINOMA

Ovarian cancer results in more deaths than all other gynecologic malignancies combined. Current estimates predict 22,220 new cases of ovarian cancer in the United States in 2005. An estimated 16,220 deaths will occur during the same period in the United States secondary to malignancy of the ovary (1). There are three histologic types of ovarian cancer; epithelial, germ cell, and sex cord stromal. Epithelial ovarian cancers are by far the most common; accounting for approximately 85% of ovarian malignancies. The risk of ovarian cancer increases with age and the disease may affect 1% or 2% of women in their ninth decade. Table 104.2 lists factors associated with an elevated and reduced risk of ovarian cancer. Standard treatment for ovarian cancer includes surgical cytoreduction in combination with

TABLE 104.2 Ovarian Carcinoma Risk Factors

Increased Risk	*Decreased Risk*
Older age	Multiparity
Late menopause	Oral contraceptive pills
Nulliparity	
Late child-bearing	
Breast-feeding	
Personal or family history of breast cancer	

platinum based chemotherapy. Although median survival for advanced ovarian cancer has improved, 5-year survival rates remain at 20% to 30%.

Signs and Symptoms

Symptoms associated with ovarian cancer are typically referred to the gastrointestinal (GI) tract and typically include increased abdominal girth, bloating, and pelvic pressure. Additional symptoms include urinary frequency, constipation, and pain. Abnormal vaginal bleeding is uncommon. These symptoms are nonspecific and are often ignored by both patient and physician. Accepted doctrine holds that symptoms associated with ovarian cancer do not develop until the disease has reached an advanced state when cure is unlikely. However, Goff et al. (22) prospectively collected presenting symptoms of women presenting to primary care facilities. The triad of abdominal bloating, increased abdominal girth, and urinary frequency was significantly associated with the diagnosis of ovarian cancer. Symptoms were reported, not only by patients with metastatic disease, but also by those with early stage disease. The presence of these symptoms especially if they are severe, frequent, and of recent onset warrants further evaluation.

An ovarian cancer patient's symptoms are typically secondary to the presence of an adnexal mass and ascites. The pelvic examination, an essential component of an annual physical examination in a woman of any age, permits evaluation of the adnexal with the potential for early detection of masses. The discovery of an adnexal mass requires further investigation. The evaluation of such a mass differs according to a patient's menstrual status.

Adnexal Mass

Premenarche Period

Approximately two thirds of ovarian tumors discovered in the prepubescent age group are benign. The most common neoplasms are *benign cystic teratoma* (dermoid), *benign simple cyst,* and *cystadenoma*. One third of tumors in this age group are classified as malignancies with 80% to

90% arising from the germ cells or gonadal stromal cells of the ovaries (23). Usually no risk factors are elucidated. The most common presenting complaint is pain, which is caused by rapid tumor growth. These neoplasms typically express a variety of serum tumor markers—lactate dehydrogenase, α-fetoprotein, human chorionic gonadotropin, and inhibin—which assist in making the diagnosis.

Reproductive Period

The majority of ovarian masses found during this period are benign functional cysts. These cysts are the result of normal, cyclic follicle maturation. Approximately every 4 weeks a mature follicle develops and ovulation occurs. At the site of ovulation, a corpus luteum forms and may occasionally become enlarged because of internal hemorrhage. If ovulation fails to occur, a unilocular cyst is formed and may reach 10 cm in diameter. Functional cysts typically resolve spontaneously within 2 to 4 weeks. In a classic study by Spanos (24), 92% of persistent adnexal masses were benign neoplasms while 6.8% were malignant. While most adnexal masses are benign, the possibility of a malignancy exists and close followup or referral is warranted.

Ovarian cysts are usually detected on routine pelvic examination or during the radiographic evaluation of a particular sign or symptom. Ultrasound is the best method to investigate and monitor ovarian cysts. Features including irregular size, the presence of septa or nodules, a solid component, and size larger than 5 cm are concerning.

If ovarian enlargement persists after 2 to 4 weeks and if it is demonstrated to be truly cystic by ultrasound, a period of suppressive therapy and observation is warranted. Oral contraceptive pills containing 35 to 50 μg of ethinyl estradiol (see Chapter 100) may be prescribed for 3 months to suppress gonadotropins. This therapy prevents future cyst formation and provides a stable hormonal milieu for the existing cyst to regress. Estrogen blocks the pituitary gonadotrophins that are the stimulus for the formation and maintenance of ovarian cysts. If the ovarian cyst persists for longer than 6 weeks despite gonadotropin suppression, the diagnosis of ovarian neoplasia should be considered strongly and a gynecologist should be consulted.

Perimenopausal and Menopausal Periods

The potential for ovarian malignancy is highest in the postmenopausal female. In the United States, a woman's lifetime risk of ovarian cancer is 1 in 70. The median age of diagnosis of epithelial ovarian cancer, the most common histologic type, is 65 years. Given the poor prognosis associated with this cancer, some investigators have proposed aggressive screening for and management of ovarian enlargement.

In 1972, Barber and Graber (25) proposed that any palpable ovary in a postmenopausal women is abnormal and requires laparotomy. They called this the *postmenopausal palpable ovary (PMPO) syndrome*. However, continued experience has demonstrated that, although evaluation is essential, a more conservative approach to management of the PMPO syndrome is warranted. Fewer 10% of patients with the PMPO syndrome have an ovarian malignancy (26).

Screening

In contrast to cervical and endometrial cancer patients, most women with ovarian cancer are diagnosed with advanced stage disease. As mentioned above, the pelvic examination is a crucial component of the annual physical examination in a woman of any age. Currently, palpation of the adnexae is the only available cost-effective method of screening for ovarian cancer. CA 125 and ultrasound do not have sufficient specificity to screen asymptomatic patients. Preliminary data concerning the use of proteomics for the early identification of ovarian cancer patients appears promising (27). However, further validation is required prior to utilizing this modality to screen the general population for ovarian cancer.

Although use of pelvic ultrasound and measurement of serum tumor markers (e.g., CA-125) is becoming more widespread for screening for ovarian cancer, the efficacy of these tests in the general population is controversial. The sensitivity of CA-125 as a single screening mechanism is low (particularly before menopause) (28). Several systems have been developed to predict the probability of ovarian malignancy based on either serial measurements of a single tumor marker such as CA 125 or a single measurement of a combination of risk factors such as patient age, tumor markers and/or radiographic findings (29–33). With the risk of ovarian cancer algorithm, serial CA-125 values are obtained from individuals in order to determine the possibility of malignancy. The risk calculation from serial CA-125 levels demonstrates a significant enhancement for the detection of early stage ovarian cancer (31–33). The risk of ovarian cancer algorithm is currently utilized by the Gynecologic Oncology Group to determine risk during longitudinal screening among women at increased genetic risk of ovarian cancer.

Prevention

Table 104.2 lists factors associated with altered ovarian cancer risk. Incessant ovulation appears to be associated with an increased risk of ovarian cancer. Exposure to progestins appears to offer protection. Pregnancy, which halts ovulation and results in prolonged progestin exposure, reduces the risk of developing epithelial ovarian cancer. Use of oral contraceptives was associated with a relative risk of

0.6 of developing ovarian cancer (34–35). The use of combined oral contraceptives can decrease the risk of ovarian by 10% to 12% with each year of use, with a 50% risk reduction after 5 years and 80%. This protective effect continued, regardless of the time of discontinuation of the combined oral contraceptives (36).

Genetic Risk

The vast majority of ovarian cancers are sporadic. Approximately 10% to 15% of cases are considered hereditary. Breast and ovarian cancer syndrome is associated with breast cancer gene 1 (BRCA 1) and breast cancer gene 2 (BRCA 2) mutations and carry a 20% to 40% risk of ovarian cancer. Women from families with hereditary nonpolyposis colorectal cancer are also at increased risk. These syndromes are inherited in an autosomal dominant fashion. Patients who give a history of multiple family members with ovarian, breast (particularly premenopausal) and/or colon cancer warrant referral to a center capable of providing appropriate genetic counseling and discussion of surveillance tactics. After completion of child-bearing, women with a known familial cancer mutation should consider prophylactic surgery. For women with BRCA mutations, who have not completed child-bearing, the use of combined oral contraceptives significantly decreases the risk of ovarian cancer (37). However, use of oral contraceptive pills (OCPs) for more than 5 years or before age 30 may be associated with an increased risk of breast cancer in women with BRCA 1 mutations (38).

Any female patient carries a significant risk of developing a malignancy of the reproductive tract. In the United States, widespread use of the Papanicolaou smear has resulted in a drastic reduction in cervical cancer rates. Prompt evaluation of postmenopausal bleeding can result in early diagnosis of endometrial cancer. Ovarian cancer continues to be typically identified at a late stage; however prompt evaluation of symptoms may result in early diagnosis. A facility with proper screening, workup, and referral of women at risk for gynecologic cancers is critical for the primary care physician.

SPECIFIC REFERENCES*

1. Jemal A, Murray T, Ward E, et al. Cancer statistics, 2005. CA Cancer J Clin 2005;55:10.
2. Basta A, Adamek K, Pitynski K. Intraepithelial neoplasia and early stage vulvar cancer. Epidemiological, clinical and virological observations. Eur J Gynaecol Oncol 1999;20:111.
3. McNally OM, Mulvany NJ, Pagano R, et al. VIN 3: a clinicopathologic review. Int J Gynecol Cancer 2002;12:490.
4. Trimble CL, Hildesheim A, Brinton LA, et al. Heterogeneous etiology of squamous carcinoma of the vulva. Obstet Gynecol 1996;76:59.
5. Hildesheim A, Han CL, Brinton LA, et al. Human papillomavirus type 16 and risk of preinvasive and invasive vulvar cancer: results from a seroepidemiological case-control study. Obstet Gynecol 1997;90:748.
6. Walboomers JM, Jacobs MV, Manos MM, et al. Human papillomavirus is a necessary cause of invasive cervical cancer worldwide. J Pathol 1999;189:12.
7. Clifford GM, Smith JS, Plummer M, et al. Human papillomavirus types in invasive cervical cancer worldwide: a meta-analysis. Br J Cancer 2003;88:63.
8. Ho GY, Bierman R, Beardsley L, et al. Natural history of cervicovaginal papillomavirus infection in young women. N Engl J Med 1998;338:423.
9. Maiman M. Management of cervical neoplasia in human immunodeficiency virus-infected women. J Natl Cancer Inst Monogr 1998(23):43.
10. Wabinga HR, Parkin DM, Wabwire-Mangen F, et al. Trends in cancer incidence in Kyadondo County, Uganda, 1960–1997. Br J Cancer 2000; 82:1585.
11. Newton R, Ziegler J, Beral V, et al. A case-control study of human immunodeficiency virus infection and cancer in adults and children residing in Kampala, Uganda. Int J Cancer 2001;92:622.
12. Nanda K, McCrory DC, Myers ER, et al. Accuracy of the Papanicolaou test in screening for and follow-up of cervical cytologic abnormalities: a systematic review. Ann Intern Med 2000;132:810.
13. Austin RM, Ramzy I. Increased detection of epithelial cell abnormalities by liquid-based gynecologic cytology preparations. A review of accumulated data. Acta Cytol 1998;42:178.
14. Vassilakos P, Saurel J, Rondez R. Direct-to-vial use of the AutoCyte PREP liquid-based preparation for cervical-vaginal specimens in three European laboratories. Acta Cytol 1999;43:65.
15. ACOG Practice Bulletin: The American College of Obstetricians and Gynecologists;2003.45.
16. Solomon D, Davey D, Kurman R, et al. The 2001 Bethesda System: terminology for reporting results of cervical cytology. JAMA 2002;287:2114.
17. Effects of hormone replacement therapy on endometrial histology in postmenopausal women. The Postmenopausal Estrogen/Progestin Interventions (PEPI) Trial. The Writing Group for the PEPI Trial. JAMA 1996;275:370.
18. Ernster VL, Bush TL, Huggins GR, et al. Benefits and risks of menopausal estrogen and/or progestin hormone use. Prev Med 1988;17:201.
19. Dijkhuizen FP, Mol BW, Brolmann HA, et al. The accuracy of endometrial sampling in the diagnosis of patients with endometrial carcinoma and hyperplasia: a meta-analysis. Cancer 2000;89:1765.
20. Guido RS, Kanbour-Shakir A, Rulin MC, et al. Pipelle endometrial sampling. Sensitivity in the detection of endometrial cancer. J Reprod Med 1995;40:553.
21. Carter J, Carson LF, Byers L, et al. Transvaginal ultrasound in gynecologic oncology. Obstet Gynecol Surv 1991;46:687.
22. Goff BA, Mandel LS, Melancon CH, et al. Frequency of symptoms of ovarian cancer in women presenting to primary care clinics. JAMA 2004;291:2705.
23. Breen JL, Maxson WS. Ovarian tumors in children and adolescents. Clin Obstet Gynecol 1977;20:607.
24. Spanos WJ. Preoperative hormonal therapy of cystic adnexal masses. Am J Obstet Gynecol 1973;116:551.
25. Barber HR, Graber EA. The PMPO syndrome (postmenopausal palpable ovary syndrome). CA Cancer J Clin 1972;22:357.
26. Goldstein SR, Subramanyam B, Snyder JR, et al. The postmenopausal cystic adnexal mass: the potential role of ultrasound in conservative management. Obstet Gynecol 1989;73:8.
27. Petricoin EF, Ardekani AM, Hitt BA, et al. Use of proteomic patterns in serum to identify ovarian cancer. Lancet 2002;359:572.
28. Eltabbakh GH, Belinson JL, Kennedy AW, et al. Serum CA-125 measurements > 65 U/mL. Clinical value. J Reprod Med 1997;42:617.
29. Twickler DM, Forte TB, Santos-Ramos R, et al. The Ovarian Tumor Index predicts risk for malignancy. Cancer 1999;86:2280.
30. Sassone AM, Timor-Tritsch IE, Artner A, et al. Transvaginal sonographic characterization of ovarian disease: evaluation of a new scoring system to predict ovarian malignancy. Obstet Gynecol 1991;78:70.
31. Skates SJ, Xu FJ, Yu YH, et al. Toward an optimal algorithm for ovarian cancer screening with longitudinal tumor markers. Cancer 1995;76:2004.
32. Jacobs IJ, Skates SJ, MacDonald N, et al. Screening for ovarian cancer: a pilot randomised controlled trial. Lancet 1999;353:1207.
33. Skates SJ, Menon U, MacDonald N, et al. Calculation of the risk of ovarian cancer from serial CA-125 values for preclinical detection in postmenopausal women. J Clin Oncol 2003; 21:206.
34. Oral contraceptive use and the risk of ovarian cancer. The Centers for Disease Control Cancer and Steroid Hormone Study. JAMA 1983; 249:1596.
35. Rosenberg L, Shapiro S, Slone D, et al. Epithelial ovarian cancer and combination oral contraceptives. JAMA 1982;247:3210.

*Bold numerals denote published controlled clinical trials, meta-analyses, or consensus-based recommendations.

36. Hankinson SE, Colditz GA, Hunter DJ, et al. A quantitative assessment of oral contraceptive use and risk of ovarian cancer. Obstet Gynecol 1992;80:708.

37. Narod SA, Risch H, Moslehi R, et al. Oral contraceptives and the risk of hereditary ovarian cancer. Hereditary Ovarian Cancer Clinical Study Group. N Engl J Med 1998;339:424.

38. Narod SA, Dube MP, Klijn J, et al. Oral contraceptives and the risk of breast cancer in BRCA1 and BRCA2 mutation carriers. J Natl Cancer Inst 2002;94:1773.

For annotated ***General References*** *and resources related to this chapter, visit www.hopkinsbayview.org/PAMreferences.*

Chapter 105

Diseases of the Breast

Rima J. Couzi and Michael J. Purtell

Breast cancer is the most commonly diagnosed cancer in women, accounting for 32% of all new cancer diagnoses. It is second only to lung cancer in cancer deaths. In 2005 alone, an estimated 211,240 women will be diagnosed with breast cancer, and 40,410 will die of the disease (1). The current cumulative lifetime risk for developing invasive breast cancer is one in seven. This statistic, although accurate, is often misinterpreted as being a constant risk at any age. The risk of developing breast cancer increases proportionally with age from 1 in 207 in women younger than 40 years to 1 in 13 in the 60 to 79 age group (1). Women tend to overestimate their risk of developing breast cancer, and breast-related complaints are a significant source of anxiety to patients, despite the fact that most of these are secondary to benign causes. Many women view breast cancer as the leading threat to their health, although statistically it ranks behind cardiovascular diseases and lung cancer as a cause of death in women (2,3). The primary caregiver must have a rational approach to the evaluation and treatment of breast complaints and breast masses. He or she implements the screening program for cancer and supervises the patient's referral. If cancer is found, the primary caregiver is the one to whom the patient initially turns for information. A reassuring patient–caregiver relationship is critical in dealing with this emotionally charged area of medicine.

NORMAL ANATOMY AND PHYSIOLOGY OF THE BREAST

The breast is a modified sweat gland that consists of a tree-like structure with 5 to 10 primary milk ducts that originate at the nipple. These branch into segmental ducts and subsegmental ducts that end in terminal duct lobular units (see Harris, at www.hopkinsbayview.org/PAMreferences). These units are embedded in loose connective tissue with a rich capillary supply. The terminal duct lobular units, which are lined by cuboidal epithelium, are sensitive to hormonal influences and are the basic lactational units of the breast. There are complex interactions between steroid hormones, peptide hormones, and growth factors that affect breast development, maturation, and differentiation. Briefly, estrogen stimulates the proliferation of ductal tissue, whereas progesterone stimulates the proliferation and differentiation of the lobules. The production of milk is regulated by prolactin. During the follicular phase of the menstrual cycle, the cuboidal epithelial cells proliferate.

In the luteal phase, the lobular stromal cells become edematous and the ductules open up with secretions from the cuboidal cells.

During pregnancy the lobular units proliferate maximally and only rarely return to normal in the postpartum period. As pregnancy proceeds, colostrum is formed from fluid accumulation and desquamation of epithelial cells. Colostrum is then released in the immediate postpartum period. In the postmenopausal years, the loss of hormonal stimulation results in a decrease in the number of lobular units and atrophy of the remaining ones. The connective tissue also becomes less cellular with an increased fat content. The dynamic changes that occur in the breast at different phases can result in a spectrum of benign breast disorders with histologic features that range from cystic and fibrous changes to ductal, lobular, and stromal proliferation. It is important to realize that anatomic changes associated with normal hormonal fluctuations during a menstrual cycle do not occur to the same degree in all areas of the breast. This accounts for the asymmetric palpatory findings in the normal breast, which is often lumpy.

SCREENING PROCEDURES

The aim of breast cancer screening is to detect breast cancer at the earliest possible stage, when effective treatments confer the greatest chances for long-term survival. There are three commonly used screening modalities for breast cancer and these are often used concurrently: mammography, clinical breast examination, and breast self examination. A main endpoint in assessing the benefit from screening is whether it decreases cancer-related mortality.

The role of screening mammography in reducing mortality from breast cancer and the age at which to start and stop screening have been a source of much debate over the years. Eight randomized controlled trials of breast cancer screening as well as several cohort and case-control studies have been conducted. A meta-analysis of 13 studies, including the eight randomized controlled screening trials, showed an overall 25% reduction in breast cancer mortality for the women who underwent screening compared with those who did not ([randomized risk] RR 0.75, 95% [confidence interval CI, 0.68 to 0.83) (4).

A re-analysis of published reports by the Cochrane Institute stirred considerable controversy in 2001 when the authors suggested that mammography is of no value for women of any age. They deemed that only two trials were methodologically sound and found no benefit from screening mammography in these trials (5,6). However there have been rebuttals of this analysis, and more recent updates of the trials appear to show that screening mammography does decrease mortality from breast cancer (7–11). The impact of news media coverage of this controversy was examined in a recent article (12).

At this time there is strong consensus among the major American medical societies that routine screening mammography, with or without clinical breast examination, should be offered to women age 50 years and older. There is less agreement on screening women age 40 to 49 years and little data on which to base recommendations for screening women older than 74 years.

The American Cancer Society, American College of Radiology, American Medical Association, the American College of Obstetrics and Gynecology, and the National Cancer Institute (NCI) all recommend routine screening starting at age 40 (13–16). This recommendation is also supported by the U.S. Preventive Services Task Force (17).

The Canadian Task Force on the Periodic Health Examination and the American College of Physicians recommend starting screening mammography at the age of 50 years (18).

In 1997, the National Institutes of Health (NIH) held a consensus conference on breast cancer screening in women age 40 to 49 years. It was concluded that there were not enough data to recommend routine mammographic screening for women in that age group, and that each woman should decide individually about screening after discussion with her health care provider. Nevertheless, the NCI recommends screening every 1 to 2 years for women 40 to 49 years of age.

The disagreement on the benefit of mammography for women age 40 to 49 years stems in part from the length of followup time needed to show a reduction in breast cancer mortality among screened women. At 11 to 16 years of followup, the Canadian National Breast Screening study in women in their forties continues to fail to show a reduction in breast cancer mortality among screened women (18). However a meta-analysis performed by the U.S. Preventive Services Task Force shows a relative risk of breast cancer mortality of 0.85 for screened women younger than 50 after 14 years of observation (9). The number of women needed to be screened to prevent one death from breast cancer was 1,792. This compares with the need to screen 838 women older than 50 years to prevent a breast cancer-related death (9). Most of the cancers found in women who begin screening in their forties are not discovered until the women are in their fifties. Some authors have suggested in the past that the incremental benefit of starting screening at 40 years of age is not worth exposing women to the emotional and physical harms of screening for an extra decade. The possibility that, for most women, the outcome would have been the same had they started screening after 50 years of age has been raised. Another concern is the lower test specificity in young women, who often have dense breasts, complicating interpretation. This leads to a much higher benign-to-malignant biopsy ratio than that found in older women. For women 40 to 49 years old or their clinicians who are considering delaying the initiation of screening, Gail and Rimer have provided risk-based recommendations that may help the primary caregiver in the counseling process and in the selection of patients who might best be served by screening mammography (19).

Whatever decision the primary caregiver makes about the usefulness of screening mammography in young women, it is important to discuss the benefits and the risks of screening with all women about to start screening. A woman needs to understand her likely experience when she goes for testing, particularly if it is her first mammogram. Patients should know that mammography may be uncomfortable because of the need for breast compression in order to obtain a good image quality. The communication plan following mammography should be worked out ahead of time to minimize the anxiety of waiting for a telephone call, although breast cancer screening centers now increasingly offer immediate film interpretation. This allows the radiologist to order additional mammographic views or breast ultrasound at the same visit, thereby lowering the recall rate and possibly patient anxiety. Young women in particular should understand the poor specificity of mammography and the high likelihood of a recommendation for intervention (biopsy or early followup), especially with the first mammogram. The patient should know that if she receives that recommendation, the chance of benign or no disease far outweighs the chance of cancer. In the United States, additional evaluation is recommended in about 11% of cases, of which 90% are ultimately proved to be benign conditions (20). False-positive mammograms can result in a heightened state of anxiety about breast cancer that can last several months (21).

There is a paucity of data to guide the recommendation on what age to stop screening, as few women older than 70 years old were enrolled in screening trials. Although the incidence of breast cancer increases with age, the benefit of screening mammography in the elderly may be offset by increasing comorbidities and reduced life expectancy. For example, detecting a clinically occult, slow growing breast cancer in an 85-year-old woman with heart failure and a short life expectancy is likely to be more harmful than beneficial. However it is reasonable to continue screening women older than 70 years if their life expectancy is not compromised by comorbid disease. Biennial mammography beyond age 65 years has been shown to be cost-effective by the U.S. preventive Task Force (22).

The independent role of clinical breast examination (CBE) in decreasing mortality from breast cancer is less well defined, but CBE is an important component of screening, as 10% to 15% of palpable breast cancers are not visualized by mammography. Breast self-examination (BSE) is often advocated, but there is no evidence that it is effective as a screening modality and it may increase the chance of having a breast biopsy for benign disease (17,23). BSE should not substitute for mammography and a CBE. However, if a woman wishes to perform BSE, she should be taught the proper technique and be instructed on how to differentiate normal breast tissue from suspicious breast lumps.

Several new screening procedures are under review but are not currently recommended for population screening. These include digital mammography, computer-assisted detection, and magnetic resonance imaging (MRI). Digital mammography is costlier than conventional mammography, but was recently found to be significantly better at detecting breast cancer in young women, premenopausal and perimenopausal women, and women with dense breasts (24). Studies have shown that breast MRI has an increased sensitivity but a reduced specificity compared with mammography. Women with breast cancer gene 1 (BRCA 1) or breast cancer gene 2 (BRCA 2) mutations have a significant lifetime risk for developing breast cancer and may benefit from breast MRI screening (25,26). However, this is an expensive screening modality and at this point it is unknown if it improves survival rates.

CLINICAL CHARACTERISTICS OF COMMON DISEASES OF THE BREAST

Benign Tumors

Breast complaints are common in primary care practice and the vast majority of these complaints are related to benign conditions. It is important to have a clear understanding of the clinical features of benign conditions and to evaluate and follow the patient in order to avoid failing to diagnose breast cancer.

The patient may be asymptomatic or present with breast pain, nonbreast pain, focal or diffuse breast lumps, or nipple discharge. Most benign breast diseases are related to the hormonal changes that occur during the three main reproductive periods. Histologically confirmed benign breast conditions may be associated with no increased risk versus a small or moderate increase in risk for subsequent development of breast cancer (27).

Fibroadenoma

Fibroadenoma is the most common cause of a unilateral discrete mass in the 15- to 35-year-old age group, with a peak incidence from 20 to 25 years of age. In 10% to 15% of cases, there are multiple tumors. These are benign tumors that contain both epithelial and stromal components, and usually remain static at 1 to 2 cm in size. The etiology of these tumors is unknown, but a hormonal relationship is postulated as the tumors can grow significantly during pregnancy, persist during the reproductive years, and regress in the postmenopausal years.

The patient with a fibroadenoma usually reports a breast mass but denies pain, nipple discharge, or other breast changes. On physical examination, the lesion is usually firm but not rock-hard; it is smooth and well circumscribed, nontender, and easily moveable. It often rolls about in the breast, mimicking a very large marble. Mammography reveals a discrete, round, well-circumscribed lesion. New or enlarging lesions need to be distinguished from cancer. Many believe that fibroadenomas also have a characteristic ultrasonographic appearance. There is some controversy about the optimal management of these lesions. Most surgeons recommend obtaining a core biopsy or fine-needle aspiration (FNA) to establish the diagnosis histologically. If the diagnosis is confirmed, close followup with CBE and imaging to assess for stability is accepted clinical practice, especially in women under 25 years. Close followup is important because of the rare possibility of simultaneous lobular carcinoma or progression to cystosarcoma phyllodes. Excisional biopsy is often recommended for women older than 25 years.

Phyllodes Tumor

Phyllodes tumor is a unique sarcomatous tumor of the breast that may arise from fibroadenoma. The mean age of presentation ranges between 44 and 50 years. Rapid growth of a breast mass is often reported. The mass is usually well-circumscribed, with a rubbery and lobulated consistency, and can be quite large at presentation. Histologically, phyllodes tumors differ from fibroadenomas in that the stromal elements have increased cellularity, pleomorphism, nuclear atypia, and mitotic figures. The tumors are classified as benign, borderline malignant, or malignant based on histological features. The malignancy rate is 20% to 30%, and approximately one third to one half of these will metastasize, primarily in a hematogenous fashion, with lung involvement the most frequent site. However, the overall metastatic rate for all phyllodes tumors is less than 5%. The current surgical practice is to perform a wide local excision with adequate clear margins. Mastectomy may be necessary for larger tumors and for repeated local recurrences (28).

Intraductal Papilloma

Intraductal papillomas often present with serosanguineous, spontaneous, recurrent, or persistent nipple discharge from a single duct. These small tumors are not palpable, but their location can usually be determined by applying pressure on various quadrants of the areolocutaneous margin and noting which quadrant produces the discharge. An intraductal papillary cancer is a possibility that must be excluded by excising a small, pie-shaped segment in the area producing the discharge.

Fibrocystic Disease

Fibrocystic changes of the breast are common and occur to some extent in most women. These changes consist of an increased number of cysts or fibrous tissue in a normal breast and are considered a normal variant. Fibrocystic disease is diagnosed when fibrocystic changes are associated with symptoms such as of breast pain, nipple discharge, or breast lumpiness. A hormonal basis is thought to be at play, and the pain is often more prominent just before the onset of menses. On physical examination the breast feels lumpy, with bilateral, diffuse, tender, easily movable ill-defined masses, usually in the upper outer quadrant of the breasts. Breast cysts can sometimes enlarge acutely and cause sudden and severe localized pain. The subareolar ducts may be dilated and spontaneous discharge of thick, gray-green fluid is common. Histologically, cyst and ductal ectasia is noted.

Because of clinical and sometimes radiological uncertainty, many patients undergo at least one biopsy to rule out cancer. Most lesions are benign; usually, the histology is either normal (70%) or shows only epithelial hyperplasia (25%). These findings are of little concern, as such patients are at low risk for development of breast cancer and do not require more vigilant followup than normal (29). In contrast, a report of hyperplasia with atypia (3% to 4% of benign biopsies) is significant, particularly if the mother or a sister of the patient has had breast cancer. In the absence of a positive family history, the finding of atypia increases the risk for breast cancer development fourfold, and in association with a positive family history this risk is increased almost 11-fold (29). These patients require careful followup, with annual mammogram and biannual physical examinations, and in selected cases, even prophylactic bilateral mastectomies may be considered, especially if the woman has a mutation of the BRCA 1 or BRCA 2 gene (30).

Premature Hyperplasia

A concentric unilateral swelling can occur beneath the nipple before puberty in girls. This commonly occurs between the ages of 7 and 9 years. The lump can be 1 to 2 cm in diameter and is usually nontender. Within a year, a contralateral lump appears and often both lumps remain static until puberty. Since a biopsy is functionally equivalent to a mastectomy in a child, it is contraindicated.

Gynecomastia

Among men with breast masses, the differential diagnosis includes gynecomastia (see Chapter 85) and male breast cancer. The latter is rare, accounting for approximately 1% of all breast cancers. Although gynecomastia has many causes, it has a characteristic presentation. Gynecomastia appears as a breast mass beneath the areola that is usually slightly tender and easily movable. It is never associated with ulceration or nipple retraction. If gynecomastia is ruled out, a breast mass in a male should be examined by biopsy.

Cancer

The widespread use of screening mammography has changed the presentation of breast cancer, with increasing detection of smaller nonpalpable lesions. Sometimes a breast lump is found by the patient or is detected by the primary caregiver during a routine examination. The classical clinical finding that raises suspicion for breast cancer is the presence of a single, often painless, hard fixed lesion measuring more than 2 cm. There may be associated subtle skin dimpling or nipple retraction. Approximately 15% of cases are locally advanced at presentation. These are associated with more significant skin dimpling with peau d'orange appearance, erythema, altered venous pattern, matted fixed axillary nodes, or a mass fixed to the chest wall.

EVALUATION OF A BREAST MASS

History: Risk Factors and Symptoms

The chance of a woman developing cancer increases with age (1). Most women who present with a breast lump will need additional testing, although most lumps will ultimately prove to be benign lesions. The evaluation starts with a careful history and physical examination. The history should elicit information on the location of the lump, how it was detected, how long it has been present, any associated complaints, whether it waxes and wanes at different times in the menstrual cycle, and if it has changed in size. The reproductive history, use of oral contraceptives or hormone replacement therapy, alcohol use, previous history of breast biopsy, and family history of breast cancer are also important components of the history.

Women are becoming increasingly sensitive to the possibility of developing breast cancer and are more aware of factors that may modulate their risk (Table 105.1). Genetic testing for breast cancer susceptibility genes (BRCA 1 and BRCA 2) has now become commercially available. Women with worrisome family histories, those who have developed breast cancer before age 40, and women of Ashkenazi Jewish descent may be candidates for such testing. These women should be referred to a specialized risk assessment clinic, usually located in an academic center, where a genetic counselor is involved in the evaluation. Counseling is provided on the risks and benefits, limitations and potential insurance implications of genetic testing. Guidelines for such testing have been published by the American Society of Clinical Oncology (31).

TABLE 105.1 Risk Factors for Carcinoma of the Breast

Factors	*Relative Risk*
Positive family history	1–5 (see text)
Early menarche and late menopause (cyclic ovarian activity >40 yr)	Slight
Nulliparity	Slight
Previous breast cancer	5
Benign disease of the breast	1–4 (see text)
Radiation	Dependent on dosage

Most breast cancers are sporadic and genetic testing is not recommended in these instances. Women tend to overestimate their breast cancer risk, and also may not realize that their risk of dying from breast cancer is one third of their chance of developing the disease. It falls on the primary caregiver to guide the patient in understanding her own risk and to counsel her as to whether her risk may justify a request for genetic testing. There are well established risk factors for breast cancer (32). For an average woman increasing age confers the highest relative risk for breast cancer. In ascertaining a woman's risk, the menstrual and reproductive history is also important. Early menarche and late menopause are associated with a slightly increased risk for development of breast cancer, whereas menopause before 35 years of age (normal or surgical) reduces the risk. The risk of breast cancer is increased in nulliparous women, whereas a full-term pregnancy before age 18 years offers some protection. It appears unlikely that the use of oral contraceptives changes a woman's risk of breast cancer (see Chapter 100), but postmenopausal estrogen replacement therapy may increase the risk by 30% (see Chapter 106). The occurrence of breast cancer in a first-degree relative (sister or mother) increases a woman's probability of developing cancer two- to fourfold. A second degree-relative with breast cancer increases the risk to a lower extent. A personal history of a breast biopsy showing atypical hyperplasia also increases the risk fourfold (29). The other major risk factor besides family history is a personal history of breast cancer, which increases the risk of contralateral breast cancer fivefold (33).

Two risk-prediction models are widely available and can be used to assess a woman's personal level of breast cancer risk. The Gail model developed for the NCI is available at http://bcra.nci.nih.gov/brc/q1.htm. This tool was used to select patients for the Breast Cancer Prevention trial discussed later in this chapter. The revised Gail model incorporates information about race. The limitations of this tool stem from not including information about second- and third-degree relatives, thereby making it unreliable for patients with a strong family history of breast cancer. For such women, the risk assessment tool developed by Claus (34) is more appropriate.

The patient should be questioned about the presence of other symptoms (e.g., pain, discharge) related to a breast mass, the duration of those symptoms if present, and whether the discovery of the mass or onset of the other symptoms was associated with changes in the menses, injury to the breast, pregnancy, or changes in medication.

After the presence of a mass, *nipple discharge* is the second most common sign of breast cancer. Nonlactational

mastectomy is 2% to 9%, with recurrence usually in the first 5 years (43,44). Among patients choosing lumpectomy and radiotherapy, more than 80% are satisfied with the cosmetic results. The treatment is accompanied by minimal, if any, postoperative breast lymphedema or impaired wound healing. The irradiated breast atrophies over a number of months and may remain tender during this period. For some patients, reduction mammoplasty of the opposite breast may need to be considered.

In summary, the patient should have the surgical choices outlined for her, and be informed of the benefits and disadvantages of the treatment options. She should be given the option of discussing neoadjuvant chemotherapy or hormonal therapy if there is doubt about the ability to perform breast conservation surgery, or if she has locally advanced disease.

Intraductal Carcinoma

With the increased use of mammography, up to 20% of all new breast cancers are noninvasive *intraductal lesions* (45). The optimal treatment for these lesions has not been defined precisely. Mastectomy is curative 99% of the time, but it is probably an overly aggressive treatment. However, a simple lumpectomy may not be sufficient. The National Surgical Adjuvant Breast Project study compared breast irradiation versus no irradiation after local excision for patients with small (<2.5 cm), intraductal (noninvasive) carcinoma (46). The study concluded that omission of breast irradiation after local excision for intraductal cancer is unacceptable because of a 16% rate of relapse at or near the biopsy site. Approximately half of these recurrences were invasive, and radiotherapy appeared to reduce their incidence by 70%. This conclusion is not universally accepted. It is unclear to what degree radiotherapy prevented or merely delayed local recurrences. Other, albeit nonrandomized, studies, suggest that, with careful patient selection, a practitioner can identify women who may not need irradiation after removal of an intraductal lesion. The following features are associated with a better prognosis: (a) a completely excised, well-differentiated tumor without comedonecrosis; (b) a tumor smaller than 2.5 cm in diameter; (c) a tumor found incidentally or detected by mammographic microcalcifications; or (d) a tumor that occurs in an older woman. The recurrence rate in such cases can be as low as 3% (47). Many believe that patients whose tumors have these characteristics can be cured by simple excision without irradiation (48). Clinical trials are ongoing to define more clearly the selection criteria to identify those patients who may not require radiotherapy.

Multimodality Treatment

Patients with locally advanced, unresectable disease, or with inflammatory disease should be considered for treatment with initial systemic chemotherapy followed by surgery, if sufficient tumor reduction occurs, or by local irradiation with or without further chemotherapy. For a select group, such an approach may allow long-term survival. Other patients who should be considered for preoperative therapy are those who desire breast conserving therapy but have tumors too large for such as option. Several cycles of chemotherapy—or, for older, less fit patients with estrogen receptor–positive tumors, a short course of an oral antiestrogen or an aromatase inhibitor—induces sufficient tumor regression to allow lumpectomy with negative margins. The aromatase inhibitors anastrozole and letrozole are associated with a higher rate of breast conservation than is tamoxifen, with 44% and 45% of patients who would have otherwise required a mastectomy becoming eligible for lumpectomy (49,50).

Prognosis, Further Therapy, and Followup

Prognosis

Current estimates of survival are based mainly on tumor size, on whether the tumor is wholly intraductal (noninvasive), and on the results of axillary node sampling. The cure rate with mastectomy approaches 100% for women whose tumor consists only of intraductal carcinoma. Axillary node involvement occurs in fewer than 3% of these patients, so node resection provides little further information and may be omitted.

A special case is *lobular carcinoma in situ* (LCIS). This diagnosis is viewed more accurately as a risk factor for breast cancer in a manner similar to the finding of hyperplasia with atypia on a biopsy. Although there continues to be some disagreement among experts about how significant a risk factor LCIS is, a reasonable estimate is that a woman with a finding of LCIS has a 15% to 30% lifetime risk of developing invasive cancer, or approximately 0.5% to 1% risk of cancer per year. It is important to realize that this risk applies to both breasts. Recommendations vary for LCIS, but most oncologists recommend close mammographic follow-up, with prophylactic bilateral mastectomies reserved for women who are psychologically unable to deal with their increased risk of breast cancer. Such women should be considered for preventive therapy with tamoxifen (see Prevention).

For women with invasive cancer, the status of the axillary lymph nodes is the best indicator of prognosis. Overall survival at 10 years is approximately 65% with no node involvement, 37% with one to three positive nodes, and 13% with four or more nodes involved (51,52). The size of the tumor is also important. Patients with tumors larger than 5 cm do somewhat worse, especially if there are positive nodes. Patients with tumors smaller than 1.0 cm, especially if less than 0.5 cm, with uninvolved nodes do better. Within these subgroups, patients whose tumor is rich in estrogen receptors and/or progesterone receptors may do better than those whose tumor lacks significant receptor content (53). However, estrogen and progesterone receptor content is more properly considered as a predictor for response to hormonal treatments rather than as a prognostic indicator. The need to determine more accurately the prognosis of individual patients is important, because prognostic category is the basis for patient selection for adjuvant therapy after treatment of the primary tumor. Patients whose tumor appears well-differentiated to the pathologist tend to survive better than those whose tumor appears poorly differentiated. The pathology report usually includes a description of the size of the tumor, the degree of differentiation of the cancer cells, a marker of proliferation such as the Ki-67 index, the estrogen, progesterone, and Her-2/Neu oncogene expression status, as well as the number of positive lymph nodes. All of these are taken into consideration when deciding which adjuvant therapy the patient should be offered.

From this discussion it is clear that axillary dissection serves mainly to obtain prognostic information and may not directly improve a patient's survival. Unfortunately, it is the disruption of the lymphatic drainage of the arm and nerve damage from this operation that result in the long-term sequelae of arm swelling, arm and shoulder pain, and hypoesthesia or hyperesthesia. In attempts to minimize this operation, techniques have been developed to identify intraoperatively the axillary lymph nodes to which a particular woman's breast cancer would first metastasize. Injection of the tumor with a radioactive colloid and/or dye (methylene blue) with diffusion of the tracer to the axilla allows the surgeon to identify the lymph nodes that initially drain the tumor. Removal and pathologic examination of these nodes can predict whether the remaining nodes will be involved with breast cancer. If the sentinel nodes prove negative, then the chance that no other nodes are involved is greater than 95% and the patient can be spared a formal axillary dissection with its consequences (54). The American Society of Clinical Oncology has recently published guidelines for the use of sentinel lymph node biopsy in early stage breast cancer (55). This technique is not recommended for >5 cm tumors, for locally advanced or inflammatory breast cancer, in the presence of clinically suspicious axillary nodal enlargement, or if the axilla has been operated on in the past.

The primary caregiver needs to be mindful of two aspects of the sentinel node approach. First, there is a necessary learning curve for this procedure. In inexperienced hands, the rate of false-negative findings may be as high as 30%. A minimum of 20 sentinel lymph node biopsy procedures in combination with axillary lymph node dissection or with mentoring is required to minimize the risk of false-negative results (55). Second, the limited number of nodes presented to the pathologist (one to three) allows them to be examined in detail. Not only are thinner slices produced, but also the pathology department has the ability to stain the slides with antibodies to the cytokeratin of breast cancer cells. These detailed procedures greatly increase the sensitivity of the examination. Microscopic nests of tumor cells that would not be found by a routine dissection can now be detected, thus upstaging the disease in approximately 10% of patients. There is controversy about whether a node containing a few tumor cells discoverable only through such detailed scrutiny should be considered positive or negative when making a decision concerning adjuvant therapy (56). Completion of axillary lymph node dissection is recommended if the sentinel lymph node is positive for cancer, as approximately 50% of the patients will have additional positive lymph nodes (55).

Adjuvant Therapy

Adjuvant systemic therapy decreases the annual predicted death rate by approximately 30% (57). Therefore, the absolute degree of benefit from adjuvant therapy increases as the predicted prognosis worsens and, conversely, may be clinically insignificant in a woman whose cure rate with primary treatment alone is high. For example, a woman with one to three positive nodes has a 50% chance of recurrence. Therefore, adjuvant therapy reduces the risk of recurrence by (50% × 30%), or 15%. However, a woman with a tumor smaller than 1.0 cm and no positive nodes has a cure rate of more than 90%. In this case, adjuvant therapy would decrease the risk of recurrence by 3% at most. Most oncologists would urge adjuvant therapy in the former case but may be more reserved in the latter case. It should be noted that in surveys, women have stated that they would accept the short-term side effects of adjuvant chemotherapy for as little as a 1% improved probability of survival. Consequently, almost all patients, particularly those with poor prognoses, should have the benefits of further treatment with chemotherapy, hormonal therapy, and radiotherapy presented to them by the medical or radiation oncologist (see Chapter 10).

Currently, patients are selected for various adjuvant therapies based on the number of axillary nodes involved, their menopausal status, and the estrogen and progesterone receptor status of the tumor. Her-2/neu positivity, either by immunohistochemical staining (3+ intensity), or amplification of the gene on fluorescent in situ hybridization (FISH), has just recently become an important factor to consider as well. Two large adjuvant chemotherapy clinical trials have shown that addition of trastuzumab, a monoclonal antibody against the extracellular domain of Her-2, to chemotherapy significantly improves outcomes in Her-2 positive early breast cancer (58,59). These reports have caused considerable excitement and have been hailed as a revolutionary development in the treatment of breast cancer (60). Systemic chemotherapy is recommended to almost all women with metastases to axillary nodes. For patients who opt for lumpectomy and radiotherapy, results seem to be better if the chemotherapy is delivered between the lumpectomy and the breast irradiation (61). For premenopausal women, a major shift in the paradigm for guiding the selection of adjuvant therapy has been the realization that both premenopausal and postmenopausal women accrue the same benefit from tamoxifen, an estrogen receptor modulator. It is now standard to treat premenopausal women whose tumors are receptor positive with tamoxifen after chemotherapy or with tamoxifen alone in selected patients with good prognoses. Additionally, because the most recent meta-analysis of adjuvant therapies suggested that oophorectomy is as effective as chemotherapy in premenopausal patients with receptor-positive tumors, there is renewed interest in medical oophorectomy using luteinizing hormone-releasing hormone (LHRH) agonists combined with tamoxifen or an aromatase inhibitor (62). Similarly, use of tamoxifen or an aromatase inhibitor is recommended for most postmenopausal women if their tumors are either estrogen or progesterone receptor positive. Recent trials have shown that the aromatase inhibitors anastrozole, letrozole, and exemestane play an important role and should be incorporated in the planning of adjuvant hormonal therapy (63). The postmenopausal patient with positive nodes whose tumor is estrogen receptor–positive may obtain a small increase in survival by the addition of chemotherapy to tamoxifen (57). Whether such treatment is warranted, given the additional toxicity, is for the individual patient to decide. Postmenopausal patients whose tumors lack estrogen receptors can benefit from chemotherapy, especially if their axillary nodes contain tumor. Patients diagnosed with only ductal carcinoma *in situ* should also be considered for tamoxifen, especially if the ductal carcinoma in situ (DCIS) is estrogen receptor positive. A clinical trial demonstrated a 44% to 52% decrease in the incidence of invasive breast cancer in the ipsilateral and contralateral breasts when tamoxifen was employed along with radiation (64). However, at this time, there is no survival advantage with adjuvant tamoxifen for DCIS.

Several adjuvant chemotherapeutic regimens are available, each differing in side effects and duration of treatment. In discussing the potential benefit of adjuvant therapy, it is important to present the data to the patient in terms of the absolute, rather than the relative benefit of therapy. A useful tool is the Adjuvant! program (www.adjuvant_online.com), which incorporates the tumor characteristics and the patient's general health status in providing estimates of the absolute benefit from chemotherapy, hormonal therapy, or combined therapy. It is also important to explain to the patient that adjuvant therapy does not assure that the tumor will not recur, but when selected appropriately, may decrease the chance of such recurrences.

Postmastectomy radiotherapy should be considered for all women with node-positive disease. Studies have shown not only a decreased local recurrence rate in women receiving postoperative radiotherapy but also an increased survival rate (65,66). Although these results are still controversial for women with fewer than four positive nodes, an NCI consensus conference recommended postmastectomy radiotherapy for women with four or more positive nodes (67). Radiation therapy should also be considered for women with tumors larger than 5 cm, even if the lymph nodes are negative for cancer.

There are uncommon long-term side effects of adjuvant therapy that must be recognized by the patient and the primary caregiver. Chemotherapy can cause premature menopause and a slight increase in the incidence of second neoplasms, mainly hematologic. Radiotherapy can lead to darkened skin, pulmonary damage, or later solid neoplasms (but not breast cancer in the unaffected breast). In 20% of patients, tamoxifen causes bothersome hot flushes that, if severe, can sometimes be ameliorated with one of the selective serotonin reuptake inhibitors (68,69). There is an increased incidence of endometrial carcinoma in women treated with tamoxifen (annual rate, 1.7 per 1000, or an approximately two and half-fold increased risk [70]. Therefore, all women taking tamoxifen should have annual gynecologic examinations and should be instructed to report any spotting. More detailed followup, such as uterine sonography, is unwarranted. The rate of cataract development is also slightly higher, so periodic eye examinations are also recommended (70). Tamoxifen also increases the risk of pulmonary embolism and deep vein thrombosis, with risk ratios of 3.0 and 1.6 respectively, relative to women who do not receive the drug (70). Tamoxifen does seem to decrease the risk of developing cancer in the unaffected breast, and it may have a bone-preserving effect in postmenopausal women. In contrast, aromatase inhibitors do not appear to increase the risk of vascular complications or endometrial cancer. They are however, associated with increased musculoskeletal complaints and a higher risk for osteopenia, osteoporosis, and osteoporotic fractures (71,72).

The selection criteria for adjuvant systemic therapy are constantly being re-examined as new information is obtained. Refining the criteria for benefit from chemotherapy is important as many women may be receiving chemotherapy unnecessarily because of a low personal risk of recurrence. For patients with node-negative, estrogen receptor–positive breast cancer, the likelihood of breast cancer recurrence can now be refined with the commercial availability of a 21-gene reverse transcriptase polymerase chain reaction (RT-PCR) assay that can be ordered on paraffin-embedded tumor tissue. A recurrence score is provided and this predicts the patient's individual chances of distant recurrence if treated with tamoxifen alone (73). The test is expensive and as yet is not covered by many insurance carriers.

Followup

The patient with breast cancer has a fivefold greater risk of developing cancer in the other breast (33). Consequently, she should be screened with routine mammography and physical examinations, as would any woman with moderately increased risk. Patients choosing lumpectomy and radiotherapy should have a biannual mammogram initially and careful examination of the irradiated breast every 3 months to look for a local, potentially curable recurrence. Patients who have had a mastectomy should have the scar examined at regular intervals, because 10% of patients with recurrences in the scar may be cured with local resection followed by radiotherapy.

At present there is little evidence to support the concept that the asymptomatic patient benefits by the early diagnosis and treatment of systemic metastases (74). No studies have demonstrated that monitoring of patients with radiography, liver function tests, or breast cancer markers at regular intervals improves survival or minimizes the morbidity of a relapse. This probably is true because there is no curative salvage therapy. If these studies are normal, they serve to reassure the patient. However, if they are abnormal, they often initiate a series of difficult management issues that mainly provoke uncertainty in the caregiver and anxiety in the patient without clear benefit to either. Therefore, followup plans can be individualized. Most women, when apprised of the lack of benefit from detailed laboratory and imaging followup, are comfortable doing without these studies.

Prevention

A large trial in the United States examined the use of tamoxifen for 5 years in women who were without known breast cancer but were considered to be at higher risk for development of the disease (70). The cohort receiving tamoxifen had a 50% odds reduction of developing breast cancer. This cohort also acquired a two-to-threefold increased risk for development of a deep vein thrombosis or uterine carcinoma. The tumors that were prevented were receptor-positive, suggesting that the effect may have been more related to early treatment than to prevention. Despite these results, many women at high risk are not receiving tamoxifen. One reason is that the absolute number of breast cancers prevented in the treated group was quite small. Additionally, two smaller European studies failed to confirm the American findings (75,76). Because a trial examining the effect of another estrogen receptor modulator, raloxifene, on osteoporosis saw a reduction in breast cancers in the treated group (77), a clinical trial is being conducted in the United States examining the effect of tamoxifen or raloxifene on breast cancer development. The primary caregiver needs to keep abreast of this field and to be aware of the results as they become available. The current recommendation would be to discuss preventive therapy using tamoxifen with any woman younger than 60 years of age who has a 1.67 or greater risk of developing breast cancer as determined by the Gail tool (http://bcra.nci.nih.gov/brc/q1.htm), as well as any woman who is older than 60 years of age or who has LCIS (see Prognosis).

Breast Cancer in the Elderly

Fifty percent of all new breast cancers occur in women 65 years of age or older. In the year 2020, it is estimated that 20% of the U.S. population will be that old (78). In patients older than 68 years of age with breast cancer, 60% of the tumors are node negative and at least 58% are estrogen receptor positive (79). Several studies have shown that older women are less likely than younger women to receive postoperative radiation or adjuvant systemic therapy (80,81). In healthier older women, such undertreatment may lead to poorer outcomes.

A major factor related to the ultimate benefits of adjuvant chemotherapy in older women is the effect of comorbidity on survival. Women with breast cancer who have three or more comorbid illnesses have a 20-fold increased risk of dying from a cause other than breast cancer when compared with women who have no comorbid conditions, even after adjustment for disease stage, type of therapy, race, and social and behavioral factors (82).

It is clear that the benefits of adjuvant therapy decrease with increasing age and comorbidity. The effect of adjuvant treatment on overall life expectancy is small for the oldest patients. Provided they are in good health and have a life expectancy of at least 5 years, women in their eighties who have estrogen receptor–positive, high-risk node-negative, or node-positive tumors should be considered for adjuvant hormonal therapy with tamoxifen or an aromatase inhibitor. Chemotherapy is unlikely to benefit these patients unless they are in excellent health and have high-risk, estrogen receptor–negative, node-positive tumors. The greatest dilemma is for women in their seventies. Comorbidity and risk of metastases must be carefully considered in each of these cases before final recommendations about treatment are made.

Older patients are clearly underrepresented in cancer clinical trials (83). Efforts are now underway to overcome this deficiency, with increasing focus on breast cancer research in older women.

SPECIFIC REFERENCES*

1. Jemal A, Murray T, Ward E, et al. Cancer statistics, 2005. CA Cancer J Clin 2005;55:10.
2. Phillips KA, Glendon G, Knight JA. Putting the risk of breast cancer in perspective. N Engl J Med 1999;340:141.
3. Black WC, Nease RF, Jr., Tosteson AN. Perceptions of breast cancer risk and screening effectiveness in women younger than 50 years of age. J Natl Cancer Inst 1995;87:720.
4. Kerlikowske K, Grady D, Rubin SM, et al. Efficacy of screening mammography. A meta-analysis. JAMA 1995;273:149.
5. Olsen O, Gotzsche PC. Cochrane review on screening for breast cancer with mammography. The Lancet 2001;358:1340.
6. Olsen O, Gotzsche PC. Screening for breast cancer with mammography. Cochrane Database Syst Rev 2001;CD001877.
7. Duffy SW. Interpretation of the breast screening trials: a commentary on the recent paper by Gotzsche and Olsen. Breast 2001;10:209.
8. Duffy SW, Tabar L, Smith RA. The mammographic screening trials: commentary on the recent work by Olsen and Gotzsche. CA Cancer J Clin 2002;52:68.
9. Humphrey LL, Helfand M, Chan BKS, et al. Breast cancer screening: A summary of the evidence for the U. S. Preventive Services Task Force. Ann Intern Med 2002;137:347.
10. Freedman DA, Petitti DB, Robins JM. On the efficacy of screening for breast cancer. Int J Epidemiol 2004;33:43.
11. Nystrom L, Andersson I, Bjurstam N, et al. Long-term effects of mammography screening: updated overview of the Swedish randomised trials. Lancet 2002;359:909.
12. Steele WR, Mebane F, Viswanath K, et al. News media coverage of a women's health controversy: how newspapers and TV outlets covered a recent debate over screening mammography. Women Health 2005;41:83.
13. Smith RA, Saslow D, Andrews Sawyer K, et al. American Cancer Society Guidelines for Breast Cancer Screening: Update 2003. CA Cancer J Clin 2003;53:141.
14. ACOG practice bulletin. Clinical management guidelines for obstetrician-gynecologists. Obstet Gynecol 2003;101:821.
15. Gordillo C. Breast cancer screening guidelines agreed on by AMA, other medically related organizations. JAMA 1989;262:1155.
16. The use of diagnostic tests for screening and evaluating breast lesions. Health and Public Policy Committee, American College of Physicians. Ann Intern Med 1985;103:143.
17. U.S. Preventative Services Taskforce. Screening for breast cancer: recommendations and rationale. Ann Intern Med 2002;137:344.
18. Miller AB, To T, Baines CJ, et al. The Canadian National Breast Screening Study-1: breast cancer mortality after 11 to 16 years of follow-up: a randomized screening trial of mammography in women age 40 to 49 years. Ann Intern Med 2002;137:305.
19. Gail M, Rimer B. Risk-based recommendations for mammographic screening for women in their forties. J Clin Oncol 1998;16:3105.
20. Elmore JG, Barton MB, Moceri VM, et al. Ten-year risk of f false positive screening mammograms and clinical breast examinations. N Engl J Med 1998;338:1089.
21. Lerman C, Trock B, Rimer BK, et al. Psychological and behavioral implications of abnormal mammograms. Ann Intern Med 1991;114:657.

*Bold numerals denote published controlled clinical trials, meta-analyses, or consensus-based recommendations.

22. Mandelblatt J, Saha S, Teutsch S, et al. The cost-effectiveness of screening mammography beyond age 65 years: a systematic review for the U.S. Preventive Services Task Force. Ann Intern Med 2003;139:835.
23. Thomas DB, Gao DL, Ray RM, et al. Randomized trial of breast self-examination in Shanghai: final results. J Natl Cancer Inst 2002;94:1445.
24. Pisano ED, Gatsonis C, Hendrick E, et al. Diagnostic performance of digital versus film mammography for breast-cancer screening. N Engl J Med 2005;353:1773.
25. Kriege M, Brekelmans CTM, Boetes C, et al. Efficacy of MRI and mammography for breast-cancer screening in women with a familial or genetic predisposition. N Engl J Med 2004;351:427.
26. Warner E, Plewes DB, Hill KA, et al. Surveillance of BRCA1 and BRCA2 mutation carriers with magnetic resonance imaging, ultrasound, mammography, and clinical breast examination. JAMA 2004;292:1317.
27. Santen RJ, Mansel R. Benign breast disorders. N Engl J Med 2005;353:275.
28. Komenaka IK, El Tamer M, Pile-Spellman E, et al. Core needle biopsy as a diagnostic tool to differentiate phyllodes tumor from fibroadenoma. Arch Surg 2003;138:987.
29. Dupont WD, Page DL. Risk factors for breast cancer in women with proliferative breast disease. N Engl J Med 1985;312:146.
30. Rebbeck TR, Friebel T, Lynch HT, et al. Bilateral prophylactic mastectomy reduces breast cancer risk in BRCA1 and BRCA2 mutation carriers: The PROSE Study Group. J Clin Oncol 2004; 22:1055.
31. American Society of Clinical Oncology. American Society of Clinical Oncology Policy Statement Update: Genetic testing for cancer susceptibility. J Clin Oncol 2003;21:2397.
32. Armstrong K, Eisen A, Weber B. Assessing the risk of breast cancer. N Engl J Med 2000;342:564.
33. Nielsen M, Christensen L, Andersen J. Contralateral cancerous breast lesions in women with clinical invasive breast carcinoma. Cancer 1986;57:897.
34. Claus EB, Risch N, Thompson WD. Autosomal dominant inheritance of early-onset breast cancer. Implications for risk prediction. Cancer 1994;73:643.
35. Gisvold JJ, Goellner JR, Grant CS, et al. Breast biopsy: a comparative study of stereotaxically guided core and excisional techniques. AJR Am J Roentgenol 1994;162:815.
36. Schmidt RA. Stereotactic breast biopsy. CA Cancer J Clin 1994;44:172.
37. Mansel RE, Wisbey JR, Hughes LE. Controlled trial of the antigonadotropin danazol in painful nodular benign breast disease. Lancet 1982; 1:928.
38. Kontostolis E, Stefanidis K, Navrozoglou I, et al. Comparison of tamoxifen with danazol for treatment of cyclical mastalgia. Gynecol Endocrinol 1997;11:393.
39. Fisher B, Anderson S, Bryant J, et al. Twenty-year follow-up of a randomized trial comparing total mastectomy, lumpectomy, and lumpectomy plus irradiation for the treatment of invasive breast cancer. N Engl J Med 2002; 347:1233.
40. Hanrahan EO, Hennessy BT, Valero V. Neoadjuvant systemic therapy for breast cancer: an overview and review of recent clinical trials. Expert Opin Pharmacother 2005;6:1477.
41. Huober J, Krainick-Strobel U, Kurek R, et al. Neoadjuvant endocrine therapy in primary breast cancer. Clin Breast Cancer 2004;5:341.
42. Galper S, Blood E, Gelman R, et al. Prognosis after local recurrence after conservative surgery and radiation for early-stage breast cancer. Int J Radiat Oncol Biol Phys 2005;61:348.
43. Lichter AS, Lippman ME, Danforth DN, Jr., et al. Mastectomy versus breast-conserving therapy in the treatment of stage I and II carcinoma of the breast: a randomized trial at the National Cancer Institute. J Clin Oncol 1992;10:976.
44. Gage I, Recht A, Gelman R, et al. Long-term outcome following breast-conserving surgery and radiation therapy. Int J Radiat Oncol Biol Phys 1995;33:245.
45. Burstein HJ, Polyak K, Wong JS, et al. Ductal carcinoma in situ of the breast. N Engl J Med 2004;350:1430.
46. Fisher B, Costantino J, Redmond C, et al. Lumpectomy compared with lumpectomy and radiation therapy for the treatment of intraductal breast Cancer. N Engl J Med 1993;328:1581.
47. Lagios MD. Duct carcinoma in situ. Pathology and treatment. Surg Clin North Am 1990;70:853.
48. Silverstein MJ. An argument against routine use of radiotherapy for ductal carcinoma in situ. Oncology (Williston Park) 2003;17:1511.
49. Smith IE, Dowsett M, Ebbs SR, et al. Neoadjuvant treatment of postmenopausal breast cancer with anastrozole, tamoxifen, or both in combination: the Immediate Preoperative Anastrozole, Tamoxifen, or Combined With Tamoxifen (IMPACT) multicenter double-blind randomized trial. J Clin Oncol 2005;23:5108.
50. Eiermann W, Paepke S, Appfelstaedt J, et al. Preoperative treatment of postmenopausal breast cancer patients with letrozole: a randomized double-blind multicenter study. Ann Oncol 2001;12:1527.
51. Fisher B, Slack N, Katrych D, et al. Ten year follow-up results of patients with carcinoma of the breast in a co-operative clinical trial evaluating surgical adjuvant chemotherapy. Surg Gynecol Obstet 1975;140:528.
52. Fisher B, Bauer M, Wickerham DL, et al. Relation of number of positive axillary nodes to the prognosis of patients with primary breast cancer. An NSABP update. Cancer 1983;52: 1551.
53. McGuire WL, Clark GM, Dressler LG, et al. Role of steroid hormone receptors as prognostic factors in primary breast cancer. NCI Monogr 1986;19.
54. Veronesi U, Paganelli G, Viale G, et al. A randomized comparison of sentinel-node biopsy with routine axillary dissection in breast cancer. N Engl J Med 2003;349:546.
55. Lyman GH, Giuliano AE, Somerfield MR, et al. American Society of Clinical Oncology guideline recommendations for sentinel lymph node biopsy in early-stage breast cancer. J Clin Oncol 2005;23:7703.
56. Rosser RJ, Giuliano A, McMasters K. Safety of sentinel lymph node dissection and significance of cytokeratin micrometastases. J Clin Oncol 2001;19:1882.
57. Early Breast Cancer Trialists' Collaborative Group. Effects of chemotherapy and hormonal therapy for early breast cancer on recurrence and 15-year survival: an overview of the randomised trials. Lancet 2005;365:1687.
58. Romond EH, Perez EA, Bryant J, et al. Trastuzumab plus adjuvant chemotherapy for operable HER2-positive breast cancer. N Engl J Med 2005;353:1673.
59. Piccart-Gebhart MJ, Procter M, Leyland-Jones B, et al. Trastuzumab after adjuvant chemotherapy in HER2-positive breast cancer. N Engl J Med 2005;353:1659.

60. Hortobagyi GN. Trastuzumab in the treatment of breast cancer. N Engl J Med 2005;353:1734.
61. Recht A, Come SE, Henderson IC, et al. The sequencing of chemotherapy and radiation therapy after conservative surgery for early-stage breast cancer. N Engl J Med 1996;334:1356.
62. Prowell TM, Davidson NE. What is the role of ovarian ablation in the management of primary and metastatic breast cancer today? Oncologist 2004;9:507.
63. Winer EP, Hudis C, Burstein HJ, et al. American Society of Clinical Oncology Technology assessment on the use of aromatase inhibitors as adjuvant therapy for postmenopausal women with hormone receptor-positive breast cancer: status report 2004. J Clin Oncol 2005;23:619.
64. Fisher B, Dignam J, Wolmark N, et al. Tamoxifen in treatment of intraductal breast cancer: National Surgical Adjuvant Breast and Bowel Project B-24 randomised controlled trial. Lancet 1999;353:1993.
65. Overgaard M, Hansen PS, Overgaard J, et al. Postoperative radiotherapy in high-risk premenopausal women with breast cancer who receive adjuvant chemotherapy. N Engl J Med 1997;337:949.
66. Ragaz J, Jackson SM, Le N, et al. Adjuvant radiotherapy and chemotherapy in node-positive premenopausal women with breast cancer. N Engl J Med 1997;337:956.
67. Eifel P, Axelson JA, Costa J, et al. National Institutes of Health Consensus Development Conference Statement: adjuvant therapy for breast cancer, November 1–3, 2000. J Natl Cancer Inst 2001;93:979.
68. Biglia N, Torta R, Roagna R, et al. Evaluation of low-dose venlafaxine hydrochloride for the therapy of hot flushes in breast cancer survivors. Maturitas 2005;52:78.
69. Treatment of menopause-associated vasomotor symptoms: position statement of The North American Menopause Society. Menopause 2004;11:11.
70. Fisher B, Costantino JP, Wickerham DL, et al. Tamoxifen for the prevention of breast cancer: current status of the National Surgical Adjuvant Breast and Bowel Project P-1 study. J Natl Cancer Inst 2005;97:1652.
71. Goss PE, Ingle JN, Martino S, et al. Randomized trial of letrozole following tamoxifen as extended adjuvant therapy in receptor-positive breast cancer: updated findings from NCIC CTG MA. 17. J Natl Cancer Inst 2005;97:1262.
72. Howell A, Cuzick J, Baum M, et al. Results of the ATAC (Arimidex, Tamoxifen, Alone or in Combination) trial after completion of 5 years' adjuvant treatment for breast cancer. Lancet 2005;365:60.
73. Paik S, Shak S, Tang G, et al. A multigene assay to predict recurrence of tamoxafine-treated node-negative breast cancer. N Engl J Med 2004;351:2817.
74. Recommended breast cancer surveillance guidelines. American Society of Clinical Oncology. J Clin Oncol 1997;15:2149.
75. Powles T, Eeles R, Ashley S, et al. Interim analysis of the incidence of breast cancer in the Royal Marsden Hospital tamoxifen randomised chemoprevention trial. Lancet 1998;352:98.
76. Veronesi U, Maisonneuve P, Costa A, et al. Prevention of breast cancer with tamoxifen: preliminary findings from the Italian randomised trial among hysterectomised women. Italian Tamoxifen Prevention Study. Lancet 1998;352:93.
77. Cummings SR, Eckert S, Krueger KA, et al. The Effect of raloxifene on risk of breast cancer in postmenopausal women: results from the MORE randomized trial. JAMA 1999;281:2189.
78. Yancik R, Ries LA. Aging and cancer in America. Demographic and epidemiologic perspectives. Hematol Oncol Clin North Am 2000;14:17.
79. Diab SG, Elledge RM, Clark GM. Tumor characteristics and clinical outcome of elderly women with breast cancer. J Natl Cancer Inst 2000;92:550.
80. Hurria A, Leung D, Trainor K, et al. Factors influencing treatment patterns of breast cancer patients age 75 and older. Crit Rev Oncol Hematol 2003;46:121.
81. Mandelblatt JS, Hadley J, Kerner JF, et al. Patterns of breast carcinoma treatment in older women: patient preference and clinical and physical influences. Cancer 2000;89:561.
82. Satariano WA, Ragland DR. The effect of comorbidity on 3-year survival of women with primary breast cancer. Ann Intern Med 1994;120:104.
83. Talarico L, Chen G, Pazdur R. Enrollment of elderly patients in clinical trials for cancer drug registration: a 7-year experience by the US Food and Drug Administration. J Clin Oncol 2004;22:4626.

For annotated **General References** *and resources related to this chapter, visit www.hopkinsbayview.org/PAMreferences.*

Chapter 106

Menopause and Beyond

Redonda G. Miller

Each year more than 31 million women in the United States experience menopause. These women frequently present to primary care clinicians with a number of symptoms related to estrogen deficiency, as well as with the need to deal with the psychosocial issues related to midlife changes in family and social relationships. Menopause occurs on average at age 51 years, but may occur earlier in smokers (1). Given the increasing life expectancy in the United States, the average woman can expect to spend more than one third of her life in the postmenopausal years.

Because several chronic diseases associated with aging are first manifested at menopause, this is an opportune time for the primary care clinician and patient to assess risk and initiate preventive strategies for cardiovascular disease, osteoporosis, and cancer, in addition to addressing the symptoms of menopause. That assessment has been made more difficult by recent studies that have suggested that some of these diseases might be adversely affected in some women by hormone therapy (HT), the most effective treatment for menopausal vasomotor symptoms (see www.hopkinsbayview.org/PAMreferences). These issues are discussed below.

DEFINITION AND PHYSIOLOGY

The menopause is defined as the *last* menses. This is a clinical diagnosis that can be determined with certainty only when menses have been absent for 12 months. *Perimenopause* is the span of time that encompasses the period of initial menstrual irregularity, typically 2 to 8 years before menopause, the menopause itself, and the year subsequent to the menopause. Perimenopause usually begins in the forties, but it is not uncommon for women to experience symptoms as early as their thirties.

During perimenopause, a host of hormonal changes occur. Ovarian follicles undergo progressive atresia over the course of a woman's lifetime, with a consequent gradual fall in circulating estradiol. There is also a loss of production of the glycoprotein inhibin by the ovaries. Inhibin provides negative feedback to the pituitary gland, and, in its absence, pituitary production of follicle-stimulating hormone (FSH) and luteinizing hormone (LH) increases. An FSH level greater than 30 mIU may support the diagnosis of menopause, but the level tends to fluctuate significantly throughout the perimenopause and is not reliably diagnostic. Routine measurement of FSH, therefore, is not recommended. On the other hand, FSH measurement is useful in certain situations, such as in a hysterectomized woman without classic vasomotor symptoms or a woman who may be experiencing premature ovarian failure.

Because both estradiol and FSH have large fluctuations during this period, the diagnosis of perimenopause is often made clinically, with the onset of menstrual cycle irregularity in a woman with previously regular menstrual cycles. Menstrual irregularity can take the form of shortened cycles, missed cycles, or irregular spotting. Some patients have regular cycles up until the point of menopause. A perimenopausal woman should be cautioned that pregnancy is a possibility until she has been amenorrheic for more than 1 year or until FSH levels have consistently been greater than 30 mIU.

Women may consult their primary care clinicians during this period for concerns about abnormal uterine bleeding or amenorrhea. Patients with abnormal vaginal bleeding (see Chapter 101) should be referred immediately for evaluation. Amenorrhea in women younger than 50 years of age should be evaluated with a pregnancy test. Thyroid dysfunction can also affect the menstrual cycle and should be assessed by screening tests in women who present with menstrual irregularities.

TABLE 106.1 Office Evaluation of the Perimenopausal Patient

Assess Current Symptoms
Hot flashes
Menstrual irregularity: abnormal bleeding, amenorrhea
Symptoms of pelvic floor relaxation; bladder dysfunction
Sexual function (e.g., loss of libido, dyspareunia)
Sleep disturbances
Assess Risk of Osteoporosis, Breast Cancer, Endometrial Cancer, Cardiovascular Disease
Reproductive history: menarche, parity, contraception, surgical history
Physical activity, use of tobacco
Dietary history (e.g., intake of vitamin D and calcium)
History of hormone therapy (HT)
Family history of osteoporosis, cancer, heart disease
History of fractures, loss of height
Assess Psychosocial Status
Mood changes, difficulty with concentration
Expectations of menopause
Family and work
Assess Chronic Medical Conditions That May Affect HT Decision
Hypertension
Diabetes mellitus
Hyperlipidemia
Gallbladder disease
Thromboembolic disease
Physical Examination, to Include
Weight, height, body mass index
Posture
Vision and hearing screens
Breast examination
Pelvic and rectal examination
Laboratory Testing, to Include
Lipid profile
Serum thyroid-stimulating hormone, if indicated
Serum follicle-stimulating hormone, if indicated
Bone mineral density, if indicated (see Chapter 103)
Screening protocols for mammography, colon cancer, and cervical cancer (see Chapter 1)
Counseling and Patient Education
Exercise prescription
Nutrition and weight management
Vitamin D and calcium supplementation
Avoidance of triggers for hot flushes
Benefits and risks of HT
Alternatives to HT therapy

CLINICAL CONSIDERATIONS

Clinical guidelines (see www.hopkinsbayview.org/PAM references) for management of menopause generally recommend that the office evaluation of the menopausal patient include a comprehensive risk assessment and screening, as well as attention to the common symptoms of estrogen deficiency (Table 106.1).

The severity of menopausal symptoms is highly variable and is related to both physiologic and cultural factors. Some women are quite debilitated, whereas others have minimal or no symptoms. As an example, a prospective study of 478 Australian women from premenopause to postmenopause found that the number of women reporting five or more symptoms increased by 14% from early to late menopause. Lower estrogen levels, smoking, and a history of no occupation predicted vasomotor symptoms. Insomnia, which increased throughout the menopause, was related not only to hot flashes but also to psychosocial factors (2).

Regardless of initial symptom severity, there are many long-term effects of estrogen deficiency on bone, heart, and breast, which should be evaluated in every patient.

Vasomotor Symptoms

Vasomotor symptoms are the most common reason women seek medical care during perimenopause. These symptoms are usually most common in the first 2 to 3 years of perimenopause and then taper off gradually. The prevalence varies by culture. Up to 75% of women in the United States and Europe experience hot flashes, whereas only 20% of Asian women do. In migration studies of Japanese women, the incidence of hot flashes approached the overall U.S. incidence within one or two generations, which implicates nongenetic factors, such as diet (3). The intensity and frequency of hot flashes are also variable and are usually more severe in women who undergo surgical menopause.

The hot flash is a sensation of heat that typically develops in the head and neck region and then slowly spreads down the arms and across the chest. Intense diaphoresis and visible flushing may accompany the hot flash. Occasionally women may experience a prodrome of nausea, light-headedness, or palpitations. The episode may end with chills and a feeling of coldness. The entire event usually lasts between 30 seconds and 5 minutes. Hot flashes frequently occur at night, leading to lack of sleep and subsequent daytime fatigue and irritability. Other triggers of hot flashes include spicy food, caffeine, alcohol, stress, humid environments, and sexual activity. In a study of African American and Caucasian women, significant predictors of hot flashes were higher FSH levels, anxiety, alcohol use, body mass index, and parity; there was no difference by race (4).

The exact cause of hot flashes is unknown, but they may be related to alterations in the hypothalamic thermoregulatory center that are precipitated by a lack of estrogen and increasing gonadotropin levels. Documented increases in skin conductance and peripheral temperature and a subsequent fall in core temperature coincide with the flash (5). Studies using an ingested telemetry pill found that the thermoneutral zone, that is, the range of core body temperature within which sweating, peripheral vasodilatation, and shivering do not occur, is virtually nonexistent in symptomatic women but normal in asymptomatic women (6). Central sympathetic activation is increased in symptomatic women and also reduces the thermoneutral zone in animals. The beneficial effect of clonidine for hot flashes may relate to its reduction of central sympathetic activation.

Treatment

Simple measures can help women cope with hot flashes. Wearing layered clothing permits adjustments for temperature. Regular exercise and avoidance of known triggers can help with prevention. Table 106.2 lists common therapies for vasomotor symptoms, of which estrogen replacement is the most effective. It has been shown to decrease hot flashes by >90% and improve night-time insomnia. Both oral and transdermal estrogens (see later discussion)

TABLE 106.2 Therapies for Menopausal Vasomotor Symptoms

Agent	Dose	Side Effects
Estrogen	Variable (see Table 106.5)	Breast tenderness, vaginal spotting, headaches
Progestins		
Medroxyprogesterone acetate	Oral: 5–10 mg PO q.d. Depot: 50–150 mg every month Transdermal: 20 mg PO q.d.	Breast tenderness, irritability, depression, headaches
Levonorgestrel	Intrauterine device, 20 μg q.d.	
α_2-Adrenergic Agents		
Clonidine	Oral: 0.1–0.3 mg PO t.i.d.	Fatigue, dizziness, dry mouth, constipation
Methyldopa	500 mg PO b.i.d.	Headache, somnolence, gastrointestinal upset
Serotonin reuptake inhibitors		
Paroxetine CR	12.5–25 mg q.d.	Somnolence, dry mouth, decreased appetite, nausea, constipation
Venlafaxine	37.5–150 mg q.d.	
Fluoxetine	20 mg q.d.	
Gabapentin	300 mg t.i.d.	Drowsiness, lethargy
Herbals		
Soy protein	Variable	Gastrointestinal upset
Black cohosh		

are effective and work within 1 to 4 weeks. Newer options for estrogen delivery that are effective in reducing hot flashes include a topical emulsion applied daily and an intravaginal estradiol ring inserted by the patient every 3 months (7). Most women respond to standard doses, but occasionally higher doses are required (often in women with an abrupt, surgical menopause). Lower doses of estrogens, now more popular in the wake of recent concern about the adverse effects of estrogen, have demonstrated efficacy for the treatment of hot flashes (8).

For women who are unable or unwilling to take estrogen, other alternatives are available, but none is as effective as estrogen. Progestins alone by oral, topical, or injectable routes may provide effective relief, but often with undesirable consequences such as weight gain. Furthermore, long-term safety of progestational agents for treatment of hot flashes has not been established. The antihypertensive agents clonidine and methyldopa are moderately effective in controlling vasomotor symptoms, but side effects of drowsiness, constipation, and dry mouth may be limiting. Estrogen's interaction with serotonergic and dopaminergic neurotransmitters has led to the use of one class of antidepressants, selective serotonin reuptake inhibitors (SSRIs) (see Chapter 24). Clinical trials of paroxetine, venlafaxine, and fluoxetine found reductions in hot flash scores of 50% to 60%, with associated improvement in sleep and depression (9–11). Gabapentin, a gamma-aminobutyric acid analog used for the treatment of seizures, has also been shown to be efficacious for vasomotor symptoms, possibly through its effect on hypothalamic tachykinin activity. A dose of 900 mg/day resulted in a 54% reduction in hot flush score (12). Gradual titration of dose is necessary to prevent side effects (see Table 106.2).

Finally, herbal preparations may provide a benefit in the treatment of vasomotor symptoms. Many women prefer herbals as a more natural alternative than prescription medication, and food supplements are being heavily marketed in the United States. The most studied agents are black cohosh and soy protein.

Black cohosh (*Actaea racemosa*) is a North American herb used by Native Americans and thought to have estrogenic properties. As with many herbal preparations, the safety and efficacy of this substance are not well established (see Chapter 5). A systematic review (13) yielded mixed results, and one randomized controlled trial in breast cancer patients found no benefit of black cohosh over placebo for treatment of hot flashes (14). A standardized extract of black cohosh is marketed as Remifemin and frequently prescribed in Europe.

Phytoestrogens are plant steroids that bind to estrogen receptors, although with much less affinity than human estrogen. They exhibit both estrogenic and antiestrogenic effects. Isoflavones, one of three types of phytoestrogens, are thought to have the most estrogenic activity. Isoflavones are found in soy, chickpeas, lentils, and beans. There appears to be individual variation in the physiologic response to ingestion of isoflavones, but they are relatively well tolerated except for moderate gastrointestinal distress. Although some small studies of soy protein found statistically significant reductions of hot flushes with supplementation, the clinical significance was small, approximately one hot flash per day (15,16). Larger, placebo-controlled trials have not documented any benefit (17,18). Isoflavones may favorably affect the lipid profile by increasing high-density lipoprotein (HDL) and decreasing low-density lipoprotein (LDL) cholesterol levels, but recent studies have suggested no improvements in bone mineral density (19) and a possible risk of long-term endometrial hyperplasia with use over 5 years (20). Therefore, it is difficult to endorse long-term use of these agents.

Urogenital Symptoms

After menopause, the urogenital tract undergoes significant changes and atrophy. Although the exact role of estrogen is unknown, estrogen receptors are located throughout the urogenital tract, and the decline in estrogen levels often correlates with the development of symptoms. Symptoms can be highly variable in character and onset. Some women experience vaginal dryness, itching, and burning. Dyspareunia and loss of libido may be sequelae. Up to one third of women develop urinary incontinence, usually with a stress pattern (see Chapter 54). Estrogen receptors are also found on the pelvic musculature and ligaments, and the decline in estrogen may lead to uterine and bladder prolapse. Other factors that further increase the risk of prolapse include advancing age and history of multiple births. Finally, estrogen plays a role in maintaining vaginal acidity by allowing lactic acid–producing bacilli to flourish. Without estrogen, the flora may shift to bacteria such as *Escherichia coli*, leading to more frequent urinary tract infections (UTIs). All of these symptoms may occur within the perimenopause or may take up to 10 years to manifest. Many women never approach their primary care provider about this problem because of embarrassment or the misconception that these symptoms cannot be treated.

Treatment

Estrogen is effective in alleviating many of the urogenital symptoms. It improves vaginal dryness, atrophic vaginitis, and dyspareunia. Estrogen has also been shown to lessen the symptoms of urinary incontinence in perimenopausal women (21), but seems to have no benefit and possibly worsens urinary incontinence in older women (22) (see Chapter 54). Postmenopausal women with recurrent UTIs can prolong time to recurrence by using estrogen (23).

Lower doses of estrogen are needed for the relief of genitourinary symptoms than for vasomotor symptoms (Table 106.3). Local delivery of estrogen can result in high tissue

TABLE 106.3 Therapies for Vaginal Dryness and Genitourinary Symptoms

Preparation	*Estrogen (Brand)*	*Dose*
Lubricants	No estrogen (Replens)	Use liberally as needed with intercourse
Cream	Conjugated estrogens (Premarin)	0.5–2.0 g q.d. for 3 weeks each month
	Estradiol (Estrace)	2–4 g q.d. × 2 wk then ↓ dose
	Estropipate (Ogen)	2–4 g q.d. for 3 wk each month
	Dienestrol (Ortho Dienestrol)	1–2 applicators q.d. for 1–2 wk then ↓ dose
Ring	Estradiol (Estring, Femring)	Insert and replace every 90 d
Tablet	Estradiol (Vagifem)	1 tablet vaginally q.d. × 2 wk, then 1 tablet twice weekly

levels and is often adequate. Numerous preparations of local estrogen therapy are available today. They include creams (conjugated equine estrogens, estradiol, and diethylstilbestrol), estriol pessaries, and estradiol rings and tablets. All seem comparable in effectiveness, so patient preference plays a large role in choice. Both creams and pessaries, however, can be messy to administer and result in discharge. On the other hand, the vaginal ring and estrogen tablets are well tolerated and only rarely result in mild leukorrhea. Given the low doses used, local estrogen administration is relatively safe and does not seem to result in endometrial hypertrophy. Most preparations do not, however, confer the added benefit on vasomotor symptoms, lipid profile, and bone density that systemic administration does.

Cognition and Depression

Women may experience many cognitive symptoms during the perimenopause. Many women describe difficulty with concentration, poor memory, and feelings of sadness or depression. It remains controversial whether these symptoms are truly related to menopause or perhaps are related to the loss of sleep and fatigue associated with nocturnal hot flashes. Another possibility is that they are a reaction to the changes in a woman's cultural roles that may be associated with menopause. Data supporting these hypotheses are conflicting. One longitudinal analysis of more than 2,500 women found no relationship between menopause and depression (24), but another large, cross-sectional study suggested that postmenopausal women using estrogen alone were at decreased risk for depression (25). The second study, however, found no decrease in risk of depression risk among women using *both* estrogen and progestin.

Sexual Dysfunction

A loss of libido is another frequent concern described by perimenopausal and menopausal women. The lack of interest in sex is probably multifactorial. Depression and low self-esteem, vaginal dryness and dyspareunia, and a decline in testosterone levels may all play a role. Some experts promote the addition of androgens to estrogen therapy to improve libido (26). Testosterone can be delivered as methyltestosterone, 1.25 to 2.5 mg/day; as micronized testosterone, 2.5 to 5.0 mg/day; or with a transdermal patch, 150 to 300 μg/day. Androgens can also prevent postmenopausal bone loss. The side effects of excessive androgen use include acne, hirsutism, alopecia, and voice deepening. Androgens may lower HDL levels, potentially worsening cardiovascular risk. The American Association of Clinical Endocrinologists practice guidelines (27) suggest four situations in which androgen plus estrogen therapy may be considered: (a) oophorectomized women, (b) women who have experienced inadequate relief of vasomotor symptoms with estrogen, (c) women who are at risk for osteoporosis and unable to take other therapies, and (d) women with unsatisfactory sexual function, especially loss of libido. The North American Menopause Society (NAMS) in 2005 concluded that the only indication for testosterone therapy in postmenopausal women is to treat decreased sexual desire in women, finding no other use supported by the evidence (28). In addition to the concerns noted above, the NAMS recommends that clinicians who use testosterone for this indication understand that dosage forms used to treat men have not been tested in women and may be supraphysiologic. For that reason, smaller dosages should be used and blood testosterone levels monitored. Large, randomized trials examining the benefits of adding androgen therapy to estrogen in postmenopausal women do not yet exist. Chapter 101 discusses female sexual dysfunction.

Cardiovascular Changes

The leading cause of death among American women is coronary heart disease (CHD). Before menopause, the rate of myocardial infarction in women is much lower than in men, but by the eighth decade the rates have equalized. Much of the premenopausal protection from CHD in women has been attributed to estrogen.

There are several effects of estrogen on the cardiovascular system. The most obvious effect is on the lipid profile. Within 6 months of the menopause, total cholesterol and LDL cholesterol begin to increase. HDL cholesterol levels fall as a result of the estrogen deficiency. This is particularly important in women, because low HDL seems to be a stronger predictor of CHD death in women than in men. Other changes that take place with menopause are increased levels of plasminogen activator inhibitor type 1 (PAI-1), lipoprotein(a), and homocysteine. Each of these is thought to be an independent risk factor for CHD.

Observational studies have demonstrated a protective effect of estrogen on cardiovascular disease. Estrogen appears to decrease the risk of CHD and CHD death in postmenopausal women by 40% to 60% (29). Estrogen may exert much of its protective effect through changes in the lipid profile. Oral estrogen increases HDL cholesterol by roughly 15% and decreases LDL cholesterol by up to 19% (30,31). Triglycerides are also increased, but usually not to a large degree. Addition of a progestin, such as medroxyprogesterone acetate, to estrogen attenuates the beneficial effects on lipids but does not eliminate them (31). With norethindrone acetate use, LDL is still lowered, but there does not seem to be a beneficial increase in HDL. Micronized progestin may be least detrimental on the lipid profile. Estrogen may have other favorable effects on the cardiovascular system. Evidence suggests that it decreases levels of PAI-1, lipoprotein(a), and homocysteine. There is also literature to support a direct vasodilatory effect of estrogen on the coronary vasculature.

The role of estrogen replacement therapy in secondary prevention of CHD was not supported by clinical trials. In the first randomized, controlled trial, the Heart and Estrogen/Progestin Replacement Study (HERS), postmenopausal women with established CHD had similar rates of MI and CHD death whether they were treated with hormone replacement or not (32). Analysis of time trends in the study revealed an excess of events in the estrogen-treated group in year 1 but fewer events in years 4 and 5. This may represent a manifestation of the early prothrombotic effects of estrogen (with increased early events) followed by more long-term beneficial changes. Alternatively, high-risk women may have cardiac events early, leaving only lower risk women in the study. These findings were further backed by the Women's Health Initiative Study. In over 16,000 women with an average age of 63 years, conjugated equine estrogen (CEE) + medroxyprogesterone (MPA) did not confer protection against cardiac events (33). Likewise, CEE alone did not reduce cardiac outcomes in the estrogen-only arm (34). Speculation exists about whether these patients already had subclinical atherosclerotic disease given their age or whether the duration of the study (5.2 years) was insufficient to show a benefit; furthermore, it is unclear how to apply these findings from an older population roughly 12 years past menopause to younger, perimenopausal women. Regardless, the American Heart Association (AHA) has concluded that HT should not be initiated for the secondary prevention of cardiovascular disease and that there is insufficient evidence for its use in primary prevention (35).

Osteoporosis

Osteoporosis is a large health problem that remains underdiagnosed. An average 50-year-old white woman has up to a 50% chance of sustaining an osteoporotic fracture in her lifetime (36). Hip fractures alone are associated with a significant mortality rate of 20% at 1 year. Other sequelae of fracture include difficulty with ambulation, dependence on assisted living, chronic pain, and loss of quality of life. The most rapid loss of bone mineralization occurs in the years after menopause. After 30 years of age, most women experience a loss of approximately 0.5% to 1.0% of their bone density per year. In the first 5 years after menopause, the rate accelerates to 3% to 5% per year before returning to the baseline rate. Prevention of perimenopausal bone loss is therefore crucial. Serial yearly height measurements in the office may provide an early clue to the development of osteoporosis. The loss of 1 inch or more in height is highly suggestive of the disease.

All perimenopausal women should be counseled regarding proper dietary calcium intake. The National Osteoporosis Foundation recommends that postmenopausal women consume at least 1,200 mg/day, or 1,500 mg/day if frank osteoporosis is present. Women also should be encouraged to pursue weight-bearing exercise, as this has been shown to be helpful in bone density preservation. Chapter 103 discusses osteoporosis and its management more thoroughly.

SUMMARY OF THERAPEUTIC OPTIONS

Hormone Therapy

HT is not for every woman. The enthusiasm for use of HT for prevention of chronic diseases has been tempered by the sobering results of recent data from the Women's Health Initiative (WHI), the first large, randomized controlled trial of HT in postmenopausal women.

Advantages of Hormone Therapy

Many advantages of estrogen have been discussed. One of the most rapid benefits a woman taking HT experiences is significant relief of vasomotor symptoms. Hot flashes diminish within days to weeks, and no other therapy is as efficacious. Vaginal dryness improves, leading to improved ability to have intercourse. UTIs are less frequent as well.

Estrogen plays a significant role in the prevention of osteoporosis and fracture. Use of estrogen at menopause allows a woman to preserve bone density and aids in the prevention of osteoporosis. In women who are already osteopenic or osteoporotic, estrogen serves to increase bone density and decrease the fracture rate by up to 40% to 60%. In the WHI, use of either CEE + MPA or CEE alone resulted in a significant reduction in both vertebral and hip fractures in healthy women who were not necessarily osteoporotic (33,34). More recently, ultra-low doses of estradiol 2.5 mg/day were demonstrated to increase bone mineral density in healthy women older than age 65 years (37).

Estrogen therapy (ET) has also been linked to a decreased rate of colon cancer, perhaps via its effects on bile acids (38). Data from the WHI confirmed a protective effect in both combination and estrogen-only arms (33,34). Other purported but not proven roles of HT include prevention of macular degeneration, lens opacities, tooth loss, age-related hypertension, and skin aging.

Disadvantages of Hormone Therapy

Some of the more prevalent disadvantages of estrogen therapy are the non–life-threatening side effects. Menopausal women starting HT may experience breast tenderness or vaginal spotting. These symptoms tend to resolve within 2 months in most women. Low-dose oral bromocriptine (2.5 mg twice daily) may be helpful in alleviating the breast tenderness on a short-term basis, as may prescribing an estrogen-free period a few days each month. Contrary to popular belief, postmenopausal doses of estrogen are not associated with weight gain.

The biggest fear shared by many women is that estrogen may cause breast cancer. These fears are not unfounded, and many studies have unsuccessfully attempted to put the issue to rest. Given the observational nature of most of these studies, they are confounded by selection and lead-time bias. Two studies are often cited. The Nurses' Health Study monitored almost 70,000 postmenopausal women and found a relative risk for development of breast cancer of 1.3 to 1.4 among current users of estrogen (39). Duration of use greater than 10 years was highly correlated with the development of breast cancer, and former use was not. Conversely, the Iowa study of high-risk women with positive family histories showed no increased risk, even with use lasting longer than 5 years (40). The WHI has not clarified the issue as much as had been hoped. Women assigned to CEE + MPA had a small increased risk of breast cancer compared to patients taking placebo (HR = 1.24) (33), but women in the CEE-only arm developed fewer cases of breast cancer than did women in the placebo arm (34). No study has definitively shown increased mortality due to breast cancer, leading some experts to postulate that estrogen use may result in "better-differentiated" and less aggressive tumors. Another possibility is that women who use estrogen are more compliant with mammography and more likely to have cancers detected earlier or perhaps it is the use of progestational agents that increase a woman's risk rather than the estrogen component. Estrogen's exact role in the development of breast cancer, therefore, remains controversial.

Studies have repetitively linked endometrial adenocarcinoma to the use of unopposed estrogen in women with an intact uterus. The risk is roughly 2.3 times that of women who do not use estrogen. Risk is related to duration of use. In women using unopposed estrogen for longer than 10 years, the relative risk rises to 9.5 (41). If estrogen is combined with a progestin, the risk is not elevated above that of nonusers. Therefore, use of a progestin *with* estrogen in nonhysterectomized women should be considered the standard of care. The progestin may be given continuously or cyclically with the same protective benefit. Given that many women will experience some mild vaginal spotting with the institution of HT, one must distinguish this fairly common side effect from a more serious problem. If vaginal bleeding is mild and occurs immediately in an otherwise healthy woman initiating HT, watchful waiting is appropriate. Temporarily increasing the dose of progestin may help alleviate this bleeding. If the bleeding persists beyond 6 months, is particularly heavy, or starts months to years *after* the initiation of HT, the patient should be further evaluated. A transvaginal ultrasound examination may be helpful in assessing the thickness of the uterine lining and detecting fibroids. Referral to a gynecologist and probable endometrial biopsy is also warranted.

Estrogen therapy has been undisputedly linked to an increased risk of venous thromboembolic disease, and recent WHI data support this association (31,33,34,42). Users tend to have 2.5 to 3.5 times the risk of nonusers. This is less than the risk associated with oral contraceptive use, probably because postmenopausal doses of estrogen are considerably lower than those in oral contraceptives. Estrogen also increases the risk of gallbladder disease in women, albeit only modestly (32). In the liver, estrogen can increase the metabolism and turnover of cholesterol, leading to increased excretion in the bile and subsequent stone formation. This side effect has not been associated with higher mortality.

The absolute contraindications to estrogen are relatively few. Most experts would agree that a personal history of breast cancer and acute thromboembolic disease fall into this category (Table 106.4). Many of the disadvantages listed previously must be taken in context with the patient's individual risks and may be considered relative contraindications, depending on the clinical setting. Some of the relative contraindications can be addressed by alternative delivery; transdermal estrogen avoids the first-pass effect and has some advantages in specific situations (see Available Formulations section).

SPECIFIC REFERENCES*

1. McKinlay SM, Bifano NL, McKinlay JB. Smoking and age at menopause. Ann Intern Med 1985;103:350.
2. Dennerstein L, Dudley EC, Hopper JL, et al. A prospective population-based study of menopausal symptoms. Obstet Gynecol 2000; 96:351.
3. Kolonel LW, Hankin JH, Nomura A. Multiethnic studies of diet, nutrition and cancer in Hawaii. In: Hayashi Y, Nagao M, Sugimura T, et al., eds. Nutrition and cancer. Tokyo: Japanese Science Society Press; 1986: 29.
4. Freeman EW, Sammel MD, Grisso JA, et al. Hot flushes in the late reproductive years: risk factors for African-American and Caucasian women. J Womens Health Gend Based Med 2001;10:67.
5. Tataryn IV, Lomax P, Meldrum DR, et al. Objective techniques for the assessment of postmenopausal hot flushes. Obstet Gynecol 1981;57:340.
6. Freedman RR. Physiology of hot flushes. Am J Human Biol 2001;13:453.
7. Speroff L. Efficacy and tolerability of a novel estradiol vaginal ring for relief of menopausal symptoms. Obstet Gynecol 2003;102:823.
8. Utian WH, Shoupe D, Bachmann G, et al. Relief of vasomotor symptoms and vaginal atrophy with lower doses of conjugated equine estrogen and medroxyprogesterone acetate. Fertil Steril 2001;75:1065.
9. Stearns V, Beebe KL, Iyengar M, Dube E. Paroxetine controlled release in the treatment of menopausal hot flashes. JAMA 2003;289:2827.
10. Loprinzi CL, Kugler JW, Sloan JA, et al. Venlafaxine in management of hot flushes in survivors of breast cancer: a randomised controlled trial. Lancet 2000;356:2059.
11. Loprinzi CL, Sloan JA, Perez EA, et al. Phase III evaluation of fluoxetine for treatment of hot flashes. J Clin Oncol 2002;20:1578.
12. Guttuso Jr, T, Kurlan R, McDermott MP, et al. Gabapentin's effects on hot flashes in postmenopausal women: a randomized controlled trial. Obstet Gynecol 2003;101:337.
13. Huntley AL, Ernst E. A systematic review of herbal medicinal products for the treatment of menopausal symptoms. Menopause 2003; 10:465.
14. Jacobson JS, Troxel AB, Evans J, et al. Randomized trial of black cohosh for the treatment of hot flushes among women with a history of breast cancer. J Clin Oncol 2001;19: 2739.
15. Washburn S, Burke GL, Morgan T, et al. Effect of soy protein supplementation on serum lipoproteins, blood pressure, and menopausal symptoms in perimenopausal women. Menopause 1999;6:7.
16. Albertazzi P, Pansini F, Bonaccorsi G, et al. The effect of dietary soy supplementation on hot flushes. Obstet Gynecol 1998;91:6.
17. Burke GL, Legault C, Anthony M, et al. Soy protein and isoflavone effects on vasomotor symptoms in peri- and postmenopausal women: the Soy Estrogen Alternative Study. Menopause 2003;10:147.
18. Tice JA, Ettinger B, Ensrud K, et al. Phytoestrogen supplements for the treatment of hot flashes: the isoflavone clover extract (ICE) study. JAMA 2003;290:207.
19. Alexandersen P, Toussaint A, Christiansen C, et al. Ipriflavone in the treatment of postmenopausal osteoporosis: a randomized controlled trial. JAMA 2001;285:1482.
20. Unfer V, Casini ML, Costabile L, et al. Endometrial effects of long-term treatment with phytoestrogens: a randomized, double-blind, placebo-controlled study. Fertil Steril 2004;82: 145.
21. Fantl JA, Cardozo L, McClish DK. Estrogen therapy in the management of urinary incontinence in postmenopausal women: a meta-analysis. First report of the Hormones and Urogenital Therapy Committee. Obstet Gynecol 1994;83:12.
22. Hendrix SL, Cochrane BB, Nygaard IE, et al. Effects of estrogen with and without progestin on urinary incontinence. JAMA 2005;293:935.
23. Eriksen B. A randomized, open, parallel-group study on the preventive effect of an estradiol vaginal ring (Estring) on recurrent urinary infections in postmenopausal women. Am J Obstet Gynecol 1999;180:1072.
24. Avis NE, Brambilla D, McKinlay SM, et al. A longitudinal analysis of the association between menopause and depression: results from the Massachusetts women's health study. Ann Epidemiol 1994;4:214.
25. Whooley MA, Grady D, Cauley JA, et al. Postmenopausal estrogen therapy and depressive symptoms in older women. J Gen Intern Med 2000;15:535.
26. Davis SR, McCloud P, Strauss BJ, et al. Testosterone enhances estradiol's effects on postmenopausal bone density and sexuality. Maturitas 1995;21:227.
27. American Assoication of Clinical Enocrinologists. AACE Medical Guidelines for Clinical Practice for Management of Menopause. Endocr Practice 1999;5:355.
28. The North American Menopause Society. The role of testosterone therapy in postmenopausal women: position statement of the North American Menopause Society. Menopause 2005;12:497.
29. Grodstein F, Stampfer MJ, Manson JE, et al. Postmenopausal estrogen and progestin use and the risk of cardiovascular disease. N Engl J Med 1996;335:453.
30. Walsh BW, Schiff I, Rosner B, et al. Effects of postmenopausal estrogen replacement on the concentrations and metabolism of plasma lipoproteins. N Engl J Med 1991;325:1196.
31. The Writing Group for the PEPI Trial. Effects of estrogen or estrogen/progestin regimens on heart disease risk factors in postmenopausal women. JAMA 1995;273:199.
32. Hulley S, Grady D, Bush T, et al. Randomized trial of estrogen plus progestin for secondary prevention of coronary heart disease in postmenopausal women. JAMA 1998;280:605.
33. Women's Health Initiative Investigators. Risks and benefits of estrogen plus progestin in healthy postmenopausal women: principal results from the Women's Health Initiative randomized controlled trial. JAMA 2002;288:321.
34. The Women's Health Initiative Steering Committee. Effects of conjugated equine estrogen in postmenopausal women with hysterectomy. The Women's Health Initiative randomized controlled trial. JAMA 2004;291: 1701.
35. Mosca L, Collins P, Herrington DM, et al. Hormone replacement therapy and cardiovascular disease. Circulation 2001;104: 499.
36. Chrischilles EA, Butler CD, Davis CS, et al. A model of lifetime osteoporosis impact. Arch Intern Med 1991;151:2026.
37. Prestwood KM, Kenny AM, Kleppinger A, et al. Ultralow-dose micronized 17beta-estradiol and bone density and bone metabolism in older women: a randomized controlled trial. JAMA 2003;290:1042.
38. Nanda K, Bastian LA, Hasselblad V, et al. Hormone replacement therapy and the risk of colorectal cancer: a meta-analysis. Obstet Gynecol 1999;93:880.
39. Colditz GA, Hankinson SE, Hunter DJ, et al. The use of estrogens and progestins and the risk of breast cancer in postmenopausal women. N Engl J Med 1995;332:1589.
40. Sellers TA, Mink PJ, Cerhan JR, et al. The role of hormone replacement therapy in the risk for breast cancer and total mortality in women with a family history of breast cancer. Ann Intern Med 1997;127:973.
41. Grady D, Gebretsadik T, Kerlikowske K, et al. Hormone replacement therapy and endometrial cancer risk: a meta-analysis. Obstet Gynecol 1995;85:304.
42. Daly E, Vassey MP, Hawkins MM, et al. Risk of venous thromboembolism in users of hormone replacement therapy. Lancet 1996;348:977.
43. Yaffe K, Sawaya G, Lieberburg I, et al. Estrogen therapy in postmenopausal women: effects on cognitive function and dementia. JAMA 1998;279:688.
44. Henderson VW, Paganini-Hill A, Miller BL, et al. Estrogen for Alzheimer's disease in women: randomized, double-blind, placebo-controlled trial. Neurology 2000;54:295.
45. Mulnard RA, Cotman CW, Kawas C, et al. Estrogen replacement therapy for treatment of mild to moderate Alzheimer's disease: a randomized controlled trial. JAMA 2000;283:1007.
46. Shumaker SA, Legault C, Rapp SR, et al. Estrogen plus progestin and the incidence of dementia and mild cognitive impairment in postmenopausal women. JAMA 2003;289:2651.
47. Shumaker SA, Legault C, Kuller L, et al. Conjugated equine estrogens and incidence of probable dementia and mild cognitive impairment in postmenopausal women. JAMA 2004;291:2947.
48. Rodriguez C, Patel AV, Calle EE, et al. Estrogen replacement therapy and ovarian cancer mortality in a large prospective study of US women. JAMA 2001;285:1460.
49. Miller RG, Ashar BH. Managing menopause: Current therapeutic options for vasomotor symptoms. Adv Stud Med 2004;4:484.
50. Lindsay R, Gallagher JC, Kleerekoper M, et al. Effect of lower doses of conjugated equine estrogens with and without medroxyprogesterone acetate in early postmenopausal women. JAMA 2002;287:2668.
51. Scarabin PY, Oger E, Plu-Bureau G. Differential association of oral and transdermal oestrogen-replacement therapy with venous thromboembolism risk. Lancet 2003;362:428.
52. Speroff L, Rowan J, Symons J, et al. The comparative effect on bone density, endometrium, and lipids of continuous hormones as replacement therapy (CHART study): a randomized controlled trial. JAMA 1996;276:1397.
53. Antoniou G, Kaligura D, Karakitsos P, et al. Transdermal estrogen with a levonorgestrel-releasing intrauterine device for climacteric complaints versus estradiol-releasing vaginal ring with a vaginal progesterone suppository: clinical and endometrial responses. Maturitas 1997;26:103.
54. Miller RG, Chang KK. Management of the menopausal patient. Primary Care Reports 2000;6:39.
55. Delmas PD, Bjarnason NH, Mitlak BH, et al. Effects of raloxifene on bone mineral density, serum cholesterol concentrations, and uterine endometrium in postmenopausal women. N Engl J Med 1997;337:1641.

*Bold numerals denote published controlled clinical trials, meta-analyses, or consensus-based recommendations.

56. Cummings SR, Eckert S, Krueger KA, et al. The effect of raloxifene on risk of breast cancer in postmenopausal women: results from the MORE randomized trial. Multiple Outcomes of Raloxifene Evaluation. JAMA 1999;282:2189.
57. Johannes CB, Crawford SL, Posner JG, et al. Longitudinal patterns and correlates of hormone replacement therapy use in middle-aged women. Am J Epidemiol 1994;140:439.
58. Grady D, Ettinger B, Tosteson AN, et al. Predictors of difficulty when discontinuing postmenopausal hormone therapy. Obstet Gynecol 2003;102:1233.
59. NIH State-of-the-Science Panel. National Institutes of Health State-of-the-Science Conference Statement: management of Menopause-related symptoms. Ann Intern Med 2005;142:1003.
60. Treatment of menopause-associated vasomotor symptoms: position statement of The North American Menopause Society. Menopause 2004;11:11.
61. U.S. Preventive Services Task Force. Hormone therapy for prevention of chronic conditions in postmenopausal women: recommendations from the U.S. Preventive Services Task Force. Ann Intern Med 2005;142:855
62. Col NF, Weber G, Stiggelbout A, et al. Short-term menopausal hormone therapy for symptom relief: an updated decision model. Arch Intern Med 2004;164:1634.

*For annotated **General References** and resources related to this chapter, visit www.hopkinsbayview.org/PAMreferences.*

SECTION 15

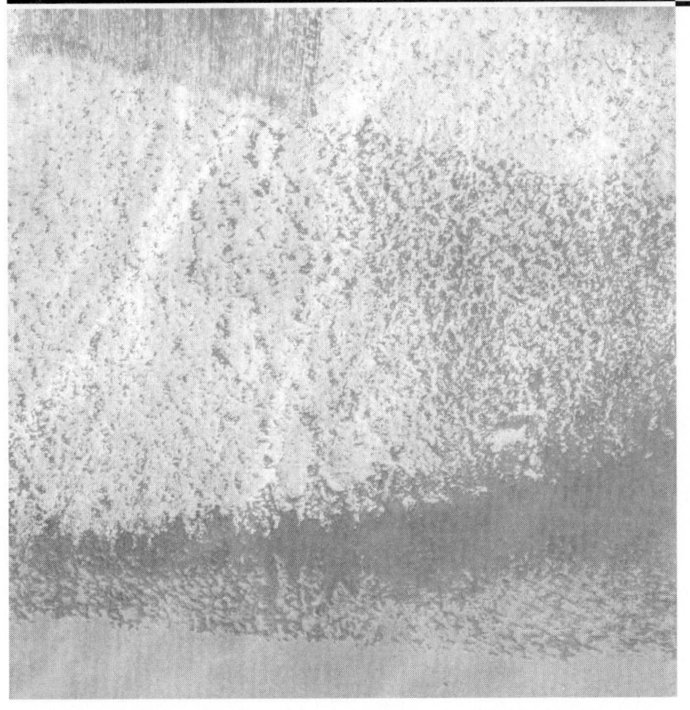

Selected Problems of the Eyes

Chapter 107

Common Problems Associated with Impaired Vision: Refractive Errors and Laser Refractive Surgery, Cataracts, and Age-Related Macular Degeneration

*Nada S. Jabbur and Sharon D. Solomon**

*In previous editions, Andrew Schachat, MD, contributed to this chapter.

REFRACTIVE ERRORS AND CORRECTIVE SURGERY

Anatomy and Types of Refractive Errors

Refractive errors of the eye include myopia, hyperopia and astigmatism. A myopic eye is nearsighted and needs diverging (minus) corrective lenses to be able to see at distance. A hyperopic eye is weaker for near vision and can see better at distance when uncorrected; it requires converging (plus) lenses to improve vision. Both myopia and hyperopia may be congenital; the curvature of the cornea and anteroposterior length of the eyeball often explain the amount and type of refractive error (e.g., a longer than average eye will be more myopic). Acquired myopia may be due to progression of a cataract or elongation of the eye after retinal detachment repair. Acquired hyperopia may be due to latent hyperopia that becomes manifest later in adulthood, or may be related to swelling in the retina. Astigmatism is generally caused by irregularities of the cornea or crystalline lens and causes distortion of vision and difficulty with night vision when uncorrected. It is rarely an isolated condition and is generally associated with myopia or hyperopia. Presbyopia is an age-related condition that affects everyone, in which the crystalline lens progressively loses its elasticity or ability to accommodate. Individuals approaching the age of 40 may begin to depend on magnifying glasses to improve their near vision activities, including reading. Those individuals who are hyperopic will notice their presbyopia before the age of 40, while those who are nearsighted can use their myopia to read without glasses.

The cornea is the transparent avascular anterior portion of the eye, typically 540 microns thick centrally and closer to 1,000 microns in the periphery. The cornea contributes 43.25 diopters or 74% of the focusing power of the eye; in addition it is usually responsible for most astigmatism in the eye. The remaining focusing power of the eye is provided by the lens. When patients undergo cataract surgery, refractive surgery is being performed and the power of the monofocal intraocular lens can be chosen to improve distance and/or near vision. When there is no abnormality of the lens, and in most young patients, refractive surgery may performed on the cornea to improve vision, if a patient is found to be a good candidate for such an elective surgery.

Refractive Surgery Techniques

Radial Keratotomy

In the 1980s, radial keratotomy (RK) was a popular incisional surgery. This involved making peripheral pupil sparing radial corneal incisions (typically 4 to 8) to flatten the central curvature of the cornea, thereby reducing myopia. This was often associated with smaller peripheral arcuate corneal incisions to treat any associated astigmatism. This type of surgery was often successful initially, but a long-term followup study revealed that the stability of the surgery was lacking and that there was a tendency for a hyperopic shift because of a continued long term flattening effect, especially in those who were initially more myopic (1). In addition, some patients had night vision disturbances because of the proximity of the incisions to the physiologically dilated pupil in dim light conditions. Finally, patients who have undergone RK are prone to traumatic rupture of the globe through the incisions when subject to trauma to the face and eye.

Excimer Laser and Wavefront Technology

RK was superseded by excimer laser vision correction when the U.S. Food and Drug Administration (FDA) approved the first such laser to reshape the cornea and treat myopia in 1995. Since then, excimer lasers have been developed with newer software and features and are now employed in the treatment of moderate farsightedness, nearsightedness, and mixed astigmatism (2,3). Excimer lasers work in the ultraviolet range and ablate corneal tissue, under topical anesthesia (numbing drops), by breaking molecular bonds of the corneal molecules that they are focused on. Myopic ablations thin the cornea centrally and hyperopic revisions are midperipheral ablations that flatten the cornea in a ring fashion, thereby steepening the central cornea. Conventional excimer lasers correct the spherical as well as the astigmatic component of a refraction; these are known as lower order aberrations. With the advent of wavefront technology, adapted from astronomy, higher order aberrations or irregularities of the eye can be treated to improve the quality of vision, especially under low light conditions. This is especially beneficial in persons with larger pupils, in dim light, or low contrast conditions. An image of the eye, measuring both higher and lower order aberrations, is taken and entered digitally into the computer of the laser. Customized algorithms direct the laser surgery, but require a deeper corneal ablation and may not be an option in patients with thinner central corneas.

Surface Ablations: PRK, LASIK, LASEK

Excimer lasers reshape the cornea superficially in a procedure known as surface ablation. In surface ablations, the epithelial layer of the cornea is removed so that the superficial stroma can be exposed and ablated to achieve the desired refraction. When the epithelium is discarded prior to the stromal ablation, the procedure is known as photorefractive keratectomy (PRK), and the patient will require a bandage contact lens for the first week while healing occurs. When there is an attempt to preserve the epithelium, this is known as a lamellar surgery, in which a superficial corneal flap is created. In LASIK (laser-assisted in situ keratomileusis), the flap is composed of epithelium and a thin layer of the underlying stroma. LASEK, or e-LASIK, is a modification of this technique in which the flap consists only of epithelium. Surface ablations are typically chosen when patients have thinner corneas, or have problems with the corneal epithelium. Whether to use PRK or LASIK techniques is determined by the ophthalmologist.

LASIK is currently the most common refractive procedure performed. It has the dual advantage of a shorter recovery period and reduced perioperative discomfort. The energy of the excimer laser is typically applied to the superficial area of the stroma after creating a 100- to 160-micron-deep anterior corneal flap (this typically includes approximately 50 microns of epithelium and the remainder is superficial stromal tissue). The corneal flaps are created using a microkeratome, a mechanical device which cuts the cornea using a blade, or by using an infrared femtosecond laser, which gives a more precise thickness of flap and has a reduced chance of complications such as an incomplete or very thin flap (4).

Correction of Presbyopia

There is no corneal procedure available in the United States that can improve reading vision without affecting distance acuity in the same eye. *Monovision* is an approach in which the dominant eye is corrected for distance vision and the non-dominant eye is corrected for improved near vision. This technique may be tried first with contact lenses and when successful, can be adapted surgically. *Conductive keratoplasty* (CK) is a surgical technique that can improve presbyopia temporarily. It uses radiofrequency energy applied to the periphery of the cornea, where consequent shrinking of the corneal tissue leads to steepening of the central cornea. Patients may need multiple enhancements of the surgery as the effect regresses, and some patients have induced astigmatism (5). Multifocal intraocular lenses at the time of cataract surgery are being introduced to improve distance, intermediate, and near vision (presbyopia). These lenses are not yet the standard of care for intraocular lens implantation, and 5% of patients may experience severe halos at night. In the future, multifocal corneal ablations may allow simultaneous bilateral improvement of distance vision and presbyopia.

Patient Selection and Evaluation

In spite of multiple advances in technology, some patients are not candidates for excimer laser vision correction. Contraindications to laser vision correction may be elicited upon a review of systems and a thorough ophthalmologic exam. Patients in whom refractive surgery is not indicated include those with unstable vision, dry eyes, thin corneas, corneal scars, and autoimmune diseases, as well as patients taking amiodarone or isotretinoin (Accutane) or who are pregnant or nursing. Keratoconus, a progressive condition which causes steepening of the cornea is another contraindication to refractive surgery; early forms are diagnosed by mapping of the corneal surface, a procedure known as corneal topography. Patients with extreme degrees of myopia and hyperopia also are not good candidates for laser surgery. Some highly myopic patients may be candidates for an intraocular procedure in which an intraocular lens is inserted in addition to the normal crystalline lens of the eye (phakic intraocular lens [IOL]).

Patients interested in being evaluated for refractive surgery should not wear contact lenses for at least 2 to 3 weeks prior to the evaluation and surgery. Contact lens wear can cause a reversible change in the cornea, known as corneal warpage, that needs to be differentiated from an early form of keratoconus.

Patient Experience and Outcomes

Corneal refractive surgery is performed under topical anesthesia. Some patients require an anxiolytic agent since patient cooperation for laser centration is essential. Patients will experience mild discomfort 30 minutes after the numbing effect wears off and are advised to refrain from work the rest of the day and avoid activities that increase the risk of flap dislocation (e.g., contact sports) or infection (e.g., no swimming for a month). Topical medications including an antibiotic and an anti-inflammatory agent are given for a short period of time. Patients who undergo lamellar surgeries such as LASIK tend to have a quicker recovery, and more than 80% of patients find that they may drive the following day without distance glasses. Other patients who undergo surface ablations may take 1 to 2 weeks to recover. Most patients will experience mildly dry eyes in the first month postoperatively. Patients with a larger refractive error to be corrected may experience more fluctuations in comfort and vision postoperatively; this is discussed on an individual basis with the ophthalmologist. Patients in the presbyopic age group are warned about needing near vision aids.

Approximately 90% of patients obtain vision in the 20/25 to 20/20 range and more than 95% of patients obtain 20/40 or good driving vision. The ophthalmologist should discuss these likely outcomes with every patient, as well as the influence of important variables such as the age of the patient and any impairments to wound healing, the amount and type of refractive error, and the proposed surgical technique and the surgeon's experience. In the cases where the desired outcome is not obtained and if there are no contraindications, the surgeon may recommend an enhancement procedure. This is typically not done within 3 months from the initial surgery, since stability of vision is important for a good outcome. Patients who are good candidates for laser vision correction may retain their corrected vision for life (if there are no other ocular changes as they age, e.g., cataract).

Complications of Refractive Surgery

Complications are reduced when patients are screened carefully for corrective surgery, but may still occur in 5% or less. Complications of initial or enhancement surgery include fluctuations of vision and corneal ectasia, dry eyes, inflammation under the flap created in LASIK, infection, flap folds or striae, epithelial downgrowth (cells growing under the flap), flap dislocation after trauma, and permanent qualitative or quantitative changes in vision.

CATARACTS

A cataract is an opacification of the lens of the eye. Approximately 95% of people older than 60 years of age have some opacification of the lens, but most often these opacities are of no visual importance. A *significant cataract* results in interference with visual acuity and daily activities. According to the World Health Organization (WHO), cataracts are the leading cause of blindness and visual impairment in the world. The incidence of diminished visual acuity from cataracts increases steadily after 50 years, reaching almost 50% in people older than 75 years of age. Cataracts are usually bilateral, and the progression is slow and may vary between eyes. The rate of progression is not individually predictable, and there is no treatment that retards the progression. When the cataract is diagnosed, prescribing new glasses may help improve the vision and when it is advanced, the only therapy is surgery.

Anatomy and Physiology

The lens is located immediately posterior to the iris and is suspended there by radially attached zonular fibers from the ciliary body. It is a biconvex, transparent structure with an elastic capsule whose shape is altered by ciliary body contraction, permitting images to be brought into sharp

TABLE 107.1 Causes of Cataracts

Senescent	Age is the most common risk factor
Congenital	Autosomal dominant inheritance (25%); maternal malnutrition, infection (rubella, syphilis), metabolic disturbances, or the effects of maternal medications; prematurity
Traumatic	Unilateral; lens may be loose or unstable; radiation ionizing, infrared (e.g., glassblowers), ultraviolet, microwave
Metabolic	Diabetes mellitus, Wilson disease, galactosemia, hypocalcemia, myotonic dystrophy
Secondary	Associated with drug therapy: corticosteroids, phenothiazines, miotics, amiodarone, statins Associated with uveitis, skin diseases, glaucoma, degenerative ocular disorders (retinitis pigmentosa, chronic hypotony, essential iris atrophy)

focus on the retina. The lens is acellular and avascular and lacks innervation. Nourishment is provided from the surrounding aqueous and vitreous humor, and metabolic byproducts are removed by diffusion into the aqueous humor. The continued transparency of the lens requires the active metabolism of the elastic capsular epithelium, so any insult to the epithelium may result in lenticular opacities. New lenticular fibers are produced throughout life, and, because none are lost, increasing density of the fibers of the lens develops with age, which also contributes to cataract formation.

Causes

There are many causes of cataracts (Table 107.1). Although senescent cataracts—the result of the aging process just described—account for the vast majority of cataracts, the generalist occasionally sees patients with congenital or traumatic lens opacities. The mechanism of opacification in all of these instances is thought to be direct trauma or interference with metabolic activity of the capsular epithelium and with continued fiber production.

Many types of cataracts have a distinctive appearance. The ophthalmologist may therefore suggest the possibility of an underlying disorder such as myotonic dystrophy (iridescent spots) or Wilson disease (sunflower cataract). Steroid therapy, diabetes mellitus and radiation treatment are typically associated with posterior subcapsular cataracts, although these may also be idiopathic or related to numerous other conditions. Age-related cataract is significantly associated with dermatologic abnormalities and their treatment (e.g., steroid use).

Symptoms and Examination

The primary symptom of cataract is impaired vision; usually patients describe a constant fog over the eye. They may also see rings or halos around lights and objects. Objects appear more blue and yellow in color. With immature cataract formation, distant vision often is impaired to a greater extent than is near vision.

The location of the cataract within the lens determines the extent of the visual loss. Central opacities cause noticeable loss of vision and a distinct glare when the patient is in bright light. They also cause a myopic shift in the lens, thus worsening distance vision and sometimes improving near vision. Bright light constricts the pupil so that the dense portion of the lens occludes and diffuses light. Therefore the patient who has central opacities finds that vision is better in low light, when the pupil is widely dilated. In selected cases, use of dilating drops (mydriatics) is helpful and delays the need for surgery. Because there may be contraindications to the use of mydriatics (e.g., narrow-angle glaucoma attacks may be precipitated), it is best to rely on an ophthalmologist to prescribe them. Peripheral opacities cause noticeable loss of vision only late in the development of the cataract.

Cataracts are easily identified by illuminating the lens with a slit lamp, but most general physicians find that they can see a cataract easily through a moderately plus lens (such as a +2 or +3 lens on the dial) of the direct ophthalmoscope. Visual acuity should be tested in both eyes if cataracts are suspected. If the patient describes any impairment in visual acuity, the patient should be referred to an ophthalmologist. In adults, screening for cataracts is best done by a visual acuity examination with use of a Snellen chart. Additionally, other testing such as a brightness acuity test (BAT) evaluates a patient's vision with bright lights simulating situations such as night driving.

Cataract Surgery

Indications

Before surgery is indicated, new glasses for the progressive myopia associated with many nuclear cataracts may improve the vision of patients with cataracts. Also, visual aids, such as magnifying lenses and large-print materials, may be helpful. The decision to remove a cataract is determined by the visual needs of the patient, the degree of the cataract, and the presence of any other ocular abnormalities (e.g., the need to follow closely retinal pathology especially if laser treatment is required). The ophthalmologist performs a complete ocular assessment before advising the patient about surgery.

Each patient must determine his or her own visual needs based on daily activities. The ability to read, drive, cross streets safely, and perform daily routines is clearly of prime importance. For example, a patient usually requires visual acuity of at least 20/40 in the better eye to operate a motor vehicle safely or to continue moderately active daily life. Blurred vision has an important impact on a patient's functioning and well-being. Because the impact of blurred vision is so significant and the success rate for cataract surgery so high, it is not surprising how often the procedure is performed.

Surgery

Cataract surgery should be performed after thoughtful deliberation, keeping in mind that complications occur occasionally. For patients with other health problems, the generalist and the ophthalmologist should plan cataract surgery together. Cataract extraction is an elective procedure, and the patient should be in the best possible condition at the time of operation.

Approximately 2 million cataract extractions are performed yearly on Medicare beneficiaries, and cataract surgery is the most common major surgical procedure performed in the elderly in this country. Surgery involves removal of the opacified lens from the eye. Prior to 1990, the overwhelming majority of cataract surgeries were extracapsular (i.e., the posterior capsule of the lens was left intact) and used microsurgical techniques. Since then, small wound cataract surgery or phacoemulsification have greatly improved the immediate outcome of surgery and have significantly shortened the period of disability. In the small wound technique, a phacoemulsification instrument tip (2- to 3-mm wide) is introduced into the eye and emulsifies the cataract using a small vibrating piezo electrode. Cold fluid irrigates the eye to prevent any thermal injury and helps to aspirate the tiny pieces out of the eye.

Both eyes usually require an operation, but normally only one lens is extracted at a time, so that the patient has vision on the nonoperated side when the eye that has been operated on is covered by a patch for a few days after surgery. Some surgeons attempt to avoid the use of a patch, and so-called no-stitch surgery with very small incisions is popular. There is no definitive evidence that any particular extracapsular surgical approach is better than any other. For patients with bilateral cataracts, the second procedure is usually performed as early as a week after the first; once the visual result is known in the first eye.

Preoperative Evaluation

The current standard of care is a careful history and physical examination, but few if any laboratory investigations are required. A randomized trial showed that routine preoperative testing before cataract surgery did not reduce the incidence of perioperative medical complications (6). The testing evaluated in this study included electrocardiogram (ECG), complete blood count (CBC), and levels of electrolytes, urea, nitrogen, creatinine, and glucose

The history should elicit clues about bleeding tendencies. Patients who take anticoagulants, such as aspirin or aspirin-containing products or oral warfarin, should inform their ophthalmologists about these medications. If possible, aspirin should be discontinued for 7 to 14 days before the surgery, although some surgeons do not stop aspirin, given the low risk of bleeding with small-incision surgery. When anticoagulants cannot be discontinued, the surgeon will elect a clear corneal avascular incision. In adult patients, the surgery is often performed using topical and intraocular preservative-free lidocaine, supplemented in many patients with a periocular anesthetic.

The ability of the patient to lie flat should be assessed. If a patient cannot lie flat, the neck can be hyperextended and a temporal approach to the eye may be more helpful, especially if the patient has a prominent supraorbital rim. Additional support can be placed under the head and a mild Trendelenburg position can help patients with stiff necks (e.g., ankylosing spondylitis or rheumatoid arthritis). Diabetes mellitus and hypertension, if present, should be controlled. A recent myocardial infarction (within 6 months) should delay surgery.

Patient Experience. Cataract surgery is performed on an outpatient basis. After discharge from the surgical unit a patient must restrict his or her activities for several weeks to minimize the frequency of complications, although with small incisions and the newest microsurgical techniques the rehabilitation period is shorter. There are no permanent restrictions; however, caution with steps or when walking and working with machinery may be necessary if perception is seriously altered by an imbalance between the two eyes, especially while waiting to have the other eye surgery performed. Postoperative appointments with the ophthalmologist are typically on the first day after surgery, and 1 week and 4 to 6 weeks postoperatively. The primary care clinician should be aware of the following postoperative problems.

Complications

Complications may occur intraoperatively or in the early or late postoperative period. The overall rate of any complication is approximately 5% of cataract operations, and is also related to the surgeon's experience and to the patient's preexisting eye condition; in only 1 in every 5,000 eyes operated is eyesight lost because of complications.

Inflammation and Infection

All postoperative patients have some degree of traumatic intraocular inflammation. This is usually controlled effectively with topical corticosteroids. Bacterial intraocular infection, endophthalmitis, is a dangerous postoperative inflammation that must be recognized early before it devastates the eye. If a patient complains of decreased vision, pain, discharge, and redness, endophthalmitis may be present and the patient should be seen immediately by an ophthalmologist. Most infections occur within a few days after surgery; however, an operated eye is predisposed to involvement from systemic infection, so a patient with an acute red eye occurring at any time after eye surgery should be seen urgently by an ophthalmologist. Low-grade chronic inflammation is common after cataract surgery, and resultant macular edema is one of the most common causes of postoperative visual loss.

Hemorrhage

The sudden occurrence of hemorrhage in the uveal tract (the iris, the ciliary body, and the choroid) can adversely influence the final visual outcome. Although this complication is usually seen intraoperatively, it may rarely occur postoperatively. It is recognized usually by painless but precipitous change in visual acuity. Postoperative hemorrhage from the iris or an inadequately closed corneoscleral wound is more common than is vitreous hemorrhage. In all instances of hemorrhage, urgent referral to an ophthalmologist is indicated. Although anticoagulation is not an absolute contraindication to cataract extraction, it probably does increase the risk of hemorrhage. For this reason, anticoagulants and antiplatelet agents such as aspirin are stopped, if possible, before and for 1 to 2 weeks after surgery.

Retinal Detachment

The incidence of retinal detachment after cataract surgery is approximately 1% to 3%. Retinal detachment may present as suddenly decreased visual acuity, flashes of light, and the development of floaters, veils, or curtains in the visual field. Patients with symptoms of retinal detachment should be seen immediately by an ophthalmologist so that surgical reattachment of the retina may be accomplished.

Glaucoma

A rise in intraocular pressure may occur in the first few days after surgery and may present as blurred vision, a painful red eye and often nausea and vomiting. This may be due to increased inflammation or retained viscoelastic material used during surgery. Glaucoma may also appear as late as 1 to 2 years after surgery in 0.6% to 5% of patients, depending on the type of surgery. This may also result in decreased visual acuity caused by corneal edema.

Delayed Opacification of the Posterior Capsule

Approximately 20% to 50% of patients experience a gradual decrease in vision in the first few years after cataract surgery because of opacification of the posterior lens capsule. This complication can be treated effectively by a special laser instrument (yttrium-aluminum-garnet [YAG]) that opens the posterior capsule without the need for intraocular surgery. The procedure is painless and is performed in the office. However, it is performed only when the potential for visual improvement outweighs the risks, because retinal detachment and perhaps macular edema become somewhat more common (7).

Optical Correction after Cataract Extraction

The removal of a cataract improves light transmission to the retina, but vision remains blurred without corrective lenses. Three types of lenses are used: aphakic spectacles, contact lenses, and intraocular lenses. The last option is now the norm. Aphakic spectacles are discussed mainly for historical reasons. Contact lenses are used more than aphakic spectacles, but almost all patients, even children, are now candidates for intraocular lenses.

Aphakic spectacles are rarely used today. With aphakic spectacles there is a narrower field of vision, as well as considerable distortion of images, which appear rounded and three to five times larger than when the lens is present in the eye. Peripheral ring scotomata and loss of some depth perception also occur. The use of *contact lenses* after cataract extraction provides considerable improvement over spectacles. There is substantial distortion reduction and expansion of the field of vision. However, the patient must be motivated to use contact lenses and most patients as they get older become contact lens–intolerant due to dry eyes.

Because of the visual handicap experienced after cataract extraction, plastic *intraocular lenses* are inserted at the time of surgery in 95% or more of patients undergoing cataract extraction. Long-term survival of these inert prostheses is very good. The insertion of intraocular implants adds a few minutes to the operative time beyond that required for lens extraction. If the eye is otherwise healthy, more than 90% of patients undergoing this technique experience an improvement in vision to 20/40 or better. New multifocal lenses and accommodative intraocular lenses (to replace bifocals) have been approved by the FDA. Patients who drive at night frequently, who have one functional eye, or who have severe astigmatism are not good candidates for these lenses.

AGE-RELATED MACULAR DEGENERATION

The macula is the anatomic center of the retina, defined by its unique cellular configuration, pigment content, and ability to provide fine visual acuity for reading. Normal aging results in numerous changes in the macula, many of which are clinically undetectable. However, as degeneration of the outer retinal layers continues to progress, central vision loss may occur. This condition is known as age-related macular degeneration (AMD).

Epidemiology

AMD is the leading cause of severe loss of central visual acuity in people older than 65 years of age in the United States. The prevalence is strongly correlated with age, with 30% of adults age 75 years or older already affected with early AMD, and another 28% predicted to develop it over the next 5 years (8). While the occurrence of AMD increase with advancing age, a number of other risk factors are associated with this disorder. AMD is much more prevalent in populations of European descent, particularly in those with fair skin and light-colored irides (9). Studies of monozygotic twins have shown markedly similar incidences of AMD prevalence and progression, suggestive of a genetic component (10). Tobacco use has been associated with an increased risk for the development of AMD in many population-based studies, with susceptible individuals developing the disease 5 to 10 years earlier than their nonsmoking counterparts (11). Systemic hypertension has also been strongly correlated with the development of AMD (12). Although excessive exposure to light can damage the retina through the formation of reactive oxygen intermediates, clinical assessment of this potentially important factor is limited by the difficulty of quantifying light exposure over a lifetime. Thus, there are conflicting studies on the association of ultraviolet light and the development of AMD in susceptible individuals.

Clinical Features

The clinical hallmark of AMD is the presence of *drusen*, which are discrete, dull yellow deposits located in the outer retina and typically confined to the macula. Many people older than the age of 50 have some drusen. Because drusen do not always affect the function of overlying photoreceptors, not all patients with drusen develop visual symptoms. For this reason, a classification system for AMD has been developed, from population-based studies, that characterizes the number, size, and quality of drusen and their associated features. These features are predictive of an individual's risk for advanced disease and severe vision loss.

Drusen are classified morphologically as either hard (discrete, well-demarcated boundaries) or soft (amorphous, poorly demarcated boundaries). Small drusen are difficult to see with the direct ophthalmoscope, but larger or soft drusen should be apparent. Hard drusen (Fig. 107.1, see Color Plate section) are typically less than 63 μm in diameter. Patients with small numbers of hard drusen are considered to be at low-risk for the progression of AMD. Numerous hard drusen, soft drusen, especially when confluent, and intermediate size ($\geq$63 μm) and large size drusen ($\geq$125 μm) are independent risk factors for vision loss from AMD (Fig. 107.2, see Color Plate section).

Non-neovascular AMD (referred to commonly as *dry* AMD), the more common form of the disease, is less likely to account for severe vision loss in those affected. It is characterized by the presence of drusen with varying degrees of pigmentary changes and atrophy of the outer retina. The presence of drusen may lead to attenuation or atrophy of the outer layer of the retina known as the retinal pigment epithelium (RPE). Geographic atrophy of the RPE occurs when this attenuation covers a contiguous area and is associated with overlying photoreceptor loss. Consequently, geographic atrophy in AMD may be associated with severe visual loss depending on its extent and location relative to the fovea, the anatomic center of the macula (Fig. 107.3, see Color Plate section). As atrophy develops, other abnormalities of the RPE may occur. Pigment may migrate from the RPE layer to the inner photoreceptor layer, resulting in focal clumps of hyperpigmentation. Pigmentary alteration, in association with intermediate and large-sized drusen, is a risk factor for progression of the nonneovascular form of AMD.

Neovascular AMD (referred to commonly as *wet* AMD) is characterized by the growth of new blood vessels from the choroid through disturbances in Bruch membrane into the subretinal or sub-RPE space. These abnormal subretinal blood vessels form a fibrovascular network, known as choroidal neovascularization (CNV), that leaks, disturbing the integrity and function of the regional photoreceptors. The patient may present with clinically evident macular subretinal fluid, subretinal hemorrhage, and/or subretinal lipid (Fig. 107.4, see Color Plate section), signifying deterioration from the previous, often visually stable, nonneovascular state and heralding the onset of severe vision loss.

Often, the CNV itself is not directly visible on examination and must be diagnosed by a technique known as fluorescein angiography. During this procedure, fluorescein dye is injected intravenously in the antecubital fossa. Within 10 to 20 seconds, the dye can be photographed traversing the normal retinal vessels and accumulating and then leaking from the abnormal choroidal neovascularization (Fig. 107.5).

The fluorescein angiographic leakage patterns of CNV are classified as either classic or occult. Hyperfluorescence from classic CNV tends to occur early in the course of the fluorescein study, typically by 50 seconds, and is usually well-defined with progressive leakage that increases in intensity and extent (Fig. 107.6). Occult CNV is characterized angiographically by poorly-defined stippled hyperfluorescence that develops late in the course of the study (Fig. 107.7). Characterizing the type of CNV that is the source of subretinal leakage is important in determining patient prognosis. Occult choroidal neovascularization tends to be more indolent and less often associated with rapid, severe vision loss compared to its classic CNV counterpart. Approximately 30% of patients with occult leakage may maintain vision and remain relatively clinically stable for a period of months without treatment. However, occult CNV

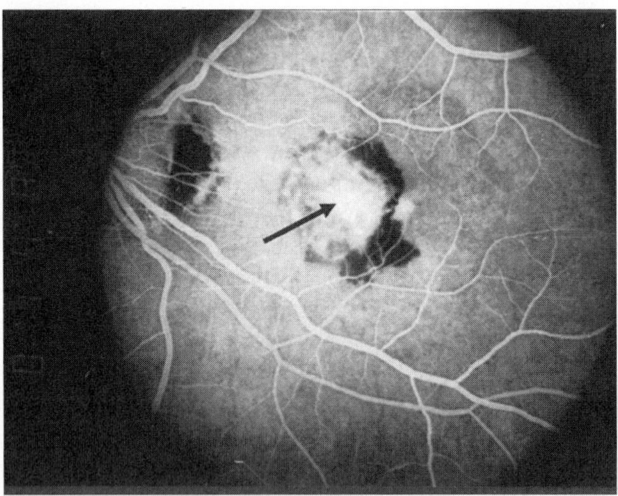

FIGURE 107.5. Fluorescein angiogram of the same eye as in Fig. 107.4. The black arrow points to an area of hyperfluorescence that represents CNV, confirming the diagnosis of neovascular AMD. The adjacent blocked fluorescence is from the subretinal hemorrhage seen in the previous photograph.

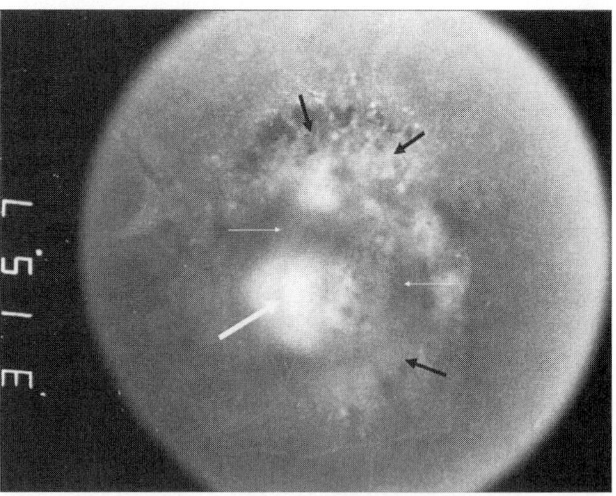

FIGURE 107.7. This fluorescein frame at 315.7 seconds shows intense hyperfluorescence in the inferior macula (white arrow) that may represent classic CNV that is actively leaking. The more superior speckled hyperfluorescence (*black arrows*) represents poorly defined late leakage consistent with occult CNV.

may deteriorate and even decompensate into classic CNV, which is typically much more aggressive, resulting in a more precipitous clinical and visual decline.

Natural History and Prevention

The probability of progression of AMD depends on the clinical morphology at baseline. The Age-Related Eye Disease Study (AREDS) followed over 3,600 participants with various stages of AMD for more than 6 years. It was observed that participants with extensive small drusen, pigmentary abnormalities, or at least one intermediate size druse in the macula had only a 1.3% probability of progression to advanced AMD by 5 years. The 5-year estimated probability of progression to advanced AMD was 18% in an eye with extensive intermediate drusen, large drusen, or noncentral geographic atrophy that was not beneath the foveal center. Participants in AREDS who already had advanced AMD in one eye or vision loss due to nonadvanced AMD in one eye had a 43% probability of progression to advanced AMD in the fellow eye at 5 years (13). In addition to characterizing the natural history of AMD, AREDS was a landmark controlled, clinical trial that demonstrated that micronutrient therapy, in the form of antioxidants plus zinc, may delay progression to advanced AMD and concomitant vision loss. Patients in AREDS with high-risk non-neovascular features, including extensive intermediate drusen, large drusen, noncentral geographic atrophy, or already advanced AMD in one eye who were randomized to oral antioxidants plus zinc, had as much as a 25% relative risk reduction in progression to advanced AMD in the fellow eye. Absolute benefits were modest; the estimated probability of significant visual loss at 5 years was 29% with placebo and 20% with antioxidants and zinc (14). The antioxidants (vitamin C 500 mg, vitamin E 400 international units, and β-carotene 15 mg) plus zinc (80 mg) are available in several commercially produced over-the-counter (OTC) supplements. Copper (2 mg) is added to the supplement to reduce the theoretical risk of zinc-induced copper deficiency anemia. Other potential adverse effects may include increased risk of urinary tract infection and prostatic hyperplasia in men and stress incontinence in women. Since previous studies have shown that β-carotene may increase lung cancer incidence and

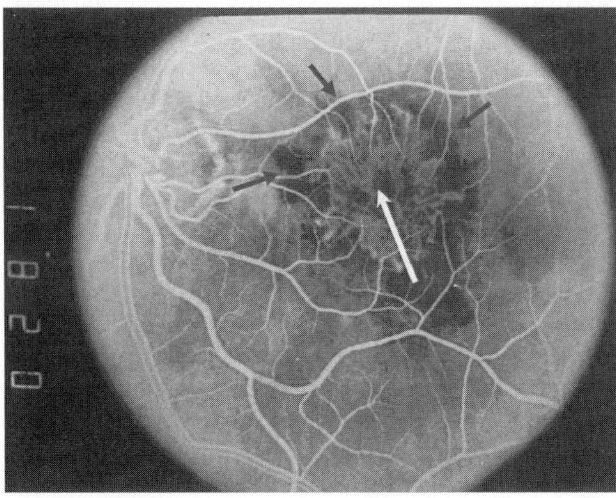

FIGURE 107.6. This fluorescein frame at 28.1 seconds shows early hyperfluorescence that is well-defined, indicative of classic CNV. The white arrow points to filling of the CNV itself with the fluorescein dye. The black arrow shows surrounding blocked fluorescence that could represent hemorrhage.

mortality in smokers, it may be advisable for smokers to avoid this combination of supplements.

A more recent epidemiologic study in a large cohort of persons age 55 or older in the Netherlands also showed that a high dietary intake of β-carotene, vitamins C and E, and zinc was associated with a 35% reduction in the incidence of AMD (15). Ophthalmologists generally counsel their patients to discuss micronutrient therapy with their primary care provider. Patients with no clinical features suggestive of AMD or with only small drusen in the macula have a low risk of progression to advanced disease and vision loss and have not been shown to derive increased benefit from micronutrient supplementation.

Adult patients older than the age of 55 years should have a dilated examination by an ophthalmologist to ascertain their risk of developing advanced AMD. Those with high-risk non-neovascular features should consider micronutrient supplementation as recommended by their retina specialist and approved by their internist. Patients should also be instructed how to monitor their vision so that they can alert their ophthalmologist immediately should they develop a central decrease in vision or central distortion of vision in one eye.

Treatment

Interventional therapies are available for patients with neovascular AMD. The Macular Photocoagulation Study (MPS) compared the benefit of thermal laser photocoagulation with that of no treatment for patients with well-defined choroidal neovascularization that was extrafoveal or outside the foveal center. After 3.5 years of followup, 62% of untreated patients had a loss of six or more lines of vision, as measured on a Snellen visual acuity chart, compared with 47% of treated patients (16). Subsequent investigations extended the treatment recommendations to include neovascular lesions closer to the foveal center, or juxtafoveal lesions, as well as subfoveal lesions. Even with this new treatment approach, only 10% of patients with neovascular AMD met the strict morphologic criteria that predicted treatment benefit. Since the thermal laser destroys not only the choroidal neovascular vessels that cause central vision loss but also the overlying healthy retina, it leaves a resultant blank spot in the area of treatment, which itself often results in decreased vision. While thermal laser photocoagulation is still the preferred treatment for well-defined extrafoveal and juxtafoveal CNV lesions, newer options for the treatment of subfoveal neovascular AMD have been developed.

Photodynamic therapy (PDT) with verteporfin (Visudyne) is a two-step process that offers a chance for clinical and visual stabilization in patients with subfoveal CNV. First, a photosensitizing drug, verteporfin, is administered intravenously and allowed to circulate in the retinal and choroidal circulation, binding preferentially to neovascular endothelial cells. In the second step, a low-power laser is used to activate the verteporfin. Toxic intermediates are produced as the cold laser shines on the macula of the affected eye, damaging the choroidal neovascular vessels while leaving the normal retinal vasculature intact. Although the abnormal vessels tend to recur after treatment, with 90% of patients showing angiographic evidence of leakage three months after their first treatment, following a series of five to six treatments over 2 years the leakage gradually stops and a small fibrovascular or disciform scar forms in the macular center. The disciform scar that forms following treatment is typically less expansive than that forming in the eye with subfoveal CNV that remains untreated, thus preserving greater central vision.

In a randomized, placebo-controlled trial involving 600 patients with subfoveal CNV lesions caused by AMD, among those with classic CNV lesions, 59% of the verteporfin-treated patients compared to 31% of placebo-treated patients lost fewer than three lines of vision at the month 24 examination (17). Another trial showed that treatment with PDT with verteporfin reduced the risk of moderate and severe vision loss compared to placebo in patients with occult CNV and evidence of recent disease progression (18).

Verteporfin has a relatively short half-life and is cleared in 48 hours. Patients must therefore remain indoors and out of sunlight for the 48 hours following treatment to avoid photosensitivity reactions, such as mild sunburn. Severe vision loss as a result of treatment occurs in approximately 2% to 4% of patients. The annual cost for photodynamic therapy with verteporfin was estimated to be at least $5,000 for three or four treatments (19).

Therapies targeting the angiogenic processes underlying CNV formation have also been developed. Vascular endothelial growth factor (VEGF) has been shown to be necessary for the development of retinal neovascularization in experimental models (20). Pegaptanib (Macugen), a peptide that binds and blocks the activity of VEGF, has been approved for the treatment of all subtypes of neovascular AMD. In a randomized controlled trial, intravitreous injections of pegaptanib or placebo were administered every 6 weeks into one eye of patients with neovascular AMD. Over a period of 54 weeks, 70% of the patients receiving intravitreous pegaptanib lost fewer than 15 letters of visual acuity compared with 55% among the controls. The risk of severe loss of visual acuity (loss of 30 letters or more) was reduced from 22% in the sham-injection group to 10% in the treatment group (21).

Among serious adverse events observed were endophthalmitis (1.3%), a serious intraocular infection, traumatic injury to the lens (0.6%), and retinal detachment (0.7%). The cost of a single injection of pegaptanib is approximately $1,000 and is reimbursed by Medicare; a series of nine treatments at 6-week intervals is recommended (19).

SPECIFIC REFERENCES*

1. Waring GO 3rd, Lynn MJ, McDonnell PJ. Results of the prospective evaluation of radial keratotomy (PERK) study 10 years after surgery. Arch Ophthalmol 1994;112:1298.
2. Sugar A, Rapuano CJ, Culbertson WW, et al. Laser in situ keratomileusis for myopia and astigmatism: safety and efficacy—ophthalmic technology assessment: key messages—a report by the American Academy of Ophthalmology. Ophthalmology 2002;109:175.
3. Varley GA, Huang D, Rapuano CJ, et al. LASIK for hyperopia, hyperopic astigmatism, and mixed astigmatism: a report by the American Academy of Ophthalmology. Ophthalmology 2004;111:1604.
4. Kezirian GM, Stonecipher KG. Comparison of the IntraLase femtosecond laser and mechanical microkeratomes for laser in situ keratomileusis. J Cataract Refract Surg 2004;30:804.
5. McDonald MB, Durrie D, Asbell P, et al. Treatment of presbyopia with conductive keratoplasy: six-month results of the 1-year United States FDA clinical trial. Cornea 2004;23:661.
6. Schein OD, Katz J, Bass EB, et al. The value of routine preoperative medical testing before cataract surgery. N Engl J Med 2000;342:168.
7. Tielsch JM, Legro MW, Cassard SD, et al. Risk factors for retinal detachment after cataract surgery: a population-based case-control study. Ophthalmology 1996;103:1537.
8. Klein R, Klein BE, Tomany SC, et al. Ten-year incidence and progression of age-related maculopathy: The Beaver Dam eye study. Ophthalmology 2002;109:1767.
9. Friedman DS, Katz J, Bressler NM, et al. Racial differences in the prevalence of age-related macular degeneration: the Baltimore Eye Survey. Ophthalmology 1999;106:1049.
10. Gottfredsdottir MS, Sverrisson T, Musch DC, et al. Age related macular degeneration in monozygotic twins and their spouses in Iceland. Acta Ophthalmol Scand 1999;77:422.
11. Mitchell P, Wang JJ, Smith W, et al. Smoking and the five-year incidence of age-related maculopathy: the Blue Mountains Eye Study. Arch Ophthalmol 2002;120:1357.
12. Hyman L, Schachat AP, He Q, et al. Hypertension, cardiovascular disease, and age-related macular degeneration. Age-related macular degeneration risk factors study group. Arch Ophthalmol 2000;118:351.
13. Age-Related Eye Disease Study Research Group. A randomized, placebo-controlled, clinical trial of high-dose supplementation with Vitamins C and E, beta carotene, and zinc for age-related macular degeneration and vision loss, AREDS Report No. 8. Arch Ophthalmol 2001;119:1417.
14. Antioxidant vitamins and zinc for macular degeneration. Med Lett Drugs Ther 2003;45:45.
15. van Leeuwen R, Boekhoorn S, Vingerling JR. Dietary intake of antioxidants and risk of age-related macular degeneration. JAMA 2005;294:3101–3107.
16. Macular Photocoagulation Study Group. Argon laser photocoagulation for neovascular maculopathy: three-year results from randomized clinical trials. Arch Ophthalmol 1986;104:694.
17. Photodynamic therapy of subfoveal choroidal neovascularization in age-related macular degeneration with verteporfin. Two-year results of 2 randomized clinical trials—Tap Report 2. Treatment of Age-Related Macular Degeneration with Photodynamic Therapy (TAP) Study Group. Arch Ophthalmol 2001;119:198.
18. Verteporfin in Photodynamic Therapy Study Group. Verteporfin therapy of subfoveal choroidal neovascularization in age-related macular degeneration: two-year results of a randomized clinical trial including lesions with occult with no classic choroidal neovascularization—Verteporfin in Photodynamic Therapy Report 2. Am J Ophthalmol 2001;131:541.
19. Pegaptanib sodium (Macugen) for macular degeneration. Med Lett Drugs Ther 2005;47:55.
20. Aiello LP, Pierce EA, Foley ED, et al. Suppression of retinal neovascularization in vivo by inhibition of vascular endothelial growth factor (VEGF) using soluble VEGF-receptor chimeric proteins. Proc Natl Acad Sci USA 1995;92:10457.
21. Gragoudas ES, Adamis AP, Cunningham ET, et al., for the VEGF Inhibition Study in Ocular Neovascularization Clinical Trial Group: pegaptanib for neovascular age-related macular degeneration. N Engl J Med 2004;351:2805.

*Bold numerals denote published controlled clinical trials, meta-analyses, or consensus-based recommendations.

*For annotated **General References** and resources related to this chapter, visit www.hopkinsbayview.org/PAMreferences.*

Chapter 108

Glaucoma

David S. Friedman

Glaucoma is a progressive disease of the optic nerve head with a characteristic appearance (and cupping). Although many persons with glaucoma have elevated intraocular pressure (IOP), virtually all population-based studies of glaucoma have found that at the initial screening half of those with glaucoma have IOPs that are less than 21 mm Hg are not considered "normal." In developed countries fewer than half of those with glaucoma know they have the disease, and in the developing world it is uncommon for persons with glaucoma to be diagnosed. Glaucoma is the second leading case of blindness in the United States, with over 2 million Americans affected. As with all chronic diseases associated with older age, glaucoma prevalence will increase in the coming decades to an estimated 3.2 million affected individuals, because of the aging of the U.S. population (1). Many more will require treatment and monitoring of high IOP.

The glaucomas are classified into primary and secondary groups (Table 108.1). Among African Americans, whites, and Hispanics, primary open-angle glaucoma accounts for 95% of all patients with glaucoma, but among other populations (e.g., Chinese and those from south India), angle-closure glaucoma accounts for almost half the cases (2–4). Secondary glaucomas occur when IOP is elevated because of a known cause such as trauma or intraocular inflammation and is far less common than primary open-angle and primary angle-closure glaucoma.

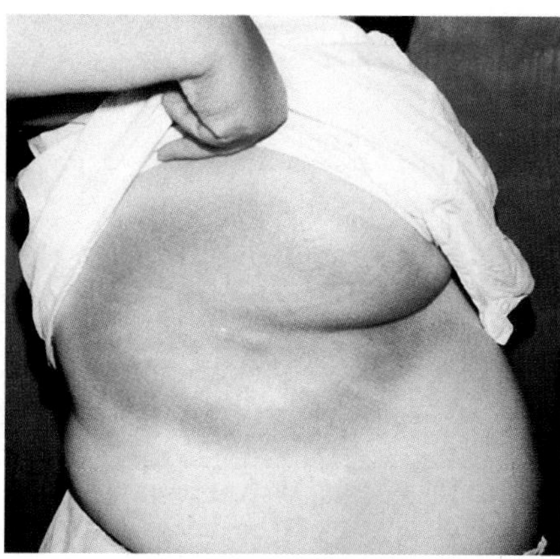

FIGURE 38.2. Classic erythema migrans rash of early Lyme disease with bright red border and partial central clearing, the so-called "bull's-eye" rash. (Photograph courtesy of Paul Auwaerter, M.D.)

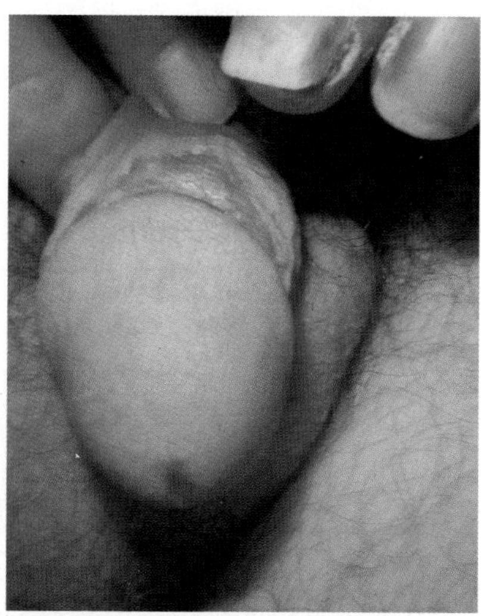

FIGURE 78.5. Moist shallow circular lesions characteristic of circinate balanitis. From: John A. Flynn, MD, MBA.

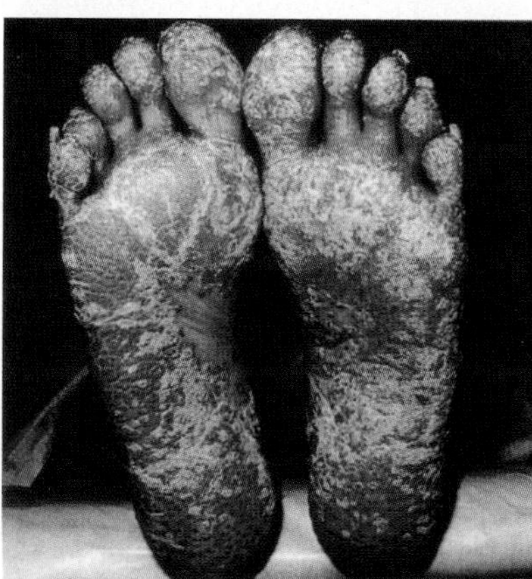

FIGURE 78.6. Extensive keratoderma blennorrhagica involving the soles (with permission from Provost TT, Flynn JA. Cutaneous Medicine: Cutaneous Manifestations of Systemic Disease, 2001). From: John A. Flynn, MD, MBA.

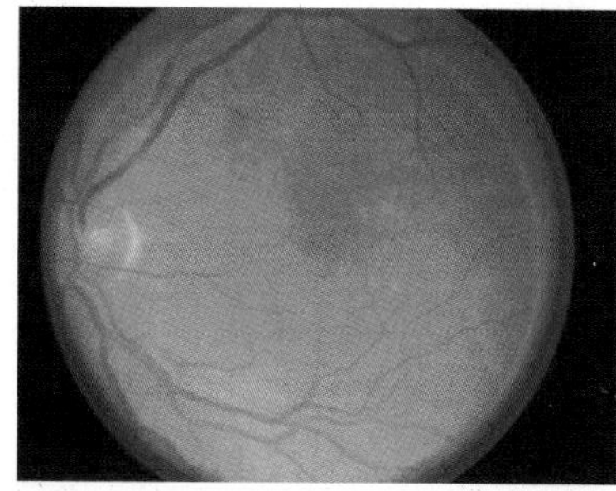

FIGURE 107.1. Left eye of a patient with small, hard drusen in the macula. Drusen are the barley visible tiny yellow deposits around the foveal center.

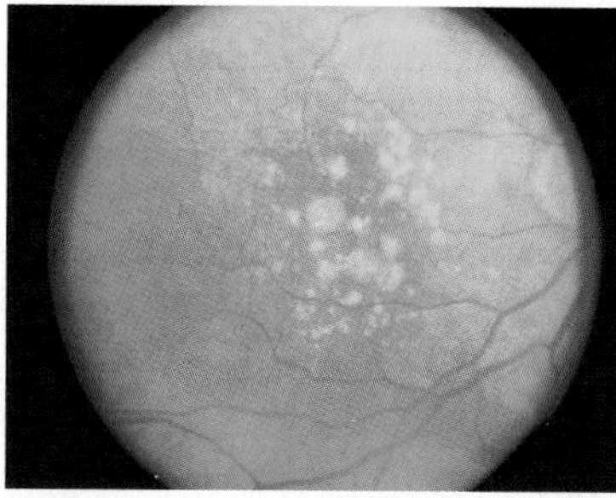

FIGURE 107.2. Right eye of a patient with a myriad of large drusen in and around the foveal center. This eye is at high risk for progression of AMD.

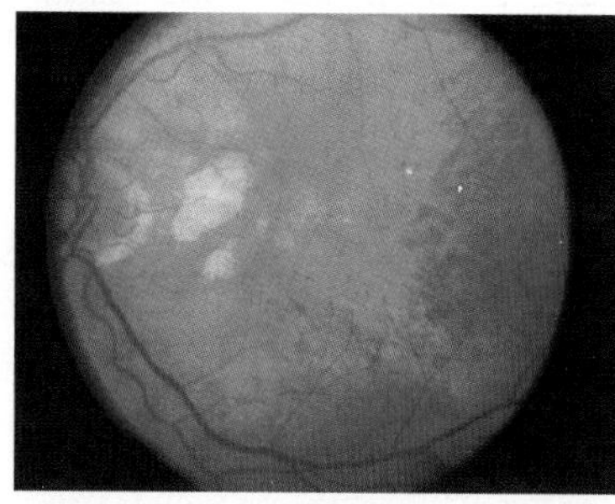

FIGURE 107.3. Left eye of a patient with central (extending beneath the fovea) GA. Note the hypopigmented well-circumscribed area that represents a loss of retinal tissue and underlying retinal pigment epithelium. The choroidal vessels can be seen through the area of atrophy.

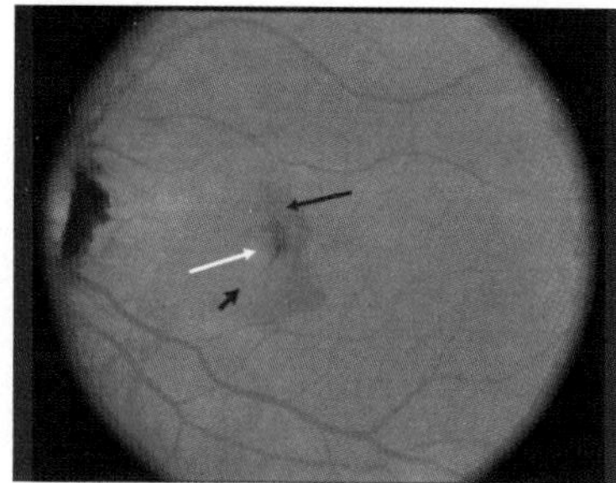

FIGURE 107.4. Left eye of a patient with subretinal hemorrhage (black arrow) and subretinal fluid (white arrow) that extend beneath the foveal center. This eye has the neovascular form of AMD.

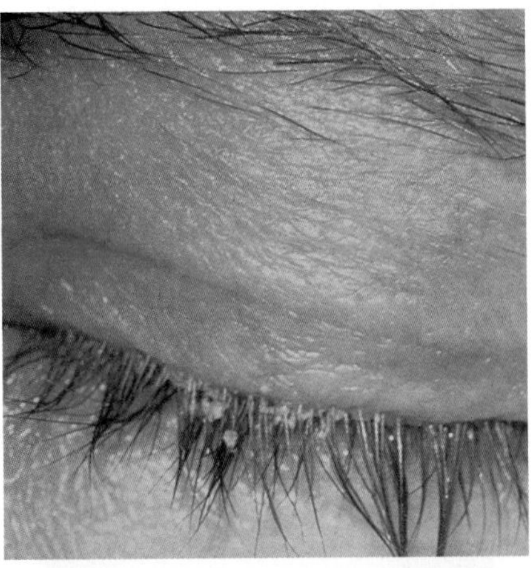

FIGURE 109.2. Seborrheic blepharitis. Note the oil debris, scurf on the lashes, but no broken or missing lashes.

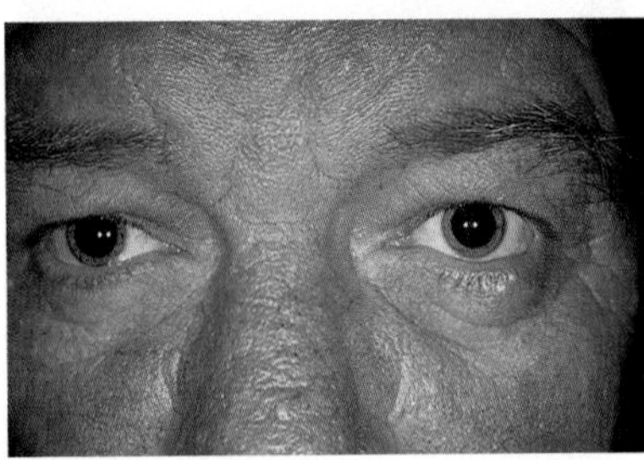

FIGURE 109.3. Acne rosacea with hordeolum. Man with rhinophyma, oily skin, and acute localized painful swelling (hordeolum) on the left lower eyelid.

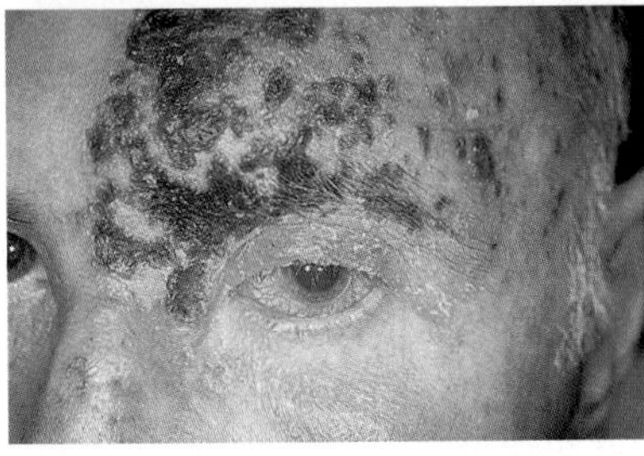

FIGURE 109.4. Herpes zoster. Note the crusting lesions on the forehead and scaling of the upper eyelid with conjunctival injection.

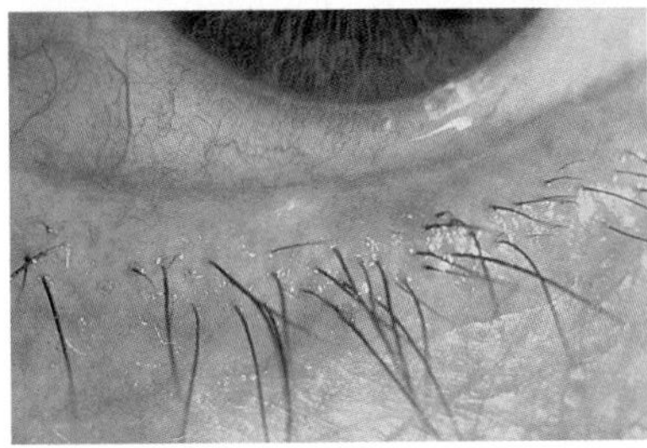

FIGURE 109.5. Staphylococcal blepharitis. Note that the lashes are sparse, misdirected, and of varying lengths. The lid margin shows ulceration.

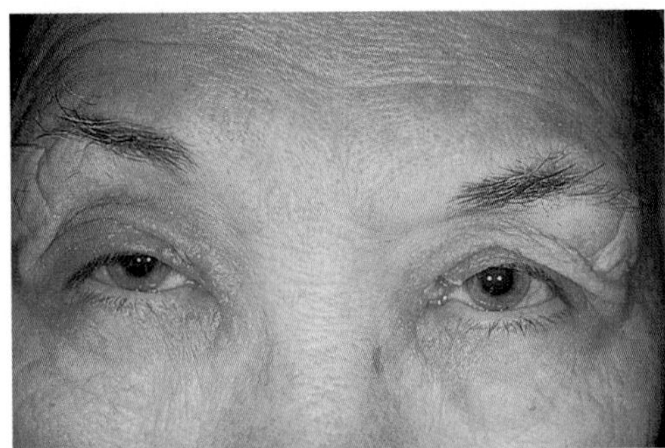

FIGURE 109.6. Blepharitis. Woman with morning discharge and crusting in both eyes. Note the redness and swelling of the eyelids.

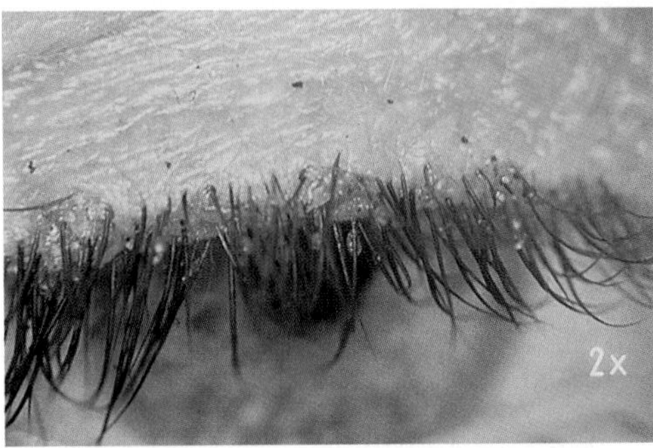

FIGURE 109.7. Parasitic blepharitis. Note the adult lice and nits on the lashes of a patient with *Pediculosis pubis*.

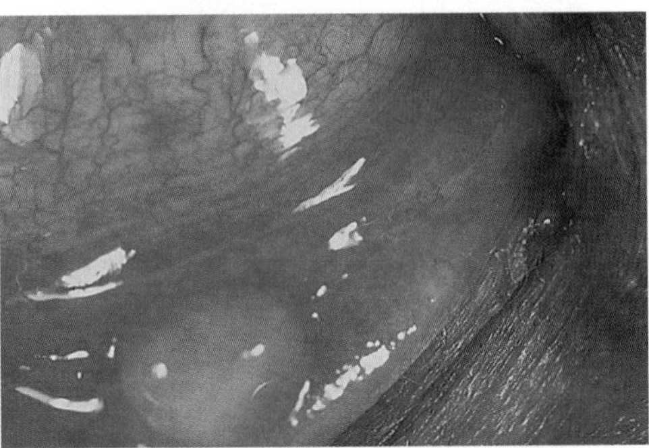

FIGURE 109.8. Chalazion. Note the localized swelling of the inferior tarsal conjunctiva in a patient with chronic blepharitis. The lower lid is retracted inferiorly.

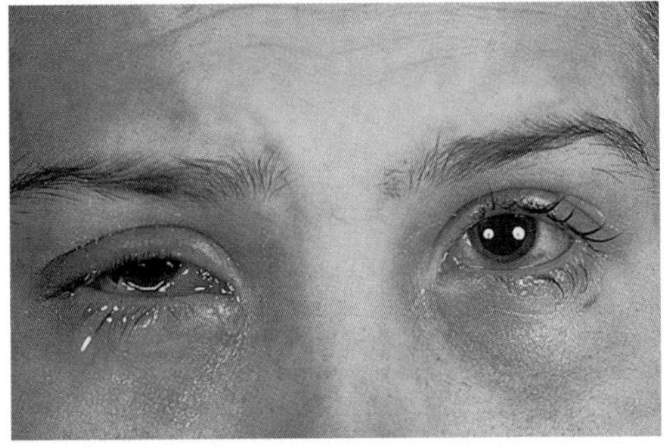

FIGURE 109.9. Hyperacute purulent conjunctivitis. Note the severe degree of injection, swelling, and purulent discharge.

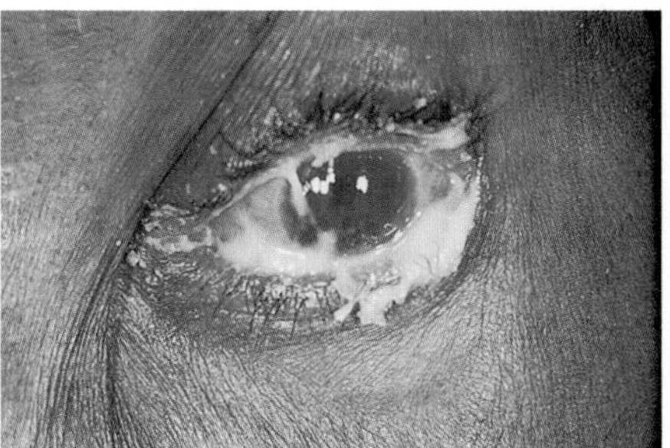

FIGURE 109.10. Acute bacterial conjunctivitis (severe example). Note the marked erythema, pus, and edema.

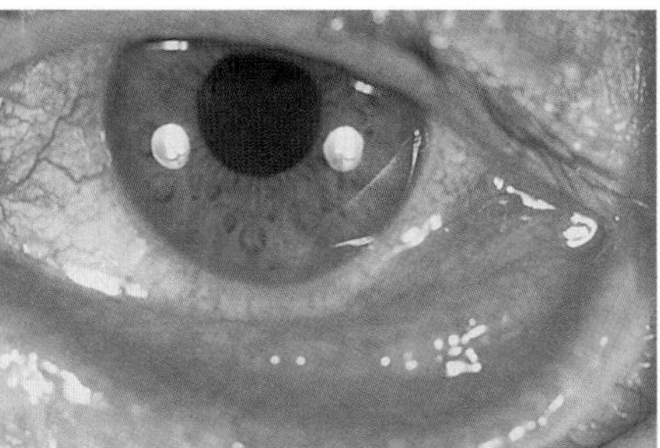

FIGURE 109.11. Viral conjunctivitis. Note the watery conjunctival discharge and conjunctival hyperemia. The lower lid is retracted inferiorly, demonstrating tarsal conjunctival edema and injection.

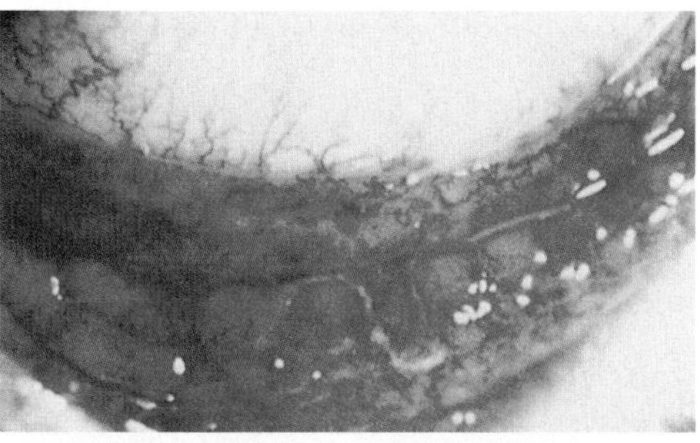

FIGURE 109.12. Inclusion conjunctivitis. Note the redness, edema of the lid and co njunctiva, and the many small follicles appearing as pale mounds.

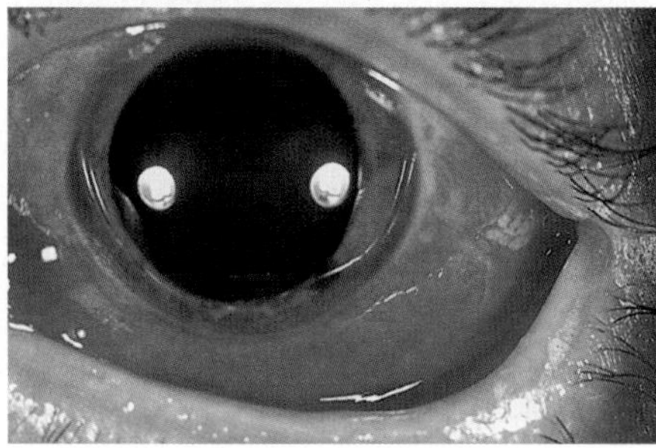

FIGURE 109.13. Subconjunctival hemorrhage (severe example). Note the diffuse conjunctival redness. (Pupil has been pharmacologically dilated.)

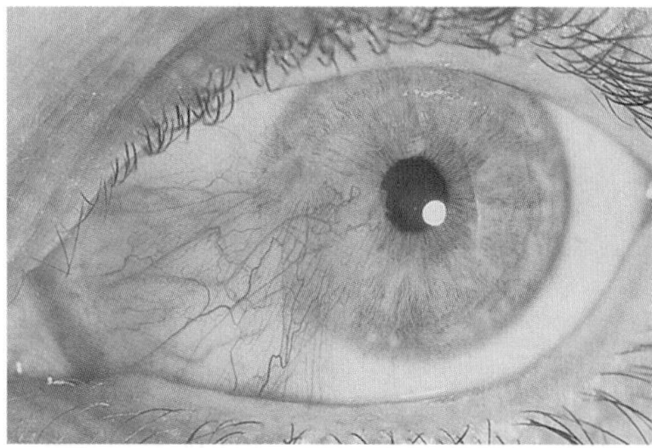

FIGURE 109.14. Pterygium. Note the localized conjunctival injection with extension of blood vessels into the cornea.

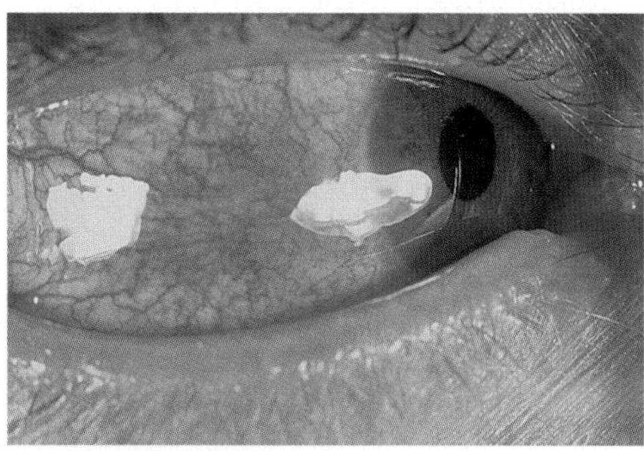

FIGURE 109.15. Episcleritis. Note the localized redness without discharge. (Light reflexes artifacts are present on the surface of the eye.)

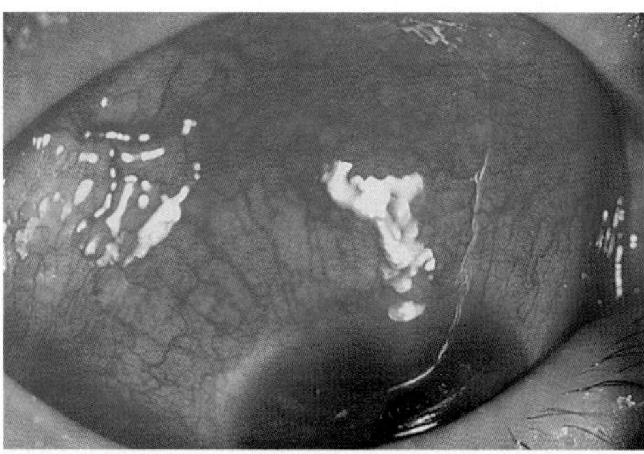

FIGURE 109.16. Scleritis. Note the diffuse intense redness without discharge. (Patient with rheumatoid arthritis.)

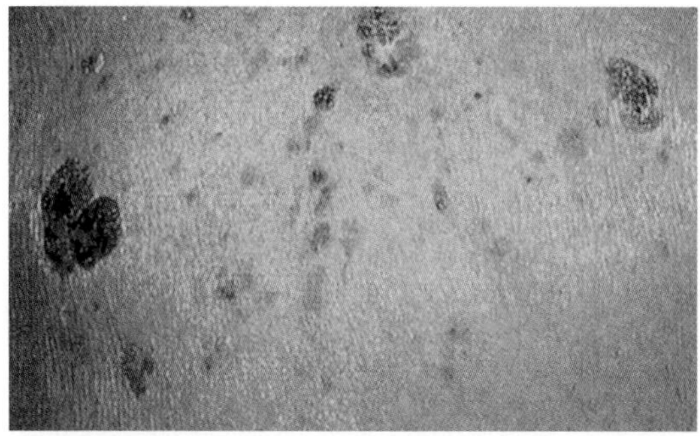

FIGURE 113.1. Multiple seborrheic keratoses (upper back). "Stuck-on," sharply circumscribed, tan to deep brown, finely papillated to verrucous flat-topped papules and plaques.

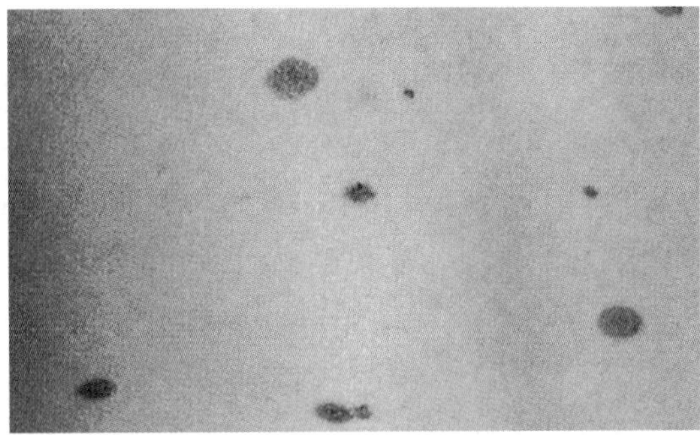

FIGURE 114.1. Atypical moles (dysplastic nevi). Multiple lesions, showing one to four of the ABCDs: asymmetry, border irregularity, color variegation, diameter 6 mm or greater.

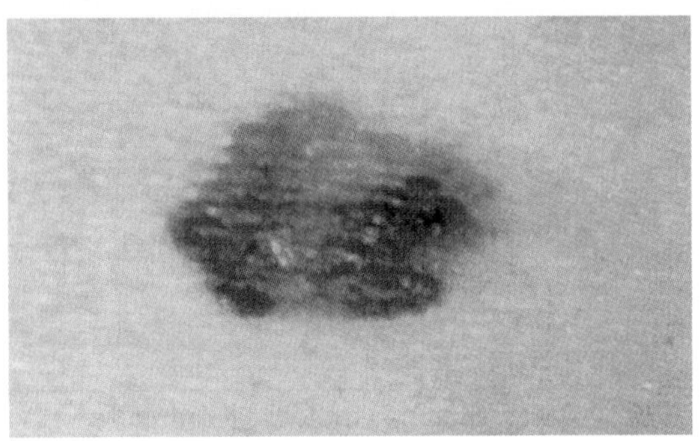

FIGURE 114.2. Superficial spreading malignant melanoma.

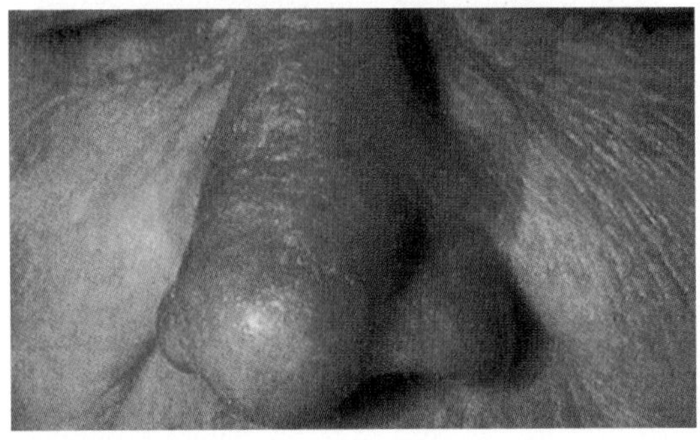

FIGURE 114.3. Actinic keratosis, nose.

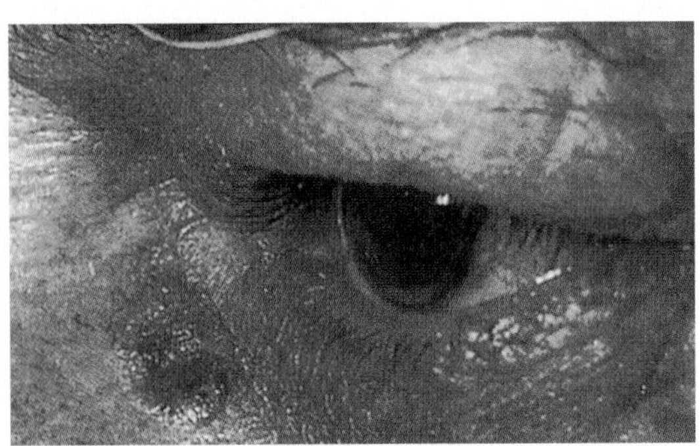

FIGURE 114.4. Basal cell carcinoma.

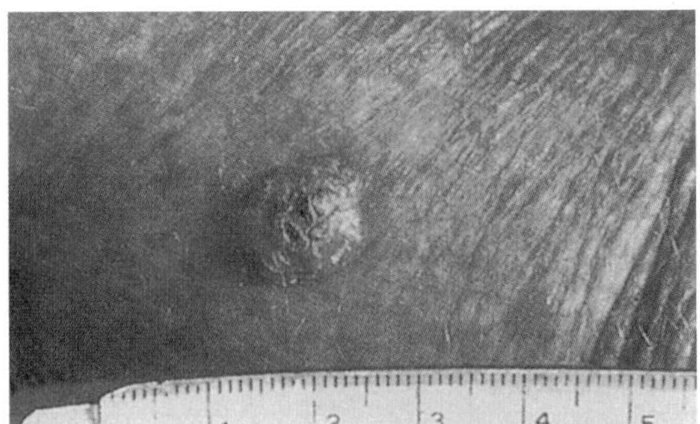

FIGURE 114.5. Squamous cell carcinoma.

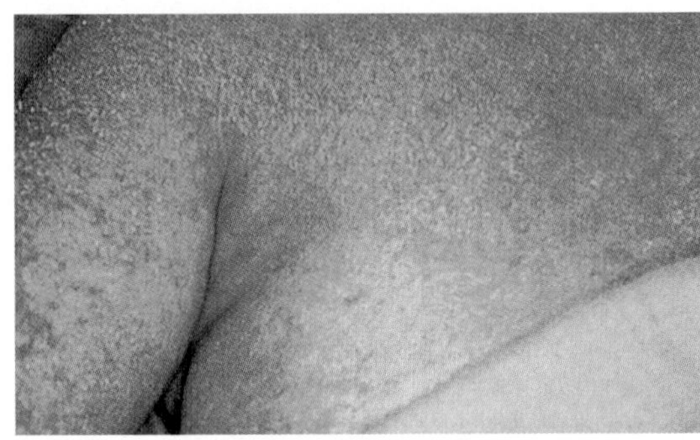

FIGURE 116.1. Asteatotic dermatitis (upper back and arm). Reticulate erythema highlighting minute cracks in the skin, diffuse dryness (asteatosis), and scale.

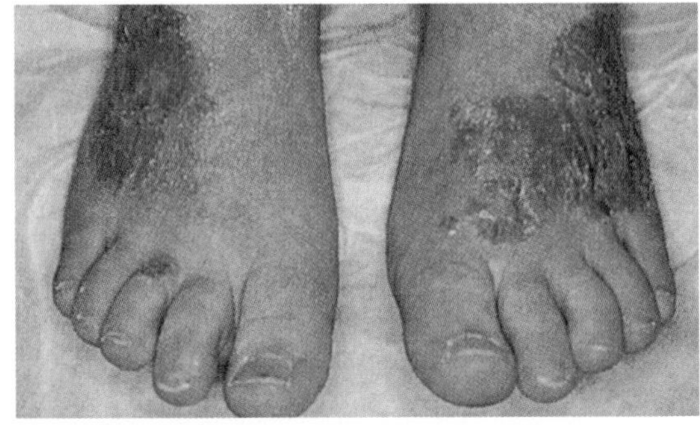

FIGURE 116.2. Acute contact dermatitis from shoes.

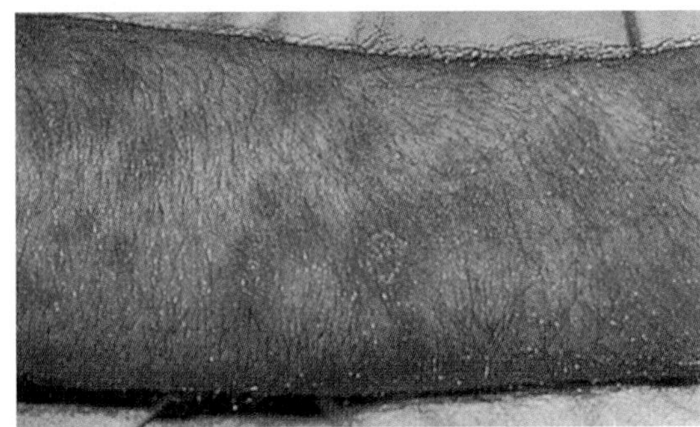

FIGURE 118.1. Erythema multiforme (extensor arm). Erythematous macules with dusky central area ("target") with focal areas of fine scale.

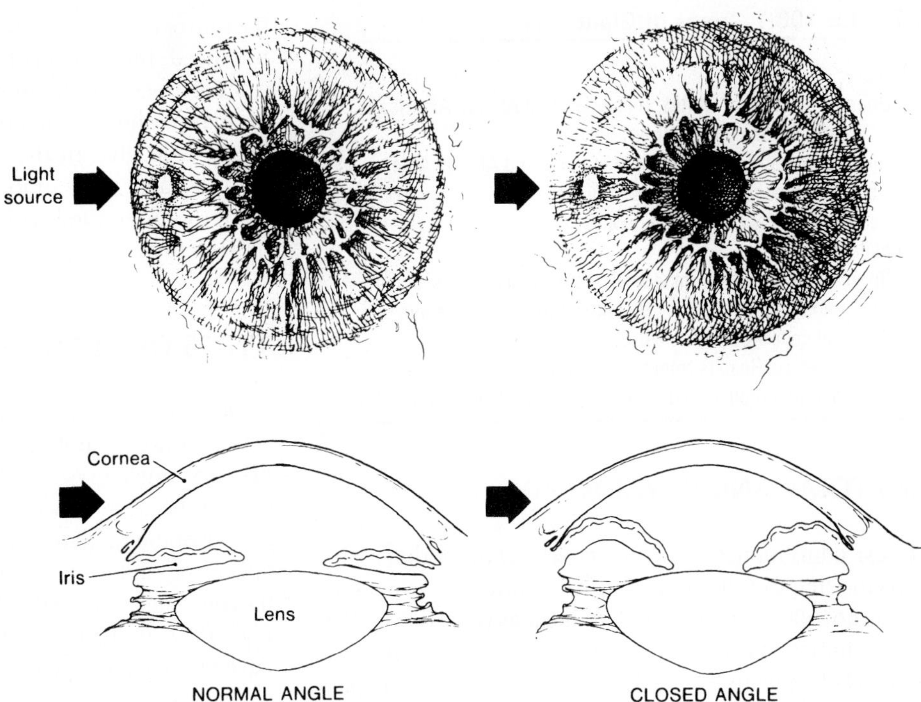

FIGURE 108.2. Illustration showing a shadow cast on the nasal side of the iris resultant from the bowed iris in angle-closure glaucoma (*right*). In open-angle glaucoma, the iris is not bowed, so the shadow is not cast (*left*).

ersons of European descent older than the age of 40 is around 2%, while nearly 6% of African Americans in this age range are affected (6–9).

Prevalence increases substantially with age, approaching 10% for whites older than 75 years of age and 20% for blacks (2). Hispanics appear to have rates intermediate between whites and blacks. Indeed, because open-angle glaucoma is so prevalent, is asymptomatic, and is treatable, open-angle glaucoma is the primary reason behind the recommendation for annual eye examination for people 65 years and older. Primary open-angle glaucoma causes 15% to 20% of all blindness in this country (10). Men and women are affected equally, but African Americans are affected at a higher frequency and at an earlier age, and open-angle glaucoma is the leading cause of blindness in African Americans. Recent research in Hispanics in Arizona and Los Angeles indicates that Hispanics have rates similar to whites until their sixties, when rates increase dramatically and are closer to those of blacks (11–12).

Open-angle glaucoma is familiar, but the pattern of inheritance is not yet known. Siblings of affected individuals are at 10 times the risk of having open-angle glaucoma (13). An association between open-angle glaucoma and both diabetes mellitus (DM) and elevated blood pressure has been proposed, but these hypotheses are uncertain and more research is necessary to define such relationships. Patients who have high degrees of myopia (near vision) likely are at higher risk of open-angle glaucoma, but this hypothesis is uncertain as well (14). Glaucoma risk may also be increased with prolonged use of oral and nasal glucocorticoid inhalers, especially in individuals with a family history of glaucoma (15,16).

Manifestations and Physical Examination

Open-angle glaucoma is typically asymptomatic until its latest stages. When symptoms do occur, damage to the optic nerve is present and may be substantial. Central vision and the ability to recognize forms on a vision test chart are preserved until very late. For this reason, testing of visual acuity is not a reliable method to screen for glaucoma. Occasionally, a patient with open-angle glaucoma may notice halos around lights and blurring of vision if there is a sudden rise in IOP. Patients with this history should be referred urgently to an ophthalmologist. Patients with open-angle glaucoma rarely complain of headache that can be attributed to increased IOP.

The ocular pressure may be elevated for years before any change in the optic disk is noted. The change in the optic disk is revealed by increasing excavation of the central physiologic disk cup, visible on funduscopic examination (Fig. 108.3). This is most easily seen by use of the direct ophthalmoscope, and by the ophthalmologist using a slit lamp and a handheld lens (which allows for stereoscopic viewing). Over years the pink color of the disk fades and becomes pale, and vessels coursing over the disk show a sharp bend at the rim. Patients thought to have an enlarged optic cup (cup-to-disk ratio $\geq$0.7) should be referred to an ophthalmologist within a month.

TABLE 108.1 Types of Glaucoma

Primary
- Open angle: 90% of whites, Hispanics, and African Americans, 50% of Chinese and southern Indians
- Angle closure: 10% of whites, Hispanics, and African Americans, 50% of Chinese and southern Indians
- Congenital: infant and juvenile onset

Secondary
- Open angle: Results from topical or systemic steroids, ocular inflammation, or obstructed venous return from the eye (e.g., carotid cavernous sinus fistula)
- Angle closure: Results from trauma, neovascular change in the iris, ocular neoplasia, cataract surgery, and iris abnormalities

ANATOMY AND PHYSIOLOGY

The eye continuously circulates *aqueous humor* that maintains the shape of the eye and provides nutrition to avascular intraocular structures such as the lens (Fig. 108.1). IOP is maintained in a steady state by ongoing production and removal of aqueous humor. Elevated eye pressure is in part caused by obstruction to the outflow of aqueous humor at the level of the trabecular meshwork. The aqueous humor is a clear ultrafiltrate of the blood and occupies part of the posterior and anterior chambers of the eye. It is produced both by secretion and ultrafiltration at the level of the epithelium of the ciliary body. At least two enzymes have been implicated in aqueous formation: sodium/potassium-activated adenosine triphosphatase (ATPase) and carbonic anhydrase. Antagonists of these enzymes appear to reduce the rate of aqueous formation and thereby low produced, the aqueous humor circulates fro rior chamber into the anterior chamber of the becular meshwork, an intricate system of conn fibers, is located in the periphery of the ant ber. The aqueous humor percolates through work to be reunited with the venous blood v of Schlemm.

TYPES OF GLAUCOMA

Table 108.1 outlines the major types and cau coma. However, only primary open-angle gla primary angle-closure glaucoma are discus chapter because they are the types likely to be arly. Open-angle glaucoma takes its name from appearing anterior chamber angle, a cont narrow angle of angle-closure glaucoma, as Fig. 108.2. Individuals with *normal-tension gl* have similarly to those with higher pressure glaucoma, and research has shown that IC therapy can prevent progression of the disea individuals (5).

Primary Open-Angle Glaucoma

Prevalence and Risk Factors

Primary open-angle glaucoma is by far the mo cause of glaucoma in the United States; the pre

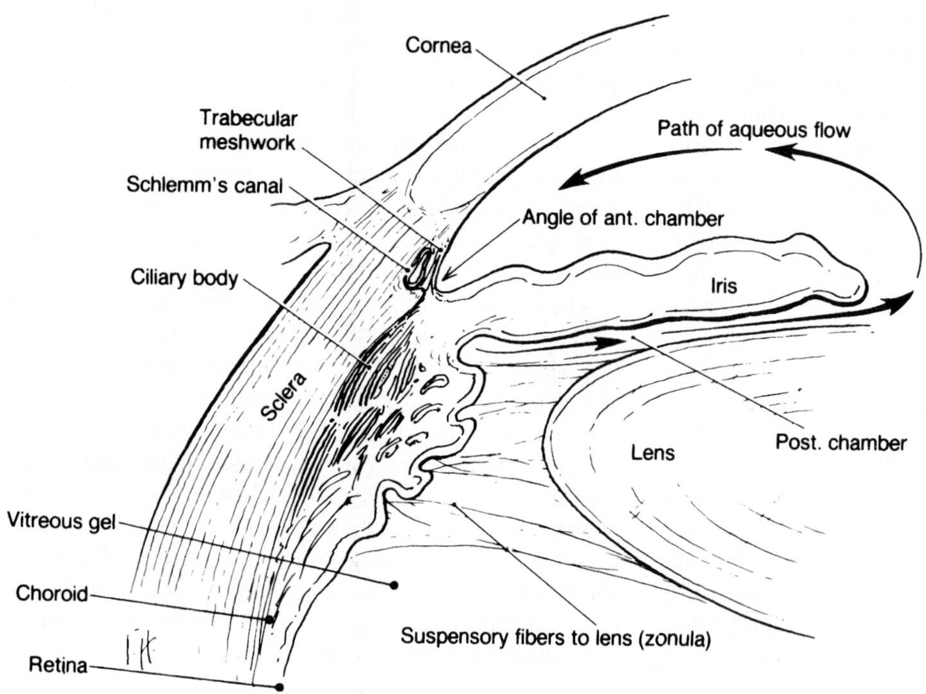

FIGURE 108.1. Anato eye: cross-section of th (Modified from Basm Grant's method of 8th ed. Baltimore: Wi Wilkins, 1971:543.)

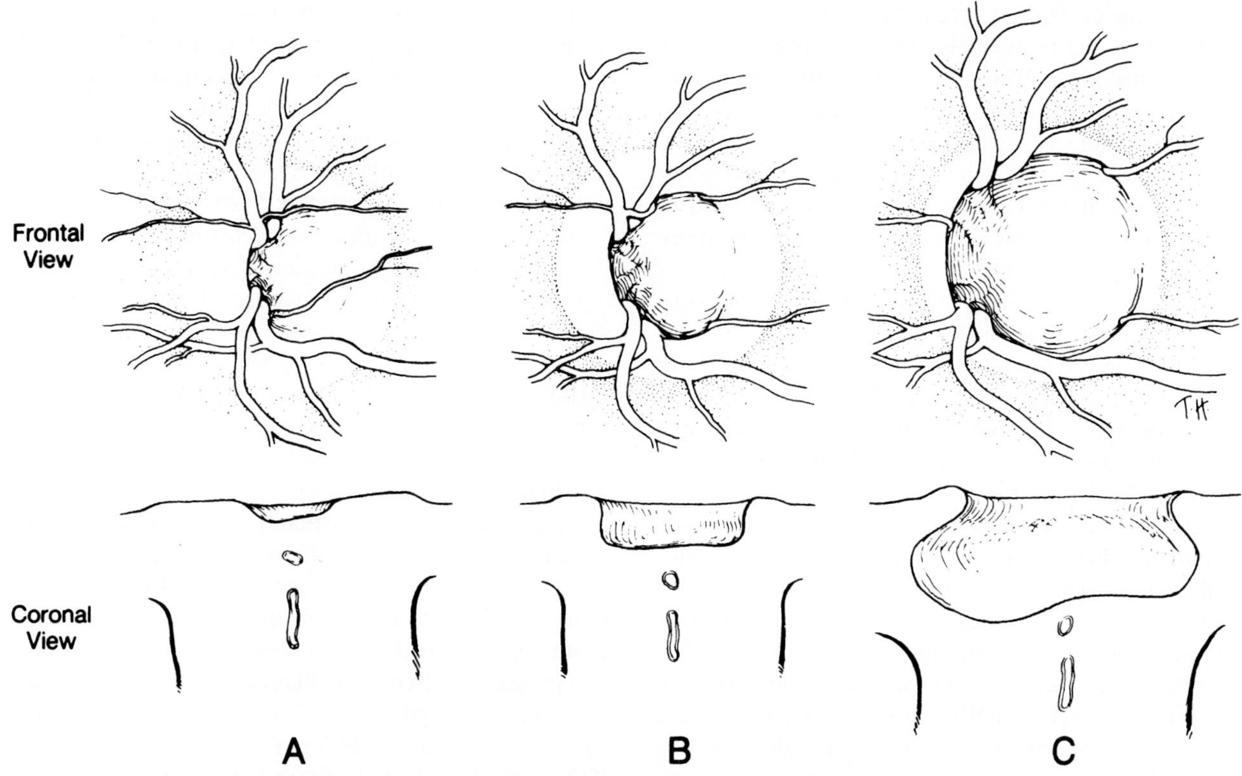

FIGURE 108.3. Changes in the optic disk with increasing intraocular pressure showing on both the frontal and coronal views: **(A)** normal, **(B)** early change, and **series (C)** late change.

One should assume that open-angle glaucoma has no symptoms until the patient is on the verge of blindness. Detection must be accomplished based on knowledge of risk factors (age, race, and family history) and examination findings. The diagnosis is then confirmed after referral to an ophthalmologist.

In evaluating the patient with suspicion for glaucoma, the ophthalmologist typically measures the eye pressure, visualizes the angle of the anterior chamber and the fundus, and assesses the visual fields.

Screening for Open-Angle Glaucoma

The ideal method for screening for primary open-angle glaucoma is controversial, and false positive and false negative detection rates are high. Population-based screening for glaucoma remains difficult because of the lack of an ideal screening device, the relatively high cost of screening and referral, and the limited data on treatment efficacy. However, recent developments have increased the evidence in support of wider screening, and the Center for Medicare and Medical Services recently added a benefit for glaucoma screening to Medicare beneficiaries with known risk factors. A new screening device, the frequency doubling technology perimeter, has demonstrated sensitivity and specificity over 90% in several reports, but widespread effectiveness has not been tested (17,18). Additionally, two large clinical trials indicate that lowering eye pressure is associated with slower progression of glaucoma (5,19), and one multi-center study demonstrated that lowering IOP decreases the likelihood of developing glaucoma in individuals with elevated IOP who do not have optic nerve damage (20).

Screening for glaucoma involves one of three different approaches: tonometry, funduscopic assessment or imaging of the optic cup and nerve fiber layer, and visual field assessment. For years it was recommended that primary care clinicians screen high-risk patients for glaucoma by measuring eye pressure directly with a Schiotz tonometer. This approach is too insensitive and nonspecific to be of value. IOP screening, even with ideal instruments, has poor screening characteristics, because half of all individuals with glaucoma will have eye pressures in the normal range on a single IOP screen. New digital imaging devices show promise for detecting glaucoma by assessing the optic nerve head appearance. These instruments can collect data through an undilated pupil in under 1 minute and may be more widely used in the future (21). Finally, functional tests such as the perimeter described above show promise as screening devices. They obtain results in under 2 minutes per eye, are portable and inexpensive, and could conceivably be used in public settings such as departments of motor vehicles. Others have adapted this approach to the Internet so that individuals can test themselves. More research is needed, however, to study the performance of each of these devices in community-based populations. Because ophthalmologists generally do all three evaluations, the ideal screening approach at present is a complete eye examination. Primary care clinicians are encouraged to advise white and Hispanic patients age 65 and older (those at higher risk) to be referred to an eye specialist every 1 or 2 years glaucoma screening, whereas African Americans should be referred at an earlier age, perhaps even age 50.

Patients referred to an ophthalmologist generally have an evaluation consisting of several observations: determination of the IOP by applanation tonometry; funduscopic assessment of the optic disk and retina through the dilated pupil; visual field assessment, usually with a computerized perimeter; and gonioscopic examination, which permits the ophthalmologist to visualize the angle of the anterior chamber by using an instrument containing a contact lens and mirror. The patient usually experiences minimal or no discomfort during these procedures.

Approximately one fifth of patients found to have asymptomatic increased IOP on preliminary screening are shown to have glaucoma after thorough evaluation. Approximately 30% may be found not to have elevated pressures on reassessment, and about 50% have "ocular hypertension" without glaucoma. A large National Institutes of Health (NIH)-funded trial recently documented that individuals with elevated IOP have about a 10% risk of developing early glaucoma over 5 years of followup, and this risk can be reduced by half with lowering of IOP (20). Furthermore, important risk factors were identified in that trial to help determine which individuals with elevated IOP require treatment (22). Important risk factors included higher IOP, larger cup-to-disc ratio, and a thin central cornea. Individuals with certain combinations of these characteristics had over a 30% risk of developing glaucoma over 5 years, while those in the lower risk groups had about a 2% risk. Risk assessment is therefore an important aspect of the management of ocular hypertension.

Treatment

When the ophthalmologist establishes the diagnosis of open-angle glaucoma, treatment is prescribed based on the level of IOP, the degree of visual field loss, and the amount of optic nerve damage. As stated above, lowering IOP in individuals with open-angle glaucoma has recently been proven to slow the rate of progression of the disease. IOP lowering can be achieved by three different approaches: medical therapy, laser treatment, and surgical procedures.

Most ophthalmologists initially treat open-angle glaucoma with medicines, although the American Academy of Ophthalmology Preferred Practice Pattern recommends that all three approaches be discussed and considered as potential primary treatments. While a recent NIH-sponsored multicenter clinical trial comparing surgery to medications as first-line therapy showed no difference in outcomes at 5 years, most ophthalmologists do not recommend surgery until later in the disease course given the potential for poor outcomes that exists.

The options for *medical treatments* have increased over the last decade with the addition of topical prostaglandins, α-agonists, and carbonic anhydrase inhibitors (CAIs). IOP-lowering drugs work by one of three mechanisms: they decrease aqueous production (β-blockers, α-agonists, and CAIs), increase outflow through the trabecular meshwork (miotics, prostaglandins, and α-agonists), or increase outflow through alternative pathways (uveoscleral outflow, prostaglandins).

The aim of therapy is to maintain the IOP at a level that does not lead to further optic nerve damage. Target pressures are chosen based on the IOP at which the patient sustained damage and the severity of the glaucoma. For example, an individual who presents with severe damage at a pressure of 20 mm Hg likely needs a pressure around 14 mm Hg to be safe, whereas an individual with mild disease and a pressure of 30 mm Hg might be followed at an IOP of 24 mm Hg. The relatively low rate of side effects and effective IOP-lowering with prostaglandins has led to wide use of these compounds, and they are now the most frequently prescribed first-line therapy for glaucoma. Furthermore, prostaglandins are used once a day, resulting in greater patient compliance. No definite systemic side effects have been shown to be caused by prostaglandins. Ocular side effects include changing blue or hazel eyes to brown in a significant proportion of individuals. These agents also increase eyelashes in number and length. β-Blockers are still frequently prescribed for glaucoma either as primary or secondary therapy. α-Agonists and topical CAIs are less frequently prescribed, and appear slightly less effective than prostaglandins and β-blockers. Combination drops are also available, with a combination β-blocker and topical CAI widely used. Miotics, which were the mainstay of therapy for many years, are now rarely used because they cause miosis and dim vision. Eye drops enter the bloodstream directly through the nasal mucosa without any first pass through the liver, resulting in relatively high drug levels in the blood. β-Blocking agents can exacerbate congestive heart failure, can cause shortness of breath in otherwise healthy elderly individuals (23), lead to depression, and raise low-density lipoprotein (LDL) cholesterol. α-Agonists can cause dry mouth and, in up to 10% of patients, significant lethargy. All individuals on these agents should be questioned about this side effect, because many may not identify the association with the eye drops they are taking. α-Agonists can also lead to systemic hypotension. Topical CAIs are usually well tolerated with no reports of aplastic anemia or kidney stones caused

TABLE 108.2 Systemic Effects of Medications Used to Treat Glaucoma

Considerable absorption of drug may occur through the nasal mucosa via flow through the lacrimal duct. Closing the eye for 2 minutes after instillation or pressing on the nasal lacrimal duct decreases the systemic uptake of eyedrops.

β-Adrenergic blocking agents
- Pulmonary: bronchospasm (the incidence is decreased with selective β-blockers such as betaxolol)
- Cardiovascular: bradycardia, hypotension, decreased cardiac contractility
- Central nervous system: fatigue, depression, memory loss, impotence

Miotics (e.g., Pilocarpine)
- Unstable refractive error, decreased night vision especially in those with cataracts, ciliary muscle spasms, ocular burning; long-acting agents such as phospholine iodide because of irreversible depletion of cholinesterase may make general anesthesia dangerous.

α-Agonists
- Systemic hypotension, somnolence, dry mouth, dizziness

Oral carbonic anhydrase inhibitor
- Malaise, fatigue, anorexia, depression, decreased libido, systemic acidosis (especially a risk in those with severe respiratory disease or those taking large dosages of salicylates), nausea, vomiting, diarrhea, alterations in taste of carbonated beverages. Topical carbonic anhydrase inhibitors do not appear to produce these side effects.

Data from Everitt DE, Avorn J. Systemic effects of medications used to treat glaucoma. Ann Intern Med 1990;112:120.

by these agents since they were released nearly 10 years ago.

Oral CAIs are now rarely prescribed for glaucoma. Topical CAIs are used first, but in rare patients, oral CAIs can significantly drop the eye pressure when topical therapy is inadequate. Oral CAIs have myriad side effects (Table 108.2) and are therefore only used as a last resort.

Topical agents for glaucoma are usually tested in a one-eyed trial to see if they are effective for the patient. Once effectiveness and tolerability is determined, the agents are typically used bilaterally unless there is no evidence of disease in the contralateral eye. Once the target IOP has been attained, the ophthalmologist usually examines the patient two to four times per year for assessment of visual fields, measurement of IOP, funduscopic examination, and gonioscopy.

Argon laser trabeculoplasty is an alternative approach to lowering IOP for individuals with glaucoma and ocular hypertension and is considered a reasonable first-line therapy. This office procedure requires only topical anesthesia and can result in a significant reduction in ocular pressure in close to 90% of patients. However, this effect is frequently transient, with about 50% of treatments still effective 5 years after initial treatment (24). The safety of this treatment is well documented in two large NIH-sponsored clinical trials (24,25). The mechanism by which laser trabeculoplasty exerts its beneficial effects is uncertain but is most likely due to the release of chemical mediators in the trabecular meshwork at the time treatment. A modification of this procedure using a different laser may allow for more repeat laser treatments than is currently possible using the argon laser, but data remain limited as to whether or not multiple treatments are effective.

Surgery in primary open-angle glaucoma is designed to construct outflow channels for the aqueous humor or, in the some severe cases, to destroy the ciliary body in order to decrease aqueous production. Surgery lowers pressure more than medicines or lasers but has more potential adverse consequences. In the last few years, tremendous advances have been made in glaucoma filtering surgery. The major problem with the procedure, which makes a hole in the eye to allow aqueous drainage into the subconjunctival space, is the tendency for healing, which closes the hole and results in failure to control IOP. Topical antimetabolites used at the time of surgery are associated with a substantial increase in the success rate by preventing scarring of the new channel. There is concern about late infections in all patients who have had glaucoma filtering surgery, and late infections may be more common in these antimetabolite procedures. Currently, unless results from new trials recommend otherwise, surgical procedures are reserved for patients in whom medical management fails. Medications may still be required after surgery. New nonpenetrating procedures, in which the aqueous fluid percolates through a very thin membrane of tissue that is left at the time of surgery, are under investigation and show promise. These appear to have a safer profile than standard filtration procedures, but do not lower IOP as much as the more standard glaucoma procedure ("trabeculectomy"). Another significant improvement on the horizon is the use of more specific agents to modulate wound healing. These drugs may lead to more healthy tissue after surgery and may reduce the likelihood of eye infections in operated eyes.

Monitoring

The patient with open-angle glaucoma must receive regular ophthalmologic followup, but claims data indicate that a substantial proportion drop out from care. The generalist can remind patients of the need for regular examinations if they carry a glaucoma diagnosis. In addition, the primary care clinician should be alert to any side effects from the drugs prescribed by the ophthalmologist (Table 108.2).

There has been concern about the impact of systemic medications on glaucoma, particularly anticholinergics, adrenergics, hypnotics, and corticosteroids. Except for corticosteroids, none of these drugs is contraindicated in open-angle glaucoma. The concern raised by these medications is that they can cause acute angle-closure glaucoma in susceptible individuals, but angle-closure glaucoma is relatively rare among most U.S. populations, and individuals with angle-closure who are diagnosed are routinely treated with iridotomy which removes the risk from most of these medications. Systemic corticosteroids (including inhaled steroids) and, in particular, corticosteroids applied to the eye may raise IOP and are relatively contraindicated in open-angle glaucoma.

Primary Angle-Closure Glaucoma

The basic defect in primary angle-closure glaucoma is the inability of aqueous humor to reach the filtration apparatus. When the pupil is in a mid-dilated position, the iris is bowed forward and blocks the outflow of aqueous humor (Fig. 108.2). The primary site of aqueous blockage is at the iris–lens interface. The iris moves forward as the pressure rises behind it, and physically blocks the trabecular meshwork. Chronic forms of angle closure also exist.

Although angle-closure glaucoma is far less common than open-angle glaucoma in the United States, one must be aware of the possibility of acute angle-closure attacks. These can occur spontaneously, or they may be precipitated by the use of mydriatics, sympathomimetics, hypnotics, and in several instances, topiramate (an antiseizure medicine); if this occurs, urgent recognition and treatment are mandatory to prevent damage to the eye. Additionally, cases of angle-closure glaucoma can be misdiagnosed as possible neurosurgical or gastrointestinal conditions (because of symptoms such as headaches and nausea and vomiting), so recognition of the condition is important. Patients may have a positive family history, women are affected more than men, and the condition is far more common among Asians and those from the Indian subcontinent than among whites, African Americans, and Hispanics.

Patients who have smaller eyes with shallow anterior chambers are predisposed to primary angle-closure glaucoma. Patients with these predispositions can develop either acute attacks of angle-closure glaucoma, with extremely elevated eye pressure and pain, or can develop a silent form of the disease known as chronic angle-closure glaucoma. The probability of inducing acute angle-closure glaucoma through dilation of the pupils in older blacks and whites is less than 1 in 3,000, so one should use mydriatic eyedrops for individuals in need of a detailed examination of the eye whenever medically necessary. If an acute attack develops in such a circumstance, it can often be treated rapidly with minimal adverse sequelae.

Diagnosis

Early diagnosis of an acute angle closure crisis is critical because blindness may ensue and virtually every case is surgically curable if diagnosed early. Cure is increasingly less likely if repeated attacks have occurred and have resulted in scarring of the trabecular meshwork. Although many acute attacks occur without any prodromal symptoms, some may experience episodes of ocular pain (usually located in the periocular or supraocular region), episodes of blurred vision, and seeing halos around lights at night before the initial attack. These symptoms occur because of corneal epithelial edema that has developed as a result of the increased IOP. Often patients find relief in well-lighted rooms or outdoors, where daylight causes constriction of the pupil and opening of the anterior chamber angle.

Examination during an acute attack usually reveals marked elevation of IOP, from 25 to as high as 90 mm Hg. The eye is red and painful, although rarely the patient complains of abdominal pain or headache only. Frequently there is tearing and photophobia. Corneal edema is present during an acute attack, and the anterior chamber may appear cloudy because of inflammation.

In patients predisposed to angle-closure glaucoma, the anterior chamber is shallow. This may be seen by illuminating the eye with a flashlight from the side and showing a shadow resulting from the bowed iris over the nasal portion of the eye (Fig. 108.2). This penlight test does not appear to separate well individuals with occludable angles from those with open angles, and is of questionable value in a general practitioner's office. Examination of the anterior chamber angle with a gonioscopic lens may reveal scarring of the trabecular meshwork and peripheral anterior synechiae.

Differential Diagnosis

The patient who has acute angle-closure glaucoma may present with an acute red eye. Initially, angle-closure glaucoma should be differentiated from acute iritis, acute conjunctivitis, and iridocyclitis. Chapter 109 discusses this differential diagnosis.

Treatment

Severe attacks of angle-closure glaucoma may cause blindness in 2 to 3 days or less depending on the level of IOP and the sensitivity of the optic nerve to ischemia. In some instances, ciliary ischemia stops aqueous production before blindness occurs. However, untreated acute attacks typically result in severe blinding glaucoma.

If the diagnosis of acute angle-closure glaucoma is suspected, an urgent referral to an ophthalmologist is indicated. The ophthalmologist probably will initiate treatment with immediate administration of acetazolamide (Diamox) 500 mg orally and instillation of pressure-lowering eye drops. If it will take hours to reach an ophthalmologist, therapy should be initiated in advance. In severe cases, the ingestion of hyperosmotic glycerol—1 mL/kg mixed as a 50% solution with chilled juice—almost always interrupts an acute attack. Hyperosmotic agents such as glycerol or intravenous mannitol dehydrate the vitreous and lower eye pressure. Practitioners who use mydriatics for funduscopic examination or who have patients with narrow anterior ocular chambers may want to have an angle-closure kit consisting of glycerol (glycerin, available as generic), acetazolamide (Diamox), and a β-blocker eye drop for use if an acute attack develops. Other possible treatments for an acute angle-closure crisis include laser iridoplasty and paracentesis, but these are generally carried out by an ophthalmologist.

Patients found to have a shallow anterior chamber even if they have not had a symptomatic attack of glaucoma should be referred to an ophthalmologist for evaluation, for education regarding specific manifestations of an acute attack, and for their initial treatment, usually prophylactic argon laser iridotomy.

The definitive treatment of acute primary angle-closure glaucoma is essentially surgical. If the diagnosis is made early enough in the course of the disease, a peripheral iridotomy can be done to relieve the pupillary block and allow the IOP to return to normal. In some acute cases, the trabecular meshwork remains permanently damaged or the filtering angle is scarred closed. Chronic medical therapy or even surgery may be required to prevent progressive optic nerve damage in these cases. Laser peripheral iridotomy under topical anesthesia has little risk and results in cure in most cases. Surgical iridectomy may also be performed. The laser iridotomy in the attack eye is performed as soon as the view is clear enough to do so. Generally, the laser iridotomy in the contralateral eye is performed soon after the attack, within 1 or 2 days. Followup care by the ophthalmologist after laser iridotomy is necessary to confirm that IOP control has been achieved.

When a patient has a shallow anterior chamber or is under treatment for angle-closure glaucoma, there should be concern about the use of certain medications. Systemic anticholinergics and adrenergic drugs may rarely precipitate an acute attack by causing dilation of the pupils. Hypnotics have also been implicated in causing acute attacks. Corticosteroids or vasodilating drugs are not contraindicated in patients with angle-closure glaucoma.

SPECIFIC REFERENCES

1. Friedman DS, Wolfs RC, O'Colmain BJ, et al. Eye Diseases Prevalence Research Group. Prevalence of open-angle glaucoma among adults in the United States. Arch Ophthalmol 2004;122:532.
2. Tielsch JM, Sommer A, Katz J, et al. Racial variations in the prevalence of primary open-angle glaucoma. The Baltimore Eye Survey. JAMA 1991;266:369.
3. Foster PJ, Oen FT, Machin D, et al. The prevalence of glaucoma in Chinese residents of Singapore: a cross-sectional population survey of the Tanjong Pagar district. Arch Ophthalmol 2000;118:1105.
4. Dandona L, Dandona R, Mandal P, et al. Angle-closure glaucoma in an urban population in southern India. The Andhra Pradesh eye disease study. Ophthalmol 2000;107:1710.
5. Collaborative Normal-Tension Glaucoma Study Group. The effectiveness of intraocular pressure reduction in the treatment of normal-tension glaucoma. Am J Ophthalmol 1998;126:498.
6. Mitchell P, Smith W, Attebo K, et al. Prevalence of open-angle glaucoma in Australia. The Blue Mountains Eye Study. Ophthalmol 1996;103:1661.
7. Coffey M, Reidy A, Wormald R, et al. Prevalence of glaucoma in the west of Ireland. Br J Ophthalmol 1993;77:17.
8. Dielemans I, Vingerling JR, Wolfs RC, et al. The prevalence of primary open-angle glaucoma in a population-based study in the Netherlands: The Rotterdam Study. Ophthalmol 1994;101:1851.
9. Wensor MD, McCarty CA, Stanislavsky YL, et al. The prevalence of glaucoma in the Melbourne Visual Impairment Project. Ophthalmol 1998;105:733.
10. Congdon N, O'Colmain B, Klaver CC, et al. Eye Diseases Prevalence Research Group. Causes and prevalence of visual impairment among adults in the United States. Arch Ophthalmol 2004;122:477.
11. Varma R, Ying-Lai M, Francis BA, et al. Los Angeles Latino Eye Study Group. Prevalence of open-angle glaucoma and ocular hypertension in Latinos: the Los Angeles Latino Eye Study. Ophthalmol 2004;111:1439.
12. Quigley HA, West SK, Rodriguez J, et al. The prevalence of glaucoma in a population-based study of Hispanic subjects: Proyecto VER. Arch Ophthalmol 2001;119:1819.
13. Wolfs RC, Klaver CC, Ramrattan RS, et al. Genetic risk of primary open-angle glaucoma. Population-based familial aggregation study. Arch Ophthalmol 1998;116:1640.
14. Mitchell P, Hourihan F, Sandbach J, et al. The relationship between glaucoma and myopia: the Blue Mountains Eye Study. Ophthalmol 1999;106:2010.
15. Garbe E, LeLorier J, Boivin JF, et al. Inhaled and nasal glucocorticoids and the risks of ocular hypertension or open-angle glaucoma. JAMA 1997;277:722.
16. Mitchell P, Cumming RG, Mackey DA. Inhaled corticosteroids, family history, and risk of glaucoma. Ophthalmol 1999;106:2301.
17. Quigley HA. Identification of glaucoma-related visual field abnormality with the screening protocol of frequency doubling technology. Am J Ophthalmol 1998;125:819.
18. Patel SC, Friedman DS, Varadkar P, et al. Algorithm for interpreting the results of frequency doubling perimetry. Am J Ophthalmol 2000;129:323.
19. The AGIS Investigators. The advanced glaucoma intervention study (AGIS). 7. The relationship between control of intraocular pressure and visual field deterioration. Am J Ophthalmol 2000;130:429.
20. Kass MA, Heuer DK, Higginbotham EJ, et al. The Ocular Hypertension Treatment Study: a randomized trial determines that topical ocular hypotensive medication delays or prevents the onset of primary open-angle glaucoma. Arch Ophthalmol 2002;120:701.
21. Wollstein G, Garway-Heath DF, Fontana L, et al. Identifying early glaucomatous changes. Comparison between expert clinical assessment of optic disc photographs and confocal scanning ophthalmoscopy. Ophthalmol 2000;107:2272.
22. Gordon MO, Beiser JA, Brandt JD, et al. The Ocular Hypertension Treatment Study: baseline factors that predict the onset of primary open-angle glaucoma. Arch Ophthalmol 2002; 120:714.
23. Diggory P, Heyworth P, Chau G, et al. Unsuspected bronchospasm in association with topical timolol—a common problem in elderly people: can we easily identify those affected and do cardioselective agents lead to improvement? Age Ageing 1994;23:17.
24. Anonymous. The advanced glaucoma intervention study (AGIS). 4. Comparison of treatment outcomes within race. Ophthalmol 1998;105:1146.
25. Glaucoma Laser Trial Research Group. The Glaucoma Laser Trial (GLT) and glaucoma laser trial follow-up study. Am J Ophthalmol 1995; 120:718.

*For annotated **General References** and resources related to this chapter, visit www.hopkinsbayview.org/PAMreferences.*

Chapter 109

Diseases of the Eyelid, Conjunctiva, and Anterior Segment of the Eye

Robert S. Weinberg

Patients with eye problems often present for care initially to their primary care provider. It is important, therefore, to recognize the nature and severity of a patient's ocular complaint and to formulate a logical approach to the evaluation and treatment. A few problems require urgent ophthalmic attention, but many may be initially managed by the primary care provider.

With a systematic approach to the patient, beginning with the history and proceeding with examination of the parts of the eye suggested by the history, one should be able to recognize what external ocular problems may be safely managed. When referral to an ophthalmologist is indicated, one should understand whether that referral should be on an emergent, urgent, or routine basis and what should be expected from the consultation.

Often, discussions about eye problems for the generalist center around the *red eye,* a dramatic presentation, frequently causing a patient to seek medical attention. Although the approach to the red eye is covered in this chapter, it is only one of many presenting complaints.

APPROACH TO THE PATIENT

Even with a problem that appears limited to the eye and the visual system, obtaining an accurate history is most important in suggesting a diagnosis. History should include information about the duration and severity, whether or not there is any perceived change in vision, and whether the problem is unilateral or bilateral. Other complaints peculiar to the eye include photophobia, pain or foreign body sensation, and redness or discharge. The time of day that symptoms occur may be important because some conditions are worse on awakening whereas others worsen as the day progresses. Because there is a relationship between skin disease and eye disease, awareness of a previously diagnosed dermatologic problem such as acne rosacea or atopic dermatitis is important. Because there is a perception by lay people that eye drops are not medicines and because some eye preparations are available over the counter (OTC), one should ask the patient if they have tried to care for the problem using drops or ointments. Also, patients may not make the connection of current symptoms with recent or past ocular surgery, and therefore this history must be solicited. Because patients who wear contact lenses, even occasionally, may have specific related problems, that history too should be obtained.

EXAMINATION AND ANATOMY

All conditions discussed in this chapter involve the parts of the eye visible with normal room illumination or with the aid of a flashlight and without additional magnification. Figure 109.1 shows the pertinent anatomy of those parts of the anterior segment of the eye visible with room illumination or with a handheld light.

Visual Acuity

Examination of the eye should always begin with a measurement of visual acuity. This should be done one eye at a time and with glasses, if the patient wears them. Although an eye chart may be used, simply having the patient cover one eye at a time and look at an object in the examination room will provide information about whether or not there is any subjective difference in vision between the two eyes. If the perceived change is new, ophthalmology referral is indicated without regard to the cause of the problem.

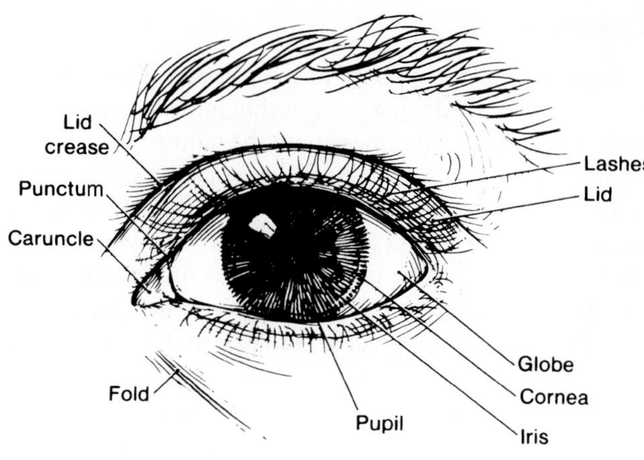

FIGURE 109.1. External landmarks of the eye.

Systematic Examination of the External Eye

The examiner should begin the evaluation by judging the patient's face for redness, scaling dermatoses, or telangiectasias on the cheeks, nose, and eyelids. Examination of the *eyelids* begins with an assessment of the position of the lids. Asymmetry of lid position, either ptosis or lid retraction, may suggest an orbital abnormality, such as thyroid ophthalmopathy. Periorbital edema, or swelling of the lids, may be present. The lids should be examined for lesions distorting the normal contour. Normal *eyelashes* are roughly parallel and of equal length, with none missing or broken and without discharge. Even without the aid of a slit lamp, the *tear film* is visible as a thin layer of liquid above the lower eyelid. Quantitative measurement of the tear film, *Schirmer test,* usually done by an ophthalmologist, can confirm an impression of dry eye or tear dysfunction. Even without a Schirmer test, close inspection of the external eye can provide an indication of a dry eye. Alternatively, tearing, or *epiphora,* may in itself be a presenting complaint or a secondary sign of ocular inflammation.

The space between the upper and lower eyelids when the eye is open is the *palpebral fissure*. The *conjunctiva* is the mucous membrane lining the eyelids and covering the globe. The normal conjunctiva is lustrous, secondary to the moisture of the tear film. Small conjunctival vessels are present. Although the conjunctiva appears white, it is actually translucent, with the white color that of the underlying sclera. The *episclera* is vascularized connective tissue deep to the conjunctiva and superficial to the sclera. The *sclera,* relatively rigid connective tissue, is normally white to pale yellow in color. The sclera begins at the limbus, the peripheral margin of the cornea, and extends posteriorly to the optic nerve. Areas of scleral thinning or translucency may be seen normally within the palpebral fissure, anterior to the insertions of the horizontal rectus muscles. The *cornea* is thin, 500 to 600 μm, and transparent. The normal cornea is 11 mm in diameter. The *anterior chamber* is the optically clear space, filled with aqueous humor, between the cornea and the iris. Anterior chamber depth may be approximated by shining a hand light at the lateral limbus. If a shadow is seen on the nasal iris, the anterior chamber is shallow (see Chapter 108). The *iris* is a vascular pigmented structure, which is referred to when describing the color of the eye. Iris color is variable, and focal areas of hyperpigmentation, iris nevi, are common.

SKIN AND EYE

The patient with a chronic skin disease may present with ocular complaints of itching or scaling associated with that dermatologic disorder. The patient with an acute skin disease may seek medical attention because of dermatitis involving the eyelids or periorbital area. Pain can be the presenting complaint of herpes zoster ophthalmicus, even before the development of cutaneous vesicles. Redness of the eye may be secondary to eyelid disease. Examination of the eyes should begin with a general observation of the skin of the face. Special attention should be given to the eyelids and eyelashes.

Scaling Dermatoses and Atopic Dermatitis

Patients complain of itching but may have pain if there is associated bacterial blepharitis. Examination usually reveals scaling and redness of the eyelids. Patients with atopic dermatitis may have a combination of staphylococcal blepharitis and herpes simplex blepharitis or keratitis. Atopic dermatitis is one of the few diseases associated with bilateral herpes simplex keratitis (1).

Seborrheic dermatitis is extremely common. In addition to dandruff, there may be scaling of the nose and face and eyelids. Redness of the eyes and morning discharge often occurs. Seborrheic blepharitis with oily debris along the eyelid margin, scurf, is a sign of seborrheic blepharitis (Fig. 109.2, Color Plate section).

Acne rosacea is a common cause of ocular problems. Ocular problems may actually be the presenting complaint for a patient with acne rosacea. A sty in an adult should prompt one to consider that that patient may have acne rosacea. Early in the course of acne rosacea, telangiectases on the cheeks and nose and eyelids may be difficult to see without magnification, perhaps the reason that an ophthalmologist, with the aid of a slit-lamp instrument, may suggest the diagnosis in an early stage (Fig. 109.3, Color Plate section).

Herpes zoster may affect any dermatome. Between 9% and 16% of patients with herpes zoster have involvement of the skin innervated by the trigeminal nerve (2). Unilateral headache or eye pain may be the presenting complaint, hours to days before vesicles appear. Ocular involvement may be in the form of blepharitis, with swelling of the eyelids and vesicles on the skin, or as acute uveitis, with blurred vision, pain, redness, and photophobia (Fig. 109.4, Color Plate section).

Management

When a patient with an acute or chronic skin problem complains of eye problems, whether it is itching, discharge, or pain, urgent referral to an ophthalmologist is appropriate.

EYELIDS

Disorders of the eyelids are a frequent cause of ocular problems. Patients complain of redness of the eyes, with discharge and discomfort, but no change in vision. Blepharitis, inflammation of the eyelids, causes discharge, which tends to be worse in the morning upon awakening.

History

Eyelid disorders tend to become chronic. Symptoms often are worse in the morning upon awakening. If there is discharge, noting that the discharge occurs in the morning should strongly suggest the diagnosis of blepharitis.

Examination

Patients with blepharitis may notice redness of the eyes, with conjunctival injection secondary to inflammation of the eyelids. Redness of the eyes can be caused by irritation from the discharge on the eyelids or from changes in the tear film, associated with meibomian gland congestion. When there is meibomian gland congestion in blepharitis, there is less oil in the tear film, allowing for more rapid evaporation of the aqueous component of the tears and causing dryness of the eye. Tear dysfunction with an abnormality of the tear film occurs frequently in patients with blepharitis. Eyelid swelling and ptosis also may be present.

Abnormalities in *eyelid position* may present with redness of the eye or foreign body sensation. Normally, the eyelid margin touches the globe. Ectropion, outward turning of the lid margin, is associated with exposure of the tarsal conjunctiva, and may be accompanied by incomplete eyelid closure. Eyelids with ectropion appear red. Entropion, inward turning of the lid margin, is associated with redness and foreign body sensation. When the lid margin turns in, eyelashes may rub against the eye. Both ectropion and entropion may be cicatricial, secondary most commonly to a thermal or chemical burn, or may be secondary to age-related decreases in eyelid skin elasticity. Both entropion and ectropion should be evaluated and managed by an ophthalmologist.

Eyelashes

Examination of the eyelashes can be done with room illumination or with the use of a flashlight. Attention to the eyelashes may provide clues about the nature of a patient's ocular complaints. Normally, the lashes are roughly equal in length and have a uniform distribution, with no areas of the lid margin devoid of lashes. A history of loss of lashes, sparse lashes, or discharge on the lashes suggests blepharitis. Inwardly directed lashes, trichiasis, can be a cause of foreign body sensation, corneal irritation, and redness of the eye.

Edema

Systemic diseases may cause swelling of the eyelids. Patients with thyroid dysfunction can have eyelid swelling. Because the skin of the lids is especially thin, conditions with fluid retention, such as congestive heart failure or renal failure, may cause fluid to be retained in the eyelids. Allergic conjunctivitis (see Table 109.3) is frequently associated with eyelid swelling.

Blepharitis

Blepharitis may be infectious or noninfectious. Infectious blepharitis is common and most frequently caused by coagulase-negative staphylococcal species. *Staphylococcus aureus* is perhaps the next most common bacterial cause of blepharitis. Other bacteria, such as *Streptococcus* species, and various gram-negative organisms, such as *Pseudomonas* species, *Klebsiella pneumonia,* and *Escherichia coli,* may also cause blepharitis. Specific signs in blepharitis caused by staphylococcal species include lid margin ulcerations, broken and missing eyelashes, and collarettes or fibrin on the base of lashes (Fig. 109.5, Color Plate section).

Seborrheic blepharitis, associated with seborrheic dermatitis, causes oily debris, scurf, on the eyelid margins. Mixed blepharitis refers to the simultaneous coexistence of staphylococcal blepharitis and seborrheic blepharitis. Viral blepharitis is less common than bacterial blepharitis but presents with vesicles on the eyelids (Fig. 109.6, Color Plate section). Herpes zoster and herpes simplex both can cause viral blepharitis. In the past, vaccinia vesicular dermatitis after smallpox vaccination was a more frequent cause of viral blepharitis, with inoculation of the eyelids by a patient's hands touching their recent smallpox vaccination site. Parasitic blepharitis occurs most commonly associated with infection by *Phthirus pubis.* Pubic hair and eyelashes are strong enough and far enough apart to allow the parasites to grow (Fig. 109.7, Color Plate section). Patients with parasitic blepharitis complain of itching of the eyes. Adult lice and nits are visible on the eyelashes.

The lid margins, surrounding skin, conjunctiva, and cornea may be involved singly or collectively. The skin may also show changes of seborrheic dermatitis or it may be excoriated and macerated, especially at the lateral canthus. Crusting is noted at the bases of the eyelashes. The conjunctiva may show changes of papillary hyperplasia (multiple conjunctival mounds with a central single vessel). Corneal changes occur after months of inflammation and are manifest as fine discrete peripheral defects. There may also be ulceration, clouding, and vascularization of the margins of the cornea. The diagnosis of conjunctival involvement in blepharitis is made by examination and, in cases in doubt, by scraping the conjunctivae and the margins of the eyelids and by culturing the exudate.

Treatment should be continued for at least 3 weeks. Daily cleansing of the eyelashes with a neutral soap (e.g., dilute Johnson's Baby Shampoo) followed by the application of an antibiotic ointment (erythromycin, bacitracin, or sulfacetamide) to the eyelashes at bedtime for several weeks reduces the bacterial count, cleanses the lids, and minimizes recurrences. Patients with blepharitis are often best served by an ophthalmologist to guide their long-term management.

Hordeolum

A hordeolum (Fig. 109.3, Color Plate section) is a common infection in the glands of the eyelid caused by *S. aureus*. It is characterized by the sudden onset of localized pain, swelling, redness, and often purulent discharge. The infected gland may be a meibomian gland just under the conjunctival side of the eyelid, and this is called an *internal hordeolum*. An internal hordeolum may be large and may point to either the skin or the conjunctival side of the lid. Also, a smaller gland associated with an eyelash follicle under the skin side of the lid may be infected, and this is called an *external hordeolum* or *sty*. A sty usually is smaller than an internal hordeolum but is easily recognized in that it always points to the skin side of the lid.

The differential diagnosis includes tumors of the lid margin (see Lid Margin Tumors section) and other localized inflammatory lesions of the eyelid, such as *Molluscum contagiosum* or herpes simplex, before vesicles develop. Patients with sties or hordeola have blepharitis, so the history of morning discharge and redness and the observation of irregular, missing, or broken eyelashes supports the diagnosis. Many adult patients have acne rosacea with blepharitis and develop recurrent sties.

Management should not only be aimed at treating the acute problem, the hordeolum, but also at handling the pre-existing chronic problem, the blepharitis. Both types of hordeolum may be treated without obtaining a culture. Initial management consists of hot compresses, applied for 5 minutes or more at least two to four times a day, and topical ophthalmic antibiotic ointment, such as erythromycin, bacitracin, or sulfacetamide 10%, applied at bedtime. Systemic antibiotics are not indicated, unless there is evidence of cellulitis. Because most hordeola resolve with conservative management, and to avoid initiating increased inflammation, incision and drainage by the ophthalmologist is generally not done for 3 or more weeks.

Chalazion

A chalazion is a sterile lipogranulomatous inflammation of a meibomian gland secondary to chronic inflammation (Fig. 109.8, Color Plate section). A chalazion can develop from an internal hordeolum that does not resolve. The swelling may appear anywhere on the eyelid (although the upper lid is a more common location), and it usually points toward the conjunctival side. Chalazia are frequently seen in patients with acne rosacea. The presence of blepharitis, with or without acne rosacea, confirms the diagnosis. The differential diagnosis includes various lid margin tumors. However, these are rare, whereas chalazia are common. A chalazion is not painful but may cause discomfort or a feeling of fullness in the lid. Visual acuity may rarely be affected if the chalazion is large enough to cause pressure on the cornea and induce astigmatism. Some chalazia do resolve over periods of months. Incision and drainage by the ophthalmologist is frequently recommended if the patient is not willing to wait for the possibility of gradual slow resorption over time. Therefore, an ophthalmologist should be consulted if there is doubt about the diagnosis or treatment.

Lid Margin Tumors

Sties and chalazia are very common, but they must be differentiated from lid margin tumors, which occur rarely. Lid margin tumors are usually slow growing, not painful, and not associated with underlying blepharitis. Chronic irritation of the eye with redness may be caused by lid margin tumors, which prevent complete lid closure. Both squamous and basal cell carcinomas can occur on the eyelids, as can malignant melanomas. Patients suspected of such lesions should be referred to an ophthalmologist.

THE DRY EYE AND TEAR DYSFUNCTION

The *tear film* provides nutrition and protection to the cornea and the conjunctiva. The terms "dry eye," decreased tear production, and keratitis sicca are synonymous but are more appropriately included in the term *tear dysfunction*. Tear dysfunction is a frequent cause of chronically red eyes.

The tear film consists of three layers. The outer layer of the tear film, the oily layer, is produced by the oil glands of the lids and serves to prevent evaporation of the aqueous layer. Patients with acne rosacea may have rapid evaporation of tears because the oily secretions of the meibomian glands are so viscous that there is insufficient oil in the tear film. The middle layer of the tear film, the aqueous layer, is produced by the lacrimal gland and accessory lacrimal glands. The aqueous layer of the tear film provides oxygen to the cornea. The inner layer of the tear film, the mucous layer, is produced by the goblet cells of the conjunctiva. The mucous layer allows the aqueous layer of the tear film to adhere to the cornea. Although patients with red eyes may have problems with any layer of the tear film, the term "dry eye" generally refers to a decrease in the aqueous component of the tear film. The term "tear dysfunction" means an abnormality of the tear film, whether causing rapid evaporation, insufficient mucus, or inadequate aqueous production in patients with, as examples, acne rosacea, pemphigoid, or a connective tissue disorder, respectively.

History

Patients with tear dysfunction usually have complaints of redness and burning, itching and foreign body sensation, or blurring and decreased vision. The redness and most other complaints associated with decreased tear production are generally worse as the day progresses, with normal activity allowing progressive evaporation of tears and more and more drying. Symptoms in patients with tear dysfunction tend to be less on awakening, because the eyes have been closed during sleep and drying does not occur when the eyes are closed.

Examination

Although it is easy for an ophthalmologist to assess the status of the tear film with the use of fluorescein staining and slit-lamp biomicroscopy, close inspection of the tear meniscus, the layer of tears above the lower lid margin, can be done with flashlight illumination. A layer of moisture, approximately 1 to 2 mm high, is normally visible above the lower lid. The normally lustrous cornea often appears dull or with certainly less luster in a patient who has dry eyes.

Causes

Ocular conditions that cause tear dysfunction include blepharitis; acne rosacea; exophthalmos (with decreased blinking and a larger area from which tears can evaporate); and cicatrizing conjunctivitis (such as that seen with chemical burns), Stevens-Johnson syndrome, or mucous membrane pemphigoid (with loss of normal goblet cells).

Many patients have tear dysfunction as part of a *systemic disease*. Sjögren syndrome with an associated dry mouth and dry eye is frequently seen with connective tissue disease or sarcoidosis.

Both *topical and systemic medications* may alter tear production. Among the most commonly used medications that can cause tear dysfunction are β-blockers, diuretics, and some psychoactive drugs.

Management

Although the initial treatment of tear dysfunction may simply involve the frequent use of artificial tears, routine nonurgent referral to an ophthalmologist often is indicated because of the chronic and often therapeutically frustrating nature of this problem. If systemic medications are implicated in causation of tear dysfunction, selection of medications that do not cause dry eye may be advisable.

Topical cyclosporine 0.05% is approved for treating the inflammation associated with tear dysfunction. Topical cyclosporine, used twice daily, can improve ocular comfort, but patients should be advised that it may take 3 to 6 weeks for an effect to be noted. These drops may burn initially. Artificial tears should be continued with topical cyclosporine, but may be needed less often after topical cyclosporine is used.

CONJUNCTIVA

The conjunctiva is a mucous membrane, which is the inner lining of the eyelids (palpebral conjunctiva), and the outer coating of the globe (bulbar conjunctiva).

History

Patients with conjunctival disease complain of redness and usually discharge. There may also be irritation or foreign body sensation, but there is no pain (unless severe, e.g., in hyperacute forms, see Hyperacute Bacterial Conjunctivitis) nor change in vision with isolated conjunctivitis.

Examination

Normally, the conjunctiva is translucent, allowing the *color* of the underlying white or off-white color of the sclera to be seen. Yellow coloration of the conjunctiva is seen in patients with jaundice or in patients who have had a subconjunctival hemorrhage in which the blood is being resorbed. The conjunctiva is normally lustrous, shiny, and reflecting light. Decreased conjunctival *luster* can be a sign of a dry eye and may be seen in patients with tear dysfunction, conjunctival cicatrization, or vitamin A deficiency. Hyperemia of the conjunctiva has many causes such as polycythemia, acne rosacea, and conditions with venous obstruction (superior vena cava syndrome), as well as conjunctivitis.

Conjunctivitis

The diagnosis and management of conjunctivitis can be confusing, considering the variety of ocular infections. Conjunctivitis is usually not painful, but often there is mild discomfort, burning, discharge, tearing, itching, and lid swelling. Vision is well preserved. Conjunctivitis tends to cause diffuse conjunctival redness; it is usually bilateral but may present initially in one eye. Examination of the conjunctiva with a flashlight will show if a discharge is present.

Most instances of conjunctivitis in adults are not emergencies, and often they are self-limited. However, conjunctivitis may lead to serious complications such as corneal scarring, lid damage, or, in cases in which the patient has had previous glaucoma filtration surgery, endophthalmitis. If a conjunctival filtering bleb is present, indicating successful filtration surgery, bacteria may enter the eye through that scleral opening. In the normal eye, an intact sclera prevents access of bacteria to the vitreous of the eye.

Conjunctival Flora

Under normal conditions the conjunctival sac has a bacterial flora composed of several species. The most commonly encountered organism is *S. albus,* followed by corynebacteria, *S. aureus,* and *Streptococcus* species. Some normal patients harbor *Pseudomonas* species and fungi. This complex flora complicates the establishment of a specific cause in a patient with infectious conjunctivitis and is the reason that routine culture of the conjunctival discharge is not recommended.

Laboratory Diagnosis

Occasionally, there may be doubt about the diagnosis of conjunctivitis. In this uncommon situation, a simple culture or staining by the laboratory of the conjunctival material helps in determining the cause and subsequent management of the condition. The eyes and conjunctivae are not sterile, and organisms, even pathogens, may be cultured from normal subjects (see Conjunctival Flora). A positive culture does not necessarily mean there is a clinical infection. Most often, however, an adequate diagnosis can be made from the appearance of the conjunctiva, and a culture is unnecessary. Immunologic tests are available and permit immediate diagnosis of some causes of infectious conjunctivitis, especially chlamydia. The availability of these tests varies from community to community. Therefore, one not familiar with their use should consult an ophthalmologist for a recommendation.

In the occasional instance that culture is initiated, specimens should be obtained with a sterile swab by everting the eyelid and wiping the conjunctival sac. This material should be obtained without topical anesthesia because the preservatives in the anesthetic solution inhibit the growth of organisms. The specimen must be transferred immediately into transport media or delivered immediately to the laboratory for culturing. Each eye should be cultured separately, even if there is only monocular involvement, so that the apparently uninfected eye provides information about the nature of the normal flora.

TABLE 109.1 Diagnosis Based on Cells in Material Scraped from Conjunctiva

Cells	*Significance*
Polymorphonuclear leukocytes	Bacterial, fungal, chlamydial (inclusion conjunctivitis), trachoma, Stevens-Johnson syndrome
Mononuclear cells	Viral
Eosinophils	Allergy, ocular pemphigoid
Epithelial metaplasia (atypical, large cells)	*Chlamydia,* herpes simplex

Scraping is recommended in the evaluation of patients with conjunctivitis only when the diagnosis is uncertain. Referral to an ophthalmologist in situations in which scrapings are considered is recommended if one is not experienced in this technique.

After culture (if done), a topical anesthetic (e.g., proparacaine [Ophthaine]) should be instilled, and scrapings of the conjunctiva, well away from the cornea, should be obtained. A sterile platinum spatula (available from medical supply stores) or the dull side of a sterile scalpel blade can be used to scrape the conjunctiva. The material obtained by this method is smeared on a glass slide and sent to the laboratory to be stained with Gram or Giemsa stain. The appearance of the cells found in these scrapings is helpful in determining the diagnosis. Table 109.1 lists the differential findings, which are also discussed in the following sections below.

Hyperacute Bacterial Conjunctivitis

The name of this condition reflects its onset and the very thick exudate associated with it (Fig. 109.9, Color Plate section). Typically, the discharge is so copious that it accumulates in the lashes or runs down the patient's cheek. One eye is usually involved before the other, but within several days the second eye becomes involved through autoinoculation. The infection quickly involves the surrounding structures and is associated with aching discomfort, swelling of the lid, and tenderness of the eye. Enlarged preauricular lymph nodes are often present. Early in the course of the infection the cornea is not involved, but as the conjunctival swelling and tissue reaction increase, a peripheral corneal ring ulcer may develop because of compression of the peripheral corneal circulation.

Neisseria gonorrhoeae or *N. meningitidis* is usually implicated in this hyperacute form of infection. Inoculation is a result of spread by autoinoculation from infected genitalia. The gonococcus has the ability to penetrate the intact corneal epithelium, so central corneal ulceration and endophthalmitis may also occur. Meningococcal conjunctivitis is indistinguishable from gonococcal conjunctivitis, although the former occurs more often in younger patients, may be bilateral at the onset, and can proceed to metastatic meningitis or meningococcemia.

If needed in establishing the diagnosis of hyperacute conjunctivitis, conjunctival scrapings reveal an overwhelming number of polymorphonuclear leukocytes and intracellular gram-negative diplococci. Culture should be obtained on Thayer-Martin selective medium or should be sent to the laboratory on Transgrow medium. The differentiation between gonococcus and meningococcus requires special bacteriologic studies.

Therapy of hyperacute conjunctivitis must be prompt to avoid corneal damage or systemic spread and should include the administration of both systemic and topical antibiotics. Because of the seriousness of this condition, an ophthalmologist should be consulted immediately. Institution of appropriate antibiotics by the ophthalmologist should result in the disappearance of the discharge within 24 to 48 hours, although lid swelling and conjunctival reaction do not abate for several days. If a corneal ulcer occurs, it takes time, often weeks, to heal; if the cornea has been scarred, visual acuity may be affected. In rare cases endophthalmitis may occur, and blindness is possible.

Acute Bacterial Conjunctivitis

Acute bacterial conjunctivitis, like hyperacute bacterial conjunctivitis, has an abrupt onset but is characterized by a less thick often mucopurulent discharge. This form of conjunctivitis is often called catarrh or *pink eye* (Fig. 109.10, Color Plate section); it is seen at all ages and at any time of year. Pink eye is a nonspecific term applied to almost any minor infectious conjunctivitis, especially bacterial and viral forms. The most common cause of bacterial conjunctivitis is *S. aureus* infection. *Pneumococcus* and *Haemophilus* species also cause the problem, but infections with these organisms have a more restricted geographic distribution than do staphylococcal infections; pneumococcal infections occur primarily in the northern states during the colder months, and *Haemophilus infections* occur more commonly in the warmer regions of the United States throughout the year. Also, pneumococcal or *Haemophilus conjunctivitis* is more common in younger patients than is staphylococcal conjunctivitis. Rarely, other bacteria, such as *Moraxella lacunata, Escherichia coli,* or *Proteus* species, cause this form of conjunctivitis.

Patients complain of eye irritation and watering, and typically the eyelids stick together after sleep. The infection starts unilaterally, but very often, because of autoinoculation, the contralateral eye becomes involved in 1 or 2 days. Examination reveals hyperemia of the palpebral conjunctiva; bulbar conjunctival petechiae, characteristic of *Haemophilus* infection, may be seen.

Acute bacterial conjunctivitis is usually self-limited and generally lasts 7 to 14 days, although *Haemophilus* infections may last somewhat longer. The diagnosis is suspected by the examination; however, with the unusual situation of doubt, the diagnosis could be confirmed by examination of the scrapings of the conjunctiva and by culturing the exudate.

Topical treatment usually results in the resolution of symptoms in a day or two. A number of effective topical antibiotics are available, and one should be used for 5 to 6 days. Sodium sulfacetamide (Sulamyd-10%)—either the solution (two drops in the eye every 3 hours while awake) or the ointment (a small amount applied to the lower conjunctival sac four times a day and at bedtime)—is generally satisfactory. If there is an allergy to sulfa drugs, erythromycin or bacitracin ophthalmic ointment, or a topical fluoroquinolone solution, four times a day and at bedtime may be used. Topical aminoglycosides occasionally may be indicated for a specific infection, but they may cause redness, irritation, and *conjunctivitis medicamentosa.* Therefore, topical aminoglycosides should be limited and generally left to an ophthalmologist to prescribe. Cool compresses several times a day may provide comfort and diminish matting.

Chronic Bacterial Conjunctivitis

S. aureus causes most cases of chronic bacterial conjunctivitis, but occasionally it is caused by other agents, such as *S. epidermidis, Moraxella lacunata, Corynebacterium diphtheriae,* or *Streptococcus pyogenes. S. aureus* colonizes the margin of the eyelid and the follicles containing the eyelashes. Both *S. aureus* and *S. epidermidis* elaborate an exotoxin that injures the conjunctiva and cornea, and this toxin is responsible for the chronic inflammation.

Patients with chronic bacterial conjunctivitis complain of a sensation of a foreign body in the eye and redness and itching; often eyelids stick together after sleep. There is often a history of recurrent styes (see Hordeolum and Chalazion sections) and loss of eyelashes. Examination shows erythema of the lid margin, and sometimes a minimal exudate is present. Occasionally, mucous strands may be found in the conjunctival fornices (the space between the bulbar and palpebral conjunctiva), and the eyelids may appear thickened and red.

The lid margins, surrounding skin, conjunctiva, and cornea may be involved singularly or collectively. The skin may also show changes of seborrheic dermatitis or it may be excoriated and macerated, especially at the lateral canthal margin. Crusting is noted at the bases of the eyelashes. The conjunctiva may show changes of papillary hyperplasia (multiple conjunctival mounds with a central single vessel). Corneal changes occur after months of inflammation and are manifest as fine discrete peripheral defects. There may also be ulceration, clouding, and vascularization of the margins of the cornea. The diagnosis is made by examination and, in the occasional situation of doubt, by scraping the conjunctivae and the margins of the eyelids and by culturing the exudate or by referring the patient to an ophthalmologist.

Usually, a topical fluoroquinolone or sulfacetamide, one or two drops or a small amount of ointment every 4 hours while awake, or erythromycin ointment every 4 hours while awake, is effective. Treatment should be continued for 2 weeks. Daily cleansing of the eyelashes with a neutral soap (e.g., Johnson's Baby Shampoo) followed by the application of the topical reduces the bacterial count, cleanses the lids, and minimizes recurrences.

Viral Conjunctivitis

Viral conjunctivitis, also known as acute follicular conjunctivitis, is common. It is caused by a variety of agents. The onset is abrupt and unilateral, but contralateral involvement in a day or 2 from autoinoculation is very common. Excessive tearing is often the major complaint, and there is no purulent discharge. The conjunctiva nearly always shows hyperemia, which may be diffuse or segmental (Fig. 109.11, Color Plate section). Viral conjunctivitis may be accompanied by tender preauricular lymphadenopathy. Often, the lymphoid tissue of the eyelid becomes edematous in response to the infection and may appear as elevated palpebral and bulbar conjunctival lesions. When there is doubt about the diagnosis, examination of the conjunctival scrapings shows mononuclear cells. Viral cultures are expensive but are occasionally used by ophthalmologists in special circumstances.

The disease is self-limited, lasting usually less than one week, and treatment is therefore supportive. Vasoconstrictive drops (two drops four times a day for a few days) containing naphazoline (e.g., over the counter agents Albalon, Naphcon-A, or Vasocon-A) are helpful in relieving conjunctival congestion and hyperemia, and cool compresses as needed also provide relief. Sulfacetamide (Sulamyd) or erythromycin (Ilotycin), as described above, may be used if symptoms have not been controlled in a few days with topical vasoconstrictive drops; in this instance bacterial conjunctivitis may have developed.

Rarely, corneal inflammation may develop and cause an opacity in the cornea. When corneal opacification is noted, an ophthalmologist should be consulted urgently because loss of vision may occur. Some types of viral conjunctivitis *(epidemic keratoconjunctivitis)* are highly contagious. The examiner should take care not to become infected or to infect other patients; all instruments should be cleansed, and thorough hand washing is critical. The family should be instructed that disease transmission is via tear droplets, so towels and washcloths should not be shared. Because epidemic keratoconjunctivitis is so contagious, the patient should stay away, for about 10 to 12 days, from school or jobs where individuals are aggregated in one space. Often referral to an ophthalmologist is appropriate if there is doubt about the diagnosis or if there is concern about the spread of the disease to others.

Inclusion Conjunctivitis

Inclusion conjunctivitis (inclusion blennorrhea) is common in sexually active young adults. The disease is caused by a species of *Chlamydia* and is a result of contamination of the eye from the urethra after a sexual contact.

The problem is usually characterized by the abrupt onset of ocular discomfort, with varying degrees of diffuse conjunctival hyperemia and sometimes mucopurulent discharge that may result in matting of the eyelashes. The eyelids appear swollen, and inspection of the palpebral conjunctiva, especially of the lower lid, shows many small follicles (raised pale mounds of varying size) (Fig. 109.12, Color Plate section). Occasionally, preauricular lymphadenopathy develops. Without treatment, the disease becomes chronic and remitting, and in 2 or 3 weeks a superficial corneal inflammation (keratitis) may appear. This may be identified with the naked eye as dots or cloudy streaks on the superior portion of the cornea. Also at this stage, there may be an associated iritis manifested by photophobia and blurring of vision.

This syndrome may occur in association with urethritis in men or with cervicitis and a vaginal discharge in women. Most often, however, there are no genitourinary symptoms, although *Chlamydia* species can be cultured from the urethra in men or the endocervical canal in women. Highly specific and sensitive tests for the detection of *Chlamydia* (see Chapter 37) are available commercially, and these appear to be diagnostic in patients with conjunctivitis. In some cases, reactive arthritis is present (see Chapter 78).

The diagnosis is suggested by the history and appearance, but if there is doubt it may be confirmed by the direct slide test of the conjunctiva or examination of the material obtained from conjunctival scraping. This material, when stained by the laboratory with Giemsa stain, shows large basophilic cytoplasmic inclusion bodies. Gram stain does not reveal these bodies but shows many polymorphonuclear leukocytes.

Therapy is effective but must be systemic. Oral tetracycline, 250 mg four times daily for 21 days, is the preferable regimen; when tetracycline cannot be given, good results may be achieved with erythromycin, 250 mg four times daily for 21 days, or trimethoprim– sulfamethoxazole (e.g., Bactrim DS or Septra DS), 1 tablet twice daily for 21 days. It may take several months for the follicular hyperplasia to resolve, but the patient should experience symptomatic improvement within several days. The application of cool compresses for 20 minutes several times a day also provides comfort in the first few days of treatment. Because this disease is difficult to diagnose, referral to an ophthalmologist is appropriate.

Because the disease must be assumed to be sexually transmitted, the sexual partner should be similarly treated. Other venereal diseases should be sought, and a condom should be used until therapy has been completed.

Allergic Conjunctivitis

Allergic conjunctivitis is a common and mild conjunctivitis often encountered in patients with allergic rhinitis (see Chapter 30). Often the patient describes a history of allergy to grasses, pollens, and other agents and usually complains of itching and tearing. Often, there is marked swelling of the conjunctiva and slight to moderate redness of the eye, and at times there is serous crusting in the morning.

When there is doubt about the diagnosis, conjunctival scrapings (see Table 109.1) may be examined. A finding of many eosinophils is diagnostic. When conjunctivitis is associated with allergic rhinitis, it usually parallels the rhinitis in severity and duration. When it occurs as an isolated problem, it is short-lived and treatment is symptomatic. An over the counter topical astringent solution (e.g., Albalon, Naphcon-A, or Vasocon-A, using one to two drops four times daily for 1 to 2 days) and cool compresses as needed are very effective. Occasionally, symptoms are severe, and oral antihistamines may relieve itching.

Topical antihistamine solutions (e.g., Naphcon-A, over the counter) and topical mast cell stabilizers (e.g., pemirolast [Alamast], which requires a prescription) are effective for chronic or seasonal allergic conjunctivitis. Corticosteroid eye drops (e.g., HMS Liquifilm or FML Liquifilm) are also very effective for this condition, but they must be used cautiously because their use is associated with corneal ulceration and perforation in the presence of herpes simplex infection, the development of fungal infection, and, when used chronically, the development in some patients of open-angle glaucoma and, rarely, cataract formation. For these reasons, topical corticosteroids are not recommended without at least a telephone consultation with an ophthalmologist.

Chemical Conjunctivitis

Many agents may enter the conjunctiva and produce inflammation. Irritation from such agents as smoke, smog, sprays, chlorinated water, hairspray, makeup, and industrial dust is common. The history of the exposure makes the diagnosis obvious. The patient should thoroughly rinse the conjunctival sac with water as soon as contamination with a chemical has occurred. The patient will also benefit from cool compresses for 15 to 20 minutes several times a day, and occasionally the use of an over-the-counter topical vasoconstrictor solution (Albalon, Naphcon-A, or Vasocon-A) as necessary.

Conjunctivitis medicamentosa is conjunctival injection secondary to use of eye drops, which may be irritating to the conjunctiva. This condition can occur usually after several days to weeks of instillation of almost any type of eye drop. Patients complain of redness, discomfort and tearing, or itching. Generally there is no discharge. The history of eye drop or ointment use is essential to establishing the diagnosis. Topical aminoglycosides and some antiglaucoma agents are frequent causes of conjunctivitis medicamentosa. Treatment consists of stopping the inciting agent and using artificial tears for comfort. Because either the preservative or the active ingredient of the eye drop may be the inciting agent, preservative-free artificial tears may be indicated.

In the case of an injury from an acid or alkali, serious permanent damage may occur, and this problem is a true ophthalmologic emergency. Patients should be advised to irrigate the conjunctival sac with copious amounts of water and to see an ophthalmologist immediately. If the patient presents first to the primary practitioner's office, irrigation should be repeated promptly and the patient should then be sent immediately to an ophthalmologist. Overirrigation may increase irritation slightly, but underirrigation may make blindness more likely. Therefore, when in doubt, one should always irrigate. Normal saline stings less than water, but one should use whatever is immediately available.

Subconjunctival Hemorrhage

The conjunctiva is thin and transparent. Subconjunctival hemorrhage is an accumulation of blood under the conjunctiva (Fig. 109.13, Color Plate section). Acutely, a subconjunctival hemorrhage presents as a localized, usually unilateral, bright red area within the palpebral fissure. Subconjunctival hemorrhages are not painful and do not affect vision. A patient may be unaware of a subconjunctival hemorrhage until looking in the mirror or until someone else notices that one eye is bright red. Subconjunctival hemorrhages may occur spontaneously, especially in older individuals with dry eyes, but can be associated with minor eye rubbing or trauma, or with Valsalva maneuver associated with straining at stool, vomiting, coughing, or sneezing. Subconjunctival hemorrhage may occur during uncomplicated eye surgery, especially if subconjunctival injections are given at the time of surgery. Anticoagulants may be associated with subconjunctival hemorrhages, especially if doses are excessive. Uncommonly, topical corticosteroid eye drops, which cause increased capillary fragility, can be a cause of subconjunctival hemorrhage.

Only rarely a subconjunctival hemorrhage may be indicative of a bleeding diathesis. Therefore, workup is generally not indicated unless there are signs of bleeding or easy bruisability elsewhere. There is no specific treatment. Artificial tears may be recommended if there is discomfort.

Pterygium and Scarring

A *pterygium* is localized fibrovascular tissue (Fig. 109.14, Color Plate section), which is most frequently present within the interpalpebral fissure, at the three or nine o'clock position. A pterygium begins with localized conjunctival swelling and is termed a *pinguecula* when it does not extend onto the cornea. Once fibrovascular tissue extends onto the cornea, the lesion is called a pterygium. Occasionally, both pinguecula and pterygia can become inflamed, causing local redness. There is no discharge or change in vision. Discomfort, if present, is minimal. Both pingueculae and pterygia are caused by chronic exposure to ultraviolet light. Long-term exposure to dust and wind may also be contributory. Acute conjunctival injection may be managed with lubrication with artificial tears. Rarely are topical anti-inflammatory agents necessary. Patients believed to have pterygia or pinguecula should be referred to an ophthalmologist for evaluation and continuing care.

Normally, there is no *scarring* of the conjunctiva. Conditions characterized by conjunctival cicatrization frequently present with shortening of the inferior fornix, seen as *symblepharon*, bands of scar tissue between the tarsal and bulbar conjunctiva. Such scarring can follow chemical conjunctivitis or Stevens-Johnson syndrome but may be the initial manifestation of mucous membrane pemphigoid, a systemic disease occurring in the elderly (see Chapter 117).

EPISCLERA AND EPISCLERITIS

The episclera is vascularized connective tissue deep to the conjunctiva and above the sclera. Normally, episcleral vessels are barely visible without the magnification of a slit-lamp biomicroscope.

Patients with episcleritis complain of the sudden or gradual onset of localized redness, with mild discomfort, but no change in vision. Although most patients with episcleritis have no underlying systemic disease, approximately 25% of patients do. Of these, connective tissue disease, rheumatoid arthritis, syndromes with human leukocyte antigen (HLA-B27) (ankylosing spondylitis, inflammatory bowel disease, reactive arthritis, and psoriatic arthritis), systemic lupus erythematosus (SLE), and polyarteritis are the most common. In the patient with inflammatory bowel disease, acute episcleritis may be a problem, which heralds a flare-up of the bowel inflammation. Patients with acne rosacea may have episcleritis. Gout is a rare cause of episcleritis.

Episcleritis is characterized by localized redness, usually of one eye. There is no discharge. Tenderness may be present, but discomfort is generally mild and pain unusual.

There are two main types of *episcleritis*: diffuse and nodular. Diffuse episcleritis is more common and less frequently associated with systemic disease. Nodular episcleritis is characterized by localized swelling on the surface of the eye (Fig. 109.15, Color Plate section). This form of episcleritis is usually associated with connective tissue disease and may be either an initial or a late manifestation.

Management

Patients with episcleritis generally should be referred to an ophthalmologist for confirmation of the diagnosis and to be certain that scleritis is not present (see next section). Episcleritis is not vision threatening. Because episcleritis tends to be self-limited, clearing spontaneously within 7 to 10 days, treatment may not be necessary. However, because episcleritis responds well to topical corticosteroid drops, they frequently are prescribed to shorten the course of the condition. The generalist in the care of patient's with episcleritis is usually focused on the search for a systemic cause for the condition.

SCLERA AND SCLERITIS

The sclera is connective tissue deep to the conjunctiva and episclera and external to the retina. Composed of interlaced collagen fibrils, the sclera is similar in structure to cartilage, begins at the periphery of the cornea (the limbus), and extends circumferentially to the optic nerve.

Scleritis is inflammation of the sclera, and it may be unilateral or bilateral. Scleritis characteristically causes severe pain. That pain may be interpreted by the patient as ocular, but a history of severe unilateral headache, accompanied by nausea and vomiting is not unusual. Scleritis should be considered in a patient who has headache, nausea, and vomiting, and redness of the eyes. There is no discharge, but there may be complaints of decreased vision, photophobia, and pain on eye movement.

Ocular redness in scleritis may be diffuse or localized and unilateral or bilateral (Fig. 109.16, Color Plate section). The redness is darker than the bright red color of an acute subconjunctival hemorrhage and generally darker than the redness of episcleritis. There is no discharge, but tearing may be copious. Differentiation from episcleritis can be difficult without the use of a slit-lamp biomicroscope. However, the instillation by an ophthalmologist of 2.5% phenylephrine hydrochloride ophthalmic solution can blanch vessels in most instances of episcleritis but has no effect on the redness in scleritis.

Approximately 75% of patients with scleritis have an associated systemic disease. Systemic causes of scleritis are similar to those of episcleritis. Rheumatoid arthritis is the most common.

Management

Because of the severity of the pain experienced by patients with scleritis, urgent referral to an ophthalmologist is indicated. The primary care provider plays an important role in directing the diagnostic search for an underlying systemic cause and in collaborating with the ophthalmologist in the medical management of the condition. The treatment of scleritis requires the use of systemic medications. Corticosteroids, frequently in high oral or intravenous doses, are the initial therapeutic choice. But for patients either unresponsive to high dose corticosteroids (doses greater than 60 to 80 mg/day of prednisone) or in whom high dose corticosteroids are contraindicated, oral cyclophosphamide (Cytoxan) is frequently necessary. Treatment of scleritis is aimed at control of pain and cessation of tissue destruction, and weeks or months of therapy may be necessary to control the disease. An ophthalmologist should be consulted urgently to confirm the diagnosis and help in the management.

CORNEA

The cornea normally is crystal clear, and it is highly innervated. Corneal disease causes decreased vision, pain, foreign body sensation, and redness. If the symptoms are acute, the differential diagnosis includes corneal abrasions, corneal foreign bodies, and corneal ulceration. *Corneal injury* is usually recognized easily because of intense pain localized to the cornea after trauma and because of identification of a corneal lesion. Hand light examination can demonstrate irregularity of the corneal surface and may show a foreign body, corneal opacity, or corneal edema.

If the injury is secondary to minor trauma (corneal abrasion) from a foreign body, the foreign body should be removed and a patch placed over the eye for 24 hours; the use of a topical antiprostaglandin agent without patching is also considered an acceptable treatment. On the other hand, if an extensive epithelial defect (as revealed by fluorescein staining) is present, urgent ophthalmologic referral is indicated.

Fluorescein staining is easily accomplished by moistening a sterile fluorescein strip in the lower conjunctival sac and waiting a moment for the fluorescein to diffuse into the tears. The epithelial defect stains a brilliant green. A penlight with a cobalt blue filter (e.g., Blu-Spot no. 2015, available from medical supply companies) is inexpensive and highlights fluorescein staining. Corneal ulcers also stain with fluorescein, but staining appears to be deeper, indicating subepithelial corneal involvement. Corneal ulceration can lead to blindness, and patients suspected of having this condition should see an ophthalmologist emergently.

Patients with *corneal abrasions* most often will provide a history of trauma. That trauma may be relatively minor, such as eye rubbing, or may be more severe, with a history of a scratch by a sharp object. Frequently, patients with corneal abrasions have difficulty keeping their eyes open and, in addition to redness of the involved eye, have copious tearing.

With a *corneal foreign body* there is a history of the sudden onset of severe sensation of an object in the eye, accompanied by tearing, redness, and blurred vision. There is often a history of working with tools, especially those that are power driven, but there may be a history of exposure to wind or a dusty environment.

Foreign bodies often lodge in the conjunctiva or cornea. Most often they can be visualized with the naked eye; if not, sterile fluorescein staining (see above) may outline an area of corneal epithelial damage. Foreign bodies may be removed by irrigation of the conjunctival sac with a sterile solution of physiologic saline or eyewash. If they are not rinsed away, mechanical removal is indicated. Embedded corneal foreign bodies should be removed by an ophthalmologist, because the depth of penetration of the foreign body into the cornea should be determined by slit-lamp biomicroscopy. If a foreign body is deeply embedded in the cornea, surgical removal may be indicated to allow for suturing of the entry site if there is a full thickness corneal penetration. Superficial corneal foreign bodies may be removed at the slit lamp biomicroscope, after placing in the eye a drop of topical anesthetic (e.g., Ophthaine) and removing the foreign body with a sterile needle.

A cotton swab should *not* be used to remove a foreign body from the cornea because often it is irritating to the structure and thus delays healing. If the foreign body is not on the cornea, removal is easier and usually does not require anesthesia. After removal, it is wise to instill an antibiotic (e.g., sulfacetamide 10% or bacitracin) and cover the eye with a patch for 24 hours. The eye patch should be applied tightly enough to prevent the eyelids from moving. If the patch falls off before the 24 hours, the patient should not try to reapply it because often this may cause more irritation. Recently, ophthalmologists have begun using patching for corneal abrasions less often so that the patient can still see with the injured eye. When the eye is not patched, a topical antiprostaglandin, such as diclofenac or ketorolac, may be used for a day or two for comfort.

If the offending material is a piece of metal, rust rings surrounding the area of the epithelial defect may be observed. These rings are not harmful; although they may lead to later inflammation, only the foreign body should be removed. In any instance when the foreign body is not easily removed or if symptoms persist beyond a day after removal of a foreign body, an ophthalmologist should see the patient urgently.

With *corneal ulcer,* often the patient who uses contact lenses will complain of the sudden onset of pain, redness, and discharge.

Corneal edema when acute is associated with blurred vision and conjunctival redness, sometimes associated with nausea and vomiting. This is usually caused by sudden and marked elevation of intraocular pressure. The edema is secondary to the aqueous humor being forced into the cornea. Angle-closure glaucoma is the usual cause; therefore, a positive family history, a past history of haloes around lights, and the presence of hyperopia or farsightedness often are present (see Chapter 108).

When there is a chronic history of blurred vision not accompanied by pain and associated with decreased corneal clarity, on examination there may be chronic corneal edema present. Corneal problems of this type should be referred to an ophthalmologist.

ANTERIOR CHAMBER: IRITIS

The anterior chamber is the optically clear space between the cornea and the iris.

Patients with anterior chamber inflammation complain of pain, redness, and sensitivity to light. Symptoms may be acute. If there is a history of blunt trauma, bleeding into the anterior chamber (hyphema) or traumatic iritis should be suspected. On examination, it is important to look for the depth and clarity of the anterior chamber.

Acute iritis presents with pain, photophobia, and redness. Although acute iritis may arise spontaneously, blunt trauma to the eye can cause iritis (traumatic iritis). There is no discharge, but vision may be blurred. The redness in acute iritis is diffuse. Slit-lamp biomicroscopy is necessary to fully evaluate the amount of anterior segment inflammation. Patients suspected of having acute iritis should be urgently referred to an ophthalmologist for diagnosis and management.

Hyphema

Hyphema is the accumulation of blood in the anterior chamber of the eye. A hyphema, if large enough, can be seen with room illumination or with a flashlight. Hyphemas are most often preceded by blunt trauma directly to the eye but can occur without trauma in rare patients with a bleeding disorder.

Hypopyon

Hypopyon is the accumulation of white blood cells in the anterior chamber of the eye. Corneal ulceration (see above) is the most common cause of hypopyon. Patients complain of severe pain, redness, decreased vision, and discharge. Other causes of hypopyon include endophthalmitis and severe iritis.

Patients suspected of having anterior chamber disorders should be referred emergently to an ophthalmologist.

APPROACH TO THE RED EYE

A complaint by a patient of a red eye is common in an ambulatory practice. Many of the conditions discussed in this chapter can cause redness of the eye. A red eye is usually caused by an infection and most often is self-limited; however, there are serious considerations in the differential diagnosis of this infection that must be recognized so that an urgent ophthalmologic consultation can be obtained. *Hyperacute conjunctivitis, keratitis* (corneal inflammation), *iritis* or *uveitis* (inflammation of the uveal tract), *scleritis,* and *acute glaucoma* are important vision-threatening conditions that cause a red eye; patients suspected of having one of these conditions should be referred to an ophthalmologist (Table 109.2).

TABLE 109.2 Major Causes of a Red Eye

Conditions that require referral to an ophthalmologist
Acute glaucoma
Acute iritis
Acute corneal tear or infection (keratitis)
Acute scleritis or episcleritis
Bacterial conjunctivitis (hyperacute)
Conditions that usually can be managed by a generalist
Bacterial conjunctivitis (acute and chronic)
Viral conjunctivitis
Inclusion conjunctivitis
Allergic conjunctivitis
Chemical conjunctivitis
Foreign body
Subconjunctival hemorrhage

Several important features of the history and physical examination (Table 109.3) may suggest a specific diagnosis. The patient should be asked specifically whether treatment for an ocular disorder has been given, whether pain in one or both eyes has been experienced, and whether there is visual loss or photophobia (light sensitivity). When the eyes are examined, it is essential to evaluate the following features: Visual acuity, the nature of the discharge, the appearance of the cornea, the size and reactivity of the pupil, and the extent of the redness. When evaluating the extent of redness, an attempt should be made to determine whether there is simply conjunctival injection or whether there is ciliary injection as well. The ciliary vessels run in the sclera beneath the conjunctiva. Ciliary injection usually causes a purplish or violaceous zone of injection around the cornea. Unlike the conjunctival vessels, ciliary vessels do not constrict after the administration of a weak solution of a mydriatic such as 2.5% phenylephrine (Neo-Synephrine). The conjunctival vessels move with the conjunctiva when the conjunctiva is touched with a cotton swab. Ciliary vessels do not. Glaucoma, keratitis, and scleritis are characterized in most cases by ciliary injection. In selected patients, special assessments, such as measurement of ocular tension or inspection of the eye after fluorescein staining, are necessary to establish a diagnosis.

TABLE 109.3 Important Observations in Evaluation of a Patient with a Red Eye

	Glaucoma	*Iritis*	*Corneal Injury*	*Scleritis*	*Episcleritis*	*Bacterial Conjunctivitis*	*Inclusion Conjunctivitis*	*Viral Conjunctivitis*	*Keratitis*	*Allergic Conjunctivitis*
History of previous ocular disorder or condition predisposing to an ocular disorder	+/−	+/−	−	+	−	−	−	−	Often	Previous history of allergies
Pain[a]	+	+	+	+	+	Mild discomfort or burning	Mild discomfort or burning	Mild discomfort or burning	+	−
Visual acuity	Diminished and blurred	Blurred	Usually diminished	Normal	Normal	Normal	Occasionally blurred, if chronic	Normal	Diminished	Usually normal
Discharge	None	None	Usually none	None	None	Present: thick or thin	None or mucopurulent	Watery	Usually some	Mild or none
Appearance of cornea	May be hazy	Normal	May be streaky	Normal	Normal	Normal	Normal except if late when superior dots or streaking may be seen	Normal	Corneal opacity	Normal
Pupil	Often dilated, mid-dilated, or fixed	Small and different from opposite side	Normal	Normal	Normal	Normal	Normal	Normal	Normal	Normal
Redness	Around cornea	Around cornea	Localized or diffuse	Localized or diffuse	Localized	Diffuse	Diffuse (variable)	Segmental or diffuse	Around cornea	Diffuse
Selected evaluations	Ocular pressure[b] in eye is high (see Chapter 108)	Normal	Fluorescein stain[c] shows epithelial defect as brilliant green	A drop of phenylephrine 21/2% on the conjunctiva will constrict superficial but not deep vessels (see the text)	None	None	None	None	A diagnostic scraping may be performed by an ophthalmologist	None

[a] Photophobia in addition to pain may be seen in varying degrees with nearly any of theses conditions, but its presence is neither universal nor diagnostic.
[b] Should not be measured if a discharge is present or a corneal ulceration in seen.
[c] Use individually packaged sterile fluorescein strips.

Before making the decision to treat a patient without obtaining ophthalmology consultation, one should answer the following questions:

- Has a thorough ocular examination been performed?
- Is impaired vision present and, if so, has an explanation been identified?
- Is the natural history of the condition known or is the usual response to treatment known?
- Has the appropriate followup arrangement been made to confirm that the condition is self-limited and improving?

Conjunctival infections, allergies, eyelid inflammation, and irritation are the most common causes of red or irritated eyes, as discussed in detail above. Most patients with these problems can be managed without consulting and ophthalmologist.

SPECIFIC REFERENCES

1. Pavan-Langston D. Viral disease of the cornea and external eye. In: Albert DM, Jakobiec FA, eds. Principles and practice of ophthalmology. 2nd ed. Philadelphia: WB Saunders, 2000: 846.
2. Womack L, Liesegant T. Complications of herpes zoster ophthalmicus. Arch Ophthalmol 1983;101:42.

For annotated ***General References*** *and resources related to this chapter, visit www.hopkinsbayview.org/PAMreferences.*

SECTION 16

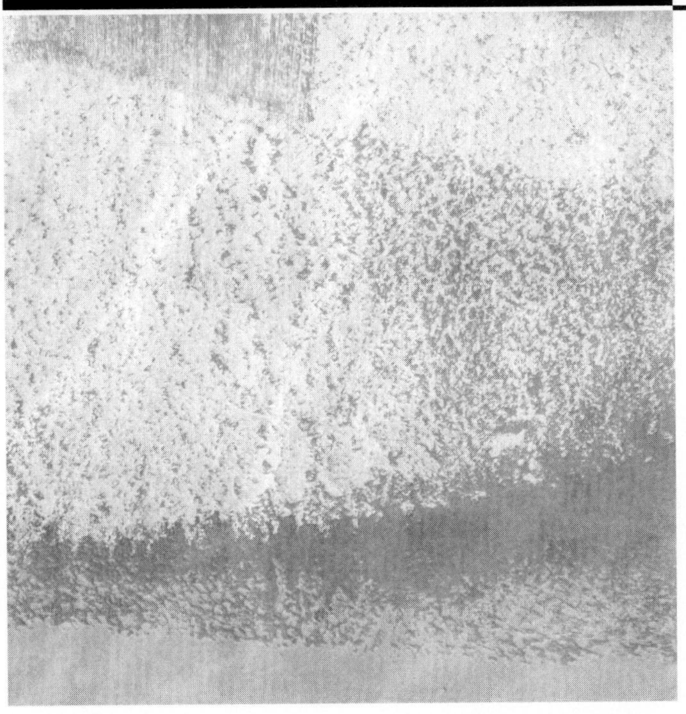

Selected Problems of the Ears, Nose, Throat, and Oral Cavity

Chapter 110

Hearing Loss and Associated Problems

John K. Niparko, Sara Love-Schlessman, and Howard W. Francis

In the United States, an estimated one in nine people develops a permanent hearing impairment that diminishes the ability to carry out everyday communication. Hearing loss is especially common in the elderly, who account for 40% of the hearing impaired. In fact, the only chronic disorders that are more prevalent are hypertension and arthritis. Many causes of hearing impairment are preventable. Early detection and intervention can often ameliorate an acquired hearing impairment.

When evaluating a patient with hearing loss, the practitioner should determine the mechanism of loss (conductive or sensorineural), the likely cause, and the need for referral to an otolaryngologist for further evaluation. This chapter includes a brief review of the anatomy and physiology of the auditory system that will help in understanding auditory pathology, and details strategies of diagnosis and early treatment.

EAR STRUCTURE AND FUNCTION

The *external ear* (Fig. 110.1) is composed of the auricle, the auditory meatus, and the external ear canal. The outer portion of the canal is cartilaginous and is covered by thick skin that contains hair follicles and the cerumen-secreting glands; cerumen protects the epithelium and captures foreign particles entering the canal. The inner portion of the canal is bony and is covered by squamous epithelium without hair follicles or cerumen glands.

The *middle ear* (Fig. 110.1) consists of the tympanic membrane, the air space behind it, and the three linked ossicles: the malleus, incus, and stapes. The malleus is attached to the tympanic membrane and is linked to the stapes by the incus. The stapes makes contact with the inner ear via the stapes footplate at the oval window. The middle ear is lined with a mucus-secreting epithelium similar to that which lines the nose. The middle ear communicates with the nasopharynx via the eustachian tube and posteriorly with the mastoid air cells. Intermittent opening of the eustachian tube ensures equal pressure on either side of the tympanic membrane, which facilitates the transmission of sound from the tympanic membrane to the oval window.

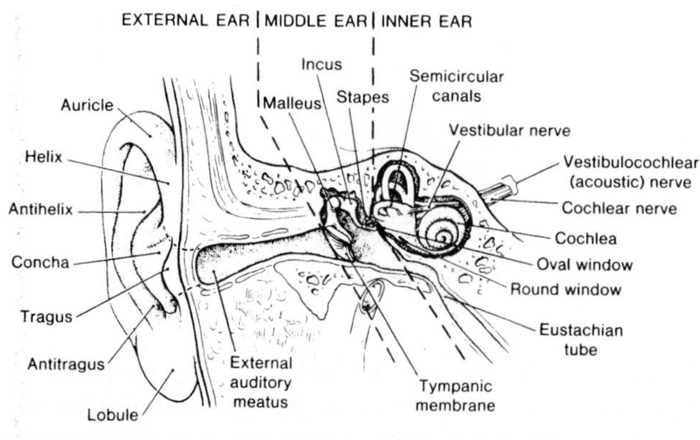

FIGURE 110.1. Normal structures of the ear.

The *inner ear* (Fig. 110.1) lies within the temporal bone of the lateral skull base and is encased in the compact otic capsule and is fluid filled. It consists of sensory organs for hearing (*cochlea*) and balance (*vestibular labyrinth*). Nerves from the cochlea and vestibular labyrinth unite to form the eighth cranial nerve.

Cranial nerve VII (facial) traverses the temporal bone in close association with the middle and inner ear structures. For this reason, facial muscle paresis and paresthesias of the anterior two-thirds of the tongue and soft palate may manifest from pathologic processes of the middle and inner ear.

Sound is funneled through the auricle into the external ear canal, vibrating the tympanic membrane; the vibration is transferred across the ossicular chain. The large surface area of the vibrating tympanic membrane, and the lever action of the ossicles improve sound transmission to the inner ear, where vibrations of the stapes footplate create a fluid wave in the cochlea. This wave stimulates the hair cells that translate vibratory energy into action potentials that trigger auditory neurons.

DETERMINING SEVERITY AND MECHANISM OF HEARING LOSS

Regardless of the specific cause of hearing loss, the approximate severity of the impairment and the probable cause can often be determined in the office. This determination can be made from a combination of the history, the patient's ability to hear the spoken voice, and testing with a tuning fork.

Suggested Questions for History

To help establish a differential diagnosis for the possible causes of hearing loss, the following information should be acquired:

- Is one ear involved or both? Is speech better understood on the telephone in one ear compared to the other?
- Was the onset of hearing loss abrupt or gradual? Has it progressed rapidly? Has hearing acuity fluctuated?
- Does the patient have associated tinnitus, vertigo, otalgia, otorrhea, or facial weakness?
- Is there a family history of hearing loss?
- Has the patient a history of noise exposure?
- Are there related causes of hearing loss such as syphilis, diabetes mellitus (DM), hypothyroidism, head trauma, or autoimmune disease?
- Has the patient been exposed to ototoxic agents such as aminoglycosides, diuretics, aspirin, or chemotherapeutic agents?

Evaluating the Severity and Range of Hearing Impairment

A practical method for evaluating the *severity of hearing impairment* includes a historical estimate of speech recognition impairment in noisy settings and an assessment of response to voice testing in the office; these two findings can be equated with various levels of abnormality in the audiogram (Table 110.1). *Slight* impairment indicates difficulty in hearing distant speech in noise (e.g., group meetings, social gatherings, or the theater). *Moderate impairment* includes some difficulty with short-distance speech and conversation. *Severe impairment* indicates no understanding of the conversational voice but understanding of the amplified voice. Amplification may be achieved by raising the voice or electronically by use of a hearing aid (see Hearing Aids). *Profound* (or total) impairment indicates inability to hear and understand the spoken voice despite maximal

TABLE 110.1 A Practical Method for Approximating the Severity of Hearing Loss in the Office

Severity of Hearing Loss	*Social Difficulty*	*Office Voice Test*	*Pure-Tone Audiogram*
Normal hearing	None	18 ft or more using normal voice	No loss over 10 dB
Slight hearing loss	Long-distance speech	Not over 12 ft using normal voice	10–30 dB loss
Moderate hearing loss	Short-distance speech	Not over 3 ft using normal voice	Up to 60 dB loss
Severe hearing loss	All unamplified voices	Raised voice at meatus	Over 60 dB loss
Profound hearing loss	Voices never heard	All speech and sound	Over 90 dB loss

Adapted from Mawson SP. Disease of the ear. Baltimore: Williams & Wilkins, 1974.

amplification. This also may be summarized by recalling that a soft whisper is about 25 decibels (dB), a moderate whisper is about 40 dB, and conversational speech is about 60 dB. In the office, ambient sound can markedly affect the ability of a patient with hearing impairment to respond to this cursory assessment of audition. Therefore as quiet an environment as possible is advised.

In the patient with significant hearing impairment, the *frequency range* can be approximated in the office by testing recognition of words containing the sound "ah" (low frequency, vowel sound), such as *apple, hot dog,* and *airplane,* and the sounds "s" (high frequency, consonant), such as *ice cream, stairway, baseball,* and *sunset,* when these words are spoken in a medium voice about 2 feet behind the test ear, with the opposite ear covered.

Physical Findings

Otoscopy

Assessment of the External Canal and Tympanic Membrane

Complete inspection of the external ear canal and drum requires pulling the pinna in a posterosuperior direction to align the membranous and bony portions of the canal. The entire drum should be inspected (Fig. 110.2), particularly the posterosuperior aspect, where chronic inflammatory changes often occur. Cerumen accumulation in this region of the drum is unusual and may suggest an underlying problem (Fig. 110.3).

Membrane Mobility

During the otoscopic examination, it is important to assess tympanic membrane mobility with air insufflation. To do this, the examiner must seal the otoscope speculum tip with the ear canal. The absence of mobility suggests a pathologic condition such as negative pressure consequent to eustachian tube dysfunction, middle ear fluid, or a mass.

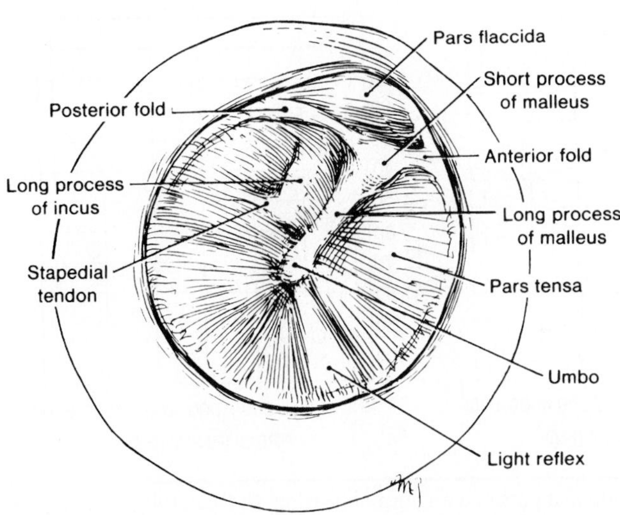

FIGURE 110.2. Right tympanic membrane, showing important landmarks.

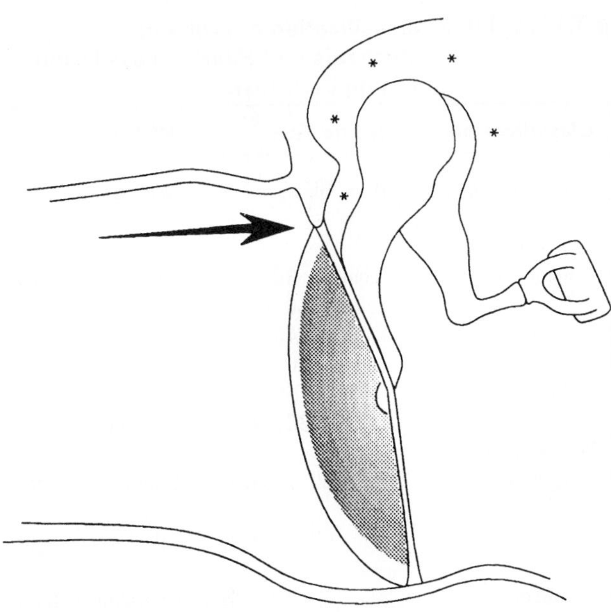

FIGURE 110.3. Cross-sectional drawing of middle ear depicted in Figure 110.1. Arrow indicates the region of the tympanic membrane that may develop a retraction. Retraction pockets may accumulate desquamated debris and extend into regions of the epitympanum depicted by asterisks.

Preliminary Hearing Testing

Tuning Fork Tests

The mechanism of hearing loss can be classified as conductive or sensorineural through use of a 512-Hz tuning fork. Conductive losses result from external or middle ear disease, whereas sensorineural losses are caused by an inner ear or auditory neuronal problem.

Weber Test

For Weber's test, the tuning fork is held against a spot in the midline of the forehead and the patient is asked in which ear it sounds louder (Table 110.2). A unilateral conductive hearing loss with normal bilateral inner ear function produces a louder sound in the affected ear. A unilateral sensorineural hearing loss produces a louder sound in the normal ear.

Rinne Test

In the Rinne test, the vibrating tuning fork stem is placed against the mastoid bone and held in place until it becomes no longer audible, then it is held about an inch away from the external meatus (Table 110.2). The Rinne test can differentiate conductive from sensorineural

TABLE 110.2 Classification of Probable Mechanism of Hearing Loss Using Tuning Fork Tests

Classification	*Rinne Test*	*Weber Test*
Normal Hearing Both ears	AC > BC	Midline
Conductive Loss[a]		
Right ear	Right ear: BC > AC Left ear: AC > BC	Lateralized to right ear
Left ear	Right ear: AC > BC Left ear: BC > AC	Lateralized to left ear
Both ears	Right ear: BC > AC Left ear: BC > AC	Lateralized to poorer ear
Sensorineural Loss		
Right ear	AC > BC bilaterally	Lateralized to left ear
Left ear	AC > BC bilaterally	Lateralized to right ear
Both ears	AC > BC bilaterally	Lateralized to better ear

[a]Because sound transmission by air is much more efficient than by bone, air conduction may remain greater than bone conduction in early or minimal conductive hearing loss.
AC, Air conduction; *BC*, bone conduction.

hearing losses. Air conduction is perceived after the bone conduction extinguishes with normal hearing and with sensorineural hearing loss, whereas the reverse is true for conductive losses. Alternatively, one can compare the perceived loudness of bone versus air conduction.

Speech Recognition Testing

In patients with sensorineural hearing loss, impaired understanding of speech may differentiate cochlear and neural (retrocochlear) deficits. In the latter condition, patients generally have a greater reduction of speech discrimination than do those who have cochlear disorders. Recruitment, a sense of ear discomfort with sudden increments in the loudness of a sound, is characteristic of cochlear dysfunction.

Audiometry

Whereas the office examination can only approximate the loss, audiometric evaluation establishes the precise level of hearing loss. Pure tone air conduction and bone conduction measurements are made for sounds of varying intensity (decibels) and frequency. Results are plotted on a graph called an audiogram in which the vertical axis shows the sounds heard in decibels and the horizontal axis shows the frequency of the stimulus in Hertz. Figure 110.4 reproduces examples of audiograms showing normal hearing, conductive hearing loss, and sensorineural hearing loss. Speech audiometry measures the subject's ability to hear and understand the spoken word.

Audiometry is performed by audiologists, some of whom have their offices in association with an otolaryngologist. Many, however, are independent. Patients can be referred directly to an audiologist from a primary care physician. The location of an accredited audiologist can be obtained by telephoning the action line of the American Speech-Language Association (ASHA) at 800-638-8255 or www.ASHA.org.

An audiogram is easily accomplished when proper testing facilities are available. The patient is comfortably seated in a soundproof room and is asked to record the sounds heard. A series of pure tones are presented to the patient. The procedure takes only about 20 to 30 minutes.

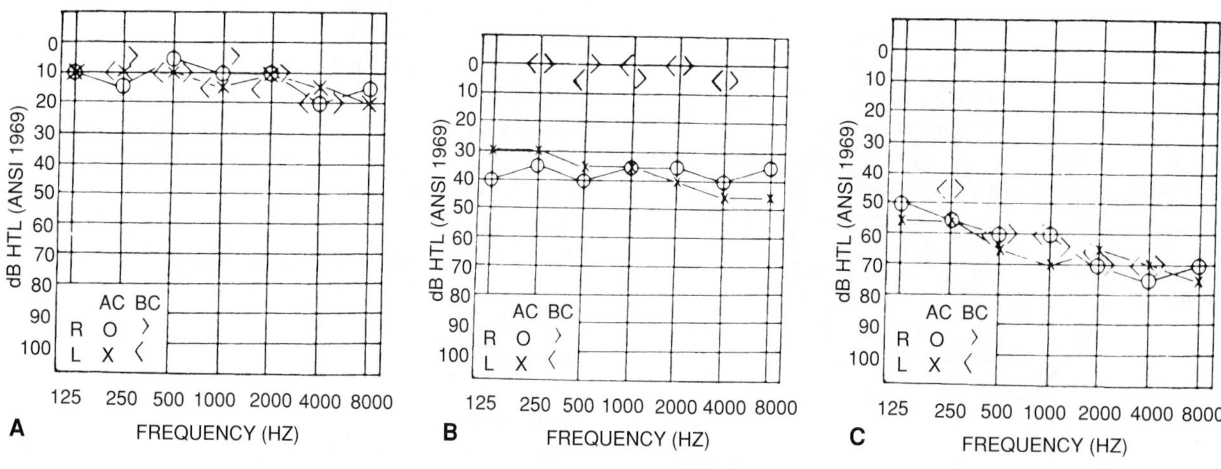

FIGURE 110.4. Examples of audiograms. **A:** Audiogram in a person with normal hearing. **B:** Bilateral conductive hearing loss (moderate). **C:** Bilateral sensorineural hearing loss (severe). (From Price LL, Snider RM. The geriatric patient: ear, nose, and throat problems. In: Reichel W, ed. Clinical aspects of aging. Baltimore: Williams & Wilkins, 1978;404.)

Small hand-held audioscopes, costing about $500, are available for use in the office by general physicians. These are useful as a rough screen of hearing impairment. Usually four pure tones are emitted in sequence. Because of masking effects, background noise can adversely affect a patient's ability to respond to test signals and the examining room must be quiet.

The lowest audible intensity for normal ears is approximately 10 to 20 dB (Fig. 110.4). Conversational speech is typically delivered at 45 to 55 dB. The ASHA has categorized hearing loss as mild (26 to 40 dB), moderate (41 to 55 dB), moderately severe (56 to 70 dB), severe (71 to 90 dB), and profound (greater than 91 dB).

An *assisted listening device* can be valuable in conversing in the office with a patient who is hearing impaired. This device is simply a system of a microphone, amplifier, and earphones. It also reduces some of the background noise in the room and amplifies the examiner's spoken word. Such devices can be obtained in electronics stores or by ordering directly from a manufacturer (e.g., Pocketalker, Williams Sound, telephone 800-328-6190; or Chorus, Audiological Engineering Corp., 800-283-4601).

After this initial evaluation, the presence or absence of hearing loss should be established. If there is hearing loss, it should be determined whether it is primarily unilateral or bilateral and whether it is primarily sensorineural or conductive. Further assessment and care for patients with moderate or severe hearing loss usually requires the assistance of an otolaryngologist. An asymmetric hearing loss should prompt a referral for more sophisticated testing (see discussion of specific conditions below).

CAUSES OF HEARING LOSS: OVERVIEW

Table 110.3 lists the major causes of hearing loss in adults. For each condition, the table indicates mechanism, onset (rapid or gradual), and whether the condition is typically unilateral or bilateral. The guidelines that follow will enable the general physician to reach a working diagnosis in most instances and to choose between primary treatment and referral for care by a specialist.

Conditions of the External Ear

Cerumen Impaction

The patient usually complains of intermittent fullness and hearing impairment on the affected side and may give a history of episodes. These symptoms may increase after showering or swimming, as moisture occludes the ear canal, or with cotton-tipped swab use. Diagnosis is made by otoscopy.

Several precautions should be kept in mind in considering cerumen removal. An only hearing ear, a postsurgical ear, and an ear that is prone to infection (as with any form of immunocompromise) should not be irrigated. If the drum is not visible, it is advisable to defer irrigation to reduce any worsening of the cerumen impaction. If the cerumen appears to be soft, it may be removed by irrigation with use of a rubber-bulb or other syringe and warm tap water, directing the water upward and backward against the wall of the canal. If painful, irrigation should be discontinued and the patient referred to an otolaryngologist. If the cerumen is hard and difficult to remove, a few drops of hydrogen peroxide (or carbamide peroxide, Debrox) should be instilled twice daily for 1 week before irrigation. An alternative approach is for the patient to use mineral oil or baby oil drops in the ear on a regular basis as both effectively liquefy cerumen.

Alternatively, a ceruminolytic agent (Cerumenex) may be used. Generally, ceruminolytic agents should be used only in the office because casual use by the patient at home increases the risk of allergic dermatitis. With the patient's head tilted laterally at a 45-degree angle, the ear is filled with ceruminolytic drops. A cotton plug is inserted for 15 to 20 minutes; the ear is then irrigated with lukewarm water and a soft rubber or other syringe. After irrigation, the tympanic membrane usually shows some injection around the handle of the malleus. Hearing impairment should be relieved after removal of cerumen. The occasional patient with an impaction may not respond to the usual measures described above and should be referred to an otolaryngologist.

Complications from ear irrigation include pain, tympanic membrane perforation, dizziness, bleeding, tinnitus, retention of water behind incompletely removed wax, and infection. Complications requiring specialist referral occur in general practice at the rate of about 1 in 1,000 ears syringed (1). Tympanic membrane rupture, ossicular rupture, round and oval window fistulae, and subluxation of the stapedial footplate have been reported after oral jet irrigation use (2).

An impaction often follows vigorous efforts by the patient to remove wax with a cotton-tipped swab. The patient should be reminded that ear wax is secreted to protect the lining of the canal and that the swab should be used only to remove cerumen in the outer portion of the canal, for cosmetic purposes.

Recurrent impactions are often caused by eczema of the skin of the external ear canal as the desquamated debris impedes cerumen movement. Often topical therapy of the skin condition (see Otitis Externa) is critical to avoiding repeated cerumen accumulation and infection.

Foreign Body

Foreign bodies in the ear canal are most often the result of accidental insertion or entrance of an insect, which is followed by fullness and hearing impairment. Foreign bodies

TABLE 110.3 Causes of Hearing Loss in Adults

Causes	Mechanism	Onset Rapid (Hours to Days) or Gradual (Months to Years)	Bilateral or Unilateral
External Auditory Canal			
Cerumen impaction	C	Either	Usually unilateral
Foreign body	C	Rapid	Unilateral
Otitis externa	C	Rapid	Unilateral
New growth	C	Gradual	Unilateral
Middle Ear			
Serous otitis media	C	Either	Either
Acute otitis media	C	Rapid	Unilateral
Barotrauma	C or SN	Rapid	Unilateral
Traumatic perforation of tympanic membrane	C	Rapid	Unilateral
Chronic otitis media	C	Gradual	Unilateral
Cholesteatoma	C or SN	Gradual	Either
Ossicular chain problem			
Adhesive otitis media	C	Gradual	Unilateral
Tympanosclerosis	C	Gradual	Either
Traumatic injury	C or SN	Rapid	Unilateral
Otosclerosis	C and/or SN	Gradual	Bilateral
New growths	C or SN	Gradual	Unilateral
Inner Ear			
Presbycusis	SN	Gradual	Bilateral
Acoustic trauma	SN	Gradual	Bilateral
Drug-induced	SN	Either	Bilateral
Meniere syndrome	SN	Rapid	Usually unilateral
Central nervous system infection			
Meningitis	SN	Rapid	Either
Syphilis	SN	Either	Either
Tuberculosis	SN	Either	Either
Acoustic neuroma	SN	Gradual	Unilateral
Mumps	SN	Rapid	Unilateral
Atraumatic sudden sensorineural hearing loss	SN	Rapid	Unilateral

C, Conductive; *SN*, sensorineural.

can be removed by the use of alligator forceps or a wax spoon. Removal by irrigation should be avoided if the foreign body is a vegetable, as water causes further swelling. Insects should first be killed by instillation of mineral oil. Hearing impairment resolves promptly after removal of a foreign body. Great care must be taken to avoid damage to the eardrum, especially in children and patients in whom the foreign body is deeply imbedded. In difficult extractions, an otolaryngologist may suggest anesthesia, either local injection or general.

Otitis Externa (Swimmer Ear)

Otitis externa is most common in the summer, when heat and moisture promote swelling and maceration of the stratum corneum of the skin. In the external canal, this process may at first cause pruritus. The patient may give a history of having scratched the ear for a few days before the onset of drainage and pain. The pain is aggravated by movement of the external ear and jaw motion. Hearing impairment occurs in patients with swelling or debris that occludes the canal. The characteristics of the skin of the canal and of the exudate may provide adequate clues to the cause, and cultures are needed only for patients who do not respond promptly to topical treatment. Copious or greenish exudate suggests *Pseudomonas aeruginosa,* the bacteria most often seen in otitis externa. Yellow crusting in the midst of a purulent exudate suggests *Staphylococcus aureus.* Canal skin that is scaling, cracked, and weeping indicates *secondary eczema.* Fluffy material resembling bread mold, varying in color from white to black, suggests a *fungal agent* (*Aspergillus* or *Candida*).

There are three general principles of treatment for all types of otitis externa: removal of all infected debris (with a suction cannula if available), acidification of the canal to inhibit bacterial and fungal growth, and instillation of an appropriate topical antimicrobial (see next paragraph). Lavage with hydrogen peroxide, commonly done in the past, is not recommended because it may be irritating to the inflamed and sensitive tissues and it is not adequately cidal to microbes.

For *bacterial infections* the patient should instill an antimicrobial-corticosteroid preparation (e.g., Cortisporin Otic Suspension, containing polymyxin B–neomycin–hydrocortisone, three or four drops three to four times daily for 5 to 7 days). Alternative topical antimicrobial agents include ofloxacin otic solution (Daiichi) and ciprofloxacin hydrochloride with hydrocortisone (Bayer), which are well tolerated. The use of Cortisporin otic solution, however may be painful to the inflamed ear and should be avoided in preference for the suspension. Gentle daily irrigation of the canal by the patient with a solution of acetic acid (50:50 white vinegar in sterile water) either alone or with steroids has the dual benefit of debriding infected material and acidifying the canal.

We emphasize that aminoglycoside preparations such as Cortisporin Otic remain the mainstay of topical antibiotic therapy for external otitis and selected cases of otitis media. This approach appears to avert intractable infection associated with microbial resistance. If potentially ototoxic antibiotics such as one containing an aminoglycoside are prescribed, the patient should be warned of the risk as well as instructed to contact their physician if dizziness, vertigo, additional hearing loss tinnitus occur. To address ototoxicity concerns, in 2004 a panel of otolaryngologists developed a consensus position for the treatment of otitic disease with topical antibiotics (3). The recommendations held that in the event of a known tympanic membrane perforation preparations free of potential ototoxicity should be used. Quinolone-containing otic topicals offer such a preparation. However, bacterial resistance to quinolones is increasingly recognized. Quinolone-resistant *Streptococcus pneumoniae* have achieved the status of "super bugs" in that there are no antibiotics available for therapy against these pathogens (4). Clearance of the bacteria under microscopic assistance with thorough cleaning of the ear canal likely reduces the risk of the emergence of resistant organisms with any topical therapy. Notwithstanding the above recommendations, otolaryngologists commonly use topical aminoglycoside preparations in practice (5,6). Clinical ototoxicity attributable to topical therapies for otitis externa has not been evident in the literature or practice, and is even rare when used in patients with otitis media with perforation (5–7).

For *fungal infections,* the canal should be thoroughly cleaned out and lightly dusted with sulfanilamide powder by the clinician. A dispenser containing sulfanilamide powder for this use can be obtained from any pharmacy. The fungal infection usually resolves after a single dusting with this powder. Clotrimazole (Lotrimin) 1% solution, three drops twice a day for 14 days, is an effective alternative. Daily irrigations with an acetic acid preparation also provide benefit. Topical steroid creams may be needed to address excessive desquamation.

For *eczema* without superimposed infection, a topical *steroid cream* is applied daily for 14 days (e.g., triamcinolone 0.1%). If satisfactory control has been achieved with the steroid, then chronic symptoms, which are very common, may be controlled by weekly and, eventually, monthly applications.

In some patients, the canal may be so swollen that topical medication does not enter the canal adequately. In this case, a cylindrical cotton wick (or a commercially available sponge wick, such as Oto-wick) should be inserted by gentle twisting into the canal until only the end is visible. The patient may then apply several drops of the medication to the wick three to four times daily, and the wick will carry it into the canal. The wick can usually be removed after 48 to 72 hours, and treatment can be continued as stated above.

Most episodes of otitis externa resolve completely after 5 to 7 days, and it is important to terminate topical treatment at this time. Topical medicines alter the canal environment and persistent treatment often leads to atopic or chemical dermatitis or fungal colonization. As a precaution against overtreatment, the prescription for eardrops should be nonrefillable, and only a small amount (10 mL) should be dispensed.

During treatment of otitis externa, moisture must be kept from entering the ear canal. During bathing, the ear should be plugged with cotton impregnated with petroleum jelly. To prevent recurrence, the patient should be warned against the future use of cotton-tipped swabs or other objects in the ear. Hearing impairment caused by otitis externa should resolve promptly when swelling recedes.

In two situations, the patient with otitis externa requires prompt referral to an otolaryngologist: patients whose findings suggest *mastoiditis* (slow response of the otitis externa to treatment and tenderness over the mastoid process); and patients whose findings suggest *malignant otitis externa*, usually diabetic or immunologically impaired patients. Malignant otitis externa is an osteitis of the bone underlying the external auditory canal, caused by *Pseudomonas.* The distinguishing features are fever, excruciating pain, and the presence of friable, reddish granulation tissue that fills a breach in the canal epithelium. Because of the propensity for rapid spread to contiguous structures, this condition is an emergency, requiring hospital admission for débridement and intravenous antibiotics.

New Growth

Malignancies of auricular and periauricular skin are both common and notoriously difficult to control (8,9), and any suspicion of a new growth should prompt urgent referral to an otolaryngologist. Cutaneous malignancies that commonly occur in these sites are *basal cell carcinomas* and *squamous cell carcinomas,* which often exhibit aggressive clinical characteristics. Moreover, multiple tissue planes and the topography of this region can confound cure (Fig. 110.5). If diagnosed late, cutaneous malignancies of the auricle, pre-auricular region and external auditory canal often extend along embryologic planes to involve deep structures such as the parotid gland, and may erode into the mastoid cortex en route to the skull base. The morbidity and mortality associated with such extensions underscore the importance of early complete initial removal of malignancies in this region. Malignancies of the external auditory canal commonly present with a history of chronic otitis externa the prolonged treatment of which results in delayed diagnosis and treatment. Early referral of patients with suspicious ear lesions and refractory otitis externa is recommended.

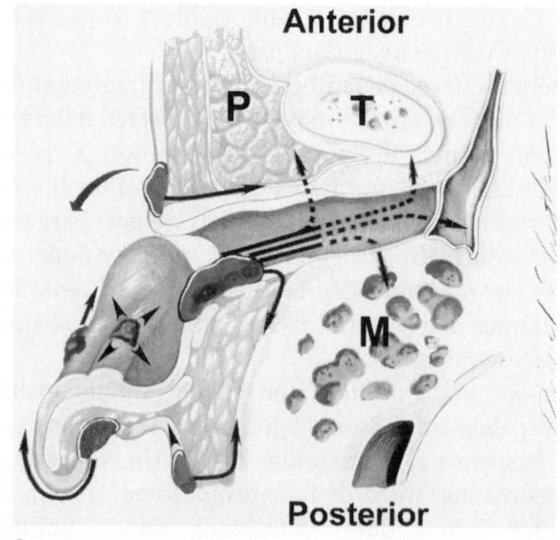

A

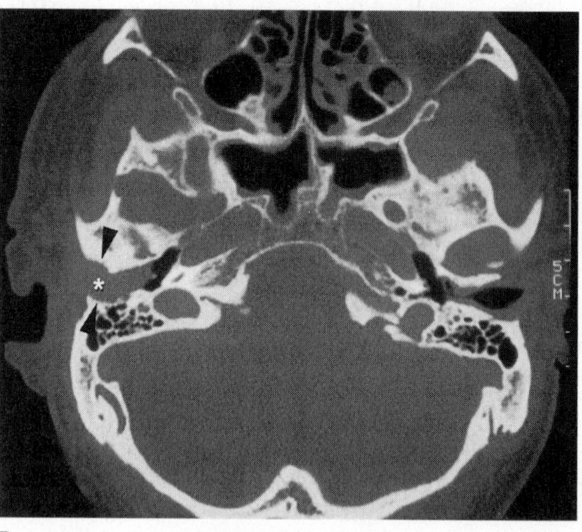

B

FIGURE 110.5. Cutaneous malignancies of the ear. **A:** Axial cross-sectional drawing of ear and temporal bone indicating potential paths of spread of cutaneous malignancies originating on the auricle, the pre-auricular region and external auditory canal. M: mastoid; P: parotid gland; T: temporomandibular joint. **B:** Axial computerized tommography of head, indicating soft-tissue obliteration of the right ear canal (*) and erosion of its bony walls (*arrowheads*).

Conditions of the Middle Ear

Conductive hearing loss is produced by conditions of the middle ear, tympanic membrane, and external ear canal. Most commonly, however, conductive hearing loss results from interference with the sound transformer mechanism of the tympanic membrane and middle ear ossicles. In addition to the history, the middle ear assessment includes otoscopic inspection for signs of acute inflammation (erythema, discharge, or bulging of the tympanic membrane), changes in the tympanic membrane not caused by acute inflammation (retraction, scarring, distortion of normal structures, perforation), cholesteatoma (squamous debris accumulation within the middle ear), and evidence of reduced middle ear aeration as indicated by diminished movement of the drum on pneumatic insufflation.

Serous Otitis Media

The patient usually complains of fullness and decreased hearing in one or both ears with minimal or no pain. There is often a history of recent viral upper respiratory infection, exacerbation of allergic or vasomotor rhinitis, or prior acute otitis media. Rarely, serous otitis media may be caused by nasopharyngeal carcinoma, and this possibility must be ruled out in adults with a new onset of serous otitis that does not resolve after appropriate management (see this section). There is otoscopic evidence of eustachian tube closure and retraction of the tympanic membrane, failure of the membrane to move on pneumatic otoscopy (a crude test of eustachian tube patency, but not always abnormal in serous otitis), or a visible air–fluid level behind the membrane. Usually the tuning fork test reveals a conductive hearing loss (see Preliminary Hearing Testing and Table 110.2).

Medical management consists first of using systemic antibiotics as chronic middle ear effusions are culture positive in up to 50% of cases. Recommended regimens include a 10-day course of amoxicillin alone or combined with clavulanate, cefuroxime axetil, cefaclor, or trimethoprim–sulfamethoxazole (10,11). Topical decongestants in the form of nasal sprays or drops are often used to relieve eustachian tube obstruction. Nasal sprays containing sympathomimetics may be obtained over the counter (e.g., Neo-Synephrine 0.25% or 0.50% spray or drops). After 3 to 4 days of topical treatment, rebound nasal mucosal hyperemia may occur. Therefore the patient should be instructed explicitly to discontinue spray (or drops) after 3 days. Systemic decongestants (e.g., pseudoephedrine) are probably not helpful (12). If serous otitis media coincides with symptoms of allergic rhinitis, Eustachian tube function and middle ear aeration may be helped by the use of a nasal steroid spray for a few weeks or the duration of the seasonal allergy alone or in combination with an antihistamine (see Chapter 30).

All patients should be reevaluated after 4 to 6 weeks. If conductive hearing loss persists beyond 6 weeks, the patient should be referred to an otolaryngologist, who will confirm and quantify the conductive hearing loss and check for other conditions that may be causing the hearing loss. Persistent effusion after 3 months of medical therapy is an indication for surgery, particularly when associated with hearing loss or tympanic membrane changes. Surgery consists of a myringotomy with placement of a ventilation tube. This procedure is usually done under local anesthesia in the office. The tube typically falls out spontaneously in several months. The results are excellent but the patient must keep moisture out of the ear (e.g., avoid swimming) until healing is complete, which usually takes 6 to 18 months.

Acute Otitis Media

Patients with acute suppurative otitis media complain of marked pain in the ear and most give a history of a recent upper respiratory infection. Drainage of purulent material from the ear indicates probable tympanic membrane perforation or concomitant otitis externa. On examination, there is injection and loss of luster of the tympanic membrane, grayish-pink coloration of the entire membrane, and, eventually, bulging of the membrane and loss of landmarks. Some patients have a conductive hearing loss demonstrated by tuning fork tests (see Preliminary Hearing Testing and Table 110.2). There may be tenderness to palpation of the mastoid bone because the mucosa lining of the mastoid cells is continuous with that of the middle ear. Evidence of otitis externa is usually not present. The most common etiologic agents are *S. pneumoniae* (Pneumococcus), *Haemophilus influenza,* and *Moraxella catarrhalis*(10,11). Although some cases are caused by viral pathogens, diagnosis of these cases is usually not practical and treatment should be the same for all patients with acute otitis media.

Medical treatment consists of systemic antimicrobials for 10 days. The antibiotic course should be completed to avoid recurrent or persistent infection and mastoiditis. Amoxicillin, 500 mg three times daily for 10 days, remains the drug of first choice. The growing prevalence of β-lactamase–producing bacteria may necessitate the use of amoxicillin–clavulanate (Augmentin 250/125 or 500/125 tablets), cefuroxime axetil (Ceftin 250 or 500 mg tablets) or clindamycin (Cleocin 300 mg tablets) as second line antimicrobial choices. For penicillin-allergic patients, erythromycin, cefuroxime axetil, and trimethoprim-sulfamethoxazole (TMP-SMX) (e.g., Bactrim, Septra, or generic) may be used. Aspirin, acetaminophen, or ibuprofen every 4 to 6 hours should be recommended for pain. If perforation with discharge occurs, Cortisporin otic suspension, four drops three times daily for 1 week, may be added to the treatment. If the tympanic membrane is bulging with pus and the patient describes severe pain or vertigo, myringotomy by an otolaryngologist is indicated to prevent extension of the infection and resultant complications.

Close followup is recommended within a week of starting therapy to ensure a normal response to treatment. Recovery from the pain of acute otitis media is usually prompt. Pain and fever should be absent by 3 days of therapy. If not, alternative antibiotics should be prescribed with followup within a few days. Within 1 to 4 weeks, hearing impairment should resolve and the tympanic membrane assumes its normal appearance. Serous otitis may be present after other signs and symptoms of acute otitis have resolved. In the patient who notes persistent otalgia, fever, or other signs of toxicity despite adequate antibiotics for 48 hours, subacute mastoiditis should be suspected, and prompt referral to an otolaryngologist is indicated. Facial nerve dysfunction, vertigo, and signs of central nervous system (CNS) infection likewise require prompt evaluation and management. Frequent recurrence of otitis media, failure of serous otitis to resolve, persistence of a tympanic membrane perforation, and significant persistent hearing loss after 4 to 6 weeks are all indications for referral so that potential serious underlying pathology can be ruled out.

Barotrauma

Barotrauma refers to symptoms and signs produced by a sudden pressure differential between the middle ear and the surrounding atmosphere. The patient gives a history of fullness, pain, and decreased hearing in one or both ears. This problem is most commonly associated with descents while flying or scuba diving. Otoscopic findings vary from mild tympanic membrane retraction to hemotympanum, with or without perforation. There may be conductive or neurosensory hearing loss. Any patient with moderate or severe unilateral hearing loss should be referred to an otolaryngologist because of the possibility of inner ear involvement. For patients with mild symptoms, topical or oral decongestants may alleviate symptoms. Prophylaxis against barotrauma consists of use of the Valsalva maneuver and chewing gum or swallowing during descent in airplanes, and management of allergic conditions involving the upper respiratory tract.

Temporal Bone Fractures

Traditional classification of the lateral skull base is based on the orientation of the fracture line in relation to the long axis of the temporal bone (petrous pyramid). Knowledge of the fracture line orientation predicts the extent of middle- and inner-ear damage and the pattern of cranial nerve injury. Eighty percent of temporal bone fractures are longitudinal, most often caused by blows to the lateral skull (13). Longitudinal fracture follow the long axis of the temporal bone coursing along at 45-degree angle from the external meatus toward the postnasal chamber. The plane of fracture extends along the external ear canal to involve the ossicular chain (to produce a conductive hearing loss) and occasionally the facial nerve. Transverse temporal bone fractures extend perpendicularly to the long axis of temporal bone, crossing the inner ear (to produce a sensorineural hearing loss) and often the facial nerve. Transverse fractures account for approximately 20% of temporal bone fractures. Evaluation of a temporal bone fracture requires a careful otoscopic and cranial nerve evaluation, supplemented by high-resolution computerized tomography (CT) scanning. Treatment is dictated by sequelae of the fracture.

Traumatic Perforation of Tympanic Membrane

A tympanic membrane perforation may be caused by a cotton-tipped swab or other object for removing wax, foreign bodies, forcefully directed water, and blast waves resulting from detonation of high explosives. Symptoms include decreased hearing, tinnitus, pain, and bleeding. Otoscopic examination reveals a perforation, commonly in the area of the pars tensa (Fig. 110.2). Air insufflation, which aids in the diagnosis, especially if a perforation is suspected but not seen, shows an immobile tympanic membrane.

The objective of treatment is the prevention of infection. Most linear tears and small perforations of the membrane heal spontaneously in several weeks. Large perforations may require grafting by an otolaryngologist. This procedure is usually done under general anesthesia as an outpatient procedure. A piece of temporal fascia is used for the patch. The results are highly successful with minimal postoperative discomfort. If there is a strong possibility that the middle ear has been contaminated at the time of injury, oral antibiotics (ampicillin or erythromycin 250 mg four times daily for 1 week) are indicated. Patients should prevent water or other contaminants from entering the ear by the insertion of a petroleum jelly-covered cotton plug. Swimming should be avoided altogether. Patients whose perforation was self-inflicted should be warned against future syringing and probing to remove cerumen.

After spontaneous closure or myringoplasty, the hearing loss caused by perforation usually resolves completely. Within a few months the perforation or surgical repair is no longer visible, although occasionally a thin area or a whitish scar remains. Tinnitus, sensorineural hearing loss, and vertigo are signs of inner ear injury and necessitate prompt referral to an otolaryngologist, who will evaluate the patient for a fistula, which requires prompt repair.

Chronic Otitis Media

Chronic otitis is present when a patient has otorrhea, either persistent or recurrent, and there is perforation of the tympanic membrane and usually some degree of conductive hearing loss. The management of this problem has two objectives: eradication of infection and restoration of hearing. When chronic otitis media is initially recognized, the patient should be referred to an otolaryngologist for evaluation (14).

Chronic otitis media can be divided into two major subgroups: inactive and active. Table 110.4 summarizes the

TABLE 110.4 Chronic Otitis Media: Features Distinguishing Inactive and Active (Cholesteatoma) Forms

Feature	*Inactive*	*Active (Cholesteatoma)*
Discharge	Mucoid or mucopurulent	Purulent, foul
Location of pathology	Middle ear; eustachian tube	Middle ear, attic, antrum, any part of temporal bone
Tympanic membrane perforation	Pars tensa (central)[a]	Pars flaccida[a] or marginal
Middle ear mucosa	Mucous membrane	Stratified squamous epithelium
Radiographs	Normal; clouding of mastoid cells	Underdevelopment or sclerosis of mastoid cells; bone destruction
Cholesteatoma formation	No	Yes
Bone erosion	No	Yes
Treatment of infection	Medical/surgical (surgery if the perforation fails to heal spontaneously)	Surgical

[a]See Figure 110.2.

clinical characteristics of these two groups. The fundamental difference in the active subgroup is the presence of, or potential for, bone destruction caused by invasion by squamous epithelium known as *cholesteatoma.* Cholesteatoma occurs when squamous epithelium of the auditory canal invades the middle ear through a preexisting perforation (acquired cholesteatoma). The cholesteatoma appears as a mass of keratinaceous debris that accumulates at the site of invasion of squamous epithelium. As the mass enlarges, it carries the potential to erode bone and promote further infection. Facial paralysis caused by cranial nerve VII involvement, meningitis, and brain abscess may occur as a complication of active cholesteatoma.

The commonly performed surgical procedures for chronic otitis media are described below.

- *Simple mastoidectomy* removes the mastoid cells and cholesteatoma, usually through a postauricular incision. The canal wall remains intact.
- In *modified radical mastoidectomy,* the mastoid cells are exteriorized to form a common cavity with the external auditory canal, draining and eradicating infection caused by cholesteatoma.
- In *myringoplasty,* the tympanic membrane perforation is closed by use of a tissue graft.
- In *tympanoplasty,* the conductive mechanism, including tympanic membrane perforation and ossicular disruptions, is repaired.

These operative procedures are usually done as outpatient surgical procedures. General anesthesia is usually required for both types of mastoidectomy, whereas the plasty procedures can most often be done with only local anesthesia. There is moderate discomfort for 2 to 3 days. However, for 4 to 6 weeks after any of these procedures, the patient must avoid heavy lifting, strenuous exercise, or any similar activity that could result in a Valsalva maneuver, which results in the increase of air pressure in the middle ear and may disrupt the repair. The success rate of all these procedures is approximately 80%.

Complications of Otitis Media

Acute or chronic suppurative otitis media may become complicated by extension of infection beyond the confines of the middle ear into bone and other surrounding structures. These complicating infections are mastoiditis, facial nerve paralysis (caused by cranial nerve VII involvement), petrositis (inflammation of the petrous portion of the sphenoid with diplopia, pain around the eye, and persistent otorrhea), labyrinthitis, brain abscess, extradural abscess, subdural abscess, lateral sinus thrombophlebitis, meningitis, and otitic hydrocephalus. Symptoms not attributable to the typical course of acute or chronic otitis media may signify the presence of one of these complications and require immediate referral and hospitalization.

Ossicular Chain Problems

The most common of these (adhesive otitis media and tympanosclerosis) occur as sequelae to otitis media. Others (ossicular injury or otosclerosis) may affect the ossicular chain in the absence of a history of or signs of prior otitis media. Ossicular chain problems may be recognized by demonstrating conductive hearing loss (usually chronic, either unilateral or bilateral). Changes of the tympanic membrane indicative of prior otitis media may or may not be present, depending on the problem. In some conditions, otoscopy may even be diagnostic. Each of these conditions requires referral to an otolaryngologist for accurate diagnosis and consideration of surgical management.

Adhesive Otitis Media

There is a history of ear infection, and the tympanic membrane is retracted and atrophic in areas of healed perforations. The eardrum is usually draped over the promontory and incudostapedial complex. Adhesive otitis media is usually a late complication seen in patients with persistent middle ear inflammation. Hearing loss is usually mild, although some patients may require ossicular reconstruction or a hearing aid (see Hearing Aids).

Tympanosclerosis

There is a history of infection, often bilateral. There is usually, but not always, a tympanic membrane perforation, and discrete plaques of dense collagen with calcified hyaline may be seen in the middle ear. In selected patients tympanic membrane and ossicular reconstruction is necessary to improve hearing.

Traumatic Ossicular Injury

There is a history of trauma (e.g., temporal bone fracture and the causes of traumatic perforation listed above) followed by unilateral hearing loss, which may be conductive or mixed. A hemotympanum (blood behind the eardrum) is usually seen, although occasionally the tympanic membrane is normal. Hearing status after surgical exploration depends on the type of injury found at surgery.

Otosclerosis

Otosclerosis is a disease of the labyrinthine capsule in which spongelike bone is laid down, causing fixation of the stapes and conductive hearing loss, usually bilateral. The history discloses a slowly progressive hearing loss. Onset is usually in the late teens to thirties, but occasionally in the forties. It is seen more commonly in females (F-to-M ratio 2:1). It is often accelerated by pregnancy. From 50% to 70% of cases are hereditary, following an autosomal dominant mode of inheritance. History is key in establishing the diagnosis because examination of the tympanic membrane is usually normal. This is the most common cause of progressive conductive hearing loss in young adults. The results of surgery, consisting of stapedectomy or stapedotomy and prosthetic replacement, are excellent.

New Growths of Middle Ear

A number of benign and malignant growths may be seen on inspection of the tympanic membrane of patients with progressive unilateral conductive hearing loss. Malignant tumors most commonly present with a history of chronic discharge, occasionally bloody.

CHRONIC SENSORINEURAL HEARING LOSS

Presbycusis

A certain degree of hearing loss, beginning in the high-frequency range, is universal among elderly people. Most do not complain of deafness, and often a family member is the first to notice the hearing deficit. Clearly, social and psychological factors are important in determining the level of reported disability. For this reason, in the general population of elderly, in whom hearing loss is common, screening of asymptomatic patients using an office audiogram is not usually recommended because obtaining a hearing aid (see Hearing Aids), the usual prescription, is expensive and cumbersome and most patients will not use one until they have perceived their hearing problem and seek a remedy on their own. Instead the U.S. Preventive Services Task Force recommends periodically questioning elderly patients about their hearing, counseling them about the availability of hearing aid devices, and making referrals for abnormalities when appropriate (http://www.ahrq.gov/clinic/uspstfix.htm).

When an older patient is first found to have moderate hearing loss, the patient and family should be counseled as outlined below (see Dealing with The Patient with Permanent Hearing Loss), and the patient offered a referral for evaluation by an audiologist (see Audiometry, above) or by an otolaryngologist (15).

Noise-Induced Hearing Loss

Noise-induced hearing loss is a form of sensorineural hearing loss commonly found in patients employed in high-noise industries or exposed to intense noise from power tools, firearms, and other sources (16). Loud rock music also may cause hearing loss, but because of the range of sound it is a slower process, often occurring 10 to 15 years after repeated exposure. Like presbycusis, it is initially a high-frequency hearing loss, eventually involving lower frequencies. Prophylaxis by wearing muffs and earplugs in high-noise settings and reducing noise levels are the best ways to prevent acoustic trauma. Established hearing loss caused by noise is usually irreversible, but progressive hearing loss can be prevented. Acute hearing loss caused by an acute episode of acoustic trauma, such as gunfire or cordless telephone ringer accidents (a loud sound or shock caused by electrical surge), is often reversible and referred to as a temporary threshold shift.

TABLE 110.5 Drugs That May Cause Sensorineural Hearing Loss

Antibiotics	Diuretics
Streptomycin	Ethacrynic acid
Neomycin	Furosemide
Gentamycin	Other Drugs
Tobramycin	Salicylates
Chloramphenicol	Quinidine
Vancomycin	Quinine
	Cisplatin

Drug-Induced Hearing Loss

A number of drugs may produce bilateral sensorineural hearing loss, and the patient's personal physician often is the first to learn of this problem (Table 110.5). For most of these drugs, ototoxicity is dose related; however, hearing impairment may occur even at therapeutic dosages. A mild hearing loss occurs in as many as 10% of patients whose serum levels of gentamicin and tobramycin are maintained within the therapeutic range (17).

The prognosis for drug-induced hearing loss varies according to the drug. Salicylates in high dosages and quinine usually produce temporary, high-frequency deafness, but permanent deafness has been reported in patients surviving salicylate poisoning and in infants of mothers who received quinine during pregnancy. Aminoglycoside ototoxicity may occur suddenly after a few doses, may be permanent, and may progress after discontinuation of the drug. Diuretic-induced ototoxicity may be seen after extremely high dosages, usually in patients with renal insufficiency. Its onset may be sudden, after intravenous (and rarely oral) administration, and the hearing deficit may be permanent.

Ménière Syndrome

Ménière syndrome is characterized by spells of a constellation of otologic symptoms. Symptoms are thought to be caused by endolymphatic hydrops manifested by excess fluid and pressure in the cochlea and vestibular labyrinth. Ménière attacks consist of fluctuant hearing loss, roaring tinnitus, aural fullness, and spontaneous peripheral-pattern vertigo (see Chapter 89). However, in many instances the disorder produces a nonclassic array of symptoms. An attack may last for minutes to an hour, often with nystagmus present on physical examination. Between attacks, tinnitus and sensorineural hearing loss often persist. Symptoms are unilateral in 70% to 80% of cases (18). The hearing loss and vertiginous episodes may occur simultaneously, or in tandem. Vertigo may be accompanied by nausea and emesis. In severe episodes, other vagal symptoms may occur, including pallor and sweating and rarely bradycardia. Audiometry demonstrates sensorineural hearing loss, predominantly in lower frequencies in early stages of the disease.

The *differential diagnosis* of Ménière syndrome includes a number of conditions that may also present with hearing loss and vertigo unrelated to position change: viral labyrinthitis, acoustic neurinoma, syphilitic vertigo, labyrinthine fistula, vestibular granuloma, temporal bone fracture, or multiple sclerosis (see Chapter 89 for details regarding vertigo).

Treatment

Patients with suspected Ménière syndrome should be referred promptly to an otolaryngologist to confirm the diagnosis and initiate treatment. Patients are placed on a low sodium diet (<2,000 mg/day) and are treated empirically with diuretics, 25 to 50 mg of hydrochlorothiazide daily or its equivalent, with attention to avoid hypokalemia (see Chapter 50). The antihistamine meclizine can be tried in a dosage of 25 mg three to four times daily, but often this fails to prevent attacks of vertigo. For nausea, the patient should take the antiemetic prochlorperazine either as a 5- or 10-mg capsule four times daily, or as a 25-mg suppository twice daily. After the acute attack has subsided, the patient should continue diuretic treatment; after 1 year without recurrence, diuretic treatment can be discontinued. For the occasional patient with severe recurrent Ménière syndrome refractory to medical treatment, several surgical procedures offer high response rates. Treatment with intratympanic injection of gentamicin can be beneficial when vertigo persists despite optimal medical management, which may be required in an estimated 10% of patients. Surgical ablation of the vestibular labyrinth is required to control vertigo symptoms in an extremely small percentage of patients (19).

Prognosis

Ménière disease tends to be chronic and progressive, but fluctuates unpredictably. Acute attacks of vertigo often increase in frequency during the first few years after presentation, then decrease in frequency and cease. Symptoms other than hearing loss improve in 60% to 80% of people irrespective of treatment (20). However, there is sustained loss of hearing. In the minority of patients who develop second ear, contralateral involvement, the disease generally manifests less severe symptoms.

ACOUSTIC NEUROMA

Acoustic neuroma, an uncommon, benign tumor, usually arises from the vestibular fibers of nerve VIII. It grows slowly, expanding within the internal auditory meatus until it is large enough to extend into the posterior fossa and compress adjacent structures of the CNS. Essentially all patients present with symptoms of eighth nerve impairment: unilateral, usually chronic hearing loss is found in the majority of patients. Most frequently, patients will note a progressive inability to discriminate speech on the telephone using the involved ear. Tinnitus and chronic, usually mild, positional vertigo or sense of imbalance occurs in many patients. Audiometry usually demonstrates significant sensorineural hearing loss with poor discrimination of speech. Neurologic examination (see Chapter 86) shows involvement of the following neurologic structures, in decreasing order of frequency: cranial nerves VIII, V, VII, VI, and cerebellum (ataxia, with tendency to fall toward the side of the lesion). Referral to an otolaryngologist for evaluation is essential whenever unilateral sensorineural hearing loss is initially found. Diagnosis of acoustic neuroma is based on a characteristic audiogram or other audiologic or vestibular findings, but must be either ruled out or confirmed with magnetic resonance imaging of the internal auditory canal and posterior fossa (Fig. 110.6) (21). The results of surgical treatment generally permit the patient to resume usual activity, but often with permanent unilateral hearing loss (22). In a few patients with good hearing preoperatively, it may be possible to preserve hearing. Stereotactic radiation of acoustic neuromas offers a treatment option that is noninvasive. Radiation is designed to induce a fibrotic response of the tumor capsule with the goal of controlling tumor growth. Treatment using radiation is generally employed for tumors in patients with medical conditions that preclude surgery.

SUDDEN SENSORINEURAL HEARING LOSS

Sudden sensorineural hearing loss, usually unilateral, is an otologic emergency. The cause is often difficult to ascertain and may include viral cochleitis, arterial occlusion (especially in patients with other evidence of arterial occlusive disease, such as embolic transient ischemic attacks), inner ear fistula, autoimmune factors (23), sudden expansion of a cerebellopontine angle tumor (e.g., a meningioma or acoustic neuroma, see Acoustic Neuroma), temporal bone fracture, and noise trauma. Symptoms, which occur over a matter of minutes to hours, include tinnitus or

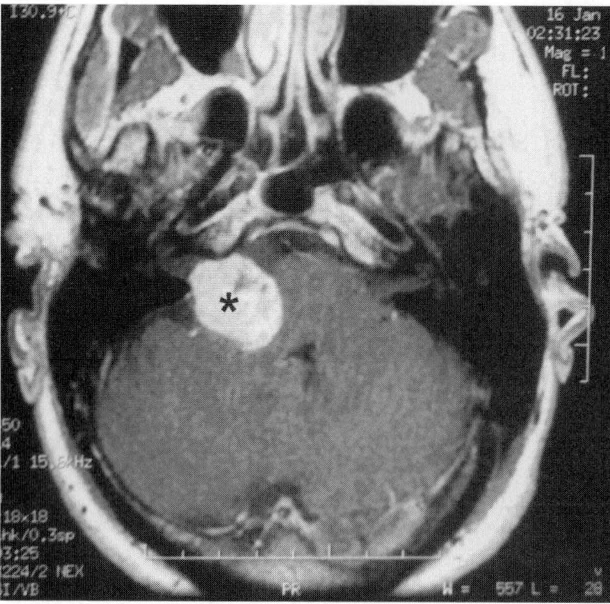

FIGURE 110.6. MRI of internal auditory canals and posterior fossa demonstrating a right-sided vestibular schwannoma (acoustic neuroma) marked with asterisk. The tumor demonstrates 2.3 cm extension from the (expanded) porous acousticus of the internal auditory canal into the cerebellopontine angle, placing the patient at risk for cranial neuropathies and increased intracranial pressure as a consequence of pontomedullary brain stem compression (T1 image with gadolinium enhancement).

hearing loss. After prompt evaluation for conductive hearing loss (including simple cerumen impaction), these patients should be referred immediately for evaluation by an otolaryngologist. A number of empirical medical therapies (e.g., corticosteroids, vasodilators, membrane-deforming agents, or anticoagulants) have been tried with varying success. Most recently, the use of intratympanic dexamethasone administered via transtympanic injection has shown promise in treating sudden, idiopathic sensorineural hearing loss, particularly if administered within days of the onset of the loss (24). For patients with suspected inner ear fistulas, surgical exploration may be necessary.

Most patients have permanent, severe unilateral hearing loss, and they and their families should be instructed about adequate noise protection for the only hearing ear, preferential seating for optimal use of the good ear, and precautions when driving to compensate for missed sound cues.

TINNITUS

Tinnitus ("ringing") is the perception of sounds in the absence of a normal sound stimulus. Intermittent tinnitus is common in the general population. Persistent tinnitus may be caused by a number of identifiable problems. Occasionally, tinnitus may be experienced only at night, in bed, when ambient noise is reduced.

Subjective Tinnitus

The term *subjective tinnitus* is used when the subject complains of noises that cannot be heard by the observer. Subjective tinnitus may be subdivided into two types.

Tympanic tinnitus usually arises as a result of a conductive lesion (all of the causes of conductive hearing loss, Table 110.3). It is thought to be caused by removal of the normal masking effect of ambient noise, with emergence of otherwise subaudible tympanic, vascular, and muscular noises. The patient often describes the tinnitus as pulsating.

Petrous tinnitus is caused by conditions affecting the cochlea or eighth nerve that lead to sensorineural hearing loss (Table 110.3). It is attributed to recognition of auditory stimuli produced by mechanical cochlear deformation or hyperirritability of the acoustic nerve. It may be intermittent or continuous with varying intensity.

After the patient's primary otologic problem has been defined, the most important requirement in helping the patient with tinnitus is reassurance because patients may believe that their tinnitus reflects a serious intracranial condition. Bedtime sedation to ensure adequate sleep is important. Some patients also find that the sound of an FM radio (FM delivers a broader range of frequencies, particularly in the higher spectrum than AM) helps them get to sleep by competing with the more distressing sounds caused by tinnitus. For patients with severe tinnitus, *masking treatment* (an apparatus that externally generates white noise and is available from an audiologist) may be helpful. Recently developed digital music players can be especially helpful for masking. The distressing nature of severe and chronic tinnitus has resulted in the development of tinnitus clinics and support groups in most large cities (25). The critical role of tricyclic antidepressants in managing patients with coexisting disabling tinnitus and depression is now well established (26).

Objective Tinnitus

Objective tinnitus is a noise audible to the examiner and originates from the region of the patient's ear. Causes include aneurysm of the internal carotid artery, benign vascular tumors of the middle ear, temporomandibular joint instability, and myoclonus of the palatal muscles. Although not audible by the examiner, a complaint of pulsatile tinnitus may also indicate benign intracranial hypertension. These patients should be referred to an otolaryngologist for a diagnostic workup. Also, patients with tinnitus that lateralizes to one ear should also be referred for further evaluation.

DEALING WITH THE PATIENT WITH PERMANENT HEARING LOSS

Communication

Counseling of the family and others who speak to the patient with moderate to severe hearing loss should emphasize the following points.

- Facilitate communication by consistently using the following adjuncts to speech: face patients, obtain their attention, use gestures, speak at a moderate pace and audibly, or move closer if the patient says that it helps. Most patients with significant hearing loss are most affected at high frequencies and have better preservation of their lower frequency hearing. Since speech frequencies are generally higher during shouting, the use of a full clear voice is more constructive.
- Ensure adequate lighting (to aid in lip reading and facial expressions) and minimize background noise, which confuses sound perception.
- Be patient and ask how you can facilitate communication.

For the patient with *profound* or *total hearing loss,* the principle governing all communication is that the patient must see the message. Most patients let the physician know the mode of communication they prefer (lip reading or writing). Whenever there is any question about the effectiveness of lip reading, written exchange of information should be used. This can be facilitated by ensuring that paper and a pen or pencil are always available to the patient. The use of a word processor program with large font is particularly helpful in facilitating communication with deaf patients. When sign language is the preferred mode of communication, arrangements should be made in advance for an interpreter to be present at appointments. Also, various devices are now available, although they are moderately expensive, that make it possible for totally deaf people to receive telephone calls (messages are entered by the sender in code on a touch-tone unit and displayed visually for the deaf receiver) and to follow television programs. Many people who are totally deaf at an early age learn sign language, and programs for learning sign language are widely available. Valuable information to help people with any level of hearing impairment may be obtained from Self-Help for Hard of Hearing People, Inc., www.SHHH.org, and The A.G. Bell Association for the Deaf and Hard of Hearing, www.AGBell.org.

Hearing Aids

Hearing aids (miniature, battery-powered microphone–amplifier–loudspeaker units) can assist the patient with sensorineural hearing loss and patients with irreversible conductive loss (27). The currently available aids include in-the-ear, delicate, and behind-the-ear units. Older devices were incorporated into eyeglasses or carried in a pocket with a wire connection to the ear mold. Hearing aids can increase the intensity of a sound by up to 70 dB. Thus, a sound of about 60 dB (the level of average conversational speech) passing through an aid may enter the ear at a level of 130 dB. This represents the maximal usable gain of an aid because sounds above this level become painful.

Federal law now prevents the sale of hearing aids to people who have not been evaluated first by a physician. Only trial and adjustment determine whether a patient referred for a hearing aid will benefit. Medicare and other third-party insurers do not pay for hearing aids and they are expensive, typically costing over 600 dollars. Most hearing aid dealers allow a 30-day trial period during which the patient pays a rental fee; some states require this by law. Currently, only a minority of people who would benefit from a hearing aid own one, usually because of the cost and the difficulty or embarrassment perceived in using it. Also, many who own units do not use them regularly because of difficulty in using them or the presence of irritating sounds, which often can be eliminated by adjustment of the device by an audiologist.

Patients may mention certain specific problems with the hearing aid to their personal physicians. There may be irritation of the conchal cartilage, infection in the external canal, or an increase in cerumen accumulation. In each of these situations, the fitting audiologist should evaluate use of the aid. A better fitting mold is needed to avoid recurrence in some patients. Others may do well by removing the aid periodically during the day.

Amplification devices have evolved considerably in the past decade. Digital hearing aids convert electronic sound information from the microphone into a digitized code, which is then processed by an amplifier consisting of microchips instead of electronic circuitry. All adjustments are programmed using computer software. Substantially more expensive, the primary advantage of digital signal processing is the greater processing power than prior analog signal processors in the hearing aid. The greater processing power represents greater decision making ability by the instrument, allowing many more adjustments and greater precision of adjustments for the listener to make according to the acoustic environment.

For selected patients, semi-implantable systems including implantable bone conduction aids and cochlear implants are now available (28). The cochlear implant is used in patients who are unable to derive significant benefit from the use of powerful hearing aids. Young deaf children who are appropriately managed with cochlear implants demonstrate an increased likelihood of gaining access to mainstream education opportunities (29). Deaf adults with previous experience with verbal language also enjoy significant changes in quality of life as a result of increased access to the spoken word (30).

SPECIFIC REFERENCES*

1. Sharp JF, Wilson JA, Ross L, et al. Ear wax removal: a survey of current practice. BMJ 1990;301:1251.
2. Dinsdale RC, Roland PS, Manning SC, et al. Catastrophic otologic injury from oral jet irrigation of the external auditory canal. Laryngoscope 1991;101:75.
3. Roland P, Stewart M, Hannley M, et al. Consensus panel on role of potentially ototoxic antibiotics for topical middle ear use: Introduction, methodology and recommendations. Arch Otolaryngol Head Neck Surg 2004;130:35:S51.
4. Hancock RE. Mechanisms of action of newer antibiotics for Gram-positive pathogens. Lancet Infect Dis 2005;5:209.
5. Lundy LB, Graham MD. Ototoxicity and ototopical medications: a survey of otolaryngologists. Am J Otol 1993;14:141.
6. Walby P, Stewart R, Kerr AG. Aminoglycoside ear drop ototoxicity: a topical dilemma. Clin Ototlaryngol 1998;23:289.
7. Pickett BP, Shinn JB, Smith MFW. Ear drop toxicity: reality or myth? Am J Otol 1997;189:782.
8. Niparko J, Swanson N, Baker S, et al. Local control of auricular and periauricular cutaneous carcinoma with Mohs surgery. Laryngoscope 1990;100:1047.
9. Gillespie MB, Francis HW, Chee N, et al. Squamous cell carcinoma of the temporal bone: a radiographic-pathologic correlation. Arch Otolaryngol Head Neck Surg 2001;127:803.

*Bold numerals denote published controlled clinical trials, meta-analyses, or consensus-based recommendations.

10. Bluestone CD, Klein JO. Otitis media, atelectasis and Eustachian tube dysfunction. In: Bluestone CD, Stool SE, eds. Pediatric Otolaryngology. 2nd ed. Philadelphia: WB Saunders, 1990: 320.
11. Hoberman A, Paradise JL. Acute otitis media: diagnosis and management in the year 2000. Pediatr Ann 2000;29:609.
12. Bluestone CD, Mandel EM, Cantekin EI, et al. Evaluation of decongestant antihistamine therapy for otitis media with effusion. Ann Otol Rhinol Laryngol 1983;92:35.
13. Backous D, Minor L, Niparko J. Trauma to the external auditory canal and temporal bone. Otolaryngol Clin North Am 1996;29:5.
14. Kemink J, Telian S, Niparko J. Evaluation and treatment of the draining ear. Modern Med 1988;56:76.
15. Miller MH. Restoring hearing to the older patient: the physician's role. Geriatrics 1986;41:75.
16. Dobie RA. Noise-induced hearing loss: the family physician's role. Am Fam Physician 1987;36:141.
17. Smith CR, Lipsky JJ, Laskin OL, et al. Double-blind comparison of the nephrotoxicity and auditory toxicity of gentamicin and tobramycin. N Engl J Med 1980;302:1106.
18. Balkany TJ, Kires B, Arenberg IK. Bilateral aspects of Meniere's disease. Otolaryngol Clin North Am 1980;13:4.
19. Minor LB, Schessel DA, Carey JP. Meniere's disease. Curr Opin Neurol 2004;17:9.
20. Torok N. Old and new in Meniere's disease. Laryngoscope 1977;87:1870.
21. Armington WG, Harnsberger HR, Smoker WR, et al. Normal and diseased acoustic pathway: evaluation with MR imaging. Radiology 1988;167:509.
22. Ojemann RG, Montgomery WW, Weiss AD. Evaluation and surgical treatment of acoustic neuroma. N Engl J Med 1972;287:895.
23. Stone JH, Francis HW. Immune-mediated inner ear disease. Curr Opin Rheumatol 2000;12:32.
24. Chandrasekhar SS. Intratympanic dexamethasone for sudden sensorineural hearing loss: clinical and laboratory evaluation. Otol Neurotol. 2001;22:18.
25. O'Connor S, Hawthorne M, Britten SR, et al. The management of a population of tinnitus sufferers in a specialized clinic: part II. Identification of psychiatric morbidity in a population of tinnitus sufferers. J Laryngol Otol 1987;101:791.
26. Sullivan M, Katon W, Russo J, et al. A randomized trial of nortriptyline for severe chronic tinnitus. Effects on depression, disability, and tinnitus symptoms. Arch Intern Med 1993;153:2251.
27. Department of Health, Education and Welfare. A report on hearing aid health care. Washington, DC: US Government Printing Office, 1974.
28. Cohen N, Waltzman S. The Department of Veterans Affairs Cochlear Implant Study Group: a prospective, randomized study of cochlear implants. N Engl J Med 1993;328:233.
29. Francis HW, Koch ME, Wyatt JR, et al. Trends in educational placement and cost benefit considerations in children with cochlear implants. Arch Otolaryngol Head Neck Surg 1999;125:499.
30. Palmer CA, Niparko JK, Wyatt JR, et al. A prospective study of the cost-utility of the multichannel cochlear implant. Arch Otolaryngol Head Neck Surg 1999;125:1221.

*For annotated **General References** and resources related to this chapter, visit www.hopkinsbayview.org/PAMreferences.*

Chapter 111

Selected Disorders of the Nose and Throat: Epistaxis, Snoring, Anosmia, Hoarseness, and Hiccups

Matthew L. Kashima

EPISTAXIS

Epistaxis is a very common occurrence, with most individuals having at least one "nosebleed" during their lifetime. Most episodes of epistaxis do not require medical attention and are usually self-limited with inconsequential loss of blood. Rarely, severe uncontrolled epistaxis may cause aspiration and substantial blood loss and may be life threatening. Estimates are that only 10% of nose bleeds are brought to the attention of a health care provider. Less than half of these require consultation with an otolaryngologist. Most patients with epistaxis are successfully managed by their primary care provider. The overall goal in the management of epistaxis is to stop the bleeding and ultimately to correct any underlying pathology that precipitated the event.

Pathophysiology

Epistaxis is defined as bleeding emanating from the nose or nasopharynx. The blood may flow anteriorly through the nares or posteriorly and may be expectorated and or swallowed. The nasal mucosa has a rich anastomosis of vessels, arising from multiple sources. The blood supply to the lateral nasal wall is derived from the internal maxillary and facial arteries from the external carotid system. The nasal septum is supplied by the anterior and posterior ethmoid arteries from the internal carotid system.

The nasal mucosa is composed of a thin stratified columnar epithelium with goblet cells supplying the mucous blanket. The nasal secretions help to protect the underlying epithelium. On the lateral nasal wall (i.e., on the turbinates), the submucosa is thickened with the presence of venous sinusoids and mucous glands. The submucosa of the nasal epithelium lining the septum can be quite thin with blood vessels in close proximity to the mucosal surface. Dryness or irritation causes mucosal disruption and bleeding from underlying vessels. These vessels will not be fully protected from rebleeding until the overlying mucosa has healed. A cycle of rebleeding may occur as local infection and inflammation initiate the formation of granulation tissue, which remains quite friable and will cause persistent bleeding. The rebleeding cycle ceases only when the underlying epithelium is regenerated and the submucosal vessels are protected.

The anterior septum is particularly prone to environmental irritation (dry air, smoke and other irritants, allergens, toxic inhalants); it is the site of approximately 90% of all episodes of epistaxis. The most frequent site of bleeding is Kiesselbach plexus or Little area, an area on the anterior portion of the nasal septum rich in capillaries. Anterior epistaxis occurs more frequently when the weather is cold and humidity low. More posteriorly, on the septum and in the lateral nasal wall, the vessels are of a larger caliber, and epistaxis from these posterior vessels is typically quite brisk. With increasing age and concomitant arteriovascular disease, posterior epistaxis becomes more prevalent. The presence of arterial disease in these vessels also compromises vascular contraction during acute epistaxis, which prolongs uncontrolled bleeding (1). The posterior nasal cavity is very difficult to access and evaluate, so posterior epistaxis can be difficult to control.

Etiology

The etiology of epistaxis usually can be readily determined (2). It is more important to ascertain the cause of the nasal

TABLE 111.1 Causes of Epistaxis

Local mucosal irritation
Trauma
Fracture
Surgery
Anatomic derangement
Septal deviation
Foreign body
Neoplasm
Hypertension (?)
Chronic renal failure
Defects of coagulation
Heredity
Medication

Adapted from Lepore ML. Epistaxis. In: Bailey BJ, ed. Head and neck surgery—otolaryngology. 1st ed. Philadelphia: JP Lippincott, 1993:8.

bleeding in refractory and recurrent cases, as opposed to isolated episodes that are self-limited and not severe. Recurrent and refractory epistaxis may point to a significant underlying medical condition. Epistaxis often is caused by a combination of factors, so it is helpful when evaluating a patient with problematic epistaxis to consider both local factors and systemic factors (Table 111.1).

Local Factors

Conditions that alter the physiology of the nasal mucosa and environmental factors, such as decreased temperature and humidity, lead to disruption of the nasal epithelium and subsequent vascular injury and hemorrhage. For example, hospital admissions for epistaxis increase during the winter months, with up to two-thirds occurring during January and February in the northern hemisphere (3). This may be related to low humidity in households with dry-air heating systems. Patients requiring oxygen supplementation either as inpatients or at home are at increased risk of having epistaxis. This is due to the drying effect of the oxygen, which is delivered via nasal cannula. The dry membranes and cannula can be sites that develop crusts and be subject to digital trauma as described below.

Local trauma is also commonly implicated in epistaxis. Any blunt force directed to the mid-face or adjacent regions can cause shearing of the nasal mucosa, which will be accompanied by brisk nasal bleeding. This can be seen in severe facial trauma or in isolated nasal fractures. More common is trauma from persistent nose picking. Patients who use their fingers to remove crusts from their nose are likely to disrupt the mucosa. Chronic digital trauma can lead to persistent ulcerations with concomitant granulation tissue formation, which can increase the frequency of bleeding. Patients with recent nosebleeds may perceive nasal obstruction due to crusting and promote rebleeding while trying to remove the crust. Local inflammation due to upper respiratory infections, chronic sinusitis, allergic rhinitis, or environmental irritants can also alter normal nasal physiology, thinning the nasal mucosa leading to dryness and crusting with subsequent vascular exposure and bleeding.

Anatomical derangements such as nasal septal deviation are also common in patients with epistaxis (4). It is not clear how septal deformities promote epistaxis. Septal deflections can cause disruption of laminar airflow. Eddies occur in these areas, which dry out, making them prone to bleeding. Intranasal foreign bodies are rare in adults but are an important cause of epistaxis in children. Foreign bodies will often present as unilateral, foul smelling rhinorrhea which is refractory to medical therapy. In adults, a nasal foreign body may be found in a victim of a recent motor vehicle accident who unknowingly had a piece of glass impacted in the nasal cavity that was not readily apparent on initial evaluation. Industrial chemical exposures, (e.g., to the fumes of chromates, ammonia, and sulfuric acid) have also been implicated in causing recurrent epistaxis (5). Cigarette smoke, including second-hand sources, is also an irritant that can promote epistaxis.

Epistaxis occasionally occurs subsequent to iatrogenic trauma (nasal and sinus surgery). Benign and malignant intranasal tumors are uncommon but can present with persistent epistaxis.

Systemic Factors

A variety of systemic factors related to either vascular fragility or clotting abnormalities may contribute to epistaxis. Long-standing hypertension may be a factor in promoting epistaxis, but it remains controversial whether there is a higher rate of arterial hypertension in epistaxis patients versus normal control subjects (1). It appears that hypertensive patients on diuretics are more susceptible to epistaxis than those taking β-blockers (6). Many patients have elevated blood pressure at the time of their treatment for epistaxis, but this may simply be a result of pain and anxiety. It is important to ascertain whether or not hypertension returns to normal after treatment, so that patients found to have underlying hypertension can receive appropriate treatment (7). Generalized vascular disease associated with hypertension may also be a factor, because underlying atherosclerotic vessels are known to have decreased elasticity and capacity to contract and assist in clot formation.

Patients with end-stage renal disease on hemodialysis are prone to recurrent epistaxis. This may be because of a decrease in platelet activity or frequent exposure to heparin (8,9). Septal perforation is noted in up to 8% of patients with chronic renal failure, and this perforation can precipitate turbulent airflow, local irritation and crusting, and recurrent hemorrhage similar to septal deviation. Alcohol abuse with associated poor nutrition and vitamin C and K deficiencies may lead to poor wound healing and poor clot formation. Additionally, liver disease secondary to alcohol abuse can cause alterations in the normal clotting mechanism, thus setting the stage for persistent and recurrent epistaxis.

Patients with hereditary coagulation abnormalities, such as hemophilia or von Willebrand disease, can have problematic and persistent epistaxis. Acquired conditions, such as thrombocytopenia from a hematologic malignancy or chemotherapy, may also be significant. Osler-Rendu-Weber disease (hereditary hemorrhagic telangiectasia) very commonly presents with recurrent epistaxis. This inherited condition results in a lack of the contractile elements in the vessel walls with formation of telangiectasias on the nasal, oral, intraoral, and gastric mucosa. These patients often have recurrent gastrointestinal (GI) bleeding as well as epistaxis, and treatment can be problematic requiring multiple treatments over the lifetime of the patient. It is not unusual to need multiple transfusions and multiple surgical interventions (e.g., cauterization, embolization).

Numerous medications are also implicated in epistaxis. Nonsteroidal anti-inflammatory drugs (NSAIDs) are commonly a factor, with as many as 75% of epistaxis patients having previously been on one of these drugs (10). It is important to determine by a careful history if these agents, including aspirin, have been used, for what length of time they were used, and the time of their last use (11). These medications interfere with normal platelet function by inhibiting the cyclooxygenase pathway and arachidonic acid metabolism. Other agents that dry the nasal mucosa, such as tricyclic antidepressants, antipsychotic agents, and antihistamines, may promote mucosal disruption and bleeding. Nasal steroid sprays may also cause epistaxis, either because of the vehicle, the medication itself, or trauma from the nasal spray applicator. With prolonged use, nasal steroids can thin the nasal mucosa, leading to an increased risk of epistaxis.

Approach to Management

Management of a patient with epistaxis should proceed at a pace congruent with the severity of bleeding and acuity of the situation. The ABCs (airway, breathing, and circulation) of resuscitation need to be followed. Patients should be assessed for hemodynamic stability and the severity of their blood loss. Intravenous access should be established in all patients who are actively bleeding.

Fortunately, most epistaxis is not accompanied by massive blood loss, and the focus is on local control of the bleeding. It is important, though, not to take a casual approach to epistaxis because fatalities, although rare, are known to occur, especially in patients with existing comorbidities such as coronary artery disease or chronic pulmonary disease. The demeanor of the health care provider can do much to ease the anxiety of the patient with epistaxis. A calm, matter of fact demeanor will help to reassure the patient that they are in good hands and the episode will be resolved. An anxious or harried interaction with the patient can serve to increase their anxiety and stress levels leading to increased pulse and blood pressure, which will make controlling the epistaxis more difficult.

The initial history should ascertain on which side the bleeding began and whether or not it was mostly isolated nasal bleeding or associated with excessive spitting up of blood, which would suggest a posterior bleeding site. The duration of the nosebleed and an estimation of blood loss are also pertinent. A history of previous epistaxis and how those episodes were treated may suggest the initial treatment in a given situation. A past medical history should ascertain whether or not hypertension, liver disease, alcoholism, cardiac disease, or renal insufficiency is present. A review of the patient's medications will determine if nonsteroidal anti-inflammatory agents, warfarin, or aspirin-containing products are contributing to clotting abnormalities.

At initial presentation, it is reasonable to obtain laboratory studies, including a complete blood count (CBC) (to determine if anemia is present), prothrombin time (PT)/partial thromboplastin time (PTT) and platelets (to assess for significant coagulopathy), and a type-and-screen to make blood available if the episode of epistaxis is intractable. Hematocrit taken at the time of presentation may not accurately reflect the severity of blood loss because of a lack of hemodilution that will occur as intravascular volume is restored.

The next step is to examine the nasal cavity. Universal precautions for all health care personnel are important, because epistaxis management can be quite bloody. Appropriate protective gear should be worn, including eyewear, gowns, gloves, and caps. The patient should be supplied with a handful of gauze or tissues and should be draped appropriately to allow comfortable examination. Strong suction is a must, preferably with a Frazier tip suction. A headlight and nasal speculum are helpful in performing intranasal examination, although an otoscope or other hand held light can be used. Intranasal examination may be aided by decongesting the nose. Topical decongestants (e.g., oxymetazoline 0.05%, two to three sprays in each nostril) will cause significant vasoconstriction and either decrease or stop the flow of blood (12). All clots should be removed from the nose, preferably through intranasal suctioning, and patients also may be asked to blow their noses to remove any clots prior to decongesting the nose. This allows for the decongestant to contact the mucosa directly to maximize its effect.

Treatment

Treatment of epistaxis should be performed in a step-like fashion to provide the least invasive means to control the episode. Because most nasal bleeding is anterior, local compression of the nose should be performed initially using the thumb and index finger to compress the cartilaginous portion of the nose. This can be initiated by instructing the patient to perform this maneuver while the other materials are being collected. This allows for a clot to form and set at the bleeding site. Fifteen minutes of direct pressure should be applied. The patient or health care providers should hold pressure while watching a clock in order to complete the entire time. If any break in holding pressure occurs, the time should be reset and 15 minutes of holding pressure begun again. During this time the patient should be instructed to sit calmly with their head held forward and their mouth open. Any draining blood will drip off the tip of the nose or be expectorated out of the mouth into an appropriate receptacle. Holding the head back as is commonly advised will encourage blood to be swallowed, which can lead to GI upset and emesis. The Valsalva will raise the venous pressure in the head and can inhibit successful clotting of a bleeding site in the nose. If compression is unsuccessful, the nose should be cleaned of clot by suctioning and vigorous nose blowing followed by the application of decongestant spray to both sides of the nose. Pressure should then be applied as described above for 15 minutes. The algorithm as described so far can be performed anywhere and does not require special equipment, medications, or specialty training and should be given as instructions to patients following an episode of epistaxis should they have a rebleed.

If bleeding persists despite the above intervention, it is imperative to visualize the bleeding site. Lighting, suction, and patience are invaluable tools to this end. If the bleeding site is seen to be anterior, a cotton ball impregnated with a decongestant and lidocaine may be used to anesthetize and further decongest the area of the bleeding vessel. Silver nitrate cautery can be used to lightly cauterize the area around the vessel. The silver nitrate stick should be used from a peripheral to central fashion around the bleeding vessel, with the stick rolled over the mucosa lightly until a gray residue appears. This technique is difficult to perform during active bleeding and often will be unsuccessful. It is important to avoid deep chemical cautery with silver nitrate, as well as bilateral septal cautery, to avoid injury to the underlying cartilage, which can lead to septal perforation. If the bleeding is controlled with this method, a cotton swab saturated with normal saline should be used to neutralize any residual silver nitrate and curtail the chemical cautery. After silver nitrate cautery, an antibiotic ointment should be applied to prevent crusting and subsequent local bacterial infection.

If the bleeding persists, the next level of intervention is anterior packing. Traditional anterior packing dictates placement of a layer of half-inch lubricated gauze coated in antibiotic ointment. This is a difficult technique to master and is now seldom performed. There are several commercially available expandable nasal tampons (Merocel, Xomed Surgical Products, Jacksonville, FL; Rapid Rhino, Applied Therapeutics, Inc Newbury, Berkshire UK) that can be as effective and are much easier to place. When using a nasal tampon, it is important to have a good idea where the site of bleeding is to determine the length of the nasal tampon to apply. The common length is up to 10 cm, which will pack the entire nose, including the posterior choana. It is also important to understand that the floor of the nose slants caudally from an anterior to posterior direction and that the tampon should be directed somewhat inferiorly as opposed to cranially. The nasal tampon can be coated with an antibacterial ointment to prevent premature expansion of the tampon by blood during the insertion and to provide an impediment to bacterial overgrowth of the packing. The packing should be left in place from 3 to 5 days to allow clotting and healing of the bleeding area. If necessary, bilateral tampons or synthetic sponge packs can be placed. The success rate is high, and minimal experience is needed for placement. Additionally, patient tolerance of this form of packing is superior to the classic layered gauze. After placing the pack, the oropharynx should be examined to determine if there is any residual bleeding. If there is bleeding noted posteriorly, the anterior tampons may be inadequate and posterior packing may be needed. After packing, an oral antibiotic such as a first-or second-generation cephalosporin (e.g., cephalexin 250 mg orally four times daily) or amoxicillin/clavulanate (Augmentin, 500 mg twice daily) with staphylococcal coverage should be used for 10 days to avoid bacterial overgrowth and to prevent toxic shock syndrome (TSS).

A downside to conventional packing is that it needs to be removed. This is usually done 3 to 5 days after the packing was placed. This is usually not an adequate length of time to allow for the site of bleeding to mucosalize. Additionally, the placement and removal of the packing material can abrade the nasal mucosa and cause bleeding. Any time packing is removed preparations should be made and materials available to repack the nose should bleeding recur. To avoid this possibility, many practitioners will use absorbable materials to pack the nose first. Several options are available (Surgicel, Johnson and Johnson, Somerville, NJ; Gelfoam, Pharmacia & Upjohn, Kalamazoo, MI; Avitene, Davol Inc., Cranston RI; Floseal, Baxter, Deerfield, IL; Thrombin, JONES PHARMA Inc., St. Louis, MO). These materials are not designed specifically for intranasal use and need to be formed to the desired size and shape. They can be applied to an identified bleeding site, active or quiescent, to stop bleeding and facilitate healing (13).

The posterior vessels are difficult to visualize and are not affected by pressure from the usual anterior nasal packing. Posterior packing is necessary in cases of a posterior site of bleeding and in situations where nasal septal deflection prohibits adequate insertion of a tampon. Although only about 5% of epistaxis originates from a posterior nasal source, it is these patients who are at most risk of complications and adverse sequelae (14). Posterior nasal packing is difficult to perform and requires a complex procedure to allow insertion of a nasal pack from the oropharynx into the nasopharynx. Commercially available balloon intranasal catheters (Epistat, Xomed Surgical Products, Jacksonville, FL) may be placed by otolaryngologists or other clinicians experienced in their use. A Foley catheter can also be used as a posterior pack. Because insertion of the posterior packing is painful, the clinician should provide mild sedation before placement. Additionally, any patient who undergoes posterior nasal packing should be admitted to the hospital for observation. Posterior packing will cause swallowing difficulty, so maintenance of hydration by administration of intravenous fluids is important. Posterior nasal packing is usually removed after about 48 to 72 hours. It can be difficult to determine whether posterior packing is necessary, and it is reasonable to proceed with anterior packing first and if this fails to control the bleeding, proceed with posterior packing.

Consideration should be given as well to hospitalization of elderly and debilitated patients who require anterior nasal packing. An otolaryngologist should be consulted if there is doubt about the management of such a patient. Bilateral, as well as posterior, nasal packing will obstruct the nasal airway and may promote hypoxia or hypercapnia (15). Also, posterior packing and the mild sedation it requires can promote decreased arterial oxygenation and hypercapnia. Continuous pulse oximetry is indicated and admission to an appropriate level unit to ensure the necessary surveillance based on the patient's age and general health. These patients are at risk for a nasal vagal response, bradycardia, hypertension, apnea, dislodged packing, aspiration, persistent bleeding, and significant hypoxia.

Surgical Interventions

If these packing procedures are ineffective, more invasive procedures may be performed by a consulting otolaryngologist, including extracranial arterial ligations, if necessary (16,17). Embolization of active nasal bleeding can be done in centers with interventional neuroradiology (18).

Special Cases

In patients with severe coagulopathy or thrombocytopenia, placement of intranasal packing can be problematic, because at the time of removal a raw nasal mucosa may continue to bleed. Transfusion of clotting factors and platelets can be helpful in stopping the bleeding temporarily, but, in some circumstances packing may still be needed. In these cases, the use of a porcine pack may be appropriate. This entails using a strip of ordinary salt pork to pack the nose. Homogenates of salt pork contain an activation factor that promotes platelet aggregation. Additionally, the porcine packing is less irritating to the nose, and upon removal there is less nasal mucosal irritation to promote bleeding (19).

Nasal bleeding associated with significant facial or head trauma can be complicated by disruption of the cribriform plate in the anterior cranial base permitting displacement of packing material into the intracranial space. Therefore, in these situations, packing and nasal instrumentation should be deferred and prompt otolaryngology consultation arranged. Arterial embolization is also an effective method for intractable nosebleeds, especially in patients who are not considered surgical candidates (19).

Followup and Patient Education

Most patients can be treated in an outpatient setting and return for packing removal. If the patient's epistaxis is recurrent and persistent, prompt otolaryngologic evaluation is appropriate, even if packing was unnecessary. Persistent and refractory epistaxis can be evaluated by testing for coagulopathy or any hematopoietic malignancies. Sinus radiographs or computed tomography (CT) can rule out an intranasal mass. Nasal endoscopy has revolutionized sinonasal evaluation; it allows a well-illuminated, magnified view of the entire nasal cavity to assess for potential bleeding sites, anatomic abnormalities and tumors. This procedure is easy to perform in the otolaryngology office setting using topical anesthesia.

Many patients with persistent epistaxis, even after determining there is no sinister underlying pathology, will have etiologic factors that cannot be modified. For example, patients may require warfarin or may have an underlying chronic medical condition that is unlikely to change. It is important to educate these individuals about conservative measures that can alleviate the cycle of epistaxis. Patients should be informed about the physiology of epistaxis, with a cycle of desiccation, crusting, mucosal disruption, and hemorrhage followed by crusting and rebleeding. It may be helpful to explain this phenomenon by analogy to a puddle of water that dries and one can then see the ground on the bottom caking and cracking. This exemplifies the nasal mucosa and its fragility and need for humidification. Patients should be instructed to avoid aspirin therapy within 2 weeks of their nosebleed to allow for a reasonable period of time for healing. Additionally, humidification of the nose should be stressed with liberal use of nasal saline spray every hour while awake and application of a nasal emollient (Vaseline, Bacitracin) twice a day to the nasal vestibule. Room humidifiers should also be used to elevate the humidification of the household air and are particularly useful while sleeping.

Patients should be instructed what to do if subsequent nosebleeds occur. This includes instructing the patient in digital compression of the anterior nose. Application of pressure to the entire soft pliable portion of the nose with the thumb and finger should be demonstrated. It is important to stress that this maneuver should be performed for at least 15 minutes by the clock without peeking to see if bleeding is continuing. Patients prone to nosebleeds should keep oxymetazoline spray (0.05%) on hand, remove any intranasal clots by blowing, and spray each nostril generously two to three times. These self-administered treatments control simple epistaxis in about two thirds of patients (12). If these methods fail, patients should be instructed to seek care from their provider or an emergency room for more definitive management.

Some patients who are prone to persistent and severe nosebleeds (e.g., those with hereditary hemorrhagic telangiectasias) have learned to self-apply anterior packing. In the situation of recurrent one-sided nosebleeds, certain anatomic abnormalities may respond to "nasal rest." This is achieved by having a patient take a small cotton ball impregnated with petroleum jelly and place it into the anterior nares to obstruct all airflow in the bleeding nasal cavity. This can be continued for several days at a time to prevent desiccation and allow for healing.

SNORING

Snoring is a significant behavioral and social problem with potentially important medical implications. Approximately 25% to 50% of men and 15% to 30% of women become chronic snorers (20). Chronic snoring may be a symptom of obstructive sleep apnea (OSA) syndrome (see Chapter 7). Although it is the cardinal symptom, snoring is not a specific marker for OSA (21). Snoring without OSA is often designated benign snoring, but a better term may be nonapneic snoring, because the medical implications of benign snoring are still being elucidated. There is no clear evidence that nonapneic snoring is a significant risk factor for the more severe medical consequences of OSA. However, nonapneic snoring may fragment sleep and result in daytime hypersomnolence and dysfunction. The personal and social impact of snoring can be substantial, such as when bed partners require alternative sleeping arrangements (22). Primary care clinicians and otolaryngologists are often called on to evaluate and treat individuals with this condition and differentiate it from other sleep disorders.

Pathophysiology

Snoring is a consequence of the elasticity of the soft tissues of the oropharynx. The snoring sound is thought to be generated by vibrations of the collapsing soft tissues of the pharynx, soft palate, uvula and, infrequently, the nasal passages. It can be difficult to determine the exact site responsible for snoring. Compared with nonsnorers, nonapneic snorers are noted to have smaller airways with higher airway compliances, but these changes are not as severe as in patients with sleep apnea (21). Airway collapsibility is deterred by sustained pharyngeal muscle tone, which is absent during rapid eye movement (REM) sleep. Thus, snoring is significantly related to the stage of sleep (23).

One of the difficulties in studying snoring and assessing appropriate management interventions is that there are few objective measures of this phenomenon. Often the clinician has to rely on snoring assessment by the bed partner, because approximately 75% of snoring patients are unaware that they snore and if they are aware of snoring it is usually because of the complaints of others (22). Common risk factors for snoring are male gender, obesity, alcohol consumption, ingestion of sedatives or muscle relaxants, and smoking. Even small amounts of alcohol can exacerbate snoring. The use of sedatives or muscle relaxants will also cause a relaxation of the pharyngeal musculature and promote snoring. Smoking may also contribute by increasing pharyngeal inflammation and edema due to the irritant effects of tobacco smoke, leading to pharyngeal narrowing and subsequent snoring. Nasal obstruction from chronic rhinitis or sinusitis may also be a contributing factor. There may also be a familial predisposition to snoring (24).

Evaluation

The office evaluation of patients with snoring should focus on their medical and sleep histories and include a general examination with emphasis on the head and neck. The main task of the evaluation is to determine how severe and disruptive the snoring is and whether further evaluation for OSA syndrome (as outlined in Chapter 7 and below) is indicated.

Sleep and Medical Histories

Patients should be queried about their awareness of snoring and whether they awake at night with a gasping or choking sensation. They should also be asked if they awake in the morning feeling rested or not and if they awake with a headache. Symptoms of daytime somnolence should be ascertained, especially interference with work, driving, or other tasks.

Because most snorers are unaware of their problem, it is helpful to talk to a bed partner or other close observer. This person should be questioned about the frequency, persistence, and severity of snoring and especially whether there are apneic periods, gasping, or choking. Initial assessment of the degree of personal and social disruption is also pertinent; for example, is the patient able to maintain a normal sleeping arrangement or must the patient or bed partner leave the room for sleep? For the reasons indicated above, it is important to inquire about recent change in weight and its effects on the snoring pattern, as well as the use of alcohol, tobacco, and prescription and over-the-counter drug use. Finally, the patient should be questioned about nasal and sinus symptoms that may be associated with snoring.

Examination

Physical examination is directed at the head and neck. Careful nasal examination should be performed to look for nasal polyps, nasal septal deviation, turbinate hypertrophy, or any evidence of anatomic nasal airway obstruction (see Chapter 33). The oral examination should focus on identifying macroglossia and tonsillar hypertrophy. Sometimes the uvula may be elongated, swollen, or inflamed from vibrations produced during snoring.

If snoring is severe or disruptive, referral to an otolaryngologist is indicated for airway assessment, usually with transnasal flexible fiberoptic laryngoscopy to rule out any anatomic obstruction. Flexible fiberoptic laryngoscopy can be performed easily with topical anesthesia, and it provides a useful evaluation of the entire upper airway.

Because OSA syndrome can have significant and preventable morbidity, it is important to consider whether it is present in patients who snore. Nevertheless, most snorers do not have OSA syndrome. There are as yet no validated clinical criteria for determining whether a patient who snores has sleep apnea; diagnosis is dependent on polysomnography. Important features associated with OSA syndrome include apneas reported by an observer, nocturnal gasping or choking reported by the patient or an observer, very loud or disruptive snoring, daytime somnolence, hypertension, nocturnal or early morning angina or palpitations, and headaches on awakening, which are characteristically brief (25). Additionally, an Epworth Sleepiness Scale can be applied to help determine if further testing is needed. If some of these features are present, and especially if one or more are severe, further testing, such as overnight pulse oximetry or formal polysomnography (sleep study), is indicated (20) (see Chapter 7).

Treatment of Nonapneic Snoring

There are two therapeutic approaches to nonapneic snoring: low-risk conservative measures and surgery, commonly directed at the soft palate. If conservative measures do not produce satisfactory results, and surgical options are considered, the patient should undergo polysomnography to rule out OSA syndrome before referral to an otolaryngologist. This will prevent future masking of OSA symptoms by the surgical intervention and unanticipated perioperative complications of existing OSA.

Nonsurgical Treatment

Conservative measures aimed at decreasing upper airway resistance include improved overall muscle tone and weight loss. This can be achieved by instituting an exercise program. For some patients, weight loss is the only nonsurgical therapy that will relieve benign snoring. Although it is unclear how much weight loss is needed to provide symptomatic improvement, achievement of ideal body weight is not necessary (21). Most patients will note a marked improvement in snoring symptoms with a 10% weight loss. Addressing sleep posture is also helpful in some patients. Bed partners will often relate that snoring is worse in certain positions and absent in others. Many patients achieve marked reduction in snoring when sleeping in the lateral decubitus or prone positions. The classic treatment of sewing a pocket in the back of the pajamas to place one or more tennis balls to force the patient to sleep on the side has anecdotal support.

The use of over-the-counter nasal dilation devices, such as an external adhesive strip (e.g., Breathe Right), may provide relief in some patients, but studies are inconclusive (26). Internal nasal dilators are much less tolerated by patients. In general, nasal devices are not effective, becasue most snoring is not caused by the nasal airway. Nasal devices will help patients with nasal valve collapse as the cause of their snoring. The use of various oromandibular splinting devices that advance the lower jaw (sleep splints) has been advocated by many dental professionals, and some efficacy has been reported (21,27). These devices, unfortunately, are often poorly tolerated and require customized fitting by a dentist or oral surgeon who is familiar with their application to achieve satisfactory results.

The use of phosphocholinamine, a tissue lubricant placed intranasally, has been found to reduce snoring frequency by about 25% in a small study (28). However, this is an oil-based agent, and there is the theoretical risk of aspiration and lipoid pneumonia. Protriptyline, a tricyclic antidepressant, has also been found to reduce snoring by as much as 30% (29) in most patients. The long-term efficacy, however, is unknown, and the anticholinergic side effects may be bothersome. If significant nasal obstruction is present, it is reasonable to treat with systemic decongestants (see Chapter 33) and intranasal steroids (see Chapter 30) to maximize the cross-sectional area of the nasal airway. Improving the nasal airway may be enough in some patients to obviate or reduce snoring. Continuous positive airway pressure (CPAP) administered via a nasal mask is commonly used to treat OSA. This device applies a pneumatic "splint" to the upper airway structures and almost invariably eliminates snoring. Nonapneic snorers are often hesitant to use the CPAP system and usually tolerate it poorly. It is not clear why nonapneic snorers are less tolerant of CPAP, but it may be because of the lack of significant symptomatic benefits compared with patients with OSA (30).

Surgical Treatments

When the snoring patient has an obvious anatomic abnormality that leads to upper airway obstruction (such as enlarged tonsils and adenoids, severely deviated nasal septum, or nasal polyps), surgical therapy may be recommended by an otolaryngologist.

Uvulopalatopharyngoplasty (UPPP) was first described in the early 1960s as a treatment for snoring (31). This technique was subsequently applied as treatment for OSA with some success. The technique entails removal of any existing tonsil tissue and partial resection of the soft palate, uvula, and anterior tonsillar pillars. The airway is thus opened, allowing for increased airflow and reducing the extent of vibratory tissue to generate snoring. Although UPPP is initially quite effective in snoring resolution, long-term success rates range only from 46% to 73% (32). This may be due to transient weight loss after surgery. Most patients will lose 5 to 15 pounds after surgery because of poor oral intake after surgery. This weight loss is often not sustained and may explain why the long term success of UPPP. UPPP is an aggressive procedure that requires an approximate 3-week postoperative convalescence. Patients often complain of severe odynophagia postoperatively, and because of this only 60% of patients indicate they would undergo the same treatment again (33). Another disadvantage of UPPP is nasopharyngeal incompetence; almost one fourth of patients complain of intermittent nasopharyngeal regurgitation for up to 1 year after surgery (34).

Because of the limitations of UPPP, there has been an ongoing search for more effective and safer palatal procedures for benign snoring. Laser or cautery-assisted uvuloplasty, in which the uvula alone is truncated in the office setting under local anesthesia, has gained popularity. Uvuloplasty is associated with fewer complications than UPPP, but the technique still entails significant post procedure pain. Uvuloplasty appears to be equally effective as UPPP for snoring treatment, but multiple office excisions are often required and up to 77% of patients abandon their course of uvuloplasty therapy because of pain (35). Uvuloplasty may rarely cause postoperative bleeding and temporary nasopharyngeal regurgitation.

Other forms of surgical therapies for snoring use laser or other modalities to produce palatal stiffening (20). A newer technique involves the delivery of radiofrequency energy (Somnoplasty, Somnus Medical Technologies) with a needle electrode into various sites of the soft palate, resulting in fibrosis and stiffening (36). Radiofrequency ablation is generally safe, minimally invasive, and has few complications (37). Postoperative pain is minimal, because there is no mucosal disruption, and acetaminophen alone is often sufficient for analgesia. Radiofrequency ablation can require three to four treatments to achieve an appropriate level of snoring cessation. Large-scale trials or systematic reviews of surgical therapies for snoring are not yet available (20). This technique can also be used to address the base of tongue to reduce tissue bulk and address snoring at this anatomic site too.

ANOSMIA

Chemosensory disorders affect up to 2 million adults in the United States (39). Unfortunately, the sense of smell is often ignored by clinicians and it is often thought of as an inconvenience rather than a disease spectrum. Anosmia can result in significant debility, especially in individuals who rely on the sense of smell for their occupation (e.g., chefs, police officers, florists). Additionally, anosmia can be dangerous because affected individuals are unable to discern gas leaks, spoiled food, or smoke. Anosmia and its often accompanying decreased sense of taste can lead to eating displeasure and poor nutritional intake.

Pathophysiology

The sense of smell depends on olfactory chemoreceptors located high in the nasal cavity along the upper septum and cribriform plate, which underlies the anterior cranial fossa. These receptors transmit impulse back to cranial nerve I, the olfactory nerve. The odorant molecules are dissolved in the nasal mucous and presented to the neurepithelium of the olfactory nerve for processing. It is not completely understood how the normally functioning olfactory system is able to process and differentiate the multitude of odors presented to it (40). The sense of taste is a more gross perception, which is mediated by taste buds located on the tongue, soft palate, and oropharynx. The sensation of taste generated by these receptors is limited to the basic qualities of salty, sour, sweet, and bitter. Most individual perceptions of flavor and taste are in fact olfactory sensations, classically evidenced by the fact that children are often convinced to take distasteful medicine by holding their nose and preventing any olfactory input. Thus, a patient who complains of a diminished taste may in fact have hyposmia or anosmia.

There is also a chemosensory sense mediated by the trigeminal nerve, cranial nerve V, which is triggered by pungent and irritant compounds, such as hot peppers, horseradish, or mustard, and perceived as burning or irritating. This pathway is independent from the other modalities of taste and smell.

Dysfunction of smell is classified as complete or partial and is referred to, respectively, as anosmia or hyposmia. Another interesting variation of smell disturbance is phantosmia, in which spontaneous and distorted olfactory hallucinations are manifest. These phantosmias are often described in association in patients with seizure activity, psychiatric illness, and Alzheimer disease (41). Dysosmia is defined as a distorted sense of smell and is often used to describe when person senses nonexistent unpleasant odors instead of the expected smell.

Etiology

As people age, the sense of smell declines naturally, and the decline may not be perceptible because it is gradual. Patients are very sensitive to an acute decrease in their sense of smell. When evaluating a patient with diminished smell or taste, it is important to determine the duration of the complaint, whether the loss was gradual or acute, and whether the sensory loss acutely followed head trauma or an upper respiratory tract infection (a more gradual progression would accompany sinusitis, nasal polyposis,

TABLE 111.2 Some Common Medications That Can Impair the Sense of Smell

β-Blockers
Ciprofloxacin
Diltiazem
Docycycline
Enalapril
Methotrexate
Nifedipine

Adapted from Ackerman BH, Kasbekar N. Disturbances of taste and smell induced by drugs. Pharmacotherapy 1997;17:482.

or an intracranial tumor). The patient's medication list should be reviewed because many medications alter the senses of taste and smell (42). Table 111.2 shows common medications that can impair the sense of smell.

Anosmia can be considered in two broad categories: sensorineural, in which the olfactory loss is constant, and conductive, whereby the patient may intermittently have olfactory function. *Sensorineural loss* signifies a loss of the neuroepithelium, damage to the olfactory nerves, or injury to the olfactory centers in the brain resulting in the inability to smell. Conductive loss is caused by the inability of odorant molecules to reach the olfactory neuroepithelium. This would be the case with an acute upper respiratory infection with nasal inflammation or nasal polyps.

Common causes of sensorineural anosmia include postviral, traumatic, and neoplastic. Postvirally induced anosmia is quite common, accounting for up to a third of anosmia cases. Patients will typically report a very severe respiratory tract infection, and as their congestion resolves they do not regain their sense of smell. The etiologic factor is damage to the olfactory neuroepithelium by the viral agent. These patients are usually not completely anosmic and have a reduced sense of smell, hyposmia. These patients also tend to be older individuals, which may suggest that the anosmia may be related to a series of viral insults throughout life, resulting in progressive anosmia.

History of head trauma including prior surgery is another important cause of anosmia. Up to 5% of patients suffering head injury will have olfactory loss, depending on the severity of the head injury (43). The mechanism of injury is typically a frontal or occipital blow, which results in stretching or sheering of the olfactory nerves as they exit the cribriform plate. Loss of consciousness, concussion, and skull fracture are not necessary to precipitate anosmia. These patients are typically younger and are often completely anosmic.

Neoplasms of the olfactory tract are uncommon causes of anosmia. Intracranial abnormalities will generally present with other symptoms and not isolated smell disturbance. Imaging studies, CT scan of the paranasal sinuses and MRI scan of the olfactory tract, can yield information about the anatomy of the olfactory tracts but infrequently discover a lesion responsible for anosmia (44). Prior radiation therapy also often results in marked dysfunction of both smell and taste (45). Rare causes include endocrine disorders such as Kallmann syndrome (hypogonadotropic hypogonadism; see Chapter 81) and Turner syndrome (46). About 20% of patients presenting with anosmia do not have evidence of the preceding causes and after a careful workup will be classified as having an idiopathic cause.

Conductive anosmia can be because of a variety of causes: chronic rhinosinusitis, nasal polyposis, nasal septal deviation, or intranasal mass. History and physical examination are keys to successful diagnosis and treatment of conductive deficits.

Evaluation

As with many disorders, a complete history and physical examination can direct the healthcare provider to a potential cause and treatment plan. Physical examination should focus on the nasal anatomy (see Chapter 33). Inspection of the anterior nasal cavities may not be adequate to completely evaluate potential causes of anosmia. If anterior anatomic abnormalities are observed or if the cause of anosmia remains unclear, referral to an otolaryngologist is indicated. Anterior rhinoscopy can miss almost half of the cases where there a conductive cause. Nasal endoscopy is more sensitive in detecting intranasal abnormalities that may be causing decreased sense of smell (43).

An appropriate next step in anosmia evaluation would be to determine if the smell disturbance is reversible. This can be done clinically by using a short course of high-dose systemic corticosteroids in a tapered fashion (e.g., oral prednisone 60 mg daily for several days, followed by tapering doses to complete a 10-day course). If the olfactory deficit results from nasal inflammation, such as allergic rhinitis or chronic rhinosinusitis, then the olfactory deficit can be temporarily reversed. If the patient does not respond to this steroid challenge, imaging studies and consultation with an otolaryngologist may be warranted, especially if the history or examination do not suggest a cause. The best initial test is a CT of the sinuses. Sinus CT will completely delineate the nasal cavity and determine if there is adequate patency of the air passages and will evaluate for associated sinusitis. CT scans are poor for evaluating soft tissue and the anterior cranial fossa. When the cause of anosmia remains obscure, a magnetic resonance image may be needed to rule out anterior cranial fossa tumors, such as meningioma, or other soft tissue neoplasms.

Olfactory Testing

Olfactory testing may be performed by an otolaryngologist to determine threshold odor identification or odor intensity. Odor identification is often tested using the University of Pennsylvania Smell Identification Test. In this test, a patient releases 40 microencapsulated odorants by rubbing designated areas on a card and answers corresponding questions about the identities of the odors. The answers are graded using normative data based on gender and age.

Treatment and Management

Inflammatory nasal disease is a common entity affecting a patient's sense of smell. Some patients will have subacute sinusitis in which the nasal symptoms (congestion, facial pain, and nasal drainage) are subtle and not appreciated, and the primary complaint of the patient is anosmia or a distorted sense of smell. CT (see Evaluation) may show chronic sinusitis, and subsequent treatment of this sinusitis (see Chapter 33) can, in many cases, restore normal olfaction. Nasal polyposis treatment either with medications or surgical removal by an otolaryngologist may restore normal olfaction, although polyps often recur and olfaction may be compromised early as polyps regrow.

The prognosis for recovery of disorders of odorant conduction (polyps, septal deviation, or rhinosinusitis) causing poor delivery of olfactants to the neuroepithelium is good if the underlying nasal pathology can be remedied. Sensorineural loss caused by damage to the olfactory neurons after trauma or viral infection has a much less favorable prognosis. Approximately 30% of patients with posttraumatic anosmia improve partially or completely within the first year, most within the first 12 weeks (47).

Vitamin A and zinc are commonly prescribed for anosmia; however, their efficacy is not well supported (48). Newer and not yet standardized approaches for disorders of olfaction, such as olfactory epithelial biopsy by an otolaryngologist, with histopathologic and electron microscopic evaluation, are being studied in some centers.

It is important to counsel patients who suffer persistent anosmia about coping maneuvers, such as having appropriate gas and smoke detectors in their home and having adequate assistance with food preparation and evaluation for spoiled foods. Detecting the need to change diapers for small children and cleaning up after pets may be problematic for patients with anosmia. In food preparation, care must be taken not to overuse salt and sugar to add flavor because these additives may precipitate other medical problems. The use of temperature (i.e., hot or cold), texture, and spices in food preparation can be helpful to make food more palatable.

HOARSENESS

Because the voice is so important to interpersonal communication, hoarseness causes a great deal of patient distress. Hoarseness is an imprecise term used to describe any alteration in a patient's normal voice quality. Otolaryngologists and speech pathologists use the term *dysphonia* to more accurately portray abnormal voice quality and localize the disease process to the laryngeal structures. Hoarseness is the symptom and dysphonia is the corresponding sign. A dysphonic patient will have a breathy, strained, rough, raspy, tremulous, or weak voice. A complaint of hoarseness should be evaluated thoughtfully, because it may represent a significant underlying pathology. Appropriate referral to an otolaryngologist for direct visualization of the laryngeal structures is warranted if hoarseness persists longer than a few weeks.

Pathophysiology

The evaluation of hoarseness depends on an understanding of the pertinent anatomy and normal physiology involved with voice production. The vocal tract can be thought of in three separate compartments: the lungs, the larynx, and the oral cavity. The lungs are the power source for voice production. The true vocal folds of the larynx are the anatomic site for sound production. Sound is generated by airflow through closely approximated vocal folds. The quality of the sound produced is determined by multiple factors, including the degree of vocal fold opposition, the tension in the laryngeal musculature, and the properties of the vocal fold epithelium itself (49). In the oral cavity and oropharynx, sound produced in the laryngeal structures is further modified by the tongue, lips, and teeth. Strictly speaking, the laryngeal phase of sound production is the site of origin of true hoarseness and dysphonia. The pulmonary portion of vocal production will determine the strength of the sound produced, and the oral cavity is primarily involved in articulation and the refinement of the sound to produce speech. An alteration in the oral phase of vocal production is more appropriately termed dysarthria.

The larynx is composed of a cartilaginous skeleton, including the epiglottis, thyroid cartilage, cricoid cartilage, and paired arytenoid cartilages. This cartilaginous framework provides for continuity of airflow from the trachea, through the glottis, to the oral tract. The soft tissue structures in the larynx are composed of laryngeal musculature, including the vocal fold abductors, adductors, and tensors. These muscular structures adjust the coaptation and tension of the vocal folds, which is a major determinant of the quality of sound production. Any alteration in the innervation or function of the laryngeal musculature will result in dysphonia. The mucosal epithelium for most of the larynx is made up of columnar epithelium and mucous-secreting goblet cells, which promote a moist environment for efficient voice production. The true vocal folds are lined with squamous epithelium, which overlies a loose lamina propria (50). This histologic arrangement allows the subglottic airflow to traverse the larynx and produce a mucosal wave in the overlying epithelium, generating sound. Increased viscosity of the loose lamina propria of the vocal folds from dehydration, inflammation, or scarring will result in the need for an increase in the pressure of the airflow through the larynx to establish the vibratory phase of the vocal folds. Adequate hydration of this gelatinous lamina propria layer and the maintenance of a lubricated mucosa of the laryngeal structures are important in determining the quality of laryngeal sound production.

Many local and systemic disorders alter these important elements of the laryngeal environment. With the exception of the cricothyroid muscle, which provides some vocal fold tension, the laryngeal muscles are innervated by the recurrent laryngeal nerves. It is an important anatomic consideration that the recurrent laryngeal nerves, after branching from the main trunks of the vagus nerves, travel in slightly different pathways to ultimately provide laryngeal innervation. The right recurrent laryngeal nerve loops around the right subclavian artery, whereas the left recurrent laryngeal nerve loops around the arch of the aorta, and both travel cephalad to enter the larynx below the thyroid cartilage. The left recurrent laryngeal nerve (but usually not the right) traverses the mediastinum and may be impacted by a variety of mediastinal lesions. Any lesion along the course of the recurrent laryngeal nerves may result in paralysis of the ipsilateral vocal fold. It is also important to know that the motor fibers of the vagus nerve originate in the nucleus ambiguous of the medulla, and any neurologic process at the brainstem level can impact vocal function (51). Sound production also requires the coordination of efforts between the expiratory thoracic musculature and laryngeal musculature.

Differential Diagnosis and Evaluation

Table 111.3 shows the differential diagnosis of hoarseness as broad. A careful history and physical examination, and sometimes visualization of the laryngeal structures (see Snoring, Evaluation, Hoarseness, and Pathophysiology), allows a diagnosis to be made in most cases.

History

Initial evaluation starts with characterizing a patient's voice complaints. A rough and raspy sound suggests a mucosal irregularity, whereas a breathiness or weakness of the voice suggests an incomplete closure of the true vocal folds (e.g., vocal fold paralysis or an endolaryngeal mass preventing apposition of the true vocal folds). It is also important to listen carefully to the patient to determine if the complaint of hoarseness is related to an articulation or resonance disturbance of the oral phase of speech or to a lack of speech volume resulting from an inadequate pulmonary phase of voice production. The duration of symptoms is important, because acute voice alteration may represent a self-limited process such as a viral upper respiratory tract infection, whereas chronic and progressive hoarseness is more concerning for an underlying condition. Fluctuation of the hoarseness implies that a fixed lesion (e.g., polyp, nodule, or tumor) is not present.

TABLE 111.3 Common Problems That Can Cause Hoarseness

Laryngitis
Acute viral
Gastroesophageal reflux
Postnasal drip/sinusitis
Benign lesions
Vocal nodules
Vocal polyps
Laryngeal papilloma
Squamous cell carcinoma
Vocal fold paralysis
Functional dysphonia
Hypothyroidism

Any inciting event, such as recent *voice abuse,* neck trauma, or intubation, should be elicited. Recent voice abuse suggests that a vocal fold hemorrhage or nodules are the cause of the persistent hoarseness. Hoarseness that develops after a single event of excessive vocal use or coughing often represents an acute vocal fold hemorrhage which will resolve over the course of weeks. Vocal fold polyps are usually pedunculated masses and are often associated with smoking. They are located on the free edge of the true vocal fold and are extremely common benign lesions causing hoarseness in the adult patient. *Neck trauma* can result in arytenoid dislocation, laryngeal fractures, or even recurrent laryngeal nerve paralysis. Recent *endotracheal intubation* can also produce persistent hoarseness from arytenoid dislocation, recurrent nerve paresis (or paralysis), traumatic laryngeal granulomas, or atrophic changes of the glottis.

Voice complaints that are worse in the morning and resolve during the day are suggestive of laryngeal irritation from *gastroesophageal reflux disease (GERD)*. Patients with laryngeal manifestations of GERD often do not have the classic symptoms of heartburn and indigestion (52). Associated symptoms should also be carefully investigated. *Dysphagia or aspiration* associated with hoarseness may indicate that a laryngeal tumor is present or that a neurologic process, such as recurrent laryngeal nerve paralysis, is the culprit. Persistent otalgia with a normal ear examination is also worrisome for referred pain from a supraglottic or glottic malignancy. Such pain is referred to the area of the ear via the vagus nerve, which, in addition to supplying the laryngeal structures, contributes to the innervation of the external ear canal. *Allergic rhinitis or chronic sinusitis* with postnasal drainage may also promote chronic laryngeal irritation and inflammation leading to hoarseness. It is important to elucidate *past surgical history,* because an endotracheal intubation may damage the larynx, and may place the recurrent laryngeal nerve at risk (Table 111.4).

Hypothyroidism may produce significant hoarseness because of edema of the laryngeal submucosal lamina propria (53). Medications also may be implicated in voice disturbances. Aspirin, nonsteroidal anti-inflammatory agents, and anticoagulants may promote vocal fold

TABLE 111.4 Surgical Procedures with a Risk of Laryngeal Denervation

Carotid endarterectomy
Anterior cervical fusion
Thyroidectomy
Esophagectomy
Tracheal surgery
Skull base surgery
Thoracic aneurysm repair
Cardiac surgery

hemorrhage. Antihistamines and diuretics may produce upper airway dryness, which also will adversely affect the voice (54).

Social history is also important in evaluating patients with hoarseness and dysphonia. Exposure to tobacco smoke, ethanol, or environmental pollutants directly causes laryngeal irritation and increases the risk for laryngeal carcinoma. Cigarette smoking and alcohol also contribute to the drying of secretions and chronic inflammation. An understanding of the patient's activities that involve the voice (e.g., a teacher, singer, or avid sports fan) is pertinent to diagnosis and to treatment. Patients who use their voice professionally often require early and aggressive intervention and specialized long-term care. The presence of a loud work environment or frequent contact with individuals who have hearing loss may require a patient to speak in an unnaturally loud voice, which can promote the formation of vocal fold nodules. Such patients should be referred to an otolaryngologist and may require therapy with a speech language pathologist.

Physical Examination

A focused head and neck examination should be performed on patients who present with a complaint of hoarseness. Otoscopic examination helps to identify whether associated ear complaints are due to otologic pathology or may be referred from a laryngeal process. Nasal examination may demonstrate abnormal secretions, polyps, or purulence, suggesting chronic rhinitis or sinusitis. Oral cavity and oropharyngeal examination may reveal "cobble stoning" or lymphoid hypertrophy of the posterior pharyngeal wall suggestive of chronic postnasal drainage. The neck should be carefully palpated for thyroid masses, diffuse thyromegaly, lymphadenopathy, or other lesions (e.g., carotid body tumor). Cranial nerve evaluation, to determine if abnormalities are present that may be associated with a vagal neuropathy, is also indicated. The presence or absence of manifestations of hypothyroidism (see Chapter 80) should be assessed.

When a current or recent upper respiratory tract infection is identified and hoarseness has been of a short duration (less than 2 weeks), it is reasonable to defer direct laryngeal examination. In this situation, hoarseness likely is a result of acute viral laryngitis, which should resolve in a few weeks. If it does not, visualization of the larynx is needed and referral to an otolaryngologist is appropriate.

Examination by an Otolaryngologist

A patient with hoarseness that has persisted for more than 2 to 3 weeks should undergo visualization of the laryngeal structures by an otolaryngologist. Any gross abnormality of the larynx, such as polyps, nodules, tumor, or vocal fold motion impairment, usually can be identified by indirect mirror examination. In approximately 15% of patients, the laryngeal structures are not fully visualized because of the patient's anatomy (e.g., an overhanging or retroflexed epiglottis) or an overactive gag reflex. In these cases, for complete visualization of laryngeal structures, the otolaryngologist will use transnasal flexible fiberoptic laryngoscopy. This procedure is easy to perform, is well tolerated, and usually lasts less than 5 minutes. This endoscopic examination may be recorded and documented by video. Occasionally, patients need to be taken to the operating room for direct laryngoscopy. This relatively brief procedure requires general endotracheal anesthesia and intubation but allows a very detailed microscopic examination of the entire larynx and biopsy of suspicious lesions.

Ancillary Testing

Thyroid function tests should be done if hypothyroidism is suspected (see Chapter 80). Video stroboscopy is a specialized examination performed by an otolaryngologist that requires a strobe light which is synchronized to the patient's voice (55). The larynx is visualized under a stroboscopic light source that displays slow motion and allows a very finely detailed examination of the mucosal wave of the true vocal fold. This examination may reveal subtle neurologic deficits with inadequate glottic closure, submucosal cysts, and mucosal abnormalities such as dysplasia or tumor. In the event that a vocal fold paralysis is noted and there is no previous surgical procedure that would put the recurrent laryngeal nerve at risk, an imaging study such as a CT or magnetic resonance image (from the skull base through the entire course of the recurrent laryngeal nerve), should be performed to rule out a neoplastic process. It is important that evaluation of left true vocal fold paralysis include the aortic arch, because this represents the course of the recurrent laryngeal nerve. If dysphagia is present, a barium swallow or esophagoscopy may be pertinent to evaluate for an esophageal neoplasm, which also may be implicated in recurrent laryngeal nerve paralysis.

Management

Treatment for hoarseness depends on its cause (Table 111.3). *Inflammatory processes and acute laryngitis* are often self-limited. It is important to note that true vocal folds have no lymphatic elements so resolution of edema and restoration of a truly normal voice may take some time. The patient should maintain adequate hydration and avoid the use of antihistamines and decongestants, which may have a drying effect and delay recovery. If the symptom persists and there is an associated sore throat, treatment for chronic or relapsing pharyngitis may be indicated (see Chapter 33).

Laryngeal complications of *gastroesophageal reflux* are best managed by use of proton pump inhibitors (PPI) in a higher dose than used for usual esophageal GERD, because this is an atypical or extraesophageal manifestation of GERD that requires more aggressive therapy (see Chapter 42). Patients should also be educated in reflux precautions: dietary modification, weight loss, smoking cessation, avoidance of activity immediately following meals, separation of the last meal from sleep by 3 to 4 hours, and elevating the head of bed. Patients will often improve after a 6- to 8-week course of PPI therapy, but a 6-month course of therapy is recommended for these symptoms to resolve completely and the laryngeal examination to normalize. Chronic laryngitis from *toxic exposure* such as cigarette smoke is best treated by smoking cessation or the elimination of other inciting agents. Vocal hygiene measures are important adjunctive treatments for all causes of hoarseness (see Vocal Hygiene).

Anatomic Lesions

The treatment of *vocal fold polyps* is simple surgical excision by suspension microlaryngoscopy. *Vocal fold nodules* often occur on the free edge of the vocal fold secondary to voice abuse. These nodules often resolve with appropriate speech therapy and voice rest. If vocal nodules progress to fibrotic lesions, they may need to be excised surgically, as resolution by conservative measures is unlikely. Postintubation lesions such as true *vocal fold granulomas* are present in the posterior glottis where the endotracheal tube was positioned. A granuloma can also form in the posterior glottis with gastroesophageal reflux or extreme vocal abuse or in patients with chronic and marked cough syndromes. These granulomas can usually be ameliorated by speech therapy and inhaled steroids combined with aggressive treatment for gastroesophageal reflux to reduce further mucosal injury. These lesions, unless they are obstructing the airway, rarely require surgical treatment. Human papilloma virus can cause recurrent respiratory *papillomatosis* that affects the glottis; although they are present in all age groups, they are usually seen in children. This viral illness has no curative medical therapy at present. The recommended therapy is frequent surgical excisions using a carbon dioxide laser, microsurgical debrider, and microlaryngeal instruments. These lesions will recur, and serial excisions are required. Rarely, papillomas can undergo malignant transformation.

Neoplastic lesions, such as laryngeal tumors, cause hoarseness from the tumor mass itself, interruption of the normal mucosal wave, or by contiguous spread and true vocal fold paresis or paralysis. These lesions are often easily detected on laryngeal examination and require operative biopsy for a tissue diagnosis. Treatment often requires surgical excision, irradiation, chemotherapy, or a combination of the three modalities.

Vocal fold paralysis with no obvious etiology (such as a previous surgical procedure that placed the recurrent nerve at risk) requires workup (see Examination by an Otolaryngologist and Ancillary Testing) to rule out an underlying neoplasm anywhere along the tract of the recurrent laryngeal nerve. If no lesions are found and the paralysis is accompanied by significant hoarseness with a harsh breathy voice or aspiration, a procedure can be performed to medialize this vocal fold toward the normal opposite side, either by an injection into the true vocal fold or by operative introduction of a spacer (medialization laryngoplasty) (56).

Vocal Hygiene

Patients with any process causing hoarseness should be educated about voice abuse. They should be advised to avoid straining their voices by using a loud voice or harsh whispering. It is important for these patients to maintain adequate hydration (e.g., six or more large glasses of water each day). Caffeine and alcohol should be avoided because of their drying and diuretic effects. Antihistamines and drugs with anticholinergic side effects should also be avoided, because they cause excessive dryness. Guaifenesin (e.g., Robitussin) may also be helpful as a mucolytic.

HICCUPS

Hiccups are a common phenomenon that affects, at some time or another, most individuals. Usually, a bout of hiccups is a mild short-lived annoyance that resolves spontaneously. When hiccups are prolonged (more than 48 hours) or intractable (more than 1 month) it is important to rule out a serious underlying medical illness. Hiccups, sometimes referred to as *singultus,* involve the involuntary spasmodic contraction of the diaphragm. This spasmodic contraction of the diaphragm begins at inspiration, which is suddenly checked by closure of the glottis, giving the characteristic sound of hiccuping (57).

Pathophysiology

For unknown reasons, persistent hiccups in men are found to be caused by a specific organic etiology in over 90% of cases, whereas specific causes are less likely to be found in women after detailed evaluation (58). The afferent portion of the hiccup reflex arc arises from the phrenic and vagus nerves and the thoracic sympathetic chain. There is no discrete central connection for this reflex arc, although it appears to be located somewhere in the spinal cord, between segments C3 and C5. The phrenic nerve provides the efferent limb of the reflex arc. Fluoroscopy reveals that hiccups are most often unilateral, with the left diaphragm being more frequently involved than the right (59). The frequency of hiccups decreases as arterial PCO_2 rises, and this is the physiologic basis for the popular hiccup treatment of breathing into a paper bag. The etiology of self-limited hiccups appears to be related mostly to ingestion of food and alcohol and gastric distention. These self-limited hiccups are thought to result from peripheral irritation of the branches of the vagus and phrenic nerve in the upper abdomen (57). Local irritation of the vagus nerve and diaphragm (e.g., by pneumonia, aortic aneurysm, pericarditis, abdominal abscesses, and various thoracic and abdominal tumors) appears to be an important mechanism for development of intractable hiccups. Additionally, central nervous system (CNS) lesions, such as multiple sclerosis, meningitis, and CNS neoplasms can also provoke hiccups. Psychogenic factors also may be the cause of intractable hiccups. Stress, conversion reaction, anxiety states, and malingering may all be psychogenic factors in the etiology of hiccups.

Evaluation

A focused history to determine the onset, precipitating factors, and duration of the hiccups is important. Associated medical events, such as trauma, surgery, or recent acute illness, should be elicited. Weight loss, fatigue, or night sweats suggest an underlying malignancy. The presence of hiccups during sleep usually indicates an underlying organic cause, whereas if the hiccups cease during sleep a psychogenic or idiopathic etiology is more likely (58). Any previous bouts of hiccups and the response to therapy should be reviewed and may suggest precipitants and effective treatments.

The head and neck, chest, and abdomen should be examined. The ears should be examined for any external auditory canal abnormality, which may trigger hiccups by irritating the vagally supplied external auditory canal skin. Pharyngitis or oropharyngeal inflammation may also be a trigger for hiccups. A cervical process, such as a thyroid tumor or malignant lymphadenopathy along the course of the recurrent laryngeal nerve in the neck, may also provide a trigger for these episodes. Examination of the chest is important to assess for infection, thoracic aortic aneurysm, pericarditis, or pulmonary or mediastinal tumor. The abdomen should be evaluated for an acute process such as bowel obstruction or abscess or an underlying neoplasm. A detailed neurologic examination should be performed, because early multiple sclerosis is thought to be one of the most frequent neurologic causes of intractable hiccups in young adults (60).

A chest radiograph may be helpful in evaluating patients with hiccups by ruling out pulmonary, mediastinal, or cardiac sources of phrenic, vagus nerve, or diaphragmatic irritation (61,62). Because hyponatremia may cause hiccups, the serum sodium concentration should be measured (63). Other studies may be indicated based on the findings identified by the history and physical examination.

Management

The most important consideration in the management of prolonged and intractable hiccups is to determine the etiology and correct any underlying pathology if possible. Once the instigating cause has resolved, the hiccup bout should also abate. In cases where the cause is idiopathic or not immediately apparent, therapies should be initiated that are specifically directed at terminating hiccups.

Initial efforts to treat hiccups usually involve physical maneuvers. These are performed in an attempt to interrupt the reflex arc. Many of these are folk remedies, such as swallowing rapidly and sequentially small sips of water or inducing a startle reaction. The previously mentioned breathing into a paper bag may also be tried. A more established maneuver that can be performed by the clinician is stimulation of the nasopharynx with a red rubber catheter; cessation rates of nearly 100% have been reported with this technique (59).

If physical maneuvers fail, then pharmacologic intervention should be attempted. Unfortunately, most studies related to the use of pharmacologic agents for hiccups have involved only small numbers of patients or relied on anecdotal clinical observations. Chlorpromazine hydrochloride is the most commonly used drug. The mechanism of action is unclear. However, a cure rate for intractable hiccups of almost 80% has been reported (64). Care must be taken when administering chlorpromazine intravenously (25 to 50 mg in 500 to 1,000 mL of normal saline over several hours) or intramuscularly (25 to 50 mg), because postural hypotension is common. If hiccup cessation is achieved with initial parenteral treatment, then 25 to 50 mg orally twice daily is recommended for 7 to 10 days (65).

Metoclopramide is the second drug of choice for intractable hiccups, with 10 mg given as an intravenous infusion over 1 to 2 minutes. If successful, an oral maintenance dose of 10 mg four times daily may be used for 7 to 10 days. Success rates of approximately 80% with metoclopramide have been reported (66). Many anticonvulsants also have been reported to be effective for treating hiccups, including phenytoin, phenobarbital, carbamazepine, and valproic acid. Phenytoin is the most efficacious in patients who have a central neurologic cause of their hiccups (67). In patients with multiple sclerosis, carbamazepine has been reported to be an effective agent for treating associated hiccups (68).

Less conventional therapies, such as hypnosis, psychotherapy, and acupuncture, may be tried if physical maneuvers and drug therapy fails (69,70). Surgical disruption of the phrenic nerve is considered only as a last resort. Before embarking on this mode of therapy, it is important for the otolaryngologist to identify which leaflet of the diaphragm is involved. An initial attempt at blocking the phrenic nerve with a local anesthetic usually should be performed to determine if phrenic nerve surgery would be fruitful.

SPECIFIC REFERENCES*

1. Jackson KR, Jackson RT. Factors associated with active, refractory epistaxis. Arch Otolaryngol Head Neck Surg 1988;114:862.
2. Alvi A, Joyner-Triplett N. Acute epistaxis: how to spot the source and stop the flow. Postgrad Med 1996;99:83.
3. Pollice PA, Yoder MG. Epistaxis: a retrospective review of hospitalized patients. Otolaryngol Head Neck Surg 1997;117:49.
4. O'Reilly BJ, Simpson DC, Dharmeratnam R. Recurrent epistaxis and nasal septal deviation in young adults. Clin Otolaryngol 1996;21:12.
5. Sessions RB. Nasal hemorrhage. Otolaryngol Clin North Am 1973;6:727.
6. Dhillons RS, East CA. Ear, nose and throat and head and neck surgery. London: Churchill Livingstone, 1994.
7. Herkner H, Laggner AN, Mullner M, et al. Hypertension in patients presenting with epistaxis. Ann Emerg Med 2000;35:126.
8. Milam SB, Cooper RL. Extensive bleeding following extractions in a patient undergoing chronic hemodialysis. Oral Surg Oral Med Oral Pathol 1983;55:14.
9. Simpson HK, Baird J, Allison M, et al. Long-term use of low molecular weight heparin tinzaparin in haemodialysis. Haemostasis 1996;26:90.
10. McGarry GW. Drug induced epistaxis? J R Soc Med 1990;83:812.
11. Akama H, Hama N, Amano K. Epistaxis induced by a non-steroidal anti-inflammatory drug? J R Soc Med 1990;83:538.
12. Krempl GA, Noorily AD. Use of oxymetazoline in the management of epistaxis. Ann Otol Rhinol Laryngol 1995;104:704.
13. Mathiasen RA, Cruz RM. Prospective, randomized, controlled clinical trial of a novel matrix hemostatic sealant in patients with acute anterior epistaxis. Laryngoscope 2005;115:899.
14. Viducich RA, Blanda MP, Gerson LW. Posterior epistaxis: clinical features and acute complications. Ann Emerg Med 1995;25:592.
15. Peretta LJ, Denslow BL, Brown CG. Emergency evaluation and management of epistaxis. Emerg Med Clin North Am 1987;5:265.
16. Shaw CB, Wax MK, Wetmore SJ. Epistaxis: a comparison of treatment. Otolaryngol Head Neck Surg 1993;109:60.
17. Small M, Moran AG. Epistaxis and arterial ligation. J Laryngol Otol 1984;98:281.
18. Ernst RJ, Bulas RV, Gaskill-Shipley M, et al. Endovascular therapy of intractable epistaxis complicated by carotid artery occlusive disease. Am J Neuroradiol 1995;16:1463.
19. Carr ME, Gabriel DA. Nasal packing with porcine fatty tissue for epistaxis complicated by qualitative platelet disorders. J Emerg Med 1985;3:449.
20. Jones TM, Ah-See KW. Surgical and non-surgical interventions used primarily for snoring. (Protocol). *The Cochrane Database of Systematic Reviews 2001*; Issue 2. Art. No.: CD003028. DOI: 10.1002/14651858.CD003028.
21. Hoffstein V. Snoring. Chest 1996;109:201.
22. Hoffstein V, Mateika S, Anderson D. Snoring: is it in the ear of the beholder? Sleep 1994;17: 522.
23. Perez-Padilla JR, West P, Kryger M. Snoring in normal young adults: prevalence in sleep stages and associated changes in oxygen saturation, heart rate, and breathing pattern. Sleep 1987;10:249.
24. Teculescu DB, Mauffret-Stephan F. Familial predispositions to snoring [Letter]. Thorax 1994;49:95.
25. Loh NK, Dinner DS, Foldvary N, et al. Do patients with obstructive sleep apnea wake up with headaches? Arch Intern Med 1999;159:1765.
26. Breathe Right nasal strips to decrease snoring. Med Lett Drugs Ther 1994;36:100.
27. O'Sullivan RA, Hillman DR, Mateljan R, et al. Mandibular advancement splint: an appliance to treat snoring and obstructive sleep apnea. Am J Respir Crit Care Med 1995;151:194.
28. Hoffstein V, Mateika S, Halko S, et al. Reduction in snoring with phosphocholinamine, a long-acting tissue-lubricating agent. Am J Otolaryngol 1987;8:236.
29. Series F, Marc I. Effects of protriptyline on snoring characteristics. Chest 1993;104:14.
30. Rauscher H, Formanek D, Zwick H. Nasal continuous positive airway pressure for nonapneic snoring? Chest 1995;107:58.
31. Fujita S, Conway W, Zorick F, et al. Surgical correction of anatomic abnormalities in obstructive sleep apnea syndrome: uvulopalatopharyngoplasty. Otolaryngol Head Neck Surg 1981;89:923.
32. Littlefield PD, Mair EA. Snoring surgery: which one is best for you? Ear Nose Throat J 1999;78:861.
33. Katsantonis GP, Friedman WH, Rosenblum BN, et al. The surgical treatment of snoring: a patient's perspective. Laryngoscope 1990;100:138.
34. Croft CB, Golding-Wood DG. Uses and complications of uvulopalatopharyngoplasty. J Laryngol Otol 1990;104:871.
35. Astor FC, Hanft KL, Benson C, et al. Analysis of short-term outcome after office-based laser-assisted uvulopalatoplasty. Otolaryngol Head Neck Surg 1998;118:478.
36. Powell NB, Riley RW, Troell RJ, et al. Radio frequency volumetric reduction of the tongue: a porcine pilot study for the treatment of obstructive sleep apnea syndrome. Chest 1997;111:1348.
37. Pazos G, Mair EA. Complications of radiofrequency ablation in the treatment of sleep-disordered breathing. Otolaryngol Head Neck Surg 2001;125:462.
38. Standards of Practice Committee of the American Sleep Disorders Association. Practice parameters for the use of laser-assisted uvulopalatoplasty. Sleep 1994;17:744.
39. Mott AE, Leopold DA. Disorders in taste and smell. Med Clin North Am 1991;75:1321.
40. Anholt RR. Molecular physiology of olfaction. Am J Physiol 1989;257:C1043.
41. Pryse-Phillips W. Disturbances in the sense of smell is psychiatric patients. Proc R Soc Med 1975;68:472.
42. Ackerman BH, Kasbekar N. Disturbances of taste and smell induced by drugs. Pharmacotherapy 1997;17:482.
43. Costanzo R, Becker DP. Smell and taste disorders in head injury and neurosurgery patients. In: Meiselman HL, Rivlin RS, eds. Clinical measurement of taste and smell. New York: Macmillan, 1986: 565.
44. Holbrook EH, Leopold DA. Anosmia: diagnosis and management. Curr Opin Otolaryngol Head Neck Surg. 2003;11:54.
45. Ophir D, Guterman A, Gross-Isseroff R. Changes in smell acuity induced by radiation exposure of the olfactory mucosa. Arch Otolaryngol Head Neck Surg 1998;114:853.
46. Smith DV. Taste and smell dysfunction. In: Paperella MM, Shumrick DA, Gluckman JL, et al., eds. Otolaryngology—head and neck. 3rd ed. Vol. 3. Philadelphia: WB Saunders, 1990: 1911.
47. Duncan JH, Seiden AM, Paik SI, et al. Differences among patients with smell impairment resulting from head trauma, nasal disease, or prior upper respiratory infection. Chem Senses 1991;16.
48. Henkin RI, Schecter PJ, Friedewald WT, et al. A double blind study of the effects of zinc sulfate on taste and smell dysfunction. Am J Med Sci 1976;272:285.
49. Jiang J, Lin E, Hanson DG. Vocal fold physiology. Otolaryngol Clin North Am 2000;33:699.
50. Hirano M. Morphological structure of the vocal cord as a vibrator and its variations. Folia Phoniatr (Basel) 1974;26:89.
51. Furstenburg AC, Magielski JG. A motor pattern in the nucleus ambiguus: its clinical significance. Ann Otol Rhinol Laryngol 1972;64:788.
52. Koufman JA. The otolaryngologic manifestations of gastroesophageal reflux disease (GERD): a clinical investigation of 225 patients using ambulatory 24-hour pH monitoring and an experimental investigation of the role of acid and pepsin in the development of laryngeal injury. Laryngoscope 1991;101[4 Pt 2 Suppl 53]:1.
53. Ritter FN. Endocrinology. In: Paparella M, Shumrick D, eds. Otolaryngology. Philadelphia: WB Saunders, 1973: 727.
54. Sataloff RT, Hawkshaw M, Rosen DC. Medications: effects and side effects in professional voice users. In: Sataloff RT, ed. Professional voice. San Diego: Singular Publishing Group, 1997: 457.
55. Sataloff RT, Spiegel JR, Hawkshaw MJ. Strobovideolaryngoscopy: results and clinical value. Ann Otol Rhinol Laryngol 1991;100:725.
56. Wanamaker JR, Netterville JL, Ossoff RH. Phonosurgery: silastic medialization for unilateral vocal fold paralysis. Op Techn Otolaryngol Head Neck Surg 1993;4:207.
57. Haubrich WS. Hiccup. In: Bockus ML, ed. Gastroenterology. 4th ed. Philadelphia: WB Saunders, 1985: 195.
58. Sovadjian JV, Cain JC. Intractable hiccups: etiologic factors in 220 cases. Postgrad Med 1968;43:72.

*Bold numerals denote published controlled clinical trials, meta-analyses, or consensus-based recommendations.

59. Salem MR, Baraka A, Rattenborg CC, et al. Treatment of hiccups by pharyngeal stimulation in anesthetized and conscious subjects. JAMA 1967;202:126.
60. Birkhead R, Friedman J. Hiccups and vomiting as initial manifestations of multiple sclerosis [Letter]. J Neurol Neurosurg Psychiatry 1987;50:232.
61. Nathan M, Leshner R, Keller A. Intractable hiccups. Laryngoscope 1980;90:1612.
62. Graham D. Esophageal motor abnormality during hiccup. Gastroenterology 1986;90:2039.
63. Jones J, Lloyd T, Cannon L. Persistent hiccups as an unusual manifestation of hyponatremia. J Emerg Med 1987;5:283.
64. Davignon A, Lauieux G, Genest J. Chlorpromazine in the treatment of persistent hiccough. Union Med Can 1955;84:282.
65. Loft LM, Ward RF. Hiccups: a case presentation and etiologic review. Arch Otolaryngol Head Neck Surg 1992;118:1115.
66. Middleton RSW. The use of metoclopramide in the elderly. Postgrad Med J 1973;49[Suppl]:90.
67. Laing T, Marariu M, Malik G, et al. Intractable hiccups and a posterior fossa arteriovenous malformation: a case report. Henry Ford Hosp Med J 1981;29:145.
68. McFarling DA, Susac JO. Hoquet diabolique: intractable hiccups as a manifestation of multiple sclerosis. Neurology 1979;29:797.
69. Smedley WP, Barnes WT. Postoperative use of hypnosis on a cardiovascular service. JAMA 1966;197:371.
70. Wensel LO. Acupuncture in medical practice. Reston, VA: Reston Publishing, 1980:200.

For annotated ***General References*** *and resources related to this chapter, visit www.hopkinsbayview.org/PAMreferences.*

Chapter 112

Common Problems of the Teeth and Oral Cavity

Douglas K. MacLeod and David E. Kern

The purpose of this chapter is to provide guidelines for recognizing, treating, and referring patients with acute dental and oral problems and to increase awareness of chronic dental and oral problems that may require referral and treatment. These types of problems are often neglected by the patient because of fear or ignorance about possible corrective treatment, anticipated pain from the procedure, or the anticipated cost of treatment.

ORAL EXAMINATION

The systematic examination of the oral cavity should include lips, cheeks (buccal mucosa), hard and soft palate, salivary ducts (parotid duct orifice in the buccal mucosa opposite the upper second molars and submandibular duct orifice beside the lingual frenulum), tonsillar area, tongue, floor of the mouth, gingiva, and teeth, noting the normal structures and any deviations from normal. A dental examination includes an evaluation of the number (20 in the primary dentition and 32 in the permanent dentition; Fig. 112.1), position, and arrangement of the teeth and a check for caries (see Dental Caries), erosions, abrasions, and fractures. It is important to examine the gingiva completely. The normal healthy gingiva is firm, pink, and nontender and does not bleed on palpation or probing. Figure 112.2 shows the parts of a tooth and its adjacent structures.

ACUTE DENTAL AND ORAL PROBLEMS

Toothaches (Pulpitis)

Presentation

Patients with toothache have a large carious lesion (see Dental Caries, below), a large restoration (filling), or a combination of both. In the early stages, there is inflammation involving a portion of the pulp tissue (the central portion of the tooth, containing vital soft tissue; Fig. 112.2A).

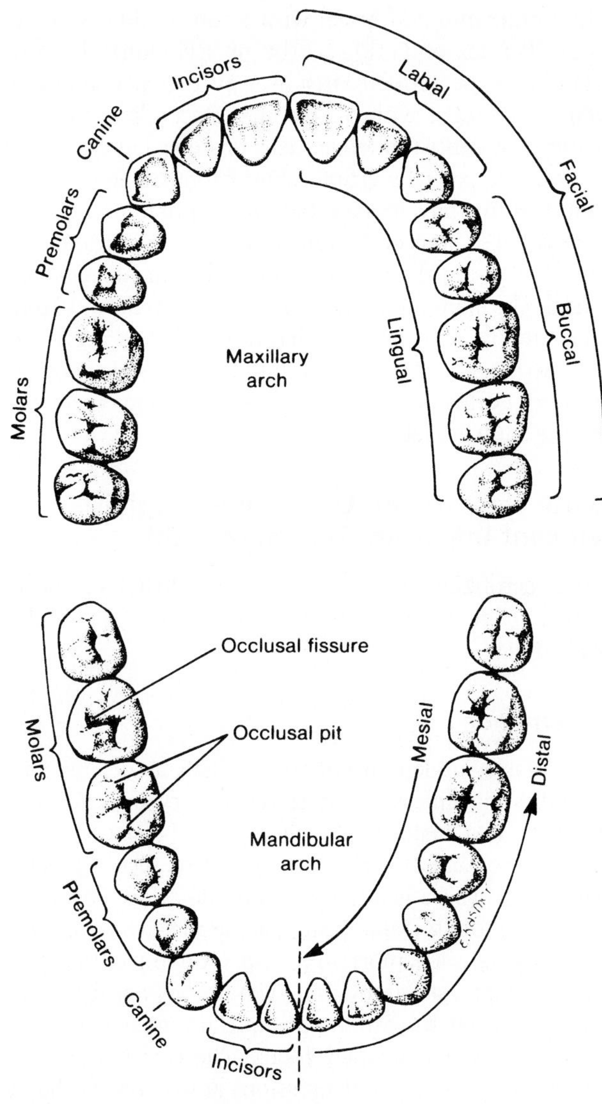

FIGURE 112.1. Permanent dentition.

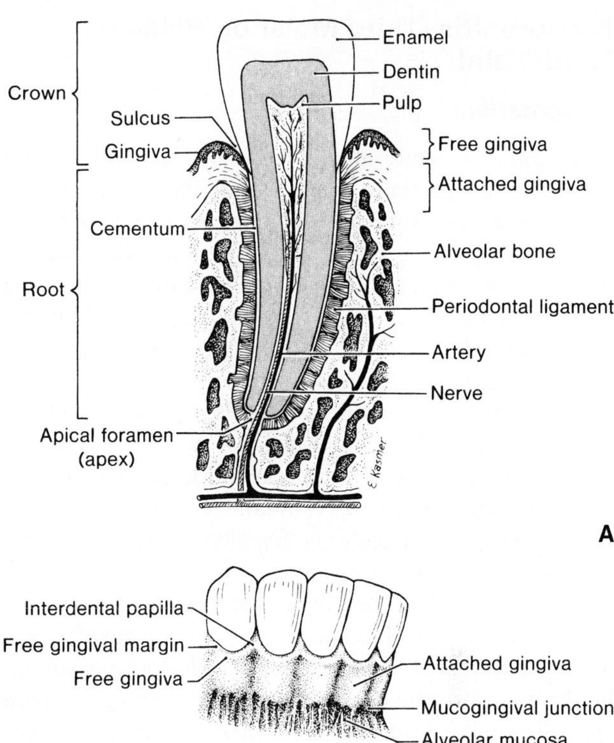

FIGURE 112.2. Structure of normal teeth and gingiva. **A:** A tooth and its parts. **B:** Teeth and gingiva.

There is severe pain in response to thermal stimuli, particularly cold, and this pain persists for longer than 15 seconds after the stimulus is removed. As the area of inflammation increases, the pain becomes more severe; it may radiate to the suborbital area, the side of the face, or the ear. When total necrosis of the pulp occurs, sensitivity to thermal stimuli is lost. If, at this point, the inflammatory exudate cannot escape into the oral cavity, the pressure is released via the root apex, and there is exquisite sensitivity to percussion of the crown of the tooth. The signs and symptoms of pulpitis may be confused with pericoronitis (wisdom teeth pain, see below, Wisdom Tooth Pain) or periodontitis (see Periodontal Disease), and without further diagnostic aids (i.e., dental x-rays) it may be difficult to differentiate between these conditions.

If pulpitis is not treated, complications may occur, ranging from a localized alveolar abscess (an abscess of the bony supporting structure of the teeth) to facial cellulitis. The rate and type of complication depends on the location of the affected tooth, host resistance, and virulence of the bacteria present.

Treatment

Depending on the situation when the patient is seen, one has three options. For patients who are afebrile and have no extraoral swelling (swelling that produces facial asymmetry) or intraoral swelling (swelling that disrupts the supporting alveolar bone and soft tissue), analgesics (acetaminophen 650 mg and/or codeine 30 mg or immediate-release oxycodone 5 mg every 4 hours) and referral within 24 hours are indicated. In this situation the value of antibiotics is unproven (1). When slight extraoral or intraoral swelling or a low-grade temperature elevation is present, antibiotics (penicillin V 250 mg or, for patients allergic to penicillin, clindamycin 300 mg every 6 hours) are recommended, and the patient should be seen by a dentist within 12 to 24 hours. Patients with temperatures greater than 101°F (38.5°C) with intraoral or extraoral swelling causing facial asymmetry need immediate consultation and treatment by a dentist. Treatment of these types of problems varies from extraction of the affected tooth, root canal therapy (endodontics), or incision and drainage to hospital admission for intravenous antibiotics for facial cellulitis.

Pericoronitis (Third Molar or Wisdom Tooth Pain)

Presentation

Pericoronitis is acute inflammation of the tissue around the crown of a partially erupted tooth. Patients with pericoronitis are usually between the ages of 15 and 25, although rarely the condition can be seen in older patients if they still have their third molars. The patient may give a history of subacute episodes of pain of the gingiva that partially covers the crown of an incompletely erupted tooth. The tooth most often affected is the mandibular third molar (wisdom tooth). The space between the crown of the tooth and the overlying gingival flap is an ideal area for the accumulation of food and bacteria; this leads to inflammation. The flap is traumatized by contact with the tooth in the opposing jaw, usually the maxillary third molar, and the inflammation is aggravated.

The patient describes pain that radiates to the ear, throat, and floor of the mouth. He or she complains of a foul taste, and there is swelling of the affected area so that he cannot close the jaw properly. In severe cases, pain spreading to the oropharynx and base of the tongue makes it difficult to swallow. The gingival tissue is markedly red, swollen, and tender (Fig. 112.3A). Occasionally, tender lymphadenopathy and systemic manifestations (fever, leukocytosis, and malaise) are present. Peritonsillar abscess, cellulitis, and Ludwig angina (cellulitis of the floor of the mouth) are possible complications.

Treatment

In afebrile patients, one needs only to make a dental referral and prescribe analgesics. Febrile patients should be treated with antibiotics (penicillin V 500 mg or, for patients allergic to penicillin, clindamycin 300 mg every 6 hours), moderate analgesics (acetaminophen 650 mg and/or codeine 30 mg or immediate-release oxycodone 5 mg every 4 to 6 hours), and chlorhexidine gluconate 0.12% oral rinse and brush with a soft toothbrush twice a day (Peridex or Periogard, by prescription); the rinse should be expectorated after use. All patients should be seen by a dentist within 24 hours. Depending on many factors, the dentist either excises or debrides the flap or removes the partially erupted lower tooth. The preferred treatment for third molars that are erupting in a position that produces poor occlusion is to remove the traumatizing maxillary third molar tooth and allow the infected flap to heal. The mandibular tooth is then removed 7 to 10 days later, after the acute infection has resolved. When pericoronitis involves eruption of third molars that are in good position for occlusion, the inflamed gingival flap is removed and the teeth are left in place.

Acute Necrotizing Ulcerative Gingivitis (Vincent Infection, Trench Mouth)

Acute necrotizing ulcerative gingivitis (ANUG) may occur at any age, but it is more common among young to middle-aged adults.

Presentation

ANUG has a sudden onset and is usually associated with a debilitating illness or acute respiratory infection. Often there is a history of a change in the patient's life, such as protracted work without rest or recent psychologic stress. There is a fetid mouth odor, and the patient describes a foul metallic taste, increased salivation, spontaneous gingival hemorrhage, and pronounced bleeding with the slightest stimulation. The lesions are extremely sensitive to touch; pain is constant and gnawing and is intensified by hot or spicy foods. The oral findings are punched-out crater-like depressions at the crest of the interdental papillae or marginal gingiva. The surface of the gingiva is covered by gray pseudomembranous slough that is demarcated from the gingiva by a pronounced linear erythema (Fig. 112.3B). Patients usually have submandibular

A 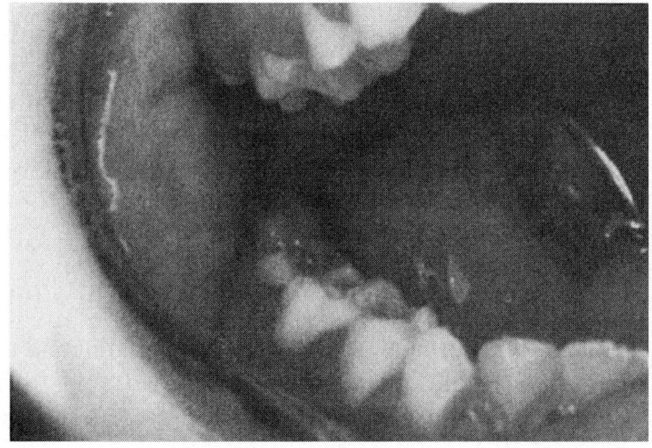

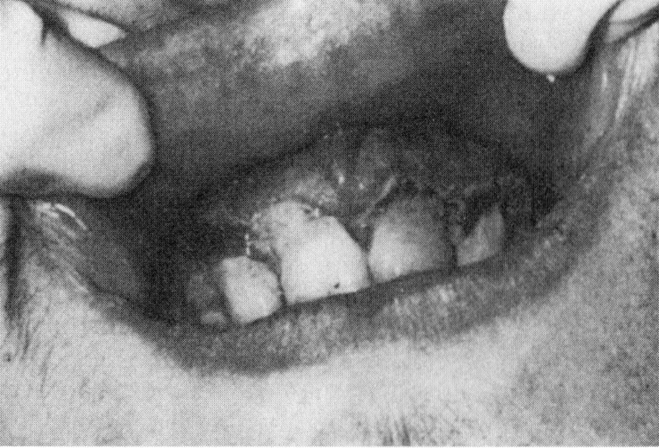 B

FIGURE 112.3. **A:** Pericoronitis of the mandibular third molar. **B:** Acute necrotizing ulcerative gingivitis.

lymphadenopathy and slight elevation in temperature; in severe cases, high fever, tachycardia, leukocytosis, loss of appetite, and malaise are seen.

Most investigators believe that ANUG is caused by two agents, which are normal oral flora: a fusiform bacillus and *Borrelia vincentii,* a spirochete. Histologically, the stratified squamous epithelium of the gingiva is ulcerated and replaced by a thick fibrinous exudate containing many polymorphonuclear leukocytes and microorganisms.

Complications include destruction of the gingiva and underlying supporting tissues, which after repeated episodes of ANUG can result in the loss of teeth. In rare cases, severe sequelae, such as noma (rapidly spreading gangrene of oral and facial tissue, which occurs in the debilitated and nutritionally deficient patient), fusospirochetal meningitis, peritonitis, pneumonia, bacteremia, and brain abscess, have been reported.

Treatment

Patients with severe ANUG need immediate hospital admission, intravenous antibiotics, and supportive care (analgesics, hydrogen peroxide mouthwashes) until systemic symptoms subside. Patients with less severe ANUG need immediate attention by a dentist. At this visit, after treatment with a topical anesthetic, a cotton pellet and carbamide peroxide solution (an oxygenating and foaming agent, such as Gly Oxide) are used to remove the pseudomembrane and surface debris. Antimicrobials are usually prescribed for a few days by the dentist. After irrigation with warm water, the superficial calculus is removed. Patients are instructed to avoid tobacco and alcohol, to rinse with warm water and chlorhexidine gluconate 0.12% twice daily, and to confine toothbrushing to the removal of surface debris. When these instructions are followed after effective removal of all irritants by the dentist, a patient usually improves markedly within 5 days. If after the acute phase the patient does not continue periodic dental care, ANUG may recur and lead to eventual tooth loss.

Recurrent Aphthous Stomatitis

Aphthous ulcers, also called *canker sores,* occur at some time in 20% to 50% of the adult population, are slightly more common in females, have familial tendencies, and occur most often during the winter and spring (2). Recurrent aphthous stomatitis (RAS) was once thought to be a recurrent infection by the herpes simplex virus (HSV), but that is not the case; the cause of the condition is still unknown.

Presentation

Aphthous stomatitis is characterized by superficial ulcerations on the mucous membranes of the lips, cheek, tongue, floor of the mouth, palate, and gingiva. This condition begins with a prodromal burning 1 to 48 hours before the appearance of discrete vesicles, which are approximately 2 to 5 mm in diameter and are painful. After 2 days, they rupture and form saucer-like ulcers that consist of a red or grayish red central portion and an elevated rim-like periphery. There may be a single lesion or multiple ulcers.

The lesions heal spontaneously within 7 to 10 days. As a rule, the lesions are larger than those seen in acute herpetic gingivostomatitis (see next section) and do not exhibit the diffuse gingival involvement or systemic symptoms seen in that condition.

RAS occurs in the following forms:

- *Occasional aphthae:* a single lesion, at intervals from months to years, that heals uneventfully
- *Acute multiple aphthae:* acute episode that persists for weeks, with lesions developing sequentially at different sites in the mouth, often associated with acute gastrointestinal disorders
- *Chronic recurrent aphthae:* one or more lesions always present for years

Treatment

Treatment of aphthae is symptomatic. There is some evidence that chlorhexidine gluconate mouth rinses or gels can reduce the severity of episodes (3). A mouthwash containing equal parts of Benadryl suspension and Kaopectate (Benadryl 5 mg/mL mixed with an equal amount of Kaopectate, prepared by a pharmacist) is helpful in reducing the pain, as is viscous Xylocaine applied by cotton-tip applicator to painful lesions. Topical corticosteroids (e.g., triamcinolone in Orabase) may decrease the duration of ulceration and symptoms (3). The Orabase aspect of this product is a paste specially designed to adhere to the surface of oral lesions.

In more severe cases, tetracycline has been successful in decreasing pain and duration of the ulcers; the patient should be instructed to empty a 250-mg capsule in 50 mL of water and to use this as a rinse, which is then swallowed, three or four times a day for 5 to 7 days. The patient should be encouraged to take sufficient amounts of nonirritating liquids or soft food to maintain hydration and nutrition. Intake may be facilitated by using a straw to prevent contact with the painful ulcers. Based on empiric experience, the amino acid L-lysine may also help reduce symptoms. The patient should be instructed to take orally 1,000 to 1,500 mg with each meal during prodromal symptoms and on the days lesions are present and then as a preventive measure, 500 mg with each meal indefinitely.

Acute Herpetic Gingivostomatitis

Acute herpetic gingivostomatitis (AHGS) occurs most often in infants and children younger than the age of 6 years, and it is equally common in males and females. It is caused by herpes simplex virus (HSV) and most oral infections are caused by HSV type 1. However, it also occurs in older patients, including (rarely) the elderly (4). Most adults have developed immunity to HSV as a result of childhood infection, usually inapparent. Although recurrent acute herpetic gingivostomatitis has been reported, it does not usually recur unless immunity has been altered by a debilitating systemic disease.

Presentation

AHGS appears as a diffuse, erythematous, shiny involvement of the gingiva and the adjacent oral mucosa, with varying degrees of edema and gingival bleeding. In the initial stage it is characterized by the presence of discrete spherical gray vesicles that may occur in the gingiva, labial and buccal mucosa, soft palate, pharynx, sublingual mucosa, and tongue. Within 24 hours the vesicles rupture and form small painful ulcers with a red, elevated, halo-like margin and a depressed yellowish or grayish white central portion. Regional lymphadenopathy, fever as high as 105°F (40.5°C), and generalized malaise are common. The course is limited to 7 to 10 days, and the ulcers heal without scarring. This condition is differentiated by the presence of diffuse gingival involvement and systemic symptoms, which are not present in RAS. Tzanck testing was positive in 77% in a series of 13 patients (4). Viral culture is considered the gold standard and most sensitive of diagnostic techniques, but is seldom required.

Treatment

AHGS usually runs a benign, self-limiting course in immunocompetent patients. In the immunocompromized patient, prompt recognition and treatment is important, because these patients are at risk for dissemination. Symptomatic treatment includes a systemic analgesic and antipyretic, such as acetominophen, and a palliative mouth rinse, such as a diphenhdramine/Kaopectate mix (see RAS, above). Antibacterial agents are not helpful, and corticosteroids are contraindicated. The use of systemic or topical antiviral therapy (acyclovir, valacyclovir, famciclovir) is uncertain. Its use is probably warranted in the management of severely infected and immunocompromized patients, although this should be done in consultation with an infectious disease specialist or a dentist (see Chapter 102 for a discussion of antiviral therapy).

Herpes Simplex Labialis

Recurrent herpes simplex infections of the lips or perioral area occur in 20% to 40% of the adult population. Evidence suggests that recurrent herpes is not a reinfection but a reactivation of virus that remains latent in the nerve tissue.

Presentation

The natural history of this problem has been well delineated. Most affected subjects have several episodes during an average year. In approximately 60% of episodes, there is prodromal tingling for a number of hours before the appearance of the first vesicles. Pain is moderate to severe during the first 24 hours after appearance of vesicles and then rapidly diminishes. After 48 hours, vesicles are usually replaced by ulcer crusts. The process usually resolves after 7 to 9 days, but lesions may persist as long as 2 weeks. Chapter 117 discusses the therapy of this condition.

Sialadenitis

Presentation

Sialadenitis is an inflammation of the salivary gland. Patients with sialadenitis experience pain and enlargement of the affected gland. In bacterial sialadenitis, the pain and swelling are not related to eating. The overlying skin may be red and tense, and the affected gland yields a purulent discharge at the duct orifice. Bacterial sialadenitis is more common in children than in adults. Obstructive sialadenitis is more common than bacterial infection of the salivary glands and is associated with salivary stones or a mucous plug. It occurs most often in middle-aged men. The involved gland is enlarged and painful, and the symptoms are more prominent before, during, and soon after eating. The submandibular gland is most often affected (75% of cases), whereas the parotid (20% of cases) and major sublingual glands (5% of cases) are less often involved. Mumps is more common in children but does occur in adults, when it often is more severe. The parotid gland is swollen and tender, and there is usually no redness, heat, or discharge. Most often both parotids are involved and, often, other salivary glands. Systemic symptoms are common.

Treatment

Treatment of bacterial sialadenitis consists of heat application (external moist heat packs to the affected gland for 15 to 20 minutes and intraoral warm rinses), analgesics (acetaminophen 650 mg and/or immediate-release oxycodone 5 to 10 mg or codeine 30 mg every 4 to 6 hours), antibiotics (penicillin V 500 mg or, for patients allergic to penicillin, clindamycin 300 mg every 6 hours for 7 days), and a liquid diet for the first 2 to 3 days.

The management of obstructive sialadenitis is more complex. When this diagnosis is suspected, the patient should be referred to a dentist or otolaryngologist. In cases in which the stone is lodged in the duct, the acute phase is managed in the same manner as is bacterial sialadenitis, and after resolution has begun a sialogram is obtained to determine the extent of the problem. Surgical removal of the stone from the duct is eventually performed to prevent recurrence. In chronic obstructive sialadenitis, surgical excision of the gland is often necessary. The likelihood of recurrence after the first episode is unknown.

Temporomandibular Joint Pain

Several studies of healthy populations have shown that symptoms of temporomandibular joint (TMJ) disorders are present at some time in 25% to 50% of people but are not considered a serious problem by most patients (5). Most (70% to 90%) patients who have these symptoms are women between the ages of 24 and 40. Multiple factors may lead to TMJ pain; there may be a history of stress, bruxism (grinding of teeth), external blows to the jaws, or whiplash injury. TMJ pain may be present at some point in 20% of patients with rheumatoid arthritis. Patients with osteoarthritis of other joints may complain of TMJ clicking and snapping, but pain is usually absent.

Presentation

TMJ disorders are characterized by pain and tenderness in the muscles of mastication and in the TMJ, by crepitus when the joint is moved, and by a decrease in range of motion. In some severe cases there is a noticeable incoordination on the opening and closing of the jaw. This appears as a unilateral shift of the chin upon opening or closing the mouth. Examination may show malocclusion caused by teeth that interfere with the normal movement of the mandible or tenderness of the muscles of mastication.

Treatment

Patients with acute TMJ pain should be managed with moderate analgesics (acetaminophen 650 mg and/or immediate-release oxycodone 5 to 10 mg or codeine 30 mg every 4 to 6 hours) and referral to a dentist within 24 to 48 hours to begin therapy. The dentist's goal is to make the patient aware of the cause of the problem through education. Depending on the severity of symptoms and the state of the patient's dentition, the dentist will prescribe one or a combination of the following: avoidance of excessive jaw motion, moist heat to affected muscles, soft diet, disengagement of upper and lower jaws with a night guard to separate the upper and lower teeth (a hard appliance constructed to fit the individual patient, which is quite costly), therapeutic exercises, and vapocoolant spray (ethyl chloride to decrease muscle pain). In atypical cases, trigger point injections of xylocaine may be used to distinguish TMJ symptoms from trigeminal neuralgia (see Chapter 87). Once the acute episode has subsided (in about 7 to 14 days) the dentist can detect and eliminate any occlusal interferences and rule out any degenerative joint disease that may have predisposed the patient to TMJ symptoms. In the past, injections of sclerosing agents into the TMJ and condylectomy were tried, but with poor success. In a 10-year study, 97 of 100 patients treated conservatively improved. Of these, 83 had permanent improvement. Of the three patients who had intractable severe symptoms, two required prolonged psychotherapy and one developed systemic arteritis (6).

Local Alveolar Osteitis (Dry Socket)

Local alveolar osteitis (dry socket) is the most common complication of tooth extraction. It occurs in approximately 5% of all tooth extractions, but it is more common after the removal of an impacted third molar. This problem results from the loss of the blood clot located at the site of the extraction. Most often this occurs when the extraction has been difficult and has resulted in considerable trauma to the socket and gum.

Patients with this problem describe intense localized pain 2 or 3 days after an extraction. This pain is caused by irritation of the sensory nerves in the dry exposed bony socket. There is often a foul odor emanating from the socket, but no suppuration is present.

One should control the pain the patient is experiencing with immediate-release oxycodone, 5 to 10 mg or codeine 30 mg every 3 to 4 hours, and acetaminophen, 650 mg three to four times per day. The patient should be referred promptly to a dentist for irrigation and the placement of a dressing. The dentist needs to see the patient every day or two for approximately 10 days until the socket becomes reepithelialized. There are no long-term sequelae.

CHRONIC DENTAL AND ORAL PROBLEMS

Periodontal Disease (Pyorrhea)

Periodontal disease is a general term used to describe diseases that destroy the gingival and bony structures that support the teeth (Figs. 112.4 and 112.5). Periodontal

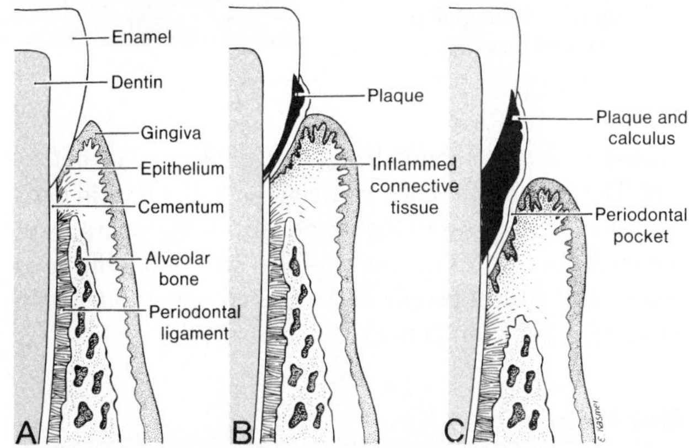

FIGURE 112.4. Dentogingival junction in health. **A:** Plaque free. **B:** Gingivitis resulting from plaque accumulation with inflammation of soft tissue. **C:** Periodontitis resulting from long-standing inflammation that has caused bone loss and tooth mobility.

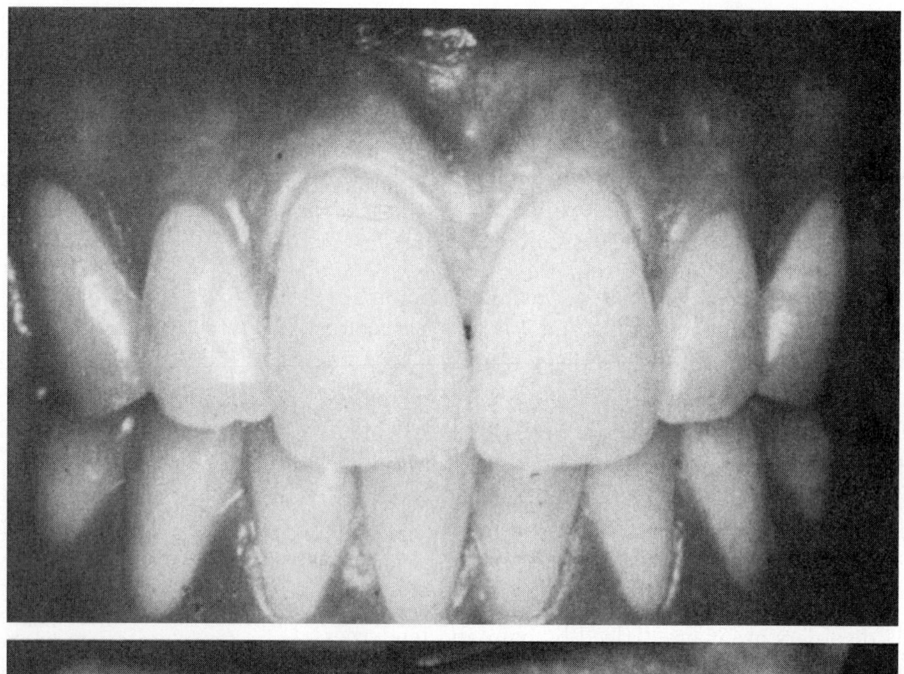

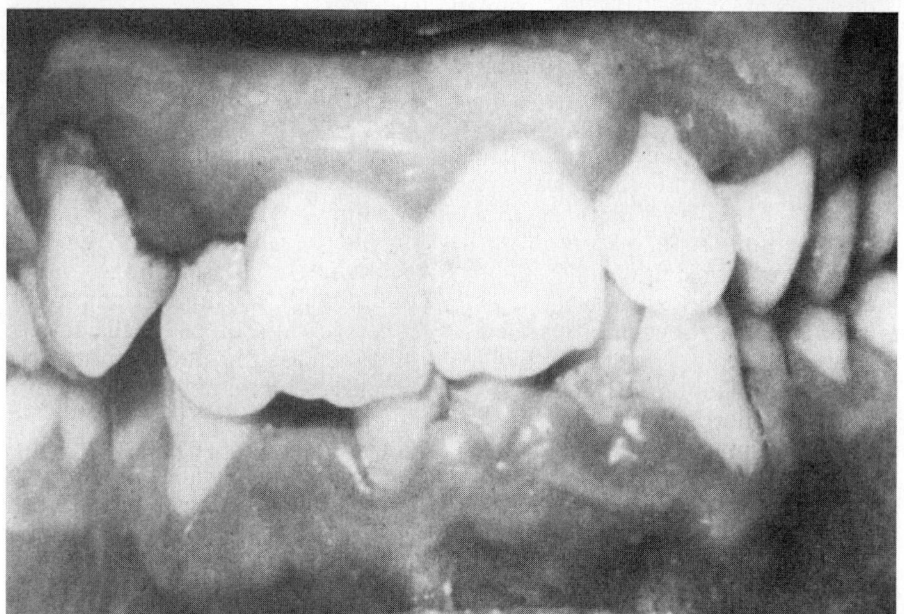

FIGURE 112.5. Normal gingiva **(A)** and chronic periodontal inflammation **(B)** showing swelling, blunting of interdental papillae, erythema, and bleeding.

disease is usually subdivided into *gingivitis* and *periodontitis*. The major difference between the two is that in periodontitis there is loss of the supporting bony apparatus of the teeth. Two thirds of young adults, 80% of middle-aged adults, and 90% of people in the United States older than 65 years suffer from periodontal disease (7).

Risk Factors

Poor oral hygiene, which permits plaque to accumulate on the teeth, is the major etiologic factor. Most periodontal disease, and therefore most loss of teeth, is preventable. Prevention consists of routine plaque control (see Treatment).

Medical problems (8) that are risk factors for periodontal disease include *smoking*, *oral tobacco use*, and *diabetes*. *Osteoporosis* increases the risk of periodontal attachement loss (9). The presence of periodontal disease is associated with an increase risk for cardiovascular disease and stroke (10,11), although it is unclear whether the relationship is causal (12).

Medications that commonly cause gingival overgrowth include *phenytoin*, *cyclosporine*, and *calcium channel blockers*. Calcium channel blocking drugs are widely used for management of cardiovascular conditions. Nifedipine is one of the most often prescribed drugs in this group and the first to be associated with gingival overgrowth.

Most other calcium channel blocking agents have been associated with gingival enlargement, although not to the same degree as nifedipine. The onset of gingival enlargement usually appears within 2 months after initiation of nifedipine therapy and is most pronounced in the anterior facial gingiva. The tendency for overgrowth occurs in approximately 15% to 20% of patients, and although it does not appear to be dose related, occasionally a decrease in enlargement after dosage reduction has been reported. The histologic, histochemical, and electron microscopic examinations of nifedipine-induced gingival enlargement closely resembles phenytoin- or cyclosporine-induced gingival overgrowth, suggesting a similar pathogenic mechanism. Chronic inflammation is always present, and an association between plaque accumulation and drug-induced overgrowth has been documented. Meticulous plaque control does not usually cause remission or consistently stop recurrence after surgical removal. Whenever gingival overgrowth develops, an alternative to nifedipine should be considered. If a calcium channel blocking agent is essential for the patient, an agent other than a dihydropyridine should be used. Examples of such agents that could be used in this situation include diltiazem and verapamil.

Patients who have had organ transplants may be taking cyclosporine, an immunosuppressant drug used extensively to suppress organ and bone marrow transplant rejection. The combination of cyclosporine and calcium channel blocking agents appears to have a synergistic effect on the gingiva. The hyperplasia produced is extreme and often recurs after surgical excision.

Gingivitis

Presentation

Gingivitis is usually seen in one of four forms: *acute,* a painful condition that has a rapid onset and is of short duration; *subacute,* which is less severe than the acute condition; *recurrent,* which reappears after being eliminated by treatment or after disappearing spontaneously; and *chronic,* the most common form, which has a slow onset, is of a long duration, and is usually painless unless complicated by acute exacerbations (Fig. 112.5).

The early signs of inflammation of the gingiva, which precede frank gingivitis, are increased gingival fluid secretion and bleeding from the gingival sulcus upon gentle probing. Healthy gingiva is usually coral pink, whereas in gingivitis the gingiva becomes bright red secondary to increased vascularity and a decrease in keratinization. These changes start in the interdental papillae and free gingiva and spread to the attached gingiva. Both acute and chronic forms produce changes in the normally firm resilient consistency of the gingiva. In acute gingivitis the gingiva has a diffuse edematous appearance, whereas in the chronic form the tissue has a fibrous appearance that pits on pressure.

The development of gingivitis is a consequence of supragingival and subgingival plaque formation (Fig. 112.4). Plaque is a transparent deposit composed primarily of bacteria and their byproducts. Gram-positive filamentous rods, mainly *Actinomyces,* appear to be of major significance. Small amounts of plaque are not visible unless they are stained. As plaque accumulates, it becomes visible as a mass that varies in color from gray to yellowish gray to yellow. Measurable amounts of plaque may form within 1 hour after a thorough cleaning of the teeth, with maximal accumulation in 30 days or less. Bacterial plaque, if left undisturbed, mineralizes and forms calculus (tartar), as shown in Fig. 112.4C. This process usually starts between the first and fourteenth day after plaque formation. Calculus is always covered by plaque. When calculus is present, the gingival tissues are unhealthy by definition. The major complication of untreated gingivitis is periodontitis, that is, the extension of the inflammation to the supporting bony structures of the teeth (see Periodontitis and Fig. 112.4C).

Treatment

Patients presenting with any one of the four forms of gingivitis usually require one to three dental visits (spread over about a 4-week period) for treatment. The mechanical removal of plaque and calculus from the affected areas of the teeth and gingiva (scaling) and smoothing of root surfaces (root planing) result in a decrease in probing depth and a decrease of attachment loss between the gingiva and tooth (13). After all the plaque and calculus have been removed by the dentist, the disease process is explained to the patient, who is then instructed in proper *plaque control measures,* including effective brushing and flossing. A soft-bristled toothbrush or a battery-powered rotating or oscillating toothbrush should be recommended. Effective brushing cleans both the teeth and gingiva and facilitates the removal of plaque. Powered toothbrushes have been shown to be more effecte than manual burshes in removing plaque and reducing gingivitis (14). Floss should be rubbed vertically up and down three to five times in each interdental space first against the one tooth and then against the adjacent one, once daily. Maintenance of the disease-free state is possible only by continued effective plaque control measures by the patient and by professional cleaning every 4 to 12 months (to remove plaque and calculus that may be missed by brushing and flossing). Topical antimicrobial mouthwashes provide modest benefit (15,16). Chlorhexidine gluconate, 0.12% oral rinse twice daily (Peridex or PerioGard, available by prescription), has been shown to be microbicidal. The rinse should be expectorated after use. Complications from its use are common and include a brown stain of the teeth, possible taste alterations, and increase in calculus formation. For these reasons a patient should not use the material without consulting a dentist. Factors that usually result in recurrence are incomplete removal of plaque and calculus, inadequate plaque control because of insufficient patient instruction, premature dismissal of the patient before competence is demonstrated, and lack of patient cooperation.

Periodontitis

Presentation

A patient with periodontitis has red and bleeding gums and an unpleasant taste in his or her mouth but is usually free of pain unless there is an acute infection superimposed on the underlying chronic process. The principal physical findings are the signs of inflammation of the gingiva described above and periodontal pockets around the teeth, from which pus may often be expressed upon gentle pressure. As periodontitis advances, the teeth loosen and spread apart, creating unattractive spaces and exposing the roots of the teeth as the bony support is lost. Mastication is impaired, and spontaneous pain and acute abscess may occur. The most important consequence of periodontitis is the destruction of the alveolar bone, which deprives the teeth of their support and is responsible for the loss of the teeth. The essential steps leading to destruction of bone are gingivitis, degeneration of collagen bundles of the periodontal ligament, and conversion of the shallow (3 mm or less) physiologic gingival sulcus to a deepened periodontal pocket (more than 3 mm). As this pocket deepens, more debris accumulates in it. Inflammation progresses further inward, and the gums recede permanently. The apically progressing inflammation eventually reaches the alveolar crest, and bone resorption begins. This process continues, resulting in continued destruction of the alveolar bone.

Treatment

Most patients with periodontitis can be treated effectively, provided the diagnosis is made before a significant amount of supporting alveolar bone is lost. The aims of treatment are to preserve the teeth by eliminating the disease, restore effective function, and prevent recurrence. When treated in the early stages, the major consequence of periodontitis (loss of bone support for the teeth) can be prevented. If proper treatment is postponed, there may be insufficient bone support once treatment is undertaken, and the natural teeth may eventually be lost. Although some patients do not seem concerned with this problem, many are subsequently disappointed when they find dentures do not function as efficiently as natural teeth.

Treatment of periodontitis is divided into two phases. Phase I is similar to the treatment of gingivitis described above; that is, removal of local irritant (plaque and calculus) and institution of effective plaque control (continual removal of the plaque). This treatment allows resolution of the inflammation. Although both topical (15,16) and systemic (17) antibiotics provide modest adjunctive benefit, their role in the treatment of periodontal disease is not well established. They are usually used in conjunction with mechanical débridement in patients with fever, lymphadenopathy, resistant or severe disease. Smoking cessation should always be counselled (see Chapter 27). The success of Phase I of therapy depends largely on the patient's ability to maintain plaque-free teeth (see Gingivitis, above). Phase II is the surgical phase, in which the goal is to improve the gingival architecture that remains despite the disease. Experience shows that patients have difficulty preventing inflammation in periodontal pockets greater than 5 mm. Surgical treatment is therefore designed to decrease the depths of the pockets.

Denture Problems

Twenty million American adults are missing all their teeth. Of these, many have obtained dentures. Additionally, many of the edentulous population have managed well without teeth, are content to remain as they are, and, regardless of the quality of dentures constructed, are unwilling or unable to adapt to using dentures.

Presentation

Often a patient who has had dentures for years, upon specific questioning, indicates the dentures are not satisfactory. The most common denture problems are looseness and discomfort. If the patient is followed at least yearly by his or her dentist, one can generally assume the present situation is the best that can be achieved. On the other hand, if the patient has tolerated the same set of loose or uncomfortable dentures without seeking help for a number of years, he or she should be encouraged to seek care promptly. Failure to remove dentures at night is the reason for denture problems in some patients. This practice can cause bony erosion with loss of conformity of the dentures to the supporting structures, mucosal ulceration, and oral candidiasis.

Treatment

Depending on the condition of the patient's oral cavity, the present dentures, and the edentulous ridges, a number of treatment modalities are available, including rebasing or relining the existing dentures (5 to 7 days), making a new set of dentures (2 to 5 weeks), and preprosthetic correction of soft and hard tissue (4 to 6 weeks of healing), followed by relining, rebasing, or remaking of dentures. In recent years, there have been marked improvements in dental implants for patients who have had trouble using dentures (especially lower dentures). The placement of implants is expensive (about \$1,600 to \$1,800 per implant, often with a reduction in price for multiple installations, and often five to six implants are used per arch) and time consuming (2 to 3 months) and requires that new dentures are made after placement of implants. The implants function as a replacement for the teeth roots the patient had previously lost through dental caries, periodontitis, or trauma. Most conservative dentists reserve implants for the patient missing at least all posterior teeth or all natural teeth.

Dental Caries

Dental caries is a disease of the calcified tissues of the teeth characterized by demineralization of the inorganic portion (enamel and dentin of the tooth; Fig. 112.2A). Dental caries is one of the most common diseases in humans. It affects all people regardless of race, location, or economic stratum, and it can occur at any age. Poor oral hygiene and a diet high in sugar promote caries, whereas routine oral hygiene and raw coarse foods tend to reduce caries. Ingestion of fluorides in drinking water reduces susceptibility to caries. The form of the tooth affects caries; that is, the deep pits and fissures on molars and premolars especially predispose these teeth to the disorder.

Presentation

Dental caries usually presents as a nonpainful, white, brown, or black spot on the enamel of a tooth. The most common location is the biting surface in conjunction with the pits and fissures of the tooth. Other locations include the smooth surfaces where the teeth come into contact with each other. Without the aid of special equipment (radiographs and hand instruments) and expertise of dental personnel, the best indicator of dental caries is the presence of brown or black spots in areas associated with lost portions of the tooth.

When a caries progresses rapidly to involve the pulp, as in children, the term *acute caries* is used. Slowly progressing caries seen in adults is called chronic caries. Occasionally, a carious lesion may cease to progress (arrested caries). This is caused by breakage of enamel walls, thereby exposing the lesion to the cleaning action of the toothbrush, saliva, fluoride, and mastication. The term *recurrent caries* is used for carious lesions that begin around the margins of defective restorations.

A carious lesion usually develops after bacterial plaque (see Gingivitis) forms on the tooth surface. The primary bacteria involved in this process are *Streptococcus mutans* and *Lactobacillus acidophilus*. These bacteria metabolize dietary fructose to produce lactic acid, which results in decalcification of the enamel. The rate of development of caries depends on the susceptibility of the enamel.

Prevention

The most cost-effective preventive approach to preventing dental caries is the fluoridation of public water supplies (18). Individual approaches that are effective in reducing tooth decay include good dental hygiene (see Gingivitis) and the use of topical flourides (toothpastes, mouthrinses, gels, or varnishes) (19).

Treatment

The treatment for most carious lesions is their removal, followed by a restoration (filling) that replaces the lost portions of the tooth. The goals are to remove the lesion, protect the pulp from irritants, and restore the tooth to function. With the advent of enamel and dentin bonding agents, a sealant (a thin plastic layer of resin) can be placed over a noncarious tooth in the deep fissures to prevent dental caries (20). In cases when caries involves a tooth already significantly affected by periodontal disease, the tooth must be removed.

The major *complication* that results from delaying treatment is acute pulpitis and its complications (see Toothaches). Additionally, delaying treatment may result in a more difficult restoration or possible loss of the involved tooth. In cases in which the existing decay process is very close to the pulp, the heat generated by the rotary instruments used to prepare the restoration may result in a transient pulpal inflammation. This inflammation results in a dull ache in the tooth for 2 to 3 days, which is usually relieved by aspirin or ibuprofen or other nonsteroidal anti-inflammatory drug (NSAID). When the restoration process leaves only a paper-thin layer of dentin covering the pulp tissue, the transient pulpitis may be converted to acute pulpitis (irreversible), which then requires tooth extraction or root canal therapy for relief of pain. Root canal therapy consists of three parts: Removal of the infected nerve tissue, débridement and preparation of the nerve canal space, and obturation (filling) of the canal space with a biologically inert material.

Angular Cheilosis

Presentation

Angular cheilosis is characterized by a feeling of dryness and a burning sensation at the corners of the mouth. The epithelium at the commissures appears wrinkled and macerated. In time, the wrinkles deepen to fissures that appear ulcerated but do not bleed, although a crust may form. These lesions stop at the junction of the mucous membranes. They show a tendency for spontaneous improvement; only rarely do the lesions completely disappear.

There are several causes for cheilosis. A number of microorganisms may cause it in otherwise healthy people: *Candida albicans*, staphylococci, and streptococci. Additionally, angular cheilosis caused by overclosure of the jaws may be seen in edentulous patients. Overclosure causes a fold to be produced at the corners of the mouth in which saliva tends to collect, inviting the growth of microorganisms. Angular cheilosis is also seen in riboflavin deficiency, which usually occurs in patients with multiple vitamin

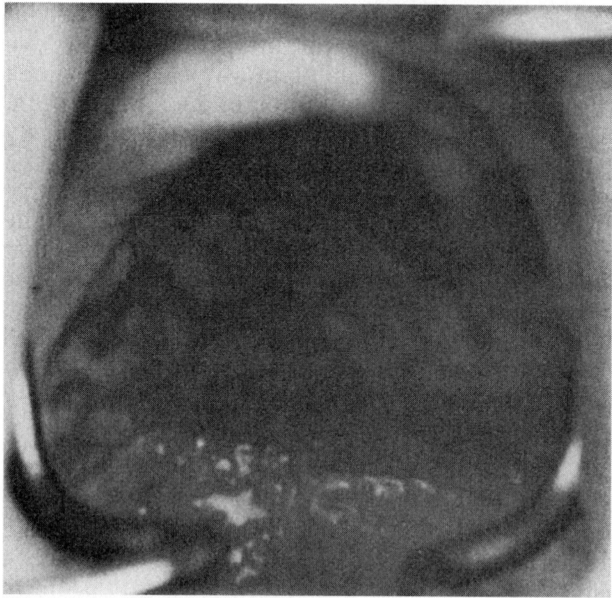

FIGURE 112.6. Candidiasis (thrush) of the hard palate.

deficiencies. The lips show fissures, painful cracks, and scaling; these changes become severe at the corners of the mouth and are similar in appearance to angular cheilosis caused by overclosure of the mandible.

Treatment

Edentulous patients troubled by angular cheilosis should be referred to a dentist, who will evaluate them for mandibular overclosure, because correction of this problem (making or remaking of dentures) may lead to remission. Treatment is otherwise symptomatic and consists of applying petrolatum-containing ointment (e.g., Vaseline, Chapstick) to the scaling area to minimize discomfort.

Thrush (Oral Candidiasis)

Presentation

The typical lesions of oral candidiasis are white curd-like plaques on an erythematous mucosa (Fig. 112.6). These plaques are loosely attached and may be scraped off the oral mucosa. They begin as pinpoint spots. Involvement may include the corners of the mouth, as noted in the previous section. The tongue is often reddened, and the patient describes a burning sensation.

Thrush may occur chronically in patients with poor oral hygiene and poor nutrition. It may also be brought on or exacerbated by debilitating systemic illness, antibiotic therapy, impaired immune system, corticosteroids, immunosuppressive agents, or dental extraction. Thrush does not appear to be more common in diabetic patients. It is common in patients with human immunodeficiency virus infection (see Chapter 39).

The white plaques of thrush may suggest hyperkeratosis or leukoplakia. In these instances, a potassium hydoxide preparation of scrapings reveals pseudo-hyphae and budding spores characterisitic of candidiasis.

Treatment

The patient should be advised to use good oral hygiene practices. Specific treatment consists of nystatin oral suspension, 4 to 6 mL held in the mouth for several minutes before swallowing, four times daily. Thrush usually resolves entirely after 1 to 2 weeks of treatment. Treatment should be continued for several days after visible lesions have disappeared. More intensive treatment is needed in patients with human immunodeficiency virus infection (see Chapter 39).

Halitosis

Presentation

Halitosis is a foul or offensive odor emanating from the oral cavity. Mouth odors originate from local or remote sites. The local causes can be retention of odoriferous food particles on or between the teeth, ANUG (see above), caries, chronic periodontal disease, dentures, tobacco smoking, medications and other causes of xerostomia (dry mouth), healing of surgical or extraction wounds, or debris accumulated between the small papilla of the tongue. Extraoral causes of halitosis include infection in adjacent structures (rhinitis, sinusitis, tonsillitis), pulmonary infections, alcoholic breath, the acetone odor of the diabetic, or the uremic breath associated with renal failure. Metabolites from certain foods that are excreted through the lungs (e.g. onions, garlic, pastrami, alcohol, meats) can also produce halitosis. Breath odor worsens with age, as regressive changes occur in the salivary gland that affect the quantity and quality of saliva.

Treatment

Local causes of this condition are treated by improvement in oral hygiene (brushing teeth and tongue) and by specific treatment of the underlying conditions by a dentist. If these measures are unsuccessful, mouthwashes (21) or breath fresheners used frequently (every 2 to 4 hours) may greatly reduce the problem. Halitosis caused by remote factors may be masked with mouthwashes and fresheners until the remote problem has been resolved. When foods or medication are a factor, dietary or medication changes may help.

Xerostomia (Dry Mouth)

Presentation

Xerostomia, or dry mouth, results from a partial or complete lack of saliva. This defect results in cracking of the lips, difficulty in swallowing, or changes in the tongue texture. The patient often increases liquid consumption to eliminate the dryness. Xerostomia may be a secondary complication of salivary gland disease (e.g., Sjögren syndrome) or radiation treatment, but medication is the most common cause. Anticholinergic, decongestant, and antihistamine drugs are the most common offenders.

The loss of saliva results in a loss of the protective coating of the mucous membranes of the oral cavity. Infections, severe dental caries, problems with dentures, and halitosis commonly result from the loss of saliva.

Treatment

Treatment of xerostomia is symptomatic. Patients should be referred to a dentist for an evaluation to identify a related problem such as caries, and for instruction in the use of daily topical fluoride to help prevent recurrence of caries. The dryness may be lessened if the patient regularly irrigates the mouth with topical methylcellulose or a saliva substitute (Glandosane, Oralube, MOI STIR, Salive Substitute [Roxane Laboratories] or Xerolube, all available without prescription). The saliva substitutes also decrease the risk of caries because they contain sodium fluoride.

Common Tongue Conditions

Geographic Tongue

Benign migratory glossitis, or geographic tongue, is an asymptomatic inflammatory condition consisting of multiple areas of desquamation of the filiform papillae of the tongue in an irregular pattern (Fig. 112.7A). The central portion of an affected area is usually denuded, and the border may be outlined by a thin yellowish white line or band. The fungiform papillae persist in the desquamated area as small, elevated, red dots. The areas of desquamation remain for a short time in one location and then

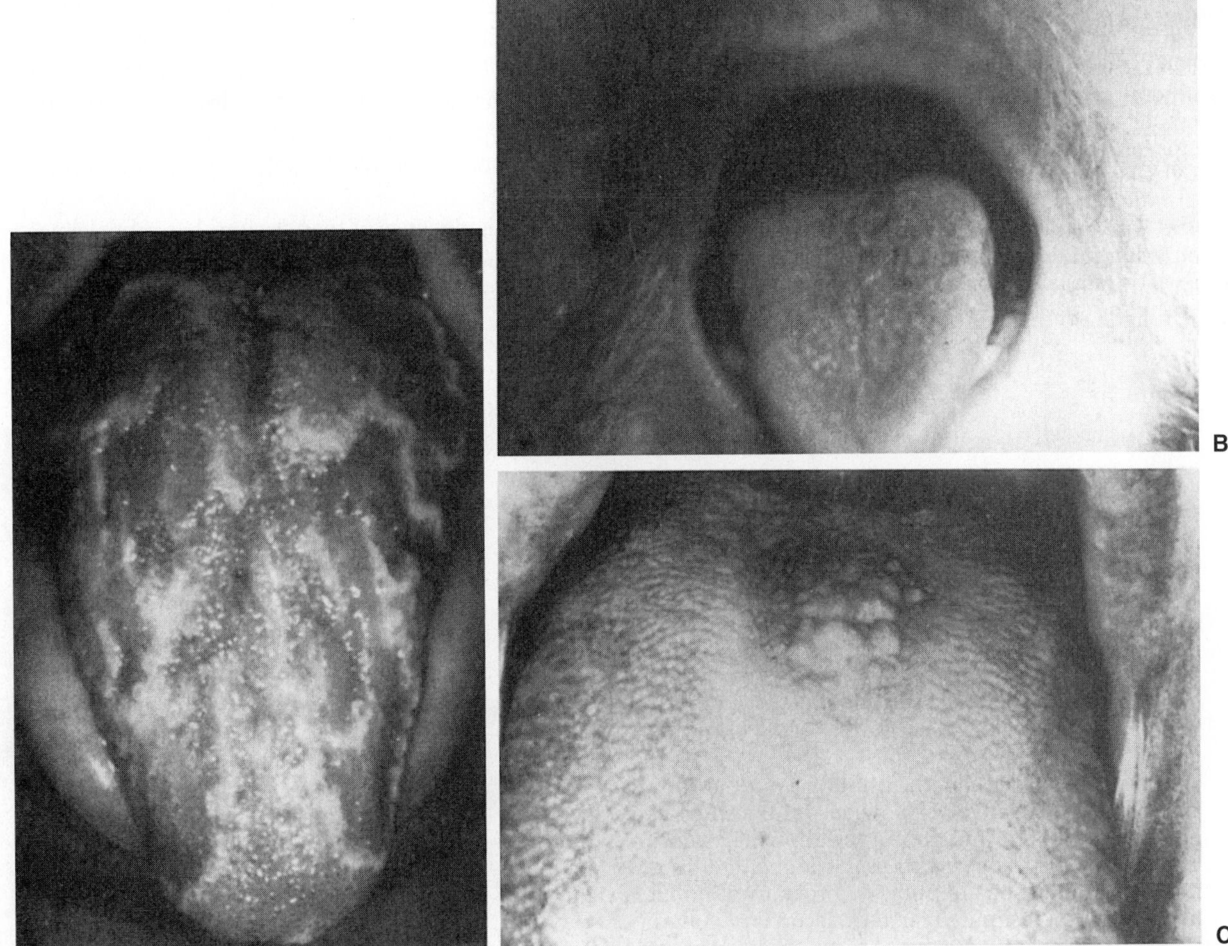

FIGURE 112.7. Common benign problems of the tongue. **A:** Geographic tongue. **B:** Hairy tongue. **C:** Median rhomboid glossitis.

heal and reappear in other locations. The condition may persist for weeks or months and then regress, only to recur at a later date. Women are affected twice as often as men, and there is no racial difference. Because the cause is unknown and the condition is benign, management consists of reassurance. Large doses of vitamins are not effective.

Hairy Tongue

Hairy tongue is a condition characterized by hypertrophy of the filiform papillae of the tongue caused by the lack of normal desquamation of the keratin layer (Fig. 112.7B). This results in a thick matted layer on the dorsum of the tongue. The color of the papillae varies from yellowish white to brown or even black depending on their staining by extrinsic factors (tobacco, foods, or medications). The hypertrophied tissue may touch the palate and produce gagging in some patients. Most patients with hairy tongue are heavy smokers, but the cause is unknown. Treatment of this benign condition consists of brushing the tongue with a tongue blade or toothbrush to promote desquamation and remove debris.

Median Rhomboid Glossitis

Median rhomboid glossitis is a congenital abnormality of the tongue that appears clinically as an ovoid-, diamond-, or rhomboid-shaped reddish patch on the dorsal surface of the tongue. On examination, there is a slightly raised or flat area that is distinctive because there are no filiform papillae (Fig. 112.7C). Despite its name, this abnormality is not inflammatory; it is caused by failure of the tuberculum impar to retract before fusion of the lateral halves of the tongue, so that a structure free of papillae is interposed. The prevalence of the abnormality is less than 1%, and there are no sex or racial differences. The only clinical significance of this innocuous condition is that it is occasionally mistaken for a carcinoma; differentiation from cancer is aided by the presence of the lesion since childhood and the fact that a carcinoma rarely develops on the dorsum of the tongue. If one is unsure of the diagnosis, the patient should be referred to a dentist.

Leukoplakia and Erythroplakia

Presentation

Leukoplakia and erythroplakia are asymptomatic conditions of the oral mucosa that may become malignant. *Leukoplakia* varies in appearance from a grayish white, flattened, scaly lesion to a thick irregularly shaped plaque (Fig. 112.8). Histologically, there is hyperkeratosis, acanthosis, and some degree of dyskeratosis. It is commonly associated with underlying inflammation caused by a chronic irritant (tobacco, alcohol, poorly constructed dentures). Leukoplakia may be found anywhere in the oral cavity but most often is found in the buccal mucosa, followed, in descending order, by the alveolar mucosa, tongue, lip, hard and soft palates, floor of the mouth, and gingiva. *Erythroplakia* refers to a lesion that is velvety red in appearance, small (2 cm or less), and with or without a hyperkeratotic component. It is found in the floor of the mouth, soft palate, and ventrolateral border of the tongue.

The significance of these lesions has been delineated in a longitudinal study of mucosal lesions (22). Of 200 white lesions examined by biopsy, only four were malignant. In the same study, an erythroplastic component was present

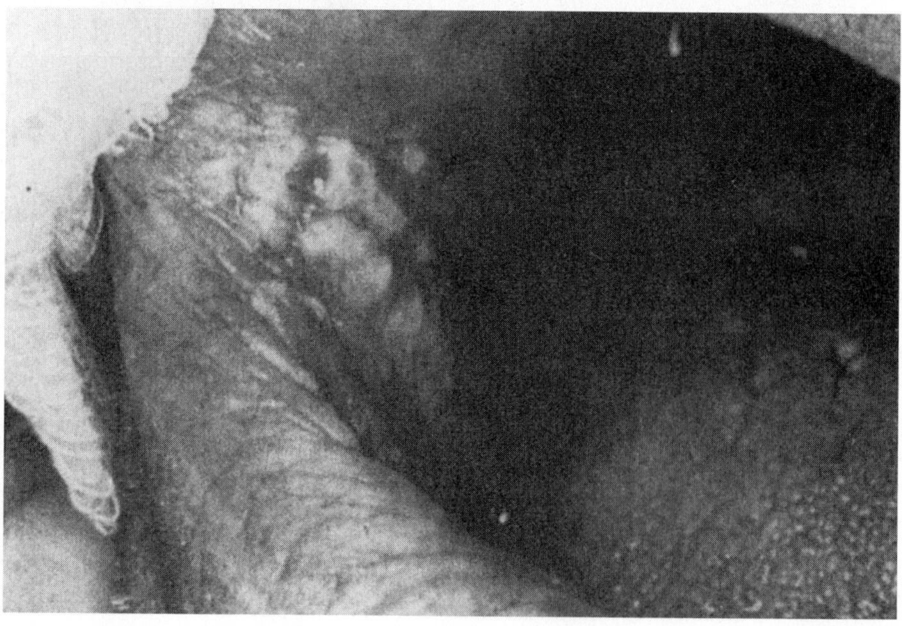

FIGURE 112.8. Leukoplakia showing early changes of epidermoid carcinoma.

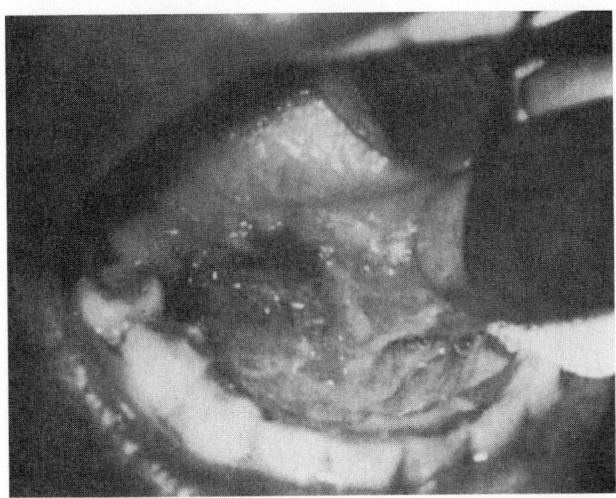

FIGURE 112.9. Squamous cell carcinoma of the floor of the mouth.

in 90% of the 158 asymptomatic squamous cell carcinomas found, suggesting, but not proving, that erythroplakia may be an important precursor of squamous cell cancer. Pathologically, erythroplakia usually is manifest as high-grade dysplasia.

Treatment

It is impossible to determine which lesion showing leukoplakia or erythroplakia will undergo malignant transformation, although erythroplakia is more likely to do so. Discontinuance of chronic irritants is recommended, followed by a 14-day observation period to allow inflammatory lesions to heal. If the lesion persists, referral to a dental surgeon for a biopsy and regular followup surveillance, even if the lesion is benign, are indicated. The biopsy procedure is as simple as having a restoration (filling) or a tooth extraction.

Other conditions that may resemble leukoplakia or erythroplakia are lichen planus, chemical burns, candidiasis (thrush), psoriasis, lupus erythematosus, and syphilitic mucous patches. Each of these has characteristic histologic features.

Squamous Cell Carcinoma

More than 90% of all malignant tumors of the oral cavity are squamous cell carcinomas. They are four times more common in men than women and are most common after the fourth decade. In the United States, oral cancer is the eighth most common form of cancer in men and the twelfth in women. Fifteen thousand new cases are found each year, and about 7500 patients die of this disease annually. Of lip carcinomas, 95% occur on the lower lip and appear as an ulcer, wart, sore, or scale (22). This lesion is more common in fair-skinned patients. Of the intraoral carcinomas, 50% occur on the tongue (usually the ventrolateral border; Fig. 112.9) and 16% on the floor of the mouth; the remaining 34% are equally distributed between the gingival mucosa, palate, and buccal mucosa. Sixty percent of intraoral carcinomas present as ulcers, 30% as growths, and the remaining 10% as white lesions or other abnormalities of the mucosa (23). Carcinoma of the tongue and floor of the mouth metastasizes early and carries a poor prognosis.

The cause of oral carcinoma is unknown. Tobacco use and alcohol abuse are the major risk factors. Certain viral infections (e.g., Epstein-Barr and human papilloma virus), radiation exposure, dietary, and genetic factors may also increase risk.

Presentation and Evaluation

Patients usually give a history of knowledge of the lesion for 6 to 18 months when they first present; for many reasons they have not sought evaluation. All patients with suspicious lesions should be referred promptly to a dental surgeon for biopsy. Biopsy is a simple procedure, not very different from having a restoration or tooth extraction. Usually it is done under local anesthesia.

Treatment

Definitive surgery is a team effort between the otolaryngologist and the dentist. The dentist's role is to evaluate, for long-term prognosis, any teeth not to be removed in the surgical field and to remove any of these teeth affected with untreatable periodontitis. This is done to avoid osteoradionecrosis, a condition seen in the postradiation patient in whom the socket of an extracted tooth fails to heal as the result of diminished blood supply. Lip tumors have the highest success rate (10-year cure rate between 80% and 92%), whereas only one-fifth of patients with tongue cancer live longer than 5 years.

SPECIFIC REFERENCES*

1. Nagle D, Reader A, Beck M, Weaver J. Effect of systemic penicillin on pain in untreated irreversible pulpitis. Oral Surg Oral Med Oral Pathol Oral Radiol Endod 2000;90:636.
2. Graykowski EA, Barile MF, Lee WB, et al. Recurrent aphthous stomatitis: clinical, therapeutic, histopathologic, and hypersensitivity aspects. JAMA 1966;196:637.
3. Porter S, Scully C. Aphthous ulcers (recurrent). Clin Evid 2005;13:1687.
4. Chauvin PJ, Ajar AH. Acute herpetic gingivostomatitis in adults: a review of 13 cases, including diagnosis and management. J Can Dent Assoc 2002;68:247.
5. Franks AS. The social character of temporomandibular joint dysfunction. Dent Pract Dent Rec 1964;15:94.
6. Apfelberg DB, Lavey E, Janetos G, et al. Temporomandibular joint disease: results of a ten year study. Postgrad Med 1979;65:167.

*Bold numerals denote published controlled clinical trials, meta-analyses, or consensus-based recommendations.

7. U.S. Department of Health, Education and Welfare, Public Health Service. Research explores pyorrhea and other gum diseases: periodontal disease (PHS Publication 1482). Washington, DC: US Government Printing Office, 1970.
8. Pihlstrom BL, Michalowicz BS, Johnson NW. Periodontal diseases. Lancet 2005;366:1809.
9. Yoshihara A, Seida Y, Hanada N, et al. A longitudinal study of the relationship between periodontal disease and bone mineral density in community-dwelling older adults. J Clin Periodontol 2004;31:680.
10. Janket SJ, Baird AE, Chuang SK, et al. Meta-analysis of periodontal disease and risk of coronary heart disease and stroke. Oral Surg Oral Med Oral Pathol Oral Radiol Endod 2003;95:559.
11. Joshipura KJ, Hung HC, Rimm EB, et al. Periodontal disease, tooth loss, and incidence of ischemic stroke. Stroke 2003;34:47.
12. Hujoel PP, Drangsholt M, Spiekerman C, et al. Examining the link between coronary heart disease and the elimination of chronic dental infections. J Am Dent Assoc 2001;132:883.
13. Hung HC, Douglass CW. Meta-analysis of the effects of scaling and root planing, surgical treatment, and antibiotic therapies on periodontal probing depth and attachment loss. J Clin Periodontol 2002;29:975.
14. Robinson PG, Deacon SA, Deery C, et al. Manual versus powered toothbrushing for oral health. Cochrane Database System Rev 2005;2:CD002281.
15. Hanes PJ, Pruvis JP. Local anti-infective therapy: pharmacological agents: a systematic review. Ann Periodontol 2003;8:79.
16. Bonito AJ, Lux L, Lohr KN. Impact of local adjuncts to scaling and root planing in periodontal disease therapy: a systematic review. J Periodontol 2005;76:1227.
17. Haffajee AD, Socransky SS, Gunsolley JC. Systematic anti-infective periodontal therapy: a systematic review. Ann Periodontol 2003;8:115.
18. McDonagh MS, Whiting PF, Wilson PM, et al. Systematic review of water fluoridation. BMJ 2000;321:855.
19. Marinho VCC, Higgins JPT, Logan S, et al. Topical fluoride (toothpastes, mouthrinses, gels or varnishes) for preventing dental caries in children and adolescents. Cochrane Database System Rev 2003;4:CD002782.
20. Ahovuo-Saloranta A, Hiiri A, Nordblad A, et al. Pit and fissure sealants for preventing dental decay in the permanent teeth of children and adolescents. Cochrane Database System Rev 2004;3:CD001830.
21. Scully C, Porter S. Halitosis. BMJ, 2006. Available at: http://www.clinicalevidence.com/ceweb/conditions/index.jsp.
22. Mashberg A, Morrissey JB, Garfinkel L. A study of the appearance of early asymptomatic oral squamous cell carcinoma. Cancer (Philadelphia) 1973;32:1436.
23. Bhaskar SN. Synopsis of oral pathology. 4th ed. St. Louis: CV Mosby, 1973:463.

*For annotated **General References** and resources related to this chapter, visit www.hopkinsbayview.org/PAMreferences.*

SECTION 17

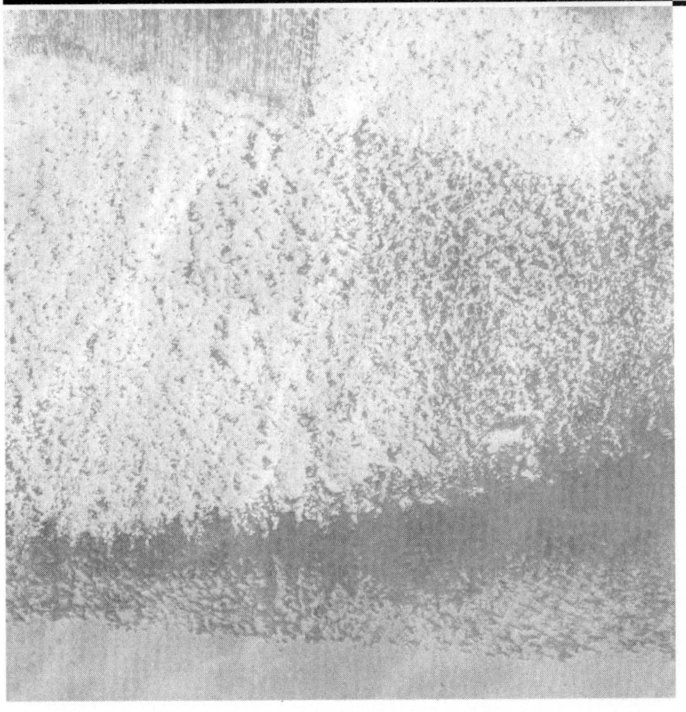

Common Disorders of the Skin

Chapter 113

Diagnoses and Treatment of Skin Disorders

S. Elizabeth Whitmore

SKIN EXAMINATION AND DEFINITIONS

The primary goal of the skin examination is to define the *morphology* (appearance) of the lesion and the extent of disease. The former allows the correct diagnosis to be made and the latter aids in the determination of prognosis and treatment. The examination of the lesion or eruption of concern is ideally followed by a complete skin examination. This latter may reveal findings helpful in diagnosis or may expose a previously unrecognized skin disease. The examination is most easily done in a systematic fashion, starting at the top with the scalp, face, and oral mucosa and then moving to the anterior then posterior aspect of the body. Good lighting is essential.

Mastering the definitions of commonly used dermatologic terms should aid in both diagnosis and communication with other physicians:

- *Atrophy:* Thinning of the epidermis or dermis causing fine wrinkling or depression of the skin (e.g., discoid lupus erythematosus, steroid-induced atrophy, normal aging).
- *Bulla:* A blister, similar to a vesicle but larger than 5 mm in diameter, filled with serous or serosanguinous fluid (e.g., friction blister, bullous pemphigoid).
- *Burrow:* A linear thread-like elevation of the skin, typically a few millimeters long (pathognomonic for scabies).
- *Comedone:* A plugged pilosebaceous follicle (e.g., a closed comedone or "whitehead" seen in acne).
- *Crust:* Yellowish-brown sticky debris consisting of dried serum, scale, and usually bacteria (e.g., impetigo, impetiginized eczema).
- *Cyst:* A circumscribed, firm, yet often slightly compressible, spherical lesion, fixed in the dermis (e.g., epidermal inclusion cyst).
- *Erosion:* A focal loss of a portion of the epidermis, nonscarring (e.g., candidiasis in the inframammary crease with a moist surface, impetigo).
- *Excoriation:* A self-inflicted disruption of the epidermis.
- *Fissure:* A vertical cut extending into the dermis (e.g., angular cheilitis or "cracks at the angle of the mouth" caused by *Candida*, salivary enzymes, or a vitamin deficiency).
- *Hive:* See *Wheal.*
- *Hyperkeratotic:* Heaped up or stacked scale (e.g., hypertrophic actinic keratosis, squamous cell carcinoma, wart).
- *Macule* or *macular:* A flat color change (e.g., freckle, café-au-lait spot, junctional nevus, or "flat brown mole").
- *Morphology:* Shape of the primary lesion (e.g., stellate, linear, round, or diffuse).
- *Nodule:* A solid lesion up to 2 cm in diameter with an appreciable deep (dermal or subcutaneous) component (e.g., dermatofibroma, nodular melanoma, erythema nodosum, lipoma).
- *Papule:* An elevated often dome-shaped bump up to 10 mm in diameter, (e.g., intradermal nevus or "skin-colored mole," molluscum contagiosum).
- *Plaque:* A flat-topped elevated area of skin, the surface area of which is much greater than the thickness (e.g., psoriasis, cutaneous T-cell lymphoma, or "mycosis fungoides").
- *Pustule:* A circumscribed lesion visibly filled with purulent material (e.g., folliculitis, acne pustule, pustular psoriasis).

- *Scale:* Surface alteration resulting in a flaky surface, caused by abnormal proliferation or desquamation of the outermost epidermal layer, the stratum corneum (e.g., psoriasis, seborrheic dermatitis, tinea).
- *Sclerosis:* Scar-like induration (e.g., systemic sclerosis, localized scleroderma or "morphea").
- *Secondary changes:* Changes that occur as a result of the natural development or external manipulation of the primary lesion.
- *Telangiectasia:* A dilated superficial capillary or venule; may be linear, spider-like, or mat-like (e.g., starburst leg telangiectasias, telangiectasias in a basal cell carcinoma or in an area of steroid- or lupus-induced atrophy).
- *Tumor:* A large mass, greater than 2 cm in diameter, with significant thickness (e.g., neglected squamous cell carcinoma, cutaneous lymphoma).
- *Ulcer:* A loss of skin extending into the dermis that always heals with scarring (any loss that penetrates the dermal–epidermal junction scars; e.g., venous stasis ulcer, pyoderma gangrenosum).
- *Urticarial:* Adjective describing plaques that are edematous, erythematous, or blanched (e.g., urticaria or "wheals" or "hives," urticarial vasculitis, Sweet syndrome, or "acute febrile neutrophilic dermatosis").
- *Vesicle:* A blister up to 5 mm in diameter filled with serous or serosanguinous fluid (e.g., herpes simplex infection, vesicular hand dermatitis).
- *Wheal or hive:* An erythematous or blanched edematous plaque with no surface change, *present for no more than 24 hours* (urticaria, by definition).

Based on the morphology of the observed skin changes, a differential diagnosis or diagnosis of the skin lesion or eruption may be made, which may or may not require biopsy for confirmation. Table 113.1 provides a summary of selected disorders categorized by morphology and pathophysiology of disease. Those conditions that are common, diagnostically difficult, and therapeutically complicated are discussed in detail in the chapters that follow.

TOPICAL THERAPEUTICS

Topical Corticosteroids

Topical corticosteroids are categorized based on the degree of vasoconstriction produced upon application to the skin, with superpotent products producing the most vasoconstriction. Vasoconstriction correlates well with biologic activity, therapeutic efficacy, and undesirable side effects. The latter include local effects such as acne, rosacea, striae, atrophy (cigarette paper-like wrinkling of the skin), and increased risk of fungal infection. In addition, systemic effects, as evidenced by hypothalamic–pituitary–adrenal axis suppression, may occur with the use of potent corticosteroids over large areas.

Although there are over 20 different preparations, it is easiest to become familiar with and prescribe just four different corticosteroids based on the strength needed. All topical corticosteroids except 0.5% and 1% hydrocortisone are by prescription only. Examples include:

- Low potency: hydrocortisone 1% or 2.5%;
- Mid-potency: triamcinolone (acetonide) 0.1%;
- High potency: fluocinonide;
- Super potency: clobetasol (propionate).

Generally, only low-potency preparations should be used on the face and in areas of thin skin (e.g., folds and genitalia). Unless a drying effect is desired, ointments are preferred as they aid most in restoring the skin barrier.

An accurate estimation of the amount of corticosteroid needed is important because of the cost of these preparations. Dermatoses are generally treated until clear, and the application is repeated for recurrences. Acute and subacute dermatitis generally clear in 1 to 2 weeks; chronic dermatitis may require chronic intermittent therapy. One gram covers a 10 × 10-cm area: 2 g covers the hands, head, face, or anogenital area; 3 g covers the anterior or posterior trunk or an arm; 4 g covers a single lower extremity; and 30 g covers the entire skin surface. Therefore, for a 1-week two times daily application for each of these areas, 30 g, 45 g, 60 g, and 420 g, respectively, should be prescribed. Most corticosteroids come in 15-, 30-, 60-, and 120-g tubes. Additionally, 1-pound jars of hydrocortisone or 0.1% triamcinolone cream or ointment may be requested.

Emollients (Skin Moisturizers)

Very simply, emollients may be classified as *oil in water* (mostly water), *water in oil* (mostly oil), and *oil* preparations. Because the purpose of emollients is to trap moisture after hydrating the skin with a warm bath or shower, occlusive substances are most efficient. Unfortunately, not all patients are amenable to putting petroleum jelly on their skin one or two times a day. A good compromise is Eucerin Original lotion or Nivea moisturizing cream (water in oil). Still lighter oil-in-water moisturizers include Lubriderm, Moisturel, Curel, Vaseline Intensive Care, and Keri lotions. Formulations that contain α-hydroxy acids aid in normal desquamation of the skin, making it softer and smoother (e.g., Am-Lacten, Eucerin Plus, and AquaGlycolic lotion). Although they are useful, patients who have "sensitive" or irritated skin may experience stinging and develop an irritant contact dermatitis from the added α-hydroxy acid. A good rule to follow is that if it burns or stings, it should not be used.

Topical Antifungal Agents

Several topical antifungal agents are available (see Chapter 117). *Polyenes* such as nystatin (cream, ointment, and

TABLE 113.1 Selected Skin Disorders Based on Morphology

Disorder	Description	Common Presentation	Possible Systemic Associations	Risks	Recommendations	Differential Diagnosis	Key to Diagnosis
HYPOPIGMENTED AND DEPIGMENTED MACULES AND PATCHES							
Vitiligo	Depigmented patches caused by loss of melanocytes, immunologically mediated; favors periorificial and "tip" areas	New-onset stark white skin around the eyes, lips, fingertips, and penis	Autoimmune thyroiditis, pernicious anemia, Addison disease, diabetes mellitus	Skin cancer	Sunscreens	Postinflammatory hypopigmentation, albinism, chemical leukoderma	Acquired depigmentation without a history of exposure to phenolic compounds which may cause depigmentation
Idiopathic guttate hypomelanosis, "snowflakes"	Hypopigmented 3- to 8-mm macules caused by focal loss of melanin production	Asymptomatic whitish macules on the pretibial and extensor forearm surfaces	None	None	Sunscreens	Vitiligo	Small macules of hypopigmentation on sun-damaged skin
Tinea versicolor	See Chapter 117						
Halo nevus	Symmetric depigmented halo around a nevus	Small symmetric halo surrounding an evenly pigmented brown papule in a young individual	In adults and those with a history of melanoma, suspect melanloma or associated metastatic melanoma	Misdiagnosis	If halo is asymmetric or nevus is abnormal by the ABCDs, biopsy to rule out melanoma	Melanoma with regression, dysplastic nevus	Symmetric mole with symmetric halo of depigmentation
HYPERPIGMENTED MACULES AND PATCHES							
Junctional nevus	Light to dark macule of uniform shape and brown color, may develop from early childhood to early thirties; formed by nests of melanocytes at the dermal–epidermal junction	2- to 6-mm sharply circumscribed, evenly pigmented, brown macule	None	People with >40 to 50 nevi have an increased risk of melanoma	Monthly self-examinations; intermittent physican examination	Lentigo simplex, freckle	May be difficult to clinically distinguish from lentigo and freckles; however, all three are benign
Solar lentigo	"Liver spot"; brown, 2-mm to 2-cm macule occurring on a background of chronic sun-damaged skin	Multiple hyperpigmented 3- to 8-mm brown macules on the face and dorsal hands	None	None	Prevention: sunscreen use; elective treatment: cryosurgery, laser surgery, hydroquinone creams	Lentigo simplex, lentigo maligna (i.e., melanoma *in situ*)	Homogeneous pigmentation on background of sun-damaged skin

(continued)

TABLE 113.1 (Continued) Selected Skin Disorders Based on Morphology

Disorder	Description	Common Presentation	Possible Systemic Associations	Risks	Recommendations	Differential Diagnosis	Key to Diagnosis
			HYPERPIGMENTED MACULES AND PATCHES				
Café-au-lait spot	Evenly pigmented, light to medium brown, 1- to several cm macule; noted at birth or in early childhood	Tan brown macule	Neurofibromatosis: Presence of six café-au-lait spots greater than 1.5 cm often with axillary freckling; may have tumors, e.g., CNS neoplasms, pheochromocytoma Albright syndrome: large, unilateral, pigmented macule with an irregular border, polyostotic fibrous dysplasia and precocious puberty Tuberous sclerosis: cafe-au-lait spots, seizures, adenoma sebaceum (perinasal skin colored papules), and ash leaf macules (hypopigmented macules)		Lightening or removal may be attempted with laser surgery	Junctional nevus	Macular pigmentation with no surface change (i.e., no epidermal alteration)
Melasma	Irregular tan to brown pigmentation; favors cheeks, forehead and upper lip	Patchy brown discoloration on central forehead and cheeks	Pregnancy and exogenous estrogens	N/A	Sunscreens and avoidance of sun exposure, hydroquinone cream, or elective laser surgery	Hydroquinone induced in "pseudo-ochronosis"	Female, facial location, intensifies in the summer
Xanthelasma	See Chapter 82						
Xanthoma	See Chapter 82						

			PAPULES				
Warts, tumors	See Chapter 117						
Compound nevus	Tan to dark brown, 2- to 6-mm dome-shaped papule, formed by nests of melanocytes, both at the dermal epidermal junction and in the dermis	Stable brown "mole"	None	None	Patient self-examinations for changes, as with all nevi; biopsy if diagnosis is in question	Melanoma, intradermal nevus, dermatofibroma, neurofibroma	Soft, circumscribed, symmetric, evenly colored papule
Intradermal nevus	Skin color to light brown, generally 2- to 6-mm fleshy papule; consists of nests of melanocytes confined to the dermis	Dome shaped, skin-colored papule	None	None	Biopsy if diagnosis is in question	Amelanotic melanoma, dermatofibroma, neurofibroma	Soft, circumscribed, symmetric, skin colored papule
Seborrheic keratosis (Fig. 113.1)	"Stuck on" appearing tan, yellowish-brown to black-brown plaque with a friable, fine papulated, or smooth surface studded with tiny white flecks of keratin; caused by local proliferation of the epidermis; common after age 30	Tan to dark brown finely papulated "stuck on" flat topped papules over the trunk	"Sudden" eruption of many inflamed seborrheic keratoses; may herald a malignancy, most often with adenocarcinoma	None	Liquid nitrogen cryosurgery or curettage may be used on pruritic or troublesome lesions; biopsy, never destroy, if diagnosis is in question	Wart, squamous cell carcinoma, basal cell carcinoma, melanoma	Characteristic "stuck on" appearance
Cherry angioma	"Cherry red" 0.5- to 6-mm dome-shaped nonblanching papules which favor the trunk, formed by dilated capillaries; common after age 30	Minute to 4-mm red to purple dome-shaped papules	Hereditary hemorrhagic telangiectasia: autosomal dominant, punctate telangiectasias on the oral mucosa and fingers +/− AV malformations in the GI tract, lungs, and CNS CREST: sclerodactyly with punctate and matlike telangiectasias on the face and fingers	None	Cauterize if traumatized or if desired for cosmesis	Hemangioma	Characteristic size and cherry red appearance

(continued)

TABLE 113.1 (Continued) Selected Skin Disorders Based on Morphology

Disorder	*Description*	*Common Presentation*	*Possible Systemic Associations*	*Risks*	*Recommendations*	*Differential Diagnosis*	*Key to Diagnosis*
Dermatofibroma	Smooth, circumscribed, 3- to 10-mm papule in the skin; feels like a "pea in the skin"; composed of fibroblasts	Small, brownish ill-defined macule with underlying papule		None	Biopsy if diagnosis is in question	Nodular melanoma, nevus	Characteristic "pea-like" dermal papule without surface change
Condyloma acuminatum	See Chapter 117						
Molluscum contagiosum	See Chapter 117						
Basal cell carcinoma	See Chapter 114						
Squamous cell carcinoma	See Chapter 114						
Kaposi sarcoma	See Chapter 39						
			PLAQUES				
Psoriasis	See Chapter 116						
Seborrheic dermatitis	See Chapter 116						
Atopic dermatitis	See Chapter 116						
Nummular dermatitis	See Chapter 116						
Secondary syphilis	See Chapter 37						
Contact dermatitis	See Chapter 116						
Tinea	See Chapter 117						
Xanthoma	See Chapter 82						

				PLAQUES			
Pityriasis rosea	Self-limited eruption, lasting several weeks, initial lesion: herald patch; >1-cm erythematous oval plaque with fine peripheral scale, usually on the chest, followed in 7–14 days by an eruption of smaller plaques over the trunk; pruritus	1- to 3-cm oval plaque, followed by a shower of 25–100 similar 3- to 15-mm papules and plaques on the trunk, with the long axes of the lesions oriented along the skin lines in a "Christmas tree" pattern	None	None	If pruritic, midpotency topical corticosteroids; if extremely pruritic, consider phototherapy	Secondary syphilis, primary HIV exanthem, tinea corporis, tinea versicolor, psoriasis	Herald patch, negative test for syphilis
Pityriasis alba	A mild form of dermatitis, in young patients; hypopigmented, slightly scaly, up to several cm macules or minimally elevated plaques; occasionally pruritic	Asymptomatic scaly patches over the arms and legs	More common in patients with atopy	None	Emollients, hydrocortisone; phototherapy	Tinea versicolor, hypopigmented mycosis fungoides, sarcoidosis	May be difficult to exclude other diagnoses without further evaluation (i.e., KOH +/− biopsy)
Mycosis fungoides	Cutaneous T-cell lymphoma most often affects patients older than age 40; however, any age may be affected; erythematous to brawny patches, plaques, or tumors; may assume bizarre irregular shapes; asymptomatic or pruritic	Several-year history of scaly reddish plaques gradually increasing in number over the trunk	None	Although a lymphoma, evidence of systemic involvement with simple testing is usually absent unless the disease progresses; poor prognosis is associated with greater than 10% body surface area involvement, tumor, and lymphadenopathy (the latter requires biopsy to determine reactive vs. neoplastic)	Treatment varies with the stage of the disease and age of patient; PUVA, electron beam, topical nitrogen mustard, interferon-γ, observation	Parapsoriasis, psoriasis, sarcoidosis, pityriasis alba	Biopsy required

(continued)

TABLE 113.1 (Continued) Selected Skin Disorders Based on Morphology

Disorder	Description	Common Presentation	Possible Systemic Associations	Risks	Recommendations	Differential Diagnosis	Key to Diagnosis
Erythema nodosum	Hypersensitivity reaction to some antigen, erythematous, tender nodules most often on the pretibial legs; develop in crops and involute over 2–3 weeks, resolve with a local bruise, never suppurate and drain; caused by a localized inflammatory infiltrate in the septum surrounding fat lobules	Acute onset of erythematous nodules over the pretibial area associated with mild arthralgias	More common associations include streptococcal infection, vaginal candidiasis, tuberculosis, viral hepatitis, coccidioidomycosis, histoplasmosis, lymphogranuloma venereum, *Yersinia enterocolitica*; inflammatory bowel disease, or reaction to sulfonamides, barbiturates, various antibiotics, salicylates, oral contraceptives, or pregnancy	None	Evaluation to exclude possible associations; review of Rx and OTC medications, throat culture, ASO titer, chest radiograph, PPD; complete viral hepatitis screen; additional workup based on clinical findings; reassess chronic disease with a search for "occult infection" (dental, sinus, gallbladder, other gastrointestional, etc.)	Other forms of panniculitis and polyarteritis nodosa	Tender nodules on the pretibial legs that resolve over a few weeks without ever ulcerating
Lipoma	Benign fatty tumor, often solitary, on the trunk	Asymptomatic rubbery nodule, movable under the skin	None	None	Excision if desired or diagnosis is in question	Cyst, neurofibroma, soft tissue malignancies	Soft nodule, freely movable under the skin

CNS, central nervous system; AV, atrioventricular; GI, gastrointestinal; CREST, *c*alcinosis, *R*aynaud phenomenon, *e*sophageal motility disorders, *s*clerodactyly, and *t*elangiectasia; HIV, human immunodeficiency virus; OTC, over the counter; ASO, antistreptolysin; PPD, purified protein derivative of tuberculin.

powder, by prescription) are used only for candida. In contrast, topicals that may be used for both candida and dermatophytes include *imidazoles,* such as clotrimazole (Mycelex OTC and Lotrimin AF cream, lotion, and solution, all over the counter), sulconazole (Exelderm 1% cream or solution, by prescription), and ketoconazole (Nizoral cream or 2% shampoo, by prescription), which are fungistatic. Finally, for dermatophyte but not *Candida* infections, *allylamines,* such as terbinafine, may be used and are fungicidal (Lamisil cream, lotion, or spray, over-the-counter).

Creams are applied one or two times per day and should be continued for 2 weeks after clinical resolution of the infection, and as needed for recurrences. Nizoral shampoo is intended for treatment of scalp seborrheic dermatitis, but it may also be used for tinea versicolor. For the former, it is lathered on the scalp and rinsed after 3 minutes, two or three times per week; for the latter, it is applied to the trunk from the neck to the waistline, left 5 minutes, then lathered and rinsed, daily for 10 to 14 days, with a single application repeated every 1 to 2 weeks to prevent recurrences.

Compresses and Baths

Compresses are used to dry and débride localized areas of acute dermatitis, characterized by moist, erythematous, edematous papules, plaques, and vesicles or bullae with serous discharge. Several solutions dry by precipitating protein (Burow aluminum acetate solution, 1:20 dilution; Domeboro aluminum sulfate and calcium acetate solution, 1:20 dilution; Aveeno Colloidal Oatmeal Packet). Some act as germicidals (silver nitrate 0.1% to 0.5% solution, acetic acid 1% to 5% solution). All, including saline made by adding 2 teaspoons salt per 1 L of water, promote drying through evaporation and remove devitalized tissue through physical softening, allowing mechanical removal upon lifting the damp ("wet to damp") or dry ("wet to dry") dressing.

Compresses may be gauze or cotton sheeting. For the latter, a clean sheet should be cut and folded into six to eight layers to approximate the area of affected skin. This is immersed in the soaking solution and squeezed just short of dripping wet. It is placed on the site for 15 to 30 minutes, three or four times per day, and is rewetted every 15 minutes for a "wet to damp" dressing.

When more than one third of the body surface area is affected by acute dermatitis or impetiginization, compresses are not only impractical but may cause hypothermia. Warm *baths* are used instead. Preferred drying and soothing additives include Aveeno Oatmeal Packet, sodium bicarbonate (baking soda, 3 cups), hydrolyzed starch (Lint, 4 cups mixed with water in a large mixing bowl and then added to the bath water), and a mix of half of each of the bicarbonate and starch mixtures.

Baths are also useful for generalized dry pruritic dermatoses such as atopic dermatitis, generalized psoriasis, morbilliform drug eruptions, and erythroderma. Instead of drying additives, oil (one eighth cup bath oil or Aveeno Oilated Oatmeal Packet) is added to the bath water to help trap moisture in the skin. Patients must be warned about oil making the bathtub slippery and should be advised to purchase secure bath mats for the tub and for the floor outside the tub. Unsteady or frail patients should not use bath oil. Baths should be taken three or four times a day for 20 minutes and a heavy moisturizer (e.g., Vaseline jelly, Aquaphor ointment, Eucerin Original Lotion) must be reapplied immediately after lightly patting dry, leaving some moisture on the skin.

SKIN BIOPSY

Skin biopsy for histologic examination of the skin is required to confirm the diagnosis of many skin conditions. Types of biopsies that may be used include *punch, ellipse,* and *shave.* They may be *incisional* (sampling a portion of the lesion) or *excisional* (removing the entire lesion). Skin biopsy is a simple and invaluable procedure that may be easily mastered with the help of a skilled instructor and practice.

GENERAL REFERENCES

Ackerman BA, Kerl H, Sanchez J. A clinical atlas of 101 common skin diseases with histopathologic correlation. New York: Ardor Scribendi, 2000.

Fitzpatrick TP, Johnson RA, Wolff K, et al. Color atlas and synopsis of clinical dermatology. 3rd ed. New York: McGraw-Hill, 1997.
A concise disease discussion, with excellent photographs.

Habib TP, Quitadamo MJ, Campbell JL, et al. Skin disease: diagnosis and treatment. St. Louis: Mosby, 2001.
An excellent text of clinical diagnosis and therapy.

Kazin, RA, Lowitt NR, Lowitt MH. Update in dermatology. Ann Intern Med 2001;135:124.
Highlights 10 articles of interest to the generalist.

Lamberg SI. The little black book of dermatology. Malden, MA: Blackwell, 2000.
A comprehensive clinical handbook organized by chief complaint, body part affected, or associated condition.

Lookingbill DP, Marks JG Jr. Principals of dermatology. 3rd ed. Philadelphia, PA: WB Saunders, 2000.

Websites

American Cancer Society website; also telephone 800-ACS-2345). Available at: http://www.cancer.org.
An excellent resource for educational materials on skin cancer for physicians and patients.

American Academy of Dermatology website. Available at: http://www.aad.org.

National Psoriasis Foundation website. Available at: http://www.psoriasis.org.

University of Iowa. Available at: http://tray.dermatology.uiowa.edu/home.html.

University of Iowa Website with over 300 clinical photographs; also resource for dermatology patient support group.)

Available at: http://www.med.jhu.edu/peds/dermatlas. Last accessed DATE.

Also see review: Lamberg L. Internet dermatology atlas aids physicians and parents. JAMA 2001;25:2065.

Chapter 114

Atypical Moles and Common Cancers of the Skin

S. Elizabeth Whitmore

The three most common types of skin cancer have a definite relationship to natural and artificial ultraviolet radiation (UVR) exposure in non-Hispanic white individuals (1,2). Despite this generally known association, Americans still tend to be "sun seekers," commonly vacationing in UVR rich locations such as the oceanside, ski slopes, and Disney World. A collection of statistics from sources including the American Academy of Dermatology, the American Cancer Society, and peer-reviewed journals sum up the next generation's UVR exposure activities (3):

1. Four out of 5 children age 12 to 17 years are aware of the potential dangers of tanning, but 60% of the same age group experience sunburn at least once a summer.
2. Fifty-three percent of girls between 12 and 17 years of age wear sunscreen, versus only about one third of boys in the same age group.
3. Persons who have used a tanning bed are 2.5 times more likely than other persons who have not to develop squamous cell carcinoma.
4. Regular use of a tanning bed is associated with an eightfold increase in melanoma risk; even casual use is associated with a threefold increase.
5. More than one third of teen girls and 11% of teen boys have used a tanning bed at least once in their lives.
6. Approximately 28% of female adolescents and 7% of male adolescents have used a tanning facility three or more times.
7. In all, more than one million people make use of a tanning salon, booth, or bed every day.

Despite the widely recognized morbidity and mortality associated with skin cancer, it seems that our risk taking through UVR exposure will probably not change until a tan is no longer deemed "fashionable."

ATYPICAL MOLES

Atypical moles (dysplastic nevi) affect 10% to 30% of the general population. These acquired lesions have clinical and histologic features that differ from common moles (melanocytic nevi). Common moles are tan to dark brown in color, sharply circumscribed, 2- to 6-mm macules or papules that develop in childhood or early adulthood; the average adult has 20 common moles. In contrast, *atypical moles or dysplastic nevi are often larger than 6 mm, irregular or ill-defined, variegated in color* (Fig. 114.1, Color Plate section), and *may continue to appear after age 35.* Because of these atypical features, biopsy may be required to exclude the possible diagnosis of melanoma.

Patients with a few nonfamilial atypical moles and no personal history of melanoma are at increased risk for melanoma when compared with the general population, with a relative risk somewhere between 2 and 8 (4). With the goal of detecting melanomas as early as possible, these patients are asked to perform monthly self-examinations, looking for any change in the appearance of a mole, and to have physician skin examinations done every 6 to 12 months. Full body photography is very useful, aiding both patients and physicians in the detection of new or changing moles, hopefully allowing melanoma to be diagnosed at the earliest stages should it develop (5).

The *familial atypical mole and melanoma (FAMM) syndrome,* formerly called the dysplastic nevus syndrome, is associated with an extremely high risk of melanoma. Although the prevalence is probably greatly underestimated, it is said to affect at least 300,000 people. These individuals begin to develop atypical lesions at puberty and continue to develop new lesions throughout their lives. Patients with this syndrome have a family history of melanoma in at least one first- or second-degree relative and many nevi, often more than 50, some or many of which are atypical. Patients with the FAMM syndrome have a lifetime risk of developing melanoma approaching 100%. Patients with sporadic atypical mole syndrome with a mole pattern similar to that of the FAMM syndrome also have a significantly increased risk of developing melanoma. All these patients should perform monthly self-examinations, with the aid of baseline full body photographs, as noted above, looking for any changes in the appearance of their moles. Additionally, they should be examined at 3- to 12-month intervals by a dermatologist. Patients should be counseled on methods of self-examination (using their photographs placed in an photoalbum to facilitate a systematic full skin examination) and means of sun protection (avoidance of exposure during peak sun intensity hours, use of high sun-protection factor sunscreen, and appropriate protective clothing) because sun exposure increases the risk of malignancy. Also, because early detection saves lives, it should be made clear that other family members may be similarly affected and advised.

MELANOMA

Cutaneous malignant melanoma is the third most common type of skin cancer and the leading cause of death from skin disease (4,6). Excluding the "nonmelanoma skin cancers" (basal and squamous cell carcinomas), in the United States, melanoma ranks as the fifth and seventh most common cancer in men and women, respectively. In this country, an estimated 55,000 persons were diagnosed with melanoma and 7,900 persons died because of melanoma in 2004. Comparing melanoma statistics from 1950 to 2000, there has been a 619% increase in annual diagnosis and 165% increase in annual mortality. Melanoma remains the most common cancer diagnosed in women from 20 to 29 years of age (6).

Although melanoma occurs with greatest frequency within a small subpopulation of persons having the FAMM syndrome or nonfamilial atypical moles, most patients who develop melanoma have neither of these relatively uncommon risk factors. Six much more common independent risk factors for melanoma include family history of melanoma, blond or red hair, marked freckling on the upper back, three or more blistering sunburns before age 20, three or more summers spent outside working as a teen, and the presence of actinic keratoses. Having one or two of these risk factors increases risk by 3.5-fold and having three or more risk factors increases risk by 20-fold. Although rare in African Americans, melanomas are most often found on the hands and feet, where incidence is similar among various races. Although the cause of melanoma is unknown, ultraviolet radiation is an important risk factor. Evidence for this includes the greater incidence of melanoma found in persons living closer to the equator, persons having a history of blistering sunburns, and persons with a history of basal or squamous cell carcinoma (7).

As a general rule, all pigmented lesions should be scrutinized for atypical features that may suggest melanoma. These include the *ABCDs: asymmetry, border irregularity, color variegation* (variable degrees of brown, tan, black, red, white, or blue), and *diameter greater than 6 mm.* Although one or more of these features may be present in a given melanoma, they may be absent. Adding *"E"* to denote *"evolving"* has been proposed to aid in the diagnosis of melanomas lacking the "ABCD" features. Evolving, as defined by its proponents, may designate such things as changes in size, shape, and shades of color, itching, tenderness, and bleeding (8). The utility of this addition is easily seen in the case of a nodular melanoma. This cancer characteristically presents as a symmetric, dome-shaped, deeply but evenly pigmented, rapidly *growing* (evolving) papule or nodule, exhibiting none of the ABCDs.

Excisional biopsy of *changing* or *atypical* moles should generally be performed, and ongoing close surveillance of patients with many remaining moles or the sporadic or familial atypical mole syndrome by a dermatologist or practitioner skilled in the area should be recommended. Finally, patient education is of key importance, with focus on the appearance of atypical moles and melanomas using the ABCDEs, monthly or bimonthly self-examination, protection from the sun (sun avoidance, sunscreen use, and protective clothing), and awareness of the possible familial link (i.e., patients with atypical moles or melanoma should most certainly inform relatives of the possible genetic link and the need for skin examination).

There are four common subtypes of melanoma: superficial spreading, nodular, lentigo maligna, and acral lentiginous melanoma (9,10). Fortunately, the characteristically difficult to diagnose amelanotic melanoma, which is usually white, pink, or red, is relatively rare. Table 114.1 shows the characteristics of these melanoma subtypes.

Superficial spreading melanoma arises from a pre-existing nevus in approximately 25% to 50% of cases. Typically, radial or outward growth occurs over a period of months to years. Clinical changes caused by this malignant transformation are generally seen as a change in diameter and border irregularity. With time, growth descends vertically from the epidermal–dermal junction and the surface becomes papular. This vertical growth creates the potential for metastasis. Figure 114.2 shows a superficial spreading melanoma (see Color Plate section).

Nodular melanoma usually does not manifest any of the ABCDs, but does exhibit the "E" (evolution) of atypical pigmented lesions, as it generally has no radial but only a vertical growth phase. This type of melanoma is usually a dome-shaped or polypoid, symmetric, deeply pigmented papule. It may develop *de novo* or arise within a pre-existing nevus. Nodular melanoma tends to grow rapidly over weeks to months.

Lentigo maligna melanoma occurs on sun-exposed skin, most commonly on the face. It arises from a pre-existing

TABLE 114.1 Features of the Subtypes of Melanoma

Melanoma Subtype[a]	*Approximate Frequency (%)*	*Clinical Appearance*	*Location*	*Age Group Most Often Affected*	*Differential Diagnosis*
Superficial spreading	70	Usually brown but may be variably colored brown, black, blue, red, and white; flattish papule, plaque, or maculopapule, usually over 6 mm in diameter; usually showing 1 or more of the ABCDs[b] of atypical moles and melanoma	Anywhere, often on the back in men and on the legs in women	30–40 yr	Nevus, seborrheic keratosis
Nodular	16	Colored as above or amelantoic, dome-shaped or polypoid papule or nodule; typically symmetric and uniform	Anywhere	40–50 yr	Nevus, thrombosed capillary hemangioma, pyogenic granuloma
Lentigo maligna	5	Tan or brown, less often black, blue, or red, irregular macule with focal surface elevation; later may develop distinct papules and nodules within	Face most often; other sun-exposed surfaces	50–70 yr	Solar lentigo (liver spot)
Acral lentiginous	<5	Similar in appearance to lentigo maligna melanoma; when it occurs as a pigmented streak in the nail with extension onto the nail fold skin, it is called *Hutchinson sign* (see text); seen most often in African Americans and Asians	Palms, soles, phalanges	All ages	Nevus, postinflammatory or drug-induced hyperpigmentation, fungal infection-induced nail dystrophy; pyogenic granuloma

[a]Other rare types combined make up less than 5% of melanoma.
[b]ABCDs, see text p. 1735.

lentigo maligna, which is a tan, brown, or brown/black, typically irregularly outlined macule on a sun-exposed site, usually present for many years. In fact, the term lentigo means freckle. Lentigo maligna melanoma has a radial growth phase like that of superficial spreading melanoma and therefore commonly shows the ABCDs of atypical pigmented lesions.

Acral lentiginous melanoma occurs with equal frequency in both light and deeply pigmented persons. This is in contrast to all other types of melanomas, which are rare in deeply pigmented persons. It is the most frequent type of melanoma occurring in African Americans and Asians. It presents on the peripheral parts (hence the name), especially the palms, soles, or subungually (underneath the nail plate) within the nail unit, and usually displays some of the ABCDs of atypical pigmented lesions. *Hutchinson sign* marked by pigment extending onto the skin of the nailfold in association with a subungual pigmented lesion is highly suggestive of melanoma, and biopsy is mandatory. Acral lentiginous melanoma frequently has a poor prognosis because diagnosis is often delayed. Up to 50% of patients with acral lentiginous melanoma give a history of preceding trauma of the skin in the area of the lesion. This history and the mistaken acceptance by the patient and physician that the pigment change or nail dystrophy is the result of trauma often contributes to a delay in biopsy and diagnosis.

Although the U.S. Preventive Services Task Force has not found sufficient evidence to recommend routine full body skin examination for melanoma, an argument can be made that early detection and excision is associated with a lower incidence of melanoma associated morbidity and mortality. With the latter in mind, our urgent aim is to detect melanoma as early in evolution as possible. At present, this seems best facilitated through public and professional education. A study involving 102 patients (47 male, 55 female) diagnosed with melanoma seen at one institution between 1995 and 1997 found that 55% of malignancies were self-detected, whereas 24% were detected by the health care provider. Those detected by professionals were thinner than those detected by patients (0.23 mm versus 0.9 mm, $p < .001$). These data should motivate continued patient and professional education (11).

Patients with suspicious lesions should be referred to a dermatologist or surgeon for evaluation for possible melanoma. In contrast to patients with suspected basal cell carcinoma (BCC) or squamous cell carcinoma (SCC) in whom a delay of 4 to 6 weeks is acceptable, patients with melanoma should be seen within a week or two. The suspected lesion will likely be fully excised for diagnosis. When full excision of the lesion is not possible because of anatomic location or size, an incisional biopsy of the most atypical and elevated area of the lesion is performed. If the diagnosis of melanoma is confirmed histologically, re-excision with an appropriate margin of normal surrounding tissue, as dictated by the vertical thickness of the melanoma, is necessary: 0.5 cm for melanoma *in situ*; 1 to 2 cm for melanoma 1 to 2 mm in thickness; and at least 2 cm for melanoma 2 mm or more in thickness. The exact optimal re-excision margin in this last case (melanoma thickness of 2 mm or greater) is felt "yet to be determined" (12). Simultaneous sentinel lymph node excision or elective lymph node dissection in patients with melanoma clinically limited to the skin remains controversial. Although data are still being gathered regarding the use of sentinel lymph node biopsy, many centers routinely perform sentinel lymph node biopsies for melanomas 1 mm or greater in thickness (6,13).

In otherwise asymptomatic patients, followup surveillance for Stage I melanoma (thickness up to 2 mm without ulceration and no nodal or distant spread) entails yearly, or more frequent, full skin and lymph node examination. Surveillance for Stage II (excluding Stage I melanoma, any thickness, with or without ulceration, and again, no evidence of nodal or distant spread) is similar. Surveillance testing such as serum lactate dehydrogenase (LDH), chest radiograph, and other imaging studies are not generally recommended. For patients with greater risk for additional melanomas, such as those with atypical moles, full skin examination is often recommended at 3- to 6-month intervals (6). Full-body photography to aid in ongoing self and physician skin examination (as above, placing these photographs in an orderly fashion in a photoalbum to facilitate a systematic full body skin examination) for changing or new "moles" (or melanoma!) is believed to aid in the diagnosis of melanoma (5). Finally, the need for ocular examination for melanocytic lesions in person with cutaneous melanoma is debated. Data seem to be stronger for the converse of this (i.e., skin examination in persons with a history of ocular melanoma) (14).

The prognosis for a patient after excision of a primary cutaneous melanoma depends on the thickness of the melanoma and whether there is evidence of spread to lymph nodes or distant metastases. Ten-year survival rates, based on melanoma thickness, are as follows: $\leq$1 mm, 88%; >1 to 2 mm, 79%; >2 to 4.0 mm, 64%; >4 mm, 54%. If ulceration is present, 10-year survival rates decrease to 83%, 64%, 51%, and 32%, respectively. In patients with microscopic metastases to the regional lymph nodes, the 5-year median survival *is less* than 70%; with macroscopic lymph node metastases, *less than* 60%; and with noncutanous or subcutaneous distant metastases, *less than* 10% (15).

Adjuvant therapy for persons at "high risk" for recurrence and mortality after definitive surgery is controversial. High dose interferon α-2b, approved by the U.S. Food and Drug Administration (FDA), may be considered for those with Stage IIB or IIC (melanoma without evidence of spread and "thicker than 2 mm with ulceration" or "thicker than 4 mm with or without ulceration") and Stage III (melanoma associated with spread limited to regional lymph nodes). High-dose interferon causes unpleasant and sometimes intolerable side effects including flu like symptoms with fatigue, fever, headache, and nausea, as well as weight loss, depression, and also possible myelosuppression, and is associated with only modest efficacy. It is best reserved for eligible patients who are otherwise healthy with an expected life expectancy of greater than 10 years in whom the chance of recurrence is believed to be greatest (6). Therapeutic melanoma vaccines hold promise but are still investigational (6).

ACTINIC KERATOSIS AND NONMELANOMA SKIN CANCER

Actinic Keratosis

Actinic keratoses are sun-induced precancers or focal areas of epidermal dysplasia (Table 114.2). Although occasionally seen in teenagers, they generally begin to develop

TABLE 114.2 Nonmelanoma Skin Cancers, Keratoacanthomas, and Actinic Keratoses

Neoplasm	Clinical Type	Presentation	Key Features	Differential Diagnosis
Actinic keratosis		Erythematous, scaly to hyperkeratotic macules; ill-defined border; usually multiple; always on sun-damage skin	Scaly, ill-defined lesion on sun-damaged skin	Bowen disease, superficial BCC, SCC, dermatitis, tinea
Keratoacanthoma		Firm to hard, volcano-like crater with a central keratin plug	Keratin-filled "crater"	SCC, prurigo nodularis
Basal cell carcinoma (BCC)	Noduloulcerative	Small, firm, waxy papule often with telangiectasias; may ulcerate, often on the face	Waxy papule	Intradermal nevus, fibrous papule, folliculitis, seborrheic keratosis
	Superficial	Erythematous, sharply circumscribed, scaly macule border or thin plaque with a fine thready border, often on the trunk	Thread-like border	Actinic keratosis, Bowen disease, nummular dermatitis, contact dermatitis, tinea
	Morpheaform	Spontaneous scar-like lesion; whitish yellow, smooth, shiny scar surface	"Spontaneous" scar	Scar, granuloma annulare, sarcoid, localized scleroderma
	Pigmented	Blue, brown, or black waxy papule; mostly found in deeply pigmented white, Asian, or African American people	Pigmented waxy papule	Seborrheic keratosis, nevus, melanoma
Squamous cell carcinoma (SCC)	Common SCC	Firm to hard, erythematous, hyperkeratotic nodule, or ulcerated nodule; especially on the dorsal hands, forearms, and face	Firm/hard keratotic nodule	Keratoacanthoma, hypertrophic actinic keratosis, seborrheic keratosis, prurigo nodularis
	Bowen disease, SCC *in situ*	Erythematous, sharply circumscribed, scaly macule or thin plaque	Circumscribed scaly erythema	Actinic keratosis, superficial BCC, dermatitis, tinea

in the fourth or fifth decades of life in fair-skinned persons with other evidence of sun damage, such as freckling or solar lentigines (liver spots). Lesions appear as ill-defined erythematous, generally 2- to 8-mm scaly macules or minimally elevated hyperkeratotic papules on sun-exposed sites (Fig. 114.3, Color Plate section). They are most easily detected by gently running the fingertips over the area because they feel like islands of fine sandpaper. Although precancerous, less than 1% progress to invasive SCC.

Options for treatment of actinic keratoses include topical 5-fluorouracil cream (Carac, Fluoroplex, Efudex), imiquimod cream (Aldara) (16), or cryotherapy using liquid nitrogen to destroy the abnormal epidermis. With cryotherapy, the treated area may blister, crust, and then heal in 1 to 2 weeks without scarring. However, postinflammatory hypopigmentation or depigmentation, leaving a whitish macule, is not uncommon. If one is unfamiliar with either of these forms of therapy, referral to a dermatologist is appropriate. New lesions are likely to occur, and patients with actinic keratoses should be examined every 6 to 12 months.

Nonmelanoma Skin Cancers

The two most common skin cancers and the most common cancers in humans, *BCC* and *SCC*, make up 95% of the estimated 1.3 million skin cancers expected in 2001 in the United States. The anticipated ratio of BCC to SCC is 4:1 (17,18).

The most important risk factors for nonmelanoma skin cancers (NMSCs) include cumulative sun exposure (for most Americans, over 80% of the lifetime sun exposure occurs before age 18), fair skin color, and older age. Less well-established but important risk factors for SCC include tobacco smoking and sunlamp or suntan parlor use.

TABLE 115.1 Acne Therapy

Type of Acne	*Clinical Appearance*	*General Hygiene*	*Initial Therapy*	*Re-Evaluate*	*Therapy if Not Responding*[b]	*Therapy Change if Responding Nicely*
Comedonal acne	Open and closed comedones (blackheads and whiteheads)	*Gently* wash face with fingertips two times/day using antibacterial soap	Retin A 0.01% gel or 0.05% cream daily	8 wk	Increase Retin A to twice daily or change to 0.025% gel or 0.1% cream	No change
Inflammatory acne	Comedones and inflammatory papules and pustules	As above	Retin A, p.m. Benzoyl peroxide (BPO) gel a.m. or as tolerated[c] or sulfur/ sufacetamide lotion or clindamycin 1% solution or gel two times/day	8 wk	Add oral antibiotics; tetracycline 500 mg two times per day or doxycyline 100 mg two times a day; if no response after 8 wk, refer	Decrease oral antibiotics by one tablet each month; if flare occurs, increase by one tablet and hold for several months; then decrease again and re-evaluate
Cystic acne	As above plus cystic or nodular lesions	As above	Retin A and BPO or topical antibiotic,[d] plus oral antibiotics as above	8 wk	Accutane[e] (*cis*-retinoic acid) administered by a physician with experience using this teratogenic drug	
Scarring inflammatory acne[e]	Inflammatory acne with resultant scarring					

[a]A good review of acne therapy is provided in Leyden JJ. Therapy for acne vulgaris. N Engl J Med 1997;336:1156.
[b]If not responding, always review patient's regimen; the patient may be noncompliant or just unintentionally using medications incorrectly.
[c]BPOs (benzoyl peroxide), such as OTC Oxy or Rx Brevoxyl 4%, Benzac AC 5%, Desquam E 5%. The advantage of BPO over topical antibiotic is that BPOs are bacteriocidal for *Propionibacterium acnes,* so there is less chance for bacterial resistance. Patients should be instructed to use these drying medications as tolerated and as limited by irritation.
[d]Topical clindamycin solution or T gel.
[e]Scarring inflammatory acne is not an FDA-approved indication for Accutane; recommend referral to a dermatologist who is interested in treating this challenging form of acne to prevent further permanent disfiguring scarring.

as tretinoin (Retin A and Avita), adapalene (Differin), or tazarotene (Tazorac). Although all these agents work through a similar mechanism, they vary in their therapeutic effects and irritancy effects. A mild agent is tretinoin cream 0.025% and a very strong agent is tazarotene gel 0.1%.

When prescribing topical retinoids, patients should be instructed in the following fashion: carefully read and follow the medication instructions included with the product; expect mild irritation; and titrate to tolerance, that is, if daily application is excessively irritating, reduce the frequency of application to two, three, or four times per week, as tolerated. Patients need to know that dosing frequency is best left up to them and that it may vary over time (e.g., twice weekly application in the dry, cold winter months versus daily application in the hot, humid summer months). Because all retinoids are teratogenic, topical retinoids should not be used in persons presently pregnant or considering conception. Specifically, tazarotene is included with Pregnancy Category X medications and thus proper testing to exclude pregnancy when starting therapy and adequate birth control measures to prevent pregnancy *must* be used in conjunction with therapy. The remaining topical retinoids are Pregnancy Category C medications. Caution is also recommended regarding use in lactating women. The clinician not familiar with these agents should read the manufacturers' summaries before prescribing topical synthetic vitamin A derivatives.

INFLAMMATORY ACNE

Mild inflammatory acne consisting of comedones and erythematous papules with or without pustules (usually up to 15 papules) may be treated with a combination of a comedolytic agent (see above) and a topical antibacterial directed at *P. acnes.* Appropriate antibacterial agents for this condition are topical benzoyl peroxide (uniquely free of problems with the development of bacterial resistance), sulfacetamide/sulfur, and clindamycin preparations. Benzoyl peroxide is a primary irritant, so low concentrations are best (2.5% to 5%) in all patients, except those with exceptionally excessive sebum, in whom a more concentrated gel (8% to 10%) is helpful because of its drying effect. Benzoyl peroxide as a leave-on gel or wash-off cleanser is available over-the-counter (e.g., Oxy Sensitive Skin Treatment 2.5% gel or Oxy 10 Acne Treatment 10% gel; Oxy Clean Moisturizing Face Wash or Medicated Cleansing Bar) and by prescription (e.g., Brevoxyl 4% or 8% Gel, Cleansing Lotion or Creamy Wash, Benzac AC 2.5%, 5%, or 10% Gel). Daily or less frequent use as tolerated is recommended, to be adjusted by the patient. If intolerance or allergy occurs with benzoyl peroxide use, topical sodium sulfacetamide and/or sulfur cream or lotion (e.g., Acnomel cream [OTC] or Klaron lotion) or clindamycin 1% (e.g., Cleocin T Pledgets, Cleocin T Gel) may be substituted. Benzoyl peroxide and tretinoin should not be applied simultaneously because of resultant oxidation of the latter; therefore, one is used in the morning and the other at night. Topical antibiotics and tretinoin may be applied together. The patient may use medicated (as mentioned under comedonal acne) or nonmedicated makeup, as long as it is oil free.

For females interested in possible hormonal therapy, an oral contraceptive pill (OCP) may be offered if not otherwise contraindicated. In teenagers younger than 18, this discussion must always include a parent or guardian. Because of the moral issues that arise for some families regarding an OCP, a physician should never be insistent on this therapy. The effects of estrogen-containing OCPs, which are believed to lead to improvement in acne are reduced ovarian androgen production and enhanced sex hormone-binding globulin (SHBG) synthesis, leading to decreased free testosterone. Although Ortho-Tri-Cyclen (35 μg ethinyl estradiol and 0.180-, 0.215-, 0.250-mg norgestimate) has the U.S. Food and Drug Administration (FDA)-approved indication for acne therapy, Yasmin (30 μg ethinyl estradiol and 3 mg drospirenone) may be more effective because of its unique progestin component which is an analog of spironalactone and, like spironalactone, acts to block androgen receptors. A randomized, double-blind, multicenter trial of women with mild to moderate acne vulgaris given Yasmin ($n = 568$) or Ortho Tri-Cyclen ($n = 586$) for six cycles found Yasmin to be modestly superior in effecting total lesion count reduction and in the resultant investigator's and subject's assessment of the therapeutic effect ($p \leq 0.02$) (11). Generally, OCPs containing norgestrel and levonorgestrel (e.g., Lo/Ovral, Triphasil) are probably best avoided, as other progestins are available with lesser androgenic effects. Finally, low-dose estrogen OCPs (20 μg ethinyl estradiol) would not be expected to be as beneficial as those containing 30 μg because of lesser effects on SHBG synthesis and thus free testosterone levels.

Although a recent study has suggested that oral antibiotics alone (oxytetracycline 1 g/day or minocycline 100 mg per day) are no more effective for "mild to moderate inflammatory acne" than topical benzoyl peroxide alone (12), dermatologists generally use oral antibiotics *in combination with topical agents* (especially important is topical benzoyl peroxide to prevent the development of resistant *P. acnes*) in patients who do not respond to topical benzoyl peroxide and tretinoin. Generally, if inflammatory acne does not improve after 6 to 8 weeks of topical therapy or if a patient *initially* presents with moderate or severe inflammatory acne or inflammatory acne of any severity that is negatively affecting self-esteem, treatment traditionally includes an oral antibiotic, such as tetracycline 500 mg two times a day (if nausea develops, a reduced dose of 250 mg two times a day may be tried), doxycycline 100 mg two times per day (patients must be cautioned about associated photosensitivity), or minocycline 100 mg once to twice daily. Especially with extremely determined and/or compliant acne patients, it should be made clear that if the medication is making them feel nauseated (due to tetracycline most often), "not so good," depressed (due to minocycline most often), or causing headache (due to minocycline most often) or severe headache (as in pseudotumor cerebri, which requires immediate attention, and is possible with any of the tetracyclines), the antibiotic should be stopped and another substituted. Also, cautioning the patient about these potential side effects, including depression, may open yet another door for her or him reveal depressive symptoms, if present. Oral antibiotics are always used in combination with topicals, in anticipation of tapering or discontinuing oral therapy after several weeks or months while continuing topicals alone (Table 115.1). Patients should be told that antibiotics only suppress and do not cure acne. Therefore, as long as a patient is still in his or her "acne years" (the duration of which is always difficult to predict), ongoing treatment is necessary. Patients on long-term oral or topical antibiotic therapy should be watched for the development of *P. acnes* antibiotic resistance, characterized by worsening or flaring of previously well-controlled acne (13).

Other possible causes of sudden worsening or lack of improvement with oral antibiotic therapy include secondary folliculitis because of resistant *Staphylococcus aureus*, gram-negative bacteria, and yeast (pityrosporum). An additional possible exacerbating factor to consider in females includes androgen excess; despite initial evaluation for this, clearly a patient could develop an excess or manifestations thereof at some point after initially seeking treatment; thus, repeated clinical and laboratory evaluation should be considered. Yet another cause for worsening or nonresponsive acne in male and female teens and adults is anabolic steroids use; change in body physique, androgenic alopecia (male and female patterned hair loss), and striae in both genders, gynecomastia in males, and reduction in breast size, change in vocal tone, and hirsutism in females may also be present.

CYSTIC ACNE

Cystic acne, characterized by deep-seated, inflammatory, nodular cysts, should always be treated aggressively to prevent permanent scarring. If patients do not respond to oral antibiotics in combination with topical agents in 6 to 8 weeks, referral to a dermatologist should be made. Although the dermatologist may prescribe an alternative nonretinoid therapy, it is likely that the systemic retinoid isotretinoin (13- *cis*-retinoic acid, Accutane) will be needed. Isotretinoin is "curative" in approximately 70% of patients, although the basis for this is unknown. The greatest concern with isotretinoin is its teratogenic potential. It may produce fetal anomalies involving the central nervous system, heart, bones, and thymus in 30% to 40% of exposed fetuses. All women of child-bearing age must be counseled on the use of two concurrent forms of contraception (see Chapter 100). In the very unlikely event that pregnancy develops, an abortion is usually recommended. It is wise to establish whether a patient is morally against abortion before beginning therapy. If this is the case, to guarantee the risk of pregnancy is zero, this individual should remain abstinent from sexual intercourse for the 20- to 28-week period of treatment, as well as for 1 month before and after treatment, or forego isotretinoin therapy. The maker of isotretinoin (Roche Dermatologics) has developed a patient instruction/consent form packet that is critical for both the clinician and the patient to review carefully.

Some side effects with isotretinoin therapy are essentially inescapable. These include dry skin, lips, nose, and eyes. Mild elevations of triglyceride, cholesterol, and liver enzymes are seen in approximately 25% of patients. Infrequent or unusual side effects include hair loss, musculoskeletal aches, *S. aureus* folliculitis and ocular keratitis, reduced night vision, marked elevation of triglyceride with the potential for an associated acute pancreatitis, marked elevation of cholesterol and liver enzymes, leukopenia, and pseudotumor cerebri.

Some patients developing triglyceride elevations may have an inherited familial lipid disorder (14) and a useful patient summary regarding this unusual side effect of isotretinoin therapy is available (15).

ROSACEA (ACNE ROSACEA)

Acne rosacea, usually referred to as *"rosacea,"* is a chronic inflammatory disorder favoring the central portion of the face. It occurs most commonly in fair-skinned whites with blue eyes. Affected patients usually develop initial signs of the disease in their twenties or thirties with central facial erythema, exaggerated flushing, telangiectasias, and intermittent erythematous follicular papules and pustules and edema. Rarely, patients may develop associated *rhinophyma*; this bulbous nose enlargement is seen more often in men than in women and is caused by hyperplasia of the sebaceous glands. Rosacea does not cause comedones and therefore can be differentiated from acne vulgaris. However, occasionally patients have both rosacea and acne.

Rosacea may also involve the eyes, causing a mild inflammation of the lid margins manifest by mild erythema and causing the sensation of dry or scratchy eyes. Other slightly or somewhat less common changes include conjunctivitis, blepharitis, episcleritis, and recurrent chalazion and hordeolum (see Chapter 109). Less than 5% of patients with rosacea develop a painful and vision-threatening condition of the cornea, *rosacea keratitis.*

Although the cause of rosacea remains unknown, the condition is characteristically so well controlled with antibiotics that lack of a clinical response should raise a question about the diagnosis. Mild disease is generally treated with topical therapy alone. However, for patients with ocular symptoms, a moderate number of papules, or with burning and stinging, systemic treatment is preferred: tetracycline 500 mg, doxycycline (photosensitizing) 100 mg, or minocycline 100 mg, once to twice daily. If a good response is seen, the dose may be reduced at 1 and 2 months and then the drug discontinued at 3 months, switching over to topical therapy alone. If a flare occurs, the oral antibiotic may be restarted and tapered again. Although some patients can discontinue therapy after several months, most flare without some therapy. For long-term treatment, topical therapies are generally preferred and include metronidazole gel, lotion, or cream (MetroGel, -Lotion, -Cream, or Noritate Cream), sodium sulfacetamide and or sulfur products (e.g., Rosac cream, Klaron lotion, and Acnomel cream [OTC]), and azelaic acid (Finacea gel) applied to the affected central face once to twice daily after washing.

HIDRADENITIS SUPPURATIVA

Hidradenitis suppurativa is characterized by inflammation and occlusion of follicles in areas where apocrine glands are found. Onset is usually in the late teens or early adult years, and disease may persist for decades. Sites where apocrine glands are normally present, or, where ectopic apocrine glands are sporadically present, are affected. These sites include the axillae, perineum, inguinal folds, pubic region, and often the umbilicus, breasts, postauricular area, scalp, and back. Affected areas are studded with large comedones, inflammatory papules, pustules, and cysts. Sinus tracts form when cysts rupture and may drain serum, blood, or purulent material. Patients may also have cystic facial acne and scarring scalp folliculitis.

Complications of and associations with hidradenitis suppurativa may include secondary amyloidosis, anemia of chronic disease, sacroiliitis, and depression. Finally, patients are at risk for episodes of acute bacterial cellulitis and, after many years, squamous cell carcinoma (SCC) in this chronically inflamed tissue.

The differential diagnosis of hidradenitis suppurativa includes recurrent bacterial folliculitis and furunculosis (see Chapter 32), scrofuloderma (*Mycobacterium tuberculosis* infection with an ulcerated draining lymph node), granuloma inguinale (*Calymmatobacterium granulomatis*, a sexually transmitted disease (STD) characterized by genital and inguinal sinuses and hypertrophic scars), lymphogranuloma venereum (see Chapter 37), Crohn disease (see Chapter 45), and a pilonidal cyst. The diagnosis of hidradenitis suppurativa is made by recognizing comedones, which are not present in these other disorders. Skin biopsies for histopathology and tissue cultures may be required to exclude other diagnoses.

The pathogenesis of this disorder is not well understood. It is debated whether infection in these patients is a primary or secondary event. Treatment consists of short courses of antibiotics for acute secondary infection. Specific antibiotic therapy should be based on the results of culture taken from draining lesions. Chronic ongoing therapy may include oral tetracyclines (e.g., doxycycline 100 mg twice daily), chosen for their anti-inflammatory and antibacterial effects, and topical benzoyl peroxide to reduce the risk of bacterial resistance, in a regimen similar to that used in acne (see Inflammatory Acne). Adjunctive oral contraceptive therapy may be beneficial in some women. Surgical therapy ranging from tract marsupialization to deep wide excision should be considered for patients with severe disease. Although investigational, there have been several case reports and one case series reporting improvement in patients treated with infliximab (alone or in combination with other therapies) (16); controlled trials are clearly needed to determine whether this is an acceptable therapeutic option for this debilitating and very difficult to treat chronic condition.

MILIARIA

Miliaria is a disorder of sweat retention caused by occlusion of the ducts of the eccrine glands. Unlike the sebaceous and apocrine glands, which secrete through the hair follicles to the skin surface, eccrine glands are separate from hair follicles. They are directly connected to the surface of the skin through eccrine ducts. Although it is not a follicular disorder, as are acne and folliculitis, it may mimic these disorders. Miliaria occurs most often in active people who are perspiring heavily and who are wearing occlusive clothing or are confined to bed for extended periods.

The eruption almost always occurs on the trunk. When the sweat duct is occluded very superficially, asymptomatic, noninflammatory, 1- to 2-mm vesicles that easily rupture are seen in the upper central chest or back (*miliaria crystallina*), creating a distinctive appearance. When the duct is occluded deeper in the skin, pruritic, nonfollicular, erythematous papules occur over the chest and back (*miliaria rubra*). Lesions may be few to many in number.

The differential diagnosis of miliaria rubra includes infectious and noninfectious folliculitis. These forms of folliculitis are distinguished by their involvement of hair follicles as opposed to the eccrine ducts.

The treatment of miliaria includes providing a cool environment, removing occlusive clothing, and modifying positioning in bedridden persons. Cool baths and topical antipruritic lotions containing menthol or phenol (e.g., Sarna lotion) may reduce pruritus when present. Drying lotions (e.g., Zeasorb AF lotion/powder) may also be helpful.

NONINFECTIOUS ALOPECIA: NONSCARRING AND SCARRING

When assessing the chief complaint of hair loss, it is helpful to understand normal hair physiology. Every individual hair may be classified based on whether it is growing, transitional, or resting. These phases are *anagen* (lasting 2 to 6 years), *catagen* (lasting 2 to 3 weeks), and *telogen* (lasting 2 to 3 months), respectively (17). Scalp hair loss in excess of normal shedding or *alopecia* involving the scalp may be *nonscarring* or *scarring*; fortunately, nonscarring alopecia is far more common.

Nonscarring Alopecia

Nonscarring alopecia is so designated because the affected hair follicles are not permanently lost or damaged. Clinically, noninflammatory and nonscarring alopecia (hair loss without visible changes of erythema, scale, scarring) is characteristic of male and female pattern hair loss (androgenetic alopecia), alopecia areata (histologically inflammatory), telogen effluvium, anagen effluvium, and various systemic causes of diffuse hair thinning, including thyroid disease, systemic lupus erythematosus, and drug-induced hair loss.

Androgenetic alopecia is common in both men and women. Typically, men experience a frontal and vertex type of thinning, variably followed by confluence over the entire crown (top of the head); in contrast, women experience mild to moderate thinning over the entire crown with notable sparing of the frontal hair margin. In both genders, the onset of androgenetic alopecia may be as early as the late teens. Rarely, women show a male pattern of hair loss. In all women with hair loss, regardless of the pattern, one should look for signs of virilization (e.g., facial, upper chest, upper back, and upper abdomen hair growth; clitoral hypertrophy; deepening voice; and muscular body habitus). Appropriate evaluation should be performed to exclude hyperandrogenemia caused by adrenal hyperplasia, polycystic ovary disease, insulin resistance (18) that is often accompanied by acanthosis nigricans, a velvety hyperpigmentation around the base of the neck and axillae, and various adrenal and ovarian tumors (see Chapter 101). Additionally, women who are taking testosterone (e.g., Estratest), progestational drugs with greater androgen effects (e.g., levonorgestrol), or over-the-counter dehydroepiandrosterone should be told that these agents aggravate androgenetic alopecia and are best stopped.

Treatment options in patients who desire more hair include oral finasteride (Propecia, 1-mg tablets) for men and topical *minoxidil, hair transplants,* and various *hair prostheses*, varying from woven-in individual hairs to full-scalp wigs, for both women and men. Each of these treatments has its disadvantages. OTC topical *minoxidil* 2% solution (Rogaine) produces significant hair growth in only approximately 20% of patients; however, a greater percentage of patients have a reduction in further hair loss. Rogaine Extra Strength for Men (minoxidil 5% solution) is also available over-the-counter and is said to grow 45% more hair than the 2% Rogaine. Oral finasteride or topical minoxidil therapy must be ongoing to maintain hair growth, at a cost of $20 to $60 per month. In contrast, hair *transplants* are permanent. Many patients are very pleased with the results. Hair weaves in which natural or synthetic hair is woven into the patient's own hair must be repeated as the hair grows out. Finally, although some people do well with a wig, they may be uncomfortable, difficult to manage, and costly.

Telogen effluvium is a common disorder in which patients experience shedding of telogen hairs diffusely over the scalp. The percentage of telogen or resting hairs may shift upward to approach 20% (versus normal 10%) of the scalp hair. This amount of hair loss is usually evident only to the patient, who notes excessive hair coming out on shampooing and combing. Telogen effluvium may begin 2 to 3 months after such events as childbirth, general anesthesia, and catabolic states such as high fever for many days, rapid weight loss, and protein malnutrition. This form of alopecia is self-limited; however, several months may elapse before hair loss stops and new anagen hair growth begins. Because (anagen) hair grows approximately 1 cm per month, depending on the individual's chosen hair length, return to the "pretelogen effluvium" appearance may take a year or so. Reassurance of this expected ultimate outcome is extremely important.

Numerous nonchemotherapeutic drugs have been reported to cause hair loss through a variety of mechanisms, primarily affecting telogen hairs (10% to 20% of the scalp hairs), therefore producing a chronic telogen effluvium that is usually appreciable only to the patient. The most common of these drugs are anticoagulants, anticonvulsants, and cholesterol-lowering agents. This hair loss is reversible with discontinuance of the causative medication. If the medication cannot be eliminated, patients should be reassured of the self-limited nature of this side effect.

Anagen effluvium may be caused by chemotherapeutic agents and ionizing irradiation. Patients have shedding of the actively growing hairs in the scalp, which constitute approximately 90% of the total scalp hair. Hairs are shed rapidly over a matter of days, and patients typically have no or only very sparse hairs left on the scalp (the remaining telogen hairs). With the occasional exception of ionizing radiation-induced effluvium, this hair loss is temporary.

Alopecia areata is an immunologically mediated form of hair loss that typically presents with one to a few coin-shaped areas of hair loss. Although yet to be determined, it is believed that a certain genetic constitution and triggering factors are necessary for disease expression. Infrequently, patients may have total scalp hair loss (*alopecia totalis*) or total body hair loss (*alopecia universalis*). Most patients with just one or two patches of alopecia will have spontaneous hair regrowth within 1 year; however, recurrences in the same or new sites are common. Although most patients with alopecia areata do not have any associated disorders, alopecia areata is associated with an increased lifetime risk of autoimmune conditions, such as thyroid disease, pernicious anemia, and Addison disease. Initial treatment of patients with alopecia areata usually consists of topical corticosteroid solutions (e.g., clobetasol or fluocinonide solution, three to four drops applied to each quarter-sized area, including 0.5 cm of radially encircling normal scalp) or corticosteroid scalp injections. Other treatments (e.g., topical minoxidil, topical irritants, topical sensitizers, photochemotherapy) may be helpful in some patients, but, as with topical and intralesional corticosteroids, well-controlled studies demonstrating efficacy are limited or lacking.

Although still other disorders may cause variable degrees of nonscarring alopecia, the alopecia is merely secondary to the primary inflammatory process or because of trauma. Examples of the former include tinea capitis and seborrheic dermatitis and the latter include prolonged pressure-associated ischemia-induced alopecia (e.g., prolonged unrecognized unconscious state, prolonged surgery) and trichotillomania (self-inflicted alopecia).

Scarring Alopecia

Scarring alopecia is relatively uncommon. It is characterized by focal scarring with a loss of hair and visible hair follicles. One of the most common forms of scarring alopecia seen occurs primarily in African American women (19).

After years of chemical permanent solutions and traction, a resultant permanent hair loss favoring the crown and temporal scalp may develop. Similar to our paradigm for the development of nonmelanoma skin cancer with repeated sun exposures beginning in childhood eventuating in skin cancer after the third or fourth decade, the same model may be applied to this externally induced scarring hair loss. As with skin cancer, education to prevent disease must begin in school children.

Causes of scarring alopecia that are independent of external factors are discoid lupus erythematosus, folliculitis decalvans, cicatricial pemphigoid, lichen planopilaris, and pseudopelade (idiopathic scarring alopecia). Scarring alopecia is irreversible in most instances because the scarred follicles are incapable of producing new anagen hairs. Patients suspected of having scarring alopecia should be referred as early as possible to a dermatologist in hopes of preventing further permanent hair loss.

SPECIFIC REFERENCES

1. Cordain L, Lindeberg S, Hurtado M, et al. Acne vulgaris: A disease of western civilization. Arch Dermatol 2002;138:1584.
2. Lehmann H, Andrews JP, Robinson KA, et al. Evidence report/technology assessment number 17. Management of acne. Johns Hopkins Evidence Based Practice Centre, September 2000. Available at: http://www.ahcpr.gov/clinic/epcsums/acnesum.htm.
3. Shalita AR, Pochi PE, Leyden JJ, et al. Acne therapy in the '90s. J Int Postgrad Med 1991;4:1.
4. Kligman AM. Postadolescent acne in women. Cutis 1991;48:75.
5. Goulden V, Stables I, Cunliffe WJ. Prevalence of facial acne in adults. J Am Acad Dermatol 1999; 41:577.
6. Jick SS, Kremers HM, Vasilakis-Scaramozza C. Isotretinoin use and risk of depression, psychotic symptoms, suicide, and attempted suicide. Arch Dermatol 2000;36:1231.
7. Wysowski DK, Pitts M, Beitz J. Depression and suicide in patients treated with isotretinoin. N Engl J Med 2001;344:460.
8. Chia CY, Lane W, Chibnall J, et al. Isotretinoin therapy and mood changes in adolescents with moderate to severe acne. Arch Dermatol 2005; 141:557.
9. Sherertz EF. Acneiform eruption due to megadose vitamins B_6 and B_{12}. Cutis 1991;48: 119.
10. Lucky AW. Hormonal correlates of acne and hirsutism. Proceedings of a symposium, NICHD conference: androgens and women's health. Am J Med 1995;98:89S.
11. Thorneycroft IH, Golnick H, Schellschmidt I. Superiority of a combined contraceptive containing drospirenone to a triphasic preparation containing norgestimate in acne treatment. Cutis 2004;74:123.
12. Ozolins M, Eady EA, Avery AJ, et al. . Comparison of five antimicrobial regimens for treatment of mild to moderate inflammatory facial acne vulgaris in the community: randomised controlled trial. Lancet 2004;364: 2188.
13. Coates P, Vyakrnam S, Eady EA, et al. Prevalence of antibiotic-resistant propionibacteria on the skin of acne patients: 10-year surveillance data and snapshot distribution study. Br J Dermatol 2002;146:840.
14. Rodondi N, Darioli R, Ramelet AA, et al. High risk for hyperlipidemia and the metabolic syndrome after an episode of hypertriglyceridemia during 13-cis retinoic acid therapy for acne: a pharmacogenetic study. Ann Intern Med 2002;136:582.
15. Anonymous. An unusual "side effect" of an acne drug. Ann Intern Med 2002;136:38(I–38).
16. Sullivan TP, Welsh E, Kerdel FA, et al. Infliximab for hidradenitis suppurativa. Br J Dermatol 2003;149:1046.
17. Price VH. Treatment of hair loss. N Engl J Med 1999;341:964.
18. Beatty OL, Harper R, Sheridan B, et al. Insulin resistance in offspring of hypertensive parents. BMJ 1993;10:92.
19. Ackerman AB, Walton NW, Jones RE, et al. Hot comb alopecia/follicular degeneration syndrome in African-American women is traction alopecia! Dermatopathol Pract Concept 2000;6:320.

*For annotated **General References** and resources related to this chapter, visit www.hopkinsbayview.org/PAMreferences.*

Chapter 116

Dermatitis and Psoriasis

S. Elizabeth Whitmore

DERMATITIS

Dermatitis, or *eczema*, is a nonspecific term indicating inflammatory changes visible in the epidermal surface of the skin. No matter what the specific "subtype" of dermatitis, acute, subacute, and/or chronic changes may be seen. In *acute dermatitis*, changes consist of edema, papules, vesicles, serous discharge, crusting, scaling, and erythema. In *subacute dermatitis*, lesions are erythematous and scaly and may be edematous, but serous discharge and crusting are absent. In *chronic dermatitis*, changes consist of a scaly thickening of the skin, giving a washboard or tree bark appearance called *lichenification*. The phase, acute, subacute, or chronic, generally determines the prescribed treatment. Table 116.1 summarizes the features, treatment, and prognosis of several specific types of dermatitis. The different types of dermatitis are traditionally categorized based on associated manifestations, as with "atopic" dermatitis; mechanism, as with "contact" dermatitis; morphology, as with "nummular" dermatitis; and location, as with "hand" dermatitis. Dermatitis can be viewed as primarily caused by endogenous (e.g., atopy) or exogenous (e.g., external contact) factors, although both factors are eventually involved.

Atopic Dermatitis

Atopic dermatitis is considered an endogenous dermatitis. Affected patients will usually confirm the validity of the quote, "atopic dermatitis is the itch that rashes." Patients typically have associated atopic diseases, such as allergic rhinitis or allergic asthma, and 70% give a family history of atopy. Atopic diseases are characterized by an imbalance in the normal T helper cell immune response, with T_H2 cells infiltrating the affected tissues. This dominant T_H2 response with a predominance of T_H2-derived cytokines (e.g., interleukin-4, -5, and -13) over T_H1 cytokines (e.g., interferon-γ and interleukin-12) is believed to play a key role in the pathogenesis of disease (1). Other immunologic alterations, including elevated serum immunoglobulin E (IgE) levels, a reduced delayed hypersensitivity response, decreased numbers of T-suppressor lymphocytes, increased percentage of B lymphocytes with surface-bound IgE-1, and decreased number or activity of natural killer lymphocytes, may be seen. However, not all patients with atopic dermatitis express these abnormalities, and their role in the development of atopic dermatitis is unclear.

Atopic dermatitis may be divided into subsets based on age of onset: *infantile*, with onset between 2 months and 2 years; *childhood*, with onset between 2 years and adolescence, and *adult*, with onset in adulthood. Areas of involvement are typically those that patients can scratch. Therefore, affected sites include the cheeks and extensor surface of the arms and legs in infants; the flexural surface of the arms, legs, neck, wrists, and ankles in children; and these same sites and often also (or only) the hands or face in adults. The morphology of the lesions varies based on duration and external trauma (e.g., rubbing and scratching). *Acute lesions* consist of erythema, edema, papules, vesicles, erosions, crusts, and scale, whereas *chronic lesions* consist of scaly papules coalescing into lichenified plaques, often with focal excoriations.

Treatment depends on the patient's age and the location of the dermatitis. For all ages, facial dermatitis is usually treated with over-the-counter (0.5% or 1%) hydrocortisone ointment or cream. In children, hydrocortisone or slightly more potent prescription steroids (e.g., hydrocortisone butyrate) are used on nonfacial sites. In teens and in adults, fluorinated mid-potency (e.g., triamcinolone acetonide, betamethasone valerate) to high-potency (e.g., fluocinonide, betamethasone dipropionate) corticosteroids are used on nonfacial sites. Care must be taken to avoid local and systemic side effects. Corticosteroids applied to large body surface areas may produce hypercortisolism and hypothalamic–pituitary–adrenal axis suppression in the same way that orally administered steroids may. Topical

TABLE 116.1 Summary of the Diagnostic, Therapeutic, and Prognostic Features of the Phases of Dermatitis

Phase	Typical Morphology	Primary Treatment of Dermatitis	Indicators of Colonization or Secondary Infection Requiring Therapy	Treatment of Infection	Second-Line Treatment for Unresponsive Dermatitis, or First-Line Treatment for Very Severe Dermatitis	General Prognosis
Acute dermatitis	Papules, papulovesicles, erythema, serous discharge, and crusting	Saline compresses four times per day, switching when dry to corticosteroid creams[a] two times/day (high potency) and emollients with antipruritic agents	Moderate to severe crusting representing impetiginization or erythema representing erysipelas or cellulitis	Oral antistaphylococcal antibiotics except in cases of erysipelas or cellulitis, which typically require i.v. antibiotics (see Chapter 32)	Prednisone 0.7 to 1 mg/kg/day tapered over approximately 2 wk	Usually excellent
Subacute dermatitis	Erythema, edema, papules, and scale	Topical corticosteroid (high-potency) ointments[a] and emollients[b]	As above or numerous excoriations	As above	Phototherapy or photochemotherapy with UVB or PUVA, respectively	Usually good, but recurrences are not uncommon
Chronic dermatitis	Lichenified or thickened papules and plaques	As above	As above or nonhealing fissures	As above	As above	Treatment is difficult, recurrences very common

[a]Only low-potency corticosteroids should be used on the face; elsewhere, when using super-, high-, or mid-potency corticosteroids, side effects such as atrophy, telangiectasia, striae, or systemic absorption with hypercortisolism and hypothalamic–pituitary–adrenal axis suppression are possible.
[b]Corticosteroids and emollients are discussed in detail in "Topical Therapeutics," Chapter 113.
UVB, ultraviolet B; PUVA, phototherapy light unit.

corticosteroids should always be used in combination with emollients, such as simple oil or water and oil moisturizing creams and lotions; see Chapter 113. Emollients protect, hydrate, and permit the skin to repair, thereby restoring the barrier between the body and the environment. Topical steroid use should be discontinued as soon as the lesions have cleared and should be restarted as needed. Not infrequently, patients with atopic dermatitis may require intermittent oral antibiotics for recurrent infection, or "dermatitis-triggering" colonization with *Staphylococcus aureus*.

Alternative nonsteroidal anti-inflammatory agents, tacrolimus (Protopic ointment, 0.03% and 0.1%), which for many years has been used systemically to prevent organ transplant rejection, and pimecrolimus (Elidel cream) may be used if topical corticosteroids cannot be used or are ineffective. The U.S. Food and Drug Administration (FDA) has recommended their use "only as second-line agents for short term and intermittent treatment of atopic dermatitis in patients unresponsive or intolerant of other treatments." This recommendation and "black-box" warning was prompted by animal studies and a small number of reports of cancer in patients treated with either of these topicals. Although it is known that systemic administration of tacrolimus may be associated with an increased risk of malignancy, especially lymphoma (pimecrolimus is not available for systemic use), any causative association with noncutaneous malignancies has been disputed by many because of the limited "case report evidence" as well as the fact that drug absorption with proper use is quite limited (2). On the other hand, concerns truly exist about local effects of these topicals, particularly in sun exposed sites, and include local immune suppression and alteration of normal deoxyribonucleic acid (DNA) repair capacity, possibly increasing the risk of infections and skin cancer (3). Until more data are available, use of these two topical agents should follow the recommendations of the FDA.

For patients unresponsive to these therapies, a consulting dermatologist would consider in-office phototherapy using ultraviolet (UV)-B radiation or photochemotherapy with psoralen and UV-A radiation (psoralen plus ultraviolet light of A wavelength [PUVA]). Because systemic corticosteroid therapy is associated with numerous long-term unacceptable side effects, it should be avoided in the treatment of atopic dermatitis. Alternative systemic immune modulating therapies, such as cyclosporine, interferon-γ, mycophenolate mofetil, and various immune modulating monoclonal antibodies, are still under investigation in the treatment of recalcitrant atopic dermatitis.

The generalist should be familiar with the nonpharmacologic measures to aid patients with atopic dermatitis. Measures that reduce anxiety, such as adjunctive massage therapy administered by the parents, may be helpful in children with atopic dermatitis (4). Also, although most patients with chronic atopic dermatitis have discovered which products to use and which to avoid, review of exacerbating factors may be helpful (e.g., irritating harsh soaps, recurrent wetting and drying, and coarse fabrics).

As a point of information, the generalist should inform patients with respiratory allergies that although desensitization immunotherapy may be helpful for allergic rhinitis and conjunctivitis, it will have no effect on the course of their atopic dermatitis. In contrast, addressing food allergies with appropriate dietary elimination is helpful in some children (5). Dietary modifications, especially in children, should be supervised by a qualified dietitian. Occasionally, adults may find certain foods exacerbate their dermatitis (e.g., gluten, milk). In these instances, as long as a balanced diet is maintained, a trial elimination of suspected triggers for 6 to 8 weeks should be encouraged. An occasional patient thought to have atopic dermatitis may instead have dermatitis herpetiformis. This is an extremely pruritic papulovesicular eruption on the extensor surfaces and lower back. Affected individuals have a gluten sensitivity with antigliadin antibodies or antiendomysial antibodies. The diagnosis is made by skin biopsy for routine histology and direct immunofluorescence; the latter will reveal IgA deposited in the dermal papillae.

Nummular Dermatitis

Nummular dermatitis is an idiopathic dermatosis seen most often in adults. Lesions consist of pruritic, sharply circumscribed, 1- to 2-cm, vesicular (acute) to lichenified (chronic), erythematous plaques favoring the extremities. Lesions may be mistaken for tinea corporis or impetigo because of their annular shape. Tinea is ruled out with a negative potassium hydroxide preparation (see Chapter 117), and impetigo is excluded based on the lack of honeycomb-like surface crust.

Treatment for nummular dermatitis is similar to that for atopic dermatitis. Emollients in combination with mid-to high-potency corticosteroids generally clear the lesions. To prevent recurrences after clearing, the topical corticosteroid should be tapered over 2 weeks with one application every other or every third day. Patients with unresponsive dermatitis may have misunderstood the importance of the topical steroid application or instead may have a secondary staphylococcal infection that requires specific treatment (Table 116.1).

Asteatotic Dermatitis

Asteatotic, xerotic, or *dry skin* dermatitis is most often seen in the wintertime in people living in low-humidity environments. Factors associated with decreased sebum oil production such as slowly declining testosterone levels in men and women after the sixth decade, cholesterol lowering medications, and any medications that reduce the production or effects of androgens (e.g., chemotherapeutic drugs and antiandrogens that suppress gonadal function or block androgen effects) may predispose patients to asteatotic dermatitis. Diminished epidermal and sebaceous gland sebum production allows loss of normally retained moisture in the stratum corneum. Skin changes typically begin with dryness in the early fall, which then progresses to patches of faint erythema appearing *cracked* or superficially fissured (Fig. 116.1, Color Plate section). Patients complain of a stinging, tight feeling to their skin with or without associated pruritus.

Treatment involves hydration of the skin with warm baths or showers using oilated soaps (e.g., Oil of Olay Body Wash, Dove, Oilatum, or Aveeno Oilated Oatmeal Soap) followed by *patting dry,* leaving some moisture on the skin. A mid-potency corticosteroid ointment (as opposed to a cream) is then applied to the erythema, with a *top coat* of an emollient (see Chapter 113) to these and all areas of the skin. Extremely hot showers, which strip natural body oils; drying soaps; and stiff large-fiber clothing (e.g., wool) should be avoided. When the dermatitis has cleared, only the topical corticosteroid is discontinued; all other measures must be continued as long as the dry environmental exposure or sebum-reducing medication continues.

Contact Dermatitis

Contact dermatitis may be either *irritant* or *allergic* in nature. Irritant contact dermatitis may develop in anyone, whereas allergic contact dermatitis occurs only in people immunologically capable of recognizing and reacting to a particular allergen.

Irritant contact dermatitis to harsh chemicals results in a scalded, erythematous, moist appearance of the skin with peeling of the most superficial epidermis, leaving a lacy border. This is often caused by substances with extremes of pH, such as harsh alkaline cleansers and strong acid solutions. In contrast, mild irritants produce macular erythema that, with chronic exposure, may evolve into scaly plaques. With all forms of contact dermatitis, the eruption is limited to the area of contact. It is often the localized distribution and shape of the lesion that suggests the diagnosis, for example, irritant contact dermatitis at the forearm site of a solvent spill and allergic contact dermatitis on the earlobes bearing gold-colored earrings.

Allergic contact dermatitis (Fig. 116.2, Color Plate section) is caused by a delayed hypersensitivity reaction. Sensitization, if and when it develops, takes place through cutaneous exposure and requires approximately 1 week. A substance containing an allergen (hapten) is applied to the skin; the hapten binds to a protein to form a complete allergen, which is processed by the Langerhans cell, the resident antigen-presenting cell in the epidermis. As sensitization proceeds, the Langerhans cell moves into the dermis and through the lymphatics to the local lymph nodes, where it stimulates a lymphocyte clone that recognizes the antigen. If the substance is still in the skin 1 week after initial application or when subsequent re-exposure takes place, the Langerhans cells within the epidermis present the allergen to the memory T cells. These T cells secrete cytokines and other soluble mediators, which lead to recruitment of additional inflammatory cells (e.g., monocytes, neutrophils), resulting in the clinical picture of an acute dermatitis.

The most common cause of allergic contact dermatitis is a *plant dermatitis,* caused by the *Rhus* genus, which includes *poison ivy, oak, and sumac.* In sensitized persons, a minute amount of the oleoresin (oil) from these plants will produce a vesiculobullous eruption in the areas of contact, beginning 6 to 72 hours after exposure. Patients often note that new blisters continue to develop over many days and assume that their scratching is causing the rash to "spread." However, this is not the case; once the allergen is flushed from the skin, spreading cannot occur. The reason that new lesions may continue to develop for many days is because lesions take longer to evolve on skin that is thicker and penetration is slower (e.g., the palm) or where lesser amounts of oleoresin have contacted the skin. Also, continued unrecognized exposure to the oleoresin that may persist on clothing, tools, sports equipment, or the fur of pets may lead to "chronic poison ivy." Allergens other than *Rhus* are less common sensitizers and typically produce a less pronounced dermatitis with erythema, edema, and mild or no vesiculation. Such allergens include nickel (commonly found in gold-colored costume jewelry); neomycin, benzocaine, and merthiolate in topical medicinals; fragrances and preservatives in cosmetics and personal products; and preservatives in ophthalmologic, otic, and dermatologic prescription and nonprescription medications. Various common *occupational exposures* may also cause allergic contact dermatitis. More common allergens include potassium dichromate in cement, dyes, or textiles; epoxy resins in adhesives, finishing products, and casings for electrical devices; natural rosin in adhesive materials; thiuram, mercaptobenzothiazole, and carbamates in rubber products; glyceryl monothioglycolate and paraphenylenediamine in hair wave and dye formulations; and acrylates in methylmethacrylate used in orthopedic surgery, dentistry, and nail sculpturing.

Allergic contact dermatitis characteristically develops unexpectedly, appearing "out of the blue" after months or years of unremarkable exposures. Evaluation for possible allergic contact dermatitis requires a detailed history of personal product use, occupational exposures, and avocational exposures followed by patch testing with standardized common and suspected allergens to confirm the diagnosis and identify the causative allergen. When the diagnosis appears to be allergic contact dermatitis but no direct exposure is uncovered, unrecognized exposures should be sought. For example, occasionally the allergen exposure occurs through contact with the "nonallergic" spouses' personal products or work clothes.

The prevention of irritant and allergic contact dermatitis involves the recognition of irritants or allergens and elimination or minimization of exposure. Topical treatment is similar to that used for atopic dermatitis with emollients in combination with mid- to high-potency topical corticosteroids (Table 116.1). In cases of vesiculobullous dermatitis or dermatitis involving the face, hands, or genitalia, oral corticosteroids may be administered if no contraindications exist. Treatment should begin with 0.7 mg/kg/day of prednisone tapered over 2 weeks (e.g., 40 to 60 mg for 4 days, 30 to 40 mg for 5 days, and 20 mg for 5 days).

Contact Urticaria

Contact urticaria, although not a form of dermatitis, is a contact reaction. It may be caused by a histamine releasing nonimmunologic substance or an allergen-induced IgE-mediated immunologic reaction. The most common cause of immune mediated contact urticaria is *latex protein* (6,7). It is estimated that 10% of health care workers have been sensitized to natural rubber latex. Latex is ubiquitous in our environment, being present in over 40,000 medical and nonmedical devices and products. Childhood exposure to latex during surgical procedures greatly increases the risk for development of latex allergy. In fact, in one study of children who have experienced at least three surgical procedures, the prevalence of latex allergy was 34% (8).

Health care workers with latex contact urticaria typically present with a history of itching and hives in areas of contact with gloves. Identification of this allergy is important because, in addition to local reaction, latex exposure may cause generalized urticaria and even anaphylaxis, depending on how much histamine reaches the systemic circulation. Anaphylaxis is more likely to occur with oral, vaginal, rectal, or invasive intracorporeal latex contact. Diagnosis is made by *in vitro* latex IgE radioallergosorbent assay test (RAST) or *in vivo* patch, prick, or scratch testing. The former is preferred, because *in vivo* testing may cause anaphylaxis. However, RAST testing is not 100% sensitive; therefore, when allergy is strongly suspected and RAST testing is negative, referral to an allergist for skin testing is appropriate. Patients with latex allergy and all their health care providers must be educated about the potential life-threatening nature of this product and should be counseled on avoidance of all latex items, including latex gloves, balloons, condoms, and medical devices such as latex tubing, dental dams, surgeons' gloves, and catheters. A Medic Alert bracelet should be worn and an epinephrine-containing autoinjector (Epi-Pen) should be prescribed and carried by the patient at all times for an emergency (see Chapter 30).

Hand Dermatitis

Hand dermatitis is a very broad term encompassing conditions that affect the hands exclusively, such as *dyshidrotic hand dermatitis*, also known as *vesicular hand dermatitis*, and several forms of dermatitis that may affect any area, including the hands (e.g., atopic hand dermatitis, nummular hand dermatitis, and contact hand dermatitis). *Dyshidrotic or vesicular hand dermatitis* is an idiopathic condition in which pinpoint to 2-mm vesicles develop on the sides of the fingers and often the palms. The lesions are intensely pruritic and usually cycle over 1 to 2 weeks, with cycles recurring at variable intervals every several weeks to several months. As each cycle resolves, there is focal desquamation (peeling) of the affected skin.

Hand dermatitis is idiopathic. Although this disorder is called dyshidrotic, there is actually no consistently identified abnormality in eccrine gland function (sweating). Similarly, the inflammation is not because of a contact allergy. However, because allergic contact dermatitis may occasionally mimic this condition (depending on mode of contact), any suspicion of allergic contact dermatitis should be investigated with patch testing. Treatment for vesicular hand dermatitis includes frequent emollient application and a high potency topical corticosteroid cream or ointment (e.g., fluocinonide) used for flares of disease. Followup visits should include examination for the steroid-induced side effect of skin atrophy (evidenced by shiny thin-appearing skin, loss of skin lines, or increased visibility of dermal vessels). Patients with recalcitrant dermatitis should be referred to a dermatologist for alternative therapies (e.g., phototherapy or photochemotherapy).

Infectious Eczematoid Dermatitis

Infectious eczematoid dermatitis is a secondary change within a primary form of dermatitis. Patients become infected with *S. aureus* and other organisms (usually gram-positive bacteria) and show extensive crusting and exudation within their primary dermatitis. Treatment includes systemic antistaphylococcal antibiotics. If methicillin resistant *Staphylococcal aureus* infection is suspected, bacterial culture and antibiotic sensitivity of the affected skin (swabbing the area) should be performed to direct the choice of antibiotic. Finally, treatment of the primary dermatitis should include soaks, topical corticosteroids, and emollients.

Intertriginous Dermatitis (Intertrigo)

Intertriginous dermatitis occurs in skin folds, such as the inframammary creases, abdominal folds, inguinal folds, gluteal cleft, finger and toe webs, and angles of the mouth. Patients develop moist erythema and, at times, fissures with weeping of serous fluid. Such skin changes provide a very hospitable environment for yeast and bacterial growth. The affected areas typically burn, sting, and itch.

The differential diagnosis of intertrigo includes primary *Candida* infection, *seborrheic dermatitis*, and *psoriasis*. *Candida* infection is diagnosed with a positive potassium hydroxide preparation (see Chapter 117) or, if unavailable, "swab" culturette submitted for fungal culture. Seborrheic dermatitis and psoriasis are usually diagnosed by identifying skin lesions elsewhere. When presumed intertrigo does not respond to therapy, unusual diagnoses such as *Bowen disease* (squamous cell carcinoma [SCC] *in situ*), *extramammary Paget disease*, *Langerhans cell histiocytosis*, and *glucagonoma syndrome* must be considered and a biopsy should be taken.

Therapy for intertrigo is directed at keeping the affected areas dry. Gauze may be placed in skin folds where appropriate, and a powder (e.g., Zeasorb or Zeasorb-AF, which contains an antifungal agent) or plain talc or baby powder should be applied frequently to dry the skin and reduce yeast colonization or infection. If obesity is the cause of the problem (e.g., abdominal or inguinal folds), weight reduction should be discussed with the patient (see Chapter 83). A cool environment is also beneficial. In edentulous patients with intertriginous dermatitis at the angles of the mouth because of overlapping skin, appropriate treatment for possible oral candidiasis and denture refitting should be prescribed. If these measures are ineffective, referral to a dermatologist for consideration of collagen injections may be considered. Collagen is injected into the crease formed by the opposing folds of skin. Although collagen injections must be repeated every 6 to 12 months, they may be a very worthwhile treatment for this chronic painful fissuring.

Seborrheic Dermatitis

Seborrheic dermatitis is a common condition present in approximately 3% to 5% of the population. Onset of seborrheic dermatitis is usually in early adulthood, and the course is characterized by frequent spontaneous remissions and exacerbations. In this disorder, an inflammatory epidermal hyperproliferation affects the areas the body more heavily populated with sebaceous glands, favoring the scalp and facial hair-bearing areas, central face (glabellar area and nasal folds), ears, presternal chest, axillae, umbilicus, inguinal folds, gluteal cleft, and perianal skin. Pruritus is variably present. *Dandruff*, a term commonly used synonymously with seborrheic dermatitis, is generally considered a noninflammatory (nonerythematous) scaling of the scalp skin.

Although the cause of seborrheic dermatitis is unknown, several observations have been made and hypotheses proposed over the years. *Pityrosporum*, a lipophilic yeast normally present on the skin, has been suggested as the cause of seborrheic dermatitis in that the yeast stimulates an immune response with resultant cutaneous inflammation. Although seborrheic dermatitis may occur in any individual, it occurs for unknown reasons with increased frequency and severity in patients with acquired immunodeficiency syndrome and Parkinson disease.

The treatment of seborrheic dermatitis is directed at decreasing epidermal hyperproliferation, inflammation, and *Pityrosporum* yeast using, respectively, topical tars, hydrocortisone, and ketoconazole. For the scalp, ketoconazole, selenium sulfide, zinc pyrithione, or tar shampoos and clear nongreasy mid- to high-potency corticosteroid solutions are preferred. Specifically, treatment for the scalp may include a medicated shampoo used every other night for 1 month, followed by prophylactic use once to twice weekly. If this alone is not effective, a fluorinated corticosteroid solution (e.g., Cormax Scalp Application, Lidex Solution) applied after shampooing should be added (two to three drops massaged into each quarter-sized of the affected scalp). Once under control, the corticosteroid is discontinued and repeated for recurrences only. For facial and body seborrheic dermatitis, hydrocortisone 1% cream (solution for the beard, mustache, eyebrows, outer auditory canal) may be used up to two times a day to control redness and scaling. Alternatively, ketoconazole cream (e.g., Nizoral 2% cream) may be used twice daily in a similar fashion. However, unlike hydrocortisone, ketoconazole cream may be continued after clearance to prevent recurrences.

Perioral Dermatitis

Perioral and sometimes *periorificial dermatitis* is an eruption of minute papules and pustules on a background of erythema and scant scale in a perioral or periorificial (mouth, eyes, and nares) location. Although it may occur at any age, it is most common in young women. It is uncommon and may be differentiated from acne by the lack of comedones and from contact dermatitis by the fact that it always spares the vermilion border, beginning 2 to 3 mm from the lip margin. Unlike allergic contact dermatitis, the most common symptoms are burning and stinging but not itching. *Perioral/periorificial dermatitis*, especially in the perinasal area, is a frequent precursor of acne in adolescent children and also frequently overlaps with perinasal seborrheic dermatitis and rosacea in adults.

The cause of *perioral dermatitis* is not known, but it has been associated with topical and aerosolized inhaled fluorinated corticosteroids and fluorinated toothpastes. Initial treatment is similar to that used for acne rosacea (see Chapter 115), but medications can usually be stopped in 4 to 8 weeks, often without a recurrence. If recurrences do occur, treatment is simply repeated.

PSORIASIS

Definition and Prevalence

Psoriasis is an idiopathic benign epidermal hyperproliferation that affects 2% of the population (9,10). It is believed to be of multifactorial inheritance, with multiple genetic and environmental factors required for expression. Although the average age at onset of psoriasis is approximately 30 years, more than one third of patients develop the disease before age 20 years. Most patients who develop psoriasis have lifelong disease with periods of remission and exacerbation. Factors associated with exacerbation include sunlight/UV radiation deprivation (likely because of lack of beneficial UV radiation effects on psoriasis lesions but possibly also due to reduced serum levels of vitamin D), infections, certain drugs including lithium and antimalarials, local cutaneous trauma, alcohol ingestion, and physical and psychological stress.

Psoriasis may have a significant negative impact on many important aspects of life. Unlike other chronic diseases that may be easily concealed, psoriasis may be obvious because of thickened crumbly nails, heavy scalp scale, or hand, elbow, or knee involvement. The effect of the disease on the quality of life in patients with psoriasis has been compared with patients having other chronic diseases. When asked how many years of life patients would be willing to give up or how willing they would be to risk their lives to be free of their disease, patients with moderate psoriasis responded similarly to patients having had a kidney transplant. Patients with severe psoriasis responded similarly to those undergoing hospital-based dialysis (9). Patients with psoriasis involving exposed areas may also experience social rejection by people who believe that the disease is contagious or represents a manifestation of a disease or disorder they irrationally fear, such as acquired immunodeficiency syndrome (AIDS). Psoriasis may be a devastating financial burden also. It may cause physical and occupational disability, particularly when it affects the hands or feet or causes incapacitating psoriatic arthritis.

Clinical Presentation

Psoriasis may be divided into four major subtypes depending on the appearance of lesions: plaque, guttate, erythrodermic, or pustular. *Chronic plaque psoriasis* is the most common type of psoriasis. Patients exhibit one to many deeply erythematous, sharply demarcated, oval plaques several centimeters in diameter, with moderate to heavy silvery white surface scale, commonly on the scalp and over one or more extensor surfaces. Intertriginous plaques may also be present in the axillary, inframammary, umbilical, abdominal, inguinal, gluteal, and popliteal fossae. These fold area lesions have little or no scale and instead are moist and intensely erythematous. Patients who have numerous widespread plaques have *generalized plaque psoriasis.*

Guttate psoriasis is the next most common type of psoriasis. Approximately one third of patients have a sibling or parent with psoriasis (versus about 8% of the general population with such a family history) (11). Guttate psoriasis is characterized by an acute exanthem-like eruption of guttate (drop-like) erythematous, scaly papules, generally 1 mm to 1 cm in diameter. Although lesions are typically on the trunk and proximal extremities, the eruption may be widespread, involving the face, scalp, hands, and feet. Guttate psoriasis is often triggered by an infection, most often a streptococcal pharyngitis or a viral upper respiratory tract infection (URTI).

Erythrodermic psoriasis and *pustular psoriasis* are rare. In both types, a generalized exfoliative erythroderma (a scaly erythema) is present. In pustular psoriasis, crops of tiny, superficial, nonfollicular pustules develop, coalesce into "lakes of pus," and then desquamate in waves of lacy scale. Erythrodermic and pustular psoriasis are severe diseases, particularly in patients with other chronic illnesses. Potential complications include high-output congestive heart failure, sepsis, intravascular volume depletion, and vitamin and nutrient deficiencies caused by increased requirements and losses.

Nail involvement is seen in 30% of patients. Although not pathognomonic, the most commonly noted changes are pitting (ice pick-like marks in the nail plate, Fig. 116.3), *onycholysis* (separation of the nail plate from the nail bed, with resultant white color caused by air between the plate and bed), and *subungual hyperkeratosis* (crumbly scale between the plate and bed). The latter may be very distressing because it is both obvious on casual observation and often difficult to adequately treat.

Extracutaneous Disease

Arthritis has been said to affect less than 5% to nearly one third of patients with psoriasis. Although it is generally believed that psoriasis and psoriatic arthritis are one disease involving two organ systems, it has been suggested that the two are separate entities occurring together by chance and that the activity of the psoriasis may modify or enhance the activity of simultaneously occurring joint disease (12). Regardless of cause, any patient with psoriasis and debilitating or destructive arthritis should be treated aggressively to prevent disease progression and disability.

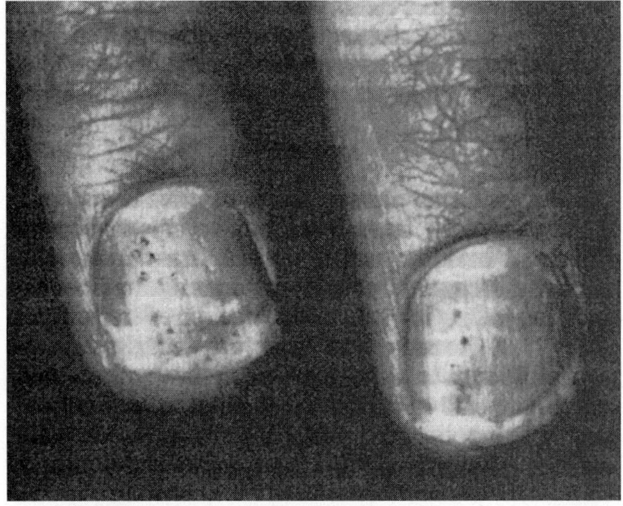

FIGURE 116.3. Minute pits are commonly seen on the surface of nails in patients with psoriasis.

Pathogenesis

Skin affected by psoriasis exhibits an accelerated rate of epidermal cell replication and a dysfunction of normal keratinocyte-to-keratinocyte inhibition of uncontrolled proliferation. Although not to the same degree, normal-appearing skin shows mildly accelerated proliferation. A basic issue that is still not fully understood is whether the primary defect triggering defective epidermal turnover resides in cytotoxic T cells, keratinocytes, locally produced cytokines, or other factors.

Treatment

Therapy for psoriasis depends on the degree of body surface area involvement and the clinical subtype of disease and prior response to therapy (10). One caveat should be noted by all clinicians prescribing any medications for patients with psoriasis, even mild psoriasis. Although systemic corticosteroids dramatically improve psoriasis acutely and in years past may have been used to treat psoriasis, systemic corticosteroids should be avoided. First, systemic corticosteroids would not be appropriate for psoriasis because it is a chronic disease requiring chronic therapy and, second, eventual corticosteroid withdrawal or dosage tapering may precipitate erythrodermic or pustular psoriasis.

Localized chronic plaque psoriasis is treated with bland emollients alone or combined with keratolytics (e.g., U-Lactin lotion, over the counter; AmLactin lotion, over the counter; Lac-Hydrin cream 12%, by prescription), topical corticosteroids, calcipotriene (Dovonex ointment or cream, a topical vitamin D derivative), or tazarotene (Tazorac 0.05% and 0.1% gel, a synthetic topical vitamin A derivative, *nota bene*: teratogen, Pregnancy Category X) applied twice daily. Although generic formulations of topical steroids tend to be relatively inexpensive, the vitamin D and vitamin A derivatives are very expensive. If these products made psoriasis vanish forever, patients would probably be happy to pay any price. But because this is not the case, patients who sacrifice to purchase them are likely to be disappointed. Topical steroids and vitamin D and vitamin A derivatives appear to be of similar efficacy in clinical trials; however, in a given patient one treatment may be much more effective than another. To achieve the best possible response, often some combination of a vitamin D or A topical and a corticosteroid is sought, requiring both a motivated patient and an empathetic clinician. A potential side effect of potent topical corticosteroids is atrophy (cigarette paper wrinkling or striae when severe). Side effects common to calcipotriene and vitamin A derivatives are irritation and stinging.

Generalized plaque psoriasis is difficult, time consuming, and expensive to treat with topical preparations. Also, the greater volume of topical corticosteroid needed to cover all the areas of psoriasis may ultimately produce effects similar to systemic corticosteroid administration. For these reasons, patients with generalized plaque psoriasis are frequently treated with phototherapy using broadband UVB radiation (UV radiation 290 to 320 nm wavelength; used since the 1920s), more recently introduced narrowband UVB (peak 311 nm wavelength; in contrast to broadband UVB, provides the optimal therapeutic wavlength), or photochemotherapy with the phototoxic agent 8-methoxypsoralen (Oxsoralen Ultra) orally in combination with controlled UVA radiation (UV radiation 320 to 400 nm wavelength) given in a PUVA. Patients are generally treated three times a week until clearance occurs and then may receive maintenance light treatments (PUVA only; UVB maintenance should not be used because of the risk of sunburn) or may discontinue treatments until the next flare of psoriasis occurs. A patient should never be given 8-methoxypsoralen to be used with natural sunlight or in a suntan parlor because severe burns and even death may occur. Also, self-administered light treatment even without a phototoxic agent is best avoided because careful monitoring is difficult and severe burning may result. Over a long period, PUVA therapy increases a patient's risk of skin cancer, both nonmelanoma and likely also melanoma skin cancer. Therefore, patients treated with PUVA should be followed throughout their lives, preferably with yearly full skin examinations. Alternative therapies to phototherapy and photochemotherapy include methotrexate, acitretin, cyclosporine (12,13), and *"the biologics."*

Guttate psoriasis, particularly with the initial episode, is usually very responsive to most treatments. Sunlight or in-office UVB phototherapy combined with emollients and low-potency topical corticosteroids often work well. Additionally, because triggering infections, especially streptococcal pharyngitis, may precipitate guttate psoriasis, appropriate evaluation should be performed.

Erythrodermic and pustular psoriasis may cause severe and even life-threatening illness, particularly in elderly patients with cardiovascular disease. Depending on the severity of the psoriasis and underlying medical problems, patients may require hospitalization, warm baths, bland emollients, and systemic therapy with acitretin (a synthetic retinoid), weekly low-dose methotrexate, or cyclosporine. Patients without infection may have signs and symptoms identical to those seen with sepsis, with cyclic fevers up to 104°F (40°C) and an increase in white blood cell count up to 40,000 cells per cubic millimeter with neutrophilia, tachycardia, and orthostatic hypotension, so that possible sepsis must be excluded with blood and urine cultures and other appropriate testing. The hemodynamic instability seen is caused by marked vasodilation and increased cardiac output and is particularly problematic in the setting of pre-existent cardiovascular disease or volume depletion. In addition, vitamin and nutrient deficiencies may result from the accelerated epidermal turnover rate. After all the acute cutaneous and systemic problems have been addressed and the patient's cutaneous disease is controlled, the systemic therapy for psoriasis generally must be continued or PUVA substituted to prevent severe flares.

Patients requiring systemic therapies for psoriasis are probably best cared for with the consultation of a dermatologist. Those receiving methotrexate, acitretin, or cyclosporine must be monitored closely. Methotrexate and cyclosporine yield comparable response rates in most types of moderate to severe psoriasis (12), whereas acitretin is extremely useful in treatment of pustular psoriasis. Methotrexate is an abortifacient and must not be taken by either men or women within 3 months of planned conception. The most important side effects of methotrexate are acute cytopenias and chronic hepatitis and cirrhosis. Acitretin is teratogenic. Women taking acitretin must abstain from alcohol and wait 2 years after drug cessation to begin to try to conceive. For this reason, it may be best to avoid this medication totally in women of child-bearing potential. Important potential side effects of acitretin include hypertriglyceridemia and hypercholesterolemia, hepatitis, pseudotumor cerebri, bony hyperostosis, hair loss, fragile skin, painful palmar and plantar desquamation, and arthralgias. Cyclosporine has many notable side effects, including hypertension, decreased renal blood flow, glomerular and tubular toxicity, paresthesias, and anergy (13). Whether cyclosporine is associated with an increased risk of cutaneous or lymphoproliferative malignancies in nontransplant patients is unclear (14).

The most recently introduced systemic therapies for psoriasis are the *"biologics."* These agents are targeted at the immunologic alterations found in psoriasis. Like all systemic therapies, they are reserved for moderate to severe psoriasis. As they have not been in clinical use for 20 or 30 years, potential long-term side effects are not known, something both clinicians and patients must understand and accept prior to going forth with therapy. The FDA has approved three parenteral agents for treatment of moderate to severe psoriasis: alefacept (LFA3TIP) and efalizumab (anti CD11a) are both inhibitors of T-cell activation while etanercept is an inhibitor of tumor necrosis factor-α (TNF-α). These agents have been shown to be more effective than placebo in studies of 3 months or longer. Etanercept has also been FDA-approved for the treatment of psoriatic arthritis. In the short term, these agents appear relatively safe; alefacept requires monitoring of T-lymphocyte counts, efalizumab requires monitoring of platelet counts, while etanercept therapy should include baseline tuberculin skin testing and observation during therapy for signs or symptoms of infection, lupus-like syndromes, neurologic events (especially new onset of demyelinating disease), and heart failure. In general, etanercept should not be used in persons with demyelinating diseases or congestive heart failure (15).

Although these medications are generally well tolerated during therapy, the greatest concern is the unknown long term risk for malignancy and lymphoproliferative disorders. Note should be made that a recent study in patients with rheumatoid arthritis treated with TNF-α inhibitors, compared with those patients not so treated, followed for less than 4 years found a relative risk of 4.9 for the development of lymphoma (16). One other factor regarding the biologics is their cost. Regardless of "who" is paying for them, ultimately the expense may impact individual patients in the form of higher insurance rates or even difficulty in getting insurance given their diagnosis of psoriasis. It has been estimated that although the cost of 3 months of treatment with one of the biologics is $16,000 and upward, given response rates of less than 50%, "successful treatment" is $35,000 and upward (17,18). It should also be realized that most patients on one of the biologics receive more than 3 months of biologic therapy per year. These costs compare with similar estimates of "successful treatment" costs (taking into consideration expected response rates for other therapies) of other therapies, including: methotrexate—$5,400; cyclosporine—$14,200; acitretin—$17,300; PUVA—$5,700; and UVB—$5,100 (17). It seems clear that the biologics are a wonderful addition to the therapeutic armamentarium for psoriasis, especially in patients with severe disease who have exhausted other possible therapies, however, as should be said about innumerable medications, thoughtful consideration of options, long-term toxicities, and implications of biologic therapy should be undertaken before initiating therapy.

Other investigational therapies may eventually prove useful. Among these are thiazolidinediones (e.g., pioglitazone), particularly attractive for patients also requiring oral hypoglycemic agents. Thiazolidinediones are insulin sensitizing agents that act as ligands for the peroxisome proliferator-activated receptor-γ, a member of the nuclear hormone receptor superfamily that includes the retinoic acid receptor and the vitamin D receptor (notably, both these receptors are targets of presently available FDA-approved topical and systemic psoriasis therapies). The potential beneficial effect is believed to occur through inhibition of cell proliferation and promotion of cell differentiation (19,20). Although the data are limited, a 10-week, double-blind, randomized, placebo-controlled, parallel group study of 70 nondiabetic patients with moderate to severe psoriasis treated with 15 mg, 30 mg, or placebo showed clearing or near clearing of psoriasis in 40% of treated patients compared with 12.5% of patients receiving placebo (21). Hopefully, additional studies will reveal whether thiazolidinediones will be useful in the treatment of psoriasis. Finally, the possible role of gluten sensitivity in psoriasis and psoriatic arthritis has yet to fully elucidated. Notably, it has been reported that patients having elevated serum gliadin antibodies see improvement in their psoriasis with the institution of a gluten-free diet (22–24).

SPECIFIC REFERENCES*

1. Kay AB. Allergy and allergic diseases. First of two parts. N Engl J Med 2001;344:30.
2. Topical pimecrolimuus, tacrolimus, and the risk for cancer: An expert interview with Lawrence Eichenfield, MD. Medscape Dermatology 2005;7(1). Available at: http://www.medscape.com/viewarticle/502337.
3. Yarosh DB, Canning MT, Teicher D, et al. After sun reversal of DNA damage: enhancing skin repair. Mutat Res 2005;571:57.
4. Schachner L, Field T, Hernandez-Reif M, et al. Atopic dermatitis symptoms decreased in children following massage therapy. Ped Derm 1998;5:390.
5. Burks AW, James JM, Hiegel A, et al. Atopic dermatitis and food hypersensitivity reactions. J Pediatr, 1998;132:132.
6. Bubak ME, Reed CE, Fransway AF. Allergic reactions to latex among health-care workers. Mayo Clin Proc 1992;67:1075.
7. Sussman GL, Tarlo S, Dolovich J. The spectrum of IgE-moderated responses to latex. JAMA 1991;265:2844.
8. Brehler R, Kütting B. Natural rubber latex allergy: a problem of interdisciplinary concern in medicine. Arch Intern Med 2001;161:1057.
9. Baughman RD. A 61-year-old man with psoriasis. JAMA 1996; 276:1421.
10. Greaves MW, Weinstein GD. Treatment of psoriasis. N Engl J Med 1995;332:581.
11. Naldi L, Peli L, Parazzini F, et al. Family history of psoriasis, stressful life events, and recent infectious disease are risk factors for a first episode of acute guttate psoriasis: results of a case-control study. J Am Acad Dermatol 2001; 44:433.
12. Heydendael VMR, Spuls PI, Opmeer BC, et al. Methotrexate versus cyclosporine in moderate-to-severe chronic plaque psoriasis. N Engl J Med 2003;349:658.
13. Ellis CN, Fradin MS, Messana JM, et al. Cyclosporine for plaque type psoriasis. N Engl J Med 1991;324:277.
14. Zacharie H, Kragballe K. Cyclosporine versus methotrexate toxicity in psoriasis. Lancet 1990; 335:924.

*Bold numerals denote published controlled clinical trials, meta-analyses, or consensus-based recommendations.

15. Kipnis CD, Myers WA, Opeola M, et al. Biologic treatments for psoriasis. J Am Acad Dermatol 2005: 52:671.
16. Geborek P, Bladstrom A, Turesson C, et al. Tumor necrosis factor blockers do not increase overall tumor risk in patients with rheumatoid arthritis, but may be associated with an increased risk of lymphomas. Ann Rheum Dis 2005;64:699.
17. Koo J. In the age of the biologics, is phototherapy obsolete? Cosmetic Dermatol 2004;17:3.
18. Whitmore SE. Appropriate use of alefacept therapy for psoriasis. Arch Dermatol 2004;140:239.
19. Ellis CN, Varani J, Fisher GJ, et al. Troglitazone improves psoriasis and normalizes models of proliferative skin disease. Arch Dermatol 2000;136:609.
20. King AB. A comparison in the clinical setting of efficacy and side effects of three thiazolidinediones. Diabetes Care 2000;23:557.
21. Shafiq N, Malhotra S, Pandhi P, et al. Pilot trial: Pioglitazone versus placebo in patients with plaque psoriasis (the P6). Int J Dermatol 2004;44:328.
22. Michaëlsson G, Gerden B, Hagforsen E, et al. Psoriasis patients with antibodies to gliadin can be improved with gluten-free diet. Br J Dermatol 2000;142:44.
23. Michaelsson G, Ahs S, Hammarstrom I, et al. Gluten-free diet in psoriasis patients with antibodies to gliadin results in decreased expression of tissue transglutaminase and fewer Ki67+ cells in the dermis. Acta Derm Venereol 2003;83:425.
24. Lindqvist U, Rudsander A, Bostrom A, et al. IgA antibodies to gliadin and celiac disease in psoriatic arthritis. Rheum 2002;41:31.

For annotated General References and resources related to this chapter, visit www.hopkinsbayview.org/PAMreferences.

Chapter 117

Primary Superficial Fungal and Viral Infections and Infestations

S. Elizabeth Whitmore

DERMATOPHYTE INFECTIONS

Dermatophyte infections are caused by fungi that penetrate the hair, nails, and stratum corneum of the skin. Symptoms of fungal infections, regardless of location, are usually pruritus or stinging. Although transmission of infection may occur through direct contact, indirect transmission is more common with exposure to dermatophyte-laden caps, pillow cases, towels, and clothing, as well as baths, showers, pool decks, and gymnasium floors.

Tinea Capitis

Tinea capitis (scalp infection) is seen primarily in preadolescent children 4 to 12 years old. Rarely, healthy adults and occasionally immunosuppressed individuals develop this infection. In the United States, tinea capitis is caused usually by *Trichophyton tonsurans.* Within well-defined scaly patches of the scalp, broken hairs, flush with the scalp up to a few millimeters in length, are seen. In contrast to seborrheic dermatitis, lymphadenopathy is usually present (1). The most severe complication of tinea capitis is *kerion formation,* in which boggy, inflammatory, pustular plaques of potentially scarring hair loss develop. If this is not treated early and aggressively with antifungals in combination with intralesional or oral corticosteroids, it generally causes a disfiguring permanent scarring in the scalp. Tinea capitis is diagnosed with a positive potassium hydroxide (KOH) preparation (see Yeast Infections) or fungal swab culture (2). With a kerion, the KOH preparation and fungal culture may be negative because of the intense host response.

When the diagnosis of kerion is suspected, treatment should be given as soon as possible in an attempt to prevent irreversible scarring alopecia. This includes selenium sulfide or ketoconazole shampoo to reduce spore shedding and oral griseofulvin to eradicate the fungus. Griseofulvin is not only teratogenic but may also reduce the effectiveness of oral contraceptive pills (OCPs). Young women who are sexually active must be instructed on the use of two forms of birth control when prescribed griseofulvin, and a pregnancy test must also be performed before institution of therapy if there is any question of pregnancy. Common side effects of griseofulvin include mild diarrhea and headache limited to the first several days of treatment. If these symptoms persist more than a few days, dosage reduction or initiation of another antifungal (e.g., fluconazole once weekly treatments for 2 months [3], itraconazole, or terbinafine [4]) may be substituted but it is best to consult, at least by telephone, with a dermatologist because newer drugs do not yet have U.S. Food and Drug Administration (FDA) approval and certain contraindications may exist. After 4 to 6 weeks of therapy, fungal culture is repeated; if results are negative 2 weeks later, treatment is stopped at that time.

Tinea Faciei

Tinea faciei is often misdiagnosed as rosacea or cutaneous lupus. Lesions tend to appear less "ringworm-like" (less sharp and clearly annular) than fungal infections elsewhere on the body. Patients often note that lesions flare with sun exposure, again suggesting diagnoses such as lupus erythematosus and acne rosacea instead of tinea. Lesions vary from erythematous, ill-defined, scaly plaques to the more classic sharply circumscribed plaques with leading edge scale and central clearing. Diagnosis may be made with a positive KOH preparation; however, on the face, false-negative KOH preparations are common with tinea faciei, and diagnosis may require culture or biopsy. Treatment is generally an oral antifungal (e.g., griseofulvin, itraconazole, fluconazole) because topical therapy may fail to clear this infection.

Tinea Corporis

Tinea corporis indicates a tinea infection outside of the head, face, groin, hands, and feet. Classic lesions are annular (ring-like) plaques that show a delicate scale at the advancing margin. KOH preparation from these lesions is usually positive. Treatment usually consists of topical imidazole antifungals (see Chapter 113) for 1 month with systemic therapy reserved for patients with a great number of lesions or unresponsive to prior topical treatment.

Tinea Cruris

Tinea cruris is predominantly seen in men. Lesions are semicircular scaly plaques on the superior medial thighs extending into the inguinal folds and onto the perineum. Diagnosis is based on a positive KOH preparation. Treatment with topical imidazoles (see Chapter 113) for a few to several weeks is usually adequate to control the problem.

Tinea Pedis

Tinea pedis is exceedingly common, eventually affecting up to 80% of men. Patients may have interdigital and plantar involvement with absent or moderate erythema, scale, and focal maceration. Less commonly seen is acute onset "oozing and blistering" on the plantar feet. Occasionally, interdigital tinea pedis with interdigital fissures may provide a point of entry for *Streptococcus*, which may ascend and cause recurrent streptococcal erysipelas cellulitis of the leg (5). Diagnosis is made with a positive KOH preparation, and treatment may be initiated with topical imidazoles. When plantar involvement is present, topical therapy may be unsuccessful and requires oral therapy for complete clearance. If treatment failure occurs in a patient at risk for leg cellulitis (e.g., history of prior leg erysipelas or cellulitis, venous stasis, or deep or superficial venous thrombosis), oral therapy should be prescribed to decrease the risk of recurrent ascending bacterial streptococcal cellulitis (6).

Tinea Manum

Tinea manum (tinea of the palmar skin) is uncommon. When seen, it often manifests as "two feet, one hand" syndrome, with areas of involvement as the name implies. The palm shows diffuse usually noninflammatory scaling, and the KOH preparation or fungal culture is positive. Treatment typically requires systemic therapy, but topical imidazoles (see Chapter 113) may initially be tried for 6 to 8 weeks. If topical therapy is unsuccessful or if nail involvement is present, oral itraconazole or terbinafine may be prescribed.

Tinea Unguium (Onychomycosis)

Tinea unguium of the toenails is very common, whereas fingernail infection is relatively rare. Although the incidence of tinea unguium is from 2% to 13% of the general population, the prevalence in the older male population is much higher. Tinea unguium represents approximately 30% of all mycotic infections of the skin and nails. Changes include white discoloration, subungual crumbly debris, and thickening of the nails. Patients are typically asymptomatic unless the toenails become ingrown or secondary bacterial infection occurs. Treatment is notoriously difficult. Although topical therapy is an option (e.g., Penlac Nail Lacquer, Mycocide NS [OTC], Fungi-Nail [OTC]), it generally is only useful in reducing the extent of infection with resultant improvement in the appearance of the nails. True cure rates with topical therapy are generally about 10%.

When patients desiring systemic therapy understand the expense, potential side effects, and required laboratory studies (baseline liver function test[s], generally repeated monthly when dosing is continuous), itraconazole or terbinafine may be used. Cure rates several months after completion of a 3-month course of therapy vary from 50% to more than 70%. Because these drugs are retained in the nail for many months after drug discontinuance, patients should not be evaluated until several months after completion of therapy. If they are not clear, another 3-month course of therapy may be initiated. An alternative dosing regimen has been described for terbinafine therapy which shows promise. Investigators studying 59 consecutive patients receiving one week in duration "pulse" dosing at various intervals found a greater than 60% cure rate when the pulsing interval was 3 months or less, i.e., similar to the response seen with 3 months of daily therapy. The optimal regimen (to minimize medication required, yet yield this 60% cure rate) was 4 pulses of terbinafine 250 milligrams per day for 7 days every 3 months. This regimen reduces both drug exposure and expense, i.e., 28 tablets versus 90 tablets ingested; hopefully, these results will be confirmed in randomized, double-blind, placebo controlled trials in the near future (7). After completion of systemic therapy, discarding old footwear or replacement of shoe insoles, as well as ongoing topical prophylactic antifungal preparations may help reduce recurrence rates.

YEAST INFECTIONS

Candidiasis

Candida albicans and other *Candida* species are yeast-like fungi that most often cause superficial cutaneous infections; however, in immunocompromised patients, *Candida* may cause systemic infections, including septicemia. *Candida* infection presents most often as a diaper rash in infants, summertime inframammary rash in women, vaginitis in premenopausal women, oral candidiasis in endogenously or exogenously immunosuppressed patients, and buttock and perineal rash in incontinent patients. The cutaneous changes are similar in most areas and appear as erythematous, slick, shiny patches with an irregular border of delicate scale and often satellite papules and pustules. The diagnosis can be confirmed with a KOH preparation or a swab culture.

Candidiasis may be treated with topical nystatin cream or an imidazole cream (see Chapter 113). Topicals should be applied two times a day and are continued for 1 to 2 weeks after clearing is seen. For infections unresponsive to topical therapy and when benefit outweighs risks, expense, and required testing, oral itraconazole or fluconazole for 10 to 14 days may be used. Pretreatment liver function tests are prudent in patients with multiple medical problems, and all patients should be instructed to report any signs or symptoms of hepatotoxicity during treatment. Topical nystatin powder or simple body powder may be helpful in preventing recurrences.

Tinea Versicolor

Tinea versicolor is a chronically recurring superficial yeast infection of the skin caused by *Pityrosporum orbiculare,* also known as *Malassezia furfur.* Tinea versicolor is seen most often in teens and young adults. It is common year-round in tropical climates and during the warm months in temperate climates.

Tinea versicolor appears as round to oval, scaly hypopigmented, hyperpigmented, or salmon colored macules that coalesce to form large confluent patches over the upper trunk and shoulders and, less often, on the face, scalp, genitalia, arms, and thighs. Although usually asymptomatic, some patients may have significant pruritus, particularly when perspiring during and after exercising. Diagnosis is made with a positive KOH preparation showing pseudohyphae and spores (Fig. 117.1). A simple and usually effective 5-day therapy is daily ketoconazole shampoo (prescription Nizoral 2% or over-the-counter Nizoral AD 1%) applied undiluted as a lotion and left on for 5 minutes before being rinsed. Once-weekly applications may be useful in preventing recurrences. Although not yet an FDA-approved indication, oral itraconazole 200 mg daily for 1 week in a controlled trial appears effective (8); however, recurrence is common.

In contrast to the superficial "epidermal" fungal infections mentioned above, deep fungal infections of the skin involve the underlying dermis. Excluding sporotrichosis,

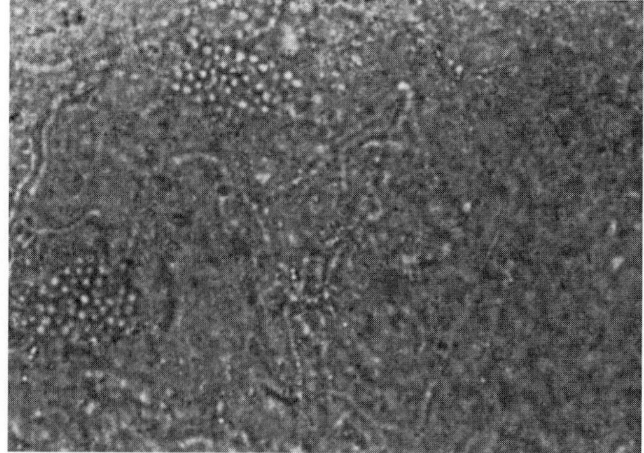

FIGURE 117.1. Short hyphae and spores of *Malassezia furfur* seen in tinea versicolor (potassium hydroxide preparation, ×400).

TABLE 117.1 Selected Deep Fungal Infections

Fungus	Endemic Area in the United States/Source	Usual Site of Primary Infection/Associated Cutaneous Hypersensitivity Reactions	Primary Cutaneous Inoculation[a]	Cutaneous Lesions Caused by Organisms
Blastomyces dermatitidis	Mississippi River basin, Great Lakes region, Southeast United States/bird excreta, wood	Pulmonary/rare erythema nodosum	Rare	Present in 70%; centrifugally enlarging plaques with a verrucous, pustular border; also, pustular ulcerations, subcutaneous abscesses, widespread or acral pustules
Coccidioides immitis	Southwest United States/soil	Pulmonary/50% of symptomatic infections with toxic erythema: diffuse exanthem, erythema multiforme, erythema nodosum	Rare	Verrucous plaque or granulomatous nodule (especially face); also, papules, pustules, nodules, subcutaneous
Histoplasma capsulatum	Central and southeast United States/bird and bat excreta, especially chicken coops	Pulmonary/rare erythema nodosum	Rare	Nasal or oral mucosal lesions in 50%; also, 6% with variable cutaneous lesions; ulcerating papules, nodules, plaques; ulcers, erythroderma[b]
Sporothrix schenckii	Ubiquitous, humidity favors growth/decaying vegetable matter, wood ("splinters")	Cutaneous (pulmonary possible)	Common	A papule that enlarges into an ulcerated nodule, usually with associated regional lymphangitis and lymphadenopathy
Cryptococcus neoformans	Ubiquitous/pigeon excreta, soil, some fruits	Pulmonary	Rare	Papules, pustules, ulcerating nodules, ulcers, abscesses, acneiform lesions, cellulitis, ecchymoses, vasculitis[b]
Candida albicans and *Candida tropicalis*	Ubiquitous	Oral mucosa, then esophagus most often	Rare	Erythematous to purpuric 0.5- to 1-cm papulonodules commonly on the trunk and proximal extremities, with associated fever and myalgia; also cellulitis, ecthyma gangrenosumlike eschar, nodular folliculitis and abscesses, purpura

[a]Nodule or chancriform ulcer with or without lymphangitis or lymphadenopathy.
[b]In human immunodeficiency virus–infected patients, may develop molluscum contagiosum-like lesions.

cutaneous infection usually results from seeding of the skin from a distant visceral organ infection (e.g., pulmonary). Table 117.1 summarizes some of the more common deep fungal infections.

Potassium Hydroxide Wet Mount Preparation

Dermatophyte and yeast infections of the skin are diagnosed with microscopic examination of surface skin scale. For this examination, scale is scraped from the advancing margin of an active lesion using a no. 15 surgical blade held at a slightly less than 90-degree angle to the skin surface. The scale is placed on a glass slide, one to two drops of KOH 20% added, and a coverslip applied. This is gently heated with a low flame, avoiding boiling, which, if it occurs, will result in crystallization and invalidation of the procedure. With light microscopy, the slide is scanned with the 10× objective and then examined more closely with the 40× objective. Dermatophyte hyphae are seen as refractile rod-shaped filaments of uniform width with characteristic branching (Fig. 117.2A). These hyphae traverse several normal cells and therefore can be distinguished from cell membranes. In contrast, *Candida* and *Pityrosporum* appear as nonbranching pseudohyphae and clusters of budding spores (Fig. 117.2B). Occasionally, *Candida* may show branching hyphae.

Fungal Culture

When the diagnosis of a fungal infection is strongly suspected despite a negative KOH preparation, when KOH examination is not available, and when the identification of a specific dermatophyte is important, a fungal culture should be done. Depending on the site of suspected infection, scale is taken from the advancing margin of the skin lesion, under the nail, or the scalp. The latter sample should also include several "broken off" hairs extracted with tweezers or forceps. Specimens may be placed

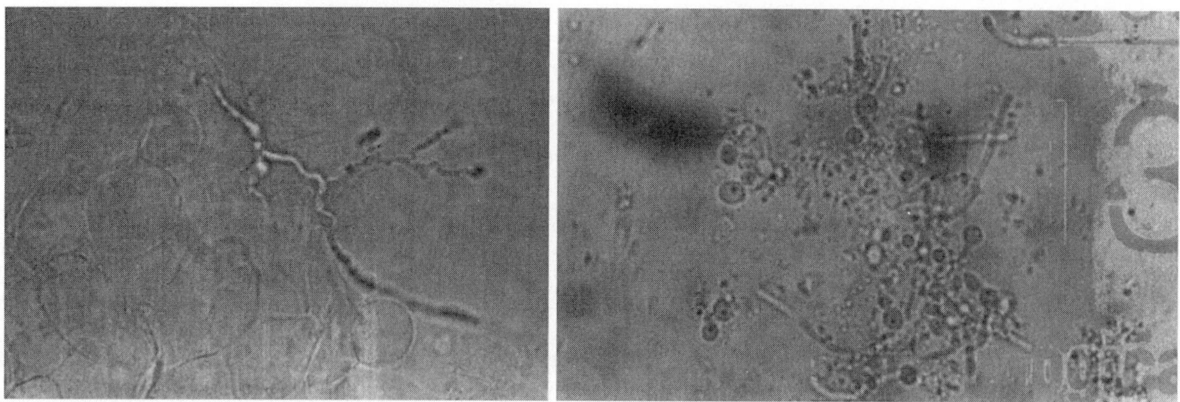

FIGURE 117.2. **A:** Hyphae of *tinea* (potassium hydroxide preparation, ×400). **B:** Pseudohyphae of *Candida* (potassium hydroxide preparation, ×400). (Courtesy of William G. Merz, PhD.)

between two glass slides, taped together, and sent in a sterile cup to the laboratory. Alternatively, particularly when the patient is not able to hold still and using a no. 15 blade may be dangerous, a culturette swab firmly rubbed over the area may be used.

LOCALIZED VIRAL INFECTIONS OF THE SKIN

Warts

Warts, also known as *verrucae,* are benign proliferations of the epidermis caused by human papilloma virus (HPV) infection. Warts are most common in children and immunocompromised patients. Three clinical features of all forms of warts include disruption of normal skin lines, surface pinpoint black dots (thrombosed capillaries), and appearance at sites of contact or trauma.

Common warts (*verrucae vulgaris*) may be noted initially as smooth, skin-colored, <1-mm papules that gradually enlarge to several millimeters with a rough, finely papulated, or hyperkeratotic (warty) surface. Warts may coalesce to form large plaques. Common warts are most often found on the hands.

Flat warts (*verrucae plana*) are skin-colored to pink flat-topped papules usually less than a few millimeters in diameter. They occur most commonly on the dorsal aspect of the hands, face, and, in women, the legs.

Genital warts (*condylomata acuminata*) begin as minute flat papules that often become verrucous on the external genitalia, vagina, cervix, perirectal, and/or anal canal. This HPV infection of the cervix or anorectal area predisposes to intraepithelial neoplasia. Immunosuppression, for example, from immunosuppressive therapy in an organ transplant recipient to a patient infected with human immunodeficiency virus (HIV), may increase the risk of anal intraepithelial neoplasia when genital warts are present.

Plantar warts (*verrucae plantaris*) appear as circumscribed, thickened, barely elevated papules with surface callous. Extensive infection with HPV may manifest as warts covering the entire heel or plantar aspect of the foot. Plantar warts are often confused with corns or clavi. Warts can be distinguished from corns by paring the surface with a no. 15 surgical blade as the typical minute black dots (thrombosed capillaries) should become visible. In contrast, paring of corns reveals a central core that is easily removed with the paring blade.

Treatment

Two precepts should be remembered when treating warts: There are no guarantees in the success of any treatment and the lesions themselves are benign and should not be treated with modalities that result in harm or scarring, such as ionizing irradiation, deep surgical excision, or deep destructive therapies (extending into the dermis).

Treatment of common, flat, and plantar warts is typically daily self-application of *topical 17% salicylic acid solution* (e.g., Occlusal or Duofilm) or a 40% salicylic acid patch (MediPlast), all available over the counter. Before application, the wart may be soaked in warm water for several minutes and then filed to remove the white macerated surface with a nail file or pumice stone (available in pharmacies). Because of the risk of infection transmission, whatever instrument is used it must not be used elsewhere or by others. If after 6 weeks of daily therapy the wart is still present, weekly or biweekly *liquid nitrogen cryotherapy* may be started. Patients should be warned that although liquid nitrogen should not cause scarring, it may cause blistering and, upon healing, permanent depigmentation of the skin, particularly important with face and hand warts, and, rarely, superficial nerve damage (usually on the lateral surface of the digits). If after several cryotherapy sessions warts are still present, other options should be considered, such as "watchful waiting," laser vaporization, and curette and desiccation. Patients should be warned that these latter treatments may cause scarring.

Initial treatment of condyloma acuminatum may be administered by the patient. Two options are available. Podofilox 0.5% (Condylox gel or solution) is a patient-applied podophyllin derivative that is applied two times a day for 3 consecutive days each week. After several weeks of treatment, clearance rates are 30% to 50%. Another patient-applied medication is imiquimod 5% cream (Aldara). This agent causes local endogenous cytokine release that is believed to lead to a host effected clearance of HPV. Imiquimod cream is applied three times per week for up to 4 months. Both of these medications require a prescription. If these medications are ineffective, liquid nitrogen cryotherapy may be used in the same manner as outlined for other warts. Additional alternative therapies, which may be considered by a consulting dermatologist, include laser vaporization, curette and desiccation, and scalpel excision.

Molluscum Contagiosum

Molluscum contagiosum is common in young children and HIV-infected patients. Lesions are caused by the pox virus, a DNA virus. The lesions are umbilicated, skin-colored to whitish, 1- to 4-mm papules, typically on the neck, trunk, genital, and eyelid areas. The central umbilicated depression contains molluscum bodies, which are enlarged degrading keratinocytes, packed with viral material. The diagnosis is made by obtaining a curette of the molluscum for KOH preparation. With light microscopy, the round, homogeneous, 25-μm molluscum bodies are easily seen.

In children, simple nonthreatening treatments are best. Scotch tape stripping (tape quickly and firmly applied and immediately removed a dozen times) once to twice daily for several weeks may suffice by unroofing the lesion and stimulating a host response through the mild local trauma. Alternatively, topical salicylic acid 17% preparations (as for warts; see above) or topical tretinoin (Retin-A 0.025% gel) applied directly to the lesion twice a day may be tried for 6 weeks. If lesions persist, either curettage or liquid nitrogen cryotherapy may be used, remembering that the latter may cause permanent depigmentation.

HERPES INFECTION

Herpes Simplex

Herpes simplex virus (HSV) infection may be caused by HSV type I or II, typically with type I causing *herpes labialis* and type II causing *herpes genitalis*. HSV is commonly present in asymptomatic individuals. For example, a study of randomly selected patients in a family medicine clinic found 56% seropositivity for HSV I, 23% seropositivity for HSV II, 12% seropositivity for both HSV I and II, and 33% seronegativity (9). Active infection results in a recurrent localized clustered (herpetic) blistering of the skin. After a primary infection has occurred, the virus remains dormant in the cranial nerve or dorsal root nerve ganglia innervating the region of cutaneous infection. Lesions may recur at any time, often being triggered by sun exposure, illness, menses, local trauma, and physical and psychologic stress. Transmission occurs through direct contact with an infected person actively shedding virus. The virus may live on fomites, but unlike HPV, HSV quickly dies on drying (30 minutes), making fomite transmission unlikely.

Primary herpes infection in the oral cavity causes the painful febrile illness acute herpetic gingivostomatitis (see Chapter 112). After healing the virus remains latent, and subsequent reactivation causes herpes labialis, manifest as clustered vesicles on or about the lips. Notably, most patients with recurrent herpes labialis have no history of primary acute herpetic gingivostomatitis or herpetic infection elsewhere and therefore are presumed to have had an asymptomatic primary oral infection. Lesions heal in approximately 1 to 2 weeks, with a typical sequence of rupture, crusting, and desquamation. The lesions are infectious as long as the skin is not intact. The importance of asymptomatic viral shedding in viral transmission, as is known to occur with genital herpes and with exceptionally high frequency in patients with acquired immunodeficiency syndrome (AIDS), is not known, although in one prospective study of couples with one infected partner, 70% of partner infections occurred during periods of asymptomatic shedding (10). Genital herpes, the most common cause of genital ulcers, is discussed in Chapter 37.

Herpes simplex infection may occur anywhere on the body; a common site in health care workers is on the finger (*herpetic whitlow*), acquired through exposure to a patient with active herpes infection. Viral transmission has been reported to occur through vinyl gloves, so one is wise to double glove if touching herpes lesions is required during an examination or in the provision of care.

Chronic herpetic infections in immunocompromised patients appear as chronic punched-out ulcers that may be solitary or multiple. The expanded AIDS surveillance case definition for AIDS diagnosis includes a chronic herpes simplex ulcer present for 1 month or longer in a patient infected with HIV.

Fortunately, *cutaneous complications* of HSV infection are rare. These complications include *cutaneous dissemination* in patients with generalized atopic dermatitis and *recurrent erythema multiforme* as a hypersensitivity response. A history of the latter is an indication for ongoing prophylactic antiviral therapy (see Chapters 102, 112, and

118). Ocular complications include *herpetic keratitis,* a primary or secondary infection that involves the cornea of the eye and is best managed emergently by an ophthalmologist because of the potential for permanent corneal scarring and loss of vision. Albeit rare, the most common systemic complication is Bell palsy (11). Other serious and systemic complications that are rare complications of HSV include acute ascending necrotizing myelopathy and necrotizing lymphadenitis associated with herpes genitalis (12) and recurrent lymphocytic meningitis (13).

Treatment

Although no treatment is necessary for recurrent facial HSV, an FDA-approved regimen of valacyclovir, 2 g twice a day, may abort or reduce the duration of lesions when taken at the first signs of recurrence (i.e., optimally, with the onset of premonitory dysesthesia in individuals who experience this symptom). Antiviral prophylaxis (e.g., valacyclovir 500 mg daily) should be given when HSV recurrences may complicate any facial cutaneous surgery, oral surgery, or other dental work. Prophylaxis may also be welcomed by patients when recurrences may be anticipated, such as ski trips (oral antiviral and topical high SPF sunscreen), or important ceremonial social events (14).

Novel treatments appear to have promise for HSV. In a randomized, double-blind, placebo-controlled, pilot study, stannous fluoride 0.4% gel applied twice daily at the onset of prodromal symptoms prevented blisters from developing in most individuals, and in those who developed lesions, it decreased their duration significantly (15). Also, aspirin initiated at the onset of recurrent HSV, at a dose of 125 mg, decrease the duration of lesions by almost 50%, whereas a dose of aspirin of 250 mg/day did not show this benefit (16).

Herpes Zoster (Shingles)

Herpes zoster represents a reactivation of the varicella–zoster virus. After initial varicella (chickenpox) infection, the virus resides in a dorsal root or cranial nerve ganglia. At any point thereafter, latent virus may be reactivated and produce multiple erythematous plaques surmounted by clustered vesicles, in a dermatomal or zosteriform distribution. In an immunocompetent patient, lesions begin with vesicles that become turbid in 3 days, dry and crust in 7 to 10 days, and clear within 2 to 3 weeks. New lesions may continue to appear for up to 1 week. Herpes zoster affects a thoracic dermatome in 50%, a cervical dermatome in 20%, the trigeminal dermatome in 15%, and a lumbosacral dermatome in 10% of patients. Of patients with herpes zoster, two thirds are older than 50 years of age and about 10% are younger than 20 years of age (17).

Often, patients who have herpes zoster develop a prodrome of pain in the affected dermatome. Occasionally, this painful prodrome is misdiagnosed as an acute painful disease such as pleurisy, myocardial infarction, cholecystitis, appendicitis, renal colic, or a ruptured intervertebral disk. Rarely, patients may experience acute segmental neuralgia with a concurrent rise in varicella virus antibodies without developing skin lesions. This is called zoster sine herpete.

There are several very significant potential complications of zoster. When the trigeminal dermatome is affected, involvement of the second branch may be associated with involvement of the eye. Affected patients should be evaluated emergently by an ophthalmologist because keratitis, uveitis, secondary glaucoma, iridocyclitis, or rarely panophthalmitis may develop. *Ramsay-Hunt* syndrome is the constellation of herpes zoster affecting the facial and auditory nerves, causing facial palsy with cutaneous zoster of the external ear or tympanic membrane with associated tinnitus, vertigo, and/or hearing deficit. Among all patients with herpes zoster, motor nerve involvement occurs in only 5%. The incidence is probably understated because mild or partial deficits likely go undetected. Weakness or paralysis usually begins within weeks of the onset of the rash and may involve the muscle groups outside of the affected dermatome. Full recovery from this weakness or paralysis occurs spontaneously in only about half of patients who are so affected (18). Meningoencephalitis may develop with cranial nerve herpes zoster in immunocompromised patients, most often in association with cutaneous dissemination. *Granulomatous angiitis* of cerebral arteries is an unusual complication of ophthalmic zoster that may lead to a syndrome of delayed contralateral hemiplegia occurring weeks to a few months after an episode of zoster. Such patients are usually diagnosed as having a typical cerebrovascular accident, but arteriograms reveal segmental narrowing or occlusion of cerebral arteries ipsilateral to the site of the ophthalmic zoster. Finally, *disseminated herpes zoster,* defined as more than 20 vesicles at a distance from the primary dermatome, occurs almost exclusively in immunocompromised patients. Such patients should be hospitalized for intravenous acyclovir therapy and isolated as appropriate to protect those not immune to the virus. Approximately 10% of patients with disseminated cutaneous lesions develop widespread often fatal visceral infection, particularly of the lungs, liver, and brain.

The presumptive diagnosis of herpes zoster is made clinically. A *Tzanck smear,* done when there is doubt about the diagnosis, shows multinucleated giant cells (see page 1921). Such a positive smear confirms that the eruption is herpes zoster or herpes simplex and rules out other blistering disorders such as impetigo, erythema multiforme, and pemphigus, which occasionally may be confused with herpes infection. Herpes simplex can occur in a dermatomal pattern, so any case of "recurrent" herpes zoster should be cultured because the correct diagnosis is more likely recurrent dermatomal HSV infection. It is important to confirm this infection because recurrent zoster (as opposed to HSV) raises the possibility of an associated illness causing immunosuppression and should prompt further evaluation of immune function.

The early treatment of acute herpes zoster reduces the severity, shortens the duration of the infection, and potentially reduces the incidence of post herpetic neuralgia. Kost and Straus (19) put forth a useful algorithm for treatment and prevention of acute herpes zoster and postherpetic neuralgia (PHN). Antiviral therapy affects the course of disease if initiated within 48 to 72 hours of its onset. A 1-week course of an oral antiviral (e.g., acyclovir [Zovirax] 800 mg five times a day, valacyclovir [Valtrex] 1,000 mg three times a day, famciclovir [Famvir] 500 mg three times a day) is used in immunocompetent patients. Acyclovir has been shown to reduce zoster-associated acute pain and new lesion formation, and both valacyclovir and famciclovir reduce acute pain and speed healing (20,21).

Topical therapy will ease the pain from open lesions. Wet to damp dressings promote drying of the lesions, and a topical ointment (e.g., plain petrolatum or antibiotic ointment with caution given the potential development of allergic contact dermatitis if Neosporin or bacitracin are used) generously applied promotes healing, prevents secondary infection, and reduces the pain caused by air contacting the denuded skin. If acute neuralgia is present, nonsteroidal anti-inflammatory drugs, amitriptyline, or narcotics may be needed to provide comfort. These must be used with caution, particularly in persons living alone, those on multiple medications, and the elderly.

In hospitalized patients with even routine, nondisseminated zoster, contact and respiratory precautions should be instituted. With the advent of polymerase chain reaction technology, it has been shown that viral shedding does occur in patients with herpes zoster; in one report, detectable varicella zoster virus was found at distant sites within an otherwise healthy affected patient's room, including the surface of the room air conditioner filter, consistent with aerosolized spread (22).

PHN, or pain after the cutaneous lesions have resolved, is most commonly seen in patients older than 50 years. Other predictors of the development of PHN include a greater number of health care encounters in the 6 months before zoster, baseline conditions causing immunosuppression, treatment with steroids in the 6 months before zoster, and zoster associated prodromal symptoms, discomfort severe enough to interfere with daily living, and prolonged time to crusting of skin lesions (23). Both valacyclovir and famciclovir have been shown to reduce the incidence and duration of PHN (20,21). Its been estimated that six patients need to be treated with antivirals to prevent one case of PHN (24). The utility of supplemental corticosteroids in the prevention of PHN remains controversial (25,26) and therefore is not recommended. A small study found that amitriptyline 10 to 25 mg nightly initiated at the time of diagnosis of acute zoster reduced the incidence of PHN by 50% (27). If larger studies ultimately show this same benefit, amitriptyline (with appropriate caution; see Chapters 12 and 24) would seem to be an ideal treatment for persons with painful acute herpes zoster.

Once developed, treatment of PHN may be very difficult. Some success has been reported with topical capsaicin cream (Zostrix 0.025% and Zostrix HP 0.075%), applied four times a day. Capsaicin depletes substance P in peripheral sensory nerves and may alleviate pain. Not infrequently, there is a delay of several weeks before an effect is appreciated. Patients must be cautioned that about four applications are needed to fully deplete the substance contributing to pain (substance P), so the first few applications (typically, three) when substance P is being released produce local burning and stinging. However, with subsequent *consistent* applications, the pain should not recur. Alternatively or in conjunction with capsaicin, anesthetic over the counter LidoDerm topical patches and over the counter ELA-Max cream may be tried. Unfortunately, both are quite expensive for long-term use. For some patients, systemic treatment with amitriptyline (as opposed to prevention) is appropriate initial therapy for PHN. Oral amitriptyline in dosages of 12.5 to 150 mg/day (27) may decrease the discomfort of PHN (see Chapters 12 and 24). Gabapentin studied over a 2-month treatment period in a multicenter, double-blind, randomized, placebo-controlled study also was found to be effective in reducing pain and sleep disturbance and improving mood and quality of life (28). PHN most often remits spontaneously within 6 months; however, when this is not the case and the pain cannot be controlled, referral to a pain specialist is appropriate. Although still investigational (29), intrathecal methylprednisolone may prove to be helpful for intractable PHN.

Tzanck Smear

The sensitivity of a *Tzanck smear* in detecting herpetic changes is greatest when a specimen is taken from the intact vesicle. A chosen vesicle is unroofed, and the base is firmly scraped with a no. 15 surgical blade and smeared onto a glass slide. When vesicles are not present, an early crusted papule is sampled by removing the surface crust and scraping the base. Immediate tissue smear staining is performed with the commercially available Tzanck stain (Dif-Quik Stain, Baxter Scientific Products, McGraw Park, IL), which is a three-step immediate stain. Alternatively, a Giemsa stain may be done by combining 0.5 mL water with 0.5 mL Giemsa tissue stain in a small syringe and flooding over the specimen and then thoroughly rinsing with tap water after 30 seconds. Although the slide may be viewed directly, covering with mounting medium and a coverslip greatly improves resolution. The slide is searched for giant

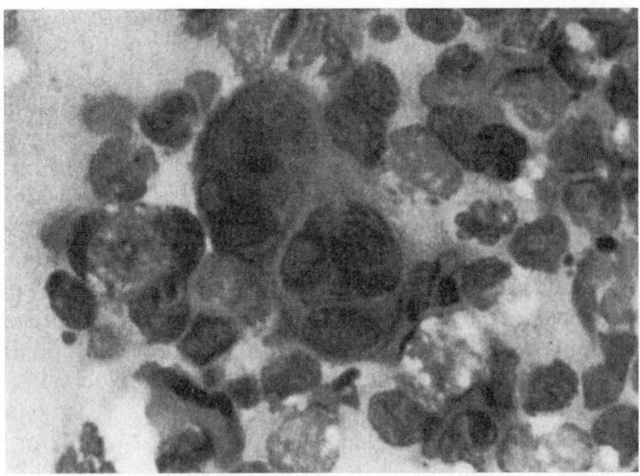

FIGURE 117.3. Tzanck smear: gentle scraping from the base of a vesicle and stained with Wright or Giemsa stain. Multinucleated cells from herpes simplex are shown (×400).

cells containing multiple syncytial nuclei (nuclei that mold together in a jigsaw puzzle-like fashion) (Fig. 117.3). The Tzanck smear preparation should be positive when performed on lesions of herpes simplex, varicella, and herpes zoster eruptions (Fig. 117.3). If the Tzanck smear is nondiagnostic, biopsy of a papule, vesicle, or crusted papule for routine histopathology (results available in 2 to 4 days) should reveal diagnostic herpetic changes of balloon cells and multinucleated giant cells.

INFESTATIONS

Scabies

Human scabies is caused by infestation with the mite *Sarcoptes scabiei* var. *hominis*. Infestation causes an intense intractable pruritus that is classically most disturbing at night, when competing external stimuli are minimal. The signs and symptoms of scabies infestation are caused by the host's immune response to the mite and its eggs and feces. Generally, this response is delayed, so patients become itchy approximately 10 days to 2 weeks after exposure and infestation. Scabies is seen most often in children, and the pathognomonic lesions are burrows, which are thread-like linear ridges a few millimeters in length with a minute black dot at one end. Burrows occur most often on the hands, wrists, soles, waist, penis, nipples, axillae, and gluteal cleft. Depending on the duration of infestation, patients may have few to innumerable scratches, excoriations, crusts, and eczematous papules and plaques. Less often, small nodules may develop, tending to favor the scrotum, axillae, and buttocks.

Scabies infestation is confirmed by identifying the mite, eggs, or feces in the superficial skin. This often can be done by scraping the black dot at one end of a burrow using a no. 15 surgical blade. If a black dot is not seen, both ends of the burrow are scraped. The sample is prepared on a glass slide with a drop of mineral oil and a coverslip and then viewed with light microscopy. The mite is an approximately 0.2 mm with eight short legs; eggs are smaller and oval and feces are still smaller round pellets.

Patients and family members should be treated with an overnight application of prescription lindane lotion (Kwell lotion, 30 mL per single application) or permethrin cream (Elimite cream, 30 g per single application, 60-g tube). Either is applied from the neck down, using an old toothbrush to get under the finger and toenails and showered off 8 to 12 hours later. After this is completed, patients often require emollients and a mid-potency corticosteroid (e.g., triamcinolone 0.1% ointment) after using the scabicides to suppress the "hyperreactivity" caused by the mites (see Chapter 113). Although both lindane and permethrin are neurotoxins, systemic absorption of lindane is greater (30) so it should be avoided in infants, pregnant and lactating women, and patients with seizure disorders. It should also be avoided when enhanced systemic absorption is possible, such as in patients with extensive secondary excoriations and dermatitis or with widespread skin diseases (e.g., generalized atopic dermatitis, widespread psoriasis). All bed clothing, linens, unwashed clothing, and stuffed animals should be washed and dried in a hot dryer. The latter is necessary, because it is the temperature of the hot dryer that kills the mite. Alternatively, the mites and eggs may be killed by placing the items in airtight plastic bags for 2 weeks.

An alternative treatment now available in this country in patients resistant to topical scabicidal therapy is ivermectin (3-mg tablets) (31,32). If used, the Centers for Disease Control and Prevention (CDC) recommends a dose of ivermectin 0.2 mg/kg (e.g., a single dose of four tablets for a 60-kg adult), repeated in 2 weeks as an alternative to topical permethrin cream (33).

Pediculosis

Infestation with the human louse (*Pediculus humanus capitis* and *corporis, Phthirus pubis*) affects different areas of the body and is called *pediculosis capitis, corporis,* and *pubis*. *Pediculosis capitis* is most common in children. Patients with lice often have intense pruritus, scalp and posterior neck excoriations, and often secondary bacterial infection with pustules, crusting, and adenopathy. *Pediculosis corporis* is seen most often in patients exposed to others who, like themselves, are unable to maintain good hygiene. *Pediculosis pubis* (pubic lice) is usually a sexually transmitted disorder.

Patients with pediculosis usually have nits firmly attached to head, body, or pubic hairs (Fig. 117.4). Nits are less than 1-mm-long "shells" that may or may not still

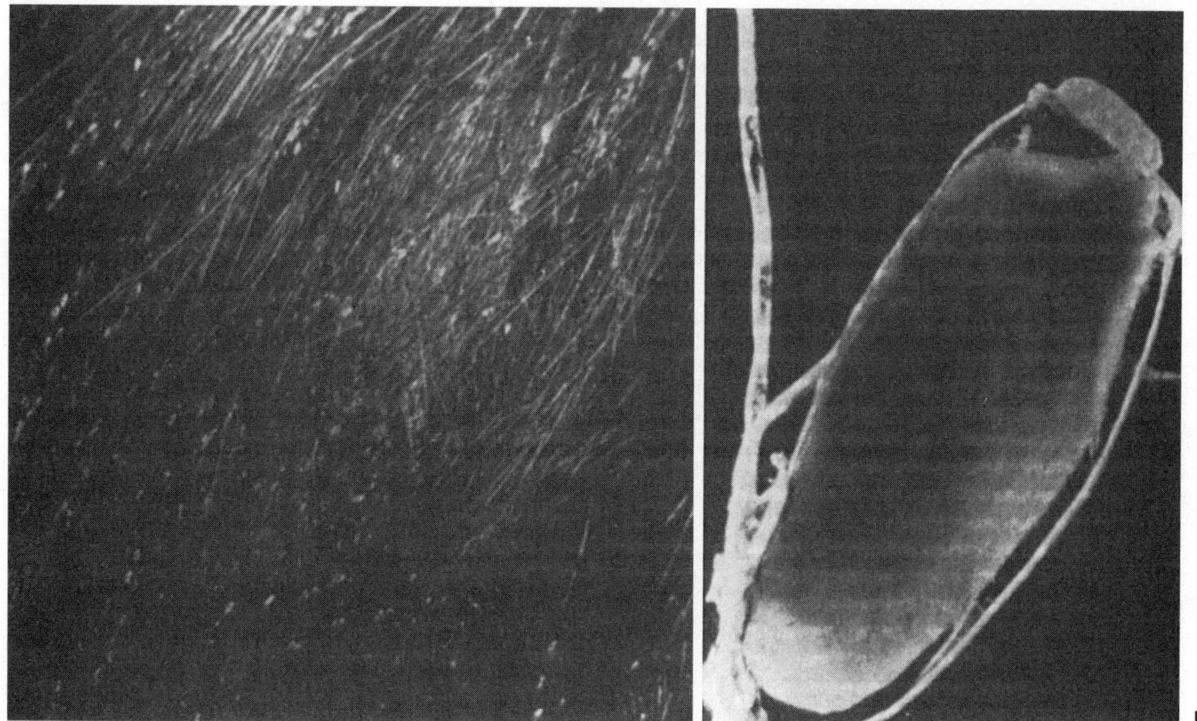

FIGURE 117.4. *Pediculus humanus* var. *capitis* (head louse). **A:** Gross appearance of nits on the hair shaft. **B:** Microscopic appearance (×100). (Courtesy of Reed and Carnrick, Kenilworth, NJ.)

contain an egg. Lice hatch from these eggs and are visible, being less than 2 mm long with three pairs of legs that terminate in sharp claws. They are found in the hair or adjacent skin and, specifically in pediculosis corporis, in the seams of clothing. Treatment should be initiated with pyrethrin shampoo (RID, OTC), lindane shampoo or lotion (Kwell), or malathion lotion (Ovide) for pediculosis capitis and pubis (note, Ovide is only labeled for scalp treatment and is contraindicated in neonates and infants) and lindane lotion for pediculosis corporis. The shampoos are left on for 5 to 10 minutes and then washed off; the lotions are left on overnight. Because no pediculicides are 100% ovicidal, nits that potentially contain living eggs and will remain attached to the hair after treatment must be removed with a fine-tooth comb after undiluted white vinegar is applied to the hair for 15 minutes. Close contacts should be treated in a similar fashion, and bed clothing and linens and unwashed clothes should be washed and put through a hot dryer cycle to destroy the lice and eggs. Alternatively, these items may be sealed in an airtight plastic bag for 2 weeks.

SPECIFIC REFERENCES*

1. Hubbard TW. The predictive value of symptoms in diagnosing childhood tinea capitis. Arch Pediatr Adolesc Med 1999;153:1150.
2. Friedlander S, Pickering B, Cunningham BB, et al. The utility of the cotton swab method in the diagnosis of tinea capitis. Pediatrics 1999; 104:276.
3. Gupta AK, Dlova N, Taborda P, et al. Once weekly fluconazole is effective in children in the treatment of tinea capitis: a prospective, multicentre study. Br J Dermatol 2000;142:965.
4. Haroon TS, Hussain I, Aman S, et al. A randomized double-blind comparative study of terbinafine for 1, 2 and 4 weeks in tinea capitis. Br J Dermatol 1996;135:86.
5. Semel JD, Goldin H. Association of athlete's foot with cellulitis of the lower extremities: diagnostic value of bacterial cultures of ipsilateral interdigital space samples. Clin Infect Dis 1996;23:1162.
6. Eriksson B, Jorup-Rönström C, Karkkonen K, et al. Erysipelas: clinical and bacteriologic spectrum and serological aspects. Clin Infect Dis 1996;23:1091.
7. Zaias N, Rebell G. The successful treatment of *Trichophyton rubrum* nail bed (distal subungual) onychomycosis with intermittent pulse-dosed terbinafine. Arch Dermatol 2004;140:691.
8. Nickman JG. A double-blinded, randomized placebo controlled evaluation of short term treatment with oral itraconazole in patients with tinea versicolor. J Am Acad Dermatol 1996;34: 785.
9. Oliver L, Wald A, Kim M, et al. Seroprevalence of herpes simplex virus infection in a family medicine clinic. Arch Fam Med 1995;4:228.
10. Mertz GJ, Benedetti J, Ashley R, et. al. Risk factors for the sexual transmission of genital herpes. Ann Intern Med 1992;116:197–202.
11. Murakami S, Mizobuchi M, Nakashiro Y, et al. Bell's palsy and herpes simplex virus: identification of viral DNA in endoneurial fluid and muscle. Ann Intern Med 1996;124:27.
12. Wiley CA, VanPatten PD, Carpenter PM, et al. Acute ascending necrotizing myelopathy caused by herpes simplex virus type II. Neurology 1987;37:1791.
13. Tedder DG, Ashley R, Tyler KL, et al. Herpes simplex virus infection as cause of benign recurrent lymphocytic meningitis. Ann Intern Med 1994;121:334.
14. Rooney JF, Strauss SE, Mannix ML, et al. Oral acyclovir to suppress frequently recurrent herpes labialis. Ann Intern Med 1993;118:268.
15. Embro WJ. Treatment of herpes simplex labialis

*Bold numerals denote published controlled clinical trials, meta-analyses, or consensus-based recommendations.

with stannous fluoride gel. Cosmetic Dermatol 1999;39.
16. Karadi I, Karpati S, Romics L. Aspirin in the management of recurrent herpes simplex virus infection. Ann Intern Med 1998;128:696.
17. Oxman MN, Strauss SE. Varicella and herpes zoster. In: Freedberg IM, Eisen AZ, Wolff K, et al., eds. Fitzpatrick's dermatology in general medicine. 5th ed. New York: McGraw-Hill, 1999: 2436.
18. Akiyama N. Herpes zoster infection complicated by motor paralysis. J Dermatol 2000;27:252.
19. Kost RG, Straus SE. Postherpetic neuralgia: pathogenesis, treatment, and prevention. N Engl J Med 1996;335:32.
20. Tyring S, Barbarash RA, Nahlik JE, et al. Famciclovir for the treatment of acute herpes zoster: effects on acute disease and postherpetic neuralgia. A randomized, double-blind, placebo-controlled trial. Collaborative Famciclovir Herpes Zoster Study Group. Ann Intern Med 1995;123:89.
21. Tyring SK, Beutner KR Tucker BA, et. al. Antiviral therapy for herpes zoster: randomized, controlled clinical trial of valacylovir and famciclovir therapy in immunocompetent patients 50 years and older. Arch Fam Med, 2000;9:863–9.
22. Yoshikawa T, Khira M, Suzuki K, et al. Rapid contamination of the environments with varicella zoster virus DNA from a patient with herpes zoster. J Med Virol 2001;63:64.
23. Choo PW, Galil K, Donahue JG, et al. Risk factors for postherpetic neuralgia. Arch Intern Med 1997;157:1217.
24. Jackson JL, Gibbons R, Meyer G, et al. The effect of treating herpes zoster with oral acyclovir in preventing postherpetic neuralgia: a meta-analysis. Arch Intern Med 1997;157:909.
25. Whitley RJ, Weiss H, Gnann JW, et al. Acyclovir with and without prednisone for the treatment of herpes zoster. A randomized, placebo-controlled trial. Ann Intern Med 1996;125: 376.
26. Wood MJ, Johnson RW, McKendrick MW, et al. A randomized trial of acyclovir for 7 days or 21 days with and without prednisolone for treatment of acute herpes zoster. N Engl J Med 1994;330:896.
27. Max MB, Schafer SC, Culnane M, et al. Amitriptyline, but not lorazepam, relieves post-herpetic neuralgia. Neurology 1988;38:1427.
28. Rowbotham M, Hardern N, Stacey B, et al, for the Gabapentin Postherpetic Neuralgia Study Group. Gabapentin for the treatment of postherpetic neuralgia. JAMA 1998;280:187.
29. Kotani N, Matsuki A, Watson CPN. Correspondence regarding intrathecal methylprednisolone for intractable postherpetic neuralgia. N Engl J Med 2000;344:1019.
30. Meinking TL, Taplin D. Safety of permethrin versus lindane for the treatment of scabies. Arch Dermatol 1996;132:959.
31. Meinking TL, Taplin D, Hermida JL, et al. The treatment of scabies with ivermectin. N Engl J Med 1995;333:26.
32. Usa V, Gopalakrishnan Nair TV. A comparative study of oral ivermectin and topical permethrin cream in the treatment of scabies. J Am Acad Dermatol 2000;42:236–40.
33. Centers for Disease Control. Sexually Transmitted Diseases Treatment Guidelines 2002. Accessed at http://www.cdc.gov.

For annotated ***General References*** *and resources related to this chapter, visit www.hopkinsbayview.org/PAMreferences.*

Chapter 118

Autoimmune Blistering Diseases, Photosensitive Eruptions, and Drug Eruptions

S. Elizabeth Whitmore

AUTOIMMUNE BLISTERING DISORDERS

Primary bullous dermatoses associated with autoantibodies to various components of the epidermis and underlying basement membrane zone of the skin (1) include bullous pemphigoid, pemphigus vulgaris, bullous lupus erythematosus, acquired epidermolysis bullosa acquisita, linear immunoglobulin A (IgA) bullous dermatosis, vancomycin and other drug-induced linear IgA dermatoses, and paraneoplastic pemphigus. Patients with these conditions have flaccid to tense bullae, with or without an erythematous, urticarial base, distributed in a localized or generalized fashion on the skin and mucosal surfaces. Because some of these disorders may be associated with significant morbidity and mortality, patients suspected of having an autoimmune blistering disorder should undergo skin biopsy for routine histologic and special staining (direct immunofluorescence to identify the site of deposited immunoglobulin within the epidermis). Particularly in the treatment of pemphigus vulgaris, very aggressive therapies, including prednisone, cytotoxic agents, and plasmapheresis, may be required (2). The various patterns of these disorders are as follows.

Bullous pemphigoid typically includes mild asymptomatic oral involvement and tense skin blisters on an urticarial base; affected patients are usually older than age 60. Herpes gestationis is similar to bullous pemphigoid, but it occurs in association with pregnancy. *Pemphigus vulgaris* is associated with extensive oral lesions and flaccid cutaneous blisters that exhibit a positive *Nikolsky* sign in which pressure applied to a blister causes the blister to enlarge by spreading outward into the adjacent skin.

Bullous diseases associated with systemic disease or medications include paraneoplastic pemphigus, bullous lupus erythematosus, and drug-induced linear IgA dermatosis. *Paraneoplastic pemphigus* (PNP) (3), like pemphigus vulgaris, is associated with extensive oral lesions but, unlike pemphigus vulgaris, cutaneous lesions are variable and may include bullous pemphigoid-like lesions with tense vesiculobullae, erythema multiforme-like lesions with targetoid "bulls eye" lesions, and lichen planus-like lesions with violaceous flat topped papules and plaques, usually with an upper body predominance. A recent review has summarized the malignancies and frequencies thereof associated with PNP: over 80% of neoplasms are hematologic-related malignancies and include non-Hodgkins lymphoma (39%), chronic lymphocytic leukemia (18%), Castleman disease (18%); associated non-hematologic associated malignancies include epithelial-origin-carcinoma (9%), mesenchymal origin-sarcoma (6%), and melanoma (<1%) (4). *Bullous lupus erythematosus* occurs in the setting of systemic lupus erythematosus; lesions may resemble those seen in bullous pemphigoid with vesiculobullous lesions on an urticarial base or may appear more erythema multiforme-like with targetoid, hemorrhagic blisters. Vancomycin and other drug-induced linear IgA dermatoses appear similar to bullous pemphigoid. The eruption typically clears within weeks of withdrawal of the inciting drug, however occasionally the eruption persists, thereby defining idiopathic linear IgA disease, unmasked by a drug. In general, one will want to consult with a dermatologist if there is any doubt about the diagnosis or treatment of a patient suspected of having a form of autoimmune blistering disorder.

PHOTOSENSITIVITY

Photosensitivity is an abnormal response to natural sunlight or artificial ultraviolet (UV) radiation or visible light. It manifests as a diffuse macular erythema (*phototoxic reaction*) or a papular or papulovesicular erythema (e.g., *photoallergic reaction*) on the exposed surfaces. The phototoxic or sunburn-like reaction is caused by phototoxic drugs such as sulfonamides, quinolones, doxycycline, phenothiazines, nonsteroidal anti-inflammatory drugs (NSAIDs), porphyrin precursors, and psoralens. Just like a sunburn, it is either asymptomatic or painful. This is a nonimmunologic toxic reaction that occurs in any patient who has a sufficiently high serum level of a photoactivated drug and sufficient UVA (wavelength from 320 to 400 mm) radiation exposure. Besides the usual summer sunlight, other significant UVA exposures should be remembered: wintertime sunlight, most intense on highly reflective snow covered high altitude places like ski slopes, sunlight passing through car windows (unlike UVB, spanning wavelengths from 290 to 320 mm, longer wavelength UVA does pass through glass), and tanning salon sessions. Although any of these drugs may cause severe phototoxicity, the most frightening reaction and outcome results when psoralen is taken before tanning salon or natural sunlight exposure. Indeed, death from burns has occurred with tanning salon exposure after taking psoralen. Patients may unknowingly receive a severe phototoxic reaction if they take any of these drugs and attend a tanning salon session or sun bathe.

Sun-exposed site pruritic, papular, or papulovesicular erythema may represent a *drug-induced photoallergic eruption*, *polymorphous light eruption*, or *cutaneous lupus erythematosus*. The drug-induced photoallergic eruption is a cell-mediated immune reaction that is most often caused by thiazides, NSAIDs, sulfonamides and sulfonylureas, oral contraceptives, and quinidine. *Polymorphous light eruption* is a common idiopathic disorder in which patients develop a pruritic papular eruption on the extensor surface of the arms and other sun-exposed sites, typically sparing the chronically sun-exposed ("hardened") face. The eruption typically occurs with each of the first several beach, pool, or picnic sun exposures in the late spring or summer months. After these two or three exposure-associated rashes, patients usually become hardened on the sites of the prior eruption, showing a tan, and have no further problems until the next spring or summer. When the diagnosis of photoallergic drug eruption or polymorphous light eruption cannot be made based on the patient's appearance and clinical course (photoallergy should resolve with drug withdrawal and polymorphous light eruption should resolve with continued sun exposure), further evaluation for possible lupus erythematosus, including *skin biopsy*, should be done. A dermatologist should be consulted if there is doubt about the diagnosis.

In all patients with photosensitive disorders, appropriate protective sun-blocking clothing and high sun protection factor (e.g., sun protection factor [SPF] 30) sunscreens should be used. These eruptions are caused primarily by UVA radiation in the case of drug eruptions and UVB and UVA radiation in the case of polymorphous light eruption and lupus erythematosus. UVA passes through window glass and patients who are photosensitive or on photosensitizing drugs should be made aware to avoid sunlight received through glass.

Sunscreens and Sunblocks

Sunscreens or sunblocks and physical protection should be recommended not only for people with photosensitivity, but also for all individuals receiving significant ultraviolet radiation exposure, regardless of whether it is "sunny or overcast." Albeit undesirable, when sunburn does occur, it serves as a great reminder to use protection in the future. Sunburn is not reversible, thus treatment is palliative (oral analgesics, tepid water baths, and appropriate hydration); corticosteroids have no effect on sunburn. Suntanning should be discouraged not only because it may cause sunburn, "liver spots" (solar lentigos), leathery skin and wrinkling, but, most impotantly because both UVB and UVA are known carcinogens which cause skin cancer.

Although there have been conflicting reports about a possible causative association between sunscreen use and melanoma, a meta-analysis of studies identified through a MEDLINE search of publications between the years 1966 and 2003, which examined sunscreen use prior to the development of melanoma, found no association between sunscreen use and melanoma. Although this analysis did not find a protective effect of sunscreen use, the authors commented that this lack of an association may have been because of the fact that the studies analyzed may have failed to control for significant confounders (5). Regardless, we can assure patients that sunscreens may be used safely in combination with appropriate physical protection (clothing, hats, sunglasses, umbrellas) and minimization of exposure during of peak UV radiation (UVR) hours surrounding noontime.

Sunscreens contain chemicals that absorb UVR. Adverse reactions to any sunscreen may occur. These chemicals are altered by radiation, and this is believed to be the cause of burning and stinging that may occur with higher SPF sunscreens, particularly when used on the face. Such reactions are most common in fair-skinned women especially if also using α-hydroxy acid or retinoic acid-based (e.g., Renova, Retin-A) facial creams. The alternative to sunscreens for people who experience either stinging or true allergic reactions are *sunblocks*. These block rather than absorb UVR and include plain zinc oxide (visibly white) and micronized zinc oxide and titanium dioxide (translucent when applied). Sunblocks tend to be less cosmetically acceptable because they have a chalky feel; however, they effectively block both UVB and UVA.

Sunscreens and sunblocks are given an *SPF* rating, which is the ratio of time needed for UV- radiation to cause minimal erythema (redness) when using versus not using the sunscreen. In the laboratory, an SPF of 15 screens 92% of UVB, and an SPF of 30 screens 96% of UVB. However, most sunscreen users apply significantly less than 50% of the amount of lotion needed for this protection, turning an SPF 30 product effectively into an SPF 15 product, at best. For this reason, it is best to recommend an SPF 30 sunscreen. Finally, because some people may ordinarily obtain some or all of their vitamin D from the sun instead of through their daily diet or by taking supplemental vitamins, the recommendation for sunscreens and sun avoidance should also include a recommendation for adequate daily vitamin D ingestion (see Chapter 103).

DRUG ERUPTIONS

Numerous prescription and nonprescription medications may cause a wide array of cutaneous abnormalities and aggravate pre-existing dermatoses (Table 118.1). It has been estimated that in hospitalized patients, 1% to 3% have adverse cutaneous drug reactions and 2% of these reactions are severe, being associated with significant morbidity and potential mortality (6,7). A systematic review of the MEDLINE database from 1966 to 2000 identified nine large studies containing primary data on the rates of cutaneous reactions to drugs. Analysis of these studies revealed "remarkable agreement" between the studies on reaction rates to drugs, with antibiotics causing most reactions (8). Although this is a large body of data, one might question the accuracy of diagnoses of drug reactions when not systematically confirmed. An interesting addition to this data is a prospective survey of cutaneous drug reactions occurring in a single hospital in Paris, France over a 6-month period. In this study, criteria for diagnosis were quite strict; patients were examined by a dermatologist and a group of dermatologists and pharmacologists evaluated "the drug imputability and preventability" after reviewing the patient's history, timing of medications, and appearance and timing of the eruption. The calculated prevalence of cutaneous drug reactions in these hospitalized patients was 3.6 per 1000, significantly less than the above stated rates of "1% to 3%." Similar to past studies, the majority of the eruptions were attributable to antibiotics (mostly penicillins). Fifteen percent of reactions were judged to be preventable. Interestingly, 31% of the patients with reactions had a history of a prior immunologic reaction to a drug, suggesting a possible genetic susceptibility for drug reactions. It should be noted that in these patients diagnosed with reactions, imputability was "definitive" in only 44% and "probable" in the remaining 56%, thereby highlighting the difficulty in defining rates of drug reactions *even* when systematic evaluation is performed (9). Excluding urticaria (Coombs and Type I immunologic reaction) and vasculitis (Type III immunologic reaction), cutaneous drug reactions are considered "delayed hypersensitivity reactions" (Type IV immunologic reactions), mediated by activated T cells with activation of different T-cell subsets leading to varied reactions, including exanthems (e.g., macular and papular exanthem), eczema (e.g., systemic allergic contact dermatitis), bullous reactions (e.g., bullous fixed drug eruption, erythema multiforme, toxic epidermal necrolysis, linear IgA bullous drug eruption), and pustular eruptions (pustular exanthem) (10).

Urticaria

Chapter 30 discusses urticaria.

Exanthems

The most commonly seen acute drug-induced eruption is a pruritic exanthem. This is usually macular and papular (morbilliform) but may be a purely macular erythema, exfoliative erythroderma, or scarlatiniform eruption.

TABLE 118.1 Adverse Cutaneous Drug Reactions and Some Common Causative Drugs

Acne
- Androgenic hormones
- Corticosteroids
- Halogens (bromides, iodides)
- Anticonvulsants
- Tuberculostatic drugs
- Lithium
- Cyclosporin
- Vitamin B_{12}
- Oral contraceptives

Alopecia
- Cytostatic drugs
- Anticoagulants
- Androgenic hormones
- Phenytoin
- Cholesterol-lowering agents
- Colchicine

"DRESS"[1]
- Phenytoin
- Phenobarbital
- Carbamazepine
- Lamotrigine
- Allopurinol
- Isoniazide
- Minocycline
- Terbinafine
- Sulfasalazine
- Hydrochlorothaizide
- Cyclosporine
- Nevirapine

Drug-induced cutaneious lupus erythematosus[2]
- Hydrochlorothiazide
- ACE inhibitors
- Calcium channel blockers
- Interferons
- Statins

Erythema multiforme and toxic epidermal necrolysis
- Sulfonamides
- Penicillins
- Nonsteroidal anti-inflammatory drugs
- Anticonvulsants

Exanthematous eruptions (see text)
- Penicillins
- Sulfonamides
- Barbiturates
- Phenytoin
- Carbamazepine
- Allopurinol
- Gold salts
- Phenothiazines

Fixed drug eruptions[a]
- Phenolphthalein
- Tetracyclines
- Sulfonamides
- Barbiturates
- Penicillins

Pityriasis rosea-like eruptions (see Table 113.1; pityriasis rosea)
- Barbiturates
- Gold
- Metronidazole
- Bismuth
- Captopril
- Clonidine
- Metoprolol

Photosensitivity
- Tetracycline
- Demeclocycline
- Doxycycline
- Sulfonamides
- Nonsteroidal anti-inflammatory drugs
- Phenothiazines
- Thiazide diuretics
- Calcium channel blocker
- Psoralens

Porhyria cutanea tarda[c]
- Estrogens
- Androgens
- Alcohol
- Antimalarials
- Sulfonamides
- Sulfonylureas
- Rifampicin
- Quinidine
- Quinine

Acute intermittent porphyria[c]
- Estrogens
- Androgens
- Alcohol
- Antimalarials
- Sulfonamides
- Sulfonylureas
- Barbiturates

Urticaria/angioedema
- Opiates
- Penicillins
- Sulfonamides
- Aspirin
- Quinine
- Nonsteroidal anti-inflammatory drugs
- ACE inhibitors
- Radiocontrast media
- Hyperosmolar solutions
- Amphetamines
- Azodyes and benzoates in drugs

Eczematous eruptions
- β-Blockers
- Diuretics
- Sulfonylureas
- Phenothiazines
- Penicillins
- Sulfonamides

(continued)

TABLE 118.1 (Continued) Adverse Cutaneous Drug Reactions and Some Common Causative Drugs

Nonpigmenting fixed drug eruption[b]	Pruritus
Acetaminophen	Opiates
Pseudoephedrine	Aspirin
Radiocontrast media	Antidepressants
Leukocytoclastic vasculitis	Belladonna alkaloids
Sulfonamides	Barbiturates
Phenytoin	CNS stimulants
Allopurinol	Estrogens
Papulosquamous eruptions (psoriasislike eruptions or exacerbation of psoriasis)	Hepatotoxic drugs
Antimalarials	
Lithium	
β-Blockers	
ACE inhibitors	
Sulfonamides	
Lichen planus-like eruptions	
Gold	
Captopril	
Furosemide	
β-Blockers	
Quinidine	
Quinine	
Sulfonylureas	
Thiazides	

[a]One or more, 1–4 cm, asymmetrically distributed erythematous patches that resolve with hyperpigmentation and become acutely inflamed again with drug readministration.
[b]One or more, 1–4 cm, erythematous macules that fade completely and become acutely inflamed with drug readministration.
[c]Not described in this textbook.
ACE, angiotensin-converting enzyme; CNS, central nervous system.
[1]Drug rash with eosinophilia and systemic symptoms, i.e., drug hypersensitivity syndrome.
[2]Arch Dermatol 2003;139:45 (Ref #15).

Although innumerable drugs may cause this eruption, the most commonly implicated drugs include penicillins and semisynthetic penicillins, cephalosporins, sulfonamides, quinidine, cimetidine, allopurinol, carbamazepine, phenytoin, isoniazid, and nitrofurantoin.

Although data suggest that patient-reported history regarding drug allergy, particularly penicillin allergy, may be incorrect (11), it should always be presumed to be accurate, and if the decision is made to administer the drug, a reaction must be anticipated. When the question of possible immediate reaction (IgE, anaphylaxis) to penicillins and cephalosporins arises, testing may be done to confirm or exclude an IgE mediated allergy (see Chapter 30). Unfortunately, such testing is not available for other drugs or for other types of immune reactions.

Eruptions may begin at any time but usually occur at one of two periods of drug administration: after 2 to 3 days or after 9 to 10 days. The early form is seen in patients who have previously been sensitized to the drug. With this prior sensitization, an exanthem may or may not have occurred, depending on the timing of sensitization and how soon the drug was stopped. The more delayed reaction occurring 9 to 10 days after drug initiation occurs in patients not previously sensitized to the drug. Systemic manifestations of drug sensitivity are absent. In contrast, when visceral hypersensitivity occurs (i.e., "drug hypersensitivity *syndrome*" or drug rash with eosinophilia and systemic symptoms [DRESS]), onset is usually 2 to 8 weeks after initiation of the offending drug, however, onset may be more delayed (e.g., as seen in minocycline hypersensitivity syndrome). Eosinophilia occurs in combination with variable organ involvement, which may include the lymph nodes, kidneys, liver, spleen, lungs, gastrointestinal tract, pancreas, heart, thyroid gland, peripheral nerves, parotid and salivary glands, and bone marrow. Hypersensivity syndromes are most commonly due to anticonvulsants (phenytoin, phenobarbital, carbamazepine, lamotrigine), allopurinol, isoniazid, and minocycline, but have also been reported with several drugs (e.g., terbinafine, sulfasalazine, hydrochlorothiazide, cyclosporine, nevirapine) (10,12,13). Rarely, an exanthem may be complicated by the subsequent development of yet another immunologic reaction, e.g., toxic epidermal necrolysis (see Toxic Epidermal Necrolysis below).

With uncomplicated nonbullous cutaneous eruptions, the suspected causative drug should be stopped if possible, and topical treatment begun to reduce pruritus. Such treatment includes frequent application of bland, topical, over-the-counter preparations containing menthol or phenol such as Sarna or Sarna HC (with 1% hydrocortisone) lotion or Aveeno Anti-Itch cream. In contrast, systemic drug hypersensitivity syndromes require immediate intervention with prompt discontinuation of all suspected drugs and close observation (7).

Erythema Multiforme

Erythema multiforme is a mucocutaneous hypersensitivity syndrome caused most commonly by a drug or infection. It is divided into erythema multiforme minor and erythema multiforme major, depending on whether it affects one or more than one mucosal surface, respectively (7,14). Although the pathogenesis of erythema multiforme is unknown, it is believed that an infection or a drug leads to a cell-mediated cytotoxic reaction in the epidermis.

Erythema multiforme major, which accounts for approximately 20% of cases of erythema multiforme, may cause morbidity and even mortality. It is associated with drugs more often than erythema multiforme minor, but similar infections may cause both forms. Patients usually have a prodrome of malaise, myalgia, fever, and sometimes upper respiratory symptoms. The eruption develops rapidly, is generally widespread, and involves at least two mucosal surfaces, usually the conjunctiva and the oral mucosa. Cutaneous lesions evolve quickly from macules into target-like plaques with dusky centers (Fig. 118.1, Color Plate section), often surmounted by blisters and often confluent over large areas. Usually, the lips are covered with hemorrhagic crusts and the mucosa shows diffuse pseudomembranous denudation, and the eyes show conjunctival injection, erosions, or exudate. Less often the nasal, genital, esophageal, and, rarely, the respiratory mucosae are involved.

The most common and significant acute complication of erythema multiforme major is secondary bacterial infection and sepsis; the most devastating long-term complication is ocular scarring and vision loss. Patients with erythema multiforme major must be hospitalized and, depending on the extent of disease, may benefit from care in a burn unit. Ophthalmologic consultation should be obtained immediately.

Erythema multiforme minor causes 80% of all cases of erythema multiforme. It is seen in patients of all ages but is more common in patients who are between the ages of 20 and 40 years. Most cases of erythema multiforme minor are caused by a preceding herpes simplex virus infection. Most patients with recurrent erythema multiforme minor, even those without a history of HSV infection, have detectable HSV deoxyribonucleic acid (DNA) in the lesions. Causes of erythema multiforme minor other than herpes simplex infection include other viral infections, *Mycoplasma pneumoniae*, other bacterial infections, and drugs (most commonly sulfonamides, penicillins, NSAIDs, and anticonvulsants).

Erythema multiforme minor begins with asymptomatic to tender erythematous to violaceous macules that evolve into papules with an expanding border, leaving a non-blanchable, dusky, slightly depressed center, creating an iris or target lesion. Lesions may coalesce into plaques or become bullous (*bullous erythema multiforme*). The eruption favors the palms and soles, dorsal hands and feet, and knees and elbows, but may be widely distributed. Approximately 20% of patients have mucosal lesions with mild to extensive flaccid bullae and deep erosions of the lips, buccal mucosa, and gingiva. Erythema multiforme is occasionally limited to the mouth without cutaneous lesions. Patients may have associated fever and malaise. If the diagnosis cannot be made on clinical grounds, skin biopsy should be done and will show necrotic keratinocytes, epidermal and dermal edema, and a mononuclear cell infiltrate. The treatment of erythema multiforme minor involves identification of the causative drug or infection and withdrawal of any suspected offending drug. Although necessary, treatment of a causative infection does not change the course of the erythema multiforme. For symptomatic relief, the oral lesions may be treated with an oral suspension containing diphenhydramine and antacid (e.g., Benadryl Elixir and Maalox in equal parts; swish for 1 minute and expectorate, four to six times per day) or sucralfate (e.g., Carafate 16 g [16 tabs] in 60 mL water; add to 180 mL 70% sorbitol; paint on erosions with finger as needed) in combination with 3% hydrogen peroxide washes (swish for 15 seconds and expectorate or swab with dental sponge four to six times per day). Topical anesthetics (Xylocaine gel) may be applied to individual painful lesions before meals. The use of systemic corticosteroids is controversial, and consultation with a dermatologist is recommended. One should note that if used, corticosteroid therapy should be given early in the course of the disease. If given after the eruption has fully evolved, one would not be expected to alter the severity of erythema multiforme and use of corticosteroids may increase the risk of secondary infection and even impair healing. In cases of recurrent erythema multiforme minor triggered by HSV, prophylactic acyclovir should be given to prevent HSV recurrences.

Toxic Epidermal Necrolysis

Toxic epidermal necrolysis (TEN), fortunately uncommon, is associated with a 25% to more than 40% mortality rate. Because it has many features in common with erythema multiforme major, these reactions are believed to represent a continuum of one disease. TEN is most often caused by drugs, especially sulfonamides, anticonvulsants, NSAIDs, allopurinol, colchicine, cephalosporins, quinolones, and aminopenicillins (14).

Similar to a sunburn, TEN typically begins with a diffuse painful erythema, often first noted on the trunk. Rapidly, patchy, and then coalescing areas of dusky epidermal necrosis and skin sloughing develop. Oral and ocular manifestations are similar to the changes seen in erythema multiforme major. Although the diagnosis is made presumptively and appropriate management initiated, biopsy should be done to confirm the diagnosis if there is any question. Routine histopathology reveals epidermal necrosis with sloughing of the epidermis from the dermis and a sparse mononuclear perivascular dermal infiltrate.

Patients with TEN are critically ill and may develop a number of associated problems, including cytopenias, hepatitis, hypoalbuminemia, hypophosphatemia, prerenal azotemia, disseminated intravascular coagulation, and pancreatitis (7). These patients should urgently be admitted to a hospital and for intensive care, ideally in a burn unit. Urgent consultation with a burn unit or medical intensivist, a dermatologist or plastic surgeon, and an ophthalmologist should be obtained. Debate is ongoing as to whether high-dose intravenous immunoglobulin (IVIG) therapy is useful in patients with TEN, as some retrospective analyses have demonstrated reduced mortality rates while others have not (15,16). In a recent "negative" retrospective analysis of 16 patients treated with IVIG and 16 not so treated, mortality rates were 25% and 38%, respectively, but this appreciable difference in mortality did not reach "statistical significance" as the number of patients studied was small. Unfortunately, or fortunately, large studies of TEN patients are common because of the relative rarity of TEN (16). Until randomized, double-blind placebo controlled studies are available, some treatment centers have begun administering IVIG to patients with TEN, as the natural history of this disorder is associated with such a high mortality rate and the risk of IVIG therapy is low. Regardless of treatment, mortality is most often the result of sepsis, whereas chronic morbidity in survivors is most often caused by cutaneous and ocular scarring, with the latter potentially leading to severe vision loss.

Nonspecific Eruptions Secondary to Drugs

Toxicity in the Elderly

Drug toxicity is an important cause of cutaneous eruptions in patients with declining renal or hepatic function, particularly when they are on multiple drugs that compete for hepatic metabolism or renal secretion. Such situations are typical of the elderly, who are most at risk for drug reactions in general (see Chapter 12).

Toxic drug eruptions may occur at any time while the patient is taking a drug. When an eruption occurs months or even years after the start of a drug, a toxic drug reaction is often not considered. Such instances of toxicity after many months of drug administration may result in pruritus with an associated or resultant dermatitis and possibly exacerbation of previously existing skin diseases (e.g., psoriasis, atopic dermatitis). Drug withdrawal in this situation usually leads to a slow improvement over several weeks. Toxic drug reactions should be considered in patients complaining of new, usually symmetric, dermatoses or exacerbation of previously stable skin conditions, even if a patient has been on a drug for months or years. Whenever possible, such drugs should be eliminated or reduced in dosage (17–19).

SPECIFIC REFERENCES*

1. Yancey KB. The pathophysiology of autoimmune blistering diseases. J Clin Invest 2005;115:825.
2. Minouni D, Nousari CH, Cummins DL, et al. Differences and similarities among expert opinions on the diagnosis and treatment of pemphigus vulgaris. J Am Acad Dermatol 2003;49:1059.
3. Anhalt GJ, Kim SC, Stanley JR, et al. Paraneoplastic pemphigus. An autoimmune mucocutaneous disease associated with neoplasia. N Engl J Med 1990;323:1729.
4. Kaplan I, Hodak E, Ackerman L, et al. Neoplasms associated with paraneoplastic pemphigus: a review with emphasis on non-hematologic malignancy and oral mucosal manifestations. Oral Oncol 2004;40:553.
5. Dennis LK, Freeman LEB, VanBeek MJ. Sunsreen use and risk for melanoma: a quantitative review. Ann Intern Med 2003;139:966.
6. Svensson CK, Cowen EW, Gaspari AA. Cutaneous drug reactions. Pharmacol Rev 2001;53:357–79.
7. Roujeau JC, Stern RS. Severe adverse cutaneous reactions to drugs. N Engl J Med 1994;331:1272.
8. Bigby M. Rates of cutaneous reactions to drugs. Arch Dermatol 2001;137:765.
9. Fiszenson-Albala F, Auzerie V, Mahe E, et al. A 6-month prospective survey of cutaneous drug reactions in a hospital setting. Br J Dermatol 2003;149:1018.
10. Pichler WM. Delayed drug hypersensitivity reactions (review). Ann Intern Med 2003;139:683.
11. Salkind AR, Cuddy PG, Foxworth JW. Is this patient allergic to penicillin? An evidence-based study analysis of the likelihood of penicillin allergy. JAMA 2001;285:2498.
12. Michel F, Navellou JC, Ferraud D, et al. DRESS syndrome in a patient on sulfasalazine for rheumatoid arthritis. Joint Bone Spine 2005;72:82.
13. Abecassis S, Roujeau JC, Bocquet H, et al. Severe sialadenitis: a new complication of drug reaction with eosinophilia and systemic symptoms. J Am Acad Dermatol 2004;51:827.
14. Roujeau JC, Kelly JP, Naldi L, et al. Medication use and the risk of Stevens–Johnson syndrome or toxic epidermal necrolysis. N Engl J Med 1995;333:1600.
15. Wolff K, Tappeiner G. Treatment of toxic epidermal necrolysis: the uncertainty persists but the fog is dispersing. Arch Dermatol 2003;139:85.
16. Shortt R, Gomez M, Mittman N, et al. Intravenous immunoglobulin does not improve outcome in toxic epidermal necrolysis. J Burn Care Rehabil 2004;25:246.
17. Gilleaudeau P, Vallat VP, Carter DM, et al. Angiotensin-converting enzyme inhibitors as possible exacerbating drugs in psoriasis. J Am Acad Dermatol 1993;28:490.
18. Cohen AD, Kagen M, Friger M, et al. Calcium channel blockers intake and psoriasis: a case control study. Acta Derm Venereol 2001;81:347.
19. Carrington PR, Sanusi ID, Zahradka S, et al. Enalapril-associated erythema and vasculitis. Cutis 1993;51:121.

*Bold numerals denote published controlled clinical trials, meta-analyses, or consensus-based recommendations.

For annotated ***General References*** *and resources related to this chapter, visit www.hopkinsbayview.org/PAMreferences.*

INDEX

Page numbers followed by *t* and *f* indicate tables and figures, respectively.

B

H

I

M